OPTUM360°™

Simplify your ordering. Magnify your savings.

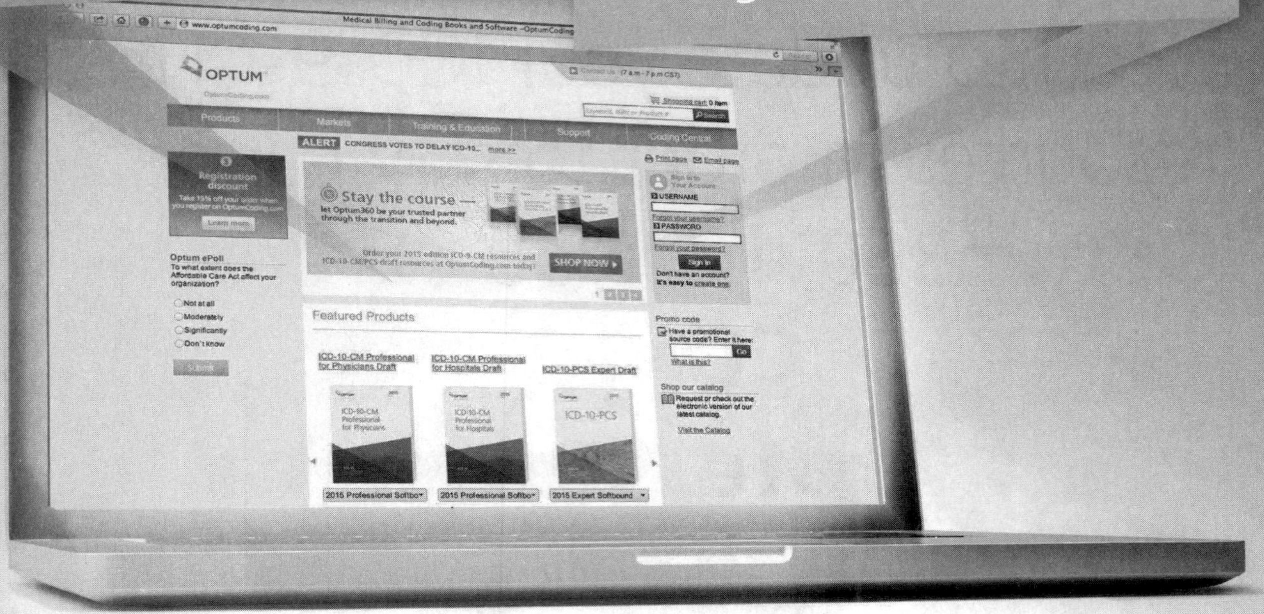

1 Click.

Visit optumcoding.com

- Find the products you need quickly and easily.
- View all available formats and edition years on the same page.
- Chat live with a customer service representative.
- Visit Coding Central for expert resources including articles, *Inside Track to ICD-10* and coding scenarios to test your knowledge.
- View our catalog online. Utilize our interactive online catalog features to view product information quickly and easily.

2 Register.

By registering, you'll be able to:

- Enjoy special promotions, discounts and automatic rewards.
- Get recommendations based on your order history.
- Check on shipment status and tracking.
- View order and payment history.
- Pay invoices.
- Manage your address book and ship orders to multiple locations.
- Renew your order with a single click.
- Compile a wish list of the products you want and purchase when you're ready.

3 Save.

Get 15% off your next order

Register for an account and receive a coupon via email for 15% off your next order.

Plus, save even more with our no-cost eRewards program.

OptumCoding.com eRewards program

Register for an account and you're automatically enrolled in our eRewards program, where you'll get a $50 coupon for every $500 you spend*. When logged in at optumcoding.com, the eRewards meter keeps track of purchases toward your next reward.

Visit us at optumcoding.com to register today!

*Offer valid only for customers who are NOT part of our Medallion or Partner Account programs. You must be registered at optumcoding.com to have your online purchases tracked for rewards purposes. Shipping charges and taxes still apply and cannot be used for rewards. Optum Coding eReward offers valid online only.
OPTPRJ5482 SPRJ1691

OPTUM™

ICD-10-CM Professional for Hospitals

The Complete Official Draft Code Set

2015

Publisher's Notice

The *ICD-10-CM Professional for Hospitals: The Complete Official Draft Code Set* is designed to be an accurate and authoritative source regarding coding and every reasonable effort has been made to ensure accuracy and completeness of the content. However, Optum makes no guarantee, warranty, or representation that this publication is accurate, complete, or without errors. It is understood that Optum is not rendering any legal or other professional services or advice in this publication and that Optum bears no liability for any results or consquences that may arise from the use of this book.

Our Commitment to Accuracy

Optum is committed to producing accurate and reliable materials.

To report corrections, please visit www.optumcoding.com/accuracy or email accuracy@optum.com. You can also reach customer service by calling 1.800.464.3649, option 1.

Acknowledgments

Lauri Gray, RHIT, CPC, AHIMA-Approved ICD-10-CM/PCS Trainer, *Product Manager*
Karen Schmidt, BSN, *Technical Director*
Stacy Perry, *Manager, Desktop Publishing*
Anita Schmidt, BS, RHIT, *Clinical Technical Editor*
Peggy Willard, CCS, AHIMA-Approved ICD-10-CM/PCS Trainer, *Clinical Technical Editor*
Lisa Singley, *Project Manager*
Tracy Betzler, *Senior Desktop Publishing Specialist*
Hope M. Dunn, *Senior Desktop Publishing Specialist*
Katie Russell, *Desktop Publishing Specialist*
Kate Holden, *Editor*

Copyright

Made in the USA
ISBN 978-1-62254-036-5

Anita Schmidt, BS, RHIT

Ms. Schmidt has expertise in Level I Adult and Pediatric Trauma hospital coding, specializing in ICD-9-CM, DRG, and CPT coding. Her experience includes analysis of medical record documentation and assignment of ICD-9-CM codes and DRGs, and CPT code assignments for same-day surgery cases. She has conducted coding training and auditing inclusive of DRG validation, conducted electronic health record training, and worked with clinical documentation specialists to identify documentation needs and potential areas for physician education. Ms. Schmidt is an active member of the American Health Information Management Association (AHIMA) and the Minnesota Health Information Management Association (MHIMA).

Karen Schmidt, BSN

Ms. Schmidt has more than 25 years of health care experience beginning with a strong clinical background in critical care nursing and later functioning as director of case management, including the components of quality assurance, utilization management, concurrent coding, case-mix analysis, and discharge planning. Her areas of expertise include ICD-9-CM/DRG coding, outpatient observation, billing compliance, implementation of concurrent coding methodology, and physician documentation education. She is an active member of the American Health Information Management Association (AHIMA).

Peggy Willard, CCS, AHIMA-Approved ICD-10-CM/PCS Trainer

Ms. Willard has several years of experience in Level I Adult and Pediatric Trauma hospital coding, specializing in ICD-9-CM, DRG, and CPT coding. She has been extensively trained in ICD-10-CM and PCS. Her recent experience includes in-depth analysis of medical record documentation, ICD-10-CM code assignment, and DRG shifts based on ICD-10-CM code assignment. Ms. Willard's expertise includes conducting coding audits, conducting coding training for coding staff and clinical documentation specialists, and creating internal ICD-10-CM coding guidelines/tips. Ms. Willard is an active member of the American Health Information Management Association (AHIMA) and the Minnesota Health Information Management Association (MHIMA).

Contents

Preface

ICD-10-CM Official Preface

This 2015 update of the International Classification of Diseases, 10th revision, Clinical Modification (ICD-10-CM) is being published by the United States government in recognition of its responsibility to promulgate this classification throughout the United States for morbidity coding. The International Statistical Classification of Diseases and Related Health Problems, 10th Revision (ICD-10), published by the World Health Organization (WHO), is the foundation of ICD-10-CM. ICD-10 continues to be the classification used in cause-of-death coding in the United States. The ICD-10-CM is comparable with the ICD-10. The WHO Collaborating Center for the Family of International Classifications in North America, housed at the National Center for Health Statistics (NCHS), has responsibility for the implementation of ICD and other WHO-FIC classifications and serves as a liaison with the WHO, fulfilling international obligations for comparable classifications and the national health data needs of the United States. The historical background of ICD and ICD-10 can be found in the Introduction to the International Classification of Diseases and Related Health Problems (ICD-10), 2008, World Health Organization, Geneva, Switzerland.

ICD-10-CM is the United States' clinical modification of the World Health Organization's ICD-10. The term clinical is used to emphasize the modification's intent: to serve as a useful tool in the area of classification of morbidity data for indexing of medical records, medical care review, and ambulatory and other medical care programs, as well as for basic health statistics. To describe the clinical picture of the patient the codes must be more precise than those needed only for statistical groupings and trend analysis.

Characteristics of ICD-10-CM

ICD-10-CM far exceeds its predecessors in the number of concepts and codes provided. The disease classification has been expanded to include health-related conditions and to provide greater specificity at the 6th and 7th character level. The 6th and 7th characters are not optional and are intended for use in recording the information documented in the clinical record.

Introduction

History and Future of ICD-1Ø-CM

The ICD-1Ø-CM classification system was developed by the National Center for Health Statistics (NCHS) as a clinical modification to the ICD-1Ø system developed by the World Health Organization (WHO), primarily as a unique system for use in the United States for morbidity and mortality reporting. Although ICD-1Ø-CM has not yet been implemented for use in the United States, ICD-1Ø has been adopted for use in the coding and classification of mortality data from death certificates. ICD-1Ø replaced ICD-9 for this purpose as of January 1, 1999. Upon legislative approval, ICD-1Ø-CM is planned as the replacement for ICD-9-CM, volumes 1 and 2.

ICD-1Ø is the copyrighted product of the World Health Organization (WHO), which has authorized the development of a clinical modification (CM) of ICD-1Ø for use in the United States. However, all modifications to the ICD-1Ø must conform to WHO conventions for ICD. The development of ICD-1Ø-CM included comprehensive evaluation by a Technical Advisory Panel and extensive consultation with physician groups, clinical coders, and other industry experts.

The ICD-1Ø-CM draft and crosswalk between ICD-9-CM and ICD-1Ø-CM were made available on the Centers for Medicare and Medicaid Services (CMS) website for public comment. The initial public comment period extended from December 1997 through February 1998. A field test for ICD-1Ø-CM was conducted in the summer of 2ØØ3 jointly by The American Hospital Association (AMA) and the American Health Information Management Association (AHIMA). Public comments and suggestions were reviewed and additional modifications to ICD-1Ø-CM were made. Revisions were made to ICD-1Ø-CM based on the established update process for ICD-9-CM (the ICD-9-CM Coordination and Maintenance Committee) and the World Health Organization's ICD-1Ø (the Update and Revision Committee).

These revisions to ICD-1Ø-CM have included:

- information relevant to ambulatory and managed care encounters
- expanded injury codes
- creation of combination diagnosis/symptom codes to reduce the number of codes needed to fully describe a condition
- the addition of 6th and 7th character classifications
- incorporation of common 4th and 5th character classifications
- classifications specific to laterality
- classification refinement for increased data granularity

This new structure allows for further expansion than was possible with the ICD-9-CM classification system.

This new 2Ø15 draft update release is available for public viewing. ICD-1Ø-CM codes are not currently valid for any purpose or use other than the reporting of mortality data for death certificates.

The Department of Health and Human Services (HHS) published the final rule regarding the adoption of both ICD-1Ø-CM and ICD-1Ø-PCS in the January 16, 2ØØ9, Federal Register (45 CFR part 162 [CMS—ØØ13—F]). The initial compliance date for implementation of ICD-1Ø-CM and ICD-1Ø-PCS as a replacement for ICD-9-CM was set at October 1, 2Ø13. On April 17, 2Ø12, the Department of Health and Human Services (HHS) released a notice to postpone the date by which certain health care entities have to comply with International Classification of Diseases, 1Øth Revision diagnosis and procedure codes (ICD-1Ø). The compliance date for implementation of ICD-1Ø-CM and ICD-1Ø-PCS as a replacement for ICD-9-CM was changed to October 1, 2Ø14. On April 1, 2Ø14, Congress enacted the Protecting Access to Medicare Act of 2Ø14, which contained a provision to delay the implementation of ICD-1Ø-CM/PCS by a least one year. The act prohibits the Department of Health and Human Services (HHS) from adopting the ICD-1Ø-CM/PCS code sets as the mandatory standard until at least October 1, 2Ø15.

ICD-1Ø-CM for Hospitals: The Complete Official Draft Code Set

ICD-10-CM for Hospitals: The Complete Official Draft Code Set 2015 includes many of the enhancements described below in direct response to requests from our subscribers. Many of these enhancements were introduced in the Optum *ICD-9-CM for Hospitals* and users will find many of the conventions, icons, color bars, and other enhancements familiar since many of these features are similar to the hallmark color coding and symbols of our ICD-9-CM code books.

As you review the content, you will find the following:

- Optum Exclusive feature—Check XTension Alert symbol, indicating the need for one or more "filler" x character assignments in the 5th and/or 6th character position to appropriately assign a required character in the 7th character position
- Optum Exclusive feature—Key word differentiation by the use of a green font that highlights the differentiating terms in similar code descriptions in a given category
- Optum Exclusive feature — Exclusive *following* references and Check Additional Character symbol in the indexes. The *following* references (designed and used exclusively by Optum) help coders locate those alphanumeric codes that are out of sequence in the tabular section.
- Optum Exclusive feature — Exclusive shaded guides in the index help users easily follow the indent levels for the subterms under a main term.
- Illustrations at the back of the book feature anatomy and terminology included in the ICD-1Ø-CM classification system
- The complete ICD-1Ø-CM official guidelines for coding and reporting, published by the U.S. Department of Health and Human Services and approved by the cooperating parties (American Health Information Management Association, National Center for Health Statistics, Centers for Medicare and Medicaid Services, American Hospital Association)
- Exclusive color coding, symbols, and footnotes that alert coders to coding and reimbursement issues, including the majority of the Medicare code edits and identification of conditions that significantly affect DRG assignment
- The complication and comorbidity (CC) exclusion list, integrated beneath the applicable codes, which makes it easier to determine complications and comorbidities excluded with a particular principal diagnosis
- All official ICD-1Ø-CM codes, indexes, notes, footnotes, and symbols
- Icons and definitions to differentiate between the two types of Excludes notes
- Check 4th, 5th, 6th, and 7th character symbols identify codes that require the addition of a 4th, 5th, 6th, or 7th character for code specificity and validity
- Color coding and symbol legend at the bottom of each page

Please review "How to Use *ICD-10-CM for Hospitals*" in this manual to learn about the features that will help you assign and report correct codes, ensuring appropriate reimbursement.

How to Use ICD-10-CM for Hospitals (Draft 2015)

This draft of the International Classification of Diseases, 10th Revision, Clinical Modification (ICD-10-CM) is being published by the United States Government in recognition of its responsibility to promulgate this classification throughout the United States for morbidity coding. This code book represents an adaptation of ICD-10 which was created specifically for use in the United States. Future revisions to ICD-10-CM will be made based on the established update process for ICD-9-CM (the ICD-9-CM Coordination and Maintenance Committee) and the World Health Organization's ICD-10 (the Update and Revision Committee). ICD-10-CM has been approved for implementation on October 1, 2015.

Steps to Correct Coding

1. Before beginning to use this code book, review section 1.A., "Conventions for the ICD-10-CM" and section 1.B., "General Coding Guidelines" of the ICD-10-CM Draft Official Guidelines for Coding and Reporting 2014.
2. Look up the main term in the alphabetic index and scan the subterm entries as appropriate. Review continued lines and additional subterms that may appear in the next column or on the next page.
3. Note all parenthetical terms (nonessential modifiers) that help in code selection but do not affect code assignment. Shaded vertical guidelines in the Index are provided to help determine the indentation level for each subterm in relation to the main terms.
4. Pay close attention to the following instructions in the Index:
   - "see," "see also," and "see category" cross-references
   - "with"/"without" notes
   - omit code" notes
   - due to" subterms
   - other instructions found in note boxes, such as "code by site"
   - *Following* references and Check Additional Character symbol in the indexes. The *following* references (designed and used exclusively by Optum) help coders locate those alphanumeric codes that are out of sequence in the tabular section.
5. Do not code from the alphabetic index without verifying the accuracy of the code in the tabular list. Locate the code in the alphanumerically arranged tabular list.
6. To determine the appropriateness of the code selection and proper coding, read all instructional material:
   - "includes" and both types of "excludes" notes
   - "use additional code" and "code first underlying disease"
   - instructions
   - code also"
   - 4th, 5th, and 6thcharacter requirements and 7th character extension requirements
   - CC Exclusions
   - age and sex symbols
7. Consult the official draft ICD-10-CM guidelines, which govern the use of specific codes. These guidelines provide both general and chapter-specific coding guidance.
8. Confirm and assign the correct code.

Organization

This book is organized in the following manner:

Introduction

The introductory material in this book includes the ICD-10-CM Official Preface, the history and future of ICD-10-CM as well as an overview of the classification system.

Draft Official ICD-10-CM Conventions and Guidelines

This section provides an explanation of the conventions and guidelines regulating the appropriate assignment and reporting of ICD-10-CM codes. This coding guidance is presented by the National Center for Health Statistics (NCHS), a governmental agency of the Centers for Disease Control and Prevention (CDC), within the United States Department of Health and Human Services (DHHS).

Alphabetic Index to Diseases

The alphabetic index to diseases is arranged in alphabetic order by disease — by specific illness, injury, eponym, abbreviation, or other descriptive diagnostic term. The Index also lists diagnostic terms for other reasons for encounters with health care professionals.

Neoplasm Table

The Neoplasm Table provides the proper code based upon histology of the neoplasm and site.

Table of Drugs and Chemicals

The Table of Drugs and Chemicals is also included within the Alphabetic Index.

The Table of Drugs and Chemicals lists the drug and the specific codes that identify the drug and the intent. No additional external cause of injury and poisoning code is assigned in ICD-10-CM.

Index to External Causes

The alphabetic index to External Causes of injuries is arranged in alphabetic order by main term indicating the event.

Tabular List of Diseases

ICD-10-CM codes and descriptors are arranged numerically within the tabular list of diseases within 21 separate chapters according to body system or nature of injury and disease. Classifications which were previously considered supplemental to ICD-9-CM (e.g., V codes and E codes) are incorporated into the tabular listing of ICD-10-CM as individual chapters. Chapters 20 External Causes of Morbidity and 21 Factors Influencing Health Status and Contact with Health Services include chapter-specific guidelines.

Illustrations

This section includes illustrations of normal anatomy with ICD-10-CM specific terminology.

Use of Official Sources

The *ICD-10-CM for Hospitals* contains the official U.S. Department of Health and Human Services, Tenth Revision, Clinical Modification (ICD-10-CM) codes, effective for the current year.

The color coding, footnotes, and symbols, which identify coding and reimbursement issues, are derived from official federal government sources, including the Medicare Code Edits (MCE), version 31R.

ICD-10-CM Draft Official Conventions

The ICD-10-CM conventions are general rules for the use of the classification system, independent of the guidelines. These conventions are incorporated within the Index and tabular list as instructional notes and are applicable regardless of the health care setting.

Format

ICD-10-CM is divided into two main parts: the Index, an alphabetical list of terms and their corresponding code, and the tabular list, a sequential, alphanumeric list of codes divided into chapters based on body system or condition. The Index contains the Index to Diseases and Injuries (main index) and the Index to External Causes of Injury. Also included in the main Index is the Neoplasm Table and a Table of Drugs and Chemicals.

The tabular list contains categories, subcategories, and valid codes.

ICD-10-CM is an alphanumeric classification system. The 1st character of a three-character category is a letter. The 2nd and 3rd characters may be numbers or alpha characters. A three-character category without further subclassification is equivalent to a valid three-character code. Subcategories are either four or five characters. Subcategory characters include either letters or numbers. Codes may be four, five, or six characters in length, in which each level of subdivision after a category is a subcategory. The final level of subdivision is a valid code. The final character in a code may be either a letter or a number.

The ICD-10-CM uses the letter "X" as a place-holder. A placeholder "X" is used as a 5th character place-holder at certain six-character codes to allow for future expansion, without disturbing the 6th character structure. For instance, an initial encounter for accidental poisoning by penicillin is coded to T36.0X1A. The "X" in the 5th character position is a place-holder, or filler character.

Similarly, certain categories have applicable 7th character extensions. In these cases, the 7th character extension is required for all codes within the category, or as otherwise instructed in the tabular list notations. 7th character extensions must always be the last character in the data field. If a code is not a full six characters in length, a dummy place-holder "X" must be used to fill in the empty characters when a 7th character extension is required.

Punctuation

[ ] In the tabular list, brackets are used to enclose synonyms, alternative wording, or explanatory phrases. In the Index, brackets are used to identify manifestation codes.

( ) Parentheses are used in both the Index and tabular list to enclose nonessential modifiers; supplementary words that may be present or absent in the statement of a disease or procedure without affecting the code number to which it is assigned.

: Colons are used in the tabular list after an incomplete term that needs one or more of the modifiers following the colon to make it assignable to a given category.

Abbreviations

NEC

The abbreviation NEC, "Not elsewhere classifiable" represents "other specified" in the ICD-10-CM. An index entry that states NEC directs the coder to an "other specified" code in the tabular list. Codes titled "Other" or "Other specified" in the tabular list (usually a code with a 4th or 6th character 8 and 5th character 9) are for use when the information in the medical record provides detail for which a specific code does not exist.

NOS

The abbreviation NOS, "Not otherwise specified," in the tabular list may be interpreted as "unspecified." Codes in the tabular list with "Unspecified" in the title (usually a code with a 4th or 6th character 9 and 5th character 0) are for use when the information in the medical record is insufficient to assign a more specific code.

Typeface

Boldface

Boldface type is used for main term entries in the alphabetic index, and all codes and descriptions in the tabular list.

Italicized

Italicized type is used for all exclusion notes and to identify manifestation codes, those codes that should not be reported as first-listed (principal) diagnoses.

General Notes

The following conventions and notes appear only in the tabular list of Diseases:

Includes Notes

The word "Includes" appears immediately under certain categories to further define, clarify, or give examples of the content of a code category.

Inclusion Terms

Lists of inclusion terms are included under certain codes. These terms indicate some of the conditions for which that code number may be used. Inclusion terms may be synonyms with the code title, or, in the case of "other specified" codes, the terms may also provide a list of various conditions included within a classification code. The inclusion terms are not exhaustive. The Index may provide additional terms that may also be assigned to a given code.

Excludes Notes

ICD-10-CM has two types of excludes notes. Each note has a different definition for use. However, they are similar in that they both indicate that codes excluded from each other are independent of each other.

Excludes 1

An Excludes 1 note is a "pure" excludes. It means "NOT CODED HERE!" An Excludes 1 note indicates mutually exclusive codes; two conditions that cannot be reported together. For example, a congenital form of a disease may not be reported with the acquired form of the same condition. The code excluded should never be reported with the applicable codes listed above the excludes notation.

Excludes 2

An Excludes 2 note means "NOT INCLUDED HERE." An Excludes 2 note indicates that although the excluded condition is not part of the condition it is excluded from, a patient may have both conditions at the same time. Therefore, when an Excludes 2 note appears under a code, it may be acceptable to use both the code and the excluded code together if supported by the medical documentation.

Default Codes

In the index, the default code is the code listed next to the main term. The default code represents the condition most commonly associated with the main term. This code may be assigned when documentation does not facilitate reporting a more specific code. Alternately, it may provide an unspecified code for the condition.

Syndromes

Follow the alphabetic index guidance when coding syndromes. In the absence of index guidance, assign codes for the documented manifestations of the syndrome.

And

When the term "and" is used in a narrative statement it may be interpreted as "and/or."

With/Without

When "with" and "without" are the two options for the final character of a set of codes, the default is always "without." For five-character codes, a "Ø" as the 5th position character represents "without," and "1" represents "with." For six-character codes, the 6th position character "1" represents "with" and "9" represents "without."

Instructional Notes Used in the Tabular List

In the tabular section, the following instructional notes appear in red type for emphasis:

Code First/Use additional code:

These instructional notes are in red type and provide sequencing instruction. They may appear independently of each other or to designate certain etiology/manifestation paired codes. These instructions signal the coder that an additional code should be reported to provide a more complete picture of that diagnosis.

In etiology/manifestation coding, ICD-1Ø-CM requires the underlying condition to be sequenced first, followed by the manifestation. In these situations, codes with "In diseases classified elsewhere" in the code description are never permitted as a first-listed or principal diagnosis code and must be sequenced following the underlying condition code.

Code Also:

A code also note alerts the coder that more than one code may be required to fully describe the condition. Code sequencing is discretionary. Factors that may determine sequencing include severity and reason for the encounter. These coding notes appear in red type.

Additional Conventions

Color-coding and symbols are included to alert the coder to important reimbursement issues affected by the diagnosis code assignment. Some codes may carry more than one color and/or symbol. For a quick reference to the color codes and their meanings, refer to the color/symbol legend located at the bottom of each page in the tabular listing.

Additional Characters Required

√4th This symbol indicates that the code requires a 4th character.

√5th This symbol indicates that the code requires a 5th character.

√6th This symbol indicates that the code requires a 6th character.

√7th This symbol indicates that the code requires a 7th character.

√x7th This symbol indicates that the code requires a 7th character following the placeholder "X". Codes with fewer than six characters that require a 7th character must contain placeholder "X" to fill in the empty character(s).

Boldface

Note

The term "Note" appears enclosed within a red icon and precedes the instructional information. These notes function as an alert, to highlight coding instruction within the text.

Key Word

Green font is used throughout the tabular list of Diseases to differentiate the key words that appear in similar code descriptions in a given category or subcategory.

For example, refer to the list of codes below from category C7A:

C7A.Ø2Ø Malignant carcinoid tumor of the **appendix**

C7A.Ø21 Malignant carcinoid tumor of the **cecum**

C7A.Ø22 Malignant carcinoid tumor of the **ascending colon**

C7A.Ø23 Malignant carcinoid tumor of the **transverse colon**

C7A.Ø24 Malignant carcinoid tumor of the **descending colon**

C7A.Ø25 Malignant carcinoid tumor of the **sigmoid colon**

C7A.Ø29 Malignant carcinoid tumor of the large intestine, **unspecified portion**

The portion of the code description that appears in bold font above appears in green font in the tabular list, to assist the coder in quickly identifying the key terms and in identifying the correct code. This convention is especially useful when the codes describe laterality, such as the following codes from category H4Ø.22:

H4Ø.221 Chronic angle-closure glaucoma, **right** eye

H4Ø.222 Chronic angle-closure glaucoma, **left** eye

H4Ø.223 Chronic angle-closure glaucoma, **bilateral**

H4Ø.229 Chronic angle-closure glaucoma, **unspecified** eye

The key word convention is only used in those categories in which there are multiple codes with very similar descriptions with only a few words that differentiate them.

Color Coding—Medicare Code Edits

Medicare Administrative Contractors (MACs) and many payers use Medicare code edits to check the coding accuracy on claims. The coding edit information in this manual is effective from October 1, 2Ø14, to September 3Ø, 2Ø15, and reflects those edits used for acute care hospital inpatient admission. This ICD-1Ø version of the Medicare Code Editor (MCE) is version 31R. However, the MCE is not intended to be used to process claims because the ICD-1Ø code set will not be mandated for use until the implementation of ICD-1Ø beginning no sooner than October 1, 2Ø15.

The Medicare code edits are listed below:

- Invalid diagnosis or procedure code
- External causes of morbidity codes as principal diagnosis
- Duplicate of PDx
- *Age conflict
- *Sex conflict
- *Manifestation code as principal diagnosis
- Nonspecific principal diagnosis (Discontinued as of 1Ø/1/Ø7)
- *Questionable principal diagnosis
- *Unacceptable principal diagnosis
- Nonspecific O.R. procedure (Discontinued as of 1Ø/1/Ø7)
- Noncovered procedure
- Open biopsy check (Discontinued as of 1Ø/1/1Ø)
- Bilateral procedure (Discontinued as of ICD-1Ø implementation)
- Invalid age
- Invalid sex
- Invalid discharge status
- Limited coverage
- *Wrong procedure performed

Starred edits above that are related to diagnosis issues are identified in this manual by color bars, symbols, or footnotes as described below.

Age and Sex Edit Symbols

The age edits below are used to detect inconsistencies between the patient's age and diagnosis. The following edit symbols appear in the tabular list of diseases to the right of the code description.

Newborn Age: 0 N

These diagnoses are intended for newborns and neonates and the patient's age must be Ø years.

Pediatric Age: 0-17 P

These diagnoses are intended for children and the patient's age must between Ø and 17 years.

Maternity Age: 12-55 M

These diagnoses are intended for childbearing patients between the age of 12 and 55 years.

Adult Age: 15-124 A

These diagnoses are intended for the patients between the age of 15 and 124 years.

The sex symbols below are used to detect inconsistencies between the patient's sex and diagnosis. These symbols appear in the tabular list of diseases to the right of the code description.

♂ **Male diagnosis only**

This symbol appears to the right of the code description. This reference appears in the disease and procedure tabular list.

♀ **Female diagnosis only**

This symbol appears to the right of the code description. This reference appears in the disease and procedure tabular list.

Manifestation Code

These codes appear in italic type, with a blue color bar over the title. A manifestation code cannot be reported as a first-listed or principal diagnosis. By definition, a manifestation code represents a demonstration of some aspect of an underlying disease, which is separately classifiable. In the alphabetic index, these codes are listed as the secondary code in brackets. The underlying disease code is listed first.

Unacceptable PDx

These codes will appear with a gray color bar over the code title. These codes do not describe a current illness or injury, but a circumstance which influences a patient's health status. They are considered an unacceptable principal diagnosis for *inpatient* admission.

Questionable admission diagnoses will also appear with a gray color bar over the code title along with a reference to footnote 13. These codes, although not unacceptable as a PDx, may be considered a "questionable admission" when used as PDx in an acute care hospital.

Hospital Acquired Condition (HAC)

These codes will appear with a yellow color bar over the code title. These codes identify conditions that are high cost or high volume or both, are either a complication or comorbidity (CC) or major complication or comorbidity (MCC) that as a secondary diagnosis results in assignment of a case to a higher-paying MS-DRG. These conditions are reasonably preventable through the application of evidence-based guidelines. If the condition is not present on admission (meaning it developed during the hospital admission), the case will not group to the higher-paying MS-DRG based solely upon the reporting of the HAC code. Many of these HACs are conditional, and are based on reporting the specific diagnosis code(s) in combination with certain procedure codes, notated in footnotes.

Wrong Procedure Performed Edit

The Wrong Surgery Edit was created to identify cases in which wrong surgeries occurred. Any claim with a code from the Y65.51-Y65.53 will be denied and returned to the provider. A surgical or other invasive procedure is considered to be a wrong procedure if:

- The procedure was performed on the wrong site
- The procedure was performed on the wrong patient, or
- The incorrect procedure was performed on a patient.

Other Notations in the Tabular

CC CC Condition

This symbol designates a complication or comorbidity diagnosis that may affect DRG assignment. A complication or comorbidity diagnosis, CC condition, is defined as a significant acute disease, a significant acute manifestation of a chronic disease, an advanced or end stage chronic disease, or a chronic disease associated with systemic physiological decompensation and debility that have consistently greater impact on hospital resources.

A CC icon most often appears to the right of the code description.

MCC MCC Condition

This symbol designates a major complication or comorbidity diagnosis that may affect DRG assignment. An MCC condition meets the same criteria as a CC condition but is associated with a higher acuity level and hospital resource consumption is expected to be higher than that for a CC condition. There are fewer conditions that meet the criteria as an MCC than those for a CC condition.

Similar to a CC icon, an MCC icon appears to the right of the code description.

CC Excludes Notations

Many distinct CC Excludes notations appear directly below the code to which they relate. However, in some cases the CC Excludes information is identical for all codes within a category or subcategory. In those cases, the CC Excludes notation is listed once, at the beginning of the category or subcategory. For example:

G43.6 Persistent migraine aura with cerebral infarction
CC Excl: For CC codes in subcategory G43.6, unless otherwise noted: G43.6Ø1-G43.619, I63.ØØ-I66.9

There are four codes with a CC designation in subcategory G43.6; the CC Excludes notation above applies to all four codes.

Optum ICD-1Ø-CM coding manuals include references to a previously designated CC Excludes notation, and those CC or MCC codes for which there are no excluded conditions. Refer to examples below:

K67 Disorders of peritoneum in infectious diseases classified elsewhere
CC Excl: See code: K65

A17.83 Tuberculosis neuritis
CC Excl: No Excl

By definition of being a condition which acts as its own CC or MCC, PDxCC or PDxMCC, the CC exclusion concept (the two conditions being too interrelated) does not apply. However, if a condition carries separate PDxCC/PDxMCC and MCC/CC designations, a CC excludes notation will appear for the CC or MCC designation.

PDx CC PDx MCC PDxCC or PDxMCC Condition

When the MS-DRG system was translated from ICD-9-CM to ICD-1Ø-CM, some significant differences existed. One involved the assignment of two codes in ICD-9-CM, one for an underlying condition, and one for a related acute manifestation. In ICD-1Ø-CM, only one combination code was necessary to replicate the same clinical concept. However, in ICD-9-CM, one of the two codes acted as a CC or MCC for the other. To address this situation, CMS has introduced the concept of certain ICD-1Ø-CM diagnosis codes acting as their own CC or MCC when sequenced as a principal diagnosis. For example, refer to the table below:

ICD-9 PDx	ICD-9 SDx	CC Level	ICD-1Ø Code with CC or MCC
415.19 Other pulm embolism	415.Ø Acute cor pulmonale	MCC	I26.Ø9 Other pulm embolism with acute cor pulmonale

In the ICD-9-CM MS-DRG system, diagnosis code 415.Ø acts as an MCC for code 415.19, grouping the case to the highest weighted DRG in its subgroup. In the ICD-1Ø-CM MS-DRG system, the same clinical concept, represented by code I26.Ø9 is sequenced as the principal diagnosis and the code functions as its own MCC. Codes which function as their own CC or MCC when sequenced as a principal diagnosis are designated with the PDxCC or PDxMCC icon to the right of the code description.

HIV HIV

This symbol indicates that the condition is considered a major HIV related diagnosis. When the condition is coded in combination with a diagnosis of human immunodeficiency virus (HIV), code B2Ø, the case will move from MS-DRG 977 to MS-DRGs 974-976.

Bracketed Codes

Some of the ICD-1Ø-CM or ICD-1Ø-PCS referenced codes that appear in this manual use bracketing as a space-saving convention. The numbers or letters within the brackets correspond to all appropriate, valid characters for the character position where the bracket appears. For example:

SØ4.Ø1[1,2,9] Injury of optic nerve, [right, left, unspecified] eye

The bracketed code above represents three distinct codes:

SØ4.Ø11 Injury of optic nerve, right eye

SØ4.Ø12 Injury of optic nerve, left eye

SØ4.Ø19 Injury of optic nerve, unspecified eye

Similarly, ICD-1Ø-PCS codes may be represented in the same way:

OSU[A,E,R,S] ØBZ Supplement [Right, Left Hip Joint; Acetabular, Femoral Surface] with Resurfacing Device, Open Approach

The bracketed code above represents four distinct codes:

ØSUAØBZ Supplement Right Hip Joint, Acetabular Surface with Resurfacing Device, Open Approach

ØSUEØBZ Supplement Left Hip Joint, Acetabular Surface with Resurfacing Device, Open Approach

ØSURØBZ Supplement Right Hip Joint, Femoral Surface with Resurfacing Device, Open Approach

ØSUSØBZ Supplement Left Hip Joint, Femoral Surface with Resurfacing Device, Open Approach

Bracketed codes are most often found in CC Excludes notations, as well as in footnotes related to Hospital Acquired Conditions (HACs).

Footnotes

All footnotes are identified by a numerical superscript that appears to the upper left of the code. For example:

10 I49.Ø1 Ventricular fibrillation

The footnote 1Ø indicates "MCC = Only if patient is discharged alive." This means that ventricular fibrillation is considered a major complication or comorbidity that may affect DRG assignment only if the patient is discharged alive. Otherwise ventricular fibrillation is assigned as a non-MCC condition.

The following list identifies the meaning of each footnote number in the tabular list of diseases:

1 [HAC Ø6: Catheter-Associated Urinary Tract Infection (UTI)] This condition represents a hospital acquired condition (HAC) when reported as a secondary diagnosis along with a secondary diagnosis of T83.51XA (Infection and inflammatory reaction due to indwelling urinary catheter, initial encounter) and neither are present on admission.

2 [HAC 11: Surgical Site Infection Following Bariatric Surgery] This condition represents a hospital acquired condition (HAC) when reported as the principal diagnosis along with a secondary diagnosis of K68.11 or K95.Ø1 or K95.81 (surgical site infection) or T81.4XXA (Infection following a procedure, initial encounter) and in combination with one of the following procedure codes, which represent bariatric procedures: ØD16[Ø,4,8][7,J,K,Z][9,A,B,L] or ØDV64CZ. The secondary diagnosis code is not present on admission.

3 [HAC 1Ø: Deep Vein Thrombosis (DVT)/Pulmonary Embolism (PE) with Total Knee or Hip Replacement] This condition represents a hospital acquired condition (HAC) when reported as a secondary diagnosis in combination with one of the following procedural codes that represent total knee or hip replacement: ØSR[9,B]Ø[1,2,3,4,J][9,A,Z]; ØSR[9,B]Ø[7,K]Z; ØSR[A,E]Ø[Ø,1,3,J][9,A,Z]; ØSR[A,E]Ø[7,K]Z; ØSR[C,D,T,U,V,W]Ø[7,K]Z; ØSR[C,D,T,U,V,W]ØJ[9,A,Z]; ØSR[R,S]Ø[1,3,J][9,A,Z]; ØSR[R,S]Ø[7,K]Z; ØSU[9,B]ØBZ; ØSU[A,E,R,S]ØBZ. The secondary diagnosis code is not present on admission.

4 [HAC 11: Surgical Site Infection Following Bariatric Surgery] This condition represents a hospital acquired condition (HAC) when reported as a secondary diagnosis along with PDx E66.Ø1 (Morbid obesity) and in combination with one of the following procedure codes, which represent bariatric procedures: ØD16[Ø,4,8][7,J,K,Z][9,A,B,L] or ØDV64CZ. The secondary diagnosis code is not present on admission.

5 [HAC Ø8: Surgical Site Infection — Mediastinitis after Coronary Bypass Graft (CABG)] This condition represents a hospital acquired condition (HAC) when reported as a secondary diagnosis in combination with one of the following procedure codes, which represent Coronary Bypass Graft (CABG): Ø21[Ø,1,2,3][Ø,4][9,A,J,K][3,8,9,C,F,W]; Ø21[Ø,1,2,3][Ø,4]Z[3,8,9,C,F]. The secondary diagnosis code is not present on admission.

6 [HAC 12: Surgical Site Infection — Certain Orthopedic Procedures of Spine, Shoulder and Elbow] This condition represents a hospital acquired condition (HAC) when reported as a secondary diagnosis in combination with one of the following procedure codes, which represent spine, shoulder, and elbow procedures: ØRG[Ø,1,2,4,6,7,8,A][Ø,3,4][7,A,J,K,Z][Ø,1,J]; ØRG[E,F,G,H,J,K][Ø,3,4][4,7,J,K,Z]Z; ØRG[L,M][Ø,3,4][4,5,7,J,K,Z]Z; ØRQ[E,F,G,H,J,K,L,M][Ø,3,4,X]ZZ; ØRU[E,F,G,H,J,K,L,M][Ø,3,4][7,J,K]Z; ØSG[Ø,1,3][Ø,3,4][7,A,J,K,Z][Ø,1,J]; ØSG[7,8][Ø,3,4[4,7,J,K,Z]Z. The secondary diagnosis code is not present on admission.

7 This condition represents a hospital acquired condition (HAC) only when reported as the initial encounter (7th character A, B, or C) and the diagnosis is not present upon admission.

8 [HAC 13: Surgical Site Infection (SSI) Following Cardiac Implantable Electronic Device (CIED) Procedures] This condition represents a hospital acquired condition (HAC) when reported as a secondary diagnosis in combination with one of the following procedure codes: Ø2H43[J,K,M]Z; Ø2H[6,7]3[J,M]Z; Ø2H[K,L]3JZ; Ø2HN[Ø,3,4][J,M]Z; Ø2PA[Ø,3,4]MZ; Ø2PAXMZ; Ø2WA[Ø,3,4]MZ; ØJH[6,8][Ø,3][4,5,6,7,8,9,P]Z; ØJ[P,W]T[Ø,3]PZ. The secondary diagnosis is not present upon admission.

9 [HAC 14: Iatrogenic Pneumothorax w/ Venous Catheterization] This condition represents a hospital acquired condition (HAC) when reported as a secondary diagnosis in combination with one of the following procedure codes: Ø5H[M,N,P,Q]33Z or ØJH63XZ. The secondary diagnosis is not present upon admission.

1Ø These codes are considered major complication/comorbidity (MCC) conditions and may affect MS-DRG assignment only if the patient is discharged alive.

11 These codes indicate that the wrong procedure was performed on the patient and reimbursement may be affected.

12 This condition represents an unacceptable PDx only when reported as the initial encounter (7th character A).

13 These codes, although not unacceptable as PDx, would be considered questionable as a PDx for acute care hospital admissions.

Other Notations in the Index

Following References

The index includes *following* references to assist in locating "out-of-sequence" codes in the tabular list. "Out-of-sequence" codes contain an alphabetic character (letter) in the 3rd or 4th character position. These codes are placed according to the classification rules — the placement of the codes according to condition — not according to alphabetic or numeric sequencing rules.

Example:

Carcinoma (malignant) (*see also* Neoplasm, by site, malignant)neuroendocrine (*see also* Tumor, neuroendocrine)
  high grade, any site C7A.1 (*following* C75)
  poorly differentiated, any site C7A.1 (*following* C75)

In the tabular rubric, C7A is included after rubric C75 and before C76.

Gout, chronic (*see also* Gout, gouty) M1A.9
  drug-induced M1A.2Ø (*following* MØ8)
    ankle M1A.27-(*following* MØ8)
    elbow M1A.22-(*following* MØ8)

In the tabular rubric, MIA is included after rubric MØ8 and before M1Ø.

ICD-10-CM Draft Official Guidelines for Coding and Reporting 2014

Narrative changes appear in **bold** text.

Items underlined have been moved within the guidelines since the 2013 version.

Italics are used to indicate revisions to heading changes.

The Centers for Medicare and Medicaid Services (CMS) and the National Center for Health Statistics (NCHS), two departments within the U.S. Federal Government's Department of Health and Human Services (DHHS) provide the following guidelines for coding and reporting using the International Classification of Diseases, 10th Revision, Clinical Modification (ICD-10-CM). These guidelines should be used as a companion document to the official version of the ICD-10-CM as published on the NCHS website. The ICD-10-CM is a morbidity classification published by the United States for classifying diagnoses and reason for visits in all health care settings. The ICD-10-CM is based on the ICD-10, the statistical classification of disease published by the World Health Organization (WHO).

These guidelines have been approved by the four organizations that make up the Cooperating Parties for the ICD-10-CM: the American Hospital Association (AHA), the American Health Information Management Association (AHIMA), CMS, and NCHS.

These guidelines are a set of rules that have been developed to accompany and complement the official conventions and instructions provided within the ICD-10-CM itself. The instructions and conventions of the classification take precedence over guidelines. These guidelines are based on the coding and sequencing instructions in the Tabular List and Alphabetic Index of ICD-10-CM, but provide additional instruction. Adherence to these guidelines when assigning ICD-10-CM diagnosis codes is required under the Health Insurance Portability and Accountability Act (HIPAA). The diagnosis codes (Tabular List and Alphabetic Index) have been adopted under HIPAA for all healthcare settings. A joint effort between the healthcare provider and the coder is essential to achieve complete and accurate documentation, code assignment, and reporting of diagnoses and procedures. These guidelines have been developed to assist both the healthcare provider and the coder in identifying those diagnoses and procedures that are to be reported. The importance of consistent, complete documentation in the medical record cannot be overemphasized. Without such documentation accurate coding cannot be achieved. The entire record should be reviewed to determine the specific reason for the encounter and the conditions treated.

The term encounter is used for all settings, including hospital admissions. In the context of these guidelines, the term provider is used throughout the guidelines to mean physician or any qualified health care practitioner who is legally accountable for establishing the patient's diagnosis. Only this set of guidelines, approved by the Cooperating Parties, is official.

The guidelines are organized into sections. Section I includes the structure and conventions of the classification and general guidelines that apply to the entire classification, and chapter-specific guidelines that correspond to the chapters as they are arranged in the classification. Section II includes guidelines for selection of principal diagnosis for non-outpatient settings. Section III includes guidelines for reporting additional diagnoses in non-outpatient settings. Section IV is for outpatient coding and reporting. It is necessary to review all sections of the guidelines to fully understand all of the rules and instructions needed to code properly.

Section I. Conventions, general coding guidelines and chapter specific guidelines

The conventions, general guidelines and chapter-specific guidelines are applicable to all health care settings unless otherwise indicated. The conventions and instructions of the classification take precedence over guidelines.

A. Conventions for the ICD-10-CM

The conventions for the ICD-10-CM are the general rules for use of the classification independent of the guidelines. These conventions are incorporated within the Alphabetic Index and Tabular List of the ICD-10-CM as instructional notes.

1. The Alphabetic Index and Tabular List

The ICD-10-CM is divided into the Alphabetic Index, an alphabetical list of terms and their corresponding code, and the Tabular List, a structured chronological list of codes divided into chapters based on body system or condition. The Alphabetic Index consists of the following parts: the Index of Diseases and Injury, the Index of External Causes of Injury, the Table of Neoplasms and the Table of Drugs and Chemicals.

See Section I.C2. General guidelines

See Section I.C.19. Adverse effects, poisoning, underdosing and toxic effects

2. Format and Structure

The ICD-10-CM Tabular List contains categories, subcategories and codes. Characters for categories, subcategories and codes may be either a letter or a number. All categories are 3 characters. A three-character category that has no further subdivision is equivalent to a code. Subcategories are either 4 or 5 characters. Codes may be 3, 4, 5, 6 or 7 characters. That is, each level of subdivision after a category is a subcategory. The final level of subdivision is a code. Codes that have applicable 7th characters are still referred to as codes, not subcategories. A code that has an applicable 7th character is considered invalid without the 7th character.

The ICD-10-CM uses an indented format for ease in reference.

3. Use of codes for reporting purposes

For reporting purposes only codes are permissible, not categories or subcategories, and any applicable 7th character is required.

4. Placeholder character

The ICD-10-CM utilizes a placeholder character "X". The "X" is used as a placeholder at certain codes to allow for future expansion. An example of this is at the poisoning, adverse effect and underdosing codes, categories T36-T50.

Where a placeholder exists, the X must be used in order for the code to be considered a valid code.

5. 7th Characters

Certain ICD-10-CM categories have applicable 7th characters. The applicable 7th character is required for all codes within the category, or as the notes in the Tabular List instruct. The 7th character must always be the 7th character in the data field. If a code that requires a 7th character is not 6 characters, a placeholder X must be used to fill in the empty characters.

6. Abbreviations

a. Alphabetic Index abbreviations

NEC "Not elsewhere classifiable"

This abbreviation in the Alphabetic Index represents "other specified". When a specific code is not available for a condition, the Alphabetic Index directs the coder to the "other specified" code in the Tabular List.

NOS "Not otherwise specified"

This abbreviation is the equivalent of unspecified.

b. Tabular List abbreviations

NEC "Not elsewhere classifiable"

This abbreviation in the Tabular List represents "other specified". When a specific code is not available for a condition the Tabular List includes an NEC entry under a code to identify the code as the "other specified" code.

NOS "Not otherwise specified"

This abbreviation is the equivalent of unspecified.

7. Punctuation

[ ] Brackets are used in the Tabular List to enclose synonyms, alternative wording or explanatory phrases. Brackets are used in the Alphabetic Index to identify manifestation codes.

( ) Parentheses are used in both the Alphabetic Index and Tabular List to enclose supplementary words that may be present or absent in the statement of a disease or procedure without affecting the code number to which it is assigned. The terms within the parentheses are referred to as nonessential modifiers. **The nonessential modifiers in the Alphabetic Index to Diseases apply to subterms following a main term except when a nonessential modifier and a subentry are mutually exclusive, the subentry takes precedence. For example, in the ICD-10-CM Alphabetic Index under the main term Enteritis, "acute" is a nonessential modifier and "chronic" is a subentry. In this case, the nonessential modifier "acute" does not apply to the subentry "chronic".**

: Colons are used in the Tabular List after an incomplete term which needs one or more of the modifiers following the colon to make it assignable to a given category.

8. Use of "and"

See Section I.A.14. Use of the term "And"

9. Other and Unspecified codes

a. "Other" codes

Codes titled "other" or "other specified" are for use when the information in the medical record provides detail for which a specific code does not exist. Alphabetic Index entries with NEC in the line designate "other" codes in the Tabular List. These Alphabetic Index entries represent specific disease entities for which no specific code exists so the term is included within an "other" code.

b. "Unspecified" codes

Codes titled "unspecified" are for use when the information in the medical record is insufficient to assign a more specific code. For those categories for which an unspecified code is not provided, the "other specified" code may represent both other and unspecified.

See Section I.B.18 Use of Signs/Symptom/Unspecified Codes

10. Includes Notes

This note appears immediately under a three character code title to further define, or give examples of, the content of the category.

11. Inclusion Terms

List of terms is included under some codes. These terms are the conditions for which that code is to be used. The terms may be synonyms of the code title, or, in the case of "other specified" codes, the terms are a list of the various conditions assigned to that code. The inclusion terms are not necessarily exhaustive. Additional terms found only in the Alphabetic Index may also be assigned to a code.

12. Excludes Notes

The ICD-10-CM has two types of excludes notes. Each type of note has a different definition for use but they are all similar in that they indicate that codes excluded from each other are independent of each other.

a. Excludes1

A type 1 Excludes note is a pure excludes note. It means "NOT CODED HERE!" An Excludes1 note indicates that the code excluded should never be used at the same time as the code above the Excludes1 note. An Excludes1 is used when two conditions cannot occur together, such as a congenital form versus an acquired form of the same condition.

b. Excludes2

A type 2 Excludes note represents "Not included here". An excludes2 note indicates that the condition excluded is not part of the condition represented by the code, but a patient may have both conditions at the same time. When an Excludes2 note appears under a code, it is acceptable to use both the code and the excluded code together, when appropriate.

13. Etiology/manifestation convention ("code first", "use additional code" and "in diseases classified elsewhere" notes)

Certain conditions have both an underlying etiology and multiple body system manifestations due to the underlying etiology. For such conditions, the ICD-10-CM has a coding convention that requires the underlying condition be sequenced first followed by the manifestation.

Wherever such a combination exists, there is a "use additional code" note at the etiology code, and a "code first" note at the manifestation code. These instructional notes indicate the proper sequencing order of the codes, etiology followed by manifestation.

In most cases the manifestation codes will have in the code title, "in diseases classified elsewhere." Codes with this title are a component of the etiology/ manifestation convention. The code title indicates that it is a manifestation code. "In diseases classified elsewhere" codes are never permitted to be used as first-listed or principal diagnosis codes. They must be used in conjunction with an underlying condition code and they must be listed following the underlying condition. See category FØ2, Dementia in other diseases classified elsewhere, for an example of this convention.

There are manifestation codes that do not have "in diseases classified elsewhere" in the title. For such codes, there is a "use additional code" note at the etiology code and a "code first" note at the manifestation code and the rules for sequencing apply.

In addition to the notes in the Tabular List, these conditions also have a specific Alphabetic Index entry structure. In the Alphabetic Index both conditions are listed together with the etiology code first followed by the manifestation codes in brackets. The code in brackets is always to be sequenced second.

An example of the etiology/manifestation convention is dementia in Parkinson's disease. In the Alphabetic Index, code G2Ø is listed first, followed by code FØ2.8Ø or FØ2.81 in brackets. Code G2Ø represents the underlying etiology, Parkinson's disease, and must be sequenced first, whereas codes FØ2.8Ø and FØ2.81 represent the manifestation of dementia in diseases classified elsewhere, with or without behavioral disturbance.

"Code first" and "Use additional code" notes are also used as sequencing rules in the classification for certain codes that are not part of an etiology/ manifestation combination.

See Section I.B.7. Multiple coding for a single condition.

14. "And"

The word "and" should be interpreted to mean either "and" or "or" when it appears in a title.

For example, cases of "tuberculosis of bones", "tuberculosis of joints" and "tuberculosis of bones and joints" are classified to subcategory A18.Ø, Tuberculosis of bones and joints.

15. "With"

The word "with" should be interpreted to mean "associated with" or "due to" when it appears in a code title, the Alphabetic Index, or an instructional note in the Tabular List.

The word "with" in the Alphabetic Index is sequenced immediately following the main term, not in alphabetical order.

16. "See" and "See Also"

The "see" instruction following a main term in the Alphabetic Index indicates that another term should be referenced. It is necessary to go to the main term referenced with the "see" note to locate the correct code.

A "see also" instruction following a main term in the Alphabetic Index instructs that there is another main term that may also be referenced that may provide additional Alphabetic Index entries that may be useful. It is not necessary to follow the "see also" note when the original main term provides the necessary code.

17. "Code also note"

A "code also" note instructs that two codes may be required to fully describe a condition, but this note does not provide sequencing direction.

18. Default codes

A code listed next to a main term in the ICD-1Ø-CM Alphabetic Index is referred to as a default code. The default code represents that condition that is most commonly associated with the main term, or is the unspecified code for the condition. If a condition is documented in a medical record (for example, appendicitis) without any additional information, such as acute or chronic, the default code should be assigned.

B. General Coding Guidelines

1. Locating a code in the ICD-1Ø-CM

To select a code in the classification that corresponds to a diagnosis or reason for visit documented in a medical record, first locate the term in the Alphabetic Index, and then verify the code in the Tabular List. Read and be guided by instructional notations that appear in both the Alphabetic Index and the Tabular List.

It is essential to use both the Alphabetic Index and Tabular List when locating and assigning a code. The Alphabetic Index does not always provide the full code. Selection of the full code, including laterality and any applicable 7th character can only be done in the Tabular List. A dash (-) at the end of an Alphabetic Index entry indicates that additional characters are required. Even if a dash is not included at the Alphabetic Index entry, it is necessary to refer to the Tabular List to verify that no 7th character is required.

2. Level of Detail in Coding

Diagnosis codes are to be used and reported at their highest number of characters available.

ICD-1Ø-CM diagnosis codes are composed of codes with 3, 4, 5, 6 or 7 characters. Codes with three characters are included in ICD-1Ø-CM as the heading of a category of codes that may be further subdivided by the use of fourth and/or fifth characters and/or sixth characters, which provide greater detail.

A three-character code is to be used only if it is not further subdivided. A code is invalid if it has not been coded to the full number of characters required for that code, including the 7th character, if applicable.

3. Code or codes from AØØ.Ø through T88.9, ZØØ-Z99.8

The appropriate code or codes from AØØ.Ø through T88.9, ZØØ-Z99.8 must be used to identify diagnoses, symptoms, conditions, problems, complaints or other reason(s) for the encounter/visit.

4. Signs and symptoms

Codes that describe symptoms and signs, as opposed to diagnoses, are acceptable for reporting purposes when a related definitive diagnosis has not been established (confirmed) by the provider. Chapter 18 of ICD-1Ø-CM, Symptoms, Signs, and Abnormal Clinical and Laboratory Findings, Not Elsewhere Classified (codes RØØ.Ø - R99) contains many, but not all codes for symptoms.

See Section I.B.18 Use of Signs/Symptom/Unspecified Codes

5. Conditions that are an integral part of a disease process

Signs and symptoms that are associated routinely with a disease process should not be assigned as additional codes, unless otherwise instructed by the classification.

6. Conditions that are not an integral part of a disease process

Additional signs and symptoms that may not be associated routinely with a disease process should be coded when present.

7. Multiple coding for a single condition

In addition to the etiology/manifestation convention that requires two codes to fully describe a single condition that affects multiple body systems, there are other single conditions that also require more than one code. "Use additional code" notes are found in the Tabular List at codes that are not part of an etiology/manifestation pair where a secondary code is useful to fully describe a condition. The sequencing rule is the same as the etiology/manifestation pair, "use additional code" indicates that a secondary code should be added.

For example, for bacterial infections that are not included in chapter 1, a secondary code from category B95, Streptococcus, Staphylococcus, and Enterococcus, as the cause of diseases classified elsewhere, or B96, Other bacterial agents as the cause of diseases classified elsewhere, may be required to identify the bacterial organism causing the infection. A "use additional code" note will normally be found at the infectious disease code, indicating a need for the organism code to be added as a secondary code.

"Code first" notes are also under certain codes that are not specifically manifestation codes but may be due to an underlying cause. When there is a "code first" note and an underlying condition is present, the underlying condition should be sequenced first.

"Code, if applicable, any causal condition first", notes indicate that this code may be assigned as a principal diagnosis when the causal condition is unknown or not applicable. If a causal condition is known, then the code for that condition should be sequenced as the principal or first-listed diagnosis.

Multiple codes may be needed for sequela, complication codes and obstetric codes to more fully describe a condition. See the specific guidelines for these conditions for further instruction.

8. Acute and Chronic Conditions

If the same condition is described as both acute (subacute) and chronic, and separate subentries exist in the Alphabetic Index at the same indentation level, code both and sequence the acute (subacute) code first.

9. Combination Code

A combination code is a single code used to classify:

Two diagnoses, or

A diagnosis with an associated secondary process (manifestation)

A diagnosis with an associated complication

Combination codes are identified by referring to subterm entries in the Alphabetic Index and by reading the inclusion and exclusion notes in the Tabular List.

Assign only the combination code when that code fully identifies the diagnostic conditions involved or when the Alphabetic Index so directs. Multiple coding should not be used when the classification provides a combination code that clearly identifies all of the elements documented in the diagnosis. When the combination code lacks necessary specificity in describing the manifestation or complication, an additional code should be used as a secondary code.

10. Sequela (Late Effects)

A sequela is the residual effect (condition produced) after the acute phase of an illness or injury has terminated. There is no time limit on when a sequela code can be used. The residual may be apparent early, such as in cerebral infarction, or it may occur months or years later, such as that due to a previous injury. Coding of sequela generally requires two codes sequenced in the following order: The condition or nature of the sequela is sequenced first. The sequela code is sequenced second.

An exception to the above guidelines are those instances where the code for the sequela is followed by a manifestation code identified in the Tabular List and title, or the sequela code has been expanded (at the fourth, fifth or sixth character levels) to include the manifestation(s). The code for the acute phase of an illness or injury that led to the sequela is never used with a code for the late effect.

See Section I.C.9. Sequelae of cerebrovascular disease

See Section I.C.15. Sequelae of complication of pregnancy, childbirth and the puerperium

See Section I.C.19. Application of 7th characters for Chapter 19

11. Impending or Threatened Condition

Code any condition described at the time of discharge as "impending" or "threatened" as follows:

If it did occur, code as confirmed diagnosis.

If it did not occur, reference the Alphabetic Index to determine if the condition has a subentry term for "impending" or "threatened" and also reference main term entries for "Impending" and for "Threatened."

If the subterms are listed, assign the given code.

If the subterms are not listed, code the existing underlying condition(s) and not the condition described as impending or threatened.

12. Reporting Same Diagnosis Code More than Once

Each unique ICD-10-CM diagnosis code may be reported only once for an encounter. This applies to bilateral conditions when there are no distinct codes identifying laterality or two different conditions classified to the same ICD-10-CM diagnosis code.

13. Laterality

Some ICD-10-CM codes indicate laterality, specifying whether the condition occurs on the left, right or is bilateral. If no bilateral code is provided and the condition is bilateral, assign separate codes for both the left and right side. If the side is not identified in the medical record, assign the code for the unspecified side.

14. Documentation for BMI, Non-pressure Ulcers and Pressure Ulcer Stages

For the Body Mass Index (BMI), depth of non-pressure chronic ulcers and pressure ulcer stage codes, code assignment may be based on medical record documentation from clinicians who are not the patient's provider (i.e., physician or other qualified healthcare practitioner legally accountable for establishing the patient's diagnosis), since this information is typically documented by other clinicians involved in the care of the patient (e.g., a dietitian often documents the BMI and nurses often documents the pressure ulcer stages). However, the associated diagnosis (such as overweight, obesity, or pressure ulcer) must be documented by the patient's provider. If there is conflicting medical record documentation, either from the same clinician or different clinicians, the patient's attending provider should be queried for clarification.

The BMI codes should only be reported as secondary diagnoses. As with all other secondary diagnosis codes, the BMI codes should only be assigned when they meet the definition of a reportable additional diagnosis (see Section III, Reporting Additional Diagnoses).

15. Syndromes

Follow the Alphabetic Index guidance when coding syndromes. In the absence of Alphabetic Index guidance, assign codes for the documented manifestations of the syndrome.

Additional codes for manifestations that are not an integral part of the disease process may also be assigned when the condition does not have a unique code.

16. Documentation of Complications of Care

Code assignment is based on the provider's documentation of the relationship between the condition and the care or procedure. The guideline extends to any complications of care, regardless of the chapter the code is located in. It is important to note that not all conditions that occur during or following medical care or surgery are classified as complications. There must be a cause-and-effect relationship between the care provided and the condition, and an indication in the documentation that it is a complication. Query the provider for clarification, if the complication is not clearly documented.

17. Borderline Diagnosis

If the provider documents a "borderline" diagnosis at the time of discharge, the diagnosis is coded as confirmed, unless the classification provides a specific entry (e.g., borderline diabetes). If a borderline condition has a specific index entry in ICD-10-CM, it should be coded as such. Since borderline conditions are not uncertain diagnoses, no distinction is made between the care setting (inpatient versus outpatient). Whenever the documentation is unclear regarding a borderline condition, coders are encouraged to query for clarification.

18. Use of Sign/Symptom/Unspecified Codes

Sign/symptom and "unspecified" codes have acceptable, even necessary, uses. While specific diagnosis codes should be reported when they are supported by the available medical record documentation and clinical knowledge of the patient's health condition, there are instances when signs/symptoms or unspecified codes are the best choices for accurately reflecting the healthcare encounter. Each healthcare encounter should be coded to the level of certainty known for that encounter.

If a definitive diagnosis has not been established by the end of the encounter, it is appropriate to report codes for sign(s) and/or symptom(s) in lieu of a definitive diagnosis. When sufficient clinical information isn't known or available about a particular health condition to assign a more specific code, it is acceptable to report the appropriate "unspecified" code (e.g., a diagnosis of pneumonia has been determined, but not the specific type). Unspecified codes should be reported when they are the codes that most accurately reflects what is known about the patient's condition at the time of that particular encounter. It would be inappropriate to select a specific code that is not supported by the medical record documentation or conduct medically unnecessary diagnostic testing in order to determine a more specific code.

C. Chapter-Specific Coding Guidelines

In addition to general coding guidelines, there are guidelines for specific diagnoses and/or conditions in the classification. Unless otherwise indicated, these guidelines apply to all health care settings. Please refer to Section II for guidelines on the selection of principal diagnosis.

1. Chapter 1: Certain Infectious and Parasitic Diseases (AØØ-B99)

a. Human immunodeficiency virus (HIV) infections

1) Code only confirmed cases

Code only confirmed cases of HIV infection/illness. This is an exception to the hospital inpatient guideline Section II, H.

In this context, "confirmation" does not require documentation of positive serology or culture for HIV; the provider's diagnostic statement that the patient is HIV positive, or has an HIV-related illness is sufficient.

2) Selection and sequencing of HIV codes

(a) Patient admitted for HIV-related condition

If a patient is admitted for an HIV-related condition, the principal diagnosis should be B2Ø, Human immunodeficiency virus [HIV] disease followed by additional diagnosis codes for all reported HIV-related conditions.

(b) Patient with HIV disease admitted for unrelated condition

If a patient with HIV disease is admitted for an unrelated condition (such as a traumatic injury), the code for the unrelated condition (e.g., the nature of injury code) should be the principal diagnosis. Other diagnoses would be B2Ø followed by additional diagnosis codes for all reported HIV-related conditions.

(c) Whether the patient is newly diagnosed

Whether the patient is newly diagnosed or has had previous admissions/encounters for HIV conditions is irrelevant to the sequencing decision.

(d) Asymptomatic human immunodeficiency virus

Z21, Asymptomatic human immunodeficiency virus [HIV] infection status, is to be applied when the patient without any documentation of symptoms is listed as being "HIV positive," "known HIV," "HIV test positive," or similar terminology. Do not use this code if the term "AIDS" is used or if the patient is treated for any HIV-related illness or is described as having any condition(s) resulting from his/her HIV positive status; use B2Ø in these cases.

(e) Patients with inconclusive HIV serology

Patients with inconclusive HIV serology, but no definitive diagnosis or manifestations of the illness, may be assigned code R75, Inconclusive laboratory evidence of human immunodeficiency virus [HIV].

(f) Previously diagnosed HIV-related illness

Patients with any known prior diagnosis of an HIV-related illness should be coded to B2Ø. Once a patient has developed an HIV-related illness, the patient should always be assigned code B2Ø on every subsequent admission/encounter. Patients previously diagnosed with any HIV illness (B2Ø) should never be assigned to R75 or Z21, Asymptomatic human immunodeficiency virus [HIV] infection status.

(g) HIV infection in pregnancy, childbirth and the puerperium

During pregnancy, childbirth or the puerperium, a patient admitted (or presenting for a health care encounter) because of an HIV-related illness should receive a principal diagnosis code of O98.7-, Human immunodeficiency [HIV] disease complicating pregnancy, childbirth and the puerperium, followed by B2Ø and the code(s) for the HIV-related illness(es). Codes from Chapter 15 always take sequencing priority.

Patients with asymptomatic HIV infection status admitted (or presenting for a health care encounter) during pregnancy, childbirth, or the puerperium should receive codes of O98.7- and Z21.

(h) Encounters for testing for HIV

If a patient is being seen to determine his/her HIV status, use code Z11.4, Encounter for screening for human immunodeficiency virus [HIV]. Use additional codes for any associated high risk behavior.

If a patient with signs or symptoms is being seen for HIV testing, code the signs and symptoms. An additional counseling code Z71.7, Human immunodeficiency virus [HIV] counseling, may be used if counseling is provided during the encounter for the test.

When a patient returns to be informed of his/her HIV test results and the test result is negative, use code Z71.7, Human immunodeficiency virus [HIV] counseling.

If the results are positive, see previous guidelines and assign codes as appropriate.

b. Infectious agents as the cause of diseases classified to other chapters

Certain infections are classified in chapters other than Chapter 1 and no organism is identified as part of the infection code. In these instances, it is necessary to use an additional code from Chapter 1 to identify the organism. A code from category B95, Streptococcus, Staphylococcus, and Enterococcus as the cause of diseases classified to other chapters, B96, Other bacterial agents as the cause of diseases classified to other chapters, or B97, Viral agents as the cause of diseases classified to other chapters, is to be used as an additional code to identify the organism. An instructional note will be found at the infection code advising that an additional organism code is required.

c. Infections resistant to antibiotics

Many bacterial infections are resistant to current antibiotics. It is necessary to identify all infections documented as antibiotic resistant. Assign a code from category Z16, Resistance to antimicrobial drugs, following the infection code only if the infection code does not identify drug resistance.

d. Sepsis, severe sepsis, and septic shock

1) Coding of sepsis and severe sepsis

(a) Sepsis

For a diagnosis of sepsis, assign the appropriate code for the underlying systemic infection. If the type of infection or causal organism is not further specified, assign code A41.9, Sepsis, unspecified organism.

A code from subcategory R65.2, Severe sepsis, should not be assigned unless severe sepsis or an associated acute organ dysfunction is documented.

(i) Negative or inconclusive blood cultures and sepsis

Negative or inconclusive blood cultures do not preclude a diagnosis of sepsis in patients with clinical evidence of the condition, however, the provider should be queried.

(ii) Urosepsis

The term urosepsis is a nonspecific term. It is not to be considered synonymous with sepsis. It has no default code in the Alphabetic Index. Should a provider use this term, he/she must be queried for clarification.

(iii) Sepsis with organ dysfunction

If a patient has sepsis and associated acute organ dysfunction or multiple organ dysfunction (MOD), follow the instructions for coding severe sepsis.

(iv) Acute organ dysfunction that is not clearly associated with the sepsis

If a patient has sepsis and an acute organ dysfunction, but the medical record documentation indicates that the acute organ dysfunction is related to a medical condition other than the sepsis, do not assign a code from subcategory R65.2, Severe sepsis. An acute organ dysfunction must be associated with the sepsis in order to assign the severe sepsis code. If the documentation is not clear as to whether an acute organ dysfunction is related to the sepsis or another medical condition, query the provider.

(b) **Severe sepsis**

The coding of severe sepsis requires a minimum of 2 codes: first a code for the underlying systemic infection, followed by a code from subcategory R65.2, Severe sepsis. If the causal organism is not documented, assign code A41.9, Sepsis, unspecified organism, for the infection. Additional code(s) for the associated acute organ dysfunction are also required.

Due to the complex nature of severe sepsis, some cases may require querying the provider prior to assignment of the codes.

2) **Septic shock**

(a) Septic shock generally refers to circulatory failure associated with severe sepsis, and therefore, it represents a type of acute organ dysfunction.

For cases of septic shock, the code for the systemic infection should be sequenced first, followed by code R65.21, Severe sepsis with septic shock or code T81.12, Postprocedural septic shock. Any additional codes for the other acute organ dysfunctions should also be assigned. As noted in the sequencing instructions in the Tabular List, the code for septic shock cannot be assigned as a principal diagnosis.

3) **Sequencing of severe sepsis**

If severe sepsis is present on admission, and meets the definition of principal diagnosis, the underlying systemic infection should be assigned as principal diagnosis followed by the appropriate code from subcategory R65.2 as required by the sequencing rules in the Tabular List. A code from subcategory R65.2 can never be assigned as a principal diagnosis.

When severe sepsis develops during an encounter (it was not present on admission) the underlying systemic infection and the appropriate code from subcategory R65.2 should be assigned as secondary diagnoses.

Severe sepsis may be present on admission but the diagnosis may not be confirmed until sometime after admission. If the documentation is not clear whether severe sepsis was present on admission, the provider should be queried.

4) **Sepsis and severe sepsis with a localized infection**

If the reason for admission is both sepsis or severe sepsis and a localized infection, such as pneumonia or cellulitis, a code(s) for the underlying systemic infection should be assigned first and the code for the localized infection should be assigned as a secondary diagnosis. If the patient has severe sepsis, a code from subcategory R65.2 should also be assigned as a secondary diagnosis. If the patient is admitted with a localized infection, such as pneumonia, and sepsis/severe sepsis doesn't develop until after admission, the localized infection should be assigned first, followed by the appropriate sepsis/severe sepsis codes.

5) **Sepsis due to a postprocedural infection**

(a) **Documentation of causal relationship**

As with all postprocedural complications, code assignment is based on the provider's documentation of the relationship between the infection and the procedure.

(b) **Sepsis due to a postprocedural infection**

For such cases, the postprocedural infection code, such as, T80.2, Infections following infusion, transfusion, and therapeutic injection, T81.4, Infection following a procedure, T88.0, Infection following immunization, or O86.0, Infection of obstetric surgical wound, should be coded first, followed by the code for the specific infection. If the patient has severe sepsis the appropriate code from subcategory R65.2 should also be assigned with the additional code(s) for any acute organ dysfunction.

(c) **Postprocedural infection and postprocedural septic shock**

In cases where a postprocedural infection has occurred and has resulted in severe sepsis and postprocedural septic shock, the code for the precipitating complication such as code T81.4, Infection following a procedure, or O86.0, Infection of obstetrical surgical wound should be coded first followed by code R65.21, Severe sepsis with septic shock and a code for the systemic infection.

6) **Sepsis and severe sepsis associated with a noninfectious process (condition)**

In some cases a noninfectious process (condition), such as trauma, may lead to an infection which can result in sepsis or severe sepsis. If sepsis or severe sepsis is documented as associated with a noninfectious condition, such as a burn or serious injury, and this condition meets the definition for principal diagnosis, the code for the noninfectious condition should be sequenced first, followed by the code for the resulting infection. If severe sepsis, is present a code from subcategory R65.2 should also be assigned with any associated organ dysfunction(s) codes. It is not necessary to assign a code from subcategory R65.1, Systemic inflammatory response syndrome (SIRS) of non-infectious origin, for these cases.

If the infection meets the definition of principal diagnosis it should be sequenced before the non-infectious condition. When both the associated non-infectious condition and the infection meet the definition of principal diagnosis either may be assigned as principal diagnosis.

Only one code from category R65, Symptoms and signs specifically associated with systemic inflammation and infection, should be assigned. Therefore, when a non-infectious condition leads to an infection resulting in severe sepsis, assign the appropriate code from subcategory R65.2, Severe sepsis. Do not additionally assign a code from subcategory R65.1, Systemic inflammatory response syndrome (SIRS) of non-infectious origin.

See Section I.C.18. SIRS due to non-infectious process

7) **Sepsis and septic shock complicating abortion, pregnancy, childbirth, and the puerperium**

See Section I.C.15. Sepsis and septic shock complicating abortion, pregnancy, childbirth and the puerperium

8) **Newborn sepsis**

See Section I.C.16. f. Bacterial sepsis of Newborn

e. **Methicillin resistant *Staphylococcus aureus* (MRSA) conditions**

1) **Selection and sequencing of MRSA codes**

(a) **Combination codes for MRSA infection**

When a patient is diagnosed with an infection that is due to methicillin resistant *Staphylococcus aureus* (MRSA), and that infection has a combination code that includes the causal organism (e.g., sepsis, pneumonia) assign the appropriate combination code for the condition (e.g., code A41.02, Sepsis due to Methicillin resistant *Staphylococcus aureus* or code J15.212, Pneumonia due to Methicillin resistant *Staphylococcus aureus*). Do not assign code B95.62, Methicillin resistant *Staphylococcus aureus* infection as the cause of diseases classified elsewhere, as an additional code because the combination code includes the type of infection and the MRSA organism. Do not assign a code from subcategory Z16.11, Resistance to penicillins, as an additional diagnosis.

See Section C.1. for instructions on coding and sequencing of sepsis and severe sepsis.

(b) **Other codes for MRSA infection**

When there is documentation of a current infection (e.g., wound infection, stitch abscess, urinary tract infection) due to MRSA, and that infection does not have a combination code that includes the causal organism, assign the appropriate code to identify the condition along with code B95.62, Methicillin resistant *Staphylococcus aureus* infection as the cause of diseases classified elsewhere for the MRSA infection. Do not assign a code from subcategory Z16.11, Resistance to penicillins.

(c) **Methicillin susceptible *Staphylococcus aureus* (MSSA) and MRSA colonization**

The condition or state of being colonized or carrying MSSA or MRSA is called colonization or carriage, while an individual person is described as being colonized or being a carrier. Colonization means that MSSA or MSRA is present on or in the body without necessarily causing illness. A positive MRSA colonization test might be documented by the provider as "MRSA screen positive" or "MRSA nasal swab positive".

Assign code Z22.322, Carrier or suspected carrier of Methicillin resistant *Staphylococcus aureus*, for patients documented as having MRSA colonization. Assign code Z22.321, Carrier or suspected carrier of Methicillin susceptible *Staphylococcus aureus*, for patient documented as having MSSA colonization. Colonization is not necessarily indicative of a disease process or as the cause of a specific condition the patient may have unless documented as such by the provider.

(d) MRSA colonization and infection

If a patient is documented as having both MRSA colonization and infection during a hospital admission, code Z22.322, Carrier or suspected carrier of Methicillin resistant *Staphylococcus aureus*, and a code for the MRSA infection may both be assigned.

2. Chapter 2: Neoplasms (CØØ-D49)

General guidelines

Chapter 2 of the ICD-1Ø-CM contains the codes for most benign and all malignant neoplasms. Certain benign neoplasms, such as prostatic adenomas, may be found in the specific body system chapters. To properly code a neoplasm it is necessary to determine from the record if the neoplasm is benign, in-situ, malignant, or of uncertain histologic behavior. If malignant, any secondary (metastatic) sites should also be determined.

Primary malignant neoplasms overlapping site boundaries

A primary malignant neoplasm that overlaps two or more contiguous (next to each other) sites should be classified to the subcategory/code .8 ('overlapping lesion'), unless the combination is specifically indexed elsewhere. For multiple neoplasms of the same site that are not contiguous such as tumors in different quadrants of the same breast, codes for each site should be assigned.

Malignant neoplasm of ectopic tissue

Malignant neoplasms of ectopic tissue are to be coded to the site of origin mentioned, e.g., ectopic pancreatic malignant neoplasms involving the stomach are coded to pancreas, unspecified (C25.9).

The neoplasm table in the Alphabetic Index should be referenced first. However, if the histological term is documented, that term should be referenced first, rather than going immediately to the Neoplasm Table, in order to determine which column in the Neoplasm Table is appropriate. For example, if the documentation indicates "adenoma," refer to the term in the Alphabetic Index to review the entries under this term and the instructional note to "see also neoplasm, by site, benign." The table provides the proper code based on the type of neoplasm and the site. It is important to select the proper column in the table that corresponds to the type of neoplasm. The Tabular List should then be referenced to verify that the correct code has been selected from the table and that a more specific site code does not exist.

See Section I.C.21. Factors influencing health status and contact with health services, Status, for information regarding Z15.Ø, codes for genetic susceptibility to cancer.

a. Treatment directed at the malignancy

If the treatment is directed at the malignancy, designate the malignancy as the principal diagnosis.

The only exception to this guideline is if a patient admission/encounter is solely for the administration of chemotherapy, immunotherapy or radiation therapy, assign the appropriate Z51.- code as the first-listed or principal diagnosis, and the diagnosis or problem for which the service is being performed as a secondary diagnosis.

b. Treatment of secondary site

When a patient is admitted because of a primary neoplasm with metastasis and treatment is directed toward the secondary site only, the secondary neoplasm is designated as the principal diagnosis even though the primary malignancy is still present.

c. Coding and sequencing of complications

Coding and sequencing of complications associated with the malignancies or with the therapy thereof are subject to the following guidelines:

1) Anemia associated with malignancy

When admission/encounter is for management of an anemia associated with the malignancy, and the treatment is only for anemia, the appropriate code for the malignancy is sequenced as the principal or first-listed diagnosis followed by the appropriate code for the anemia (such as code D63.Ø, Anemia in neoplastic disease).

2) Anemia associated with chemotherapy, immunotherapy and radiation therapy

When the admission/encounter is for management of an anemia associated with an adverse effect of the administration of chemotherapy or immunotherapy and the only treatment is for the anemia, the anemia code is sequenced first followed by the appropriate codes for the neoplasm and the adverse effect (T45.1X5, Adverse effect of antineoplastic and immunosuppressive drugs).

When the admission/encounter is for management of an anemia associated with an adverse effect of radiotherapy, the anemia code should be sequenced first, followed by the appropriate neoplasm code and code Y84.2, Radiological procedure and radiotherapy as the cause of abnormal reaction of the patient, or of later complication, without mention of misadventure at the time of the procedure.

3) Management of dehydration due to the malignancy

When the admission/encounter is for management of dehydration due to the malignancy and only the dehydration is being treated (intravenous rehydration), the dehydration is sequenced first, followed by the code(s) for the malignancy.

4) Treatment of a complication resulting from a surgical procedure

When the admission/encounter is for treatment of a complication resulting from a surgical procedure, designate the complication as the principal or first-listed diagnosis if treatment is directed at resolving the complication.

d. Primary malignancy previously excised

When a primary malignancy has been previously excised or eradicated from its site and there is no further treatment directed to that site and there is no evidence of any existing primary malignancy, a code from category Z85, Personal history of malignant neoplasm, should be used to indicate the former site of the malignancy. Any mention of extension, invasion, or metastasis to another site is coded as a secondary malignant neoplasm to that site. The secondary site may be the principal or first-listed with the Z85 code used as a secondary code.

e. Admissions/Encounters involving chemotherapy, immunotherapy and radiation therapy

1) Episode of care involves surgical removal of neoplasm

When an episode of care involves the surgical removal of a neoplasm, primary or secondary site, followed by adjunct chemotherapy or radiation treatment during the same episode of care, the code for the neoplasm should be assigned as principal or first-listed diagnosis.

2) Patient admission/encounter solely for administration of chemotherapy, immunotherapy and radiation therapy

If a patient admission/encounter is solely for the administration of chemotherapy, immunotherapy or radiation therapy assign code Z51.Ø, Encounter for antineoplastic radiation therapy, or Z51.11, Encounter for antineoplastic chemotherapy, or Z51.12, Encounter for antineoplastic immunotherapy as the first-listed or principal diagnosis. If a patient receives more than one of these therapies during the same admission more than one of these codes may be assigned, in any sequence.

The malignancy for which the therapy is being administered should be assigned as a secondary diagnosis.

3) Patient admitted for radiation therapy, chemotherapy or immunotherapy and develops complications
When a patient is admitted for the purpose of radiotherapy, immunotherapy or chemotherapy and develops complications such as uncontrolled nausea and vomiting or dehydration, the principal or first-listed diagnosis is Z51.0, Encounter for antineoplastic radiation therapy, or Z51.11, Encounter for antineoplastic chemotherapy, or Z51.12, Encounter for antineoplastic immunotherapy followed by any codes for the complications.

f. Admission/encounter to determine extent of malignancy
When the reason for admission/encounter is to determine the extent of the malignancy, or for a procedure such as paracentesis or thoracentesis, the primary malignancy or appropriate metastatic site is designated as the principal or first-listed diagnosis, even though chemotherapy or radiotherapy is administered.

g. Symptoms, signs, and abnormal findings listed in Chapter 18 associated with neoplasms
Symptoms, signs, and ill-defined conditions listed in Chapter 18 characteristic of, or associated with, an existing primary or secondary site malignancy cannot be used to replace the malignancy as principal or first-listed diagnosis, regardless of the number of admissions or encounters for treatment and care of the neoplasm.

See section I.C.21. Factors influencing health status and contact with health services, Encounter for prophylactic organ removal.

h. Admission/encounter for pain control/management
See Section I.C.6. for information on coding admission/encounter for pain control/management.

i. Malignancy in two or more noncontiguous sites
A patient may have more than one malignant tumor in the same organ. These tumors may represent different primaries or metastatic disease, depending on the site. Should the documentation be unclear, the provider should be queried as to the status of each tumor so that the correct codes can be assigned.

j. Disseminated malignant neoplasm, unspecified
Code C80.0, Disseminated malignant neoplasm, unspecified, is for use only in those cases where the patient has advanced metastatic disease and no known primary or secondary sites are specified. It should not be used in place of assigning codes for the primary site and all known secondary sites.

k. Malignant neoplasm without specification of site
Code C80.1, Malignant (primary) neoplasm, unspecified, equates to Cancer, unspecified. This code should only be used when no determination can be made as to the primary site of a malignancy. This code should rarely be used in the inpatient setting.

l. Sequencing of neoplasm codes

1) Encounter for treatment of primary malignancy
If the reason for the encounter is for treatment of a primary malignancy, assign the malignancy as the principal/first-listed diagnosis. The primary site is to be sequenced first, followed by any metastatic sites.

2) Encounter for treatment of secondary malignancy
When an encounter is for a primary malignancy with metastasis and treatment is directed toward the metastatic (secondary) site(s) only, the metastatic site(s) is designated as the principal/first-listed diagnosis. The primary malignancy is coded as an additional code.

3) Malignant neoplasm in a pregnant patient
When a pregnant woman has a malignant neoplasm, a code from subcategory O9A.1-, Malignant neoplasm complicating pregnancy, childbirth, and the puerperium, should be sequenced first, followed by the appropriate code from Chapter 2 to indicate the type of neoplasm.

4) Encounter for complication associated with a neoplasm
When an encounter is for management of a complication associated with a neoplasm, such as dehydration, and the treatment is only for the complication, the complication is coded first, followed by the appropriate code(s) for the neoplasm.

The exception to this guideline is anemia. When the admission/encounter is for management of an anemia associated with the malignancy, and the treatment is only for anemia, the appropriate code for the malignancy is sequenced as the principal or first-listed diagnosis followed by code D63.0, Anemia in neoplastic disease.

5) Complication from surgical procedure for treatment of a neoplasm
When an encounter is for treatment of a complication resulting from a surgical procedure performed for the treatment of the neoplasm, designate the complication as the principal/first-listed diagnosis. See guideline regarding the coding of a current malignancy versus personal history to determine if the code for the neoplasm should also be assigned.

6) Pathologic fracture due to a neoplasm
When an encounter is for a pathological fracture due to a neoplasm, and the focus of treatment is the fracture, a code from subcategory M84.5, Pathological fracture in neoplastic disease, should be sequenced first, followed by the code for the neoplasm.

If the focus of treatment is the neoplasm with an associated pathological fracture, the neoplasm code should be sequenced first, followed by a code from M84.5 for the pathological fracture.

m. Current malignancy versus personal history of malignancy
When a primary malignancy has been excised but further treatment, such as an additional surgery for the malignancy, radiation therapy or chemotherapy is directed to that site, the primary malignancy code should be used until treatment is completed.

When a primary malignancy has been previously excised or eradicated from its site, there is no further treatment (of the malignancy) directed to that site, and there is no evidence of any existing primary malignancy, a code from category Z85, Personal history of malignant neoplasm, should be used to indicate the former site of the malignancy.

See Section I.C.21. Factors influencing health status and contact with health services, History (of)

n. Leukemia, multiple myeloma, and malignant plasma cell neoplasms in remission versus personal history
The categories for leukemia, and category C90, Multiple myeloma and malignant plasma cell neoplasms, have codes indicating whether or not the leukemia has achieved remission. There are also codes Z85.6, Personal history of leukemia, and Z85.79, Personal history of other malignant neoplasms of lymphoid, hematopoietic and related tissues. If the documentation is unclear, as to whether the leukemia has achieved remission, the provider should be queried.

See Section I.C.21. Factors influencing health status and contact with health services, History (of)

o. Aftercare following surgery for neoplasm
See Section I.C.21. Factors influencing health status and contact with health services, Aftercare

p. Follow-up care for completed treatment of a malignancy
See Section I.C.21. Factors influencing health status and contact with health services, Follow-up

q. Prophylactic organ removal for prevention of malignancy
See Section I.C. 21, Factors influencing health status and contact with health services, Prophylactic organ removal

r. Malignant neoplasm associated with transplanted organ
A malignant neoplasm of a transplanted organ should be coded as a transplant complication. Assign first the appropriate code from category T86.-, Complications of transplanted organs and tissue, followed by code C80.2, Malignant neoplasm associated with transplanted organ. Use an additional code for the specific malignancy.

3. Chapter 3: Disease of the Blood and Blood-forming Organs and Certain Disorders Involving the Immune Mechanism (D50-D89)
Reserved for future guideline expansion

4. Chapter 4: Endocrine, Nutritional, and Metabolic Diseases (E00-E89)

a. Diabetes mellitus

The diabetes mellitus codes are combination codes that include the type of diabetes mellitus, the body system affected, and the complications affecting that body system. As many codes within a particular category as are necessary to describe all of the complications of the disease may be used. They should be sequenced based on the reason for a particular encounter. Assign as many codes from categories E08 – E13 as needed to identify all of the associated conditions that the patient has.

1) Type of diabetes

The age of a patient is not the sole determining factor, though most type 1 diabetics develop the condition before reaching puberty. For this reason type 1 diabetes mellitus is also referred to as juvenile diabetes.

2) Type of diabetes mellitus not documented

If the type of diabetes mellitus is not documented in the medical record the default is E11.-, Type 2 diabetes mellitus.

3) Diabetes mellitus and the use of insulin

If the documentation in a medical record does not indicate the type of diabetes but does indicate that the patient uses insulin, code E11, Type 2 diabetes mellitus, should be assigned. Code Z79.4, Long-term (current) use of insulin, should also be assigned to indicate that the patient uses insulin. Code Z79.4 should not be assigned if insulin is given temporarily to bring a type 2 patient's blood sugar under control during an encounter.

4) Diabetes mellitus in pregnancy and gestational diabetes

See Section I.C.15. Diabetes mellitus in pregnancy.

See Section I.C.15. Gestational (pregnancy induced) diabetes

5) Complications due to insulin pump malfunction

(a) Underdose of insulin due to insulin pump failure

An underdose of insulin due to an insulin pump failure should be assigned to a code from subcategory T85.6, Mechanical complication of other specified internal and external prosthetic devices, implants and grafts, that specifies the type of pump malfunction, as the principal or first-listed code, followed by code T38.3x6-, Underdosing of insulin and oral hypoglycemic [antidiabetic] drugs. Additional codes for the type of diabetes mellitus and any associated complications due to the underdosing should also be assigned.

(b) Overdose of insulin due to insulin pump failure

The principal or first-listed code for an encounter due to an insulin pump malfunction resulting in an overdose of insulin, should also be T85.6-, Mechanical complication of other specified internal and external prosthetic devices, implants and grafts, followed by code T38.3X1-, Poisoning by insulin and oral hypoglycemic [antidiabetic] drugs, accidental (unintentional).

6) Secondary diabetes mellitus

Codes under categories E08, Diabetes mellitus due to underlying condition, E09, Drug or chemical induced diabetes mellitus, and E13, Other specified diabetes mellitus, identify complications/manifestations associated with secondary diabetes mellitus. Secondary diabetes is always caused by another condition or event (e.g., cystic fibrosis, malignant neoplasm of pancreas, pancreatectomy, adverse effect of drug, or poisoning).

(a) Secondary diabetes mellitus and the use of insulin

For patients who routinely use insulin, code Z79.4, Long-term (current) use of insulin, should also be assigned. Code Z79.4 should not be assigned if insulin is given temporarily to bring a patient's blood sugar under control during an encounter.

(b) Assigning and sequencing secondary diabetes codes and its causes

The sequencing of the secondary diabetes codes in relationship to codes for the cause of the diabetes is based on the Tabular List instructions for categories E08, E09 and E13.

(i) Secondary diabetes mellitus due to pancreatectomy

For postpancreatectomy diabetes mellitus (lack of insulin due to the surgical removal of all or part of the pancreas), assign code E89.1, Postprocedural hypoinsulinemia. Assign a code from category E13 and a code from subcategory Z90.41-, Acquired absence of pancreas, as additional codes.

(ii) Secondary diabetes due to drugs

Secondary diabetes may be caused by an adverse effect of correctly administered medications, poisoning or sequela of poisoning.

See section I.C.19.e for coding of adverse effects and poisoning, and section I.C.20 for external cause code reporting.

5. Chapter 5: Mental, Behavioral and Neurodevelopmental Disorders (F01 – F99)

a. Pain disorders related to psychological factors

Assign code F45.41, for pain that is exclusively related to psychological disorders. As indicated by the Excludes 1 note under category G89, a code from category G89 should not be assigned with code F45.41

Code F45.42, Pain disorders with related psychological factors, should be used with a code from category G89, Pain, not elsewhere classified, if there is documentation of a psychological component for a patient with acute or chronic pain.

See Section I.C.6. Pain

b. Mental and behavioral disorders due to psychoactive substance use

1) In remission

Selection of codes for "in remission" for categories F10-F19, Mental and behavioral disorders due to psychoactive substance use (categories F10-F19 with -.21) requires the provider's clinical judgment. The appropriate codes for "in remission" are assigned only on the basis of provider documentation (as defined in the Official Guidelines for Coding and Reporting).

2) Psychoactive substance use, abuse and dependence

When the provider documentation refers to use, abuse and dependence of the same substance (e.g. alcohol, opioid, cannabis, etc.), only one code should be assigned to identify the pattern of use based on the following hierarchy:

- If both use and abuse are documented, assign only the code for abuse
- If both abuse and dependence are documented, assign only the code for dependence
- If use, abuse and dependence are all documented, assign only the code for dependence
- If both use and dependence are documented, assign only the code for dependence.

3) Psychoactive substance use

As with all other diagnoses, the codes for psychoactive substance use (F10.9-, F11.9-, F12.9-, F13.9-, F14.9-, F15.9-, F16.9-) should only be assigned based on provider documentation and when they meet the definition of a reportable diagnosis (see Section III, Reporting Additional Diagnoses). The codes are to be used only when the psychoactive substance use is associated with a mental or behavioral disorder, and such a relationship is documented by the provider.

6. Chapter 6: Diseases of Nervous System (G00-G99)

a. Dominant/nondominant side

Codes from category G81, Hemiplegia and hemiparesis, and subcategories, G83.1, Monoplegia of lower limb, G83.2, Monoplegia of upper limb, and G83.3, Monoplegia, unspecified, identify whether the dominant or nondominant side is affected. Should the affected side be documented, but not specified as dominant or nondominant, and the classification system does not indicate a default, code selection is as follows:

- For ambidextrous patients, the default should be dominant.
- If the left side is affected, the default is non-dominant.

- If the right side is affected, the default is dominant.

b. Pain - Category G89

1) General coding information

Codes in category G89, Pain, not elsewhere classified, may be used in conjunction with codes from other categories and chapters to provide more detail about acute or chronic pain and neoplasm-related pain, unless otherwise indicated below.

If the pain is not specified as acute or chronic, post-thoracotomy, postprocedural, or neoplasm-related, do not assign codes from category G89.

A code from category G89 should not be assigned if the underlying (definitive) diagnosis is known, unless the reason for the encounter is pain control/ management and not management of the underlying condition.

When an admission or encounter is for a procedure aimed at treating the underlying condition (e.g., spinal fusion, kyphoplasty), a code for the underlying condition (e.g., vertebral fracture, spinal stenosis) should be assigned as the principal diagnosis. No code from category G89 should be assigned.

(a) Category G89 codes as principal or first-listed diagnosis

Category G89 codes are acceptable as principal diagnosis or the first-listed code:

- When pain control or pain management is the reason for the admission/encounter (e.g., a patient with displaced intervertebral disc, nerve impingement and severe back pain presents for injection of steroid into the spinal canal). The underlying cause of the pain should be reported as an additional diagnosis, if known.
- When a patient is admitted for the insertion of a neurostimulator for pain control, assign the appropriate pain code as the principal or first-listed diagnosis. When an admission or encounter is for a procedure aimed at treating the underlying condition and a neurostimulator is inserted for pain control during the same admission/encounter, a code for the underlying condition should be assigned as the principal diagnosis and the appropriate pain code should be assigned as a secondary diagnosis.

(b) Use of category G89 codes in conjunction with site specific pain codes

(i) Assigning category G89 and site-specific pain codes

Codes from category G89 may be used in conjunction with codes that identify the site of pain (including codes from chapter 18) if the category G89 code provides additional information. For example, if the code describes the site of the pain, but does not fully describe whether the pain is acute or chronic, then both codes should be assigned.

(ii) Sequencing of category G89 codes with site-specific pain codes

The sequencing of category G89 codes with site-specific pain codes (including chapter 18 codes), is dependent on the circumstances of the encounter/admission as follows:

- If the encounter is for pain control or pain management, assign the code from category G89 followed by the code identifying the specific site of pain (e.g., encounter for pain management for acute neck pain from trauma is assigned code G89.11, Acute pain due to trauma, followed by code M54.2, Cervicalgia, to identify the site of pain).
- If the encounter is for any other reason except pain control or pain management, and a related definitive diagnosis has not been established (confirmed) by the provider, assign the code for the specific site of pain first, followed by the appropriate code from category G89.

2) Pain due to devices, implants and grafts

See Section I.C.19. Pain due to medical devices

3) Postoperative pain

The provider's documentation should be used to guide the coding of postoperative pain, as well as *Section III. Reporting Additional Diagnoses* and *Section IV. Diagnostic Coding and Reporting in the Outpatient Setting.*

The default for post-thoracotomy and other postoperative pain not specified as acute or chronic is the code for the acute form.

Routine or expected postoperative pain immediately after surgery should not be coded.

(a) Postoperative pain not associated with specific postoperative complication

Postoperative pain not associated with a specific postoperative complication is assigned to the appropriate postoperative pain code in category G89.

(b) Postoperative pain associated with specific postoperative complication

Postoperative pain associated with a specific postoperative complication (such as painful wire sutures) is assigned to the appropriate code(s) found in Chapter 19, Injury, poisoning, and certain other consequences of external causes. If appropriate, use additional code(s) from category G89 to identify acute or chronic pain (G89.18 or G89.28).

4) Chronic pain

Chronic pain is classified to subcategory G89.2. There is no time frame defining when pain becomes chronic pain. The provider's documentation should be used to guide use of these codes.

5) Neoplasm related pain

Code G89.3 is assigned to pain documented as being related, associated or due to cancer, primary or secondary malignancy, or tumor. This code is assigned regardless of whether the pain is acute or chronic.

This code may be assigned as the principal or first-listed code when the stated reason for the admission/encounter is documented as pain control/pain management. The underlying neoplasm should be reported as an additional diagnosis.

When the reason for the admission/encounter is management of the neoplasm and the pain associated with the neoplasm is also documented, code G89.3 may be assigned as an additional diagnosis. It is not necessary to assign an additional code for the site of the pain.

See Section I.C.2 for instructions on the sequencing of neoplasms for all other stated reasons for the admission/encounter (except for pain control/pain management).

6) Chronic pain syndrome

Central pain syndrome (G89.Ø) and chronic pain syndrome (G89.4) are different than the term "chronic pain," and therefore codes should only be used when the provider has specifically documented this condition.

See Section I.C.5. Pain disorders related to psychological factors

7. Chapter 7: Diseases of Eye and Adnexa (HØØ-H59)

a. Glaucoma

1) Assigning glaucoma codes

Assign as many codes from category H4Ø, Glaucoma, as needed to identify the type of glaucoma, the affected eye, and the glaucoma stage.

2) Bilateral glaucoma with same type and stage

When a patient has bilateral glaucoma and both eyes are documented as being the same type and stage, and there is a code for bilateral glaucoma, report only the code for the type of glaucoma, bilateral, with the seventh character for the stage.

When a patient has bilateral glaucoma and both eyes are documented as being the same type and stage, and the classification does not provide a code for bilateral glaucoma (i.e. subcategories H4Ø.1Ø, H4Ø.11 and H4Ø.2Ø) report only one code for the type of glaucoma with the appropriate seventh character for the stage.

3) **Bilateral glaucoma stage with different types or stages**
When a patient has bilateral glaucoma and each eye is documented as having a different type or stage, and the classification distinguishes laterality, assign the appropriate code for each eye rather than the code for bilateral glaucoma.

When a patient has bilateral glaucoma and each eye is documented as having a different type, and the classification does not distinguish laterality (i.e. subcategories H4Ø.1Ø, H4Ø.11 and H4Ø.2Ø), assign one code for each type of glaucoma with the appropriate seventh character for the stage.

When a patient has bilateral glaucoma and each eye is documented as having the same type, but different stage, and the classification does not distinguish laterality (i.e. subcategories H4Ø.1Ø, H4Ø.11 and H4Ø.2Ø), assign a code for the type of glaucoma for each eye with the seventh character for the specific glaucoma stage documented for each eye.

4) **Patient admitted with glaucoma and stage evolves during the admission**
If a patient is admitted with glaucoma and the stage progresses during the admission, assign the code for highest stage documented.

5) **Indeterminate stage glaucoma**
Assignment of the seventh character "4" for "indeterminate stage" should be based on the clinical documentation. The seventh character "4" is used for glaucomas whose stage cannot be clinically determined. This seventh character should not be confused with the seventh character "Ø", unspecified, which should be assigned when there is no documentation regarding the stage of the glaucoma.

8. **Chapter 8: Diseases of Ear and Mastoid Process (H6Ø-H95)**
Reserved for future guideline expansion

9. **Chapter 9: Diseases of Circulatory System (IØØ-I99)**

a. **Hypertension**

1) **Hypertension with heart disease**
Heart conditions classified to I5Ø.- or I51.4-I51.9, are assigned to, a code from category I11, Hypertensive heart disease, when a causal relationship is stated (due to hypertension) or implied (hypertensive). Use an additional code from category I5Ø, Heart failure, to identify the type of heart failure in those patients with heart failure.

The same heart conditions (I5Ø.-, I51.4-I51.9) with hypertension, but without a stated causal relationship, are coded separately. Sequence according to the circumstances of the admission/encounter.

2) **Hypertensive chronic kidney disease**
Assign codes from category I12, Hypertensive chronic kidney disease, when both hypertension and a condition classifiable to category N18, Chronic kidney disease (CKD), are present. Unlike hypertension with heart disease, ICD-1Ø-CM presumes a cause-and-effect relationship and classifies chronic kidney disease with hypertension as hypertensive chronic kidney disease.

The appropriate code from category N18 should be used as a secondary code with a code from category I12 to identify the stage of chronic kidney disease.

See Section I.C.14. Chronic kidney disease.

If a patient has hypertensive chronic kidney disease and acute renal failure, an additional code for the acute renal failure is required.

3) **Hypertensive heart and chronic kidney disease**
Assign codes from combination category I13, Hypertensive heart and chronic kidney disease, when both hypertensive kidney disease and hypertensive heart disease are stated in the diagnosis. Assume a relationship between the hypertension and the chronic kidney disease, whether or not the condition is so designated. If heart failure is present, assign an additional code from category I5Ø to identify the type of heart failure.

The appropriate code from category N18, Chronic kidney disease, should be used as a secondary code with a code from category I13 to identify the stage of chronic kidney disease.

See Section I.C.14. Chronic kidney disease.

The codes in category I13, Hypertensive heart and chronic kidney disease, are combination codes that include hypertension, heart disease and chronic kidney disease. The Includes note at I13 specifies that the conditions included at I11 and I12 are included together in I13. If a patient has hypertension, heart disease and chronic kidney disease then a code from I13 should be used, not individual codes for hypertension, heart disease and chronic kidney disease, or codes from I11 or I12.

For patients with both acute renal failure and chronic kidney disease an additional code for acute renal failure is required.

4) **Hypertensive cerebrovascular disease**
For hypertensive cerebrovascular disease, first assign the appropriate code from categories I6Ø-I69, followed by the appropriate hypertension code.

5) **Hypertensive retinopathy**
Subcategory H35.Ø, Background retinopathy and retinal vascular changes, should be used with a code from category I1Ø – I15, Hypertensive disease to include the systemic hypertension. The sequencing is based on the reason for the encounter.

6) **Hypertension, secondary**
Secondary hypertension is due to an underlying condition. Two codes are required: one to identify the underlying etiology and one from category I15 to identify the hypertension. Sequencing of codes is determined by the reason for admission/encounter.

7) **Hypertension, transient**
Assign code RØ3.Ø, Elevated blood pressure reading without diagnosis of hypertension, unless patient has an established diagnosis of hypertension. Assign code O13.-, Gestational [pregnancy-induced] hypertension without significant proteinuria, or O14.-, Pre-eclampsia, for transient hypertension of pregnancy.

8) **Hypertension, controlled**
This diagnostic statement usually refers to an existing state of hypertension under control by therapy. Assign the appropriate code from categories I1Ø-I15, Hypertensive diseases.

9) **Hypertension, uncontrolled**
Uncontrolled hypertension may refer to untreated hypertension or hypertension not responding to current therapeutic regimen. In either case, assign the appropriate code from categories I1Ø-I15, Hypertensive diseases.

b. **Atherosclerotic coronary artery disease and angina**
ICD-1Ø-CM has combination codes for atherosclerotic heart disease with angina pectoris. The subcategories for these codes are I25.11, Atherosclerotic heart disease of native coronary artery with angina pectoris and I25.7, Atherosclerosis of coronary artery bypass graft(s) and coronary artery of transplanted heart with angina pectoris.

When using one of these combination codes it is not necessary to use an additional code for angina pectoris. A causal relationship can be assumed in a patient with both atherosclerosis and angina pectoris, unless the documentation indicates the angina is due to something other than the atherosclerosis.

If a patient with coronary artery disease is admitted due to an acute myocardial infarction (AMI), the AMI should be sequenced before the coronary artery disease.

See Section I.C.9. Acute myocardial infarction (AMI)

c. **Intraoperative and postprocedural cerebrovascular accident**
Medical record documentation should clearly specify the cause-and-effect relationship between the medical intervention and the cerebrovascular accident in order to assign a code for intraoperative or postprocedural cerebrovascular accident.

Proper code assignment depends on whether it was an infarction or hemorrhage and whether it occurred intraoperatively or postoperatively. If it was a cerebral hemorrhage, code assignment depends on the type of procedure performed.

d. Sequelae of cerebrovascular disease

1) Category I69, sequelae of cerebrovascular disease

Category I69 is used to indicate conditions classifiable to categories I60-I67 as the causes of sequela (neurologic deficits), themselves classified elsewhere. These "late effects" include neurologic deficits that persist after initial onset of conditions classifiable to categories I60-I67. The neurologic deficits caused by cerebrovascular disease may be present from the onset or may arise at any time after the onset of the condition classifiable to categories I60-I67.

Codes from category I69, Sequelae of cerebrovascular disease, that specify hemiplegia, hemiparesis and monoplegia identify whether the dominant or nondominant side is affected. Should the affected side be documented, but not specified as dominant or nondominant, and the classification system does not indicate a default, code selection is as follows:

- For ambidextrous patients, the default should be dominant.
- If the left side is affected, the default is non-dominant.
- If the right side is affected, the default is dominant.

2) Codes from category I69 with codes from I60-I67

Codes from category I69 may be assigned on a health care record with codes from I60-I67, if the patient has a current cerebrovascular disease and deficits from an old cerebrovascular disease.

3) Codes from category I69 and Personal history of transient ischemic attack (TIA) and cerebral infarction (Z86.73)

Codes from category I69 should not be assigned if the patient does not have neurologic deficits.

See Section I.C.21. 4. History (of) for use of personal history codes

e. Acute myocardial infarction (AMI)

1) ST elevation myocardial infarction (STEMI) and non ST elevation myocardial infarction (NSTEMI)

The ICD-10-CM codes for acute myocardial infarction (AMI) identify the site, such as anterolateral wall or true posterior wall. Subcategories I21.0-I21.2 and code I21.3 are used for ST elevation myocardial infarction (STEMI). Code I21.4, Non-ST elevation (NSTEMI) myocardial infarction, is used for non ST elevation myocardial infarction (NSTEMI) and nontransmural MIs.

If NSTEMI evolves to STEMI, assign the STEMI code. If STEMI converts to NSTEMI due to thrombolytic therapy, it is still coded as STEMI.

For encounters occurring while the myocardial infarction is equal to, or less than, four weeks old, including transfers to another acute setting or a postacute setting, and the patient requires continued care for the myocardial infarction, codes from category I21 may continue to be reported. For encounters after the 4 week time frame and the patient is still receiving care related to the myocardial infarction, the appropriate aftercare code should be assigned, rather than a code from category I21. For old or healed myocardial infarctions not requiring further care, code I25.2, Old myocardial infarction, may be assigned.

2) Acute myocardial infarction, unspecified

Code I21.3, ST elevation (STEMI) myocardial infarction of unspecified site, is the default for the unspecified term acute myocardial infarction. If only STEMI or transmural MI without the site is documented, query the provider as to the site, or assign code I21.3.

3) AMI documented as nontransmural or subendocardial but site provided

If an AMI is documented as nontransmural or subendocardial, but the site is provided, it is still coded as a subendocardial AMI.

See Section I.C.21.3 for information on coding status post administration of tPA in a different facility within the last 24 hrs.

4) Subsequent acute myocardial infarction

A code from category I22, Subsequent ST elevation (STEMI) and non ST elevation (NSTEMI) myocardial infarction, is to be used when a patient who has suffered an AMI has a new AMI within the 4 week time frame of the initial AMI. A code from category I22 must be used in conjunction with a code from category I21. The sequencing of the I22 and I21 codes depends on the circumstances of the encounter.

10. Chapter 10: Diseases of the Respiratory System (J00-J99)

a. Chronic Obstructive Pulmonary Disease [COPD] and Asthma

1) Acute exacerbation of chronic obstructive bronchitis and asthma

The codes in categories J44 and J45 distinguish between uncomplicated cases and those in acute exacerbation. An acute exacerbation is a worsening or a decompensation of a chronic condition. An acute exacerbation is not equivalent to an infection superimposed on a chronic condition, though an exacerbation may be triggered by an infection.

b. Acute Respiratory Failure

1) Acute respiratory failure as principal diagnosis

A code from subcategory J96.0, Acute respiratory failure, or subcategory J96.2, Acute and chronic respiratory failure, may be assigned as a principal diagnosis when it is the condition established after study to be chiefly responsible for occasioning the admission to the hospital, and the selection is supported by the Alphabetic Index and Tabular List. However, chapter-specific coding guidelines (such as obstetrics, poisoning, HIV, newborn) that provide sequencing direction take precedence.

2) Acute respiratory failure as secondary diagnosis

Respiratory failure may be listed as a secondary diagnosis if it occurs after admission, or if it is present on admission, but does not meet the definition of principal diagnosis.

3) Sequencing of acute respiratory failure and another acute condition

When a patient is admitted with respiratory failure and another acute condition, (e.g., myocardial infarction, cerebrovascular accident, aspiration pneumonia), the principal diagnosis will not be the same in every situation. This applies whether the other acute condition is a respiratory or nonrespiratory condition. Selection of the principal diagnosis will be dependent on the circumstances of admission. If both the respiratory failure and the other acute condition are equally responsible for occasioning the admission to the hospital, and there are no chapter-specific sequencing rules, the guideline regarding two or more diagnoses that equally meet the definition for principal diagnosis (Section II, C.) may be applied in these situations.

If the documentation is not clear as to whether acute respiratory failure and another condition are equally responsible for occasioning the admission, query the provider for clarification.

c. Influenza due to certain identified influenza viruses

Code only confirmed cases of influenza due to certain identified influenza viruses (category J09), and due to other identified influenza virus (category J10). This is an exception to the hospital inpatient guideline Section II, H. (Uncertain Diagnosis).

In this context, "confirmation" does not require documentation of positive laboratory testing specific for avian or other novel influenza A or other identified influenza virus. However, coding should be based on the provider's diagnostic statement that the patient has avian influenza, or other novel influenza A, for category J09, or has another particular identified strain of influenza, such as H1N1 or H3N2, but not identified as novel or variant, for category J10.

If the provider records "suspected" or "possible" or "probable" avian influenza, or novel influenza, or other identified influenza, then the appropriate influenza code from category J11, Influenza due to unidentified influenza virus, should be assigned. A code from category J09, Influenza due to certain identified influenza viruses, should not be assigned nor should a code from category J10, Influenza due to other identified influenza virus.

d. Ventilator associated pneumonia

1) Documentation of ventilator associated pneumonia

As with all procedural or postprocedural complications, code assignment is based on the provider's documentation of the relationship between the condition and the procedure.

Code J95.851, Ventilator associated pneumonia, should be assigned only when the provider has documented ventilator associated pneumonia (VAP). An additional code to identify the organism (e.g., Pseudomonas aeruginosa, code B96.5) should also be assigned. Do not assign an additional code from categories J12-J18 to identify the type of pneumonia.

Code J95.851 should not be assigned for cases where the patient has pneumonia and is on a mechanical ventilator and the provider has not specifically stated that the pneumonia is ventilator-associated pneumonia. If the documentation is unclear as to whether the patient has a pneumonia that is a complication attributable to the mechanical ventilator, query the provider.

2) Ventilator associated pneumonia develops after admission

A patient may be admitted with one type of pneumonia (e.g., code J13, Pneumonia due to Streptococcus pneumonia) and subsequently develop VAP. In this instance, the principal diagnosis would be the appropriate code from categories J12-J18 for the pneumonia diagnosed at the time of admission. Code J95.851, Ventilator associated pneumonia, would be assigned as an additional diagnosis when the provider has also documented the presence of ventilator associated pneumonia.

11. Chapter 11: Diseases of the Digestive System (KØØ-K95)

Reserved for future guideline expansion

12. Chapter 12: Diseases of the Skin and Subcutaneous Tissue (LØØ-L99)

a. Pressure ulcer stage codes

1) Pressure ulcer stages

Codes from category L89, Pressure ulcer, are combination codes that identify the site of the pressure ulcer as well as the stage of the ulcer.

The ICD-1Ø-CM classifies pressure ulcer stages based on severity, which is designated by stages 1-4, unspecified stage and unstageable.

Assign as many codes from category L89 as needed to identify all the pressure ulcers the patient has, if applicable.

2) Unstageable pressure ulcers

Assignment of the code for unstageable pressure ulcer (L89.--Ø) should be based on the clinical documentation. These codes are used for pressure ulcers whose stage cannot be clinically determined (e.g., the ulcer is covered by eschar or has been treated with a skin or muscle graft) and pressure ulcers that are documented as deep tissue injury but not documented as due to trauma. This code should not be confused with the codes for unspecified stage (L89.--9). When there is no documentation regarding the stage of the pressure ulcer, assign the appropriate code for unspecified stage (L89.--9).

3) Documented pressure ulcer stage

Assignment of the pressure ulcer stage code should be guided by clinical documentation of the stage or documentation of the terms found in the Alphabetic Index. For clinical terms describing the stage that are not found in the Alphabetic Index, and there is no documentation of the stage, the provider should be queried.

4) Patients admitted with pressure ulcers documented as healed

No code is assigned if the documentation states that the pressure ulcer is completely healed.

5) Patients admitted with pressure ulcers documented as healing

Pressure ulcers described as healing should be assigned the appropriate pressure ulcer stage code based on the documentation in the medical record. If the documentation does not provide information about the stage of the healing pressure ulcer, assign the appropriate code for unspecified stage.

If the documentation is unclear as to whether the patient has a current (new) pressure ulcer or if the patient is being treated for a healing pressure ulcer, query the provider.

6) Patient admitted with pressure ulcer evolving into another stage during the admission

If a patient is admitted with a pressure ulcer at one stage and it progresses to a higher stage, assign the code for the highest stage reported for that site.

13. Chapter 13: Diseases of the Musculoskeletal System and Connective Tissue (MØØ-M99)

a. Site and laterality

Most of the codes within Chapter 13 have site and laterality designations. The site represents the bone, joint or the muscle involved. For some conditions where more than one bone, joint or muscle is usually involved, such as osteoarthritis, there is a "multiple sites" code available. For categories where no multiple site code is provided and more than one bone, joint or muscle is involved, multiple codes should be used to indicate the different sites involved.

1) Bone versus joint

For certain conditions, the bone may be affected at the upper or lower end, (e.g., avascular necrosis of bone, M87, Osteoporosis, M8Ø, M81). Though the portion of the bone affected may be at the joint, the site designation will be the bone, not the joint.

b. Acute traumatic versus chronic or recurrent musculoskeletal conditions

Many musculoskeletal conditions are a result of previous injury or trauma to a site, or are recurrent conditions. Bone, joint or muscle conditions that are the result of a healed injury are usually found in chapter 13. Recurrent bone, joint or muscle conditions are also usually found in chapter 13. Any current, acute injury should be coded to the appropriate injury code from chapter 19. Chronic or recurrent conditions should generally be coded with a code from chapter 13. If it is difficult to determine from the documentation in the record which code is best to describe a condition, query the provider.

c. Coding of Pathologic Fractures

7th character A is for use as long as the patient is receiving active treatment for the fracture. Examples of active treatment are: surgical treatment, emergency department encounter, evaluation and treatment by a new physician. 7th character, D is to be used for encounters after the patient has completed active treatment. The other 7th characters, listed under each subcategory in the Tabular List, are to be used for subsequent encounters for treatment of problems associated with the healing, such as malunions, nonunions, and sequelae.

Care for complications of surgical treatment for fracture repairs during the healing or recovery phase should be coded with the appropriate complication codes.

See Section I.C.19. Coding of traumatic fractures.

d. Osteoporosis

Osteoporosis is a systemic condition, meaning that all bones of the musculoskeletal system are affected. Therefore, site is not a component of the codes under category M81, Osteoporosis without current pathological fracture. The site codes under category M8Ø, Osteoporosis with current pathological fracture, identify the site of the fracture, not the osteoporosis.

1) Osteoporosis without pathological fracture

Category M81, Osteoporosis without current pathological fracture, is for use for patients with osteoporosis who do not currently have a pathologic fracture due to the osteoporosis, even if they have had a fracture in the past. For patients with a history of osteoporosis fractures, status code Z87.31Ø, Personal history of (healed) osteoporosis fracture, should follow the code from M81.

2) Osteoporosis with current pathological fracture

Category M8Ø, Osteoporosis with current pathological fracture, is for patients who have a current pathologic fracture at the time of an encounter. The codes under M8Ø identify the site of the fracture. A code from category M8Ø, not a traumatic fracture code, should be used for any patient with known osteoporosis who suffers a fracture, even if the patient had a minor fall or trauma, if that fall or trauma would not usually break a normal, healthy bone.

14. **Chapter 14: Diseases of Genitourinary System (N00-N99)**

a. **Chronic kidney disease**

1) **Stages of chronic kidney disease (CKD)**

The ICD-10-CM classifies CKD based on severity. The severity of CKD is designated by stages 1-5. Stage 2, code N18.2, equates to mild CKD; stage 3, code N18.3, equates to moderate CKD; and stage 4, code N18.4, equates to severe CKD. Code N18.6, End stage renal disease (ESRD), is assigned when the provider has documented end-stage-renal disease (ESRD).

If both a stage of CKD and ESRD are documented, assign code N18.6 only.

2) **Chronic kidney disease and kidney transplant status**

Patients who have undergone kidney transplant may still have some form of chronic kidney disease (CKD) because the kidney transplant may not fully restore kidney function. Therefore, the presence of CKD alone does not constitute a transplant complication. Assign the appropriate N18 code for the patient's stage of CKD and code Z94.0, Kidney transplant status. If a transplant complication such as failure or rejection or other transplant complication is documented, see section I.C.19.g for information on coding complications of a kidney transplant. If the documentation is unclear as to whether the patient has a complication of the transplant, query the provider.

3) **Chronic kidney disease with other conditions**

Patients with CKD may also suffer from other serious conditions, most commonly diabetes mellitus and hypertension. The sequencing of the CKD code in relationship to codes for other contributing conditions is based on the conventions in the Tabular List.

See I.C.9. Hypertensive chronic kidney disease.

See I.C.19. Chronic kidney disease and kidney transplant complications.

15. **Chapter 15: Pregnancy, Childbirth, and the Puerperium (O00-O9A)**

a. **General Rules for Obstetric Cases**

1) **Codes from chapter 15 and sequencing priority**

Obstetric cases require codes from chapter 15, codes in the range O00-O9A, Pregnancy, Childbirth, and the Puerperium. Chapter 15 codes have sequencing priority over codes from other chapters. Additional codes from other chapters may be used in conjunction with chapter 15 codes to further specify conditions. Should the provider document that the pregnancy is incidental to the encounter, then code Z33.1, Pregnant state, incidental, should be used in place of any chapter 15 codes. It is the provider's responsibility to state that the condition being treated is not affecting the pregnancy.

2) **Chapter 15 codes used only on the maternal record**

Chapter 15 codes are to be used only on the maternal record, never on the record of the newborn.

3) **Final character for trimester**

The majority of codes in Chapter 15 have a final character indicating the trimester of pregnancy. The timeframes for the trimesters are indicated at the beginning of the chapter. If trimester is not a component of a code it is because the condition always occurs in a specific trimester, or the concept of trimester of pregnancy is not applicable. Certain codes have characters for only certain trimesters because the condition does not occur in all trimesters, but it may occur in more than just one.

Assignment of the final character for trimester should be based on the provider's documentation of the trimester (or number of weeks) for the current admission/encounter. This applies to the assignment of trimester for pre-existing conditions as well as those that develop during or are due to the pregnancy. The provider's documentation of the number of weeks may be used to assign the appropriate code identifying the trimester.

Whenever delivery occurs during the current admission, and there is an "in childbirth" option for the obstetric complication being coded, the "in childbirth" code should be assigned.

4) **Selection of trimester for inpatient admissions that encompass more than one trimesters**

In instances when a patient is admitted to a hospital for complications of pregnancy during one trimester and remains in the hospital into a subsequent trimester, the trimester character for the antepartum complication code should be assigned on the basis of the trimester when the complication developed, not the trimester of the discharge. If the condition developed prior to the current admission/encounter or represents a pre-existing condition, the trimester character for the trimester at the time of the admission/encounter should be assigned.

5) **Unspecified trimester**

Each category that includes codes for trimester has a code for "unspecified trimester." The "unspecified trimester" code should rarely be used, such as when the documentation in the record is insufficient to determine the trimester and it is not possible to obtain clarification.

6) **7th character for fetus identification**

Where applicable, a 7th character is to be assigned for certain categories (O31, O32, O33.3 - O33.6, O35, O36, O40, O41, O60.1, O60.2, O64, and O69) to identify the fetus for which the complication code applies.

Assign 7th character "0":

- For single gestations
- When the documentation in the record is insufficient to determine the fetus affected and it is not possible to obtain clarification.
- When it is not possible to clinically determine which fetus is affected.

b. **Selection of OB principal or first-listed diagnosis**

1) **Routine outpatient prenatal visits**

For routine outpatient prenatal visits when no complications are present, a code from category Z34, Encounter for supervision of normal pregnancy, should be used as the first-listed diagnosis. These codes should not be used in conjunction with chapter 15 codes.

2) **Prenatal outpatient visits for high-risk patients**

For routine prenatal outpatient visits for patients with high-risk pregnancies, a code from category O09, Supervision of high-risk pregnancy, should be used as the first-listed diagnosis. Secondary chapter 15 codes may be used in conjunction with these codes if appropriate.

3) **Episodes when no delivery occurs**

In episodes when no delivery occurs, the principal diagnosis should correspond to the principal complication of the pregnancy which necessitated the encounter. Should more than one complication exist, all of which are treated or monitored, any of the complications codes may be sequenced first.

4) **When a delivery occurs**

When a delivery occurs, the principal diagnosis should correspond to the main circumstances or complication of the delivery. In cases of cesarean delivery, the selection of the principal diagnosis should be the condition established after study that was responsible for the patient's admission. If the patient was admitted with a condition that resulted in the performance of a cesarean procedure, that condition should be selected as the principal diagnosis. If the reason for the admission/encounter was unrelated to the condition resulting in the cesarean delivery, the condition related to the reason for the admission/encounter should be selected as the principal diagnosis.

5) **Outcome of delivery**

A code from category Z37, Outcome of delivery, should be included on every maternal record when a delivery has occurred. These codes are not to be used on subsequent records or on the newborn record.

c. **Pre-existing conditions versus conditions due to the pregnancy**

Certain categories in Chapter 15 distinguish between conditions of the mother that existed prior to pregnancy (pre-existing) and those that are a direct result of pregnancy. When assigning codes from Chapter 15, it is important to assess if a condition was pre-existing prior to pregnancy or developed during or due to the pregnancy in order to assign the correct code.

Categories that do not distinguish between pre-existing and pregnancy-related conditions may be used for either. It is acceptable to use codes specifically for the puerperium with codes complicating pregnancy and childbirth if a condition arises postpartum during the delivery encounter.

d. **Pre-existing hypertension in pregnancy**

Category O1Ø, Pre-existing hypertension complicating pregnancy, childbirth and the puerperium, includes codes for hypertensive heart and hypertensive chronic kidney disease. When assigning one of the O1Ø codes that includes hypertensive heart disease or hypertensive chronic kidney disease, it is necessary to add a secondary code from the appropriate hypertension category to specify the type of heart failure or chronic kidney disease.

See Section I.C.9. Hypertension.

e. **Fetal conditions affecting the management of the mother**

1) **Codes from categories O35 and O36**

Codes from categories O35, Maternal care for known or suspected fetal abnormality and damage, and O36, Maternal care for other fetal problems, are assigned only when the fetal condition is actually responsible for modifying the management of the mother, i.e., by requiring diagnostic studies, additional observation, special care, or termination of pregnancy. The fact that the fetal condition exists does not justify assigning a code from this series to the mother's record.

2) **In utero surgery**

In cases when surgery is performed on the fetus, a diagnosis code from category O35, Maternal care for known or suspected fetal abnormality and damage, should be assigned identifying the fetal condition. Assign the appropriate procedure code for the procedure performed.

No code from Chapter 16, the perinatal codes, should be used on the mother's record to identify fetal conditions. Surgery performed in utero on a fetus is still to be coded as an obstetric encounter.

f. **HIV Infection in pregnancy, childbirth and the puerperium**

During pregnancy, childbirth or the puerperium, a patient admitted because of an HIV-related illness should receive a principal diagnosis from subcategory O98.7-, Human immunodeficiency [HIV] disease complicating pregnancy, childbirth and the puerperium, followed by the code(s) for the HIV-related illness(es).

Patients with asymptomatic HIV infection status admitted during pregnancy, childbirth, or the puerperium should receive codes of O98.7- and Z21, Asymptomatic human immunodeficiency virus [HIV] infection status.

g. **Diabetes mellitus in pregnancy**

Diabetes mellitus is a significant complicating factor in pregnancy. Pregnant women who are diabetic should be assigned a code from category O24, Diabetes mellitus in pregnancy, childbirth, and the puerperium, first, followed by the appropriate diabetes code(s) (EØ8-E13) from Chapter 4.

h. **Long term use of insulin**

Code Z79.4, Long-term (current) use of insulin, should also be assigned if the diabetes mellitus is being treated with insulin.

i. **Gestational (pregnancy induced) diabetes**

Gestational (pregnancy induced) diabetes can occur during the second and third trimester of pregnancy in women who were not diabetic prior to pregnancy. Gestational diabetes can cause complications in the pregnancy similar to those of pre-existing diabetes mellitus. It also puts the woman at greater risk of developing diabetes after the pregnancy. Codes for gestational diabetes are in subcategory O24.4, Gestational diabetes mellitus. No other code from category O24, Diabetes mellitus in pregnancy, childbirth, and the puerperium, should be used with a code from O24.4.

The codes under subcategory O24.4 include diet controlled and insulin controlled. If a patient with gestational diabetes is treated with both diet and insulin, only the code for insulin-controlled is required.

Code Z79.4, Long-term (current) use of insulin, should not be assigned with codes from subcategory O24.4.

An abnormal glucose tolerance in pregnancy is assigned a code from subcategory O99.81, Abnormal glucose complicating pregnancy, childbirth, and the puerperium.

j. **Sepsis and septic shock complicating abortion, pregnancy, childbirth and the puerperium**

When assigning a chapter 15 code for sepsis complicating abortion, pregnancy, childbirth, and the puerperium, a code for the specific type of infection should be assigned as an additional diagnosis. If severe sepsis is present, a code from subcategory R65.2, Severe sepsis, and code(s) for associated organ dysfunction(s) should also be assigned as additional diagnoses.

k. **Puerperal sepsis**

Code O85, Puerperal sepsis, should be assigned with a secondary code to identify the causal organism (e.g., for a bacterial infection, assign a code from category B95-B96, Bacterial infections in conditions classified elsewhere). A code from category A4Ø, Streptococcal sepsis, or A41, Other sepsis, should not be used for puerperal sepsis. If applicable, use additional codes to identify severe sepsis (R65.2-) and any associated acute organ dysfunction.

l. **Alcohol and tobacco use during pregnancy, childbirth and the puerperium**

1) **Alcohol use during pregnancy, childbirth and the puerperium**

Codes under subcategory O99.31, Alcohol use complicating pregnancy, childbirth, and the puerperium, should be assigned for any pregnancy case when a mother uses alcohol during the pregnancy or postpartum. A secondary code from category F1Ø, Alcohol related disorders, should also be assigned to identify manifestations of the alcohol use.

2) **Tobacco use during pregnancy, childbirth and the puerperium**

Codes under subcategory O99.33, Smoking (tobacco) complicating pregnancy, childbirth, and the puerperium, should be assigned for any pregnancy case when a mother uses any type of tobacco product during the pregnancy or postpartum. A secondary code from category F17, Nicotine dependence, or code Z72.Ø, Tobacco use, should also be assigned to identify the type of nicotine dependence.

m. **Poisoning, toxic effects, adverse effects and underdosing in a pregnant patient**

A code from subcategory O9A.2, Injury, poisoning and certain other consequences of external causes complicating pregnancy, childbirth, and the puerperium, should be sequenced first, followed by the appropriate injury, poisoning, toxic effect, adverse effect or underdosing code, and then the additional code(s) that specifies the condition caused by the poisoning, toxic effect, adverse effect or underdosing.

See Section I.C.19. Adverse effects, poisoning, underdosing and toxic effects.

n. **Normal delivery, code O8Ø**

1) **Encounter for full term uncomplicated delivery**

Code O8Ø should be assigned when a woman is admitted for a full-term normal delivery and delivers a single, healthy infant without any complications antepartum, during the delivery, or postpartum during the delivery episode. Code O8Ø is always a principal diagnosis. It is not to be used if any other code from chapter 15 is needed to describe a current complication of the antenatal, delivery, or perinatal period. Additional codes from other chapters may be used with code O8Ø if they are not related to or are in any way complicating the pregnancy.

2) **Uncomplicated delivery with resolved antepartum complication**
Code O80 may be used if the patient had a complication at some point during the pregnancy, but the complication is not present at the time of the admission for delivery.

3) **Outcome of delivery for O80**
Z37.0, Single live birth, is the only outcome of delivery code appropriate for use with O80.

o. **The peripartum and postpartum periods**

1) **Peripartum and postpartum periods**
The postpartum period begins immediately after delivery and continues for six weeks following delivery. The peripartum period is defined as the last month of pregnancy to five months postpartum.

2) **Peripartum and postpartum complication**
A postpartum complication is any complication occurring within the six-week period.

3) **Pregnancy-related complications after 6 week period**
Chapter 15 codes may also be used to describe pregnancy-related complications after the peripartum or postpartum period if the provider documents that a condition is pregnancy related.

4) **Admission for routine postpartum care following delivery outside hospital**
When the mother delivers outside the hospital prior to admission and is admitted for routine postpartum care and no complications are noted, code Z39.0, Encounter for care and examination of mother immediately after delivery, should be assigned as the principal diagnosis.

5) **Pregnancy associated cardiomyopathy**
Pregnancy associated cardiomyopathy, code O90.3, is unique in that it may be diagnosed in the third trimester of pregnancy but may continue to progress months after delivery. For this reason, it is referred to as peripartum cardiomyopathy. Code O90.3 is only for use when the cardiomyopathy develops as a result of pregnancy in a woman who did not have pre-existing heart disease.

p. **Code O94, Sequelae of complication of pregnancy, childbirth, and the puerperium**

1) **Code O94**
Code O94, Sequelae of complication of pregnancy, childbirth, and the puerperium, is for use in those cases when an initial complication of a pregnancy develops a sequelae requiring care or treatment at a future date.

2) **After the initial postpartum period**
This code may be used at any time after the initial postpartum period.

3) **Sequencing of code O94**
This code, like all late effect codes, is to be sequenced following the code describing the sequelae of the complication.

q. **Termination of Pregnancy and Spontaneous Abortions**

1) **Abortion with liveborn fetus**
When an attempted termination of pregnancy results in a liveborn fetus, assign code Z33.2, Encounter for elective termination of pregnancy and a code from category Z37, Outcome of Delivery.

2) **Retained products of conception following an abortion**
Subsequent encounters for retained products of conception following a spontaneous abortion or elective termination of pregnancy are assigned the appropriate code from category O03, Spontaneous abortion, or codes O07.4, Failed attempted termination of pregnancy without complication and Z33.2, Encounter for elective termination of pregnancy. This advice is appropriate even when the patient was discharged previously with a discharge diagnosis of complete abortion.

3) **Complications leading to abortion**
Codes from Chapter 15 may be used as additional codes to identify any documented complications of the pregnancy in conjunction with codes in categories in O07 and O08.

r. **Abuse in a pregnant patient**
For suspected or confirmed cases of abuse of a pregnant patient, a code(s) from subcategories O9A.3, Physical abuse complicating pregnancy, childbirth, and the puerperium, O9A.4, Sexual abuse complicating pregnancy, childbirth, and the puerperium, and O9A.5, Psychological abuse complicating pregnancy, childbirth, and the puerperium, should be sequenced first, followed by the appropriate codes (if applicable) to identify any associated current injury due to physical abuse, sexual abuse, and the perpetrator of abuse.

See Section I.C.19.f. Adult and child abuse, neglect and other maltreatment.

16. Chapter 16: Certain Conditions Origination in the Perinatal Period (P00-P96)

For coding and reporting purposes the perinatal period is defined as before birth through the 28th day following birth. The following guidelines are provided for reporting purposes

a. **General Perinatal Rules**

1) **Use of Chapter 16 codes**
Codes in this chapter are never for use on the maternal record. Codes from Chapter 15, the obstetric chapter, are never permitted on the newborn record. Chapter 16 codes may be used throughout the life of the patient if the condition is still present.

2) **Principal diagnosis for birth record**
When coding the birth episode in a newborn record, assign a code from category Z38, Liveborn infants according to place of birth and type of delivery, as the principal diagnosis. A code from category Z38 is assigned only once, to a newborn at the time of birth. If a newborn is transferred to another institution, a code from category Z38 should not be used at the receiving hospital.

A code from category Z38 is used only on the newborn record, not on the mother's record.

3) **Use of codes from other chapters with codes from Chapter 16**
Codes from other chapters may be used with codes from chapter 16 if the codes from the other chapters provide more specific detail. Codes for signs and symptoms may be assigned when a definitive diagnosis has not been established. If the reason for the encounter is a perinatal condition, the code from chapter 16 should be sequenced first.

4) **Use of Chapter 16 codes after the perinatal period**
Should a condition originate in the perinatal period, and continue throughout the life of the patient, the perinatal code should continue to be used regardless of the patient's age.

5) **Birth process or community acquired conditions**
If a newborn has a condition that may be either due to the birth process or community acquired and the documentation does not indicate which it is, the default is due to the birth process and the code from Chapter 16 should be used. If the condition is community-acquired, a code from Chapter 16 should not be assigned.

6) **Code all clinically significant conditions**
All clinically significant conditions noted on routine newborn examination should be coded. A condition is clinically significant if it requires:

- clinical evaluation; or
- therapeutic treatment; or
- diagnostic procedures; or
- extended length of hospital stay; or
- increased nursing care and/or monitoring; or
- has implications for future health care needs

Note: The perinatal guidelines listed above are the same as the general coding guidelines for "additional diagnoses", except for the final point regarding implications for future health care needs. Codes should be assigned for conditions that have been specified by the provider as having implications for future health care needs.

b. Observation and evaluation of newborns for suspected conditions not found
Reserved for future expansion

c. Coding Additional Perinatal Diagnoses

1) Assigning codes for conditions that require treatment
Assign codes for conditions that require treatment or further investigation, prolong the length of stay, or require resource utilization.

2) Codes for conditions specified as having implications for future health care needs
Assign codes for conditions that have been specified by the provider as having implications for future health care needs.

Note: This guideline should not be used for adult patients.

d. Prematurity and fetal growth retardation
Providers utilize different criteria in determining prematurity. A code for prematurity should not be assigned unless it is documented. Assignment of codes in categories PØ5, Disorders of newborn related to slow fetal growth and fetal malnutrition, and PØ7, Disorders of newborn related to short gestation and low birth weight, not elsewhere classified, should be based on the recorded birth weight and estimated gestational age. Codes from category PØ5 should not be assigned with codes from category PØ7.

When both birth weight and gestational age are available, two codes from category PØ7 should be assigned, with the code for birth weight sequenced before the code for gestational age.

e. Low birth weight and immaturity status
Codes from category PØ7, Disorders of newborn related to short gestation and low birth weight, not elsewhere classified, are for use for a child or adult who was premature or had a low birth weight as a newborn and this is affecting the patient's current health status.

See Section I.C.21. Factors influencing health status and contact with health services, Status.

f. Bacterial sepsis of newborn
Category P36, Bacterial sepsis of newborn, includes congenital sepsis. If a perinate is documented as having sepsis without documentation of congenital or community acquired, the default is congenital and a code from category P36 should be assigned. If the P36 code includes the causal organism, an additional code from category B95, Streptococcus, Staphylococcus, and Enterococcus as the cause of diseases classified elsewhere, or B96, Other bacterial agents as the cause of diseases classified elsewhere, should not be assigned. If the P36 code does not include the causal organism, assign an additional code from category B96. If applicable, use additional codes to identify severe sepsis (R65.2-) and any associated acute organ dysfunction.

g. Stillbirth
Code P95, Stillbirth, is only for use in institutions that maintain separate records for stillbirths. No other code should be used with P95. Code P95 should not be used on the mother's record.

17. Chapter 17: Congenital Malformations, Deformations, and Chromosomal Abnormalities (QØØ-Q99)
Assign an appropriate code(s) from categories QØØ-Q99, Congenital malformations, deformations, and chromosomal abnormalities when a malformation/deformation or chromosomal abnormality is documented. A malformation/deformation/or chromosomal abnormality may be the principal/first-listed diagnosis on a record or a secondary diagnosis.

When a malformation/deformation/or chromosomal abnormality does not have a unique code assignment, assign additional code(s) for any manifestations that may be present.

When the code assignment specifically identifies the malformation/deformation/or chromosomal abnormality, manifestations that are an inherent component of the anomaly should not be coded separately. Additional codes should be assigned for manifestations that are not an inherent component.

Codes from Chapter 17 may be used throughout the life of the patient. If a congenital malformation or deformity has been corrected, a personal history code should be used to identify the history of the malformation or deformity. Although present at birth, malformation/deformation/or chromosomal abnormality may not be identified until later in life. Whenever the condition is diagnosed by the physician, it is appropriate to assign a code from codes QØØ-Q99.

For the birth admission, the appropriate code from category Z38, Liveborn infants, according to place of birth and type of delivery, should be sequenced as the principal diagnosis, followed by any congenital anomaly codes, QØØ- Q99.

18. Chapter 18: Symptoms, Signs, and Abnormal Clinical and Laboratory Findings, Not Elsewhere Classified (RØØ-R99)
Chapter 18 includes symptoms, signs, abnormal results of clinical or other investigative procedures, and ill-defined conditions regarding which no diagnosis classifiable elsewhere is recorded. Signs and symptoms that point to a specific diagnosis have been assigned to a category in other chapters of the classification.

a. Use of symptom codes
Codes that describe symptoms and signs are acceptable for reporting purposes when a related definitive diagnosis has not been established (confirmed) by the provider.

b. Use of a symptom code with a definitive diagnosis code
Codes for signs and symptoms may be reported in addition to a related definitive diagnosis when the sign or symptom is not routinely associated with that diagnosis, such as the various signs and symptoms associated with complex syndromes. The definitive diagnosis code should be sequenced before the symptom code.

Signs or symptoms that are associated routinely with a disease process should not be assigned as additional codes, unless otherwise instructed by the classification.

c. Combination codes that include symptoms
ICD-1Ø-CM contains a number of combination codes that identify both the definitive diagnosis and common symptoms of that diagnosis. When using one of these combination codes, an additional code should not be assigned for the symptom.

d. Repeated falls
Code R29.6, Repeated falls, is for use for encounters when a patient has recently fallen and the reason for the fall is being investigated.

Code Z91.81, History of falling, is for use when a patient has fallen in the past and is at risk for future falls. When appropriate, both codes R29.6 and Z91.81 may be assigned together.

e. Coma scale
The coma scale codes (R4Ø.2-) can be used in conjunction with traumatic brain injury codes, acute cerebrovascular disease or sequelae of cerebrovascular disease codes. These codes are primarily for use by trauma registries, but they may be used in any setting where this information is collected. The coma scale codes should be sequenced after the diagnosis code(s).

These codes, one from each subcategory, are needed to complete the scale. The 7th character indicates when the scale was recorded. The 7th character should match for all three codes.

At a minimum, report the initial score documented on presentation at your facility. This may be a score from the emergency medicine technician (EMT) or in the emergency department. If desired, a facility may choose to capture multiple Glasgow coma scale scores.

Assign code R4Ø.24, Glasgow coma scale, total score, when only the total score is documented in the medical record and not the individual score(s).

f. Functional quadriplegia
Functional quadriplegia (code R53.2) is the lack of ability to use one's limbs or to ambulate due to extreme debility. It is not associated with neurologic deficit or injury, and code R53.2 should not be used for cases of neurologic quadriplegia. It should only be assigned if functional quadriplegia is specifically documented in the medical record.

g. SIRS due to non-infectious process
The systemic inflammatory response syndrome (SIRS) can develop as a result of certain non-infectious disease processes, such as trauma, malignant neoplasm, or pancreatitis. When SIRS is documented with a noninfectious condition, and no subsequent infection is documented, the code for the underlying condition, such as an injury, should be assigned, followed by code R65.1Ø, Systemic inflammatory response syndrome (SIRS) of non-infectious origin without acute organ dysfunction, or code R65.11, Systemic inflammatory response syndrome (SIRS) of non-infectious origin

with acute organ dysfunction. If an associated acute organ dysfunction is documented, the appropriate code(s) for the specific type of organ dysfunction(s) should be assigned in addition to code R65.11. If acute organ dysfunction is documented, but it cannot be determined if the acute organ dysfunction is associated with SIRS or due to another condition (e.g., directly due to the trauma), the provider should be queried.

h. Death NOS

Code R99, Ill-defined and unknown cause of mortality, is only for use in the very limited circumstance when a patient who has already died is brought into an emergency department or other healthcare facility and is pronounced dead upon arrival. It does not represent the discharge disposition of death.

19. Chapter 19: Injury, Poisoning, and Certain Other Consequences of External Causes (S00-T88)

a. Application of 7th Characters in Chapter 19

Most categories in chapter 19 have a 7th character requirement for each applicable code. Most categories in this chapter have three 7th character values (with the exception of fractures): A, initial encounter, D, subsequent encounter and S, sequela. Categories for traumatic fractures have additional 7th character values.

7th character "A", initial encounter is used while the patient is receiving active treatment for the condition. Examples of active treatment are: surgical treatment, emergency department encounter, and evaluation and treatment by a new physician.

7th character "D" subsequent encounter is used for encounters after the patient has received active treatment of the condition and is receiving routine care for the condition during the healing or recovery phase. Examples of subsequent care are: cast change or removal, removal of external or internal fixation device, medication adjustment, other aftercare and follow up visits following treatment of the injury or condition.

The aftercare Z codes should not be used for aftercare for conditions such as injuries or poisonings, where 7th characters are provided to identify subsequent care. For example, for aftercare of an injury, assign the acute injury code with the 7th character "D" (subsequent encounter).

7th character "S", sequela, is for use for complications or conditions that arise as a direct result of a condition, such as scar formation after a burn. The scars are sequelae of the burn. When using 7th character "S", it is necessary to use both the injury code that precipitated the sequela and the code for the sequela itself. The "S" is added only to the injury code, not the sequela code. The 7th character "S" identifies the injury responsible for the sequela. The specific type of sequela (e.g. scar) is sequenced first, followed by the injury code.

b. Coding of injuries

When coding injuries, assign separate codes for each injury unless a combination code is provided, in which case the combination code is assigned. Code T07, Unspecified multiple injuries should not be assigned in the inpatient setting unless information for a more specific code is not available. Traumatic injury codes (S00-T14.9) are not to be used for normal, healing surgical wounds or to identify complications of surgical wounds.

The code for the most serious injury, as determined by the provider and the focus of treatment, is sequenced first.

1) Superficial injuries

Superficial injuries such as abrasions or contusions are not coded when associated with more severe injuries of the same site.

2) Primary injury with damage to nerves/blood vessels

When a primary injury results in minor damage to peripheral nerves or blood vessels, the primary injury is sequenced first with additional code(s) for injuries to nerves and spinal cord (such as category S04), and/or injury to blood vessels (such as category S15). When the primary injury is to the blood vessels or nerves, that injury should be sequenced first.

c. Coding of traumatic fractures

The principles of multiple coding of injuries should be followed in coding fractures. Fractures of specified sites are coded individually by site in accordance with both the provisions within categories S02, S12, S22, S32, S42, S49, S52, S59, S62, S72, S79, S82, S89, S92 and the level of detail furnished by medical record content.

A fracture not indicated as open or closed should be coded to closed. A fracture not indicated whether displaced or not displaced should be coded to displaced.

More specific guidelines are as follows:

1) Initial vs. subsequent encounter for fractures

Traumatic fractures are coded using the appropriate 7th character extension for initial encounter (A, B, C) while the patient is receiving active treatment for the fracture. Examples of active treatment are: surgical treatment, emergency department encounter, and evaluation and treatment by a new physician. The appropriate 7th character for initial encounter should also be assigned for a patient who delayed seeking treatment for the fracture or nonunion.

Fractures are coded using the appropriate 7th character extension for subsequent care for encounters after the patient has completed active treatment of the fracture and is receiving routine care for the fracture during the healing or recovery phase. Examples of fracture aftercare are: cast change or removal, removal of external or internal fixation device, medication adjustment, and follow-up visits following fracture treatment.

Care for complications of surgical treatment for fracture repairs during the healing or recovery phase should be coded with the appropriate complication codes.

Care of complications of fractures, such as malunion and nonunion, should be reported with the appropriate 7th character extensions for subsequent care with nonunion (K, M, N,) or subsequent care with malunion (P, Q, R).

A code from category M80, not a traumatic fracture code, should be used for any patient with known osteoporosis who suffers a fracture, even if the patient had a minor fall or trauma, if that fall or trauma would not usually break a normal, healthy bone.

See Section I.C.13. Osteoporosis.

The aftercare Z codes should not be used for aftercare for traumatic fractures. For aftercare of a traumatic fracture, assign the acute fracture code with the appropriate 7th character.

2) Multiple fractures sequencing

Multiple fractures are sequenced in accordance with the severity of the fracture.

d. Coding of burns and corrosions

The ICD-10-CM makes a distinction between burns and corrosions. The burn codes are for thermal burns, except sunburns, that come from a heat source, such as a fire or hot appliance. The burn codes are also for burns resulting from electricity and radiation. Corrosions are burns due to chemicals. The guidelines are the same for burns and corrosions.

Current burns (T20-T25) are classified by depth, extent and by agent (X code). Burns are classified by depth as first degree (erythema), second degree (blistering), and third degree (full-thickness involvement). Burns of the eye and internal organs (T26-T28) are classified by site, but not by degree.

1) Sequencing of burn and related condition codes

Sequence first the code that reflects the highest degree of burn when more than one burn is present.

a. When the reason for the admission or encounter is for treatment of external multiple burns, sequence first the code that reflects the burn of the highest degree.

b. When a patient has both internal and external burns, the circumstances of admission govern the selection of the principal diagnosis or first-listed diagnosis.

c. When a patient is admitted for burn injuries and other related conditions such as smoke inhalation and/or respiratory failure, the circumstances of admission govern the selection of the principal or first-listed diagnosis.

2) **Burns of the same local site**
Classify burns of the same local site (three-character category level, T20-T28) but of different degrees to the subcategory identifying the highest degree recorded in the diagnosis.

3) **Non-healing burns**
Non-healing burns are coded as acute burns.

Necrosis of burned skin should be coded as a non-healed burn.

4) **Infected burn**
For any documented infected burn site, use an additional code for the infection.

5) **Assign separate codes for each burn site**
When coding burns, assign separate codes for each burn site. Category T30, Burn and corrosion, body region unspecified is extremely vague and should rarely be used.

6) **Burns and corrosions classified according to extent of body surface involved**
Assign codes from category T31, Burns classified according to extent of body surface involved, or T32, Corrosions classified according to extent of body surface involved, when the site of the burn is not specified or when there is a need for additional data. It is advisable to use category T31 as additional coding when needed to provide data for evaluating burn mortality, such as that needed by burn units. It is also advisable to use category T31 as an additional code for reporting purposes when there is mention of a third-degree burn involving 20 percent or more of the body surface.

Categories T31 and T32 are based on the classic "rule of nines" in estimating body surface involved: head and neck are assigned nine percent, each arm nine percent, each leg 18 percent, the anterior trunk 18 percent, posterior trunk 18 percent, and genitalia one percent. Providers may change these percentage assignments where necessary to accommodate infants and children who have proportionately larger heads than adults, and patients who have large buttocks, thighs, or abdomen that involve burns.

7) **Encounters for treatment of sequela of burns**
Encounters for the treatment of the late effects of burns or corrosions (i.e., scars or joint contractures) should be coded with a burn or corrosion code with the 7th character "S" for sequela.

8) **Sequelae with a late effect code and current burn**
When appropriate, both a code for a current burn or corrosion with 7th character "A" or "D" and a burn or corrosion code with 7th character "S" may be assigned on the same record (when both a current burn and sequelae of an old burn exist). Burns and corrosions do not heal at the same rate and a current healing wound may still exist with sequela of a healed burn or corrosion.

9) **Use of an external cause code with burns and corrosions**
An external cause code should be used with burns and corrosions to identify the source and intent of the burn, as well as the place where it occurred.

e. Adverse effects, poisoning, underdosing and toxic effects
Codes in categories T36-T65 are combination codes that include the substance that was taken as well as the intent. No additional external cause code is required for poisonings, toxic effects, adverse effects and underdosing codes.

1) **Do not code directly from the Table of Drugs**
Do not code directly from the Table of Drugs and Chemicals. Always refer back to the Tabular List.

2) **Use as many codes as necessary to describe**
Use as many codes as necessary to describe completely all drugs, medicinal or biological substances.

3) **If the same code would describe the causative agent**
If the same code would describe the causative agent for more than one adverse reaction, poisoning, toxic effect or underdosing, assign the code only once.

4) **If two or more drugs, medicinal or biological substances**
If two or more drugs, medicinal or biological substances are reported, code each individually unless a combination code is listed in the Table of Drugs and Chemicals.

5) **The occurrence of drug toxicity is classified in ICD-10-CM as follows:**

(a) **Adverse effect**
When coding an adverse effect of a drug that has been correctly prescribed and properly administered, assign the appropriate code for the nature of the adverse effect followed by the appropriate code for the adverse effect of the drug (T36-T50). The code for the drug should have a 5th or 6th character "5" (for example T36.0X5-) Examples of the nature of an adverse effect are tachycardia, delirium, gastrointestinal hemorrhaging, vomiting, hypokalemia, hepatitis, renal failure, or respiratory failure.

(b) **Poisoning**
When coding a poisoning or reaction to the improper use of a medication (e.g., overdose, wrong substance given or taken in error, wrong route of administration), first assign the appropriate code from categories T36-T50. The poisoning codes have an associated intent as their 5th or 6th character (accidental, intentional self-harm, assault and undetermined. Use additional code(s) for all manifestations of poisonings.

If there is also a diagnosis of abuse or dependence of the substance, the abuse or dependence is assigned as an additional code.

Examples of poisoning include:

(i) Error was made in drug prescription
Errors made in drug prescription or in the administration of the drug by provider, nurse, patient, or other person.

(ii) Overdose of a drug intentionally taken
If an overdose of a drug was intentionally taken or administered and resulted in drug toxicity, it would be coded as a poisoning.

(iii) Nonprescribed drug taken with correctly prescribed and properly administered drug
If a nonprescribed drug or medicinal agent was taken in combination with a correctly prescribed and properly administered drug, any drug toxicity or other reaction resulting from the interaction of the two drugs would be classified as a poisoning.

(iv) Interaction of drug(s) and alcohol
When a reaction results from the interaction of a drug(s) and alcohol, this would be classified as poisoning.

See Section I.C.4. if poisoning is the result of insulin pump malfunctions.

(c) **Underdosing**
Underdosing refers to taking less of a medication than is prescribed by a provider or a manufacturer's instruction. For underdosing, assign the code from categories T36-T50 (fifth or sixth character "6").

Codes for underdosing should never be assigned as principal or first-listed codes. If a patient has a relapse or exacerbation of the medical condition for which the drug is prescribed because of the reduction in dose, then the medical condition itself should be coded.

Noncompliance (Z91.12-, Z91.13-) or complication of care (Y63.6-Y63.9) codes are to be used with an underdosing code to indicate intent, if known.

(d) **Toxic effects**
When a harmful substance is ingested or comes in contact with a person, this is classified as a toxic effect. The toxic effect codes are in categories T51-T65.

Toxic effect codes have an associated intent: accidental, intentional self-harm, assault and undetermined.

f. Adult and child abuse, neglect and other maltreatment

Sequence first the appropriate code from categories T74.- (Adult and child abuse, neglect and other maltreatment, confirmed) or T76.- (Adult and child abuse, neglect and other maltreatment, suspected) for abuse, neglect and other maltreatment, followed by any accompanying mental health or injury code(s).

If the documentation in the medical record states abuse or neglect it is coded as confirmed (T74.-). It is coded as suspected if it is documented as suspected (T76.-).

For cases of confirmed abuse or neglect an external cause code from the assault section (X92-Y08) should be added to identify the cause of any physical injuries. A perpetrator code (Y07) should be added when the perpetrator of the abuse is known. For suspected cases of abuse or neglect, do not report external cause or perpetrator code.

If a suspected case of abuse, neglect or mistreatment is ruled out during an encounter code Z04.71, Encounter for examination and observation following alleged physical adult abuse, ruled out, or code Z04.72, Encounter for examination and observation following alleged child physical abuse, ruled out, should be used, not a code from T76.

If a suspected case of alleged rape or sexual abuse is ruled out during an encounter code Z04.41, Encounter for examination and observation following alleged physical adult abuse, ruled out, or code Z04.42, Encounter for examination and observation following alleged rape or sexual abuse, ruled out, should be used, not a code from T76.

See Section I.C.15. Abuse in a pregnant patient.

g. Complications of care

1) General guidelines for complications of care

(a) Documentation of complications of care

See Section I.B.16. for information on documentation of complications of care.

2) Pain due to medical devices

Pain associated with devices, implants or grafts left in a surgical site (for example painful hip prosthesis) is assigned to the appropriate code(s) found in Chapter 19, Injury, poisoning, and certain other consequences of external causes. Specific codes for pain due to medical devices are found in the T code section of the ICD-10-CM. Use additional code(s) from category G89 to identify acute or chronic pain due to presence of the device, implant or graft (G89.18 or G89.28).

3) Transplant complications

(a) Transplant complications other than kidney

Codes under category T86, Complications of transplanted organs and tissues, are for use for both complications and rejection of transplanted organs. A transplant complication code is only assigned if the complication affects the function of the transplanted organ. Two codes are required to fully describe a transplant complication: the appropriate code from category T86 and a secondary code that identifies the complication.

Pre-existing conditions or conditions that develop after the transplant are not coded as complications unless they affect the function of the transplanted organs.

See I.C.21. for transplant organ removal status

See I.C.2. for malignant neoplasm associated with transplanted organ.

(b) Kidney transplant complications

Patients who have undergone kidney transplant may still have some form of chronic kidney disease (CKD) because the kidney transplant may not fully restore kidney function. Code T86.1- should be assigned for documented complications of a kidney transplant, such as transplant failure or rejection or other transplant complication. Code T86.1- should not be assigned for post kidney transplant patients who have chronic kidney (CKD) unless a transplant complication such as transplant failure or rejection is documented. If the documentation is unclear as to whether the patient has a complication of the transplant, query the provider.

Conditions that affect the function of the transplanted kidney, other than CKD, should be assigned a code from subcategory T86.1, Complications of transplanted organ, Kidney, and a secondary code that identifies the complication.

For patients with CKD following a kidney transplant, but who do not have a complication such as failure or rejection, *see section I.C.14. Chronic kidney disease and kidney transplant status.*

4) Complication codes that include the external cause

As with certain other T codes, some of the complications of care codes have the external cause included in the code. The code includes the nature of the complication as well as the type of procedure that caused the complication. No external cause code indicating the type of procedure is necessary for these codes.

5) Complications of care codes within the body system chapters

Intraoperative and postprocedural complication codes are found within the body system chapters with codes specific to the organs and structures of that body system. These codes should be sequenced first, followed by a code(s) for the specific complication, if applicable.

20. Chapter 20: External Causes of Morbidity (V00-Y99)

The external causes of morbidity codes should never be sequenced as the first-listed or principal diagnosis.

External cause codes are intended to provide data for injury research and evaluation of injury prevention strategies. These codes capture how the injury or health condition happened (cause), the intent (unintentional or accidental; or intentional, such as suicide or assault), the place where the event occurred the activity of the patient at the time of the event, and the person's status (e.g., civilian, military).

There is no national requirement for mandatory ICD-10-CM external cause code reporting. Unless a provider is subject to a state-based external cause code reporting mandate or these codes are required by a particular payer, reporting of ICD-10-CM codes in Chapter 20, External Causes of Morbidity, is not required. In the absence of a mandatory reporting requirement, providers are encouraged to voluntarily report external cause codes, as they provide valuable data for injury research and evaluation of injury prevention strategies.

a. General external cause coding guidelines

1) Used with any code in the range of A00.0-T88.9, Z00-Z99

An external cause code may be used with any code in the range of A00.0-T88.9, Z00-Z99, classification that is a health condition due to an external cause. Though they are most applicable to injuries, they are also valid for use with such things as infections or diseases due to an external source, and other health conditions, such as a heart attack that occurs during strenuous physical activity.

2) External cause code used for length of treatment

Assign the external cause code, with the appropriate 7th character (initial encounter, subsequent encounter or sequela) for each encounter for which the injury or condition is being treated.

3) Use the full range of external cause codes

Use the full range of external cause codes to completely describe the cause, the intent, the place of occurrence, and if applicable, the activity of the patient at the time of the event, and the patient's status, for all injuries, and other health conditions due to an external cause.

4) Assign as many external cause codes as necessary

Assign as many external cause codes as necessary to fully explain each cause. If only one external code can be recorded, assign the code most related to the principal diagnosis.

5) The selection of the appropriate external cause code

The selection of the appropriate external cause code is guided by the Alphabetic Index of External Causes and by Inclusion and Exclusion notes in the Tabular List.

6) **External cause code can never be a principal diagnosis**
An external cause code can never be a principal (first-listed) diagnosis.

7) **Combination external cause codes**
Certain of the external cause codes are combination codes that identify sequential events that result in an injury, such as a fall which results in striking against an object. The injury may be due to either event or both. The combination external cause code used should correspond to the sequence of events regardless of which caused the most serious injury.

8) **No external cause code needed in certain circumstances**
No external cause code from Chapter 20 is needed if the external cause and intent are included in a code from another chapter (e.g. T36.0x1- Poisoning by penicillins, accidental (unintentional)).

b. **Place of occurrence guideline**
Codes from category Y92, Place of occurrence of the external cause, are secondary codes for use after other external cause codes to identify the location of the patient at the time of injury or other condition.

A place of occurrence code is used only once, at the initial encounter for treatment. No 7th characters are used for Y92. Only one code from Y92 should be recorded on a medical record.

Do not use place of occurrence code Y92.9 if the place is not stated or is not applicable.

c. **Activity code**
Assign a code from category Y93, Activity code, to describe the activity of the patient at the time the injury or other health condition occurred.

An activity code is used only once, at the initial encounter for treatment. Only one code from Y93 should be recorded on a medical record.

The activity codes are not applicable to poisonings, adverse effects, misadventures or sequela.

Do not assign Y93.9, Unspecified activity, if the activity is not stated.

A code from category Y93 is appropriate for use with external cause and intent codes if identifying the activity provides additional information about the event.

d. **Place of occurrence, activity, and status codes used with other external cause code**
When applicable, place of occurrence, activity, and external cause status codes are sequenced after the main external cause code(s). Regardless of the number of external cause codes assigned, there should be only one place of occurrence code, one activity code, and one external cause status code assigned to an encounter.

e. **If the reporting format limits the number of external cause codes**
If the reporting format limits the number of external cause codes that can be used in reporting clinical data, report the code for the cause/intent most related to the principal diagnosis. If the format permits capture of additional external cause codes, the cause/intent, including medical misadventures, of the additional events should be reported rather than the codes for place, activity, or external status.

f. **Multiple external cause coding guidelines**
More than one external cause code is required to fully describe the external cause of an illness or injury. The assignment of external cause codes should be sequenced in the following priority:

If two or more events cause separate injuries, an external cause code should be assigned for each cause. The first-listed external cause code will be selected in the following order:

External codes for child and adult abuse take priority over all other external cause codes.

See Section I.C.19., Child and Adult abuse guidelines.

External cause codes for terrorism events take priority over all other external cause codes except child and adult abuse.

External cause codes for cataclysmic events take priority over all other external cause codes except child and adult abuse and terrorism.

External cause codes for transport accidents take priority over all other external cause codes except cataclysmic events, child and adult abuse and terrorism.

Activity and external cause status codes are assigned following all causal (intent) external cause codes.

The first-listed external cause code should correspond to the cause of the most serious diagnosis due to an assault, accident, or self-harm, following the order of hierarchy listed above.

g. **Child and adult abuse guideline**
Adult and child abuse, neglect and maltreatment are classified as assault. Any of the assault codes may be used to indicate the external cause of any injury resulting from the confirmed abuse.

For confirmed cases of abuse, neglect and maltreatment, when the perpetrator is known, a code from Y07, Perpetrator of maltreatment and neglect, should accompany any other assault codes.

See Section I.C.19. Adult and child abuse, neglect and other maltreatment

h. **Unknown or undetermined intent guideline**
If the intent (accident, self-harm, assault) of the cause of an injury or other condition is unknown or unspecified, code the intent as accidental intent. All transport accident categories assume accidental intent.

1) **Use of undetermined intent**
External cause codes for events of undetermined intent are only for use if the documentation in the record specifies that the intent cannot be determined.

i. **Sequelae (Late Effects) of external cause guidelines**

1) **Sequelae external cause codes**
Sequela are reported using the external cause code with the 7th character extension "S" for sequela. These codes should be used with any report of a late effect or sequela resulting from a previous injury.

2) **Sequela external cause code with a related current injury**
A sequela external cause code should never be used with a related current nature of injury code.

3) **Use of sequela external cause codes for subsequent visits**
Use a late effect external cause code for subsequent visits when a late effect of the initial injury is being treated. Do not use a late effect external cause code for subsequent visits for follow-up care (e.g., to assess healing, to receive rehabilitative therapy) of the injury when no late effect of the injury has been documented.

j. **Terrorism guidelines**

1) **Cause of injury identified by the Federal Government (FBI) as terrorism**
When the cause of an injury is identified by the Federal Government (FBI) as terrorism, the first-listed external cause code should be a code from category Y38, Terrorism. The definition of terrorism employed by the FBI is found at the inclusion note at the beginning of category Y38. Use additional code for place of occurrence (Y92.-). More than one Y38 code may be assigned if the injury is the result of more than one mechanism of terrorism.

2) **Cause of an injury is suspected to be the result of terrorism**
When the cause of an injury is suspected to be the result of terrorism a code from category Y38 should not be assigned. Suspected cases should be classified as assault.

3) **Code Y38.9, terrorism, secondary effects**
Assign code Y38.9, Terrorism, secondary effects, for conditions occurring subsequent to the terrorist event. This code should not be assigned for conditions that are due to the initial terrorist act.

It is acceptable to assign code Y38.9 with another code from Y38 if there is an injury due to the initial terrorist event and an injury that is a subsequent result of the terrorist event.

k. **External cause status**
A code from category Y99, External cause status, should be assigned whenever any other external cause code is assigned for an encounter, including an Activity code, except for the events noted below. Assign a code from category Y99, External cause status, to

indicate the work status of the person at the time the event occurred. The status code indicates whether the event occurred during military activity, whether a non-military person was at work, whether an individual including a student or volunteer was involved in a non-work activity at the time of the causal event.

A code from Y99, External cause status, should be assigned, when applicable, with other external cause codes, such as transport accidents and falls. The external cause status codes are not applicable to poisonings, adverse effects, misadventures or late effects.

Do not assign a code from category Y99 if no other external cause codes (cause, activity) are applicable for the encounter.

An external cause status code is used only once, at the initial encounter for treatment. Only one code from Y99 should be recorded on a medical record.

Do not assign code Y99.9, Unspecified external cause status, if the status is not stated.

21. Chapter 21: Factors Influencing Health Status and Contact with Health Services (ZØØ-Z99)

Note: The chapter specific guidelines provide additional information about the use of Z codes for specified encounters.

a. Use of Z codes in any healthcare setting

Z codes are for use in any healthcare setting. Z codes may be used as either a first-listed (principal diagnosis code in the inpatient setting) or secondary code, depending on the circumstances of the encounter. Certain Z codes may only be used as first-listed or principal diagnosis.

b. Z Codes indicate a reason for an encounter

Z codes are not procedure codes. A corresponding procedure code must accompany a Z code to describe any procedure performed.

c. Categories of Z codes

1) Contact/exposure

Category Z2Ø indicates contact with, and suspected exposure to, communicable diseases. These codes are for patients who do not show any sign or symptom of a disease but are suspected to have been exposed to it by close personal contact with an infected individual or are in an area where a disease is epidemic.

Category Z77, indicates contact with and suspected exposures hazardous to health.

Contact/exposure codes may be used as a first-listed code to explain an encounter for testing, or, more commonly, as a secondary code to identify a potential risk.

2) Inoculations and vaccinations

Code Z23 is for encounters for inoculations and vaccinations. It indicates that a patient is being seen to receive a prophylactic inoculation against a disease. Procedure codes are required to identify the actual administration of the injection and the type(s) of immunizations given. Code Z23 may be used as a secondary code if the inoculation is given as a routine part of preventive health care, such as a well-baby visit.

3) Status

Status codes indicate that a patient is either a carrier of a disease or has the sequelae or residual of a past disease or condition. This includes such things as the presence of prosthetic or mechanical devices resulting from past treatment. A status code is informative, because the status may affect the course of treatment and its outcome. A status code is distinct from a history code. The history code indicates that the patient no longer has the condition.

A status code should not be used with a diagnosis code from one of the body system chapters, if the diagnosis code includes the information provided by the status code. For example, code Z94.1, Heart transplant status, should not be used with a code from subcategory T86.2, Complications of heart transplant. The status code does not provide additional information. The complication code indicates that the patient is a heart transplant patient.

For encounters for weaning from a mechanical ventilator, assign a code from subcategory J96.1, Chronic respiratory failure, followed by code Z99.11, Dependence on respirator [ventilator] status.

The status Z codes/categories are:

Z14 Genetic carrier

Genetic carrier status indicates that a person carries a gene, associated with a particular disease, which may be passed to offspring who may develop that disease. The person does not have the disease and is not at risk of developing the disease.

Z15 Genetic susceptibility to disease

Genetic susceptibility indicates that a person has a gene that increases the risk of that person developing the disease.

Codes from category Z15 should not be used as principal or first-listed codes. If the patient has the condition to which he/she is susceptible, and that condition is the reason for the encounter, the code for the current condition should be sequenced first. If the patient is being seen for follow-up after completed treatment for this condition, and the condition no longer exists, a follow-up code should be sequenced first, followed by the appropriate personal history and genetic susceptibility codes. If the purpose of the encounter is genetic counseling associated with procreative management, code Z31.5, Encounter for genetic counseling, should be assigned as the first-listed code, followed by a code from category Z15. Additional codes should be assigned for any applicable family or personal history.

Z16 Resistance to antimicrobial drugs

This code indicates that a patient has a condition that is resistant to antimicrobial drug treatment. Sequence the infection code first.

Z17 Estrogen receptor status

Z18 Retained foreign body fragments

Z21 Asymptomatic HIV infection status

This code indicates that a patient has tested positive for HIV but has manifested no signs or symptoms of the disease.

Z22 Carrier of infectious disease

Carrier status indicates that a person harbors the specific organisms of a disease without manifest symptoms and is capable of transmitting the infection.

Z28.3 Underimmunization status

Z33.1 Pregnant state, incidental

This code is a secondary code only for use when the pregnancy is in no way complicating the reason for visit. Otherwise, a code from the obstetric chapter is required.

Z66 Do not resuscitate

This code may be used when it is documented by the provider that a patient is on do not resuscitate status at any time during the stay.

Z67 Blood type

Z68 Body mass index (BMI)

Z74.Ø1 Bed confinement status

Z76.82 Awaiting organ transplant status

Z78 Other specified health status

Code Z78.1, Physical restraint status, may be used when it is documented by the provider that a patient has been put in restraints during the current encounter. Please note that this code should not be reported when it is documented by the provider that a patient is temporarily restrained during a procedure.

Z79 Long-term (current) drug therapy

Codes from this category indicate a patient's continuous use of a prescribed drug (including such things as aspirin therapy) for the long-term treatment of a condition or for prophylactic use. It is not for use for patients who have addictions to drugs. This subcategory is not for use of medications for detoxification or maintenance programs to prevent withdrawal symptoms in patients with drug dependence (e.g., methadone maintenance for opiate dependence). Assign the appropriate code for the drug dependence instead.

Assign a code from Z79 if the patient is receiving a medication for an extended period as a prophylactic measure (such as for the prevention of deep vein thrombosis) or as treatment of a chronic condition (such as arthritis) or a disease requiring a lengthy course of treatment (such as cancer). Do not assign a code from category Z79 for medication being administered for a brief period of time to treat an acute illness or injury (such as a course of antibiotics to treat acute bronchitis).

Z88 Allergy status to drugs, medicaments and biological substances

Except: Z88.9, Allergy status to unspecified drugs, medicaments and biological substances status

Z89 Acquired absence of limb

Z9Ø Acquired absence of organs, not elsewhere classified

Z91.Ø- Allergy status, other than to drugs and biological substances

Z92.82 Status post administration of tPA (rtPA) in a different facility within the last 24 hours prior to admission to a current facility

Assign code Z92.82, Status post administration of tPA (rtPA) in a different facility within the last 24 hours prior to admission to current facility, as a secondary diagnosis when a patient is received by transfer into a facility and documentation indicates they were administered tissue plasminogen activator (tPA) within the last 24 hours prior to admission to the current facility.

This guideline applies even if the patient is still receiving the tPA at the time they are received into the current facility.

The appropriate code for the condition for which the tPA was administered (such as cerebrovascular disease or myocardial infarction) should be assigned first.

Code Z92.82 is only applicable to the receiving facility record and not to the transferring facility record.

Z93 Artificial opening status

Z94 Transplanted organ and tissue status

Z95 Presence of cardiac and vascular implants and grafts

Z96 Presence of other functional implants

Z97 Presence of other devices

Z98 Other postprocedural states

Assign code Z98.85, Transplanted organ removal status, to indicate that a transplanted organ has been previously removed. This code should not be assigned for the encounter in which the transplanted organ is removed. The complication necessitating removal of the transplant organ should be assigned for that encounter.

See section I.C19.g.3. for information on the coding of organ transplant complications.

Z99 Dependence on enabling machines and devices, not elsewhere classified

Note: Categories Z89-Z9Ø and Z93-Z99 are for use only if there are no complications or malfunctions of the organ or tissue replaced, the amputation site or the equipment on which the patient is dependent.

4) History (of)

There are two types of history Z codes, personal and family. Personal history codes explain a patient's past medical condition that no longer exists and is not receiving any treatment, but that has the potential for recurrence, and therefore may require continued monitoring.

Family history codes are for use when a patient has a family member(s) who has had a particular disease that causes the patient to be at higher risk of also contracting the disease.

Personal history codes may be used in conjunction with follow-up codes and family history codes may be used in conjunction with screening codes to explain the need for a test or procedure. History codes are also acceptable on any medical record regardless of the reason for visit. A history of an illness, even if no longer present, is important information that may alter the type of treatment ordered.

The history Z code categories are:

Z8Ø Family history of primary malignant neoplasm

Z81 Family history of mental and behavioral disorders

Z82 Family history of certain disabilities and chronic diseases (leading to disablement)

Z83 Family history of other specific disorders

Z84 Family history of other conditions

Z85 Personal history of malignant neoplasm

Z86 Personal history of certain other diseases

Z87 Personal history of other diseases and conditions

Z91.4- Personal history of psychological trauma, not elsewhere classified

Z91.5 Personal history of self-harm

Z91.8- Other specified personal risk factors, not elsewhere classified

Exception: Z91.83, Wandering in diseases classified elsewhere

Z92 Personal history of medical treatment

Except: Z92.Ø, Personal history of contraception

Except: Z92.82, Status post administration of tPA (rtPA) in a different facility within the last 24 hours prior to admission to a current facility

5) Screening

Screening is the testing for disease or disease precursors in seemingly well individuals so that early detection and treatment can be provided for those who test positive for the disease (e.g., screening mammogram).

The testing of a person to rule out or confirm a suspected diagnosis because the patient has some sign or symptom is a diagnostic examination, not a screening. In these cases, the sign or symptom is used to explain the reason for the test.

A screening code may be a first-listed code if the reason for the visit is specifically the screening exam. It may also be used as an additional code if the screening is done during an office visit for other health problems. A screening code is not necessary if the screening is inherent to a routine examination, such as a pap smear done during a routine pelvic examination.

Should a condition be discovered during the screening then the code for the condition may be assigned as an additional diagnosis.

The Z code indicates that a screening exam is planned. A procedure code is required to confirm that the screening was performed.

The screening Z codes/categories:

Z11 Encounter for screening for infectious and parasitic diseases

Z12 Encounter for screening for malignant neoplasms

Z13 Encounter for screening for other diseases and disorders

Except: Z13.9, Encounter for screening, unspecified

Z36 Encounter for antenatal screening for mother

6) Observation

There are two observation Z code categories. They are for use in very limited circumstances when a person is being observed for a suspected condition that is ruled out. The observation codes are not for use if an injury or illness or any signs or symptoms related to the suspected condition are present. In such cases the diagnosis/symptom code is used with the corresponding external cause code.

The observation codes are to be used as principal diagnosis only. Additional codes may be used in addition to the observation code but only if they are unrelated to the suspected condition being observed.

Codes from subcategory Z03.7, Encounter for suspected maternal and fetal conditions ruled out, may either be used as a first-listed or as an additional code assignment depending on the case. They are for use in very limited circumstances on a maternal record when an encounter is for a suspected maternal or fetal condition that is ruled out during that encounter (for example, a maternal or fetal condition may be suspected due to an abnormal test result). These codes should not be used when the condition is confirmed. In those cases, the confirmed condition should be coded. In addition, these codes are not for use if an illness or any signs or symptoms related to the suspected condition or problem are present. In such cases the diagnosis/symptom code is used.

Additional codes may be used in addition to the code from subcategory Z03.7, but only if they are unrelated to the suspected condition being evaluated.

Codes from subcategory Z03.7 may not be used for encounters for antenatal screening of mother. *See Section I.C.21.c.5, Screening.*

For encounters for suspected fetal condition that are inconclusive following testing and evaluation, assign the appropriate code from category O35, O36, O40 or O41.

The observation Z code categories:

Z03 Encounter for medical observation for suspected diseases and conditions ruled out

Z04 Encounter for examination and observation for other reasons

Except: Z04.9, Encounter for examination and observation for unspecified reason

7) Aftercare

Aftercare visit codes cover situations when the initial treatment of a disease has been performed and the patient requires continued care during the healing or recovery phase, or for the long-term consequences of the disease. The aftercare Z code should not be used if treatment is directed at a current, acute disease. The diagnosis code is to be used in these cases. Exceptions to this rule are codes Z51.0, Encounter for antineoplastic radiation therapy, and codes from subcategory Z51.1, Encounter for antineoplastic chemotherapy and immunotherapy. These codes are to be first-listed, followed by the diagnosis code when a patient's encounter is solely to receive radiation therapy, chemotherapy, or immunotherapy for the treatment of a neoplasm. If the reason for the encounter is more than one type of antineoplastic therapy, code Z51.0 and a code from subcategory Z51.1 may be assigned together, in which case one of these codes would be reported as a secondary diagnosis.

The aftercare Z codes should also not be used for aftercare for injuries. For aftercare of an injury, assign the acute injury code with the appropriate 7th character (for subsequent encounter).

The aftercare codes are generally first-listed to explain the specific reason for the encounter. An aftercare code may be used as an additional code when some type of aftercare is provided in addition to the reason for admission and no diagnosis code is applicable. An example of this would be the closure of a colostomy during an encounter for treatment of another condition.

Aftercare codes should be used in conjunction with other aftercare codes or diagnosis codes to provide better detail on the specifics of an aftercare encounter visit, unless otherwise directed by the classification. Should a patient receive multiple types of antineoplastic therapy during the same encounter, code Z51.0, Encounter for antineoplastic radiation therapy, and codes from subcategory Z51.1, Encounter for antineoplastic chemotherapy and immunotherapy, may be used together on a record. The sequencing of multiple aftercare codes depends on the circumstances of the encounter.

Certain aftercare Z code categories need a secondary diagnosis code to describe the resolving condition or sequelae. For others, the condition is included in the code title.

Additional Z code aftercare category terms include fitting and adjustment, and attention to artificial openings.

Status Z codes may be used with aftercare Z codes to indicate the nature of the aftercare. For example code Z95.1, Presence of aortocoronary bypass graft, may be used with code Z48.812, Encounter for surgical aftercare following surgery on the circulatory system, to indicate the surgery for which the aftercare is being performed. A status code should not be used when the aftercare code indicates the type of status, such as using Z43.0, Encounter for attention to tracheostomy, with Z93.0, Tracheostomy status.

The aftercare Z category/codes:

Z42 Encounter for plastic and reconstructive surgery following medical procedure or healed injury

Z43 Encounter for attention to artificial openings

Z44 Encounter for fitting and adjustment of external prosthetic device

Z45 Encounter for adjustment and management of implanted device

Z46 Encounter for fitting and adjustment of other devices

Z47 Orthopedic aftercare

Z48 Encounter for other postprocedural aftercare

Z49 Encounter for care involving renal dialysis

Z51 Encounter for other aftercare

8) Follow-up

The follow-up codes are used to explain continuing surveillance following completed treatment of a disease, condition, or injury. They imply that the condition has been fully treated and no longer exists. They should not be confused with aftercare codes, or injury codes with a 7th character for subsequent encounter, that explain ongoing care of a healing condition or its sequelae. Follow-up codes may be used in conjunction with history codes to provide the full picture of the healed condition and its treatment. The follow-up code is sequenced first, followed by the history code.

A follow-up code may be used to explain multiple visits. Should a condition be found to have recurred on the follow-up visit, then the diagnosis code for the condition should be assigned in place of the follow-up code.

The follow-up Z code categories:

Z08 Encounter for follow-up examination after completed treatment for malignant neoplasm

Z09 Encounter for follow-up examination after completed treatment for conditions other than malignant neoplasm

Z39 Encounter for maternal postpartum care and examination

9) Donor

Codes in category Z52, Donors of organs and tissues, are used for living individuals who are donating blood or other body tissue. These codes are only for individuals donating for others, not for self-donations. They are not used to identify cadaveric donations.

10) Counseling

Counseling Z codes are used when a patient or family member receives assistance in the aftermath of an illness or injury, or when support is required in coping with family or social problems. They are not used in conjunction with a diagnosis code when the counseling component of care is considered integral to standard treatment.

The counseling Z codes/categories:

Z30.0- Encounter for general counseling and advice on contraception

- Z31.5 Encounter for genetic counseling
- Z31.6- Encounter for general counseling and advice on procreation
- Z32.2 Encounter for childbirth instruction
- Z32.3 Encounter for childcare instruction
- Z69 Encounter for mental health services for victim and perpetrator of abuse
- Z7Ø Counseling related to sexual attitude, behavior and orientation
- Z71 Persons encountering health services for other counseling and medical advice, not elsewhere classified
- Z76.81 Expectant mother prebirth pediatrician visit

11) Encounters for obstetrical and reproductive services

See Section I.C.15. Pregnancy, Childbirth, and the Puerperium, for further instruction on the use of these codes.

Z codes for pregnancy are for use in those circumstances when none of the problems or complications included in the codes from the Obstetrics chapter exist (a routine prenatal visit or postpartum care). Codes in category Z34, Encounter for supervision of normal pregnancy, are always first-listed and are not to be used with any other code from the OB chapter.

Codes in category Z3A, Weeks of gestation, may be assigned to provide additional information about the pregnancy. **The date of the admission should be used to determine weeks of gestation for inpatient admissions that encompass more than one gestational week.**

The outcome of delivery, category Z37, should be included on all maternal delivery records. It is always a secondary code. Codes in category Z37 should not be used on the newborn record.

Z codes for family planning (contraceptive) or procreative management and counseling should be included on an obstetric record either during the pregnancy or the postpartum stage, if applicable.

Z codes/categories for obstetrical and reproductive services:

- Z3Ø Encounter for contraceptive management
- Z31 Encounter for procreative management
- Z32.2 Encounter for childbirth instruction
- Z32.3 Encounter for childcare instruction
- Z33 Pregnant state
- Z34 Encounter for supervision of normal pregnancy
- Z36 Encounter for antenatal screening of mother
- Z3A Weeks of gestation
- Z37 Outcome of delivery
- Z39 Encounter for maternal postpartum care and examination
- Z76.81 Expectant mother prebirth pediatrician visit

12) Newborns and Infants

See Section I.C.16. Newborn (Perinatal) Guidelines, for further instruction on the use of these codes.

Newborn Z codes/categories:

- Z76.1 Encounter for health supervision and care of foundling
- ZØØ.1- Encounter for routine child health examination
- Z38 Liveborn infants according to place of birth and type of delivery

13) Routine and administrative examinations

The Z codes allow for the description of encounters for routine examinations, such as, a general check-up, or, examinations for administrative purposes, such as, a pre-employment physical. The codes are not to be used if the examination is for diagnosis of a suspected condition or for treatment purposes. In such cases the diagnosis code is used. During a routine exam, should a diagnosis or condition be discovered, it should be coded as an additional code. Pre-existing and chronic conditions and history codes may also be included as additional codes as long as the examination is for administrative purposes and not focused on any particular condition.

Some of the codes for routine health examinations distinguish between "with" and "without" abnormal findings. Code assignment depends on the information that is known at the time the encounter is being coded. For example, if no abnormal findings were found during the examination, but the encounter is being coded before test results are back, it is acceptable to assign the code for "without abnormal findings." When assigning a code for "with abnormal findings," additional code(s) should be assigned to identify the specific abnormal finding(s).

Pre-operative examination and pre-procedural laboratory examination Z codes are for use only in those situations when a patient is being cleared for a procedure or surgery and no treatment is given.

The Z codes/categories for routine and administrative examinations:

- ZØØ Encounter for general examination without complaint, suspected or reported diagnosis
- ZØ1 Encounter for other special examination without complaint, suspected or reported diagnosis
- ZØ2 Encounter for administrative examination
  Except: ZØ2.9, Encounter for administrative examinations, unspecified
- Z32.Ø- Encounter for pregnancy test

14) Miscellaneous Z codes

The miscellaneous Z codes capture a number of other health care encounters that do not fall into one of the other categories. Certain of these codes identify the reason for the encounter; others are for use as additional codes that provide useful information on circumstances that may affect a patient's care and treatment.

Prophylactic Organ Removal

For encounters specifically for prophylactic removal of an organ (such as prophylactic removal of breasts due to a genetic susceptibility to cancer or a family history of cancer), the principal or first-listed code should be a code from category Z4Ø, Encounter for prophylactic surgery, followed by the appropriate codes to identify the associated risk factor (such as genetic susceptibility or family history).

If the patient has a malignancy of one site and is having prophylactic removal at another site to prevent either a new primary malignancy or metastatic disease, a code for the malignancy should also be assigned in addition to a code from subcategory Z4Ø.Ø, Encounter for prophylactic surgery for risk factors related to malignant neoplasms. A Z4Ø.Ø code should not be assigned if the patient is having organ removal for treatment of a malignancy, such as the removal of the testes for the treatment of prostate cancer.

Miscellaneous Z codes/categories:

- Z28 Immunization not carried out
  Except: Z28.3, Underimmunization status
- Z4Ø Encounter for prophylactic surgery
- Z41 Encounter for procedures for purposes other than remedying health state
  Except: Z41.9, Encounter for procedure for purposes other than remedying health state, unspecified
- Z53 Persons encountering health services for specific procedures and treatment, not carried out
- Z55 Problems related to education and literacy
- Z56 Problems related to employment and unemployment
- Z57 Occupational exposure to risk factors
- Z58 Problems related to physical environment
- Z59 Problems related to housing and economic circumstances
- Z6Ø Problems related to social environment
- Z62 Problems related to upbringing
- Z63 Other problems related to primary support group, including family circumstances

Z64 Problems related to certain psychosocial circumstances
Z65 Problems related to other psychosocial circumstances
Z72 Problems related to lifestyle
Z73 Problems related to life management difficulty
Z74 Problems related to care provider dependency
Except: Z74.01, Bed confinement status
Z75 Problems related to medical facilities and other health care
Z76.0 Encounter for issue of repeat prescription
Z76.3 Healthy person accompanying sick person
Z76.4 Other boarder to healthcare facility
Z76.5 Malingerer [conscious simulation]
Z91.1- Patient's noncompliance with medical treatment and regimen
Z91.83 Wandering in diseases classified elsewhere
Z91.89 Other specified personal risk factors, not elsewhere classified

15) Nonspecific Z codes

Certain Z codes are so non-specific, or potentially redundant with other codes in the classification, that there can be little justification for their use in the inpatient setting. Their use in the outpatient setting should be limited to those instances when there is no further documentation to permit more precise coding. Otherwise, any sign or symptom or any other reason for visit that is captured in another code should be used.

Nonspecific Z codes/categories:

Z02.9 Encounter for administrative examinations, unspecified
Z04.9 Encounter for examination and observation for unspecified reason
Z13.9 Encounter for screening, unspecified
Z41.9 Encounter for procedure for purposes other than remedying health state, unspecified
Z52.9 Donor of unspecified organ or tissue
Z86.59 Personal history of other mental and behavioral disorders
Z88.9 Allergy status to unspecified drugs, medicaments and biological substances status
Z92.0 Personal history of contraception

16) Z codes that may only be principal/first-listed diagnosis

The following Z codes/categories may only be reported as the principal/first-listed diagnosis, except when there are multiple encounters on the same day and the medical records for the encounters are combined:

Z00 Encounter for general examination without complaint, suspected or reported diagnosis
Z01 Encounter for other special examination without complaint, suspected or reported diagnosis
Z02 Encounter for administrative examination
Z03 Encounter for medical observation for suspected diseases and conditions ruled out
Z04 Encounter for examination and observation for other reasons
Z31.81 Encounter for male factor infertility in female patient
Z31.82 Encounter for Rh incompatibility status
Z31.83 Encounter for assisted reproductive fertility procedure cycle
Z31.84 Encounter for fertility preservation procedure
Z33.2 Encounter for elective termination of pregnancy
Z34 Encounter for supervision of normal pregnancy
Z38 Liveborn infants according to place of birth and type of delivery
Z39 Encounter for maternal postpartum care and examination
Z42 Encounter for plastic and reconstructive surgery following medical procedure or healed injury
Z51.0 Encounter for antineoplastic radiation therapy
Z51.1- Encounter for antineoplastic chemotherapy and immunotherapy
Z52 Donors of organs and tissues
Except: Z52.9, Donor of unspecified organ or tissue
Z76.1 Encounter for health supervision and care of foundling
Z76.2 Encounter for health supervision and care of other healthy infant and child
Z99.12 Encounter for respirator [ventilator] dependence during power failure

Section II. Selection of Principal Diagnosis

The circumstances of inpatient admission always govern the selection of principal diagnosis. The principal diagnosis is defined in the Uniform Hospital Discharge Data Set (UHDDS) as "that condition established after study to be chiefly responsible for occasioning the admission of the patient to the hospital for care."

The UHDDS definitions are used by hospitals to report inpatient data elements in a standardized manner. These data elements and their definitions can be found in the July 31, 1985, Federal Register (Vol. 50, No, 147), pp. 31038-40.

Since that time the application of the UHDDS definitions has been expanded to include all non-outpatient settings (acute care, short term, long term care and psychiatric hospitals; home health agencies; rehab facilities; nursing homes, etc).

In determining principal diagnosis the coding conventions in the ICD-10-CM, the Tabular List and Alphabetic Index take precedence over these official coding guidelines.

(See Section I.A., Conventions for the ICD-10-CM)

The importance of consistent, complete documentation in the medical record cannot be overemphasized. Without such documentation the application of all coding guidelines is a difficult, if not impossible, task.

A. Codes for symptoms, signs, and ill-defined conditions

Codes for symptoms, signs, and ill-defined conditions from Chapter 18 are not to be used as principal diagnosis when a related definitive diagnosis has been established.

B. Two or more interrelated conditions, each potentially meeting the definition for principal diagnosis

When there are two or more interrelated conditions (such as diseases in the same ICD-10-CM chapter or manifestations characteristically associated with a certain disease) potentially meeting the definition of principal diagnosis, either condition may be sequenced first, unless the circumstances of the admission, the therapy provided, the Tabular List, or the Alphabetic Index indicate otherwise.

C. Two or more diagnoses that equally meet the definition for principal diagnosis

In the unusual instance when two or more diagnoses equally meet the criteria for principal diagnosis as determined by the circumstances of admission, diagnostic workup and/or therapy provided, and the Alphabetic Index, Tabular List, or another coding guidelines does not provide sequencing direction, any one of the diagnoses may be sequenced first.

D. Two or more comparative or contrasting conditions

In those rare instances when two or more contrasting or comparative diagnoses are documented as "either/or" (or similar terminology), they are coded as if the diagnoses were confirmed and the diagnoses are sequenced according to the circumstances of the admission. If no further determination can be made as to which diagnosis should be principal, either diagnosis may be sequenced first.

E. A symptom(s) followed by contrasting/comparative diagnoses

When a symptom(s) is followed by contrasting/comparative diagnoses, the symptom code is sequenced first. **However, if the symptom code is integral to the conditions listed, no code for the symptom is reported.** All the contrasting/comparative diagnoses should be coded as additional diagnoses.

F. Original treatment plan not carried out

Sequence as the principal diagnosis the condition, which after study occasioned the admission to the hospital, even though treatment may not have been carried out due to unforeseen circumstances.

G. Complications of surgery and other medical care

When the admission is for treatment of a complication resulting from surgery or other medical care, the complication code is sequenced as the principal diagnosis. If the complication is classified to the T8Ø-T88 series and the code lacks the necessary specificity in describing the complication, an additional code for the specific complication should be assigned.

H. Uncertain diagnosis

If the diagnosis documented at the time of discharge is qualified as "probable", "suspected", "likely", "questionable", "possible", or "still to be ruled out", or other similar terms indicating uncertainty, code the condition as if it existed or was established. The bases for these guidelines are the diagnostic workup, arrangements for further workup or observation, and initial therapeutic approach that correspond most closely with the established diagnosis.

Note: This guideline is applicable only to inpatient admissions to short-term, acute, long-term care and psychiatric hospitals.

I. Admission from observation unit

1. **Admission Following Medical Observation**
   When a patient is admitted to an observation unit for a medical condition, which either worsens or does not improve, and is subsequently admitted as an inpatient of the same hospital for this same medical condition, the principal diagnosis would be the medical condition which led to the hospital admission.
2. **Admission Following Post-Operative Observation**
   When a patient is admitted to an observation unit to monitor a condition (or complication) that develops following outpatient surgery, and then is subsequently admitted as an inpatient of the same hospital, hospitals should apply the Uniform Hospital Discharge Data Set (UHDDS) definition of principal diagnosis as "that condition established after study to be chiefly responsible for occasioning the admission of the patient to the hospital for care."

J. Admission from outpatient surgery

When a patient receives surgery in the hospital's outpatient surgery department and is subsequently admitted for continuing inpatient care at the same hospital, the following guidelines should be followed in selecting the principal diagnosis for the inpatient admission:

- If the reason for the inpatient admission is a complication, assign the complication as the principal diagnosis.
- If no complication, or other condition, is documented as the reason for the inpatient admission, assign the reason for the outpatient surgery as the principal diagnosis.
- If the reason for the inpatient admission is another condition unrelated to the surgery, assign the unrelated condition as the principal diagnosis.

K. Admissions/Encounters for Rehabilitation

When the purpose for the admission/encounter is rehabilitation, sequence first the code for the condition for which the service is being performed. For example, for an admission/encounter for rehabilitation for right-sided dominant hemiplegia following a cerebrovascular infarction, report code I69.351, Hemiplegia and hemiparesis following cerebral infarction affecting right dominant side, as the first-listed or principal diagnosis.

If the condition for which the rehabilitation service is no longer present, report the appropriate aftercare code as the first-listed or principal diagnosis. For example, if a patient with severe degenerative osteoarthritis of the hip, underwent hip replacement and the current encounter/admission is for rehabilitation, report code Z47.1, Aftercare following joint replacement surgery, as the first-listed or principal diagnosis.

See Section I.C.21.c.7, Factors influencing health states and contact with health services, Aftercare.

Section III. Reporting Additional Diagnoses

GENERAL RULES FOR OTHER (ADDITIONAL) DIAGNOSES

For reporting purposes the definition for "other diagnoses" is interpreted as additional conditions that affect patient care in terms of requiring:

clinical evaluation; or

therapeutic treatment; or

diagnostic procedures; or

extended length of hospital stay; or

increased nursing care and/or monitoring.

The UHDDS item #11-b defines Other Diagnoses as "all conditions that coexist at the time of admission, that develop subsequently, or that affect the treatment received and/or the length of stay. Diagnoses that relate to an earlier episode which have no bearing on the current hospital stay are to be excluded." UHDDS definitions apply to inpatients in acute care, short-term, long term care and psychiatric hospital setting. The UHDDS definitions are used by acute care short-term hospitals to report inpatient data elements in a standardized manner. These data elements and their definitions can be found in the July 31, 1985, Federal Register (Vol. 5Ø, No, 147), pp. 31Ø38-4Ø.

Since that time the application of the UHDDS definitions has been expanded to include all non-outpatient settings (acute care, short term, long term care and psychiatric hospitals; home health agencies; rehab facilities; nursing homes, etc).

The following guidelines are to be applied in designating "other diagnoses" when neither the Alphabetic Index nor the Tabular List in ICD-1Ø-CM provide direction. The listing of the diagnoses in the patient record is the responsibility of the attending provider.

A. **Previous conditions**
   If the provider has included a diagnosis in the final diagnostic statement, such as the discharge summary or the face sheet, it should ordinarily be coded. Some providers include in the diagnostic statement resolved conditions or diagnoses and status-post procedures from previous admission that have no bearing on the current stay. Such conditions are not to be reported and are coded only if required by hospital policy.

   However, history codes (categories Z8Ø-Z87) may be used as secondary codes if the historical condition or family history has an impact on current care or influences treatment.

B. **Abnormal findings**
   Abnormal findings (laboratory, x-ray, pathologic, and other diagnostic results) are not coded and reported unless the provider indicates their clinical significance. If the findings are outside the normal range and the attending provider has ordered other tests to evaluate the condition or prescribed treatment, it is appropriate to ask the provider whether the abnormal finding should be added.

   Please note: This differs from the coding practices in the outpatient setting for coding encounters for diagnostic tests that have been interpreted by a provider.

C. **Uncertain Diagnosis**
   If the diagnosis documented at the time of discharge is qualified as "probable", "suspected", "likely", "questionable", "possible", or "still to be ruled out" or other similar terms indicating uncertainty, code the condition as if it existed or was established. The bases for these guidelines are the diagnostic workup, arrangements for further workup or observation, and initial therapeutic approach that correspond most closely with the established diagnosis.

   Note: This guideline is applicable only to inpatient admissions to short-term, acute, long-term care and psychiatric hospitals.

Section IV. Diagnostic Coding and Reporting Guidelines for Outpatient Services

These coding guidelines for outpatient diagnoses have been approved for use by hospitals/ providers in coding and reporting hospital-based outpatient services and provider-based office visits.

Information about the use of certain abbreviations, punctuation, symbols, and other conventions used in the ICD-1Ø-CM Tabular List (code numbers and titles), can be found in Section IA of these guidelines, under "Conventions Used in the Tabular List." **Section I.B. contains general guidelines that apply to the entire classification. Section I.C. contains chapter-specific guidelines that correspond to the chapters as they are arranged in the classification.** Information about the correct sequence to use in finding a code is also described in Section I.

The terms encounter and visit are often used interchangeably in describing outpatient service contacts and, therefore, appear together in these guidelines without distinguishing one from the other.

Though the conventions and general guidelines apply to all settings, coding guidelines for outpatient and provider reporting of diagnoses will vary in a number of instances from those for inpatient diagnoses, recognizing that:

The Uniform Hospital Discharge Data Set (UHDDS) definition of principal diagnosis applies only to inpatients in acute, short-term, long-term care and psychiatric hospitals.

Coding guidelines for inconclusive diagnoses (probable, suspected, rule out, etc.) were developed for inpatient reporting and do not apply to outpatients.

A. Selection of first-listed condition

In the outpatient setting, the term first-listed diagnosis is used in lieu of principal diagnosis.

In determining the first-listed diagnosis the coding conventions of ICD-1Ø-CM, as well as the general and disease specific guidelines take precedence over the outpatient guidelines.

Diagnoses often are not established at the time of the initial encounter/visit. It may take two or more visits before the diagnosis is confirmed.

The most critical rule involves beginning the search for the correct code assignment through the Alphabetic Index. Never begin searching initially in the Tabular List as this will lead to coding errors.

1. Outpatient surgery

When a patient presents for outpatient surgery (same day surgery), code the reason for the surgery as the first-listed diagnosis (reason for the encounter), even if the surgery is not performed due to a contraindication.

2. Observation stay

When a patient is admitted for observation for a medical condition, assign a code for the medical condition as the first-listed diagnosis.

When a patient presents for outpatient surgery and develops complications requiring admission to observation, code the reason for the surgery as the first reported diagnosis (reason for the encounter), followed by codes for the complications as secondary diagnoses.

B. Codes from AØØ.Ø through T88.9, ZØØ-Z99

The appropriate code(s) from AØØ.Ø through T88.9, ZØØ-Z99 must be used to identify diagnoses, symptoms, conditions, problems, complaints, or other reason(s) for the encounter/visit.

C. Accurate reporting of ICD-1Ø-CM diagnosis codes

For accurate reporting of ICD-1Ø-CM diagnosis codes, the documentation should describe the patient's condition, using terminology which includes specific diagnoses as well as symptoms, problems, or reasons for the encounter. There are ICD-1Ø-CM codes to describe all of these.

D. Codes that describe symptoms and signs

Codes that describe symptoms and signs, as opposed to diagnoses, are acceptable for reporting purposes when a diagnosis has not been established (confirmed) by the provider. Chapter 18 of ICD-1Ø-CM, Symptoms, Signs, and Abnormal Clinical and Laboratory Findings Not Elsewhere Classified (codes RØØ-R99) contain many, but not all codes for symptoms.

E. Encounters for circumstances other than a disease or injury

ICD-1Ø-CM provides codes to deal with encounters for circumstances other than a disease or injury. The Factors Influencing Health Status and Contact with Health Services codes (ZØØ-Z99) are provided to deal with occasions when circumstances other than a disease or injury are recorded as diagnosis or problems.

See Section I.C.21. Factors influencing health status and contact with health services.

F. Level of Detail in Coding

1. ICD-1Ø-CM codes with 3, 4, 5, 6 or 7 characters

ICD-1Ø-CM is composed of codes with 3, 4, 5, 6 or 7 characters. Codes with three characters are included in ICD-1Ø-CM as the heading of a category of codes that may be further subdivided by the use of fourth, fifth, sixth or seventh characters to provide greater specificity.

2. Use of full number of characters required for a code

A three-character code is to be used only if it is not further subdivided. A code is invalid if it has not been coded to the full number of characters required for that code, including the 7th character extension, if applicable.

G. ICD-1Ø-CM code for the diagnosis, condition, problem, or other reason for encounter/visit

List first the ICD-1Ø-CM code for the diagnosis, condition, problem, or other reason for encounter/visit shown in the medical record to be chiefly responsible for the services provided. List additional codes that describe any coexisting conditions. In some cases the first-listed diagnosis may be a symptom when a diagnosis has not been established (confirmed) by the physician.

H. Uncertain diagnosis

Do not code diagnoses documented as "probable", "suspected," "questionable," "rule out," or "working diagnosis" or other similar terms indicating uncertainty. Rather, code the condition(s) to the highest degree of certainty for that encounter/visit, such as symptoms, signs, abnormal test results, or other reason for the visit.

Please note: This differs from the coding practices used by short-term, acute care, long-term care and psychiatric hospitals.

I. Chronic diseases

Chronic diseases treated on an ongoing basis may be coded and reported as many times as the patient receives treatment and care for the condition(s)

J. Code all documented conditions that coexist

Code all documented conditions that coexist at the time of the encounter/visit, and require or affect patient care treatment or management. Do not code conditions that were previously treated and no longer exist. However, history codes (categories Z8Ø-Z87) may be used as secondary codes if the historical condition or family history has an impact on current care or influences treatment.

K. Patients receiving diagnostic services only

For patients receiving diagnostic services only during an encounter/visit, sequence first the diagnosis, condition, problem, or other reason for encounter/visit shown in the medical record to be chiefly responsible for the outpatient services provided during the encounter/visit. Codes for other diagnoses (e.g., chronic conditions) may be sequenced as additional diagnoses.

For encounters for routine laboratory/radiology testing in the absence of any signs, symptoms, or associated diagnosis, assign ZØ1.89, Encounter for other specified special examinations. If routine testing is performed during the same encounter as a test to evaluate a sign, symptom, or diagnosis, it is appropriate to assign both the Z code and the code describing the reason for the non-routine test.

For outpatient encounters for diagnostic tests that have been interpreted by a physician, and the final report is available at the time of coding, code any confirmed or definitive diagnosis(es) documented in the interpretation. Do not code related signs and symptoms as additional diagnoses.

Please note: This differs from the coding practice in the hospital inpatient setting regarding abnormal findings on test results.

L. Patients receiving therapeutic services only

For patients receiving therapeutic services only during an encounter/visit, sequence first the diagnosis, condition, problem, or other reason for encounter/visit shown in the medical record to be chiefly responsible for the outpatient services provided during the encounter/visit. Codes for other diagnoses (e.g., chronic conditions) may be sequenced as additional diagnoses.

The only exception to this rule is that when the primary reason for the admission/encounter is chemotherapy or radiation therapy, the appropriate Z code for the service is listed first, and the diagnosis or problem for which the service is being performed listed second.

M. Patients receiving preoperative evaluations only

For patients receiving preoperative evaluations only, sequence first a code from subcategory ZØ1.81, Encounter for pre-procedural examinations, to describe the pre-op consultations. Assign a code for the condition to describe the reason for the surgery as an additional diagnosis. Code also any findings related to the pre-op evaluation.

N. Ambulatory surgery

For ambulatory surgery, code the diagnosis for which the surgery was performed. If the postoperative diagnosis is known to be different from the preoperative diagnosis at the time the diagnosis is confirmed, select the postoperative diagnosis for coding, since it is the most definitive.

O. Routine outpatient prenatal visits

See Section I.C.15. Routine outpatient prenatal visits.

P. Encounters for general medical examinations with abnormal findings

The subcategories for encounters for general medical examinations, ZØØ.Ø-, provide codes for with and without abnormal findings. Should a general medical examination result in an abnormal finding, the code for general medical examination with abnormal finding should be assigned as the first-listed diagnosis. A secondary code for the abnormal finding should also be coded.

Q. Encounters for routine health screenings

See Section I.C.21. Factors influencing health status and contact with health services, Screening

Appendix I. Present on Admission Reporting Guidelines

Introduction

These guidelines are to be used as a supplement to the *ICD-1Ø-CM Official Guidelines for Coding and Reporting* to facilitate the assignment of the Present on Admission (POA) indicator for each diagnosis and external cause of injury code reported on claim forms (UB-Ø4 and 837 Institutional).

These guidelines are not intended to replace any guidelines in the main body of the *ICD-1Ø-CM Official Guidelines for Coding and Reporting.* The POA guidelines are not intended to provide guidance on when a condition should be coded, but rather, how to apply the POA indicator to the final set of diagnosis codes that have been assigned in accordance with Sections I, II, and III of the official coding guidelines. Subsequent to the assignment of the ICD-1Ø-CM codes, the POA indicator should then be assigned to those conditions that have been coded.

As stated in the Introduction to the *ICD-1Ø-CM Official Guidelines for Coding and Reporting,* a joint effort between the healthcare provider and the coder is essential to achieve complete and accurate documentation, code assignment, and reporting of diagnoses and procedures. The importance of consistent, complete documentation in the medical record cannot be overemphasized. Medical record documentation from any provider involved in the care and treatment of the patient may be used to support the determination of whether a condition was present on admission or not. In the context of the official coding guidelines, the term "provider" means a physician or any qualified healthcare practitioner who is legally accountable for establishing the patient's diagnosis.

These guidelines are not a substitute for the provider's clinical judgment as to the determination of whether a condition was/was not present on admission. The provider should be queried regarding issues related to the linking of signs/symptoms, timing of test results, and the timing of findings.

General Reporting Requirements

All claims involving inpatient admissions to general acute care hospitals or other facilities that are subject to a law or regulation mandating collection of present on admission information.

Present on admission is defined as present at the time the order for inpatient admission occurs -- conditions that develop during an outpatient encounter, including emergency department, observation, or outpatient surgery, are considered as present on admission.

POA indicator is assigned to principal and secondary diagnoses (as defined in Section II of the Official Guidelines for Coding and Reporting) and the external cause of injury codes.

Issues related to inconsistent, missing, conflicting or unclear documentation must still be resolved by the provider.

If a condition would not be coded and reported based on UHDDS definitions and current official coding guidelines, then the POA indicator would not be reported.

Reporting Options

Y – Yes

N – No

U – Unknown

W – Clinically undetermined

Unreported/Not used (or "1" for Medicare usage) – (Exempt from POA reporting)

Reporting Definitions

Y – present at the time of inpatient admission

N – not present at the time of inpatient admission

U – documentation is insufficient to determine if condition is present on admission

W – provider is unable to clinically determine whether condition was present on admission or not

Timeframe for POA Identification and Documentation

There is no required timeframe as to when a provider (per the definition of "provider" used in these guidelines) must identify or document a condition to be present on admission. In some clinical situations, it may not be possible for a provider to make a definitive diagnosis (or a condition may not be recognized or reported by the patient) for a period of time after admission. In some cases it may be several days before the provider arrives at a definitive diagnosis. This does not mean that the condition was not present on admission. Determination of whether the condition was present on admission or not will be based on the applicable POA guideline as identified in this document, or on the provider's best clinical judgment.

If at the time of code assignment the documentation is unclear as to whether a condition was present on admission or not, it is appropriate to query the provider for clarification.

Assigning the POA Indicator

Condition is on the "Exempt from Reporting" list

Leave the "present on admission" field blank if the condition is on the list of ICD-1Ø-CM codes for which this field is not applicable. This is the only circumstance in which the field may be left blank.

POA Explicitly Documented

Assign "Y" for any condition the provider explicitly documents as being present on admission.

Assign "N" for any condition the provider explicitly documents as not present at the time of admission.

Conditions diagnosed prior to inpatient admission

Assign "Y" for conditions that were diagnosed prior to admission (example: hypertension, diabetes mellitus, asthma).

Conditions diagnosed during the admission but clearly present before admission

Assign "Y" for conditions diagnosed during the admission that were clearly present but not diagnosed until after admission occurred.

Diagnoses subsequently confirmed after admission are considered present on admission if at the time of admission they are documented as suspected, possible, rule out, differential diagnosis, or constitute an underlying cause of a symptom that is present at the time of admission.

Condition develops during outpatient encounter prior to inpatient admission

Assign "Y" for any condition that develops during an outpatient encounter prior to a written order for inpatient admission.

Documentation does not indicate whether condition was present on admission

Assign "U" when the medical record documentation is unclear as to whether the condition was present on admission. "U" should not be routinely assigned and used only in very limited circumstances. Coders are encouraged to query the providers when the documentation is unclear.

Documentation states that it cannot be determined whether the condition was or was not present on admission

Assign "W" when the medical record documentation indicates that it cannot be clinically determined whether or not the condition was present on admission.

Chronic condition with acute exacerbation during the admission

If a single code identifies both the chronic condition and the acute exacerbation, see POA guidelines pertaining to combination codes.

If a single code only identifies the chronic condition and not the acute exacerbation (e.g., acute exacerbation of chronic leukemia), assign "Y."

Conditions documented as possible, probable, suspected, or rule out at the time of discharge

If the final diagnosis contains a possible, probable, suspected, or rule out diagnosis, and this diagnosis was based on signs, symptoms or clinical findings suspected at the time of inpatient admission, assign "Y."

If the final diagnosis contains a possible, probable, suspected, or rule out diagnosis, and this diagnosis was based on signs, symptoms or clinical findings that were not present on admission, assign "N".

Conditions documented as impending or threatened at the time of discharge

If the final diagnosis contains an impending or threatened diagnosis, and this diagnosis is based on symptoms or clinical findings that were present on admission, assign "Y".

If the final diagnosis contains an impending or threatened diagnosis, and this diagnosis is based on symptoms or clinical findings that were not present on admission, assign "N".

Acute and Chronic Conditions

Assign "Y" for acute conditions that are present at time of admission and N for acute conditions that are not present at time of admission.

Assign "Y" for chronic conditions, even though the condition may not be diagnosed until after admission.

If a single code identifies both an acute and chronic condition, see the POA guidelines for combination codes.

Combination Codes

Assign "N" if any part of the combination code was not present on admission (e.g., COPD with acute exacerbation and the exacerbation was not present on admission; gastric ulcer that does not start bleeding until after admission; asthma patient develops status asthmaticus after admission).

Assign "Y" if all parts of the combination code were present on admission (e.g., patient with acute prostatitis admitted with hematuria).

If the final diagnosis includes comparative or contrasting diagnoses, and both were present, or suspected, at the time of admission, assign "Y".

For infection codes that include the causal organism, assign "Y" if the infection (or signs of the infection) was present on admission, even though the culture results may not be known until after admission (e.g., patient is admitted with pneumonia and the provider documents pseudomonas as the causal organism a few days later).

Same Diagnosis Code for Two or More Conditions

When the same ICD-10-CM diagnosis code applies to two or more conditions during the same encounter (e.g. two separate conditions classified to the same ICD-10-CM diagnosis code):

> Assign "Y" if all conditions represented by the single ICD-10-CM code were present on admission (e.g. bilateral unspecified age-related cataracts).
>
> Assign "N" if any of the conditions represented by the single ICD-10-CM code was not present on admission (e.g. traumatic secondary and recurrent hemorrhage and seroma is assigned to a single code T79.2, but only one of the conditions was present on admission).

Obstetrical conditions

Whether or not the patient delivers during the current hospitalization does not affect assignment of the POA indicator. The determining factor for POA assignment is whether the pregnancy complication or obstetrical condition described by the code was present at the time of admission or not.

If the pregnancy complication or obstetrical condition was present on admission (e.g., patient admitted in preterm labor), assign "Y".

If the pregnancy complication or obstetrical condition was not present on admission (e.g., 2nd degree laceration during delivery, postpartum hemorrhage that occurred during current hospitalization, fetal distress develops after admission), assign "N".

If the obstetrical code includes more than one diagnosis and any of the diagnoses identified by the code were not present on admission assign "N". (e.g., Category O11, Pre-existing hypertension with pre-eclampsia).

Perinatal conditions

Newborns are not considered to be admitted until after birth. Therefore, any condition present at birth or that developed in utero is considered present at admission and should be assigned "Y". This includes conditions that occur during delivery (e.g., injury during delivery, meconium aspiration, exposure to streptococcus B in the vaginal canal).

Congenital conditions and anomalies

Assign "Y" for congenital conditions and anomalies except for categories Q00-Q99, Congenital anomalies, which are on the exempt list. Congenital conditions are always considered present on admission.

External cause of injury codes

Assign "Y" for any external cause code representing an external cause of morbidity that occurred prior to inpatient admission (e.g., patient fell out of bed at home, patient fell out of bed in emergency room prior to admission).

Assign "N" for any external cause code representing an external cause of morbidity that occurred during inpatient hospitalization (e.g., patient fell out of hospital bed during hospital stay, patient experienced an adverse reaction to a medication administered after inpatient admission).

Categories and Codes Exempt from Diagnosis Present on Admission Requirement

Note: "Diagnosis present on admission" for these code categories are exempt because they represent circumstances regarding the healthcare encounter or factors influencing health status that do not represent a current disease or injury or are always present on admission.

B90–B94	Sequelae of infectious and parasitic diseases
E64	Sequelae of malnutrition and other nutritional deficiences
I25.2	Old myocardial infarction
I69	Sequelae of cerebrovascular disease
O09	Supervision of high risk pregnancy
O66.5	Attempted application of vacuum extractor and forceps
O80	Encounter for full-term uncomplicated delivery
O94	Sequelae of complication of pregnancy, childbirth, and the puerperium
P00	Newborn (suspected to be) affected by maternal conditions that may be unrelated to present pregnancy
Q00 – Q99	Congenital malformations, deformations and chromosomal abnormalities
S00-T88.9	Injury, poisoning and certain other consequences of external causes with 7th character representing subsequent encounter or sequela
V00- V09	Pedestrian injured in transport accident Except: V00.81-, Accident with wheelchair (powered) V00.83-, Accident with motorized mobility scooter
V10-V19	Pedal cycle rider injured in transport accident
V20-V29	Motorcycle rider injured in transport accident

V3Ø-V39	Occupant of three-wheeled motor vehicle injured in transport accident
V4Ø-V49	Car occupant injured in transport accident
V5Ø-V59	Occupant of pick-up truck or van injured in transport accident
V6Ø-V69	Occupant of heavy transport vehicle injured in transport accident
V7Ø-V79	Bus occupant injured in transport accident
V8Ø-V89	Other land transport accidents
V9Ø-V94	Water transport accidents
V95-V97	Air and space transport accidents
V98-V99	Other and unspecified transport accidents
WØ9	Fall on and from playground equipment
W14	Fall from tree
W15	Fall from cliff
W17.Ø	Fall into well
W17.1	Fall into storm drain or manhole
W18.Ø1	Striking against sports equipment with subsequent fall
W21	Striking against or struck by sports equipment
W3Ø	Contact with agricultural machinery
W31	Contact with other and unspecified machinery
W32-W34	Accidental handgun discharge and malfunction
W35- W4Ø	Exposure to inanimate mechanical forces
W52	Crushed, pushed or stepped on by crowd or human stampede
W56	Contact with nonvenomous marine animal
W58	Contact with crocodile or alligator
W61	Contact with birds (domestic) (wild)
W62	Contact with nonvenomous amphibians
W89	Exposure to man-made visible and ultraviolet light
XØ2	Exposure to controlled fire in building or structure
XØ3	Exposure to controlled fire, not in building or structure
XØ4	Exposure to ignition of highly flammable material
X52	Prolonged stay in weightless environment
X71	Intentional self-harm by drowning and submersion Except: X71.Ø-, Intentional self-harm by drowning and submersion while in bath tub
X72	Intentional self-harm by handgun discharge
X73	Intentional self-harm by rifle, shotgun and larger firearm discharge
X74	Intentional self-harm by other and unspecified firearm and gun discharge
X75	Intentional self-harm by explosive material
X76	Intentional self-harm by smoke, fire and flames
X77	Intentional self-harm by steam, hot vapors and hot objects
X81	Intentional self-harm by jumping or lying in front of moving object
X82	Intentional self-harm by crashing of motor vehicle
X83	Intentional self-harm by other specified means
YØ3	**Assault by crashing of motor vehicle**
YØ7	**Perpetrator of assault, maltreatment and neglect**
YØ8.8	**Assault by strike by sports equipment**
Y21	Drowning and submersion, undetermined intent
Y22	Handgun discharge, undetermined intent
Y23	Rifle, shotgun and larger firearm discharge, undetermined intent
Y24	Other and unspecified firearm discharge, undetermined intent
Y3Ø	Falling, jumping or pushed from a high place, undetermined intent
Y32	**Assault by crashing of motor vehicle, undetermined intent**
Y36	Operations of war
Y37	Military operations
Y92	Place of occurrence of the external cause
Y93	Activity code
Y99	External cause status
ZØØ	Encounter for general examination without complaint, suspected or reported diagnosis
ZØ1	Encounter for other special examination without complaint, suspected or reported diagnosis
ZØ2	Encounter for administrative examination
ZØ3	Encounter for medical observation for suspected diseases and conditions ruled out
ZØ8	Encounter for follow-up examination following completed treatment for malignant neoplasm
ZØ9	Encounter for follow-up examination after completed treatment for conditions other than malignant neoplasm
Z11	Encounter for screening for infectious and parasitic diseases
Z11.8	Encounter for screening for other infectious and parasitic diseases
Z12	Encounter for screening for malignant neoplasms
Z13	Encounter for screening for other diseases and disorders
Z13.4	Encounter for screening for certain developmental disorders in childhood
Z13.5	Encounter for screening for eye and ear disorders
Z13.6	Encounter for screening for cardiovascular disorders
Z13.83	Encounter for screening for respiratory disorder NEC
Z13.89	Encounter for screening for other disorder
Z14	Genetic carrier
Z15	Genetic susceptibility to disease
Z17	Estrogen receptor status
Z18	Retained foreign body fragments
Z22	Carrier of infectious disease
Z23	Encounter for immunization
Z28	Immunization not carried out and underimmunization status
Z28.3	Underimmunization status
Z3Ø	Encounter for contraceptive management
Z31	Encounter for procreative management
Z34	Encounter for supervision of normal pregnancy
Z36	Encounter for antenatal screening of mother
Z37	Outcome of delivery
Z38	Liveborn infants according to place of birth and type of delivery
Z39	Encounter for maternal postpartum care and examination
Z41	Encounter for procedures for purposes other than remedying health state
Z42	Encounter for plastic and reconstructive surgery following medical procedure or healed injury
Z43	Encounter for attention to artificial openings
Z44	Encounter for fitting and adjustment of external prosthetic device
Z45	Encounter for adjustment and management of implanted device
Z46	Encounter for fitting and adjustment of other devices
Z47.8	Encounter for other orthopedic aftercare
Z49	Encounter for care involving renal dialysis
Z51	Encounter for other aftercare
Z51.5	Encounter for palliative care
Z51.8	Encounter for other specified aftercare
Z52	Donors of organs and tissues
Z59	Problems related to housing and economic circumstances
Z63	Other problems related to primary support groupincluding family circumstances
Z65	Problems related to other psychosocial circumstances
Z65.8	Other specified problems related to psychosocial circumstances
Z67.1-Z67.9	Blood type
Z68	Body mass index (BMI)
Z72	Problems related to lifestyle
Z74.Ø1	Bed confinement status
Z76	Persons encountering health services in other circumstances
Z77.11Ø-Z77.128	Environmental pollution and hazards in the physical environment
Z78	Other specified health status
Z79	Long term (current) drug therapy
Z8Ø	Family history of primary malignant neoplasm
Z81	Family history of mental and behavioral disorders
Z82	Family history of certain disabilities and chronic diseases (leading to disablement)
Z83	Family history of other specific disorders
Z84	Family history of other conditions
Z85	Personal history of primary malignant neoplasm
Z86	Personal history of certain other diseases
Z87	Personal history of other diseases and conditions
Z87.828	Personal history of other (healed) physical injury and trauma
Z87.891	Personal history of nicotine dependence

Z88	Allergy status to drugs, medicaments and biological substances
Z89	Acquired absence of limb
Z90.710	Acquired absence of both cervix and uterus
Z91.0	Allergy status, other than to drugs and biological substances
Z91.4	Personal history of psychological trauma, not elsewhere classified
Z91.5	Personal history of self-harm
Z91.8	Other specified risk factors, not elsewhere classified
Z92	Personal history of medical treatment
Z93	Artificial opening status
Z94	Transplanted organ and tissue status
Z95	Presence of cardiac and vascular implants and grafts
Z97	Presence of other devices
Z98	Other postprocedural states
Z99	Dependence on enabling machines and devices, not elsewhere classified

ICD-1Ø-CM Index to Diseases and Injuries

A

- **Aarskog's syndrome** Q87.1
- **Abandonment** — *see* Maltreatment
- **Abasia** (-astasia) (hysterical) F44.4
- **Abderhalden-Kaufmann-Lignac syndrome** (cystinosis) E72.Ø4
- **Abdomen, abdominal** (*see also* condition)
  - acute R1Ø.Ø
  - angina K55.1
  - muscle deficiency syndrome Q79.4
- **Abdominalgia** — *see* Pain, abdominal
- **Abduction contracture, hip or other joint** — *see* Contraction, joint
- **Aberrant** (congenital) (*see also* Malposition, congenital)
  - adrenal gland Q89.1
  - artery (peripheral) Q27.8
    - basilar NEC Q28.1
    - cerebral Q28.3
    - coronary Q24.5
    - digestive system Q27.8
    - eye Q15.8
    - lower limb Q27.8
    - precerebral Q28.1
    - pulmonary Q25.79
    - renal Q27.2
    - retina Q14.1
    - specified site NEC Q27.8
    - subclavian Q27.8
    - upper limb Q27.8
    - vertebral Q28.1
  - breast Q83.8
  - endocrine gland NEC Q89.2
  - hepatic duct Q44.5
  - pancreas Q45.3
  - parathyroid gland Q89.2
  - pituitary gland Q89.2
  - sebaceous glands, mucous membrane, mouth, congenital Q38.6
  - spleen Q89.Ø9
  - subclavian artery Q27.8
  - thymus (gland) Q89.2
  - thyroid gland Q89.2
  - vein (peripheral) NEC Q27.8
    - cerebral Q28.3
    - digestive system Q27.8
    - lower limb Q27.8
    - precerebral Q28.1
    - specified site NEC Q27.8
    - upper limb Q27.8
- **Aberration**
  - distantial — *see* Disturbance, visual
  - mental F99
- **Abetalipoproteinemia** E78.6
- **Abiotrophy** R68.89
- **Ablatio, ablation**
  - retinae — *see* Detachment, retina
- **Ablepharia, ablepharon** Q1Ø.3
- **Abnormal, abnormality, abnormalities** (*see also* Anomaly)
  - acid-base balance (mixed) E87.4
  - albumin R77.Ø
  - alphafetoprotein R77.2
  - alveolar ridge KØ8.9
  - anatomical relationship Q89.9
  - apertures, congenital, diaphragm Q79.1
  - auditory perception H93.29- ☑
    - diplacusis — *see* Diplacusis
    - hyperacusis — *see* Hyperacusis
    - recruitment — *see* Recruitment, auditory
    - threshold shift — *see* Shift, auditory threshold
  - autosomes Q99.9
    - fragile site Q95.5
  - basal metabolic rate R94.8
  - biosynthesis, testicular androgen E29.1
  - bleeding time R79.1
  - blood level (of)
    - cobalt R79.Ø
    - copper R79.Ø
    - iron R79.Ø
    - lithium R78.89

- **Abnormal, abnormality, abnormalities** — *continued*
  - blood level — *continued*
    - magnesium R79.Ø
    - mineral NEC R79.Ø
    - zinc R79.Ø
  - blood pressure
    - elevated RØ3.Ø
    - low reading (nonspecific) RØ3.1
  - blood sugar R73.Ø9
  - blood-gas level R79.81
  - bowel sounds R19.15
    - absent R19.11
    - hyperactive R19.12
  - brain scan R94.Ø2
  - breathing RØ6.9
  - caloric test R94.138
  - cerebrospinal fluid R83.9
    - cytology R83.6
    - drug level R83.2
    - enzyme level R83.Ø
    - hormones R83.1
    - immunology R83.4
    - microbiology R83.5
    - nonmedicinal level R83.3
    - specified type NEC R83.8
  - chemistry, blood R79.9
    - C-reactive protein R79.82
    - drugs — *see* Findings, abnormal, in blood
    - gas level R79.81
    - minerals R79.Ø
    - pancytopenia D61.818
    - PTT R79.1
    - specified NEC R79.89
    - toxins — *see* Findings, abnormal, in blood
  - chest sounds (friction) (rales) RØ9.89
  - chromosome, chromosomal Q99.9
    - with more than three X chromosomes, female Q97.1
    - analysis result R89.8
      - bronchial washings R84.8
      - cerebrospinal fluid R83.8
      - cervix uteri NEC R87.89
      - nasal secretions R84.8
      - nipple discharge R89.8
      - peritoneal fluid R85.89
      - pleural fluid R84.8
      - prostatic secretions R86.8
      - saliva R85.89
      - seminal fluid R86.8
      - sputum R84.8
      - synovial fluid R89.8
      - throat scrapings R84.8
      - vagina R87.89
      - vulva R87.89
      - wound secretions R89.8
    - dicentric replacement Q93.2
    - ring replacement Q93.2
    - sex Q99.8
      - female phenotype Q97.9
        - specified NEC Q97.8
      - male phenotype Q98.9
        - specified NEC Q98.8
      - structural male Q98.6
    - specified NEC Q99.8
  - clinical findings NEC R68.89
  - coagulation D68.9
    - newborn, transient P61.6
    - profile R79.1
    - time R79.1
  - communication — *see* Fistula
  - conjunctiva, vascular H11.41- ☑
  - coronary artery Q24.5
  - cortisol-binding globulin E27.8
  - course, eustachian tube Q17.8
  - creatinine clearance R94.4
  - cytology
    - anus R85.619
      - atypical squamous cells cannot exclude high grade squamous intraepithelial lesion (ASC-H) R85.611
      - atypical squamous cells of undetermined significance (ASC-US) R85.61Ø

- **Abnormal, abnormality, abnormalities** — *continued*
  - cytology — *continued*
    - anus — *continued*
      - cytologic evidence of malignancy R85.614
      - high grade squamous intraepithelial lesion (HGSIL) R85.613
      - human papillomavirus (HPV) DNA test
        - high risk positive R85.81
        - low risk postive R85.82
      - inadequate smear R85.615
      - low grade squamous intraepithelial lesion (LGSIL) R85.612
      - satisfactory anal smear but lacking transformation zone R85.616
      - specified NEC R85.618
      - unsatisfactory smear R85.615
    - female genital organs — *see* Abnormal, Papanicolaou (smear)
  - dark adaptation curve H53.61
  - dentofacial NEC — *see* Anomaly, dentofacial
  - development, developmental Q89.9
    - central nervous system QØ7.9
  - diagnostic imaging
    - abdomen, abdominal region NEC R93.5
    - biliary tract R93.2
    - breast R92.8
    - central nervous system NEC R9Ø.89
    - cerebrovascular NEC R9Ø.89
    - coronary circulation R93.1
    - digestive tract NEC R93.3
    - gastrointestinal (tract) R93.3
    - genitourinary organs R93.8
    - head R93.Ø
    - heart R93.1
    - intrathoracic organ NEC R93.8
    - limbs R93.6
    - liver R93.2
    - lung (field) R91.8
    - musculoskeletal system NEC R93.7
    - retroperitoneum R93.5
    - site specified NEC R93.8
    - skin and subcutaneous tissue R93.8
    - skull R93.Ø
    - urinary organs R93.4
  - direction, teeth, fully erupted M26.3Ø
  - ear ossicles, acquired NEC H74.39- ☑
    - ankylosis — *see* Ankylosis, ear ossicles
    - discontinuity — *see* Discontinuity, ossicles, ear
    - partial loss — *see* Loss, ossicles, ear (partial)
  - Ebstein Q22.5
  - echocardiogram R93.1
  - echoencephalogram R9Ø.81
  - echogram — *see* Abnormal, diagnostic imaging
  - electrocardiogram [ECG] [EKG] R94.31
  - electroencephalogram [EEG] R94.Ø1
  - electrolyte — *see* Imbalance, electrolyte
  - electromyogram [EMG] R94.131
  - electro-oculogram [EOG] R94.11Ø
  - electrophysiological intracardiac studies R94.39
  - electroretinogram [ERG] R94.111
  - erythrocytes
    - congenital, with perinatal jaundice D58.9
  - feces (color) (contents) (mucus) R19.5
  - finding — *see* Findings, abnormal, without diagnosis
  - fluid
    - amniotic — *see* Abnormal, specimen, specified
    - cerebrospinal — *see* Abnormal, cerebrospinal fluid
    - peritoneal — *see* Abnormal, specimen, digestive organs
    - pleural — *see* Abnormal, specimen, respiratory organs
    - synovial — *see* Abnormal, specimen, specified
    - thorax (bronchial washings) (pleural fluid) — *see* Abnormal, specimen, respiratory organs
    - vaginal — *see* Abnormal, specimen, female genital organs
  - form
    - teeth KØØ.2
    - uterus — *see* Anomaly, uterus
  - function studies
    - auditory R94.12Ø
    - bladder R94.8

Abnormal, abnormality, abnormalities — *continued*
- function studies — *continued*
  - brain R94.Ø9
  - cardiovascular R94.3Ø
  - ear R94.128
  - endocrine NEC R94.7
  - eye NEC R94.118
  - kidney R94.4
  - liver R94.5
  - nervous system
    - central NEC R94.Ø9
    - peripheral NEC R94.138
  - pancreas R94.8
  - placenta R94.8
  - pulmonary R94.2
  - special senses NEC R94.128
  - spleen R94.8
  - thyroid R94.6
  - vestibular R94.121
- gait — *see* Gait
  - hysterical F44.4
- gastrin secretion E16.4
- globulin R77.1
  - cortisol-binding E27.8
  - thyroid-binding EØ7.89
- glomerular, minor (*see also* NØØ-NØ7 with fourth character .Ø) NØ5.Ø
- glucagon secretion E16.3
- glucose tolerance (test) (non-fasting) R73.Ø9
- gravitational (G) forces or states (effect of) T75.81 ☑
- hair (color) (shaft) L67.9
  - specified NEC L67.8
- hard tissue formation in pulp (dental) KØ4.3
- head movement R25.Ø
- heart
  - rate RØØ.9
    - specified NEC RØØ.8
  - shadow R93.1
  - sounds NEC RØ1.2
- hemoglobin (disease) (*see also* Disease, hemoglobin) D58.2
  - trait — *see* Trait, hemoglobin, abnormal
- histology NEC R89.7
- immunological findings R89.4
  - in serum R76.9
    - specified NEC R76.8
- increase in appetite R63.2
- involuntary movement — *see* Abnormal, movement, involuntary
- jaw closure M26.51
- karyotype R89.8
- kidney function test R94.4
- knee jerk R29.2
- leukocyte (cell) (differential) NEC D72.9
- liver
- loss of
  - height R29.89Ø
  - weight R63.4
- mammogram NEC R92.8
  - calcification (calculus) R92.1
  - microcalcification R92.Ø
- Mantoux test R76.11
- movement (disorder) (*see also* Disorder, movement)
  - head R25.Ø
  - involuntary R25.9
    - fasciculation R25.3
    - of head R25.Ø
    - spasm R25.2
    - specified type NEC R25.8
    - tremor R25.1
- myoglobin (Aberdeen) (Annapolis) R89.7
- neonatal screening PØ9
- oculomotor study R94.113
- palmar creases Q82.8
- Papanicolaou (smear)
  - anus R85.619
    - atypical squamous cells cannot exclude high grade squamous intraepithelial lesion (ASC-H) R85.611
    - atypical squamous cells of undetermined significance (ASC-US) R85.61Ø
    - cytologic evidence of malignancy R85.614
    - high grade squamous intraepithelial lesion (HGSIL) R85.613
    - human papillomavirus (HPV) DNA test
      - high risk positive R85.81
      - low risk postive R85.82

Abnormal, abnormality, abnormalities — *continued*
- Papanicolaou — *continued*
  - anus — *continued*
    - inadequate smear R85.615
    - low grade squamous intraepithelial lesion (LGSIL) R85.612
    - satisfactory anal smear but lacking transformation zone R85.616
    - specified NEC R85.618
    - unsatisfactory smear R85.615
  - bronchial washings R84.6
  - cerebrospinal fluid R83.6
  - cervix R87.619
    - atypical squamous cells cannot exclude high grade squamous intraepithelial lesion (ASC-H) R87.611
    - atypical squamous cells of undetermined significance (ASC-US) R87.61Ø
    - cytologic evidence of malignancy R87.614
    - high grade squamous intraepithelial lesion (HGSIL) R87.613
    - inadequate smear R87.615
    - low grade squamous intraepithelial lesion (LGSIL) R87.612
    - non-atypical endometrial cells R87.618
    - satisfactory cervical smear but lacking transformation zone R87.616
    - specified NEC R87.618
    - thin preparaton R87.619
    - unsatisfactory smear R87.615
  - nasal secretions R84.6
  - nipple discharge R89.6
  - peritoneal fluid R85.69
  - pleural fluid R84.6
  - prostatic secretions R86.6
  - saliva R85.69
  - seminal fluid R86.6
  - sites NEC R89.6
  - sputum R84.6
  - synovial fluid R89.6
  - throat scrapings R84.6
  - vagina R87.629
    - atypical squamous cells cannot exclude high grade squamous intraepithelial lesion (ASC-H) R87.621
    - atypical squamous cells of undetermined significance (ASC-US) R87.62Ø
    - cytologic evidence of malignancy R87.624
    - high grade squamous intraepithelial lesion (HGSIL) R87.623
    - inadequate smear R87.625
    - low grade squamous intraepithelial lesion (LGSIL) R87.622
    - specified NEC R87.628
    - thin preparation R87.629
    - unsatisfactory smear R87.625
  - vulva R87.69
  - wound secretions R89.6
- partial thromboplastin time (PTT) R79.1
- pelvis (bony) — *see* Deformity, pelvis
- percussion, chest (tympany) RØ9.89
- periods (grossly) — *see* Menstruation
- phonocardiogram R94.39
- plantar reflex R29.2
- plasma
  - protein R77.9
    - specified NEC R77.8
  - viscosity R7Ø.1
- pleural (folds) Q34.Ø
- posture R29.3
- product of conception OØ2.9
  - specified type NEC OØ2.89
- prothrombin time (PT) R79.1
- pulmonary
  - artery, congenital Q25.79
  - function, newborn P28.89
  - test results R94.2
- pulsations in neck RØØ.2
- pupillary H21.56- ☑
  - function (reaction) (reflex) — *see* Anomaly, pupil, function
- radiological examination — *see* Abnormal, diagnostic imaging
- red blood cell(s) (morphology) (volume) R71.8
- reflex — *see* Reflex
- renal function test R94.4
- response to nerve stimulation R94.13Ø

Abnormal, abnormality, abnormalities — *continued*
- retinal correspondence H53.31
- retinal function study R94.111
- rhythm, heart (*see also* Arrhythmia)
- saliva — *see* Abnormal, specimen, digestive organs
- scan
  - kidney R94.4
  - liver R93.2
  - thyroid R94.6
- secretion
  - gastrin E16.4
  - glucagon E16.3
- semen, seminal fluid — *see* Abnormal, specimen, male genital organs
- serum level (of)
  - acid phosphatase R74.8
  - alkaline phosphatase R74.8
  - amylase R74.8
  - enzymes R74.9
    - specified NEC R74.8
  - lipase R74.8
  - triacylglycerol lipase R74.8
- shape
  - gravid uterus — *see* Anomaly, uterus
- sinus venosus Q21.1
- size, tooth, teeth KØØ.2
- spacing, tooth, teeth, fully erupted M26.3Ø
- specimen
  - digestive organs (peritoneal fluid) (saliva) R85.9
    - cytology R85.69
    - drug level R85.2
    - enzyme level R85.Ø
    - histology R85.7
    - hormones R85.1
    - immunology R85.4
    - microbiology R85.5
    - nonmedicinal level R85.3
    - specified type NEC R85.89
  - female genital organs (secretions) (smears) R87.9
    - cytology R87.69
      - cervix R87.619
        - human papillomavirus (HPV) DNA test
          - high risk positive R87.81Ø
          - low risk positive R87.82Ø
        - inadequate (unsatisfactory) smear R87.615
        - non-atypical endometrial cells R87.618
        - specified NEC R87.618
      - vagina R87.629
        - human papillomavirus (HPV) DNA test
          - high risk positive R87.811
          - low risk positive R87.821
        - inadequate (unsatisfactory) smear R87.625
      - vulva R87.69
    - drug level R87.2
    - enzyme level R87.Ø
    - histological R87.7
    - hormones R87.1
    - immunology R87.4
    - microbiology R87.5
    - nonmedicinal level R87.3
    - specified type NEC R87.89
  - male genital organs (prostatic secretions) (semen) R86.9
    - cytology R86.6
    - drug level R86.2
    - enzyme level R86.Ø
    - histological R86.7
    - hormones R86.1
    - immunology R86.4
    - microbiology R86.5
    - nonmedicinal level R86.3
    - specified type NEC R86.8
  - nipple discharge — *see* Abnormal, specimen, specified
  - respiratory organs (bronchial washings) (nasal secretions) (pleural fluid) (sputum) R84.9
    - cytology R84.6
    - drug level R84.2
    - enzyme level R84.Ø
    - histology R84.7
    - hormones R84.1
    - immunology R84.4
    - microbiology R84.5
    - nonmedicinal level R84.3
    - specified type NEC R84.8

- **Abnormal, abnormality, abnormalities** — *continued*
  - specimen — *continued*
    - specified organ, system and tissue NOS R89.9
      - cytology R89.6
      - drug level R89.2
      - enzyme level R89.Ø
      - histology R89.7
      - hormones R89.1
      - immunology R89.4
      - microbiology R89.5
      - nonmedicinal level R89.3
      - specified type NEC R89.8
    - synovial fluid — *see* Abnormal, specimen, specified
    - thorax (bronchial washings) (pleural fluids) — *see* Abnormal, specimen, respiratory organs
    - vagina (secretion) (smear) R87.629
    - vulva (secretion) (smear) R87.69
    - wound secretion — *see* Abnormal, specimen, specified
  - spermatozoa — *see* Abnormal, specimen, male genital organs
  - sputum (amount) (color) (odor) RØ9.3
  - stool (color) (contents) (mucus) R19.5
    - bloody K92.1
    - guaiac positive R19.5
  - synchondrosis Q78.8
  - thermography (*see also* Abnormal, diagnostic imaging) R93.8
  - thyroid-binding globulin EØ7.89
  - tooth, teeth (form) (size) KØØ.2
  - toxicology (findings) R78.9
  - transport protein E88.Ø9
  - tumor marker NEC R97.8
  - ultrasound results — *see* Abnormal, diagnostic imaging
  - umbilical cord complicating delivery O69.9 ☑
  - urination NEC R39.19
  - urine (constituents) R82.9Ø
    - bile R82.2
    - cytological examination R82.8
    - drugs R82.5
    - fat R82.Ø
    - glucose R81
    - heavy metals R82.6
    - hemoglobin R82.3
    - histological examination R82.8
    - ketones R82.4
    - microbiological examination (culture) R82.7
    - myoglobin R82.1
    - positive culture R82.7
    - protein — *see* Proteinuria
    - specified substance NEC R82.99
      - chromoabnormality NEC R82.91
    - substances nonmedical R82.6
  - uterine hemorrhage — *see* Hemorrhage, uterus
  - vectorcardiogram R94.39
  - visually evoked potential (VEP) R94.112
  - white blood cells D72.9
    - specified NEC D72.89
  - X-ray examination — *see* Abnormal, diagnostic imaging
- **Abnormity** (any organ or part) — *see* Anomaly
- **Abocclusion** M26.29
  - hemolytic disease (newborn) P55.1
  - incompatibility reaction ABO — *see* Complication(s), transfusion, incompatibility reaction, ABO
- **Abolition, language** R48.8
- **Aborter, habitual or recurrent** — *see* Loss (of), pregnancy, recurrent
- **Abortion** (complete) (spontaneous) OØ3.9
  - with
    - retained products of conception — *see* Abortion, incomplete
  - attempted (elective) (failed) OØ7.4
    - complicated by OØ7.3Ø
      - afibrinogenemia OØ7.1
      - cardiac arrest OØ7.36
      - chemical damage of pelvic organ(s) OØ7.34
      - circulatory collapse OØ7.31
      - cystitis OØ7.38
      - defibrination syndrome OØ7.1
      - electrolyte imbalance OØ7.33
      - embolism (air) (amniotic fluid) (blood clot) (fat) (pulmonary) (septic) (soap) OØ7.2
      - endometritis OØ7.Ø
      - genital tract and pelvic infection OØ7.Ø
      - hemolysis OØ7.1

- **Abortion** — *continued*
  - attempted — *continued*
    - complicated by — *continued*
      - hemorrhage (delayed) (excessive) OØ7.1
      - infection
        - genital tract or pelvic OØ7.Ø
        - urinary tract tract OØ7.38
      - intravascular coagulation OØ7.1
      - laceration of pelvic organ(s) OØ7.34
      - metabolic disorder OØ7.33
      - oliguria OØ7.32
      - oophoritis OØ7.Ø
      - parametritis OØ7.Ø
      - pelvic peritonitis OØ7.Ø
      - perforation of pelvic organ(s) OØ7.34
      - renal failure or shutdown OØ7.32
      - salpingitis or salpingo-oophoritis OØ7.Ø
      - sepsis OØ7.37
      - shock OØ7.31
      - specified condition NEC OØ7.39
      - tubular necrosis (renal) OØ7.32
      - uremia OØ7.32
      - urinary tract infection OØ7.38
      - venous complication NEC OØ7.35
        - embolism (air) (amniotic fluid) (blood clot) (fat) (pulmonary) (septic) (soap) OØ7.2
  - complicated (by) (following) OØ3.8Ø
    - afibrinogenemia OØ3.6
    - cardiac arrest OØ3.86
    - chemical damage of pelvic organ(s) OØ3.84
    - circulatory collapse OØ3.81
    - cystitis OØ3.88
    - defibrination syndrome OØ3.6
    - electrolyte imbalance OØ3.83
    - embolism (air) (amniotic fluid) (blood clot) (fat) (pulmonary) (septic) (soap) OØ3.7
    - endometritis OØ3.5
    - genital tract and pelvic infection OØ3.5
    - hemolysis OØ3.6
    - hemorrhage (delayed) (excessive) OØ3.6
    - infection
      - genital tract or pelvic OØ3.5
      - urinary tract OØ3.88
    - intravascular coagulation OØ3.6
    - laceration of pelvic organ(s) OØ3.84
    - metabolic disorder OØ3.83
    - oliguria OØ3.82
    - oophoritis OØ3.5
    - parametritis OØ3.5
    - pelvic peritonitis OØ3.5
    - perforation of pelvic organ(s) OØ3.84
    - renal failure or shutdown OØ3.82
    - salpingitis or salpingo-oophoritis OØ3.5
    - sepsis OØ3.87
    - shock OØ3.81
    - specified condition NEC OØ3.89
    - tubular necrosis (renal) OØ3.82
    - uremia OØ3.82
    - urinary tract infection OØ3.88
    - venous complication NEC OØ3.85
      - embolism (air) (amniotic fluid) (blood clot) (fat) (pulmonary) (septic) (soap) OØ3.7
  - failed — *see* Abortion, attempted
  - habitual or recurrent N96
    - with current abortion — *see* categories OØ3-OØ6
    - without current pregnancy N96
    - care in current pregnancy O26.2- ☑
  - incomplete (spontaneous) OØ3.4
    - complicated (by) (following) OØ3.3Ø
      - afibrinogenemia OØ3.1
      - cardiac arrest OØ3.36
      - chemical damage of pelvic organ(s) OØ3.34
      - circulatory collapse OØ3.31
      - cystitis OØ3.38
      - defibrination syndrome OØ3.1
      - electrolyte imbalance OØ3.33
      - embolism (air) (amniotic fluid) (blood clot) (fat) (pulmonary) (septic) (soap) OØ3.2
      - endometritis OØ3.Ø
      - genital tract and pelvic infection OØ3.Ø
      - hemolysis OØ3.1
      - hemorrhage (delayed) (excessive) OØ3.1
      - infection
        - genital tract or pelvic OØ3.Ø
        - urinary tract OØ3.38
      - intravascular coagulation OØ3.1
      - laceration of pelvic organ(s) OØ3.34
      - metabolic disorder OØ3.33

- **Abortion** — *continued*
  - incomplete — *continued*
    - complicated — *continued*
      - oliguria OØ3.32
      - oophoritis OØ3.Ø
      - parametritis OØ3.Ø
      - pelvic peritonitis OØ3.Ø
      - perforation of pelvic organ(s) OØ3.34
      - renal failure or shutdown OØ3.32
      - salpingitis or salpingo-oophoritis OØ3.Ø
      - sepsis OØ3.37
      - shock OØ3.31
      - specified condition NEC OØ3.39
      - tubular necrosis (renal) OØ3.32
      - uremia OØ3.32
      - urinary infection OØ3.38
      - venous complication NEC OØ3.35
        - embolism (air) (amniotic fluid) (blood clot) (fat) (pulmonary) (septic) (soap) OØ3.2
  - induced (encounter for) Z33.2
    - complicated by OØ4.8Ø
      - afibrinogenemia OØ4.6
      - cardiac arrest OØ4.86
      - chemical damage of pelvic organ(s) OØ4.84
      - circulatory collapse OØ4.81
      - cystitis OØ4.88
      - defibrination syndrome OØ4.6
      - electrolyte imbalance OØ4.83
      - embolism (air) (amniotic fluid) (blood clot) (fat) (pulmonary) (septic) (soap) OØ4.7
      - endometritis OØ4.5
      - genital tract and pelvic infection OØ4.5
      - hemolysis OØ4.6
      - hemorrhage (delayed) (excessive) OØ4.6
      - infection
        - genital tract or pelvic OØ4.5
        - urinary tract OØ4.88
      - intravascular coagulation OØ4.6
      - laceration of pelvic organ(s) OØ4.84
      - metabolic disorder OØ4.83
      - oliguria OØ4.82
      - oophoritis OØ4.5
      - parametritis OØ4.5
      - pelvic peritonitis OØ4.5
      - perforation of pelvic organ(s) OØ4.84
      - renal failure or shutdown OØ4.82
      - salpingitis or salpingo-oophoritis OØ4.5
      - sepsis OØ4.87
      - shock OØ4.81
      - specified condition NEC OØ4.89
      - tubular necrosis (renal) OØ4.82
      - uremia OØ4.82
      - urinary tract infection OØ4.88
      - venous complication NEC OØ4.85
        - embolism (air) (amniotic fluid) (blood clot) (fat) (pulmonary) (septic) (soap) OØ4.7
  - missed OØ2.1
  - spontaneous — *see* Abortion (complete) (spontaneous)
    - threatened O2Ø.Ø
  - threatened (spontaneous) O2Ø.Ø
  - tubal OØØ.1
- **Abortus fever** A23.1
- **Aboulomania** F6Ø.7
- **Abrami's disease** D59.8
- **Abramov-Fiedler myocarditis** (acute isolated myocarditis) I4Ø.1
- **Abrasion** T14.8
  - abdomen, abdominal (wall) S3Ø.811 ☑
  - alveolar process SØØ.512 ☑
  - ankle S9Ø.51- ☑
  - antecubital space — *see* Abrasion, elbow
  - anus S3Ø.817 ☑
  - arm (upper) S4Ø.81- ☑
  - auditory canal — *see* Abrasion, ear
  - auricle — *see* Abrasion, ear
  - axilla — *see* Abrasion, arm
  - back, lower S3Ø.81Ø ☑
  - breast S2Ø.11- ☑
  - brow SØØ.81 ☑
  - buttock S3Ø.81Ø ☑
  - calf — *see* Abrasion, leg
  - canthus — *see* Abrasion, eyelid
  - cheek SØØ.81 ☑
    - internal SØØ.512 ☑
  - chest wall — *see* Abrasion, thorax
  - chin SØØ.81 ☑
  - clitoris S3Ø.814 ☑

- **Abrasion** — *continued*
  - cornea S05.Ø- ☑
  - costal region — *see* Abrasion, thorax
  - dental KØ3.1
  - digit(s)
    - foot — *see* Abrasion, toe
    - hand — *see* Abrasion, finger
  - ear SØØ.41- ☑
  - elbow S5Ø.31- ☑
  - epididymis S3Ø.813 ☑
  - epigastric region S3Ø.811 ☑
  - epiglottis S1Ø.11 ☑
  - esophagus (thoracic) S27.818 ☑
    - cervical S1Ø.11 ☑
  - eyebrow — *see* Abrasion, eyelid
  - eyelid SØØ.21- ☑
  - face SØØ.81 ☑
  - finger(s) S6Ø.41- ☑
    - index S6Ø.41- ☑
    - little S6Ø.41- ☑
    - middle S6Ø.41- ☑
    - ring S6Ø.41- ☑
  - flank S3Ø.811 ☑
  - foot (except toe(s) alone) S9Ø.81- ☑
    - toe — *see* Abrasion, toe
  - forearm S5Ø.81- ☑
    - elbow only — *see* Abrasion, elbow
  - forehead SØØ.81 ☑
  - genital organs, external
    - female S3Ø.816 ☑
    - male S3Ø.815 ☑
  - groin S3Ø.811 ☑
  - gum SØØ.512 ☑
  - hand S6Ø.51- ☑
  - head SØØ.91 ☑
    - ear — *see* Abrasion, ear
    - eyelid — *see* Abrasion, eyelid
    - lip SØØ.511 ☑
    - nose SØØ.31 ☑
    - oral cavity SØØ.512 ☑
    - scalp SØØ.Ø1 ☑
    - specified site NEC SØØ.81 ☑
  - heel — *see* Abrasion, foot
  - hip S7Ø.21- ☑
  - inguinal region S3Ø.811 ☑
  - interscapular region S2Ø.419 ☑
  - jaw SØØ.81 ☑
  - knee S8Ø.21- ☑
  - labium (majus) (minus) S3Ø.814 ☑
  - larynx S1Ø.11 ☑
  - leg (lower) S8Ø.81- ☑
    - knee — *see* Abrasion, knee
    - upper — *see* Abrasion, thigh
  - lip SØØ.511 ☑
  - lower back S3Ø.81Ø ☑
  - lumbar region S3Ø.81Ø ☑
  - malar region SØØ.81 ☑
  - mammary — *see* Abrasion, breast
  - mastoid region SØØ.81 ☑
  - mouth SØØ.512 ☑
  - nail
    - finger — *see* Abrasion, finger
    - toe — *see* Abrasion, toe
  - nape S1Ø.81 ☑
  - nasal SØØ.31 ☑
  - neck S1Ø.91 ☑
    - specified site NEC S1Ø.81 ☑
    - throat S1Ø.11 ☑
  - nose SØØ.31 ☑
  - occipital region SØØ.Ø1 ☑
  - oral cavity SØØ.512 ☑
  - orbital region — *see* Abrasion, eyelid
  - palate SØØ.512 ☑
  - palm — *see* Abrasion, hand
  - parietal region SØØ.Ø1 ☑
  - pelvis S3Ø.81Ø ☑
  - penis S3Ø.812 ☑
  - perineum
    - female S3Ø.814 ☑
    - male S3Ø.81Ø ☑
  - periocular area — *see* Abrasion, eyelid
  - phalanges
    - finger — *see* Abrasion, finger
    - toe — *see* Abrasion, toe
  - pharynx S1Ø.11 ☑
  - pinna — *see* Abrasion, ear
  - popliteal space — *see* Abrasion, knee
  - prepuce S3Ø.812 ☑
  - pubic region S3Ø.81Ø ☑
  - pudendum
    - female S3Ø.816 ☑
    - male S3Ø.815 ☑
  - sacral region S3Ø.81Ø ☑
  - scalp SØØ.Ø1 ☑
  - scapular region — *see* Abrasion, shoulder
  - scrotum S3Ø.813 ☑
  - shin — *see* Abrasion, leg
  - shoulder S4Ø.21- ☑
  - skin NEC T14.8
  - sternal region S2Ø.319 ☑
  - submaxillary region SØØ.81 ☑
  - submental region SØØ.81 ☑
  - subungual
    - finger(s) — *see* Abrasion, finger
    - toe(s) — *see* Abrasion, toe
  - supraclavicular fossa S1Ø.81 ☑
  - supraorbital SØØ.81 ☑
  - temple SØØ.81 ☑
  - temporal region SØØ.81 ☑
  - testis S3Ø.813 ☑
  - thigh S7Ø.31- ☑
  - thorax, thoracic (wall) S2Ø.91 ☑
    - back S2Ø.41- ☑
    - front S2Ø.31- ☑
  - throat S1Ø.11 ☑
  - thumb S6Ø.31- ☑
  - toe(s) (lesser) S9Ø.416 ☑
    - great S9Ø.41- ☑
  - tongue SØØ.512 ☑
  - tooth, teeth (dentifrice) (habitual) (hard tissues) (occupational) (ritual) (traditional) KØ3.1
  - trachea S1Ø.11 ☑
  - tunica vaginalis S3Ø.813 ☑
  - tympanum, tympanic membrane — *see* Abrasion, ear
  - uvula SØØ.512 ☑
  - vagina S3Ø.814 ☑
  - vocal cords S1Ø.11 ☑
  - vulva S3Ø.814 ☑
  - wrist S6Ø.81- ☑
- **Abrism** — *see* Poisoning, food, noxious, plant
- **Abruptio placentae** O45.9- ☑
  - with
    - afibrinogenemia O45.Ø1- ☑
    - coagulation defect O45.ØØ- ☑
      - specified NEC O45.Ø9- ☑
    - disseminated intravascular coagulation O45.Ø2- ☑
    - hypofibrinogenemia O45.Ø1- ☑
  - specified NEC O45.8- ☑
- **Abruption, placenta** — *see* Abruptio placentae
- **Abscess** (connective tissue) (embolic) (fistulous) (infective) (metastatic) (multiple) (pernicious) (pyogenic) (septic) LØ2.91
  - with
    - diverticular disease (intestine) K57.8Ø
      - with bleeding K57.81
      - large intestine K57.2Ø
        - with
          - bleeding K57.21
          - small intestine K57.4Ø
            - with bleeding K57.41
      - small intestine K57.ØØ
        - with
          - bleeding K57.Ø1
          - large intestine K57.4Ø
            - with bleeding K57.41
    - lymphangitis — *code by* site under Abscess
  - abdomen, abdominal
    - cavity K65.1
    - wall LØ2.211
  - abdominopelvic K65.1
  - accessory sinus — *see* Sinusitis
  - adrenal (capsule) (gland) E27.8
  - alveolar KØ4.7
    - with sinus KØ4.6
  - amebic AØ6.4
    - brain (and liver or lung abscess) AØ6.6
    - genitourinary tract AØ6.82
    - liver (without mention of brain or lung abscess) AØ6.4
    - lung (and liver) (without mention of brain abscess) AØ6.5
    - specified site NEC AØ6.89
- **Abscess** — *continued*
  - amebic — *continued*
    - spleen AØ6.89
  - anerobic A48.Ø
  - ankle — *see* Abscess, lower limb
  - anorectal K61.2
  - antecubital space — *see* Abscess, upper limb
  - antrum (chronic) (Highmore) — *see* Sinusitis, maxillary
  - anus K61.Ø
  - apical (tooth) KØ4.7
    - with sinus (alveolar) KØ4.6
  - appendix K35.3
  - areola (acute) (chronic) (nonpuerperal) N61
    - puerperal, postpartum or gestational — *see* Infection, nipple
  - arm (any part) — *see* Abscess, upper limb
  - artery (wall) I77.89
  - atheromatous I77.2
  - auricle, ear — *see* Abscess, ear, external
  - axilla (region) LØ2.41- ☑
    - lymph gland or node LØ4.2
  - back (any part, except buttock) LØ2.212
  - Bartholin's gland N75.1
    - with
      - abortion — *see* Abortion, by type complicated by, sepsis
      - ectopic or molar pregnancy OØ8.Ø
    - following ectopic or molar pregnancy OØ8.Ø
  - Bezold's — *see* Mastoiditis, acute
  - bilharziasis B65.1
  - bladder (wall) — *see* Cystitis, specified type NEC
  - bone (subperiosteal) (*see also* Osteomyelitis, specified type NEC)
    - accessory sinus (chronic) — *see* Sinusitis
    - chronic or old — *see* Osteomyelitis, chronic
    - jaw (lower) (upper) M27.2
    - mastoid — *see* Mastoiditis, acute, subperiosteal
    - petrous — *see* Petrositis
    - spinal (tuberculous) A18.Ø1
      - nontuberculous — *see* Osteomyelitis, vertebra
  - bowel K63.Ø
  - brain (any part) (cystic) (otogenic) GØ6.Ø
    - amebic (with abscess of any other site) AØ6.6
    - gonococcal A54.82
    - pheomycotic (chromomycotic) B43.1
    - tuberculous A17.81
  - breast (acute) (chronic) (nonpuerperal) N61
    - newborn P39.Ø
    - puerperal, postpartum, gestational — *see* Mastitis, obstetric, purulent
  - broad ligament N73.2
    - acute N73.Ø
    - chronic N73.1
  - Brodie's (localized) (chronic) M86.8X- ☑
  - bronchi J98.Ø9
  - buccal cavity K12.2
  - bulbourethral gland N34.Ø
  - bursa M71.ØØ
    - ankle M71.Ø7- ☑
    - elbow M71.Ø2- ☑
    - foot M71.Ø7- ☑
    - hand M71.Ø4- ☑
    - hip M71.Ø5- ☑
    - knee M71.Ø6- ☑
    - multiple sites M71.Ø9
    - pharyngeal J39.1
    - shoulder M71.Ø1- ☑
    - specified site NEC M71.Ø8
    - wrist M71.Ø3- ☑
  - buttock LØ2.31
  - canthus — *see* Blepharoconjunctivitis
  - cartilage — *see* Disorder, cartilage, specified type NEC
  - cecum K35.3
  - cerebellum, cerebellar GØ6.Ø
    - sequelae GØ9
  - cerebral (embolic) GØ6.Ø
    - sequelae GØ9
  - cervical (meaning neck) LØ2.11
    - lymph gland or node LØ4.Ø
  - cervix (stump) (uteri) — *see* Cervicitis
  - cheek (external) LØ2.Ø1
    - inner K12.2
  - chest J86.9
    - with fistula J86.Ø
    - wall LØ2.213
  - chin LØ2.Ø1
  - choroid — *see* Inflammation, chorioretinal

Abscess — *continued*
- circumtonsillar J36
- cold (lung) (tuberculous) (*see also* Tuberculosis, abscess, lung)
  - articular — *see* Tuberculosis, joint
- colon (wall) K63.Ø
- colostomy K94.Ø2
- conjunctiva — *see* Conjunctivitis, acute
- cornea H16.31- ☑
- corpus
  - cavernosum N48.21
  - luteum — *see* Oophoritis
- Cowper's gland N34.Ø
- cranium GØ6.Ø
- cul-de-sac (Douglas') (posterior) — *see* Peritonitis, pelvic, female
- cutaneous — *see* Abscess, by site
- dental KØ4.7
  - with sinus (alveolar) KØ4.6
- dentoalveolar KØ4.7
  - with sinus KØ4.6
- diaphragm, diaphragmatic K65.1
- Douglas' cul-de-sac or pouch — *see* Peritonitis, pelvic, female
- Dubois A5Ø.59
- ear (middle) (*see also* Otitis, media, suppurative)
  - acute — *see* Otitis, media, suppurative, acute
  - external H6Ø.Ø- ☑
- entamebic — *see* Abscess, amebic
- enterostomy K94.12
- epididymis N45.4
- epidural GØ6.2
  - brain GØ6.Ø
  - spinal cord GØ6.1
- epiglottis J38.7
- epiploon, epiploic K65.1
- erysipelatous — *see* Erysipelas
- esophagus K2Ø.8
- ethmoid (bone) (chronic) (sinus) J32.2
- external auditory canal — *see* Abscess, ear, external
- extradural GØ6.2
  - brain GØ6.Ø
    - sequelae GØ9
  - spinal cord GØ6.1
- extraperitoneal K68.19
- eye — *see* Endophthalmitis, purulent
- eyelid HØØ.Ø3- ☑
- face (any part, except ear, eye and nose) LØ2.Ø1
- fallopian tube — *see* Salpingitis
- fascia M72.8
- fauces J39.1
- fecal K63.Ø
- femoral (region) — *see* Abscess, lower limb
- filaria, filarial — *see* Infestation, filarial
- finger (any) (*see also* Abscess, hand)
  - nail — *see* Cellulitis, finger
- foot LØ2.61- ☑
- forehead LØ2.Ø1
- frontal sinus (chronic) J32.1
- gallbladder K81.Ø
- genital organ or tract
  - female (external) N76.4
  - male N49.9
    - multiple sites N49.8
    - specified NEC N49.8
- gestational mammary O91.11- ☑
- gestational subareolar O91.11- ☑
- gingival KØ5.21
- gland, glandular (lymph) (acute) — *see* Lymphadenitis, acute
- gluteal (region) LØ2.31
- gonorrheal — *see* Gonococcus
- groin LØ2.214
- gum KØ5.21
- hand LØ2.51- ☑
- head NEC LØ2.811
  - face (any part, except ear, eye and nose) LØ2.Ø1
- heart — *see* Carditis
- heel — *see* Abscess, foot
- helminthic — *see* Infestation, helminth
- hepatic (cholangitic) (hematogenic) (lymphogenic) (pylephlebitic) K75.Ø
  - amebic AØ6.4
- hip (region) — *see* Abscess, lower limb
- ileocecal K35.3
- ileostomy (bud) K94.12
- iliac (region) LØ2.214

Abscess — *continued*
- iliac — *continued*
  - fossa K35.3
- infraclavicular (fossa) — *see* Abscess, upper limb
- inguinal (region) LØ2.214
  - lymph gland or node LØ4.1
- intestine, intestinal NEC K63.Ø
  - rectal K61.1
- intra-abdominal (*see also* Abscess, peritoneum) K65.1
  - postoperative T81.4 ☑
    - retroperitoneal K68.11
- intracranial GØ6.Ø
- intramammary — *see* Abscess, breast
- intraorbital — *see* Abscess, orbit
- intraperitoneal K65.1
- intrasphincteric (anus) K61.4
- intraspinal GØ6.1
- intratonsillar J36
- ischiorectal (fossa) K61.3
- jaw (bone) (lower) (upper) M27.2
- joint — *see* Arthritis, pyogenic or pyemic
  - spine (tuberculous) A18.Ø1
    - nontuberculous — *see* Spondylopathy, infective
- kidney N15.1
  - with calculus N2Ø.Ø
    - with hydronephrosis N13.6
  - puerperal (postpartum) O86.21
- knee (*see also* Abscess, lower limb)
  - joint MØØ.9
- labium (majus) (minus) N76.4
- lacrimal
  - caruncle — *see* Inflammation, lacrimal, passages, acute
  - gland — *see* Dacryoadenitis
  - passages (duct) (sac) — *see* Inflammation, lacrimal, passages, acute
- lacunar N34.Ø
- larynx J38.7
- lateral (alveolar) KØ4.7
  - with sinus KØ4.6
- leg (any part) — *see* Abscess, lower limb
- lens H27.8
- lingual K14.Ø
  - tonsil J36
- lip K13.Ø
- Littre's gland N34.Ø
- liver (cholangitic) (hematogenic) (lymphogenic) (pylephlebitic) (pyogenic) K75.Ø
  - amebic (due to Entamoeba histolytica) (dysenteric) (tropical) AØ6.4
    - with
      - brain abscess (and liver or lung abscess) AØ6.6
      - lung abscess AØ6.5
- loin (region) LØ2.211
- lower limb LØ2.41- ☑
- lumbar (tuberculous) A18.Ø1
  - nontuberculous LØ2.212
- lung (miliary) (putrid) J85.2
  - with pneumonia J85.1
    - due to specified organism (see Pneumonia, in (due to))
  - amebic (with liver abscess) AØ6.5
    - with
      - brain abscess AØ6.6
      - pneumonia AØ6.5
- lymph, lymphatic, gland or node (acute) (*see also* Lymphadenitis, acute)
  - mesentery I88.Ø
- malar M27.2
- mammary gland — *see* Abscess, breast
- marginal, anus K61.Ø
- mastoid — *see* Mastoiditis, acute
- maxilla, maxillary M27.2
  - molar (tooth) KØ4.7
    - with sinus KØ4.6
  - premolar KØ4.7
  - sinus (chronic) J32.Ø
- mediastinum J85.3
- meibomian gland — *see* Hordeolum
- meninges GØ6.2
- mesentery, mesenteric K65.1
- mesosalpinx — *see* Salpingitis
- mons pubis LØ2.215
- mouth (floor) K12.2
- muscle — *see* Myositis, infective
- myocardium I4Ø.Ø

Abscess — *continued*
- nabothian (follicle) — *see* Cervicitis
- nasal J32.9
- nasopharyngeal J39.1
- navel LØ2.216
  - newborn P38.9
    - with mild hemorrhage P38.1
    - without hemorrhage P38.9
- neck (region) LØ2.11
  - lymph gland or node LØ4.Ø
- nephritic — *see* Abscess, kidney
- nipple N61
  - associated with
    - lactation — *see* Pregnancy, complicated by,
    - pregnancy — *see* Pregnancy, complicated by
- nose (external) (fossa) (septum) J34.Ø
  - sinus (chronic) — *see* Sinusitis
- omentum K65.1
- operative wound T81.4 ☑
- orbit, orbital — *see* Cellulitis, orbit
- otogenic GØ6.Ø
- ovary, ovarian (corpus luteum) — *see* Oophoritis
- oviduct — *see* Oophoritis
- palate (soft) K12.2
  - hard M27.2
- palmar (space) — *see* Abscess, hand
- pancreas (duct) — *see* Pancreatitis, acute
- parafrenal N48.21
- parametric, parametrium N73.2
  - acute N73.Ø
  - chronic N73.1
- paranephric N15.1
- parapancreatic — *see* Pancreatitis, acute
- parapharyngeal J39.Ø
- pararectal K61.1
- parasinus — *see* Sinusitis
- parauterine (*see also* Disease, pelvis, inflammatory) N73.2
- paravaginal — *see* Vaginitis
- parietal region (scalp) LØ2.811
- parodontal KØ5.21
- parotid (duct) (gland) K11.3
  - region K12.2
- pectoral (region) LØ2.213
- pelvis, pelvic
  - female — *see* Disease, pelvis, inflammatory
  - male, peritoneal K65.1
- penis N48.21
  - gonococcal (accessory gland) (periurethral) A54.1
- perianal K61.Ø
- periapical KØ4.7
  - with sinus (alveolar) KØ4.6
- periappendicular K35.3
- pericardial I3Ø.1
- pericecal K35.3
- pericemental KØ5.21
- pericholecystic — *see* Cholecystitis, acute
- pericoronal KØ5.21
- peridental KØ5.21
- perimetric (*see also* Disease, pelvis, inflammatory) N73.2
- perinephric, perinephritic — *see* Abscess, kidney
- perineum, perineal (superficial) LØ2.215
  - urethra N34.Ø
- periodontal (parietal) KØ5.21
  - apical KØ4.7
- periosteum, periosteal (*see also* Osteomyelitis, specified type NEC)
  - with osteomyelitis (*see also* Osteomyelitis, specified type NEC)
    - acute — *see* Osteomyelitis, acute
    - chronic — *see* Osteomyelitis, chronic
- peripharyngeal J39.Ø
- peripleuritic J86.9
  - with fistula J86.Ø
- periprostatic N41.2
- perirectal K61.1
- perirenal (tissue) — *see* Abscess, kidney
- perisinuous (nose) — *see* Sinusitis
- peritoneum, peritoneal (perforated) (ruptured) K65.1
  - with appendicitis K35.3
  - pelvic
    - female — *see* Peritonitis, pelvic, female
    - male K65.1
  - postoperative T81.4 ☑
  - puerperal, postpartum, childbirth O85
  - tuberculous A18.31
- peritonsillar J36

Abscess — *continued*
- perityphlic K35.3
- periureteral N28.89
- periurethral N34.Ø
  - gonococcal (accessory gland) (periurethral) A54.1
- periuterine (*see also* Disease, pelvis, inflammatory) N73.2
- perivesical — *see* Cystitis, specified type NEC
- petrous bone — *see* Petrositis
- phagedenic NOS LØ2.91
  - chancroid A57
- pharynx, pharyngeal (lateral) J39.1
- pilonidal LØ5.Ø1
- pituitary (gland) E23.6
- pleura J86.9
  - with fistula J86.Ø
- popliteal — *see* Abscess, lower limb
- postcecal K35.3
- postlaryngeal J38.7
- postnasal J34.Ø
- postoperative (any site) T81.4 ☑
  - retroperitoneal K68.11
- postpharyngeal J39.Ø
- posttonsillar J36
- post-typhoid AØ1.Ø9
- pouch of Douglas — *see* Peritonitis, pelvic, female
- premammary — *see* Abscess, breast
- prepatellar — *see* Abscess, lower limb
- prostate N41.2
  - gonococcal (acute) (chronic) A54.22
- psoas muscle K68.12
- puerperal — *code by* site under Puerperal, abscess
- pulmonary — *see* Abscess, lung
- pulp, pulpal (dental) KØ4.Ø
- rectovaginal septum K63.Ø
- rectovesical — *see* Cystitis, specified type NEC
- rectum K61.1
- renal — *see* Abscess, kidney
- retina — *see* Inflammation, chorioretinal
- retrobulbar — *see* Abscess, orbit
- retrocecal K65.1
- retrolaryngeal J38.7
- retromammary — *see* Abscess, breast
- retroperitoneal NEC K68.19
  - postprocedural K68.11
- retropharyngeal J39.Ø
- retrouterine — *see* Peritonitis, pelvic, female
- retrovesical — *see* Cystitis, specified type NEC
- root, tooth KØ4.7
  - with sinus (alveolar) KØ4.6
- round ligament (*see also* Disease, pelvis, inflammatory) N73.2
- rupture (spontaneous) NOS LØ2.91
- sacrum (tuberculous) A18.Ø1
  - nontuberculous M46.28
- salivary (duct) (gland) K11.3
- scalp (any part) LØ2.811
- scapular — *see* Osteomyelitis, specified type NEC
- sclera — *see* Scleritis
- scrofulous (tuberculous) A18.2
- scrotum N49.2
- seminal vesicle N49.Ø
- septal, dental KØ4.7
  - with sinus (alveolar) KØ4.6
- serous — *see* Periostitis
- shoulder (region) — *see* Abscess, upper limb
- sigmoid K63.Ø
- sinus (accessory) (chronic) (nasal) (*see also* Sinusitis)
  - intracranial venous (any) GØ6.Ø
- Skene's duct or gland N34.Ø
- skin — *see* Abscess, by site
- specified site NEC LØ2.818
- spermatic cord N49.1
- sphenoidal (sinus) (chronic) J32.3
- spinal cord (any part) (staphylococcal) GØ6.1
  - tuberculous A17.81
- spine (column) (tuberculous) A18.Ø1
  - epidural GØ6.1
  - nontuberculous — *see* Osteomyelitis, vertebra
- spleen D73.3
  - amebic AØ6.89
- stitch T81.4 ☑
- subarachnoid GØ6.2
  - brain GØ6.Ø
  - spinal cord GØ6.1
- subareolar — *see* Abscess, breast
- subcecal K35.3
- subcutaneous (*see also* Abscess, by site)

Abscess — *continued*
- subcutaneous (*see also* Abscess, by site) — *continued*
  - pheomycotic (chromomycotic) B43.2
- subdiaphragmatic K65.1
- subdural GØ6.2
  - brain GØ6.Ø
    - sequelae GØ9
  - spinal cord GØ6.1
- subgaleal LØ2.811
- subhepatic K65.1
- sublingual K12.2
  - gland K11.3
- submammary — *see* Abscess, breast
- submandibular (region) (space) (triangle) K12.2
  - gland K11.3
- submaxillary (region) LØ2.Ø1
  - gland K11.3
- submental LØ2.Ø1
  - gland K11.3
- subperiosteal — *see* Osteomyelitis, specified type NEC
- subphrenic K65.1
  - postoperative T81.4 ☑
- suburethral N34.Ø
- sudoriparous L75.8
- supraclavicular (fossa) — *see* Abscess, upper limb
- suprapelvic, acute N73.Ø
- suprarenal (capsule) (gland) E27.8
- sweat gland L74.8
- tear duct — *see* Inflammation, lacrimal, passages, acute
- temple LØ2.Ø1
- temporal region LØ2.Ø1
- temporosphenoidal GØ6.Ø
- tendon (sheath) M65.ØØ
  - ankle M65.Ø7- ☑
  - foot M65.Ø7- ☑
  - forearm M65.Ø3- ☑
  - hand M65.Ø4- ☑
  - lower leg M65.Ø6- ☑
  - pelvic region M65.Ø5- ☑
  - shoulder region M65.Ø1- ☑
  - specified site NEC M65.Ø8
  - thigh M65.Ø5- ☑
  - upper arm M65.Ø2- ☑
- testis N45.4
- thigh — *see* Abscess, lower limb
- thorax J86.9
  - with fistula J86.Ø
- throat J39.1
- thumb (*see also* Abscess, hand)
  - nail — *see* Cellulitis, finger
- thymus (gland) E32.1
- thyroid (gland) EØ6.Ø
- toe (any) (*see also* Abscess, foot)
  - nail — *see* Cellulitis, toe
- tongue (staphylococcal) K14.Ø
- tonsil(s) (lingual) J36
- tonsillopharyngeal J36
- tooth, teeth (root) KØ4.7
  - with sinus (alveolar) KØ4.6
  - supporting structures NEC KØ5.21
- trachea J39.8
- trunk LØ2.219
  - abdominal wall LØ2.211
  - back LØ2.212
  - chest wall LØ2.213
  - groin LØ2.214
  - perineum LØ2.215
  - umbilicus LØ2.216
- tubal — *see* Salpingitis
- tuberculous — *see* Tuberculosis, abscess
- tubo-ovarian — *see* Salpingo-oophoritis
- tunica vaginalis N49.1
- umbilicus LØ2.216
- upper
  - limb LØ2.41- ☑
  - respiratory J39.8
- urethral (gland) N34.Ø
- urinary N34.Ø
- uterus, uterine (wall) (*see also* Endometritis)
  - ligament (*see also* Disease, pelvis, inflammatory) N73.2
  - neck — *see* Cervicitis
- uvula K12.2
- vagina (wall) — *see* Vaginitis
- vaginorectal — *see* Vaginitis

Abscess — *continued*
- vas deferens N49.1
- vermiform appendix K35.3
- vertebra (column) (tuberculous) A18.Ø1
  - nontuberculous — *see* Osteomyelitis, vertebra
- vesical — *see* Cystitis, specified type NEC
- vesico-uterine pouch — *see* Peritonitis, pelvic, female
- vitreous (humor) — *see* Endophthalmitis, purulent
- vocal cord J38.3
- von Bezold's — *see* Mastoiditis, acute
- vulva N76.4
- vulvovaginal gland N75.1
- web space — *see* Abscess, hand
- wound T81.4 ☑
- wrist — *see* Abscess, upper limb

Absence (of) (organ or part) (complete or partial)
- adrenal (gland) (congenital) Q89.1
  - acquired E89.6
- albumin in blood E88.Ø9
- alimentary tract (congenital) Q45.8
  - upper Q4Ø.8
- alveolar process (acquired) — *see* Anomaly, alveolar
- ankle (acquired) Z89.44- ☑
- anus (congenital) Q42.3
  - with fistula Q42.2
- aorta (congenital) Q25.4
- appendix, congenital Q42.8
- arm (acquired) Z89.2Ø- ☑
  - above elbow Z89.22- ☑
    - congenital (with hand present) — *see* Agenesis, arm, with hand present
      - and hand — *see* Agenesis, forearm, and hand
  - below elbow Z89.21- ☑
    - congenital (with hand present) — *see* Agenesis, arm, with hand present
      - and hand — *see* Agenesis, forearm, and hand
  - congenital — *see* Defect, reduction, upper limb
  - shoulder (following explantation of shoulder joint prosthesis) (joint) (with or without presence of antibiotic-impregnated cement spacer) Z89.23- ☑
    - congenital (with hand present) — *see* Agenesis, arm, with hand present
- artery (congenital) (peripheral) Q27.8
  - brain Q28.3
  - coronary Q24.5
  - pulmonary Q25.79
  - specified NEC Q27.8
  - umbilical Q27.Ø
- atrial septum (congenital) Q21.1
- auditory canal (congenital) (external) Q16.1
- auricle (ear), congenital Q16.Ø
- bile, biliary duct, congenital Q44.5
- bladder (acquired) Z9Ø.6
  - congenital Q64.5
- bowel sounds R19.11
- brain QØØ.Ø
  - part of QØ4.3
- breast(s) (and nipple(s)) (acquired) Z9Ø.1- ☑
  - congenital Q83.8
- broad ligament Q5Ø.6
- bronchus (congenital) Q32.4
- canaliculus lacrimalis, congenital Q1Ø.4
- cerebellum (vermis) QØ4.3
- cervix (acquired) (with uterus) Z9Ø.71Ø
  - with remaining uterus Z9Ø.712
  - congenital Q51.5
- chin, congenital Q18.8
- cilia (congenital) Q1Ø.3
  - acquired — *see* Madarosis
- clitoris (congenital) Q52.6
- coccyx, congenital Q76.49
- cold sense R2Ø.8
- congenital
  - lumen — *see* Atresia
  - organ or site NEC — *see* Agenesis
  - septum — *see* Imperfect, closure
- corpus callosum QØ4.Ø
- cricoid cartilage, congenital Q31.8
- diaphragm (with hernia), congenital Q79.1
- digestive organ(s) or tract, congenital Q45.8
  - acquired NEC Z9Ø.49
  - upper Q4Ø.8
- ductus arteriosus Q28.8
- duodenum (acquired) Z9Ø.49
  - congenital Q41.Ø

Absence — *continued*
- ear, congenital Q16.9
  - acquired H93.8- ☑
  - auricle Q16.Ø
  - external Q16.Ø
  - inner Q16.5
  - lobe, lobule Q17.8
  - middle, except ossicies Q16.4
    - ossicles Q16.3
  - ossicles Q16.3
- ejaculatory duct (congenital) Q55.4
- endocrine gland (congenital) NEC Q89.2
  - acquired E89.89
- epididymis (congenital) Q55.4
  - acquired Z9Ø.79
- epiglottis, congenital Q31.8
- esophagus (congenital) Q39.8
  - acquired (partial) Z9Ø.49
- eustachian tube (congenital) Q16.2
- extremity (acquired) Z89.9
  - congenital Q73.Ø
  - knee (following explantation of knee joint prosthesis) (joint) (with or without presence of antibiotic-impregnated cement spacer) Z89.52- ☑
  - lower (above knee) Z89.619
    - below knee Z89.51- ☑
  - upper — *see* Absence, arm
- eye (acquired) Z9Ø.Ø1
  - congenital Q11.1
  - muscle (congenital) Q1Ø.3
- eyeball (acquired) Z9Ø.Ø1
- eyelid (fold) (congenital) Q1Ø.3
  - acquired Z9Ø.Ø1
- face, specified part NEC Q18.8
- fallopian tube(s) (acquired) Z9Ø.79
  - congenital Q5Ø.6
- family member (causing problem in home) NEC (*see also* Disruption, family) Z63.32
- femur, congenital — *see* Defect, reduction, lower limb, longitudinal, femur
- fibrinogen (congenital) D68.2
  - acquired D65
- finger(s) (acquired) Z89.Ø2- ☑
  - congenital — *see* Agenesis, hand
- foot (acquired) Z89.43- ☑
  - congenital — *see* Agenesis, foot
- forearm (acquired) — *see* Absence, arm, below elbow
- gallbladder (acquired) Z9Ø.49
  - congenital Q44.Ø
- gamma globulin in blood D8Ø.1
  - hereditary D8Ø.Ø
- genital organs
  - acquired (female) (male) Z9Ø.79
  - female, congenital Q52.8
    - external Q52.71
    - internal NEC Q52.8
  - male, congenital Q55.8
- genitourinary organs, congenital NEC
  - female Q52.8
  - male Q55.8
- globe (acquired) Z9Ø.Ø1
  - congenital Q11.1
- glottis, congenital Q31.8
- hand and wrist (acquired) Z89.11- ☑
  - congenital — *see* Agenesis, hand
- head, part (acquired) NEC Z9Ø.Ø9
- heat sense R2Ø.8
- hip (following explantation of hip joint prosthesis) (joint) (with or without presence of antibiotic-impregnated cement spacer) Z89.62- ☑
- hymen (congenital) Q52.4
- ileum (acquired) Z9Ø.49
  - congenital Q41.2
- immunoglobulin, isolated NEC D8Ø.3
  - IgA D8Ø.2
  - IgG D8Ø.3
  - IgM D8Ø.4
- incus (acquired) — *see* Loss, ossicles, ear
  - congenital Q16.3
- inner ear, congenital Q16.5
- intestine (acquired) (small) Z9Ø.49
  - congenital Q41.9
    - specified NEC Q41.8
  - large Z9Ø.49
    - congenital Q42.9
      - specified NEC Q42.8
- iris, congenital Q13.1

Absence — *continued*
- jejunum (acquired) Z9Ø.49
  - congenital Q41.1
- joint
  - acquired
    - hip (following explantation of hip joint prosthesis) (with or without presence of antibiotic-impregnated cement spacer) Z89.62- ☑
    - knee (following explantation of knee joint prosthesis) (with or without presence of antibiotic-impregnated cement spacer) Z89.52- ☑
    - shoulder (following explantation of shoulder joint prosthesis) (with or without presence of antibiotic-impregnated cement spacer) Z89.23- ☑
  - congenital NEC Q74.8
- kidney(s) (acquired) Z9Ø.5
  - congenital Q6Ø.2
    - bilateral Q6Ø.1
    - unilateral Q6Ø.Ø
- knee (following explantation of knee joint prosthesis) (joint) (with or without presence of antibiotic-impregnated cement spacer) Z89.52- ☑
- labyrinth, membranous Q16.5
- larynx (congenital) Q31.8
  - acquired Z9Ø.Ø2
- leg (acquired) (above knee) Z89.61- ☑
  - below knee (acquired) Z89.51- ☑
  - congenital — *see* Defect, reduction, lower limb
- lens (acquired) (*see also* Aphakia)
  - congenital Q12.3
  - post cataract extraction Z98.4- ☑
- limb (acquired) — *see* Absence, extremity
- lip Q38.6
- liver (congenital) Q44.7
- lung (fissure) (lobe) (bilateral) (unilateral) (congenital) Q33.3
  - acquired (any part) Z9Ø.2
- menstruation — *see* Amenorrhea
- muscle (congenital) (pectoral) Q79.8
  - ocular Q1Ø.3
- neck, part Q18.8
- neutrophil — *see* Agranulocytosis
- nipple(s) (with breast(s)) (acquired) Z9Ø.1- ☑
  - congenital Q83.2
- nose (congenital) Q3Ø.1
  - acquired Z9Ø.Ø9
- organ
  - of Corti, congenital Q16.5
  - or site, congenital NEC Q89.8
    - acquired NEC Z9Ø.89
- osseous meatus (ear) Q16.4
- ovary (acquired)
  - bilateral Z9Ø.722
  - congenital
    - bilateral Q5Ø.Ø2
    - unilateral Q5Ø.Ø1
  - unilateral Z9Ø.721
- oviduct (acquired)
  - bilateral Z9Ø.722
  - congenital Q5Ø.6
  - unilateral Z9Ø.721
- pancreas (congenital) Q45.Ø
  - acquired Z9Ø.41Ø
    - complete Z9Ø.41Ø
    - partial Z9Ø.411
    - total Z9Ø.41Ø
- parathyroid gland (acquired) E89.2
  - congenital Q89.2
- patella, congenital Q74.1
- penis (congenital) Q55.5
  - acquired Z9Ø.79
- pericardium (congenital) Q24.8
- pituitary gland (congenital) Q89.2
  - acquired E89.3
- prostate (acquired) Z9Ø.79
  - congenital Q55.4
- pulmonary valve Q22.Ø
- punctum lacrimale (congenital) Q1Ø.4
- radius, congenital — *see* Defect, reduction, upper limb, longitudinal, radius
- rectum (congenital) Q42.1
  - with fistula Q42.Ø
  - acquired Z9Ø.49
- respiratory organ NOS Q34.9
- rib (acquired) Z9Ø.89

Absence — *continued*
- rib — *continued*
  - congenital Q76.6
- sacrum, congenital Q76.49
- salivary gland(s), congenital Q38.4
- scrotum, congenital Q55.29
- seminal vesicles (congenital) Q55.4
  - acquired Z9Ø.79
- septum
  - atrial (congenital) Q21.1
  - between aorta and pulmonary artery Q21.4
  - ventricular (congenital) Q2Ø.4
- sex chromosome
  - female phenotype Q97.8
  - male phenotype Q98.8
- skull bone (congenital) Q75.8
  - with
    - anencephaly QØØ.Ø
    - encephalocele — *see* Encephalocele
    - hydrocephalus QØ3.9
      - with spina bifida — *see* Spina bifida, by site, with hydrocephalus
    - microcephaly QØ2
- spermatic cord, congenital Q55.4
- spine, congenital Q76.49
- spleen (congenital) Q89.Ø1
  - acquired Z9Ø.81
- sternum, congenital Q76.7
- stomach (acquired) (partial) Z9Ø.3
  - congenital Q4Ø.2
- superior vena cava, congenital Q26.8
- teeth, tooth (congenital) KØØ.Ø
  - acquired (complete) KØ8.1Ø9
    - class I KØ8.1Ø1
    - class II KØ8.1Ø2
    - class III KØ8.1Ø3
    - class IV KØ8.1Ø4
    - due to
      - caries KØ8.139
        - class I KØ8.131
        - class II KØ8.132
        - class III KØ8.133
        - class IV KØ8.134
      - periodontal disease KØ8.129
        - class I KØ8.121
        - class II KØ8.122
        - class III KØ8.123
        - class IV KØ8.124
      - specified NEC KØ8.199
        - class I KØ8.191
        - class II KØ8.192
        - class III KØ8.193
        - class IV KØ8.194
      - trauma KØ8.119
        - class I KØ8.111
        - class II KØ8.112
        - class III KØ8.113
        - class IV KØ8.114
    - partial KØ8.4Ø9
      - class I KØ8.4Ø1
      - class II KØ8.4Ø2
      - class III KØ8.4Ø3
      - class IV KØ8.4Ø4
      - due to
        - caries KØ8.439
          - class I KØ8.431
          - class II KØ8.432
          - class III KØ8.433
          - class IV KØ8.434
        - periodontal disease KØ8.429
          - class I KØ8.421
          - class II KØ8.422
          - class III KØ8.423
          - class IV KØ8.424
        - specified NEC KØ8.499
          - class I KØ8.491
          - class II KØ8.492
          - class III KØ8.493
          - class IV KØ8.494
        - trauma KØ8.419
          - class I KØ8.411
          - class II KØ8.412
          - class III KØ8.413
          - class IV KØ8.414
- tendon (congenital) Q79.8
- testis (congenital) Q55.Ø
  - acquired Z9Ø.79
- thumb (acquired) Z89.Ø1- ☑

Abuse — *continued*
- drug — *continued*
  - solvent — *see* Abuse, drug, inhalant
  - steroids F55.3
  - stimulant NEC F15.1Ø
    - with
      - anxiety disorder F15.18Ø
      - intoxication F15.129
        - with
          - delirium F15.121
          - perceptual disturbance F15.122
        - uncomplicated F15.12Ø
      - mood disorder F15.14
      - other specified disorder F15.188
      - psychosis F15.159
        - delusions F15.15Ø
        - hallucinations F15.151
      - sexual dysfunction F15.181
      - sleep disorder F15.182
      - unspecified disorder F15.19
  - tranquilizers — *see* Abuse, drug, sedative
  - vitamins F55.4
- hallucinogens — *see* Abuse, drug, hallucinogen
- hashish — *see* Abuse, drug, cannabis
- herbal or folk remedies F55.1
- hormones F55.3
- hypnotic — *see* Abuse, drug, sedative
- inhalant — *see* Abuse, drug, inhalant
- laxatives F55.2
- LSD — *see* Abuse, drug, hallucinogen
- marihuana — *see* Abuse, drug, cannabis
- morphine type (opioids) — *see* Abuse, drug, opioid
- non-psychoactive substance NEC F55.8
  - antacids F55.Ø
  - folk remedies F55.1
  - herbal remedies F55.1
  - hormones F55.3
  - laxatives F55.2
  - steroids F55.3
  - vitamins F55.4
- opioids — *see* Abuse, drug, opioid
- PCP (phencyclidine) (or related substance) — *see* Abuse, drug, hallucinogen
- physical (adult) (child) — *see* Maltreatment
- psychoactive substance — *see* Abuse, drug, psychoactive NEC
- psychological (adult) (child) — *see* Maltreatment
- sedative — *see* Abuse, drug, sedative
- sexual — *see* Maltreatment
- solvent — *see* Abuse, drug, inhalant
- steroids F55.3
- vitamins F55.4

Acalculia R48.8
- developmental F81.2

Acanthamebiasis (with) B6Ø.1Ø
- conjunctiva B6Ø.12
- keratoconjunctivitis B6Ø.13
- meningoencephalitis B6Ø.11
- other specified B6Ø.19

Acanthocephaliasis B83.8
Acanthocheilonemiasis B74.4
Acanthocytosis E78.6
Acantholysis L11.9
Acanthosis (acquired) (nigricans) L83
- benign Q82.8
- congenital Q82.8
- seborrheic L82.1
  - inflamed L82.Ø
- tongue K14.3

Acapnia E87.3
Acarbia E87.2
Acardia, acardius Q89.8
Acardiacus amorphus Q89.8
Acardiotrophia I51.4
Acariasis B88.Ø
- scabies B86

Acarodermatitis (urticarioides) B88.Ø
Acarophobia F4Ø.218
Acatalasemia, acatalasia E8Ø.3
Acathisia (drug induced) G25.71
Accelerated atrioventricular conduction I45.6
Accentuation of personality traits (type A) Z73.1
Accessory (congenital)
- adrenal gland Q89.1
- anus Q43.4
- appendix Q43.4
- atrioventricular conduction I45.6

Accessory — *continued*
- auditory ossicles Q16.3
- auricle (ear) Q17.Ø
- biliary duct or passage Q44.5
- bladder Q64.79
- blood vessels NEC Q27.9
  - coronary Q24.5
- bone NEC Q79.8
- breast tissue, axilla Q83.1
- carpal bones Q74.Ø
- cecum Q43.4
- chromosome(s) NEC (nonsex) Q92.9
  - with complex rearrangements NEC Q92.5
    - seen only at prometaphase Q92.8
  - 13 — *see* Trisomy, 13
  - 18 — *see* Trisomy, 18
  - 21 — *see* Trisomy, 21
  - partial Q92.9
  - sex
    - female phenotype Q97.8
- coronary artery Q24.5
- cusp(s), heart valve NEC Q24.8
  - pulmonary Q22.3
- cystic duct Q44.5
- digit(s) Q69.9
- ear (auricle) (lobe) Q17.Ø
- endocrine gland NEC Q89.2
- eye muscle Q1Ø.3
- eyelid Q1Ø.3
- face bone(s) Q75.8
- fallopian tube (fimbria) (ostium) Q5Ø.6
- finger(s) Q69.Ø
- foreskin N47.8
- frontonasal process Q75.8
- gallbladder Q44.1
- genital organ(s)
  - female Q52.8
    - external Q52.79
    - internal NEC Q52.8
  - male Q55.8
- genitourinary organs NEC Q89.8
  - female Q52.8
  - male Q55.8
- hallux Q69.2
- heart Q24.8
  - valve NEC Q24.8
    - pulmonary Q22.3
- hepatic ducts Q44.5
- hymen Q52.4
- intestine (large) (small) Q43.4
- kidney Q63.Ø
- lacrimal canal Q1Ø.6
- leaflet, heart valve NEC Q24.8
- ligament, broad Q5Ø.6
- liver Q44.7
  - duct Q44.5
- lobule (ear) Q17.Ø
- lung (lobe) Q33.1
- muscle Q79.8
- navicular of carpus Q74.Ø
- nervous system, part NEC QØ7.8
- nipple Q83.3
- nose Q3Ø.8
- organ or site not listed — *see* Anomaly, by site
- ovary Q5Ø.31
- oviduct Q5Ø.6
- pancreas Q45.3
- parathyroid gland Q89.2
- parotid gland (and duct) Q38.4
- pituitary gland Q89.2
- preauricular appendage Q17.Ø
- prepuce N47.8
- renal arteries (multiple) Q27.2
- rib Q76.6
  - cervical Q76.5
- roots (teeth) KØØ.2
- salivary gland Q38.4
- sesamoid bones Q74.8
  - foot Q74.2
  - hand Q74.Ø
- skin tags Q82.8
- spleen Q89.Ø9
- sternum Q76.7
- submaxillary gland Q38.4
- tarsal bones Q74.2
- teeth, tooth KØØ.1
- tendon Q79.8
- thumb Q69.1

Accessory — *continued*
- thymus gland Q89.2
- thyroid gland Q89.2
- toes Q69.2
- tongue Q38.3
- tooth, teeth KØØ.1
- tragus Q17.Ø
- ureter Q62.5
- urethra Q64.79
- urinary organ or tract NEC Q64.8
- uterus Q51.2
- vagina Q52.1Ø
- valve, heart NEC Q24.8
  - pulmonary Q22.3
- vertebra Q76.49
- vocal cords Q31.8
- vulva Q52.79

Accident
- birth — *see* Birth, injury
- cardiac — *see* Infarct, myocardium
- cerebral I63.9
- cerebrovascular (embolic) (ischemic) (thrombotic) I63.9
  - aborted I63.9
  - hemorrhagic — *see* Hemorrhage, intracranial, intracerebral
  - old (without sequelae) Z86.73
    - with sequelae (of) — *see* Sequelae, infarction, cerebral
- coronary — *see* Infarct, myocardium
- craniovascular I63.9
- vascular, brain I63.9

Accidental — *see* condition
Accommodation (disorder) (*see also* condition)
- hysterical paralysis of F44.89
- insufficiency of H52.4
- paresis — *see* Paresis, of accommodation
- spasm — *see* Spasm, of accommodation

Accouchement — *see* Delivery
Accreta placenta O43.21- ☑
Accretio cordis (nonrheumatic) I31.Ø
Accretions, tooth, teeth KØ3.6
Acculturation difficulty Z6Ø.3
Accumulation secretion, prostate N42.89
Acephalia, acephalism, acephalus, acephaly QØØ.Ø
Acephalobrachia monster Q89.8
Acephalochirus monster Q89.8
Acephalogaster Q89.8
Acephalostomus monster Q89.8
Acephalothorax Q89.8
Acerophobia F4Ø.298
Acetonemia R79.89
- in Type 1 diabetes E1Ø.1Ø
  - with coma E1Ø.11

Acetonuria R82.4
Achalasia (cardia) (esophagus) K22.Ø
- congenital Q39.5
- pylorus Q4Ø.Ø
- sphincteral NEC K59.8

Ache(s) — *see* Pain
Acheilia Q38.6
Achillobursitis — *see* Tendinitis, Achilles
Achillodynia — *see* Tendinitis, Achilles
Achlorhydria, achlorhydric (neurogenic) K31.83
- anemia D5Ø.8
- diarrhea K31.83
- psychogenic F45.8
- secondary to vagotomy K91.1

Achluophobia F4Ø.228
Acholia K82.8
Acholuric jaundice (familial) (splenomegalic) (*see also* Spherocytosis)
- acquired D59.8

Achondrogenesis Q77.Ø
Achondroplasia (osteosclerosis congenita) Q77.4
Achroma, cutis L8Ø
Achromat (ism), achromatopsia (acquired) (congenital) H53.51
Achromia, congenital — *see* Albinism
Achromia parasitica B36.Ø
Achylia gastrica K31.89
- psychogenic F45.8

Acid
- burn — *see* Corrosion
- deficiency
  - amide nicotinic E52
  - ascorbic E54
  - folic E53.8

- **Acid** — *continued*
  - deficiency — *continued*
    - nicotinic E52
    - pantothenic E53.8
  - intoxication E87.2
  - peptic disease K3Ø
  - phosphatase deficiency E83.39
  - stomach K3Ø
    - psychogenic F45.8
- **Acidemia** E87.2
  - argininosuccinic E72.22
  - isovaleric E71.11Ø
  - metabolic (newborn) P19.9
    - first noted before onset of labor P19.Ø
    - first noted during labor P19.1
    - noted at birth P19.2
  - methylmalonic E71.12Ø
  - pipecolic E72.3
  - propionic E71.121
- **Acidity, gastric** (high) K3Ø
  - psychogenic F45.8
- **Acidocytopenia** — *see* Agranulocytosis
- **Acidocytosis** D72.1
- **Acidopenia** — *see* Agranulocytosis
- **Acidosis** (lactic) (respiratory) E87.2
  - in Type 1 diabetes E1Ø.1Ø
    - with coma E1Ø.11
  - kidney, tubular N25.89
  - lactic E87.2
  - metabolic NEC E87.2
    - with respiratory acidosis E87.4
    - late, of newborn P74.Ø
  - mixed metabolic and respiratory, newborn P84
  - newborn P84
  - renal (hyperchloremic) (tubular) N25.89
  - respiratory E87.2
    - complicated by
      - metabolic
        - acidosis E87.4
        - alkalosis E87.4
- **Aciduria**
  - argininosuccinic E72.22
  - glutaric (type I) E72.3
    - type II E71.313
    - type III E71.5- ☑
  - orotic (congenital) (hereditary) (pyrimidine deficiency) E79.8
    - anemia D53.Ø
- **Acladiosis** (skin) B36.Ø
- **Aclasis, diaphyseal** Q78.6
- **Acleistocardia** Q21.1
- **Aclusion** — *see* Anomaly, dentofacial, malocclusion
- **Acne** L7Ø.9
  - artificialis L7Ø.8
  - atrophica L7Ø.2
  - cachecticorum (Hebra) L7Ø.8
  - conglobata L7Ø.1
  - cystic L7Ø.Ø
  - decalvans L66.2
  - excoriée des jeunes filles L7Ø.5
  - frontalis L7Ø.2
  - indurata L7Ø.Ø
  - infantile L7Ø.4
  - keloid L73.Ø
  - lupoid L7Ø.2
  - necrotic, necrotica (miliaris) L7Ø.2
  - neonatal L7Ø.4
  - nodular L7Ø.Ø
  - occupational L7Ø.8
  - picker's L7Ø.5
  - pustular L7Ø.Ø
  - rodens L7Ø.2
  - rosacea L71.9
  - specified NEC L7Ø.8
  - tropica L7Ø.3
  - varioliformis L7Ø.2
  - vulgaris L7Ø.Ø
- **Acnitis** (primary) A18.4
- **Acosta's disease** T7Ø.29 ☑
- **Acoustic** — *see* condition
- **Acousticophobia** F4Ø.298
- **Acquired** (*see also* condition)
  - immunodeficiency syndrome (AIDS) B2Ø
- **Acrania** QØØ.Ø
- **Acroangiodermatitis** I78.9
- **Acroasphyxia, chronic** I73.89
- **Acrobystitis** N47.7
- **Acrocephalopolysyndactyly** Q87.Ø
- **Acrocephalosyndactyly** Q87.Ø
- **Acrocephaly** Q75.Ø
- **Acrochondrohyperplasia** — *see* Syndrome, Marfan's
- **Acrocyanosis** I73.8 ☑
  - newborn P28.2
    - meaning transient blue hands and feet — *omit code*
- **Acrodermatitis** L3Ø.8
  - atrophicans (chronica) L9Ø.4
  - continua (Hallopeau) L4Ø.2
  - enteropathica (hereditary) E83.2
  - Hallopeau's L4Ø.2
  - infantile papular L44.4
  - perstans L4Ø.2
  - pustulosa continua L4Ø.2
  - recalcitrant pustular L4Ø.2
- **Acrodynia** — *see* Poisoning, mercury
- **Acromegaly, acromegalia** E22.Ø
- **Acromelalgia** I73.81
- **Acromicria, acromikria** Q79.8
- **Acronyx** L6Ø.Ø
- **Acropachy, thyroid** — *see* Thyrotoxicosis
- **Acroparesthesia** (simple) (vasomotor) I73.89
- **Acropathy, thyroid** — *see* Thyrotoxicosis
- **Acrophobia** F4Ø.241
- **Acroposthitis** N47.7
- **Acroscleriasis, acroscleroderma, acrosclerosis** — *see* Sclerosis, systemic
- **Acrosphacelus** I96
- **Acrospiroma, eccrine** — *see* Neoplasm, skin, benign
- **Acrostealgia** — *see* Osteochondropathy
- **Acrotrophodynia** — *see* Immersion
- **ACTH ectopic syndrome** E24.3
- **Actinic** — *see* condition
- **Actinobacillosis, actinobacillus** A28.8
  - mallei A24.Ø
  - muris A25.1
- **Actinomyces israelii** (infection) — *see* Actinomycosis
- **Actinomycetoma** (foot) B47.1
- **Actinomycosis, actinomycotic** A42.9
  - with pneumonia A42.Ø
  - abdominal A42.1
  - cervicofacial A42.2
  - cutaneous A42.89
  - gastrointestinal A42.1
  - pulmonary A42.Ø
  - sepsis A42.7
  - specified site NEC A42.89
- **Actinoneuritis** G62.82
- **Action, heart**
  - disorder I49.9
  - irregular I49.9
    - psychogenic F45.8
- **Activated protein C resistance** D68.51
- **Active** — *see* condition
- **Acute** (*see also* condition)
  - abdomen R1Ø.Ø
  - gallbladder — *see* Cholecystitis, acute
- **Acyanotic heart disease** (congenital) Q24.9
- **Acystia** Q64.5
- **Adair-Dighton syndrome** (brittle bones and blue sclera, deafness) Q78.Ø
- **Adamantinoblastoma** — *see* Ameloblastoma
- **Adamantinoma** (*see also* Cyst, calcifying odontogenic)
  - long bones C4Ø.9Ø
    - lower limb C4Ø.2- ☑
    - upper limb C4Ø.Ø- ☑
  - malignant C41.1
    - jaw (bone) (lower) C41.1
      - upper C41.Ø
  - tibial C4Ø.2- ☑
- **Adamantoblastoma** — *see* Ameloblastoma
- **Adams-Stokes** (-Morgagni) disease or syndrome I45.9
- **Adaption reaction** — *see* Disorder, adjustment
- **Addiction** (*see also* Dependence) F19.2Ø
  - alcohol, alcoholic (ethyl) (methyl) (wood) (without remission) F1Ø.2Ø
    - with remission F1Ø.21
  - drug — *see* Dependence, drug
  - ethyl alcohol (without remission) F1Ø.2Ø
    - with remission F1Ø.21
  - heroin — *see* Dependence, drug, opioid
  - methyl alcohol (without remission) F1Ø.2Ø
    - with remission F1Ø.21
  - methylated spirit (without remission) F1Ø.2Ø
    - with remission F1Ø.21
- **Addiction** — *continued*
  - morphine (-like substances) — *see* Dependence, drug, opioid
  - nicotine — *see* Dependence, drug, nicotine
  - opium and opioids — *see* Dependence, drug, opioid
  - tobacco — *see* Dependence, drug, nicotine
- **Addison-Biermer anemia** (pernicious) D51.Ø
- **Addisonian crisis** E27.2
- **Addison's**
  - anemia (pernicious) D51.Ø
  - disease (bronze) or syndrome E27.1
    - tuberculous A18.7
  - keloid L94.Ø
- **Addison-Schilder complex** E71.528
- **Additional** (*see also* Accessory)
  - chromosome(s) Q99.8
    - 21 — *see* Trisomy, 21
    - sex — *see* Abnormal, chromosome, sex
- **Adduction contracture, hip or other joint** — *see* Contraction, joint
- **Adenitis** (*see also* Lymphadenitis)
  - acute, unspecified site LØ4.9
  - axillary I88.9
    - acute LØ4.2
    - chronic or subacute I88.1
  - Bartholin's gland N75.8
  - bulbourethral gland — *see* Urethritis
  - cervical I88.9
    - acute LØ4.Ø
    - chronic or subacute I88.1
  - chancroid (Hemophilus ducreyi) A57
  - chronic, unspecified site I88.1
  - Cowper's gland — *see* Urethritis
  - due to Pasteurella multocida (p. septica) A28.Ø
  - epidemic, acute B27.Ø9
  - gangrenous LØ4.9
  - gonorrheal NEC A54.89
  - groin I88.9
    - acute LØ4.1
    - chronic or subacute I88.1
  - infectious (acute) (epidemic) B27.Ø9
  - inguinal I88.9
    - acute LØ4.1
    - chronic or subacute I88.1
  - lymph gland or node, except mesenteric I88.9
    - acute — *see* Lymphadenitis, acute
    - chronic or subacute I88.1
  - mesenteric (acute) (chronic) (nonspecific) (subacute) I88.Ø
  - parotid gland (suppurative) — *see* Sialoadenitis
  - salivary gland (any) (suppurative) — *see* Sialoadenitis
  - scrofulous (tuberculous) A18.2
  - Skene's duct or gland — *see* Urethritis
  - strumous, tuberculous A18.2
  - subacute, unspecified site I88.1
  - sublingual gland (suppurative) — *see* Sialoadenitis
  - submandibular gland (suppurative) — *see* Sialoadenitis
  - submaxillary gland (suppurative) — *see* Sialoadenitis
  - tuberculous — *see* Tuberculosis, lymph gland
  - urethral gland — *see* Urethritis
  - Wharton's duct (suppurative) — *see* Sialoadenitis
- **Adenoacanthoma** — *see* Neoplasm, malignant, by site
- **Adenoameloblastoma** — *see* Cyst, calcifying odontogenic
- **Adenocarcinoid** (tumor) — *see* Neoplasm, malignant, by site
- **Adenocarcinoma** (*see also* Neoplasm, malignant, by site)
  - acidophil
    - specified site — *see* Neoplasm, malignant, by site
    - unspecified site C75.1
  - adrenal cortical C74.Ø- ☑
  - alveolar — *see* Neoplasm, lung, malignant
  - apocrine
    - breast — *see* Neoplasm, breast, malignant
    - in situ
      - breast DØ5.8- ☑
      - specified site NEC — *see* Neoplasm, skin, in situ
      - unspecified site DØ4.9
    - specified site NEC — *see* Neoplasm, skin, malignant
    - unspecified site C44.99
  - basal cell
    - specified site — *see* Neoplasm, skin, malignant
    - unspecified site CØ8.9
  - basophil
    - specified site — *see* Neoplasm, malignant, by site

Index

Adenocarcinoma — Adenoma

DRAFT

Adenoma — *continued*
- liver cell D13.4
- macrofollicular
  - specified site — *see* Neoplasm, benign, by site
  - unspecified site D34
- malignant, malignum — *see* Neoplasm, malignant, by site
- microcystic
  - pancreas D13.7
  - specified site NEC — *see* Neoplasm, benign, by site
  - unspecified site D13.7
- microfollicular
  - specified site — *see* Neoplasm, benign, by site
  - unspecified site D34
- mucoid cell
  - specified site — *see* Neoplasm, benign, by site
  - unspecified site D35.2
- multiple endocrine
  - single specified site — *see* Neoplasm, uncertain behavior, by site
  - two or more specified sites D44- ☑
  - unspecified site D44.9
- nipple D24- ☑
- papillary (*see also* Neoplasm, benign, by site)
  - eccrine — *see* Neoplasm, skin, benign, by site
- Pick's tubular
  - specified site — *see* Neoplasm, benign, by site
  - unspecified site
    - female D27.9
    - male D29.2Ø
- pleomorphic
  - carcinoma in — *see* Neoplasm, salivary gland, malignant
    - specified site — *see* Neoplasm, malignant, by site
    - unspecified site CØ8.9
- polypoid (*see also* Neoplasm, benign)
  - adenocarcinoma in — *see* Neoplasm, malignant, by site
  - adenocarcinoma in situ — *see* Neoplasm, in situ, by site
- prostate — *see* Neoplasm, benign, prostate
- rete cell D29.2Ø
- sebaceous — *see* Neoplasm, skin, benign
- Sertoli cell
  - specified site — *see* Neoplasm, benign, by site
  - unspecified site
    - female D27.9
    - male D29.2Ø
- skin appendage — *see* Neoplasm, skin, benign
- sudoriferous gland — *see* Neoplasm, skin, benign
- sweat gland — *see* Neoplasm, skin, benign
- testicular
  - specified site — *see* Neoplasm, benign, by site
  - unspecified site
    - female D27.9
    - male D29.2Ø
- tubular (*see also* Neoplasm, benign, by site)
  - adenocarcinoma in — *see* Neoplasm, malignant, by site
  - adenocarcinoma in situ — *see* Neoplasm, in situ, by site
  - Pick's
    - specified site — *see* Neoplasm, benign, by site
    - unspecified site
      - female D27.9
      - male D29.2Ø
- tubulovillous (*see also* Neoplasm, benign, by site)
  - adenocarcinoma in — *see* Neoplasm, malignant, by site
  - adenocarcinoma in situ — *see* Neoplasm, in situ, by site
- villous — *see* Neoplasm, uncertain behavior, by site
  - adenocarcinoma in — *see* Neoplasm, malignant, by site
  - adenocarcinoma in situ — *see* Neoplasm, in situ, by site
- water-clear cell D35.1

Adenomatosis
- endocrine (multiple) E31.2Ø
  - single specified site — *see* Neoplasm, uncertain behavior, by site
- erosive of nipple D24- ☑
- pluriendocrine — *see* Adenomatosis, endocrine
- pulmonary D38.1
  - malignant — *see* Neoplasm, lung, malignant
- specified site — *see* Neoplasm, benign, by site

Adenomatosis — *continued*
- unspecified site D12.6

Adenomatous
- goiter (nontoxic) EØ4.9
  - with hyperthyroidism — *see* Hyperthyroidism, with, goiter, nodular
  - toxic — *see* Hyperthyroidism, with, goiter, nodular

Adenomyoma (*see also* Neoplasm, benign, by site)
- prostate — *see* Enlarged, prostate

Adenomyometritis N8Ø.Ø

Adenomyosis N8Ø.Ø

Adenopathy (lymph gland) R59.9
- generalized R59.1
- inguinal R59.Ø
- localized R59.Ø
- mediastinal R59.Ø
- mesentery R59.Ø
- syphilitic (secondary) A51.49
- tracheobronchial R59.Ø
  - tuberculous A15.4
    - primary (progressive) A15.7
- tuberculous (*see also* Tuberculosis, lymph gland)
  - tracheobronchial A15.4
    - primary (progressive) A15.7

Adenosalpingitis — *see* Salpingitis

Adenosarcoma — *see* Neoplasm, malignant, by site

Adenosclerosis I88.8

Adenosis (sclerosing) breast — *see* Fibroadenosis, breast

Adenovirus, as cause of disease classified elsewhere B97.Ø

Adentia (complete) (partial) — *see* Absence, teeth

Adherent (*see also* Adhesions)
- labia (minora) N9Ø.89
- pericardium (nonrheumatic) I31.Ø
  - rheumatic IØ9.2
- placenta (with hemorrhage) O72.Ø
  - without hemorrhage O73.Ø
- prepuce, newborn N47.Ø
- scar (skin) L9Ø.5
- tendon in scar L9Ø.5

Adhesions, adhesive (postinfective) K66.Ø
- with intestinal obstruction K56.5
- abdominal (wall) — *see* Adhesions, peritoneum
- appendix K38.8
- bile duct (common) (hepatic) K83.8
- bladder (sphincter) N32.89
- bowel — *see* Adhesions, peritoneum
- cardiac I31.Ø
  - rheumatic IØ9.2
- cecum — *see* Adhesions, peritoneum
- cervicovaginal N88.1
  - congenital Q52.8
  - postpartal O9Ø.89
    - old N88.1
- cervix N88.1
- ciliary body NEC — *see* Adhesions, iris
- clitoris N9Ø.89
- colon — *see* Adhesions, peritoneum
- common duct K83.8
- congenital (*see also* Anomaly, by site)
  - fingers — *see* Syndactylism, complex, fingers
  - omental, anomalous Q43.3
  - peritoneal Q43.3
  - tongue (to gum or roof of mouth) Q38.3
- conjunctiva (acquired) H11.21- ☑
  - congenital Q15.8
- cystic duct K82.8
- diaphragm — *see* Adhesions, peritoneum
- due to foreign body — *see* Foreign body
- duodenum — *see* Adhesions, peritoneum
- ear
  - middle H74.1- ☑
- epididymis N5Ø.8
- epidural — *see* Adhesions, meninges
- epiglottis J38.7
- eyelid HØ2.59
- female pelvis N73.6
- gallbladder K82.8
- globe H44.89
- heart I31.Ø
  - rheumatic IØ9.2
- ileocecal (coil) — *see* Adhesions, peritoneum
- ileum — *see* Adhesions, peritoneum
- intestine (*see also* Adhesions, peritoneum)
  - with obstruction K56.5
- intra-abdominal — *see* Adhesions, peritoneum
- iris H21.5Ø- ☑

Adhesions, adhesive — *continued*
- iris — *continued*
  - anterior H21.51- ☑
  - goniosynechiae H21.52- ☑
  - posterior H21.54- ☑
  - to corneal graft T85.89 ☑
- joint — *see* Ankylosis
  - knee M23.8X ☑
  - temporomandibular M26.61
- labium (majus) (minus), congenital Q52.5
- liver — *see* Adhesions, peritoneum
- lung J98.4
- mediastinum J98.5
- meninges (cerebral) (spinal) G96.12
  - congenital QØ7.8
  - tuberculous (cerebral) (spinal) A17.Ø
- mesenteric — *see* Adhesions, peritoneum
- nasal (septum) (to turbinates) J34.89
- ocular muscle — *see* Strabismus, mechanical
- omentum — *see* Adhesions, peritoneum
- ovary N73.6
  - congenital (to cecum, kidney or omentum) Q5Ø.39
- paraovarian N73.6
- pelvic (peritoneal)
  - female N73.6
    - postprocedural N99.4
  - male — *see* Adhesions, peritoneum
  - postpartal (old) N73.6
  - tuberculous A18.17
- penis to scrotum (congenital) Q55.8
- periappendiceal (*see also* Adhesions, peritoneum)
- pericardium (nonrheumatic) I31.Ø
  - focal I31.8
  - rheumatic IØ9.2
  - tuberculous A18.84
- pericholecystic K82.8
- perigastric — *see* Adhesions, peritoneum
- periovarian N73.6
- periprostatic N42.89
- perirectal — *see* Adhesions, peritoneum
- perirenal N28.89
- peritoneum, peritoneal (postinfective) (postprocedural) K66.Ø
  - with obstruction (intestinal) K56.5
  - congenital Q43.3
  - pelvic, female N73.6
    - postprocedural N99.4
  - postpartal, pelvic N73.6
  - to uterus N73.6
- peritubal N73.6
- periureteral N28.89
- periuterine N73.6
- perivesical N32.89
- perivesicular (seminal vesicle) N5Ø.8
- pleura, pleuritic J94.8
  - tuberculous NEC A15.6
- pleuropericardial J94.8
- postoperative (gastrointestinal tract) K66.Ø
  - with obstruction K91.3
  - due to foreign body accidentally left in wound — *see* Foreign body, accidentally left during a procedure
  - pelvic peritoneal N99.4
  - urethra — *see* Stricture, urethra, postprocedural
  - vagina N99.2
- postpartal, old (vulva or perineum) N9Ø.89
- preputial, prepuce N47.5
- pulmonary J98.4
- pylorus — *see* Adhesions, peritoneum
- sciatic nerve — *see* Lesion, nerve, sciatic
- seminal vesicle N5Ø.8
- shoulder (joint) — *see* Capsulitis, adhesive
- sigmoid flexure — *see* Adhesions, peritoneum
- spermatic cord (acquired) N5Ø.8
  - congenital Q55.4
- spinal canal G96.12
- stomach — *see* Adhesions, peritoneum
- subscapular — *see* Capsulitis, adhesive
- temporomandibular M26.61
- tendinitis (*see also* Tenosynovitis, specified type NEC)
  - shoulder — *see* Capsulitis, adhesive
- testis N44.8
- tongue, congenital (to gum or roof of mouth) Q38.3
  - acquired K14.8
- trachea J39.8
- tubo-ovarian N73.6
- tunica vaginalis N44.8
- uterus N73.6

- **Adhesions, adhesive** — *continued*
  - uterus — *continued*
    - internal N85.6
    - to abdominal wall N73.6
  - vagina (chronic) N89.5
    - postoperative N99.2
  - vitreomacular H43.82- ☑
  - vitreous H43.89
  - vulva N90.89
- **Adiaspiromycosis** B48.8
- **Adie** (-Holmes) **pupil or syndrome** — *see* Anomaly, pupil, function, tonic pupil
- **Adiponecrosis neonatorum** P83.8
- **Adiposis** (*see also* Obesity)
  - cerebralis E23.6
  - dolorosa E88.2
- **Adiposity** (*see also* Obesity)
  - heart — *see* Degeneration, myocardial
  - localized E65
- **Adiposogenital dystrophy** E23.6
- **Adjustment**
  - disorder — *see* Disorder, adjustment
  - implanted device — *see* Encounter (for), adjustment (of)
  - prosthesis, external — *see* Fitting
  - reaction — *see* Disorder, adjustment
- **Administration of tPA** (rtPA) in a different facility within the last 24 hours prior to admission to current facility Z92.82
- **Admission** (for) (*see also* Encounter (for))
  - adjustment (of)
    - artificial
      - arm Z44.00- ☑
        - complete Z44.01- ☑
        - partial Z44.02- ☑
      - eye Z44.2 ☑
      - leg Z44.10- ☑
        - complete Z44.11- ☑
        - partial Z44.12- ☑
    - brain neuropacemaker Z46.2
      - implanted Z45.42
    - breast
      - implant Z45.81 ☑
      - prosthesis (external) Z44.3 ☑
    - colostomy belt Z46.89
    - contact lenses Z46.0
    - cystostomy device Z46.6
    - dental prosthesis Z46.3
    - device NEC
      - abdominal Z46.89
      - implanted Z45.89
        - cardiac Z45.09
          - defibrillator (with synchronous cardiace pacemaker) Z45.02
          - pacemaker Z45.018
            - pulse generator Z45.010
        - hearing device Z45.328
          - bone conduction Z45.320
          - cochlear Z45.321
        - infusion pump Z45.1
        - nervous system Z45.49
          - CSF drainage Z45.41
          - hearing device — *see* Admission, adjustment, device, implanted, hearing device
          - neuropacemaker Z45.42
          - visual substitution Z45.31
        - specified NEC Z45.89
        - vascular access Z45.2
        - visual substitution Z45.31
      - nervous system Z46.2
        - implanted — *see* Admission, adjustment, device, implanted, nervous system
      - orthodontic Z46.4
      - prosthetic Z44.9
        - arm — *see* Admission, adjustment, artificial, arm
        - breast Z44.3 ☑
        - dental Z46.3
        - eye Z44.2 ☑
        - leg — *see* Admission, adjustment, artificial, leg
        - specified type NEC Z44.8
      - substitution
        - auditory Z46.2

- **Admission** — *continued*
  - adjustment — *continued*
    - device — *continued*
      - substitution — *continued*
        - auditory — *continued*
          - implanted — *see* Admission, adjustment, device, implanted, hearing device
        - nervous system Z46.2
          - implanted — *see* Admission, adjustment, device, implanted, nervous system
        - visual Z46.2
          - implanted Z45.31
      - urinary Z46.6
    - hearing aid Z46.1
      - implanted — *see* Admission, adjustment, device, implanted, hearing device
    - ileostomy device Z46.89
    - intestinal appliance or device NEC Z46.89
    - neuropacemaker (brain) (peripheral nerve) (spinal cord) Z46.2
      - implanted Z45.42
    - orthodontic device Z46.4
    - orthopedic (brace) (cast) (device) (shoes) Z46.89
    - pacemaker
      - cardiac Z45.018
        - pulse generator Z45.010
      - nervous system Z46.2
        - implanted Z45.42
    - portacath (port-a-cath) Z45.2
    - prosthesis Z44.9
      - arm — *see* Admission, adjustment, artificial, arm
      - breast Z44.3 ☑
      - dental Z46.3
      - eye Z44.2 ☑
      - leg — *see* Admission, adjustment, artificial, leg
      - specified NEC Z44.8
    - spectacles Z46.0
  - aftercare (*see also* Aftercare) Z51.89
    - postpartum
      - immediately after delivery Z39.0
      - routine follow-up Z39.2
    - radiation therapy (antineoplastic) Z51.0
  - attention to artificial opening (of) Z43.9
    - artificial vagina Z43.7
    - colostomy Z43.3
    - cystostomy Z43.5
    - enterostomy Z43.4
    - gastrostomy Z43.1
    - ileostomy Z43.2
    - jejunostomy Z43.4
    - nephrostomy Z43.6
    - specified site NEC Z43.8
      - intestinal tract Z43.4
      - urinary tract Z43.6
    - tracheostomy Z43.0
    - ureterostomy Z43.6
    - urethrostomy Z43.6
  - breast augmentation or reduction Z41.1
  - breast reconstruction following mastectomy Z42.1
  - change of
    - dressing (nonsurgical) Z48.00
    - neuropacemaker device (brain) (peripheral nerve) (spinal cord) Z46.2
      - implanted Z45.42
    - surgical dressing Z48.01
  - circumcision, ritual or routine (in absence of diagnosis) Z41.2
  - clinical research investigation (control) (normal comparison) (participant) Z00.6
  - contraceptive management Z30.9
  - cosmetic surgery NEC Z41.1
  - counseling (*see also* Counseling)
    - dietary Z71.3
    - HIV Z71.7
    - human immunodeficiency virus Z71.7
    - nonattending third party Z71.0
    - procreative management NEC Z31.69
  - delivery, full-term, uncomplicated O80
    - cesarean, without indication O82
  - dietary surveillance and counseling Z71.3
  - ear piercing Z41.3
  - examination at health care facility (adult) (*see also* Examination) Z00.00
    - with abnormal findings Z00.01

- **Admission** — *continued*
  - examination at health care facility (*see also* Examination) — *continued*
    - clinical research investigation (control) (normal comparison) (participant) Z00.6
    - dental Z01.20
      - with abnormal findings Z01.21
    - donor (potential) Z00.5
    - ear Z01.10
      - with abnormal findings NEC Z01.118
    - eye Z01.00
      - with abnormal findings Z01.01
    - general, specified reason NEC Z00.8
    - hearing Z01.10
      - with abnormal findings NEC Z01.118
    - postpartum checkup Z39.2
    - psychiatric (general) Z00.8
      - requested by authority Z04.6
    - vision Z01.00
      - with abnormal findings Z01.01
  - fitting (of)
    - artificial
      - arm — *see* Admission, adjustment, artificial, arm
      - eye Z44.2 ☑
      - leg — *see* Admission, adjustment, artificial, leg
    - brain neuropacemaker Z46.2
      - implanted Z45.42
    - breast prosthesis (external) Z44.3 ☑
    - colostomy belt Z46.89
    - contact lenses Z46.0
    - cystostomy device Z46.6
    - dental prosthesis Z46.3
    - dentures Z46.3
    - device NEC
      - abdominal Z46.89
      - nervous system Z46.2
        - implanted — *see* Admission, adjustment, device, implanted, nervous system
      - orthodontic Z46.4
      - prosthetic Z44.9
        - breast Z44.3 ☑
        - dental Z46.3
        - eye Z44.2 ☑
      - substitution
        - auditory Z46.2
          - implanted — *see* Admission, adjustment, device, implanted, hearing device
        - nervous system Z46.2
          - implanted — *see* Admission, adjustment, device, implanted, nervous system
        - visual Z46.2
          - implanted Z45.31
    - hearing aid Z46.1
    - ileostomy device Z46.89
    - intestinal appliance or device NEC Z46.89
    - neuropacemaker (brain) (peripheral nerve) (spinal cord) Z46.2
      - implanted Z45.42
    - orthodontic device Z46.4
    - orthopedic device (brace) (cast) (shoes) Z46.89
    - prosthesis Z44.9
      - arm — *see* Admission, adjustment, artificial, arm
      - breast Z44.3 ☑
      - dental Z46.3
      - eye Z44.2 ☑
      - leg — *see* Admission, adjustment, artificial, leg
      - specified type NEC Z44.8
    - spectacles Z46.0
  - follow-up examination Z09
  - intrauterine device management Z30.431
    - initial prescription Z30.014
  - mental health evaluation Z00.8
    - requested by authority Z04.6
  - observation — *see* Observation
  - Papanicolaou smear, cervix Z12.4
    - for suspected malignant neoplasm Z12.4
  - plastic and reconstructive surgery following medical procedure or healed injury NEC Z42.8
  - plastic surgery, cosmetic NEC Z41.1
  - postpartum observation
    - immediately after delivery Z39.0
    - routine follow-up Z39.2
  - poststerilization (for restoration) Z31.0
    - aftercare Z31.42

Admission — *continued*
procreative management Z31.9
prophylactic (measure)
organ removal Z4Ø.ØØ
breast Z4Ø.Ø1
ovary Z4Ø.Ø2
specified organ NEC Z4Ø.Ø9
testes Z4Ø.Ø9
vaccination Z23
psychiatric examination (general) ZØØ.8
requested by authority ZØ4.6
radiation therapy (antineoplastic) Z51.Ø
reconstructive surgery following medical procedure or healed injury NEC Z42.8
removal of
cystostomy catheter Z43.5
drains Z48.Ø3
dressing (nonsurgical) Z48.ØØ
intrauterine contraceptive device Z3Ø.432
neuropacemaker (brain) (peripheral nerve) (spinal cord) Z46.2
implanted Z45.42
staples Z48.Ø2
surgical dressing Z48.Ø1
sutures Z48.Ø2
ureteral stent Z46.6
respirator [ventilator] use during power failure Z99.12
restoration of organ continuity (poststerilization) Z31.Ø
aftercare Z31.42
sensitivity test (*see also* Test, skin)
allergy NEC ZØ1.82
Mantoux Z11.1
tuboplasty following previous sterilization Z31.Ø
aftercare Z31.42
vasoplasty following previous sterilization Z31.Ø
aftercare Z31.42
vision examination ZØ1.ØØ
with abnormal findings ZØ1.Ø1
waiting period for admission to other facility Z75.1
Adnexitis (suppurative) — *see* Salpingo-oophoritis
Adolescent X-linked adrenoleukodystrophy E71.521
Adrenal (gland) — *see* condition
Adrenalism, tuberculous A18.7
Adrenalitis, adrenitis E27.8
autoimmune E27.1
meningococcal, hemorrhagic A39.1
Adrenarche, premature E27.Ø
Adrenocortical syndrome — *see* Cushing's, syndrome
Adrenogenital syndrome E25.9
acquired E25.8
congenital E25.Ø
salt loss E25.Ø
Adrenogenitalism, congenital E25.Ø
Adrenoleukodystrophy E71.529
neonatal E71.511
X-linked E71.529
Addison only phenotype E71.528
Addison-Schilder E71.528
adolescent E71.521
adrenomyeloneuropathy E71.522
childhood cerebral E71.52Ø
other specified E71.528
Adrenomyeloneuropathy E71.522
Adventitious bursa — *see* Bursopathy, specified type NEC
Adverse effect — *see* Table of Drugs and Chemicals, categories T36-T5Ø, with 6th character 5
Advice — *see* Counseling
Adynamia (episodica) (hereditary) (periodic) G72.3
Aeration lung imperfect, newborn — *see* Atelectasis
Aerobullosis T7Ø.3 ☑
Aerocele — *see* Embolism, air
Aerodermectasia
subcutaneous (traumatic) T79.7 ☑
Aerodontalgia T7Ø.29 ☑
Aeroembolism T7Ø.3 ☑
Aerogenes capsulatus infection A48.Ø
Aero-otitis media T7Ø.Ø ☑
Aerophagy, aerophagia (psychogenic) F45.8
Aerophobia F4Ø.228
Aerosinusitis T7Ø.1 ☑
Aerotitis T7Ø.Ø ☑
Affection — *see* Disease
Afibrinogenemia (*see also* Defect, coagulation) D68.8
acquired D65
congenital D68.2
following ectopic or molar pregnancy OØ8.1

Afibrinogenemia — *continued*
in abortion — *see* Abortion, by type, complicated by, afibrinogenemia
puerperal O72.3
African
sleeping sickness B56.9
tick fever A68.1
trypanosomiasis B56.9
gambian B56.Ø
rhodesian B56.1
Aftercare (*see also* Care) Z51.89
following surgery (for) (on)
amputation Z47.81
attention to
drains Z48.Ø3
dressings (nonsurgical) Z48.ØØ
surgical Z48.Ø1
sutures Z48.Ø2
circulatory system Z48.812
delayed (planned) wound closure Z48.1
digestive system Z48.815
explantation of joint prosthesis (staged procedure)
hip Z47.32
knee Z47.33
shoulder Z47.31
genitourinary system Z48.816
joint replacement Z47.1
neoplasm Z48.3
nervous system Z48.811
oral cavity Z48.814
organ transplant
bone marrow Z48.29Ø
heart Z48.21
heart-lung Z48.28Ø
kidney Z48.22
liver Z48.23
lung Z48.24
multiple organs NEC Z48.288
specified NEC Z48.298
orthopedic NEC Z47.89
planned wound closure Z48.1
removal of internal fixation device Z47.2
respiratory system Z48.813
scoliosis Z47.82
sense organs Z48.81Ø
skin and subcutaneous tissue Z48.817
specified body system
circulatory Z48.812
digestive Z48.815
genitourinary Z48.816
nervous Z48.811
oral cavity Z48.814
respiratory Z48.813
sense organs Z48.81Ø
skin and subcutaneous tissue Z48.817
teeth Z48.814
specified NEC Z48.89
spinal Z48.89
teeth Z48.814
fracture — *code to* fracture with seventh character D
involving
removal of
drains Z48.Ø3
dressings (nonsurgical) Z48.ØØ
staples Z48.Ø2
surgical dressings Z48.Ø1
sutures Z48.Ø2
neuropacemaker (brain) (peripheral nerve) (spinal cord) Z46.2
implanted Z45.42
orthopedic NEC Z47.89
postprocedural — *see* Aftercare, following surgery
After-cataract — *see* Cataract, secondary
Agalactia (primary) O92.3
elective, secondary or therapeutic O92.5
Agammaglobulinemia (acquired (secondary)) (nonfamilial) D8Ø.1
with
immunoglobulin-bearing B-lymphocytes D8Ø.1
lymphopenia D81.9
autosomal recessive (Swiss type) D8Ø.Ø
Bruton's X-linked D8Ø.Ø
common variable (CVAgamma) D8Ø.1
congenital sex-linked D8Ø.Ø
hereditary D8Ø.Ø
lymphopenic D81.9
Swiss type (autosomal recessive) D8Ø.Ø

Agammaglobulinemia — *continued*
X-linked (with growth hormone deficiency)(Bruton) D8Ø.Ø
Aganglionosis (bowel) (colon) Q43.1
Age (old) — *see* Senility
Agenesis
adrenal (gland) Q89.1
alimentary tract (complete) (partial) NEC Q45.8
upper Q4Ø.8
anus, anal (canal) Q42.3
with fistula Q42.2
aorta Q25.4
appendix Q42.8
arm (complete) Q71.Ø- ☑
with hand present Q71.1- ☑
artery (peripheral) Q27.9
brain Q28.3
coronary Q24.5
pulmonary Q25.79
specified NEC Q27.8
umbilical Q27.Ø
auditory (canal) (external) Q16.1
auricle (ear) Q16.Ø
bile duct or passage Q44.5
bladder Q64.5
bone Q79.9
brain QØØ.Ø
part of QØ4.3
breast (with nipple present) Q83.8
with absent nipple Q83.Ø
bronchus Q32.4
canaliculus lacrimalis Q1Ø.4
carpus — *see* Agenesis, hand
cartilage Q79.9
cecum Q42.8
cerebellum QØ4.3
cervix Q51.5
chin Q18.8
cilia Q1Ø.3
circulatory system, part NOS Q28.9
clavicle Q74.Ø
clitoris Q52.6
coccyx Q76.49
colon Q42.9
specified NEC Q42.8
corpus callosum QØ4.Ø
cricoid cartilage Q31.8
diaphragm (with hernia) Q79.1
digestive organ(s) or tract (complete) (partial) NEC Q45.8
upper Q4Ø.8
ductus arteriosus Q28.8
duodenum Q41.Ø
ear Q16.9
auricle Q16.Ø
lobe Q17.8
ejaculatory duct Q55.4
endocrine (gland) NEC Q89.2
epiglottis Q31.8
esophagus Q39.8
eustachian tube Q16.2
eye Q11.1
adnexa Q15.8
eyelid (fold) Q1Ø.3
face
bones NEC Q75.8
specified part NEC Q18.8
fallopian tube Q5Ø.6
femur — *see* Defect, reduction, lower limb, longitudinal, femur
fibula — *see* Defect, reduction, lower limb, longitudinal, fibula
finger (complete) (partial) — *see* Agenesis, hand
foot (and toes) (complete) (partial) Q72.3- ☑
forearm (with hand present) — *see* Agenesis, arm, with hand present
and hand Q71.2- ☑
gallbladder Q44.Ø
gastric Q4Ø.2
genitalia, genital (organ(s))
female Q52.8
external Q52.71
internal NEC Q52.8
male Q55.8
glottis Q31.8
hair Q84.Ø
hand (and fingers) (complete) (partial) Q71.3- ☑
heart Q24.8

- **Alcohol, alcoholic, alcohol-induced** — *continued*
  - dementia F10.97
    - with dependence F10.27
  - deterioration F10.97
    - with dependence F10.27
  - hallucinosis (acute) F10.951
    - in
      - abuse F10.151
      - dependence F10.251
  - insanity F10.959
  - intoxication (acute) (without dependence) F10.129
    - with
      - delirium F10.121
      - dependence F10.229
        - with delirium F10.221
        - uncomplicated F10.220
    - uncomplicated F10.120
  - jealousy F10.988
  - Korsakoff's, Korsakov's, Korsakow's F10.26
  - liver K70.9
    - acute — *see* Disease, liver, alcoholic, hepatitis
  - mania (acute) (chronic) F10.959
  - paranoia, paranoid (type) psychosis F10.950
  - pellagra E52
  - poisoning, accidental (acute) NEC — *see* Table of Drugs and Chemicals, alcohol, poisoning
  - psychosis — *see* Psychosis, alcoholic
  - withdrawal (without convulsions) F10.239
    - with delirium F10.231
- **Alcoholism** (chronic) (without remission) F10.20
  - with
    - psychosis — *see* Psychosis, alcoholic
    - remission F10.21
  - Korsakov's F10.96
    - with dependence F10.26
- **Alder** (-Reilly) **anomaly or syndrome** (leukocyte granulation) D72.0
- **Aldosteronism** E26.9
  - familial (type I) E26.02
  - glucocorticoid-remediable E26.02
  - primary (due to (bilateral) adrenal hyperplasia) E26.09
  - primary NEC E26.09
  - secondary E26.1
  - specified NEC E26.89
- **Aldosteronoma** D44.10
- **Aldrich** (-Wiskott) **syndrome** (eczema-thrombocytopenia) D82.0
- **Alektorophobia** F40.218
- **Aleppo boil** B55.1
- **Aleukemic** — *see* condition
- **Aleukia**
  - congenital D70.0
  - hemorrhagica D61.9
    - congenital D61.09
  - splenica D73.1
- **Alexia** R48.0
  - developmental F81.0
  - secondary to organic lesion R48.0
- **Algoneurodystrophy** M89.00
  - ankle M89.07- ☑
  - foot M89.07- ☑
  - forearm M89.03- ☑
  - hand M89.04- ☑
  - lower leg M89.06- ☑
  - multiple sites M89.0- ☑
  - shoulder M89.01- ☑
  - specified site NEC M89.08
  - thigh M89.05- ☑
  - upper arm M89.02- ☑
- **Algophobia** F40.298
- **Alienation, mental** — *see* Psychosis
- **Alkalemia** E87.3
- **Alkalosis** E87.3
  - metabolic E87.3
    - with respiratory acidosis E87.4
  - respiratory E87.3
- **Alkaptonuria** E70.29
- **Allen-Masters syndrome** N83.8
- **Allergy, allergic** (reaction) (to) T78.40 ☑
  - air-borne substance NEC (rhinitis) J30.89
  - alveolitis (extrinsic) J67.9
    - due to
      - Aspergillus clavatus J67.4
      - Cryptostroma corticale J67.6
      - organisms (fungal, thermophilic actinomycete) growing in ventilation (air conditioning) systems J67.7
- **Allergy, allergic** — *continued*
  - alveolitis — *continued*
    - specified type NEC J67.8
  - anaphylactic reaction or shock T78.2 ☑
  - angioneurotic edema T78.3 ☑
  - animal (dander) (epidermal) (hair) (rhinitis) J30.81
  - bee sting (anaphylactic shock) — *see* Toxicity, venom, arthropod, bee
  - biological — *see* Allergy, drug
  - colitis K52.2
  - dander (animal) (rhinitis) J30.81
  - dandruff (rhinitis) J30.81
  - dental restorative material (existing) K08.55
  - dermatitis — *see* Dermatitis, contact, allergic
  - diathesis — *see* History, allergy
  - drug, medicament & biological (any) (external) (internal) T78.40 ☑
    - correct substance properly administered — *see* Table of Drugs and Chemicals, by drug, adverse effect
    - wrong substance given or taken NEC (by accident) — *see* Table of Drugs and Chemicals, by drug, poisoning
  - due to pollen J30.1
  - dust (house) (stock) (rhinitis) J30.89
    - with asthma — *see* Asthma, allergic extrinsic
  - eczema — *see* Dermatitis, contact, allergic
  - epidermal (animal) (rhinitis) J30.81
  - feathers (rhinitis) J30.89
  - food (any) (ingested) NEC T78.1 ☑
    - anaphylactic shock — *see* Shock, anaphylactic, due to food
    - dermatitis — *see* Dermatitis, due to, food
    - dietary counseling and surveillance Z71.3
    - in contact with skin L23.6
    - rhinitis J30.5
    - status (without reaction) Z91.018
      - eggs Z91.012
      - milk products Z91.011
      - peanuts Z91.010
      - seafood Z91.013
      - specified NEC Z91.018
  - gastrointestinal K52.2
  - grain J30.1
  - grass (hay fever) (pollen) J30.1
    - asthma — *see* Asthma, allergic extrinsic
  - hair (animal) (rhinitis) J30.81
  - history (of) — *see* History, allergy
  - horse serum — *see* Allergy, serum
  - inhalant (rhinitis) J30.89
    - pollen J30.1
  - kapok (rhinitis) J30.89
  - medicine — *see* Allergy, drug
  - milk protein K52.2
  - nasal, seasonal due to pollen J30.1
  - pneumonia J82
  - pollen (any) (hay fever) J30.1
    - asthma — *see* Asthma, allergic extrinsic
  - primrose J30.1
  - primula J30.1
  - purpura D69.0
  - ragweed (hay fever) (pollen) J30.1
    - asthma — *see* Asthma, allergic extrinsic
  - rose (pollen) J30.1
  - seasonal NEC J30.2
  - Senecio jacobae (pollen) J30.1
  - serum (*see also* Reaction, serum) T80.69 ☑
    - anaphylactic shock T80.59 ☑
  - shock (anaphylactic) T78.2 ☑
    - due to
      - administration of blood and blood products T80.51 ☑
      - adverse effect of correct medicinal substance properly administered T88.6 ☑
      - immunization T80.52 ☑
      - serum NEC T80.59 ☑
      - vaccination T80.52 ☑
  - specific NEC T78.49 ☑
  - tree (any) (hay fever) (pollen) J30.1
    - asthma — *see* Asthma, allergic extrinsic
  - upper respiratory J30.9
  - urticaria L50.0
  - vaccine — *see* Allergy, serum
  - wheat — *see* Allergy, food
- **Allescheriasis** B48.2
- **Alligator skin disease** Q80.9
- **Allocheiria, allochiria** R20.8
- **Almeida's disease** — *see* Paracoccidioidomycosis
- **Alopecia** (hereditaria) (seborrheica) L65.9
  - androgenic L64.9
    - drug-induced L64.0
    - specified NEC L64.8
  - areata L63.9
    - ophiasis L63.2
    - specified NEC L63.8
    - totalis L63.0
    - universalis L63.1
  - cicatricial L66.9
    - specified NEC L66.8
  - circumscripta L63.9
  - congenital, congenitalis Q84.0
  - due to cytotoxic drugs NEC L65.8
  - mucinosa L65.2
  - postinfective NEC L65.8
  - postpartum L65.0
  - premature L64.8
  - specific (syphilitic) A51.32
  - specified NEC L65.8
  - syphilitic (secondary) A51.32
  - totalis (capitis) L63.0
  - universalis (entire body) L63.1
  - X-ray L58.1
- **Alpers' disease** G31.81
- **Alpine sickness** T70.29 ☑
- **Alport syndrome** Q87.81
- **ALTE** (apparent life threatening event) **in newborn and infant** R68.13
- **Alteration** (of), **Altered**
  - awareness, transient R40.4
  - mental status R41.82
  - pattern of family relationships affecting child Z62.898
  - sensation
    - following
      - cerebrovascular disease I69.998
        - cerebral infarction I69.398
        - intracerebral hemorrhage I69.198
        - nontraumatic intracranial hemorrhage NEC I69.298
        - specified disease NEC I69.898
        - subarachnoid hemorrhage I69.098
- **Alternating** — *see* condition
- **Altitude, high** (effects) — *see* Effect, adverse, high altitude
- **Aluminosis** (of lung) J63.0
- **Alveolitis**
  - allergic (extrinsic) — *see* Pneumonitis, hypersensitivity
  - due to
    - Aspergillus clavatus J67.4
    - Cryptostroma corticale J67.6
  - fibrosing (cryptogenic) (idiopathic) J84.112
  - jaw M27.3
  - sicca dolorosa M27.3
- **Alveolus, alveolar** — *see* condition
- **Alymphocytosis** D72.810
  - thymic (with immunodeficiency) D82.1
- **Alymphoplasia, thymic** D82.1
- **Alzheimer's disease or sclerosis** — *see* Disease, Alzheimer's
- **Amastia** (with nipple present) Q83.8
  - with absent nipple Q83.0
- **Amathophobia** F40.228
- **Amaurosis** (acquired) (congenital) (*see also* Blindness)
  - fugax G45.3
  - hysterical F44.6
  - Leber's congenital H35.50
  - uremic — *see* Uremia
- **Amaurotic idiocy** (infantile) (juvenile) (late) E75.4
- **Amaxophobia** F40.248
- **Ambiguous genitalia** Q56.4
- **Amblyopia** (congenital) (ex anopsia) (partial) (suppression) H53.00- ☑
  - anisometropic — *see* Amblyopia, refractive
  - deprivation H53.01- ☑
  - hysterical F44.6
  - nocturnal (*see also* Blindness, night)
    - vitamin A deficiency E50.5
  - refractive H53.02- ☑
  - strabismic H53.03- ☑
  - tobacco H53.8
  - toxic NEC H53.8
  - uremic — *see* Uremia
- **Ameba, amebic** (histolytica) (*see also* Amebiasis)
  - abscess (liver) A06.4
- **Amebiasis** A06.9

- **Amebiasis** — *continued*
  - with abscess — *see* Abscess, amebic
  - acute AØ6.Ø
  - chronic (intestine) AØ6.1
    - with abscess — *see* Abscess, amebic
  - cutaneous AØ6.7
  - cutis AØ6.7
  - cystitis AØ6.81
  - genitourinary tract NEC AØ6.82
  - hepatic — *see* Abscess, liver, amebic
  - intestine AØ6.Ø
  - nondysenteric colitis AØ6.2
  - skin AØ6.7
  - specified site NEC AØ6.89
- **Ameboma** (of intestine) AØ6.3
- **Amelia** Q73.Ø
  - lower limb — *see* Agenesis, leg
  - upper limb — *see* Agenesis, arm
- **Ameloblastoma** (*see also* Cyst, calcifying odontogenic)
  - long bones C4Ø.9- ☑
    - lower limb C4Ø.2- ☑
    - upper limb C4Ø.Ø- ☑
  - malignant C41.1
    - jaw (bone) (lower) C41.1
      - upper C41.Ø
  - tibial C4Ø.2- ☑
- **Amelogenesis imperfecta** KØØ.5
  - nonhereditaria (segmentalis) KØØ.4
- **Amenorrhea** N91.2
  - hyperhormonal E28.8
  - primary N91.Ø
  - secondary N91.1
- **Amentia** — *see* Disability, intellectual
  - Meynert's (nonalcoholic) FØ4
- **American**
  - leishmaniasis B55.2
  - mountain tick fever A93.2
- **Ametropia** — *see* Disorder, refraction
- **Amianthosis** J61
- **Amimia** R48.8
- **Amino-acid disorder** E72.9
  - anemia D53.Ø
- **Aminoacidopathy** E72.9
- **Aminoaciduria** E72.9
- **Amnesia** R41.3
  - anterograde R41.1
  - auditory R48.8
  - dissociative F44.Ø
  - hysterical F44.Ø
  - postictal in epilepsy — *see* Epilepsy
  - psychogenic F44.Ø
  - retrograde R41.2
  - transient global G45.4
- **Amnes(t)ic syndrome** (post-traumatic) FØ4
  - induced by
    - alcohol F1Ø.96
      - with dependence F1Ø.26
    - psychoactive NEC F19.96
      - with
        - abuse F19.16
        - dependence F19.26
    - sedative F13.96
      - with dependence F13.26
- **Amnion, amniotic** — *see* condition
- **Amnionitis** — *see* Pregnancy, complicated by
- **Amok** F68.8
- **Amoral traits** F6Ø.89
- **Ampulla**
  - lower esophagus K22.8
  - phrenic K22.8
- **Amputation** (*see also* Absence, by site, acquired)
  - neuroma (postoperative) (traumatic) — *see* Complications, amputation stump, neuroma
  - stump (surgical)
    - abnormal, painful, or with complication (late) — *see* Complications, amputation stump
    - healed or old NOS Z89.9
  - traumatic (complete) (partial)
    - arm (upper) (complete) S48.91- ☑
      - at
        - elbow S58.Ø1- ☑
          - partial S58.Ø2- ☑
        - shoulder joint (complete) S48.Ø1- ☑
          - partial S48.Ø2- ☑
      - between
        - elbow and wrist (complete) S58.11- ☑
          - partial S58.12- ☑
- **Amputation** — *continued*
  - traumatic — *continued*
    - arm — *continued*
      - between — *continued*
        - shoulder and elbow (complete) S48.11- ☑
          - partial S48.12- ☑
      - partial S48.92- ☑
    - breast (complete) S28.21- ☑
      - partial S28.22- ☑
    - clitoris (complete) S38.211 ☑
      - partial S38.212 ☑
    - ear (complete) SØ8.11- ☑
      - partial SØ8.12- ☑
    - finger (complete) (metacarpophalangeal) S68.11- ☑
      - index S68.11- ☑
      - little S68.11- ☑
      - middle S68.11- ☑
      - partial S68.12- ☑
        - index S68.12- ☑
        - little S68.12- ☑
        - middle S68.12- ☑
        - ring S68.12- ☑
      - ring S68.11- ☑
      - thumb — *see* Amputation, traumatic, thumb
      - transphalangeal (complete) S68.61- ☑
        - index S68.61- ☑
        - little S68.61- ☑
        - middle S68.61- ☑
        - partial S68.62- ☑
          - index S68.62- ☑
          - little S68.62- ☑
          - middle S68.62- ☑
          - ring S68.62- ☑
        - ring S68.61- ☑
    - foot (complete) S98.91- ☑
      - at ankle level S98.Ø1- ☑
        - partial S98.Ø2- ☑
      - midfoot S98.31- ☑
        - partial S98.32- ☑
      - partial S98.92- ☑
    - forearm (complete) S58.91- ☑
      - at elbow level (complete) S58.Ø1- ☑
        - partial S58.Ø2- ☑
      - between elbow and wrist (complete) S58.11- ☑
        - partial S58.12- ☑
      - partial S58.92- ☑
    - genital organ(s) (external)
      - female (complete) S38.211 ☑
        - partial S38.212 ☑
      - male
        - penis (complete) S38.221 ☑
          - partial S38.222 ☑
        - scrotum (complete) S38.231 ☑
          - partial S38.232 ☑
        - testes (complete) S38.231 ☑
          - partial S38.232 ☑
    - hand (complete) (wrist level) S68.41- ☑
      - finger(s) alone — *see* Amputation, traumatic, finger
      - partial S68.42- ☑
      - thumb alone — *see* Amputation, traumatic, thumb
      - transmetacarpal (complete) S68.71- ☑
        - partial S68.72- ☑
    - head
      - ear — *see* Amputation, traumatic, ear
      - nose (partial) SØ8.812 ☑
        - complete SØ8.811 ☑
      - part SØ8.89 ☑
        - scalp SØ8.Ø ☑
    - hip (and thigh) (complete) S78.91- ☑
      - at hip joint (complete) S78.Ø1- ☑
        - partial S78.Ø2- ☑
      - between hip and knee (complete) S78.11- ☑
        - partial S78.12- ☑
      - partial S78.92- ☑
    - labium (majus) (minus) (complete) S38.21- ☑
      - partial S38.21- ☑
    - leg (lower) S88.91- ☑
      - at knee level S88.Ø1- ☑
        - partial S88.Ø2- ☑
      - between knee and ankle S88.11- ☑
        - partial S88.12- ☑
      - partial S88.92- ☑
    - nose (partial) SØ8.812 ☑
- **Amputation** — *continued*
  - traumatic — *continued*
    - nose — *continued*
      - complete SØ8.811 ☑
    - penis (complete) S38.221 ☑
      - partial S38.222 ☑
    - scrotum (complete) S38.231 ☑
      - partial S38.232 ☑
    - shoulder — *see* Amputation, traumatic, arm
      - at shoulder joint — *see* Amputation, traumatic, arm, at shoulder joint
    - testes (complete) S38.231 ☑
      - partial S38.232 ☑
    - thigh — *see* Amputation, traumatic, hip
    - thorax, part of S28.1 ☑
      - breast — *see* Amputation, traumatic, breast
    - thumb (complete) (metacarpophalangeal) S68.Ø1- ☑
      - partial S68.Ø2- ☑
      - transphalangeal (complete) S68.51- ☑
        - partial S68.52- ☑
    - toe (lesser) S98.13- ☑
      - great S98.11- ☑
        - partial S98.12- ☑
      - more than one S98.21- ☑
        - partial S98.22- ☑
      - partial S98.14- ☑
    - vulva (complete) S38.211 ☑
      - partial S38.212 ☑
- **Amputee** (bilateral) (old) Z89.9
- **Amsterdam dwarfism** Q87.1
- **Amusia** R48.8
  - developmental F8Ø.89
- **Amyelencephalus, amyelencephaly** QØØ.Ø
- **Amyelia** QØ6.Ø
- **Amygdalitis** — *see* Tonsillitis
- **Amygdalolith** J35.8
- **Amyloid heart** (disease) E85.4 [I43]
- **Amyloidosis** (generalized) (primary) E85.9
  - with lung involvement E85.4 [J99]
  - familial E85.2
  - genetic E85.2
  - heart E85.4 [I43]
  - hemodialysis-associated E85.3
  - liver E85.4 [K77]
  - localized E85.4
  - neuropathic heredofamilial E85.1
  - non-neuropathic heredofamilial E85.Ø
  - organ limited E85.4
  - Portuguese E85.1
  - pulmonary E85.4 [J99]
  - secondary systemic E85.3
  - skin (lichen) (macular) E85.4 [L99]
  - specified NEC E85.8
  - subglottic E85.4 [J99]
- **Amylopectinosis** (brancher enzyme deficiency) E74.Ø3
- **Amylophagia** — *see* Pica
- **Amyoplasia congenita** Q79.8
- **Amyotonia** M62.89
  - congenita G7Ø.2
- **Amyotrophia, amyotrophy, amyotrophic** G71.8
  - congenita Q79.8
  - diabetic — *see* Diabetes, amyotrophy
  - lateral sclerosis G12.21
  - neuralgic G54.5
  - spinal progressive G12.21
- **Anacidity, gastric** K31.83
  - psychogenic F45.8
- **Anaerosis of newborn** P28.89
- **Analbuminemia** E88.Ø9
- **Analgesia** — *see* Anesthesia
- **Analphalipoproteinemia** E78.6
- **Anaphylactic**
  - purpura D69.Ø
  - shock or reaction — *see* Shock, anaphylactic
- **Anaphylactoid shock or reaction** — *see* Shock, anaphylactic
- **Anaphylactoid syndrome of pregnancy** O88.Ø1- ☑
- **Anaphylaxis** — *see* Shock, anaphylactic
- **Anaplasia cervix** (*see also* Dysplasia, cervix) N87.9
- **Anaplasmosis, human** A77.49
- **Anarthria** R47.1
- **Anasarca** R6Ø.1
  - cardiac — *see* Failure, heart, congestive
  - lung J18.2
  - newborn P83.2
  - nutritional E43

- **Anasarca** — *continued*
  - pulmonary J18.2
  - renal NØ4.9
- **Anastomosis**
  - aneurysmal — *see* Aneurysm
  - arteriovenous ruptured brain I6Ø.8
  - intestinal K63.89
    - complicated NEC K91.89
      - involving urinary tract N99.89
  - retinal and choroidal vessels (congenital) Q14.8
- **Anatomical narrow angle** H4Ø.Ø3- ☑
- **Ancylostoma, ancylostomiasis** (braziliense) (caninum) (ceylanicum) (duodenale) B76.Ø
  - Necator americanus B76.1
- **Andersen's disease** (glycogen storage) E74.Ø9
- **Anderson-Fabry disease** E75.21
- **Andes disease** T7Ø.29 ☑
- **Andrews' disease** (bacterid) LØ8.89
- **Androblastoma**
  - benign
    - specified site — *see* Neoplasm, benign, by site
    - unspecified site
      - female D27.9
      - male D29.2Ø
  - malignant
    - specified site — *see* Neoplasm, malignant, by site
    - unspecified site
      - female C56.9
      - male C62.9Ø
  - specified site — *see* Neoplasm, uncertain behavior, by site
  - tubular
    - with lipid storage
      - specified site — *see* Neoplasm, benign, by site
      - unspecified site
        - female D27.9
        - male D29.2Ø
    - specified site — *see* Neoplasm, benign, by site
    - unspecified site
      - female D27.9
      - male D29.2Ø
  - unspecified site
    - female D39.1Ø
    - male D4Ø.1Ø
- **Androgen insensitivity syndrome** (*see also* Syndrome, androgen insensitivity) E34.5Ø
- **Androgen resistance syndrome** (*see also* Syndrome, androgen insensitivity) E34.5Ø
- **Android pelvis** Q74.2
  - with disproportion (fetopelvic) O33.3 ☑
    - causing obstructed labor O65.3
- **Androphobia** F4Ø.29Ø
- **Anectasis, pulmonary** (newborn) — *see* Atelectasis
- **Anemia** (essential) (general) (hemoglobin deficiency) (infantile) (primary) (profound) D64.9
  - with (due to) (in)
    - disorder of
      - anaerobic glycolysis D55.2
      - pentose phosphate pathway D55.1
    - koilonychia D5Ø.9
  - achlorhydric D5Ø.8
  - achrestic D53.1
  - Addison (-Biermer) (pernicious) D51.Ø
  - agranulocytic — *see* Agranulocytosis
  - amino-acid-deficiency D53.Ø
  - aplastic D61.9
    - congenital D61.Ø9
    - drug-induced D61.1
    - due to
      - drugs D61.1
      - external agents NEC D61.2
      - infection D61.2
      - radiation D61.2
    - idiopathic D61.3
    - red cell (pure) D6Ø.9
      - chronic D6Ø.Ø
      - congenital D61.Ø1
      - specified type NEC D6Ø.8
      - transient D6Ø.1
    - specified type NEC D61.89
    - toxic D61.2
  - aregenerative
    - congenital D61.Ø9
  - asiderotic D5Ø.9
  - atypical (primary) D64.9
  - Baghdad spring D55.Ø
  - Balantidium coli AØ7.Ø
  - Biermer's (pernicious) D51.Ø

- **Anemia** — *continued*
  - blood loss (chronic) D5Ø.Ø
    - acute D62
  - bothriocephalus B7Ø.Ø [D63.8]
  - brickmaker's B76.9 [D63.8]
  - cerebral I67.89
  - childhood D58.9
  - chlorotic D5Ø.8
  - chronic
    - blood loss D5Ø.Ø
    - hemolytic D58.9
      - idiopathic D59.9
    - simple D53.9
  - chronica congenita aregenerativa D61.Ø9
  - combined system disease NEC D51.Ø [G32.Ø]
    - due to dietary vitamin B12 deficiency D51.3 [G32.Ø]
  - complicating pregnancy, childbirth or puerperium — *see* Pregnancy, complicated by (management affected by), anemia
  - congenital P61.4
    - aplastic D61.Ø9
    - due to isoimmunization NOS P55.9
    - dyserythropoietic, dyshematopoietic D64.4
    - following fetal blood loss P61.3
    - Heinz body D58.2
    - hereditary hemolytic NOS D58.9
    - pernicious D51.Ø
    - spherocytic D58.Ø
  - Cooley's (erythroblastic) D56.1
  - cytogenic D51.Ø
  - deficiency D53.9
    - 6-PGD D55.1
    - 2, 3 diphosphoglycurate mutase D55.2
    - 2, 3 PG D55.2
    - 6 phosphogluconate dehydrogenase D55.1
    - amino-acid D53.Ø
    - combined B12 and folate D53.1
    - enzyme D55.9
      - drug-induced (hemolytic) D59.2
      - glucose-6-phosphate dehydrogenase (G6PD) D55.Ø
      - glycolytic D55.2
      - nucleotide metabolism D55.3
      - related to hexose monophosphate (HMP) shunt pathway NEC D55.1
      - specified type NEC D55.8
    - erythrocytic glutathione D55.1
    - folate D52.9
      - dietary D52.Ø
      - drug-induced D52.1
    - folic acid D52.9
      - dietary D52.Ø
      - drug-induced D52.1
    - G SH D55.1
    - G6PD D55.Ø
    - GGS-R D55.1
    - glucose-6-phosphate dehydrogenase D55.Ø
    - glutathione reductase D55.1
    - glyceraldehyde phosphate dehydrogenase D55.2
    - hexokinase D55.2
    - iron D5Ø.9
      - secondary to blood loss (chronic) D5Ø.Ø
    - nutritional D53.9
      - with
        - poor iron absorption D5Ø.8
        - specified deficiency NEC D53.8
    - phosphofructo-aldolase D55.2
    - phosphoglycerate kinase D55.2
    - PK D55.2
    - protein D53.Ø
    - pyruvate kinase D55.2
    - transcobalamin II D51.2
    - triose-phosphate isomerase D55.2
    - vitamin B12 NOS D51.9
      - dietary D51.3
      - due to
        - intrinsic factor deficiency D51.Ø
        - selective vitamin B12 malabsorption with proteinuria D51.1
      - pernicious D51.Ø
      - specified type NEC D51.8
  - Diamond-Blackfan (congenital hypoplastic) D61.Ø1
  - dibothriocephalus B7Ø.Ø [D63.8]
  - dimorphic D53.1
  - diphasic D53.1
  - Diphyllobothrium (Dibothriocephalus) B7Ø.Ø [D63.8]
  - due to (in) (with)
    - antineoplastic chemotherapy D64.81

- **Anemia** — *continued*
  - due to — *continued*
    - blood loss (chronic) D5Ø.Ø
      - acute D62
    - chemotherapy, antineoplastic D64.81
    - chronic disease classified elsewhere NEC D63.8
    - chronic kidney disease D63.1
    - deficiency
      - amino-acid D53.Ø
      - copper D53.8
      - folate (folic acid) D52.9
        - dietary D52.Ø
        - drug-induced D52.1
      - molybdenum D53.8
      - protein D53.Ø
      - zinc D53.8
    - dietary vitamin B12 deficiency D51.3
    - disorder of
      - glutathione metabolism D55.1
      - nucleotide metabolism D55.3
    - drug — *see* Anemia, by type (*see also* Table of Drugs and Chemicals)
    - end stage renal disease D63.1
    - enzyme disorder D55.9
    - fetal blood loss P61.3
    - fish tapeworm (D.latum) infestation B7Ø.Ø [D63.8]
    - hemorrhage (chronic) D5Ø.Ø
      - acute D62
    - impaired absorption D5Ø.9
    - loss of blood (chronic) D5Ø.Ø
      - acute D62
    - myxedema EØ3.9 [D63.8]
    - Necator americanus B76.1 [D63.8]
    - prematurity P61.2
    - selective vitamin B12 malabsorption with proteinuria D51.1
    - transcobalamin II deficiency D51.2
  - Dyke-Young type (secondary) (symptomatic) D59.1
  - dyserythropoietic (congenital) D64.4
  - dyshematopoietic (congenital) D64.4
  - Egyptian B76.9 [D63.8]
  - elliptocytosis — *see* Elliptocytosis
  - enzyme-deficiency, drug-induced D59.2
  - epidemic (*see also* Ancylostomiasis) B76.9 [D63.8]
  - erythroblastic
    - familial D56.1
    - newborn (*see also* Disease, hemolytic) P55.9
    - of childhood D56.1
  - erythrocytic glutathione deficiency D55.1
  - erythropoietin-resistant anemia (EPO resistant anemia) D63.1
  - Faber's (achlorhydric anemia) D5Ø.9
  - factitious (self-induced blood letting) D5Ø.Ø
  - familial erythroblastic D56.1
  - Fanconi's (congenital pancytopenia) D61.Ø9
  - favism D55.Ø
  - fish tapeworm (D. latum) infestation B7Ø.Ø [D63.8]
  - folate (folic acid) deficiency D52.9
  - glucose-6-phosphate dehydrogenase (G6PD) deficiency D55.Ø
  - glutathione-reductase deficiency D55.1
  - goat's milk D52.Ø
  - granulocytic — *see* Agranulocytosis
  - Heinz body, congenital D58.2
  - hemolytic D58.9
    - acquired D59.9
      - with hemoglobinuria NEC D59.6
      - autoimmune NEC D59.1
      - infectious D59.4
      - specified type NEC D59.8
      - toxic D59.4
    - acute D59.9
      - due to enzyme deficiency specified type NEC D55.8
      - Lederer's D59.1
    - autoimmune D59.1
      - drug-induced D59.Ø
    - chronic D58.9
      - idiopathic D59.9
    - cold type (secondary) (symptomatic) D59.1
    - congenital (spherocytic) — *see* Spherocytosis
    - due to
      - cardiac conditions D59.4
      - drugs (nonautoimmune) D59.2
        - autoimmune D59.Ø
      - enzyme disorder D55.9
        - drug-induced D59.2

- **Anemia** — *continued*
  - hemolytic — *continued*
    - due to — *continued*
      - presence of shunt or other internal prosthetic device D59.4
    - familial D58.9
    - hereditary D58.9
      - due to enzyme disorder D55.9
        - specified type NEC D55.8
      - specified type NEC D58.8
    - idiopathic (chronic) D59.9
    - mechanical D59.4
    - microangiopathic D59.4
    - nonautoimmune D59.4
      - drug-induced D59.2
    - nonspherocytic
      - congenital or hereditary NEC D55.8
        - glucose-6-phosphate dehydrogenase deficiency D55.Ø
        - pyruvate kinase deficiency D55.2
        - type
          - I D55.1
          - II D55.2
      - type
        - I D55.1
        - II D55.2
    - secondary D59.4
      - autoimmune D59.1
    - specified (hereditary) type NEC D58.8
    - Stransky-Regala type (*see also* Hemoglobinopathy) D58.8
    - symptomatic D59.4
      - autoimmune D59.1
    - toxic D59.4
    - warm type (secondary) (symptomatic) D59.1
  - hemorrhagic (chronic) D5Ø.Ø
    - acute D62
  - Herrick's D57.1
  - hexokinase deficiency D55.2
  - hookworm B76.9 [D63.8]
  - hypochromic (idiopathic) (microcytic) (normoblastic) D5Ø.9
    - due to blood loss (chronic) D5Ø.Ø
      - acute D62
    - familial sex-linked D64.Ø
    - pyridoxine-responsive D64.3
    - sideroblastic, sex-linked D64.Ø
  - hypoplasia, red blood cells D61.9
    - congenital or familial D61.Ø1
  - hypoplastic (idiopathic) D61.9
    - congenital or familial (of childhood) D61.Ø1
  - hypoproliferative (refractive) D61.9
  - idiopathic D64.9
    - aplastic D61.3
    - hemolytic, chronic D59.9
  - in (due to) (with)
    - chronic kidney disease D63.1
    - end stage renal disease D63.1
    - failure, kidney (renal) D63.1
    - neoplastic disease (*see also* Neoplasm) D63.Ø
  - intertropical (*see also* Ancylostomiasis) D63.8
  - iron deficiency D5Ø.9
    - secondary to blood loss (chronic) D5Ø.Ø
      - acute D62
    - specified type NEC D5Ø.8
  - Joseph-Diamond-Blackfan (congenital hypoplastic) D61.Ø1
  - Lederer's (hemolytic) D59.1
  - leukoerythroblastic D61.82
  - macrocytic D53.9
    - nutritional D52.Ø
    - tropical D52.8
  - malarial (*see also* Malaria) B54 [D63.8]
  - malignant (progressive) D51.Ø
  - malnutrition D53.9
  - marsh (*see also* Malaria) B54 [D63.8]
  - Mediterranean (with other hemoglobinopathy) D56.9
  - megaloblastic D53.1
    - combined B12 and folate deficiency D53.1
    - hereditary D51.1
    - nutritional D52.Ø
    - orotic aciduria D53.Ø
    - refractory D53.1
    - specified type NEC D53.1
  - megalocytic D53.1
  - microcytic (hypochromic) D5Ø.9
    - due to blood loss (chronic) D5Ø.Ø
      - acute D62
- **Anemia** — *continued*
  - microcytic — *continued*
    - familial D56.8
  - microdrepanocytosis D57.4Ø
  - microelliptopoikilocytic (Rietti-Greppi- Micheli) D56.9
  - miner's B76.9 [D63.8]
  - myelodysplastic D46.9
  - myelofibrosis D75.81
  - myelogenous D64.89
  - myelopathic D64.89
  - myelophthisic D61.82
  - myeloproliferative D47.Z9 (*following* D47.4)
  - newborn P61.4
    - due to
      - ABO (antibodies, isoimmunization, maternal/fetal incompatibility) P55.1
      - Rh (antibodies, isoimmunization, maternal/fetal incompatibility) P55.Ø
    - following fetal blood loss P61.3
    - posthemorrhagic (fetal) P61.3
  - nonspherocytic hemolytic — *see* Anemia, hemolytic, nonspherocytic
  - normocytic (infectional) D64.9
    - due to blood loss (chronic) D5Ø.Ø
      - acute D62
    - myelophthisic D61.82
  - nutritional (deficiency) D53.9
    - with
      - poor iron absorption D5Ø.8
      - specified deficiency NEC D53.8
    - megaloblastic D52.Ø
  - of prematurity P61.2
  - orotaciduric (congenital) (hereditary) D53.Ø
  - osteosclerotic D64.89
  - ovalocytosis (hereditary) — *see* Elliptocytosis
  - paludal (*see also* Malaria) B54 [D63.8]
  - pernicious (congenital) (malignant) (progressive) D51.Ø
  - pleochromic D64.89
    - of sprue D52.8
  - posthemorrhagic (chronic) D5Ø.Ø
    - acute D62
    - newborn P61.3
  - postoperative (postprocedural)
    - due to (acute) blood loss D62
      - chronic blood loss D5Ø.Ø
    - specified NEC D64.9
  - postpartum O9Ø.81
  - pressure D64.89
  - progressive D64.9
    - malignant D51.Ø
    - pernicious D51.Ø
  - protein-deficiency D53.Ø
  - pseudoleukemica infantum D64.89
  - pure red cell D6Ø.9
    - congenital D61.Ø1
  - pyridoxine-responsive D64.3
  - pyruvate kinase deficiency D55.2
  - refractory D46.4
    - with
      - excess of blasts D46.2Ø
        - 1 (RAEB 1) D46.21
        - 2 (RAEB 2) D46.22
        - in transformation (RAEB T) — *see* Leukemia, acute myeloblastic
      - hemochromatosis D46.1
      - sideroblasts (ring) (RARS) D46.1
    - without ring sideroblasts, so stated D46.Ø
    - without sideroblasts without excess of blasts D46.Ø
    - megaloblastic D53.1
    - sideroblastic D46.1
    - sideropenic D5Ø.9
  - Rietti-Greppi-Micheli D56.9
  - scorbutic D53.2
  - secondary to
    - blood loss (chronic) D5Ø.Ø
      - acute D62
    - hemorrhage (chronic) D5Ø.Ø
      - acute D62
  - semiplastic D61.89
  - sickle-cell — *see* Disease, sickle-cell
  - sideroblastic D64.3
    - hereditary D64.Ø
    - hypochromic, sex-linked D64.Ø
    - pyridoxine-responsive NEC D64.3
    - refractory D46.1
    - secondary (due to)
      - disease D64.1
      - drugs and toxins D64.2
- **Anemia** — *continued*
  - sideroblastic — *continued*
    - specified type NEC D64.3
  - sideropenic (refractory) D5Ø.9
    - due to blood loss (chronic) D5Ø.Ø
      - acute D62
  - simple chronic D53.9
  - specified type NEC D64.89
  - spherocytic (hereditary) — *see* Spherocytosis
  - splenic D64.89
  - splenomegalic D64.89
  - stomatocytosis D58.8
  - syphilitic (acquired) (late) A52.79 [D63.8]
  - target cell D64.89
  - thalassemia D56.9
  - thrombocytopenic — *see* Thrombocytopenia
  - toxic D61.2
  - tropical B76.9 [D63.8]
    - macrocytic D52.8
  - tuberculous A18.89 [D63.8]
  - vegan D51.3
  - vitamin
    - B6-responsive D64.3
    - B12 deficiency (dietary) pernicious D51.Ø
  - von Jaksch's D64.89
  - Witts' (achlorhydric anemia) D5Ø.8
- **Anemophobia** F4Ø.228
- **Anencephalus, anencephaly** QØØ.Ø
- **Anergasia** — *see* Psychosis, organic
- **Anesthesia, anesthetic** R2Ø.Ø
  - complication or reaction NEC (*see also* Complications, anesthesia) T88.59 ☑
    - due to
      - correct substance properly administered — *see* Table of Drugs and Chemicals, by drug, adverse effect
      - overdose or wrong substance given — *see* Table of Drugs and Chemicals, by drug, poisoning
  - cornea H18.81- ☑
  - dissociative F44.6
  - functional (hysterical) F44.6
  - hyperesthetic, thalamic G89.Ø
  - hysterical F44.6
  - local skin lesion R2Ø.Ø
  - sexual (psychogenic) F52.1
  - shock (due to) T88.2 ☑
  - skin R2Ø.Ø
  - testicular N5Ø.9
- **Anetoderma** (maculosum) (of) L9Ø.8
  - Jadassohn-Pellizzari L9Ø.2
  - Schweniger-Buzzi L9Ø.1
- **Aneurin deficiency** E51.9
- **Aneurysm** (anastomotic) (artery) (cirsoid) (diffuse) (false) (fusiform) (multiple) (saccular) I72.9
  - abdominal (aorta) I71.4
    - ruptured I71.3
    - syphilitic A52.Ø1
  - aorta, aortic (nonsyphilitic) I71.9
    - abdominal I71.4
      - ruptured I71.3
    - arch I71.2
      - ruptured I71.1
    - arteriosclerotic I71.9
      - ruptured I71.8
    - ascending I71.2
      - ruptured I71.1
    - congenital Q25.4
    - descending I71.9
      - abdominal I71.4
        - ruptured I71.3
      - ruptured I71.8
      - thoracic I71.2
        - ruptured I71.1
    - ruptured I71.8
    - sinus, congenital Q25.4
    - syphilitic A52.Ø1
    - thoracic I71.2
      - ruptured I71.1
    - thoracoabdominal I71.6
      - ruptured I71.5
    - thorax, thoracic (arch) I71.2
      - ruptured I71.1
    - transverse I71.2
      - ruptured I71.1
    - valve (heart) (*see also* Endocarditis, aortic) I35.8
  - arteriosclerotic I72.9
    - cerebral I67.1

- **Aneurysm** — *continued*
  - arteriosclerotic — *continued*
    - cerebral — *continued*
      - ruptured — *see* Hemorrhage, intracranial, subarachnoid
  - arteriovenous (congenital) (*see also* Malformation, arteriovenous)
    - acquired I77.Ø
      - brain I67.1
      - coronary I25.41
      - pulmonary I28.Ø
    - brain Q28.2
      - ruptured I6Ø.8
    - peripheral — *see* Malformation, arteriovenous, peripheral
    - precerebral vessels Q28.Ø
    - specified site NEC (*see also* Malformation, arteriovenous)
      - acquired I77.Ø
  - basal — *see* Aneurysm, brain
  - berry (congenital) (nonruptured) I67.1
    - ruptured I6Ø.7
  - brain I67.1
    - arteriosclerotic I67.1
      - ruptured — *see* Hemorrhage, intracranial, subarachnoid
    - arteriovenous (congenital) (nonruptured) Q28.2
      - acquired I67.1
        - ruptured I6Ø.8
      - ruptured I6Ø.8
    - berry (congenital) (nonruptured) I67.1
      - ruptured (*see also* Hemorrhage, intracranial, subarachnoid) I6Ø.7
    - congenital Q28.3
      - ruptured I6Ø.7
    - meninges I67.1
      - ruptured I6Ø.8
    - miliary (congenital) (nonruptured) I67.1
      - ruptured (*see also* Hemorrhage, intracranial, subarachnoid) I6Ø.7
    - mycotic I33.Ø
    - ruptured — *see* Hemorrhage, intracranial, subarachnoid
    - syphilitic (hemorrhage) A52.Ø5
  - cardiac (false) (*see also* Aneurysm, heart) I25.3
  - carotid artery (common) (external) I72.Ø
    - internal (intracranial) I67.1
      - extracranial portion I72.Ø
    - ruptured into brain I6Ø.Ø- ☑
    - syphilitic A52.Ø9
      - intracranial A52.Ø5
  - cavernous sinus I67.1
    - arteriovenous (congenital) (nonruptured) Q28.3
      - ruptured I6Ø.8
  - celiac I72.8
  - central nervous system, syphilitic A52.Ø5
  - cerebral — *see* Aneurysm, brain
  - chest — *see* Aneurysm, thorax
  - circle of Willis I67.1
    - congenital Q28.3
      - ruptured I6Ø.6
    - ruptured I6Ø.6
  - common iliac artery I72.3
  - congenital (peripheral) Q27.8
    - brain Q28.3
      - ruptured I6Ø.7
    - coronary Q24.5
    - digestive system Q27.8
    - lower limb Q27.8
    - pulmonary Q25.79
    - retina Q14.1
    - specified site NEC Q27.8
    - upper limb Q27.8
  - conjunctiva — *see* Abnormality, conjunctiva, vascular
  - conus arteriosus — *see* Aneurysm, heart
  - coronary (arteriosclerotic) (artery) I25.41
    - arteriovenous, congenital Q24.5
    - congenital Q24.5
    - ruptured — *see* Infarct, myocardium
    - syphilitic A52.Ø6
    - vein I25.89
  - cylindroid (aorta) I71.9
    - ruptured I71.8
    - syphilitic A52.Ø1
  - ductus arteriosus Q25.Ø
  - endocardial, infective (any valve) I33.Ø
  - femoral (artery) (ruptured) I72.4
  - gastroduodenal I72.8

- **Aneurysm** — *continued*
  - gastroepiploic I72.8
  - heart (wall) (chronic or with a stated duration of over 4 weeks) I25.3
    - valve — *see* Endocarditis
  - hepatic I72.8
  - iliac (common) (artery) (ruptured) I72.3
  - infective I72.9
    - endocardial (any valve) I33.Ø
  - innominate (nonsyphilitic) I72.8
    - syphilitic A52.Ø9
  - interauricular septum — *see* Aneurysm, heart
  - interventricular septum — *see* Aneurysm, heart
  - intrathoracic (nonsyphilitic) I71.2
    - ruptured I71.1
    - syphilitic A52.Ø1
  - lower limb I72.4
  - lung (pulmonary artery) I28.1
  - mediastinal (nonsyphilitic) I72.8
    - syphilitic A52.Ø9
  - miliary (congenital) I67.1
    - ruptured — *see* Hemorrhage, intracerebral, subarachnoid, intracranial
  - mitral (heart) (valve) I34.8
  - mural — *see* Aneurysm, heart
  - mycotic I72.9
    - endocardial (any valve) I33.Ø
    - ruptured, brain — *see* Hemorrhage, intracerebral, subarachnoid
  - myocardium — *see* Aneurysm, heart
  - neck I72.Ø
  - pancreaticoduodenal I72.8
  - patent ductus arteriosus Q25.Ø
  - peripheral NEC I72.8
    - congenital Q27.8
      - digestive system Q27.8
      - lower limb Q27.8
      - specified site NEC Q27.8
      - upper limb Q27.8
  - popliteal (artery) (ruptured) I72.4
  - precerebral, congenital (nonruptured) Q28.1
  - pulmonary I28.1
    - arteriovenous Q25.72
      - acquired I28.Ø
    - syphilitic A52.Ø9
    - valve (heart) — *see* Endocarditis, pulmonary
  - racemose (peripheral) I72.9
    - congenital — *see* Aneurysm, congenital
  - radial I72.1
  - Rasmussen NEC A15.Ø
  - renal (artery) I72.2
  - retina (*see also* Disorder, retina, microaneurysms)
    - congenital Q14.1
    - diabetic — *see* Diabetes, microaneurysms, retinal
  - sinus of Valsalva Q25.4
  - specified NEC I72.8
  - spinal (cord) I72.8
    - syphilitic (hemorrhage) A52.Ø9
  - splenic I72.8
  - subclavian (artery) (ruptured) I72.8
    - syphilitic A52.Ø9
  - superior mesenteric I72.8
  - syphilitic (aorta) A52.Ø1
    - central nervous system A52.Ø5
    - congenital (late) A5Ø.54 [I79.Ø]
    - spine, spinal A52.Ø9
  - thoracoabdominal (aorta) I71.6
    - ruptured I71.5
    - syphilitic A52.Ø1
  - thorax, thoracic (aorta) (arch) (nonsyphilitic) I71.2
    - ruptured I71.1
    - syphilitic A52.Ø1
  - traumatic (complication) (early), specified site — *see* Injury, blood vessel
  - tricuspid (heart) (valve) IØ7.8
  - ulnar I72.1
  - upper limb (ruptured) I72.1
  - valve, valvular — *see* Endocarditis
  - venous (*see also* Varix) I86.8
    - congenital Q27.8
      - digestive system Q27.8
      - lower limb Q27.8
      - specified site NEC Q27.8
      - upper limb Q27.8
  - ventricle — *see* Aneurysm, heart
  - visceral NEC I72.8
- **Angelman syndrome** Q93.5
- **Anger** R45.4
- **Angiectasis, angiectopia** I99.8
- **Angiitis** I77.6
  - allergic granulomatous M3Ø.1
  - hypersensitivity M31.Ø
  - necrotizing M31.9
    - specified NEC M31.8
  - nervous system, granulomatous I67.7
- **Angina** (attack) (cardiac) (chest) (heart) (pectoris) (syndrome) (vasomotor) I2Ø.9
  - with
    - atherosclerotic heart disease — *see* Arteriosclerosis, coronary (artery),
    - documented spasm I2Ø.1
  - abdominal K55.1
  - accelerated — *see* Angina, unstable
  - agranulocytic — *see* Agranulocytosis
  - angiospastic — *see* Angina, with documented spasm
  - aphthous BØ8.5
  - crescendo — *see* Angina, unstable
  - croupous JØ5.Ø
  - cruris I73.9
  - de novo effort — *see* Angina, unstable
  - diphtheritic, membranous A36.Ø
  - equivalent I2Ø.8
  - exudative, chronic J37.Ø
  - following acute myocardial infarction I23.7
  - gangrenous diphtheritic A36.Ø
  - intestinal K55.1
  - Ludovici K12.2
  - Ludwig's K12.2
  - malignant diphtheritic A36.Ø
  - membranous JØ5.Ø
    - diphtheritic A36.Ø
    - Vincent's A69.1
  - mesenteric K55.1
  - monocytic — *see* Mononucleosis, infectious
  - of effort — *see* Angina, specified NEC
  - phlegmonous J36
    - diphtheritic A36.Ø
  - post-infarctional I23.7
  - pre-infarctional — *see* Angina, unstable
  - Prinzmetal — *see* Angina, with documented spasm
  - progressive — *see* Angina, unstable
  - pseudomembranous A69.1
  - pultaceous, diphtheritic A36.Ø
  - spasm-induced — *see* Angina, with documented spasm
  - specified NEC I2Ø.8
  - stable I2Ø.9
  - stenocardia — *see* Angina, specified NEC
  - stridulous, diphtheritic A36.2
  - tonsil J36
  - trachealis JØ5.Ø
  - unstable I2Ø.Ø
  - variant — *see* Angina, with documented spasm
  - Vincent's A69.1
  - worsening effort — *see* Angina, unstable
- **Angioblastoma** — *see* Neoplasm, connective tissue, uncertain behavior
- **Angiocholecystitis** — *see* Cholecystitis, acute
- **Angiocholitis** (*see also* Cholecystitis, acute) K83.Ø
- **Angiodysgenesis spinalis** G95.19
- **Angiodysplasia** (cecum) (colon) K55.2Ø
  - with bleeding K55.21
  - duodenum (and stomach) K31.819
    - with bleeding K31.811
  - stomach (and duodenum) K31.819
    - with bleeding K31.811
- **Angioedema** (allergic) (any site) (with urticaria) T78.3 ☑
  - hereditary D84.1
- **Angioendothelioma** — *see* Neoplasm, uncertain behavior, by site
  - benign D18.ØØ
    - intra-abdominal D18.Ø3
    - intracranial D18.Ø2
    - skin D18.Ø1
    - specified site NEC D18.Ø9
  - bone — *see* Neoplasm, bone, malignant
  - Ewing's — *see* Neoplasm, bone, malignant
- **Angioendotheliomatosis** C85.8- ☑
- **Angiofibroma** (*see also* Neoplasm, benign, by site)
  - juvenile
    - specified site — *see* Neoplasm, benign, by site
    - unspecified site D1Ø.6
- **Angiohemophilia** (A) (B) D68.Ø
- **Angioid streaks** (choroid) (macula) (retina) H35.33
- **Angiokeratoma** — *see* Neoplasm, skin, benign

- **Angiokeratoma** — *continued*
  - corporis diffusum E75.21
- **Angioleiomyoma** — *see* Neoplasm, connective tissue, benign
- **Angiolipoma** (*see also* Lipoma)
  - infiltrating — *see* Lipoma
- **Angioma** (*see also* Hemangioma, by site)
  - capillary I78.1
  - hemorrhagicum hereditaria I78.Ø
  - intra-abdominal D18.Ø3
  - intracranial D18.Ø2
  - malignant — *see* Neoplasm, connective tissue, malignant
  - plexiform D18.ØØ
    - intra-abdominal D18.Ø3
    - intracranial D18.Ø2
    - skin D18.Ø1
    - specified site NEC D18.Ø9
  - senile I78.1
  - serpiginosum L81.7
  - skin D18.Ø1
  - specified site NEC D18.Ø9
  - spider I78.1
  - stellate I78.1
  - venous Q28.3
- **Angiomatosis** Q82.8
  - bacillary A79.89
  - encephalotrigeminal Q85.8
  - hemorrhagic familial I78.Ø
  - hereditary familial I78.Ø
  - liver K76.4
- **Angiomyolipoma** — *see* Lipoma
- **Angiomyoliposarcoma** — *see* Neoplasm, connective tissue, malignant
- **Angiomyoma** — *see* Neoplasm, connective tissue, benign
- **Angiomyosarcoma** — *see* Neoplasm, connective tissue, malignant
- **Angiomyxoma** — *see* Neoplasm, connective tissue, uncertain behavior
- **Angioneurosis** F45.8
- **Angioneurotic edema** (allergic) (any site) (with urticaria) T78.3 ☑
  - hereditary D84.1
- **Angiopathia, angiopathy** I99.9
  - cerebral I67.9
    - amyloid E85.4 [I68.Ø]
  - diabetic (peripheral) — *see* Diabetes, angiopathy
  - peripheral I73.9
    - diabetic — *see* Diabetes, angiopathy
    - specified type NEC I73.89
  - retinae syphilitica A52.Ø5
  - retinalis (juvenilis)
    - diabetic — *see* Diabetes, retinopathy
    - proliferative — *see* Retinopathy, proliferative
- **Angiosarcoma** (*see also* Neoplasm, connective tissue, malignant)
  - liver C22.3
- **Angiosclerosis** — *see* Arteriosclerosis
- **Angiospasm** (peripheral) (traumatic) (vessel) I73.9
  - brachial plexus G54.Ø
  - cerebral G45.9
  - cervical plexus G54.2
  - nerve
    - arm — *see* Mononeuropathy, upper limb
      - axillary G54.Ø
      - median — *see* Lesion, nerve, median
      - ulnar — *see* Lesion, nerve, ulnar
    - axillary G54.Ø
    - leg — *see* Mononeuropathy, lower limb
    - median — *see* Lesion, nerve, median
    - plantar — *see* Lesion, nerve, plantar
    - ulnar — *see* Lesion, nerve, ulnar
- **Angiospastic disease or edema** I73.9
- **Angiostrongyliasis**
  - due to
    - Parastrongylus
      - cantonensis B83.2
      - costaricensis B81.3
  - intestinal B81.3
- **Anguillulosis** — *see* Strongyloidiasis
- **Angulation**
  - cecum — *see* Obstruction, intestine
  - coccyx (acquired) (*see also* subcategory) M43.8 ☑
    - congenital NEC Q76.49
  - femur (acquired) (*see also* Deformity, limb, specified type NEC, thigh)
- **Angulation** — *continued*
  - femur (*see also* Deformity, limb, specified type, thigh) — *continued*
    - congenital Q74.2
  - intestine (large) (small) — *see* Obstruction, intestine
  - sacrum (acquired) (*see also* subcategory) M43.8 ☑
    - congenital NEC Q76.49
  - sigmoid (flexure) — *see* Obstruction, intestine
  - spine — *see* Dorsopathy, deforming, specified NEC
  - tibia (acquired) (*see also* Deformity, limb, specified type NEC, lower leg)
    - congenital Q74.2
  - ureter N13.5
    - with infection N13.6
  - wrist (acquired) (*see also* Deformity, limb, specified type NEC, forearm)
    - congenital Q74.Ø
- **Angulus infectiosus** (lips) K13.Ø
- **Anhedonia** R45.84
- **Anhidrosis** L74.4
- **Anhydration, anhydremia** E86.Ø
  - with
    - hypernatremia E87.Ø
    - hyponatremia E87.1
- **Anhydremia** E86.Ø
  - with
    - hypernatremia E87.Ø
    - hyponatremia E87.1
- **Anidrosis** L74.4
- **Aniridia** (congenital) Q13.1
- **Anisakiasis** (infection) (infestation) B81.Ø
- **Anisakis larvae infestation** B81.Ø
- **Aniseikonia** H52.32
- **Anisocoria** (pupil) H57.Ø2
  - congenital Q13.2
- **Anisocytosis** R71.8
- **Anisometropia** (congenital) H52.31
- **Ankle** — *see* condition
- **Ankyloblepharon** (eyelid) (acquired) (*see also* Blepharophimosis)
  - filiforme (adnatum) (congenital) Q1Ø.3
  - total Q1Ø.3
- **Ankyloglossia** Q38.1
- **Ankylosis** (fibrous) (osseous) (joint) M24.6Ø
  - ankle M24.67- ☑
  - arthrodesis status Z98.1
  - cricoarytenoid (cartilage) (joint) (larynx) J38.7
  - dental KØ3.5
  - ear ossicles H74.31- ☑
  - elbow M24.62- ☑
  - foot M24.67- ☑
  - hand M24.64- ☑
  - hip M24.65- ☑
  - incostapedial joint (infectional) — *see* Ankylosis, ear ossicles
  - jaw (temporomandibular) M26.61
  - knee M24.66- ☑
  - lumbosacral (joint) M43.27
  - postoperative (status) Z98.1
  - produced by surgical fusion, status Z98.1
  - sacro-iliac (joint) M43.28
  - shoulder M24.61- ☑
  - spine (joint) (*see also* Fusion, spine)
    - spondylitic — *see* Spondylitis, ankylosing
  - surgical Z98.1
  - temporomandibular M26.61
  - tooth, teeth (hard tissues) KØ3.5
  - wrist M24.63- ☑
- **Ankylostoma** — *see* Ancylostoma
- **Ankylostomiasis** — *see* Ancylostomiasis
- **Ankylurethria** — *see* Stricture, urethra
- **Annular** (*see also* condition)
  - detachment, cervix N88.8
  - organ or site, congenital NEC — *see* Distortion
  - pancreas (congenital) Q45.1
- **Anodontia** (complete) (partial) (vera) KØØ.Ø
  - acquired KØ8.1Ø ☑
- **Anomaly, anomalous** (congenital) (unspecified type) Q89.9
  - abdominal wall NEC Q79.59
  - acoustic nerve QØ7.8
  - adrenal (gland) Q89.1
  - Alder (-Reilly) (leukocyte granulation) D72.Ø
  - alimentary tract Q45.9
    - upper Q4Ø.9
  - alveolar M26.7Ø
    - hyperplasia M26.79
- **Anomaly, anomalous** — *continued*
  - alveolar — *continued*
    - hyperplasia — *continued*
      - mandibular M26.72
      - maxillary M26.71
    - hypoplasia M26.79
      - mandibular M26.74
      - maxillary M26.73
    - ridge (process) M26.79
    - specified NEC M26.79
  - ankle (joint) Q74.2
  - anus Q43.9
  - aorta (arch) NEC Q25.4
    - coarctation (preductal) (postductal) Q25.1
  - aortic cusp or valve Q23.9
  - appendix Q43.8
  - apple peel syndrome Q41.1
  - aqueduct of Sylvius QØ3.Ø
    - with spina bifida — *see* Spina bifida, with hydrocephalus
  - arm Q74.Ø
  - arteriovenous NEC
    - coronary Q24.5
    - gastrointestinal Q27.33
      - acquired — *see* Angiodysplasia
  - artery (peripheral) Q27.9
    - basilar NEC Q28.1
    - cerebral Q28.3
    - coronary Q24.5
    - digestive system Q27.8
    - eye Q15.8
    - great Q25.9
      - specified NEC Q25.8
    - lower limb Q27.8
    - peripheral Q27.9
      - specified NEC Q27.8
    - pulmonary NEC Q25.79
    - renal Q27.2
    - retina Q14.1
    - specified site NEC Q27.8
    - subclavian Q27.8
    - umbilical Q27.Ø
    - upper limb Q27.8
    - vertebral NEC Q28.1
  - aryteno-epiglottic folds Q31.8
  - atrial
    - bands or folds Q2Ø.8
    - septa Q21.1
  - atrioventricular
    - excitation I45.6
    - septum Q21.Ø
  - auditory canal Q17.8
  - auricle
    - ear Q17.8
      - causing impairment of hearing Q16.9
    - heart Q2Ø.8
  - Axenfeld's Q15.Ø
  - back Q89.9
  - band
    - atrial Q2Ø.8
    - heart Q24.8
    - ventricular Q24.8
  - Bartholin's duct Q38.4
  - biliary duct or passage Q44.5
  - bladder Q64.7Ø
    - absence Q64.5
    - diverticulum Q64.6
    - exstrophy Q64.1Ø
      - cloacal Q64.12
      - extroversion Q64.19
      - specified type NEC Q64.19
      - supravesical fissure Q64.11
    - neck obstruction Q64.31
    - specified type NEC Q64.79
  - bone Q79.9
    - arm Q74.Ø
    - face Q75.9
    - leg Q74.2
    - pelvic girdle Q74.2
    - shoulder girdle Q74.Ø
    - skull Q75.9
      - with
        - anencephaly QØØ.Ø
        - encephalocele — *see* Encephalocele
        - hydrocephalus QØ3.9
          - with spina bifida — *see* Spina bifida, by site, with hydrocephalus
        - microcephaly QØ2

- **Anomaly, anomalous** — *continued*
  - brain (multiple) QØ4.9
    - vessel Q28.3
  - breast Q83.9
  - broad ligament Q5Ø.6
  - bronchus Q32.4
  - bulbus cordis Q21.9
  - bursa Q79.9
  - canal of Nuck Q52.4
  - canthus Q1Ø.3
  - capillary Q27.9
  - cardiac Q24.9
    - chambers Q2Ø.9
      - specified NEC Q2Ø.8
    - septal closure Q21.9
      - specified NEC Q21.8
    - valve NEC Q24.8
      - pulmonary Q22.3
  - cardiovascular system Q28.8
  - carpus Q74.Ø
  - caruncle, lacrimal Q1Ø.6
  - cascade stomach Q4Ø.2
  - cauda equina QØ6.3
  - cecum Q43.9
  - cerebral QØ4.9
    - vessels Q28.3
  - cervix Q51.9
  - Chédiak-Higashi (-Steinbrinck) (congenital gigantism of peroxidase granules) E7Ø.33Ø
  - cheek Q18.9
  - chest wall Q67.8
    - bones Q76.9
  - chin Q18.9
  - chordae tendineae Q24.8
  - choroid Q14.3
    - plexus QØ7.8
  - chromosomes, chromosomal Q99.9
    - D (1) — *see* condition, chromosome 13
    - E (3) — *see* condition, chromosome 18
    - G — *see* condition, chromosome 21
    - sex
      - female phenotype Q97.8
      - gonadal dysgenesis (pure) Q99.1
      - Klinefelter's Q98.4
      - male phenotype Q98.9
      - Turner's Q96.9
    - specified NEC Q99.8
  - cilia Q1Ø.3
  - circulatory system Q28.9
  - clavicle Q74.Ø
  - clitoris Q52.6
  - coccyx Q76.49
  - colon Q43.9
  - common duct Q44.5
  - communication
    - coronary artery Q24.5
    - left ventricle with right atrium Q21.Ø
  - concha (ear) Q17.3
  - connection
    - portal vein Q26.5
    - pulmonary venous Q26.4
      - partial Q26.3
      - total Q26.2
    - renal artery with kidney Q27.2
  - cornea (shape) Q13.4
  - coronary artery or vein Q24.5
  - cranium — *see* Anomaly, skull
  - cricoid cartilage Q31.8
  - cystic duct Q44.5
  - dental
    - alveolar — *see* Anomaly, alveolar
    - arch relationship M26.2Ø
      - specified NEC M26.29
  - dentofacial M26.9
    - alveolar — *see* Anomaly, alveolar
    - dental arch relationship M26.2Ø
      - specified NEC M26.29
    - functional M26.5Ø
      - specified NEC M26.59
    - jaw size M26.ØØ
      - macrogenia M26.Ø5
      - mandibular
        - hyperplasia M26.Ø3
        - hypoplasia M26.Ø4
      - maxillary
        - hyperplasia M26.Ø1
        - hypoplasia M26.Ø2
      - microgenia M26.Ø6

- **Anomaly, anomalous** — *continued*
  - dentofacial — *continued*
    - jaw size — *continued*
      - specified type NEC M26.Ø9
    - jaw-cranial base relationship M26.1Ø
      - asymmetry M26.12
        - maxillary M26.11
      - specified type NEC M26.19
    - malocclusion M26.4
      - dental arch relationship NEC M26.29
      - jaw size — *see* Anomaly, dentofacial, jaw size
      - jaw-cranial base relationship — *see* Anomaly, dentofacial, jaw-cranial base relationship
    - specified type NEC M26.89
    - temporomandibular joint M26.6Ø
      - adhesions M26.61
      - ankylosis M26.61
      - arthralgia M26.62
      - articular disc M26.63
      - specified type NEC M26.69
    - tooth position, fully erupted M26.3Ø
      - specified NEC M26.39
  - dermatoglyphic Q82.8
  - diaphragm (apertures) NEC Q79.1
  - digestive organ(s) or tract Q45.9
    - lower Q43.9
    - upper Q4Ø.9
  - distance, interarch (excessive) (inadequate) M26.25
  - distribution, coronary artery Q24.5
  - ductus
    - arteriosus Q25.Ø
    - botalli Q25.Ø
  - duodenum Q43.9
  - dura (brain) QØ4.9
    - spinal cord QØ6.9
  - ear (external) Q17.9
    - causing impairment of hearing Q16.9
    - inner Q16.5
    - middle (causing impairment of hearing) Q16.4
    - ossicles Q16.3
  - Ebstein's (heart) (tricuspid valve) Q22.5
  - ectodermal Q82.9
  - Eisenmenger's (ventricular septal defect) Q21.8
  - ejaculatory duct Q55.4
  - elbow Q74.Ø
  - endocrine gland NEC Q89.2
  - epididymis Q55.4
  - epiglottis Q31.8
  - esophagus Q39.9
  - eustachian tube Q17.8
  - eye Q15.9
    - anterior segment Q13.9
      - specified NEC Q13.89
    - posterior segment Q14.9
      - specified NEC Q14.8
    - ptosis (eyelid) Q1Ø.Ø
    - specified NEC Q15.8
  - eyebrow Q18.8
  - eyelid Q1Ø.3
    - ptosis Q1Ø.Ø
  - face Q18.9
    - bone(s) Q75.9
  - fallopian tube Q5Ø.6
  - fascia Q79.9
  - femur NEC Q74.2
  - fibula NEC Q74.2
  - finger Q74.Ø
  - fixation, intestine Q43.3
  - flexion (joint) NOS Q74.9
    - hip or thigh Q65.89
  - foot NEC Q74.2
    - varus (congenital) Q66.3
  - foramen
    - Botalli Q21.1
    - ovale Q21.1
  - forearm Q74.Ø
  - forehead Q75.8
  - form, teeth KØØ.2
  - fovea centralis Q14.1
  - frontal bone — *see* Anomaly, skull
  - gallbladder (position) (shape) (size) Q44.1
  - Gartner's duct Q52.4
  - gastrointestinal tract Q45.9
  - genitalia, genital organ(s) or system
    - female Q52.9
      - external Q52.7Ø
      - internal NOS Q52.9
    - male Q55.9

- **Anomaly, anomalous** — *continued*
  - genitalia, genital organ(s) or system — *continued*
    - male — *continued*
      - hydrocele P83.5
      - specified NEC Q55.8
  - genitourinary NEC
    - female Q52.9
    - male Q55.9
  - Gerbode Q21.Ø
  - glottis Q31.8
  - granulation or granulocyte, genetic (constitutional) (leukocyte) D72.Ø
  - gum Q38.6
  - gyri QØ7.9
  - hair Q84.2
  - hand Q74.Ø
  - hard tissue formation in pulp KØ4.3
  - head — *see* Anomaly, skull
  - heart Q24.9
    - auricle Q2Ø.8
    - bands or folds Q24.8
    - fibroelastosis cordis I42.4
    - obstructive NEC Q22.6
    - patent ductus arteriosus (Botalli) Q25.Ø
    - septum Q21.9
      - auricular Q21.1
      - interatrial Q21.1
      - interventricular Q21.Ø
        - with pulmonary stenosis or atresia, dextra-position of aorta and hypertrophy of right ventricle Q21.3
      - specified NEC Q21.8
      - ventricular Q21.Ø
        - with pulmonary stenosis or atresia, dextra-position of aorta and hypertrophy of right ventricle Q21.3
    - tetralogy of Fallot Q21.3
    - valve NEC Q24.8
      - aortic
        - bicuspid valve Q23.1
        - insufficiency Q23.1
        - stenosis Q23.Ø
          - subaortic Q24.4
      - mitral
        - insufficiency Q23.3
        - stenosis Q23.2
      - pulmonary Q22.3
        - atresia Q22.Ø
        - insufficiency Q22.2
        - stenosis Q22.1
          - infundibular Q24.3
          - subvalvular Q24.3
      - tricuspid
        - atresia Q22.4
        - stenosis Q22.4
    - ventricle Q2Ø.8
  - heel NEC Q74.2
  - Hegglin's D72.Ø
  - hemianencephaly QØØ.Ø
  - hemicephaly QØØ.Ø
  - hemicrania QØØ.Ø
  - hepatic duct Q44.5
  - hip NEC Q74.2
  - hourglass stomach Q4Ø.2
  - humerus Q74.Ø
  - hydatid of Morgagni
    - female Q5Ø.5
    - male (epididymal) Q55.4
      - testicular Q55.29
  - hymen Q52.4
  - hypersegmentation of neutrophils, hereditary D72.Ø
  - hypophyseal Q89.2
  - ileocecal (coil) (valve) Q43.9
  - ileum Q43.9
  - ilium NEC Q74.2
  - integument Q84.9
    - specified NEC Q84.8
  - interarch distance (excessive) (inadequate) M26.25
  - intervertebral cartilage or disc Q76.49
  - intestine (large) (small) Q43.9
    - with anomalous adhesions, fixation or malrotation Q43.3
  - iris Q13.2
  - ischium NEC Q74.2
  - jaw — *see* Anomaly, dentofacial
    - alveolar — *see* Anomaly, alveolar
    - jaw-cranial base relationship — *see* Anomaly, dentofacial, jaw-cranial base relationship

Anomaly, anomalous — *continued*
- jejunum Q43.8
- joint Q74.9
  - specified NEC Q74.8
- Jordan's D72.Ø
- kidney(s) (calyx) (pelvis) Q63.9
  - artery Q27.2
  - specified NEC Q63.8
- Klippel-Feil (brevicollis) Q76.1
- knee Q74.1
- labium (majus) (minus) Q52.7Ø
- labyrinth, membranous Q16.5
- lacrimal apparatus or duct Q1Ø.6
- larynx, laryngeal (muscle) Q31.9
  - web (bed) Q31.Ø
- lens Q12.9
- leukocytes, genetic D72.Ø
  - granulation (constitutional) D72.Ø
- lid (fold) Q1Ø.3
- ligament Q79.9
  - broad Q5Ø.6
  - round Q52.8
- limb Q74.9
  - lower NEC Q74.2
    - reduction deformity — *see* Defect, reduction, lower limb
  - upper Q74.Ø
- lip Q38.Ø
- liver Q44.7
  - duct Q44.5
- lower limb NEC Q74.2
- lumbosacral (joint) (region) Q76.49
  - kyphosis — *see* Kyphosis, congenital
  - lordosis — *see* Lordosis, congenital
- lung (fissure) (lobe) Q33.9
- mandible — *see* Anomaly, dentofacial
- maxilla — *see* Anomaly, dentofacial
- May (-Hegglin) D72.Ø
- meatus urinarius NEC Q64.79
- meningeal bands or folds QØ7.9
  - constriction of QØ7.8
  - spinal QØ6.9
- meninges QØ7.9
  - cerebral QØ4.8
  - spinal QØ6.9
- meningocele QØ5.9
- mesentery Q45.9
- metacarpus Q74.Ø
- metatarsus NEC Q74.2
- middle ear Q16.4
  - ossicles Q16.3
- mitral (leaflets) (valve) Q23.9
  - insufficiency Q23.3
  - specified NEC Q23.8
  - stenosis Q23.2
- mouth Q38.6
- Müllerian (*see also* Anomaly, by site)
  - uterus NEC Q51.818
- multiple NEC Q89.7
- muscle Q79.9
  - eyelid Q1Ø.3
- musculoskeletal system, except limbs Q79.9
- myocardium Q24.8
- nail Q84.6
- narrowness, eyelid Q1Ø.3
- nasal sinus (wall) Q3Ø.8
- neck (any part) Q18.9
- nerve QØ7.9
  - acoustic QØ7.8
  - optic QØ7.8
- nervous system (central) QØ7.9
- nipple Q83.9
- nose, nasal (bones) (cartilage) (septum) (sinus) Q3Ø.9
  - specified NEC Q3Ø.8
- ocular muscle Q15.8
- omphalomesenteric duct Q43.Ø
- opening, pulmonary veins Q26.4
- optic
  - disc Q14.2
  - nerve QØ7.8
- opticociliary vessels Q13.2
- orbit (eye) Q1Ø.7
- organ Q89.9
  - of Corti Q16.5
- origin
  - artery
    - innominate Q25.8
    - pulmonary Q25.79

Anomaly, anomalous — *continued*
- origin — *continued*
  - artery — *continued*
    - renal Q27.2
    - subclavian Q25.8
- osseous meatus (ear) Q16.1
- ovary Q5Ø.39
- oviduct Q5Ø.6
- palate (hard) (soft) NEC Q38.5
- pancreas or pancreatic duct Q45.3
- papillary muscles Q24.8
- parathyroid gland Q89.2
- paraurethral ducts Q64.79
- parotid (gland) Q38.4
- patella Q74.1
- Pelger-Huët (hereditary hyposegmentation) D72.Ø
- pelvic girdle NEC Q74.2
- pelvis (bony) NEC Q74.2
  - rachitic E64.3
- penis (glans) Q55.69
- pericardium Q24.8
- peripheral vascular system Q27.9
- Peter's Q13.4
- pharynx Q38.8
- pigmentation L81.9
  - congenital Q82.8
- pituitary (gland) Q89.2
- pleural (folds) Q34.Ø
- portal vein Q26.5
  - connection Q26.5
- position, tooth, teeth, fully erupted M26.3Ø
  - specified NEC M26.39
- precerebral vessel Q28.1
- prepuce Q55.69
- prostate Q55.4
- pulmonary Q33.9
  - artery NEC Q25.79
  - valve Q22.3
    - atresia Q22.Ø
    - insufficiency Q22.2
    - specified type NEC Q22.3
    - stenosis Q22.1
      - infundibular Q24.3
      - subvalvular Q24.3
  - venous connection Q26.4
    - partial Q26.3
    - total Q26.2
- pupil Q13.2
  - function H57.ØØ
    - anisocoria H57.Ø2
    - Argyll Robertson pupil H57.Ø1
    - miosis H57.Ø3
    - mydriasis H57.Ø4
    - specified type NEC H57.Ø9
    - tonic pupil H57.Ø5- ☑
- pylorus Q4Ø.3
- radius Q74.Ø
- rectum Q43.9
- reduction (extremity) (limb)
  - femur (longitudinal) — *see* Defect, reduction, lower limb, longitudinal, femur
  - fibula (longitudinal) — *see* Defect, reduction, lower limb, longitudinal, fibula
  - lower limb — *see* Defect, reduction, lower limb
  - radius (longitudinal) — *see* Defect, reduction, upper limb, longitudinal, radius
  - tibia (longitudinal) — *see* Defect, reduction, lower limb, longitudinal, tibia
  - ulna (longitudinal) — *see* Defect, reduction, upper limb, longitudinal, ulna
  - upper limb — *see* Defect, reduction, upper limb
- refraction — *see* Disorder, refraction
- renal Q63.9
  - artery Q27.2
  - pelvis Q63.9
    - specified NEC Q63.8
- respiratory system Q34.9
  - specified NEC Q34.8
- retina Q14.1
- rib Q76.6
  - cervical Q76.5
- Rieger's Q13.81
- rotation — *see* Malrotation
  - hip or thigh Q65.89
- round ligament Q52.8
- sacroiliac (joint) NEC Q74.2
- sacrum NEC Q76.49
  - kyphosis — *see* Kyphosis, congenital

Anomaly, anomalous — *continued*
- sacrum — *continued*
  - lordosis — *see* Lordosis, congenital
- saddle nose, syphilitic A5Ø.57
- salivary duct or gland Q38.4
- scapula Q74.Ø
- scrotum — *see* Malformation, testis and scrotum
- sebaceous gland Q82.9
- seminal vesicles Q55.4
- sense organs NEC QØ7.8
- sex chromosomes NEC (*see also* Anomaly, chromosomes)
  - female phenotype Q97.8
  - male phenotype Q98.9
- shoulder (girdle) (joint) Q74.Ø
- sigmoid (flexure) Q43.9
- simian crease Q82.8
- sinus of Valsalva Q25.4
- skeleton generalized Q78.9
- skin (appendage) Q82.9
- skull Q75.9
  - with
    - anencephaly QØØ.Ø
    - encephalocele — *see* Encephalocele
    - hydrocephalus QØ3.9
      - with spina bifida — *see* Spina bifida, by site, with hydrocephalus
    - microcephaly QØ2
- specified organ or site NEC Q89.8
- spermatic cord Q55.4
- spine, spinal NEC Q76.49
  - column NEC Q76.49
    - kyphosis — *see* Kyphosis, congenital
    - lordosis — *see* Lordosis, congenital
  - cord QØ6.9
  - nerve root QØ7.8
- spleen Q89.Ø9
  - agenesis Q89.Ø1
- stenonian duct Q38.4
- sternum NEC Q76.7
- stomach Q4Ø.3
- submaxillary gland Q38.4
- tarsus NEC Q74.2
- tendon Q79.9
- testis — *see* Malformation, testis and scrotum
- thigh NEC Q74.2
- thorax (wall) Q67.8
  - bony Q76.9
- throat Q38.8
- thumb Q74.Ø
- thymus gland Q89.2
- thyroid (gland) Q89.2
  - cartilage Q31.8
- tibia NEC Q74.2
  - saber A5Ø.56
- toe Q74.2
- tongue Q38.3
- tooth, teeth KØØ.9
  - eruption KØØ.6
  - position, fully erupted M26.3Ø
  - spacing, fully erupted M26.3Ø
- trachea (cartilage) Q32.1
- tragus Q17.9
- tricuspid (leaflet) (valve) Q22.9
  - atresia or stenosis Q22.4
  - Ebstein's Q22.5
- Uhl's (hypoplasia of myocardium, right ventricle) Q24.8
- ulna Q74.Ø
- umbilical artery Q27.Ø
- union
  - cricoid cartilage and thyroid cartilage Q31.8
  - thyroid cartilage and hyoid bone Q31.8
  - trachea with larynx Q31.8
- upper limb Q74.Ø
- urachus Q64.4
- ureter Q62.8
  - obstructive NEC Q62.39
    - cecoureterocele Q62.32
    - orthotopic ureterocele Q62.31
- urethra Q64.7Ø
  - absence Q64.5
  - double Q64.74
  - fistula to rectum Q64.73
  - obstructive Q64.39
    - stricture Q64.32
  - prolapse Q64.71
  - specified type NEC Q64.79
- urinary tract Q64.9

- **Anomaly, anomalous** — *continued*
  - uterus Q51.9
    - with only one functioning horn Q51.4
  - uvula Q38.5
  - vagina Q52.4
  - valleculae Q31.8
  - valve (heart) NEC Q24.8
    - coronary sinus Q24.5
    - inferior vena cava Q24.8
    - pulmonary Q22.3
    - sinus coronario Q24.5
    - venae cavae inferioris Q24.8
  - vas deferens Q55.4
  - vascular Q27.9
    - brain Q28.3
    - ring Q25.4
  - vein(s) (peripheral) Q27.9
    - brain Q28.3
    - cerebral Q28.3
    - coronary Q24.5
    - developmental Q28.3
    - great Q26.9
      - specified NEC Q26.8
  - vena cava (inferior) (superior) Q26.9
  - venous — *see* Anomaly, vein(s)
  - venous return Q26.8
  - ventricular
    - bands or folds Q24.8
    - septa Q21.Ø
  - vertebra Q76.49
    - kyphosis — *see* Kyphosis, congenital
    - lordosis — *see* Lordosis, congenital
  - vesicourethral orifice Q64.79
  - vessel(s) Q27.9
    - optic papilla Q14.2
    - precerebral Q28.1
  - vitelline duct Q43.Ø
  - vitreous body or humor Q14.Ø
  - vulva Q52.7Ø
  - wrist (joint) Q74.Ø
- **Anomia** R48.8
- **Anonychia** (congenital) Q84.3
  - acquired L6Ø.8
- **Anophthalmos, anophthalmus** (congenital) (globe) Q11.1
  - acquired Z9Ø.Ø1
- **Anopia, anopsia** H53.46- ☑
  - quadrant H53.46- ☑
- **Anorchia, anorchism, anorchidism** Q55.Ø
- **Anorexia** R63.Ø
  - hysterical F44.89
  - nervosa F5Ø.ØØ
    - atypical F5Ø.9
    - binge-eating type F5Ø.2
      - with purging F5Ø.Ø2
    - restricting type F5Ø.Ø1
- **Anorgasmy, psychogenic** (female) F52.31
  - male F52.32
- **Anosmia** R43.Ø
  - hysterical F44.6
  - postinfectional J39.8
- **Anosognosia** R41.89
- **Anosteoplasia** Q78.9
- **Anovulatory cycle** N97.Ø
- **Anoxemia** RØ9.Ø2
  - newborn P84
- **Anoxia** (pathological) RØ9.Ø2
  - altitude T7Ø.29 ☑
  - cerebral G93.1
    - complicating
      - anesthesia (general) (local) or other sedation T88.59 ☑
        - in labor and delivery O74.3
        - in pregnancy O29.21- ☑
        - postpartum, puerperal O89.2
      - delivery (cesarean) (instrumental) O75.4
    - during a procedure G97.81
    - newborn P84
    - resulting from a procedure G97.82
  - due to
    - drowning T75.1 ☑
    - high altitude T7Ø.29 ☑
  - heart — *see* Insufficiency, coronary
  - intrauterine P84
  - myocardial — *see* Insufficiency, coronary
  - newborn P84
  - spinal cord G95.11
- **Anoxia** — *continued*
  - systemic (by suffocation) (low content in atmosphere) — *see* Asphyxia, traumatic
- **Anteflexion** — *see* Anteversion
- **Antenatal**
  - care (normal pregnancy) Z34.9Ø
  - screening (encounter for) of mother Z36
- **Antepartum** — *see* condition
- **Anterior** — *see* condition
- **Antero-occlusion** M26.22Ø
- **Anteversion**
  - cervix — *see* Anteversion, uterus
  - femur (neck), congenital Q65.89
  - uterus, uterine (cervix) (postinfectional) (postpartal, old) N85.4
    - congenital Q51.818
    - in pregnancy or childbirth — *see* Pregnancy, complicated by
- **Anthophobia** F4Ø.228
- **Anthracosilicosis** J6Ø
- **Anthracosis** (lung) (occupational) J6Ø
  - lingua K14.3
- **Anthrax** A22.9
  - with pneumonia A22.1
  - cerebral A22.8
  - colitis A22.2
  - cutaneous A22.Ø
  - gastrointestinal A22.2
  - inhalation A22.1
  - intestinal A22.2
  - meningitis A22.8
  - pulmonary A22.1
  - respiratory A22.1
  - sepsis A22.7
  - specified manifestation NEC A22.8
- **Anthropoid pelvis** Q74.2
  - with disproportion (fetopelvic) O33.Ø
- **Anthropophobia** F4Ø.1Ø
  - generalized F4Ø.11
- **Antibodies, maternal** (blood group) — *see* Isoimmunization, affecting management of pregnancy
  - anti-D — *see* Isoimmunization, affecting management of pregnancy, Rh
  - newborn P55.Ø
- **Antibody**
  - anticardiolipin R76.Ø
    - with
      - hemorrhagic disorder D68.312
      - hypercoagulable state D68.61
  - antiphosphatidylglycerol R76.Ø
    - with
      - hemorrhagic disorder D68.312
      - hypercoagulable state D68.61
  - antiphosphatidylinositol R76.Ø
    - with
      - hemorrhagic disorder D68.312
      - hypercoagulable state D68.61
  - antiphosphatidylserine R76.Ø
    - with
      - hemorrhagic disorder D68.312
      - hypercoagulable state D68.61
  - antiphospholipid R76.Ø
    - with
      - hemorrhagic disorder D68.312
      - hypercoagulable state D68.61
- **Anticardiolipin syndrome** D68.61
- **Anticoagulant, circulating** (intrinsic) (*see also* Disorder, hemorrhagic) D68.318
  - drug-induced (extrinsic) (*see also* Disorder, hemorrhagic) D68.32
- **Antidiuretic hormone syndrome** E22.2
- **Antimonial cholera** — *see* Poisoning, antimony
- **Antiphospholipid**
  - antibody
    - with hemorrhagic disorder D68.312
    - syndrome D68.61
- **Antisocial personality** F6Ø.2
- **Antithrombinemia** — *see* Circulating anticoagulants
- **Antithromboplastinemia** D68.318
- **Antithromboplastinogenemia** D68.318
- **Antitoxin complication or reaction** — *see* Complications, vaccination
- **Antlophobia** F4Ø.228
- **Antritis** J32.Ø
  - maxilla J32.Ø
    - acute JØ1.ØØ
      - recurrent JØ1.Ø1
  - stomach K29.6Ø
- **Antritis** — *continued*
  - stomach — *continued*
    - with bleeding K29.61
- **Antrum, antral** — *see* condition
- **Anuria** R34
  - calculous (impacted) (recurrent) (*see also* Calculus, urinary) N2Ø.9
  - following
    - abortion — *see* Abortion by type complicated by, renal failure
    - ectopic or molar pregnancy OØ8.4
  - newborn P96.Ø
  - postprocedural N99.Ø
  - postrenal N13.8
  - traumatic (following crushing) T79.5 ☑
- **Anus, anal** — *see* condition
- **Anusitis** K62.89
- **Anxiety** F41.9
  - depression F41.8
  - episodic paroxysmal F41.Ø
  - generalized F41.1
  - hysteria F41.8
  - neurosis F41.1
  - panic type F41.Ø
  - reaction F41.1
  - separation, abnormal (of childhood) F93.Ø
  - specified NEC F41.8
  - state F41.1
- **Aorta, aortic** — *see* condition
- **Aortectasia** — *see* Ectasia, aorta
  - with aneurysm — *see* Aneurysm, aorta
- **Aortitis** (nonsyphilitic) (calcific) I77.6
  - arteriosclerotic I7Ø.Ø
  - Doehle-Heller A52.Ø2
  - luetic A52.Ø2
  - rheumatic — *see* Endocarditis, acute, rheumatic
  - specific (syphilitic) A52.Ø2
  - syphilitic A52.Ø2
    - congenital A5Ø.54 [I79.1]
- **Apathetic thyroid storm** — *see* Thyrotoxicosis
- **Apathy** R45.3
- **Apeirophobia** F4Ø.228
- **Apepsia** K3Ø
  - psychogenic F45.8
- **Aperistalsis, esophagus** K22.Ø
- **Apertognathia** M26.29
- **Apert's syndrome** Q87.Ø
- **Aphagia** R13.Ø
  - psychogenic F5Ø.9
- **Aphakia** (acquired) (postoperative) H27.Ø- ☑
  - congenital Q12.3
- **Aphasia** (amnestic) (global) (nominal) (semantic) (syntactic) R47.Ø1
  - acquired, with epilepsy (Landau-Kleffner syndrome) — *see* Epilepsy, specified NEC
  - auditory (developmental) F8Ø.2
  - developmental (receptive type) F8Ø.2
    - expressive type F8Ø.1
    - Wernicke's F8Ø.2
  - following
    - cerebrovascular disease I69.92Ø
      - cerebral infarction I69.32Ø
      - intracerebral hemorrhage I69.12Ø
      - nontraumatic intracranial hemorrhage NEC I69.22Ø
      - specified disease NEC I69.82Ø
      - subarachnoid hemorrhage I69.Ø2Ø
  - primary progressive G31.Ø1 [FØ2.8Ø]
    - with behavioral disturbance G31.Ø1 [FØ2.81]
  - progressive isolated G31.Ø1 [FØ2.8Ø]
    - with behavioral disturbance G31.Ø1 [FØ2.81]
  - sensory F8Ø.2
  - syphilis, tertiary A52.19
  - Wernicke's (developmental) F8Ø.2
- **Aphonia** (organic) R49.1
  - hysterical F44.4
  - psychogenic F44.4
- **Aphthae, aphthous** (*see also* condition)
  - Bednar's K12.Ø
  - cachectic K14.Ø
  - epizootic BØ8.8
  - fever BØ8.8
  - oral (recurrent) K12.Ø
  - stomatitis (major) (minor) K12.Ø
  - thrush B37.Ø
  - ulcer (oral) (recurrent) K12.Ø
    - genital organ(s) NEC
      - female N76.6

- **Aphthae, aphthous** — *continued*
  - ulcer — *continued*
    - genital organ(s) — *continued*
      - male N5Ø.8
    - larynx J38.7
- **Apical** — *see* condition
- **Apiphobia** F4Ø.218
- **Aplasia** (*see also* Agenesis)
  - abdominal muscle syndrome Q79.4
  - alveolar process (acquired) — *see* Anomaly, alveolar
    - congenital Q38.6
  - aorta (congenital) Q25.4
  - axialis extracorticalis (congenita) E75.29
  - bone marrow (myeloid) D61.9
    - congenital D61.Ø1
  - brain QØØ.Ø
    - part of QØ4.3
  - bronchus Q32.4
  - cementum KØØ.4
  - cerebellum QØ4.3
  - cervix (congenital) Q51.5
  - congenital pure red cell D61.Ø1
  - corpus callosum QØ4.Ø
  - cutis congenita Q84.8
  - erythrocyte congenital D61.Ø1
  - extracortical axial E75.29
  - eye Q11.1
  - fovea centralis (congenital) Q14.1
  - gallbladder, congenital Q44.Ø
  - iris Q13.1
  - labyrinth, membranous Q16.5
  - limb (congenital) Q73.8
    - lower — *see* Defect, reduction, lower limb
    - upper — *see* Agenesis, arm
  - lung, congenital (bilateral) (unilateral) Q33.3
  - pancreas Q45.Ø
  - parathyroid-thymic D82.1
  - Pelizaeus-Merzbacher E75.29
  - penis Q55.5
  - prostate Q55.4
  - red cell (with thymoma) D6Ø.9
    - acquired D6Ø.9
      - due to drugs D6Ø.9
    - adult D6Ø.9
    - chronic D6Ø.Ø
    - congenital D61.Ø1
    - constitutional D61.Ø1
    - due to drugs D6Ø.9
    - hereditary D61.Ø1
    - of infants D61.Ø1
    - primary D61.Ø1
    - pure D61.Ø1
      - due to drugs D6Ø.9
    - specified type NEC D6Ø.8
    - transient D6Ø.1
  - round ligament Q52.8
  - skin Q84.8
  - spermatic cord Q55.4
  - spleen Q89.Ø1
  - testicle Q55.Ø
  - thymic, with immunodeficiency D82.1
  - thyroid (congenital) (with myxedema) EØ3.1
  - uterus Q51.Ø
  - ventral horn cell QØ6.1
- **Apnea, apneic** (of) (spells) RØ6.81
  - newborn NEC P28.4
    - obstructive P28.4
    - sleep (central) (obstructive) (primary) P28.3
  - prematurity P28.4
  - sleep G47.3Ø
    - central (primary) G47.31
      - in conditions classified elsewhere G47.37
    - obstructive (adult) (pediatric) G47.33
    - primary central G47.31
    - specified NEC G47.39
- **Apneumatosis, newborn** P28.Ø
- **Apocrine metaplasia** (breast) — *see* Dysplasia, mammary, specified type NEC
- **Apophysitis** (bone) (*see also* Osteochondropathy)
  - calcaneus M92.8
  - juvenile M92.9
- **Apoplectiform convulsions** (cerebral ischemia) I67.82
- **Apoplexia, apoplexy, apoplectic**
  - adrenal A39.1
  - heart (auricle) (ventricle) — *see* Infarct, myocardium
  - heat T67.Ø ☑
  - hemorrhagic (stroke) — *see* Hemorrhage, intracranial
- **Apoplexia, apoplexy, apoplectic** — *continued*
  - meninges, hemorrhagic — *see* Hemorrhage, intracranial, subarachnoid
  - uremic N18.9 [I68.8]
- **Appearance**
  - bizarre R46.1
  - specified NEC R46.89
  - very low level of personal hygiene R46.Ø
- **Appendage**
  - epididymal (organ of Morgagni) Q55.4
  - intestine (epiploic) Q43.8
  - preauricular Q17.Ø
  - testicular (organ of Morgagni) Q55.29
- **Appendicitis** (pneumococcal) (retrocecal) K37
  - with
    - perforation or rupture K35.2
    - peritoneal abscess K35.3
    - peritonitis NEC K35.3
      - generalized (with perforation or rupture) K35.2
      - localized (with perforation or rupture) K35.3
  - acute (catarrhal) (fulminating) (gangrenous) (obstructive) (retrocecal) (suppurative) K35.8Ø
    - with
      - peritoneal abscess K35.3
      - peritonitis NEC K35.3
        - generalized (with perforation or rupture) K35.2
        - localized (with perforation or rupture) K35.3
    - specified NEC K35.89
  - amebic AØ6.89
  - chronic (recurrent) K36
  - exacerbation — *see* Appendicitis, acute
  - gangrenous — *see* Appendicitis, acute
  - healed (obliterative) K36
  - interval K36
  - neurogenic K36
  - obstructive K36
  - recurrent K36
  - relapsing K36
  - subacute (adhesive) K36
  - subsiding K36
  - suppurative — *see* Appendicitis, acute
  - tuberculous A18.32
- **Appendicopathia oxyurica** B8Ø
- **Appendix, appendicular** (*see also* condition)
  - epididymis Q55.4
  - Morgagni
    - female Q5Ø.5
    - male (epididymal) Q55.4
      - testicular Q55.29
  - testis Q55.29
- **Appetite**
  - depraved — *see* Pica
  - excessive R63.2
  - lack or loss (*see also* Anorexia) R63.Ø
    - nonorganic origin F5Ø.8
    - psychogenic F5Ø.8
  - perverted (hysterical) — *see* Pica
- **Apple peel syndrome** Q41.1
- **Apprehension state** F41.1
- **Apprehensiveness, abnormal** F41.9
- **Approximal wear** KØ3.Ø
- **Apraxia** (classic) (ideational) (ideokinetic) (ideomotor) (motor) (verbal) R48.2
  - following
    - cerebrovascular disease I69.99Ø
      - cerebral infarction I69.39Ø
      - intracerebral hemorrhage I69.19Ø
      - nontraumatic intracranial hemorrhage NEC I69.29Ø
      - specified disease NEC I69.89Ø
      - subarachnoid hemorrhage I69.Ø9Ø
  - oculomotor, congenital H51.8
- **Aptyalism** K11.7
- **Apudoma** — *see* Neoplasm, uncertain behavior, by site
- **Aqueous misdirection** H4Ø.83- ☑
- **Arabicum elephantiasis** — *see* Infestation, filarial
- **Arachnitis** — *see* Meningitis
- **Arachnodactyly** — *see* Syndrome, Marfan's
- **Arachnoiditis** (acute) (adhesive) (basal) (brain) (cerebrospinal) — *see* Meningitis
- **Arachnophobia** F4Ø.21Ø
- **Arboencephalitis, Australian** A83.4
- **Arborization block** (heart) I45.5
- **ARC** (AIDS-related complex) B2Ø
- **Arches** — *see* condition
- **Arcuate uterus** Q51.81Ø
- **Arcuatus uterus** Q51.81Ø
- **Arcus** (cornea) senilis — *see* Degeneration, cornea, senile
- **Arc-welder's lung** J63.4
- **Areflexia** R29.2
- **Areola** — *see* condition
- **Argentaffinoma** (*see also* Neoplasm, uncertain behavior, by site)
  - malignant — *see* Neoplasm, malignant, by site
  - syndrome E34.Ø
- **Argininemia** E72.21
- **Arginosuccinic aciduria** E72.22
- **Argyll Robertson phenomenon, pupil or syndrome** (syphilitic) A52.19
  - atypical H57.Ø9
  - nonsyphilitic H57.Ø9
- **Argyria, argyriasis**
  - conjunctival H11.13- ☑
  - from drug or medicament — *see* Table of Drugs and Chemicals, by substance
- **Argyrosis, conjunctival** H11.13- ☑
- **Arhinencephaly** QØ4.1
- **Ariboflavinosis** E53.Ø
- **Arm** — *see* condition
- **Arnold-Chiari disease, obstruction or syndrome** (type II) QØ7.ØØ
  - with
    - hydrocephalus QØ7.Ø2
      - with spina bifida QØ7.Ø3
    - spina bifida QØ7.Ø1
      - with hydrocephalus QØ7.Ø3
  - type III — *see* Encephalocele
  - type IV QØ4.8
- **Aromatic amino-acid metabolism disorder** E7Ø.9
  - specified NEC E7Ø.8
- **Arousals, confusional** G47.51
- **Arrest, arrested**
  - cardiac I46.9
    - complicating
      - abortion — *see* Abortion, by type, complicated by, cardiac arrest
      - anesthesia (general) (local) or other sedation — *see* Table of Drugs and Chemicals, by drug
        - in labor and delivery O74.2
        - in pregnancy O29.11- ☑
        - postpartum, puerperal O89.1
      - delivery (cesarean) (instrumental) O75.4
    - due to
      - cardiac condition I46.2
      - specified condition NEC I46.8
    - intraoperative I97.71- ☑
    - newborn P29.81
    - postprocedural I97.12- ☑
      - obstetric procedure O75.4
  - cardiorespiratory — *see* Arrest, cardiac
  - circulatory — *see* Arrest, cardiac
  - deep transverse O64.Ø ☑
  - development or growth
    - bone — *see* Disorder, bone, development or growth
    - child R62.5Ø
    - tracheal rings Q32.1
  - epiphyseal
    - complete
      - femur M89.15- ☑
      - humerus M89.12- ☑
      - tibia M89.16- ☑
      - ulna M89.13- ☑
    - forearm M89.13- ☑
      - specified NEC M89.13- ☑
      - ulna — *see* Arrest, epiphyseal, by type, ulna
    - lower leg M89.16- ☑
      - specified NEC M89.168
      - tibia — *see* Arrest, epiphyseal, by type, tibia
    - partial
      - femur M89.15- ☑
      - humerus M89.12- ☑
      - tibia M89.16- ☑
      - ulna M89.13- ☑
    - specified NEC M89.18
  - granulopoiesis — *see* Agranulocytosis
  - growth plate — *see* Arrest, epiphyseal
  - heart — *see* Arrest, cardiac
  - legal, anxiety concerning Z65.3
  - physeal — *see* Arrest, epiphyseal
  - respiratory RØ9.2
    - newborn P28.81

Arrest, arrested — *continued*
sinus I45.5
spermatogenesis (complete) — *see* Azoospermia
incomplete — *see* Oligospermia
transverse (deep) O64.0 ☑
Arrhenoblastoma
benign
specified site — *see* Neoplasm, benign, by site
unspecified site
female D27.9
male D29.20
malignant
specified site — *see* Neoplasm, malignant, by site
unspecified site
female C56.9
male C62.90
specified site — *see* Neoplasm, uncertain behavior, by site
unspecified site
female D39.10
male D40.10
Arrhythmia (auricle) (cardiac) (juvenile) (nodal) (reflex) (sinus) (supraventricular) (transitory) (ventricle) I49.9
block I45.9
extrasystolic I49.49
newborn
bradycardia P29.12
occurring before birth P03.819
before onset of labor P03.810
during labor P03.811
tachycardia P29.11
psychogenic F45.8
specified NEC I49.8
vagal R55
ventricular re-entry I47.0
Arrillaga-Ayerza syndrome (pulmonary sclerosis with pulmonary hypertension) I27.0
Arsenical pigmentation L81.8
from drug or medicament — *see* Table of Drugs and Chemicals
Arsenism — *see* Poisoning, arsenic
Arterial — *see* condition
Arteriofibrosis — *see* Arteriosclerosis
Arteriolar sclerosis — *see* Arteriosclerosis
Arteriolith — *see* Arteriosclerosis
Arteriolitis I77.6
necrotizing, kidney I77.5
renal — *see* Hypertension, kidney
Arteriolosclerosis — *see* Arteriosclerosis
Arterionephrosclerosis — *see* Hypertension, kidney
Arteriopathy I77.9
Arteriosclerosis, arteriosclerotic (diffuse) (obliterans) (of) (senile) (with calcification) I70.90
aorta I70.0
arteries of extremities — *see* Arteriosclerosis, extremities
brain I67.2
bypass graft
coronary — *see* Arteriosclerosis, coronary, bypass graft
extremities — *see* Arteriosclerosis, extremities, bypass graft
cardiac — *see* Disease, heart, ischemic, atherosclerotic
cardiopathy — *see* Disease, heart, ischemic, atherosclerotic
cardiorenal — *see* Hypertension, cardiorenal
cardiovascular — *see* Disease, heart, ischemic, atherosclerotic
carotid (*see also* Occlusion, artery, carotid) I65.2- ☑
central nervous system I67.2
cerebral I67.2
cerebrovascular I67.2
coronary (artery) I25.10
bypass graft I25.810
with
angina pectoris I25.709
with documented spasm I25.701
specified type NEC I25.708
unstable I25.700
ischemic chest pain I25.709
autologous artery I25.810
with
angina pectoris I25.729
with documented spasm I25.721
specified type I25.728
unstable I25.720
ischemic chest pain I25.729
autologous vein I25.810

Arteriosclerosis, arteriosclerotic — *continued*
coronary — *continued*
bypass graft — *continued*
autologous vein — *continued*
with
angina pectoris I25.719
with documented spasm I25.711
specified type I25.718
unstable I25.710
ischemic chest pain I25.719
nonautologous biological I25.810
with
angina pectoris I25.739
with documented spasm I25.731
specified type I25.738
unstable I25.730
ischemic chest pain I25.739
specified type NEC I25.810
with
angina pectoris I25.799
with documented spasm I25.791
specified type I25.798
unstable I25.790
ischemic chest pain I25.799
due to
calcified coronary lesion (severely) I25.84
lipid rich plaque I25.83
native vessel
with
angina pectoris I25.119
with documented spasm I25.111
specified type NEC I25.118
unstable I25.110
ischemic chest pain I25.119
transplanted heart I25.811
bypass graft I25.812
with
angina pectoris I25.769
with documented spasm I25.761
specified type I25.768
unstable I25.760
ischemic chest pain I25.769
native coronary artery I25.811
with
angina pectoris I25.759
with documented spasm I25.751
specified type I25.758
unstable I25.750
ischemic chest pain I25.759
extremities (native arteries) I70.209
bypass graft I70.309
autologous vein graft I70.409
leg I70.409
with
gangrene (and intermittent claudication, rest pain and ulcer) I70.469
intermittent claudication I70.419
rest pain (and intermittent claudication) I70.429
bilateral I70.403
with
gangrene (and intermittent claudication, rest pain and ulcer) I70.463
intermittent claudication I70.463
rest pain (and intermittent claudication) I70.423
specified type NEC I70.493
left I70.402
with
gangrene (and intermittent claudication, rest pain and ulcer) I70.462
intermittent claudication I70.412
rest pain (and intermittent claudication) I70.422
ulceration (and intermittent claudication and rest pain) I70.449
ankle I70.443
calf I70.442
foot site NEC I70.445
heel I70.444
lower leg NEC I70.448
midfoot I70.444
thigh I70.441
specified type NEC I70.492

Arteriosclerosis, arteriosclerotic — *continued*
extremities — *continued*
bypass graft — *continued*
autologous vein graft — *continued*
leg — *continued*
right I70.401
with
gangrene (and intermittent claudication, rest pain and ulcer) I70.461
intermittent claudication I70.411
rest pain (and intermittent claudication) I70.421
ulceration (and intermittent claudication and rest pain) I70.439
ankle I70.433
calf I70.432
foot site NEC I70.435
heel I70.434
lower leg NEC I70.438
midfoot I70.434
thigh I70.431
specified type NEC I70.491
specified type NEC I70.499
specified NEC I70.408
with
gangrene (and intermittent claudication, rest pain and ulcer) I70.468
intermittent claudication I70.418
rest pain (and intermittent claudication) I70.428
ulceration (and intermittent claudication and rest pain) I70.45
specified type NEC I70.498
leg I70.309
with
gangrene (and intermittent claudication, rest pain and ulcer) I70.369
intermittent claudication I70.319
rest pain (and intermittent claudication) I70.329
bilateral I70.303
with
gangrene (and intermittent claudication, rest pain and ulcer) I70.363
intermittent claudication I70.313
rest pain (and intermittent claudication) I70.323
specified type NEC I70.393
left I70.302
with
gangrene (and intermittent claudication, rest pain and ulcer) I70.362
intermittent claudication I70.312
rest pain (and intermittent claudication) I70.322
ulceration (and intermittent claudication and rest pain) I70.349
ankle I70.343
calf I70.342
foot site NEC I70.345
heel I70.344
lower leg NEC I70.348
midfoot I70.344
thigh I70.341
specified type NEC I70.392
right I70.301
with
gangrene (and intermittent claudication, rest pain and ulcer) I70.361
intermittent claudication I70.311
rest pain (and intermittent claudication) I70.321
ulceration (and intermittent claudication and rest pain I70.339
ankle I70.333
calf I70.332
foot site NEC I70.335
heel I70.334
lower leg NEC I70.338
midfoot I70.334
thigh I70.331
specified type NEC I70.391

Arteriosclerosis, arteriosclerotic — *continued*
- extremities — *continued*
  - leg — *continued*
    - left — *continued*
      - with — *continued*
        - ulceration — *continued*
          - midfoot I7Ø.244
          - thigh I7Ø.241
      - specified type NEC I7Ø.292
    - right I7Ø.2Ø1
      - with
        - gangrene (and intermittent claudication, rest pain and ulcer) I7Ø.261
        - intermittent claudication I7Ø.211
        - rest pain (and intermittent claudication) I7Ø.221
        - ulceration (and intermittent claudication and rest pain) I7Ø.239
          - ankle I7Ø.233
          - calf I7Ø.232
          - foot site NEC I7Ø.235
          - heel I7Ø.234
          - lower leg NEC I7Ø.238
          - midfoot I7Ø.234
          - thigh I7Ø.231
      - specified type NEC I7Ø.291
    - specified type NEC I7Ø.299
  - specified site NEC I7Ø.2Ø8
    - with
      - gangrene (and intermittent claudication, rest pain and ulcer) I7Ø.268
      - intermittent claudication I7Ø.218
      - rest pain (and intermittent claudication) I7Ø.228
      - ulceration (and intermittent claudication and rest pain) I7Ø.25
    - specified type NEC I7Ø.298
- generalized I7Ø.91
- heart (disease) — *see* Arteriosclerosis, coronary (artery),
- kidney — *see* Hypertension, kidney
- medial — *see* Arteriosclerosis, extremities
- mesenteric (artery) K55.1
- Mönckeberg's — *see* Arteriosclerosis, extremities
- myocarditis I51.4
- peripheral (of extremities) — *see* Arteriosclerosis, extremities
- pulmonary (idiopathic) I27.Ø
- renal (arterioles) (*see also* Hypertension, kidney) artery I7Ø.1
- retina (vascular) I7Ø.8 [H35.Ø-] ☑
- specified artery NEC I7Ø.8
- spinal (cord) G95.19
- vertebral (artery) I67.2

Arteriospasm I73.9

Arteriovenous — *see* condition

Arteritis I77.6
- allergic M31.Ø
- aorta (nonsyphilitic) I77.6
  - syphilitic A52.Ø2
- aortic arch M31.4
- brachiocephalic M31.4
- brain I67.7
  - syphilitic A52.Ø4
- cerebral I67.7
  - in systemic lupus erythematosus M32.19
  - listerial A32.89
  - syphilitic A52.Ø4
  - tuberculous A18.89
- coronary (artery) I25.89
  - rheumatic IØ1.8
    - chronic IØ9.89
  - syphilitic A52.Ø6
- cranial (left) (right), giant cell M31.6
- deformans — *see* Arteriosclerosis
- giant cell NEC M31.6
  - with polymyalgia rheumatica M31.5
- necrosing or necrotizing M31.9
  - specified NEC M31.8
- nodosa M3Ø.Ø
- obliterans — *see* Arteriosclerosis
- pulmonary I28.8
- rheumatic — *see* Fever, rheumatic
- senile — *see* Arteriosclerosis
- suppurative I77.2
- syphilitic (general) A52.Ø9
  - brain A52.Ø4
  - coronary A52.Ø6

Arteritis — *continued*
- syphilitic — *continued*
  - spinal A52.Ø9
- temporal, giant cell M31.6
- young female aortic arch syndrome M31.4

Artery, arterial (*see also* condition)
- abscess I77.89
- single umbilical Q27.Ø

Arthralgia (allergic) (*see also* Pain, joint)
- in caisson disease T7Ø.3 ☑
- temporomandibular M26.62

Arthritis, arthritic (acute) (chronic) (nonpyogenic) (subacute) M19.9Ø
- allergic — *see* Arthritis, specified form NEC
- ankylosing (crippling) (spine) (*see also* Spondylitis, ankylosing)
  - sites other than spine — *see* Arthritis, specified form NEC
- atrophic — *see* Osteoarthritis
  - spine — *see* Spondylitis, ankylosing
- back — *see* Spondylopathy, inflammatory
- blennorrhagic (gonococcal) A54.42
- Charcot's — *see* Arthropathy, neuropathic
  - diabetic — *see* Diabetes, arthropathy, neuropathic
  - syringomyelic G95.Ø
- chylous (filarial) (*see also* category MØ1) B74.9
- climacteric (any site) NEC — *see* Arthritis, specified form NEC
- crystal (-induced) — *see* Arthritis, in, crystals
- deformans — *see* Osteoarthritis
- degenerative — *see* Osteoarthritis
- due to or associated with
  - acromegaly E22.Ø
  - brucellosis — *see* Brucellosis
  - caisson disease T7Ø.3 ☑
  - diabetes — *see* Diabetes, arthropathy
  - dracontiasis (*see also* category MØ1) B72
  - enteritis NEC
    - regional — *see* Enteritis, regional
  - erysipelas (*see also* category MØ1) A46
  - erythema
    - epidemic A25.1
    - nodosum L52
  - filariasis NOS B74.9
  - glanders A24.Ø
  - helminthiasis (*see also* category MØ1) B83.9
  - hemophilia D66 [M36.2]
  - Henoch- (Schönlein) purpura D69.Ø [M36.4]
  - human parvovirus (*see also* category MØ1) B97.6
  - infectious disease NEC MØ1 ☑
  - leprosy (see also category MØ1) (*see also* Leprosy) A3Ø.9
  - Lyme disease A69.23
  - mycobacteria (*see also* category MØ1) A31.8
  - parasitic disease NEC (*see also* category MØ1) B89
  - paratyphoid fever (see also category MØ1) (*see also* Fever, paratyphoid) AØ1.4
  - rat bite fever (*see also* category MØ1) A25.1
  - regional enteritis — *see* Enteritis, regional
  - respiratory disorder NOS J98.9
  - serum sickness (*see also* Reaction, serum) T8Ø.69 ☑
  - syringomyelia G95.Ø
  - typhoid fever AØ1.Ø4
- epidemic erythema A25.1
- febrile — *see* Fever, rheumatic
- gonococcal A54.42
- gouty (acute) — *see* Gout, idiopathic
- in (due to)
  - acromegaly (*see also* subcategory M14.8-) E22.Ø
  - amyloidosis (*see also* subcategory M14.8-) E85.4
  - bacterial disease (*see also* subcategory MØ1) A49.9
  - Behçet's syndrome M35.2
  - caisson disease (*see also* subcategory M14.8-) T7Ø.3 ☑
  - coliform bacilli (Escherichia coli) — *see* Arthritis, in, pyogenic organism NEC
  - crystals M11.9
    - dicalcium phosphate — *see* Arthritis, in, crystals, specified type NEC
    - hydroxyapatite M11.Ø- ☑
    - pyrophosphate — *see* Arthritis, in, crystals, specified type NEC
    - specified type NEC M11.8Ø
      - ankle M11.87- ☑
      - elbow M11.82- ☑
      - foot joint M11.87- ☑
      - hand joint M11.84- ☑

Arthritis, arthritic — *continued*
- in — *continued*
  - crystals — *continued*
    - specified type — *continued*
      - hip M11.85- ☑
      - knee M11.86- ☑
      - multiple sites M11.8- ☑
      - shoulder M11.81- ☑
      - vertebrae M11.88
      - wrist M11.83- ☑
  - dermatoarthritis, lipoid E78.81
  - dracontiasis (dracunculiasis) (*see also* category MØ1) B72
  - endocrine disorder NEC (*see also* subcategory M14.8-) E34.9
  - enteritis, infectious NEC (*see also* category MØ1) AØ9
    - specified organism NEC (*see also* category MØ1) AØ8.8
  - erythema
    - multiforme (*see also* subcategory M14.8-) L51.9
    - nodosum (*see also* subcategory M14.8-) L52
  - gout — *see* Gout, idiopathic
  - helminthiasis NEC (*see also* category MØ1) B83.9
  - hemochromatosis (*see also* subcategory M14.8-) E83.118
  - hemoglobinopathy NEC D58.2 [M36.3]
  - hemophilia NEC D66 [M36.2]
  - Hemophilus influenzae MØØ.8- ☑ [B96.3]
  - Henoch (-Schönlein) purpura D69.Ø [M36.4]
  - hyperparathyroidism NEC (*see also* subcategory M14.8-) E21.3
  - hypersensitivity reaction NEC T78.49 ☑ [M36.4]
  - hypogammaglobulinemia (*see also* subcategory M14.8-) D8Ø.1
  - hypothyroidism NEC (*see also* subcategory M14.8-) EØ3.9
  - infection — *see* Arthritis, pyogenic or pyemic
    - spine — *see* Spondylopathy, infective
  - infectious disease NEC MØ1 ☑
  - leprosy (*see also* category MØ1) A3Ø.9
  - leukemia NEC C95.9- ☑ [M36.1]
  - lipoid dermatoarthritis E78.81
  - Lyme disease A69.23
  - Mediterranean fever, familial (*see also* subcategory M14.8-) E85.Ø
  - Meningococcus A39.83
  - metabolic disorder NEC (*see also* subcategory M14.8-) E88.9
  - multiple myelomatosis C9Ø.Ø- ☑ [M36.1]
  - mumps B26.85
  - mycosis NEC (*see also* category MØ1) B49
  - myelomatosis (multiple) C9Ø.Ø- ☑ [M36.1]
  - neurological disorder NEC G98.Ø
  - ochronosis (*see also* subcategory M14.8-) E7Ø.29
  - O'nyong-nyong (*see also* category MØ1) A92.1
  - parasitic disease NEC (*see also* category MØ1) B89
  - paratyphoid fever (*see also* category MØ1) AØ1.4
  - Pseudomonas — *see* Arthritis, pyogenic, bacterial NEC
  - psoriasis L4Ø.5Ø
  - pyogenic organism NEC — *see* Arthritis, pyogenic, bacterial NEC
  - Reiter's disease — *see* Reiter's disease
  - respiratory disorder NEC (*see also* subcategory M14.8-) J98.9
  - reticulosis, malignant (*see also* subcategory M14.8-) C86.Ø
  - rubella BØ6.82
  - Salmonella (arizonae) (cholerae-suis) (enteritidis) (typhimurium) AØ2.23
  - sarcoidosis D86.86
  - specified bacteria NEC — *see* Arthritis, pyogenic, bacterial NEC
  - sporotrichosis B42.82
  - syringomyelia G95.Ø
  - thalassemia NEC D56.9 [M36.3]
  - tuberculosis — *see* Tuberculosis, arthritis
  - typhoid fever AØ1.Ø4
  - urethritis, Reiter's — *see* Reiter's disease
  - viral disease NEC (*see also* category MØ1) B34.9
- infectious or infective (*see also* Arthritis, pyogenic or pyemic)
  - spine — *see* Spondylopathy, infective
- juvenile MØ8.9Ø
  - with systemic onset — *see* Still's disease
  - ankle MØ8.97- ☑

- **Arthritis, arthritic** — *continued*
  - juvenile — *continued*
    - elbow MØ8.92- ☑
    - foot joint MØ8.97- ☑
    - hand joint MØ8.94- ☑
    - hip MØ8.95- ☑
    - knee MØ8.96- ☑
    - multiple site MØ8.99
    - pauciarticular MØ8.4Ø
      - ankle MØ8.47- ☑
      - elbow MØ8.42- ☑
      - foot joint MØ8.47- ☑
      - hand joint MØ8.44- ☑
      - hip MØ8.45- ☑
      - knee MØ8.46- ☑
      - shoulder MØ8.41- ☑
      - vertebrae MØ8.48
      - wrist MØ8.43- ☑
    - psoriatic L4Ø.54
    - rheumatoid — *see* Arthritis, rheumatoid, juvenile
    - shoulder MØ8.91- ☑
    - specified type NEC MØ8.8Ø
      - ankle MØ8.87- ☑
      - elbow MØ8.82- ☑
      - foot joint MØ8.87- ☑
      - hand joint MØ8.84- ☑
      - hip MØ8.85- ☑
      - knee MØ8.86- ☑
      - multiple site MØ8.89
      - shoulder MØ8.81- ☑
      - specified joint NEC MØ8.88
      - vertebrae MØ8.88
      - wrist MØ8.83- ☑
    - wrist MØ8.93- ☑
  - meaning osteoarthritis — *see* Osteoarthritis
  - meningococcal A39.83
  - menopausal (any site) NEC — *see* Arthritis, specified form NEC
  - mutilans (psoriatic) L4Ø.52
  - mycotic NEC (*see also* category MØ1) B49
  - neuropathic (Charcot) — *see* Arthropathy, neuropathic
    - diabetic — *see* Diabetes, arthropathy, neuropathic
    - nonsyphilitic NEC G98.Ø
    - syringomyelic G95.Ø
  - ochronotic (*see also* subcategory M14.8-) E7Ø.29
  - palindromic (any site) — *see* Rheumatism, palindromic
  - pneumococcal MØØ.1Ø
    - ankle MØØ.17- ☑
    - elbow MØØ.12- ☑
    - foot joint — *see* Arthritis, pneumococcal, ankle
    - hand joint MØØ.14- ☑
    - hip MØØ.15- ☑
    - knee MØØ.16- ☑
    - multiple site MØØ.19
    - shoulder MØØ.11- ☑
    - vertebra MØØ.18
    - wrist MØØ.13- ☑
  - postdysenteric — *see* Arthropathy, postdysenteric
  - postmeningococcal A39.84
  - postrheumatic, chronic — *see* Arthropathy, postrheumatic, chronic
  - primary progressive (*see also* Arthritis, specified form NEC)
    - spine — *see* Spondylitis, ankylosing
  - psoriatic L4Ø.5Ø
  - purulent (any site except spine) — *see* Arthritis, pyogenic or pyemic
    - spine — *see* Spondylopathy, infective
  - pyogenic or pyemic (any site except spine) MØØ.9
    - bacterial NEC MØØ.8Ø
      - ankle MØØ.87- ☑
      - elbow MØØ.82- ☑
      - foot joint — *see* Arthritis, pyogenic, bacterial NEC, ankle
      - hand joint MØØ.84- ☑
      - hip MØØ.85- ☑
      - knee MØØ.86- ☑
      - multiple site MØØ.89
      - shoulder MØØ.81- ☑
      - vertebra MØØ.88
      - wrist MØØ.83- ☑
    - pneumococcal — *see* Arthritis, pneumococcal
    - spine — *see* Spondylopathy, infective
    - staphylococcal — *see* Arthritis, staphylococcal
    - streptococcal — *see* Arthritis, streptococcal NEC
      - pneumococcal — *see* Arthritis, pneumococcal

- **Arthritis, arthritic** — *continued*
  - reactive — *see* Reiter's disease
  - rheumatic (*see also* Arthritis, rheumatoid)
    - acute or subacute — *see* Fever, rheumatic
  - rheumatoid MØ6.9
    - with
      - carditis — *see* Rheumatoid, carditis
      - endocarditis — *see* Rheumatoid, carditis
      - heart involvement NEC — *see* Rheumatoid, carditis
      - lung involvement — *see* Rheumatoid, lung
      - myocarditis — *see* Rheumatoid, carditis
      - myopathy — *see* Rheumatoid, myopathy
      - pericarditis — *see* Rheumatoid, carditis
      - polyneuropathy — *see* Rheumatoid, polyneuropathy
      - rheumatoid factor — *see* Arthritis, rheumatoid, seropositive
      - splenoadenomegaly and leukopenia — *see* Felty's syndrome
      - vasculitis — *see* Rheumatoid, vasculitis
      - visceral involvement NEC — *see* Rheumatoid, arthritis, with involvement of organs NEC
    - juvenile (with or without rheumatoid factor) MØ8.ØØ
      - ankle MØ8.Ø7- ☑
      - elbow MØ8.Ø2- ☑
      - foot joint MØ8.Ø7- ☑
      - hand joint MØ8.Ø4- ☑
      - hip MØ8.Ø5- ☑
      - knee MØ8.Ø6- ☑
      - multiple site MØ8.Ø9
      - shoulder MØ8.Ø1- ☑
      - vertebra MØ8.Ø8
      - wrist MØ8.Ø3- ☑
    - seronegative MØ6.ØØ
      - ankle MØ6.Ø7- ☑
      - elbow MØ6.Ø2- ☑
      - foot joint MØ6.Ø7- ☑
      - hand joint MØ6.Ø4- ☑
      - hip MØ6.Ø5- ☑
      - knee MØ6.Ø6- ☑
      - multiple site MØ6.Ø9
      - shoulder MØ6.Ø1- ☑
      - vertebra MØ6.Ø8
      - wrist MØ6.Ø3- ☑
    - seropositive MØ5.9
      - without organ involvement MØ5.7Ø
        - ankle MØ5.77- ☑
        - elbow MØ5.72- ☑
        - foot joint MØ5.77- ☑
        - hand joint MØ5.74- ☑
        - hip MØ5.75- ☑
        - knee MØ5.76- ☑
        - multiple sites MØ5.79
        - shoulder MØ5.71- ☑
        - vertebra — *see* Spondylitis, ankylosing
        - wrist MØ5.73- ☑
      - specified NEC MØ5.8Ø
        - ankle MØ5.87- ☑
        - elbow MØ5.82- ☑
        - foot joint MØ5.87- ☑
        - hand joint MØ5.84- ☑
        - hip MØ5.85- ☑
        - knee MØ5.86- ☑
        - multiple sites MØ5.89
        - shoulder MØ5.81- ☑
        - vertebra — *see* Spondylitis, ankylosing
        - wrist MØ5.83- ☑
    - specified type NEC MØ6.8Ø
      - ankle MØ6.87- ☑
      - elbow MØ6.82- ☑
      - foot joint MØ6.87- ☑
      - hand joint MØ6.84- ☑
      - hip MØ6.85- ☑
      - knee MØ6.86- ☑
      - multiple site MØ6.89
      - shoulder MØ6.81- ☑
      - vertebra MØ6.88
      - wrist MØ6.83- ☑
    - spine — *see* Spondylitis, ankylosing
  - rubella BØ6.82
  - scorbutic (*see also* subcategory M14.8-) E54
  - senile or senescent — *see* Osteoarthritis
  - septic (any site except spine) — *see* Arthritis, pyogenic or pyemic

- **Arthritis, arthritic** — *continued*
  - septic — *see* Arthritis, pyogenic or pyemic — *continued*
    - spine — *see* Spondylopathy, infective
  - serum (nontherapeutic) (therapeutic) — *see* Arthropathy, postimmunization
  - specified form NEC M13.8Ø
    - ankle M13.87- ☑
    - elbow M13.82- ☑
    - foot joint M13.87- ☑
    - hand joint M13.84- ☑
    - hip M13.85- ☑
    - knee M13.86- ☑
    - multiple site M13.89
    - shoulder M13.81- ☑
    - specified joint NEC M13.88
    - wrist M13.83- ☑
  - spine (*see also* Spondylopathy, inflammatory)
    - infectious or infective NEC — *see* Spondylopathy, infective
    - Marie-Strümpell — *see* Spondylitis, ankylosing
    - pyogenic — *see* Spondylopathy, infective
    - rheumatoid — *see* Spondylitis, ankylosing
    - traumatic (old) — *see* Spondylopathy, traumatic
    - tuberculous A18.Ø1
  - staphylococcal MØØ.ØØ
    - ankle MØØ.Ø7- ☑
    - elbow MØØ.Ø2- ☑
    - foot joint — *see* Arthritis, staphylococcal, ankle
    - hand joint MØØ.Ø4- ☑
    - hip MØØ.Ø5- ☑
    - knee MØØ.Ø6- ☑
    - multiple site MØØ.Ø9
    - shoulder MØØ.Ø1- ☑
    - vertebra MØØ.Ø8
    - wrist MØØ.Ø3- ☑
  - streptococcal NEC MØØ.2Ø
    - ankle MØØ.27- ☑
    - elbow MØØ.22- ☑
    - foot joint — *see* Arthritis, streptococcal, ankle
    - hand joint MØØ.24- ☑
    - hip MØØ.25- ☑
    - knee MØØ.26- ☑
    - multiple site MØØ.29
    - shoulder MØØ.21- ☑
    - vertebra MØØ.28
    - wrist MØØ.23- ☑
  - suppurative — *see* Arthritis, pyogenic or pyemic
  - syphilitic (late) A52.16
    - congenital A5Ø.55 [M12.8Ø]
  - syphilitica deformans (Charcot) A52.16
  - temporomandibular M26.69
  - toxic of menopause (any site) — *see* Arthritis, specified form NEC
  - transient — *see* Arthropathy, specified form NEC
  - traumatic (chronic) — *see* Arthropathy, traumatic
  - tuberculous A18.Ø2
    - spine A18.Ø1
  - uratic — *see* Gout, idiopathic
  - urethritica (Reiter's) — *see* Reiter's disease
  - vertebral — *see* Spondylopathy, inflammatory
  - villous (any site) — *see* Arthropathy, specified form NEC
- **Arthrocele** — *see* Effusion, joint
- **Arthrodesis status** Z98.1
- **Arthrodynia** (*see also* Pain, joint)
- **Arthrodysplasia** Q74.9
- **Arthrofibrosis, joint** — *see* Ankylosis
- **Arthrogryposis** (congenital) Q68.8
  - multiplex congenita Q74.3
- **Arthrokatadysis** M24.7
- **Arthropathy** (*see also* Arthritis) M12.9
  - Charcot's — *see* Arthropathy, neuropathic
    - diabetic — *see* Diabetes, arthropathy, neuropathic
    - syringomyelic G95.Ø
  - cricoarytenoid J38.7
  - crystal (-induced) — *see* Arthritis, in, crystals
  - diabetic NEC — *see* Diabetes, arthropathy
  - distal interphalangeal, psoriatic L4Ø.51
  - enteropathic MØ7.6Ø
    - ankle MØ7.67- ☑
    - elbow MØ7.62- ☑
    - foot joint MØ7.67- ☑
    - hand joint MØ7.64- ☑
    - hip MØ7.65- ☑
    - knee MØ7.66- ☑

- **Asphyxia, asphyxiation** — *continued*
  - antenatal P84
  - birth P84
  - bunny bag — *see* Asphyxia, due to, mechanical threat to breathing, trapped in bed clothes
  - crushing S28.Ø ☑
  - drowning T75.1 ☑
  - gas, fumes, or vapor — *see* Table of Drugs and Chemicals
  - inhalation — *see* Inhalation
  - intrauterine P84
  - local I73.ØØ
    - with gangrene I73.Ø1
  - mucus (*see also* Foreign body, respiratory tract, causing asphyxia)
  - newborn P84
  - pathological RØ9.Ø1
  - postnatal P84
    - mechanical — *see* Asphyxia, due to, mechanical threat to breathing
  - prenatal P84
  - reticularis R23.1
  - strangulation — *see* Asphyxia, due to, mechanical threat to breathing
  - submersion T75.1 ☑
  - traumatic T71.9 ☑
    - due to
      - crushed chest S28.Ø ☑
      - foreign body (in) — *see* Foreign body, respiratory tract, causing asphyxia
      - low oxygen content of ambient air T71.2Ø ☑
        - due to
          - being trapped in
            - low oxygen environment T71.29 ☑
              - in car trunk T71.221 ☑
                - circumstances undetermined T71.224 ☑
                - done with intent to harm by
                  - another person T71.223 ☑
                  - self T71.222 ☑
              - in refrigerator T71.231 ☑
                - circumstances undetermined T71.234 ☑
                - done with intent to harm by
                  - another person T71.233 ☑
                  - self T71.232 ☑
          - cave-in T71.21 ☑
      - mechanical threat to breathing (accidental) T71.191 ☑
        - circumstances undetermined T71.194 ☑
        - done with intent to harm by
          - another person T71.193 ☑
          - self T71.192 ☑
        - hanging T71.161 ☑
          - circumstances undetermined T71.164 ☑
          - done with intent to harm by
            - another person T71.163 ☑
            - self T71.162 ☑
        - plastic bag T71.121 ☑
          - circumstances undetermined T71.124 ☑
          - done with intent to harm by
            - another person T71.123 ☑
            - self T71.122 ☑
        - smothering
          - in furniture T71.151 ☑
            - circumstances undetermined T71.154 ☑
            - done with intent to harm by
              - another person T71.153 ☑
              - self T71.152 ☑
          - under
            - another person's body T71.141 ☑
              - circumstances undetermined T71.144 ☑
              - done with intent to harm T71.143 ☑
            - pillow T71.111 ☑
              - circumstances undetermined T71.114 ☑
              - done with intent to harm by
                - another person T71.113 ☑
                - self T71.112 ☑
        - trapped in bed clothes T71.131 ☑
          - circumstances undetermined T71.134 ☑
          - done with intent to harm by
            - another person T71.133 ☑
            - self T71.132 ☑
- **Asphyxia, asphyxiation** — *continued*
  - vomiting, vomitus — *see* Foreign body, respiratory tract, causing asphyxia
- **Aspiration**
  - amniotic (clear) fluid (newborn) P24.1Ø
    - with
      - pneumonia (pneumonitis) P24.11
      - respiratory symptoms P24.11
  - blood
    - newborn (without respiratory symptoms) P24.2Ø
      - with
        - pneumonia (pneumonitis) P24.21
        - respiratory symptoms P24.21
    - specified age NEC — *see* Foreign body, respiratory tract
  - bronchitis J69.Ø
  - food or foreign body (with asphyxiation) — *see* Asphyxia, food
  - liquor (amnii) (newborn) P24.1Ø
    - with
      - pneumonia (pneumonitis) P24.11
      - respiratory symptoms P24.11
  - meconium (newborn) (without respiratory symptoms) P24.ØØ
    - with
      - pneumonitis (pneumonitis) P24.Ø1
      - respiratory symptoms P24.Ø1
  - milk (newborn) (without respiratory symptoms) P24.3Ø
    - with
      - pneumonia (pneumonitis) P24.31
      - respiratory symptoms P24.31
    - specified age NEC — *see* Foreign body, respiratory tract
  - mucus (*see also* Foreign body, by site, causing asphyxia)
    - newborn P24.1Ø
      - with
        - pneumonia (pneumonitis) P24.11
        - respiratory symptoms P24.11
  - neonatal P24.9
    - specific NEC (without respiratory symptoms) P24.8Ø
      - with
        - pneumonia (pneumonitis) P24.81
        - respiratory symptoms P24.81
  - newborn P24.9
    - specific NEC (without respiratory symptoms) P24.8Ø
      - with
        - pneumonia (pneumonitis) P24.81
        - respiratory symptoms P24.81
  - pneumonia J69.Ø
  - pneumonitis J69.Ø
  - syndrome of newborn — *see* Aspiration, by substance, with pneumonia
  - vernix caseosa (newborn) P24.8Ø
    - with
      - pneumonia (pneumonitis) P24.81
      - respiratory symptoms P24.81
  - vomitus (*see also* Foreign body, respiratory tract)
    - newborn (without respiratory symptoms) P24.3Ø
      - with
        - pneumonia (pneumonitis) P24.31
        - respiratory symptoms P24.31
- **Asplenia** (congenital) Q89.Ø1
  - postsurgical Z9Ø.81
- **Assam fever** B55.Ø
- **Assault, sexual** — *see* Maltreatment
- **Assmann's focus NEC** A15.Ø
- **Astasia** (-abasia) (hysterical) F44.4
- **Asteatosis cutis** L85.3
- **Astereognosia, astereognosis** R48.1
- **Asterixis** R27.8
  - in liver disease K71.3
- **Asteroid hyalitis** — *see* Deposit, crystalline
- **Asthenia, asthenic** R53.1
  - cardiac (*see also* Failure, heart) I5Ø.9
    - psychogenic F45.8
  - cardiovascular (*see also* Failure, heart) I5Ø.9
    - psychogenic F45.8
  - heart (*see also* Failure, heart) I5Ø.9
    - psychogenic F45.8
  - hysterical F44.4
  - myocardial (*see also* Failure, heart) I5Ø.9
    - psychogenic F45.8
  - nervous F48.8
  - neurocirculatory F45.8
  - neurotic F48.8
  - psychogenic F48.8
  - psychoneurotic F48.8
- **Asthenia, asthenic** — *continued*
  - psychophysiologic F48.8
  - reaction (psychophysiologic) F48.8
  - senile R54
- **Asthenopia** (*see also* Discomfort, visual)
  - hysterical F44.6
  - psychogenic F44.6
- **Asthenospermia** — *see* Abnormal, specimen, male genital organs
- **Asthma, asthmatic** (bronchial) (catarrh) (spasmodic) J45.9Ø9
  - with
    - chronic obstructive bronchitis J44.9
      - with
        - acute lower respiratory infection J44.Ø
        - exacerbation (acute) J44.1
    - chronic obstructive pulmonary disease J44.9
      - with
        - acute lower respiratory infection J44.Ø
        - exacerbation (acute) J44.1
    - exacerbation (acute) J45.9Ø1
    - hay fever — *see* Asthma, allergic extrinsic
    - rhinitis, allergic — *see* Asthma, allergic extrinsic
    - status asthmaticus J45.9Ø2
  - allergic extrinsic J45.9Ø9
    - with
      - exacerbation (acute) J45.9Ø1
      - status asthmaticus J45.9Ø2
  - atopic — *see* Asthma, allergic extrinsic
  - cardiac — *see* Failure, ventricular, left
  - cardiobronchial I5Ø.1
  - childhood J45.9Ø9
    - with
      - exacerbation (acute) J45.9Ø1
      - status asthmaticus J45.9Ø2
  - chronic obstructive J44.9
    - with
      - acute lower respiratory infection J44.Ø
      - exacerbation (acute) J44.1
  - collier's J6Ø
  - cough variant J45.991
  - detergent J69.8
  - due to
    - detergent J69.8
    - inhalation of fumes J68.3
  - eosinophilic J82
  - extrinsic, allergic — *see* Asthma, allergic extrinsic
  - grinder's J62.8
  - hay — *see* Asthma, allergic extrinsic
  - heart I5Ø.1
  - idiosyncratic — *see* Asthma, nonallergic
  - intermittent (mild) J45.2Ø
    - with
      - exacerbation (acute) J45.21
      - status asthmaticus J45.22
  - intrinsic, nonallergic — *see* Asthma, nonallergic
  - Kopp's E32.8
  - late-onset J45.9Ø9
    - with
      - exacerbation (acute) J45.9Ø1
      - status asthmaticus J45.9Ø2
  - mild intermittent J45.2Ø
    - with
      - exacerbation (acute) J45.21
      - status asthmaticus J45.22
  - mild persistent J45.3Ø
    - with
      - exacerbation (acute) J45.31
      - status asthmaticus J45.32
  - Millar's (laryngismus stridulus) J38.5
  - miner's J6Ø
  - mixed J45.9Ø9
    - with
      - exacerbation (acute) J45.9Ø1
      - status asthmaticus J45.9Ø2
  - moderate persistent J45.4Ø
    - with
      - exacerbation (acute) J45.41
      - status asthmaticus J45.42
  - nervous — *see* Asthma, nonallergic
  - nonallergic (intrinsic) J45.9Ø9
    - with
      - exacerbation (acute) J45.9Ø1
      - status asthmaticus J45.9Ø2
  - persistent
    - mild J45.3Ø
      - with
        - exacerbation (acute) J45.31

- **Asthma, asthmatic** — *continued*
  - persistent — *continued*
    - mild — *continued*
      - with — *continued*
        - status asthmaticus J45.32
    - moderate J45.4Ø
      - with
        - exacerbation (acute) J45.41
        - status asthmaticus J45.42
    - severe J45.5Ø
      - with
        - exacerbation (acute) J45.51
        - status asthmaticus J45.52
  - platinum J45.998
  - pneumoconiotic NEC J64
  - potter's J62.8
  - predominantly allergic J45.9Ø9
  - psychogenic F54
  - pulmonary eosinophilic J82
  - red cedar J67.8
  - Rostan's I5Ø.1
  - sandblaster's J62.8
  - sequoiosis J67.8
  - severe persistent J45.5Ø
    - with
      - exacerbation (acute) J45.51
      - status asthmaticus J45.52
  - specified NEC J45.998
  - stonemason's J62.8
  - thymic E32.8
  - tuberculous — *see* Tuberculosis, pulmonary
  - Wichmann's (laryngismus stridulus) J38.5
  - wood J67.8
- **Astigmatism** (compound) (congenital) H52.2Ø- ☑
  - irregular H52.21- ☑
  - regular H52.22- ☑
- **Astraphobia** F4Ø.22Ø
- **Astroblastoma**
  - specified site — *see* Neoplasm, malignant, by site
  - unspecified site C71.9
- **Astrocytoma** (cystic)
  - anaplastic
    - specified site — *see* Neoplasm, malignant, by site
    - unspecified site C71.9
  - fibrillary
    - specified site — *see* Neoplasm, malignant, by site
    - unspecified site C71.9
  - fibrous
    - specified site — *see* Neoplasm, malignant, by site
    - unspecified site C71.9
  - gemistocytic
    - specified site — *see* Neoplasm, malignant, by site
    - unspecified site C71.9
  - juvenile
    - specified site — *see* Neoplasm, malignant, by site
    - unspecified site C71.9
  - pilocytic
    - specified site — *see* Neoplasm, malignant, by site
    - unspecified site C71.9
  - piloid
    - specified site — *see* Neoplasm, malignant, by site
    - unspecified site C71.9
  - protoplasmic
    - specified site — *see* Neoplasm, malignant, by site
    - unspecified site C71.9
  - specified site NEC — *see* Neoplasm, malignant, by site
  - subependymal D43.2
    - giant cell
      - specified site — *see* Neoplasm, uncertain behavior, by site
      - unspecified site D43.2
    - specified site — *see* Neoplasm, uncertain behavior, by site
    - unspecified site D43.2
  - unspecified site C71.9
- **Astroglioma**
  - specified site — *see* Neoplasm, malignant, by site
  - unspecified site C71.9
- **Asymbolia** R48.8
- **Asymmetry** (*see also* Distortion)
  - between native and reconstructed breast N65.1
  - face Q67.Ø
  - jaw (lower) — *see* Anomaly, dentofacial, jaw-cranial base relationship, asymmetry
- **Asynergia, asynergy** R27.8
  - ventricular I51.89
- **Asystole** (heart) — *see* Arrest, cardiac
- **At risk**
  - for falling Z91.81
- **Ataxia, ataxy, ataxic** R27.Ø
  - acute R27.8
  - brain (hereditary) G11.9
  - cerebellar (hereditary) G11.9
    - with defective DNA repair G11.3
    - alcoholic G31.2
    - early-onset G11.1
    - in
      - alcoholism G31.2
      - myxedema EØ3.9 [G13.2]
      - neoplastic disease (*see also* Neoplasm) D49.9 [G13.1]
      - specified disease NEC G32.81
    - late-onset (Marie's) G11.2
  - cerebral (hereditary) G11.9
  - congenital nonprogressive G11.Ø
  - family, familial — *see* Ataxia, hereditary
  - following
    - cerebrovascular disease I69.993
      - cerebral infarction I69.393
      - intracerebral hemorrhage I69.193
      - nontraumatic intracranial hemorrhage NEC I69.293
      - specified disease NEC I69.893
      - subarachnoid hemorrhage I69.Ø93
  - Friedreich's (heredofamilial) (cerebellar) (spinal) G11.1
  - gait R26.Ø
    - hysterical F44.4
  - general R27.8
  - gluten M35.9 [G32.81]
    - with celiac disease K9Ø.Ø [G32.81]
  - hereditary G11.9
    - with neuropathy G6Ø.2
    - cerebellar — *see* Ataxia, cerebellar
    - spastic G11.4
    - specified NEC G11.8
    - spinal (Friedreich's) G11.1
  - heredofamilial — *see* Ataxia, hereditary
  - Hunt's G11.1
  - hysterical F44.4
  - locomotor (progressive) (syphilitic) (partial) (spastic) A52.11
    - diabetic — *see* Diabetes, ataxia
  - Marie's (cerebellar) (heredofamilial) (late- onset) G11.2
  - nonorganic origin F44.4
  - nonprogressive, congenital G11.Ø
  - psychogenic F44.4
  - Roussy-Lévy G6Ø.Ø
  - Sanger-Brown's (hereditary) G11.2
  - spastic hereditary G11.4
  - spinal
    - hereditary (Friedreich's) G11.1
    - progressive (syphilitic) A52.11
  - spinocerebellar, X-linked recessive G11.1
  - telangiectasia (Louis-Bar) G11.3
- **Ataxia-telangiectasia** (Louis-Bar) G11.3
- **Atelectasis** (massive) (partial) (pressure) (pulmonary) J98.11
  - newborn P28.1Ø
    - due to resorption P28.11
    - partial P28.19
    - primary P28.Ø
    - secondary P28.19
  - primary (newborn) P28.Ø
  - tuberculous — *see* Tuberculosis, pulmonary
- **Atelocardia** Q24.9
- **Atelomyelia** QØ6.1
- **Atheroembolism**
  - of
    - extremities
      - lower I75.Ø2- ☑
      - upper I75.Ø1- ☑
    - kidney I75.81
    - specified NEC I75.89
- **Atheroma, atheromatous** (*see also* Arteriosclerosis) I7Ø.9Ø
  - aorta, aortic I7Ø.Ø
    - valve (*see also* Endocarditis, aortic) I35.8
  - aorto-iliac I7Ø.Ø
  - artery — *see* Arteriosclerosis
  - basilar (artery) I67.2
  - carotid (artery) (common) (internal) I67.2
  - cerebral (arteries) I67.2
  - coronary (artery) I25.1Ø
    - with angina pectoris — *see* Arteriosclerosis, coronary (artery),
- **Atheroma, atheromatous** — *continued*
  - degeneration — *see* Arteriosclerosis
  - heart, cardiac — *see* Disease, heart, ischemic, atherosclerotic
  - mitral (valve) I34.8
  - myocardium, myocardial — *see* Disease, heart, ischemic, atherosclerotic
  - pulmonary valve (heart) (*see also* Endocarditis, pulmonary) I37.8
  - tricuspid (heart) (valve) I36.8
  - valve, valvular — *see* Endocarditis
  - vertebral (artery) I67.2
- **Atheromatosis** — *see* Arteriosclerosis
- **Atherosclerosis** (*see also* Arteriosclerosis)
  - coronary
    - artery I25.1Ø
      - with angina pectoris — *see* Arteriosclerosis, coronary (artery),
      - due to
        - calcified coronary lesion (severely) I25.84
        - lipid rich plaque I25.83
  - transplanted heart I25.811
    - bypass graft I25.812
      - with angina pectoris — *see* Arteriosclerosis, coronary (artery),
    - native coronary artery I25.811
      - with angina pectoris — *see* Arteriosclerosis, coronary (artery),
- **Athetosis** (acquired) R25.8
  - bilateral (congenital) G8Ø.3
  - congenital (bilateral) (double) G8Ø.3
  - double (congenital) G8Ø.3
  - unilateral R25.8
- **Athlete's**
  - foot B35.3
  - heart I51.7
- **Athrepsia** E41
- **Athyrea** (acquired) (*see also* Hypothyroidism)
  - congenital EØ3.1
- **Atonia, atony, atonic**
  - bladder (sphincter) (neurogenic) N31.2
  - capillary I78.8
  - cecum K59.8
    - psychogenic F45.8
  - colon — *see* Atony, intestine
  - congenital P94.2
  - esophagus K22.8
  - intestine K59.8
    - psychogenic F45.8
  - stomach K31.89
    - neurotic or psychogenic F45.8
  - uterus (during labor) O62.2
    - with hemorrhage (postpartum) O72.1
    - postpartum (with hemorrhage) O72.1
      - without hemorrhage O75.89
- **Atopy** — *see* History, allergy
- **Atransferrinemia, congenital** E88.Ø9
- **Atresia, atretic**
  - alimentary organ or tract NEC Q45.8
    - upper Q4Ø.8
  - ani, anus, anal (canal) Q42.3
    - with fistula Q42.2
  - aorta (arch) (ring) Q25.2
  - aortic (orifice) (valve) Q23.Ø
    - arch Q25.2
    - congenital with hypoplasia of ascending aorta and defective development of left ventricle (with mitral stenosis) Q23.4
    - in hypoplastic left heart syndrome Q23.4
  - aqueduct of Sylvius QØ3.Ø
    - with spina bifida — *see* Spina bifida, with hydrocephalus
  - artery NEC Q27.8
    - cerebral Q28.3
    - coronary Q24.5
    - digestive system Q27.8
    - eye Q15.8
    - lower limb Q27.8
    - pulmonary Q25.5
    - specified site NEC Q27.8
    - umbilical Q27.Ø
    - upper limb Q27.8
  - auditory canal (external) Q16.1
  - bile duct (common) (congenital) (hepatic) Q44.2
    - acquired — *see* Obstruction, bile duct
  - bladder (neck) Q64.39
    - obstruction Q64.31
  - bronchus Q32.4

Atresia, atretic — *continued*
  cecum Q42.8
  cervix (acquired) N88.2
    congenital Q51.828
    in pregnancy or childbirth — *see* Anomaly, cervix, in pregnancy or childbirth
      causing obstructed labor O65.5
  choana Q30.0
  colon Q42.9
    specified NEC Q42.8
  common duct Q44.2
  cricoid cartilage Q31.8
  cystic duct Q44.2
    acquired K82.8
      with obstruction K82.0
  digestive organs NEC Q45.8
  duodenum Q41.0
  ear canal Q16.1
  ejaculatory duct Q55.4
  epiglottis Q31.8
  esophagus Q39.0
    with tracheoesophageal fistula Q39.1
  eustachian tube Q17.8
  fallopian tube (congenital) Q50.6
    acquired N97.1
  follicular cyst N83.0
  foramen of
    Luschka Q03.1
      with spina bifida — *see* Spina bifida, with hydrocephalus
    Magendie Q03.1
      with spina bifida — *see* Spina bifida, with hydrocephalus
  gallbladder Q44.1
  genital organ
    external
      female Q52.79
      male Q55.8
    internal
      female Q52.8
      male Q55.8
  glottis Q31.8
  gullet Q39.0
    with tracheoesophageal fistula Q39.1
  heart valve NEC Q24.8
    pulmonary Q22.0
    tricuspid Q22.4
  hymen Q52.3
    acquired (postinfective) N89.6
  ileum Q41.2
  intestine (small) Q41.9
    large Q42.9
      specified NEC Q42.8
  iris, filtration angle Q15.0
  jejunum Q41.1
  lacrimal apparatus Q10.4
  larynx Q31.8
  meatus urinarius Q64.33
  mitral valve Q23.2
    in hypoplastic left heart syndrome Q23.4
  nares (anterior) (posterior) Q30.0
  nasopharynx Q34.8
  nose, nostril Q30.0
    acquired J34.89
  organ or site NEC Q89.8
  osseous meatus (ear) Q16.1
  oviduct (congenital) Q50.6
    acquired N97.1
  parotid duct Q38.4
    acquired K11.8
  pulmonary (artery) Q25.5
    valve Q22.0
  pulmonic Q22.0
  pupil Q13.2
  rectum Q42.1
    with fistula Q42.0
  salivary duct Q38.4
    acquired K11.8
  sublingual duct Q38.4
    acquired K11.8
  submandibular duct Q38.4
    acquired K11.8
  submaxillary duct Q38.4
    acquired K11.8
  thyroid cartilage Q31.8
  trachea Q32.1
  tricuspid valve Q22.4
  ureter Q62.10

Atresia, atretic — *continued*
  ureter — *continued*
    pelvic junction Q62.11
    vesical orifice Q62.12
  ureteropelvic junction Q62.11
  ureterovesical orifice Q62.12
  urethra (valvular) Q64.39
    stricture Q64.32
  urinary tract NEC Q64.8
  uterus Q51.818
    acquired N85.8
  vagina (congenital) Q52.4
    acquired (postinfectional) (senile) N89.5
  vas deferens Q55.3
  vascular NEC Q27.8
    cerebral Q28.3
    digestive system Q27.8
    lower limb Q27.8
    specified site NEC Q27.8
    upper limb Q27.8
  vein NEC Q27.8
    digestive system Q27.8
    great Q26.8
    lower limb Q27.8
    portal Q26.5
    pulmonary Q26.3
    specified site NEC Q27.8
    upper limb Q27.8
  vena cava (inferior) (superior) Q26.8
  vesicourethral orifice Q64.31
  vulva Q52.79
    acquired N90.5

Atrichia, atrichosis — *see* Alopecia

Atrophia (*see also* Atrophy)
  cutis senilis L90.8
    due to radiation L57.8
  gyrata of choroid and retina H31.23
  senilis R54
    dermatological L90.8
      due to radiation (nonionizing) (solar) L57.8
  unguium L60.3
    congenita Q84.6

Atrophie blanche (en plaque) (de Milian) L95.0

Atrophoderma, atrophodermia (of) L90.9
  diffusum (idiopathic) L90.4
  maculatum L90.8
    et striatum L90.8
      due to syphilis A52.79
    syphilitic A51.39
  neuriticum L90.8
  Pasini and Pierini L90.3
  pigmentosum Q82.1
  reticulatum symmetricum faciei L66.4
  senile L90.8
    due to radiation (nonionizing) (solar) L57.8
  vermiculata (cheeks) L66.4

Atrophy, atrophic (of)
  adrenal (capsule) (gland) E27.49
    primary (autoimmune) E27.1
  alveolar process or ridge (edentulous) K08.20
  anal sphincter (disuse) N81.84
  appendix K38.8
  arteriosclerotic — *see* Arteriosclerosis
  bile duct (common) (hepatic) K83.8
  bladder N32.89
    neurogenic N31.8
  blanche (en plaque) (of Milian) L95.0
  bone (senile) NEC (*see also* Disorder, bone, specified type NEC)
    due to
      tabes dorsalis (neurogenic) A52.11
  brain (cortex) (progressive) G31.9
    frontotemporal circumscribed G31.01 [F02.80]
      with behavioral disturbance G31.01 [F02.81]
    senile NEC G31.1
  breast N64.2
    obstetric — *see* Disorder, breast, specified type NEC
  buccal cavity K13.79
  cardiac — *see* Degeneration, myocardial
  cartilage (infectional) (joint) — *see* Disorder, cartilage, specified NEC
  cerebellar — *see* Atrophy, brain
  cerebral — *see* Atrophy, brain
  cervix (mucosa) (senile) (uteri) N88.8
    menopausal N95.8
  Charcot-Marie-Tooth G60.0
  choroid (central) (macular) (myopic) (retina) H31.10- ☑

Atrophy, atrophic — *continued*
  choroid — *continued*
    diffuse secondary H31.12- ☑
    gyrate H31.23
    senile H31.11- ☑
  ciliary body — *see* Atrophy, iris
  conjunctiva (senile) H11.89
  corpus cavernosum N48.89
  cortical — *see* Atrophy, brain
  cystic duct K82.8
  Déjérine-Thomas G23.8
  disuse NEC — *see* Atrophy, muscle
  Duchenne-Aran G12.21
  ear H93.8- ☑
  edentulous alveolar ridge K08.20
  endometrium (senile) N85.8
    cervix N88.8
  enteric K63.89
  epididymis N50.8
  eyeball — *see* Disorder, globe, degenerated condition, atrophy
  eyelid (senile) — *see* Disorder, eyelid, degenerative
  facial (skin) L90.9
  fallopian tube (senile) N83.32
    with ovary N83.33
  fascioscapulohumeral (Landouzy- Déjérine) G71.0
  fatty, thymus (gland) E32.8
  gallbladder K82.8
  gastric K29.40
    with bleeding K29.41
  gastrointestinal K63.89
  glandular I89.8
  globe H44.52- ☑
  gum K06.0
  hair L67.8
  heart (brown) — *see* Degeneration, myocardial
  hemifacial Q67.4
    Romberg G51.8
  infantile E41
    paralysis, acute — *see* Poliomyelitis, paralytic
  intestine K63.89
  iris (essential) (progressive) H21.26- ☑
    specified NEC H21.29
  kidney (senile) (terminal) (*see also* Sclerosis, renal) N26.1
    congenital or infantile Q60.5
      bilateral Q60.4
      unilateral Q60.3
    hydronephrotic — *see* Hydronephrosis
  lacrimal gland (primary) H04.14- ☑
    secondary H04.15- ☑
  Landouzy-Déjérine G71.0
  laryngitis, infective J37.0
  larynx J38.7
  Leber's optic (hereditary) H47.22
  lip K13.0
  liver (yellow) K72.90
    with coma K72.91
    acute, subacute K72.00
      with coma K72.01
    chronic K72.10
      with coma K72.11
  lung (senile) J98.4
  macular (dermatological) L90.8
    syphilitic, skin A51.39
      striated A52.79
  mandible (edentulous) K08.20
    minimal K08.21
    moderate K08.22
    severe K08.23
  maxilla K08.20
    minimal K08.24
    moderate K08.25
    severe K08.26
  muscle, muscular (diffuse) (general) (idiopathic) (primary) M62.50
    ankle M62.57- ☑
    Duchenne-Aran G12.21
    foot M62.57- ☑
    forearm M62.53- ☑
    hand M62.54- ☑
    infantile spinal G12.0
    lower leg M62.56- ☑
    multiple sites M62.59
    myelopathic — *see* Atrophy, muscle, spinal
    myotonic G71.11
    neuritic G58.9
    neuropathic (peroneal) (progressive) G60.0

- **Atrophy, atrophic** — *continued*
  - muscle, muscular — *continued*
    - pelvic (disuse) N81.84
    - peroneal G6Ø.Ø
    - progressive (bulbar) G12.21
      - adult G12.1
      - infantile (spinal) G12.Ø
      - spinal G12.9
        - adult G12.1
        - infantile G12.Ø
    - pseudohypertrophic G71.Ø
    - shoulder region M62.51- ☑
    - specified site NEC M62.58
    - spinal G12.9
      - adult form G12.1
      - Aran-Duchenne G12.21
      - childhood form, type II G12.1
      - distal G12.1
      - hereditary NEC G12.1
      - infantile, type I (Werdnig-Hoffmann) G12.Ø
      - juvenile form, type III (Kugelberg- Welander) G12.1
      - progressive G12.21
      - scapuloperoneal form G12.1
      - specified NEC G12.8
    - syphilitic A52.78
    - thigh M62.55- ☑
    - upper arm M62.52- ☑
  - myocardium — *see* Degeneration, myocardial
  - myometrium (senile) N85.8
    - cervix N88.8
  - myopathic NEC — *see* Atrophy, muscle
  - myotonia G71.11
  - nail L6Ø.3
  - nasopharynx J31.1
  - nerve (*see also* Disorder, nerve)
    - abducens — *see* Strabismus, paralytic, sixth nerve
    - accessory G52.8
    - acoustic or auditory H93.3 ☑
    - cranial G52.9
      - eighth (auditory) H93.3 ☑
      - eleventh (accessory) G52.8
      - fifth (trigeminal) G5Ø.8
      - first (olfactory) G52.Ø
      - fourth (trochlear) — *see* Strabismus, paralytic, fourth nerve
      - second (optic) H47.2Ø
      - sixth (abducens) — *see* Strabismus, paralytic, sixth nerve
      - tenth (pneumogastric) (vagus) G52.2
      - third (oculomotor) — *see* Strabismus, paralytic, third nerve
      - twelfth (hypoglossal) G52.3
    - hypoglossal G52.3
    - oculomotor — *see* Strabismus, paralytic, third nerve
    - olfactory G52.Ø
    - optic (papillomacular bundle)
      - syphilitic (late) A52.15
        - congenital A5Ø.44
    - pneumogastric G52.2
    - trigeminal G5Ø.8
    - trochlear — *see* Strabismus, paralytic, fourth nerve
    - vagus (pneumogastric) G52.2
  - neurogenic, bone, tabetic A52.11
  - nutritional E41
  - old age R54
  - olivopontocerebellar G23.8
  - optic (nerve) H47.2Ø
    - glaucomatous H47.23- ☑
    - hereditary H47.22
    - primary H47.21- ☑
    - specified type NEC H47.29- ☑
    - syphilitic (late) A52.15
      - congenital A5Ø.44
  - orbit HØ5.31- ☑
  - ovary (senile) N83.31
    - with fallopian tube N83.33
  - oviduct (senile) — *see* Atrophy, fallopian tube
  - palsy, diffuse (progressive) G12.22
  - pancreas (duct) (senile) K86.8
  - parotid gland K11.Ø
  - pelvic muscle N81.84
  - penis N48.89
  - pharynx J39.2
  - pluriglandular E31.8
    - autoimmune E31.Ø
  - polyarthritis M15.9

- **Atrophy, atrophic** — *continued*
  - prostate N42.89
  - pseudohypertrophic (muscle) G71.Ø
  - renal (*see also* Sclerosis, renal) N26.1
  - retina, retinal (postinfectional) H35.89
  - rhinitis J31.Ø
  - salivary gland K11.Ø
  - scar L9Ø.5
  - sclerosis, lobar (of brain) G31.Ø9 [FØ2.8Ø]
    - with behavioral disturbance G31.Ø9 [FØ2.81]
  - scrotum N5Ø.8
  - seminal vesicle N5Ø.8
  - senile R54
    - due to radiation (nonionizing) (solar) L57.8
  - skin (patches) (spots) L9Ø.9
    - degenerative (senile) L9Ø.8
    - due to radiation (nonionizing) (solar) L57.8
    - senile L9Ø.8
  - spermatic cord N5Ø.8
  - spinal (acute) (cord) G95.89
    - muscular — *see* Atrophy, muscle, spinal
    - paralysis G12.2Ø
      - acute — *see* Poliomyelitis, paralytic
        - meaning progressive muscular atrophy G12.21
  - spine (column) — *see* Spondylopathy, specified NEC
  - spleen (senile) D73.Ø
  - stomach K29.4Ø
    - with bleeding K29.41
  - striate (skin) L9Ø.6
    - syphilitic A52.79
  - subcutaneous L9Ø.9
  - sublingual gland K11.Ø
  - submandibular gland K11.Ø
  - submaxillary gland K11.Ø
  - Sudeck's — *see* Algoneurodystrophy
  - suprarenal (capsule) (gland) E27.49
    - primary E27.1
  - systemic affecting central nervous system
    - in
      - myxedema EØ3.9 [G13.2]
      - neoplastic disease (*see also* Neoplasm) D49.9 [G13.1]
      - specified disease NEC G13.8
  - tarso-orbital fascia, congenital Q1Ø.3
  - testis N5Ø.Ø
  - thenar, partial — *see* Syndrome, carpal tunnel
  - thymus (fatty) E32.8
  - thyroid (gland) (acquired) EØ3.4
    - with cretinism EØ3.1
    - congenital (with myxedema) EØ3.1
  - tongue (senile) K14.8
    - papillae K14.4
  - trachea J39.8
  - tunica vaginalis N5Ø.8
  - turbinate J34.89
  - tympanic membrane (nonflaccid) H73.82- ☑
    - flaccid H73.81- ☑
  - upper respiratory tract J39.8
  - uterus, uterine (senile) N85.8
    - cervix N88.8
    - due to radiation (intended effect) N85.8
      - adverse effect or misadventure N99.89
  - vagina (senile) N95.2
  - vas deferens N5Ø.8
  - vascular I99.8
  - vertebra (senile) — *see* Spondylopathy, specified NEC
  - vulva (senile) N9Ø.5
  - Werdnig-Hoffmann G12.Ø
  - yellow — *see* Failure, hepatic
- **Attack, attacks**
  - with alteration of consciousness (with automatisms) — *see* Epilepsy, localization-related, symptomatic, with complex partial seizures
  - without alteration of consciousness — *see* Epilepsy, localization-related, symptomatic, with simple partial seizures
  - Adams-Stokes I45.9
  - akinetic — *see* Epilepsy, generalized, specified NEC
  - angina — *see* Angina
  - atonic — *see* Epilepsy, generalized, specified NEC
  - benign shuddering G25.83
  - cataleptic — *see* Catalepsy
  - coronary — *see* Infarct, myocardium
  - cyanotic, newborn P28.2
  - drop NEC R55
  - epileptic — *see* Epilepsy
  - heart — *see* infarct, myocardium
  - hysterical F44.9

- **Attack, attacks** — *continued*
  - jacksonian — *see* Epilepsy, localization-related, symptomatic, with simple partial seizures
  - myocardium, myocardial — *see* Infarct, myocardium
  - myoclonic — *see* Epilepsy, generalized, specified NEC
  - panic F41.Ø
  - psychomotor — *see* Epilepsy, localization-related, symptomatic, with complex partial seizures
  - salaam — *see* Epilepsy, spasms
  - schizophreniform, brief F23
  - shuddering, benign G25.83
  - Stokes-Adams I45.9
  - syncope R55
  - transient ischemic (TIA) G45.9
    - specified NEC G45.8
  - unconsciousness R55
    - hysterical F44.89
  - vasomotor R55
  - vasovagal (paroxysmal) (idiopathic) R55
- **Attention** (to)
  - artificial
    - opening (of) Z43.9
      - digestive tract NEC Z43.4
        - colon Z43.3
        - ilium Z43.2
        - stomach Z43.1
      - specified NEC Z43.8
      - trachea Z43.Ø
      - urinary tract NEC Z43.6
        - cystostomy Z43.5
        - nephrostomy Z43.6
        - ureterostomy Z43.6
        - urethrostomy Z43.6
    - vagina Z43.7
  - colostomy Z43.3
  - cystostomy Z43.5
  - deficit disorder or syndrome F98.8
    - with hyperactivity — *see* Disorder, attention-deficit hyperactivity
  - gastrostomy Z43.1
  - ileostomy Z43.2
  - jejunostomy Z43.4
  - nephrostomy Z43.6
  - surgical dressings Z48.Ø1
  - sutures Z48.Ø2
  - tracheostomy Z43.Ø
  - ureterostomy Z43.6
  - urethrostomy Z43.6
- **Attrition**
  - gum KØ6.Ø
  - tooth, teeth (excessive) (hard tissues) KØ3.Ø
- **Atypical, atypism** (*see also* condition)
  - cells (on cytolgocial smear) (endocervical) (endometrial) (glandular)
    - cervix R87.619
    - vagina R87.629
  - cervical N87.9
  - endometrium N85.9
    - hyperplasia N85.ØØ
  - parenting situation Z62.9
- **Auditory** — *see* condition
- **Aujeszky's disease** B33.8
- **Aurantiasis, cutis** E67.1
- **Auricle, auricular** (*see also* condition)
  - cervical Q18.2
- **Auriculotemporal syndrome** G5Ø.8
- **Austin Flint murmur** (aortic insufficiency) I35.1
- **Australian**
  - Q fever A78
  - X disease A83.4
- **Autism, autistic** (childhood) (infantile) F84.Ø
  - atypical F84.9
- **Autodigestion** R68.89
- **Autoerythrocyte sensitization** (syndrome) D69.2
- **Autographism** L5Ø.3
- **Autoimmune**
  - disease (systemic) M35.9
  - inhibitors to clotting factors D68.311
  - lymphoproliferative syndrome [ALPS] D89.82
  - thyroiditis EØ6.3
- **Autointoxication** R68.89
- **Automatism** G93.89
  - with temporal sclerosis G93.81
  - epileptic — *see* Epilepsy, localization-related, symptomatic, with complex partial seizures
  - paroxysmal, idiopathic — *see* Epilepsy, localization-related, symptomatic, with complex partial seizures

Autonomic, autonomous
  - bladder (neurogenic) N31.2
  - hysteria seizure F44.5

Autosensitivity, erythrocyte D69.2
Autosensitization, cutaneous L3Ø.2
Autosome — *see* condition by chromosome involved
Autotopagnosia R48.1
Autotoxemia R68.89
Autumn — *see* condition
Avellis' syndrome G46.8
Aversion
  - oral R63.3
    - newborn P92.- ☑
    - nonorganic origin F98.2 ☑
  - sexual F52.1

Aviator's
  - disease or sickness — *see* Effect, adverse, high altitude
  - ear T7Ø.Ø ☑

Avitaminosis (multiple) (*see also* Deficiency, vitamin) E56.9
  - B E53.9
    - with
      - beriberi E51.11
      - pellagra E52
  - B2 E53.Ø
  - B6 E53.1
  - B12 E53.8
  - D E55.9
    - with rickets E55.Ø
  - G E53.Ø
  - K E56.1
  - nicotinic acid E52

AVNRT (atrioventricular nodal re-entrant tachycardia) I47.1
AVRT (atrioventricular nodal re-entrant tachycardia) I47.1
Avulsion (traumatic)
  - blood vessel — *see* Injury, blood vessel
  - bone — *see* Fracture, by site
  - cartilage (*see also* Dislocation, by site)
    - symphyseal (inner), complicating delivery O71.6
  - external site other than limb — *see* Wound, open, by site
  - eye SØ5.7- ☑
  - head (intracranial)
    - external site NEC SØ8.89 ☑
    - scalp SØ8.Ø ☑
  - internal organ or site — *see* Injury, by site
  - joint (*see also* Dislocation, by site)
    - capsule — *see* Sprain, by site
  - kidney S37.Ø6- ☑
  - ligament — *see* Sprain, by site
  - limb (*see also* Amputation, traumatic, by site)
    - skin and subcutaneous tissue — *see* Wound, open, by site
  - muscle — *see* Injury, muscle
  - nerve (root) — *see* Injury, nerve
  - scalp SØ8.Ø ☑
  - skin and subcutaneous tissue — *see* Wound, open, by site
  - spleen S36.Ø32 ☑
  - symphyseal cartilage (inner), complicating delivery O71.6
  - tendon — *see* Injury, muscle
  - tooth SØ3.2 ☑

Awareness of heart beat RØØ.2
Axenfeld's
  - anomaly or syndrome Q15.Ø
  - degeneration (calcareous) Q13.4

Axilla, axillary (*see also* condition)
  - breast Q83.1

Axonotmesis — *see* Injury, nerve
Ayerza's disease or syndrome (pulmonary artery sclerosis with pulmonary hypertension) I27.Ø
Azoospermia (organic) N46.Ø1
  - due to
    - drug therapy N46.Ø21
    - efferent duct obstruction N46.Ø23
    - infection N46.Ø22
    - radiation N46.Ø24
    - specified cause NEC N46.Ø29
    - systemic disease N46.Ø25

Azotemia R79.89
  - meaning uremia N19

Aztec ear Q17.3
Azygos
  - continuation inferior vena cava Q26.8
  - lobe (lung) Q33.1

B

Baastrup's disease — *see* Kissing spine
Babesiosis B6Ø.Ø
Babington's disease (familial hemorrhagic telangiectasia) I78.Ø
Babinski's syndrome A52.79
Baby
  - crying constantly R68.11
  - floppy (syndrome) P94.2

Bacillary — *see* condition
Bacilluria N39.Ø
Bacillus (*see also* Infection, bacillus)
  - abortus infection A23.1
  - anthracis infection A22.9
  - coli infection (*see also* Escherichia coli) B96.2Ø
  - Flexner's AØ3.1
  - mallei infection A24.Ø
  - Shiga's AØ3.Ø
  - suipestifer infection — *see* Infection, salmonella

Back — *see* condition
Backache (postural) M54.9
  - sacroiliac M53.3
  - specified NEC M54.89

Backflow — *see* Reflux
Backward reading (dyslexia) F81.Ø
Bacteremia R78.81
  - with sepsis — *see* Sepsis

Bactericholia — *see* Cholecystitis, acute
Bacterid, bacteride (pustular) L4Ø.3
Bacterium, bacteria, bacterial
  - agent NEC, as cause of disease classified elsewhere B96.89
  - in blood — *see* Bacteremia
  - in urine — *see* Bacteriuria

Bacteriuria, bacteruria N39.Ø
  - asymptomatic N39.Ø

Bacteroides
  - fragilis, as cause of disease classified elsewhere B96.6

Bad
  - heart — *see* Disease, heart
  - trip
    - due to drug abuse — *see* Abuse, drug, hallucinogen
    - due to drug dependence — *see* Dependence, drug, hallucinogen

Baelz's disease (cheilitis glandularis apostematosa) K13.Ø
Baerensprung's disease (eczema marginatum) B35.6
Bagasse disease or pneumonitis J67.1
Bagassosis J67.1
Baker's cyst — *see* Cyst, Baker's
Bakwin-Krida syndrome (craniometaphyseal dysplasia) Q78.5
Balancing side interference M26.56
Balanitis (circinata) (erosiva) (gangrenosa) (phagedenic) (vulgaris) N48.1
  - amebic AØ6.82
  - candidal B37.42
  - due to Haemophilus ducreyi A57
  - gonococcal (acute) (chronic) A54.Ø9
  - xerotica obliterans N48.Ø

Balanoposthitis N47.6
  - gonococcal (acute) (chronic) A54.Ø9
  - ulcerative (specific) A63.8

Balanorrhagia — *see* Balanitis
Balantidiasis, balantidiosis AØ7.Ø
Bald tongue K14.4
Baldness (*see also* Alopecia)
  - male-pattern — *see* Alopecia, androgenic

Balkan grippe A78
Balloon disease — *see* Effect, adverse, high altitude
Balo's disease (concentric sclerosis) G37.5
Bamberger-Marie disease — *see* Osteoarthropathy, hypertrophic, specified type NEC
Bancroft's filariasis B74.Ø
Band(s)
  - adhesive — *see* Adhesions, peritoneum
  - anomalous or congenital (*see also* Anomaly, by site)
    - heart (atrial) (ventricular) Q24.8
    - intestine Q43.3
    - omentum Q43.3
  - cervix N88.1
  - constricting, congenital Q79.8
  - gallbladder (congenital) Q44.1
  - intestinal (adhesive) — *see* Adhesions, peritoneum

Band(s) — *continued*
  - obstructive
    - intestine K56.5
    - peritoneum K56.5
  - periappendiceal, congenital Q43.3
  - peritoneal (adhesive) — *see* Adhesions, peritoneum
  - uterus N73.6
    - internal N85.6
  - vagina N89.5

Bandemia D72.825
Bandl's ring (contraction), complicating delivery O62.4
Bangkok hemorrhagic fever A91
Bang's disease (brucella abortus) A23.1
Bankruptcy, anxiety concerning Z59.8
Bannister's disease T78.3 ☑
  - hereditary D84.1

Banti's disease or syndrome (with cirrhosis) (with portal hypertension) K76.6
Bar, median, prostate — *see* Enlargement, enlarged, prostate
Barcoo disease or rot — *see* Ulcer, skin
Barlow's disease E54
Barodontalgia T7Ø.29 ☑
Baron Münchausen syndrome — *see* Disorder, factitious
Barosinusitis T7Ø.1 ☑
Barotitis T7Ø.Ø ☑
Barotrauma T7Ø.29 ☑
  - odontalgia T7Ø.29 ☑
  - otitic T7Ø.Ø ☑
  - sinus T7Ø.1 ☑

Barraquer (-Simons) **disease or syndrome** (progressive lipodystrophy) E88.1
Barré-Guillain disease or syndrome G61.Ø
Barrel chest M95.4
Barré-Liéou syndrome (posterior cervical sympathetic) M53.Ø
Barrett's
  - disease — *see* Barrett's, esophagus
  - esophagus K22.7Ø
    - with dysplasia K22.719
      - high grade K22.711
      - low grade K22.71Ø
    - without dysplasia K22.7Ø
  - syndrome — *see* Barrett's, esophagus
  - ulcer K22.1Ø
    - with bleeding K22.11
    - without bleeding K22.1Ø

Bársony (-Polgár) (-Teschendorf) **syndrome** (corkscrew esophagus) K22.4
Barth syndrome E78.71
Bartholinitis (suppurating) N75.8
  - gonococcal (acute) (chronic) (with abscess) A54.1

Bartonellosis A44.9
  - cutaneous A44.1
  - mucocutaneous A44.1
  - specified NEC A44.8
  - systemic A44.Ø

Barton's fracture S52.56- ☑
Bartter's syndrome E26.81
Basal — *see* condition
Basan's (hidrotic) ectodermal dysplasia Q82.4
Baseball finger — *see* Dislocation, finger
Basedow's disease (exophthalmic goiter) — *see* Hyperthyroidism, with, goiter
Basic — *see* condition
Basilar — *see* condition
Bason's (hidrotic) ectodermal dysplasia Q82.4
Basopenia — *see* Agranulocytosis
Basophilia D72.824
Basophilism (cortico-adrenal) (Cushing's) (pituitary) E24.Ø
Bassen-Kornzweig disease or syndrome E78.6
Bat ear Q17.5
Bateman's
  - disease BØ8.1
  - purpura (senile) D69.2

Bathing cramp T75.1 ☑
Bathophobia F4Ø.248
Batten (-Mayou) **disease** E75.4
  - retina E75.4 [H36]

Batten-Steinert syndrome G71.11
Battered — *see* Maltreatment
Battey Mycobacterium infection A31.Ø
Battle exhaustion F43.Ø
Battledore placenta O43.19- ☑

Birth — *continued*
  injury — *continued*
    tentorial tear P1Ø.4
    testes P15.5
    vulva P15.5
  lack of care, at or after — *see* Maltreatment, child, neglect
  neglect, at or after — *see* Maltreatment, child, neglect
  palsy or paralysis, newborn, NOS (birth injury) P14.9
  premature (infant) — *see* Preterm, newborn
  shock, newborn P96.89
  trauma — *see* Birth, injury
  weight
    4ØØØ grams to 4499 grams PØ8.1
    45ØØ grams or more PØ8.Ø
    low (2499 grams or less) — *see* Low, birthweight
      extremely (999 grams or less) — *see* Low, birthweight, extreme
Birthmark Q82.5
Birt-Hogg-Dube syndrome Q87.89
Bisalbuminemia E88.Ø9
Biskra's button B55.1
Bite(s) (animal) (human)
  abdomen, abdominal
    wall S31.159 ☑
      with penetration into peritoneal cavity S31.659 ☑
      epigastric region S31.152 ☑
        with penetration into peritoneal cavity S31.652 ☑
      left
        lower quadrant S31.154 ☑
          with penetration into peritoneal cavity S31.654 ☑
        upper quadrant S31.151 ☑
          with penetration into peritoneal cavity S31.651 ☑
      periumbilic region S31.155 ☑
        with penetration into peritoneal cavity S31.655 ☑
      right
        lower quadrant S31.153 ☑
          with penetration into peritoneal cavity S31.653 ☑
        upper quadrant S31.15Ø ☑
          with penetration into peritoneal cavity S31.65Ø ☑
      superficial NEC S3Ø.871 ☑
        insect S3Ø.861 ☑
  alveolar (process) — *see* Bite, oral cavity
  amphibian (venomous) — *see* Venom, bite, amphibian
  animal (*see also* Bite, by site)
    venomous — *see* Venom
  ankle S91.Ø5- ☑
    superficial NEC S9Ø.57- ☑
      insect S9Ø.56- ☑
  antecubital space — *see* Bite, elbow
  anus S31.835 ☑
    superficial NEC S3Ø.877 ☑
      insect S3Ø.867 ☑
  arm (upper) S41.15- ☑
    lower — *see* Bite, forearm
    superficial NEC S4Ø.87- ☑
      insect S4Ø.86- ☑
  arthropod NEC — *see* Venom, bite, arthropod
  auditory canal (external) (meatus) — *see* Bite, ear
  auricle, ear — *see* Bite, ear
  axilla — *see* Bite, arm
  back (*see also* Bite, thorax, back)
    lower S31.Ø5Ø ☑
      with penetration into retroperitoneal space S31.Ø51 ☑
      superficial NEC S3Ø.87Ø ☑
        insect S3Ø.86Ø ☑
  bedbug — *see* Bite(s), by site, superficial, insect
  breast S21.Ø5- ☑
    superficial NEC S2Ø.17- ☑
      insect S2Ø.16- ☑
  brow — *see* Bite, head, specified site NEC
  buttock S31.8Ø5 ☑
    left S31.825 ☑
    right S31.815 ☑
    superficial NEC S3Ø.87Ø ☑
      insect S3Ø.86Ø ☑
  calf — *see* Bite, leg
  canaliculus lacrimalis — *see* Bite, eyelid

Bite(s) — *continued*
  canthus, eye — *see* Bite, eyelid
  centipede — *see* Toxicity, venom, arthropod, centipede
  cheek (external) SØ1.45- ☑
    internal — *see* Bite, oral cavity
    superficial NEC SØØ.87 ☑
      insect SØØ.86 ☑
  chest wall — *see* Bite, thorax
  chigger B88.Ø
  chin — *see* Bite, head, specified site NEC
  clitoris — *see* Bite, vulva
  costal region — *see* Bite, thorax
  digit(s)
    hand — *see* Bite, finger
    toe — *see* Bite, toe
  ear (canal) (external) SØ1.35- ☑
    superficial NEC SØØ.47- ☑
      insect SØØ.46- ☑
  elbow S51.Ø5- ☑
    superficial NEC S5Ø.37- ☑
      insect S5Ø.36- ☑
  epididymis — *see* Bite, testis
  epigastric region — *see* Bite, abdomen
  epiglottis — *see* Bite, neck, specified site NEC
  esophagus, cervical S11.25 ☑
    superficial NEC S1Ø.17 ☑
      insect S1Ø.16 ☑
  eyebrow — *see* Bite, eyelid
  eyelid SØ1.15- ☑
    superficial NEC SØØ.27- ☑
      insect SØØ.26- ☑
  face NEC — *see* Bite, head, specified site NEC
  finger(s) S61.259 ☑
    with
      damage to nail S61.359 ☑
    index S61.258 ☑
      with
        damage to nail S61.358 ☑
      left S61.251 ☑
        with
          damage to nail S61.351 ☑
      right S61.25Ø ☑
        with
          damage to nail S61.35Ø ☑
      superficial NEC S6Ø.478 ☑
        insect S6Ø.46- ☑
    little S61.25- ☑
      with
        damage to nail S61.35- ☑
      superficial NEC S6Ø.47- ☑
        insect S6Ø.46- ☑
    middle S61.25- ☑
      with
        damage to nail S61.35- ☑
      superficial NEC S6Ø.47- ☑
        insect S6Ø.46- ☑
    ring S61.25- ☑
      with
        damage to nail S61.35- ☑
      superficial NEC S6Ø.47- ☑
        insect S6Ø.46- ☑
    superficial NEC S6Ø.479 ☑
      insect S6Ø.469 ☑
    thumb — *see* Bite, thumb
  flank — *see* Bite, abdomen, wall
  flea — *see* Bite, by site, superficial, insect
  foot (except toe(s) alone) S91.35- ☑
    superficial NEC S9Ø.87- ☑
      insect S9Ø.86- ☑
    toe — *see* Bite, toe
  forearm S51.85- ☑
    elbow only — *see* Bite, elbow
    superficial NEC S5Ø.87- ☑
      insect S5Ø.86- ☑
  forehead — *see* Bite, head, specified site NEC
  genital organs, external
    female S31.552 ☑
      superficial NEC S3Ø.876 ☑
        insect S3Ø.866 ☑
      vagina and vulva — *see* Bite, vulva
    male S31.551 ☑
      penis — *see* Bite, penis
      scrotum — *see* Bite, scrotum
      superficial NEC S3Ø.875 ☑
        insect S3Ø.865 ☑

Bite(s) — *continued*
  genital organs, external — *continued*
    male — *continued*
      testes — *see* Bite, testis
  groin — *see* Bite, abdomen, wall
  gum — *see* Bite, oral cavity
  hand S61.45- ☑
    finger — *see* Bite, finger
    superficial NEC S6Ø.57- ☑
      insect S6Ø.56- ☑
    thumb — *see* Bite, thumb
  head SØ1.95 ☑
    cheek — *see* Bite, cheek
    ear — *see* Bite, ear
    eyelid — *see* Bite, eyelid
    lip — *see* Bite, lip
    nose — *see* Bite, nose
    oral cavity — *see* Bite, oral cavity
    scalp — *see* Bite, scalp
    specified site NEC SØ1.85 ☑
      superficial NEC SØØ.87 ☑
        insect SØØ.86 ☑
    superficial NEC SØØ.97 ☑
      insect SØØ.96 ☑
    temporomandibular area — *see* Bite, cheek
  heel — *see* Bite, foot
  hip S71.Ø5- ☑
    superficial NEC S7Ø.27- ☑
      insect S7Ø.26- ☑
  hymen S31.45 ☑
  hypochondrium — *see* Bite, abdomen, wall
  hypogastric region — *see* Bite, abdomen, wall
  inguinal region — *see* Bite, abdomen, wall
  insect — *see* Bite, by site, superficial, insect
  instep — *see* Bite, foot
  interscapular region — *see* Bite, thorax, back
  jaw — *see* Bite, head, specified site NEC
  knee S81.Ø5- ☑
    superficial NEC S8Ø.27- ☑
      insect S8Ø.26- ☑
  labium (majus) (minus) — *see* Bite, vulva
  lacrimal duct — *see* Bite, eyelid
  larynx S11.Ø15 ☑
    superficial NEC S1Ø.17 ☑
      insect S1Ø.16 ☑
  leg (lower) S81.85- ☑
    ankle — *see* Bite, ankle
    foot — *see* Bite, foot
    knee — *see* Bite, knee
    superficial NEC S8Ø.87- ☑
      insect S8Ø.86- ☑
    toe — *see* Bite, toe
    upper — *see* Bite, thigh
  lip SØ1.551 ☑
    superficial NEC SØØ.571 ☑
      insect SØØ.561 ☑
  lizard (venomous) — *see* Venom, bite, reptile
  loin — *see* Bite, abdomen, wall
  lower back — *see* Bite, back, lower
  lumbar region — *see* Bite, back, lower
  malar region — *see* Bite, head, specified site NEC
  mammary — *see* Bite, breast
  marine animals (venomous) — *see* Toxicity, venom, marine animal
  mastoid region — *see* Bite, head, specified site NEC
  mouth — *see* Bite, oral cavity
  nail
    finger — *see* Bite, finger
    toe — *see* Bite, toe
  nape — *see* Bite, neck, specified site NEC
  nasal (septum) (sinus) — *see* Bite, nose
  nasopharynx — *see* Bite, head, specified site NEC
  neck S11.95 ☑
    involving
      cervical esophagus — *see* Bite, esophagus, cervical
      larynx — *see* Bite, larynx
      pharynx — *see* Bite, pharynx
      thyroid gland S11.15 ☑
      trachea — *see* Bite, trachea
    specified site NEC S11.85 ☑
      superficial NEC S1Ø.87 ☑
        insect S1Ø.86 ☑
    superficial NEC S1Ø.97 ☑
      insect S1Ø.96 ☑
    throat S11.85 ☑

- **Bite**(s) — *continued*
  - neck — *continued*
    - throat — *continued*
      - superficial NEC S1Ø.17 ☑
        - insect S1Ø.16 ☑
  - nose (septum) (sinus) SØ1.25 ☑
    - superficial NEC SØØ.37 ☑
      - insect SØØ.36 ☑
  - occipital region — *see* Bite, scalp
  - oral cavity SØ1.552 ☑
    - superficial NEC SØØ.572 ☑
      - insect SØØ.562 ☑
  - orbital region — *see* Bite, eyelid
  - palate — *see* Bite, oral cavity
  - palm — *see* Bite, hand
  - parietal region — *see* Bite, scalp
  - pelvis S31.Ø5Ø ☑
    - with penetration into retroperitoneal space S31.Ø51 ☑
    - superficial NEC S3Ø.87Ø ☑
      - insect S3Ø.86Ø ☑
  - penis S31.25 ☑
    - superficial NEC S3Ø.872 ☑
      - insect S3Ø.862 ☑
  - perineum
    - female — *see* Bite, vulva
    - male — *see* Bite, pelvis
  - periocular area (with or without lacrimal passages) — *see* Bite, eyelid
  - phalanges
    - finger — *see* Bite, finger
    - toe — *see* Bite, toe
  - pharynx S11.25 ☑
    - superficial NEC S1Ø.17 ☑
      - insect S1Ø.16 ☑
  - pinna — *see* Bite, ear
  - poisonous — *see* Venom
  - popliteal space — *see* Bite, knee
  - prepuce — *see* Bite, penis
  - pubic region — *see* Bite, abdomen, wall
  - rectovaginal septum — *see* Bite, vulva
  - red bug B88.Ø
  - reptile NEC (*see also* Venom, bite, reptile)
    - nonvenomous — *see* Bite, by site
    - snake — *see* Venom, bite, snake
  - sacral region — *see* Bite, back, lower
  - sacroiliac region — *see* Bite, back, lower
  - salivary gland — *see* Bite, oral cavity
  - scalp SØ1.Ø5 ☑
    - superficial NEC SØØ.Ø7 ☑
      - insect SØØ.Ø6 ☑
  - scapular region — *see* Bite, shoulder
  - scrotum S31.35 ☑
    - superficial NEC S3Ø.873 ☑
      - insect S3Ø.863 ☑
  - sea-snake (venomous) — *see* Toxicity, venom, snake, sea snake
  - shin — *see* Bite, leg
  - shoulder S41.Ø5- ☑
    - superficial NEC S4Ø.27- ☑
      - insect S4Ø.26- ☑
  - snake (*see also* Venom, bite, snake)
    - nonvenomous — *see* Bite, by site
  - spermatic cord — *see* Bite, testis
  - spider (venomous) — *see* Toxicity, venom, spider
    - nonvenomous — *see* Bite, by site, superficial, insect
  - sternal region — *see* Bite, thorax, front
  - submaxillary region — *see* Bite, head, specified site NEC
  - submental region — *see* Bite, head, specified site NEC
  - subungual
    - finger(s) — *see* Bite, finger
    - toe — *see* Bite, toe
  - superficial — *see* Bite, by site, superficial
  - supraclavicular fossa S11.85 ☑
  - supraorbital — *see* Bite, head, specified site NEC
  - temple, temporal region — *see* Bite, head, specified site NEC
  - temporomandibular area — *see* Bite, cheek
  - testis S31.35 ☑
    - superficial NEC S3Ø.873 ☑
      - insect S3Ø.863 ☑
  - thigh S71.15- ☑
    - superficial NEC S7Ø.37- ☑
      - insect S7Ø.36- ☑
  - thorax, thoracic (wall) S21.95 ☑

- **Bite**(s) — *continued*
  - thorax, thoracic — *continued*
    - back S21.25- ☑
      - with penetration into thoracic cavity S21.45- ☑
    - breast — *see* Bite, breast
    - front S21.15- ☑
      - with penetration into thoracic cavity S21.35- ☑
    - superficial NEC S2Ø.97 ☑
      - back S2Ø.47- ☑
      - front S2Ø.37- ☑
      - insect S2Ø.96 ☑
        - back S2Ø.46- ☑
        - front S2Ø.36- ☑
  - throat — *see* Bite, neck, throat
  - thumb S61.Ø5- ☑
    - with
      - damage to nail S61.15- ☑
    - superficial NEC S6Ø.37- ☑
      - insect S6Ø.36- ☑
  - thyroid S11.15 ☑
    - superficial NEC S1Ø.87 ☑
      - insect S1Ø.86 ☑
  - toe(s) S91.15- ☑
    - with
      - damage to nail S91.25- ☑
    - great S91.15- ☑
      - with
        - damage to nail S91.25- ☑
    - lesser S91.15- ☑
      - with
        - damage to nail S91.25- ☑
    - superficial NEC S9Ø.47- ☑
      - great S9Ø.47- ☑
      - insect S9Ø.46- ☑
        - great S9Ø.46- ☑
  - tongue SØ1.552 ☑
  - trachea S11.Ø25 ☑
    - superficial NEC S1Ø.17 ☑
      - insect S1Ø.16 ☑
  - tunica vaginalis — *see* Bite, testis
  - tympanum, tympanic membrane — *see* Bite, ear
  - umbilical region S31.155 ☑
  - uvula — *see* Bite, oral cavity
  - vagina — *see* Bite, vulva
  - venomous — *see* Venom
  - vocal cords S11.Ø35 ☑
    - superficial NEC S1Ø.17 ☑
      - insect S1Ø.16 ☑
  - vulva S31.45 ☑
    - superficial NEC S3Ø.874 ☑
      - insect S3Ø.864 ☑
  - wrist S61.55- ☑
    - superficial NEC S6Ø.87- ☑
      - insect S6Ø.86- ☑
- **Biting, cheek or lip** K13.1
- **Biventricular failure** (heart) I5Ø.9
- **Björck** (-Thorson) **syndrome** (malignant carcinoid) E34.Ø
- **Black**
  - death A2Ø.9
  - eye SØØ.1- ☑
  - hairy tongue K14.3
  - heel (foot) S9Ø.3- ☑
  - lung (disease) J6Ø
  - palm (hand) S6Ø.22- ☑
- **Blackfan-Diamond anemia or syndrome** (congenital hypoplastic anemia) D61.Ø1
- **Blackhead** L7Ø.Ø
- **Blackout** R55
- **Bladder** — *see* condition
- **Blast** (air) (hydraulic) (immersion) (underwater)
  - blindness SØ5.8X- ☑
  - injury
    - abdomen or thorax — *see* Injury, by site
    - ear (acoustic nerve trauma) — *see* Injury, nerve, acoustic, specified type NEC
  - syndrome NEC T7Ø.8 ☑
- **Blastoma** — *see* Neoplasm, malignant, by site
  - pulmonary — *see* Neoplasm, lung, malignant
- **Blastomycosis, blastomycotic** B4Ø.9
  - Brazilian — *see* Paracoccidioidomycosis
  - cutaneous B4Ø.3
  - disseminated B4Ø.7
  - European — *see* Cryptococcosis
  - generalized B4Ø.7
  - keloidal B48.Ø
  - North American B4Ø.9

- **Blastomycosis, blastomycotic** — *continued*
  - primary pulmonary B4Ø.Ø
  - pulmonary B4Ø.2
    - acute B4Ø.Ø
    - chronic B4Ø.1
  - skin B4Ø.3
  - South American — *see* Paracoccidioidomycosis
  - specified NEC B4Ø.89
- **Bleb**(s) R23.8
  - emphysematous (lung) (solitary) J43.9
  - endophthalmitis H59.43
  - filtering (vitreous), after glaucoma surgery Z98.83
  - inflammed (infected), postprocedural H59.4Ø
    - stage 1 H59.41
    - stage 2 H59.42
    - stage 3 H59.43
  - lung (ruptured) J43.9
    - congenital — *see* Atelectasis
    - newborn P25.8
  - subpleural (emphysematous) J43.9
- **Blebitis, postprocedural** H59.4Ø
  - stage 1 H59.41
  - stage 2 H59.42
  - stage 3 H59.43
- **Bleeder** (familial) (hereditary) — *see* Hemophilia
- **Bleeding** (*see also* Hemorrhage)
  - anal K62.5
  - anovulatory N97.Ø
  - atonic, following delivery O72.1
  - capillary I78.8
    - puerperal O72.2
  - contact (postcoital) N93.Ø
  - due to uterine subinvolution N85.3
  - ear — *see* Otorrhagia
  - excessive, associated with menopausal onset N92.4
  - familial — *see* Defect, coagulation
  - following intercourse N93.Ø
  - gastrointestinal K92.2
  - hemorrhoids — *see* Hemorrhoids
  - intermenstrual (regular) N92.3
    - irregular N92.1
  - intraoperative — *see* Complication, intraoperative, hemorrhage
  - irregular N92.6
  - menopausal N92.4
  - newborn, intraventricular — *see* Newborn, affected by, hemorrhage, intraventricular
  - nipple N64.59
  - nose RØ4.Ø
  - ovulation N92.3
  - postclimacteric N95.Ø
  - postcoital N93.Ø
  - postmenopausal N95.Ø
  - postoperative — *see* Complication, postprocedural, hemorrhage
  - preclimacteric N92.4
  - puberty (excessive, with onset of menstrual periods) N92.2
  - rectum, rectal K62.5
    - newborn P54.2
  - tendencies — *see* Defect, coagulation
  - throat RØ4.1
  - tooth socket (post-extraction) K91.84Ø
  - umbilical stump P51.9
  - uterus, uterine NEC N93.9
    - climacteric N92.4
    - dysfunctional of functional N93.8
    - menopausal N92.4
    - preclimacteric or premenopausal N92.4
    - unrelated to menstrual cycle N93.9
  - vagina, vaginal (abnormal) N93.9
    - dysfunctional or functional N93.8
    - newborn P54.6
  - vicarious N94.89
- **Blennorrhagia, blennorrhagic** — *see* Gonorrhea
- **Blennorrhea** (acute) (chronic) (*see also* Gonorrhea)
  - inclusion (neonatal) (newborn) P39.1
  - lower genitourinary tract (gonococcal) A54.ØØ
  - neonatorum (gonococcal ophthalmia) A54.31
- **Blepharelosis** — *see* Entropion
- **Blepharitis** (angularis) (ciliaris) (eyelid) (marginal) (nonulcerative) HØ1.ØØ9
  - herpes zoster BØ2.39
  - left HØ1.ØØ6
    - lower HØ1.ØØ5
    - upper HØ1.ØØ4
  - right HØ1.ØØ3
    - lower HØ1.ØØ2

- **Blepharitis** — *continued*
  - right — *continued*
    - upper H01.001
  - squamous H01.029
    - left H01.026
      - lower H01.025
      - upper H01.024
    - right H01.023
      - lower H01.022
      - upper H01.021
  - ulcerative H01.019
    - left H01.016
      - lower H01.015
      - upper H01.014
    - right H01.013
      - lower H01.012
      - upper H01.011
- **Blepharochalasis** H02.30
  - congenital Q10.0
  - left H02.36
    - lower H02.35
    - upper H02.34
  - right H02.33
    - lower H02.32
    - upper H02.31
- **Blepharoclonus** H02.59
- **Blepharoconjunctivitis** H10.50- ☑
  - angular H10.52- ☑
  - contact H10.53- ☑
  - ligneous H10.51- ☑
- **Blepharophimosis** (eyelid) H02.529
  - congenital Q10.3
  - left H02.526
    - lower H02.525
    - upper H02.524
  - right H02.523
    - lower H02.522
    - upper H02.521
- **Blepharoptosis** H02.40- ☑
  - congenital Q10.0
  - mechanical H02.41- ☑
  - myogenic H02.42- ☑
  - neurogenic H02.43- ☑
  - paralytic H02.43- ☑
- **Blepharopyorrhea, gonococcal** A54.39
- **Blepharospasm** G24.5
  - drug induced G24.01
- **Blighted ovum** O02.0
- **Blind** (*see also* Blindness)
  - bronchus (congenital) Q32.4
  - loop syndrome K90.2
    - congenital Q43.8
  - sac, fallopian tube (congenital) Q50.6
  - spot, enlarged — *see* Defect, visual field, localized, scotoma, blind spot area
  - tract or tube, congenital NEC — *see* Atresia, by site
- **Blindness** (acquired) (congenital) (both eyes) H54.0
  - blast S05.8X- ☑
  - color — *see* Deficiency, color vision
  - concussion S05.8X- ☑
  - cortical H47.619
    - left brain H47.612
    - right brain H47.611
  - day H53.11
  - due to injury (current episode) S05.9- ☑
    - sequelae — *code to* injury with seventh character S
  - eclipse (total) — *see* Retinopathy, solar
  - emotional (hysterical) F44.6
  - face H53.16
  - hysterical F44.6
  - legal (both eyes) (USA definition) H54.8
  - mind R48.8
  - night H53.60
    - abnormal dark adaptation curve H53.61
    - acquired H53.62
    - congenital H53.63
    - specified type NEC H53.69
    - vitamin A deficiency E50.5
  - one eye (other eye normal) H54.40
    - left (normal vision on right) H54.42
      - low vision on right H54.12
    - low vision, other eye H54.10
    - right (normal vision on left) H54.41
      - low vision on left H54.11
  - psychic R48.8
  - river B73.01
  - snow — *see* Photokeratitis
- **Blindness** — *continued*
  - sun, solar — *see* Retinopathy, solar
  - transient — *see* Disturbance, vision, subjective, loss, transient
  - traumatic (current episode) S05.9- ☑
  - word (developmental) F81.0
    - acquired R48.0
    - secondary to organic lesion R48.0
- **Blister** (nonthermal)
  - abdominal wall S30.821 ☑
  - alveolar process S00.522 ☑
  - ankle S90.52- ☑
  - antecubital space — *see* Blister, elbow
  - anus S30.827 ☑
  - arm (upper) S40.82- ☑
  - auditory canal — *see* Blister, ear
  - auricle — *see* Blister, ear
  - axilla — *see* Blister, arm
  - back, lower S30.820 ☑
  - beetle dermatitis L24.89
  - breast S20.12- ☑
  - brow S00.82 ☑
  - calf — *see* Blister, leg
  - canthus — *see* Blister, eyelid
  - cheek S00.82 ☑
    - internal S00.522 ☑
  - chest wall — *see* Blister, thorax
  - chin S00.82 ☑
  - costal region — *see* Blister, thorax
  - digit(s)
    - foot — *see* Blister, toe
    - hand — *see* Blister, finger
  - due to burn — *see* Burn, by site, second degree
  - ear S00.42- ☑
  - elbow S50.32- ☑
  - epiglottis S10.12 ☑
  - esophagus, cervical S10.12 ☑
  - eyebrow — *see* Blister, eyelid
  - eyelid S00.22- ☑
  - face S00.82 ☑
  - fever B00.1
  - finger(s) S60.429 ☑
    - index S60.42- ☑
    - little S60.42- ☑
    - middle S60.42- ☑
    - ring S60.42- ☑
  - foot (except toe(s) alone) S90.82- ☑
    - toe — *see* Blister, toe
  - forearm S50.82- ☑
    - elbow only — *see* Blister, elbow
  - forehead S00.82 ☑
  - fracture — *omit code*
  - genital organ
    - female S30.826 ☑
    - male S30.825 ☑
  - gum S00.522 ☑
  - hand S60.52- ☑
  - head S00.92 ☑
    - ear — *see* Blister, ear
    - eyelid — *see* Blister, eyelid
    - lip S00.521 ☑
    - nose S00.32 ☑
    - oral cavity S00.522 ☑
    - scalp S00.02 ☑
    - specified site NEC S00.82 ☑
  - heel — *see* Blister, foot
  - hip S70.22- ☑
  - interscapular region S20.429 ☑
  - jaw S00.82 ☑
  - knee S80.22- ☑
  - larynx S10.12 ☑
  - leg (lower) S80.82- ☑
    - knee — *see* Blister, knee
    - upper — *see* Blister, thigh
  - lip S00.521 ☑
  - malar region S00.82 ☑
  - mammary — *see* Blister, breast
  - mastoid region S00.82 ☑
  - mouth S00.522 ☑
  - multiple, skin, nontraumatic R23.8
  - nail
    - finger — *see* Blister, finger
    - toe — *see* Blister, toe
  - nasal S00.32 ☑
  - neck S10.92 ☑
    - specified site NEC S10.82 ☑
- **Blister** — *continued*
  - neck — *continued*
    - throat S10.12 ☑
  - nose S00.32 ☑
  - occipital region S00.02 ☑
  - oral cavity S00.522 ☑
  - orbital region — *see* Blister, eyelid
  - palate S00.522 ☑
  - palm — *see* Blister, hand
  - parietal region S00.02 ☑
  - pelvis S30.820 ☑
  - penis S30.822 ☑
  - periocular area — *see* Blister, eyelid
  - phalanges
    - finger — *see* Blister, finger
    - toe — *see* Blister, toe
  - pharynx S10.12 ☑
  - pinna — *see* Blister, ear
  - popliteal space — *see* Blister, knee
  - scalp S00.02 ☑
  - scapular region — *see* Blister, shoulder
  - scrotum S30.823 ☑
  - shin — *see* Blister, leg
  - shoulder S40.22- ☑
  - sternal region S20.329 ☑
  - submaxillary region S00.82 ☑
  - submental region S00.82 ☑
  - subungual
    - finger(s) — *see* Blister, finger
    - toe(s) — *see* Blister, toe
  - supraclavicular fossa S10.82 ☑
  - supraorbital S00.82 ☑
  - temple S00.82 ☑
  - temporal region S00.82 ☑
  - testis S30.823 ☑
  - thermal — *see* Burn, second degree, by site
  - thigh S70.32- ☑
  - thorax, thoracic (wall) S20.92 ☑
    - back S20.42- ☑
    - front S20.32- ☑
  - throat S10.12 ☑
  - thumb S60.32- ☑
  - toe(s) S90.42- ☑
    - great S90.42- ☑
  - tongue S00.522 ☑
  - trachea S10.12 ☑
  - tympanum, tympanic membrane — *see* Blister, ear
  - upper arm — *see* Blister, arm (upper)
  - uvula S00.522 ☑
  - vagina S30.824 ☑
  - vocal cords S10.12 ☑
  - vulva S30.824 ☑
  - wrist S60.82- ☑
- **Bloating** R14.0
- **Bloch-Sulzberger disease or syndrome** Q82.3
- **Block, blocked**
  - alveolocapillary J84.10
  - arborization (heart) I45.5
  - arrhythmic I45.9
  - atrioventricular (incomplete) (partial) I44.30
    - with atrioventricular dissociation I44.2
    - complete I44.2
      - congenital Q24.6
    - congenital Q24.6
    - first degree I44.0
    - second degree (types I and II) I44.1
    - specified NEC I44.39
    - third degree I44.2
    - types I and II I44.1
  - auriculoventricular — *see* Block, atrioventricular
  - bifascicular (cardiac) I45.2
  - bundle-branch (complete) (false) (incomplete) I45.4
    - bilateral I45.2
    - left I44.7
      - with right bundle branch block I45.2
      - hemiblock I44.60
        - anterior I44.4
        - posterior I44.5
      - incomplete I44.7
        - with right bundle branch block I45.2
    - right I45.10
      - with
        - left bundle branch block I45.2
        - left fascicular block I45.2
      - specified NEC I45.19
    - Wilson's type I45.19
  - cardiac I45.9

- **Block, blocked** — *continued*
  - conduction I45.9
    - complete I44.2
  - fascicular (left) I44.6Ø
    - anterior I44.4
    - posterior I44.5
    - right I45.Ø
    - specified NEC I44.69
  - foramen Magendie (acquired) G91.1
    - congenital QØ3.1
      - with spina bifida — *see* Spina bifida, by site, with hydrocephalus
  - heart I45.9
    - bundle branch I45.4
      - bilateral I45.2
    - complete (atrioventricular) I44.2
    - congenital Q24.6
    - first degree (atrioventricular) I44.Ø
    - second degree (atrioventricular) I44.1
    - specified type NEC I45.5
    - third degree (atrioventricular) I44.2
  - hepatic vein I82.Ø
  - intraventricular (nonspecific) I45.4
    - bundle branch
      - bilateral I45.2
  - kidney N28.9
    - postcystoscopic or postprocedural N99.Ø
  - Mobitz (types I and II) I44.1
  - myocardial — *see* Block, heart
  - nodal I45.5
  - organ or site, congenital NEC — *see* Atresia, by site
  - portal (vein) I81
  - second degree (types I and II) I44.1
  - sinoatrial I45.5
  - sinoauricular I45.5
  - third degree I44.2
  - trifascicular I45.3
  - tubal N97.1
  - vein NOS I82.9Ø
  - Wenckebach (types I and II) I44.1
- **Blockage** — *see* Obstruction
- **Blocq's disease** F44.4
- **Blood**
  - constituents, abnormal R78.9
  - disease D75.9
  - donor — *see* Donor, blood
  - dyscrasia D75.9
    - with
      - abortion — *see* Abortion, by type, complicated by, hemorrhage
      - ectopic pregnancy OØ8.1
      - molar pregnancy OØ8.1
    - following ectopic or molar pregnancy OØ8.1
    - newborn P61.9
    - puerperal, postpartum O72.3
  - flukes NEC — *see* Schistosomiasis
  - in
    - feces K92.1
      - occult R19.5
    - urine — *see* Hematuria
  - mole OØ2.Ø
  - occult in feces R19.5
  - pressure
    - decreased, due to shock following injury T79.4 ☑
    - examination only ZØ1.3Ø
    - fluctuating I99.8
    - high — *see* Hypertension
      - borderline RØ3.Ø
      - incidental reading, without diagnosis of hypertension RØ3.Ø
    - low (*see also* Hypotension)
      - incidental reading, without diagnosis of hypotension RØ3.1
  - spitting — *see* Hemoptysis
  - staining cornea — *see* Pigmentation, cornea, stromal
  - transfusion
    - reaction or complication — *see* Complications, transfusion
  - type
    - A (Rh positive) Z67.1Ø
      - Rh negative Z67.11
    - AB (Rh positive) Z67.3Ø
      - Rh negative Z67.31
    - B (Rh positive) Z67.2Ø
      - Rh negative Z67.21
    - O (Rh positive) Z67.4Ø
      - Rh negative Z67.41
    - Rh (positive) Z67.9Ø
- **Blood** — *continued*
  - type — *continued*
    - Rh — *continued*
      - negative Z67.91
  - vessel rupture — *see* Hemorrhage
  - vomiting — *see* Hematemesis
- **Blood-forming organs, disease** D75.9
- **Bloodgood's disease** — *see* Mastopathy, cystic
- **Bloom** (-Machacek)(-Torre) **syndrome** Q82.8
- **Blount's disease or osteochondrosis** — *see* Osteochondrosis, juvenile, tibia
- **Blue**
  - baby Q24.9
  - diaper syndrome E72.Ø9
  - dome cyst (breast) — *see* Cyst, breast
  - dot cataract Q12.Ø
  - nevus D22.9
  - sclera Q13.5
    - with fragility of bone and deafness Q78.Ø
  - toe syndrome I75.Ø2- ☑
- **Blueness** — *see* Cyanosis
- **Blues, postpartal** O9Ø.6
  - baby O9Ø.6
- **Blurring, visual** H53.8
- **Blushing** (abnormal) (excessive) R23.2
- **BMI** — *see* Body, mass index
- **Boarder, hospital NEC** Z76.4
  - accompanying sick person Z76.3
  - healthy infant or child Z76.2
    - foundling Z76.1
- **Bockhart's impetigo** LØ1.Ø2
- **Bodechtel-Guttman disease** (subacute sclerosing panencephalitis) A81.1
- **Boder-Sedgwick syndrome** (ataxia-telangiectasia) G11.3
- **Body, bodies**
  - Aschoff's — *see* Myocarditis, rheumatic
  - asteroid, vitreous — *see* Deposit, crystalline
  - cytoid (retina) — *see* Occlusion, artery, retina
  - drusen (degenerative) (macula) (retinal) (*see also* Degeneration, macula, drusen)
    - optic disc — *see* Drusen, optic disc
  - foreign — *see* Foreign body
  - loose
    - joint, except knee — *see* Loose, body, joint
      - knee M23.4- ☑
    - sheath, tendon — *see* Disorder, tendon, specified type NEC
  - mass index (BMI)
    - adult
      - 19 or less Z68.1
      - 2Ø.Ø-2Ø.9 Z68.2Ø
      - 21.Ø-21.9 Z68.21
      - 22.Ø-22.9 Z68.22
      - 23.Ø-23.9 Z68.23
      - 24.Ø-24.9 Z68.24
      - 25.Ø-25.9 Z68.25
      - 26.Ø-26.9 Z68.26
      - 27.Ø-27.9 Z68.27
      - 28.Ø-28.9 Z68.28
      - 29.Ø-29.9 Z68.29
      - 3Ø.Ø-3Ø.9 Z68.3Ø
      - 31.Ø-31.9 Z68.31
      - 32.Ø-32.9 Z68.32
      - 33.Ø-33.9 Z68.33
      - 34.Ø-34.9 Z68.34
      - 35.Ø-35.9 Z68.35
      - 36.Ø-36.9 Z68.36
      - 37.Ø-37.9 Z68.37
      - 38.Ø-38.9 Z68.38
      - 39.Ø-39.9 Z68.39
      - 4Ø.Ø-44.9 Z68.41
      - 45.Ø-49.9 Z68.42
      - 5Ø.Ø-59.9 Z68.43
      - 6Ø.Ø-69.9 Z68.44
      - 7Ø and over Z68.45
    - pediatric
      - 5th percentile to less than 85th percentile for age Z68.52
      - 85th percentile to less than 95th percentile for age Z68.53
      - less than fifth percentile for age Z68.51
      - greater than or equal to ninety-fifth percentile for age Z68.54
  - Mooser's A75.2
  - rice (*see also* Loose, body, joint)
    - knee M23.4- ☑
  - rocking F98.4
- **Boeck's**
  - disease or sarcoid — *see* Sarcoidosis
  - lupoid (miliary) D86.3
- **Boerhaave's syndrome** (spontaneous esophageal rupture) K22.3
- **Boggy**
  - cervix N88.8
  - uterus N85.8
- **Boil** (*see also* Furuncle, by site)
  - Aleppo B55.1
  - Baghdad B55.1
  - Delhi B55.1
  - lacrimal
    - gland — *see* Dacryoadenitis
    - passages (duct) (sac) — *see* Inflammation, lacrimal, passages, acute
  - Natal B55.1
  - orbit, orbital — *see* Abscess, orbit
  - tropical B55.1
- **Bold hives** — *see* Urticaria
- **Bombé, iris** — *see* Membrane, pupillary
- **Bone** — *see* condition
- **Bonnevie-Ullrich syndrome** Q87.1
- **Bonnier's syndrome** H81.8 ☑
- **Bonvale dam fever** T73.3 ☑
- **Bony block of joint** — *see* Ankylosis
- **BOOP** (bronchiolitis obliterans organized pneumonia) J84.89
- **Borderline**
  - diabetes mellitus R73.Ø9
  - hypertension RØ3.Ø
  - osteopenia M85.8- ☑
  - pelvis, with obstruction during labor O65.1
  - personality F6Ø.3
- **Borna disease** A83.9
- **Bornholm disease** B33.Ø
- **Boston exanthem** A88.Ø
- **Botalli, ductus** (patent) (persistent) Q25.Ø
- **Bothriocephalus latus infestation** B7Ø.Ø
- **Botulism** (foodborne intoxication) AØ5.1
  - infant A48.51
  - non-foodborne A48.52
  - wound A48.52
- **Bouba** — *see* Yaws
- **Bouchard's nodes** (with arthropathy) M15.2
- **Bouffée délirante** F23
- **Bouillaud's disease or syndrome** (rheumatic heart disease) IØ1.9
- **Bourneville's disease** Q85.1
- **Boutonniere deformity** (finger) — *see* Deformity, finger, boutonniere
- **Bouveret** (-Hoffmann) **syndrome** (paroxysmal tachycardia) I47.9
- **Bovine heart** — *see* Hypertrophy, cardiac
- **Bowel** — *see* condition
- **Bowen's**
  - dermatosis (precancerous) — *see* Neoplasm, skin, in situ
  - disease — *see* Neoplasm, skin, in situ
  - epithelioma — *see* Neoplasm, skin, in situ
  - type
    - epidermoid carcinoma-in-situ — *see* Neoplasm, skin, in situ
    - intraepidermal squamous cell carcinoma — *see* Neoplasm, skin, in situ
- **Bowing**
  - femur (*see also* Deformity, limb, specified type NEC, thigh)
    - congenital Q68.3
  - fibula (*see also* Deformity, limb, specified type NEC, lower leg)
    - congenital Q68.4
  - forearm — *see* Deformity, limb, specified type NEC, forearm
  - leg(s), long bones, congenital Q68.5
  - radius — *see* Deformity, limb, specified type NEC, forearm
  - tibia (*see also* Deformity, limb, specified type NEC, lower leg)
    - congenital Q68.4
- **Bowleg**(s) (acquired) M21.16- ☑
  - congenital Q68.5
  - rachitic E64.3
- **Boyd's dysentery** AØ3.2
- **Brachial** — *see* condition
- **Brachycardia** RØØ.1
- **Brachycephaly** Q75.Ø

Bradley's disease A08.19
Bradyarrhythmia, cardiac I49.8
Bradycardia (sinoatrial) (sinus) (vagal) R00.1
- neonatal P29.12
- reflex G90.09
- tachycardia syndrome I49.5

Bradykinesia R25.8
Bradypnea R06.89
Bradytachycardia I49.5
Brailsford's disease or osteochondrosis — *see* Osteochondrosis, juvenile, radius
Brain (*see also* condition)
- death G93.82
- syndrome — *see* Syndrome, brain

Branched-chain amino-acid disorder E71.2
Branchial — *see* condition
- cartilage, congenital Q18.2

Branchiogenic remnant (in neck) Q18.0
Brandt's syndrome (acrodermatitis enteropathica) E83.2
Brash (water) R12
Bravais-jacksonian epilepsy — *see* Epilepsy, localization-related, symptomatic, with simple partial seizures
Braxton Hicks contractions — *see* False, labor
Brazilian leishmaniasis B55.2
BRBPR K62.5
Break, retina (without detachment) H33.30- ☑
- with retinal detachment — *see* Detachment, retina
- horseshoe tear H33.31- ☑
- multiple H33.33- ☑
- round hole H33.32- ☑

Breakdown
- device, graft or implant (*see also* Complications, by site and type, mechanical) T85.618 ☑
  - arterial graft NEC — *see* Complication, cardiovascular device, mechanical, vascular
  - breast (implant) T85.41 ☑
  - catheter NEC T85.618 ☑
    - cystostomy T83.010 ☑
    - dialysis (renal) T82.41 ☑
      - intraperitoneal T85.611 ☑
    - infusion NEC T82.514 ☑
      - spinal (epidural) (subdural) T85.610 ☑
    - urinary (indwelling) T83.018 ☑
  - electronic (electrode) (pulse generator) (stimulator)
    - bone T84.310 ☑
    - cardiac T82.119 ☑
      - electrode T82.110 ☑
      - pulse generator T82.111 ☑
      - specified type NEC T82.118 ☑
    - nervous system — *see* Complication, prosthetic device, mechanical, electronic nervous system stimulator
    - urinary — *see* Complication, genitourinary, device, urinary, mechanical
  - fixation, internal (orthopedic) NEC — *see* Complication, fixation device, mechanical
  - gastrointestinal — *see* Complications, prosthetic device, mechanical, gastrointestinal device
  - genital NEC T83.418 ☑
    - intrauterine contraceptive device T83.31 ☑
    - penile prosthesis T83.410 ☑
  - heart NEC — *see* Complication, cardiovascular device, mechanical
  - joint prosthesis — *see* Complications..., joint prosthesis,internal, mechanical, by site
  - ocular NEC — *see* Complications, prosthetic device, mechanical, ocular device
  - orthopedic NEC — *see* Complication, orthopedic, device, mechanical
  - specified NEC T85.618 ☑
  - sutures, permanent T85.612 ☑
    - used in bone repair — *see* Complications, fixation device, internal (orthopedic), mechanical
  - urinary NEC (*see also* Complication, genitourinary, device, urinary, mechanical)
    - graft T83.21 ☑
  - vascular NEC — *see* Complication, cardiovascular device, mechanical
  - ventricular intracranial shunt T85.01 ☑
- nervous F48.8
- perineum O90.1
- respirator J95.850
  - specified NEC J95.859
- ventilator J95.850

Breakdown — *continued*
- ventilator — *continued*
  - specified NEC J95.859

Breast (*see also* condition)
- buds E30.1
  - in newborn P96.89
- dense R92.2
- nodule N63

Breath
- foul R19.6
- holder, child R06.89
- holding spell R06.89
- shortness R06.02

Breathing
- labored — *see* Hyperventilation
- mouth R06.5
  - causing malocclusion M26.5 ☑
- periodic R06.3
  - high altitude G47.32

Breathlessness R06.81
Breda's disease — *see* Yaws
Breech presentation (mother) O32.1 ☑
- causing obstructed labor O64.1 ☑
- footling O32.8 ☑
  - causing obstructed labor O64.8 ☑
- incomplete O32.8 ☑
  - causing obstructed labor O64.8 ☑

Breisky's disease N90.4
Brennemann's syndrome I88.0
Brenner
- tumor (benign) D27.9
  - borderline malignancy D39.1- ☑
  - malignant C56 ☑
  - proliferating D39.1- ☑

Bretonneau's disease or angina A36.0
Breus' mole O02.0
Brevicollis Q76.49
Brickmakers' anemia B76.9 [D63.8]
Bridge, myocardial Q24.5
Bright red blood per rectum (BRBPR) K62.5
Bright's disease (*see also* Nephritis)
- arteriosclerotic — *see* Hypertension, kidney

Brill (-Zinsser) **disease** (recrudescent typhus) A75.1
- flea-borne A75.2
- louse-borne A75.1

Brill-Symmers' disease C82.90
Brion-Kayser disease — *see* Fever, parathyroid
Briquet's disorder or syndrome F45.0
Brissaud's
- infantilism or dwarfism E23.0
- motor-verbal tic F95.2

Brittle
- bones disease Q78.0
- nails L60.3
  - congenital Q84.6

Broad (*see also* condition)
- beta disease E78.2
- ligament laceration syndrome N83.8

Broad- or floating-betalipoproteinemia E78.2
Brock's syndrome (atelectasis due to enlarged lymph nodes) J98.19
Brocq-Duhring disease (dermatitis herpetiformis) L13.0
Brodie's abscess or disease M86.8X- ☑
Broken
- arches (*see also* Deformity, limb, flat foot)
- arm (meaning upper limb) — *see* Fracture, arm
- back — *see* Fracture, vertebra
- bone — *see* Fracture
- implant or internal device — *see* Complications, by site and type, mechanical
- leg (meaning lower limb) — *see* Fracture, leg
- nose S02.2 ☑
- tooth, teeth — *see* Fracture, tooth

Bromhidrosis, bromidrosis L75.0
Bromidism, bromism G92
- chronic (dependence) F13.20
- due to
  - correct substance properly administered — *see* Table of Drugs and Chemicals, by drug, adverse effect
  - overdose or wrong substance given or taken — *see* Table of Drugs and Chemicals, by drug, poisoning

Bromidrosiphobia F40.298
Bronchi, bronchial — *see* condition
Bronchiectasis (cylindrical) (diffuse) (fusiform) (localized) (saccular) J47.9

Bronchiectasis — *continued*
- with
  - acute
    - bronchitis J47.0
    - lower respiratory infection J47.0
  - exacerbation (acute) J47.1
- congenital Q33.4
- tuberculous NEC — *see* Tuberculosis, pulmonary

Bronchiolectasis — *see* Bronchiectasis
Bronchiolitis (acute) (infective) (subacute) J21.9
- with
  - bronchospasm or obstruction J21.9
  - influenza, flu or grippe — *see* Influenza, with, respiratory manifestations NEC
- chemical (chronic) J68.4
  - acute J68.0
- chronic (fibrosing) (obliterative) J44.9
- due to
  - external agent — *see* Bronchitis, acute, due to
  - human metapneumovirus J21.1
  - respiratory syncytial virus J21.0
  - specified organism NEC J21.8
- fibrosa obliterans J44.9
- influenzal — *see* Influenza, with, respiratory manifestations NEC
- obliterans J42
  - with organizing pneumonia (BOOP) J84.89
- obliterative (chronic) (subacute) J44.9
  - due to chemicals, gases, fumes or vapors (inhalation) J68.4
  - due to fumes or vapors J68.4
- respiratory, interstitial lung disease J84.115

Bronchitis (diffuse) (fibrinous) (hypostatic) (infective) (membranous) J40
- with
  - influenza, flu or grippe — *see* Influenza, with, respiratory manifestations NEC
  - obstruction (airway) (lung) J44.9
  - tracheitis (15 years of age and above) J40
    - acute or subacute J20.9
    - chronic J42
    - under 15 years of age J20.9
- acute or subacute (with bronchospasm or obstruction) J20.9
  - with
    - bronchiectasis J47.0
    - chronic obstructive pulmonary disease J44.0
  - chemical (due to gases, fumes or vapors) J68.0
  - due to
    - fumes or vapors J68.0
    - Haemophilus influenzae J20.1
    - Mycoplasma pneumoniae J20.0
    - radiation J70.0
    - specified organism NEC J20.8
    - Streptococcus J20.2
    - virus
      - coxsackie J20.3
      - echovirus J20.7
      - parainfluenzae J20.4
      - respiratory syncytial J20.5
      - rhinovirus J20.6
  - viral NEC J20.8
- allergic (acute) J45.909
  - with
    - exacerbation (acute) J45.901
    - status asthmaticus J45.902
- arachidic T17.528 ☑
- aspiration (due to fumes or vapors) J68.0
- asthmatic J45.9 ☑
  - chronic J44.9
    - with
      - acute lower respiratory infection J44.0
      - exacerbation (acute) J44.1
- capillary — *see* Pneumonia, broncho
- caseous (tuberculous) A15.5
- Castellani's A69.8
- catarrhal (15 years of age and above) J40
  - acute — *see* Bronchitis, acute
  - chronic J41.0
  - under 15 years of age J20.9
- chemical (acute) (subacute) J68.0
  - chronic J68.4
  - due to fumes or vapors J68.0
    - chronic J68.4
- chronic J42
  - with
    - airways obstruction J44.9
    - tracheitis (chronic) J42

Bronchitis — *continued*
- chronic — *continued*
  - asthmatic (obstructive) J44.9
  - catarrhal J41.Ø
  - chemical (due to fumes or vapors) J68.4
  - due to
    - chemicals, gases, fumes or vapors (inhalation) J68.4
    - radiation J7Ø.1
    - tobacco smoking J41.Ø
  - emphysematous J44.9
  - mucopurulent J41.1
  - non-obstructive J41.Ø
  - obliterans J44.9
  - obstructive J44.9
  - purulent J41.1
  - simple J41.Ø
- croupous — *see* Bronchitis, acute
- due to gases, fumes or vapors (chemical) J68.Ø
- emphysematous (obstructive) J44.9
- exudative — *see* Bronchitis, acute
- fetid J41.1
- grippal — *see* Influenza, with, respiratory manifestations NEC
- in those under 15 years age — *see* Bronchitis, acute
  - chronic — *see* Bronchitis, chronic
- influenzal — *see* Influenza, with, respiratory manifestations NEC
- mixed simple and mucopurulent J41.8
- moulder's J62.8
- mucopurulent (chronic) (recurrent) J41.1
  - acute or subacute J2Ø.9
  - simple (mixed) J41.8
- obliterans (chronic) J44.9
- obstructive (chronic) (diffuse) J44.9
- pituitous J41.1
- pneumococcal, acute or subacute J2Ø.2
- pseudomembranous, acute or subacute — *see* Bronchitis, acute
- purulent (chronic) (recurrent) J41.1
  - acute or subacute — *see* Bronchitis, acute
- putrid J41.1
- senile (chronic) J42
- simple and mucopurulent (mixed) J41.8
- smokers' J41.Ø
- spirochetal NEC A69.8
- subacute — *see* Bronchitis, acute
- suppurative (chronic) J41.1
  - acute or subacute — *see* Bronchitis, acute
- tuberculous A15.5
- under 15 years of age — *see* Bronchitis, acute
  - chronic — *see* Bronchitis, chronic
- viral NEC, acute or subacute (*see also* Bronchitis, acute) J2Ø.8

Bronchoalveolitis J18.Ø

Bronchoaspergillosis B44.1

Bronchocele meaning goiter EØ4.Ø

Broncholithiasis J98.Ø9
- tuberculous NEC A15.5

Bronchomalacia J98.Ø9
- congenital Q32.2

Bronchomycosis NOS B49 [J99]
- candidal B37.1

Bronchopleuropneumonia — *see* Pneumonia, broncho

Bronchopneumonia — *see* Pneumonia, broncho

Bronchopneumonitis — *see* Pneumonia, broncho

Bronchopulmonary — *see* condition

Bronchopulmonitis — *see* Pneumonia, broncho

Bronchorrhagia (see Hemoptysis)

Bronchorrhea J98.Ø9
- acute J2Ø.9
- chronic (infective) (purulent) J42

Bronchospasm (acute) J98.Ø1
- with
  - bronchiolitis, acute J21.9
  - bronchitis, acute (conditions in J2Ø) — *see* Bronchitis, acute
- due to external agent — *see* condition, respiratory, acute, due to
- exercise induced J45.99Ø

Bronchospirochetosis A69.8
- Castellani A69.8

Bronchostenosis J98.Ø9

Bronchus — *see* condition

Brontophobia F4Ø.22Ø

Bronze baby syndrome P83.8

Brooke's tumor — *see* Neoplasm, skin, benign

Brown enamel of teeth (hereditary) KØØ.5

Brown's sheath syndrome H5Ø.61- ☑

Brown-Séquard disease, paralysis or syndrome G83.81

Bruce sepsis A23.Ø

Brucellosis (infection) A23.9
- abortus A23.1
- canis A23.3
- dermatitis A23.9
- melitensis A23.Ø
- mixed A23.8
- sepsis A23.9
  - melitensis A23.Ø
  - specified NEC A23.8
- suis A23.2

Bruck-de Lange disease Q87.1

Bruck's disease — *see* Deformity, limb

Brugsch's syndrome Q82.8

Bruise (skin surface intact) (*see also* Contusion)
- with
  - open wound — *see* Wound, open
- internal organ — *see* Injury, by site
- newborn P54.5
- scalp, due to birth injury, newborn P12.3
- umbilical cord O69.5 ☑

Bruit (arterial) RØ9.89
- cardiac RØ1.1

Brush burn — *see* Abrasion, by site

Bruton's X-linked agammaglobulinemia D8Ø.Ø

Bruxism
- psychogenic F45.8
- sleep related G47.63

Bubbly lung syndrome P27.Ø

Bubo I88.8
- blennorrhagic (gonococcal) A54.89
- chancroidal A57
- climatic A55
- due to Haemophilus ducreyi A57
- gonococcal A54.89
- indolent (nonspecific) I88.8
- inguinal (nonspecific) I88.8
  - chancroidal A57
  - climatic A55
  - due to H. ducreyi A57
  - infective I88.8
- scrofulous (tuberculous) A18.2
- soft chancre A57
- suppurating — *see* Lymphadenitis, acute
- syphilitic (primary) A51.Ø
  - congenital A5Ø.Ø7
- tropical A55
- virulent (chancroidal) A57

Bubonic plague A2Ø.Ø

Bubonocele — *see* Hernia, inguinal

Buccal — *see* condition

Buchanan's disease or osteochondrosis M91.Ø

Buchem's syndrome (hyperostosis corticalis) M85.2

Bucket-handle fracture or tear (semilunar cartilage) — *see* Tear, meniscus

Budd-Chiari syndrome (hepatic vein thrombosis) I82.Ø

Budgerigar fancier's disease or lung J67.2

Buds
- breast E3Ø.1
  - in newborn P96.89

Buerger's disease (thromboangiitis obliterans) I73.1

Bulbar — *see* condition

Bulbus cordis (left ventricle) (persistent) Q21.8

Bulimia (nervosa) F5Ø.2
- atypical F5Ø.9
- normal weight F5Ø.9

Bulky
- stools R19.5
- uterus N85.2

Bulla (e) R23.8
- lung (emphysematous) (solitary) J43.9
  - newborn P25.8

Bullet wound (*see also* Wound, open)
- fracture — *code as* Fracture, by site
- internal organ — *see* Injury, by site

Bundle
- branch block (complete) (false) (incomplete) — *see* Block, bundle-branch
- of His — *see* condition

Bunion — *see* Deformity, toe, hallux valgus

Buphthalmia, buphthalmos (congenital) Q15.Ø

Burdwan fever B55.Ø

Bürger-Grütz disease or syndrome E78.3

Buried
- penis (congenital) Q55.64
  - acquired N48.83
- roots KØ8.3

Burke's syndrome K86.8

Burkitt
- cell leukemia C91.Ø- ☑
- lymphoma (malignant) C83.7- ☑
  - small noncleaved, diffuse C83.7- ☑
  - spleen C83.77
  - undifferentiated C83.7- ☑
- tumor C83.7- ☑
- type
  - acute lymphoblastic leukemia C91.Ø- ☑
  - undifferentiated C83.7- ☑

Burn (electricity) (flame) (hot gas, liquid or hot object) (radiation) (steam) (thermal) T3Ø.Ø
- abdomen, abdominal (muscle) (wall) T21.Ø2 ☑
  - first degree T21.12 ☑
  - second degree T21.22 ☑
  - third degree T21.32 ☑
- above elbow T22.Ø39 ☑
  - first degree T22.139 ☑
  - left T22.Ø32 ☑
    - first degree T22.132 ☑
    - second degree T22.232 ☑
    - third degree T22.332 ☑
  - right T22.Ø31 ☑
    - first degree T22.131 ☑
    - second degree T22.231 ☑
    - third degree T22.331 ☑
  - second degree T22.239 ☑
  - third degree T22.339 ☑
- acid (caustic) (external) (internal) — *see* Corrosion, by site
- alimentary tract NEC T28.2 ☑
  - esophagus T28.1 ☑
  - mouth T28.Ø ☑
  - pharynx T28.Ø ☑
- alkaline (caustic) (external) (internal) — *see* Corrosion, by site
- ankle T25.Ø19 ☑
  - first degree T25.119 ☑
  - left T25.Ø12 ☑
    - first degree T25.112 ☑
    - second degree T25.212 ☑
    - third degree T25.312 ☑
  - multiple with foot — *see* Burn, lower, limb, multiple, ankle and foot
  - right T25.Ø11 ☑
    - first degree T25.111 ☑
    - second degree T25.211 ☑
    - third degree T25.311 ☑
  - second degree T25.219 ☑
  - third degree T25.319 ☑
- anus — *see* Burn, buttock
- arm (lower) (upper) — *see* Burn, upper, limb
- axilla T22.Ø49 ☑
  - first degree T22.149 ☑
  - left T22.Ø42 ☑
    - first degree T22.142 ☑
    - second degree T22.242 ☑
    - third degree T22.342 ☑
  - right T22.Ø41 ☑
    - first degree T22.141 ☑
    - second degree T22.241 ☑
    - third degree T22.341 ☑
  - second degree T22.249 ☑
  - third degree T22.349 ☑
- back (lower) T21.Ø4 ☑
  - first degree T21.14 ☑
  - second degree T21.24 ☑
  - third degree T21.34 ☑
  - upper T21.Ø3 ☑
    - first degree T21.13 ☑
    - second degree T21.23 ☑
    - third degree T21.33 ☑
- blisters — *code as* Burn, second degree, by site
- breast(s) — *see* Burn, chest wall
- buttock(s) T21.Ø5 ☑
  - first degree T21.15 ☑
  - second degree T21.25 ☑
  - third degree T21.35 ☑
- calf T24.Ø39 ☑
  - first degree T24.139 ☑
  - left T24.Ø32 ☑

- **Burn** — *continued*
  - calf — *continued*
    - left — *continued*
      - first degree T24.132 ☑
      - second degree T24.232 ☑
      - third degree T24.332 ☑
    - right T24.031 ☑
      - first degree T24.131 ☑
      - second degree T24.231 ☑
      - third degree T24.331 ☑
    - second degree T24.239 ☑
    - third degree T24.339 ☑
  - canthus (eye) — *see* Burn, eyelid
  - caustic acid or alkaline — *see* Corrosion, by site
  - cervix T28.3 ☑
  - cheek T20.06 ☑
    - first degree T20.16 ☑
    - second degree T20.26 ☑
    - third degree T20.36 ☑
  - chemical (acids) (alkalines) (caustics) (external) (internal) — *see* Corrosion, by site
  - chest wall T21.01 ☑
    - first degree T21.11 ☑
    - second degree T21.21 ☑
    - third degree T21.31 ☑
  - chin T20.03 ☑
    - first degree T20.13 ☑
    - second degree T20.23 ☑
    - third degree T20.33 ☑
  - colon T28.2 ☑
  - conjunctiva (and cornea) — *see* Burn, cornea
  - cornea (and conjunctiva) T26.1- ☑
    - chemical — *see* Corrosion, cornea
  - corrosion (external) (internal) — *see* Corrosion, by site
  - deep necrosis of underlying tissue — *code as* Burn, third degree, by site
  - dorsum of hand T23.069 ☑
    - first degree T23.169 ☑
    - left T23.062 ☑
      - first degree T23.162 ☑
      - second degree T23.262 ☑
      - third degree T23.362 ☑
    - right T23.061 ☑
      - first degree T23.161 ☑
      - second degree T23.261 ☑
      - third degree T23.361 ☑
    - second degree T23.269 ☑
    - third degree T23.369 ☑
  - due to ingested chemical agent — *see* Corrosion, by site
  - ear (auricle) (external) (canal) T20.01 ☑
    - first degree T20.11 ☑
    - second degree T20.21 ☑
    - third degree T20.31 ☑
  - elbow T22.029 ☑
    - first degree T22.129 ☑
    - left T22.022 ☑
      - first degree T22.122 ☑
      - second degree T22.222 ☑
      - third degree T22.322 ☑
    - right T22.021 ☑
      - first degree T22.121 ☑
      - second degree T22.221 ☑
      - third degree T22.321 ☑
    - second degree T22.229 ☑
    - third degree T22.329 ☑
  - epidermal loss — *code as* Burn, second degree, by site
  - erythema, erythematous — *code as* Burn, first degree, by site
  - esophagus T28.1 ☑
  - extent (percentage of body surface)
    - less than 10 percent T31.0
    - 10-19 percent T31.10
      - with 0-9 percent third degree burns T31.10
      - with 10-19 percent third degree burns T31.11
    - 20-29 percent T31.20
      - with 0-9 percent third degree burns T31.20
      - with 10-19 percent third degree burns T31.21
      - with 20-29 percent third degree burns T31.22
    - 30-39 percent T31.30
      - with 0-9 percent third degree burns T31.30
      - with 10-19 percent third degree burns T31.31
      - with 20-29 percent third degree burns T31.32
      - with 30-39 percent third degree burns T31.33
    - 40-49 percent T31.40
      - with 0-9 percent third degree burns T31.40

- **Burn** — *continued*
  - extent — *continued*
    - 40-49 percent — *continued*
      - with 10-19 percent third degree burns T31.41
      - with 20-29 percent third degree burns T31.42
      - with 30-39 percent third degree burns T31.43
      - with 40-49 percent third degree burns T31.44
    - 50-59 percent T31.50
      - with 0-9 percent third degree burns T31.50
      - with 10-19 percent third degree burns T31.51
      - with 20-29 percent third degree burns T31.52
      - with 30-39 percent third degree burns T31.53
      - with 40-49 percent third degree burns T31.54
      - with 50-59 percent third degree burns T31.55
    - 60-69 percent T31.60
      - with 0-9 percent third degree burns T31.60
      - with 10-19 percent third degree burns T31.61
      - with 20-29 percent third degree burns T31.62
      - with 30-39 percent third degree burns T31.63
      - with 40-49 percent third degree burns T31.64
      - with 50-59 percent third degree burns T31.65
      - with 60-69 percent third degree burns T31.66
    - 70-79 percent T31.70
      - with 0-9 percent third degree burns T31.70
      - with 10-19 percent third degree burns T31.71
      - with 20-29 percent third degree burns T31.72
      - with 30-39 percent third degree burns T31.73
      - with 40-49 percent third degree burns T31.74
      - with 50-59 percent third degree burns T31.75
      - with 60-69 percent third degree burns T31.76
      - with 70-79 percent third degree burns T31.77
    - 80-89 percent T31.80
      - with 0-9 percent third degree burns T31.80
      - with 10-19 percent third degree burns T31.81
      - with 20-29 percent third degree burns T31.82
      - with 30-39 percent third degree burns T31.83
      - with 40-49 percent third degree burns T31.84
      - with 50-59 percent third degree burns T31.85
      - with 60-69 percent third degree burns T31.86
      - with 70-79 percent third degree burns T31.87
      - with 80-89 percent third degree burns T31.88
    - 90 percent or more T31.90
      - with 0-9 percent third degree burns T31.90
      - with 10-19 percent third degree burns T31.91
      - with 20-29 percent third degree burns T31.92
      - with 30-39 percent third degree burns T31.93
      - with 40-49 percent third degree burns T31.94
      - with 50-59 percent third degree burns T31.95
      - with 60-69 percent third degree burns T31.96
      - with 70-79 percent third degree burns T31.97
      - with 80-89 percent third degree burns T31.98
      - with 90 percent or more third degree burns T31.99
  - extremity — *see* Burn, limb
  - eye(s) and adnexa T26.4- ☑
    - with resulting rupture and destruction of eyeball T26.2- ☑
    - conjunctival sac — *see* Burn, cornea
    - cornea — *see* Burn, cornea
    - lid — *see* Burn, eyelid
    - periocular area — *see* Burn, eyelid
    - specified site NEC T26.3- ☑
  - eyeball — *see* Burn, eye
  - eyelid(s) T26.0- ☑
    - chemical — *see* Corrosion, eyelid
  - face — *see* Burn, head
  - finger T23.029 ☑
    - first degree T23.129 ☑
    - left T23.022 ☑
      - first degree T23.122 ☑
      - second degree T23.222 ☑
      - third degree T23.322 ☑
    - multiple sites (without thumb) T23.039 ☑
      - with thumb T23.049 ☑
        - first degree T23.149 ☑
        - left T23.042 ☑
          - first degree T23.142 ☑
          - second degree T23.242 ☑
          - third degree T23.342 ☑
        - right T23.041 ☑
          - first degree T23.141 ☑
          - second degree T23.241 ☑
          - third degree T23.341 ☑
        - second degree T23.249 ☑
        - third degree T23.349 ☑
      - first degree T23.139 ☑
      - left T23.032 ☑

- **Burn** — *continued*
  - finger — *continued*
    - multiple sites — *continued*
      - left — *continued*
        - first degree T23.132 ☑
        - second degree T23.232 ☑
        - third degree T23.332 ☑
      - right T23.031 ☑
        - first degree T23.131 ☑
        - second degree T23.231 ☑
        - third degree T23.331 ☑
      - second degree T23.239 ☑
      - third degree T23.339 ☑
    - right T23.021 ☑
      - first degree T23.121 ☑
      - second degree T23.221 ☑
      - third degree T23.321 ☑
    - second degree T23.229 ☑
    - third degree T23.329 ☑
  - flank — *see* Burn, abdominal wall
  - foot T25.029 ☑
    - first degree T25.129 ☑
    - left T25.022 ☑
      - first degree T25.122 ☑
      - second degree T25.222 ☑
      - third degree T25.322 ☑
    - multiple with ankle — *see* Burn, lower, limb, multiple, ankle and foot
    - right T25.021 ☑
      - first degree T25.121 ☑
      - second degree T25.221 ☑
      - third degree T25.321 ☑
    - second degree T25.229 ☑
    - third degree T25.329 ☑
  - forearm T22.019 ☑
    - first degree T22.119 ☑
    - left T22.012 ☑
      - first degree T22.112 ☑
      - second degree T22.212 ☑
      - third degree T22.312 ☑
    - right T22.011 ☑
      - first degree T22.111 ☑
      - second degree T22.211 ☑
      - third degree T22.311 ☑
    - second degree T22.219 ☑
    - third degree T22.319 ☑
  - forehead T20.06 ☑
    - first degree T20.16 ☑
    - second degree T20.26 ☑
    - third degree T20.36 ☑
  - fourth degree — *code as* Burn, third degree, by site
  - friction — *see* Burn, by site
  - from swallowing caustic or corrosive substance NEC — *see* Corrosion, by site
  - full thickness skin loss — *code as* Burn, third degree, by site
  - gastrointestinal tract NEC T28.2 ☑
    - from swallowing caustic or corrosive substance T28.7 ☑
  - genital organs
    - external
      - female T21.07 ☑
        - first degree T21.17 ☑
        - second degree T21.27 ☑
        - third degree T21.37 ☑
      - male T21.06 ☑
        - first degree T21.16 ☑
        - second degree T21.26 ☑
        - third degree T21.36 ☑
    - internal T28.3 ☑
      - from caustic or corrosive substance T28.8 ☑
  - groin — *see* Burn, abdominal wall
  - hand(s) T23.009 ☑
    - back — *see* Burn, dorsum of hand
    - finger — *see* Burn, finger
    - first degree T23.109 ☑
    - left T23.002 ☑
      - first degree T23.102 ☑
      - second degree T23.202 ☑
      - third degree T23.302 ☑
    - multiple sites with wrist T23.099 ☑
      - first degree T23.199 ☑
      - left T23.092 ☑
        - first degree T23.192 ☑
        - second degree T23.292 ☑
        - third degree T23.392 ☑

- **Burn** — *continued*
  - trunk — *continued*
    - abdominal wall — *see* Burn, abdominal wall
    - anus — *see* Burn, buttock
    - axilla — *see* Burn, upper limb
    - back — *see* Burn, back
    - breast — *see* Burn, chest wall
    - buttock — *see* Burn, buttock
    - chest wall — *see* Burn, chest wall
    - first degree T21.10 ☑
    - flank — *see* Burn, abdominal wall
    - genital
      - female — *see* Burn, genital organs, external, female
      - male — *see* Burn, genital organs, external, male
    - groin — *see* Burn, abdominal wall
    - interscapular region — *see* Burn, back, upper
    - labia — *see* Burn, genital organs, external, female
    - lower back — *see* Burn, back
    - penis — *see* Burn, genital organs, external, male
    - perineum
      - female — *see* Burn, genital organs, external, female
      - male — *see* Burn, genital organs, external, male
    - scapula region — *see* Burn, scapular region
    - scrotum — *see* Burn, genital organs, external, male
    - second degree T21.20 ☑
    - specified site NEC T21.09 ☑
      - first degree T21.19 ☑
      - second degree T21.29 ☑
      - third degree T21.39 ☑
    - testes — *see* Burn, genital organs, external, male
    - third degree T21.30 ☑
    - upper back — *see* Burn, back, upper
    - vulva — *see* Burn, genital organs, external, female
  - unspecified site with extent of body surface involved specified
    - less than 10 percent T31.0
    - 10-19 percent (0-9 percent third degree) T31.10
      - with 10-19 percent third degree T31.11
    - 20-29 percent (0-9 percent third degree) T31.20
      - with
        - 10-19 percent third degree T31.21
        - 20-29 percent third degree T31.22
    - 30-39 percent (0-9 percent third degree) T31.30
      - with
        - 10-19 percent third degree T31.31
        - 20-29 percent third degree T31.32
        - 30-39 percent third degree T31.33
    - 40-49 percent (0-9 percent third degree) T31.40
      - with
        - 10-19 percent third degree T31.41
        - 20-29 percent third degree T31.42
        - 30-39 percent third degree T31.43
        - 40-49 percent third degree T31.44
    - 50-59 percent (0-9 percent third degree) T31.50
      - with
        - 10-19 percent third degree T31.51
        - 20-29 percent third degree T31.52
        - 30-39 percent third degree T31.53
        - 40-49 percent third degree T31.54
        - 50-59 percent third degree T31.55
    - 60-69 percent (0-9 percent third degree) T31.60
      - with
        - 10-19 percent third degree T31.61
        - 20-29 percent third degree T31.62
        - 30-39 percent third degree T31.63
        - 40-49 percent third degree T31.64
        - 50-59 percent third degree T31.65
        - 60-69 percent third degree T31.66
    - 70-79 percent (0-9 percent third degree) T31.70
      - with
        - 10-19 percent third degree T31.71
        - 20-29 percent third degree T31.72
        - 30-39 percent third degree T31.73
        - 40-49 percent third degree T31.74
        - 50-59 percent third degree T31.75
        - 60-69 percent third degree T31.76
        - 70-79 percent third degree T31.77
    - 80-89 percent (0-9 percent third degree) T31.80
      - with
        - 10-19 percent third degree T31.81
        - 20-29 percent third degree T31.82
        - 30-39 percent third degree T31.83
        - 40-49 percent third degree T31.84
        - 50-59 percent third degree T31.85
        - 60-69 percent third degree T31.86
        - 70-79 percent third degree T31.87

- **Burn** — *continued*
  - unspecified site with extent of body surface involved specified — *continued*
    - 80-89 percent — *continued*
      - with — *continued*
        - 80-89 percent third degree T31.88
    - 90 percent or more (0-9 percent third degree) T31.90
      - with
        - 10-19 percent third degree T31.91
        - 20-29 percent third degree T31.92
        - 30-39 percent third degree T31.93
        - 40-49 percent third degree T31.94
        - 50-59 percent third degree T31.95
        - 60-69 percent third degree T31.96
        - 70-79 percent third degree T31.97
        - 80-89 percent third degree T31.98
        - 90-99 percent third degree T31.99
  - upper limb T22.00 ☑
    - above elbow — *see* Burn, above elbow
    - axilla — *see* Burn, axilla
    - elbow — *see* Burn, elbow
    - first degree T22.10 ☑
    - forearm — *see* Burn, forearm
    - hand — *see* Burn, hand
    - interscapular region — *see* Burn, back, upper
    - multiple sites T22.099 ☑
      - first degree T22.199 ☑
      - left T22.092 ☑
        - first degree T22.192 ☑
        - second degree T22.292 ☑
        - third degree T22.392 ☑
      - right T22.091 ☑
        - first degree T22.191 ☑
        - second degree T22.291 ☑
        - third degree T22.391 ☑
      - second degree T22.299 ☑
      - third degree T22.399 ☑
    - scapular region — *see* Burn, scapular region
    - second degree T22.20 ☑
    - shoulder — *see* Burn, shoulder
    - third degree T22.30 ☑
    - wrist — *see* Burn, wrist
  - uterus T28.3 ☑
  - vagina T28.3 ☑
  - vulva — *see* Burn, genital organs, external, female
  - wrist T23.079 ☑
    - first degree T23.179 ☑
    - left T23.072 ☑
      - first degree T23.172 ☑
      - second degree T23.272 ☑
      - third degree T23.372 ☑
    - multiple sites with hand T23.099 ☑
      - first degree T23.199 ☑
      - left T23.092 ☑
        - first degree T23.192 ☑
        - second degree T23.292 ☑
        - third degree T23.392 ☑
      - right T23.091 ☑
        - first degree T23.191 ☑
        - second degree T23.291 ☑
        - third degree T23.391 ☑
      - second degree T23.299 ☑
      - third degree T23.399 ☑
    - right T23.071 ☑
      - first degree T23.171 ☑
      - second degree T23.271 ☑
      - third degree T23.371 ☑
    - second degree T23.279 ☑
    - third degree T23.379 ☑
- **Burnett's syndrome** E83.52
- **Burning**
  - feet syndrome E53.9
  - sensation R20.8
  - tongue K14.6
- **Burn-out** (state) Z73.0
- **Burns' disease or osteochondrosis** — *see* Osteochondrosis, juvenile, ulna
- **Bursa** — *see* condition
- **Bursitis** M71.9
  - Achilles — *see* Tendinitis, Achilles
  - adhesive — *see* Bursitis, specified NEC
  - ankle — *see* Enthesopathy, lower limb, ankle, specified type NEC
  - calcaneal — *see* Enthesopathy, foot, specified type NEC

- **Bursitis** — *continued*
  - collateral ligament, tibial — *see* Bursitis, tibial collateral
  - due to use, overuse, pressure (*see also* Disorder, soft tissue, due to use, specified type NEC)
    - specified NEC — *see* Disorder, soft tissue, due to use, specified NEC
  - Duplay's M75.0 ☑
  - elbow NEC M70.3- ☑
    - olecranon M70.2- ☑
  - finger — *see* Disorder, soft tissue, due to use, specified type NEC, hand
  - foot — *see* Enthesopathy, foot, specified type NEC
  - gonococcal A54.49
  - gouty — *see* Gout, idiopathic
  - hand M70.1- ☑
  - hip NEC M70.7- ☑
    - trochanteric M70.6- ☑
  - infective NEC M71.10
    - abscess — *see* Abscess, bursa
    - ankle M71.17- ☑
    - elbow M71.12- ☑
    - foot M71.17- ☑
    - hand M71.14- ☑
    - hip M71.15- ☑
    - knee M71.16- ☑
    - multiple sites M71.19
    - shoulder M71.11- ☑
    - specified site NEC M71.18
    - wrist M71.13- ☑
  - ischial — *see* Bursitis, hip
  - knee NEC M70.5- ☑
    - prepatellar M70.4- ☑
  - occupational NEC (*see also* Disorder, soft tissue, due to, use)
  - olecranon — *see* Bursitis, elbow, olecranon
  - pharyngeal J39.1
  - popliteal — *see* Bursitis, knee
  - prepatellar M70.4- ☑
  - radiohumeral M77.8
  - rheumatoid M06.20
    - ankle M06.27- ☑
    - elbow M06.22- ☑
    - foot joint M06.27- ☑
    - hand joint M06.24- ☑
    - hip M06.25- ☑
    - knee M06.26- ☑
    - multiple site M06.29
    - shoulder M06.21- ☑
    - vertebra M06.28
    - wrist M06.23- ☑
  - scapulohumeral — *see* Bursitis, shoulder
  - semimembranous muscle (knee) — *see* Bursitis, knee
  - shoulder M75.5- ☑
    - adhesive — *see* Capsulitis, adhesive
  - specified NEC M71.50
    - ankle M71.57- ☑
    - due to use, overuse or pressure — *see* Disorder, soft tissue, due to, use
    - elbow M71.52- ☑
    - foot M71.57- ☑
    - hand M71.54- ☑
    - hip M71.55- ☑
    - knee M71.56- ☑
    - shoulder — *see* Bursitis, shoulder
    - specified site NEC M71.58
    - tibial collateral M76.4- ☑
    - wrist M71.53- ☑
  - subacromial — *see* Bursitis, shoulder
  - subcoracoid — *see* Bursitis, shoulder
  - subdeltoid — *see* Bursitis, shoulder
  - syphilitic A52.78
  - Thornwaldt, Tornwaldt J39.2
  - tibial collateral — *see* Bursitis, tibial collateral
  - toe — *see* Enthesopathy, foot, specified type NEC
  - trochanteric (area) — *see* Bursitis, hip, trochanteric
  - wrist — *see* Bursitis, hand
- **Bursopathy** M71.9
  - specified type NEC M71.80
    - ankle M71.87- ☑
    - elbow M71.82- ☑
    - foot M71.87- ☑
    - hand M71.84- ☑
    - hip M71.85- ☑
    - knee M71.86- ☑
    - multiple sites M71.89
    - shoulder M71.81- ☑

- **Bursopathy** — *continued*
  - specified type — *continued*
    - specified site NEC M71.88
    - wrist M71.83- ☑
- **Burst stitches or sutures** (complication of surgery) T81.31 ☑
  - external operation wound T81.31 ☑
  - internal operation wound T81.32 ☑
- **Buruli ulcer** A31.1
- **Bury's disease** L95.1
- **Buschke's**
  - disease B45.3
  - scleredema — *see* Sclerosis, systemic
- **Busse-Buschke disease** B45.3
- **Buttock** — *see* condition
- **Button**
  - Biskra B55.1
  - Delhi B55.1
  - oriental B55.1
- **Buttonhole deformity** (finger) — *see* Deformity, finger, boutonniere
- **Bwamba fever** A92.8
- **Byssinosis** J66.Ø
- **Bywaters' syndrome** T79.5 ☑

C

- **Cachexia** R64
  - cancerous R64
  - cardiac — *see* Disease, heart
  - dehydration E86.Ø
    - with
      - hypernatremia E87.Ø
      - hyponatremia E87.1
  - due to malnutrition R64
  - exophthalmic — *see* Hyperthyroidism
  - heart — *see* Disease, heart
  - hypophyseal E23.Ø
  - hypopituitary E23.Ø
  - lead — *see* Poisoning, lead
  - malignant R64
  - marsh — *see* Malaria
  - nervous F48.8
  - old age R54
  - paludal — *see* Malaria
  - pituitary E23.Ø
  - renal N28.9
  - saturnine — *see* Poisoning, lead
  - senile R54
  - Simmonds' E23.Ø
  - splenica D73.Ø
  - strumipriva EØ3.4
  - tuberculous NEC — *see* Tuberculosis
- **Café, au lait spots** L81.3
- **Caffey's syndrome** Q78.8
- **Caisson disease** T70.3 ☑
- **Cake kidney** Q63.1
- **Caked breast** (puerperal, postpartum) O92.79
- **Calabar swelling** B74.3
- **Calcaneal spur** — *see* Spur, bone, calcaneal
- **Calcaneo-apophysitis** M92.8
- **Calcareous** — *see* condition
- **Calcicosis** J62.8
- **Calciferol** (vitamin D) deficiency E55.9
  - with rickets E55.Ø
- **Calcification**
  - adrenal (capsule) (gland) E27.49
    - tuberculous E35 [B9Ø.8]
  - aorta I7Ø.Ø
  - artery (annular) — *see* Arteriosclerosis
  - auricle (ear) — *see* Disorder, pinna, specified type NEC
  - basal ganglia G23.8
  - bladder N32.89
    - due to Schistosoma hematobium B65.Ø
  - brain (cortex) — *see* Calcification, cerebral
  - bronchus J98.Ø9
  - bursa M71.4Ø
    - ankle M71.47- ☑
    - elbow M71.42- ☑
    - foot M71.47- ☑
    - hand M71.44- ☑
    - hip M71.45- ☑
    - knee M71.46- ☑
    - multiple sites M71.49
    - shoulder M75.3- ☑
    - specified site NEC M71.48
    - wrist M71.43- ☑

- **Calcification** — *continued*
  - cardiac — *see* Degeneration, myocardial
  - cerebral (cortex) G93.89
    - artery I67.2
  - cervix (uteri) N88.8
  - choroid plexus G93.89
  - conjunctiva — *see* Concretion, conjunctiva
  - corpora cavernosa (penis) N48.89
  - cortex (brain) — *see* Calcification, cerebral
  - dental pulp (nodular) KØ4.2
  - dentinal papilla KØØ.4
  - fallopian tube N83.8
  - falx cerebri G96.19
  - gallbladder K82.8
  - general E83.59
  - heart (*see also* Degeneration, myocardial)
    - valve — *see* Endocarditis
  - idiopathic infantile arterial (IIAC) Q28.8
  - intervertebral cartilage or disc (postinfective) — *see* Disorder, disc, specified NEC
  - intracranial — *see* Calcification, cerebral
  - joint — *see* Disorder, joint, specified type NEC
  - kidney N28.89
    - tuberculous N29 [B9Ø.1]
  - larynx (senile) J38.7
  - lens — *see* Cataract, specified NEC
  - lung (active) (postinfectional) J98.4
    - tuberculous B9Ø.9
  - lymph gland or node (postinfectional) I89.8
    - tuberculous (*see also* Tuberculosis, lymph gland) B9Ø.8
  - mammographic R92.1
  - massive (paraplegic) — *see* Myositis, ossificans, in, quadriplegia
  - medial — *see* Arteriosclerosis, extremities
  - meninges (cerebral) (spinal) G96.19
  - metastatic E83.59
  - Mönckeberg's — *see* Arteriosclerosis, extremities
  - muscle M61.9
    - due to burns — *see* Myositis, ossificans, in, burns
    - paralytic — *see* Myositis, ossificans, in, quadriplegia
    - specified type NEC M61.4Ø
      - ankle M61.47- ☑
      - foot M61.47- ☑
      - forearm M61.43- ☑
      - hand M61.44- ☑
      - lower leg M61.46- ☑
      - multiple sites M61.49
      - pelvic region M61.45- ☑
      - shoulder region M61.41- ☑
      - specified site NEC M61.48
      - thigh M61.45- ☑
      - upper arm M61.42- ☑
  - myocardium, myocardial — *see* Degeneration, myocardial
  - ovary N83.8
  - pancreas K86.8
  - penis N48.89
  - periarticular — *see* Disorder, joint, specified type NEC
  - pericardium (*see also* Pericarditis) I31.1
  - pineal gland E34.8
  - pleura J94.8
    - postinfectional J94.8
    - tuberculous NEC B9Ø.9
  - pulpal (dental) (nodular) KØ4.2
  - sclera H15.89
  - spleen D73.89
  - subcutaneous L94.2
  - suprarenal (capsule) (gland) E27.49
  - tendon (sheath) (*see also* Tenosynovitis, specified type NEC)
    - with bursitis, synovitis or tenosynovitis — *see* Tendinitis, calcific
  - trachea J39.8
  - ureter N28.89
  - uterus N85.8
  - vitreous — *see* Deposit, crystalline
- **Calcified** — *see* Calcification
- **Calcinosis** (interstitial) (tumoral) (universalis) E83.59
  - with Raynaud's phenomenon, esophageal dysfunction, sclerodactyly, telangiectasia (CREST syndrome) M34.1
  - circumscripta (skin) L94.2
  - cutis L94.2
- **Calciphylaxis** (*see also* Calcification, by site) E83.59
- **Calcium**
  - deposits — *see* Calcification, by site

- **Calcium** — *continued*
  - metabolism disorder E83.5Ø
  - salts or soaps in vitreous — *see* Deposit, crystalline
- **Calciuria** R82.99
- **Calculi** — *see* Calculus
- **Calculosis, intrahepatic** — *see* Calculus, bile duct
- **Calculus, calculi, calculous**
  - ampulla of Vater — *see* Calculus, bile duct
  - anuria (impacted) (recurrent) (*see also* Calculus, urinary) N2Ø.9
  - appendix K38.1
  - bile duct (common) (hepatic) K8Ø.5Ø
    - with
      - calculus of gallbladder — *see* Calculus, gallbladder and bile duct
      - cholangitis K8Ø.3Ø
        - with
          - cholecystitis — *see* Calculus, bile duct, with cholecystitis
          - obstruction K8Ø.31
        - acute K8Ø.32
          - with
            - chronic cholangitis K8Ø.36
              - with obstruction K8Ø.37
            - obstruction K8Ø.33
        - chronic K8Ø.34
          - with
            - acute cholangitis K8Ø.36
              - with obstruction K8Ø.37
            - obstruction K8Ø.35
      - cholecystitis (with cholangitis) K8Ø.4Ø
        - with obstruction K8Ø.41
        - acute K8Ø.42
          - with
            - chronic cholecystitis K8Ø.46
              - with obstruction K8Ø.47
            - obstruction K8Ø.43
        - chronic K8Ø.44
          - with
            - acute cholecystitis K8Ø.46
              - with obstruction K8Ø.47
            - obstruction K8Ø.45
      - obstruction K8Ø.51
  - biliary (*see also* Calculus, gallbladder)
    - specified NEC K8Ø.8Ø
      - with obstruction K8Ø.81
  - bilirubin, multiple — *see* Calculus, gallbladder
  - bladder (encysted) (impacted) (urinary) (diverticulum) N21.Ø
  - bronchus J98.Ø9
  - calyx (kidney) (renal) — *see* Calculus, kidney
  - cholesterol (pure) (solitary) — *see* Calculus, gallbladder
  - common duct (bile) — *see* Calculus, bile duct
  - conjunctiva — *see* Concretion, conjunctiva
  - cystic N21.Ø
    - duct — *see* Calculus, gallbladder
  - dental (subgingival) (supragingival) KØ3.6
  - diverticulum
    - bladder N21.Ø
    - kidney N2Ø.Ø
  - epididymis N5Ø.8
  - gallbladder K8Ø.2Ø
    - with
      - bile duct calculus — *see* Calculus, gallbladder and bile duct
      - cholecystitis K8Ø.1Ø
        - with obstruction K8Ø.11
        - acute K8Ø.ØØ
          - with
            - chronic cholecystitis K8Ø.12
              - with obstruction K8Ø.13
            - obstruction K8Ø.Ø1
        - chronic K8Ø.1Ø
          - with
            - acute cholecystitis K8Ø.12
              - with obstruction K8Ø.13
            - obstruction K8Ø.11
        - specified NEC K8Ø.18
          - with obstruction K8Ø.19
      - obstruction K8Ø.21
  - gallbladder and bile duct K8Ø.7Ø
    - with
      - cholecystitis K8Ø.6Ø
        - with obstruction K8Ø.61
        - acute K8Ø.62
          - with
            - chronic cholecystitis K8Ø.66
              - with obstruction K8Ø.67

- **Calculus, calculi, calculous** — *continued*
  - gallbladder and bile duct — *continued*
    - with — *continued*
      - cholecystitis — *continued*
        - acute — *continued*
          - with — *continued*
            - obstruction K8Ø.63
        - chronic K8Ø.64
          - with
            - acute cholecystitis K8Ø.66
              - with obstruction K8Ø.67
            - obstruction K8Ø.65
      - obstruction K8Ø.71
  - hepatic (duct) — *see* Calculus, bile duct
  - ileal conduit N21.8
  - intestinal (impaction) (obstruction) K56.49
  - kidney (impacted) (multiple) (pelvis) (recurrent) (staghorn) N2Ø.Ø
    - with calculus, ureter N2Ø.2
    - congenital Q63.8
  - lacrimal passages — *see* Dacryolith
  - liver (impacted) — *see* Calculus, bile duct
  - lung J98.4
  - mammographic R92.1
  - nephritic (impacted) (recurrent) — *see* Calculus, kidney
  - nose J34.89
  - pancreas (duct) K86.8
  - parotid duct or gland K11.5
  - pelvis, encysted — *see* Calculus, kidney
  - prostate N42.Ø
  - pulmonary J98.4
  - pyelitis (impacted) (recurrent) N2Ø.Ø
    - with hydronephrosis N13.2
  - pyelonephritis (impacted) (recurrent) N2Ø ☑
    - with hydronephrosis N13.2
  - renal (impacted) (recurrent) — *see* Calculus, kidney
  - salivary (duct) (gland) K11.5
  - seminal vesicle N5Ø.8
  - staghorn — *see* Calculus, kidney
  - Stensen's duct K11.5
  - stomach K31.89
  - sublingual duct or gland K11.5
    - congenital Q38.4
  - submandibular duct, gland or region K11.5
  - submaxillary duct, gland or region K11.5
  - suburethral N21.8
  - tonsil J35.8
  - tooth, teeth (subgingival) (supragingival) KØ3.6
  - tunica vaginalis N5Ø.8
  - ureter (impacted) (recurrent) N2Ø.1
    - with calculus, kidney N2Ø.2
      - with hydronephrosis N13.2
        - with infection N13.6
  - urethra (impacted) N21.1
  - urinary (duct) (impacted) (passage) (tract) N2Ø.9
    - with hydronephrosis N13.2
      - with infection N13.6
    - in (due to)
    - lower N21.9
      - specified NEC N21.8
  - vagina N89.8
  - vesical (impacted) N21.Ø
  - Wharton's duct K11.5
  - xanthine E79.8 [N22]
- **Calicectasis** N28.89
- **Caliectasis** N28.89
- **California**
  - disease B38.9
  - encephalitis A83.5
- **Caligo cornea** — *see* Opacity, cornea, central
- **Callositas, callosity** (infected) L84
- **Callus** (infected) L84
  - bone — *see* Osteophyte
    - excessive, following fracture — *code as* Sequelae of fracture
- **Calorie deficiency or malnutrition** (*see also* Malnutrition) E46
- **Calvé-Perthes disease** — *see* Legg-Calvé-Perthes disease
- **Calvé's disease** — *see* Osteochondrosis, juvenile, spine
- **Calvities** — *see* Alopecia, androgenic
- **Cameroon fever** — *see* Malaria
- **Camptocormia** (hysterical) F44.4
- **Camurati-Engelmann syndrome** Q78.3
- **Canal** (*see also* condition)
  - atrioventricular common Q21.2
- **Canaliculitis** (lacrimal) (acute) (subacute) HØ4.33- ☑
  - Actinomyces A42.89
- **Canaliculitis** — *continued*
  - chronic HØ4.42- ☑
- **Canavan's disease** E75.29
- **Canceled procedure** (surgical) Z53.9
  - because of
    - contraindication Z53.Ø9
      - smoking Z53.Ø1
    - left against medical advice (AMA) Z53.21
    - patient's decision Z53.2Ø
      - for reasons of belief or group pressure Z53.1
      - specified reason NEC Z53.29
    - specified reason NEC Z53.8
- **Cancer** (*see also* Neoplasm, by site, malignant)
  - bile duct type liver C22.1
  - blood — *see* Leukemia
  - breast (*see also* Neoplasm, breast, malignant) C5Ø.91- ☑
  - hepatocellular C22.Ø
  - lung (*see also* Neoplasm, lung, malignant) C34.9Ø
  - ovarian (*see also* Neoplasm ovary, malignant) C56.9
  - unspecified site (primary) C8Ø.1
- **Cancer (o)phobia** F45.29
- **Cancerous** — *see* Neoplasm, malignant, by site
- **Cancrum oris** A69.Ø
- **Candidiasis, candidal** B37.9
  - balanitis B37.42
  - bronchitis B37.1
  - cheilitis B37.83
  - congenital P37.5
  - cystitis B37.41
  - disseminated B37.7
  - endocarditis B37.6
  - enteritis B37.82
  - esophagitis B37.81
  - intertrigo B37.2
  - lung B37.1
  - meningitis B37.5
  - mouth B37.Ø
  - nails B37.2
  - neonatal P37.5
  - onychia B37.2
  - oral B37.Ø
  - osteomyelitis B37.89
  - otitis externa B37.84
  - paronychia B37.2
  - perionyxis B37.2
  - pneumonia B37.1
  - proctitis B37.82
  - pulmonary B37.1
  - pyelonephritis B37.49
  - sepsis B37.7
  - skin B37.2
  - specified site NEC B37.89
  - stomatitis B37.Ø
  - systemic B37.7
  - urethritis B37.41
  - urogenital site NEC B37.49
  - vagina B37.3
  - vulva B37.3
  - vulvovaginitis B37.3
- **Candidid** L3Ø.2
- **Candidosis** — *see* Candidiasis
- **Candiru infection or infestation** B88.8
- **Canities** (premature) L67.1
  - congenital Q84.2
- **Canker** (mouth) (sore) K12.Ø
  - rash A38.9
- **Cannabinosis** J66.2
- **Canton fever** A75.9
- **Cantrell's syndrome** Q87.89
- **Capillariasis** (intestinal) B81.1
  - hepatic B83.8
- **Capillary** — *see* condition
- **Caplan's syndrome** — *see* Rheumatoid, lung
- **Capsule** — *see* condition
- **Capsulitis** (joint) (*see also* Enthesopathy)
  - adhesive (shoulder) M75.Ø- ☑
  - hepatic K65.8
  - labyrinthine — *see* Otosclerosis, specified NEC
  - thyroid EØ6.9
- **Caput**
  - crepitus Q75.8
  - medusae I86.8
  - succedaneum P12.81
- **Car sickness** T75.3 ☑
- **Carapata** (disease) A68.Ø
- **Carate** — *see* Pinta
- **Carbon lung** J6Ø
- **Carbuncle** LØ2.93
  - abdominal wall LØ2.231
  - anus K61.Ø
  - auditory canal, external — *see* Abscess, ear, external
  - auricle ear — *see* Abscess, ear, external
  - axilla LØ2.43- ☑
  - back (any part) LØ2.232
  - breast N61
  - buttock LØ2.33
  - cheek (external) LØ2.Ø3
  - chest wall LØ2.233
  - chin LØ2.Ø3
  - corpus cavernosum N48.21
  - ear (any part) (external) (middle) — *see* Abscess, ear, external
  - external auditory canal — *see* Abscess, ear, external
  - eyelid — *see* Abscess, eyelid
  - face NEC LØ2.Ø3
  - femoral (region) — *see* Carbuncle, lower limb
  - finger — *see* Carbuncle, hand
  - flank LØ2.231
  - foot LØ2.63- ☑
  - forehead LØ2.Ø3
  - genital — *see* Abscess, genital
  - gluteal (region) LØ2.33
  - groin LØ2.234
  - hand LØ2.53- ☑
  - head NEC LØ2.831
  - heel — *see* Carbuncle, foot
  - hip — *see* Carbuncle, lower limb
  - kidney — *see* Abscess, kidney
  - knee — *see* Carbuncle, lower limb
  - labium (majus) (minus) N76.4
  - lacrimal
    - gland — *see* Dacryoadenitis
    - passages (duct) (sac) — *see* Inflammation, lacrimal, passages, acute
  - leg — *see* Carbuncle, lower limb
  - lower limb LØ2.43- ☑
  - malignant A22.Ø
  - navel LØ2.236
  - neck LØ2.13
  - nose (external) (septum) J34.Ø
  - orbit, orbital — *see* Abscess, orbit
  - palmar (space) — *see* Carbuncle, hand
  - partes posteriores LØ2.33
  - pectoral region LØ2.233
  - penis N48.21
  - perineum LØ2.235
  - pinna — *see* Abscess, ear, external
  - popliteal — *see* Carbuncle, lower limb
  - scalp LØ2.831
  - seminal vesicle N49.Ø
  - shoulder — *see* Carbuncle, upper limb
  - specified site NEC LØ2.838
  - temple (region) LØ2.Ø3
  - thumb — *see* Carbuncle, hand
  - toe — *see* Carbuncle, foot
  - trunk LØ2.239
    - abdominal wall LØ2.231
    - back LØ2.232
    - chest wall LØ2.233
    - groin LØ2.234
    - perineum LØ2.235
    - umbilicus LØ2.236
  - umbilicus LØ2.236
  - upper limb LØ2.43- ☑
  - urethra N34.Ø
  - vulva N76.4
- **Carbunculus** — *see* Carbuncle
- **Carcinoid** (tumor) — *see* Tumor, carcinoid
- **Carcinoidosis** E34.Ø
- **Carcinoma** (malignant) (*see also* Neoplasm, by site, malignant)
  - acidophil
    - specified site — *see* Neoplasm, malignant, by site
    - unspecified site C75.1
  - acidophil-basophil, mixed
    - specified site — *see* Neoplasm, malignant, by site
    - unspecified site C75.1
  - adnexal (skin) — *see* Neoplasm, skin, malignant
  - adrenal cortical C74.Ø- ☑
  - alveolar — *see* Neoplasm, lung, malignant
    - cell — *see* Neoplasm, lung, malignant
  - ameloblastic C41.1
    - upper jaw (bone) C41.Ø

Carcinoma — *continued*
- apocrine
  - breast — *see* Neoplasm, breast, malignant
  - specified site NEC — *see* Neoplasm, skin, malignant
  - unspecified site C44.99
- basal cell (pigmented) (*see also* Neoplasm, skin, malignant) C44.91
  - fibro-epithelial — *see* Neoplasm, skin, malignant
  - morphea — *see* Neoplasm, skin, malignant
  - multicentric — *see* Neoplasm, skin, malignant
- basaloid
- basal-squamous cell, mixed — *see* Neoplasm, skin, malignant
- basophil
  - specified site — *see* Neoplasm, malignant, by site
  - unspecified site C75.1
- basophil-acidophil, mixed
  - specified site — *see* Neoplasm, malignant, by site
  - unspecified site C75.1
- basosquamous — *see* Neoplasm, skin, malignant
- bile duct
  - with hepatocellular, mixed C22.Ø
  - liver C22.1
  - specified site NEC — *see* Neoplasm, malignant, by site
  - unspecified site C22.1
- branchial or branchiogenic C1Ø.4
- bronchial or bronchogenic — *see* Neoplasm, lung, malignant
- bronchiolar — *see* Neoplasm, lung, malignant
- bronchioloalveolar — *see* Neoplasm, lung, malignant
- C cell
  - specified site — *see* Neoplasm, malignant, by site
  - unspecified site C73
- ceruminous C44.29- ☑
- cervix uteri
  - in situ DØ6.9
    - endocervix DØ6.Ø
    - exocervix DØ6.1
    - specified site NEC DØ6.7
- chorionic
  - specified site — *see* Neoplasm, malignant, by site
  - unspecified site
    - female C58
    - male C62.9Ø
- chromophobe
  - specified site — *see* Neoplasm, malignant, by site
  - unspecified site C75.1
- cloacogenic
  - specified site — *see* Neoplasm, malignant, by site
  - unspecified site C21.2
- diffuse type
  - specified site — *see* Neoplasm, malignant, by site
  - unspecified site C16.9
- duct (cell)
  - with Paget's disease — *see* Neoplasm, breast, malignant
  - infiltrating
    - with lobular carcinoma (in situ)
      - specified site — *see* Neoplasm, malignant, by site
      - unspecified site (female) C5Ø.91- ☑
        - male C5Ø.92- ☑
    - specified site — *see* Neoplasm, malignant, by site
    - unspecified site (female) C5Ø.91- ☑
      - male C5Ø.92- ☑
- ductal
  - with lobular
    - specified site — *see* Neoplasm, malignant, by site
    - unspecified site (female) C5Ø.91- ☑
      - male C5Ø.92- ☑
- ductular, infiltrating
  - specified site — *see* Neoplasm, malignant, by site
  - unspecified site (female) C5Ø.91- ☑
    - male C5Ø.92- ☑
- embryonal
  - liver C22.7
- endometrioid
  - specified site — *see* Neoplasm, malignant, by site
  - unspecified site
    - female C56.9
    - male C61
- eosinophil
  - specified site — *see* Neoplasm, malignant, by site
  - unspecified site C75.1

Carcinoma — *continued*
- epidermoid (*see also* Neoplasm, skin, malignant)
  - in situ, Bowen's type — *see* Neoplasm, skin, in situ
- fibroepithelial, basal cell — *see* Neoplasm, skin, malignant
- follicular
  - with papillary (mixed) C73
  - moderately differentiated C73
  - pure follicle C73
  - specified site — *see* Neoplasm, malignant, by site
  - trabecular C73
  - unspecified site C73
  - well differentiated C73
- generalized, with unspecified primary site C8Ø.Ø
- glycogen-rich — *see* Neoplasm, breast, malignant
- granulosa cell C56- ☑
- hepatic cell C22.Ø
- hepatocellular C22.Ø
  - with bile duct, mixed C22.Ø
  - fibrolamellar C22.Ø
- hepatocholangiolitic C22.Ø
- Hurthle cell C73
- in
  - adenomatous
    - polyposis coli C18.9
  - pleomorphic adenoma — *see* Neoplasm, salivary glands, malignant
  - situ — *see* Carcinoma-in-situ
- infiltrating
  - duct
    - with lobular
      - specified site — *see* Neoplasm, malignant, by site
      - unspecified site (female) C5Ø.91- ☑
        - male C5Ø.92- ☑
    - with Paget's disease — *see* Neoplasm, breast, malignant
    - specified site — *see* Neoplasm, malignant
    - unspecified site (female) C5Ø.91- ☑
      - male C5Ø.92- ☑
  - ductular
    - specified site — *see* Neoplasm, malignant
    - unspecified site (female) C5Ø.91- ☑
      - male C5Ø.92- ☑
  - lobular
    - specified site — *see* Neoplasm, malignant
    - unspecified site (female) C5Ø.91- ☑
      - male C5Ø.92- ☑
- inflammatory
  - specified site — *see* Neoplasm, malignant
  - unspecified site (female) C5Ø.91- ☑
    - male C5Ø.92- ☑
- intestinal type
  - specified site — *see* Neoplasm, malignant, by site
  - unspecified site C16.9
- intracystic
  - noninfiltrating — *see* Neoplasm, in situ, by site
- intraductal (noninfiltrating)
  - with Paget's disease — *see* Neoplasm, breast, malignant
  - breast DØ5.1- ☑
  - papillary
    - with invasion
      - specified site — *see* Neoplasm, malignant, by site
      - unspecified site (female) C5Ø.91- ☑
        - male C5Ø.92- ☑
    - breast DØ5.1- ☑
    - specified site NEC — *see* Neoplasm, in situ, by site
    - unspecified site (female) DØ5.1- ☑
  - specified site NEC — *see* Neoplasm, in situ, by site
  - unspecified site (female) DØ5.1- ☑
- intraepidermal — *see* Neoplasm, in situ
  - squamous cell, Bowen's type — *see* Neoplasm, skin, in situ
- intraepithelial — *see* Neoplasm, in situ, by site
  - squamous cell — *see* Neoplasm, in situ, by site
- intraosseous C41.1
  - upper jaw (bone) C41.Ø
- islet cell
  - with exocrine, mixed
    - specified site — *see* Neoplasm, malignant, by site
    - unspecified site C25.9
  - pancreas C25.4

Carcinoma — *continued*
- islet cell — *continued*
  - specified site NEC — *see* Neoplasm, malignant, by site
  - unspecified site C25.4
- juvenile, breast — *see* Neoplasm, breast, malignant
- large cell
  - small cell
    - specified site — *see* Neoplasm, malignant, by site
    - unspecified site C34.9Ø
- Leydig cell (testis)
  - specified site — *see* Neoplasm, malignant, by site
  - unspecified site
    - female C56.9
    - male C62.9Ø
- lipid-rich (female) C5Ø.91- ☑
  - male C5Ø.92- ☑
- liver cell C22.Ø
- liver NEC C22.7
- lobular (infiltrating)
  - with intraductal
    - specified site — *see* Neoplasm, malignant, by site
    - unspecified site (female) C5Ø.91- ☑
      - male C5Ø.92- ☑
  - noninfiltrating
    - breast DØ5.Ø- ☑
    - specified site NEC — *see* Neoplasm, in situ, by site
    - unspecified site DØ5.Ø- ☑
  - specified site — *see* Neoplasm, malignant, by site
  - unspecified site (female) C5Ø.91- ☑
    - male C5Ø.92- ☑
- medullary
  - with
    - amyloid stroma
      - specified site — *see* Neoplasm, malignant, by site
      - unspecified site C73
    - lymphoid stroma
      - specified site — *see* Neoplasm, malignant, by site
      - unspecified site (female) C5Ø.91- ☑
        - male C5Ø.92- ☑
- Merkel cell C4A.9 (*following* C43)
  - anal margin C4A.51 (*following* C43)
  - anal skin C4A.51 (*following* C43)
  - canthus C4A.1- ☑ (*following* C43)
  - ear and external auricular canal C4A.2- ☑ (*following* C43)
  - external auricular canal C4A.2- ☑ (*following* C43)
  - eyelid, including canthus C4A.1- ☑ (*following* C43)
  - face C4A.3Ø (*following* C43)
    - specified NEC C4A.39 (*following* C43)
  - hip C4A.7- ☑ (*following* C43)
  - lip C4A.Ø (*following* C43)
  - lower limb, including hip C4A.7- ☑ (*following* C43)
  - neck C4A.4 (*following* C43)
  - nodal presentation C7B.1 (*following* C75)
  - nose C4A.31 (*following* C43)
  - overlapping sites C4A.8 (*following* C43)
  - perianal skin C4A.51 (*following* C43)
  - scalp C4A.4 (*following* C43)
  - secondary C7B.1 (*following* C75)
  - shoulder C4A.6- ☑ (*following* C43)
  - skin of breast C4A.52 (*following* C43)
  - trunk NEC C4A.59 (*following* C43)
  - upper limb, including shoulder C4A.6- ☑ (*following* C43)
  - visceral metastatic C7B.1 (*following* C75)
- metastatic — *see* Neoplasm, secondary, by site
- metatypical — *see* Neoplasm, skin, malignant
- morphea, basal cell — *see* Neoplasm, skin, malignant
- mucoid
  - cell
    - specified site — *see* Neoplasm, malignant, by site
    - unspecified site C75.1
- neuroendocrine (*see also* Tumor, neuroendocrine)
  - high grade, any site C7A.1 (*following* C75)
  - poorly differentiated, any site C7A.1 (*following* C75)
- nonencapsulated sclerosing C73
- noninfiltrating
  - intracystic — *see* Neoplasm, in situ, by site
  - intraductal
    - breast DØ5.1- ☑

- **Carcinoma** — *continued*
  - noninfiltrating — *continued*
    - intraductal — *continued*
      - papillary
        - breast D05.1- ☑
        - specified site NEC — *see* Neoplasm, in situ, by site
        - unspecified site D05.1- ☑
      - specified site — *see* Neoplasm, in situ, by site
      - unspecified site D05.1- ☑
    - lobular
      - breast D05.0- ☑
      - specified site NEC — *see* Neoplasm, in situ, by site
      - unspecified site (female) D05.0- ☑
  - oat cell
    - specified site — *see* Neoplasm, malignant, by site
    - unspecified site C34.90
  - odontogenic C41.1
    - upper jaw (bone) C41.0
  - papillary
    - with follicular (mixed) C73
    - follicular variant C73
    - intraductal (noninfiltrating)
      - with invasion
        - specified site — *see* Neoplasm, malignant, by site
        - unspecified site (female) C50.91- ☑
          - male C50.92- ☑
      - breast D05.1- ☑
      - specified site NEC — *see* Neoplasm, in situ, by site
      - unspecified site D05.1- ☑
    - serous
      - specified site — *see* Neoplasm, malignant, by site
      - surface
        - specified site — *see* Neoplasm, malignant, by site
        - unspecified site C56.9
      - unspecified site C56.9
  - papillocystic
    - specified site — *see* Neoplasm, malignant, by site
    - unspecified site C56.9
  - parafollicular cell
    - specified site — *see* Neoplasm, malignant, by site
    - unspecified site C73
  - pilomatrix — *see* Neoplasm, skin, malignant
  - pseudomucinous
    - specified site — *see* Neoplasm, malignant, by site
    - unspecified site C56.9
  - renal cell C64- ☑
  - Schmincke — *see* Neoplasm, nasopharynx, malignant
  - Schneiderian
    - specified site — *see* Neoplasm, malignant, by site
    - unspecified site C30.0
  - sebaceous — *see* Neoplasm, skin, malignant
  - secondary (*see also* Neoplasm, secondary, by site)
    - Merkel cell C7B.1 (*following* C75)
  - secretory, breast — *see* Neoplasm, breast, malignant
  - serous
    - papillary
      - specified site — *see* Neoplasm, malignant, by site
      - unspecified site C56.9
    - surface, papillary
      - specified site — *see* Neoplasm, malignant, by site
      - unspecified site C56.9
  - Sertoli cell
    - specified site — *see* Neoplasm, malignant, by site
    - unspecified site C62.90
      - female C56.9
      - male C62.90
  - skin appendage — *see* Neoplasm, skin, malignant
  - small cell
    - fusiform cell
      - specified site — *see* Neoplasm, malignant, by site
      - unspecified site C34.90
    - intermediate cell
      - specified site — *see* Neoplasm, malignant, by site
      - unspecified site C34.90
    - large cell
      - specified site — *see* Neoplasm, malignant, by site

- **Carcinoma** — *continued*
  - small cell — *continued*
    - large cell — *continued*
      - unspecified site C34.90
  - solid
    - with amyloid stroma
      - specified site — *see* Neoplasm, malignant, by site
      - unspecified site C73
    - microinvasive
      - specified site — *see* Neoplasm, malignant, by site
      - unspecified site C53.9
  - sweat gland — *see* Neoplasm, skin, malignant
  - theca cell C56.- ☑
  - thymic C37
  - unspecified site (primary) C80.1
  - water-clear cell C75.0
- **Carcinoma-in-situ** (*see also* Neoplasm, in situ, by site)
  - breast NOS D05.9- ☑
    - specified type NEC D05.8- ☑
  - epidermoid (*see also* Neoplasm, in situ, by site)
    - with questionable stromal invasion
      - cervix D06.9
      - specified site NEC — *see* Neoplasm, in situ, by site
      - unspecified site D06.9
    - Bowen's type — *see* Neoplasm, skin, in situ
  - intraductal
    - breast D05.1- ☑
    - specified site NEC — *see* Neoplasm, in situ, by site
    - unspecified site D05.1- ☑
  - lobular
    - with
      - infiltrating duct
        - breast (female) C50.91- ☑
          - male C50.92- ☑
        - specified site NEC — *see* Neoplasm, malignant
        - unspecified site (female) C50.91- ☑
          - male C50.92- ☑
      - intraductal
        - breast D05.8- ☑
        - specified site NEC — *see* Neoplasm, in situ, by site
        - unspecified site (female) D05.8- ☑
    - breast D05.0- ☑
    - specified site NEC — *see* Neoplasm, in situ, by site
    - unspecified site D05.0- ☑
  - squamous cell (*see also* Neoplasm, in situ, by site)
    - with questionable stromal invasion
      - cervix D06.9
      - specified site NEC — *see* Neoplasm, in situ, by site
      - unspecified site D06.9
- **Carcinomaphobia** F45.29
- **Carcinomatosis** C80.0
  - peritonei C78.6
  - unspecified site (primary) (secondary) C80.0
- **Carcinosarcoma** — *see* Neoplasm, malignant, by site
  - embryonal — *see* Neoplasm, malignant, by site
- **Cardia, cardial** — *see* condition
- **Cardiac** (*see also* condition)
  - death, sudden — *see* Arrest, cardiac
  - pacemaker
    - in situ Z95.0
    - management or adjustment Z45.018
  - tamponade I31.4
- **Cardialgia** — *see* Pain, precordial
- **Cardiectasis** — *see* Hypertrophy, cardiac
- **Cardiochalasia** K21.9
- **Cardiomalacia** I51.5
- **Cardiomegalia glycogenica diffusa** E74.02 [I43]
- **Cardiomegaly** (*see also* Hypertrophy, cardiac)
  - congenital Q24.8
  - glycogen E74.02 [I43]
  - idiopathic I51.7
- **Cardiomyoliposis** I51.5
- **Cardiomyopathy** (familial) (idiopathic) I42.9
  - alcoholic I42.6
  - amyloid E85.4 [I43]
  - arteriosclerotic — *see* Disease, heart, ischemic, atherosclerotic
  - beriberi E51.12
  - cobalt-beer I42.6
  - congenital I42.4
  - congestive I42.0

- **Cardiomyopathy** — *continued*
  - constrictive NOS I42.5
  - dilated I42.0
  - due to
    - alcohol I42.6
    - beriberi E51.12
    - cardiac glycogenosis E74.02 [I43]
    - drugs I42.7
    - external agents NEC I42.7
    - Friedreich's ataxia G11.1
    - myotonia atrophica G71.11 [I43]
    - progressive muscular dystrophy G71.0
  - glycogen storage E74.02 [I43]
  - hypertensive — *see* Hypertension, heart
  - hypertrophic (nonobstructive) I42.2
    - obstructive I42.1
      - congenital Q24.8
  - in
    - Chagas' disease (chronic) B57.2
      - acute B57.0
    - sarcoidosis D86.85
  - ischemic I25.5
  - metabolic E88.9 [I43]
    - thyrotoxic E05.90 [I43]
      - with thyroid storm E05.91 [I43]
  - newborn I42.8
    - congenital I42.4
  - nutritional E63.9 [I43]
    - beriberi E51.12
  - obscure of Africa I42.8
  - peripartum O90.3
  - postpartum O90.3
  - restrictive NEC I42.5
  - rheumatic I09.0
  - secondary I42.9
  - stress induced I51.81
  - takotsubo I51.81
  - thyrotoxic E05.90 [I43]
    - with thyroid storm E05.91 [I43]
  - toxic NEC I42.7
  - tuberculous A18.84
  - viral B33.24
- **Cardionephritis** — *see* Hypertension, cardiorenal
- **Cardionephropathy** — *see* Hypertension, cardiorenal
- **Cardionephrosis** — *see* Hypertension, cardiorenal
- **Cardiopathia nigra** I27.0
- **Cardiopathy** (*see also* Disease, heart) I51.9
  - idiopathic I42.9
  - mucopolysaccharidosis E76.3 [I52]
- **Cardiopericarditis** — *see* Pericarditis
- **Cardiophobia** F45.29
- **Cardiorenal** — *see* condition
- **Cardiorrhexis** — *see* Infarct, myocardium
- **Cardiosclerosis** — *see* Disease, heart, ischemic, atherosclerotic
- **Cardiosis** — *see* Disease, heart
- **Cardiospasm** (esophagus) (reflex) (stomach) K22.0
  - congenital Q39.5
    - with megaesophagus Q39.5
- **Cardiostenosis** — *see* Disease, heart
- **Cardiosymphysis** I31.0
- **Cardiovascular** — *see* condition
- **Carditis** (acute) (bacterial) (chronic) (subacute) I51.89
  - meningococcal A39.50
  - rheumatic — *see* Disease, heart, rheumatic
  - rheumatoid — *see* Rheumatoid, carditis
  - viral B33.20
- **Care** (of) (for) (following)
  - child (routine) Z76.2
  - family member (handicapped) (sick)
    - creating problem for family Z63.6
    - provided away from home for holiday relief Z75.5
    - unavailable, due to
      - absence (person rendering care) (sufferer) Z74.2
      - inability (any reason) of person rendering care Z74.2
  - foundling Z76.1
  - holiday relief Z75.5
  - improper — *see* Maltreatment
  - lack of (at or after birth) (infant) — *see* Maltreatment, child, neglect
  - lactating mother Z39.1
  - palliative Z51.5
  - postpartum
    - immediately after delivery Z39.0
    - routine follow-up Z39.2
  - respite Z75.5

- **Care** — *continued*
  - unavailable, due to
    - absence of person rendering care Z74.2
    - inability (any reason) of person rendering care Z74.2
  - well-baby Z76.2
- **Caries**
  - bone NEC A18.Ø3
  - dental KØ2.9
    - arrested (coronal) (root) KØ2.3
    - chewing surface
      - limited to enamel KØ2.51
      - penetrating into dentin KØ2.52
      - penetrating into pulp KØ2.53
    - coronal surface
      - chewing surface
        - limited to enamel KØ2.51
        - penetrating into dentin KØ2.52
        - penetrating into pulp KØ2.53
      - pit and fissure surface
        - limited to enamel KØ2.51
        - penetrating into dentin KØ2.52
        - penetrating into pulp KØ2.53
      - smooth surface
        - limited to enamel KØ2.61
        - penetrating into dentin KØ2.62
        - penetrating into pulp KØ2.63
    - pit and fissure surface
      - limited to enamel KØ2.51
      - penetrating into dentin KØ2.52
      - penetrating into pulp KØ2.53
    - root KØ2.7
    - smooth surface
      - limited to enamel KØ2.61
      - penetrating into dentin KØ2.62
      - penetrating into pulp KØ2.63
  - external meatus — *see* Disorder, ear, external, specified type NEC
  - hip (tuberculous) A18.Ø2
  - initial (tooth)
    - chewing surface KØ2.51
    - pit and fissure surface KØ2.51
    - smooth surface KØ2.61
  - knee (tuberculous) A18.Ø2
  - labyrinth H83.8 ☑
  - limb NEC (tuberculous) A18.Ø3
  - mastoid process (chronic) — *see* Mastoiditis, chronic
    - tuberculous A18.Ø3
  - middle ear H74.8 ☑
  - nose (tuberculous) A18.Ø3
  - orbit (tuberculous) A18.Ø3
  - ossicles, ear — *see* Abnormal, ear ossicles
  - petrous bone — *see* Petrositis
  - root (dental) (tooth) KØ2.7
  - sacrum (tuberculous) A18.Ø1
  - spine, spinal (column) (tuberculous) A18.Ø1
  - syphilitic A52.77
    - congenital (early) A5Ø.Ø2 [M9Ø.8Ø]
  - tooth, teeth — *see* Caries, dental
  - tuberculous A18.Ø3
  - vertebra (column) (tuberculous) A18.Ø1
- **Carious teeth** — *see* Caries, dental
- **Carneous mole** OØ2.Ø
- **Carnitine insufficiency** E71.4Ø
- **Carotid body or sinus syndrome** G9Ø.Ø1
- **Carotidynia** G9Ø.Ø1
- **Carotinemia** (dietary) E67.1
- **Carotinosis** (cutis) (skin) E67.1
- **Carpal tunnel syndrome** — *see* Syndrome, carpal tunnel
- **Carpenter's syndrome** Q87.Ø
- **Carpopedal spasm** — *see* Tetany
- **Carr-Barr-Plunkett syndrome** Q97.1
- **Carrier** (suspected) of
  - amebiasis Z22.1
  - bacterial disease NEC Z22.39
    - diphtheria Z22.2
    - intestinal infectious NEC Z22.1
      - typhoid Z22.Ø
    - meningococcal Z22.31
    - sexually transmitted Z22.4
    - specified NEC Z22.39
    - staphylococcal (Methicillin susceptible) Z22.321
      - Methicillin resistant Z22.322
    - streptococcal Z22.338
      - group B Z22.33Ø
    - typhoid Z22.Ø
  - cholera Z22.1
  - diphtheria Z22.2
- **Carrier** of — *continued*
  - gastrointestinal pathogens NEC Z22.1
  - genetic Z14.8
    - cystic fibrosis Z14.1
    - hemophilia A (asymptomatic) Z14.Ø1
      - symptomatic Z14.Ø2
  - gonorrhea Z22.4
  - HAA (hepatitis Australian-antigen) Z22.59
  - HB (c)(s)-AG Z22.51
  - hepatitis (viral) Z22.5Ø
    - Australia-antigen (HAA) Z22.59
    - B surface antigen (HBsAg) Z22.51
      - with acute delta- (super)infection B17.Ø
    - C Z22.52
    - specified NEC Z22.59
  - human T-cell lymphotropic virus type-1 (HTLV-1) infection Z22.6
  - infectious organism Z22.9
    - specified NEC Z22.8
  - meningococci Z22.31
  - Salmonella typhosa Z22.Ø
  - serum hepatitis — *see* Carrier, hepatitis
  - staphylococci (Methicillin susceptible) Z22.321
    - Methicillin resistant Z22.322
  - streptococci Z22.338
    - group B Z22.33Ø
  - syphilis Z22.4
  - typhoid Z22.Ø
  - venereal disease NEC Z22.4
- **Carrion's disease** A44.Ø
- **Carter's relapsing fever** (Asiatic) A68.1
- **Cartilage** — *see* condition
- **Caruncle** (inflamed)
  - conjunctiva (acute) — *see* Conjunctivitis, acute
  - labium (majus) (minus) N9Ø.89
  - lacrimal — *see* Inflammation, lacrimal, passages
  - myrtiform N89.8
  - urethral (benign) N36.2
- **Cascade stomach** K31.2
- **Caseation lymphatic gland** (tuberculous) A18.2
- **Cassidy** (-Scholte) syndrome (malignant carcinoid) E34.Ø
- **Castellani's disease** A69.8
- **Castration, traumatic, male** S38.231 ☑
- **Casts in urine** R82.99
- **Cat**
  - cry syndrome Q93.4
  - ear Q17.3
  - eye syndrome Q92.8
- **Catabolism, senile** R54
- **Catalepsy** (hysterical) F44.2
  - schizophrenic F2Ø.2
- **Cataplexy** (idiopathic) — *see* Narcolepsy
- **Cataract** (cortical) (immature) (incipient) H26.9
  - with
    - neovascularization — *see* Cataract, complicated
  - age-related — *see* Cataract, senile
  - anterior
    - and posterior axial embryonal Q12.Ø
    - pyramidal Q12.Ø
  - associated with
    - galactosemia E74.21 [H28]
    - myotonic disorders G71.19 [H28]
  - blue Q12.Ø
  - central Q12.Ø
  - cerulean Q12.Ø
  - complicated H26.2Ø
    - with
      - neovascularization H26.21- ☑
      - ocular disorder H26.22- ☑
    - glaucomatous flecks H26.23- ☑
  - congenital Q12.Ø
  - coraliform Q12.Ø
  - coronary Q12.Ø
  - crystalline Q12.Ø
  - diabetic — *see* Diabetes, cataract
  - drug-induced H26.3- ☑
  - due to
    - ocular disorder — *see* Cataract, complicated
    - radiation H26.8
  - electric H26.8
  - extraction status Z98.4- ☑
  - glass-blower's H26.8
  - heat ray H26.8
  - heterochromic — *see* Cataract, complicated
  - hypermature — *see* Cataract, senile, morgagnian type
  - in (due to)
    - chronic iridocyclitis — *see* Cataract, complicated
- **Cataract** — *continued*
  - in — *continued*
    - diabetes — *see* Diabetes, cataract
    - endocrine disease E34.9 [H28]
    - eye disease — *see* Cataract, complicated
    - hypoparathyroidism E2Ø.9 [H28]
    - malnutrition-dehydration E46 [H28]
    - metabolic disease E88.9 [H28]
    - myotonic disorders G71.19 [H28]
    - nutritional disease E63.9 [H28]
  - infantile — *see* Cataract, presenile
  - irradiational — *see* Cataract, specified NEC
  - juvenile — *see* Cataract, presenile
  - malnutrition-dehydration E46 [H28]
  - morgagnian — *see* Cataract, senile, morgagnian type
  - myotonic G71.19 [H28]
  - myxedema EØ3.9 [H28]
  - nuclear
    - embryonal Q12.Ø
    - sclerosis — *see* Cataract, senile, nuclear
  - presenile H26.ØØ- ☑
    - combined forms H26.Ø6- ☑
    - cortical H26.Ø1- ☑
    - lamellar — *see* Cataract, presenile, cortical
    - nuclear H26.Ø3- ☑
    - specified NEC H26.Ø9
    - subcapsular polar (anterior) H26.Ø4- ☑
      - posterior H26.Ø5- ☑
    - zonular — *see* Cataract, presenile, cortical
  - secondary H26.4Ø
    - Soemmering's ring H26.41- ☑
    - specified NEC H26.49- ☑
    - to eye disease — *see* Cataract, complicated
  - senile H25.9
    - brunescens — *see* Cataract, senile, nuclear
    - combined forms H25.81- ☑
    - coronary — *see* Cataract, senile, incipient
    - cortical H25.Ø1- ☑
    - hypermature — *see* Cataract, senile, morgagnian type
    - incipient (mature) (total) H25.Ø9- ☑
      - cortical — *see* Cataract, senile, cortical
      - subcapsular — *see* Cataract, senile, subcapsular
    - morgagnian type (hypermature) H25.2- ☑
    - nuclear (sclerosis) H25.1- ☑
    - polar subcapsular (anterior) (posterior) — *see* Cataract, senile, incipient
    - punctate — *see* Cataract, senile, incipient
    - specified NEC H25.89
    - subcapsular polar (anterior) H25.Ø3- ☑
      - posterior H25.Ø4- ☑
  - snowflake — *see* Diabetes, cataract
  - specified NEC H26.8
  - toxic — *see* Cataract, drug-induced
  - traumatic H26.1Ø- ☑
    - localized H26.11- ☑
    - partially resolved H26.12- ☑
    - total H26.13- ☑
  - zonular (perinuclear) Q12.Ø
- **Cataracta** (*see also* Cataract)
  - brunescens — *see* Cataract, senile, nuclear
  - centralis pulverulenta Q12.Ø
  - cerulea Q12.Ø
  - complicata — *see* Cataract, complicated
  - congenita Q12.Ø
  - coralliformis Q12.Ø
  - coronaria Q12.Ø
  - diabetic — *see* Diabetes, cataract
  - membranacea
    - accreta — *see* Cataract, secondary
    - congenita Q12.Ø
  - nigra — *see* Cataract, senile, nuclear
  - sunflower — *see* Cataract, complicated
- **Catarrh, catarrhal** (acute) (febrile) (infectious) (inflammation) (*see also* condition) JØØ
  - bronchial — *see* Bronchitis
  - chest — *see* Bronchitis
  - chronic J31.Ø
  - due to congenital syphilis A5Ø.Ø3
  - enteric — *see* Enteritis
  - eustachian H68.ØØ9
  - fauces — *see* Pharyngitis
  - gastrointestinal — *see* Enteritis
  - gingivitis KØ5.ØØ
    - nonplaque induced KØ5.Ø1
    - plaque induced KØ5.ØØ
  - hay — *see* Fever, hay

- **Catarrh, catarrhal** — *continued*
  - intestinal — *see* Enteritis
  - larynx, chronic J37.Ø
  - liver B15.9
    - with hepatic coma B15.Ø
  - lung — *see* Bronchitis
  - middle ear, chronic — *see* Otitis, media, nonsuppurative, chronic, serous
  - mouth K12.1
  - nasal (chronic) — *see* Rhinitis
  - nasobronchial J31.1
  - nasopharyngeal (chronic) J31.1
    - acute JØØ
  - pulmonary — *see* Bronchitis
  - spring (eye) (vernal) — *see* Conjunctivitis, acute, atopic
  - summer (hay) — *see* Fever, hay
  - throat J31.2
  - tubotympanal (*see also* Otitis, media, nonsuppurative)
    - chronic — *see* Otitis, media, nonsuppurative, chronic, serous
- **Catatonia** (schizophrenic) F2Ø.2
- **Catatonic**
  - disorder due to known physiologic condition FØ6.1
  - schizophrenia F2Ø.2
  - stupor R4Ø.1
- **Cat-scratch** (*see also* Abrasion)
  - disease or fever A28.1
- **Cauda equina** — *see* condition
- **Cauliflower ear** M95.1- ☑
- **Causalgia** (upper limb) G56.4- ☑
  - lower limb G57.7- ☑
- **Cause**
  - external, general effects T75.89 ☑
- **Caustic burn** — *see* Corrosion, by site
- **Cavare's disease** (familial periodic paralysis) G72.3
- **Cave-in, injury**
  - crushing (severe) — *see* Crush
  - suffocation — *see* Asphyxia, traumatic, due to low oxygen, due to cave-in
- **Cavernitis** (penis) N48.29
- **Cavernositis** N48.29
- **Cavernous** — *see* condition
- **Cavitation of lung** (*see also* Tuberculosis, pulmonary)
  - nontuberculous J98.4
- **Cavities, dental** — *see* Caries, dental
- **Cavity**
  - lung — *see* Cavitation of lung
  - optic papilla Q14.2
  - pulmonary — *see* Cavitation of lung
- **Cavovarus foot, congenital** Q66.1
- **Cavus foot** (congenital) Q66.7
  - acquired — *see* Deformity, limb, foot, specified NEC
- **Cazenave's disease** L1Ø.2
- **Cecitis** K52.9
  - with perforation, peritonitis, or rupture K65.8
- **Cecum** — *see* condition
- **Celiac**
  - artery compression syndrome I77.4
  - disease K9Ø.Ø
  - infantilism K9Ø.Ø
- **Cell**(s), **cellular** (*see also* condition)
  - in urine R82.99
- **Cellulitis** (diffuse) (phlegmonous) (septic) (suppurative) LØ3.9Ø
  - abdominal wall LØ3.311
  - anaerobic A48.Ø
  - ankle — *see* Cellulitis, lower limb
  - anus K61.Ø
  - arm — *see* Cellulitis, upper limb
  - auricle (ear) — *see* Cellulitis, ear
  - axilla LØ3.11- ☑
  - back (any part) LØ3.312
  - broad ligament
    - acute N73.Ø
  - buttock LØ3.317
  - cervical (meaning neck) LØ3.221
  - cervix (uteri) — *see* Cervicitis
  - cheek (external) LØ3.211
    - internal K12.2
  - chest wall LØ3.313
  - chronic LØ3.9Ø
  - clostridial A48.Ø
  - corpus cavernosum N48.22
  - digit
    - finger — *see* Cellulitis, finger
    - toe — *see* Cellulitis, toe
- **Cellulitis** — *continued*
  - Douglas' cul-de-sac or pouch
    - acute N73.Ø
  - drainage site (following operation) T81.4 ☑
  - ear (external) H6Ø.1- ☑
  - eosinophilic (granulomatous) L98.3
  - erysipelatous — *see* Erysipelas
  - external auditory canal — *see* Cellulitis, ear
  - eyelid — *see* Abscess, eyelid
  - face NEC LØ3.211
  - finger (intrathecal) (periosteal) (subcutaneous) (subcuticular) LØ3.Ø1- ☑
  - foot — *see* Cellulitis, lower limb
  - gangrenous — *see* Gangrene
  - genital organ NEC
    - female (external) N76.4
    - male N49.9
      - multiple sites N49.8
      - specified NEC N49.8
  - gluteal (region) LØ3.317
  - gonococcal A54.89
  - groin LØ3.314
  - hand — *see* Cellulitis, upper limb
  - head NEC LØ3.811
    - face (any part, except ear, eye and nose) LØ3.211
  - heel — *see* Cellulitis, lower limb
  - hip — *see* Cellulitis, lower limb
  - jaw (region) LØ3.211
  - knee — *see* Cellulitis, lower limb
  - labium (majus) (minus) — *see* Vulvitis
  - lacrimal passages — *see* Inflammation, lacrimal, passages
  - larynx J38.7
  - leg — *see* Cellulitis, lower limb
  - lip K13.Ø
  - lower limb LØ3.11- ☑
    - toe — *see* Cellulitis, toe
  - mouth (floor) K12.2
  - multiple sites, so stated LØ3.9Ø
  - nasopharynx J39.1
  - navel LØ3.316
    - newborn P38.9
      - with mild hemorrhage P38.1
      - without hemorrhage P38.9
  - neck (region) LØ3.221
  - nose (septum) (external) J34.Ø
  - orbit, orbital HØ5.Ø1- ☑
  - palate (soft) K12.2
  - pectoral (region) LØ3.313
  - pelvis, pelvic (chronic)
    - female (*see also* Disease, pelvis, inflammatory) N73.2
      - acute N73.Ø
    - following ectopic or molar pregnancy OØ8.Ø
    - male K65.Ø
  - penis N48.22
  - perineal, perineum LØ3.315
  - perirectal K61.1
  - peritonsillar J36
  - periurethral N34.Ø
  - periuterine (*see also* Disease, pelvis, inflammatory) N73.2
    - acute N73.Ø
  - pharynx J39.1
  - rectum K61.1
  - retroperitoneal K68.9
  - round ligament
    - acute N73.Ø
  - scalp (any part) LØ3.811
  - scrotum N49.2
  - seminal vesicle N49.Ø
  - shoulder — *see* Cellulitis, upper limb
  - specified site NEC LØ3.818
  - submandibular (region) (space) (triangle) K12.2
    - gland K11.3
  - submaxillary (region) K12.2
    - gland K11.3
  - thigh — *see* Cellulitis, lower limb
  - thumb (intrathecal) (periosteal) (subcutaneous) (subcuticular) — *see* Cellulitis, finger
  - toe (intrathecal) (periosteal) (subcutaneous) (subcuticular) LØ3.Ø3- ☑
  - tonsil J36
  - trunk LØ3.319
    - abdominal wall LØ3.311
    - back (any part) LØ3.312
    - buttock LØ3.317
    - chest wall LØ3.313
- **Cellulitis** — *continued*
  - trunk — *continued*
    - groin LØ3.314
    - perineal, perineum LØ3.315
    - umbilicus LØ3.316
  - tuberculous (primary) A18.4
  - umbilicus LØ3.316
  - upper limb LØ3.11- ☑
    - axilla — *see* Cellulitis, axilla
    - finger — *see* Cellulitis, finger
    - thumb — *see* Cellulitis, finger
  - vaccinal T88.Ø ☑
  - vocal cord J38.3
  - vulva — *see* Vulvitis
  - wrist — *see* Cellulitis, upper limb
- **Cementoblastoma, benign** — *see* Cyst, calcifying odontogenic
- **Cementoma** — *see* Cyst, calcifying odontogenic
- **Cementoperiostitis** — *see* Periodontitis
- **Cementosis** KØ3.4
- **Central auditory processing disorder** H93.25
- **Central pain syndrome** G89.Ø
- **Cephalematocele, cephal** (o)hematocele
  - newborn P52.8
    - birth injury P1Ø.8
  - traumatic — *see* Hematoma, brain
- **Cephalematoma, cephalhematoma** (calcified)
  - newborn (birth injury) P12.Ø
  - traumatic — *see* Hematoma, brain
- **Cephalgia, cephalalgia** (*see also* Headache)
  - histamine G44.ØØ9
    - intractable G44.ØØ1
    - not intractable G44.ØØ9
  - trigeminal autonomic (TAC) NEC G44.Ø99
    - intractable G44.Ø91
    - not intractable G44.Ø99
- **Cephalic** — *see* condition
- **Cephalitis** — *see* Encephalitis
- **Cephalocele** — *see* Encephalocele
- **Cephalomenia** N94.89
- **Cephalopelvic** — *see* condition
- **Cerclage** (with cervical incompetence) in pregnancy — *see* Incompetence, cervix, in pregnancy
- **Cerebellitis** — *see* Encephalitis
- **Cerebellum, cerebellar** — *see* condition
- **Cerebral** — *see* condition
- **Cerebritis** — *see* Encephalitis
- **Cerebro-hepato-renal syndrome** Q87.89
- **Cerebromalacia** — *see* Softening, brain
  - sequelae of cerebrovascular disease I69.398
- **Cerebroside lipidosis** E75.22
- **Cerebrospasticity** (congenital) G8Ø.1
- **Cerebrospinal** — *see* condition
- **Cerebrum** — *see* condition
- **Ceroid-lipofuscinosis, neuronal** E75.4
- **Cerumen** (accumulation) (impacted) H61.2- ☑
- **Cervical** (*see also* condition)
  - auricle Q18.2
  - dysplasia in pregnancy — *see* Abnormal, cervix, in pregnancy or childbirth
  - erosion in pregnancy — *see* Abnormal, cervix, in pregnancy or childbirth
  - fibrosis in pregnancy — *see* Abnormal, cervix, in pregnancy or childbirth
  - fusion syndrome Q76.1
  - rib Q76.5
  - shortening (complicating pregnancy) O26.87- ☑
- **Cervicalgia** M54.2
- **Cervicitis** (acute) (chronic) (nonvenereal) (senile (atrophic)) (subacute) (with ulceration) N72
  - with
    - abortion — *see* Abortion, by type complicated by genital tract and pelvic infection
    - ectopic pregnancy OØ8.Ø
    - molar pregnancy OØ8.Ø
  - chlamydial A56.Ø9
  - gonococcal A54.Ø3
  - herpesviral A6Ø.Ø3
  - puerperal (postpartum) O86.11
  - syphilitic A52.76
  - trichomonal A59.Ø9
  - tuberculous A18.16
- **Cervicocolpitis** (emphysematosa) (see also Cervicitis) N72
- **Cervix** — *see* condition
- **Cesarean delivery, previous, affecting management of pregnancy** O34.21

Chlorosis — *continued*
Egyptian B76.9 [D63.8]
miner's B76.9 [D63.8]
Chlorotic anemia D5Ø.8
Chocolate cyst (ovary) N8Ø.1
Choked
disc or disk — *see* Papilledema
on food, phlegm, or vomitus NOS — *see* Foreign body, by site
while vomiting NOS — *see* Foreign body, by site
Chokes (resulting from bends) T7Ø.3 ☑
Choking sensation RØ9.89
Cholangiectasis K83.8
Cholangiocarcinoma
with hepatocellular carcinoma, combined C22.Ø
liver C22.1
specified site NEC — *see* Neoplasm, malignant, by site
unspecified site C22.1
Cholangiohepatitis K83.8
due to fluke infestation B66.1
Cholangiohepatoma C22.Ø
Cholangiolitis (acute) (chronic) (extrahepatic) (gangrenous) (intrahepatic) K83.Ø
paratyphoidal — *see* Fever, paratyphoid
typhoidal AØ1.Ø9
Cholangioma D13.4
malignant — *see* Cholangiocarcinoma
Cholangitis (ascending) (primary) (recurrent) (sclerosing) (secondary) (stenosing) (suppurative) K83.Ø
with calculus, bile duct — *see* Calculus, bile duct, with cholangitis
chronic nonsuppurative destructive K74.3
Cholecystectasia K82.8
Cholecystitis K81.9
with
calculus, stones in
bile duct (common) (hepatic) — *see* Calculus, bile duct, with cholecystitis
cystic duct — *see* Calculus, gallbladder, with cholecystitis
gallbladder — *see* Calculus, gallbladder, with cholecystitis
choledocholithiasis — *see* Calculus, bile duct, with cholecystitis
cholelithiasis — *see* Calculus, gallbladder, with cholecystitis
acute (emphysematous) (gangrenous) (suppurative) K81.Ø
with
calculus, stones in
cystic duct — *see* Calculus, gallbladder, with cholecystitis, acute
gallbladder — *see* Calculus, gallbladder, with cholecystitis, acute
choledocholithiasis — *see* Calculus, bile duct, with cholecystitis, acute
cholelithiasis — *see* Calculus, gallbladder, with cholecystitis, acute
chronic cholecystitis K81.2
with gallbladder calculus K8Ø.12
with obstruction K8Ø.13
chronic K81.1
with acute cholecystitis K81.2
with gallbladder calculus K8Ø.12
with obstruction K8Ø.13
emphysematous (acute) — *see* Cholecystitis, acute
gangrenous — *see* Cholecystitis, acute
paratyphoidal, current AØ1.4
suppurative — *see* Cholecystitis, acute
typhoidal AØ1.Ø9
Cholecystolithiasis — *see* Calculus, gallbladder
Choledochitis (suppurative) K83.Ø
Choledocholith — *see* Calculus, bile duct
Choledocholithiasis (common duct) (hepatic duct) — *see* Calculus, bile duct
cystic — *see* Calculus, gallbladder
typhoidal AØ1.Ø9
Cholelithiasis (cystic duct) (gallbladder) (impacted) (multiple) — *see* Calculus, gallbladder
bile duct (common) (hepatic) — *see* Calculus, bile duct
hepatic duct — *see* Calculus, bile duct
specified NEC K8Ø.8Ø
with obstruction K8Ø.81
Cholemia (*see also* Jaundice)
familial (simple) (congenital) E8Ø.4
Gilbert's E8Ø.4
Choleperitoneum, choleperitonitis K65.3
Cholera (Asiatic) (epidemic) (malignant) AØØ.9
antimonial — *see* Poisoning, antimony
classical AØØ.Ø
due to Vibrio cholerae Ø1 AØØ.9
biovar cholerae AØØ.Ø
biovar eltor AØØ.1
el tor AØØ.1
el tor AØØ.1
Cholerine — *see* Cholera
Cholestasis NEC K83.1
with hepatocyte injury K71.Ø
due to total parenteral nutrition (TPN) K76.89
pure K71.Ø
Cholesteatoma (ear) (middle) (with reaction) H71.9- ☑
attic H71.Ø- ☑
external ear (canal) H6Ø.4- ☑
mastoid H71.2- ☑
postmastoidectomy cavity (recurrent) — *see* Complications, postmastoidectomy, recurrent cholesteatoma
recurrent (postmastoidectomy) — *see* Complications, postmastoidectomy, recurrent cholesteatoma
tympanum H71.1- ☑
Cholesteatosis, diffuse H71.3- ☑
Cholesteremia E78.Ø
Cholesterin in vitreous — *see* Deposit, crystalline
Cholesterol
deposit
retina H35.89
vitreous — *see* Deposit, crystalline
elevated (high) E78.Ø
with elevated (high) triglycerides E78.2
screening for Z13.22Ø
imbibition of gallbladder K82.4
Cholesterolemia (essential) (familial) (hereditary) (pure) E78.Ø
Cholesterolosis, cholesterosis (gallbladder) K82.4
cerebrotendinous E75.5
Cholocolic fistula K82.3
Choluria R82.2
Chondritis M94.8X9
aurical H61.Ø3- ☑
costal (Tietze's) M94.Ø
external ear H61.Ø3- ☑
patella, posttraumatic — *see* Chondromalacia, patella
pinna H61.Ø3- ☑
purulent M94.8X- ☑
tuberculous NEC A18.Ø2
intervertebral A18.Ø1
Chondroblastoma (*see also* Neoplasm, bone, benign)
malignant — *see* Neoplasm, bone, malignant
Chondrocalcinosis M11.2Ø
ankle M11.27- ☑
elbow M11.22- ☑
familial M11.1Ø
ankle M11.17- ☑
elbow M11.12- ☑
foot joint M11.17- ☑
hand joint M11.14- ☑
hip M11.15- ☑
knee M11.16- ☑
multiple site M11.19
shoulder M11.11- ☑
vertebrae M11.18
wrist M11.13- ☑
foot joint M11.27- ☑
hand joint M11.24- ☑
hip M11.25- ☑
knee M11.26- ☑
multiple site M11.29
shoulder M11.21- ☑
specified type NEC M11.2Ø
ankle M11.27- ☑
elbow M11.22- ☑
foot joint M11.27- ☑
hand joint M11.24- ☑
hip M11.25- ☑
knee M11.26- ☑
multiple site M11.29
shoulder M11.21- ☑
vertebrae M11.28
wrist M11.23- ☑
vertebrae M11.28
wrist M11.23- ☑
Chondrodermatitis nodularis helicis or anthelicis — *see* Perichondritis, ear
Chondrodysplasia Q78.9
with hemangioma Q78.4
calcificans congenita Q77.3
fetalis Q77.4
metaphyseal (Jansen's) (McKusick's) (Schmid's) Q78.5
punctata Q77.3
Chondrodystrophy, chondrodystrophia (familial) (fetalis) (hypoplastic) Q78.9
calcificans congenita Q77.3
myotonic (congenital) G71.13
punctata Q77.3
Chondroectodermal dysplasia Q77.6
Chondrogenesis imperfecta Q77.4
Chondrolysis M94.35- ☑
Chondroma (*see also* Neoplasm, cartilage, benign)
juxtacortical — *see* Neoplasm, bone, benign
periosteal — *see* Neoplasm, bone, benign
Chondromalacia (systemic) M94.2Ø
acromioclavicular joint M94.21- ☑
ankle M94.27- ☑
elbow M94.22- ☑
foot joint M94.27- ☑
glenohumeral joint M94.21- ☑
hand joint M94.24- ☑
hip M94.25- ☑
knee M94.26- ☑
patella M22.4- ☑
multiple sites M94.29
patella M22.4- ☑
rib M94.28
sacroiliac joint M94.259
shoulder M94.21- ☑
sternoclavicular joint M94.21- ☑
vertebral joint M94.28
wrist M94.23- ☑
Chondromatosis (*see also* Neoplasm, cartilage, uncertain behavior)
internal Q78.4
Chondromyxosarcoma — *see* Neoplasm, cartilage, malignant
Chondro-osteodysplasia (Morquio-Brailsford type) E76.219
Chondro-osteodystrophy E76.29
Chondro-osteoma — *see* Neoplasm, bone, benign
Chondropathia tuberosa M94.Ø
Chondrosarcoma — *see* Neoplasm, cartilage, malignant
juxtacortical — *see* Neoplasm, bone, malignant
mesenchymal — *see* Neoplasm, connective tissue, malignant
myxoid — *see* Neoplasm, cartilage, malignant
Chordee (nonvenereal) N48.89
congenital Q54.4
gonococcal A54.Ø9
Chorditis (fibrinous) (nodosa) (tuberosa) J38.2
Chordoma — *see* Neoplasm, vertebral (column), malignant
Chorea (chronic) (gravis) (posthemiplegic) (senile) (spasmodic) G25.5
with
heart involvement IØ2.Ø
active or acute (conditions in IØ1-) IØ2.Ø
rheumatic IØ2.9
with valvular disorder IØ2.Ø
rheumatic heart disease (chronic) (inactive)(quiescent) — *code to* rheumatic heart condition involved
drug-induced G25.4
habit F95.8
hereditary G1Ø
Huntington's G1Ø
hysterical F44.4
minor IØ2.9
with heart involvement IØ2.Ø
progressive G25.5
hereditary G1Ø
rheumatic (chronic) IØ2.9
with heart involvement IØ2.Ø
Sydenham's IØ2.9
with heart involvement — *see* Chorea, with rheumatic heart disease
nonrheumatic G25.5
Choreoathetosis (paroxysmal) G25.5
Chorioadenoma (destruens) D39.2
Chorioamnionitis O41.12- ☑
Chorioangioma D26.7
Choriocarcinoma — *see* Neoplasm, malignant, by site
combined with

- **Claudication, intermittent** I73.9
  - cerebral (artery) G45.9
  - spinal cord (arteriosclerotic) G95.19
    - syphilitic A52.Ø9
  - venous (axillary) I87.8
- **Claustrophobia** F4Ø.24Ø
- **Clavus** (infected) L84
- **Clawfoot** (congenital) Q66.89
  - acquired — *see* Deformity, limb, clawfoot
- **Clawhand** (acquired) (*see also* Deformity, limb, clawhand)
  - congenital Q68.1
- **Clawtoe** (congenital) Q66.89
  - acquired — *see* Deformity, toe, specified NEC
- **Clay eating** — *see* Pica
- **Cleansing of artificial opening** — *see* Attention to, artificial, opening
- **Cleft** (congenital) (*see also* Imperfect, closure)
  - alveolar process M26.79
  - branchial (cyst) (persistent) Q18.2
  - cricoid cartilage, posterior Q31.8
  - lip (unilateral) Q36.9
    - with cleft palate Q37.9
      - hard Q37.1
        - with soft Q37.5
      - soft Q37.3
        - with hard Q37.5
    - bilateral Q36.Ø
      - with cleft palate Q37.8
        - hard Q37.Ø
          - with soft Q37.4
        - soft Q37.2
          - with hard Q37.4
    - median Q36.1
  - nose Q3Ø.2
  - palate Q35.9
    - with cleft lip (unilateral) Q37.9
      - bilateral Q37.8
    - hard Q35.1
      - with
        - cleft lip (unilateral) Q37.1
          - bilateral Q37.Ø
        - soft Q35.5
          - with cleft lip (unilateral) Q37.5
            - bilateral Q37.4
    - medial Q35.5
    - soft Q35.3
      - with
        - cleft lip (unilateral) Q37.3
          - bilateral Q37.2
        - hard Q35.5
          - with cleft lip (unilateral) Q37.5
            - bilateral Q37.4
  - penis Q55.69
  - scrotum Q55.29
  - thyroid cartilage Q31.8
  - uvula Q35.7
- **Cleidocranial dysostosis** Q74.Ø
- **Cleptomania** F63.2
- **Clicking hip** (newborn) R29.4
- **Climacteric** (female) (*see also* Menopause)
  - arthritis (any site) NEC — *see* Arthritis, specified form NEC
  - depression (single episode) F32.8
  - male (symptoms) (syndrome) NEC N5Ø.8
  - paranoid state F22
  - polyarthritis NEC — *see* Arthritis, specified form NEC
  - symptoms (female) N95.1
- **Clinical research investigation** (clinical trial) (control subject) (normal comparison) (participant) ZØØ.6
- **Clitoris** — *see* condition
- **Cloaca** (persistent) Q43.7
- **Clonorchiasis, clonorchis infection** (liver) B66.1
- **Clonus** R25.8
- **Closed bite** M26.29
- **Clostridium** (C.) **perfringens, as cause of disease classified elsewhere** B96.7
- **Closure**
  - congenital, nose Q3Ø.Ø
  - cranial sutures, premature Q75.Ø
  - defective or imperfect NEC — *see* Imperfect, closure
  - fistula, delayed — *see* Fistula
  - foramen ovale, imperfect Q21.1
  - hymen N89.6
  - interauricular septum, defective Q21.1
  - interventricular septum, defective Q21.Ø
  - lacrimal duct (*see also* Stenosis, lacrimal, duct)
    - congenital Q1Ø.5
  - nose (congenital) Q3Ø.Ø
- **Closure** — *continued*
  - nose — *continued*
    - acquired M95.Ø
  - of artificial opening — *see* Attention to, artificial, opening
  - vagina N89.5
  - valve — *see* Endocarditis
  - vulva N9Ø.5
- **Clot** (blood) (*see also* Embolism)
  - artery (obstruction) (occlusion) — *see* Embolism
  - bladder N32.89
  - brain (intradural or extradural) — *see* Occlusion, artery, cerebral
  - circulation I74.9
  - heart (*see also* Infarct, myocardium)
    - not resulting in infarction I24.Ø
  - vein — *see* Thrombosis
- **Clouded state** R4Ø.1
  - epileptic — *see* Epilepsy, specified NEC
  - paroxysmal — *see* Epilepsy, specified NEC
- **Cloudy antrum, antra** J32.Ø
- **Clouston's** (hidrotic) **ectodermal dysplasia** Q82.4
- **Clubbed nail pachydermoperiostosis** M89.4Ø [L62]
- **Clubbing of finger**(s) (nails) R68.3
- **Clubfinger** R68.3
  - congenital Q68.1
- **Clubfoot** (congenital) Q66.89
  - acquired — *see* Deformity, limb, clubfoot
  - equinovarus Q66.Ø
  - paralytic — *see* Deformity, limb, clubfoot
- **Clubhand** (congenital) (radial) Q71.4- ☑
  - acquired — *see* Deformity, limb, clubhand
- **Clubnail** R68.3
  - congenital Q84.6
- **Clump, kidney** Q63.1
- **Clumsiness, clumsy child syndrome** F82
- **Cluttering** F8Ø.81
- **Clutton's joints** A5Ø.51 [M12.8Ø]
- **Coagulation, intravascular** (diffuse) (disseminated) (*see also* Defibrination syndrome)
  - complicating abortion — *see* Abortion, by type, complicated by, intravascular coagulation
  - following ectopic or molar pregnancy OØ8.1
- **Coagulopathy** (*see also* Defect, coagulation)
  - consumption D65
  - intravascular D65
    - newborn P6Ø
- **Coalition**
  - calcaneo-scaphoid Q66.89
  - tarsal Q66.89
- **Coalminer's**
  - elbow — *see* Bursitis, elbow, olecranon
  - lung or pneumoconiosis J6Ø
- **Coalworker's lung or pneumoconiosis** J6Ø
- **Coarctation**
  - aorta (preductal) (postductal) Q25.1
  - pulmonary artery Q25.71
- **Coated tongue** K14.3
- **Coats' disease** (exudative retinopathy) — *see* Retinopathy, exudative
- **Cocainism** — *see* Dependence, drug, cocaine
- **Coccidioidomycosis** B38.9
  - cutaneous B38.3
  - disseminated B38.7
  - generalized B38.7
  - meninges B38.4
  - prostate B38.81
  - pulmonary B38.2
    - acute B38.Ø
    - chronic B38.1
  - skin B38.3
  - specified NEC B38.89
- **Coccidioidosis** — *see* Coccidioidomycosis
- **Coccidiosis** (intestinal) AØ7.3
- **Coccydynia, coccygodynia** M53.3
- **Coccyx** — *see* condition
- **Cochin-China diarrhea** K9Ø.1
- **Cockayne's syndrome** Q87.1
- **Cocked up toe** — *see* Deformity, toe, specified NEC
- **Cock's peculiar tumor** L72.3
- **Codman's tumor** — *see* Neoplasm, bone, benign
- **Coenurosis** B71.8
- **Coffee-worker's lung** J67.8
- **Cogan's syndrome** H16.32- ☑
  - oculomotor apraxia H51.8
- **Coitus, painful** (female) N94.1
  - male N53.12
- **Coitus, painful** — *continued*
  - psychogenic F52.6
- **Cold** JØØ
  - with influenza, flu, or grippe — *see* Influenza, with, respiratory manifestations NEC
  - agglutinin disease or hemoglobinuria (chronic) D59.1
  - bronchial — *see* Bronchitis
  - chest — *see* Bronchitis
  - common (head) JØØ
  - effects of T69.9 ☑
    - specified effect NEC T69.8 ☑
  - excessive, effects of T69.9 ☑
    - specified effect NEC T69.8 ☑
  - exhaustion from T69.8 ☑
  - exposure to T69.9 ☑
    - specified effect NEC T69.8 ☑
  - head JØØ
  - injury syndrome (newborn) P8Ø.Ø
  - on lung — *see* Bronchitis
  - rose J3Ø.1
  - sensitivity, auto-immune D59.1
  - virus JØØ
- **Coldsore** BØØ.1
- **Colibacillosis** A49.8
  - as the cause of other disease (*see also* Escherichia coli) B96.2Ø
  - generalized A41.5Ø
- **Colic** (bilious) (infantile) (intestinal) (recurrent) (spasmodic) R1Ø.83
  - abdomen R1Ø.83
    - psychogenic F45.8
  - appendix, appendicular K38.8
  - bile duct — *see* Calculus, bile duct
  - biliary — *see* Calculus, bile duct
  - common duct — *see* Calculus, bile duct
  - cystic duct — *see* Calculus, gallbladder
  - Devonshire NEC — *see* Poisoning, lead
  - gallbladder — *see* Calculus, gallbladder
  - gallstone — *see* Calculus, gallbladder
    - gallbladder or cystic duct — *see* Calculus, gallbladder
  - hepatic (duct) — *see* Calculus, bile duct
  - hysterical F45.8
  - kidney N23
  - lead NEC — *see* Poisoning, lead
  - mucous K58.9
    - with diarrhea K58.Ø
    - psychogenic F54
  - nephritic N23
  - painter's NEC — *see* Poisoning, lead
  - pancreas K86.8
  - psychogenic F45.8
  - renal N23
  - saturnine NEC — *see* Poisoning, lead
  - ureter N23
  - urethral N36.8
    - due to calculus N21.1
  - uterus NEC N94.89
    - menstrual — *see* Dysmenorrhea
  - worm NOS B83.9
- **Colicystitis** — *see* Cystitis
- **Colitis** (acute) (catarrhal) (chronic) (noninfective) (hemorrhagic) (*see also* Enteritis) K52.9
  - allergic K52.2
  - amebic (acute) (*see also* Amebiasis) AØ6.Ø
    - nondysenteric AØ6.2
  - anthrax A22.2
  - bacillary — *see* Infection, Shigella
  - balantidial AØ7.Ø
  - Clostridium difficile AØ4.7
  - coccidial AØ7.3
  - collagenous K52.89
  - cystica superficialis K52.89
  - dietary counseling and surveillance (for) Z71.3
  - dietetic K52.2
  - drug-induced K52.1
  - due to radiation K52.Ø
  - eosinophilic K52.82
  - food hypersensitivity K52.2
  - giardial AØ7.1
  - granulomatous — *see* Enteritis, regional, large intestine
  - infectious — *see* Enteritis, infectious
  - ischemic K55.9
    - acute (fulminant) (subacute) K55.Ø
    - chronic K55.1
    - due to mesenteric artery insufficiency K55.1

Colitis — *continued*
- ischemic — *continued*
  - fulminant (acute) K55.Ø
- left sided K51.5Ø
  - with
    - abscess K51.514
    - complication K51.519
      - specified NEC K51.518
    - fistula K51.513
    - obstruction K51.512
    - rectal bleeding K51.511
- lymphocytic K52.89
- membranous
  - psychogenic F54
- microscopic (collagenous) (lymphocytic) K52.89
- mucous — *see* Syndrome, irritable, bowel
  - psychogenic F54
- noninfective K52.9
  - specified NEC K52.89
- polyposa — *see* Polyp, colon, inflammatory
- protozoal AØ7.9
- pseudomembranous AØ4.7
- pseudomucinous — *see* Syndrome, irritable, bowel
- regional — *see* Enteritis, regional, large intestine
- segmental — *see* Enteritis, regional, large intestine
- septic — *see* Enteritis, infectious
- spastic K58.9
  - with diarrhea K58.Ø
  - psychogenic F54
- staphylococcal AØ4.8
  - foodborne AØ5.Ø
- subacute ischemic K55.Ø
- thromboulcerative K55.Ø
- toxic NEC K52.1
  - due to Clostridium difficile AØ4.7
- transmural — *see* Enteritis, regional, large intestine
- trichomonal AØ7.8
- tuberculous (ulcerative) A18.32
- ulcerative (chronic) K51.9Ø
  - with
    - complication K51.919
      - abscess K51.914
      - fistula K51.913
      - obstruction K51.912
      - rectal bleeding K51.911
      - specified complication NEC K51.918
  - enterocolitis — *see* Enterocolitis, ulcerative
  - ileocolitis — *see* Ileocolitis, ulcerative
  - mucosal proctocolitis — *see* Proctocolitis, mucosal
  - proctitis — *see* Proctitis, ulcerative
  - pseudopolyposis — *see* Polyp, colon, inflammatory
  - psychogenic F54
  - rectosigmoiditis — *see* Rectosigmoiditis, ulcerative
  - specified type NEC K51.8Ø
    - with
      - complication K51.819
        - abscess K51.814
        - fistula K51.813
        - obstruction K51.812
        - rectal bleeding K51.811
        - specified complication NEC K51.818

Collagenosis, collagen disease (nonvascular) (vascular) M35.9
- cardiovascular I42.8
- reactive perforating L87.1
- specified NEC M35.8

Collapse R55
- adrenal E27.2
- cardiorespiratory R57.Ø
- cardiovascular R57.Ø
  - newborn P29.89
- circulatory (peripheral) R57.9
  - during or after labor and delivery O75.1
  - following ectopic or molar pregnancy OØ8.3
  - newborn P29.89
- during or
  - after labor and delivery O75.1
  - resulting from a procedure, not elsewhere classified T81.1Ø ☑
- external ear canal — *see* Stenosis, external ear canal
- general R55
- heart — *see* Disease, heart
- heat T67.1 ☑
- hysterical F44.89
- labyrinth, membranous (congenital) Q16.5
- lung (massive) (*see also* Atelectasis) J98.19
  - pressure due to anesthesia (general) (local) or other sedation T88.2 ☑

Collapse — *continued*
- lung (*see also* Atelectasis) — *continued*
  - pressure due to anesthesia or other sedation — *continued*
    - during labor and delivery O74.1
    - in pregnancy O29.Ø2- ☑
    - postpartum, puerperal O89.Ø9
- myocardial — *see* Disease, heart
- nervous F48.8
- neurocirculatory F45.8
- nose M95.Ø
- postoperative T81.1Ø ☑
- pulmonary (*see also* Atelectasis) J98.19
  - newborn — *see* Atelectasis
- trachea J39.8
- tracheobronchial J98.Ø9
- valvular — *see* Endocarditis
- vascular (peripheral) R57.9
  - during or after labor and delivery O75.1
  - following ectopic or molar pregnancy OØ8.3
  - newborn P29.89
- vertebra M48.5Ø- ☑
  - cervical region M48.52- ☑
  - cervicothoracic region M48.53- ☑
  - in (due to)
    - metastasis — *see* Collapse, vertebra, in, specified disease NEC
    - osteoporosis (*see also* Osteoporosis) M8Ø.88 ☑
      - cervical region M8Ø.88 ☑
      - cervicothoracic region M8Ø.88 ☑
      - lumbar region M8Ø.88 ☑
      - lumbosacral region M8Ø.88 ☑
      - multiple sites M8Ø.88 ☑
      - occipito-atlanto-axial region M8Ø.88 ☑
      - sacrococcygeal region M8Ø.88 ☑
      - thoracic region M8Ø.88 ☑
      - thoracolumbar region M8Ø.88 ☑
    - specified disease NEC M48.5Ø- ☑
      - cervical region M48.52- ☑
      - cervicothoracic region M48.53- ☑
      - lumbar region M48.56- ☑
      - lumbosacral region M48.57- ☑
      - occipito-atlanto-axial region M48.51- ☑
      - sacrococcygeal region M48.58- ☑
      - thoracic region M48.54- ☑
      - thoracolumbar region M48.55- ☑
  - lumbar region M48.56- ☑
  - lumbosacral region M48.57- ☑
  - occipito-atlanto-axial region M48.51- ☑
  - sacrococcygeal region M48.58- ☑
  - thoracic region M48.54- ☑
  - thoracolumbar region M48.55- ☑

Collateral (*see also* condition)
- circulation (venous) I87.8
- dilation, veins I87.8

Colles' fracture S52.53- ☑

Collet (-Sicard) syndrome G52.7

Collier's asthma or lung J6Ø

Collodion baby Q8Ø.2

Colloid nodule (of thyroid) (cystic) EØ4.1

Coloboma (iris) Q13.Ø
- eyelid Q1Ø.3
- fundus Q14.8
- lens Q12.2
- optic disc (congenital) Q14.2
  - acquired H47.31- ☑

Coloenteritis — *see* Enteritis

Colon — *see* condition

Colonization
- MRSA (Methicillin resistant Staphylococcus aureus) Z22.322
- MSSA (Methicillin susceptible Staphylococcus aureus) Z22.321
- status — *see* Carrier (suspected) of

Coloptosis K63.4

Color blindness — *see* Deficiency, color vision

Colostomy
- attention to Z43.3
- fitting or adjustment Z46.89
- malfunctioning K94.Ø3
- status Z93.3

Colpitis (acute) — *see* Vaginitis

Colpocele N81.5

Colpocystitis — *see* Vaginitis

Colpospasm N94.2

Column, spinal, vertebral — *see* condition

Coma R4Ø.2Ø
- with
  - motor response (none) R4Ø.231 ☑
    - abnormal R4Ø.233 ☑
    - extension R4Ø.232 ☑
    - flexion withdrawal R4Ø.234 ☑
    - localizes pain R4Ø.235 ☑
    - obeys commands R4Ø.236 ☑
  - opening of eyes (never) R4Ø.211 ☑
    - in response to
      - pain R4Ø.212 ☑
      - sound R4Ø.213 ☑
    - spontaneous R4Ø.214 ☑
  - verbal response (none) R4Ø.221 ☑
    - confused conversation R4Ø.224 ☑
    - inappropriate words R4Ø.223 ☑
    - incomprehensible words R4Ø.222 ☑
    - oriented R4Ø.225 ☑
- eclamptic — *see* Eclampsia
- epileptic — *see* Epilepsy
- Glasgow, scale score — *see* Glasgow coma scale
- hepatic — *see* Failure, hepatic, by type, with coma
- hyperglycemic (diabetic) — *see* Diabetes, coma
- hyperosmolar (diabetic) — *see* Diabetes, coma
- hypoglycemic (diabetic) — *see* Diabetes, coma, hypoglycemic
  - nondiabetic E15
- in diabetes — *see* Diabetes, coma
- insulin-induced — *see* Coma, hypoglycemic
- myxedematous EØ3.5
- newborn P91.5
- persistent vegetative state R4Ø.3
- specified NEC, without documented Glasgow coma scale score, or with partial Glasgow coma scale score reported R4Ø.244

Comatose — *see* Coma

Combat fatigue F43.Ø

Combined — *see* condition

Comedo, comedones (giant) L7Ø.Ø

Comedocarcinoma (*see also* Neoplasm, breast, malignant)
- noninfiltrating
  - breast DØ5.8- ☑
  - specified site — *see* Neoplasm, in situ, by site
  - unspecified site DØ5.8- ☑

Comedomastitis — *see* Ectasia, mammary duct

Comminuted fracture — *code as* Fracture, closed

Common
- arterial trunk Q2Ø.Ø
- atrioventricular canal Q21.2
- atrium Q21.1
- cold (head) JØØ
- truncus (arteriosus) Q2Ø.Ø
- variable immunodeficiency — *see* Immunodeficiency, common variable
- ventricle Q2Ø.4

Commotio, commotion (current)
- brain — *see* Injury, intracranial, concussion
- cerebri — *see* Injury, intracranial, concussion
- retinae SØ5.8X- ☑
- spinal cord — *see* Injury, spinal cord, by region
- spinalis — *see* Injury, spinal cord, by region

Communication
- between
  - base of aorta and pulmonary artery Q21.4
  - left ventricle and right atrium Q2Ø.5
  - pericardial sac and pleural sac Q34.8
  - pulmonary artery and pulmonary vein, congenital Q25.72
- congenital between uterus and digestive or urinary tract Q51.7

Compartment syndrome (deep) (posterior) (traumatic) T79.AØ ☑ (*following* T79.7)
- abdomen T79.A3 ☑ (*following* T79.7)
- lower extremity (hip, buttock, thigh, leg, foot, toes) T79.A2 ☑ (*following* T79.7)
- nontraumatic
  - abdomen M79.A3 (*following* M79.7)
  - lower extremity (hip, buttock, thigh, leg, foot, toes) M79.A2- ☑ (*following* M79.7)
  - specified site NEC M79.A9 (*following* M79.7)
  - upper extremity (shoulder, arm, forearm, wrist, hand, fingers) M79.A1- ☑ (*following* M79.7)
- specified site NEC T79.A9 ☑ (*following* T79.7)
- upper extremity (shoulder, arm, forearm, wrist, hand, fingers) T79.A1- ☑ (*following* T79.7)

- **Complication**(s) — *continued*
  - bone — *continued*
    - device — *continued*
      - fibrosis T84.82 ☑
      - hemorrhage T84.83 ☑
      - infection or inflammation T84.7 ☑
      - mechanical
        - breakdown T84.318 ☑
        - displacement T84.328 ☑
        - malposition T84.328 ☑
        - obstruction T84.398 ☑
        - perforation T84.398 ☑
        - protrusion T84.398 ☑
      - pain T84.84 ☑
      - specified type NEC T84.89 ☑
      - stenosis T84.85 ☑
      - thrombosis T84.86 ☑
    - graft — *see* Complications, graft, bone
    - growth stimulator (electrode) — *see* Complications, electronic stimulator device, bone
    - marrow transplant — *see* Complications, transplant, bone, marrow
  - brain neurostimulator (electrode) — *see* Complications, electronic stimulator device, brain
  - breast implant (prosthetic) T85.9 ☑
    - capsular contracture T85.44 ☑
    - embolism T85.81 ☑
    - fibrosis T85.82 ☑
    - hemorrhage T85.83 ☑
    - infection and inflammation T85.79 ☑
    - mechanical
      - breakdown T85.41 ☑
      - displacement T85.42 ☑
      - leakage T85.43 ☑
      - malposition T85.42 ☑
      - obstruction T85.49 ☑
      - perforation T85.49 ☑
      - protrusion T85.49 ☑
      - specified NEC T85.49 ☑
    - pain T85.84 ☑
    - specified type NEC T85.89 ☑
    - stenosis T85.85 ☑
    - thrombosis T85.86 ☑
  - bypass (*see also* Complications, prosthetic device or implant)
    - aortocoronary — *see* Complications, coronary artery (bypass) graft
    - arterial (*see also* Complications, graft, vascular)
      - extremity — *see* Complications, extremity artery (bypass) graft
  - cardiac (*see also* Disease, heart)
    - device, implant or graft T82.9 ☑
      - embolism T82.817 ☑
      - fibrosis T82.827 ☑
      - hemorrhage T82.837 ☑
      - infection or inflammation T82.7 ☑
        - valve prosthesis T82.6 ☑
      - mechanical
        - breakdown T82.519 ☑
          - specified device NEC T82.518 ☑
        - displacement T82.529 ☑
          - specified device NEC T82.528 ☑
        - leakage T82.539 ☑
          - specified device NEC T82.538 ☑
        - malposition T82.529 ☑
          - specified device NEC T82.528 ☑
        - obstruction T82.599 ☑
          - specified device NEC T82.598 ☑
        - perforation T82.599 ☑
          - specified device NEC T82.598 ☑
        - protrusion T82.599 ☑
          - specified device NEC T82.598 ☑
      - pain T82.847 ☑
      - specified type NEC T82.897 ☑
      - stenosis T82.857 ☑
      - thrombosis T82.867 ☑
  - cardiovascular device, graft or implant T82.9 ☑
    - aortic graft — *see* Complications, graft, vascular
    - arteriovenous
      - fistula, artificial — *see* Complication, arteriovenous, fistula, surgically created
      - shunt — *see* Complication, arteriovenous, shunt, surgically created
    - artificial heart — *see* Complication, artificial, heart
    - balloon (counterpulsation) device — *see* Complication, balloon implant, vascular

- **Complication**(s) — *continued*
  - cardiovascular device, graft or implant — *continued*
    - carotid artery graft — *see* Complications, graft, vascular
    - coronary bypass graft — *see* Complication, coronary artery (bypass) graft
    - dialysis catheter (vascular) — *see* Complication, catheter, dialysis
    - electronic T82.9 ☑
      - electrode T82.9 ☑
        - embolism T82.817 ☑
        - fibrosis T82.827 ☑
        - hemorrhage T82.837 ☑
        - infection T82.7 ☑
        - mechanical
          - breakdown T82.110 ☑
          - displacement T82.120 ☑
          - leakage T82.190 ☑
          - obstruction T82.190 ☑
          - perforation T82.190 ☑
          - protrusion T82.190 ☑
          - specified type NEC T82.190 ☑
        - pain T82.847 ☑
        - specified NEC T82.897 ☑
        - stenosis T82.857 ☑
        - thrombosis T82.867 ☑
      - embolism T82.817 ☑
      - fibrosis T82.827 ☑
      - hemorrhage T82.837 ☑
      - infection T82.7 ☑
      - mechanical
        - breakdown T82.119 ☑
        - displacement T82.129 ☑
        - leakage T82.199 ☑
        - obstruction T82.199 ☑
        - perforation T82.199 ☑
        - protrusion T82.199 ☑
        - specified type NEC T82.199 ☑
      - pain T82.847 ☑
      - pulse generator T82.9 ☑
        - embolism T82.817 ☑
        - fibrosis T82.827 ☑
        - hemorrhage T82.837 ☑
        - infection T82.7 ☑
        - mechanical
          - breakdown T82.111 ☑
          - displacement T82.121 ☑
          - leakage T82.191 ☑
          - obstruction T82.191 ☑
          - perforation T82.191 ☑
          - protrusion T82.191 ☑
          - specified type NEC T82.191 ☑
        - pain T82.847 ☑
        - specified NEC T82.897 ☑
        - stenosis T82.857 ☑
        - thrombosis T82.867 ☑
      - specified condition NEC T82.897 ☑
      - specified device NEC T82.9 ☑
        - embolism T82.817 ☑
        - fibrosis T82.827 ☑
        - hemorrhage T82.837 ☑
        - infection T82.7 ☑
        - mechanical
          - breakdown T82.118 ☑
          - displacement T82.128 ☑
          - leakage T82.198 ☑
          - obstruction T82.198 ☑
          - perforation T82.198 ☑
          - protrusion T82.198 ☑
          - specified type NEC T82.198 ☑
        - pain T82.847 ☑
        - specified NEC T82.897 ☑
        - stenosis T82.857 ☑
        - thrombosis T82.867 ☑
      - stenosis T82.857 ☑
      - thrombosis T82.867 ☑
    - extremity artery graft — *see* Complication, extremity artery (bypass) graft
    - femoral artery graft — *see* Complication, extremity artery (bypass) graft
    - heart
      - transplant — *see* Complication, transplant, heart
      - valve — *see* Complication, prosthetic device, heart valve

- **Complication**(s) — *continued*
  - cardiovascular device, graft or implant — *continued*
    - heart — *continued*
      - valve — *see* Complication, prosthetic device, heart valve — *continued*
        - graft — *see* Complication, heart, valve, graft
    - heart-lung transplant — *see* Complication, transplant, heart, with lung
    - infection or inflammation T82.7 ☑
    - umbrella device — *see* Complication, umbrella device, vascular
    - vascular graft (or anastomosis) — *see* Complication, graft, vascular
  - carotid artery (bypass) graft — *see* Complications, graft, vascular
  - catheter (device) NEC (*see also* Complications, prosthetic device or implant)
    - cystostomy T83.9 ☑
      - embolism T83.81 ☑
      - fibrosis T83.82 ☑
      - hemorrhage T83.83 ☑
      - infection and inflammation T83.59 ☑
      - mechanical
        - breakdown T83.010 ☑
        - displacement T83.020 ☑
        - leakage T83.030 ☑
        - malposition T83.020 ☑
        - obstruction T83.090 ☑
        - perforation T83.090 ☑
        - protrusion T83.090 ☑
        - specified NEC T83.090 ☑
      - pain T83.84 ☑
      - specified type NEC T83.89 ☑
      - stenosis T83.85 ☑
      - thrombosis T83.86 ☑
    - dialysis (vascular) T82.9 ☑
      - embolism T82.818 ☑
      - fibrosis T82.828 ☑
      - hemorrhage T82.838 ☑
      - infection and inflammation T82.7 ☑
      - intraperitoneal — *see* Complications, catheter, intraperitoneal
      - mechanical
        - breakdown T82.41 ☑
        - displacement T82.42 ☑
        - leakage T82.43 ☑
        - malposition T82.42 ☑
        - obstruction T82.49 ☑
        - perforation T82.49 ☑
        - protrusion T82.49 ☑
      - pain T82.848 ☑
      - specified type NEC T82.898 ☑
      - stenosis T82.858 ☑
      - thrombosis T82.868 ☑
    - epidural infusion T85.9 ☑
      - embolism T85.81 ☑
      - fibrosis T85.82 ☑
      - hemorrhage T85.83 ☑
      - infection and inflammation T85.79 ☑
      - mechanical
        - breakdown T85.610 ☑
        - displacement T85.620 ☑
        - leakage T85.630 ☑
        - malfunction T85.610 ☑
        - malposition T85.620 ☑
        - obstruction T85.690 ☑
        - perforation T85.690 ☑
        - protrusion T85.690 ☑
        - specified NEC T85.690 ☑
      - pain T85.84 ☑
      - specified type NEC T85.89 ☑
      - stenosis T85.85 ☑
      - thrombosis T85.86 ☑
    - intraperitoneal dialysis T85.9 ☑
      - embolism T85.81 ☑
      - fibrosis T85.82 ☑
      - hemorrhage T85.83 ☑
      - infection and inflammation T85.71 ☑
      - mechanical
        - breakdown T85.611 ☑
        - displacement T85.621 ☑
        - leakage T85.631 ☑
        - malfunction T85.611 ☑
        - malposition T85.621 ☑
        - obstruction T85.691 ☑

- **Complication**(s) — *continued*
  - following — *continued*
    - acute myocardial infarction — *continued*
      - ventricular
        - septal defect I23.2
        - thrombosis I23.6
    - ectopic or molar pregnancy O08.9
      - cardiac arrest O08.81
      - sepsis O08.82
      - specified type NEC O08.89
      - urinary tract infection O08.83
    - termination of pregnancy — *see* Abortion
  - gastrointestinal K92.9
    - bile duct prosthesis — *see* Complications, bile duct implant
    - esophageal anti-reflux device — *see* Complications, esophageal anti-reflux device
    - postoperative
      - colostomy — *see* Complications, colostomy
      - dumping syndrome K91.1
      - enterostomy — *see* Complications, enterostomy
      - gastrostomy — *see* Complications, gastrostomy
      - malabsorption NEC K91.2
      - obstruction K91.3
      - postcholecystectomy syndrome K91.5
      - specified NEC K91.89
      - vomiting after GI surgery K91.Ø
    - prosthetic device or implant
      - bile duct prosthesis — *see* Complications, bile duct implant
      - esophageal anti-reflux device — *see* Complications, esophageal anti-reflux device
      - specified type NEC
        - embolism T85.81 ☑
        - fibrosis T85.82 ☑
        - hemorrhage T85.83 ☑
        - mechanical
          - breakdown T85.518 ☑
          - displacement T85.528 ☑
          - malfunction T85.518 ☑
          - malposition T85.528 ☑
          - obstruction T85.598 ☑
          - perforation T85.598 ☑
          - protrusion T85.598 ☑
          - specified NEC T85.598 ☑
        - pain T85.84 ☑
        - specified complication NEC T85.89 ☑
        - stenosis T85.85 ☑
        - thrombosis T85.86 ☑
  - gastrostomy (stoma) K94.2Ø
    - hemorrhage K94.21
    - infection K94.22
    - malfunction K94.23
    - mechanical K94.23
    - specified complication NEC K94.29
  - genitourinary
    - device or implant T83.9 ☑
      - genital tract T83.9 ☑
        - infection or inflammation T83.6 ☑
        - intrauterine contraceptive device — *see* Complications, intrauterine, contraceptive device
        - mechanical — *see* Complications, by device, mechanical
        - mesh — *see* Complications, mesh
        - penile prosthesis — *see* Complications, prosthetic device, penile
        - specified type NEC T83.89 ☑
          - embolism T83.81 ☑
          - fibrosis T83.82 ☑
          - hemorrhage T83.83 ☑
          - pain T83.84 ☑
          - specified complication NEC T83.89 ☑
          - stenosis T83.85 ☑
          - thrombosis T83.86 ☑
        - vaginal mesh — *see* Complications, mesh
      - urinary system T83.9 ☑
        - cystostomy catheter — *see* Complication, catheter, cystostomy
        - electronic stimulator — *see* Complications, electronic stimulator device, urinary
        - indwelling urethral catheter — *see* Complications, catheter, urethral, indwelling
        - infection or inflammation T83.59 ☑
          - indwelling urinary catheter T83.51 ☑

- **Complication**(s) — *continued*
  - genitourinary — *continued*
    - device or implant — *continued*
      - urinary system — *continued*
        - kidney transplant — *see* Complication, transplant, kidney
        - organ graft — *see* Complication, graft, urinary organ
        - specified type NEC T83.89 ☑
          - embolism T83.81 ☑
          - fibrosis T83.82 ☑
          - hemorrhage T83.83 ☑
          - mechanical T83.198 ☑
            - breakdown T83.118 ☑
            - displacement T83.128 ☑
            - malfunction T83.118 ☑
            - malposition T83.128 ☑
            - obstruction T83.198 ☑
            - perforation T83.198 ☑
            - protrusion T83.198 ☑
            - specified NEC T83.198 ☑
          - pain T83.84 ☑
          - specified complication NEC T83.89 ☑
          - stenosis T83.85 ☑
          - thrombosis T83.86 ☑
        - sphincter implant — *see* Complications, implant, urinary sphincter
    - postprocedural
      - pelvic peritoneal adhesions N99.4
      - renal failure N99.Ø
      - specified NEC N99.89
      - stoma — *see* Complications, stoma, urinary tract
      - urethral stricture — *see* Stricture, urethra, postprocedural
      - vaginal
        - adhesions N99.2
        - vault prolapse N99.3
  - graft (bypass) (patch) (*see also* Complications, prosthetic device or implant)
    - aorta — *see* Complications, graft, vascular
    - arterial — *see* Complication, graft, vascular
    - bone T86.839
      - failure T86.831
      - infection T86.832
      - mechanical T84.318 ☑
        - breakdown T84.318 ☑
        - displacement T84.328 ☑
        - protrusion T84.398 ☑
        - specified type NEC T84.398 ☑
      - rejection T86.83Ø
      - specified type NEC T86.838
    - carotid artery — *see* Complications, graft, vascular
    - cornea T86.849
      - failure T86.841
      - infection T86.842
      - mechanical T85.398 ☑
        - breakdown T85.318 ☑
        - displacement T85.328 ☑
        - protrusion T85.398 ☑
        - specified type NEC T85.398 ☑
      - rejection T86.84Ø
      - retroprosthetic membrane T85.398 ☑
      - specified type NEC T86.848
    - femoral artery (bypass) — *see* Complication, extremity artery (bypass) graft
    - genital organ or tract — *see* Complications, genitourinary, device or implant, genital tract
    - muscle T84.9 ☑
      - breakdown T84.41Ø ☑
      - displacement T84.42Ø ☑
      - embolism T84.81 ☑
      - fibrosis T84.82 ☑
      - hemorrhage T84.83 ☑
      - infection and inflammation T84.7 ☑
      - mechanical NEC T84.49Ø ☑
      - pain T84.84 ☑
      - specified type NEC T84.89 ☑
      - stenosis T84.85 ☑
      - thrombosis T84.86 ☑
    - nerve — *see* Complication, prosthetic device or implant, specified NEC
    - skin — *see* Complications, prosthetic device or implant, skin graft
    - tendon T84.9 ☑
      - breakdown T84.41Ø ☑

- **Complication**(s) — *continued*
  - graft (*see also* Complications, prosthetic device or implant) — *continued*
    - tendon — *continued*
      - displacement T84.42Ø ☑
      - embolism T84.81 ☑
      - fibrosis T84.82 ☑
      - hemorrhage T84.83 ☑
      - infection and inflammation T84.7 ☑
      - mechanical NEC T84.49Ø ☑
      - pain T84.84 ☑
      - specified type NEC T84.89 ☑
      - stenosis T84.85 ☑
      - thrombosis T84.86 ☑
    - urinary organ T83.9 ☑
      - embolism T83.81 ☑
      - fibrosis T83.82 ☑
      - hemorrhage T83.83 ☑
      - infection and inflammation T83.59 ☑
        - indwelling urinary catheter T83.51 ☑
      - mechanical
        - breakdown T83.21 ☑
        - displacement T83.22 ☑
        - leakage T83.23 ☑
        - malposition T83.22 ☑
        - obstruction T83.29 ☑
        - perforation T83.29 ☑
        - protrusion T83.29 ☑
        - specified NEC T83.29 ☑
      - pain T83.84 ☑
      - specified type NEC T83.89 ☑
      - stenosis T83.85 ☑
      - thrombosis T83.86 ☑
    - vascular T82.9 ☑
      - embolism T82.818 ☑
      - femoral artery — *see* Complication, extremity artery (bypass) graft
      - fibrosis T82.828 ☑
      - hemorrhage T82.838 ☑
      - mechanical
        - breakdown T82.319 ☑
          - aorta (bifurcation) T82.31Ø ☑
          - carotid artery T82.311 ☑
          - specified vessel NEC T82.318 ☑
        - displacement T82.329 ☑
          - aorta (bifurcation) T82.32Ø ☑
          - carotid artery T82.321 ☑
          - specified vessel NEC T82.328 ☑
        - leakage T82.339 ☑
          - aorta (bifurcation) T82.33Ø ☑
          - carotid artery T82.331 ☑
          - specified vessel NEC T82.338 ☑
        - malposition T82.329 ☑
          - aorta (bifurcation) T82.32Ø ☑
          - carotid artery T82.321 ☑
          - specified vessel NEC T82.328 ☑
        - obstruction T82.399 ☑
          - aorta (bifurcation) T82.39Ø ☑
          - carotid artery T82.391 ☑
          - specified vessel NEC T82.398 ☑
        - perforation T82.399 ☑
          - aorta (bifurcation) T82.39Ø ☑
          - carotid artery T82.391 ☑
          - specified vessel NEC T82.398 ☑
        - protrusion T82.399 ☑
          - aorta (bifurcation) T82.39Ø ☑
          - carotid artery T82.391 ☑
          - specified vessel NEC T82.398 ☑
      - pain T82.848 ☑
      - specified complication NEC T82.898 ☑
      - stenosis T82.858 ☑
      - thrombosis T82.868 ☑
  - heart I51.9
    - assist device
      - infection and inflammation T82.7 ☑
    - following acute myocardial infarction — *see* Complications, following, acute myocardial infarction
    - postoperative — *see* Complications, circulatory system
    - transplant — *see* Complication, transplant, heart
      - and lung(s) — *see* Complications, transplant, heart, with lung
    - valve
      - graft (biological) T82.9 ☑
        - embolism T82.817 ☑

- **Complication**(s) — *continued*
  - postmastoidectomy NEC H95.19- ☑
    - cyst, mucosal H95.13- ☑
    - granulation H95.12- ☑
    - inflammation, chronic H95.11- ☑
    - recurrent cholesteatoma H95.Ø- ☑
  - postoperative — *see* Complications, postprocedural
    - circulatory — *see* Complications, circulatory system
    - ear — *see* Complications, ear
    - endocrine — *see* Complications, endocrine
    - eye — *see* Complications, eye
    - lumbar puncture G97.1
      - cerebrospinal fluid leak G97.Ø
    - nervous system (central) (peripheral) — *see* Complications, nervous system
    - respiratory system — *see* Complications, respiratory system
  - postprocedural (*see also* Complications, surgical procedure)
    - cardiac arrest
      - following cardiac surgery I97.12Ø
      - following other surgery I97.121
    - cardiac functional disturbance NEC
      - following cardiac surgery I97.19Ø
      - following other surgery I97.191
    - cardiac insufficiency
      - following cardiac surgery I97.11Ø
      - following other surgery I97.111
    - chorioretinal scars following retinal surgery H59.81- ☑
    - following cataract surgery
      - cataract (lens) fragments H59.Ø2- ☑
      - cystoid macular edema H59.Ø3- ☑
      - specified NEC H59.Ø9- ☑
      - vitreous (touch) syndrome H59.Ø1- ☑
    - heart failure
      - following cardiac surgery I97.13Ø
      - following other surgery I97.131
    - hemorrhage (hematoma) (of)
      - circulatory system organ or structure
        - following a cardiac bypass I97.611
        - following a cardiac catheterization I97.61Ø
        - following other circulatory system procedure I97.618
        - following other procedure I97.62
      - digestive system
        - following procedure on digestive system K91.84Ø
        - following procedure on other organ K91.841
      - ear
        - following other procedure H95.42
        - following procedure on ear and mastoid process H95.41
      - endocrine system
        - following endocrine system procedure E89.81Ø
        - following other procedure E89.811
      - eye and adnexa
        - following ophthalmic procedure H59.31- ☑
        - following other procedure H59.32- ☑
      - genitourinary organ or structure
        - following procedure on genitourinary organ or structure N99.82Ø
        - following procedure on other organ N99.821
      - mastoid process
        - following other procedure H95.42
        - following procedure on ear and mastoid process H95.41
      - musculoskeletal structure
        - following musculoskeletal surgery M96.83Ø
        - following non-orthopedic surgery M96.831
        - following orthopedic surgery M96.83Ø
      - nervous system
        - following a nervous system procedure G97.51
        - following other procedure G97.52
      - respiratory system
        - following a respiratory system procedure J95.83Ø
        - following other procedure J95.831
      - skin and subcutaneous tissue
        - following a dermatologic procedure L76.21
        - following a procedure on other organ L76.22
      - spleen
        - following procedure on other organ D78.22
        - following procedure on the spleen D78.21

- **Complication**(s) — *continued*
  - postprocedural (*see also* Complications, surgical procedure) — *continued*
    - specified NEC
      - circulatory system I97.89
      - digestive K91.89
      - ear H95.89
      - endocrine E89.89
      - eye and adnexa H59.89
      - genitourinary N99.89
      - mastoid process H95.89
      - metabolic E89.89
      - musculoskeletal structure M96.89
      - nervous system G97.82
      - respiratory system J95.89
      - skin and subcutaneous tissue L76.82
      - spleen D78.89
  - pregnancy NEC — *see* Pregnancy, complicated by
  - prosthetic device or implant T85.9 ☑
    - bile duct — *see* Complications, bile duct implant
    - breast — *see* Complications, breast implant
    - cardiac and vascular NEC — *see* Complications, cardiovascular device or implant
    - corneal transplant — *see* Complications, graft, cornea
    - electronic nervous system stimulator — *see* Complications, electronic stimulator device
    - epidural infusion catheter — *see* Complications, catheter, epidural
    - esophageal anti-reflux device — *see* Complications, esophageal anti-reflux device
    - genital organ or tract — *see* Complications, genitourinary, device or implant, genital tract
    - heart valve — *see* Complications, heart, valve, prosthesis
    - infection or inflammation T85.79 ☑
      - intestine transplant T86.892
      - liver transplant T86.43
      - lung transplant T86.812
      - pancreas transplant T86.892
      - skin graft T86.822
    - intraocular lens — *see* Complications, intraocular lens
    - intraperitoneal (dialysis) catheter — *see* Complications, catheter, intraperitoneal
    - joint — *see* Complications, joint prosthesis, internal
    - mechanical NEC T85.698 ☑
      - dialysis catheter (vascular) (*see also* Complication, catheter, dialysis, mechanical)
        - peritoneal — *see* Complication, catheter, intraperitoneal, mechanical
      - gastrointestinal device T85.598 ☑
      - ocular device T85.398 ☑
      - subdural (infusion) catheter T85.69Ø ☑
      - suture, permanent T85.692 ☑
        - that for bone repair — *see* Complications, fixation device, internal (orthopedic), mechanical
      - ventricular shunt
        - breakdown T85.Ø1 ☑
        - displacement T85.Ø2 ☑
        - leakage T85.Ø3 ☑
        - malposition T85.Ø2 ☑
        - obstruction T85.Ø9 ☑
        - perforation T85.Ø9 ☑
        - protrusion T85.Ø9 ☑
        - specified NEC T85.Ø9 ☑
    - mesh
      - erosion (to surrounding organ or tissue) T83.718 ☑
        - vaginal (into pelvic floor muscles) T83.711 ☑
      - exposure (into surrounding organ or tissue) T83.728 ☑
        - vaginal (into vagina) (through vaginal wall) T83.721 ☑
    - orbital — *see* Complications, orbital prosthesis
    - penile T83.9 ☑
      - embolism T83.81 ☑
      - fibrosis T83.82 ☑
      - hemorrhage T83.83 ☑
      - infection and inflammation T83.6 ☑
      - mechanical
        - breakdown T83.41Ø ☑
        - displacement T83.42Ø ☑
        - leakage T83.49Ø ☑
        - malposition T83.42Ø ☑

- **Complication**(s) — *continued*
  - prosthetic device or implant — *continued*
    - penile — *continued*
      - mechanical — *continued*
        - obstruction T83.49Ø ☑
        - perforation T83.49Ø ☑
        - protrusion T83.49Ø ☑
        - specified NEC T83.49Ø ☑
      - pain T83.84 ☑
      - specified type NEC T83.89 ☑
      - stenosis T83.85 ☑
      - thrombosis T83.86 ☑
    - prosthetic materials NEC
      - erosion (to surrounding organ or tissue) T83.718 ☑
        - vaginal (into pelvic floor muscles) T83.711 ☑
      - exposure (into surrounding organ or tissue) T83.728 ☑
        - vaginal (into vagina) (through vaginal wall) T83.721 ☑
    - skin graft T86.829
      - artificial skin or decellularized allodermis
        - embolism T85.81 ☑
        - fibrosis T85.82 ☑
        - hemorrhage T85.83 ☑
        - infection and inflammation T85.79 ☑
        - mechanical
          - breakdown T85.613 ☑
          - displacement T85.623 ☑
          - malfunction T85.613 ☑
          - malposition T85.623 ☑
          - obstruction T85.693 ☑
          - perforation T85.693 ☑
          - protrusion T85.693 ☑
          - specified NEC T85.693 ☑
        - pain T85.84 ☑
        - specified type NEC T85.89 ☑
        - stenosis T85.85 ☑
        - thrombosis T85.86 ☑
      - failure T86.821
      - infection T86.822
      - rejection T86.82Ø
      - specified NEC T86.828
    - specified NEC T85.9 ☑
      - embolism T85.81 ☑
      - fibrosis T85.82 ☑
      - hemorrhage T85.83 ☑
      - infection and inflammation T85.79 ☑
      - mechanical
        - breakdown T85.618 ☑
        - displacement T85.628 ☑
        - leakage T85.638 ☑
        - malfunction T85.618 ☑
        - malposition T85.628 ☑
        - obstruction T85.698 ☑
        - perforation T85.698 ☑
        - protrusion T85.698 ☑
        - specified NEC T85.698 ☑
      - pain T85.84 ☑
      - specified type NEC T85.89 ☑
      - stenosis T85.85 ☑
      - thrombosis T85.86 ☑
    - subdural infusion catheter — *see* Complications, catheter, subdural
    - sutures — *see* Complications, sutures
    - urinary organ or tract NEC — *see* Complications, genitourinary, device or implant, urinary system
    - vascular — *see* Complications, cardiovascular device or implant
    - ventricular shunt — *see* Complications, ventricular shunt (device)
  - puerperium — *see* Puerperal
  - puncture, spinal G97.1
    - cerebrospinal fluid leak G97.Ø
    - headache or reaction G97.1
  - pyelogram N99.89
  - radiation
    - kyphosis M96.2
    - scoliosis M96.5
  - reattached
    - extremity (infection) (rejection)
      - lower T87.1X- ☑
      - upper T87.ØX- ☑
    - specified body part NEC T87.2

Complication(s) — *continued*
- reconstructed breast
  - asymmetry between native and reconstructed breast N65.1
  - deformity N65.Ø
  - disproportion between native and reconstructed breast N65.1
  - excess tissue N65.Ø
  - misshappen N65.Ø
- reimplant NEC (*see also* Complications, prosthetic device or implant)
  - limb (infection) (rejection) — *see* Complications, reattached, extremity
  - organ (partial) (total) — *see* Complications, transplant
  - prosthetic device NEC — *see* Complications, prosthetic device
- renal N28.9
  - allograft — *see* Complications, transplant, kidney
  - dialysis — *see* Complications, dialysis
- respirator
  - mechancial J95.85Ø
    - specified NEC J95.859
- respiratory system J98.9
  - device, implant or graft — *see* Complication, prosthetic device or implant, specified NEC
  - lung transplant — *see* Complications, prosthetic device or implant, lung transplant
  - postoperative J95.89
    - air leak J95.812
    - Mendelson's syndrome (chemical pneumonitis) J95.4
    - pneumothorax J95.811
    - pulmonary insufficiency (acute) (after nonthoracic surgery) J95.2
      - chronic J95.3
      - following thoracic surgery J95.1
    - respiratory failure (acute) J95.821
      - acute and chronic J95.822
    - specified NEC J95.89
    - subglottic stenosis J95.5
    - tracheostomy complication — *see* Complications, tracheostomy
  - therapy T81.89 ☑
- sedation during labor and delivery O74.9
  - cardiac O74.2
  - central nervous system O74.3
  - pulmonary NEC O74.1
- shunt (*see also* Complications, prosthetic device or implant)
  - arteriovenous — *see* Complications, arteriovenous, shunt
  - ventricular (communicating) — *see* Complications, ventricular shunt
- skin
  - graft T86.829
    - failure T86.821
    - infection T86.822
    - rejection T86.82Ø
    - specified type NEC T86.828
- spinal
  - anesthesia — *see* Complications, anesthesia, spinal
  - catheter (epidural) (subdural) — *see* Complications, catheter
  - puncture or tap G97.1
    - cerebrospinal fluid leak G97.Ø
    - headache or reaction G97.1
- stent
  - bile duct — *see* Complications, bile duct prosthesis
  - urinary T83.9 ☑
    - embolism T83.81 ☑
    - fibrosis T83.82 ☑
    - hemorrhage T83.83 ☑
    - infection and inflammation T83.59 ☑
    - mechanical
      - breakdown T83.112 ☑
      - displacement T83.122 ☑
      - leakage T83.192 ☑
      - malposition T83.122 ☑
      - obstruction T83.192 ☑
      - perforation T83.192 ☑
      - protrusion T83.192 ☑
      - specified NEC T83.192 ☑
    - pain T83.84 ☑
    - specified type NEC T83.89 ☑
    - stenosis T83.85 ☑
    - thrombosis T83.86 ☑

Complication(s) — *continued*
- stoma
  - digestive tract
    - colostomy — *see* Complications, colostomy
    - enterostomy — *see* Complications, enterostomy
    - esophagostomy — *see* Complications, esophagostomy
    - gastrostomy — *see* Complications, gastrostomy
  - urinary tract N99.538
    - cystostomy — *see* Complications, cystostomy
    - external NOS N99.528
      - hemorrhage N99.52Ø
      - infection N99.521
      - malfunction N99.522
      - specified type NEC N99.528
    - hemorrhage N99.53Ø
    - infection N99.531
    - malfunction N99.532
    - specified type NEC N99.538
- stomach banding — *see* Complication(s), bariatric procedure
- stomach stapling — *see* Complication(s), bariatric procedure
- surgical material, nonabsorbable — *see* Complication, suture, permanent
- surgical procedure (on) T81.9 ☑
  - amputation stump (late) — *see* Complications, amputation stump
  - cardiac — *see* Complications, circulatory system
  - cholesteatoma, recurrent — *see* Complications, postmastoidectomy, recurrent cholesteatoma
  - circulatory (early) — *see* Complications, circulatory system
  - digestive system — *see* Complications, gastrointestinal
  - dumping syndrome (postgastrectomy) K91.1
  - ear — *see* Complications, ear
  - elephantiasis or lymphedema I97.89
    - postmastectomy I97.2
  - emphysema (surgical) T81.82 ☑
  - endocrine — *see* Complications, endocrine
  - eye — *see* Complications, eye
  - fistula (persistent postoperative) T81.83 ☑
  - foreign body inadvertently left in wound (sponge) (suture) (swab) — *see* Foreign body, accidentally left during a procedure
  - gastrointestinal — *see* Complications, gastrointestinal
  - genitourinary NEC N99.89
  - hematoma
    - intraoperative — *see* Complication, intraoperative, hemorrhage
    - postprocedural — *see* Complication, postprocedural, hemorrhage
  - hemorrhage
    - intraoperative — *see* Complication, intraoperative, hemorrhage
    - postprocedural — *see* Complication, postprocedural, hemorrhage
  - hepatic failure K91.82
  - hyperglycemia (postpancreatectomy) E89.1
  - hypoinsulinemia (postpancreatectomy) E89.1
  - hypoparathyroidism (postparathyroidectomy) E89.2
  - hypopituitarism (posthypophysectomy) E89.3
  - hypothyroidism (post-thyroidectomy) E89.Ø
  - intestinal obstruction K91.3
  - intracranial hypotension following ventricular shunting (ventriculostomy) G97.2
  - lymphedema I97.89
    - postmastectomy I97.2
  - malabsorption (postsurgical) NEC K91.2
    - osteoporosis — *see* Osteoporosis, postsurgical malabsorption
  - mastoidectomy cavity NEC — *see* Complications, postmastoidectomy
  - metabolic E89.89
    - specified NEC E89.89
  - musculoskeletal — *see* Complications, musculoskeletal system
  - nervous system (central) (peripheral) — *see* Complications, nervous system
  - ovarian failure E89.4Ø
    - asymptomatic E89.4Ø
    - symptomatic E89.41

Complication(s) — *continued*
- surgical procedure — *continued*
  - peripheral vascular — *see* Complications, surgical procedure, vascular
  - postcardiotomy syndrome I97.Ø
  - postcholecystectomy syndrome K91.5
  - postcommissurotomy syndrome I97.Ø
  - postgastrectomy dumping syndrome K91.1
  - postlaminectomy syndrome NEC M96.1
    - kyphosis M96.3
  - postmastectomy lymphedema syndrome I97.2
  - postmastoidectomy cholesteatoma — *see* Complications, postmastoidectomy, recurrent cholesteatoma
  - postvagotomy syndrome K91.1
  - postvalvulotomy syndrome I97.Ø
  - pulmonary insufficiency (acute) J95.2
    - chronic J95.3
    - following thoracic surgery J95.1
  - reattached body part — *see* Complications, reattached
  - respiratory — *see* Complications, respiratory system
  - shock (hypovolemic) T81.19 ☑
  - spleen (postoperative) D78.89
    - intraoperative D78.81
  - stitch abscess T81.4 ☑
  - subglottic stenosis (postsurgical) J95.5
  - testicular hypofunction E89.5
  - transplant — *see* Complications, organ or tissue transplant
  - urinary NEC N99.89
  - vaginal vault prolapse (posthysterectomy) N99.3
  - vascular (peripheral)
    - artery T81.719 ☑
      - mesenteric T81.71Ø ☑
      - renal T81.711 ☑
      - specified NEC T81.718 ☑
    - vein T81.72 ☑
  - wound infection T81.4 ☑
- suture, permanent (wire) NEC T85.9 ☑
  - with repair of bone — *see* Complications, fixation device, internal
  - embolism T85.81 ☑
  - fibrosis T85.82 ☑
  - hemorrhage T85.83 ☑
  - infection and inflammation T85.79 ☑
  - mechanical
    - breakdown T85.612 ☑
    - displacement T85.622 ☑
    - malfunction T85.612 ☑
    - malposition T85.622 ☑
    - obstruction T85.692 ☑
    - perforation T85.692 ☑
    - protrusion T85.692 ☑
    - specified NEC T85.692 ☑
  - pain T85.84 ☑
  - specified type NEC T85.89 ☑
  - stenosis T85.85 ☑
  - thrombosis T85.86 ☑
- tracheostomy J95.ØØ
  - granuloma J95.Ø9
  - hemorrhage J95.Ø1
  - infection J95.Ø2
  - malfunction J95.Ø3
  - mechanical J95.Ø3
  - obstruction J95.Ø3
  - specified type NEC J95.Ø9
  - tracheo-esophageal fistula J95.Ø4
- transfusion (blood) (lymphocytes) (plasma) T8Ø.92 ☑
  - air emblism T8Ø.Ø ☑
  - circulatory overload E87.71
  - febrile nonhemolytic transfusion reaction R5Ø.84
  - hemochromatosis E83.111
  - hemolysis T8Ø.89 ☑
  - hemolytic reaction (antigen unspecified) T8Ø.919 ☑
  - incompatibility reaction (antigen unspecified) T8Ø.919 ☑
    - ABO T8Ø.3Ø ☑
      - delayed serologic (DSTR) T8Ø.39 ☑
      - hemolytic transfusion reaction (HTR) (unspecified time after transfusion) T8Ø.319 ☑
        - acute (AHTR) (less than 24 hours after transfusion) T8Ø.31Ø ☑

- **Complication**(s) — *continued*
  - transfusion — *continued*
    - incompatibility reaction — *continued*
      - ABO — *continued*
        - hemolytic transfusion reaction — *continued*
          - delayed (DHTR) (24 hours or more after transfusion) T80.311 ☑
        - specified NEC T80.39 ☑
      - acute (antigen unspecified) T80.910 ☑
      - delayed (antigen unspecified) T80.911 ☑
      - delayed serologic (DSTR) T80.89 ☑
      - non-ABO (minor antigens (Duffy) (Kell) (Kidd) (Lewis) (M) (N) (P) (S)) T80.A0 ☑ (*following* T80.4)
        - delayed serologic (DSTR) T80.A9 ☑ (*following* T80.4)
        - hemolytic transfusion reaction (HTR) (unspecified time after transfusion) T80.A19 ☑ (*following* T80.4)
          - acute (AHTR) (less than 24 hours after transfusion) T80.A10 ☑ (*following* T80.4)
          - delayed (DHTR) (24 hours or more after transfusion) T80.A11 ☑ (*following* T80.4)
        - specified NEC T80.A9 ☑ (*following* T80.4)
      - Rh (antigens (C) (c) (D) (E) (e)) (factor) T80.40 ☑
        - delayed serologic (DSTR) T80.49 ☑
        - hemolytic transfusion reaction (HTR) (unspecified time after transfusion) T80.419 ☑
          - acute (AHTR) (less than 24 hours after transfusion) T80.410 ☑
          - delayed (DHTR) (24 hours or more after transfusion) T80.411 ☑
        - specified NEC T80.49 ☑
    - infection T80.29 ☑
    - reaction NEC T80.89 ☑
    - sepsis T80.29 ☑
    - shock T80.89 ☑
  - transplant T86.90
    - bone T86.839
      - failure T86.831
      - infection T86.832
      - rejection T86.830
      - specified type NEC T86.838
    - bone marrow T86.00
      - failure T86.02
      - infection T86.03
      - rejection T86.01
      - specified type NEC T86.09
    - cornea T86.849
      - failure T86.841
      - infection T86.842
      - rejection T86.840
      - specified type NEC T86.848
    - failure T86.92
    - heart T86.20
      - with lung T86.30
      - cardiac allograft vasculopathy T86.290
        - failure T86.32
        - infection T86.33
        - rejection T86.31
        - specified type NEC T86.39
      - failure T86.22
      - infection T86.23
      - rejection T86.21
      - specified type NEC T86.298
    - infection T86.93
    - intestine T86.859
      - failure T86.851
      - infection T86.852
      - rejection T86.850
      - specified type NEC T86.858
    - kidney T86.10
      - failure T86.12
      - infection T86.13
      - rejection T86.11
      - specified type NEC T86.19
    - liver T86.40
      - failure T86.42
      - infection T86.43
      - rejection T86.41
      - specified type NEC T86.49
    - lung T86.819
      - with heart T86.30
        - failure T86.32

- **Complication**(s) — *continued*
  - transplant — *continued*
    - lung — *continued*
      - with heart — *continued*
        - infection T86.33
        - rejection T86.31
        - specified type NEC T86.39
      - failure T86.811
      - infection T86.812
      - rejection T86.810
      - specified type NEC T86.818
    - malignant neoplasm C80.2
    - pancreas T86.899
      - failure T86.891
      - infection T86.892
      - rejection T86.890
      - specified type NEC T86.898
    - peripheral blood stem cells T86.5
    - post-transplant lymphoproliferative disorder (PTLD) D47.Z1 (*following* D47.4)
    - rejection T86.91
    - skin T86.829
      - failure T86.821
      - infection T86.822
      - rejection T86.820
      - specified type NEC T86.828
    - specified
      - tissue T86.899
        - failure T86.891
        - infection T86.892
        - rejection T86.890
        - specified type NEC T86.898
      - type NEC T86.99
    - stem cell (from peripheral blood) (from umbilical cord) T86.5
    - umbilical cord stem cells T86.5
  - trauma (early) T79.9 ☑
    - specified NEC T79.8 ☑
  - ultrasound therapy NEC T88.9 ☑
  - umbilical cord NEC
    - complicating delivery O69.9 ☑
      - specified NEC O69.89 ☑
  - umbrella device, vascular T82.9 ☑
    - embolism T82.818 ☑
    - fibrosis T82.828 ☑
    - hemorrhage T82.838 ☑
    - infection or inflammation T82.7 ☑
    - mechanical
      - breakdown T82.515 ☑
      - displacement T82.525 ☑
      - leakage T82.535 ☑
      - malposition T82.525 ☑
      - obstruction T82.595 ☑
      - perforation T82.595 ☑
      - protrusion T82.595 ☑
    - pain T82.848 ☑
    - specified type NEC T82.898 ☑
    - stenosis T82.858 ☑
    - thrombosis T82.868 ☑
  - urethral catheter — *see* Complications, catheter, urethral, indwelling
  - vaccination T88.1 ☑
    - anaphylaxis NEC T80.52 ☑
    - arthropathy — *see* Arthropathy, postimmunization
    - cellulitis T88.0 ☑
    - encephalitis or encephalomyelitis G04.02
    - infection (general) (local) NEC T88.0 ☑
    - meningitis G03.8
    - myelitis G04.89
    - protein sickness T80.62 ☑
    - rash T88.1 ☑
    - reaction (allergic) T88.1 ☑
      - serum T80.62 ☑
    - sepsis T88.0 ☑
    - serum intoxication, sickness, rash, or other serum reaction NEC T80.62 ☑
      - anaphylactic shock T80.52 ☑
    - shock (allergic) (anaphylactic) T80.52 ☑
    - vaccinia (generalized) (localized) T88.1 ☑
  - vas deferens device or implant — *see* Complications, genitourinary, device or implant, genital tract
  - vascular I99.9
    - device or implant T82.9 ☑
      - embolism T82.818 ☑
      - fibrosis T82.828 ☑
      - hemorrhage T82.838 ☑
      - infection or inflammation T82.7 ☑

- **Complication**(s) — *continued*
  - vascular — *continued*
    - device or implant — *continued*
      - mechanical
        - breakdown T82.519 ☑
          - specified device NEC T82.518 ☑
        - displacement T82.529 ☑
          - specified device NEC T82.528 ☑
        - leakage T82.539 ☑
          - specified device NEC T82.538 ☑
        - malposition T82.529 ☑
          - specified device NEC T82.528 ☑
        - obstruction T82.599 ☑
          - specified device NEC T82.598 ☑
        - perforation T82.599 ☑
          - specified device NEC T82.598 ☑
        - protrusion T82.599 ☑
          - specified device NEC T82.598 ☑
      - pain T82.848 ☑
      - specified type NEC T82.898 ☑
      - stenosis T82.858 ☑
      - thrombosis T82.868 ☑
    - dialysis catheter — *see* Complication, catheter, dialysis
    - following infusion, therapeutic injection or transfusion T80.1 ☑
    - graft T82.9 ☑
      - embolism T82.818 ☑
      - fibrosis T82.828 ☑
      - hemorrhage T82.838 ☑
      - mechanical
        - breakdown T82.319 ☑
          - aorta (bifurcation) T82.310 ☑
          - carotid artery T82.311 ☑
          - specified vessel NEC T82.318 ☑
        - displacement T82.329 ☑
          - aorta (bifurcation) T82.320 ☑
          - carotid artery T82.321 ☑
          - specified vessel NEC T82.328 ☑
        - leakage T82.339 ☑
          - aorta (bifurcation) T82.330 ☑
          - carotid artery T82.331 ☑
          - specified vessel NEC T82.338 ☑
        - malposition T82.329 ☑
          - aorta (bifurcation) T82.320 ☑
          - carotid artery T82.321 ☑
          - specified vessel NEC T82.328 ☑
        - obstruction T82.399 ☑
          - aorta (bifurcation) T82.390 ☑
          - carotid artery T82.391 ☑
          - specified vessel NEC T82.398 ☑
        - perforation T82.399 ☑
          - aorta (bifurcation) T82.390 ☑
          - carotid artery T82.391 ☑
          - specified vessel NEC T82.398 ☑
        - protrusion T82.399 ☑
          - aorta (bifurcation) T82.390 ☑
          - carotid artery T82.391 ☑
          - specified vessel NEC T82.398 ☑
      - pain T82.848 ☑
      - specified complication NEC T82.898 ☑
      - stenosis T82.858 ☑
      - thrombosis T82.868 ☑
    - postoperative — *see* Complications, postoperative, circulatory
  - vena cava device (filter) (sieve) (umbrella) — *see* Complications, umbrella device, vascular
  - ventilation therapy NEC T81.81 ☑
  - ventilator
    - mechanical J95.850
      - specified NEC J95.859
  - ventricular (communicating) shunt (device) T85.9 ☑
    - embolism T85.81 ☑
    - fibrosis T85.82 ☑
    - hemorrhage T85.83 ☑
    - infection and inflammation T85.79 ☑
    - mechanical
      - breakdown T85.01 ☑
      - displacement T85.02 ☑
      - leakage T85.03 ☑
      - malposition T85.02 ☑
      - obstruction T85.09 ☑
      - perforation T85.09 ☑
      - protrusion T85.09 ☑
      - specified NEC T85.09 ☑
    - pain T85.84 ☑

- **Complication**(s) — *continued*
  - ventricular shunt — *continued*
    - specified type NEC T85.89 ☑
    - stenosis T85.85 ☑
    - thrombosis T85.86 ☑
  - wire suture, permanent (implanted) — *see* Complications, suture, permanent
- **Compressed air disease** T70.3 ☑
- **Compression**
  - with injury — *code by* Nature of injury
  - artery I77.1
    - celiac, syndrome I77.4
  - brachial plexus G54.0
  - brain (stem) G93.5
    - due to
      - contusion (diffuse) — *see* Injury, intracranial, diffuse
        - focal — *see* Injury, intracranial, focal
      - injury NEC — *see* Injury, intracranial, diffuse
    - traumatic — *see* Injury, intracranial, diffuse
  - bronchus J98.09
  - cauda equina G83.4
  - celiac (artery) (axis) I77.4
  - cerebral — *see* Compression, brain
  - cervical plexus G54.2
  - cord
    - spinal — *see* Compression, spinal
    - umbilical — *see* Compression, umbilical cord
  - cranial nerve G52.9
    - eighth H93.3 ☑
    - eleventh G52.8
    - fifth G50.8
    - first G52.0
    - fourth — *see* Strabismus, paralytic, fourth nerve
    - ninth G52.1
    - second — *see* Disorder, nerve, optic
    - seventh G52.8
    - sixth — *see* Strabismus, paralytic, sixth nerve
    - tenth G52.2
    - third — *see* Strabismus, paralytic, third nerve
    - twelfth G52.3
  - diver's squeeze T70.3 ☑
  - during birth (newborn) P15.9
  - esophagus K22.2
  - eustachian tube — *see* Obstruction, eustachian tube, cartilaginous
  - facies Q67.1
  - fracture — *see* Fracture
  - heart — *see* Disease, heart
  - intestine — *see* Obstruction, intestine
  - laryngeal nerve, recurrent G52.2
    - with paralysis of vocal cords and larynx J38.00
      - bilateral J38.02
      - unilateral J38.01
  - lumbosacral plexus G54.1
  - lung J98.4
  - lymphatic vessel I89.0
  - medulla — *see* Compression, brain
  - nerve (*see also* Disorder, nerve) G58.9
    - arm NEC — *see* Mononeuropathy, upper limb
    - axillary G54.0
    - cranial — *see* Compression, cranial nerve
    - leg NEC — *see* Mononeuropathy, lower limb
    - median (in carpal tunnel) — *see* Syndrome, carpal tunnel
    - optic — *see* Disorder, nerve, optic
    - plantar — *see* Lesion, nerve, plantar
    - posterior tibial (in tarsal tunnel) — *see* Syndrome, tarsal tunnel
    - root or plexus NOS (in) G54.9
      - intervertebral disc disorder NEC — *see* Disorder, disc, with, radiculopathy
        - with myelopathy — *see* Disorder, disc, with, myelopathy
      - neoplastic disease (*see also* Neoplasm) D49.9 [G55]
      - spondylosis — *see* Spondylosis, with radiculopathy
    - sciatic (acute) — *see* Lesion, nerve, sciatic
    - sympathetic G90.8
    - traumatic — *see* Injury, nerve
    - ulnar — *see* Lesion, nerve, ulnar
    - upper extremity NEC — *see* Mononeuropathy, upper limb
  - spinal (cord) G95.20
    - by displacement of intervertebral disc NEC (*see also* Disorder, disc, with, myelopathy)
    - nerve root NOS G54.9
      - due to displacement of intervertebral disc NEC — *see* Disorder, disc, with, radiculopathy
        - with myelopathy — *see* Disorder, disc, with, myelopathy
    - specified NEC G95.29
    - spondylogenic (cervical) (lumbar, lumbosacral) (thoracic) — *see* Spondylosis, with myelopathy NEC
      - anterior — *see* Syndrome, anterior, spinal artery, compression
    - traumatic — *see* Injury, spinal cord, by region
  - subcostal nerve (syndrome) — *see* Mononeuropathy, upper limb, specified NEC
  - sympathetic nerve NEC G90.8
  - syndrome T79.5 ☑
  - trachea J39.8
  - ulnar nerve (by scar tissue) — *see* Lesion, nerve, ulnar
  - umbilical cord
    - complicating delivery O69.2 ☑
      - cord around neck O69.1 ☑
      - prolapse O69.0 ☑
      - specified NEC O69.2 ☑
  - ureter N13.5
  - vein I87.1
  - vena cava (inferior) (superior) I87.1
- **Compulsion, compulsive**
  - gambling F63.0
  - neurosis F42
  - personality F60.5
  - states F42
  - swearing F42
    - in Gilles de la Tourette's syndrome F95.2
  - tics and spasms F95.9
- **Concato's disease** (pericardial polyserositis) A19.9
  - nontubercular I31.1
  - pleural — *see* Pleurisy, with effusion
- **Concavity chest wall** M95.4
- **Concealed penis** Q55.69
- **Concern** (normal) **about sick person in family** Z63.6
- **Concrescence** (teeth) K00.2
- **Concretio cordis** I31.1
  - rheumatic I09.2
- **Concretion** (*see also* Calculus)
  - appendicular K38.1
  - canaliculus — *see* Dacryolith
  - clitoris N90.89
  - conjunctiva H11.12- ☑
  - eyelid — *see* Disorder, eyelid, specified type NEC
  - lacrimal passages — *see* Dacryolith
  - prepuce (male) N47.8
  - salivary gland (any) K11.5
  - seminal vesicle N50.8
  - tonsil J35.8
- **Concussion** (brain) (cerebral) (current) S06.0X- ☑
  - blast (air) (hydraulic) (immersion) (underwater)
    - abdomen or thorax — *see* Injury, blast, by site
    - ear with acoustic nerve injury — *see* Injury, nerve, acoustic, specified type NEC
  - cauda equina S34.3 ☑
  - conus medullaris S34.02 ☑
  - ocular S05.8X- ☑
  - spinal (cord)
    - cervical S14.0 ☑
    - lumbar S34.01 ☑
    - sacral S34.02 ☑
    - thoracic S24.0 ☑
  - syndrome F07.81
- **Condition** — *see* Disease
- **Conditions arising in the perinatal period** — *see* Newborn, affected by
- **Conduct disorder** — *see* Disorder, conduct
- **Condyloma** A63.0
  - acuminatum A63.0
  - gonorrheal A54.09
  - latum A51.31
  - syphilitic A51.31
    - congenital A50.07
  - venereal, syphilitic A51.31
- **Conflagration** (*see also* Burn)
  - asphyxia (by inhalation of gases, fumes or vapors) (*see also* Table of Drugs and Chemicals) T59.9- ☑
- **Conflict** (with) (*see also* Discord)
  - family Z73.9
  - marital Z63.0
    - involving divorce or estrangement Z63.5
  - parent-child Z62.820
    - parent-adopted child Z62.821
    - parent-biological child Z62.820
    - parent-foster child Z62.822
  - social role NEC Z73.5
- **Confluent** — *see* condition
- **Confusion, confused** R41.0
  - epileptic F05
  - mental state (psychogenic) F44.89
  - psychogenic F44.89
  - reactive (from emotional stress, psychological trauma) F44.89
- **Confusional arousals** G47.51
- **Congelation** T69.9 ☑
- **Congenital** (*see also* condition)
  - aortic septum Q25.4
  - intrinsic factor deficiency D51.0
  - malformation — *see* Anomaly
- **Congestion, congestive**
  - bladder N32.89
  - bowel K63.89
  - brain G93.89
  - breast N64.59
  - bronchial J98.09
  - catarrhal J31.0
  - chest R09.89
  - chill, malarial — *see* Malaria
  - circulatory NEC I99.8
  - duodenum K31.89
  - eye — *see* Hyperemia, conjunctiva
  - facial, due to birth injury P15.4
  - general R68.89
  - glottis J37.0
  - heart — *see* Failure, heart, congestive
  - hepatic K76.1
  - hypostatic (lung) — *see* Edema, lung
  - intestine K63.89
  - kidney N28.89
  - labyrinth H83.8 ☑
  - larynx J37.0
  - liver K76.1
  - lung R09.89
    - active or acute — *see* Pneumonia
  - malaria, malarial — *see* Malaria
  - nasal R09.81
  - nose R09.81
  - orbit, orbital (*see also* Exophthalmos)
    - inflammatory (chronic) — *see* Inflammation, orbit
  - ovary N83.8
  - pancreas K86.8
  - pelvic, female N94.89
  - pleural J94.8
  - prostate (active) N42.1
  - pulmonary — *see* Congestion, lung
  - renal N28.89
  - retina H35.81
  - seminal vesicle N50.1
  - spinal cord G95.19
  - spleen (chronic) D73.2
  - stomach K31.89
  - trachea — *see* Tracheitis
  - urethra N36.8
  - uterus N85.8
    - with subinvolution N85.3
  - venous (passive) I87.8
  - viscera R68.89
- **Congestive** — *see* Congestion
- **Conical**
  - cervix (hypertrophic elongation) N88.4
  - cornea — *see* Keratoconus
  - teeth K00.2
- **Conjoined twins** Q89.4
- **Conjugal maladjustment** Z63.0
  - involving divorce or estrangement Z63.5
- **Conjunctiva** — *see* condition
- **Conjunctivitis** (staphylococcal) (streptococcal) NOS H10.9
  - Acanthamoeba B60.12
  - acute H10.3- ☑
    - atopic H10.1- ☑
    - chemical (*see also* Corrosion, cornea) H10.21- ☑
    - mucopurulent H10.02- ☑
      - follicular H10.01- ☑
    - pseudomembranous H10.22- ☑

Conjunctivitis — *continued*
- acute — *continued*
  - serous except viral H1Ø.23- ☑
    - viral — *see* Conjunctivitis, viral
  - toxic H1Ø.21- ☑
- adenoviral (acute) (follicular) B3Ø.1
- allergic (acute) — *see* Conjunctivitis, acute, atopic
  - chronic H1Ø.45
    - vernal H1Ø.44
- anaphylactic — *see* Conjunctivitis, acute, atopic
- Apollo B3Ø.3
- atopic (acute) — *see* Conjunctivitis, acute, atopic
- Béal's B3Ø.2
- blennorrhagic (gonococcal) (neonatorum) A54.31
- chemical (acute) (*see also* Corrosion, cornea) H1Ø.21- ☑
- chlamydial A74.Ø
  - due to trachoma A71.1
  - neonatal P39.1
- chronic (nodosa) (petrificans) (phlyctenular) H1Ø.4Ø- ☑
  - allergic H1Ø.45
    - vernal H1Ø.44
  - follicular H1Ø.43- ☑
  - giant papillary H1Ø.41- ☑
  - simple H1Ø.42- ☑
  - vernal H1Ø.44
- coxsackievirus 24 B3Ø.3
- diphtheritic A36.86
- due to
  - dust — *see* Conjunctivitis, acute, atopic
  - filariasis B74.9
  - mucocutaneous leishmaniasis B55.2
- enterovirus type 7Ø (hemorrhagic) B3Ø.3
- epidemic (viral) B3Ø.9
  - hemorrhagic B3Ø.3
- gonococcal (neonatorum) A54.31
- granular (trachomatous) A71.1
  - sequelae (late effect) B94.Ø
- hemorrhagic (acute) (epidemic) B3Ø.3
- herpes zoster BØ2.31
- in (due to)
  - Acanthamoeba B6Ø.12
  - adenovirus (acute) (follicular) B3Ø.1
  - Chlamydia A74.Ø
  - coxsackievirus 24 B3Ø.3
  - diphtheria A36.86
  - enterovirus type 7Ø (hemorrhagic) B3Ø.3
  - filariasis B74.9
  - gonococci A54.31
  - herpes (simplex) virus BØØ.53
    - zoster BØ2.31
  - infectious disease NEC B99 ☑
  - meningococci A39.89
  - mucocutaneous leishmaniasis B55.2
  - rosacea L71.9
  - syphilis (late) A52.71
  - zoster BØ2.31
- inclusion A74.Ø
- infantile P39.1
  - gonococcal A54.31
- Koch-Weeks' — *see* Conjunctivitis, acute, mucopurulent
- light — *see* Conjunctivitis, acute, atopic
- ligneous — *see* Blepharoconjunctivitis, ligneous
- meningococcal A39.89
- mucopurulent — *see* Conjunctivitis, acute, mucopurulent
- neonatal P39.1
  - gonococcal A54.31
- Newcastle B3Ø.8
- of Béal B3Ø.2
- parasitic
  - filariasis B74.9
  - mucocutaneous leishmaniasis B55.2
- Parinaud's H1Ø.89
- petrificans H1Ø.89
- rosacea L71.9
- specified NEC H1Ø.89
- swimming-pool B3Ø.1
- trachomatous A71.1
  - acute A71.Ø
  - sequelae (late effect) B94.Ø
- traumatic NEC H1Ø.89
- tuberculous A18.59
- tularemic A21.1
- tularensis A21.1
- viral B3Ø.9

Conjunctivitis — *continued*
- viral — *continued*
  - due to
    - adenovirus B3Ø.1
    - enterovirus B3Ø.3
  - specified NEC B3Ø.8

Conjunctivochalasis H11.82- ☑

Connective tissue — *see* condition

Conn's syndrome E26.Ø1

Conradi (-Hunermann) **disease** Q77.3

Consanguinity Z84.3
- counseling Z71.89

Conscious simulation (of illness) Z76.5

Consecutive — *see* condition

Consolidation lung (base) — *see* Pneumonia, lobar

Constipation (atonic) (neurogenic) (simple) (spastic) K59.ØØ
- drug-induced — *see* Table of Drugs and Chemicals
- outlet dysfunction K59.Ø2
- psychogenic F45.8
- slow transit K59.Ø1
- specified NEC K59.Ø9

Constitutional (*see also* condition)
- substandard F6Ø.7

Constitutionally substandard F6Ø.7

Constriction (*see also* Stricture)
- auditory canal — *see* Stenosis, external ear canal
- bronchial J98.Ø9
- duodenum K31.5
- esophagus K22.2
- external
  - abdomen, abdominal (wall) S3Ø.841 ☑
  - alveolar process SØØ.542 ☑
  - ankle S9Ø.54- ☑
  - antecubital space — *see* Constriction, external, forearm
  - arm (upper) S4Ø.84- ☑
  - auricle — *see* Constriction, external, ear
  - axilla — *see* Constriction, external, arm
  - back, lower S3Ø.84Ø ☑
  - breast S2Ø.14- ☑
  - brow SØØ.84 ☑
  - buttock S3Ø.84Ø ☑
  - calf — *see* Constriction, external, leg
  - canthus — *see* Constriction, external, eyelid
  - cheek SØØ.84 ☑
    - internal SØØ.542 ☑
  - chest wall — *see* Constriction, external, thorax
  - chin SØØ.84 ☑
  - clitoris S3Ø.844 ☑
  - costal region — *see* Constriction, external, thorax
  - digit(s)
    - foot — *see* Constriction, external, toe
    - hand — *see* Constriction, external, finger
  - ear SØØ.44- ☑
  - elbow S5Ø.34- ☑
  - epididymis S3Ø.843 ☑
  - epigastric region S3Ø.841 ☑
  - esophagus, cervical S1Ø.14 ☑
  - eyebrow — *see* Constriction, external, eyelid
  - eyelid SØØ.24- ☑
  - face SØØ.84 ☑
  - finger(s) S6Ø.44- ☑
    - index S6Ø.44- ☑
    - little S6Ø.44- ☑
    - middle S6Ø.44- ☑
    - ring S6Ø.44- ☑
  - flank S3Ø.841 ☑
  - foot (except toe(s) alone) S9Ø.84- ☑
    - toe — *see* Constriction, external, toe
  - forearm S5Ø.84- ☑
    - elbow only — *see* Constriction, external, elbow
  - forehead SØØ.84 ☑
  - genital organs, external
    - female S3Ø.846 ☑
    - male S3Ø.845 ☑
  - groin S3Ø.841 ☑
  - gum SØØ.542 ☑
  - hand S6Ø.54- ☑
  - head SØØ.94 ☑
    - ear — *see* Constriction, external, ear
    - eyelid — *see* Constriction, external, eyelid
    - lip SØØ.541 ☑
    - nose SØØ.34 ☑
    - oral cavity SØØ.542 ☑
    - scalp SØØ.Ø4 ☑

Constriction — *continued*
- external — *continued*
  - head — *continued*
    - specified site NEC SØØ.84 ☑
  - heel — *see* Constriction, external, foot
  - hip S7Ø.24- ☑
  - inguinal region S3Ø.841 ☑
  - interscapular region S2Ø.449 ☑
  - jaw SØØ.84 ☑
  - knee S8Ø.24- ☑
  - labium (majus) (minus) S3Ø.844 ☑
  - larynx S1Ø.14 ☑
  - leg (lower) S8Ø.84- ☑
    - knee — *see* Constriction, external, knee
    - upper — *see* Constriction, external, thigh
  - lip SØØ.541 ☑
  - lower back S3Ø.84Ø ☑
  - lumbar region S3Ø.84Ø ☑
  - malar region SØØ.84 ☑
  - mammary — *see* Constriction, external, breast
  - mastoid region SØØ.84 ☑
  - mouth SØØ.542 ☑
  - nail
    - finger — *see* Constriction, external, finger
    - toe — *see* Constriction, external, toe
  - nasal SØØ.34 ☑
  - neck S1Ø.94 ☑
    - specified site NEC S1Ø.84 ☑
    - throat S1Ø.14 ☑
  - nose SØØ.34 ☑
  - occipital region SØØ.Ø4 ☑
  - oral cavity SØØ.542 ☑
  - orbital region — *see* Constriction, external, eyelid
  - palate SØØ.542 ☑
  - palm — *see* Constriction, external, hand
  - parietal region SØØ.Ø4 ☑
  - pelvis S3Ø.84Ø ☑
  - penis S3Ø.842 ☑
  - perineum
    - female S3Ø.844 ☑
    - male S3Ø.84Ø ☑
  - periocular area — *see* Constriction, external, eyelid
  - phalanges
    - finger — *see* Constriction, external, finger
    - toe — *see* Constriction, external, toe
  - pharynx S1Ø.14 ☑
  - pinna — *see* Constriction, external, ear
  - popliteal space — *see* Constriction, external, knee
  - prepuce S3Ø.842 ☑
  - pubic region S3Ø.84Ø ☑
  - pudendum
    - female S3Ø.846 ☑
    - male S3Ø.845 ☑
  - sacral region S3Ø.84Ø ☑
  - scalp SØØ.Ø4 ☑
  - scapular region — *see* Constriction, external, shoulder
  - scrotum S3Ø.843 ☑
  - shin — *see* Constriction, external, leg
  - shoulder S4Ø.24- ☑
  - sternal region S2Ø.349 ☑
  - submaxillary region SØØ.84 ☑
  - submental region SØØ.84 ☑
  - subungual
    - finger(s) — *see* Constriction, external, finger
    - toe(s) — *see* Constriction, external, toe
  - supraclavicular fossa S1Ø.84 ☑
  - supraorbital SØØ.84 ☑
  - temple SØØ.84 ☑
  - temporal region SØØ.84 ☑
  - testis S3Ø.843 ☑
  - thigh S7Ø.34- ☑
  - thorax, thoracic (wall) S2Ø.94 ☑
    - back S2Ø.44- ☑
    - front S2Ø.34- ☑
  - throat S1Ø.14 ☑
  - thumb S6Ø.34- ☑
  - toe(s) (lesser) S9Ø.44- ☑
    - great S9Ø.44- ☑
  - tongue SØØ.542 ☑
  - trachea S1Ø.14 ☑
  - tunica vaginalis S3Ø.843 ☑
  - uvula SØØ.542 ☑
  - vagina S3Ø.844 ☑
  - vulva S3Ø.844 ☑
  - wrist S6Ø.84- ☑

- **Contusion** — *continued*
  - sacral region S30.0 ☑
  - scalp S00.03 ☑
    - due to birth injury P12.3
  - scapular region — *see* Contusion, shoulder
  - sclera — *see* Contusion, eyeball
  - scrotum S30.22 ☑
  - seminal vesicle S37.892 ☑
  - shoulder S40.01- ☑
  - skin NEC T14.8
  - small intestine — *see* Injury, intestine, small, contusion
  - spermatic cord S30.22 ☑
  - spinal cord — *see* Injury, spinal cord, by region
    - cauda equina S34.3 ☑
    - conus medullaris S34.139 ☑
  - spleen S36.029 ☑
    - major S36.021 ☑
    - minor S36.020 ☑
  - sternal region S20.219 ☑
  - stomach S36.32 ☑
  - subconjunctival S05.1- ☑
  - subcutaneous NEC T14.8
  - submaxillary region S00.83 ☑
  - submental region S00.83 ☑
  - subperiosteal NEC T14.8
  - subungual
    - finger — *see* Contusion, finger, with damage to nail
    - toe — *see* Contusion, toe, with damage to nail
  - supraclavicular fossa S10.83 ☑
  - supraorbital S00.83 ☑
  - suprarenal gland S37.812 ☑
  - temple (region) S00.83 ☑
  - temporal
    - lobe (brain) — *see* Injury, intracranial, diffuse
      - focal — *see* Injury, intracranial, focal
    - region S00.83 ☑
  - testis S30.22 ☑
  - thigh S70.1- ☑
  - thorax (wall) S20.20 ☑
    - back S20.22- ☑
    - front S20.21- ☑
  - throat S10.0 ☑
  - thumb S60.01- ☑
    - with damage to nail S60.11- ☑
  - toe(s) (lesser) S90.12- ☑
    - with damage to nail S90.22- ☑
    - great S90.11- ☑
      - with damage to nail S90.21- ☑
      - specified type NEC S90.221 ☑
  - tongue S00.532 ☑
  - trachea (cervical) S10.0 ☑
    - thoracic S27.52 ☑
  - tunica vaginalis S30.22 ☑
  - tympanum, tympanic membrane — *see* Contusion, ear
  - ureter S37.12 ☑
  - urethra S37.32 ☑
  - urinary organ NEC S37.892 ☑
  - uterus S37.62 ☑
  - uvula S00.532 ☑
  - vagina S30.23 ☑
  - vas deferens S37.892 ☑
  - vesical S37.22 ☑
  - vocal cord(s) S10.0 ☑
  - vulva S30.23 ☑
  - wrist S60.21- ☑
- **Conus** (congenital) (any type) Q14.8
  - cornea — *see* Keratoconus
  - medullaris syndrome G95.81
- **Conversion hysteria, neurosis or reaction** F44.9
- **Converter, tuberculosis** (test reaction) R76.11
- **Conviction** (legal), **anxiety concerning** Z65.0
  - with imprisonment Z65.1
- **Convulsions** (idiopathic) (*see also* Seizure(s)) R56.9
  - apoplectiform (cerebral ischemia) I67.82
  - benign neonatal (familial) — *see* Epilepsy, generalized, idiopathic
  - dissociative F44.5
  - epileptic — *see* Epilepsy
  - epileptiform, epileptoid — *see* Seizure, epileptiform
  - ether (anesthetic) — *see* Table of Drugs and Chemicals, by drug
  - febrile R56.00
    - with status epilepticus G40.901
    - complex R56.01
- **Convulsions** — *continued*
  - febrile — *continued*
    - complex — *continued*
      - with status epilepticus G40.901
    - simple R56.00
  - hysterical F44.5
  - infantile P90
    - epilepsy — *see* Epilepsy
  - jacksonian — *see* Epilepsy, localization-related, symptomatic, with simple partial seizures
  - myoclonic G25.3
  - neonatal, benign (familial) — *see* Epilepsy, generalized, idiopathic
  - newborn P90
  - obstetrical (nephritic) (uremic) — *see* Eclampsia
  - paretic A52.17
  - post traumatic R56.1
  - psychomotor — *see* Epilepsy, localization-related, symptomatic, with complex partial seizures
  - recurrent R56.9
  - reflex R25.8
  - scarlatinal A38.8
  - tetanus, tetanic — *see* Tetanus
  - thymic E32.8
- **Convulsive** (*see also* Convulsions)
- **Cooley's anemia** D56.1
- **Coolie itch** B76.9
- **Cooper's**
  - disease — *see* Mastopathy, cystic
  - hernia — *see* Hernia, abdomen, specified site NEC
- **Copra itch** B88.0
- **Coprophagy** F50.8
- **Coprophobia** F40.298
- **Coproporphyria, hereditary** E80.29
- **Cor**
  - biloculare Q20.8
  - bovis, bovinum — *see* Hypertrophy, cardiac
  - pulmonale (chronic) I27.81
    - acute I26.09
  - triatriatum, triatrium Q24.2
  - triloculare Q20.8
    - biatrium Q20.4
    - biventriculare Q21.1
- **Corbus' disease** (gangrenous balanitis) N48.1
- **Cord** (*see also* condition)
  - around neck (tightly) (with compression)
    - complicating delivery O69.1 ☑
  - bladder G95.89
    - tabetic A52.19
- **Cordis ectopia** Q24.8
- **Corditis** (spermatic) N49.1
- **Corectopia** Q13.2
- **Cori's disease** (glycogen storage) E74.03
- **Corkhandler's disease or lung** J67.3
- **Corkscrew esophagus** K22.4
- **Corkworker's disease or lung** J67.3
- **Corn** (infected) L84
- **Cornea** (*see also* condition)
  - donor Z52.5
  - plana Q13.4
- **Cornelia de Lange syndrome** Q87.1
- **Cornu cutaneum** L85.8
- **Cornual gestation or pregnancy** O00.8
- **Coronary** (artery) — *see* condition
- **Coronavirus, as cause of disease classified elsewhere** B97.29
  - SARS-associated B97.21
- **Corpora** (*see also* condition)
  - amylacea, prostate N42.89
  - cavernosa — *see* condition
- **Corpulence** — *see* Obesity
- **Corpus** — *see* condition
- **Corrected transposition** Q20.5
- **Corrosion** (injury) (acid) (caustic) (chemical) (lime) (external) (internal) T30.4
  - abdomen, abdominal (muscle) (wall) T21.42 ☑
    - first degree T21.52 ☑
    - second degree T21.62 ☑
    - third degree T21.72 ☑
  - above elbow T22.439 ☑
    - first degree T22.539 ☑
    - left T22.432 ☑
      - first degree T22.532 ☑
      - second degree T22.632 ☑
      - third degree T22.732 ☑
    - right T22.431 ☑
      - first degree T22.531 ☑
- **Corrosion** — *continued*
  - above elbow — *continued*
    - right — *continued*
      - second degree T22.631 ☑
      - third degree T22.731 ☑
    - second degree T22.639 ☑
    - third degree T22.739 ☑
  - alimentary tract NEC T28.7 ☑
  - ankle T25.419 ☑
    - first degree T25.519 ☑
    - left T25.412 ☑
      - first degree T25.512 ☑
      - second degree T25.612 ☑
      - third degree T25.712 ☑
    - multiple with foot — *see* Corrosion, lower, limb, multiple, ankle and foot
    - right T25.411 ☑
      - first degree T25.511 ☑
      - second degree T25.611 ☑
      - third degree T25.711 ☑
    - second degree T25.619 ☑
    - third degree T25.719 ☑
  - anus — *see* Corrosion, buttock
  - arm(s) (meaning upper limb(s)) — *see* Corrosion, upper limb
  - axilla T22.449 ☑
    - first degree T22.549 ☑
    - left T22.442 ☑
      - first degree T22.542 ☑
      - second degree T22.642 ☑
      - third degree T22.742 ☑
    - right T22.441 ☑
      - first degree T22.541 ☑
      - second degree T22.641 ☑
      - third degree T22.741 ☑
    - second degree T22.649 ☑
    - third degree T22.749 ☑
  - back (lower) T21.44 ☑
    - first degree T21.54 ☑
    - second degree T21.64 ☑
    - third degree T21.74 ☑
    - upper T21.43 ☑
      - first degree T21.53 ☑
      - second degree T21.63 ☑
      - third degree T21.73 ☑
  - blisters — *code as* Corrosion, second degree, by site
  - breast(s) — *see* Corrosion, chest wall
  - buttock(s) T21.45 ☑
    - first degree T21.55 ☑
    - second degree T21.65 ☑
    - third degree T21.75 ☑
  - calf T24.439 ☑
    - first degree T24.539 ☑
    - left T24.432 ☑
      - first degree T24.532 ☑
      - second degree T24.632 ☑
      - third degree T24.732 ☑
    - right T24.431 ☑
      - first degree T24.531 ☑
      - second degree T24.631 ☑
      - third degree T24.731 ☑
    - second degree T24.639 ☑
    - third degree T24.739 ☑
  - canthus (eye) — *see* Corrosion, eyelid
  - cervix T28.8 ☑
  - cheek T20.46 ☑
    - first degree T20.56 ☑
    - second degree T20.66 ☑
    - third degree T20.76 ☑
  - chest wall T21.41 ☑
    - first degree T21.51 ☑
    - second degree T21.61 ☑
    - third degree T21.71 ☑
  - chin T20.43 ☑
    - first degree T20.53 ☑
    - second degree T20.63 ☑
    - third degree T20.73 ☑
  - colon T28.7 ☑
  - conjunctiva (and cornea) — *see* Corrosion, cornea
  - cornea (and conjunctiva) T26.6- ☑
  - deep necrosis of underlying tissue — *code as* Corrosion, third degree, by site
  - dorsum of hand T23.469 ☑
    - first degree T23.569 ☑
    - left T23.462 ☑

- **Corrosion** — *continued*
  - dorsum of hand — *continued*
    - left — *continued*
      - first degree T23.562 ☑
      - second degree T23.662 ☑
      - third degree T23.762 ☑
    - right T23.461 ☑
      - first degree T23.561 ☑
      - second degree T23.661 ☑
      - third degree T23.761 ☑
    - second degree T23.669 ☑
    - third degree T23.769 ☑
  - ear (auricle) (external) (canal) T20.41 ☑
    - drum T28.91 ☑
    - first degree T20.51 ☑
    - second degree T20.61 ☑
    - third degree T20.71 ☑
  - elbow T22.429 ☑
    - first degree T22.529 ☑
    - left T22.422 ☑
      - first degree T22.522 ☑
      - second degree T22.622 ☑
      - third degree T22.722 ☑
    - right T22.421 ☑
      - first degree T22.521 ☑
      - second degree T22.621 ☑
      - third degree T22.721 ☑
    - second degree T22.629 ☑
    - third degree T22.729 ☑
  - entire body — *see* Corrosion, multiple body regions
  - epidermal loss — *code as* Corrosion, second degree, by site
  - epiglottis T27.4 ☑
  - erythema, erythematous — *code as* Corrosion, first degree, by site
  - esophagus T28.6 ☑
  - extent (percentage of body surface)
    - less than 10 percent T32.0
    - 10-19 percent (0-9 percent third degree) T32.10
      - with 10-19 percent third degree T32.11
    - 20-29 percent (0-9 percent third degree) T32.20
      - with
        - 10-19 percent third degree T32.21
        - 20-29 percent third degree T32.22
    - 30-39 percent (0-9 percent third degree) T32.30
      - with
        - 10-19 percent third degree T32.31
        - 20-29 percent third degree T32.32
        - 30-39 percent third degree T32.33
    - 40-49 percent (0-9 percent third degree) T32.40
      - with
        - 10-19 percent third degree T32.41
        - 20-29 percent third degree T32.42
        - 30-39 percent third degree T32.43
        - 40-49 percent third degree T32.44
    - 50-59 percent (0-9 percent third degree) T32.50
      - with
        - 10-19 percent third degree T32.51
        - 20-29 percent third degree T32.52
        - 30-39 percent third degree T32.53
        - 40-49 percent third degree T32.54
        - 50-59 percent third degree T32.55
    - 60-69 percent (0-9 percent third degree) T32.60
      - with
        - 10-19 percent third degree T32.61
        - 20-29 percent third degree T32.62
        - 30-39 percent third degree T32.63
        - 40-49 percent third degree T32.64
        - 50-59 percent third degree T32.65
        - 60-69 percent third degree T32.66
    - 70-79 percent (0-9 percent third degree) T32.70
      - with
        - 10-19 percent third degree T32.71
        - 20-29 percent third degree T32.72
        - 30-39 percent third degree T32.73
        - 40-49 percent third degree T32.74
        - 50-59 percent third degree T32.75
        - 60-69 percent third degree T32.76
        - 70-79 percent third degree T32.77
    - 80-89 percent (0-9 percent third degree) T32.80
      - with
        - 10-19 percent third degree T32.81
        - 20-29 percent third degree T32.82
        - 30-39 percent third degree T32.83
        - 40-49 percent third degree T32.84
        - 50-59 percent third degree T32.85
        - 60-69 percent third degree T32.86

- **Corrosion** — *continued*
  - extent — *continued*
    - 80-89 percent — *continued*
      - with — *continued*
        - 70-79 percent third degree T32.87
        - 80-89 percent third degree T32.88
    - 90 percent or more (0-9 percent third degree) T32.90
      - with
        - 10-19 percent third degree T32.91
        - 20-29 percent third degree T32.92
        - 30-39 percent third degree T32.93
        - 40-49 percent third degree T32.94
        - 50-59 percent third degree T32.95
        - 60-69 percent third degree T32.96
        - 70-79 percent third degree T32.97
        - 80-89 percent third degree T32.98
        - 90-99 percent third degree T32.99
  - extremity — *see* Corrosion, limb
  - eye(s) and adnexa T26.9- ☑
    - with resulting rupture and destruction of eyeball T26.7- ☑
    - conjunctival sac — *see* Corrosion, cornea
    - cornea — *see* Corrosion, cornea
    - lid — *see* Corrosion, eyelid
    - periocular area — *see* Corrosion eyelid
    - specified site NEC T26.8- ☑
  - eyeball — *see* Corrosion, eye
  - eyelid(s) T26.5- ☑
  - face — *see* Corrosion, head
  - finger T23.429 ☑
    - first degree T23.529 ☑
    - left T23.422 ☑
      - first degree T23.522 ☑
      - second degree T23.622 ☑
      - third degree T23.722 ☑
    - multiple sites (without thumb) T23.439 ☑
      - with thumb T23.449 ☑
        - first degree T23.549 ☑
        - left T23.442 ☑
          - first degree T23.542 ☑
          - second degree T23.642 ☑
          - third degree T23.742 ☑
        - right T23.441 ☑
          - first degree T23.541 ☑
          - second degree T23.641 ☑
          - third degree T23.741 ☑
        - second degree T23.649 ☑
        - third degree T23.749 ☑
      - first degree T23.539 ☑
      - left T23.432 ☑
        - first degree T23.532 ☑
        - second degree T23.632 ☑
        - third degree T23.732 ☑
      - right T23.431 ☑
        - first degree T23.531 ☑
        - second degree T23.631 ☑
        - third degree T23.731 ☑
      - second degree T23.639 ☑
      - third degree T23.739 ☑
    - right T23.421 ☑
      - first degree T23.521 ☑
      - second degree T23.621 ☑
      - third degree T23.721 ☑
    - second degree T23.629 ☑
    - third degree T23.729 ☑
  - flank — *see* Corrosion, abdomen
  - foot T25.429 ☑
    - first degree T25.529 ☑
    - left T25.422 ☑
      - first degree T25.522 ☑
      - second degree T25.622 ☑
      - third degree T25.722 ☑
    - multiple with ankle — *see* Corrosion, lower, limb, multiple, ankle and foot
    - right T25.421 ☑
      - first degree T25.521 ☑
      - second degree T25.621 ☑
      - third degree T25.721 ☑
    - second degree T25.629 ☑
    - third degree T25.729 ☑
  - forearm T22.419 ☑
    - first degree T22.519 ☑
    - left T22.412 ☑
      - first degree T22.512 ☑
      - second degree T22.612 ☑

- **Corrosion** — *continued*
  - forearm — *continued*
    - left — *continued*
      - third degree T22.712 ☑
    - right T22.411 ☑
      - first degree T22.511 ☑
      - second degree T22.611 ☑
      - third degree T22.711 ☑
    - second degree T22.619 ☑
    - third degree T22.719 ☑
  - forehead T20.46 ☑
    - first degree T20.56 ☑
    - second degree T20.66 ☑
    - third degree T20.76 ☑
  - fourth degree — *code as* Corrosion, third degree, by site
  - full thickness skin loss — *code as* Corrosion, third degree, by site
  - gastrointestinal tract NEC T28.7 ☑
  - genital organs
    - external
      - female T21.47 ☑
        - first degree T21.57 ☑
        - second degree T21.67 ☑
        - third degree T21.77 ☑
      - male T21.46 ☑
        - first degree T21.56 ☑
        - second degree T21.66 ☑
        - third degree T21.76 ☑
    - internal T28.8 ☑
  - groin — *see* Corrosion, abdominal wall
  - hand(s) T23.409 ☑
    - back — *see* Corrosion, dorsum of hand
    - finger — *see* Corrosion, finger
    - first degree T23.509 ☑
    - left T23.402 ☑
      - first degree T23.502 ☑
      - second degree T23.602 ☑
      - third degree T23.702 ☑
    - multiple sites with wrist T23.499 ☑
      - first degree T23.599 ☑
      - left T23.492 ☑
        - first degree T23.592 ☑
        - second degree T23.692 ☑
        - third degree T23.792 ☑
      - right T23.491 ☑
        - first degree T23.591 ☑
        - second degree T23.691 ☑
        - third degree T23.791 ☑
      - second degree T23.699 ☑
      - third degree T23.799 ☑
    - palm — *see* Corrosion, palm
    - right T23.401 ☑
      - first degree T23.501 ☑
      - second degree T23.601 ☑
      - third degree T23.701 ☑
    - second degree T23.609 ☑
    - third degree T23.709 ☑
    - thumb — *see* Corrosion, thumb
  - head (and face) (and neck) T20.40 ☑
    - cheek — *see* Corrosion, cheek
    - chin — *see* Corrosion, chin
    - ear — *see* Corrosion, ear
    - eye(s) only — *see* Corrosion, eye
    - first degree T20.50 ☑
    - forehead — *see* Corrosion, forehead
    - lip — *see* Corrosion, lip
    - multiple sites T20.49 ☑
      - first degree T20.59 ☑
      - second degree T20.69 ☑
      - third degree T20.79 ☑
    - neck — *see* Corrosion, neck
    - nose — *see* Corrosion, nose
    - scalp — *see* Corrosion, scalp
    - second degree T20.60 ☑
    - third degree T20.70 ☑
  - hip(s) — *see* Corrosion, lower, limb
  - inhalation — *see* Corrosion, respiratory tract
  - internal organ(s) (*see also* Corrosion, by site) T28.90 ☑
    - alimentary tract T28.7 ☑
      - esophagus T28.6 ☑
    - esophagus T28.6 ☑
    - genitourinary T28.8 ☑
    - mouth T28.5 ☑
    - pharynx T28.5 ☑
    - specified organ NEC T28.99 ☑

- **Corrosion** — *continued*
  - interscapular region — *see* Corrosion, back, upper
  - intestine (large) (small) T28.7 ☑
  - knee T24.429 ☑
    - first degree T24.529 ☑
    - left T24.422 ☑
      - first degree T24.522 ☑
      - second degree T24.622 ☑
      - third degree T24.722 ☑
    - right T24.421 ☑
      - first degree T24.521 ☑
      - second degree T24.621 ☑
      - third degree T24.721 ☑
    - second degree T24.629 ☑
    - third degree T24.729 ☑
  - labium (majus) (minus) — *see* Corrosion, genital organs, external, female
  - lacrimal apparatus, duct, gland or sac — *see* Corrosion, eye, specified site NEC
  - larynx T27.4 ☑
    - with lung T27.5 ☑
  - leg(s) (meaning lower limb(s)) — *see* Corrosion, lower limb
  - limb(s)
    - lower — *see* Corrosion, lower, limb
    - upper — *see* Corrosion, upper limb
  - lip(s) T2Ø.42 ☑
    - first degree T2Ø.52 ☑
    - second degree T2Ø.62 ☑
    - third degree T2Ø.72 ☑
  - lower
    - back — *see* Corrosion, back
    - limb T24.4Ø9 ☑
      - ankle — *see* Corrosion, ankle
      - calf — *see* Corrosion, calf
      - first degree T24.5Ø9 ☑
      - foot — *see* Corrosion, foot
      - knee — *see* Corrosion, knee
      - left T24.4Ø2 ☑
        - first degree T24.5Ø2 ☑
        - second degree T24.6Ø2 ☑
        - third degree T24.7Ø2 ☑
      - multiple sites, except ankle and foot T24.499 ☑
        - ankle and foot T25.499 ☑
          - first degree T25.599 ☑
          - left T25.492 ☑
            - first degree T25.592 ☑
            - second degree T25.692 ☑
            - third degree T25.792 ☑
          - right T25.491 ☑
            - first degree T25.591 ☑
            - second degree T25.691 ☑
            - third degree T25.791 ☑
          - second degree T25.699 ☑
          - third degree T25.799 ☑
        - first degree T24.599 ☑
        - left T24.492 ☑
          - first degree T24.592 ☑
          - second degree T24.692 ☑
          - third degree T24.792 ☑
        - right T24.491 ☑
          - first degree T24.591 ☑
          - second degree T24.691 ☑
          - third degree T24.791 ☑
        - second degree T24.699 ☑
        - third degree T24.799 ☑
      - right T24.4Ø1 ☑
        - first degree T24.5Ø1 ☑
        - second degree T24.6Ø1 ☑
        - third degree T24.7Ø1 ☑
      - second degree T24.6Ø9 ☑
      - thigh — *see* Corrosion, thigh
      - third degree T24.7Ø9 ☑
  - lung (with larynx and trachea) T27.5 ☑
  - mouth T28.5 ☑
  - neck T2Ø.47 ☑
    - first degree T2Ø.57 ☑
    - second degree T2Ø.67 ☑
    - third degree T2Ø.77 ☑
  - nose (septum) T2Ø.44 ☑
    - first degree T2Ø.54 ☑
    - second degree T2Ø.64 ☑
    - third degree T2Ø.74 ☑
  - ocular adnexa — *see* Corrosion, eye
  - orbit region — *see* Corrosion, eyelid

- **Corrosion** — *continued*
  - palm T23.459 ☑
    - first degree T23.559 ☑
    - left T23.452 ☑
      - first degree T23.552 ☑
      - second degree T23.652 ☑
      - third degree T23.752 ☑
    - right T23.451 ☑
      - first degree T23.551 ☑
      - second degree T23.651 ☑
      - third degree T23.751 ☑
    - second degree T23.659 ☑
    - third degree T23.759 ☑
  - partial thickness — *code as* Corrosion, unspecified degree, by site
  - pelvis — *see* Corrosion, trunk
  - penis — *see* Corrosion, genital organs, external, male
  - perineum
    - female — *see* Corrosion, genital organs, external, female
    - male — *see* Corrosion, genital organs, external, male
  - periocular area — *see* Corrosion, eyelid
  - pharynx T28.5 ☑
  - rectum T28.7 ☑
  - respiratory tract T27.7 ☑
    - larynx — *see* Corrosion, larynx
    - specified part NEC T27.6 ☑
    - trachea — *see* Corrosion, larynx
  - sac, lacrimal — *see* Corrosion, eye, specified site NEC
  - scalp T2Ø.45 ☑
    - first degree T2Ø.55 ☑
    - second degree T2Ø.65 ☑
    - third degree T2Ø.75 ☑
  - scapular region T22.469 ☑
    - first degree T22.569 ☑
    - left T22.462 ☑
      - first degree T22.562 ☑
      - second degree T22.662 ☑
      - third degree T22.762 ☑
    - right T22.461 ☑
      - first degree T22.561 ☑
      - second degree T22.661 ☑
      - third degree T22.761 ☑
    - second degree T22.669 ☑
    - third degree T22.769 ☑
  - sclera — *see* Corrosion, eye, specified site NEC
  - scrotum — *see* Corrosion, genital organs, external, male
  - shoulder T22.459 ☑
    - first degree T22.559 ☑
    - left T22.452 ☑
      - first degree T22.552 ☑
      - second degree T22.652 ☑
      - third degree T22.752 ☑
    - right T22.451 ☑
      - first degree T22.551 ☑
      - second degree T22.651 ☑
      - third degree T22.751 ☑
    - second degree T22.659 ☑
    - third degree T22.759 ☑
  - stomach T28.7 ☑
  - temple — *see* Corrosion, head
  - testis — *see* Corrosion, genital organs, external, male
  - thigh T24.419 ☑
    - first degree T24.519 ☑
    - left T24.412 ☑
      - first degree T24.512 ☑
      - second degree T24.612 ☑
      - third degree T24.712 ☑
    - right T24.411 ☑
      - first degree T24.511 ☑
      - second degree T24.611 ☑
      - third degree T24.711 ☑
    - second degree T24.619 ☑
    - third degree T24.719 ☑
  - thorax (external) — *see* Corrosion, trunk
  - throat (meaning pharynx) T28.5 ☑
  - thumb(s) T23.419 ☑
    - first degree T23.519 ☑
    - left T23.412 ☑
      - first degree T23.512 ☑
      - second degree T23.612 ☑
      - third degree T23.712 ☑
    - multiple sites with fingers T23.449 ☑

- **Corrosion** — *continued*
  - thumb(s) — *continued*
    - multiple sites with fingers — *continued*
      - first degree T23.549 ☑
      - left T23.442 ☑
        - first degree T23.542 ☑
        - second degree T23.642 ☑
        - third degree T23.742 ☑
      - right T23.441 ☑
        - first degree T23.541 ☑
        - second degree T23.641 ☑
        - third degree T23.741 ☑
      - second degree T23.649 ☑
      - third degree T23.749 ☑
    - right T23.411 ☑
      - first degree T23.511 ☑
      - second degree T23.611 ☑
      - third degree T23.711 ☑
    - second degree T23.619 ☑
    - third degree T23.719 ☑
  - toe T25.439 ☑
    - first degree T25.539 ☑
    - left T25.432 ☑
      - first degree T25.532 ☑
      - second degree T25.632 ☑
      - third degree T25.732 ☑
    - right T25.431 ☑
      - first degree T25.531 ☑
      - second degree T25.631 ☑
      - third degree T25.731 ☑
    - second degree T25.639 ☑
    - third degree T25.739 ☑
  - tongue T28.5 ☑
  - tonsil(s) T28.5 ☑
  - total body — *see* Corrosion, multiple body regions
  - trachea T27.4 ☑
    - with lung T27.5 ☑
  - trunk T21.4Ø ☑
    - abdominal wall — *see* Corrosion, abdominal wall
    - anus — *see* Corrosion, buttock
    - axilla — *see* Corrosion, upper limb
    - back — *see* Corrosion, back
    - breast — *see* Corrosion, chest wall
    - buttock — *see* Corrosion, buttock
    - chest wall — *see* Corrosion, chest wall
    - first degree T21.5Ø ☑
    - flank — *see* Corrosion, abdominal wall
    - genital
      - female — *see* Corrosion, genital organs, external, female
      - male — *see* Corrosion, genital organs, external, male
    - groin — *see* Corrosion, abdominal wall
    - interscapular region — *see* Corrosion, back, upper
    - labia — *see* Corrosion, genital organs, external, female
    - lower back — *see* Corrosion, back
    - penis — *see* Corrosion, genital organs, external, male
    - perineum
      - female — *see* Corrosion, genital organs, external, female
      - male — *see* Corrosion, genital organs, external, male
    - scapular region — *see* Corrosion, upper limb
    - scrotum — *see* Corrosion, genital organs, external, male
    - second degree T21.6Ø ☑
    - shoulder — *see* Corrosion, upper limb
    - specified site NEC T21.49 ☑
      - first degree T21.59 ☑
      - second degree T21.69 ☑
      - third degree T21.79 ☑
    - testes — *see* Corrosion, genital organs, external, male
    - third degree T21.7Ø ☑
    - upper back — *see* Corrosion, back, upper
    - vagina T28.8 ☑
    - vulva — *see* Corrosion, genital organs, external, female
  - unspecified site with extent of body surface involved specified
    - less than 1Ø percent T32.Ø
    - 1Ø-19 percent (Ø-9 percent third degree) T32.1Ø
      - with 1Ø-19 percent third degree T32.11
    - 2Ø-29 percent (Ø-9 percent third degree) T32.2Ø

Corrosion — *continued*
- unspecified site with extent of body surface involved
  - specified — *continued*
    - 20-29 percent — *continued*
      - with
        - 10-19 percent third degree T32.21
        - 20-29 percent third degree T32.22
    - 30-39 percent (0-9 percent third degree) T32.30
      - with
        - 10-19 percent third degree T32.31
        - 20-29 percent third degree T32.32
        - 30-39 percent third degree T32.33
    - 40-49 percent (0-9 percent third degree) T32.40
      - with
        - 10-19 percent third degree T32.41
        - 20-29 percent third degree T32.42
        - 30-39 percent third degree T32.43
        - 40-49 percent third degree T32.44
    - 50-59 percent (0-9 percent third degree) T32.50
      - with
        - 10-19 percent third degree T32.51
        - 20-29 percent third degree T32.52
        - 30-39 percent third degree T32.53
        - 40-49 percent third degree T32.54
        - 50-59 percent third degree T32.55
    - 60-69 percent (0-9 percent third degree) T32.60
      - with
        - 10-19 percent third degree T32.61
        - 20-29 percent third degree T32.62
        - 30-39 percent third degree T32.63
        - 40-49 percent third degree T32.64
        - 50-59 percent third degree T32.65
        - 60-69 percent third degree T32.66
    - 70-79 percent (0-9 percent third degree) T32.70
      - with
        - 10-19 percent third degree T32.71
        - 20-29 percent third degree T32.72
        - 30-39 percent third degree T32.73
        - 40-49 percent third degree T32.74
        - 50-59 percent third degree T32.75
        - 60-69 percent third degree T32.76
        - 70-79 percent third degree T32.77
    - 80-89 percent (0-9 percent third degree) T32.80
      - with
        - 10-19 percent third degree T32.81
        - 20-29 percent third degree T32.82
        - 30-39 percent third degree T32.83
        - 40-49 percent third degree T32.84
        - 50-59 percent third degree T32.85
        - 60-69 percent third degree T32.86
        - 70-79 percent third degree T32.87
        - 80-89 percent third degree T32.88
    - 90 percent or more (0-9 percent third degree) T32.90
      - with
        - 10-19 percent third degree T32.91
        - 20-29 percent third degree T32.92
        - 30-39 percent third degree T32.93
        - 40-49 percent third degree T32.94
        - 50-59 percent third degree T32.95
        - 60-69 percent third degree T32.96
        - 70-79 percent third degree T32.97
        - 80-89 percent third degree T32.98
        - 90-99 percent third degree T32.99
- upper limb (axilla) (scapular region) T22.40 ☑
  - above elbow — *see* Corrosion, above elbow
  - axilla — *see* Corrosion, axilla
  - elbow — *see* Corrosion, elbow
  - first degree T22.50 ☑
  - forearm — *see* Corrosion, forearm
  - hand — *see* Corrosion, hand
  - interscapular region — *see* Corrosion, back, upper
  - multiple sites T22.499 ☑
    - first degree T22.599 ☑
    - left T22.492 ☑
      - first degree T22.592 ☑
      - second degree T22.692 ☑
      - third degree T22.792 ☑
    - right T22.491 ☑
      - first degree T22.591 ☑
      - second degree T22.691 ☑
      - third degree T22.791 ☑
    - second degree T22.699 ☑
    - third degree T22.799 ☑
  - scapular region — *see* Corrosion, scapular region
  - second degree T22.60 ☑
  - shoulder — *see* Corrosion, shoulder
  - third degree T22.70 ☑

Corrosion — *continued*
- upper limb — *continued*
  - wrist — *see* Corrosion, hand
- uterus T28.8 ☑
- vagina T28.8 ☑
- vulva — *see* Corrosion, genital organs, external, female
- wrist T23.479 ☑
  - first degree T23.579 ☑
  - left T23.472 ☑
    - first degree T23.572 ☑
    - second degree T23.672 ☑
    - third degree T23.772 ☑
  - multiple sites with hand T23.499 ☑
    - first degree T23.599 ☑
    - left T23.492 ☑
      - first degree T23.592 ☑
      - second degree T23.692 ☑
      - third degree T23.792 ☑
    - right T23.491 ☑
      - first degree T23.591 ☑
      - second degree T23.691 ☑
      - third degree T23.791 ☑
    - second degree T23.699 ☑
    - third degree T23.799 ☑
  - right T23.471 ☑
    - first degree T23.571 ☑
    - second degree T23.671 ☑
    - third degree T23.771 ☑
  - second degree T23.679 ☑
  - third degree T23.779 ☑

Corrosive burn — *see* Corrosion

Corsican fever — *see* Malaria

Cortical — *see* condition

Cortico-adrenal — *see* condition

Coryza (acute) J00
- with grippe or influenza — *see* Influenza, with, respiratory manifestations NEC
- syphilitic
  - congenital (chronic) A50.05

Costen's syndrome or complex M26.69

Costiveness — *see* Constipation

Costochondritis M94.0

Cot death R99

Cotard's syndrome F22

Cotia virus B08.8

Cotton wool spots (retinal) H35.81

Cotungo's disease — *see* Sciatica

Cough (affected) (chronic) (epidemic) (nervous) R05
- with hemorrhage — *see* Hemoptysis
- bronchial R05
  - with grippe or influenza — *see* Influenza, with, respiratory manifestations NEC
- functional F45.8
- hysterical F45.8
- laryngeal, spasmodic R05
- psychogenic F45.8
- smokers' J41.0
- tea taster's B49

Counseling (for) Z71.9
- abuse NEC
  - perpetrator Z69.82
  - victim Z69.81
- alcohol abuser Z71.41
  - family Z71.42
- child abuse
  - nonparental
    - perpetrator Z69.021
    - victim Z69.020
  - parental
    - perpetrator Z69.011
    - victim Z69.010
- consanguinity Z71.89
- contraceptive Z30.09
- dietary Z71.3
- drug abuser Z71.51
  - family member Z71.52
- family Z71.89
- fertility preservation (prior to cancer therapy) (prior to removal of gonads) Z31.62
- for non-attending third party Z71.0
  - related to sexual behavior or orientation Z70.2
- genetic NEC Z31.5
- health (advice) (education) (instruction) — *see* Counseling, medical
- human immunodeficiency virus (HIV) Z71.7
- impotence Z70.1
- insulin pump use Z46.81

Counseling — *continued*
- medical (for) Z71.9
  - boarding school resident Z59.3
  - consanguinity Z71.89
  - feared complaint and no disease found Z71.1
  - human immunodeficiency virus (HIV) Z71.7
  - institutional resident Z59.3
  - on behalf of another Z71.0
    - related to sexual behavior or orientation Z70.2
  - person living alone Z60.2
  - specified reason NEC Z71.89
- natural family planning
  - procreative Z31.61
  - to avoid pregnancy Z30.02
- perpetrator (of)
  - abuse NEC Z69.82
  - child abuse
    - non-parental Z69.021
    - parental Z69.011
  - rape NEC Z69.82
  - spousal abuse Z69.12
- procreative NEC Z31.69
  - fertility preservation (prior to cancer therapy) (prior to removal of gonads) Z31.62
  - using natural family planning Z31.61
- promiscuity Z70.1
- rape victim Z69.81
- religious Z71.81
- sex, sexual (related to) Z70.9
  - attitude(s) Z70.0
  - behavior or orientation Z70.1
  - combined concerns Z70.3
  - non-responsiveness Z70.1
  - on behalf of third party Z70.2
  - specified reason NEC Z70.8
- specified reason NEC Z71.89
- spiritual Z71.81
- spousal abuse (perpetrator) Z69.12
  - victim Z69.11
- substance abuse Z71.89
  - alcohol Z71.41
  - drug Z71.51
  - tobacco Z71.6
- tobacco use Z71.6
- use (of)
  - insulin pump Z46.81
- victim (of)
  - abuse Z69.81
  - child abuse
    - by parent Z69.010
    - non-parental Z69.020
  - rape NEC Z69.81

Coupled rhythm R00.8

Couvelaire syndrome or uterus (complicating delivery) O45.8X- ☑

Cowperitis — *see* Urethritis

Cowper's gland — *see* condition

Cowpox B08.010
- due to vaccination T88.1 ☑

Coxa
- magna M91.4- ☑
- plana M91.2- ☑
- valga (acquired) (*see also* Deformity, limb, specified type NEC, thigh)
  - congenital Q65.81
  - sequelae (late effect) of rickets E64.3
- vara (acquired) (*see also* Deformity, limb, specified type NEC, thigh)
  - congenital Q65.82
  - sequelae (late effect) of rickets E64.3

Coxalgia, coxalgic (nontuberculous) (*see also* Pain, joint, hip)
- tuberculous A18.02

Coxitis — *see* Monoarthritis, hip

Coxsackie (virus) (infection) B34.1
- as cause of disease classified elsewhere B97.11
- carditis B33.20
- central nervous system NEC A88.8
- endocarditis B33.21
- enteritis A08.39
- meningitis (aseptic) A87.0
- myocarditis B33.22
- pericarditis B33.23
- pharyngitis B08.5
- pleurodynia B33.0
- specific disease NEC B33.8

Crabs, meaning pubic lice B85.3

Crack baby P04.41

- **Cracked nipple** N64.Ø
  - associated with
    - lactation O92.13
    - pregnancy O92.11- ☑
    - puerperium O92.12
- **Cracked tooth** KØ3.81
- **Cradle cap** L21.Ø
- **Craft neurosis** F48.8
- **Cramp**(s) R25.2
  - abdominal — *see* Pain, abdominal
  - bathing T75.1 ☑
  - colic R1Ø.83
    - psychogenic F45.8
  - due to immersion T75.1 ☑
  - fireman T67.2 ☑
  - heat T67.2 ☑
  - immersion T75.1 ☑
  - intestinal — *see* Pain, abdominal
    - psychogenic F45.8
  - leg, sleep related G47.62
  - limb (lower) (upper) NEC R25.2
    - sleep related G47.62
  - linotypist's F48.8
    - organic G25.89
  - muscle (limb) (general) R25.2
    - due to immersion T75.1 ☑
    - psychogenic F45.8
  - occupational (hand) F48.8
    - organic G25.89
  - salt-depletion E87.1
  - sleep related, leg G47.62
  - stoker's T67.2 ☑
  - swimmer's T75.1 ☑
  - telegrapher's F48.8
    - organic G25.89
  - typist's F48.8
    - organic G25.89
  - uterus N94.89
    - menstrual — *see* Dysmenorrhea
  - writer's F48.8
    - organic G25.89
- **Cranial** — *see* condition
- **Craniocleidodysostosis** Q74.Ø
- **Craniofenestria** (skull) Q75.8
- **Craniolacunia** (skull) Q75.8
- **Craniopagus** Q89.4
- **Craniopathy, metabolic** M85.2
- **Craniopharyngeal** — *see* condition
- **Craniopharyngioma** D44.4
- **Craniorachischisis** (totalis) QØØ.1
- **Cranioschisis** Q75.8
- **Craniostenosis** Q75.Ø
- **Craniosynostosis** Q75.Ø
- **Craniotabes** (cause unknown) M83.8
  - neonatal P96.3
  - rachitic E64.3
  - syphilitic A5Ø.56
- **Cranium** — *see* condition
- **Craw-craw** — *see* Onchocerciasis
- **Creaking joint** — *see* Derangement, joint, specified type NEC
- **Creeping**
  - eruption B76.9
  - palsy or paralysis G12.22
- **Crenated tongue** K14.8
- **Creotoxism** AØ5.9
- **Crepitus**
  - caput Q75.8
  - joint — *see* Derangement, joint, specified type NEC
- **Crescent or conus choroid, congenital** Q14.3
- **CREST syndrome** M34.1
- **Cretin, cretinism** (congenital) (endemic) (nongoitrous) (sporadic) EØØ.9
  - pelvis
    - with disproportion (fetopelvic) O33.Ø
      - causing obstructed labor O65.Ø
  - type
    - hypothyroid EØØ.1
    - mixed EØØ.2
    - myxedematous EØØ.1
    - neurological EØØ.Ø
- **Creutzfeldt-Jakob disease or syndrome** (with dementia) A81.ØØ
  - familial A81.Ø9
  - iatrogenic A81.Ø9
  - specified NEC A81.Ø9
  - sporadic A81.Ø9

Creutzfeldt-Jakob disease or syndrome — *continued*

  - variant (vCJD) A81.Ø1
- **Crib death** R99
- **Cribriform hymen** Q52.3
- **Cri-du-chat syndrome** Q93.4
- **Crigler-Najjar disease or syndrome** E8Ø.5
- **Crime, victim of** Z65.4
- **Crimean hemorrhagic fever** A98.Ø
- **Criminalism** F6Ø.2
- **Crisis**
  - abdomen R1Ø.Ø
  - acute reaction F43.Ø
  - addisonian E27.2
  - adrenal (cortical) E27.2
  - celiac K9Ø.Ø
  - Dietl's N13.8
  - emotional (*see also* Disorder, adjustment)
    - acute reaction to stress F43.Ø
    - specific to childhood and adolescence F93.8
  - glaucomatocyclitic — *see* Glaucoma, secondary, inflammation
  - heart — *see* Failure, heart
  - nitritoid I95.2
    - correct substance properly administered — *see* Table of Drugs and Chemicals, by drug, adverse effect
    - overdose or wrong substance given or taken — *see* Table of Drugs and Chemicals, by drug, poisoning
  - oculogyric H51.8
    - psychogenic F45.8
  - Pel's (tabetic) A52.11
  - psychosexual identity F64.2
  - renal N28.Ø
  - sickle-cell D57.ØØ
    - with
      - acute chest syndrome D57.Ø1
      - splenic sequestration D57.Ø2
  - state (acute reaction) F43.Ø
  - tabetic A52.11
  - thyroid — *see* Thyrotoxicosis with thyroid storm
  - thyrotoxic — *see* Thyrotoxicosis with thyroid storm
- **Crocq's disease** (acrocyanosis) I73.89
- **Crohn's disease** — *see* Enteritis, regional
- **Crooked septum, nasal** J34.2
- **Cross syndrome** E7Ø.328
- **Crossbite** (anterior) (posterior) M26.24
- **Cross-eye** — *see* Strabismus, convergent concomitant
- **Croup, croupous** (catarrhal) (infectious) (inflammatory) (nondiphtheritic) JØ5.Ø
  - bronchial J2Ø.9
  - diphtheritic A36.2
  - false J38.5
  - spasmodic J38.5
    - diphtheritic A36.2
  - stridulous J38.5
    - diphtheritic A36.2
- **Crouzon's disease** Q75.1
- **Crowding, tooth, teeth, fully erupted** M26.31
- **CRST syndrome** M34.1
- **Cruchet's disease** A85.8
- **Cruelty in children** (*see also* Disorder, conduct)
- **Crural ulcer** — *see* Ulcer, lower limb
- **Crush, crushed, crushing** T14.8
  - abdomen S38.1 ☑
  - ankle S97.Ø- ☑
  - arm (upper) (and shoulder) S47.- ☑
  - axilla — *see* Crush, arm
  - back, lower S38.1 ☑
  - buttock S38.1 ☑
  - cheek SØ7.Ø ☑
  - chest S28.Ø ☑
  - cranium SØ7.1 ☑
  - ear SØ7.Ø ☑
  - elbow S57.Ø- ☑
  - extremity
    - lower
      - ankle — *see* Crush, ankle
      - below knee — *see* Crush, leg
      - foot — *see* Crush, foot
      - hip — *see* Crush, hip
      - knee — *see* Crush, knee
      - thigh — *see* Crush, thigh
      - toe — *see* Crush, toe
    - upper
      - below elbow S67.9- ☑

Crush, crushed, crushing — *continued*

  - extremity — *continued*
    - upper — *continued*
      - elbow — *see* Crush, elbow
      - finger — *see* Crush, finger
      - forearm — *see* Crush, forearm
      - hand — *see* Crush, hand
      - thumb — *see* Crush, thumb
      - upper arm — *see* Crush, arm
      - wrist — *see* Crush, wrist
  - face SØ7.Ø ☑
  - finger(s) S67.1- ☑
    - with hand (and wrist) — *see* Crush, hand, specified site NEC
    - index S67.19- ☑
    - little S67.19- ☑
    - middle S67.19- ☑
    - ring S67.19- ☑
    - thumb — *see* Crush, thumb
  - foot S97.8- ☑
    - toe — *see* Crush, toe
  - forearm S57.8- ☑
  - genitalia, external
    - female S38.ØØ2 ☑
      - vagina S38.Ø3 ☑
      - vulva S38.Ø3 ☑
    - male S38.ØØ1 ☑
      - penis S38.Ø1 ☑
      - scrotum S38.Ø2 ☑
      - testis S38.Ø2 ☑
  - hand (except fingers alone) S67.2- ☑
    - with wrist S67.4- ☑
  - head SØ7.9 ☑
    - specified NEC SØ7.8 ☑
  - heel — *see* Crush, foot
  - hip S77.Ø- ☑
    - with thigh S77.2- ☑
  - internal organ (abdomen, chest, or pelvis) NEC T14.8
  - knee S87.Ø- ☑
  - labium (majus) (minus) S38.Ø3 ☑
  - larynx S17.Ø ☑
  - leg (lower) S87.8- ☑
    - knee — *see* Crush, knee
  - lip SØ7.Ø ☑
  - lower
    - back S38.1 ☑
    - leg — *see* Crush, leg
  - neck S17.9 ☑
  - nerve — *see* Injury, nerve
  - nose SØ7.Ø ☑
  - pelvis S38.1 ☑
  - penis S38.Ø1 ☑
  - scalp SØ7.8 ☑
  - scapular region — *see* Crush, arm
  - scrotum S38.Ø2 ☑
  - severe, unspecified site T14.8
  - shoulder (and upper arm) — *see* Crush, arm
  - skull SØ7.1 ☑
  - syndrome (complication of trauma) T79.5 ☑
  - testis S38.Ø2 ☑
  - thigh S77.1- ☑
    - with hip S77.2- ☑
  - throat S17.8 ☑
  - thumb S67.Ø- ☑
    - with hand (and wrist) — *see* Crush, hand, specified site NEC
  - toe(s) S97.1Ø- ☑
    - great S97.11- ☑
    - lesser S97.12- ☑
  - trachea S17.Ø ☑
  - vagina S38.Ø3 ☑
  - vulva S38.Ø3 ☑
  - wrist S67.3- ☑
    - with hand S67.4- ☑
- **Crusta lactea** L21.Ø
- **Crusts** R23.4
- **Crutch paralysis** — *see* Injury, brachial plexus
- **Cruveilhier-Baumgarten cirrhosis, disease or syndrome** K74.69
- **Cruveilhier's atrophy or disease** G12.8
- **Crying** (constant) (continuous) (excessive)
  - child, adolescent, or adult R45.83
  - infant (baby) (newborn) R68.11
- **Cryofibrinogenemia** D89.2
- **Cryoglobulinemia** (essential) (idiopathic) (mixed) (primary) (purpura) (secondary) (vasculitis) D89.1

Cryoglobulinemia — *continued*
- with lung involvement D89.1 [J99]

Cryptitis (anal) (rectal) K62.89
Cryptococcosis, cryptococcus (infection) (neoformans) B45.9
- bone B45.3
- cerebral B45.1
- cutaneous B45.2
- disseminated B45.7
- generalized B45.7
- meningitis B45.1
- meningocerebralis B45.1
- osseous B45.3
- pulmonary B45.0
- skin B45.2
- specified NEC B45.8

Cryptopapillitis (anus) K62.89
Cryptophthalmos Q11.2
- syndrome Q87.0

Cryptorchid, cryptorchism, cryptorchidism Q53.9
- bilateral Q53.20
  - abdominal Q53.21
  - perineal Q53.22
- unilateral Q53.10
  - abdominal Q53.11
  - perineal Q53.12

Cryptosporidiosis A07.2
- hepatobiliary B88.8
- respiratory B88.8

Cryptostromosis J67.6
Crystalluria R82.99
Cubitus
- congenital Q68.8
- valgus (acquired) M21.0- ☑
  - congenital Q68.8
  - sequelae (late effect) of rickets E64.3
- varus (acquired) M21.1- ☑
  - congenital Q68.8
  - sequelae (late effect) of rickets E64.3

Cultural deprivation or shock Z60.3
Curling esophagus K22.4
Curling's ulcer — *see* Ulcer, peptic, acute
Curschmann (-Batten) (-Steinert) **disease or syndrome** G71.11
Curse, Ondine's — *see* Apnea, sleep
Curvature
- organ or site, congenital NEC — *see* Distortion
- penis (lateral) Q55.61
- Pott's (spinal) A18.01
- radius, idiopathic, progressive (congenital) Q74.0
- spine (acquired) (angular) (idiopathic) (incorrect) (postural) — *see* Dorsopathy, deforming
  - congenital Q67.5
  - due to or associated with
    - Charcot-Marie-Tooth disease (*see also* subcategory M49.8) G60.0
    - osteitis
      - deformans M88.88
      - fibrosa cystica (*see also* subcategory M49.8) E21.0
    - tuberculosis (Pott's curvature) A18.01
  - sequelae (late effect) of rickets E64.3
  - tuberculous A18.01

Cushingoid due to steroid therapy E24.2
- correct substance properly administered — *see* Table of Drugs and Chemicals, by drug, adverse effect
- overdose or wrong substance given or taken — *see* Table of Drugs and Chemicals, by drug, poisoning

Cushing's
- syndrome or disease E24.9
  - drug-induced E24.2
  - iatrogenic E24.2
  - pituitary-dependent E24.0
  - specified NEC E24.8
- ulcer — *see* Ulcer, peptic, acute

Cusp, Carabelli — *omit code*
Cut (external) (*see also* Laceration)
- muscle — *see* Injury, muscle

Cutaneous (*see also* condition)
- hemorrhage R23.3
- larva migrans B76.9

Cutis (*see also* condition)
- hyperelastica Q82.8
  - acquired L57.4
- laxa (hyperelastica) — *see* Dermatolysis
- marmorata R23.8

Cutis — *continued*
- osteosis L94.2
- pendula — *see* Dermatolysis
- rhomboidalis nuchae L57.2
- verticis gyrata Q82.8
  - acquired L91.8

Cyanosis R23.0
- due to
  - patent foramen botalli Q21.1
  - persistent foramen ovale Q21.1
- enterogenous D74.8
- paroxysmal digital — *see* Raynaud's disease
  - with gangrene I73.01
- retina, retinal H35.89

Cyanotic heart disease I24.9
- congenital Q24.9

Cycle
- anovulatory N97.0
- menstrual, irregular N92.6

Cyclencephaly Q04.9
Cyclical vomiting (*see also* Vomiting, cyclical) G43.A0 (*following* G43.7)
- psychogenic F50.8

Cyclitis (*see also* Iridocyclitis) H20.9
- chronic — *see* Iridocyclitis, chronic
- Fuchs' heterochromic H20.81- ☑
- granulomatous — *see* Iridocyclitis, chronic
- lens-induced — *see* Iridocyclitis, lens-induced
- posterior H30.2- ☑

Cycloid personality F34.0
Cyclophoria H50.54
Cyclopia, cyclops Q87.0
Cyclopism Q87.0
Cyclosporiasis A07.4
Cyclothymia F34.0
Cyclothymic personality F34.0
Cyclotropia H50.41- ☑
Cylindroma (*see also* Neoplasm, malignant, by site)
- eccrine dermal — *see* Neoplasm, skin, benign
- skin — *see* Neoplasm, skin, benign

Cylindruria R82.99
Cynanche
- diphtheritic A36.2
- tonsillaris J36

Cynophobia F40.218
Cynorexia R63.2
Cyphosis — *see* Kyphosis
Cyprus fever — *see* Brucellosis
Cyst (colloid) (mucous) (simple) (retention)
- adenoid (infected) J35.8
- adrenal gland E27.8
  - congenital Q89.1
- air, lung J98.4
- allantoic Q64.4
- alveolar process (jaw bone) M27.40
- amnion, amniotic O41.8X- ☑
- anterior
  - chamber (eye) — *see* Cyst, iris
  - nasopalatine K09.1
- antrum J34.1
- anus K62.89
- apical (tooth) (periodontal) K04.8
- appendix K38.8
- arachnoid, brain (acquired) G93.0
  - congenital Q04.6
- arytenoid J38.7
- Baker's M71.2- ☑
  - ruptured M66.0
  - tuberculous A18.02
- Bartholin's gland N75.0
- bile duct (common) (hepatic) K83.5
- bladder (multiple) (trigone) N32.89
- blue dome (breast) — *see* Cyst, breast
- bone (local) NEC M85.60
  - aneurysmal M85.50
    - ankle M85.57- ☑
    - foot M85.57- ☑
    - forearm M85.53- ☑
    - hand M85.54- ☑
    - jaw M27.49
    - lower leg M85.56- ☑
    - multiple site M85.59
    - neck M85.58
    - rib M85.58
    - shoulder M85.51- ☑
    - skull M85.58
    - specified site NEC M85.58

Cyst — *continued*
- bone — *continued*
  - aneurysmal — *continued*
    - thigh M85.55- ☑
    - toe M85.57- ☑
    - upper arm M85.52- ☑
    - vertebra M85.58
  - solitary M85.40
    - ankle M85.47- ☑
    - fibula M85.46- ☑
    - foot M85.47- ☑
    - hand M85.44- ☑
    - humerus M85.42- ☑
    - jaw M27.49
    - neck M85.48
    - pelvis M85.45- ☑
    - radius M85.43- ☑
    - rib M85.48
    - shoulder M85.41- ☑
    - skull M85.48
    - specified site NEC M85.48
    - tibia M85.46- ☑
    - toe M85.47- ☑
    - ulna M85.43- ☑
    - vertebra M85.48
  - specified type NEC M85.60
    - ankle M85.67- ☑
    - foot M85.67- ☑
    - forearm M85.63- ☑
    - hand M85.64- ☑
    - jaw M27.40
      - developmental (nonodontogenic) K09.1
        - odontogenic K09.0
      - latent M27.0
    - lower leg M85.66- ☑
    - multiple site M85.69
    - neck M85.68
    - rib M85.68
    - shoulder M85.61- ☑
    - skull M85.68
    - specified site NEC M85.68
    - thigh M85.65- ☑
    - toe M85.67- ☑
    - upper arm M85.62- ☑
    - vertebra M85.68
- brain (acquired) G93.0
  - congenital Q04.6
  - hydatid B67.99 [G94]
  - third ventricle (colloid), congenital Q04.6
- branchial (cleft) Q18.0
- branchiogenic Q18.0
- breast (benign) (blue dome) (pedunculated) (solitary) N60.0- ☑
  - involution — *see* Dysplasia, mammary, specified type NEC
  - sebaceous — *see* Dysplasia, mammary, specified type NEC
- broad ligament (benign) N83.8
- bronchogenic (mediastinal) (sequestration) J98.4
  - congenital Q33.0
- buccal K09.8
- bulbourethral gland N36.8
- bursa, bursal NEC M71.30
  - with rupture — *see* Rupture, synovium
  - ankle M71.37- ☑
  - elbow M71.32- ☑
  - foot M71.37- ☑
  - hand M71.34- ☑
  - hip M71.35- ☑
  - multiple sites M71.39
  - pharyngeal J39.2
  - popliteal space — *see* Cyst, Baker's
  - shoulder M71.31- ☑
  - specified site NEC M71.38
  - wrist M71.33- ☑
- calcifying odontogenic D16.5
  - upper jaw (bone) (maxilla) D16.4
- canal of Nuck (female) N94.89
  - congenital Q52.4
- canthus — *see* Cyst, conjunctiva
- carcinomatous — *see* Neoplasm, malignant, by site
- cauda equina G95.89
- cavum septi pellucidi — *see* Cyst, brain
- celomic (pericardium) Q24.8
- cerebellopontine (angle) — *see* Cyst, brain
- cerebellum — *see* Cyst, brain
- cerebral — *see* Cyst, brain

Cyst — *continued*
- cervical lateral Q18.1
- cervix NEC N88.8
  - embryonic Q51.6
  - nabothian N88.8
- chiasmal optic NEC — *see* Disorder, optic, chiasm
- chocolate (ovary) N8Ø.1
- choledochus, congenital Q44.4
- chorion O41.8X- ☑
- choroid plexus G93.Ø
- ciliary body — *see* Cyst, iris
- clitoris N9Ø.7
- colon K63.89
- common (bile) duct K83.5
- congenital NEC Q89.8
  - adrenal gland Q89.1
  - epiglottis Q31.8
  - esophagus Q39.8
  - fallopian tube Q5Ø.4
  - kidney Q61.ØØ
    - more than one (multiple) Q61.Ø2
      - specified as polycystic Q61.3
        - adult type Q61.2
        - infantile type NEC Q61.19
          - collecting duct dilation Q61.11
    - solitary Q61.Ø1
  - larynx Q31.8
  - liver Q44.6
  - lung Q33.Ø
  - mediastinum Q34.1
  - ovary Q5Ø.1
  - oviduct Q5Ø.4
  - periurethral (tissue) Q64.79
  - prepuce Q55.69
  - salivary gland (any) Q38.4
  - sublingual Q38.6
  - submaxillary gland Q38.6
  - thymus (gland) Q89.2
  - tongue Q38.3
  - ureterovesical orifice Q62.8
  - vulva Q52.79
- conjunctiva H11.44- ☑
- cornea H18.89- ☑
- corpora quadrigemina G93.Ø
- corpus
  - albicans N83.29
  - luteum (hemorrhagic) (ruptured) N83.1
- Cowper's gland (benign) (infected) N36.8
- cranial meninges G93.Ø
- craniobuccal pouch E23.6
- craniopharyngeal pouch E23.6
- cystic duct K82.8
- Cysticercus — *see* Cysticercosis
- Dandy-Walker QØ3.1
  - with spina bifida — *see* Spina bifida
- dental (root) KØ4.8
  - developmental KØ9.Ø
  - eruption KØ9.Ø
  - primordial KØ9.Ø
- dentigerous (mandible) (maxilla) KØ9.Ø
- dermoid — *see* Neoplasm, benign, by site
  - with malignant transformation C56.- ☑
  - implantation
    - external area or site (skin) NEC L72.Ø
    - iris — *see* Cyst, iris, implantation
    - vagina N89.8
    - vulva N9Ø.7
  - mouth KØ9.8
  - oral soft tissue KØ9.8
  - sacrococcygeal — *see* Cyst, pilonidal
- developmental KØ9.1
  - odontogenic KØ9.Ø
  - oral region (nonodontogenic) KØ9.1
  - ovary, ovarian Q5Ø.1
- dura (cerebral) G93.Ø
  - spinal G96.19
- ear (external) Q18.1
- echinococcal — *see* Echinococcus
- embryonic
  - cervix uteri Q51.6
  - fallopian tube Q5Ø.4
  - vagina Q51.6
- endometrium, endometrial (uterus) N85.8
  - ectopic — *see* Endometriosis
- enterogenous Q43.8
- epidermal, epidermoid (inclusion) (*see also* Cyst, skin) L72.Ø
  - mouth KØ9.8

Cyst — *continued*
- epidermal, epidermoid (*see also* Cyst, skin) — *continued*
  - oral soft tissue KØ9.8
- epididymis N5Ø.3
- epiglottis J38.7
- epiphysis cerebri E34.8
- epithelial (inclusion) L72.Ø
- epoophoron Q5Ø.5
- eruption KØ9.Ø
- esophagus K22.8
- ethmoid sinus J34.1
- external female genital organs NEC N9Ø.7
- eyelid (sebaceous) HØ2.829
  - infected — *see* Hordeolum
  - left HØ2.826
    - lower HØ2.825
    - upper HØ2.824
  - right HØ2.823
    - lower HØ2.822
    - upper HØ2.821
- eye NEC H57.8
  - congenital Q15.8
- fallopian tube N83.8
  - congenital Q5Ø.4
- fimbrial (twisted) Q5Ø.4
- fissural (oral region) KØ9.1
- follicle (graafian) (hemorrhagic) N83.Ø
  - nabothian N88.8
- follicular (atretic) (hemorrhagic) (ovarian) N83.Ø
  - dentigerous KØ9.Ø
  - odontogenic KØ9.Ø
  - skin L72.9
    - specified NEC L72.8
- frontal sinus J34.1
- gallbladder K82.8
- ganglion — *see* Ganglion
- Gartner's duct Q52.4
- gingiva KØ9.Ø
- gland of Moll — *see* Cyst, eyelid
- globulomaxillary KØ9.1
- graafian follicle (hemorrhagic) N83.Ø
- granulosal lutein (hemorrhagic) N83.1
- hemangiomatous D18.ØØ
  - intra-abdominal D18.Ø3
  - intracranial D18.Ø2
  - skin D18.Ø1
  - specified site NEC D18.Ø9
- hydatid (*see also* Echinococcus) B67.9Ø
  - brain B67.99 [G94]
  - liver (*see also* Cyst, liver, hydatid) B67.8
  - lung NEC B67.99 [J99]
  - Morgagni
    - female Q5Ø.5
    - male (epididymal) Q55.4
      - testicular Q55.29
  - specified site NEC B67.99
- hymen N89.8
  - embryonic Q52.4
- hypopharynx J39.2
- hypophysis, hypophyseal (duct) (recurrent) E23.6
  - cerebri E23.6
- implantation (dermoid)
  - external area or site (skin) NEC L72.Ø
  - iris — *see* Cyst, iris, implantation
  - vagina N89.8
  - vulva N9Ø.7
- incisive canal KØ9.1
- inclusion (epidermal) (epithelial) (epidermoid) (squamous) L72.Ø
  - not of skin — *code under* Cyst, by site
- intestine (large) (small) K63.89
- intracranial — *see* Cyst, brain
- intraligamentous (*see also* Disorder, ligament)
  - knee — *see* Derangement, knee
- intrasellar E23.6
- iris H21.3Ø9
  - exudative H21.31- ☑
  - idiopathic H21.3Ø- ☑
  - implantation H21.32- ☑
  - parasitic H21.33- ☑
  - pars plana (primary) H21.34- ☑
    - exudative H21.35- ☑
- jaw (bone) M27.4Ø
  - aneurysmal M27.49
  - developmental (odontogenic) KØ9.Ø
  - fissural KØ9.1
  - hemorrhagic M27.49

Cyst — *continued*
- jaw — *continued*
  - traumatic M27.49
- joint NEC — *see* Disorder, joint, specified type NEC
- kidney (acquired) N28.1
  - calyceal — *see* Hydronephrosis
  - congenital Q61.ØØ
  - more than one (multiple) Q61.Ø2
    - specified as polycystic Q61.3
      - adult type (autosomal dominant) Q61.2
      - infantile type (autosomal recessive) NEC Q61.19
        - collecting duct dilation Q61.11
  - pyelogenic — *see* Hydronephrosis
  - simple N28.1
  - solitary (single) Q61.Ø1
    - acquired N28.1
- labium (majus) (minus) N9Ø.7
  - sebaceous N9Ø.7
- lacrimal (*see also* Disorder, lacrimal system, specified NEC)
  - gland HØ4.13- ☑
  - passages or sac — *see* Disorder, lacrimal system, specified NEC
- larynx J38.7
- lateral periodontal KØ9.Ø
- lens H27.8
  - congenital Q12.8
- lip (gland) K13.Ø
- liver (idiopathic) (simple) K76.89
  - congenital Q44.6
  - hydatid B67.8
    - granulosus B67.Ø
    - multilocularis B67.5
- lung J98.4
  - congenital Q33.Ø
  - giant bullous J43.9
- lutein N83.1
- lymphangiomatous D18.1
- lymphoepithelial, oral soft tissue KØ9.8
- macula — *see* Degeneration, macula, hole
- malignant — *see* Neoplasm, malignant, by site
- mammary gland — *see* Cyst, breast
- mandible M27.4Ø
  - dentigerous KØ9.Ø
  - radicular KØ4.8
- maxilla M27.4Ø
  - dentigerous KØ9.Ø
  - radicular KØ4.8
- medial, face and neck Q18.8
- median
  - anterior maxillary KØ9.1
  - palatal KØ9.1
- mediastinum, congenital Q34.1
- meibomian (gland) — *see* Chalazion
  - infected — *see* Hordeolum
- membrane, brain G93.Ø
- meninges (cerebral) G93.Ø
  - spinal G96.19
- meniscus, knee — *see* Derangement, knee, meniscus, cystic
- mesentery, mesenteric K66.8
  - chyle I89.8
- mesonephric duct
  - female Q5Ø.5
  - male Q55.4
- milk N64.89
- Morgagni (hydatid)
  - female Q5Ø.5
  - male (epididymal) Q55.4
    - testicular Q55.29
- mouth KØ9.8
- Müllerian duct Q5Ø.4
  - appendix testis Q55.29
  - cervix Q51.6
  - fallopian tube Q5Ø.4
  - female Q5Ø.4
  - male Q55.29
  - prostatic utricle Q55.4
  - vagina (embryonal) Q52.4
- multilocular (ovary) D39.1Ø
  - benign — *see* Neoplasm, benign, by site
- myometrium N85.8
- nabothian (follicle) (ruptured) N88.8
- nasoalveolar KØ9.1
- nasolabial KØ9.1
- nasopalatine (anterior) (duct) KØ9.1
- nasopharynx J39.2

- **Cystadenofibroma** — *continued*
  - endometrioid — *continued*
    - borderline malignancy D39.1- ☑
    - malignant C56.- ☑
  - mucinous
    - specified site — *see* Neoplasm, benign, by site
    - unspecified site D27.9
  - serous
    - specified site — *see* Neoplasm, benign, by site
    - unspecified site D27.9
  - specified site — *see* Neoplasm, benign, by site
  - unspecified site D27.9
- **Cystadenoma** (*see also* Neoplasm, benign, by site)
  - bile duct D13.4
  - endometrioid — *see* Neoplasm, benign, by site
    - borderline malignancy — *see* Neoplasm, uncertain behavior, by site
  - malignant — *see* Neoplasm, malignant, by site
  - mucinous
    - borderline malignancy
      - ovary C56.- ☑
      - specified site NEC — *see* Neoplasm, uncertain behavior, by site
      - unspecified site C56.9
    - papillary
      - borderline malignancy
        - ovary C56.- ☑
        - specified site NEC — *see* Neoplasm, uncertain behavior, by site
        - unspecified site C56.9
      - specified site — *see* Neoplasm, benign, by site
      - unspecified site D27.9
    - specified site — *see* Neoplasm, benign, by site
    - unspecified site D27.9
  - papillary
    - borderline malignancy
      - ovary C56.- ☑
      - specified site NEC — *see* Neoplasm, uncertain behavior, by site
      - unspecified site C56.9
    - lymphomatosum
      - specified site — *see* Neoplasm, benign, by site
      - unspecified site D11.9
    - mucinous
      - borderline malignancy
        - ovary C56.- ☑
        - specified site NEC — *see* Neoplasm, uncertain behavior, by site
        - unspecified site C56.9
      - specified site — *see* Neoplasm, benign, by site
      - unspecified site D27.9
    - pseudomucinous
      - borderline malignancy
        - ovary C56.- ☑
        - specified site NEC — *see* Neoplasm, uncertain behavior, by site
        - unspecified site C56.9
      - specified site — *see* Neoplasm, benign, by site
      - unspecified site D27.9
    - serous
      - borderline malignancy
        - ovary C56.- ☑
        - specified site NEC — *see* Neoplasm, uncertain behavior, by site
        - unspecified site C56.9
      - specified site — *see* Neoplasm, benign, by site
      - unspecified site D27.9
    - specified site — *see* Neoplasm, benign, by site
    - unspecified site D27.9
  - pseudomucinous
    - borderline malignancy
      - ovary C56.- ☑
      - specified site NEC — *see* Neoplasm, uncertain behavior, by site
      - unspecified site C56.9
    - papillary
      - borderline malignancy
        - ovary C56.- ☑
        - specified site NEC — *see* Neoplasm, uncertain behavior, by site
        - unspecified site C56.9
      - specified site — *see* Neoplasm, benign, by site
      - unspecified site D27.9
    - specified site — *see* Neoplasm, benign, by site

- **Cystadenoma** — *continued*
  - pseudomucinous — *continued*
    - unspecified site D27.9
  - serous
    - borderline malignancy
      - ovary C56.- ☑
      - specified site NEC — *see* Neoplasm, uncertain behavior, by site
      - unspecified site C56.9
    - papillary
      - borderline malignancy
        - ovary C56.- ☑
        - specified site NEC — *see* Neoplasm, uncertain behavior, by site
        - unspecified site C56.9
      - specified site — *see* Neoplasm, benign, by site
      - unspecified site D27.9
    - specified site — *see* Neoplasm, benign, by site
    - unspecified site D27.9
- **Cystathionine synthase deficiency** E72.11
- **Cystathioninemia** E72.19
- **Cystathioninuria** E72.19
- **Cystic** (*see also* condition)
  - breast (chronic) — *see* Mastopathy, cystic
  - corpora lutea (hemorrhagic) N83.1
  - duct — *see* condition
  - eyeball (congenital) Q11.Ø
  - fibrosis — *see* Fibrosis, cystic
  - kidney (congenital) Q61.9
    - adult type Q61.2
    - infantile type NEC Q61.19
      - collecting duct dilatation Q61.11
    - medullary Q61.5
  - liver, congenital Q44.6
  - lung disease J98.4
    - congenital Q33.Ø
  - mastitis, chronic — *see* Mastopathy, cystic
  - medullary, kidney Q61.5
  - meniscus — *see* Derangement, knee, meniscus, cystic
  - ovary N83.2Ø
- **Cysticercosis, cysticerciasis** B69.9
  - with
    - epileptiform fits B69.Ø
    - myositis B69.81
  - brain B69.Ø
  - central nervous system B69.Ø
  - cerebral B69.Ø
  - ocular B69.1
  - specified NEC B69.89
- **Cysticercus cellulose infestation** — *see* Cysticercosis
- **Cystinosis** (malignant) E72.Ø4
- **Cystinuria** E72.Ø1
- **Cystitis** (exudative) (hemorrhagic) (septic) (suppurative) N3Ø.9Ø
  - with
    - fibrosis — *see* Cystitis, chronic, interstitial
    - hematuria N3Ø.91
    - leukoplakia — *see* Cystitis, chronic, interstitial
    - malakoplakia — *see* Cystitis, chronic, interstitial
    - metaplasia — *see* Cystitis, chronic, interstitial
    - prostatitis N41.3
  - acute N3Ø.ØØ
    - with hematuria N3Ø.Ø1
    - of trigone N3Ø.3Ø
      - with hematuria N3Ø.31
  - allergic — *see* Cystitis, specified type NEC
  - amebic AØ6.81
  - bilharzial B65.9 [N33]
  - blennorrhagic (gonococcal) A54.Ø1
  - bullous — *see* Cystitis, specified type NEC
  - calculous N21.Ø
  - chlamydial A56.Ø1
  - chronic N3Ø.2Ø
    - with hematuria N3Ø.21
    - interstitial N3Ø.1Ø
      - with hematuria N3Ø.11
    - of trigone N3Ø.3Ø
      - with hematuria N3Ø.31
    - specified NEC N3Ø.2Ø
      - with hematuria N3Ø.21
  - cystic (a) — *see* Cystitis, specified type NEC
  - diphtheritic A36.85
  - echinococcal
    - granulosus B67.39

- **Cystitis** — *continued*
  - echinococcal — *continued*
    - multilocularis B67.69
  - emphysematous — *see* Cystitis, specified type NEC
  - encysted — *see* Cystitis, specified type NEC
  - eosinophilic — *see* Cystitis, specified type NEC
  - follicular — *see* Cystitis, of trigone
  - gangrenous — *see* Cystitis, specified type NEC
  - glandularis — *see* Cystitis, specified type NEC
  - gonococcal A54.Ø1
  - incrusted — *see* Cystitis, specified type NEC
  - interstitial (chronic) — *see* Cystitis, chronic, interstitial
  - irradiation N3Ø.4Ø
    - with hematuria N3Ø.41
  - irritation — *see* Cystitis, specified type NEC
  - malignant — *see* Cystitis, specified type NEC
  - of trigone N3Ø.3Ø
    - with hematuria N3Ø.31
  - panmural — *see* Cystitis, chronic, interstitial
  - polyposa — *see* Cystitis, specified type NEC
  - prostatic N41.3
  - puerperal (postpartum) O86.22
  - radiation — *see* Cystitis, irradiation
  - specified type NEC N3Ø.8Ø
    - with hematuria N3Ø.81
  - subacute — *see* Cystitis, chronic
  - submucous — *see* Cystitis, chronic, interstitial
  - syphilitic (late) A52.76
  - trichomonal A59.Ø3
  - tuberculous A18.12
  - ulcerative — *see* Cystitis, chronic, interstitial
- **Cystocele** (-urethrocele)
  - female N81.1Ø
    - with prolapse of uterus — *see* Prolapse, uterus
    - lateral N81.12
    - midline N81.11
    - paravaginal N81.12
  - in pregnancy or childbirth O34.8- ☑
    - causing obstructed labor O65.5
  - male N32.89
- **Cystolithiasis** N21.Ø
- **Cystoma** (*see also* Neoplasm, benign, by site)
  - endometrial, ovary N8Ø.1
  - mucinous
    - specified site — *see* Neoplasm, benign, by site
    - unspecified site D27.9
  - serous
    - specified site — *see* Neoplasm, benign, by site
    - unspecified site D27.9
  - simple (ovary) N83.29
- **Cystoplegia** N31.2
- **Cystoptosis** N32.89
- **Cystopyelitis** — *see* Pyelonephritis
- **Cystorrhagia** N32.89
- **Cystosarcoma phyllodes** D48.6- ☑
  - benign D24- ☑
  - malignant — *see* Neoplasm, breast, malignant
- **Cystostomy**
  - attention to Z43.5
  - complication — *see* Complications, cystostomy
  - status Z93.5Ø
    - appendico-vesicostomy Z93.52
    - cutaneous Z93.51
    - specified NEC Z93.59
- **Cystourethritis** — *see* Urethritis
- **Cystourethrocele** (*see also* Cystocele)
  - female N81.1Ø
    - with uterine prolapse — *see* Prolapse, uterus
    - lateral N81.12
    - midline N81.11
    - paravaginal N81.12
  - male N32.89
- **Cytomegalic inclusion disease**
  - congenital P35.1
- **Cytomegalovirus infection** B25.9
- **Cytomycosis** (reticuloendothelial) B39.4
- **Cytopenia** D75.9
  - refractory
    - with multilineage dysplasia D46.A (*following* D46.2)
      - and ring sideroblasts (RCMD RS) D46.B (*following* D46.2)
- **Czerny's disease** (periodic hydrarthrosis of the knee) — *see* Effusion, joint, knee

D

- **Da Costa's syndrome** F45.8
- **Daae** (-Finsen) **disease** (epidemic pleurodynia) B33.Ø
- **Dabney's grip** B33.Ø
- **Dacryoadenitis, dacryadenitis** HØ4.ØØ- ☑
  - acute HØ4.Ø1- ☑
  - chronic HØ4.Ø2- ☑
- **Dacryocystitis** HØ4.3Ø- ☑
  - acute HØ4.32- ☑
  - chronic HØ4.41- ☑
  - neonatal P39.1
  - phlegmonous HØ4.31- ☑
  - syphilitic A52.71
    - congenital (early) A5Ø.Ø1
  - trachomatous, active A71.1
    - sequelae (late effect) B94.Ø
- **Dacryocystoblenorrhea** — *see* Inflammation, lacrimal, passages, chronic
- **Dacryocystocele** — *see* Disorder, lacrimal system, changes
- **Dacryolith, dacryolithiasis** HØ4.51- ☑
- **Dacryoma** — *see* Disorder, lacrimal system, changes
- **Dacryopericystitis** — *see* Dacryocystitis
- **Dacryops** HØ4.11- ☑
- **Dacryostenosis** (*see also* Stenosis, lacrimal)
  - congenital Q1Ø.5
- **Dactylitis**
  - bone — *see* Osteomyelitis
  - sickle-cell D57.ØØ
    - Hb C D57.219
    - Hb SS D57.ØØ
    - specified NEC D57.819
  - skin LØ8.9
  - syphilitic A52.77
  - tuberculous A18.Ø3
- **Dactylolysis spontanea** (ainhum) L94.6
- **Dactylosymphysis** Q7Ø.9
  - fingers — *see* Syndactylism, complex, fingers
  - toes — *see* Syndactylism, complex, toes
- **Damage**
  - arteriosclerotic — *see* Arteriosclerosis
  - brain (nontraumatic) G93.9
    - anoxic, hypoxic G93.1
      - resulting from a procedure G97.82
    - child NEC G8Ø.9
    - due to birth injury P11.2
  - cardiorenal (vascular) — *see* Hypertension, cardiorenal
  - cerebral NEC — *see* Damage, brain
  - coccyx, complicating delivery O71.6
  - coronary — *see* Disease, heart, ischemic
  - eye, birth injury P15.3
  - liver (nontraumatic) K76.9
    - alcoholic K7Ø.9
    - due to drugs — *see* Disease, liver, toxic
    - toxic — *see* Disease, liver, toxic
  - medication T88.7 ☑
  - pelvic
    - joint or ligament, during delivery O71.6
    - organ NEC
      - during delivery O71.5
      - following ectopic or molar pregnancy OØ8.6
  - renal — *see* Disease, renal
  - subendocardium, subendocardial — *see* Degeneration, myocardial
  - vascular I99.9
- **Dana-Putnam syndrome** (subacute combined sclerosis with pernicious anemia) — *see* Degeneration, combined
- **Danbolt** (-Cross) **syndrome** (acrodermatitis enteropathica) E83.2
- **Dandruff** L21.Ø
- **Dandy-Walker syndrome** QØ3.1
  - with spina bifida — *see* Spina bifida
- **Danlos' syndrome** Q79.6
- **Darier** (-White) **disease** (congenital) Q82.8
  - meaning erythema annulare centrifugum L53.1
- **Darier-Roussy sarcoid** D86.3
- **Darling's disease or histoplasmosis** B39.4
- **Darwin's tubercle** Q17.8
- **Dawson's** (inclusion body) **encephalitis** A81.1
- **De Beurmann** (-Gougerot) **disease** B42.1
- **De la Tourette's syndrome** F95.2
- **De Lange's syndrome** Q87.1
- **De Morgan's spots** (senile angiomas) I78.1
- **De Quervain's**
  - disease (tendon sheath) M65.4
  - syndrome E34.51
  - thyroiditis (subacute granulomatous thyroiditis) EØ6.1
- **De Toni-Fanconi** (-Debré) **syndrome** E72.Ø9
  - with cystinosis E72.Ø4
- **Dead**
  - fetus, retained (mother) O36.4 ☑
    - early pregnancy OØ2.1
  - labyrinth H83.2 ☑
  - ovum, retained OØ2.Ø
- **Deaf nonspeaking NEC** H91.3
- **Deafmutism** (acquired) (congenital) NEC H91.3
  - hysterical F44.6
  - syphilitic, congenital (*see also* subcategory) H94.8 A5Ø.Ø9
- **Deafness** (acquired) (complete) (hereditary) (partial) H91.9- ☑
  - with blue sclera and fragility of bone Q78.Ø
  - auditory fatigue — *see* Deafness, specified type NEC
  - aviation T7Ø.Ø ☑
    - nerve injury — *see* Injury, nerve, acoustic, specified type NEC
  - boilermaker's H83.3 ☑
  - central — *see* Deafness, sensorineural
  - conductive H9Ø.2
    - and sensorineural, mixed H9Ø.8
      - bilateral H9Ø.6
    - bilateral H9Ø.Ø
    - unilateral H9Ø.1- ☑
  - congenital H9Ø.5
    - with blue sclera and fragility of bone Q78.Ø
  - due to toxic agents — *see* Deafness, ototoxic
  - emotional (hysterical) F44.6
  - functional (hysterical) F44.6
  - high frequency H91.9- ☑
  - hysterical F44.6
  - low frequency H91.9- ☑
  - mental R48.8
  - mixed conductive and sensorineural H9Ø.8
    - bilateral H9Ø.6
    - unilateral H9Ø.7- ☑
  - nerve — *see* Deafness, sensorineural
  - neural — *see* Deafness, sensorineural
  - noise-induced (*see also* subcategory) H83.3 ☑
    - nerve injury — *see* Injury, nerve, acoustic, specified type NEC
  - nonspeaking H91.3
  - ototoxic H91.Ø ☑
  - perceptive — *see* Deafness, sensorineural
  - psychogenic (hysterical) F44.6
  - sensorineural H9Ø.5
    - and conductive, mixed H9Ø.8
      - bilateral H9Ø.6
    - bilateral H9Ø.3
    - unilateral H9Ø.4- ☑
  - sensory — *see* Deafness, sensorineural
  - specified type NEC H91.8 ☑
  - sudden (idiopathic) H91.2- ☑
  - syphilitic A52.15
  - transient ischemic H93.Ø1- ☑
  - traumatic — *see* Injury, nerve, acoustic, specified type NEC
  - word (developmental) H93.25
- **Death** (cause unknown) (of) (unexplained) (unspecified cause) R99
  - brain G93.82
  - cardiac (sudden) (with successful resuscitation) — *code to* underlying disease
    - family history of Z82.41
    - personal history of Z86.74
  - family member (assumed) Z63.4
- **Debility** (chronic) (general) (nervous) R53.81
  - congenital or neonatal NOS P96.9
  - nervous R53.81
  - old age R54
  - senile R54
- **Débove's disease** (splenomegaly) R16.1
- **Decalcification**
  - bone — *see* Osteoporosis
  - teeth KØ3.89
- **Decapsulation, kidney** N28.89
- **Decay**
  - dental — *see* Caries, dental
  - senile R54
  - tooth, teeth — *see* Caries, dental
- **Deciduitis** (acute)
  - following ectopic or molar pregnancy OØ8.Ø
- **Decline** (general) — *see* Debility
  - cognitive, age-associated R41.81
- **Decompensation**
  - cardiac (acute) (chronic) — *see* Disease, heart
  - cardiovascular — *see* Disease, cardiovascular
  - heart — *see* Disease, heart
  - hepatic — *see* Failure, hepatic
  - myocardial (acute) (chronic) — *see* Disease, heart
  - respiratory J98.8
- **Decompression sickness** T7Ø.3 ☑
- **Decrease** (d)
  - absolute neutrophile count — *see* Neutropenia
  - blood
    - platelets — *see* Thrombocytopenia
    - pressure RØ3.1
      - due to shock following
        - injury T79.4 ☑
        - operation T81.19 ☑
  - estrogen E28.39
    - postablative E89.4Ø
      - asymptomatic E89.4Ø
      - symptomatic E89.41
  - fragility of erythrocytes D58.8
  - function
    - lipase (pancreatic) K9Ø.3
    - ovary in hypopituitarism E23.Ø
    - parenchyma of pancreas K86.8
    - pituitary (gland) (anterior) (lobe) E23.Ø
      - posterior (lobe) E23.Ø
  - functional activity R68.89
  - glucose R73.Ø9
  - hematocrit R71.Ø
  - hemoglobin R71.Ø
  - leukocytes D72.819
    - specified NEC D72.818
  - libido R68.82
  - lymphocytes D72.81Ø
  - platelets D69.6
  - respiration, due to shock following injury T79.4 ☑
  - sexual desire R68.82
  - tear secretion NEC — *see* Syndrome, dry eye
  - tolerance
    - fat K9Ø.4
    - glucose R73.Ø9
    - pancreatic K9Ø.3
    - salt and water E87.8
  - vision NEC H54.7
  - white blood cell count D72.819
    - specified NEC D72.818
- **Decubitus** (ulcer) — *see* Ulcer, pressure, by site
  - cervix N86
- **Deepening acetabulum** — *see* Derangement, joint, specified type NEC, hip
- **Defect, defective** Q89.9
  - 3-beta-hydroxysteroid dehydrogenase E25.Ø
  - 11-hydroxylase E25.Ø
  - 21-hydroxylase E25.Ø
  - abdominal wall, congenital Q79.59
  - antibody immunodeficiency D8Ø.9
  - aorticopulmonary septum Q21.4
  - atrial septal (ostium secundum type) Q21.1
    - following acute myocardial infarction (current complication) I23.1
    - ostium primum type Q21.2
  - atrioventricular
    - canal Q21.2
    - septum Q21.2
  - auricular septal Q21.1
  - bilirubin excretion NEC E8Ø.6
  - biosynthesis, androgen (testicular) E29.1
  - bulbar septum Q21.Ø

Defect, defective — *continued*
- catalase E8Ø.3
- cell membrane receptor complex (CR3) D71
- circulation I99.9
  - congenital Q28.9
  - newborn Q28.9
- coagulation (factor) (*see also* Deficiency, factor) D68.9
  - with
    - ectopic pregnancy OØ8.1
    - molar pregnancy OØ8.1
  - acquired D68.4
  - antepartum with hemorrhage — *see* Hemorrhage, antepartum, with coagulation defect
  - due to
    - liver disease D68.4
    - vitamin K deficiency D68.4
  - hereditary NEC D68.2
  - intrapartum O67.Ø
  - newborn, transient P61.6
  - postpartum O72.3
  - specified type NEC D68.8
- complement system D84.1
- conduction (heart) I45.9
  - bone — *see* Deafness, conductive
- congenital, organ or site not listed — *see* Anomaly, by site
- coronary sinus Q21.1
- cushion, endocardial Q21.2
- degradation, glycoprotein E77.1
- dental bridge, crown, fillings — *see* Defect, dental restoration
- dental restoration KØ8.5Ø
  - specified NEC KØ8.59
- dentin (hereditary) KØØ.5
- Descemet's membrane, congenital Q13.89
- developmental (*see also* Anomaly)
  - cauda equina QØ6.3
- diaphragm
  - with elevation, eventration or hernia — *see* Hernia, diaphragm
  - congenital Q79.1
    - with hernia Q79.Ø
    - gross (with hernia) Q79.Ø
- ectodermal, congenital Q82.9
- Eisenmenger's Q21.8
- enzyme
  - catalase E8Ø.3
  - peroxidase E8Ø.3
- esophagus, congenital Q39.9
- extensor retinaculum M62.89
- fibrin polymerization D68.2
- filling
  - bladder R93.4
  - kidney R93.4
  - stomach R93.3
  - ureter R93.4
- Gerbode Q21.Ø
- glycoprotein degradation E77.1
- Hageman (factor) D68.2
- hearing — *see* Deafness
- high grade F7Ø
- interatrial septal Q21.1
- interauricular septal Q21.1
- interventricular septal Q21.Ø
  - with dextroposition of aorta, pulmonary stenosis and hypertrophy of right ventricle Q21.3
  - in tetralogy of Fallot Q21.3
- learning (specific) — *see* Disorder, learning
- lymphocyte function antigen-1 (LFA-1) D84.Ø
- lysosomal enzyme, post-translational modification E77.Ø
- major osseous M89.7Ø
  - ankle M89.77- ☑
  - carpus M89.74- ☑
  - clavicle M89.71- ☑
  - femur M89.75- ☑
  - fibula M89.76- ☑
  - fingers M89.74- ☑
  - foot M89.77- ☑
  - forearm M89.73- ☑
  - hand M89.74- ☑
  - humerus M89.72- ☑
  - lower leg M89.76- ☑
  - metacarpus M89.74- ☑
  - metatarsus M89.77- ☑
  - multiple sites M89.79
  - pelvic region M89.75- ☑
  - pelvis M89.75- ☑

Defect, defective — *continued*
- major osseous — *continued*
  - radius M89.73- ☑
  - scapula M89.71- ☑
  - shoulder region M89.71- ☑
  - specified NEC M89.78
  - tarsus M89.77- ☑
  - thigh M89.75- ☑
  - tibia M89.76- ☑
  - toes M89.77- ☑
  - ulna M89.73- ☑
- mental — *see* Disability, intellectual
- modification, lysosomal enzymes, post-translational E77.Ø
- obstructive, congenital
  - renal pelvis Q62.39
  - ureter Q62.39
    - atresia — *see* Atresia, ureter
    - cecoureterocele Q62.32
    - megaureter Q62.2
    - orthotopic ureterocele Q62.31
- osseous, major M89.7Ø
  - ankle M89.77- ☑
  - carpus M89.74- ☑
  - clavicle M89.71- ☑
  - femur M89.75- ☑
  - fibula M89.76- ☑
  - fingers M89.74- ☑
  - foot M89.77- ☑
  - forearm M89.73- ☑
  - hand M89.74- ☑
  - humerus M89.72- ☑
  - lower leg M89.76- ☑
  - metacarpus M89.74- ☑
  - metatarsus M89.77- ☑
  - multiple sites M89.9
  - pelvic region M89.75- ☑
  - pelvis M89.75- ☑
  - radius M89.73- ☑
  - scapula M89.71- ☑
  - shoulder region M89.71- ☑
  - specified NEC M89.78
  - tarsus M89.77- ☑
  - thigh M89.75- ☑
  - tibia M89.76- ☑
  - toes M89.77- ☑
  - ulna M89.73- ☑
- osteochondral NEC (*see also* Deformity) M95.8
- ostium
  - primum Q21.2
  - secundum Q21.1
- peroxidase E8Ø.3
- placental blood supply — *see* Insufficiency, placental
- platelets, qualitative D69.1
  - constitutional D68.Ø
- postural NEC, spine — *see* Dorsopathy, deforming
- reduction
  - limb Q73.8
    - lower Q72.9- ☑
      - absence — *see* Agenesis, leg
        - foot — *see* Agenesis, foot
      - longitudinal
        - femur Q72.4- ☑
        - fibula Q72.6- ☑
        - tibia Q72.5- ☑
      - specified type NEC Q72.89- ☑
      - split foot Q72.7- ☑
    - specified type NEC Q73.8
    - upper Q71.9- ☑
      - absence — *see* Agenesis, arm
        - forearm — *see* Agenesis, forearm
        - hand — *see* Agenesis, hand
      - lobster-claw hand Q71.6- ☑
      - longitudinal
        - radius Q71.4- ☑
        - ulna Q71.5- ☑
      - specified type NEC Q71.89- ☑
- renal pelvis Q63.8
  - obstructive Q62.39
- respiratory system, congenital Q34.9
- restoration, dental KØ8.5Ø
  - specified NEC KØ8.59
- retinal nerve bundle fibers H35.89
- septal (heart) NOS Q21.9
  - acquired (atrial) (auricular) (ventricular) (old) I51.Ø
  - atrial Q21.1

Defect, defective — *continued*
- septal — *continued*
  - atrial — *continued*
    - concurrent with acute myocardial infarction — *see* Infarct, myocardium
    - following acute myocardial infarction (current complication) I23.1
  - ventricular (*see also* Defect, ventricular septal) Q21.Ø
- sinus venosus Q21.1
- speech R47.9
  - developmental F8Ø.9
  - specified NEC R47.89
- Taussig-Bing (aortic transposition and overriding pulmonary artery) Q2Ø.1
- teeth, wedge KØ3.1
- vascular (local) I99.9
  - congenital Q27.9
- ventricular septal Q21.Ø
  - concurrent with acute myocardial infarction — *see* Infarct, myocardium
  - following acute myocardial infarction (current complication) I23.2
  - in tetralogy of Fallot Q21.3
- vision NEC H54.7
- visual field H53.4Ø
  - bilateral
    - heteronymous H53.47
    - homonymous H53.46- ☑
  - generalized contraction H53.48- ☑
  - localized
    - arcuate H53.43- ☑
    - scotoma (central area) H53.41- ☑
      - blind spot area H53.42- ☑
    - sector H53.43- ☑
    - specified type NEC H53.45- ☑
- voice R49.9
  - specified NEC R49.8
- wedge, tooth, teeth (abrasion) KØ3.1

Deferentitis N49.1
- gonorrheal (acute) (chronic) A54.23

Defibrination (syndrome) D65
- antepartum — *see* Hemorrhage, antepartum, with coagulation defect, disseminated intravascular coagulation
- following ectopic or molar pregnancy OØ8.1
- intrapartum O67.Ø
- newborn P6Ø
- postpartum O72.3

Deficiency, deficient
- 3-beta hydroxysteroid dehydrogenase E25.Ø
- 5-alpha reductase (with male pseudohermaphroditism) E29.1
- 11-hydroxylase E25.Ø
- 21-hydroxylase E25.Ø
- abdominal muscle syndrome Q79.4
- AC globulin (congenital) (hereditary) D68.2
  - acquired D68.4
- accelerator globulin (Ac G) (blood) D68.2
- acid phosphatase E83.39
- activating factor (blood) D68.2
- adenosine deaminase (ADA) D81.3
- aldolase (hereditary) E74.19
- alpha-1-antitrypsin E88.Ø1
- amino-acids E72.9
- anemia — *see* Anemia
- aneurin E51.9
- antibody with
  - hyperimmunoglobulinemia D8Ø.6
  - near-normal immunoglobins D8Ø.6
- antidiuretic hormone E23.2
- anti-hemophilic
  - factor (A) D66
    - B D67
    - C D68.1
  - globulin (AHG) NEC D66
- antithrombin (antithrombin III) D68.59
- ascorbic acid E54
- attention (disorder) (syndrome) F98.8
  - with hyperactivity — *see* Disorder, attention-deficit hyperactivity
- autoprothrombin
  - C D68.2
  - I D68.2
  - II D67
- beta-glucuronidase E76.29
- biotin E53.8
- biotin-dependent carboxylase D81.819

Deficiency, deficient — *continued*
- biotinidase D81.81Ø
- brancher enzyme (amylopectinosis) E74.Ø3
- C1 esterase inhibitor (C1-INH) D84.1
- calciferol E55.9
  - with
    - adult osteomalacia M83.8
    - rickets — *see* Rickets
- calcium (dietary) E58
- calorie, severe E43
  - with marasmus E41
    - and kwashiorkor E42
- cardiac — *see* Insufficiency, myocardial
- carnitine E71.4Ø
  - due to
    - hemodialysis E71.43
    - inborn errors of metabolism E71.42
    - Valproic acid therapy E71.43
  - iatrogenic E71.43
  - muscle palmityltransferase E71.314
  - primary E71.41
  - secondary E71.448
- carotene E5Ø.9
- central nervous system G96.8
- ceruloplasmin (Wilson) E83.Ø1
- choline E53.8
- Christmas factor D67
- chromium E61.4
- clotting (blood) (*see also* Deficiency, coagulation factor) D68.9
- clotting factor NEC (hereditary) (*see also* Deficiency, factor) D68.2
- coagulation NOS D68.9
  - with
    - ectopic pregnancy OØ8.1
    - molar pregnancy OØ8.1
  - acquired (any) D68.4
  - antepartum hemorrhage — *see* Hemorrhage, antepartum, with coagulation defect
  - clotting factor NEC (*see also* Deficiency, factor) D68.2
  - due to
    - hyperprothrombinemia D68.4
    - liver disease D68.4
    - vitamin K deficiency D68.4
  - newborn, transient P61.6
  - postpartum O72.3
  - specified NEC D68.8
- cognitive FØ9
- color vision H53.5Ø
  - achromatopsia H53.51
  - acquired H53.52
  - deuteranomaly H53.53
  - protanomaly H53.54
  - specified type NEC H53.59
  - tritanomaly H53.55
- combined glucocorticoid and mineralocorticoid E27.49
- contact factor D68.2
- copper (nutritional) E61.Ø
- corticoadrenal E27.4Ø
  - primary E27.1
- craniofacial axis Q75.Ø
- cyanocobalamin E53.8
- debrancher enzyme (limit dextrinosis) E74.Ø3
- dehydrogenase
  - long chain/very long chain acyl CoA E71.31Ø
  - medium chain acyl CoA E71.311
  - short chain acyl CoA E71.312
- diet E63.9
- dihydropyrimidine dehydrogenase (DPD) E88.89
- disaccharidase E73.9
- edema — *see* Malnutrition, severe
- endocrine E34.9
- energy-supply — *see* Malnutrition
- enzymes, circulating NEC E88.Ø9
- ergosterol E55.9
  - with
    - adult osteomalacia M83.8
    - rickets — *see* Rickets
- essential fatty acid (EFA) E63.Ø
- factor (*see also* Deficiency, coagulation)
  - Hageman D68.2
  - I (congenital) (hereditary) D68.2
  - II (congenital) (hereditary) D68.2
  - IX (congenital) (functional) (hereditary) (with functional defect) D67
  - multiple (congenital) D68.8
    - acquired D68.4

Deficiency, deficient — *continued*
- factor (*see also* Deficiency, coagulation) — *continued*
  - V (congenital) (hereditary) D68.2
  - VII (congenital) (hereditary) D68.2
  - VIII (congenital) (functional) (hereditary) (with functional defect) D66
    - with vascular defect D68.Ø
  - X (congenital) (hereditary) D68.2
  - XI (congenital) (hereditary) D68.1
  - XII (congenital) (hereditary) D68.2
  - XIII (congenital) (hereditary) D68.2
- femoral, proximal focal (congenital) — *see* Defect, reduction, lower limb, longitudinal, femur
- fibrinase D68.2
- fibrinogen (congenital) (hereditary) D68.2
  - acquired D65
- fibrin-stabilizing factor (congenital) (hereditary) D68.2
  - acquired D68.4
- folate E53.8
- folic acid E53.8
- foreskin N47.3
- fructokinase E74.11
- fructose 1,6-diphosphatase E74.19
- fructose-1-phosphate aldolase E74.19
- galactokinase E74.29
- galactose-1-phosphate uridyl transferase E74.29
- gammaglobulin in blood D8Ø.1
  - hereditary D8Ø.Ø
- glass factor D68.2
- glucocorticoid E27.49
  - mineralocorticoid E27.49
- glucose-6-phosphatase E74.Ø1
- glucose-6-phosphate dehydrogenase anemia D55.Ø
- glucuronyl transferase E8Ø.5
- glycogen synthetase E74.Ø9
- gonadotropin (isolated) E23.Ø
- growth hormone (idiopathic) (isolated) E23.Ø
- Hageman factor D68.2
- hemoglobin D64.9
- hepatophosphorylase E74.Ø9
- homogentisate 1,2-dioxygenase E7Ø.29
- hormone
  - anterior pituitary (partial) NEC E23.Ø
    - growth E23.Ø
  - growth (isolated) E23.Ø
  - pituitary E23.Ø
  - testicular E29.1
- hypoxanthine- (guanine)-phosphoribosyltransferase (HG- PRT) (total H-PRT) E79.1
- immunity D84.9
  - cell-mediated D84.8
    - with thrombocytopenia and eczema D82.Ø
  - combined D81.9
  - humoral D8Ø.9
  - IgA (secretory) D8Ø.2
  - IgG D8Ø.3
  - IgM D8Ø.4
- immuno — *see* Immunodeficiency
- immunoglobulin, selective
  - A (IgA) D8Ø.2
  - G (IgG) (subclasses) D8Ø.3
  - M (IgM) D8Ø.4
- inositol (B complex) E53.8
- intrinsic
  - factor (congenital) D51.Ø
  - sphincter N36.42
    - with urethral hypermobility N36.43
- iodine E61.8
  - congenital syndrome — *see* Syndrome, iodine-deficiency, congenital
- iron E61.1
  - anemia D5Ø.9
- kalium E87.6
- kappa-light chain D8Ø.8
- labile factor (congenital) (hereditary) D68.2
  - acquired D68.4
- lacrimal fluid (acquired) (*see also* Syndrome, dry eye)
  - congenital Q1Ø.6
- lactase
  - congenital E73.Ø
  - secondary E73.1
- Laki-Lorand factor D68.2
- lecithin cholesterol acyltransferase E78.6
- lipocaic K86.8
- lipoprotein (familial) (high density) E78.6
- liver phosphorylase E74.Ø9
- lysosomal alpha-1, 4 glucosidase E74.Ø2

Deficiency, deficient — *continued*
- magnesium E61.2
- major histocompatibility complex
  - class I D81.6
  - class II D81.7
- manganese E61.3
- menadione (vitamin K) E56.1
  - newborn P53
- mental (familial) (hereditary) — *see* Disability, intellectual
- methylenetetrahydrofolate reductase (MTHFR) E72.12
- mineralocorticoid E27.49
  - with glucocorticoid E27.49
- mineral NEC E61.8
- molybdenum (nutritional) E61.5
- moral F6Ø.2
- multiple nutrient elements E61.7
- muscle
  - carnitine (palmityltransferase) E71.314
  - phosphofructokinase E74.Ø9
- myoadenylate deaminase E79.2
- myocardial — *see* Insufficiency, myocardial
- myophosphorylase E74.Ø4
- NADH diaphorase or reductase (congenital) D74.Ø
- NADH-methemoglobin reductase (congenital) D74.Ø
- natrium E87.1
- niacin (amide) (-tryptophan) E52
- nicotinamide E52
- nicotinic acid E52
- number of teeth — *see* Anodontia
- nutrient element E61.9
  - multiple E61.7
  - specified NEC E61.8
- nutrition, nutritional E63.9
  - sequelae — *see* Sequelae, nutritional deficiency
  - specified NEC E63.8
- ornithine transcarbamylase E72.4
- ovarian E28.39
- oxygen — *see* Anoxia
- pantothenic acid E53.8
- parathyroid (gland) E2Ø.9
- perineum (female) N81.89
- phenylalanine hydroxylase E7Ø.1
- phosphoenolpyruvate carboxykinase E74.4
- phosphofructokinase E74.19
- phosphomannomutuse E74.8
- phosphomannose isomerase E74.8
- phosphomannosyl mutase E74.8
- phosphorylase kinase, liver E74.Ø9
- pituitary hormone (isolated) E23.Ø
- plasma thromboplastin
  - antecedent (PTA) D68.1
  - component (PTC) D67
- platelet NEC D69.1
  - constitutional D68.Ø
- polyglandular E31.8
  - autoimmune E31.Ø
- potassium (K) E87.6
- prepuce N47.3
- proaccelerin (congenital) (hereditary) D68.2
  - acquired D68.4
- proconvertin factor (congenital) (hereditary) D68.2
  - acquired D68.4
- protein (*see also* Malnutrition) E46
  - anemia D53.Ø
  - C D68.59
  - S D68.59
- prothrombin (congenital) (hereditary) D68.2
  - acquired D68.4
- Prower factor D68.2
- pseudocholinesterase E88.Ø9
- PTA (plasma thromboplastin antecedent) D68.1
- PTC (plasma thromboplastin component) D67
- purine nucleoside phosphorylase (PNP) D81.5
- pyracin (alpha) (beta) E53.1
- pyridoxal E53.1
- pyridoxamine E53.1
- pyridoxine (derivatives) E53.1
- pyruvate
  - carboxylase E74.4
  - dehydrogenase E74.4
- riboflavin (vitamin B2) E53.Ø
- salt E87.1
- secretion
  - ovary E28.39
  - salivary gland (any) K11.7
  - urine R34
- selenium (dietary) E59

Deformity — *continued*
- epiglottis — *continued*
  - acquired J38.7
- esophagus (congenital) Q39.9
  - acquired K22.8
- eustachian tube (congenital) NEC Q17.8
- eye, congenital Q15.9
- eyebrow (congenital) Q18.8
- eyelid (acquired) (i>see also</i> Disorder, eyelid, specified type NEC)
  - congenital Q1Ø.3
- face (acquired) M95.2
  - congenital Q18.9
- fallopian tube, acquired N83.8
- femur (acquired) — *see* Deformity, limb, specified type NEC, thigh
- fetal
  - with fetopelvic disproportion O33.7
  - causing obstructed labor O66.3
- finger (acquired) M2Ø.ØØ- ☑
  - boutonniere M2Ø.Ø2- ☑
  - congenital Q68.1
  - flexion contracture — *see* Contraction, joint, hand
  - mallet finger M2Ø.Ø1- ☑
  - specified NEC M2Ø.Ø9- ☑
  - swan-neck M2Ø.Ø3- ☑
- flexion (joint) (acquired) (*see also* Deformity, limb, flexion) M21.2Ø
  - congenital NOS Q74.9
    - hip Q65.89
- foot (acquired) (*see also* Deformity, limb, lower leg)
  - cavovarus (congenital) Q66.1
  - congenital NOS Q66.9
    - specified type NEC Q66.89
  - specified type NEC — *see* Deformity, limb, foot, specified NEC
  - valgus (congenital) Q66.6
    - acquired — *see* Deformity, valgus, ankle
  - varus (congenital) NEC Q66.3
    - acquired — *see* Deformity, varus, ankle
- forearm (acquired) (*see also* Deformity, limb, forearm)
  - congenital Q68.8
- forehead (acquired) M95.2
  - congenital Q75.8
- frontal bone (acquired) M95.2
  - congenital Q75.8
- gallbladder (congenital) Q44.1
  - acquired K82.8
- gastrointestinal tract (congenital) NOS Q45.9
  - acquired K63.89
- genitalia, genital organ(s) or system NEC
  - female (congenital) Q52.9
    - acquired N94.89
    - external Q52.7Ø
  - male (congenital) Q55.9
    - acquired N5Ø.8
- globe (eye) (congenital) Q15.8
  - acquired H44.89
- gum, acquired NEC KØ6.8
- hand (acquired) — *see* Deformity, limb, hand
  - congenital Q68.1
- head (acquired) M95.2
  - congenital Q75.8
- heart (congenital) Q24.9
  - septum Q21.9
    - auricular Q21.1
    - ventricular Q21.Ø
  - valve (congenital) NEC Q24.8
    - acquired — *see* Endocarditis
- heel (acquired) — *see* Deformity, foot
- hepatic duct (congenital) Q44.5
  - acquired K83.8
- hip (joint) (acquired) (*see also* Deformity, limb, thigh)
  - congenital Q65.9
  - due to (previous) juvenile osteochondrosis — *see* Coxa, plana
  - flexion — *see* Contraction, joint, hip
- hourglass — *see* Contraction, hourglass
- humerus (acquired) M21.82- ☑
  - congenital Q74.Ø
- hypophyseal (congenital) Q89.2
- ileocecal (coil) (valve) (acquired) K63.89
  - congenital Q43.9
- ileum (congenital) Q43.9
  - acquired K63.89
- ilium (acquired) M95.5
  - congenital Q74.2
- integument (congenital) Q84.9
- intervertebral cartilage or disc (acquired) — *see* Disorder, disc, specified NEC
- intestine (large) (small) (congenital) NOS Q43.9
  - acquired K63.89
- intrinsic minus or plus (hand) — *see* Deformity, limb, specified type NEC, forearm
- iris (acquired) H21.89
  - congenital Q13.2
- ischium (acquired) M95.5
  - congenital Q74.2
- jaw (acquired) (congenital) M26.9
- joint (acquired) NEC M21.9Ø
  - congenital Q68.8
  - elbow M21.92- ☑
  - hand M21.94- ☑
  - hip M21.95- ☑
  - knee M21.96- ☑
  - shoulder M21.92- ☑
  - wrist M21.93- ☑
- kidney(s) (calyx) (pelvis) (congenital) Q63.9
  - acquired N28.89
  - artery (congenital) Q27.2
    - acquired I77.89
- Klippel-Feil (brevicollis) Q76.1
- knee (acquired) NEC (*see also* Deformity, limb, lower leg)
  - congenital Q68.2
- labium (majus) (minus) (congenital) Q52.79
  - acquired N9Ø.89
- lacrimal passages or duct (congenital) NEC Q1Ø.6
  - acquired — *see* Disorder, lacrimal system, changes
- larynx (muscle) (congenital) Q31.8
  - acquired J38.7
  - web (glottic) Q31.Ø
- leg (upper) (acquired) NEC (*see also* Deformity, limb, thigh)
  - congenital Q68.8
  - lower leg — *see* Deformity, limb, lower leg
- lens (acquired) H27.8
  - congenital Q12.9
- lid (fold) (acquired) (*see also* Disorder, eyelid, specified type NEC)
  - congenital Q1Ø.3
- ligament (acquired) — *see* Disorder, ligament
  - congenital Q79.9
- limb (acquired) M21.9Ø
  - clawfoot M21.53- ☑
  - clawhand M21.51- ☑
  - clubfoot M21.54- ☑
  - clubhand M21.52- ☑
  - congenital, except reduction deformity Q74.9
  - flat foot M21.4- ☑
  - flexion M21.2Ø
    - ankle M21.27- ☑
    - elbow M21.22- ☑
    - finger M21.24- ☑
    - hip M21.25- ☑
    - knee M21.26- ☑
    - shoulder M21.21- ☑
    - toe M21.27- ☑
    - wrist M21.23- ☑
  - foot
    - claw — *see* Deformity, limb, clawfoot
    - club — *see* Deformity, limb, clubfoot
    - drop M21.37- ☑
    - flat — *see* Deformity, limb, flat foot
    - specified NEC M21.6X- ☑
  - forearm M21.93- ☑
  - hand M21.94- ☑
  - lower leg M21.96- ☑
  - specified type NEC M21.8Ø
    - forearm M21.83- ☑
    - lower leg M21.86- ☑
    - thigh M21.85- ☑
    - upper arm M21.82- ☑
  - thigh M21.95- ☑
  - unequal length M21.7Ø
    - short site is
      - femur M21.75- ☑
      - fibula M21.76- ☑
      - humerus M21.72- ☑
      - radius M21.73- ☑
      - tibia M21.76- ☑
      - ulna M21.73- ☑
  - upper arm M21.92- ☑
  - valgus — *see* Deformity, valgus

Deformity — *continued*
- limb — *continued*
  - varus — *see* Deformity, varus
  - wrist drop M21.33- ☑
- lip (acquired) NEC K13.Ø
  - congenital Q38.Ø
- liver (congenital) Q44.7
  - acquired K76.89
- lumbosacral (congenital) (joint) (region) Q76.49
  - acquired — *see* subcategory M43.8 ☑
  - kyphosis — *see* Kyphosis, congenital
  - lordosis — *see* Lordosis, congenital
- lung (congenital) Q33.9
  - acquired J98.4
- lymphatic system, congenital Q89.9
- Madelung's (radius) Q74.Ø
- mandible (acquired) (congenital) M26.9
- maxilla (acquired) (congenital) M26.9
- meninges or membrane (congenital) QØ7.9
  - cerebral QØ4.8
    - acquired G96.19
  - spinal cord (congenital) G96.19
    - acquired G96.19
- metacarpus (acquired) — *see* Deformity, limb, forearm
  - congenital Q74.Ø
- metatarsus (acquired) — *see* Deformity, foot
  - congenital Q66.9
- middle ear (congenital) Q16.4
  - ossicles Q16.3
- mitral (leaflets) (valve) IØ5.8
  - parachute Q23.2
  - stenosis, congenital Q23.2
- mouth (acquired) K13.79
  - congenital Q38.6
- multiple, congenital NEC Q89.7
- muscle (acquired) M62.89
  - congenital Q79.9
    - sternocleidomastoid Q68.Ø
- musculoskeletal system (acquired) M95.9
  - congenital Q79.9
  - specified NEC M95.8
- nail (acquired) L6Ø.8
  - congenital Q84.6
- nasal — *see* Deformity, nose
- neck (acquired) M95.3
  - congenital Q18.9
    - sternocleidomastoid Q68.Ø
- nervous system (congenital) QØ7.9
- nipple (congenital) Q83.9
  - acquired N64.89
- nose (acquired) (cartilage) M95.Ø
  - bone (turbinate) M95.Ø
  - congenital Q3Ø.9
    - bent or squashed Q67.4
  - saddle M95.Ø
    - syphilitic A5Ø.57
  - septum (acquired) J34.2
    - congenital Q3Ø.8
  - sinus (wall) (congenital) Q3Ø.8
    - acquired M95.Ø
  - syphilitic (congenital) A5Ø.57
    - late A52.73
- ocular muscle (congenital) Q1Ø.3
  - acquired — *see* Strabismus, mechanical
- opticociliary vessels (congenital) Q13.2
- orbit (eye) (acquired) HØ5.3Ø
  - atrophy — *see* Atrophy, orbit
  - congenital Q1Ø.7
  - due to
    - bone disease NEC HØ5.32- ☑
    - trauma or surgery HØ5.33- ☑
  - enlargement — *see* Enlargement, orbit
  - exostosis — *see* Exostosis, orbit
- organ of Corti (congenital) Q16.5
- ovary (congenital) Q5Ø.39
  - acquired N83.8
- oviduct, acquired N83.8
- palate (congenital) Q38.5
  - acquired M27.8
  - cleft (congenital) — *see* Cleft, palate
- pancreas (congenital) Q45.3
  - acquired K86.8
- parathyroid (gland) Q89.2
- parotid (gland) (congenital) Q38.4
  - acquired K11.8
- patella (acquired) — *see* Disorder, patella, specified NEC
- pelvis, pelvic (acquired) (bony) M95.5

Deformity — *continued*
- pelvis, pelvic — *continued*
  - with disproportion (fetopelvic) O33.Ø
    - causing obstructed labor O65.Ø
  - congenital Q74.2
  - rachitic sequelae (late effect) E64.3
- penis (glans) (congenital) Q55.69
  - acquired N48.89
- pericardium (congenital) Q24.8
  - acquired — *see* Pericarditis
- pharynx (congenital) Q38.8
  - acquired J39.2
- pinna, acquired (*see also* Disorder, pinna, deformity)
  - congenital Q17.9
- pituitary (congenital) Q89.2
- posture — *see* Dorsopathy, deforming
- prepuce (congenital) Q55.69
  - acquired N47.8
- prostate (congenital) Q55.4
  - acquired N42.89
- pupil (congenital) Q13.2
  - acquired — *see* Abnormality, pupillary
- pylorus (congenital) Q4Ø.3
  - acquired K31.89
- rachitic (acquired), old or healed E64.3
- radius (acquired) (*see also* Deformity, limb, forearm)
  - congenital Q68.8
- rectum (congenital) Q43.9
  - acquired K62.89
- reduction (extremity) (limb), congenital (*see also* condition and site) Q73.8
  - brain QØ4.3
  - lower — *see* Defect, reduction, lower limb
  - upper — *see* Defect, reduction, upper limb
- renal — *see* Deformity, kidney
- respiratory system (congenital) Q34.9
- rib (acquired) M95.4
  - congenital Q76.6
    - cervical Q76.5
- rotation (joint) (acquired) — *see* Deformity, limb, specified site NEC
  - congenital Q74.9
  - hip — *see* Deformity, limb, specified type NEC, thigh
    - congenital Q65.89
- sacroiliac joint (congenital) — *see* subcategory Q74.2
  - acquired — *see* subcategory M43.8 ☑
- sacrum (acquired) — *see* subcategory M43.8 ☑
- saddle
  - back — *see* Lordosis
  - nose M95.Ø
    - syphilitic A5Ø.57
- salivary gland or duct (congenital) Q38.4
  - acquired K11.8
- scapula (acquired) M95.8
  - congenital Q68.8
- scrotum (congenital) (*see also* Malformation, testis and scrotum)
  - acquired N5Ø.8
- seminal vesicles (congenital) Q55.4
  - acquired N5Ø.8
- septum, nasal (acquired) J34.2
- shoulder (joint) (acquired) — *see* Deformity, limb, upper arm
  - congenital Q74.Ø
  - contraction — *see* Contraction, joint, shoulder
- sigmoid (flexure) (congenital) Q43.9
  - acquired K63.89
- skin (congenital) Q82.9
- skull (acquired) M95.2
  - congenital Q75.8
    - with
      - anencephaly QØØ.Ø
      - encephalocele — *see* Encephalocele
      - hydrocephalus QØ3.9
        - with spina bifida — *see* Spina bifida, by site, with hydrocephalus
      - microcephaly QØ2
- soft parts, organs or tissues (of pelvis)
  - in pregnancy or childbirth NEC O34.8- ☑
    - causing obstructed labor O65.5
- spermatic cord (congenital) Q55.4
  - acquired N5Ø.8
    - torsion — *see* Torsion, spermatic cord
- spinal — *see* Dorsopathy, deforming
  - column (acquired) — *see* Dorsopathy, deforming
  - congenital Q67.5
  - cord (congenital) QØ6.9

Deformity — *continued*
- spinal — *see* Dorsopathy, deforming — *continued*
  - cord — *continued*
    - acquired G95.89
  - nerve root (congenital) QØ7.9
- spine (acquired) (i>see also</i> Dorsopathy, deforming)
  - congenital Q67.5
  - rachitic E64.3
  - specified NEC — *see* Dorsopathy, deforming, specified NEC
- spleen
  - acquired D73.89
  - congenital Q89.Ø9
- Sprengel's (congenital) Q74.Ø
- sternocleidomastoid (muscle), congenital Q68.Ø
- sternum (acquired) M95.4
  - congenital NEC Q76.7
- stomach (congenital) Q4Ø.3
  - acquired K31.89
- submandibular gland (congenital) Q38.4
- submaxillary gland (congenital) Q38.4
  - acquired K11.8
- talipes — *see* Talipes
- testis (congenital) (*see also* Malformation, testis and scrotum)
  - acquired N44.8
    - torsion — *see* Torsion, testis
- thigh (acquired) (i>see also</i> Deformity, limb, thigh)
  - congenital NEC Q68.8
- thorax (acquired) (wall) M95.4
  - congenital Q67.8
  - sequelae of rickets E64.3
- thumb (acquired) (*see also* Deformity, finger)
  - congenital NEC Q68.1
- thymus (tissue) (congenital) Q89.2
- thyroid (gland) (congenital) Q89.2
  - cartilage Q31.8
    - acquired J38.7
- tibia (acquired) (*see also* Deformity, limb, specified type NEC, lower leg)
  - congenital NEC Q68.8
  - saber (syphilitic) A5Ø.56
- toe (acquired) M2Ø.6- ☑
  - congenital Q66.9
  - hallux rigidus M2Ø.2- ☑
  - hallux valgus M2Ø.1- ☑
  - hallux varus M2Ø.3- ☑
  - hammer toe M2Ø.4- ☑
  - specified NEC M2Ø.5X- ☑
- tongue (congenital) Q38.3
  - acquired K14.8
- tooth, teeth KØØ.2
- trachea (rings) (congenital) Q32.1
  - acquired J39.8
- transverse aortic arch (congenital) Q25.4
- tricuspid (leaflets) (valve) IØ7.8
  - atresia or stenosis Q22.4
  - Ebstein's Q22.5
- trunk (acquired) M95.8
  - congenital Q89.9
- ulna (acquired) (*see also* Deformity, limb, forearm)
  - congenital NEC Q68.8
- urachus, congenital Q64.4
- ureter (opening) (congenital) Q62.8
  - acquired N28.89
- urethra (congenital) Q64.79
  - acquired N36.8
- urinary tract (congenital) Q64.9
  - urachus Q64.4
- uterus (congenital) Q51.9
  - acquired N85.8
- uvula (congenital) Q38.5
- vagina (acquired) N89.8
  - congenital Q52.4
- valgus NEC M21.ØØ
  - ankle M21.Ø7- ☑
  - elbow M21.Ø2- ☑
  - hip M21.Ø5- ☑
  - knee M21.Ø6- ☑
- valve, valvular (congenital) (heart) Q24.8
  - acquired — *see* Endocarditis
- varus NEC M21.1Ø
  - ankle M21.17- ☑
  - elbow M21.12- ☑
  - hip M21.15 ☑
  - knee M21.16- ☑
  - tibia — *see* Osteochondrosis, juvenile, tibia

Deformity — *continued*
- vas deferens (congenital) Q55.4
  - acquired N5Ø.8
- vein (congenital) Q27.9
  - great Q26.9
- vertebra — *see* Dorsopathy, deforming
- vertical talus (congenital) Q66.8Ø
  - left foot Q66.82
  - right foot Q66.81
- vesicourethral orifice (acquired) N32.89
  - congenital NEC Q64.79
- vessels of optic papilla (congenital) Q14.2
- visual field (contraction) — *see* Defect, visual field
- vitreous body, acquired H43.89
- vulva (congenital) Q52.79
  - acquired N9Ø.89
- wrist (joint) (acquired) (*see also* Deformity, limb, forearm)
  - congenital Q68.8
  - contraction — *see* Contraction, joint, wrist

Degeneration, degenerative
- adrenal (capsule) (fatty) (gland) (hyaline) (infectional) E27.8
- amyloid (*see also* Amyloidosis) E85.9
- anterior cornua, spinal cord G12.29
- anterior labral S43.49- ☑
- aorta, aortic I7Ø.Ø
  - fatty I77.89
- aortic valve (heart) — *see* Endocarditis, aortic
- arteriovascular — *see* Arteriosclerosis
- artery, arterial (atheromatous) (calcareous) (*see also* Arteriosclerosis)
  - cerebral, amyloid E85.4 [I68.Ø]
  - medial — *see* Arteriosclerosis, extremities
- articular cartilage NEC — *see* Derangement, joint, articular cartilage, by site
- atheromatous — *see* Arteriosclerosis
- basal nuclei or ganglia G23.9
  - specified NEC G23.8
- bone NEC — *see* Disorder, bone, specified type NEC
- brachial plexus G54.Ø
- brain (cortical) (progressive) G31.9
  - alcoholic G31.2
  - arteriosclerotic I67.2
  - childhood G31.9
    - specified NEC G31.89
  - cystic G31.89
    - congenital QØ4.6
  - in
    - alcoholism G31.2
    - beriberi E51.2
    - cerebrovascular disease I67.9
    - congenital hydrocephalus QØ3.9
      - with spina bifida (*see also* Spina bifida)
    - Fabry-Anderson disease E75.21
    - Gaucher's disease E75.22
    - Hunter's syndrome E76.1
    - lipidosis
      - cerebral E75.4
      - generalized E75.6
    - mucopolysaccharidosis — *see* Mucopolysaccharidosis
    - myxedema EØ3.9 [G32.89]
    - neoplastic disease (*see also* Neoplasm) D49.6 [G32.89]
    - Niemann-Pick disease E75.249 [G32.89]
    - sphingolipidosis E75.3 [G32.89]
    - vitamin B12 deficiency E53.8 [G32.89]
  - senile NEC G31.1
- breast N64.89
- Bruch's membrane — *see* Degeneration, choroid
- capillaries (fatty) I78.8
  - amyloid E85.8 [I79.8]
- cardiac (*see also* Degeneration, myocardial)
  - valve, valvular — *see* Endocarditis
- cardiorenal — *see* Hypertension, cardiorenal
- cardiovascular (*see also* Disease, cardiovascular)
  - renal — *see* Hypertension, cardiorenal
- cerebellar NOS G31.9
  - alcoholic G31.2
  - primary (hereditary) (sporadic) G11.9
- cerebral — *see* Degeneration, brain
- cerebrovascular I67.9
  - due to hypertension I67.4
- cervical plexus G54.2
- cervix N88.8
  - due to radiation (intended effect) N88.8
    - adverse effect or misadventure N99.89

Degeneration, degenerative — *continued*
- chamber angle H21.21- ☑
- changes, spine or vertebra — *see* Spondylosis
- chorioretinal (*see also* Degeneration, choroid)
  - hereditary H31.2Ø
- choroid (colloid) (drusen) H31.1Ø- ☑
  - atrophy — *see* Atrophy, choroidal
  - hereditary — *see* Dystrophy, choroidal, hereditary
- ciliary body H21.22- ☑
- cochlear — *see* subcategory H83.8 ☑
- combined (spinal cord) (subacute) E53.8 [G32.Ø]
  - with anemia (pernicious) D51.Ø [G32.Ø]
    - due to dietary vitamin B12 deficiency D51.3 [G32.Ø]
  - in (due to)
    - vitamin B12 deficiency E53.8 [G32.Ø]
      - anemia D51.9 [G32.Ø]
- conjunctiva H11.1Ø
  - concretions — *see* Concretion, conjunctiva
  - deposits — *see* Deposit, conjunctiva
  - pigmentations — *see* Pigmentation, conjunctiva
  - pinguecula — *see* Pinguecula
  - xerosis — *see* Xerosis, conjunctiva
- cornea H18.4Ø
  - calcerous H18.43
    - band keratopathy H18.42- ☑
  - familial, hereditary — *see* Dystrophy, cornea
  - hyaline (of old scars) H18.49
  - keratomalacia — *see* Keratomalacia
  - nodular H18.45- ☑
  - peripheral H18.46- ☑
  - senile H18.41- ☑
  - specified type NEC H18.49
- cortical (cerebellar) (parenchymatous) G31.89
  - alcoholic G31.2
  - diffuse, due to arteriopathy I67.2
- corticobasal G31.85
- cutis L98.8
  - amyloid E85.4 [L99]
- dental pulp KØ4.2
- disc disease — *see* Degeneration, intervertebral disc NEC
- dorsolateral (spinal cord) — *see* Degeneration, combined
- extrapyramidal G25.9
- eye, macular (*see also* Degeneration, macula)
  - congenital or hereditary — *see* Dystrophy, retina
- facet joints — *see* Spondylosis
- fatty
  - liver NEC K76.Ø
    - alcoholic K7Ø.Ø
- grey matter (brain) (Alpers') G31.81
- heart (*see also* Degeneration, myocardial)
  - amyloid E85.4 [I43]
  - atheromatous — *see* Disease, heart, ischemic, atherosclerotic
  - ischemic — *see* Disease, heart, ischemic
- hepatolenticular (Wilson's) E83.Ø1
- hepatorenal K76.7
- hyaline (diffuse) (generalized)
  - localized — *see* Degeneration, by site
- infrapatellar fat pad M79.4
- intervertebral disc NOS
  - with
    - myelopathy — *see* Disorder, disc, with, myelopathy
    - radiculitis or radiculopathy — *see* Disorder, disc, with, radiculopathy
  - cervical, cervicothoracic — *see* Disorder, disc, cervical, degeneration
    - with
      - myelopathy — *see* Disorder, disc, cervical, with myelopathy
      - neuritis, radiculitis or radiculopathy — *see* Disorder, disc, cervical, with neuritis
  - lumbar region M51.36
    - with
      - myelopathy M51.Ø6
      - neuritis, radiculitis, radiculopathy or sciatica M51.16
  - lumbosacral region M51.37
    - with
      - neuritis, radiculitis, radiculopathy or sciatica M51.17
  - sacrococcygeal region M53.3
  - thoracic region M51.34

Degeneration, degenerative — *continued*
- intervertebral disc — *continued*
  - thoracic region — *continued*
    - with
      - myelopathy M51.Ø4
      - neuritis, radiculitis, radiculopathy M51.14
  - thoracolumbar region M51.35
    - with
      - myelopathy M51.Ø5
      - neuritis, radiculitis, radiculopathy M51.15
- intestine, amyloid E85.4
- iris (pigmentary) H21.23- ☑
- ischemic — *see* Ischemia
- joint disease — *see* Osteoarthritis
- kidney N28.89
  - amyloid E85.4 [N29]
  - cystic, congenital Q61.9
  - fatty N28.89
  - polycystic Q61.3
    - adult type (autosomal dominant) Q61.2
    - infantile type (autosomal recessive) NEC Q61.19
      - collecting duct dilatation Q61.11
- Kuhnt-Junius (*see also* Degeneration, macula) H35.32
- lens — *see* Cataract
- lenticular (familial) (progressive) (Wilson's) (with cirrhosis of liver) E83.Ø1
- liver (diffuse) NEC K76.89
  - amyloid E85.4 [K77]
  - cystic K76.89
    - congenital Q44.6
  - fatty NEC K76.Ø
    - alcoholic K7Ø.Ø
  - hypertrophic K76.89
  - parenchymatous, acute or subacute K72.ØØ
    - with coma K72.Ø1
  - pigmentary K76.89
  - toxic (acute) K71.9
- lung J98.4
- lymph gland I89.8
  - hyaline I89.8
- macula, macular (acquired) (age-related) (senile) H35.3Ø
  - angioid streaks H35.33
  - atrophic age-related H35.31
  - congenital or hereditary — *see* Dystrophy, retina
  - cystoid H35.35- ☑
  - drusen H35.36- ☑
  - exudative H35.32
  - hole H35.34- ☑
  - nonexudative H35.31
  - puckering H35.37- ☑
  - toxic H35.38- ☑
- membranous labyrinth, congenital (causing impairment of hearing) Q16.5
- meniscus — *see* Derangement, meniscus
- mitral — *see* Insufficiency, mitral
- Mönckeberg's — *see* Arteriosclerosis, extremities
- motor centers, senile G31.1
- multi-system G9Ø.3
- mural — *see* Degeneration, myocardial
- muscle (fatty) (fibrous) (hyaline) (progressive) M62.89
  - heart — *see* Degeneration, myocardial
- myelin, central nervous system G37.9
- myocardial, myocardium (fatty) (hyaline) (senile) I51.5
  - with rheumatic fever (conditions in IØØ) IØ9.Ø
    - active, acute or subacute IØ1.2
      - with chorea IØ2.Ø
    - inactive or quiescent (with chorea) IØ9.Ø
  - hypertensive — *see* Hypertension, heart
  - rheumatic — *see* Degeneration, myocardial, with rheumatic fever
  - syphilitic A52.Ø6
- nasal sinus (mucosa) J32.9
  - frontal J32.1
  - maxillary J32.Ø
- nerve — *see* Disorder, nerve
- nervous system G31.9
  - alcoholic G31.2
  - amyloid E85.4 [G99.8]
  - autonomic G9Ø.9
  - fatty G31.89
  - specified NEC G31.89
- nipple N64.89
- olivopontocerebellar (hereditary) (familial) G23.8
- osseous labyrinth — *see* subcategory H83.8 ☑
- ovary N83.8
  - cystic N83.2Ø
  - microcystic N83.2Ø

Degeneration, degenerative — *continued*
- pallidal pigmentary (progressive) G23.Ø
- pancreas K86.8
  - tuberculous A18.83
- penis N48.89
- pigmentary (diffuse) (general)
  - localized — *see* Degeneration, by site
  - pallidal (progressive) G23.Ø
- pineal gland E34.8
- pituitary (gland) E23.6
- popliteal fat pad M79.4
- posterolateral (spinal cord) — *see* Degeneration, combined
- pulmonary valve (heart) I37.8
- pulp (tooth) KØ4.2
- pupillary margin H21.24- ☑
- renal — *see* Degeneration, kidney
- retina H35.9
  - hereditary (cerebroretinal) (congenital) (juvenile) (macula) (peripheral) (pigmentary) — *see* Dystrophy, retina
  - Kuhnt-Junius (*see also* Degeneration, macula) H35.32
  - macula (cystic) (exudative) (hole) (nonexudative) (pseudohole) (senile) (toxic) — *see* Degeneration, macula
  - peripheral H35.4Ø
    - lattice H35.41- ☑
    - microcystoid H35.42- ☑
    - paving stone H35.43- ☑
    - secondary
      - pigmentary H35.45- ☑
      - vitreoretinal H35.46- ☑
    - senile reticular H35.44- ☑
  - pigmentary (primary) (*see also* Dystrophy, retina)
    - secondary — *see* Degeneration, retina, peripheral, secondary
  - posterior pole — *see* Degeneration, macula
- saccule, congenital (causing impairment of hearing) Q16.5
- senile R54
  - brain G31.1
  - cardiac, heart or myocardium — *see* Degeneration, myocardial
  - motor centers G31.1
  - vascular — *see* Arteriosclerosis
- sinus (cystic) (*see also* Sinusitis)
  - polypoid J33.1
- skin L98.8
  - amyloid E85.4 [L99]
  - colloid L98.8
- spinal (cord) G31.89
  - amyloid E85.4 [G32.89]
  - combined (subacute) — *see* Degeneration, combined
  - dorsolateral — *see* Degeneration, combined
  - familial NEC G31.89
  - fatty G31.89
  - funicular — *see* Degeneration, combined
  - posterolateral — *see* Degeneration, combined
  - subacute combined — *see* Degeneration, combined
  - tuberculous A17.81
- spleen D73.Ø
  - amyloid E85.4 [D77]
- stomach K31.89
- striatonigral G23.2
- suprarenal (capsule) (gland) E27.8
- synovial membrane (pulpy) — *see* Disorder, synovium, specified type NEC
- tapetoretinal — *see* Dystrophy, retina
- thymus (gland) E32.8
  - fatty E32.8
- thyroid (gland) EØ7.89
- tricuspid (heart) (valve) IØ7.9
- tuberculous NEC — *see* Tuberculosis
- turbinate J34.89
- uterus (cystic) N85.8
- vascular (senile) — *see* Arteriosclerosis
  - hypertensive — *see* Hypertension
- vitreoretinal, secondary — *see* Degeneration, retina, peripheral, secondary, vitreoretinal
- vitreous (body) H43.81- ☑
- Wallerian — *see* Disorder, nerve
- Wilson's hepatolenticular E83.Ø1

- **Delivery** — *continued*
  - cesarean — *continued*
    - previous — *continued*
      - surgery — *continued*
        - gynecological NEC O34.8- ☑
        - rectum O34.7- ☑
        - uterus O34.29
        - vagina O34.6- ☑
    - prolapse
      - arm or hand O32.2 ☑
      - uterus O34.52- ☑
    - prolonged labor NOS O63.9
    - rectocele O34.8- ☑
    - retroversion
      - uterus O34.53- ☑
    - rigid
      - cervix O34.4- ☑
      - pelvic floor O34.8- ☑
      - perineum O34.7- ☑
      - vagina O34.6- ☑
      - vulva O34.7- ☑
    - sacculation, pregnant uterus O34.59- ☑
    - scar(s)
      - cervix O34.4- ☑
      - cesarean delivery O34.21
      - uterus O34.29
    - Shirodkar suture in situ O34.3- ☑
    - shoulder presentation O32.2 ☑
    - stenosis or stricture, cervix O34.4- ☑
    - streptococcus B carrier state O99.824
    - transverse presentation or lie O32.2 ☑
    - tumor, pelvic organs or tissues NEC O34.8- ☑
      - cervix O34.4- ☑
    - umbilical cord presentation or prolapse O69.Ø ☑
  - completely normal case O8Ø
  - complicated O75.9
    - by
      - abnormal, abnormality (of)
        - forces of labor O62.9
          - specified type NEC O62.8
        - glucose O99.814
        - uterine contractions NOS O62.9
      - abruptio placentae (*see also* Abruptio placentae) O45.9- ☑
      - abuse
        - physical O9A.32 (*following* O99)
        - psychological O9A.52 (*following* O99)
        - sexual O9A.42 (*following* O99)
      - adherent placenta O72.Ø
        - without hemorrhage O73.Ø
      - alcohol use O99.314
      - anemia (pre-existing) O99.Ø2
      - anesthetic death O74.8
      - annular detachment of cervix O71.3
      - atony, uterus O62.2
      - attempted vacuum extraction and forceps O66.5
      - Bandl's ring O62.4
      - bariatric surgery status O99.844
      - biliary tract disorder O26.62
      - bleeding — *see* Delivery, complicated by, hemorrhage
      - blood disorder NEC O99.12
      - cervical dystocia (hypotonic) O62.2
        - primary O62.Ø
        - secondary O62.1
      - circulatory system disorder O99.42
      - compression of cord (umbilical) NEC O69.2 ☑
      - condition NEC O99.89
      - contraction, contracted ring O62.4
      - cord (umbilical)
        - around neck
          - with compression O69.1 ☑
          - without compression O69.81 ☑
        - bruising O69.5 ☑
        - complication O69.9 ☑
          - specified NEC O69.89 ☑
        - compression NEC O69.2 ☑
        - entanglement O69.2 ☑
          - without compression O69.82 ☑
        - hematoma O69.5 ☑
        - presentation O69.Ø ☑
        - prolapse O69.Ø ☑
        - short O69.3 ☑
        - thrombosis (vessels) O69.5 ☑
        - vascular lesion O69.5 ☑
      - Couvelaire uterus O45.8X- ☑

- **Delivery** — *continued*
  - complicated — *continued*
    - by — *continued*
      - damage to (injury to) NEC
        - perineum O71.82
        - periurethral tissue O71.82
        - vulva O71.82
      - delay following rupture of membranes (spontaneous) — *see* Pregnancy, complicated by, premature rupture of membranes
      - depressed fetal heart tones O76
      - diabetes O24.92
        - gestational O24.429
          - diet controlled O24.42Ø
          - insulin controlled O24.424
        - pre-existing O24.32
          - specified NEC O24.82
          - type 1 O24.Ø2
          - type 2 O24.12
      - diastasis recti (abdominis) O71.89
      - dilatation
        - bladder O66.8
        - cervix incomplete, poor or slow O62.Ø
      - disease NEC O99.89
      - disruptio uteri — *see* Delivery, complicated by, rupture, uterus
      - drug use O99.324
      - dysfunction, uterus NOS O62.9
        - hypertonic O62.4
        - hypotonic O62.2
          - primary O62.Ø
          - secondary O62.1
        - incoordinate O62.4
      - eclampsia O15.1
      - embolism (pulmonary) — *see* Embolism, obstetric
      - endocrine, nutritional or metabolic disease NEC O99.284
      - failed
        - attempted vaginal birth after previous cesarean delivery O66.41
        - induction of labor O61.9
          - instrumental O61.1
          - mechanical O61.1
          - medical O61.Ø
          - specified NEC O61.8
          - surgical O61.1
        - trial of labor O66.4Ø
      - female genital mutilation O65.5
      - fetal
        - abnormal acid-base balance O68
        - acidemia O68
        - acidosis O68
        - alkalosis O68
        - death, early OØ2.1
        - deformity O66.3
        - heart rate or rhythm (abnormal) (non-reassuring) O76
        - hypoxia O77.8
        - stress O77.9
          - due to drug administration O77.1
          - electrocardiographic evidence of O77.8
          - specified NEC O77.8
          - ultrasound evidence of O77.8
      - fever during labor O75.2
      - gastric banding status O99.844
      - gastric bypass status O99.844
      - gastrointestinal disease NEC O99.62
      - gestational diabetes O24.429
        - diet controlled O24.42Ø
        - insulin (and diet) controlled O24.424
      - gonorrhea O98.22
      - hematoma O71.7
        - ischial spine O71.7
        - pelvic O71.7
        - vagina O71.7
        - vulva or perineum O71.7
      - hemorrhage (uterine) O67.9
        - associated with
          - afibrinogenemia O67.Ø
          - coagulation defect O67.Ø
          - hyperfibrinolysis O67.Ø
          - hypofibrinogenemia O67.Ø
        - due to
          - low-lying placenta O44.1- ☑
          - placenta previa O44.1- ☑

- **Delivery** — *continued*
  - complicated — *continued*
    - by — *continued*
      - hemorrhage — *continued*
        - due to — *continued*
          - premature separation of placenta (normally implanted) (*see also* Abruptio placentae) O45.9- ☑
          - retained placenta O72.Ø
          - uterine leiomyoma O67.8
        - placenta NEC O67.8
        - postpartum NEC (atonic) (immediate) O72.1
          - with retained or trapped placenta O72.Ø
          - delayed O72.2
          - secondary O72.2
          - third stage O72.Ø
      - hourglass contraction, uterus O62.4
      - hypertension, hypertensive (pre-existing) — *see* Hypertension, complicated by, childbirth (labor)
      - hypotension O26.5- ☑
      - incomplete dilatation (cervix) O62.Ø
      - incoordinate uterus contractions O62.4
      - inertia, uterus O62.2
        - during latent phase of labor O62.Ø
        - primary O62.Ø
        - secondary O62.1
      - infection (maternal) O98.92
        - carrier state NEC O99.834
        - gonorrhea O98.22
        - human immunodeficiency virus (HIV) O98.72
        - sexually transmitted NEC O98.32
        - specified NEC O98.82
        - syphilis O98.12
        - tuberculosis O98.Ø2
        - viral hepatitis O98.42
        - viral NEC O98.52
      - injury (to mother) (*see also* Delivery, complicated, by, damage to) O71.9
        - nonobstetric O9A.22 (*following* O99)
          - caused by abuse — *see* Delivery, complicated by, abuse
      - intrauterine fetal death, early OØ2.1
      - inversion, uterus O71.2
      - laceration (perineal) O7Ø.9
        - anus (sphincter) O7Ø.4
          - with third degree laceration O7Ø.2
            - with mucosa O7Ø.3
          - without third degree laceration O7Ø.4
        - bladder (urinary) O71.5
        - bowel O71.5
        - cervix (uteri) O71.3
        - fourchette O7Ø.Ø
        - hymen O7Ø.Ø
        - labia O7Ø.Ø
        - pelvic
          - floor O7Ø.1
          - organ NEC O71.5
        - perineum, perineal O7Ø.9
          - first degree O7Ø.Ø
          - fourth degree O7Ø.3
          - muscles O7Ø.1
          - second degree O7Ø.1
          - skin O7Ø.Ø
          - slight O7Ø.Ø
          - third degree O7Ø.2
        - peritoneum (pelvic) O71.5
        - rectovaginal (septum) (without perineal laceration) O71.4
          - with perineum O7Ø.2
            - with anal or rectal mucosa O7Ø.3
        - specified NEC O71.89
        - sphincter ani — *see* Delivery, complicated, by, laceration, anus (sphincter)
        - urethra O71.5
        - uterus O71.81
          - before labor O71.81
        - vagina, vaginal (deep) (high) (without perineal laceration) O71.4
          - with perineum O7Ø.Ø
            - muscles, with perineum O7Ø.1
        - vulva O7Ø.Ø
      - liver disorder O26.62
      - malignancy O9A.12 (*following* O99)
      - malnutrition O25.2

- **Delivery** — *continued*
  - complicated — *continued*
    - by — *continued*
      - malposition, malpresentation
        - without obstruction (*see also* Delivery, complicated by, obstruction) O32.9 ☑
          - breech O32.1 ☑
          - compound O32.6 ☑
          - face (brow) (chin) O32.3 ☑
          - footling O32.8 ☑
          - high head O32.4 ☑
          - oblique O32.2 ☑
          - specified NEC O32.8 ☑
          - transverse O32.2 ☑
          - unstable lie O32.Ø ☑
        - placenta (with hemorrhage) O44.1- ☑
          - without hemorrhage O44.Ø- ☑
        - uterus or cervix O65.5
      - meconium in amniotic fluid O77.Ø
      - mental disorder NEC O99.344
      - metrorrhexis — *see* Delivery, complicated by, rupture, uterus
      - nervous system disorder O99.354
      - obesity (pre-existing) O99.214
      - obesity surgery status O99.844
      - obstetric trauma O71.9
        - specified NEC O71.89
      - obstructed labor
        - due to
          - breech (complete) (frank) presentation O64.1 ☑
            - incomplete O64.8 ☑
          - brow presenation O64.3 ☑
          - buttock presentation O64.1 ☑
          - chin presentation O64.2 ☑
          - compound presentation O64.5 ☑
          - contracted pelvis O65.1
          - deep transverse arrest O64.Ø ☑
          - deformed pelvis O65.Ø
          - dystocia (fetal) O66.9
            - due to
              - conjoined twins O66.3
              - fetal
                - abnormality NEC O66.3
                - ascites O66.3
                - hydrops O66.3
                - meningomyelocele O66.3
                - sacral teratoma O66.3
                - tumor O66.3
              - hydrocephalic fetus O66.3
            - shoulder O66.Ø
          - face presentation O64.2 ☑
          - fetopelvic disproportion O65.4
          - footling presentation O64.8 ☑
          - impacted shoulders O66.Ø
          - incomplete rotation of fetal head O64.Ø ☑
          - large fetus O66.2
          - locked twins O66.1
          - malposition O64.9 ☑
            - specified NEC O64.8 ☑
          - malpresentation O64.9 ☑
            - specified NEC O64.8 ☑
          - multiple fetuses NEC O66.6
          - pelvic
            - abnormality (maternal) O65.9
              - organ O65.5
              - specified NEC O65.8
            - contraction
              - inlet O65.2
              - mid-cavity O65.3
              - outlet O65.3
          - persistent (position)
            - occipitoiliac O64.Ø ☑
            - occipitoposterior O64.Ø ☑
            - occipitosacral O64.Ø ☑
            - occipitotransverse O64.Ø ☑
          - prolapsed arm O64.4 ☑
          - shoulder presentation O64.4 ☑
        - specified NEC O66.8
      - pathological retraction ring, uterus O62.4
      - penetration, pregnant uterus by instrument O71.1
      - perforation — *see* Delivery, complicated by, laceration

- **Delivery** — *continued*
  - complicated — *continued*
    - by — *continued*
      - placenta, placental
        - ablatio (*see also* Abruptio placentae) O45.9- ☑
        - abnormality O43.9- ☑
          - specified NEC O43.89- ☑
        - abruptio (*see also* Abruptio placentae) O45.9- ☑
        - accreta O43.21- ☑
        - adherent (with hemorrhage) O72.Ø
          - without hemorrhage O73.Ø
        - detachment (premature) (*see also* Abruptio placentae) O45.9- ☑
        - disorder O43.9- ☑
          - specified NEC O43.89- ☑
        - hemorrhage NEC O67.8
        - increta O43.22- ☑
        - low (implantation) O44.1- ☑
          - without hemorrhage O44.Ø- ☑
        - malformation O43.1Ø- ☑
        - malposition O44.1- ☑
          - without hemorrhage O44.Ø- ☑
        - percreta O43.23- ☑
        - previa (central) (lateral) (low) (marginal) (partial) (total) O44.1- ☑
          - without hemorrhage O44.Ø- ☑
        - retained (with hemorrhage) O72.Ø
          - without hemorrhage O73.Ø
        - separation (premature) O45.9- ☑
          - specified NEC O45.8X- ☑
        - vicious insertion O44.1- ☑
      - precipitate labor O62.3
      - premature rupture, membranes (*see also* Pregnancy, complicated by, premature rupture of membranes) O42.9Ø
      - prolapse
        - arm or hand O32.2 ☑
        - cord (umbilical) O69.Ø ☑
        - foot or leg O32.8 ☑
        - uterus O34.52- ☑
      - prolonged labor O63.9
        - first stage O63.Ø
        - second stage O63.1
      - protozoal disease (maternal) O98.62
      - respiratory disease NEC O99.52
      - retained membranes or portions of placenta O72.2
        - without hemorrhage O73.1
      - retarded birth O63.9
      - retention of secundines (with hemorrhage) O72.Ø
        - without hemorrhage O73.Ø
        - partial O72.2
          - without hemorrhage O73.1
      - rupture
        - bladder (urinary) O71.5
        - cervix O71.3
        - pelvic organ NEC O71.5
        - urethra O71.5
        - uterus (during or after labor) O71.1
          - before labor O71.Ø- ☑
      - separation, pubic bone (symphysis pubis) O71.6
      - shock O75.1
      - shoulder presentation O64.4 ☑
      - skin disorder NEC O99.72
      - spasm, cervix O62.4
      - stenosis or stricture, cervix O65.5
      - streptococcus B carrier state O99.824
      - subluxation of symphysis (pubis) O26.72
      - syphilis (maternal) O98.12
      - tear — *see* Delivery, complicated by, laceration
      - tetanic uterus O62.4
      - trauma (obstetrical) (*see also* Delivery, complicated, by, damage to) O71.9
        - non-obstetric O9A.22 (*following* O99)
        - periurethral O71.82
        - specified NEC O71.89
      - tuberculosis (maternal) O98.Ø2
      - tumor, pelvic organs or tissues NEC O65.5
      - umbilical cord around neck
        - with compression O69.1 ☑
        - without compression O69.81 ☑
      - uterine inertia O62.2
        - during latent phase of labor O62.Ø
        - primary O62.Ø

- **Delivery** — *continued*
  - complicated — *continued*
    - by — *continued*
      - uterine inertia — *continued*
        - secondary O62.1
      - vasa previa O69.4 ☑
        - velamentous insertion of cord O43.12- ☑
    - specified complication NEC O75.89
  - delayed NOS O63.9
    - following rupture of membranes
      - artificial O75.5
    - second twin, triplet, etc. O63.2
  - forceps, low following failed vacuum extraction O66.5
  - missed (at or near term) O36.4 ☑
  - normal O8Ø
  - obstructed — *see* Delivery, complicated by, obstruction
  - precipitate O62.3
  - preterm (*see also* Pregnancy, complicated by, preterm labor) O6Ø.1Ø ☑
  - spontaneous O8Ø
  - term pregnancy NOS O8Ø
  - uncomplicated O8Ø
  - vaginal, following previous cesarean delivery O34.21
- **Delusions** (paranoid) — *see* Disorder, delusional
- **Dementia** (degenerative (primary)) (old age) (persisting) FØ3.9Ø
  - with
    - aggressive behavior FØ3.91
    - behavioral disturbance FØ3.91
    - combative behavior FØ3.91
    - Lewy bodies G31.83 [FØ2.8Ø]
      - with behavioral disturbance G31.83 [FØ2.81]
    - Parkinsonism G31.83 [FØ2.8Ø]
      - with behavioral disturbance G31.83 [FØ2.81]
    - Parkinson's disease G2Ø [FØ2.8Ø]
      - with behavioral disturbance G2Ø [FØ2.81]
    - violent behavior FØ3.91
  - alcoholic F1Ø.97
    - with dependence F1Ø.27
  - Alzheimer's type — *see* Disease, Alzheimer's
  - arteriosclerotic — *see* Dementia, vascular
  - atypical, Alzheimer's type — *see* Disease, Alzheimer's, specified NEC
  - congenital — *see* Disability, intellectual
  - frontal (lobe) G31.Ø9 [FØ2.8Ø]
    - with behavioral disturbance G31.Ø9 [FØ2.81]
  - frontotemporal G31.Ø9 [FØ2.8Ø]
    - with behavioral disturbance G31.Ø9 [FØ2.81]
    - specified NEC G31.Ø9 [FØ2.8Ø]
      - with behavioral disturbance G31.Ø9 [FØ2.81]
  - in (due to)
    - with behavioral disturbance G31.83 [FØ2.81]
    - alcohol F1Ø.97
      - with dependence F1Ø.27
    - Alzheimer's disease — *see* Disease, Alzheimer's
    - arteriosclerotic brain disease — *see* Dementia, vascular
    - cerebral lipidoses E75.- ☑ [FØ2.8Ø]
      - with behavioral disturbance E75.- ☑ [FØ2.81]
    - Creutzfeldt-Jakob disease (*see also* Creutzfeldt-Jakob disease or syndrome (with dementia)) A81.ØØ
    - epilepsy G4Ø.- ☑ [FØ2.8Ø]
      - with behavioral disturbance G4Ø.- ☑ [FØ2.81]
    - hepatolenticular degeneration E83.Ø1 [FØ2.8Ø]
      - with behavioral disturbance E83.Ø1 [FØ2.81]
    - human immunodeficiency virus (HIV) disease B2Ø [FØ2.8Ø]
      - with behavioral disturbance B2Ø [FØ2.81]
    - Huntington's disease or chorea G1Ø
    - hypercalcemia E83.52 [FØ2.8Ø]
      - with behavioral disturbance E83.52 [FØ2.81]
    - hypothyroidism, acquired EØ3.9 [FØ2.8Ø]
      - with behavioral disturbance EØ3.9 [FØ2.81]
      - due to iodine deficiency EØ1.8 [FØ2.8Ø]
        - with behavioral disturbance EØ1.8 [FØ2.81]
    - inhalants F18.97
      - with dependence F18.27
    - multiple
      - etiologies FØ3 ☑
      - sclerosis G35 [FØ2.8Ø]
        - with behavioral disturbance G35 [FØ2.81]
    - neurosyphilis A52.17 [FØ2.8Ø]
      - with behavioral disturbance A52.17 [FØ2.81]
      - juvenile A5Ø.49 [FØ2.8Ø]
        - with behavioral disturbance A5Ø.49 [FØ2.81]
    - niacin deficiency E52 [FØ2.8Ø]

- **Dementia** — *continued*
  - in — *continued*
    - niacin deficiency — *continued*
      - with behavioral disturbance E52 [F02.81]
    - paralysis agitans G20 [F02.80]
      - with behavioral disturbance G20 [F02.81]
    - Parkinson's disease G20 [F02.80]
    - pellagra E52 [F02.80]
      - with behavioral disturbance E52 [F02.81]
    - Pick's G31.01 [F02.80]
      - with behavioral disturbance G31.01 [F02.81]
    - polyarteritis nodosa M30.0 [F02.80]
      - with behavioral disturbance M30.0 [F02.81]
    - psychoactive drug F19.97
      - with dependence F19.27
      - inhalants F18.97
        - with dependence F18.27
      - sedatives, hypnotics or anxiolytics F13.97
        - with dependence F13.27
    - sedatives, hypnotics or anxiolytics F13.97
      - with dependence F13.27
    - systemic lupus erythematosus M32.- ☑ [F02.80]
      - with behavioral disturbance M32.- ☑ [F02.81]
    - trypanosomiasis
      - African B56.9 [F02.80]
        - with behavioral disturbance B56.9 [F02.81]
    - unknown etiology F03 ☑
    - vitamin B12 deficiency E53.8 [F02.80]
      - with behavioral disturbance E53.8 [F02.81]
    - volatile solvents F18.97
      - with dependence F18.27
  - infantile, infantilis F84.3
  - Lewy body G31.83 [F02.80]
    - with behavioral disturbance G31.83 [F02.81]
  - multi-infarct — *see* Dementia, vascular
  - paralytica, paralytic (syphilitic) A52.17 [F02.80]
    - with behavioral disturbance A52.17 [F02.81]
    - juvenilis A50.45
  - paretic A52.17
  - praecox — *see* Schizophrenia
  - presenile F03 ☑
    - Alzheimer's type — *see* Disease, Alzheimer's, early onset
  - primary degenerative F03 ☑
  - progressive, syphilitic A52.17
  - senile F03 ☑
    - with acute confusional state F05
    - Alzheimer's type — *see* Disease, Alzheimer's, late onset
    - depressed or paranoid type F03 ☑
  - vascular (acute onset) (mixed) (multi-infarct) (subcortical) F01.50
    - with behavioral disturbance F01.51
- **Demineralization, bone** — *see* Osteoporosis
- **Demodex folliculorum** (infestation) B88.0
- **Demophobia** F40.248
- **Demoralization** R45.3
- **Demyelination, demyelinization**
  - central nervous system G37.9
    - specified NEC G37.8
  - corpus callosum (central) G37.1
  - disseminated, acute G36.9
    - specified NEC G36.8
  - global G35
  - in optic neuritis G36.0
- **Dengue** (classical) (fever) A90
  - hemorrhagic A91
  - sandfly A93.1
- **Dennie-Marfan syphilitic syndrome** A50.45
- **Dens evaginatus, in dente or invaginatus** K00.2
- **Dense breasts** R92.2
- **Density**
  - increased, bone (disseminated) (generalized) (spotted) — *see* Disorder, bone, density and structure, specified type NEC
  - lung (nodular) J98.4
- **Dental** (*see also* condition)
  - examination Z01.20
    - with abnormal findings Z01.21
  - restoration
    - aesthetically inadequate or displeasing K08.56
    - defective K08.50
      - specified NEC K08.59
    - failure of marginal integrity K08.51
    - failure of periodontal anatomical integrity K08.54
- **Dentia praecox** K00.6
- **Denticles** (pulp) K04.2
- **Dentigerous cyst** K09.0
- **Dentin**
  - irregular (in pulp) K04.3
  - opalescent K00.5
  - secondary (in pulp) K04.3
  - sensitive K03.89
- **Dentinogenesis imperfecta** K00.5
- **Dentinoma** — *see* Cyst, calcifying odontogenic
- **Dentition** (syndrome) K00.7
  - delayed K00.6
  - difficult K00.7
  - precocious K00.6
  - premature K00.6
  - retarded K00.6
- **Dependence** (on) (syndrome) F19.20
  - with remission F19.21
  - alcohol (ethyl) (methyl) (without remission) F10.20
    - with
      - amnestic disorder, persisting F10.26
      - anxiety disorder F10.280
      - dementia, persisting F10.27
      - intoxication F10.229
        - with delirium F10.221
        - uncomplicated F10.220
      - mood disorder F10.24
      - psychotic disorder F10.259
        - with
          - delusions F10.250
          - hallucinations F10.251
      - remission F10.21
      - sexual dysfunction F10.281
      - sleep disorder F10.282
      - specified disorder NEC F10.288
      - withdrawal F10.239
        - with
          - delirium F10.231
          - perceptual disturbance F10.232
        - uncomplicated F10.230
    - counseling and surveillance Z71.41
  - amobarbital — *see* Dependence, drug, sedative
  - amphetamine(s) (type) — *see* Dependence, drug, stimulant NEC
  - amytal (sodium) — *see* Dependence, drug, sedative
  - analgesic NEC F55.8
  - anesthetic (agent) (gas) (general) (local) NEC — *see* Dependence, drug, psychoactive NEC
  - anxiolytic NEC — *see* Dependence, drug, sedative
  - barbital(s) — *see* Dependence, drug, sedative
  - barbiturate(s) (compounds) (drugs classifiable to T42) — *see* Dependence, drug, sedative
  - benzedrine — *see* Dependence, drug, stimulant NEC
  - bhang — *see* Dependence, drug, cannabis
  - bromide(s) NEC — *see* Dependence, drug, sedative
  - caffeine — *see* Dependence, drug, stimulant NEC
  - cannabis (sativa) (indica) (resin) (derivatives) (type) — *see* Dependence, drug, cannabis
  - chloral (betaine) (hydrate) — *see* Dependence, drug, sedative
  - chlordiazepoxide — *see* Dependence, drug, sedative
  - coca (leaf) (derivatives) — *see* Dependence, drug, cocaine
  - cocaine — *see* Dependence, drug, cocaine
  - codeine — *see* Dependence, drug, opioid
  - combinations of drugs F19.20
  - dagga — *see* Dependence, drug, cannabis
  - demerol — *see* Dependence, drug, opioid
  - dexamphetamine — *see* Dependence, drug, stimulant NEC
  - dexedrine — *see* Dependence, drug, stimulant NEC
  - dextromethorphan — *see* Dependence, drug, opioid
  - dextromoramide — *see* Dependence, drug, opioid
  - dextro-nor-pseudo-ephedrine — *see* Dependence, drug, stimulant NEC
  - dextrorphan — *see* Dependence, drug, opioid
  - diazepam — *see* Dependence, drug, sedative
  - dilaudid — *see* Dependence, drug, opioid
  - D-lysergic acid diethylamide — *see* Dependence, drug, hallucinogen
  - drug NEC F19.20
    - with sleep disorder F19.282
    - cannabis F12.20
      - with
        - anxiety disorder F12.280
        - intoxication F12.229
          - with
            - delirium F12.221
            - perceptual disturbance F12.222
          - uncomplicated F12.220

- **Dependence** — *continued*
  - drug — *continued*
    - cannabis — *continued*
      - with — *continued*
        - other specified disorder F12.288
        - psychosis F12.259
          - delusions F12.250
          - hallucinations F12.251
        - unspecified disorder F12.29
      - in remission F12.21
    - cocaine F14.20
      - with
        - anxiety disorder F14.280
        - intoxication F14.229
          - with
            - delirium F14.221
            - perceptual disturbance F14.222
          - uncomplicated F14.220
        - mood disorder F14.24
        - other specified disorder F14.288
        - psychosis F14.259
          - delusions F14.250
          - hallucinations F14.251
        - sexual dysfunction F14.281
        - sleep disorder F14.282
        - unspecified disorder F14.29
        - withdrawal F14.23
      - in remission F14.21
      - withdrawal symptoms in newborn P96.1
    - counseling and surveillance Z71.51
    - hallucinogen F16.20
      - with
        - anxiety disorder F16.280
        - flashbacks F16.283
        - intoxication F16.229
          - with delirium F16.221
          - uncomplicated F16.220
        - mood disorder F16.24
        - other specified disorder F16.288
        - perception disorder, persisting F16.283
        - psychosis F16.259
          - delusions F16.250
          - hallucinations F16.251
        - unspecified disorder F16.29
      - in remission F16.21
    - in remission F19.21
    - inhalant F18.20
      - with
        - anxiety disorder F18.280
        - dementia, persisting F18.27
        - intoxication F18.229
          - with delirium F18.221
          - uncomplicated F18.220
        - mood disorder F18.24
        - other specified disorder F18.288
        - psychosis F18.259
          - delusions F18.250
          - hallucinations F18.251
        - unspecified disorder F18.29
      - in remission F18.21
    - nicotine F17.200
      - with disorder F17.209
        - remission F17.201
        - specified disorder NEC F17.208
        - withdrawal F17.203
      - chewing tobacco F17.220
        - with disorder F17.229
          - remission F17.221
          - specified disorder NEC F17.228
          - withdrawal F17.223
      - cigarettes F17.210
        - with disorder F17.219
          - remission F17.211
          - specified disorder NEC F17.218
          - withdrawal F17.213
      - specified product NEC F17.290
        - with disorder F17.299
          - remission F17.291
          - specified disorder NEC F17.298
          - withdrawal F17.293
    - opioid F11.20
      - with
        - intoxication F11.229
          - with
            - delirium F11.221
            - perceptual disturbance F11.222
          - uncomplicated F11.220
        - mood disorder F11.24

- **Dependence** — *continued*
  - drug — *continued*
    - opioid — *continued*
      - with — *continued*
        - other specified disorder F11.288
        - psychosis F11.259
          - delusions F11.250
          - hallucinations F11.251
        - sexual dysfunction F11.281
        - sleep disorder F11.282
        - unspecified disorder F11.29
        - withdrawal F11.23
      - in remission F11.21
    - psychoactive NEC F19.20
      - with
        - amnestic disorder F19.26
        - anxiety disorder F19.280
        - dementia F19.27
        - intoxication F19.229
          - with
            - delirium F19.221
            - perceptual disturbance F19.222
          - uncomplicated F19.220
        - mood disorder F19.24
        - other specified disorder F19.288
        - psychosis F19.259
          - delusions F19.250
          - hallucinations F19.251
        - sexual dysfunction F19.281
        - sleep disorder F19.282
        - unspecified disorder F19.29
        - withdrawal F19.239
          - with
            - delirium F19.231
            - perceptual disturbance F19.232
          - uncomplicated F19.230
    - sedative, hypnotic or anxiolytic F13.20
      - with
        - amnestic disorder F13.26
        - anxiety disorder F13.280
        - dementia, persisting F13.27
        - intoxication F13.229
          - with delirium F13.221
          - uncomplicated F13.220
        - mood disorder F13.24
        - other specified disorder F13.288
        - psychosis F13.259
          - delusions F13.250
          - hallucinations F13.251
        - sexual dysfunction F13.281
        - sleep disorder F13.282
        - unspecified disorder F13.29
        - withdrawal F13.239
          - with
            - delirium F13.231
            - perceptual disturbance F13.232
          - uncomplicated F13.230
      - in remission F13.21
    - stimulant NEC F15.20
      - with
        - anxiety disorder F15.280
        - intoxication F15.229
          - with
            - delirium F15.221
            - perceptual disturbance F15.222
          - uncomplicated F15.220
        - mood disorder F15.24
        - other specified disorder F15.288
        - psychosis F15.259
          - delusions F15.250
          - hallucinations F15.251
        - sexual dysfunction F15.281
        - sleep disorder F15.282
        - unspecified disorder F15.29
        - withdrawal F15.23
      - in remission F15.21
  - ethyl
    - alcohol (without remission) F10.20
      - with remission F10.21
    - bromide — *see* Dependence, drug, sedative
    - carbamate F19.20
    - chloride F19.20
    - morphine — *see* Dependence, drug, opioid
  - ganja — *see* Dependence, drug, cannabis
  - glue (airplane) (sniffing) — *see* Dependence, drug, inhalant
  - glutethimide — *see* Dependence, drug, sedative

- **Dependence** — *continued*
  - hallucinogenics — *see* Dependence, drug, hallucinogen
  - hashish — *see* Dependence, drug, cannabis
  - hemp — *see* Dependence, drug, cannabis
  - heroin (salt) (any) — *see* Dependence, drug, opioid
  - hypnotic NEC — *see* Dependence, drug, sedative
  - Indian hemp — *see* Dependence, drug, cannabis
  - inhalants — *see* Dependence, drug, inhalant
  - khat — *see* Dependence, drug, stimulant NEC
  - laudanum — *see* Dependence, drug, opioid
  - LSD (-25) (derivatives) — *see* Dependence, drug, hallucinogen
  - luminal — *see* Dependence, drug, sedative
  - lysergic acid — *see* Dependence, drug, hallucinogen
  - maconha — *see* Dependence, drug, cannabis
  - marihuana — *see* Dependence, drug, cannabis
  - meprobamate — *see* Dependence, drug, sedative
  - mescaline — *see* Dependence, drug, hallucinogen
  - methadone — *see* Dependence, drug, opioid
  - methamphetamine(s) — *see* Dependence, drug, stimulant NEC
  - methaqualone — *see* Dependence, drug, sedative
  - methyl
    - alcohol (without remission) F10.20
      - with remission F10.21
    - bromide — *see* Dependence, drug, sedative
    - morphine — *see* Dependence, drug, opioid
    - phenidate — *see* Dependence, drug, stimulant NEC
    - sulfonal — *see* Dependence, drug, sedative
  - morphine (sulfate) (sulfite) (type) — *see* Dependence, drug, opioid
  - narcotic (drug) NEC — *see* Dependence, drug, opioid
  - nembutal — *see* Dependence, drug, sedative
  - neraval — *see* Dependence, drug, sedative
  - neravan — *see* Dependence, drug, sedative
  - neurobarb — *see* Dependence, drug, sedative
  - nicotine — *see* Dependence, drug, nicotine
  - nitrous oxide F19.20
  - nonbarbiturate sedatives and tranquilizers with similar effect — *see* Dependence, drug, sedative
- on
  - artificial heart (fully implantable) (mechanical) Z95.812
  - aspirator Z99.0
  - care provider (because of) Z74.9
    - impaired mobility Z74.09
    - need for
      - assistance with personal care Z74.1
      - continuous supervision Z74.3
    - no other household member able to render care Z74.2
    - specified reason NEC Z74.8
  - machine Z99.89
    - enabling NEC Z99.89
    - specified type NEC Z99.89
  - renal dialysis (hemodialysis) (peritoneal) Z99.2
  - respirator Z99.11
  - ventilator Z99.11
  - wheelchair Z99.3
- opiate — *see* Dependence, drug, opioid
- opioids — *see* Dependence, drug, opioid
- opium (alkaloids) (derivatives) (tincture) — *see* Dependence, drug, opioid
- oxygen (long-term) (supplemental) Z99.81
- paraldehyde — *see* Dependence, drug, sedative
- paregoric — *see* Dependence, drug, opioid
- PCP (phencyclidine) (*see also* Abuse, drug, hallucinogen) F16.20
- pentobarbital — *see* Dependence, drug, sedative
- pentobarbitone (sodium) — *see* Dependence, drug, sedative
- pentothal — *see* Dependence, drug, sedative
- peyote — *see* Dependence, drug, hallucinogen
- phencyclidine (PCP) (and related substances) (*see also* Abuse, drug, hallucinogen) F16.20
- phenmetrazine — *see* Dependence, drug, stimulant NEC
- phenobarbital — *see* Dependence, drug, sedative
- polysubstance F19.20
- psilocibin, psilocin, psilocyn, psilocyline — *see* Dependence, drug, hallucinogen
- psychostimulant NEC — *see* Dependence, drug, stimulant NEC
- secobarbital — *see* Dependence, drug, sedative
- seconal — *see* Dependence, drug, sedative

- **Dependence** — *continued*
  - sedative NEC — *see* Dependence, drug, sedative
  - specified drug NEC — *see* Dependence, drug
  - stimulant NEC — *see* Dependence, drug, stimulant NEC
  - substance NEC — *see* Dependence, drug
  - supplemental oxygen Z99.81
  - tobacco — *see* Dependence, drug, nicotine
    - counseling and surveillance Z71.6
  - tranquilizer NEC — *see* Dependence, drug, sedative
  - vitamin B6 E53.1
  - volatile solvents — *see* Dependence, drug, inhalant
- **Dependency**
  - care-provider Z74.9
  - passive F60.7
  - reactions (persistent) F60.7
- **Depersonalization** (in neurotic state) (neurotic) (syndrome) F48.1
- **Depletion**
  - extracellular fluid E86.9
  - plasma E86.1
  - potassium E87.6
    - nephropathy N25.89
  - salt or sodium E87.1
    - causing heat exhaustion or prostration T67.4 ☑
    - nephropathy N28.9
  - volume NOS E86.9
- **Deployment** (current) (military) status Z56.82
  - in theater or in support of military war, peacekeeping and humanitarian operations Z56.82
  - personal history of Z91.82
    - military war, peacekeeping and humanitarian deployment (current or past conflict) Z91.82
  - returned from Z91.82
- **Depolarization, premature** I49.40
  - atrial I49.1
  - junctional I49.2
  - specified NEC I49.49
  - ventricular I49.3
- **Deposit**
  - bone in Boeck's sarcoid D86.89
  - calcareous, calcium — *see* Calcification
  - cholesterol
    - retina H35.89
    - vitreous (body) (humor) — *see* Deposit, crystalline
  - conjunctiva H11.11- ☑
  - cornea H18.00- ☑
    - argentous H18.02- ☑
    - due to metabolic disorder H18.03- ☑
    - Kayser-Fleischer ring H18.04- ☑
    - pigmentation — *see* Pigmentation, cornea
  - crystalline, vitreous (body) (humor) H43.2- ☑
  - hemosiderin in old scars of cornea — *see* Pigmentation, cornea, stromal
  - metallic in lens — *see* Cataract, specified NEC
  - skin R23.8
  - tooth, teeth (betel) (black) (green) (materia alba) (orange) (tobacco) K03.6
  - urate, kidney — *see* Calculus, kidney
- **Depraved appetite** — *see* Pica
- **Depressed**
  - HDL cholesterol E78.6
- **Depression** (acute) (mental) F32.9
  - agitated (single episode) F32.2
  - anaclitic — *see* Disorder, adjustment
  - anxiety F41.8
    - persistent F34.1
  - arches (*see also* Deformity, limb, flat foot)
  - atypical (single episode) F32.8
  - basal metabolic rate R94.8
  - bone marrow D75.89
  - central nervous system R09.2
  - cerebral R29.818
    - newborn P91.4
  - cerebrovascular I67.9
  - chest wall M95.4
  - climacteric (single episode) F32.8
  - endogenous (without psychotic symptoms) F33.2
    - with psychotic symptoms F33.3
  - functional activity R68.89
  - hysterical F44.89
  - involutional (single episode) F32.8
  - major F32.9
    - with psychotic symptoms F32.3
    - recurrent — *see* Disorder, depressive, recurrent
  - manic-depressive — *see* Disorder, depressive, recurrent

- **Depression** — *continued*
  - masked (single episode) F32.8
  - medullary G93.89
  - menopausal (single episode) F32.8
  - metatarsus — *see* Depression, arches
  - monopolar F33.9
  - nervous F34.1
  - neurotic F34.1
  - nose M95.Ø
  - postnatal F53
  - postpartum F53
  - post-psychotic of schizophrenia F32.8
  - post-schizophrenic F32.8
  - psychogenic (reactive) (single episode) F32.9
  - psychoneurotic F34.1
  - psychotic (single episode) F32.3
    - recurrent F33.3
  - reactive (psychogenic) (single episode) F32.9
    - psychotic (single episode) F32.3
  - recurrent — *see* Disorder, depressive, recurrent
  - respiratory center G93.89
  - seasonal — *see* Disorder, depressive, recurrent
  - senile FØ3 ☑
  - severe, single episode F32.2
  - situational F43.21
  - skull Q67.4
  - specified NEC (single episode) F32.8
  - sternum M95.4
  - visual field — *see* Defect, visual field
  - vital (recurrent) (without psychotic symptoms) F33.2
    - with psychotic symptoms F33.3
    - single episode F32.2
- **Deprivation**
  - cultural Z6Ø.3
  - effects NOS T73.9 ☑
    - specified NEC T73.8 ☑
  - emotional NEC Z65.8
    - affecting infant or child — *see* Maltreatment, child, psychological
  - food T73.Ø ☑
  - protein — *see* Malnutrition
  - sleep Z72.82Ø
  - social Z6Ø.4
    - affecting infant or child — *see* Maltreatment, child, psychological
  - specified NEC T73.8 ☑
  - vitamins — *see* Deficiency, vitamin
  - water T73.1 ☑
- **Derangement**
  - ankle (internal) — *see* Derangement, joint, ankle
  - cartilage (articular) NEC — *see* Derangement, joint, articular cartilage, by site
    - recurrent — *see* Dislocation, recurrent
  - cruciate ligament, anterior, current injury — *see* Sprain, knee, cruciate, anterior
  - elbow (internal) — *see* Derangement, joint, elbow
  - hip (joint) (internal) (old) — *see* Derangement, joint, hip
  - joint (internal) M24.9
    - ankylosis — *see* Ankylosis
    - articular cartilage M24.1Ø
      - ankle M24.17- ☑
      - elbow M24.12- ☑
      - foot M24.17- ☑
      - hand M24.14- ☑
      - hip M24.15- ☑
      - knee NEC M23.9- ☑
      - loose body — *see* Loose, body
      - shoulder M24.11- ☑
      - wrist M24.13- ☑
    - contracture — *see* Contraction, joint
    - current injury (*see also* Dislocation)
      - knee, meniscus or cartilage — *see* Tear, meniscus
    - dislocation
      - pathological — *see* Dislocation, pathological
      - recurrent — *see* Dislocation, recurrent
    - knee — *see* Derangement, knee
    - ligament — *see* Disorder, ligament
    - loose body — *see* Loose, body
    - recurrent — *see* Dislocation, recurrent
    - specified type NEC M24.8Ø
      - ankle M24.87- ☑
      - elbow M24.82- ☑
      - foot joint M24.87- ☑
      - hand joint M24.84- ☑
      - hip M24.85- ☑
- **Derangement** — *continued*
  - joint — *continued*
    - specified type — *continued*
      - shoulder M24.81- ☑
      - wrist M24.83- ☑
    - temporomandibular M26.69
  - knee (recurrent) M23.9- ☑
    - ligament disruption, spontaneous M23.6Ø- ☑
      - anterior cruciate M23.61- ☑
      - capsular M23.67- ☑
      - instability, chronic M23.5- ☑
      - lateral collateral M23.64- ☑
      - medial collateral M23.63- ☑
      - posterior cruciate M23.62- ☑
    - loose body M23.4- ☑
    - meniscus M23.3Ø- ☑
      - cystic M23.ØØ- ☑
        - lateral M23.ØØ2
          - anterior horn M23.Ø4- ☑
          - posterior horn M23.Ø5- ☑
          - specified NEC M23.Ø6- ☑
        - medial M23.ØØ5
          - anterior horn M23.Ø1- ☑
          - posterior horn M23.Ø2- ☑
          - specified NEC M23.Ø3- ☑
      - degenerate — *see* Derangement, knee, meniscus, specified NEC
      - detached — *see* Derangement, knee, meniscus, specified NEC
      - due to old tear or injury M23.2Ø- ☑
        - lateral M23.2Ø- ☑
          - anterior horn M23.24- ☑
          - posterior horn M23.25- ☑
          - specified NEC M23.26- ☑
        - medial M23.2Ø- ☑
          - anterior horn M23.21- ☑
          - posterior horn M23.22- ☑
          - specified NEC M23.23- ☑
      - retained — *see* Derangement, knee, meniscus, specified NEC
      - specified NEC M23.3Ø- ☑
        - lateral M23.3Ø- ☑
          - anterior horn M23.34- ☑
          - posterior horn M23.35- ☑
          - specified NEC M23.36- ☑
        - medial M23.3Ø- ☑
          - anterior horn M23.31- ☑
          - posterior horn M23.32- ☑
          - specified NEC M23.33- ☑
    - old M23.8X- ☑
      - specified NEC — *see* subcategory M23.8 ☑
  - low back NEC — *see* Dorsopathy, specified NEC
  - meniscus — *see* Derangement, knee, meniscus
  - mental — *see* Psychosis
  - patella, specified NEC — *see* Disorder, patella, derangement NEC
  - semilunar cartilage (knee) — *see* Derangement, knee, meniscus, specified NEC
  - shoulder (internal) — *see* Derangement, joint, shoulder
- **Dercum's disease** E88.2
- **Derealization** (neurotic) F48.1
- **Dermal** — *see* condition
- **Dermaphytid** — *see* Dermatophytosis
- **Dermatitis** (eczematous) L3Ø.9
  - ab igne L59.Ø
  - acarine B88.Ø
  - actinic (due to sun) L57.8
    - other than from sun L59.8
  - allergic — *see* Dermatitis, contact, allergic
  - ambustionis, due to burn or scald — *see* Burn
  - amebic AØ6.7
  - ammonia L22
  - arsenical (ingested) L27.8
  - artefacta L98.1
    - psychogenic F54
  - atopic L2Ø.9
    - psychogenic F54
    - specified NEC L2Ø.89
  - autoimmune progesterone L3Ø.8
  - berlock, berloque L56.2
  - blastomycotic B4Ø.3
  - blister beetle L24.89
  - bullous, bullosa L13.9
    - mucosynechial, atrophic L12.1
    - seasonal L3Ø.8
- **Dermatitis** — *continued*
  - bullous, bullosa — *continued*
    - specified NEC L13.8
  - calorica L59.Ø
    - due to burn or scald — *see* Burn
  - caterpillar L24.89
  - cercarial B65.3
  - combustionis L59.Ø
    - due to burn or scald — *see* Burn
  - congelationis T69.1 ☑
  - contact (occupational) L25.9
    - allergic L23.9
      - due to
        - adhesives L23.1
        - cement L23.5
        - chemical products NEC L23.5
        - chromium L23.Ø
        - cosmetics L23.2
        - dander (cat) (dog) L23.81
        - drugs in contact with skin L23.3
        - dyes L23.4
        - food in contact with skin L23.6
        - hair (cat) (dog) L23.81
        - insecticide L23.5
        - metals L23.Ø
        - nickel L23.Ø
        - plants, non-food L23.7
        - plastic L23.5
        - rubber L23.5
        - specified agent NEC L23.89
    - due to
      - cement L25.3
      - chemical products NEC L25.3
      - cosmetics L25.Ø
      - dander (cat) (dog) L23.81
      - drugs in contact with skin L25.1
      - dyes L25.2
      - food in contact with skin L25.4
      - hair (cat) (dog) L23.81
      - plants, non-food L25.5
      - specified agent NEC L25.8
    - irritant L24.9
      - due to
        - cement L25.3
        - chemical products NEC L24.5
        - cosmetics L24.3
        - detergents L24.Ø
        - drugs in contact with skin L24.4
        - food in contact with skin L24.6
        - oils and greases L24.1
        - plants, non-food L24.7
        - solvents L24.2
        - specified agent NEC L24.89
  - contusiformis L52
  - diabetic — *see* EØ8-E13 with .62Ø
  - diaper L22
  - diphtheritica A36.3
  - dry skin L85.3
  - due to
    - acetone (contact) (irritant) L24.2
    - acids (contact) (irritant) L24.5
    - adhesive(s) (allergic) (contact) (plaster) L23.1
      - irritant L24.5
    - alcohol (irritant) (skin contact) (substances in category T51) L24.2
      - taken internally L27.8
    - alkalis (contact) (irritant) L24.5
    - arsenic (ingested) L27.8
    - carbon disulfide (contact) (irritant) L24.2
    - caustics (contact) (irritant) L24.5
    - cement (contact) L25.3
    - cereal (ingested) L27.2
    - chemical(s) NEC L25.3
      - taken internally L27.8
    - chlorocompounds L24.2
    - chromium (contact) (irritant) L24.81
    - coffee (ingested) L27.2
    - cold weather L3Ø.8
    - cosmetics (contact) L25.Ø
      - allergic L23.2
      - irritant L24.3
    - cyclohexanes L24.2
    - dander (cat) (dog) L23.81
    - Demodex species B88.Ø
    - Dermanyssus gallinae B88.Ø
    - detergents (contact) (irritant) L24.Ø
    - dichromate L24.81

Dermatopolymyositis — *continued*
- in neoplastic disease (*see also* Neoplasm) D49.9 [M36.Ø]
- juvenile M33.ØØ
  - with
    - myopathy M33.Ø2
    - respiratory involvement M33.Ø1
    - specified organ involvement NEC M33.Ø9
- specified NEC M33.1Ø
  - myopathy M33.12
  - respiratory involvement M33.11
  - specified organ involvement NEC M33.19

Dermatopolyneuritis — *see* Poisoning, mercury

Dermatorrhexis Q79.6
- acquired L57.4

Dermatosclerosis (*see also* Scleroderma)
- localized L94.Ø

Dermatosis L98.9
- Andrews' LØ8.89
- Bowen's — *see* Neoplasm, skin, in situ
- bullous L13.9
  - specified NEC L13.8
- exfoliativa L26
- eyelid (noninfectious)
  - dermatitis — *see* Dermatitis, eyelid
  - discoid lupus erythematosus — *see* Lupus, erythematosus, eyelid
  - xeroderma — *see* Xeroderma, acquired, eyelid
- factitial L98.1
- febrile neutrophilic L98.2
- gonococcal A54.89
- herpetiformis L13.Ø
  - juvenile L12.2
- linear IgA L13.8
- menstrual NEC L98.8
- neutrophilic, febrile L98.2
- occupational — *see* Dermatitis, contact
- papulosa nigra L82.1
- pigmentary L81.9
  - progressive L81.7
  - Schamberg's L81.7
- psychogenic F54
- purpuric, pigmented L81.7
- pustular, subcorneal L13.1
- transient acantholytic L11.1

Dermographia, dermographism L5Ø.3

Dermoid (cyst) (*see also* Neoplasm, benign, by site)
- with malignant transformation C56- ☑
- due to radiation (nonionizing) L57.8

Dermopathy
- infiltrative with thyrotoxicosis — *see* Thyrotoxicosis
- nephrogenic fibrosing L9Ø.8

Dermophytosis — *see* Dermatophytosis

Descemetocele H18.73- ☑

Descemet's membrane — *see* condition

Descending — *see* condition

Descensus uteri — *see* Prolapse, uterus

Desert
- rheumatism B38.Ø
- sore — *see* Ulcer, skin

Desertion (newborn) — *see* Maltreatment

Desmoid (extra-abdominal) (tumor) — *see* Neoplasm, connective tissue, uncertain behavior
- abdominal D48.1

Despondency F32.9

Desquamation, skin R23.4

Destruction, destructive (*see also* Damage)
- articular facet (*see also* Derangement, joint, specified type NEC)
  - knee M23.8X- ☑
  - vertebra — *see* Spondylosis
- bone (*see also* Disorder, bone, specified type NEC)
  - syphilitic A52.77
- joint (*see also* Derangement, joint, specified type NEC)
  - sacroiliac M53.3
- rectal sphincter K62.89
- septum (nasal) J34.89
- tuberculous NEC — *see* Tuberculosis
- tympanum, tympanic membrane (nontraumatic) — *see* Disorder, tympanic membrane, specified NEC
- vertebral disc — *see* Degeneration, intervertebral disc

Destructiveness (*see also* Disorder, conduct)
- adjustment reaction — *see* Disorder, adjustment

Desultory labor O62.2

Detachment
- cartilage — *see* Sprain

Detachment — *continued*
- cervix, annular N88.8
  - complicating delivery O71.3
- choroid (old) (postinfectional) (simple) (spontaneous) H31.4Ø- ☑
  - hemorrhagic H31.41- ☑
  - serous H31.42- ☑
- ligament — *see* Sprain
- meniscus (knee) (*see also* Derangement, knee, meniscus, specified NEC)
  - current injury — *see* Tear, meniscus
  - due to old tear or injury — *see* Derangement, knee, meniscus, due to old tear
- retina (without retinal break) (serous) H33.2- ☑
  - with retinal:
    - break H33.ØØ- ☑
      - giant H33.Ø3- ☑
      - multiple H33.Ø2- ☑
      - single H33.Ø1- ☑
    - dialysis H33.Ø4- ☑
  - pigment epithelium — *see* Degeneration, retina, separation of layers, pigment epithelium detachment
  - rhegmatogenous — *see* Detachment, retina, with retinal, break
  - specified NEC H33.8
  - total H33.Ø5- ☑
  - traction H33.4- ☑
- vitreous (body) H43.81 ☑

Detergent asthma J69.8

Deterioration
- epileptic FØ6.8
- general physical R53.81
- heart, cardiac — *see* Degeneration, myocardial
- mental — *see* Psychosis
- myocardial, myocardium — *see* Degeneration, myocardial
- senile (simple) R54

Deuteranomaly (anomalous trichromat) H53.53

Deuteranopia (complete) (incomplete) H53.53

Development
- abnormal, bone Q79.9
- arrested R62.5Ø
  - bone — *see* Arrest, development or growth, bone
  - child R62.5Ø
  - due to malnutrition E45
- defective, congenital (*see also* Anomaly, by site)
  - cauda equina QØ6.3
  - left ventricle Q24.8
    - in hypoplastic left heart syndrome Q23.4
  - valve Q24.8
    - pulmonary Q22.3
- delayed (*see also* Delay, development) R62.5Ø
  - arithmetical skills F81.2
  - language (skills) (expressive) F8Ø.1
  - learning skill F81.9
  - mixed skills F88
  - motor coordination F82
  - reading F81.Ø
  - specified learning skill NEC F81.89
  - speech F8Ø.9
  - spelling F81.81
  - written expression F81.81
- imperfect, congenital (*see also* Anomaly, by site)
  - heart Q24.9
  - lungs Q33.6
- incomplete
  - bronchial tree Q32.4
  - organ or site not listed — *see* Hypoplasia, by site
  - respiratory system Q34.9
- sexual, precocious NEC E3Ø.1
- tardy, mental (*see also* Disability, intellectual) F79

Developmental — *see* condition
- testing, child — *see* Examination, child

Devergie's disease (pityriasis rubra pilaris) L44.Ø

Deviation (in)
- conjugate palsy (eye) (spastic) H51.Ø
- esophagus (acquired) K22.8
- eye, skew H51.8
- midline (jaw) (teeth) (dental arch) M26.29
  - specified site NEC — *see* Malposition
- nasal septum J34.2
  - congenital Q67.4
- opening and closing of the mandible M26.53
- organ or site, congenital NEC — *see* Malposition, congenital
- septum (nasal) (acquired) J34.2

Deviation — *continued*
- septum — *continued*
  - congenital Q67.4
- sexual F65.9
  - bestiality F65.89
  - erotomania F52.8
  - exhibitionism F65.2
  - fetishism, fetishistic F65.Ø
    - transvestism F65.1
  - frotteurism F65.81
  - masochism F65.51
  - multiple F65.89
  - necrophilia F65.89
  - nymphomania F52.8
  - pederosis F65.4
  - pedophilia F65.4
  - sadism, sadomasochism F65.52
  - satyriasis F52.8
  - specified type NEC F65.89
  - transvestism F64.1
  - voyeurism F65.3
- teeth, midline M26.29
- trachea J39.8
- ureter, congenital Q62.61

Device
- cerebral ventricle (communicating) in situ Z98.2
- contraceptive — *see* Contraceptive, device
- drainage, cerebrospinal fluid, in situ Z98.2

Devic's disease G36.Ø

Devil's
- grip B33.Ø
- pinches (purpura simplex) D69.2

Devitalized tooth KØ4.99

Devonshire colic — *see* Poisoning, lead

Dextraposition, aorta Q2Ø.3
- in tetralogy of Fallot Q21.3

Dextrinosis, limit (debrancher enzyme deficiency) E74.Ø3

Dextrocardia (true) Q24.Ø
- with
  - complete transposition of viscera Q89.3
  - situs inversus Q89.3

Dextrotransposition, aorta Q2Ø.3

d-glycericacidemia E72.59

Dhat syndrome F48.8

Dhobi itch B35.6

Di George's syndrome D82.1

Di Guglielmo's disease C94.Ø- ☑

Diabetes, diabetic (mellitus) (sugar) E11.9
- with
  - amyotrophy E11.44
  - arthropathy NEC E11.618
  - autonomic (poly)neuropathy E11.43
  - cataract E11.36
  - Charcot's joints E11.61Ø
  - chronic kidney disease E11.22
  - circulatory complication NEC E11.59
  - complication E11.8
    - specified NEC E11.69
  - dermatitis E11.62Ø
  - foot ulcer E11.621
  - gangrene E11.52
  - gastroparesis E11.43
  - glomerulonephrosis, intracapillary E11.21
  - glomerulosclerosis, intercapillary E11.21
  - hyperglycemia E11.65
  - hyperosmolarity E11.ØØ
    - with coma E11.Ø1
  - hypoglycemia E11.649
    - with coma E11.641
  - kidney complications NEC E11.29
  - Kimmelsteil-Wilson disease E11.21
  - loss of protective sensation (LOPS) — *see* Diabetes, by type, with neuropathy
  - mononeuropathy E11.41
  - myasthenia E11.44
  - necrobiosis lipoidica E11.62Ø
  - nephropathy E11.21
  - neuralgia E11.42
  - neurologic complication NEC E11.49
  - neuropathic arthropathy E11.61Ø
  - neuropathy E11.4Ø
  - ophthalmic complication NEC E11.39
  - oral complication NEC E11.638
  - periodontal disease E11.63Ø
  - peripheral angiopathy E11.51
    - with gangrene E11.52
  - polyneuropathy E11.42

- **Diabetes, diabetic** — *continued*
  - type 1 — *continued*
    - with — *continued*
      - ophthalmic complication NEC E10.39
      - oral complication NEC E10.638
      - periodontal disease E10.630
      - peripheral angiopathy E10.51
        - with gangrene E10.52
      - polyneuropathy E10.42
      - renal complication NEC E10.29
      - renal tubular degeneration E10.29
      - retinopathy E10.319
        - with macular edema E10.311
        - nonproliferative E10.329
          - with macular edema E10.321
          - mild E10.329
            - with macular edema E10.321
          - moderate E10.339
            - with macular edema E10.331
          - severe E10.349
            - with macular edema E10.341
        - proliferative E10.359
          - with macular edema E10.351
      - skin complication NEC E10.628
      - skin ulcer NEC E10.622
  - type 2 E11.9
    - with
      - amyotrophy E11.44
      - arthropathy NEC E11.618
      - autonomic (poly)neuropathy E11.43
      - cataract E11.36
      - Charcot's joints E11.610
      - chronic kidney disease E11.22
      - circulatory complication NEC E11.59
      - complication E11.8
        - specified NEC E11.69
      - dermatitis E11.620
      - foot ulcer E11.621
      - gangrene E11.52
      - gastroparesis E11.43
      - glomerulonephrosis, intracapillary E11.21
      - glomerulosclerosis, intercapillary E11.21
      - hyperglycemia E11.65
      - hyperosmolarity E11.00
        - with coma E11.01
      - hypoglycemia E11.649
        - with coma E11.641
      - kidney complications NEC E11.29
      - Kimmelsteil-Wilson disease E11.21
      - mononeuropathy E11.41
      - myasthenia E11.44
      - necrobiosis lipoidica E11.620
      - nephropathy E11.21
      - neuralgia E11.42
      - neurologic complication NEC E11.49
      - neuropathic arthropathy E11.610
      - neuropathy E11.40
      - ophthalmic complication NEC E11.39
      - oral complication NEC E11.638
      - periodontal disease E11.630
      - peripheral angiopathy E11.51
        - with gangrene E11.52
      - polyneuropathy E11.42
      - renal complication NEC E11.29
      - renal tubular degeneration E11.29
      - retinopathy E11.319
        - with macular edema E11.311
        - nonproliferative E11.329
          - with macular edema E11.321
          - mild E11.329
            - with macular edema E11.321
          - moderate E11.339
            - with macular edema E11.331
          - severe E11.349
            - with macular edema E11.341
        - proliferative E11.359
          - with macular edema E11.351
      - skin complication NEC E11.628
      - skin ulcer NEC E11.622
- **Diacyclothrombopathia** D69.1
- **Diagnosis deferred** R69
- **Dialysis** (intermittent) (treatment)
  - noncompliance (with) Z91.15
  - renal (hemodialysis) (peritoneal), status Z99.2
  - retina, retinal — *see* Detachment, retina, with retinal, dialysis
- **Diamond-Blackfan anemia** (congenital hypoplastic) D61.01
- **Diamond-Gardener syndrome** (autoerythrocyte sensitization) D69.2
- **Diaper rash** L22
- **Diaphoresis** (excessive) R61
- **Diaphragm** — *see* condition
- **Diaphragmalgia** R07.1
- **Diaphragmatitis, diaphragmitis** J98.6
- **Diaphysial aclasis** Q78.6
- **Diaphysitis** — *see* Osteomyelitis, specified type NEC
- **Diarrhea, diarrheal** (disease) (infantile) (inflammatory) R19.7
  - achlorhydric K31.83
  - allergic K52.2
  - amebic (*see also* Amebiasis) A06.0
    - with abscess — *see* Abscess, amebic
    - acute A06.0
    - chronic A06.1
    - nondysenteric A06.2
  - bacillary — *see* Dysentery, bacillary
  - balantidial A07.0
  - cachectic NEC K52.89
  - Chilomastix A07.8
  - choleriformis A00.1
  - chronic (noninfectious) K52.9
  - coccidial A07.3
  - Cochin-China K90.1
    - strongyloidiasis B78.0
  - Dientamoeba A07.8
  - dietetic K52.2
  - drug-induced K52.1
  - due to
    - bacteria A04.9
      - specified NEC A04.8
    - Campylobacter A04.5
    - Capillaria philippinensis B81.1
    - Clostridium difficile A04.7
    - Clostridium perfringens (C) (F) A04.8
    - Cryptosporidium A07.2
    - drugs K52.1
    - Escherichia coli A04.4
      - enteroaggregative A04.4
      - enterohemorrhagic A04.3
      - enteroinvasive A04.2
      - enteropathogenic A04.0
      - enterotoxigenic A04.1
      - specified NEC A04.4
    - food hypersensitivity K52.2
    - Necator americanus B76.1
    - S. japonicum B65.2
    - specified organism NEC A08.8
      - bacterial A04.8
      - viral A08.39
    - Staphylococcus A04.8
    - Trichuris trichiuria B79
    - virus — *see* Enteritis, viral
    - Yersinia enterocolitica A04.6
  - dysenteric A09
  - endemic A09
  - epidemic A09
  - flagellate A07.9
  - Flexner's (ulcerative) A03.1
  - functional K59.1
    - following gastrointestinal surgery K91.89
    - psychogenic F45.8
  - Giardia lamblia A07.1
  - giardial A07.1
  - hill K90.1
  - infectious A09
  - malarial — *see* Malaria
  - mite B88.0
  - mycotic NEC B49
  - neonatal (noninfectious) P78.3
  - nervous F45.8
  - neurogenic K59.1
  - noninfectious K52.9
  - postgastrectomy K91.1
  - postvagotomy K91.1
  - protozoal A07.9
    - specified NEC A07.8
  - psychogenic F45.8
  - specified
    - bacterium NEC A04.8
    - virus NEC A08.39
  - strongyloidiasis B78.0
  - toxic K52.1
  - trichomonal A07.8
  - tropical K90.1
  - tuberculous A18.32
- **Diarrhea, diarrheal** — *continued*
  - viral — *see* Enteritis, viral
- **Diastasis**
  - cranial bones M84.88
    - congenital NEC Q75.8
  - joint (traumatic) — *see* Dislocation
  - muscle M62.00
    - ankle M62.07- ☑
    - congenital Q79.8
    - foot M62.07- ☑
    - forearm M62.03- ☑
    - hand M62.04- ☑
    - lower leg M62.06- ☑
    - pelvic region M62.05- ☑
    - shoulder region M62.01- ☑
    - specified site NEC M62.08
    - thigh M62.05- ☑
    - upper arm M62.02- ☑
  - recti (abdomen)
    - complicating delivery O71.89
    - congenital Q79.59
- **Diastema, tooth, teeth, fully erupted** M26.32
- **Diastematomyelia** Q06.2
- **Diataxia, cerebral** G80.4
- **Diathesis**
  - allergic — *see* History, allergy
  - bleeding (familial) D69.9
  - cystine (familial) E72.00
  - gouty — *see* Gout
  - hemorrhagic (familial) D69.9
    - newborn NEC P53
  - spasmophilic R29.0
- **Diaz's disease or osteochondrosis** (juvenile) (talus) — *see* Osteochondrosis, juvenile, tarsus
- **Dibothriocephalus, dibothriocephaliasis** (latus) (infection) (infestation) B70.0
  - larval B70.1
- **Dicephalus, dicephaly** Q89.4
- **Dichotomy, teeth** K00.2
- **Dichromat, dichromatopsia** (congenital) — *see* Deficiency, color vision
- **Dichuchwa** A65
- **Dicroceliasis** B66.2
- **Didelphia, didelphys** — *see* Double uterus
- **Didymytis** N45.1
  - with orchitis N45.3
- **Dietary**
  - inadequacy or deficiency E63.9
  - surveillance and counseling Z71.3
- **Dietl's crisis** N13.8
- **Dieulafoy lesion** (hemorrhagic)
  - duodenum K31.82
  - esophagus K22.8
  - intestine (colon) K63.81
  - stomach K31.82
- **Difficult, difficulty** (in)
  - acculturation Z60.3
  - feeding R63.3
    - newborn P92.9
      - breast P92.5
      - specified NEC P92.8
    - nonorganic (infant or child) F98.29
  - intubation, in anesthesia T88.4 ☑
  - mechanical, gastroduodenal stoma K91.89
    - causing obstruction K91.3
  - reading (developmental) F81.0
    - secondary to emotional disorders F93.9
  - spelling (specific) F81.81
    - with reading disorder F81.89
    - due to inadequate teaching Z55.8
  - swallowing — *see* Dysphagia
  - walking R26.2
  - work
    - conditions NEC Z56.5
    - schedule Z56.3
- **Diffuse** — *see* condition
- **Digestive** — *see* condition
- **Dihydropyrimidine dehydrogenase disease** (DPD) E88.89
- **Diktyoma** — *see* Neoplasm, malignant, by site
- **Dilaceration, tooth** K00.4
- **Dilatation**
  - anus K59.8
    - venule — *see* Hemorrhoids
  - aorta (focal) (general) — *see* Ectasia, aorta
    - with aneurysm — *see* Aneurysm, aorta
  - artery — *see* Aneurysm

- **Disease, diseased** — *continued*
  - connective tissue, systemic — *continued*
    - in (due to)
      - hypogammaglobulinemia D80.1 [M36.8]
      - ochronosis E70.29 [M36.8]
    - specified NEC M35.8
  - Conor and Bruch's (boutonneuse fever) A77.1
  - Cooper's — *see* Mastopathy, cystic
  - Cori's (glycogenosis III) E74.03
  - corkhandler's or corkworker's J67.3
  - cornea H18.9
    - specified NEC H18.89- ☑
  - coronary (artery) — *see* Disease, heart, ischemic, atherosclerotic
    - congenital Q24.5
    - ostial, syphilitic (aortic) (mitral) (pulmonary) A52.03
  - corpus cavernosum N48.9
    - specified NEC N48.89
  - Cotugno's — *see* Sciatica
  - coxsackie (virus) NEC B34.1
  - cranial nerve NOS G52.9
  - Creutzfeldt-Jakob — *see* Creutzfeldt-Jakob disease or syndrome
  - Crocq's (acrocyanosis) I73.89
  - Crohn's — *see* Enteritis, regional
  - Curschmann G71.11
  - cystic
    - breast (chronic) — *see* Mastopathy, cystic
    - kidney, congenital Q61.9
    - liver, congenital Q44.6
    - lung J98.4
      - congenital Q33.0
  - cytomegalic inclusion (generalized) B25.9
    - with pneumonia B25.0
    - congenital P35.1
  - cytomegaloviral B25.9
    - specified NEC B25.8
  - Czerny's (periodic hydrarthrosis of the knee) — *see* Effusion, joint, knee
  - Daae (-Finsen) (epidemic pleurodynia) B33.0
  - Darling's — *see* Histoplasmosis capsulati
  - de Quervain's (tendon sheath) M65.4
    - thyroid (subacute granulomatous thyroiditis) E06.1
  - Débove's (splenomegaly) R16.1
  - deer fly — *see* Tularemia
  - Degos' I77.89
  - demyelinating, demyelinizating (nervous system) G37.9
    - multiple sclerosis G35
    - specified NEC G37.8
  - dense deposit (*see also* N00-N07 with fourth character .6) N05.6
  - deposition, hydroxyapatite — *see* Disease, hydroxyapatite deposition
  - Devergie's (pityriasis rubra pilaris) L44.0
  - Devic's G36.0
  - diaphorase deficiency D74.0
  - diaphragm J98.6
  - diarrheal, infectious NEC A09
  - digestive system K92.9
    - specified NEC K92.89
  - disc, degenerative — *see* Degeneration, intervertebral disc
  - discogenic (*see also* Displacement, intervertebral disc NEC)
    - with myelopathy — *see* Disorder, disc, with, myelopathy
  - diverticular — *see* Diverticula
  - Dubois (thymus) A50.59 [E35]
  - Duchenne-Griesinger G71.0
  - Duchenne's
    - muscular dystrophy G71.0
    - pseudohypertrophy, muscles G71.0
  - ductless glands E34.9
  - Duhring's (dermatitis herpetiformis) L13.0
  - duodenum K31.9
    - specified NEC K31.89
  - Dupré's (meningism) R29.1
  - Dupuytren's (muscle contracture) M72.0
  - Durand-Nicholas-Favre (climatic bubo) A55
  - Duroziez's (congenital mitral stenosis) Q23.2
  - ear — *see* Disorder, ear
  - Eberth's — *see* Fever, typhoid
  - Ebola (virus) A98.4
  - Ebstein's heart Q22.5
  - Echinococcus — *see* Echinococcus
  - echovirus NEC B34.1
  - Eddowes' (brittle bones and blue sclera) Q78.0

- **Disease, diseased** — *continued*
  - edentulous (alveolar) ridge K06.9
    - specified NEC K06.8
  - Edsall's T67.2 ☑
  - Eichstedt's (pityriasis versicolor) B36.0
  - Ellis-van Creveld (chondroectodermal dysplasia) Q77.6
  - end stage renal (ESRD) N18.6
    - due to hypertension I12.0
  - endocrine glands or system NEC E34.9
  - endomyocardial (eosinophilic) I42.3
  - English (rickets) E55.0
  - enteroviral, enterovirus NEC B34.1
    - central nervous system NEC A88.8
  - epidemic B99.9
    - specified NEC B99.8
  - epididymis N50.9
  - Erb (-Landouzy) G71.0
  - Erdheim-Chester (ECD) E88.89
  - esophagus K22.9
    - functional K22.4
    - psychogenic F45.8
    - specified NEC K22.8
  - Eulenburg's (congenital paramyotonia) G71.19
  - eustachian tube — *see* Disorder, eustachian tube
  - external
    - auditory canal — *see* Disorder, ear, external
    - ear — *see* Disorder, ear, external
  - extrapyramidal G25.9
    - specified NEC G25.89
  - eye H57.9
    - anterior chamber H21.9
    - inflammatory NEC H57.8
    - muscle (external) — *see* Strabismus
    - specified NEC H57.8
    - syphilitic — *see* Oculopathy, syphilitic
  - eyeball H44.9
    - specified NEC H44.89
  - eyelid — *see* Disorder, eyelid
    - specified NEC — *see* Disorder, eyelid, specified type NEC
  - eyeworm of Africa B74.3
  - facial nerve (seventh) G51.9
    - newborn (birth injury) P11.3
  - Fahr (of brain) G23.8
  - Fahr Volhard (of kidney) I12.- ☑
  - fallopian tube (noninflammatory) N83.9
    - inflammatory — *see* Salpingo-oophoritis
    - specified NEC N83.8
  - familial periodic paralysis G72.3
  - Fanconi's (congenital pancytopenia) D61.09
  - fascia NEC (*see also* Disorder, muscle)
    - inflammatory — *see* Myositis
    - specified NEC M62.89
  - Fauchard's (periodontitis) — *see* Periodontitis
  - Favre-Durand-Nicolas (climatic bubo) A55
  - Fede's K14.0
  - Feer's — *see* Poisoning, mercury
  - female pelvic inflammatory (*see also* Disease, pelvis, inflammatory) N73.9
    - syphilitic (secondary) A51.42
    - tuberculous A18.17
  - Fernels' (aortic aneurysm) I71.9
  - fibrocaseous of lung — *see* Tuberculosis, pulmonary
  - fibrocystic — *see* Fibrocystic disease
  - Fiedler's (leptospiral jaundice) A27.0
  - fifth B08.3
  - file-cutter's — *see* Poisoning, lead
  - fish-skin Q80.9
    - acquired L85.0
  - Flajani (-Basedow) (exophthalmic goiter) — *see* Hyperthyroidism, with, goiter (diffuse)
  - flax-dresser's J66.1
  - fluke — *see* Infestation, fluke
  - foot and mouth B08.8
  - foot process N04.9
  - Forbes' (glycogenosis III) E74.03
  - Fordyce-Fox (apocrine miliaria) L75.2
  - Fordyce's (ectopic sebaceous glands) (mouth) Q38.6
  - Forestier's (rhizomelic pseudopolyarthritis) M35.3
    - meaning ankylosing hyperostosis — *see* Hyperostosis, ankylosing
  - Fothergill's
    - neuralgia — *see* Neuralgia, trigeminal
    - scarlatina anginosa A38.9
  - Fournier (gangrene) N49.3
    - female N76.89
  - fourth B08.8
  - Fox (-Fordyce) (apocrine miliaria) L75.2

- **Disease, diseased** — *continued*
  - Francis' — *see* Tularemia
  - Franklin C88.2
  - Frei's (climatic bubo) A55
  - Friedreich's
    - combined systemic or ataxia G11.1
    - myoclonia G25.3
  - frontal sinus — *see* Sinusitis, frontal
  - fungus NEC B49
  - Gaisböck's (polycythemia hypertonica) D75.1
  - gallbladder K82.9
    - calculus — *see* Calculus, gallbladder
    - cholecystitis — *see* Cholecystitis
    - cholesterolosis K82.4
    - fistula — *see* Fistula, gallbladder
    - hydrops K82.1
    - obstruction — *see* Obstruction, gallbladder
    - perforation K82.2
    - specified NEC K82.8
  - gamma heavy chain C88.2
  - Gamna's (siderotic splenomegaly) D73.2
  - Gamstorp's (adynamia episodica hereditaria) G72.3
  - Gandy-Nanta (siderotic splenomegaly) D73.2
  - ganister J62.8
  - gastric — *see* Disease, stomach
  - gastroesophageal reflux (GERD) K21.9
    - with esophagitis K21.0
  - gastrointestinal (tract) K92.9
    - amyloid E85.4
    - functional K59.9
      - psychogenic F45.8
    - specified NEC K92.89
  - Gee (-Herter) (-Heubner) (-Thaysen) (nontropical sprue) K90.0
  - genital organs
    - female N94.9
    - male N50.9
  - Gerhardt's (erythromelalgia) I73.81
  - Gibert's (pityriasis rosea) L42
  - Gierke's (glycogenosis I) E74.01
  - Gilles de la Tourette's (motor-verbal tic) F95.2
  - gingiva K06.9
    - specified NEC K06.8
  - gland (lymph) I89.9
  - Glanzmann's (hereditary hemorrhagic thrombasthenia) D69.1
  - glass-blower's (cataract) — *see* Cataract, specified NEC
    - salivary gland hypertrophy K11.1
  - Glisson's — *see* Rickets
  - globe H44.9
    - specified NEC H44.89
  - glomerular (*see also* Glomerulonephritis)
    - with edema — *see* Nephrosis
    - acute — *see* Nephritis, acute
    - chronic — *see* Nephritis, chronic
    - minimal change N05.0
    - rapidly progressive N01.9
  - glycogen storage E74.00
    - Andersen's E74.09
    - Cori's E74.03
    - Forbes' E74.03
    - generalized E74.00
    - glucose-6-phosphatase deficiency E74.01
    - heart E74.02 [I43]
    - hepatorenal E74.09
    - Hers' E74.09
    - liver and kidney E74.09
    - McArdle's E74.04
    - muscle phosphofructokinase E74.09
    - myocardium E74.02 [I43]
    - Pompe's E74.02
    - Tauri's E74.09
    - type 0 E74.09
    - type I E74.01
    - type II E74.02
    - type III E74.03
    - type IV E74.09
    - type V E74.04
    - type VI-XI E74.09
    - Von Gierke's E74.01
  - Goldstein's (familial hemorrhagic telangiectasia) I78.0
  - gonococcal NOS A54.9
  - graft-versus-host (GVH) D89.813
    - acute D89.810
    - acute on chronic D89.812
    - chronic D89.811
  - grainhandler's J67.8
  - granulomatous (childhood) (chronic) D71

Disease, diseased — *continued*
Graves' (exophthalmic goiter) — *see* Hyperthyroidism, with, goiter (diffuse)
Griesinger's — *see* Ancylostomiasis
Grisel's M43.6
Gruby's (tinea tonsurans) B35.Ø
Guillain-Barré G61.Ø
Guinon's (motor-verbal tic) F95.2
gum KØ6.9
gynecological N94.9
H (Hartnup's) E72.Ø2
Haff — *see* Poisoning, mercury
Hageman (congenital factor XII deficiency) D68.2
hair (color) (shaft) L67.9
follicles L73.9
specified NEC L73.8
Hamman's (spontaneous mediastinal emphysema) J98.2
hand, foot and mouth BØ8.4
Hansen's — *see* Leprosy
Hantavirus, with pulmonary manifestations B33.4
with renal manifestations A98.5
Harada's H3Ø.81- ☑
Hartnup (pellagra-cerebellar ataxia-renal aminoaciduria) E72.Ø2
Hart's (pellagra-cerebellar ataxia-renal aminoaciduria) E72.Ø2
Hashimoto's (struma lymphomatosa) EØ6.3
Hb — *see* Disease, hemoglobin
heart (organic) I51.9
with
pulmonary edema (acute) (*see also* Failure, ventricular, left) I5Ø.1
rheumatic fever (conditions in IØØ)
active IØ1.9
with chorea IØ2.Ø
specified NEC IØ1.8
inactive or quiescent (with chorea) IØ9.9
specified NEC IØ9.89
amyloid E85.4 [I43]
aortic (valve) I35.9
arteriosclerotic or sclerotic (senile) — *see* Disease, heart, ischemic, atherosclerotic
artery, arterial — *see* Disease, heart, ischemic, atherosclerotic
beer drinkers' I42.6
beriberi (wet) E51.12
black I27.Ø
congenital Q24.9
cyanotic Q24.9
specified NEC Q24.8
coronary — *see* Disease, heart, ischemic
cryptogenic I51.9
fibroid — *see* Myocarditis
functional I51.89
psychogenic F45.8
glycogen storage E74.Ø2 [I43]
gonococcal A54.83
hypertensive — *see* Hypertension, heart
hyperthyroid (*see also* Hyperthyroidism) EØ5.9Ø [I43]
with thyroid storm EØ5.91 [I43]
ischemic (chronic or with a stated duration of over 4 weeks) I25.9
atherosclerotic (of) I25.1Ø
with angina pectoris — *see* Arteriosclerosis, coronary (artery)
coronary artery bypass graft — *see* Arteriosclerosis, coronary (artery),
cardiomyopathy I25.5
diagnosed on ECG or other special investigation, but currently presenting no symptoms I25.6
silent I25.6
specified form NEC I25.89
kyphoscoliotic I27.1
meningococcal A39.5Ø
endocarditis A39.51
myocarditis A39.52
pericarditis A39.53
mitral IØ5.9
specified NEC IØ5.8
muscular — *see* Degeneration, myocardial
psychogenic (functional) F45.8
pulmonary (chronic) I27.9
in schistosomiasis B65.9 [I52]
specified NEC I27.89

Disease, diseased — *continued*
heart — *continued*
rheumatic (chronic) (inactive) (old) (quiescent) (with chorea) IØ9.9
active or acute IØ1.9
with chorea (acute) (rheumatic) (Sydenham's) IØ2.Ø
specified NEC IØ9.89
senile — *see* Myocarditis
syphilitic A52.Ø6
aortic A52.Ø3
aneurysm A52.Ø1
congenital A5Ø.54 [I52]
thyrotoxic (*see also* Thyrotoxicosis) EØ5.9Ø [I43]
with thyroid storm EØ5.91 [I43]
valve, valvular (obstructive) (regurgitant) (*see also* Endocarditis)
congenital NEC Q24.8
pulmonary Q22.3
vascular — *see* Disease, cardiovascular
heavy chain NEC C88.2
alpha C88.3
gamma C88.2
mu C88.2
Hebra's
pityriasis
maculata et circinata L42
rubra pilaris L44.Ø
prurigo L28.2
hematopoietic organs D75.9
hemoglobin or Hb
abnormal (mixed) NEC D58.2
with thalassemia D56.9
AS genotype D57.3
Bart's D56.Ø
C (Hb-C) D58.2
with other abnormal hemoglobin NEC D58.2
elliptocytosis D58.1
Hb-S D57.2- ☑
sickle-cell D57.2- ☑
thalassemia D56.8
Constant Spring D58.2
D (Hb-D) D58.2
E (Hb-E) D58.2
E-beta thalassemia D56.5
elliptocytosis D58.1
H (Hb-H) (thalassemia) D56.Ø
with other abnormal hemoglobin NEC D56.9
Constant Spring D56.Ø
I thalassemia D56.9
M D74.Ø
S or SS D57.1
SC D57.2- ☑
SD D57.8- ☑
SE D57.8- ☑
spherocytosis D58.Ø
unstable, hemolytic D58.2
hemolytic (newborn) P55.9
autoimmune (cold type) (warm type) D59.1
drug-induced D59.Ø
due to or with
incompatibility
ABO (blood group) P55.1
blood (group) (Duffy) (K(ell)) (Kidd) (Lewis) (M) (S) NEC P55.8
Rh (blood group) (factor) P55.Ø
Rh negative mother P55.Ø
specified type NEC P55.8
unstable hemoglobin D58.2
hemorrhagic D69.9
newborn P53
Henoch (-Schönlein) (purpura nervosa) D69.Ø
hepatic — *see* Disease, liver
hepatolenticular E83.Ø1
heredodegenerative NEC
spinal cord G95.89
herpesviral, disseminated BØØ.7
Hers' (glycogenosis VI) E74.Ø9
Herter (-Gee) (-Heubner) (nontropical sprue) K9Ø.Ø
Heubner-Herter (nontropical sprue) K9Ø.Ø
high fetal gene or hemoglobin thalassemia D56.9
Hildenbrand's — *see* Typhus
hip (joint) M25.9
congenital Q65.89
suppurative MØØ.9
tuberculous A18.Ø2
His (-Werner) (trench fever) A79.Ø
Hodgson's I71.2

Disease, diseased — *continued*
Hodgson's — *continued*
ruptured I71.1
Holla — *see* Spherocytosis
hookworm B76.9
specified NEC B76.8
host-versus-graft D89.813
acute D89.81Ø
acute on chronic D89.812
chronic D89.811
human immunodeficiency virus (HIV) B2Ø
Huntington's G1Ø
Hutchinson's (cheiropompholyx) — *see* Hutchinson's disease
hyaline (diffuse) (generalized)
membrane (lung) (newborn) P22.Ø
adult J8Ø
hydatid — *see* Echinococcus
hydroxyapatite deposition M11.ØØ
ankle M11.Ø7- ☑
elbow M11.Ø2- ☑
foot joint M11.Ø7- ☑
hand joint M11.Ø4- ☑
hip M11.Ø5- ☑
knee M11.Ø6- ☑
multiple site M11.Ø9
shoulder M11.Ø1- ☑
vertebra M11.Ø8
wrist M11.Ø3- ☑
hyperkinetic — *see* Hyperkinesia
hypertensive — *see* Hypertension
hypophysis E23.7
Iceland G93.3
I-cell E77.Ø
immune D89.9
immunoproliferative (malignant) C88.9
small intestinal C88.3
specified NEC C88.8
inclusion B25.9
salivary gland B25.9
infectious, infective B99.9
congenital P37.9
specified NEC P37.8
viral P35.9
specified type NEC P35.8
specified NEC B99.8
inflammatory
penis N48.29
abscess N48.21
cellulitis N48.22
prepuce N47.7
balanoposthitis N47.6
tubo-ovarian — *see* Salpingo-oophoritis
intervertebral disc (*see also* Disorder, disc)
with myelopathy — *see* Disorder, disc, with, myelopathy
cervical, cervicothoracic — *see* Disorder, disc, cervical
with
myelopathy — *see* Disorder, disc, cervical, with myelopathy
neuritis, radiculitis or radiculopathy — *see* Disorder, disc, cervical, with neuritis
specified NEC — *see* Disorder, disc, cervical, specified type NEC
lumbar (with)
myelopathy M51.Ø6
neuritis, radiculitis, radiculopathy or sciatica M51.16
specified NEC M51.86
lumbosacral (with)
neuritis, radiculitis, radiculopathy or sciatica M51.17
specified NEC M51.87
specified NEC — *see* Disorder, disc, specified NEC
thoracic (with)
myelopathy M51.Ø4
neuritis, radiculitis or radiculopathy M51.14
specified NEC M51.84
thoracolumbar (with)
myelopathy M51.Ø5
neuritis, radiculitis or radiculopathy M51.15
specified NEC M51.85
intestine K63.9
functional K59.9
psychogenic F45.8
specified NEC K59.8
organic K63.9

- **Disease, diseased** — *continued*
  - intestine — *continued*
    - protozoal A07.9
    - specified NEC K63.89
  - iris H21.9
    - specified NEC H21.89
  - iron metabolism or storage E83.10
  - island (scrub typhus) A75.3
  - itai-itai — *see* Poisoning, cadmium
  - Jakob-Creutzfeldt — *see* Creutzfeldt-Jakob disease or syndrome
  - jaw M27.9
    - fibrocystic M27.49
    - specified NEC M27.8
  - jigger B88.1
  - joint (*see also* Disorder, joint)
    - Charcot's — *see* Arthropathy, neuropathic (Charcot)
    - degenerative — *see* Osteoarthritis
      - multiple M15.9
      - spine — *see* Spondylosis
    - hypertrophic — *see* Osteoarthritis
    - sacroiliac M53.3
    - specified NEC — *see* Disorder, joint, specified type NEC
    - spine NEC — *see* Dorsopathy
    - suppurative — *see* Arthritis, pyogenic or pyemic
  - Jourdain's (acute gingivitis) K05.00
    - nonplaque induced K05.01
    - plaque induced K05.00
  - Kaschin-Beck (endemic polyarthritis) M12.10
    - ankle M12.17- ☑
    - elbow M12.12- ☑
    - foot joint M12.17- ☑
    - hand joint M12.14- ☑
    - hip M12.15- ☑
    - knee M12.16- ☑
    - multiple site M12.19
    - shoulder M12.11- ☑
    - vertebra M12.18
    - wrist M12.13- ☑
  - Katayama B65.2
  - Kedani (scrub typhus) A75.3
  - Keshan E59
  - kidney (functional) (pelvis) N28.9
    - chronic N18.9
      - hypertensive — *see* Hypertension, kidney
      - stage 1 N18.1
      - stage 2 (mild) N18.2
      - stage 3 (moderate) N18.3
      - stage 4 (severe) N18.4
      - stage 5 N18.5
    - complicating pregnancy — *see* Pregnancy, complicated by, renal disease
    - cystic (congenital) Q61.9
    - fibrocystic (congenital) Q61.8
    - hypertensive — *see* Hypertension, kidney
    - in (due to)
      - schistosomiasis (bilharziasis) B65.9 [N29]
    - multicystic Q61.4
    - polycystic Q61.3
      - adult type Q61.2
      - childhood type NEC Q61.19
        - collecting duct dilatation Q61.11
  - Kimmelstiel (-Wilson) (intercapillary polycystic (congenital) glomerulosclerosis) — *see* E08-E13 with .21
  - Kinnier Wilson's (hepatolenticular degeneration) E83.01
  - kissing — *see* Mononucleosis, infectious
  - Klebs' (*see also* Glomerulonephritis) N05- ☑
  - Klippel-Feil (brevicollis) Q76.1
  - Köhler-Pellegrini-Stieda (calcification, knee joint) — *see* Bursitis, tibial collateral
  - Kok Q89.8
  - König's (osteochondritis dissecans) — *see* Osteochondritis, dissecans
  - Korsakoff's (nonalcoholic) F04
    - alcoholic F10.96
      - with dependence F10.26
  - Kostmann's (infantile genetic agranulocytosis) D70.0
  - kuru A81.81
  - Kyasanur Forest A98.2
  - labyrinth, ear — *see* Disorder, ear, inner
  - lacrimal system — *see* Disorder, lacrimal system
  - Lafora's — *see* Epilepsy, generalized, idiopathic
  - Lancereaux-Mathieu (leptospiral jaundice) A27.0
  - Landry's G61.0

- **Disease, diseased** — *continued*
  - Larrey-Weil (leptospiral jaundice) A27.0
  - larynx J38.7
  - legionnaires' A48.1
    - nonpneumonic A48.2
  - Lenegre's I44.2
  - lens H27.9
    - specified NEC H27.8
  - Lev's (acquired complete heart block) I44.2
  - Lewy body (dementia) G31.83 [F02.80]
    - with behavioral disturbance G31.83 [F02.81]
  - Lichtheim's (subacute combined sclerosis with pernicious anemia) D51.0
  - Lightwood's (renal tubular acidosis) N25.89
  - Lignac's (cystinosis) E72.04
  - lip K13.0
  - lipid-storage E75.6
    - specified NEC E75.5
  - Lipschütz's N76.6
  - liver (chronic) (organic) K76.9
    - alcoholic (chronic) K70.9
      - acute — *see* Disease, liver, alcoholic, hepatitis
      - cirrhosis K70.30
        - with ascites K70.31
      - failure K70.40
        - with coma K70.41
      - fatty liver K70.0
      - fibrosis K70.2
      - hepatitis K70.10
        - with ascites K70.11
      - sclerosis K70.2
    - cystic, congenital Q44.6
    - drug-induced (idiosyncratic) (toxic) (predictable) (unpredictable) — *see* Disease, liver, toxic
    - end stage K72.90
      - due to hepatitis — *see* Hepatitis
    - fatty, nonalcoholic (NAFLD) K76.0
      - alcoholic K70.0
    - fibrocystic (congenital) Q44.6
    - fluke
      - Chinese B66.1
      - oriental B66.1
      - sheep B66.3
    - glycogen storage E74.09 [K77]
    - in (due to)
      - schistosomiasis (bilharziasis) B65.9 [K77]
    - inflammatory K75.9
      - alcoholic K70.1 ☑
      - specified NEC K75.89
    - polycystic (congenital) Q44.6
    - toxic K71.9
      - with
        - cholestasis K71.0
        - cirrhosis (liver) K71.7
        - fibrosis (liver) K71.7
        - focal nodular hyperplasia K71.8
        - hepatic granuloma K71.8
        - hepatic necrosis K71.10
          - with coma K71.11
        - hepatitis NEC K71.6
          - acute K71.2
          - chronic
            - active K71.50
              - with ascites K71.51
            - lobular K71.4
            - persistent K71.3
          - lupoid K71.50
            - with ascites K71.51
        - peliosis hepatis K71.8
        - veno-occlusive disease (VOD) of liver K71.8
    - veno-occlusive K76.5
  - Lobo's (keloid blastomycosis) B48.0
  - Lobstein's (brittle bones and blue sclera) Q78.0
  - Ludwig's (submaxillary cellulitis) K12.2
  - lumbosacral region M53.87
  - lung J98.4
    - black J60
    - congenital Q33.9
    - cystic J98.4
      - congenital Q33.0
    - fibroid (chronic) — *see* Fibrosis, lung
    - fluke B66.4
      - oriental B66.4
    - in
      - amyloidosis E85.4 [J99]
      - sarcoidosis D86.0
      - Sjögren's syndrome M35.02

- **Disease, diseased** — *continued*
  - lung — *continued*
    - in — *continued*
      - systemic
        - lupus erythematosus M32.13
        - sclerosis M34.81
    - interstitial J84.9
      - of childhood, specified NEC J84.848
      - respiratory bronchiolitis J84.115
      - specified NEC J84.89
    - obstructive (chronic) J44.9
      - with
        - acute
          - bronchitis J44.0
          - exacerbation NEC J44.1
          - lower respiratory infection J44.0
        - alveolitis, allergic J67.9
        - asthma J44.9
        - bronchiectasis J47.9
          - with
            - exacerbation (acute) J47.1
            - lower respiratory infection J47.0
        - bronchitis J44.9
          - with
            - exacerbation (acute) J44.1
            - lower respiratory infection J44.0
        - emphysema J44.9
        - hypersensitivity pneumonitis J67.9
      - decompensated J44.1
        - with
          - exacerbation (acute) J44.1
    - polycystic J98.4
      - congenital Q33.0
    - rheumatoid (diffuse) (interstitial) — *see* Rheumatoid, lung
  - Lutembacher's (atrial septal defect with mitral stenosis) Q21.1
  - Lyme A69.20
  - lymphatic (gland) (system) (channel) (vessel) I89.9
  - lymphoproliferative D47.9
    - specified NEC D47.Z9 (*following* D47.4)
    - T-gamma D47.Z9 (*following* D47.4)
    - X-linked D82.3
  - Magitot's M27.2
  - malarial — *see* Malaria
  - malignant (*see also* Neoplasm, malignant, by site)
  - Manson's B65.1
  - maple bark J67.6
  - maple-syrup-urine E71.0
  - Marburg (virus) A98.3
  - Marion's (bladder neck obstruction) N32.0
  - Marsh's (exophthalmic goiter) — *see* Hyperthyroidism, with, goiter (diffuse)
  - mastoid (process) — *see* Disorder, ear, middle
  - Mathieu's (leptospiral jaundice) A27.0
  - Maxcy's A75.2
  - McArdle (-Schmid-Pearson) (glycogenosis V) E74.04
  - mediastinum J98.5
  - medullary center (idiopathic) (respiratory) G93.89
  - Meige's (chronic hereditary edema) Q82.0
  - meningococcal — *see* Infection, meningococcal
  - mental F99
    - organic F09
  - mesenchymal M35.9
  - mesenteric embolic K55.0
  - metabolic, metabolism E88.9
    - bilirubin E80.7
  - metal-polisher's J62.8
  - metastatic (*see also* Neoplasm, secondary, by site) C79.9
  - microvascular - code to condition
  - microvillus
    - atrophy Q43.8
    - inclusion (MVD) Q43.8
  - middle ear — *see* Disorder, ear, middle
  - Mikulicz' (dryness of mouth, absent or decreased lacrimation) K11.8
  - Milroy's (chronic hereditary edema) Q82.0
  - Minamata — *see* Poisoning, mercury
  - minicore G71.2
  - Minor's G95.19
  - Minot's (hemorrhagic disease, newborn) P53
  - Minot-von Willebrand-Jürgens (angiohemophilia) D68.0
  - Mitchell's (erythromelalgia) I73.81
  - mitral (valve) I05.9
    - nonrheumatic I34.9
  - mixed connective tissue M35.1

Disease, diseased — *continued*
- moldy hay J67.Ø
- Monge's T7Ø.29 ☑
- Morgagni-Adams-Stokes (syncope with heart block) I45.9
- Morgagni's (syndrome) (hyperostosis frontalis interna) M85.2
- Morton's (with metatarsalgia) — *see* Lesion, nerve, plantar
- Morvan's G6Ø.8
- motor neuron (bulbar) (familial) (mixed type) (spinal) G12.2Ø
  - amyotrophic lateral sclerosis G12.21
  - progressive bulbar palsy G12.22
  - specified NEC G12.29
- moyamoya I67.5
- mu heavy chain disease C88.2
- multicore G71.2
- muscle (*see also* Disorder, muscle)
  - inflammatory — *see* Myositis
  - ocular (external) — *see* Strabismus
- musculoskeletal system, soft tissue — *see* also Disorder, soft tissue
  - specified NEC — *see* Disorder, soft tissue, specified type NEC
- mushroom workers' J67.5
- mycotic B49
- myelodysplastic, not classified C94.6
- myeloproliferative, not classified C94.6
  - chronic D47.1
- myocardium, myocardial (*see also* Degeneration, myocardial) I51.5
  - primary (idiopathic) I42.9
- myoneural G7Ø.9
- Naegeli's D69.1
- nails L6Ø.9
  - specified NEC L6Ø.8
- Nairobi (sheep virus) A93.8
- nasal J34.9
- nemaline body G71.2
- nerve — *see* Disorder, nerve
- nervous system G98.8
  - autonomic G9Ø.9
  - central G96.9
    - specified NEC G96.8
  - congenital QØ7.9
  - parasympathetic G9Ø.9
  - specified NEC G98.8
  - sympathetic G9Ø.9
  - vegetative G9Ø.9
- neuromuscular system G7Ø.9
- Newcastle B3Ø.8
- Nicolas (-Durand)-Favre (climatic bubo) A55
- nipple N64.9
  - Paget's C5Ø.Ø1- ☑
    - female C5Ø.Ø1- ☑
    - male C5Ø.Ø2- ☑
- Nishimoto (-Takeuchi) I67.5
- nonarthropod-borne NOS (viral) B34.9
  - enterovirus NEC B34.1
- nonautoimmune hemolytic D59.4
  - drug-induced D59.2
- Nonne-Milroy-Meige (chronic hereditary edema) Q82.Ø
- nose J34.9
- nucleus pulposus — *see* Disorder, disc
- nutritional E63.9
- oast-house-urine E72.19
  - ocular
    - herpesviral BØØ.5Ø
    - zoster BØ2.3Ø
- obliterative vascular I77.1
- Ohara's — *see* Tularemia
- Opitz's (congestive splenomegaly) D73.2
- Oppenheim-Urbach (necrobiosis lipoidica diabeticorum) — *see* EØ8-E13 with .62Ø
- optic nerve NEC — *see* Disorder, nerve, optic
- orbit — *see* Disorder, orbit
- Oriental liver fluke B66.1
- Oriental lung fluke B66.4
- Ormond's N13.5
- Oropouche virus A93.Ø
- Osler-Rendu (familial hemorrhagic telangiectasia) I78.Ø
- osteofibrocystic E21.Ø
- Otto's M24.7
- outer ear — *see* Disorder, ear, external
- ovary (noninflammatory) N83.9
  - cystic N83.2Ø
  - inflammatory — *see* Salpingo-oophoritis

Disease, diseased — *continued*
- ovary — *continued*
  - polycystic E28.2
  - specified NEC N83.8
- Owren's (congenital) — *see* Defect, coagulation
- pancreas K86.9
  - cystic K86.2
  - fibrocystic E84.9
  - specified NEC K86.8
- panvalvular IØ8.9
  - specified NEC IØ8.8
- parametrium (noninflammatory) N83.9
- parasitic B89
  - cerebral NEC B71.9 [G94]
  - intestinal NOS B82.9
  - mouth B37.Ø
  - skin NOS B88.9
  - specified type — *see* Infestation
  - tongue B37.Ø
- parathyroid (gland) E21.5
  - specified NEC E21.4
- Parkinson's G2Ø
- parodontal KØ5.6
- Parrot's (syphilitic osteochondritis) A5Ø.Ø2
- Parry's (exophthalmic goiter) — *see* Hyperthyroidism, with, goiter (diffuse)
- Parson's (exophthalmic goiter) — *see* Hyperthyroidism, with, goiter (diffuse)
- Paxton's (white piedra) B36.2
- pearl-worker's — *see* Osteomyelitis, specified type NEC
- Pellegrini-Stieda (calcification, knee joint) — *see* Bursitis, tibial collateral
- pelvis, pelvic
  - female NOS N94.9
    - specified NEC N94.89
  - gonococcal (acute) (chronic) A54.24
  - inflammatory (female) N73.9
    - acute N73.Ø
    - chronic N73.1
    - specified NEC N73.8
    - syphilitic (secondary) A51.42
      - late A52.76
    - tuberculous A18.17
  - organ, female N94.9
  - peritoneum, female NEC N94.89
- penis N48.9
  - inflammatory N48.29
    - abscess N48.21
    - cellulitis N48.22
  - specified NEC N48.89
- periapical tissues NOS KØ4.9Ø
- periodontal KØ5.6
  - specified NEC KØ5.5
- periosteum — *see* Disorder, bone, specified type NEC
- peripheral
  - arterial I73.9
  - autonomic nervous system G9Ø.9
  - nerves — *see* Polyneuropathy
  - vascular NOS I73.9
- peritoneum K66.9
  - pelvic, female NEC N94.89
  - specified NEC K66.8
- persistent mucosal (middle ear) H66.2Ø
  - left H66.22
    - with right H66.23
  - right H66.21
    - with left H66.23
- Petit's — *see* Hernia, abdomen, specified site NEC
- pharynx J39.2
  - specified NEC J39.2
- Phocas' — *see* Mastopathy, cystic
- photochromogenic (acid-fast bacilli) (pulmonary) A31.Ø
  - nonpulmonary A31.9
- Pick's G31.Ø1 [FØ2.8Ø]
  - with behavioral disturbance G31.Ø1 [FØ2.81]
- pigeon fancier's J67.2
- pineal gland E34.8
- pink — *see* Poisoning, mercury
- Pinkus' (lichen nitidus) L44.1
- pinworm B8Ø
- Piry virus A93.8
- pituitary (gland) E23.7
- pituitary-snuff-taker's J67.8
- pleura (cavity) J94.9
  - specified NEC J94.8
- pneumatic drill (hammer) T75.21 ☑

Disease, diseased — *continued*
- Pollitzer's (hidradenitis suppurativa) L73.2
- polycystic
  - kidney or renal Q61.3
    - adult type Q61.2
    - childhood type NEC Q61.19
      - collecting duct dilatation Q61.11
  - liver or hepatic Q44.6
  - lung or pulmonary J98.4
    - congenital Q33.Ø
  - ovary, ovaries E28.2
  - spleen Q89.Ø9
- polyethylene T84.Ø5- ☑
- Pompe's (glycogenosis II) E74.Ø2
- Posadas-Wernicke B38.9
- Potain's (pulmonary edema) — *see* Edema, lung
- prepuce N47.8
  - inflammatory N47.7
    - balanoposthitis N47.6
- Pringle's (tuberous sclerosis) Q85.1
- prion, central nervous system A81.9
  - specified NEC A81.89
- prostate N42.9
  - specified NEC N42.89
- protozoal B64
  - acanthamebiasis — *see* Acanthamebiasis
  - African trypanosomiasis — *see* African trypanosomiasis
  - babesiosis B6Ø.Ø
  - Chagas disease — *see* Chagas disease
  - intestine, intestinal AØ7.9
  - leishmaniasis — *see* Leishmaniasis
  - malaria — *see* Malaria
  - naegleriasis B6Ø.2
  - pneumocystosis B59
  - specified organism NEC B6Ø.8
  - toxoplasmosis — *see* Toxoplasmosis
- pseudo-Hurler's E77.Ø
- psychiatric F99
- psychotic — *see* Psychosis
- Puente's (simple glandular cheilitis) K13.Ø
- puerperal (*see also* Puerperal) O9Ø.89
- pulmonary (*see also* Disease, lung)
  - artery I28.9
  - chronic obstructive J44.9
    - with
      - acute bronchitis J44.Ø
      - exacerbation (acute) J44.1
      - lower respiratory infection (acute) J44.Ø
    - decompensated J44.1
      - with
        - exacerbation (acute) J44.1
  - heart I27.9
    - specified NEC I27.89
  - hypertensive (vascular) I27.Ø
  - valve I37.9
    - rheumatic IØ9.89
- pulp (dental) NOS KØ4.9Ø
- pulseless M31.4
- Putnam's (subacute combined sclerosis with pernicious anemia) D51.Ø
- Pyle (-Cohn) (craniometaphyseal dysplasia) Q78.5
- ragpicker's or ragsorter's A22.1
- Raynaud's — *see* Raynaud's disease
- reactive airway — *see* Asthma
- Reclus' (cystic) — *see* Mastopathy, cystic
- rectum K62.9
  - specified NEC K62.89
- Refsum's (heredopathia atactica polyneuritiformis) G6Ø.1
- renal (functional) (pelvis) (*see also* Disease, kidney) N28.9
  - with
    - edema — *see* Nephrosis
    - glomerular lesion — *see* Glomerulonephritis
      - with edema — *see* Nephrosis
    - interstitial nephritis N12
  - acute N28.9
  - chronic (*see also* Disease, kidney, chronic) N18.9
  - cystic, congenital Q61.9
  - diabetic — *see* EØ8-E13 with .22
  - end-stage (failure) N18.6
    - due to hypertension I12.Ø
  - fibrocystic (congenital) Q61.8
  - hypertensive — *see* Hypertension, kidney
  - lupus M32.14
  - phosphate-losing (tubular) N25.Ø
  - polycystic (congenital) Q61.3

Disease, diseased — *continued*
  renal (*see also* Disease, kidney) — *continued*
    polycystic — *continued*
      adult type Q61.2
      childhood type NEC Q61.19
        collecting duct dilatation Q61.11
    rapidly progressive NØ1.9
    subacute NØ1.9
  Rendu-Osler-Weber (familial hemorrhagic telangiectasia) I78.Ø
  renovascular (arteriosclerotic) — *see* Hypertension, kidney
  respiratory (tract) J98.9
    acute or subacute NOS JØ6.9
      due to
        chemicals, gases, fumes or vapors (inhalation) J68.3
        external agent J7Ø.9
          specified NEC J7Ø.8
        radiation J7Ø.Ø
        smoke inhalation J7Ø.5
      noninfectious J39.8
    chronic NOS J98.9
      due to
        chemicals, gases, fumes or vapors J68.4
        external agent J7Ø.9
          specified NEC J7Ø.8
        radiation J7Ø.1
      newborn P27.9
        specified NEC P27.8
    due to
      chemicals, gases, fumes or vapors J68.9
        acute or subacute NEC J68.3
        chronic J68.4
      external agent J7Ø.9
        specified NEC J7Ø.8
    newborn P28.9
      specified type NEC P28.89
    upper J39.9
      acute or subacute JØ6.9
      noninfectious NEC J39.8
      specified NEC J39.8
      streptococcal JØ6.9
  retina, retinal H35.9
    Batten's or Batten-Mayou E75.4 [H36]
    specified NEC H35.89
  rheumatoid — *see* Arthritis, rheumatoid
  rickettsial NOS A79.9
    specified type NEC A79.89
  Riga (-Fede) (cachectic aphthae) K14.Ø
  Riggs' (compound periodontitis) — *see* Periodontitis
  Ritter's LØØ
  Rivalta's (cervicofacial actinomycosis) A42.2
  Robles' (onchocerciasis) B73.Ø1
  Roger's (congenital interventricular septal defect) Q21.Ø
  Rosenthal's (factor XI deficiency) D68.1
  Ross River B33.1
  Rossbach's (hyperchlorhydria) K3Ø
  Rotes Quérol — *see* Hyperostosis, ankylosing
  Roth (-Bernhardt) — *see* Mononeuropathy, lower limb, meralgia paresthetica
  Runeberg's (progressive pernicious anemia) D51.Ø
  sacroiliac NEC M53.3
  salivary gland or duct K11.9
    inclusion B25.9
    specified NEC K11.8
    virus B25.9
  sandworm B76.9
  Schimmelbusch's — *see* Mastopathy, cystic
  Schmorl's — *see* Schmorl's disease or nodes
  Schönlein (-Henoch) (purpura rheumatica) D69.Ø
  Schottmüller's — *see* Fever, paratyphoid
  Schultz's (agranulocytosis) — *see* Agranulocytosis
  Schwalbe-Ziehen-Oppenheim G24.1
  Schwartz-Jampel G71.13
  sclera H15.9
    specified NEC H15.89
  scrofulous (tuberculous) A18.2
  scrotum N5Ø.9
  sebaceous glands L73.9
  semilunar cartilage, cystic (*see also* Derangement, knee, meniscus, cystic)
  seminal vesicle N5Ø.9
  serum NEC (*see also* Reaction, serum) T8Ø.69 ☑
  sexually transmitted A64
    anogenital
      herpesviral infection — *see* Herpes, anogenital

Disease, diseased — *continued*
  sexually transmitted — *continued*
    anogenital — *continued*
      warts A63.Ø
    chancroid A57
    chlamydial infection — *see* Chlamydia
    gonorrhea — *see* Gonorrhea
    granuloma inguinale A58
    specified organism NEC A63.8
    syphilis — *see* Syphilis
    trichomoniasis — *see* Trichomoniasis
  Sézary C84.1- ☑
  shimamushi (scrub typhus) A75.3
  shipyard B3Ø.Ø
  sickle-cell D57.1
    with crisis (vasoocclusive pain) D57.ØØ
      with
        acute chest syndrome D57.Ø1
        splenic sequestration D57.Ø2
    elliptocytosis D57.8- ☑
    Hb-C D57.2Ø
      with crisis (vasoocclusive pain) D57.219
        with
          acute chest syndrome D57.211
          splenic sequestration D57.212
      without crisis D57.2Ø
    Hb-SD D57.8Ø
      with crisis D57.819
        with
          acute chest syndrome D57.811
          splenic sequestration D57.812
    Hb-SE D57.8Ø
      with crisis D57.819
        with
          acute chest syndrome D57.811
          splenic sequestration D57.812
    specified NEC D57.8Ø
      with crisis D57.819
        with
          acute chest syndrome D57.811
          splenic sequestration D57.812
    spherocytosis D57.8Ø
      with crisis D57.819
        with
          acute chest syndrome D57.811
          splenic sequestration D57.812
    thalassemia D57.4Ø
      with crisis (vasoocclusive pain) D57.419
        with
          acute chest syndrome D57.411
          splenic sequestration D57.412
      without crisis D57.4Ø
  silo-filler's J68.8
    bronchitis J68.Ø
    pneumonitis J68.Ø
    pulmonary edema J68.1
  simian B BØØ.4
  Simons' (progressive lipodystrophy) E88.1
  sin nombre virus B33.4
  sinus — *see* Sinusitis
  Sirkari's B55.Ø
  sixth BØ8.2Ø
    due to human herpesvirus 6 BØ8.21
    due to human herpesvirus 7 BØ8.22
  skin L98.9
    due to metabolic disorder NEC E88.9 [L99]
    specified NEC L98.8
  slim (HIV) B2Ø
  small vessel I73.9
  Sneddon-Wilkinson (subcorneal pustular dermatosis) L13.1
  South African creeping B88.Ø
  spinal (cord) G95.9
    congenital QØ6.9
    specified NEC G95.89
  spine (*see also* Spondylopathy)
    joint — *see* Dorsopathy
    tuberculous A18.Ø1
  spinocerebellar (hereditary) G11.9
    specified NEC G11.8
  spleen D73.9
    amyloid E85.4 [D77]
    organic D73.9
    polycystic Q89.Ø9
    postinfectional D73.89
  sponge-diver's — *see* Toxicity, venom, marine animal, sea anemone
  Startle Q89.8

Disease, diseased — *continued*
  Steinert's G71.11
  Sticker's (erythema infectiosum) BØ8.3
  Stieda's (calcification, knee joint) — *see* Bursitis, tibial collateral
  Stokes' (exophthalmic goiter) — *see* Hyperthyroidism, with, goiter (diffuse)
  Stokes-Adams (syncope with heart block) I45.9
  stomach K31.9
    functional, psychogenic F45.8
    specified NEC K31.89
  stonemason's J62.8
  storage
    glycogen — *see* Disease, glycogen storage
    mucopolysaccharide — *see* Mucopolysaccharidosis
  striatopallidal system NEC G25.89
  Stuart-Prower (congenital factor X deficiency) D68.2
  Stuart's (congenital factor X deficiency) D68.2
  subcutaneous tissue — *see* Disease, skin
  supporting structures of teeth KØ8.9
    specified NEC KØ8.8
  suprarenal (capsule) (gland) E27.9
    hyperfunction E27.Ø
    specified NEC E27.8
  sweat glands L74.9
    specified NEC L74.8
  Sweeley-Klionsky E75.21
  Swift (-Feer) — *see* Poisoning, mercury
  swimming-pool granuloma A31.1
  Sylvest's (epidemic pleurodynia) B33.Ø
  sympathetic nervous system G9Ø.9
  synovium — *see* Disorder, synovium
  syphilitic — *see* Syphilis
  systemic tissue mast cell C96.2
  tanapox (virus) BØ8.71
  Tangier E78.6
  Tarral-Besnier (pityriasis rubra pilaris) L44.Ø
  Tauri's E74.Ø9
  tear duct — *see* Disorder, lacrimal system
  tendon, tendinous (*see also* Disorder, tendon)
    nodular — *see* Trigger finger
  terminal vessel I73.9
  testis N5Ø.9
  thalassemia Hb-S — *see* Disease, sickle-cell, thalassemia
  Thaysen-Gee (nontropical sprue) K9Ø.Ø
  Thomsen G71.12
  throat J39.2
    septic JØ2.Ø
  thromboembolic — *see* Embolism
  thymus (gland) E32.9
    specified NEC E32.8
  thyroid (gland) EØ7.9
    heart (*see also* Hyperthyroidism) EØ5.9Ø [I43]
      with thyroid storm EØ5.91 [I43]
    specified NEC EØ7.89
  Tietze's M94.Ø
  tongue K14.9
    specified NEC K14.8
  tonsils, tonsillar (and adenoids) J35.9
  tooth, teeth KØ8.9
    hard tissues KØ3.9
      specified NEC KØ3.89
    pulp NEC KØ4.99
    specified NEC KØ8.8
  Tourette's F95.2
  trachea NEC J39.8
  tricuspid IØ7.9
    nonrheumatic I36.9
  triglyceride-storage E75.5
  trophoblastic — *see* Mole, hydatidiform
  tsutsugamushi A75.3
  tube (fallopian) (noninflammatory) N83.9
    inflammatory — *see* Salpingitis
    specified NEC N83.8
  tuberculous NEC — *see* Tuberculosis
  tubo-ovarian (noninflammatory) N83.9
    inflammatory — *see* Salpingo-oophoritis
    specified NEC N83.8
  tubotympanic, chronic — *see* Otitis, media, suppurative, chronic, tubotympanic
  tubulo-interstitial N15.9
    specified NEC N15.8
  tympanum — *see* Disorder, tympanic membrane
  Uhl's Q24.8
  Underwood's (sclerema neonatorum) P83.Ø
  Unverricht (-Lundborg) — *see* Epilepsy, generalized, idiopathic

- **Disease, diseased** — *continued*
  - Urbach-Oppenheim (necrobiosis lipoidica diabeticorum) — *see* E08-E13 with .620
  - ureter N28.9
    - in (due to)
      - schistosomiasis (bilharziasis) B65.0 [N29]
  - urethra N36.9
    - specified NEC N36.8
  - urinary (tract) N39.9
    - bladder N32.9
      - specified NEC N32.89
    - specified NEC N39.8
  - uterus (noninflammatory) N85.9
    - infective — *see* Endometritis
    - inflammatory — *see* Endometritis
    - specified NEC N85.8
  - uveal tract (anterior) H21.9
    - posterior H31.9
  - vagabond's B85.1
  - vagina, vaginal (noninflammatory) N89.9
    - inflammatory NEC N76.89
    - specified NEC N89.8
  - valve, valvular I38
    - multiple I08.9
      - specified NEC I08.8
  - van Creveld-von Gierke (glycogenosis I) E74.01
  - vas deferens N50.9
  - vascular I99.9
    - arteriosclerotic — *see* Arteriosclerosis
    - ciliary body NEC — *see* Disorder, iris, vascular
    - hypertensive — *see* Hypertension
    - iris NEC — *see* Disorder, iris, vascular
    - obliterative I77.1
      - peripheral I73.9
    - occlusive I99.8
    - peripheral (occlusive) I73.9
      - in diabetes mellitus — *see* E08-E13 with .51
  - vasomotor I73.9
  - vasospastic I73.9
  - vein I87.9
  - venereal (*see also* Disease, sexually transmitted) A64
    - chlamydial NEC A56.8
      - anus A56.3
      - genitourinary NOS A56.2
      - pharynx A56.4
      - rectum A56.3
    - fifth A55
    - sixth A55
    - specified nature or type NEC A63.8
  - vertebra, vertebral (*see also* Spondylopathy)
    - disc — *see* Disorder, disc
  - vibration — *see* Vibration, adverse effects
  - viral, virus (*see also* Disease, by type of virus) B34.9
    - arbovirus NOS A94
    - arthropod-borne NOS A94
    - congenital P35.9
      - specified NEC P35.8
    - Hanta (with renal manifestations) (Dobrava) (Puumala) (Seoul) A98.5
      - with pulmonary manifestations (Andes) (Bayou) (Bermejo) (Black Creek Canal) (Choclo) (Juquitiba) (Laguna negra) (Lechiguanas) (New York) (Oran) (Sin nombre) B33.4
    - Hantaan (Korean hemorrhagic fever) A98.5
    - human immunodeficiency (HIV) B20
    - Kunjin A83.4
    - nonarthropod-borne NOS B34.9
    - Powassan A84.8
    - Rocio (encephalitis) A83.6
    - Sin nombre (Hantavirus) (cardio)-pulmonary syndrome) B33.4
    - Tahyna B33.8
    - vesicular stomatitis A93.8
  - vitreous H43.9
    - specified NEC H43.89
  - vocal cord J38.3
  - Volkmann's, acquired T79.6 ☑
  - von Eulenburg's (congenital paramyotonia) G71.19
  - von Gierke's (glycogenosis I) E74.01
  - von Graefe's — *see* Strabismus, paralytic, ophthalmoplegia, progressive
  - von Willebrand (-Jürgens) (angiohemophilia) D68.0
  - Vrolik's (osteogenesis imperfecta) Q78.0
  - vulva (noninflammatory) N90.9
    - inflammatory NEC N76.89
    - specified NEC N90.89
  - Wallgren's (obstruction of splenic vein with collateral circulation) I87.8

- **Disease, diseased** — *continued*
  - Wassilieff's (leptospiral jaundice) A27.0
  - wasting NEC R64
    - due to malnutrition E41
  - Waterhouse-Friderichsen A39.1
  - Wegner's (syphilitic osteochondritis) A50.02
  - Weil's (leptospiral jaundice of lung) A27.0
  - Weir Mitchell's (erythromelalgia) I73.81
  - Werdnig-Hoffmann G12.0
  - Wermer's E31.21
  - Werner-His (trench fever) A79.0
  - Werner-Schultz (neutropenic splenomegaly) D73.81
  - Wernicke-Posadas B38.9
  - whipworm B79
  - white blood cells D72.9
    - specified NEC D72.89
  - white matter R90.82
  - white-spot, meaning lichen sclerosus et atrophicus L90.0
    - penis N48.0
    - vulva N90.4
  - Wilkie's K55.1
  - Wilkinson-Sneddon (subcorneal pustular dermatosis) L13.1
  - Willis' — *see* Diabetes
  - Wilson's (hepatolenticular degeneration) E83.01
  - woolsorter's A22.1
  - yaba monkey tumor B08.72
  - yaba pox (virus) B08.72
  - zoonotic, bacterial A28.9
    - specified type NEC A28.8
- **Disfigurement** (due to scar) L90.5
- **Disgerminoma** — *see* Dysgerminoma
- **DISH** (diffuse idiopathic skeletal hyperostosis) — *see* Hyperostosis, ankylosing
- **Disinsertion, retina** — *see* Detachment, retina
- **Dislocatable hip, congenital** Q65.6
- **Dislocation** (articular)
  - with fracture — *see* Fracture
  - acromioclavicular (joint) S43.10- ☑
    - with displacement
      - 100%-200% S43.12- ☑
      - more than 200% S43.13- ☑
    - inferior S43.14- ☑
    - posterior S43.15- ☑
  - ankle S93.0- ☑
  - astragalus — *see* Dislocation, ankle
  - atlantoaxial S13.121 ☑
  - atlantooccipital S13.111 ☑
  - atloidooccipital S13.111 ☑
  - breast bone S23.29 ☑
  - capsule, joint — *code by* site under Dislocation
  - carpal (bone) — *see* Dislocation, wrist
  - carpometacarpal (joint) NEC S63.05- ☑
    - thumb S63.04- ☑
  - cartilage (joint) — *code by* site under Dislocation
  - cervical spine (vertebra) — *see* Dislocation, vertebra, cervical
  - chronic — *see* Dislocation, recurrent
  - clavicle — *see* Dislocation, acromioclavicular joint
  - coccyx S33.2 ☑
  - congenital NEC Q68.8
  - coracoid — *see* Dislocation, shoulder
  - costal cartilage S23.29 ☑
  - costochondral S23.29 ☑
  - cricoarytenoid articulation S13.29 ☑
  - cricothyroid articulation S13.29 ☑
  - dorsal vertebra — *see* Dislocation, vertebra, thoracic
  - ear ossicle — *see* Discontinuity, ossicles, ear
  - elbow S53.10- ☑
    - congenital Q68.8
    - pathological — *see* Dislocation, pathological NEC, elbow
    - radial head alone — *see* Dislocation, radial head
    - recurrent — *see* Dislocation, recurrent, elbow
    - traumatic S53.10- ☑
      - anterior S53.11- ☑
      - lateral S53.14- ☑
      - medial S53.13- ☑
      - posterior S53.12- ☑
      - specified type NEC S53.19- ☑
  - eye, nontraumatic — *see* Luxation, globe
  - eyeball, nontraumatic — *see* Luxation, globe
  - femur
    - distal end — *see* Dislocation, knee
    - proximal end — *see* Dislocation, hip

- **Dislocation** — *continued*
  - fibula
    - distal end — *see* Dislocation, ankle
    - proximal end — *see* Dislocation, knee
  - finger S63.25- ☑
    - index S63.25- ☑
    - interphalangeal S63.27- ☑
      - distal S63.29- ☑
        - index S63.29- ☑
        - little S63.29- ☑
        - middle S63.29- ☑
        - ring S63.29- ☑
      - index S63.27- ☑
      - little S63.27- ☑
      - middle S63.27- ☑
      - proximal S63.28- ☑
        - index S63.28- ☑
        - little S63.28- ☑
        - middle S63.28- ☑
        - ring S63.28- ☑
      - ring S63.27- ☑
    - little S63.25- ☑
    - metacarpophalangeal S63.26- ☑
      - index S63.26- ☑
      - little S63.26- ☑
      - middle S63.26- ☑
      - ring S63.26- ☑
    - middle S63.25- ☑
    - recurrent — *see* Dislocation, recurrent, finger
    - ring S63.25- ☑
    - thumb — *see* Dislocation, thumb
  - foot S93.30- ☑
    - recurrent — *see* Dislocation, recurrent, foot
    - specified site NEC S93.33- ☑
    - tarsal joint S93.31- ☑
    - tarsometatarsal joint S93.32- ☑
    - toe — *see* Dislocation, toe
  - fracture — *see* Fracture
  - glenohumeral (joint) — *see* Dislocation, shoulder
  - glenoid — *see* Dislocation, shoulder
  - habitual — *see* Dislocation, recurrent
  - hip S73.00- ☑
    - anterior S73.03- ☑
      - obturator S73.02- ☑
    - central S73.04- ☑
    - congenital (total) Q65.2
      - bilateral Q65.1
      - partial Q65.5
        - bilateral Q65.4
        - unilateral Q65.3- ☑
      - unilateral Q65.0- ☑
    - developmental M24.85- ☑
    - pathological — *see* Dislocation, pathological NEC, hip
    - posterior S73.01- ☑
    - recurrent — *see* Dislocation, recurrent, hip
  - humerus, proximal end — *see* Dislocation, shoulder
  - incomplete — *see* Subluxation, by site
  - incus — *see* Discontinuity, ossicles, ear
  - infracoracoid — *see* Dislocation, shoulder
  - innominate (pubic junction) (sacral junction) S33.39 ☑
    - acetabulum — *see* Dislocation, hip
  - interphalangeal (joint(s))
    - finger S63.279 ☑
      - distal S63.29- ☑
        - index S63.29- ☑
        - little S63.29- ☑
        - middle S63.29- ☑
        - ring S63.29- ☑
      - index S63.27- ☑
      - little S63.27- ☑
      - middle S63.27- ☑
      - proximal S63.28- ☑
        - index S63.28- ☑
        - little S63.28- ☑
        - middle S63.28- ☑
        - ring S63.28- ☑
      - ring S63.27- ☑
    - foot or toe — *see* Dislocation, toe
    - thumb S63.12- ☑
      - distal joint S63.14- ☑
      - proximal joint S63.13- ☑
  - jaw (cartilage) (meniscus) S03.0 ☑
  - joint prosthesis — *see* Complications, joint prosthesis, mechanical, displacement, by site
  - knee S83.106 ☑

- **Dislocation** — *continued*
  - knee — *continued*
    - cap — *see* Dislocation, patella
    - congenital Q68.2
    - old M23.8X- ☑
    - patella — *see* Dislocation, patella
    - pathological — *see* Dislocation, pathological NEC, knee
    - proximal tibia
      - anteriorly S83.11- ☑
      - laterally S83.14- ☑
      - medially S83.13- ☑
      - posteriorly S83.12- ☑
    - recurrent (*see also* Derangement, knee, specified NEC)
    - specified type NEC S83.19- ☑
  - lacrimal gland HØ4.16- ☑
  - lens (complete) H27.1Ø
    - anterior H27.12- ☑
    - congenital Q12.1
    - ocular implant — *see* Complications, intraocular lens
    - partial H27.11- ☑
    - posterior H27.13- ☑
    - traumatic SØ5.8X- ☑
  - ligament — *code by* site under Dislocation
  - lumbar (vertebra) — *see* Dislocation, vertebra, lumbar
  - lumbosacral (vertebra) (*see also* Dislocation, vertebra, lumbar)
    - congenital Q76.49
  - mandible SØ3.Ø ☑
  - meniscus (knee) — *see* Tear, meniscus
    - other sites - code by site under Dislocation
  - metacarpal (bone)
    - distal end — *see* Dislocation, finger
    - proximal end S63.Ø6- ☑
  - metacarpophalangeal (joint)
    - finger S63.26- ☑
      - index S63.26- ☑
      - little S63.26- ☑
      - middle S63.26- ☑
      - ring S63.26- ☑
    - thumb S63.11- ☑
  - metatarsal (bone) — *see* Dislocation, foot
  - metatarsophalangeal (joint(s)) — *see* Dislocation, toe
  - midcarpal (joint) S63.Ø3- ☑
  - midtarsal (joint) — *see* Dislocation, foot
  - neck S13.2Ø ☑
    - specified site NEC S13.29 ☑
    - vertebra — *see* Dislocation, vertebra, cervical
  - nose (septal cartilage) SØ3.1 ☑
  - occipitoatloid S13.111 ☑
  - old — *see* Derangement, joint, specified type NEC
  - ossicles, ear — *see* Discontinuity, ossicles, ear
  - partial — *see* Subluxation, by site
  - patella S83.ØØ6 ☑
    - congenital Q74.1
    - lateral S83.Ø1- ☑
    - recurrent (nontraumatic) M22.Ø- ☑
      - incomplete M22.1- ☑
    - specified type NEC S83.Ø9- ☑
  - pathological NEC M24.3Ø
    - ankle M24.37- ☑
    - elbow M24.32- ☑
    - foot joint M24.37- ☑
    - hand joint M24.34- ☑
    - hip M24.35- ☑
    - knee M24.36- ☑
    - lumbosacral joint — *see* subcategory M53.2 ☑
    - pelvic region — *see* Dislocation, pathological, hip
    - sacroiliac — *see* subcategory M53.2 ☑
    - shoulder M24.31- ☑
    - wrist M24.33- ☑
  - pelvis NEC S33.3Ø ☑
    - specified NEC S33.39 ☑
  - phalanx
    - finger or hand — *see* Dislocation, finger
    - foot or toe — *see* Dislocation, toe
  - prosthesis, internal — *see* Complications, prosthetic device, by site, mechanical
  - radial head S53.ØØ6 ☑
    - anterior S53.Ø1- ☑
    - posterior S53.Ø2- ☑
    - specified type NEC S53.Ø9- ☑
  - radiocarpal (joint) S63.Ø2- ☑
  - radiohumeral (joint) — *see* Dislocation, radial head

- **Dislocation** — *continued*
  - radioulnar (joint)
    - distal S63.Ø1- ☑
    - proximal — *see* Dislocation, elbow
  - radius
    - distal end — *see* Dislocation, wrist
    - proximal end — *see* Dislocation, radial head
  - recurrent M24.4Ø
    - ankle M24.47- ☑
    - elbow M24.42- ☑
    - finger M24.44- ☑
    - foot joint M24.47- ☑
    - hand joint M24.44- ☑
    - hip M24.45- ☑
    - knee M24.46- ☑
      - patella — *see* Dislocation, patella, recurrent
    - patella — *see* Dislocation, patella, recurrent
    - sacroiliac — *see* subcategory M53.2 ☑
    - shoulder M24.41- ☑
    - toe M24.47- ☑
    - vertebra (*see also* subcategory) M43.5 ☑
      - atlantoaxial M43.4
        - with myelopathy M43.3
    - wrist M24.43- ☑
  - rib (cartilage) S23.29 ☑
  - sacrococcygeal S33.2 ☑
  - sacroiliac (joint) (ligament) S33.2 ☑
    - congenital Q74.2
    - recurrent — *see* subcategory M53.2 ☑
  - sacrum S33.2 ☑
  - scaphoid (bone) (hand) (wrist) — *see* Dislocation, wrist
    - foot — *see* Dislocation, foot
  - scapula — *see* Dislocation, shoulder, girdle, scapula
  - semilunar cartilage, knee — *see* Tear, meniscus
  - septal cartilage (nose) SØ3.1 ☑
  - septum (nasal) (old) J34.2
  - sesamoid bone — *code by* site under Dislocation
  - shoulder (blade) (ligament) (joint) (traumatic) S43.ØØ6 ☑
    - acromioclavicular — *see* Dislocation, acromioclavicular
    - chronic — *see* Dislocation, recurrent, shoulder
    - congenital Q68.8
    - girdle S43.3Ø- ☑
      - scapula S43.31- ☑
      - specified site NEC S43.39- ☑
    - humerus S43.ØØ- ☑
      - anterior S43.Ø1- ☑
      - inferior S43.Ø3- ☑
      - posterior S43.Ø2- ☑
    - pathological — *see* Dislocation, pathological NEC, shoulder
    - recurrent — *see* Dislocation, recurrent, shoulder
    - specified type NEC S43.Ø8- ☑
  - spine
    - cervical — *see* Dislocation, vertebra, cervical
    - congenital Q76.49
    - due to birth trauma P11.5
    - lumbar — *see* Dislocation, vertebra, lumbar
    - thoracic — *see* Dislocation, vertebra, thoracic
  - spontaneous — *see* Dislocation, pathological
  - sternoclavicular (joint) S43.2Ø6 ☑
    - anterior S43.21- ☑
    - posterior S43.22- ☑
  - sternum S23.29 ☑
  - subglenoid — *see* Dislocation, shoulder
  - symphysis pubis S33.4 ☑
  - talus — *see* Dislocation, ankle
  - tarsal (bone(s)) (joint(s)) — *see* Dislocation, foot
  - tarsometatarsal (joint(s)) — *see* Dislocation, foot
  - temporomandibular (joint) SØ3.Ø ☑
  - thigh, proximal end — *see* Dislocation, hip
  - thorax S23.2Ø ☑
    - specified site NEC S23.29 ☑
    - vertebra — *see* Dislocation, vertebra
  - thumb S63.1Ø- ☑
    - interphalangeal joint — *see* Dislocation, interphalangeal (joint), thumb
    - metacarpophalangeal joint — *see* Dislocation, metacarpophalangeal (joint), thumb
  - thyroid cartilage S13.29 ☑
  - tibia
    - distal end — *see* Dislocation, ankle
    - proximal end — *see* Dislocation, knee
  - tibiofibular (joint)
    - distal — *see* Dislocation, ankle

- **Dislocation** — *continued*
  - tibiofibular — *continued*
    - superior — *see* Dislocation, knee
  - toe(s) S93.1Ø6 ☑
    - great S93.1Ø- ☑
      - interphalangeal joint S93.11- ☑
      - metatarsophalangeal joint S93.12- ☑
    - interphalangeal joint S93.119 ☑
    - lesser S93.1Ø6 ☑
      - interphalangeal joint S93.11- ☑
      - metatarsophalangeal joint S93.12- ☑
    - metatarsophalangeal joint S93.12- ☑
  - tooth SØ3.2 ☑
  - trachea S23.29 ☑
  - ulna
    - distal end S63.Ø7- ☑
    - proximal end — *see* Dislocation, elbow
  - ulnohumeral (joint) — *see* Dislocation, elbow
  - vertebra (articular process) (body) (traumatic)
    - cervical S13.1Ø1 ☑
      - atlantoaxial joint S13.121 ☑
      - atlantooccipital joint S13.111 ☑
      - atloidooccipital joint S13.111 ☑
      - joint between
        - CØ and C1 S13.111 ☑
        - C1 and C2 S13.121 ☑
        - C2 and C3 S13.131 ☑
        - C3 and C4 S13.141 ☑
        - C4 and C5 S13.151 ☑
        - C5 and C6 S13.161 ☑
        - C6 and C7 S13.171 ☑
        - C7 and T1 S13.181 ☑
      - occipitoatloid joint S13.111 ☑
    - congenital Q76.49
    - lumbar S33.1Ø1 ☑
      - joint between
        - L1 and L2 S33.111 ☑
        - L2 and L3 S33.121 ☑
        - L3 and L4 S33.131 ☑
        - L4 and L5 S33.141 ☑
    - nontraumatic — *see* Displacement, intervertebral disc
    - partial — *see* Subluxation, by site
    - recurrent NEC — *see* subcategory M43.5 ☑
    - thoracic S23.1Ø1 ☑
      - joint between
        - T1 and T2 S23.111 ☑
        - T2 and T3 S23.121 ☑
        - T3 and T4 S23.123 ☑
        - T4 and T5 S23.131 ☑
        - T5 and T6 S23.133 ☑
        - T6 and T7 S23.141 ☑
        - T7 and T8 S23.143 ☑
        - T8 and T9 S23.151 ☑
        - T9 and T1Ø S23.153 ☑
        - T1Ø and T11 S23.161 ☑
        - T11 and T12 S23.163 ☑
        - T12 and L1 S23.171 ☑
  - wrist (carpal bone) S63.ØØ6 ☑
    - carpometacarpal joint — *see* Dislocation, carpometacarpal (joint)
    - distal radioulnar joint — *see* Dislocation, radioulnar (joint), distal
    - metacarpal bone, proximal — *see* Dislocation, metacarpal (bone), proximal end
    - midcarpal — *see* Dislocation, midcarpal (joint)
    - radiocarpal joint — *see* Dislocation, radiocarpal (joint)
    - recurrent — *see* Dislocation, recurrent, wrist
    - specified site NEC S63.Ø9- ☑
    - ulna — *see* Dislocation, ulna, distal end
  - xiphoid cartilage S23.29 ☑
- **Disorder** (of) (*see also* Disease)
  - acantholytic L11.9
    - specified NEC L11.8
  - acute
    - psychotic — *see* Psychosis, acute
    - stress F43.Ø
  - adjustment (grief) F43.2Ø
    - with
      - anxiety F43.22
        - with depressed mood F43.23
      - conduct disturbance F43.24
        - with emotional disturbance F43.25
      - depressed mood F43.21
        - with anxiety F43.23

- **Disorder** — *continued*
  - adjustment — *continued*
    - with — *continued*
      - other specified symptom F43.29
  - adrenal (capsule) (gland) (medullary) E27.9
    - specified NEC E27.8
  - adrenogenital E25.9
    - drug-induced E25.8
    - iatrogenic E25.8
    - idiopathic E25.8
  - adult personality (and behavior) F69
    - specified NEC F68.8
  - affective (mood) — *see* Disorder, mood
  - aggressive, unsocialized F91.1
  - alcohol-related F10.99
    - with
      - amnestic disorder, persisting F10.96
      - anxiety disorder F10.980
      - dementia, persisting F10.97
      - intoxication F10.929
        - with delirium F10.921
        - uncomplicated F10.920
      - mood disorder F10.94
      - other specified F10.988
      - psychotic disorder F10.959
        - with
          - delusions F10.950
          - hallucinations F10.951
      - sexual dysfunction F10.981
      - sleep disorder F10.982
  - allergic — *see* Allergy
  - alveolar NEC J84.09
  - amino-acid
    - cystathioninuria E72.19
    - cystinosis E72.04
    - cystinuria E72.01
    - glycinuria E72.09
    - homocystinuria E72.11
    - metabolism — *see* Disturbance, metabolism, amino-acid
      - specified NEC E72.8
    - neonatal, transitory P74.8
    - renal transport NEC E72.09
    - transport NEC E72.09
  - amnesic, amnestic
    - alcohol-induced F10.96
      - with dependence F10.26
    - due to (secondary to) general medical condition F04
    - psychoactive NEC-induced F19.96
      - with
        - abuse F19.16
        - dependence F19.26
    - sedative, hypnotic or anxiolytic-induced F13.96
      - with dependence F13.26
  - anaerobic glycolysis with anemia D55.2
  - anxiety F41.9
    - due to (secondary to)
      - alcohol F10.980
      - amphetamine F15.980
        - in
          - abuse F15.180
          - dependence F15.280
      - anxiolytic F13.980
        - in
          - abuse F13.180
          - dependence F13.280
      - caffeine F15.980
        - in
          - abuse F15.180
          - dependence F15.280
      - cannabis F12.980
        - in
          - abuse F12.180
          - dependence F12.280
      - cocaine F14.980
        - in
          - abuse F14.180
          - dependence F14.180
      - general medical condition F06.4
      - hallucinogen F16.980
        - in
          - abuse F16.180
          - dependence F16.280
      - hypnotic F13.980
        - in
          - abuse F13.180
          - dependence F13.280

- **Disorder** — *continued*
  - anxiety — *continued*
    - due to — *continued*
      - inhalant F18.980
        - in
          - abuse F18.180
          - dependence F18.280
      - phencyclidine F16.980
        - in
          - abuse F16.180
          - dependence F16.280
      - psychoactive substance NEC F19.980
        - in
          - abuse F19.180
          - dependence F19.280
      - sedative F13.980
        - in
          - abuse F13.180
          - dependence F13.280
      - volatile solvents F18.980
        - in
          - abuse F18.180
          - dependence F18.280
    - generalized F41.1
    - mixed
      - with depression (mild) F41.8
      - specified NEC F41.3
    - organic F06.4
    - phobic F40.9
      - of childhood F40.8
    - specified NEC F41.8
  - aortic valve — *see* Endocarditis, aortic
  - aromatic amino-acid metabolism E70.9
    - specified NEC E70.8
  - arteriole NEC I77.89
  - artery NEC I77.89
  - articulation — *see* Disorder, joint
  - attachment (childhood)
    - disinhibited F94.2
    - reactive F94.1
  - attention-deficit hyperactivity (adolescent) (adult) (child) F90.9
    - combined type F90.2
    - hyperactive type F90.1
    - inattentive type F90.0
    - specified type NEC F90.8
  - attention-deficit without hyperactivity (adolescent) (adult) (child) F90.0
  - auditory processing (central) H93.25
  - autistic F84.0
  - autonomic nervous system G90.9
    - specified NEC G90.8
  - avoidant, child or adolescent F40.10
  - balance
    - acid-base E87.8
      - mixed E87.4
    - electrolyte E87.8
    - fluid NEC E87.8
  - behavioral (disruptive) — *see* Disorder, conduct
  - beta-amino-acid metabolism E72.8
  - bile acid and cholesterol metabolism E78.70
    - Barth syndrome E78.71
    - other specified E78.79
    - Smith-Lemli-Opitz syndrome E78.72
  - bilirubin excretion E80.6
  - binocular
    - movement H51.9
      - convergence
        - excess H51.12
        - insufficiency H51.11
      - internuclear ophthalmoplegia — *see* Ophthalmoplegia, internuclear
      - palsy of conjugate gaze H51.0
      - specified type NEC H51.8
    - vision NEC — *see* Disorder, vision, binocular
  - bipolar (I) F31.9
    - current episode
      - depressed F31.9
        - with psychotic features F31.5
        - without psychotic features F31.30
          - mild F31.31
          - moderate F31.32
          - severe (without psychotic features) F31.4
            - with psychotic features F31.5
      - hypomanic F31.0
      - manic F31.9
        - with psychotic features F31.2
        - without psychotic features F31.10

- **Disorder** — *continued*
  - bipolar — *continued*
    - current episode — *continued*
      - manic — *continued*
        - without psychotic features — *continued*
          - mild F31.11
          - moderate F31.12
          - severe (without psychotic features) F31.13
            - with psychotic features F31.2
      - mixed F31.60
        - mild F31.61
        - moderate F31.62
        - severe (without psychotic features) F31.63
          - with psychotic features F31.64
      - severe depression (without psychotic features) F31.4
        - with psychotic features F31.5
    - in remission (currently) F31.70
      - in full remission
        - most recent episode
          - depressed F31.76
          - hypomanic F31.72
          - manic F31.74
          - mixed F31.78
      - in partial remission
        - most recent episode
          - depressed F31.75
          - hypomanic F31.71
          - manic F31.73
          - mixed F31.77
    - organic F06.30
    - single manic episode F30.9
      - mild F30.11
      - moderate F30.12
      - severe (without psychotic symptoms) F30.13
        - with psychotic symptoms F30.2
    - specified NEC F31.89
  - bipolar II F31.81
  - bladder N32.9
    - functional NEC N31.9
    - in schistosomiasis B65.0 [N33]
    - specified NEC N32.89
  - bleeding D68.9
  - blood D75.9
    - in congenital early syphilis A50.09 [D77]
  - body dysmorphic F45.22
  - bone M89.9
    - continuity M84.9
      - specified type NEC M84.80
        - ankle M84.87- ☑
        - fibula M84.86- ☑
        - foot M84.87- ☑
        - hand M84.84- ☑
        - humerus M84.82- ☑
        - neck M84.88
        - pelvis M84.859
        - radius M84.83- ☑
        - rib M84.88
        - shoulder M84.81- ☑
        - skull M84.88
        - thigh M84.85- ☑
        - tibia M84.86- ☑
        - ulna M84.83- ☑
        - vertebra M84.88
    - density and structure M85.9
      - cyst (*see also* Cyst, bone, specified type NEC)
        - aneurysmal — *see* Cyst, bone, aneurysmal
        - solitary — *see* Cyst, bone, solitary
      - diffuse idiopathic skeletal hyperostosis — *see* Hyperostosis, ankylosing
      - fibrous dysplasia (monostotic) — *see* Dysplasia, fibrous, bone
      - fluorosis — *see* Fluorosis, skeletal
      - hyperostosis of skull M85.2
      - osteitis condensans — *see* Osteitis, condensans
      - specified type NEC M85.8- ☑
        - ankle M85.87- ☑
        - foot M85.87- ☑
        - forearm M85.83- ☑
        - hand M85.84- ☑
        - lower leg M85.86- ☑
        - multiple sites M85.89
        - neck M85.88
        - rib M85.88
        - shoulder M85.81- ☑
        - skull M85.88
        - thigh M85.85- ☑

Disorder — *continued*
- disc — *continued*
  - cervical — *continued*
    - with — *continued*
      - neuritis, radiculitis or radiculopathy — *continued*
        - C6-C7 M50.12
        - C7-T1 M50.13
        - cervicothoracic region M50.13
        - high cervical region M50.11
        - mid-cervical region M50.12
    - C2-C3 M50.91
    - C3-C4 M50.91
    - C4-C5 M50.92
    - C5-C6 M50.92
    - C6-C7 M50.92
    - C7-T1 M50.93
    - cervicothoracic region M50.93
    - degeneration M50.30
      - C2-C3 M50.31
      - C3-C4 M50.31
      - C4-C5 M50.32
      - C5-C6 M50.32
      - C6-C7 M50.32
      - C7-T1 M50.33
      - cervicothoracic region M50.33
      - high cervical region M50.31
      - mid-cervical region M50.32
    - displacement M50.20
      - C2-C3 M50.21
      - C3-C4 M50.21
      - C4-C5 M50.22
      - C5-C6 M50.22
      - C6-C7 M50.22
      - C7-T1 M50.23
      - cervicothoracic region M50.23
      - high cervical region M50.21
      - mid-cervical region M50.22
    - high cervical region M50.91
    - mid-cervical region M50.92
    - specified type NEC M50.80
      - C2-C3 M50.81
      - C3-C4 M50.81
      - C4-C5 M50.82
      - C5-C6 M50.82
      - C6-C7 M50.82
      - C7-T1 M50.83
      - cervicothoracic region M50.83
      - high cervical region M50.81
      - mid-cervical region M50.82
  - specified NEC
    - lumbar region M51.86
    - lumbosacral region M51.87
    - sacrococcygeal region M53.3
    - thoracic region M51.84
    - thoracolumbar region M51.85
- disinhibited attachment (childhood) F94.2
- disintegrative, childhood NEC F84.3
- disruptive behavior F98.9
- dissocial personality F60.2
- dissociative F44.9
  - affecting
    - motor function F44.4
      - and sensation F44.7
    - sensation F44.6
      - and motor function F44.7
  - brief reactive F43.0
  - due to (secondary to) general medical condition F06.8
  - mixed F44.7
  - organic F06.8
  - other specified NEC F44.89
- double heterozygous sickling — *see* Disease, sickle-cell
- dream anxiety F51.5
- drug induced hemorrhagic D68.32
- drug related F19.99
  - abuse — *see* Abuse, drug
  - dependence — *see* Dependence, drug
- dysmorphic body F45.1
- dysthymic F34.1
- ear H93.9- ☑
  - bleeding — *see* Otorrhagia
  - deafness — *see* Deafness
  - degenerative H93.09- ☑
  - discharge — *see* Otorrhea
  - external H61.9- ☑

Disorder — *continued*
- ear — *continued*
  - external — *continued*
    - auditory canal stenosis — *see* Stenosis, external ear canal
    - exostosis — *see* Exostosis, external ear canal
    - impacted cerumen — *see* Impaction, cerumen
    - otitis — *see* Otitis, externa
    - perichondritis — *see* Perichondritis, ear
    - pinna — *see* Disorder, pinna
    - specified type NEC H61.89- ☑
  - inner H83.9- ☑
    - vestibular dysfunction — *see* Disorder, vestibular function
  - middle H74.9- ☑
    - adhesive H74.1- ☑
    - ossicle — *see* Abnormal, ear ossicles
    - polyp — *see* Polyp, ear (middle)
    - specified NEC, in diseases classified elsewhere H75.8- ☑
  - postprocedural — *see* Complications, ear, procedure
  - specified NEC, in diseases classified elsewhere H94.8- ☑
- eating (adult) (psychogenic) F50.9
  - anorexia — *see* Anorexia
  - bulimia F50.2
  - child F98.29
    - pica F98.3
    - rumination disorder F98.21
  - pica F50.8
    - childhood F98.3
- electrolyte (balance) NEC E87.8
  - with
    - abortion — *see* Abortion by type complicated by specified condition NEC
    - ectopic pregnancy O08.5
    - molar pregnancy O08.5
  - acidosis (metabolic) (respiratory) E87.2
  - alkalosis (metabolic) (respiratory) E87.3
- elimination, transepidermal L87.9
  - specified NEC L87.8
- emotional (persistent) F34.9
  - of childhood F93.9
    - specified NEC F93.8
- endocrine E34.9
  - postprocedural E89.89
    - specified NEC E89.89
- erectile (male) (organic) (*see also* Dysfunction, sexual, male, erectile) N52.9
  - nonorganic F52.21
- erythematous — *see* Erythema
- esophagus K22.9
  - functional K22.4
  - psychogenic F45.8
- eustachian tube H69.9- ☑
  - infection — *see* Salpingitis, eustachian
  - obstruction — *see* Obstruction, eustachian tube
  - patulous — *see* Patulous, eustachian tube
  - specified NEC H69.8- ☑
- extrapyramidal G25.9
  - in deseases classified elsewhere — *see* category G26
  - specified type NEC G25.89
- eye H57.9
  - postprocedural — *see* Complication, postprocedural, eye
- eyelid H02.9
  - cyst — *see* Cyst, eyelid
  - degenerative H02.70
    - chloasma — *see* Chloasma, eyelid
    - madarosis — *see* Madarosis
    - specified type NEC H02.79
    - vitiligo — *see* Vitiligo, eyelid
    - xanthelasma — *see* Xanthelasma
  - dermatochalasis — *see* Dermatochalasis
  - edema — *see* Edema, eyelid
  - elephantiasis — *see* Elephantiasis, eyelid
  - foreign body, retained — *see* Foreign body, retained, eyelid
  - function H02.59
    - abnormal innervation syndrome — *see* Syndrome, abnormal innervation
    - blepharochalasis — *see* Blepharochalasis
    - blepharoclonus — *see* Blepharoclonus
    - blepharophimosis — *see* Blepharophimosis
    - blepharoptosis — *see* Blepharoptosis

Disorder — *continued*
- eyelid — *continued*
  - function — *continued*
    - lagophthalmos — *see* Lagophthalmos
    - lid retraction — *see* Retraction, lid
  - hypertrichosis — *see* Hypertrichosis, eyelid
  - specified type NEC H02.89
  - vascular H02.879
    - left H02.876
      - lower H02.875
      - upper H02.874
    - right H02.873
      - lower H02.872
      - upper H02.871
- factitious F68.10
  - with predominantly
    - physical symptoms F68.12
      - with psychological symptoms F68.13
    - psychological symptoms F68.11
      - with physical symptoms F68.13
- factor, coagulation — *see* Defect, coagulation
- fatty acid
  - metabolism E71.30
    - specified NEC E71.39
  - oxidation
    - LCAD E71.310
    - MCAD E71.311
    - SCAD E71.312
    - specified deficiency NEC E71.318
- feeding (infant or child) (*see also* Disorder, eating) R63.3
- feigned (with obvious motivation) Z76.5
  - without obvious motivation — *see* Disorder, factitious
- female
  - hypoactive sexual desire F52.0
  - orgasmic F52.31
  - sexual arousal F52.22
- fibroblastic M72.9
  - specified NEC M72.8
- fluency
  - adult onset F98.5
  - childhood onset F80.81
  - following
    - cerebral infarction I69.323
    - cerebrovascular disease I69.923
      - specified disease NEC I69.823
    - intracerebral hemorrhage I69.123
    - nontraumatic intracranial hemorrhage NEC I69.223
    - subarachnoid hemorrhage I69.023
  - in conditions classified elsewhere R47.82
- fluid balance E87.8
- follicular (skin) L73.9
  - specified NEC L73.8
- fructose metabolism E74.10
  - essential fructosuria E74.11
  - fructokinase deficiency E74.11
  - fructose-1, 6-diphosphatase deficiency E74.19
  - hereditary fructose intolerance E74.12
  - other specified E74.19
- functional polymorphonuclear neutrophils D71
- gallbladder, biliary tract and pancreas in diseases classified elsewhere K87
- gamma-glutamyl cycle E72.8
- gastric (functional) K31.9
  - motility K30
  - psychogenic F45.8
  - secretion K30
- gastrointestinal (functional) NOS K92.9
  - newborn P78.9
  - psychogenic F45.8
- gender-identity or -role F64.9
  - childhood F64.2
  - effect on relationship F66
  - of adolescence or adulthood (nontranssexual) F64.1
  - specified NEC F64.8
  - uncertainty F66
- genitourinary system
  - female N94.9
  - male N50.9
  - psychogenic F45.8
- globe H44.9
  - degenerated condition H44.50
    - absolute glaucoma H44.51- ☑
    - atrophy H44.52- ☑
    - leucocoria H44.53- ☑
  - degenerative H44.30

- **Disorder** — *continued*
  - muscle M62.9
    - attachment, spine — *see* Enthesopathy, spinal
    - in trichinellosis — *see* Trichinellosis, with muscle disorder
    - psychogenic F45.8
    - specified type NEC M62.89
    - tone, newborn P94.9
      - specified NEC P94.8
  - muscular
    - attachments (*see also* Enthesopathy)
      - spine — *see* Enthesopathy, spinal
    - urethra N36.44
  - musculoskeletal system, soft tissue — *see* Disorder, soft tissue
    - postprocedural M96.89
    - psychogenic F45.8
  - myoneural G7Ø.9
    - due to lead G7Ø.1
    - specified NEC G7Ø.89
    - toxic G7Ø.1
  - myotonic NEC G71.19
  - nail, in diseases classified elsewhere L62
  - neck region NEC — *see* Dorsopathy, specified NEC
  - nerve G58.9
    - abducent NEC — *see* Strabismus, paralytic, sixth nerve
    - accessory G52.8
    - acoustic — *see* subcategory H93.3 ☑
    - auditory — *see* subcategory H93.3 ☑
    - auriculotemporal G5Ø.8
    - axillary G54.Ø
    - cerebral — *see* Disorder, nerve, cranial
    - cranial G52.9
      - eighth — *see* subcategory H93.3 ☑
      - eleventh G52.8
      - fifth G5Ø.9
      - first G52.Ø
      - fourth NEC — *see* Strabismus, paralytic, fourth nerve
      - multiple G52.7
      - ninth G52.1
      - second NEC — *see* Disorder, nerve, optic
      - seventh NEC G51.8
      - sixth NEC — *see* Strabismus, paralytic, sixth nerve
      - specified NEC G52.8
      - tenth G52.2
      - third NEC — *see* Strabismus, paralytic, third nerve
      - twelfth G52.3
    - entrapment — *see* Neuropathy, entrapment
    - facial G51.9
      - specified NEC G51.8
    - femoral — *see* Lesion, nerve, femoral
    - glossopharyngeal NEC G52.1
    - hypoglossal G52.3
    - intercostal G58.Ø
    - lateral
      - cutaneous of thigh — *see* Mononeuropathy, lower limb, meralgia paresthetica
      - popliteal — *see* Lesion, nerve, popliteal
    - lower limb — *see* Mononeuropathy, lower limb
    - medial popliteal — *see* Lesion, nerve, popliteal, medial
    - median NEC — *see* Lesion, nerve, median
    - multiple G58.7
    - oculomotor NEC — *see* Strabismus, paralytic, third nerve
    - olfactory G52.Ø
    - optic NEC H47.Ø9- ☑
      - hemorrhage into sheath — *see* Hemorrhage, optic nerve
      - ischemic H47.Ø1- ☑
    - peroneal — *see* Lesion, nerve, popliteal
    - phrenic G58.8
    - plantar — *see* Lesion, nerve, plantar
    - pneumogastric G52.2
    - posterior tibial — *see* Syndrome, tarsal tunnel
    - radial — *see* Lesion, nerve, radial
    - recurrent laryngeal G52.2
    - root G54.9
      - cervical G54.2
      - lumbosacral G54.1
      - specified NEC G54.8
      - thoracic G54.3
    - sciatic NEC — *see* Lesion, nerve, sciatic

- **Disorder** — *continued*
  - nerve — *continued*
    - specified NEC G58.8
      - lower limb — *see* Mononeuropathy, lower limb, specified NEC
      - upper limb — *see* Mononeuropathy, upper limb, specified NEC
    - sympathetic G9Ø.9
    - tibial — *see* Lesion, nerve, popliteal, medial
    - trigeminal G5Ø.9
      - specified NEC G5Ø.8
    - trochlear NEC — *see* Strabismus, paralytic, fourth nerve
    - ulnar — *see* Lesion, nerve, ulnar
    - upper limb — *see* Mononeuropathy, upper limb
    - vagus G52.2
  - nervous system G98.8
    - autonomic (peripheral) G9Ø.9
      - specified NEC G9Ø.8
    - central G96.9
      - specified NEC G96.8
    - parasympathetic G9Ø.9
    - specified NEC G98.8
    - sympathetic G9Ø.9
    - vegetative G9Ø.9
  - neurohypophysis NEC E23.3
  - neurological NEC R29.818
  - neuromuscular G7Ø.9
    - hereditary NEC G71.9
    - specified NEC G7Ø.89
    - toxic G7Ø.1
  - neurotic F48.9
    - specified NEC F48.8
  - neutrophil, polymorphonuclear D71
  - nicotine use — *see* Dependence, drug, nicotine
  - nightmare F51.5
  - nose J34.9
    - specified NEC J34.89
  - obsessive-compulsive F42
  - odontogenesis NOS KØØ.9
  - opioid use
    - with
      - opioid-induced psychotic disorder F11.959
        - with
          - delusions F11.95Ø
          - hallucinations F11.951
    - due to drug abuse — *see* Abuse, drug, opioid
    - due to drug dependence — *see* Dependence, drug, opioid
  - oppositional defiant F91.3
  - optic
    - chiasm H47.49
      - due to
        - inflammatory disorder H47.41
        - neoplasm H47.42
        - vascular disorder H47.43
    - disc H47.39- ☑
      - coloboma — *see* Coloboma, optic disc
      - drusen — *see* Drusen, optic disc
      - pseudopapilledema — *see* Pseudopapilledema
    - radiations — *see* Disorder, visual, pathway
    - tracts — *see* Disorder, visual, pathway
  - orbit HØ5.9
    - cyst — *see* Cyst, orbit
    - deformity — *see* Deformity, orbit
    - edema — *see* Edema, orbit
    - enophthalmos — *see* Enophthalmos
    - exophthalmos — *see* Exophthalmos
    - hemorrhage — *see* Hemorrhage, orbit
    - inflammation — *see* Inflammation, orbit
    - myopathy — *see* Myopathy, extraocular muscles
    - retained foreign body — *see* Foreign body, orbit, old
    - specified type NEC HØ5.89
  - organic
    - anxiety FØ6.4
    - catatonic FØ6.1
    - delusional FØ6.2
    - dissociative FØ6.8
    - emotionally labile (asthenic) FØ6.8
    - mood (affective) FØ6.3Ø
    - schizophrenia-like FØ6.2
  - orgasmic (female) F52.31
    - male F52.32
  - ornithine metabolism E72.4
  - overanxious F41.1
    - of childhood F93.8

- **Disorder** — *continued*
  - pain
    - with related psychological factors F45.42
    - exclusively related to psychological factors F45.41
  - pancreatic internal secretion E16.9
    - specified NEC E16.8
  - panic F41.Ø
    - with agoraphobia F4Ø.Ø1
  - papulosquamous L44.9
    - in diseases classified elsewhere L45
    - specified NEC L44.8
  - paranoid F22
    - induced F24
    - shared F24
  - parathyroid (gland) E21.5
    - specified NEC E21.4
  - parietoalveolar NEC J84.Ø9
  - paroxysmal, mixed R56.9
  - patella M22.9- ☑
    - chondromalacia — *see* Chondromalacia, patella
    - derangement NEC M22.3X- ☑
    - recurrent
      - dislocation — *see* Dislocation, patella, recurrent
      - subluxation — *see* Dislocation, patella, recurrent, incomplete
    - specified NEC M22.8X- ☑
  - patellofemoral M22.2X- ☑
  - pentose phosphate pathway with anemia D55.1
  - perception, due to hallucinogens F16.983
    - in
      - abuse F16.183
      - dependence F16.283
  - peripheral nervous system NEC G64
  - peroxisomal E71.5Ø
    - biogenesis
      - neonatal adrenoleukodystrophy E71.511
      - specified disorder NEC E71.518
      - Zellweger syndrome E71.51Ø
    - rhizomelic chondrodysplasia punctata E71.54Ø
    - specified form NEC E71.548
      - group 1 E71.518
      - group 2 E71.53
      - group 3 E71.542
    - X-linked adrenoleukodystrophy E71.529
      - adolescent E71.521
      - adrenomyeloneuropathy E71.522
      - childhood E71.52Ø
      - specified form NEC E71.528
    - Zellweger-like syndrome E71.541
  - persistent
    - (somatoform) pain F45.41
    - affective (mood) F34.9
  - personality (*see also* Personality) F6Ø.9
    - affective F34.Ø
    - aggressive F6Ø.3
    - amoral F6Ø.2
    - anankastic F6Ø.5
    - antisocial F6Ø.2
    - anxious F6Ø.6
    - asocial F6Ø.2
    - asthenic F6Ø.7
    - avoidant F6Ø.6
    - borderline F6Ø.3
    - change (secondary) due to general medical condition FØ7.Ø
    - compulsive F6Ø.5
    - cyclothymic F34.Ø
    - dependent (passive) F6Ø.7
    - depressive F34.1
    - dissocial F6Ø.2
    - emotional instability F6Ø.3
    - expansive paranoid F6Ø.Ø
    - explosive F6Ø.3
    - following organic brain damage FØ7.9
    - histrionic F6Ø.4
    - hyperthymic F34.Ø
    - hypothymic F34.1
    - hysterical F6Ø.4
    - immature F6Ø.89
    - inadequate F6Ø.7
    - labile F6Ø.3
    - mixed (nonspecific) F6Ø.89
    - moral deficiency F6Ø.2
    - narcissistic F6Ø.81
    - negativistic F6Ø.89
    - obsessional F6Ø.5
    - obsessive (-compulsive) F6Ø.5
    - organic FØ7.9

- **Disorder** — *continued*
  - personality (*see also* Personality) — *continued*
    - overconscientious F6Ø.5
    - paranoid F6Ø.Ø
    - passive (-dependent) F6Ø.7
    - passive-aggressive F6Ø.89
    - pathological NEC F6Ø.9
    - pseudosocial F6Ø.2
    - psychopathic F6Ø.2
    - schizoid F6Ø.1
    - schizotypal F21
    - self-defeating F6Ø.7
    - specified NEC F6Ø.89
    - type A F6Ø.5
    - unstable (emotional) F6Ø.3
  - pervasive, developmental F84.9
  - phobic anxiety, childhood F4Ø.8
  - phosphate-losing tubular N25.Ø
  - pigmentation L81.9
    - choroid, congenital Q14.3
    - diminished melanin formation L81.6
    - iron L81.8
    - specified NEC L81.8
  - pinna (noninfective) H61.1Ø- ☑
    - deformity, acquired H61.11- ☑
    - hematoma H61.12- ☑
    - perichondritis — *see* Perichondritis, ear
    - specified type NEC H61.19- ☑
  - pituitary gland E23.7
    - iatrogenic (postprocedural) E89.3
    - specified NEC E23.6
  - platelets D69.1
  - plexus G54.9
    - specified NEC G54.8
  - polymorphonuclear neutrophils D71
  - porphyrin metabolism — *see* Porphyria
  - postconcussional FØ7.81
  - posthallucinogen perception F16.983
    - in
      - abuse F16.183
      - dependence F16.283
  - postmenopausal N95.9
    - specified NEC N95.8
  - postprocedural (postoperative) — *see* Complications, postprocedural
  - post-transplant lymphoproliferative D47.Z1 (*following* D47.4)
  - post-traumatic stress (PTSD) F43.1Ø
    - acute F43.11
    - chronic F43.12
  - premenstrual dysphoric (PMDD) N94.3
  - prepuce N47.8
  - propionic acidemia E71.121
  - prostate N42.9
    - specified NEC N42.89
  - psychogenic NOS (*see also* condition) F45.9
    - anxiety F41.8
    - appetite F5Ø.9
    - asthenic F48.8
    - cardiovascular (system) F45.8
    - compulsive F42
    - cutaneous F54
    - depressive F32.9
    - digestive (system) F45.8
    - dysmenorrheic F45.8
    - dyspneic F45.8
    - endocrine (system) F54
    - eye NEC F45.8
    - feeding — *see* Disorder, eating
    - functional NEC F45.8
    - gastric F45.8
    - gastrointestinal (system) F45.8
    - genitourinary (system) F45.8
    - heart (function) (rhythm) F45.8
    - hyperventilatory F45.8
    - hypochondriacal — *see* Disorder, hypochondriacal
    - intestinal F45.8
    - joint F45.8
    - learning F81.9
    - limb F45.8
    - lymphatic (system) F45.8
    - menstrual F45.8
    - micturition F45.8
    - monoplegic NEC F44.4
    - motor F44.4
    - muscle F45.8
    - musculoskeletal F45.8
    - neurocirculatory F45.8

- **Disorder** — *continued*
  - psychogenic (*see also* condition) — *continued*
    - obsessive F42
    - occupational F48.8
    - organ or part of body NEC F45.8
    - paralytic NEC F44.4
    - phobic F4Ø.9
    - physical NEC F45.8
    - rectal F45.8
    - respiratory (system) F45.8
    - rheumatic F45.8
    - sexual (function) F52.9
    - skin (allergic) (eczematous) F54
    - sleep F51.9
    - specified part of body NEC F45.8
    - stomach F45.8
  - psychological F99
    - associated with
      - disease classified elsewhere F54
      - sexual
        - development F66
        - relationship F66
      - uncertainty about gender identity F66
  - psychomotor NEC F44.4
    - hysterical F44.4
  - psychoneurotic (*see also* Neurosis)
    - mixed NEC F48.8
  - psychophysiologic — *see* Disorder, somatoform
  - psychosexual F65.9
    - development F66
    - identity of childhood F64.2
  - psychosomatic NOS — *see* Disorder, somatoform
    - multiple F45.Ø
    - undifferentiated F45.1
  - psychotic — *see* Psychosis
    - transient (acute) F23
  - puberty E3Ø.9
    - specified NEC E3Ø.8
  - pulmonary (valve) — *see* Endocarditis, pulmonary
  - purine metabolism E79.9
  - pyrimidine metabolism E79.9
  - pyruvate metabolism E74.4
  - reactive attachment (childhood) F94.1
  - reading R48.Ø
    - developmental (specific) F81.Ø
  - receptive language F8Ø.2
  - receptor, hormonal, peripheral (*see also* Syndrome, androgen insensitivity) E34.5Ø
  - recurrent brief depressive F33.8
  - reflex R29.2
  - refraction H52.7
    - aniseikonia H52.32
    - anisometropia H52.31
    - astigmatism — *see* Astigmatism
    - hypermetropia — *see* Hypermetropia
    - myopia — *see* Myopia
    - presbyopia H52.4
    - specified NEC H52.6
  - relationship F68.8
    - due to sexual orientation F66
  - REM sleep behavior G47.52
  - renal function, impaired (tubular) N25.9
  - resonance R49.9
    - specified NEC R49.8
  - respiratory function, impaired (*see also* Failure, respiration)
    - postprocedural — *see* Complication, postoperative, respiratory system
    - psychogenic F45.8
  - retina H35.9
    - angioid streaks H35.33
    - changes in vascular appearance H35.Ø1- ☑
    - degeneration — *see* Degeneration, retina
    - dystrophy (hereditary) — *see* Dystrophy, retina
    - edema H35.81
    - hemorrhage — *see* Hemorrhage, retina
    - ischemia H35.82
    - macular degeneration — *see* Degeneration, macula
    - microaneurysms H35.Ø4- ☑
    - microvascular abnormality NEC H35.Ø9
    - neovascularization — *see* Neovascularization, retina
    - retinopathy — *see* Retinopathy
    - separation of layers H35.7Ø
      - central serous chorioretinopathy H35.71- ☑
      - pigment epithelium detachment (serous) H35.72- ☑
        - hemorrhagic H35.73- ☑

- **Disorder** — *continued*
  - retina — *continued*
    - specified type NEC H35.89
    - telangiectasis — *see* Telangiectasis, retina
    - vasculitis — *see* Vasculitis, retina
  - retroperitoneal K68.9
  - right hemisphere organic affective FØ7.89
  - rumination (infant or child) F98.21
  - sacrum, sacrococcygeal NEC M53.3
  - schizoaffective F25.9
    - bipolar type F25.Ø
    - depressive type F25.1
    - manic type F25.Ø
    - mixed type F25.Ø
    - specified NEC F25.8
  - schizoid of childhood F84.5
  - schizophreniform F2Ø.81
    - brief F23
  - schizotypal (personality) F21
  - secretion, thyrocalcitonin EØ7.Ø
  - seizure (*see also* Epilepsy) G4Ø.9Ø9
    - intractable G4Ø.919
      - with status epilepticus G4Ø.911
  - semantic pragmatic F8Ø.89
    - with autism F84.Ø
  - sense of smell R43.1
    - psychogenic F45.8
  - separation anxiety, of childhood F93.Ø
  - sexual
    - arousal, female F52.22
    - aversion F52.1
    - function, psychogenic F52.9
    - maturation F66
    - nonorganic F52.9
    - preference (*see also* Deviation, sexual) F65.9
      - fetishistic transvestism F65.1
    - relationship F66
  - shyness, of childhood and adolescence F4Ø.1Ø
  - sibling rivalry F93.8
  - sickle-cell (sickling) (homozygous) — *see* Disease, sickle-cell
    - heterozygous D57.3
    - specified type NEC D57.8- ☑
    - trait D57.3
  - sinus (nasal) J34.9
    - specified NEC J34.89
  - skin L98.9
    - atrophic L9Ø.9
      - specified NEC L9Ø.8
    - granulomatous L92.9
      - specified NEC L92.8
    - hypertrophic L91.9
      - specified NEC L91.8
    - infiltrative NEC L98.6
    - newborn P83.9
      - specified NEC P83.8
    - psychogenic (allergic) (eczematous) F54
  - sleep G47.9
    - breathing-related — *see* Apnea, sleep
    - circadian rhythm G47.2Ø
      - advance sleep phase type G47.22
      - delayed sleep phase type G47.21
      - due to
        - alcohol
          - abuse F1Ø.182
          - dependence F1Ø.282
          - use F1Ø.982
        - amphetamines
          - abuse F15.182
          - dependence F15.282
          - use F15.982
        - caffeine
          - abuse F15.182
          - dependence F15.282
          - use F15.982
        - cocaine
          - abuse F14.182
          - dependence F14.282
          - use F14.982
        - drug NEC
          - abuse F19.182
          - dependence F19.282
          - use F19.982
        - opioid
          - abuse F11.182
          - dependence F11.282
          - use F11.982

- **Disorder** — *continued*
  - sleep — *continued*
    - circadian rhythm — *continued*
      - due to — *continued*
        - psychoactive substance
          - abuse F19.182
          - dependence F19.282
          - use F19.982
        - sedative, hypnotic, or anxiolytic
          - abuse F13.182
          - dependence F13.282
          - use F13.982
        - stimulant NEC
          - abuse F15.182
          - dependence F15.282
          - use F15.982
      - free running type G47.24
      - in conditions classified elsewhere G47.27
      - irregular sleep wake type G47.23
      - jet lag type G47.25
      - shift work type G47.26
      - specified NEC G47.29
    - due to
      - alcohol
        - abuse F10.182
        - dependence F10.282
        - use F10.982
      - amphetamine
        - abuse F15.182
        - dependence F15.282
        - use F15.982
      - anxiolytic
        - abuse F13.182
        - dependence F13.282
        - use F13.982
      - caffeine
        - abuse F15.182
        - dependence F15.282
        - use F15.982
      - cocaine
        - abuse F14.182
        - dependence F14.282
        - use F14.982
      - drug NEC
        - abuse F19.182
        - dependence F19.282
        - use F19.982
      - hypnotic
        - abuse F13.182
        - dependence F13.282
        - use F13.982
      - opioid
        - abuse F11.182
        - dependence F11.282
        - use F11.982
      - psychoactive substance NEC
        - abuse F19.182
        - dependence F19.282
        - use F19.982
      - sedative
        - abuse F13.182
        - dependence F13.282
        - use F13.982
      - stimulant NEC
        - abuse F15.182
        - dependence F15.282
        - use F15.982
    - emotional F51.9
    - excessive somnolence — *see* Hypersomnia
    - hypersomnia type — *see* Hypersomnia
    - initiating or maintaining — *see* Insomnia
    - nightmares F51.5
    - nonorganic F51.9
      - specified NEC F51.8
    - parasomnia type G47.50
    - specified NEC G47.8
    - terrors F51.4
    - walking F51.3
  - sleep-wake pattern or schedule — *see* Disorder, sleep, circadian rhythm
  - social
    - anxiety of childhood F40.10
    - functioning in childhood F94.9
      - specified NEC F94.8
  - soft tissue M79.9
    - ankle M79.9
    - due to use, overuse and pressure M70.90
      - ankle M70.97- ☑

- **Disorder** — *continued*
  - soft tissue — *continued*
    - due to use, overuse and pressure — *continued*
      - bursitis — *see* Bursitis
      - foot M70.97- ☑
      - forearm M70.93- ☑
      - hand M70.94- ☑
      - lower leg M70.96- ☑
      - multiple sites M70.99
      - pelvic region M70.95- ☑
      - shoulder region M70.91- ☑
      - specified site NEC M70.98
      - specified type NEC M70.80
        - ankle M70.87- ☑
        - foot M70.87- ☑
        - forearm M70.83- ☑
        - hand M70.84- ☑
        - lower leg M70.86- ☑
        - multiple sites M70.89
        - pelvic region M70.85- ☑
        - shoulder region M70.81- ☑
        - specified site NEC M70.88
        - thigh M70.85- ☑
        - upper arm M70.82- ☑
      - thigh M70.95- ☑
      - upper arm M70.92- ☑
    - foot M79.9
    - forearm M79.9
    - hand M79.9
    - lower leg M79.9
    - multiple sites M79.9
    - occupational — *see* Disorder, soft tissue, due to use, overuse and pressure
    - pelvic region M79.9
    - shoulder region M79.9
    - specified type NEC M79.89
    - thigh M79.9
    - upper arm M79.9
  - somatization F45.0
  - somatoform F45.9
    - pain (persistent) F45.41
    - somatization (multiple) (long-lasting) F45.0
    - specified NEC F45.8
    - undifferentiated F45.1
  - somnolence, excessive — *see* Hypersomnia
  - specific
    - arithmetical F81.2
    - developmental, of motor F82
    - reading F81.0
    - speech and language F80.9
    - spelling F81.81
    - written expression F81.81
  - speech R47.9
    - articulation (functional) (specific) F80.0
    - developmental F80.9
    - specified NEC R47.89
  - spelling (specific) F81.81
  - spine (*see also* Dorsopathy)
    - ligamentous or muscular attachments, peripheral — *see* Enthesopathy, spinal
    - specified NEC — *see* Dorsopathy, specified NEC
  - stereotyped, habit or movement F98.4
  - stomach (functional) — *see* Disorder, gastric
  - stress F43.9
    - post-traumatic F43.10
      - acute F43.11
      - chronic F43.12
  - sulfur-bearing amino-acid metabolism E72.10
  - sweat gland (eccrine) L74.9
    - apocrine L75.9
      - specified NEC L75.8
    - specified NEC L74.8
  - synovium M67.90
    - acromioclavicular M67.91- ☑
    - ankle M67.97- ☑
    - elbow M67.92- ☑
    - foot M67.97- ☑
    - forearm M67.93- ☑
    - hand M67.94- ☑
    - hip M67.95- ☑
    - knee M67.96- ☑
    - multiple sites M67.99
    - rupture — *see* Rupture, synovium
    - shoulder M67.91- ☑
    - specified type NEC M67.80
      - acromioclavicular M67.81- ☑
      - ankle M67.87- ☑

- **Disorder** — *continued*
  - synovium — *continued*
    - specified type — *continued*
      - elbow M67.82- ☑
      - foot M67.87- ☑
      - hand M67.84- ☑
      - hip M67.85- ☑
      - knee M67.86- ☑
      - multiple sites M67.89
      - wrist M67.83- ☑
    - synovitis — *see* Synovitis
    - upper arm M67.92- ☑
    - wrist M67.93- ☑
  - temperature regulation, newborn P81.9
    - specified NEC P81.8
  - temporomandibular joint — *see* Anomaly, dentofacial, temporomandibular joint
  - tendon M67.90
    - acromioclavicular M67.91- ☑
    - ankle M67.97- ☑
    - contracture — *see* Contracture, tendon
    - elbow M67.92- ☑
    - foot M67.97- ☑
    - forearm M67.93- ☑
    - hand M67.94- ☑
    - hip M67.95- ☑
    - knee M67.96- ☑
    - multiple sites M67.99
    - rupture — *see* Rupture, tendon
    - shoulder M67.91- ☑
    - specified type NEC M67.80
      - acromioclavicular M67.81- ☑
      - ankle M67.87- ☑
      - elbow M67.82- ☑
      - foot M67.87- ☑
      - hand M67.84- ☑
      - hip M67.85- ☑
      - knee M67.86- ☑
      - multiple sites M67.89
      - trunk M67.88
      - wrist M67.83- ☑
    - synovitis — *see* Synovitis
    - tendinitis — *see* Tendinitis
    - tenosynovitis — *see* Tenosynovitis
    - trunk M67.98
    - upper arm M67.92- ☑
    - wrist M67.93- ☑
  - thoracic root (nerve) NEC G54.3
  - thyrocalcitonin hypersecretion E07.0
  - thyroid (gland) E07.9
    - function NEC, neonatal, transitory P72.2
    - iodine-deficiency related E01.8
    - specified NEC E07.89
  - tic — *see* Tic
  - tooth K08.9
    - development K00.9
      - specified NEC K00.8
    - eruption K00.6
  - Tourette's F95.2
  - trance and possession F44.89
  - tricuspid (valve) — *see* Endocarditis, tricuspid
  - tryptophan metabolism E70.5
  - tubular, phosphate-losing N25.0
  - tubulo-interstitial (in)
    - brucellosis A23.9 [N16]
    - cystinosis E72.04
    - diphtheria A36.84
    - glycogen storage disease E74.00 [N16]
    - leukemia NEC C95.9- ☑ [N16]
    - lymphoma NEC C85.9- ☑ [N16]
    - mixed cryoglobulinemia D89.1 [N16]
    - multiple myeloma C90.0- ☑ [N16]
    - Salmonella infection A02.25
    - sarcoidosis D86.84
    - sepsis A41.9 [N16]
      - streptococcal A40.9 [N16]
    - systemic lupus erythematosus M32.15
    - toxoplasmosis B58.83
    - transplant rejection T86.91 [N16]
    - Wilson's disease E83.01 [N16]
  - tubulo-renal function, impaired N25.9
    - specified NEC N25.89
  - tympanic membrane H73.9- ☑
    - atrophy — *see* Atrophy, tympanic membrane
    - infection — *see* Myringitis
    - perforation — *see* Perforation, tympanum
    - specified NEC H73.89- ☑

- **Disorder** — *continued*
  - unsocialized aggressive F91.1
  - urea cycle metabolism E72.2Ø
    - argininemia E72.21
    - arginosuccinic aciduria E72.22
    - citrullinemia E72.23
    - ornithine transcarbamylase deficiency E72.4
    - other specified E72.29
  - ureter (in) N28.9
    - schistosomiasis B65.Ø [N29]
    - tuberculosis A18.11
  - urethra N36.9
    - specified NEC N36.8
  - urinary system N39.9
    - specified NEC N39.8
  - valve, heart
    - aortic — *see* Endocarditis, aortic
    - mitral — *see* Endocarditis, mitral
    - pulmonary — *see* Endocarditis, pulmonary
    - rheumatic
      - aortic — *see* Endocarditis, aortic, rheumatic
      - mitral — *see* Endocarditis, mitral
      - pulmonary — *see* Endocarditis, pulmonary, rheumatic
      - tricuspid — *see* Endocarditis, tricuspid
    - tricuspid — *see* Endocarditis, tricuspid
  - vestibular function H81.9- ☑
    - specified NEC — *see* subcategory H81.8 ☑
      - in diseases classified elsewhere H82.- ☑
    - vertigo — *see* Vertigo
  - vision, binocular H53.3Ø
    - abnormal retinal correspondence H53.31
    - diplopia H53.2
    - fusion with defective stereopsis H53.32
    - simultaneous perception H53.33
    - suppression H53.34
  - visual
    - cortex
      - blindness H47.619
        - left brain H47.612
        - right brain H47.611
      - due to
        - inflammatory disorder H47.629
          - left brain H47.622
          - right brain H47.621
        - neoplasm H47.639
          - left brain H47.632
          - right brain H47.631
        - vascular disorder H47.649
          - left brain H47.642
          - right brain H47.641
    - pathway H47.9
      - due to
        - inflammatory disorder H47.51- ☑
        - neoplasm H47.52- ☑
        - vascular disorder H47.53- ☑
      - optic chiasm — *see* Disorder, optic, chiasm
  - vitreous body H43.9
    - crystalline deposits — *see* Deposit, crystalline
    - degeneration — *see* Degeneration, vitreous
    - hemorrhage — *see* Hemorrhage, vitreous
    - opacities — *see* Opacity, vitreous
    - prolapse — *see* Prolapse, vitreous
    - specified type NEC H43.89
  - voice R49.9
    - specified type NEC R49.8
  - volatile solvent use
    - due to drug abuse — *see* Abuse, drug, inhalant
    - due to drug dependence — *see* Dependence, drug, inhalant
  - white blood cells D72.9
    - specified NEC D72.89
  - withdrawing, child or adolescent F4Ø.1Ø
- **Disorientation** R41.Ø
- **Displacement, displaced**
  - acquired traumatic of bone, cartilage, joint, tendon NEC — *see* Dislocation
  - adrenal gland (congenital) Q89.1
  - appendix, retrocecal (congenital) Q43.8
  - auricle (congenital) Q17.4
  - bladder (acquired) N32.89
    - congenital Q64.19
  - brachial plexus (congenital) QØ7.8
  - brain stem, caudal (congenital) QØ4.8
  - canaliculus (lacrimalis), congenital Q1Ø.6
  - cardia through esophageal hiatus (congenital) Q4Ø.1
  - cerebellum, caudal (congenital) QØ4.8
  - cervix — *see* Malposition, uterus

- **Displacement, displaced** — *continued*
  - colon (congenital) Q43.3
  - device, implant or graft (*see also* Complications, by site and type, mechanical) T85.628 ☑
    - arterial graft NEC — *see* Complication, cardiovascular device, mechanical, vascular
    - breast (implant) T85.42 ☑
    - catheter NEC T85.628 ☑
      - dialysis (renal) T82.42 ☑
        - intraperitoneal T85.621 ☑
      - infusion NEC T82.524 ☑
        - spinal (epidural) (subdural) T85.62Ø ☑
      - urinary (indwelling) T83.Ø28 ☑
        - cystostomy T83.Ø2Ø ☑
    - electronic (electrode) (pulse generator) (stimulator) — *see* Complication, electronic stimulator
    - fixation, internal (orthopedic) NEC — *see* Complication, fixation device, mechanical
    - gastrointestinal — *see* Complications, prosthetic device, mechanical, gastrointestinal device
    - genital NEC T83.428 ☑
      - intrauterine contraceptive device T83.32 ☑
      - penile prosthesis T83.42Ø ☑
    - heart NEC — *see* Complication, cardiovascular device, mechanical
    - joint prosthesis — *see* Complications, joint prosthesis, mechanical
    - ocular — *see* Complications, prosthetic device, mechanical, ocular device
    - orthopedic NEC — *see* Complication, orthopedic, device or graft, mechanical
    - specified NEC T85.628 ☑
    - urinary NEC (*see also* Complication, genitourinary, device, urinary, mechanical)
      - graft T83.22 ☑
    - vascular NEC — *see* Complication, cardiovascular device, mechanical
    - ventricular intracranial shunt T85.Ø2 ☑
  - electronic stimulator
    - bone T84.32Ø ☑
    - cardiac — *see* Complications, cardiac device, electronic
    - nervous system — *see* Complication, prosthetic device, mechanical, electronic nervous system stimulator
    - urinary — *see* Complications, electronic stimulator, urinary
  - esophageal mucosa into cardia of stomach, congenital Q39.8
  - esophagus (acquired) K22.8
    - congenital Q39.8
  - eyeball (acquired) (lateral) (old) — *see* Displacement, globe
    - congenital Q15.8
    - current — *see* Avulsion, eye
  - fallopian tube (acquired) N83.4
    - congenital Q5Ø.6
    - opening (congenital) Q5Ø.6
  - gallbladder (congenital) Q44.1
  - gastric mucosa (congenital) Q4Ø.2
  - globe (acquired) (old) (lateral) HØ5.21- ☑
    - current — *see* Avulsion, eye
  - heart (congenital) Q24.8
    - acquired I51.89
  - hymen (upward) (congenital) Q52.4
  - intervertebral disc NEC
    - with myelopathy — *see* Disorder, disc, with, myelopathy
    - cervical, cervicothoracic (with) M5Ø.2Ø
      - myelopathy — *see* Disorder, disc, cervical, with myelopathy
      - neuritis, radiculitis or radiculopathy — *see* Disorder, disc, cervical, with neuritis
    - due to trauma — *see* Dislocation, vertebra
    - lumbar region M51.26
      - with
        - myelopathy M51.Ø6
        - neuritis, radiculitis, radiculopathy or sciatica M51.16
    - lumbosacral region M51.27
      - with
        - neuritis, radiculitis, radiculopathy or sciatica M51.17
    - sacrococcygeal region M53.3
    - thoracic region M51.24
      - with
        - myelopathy M51.Ø4

- **Displacement, displaced** — *continued*
  - intervertebral disc — *continued*
    - thoracic region — *continued*
      - with — *continued*
        - neuritis, radiculitis, radiculopathy M51.14
    - thoracolumbar region M51.25
      - with
        - myelopathy M51.Ø5
        - neuritis, radiculitis, radiculopathy M51.15
  - intrauterine device T83.32 ☑
  - kidney (acquired) N28.83
    - congenital Q63.2
  - lachrymal, lacrimal apparatus or duct (congenital) Q1Ø.6
  - lens, congenital Q12.1
  - macula (congenital) Q14.1
  - Meckel's diverticulum Q43.Ø
    - malignant — *see* Table of Neoplasms, small intestine, malignant
  - nail (congenital) Q84.6
    - acquired L6Ø.8
  - opening of Wharton's duct in mouth Q38.4
  - organ or site, congenital NEC — *see* Malposition, congenital
  - ovary (acquired) N83.4
    - congenital Q5Ø.39
    - free in peritoneal cavity (congenital) Q5Ø.39
    - into hernial sac N83.4
  - oviduct (acquired) N83.4
    - congenital Q5Ø.6
  - parathyroid (gland) E21.4
  - parotid gland (congenital) Q38.4
  - punctum lacrimale (congenital) Q1Ø.6
  - sacro-iliac (joint) (congenital) Q74.2
    - current injury S33.2 ☑
    - old — *see* subcategory M53.2 ☑
  - salivary gland (any) (congenital) Q38.4
  - spleen (congenital) Q89.Ø9
  - stomach, congenital Q4Ø.2
  - sublingual duct Q38.4
  - tongue (downward) (congenital) Q38.3
  - tooth, teeth, fully erupted M26.3Ø
    - horizontal M26.33
    - vertical M26.34
  - trachea (congenital) Q32.1
  - ureter or ureteric opening or orifice (congenital) Q62.62
  - uterine opening of oviducts or fallopian tubes Q5Ø.6
  - uterus, uterine — *see* Malposition, uterus
  - ventricular septum Q21.Ø
    - with rudimentary ventricle Q2Ø.4
- **Disproportion**
  - between native and reconstructed breast N65.1
  - fiber-type G71.2
- **Disruptio uteri** — *see* Rupture, uterus
- **Disruption** (of)
  - ciliary body NEC H21.89
  - closure of
    - cornea T81.31 ☑
    - craniotomy T81.32 ☑
    - fascia (muscular) (superficial) T81.32 ☑
    - internal organ or tissue T81.32 ☑
    - laceration (external) (internal) T81.33 ☑
    - ligament T81.32 ☑
    - mucosa T81.31 ☑
    - muscle or muscle flap T81.32 ☑
    - ribs or rib cage T81.32 ☑
    - skin and subcutaneous tissue (full-thickness) (superficial) T81.31 ☑
    - skull T81.32 ☑
    - sternum (sternotomy) T81.32 ☑
    - tendon T81.32 ☑
    - traumatic laceration (external) (internal) T81.33 ☑
  - family Z63.8
    - due to
      - absence of family member due to military deployment Z63.31
      - absence of family member NEC Z63.32
      - alcoholism and drug addiction in family Z63.72
      - bereavement Z63.4
      - death (assumed) or disappearance of family member Z63.4
      - divorce or separation Z63.5
      - drug addiction in family Z63.72
      - return of family member from military deployment (current or past conflict) Z63.71
      - stressful life events NEC Z63.79
  - iris NEC H21.89

- **Disruption** — *continued*
  - ligament(s) (*see also* Sprain)
    - knee
      - current injury — *see* Dislocation, knee
      - old (chronic) — *see* Derangement, knee, instability
      - spontaneous NEC — *see* Derangement, knee, disruption ligament
  - ossicular chain — *see* Discontinuity, ossicles, ear
  - pelvic ring (stable) S32.810 ☑
    - unstable S32.811 ☑
  - traumatic injury wound repair T81.33 ☑
  - wound T81.30 ☑
    - episiotomy O90.1
    - operation T81.31 ☑
      - cesarean O90.0
      - external operation wound (superficial) T81.31 ☑
      - internal operation wound (deep) T81.32 ☑
    - perineal (obstetric) O90.1
    - traumatic injury repair T81.33 ☑
- **Dissatisfaction with**
  - employment Z56.9
  - school environment Z55.4
- **Dissecting** — *see* condition
- **Dissection**
  - aorta I71.00
    - abdominal I71.02
    - thoracic I71.01
    - thoracoabdominal I71.03
  - artery
    - carotid I77.71
    - cerebral (nonruptured) I67.0
      - ruptured — *see* Hemorrhage, intracranial, subarachnoid
    - coronary I25.42
    - iliac I77.72
    - renal I77.73
    - specified NEC I77.79
    - vertebral I77.74
  - traumatic — *see* Wound, open, by site
  - vascular I99.8
  - wound — *see* Wound, open
- **Disseminated** — *see* condition
- **Dissociation**
  - auriculoventricular or atrioventricular (AV) (any degree) (isorhythmic) I45.89
    - with heart block I44.2
  - interference I45.89
- **Dissociative reaction, state** F44.9
- **Dissolution, vertebra** — *see* Osteoporosis
- **Distension, distention**
  - abdomen R14.0
  - bladder N32.89
  - cecum K63.89
  - colon K63.89
  - gallbladder K82.8
  - intestine K63.89
  - kidney N28.89
  - liver K76.89
  - seminal vesicle N50.8
  - stomach K31.89
    - acute K31.0
    - psychogenic F45.8
  - ureter — *see* Dilatation, ureter
  - uterus N85.8
- **Distoma hepaticum infestation** B66.3
- **Distomiasis** B66.9
  - bile passages B66.3
  - hemic B65.9
  - hepatic B66.3
    - due to Clonorchis sinensis B66.1
  - intestinal B66.5
  - liver B66.3
    - due to Clonorchis sinensis B66.1
  - lung B66.4
  - pulmonary B66.4
- **Distomolar** (fourth molar) K00.1
- **Disto-occlusion** (Division I) (Division II) M26.212
- **Distortion**(s) (congenital)
  - adrenal (gland) Q89.1
  - arm NEC Q68.8
  - bile duct or passage Q44.5
  - bladder Q64.79
  - brain Q04.9
  - cervix (uteri) Q51.9
  - chest (wall) Q67.8
- **Distortion**(s) — *continued*
  - chest — *continued*
    - bones Q76.8
  - clavicle Q74.0
  - clitoris Q52.6
  - coccyx Q76.49
  - common duct Q44.5
  - coronary Q24.5
  - cystic duct Q44.5
  - ear (auricle) (external) Q17.3
    - inner Q16.5
    - middle Q16.4
      - ossicles Q16.3
  - endocrine NEC Q89.2
  - eustachian tube Q17.8
  - eye (adnexa) Q15.8
  - face bone(s) NEC Q75.8
  - fallopian tube Q50.6
  - femur NEC Q68.8
  - fibula NEC Q68.8
  - finger(s) Q68.1
  - foot Q66.9
  - genitalia, genital organ(s)
    - female Q52.8
      - external Q52.79
      - internal NEC Q52.8
  - gyri Q04.8
  - hand bone(s) Q68.1
  - heart (auricle) (ventricle) Q24.8
    - valve (cusp) Q24.8
  - hepatic duct Q44.5
  - humerus NEC Q68.8
  - hymen Q52.4
  - intrafamilial communications Z63.8
  - jaw NEC M26.89
  - labium (majus) (minus) Q52.79
  - leg NEC Q68.8
  - lens Q12.8
  - liver Q44.7
  - lumbar spine Q76.49
    - with disproportion O33.8
      - causing obstructed labor O65.0
  - lumbosacral (joint) (region) Q76.49
    - kyphosis — *see* Kyphosis, congenital
    - lordosis — *see* Lordosis, congenital
  - nerve Q07.8
  - nose Q30.8
  - organ
    - of Corti Q16.5
    - or site not listed — *see* Anomaly, by site
  - ossicles, ear Q16.3
  - oviduct Q50.6
  - pancreas Q45.3
  - parathyroid (gland) Q89.2
  - pituitary (gland) Q89.2
  - radius NEC Q68.8
  - sacroiliac joint Q74.2
  - sacrum Q76.49
  - scapula Q74.0
  - shoulder girdle Q74.0
  - skull bone(s) NEC Q75.8
    - with
      - anencephalus Q00.0
      - encephalocele — *see* Encephalocele
      - hydrocephalus Q03.9
        - with spina bifida — *see* Spina bifida, with hydrocephalus
      - microcephaly Q02
  - spinal cord Q06.8
  - spine Q76.49
    - kyphosis — *see* Kyphosis, congenital
    - lordosis — *see* Lordosis, congenital
  - spleen Q89.09
  - sternum NEC Q76.7
  - thorax (wall) Q67.8
    - bony Q76.8
  - thymus (gland) Q89.2
  - thyroid (gland) Q89.2
  - tibia NEC Q68.8
  - toe(s) Q66.9
  - tongue Q38.3
  - trachea (cartilage) Q32.1
  - ulna NEC Q68.8
  - ureter Q62.8
  - urethra Q64.79
    - causing obstruction Q64.39
  - uterus Q51.9
  - vagina Q52.4
- **Distortion**(s) — *continued*
  - vertebra Q76.49
    - kyphosis — *see* Kyphosis, congenital
    - lordosis — *see* Lordosis, congenital
  - visual (*see also* Disturbance, vision)
    - shape and size H53.15
  - vulva Q52.79
  - wrist (bones) (joint) Q68.8
- **Distress**
  - abdomen — *see* Pain, abdominal
  - acute respiratory (adult) (child) J80
  - epigastric R10.13
  - fetal P84
    - complicating pregnancy — *see* Stress, fetal
  - gastrointestinal (functional) K30
    - psychogenic F45.8
  - intestinal (functional) NOS K59.9
    - psychogenic F45.8
  - maternal, during labor and delivery O75.0
  - respiratory R06.00
    - adult J80
    - child J80
    - newborn P22.9
      - specified NEC P22.8
    - orthopnea R06.01
    - psychogenic F45.8
    - shortness of breath R06.02
    - specified type NEC R06.09
- **Distribution vessel, atypical** Q27.9
  - coronary artery Q24.5
  - precerebral Q28.1
- **Districhiasis** L68.8
- **Disturbance(s)** (*see also* Disease)
  - absorption K90.9
    - calcium E58
    - carbohydrate K90.4
    - fat K90.4
      - pancreatic K90.3
    - protein K90.4
    - starch K90.4
    - vitamin — *see* Deficiency, vitamin
  - acid-base equilibrium E87.8
    - mixed E87.4
  - activity and attention (with hyperkinesis) — *see* Disorder, attention-deficit hyperactivity
  - amino acid transport E72.00
  - assimilation, food K90.9
  - auditory nerve, except deafness — *see* subcategory H93.3 ☑
  - behavior — *see* Disorder, conduct
  - blood clotting (mechanism) (*see also* Defect, coagulation) D68.9
  - cerebral
    - nerve — *see* Disorder, nerve, cranial
    - status, newborn P91.9
      - specified NEC P91.8
  - circulatory I99.9
  - conduct (*see also* Disorder, conduct) F91.9
    - adjustment reaction — *see* Disorder, adjustment
    - compulsive F63.9
    - disruptive F91.9
    - hyperkinetic — *see* Disorder, attention-deficit hyperactivity
    - socialized F91.2
    - specified NEC F91.8
    - unsocialized F91.1
  - coordination R27.8
  - cranial nerve — *see* Disorder, nerve, cranial
  - deep sensibility — *see* Disturbance, sensation
  - digestive K30
    - psychogenic F45.8
  - electrolyte (*see also* Imbalance, electrolyte)
    - newborn, transitory P74.4
      - hyperammonemia P74.6
      - potassium balance P74.3
      - sodium balance P74.2
      - specified type NEC P74.4
  - emotions specific to childhood and adolescence F93.9
    - with
      - anxiety and fearfulness NEC F93.8
      - elective mutism F94.0
      - oppositional disorder F91.3
      - sensitivity (withdrawal) F40.10
      - shyness F40.10
      - social withdrawal F40.10
    - involving relationship problems F93.8
    - mixed F93.8
    - specified NEC F93.8

Disturbance(s) — *continued*
- endocrine (gland) E34.9
  - neonatal, transitory P72.9
    - specified NEC P72.8
- equilibrium R42
- fructose metabolism E74.10
- gait — *see* Gait
  - hysterical F44.4
  - psychogenic F44.4
- gastrointestinal (functional) K30
  - psychogenic F45.8
- habit, child F98.9
- hearing, except deafness and tinnitus — *see* Abnormal, auditory perception
- heart, functional (conditions in I44-I50)
  - due to presence of (cardiac) prosthesis I97.19- ☑
  - postoperative I97.89
    - cardiac surgery I97.19- ☑
- hormones E34.9
- innervation uterus (parasympathetic) (sympathetic) N85.8
- keratinization NEC
  - gingiva K05.10
    - nonplaque induced K05.11
    - plaque induced K05.10
  - lip K13.0
  - oral (mucosa) (soft tissue) K13.29
  - tongue K13.29
- learning (specific) — *see* Disorder, learning
- memory — *see* Amnesia
  - mild, following organic brain damage F06.8
- mental F99
  - associated with diseases classified elsewhere F54
- metabolism E88.9
  - with
    - abortion — *see* Abortion, by type with other specified complication
    - ectopic pregnancy O08.5
    - molar pregnancy O08.5
  - amino-acid E72.9
    - aromatic E70.9
    - branched-chain E71.2
    - straight-chain E72.8
    - sulfur-bearing E72.10
  - ammonia E72.20
  - arginine E72.21
  - arginosuccinic acid E72.22
  - carbohydrate E74.9
  - cholesterol E78.9
  - citrulline E72.23
  - cystathionine E72.19
  - general E88.9
  - glutamine E72.8
  - histidine E70.40
  - homocystine E72.19
  - hydroxylysine E72.3
  - in labor or delivery O75.89
  - iron E83.10
  - lipoid E78.9
  - lysine E72.3
  - methionine E72.19
  - neonatal, transitory P74.9
    - calcium and magnesium P71.9
      - specified type NEC P71.8
    - carbohydrate metabolism P70.9
      - specified type NEC P70.8
    - specified NEC P74.8
  - ornithine E72.4
  - phosphate E83.39
  - sodium NEC E87.8
  - threonine E72.8
  - tryptophan E70.5
  - tyrosine E70.20
  - urea cycle E72.20
- motor R29.2
- nervous, functional R45.0
- neuromuscular mechanism (eye), due to syphilis A52.15
- nutritional E63.9
  - nail L60.3
- ocular motion H51.9
  - psychogenic F45.8
- oculogyric H51.8
  - psychogenic F45.8
- oculomotor H51.9
  - psychogenic F45.8
- olfactory nerve R43.1
- optic nerve NEC — *see* Disorder, nerve, optic

Disturbance(s) — *continued*
- oral epithelium, including tongue NEC K13.29
- perceptual due to
  - alcohol withdrawal F10.232
  - amphetamine intoxication F15.922
    - in
      - abuse F15.122
      - dependence F15.222
  - anxiolytic withdrawal F13.232
  - cannabis intoxication (acute) F12.922
    - in
      - abuse F12.122
      - dependence F12.222
  - cocaine intoxication (acute) F14.922
    - in
      - abuse F14.122
      - dependence F14.222
  - hypnotic withdrawal F13.232
  - opioid intoxication (acute) F11.922
    - in
      - abuse F11.122
      - dependence F11.222
  - phencyclidine intoxication (acute) F19.922
    - in
      - abuse F19.122
      - dependence F19.222
  - sedative withdrawal F13.232
- personality (pattern) (trait) (*see also* Disorder, personality) F60.9
  - following organic brain damage F07.9
- polyglandular E31.9
  - specified NEC E31.8
- potassium balance, newborn P74.3
- psychogenic F45.9
- psychomotor F44.4
- psychophysical visual H53.16
- pupillary — *see* Anomaly, pupil, function
- reflex R29.2
- rhythm, heart I49.9
- salivary secretion K11.7
- sensation (cold) (heat) (localization) (tactile discrimination) (texture) (vibratory) NEC R20.9
  - hysterical F44.6
  - skin R20.9
    - anesthesia R20.0
    - hyperesthesia R20.3
    - hypoesthesia R20.1
    - paresthesia R20.2
    - specified type NEC R20.8
  - smell R43.9
    - and taste (mixed) R43.8
    - anosmia R43.0
    - parosmia R43.1
    - specified NEC R43.8
  - taste R43.9
    - and smell (mixed) R43.8
    - parageusia R43.2
    - specified NEC R43.8
- sensory — *see* Disturbance, sensation
- situational (transient) (*see also* Disorder, adjustment)
  - acute F43.0
- sleep G47.9
  - nonorganic origin F51.9
- smell — *see* Disturbance, sensation, smell
- sociopathic F60.2
- sodium balance, newborn P74.2
- speech R47.9
  - developmental F80.9
  - specified NEC R47.89
- stomach (functional) K31.9
- sympathetic (nerve) G90.9
- taste — *see* Disturbance, sensation, taste
- temperature
  - regulation, newborn P81.9
    - specified NEC P81.8
  - sense R20.8
    - hysterical F44.6
- tooth
  - eruption K00.6
  - formation K00.4
  - structure, hereditary NEC K00.5
- touch — *see* Disturbance, sensation
- vascular I99.9
  - arteriosclerotic — *see* Arteriosclerosis
- vasomotor I73.9
- vasospastic I73.9
- vision, visual H53.9

Disturbance(s) — *continued*
- vision, visual — *continued*
  - following
    - cerebral infarction I69.398
    - cerebrovascular disease I69.998
      - specified NEC I69.898
    - intracerebral hemorrhage I69.198
    - nontraumatic intracranial hemorrhage NEC I69.298
    - specified disease NEC I69.898
    - subarachnoid hemorrhage I69.098
  - psychophysical H53.16
  - specified NEC H53.8
  - subjective H53.10
    - day blindness H53.11
    - discomfort H53.14- ☑
    - distortions of shape and size H53.15
    - loss
      - sudden H53.13- ☑
      - transient H53.12- ☑
    - specified type NEC H53.19
- voice R49.9
  - psychogenic F44.4
  - specified NEC R49.8

Diuresis R35.8

Diver's palsy, paralysis or squeeze T70.3 ☑

Diverticulitis (acute) K57.92
- bladder — *see* Cystitis
- ileum — *see* Diverticulitis, intestine, small
- intestine K57.92
  - with
    - abscess, perforation or peritonitis K57.80
      - with bleeding K57.81
    - bleeding K57.93
  - congenital Q43.8
  - large K57.32
    - with
      - abscess, perforation or peritonitis K57.20
        - with bleeding K57.21
      - bleeding K57.33
      - small intestine K57.52
        - with
          - abscess, perforation or peritonitis K57.40
            - with bleeding K57.41
          - bleeding K57.53
  - small K57.12
    - with
      - abscess, perforation or peritonitis K57.00
        - with bleeding K57.01
      - bleeding K57.13
      - large intestine K57.52
        - with
          - abscess, perforation or peritonitis K57.40
            - with bleeding K57.41
          - bleeding K57.53

Diverticulosis K57.90
- with bleeding K57.91
- large intestine K57.30
  - with
    - bleeding K57.31
    - small intestine K57.50
      - with bleeding K57.51
- small intestine K57.10
  - with
    - bleeding K57.11
    - large intestine K57.50
      - with bleeding K57.51

Diverticulum, diverticula (multiple) K57.90
- appendix (noninflammatory) K38.2
- bladder (sphincter) N32.3
  - congenital Q64.6
- bronchus (congenital) Q32.4
  - acquired J98.09
- calyx, calyceal (kidney) N28.89
- cardia (stomach) K31.4
- cecum — *see* Diverticulosis, intestine, large
  - congenital Q43.8
- colon — *see* Diverticulosis, intestine, large
  - congenital Q43.8
- duodenum — *see* Diverticulosis, intestine, small
  - congenital Q43.8
- epiphrenic (esophagus) K22.5
- esophagus (congenital) Q39.6
  - acquired (epiphrenic) (pulsion) (traction) K22.5
- eustachian tube — *see* Disorder, eustachian tube, specified NEC

- **Duchenne's**
  - disease or syndrome
    - motor neuron disease G12.22
    - muscular dystrophy G71.Ø
  - locomotor ataxia (syphilitic) A52.11
  - paralysis
    - birth injury P14.Ø
    - due to or associated with
      - motor neuron disease G12.22
      - muscular dystrophy G71.Ø
- **Ducrey's chancre** A57
- **Duct, ductus** — *see* condition
- **Duhring's disease** (dermatitis herpetiformis) L13.Ø
- **Dullness, cardiac** (decreased) (increased) RØ1.2
- **Dumb ague** — *see* Malaria
- **Dumbness** — *see* Aphasia
- **Dumdum fever** B55.Ø
- **Dumping syndrome** (postgastrectomy) K91.1
- **Duodenitis** (nonspecific) (peptic) K29.8Ø
  - with bleeding K29.81
- **Duodenocholangitis** — *see* Cholangitis
- **Duodenum, duodenal** — *see* condition
- **Duplay's bursitis or periarthritis** — *see* Tendinitis, calcific, shoulder
- **Duplication, duplex** (*see also* Accessory)
  - alimentary tract Q45.8
  - anus Q43.4
  - appendix (and cecum) Q43.4
  - biliary duct (any) Q44.5
  - bladder Q64.79
  - cecum (and appendix) Q43.4
  - cervix Q51.82Ø
  - chromosome NEC
    - with complex rearrangements NEC Q92.5
    - seen only at prometaphase Q92.8
  - cystic duct Q44.5
  - digestive organs Q45.8
  - esophagus Q39.8
  - frontonasal process Q75.8
  - intestine (large) (small) Q43.4
  - kidney Q63.Ø
  - liver Q44.7
  - pancreas Q45.3
  - penis Q55.69
  - respiratory organs NEC Q34.8
  - salivary duct Q38.4
  - spinal cord (incomplete) QØ6.2
  - stomach Q4Ø.2
- **Dupré's disease** (meningism) R29.1
- **Dupuytren's contraction or disease** M72.Ø
- **Durand-Nicolas-Favre disease** A55
- **Durotomy** (inadvertent) (incidental) G97.41
- **Duroziez's disease** (congenital mitral stenosis) Q23.2
- **Dutton's relapsing fever** (West African) A68.1
- **Dwarfism** E34.3
  - achondroplastic Q77.4
  - congenital E34.3
  - constitutional E34.3
  - hypochondroplastic Q77.4
  - hypophyseal E23.Ø
  - infantile E34.3
  - Laron-type E34.3
  - Lorain (-Levi) type E23.Ø
  - metatropic Q77.8
  - nephrotic-glycosuric (with hypophosphatemic rickets) E72.Ø9
  - nutritional E45
  - pancreatic K86.8
  - pituitary E23.Ø
  - renal N25.Ø
  - thanatophoric Q77.1
- **Dyke-Young anemia** (secondary) (symptomatic) D59.1
- **Dysacusis** — *see* Abnormal, auditory perception
- **Dysadrenocortism** E27.9
  - hyperfunction E27.Ø
- **Dysarthria** R47.1
  - following
    - cerebral infarction I69.322
    - cerebrovascular disease I69.922
      - specified disease NEC I69.822
    - intracerebral hemorrhage I69.122
    - nontraumatic intracranial hemorrhage NEC I69.222
    - subarachnoid hemorrhage I69.Ø22
- **Dysautonomia** (familial) G9Ø.1
- **Dysbarism** T7Ø.3 ☑
- **Dysbasia** R26.2
  - angiosclerotica intermittens I73.9
  - hysterical F44.4
- **Dysbasia** — *continued*
  - lordotica (progressiva) G24.1
  - nonorganic origin F44.4
  - psychogenic F44.4
- **Dysbetalipoproteinemia** (familial) E78.2
- **Dyscalculia** R48.8
  - developmental F81.2
- **Dyschezia** K59.ØØ
- **Dyschondroplasia** (with hemangiomata) Q78.4
- **Dyschromia** (skin) L81.9
- **Dyscollagenosis** M35.9
- **Dyscranio-pygo-phalangy** Q87.Ø
- **Dyscrasia**
  - blood (with) D75.9
    - antepartum hemorrhage — *see* Hemorrhage, antepartum, with coagulation defect
    - intrapartum hemorrhage O67.Ø
    - newborn P61.9
      - specified type NEC P61.8
    - puerperal, postpartum O72.3
  - polyglandular, pluriglandular E31.9
- **Dysendocrinism** E34.9
- **Dysentery, dysenteric** (catarrhal) (diarrhea) (epidemic) (hemorrhagic) (infectious) (sporadic) (tropical) AØ9
  - abscess, liver AØ6.4
  - amebic (*see also* Amebiasis) AØ6.Ø
    - with abscess — *see* Abscess, amebic
    - acute AØ6.Ø
    - chronic AØ6.1
  - arthritis (*see also* category MØ1) AØ9
    - bacillary (*see also* category MØ1) AØ3.9
  - bacillary AØ3.9
    - arthritis (*see also* category MØ1) AØ3.9
    - Boyd AØ3.2
    - Flexner AØ3.1
    - Schmitz (-Stutzer) AØ3.Ø
    - Shiga (-Kruse) AØ3.Ø
    - Shigella AØ3.9
      - boydii AØ3.2
      - dysenteriae AØ3.Ø
      - flexneri AØ3.1
      - group A AØ3.Ø
      - group B AØ3.1
      - group C AØ3.2
      - group D AØ3.3
      - sonnei AØ3.3
      - specified type NEC AØ3.8
    - Sonne AØ3.3
    - specified type NEC AØ3.8
  - balantidial AØ7.Ø
  - Balantidium coli AØ7.Ø
  - Boyd's AØ3.2
  - candidal B37.82
  - Chilomastix AØ7.8
  - Chinese AØ3.9
  - coccidial AØ7.3
  - Dientamoeba (fragilis) AØ7.8
  - Embadomonas AØ7.8
  - Entamoeba, entamebic — *see* Dysentery, amebic
  - Flexner-Boyd AØ3.2
  - Flexner's AØ3.1
  - Giardia lamblia AØ7.1
  - Hiss-Russell AØ3.1
  - Lamblia AØ7.1
  - leishmanial B55.Ø
  - malarial — *see* Malaria
  - metazoal B82.Ø
  - monilial B37.82
  - protozoal AØ7.9
  - Salmonella AØ2.Ø
  - schistosomal B65.1
  - Schmitz (-Stutzer) AØ3.Ø
  - Shiga (-Kruse) AØ3.Ø
  - Shigella NOS — *see* Dysentery, bacillary
  - Sonne AØ3.3
  - strongyloidiasis B78.Ø
  - trichomonal AØ7.8
  - viral (*see also* Enteritis, viral) AØ8.4
- **Dysequilibrium** R42
- **Dysesthesia** R2Ø.8
  - hysterical F44.6
- **Dysfibrinogenemia** (congenital) D68.2
- **Dysfunction**
  - adrenal E27.9
    - hyperfunction E27.Ø
  - autonomic
    - due to alcohol G31.2
    - somatoform F45.8
- **Dysfunction** — *continued*
  - bladder N31.9
    - neurogenic NOS — *see* Dysfunction, bladder, neuromuscular
    - neuromuscular NOS N31.9
      - atonic (motor) (sensory) N31.2
      - autonomous N31.2
      - flaccid N31.2
      - nonreflex N31.2
      - reflex N31.1
      - specified NEC N31.8
      - uninhibited N31.Ø
  - bleeding, uterus N93.8
  - cerebral G93.89
  - colon K59.9
    - psychogenic F45.8
  - colostomy K94.Ø3
  - cystic duct K82.8
  - cystostomy (stoma) — *see* Complications, cystostomy
  - ejaculatory N53.19
    - anejaculatory orgasm N53.13
    - painful N53.12
    - premature F52.4
    - retarded N53.11
  - endocrine NOS E34.9
  - endometrium N85.8
  - enterostomy K94.13
  - gallbladder K82.8
  - gastrostomy (stoma) K94.23
  - gland, glandular NOS E34.9
  - heart I51.89
  - hemoglobin D75.89
  - hepatic K76.89
  - hypophysis E23.7
  - hypothalamic NEC E23.3
  - ileostomy (stoma) K94.13
  - jejunostomy (stoma) K94.13
  - kidney — *see* Disease, renal
  - labyrinthine — *see* subcategory H83.2 ☑
  - left ventricular, following sudden emotional stress I51.81
  - liver K76.89
  - male — *see* Dysfunction, sexual, male
  - orgasmic (female) F52.31
    - male F52.32
  - ovary E28.9
    - specified NEC E28.8
  - papillary muscle I51.89
  - parathyroid E21.4
  - physiological NEC R68.89
    - psychogenic F59
  - pineal gland E34.8
  - pituitary (gland) E23.3
  - platelets D69.1
  - polyglandular E31.9
    - specified NEC E31.8
  - psychophysiologic F59
  - psychosexual F52.9
    - with
      - dyspareunia F52.6
      - premature ejaculation F52.4
      - vaginismus F52.5
  - pylorus K31.9
  - rectum K59.9
    - psychogenic F45.8
  - reflex (sympathetic) — *see* Syndrome, pain, complex regional I
  - segmental — *see* Dysfunction, somatic
  - senile R54
  - sexual (due to) R37
    - alcohol F1Ø.981
    - amphetamine F15.981
      - in
        - abuse F15.181
        - dependence F15.281
    - anxiolytic F13.981
      - in
        - abuse F13.181
        - dependence F13.281
    - cocaine F14.981
      - in
        - abuse F14.181
        - dependence F14.281
    - excessive sexual drive F52.8
    - failure of genital response (male) F52.21
      - female F52.22
    - female N94.9
      - aversion F52.1

- **Dysplasia** — *continued*
  - anus (histologically confirmed) (mild) (moderate) K62.82
    - severe DØ1.3
  - arrhythmogenic right ventricular I42.8
  - arterial, fibromuscular I77.3
  - asphyxiating thoracic (congenital) Q77.2
  - brain QØ7.9
  - bronchopulmonary, perinatal P27.1
  - cervix (uteri) N87.9
    - mild N87.Ø
    - moderate N87.1
    - severe DØ6.9
  - chondroectodermal Q77.6
  - colon D12.6
  - craniometaphyseal Q78.5
  - dentinal KØØ.5
  - diaphyseal, progressive Q78.3
  - dystrophic Q77.5
  - ectodermal (anhidrotic) (congenital) (hereditary) Q82.4
    - hydrotic Q82.8
  - epithelial, uterine cervix — *see* Dysplasia, cervix
  - eye (congenital) Q11.2
  - fibrous
    - bone NEC (monostotic) M85.ØØ
      - ankle M85.Ø7- ☑
      - foot M85.Ø7- ☑
      - forearm M85.Ø3- ☑
      - hand M85.Ø4- ☑
      - lower leg M85.Ø6- ☑
      - multiple site M85.Ø9
      - neck M85.Ø8
      - rib M85.Ø8
      - shoulder M85.Ø1- ☑
      - skull M85.Ø8
      - specified site NEC M85.Ø8
      - thigh M85.Ø5- ☑
      - toe M85.Ø7- ☑
      - upper arm M85.Ø2- ☑
      - vertebra M85.Ø8
    - diaphyseal, progressive Q78.3
    - jaw M27.8
    - polyostotic Q78.1
  - florid osseous (*see also* Cyst, calcifying odontogenic)
  - high grade, focal D12.6
  - hip, congenital Q65.89
  - joint, congenital Q74.8
  - kidney Q61.4
    - multicystic Q61.4
  - leg Q74.2
  - lung, congenital (not associated with short gestation) Q33.6
  - mammary (gland) (benign) N6Ø.9- ☑
    - cyst (solitary) — *see* Cyst, breast
    - cystic — *see* Mastopathy, cystic
    - duct ectasia — *see* Ectasia, mammary duct
    - fibroadenosis — *see* Fibroadenosis, breast
    - fibrosclerosis — *see* Fibrosclerosis, breast
    - specified type NEC N6Ø.8- ☑
  - metaphyseal (Jansen's) (McKusick's) (Schmid's) Q78.5
  - muscle Q79.8
  - oculodentodigital Q87.Ø
  - periapical (cemental) (cemento-osseous) — *see* Cyst, calcifying odontogenic
  - periosteum — *see* Disorder, bone, specified type NEC
  - polyostotic fibrous Q78.1
  - prostate (*see also* Neoplasia, intraepithelial, prostate) N42.3
    - severe DØ7.5
  - renal Q61.4
    - multicystic Q61.4
  - retinal, congenital Q14.1
  - right ventricular, arrhythmogenic I42.8
  - septo-optic QØ4.4
  - skin L98.8
  - spinal cord QØ6.1
  - spondyloepiphyseal Q77.7
  - thymic, with immunodeficiency D82.1
  - vagina N89.3
    - mild N89.Ø
    - moderate N89.1
    - severe NEC DØ7.2
  - vulva N9Ø.3
    - mild N9Ø.Ø
    - moderate N9Ø.1
    - severe NEC DØ7.1
- **Dyspnea** (nocturnal) (paroxysmal) RØ6.ØØ
  - asthmatic (bronchial) J45.909
    - with
      - bronchitis J45.909
        - with
          - exacerbation (acute) J45.901
          - status asthmaticus J45.902
        - chronic J44.9
      - exacerbation (acute) J45.901
      - status asthmaticus J45.902
    - cardiac — *see* Failure, ventricular, left
  - cardiac — *see* Failure, ventricular, left
  - functional F45.8
  - hyperventilation RØ6.4
  - hysterical F45.8
  - newborn P28.89
  - orthopnea RØ6.Ø1
  - psychogenic F45.8
  - shortness of breath RØ6.Ø2
  - specified type NEC RØ6.Ø9
- **Dyspraxia** R27.8
  - developmental (syndrome) F82
- **Dysproteinemia** E88.Ø9
- **Dysreflexia, autonomic** G9Ø.4
- **Dysrhythmia**
  - cardiac I49.9
    - newborn
      - bradycardia P29.12
      - occurring before birth PØ3.819
        - before onset of labor PØ3.81Ø
        - during labor PØ3.811
      - tachycardia P29.11
    - postoperative I97.89
  - cerebral or cortical — *see* Epilepsy
- **Dyssomnia** — *see* Disorder, sleep
- **Dyssynergia**
  - biliary K83.8
  - bladder sphincter N36.44
  - cerebellaris myoclonica (Hunt's ataxia) G11.1
- **Dysthymia** F34.1
- **Dysthyroidism** EØ7.9
- **Dystocia** O66.9
  - affecting newborn PØ3.1
  - cervical (hypotonic) O62.2
    - affecting newborn PØ3.6
    - primary O62.Ø
    - secondary O62.1
  - contraction ring O62.4
  - fetal O66.9
    - abnormality NEC O66.3
    - conjoined twins O66.3
    - oversize O66.2
  - maternal O66.9
  - positional O64.9 ☑
  - shoulder (girdle) O66.Ø
    - causing obstructed labor O66.Ø
  - uterine NEC O62.4
- **Dystonia** G24.9
  - deformans progressiva G24.1
  - drug induced NEC G24.Ø9
    - acute G24.Ø2
    - specified NEC G24.Ø9
  - familial G24.1
  - idiopathic G24.1
    - familial G24.1
    - nonfamilial G24.2
    - orofacial G24.4
  - lenticularis G24.8
  - musculorum deformans G24.1
  - neuroleptic induced (acute) G24.Ø2
  - orofacial (idiopathic) G24.4
  - oromandibular G24.4
    - due to drug G24.Ø1
  - specified NEC G24.8
  - torsion (familial) (idiopathic) G24.1
    - acquired G24.8
    - genetic G24.1
    - symptomatic (nonfamilial) G24.2
- **Dystonic movements** R25.8
- **Dystrophy, dystrophia**
  - adiposogenital E23.6
  - Becker's type G71.Ø
  - cervical sympathetic G9Ø.2
  - choroid (hereditary) H31.2Ø
    - central areolar H31.22
    - choroideremia H31.21
    - gyrate atrophy H31.23
    - specified type NEC H31.29
- **Dystrophy, dystrophia** — *continued*
  - cornea (hereditary) H18.5Ø
    - endothelial H18.51
    - epithelial H18.52
    - granular H18.53
    - lattice H18.54
    - macular H18.55
    - specified type NEC H18.59
  - Duchenne's type G71.Ø
  - due to malnutrition E45
  - Erb's G71.Ø
  - Fuchs' H18.51
  - Gower's muscular G71.Ø
  - hair L67.8
  - infantile neuraxonal G31.89
  - Landouzy-Déjérine G71.Ø
  - Leyden-Möbius G71.Ø
  - muscular G71.Ø
    - benign (Becker type) G71.Ø
    - congenital (hereditary) (progressive) (with specific morphological abnormalities of the muscle fiber) G71.Ø
      - myotonic G71.11
    - distal G71.Ø
    - Duchenne type G71.Ø
    - Emery-Dreifuss G71.Ø
    - Erb type G71.Ø
    - facioscapulohumeral G71.Ø
    - Gower's G71.Ø
    - hereditary (progressive) G71.Ø
    - Landouzy-Déjérine type G71.Ø
    - limb-girdle G71.Ø
    - myotonic G71.11
    - progressive (hereditary) G71.Ø
      - Charcot-Marie (-Tooth) type G6Ø.Ø
    - pseudohypertrophic (infantile) G71.Ø
    - severe (Duchenne type) G71.Ø
  - myocardium, myocardial — *see* Degeneration, myocardial
  - nail L6Ø.3
    - congenital Q84.6
  - nutritional E45
  - ocular G71.Ø
  - oculocerebrorenal E72.Ø3
  - oculopharyngeal G71.Ø
  - ovarian N83.8
  - polyglandular E31.8
  - reflex (neuromuscular) (sympathetic) — *see* Syndrome, pain, complex regional I
  - retinal (hereditary) H35.5Ø
    - in
      - lipid storage disorders E75.6 [H36]
      - systemic lipidoses E75.6 [H36]
    - involving
      - pigment epithelium H35.54
      - sensory area H35.53
    - pigmentary H35.52
    - vitreoretinal H35.51
  - Salzmann's nodular — *see* Degeneration, cornea, nodular
  - scapuloperoneal G71.Ø
  - skin NEC L98.8
  - sympathetic (reflex) — *see* Syndrome, pain, complex regional I
    - cervical G9Ø.2
  - tapetoretinal H35.54
  - thoracic, asphyxiating Q77.2
  - unguium L6Ø.3
    - congenital Q84.6
  - vitreoretinal H35.51
  - vulva N9Ø.4
  - yellow (liver) — *see* Failure, hepatic
- **Dysuria** R3Ø.Ø
  - psychogenic F45.8

E

- **Eales' disease** H35.Ø6- ☑
- **Ear** (*see also* condition)
  - piercing Z41.3
  - tropical B36.8
  - wax (impacted) H61.2Ø
    - left H61.22
      - with right H61.23
    - right H61.21
      - with left H61.23
- **Earache** — *see* subcategory H92.Ø ☑
- **Early satiety** R68.81

Eaton-Lambert syndrome — *see* Syndrome, Lambert-Eaton
Eberth's disease (typhoid fever) AØ1.ØØ
Ebola virus disease A98.4
Ebstein's anomaly or syndrome (heart) Q22.5
Eccentro-osteochondrodysplasia E76.29
Ecchondroma — *see* Neoplasm, bone, benign
Ecchondrosis D48.Ø
Ecchymosis R58
- conjunctiva — *see* Hemorrhage, conjunctiva
- eye (traumatic) — *see* Contusion, eyeball
- eyelid (traumatic) — *see* Contusion, eyelid
- newborn P54.5
- spontaneous R23.3
- traumatic — *see* Contusion

Echinococciasis — *see* Echinococcus
Echinococcosis — *see* Echinococcus
Echinococcus (infection) B67.9Ø
- granulosus B67.4
  - bone B67.2
  - liver B67.Ø
  - lung B67.1
  - multiple sites B67.32
  - specified site NEC B67.39
  - thyroid B67.31 [E35]
- liver NOS B67.8
  - granulosus B67.Ø
  - multilocularis B67.5
- lung NEC B67.99
  - granulosus B67.1
  - multilocularis B67.69
- multilocularis B67.7
  - liver B67.5
  - multiple sites B67.61
  - specified site NEC B67.69
- specified site NEC B67.99
  - granulosus B67.39
  - multilocularis B67.69
- thyroid NEC B67.99
  - granulosus B67.31 [E35]
  - multilocularis B67.69 [E35]

Echinorhynchiasis B83.8
Echinostomiasis B66.8
Echolalia R48.8
Echovirus, as cause of disease classified elsewhere B97.12
Eclampsia, eclamptic (coma) (convulsions) (delirium) (with hypertension) NEC O15.9
- during labor and delivery O15.1
- postpartum O15.2
- pregnancy O15.Ø- ☑
- puerperal O15.2

Economic circumstances affecting care Z59.9
Economo's disease A85.8
Ectasia, ectasis
- annuloaortic I35.8
- aorta I77.819
  - with aneurysm — *see* Aneurysm, aorta
  - abdominal I77.811
  - thoracic I77.81Ø
  - thoracoabdominal I77.812
- breast — *see* Ectasia, mammary duct
- capillary I78.8
- cornea H18.71- ☑
- gastric antral vascular (GAVE) K31.819
  - with hemorrhage K31.811
  - without hemorrhage K31.819
- mammary duct N6Ø.4- ☑
- salivary gland (duct) K11.8
- sclera — *see* Sclerectasia

Ecthyma LØ8.Ø
- contagiosum BØ8.Ø2
- gangrenosum LØ8.Ø
- infectiosum BØ8.Ø2

Ectocardia Q24.8
Ectodermal dysplasia (anhidrotic) Q82.4
Ectodermosis erosiva pluriorificialis L51.1
Ectopic, ectopia (congenital)
- abdominal viscera Q45.8
  - due to defect in anterior abdominal wall Q79.59
- ACTH syndrome E24.3
- adrenal gland Q89.1
- anus Q43.5
- atrial beats I49.1
- beats I49.49
  - atrial I49.1
  - ventricular I49.3
- bladder Q64.1Ø
- bone and cartilage in lung Q33.5
- brain QØ4.8
- breast tissue Q83.8
- cardiac Q24.8
- cerebral QØ4.8
- cordis Q24.8
- endometrium — *see* Endometriosis
- gastric mucosa Q4Ø.2
- gestation — *see* Pregnancy, by site
- heart Q24.8
- hormone secretion NEC E34.2
- kidney (crossed) (pelvis) Q63.2
- lens, lentis Q12.1
- mole — *see* Pregnancy, by site
- organ or site NEC — *see* Malposition, congenital
- pancreas Q45.3
- pregnancy — *see* Pregnancy, ectopic
- pupil — *see* Abnormality, pupillary
- renal Q63.2
- sebaceous glands of mouth Q38.6
- spleen Q89.Ø9
- testis Q53.ØØ
  - bilateral Q53.Ø2
  - unilateral Q53.Ø1
- thyroid Q89.2
- tissue in lung Q33.5
- ureter Q62.63
- ventricular beats I49.3
- vesicae Q64.1Ø

Ectromelia Q73.8
- lower limb — *see* Defect, reduction, limb, lower, specified type NEC
- upper limb — *see* Defect, reduction, limb, upper, specified type NEC

Ectropion HØ2.1Ø9
- cervix N86
  - with cervicitis N72
- congenital Q1Ø.1
- eyelid (paralytic) HØ2.1Ø9
  - cicatricial HØ2.119
    - left HØ2.116
      - lower HØ2.115
      - upper HØ2.114
    - right HØ2.113
      - lower HØ2.112
      - upper HØ2.111
  - congenital Q1Ø.1
  - left HØ2.1Ø6
    - lower HØ2.1Ø5
    - upper HØ2.1Ø4
  - mechanical HØ2.129
    - left HØ2.126
      - lower HØ2.125
      - upper HØ2.124
    - right HØ2.123
      - lower HØ2.122
      - upper HØ2.121
  - right HØ2.1Ø3
    - lower HØ2.1Ø2
    - upper HØ2.1Ø1
  - senile HØ2.139
    - left HØ2.136
      - lower HØ2.135
      - upper HØ2.134
    - right HØ2.133
      - lower HØ2.132
      - upper HØ2.131
  - spastic HØ2.149
    - left HØ2.146
      - lower HØ2.145
      - upper HØ2.144
    - right HØ2.143
      - lower HØ2.142
      - upper HØ2.141
- iris H21.89
- lip (acquired) K13.Ø
  - congenital Q38.Ø
- urethra N36.8
- uvea H21.89

Eczema (acute) (chronic) (erythematous) (fissum) (rubrum) (squamous) (*see also* Dermatitis) L3Ø.9
- contact — *see* Dermatitis, contact
- dyshydrotic L3Ø.1
- external ear — *see* Otitis, externa, acute, eczematoid
- flexural L2Ø.82
- herpeticum BØØ.Ø
- hypertrophicum L28.Ø
- hypostatic — *see* Varix, leg, with, inflammation
- impetiginous LØ1.1
- infantile (due to any substance) L2Ø.83
  - intertriginous L21.1
  - seborrheic L21.1
- intertriginous NEC L3Ø.4
  - infantile L21.1
- intrinsic (allergic) L2Ø.84
- lichenified NEC L28.Ø
- marginatum (hebrae) B35.6
- pustular L3Ø.3
- stasis — *see* Varix, leg, with, inflammation
- vaccination, vaccinatum T88.1 ☑
- varicose — *see* Varix, leg, with, inflammation

Eczematid L3Ø.2
Eddowes (-Spurway) **syndrome** Q78.Ø
Edema, edematous (infectious) (pitting) (toxic) R6Ø.9
- with nephritis — *see* Nephrosis
- allergic T78.3 ☑
- amputation stump (surgical) (sequelae (late effect)) T87.89
- angioneurotic (allergic) (any site) (with urticaria) T78.3 ☑
  - hereditary D84.1
- angiospastic I73.9
- Berlin's (traumatic) SØ5.8X- ☑
- brain (cytotoxic) (vasogenic) G93.6
  - due to birth injury P11.Ø
  - newborn (anoxia or hypoxia) P52.4
    - birth injury P11.Ø
  - traumatic — *see* Injury, intracranial, cerebral edema
- cardiac — *see* Failure, heart, congestive
- cardiovascular — *see* Failure, heart, congestive
- cerebral — *see* Edema, brain
- cerebrospinal — *see* Edema, brain
- cervix (uteri) (acute) N88.8
  - puerperal, postpartum O9Ø.89
- chronic hereditary Q82.Ø
- circumscribed, acute T78.3 ☑
  - hereditary D84.1
- conjunctiva H11.42- ☑
- cornea H18.2- ☑
  - idiopathic H18.22- ☑
  - secondary H18.23- ☑
    - due to contact lens H18.21- ☑
- due to
  - lymphatic obstruction I89.Ø
  - salt retention E87.Ø
- epiglottis — *see* Edema, glottis
- essential, acute T78.3 ☑
  - hereditary D84.1
- extremities, lower — *see* Edema, legs
- eyelid NEC HØ2.849
  - left HØ2.846
    - lower HØ2.845
    - upper HØ2.844
  - right HØ2.843
    - lower HØ2.842
    - upper HØ2.841
- familial, hereditary Q82.Ø
- famine — *see* Malnutrition, severe
- generalized R6Ø.1
- glottis, glottic, glottidis (obstructive) (passive) J38.4
  - allergic T78.3 ☑
    - hereditary D84.1
- heart — *see* Failure, heart, congestive
- heat T67.7 ☑
- hereditary Q82.Ø
- inanition — *see* Malnutrition, severe
- intracranial G93.6
- iris H21.89
- joint — *see* Effusion, joint
- larynx — *see* Edema, glottis
- legs R6Ø.Ø
  - due to venous obstruction I87.1
  - hereditary Q82.Ø
- localized R6Ø.Ø
  - due to venous obstruction I87.1
- lower limbs — *see* Edema, legs
- lung J81.1
  - with heart condition or failure — *see* Failure, ventricular, left
  - acute J81.Ø
  - chemical (acute) J68.1
    - chronic J68.1

- **Edema, edematous** — *continued*
  - lung — *continued*
    - chronic J81.1
      - due to
        - chemicals, gases, fumes or vapors (inhalation) J68.1
        - external agent J7Ø.9
          - specified NEC J7Ø.8
        - radiation J7Ø.1
    - due to
      - chemicals, fumes or vapors (inhalation) J68.1
      - external agent J7Ø.9
        - specified NEC J7Ø.8
      - high altitude T7Ø.29 ☑
      - near drowning T75.1 ☑
      - radiation J7Ø.Ø
    - meaning failure, left ventricle I5Ø.1
  - lymphatic I89.Ø
    - due to mastectomy I97.2
  - macula H35.81
    - cystoid, following cataract surgery — *see* Complications, postprocedural, following cataract surgery
    - diabetic — *see* Diabetes, by type, with, retinopathy, with macular edema
  - malignant — *see* Gangrene, gas
  - Milroy's Q82.Ø
  - nasopharynx J39.2
  - newborn P83.3Ø
    - hydrops fetalis — *see* Hydrops, fetalis
    - specified NEC P83.39
  - nutritional (*see also* Malnutrition, severe)
    - with dyspigmentation, skin and hair E4Ø
  - optic disc or nerve — *see* Papilledema
  - orbit HØ5.22- ☑
  - pancreas K86.8
  - papilla, optic — *see* Papilledema
  - penis N48.89
  - periodic T78.3 ☑
    - hereditary D84.1
  - pharynx J39.2
  - pulmonary — *see* Edema, lung
  - Quincke's T78.3 ☑
    - hereditary D84.1
  - renal — *see* Nephrosis
  - retina H35.81
    - diabetic — *see* Diabetes, by type, with, retinopathy, with macular edema
  - salt E87.Ø
  - scrotum N5Ø.8
  - seminal vesicle N5Ø.8
  - spermatic cord N5Ø.8
  - spinal (cord) (vascular) (nontraumatic) G95.19
  - starvation — *see* Malnutrition, severe
  - stasis — *see* Hypertension, venous, (chronic)
  - subglottic — *see* Edema, glottis
  - supraglottic — *see* Edema, glottis
  - testis N44.8
  - tunica vaginalis N5Ø.8
  - vas deferens N5Ø.8
  - vulva (acute) N9Ø.89
- **Edentulism** — *see* Absence, teeth, acquired
- **Edsall's disease** T67.2 ☑
- **Educational handicap** Z55.9
  - specified NEC Z55.8
- **Edward's syndrome** — *see* Trisomy, 18
- **Effect**(s) (of) (from) — *see* Effect, adverse NEC
- **Effect, adverse**
  - abnormal gravitational (G) forces or states T75.81 ☑
  - abuse — *see* Maltreatment
  - air pressure T7Ø.9 ☑
    - specified NEC T7Ø.8 ☑
  - altitude (high) — *see* Effect, adverse, high altitude
  - anesthesia (*see also* Anesthesia) T88.59 ☑
    - in labor and delivery O74.9
    - in pregnancy NEC O29.3- ☑
    - local, toxic
      - in labor and delivery O74.4
      - postpartum, puerperal O89.3
    - postpartum, puerperal O89.9
    - specified NEC T88.59 ☑
      - in labor and delivery O74.8
      - postpartum, puerperal O89.8
    - spinal and epidural T88.59 ☑
      - headache T88.59 ☑
        - in labor and delivery O74.5
        - postpartum, puerperal O89.4

- **Effect, adverse** — *continued*
  - anesthesia (*see also* Anesthesia) — *continued*
    - spinal and epidural — *continued*
      - specified NEC
        - in labor and delivery O74.6
        - postpartum, puerperal O89.5
  - antitoxin — *see* Complications, vaccination
  - atmospheric pressure T7Ø.9 ☑
    - due to explosion T7Ø.8 ☑
    - high T7Ø.3 ☑
    - low — *see* Effect, adverse, high altitude
    - specified effect NEC T7Ø.8 ☑
  - biological, correct substance properly administered — *see* Effect, adverse, drug
  - blood (derivatives) (serum) (transfusion) — *see* Complications, transfusion
  - chemical substance — *see* Table of Drugs and Chemicals
  - cold (temperature) (weather) T69.9 ☑
    - chilblains T69.1 ☑
    - frostbite — *see* Frostbite
    - specified effect NEC T69.8 ☑
  - drugs and medicaments T88.7 ☑
    - specified drug — *see* Table of Drugs and Chemicals, by drug, adverse effect
    - specified effect — *code to* condition
  - electric current, electricity (shock) T75.4 ☑
    - burn — *see* Burn
  - exertion (excessive) T73.3 ☑
  - exposure — *see* Exposure
  - external cause NEC T75.89 ☑
  - foodstuffs T78.1 ☑
    - allergic reaction — *see* Allergy, food
      - causing anaphylaxis — *see* Shock, anaphylactic, due to food
    - noxious — *see* Poisoning, food, noxious
  - gases, fumes, or vapors T59.9- ☑
    - specified agent — *see* Table of Drugs and Chemicals
  - glue (airplane) sniffing
    - due to drug abuse — *see* Abuse, drug, inhalant
    - due to drug dependence — *see* Dependence, drug, inhalant
  - heat — *see* Heat
  - high altitude NEC T7Ø.29 ☑
    - anoxia T7Ø.29 ☑
    - on
      - ears T7Ø.Ø ☑
      - sinuses T7Ø.1 ☑
    - polycythemia D75.1
  - high pressure fluids T7Ø.4 ☑
  - hot weather — *see* Heat
  - hunger T73.Ø ☑
  - immersion, foot — *see* Immersion
  - immunization — *see* Complications, vaccination
  - immunological agents — *see* Complications, vaccination
  - infrared (radiation) (rays) NOS T66 ☑
    - dermatitis or eczema L59.8
  - infusion — *see* Complications, infusion
  - lack of care of infants — *see* Maltreatment, child
  - lightning — *see* Lightning
  - medical care T88.9 ☑
    - specified NEC T88.8 ☑
  - medicinal substance, correct, properly administered — *see* Effect, adverse, drug
  - motion T75.3 ☑
  - noise, on inner ear — *see* subcategory H83.3 ☑
  - overheated places — *see* Heat
  - psychosocial, of work environment Z56.5
  - radiation (diagnostic) (infrared) (natural source) (therapeutic) (ultraviolet) (X-ray) NOS T66 ☑
    - dermatitis or eczema — *see* Dermatitis, due to, radiation
    - fibrosis of lung J7Ø.1
    - pneumonitis J7Ø.Ø
    - pulmonary manifestations
      - acute J7Ø.Ø
      - chronic J7Ø.1
    - skin L59.9
  - radioactive substance NOS
    - dermatitis or eczema — *see* Radiodermatitis
  - reduced temperature T69.9 ☑
    - immersion foot or hand — *see* Immersion
    - specified effect NEC T69.8 ☑
  - serum NEC (*see also* Reaction, serum) T8Ø.69 ☑

- **Effect, adverse** — *continued*
  - specified NEC T78.8 ☑
    - external cause NEC T75.89 ☑
  - strangulation — *see* Asphyxia, traumatic
  - submersion T75.1 ☑
  - thirst T73.1 ☑
  - toxic — *see* Toxicity
  - transfusion — *see* Complications, transfusion
  - ultraviolet (radiation) (rays) NOS T66 ☑
    - burn — *see* Burn
    - dermatitis or eczema — *see* Dermatitis, due to, ultraviolet rays
      - acute L56.8
  - vaccine (any) — *see* Complications, vaccination
  - vibration — *see* Vibration, adverse effects
  - water pressure NEC T7Ø.9 ☑
    - specified NEC T7Ø.8 ☑
  - weightlessness T75.82 ☑
  - whole blood — *see* Complications, transfusion
  - work environment Z56.5
- **Effects, late** — *see* Sequelae
- **Effluvium**
  - anagen L65.1
  - telogen L65.Ø
- **Effort syndrome** (psychogenic) F45.8
- **Effusion**
  - amniotic fluid — *see* Pregnancy, complicated by, prematue rupture of membranes
  - brain (serous) G93.6
  - bronchial — *see* Bronchitis
  - cerebral G93.6
  - cerebrospinal (*see also* Meningitis)
    - vessel G93.6
  - chest — *see* Effusion, pleura
  - chylous, chyliform (pleura) J94.Ø
  - intracranial G93.6
  - joint M25.4Ø
    - ankle M25.47- ☑
    - elbow M25.42- ☑
    - foot joint M25.47- ☑
    - hand joint M25.44- ☑
    - hip M25.45- ☑
    - knee M25.46- ☑
    - shoulder M25.41- ☑
    - specified joint NEC M25.48
    - wrist M25.43- ☑
  - malignant pleural J91.Ø
  - meninges — *see* Meningitis
  - pericardium, pericardial (noninflammatory) I31.3
    - acute — *see* Pericarditis, acute
  - peritoneal (chronic) R18.8
  - pleura, pleurisy, pleuritic, pleuropericardial J9Ø
    - chylous, chyliform J94.Ø
    - due to systemic lupus erythematosis M32.13
    - influenzal — *see* Influenza, with, respiratory manifestations NEC
    - malignant J91.Ø
    - newborn P28.89
    - tuberculous NEC A15.6
      - primary (progressive) A15.7
  - spinal — *see* Meningitis
  - thorax, thoracic — *see* Effusion, pleura
- **Egg shell nails** L6Ø.3
  - congenital Q84.6
- **Egyptian splenomegaly** B65.1
- **Ehlers-Danlos syndrome** Q79.6
- **Ehrlichiosis** A77.4Ø
  - due to
    - E. chafeensis A77.41
    - E. sennetsu A79.81
    - specified organism NEC A77.49
- **Eichstedt's disease** B36.Ø
- **Eisenmenger's**
  - complex or syndrome I27.89
  - defect Q21.8
- **Ejaculation**
  - painful N53.12
  - premature F52.4
  - retarded N53.11
  - retrograde N53.14
  - semen, painful N53.12
    - psychogenic F52.6
- **Ekbom's syndrome** (restless legs) G25.81
- **Ekman's syndrome** (brittle bones and blue sclera) Q78.Ø
- **Elastic skin** Q82.8
  - acquired L57.4

- **Elastofibroma** — *see* Neoplasm, connective tissue, benign
- **Elastoma** (juvenile) Q82.8
  - Miescher's L87.2
- **Elastomyofibrosis** I42.4
- **Elastosis**
  - actinic, solar L57.8
  - atrophicans (senile) L57.4
  - perforans serpiginosa L87.2
  - senilis L57.4
- **Elbow** — *see* condition
- **Electric current, electricity, effects** (concussion) (fatal) (nonfatal) (shock) T75.4 ☑
  - burn — *see* Burn
- **Electric feet syndrome** E53.8
- **Electrocution** T75.4 ☑
  - from electroshock gun (taser) T75.4 ☑
- **Electrolyte imbalance** E87.8
  - with
    - abortion — *see* Abortion by type, complicated by, electrolyte imbalance
    - ectopic pregnancy OØ8.5
    - molar pregnancy OØ8.5
- **Elephantiasis** (nonfilarial) I89.Ø
  - arabicum — *see* Infestation, filarial
  - bancroftian B74.Ø
  - congenital (any site) (hereditary) Q82.Ø
  - due to
    - Brugia (malayi) B74.1
      - timori B74.2
    - mastectomy I97.2
    - Wuchereria (bancrofti) B74.Ø
  - eyelid HØ2.859
    - left HØ2.856
      - lower HØ2.855
      - upper HØ2.854
    - right HØ2.853
      - lower HØ2.852
      - upper HØ2.851
  - filarial, filariensis — *see* Infestation, filarial
  - glandular I89.Ø
  - graecorum A3Ø.9
  - lymphangiectatic I89.Ø
  - lymphatic vessel I89.Ø
    - due to mastectomy I97.2
  - scrotum (nonfilarial) I89.Ø
  - streptococcal I89.Ø
  - surgical I97.89
    - postmastectomy I97.2
  - telangiectodes I89.Ø
  - vulva (nonfilarial) N9Ø.89
- **Elevated, elevation**
  - antibody titer R76.Ø
  - basal metabolic rate R94.8
  - blood pressure (*see also* Hypertension)
    - reading (incidental) (isolated) (nonspecific), no diagnosis of hypertension RØ3.Ø
  - blood sugar R73.9
  - body temperature (of unknown origin) R5Ø.9
  - cancer antigen 125 [CA 125] R97.1
  - carcinoembryonic antigen [CEA] R97.Ø
  - cholesterol E78.Ø
    - with high triglycerides E78.2
  - conjugate, eye H51.Ø
  - C-reactive protein (CRP) R79.82
  - diaphragm, congenital Q79.1
  - erythrocyte sedimentation rate R7Ø.Ø
  - fasting glucose R73.Ø1
  - fasting triglycerides E78.1
  - finding on laboratory examination — *see* Findings, abnormal, inconclusive, without diagnosis, by type of exam
  - GFR (glomerular filtration rate) — *see* Findings, abnormal, inconclusive, without diagnosis, by type of exam
  - glucose tolerance (oral) R73.Ø2
  - immunoglobulin level R76.8
  - indoleacetic acid R82.5
  - lactic acid dehydrogenase (LDH) level R74.Ø
  - leukocytes D72.829
  - lipoprotein a level E78.8 ☑
  - liver function
    - study R94.5
    - test R79.89
      - alkaline phosphatase R74.8
      - aminotransferase R74.Ø
      - bilirubin R17
      - hepatic enzyme R74.8

- **Elevated, elevation** — *continued*
  - liver function — *continued*
    - test — *continued*
      - lactate dehydrogenase R74.Ø
  - lymphocytes D72.82Ø
  - prostate specific antigen [PSA] R97.2
  - Rh titer — *see* Complication(s), transfusion, incompatibility reaction, Rh (factor)
  - scapula, congenital Q74.Ø
  - sedimentation rate R7Ø.Ø
  - SGOT R74.Ø
  - SGPT R74.Ø
  - transaminase level R74.Ø
  - triglycerides E78.1
    - with high cholesterol E78.2
  - tumor associated antigens [TAA] NEC R97.8
  - tumor specific antigens [TSA] NEC R97.8
  - urine level of
    - 17-ketosteroids R82.5
    - catecholamine R82.5
    - indoleacetic acid R82.5
    - steroids R82.5
    - vanillylmandelic acid (VMA) R82.5
  - venous pressure I87.8
  - white blood cell count D72.829
    - specified NEC D72.828
- **Elliptocytosis** (congenital) (hereditary) D58.1
  - Hb C (disease) D58.1
  - hemoglobin disease D58.1
  - sickle-cell (disease) D57.8- ☑
    - trait D57.3
- **Ellison-Zollinger syndrome** E16.4
- **Ellis-van Creveld syndrome** (chondroectodermal dysplasia) Q77.6
- **Elongated, elongation** (congenital) (*see also* Distortion)
  - bone Q79.9
  - cervix (uteri) Q51.828
    - acquired N88.4
    - hypertrophic N88.4
  - colon Q43.8
  - common bile duct Q44.5
  - cystic duct Q44.5
  - frenulum, penis Q55.69
  - labia minora (acquired) N9Ø.6
  - ligamentum patellae Q74.1
  - petiolus (epiglottidis) Q31.8
  - tooth, teeth KØØ.2
  - uvula Q38.6
- **Eltor cholera** AØØ.1
- **Emaciation** (due to malnutrition) E41
- **Embadomoniasis** AØ7.8
- **Embedded tooth, teeth** KØ1.Ø
  - root only KØ8.3
- **Embolic** — *see* condition
- **Embolism** (multiple) (paradoxical) I74.9
  - air (any site) (traumatic) T79.Ø ☑
    - following
      - abortion — *see* Abortion by type complicated by embolism
      - ectopic pregnancy OØ8.2
      - infusion, therapeutic injection or transfusion T8Ø.Ø ☑
      - molar pregnancy OØ8.2
      - procedure NEC
        - artery T81.719 ☑
          - mesenteric T81.71Ø ☑
          - renal T81.711 ☑
          - specified NEC T81.718 ☑
        - vein T81.72 ☑
    - in pregnancy, childbirth or puerperium — *see* Embolism, obstetric
  - amniotic fluid (pulmonary) (*see also* Embolism, obstetric)
    - following
      - abortion — *see* Abortion by type complicated by embolism
      - ectopic pregnancy OØ8.2
      - molar pregnancy OØ8.2
  - aorta, aortic I74.1Ø
    - abdominal I74.Ø9
      - saddle I74.Ø1
    - bifurcation I74.Ø9
    - saddle I74.Ø1
    - thoracic I74.11
  - artery I74.9
    - auditory, internal I65.8
    - basilar — *see* Occlusion, artery, basilar

- **Embolism** — *continued*
  - artery — *continued*
    - carotid (common) (internal) — *see* Occlusion, artery, carotid
    - cerebellar (anterior inferior) (posterior inferior) (superior) I66.3
    - cerebral — *see* Occlusion, artery, cerebral
    - choroidal (anterior) I66.8
    - communicating posterior I66.8
    - coronary (*see also* Infarct, myocardium)
      - not resulting in infarction I24.Ø
    - extremity I74.4
      - lower I74.3
      - upper I74.2
    - hypophyseal I66.8
    - iliac I74.5
    - limb I74.4
      - lower I74.3
      - upper I74.2
    - mesenteric (with gangrene) K55.Ø
    - ophthalmic — *see* Occlusion, artery, retina
    - peripheral I74.4
    - pontine I66.8
    - precerebral — *see* Occlusion, artery, precerebral
    - pulmonary — *see* Embolism, pulmonary
    - renal N28.Ø
    - retinal — *see* Occlusion, artery, retina
    - septic I76
    - specified NEC I74.8
    - vertebral — *see* Occlusion, artery, vertebral
  - basilar (artery) I65.1
  - blood clot
    - following
      - abortion — *see* Abortion by type complicated by embolism
      - ectopic or molar pregnancy OØ8.2
    - in pregnancy, childbirth or puerperium — *see* Embolism, obstetric
  - brain (*see also* Occlusion, artery, cerebral)
    - following
      - abortion — *see* Abortion by type complicated by embolism
      - ectopic or molar pregnancy OØ8.2
    - puerperal, postpartum, childbirth — *see* Embolism, obstetric
  - capillary I78.8
  - cardiac (*see also* Infarct, myocardium)
    - not resulting in infarction I24.Ø
  - carotid (artery) (common) (internal) — *see* Occlusion, artery, carotid
  - cavernous sinus (venous) — *see* Embolism, intracranial venous sinus
  - cerebral — *see* Occlusion, artery, cerebral
  - cholesterol — *see* Atheroembolism
  - coronary (artery or vein) (systemic) — *see* Occlusion, coronary
  - due to device, implant or graft (*see also* Complications, by site and type, specified NEC)
    - arterial graft NEC T82.818 ☑
    - breast (implant) T85.81 ☑
    - catheter NEC T85.81 ☑
      - dialysis (renal) T82.818 ☑
        - intraperitoneal T85.81 ☑
      - infusion NEC T82.818 ☑
        - spinal (epidural) (subdural) T85.81 ☑
      - urinary (indwelling) T83.81 ☑
    - electronic (electrode) (pulse generator) (stimulator)
      - bone T84.81 ☑
      - cardiac T82.817 ☑
      - nervous system (brain) (peripheral nerve) (spinal) T85.81 ☑
      - urinary T83.81 ☑
    - fixation, internal (orthopedic) NEC T84.81 ☑
    - gastrointestinal (bile duct) (esophagus) T85.81 ☑
    - genital NEC T83.81 ☑
    - heart (graft) (valve) T82.817 ☑
    - joint prosthesis T84.81 ☑
    - ocular (corneal graft) (orbital implant) T85.81 ☑
    - orthopedic (bone graft) NEC T86.838
    - specified NEC T85.81 ☑
    - urinary (graft) NEC T83.81 ☑
    - vascular NEC T82.818 ☑
    - ventricular intracranial shunt T85.81 ☑
  - extremities
    - lower — *see* Embolism, vein, lower extremity
      - arterial I74.3
    - upper I74.2

Embolism — *continued*
  eye H34.9
  fat (cerebral) (pulmonary) (systemic) T79.1 ☑
    complicating delivery — *see* Embolism, obstetric
    following
      abortion — *see* Abortion by type complicated by embolism
      ectopic or molar pregnancy OØ8.2
  following
    abortion — *see* Abortion by type complicated by embolism
    ectopic or molar pregnancy OØ8.2
    infusion, therapeutic injection or transfusion
      air T8Ø.Ø ☑
  heart (fatty) (*see also* Infarct, myocardium)
    not resulting in infarction I24.Ø
  hepatic (vein) I82.Ø
  in pregnancy, childbirth or puerperium — *see* Embolism, obstetric
  intestine (artery) (vein) (with gangrene) K55.Ø
  intracranial (*see also* Occlusion, artery, cerebral)
    venous sinus (any) GØ8
      nonpyogenic I67.6
  intraspinal venous sinuses or veins GØ8
    nonpyogenic G95.19
  kidney (artery) N28.Ø
  lateral sinus (venous) — *see* Embolism, intracranial, venous sinus
  leg — *see* Embolism, vein, lower extremity
    arterial I74.3
  longitudinal sinus (venous) — *see* Embolism, intracranial, venous sinus
  lung (massive) — *see* Embolism, pulmonary
  meninges I66.8
  mesenteric (artery) (vein) (with gangrene) K55.Ø
  obstetric (in) (pulmonary)
    childbirth O88.82
      air O88.Ø2
      amniotic fluid O88.12
      blood clot O88.22
      fat O88.82
      pyemic O88.32
      septic O88.32
      specified type NEC O88.82
    pregnancy O88.81- ☑
      air O88.Ø1- ☑
      amniotic fluid O88.11- ☑
      blood clot O88.21- ☑
      fat O88.81- ☑
      pyemic O88.31- ☑
      septic O88.31- ☑
      specified type NEC O88.81- ☑
    puerperal O88.83
      air O88.Ø3
      amniotic fluid O88.13
      blood clot O88.23
      fat O88.83
      pyemic O88.33
      septic O88.33
      specified type NEC O88.83
  ophthalmic — *see* Occlusion, artery, retina
  penis N48.81
  peripheral artery NOS I74.4
  pituitary E23.6
  popliteal (artery) I74.3
  portal (vein) I81
  postoperative, postrpocedural
    artery T81.719 ☑
      mesenteric T81.71Ø ☑
      renal T81.711 ☑
      specified NEC T81.718 ☑
    vein T81.72 ☑
  precerebral artery — *see* Occlusion, artery, precerebral
  puerperal — *see* Embolism, obstetric
  pulmonary (acute) (artery) (vein) I26.99
    with acute cor pulmonale I26.Ø9
    chronic I27.82
    following
      abortion — *see* Abortion by type complicated by embolism
      ectopic or molar pregnancy OØ8.2
    healed or old Z86.711
    in pregnancy, childbirth or puerperium — *see* Embolism, obstetric
    personal history of Z86.711
    saddle I26.92
      with acute cor pulmonale I26.Ø2

Embolism — *continued*
  pulmonary — *continued*
    septic I26.9Ø
      with acute cor pulmonale I26.Ø1
  pyemic (multiple) I76
    following
      abortion — *see* Abortion by type complicated by embolism
      ectopic or molar pregnancy OØ8.2
    Hemophilus influenzae A41.3
    pneumococcal A4Ø.3
      with pneumonia J13
    puerperal, postpartum, childbirth (any organism) — *see* Embolism, obstetric
    specified organism NEC A41.89
    staphylococcal A41.2
    streptococcal A4Ø.9
  renal (artery) N28.Ø
    vein I82.3
  retina, retinal — *see* Occlusion, artery, retina
  saddle
    abdominal aorta I74.Ø1
    pulmonary artery I26.92
      with acute cor pulmonale I26.Ø2
  septic (arterial) I76
    complicating abortion — *see* Abortion, by type, complicated by, embolism
  sinus — *see* Embolism, intracranial, venous sinus
  soap complicating abortion — *see* Abortion, by type, complicated by, embolism
  spinal cord G95.19
    pyogenic origin GØ6.1
  spleen, splenic (artery) I74.8
  upper extremity I74.2
  vein (acute) I82.9Ø
    antecubital I82.61- ☑
      chronic I82.71- ☑
    axillary I82.A1- ☑ (*following* I82.7)
      chronic I82.A2- ☑ (*following* I82.7)
    basilic I82.61- ☑
      chronic I82.71- ☑
    brachial I82.62- ☑
      chronic I82.72- ☑
    brachiocephalic (innominate) I82.29Ø
      chronic I82.291
    cephalic I82.61- ☑
      chronic I82.71- ☑
    chronic I82.91
    deep (DVT) I82.4Ø- ☑
      calf I82.4Z- ☑
        chronic I82.5Z- ☑
      lower leg I82.4Z- ☑
        chronic I82.5Z- ☑
      thigh I82.4Y- ☑
        chronic I82.5Y- ☑
      upper leg I82.4Y ☑
        chronic I82.5Y-
    femoral I82.41- ☑
      chronic I82.51- ☑
    iliac (iliofemoral) I82.42- ☑
      chronic I82.52- ☑
    innominate I82.29Ø
      chronic I82.291
    internal jugular I82.C1- ☑ (*following* I82.7)
      chronic I82.C2- ☑ (*following* I82.7)
    lower extremity
      deep I82.4Ø- ☑
        chronic I82.5Ø- ☑
        specified NEC I82.49- ☑
          chronic NEC I82.59- ☑
      distal
        deep I82.4Z- ☑
      proximal
        deep I82.4Y- ☑
          chronic I82.5Y- ☑
      superficial I82.81- ☑
    popliteal I82.43- ☑
      chronic I82.53- ☑
    radial I82.62- ☑
      chronic I82.72- ☑
    renal I82.3
    saphenous (greater) (lesser) I82.81- ☑
    specified NEC I82.89Ø
      chronic NEC I82.891
    subclavian I82.B1- ☑ (*following* I82.7)
      chronic I82.B2- ☑ (*following* I82.7)
    thoracic NEC I82.29Ø

Embolism — *continued*
  vein — *continued*
    thoracic — *continued*
      chronic I82.291
    tibial I82.44- ☑
      chronic I82.54- ☑
    ulnar I82.62- ☑
      chronic I82.72- ☑
    upper extremity I82.6Ø- ☑
      chronic I82.7Ø- ☑
      deep I82.62- ☑
        chronic I82.72- ☑
      superficial I82.61- ☑
        chronic I82.71- ☑
  vena cava
    inferior (acute) I82.22Ø
      chronic I82.221
    superior (acute) I82.21Ø
      chronic I82.211
  venous sinus GØ8
  vessels of brain — *see* Occlusion, artery, cerebral

Embolus — *see* Embolism

Embryoma (*see also* Neoplasm, uncertain behavior, by site)
  benign — *see* Neoplasm, benign, by site
  kidney C64.- ☑
  liver C22.Ø
  malignant (*see also* Neoplasm, malignant, by site)
    kidney C64.- ☑
    liver C22.Ø
    testis C62.9- ☑
      descended (scrotal) C62.1- ☑
      undescended C62.Ø- ☑
  testis C62.9- ☑
    descended (scrotal) C62.1- ☑
    undescended C62.Ø- ☑

Embryonic
  circulation Q28.9
  heart Q28.9
  vas deferens Q55.4

Embryopathia NOS Q89.9

Embryotoxon Q13.4

Emesis — *see* Vomiting

Emotional lability R45.86

Emotionality, pathological F6Ø.3

Emotogenic disease — *see* Disorder, psychogenic

Emphysema (atrophic) (bullous) (chronic) (interlobular) (lung) (obstructive) (pulmonary) (senile) (vesicular) J43.9
  cellular tissue (traumatic) T79.7 ☑
    surgical T81.82 ☑
  centrilobular J43.2
  compensatory J98.3
  congenital (interstitial) P25.Ø
  conjunctiva H11.89
  connective tissue (traumatic) T79.7 ☑
    surgical T81.82 ☑
  due to chemicals, gases, fumes or vapors J68.4
  eyelid(s) — *see* Disorder, eyelid, specified type NEC
    surgical T81.82 ☑
    traumatic T79.7 ☑
  interstitial J98.2
    congenital P25.Ø
    perinatal period P25.Ø
  laminated tissue T79.7 ☑
    surgical T81.82 ☑
  mediastinal J98.2
    newborn P25.2
  orbit, orbital — *see* Disorder, orbit, specified type NEC
  panacinar J43.1
  panlobular J43.1
  specified NEC J43.8
  subcutaneous (traumatic) T79.7 ☑
    nontraumatic J98.2
    postprocedural T81.82 ☑
    surgical T81.82 ☑
  surgical T81.82 ☑
  thymus (gland) (congenital) E32.8
  traumatic (subcutaneous) T79.7 ☑
  unilateral J43.Ø

Empty nest syndrome Z6Ø.Ø

Empyema (acute) (chest) (double) (pleura) (supradiaphragmatic) (thorax) J86.9
  with fistula J86.Ø
  accessory sinus (chronic) — *see* Sinusitis
  antrum (chronic) — *see* Sinusitis, maxillary
  brain (any part) — *see* Abscess, brain

Empyema — *continued*
  ethmoidal (chronic) (sinus) — *see* Sinusitis, ethmoidal
  extradural — *see* Abscess, extradural
  frontal (chronic) (sinus) — *see* Sinusitis, frontal
  gallbladder K81.Ø
  mastoid (process) (acute) — *see* Mastoiditis, acute
  maxilla, maxillary M27.2
    sinus (chronic) — *see* Sinusitis, maxillary
  nasal sinus (chronic) — *see* Sinusitis
  sinus (accessory) (chronic) (nasal) — *see* Sinusitis
  sphenoidal (sinus) (chronic) — *see* Sinusitis, sphenoidal
  subarachnoid — *see* Abscess, extradural
  subdural — *see* Abscess, subdural
  tuberculous A15.6
  ureter — *see* Ureteritis
  ventricular — *see* Abscess, brain
En coup de sabre lesion L94.1
Enamel pearls KØØ.2
Enameloma KØØ.2
Enanthema, viral BØ9
Encephalitis (chronic) (hemorrhagic) (idiopathic) (nonepidemic) (spurious) (subacute) GØ4.9Ø
  acute (*see also* Encephalitis, viral) A86
    disseminated GØ4.ØØ
      infectious GØ4.Ø1
      noninfectious GØ4.81
      postimmunization (postvaccination) GØ4.Ø2
      postinfectious GØ4.Ø1
    inclusion body A85.8
    necrotizing hemorrhagic GØ4.3Ø
      postimmunization GØ4.32
      postinfectious GØ4.31
      specified NEC GØ4.39
  arboviral, arbovirus NEC A85.2
  arthropod-borne NEC (viral) A85.2
  Australian A83.4
  California (virus) A83.5
  Central European (tick-borne) A84.1
  Czechoslovakian A84.1
  Dawson's (inclusion body) A81.1
  diffuse sclerosing A81.1
  disseminated, acute GØ4.ØØ
  due to
    cat scratch disease A28.1
    human immunodeficiency virus (HIV) disease B2Ø [GØ5.3]
    malaria — *see* Malaria
    rickettsiosis — *see* Rickettsiosis
    smallpox inoculation GØ4.Ø2
    typhus — *see* Typhus
  Eastern equine A83.2
  endemic (viral) A86
  epidemic NEC (viral) A86
  equine (acute) (infectious) (viral) A83.9
    Eastern A83.2
    Venezuelan A92.2
    Western A83.1
  Far Eastern (tick-borne) A84.Ø
  following vaccination or other immunization procedure GØ4.Ø2
  herpes zoster BØ2.Ø
  herpesviral BØØ.4
    due to herpesvirus 6 B1Ø.Ø1
    due to herpesvirus 7 B1Ø.Ø9
    specified NEC B1Ø.Ø9
  Ilheus (virus) A83.8
  in (due to)
    actinomycosis A42.82
    adenovirus A85.1
    African trypanosomiasis B56.9 [GØ5.3]
    Chagas' disease (chronic) B57.42
    cytomegalovirus B25.8
    enterovirus A85.Ø
    herpes (simplex) virus BØØ.4
      due to herpesvirus 6 B1Ø.Ø1
      due to herpesvirus 7 B1Ø.Ø9
      specified NEC B1Ø.Ø9
    infectious disease NEC B99 ☑ [GØ5.3]
    influenza — *see* Influenza, with, encephalopathy
    listeriosis A32.12
    measles BØ5.Ø
    mumps B26.2
    naegleriasis B6Ø.2
    parasitic disease NEC B89 [GØ5.3]
    poliovirus A8Ø.9 [GØ5.3]
    rubella BØ6.Ø1

Encephalitis — *continued*
  in — *continued*
    syphilis
      congenital A5Ø.42
      late A52.14
    systemic lupus erythematosus M32.19
    toxoplasmosis (acquired) B58.2
      congenital P37.1
    tuberculosis A17.82
    zoster BØ2.Ø
  inclusion body A81.1
  infectious (acute) (virus) NEC A86
  Japanese (B type) A83.Ø
  La Crosse A83.5
  lead — *see* Poisoning, lead
  lethargica (acute) (infectious) A85.8
  louping ill A84.8
  lupus erythematosus, systemic M32.19
  lymphatica A87.2
  Mengo A85.8
  meningococcal A39.81
  Murray Valley A83.4
  otitic NEC H66.4Ø [GØ5.3]
  parasitic NOS B71.9
  periaxial G37.Ø
  periaxialis (concentrica) (diffuse) G37.5
  postchickenpox BØ1.11
  postexanthematous NEC BØ9
  postimmunization GØ4.Ø2
  postinfectious NEC GØ4.Ø1
  postmeasles BØ5.Ø
  postvaccinal GØ4.Ø2
  postvaricella BØ1.11
  postviral NEC A86
  Powassan A84.8
  Rasmussen GØ4.81
  Rio Bravo A85.8
  Russian
    autumnal A83.Ø
    spring-summer (taiga) A84.Ø
  saturnine — *see* Poisoning, lead
  specified NEC GØ4.81
  St. Louis A83.3
  subacute sclerosing A81.1
  summer A83.Ø
  suppurative GØ4.81
  tick-borne A84.9
  Torula, torular (cryptococcal) B45.1
  toxic NEC G92
  trichinosis B75 [GØ5.3]
  type
    B A83.Ø
    C A83.3
  van Bogaert's A81.1
  Venezuelan equine A92.2
  Vienna A85.8
  viral, virus A86
    arthropod-borne NEC A85.2
      mosquito-borne A83.9
        Australian X disease A83.4
        California virus A83.5
        Eastern equine A83.2
        Japanese (B type) A83.Ø
        Murray Valley A83.4
        specified NEC A83.8
        St. Louis A83.3
        type B A83.Ø
        type C A83.3
        Western equine A83.1
      tick-borne A84.9
        biundulant A84.1
        central European A84.1
        Czechoslovakian A84.1
        diphasic meningoencephalitis A84.1
        Far Eastern A84.Ø
        Russian spring-summer (taiga) A84.Ø
        specified NEC A84.8
    specified type NEC A85.8
  Western equine A83.1
Encephalocele QØ1.9
  frontal QØ1.Ø
  nasofrontal QØ1.1
  occipital QØ1.2
  specified NEC QØ1.8
Encephalocystocele — *see* Encephalocele
Encephaloduroarteriomyosynangiosis (EDAMS) I67.5
Encephalomalacia (brain) (cerebellar) (cerebral) — *see* Softening, brain

Encephalomeningitis — *see* Meningoencephalitis
Encephalomeningocele — *see* Encephalocele
Encephalomeningomyelitis — *see* Meningoencephalitis
Encephalomyelitis (*see also* Encephalitis) GØ4.9Ø
  acute disseminated GØ4.ØØ
    infectious GØ4.Ø1
    noninfectious GØ4.81
    postimmunization GØ4.Ø2
    postinfectious GØ4.Ø1
  acute necrotizing hemorrhagic GØ4.3Ø
    postimmunization GØ4.32
    postinfectious GØ4.31
    specified NEC GØ4.39
  benign myalgic G93.3
  equine A83.9
    Eastern A83.2
    Venezuelan A92.2
    Western A83.1
  in diseases classified elsewhere GØ5.3
  myalgic, benign G93.3
  postchickenpox BØ1.11
  postinfectious NEC GØ4.Ø1
  postmeasles BØ5.Ø
  postvaccinal GØ4.Ø2
  postvaricella BØ1.11
  rubella BØ6.Ø1
  specified NEC GØ4.81
  Venezuelan equine A92.2
Encephalomyelocele — *see* Encephalocele
Encephalomyelomeningitis — *see* Meningoencephalitis
Encephalomyelopathy G96.9
Encephalomyeloradiculitis (acute) G61.Ø
Encephalomyeloradiculoneuritis (acute) (Guillain-Barré) G61.Ø
Encephalomyeloradiculopathy G96.9
Encephalopathia hyperbilirubinemica, newborn P57.9
  due to isoimmunization (conditions in P55) P57.Ø
Encephalopathy (acute) G93.4Ø
  acute necrotizing hemorrhagic GØ4.3Ø
    postimmunization GØ4.32
    postinfectious GØ4.31
    specified NEC GØ4.39
  alcoholic G31.2
  anoxic — *see* Damage, brain, anoxic
  arteriosclerotic I67.2
  centrolobar progressive (Schilder) G37.Ø
  congenital QØ7.9
  degenerative, in specified disease NEC G32.89
  demyelinating callosal G37.1
  due to
    drugs (*see also* Table of Drugs and Chemicals) G92
  hepatic — *see* Failure, hepatic
  hyperbilirubinemic, newborn P57.9
    due to isoimmunization (conditions in P55) P57.Ø
  hypertensive I67.4
  hypoglycemic E16.2
  hypoxic — *see* Damage, brain, anoxic
  hypoxic ischemic P91.6Ø
    mild P91.61
    moderate P91.62
    severe P91.63
  in (due to) (with)
    birth injury P11.1
    hyperinsulinism E16.1 [G94]
    influenza — *see* Influenza, with, encephalopathy
    lack of vitamin (*see also* Deficiency, vitamin) E56.9 [G32.89]
    neoplastic disease (*see also* Neoplasm) D49.9 [G13.1]
    serum (*see also* Reaction, serum) T8Ø.69 ☑
    syphilis A52.17
    trauma (postconcussional) FØ7.81
      current injury — *see* Injury, intracranial
    vaccination GØ4.Ø2
  lead — *see* Poisoning, lead
  metabolic G93.41
    drug induced G92
    toxic G92
  myoclonic, early, symptomatic — *see* Epilepsy, generalized, specified NEC
  necrotizing, subacute (Leigh) G31.82
  pellagrous E52 [G32.89]
  portosystemic — *see* Failure, hepatic
  postcontusional FØ7.81
    current injury — *see* Injury, intracranial, diffuse

- **Encephalopathy** — *continued*
  - posthypoglycemic (coma) E16.1 [G94]
  - postradiation G93.89
  - saturnine — *see* Poisoning, lead
  - septic G93.41
  - specified NEC G93.49
  - spongioform, subacute (viral) A81.Ø9
  - toxic G92
    - metabolic G92
  - traumatic (postconcussional) FØ7.81
    - current injury — *see* Injury, intracranial
  - vitamin B deficiency NEC E53.9 [G32.89]
    - vitamin B1 E51.2
  - Wernicke's E51.2
- **Encephalorrhagia** — *see* Hemorrhage, intracranial, intracerebral
- **Encephalosis, posttraumatic** FØ7.81
- **Enchondroma** (*see also* Neoplasm, bone, benign)
- **Enchondromatosis** (cartilaginous) (multiple) Q78.4
- **Encopresis** R15.9
  - functional F98.1
  - nonorganic origin F98.1
  - psychogenic F98.1
- **Encounter** (with health service) (for) Z76.89
  - adjustment and management (of)
    - breast implant Z45.81 ☑
    - implanted device NEC Z45.89
    - myringotomy device (stent) (tube) Z45.82
  - administrative purpose only ZØ2.9
    - examination for
      - adoption ZØ2.82
      - armed forces ZØ2.3
      - disability determination ZØ2.71
      - driving license ZØ2.4
      - employment ZØ2.1
      - insurance ZØ2.6
      - medical certificate NEC ZØ2.79
      - paternity testing ZØ2.81
      - residential institution admission ZØ2.2
      - school admission ZØ2.Ø
      - sports ZØ2.5
    - specified reason NEC ZØ2.89
  - aftercare — *see* Aftercare
  - antenatal screening Z36
  - assisted reproductive fertility procedure cycle Z31.83
  - blood typing ZØ1.83
    - Rh typing ZØ1.83
  - breast augmentation or reduction Z41.1
  - breast implant exchange (different material) (different size) Z45.81 ☑
  - breast reconstruction following mastectomy Z42.1
  - check-up — *see* Examination
  - chemotherapy for neoplasm Z51.11
  - colonoscopy, screening Z12.11
  - counseling — *see* Counseling
  - delivery, full-term, uncomplicated O8Ø
    - cesarean, without indication O82
  - ear piercing Z41.3
  - examination — *see* Examination
  - expectant parent(s) (adoptive) pre-birth pediatrician visit Z76.81
  - fertility preservation procedure (prior to cancer therapy) (prior to removal of gonads) Z31.84
  - fitting (of) — *see* Fitting (and adjustment) (of)
  - genetic
    - counseling Z31.5
    - testing — *see* Test, genetic
  - hearing conservation and treatment ZØ1.12
  - immunotherapy for neoplasm Z51.12
  - in vitro fertilization cycle Z31.83
  - instruction (in)
    - child care (postpartal) (prenatal) Z32.3
    - childbirth Z32.2
    - natural family planning
      - procreative Z31.61
      - to avoid pregnancy Z3Ø.Ø2
  - insulin pump titration Z46.81
  - joint prosthesis insertion following prior explantation of joint prosthesis (staged procedure)
    - hip Z47.32
    - knee Z47.33
    - shoulder Z47.31
  - laboratory (as part of a general medical examination) ZØØ.ØØ
    - with abnormal findings ZØØ.Ø1
  - mental health services (for)
    - abuse NEC
      - perpetrator Z69.82

- **Encounter** — *continued*
  - mental health services — *continued*
    - abuse — *continued*
      - victim Z69.81
    - child abuse
      - nonparental
        - perpetrator Z69.Ø21
        - victim Z69.Ø2Ø
      - parental
        - perpetrator Z69.Ø11
        - victim Z69.Ø1Ø
    - spousal or partner abuse
      - perpetrator Z69.12
      - victim Z69.11
  - observation (for) (ruled out)
    - exposure to (suspected)
      - anthrax ZØ3.81Ø
      - biological agent NEC ZØ3.818
  - pediatrician visit, by expectant parent(s) (adoptive) Z76.81
  - plastic and reconstructive surgery following medical procedure or healed injury NEC Z42.8
  - pregnancy
    - supervision of — *see* Pregnancy, supervision of
    - test Z32.ØØ
      - result negative Z32.Ø2
      - result positive Z32.Ø1
  - radiation therapy (antineoplastic) Z51.Ø
  - radiological (as part of a general medical examination) ZØØ.ØØ
    - with abnormal findings ZØØ.Ø1
  - reconstructive surgery following medical procedure or healed injury NEC Z42.8
  - removal (of) (*see also* Removal)
    - artificial
      - arm Z44.ØØ- ☑
        - complete Z44.Ø1- ☑
        - partial Z44.Ø2- ☑
      - eye Z44.2- ☑
      - leg Z44.1Ø- ☑
        - complete Z44.11- ☑
        - partial Z44.12- ☑
    - breast implant Z45.81 ☑
      - tissue expander (without synchronous insertion of permanent implant) Z45.81 ☑
    - device Z46.9
      - specified NEC Z46.89
    - external
      - fixation device — *code to* fracture with seventh character D
      - prosthesis, prosthetic device Z44.9
        - breast Z44.3- ☑
        - specified NEC Z44.8
    - implanted device NEC Z45.89
    - insulin pump Z46.81
    - internal fixation device Z47.2
    - myringotomy device (stent) (tube) Z45.82
    - nervous system device NEC Z46.2
      - brain neuropacemaker Z46.2
      - visual substitution device Z46.2
        - implanted Z45.31
    - non-vascular catheter Z46.82
    - orthodontic device Z46.4
    - stent
      - ureteral Z46.6
    - urinary device Z46.6
  - repeat cervical smear to confirm findings of recent normal smear following initial abnormal smear ZØ1.42
  - respirator [ventilator] use during power failure Z99.12
  - Rh typing ZØ1.83
  - screening — *see* Screening
  - specified NEC Z76.89
  - sterilization Z3Ø.2
  - suspected condition, ruled out
    - amniotic cavity and membrane ZØ3.71
    - cervical shortening ZØ3.75
    - fetal anomaly ZØ3.73
    - fetal growth ZØ3.74
    - maternal and fetal conditions NEC ZØ3.79
    - oligohydramnios ZØ3.71
    - placental problem ZØ3.72
    - polyhydramnios ZØ3.71
  - suspected exposure (to), ruled out
    - anthrax ZØ3.81Ø
    - biological agents NEC ZØ3.818
  - termination of pregnancy, elective Z33.2
  - testing — *see* Test

- **Encounter** — *continued*
  - therapeutic drug level monitoring Z51.81
  - titration, insulin pump Z46.81
  - to determine fetal viability of pregnancy O36.8Ø ☑
  - training
    - insulin pump Z46.81
  - X-ray of chest (as part of a general medical examination) ZØØ.ØØ
    - with abnormal findings ZØØ.Ø1
- **Encystment** — *see* Cyst
- **Endarteritis** (bacterial, subacute) (infective) I77.6
  - brain I67.7
  - cerebral or cerebrospinal I67.7
  - deformans — *see* Arteriosclerosis
  - embolic — *see* Embolism
  - obliterans (*see also* Arteriosclerosis)
    - pulmonary I28.8
  - pulmonary I28.8
  - retina — *see* Vasculitis, retina
  - senile — *see* Arteriosclerosis
  - syphilitic A52.Ø9
    - brain or cerebral A52.Ø4
    - congenital A5Ø.54 [I79.8]
  - tuberculous A18.89
- **Endemic** — *see* condition
- **Endocarditis** (chronic) (marantic) (nonbacterial) (thrombotic) (valvular) I38
  - with rheumatic fever (conditions in IØØ)
    - active — *see* Endocarditis, acute, rheumatic
    - inactive or quiescent (with chorea) IØ9.1
  - acute or subacute I33.9
    - infective I33.Ø
    - rheumatic (aortic) (mitral) (pulmonary) (tricuspid) IØ1.1
      - with chorea (acute) (rheumatic) (Sydenham's) IØ2.Ø
  - aortic (heart) (nonrheumatic) (valve) I35.8
    - with
      - mitral disease IØ8.Ø
        - with tricuspid (valve) disease IØ8.3
        - active or acute IØ1.1
          - with chorea (acute) (rheumatic) (Sydenham's) IØ2.Ø
      - rheumatic fever (conditions in IØØ)
        - active — *see* Endocarditis, acute, rheumatic
        - inactive or quiescent (with chorea) IØ6.9
      - tricuspid (valve) disease IØ8.2
        - with mitral (valve) disease IØ8.3
    - acute or subacute I33.9
    - arteriosclerotic I35.8
    - rheumatic IØ6.9
      - with mitral disease IØ8.Ø
        - with tricuspid (valve) disease IØ8.3
        - active or acute IØ1.1
          - with chorea (acute) (rheumatic) (Sydenham's) IØ2.Ø
      - active or acute IØ1.1
        - with chorea (acute) (rheumatic) (Sydenham's) IØ2.Ø
      - specified NEC IØ6.8
    - specified cause NEC I35.8
    - syphilitic A52.Ø3
  - arteriosclerotic I38
  - atypical verrucous (Libman-Sacks) M32.11
  - bacterial (acute) (any valve) (subacute) I33.Ø
  - candidal B37.6
  - congenital Q24.8
  - constrictive I33.Ø
  - Coxiella burnetii A78 [I39]
  - Coxsackie B33.21
  - due to
    - prosthetic cardiac valve T82.6 ☑
    - Q fever A78 [I39]
    - Serratia marcescens I33.Ø
    - typhoid (fever) AØ1.Ø2
  - gonococcal A54.83
  - infectious or infective (acute) (any valve) (subacute) I33.Ø
  - lenta (acute) (any valve) (subacute) I33.Ø
  - Libman-Sacks M32.11
  - listerial A32.82
  - Löffler's I42.3
  - malignant (acute) (any valve) (subacute) I33.Ø
  - meningococcal A39.51
  - mitral (chronic) (double) (fibroid) (heart) (inactive) (valve) (with chorea) IØ5.9
    - with
      - aortic (valve) disease IØ8.Ø

Endocarditis — *continued*
- mitral — *continued*
  - with — *continued*
    - aortic disease — *continued*
      - with tricuspid (valve) disease IØ8.3
      - active or acute IØ1.1
        - with chorea (acute) (rheumatic) (Sydenham's) IØ2.Ø
    - rheumatic fever (conditions in IØØ)
      - active — *see* Endocarditis, acute, rheumatic
      - inactive or quiescent (with chorea) IØ5.9
    - tricuspid (valve) disease IØ8.1
      - with aortic (valve) disease IØ8.3
  - active or acute IØ1.1
    - with chorea (acute) (rheumatic) (Sydenham's) IØ2.Ø
  - bacterial I33.Ø
  - arteriosclerotic I34.8
  - nonrheumatic I34.8
    - acute or subacute I33.9
  - specified NEC IØ5.8
- monilial B37.6
- multiple valves IØ8.9
  - specified disorders IØ8.8
- mycotic (acute) (any valve) (subacute) I33.Ø
- pneumococcal (acute) (any valve) (subacute) I33.Ø
- pulmonary (chronic) (heart) (valve) I37.8
  - with rheumatic fever (conditions in IØØ)
    - active — *see* Endocarditis, acute, rheumatic
    - inactive or quiescent (with chorea) IØ9.89
      - with aortic, mitral or tricuspid disease IØ8.8
  - acute or subacute I33.9
    - rheumatic IØ1.1
      - with chorea (acute) (rheumatic) (Sydenham's) IØ2.Ø
  - arteriosclerotic I37.8
  - congenital Q22.2
  - rheumatic (chronic) (inactive) (with chorea) IØ9.89
    - active or acute IØ1.1
      - with chorea (acute) (rheumatic) (Sydenham's) IØ2.Ø
  - syphilitic A52.Ø3
- purulent (acute) (any valve) (subacute) I33.Ø
- Q fever A78 [I39]
- rheumatic (chronic) (inactive) (with chorea) IØ9.1
  - active or acute (aortic) (mitral) (pulmonary) (tricuspid) IØ1.1
    - with chorea (acute) (rheumatic) (Sydenham's) IØ2.Ø
- rheumatoid — *see* Rheumatoid, carditis
- septic (acute) (any valve) (subacute) I33.Ø
- streptococcal (acute) (any valve) (subacute) I33.Ø
- subacute — *see* Endocarditis, acute
- suppurative (acute) (any valve) (subacute) I33.Ø
- syphilitic A52.Ø3
- toxic I33.9
- tricuspid (chronic) (heart) (inactive) (rheumatic) (valve) (with chorea) IØ7.9
  - with
    - aortic (valve) disease IØ8.2
      - mitral (valve) disease IØ8.3
    - mitral (valve) disease IØ8.1
      - aortic (valve) disease IØ8.3
    - rheumatic fever (conditions in IØØ)
      - active — *see* Endocarditis, acute, rheumatic
      - inactive or quiescent (with chorea) IØ7.8
  - active or acute IØ1.1
    - with chorea (acute) (rheumatic) (Sydenham's) IØ2.Ø
  - arteriosclerotic I36.8
  - nonrheumatic I36.8
    - acute or subacute I33.9
  - specified cause, except rheumatic I36.8
- tuberculous — *see* Tuberculosis, endocarditis
- typhoid AØ1.Ø2
- ulcerative (acute) (any valve) (subacute) I33.Ø
- vegetative (acute) (any valve) (subacute) I33.Ø
- verrucous (atypical) (nonbacterial) (nonrheumatic) M32.11

Endocardium, endocardial (*see also* condition)
- cushion defect Q21.2

Endocervicitis (*see also* Cervicitis)
- due to intrauterine (contraceptive) device T83.6 ☑
- hyperplastic N72

Endocrine — *see* condition

Endocrinopathy, pluriglandular E31.9

Endodontic
- overfill M27.52

Endodontic — *continued*
- underfill M27.53

Endodontitis KØ4.Ø

Endomastoiditis — *see* Mastoiditis

Endometrioma N8Ø.9

Endometriosis N8Ø.9
- appendix N8Ø.5
- bladder N8Ø.8
- bowel N8Ø.5
- broad ligament N8Ø.3
- cervix N8Ø.Ø
- colon N8Ø.5
- cul-de-sac (Douglas') N8Ø.3
- exocervix N8Ø.Ø
- fallopian tube N8Ø.2
- female genital organ NEC N8Ø.8
- gallbladder N8Ø.8
- in scar of skin N8Ø.6
- internal N8Ø.Ø
- intestine N8Ø.5
- lung N8Ø.8
- myometrium N8Ø.Ø
- ovary N8Ø.1
- parametrium N8Ø.3
- pelvic peritoneum N8Ø.3
- peritoneal (pelvic) N8Ø.3
- rectovaginal septum N8Ø.4
- rectum N8Ø.5
- round ligament N8Ø.3
- skin (scar) N8Ø.6
- specified site NEC N8Ø.8
- stromal D39.Ø
- umbilicus N8Ø.8
- uterus (internal) N8Ø.Ø
- vagina N8Ø.4
- vulva N8Ø.8

Endometritis (decidual) (nonspecific) (purulent) (senile) (atrophic) (suppurative) N71.9
- with ectopic pregnancy OØ8.Ø
- acute N71.Ø
- blenorrhagic (gonococcal) (acute) (chronic) A54.24
- cervix, cervical (with erosion or ectropion) (*see also* Cervicitis)
  - hyperplastic N72
- chlamydial A56.11
- chronic N71.1
- following
  - abortion — *see* Abortion by type complicated by genital infection
  - ectopic or molar pregnancy OØ8.Ø
- gonococcal, gonorrheal (acute) (chronic) A54.24
- hyperplastic (*see also* Hyperplasia, endometrial) N85.ØØ
  - cervix N72
- puerperal, postpartum, childbirth O86.12
- subacute N71.Ø
- tuberculous A18.17

Endometrium — *see* condition

Endomyocardiopathy, South African I42.3

Endomyocarditis — *see* Endocarditis

Endomyofibrosis I42.3

Endomyometritis — *see* Endometritis

Endopericarditis — *see* Endocarditis

Endoperineuritis — *see* Disorder, nerve

Endophlebitis — *see* Phlebitis

Endophthalmia — *see* Endophthalmitis, purulent

Endophthalmitis (acute) (infective) (metastatic) (subacute) H44.ØØ9
- bleb associated (*see also* Bleb, inflammed (infected), postprocedural H59.4 ☑
- gonorrheal A54.39
- in (due to)
  - cysticercosis B69.1
  - onchocerciasis B73.Ø1
  - toxocariasis B83.Ø
- panuveitis — *see* Panuveitis
- parasitic H44.12- ☑
- purulent H44.ØØ- ☑
  - panophthalmitis — *see* Panophthalmitis
  - vitreous abscess H44.Ø2- ☑
- specified NEC H44.19
- sympathetic — *see* Uveitis, sympathetic

Endosalpingioma D28.2

Endosalpingiosis N94.89

Endosteitis — *see* Osteomyelitis

Endothelioma, bone — *see* Neoplasm, bone, malignant

Endotheliosis (hemorrhagic infectional) D69.8

Endotoxemia — code to condition

Endotrachelitis — *see* Cervicitis

Engelmann (-Camurati) **syndrome** Q78.3

English disease — *see* Rickets

Engman's disease L3Ø.3

Engorgement
- breast N64.59
  - newborn P83.4
  - puerperal, postpartum O92.79
- lung (passive) — *see* Edema, lung
- pulmonary (passive) — *see* Edema, lung
- stomach K31.89
- venous, retina — *see* Occlusion, retina, vein, engorgement

Enlargement, enlarged (*see also* Hypertrophy)
- adenoids J35.2
  - with tonsils J35.3
- alveolar ridge KØ8.8
  - congenital — *see* Anomaly, alveolar
- apertures of diaphragm (congenital) Q79.1
- gingival KØ6.1
- heart, cardiac — *see* Hypertrophy, cardiac
- lacrimal gland, chronic HØ4.Ø3- ☑
- liver — *see* Hypertrophy, liver
- lymph gland or node R59.9
  - generalized R59.1
  - localized R59.Ø
- orbit HØ5.34- ☑
- organ or site, congenital NEC — *see* Anomaly, by site
- parathyroid (gland) E21.Ø
- pituitary fossa R93.Ø
- prostate N4Ø.Ø
  - with lower urinary tract symptoms (LUTS) N4Ø.1
  - without lower urinary tract symtpoms (LUTS) N4Ø.Ø
- sella turcica R93.Ø
- spleen — *see* Splenomegaly
- thymus (gland) (congenital) E32.Ø
- thyroid (gland) — *see* Goiter
- tongue K14.8
- tonsils J35.1
  - with adenoids J35.3
- uterus N85.2

Enophthalmos HØ5.4Ø- ☑
- due to
  - orbital tissue atrophy HØ5.41- ☑
  - trauma or surgery HØ5.42- ☑

Enostosis M27.8

Entamebic, entamebiasis — *see* Amebiasis

Entanglement
- umbilical cord(s) O69.2 ☑
  - with compression O69.2 ☑
    - without compression O69.82 ☑
  - around neck (with compression) O69.1 ☑
    - without compression O69.81 ☑
  - of twins in monoamniotic sac O69.2 ☑

Enteralgia — *see* Pain, abdominal

Enteric — *see* condition

Enteritis (acute) (diarrheal) (hemorrhagic) (noninfective) (septic) K52.9
- adenovirus AØ8.2
- aertrycke infection AØ2.Ø
- allergic K52.2
- amebic (acute) AØ6.Ø
  - with abscess — *see* Abscess, amebic
  - chronic AØ6.1
    - with abscess — *see* Abscess, amebic
    - nondysenteric AØ6.2
  - nondysenteric AØ6.2
- astrovirus AØ8.32
- bacillary NOS AØ3.9
- bacterial AØ4.9
  - specified NEC AØ4.8
- calicivirus AØ8.31
- candidal B37.82
- Chilomastix AØ7.8
- choleriformis AØØ.1
- chronic (noninfectious) K52.9
  - ulcerative — *see* Colitis, ulcerative
- cicatrizing (chronic) — *see* Enteritis, regional, small intestine
- Clostridium
  - botulinum (food poisoning) AØ5.1
  - difficile AØ4.7
- coccidial AØ7.3
- coxsackie virus AØ8.39
- dietetic K52.2
- drug-induced K52.1

- **Enteritis** — *continued*
  - due to
    - astrovirus A08.32
    - calicivirus A08.31
    - coxsackie virus A08.39
    - drugs K52.1
    - echovirus A08.39
    - enterovirus NEC A08.39
    - food hypersensitivity K52.2
    - infectious organism (bacterial) (viral) — *see* Enteritis, infectious
    - torovirus A08.39
    - Yersinia enterocolitica A04.6
  - echovirus A08.39
  - eltor A00.1
  - enterovirus NEC A08.39
  - eosinophilic K52.81
  - epidemic (infectious) A09
  - fulminant K55.0
  - gangrenous — *see* Enteritis, infectious
  - giardial A07.1
  - infectious NOS A09
    - due to
      - adenovirus A08.2
      - Aerobacter aerogenes A04.8
      - Arizona (bacillus) A02.0
      - bacteria NOS A04.9
        - specified NEC A04.8
      - Campylobacter A04.5
      - Clostridium difficile A04.7
      - Clostridium perfringens A04.8
      - Enterobacter aerogenes A04.8
      - enterovirus A08.39
      - Escherichia coli A04.4
        - enteroaggregative A04.4
        - enterohemorrhagic A04.3
        - enteroinvasive A04.2
        - enteropathogenic A04.0
        - enterotoxigenic A04.1
        - specified NEC A04.4
      - specified
        - bacteria NEC A04.8
        - virus NEC A08.39
      - Staphylococcus A04.8
      - virus NEC A08.4
        - specified type NEC A08.39
      - Yersinia enterocolitica A04.6
    - specified organism NEC A08.8
  - influenzal — *see* Influenza, with, digestive manifestations
  - ischemic K55.9
    - acute K55.0
    - chronic K55.1
  - microsporidial A07.8
  - mucomembranous, myxomembranous — *see* Syndrome, irritable bowel
  - mucous — *see* Syndrome, irritable bowel
  - necroticans A05.2
  - necrotizing of newborn — *see* Enterocolitis, necrotizing, in newborn
  - neurogenic — *see* Syndrome, irritable bowel
  - newborn necrotizing — *see* Enterocolitis, necrotizing, in newborn
  - noninfectious K52.9
  - norovirus A08.11
  - parasitic NEC B82.9
  - paratyphoid (fever) — *see* Fever, paratyphoid
  - protozoal A07.9
    - specified NEC A07.8
  - radiation K52.0
  - regional (of) K50.90
    - with
      - complication K50.919
        - abscess K50.914
        - fistula K50.913
        - intestinal obstruction K50.912
        - rectal bleeding K50.911
        - specified complication NEC K50.918
    - colon — *see* Enteritis, regional, large intestine
    - duodenum — *see* Enteritis, regional, small intestine
    - ileum — *see* Enteritis, regional, small intestine
    - jejunum — *see* Enteritis, regional, small intestine
    - large bowel — *see* Enteritis, regional, large intestine
    - large intestine (colon) (rectum) K50.10
      - with
        - complication K50.119
          - abscess K50.114

- **Enteritis** — *continued*
  - regional — *continued*
    - large intestine — *continued*
      - with — *continued*
        - complication — *continued*
          - fistula K50.113
          - intestinal obstruction K50.112
          - rectal bleeding K50.111
          - small intestine (duodenum) (ileum) (jejunum) involvement K50.80
            - with
              - complication K50.819
                - abscess K50.814
                - fistula K50.813
                - intestinal obstruction K50.812
                - rectal bleeding K50.811
                - specified complication NEC K50.818
          - specified complication NEC K50.118
    - rectum — *see* Enteritis, regional, large intestine
    - small intestine (duodenum) (ileum) (jejunum) K50.00
      - with
        - complication K50.019
          - abscess K50.014
          - fistula K50.013
          - intestinal obstruction K50.012
          - large intestine (colon) (rectum) involvement K50.80
            - with
              - complication K50.819
                - abscess K50.814
                - fistula K50.813
                - intestinal obstruction K50.812
                - rectal bleeding K50.811
                - specified complication NEC K50.818
          - rectal bleeding K50.011
          - specified complication NEC K50.018
  - rotaviral A08.0
  - Salmonella, salmonellosis (arizonae) (cholerae-suis) (enteritidis) (typhimurium) A02.0
  - segmental — *see* Enteritis, regional
  - septic A09
  - Shigella — *see* Infection, Shigella
  - small round structured NEC A08.19
  - spasmodic, spastic — *see* Syndrome, irritable bowel
  - staphylococcal A04.8
    - due to food A05.0
  - torovirus A08.39
  - toxic NEC K52.1
    - due to Clostridium difficile A04.7
  - trichomonal A07.8
  - tuberculous A18.32
  - typhosa A01.00
  - ulcerative (chronic) — *see* Colitis, ulcerative
  - viral A08.4
    - adenovirus A08.2
    - enterovirus A08.39
    - Rotavirus A08.0
    - small round structured NEC A08.19
    - specified NEC A08.39
    - virus specified NEC A08.39
- **Enterobiasis** B80
- **Enterobius vermicularis** (infection) (infestation) B80
- **Enterocele** (*see also* Hernia, abdomen)
  - pelvic, pelvis (acquired) (congenital) N81.5
  - vagina, vaginal (acquired) (congenital) NEC N81.5
- **Enterocolitis** (*see also* Enteritis) K52.9
  - due to Clostridium difficile A04.7
  - fulminant ischemic K55.0
  - granulomatous — *see* Enteritis, regional
  - hemorrhagic (acute) K55.0
    - chronic K55.1
  - infectious NEC A09
  - ischemic K55.9
  - necrotizing
    - due to Clostridium difficile A04.7
    - in newborn P77.9
      - stage 1 (without pneumatosis, without perforation) P77.1
      - stage 2 (with pneumatosis, without perforation) P77.2
      - stage 3 (with pneumatosis, with perforation) P77.3
  - noninfectious K52.9
    - newborn — *see* Enterocolitis, necrotizing, in newborn

- **Enterocolitis** — *continued*
  - pseudomembranous (newborn) A04.7
  - radiation K52.0
    - newborn — *see* Enterocolitis, necrotizing, in newborn
  - ulcerative (chronic) — *see* Pancolitis, ulcerative (chronic)
- **Enterogastritis** — *see* Enteritis
- **Enteropathy** K63.9
  - gluten-sensitive K90.0
  - hemorrhagic, terminal K55.0
  - protein-losing K90.4
- **Enteroperitonitis** — *see* Peritonitis
- **Enteroptosis** K63.4
- **Enterorrhagia** K92.2
- **Enterospasm** (*see also* Syndrome, irritable, bowel)
  - psychogenic F45.8
- **Enterostenosis** (*see also* Obstruction, intestine) K56.69
- **Enterostomy**
  - complication — *see* Complication, enterostomy
  - status Z93.4
- **Enterovirus, as cause of disease classified elsewhere** B97.10
  - coxsackievirus B97.11
  - echovirus B97.12
  - other specified B97.19
- **Enthesopathy** (peripheral) M77.9
  - Achilles tendinitis — *see* Tendinitis, Achilles
  - ankle and tarsus M77.9
    - specified type NEC — *see* Enthesopathy, foot, specified type NEC
  - anterior tibial syndrome M76.81- ☑
  - calcaneal spur — *see* Spur, bone, calcaneal
  - elbow region M77.8
    - lateral epicondylitis — *see* Epicondylitis, lateral
    - medial epicondylitis — *see* Epicondylitis, medial
  - foot NEC M77.9
    - metatarsalgia — *see* Metatarsalgia
    - specified type NEC M77.5- ☑
  - forearm M77.9
  - gluteal tendinitis — *see* Tendinitis, gluteal
  - hand M77.9
  - hip — *see* Enthesopathy, lower limb, specified type NEC
  - iliac crest spur — *see* Spur, bone, iliac crest
  - iliotibial band syndrome — *see* Syndrome, iliotibial band
  - knee — *see* Enthesopathy, lower limb, lower leg, specified type NEC
  - lateral epicondylitis — *see* Epicondylitis, lateral
  - lower limb (excluding foot) M76.9
    - Achilles tendinitis — *see* Tendinitis, Achilles
    - anterior tibial syndrome M76.81- ☑
    - gluteal tendinitis — *see* Tendinitis, gluteal
    - iliac crest spur — *see* Spur, bone, iliac crest
    - iliotibial band syndrome — *see* Syndrome, iliotibial band
    - patellar tendinitis — *see* Tendinitis, patellar
    - pelvic region — *see* Enthesopathy, lower limb, specified type NEC
    - peroneal tendinitis — *see* Tendinitis, peroneal
    - posterior tibial syndrome M76.82- ☑
    - psoas tendinitis — *see* Tendinitis, psoas
    - shoulder M77.9
    - specified type NEC M76.89- ☑
    - tibial collateral bursitis — *see* Bursitis, tibial collateral
  - medial epicondylitis — *see* Epicondylitis, medial
  - metatarsalgia — *see* Metatarsalgia
  - multiple sites M77.9
  - patellar tendinitis — *see* Tendinitis, patellar
  - pelvis M77.9
  - periarthritis of wrist — *see* Periarthritis, wrist
  - peroneal tendinitis — *see* Tendinitis, peroneal
  - posterior tibial syndrome M76.82- ☑
  - psoas tendinitis — *see* Tendinitis, psoas
  - shoulder region — *see* Lesion, shoulder
  - specified site NEC M77.9
  - specified type NEC M77.8
  - spinal M46.00
    - cervical region M46.02
    - cervicothoracic region M46.03
    - lumbar region M46.06
    - lumbosacral region M46.07
    - multiple sites M46.09
    - occipito-atlanto-axial region M46.01
    - sacrococcygeal region M46.08

- **Enthesopathy** — *continued*
  - spinal — *continued*
    - thoracic region M46.Ø4
    - thoracolumbar region M46.Ø5
  - tibial collateral bursitis — *see* Bursitis, tibial collateral
  - upper arm M77.9
  - wrist and carpus NEC M77.8
    - calcaneal spur — *see* Spur, bone, calcaneal
    - periarthritis of wrist — *see* Periarthritis, wrist
- **Entomophobia** F4Ø.218
- **Entomophthoromycosis** B46.8
- **Entrance, air into vein** — *see* Embolism, air
- **Entrapment, nerve** — *see* Neuropathy, entrapment
- **Entropion** (eyelid) (paralytic) HØ2.ØØ9
  - cicatricial HØ2.Ø19
    - left HØ2.Ø16
      - lower HØ2.Ø15
      - upper HØ2.Ø14
    - right HØ2.Ø13
      - lower HØ2.Ø12
      - upper HØ2.Ø11
  - congenital Q1Ø.2
  - left HØ2.ØØ6
    - lower HØ2.ØØ5
    - upper HØ2.ØØ4
  - mechanical HØ2.Ø29
    - left HØ2.Ø26
      - lower HØ2.Ø25
      - upper HØ2.Ø24
    - right HØ2.Ø23
      - lower HØ2.Ø22
      - upper HØ2.Ø21
  - right HØ2.ØØ3
    - lower HØ2.ØØ2
    - upper HØ2.ØØ1
  - senile HØ2.Ø39
    - left HØ2.Ø36
      - lower HØ2.Ø35
      - upper HØ2.Ø34
    - right HØ2.Ø33
      - lower HØ2.Ø32
      - upper HØ2.Ø31
  - spastic HØ2.Ø49
    - left HØ2.Ø46
      - lower HØ2.Ø45
      - upper HØ2.Ø44
    - right HØ2.Ø43
      - lower HØ2.Ø42
      - upper HØ2.Ø41
- **Enucleated eye** (traumatic, current) SØ5.7- ☑
- **Enuresis** R32
  - functional F98.Ø
  - habit disturbance F98.Ø
  - nocturnal N39.44
    - psychogenic F98.Ø
  - nonorganic origin F98.Ø
  - psychogenic F98.Ø
- **Eosinopenia** — *see* Agranulocytosis
- **Eosinophilia** (allergic) (hereditary) (idiopathic) (secondary) D72.1
  - with
    - angiolymphoid hyperplasia (ALHE) D18.Ø1
  - infiltrative J82
  - Löffler's J82
  - peritoneal — *see* Peritonitis, eosinophilic
  - pulmonary NEC J82
  - tropical (pulmonary) J82
- **Eosinophilia-myalgia syndrome** M35.8
- **Ependymitis** (acute) (cerebral) (chronic) (granular) — *see* Encephalomyelitis
- **Ependymoblastoma**
  - specified site — *see* Neoplasm, malignant, by site
  - unspecified site C71.9
- **Ependymoma** (epithelial) (malignant)
  - anaplastic
    - specified site — *see* Neoplasm, malignant, by site
    - unspecified site C71.9
  - benign
    - specified site — *see* Neoplasm, benign, by site
    - unspecified site D33.2
  - myxopapillary D43.2
    - specified site — *see* Neoplasm, uncertain behavior, by site
    - unspecified site D43.2
  - papillary D43.2
    - specified site — *see* Neoplasm, uncertain behavior, by site
    - unspecified site D43.2
- **Ependymoma** — *continued*
  - specified site — *see* Neoplasm, malignant, by site
  - unspecified site C71.9
- **Ependymopathy** G93.89
- **Ephelis, ephelides** L81.2
- **Epiblepharon** (congenital) Q1Ø.3
- **Epicanthus, epicanthic fold** (eyelid) (congenital) Q1Ø.3
- **Epicondylitis** (elbow)
  - lateral M77.1- ☑
  - medial M77.Ø- ☑
- **Epicystitis** — *see* Cystitis
- **Epidemic** — *see* condition
- **Epidermidalization, cervix** — *see* Dysplasia, cervix
- **Epidermis, epidermal** — *see* condition
- **Epidermodysplasia verruciformis** BØ7.8
- **Epidermolysis**
  - bullosa (congenital) Q81.9
    - acquired L12.3Ø
      - drug-induced L12.31
      - specified cause NEC L12.35
    - dystrophica Q81.2
    - letalis Q81.1
    - simplex Q81.Ø
    - specified NEC Q81.8
  - necroticans combustiformis L51.2
    - due to drug — *see* Table of Drugs and Chemicals, by drug
- **Epidermophytid** — *see* Dermatophytosis
- **Epidermophytosis** (infected) — *see* Dermatophytosis
- **Epididymis** — *see* condition
- **Epididymitis** (acute) (nonvenereal) (recurrent) (residual) N45.1
  - with orchitis N45.3
  - blennorrhagic (gonococcal) A54.23
  - caseous (tuberculous) A18.15
  - chlamydial A56.19
  - filarial (*see also* Infestation, filarial) B74.9 [N51]
  - gonococcal A54.23
  - syphilitic A52.76
  - tuberculous A18.15
- **Epididymo-orchitis** (*see also* Epididymitis) N45.3
- **Epidural** — *see* condition
- **Epigastrium, epigastric** — *see* condition
- **Epigastrocele** — *see* Hernia, ventral
- **Epiglottis** — *see* condition
- **Epiglottitis, epiglottiditis** (acute) JØ5.1Ø
  - with obstruction JØ5.11
  - chronic J37.Ø
- **Epignathus** Q89.4
- **Epilepsia partialis continua** (*see also* Kozhevnikof's epilepsy) G4Ø.1- ☑
- **Epilepsy, epileptic, epilepsia** (attack) (cerebral) (convulsion) (fit) (seizure) G4Ø.9Ø9

> *Note: the following terms are to be considered equivalent to intractable: pharmacoresistant (pharmacologically resistant), treatment resistant, refractory (medically) and poorly controlled*

  - with
    - complex partial seizures — *see* Epilepsy, localization-related, symptomatic, with complex partial seizures
    - grand mal seizures on awakening — *see* Epilepsy, generalized, specified NEC
    - myoclonic absences — *see* Epilepsy, generalized, specified NEC
    - myoclonic-astatic seizures — *see* Epilepsy, generalized, specified NEC
    - simple partial seizures — *see* Epilepsy, localization-related, symptomatic, with simple partial seizures
  - akinetic — *see* Epilepsy, generalized, specified NEC
  - benign childhood with centrotemporal EEG spikes — *see* Epilepsy, localization-related, idiopathic
  - benign myoclonic in infancy G4Ø.8Ø- ☑
  - Bravais-jacksonian — *see* Epilepsy, localization-related, symptomatic, with simple partial seizures
  - childhood
    - with occipital EEG paroxysms — *see* Epilepsy, localization-related, idiopathic
    - absence G4Ø.AØ9 (*following* G4Ø.3)
      - intractable G4Ø.A19 (*following* G4Ø.3)
        - with status epilepticus G4Ø.A11 (*following* G4Ø.3)
        - without status epilepticus G4Ø.A19 (*following* G4Ø.3)
      - not intractable G4Ø.AØ9 (*following* G4Ø.3)
- **Epilepsy, epileptic, epilepsia** — *continued*
  - childhood — *continued*
    - absence — *continued*
      - not intractable — *continued*
        - with status epilepticus G4Ø.AØ1 (*following* G4Ø.3)
        - without status epilepticus G4Ø.AØ9 (*following* G4Ø.3)
  - climacteric — *see* Epilepsy, specified NEC
  - cysticercosis B69.Ø
  - deterioration (mental) FØ6.8
  - due to syphilis A52.19
  - focal — *see* Epilepsy, localization-related, symptomatic, with simple partial seizures
  - generalized
    - idiopathic G4Ø.3Ø9
      - intractable G4Ø.319
        - with status epilepticus G4Ø.311
        - without status epilepticus G4Ø.319
      - not intractable G4Ø.3Ø9
        - with status epilepticus G4Ø.3Ø1
        - without status epilepticus G4Ø.3Ø9
    - specified NEC G4Ø.4Ø9
      - intractable G4Ø.419
        - with status epilepticus G4Ø.411
        - without status epilepticus G4Ø.419
      - not intractable G4Ø.4Ø9
        - with status epilepticus G4Ø.4Ø1
        - without status epilepticus G4Ø.4Ø9
  - impulsive petit mal — *see* Epilepsy, juvenile myoclonic
  - intractable G4Ø.919
    - with status epilepticus G4Ø.911
    - without status epilepticus G4Ø.919
  - juvenile absence G4Ø.AØ9 (*following* G4Ø.3)
    - intractable G4Ø.A19 (*following* G4Ø.3)
      - with status epilepticus G4Ø.A11 (*following* G4Ø.3)
      - without status epilepticus G4Ø.A19 (*following* G4Ø.3)
    - not intractable G4Ø.AØ9 (*following* G4Ø.3)
      - with status epilepticus G4Ø.AØ1 (*following* G4Ø.3)
      - without status epilepticus G4Ø.AØ9 (*following* G4Ø.3)
  - juvenile myoclonic G4Ø.BØ9 (*following* G4Ø.3)
    - intractable G4Ø.B19 (*following* G4Ø.3)
      - with status epilepticus G4Ø.B11 (*following* G4Ø.3)
      - without status epilepticus G4Ø.B19 (*following* G4Ø.3)
    - not intractable G4Ø.BØ9 (*following* G4Ø.3)
      - with status epilepticus G4Ø.BØ1 (*following* G4Ø.3)
      - without status epilepticus G4Ø.BØ9 (*following* G4Ø.3)
  - localization-related (focal) (partial)
    - idiopathic G4Ø.ØØ9
      - with seizures of localized onset G4Ø.ØØ9
        - intractable G4Ø.Ø19
          - with status epilepticus G4Ø.Ø11
          - without status epilepticus G4Ø.Ø19
        - not intractable G4Ø.ØØ9
          - with status epilepticus G4Ø.ØØ1
          - without status epilepticus G4Ø.ØØ9
    - symptomatic
      - with complex partial seizures G4Ø.2Ø9
        - intractable G4Ø.219
          - with status epilepticus G4Ø.211
          - without status epilepticus G4Ø.219
        - not intractable G4Ø.2Ø9
          - with status epilepticus G4Ø.2Ø1
          - without status epilepticus G4Ø.2Ø9
      - with simple partial seizures G4Ø.1Ø9
        - intractable G4Ø.119
          - with status epilepticus G4Ø.111
          - without status epilepticus G4Ø.119
        - not intractable G4Ø.1Ø9
          - with status epilepticus G4Ø.1Ø1
          - without status epilepticus G4Ø.1Ø9
  - myoclonus, myoclonic (progressive) — *see* Epilepsy, generalized, specified NEC
  - not intractable G4Ø.9Ø9
    - with status epilepticus G4Ø.9Ø1
    - without status epilepticus G4Ø.9Ø9
  - on awakening — *see* Epilepsy, generalized, specified NEC
  - parasitic NOS B71.9 [G94]

Epilepsy, epileptic, epilepsia — *continued*
- partialis continua (*see also* Kozhevnikof's epilepsy) G40.1- ☑
- peripheral — *see* Epilepsy, specified NEC
- procursiva — *see* Epilepsy, localization-related, symptomatic, with simple partial seizures
- progressive (familial) myoclonic — *see* Epilepsy, generalized, idiopathic
- reflex — *see* Epilepsy, specified NEC
- related to
  - alcohol G40.509
    - not intractable G40.509
      - with status epilepticus G40.501
      - without status epliepticus G40.509
  - drugs G40.509
    - not intractable G40.509
      - with status epilepticus G40.501
      - without status epliepticus G40.509
  - external causes G40.509
    - not intractable G40.509
      - with status epilepticus G40.501
      - without status epliepticus G40.509
  - hormonal changes G40.509
    - not intractable G40.509
      - with status epilepticus G40.501
      - without status epliepticus G40.509
  - sleep deprivation G40.509
    - not intractable G40.509
      - with status epilepticus G40.501
      - without status epliepticus G40.509
  - stress G40.509
    - not intractable G40.509
      - with status epilepticus G40.501
      - without status epliepticus G40.509
- somatomotor — *see* Epilepsy, localization-related, symptomatic, with simple partial seizures
- somatosensory — *see* Epilepsy, localization-related, symptomatic, with simple partial seizures
- spasms G40.822
  - intractable G40.824
    - with status epilepticus G40.823
    - without status epilepticus G40.824
  - not intractable G40.822
    - with status epilepticus G40.821
    - without status epilepticus G40.822
- specified NEC G40.802
  - intractable G40.804
    - with status epilepticus G40.803
    - without status epilepticus G40.804
  - not intractable G40.802
    - with status epilepticus G40.801
    - without status epilepticus G40.802
- syndromes
  - generalized
    - idiopathic G40.309
      - intractable G40.319
        - with status epilepticus G40.311
        - without status epilepticus G40.319
      - not intractable G40.309
        - with status epilepticus G40.301
        - without status epilepticus G40.309
    - specified NEC G40.409
      - intractable G40.419
        - with status epilepticus G40.411
        - without status epilepticus G40.419
      - not intractable G40.409
        - with status epilepticus G40.401
        - without status epilepticus G40.409
  - localization-related (focal) (partial)
    - idiopathic G40.009
      - with seizures of localized onset G40.009
        - intractable G40.019
          - with status epilepticus G40.011
          - without status epilepticus G40.019
        - not intractable G40.009
          - with status epilepticus G40.001
          - without status epilepticus G40.009
    - symptomatic
      - with complex partial seizures G40.209
        - intractable G40.219
          - with status epilepticus G40.211
          - without status epilepticus G40.219
        - not intractable G40.209
          - with status epilepticus G40.201
          - without status epilepticus G40.209
      - with simple partial seizures G40.109
        - intractable G40.119
          - with status epilepticus G40.111

Epilepsy, epileptic, epilepsia — *continued*
- syndromes — *continued*
  - localization-related — *continued*
    - symptomatic — *continued*
      - with simple partial seizures — *continued*
        - intractable — *continued*
          - without status epilepticus G40.119
        - not intractable G40.109
          - with status epilepticus G40.101
          - without status epilepticus G40.109
  - specified NEC G40.802
    - intractable G40.804
      - with status epilepticus G40.803
      - without status epilepticus G40.804
    - not intractable G40.802
      - with status epilepticus G40.801
      - without status epilepticus G40.802
- tonic (-clonic) — *see* Epilepsy, generalized, specified NEC
- twilight F05
- uncinate (gyrus) — *see* Epilepsy, localization-related, symptomatic, with complex partial seizures
- Unverricht (-Lundborg) (familial myoclonic) — *see* Epilepsy, generalized, idiopathic
- visceral — *see* Epilepsy, specified NEC
- visual — *see* Epilepsy, specified NEC

Epiloia Q85.1

Epimenorrhea N92.0

Epipharyngitis — *see* Nasopharyngitis

Epiphora H04.20- ☑
- due to
  - excess lacrimation H04.21- ☑
  - insufficient drainage H04.22- ☑

Epiphyseal arrest — *see* Arrest, epiphyseal

Epiphyseolysis, epiphysiolysis — *see* Osteochondropathy

Epiphysitis (*see also* Osteochondropathy)
- juvenile M92.9
- syphilitic (congenital) A50.02

Epiplocele — *see* Hernia, abdomen

Epiploitis — *see* Peritonitis

Epiplosarcomphalocele — *see* Hernia, umbilicus

Episcleritis (suppurative) H15.10- ☑
- in (due to)
  - syphilis A52.71
  - tuberculosis A18.51
- nodular H15.12- ☑
- periodica fugax H15.11- ☑
  - angioneurotic — *see* Edema, angioneurotic
- syphilitic (late) A52.71
- tuberculous A18.51

Episode
- affective, mixed F39
- depersonalization (in neurotic state) F48.1
- depressive F32.9
  - major F32.9
    - mild F32.0
    - moderate F32.1
    - severe (without psychotic symptoms) F32.2
      - with psychotic symptoms F32.3
  - recurrent F33.9
    - brief F33.8
  - specified NEC F32.8
- hypomanic F30.8
- manic F30.9
  - with
    - psychotic symptoms F30.2
    - remission (full) F30.4
      - partial F30.3
  - without psychotic symptoms F30.10
    - mild F30.11
    - moderate F30.12
    - severe (without psychotic symptoms) F30.13
      - with psychotic symptoms F30.2
  - other specified F30.8
  - recurrent F31.89
- psychotic F23
  - organic F06.8
- schizophrenic (acute) NEC, brief F23

Epispadias (female) (male) Q64.0

Episplenitis D73.89

Epistaxis (multiple) R04.0
- hereditary I78.0
- vicarious menstruation N94.89

Epithelioma (malignant) (*see* also Neoplasm, malignant, by site)
- adenoides cysticum — *see* Neoplasm, skin, benign
- basal cell — *see* Neoplasm, skin, malignant

Epithelioma — *continued*
- benign — *see* Neoplasm, benign, by site
- Bowen's — *see* Neoplasm, skin, in situ
- calcifying, of Malherbe — *see* Neoplasm, skin, benign
- external site — *see* Neoplasm, skin, malignant
- intraepidermal, Jadassohn — *see* Neoplasm, skin, benign
- squamous cell — *see* Neoplasm, malignant, by site

Epitheliomatosis pigmented Q82.1

Epitheliopathy, multifocal placoid pigment H30.14- ☑

Epithelium, epithelial — *see* condition

Epituberculosis (with atelectasis) (allergic) A15.7

Eponychia Q84.6

Epstein's
- nephrosis or syndrome — *see* Nephrosis
- pearl K09.8

Epulis (gingiva) (fibrous) (giant cell) K06.8

Equinia A24.0

Equinovarus (congenital) (talipes) Q66.0
- acquired — *see* Deformity, limb, clubfoot

Equivalent
- convulsive (abdominal) — *see* Epilepsy, specified NEC
- epileptic (psychic) — *see* Epilepsy, localization-related, symptomatic, with complex partial seizures

Erb (-Duchenne) **paralysis** (birth injury) (newborn) P14.0

Erb-Goldflam disease or syndrome G70.00
- with exacerbation (acute) G70.01
- in crisis G70.01

Erb's
- disease G71.0
- palsy, paralysis (brachial) (birth) (newborn) P14.0
  - spinal (spastic) syphilitic A52.17
- pseudohypertrophic muscular dystrophy G71.0

Erdheim's syndrome (acromegalic macrospondylitis) E22.0

Erection, painful (persistent) — *see* Priapism

Ergosterol deficiency (vitamin D) E55.9
- with
  - adult osteomalacia M83.8
  - rickets — *see* Rickets

Ergotism (*see also* Poisoning, food, noxious, plant)
- from ergot used as drug (migraine therapy) — *see* Table of Drugs and Chemicals

Erosio interdigitalis blastomycetica B37.2

Erosion
- artery I77.2
  - without rupture I77.89
- bone — *see* Disorder, bone, density and structure, specified NEC
- bronchus J98.09
- cartilage (joint) — *see* Disorder, cartilage, specified type NEC
- cervix (uteri) (acquired) (chronic) (congenital) N86
  - with cervicitis N72
- cornea (nontraumatic) — *see* Ulcer, cornea
  - recurrent H18.83- ☑
  - traumatic — *see* Abrasion, cornea
- dental (idiopathic) (occupational) (due to diet, drugs or vomiting) K03.2
- duodenum, postpyloric — *see* Ulcer, duodenum
- esophagus K22.10
  - with bleeding K22.11
- gastric — *see* Ulcer, stomach
- gastrojejunal — *see* Ulcer, gastrojejunal
- implanted mesh — *see* Complications, mesh
- intestine K63.3
- lymphatic vessel I89.8
- pylorus, pyloric (ulcer) — *see* Ulcer, stomach
- spine, aneurysmal A52.09
- stomach — *see* Ulcer, stomach
- teeth (idiopathic) (occupational) (due to diet, drugs or vomiting) K03.2
- urethra N36.8
- uterus N85.8

Erotomania F52.8

Error
- metabolism, inborn — *see* Disorder, metabolism
- refractive — *see* Disorder, refraction

Eructation R14.2
- nervous or psychogenic F45.8

Eruption
- creeping B76.9
- drug (generalized) (taken internally) L27.0
  - fixed L27.1
  - in contact with skin — *see* Dermatitis, due to drugs
  - localized L27.1

Eruption — *continued*
- Hutchinson, summer L56.4
- Kaposi's varicelliform BØØ.Ø
- napkin L22
- polymorphous light (sun) L56.4
- recalcitrant pustular L13.8
- ringed R23.8
- skin (nonspecific) R21
  - creeping (meaning hookworm) B76.9
  - due to inoculation/vaccination (generalized) (*see also* Dermatitis, due to, vaccine) L27.Ø
    - localized L27.1
  - erysipeloid A26.Ø
  - feigned L98.1
  - Kaposi's varicelliform BØØ.Ø
  - lichenoid L28.Ø
  - meaning dermatitis — *see* Dermatitis
  - toxic NEC L53.Ø
- tooth, teeth, abnormal (incomplete) (late) (premature) (sequence) KØØ.6
- vesicular R23.8

Erysipelas (gangrenous) (infantile) (newborn) (phlegmonous) (suppurative) A46
- external ear A46 [H62.4Ø]
- puerperal, postpartum O86.89

Erysipeloid A26.9
- cutaneous (Rosenbach's) A26.Ø
- disseminated A26.8
- sepsis A26.7
- specified NEC A26.8

Erythema, erythematous (infectional) (inflammation) L53.9
- ab igne L59.Ø
- annulare (centrifugum) (rheumaticum) L53.1
- arthriticum epidemicum A25.1
- brucellum — *see* Brucellosis
- chronic figurate NEC L53.3
- chronicum migrans (Borrelia burgdorferi) A69.2Ø
- diaper L22
- due to
  - chemical NEC L53.Ø
    - in contact with skin L24.5
  - drug (internal use) — *see* Dermatitis, due to, drugs
- elevatum diutinum L95.1
- endemic E52
- epidemic, arthritic A25.1
- figuratum perstans L53.3
- gluteal L22
- heat — *code by site under* Burn, first degree
- ichthyosiforme congenitum bullous Q8Ø.3
- in diseases classified elsewhere L54
- induratum (nontuberculous) L52
  - tuberculous A18.4
- infectiosum BØ8.3
- intertrigo L3Ø.4
- iris L51.9
- marginatum L53.2
  - in (due to) acute rheumatic fever IØØ
- medicamentosum — *see* Dermatitis, due to, drugs
- migrans A26.Ø
  - chronicum A69.2Ø
  - tongue K14.1
- multiforme (major) (minor) L51.9
  - bullous, bullosum L51.1
  - conjunctiva L51.1
  - nonbullous L51.Ø
  - pemphigoides L12.Ø
  - specified NEC L51.8
- napkin L22
- neonatorum P83.8
  - toxic P83.1
- nodosum L52
  - tuberculous A18.4
- palmar L53.8
- pernio T69.1 ☑
- rash, newborn P83.8
- scarlatiniform (recurrent) (exfoliative) L53.8
- solare L55.Ø
- specified NEC L53.8
- toxic, toxicum NEC L53.Ø
  - newborn P83.1
- tuberculous (primary) A18.4

Erythematous, erythematosus — *see* condition

Erythermalgia (primary) I73.81

Erythralgia I73.81

Erythrasma LØ8.1

Erythredema (polyneuropathy) — *see* Poisoning, mercury

Erythremia (acute) C94.Ø- ☑
- chronic D45
- secondary D75.1

Erythroblastopenia (*see also* Aplasia, red cell) D6Ø.9
- congenital D61.Ø1

Erythroblastophthisis D61.Ø9

Erythroblastosis (fetalis) (newborn) P55.9
- due to
  - ABO (antibodies) (incompatibility) (isoimmunization) P55.1
  - Rh (antibodies) (incompatibility) (isoimmunization) P55.Ø

Erythrocyanosis (crurum) I73.89

Erythrocythemia — *see* Erythremia

Erythrocytosis (megalosplenic) (secondary) D75.1
- familial D75.Ø
- oval, hereditary — *see* Elliptocytosis
- secondary D75.1
- stress D75.1

Erythroderma (secondary) (*see also* Erythema) L53.9
- bullous ichthyosiform, congenital Q8Ø.3
- desquamativum L21.1
- ichthyosiform, congenital (bullous) Q8Ø.3
- neonatorum P83.8
- psoriaticum L4Ø.8

Erythrodysesthesia, palmar plantar (PPE) L27.1

Erythrogenesis imperfecta D61.Ø9

Erythroleukemia C94.Ø- ☑

Erythromelalgia I73.81

Erythrophagocytosis D75.89

Erythrophobia F4Ø.298

Erythroplakia, oral epithelium, and tongue K13.29

Erythroplasia (Queyrat) DØ7.4
- specified site — *see* Neoplasm, skin, in situ
- unspecified site DØ7.4

Escherichia coli (E. coli), **as cause of disease classified elsewhere** B96.2Ø
- non-O157 Shiga toxin-producing (with known O group) B96.22
- non-Shiga toxin-producing B96.29
- O157 B96.21
- O157 with confirmation of Shiga toxin when H antigen is unknown, or is not H7 B96.21
- O157:H- (nonmotile) with confirmation of Shiga toxin B96.21
- O157:H7 with or without confirmation of Shiga toxin-production B96.21
  - specified NEC B96.22
- Shiga toxin-producing (with unspecified O group) (STEC) B96.23
- specified NEC B96.29

Esophagismus K22.4

Esophagitis (acute) (alkaline) (chemical) (chronic) (infectional) (necrotic) (peptic) (postoperative) K2Ø.9
- candidal B37.81
- due to gastrointestinal reflux disease K21.Ø
- eosinophilic K2Ø.Ø
- reflux K21.Ø
- specified NEC K2Ø.8
- tuberculous A18.83
- ulcerative K22.1Ø
  - with bleeding K22.11

Esophagocele K22.5

Esophagomalacia K22.8

Esophagospasm K22.4

Esophagostenosis K22.2

Esophagostomiasis B81.8

Esophagotracheal — *see* condition

Esophagus — *see* condition

Esophoria H5Ø.51
- convergence, excess H51.12
- divergence, insufficiency H51.8

Esotropia — *see* Strabismus, convergent concomitant

Espundia B55.2

Essential — *see* condition

Esthesioneuroblastoma C3Ø.Ø

Esthesioneurocytoma C3Ø.Ø

Esthesioneuroepithelioma C3Ø.Ø

Esthiomene A55

Estivo-autumnal malaria (fever) B5Ø.9

Estrangement (marital) Z63.5
- parent-child NEC Z62.89Ø

Estriasis — *see* Myiasis

Ethanolism — *see* Alcoholism

Etherism — *see* Dependence, drug, inhalant

Ethmoid, ethmoidal — *see* condition

Ethmoiditis (chronic) (nonpurulent) (purulent) (*see also* Sinusitis, ethmoidal)
- influenzal — *see* Influenza, with, respiratory manifestations NEC
- Woakes' J33.1

Ethylism — *see* Alcoholism

Eulenburg's disease (congenital paramyotonia) G71.19

Eumycetoma B47.Ø

Eunuchoidism E29.1
- hypogonadotropic E23.Ø

European blastomycosis — *see* Cryptococcosis

Eustachian — *see* condition

Evaluation (for) (of)
- development state
  - adolescent ZØØ.3
  - period of
    - delayed growth in childhood ZØØ.7Ø
      - with abnormal findings ZØØ.71
    - rapid growth in childhood ZØØ.2
  - puberty ZØØ.3
- growth and developmental state (period of rapid growth) ZØØ.2
  - delayed growth ZØØ.7Ø
    - with abnormal findings ZØØ.71
- mental health (status) ZØØ.8
  - requested by authority ZØ4.6
- period of
  - delayed growth in childhood ZØØ.7Ø
    - with abnormal findings ZØØ.71
  - rapid growth in childhood ZØØ.2
- suspected condition — *see* Observation

Evans syndrome D69.41

Event, apparent life threatening in newborn and infant (ALTE) R68.13

Eventration (*see also* Hernia, ventral)
- colon into chest — *see* Hernia, diaphragm
- diaphragm (congenital) Q79.1

Eversion
- bladder N32.89
- cervix (uteri) N86
  - with cervicitis N72
- foot NEC (*see also* Deformity, valgus, ankle)
  - congenital Q66.6
- punctum lacrimale (postinfectional) (senile) HØ4.52- ☑
- ureter (meatus) N28.89
- urethra (meatus) N36.8
- uterus N81.4

Evidence
- cytologic
  - of malignancy on anal smear R85.614
  - of malignancy on cervical smear R87.614
  - of malignancy on vaginal smear R87.624

Evisceration
- birth injury P15.8
- traumatic NEC
  - eye — *see* Enucleated eye

Evulsion — *see* Avulsion

Ewing's sarcoma or tumor — *see* Neoplasm, bone, malignant

Examination (for) (following) (general) (of) (routine) ZØØ.ØØ
- with abnormal findings ZØØ.Ø1
- abuse, physical (alleged), ruled out
  - adult ZØ4.71
  - child ZØ4.72
- adolescent (development state) ZØØ.3
- alleged rape or sexual assault (victim), ruled out
  - adult ZØ4.41
  - child ZØ4.42
- allergy ZØ1.82
- annual (adult) (periodic) (physical) ZØØ.ØØ
  - with abnormal findings ZØØ.Ø1
  - gynecological ZØ1.419
    - with abnormal findings ZØ1.411
- antibody response ZØ1.84
- blood — *see* Examination, laboratory
- blood pressure ZØ1.3Ø
  - with abnormal findings ZØ1.31
- cancer staging — *see* Neoplasm, malignant, by site
- cervical Papanicolaou smear Z12.4
  - as part of routine gynecological examination ZØ1.419
    - with abnormal findings ZØ1.411
- child (over 28 days old) ZØØ.129
  - with abnormal findings ZØØ.121
  - under 28 days old — *see* Newborn, examination
- clinical research control or normal comparison (control) (participant) ZØØ.6

Exhaustion, exhaustive — *continued*
- due to
  - cold T69.8 ☑
  - excessive exertion T73.3 ☑
  - exposure T73.2 ☑
  - neurasthenia F48.8
- heart — *see* Failure, heart
- heat (*see also* Heat, exhaustion) T67.5 ☑
  - due to
    - salt depletion T67.4 ☑
    - water depletion T67.3 ☑
- maternal, complicating delivery O75.81
- mental F48.8
- myocardium, myocardial — *see* Failure, heart
- nervous F48.8
- old age R54
- psychogenic F48.8
- psychosis F43.Ø
- senile R54
- vital NEC Z73.Ø

Exhibitionism F65.2

Exocervicitis — *see* Cervicitis

Exomphalos Q79.2
- meaning hernia — *see* Hernia, umbilicus

Exophoria H5Ø.52
- convergence, insufficiency H51.11
- divergence, excess H51.8

Exophthalmos HØ5.2- ☑
- congenital Q15.8
- constant NEC HØ5.24- ☑
- displacement, globe — *see* Displacement, globe
- due to thyrotoxicosis (hyperthyroidism) — *see* Hyperthyroidism, with, goiter (diffuse)
- dysthyroid — *see* Hyperthyroidism, with, goiter (diffuse)
- goiter — *see* Hyperthyroidism, with, goiter (diffuse)
- intermittent NEC HØ5.25- ☑
- malignant — *see* Hyperthyroidism, with, goiter (diffuse)
- orbital
  - edema — *see* Edema, orbit
  - hemorrhage — *see* Hemorrhage, orbit
- pulsating NEC HØ5.26- ☑
- thyrotoxic, thyrotropic — *see* Hyperthyroidism, with, goiter (diffuse)

Exostosis (*see also* Disorder, bone)
- cartilaginous — *see* Neoplasm, bone, benign
- congenital (multiple) Q78.6
- external ear canal H61.81- ☑
- gonococcal A54.49
- jaw (bone) M27.8
- multiple, congenital Q78.6
- orbit HØ5.35- ☑
- osteocartilaginous — *see* Neoplasm, bone, benign
- syphilitic A52.77

Exotropia — *see* Strabismus, divergent concomitant

Explanation of
- investigation finding Z71.2
- medication Z71.89

Exposure (to) (*see also* Contact, with) T75.89 ☑
- acariasis Z2Ø.7
- AIDS virus Z2Ø.6
- air pollution Z77.11Ø
- algae and algae toxins Z77.121
- algae bloom Z77.121
- anthrax Z2Ø.81Ø
- aromatic amines Z77.Ø2Ø
- aromatic (hazardous) compounds NEC Z77.Ø28
- aromatic dyes NOS Z77.Ø28
- arsenic Z77.Ø1Ø
- asbestos Z77.Ø9Ø
- bacterial disease NEC Z2Ø.818
- benzene Z77.Ø21
- blue-green algae bloom Z77.121
- body fluids (potentially hazardous) Z77.21
- brown tide Z77.121
- chemicals (chiefly nonmedicinal) (hazardous) NEC Z77.Ø98
- cholera Z2Ø.Ø9
- chromium compounds Z77.Ø18
- cold, effects of T69.9 ☑
  - specified effect NEC T69.8 ☑
- communicable disease Z2Ø.9
  - bacterial NEC Z2Ø.818
  - specified NEC Z2Ø.89
  - viral NEC Z2Ø.828
- cyanobacteria bloom Z77.121

Exposure — *continued*
- disaster Z65.5
- discrimination Z6Ø.5
- dyes Z77.Ø98
- effects of T73.9 ☑
- environmental tobacco smoke (acute) (chronic) Z77.22
- Escherichia coli (E. coli) Z2Ø.Ø1
- exhaustion due to T73.2 ☑
- fiberglass — *see* Table of Drugs and Chemicals, fiberglass
- German measles Z2Ø.4
- gonorrhea Z2Ø.2
- hazardous metals NEC Z77.Ø18
- hazardous substances NEC Z77.29
- hazards in the physical environment NEC Z77.128
- hazards to health NEC Z77.9
- human immunodeficiency virus (HIV) Z2Ø.6
- human T-lymphotropic virus type-1 (HTLV-1) Z2Ø.89
- implanted
  - mesh — *see* Complications, mesh
  - prosthetic materials NEC — *see* Complications, prosthetic materials NEC
- infestation (parasitic) NEC Z2Ø.7
- intestinal infectious disease NEC Z2Ø.Ø9
  - Escherichia coli (E. coli) Z2Ø.Ø1
- lead Z77.Ø11
- meningococcus Z2Ø.811
- mold (toxic) Z77.12Ø
- nickel dust Z77.Ø18
- noise Z77.122
- occupational
  - air contaminants NEC Z57.39
  - dust Z57.2
  - environmental tobacco smoke Z57.31
  - extreme temperature Z57.6
  - noise Z57.Ø
  - radiation Z57.1
  - risk factors Z57.9
    - specified NEC Z57.8
  - toxic agents (gases) (liquids) (solids) (vapors) in agriculture Z57.4
  - toxic agents (gases) (liquids) (solids) (vapors) in industry NEC Z57.5
  - vibration Z57.7
- parasitic disease NEC Z2Ø.7
- pediculosis Z2Ø.7
- persecution Z6Ø.5
- pfiesteria piscicida Z77.121
- poliomyelitis Z2Ø.89
- pollution
  - air Z77.11Ø
  - environmental NEC Z77.118
  - soil Z77.112
  - water Z77.111
- polycyclic aromatic hydrocarbons Z77.Ø28
- prenatal (drugs) (toxic chemicals) — *see* Newborn, affected by (suspected to be), noxious substances transmitted via placenta or breast milk
- rabies Z2Ø.3
- radiation, naturally occurring NEC Z77.123
- radon Z77.123
- red tide (Florida) Z77.121
- rubella Z2Ø.4
- second hand tobacco smoke (acute) (chronic) Z77.22
  - in the perinatal period P96.81
- sexually-transmitted disease Z2Ø.2
- smallpox (laboratory) Z2Ø.89
- syphilis Z2Ø.2
- terrorism Z65.4
- torture Z65.4
- tuberculosis Z2Ø.1
- uranium Z77.Ø12
- varicella Z2Ø.82Ø
- venereal disease Z2Ø.2
- viral disease NEC Z2Ø.828
- war Z65.5
- water pollution Z77.111

Exsanguination — *see* Hemorrhage

Exstrophy
- abdominal contents Q45.8
- bladder Q64.1Ø
  - cloacal Q64.12
  - specified type NEC Q64.19
  - supravesical fissure Q64.11

Extensive — *see* condition

Extra (*see also* Accessory)
- marker chromosomes (normal individual) Q92.61
  - in abnormal individual Q92.62

Extra — *continued*
- rib Q76.6
  - cervical Q76.5

Extrasystoles (supraventricular) I49.49
- atrial I49.1
- auricular I49.1
- junctional I49.2
- ventricular I49.3

Extrauterine gestation or pregnancy — *see* Pregnancy, by site

Extravasation
- blood R58
- chyle into mesentery I89.8
- pelvicalyceal N13.8
- pyelosinus N13.8
- urine (from ureter) R39.Ø
- vesicant agent
  - antineoplastic chemotherapy T8Ø.81Ø ☑
  - other agent NEC T8Ø.818 ☑

Extremity — *see* condition, limb

Extrophy — *see* Exstrophy

Extroversion
- bladder Q64.19
- uterus N81.4
  - complicating delivery O71.2
  - postpartal (old) N81.4

Extruded tooth (teeth) M26.34

Extrusion
- breast implant (prosthetic) T85.42 ☑
- eye implant (globe) (ball) T85.328 ☑
- intervertebral disc — *see* Displacement, intervertebral disc
- ocular lens implant (prosthetic) — *see* Complications, intraocular lens
- vitreous — *see* Prolapse, vitreous

Exudate
- pleural — *see* Effusion, pleura
- retina H35.89

Exudative — *see* condition

Eye, eyeball, eyelid — *see* condition

Eyestrain — *see* Disturbance, vision, subjective

Eyeworm disease of Africa B74.3

F

Faber's syndrome (achlorhydric anemia) D5Ø.9

Fabry (-Anderson) **disease** E75.21

Faciocephalalgia, autonomic (*see also* Neuropathy, peripheral, autonomic) G9Ø.Ø9

Factor(s)
- psychic, associated with diseases classified elsewhere F54
- psychological
  - affecting physical conditions F54
  - or behavioral
    - affecting general medical condition F54
    - associated with disorders or diseases classified elsewhere F54

Fahr disease (of brain) G23.8

Fahr Volhard disease (of kidney) I12.- ☑

Failure, failed
- abortion — *see* Abortion, attempted
- aortic (valve) I35.8
  - rheumatic IØ6.8
- attempted abortion — *see* Abortion, attempted
- biventricular I5Ø.9
- bone marrow — *see* Anemia, aplastic
- cardiac — *see* Failure, heart
- cardiorenal (chronic) I5Ø.9
  - hypertensive I13.2
- cardiorespiratory (*see also* Failure, heart) RØ9.2
- cardiovascular (chronic) — *see* Failure, heart
- cerebrovascular I67.9
- cervical dilatation in labor O62.Ø
- circulation, circulatory (peripheral) R57.9
  - newborn P29.89
- compensation — *see* Disease, heart
- compliance with medical treatment or regimen — *see* Noncompliance
- congestive — *see* Failure, heart, congestive
- dental implant (endosseous) M27.69
  - due to
    - failure of dental prosthesis M27.63
    - lack of attached gingiva M27.62
    - occlusal trauma (poor prosthetic design) M27.62
    - parafunctional habits M27.62

- **Failure, failed** — *continued*
  - dental implant — *continued*
    - due to — *continued*
      - periodontal infection (peri-implantitis) M27.62
      - poor oral hygiene M27.62
    - osseointegration M27.61
      - due to
        - complications of systemic disease M27.61
        - poor bone quality M27.61
      - iatrogenic M27.61
    - post-osseointegration
      - biological M27.62
      - due to complications of systemic disease M27.62
      - iatrogenic M27.62
      - mechanical M27.63
    - pre-integration M27.61
    - pre-osseointegration M27.61
    - specified NEC M27.69
  - descent of head (at term) of pregnancy (mother) O32.4 ☑
  - endosseous dental implant — *see* Failure, dental implant
  - engagement of head (term of pregnancy) (mother) O32.4 ☑
  - erection (penile) (*see also* Dysfunction, sexual, male, erectile) N52.9
    - nonorgqanic F52.21
  - examination(s), anxiety concerning Z55.2
  - expansion terminal respiratory units (newborn) (primary) P28.0
  - forceps NOS (with subsequent cesarean delivery) O66.5
  - gain weight (child over 28 days old) R62.51
    - adult R62.7
    - newborn P92.6
  - genital response (male) F52.21
    - female F52.22
  - heart (acute) (senile) (sudden) I50.9
    - with
      - acute pulmonary edema — *see* Failure, ventricular, left
      - decompensation — *see* Failure, heart, congestive
      - dilatation — *see* Disease, heart
    - arteriosclerotic I70.90
    - biventricular I50.9
    - combined left-right sided I50.9
    - compensated I50.9
    - complicating
      - anesthesia (general) (local) or other sedation
        - in labor and delivery O74.2
        - in pregnancy O29.12- ☑
        - postpartum, puerperal O89.1
      - delivery (cesarean) (instrumental) O75.4
    - congestive (compensated) (decompensated) I50.9
      - with rheumatic fever (conditions in I00)
        - active I01.8
        - inactive or quiescent (with chorea) I09.81
      - newborn P29.0
      - rheumatic (chronic) (inactive) (with chorea) I09.81
        - active or acute I01.8
          - with chorea I02.0
    - decompensated I50.9
    - degenerative — *see* Degeneration, myocardial
    - diastolic (congestive) I50.30
      - acute (congestive) I50.31
        - and (on) chronic (congestive) I50.33
      - chronic (congestive) I50.32
        - and (on) acute (congestive) I50.33
      - combined with systolic (congestive) I50.40
        - acute (congestive) I50.41
          - and (on) chronic (congestive) I50.43
        - chronic (congestive) I50.42
          - and (on) acute (congestive) I50.43
    - due to presence of cardiac prosthesis I97.13- ☑
    - following cardiac surgery I97.13- ☑
    - high output NOS I50.9
    - hypertensive — *see* Hypertension, heart
    - left (ventricular) — *see* Failure, ventricular, left
    - low output (syndrome) NOS I50.9
    - newborn P29.0
    - organic — *see* Disease, heart
    - peripartum O90.3
    - postprocedural I97.13- ☑
    - rheumatic (chronic) (inactive) I09.9
    - right (ventricular) (secondary to left heart failure) — *see* Failure, heart, congestive

- **Failure, failed** — *continued*
  - heart — *continued*
    - systolic (congestive) I50.20
      - acute (congestive) I50.21
        - and (on) chronic (congestive) I50.23
      - chronic (congestive) I50.22
        - and (on) acute (congestive) I50.23
      - combined with diastolic (congestive) I50.40
        - acute (congestive) I50.41
          - and (on) chronic (congestive) I50.43
        - chronic (congestive) I50.42
          - and (on) acute (congestive) I50.43
    - thyrotoxic (*see also* Thyrotoxicosis) E05.90 [I43]
      - with thyroid storm E05.91 [I43]
    - valvular — *see* Endocarditis
  - hepatic K72.90
    - with coma K72.91
    - acute or subacute K72.00
      - with coma K72.01
      - due to drugs K71.10
        - with coma K71.11
    - alcoholic (acute) (chronic) (subacute) K70.40
      - with coma K70.41
    - chronic K72.10
      - with coma K72.11
      - due to drugs (acute) (subacute) (chronic) K71.10
        - with coma K71.11
    - due to drugs (acute) (subacute) (chronic) K71.10
      - with coma K71.11
    - postprocedural K91.82
  - hepatorenal K76.7
  - induction (of labor) O61.9
    - abortion — *see* Abortion, attempted
    - by
      - oxytocic drugs O61.0
      - prostaglandins O61.0
    - instrumental O61.1
    - mechanical O61.1
    - medical O61.0
    - specified NEC O61.8
    - surgical O61.1
  - intubation during anesthesia T88.4 ☑
    - in pregnancy O29.6- ☑
    - labor and delivery O74.7
    - postpartum, puerperal O89.6
  - involution, thymus (gland) E32.0
  - kidney (*see also* Disease, kidney, chronic) N19
    - acute (*see also* Failure, renal, acute) N17.9
  - lactation (complete) O92.3
    - partial O92.4
  - Leydig's cell, adult E29.1
  - liver — *see* Failure, hepatic
  - menstruation at puberty N91.0
  - mitral I05.8
  - myocardial, myocardium (*see also* Failure, heart) I50.9
    - chronic (*see also* Failure, heart, congestive) I50.9
    - congestive (*see also* Failure, heart, congestive) I50.9
  - orgasm (female) (psychogenic) F52.31
    - male F52.32
  - ovarian (primary) E28.39
    - iatrogenic E89.40
      - asymptomatic E89.40
      - symptomatic E89.41
    - postprocedural (postablative) (postirradiation) (postsurgical) E89.40
      - asymptomatic E89.40
      - symptomatic E89.41
  - ovulation causing infertility N97.0
  - polyglandular, autoimmune E31.0
  - prosthetic joint implant — *see* Complications, joint prosthesis, mechanical, breakdown, by site
  - renal N19
    - with
      - tubular necrosis (acute) N17.0
    - acute N17.9
      - with
        - cortical necrosis N17.1
        - medullary necrosis N17.2
        - tubular necrosis N17.0
      - specified NEC N17.8
    - chronic N18.9
      - hypertensive — *see* Hypertension, kidney
    - congenital P96.0
    - end stage (chronic) N18.6
      - due to hypertension I12.0
    - following
      - abortion — *see* Abortion by type complicated by specified condition NEC

- **Failure, failed** — *continued*
  - renal — *continued*
    - following — *continued*
      - crushing T79.5 ☑
      - ectopic or molar pregnancy O08.4
      - labor and delivery (acute) O90.4
    - hypertensive — *see* Hypertension, kidney
    - postprocedural N99.0
  - respiration, respiratory J96.90
    - with
      - hypercapnia J96.92
      - hypoxia J96.91
    - acute J96.00
      - with
        - hypercapnia J96.02
        - hypoxia J96.01
    - acute and (on) chronic J96.20
      - with
        - hypercapnia J96.22
        - hypoxia J96.21
    - center G93.89
    - chronic J96.10
      - with
        - hypercapnia J96.12
        - hypoxia J96.11
    - newborn P28.5
    - postprocedural (acute) J95.821
      - acute and chronic J95.822
  - rotation
    - cecum Q43.3
    - colon Q43.3
    - intestine Q43.3
    - kidney Q63.2
  - sedation (conscious) (moderate) during procedure T88.52 ☑
    - history of Z92.83
  - segmentation (*see also* Fusion)
    - fingers — *see* Syndactylism, complex, fingers
    - vertebra Q76.49
      - with scoliosis Q76.3
  - seminiferous tubule, adult E29.1
  - senile (general) R54
  - sexual arousal (male) F52.21
    - female F52.22
  - testicular endocrine function E29.1
  - to thrive (child over 28 days old) R62.51
    - adult R62.7
    - newborn P92.6
  - transplant T86.92
    - bone T86.831
      - marrow T86.02
    - cornea T86.841
    - heart T86.22
      - with lung(s) T86.32
    - intestine T86.851
    - kidney T86.12
    - liver T86.42
    - lung(s) T86.811
      - with heart T86.32
    - pancreas T86.891
    - skin (allograft) (autograft) T86.821
    - specified organ or tissue NEC T86.891
    - stem cell (peripheral blood) (umbilical cord) T86.5
  - trial of labor (with subsequent cesarean delivery) O66.40
    - following previous cesarean delivery O66.41
  - tubal ligation N99.89
  - urinary — *see* Disease, kidney, chronic
  - vacuum extraction NOS (with subsequent cesarean delivery) O66.5
  - vasectomy N99.89
  - ventouse NOS (with subsequent cesarean delivery) O66.5
  - ventricular (*see also* Failure, heart) I50.9
    - left I50.1
      - with rheumatic fever (conditions in I00)
        - active I01.8
          - with chorea I02.0
        - inactive or quiescent (with chorea) I09.81
      - rheumatic (chronic) (inactive) (with chorea) I09.81
        - active or acute I01.8
          - with chorea I02.0
    - right (*see also* Failure, heart, congestive) I50.9
  - vital centers, newborn P91.8
- **Fainting** (fit) R55
- **Fallen arches** — *see* Deformity, limb, flat foot
- **Falling, falls** (repeated) R29.6

- **Falling, falls** — *continued*
  - any organ or part — *see* Prolapse
- **Fallopian**
  - insufflation Z31.41
  - tube — *see* condition
- **Fallot's**
  - pentalogy Q21.8
  - tetrad or tetralogy Q21.3
  - triad or trilogy Q22.3
- **False** (*see also* condition)
  - croup J38.5
  - joint — *see* Nonunion, fracture
  - labor (pains) O47.9
    - at or after 37 completed weeks of gestation O47.1
    - before 37 completed weeks of gestation O47.Ø- ☑
  - passage, urethra (prostatic) N36.5
  - pregnancy F45.8
- **Family, familial** (*see also* condition)
  - disruption Z63.8
    - involving divorce or separation Z63.5
  - Li-Fraumeni (syndrome) Z15.Ø1
  - planning advice Z3Ø.Ø9
  - problem Z63.9
    - specified NEC Z63.8
  - retinoblastoma C69.2- ☑
- **Famine** (effects of) T73.Ø ☑
  - edema — *see* Malnutrition, severe
- **Fanconi** (-de Toni)(-Debré) **syndrome** E72.Ø9
  - with cystinosis E72.Ø4
- **Fanconi's anemia** (congenital pancytopenia) D61.Ø9
- **Farber's disease or syndrome** E75.29
- **Farcy** A24.Ø
- **Farmer's**
  - lung J67.Ø
  - skin L57.8
- **Farsightedness** — *see* Hypermetropia
- **Fascia** — *see* condition
- **Fasciculation** R25.3
- **Fasciitis** M72.9
  - diffuse (eosinophilic) M35.4
  - infective M72.8
    - necrotizing M72.6
  - necrotizing M72.6
  - nodular M72.4
  - perirenal (with ureteral obstruction) N13.5
    - with infection N13.6
  - plantar M72.2
  - specified NEC M72.8
  - traumatic (old) M72.8
    - current — *code by* site under Sprain
- **Fascioliasis** B66.3
- **Fasciolopsis, fasciolopsiasis** (intestinal) B66.5
- **Fascioscapulohumeral myopathy** G71.Ø
- **Fast pulse** RØØ.Ø
- **Fat**
  - embolism — *see* Embolism, fat
  - excessive (*see also* Obesity)
    - in heart — *see* Degeneration, myocardial
  - in stool R19.5
  - localized (pad) E65
    - heart — *see* Degeneration, myocardial
    - knee M79.4
    - retropatellar M79.4
  - necrosis
    - breast N64.1
    - mesentery K65.4
    - omentum K65.4
  - pad E65
    - knee M79.4
- **Fatigue** R53.83
  - auditory deafness — *see* Deafness
  - chronic R53.82
  - combat F43.Ø
  - general R53.83
    - psychogenic F48.8
  - heat (transient) T67.6 ☑
  - muscle M62.89
  - myocardium — *see* Failure, heart
  - neoplasm-related R53.Ø
  - nervous, neurosis F48.8
  - operational F48.8
  - psychogenic (general) F48.8
  - senile R54
  - voice R49.8
- **Fatness** — *see* Obesity
- **Fatty** (*see also* condition)
  - apron E65
- **Fatty** — *continued*
  - degeneration — *see* Degeneration, fatty
  - heart (enlarged) — *see* Degeneration, myocardial
  - liver NEC K76.Ø
    - alcoholic K7Ø.Ø
    - nonalcoholic K76.Ø
  - necrosis — *see* Degeneration, fatty
- **Fauces** — *see* condition
- **Fauchard's disease** (periodontitis) — *see* Periodontitis
- **Faucitis** JØ2.9
- **Favism** (anemia) D55.Ø
- **Favus** — *see* Dermatophytosis
- **Fazio-Londe disease or syndrome** G12.1
- **Fear complex or reaction** F4Ø.9
- **Fear of** — *see* Phobia
- **Feared complaint unfounded** Z71.1
- **Febris, febrile** (*see also* Fever)
  - flava (*see also* Fever, yellow) A95.9
  - melitensis A23.Ø
  - pestis — *see* Plague
  - recurrens — *see* Fever, relapsing
  - rubra A38.9
- **Fecal**
  - incontinence R15.9
  - smearing R15.1
  - soiling R15.1
  - urgency R15.2
- **Fecalith** (impaction) K56.41
  - appendix K38.1
  - congenital P76.8
- **Fede's disease** K14.Ø
- **Feeble rapid pulse due to shock following injury** T79.4 ☑
- **Feeble-minded** F7Ø
- **Feeding**
  - difficulties R63.3
  - problem R63.3
    - newborn P92.9
      - specified NEC P92.8
    - nonorganic (adult) — *see* Disorder, eating
- **Feeling** (of)
  - foreign body in throat RØ9.89
- **Feer's disease** — *see* Poisoning, mercury
- **Feet** — *see* condition
- **Feigned illness** Z76.5
- **Feil-Klippel syndrome** (brevicollis) Q76.1
- **Feinmesser's** (hidrotic) **ectodermal dysplasia** Q82.4
- **Felinophobia** F4Ø.218
- **Felon** (*see also* Cellulitis, digit)
  - with lymphangitis — *see* Lymphangitis, acute, digit
- **Felty's syndrome** MØ5.ØØ
  - ankle MØ5.Ø7- ☑
  - elbow MØ5.Ø2- ☑
  - foot joint MØ5.Ø7- ☑
  - hand joint MØ5.Ø4- ☑
  - hip MØ5.Ø5- ☑
  - knee MØ5.Ø6- ☑
  - multiple site MØ5.Ø9
  - shoulder MØ5.Ø1- ☑
  - vertebra — *see* Spondylitis, ankylosing
  - wrist MØ5.Ø3- ☑
- **Female genital cutting status** — *see* Female genital mutilation status (FGM)
- **Female genital mutilation status** (FGM) N9Ø.81Ø
  - specified NEC N9Ø.818
  - type I (clitorectomy status) N9Ø.811
  - type II (clitorectomy with excision of labia minora status) N9Ø.812
  - type III (infibulation status) N9Ø.813
  - type IV N9Ø.818
- **Femur, femoral** — *see* condition
- **Fenestration, fenestrated** (*see also* Imperfect, closure)
  - aortico-pulmonary Q21.4
  - cusps, heart valve NEC Q24.8
    - pulmonary Q22.3
  - pulmonic cusps Q22.3
- **Fernell's disease** (aortic aneurysm) I71.9
- **Fertile eunuch syndrome** E23.Ø
- **Fetid**
  - breath R19.6
  - sweat L75.Ø
- **Fetishism** F65.Ø
  - transvestic F65.1
- **Fetus, fetal** (*see also* condition)
  - alcohol syndrome (dysmorphic) Q86.Ø
  - compressus O31.Ø- ☑
  - hydantoin syndrome Q86.1
- **Fetus, fetal** — *continued*
  - lung tissue P28.Ø
  - papyraceous O31.Ø- ☑
- **Fever** (inanition) (of unknown origin) (persistent) (with chills) (with rigor) R5Ø.9
  - abortus A23.1
  - Aden (dengue) A9Ø
  - African tick-borne A68.1
  - American
    - mountain (tick) A93.2
    - spotted A77.Ø
  - aphthous BØ8.8
  - arbovirus, arboviral A94
    - hemorrhagic A94
    - specified NEC A93.8
  - Argentinian hemorrhagic A96.Ø
  - Assam B55.Ø
  - Australian Q A78
  - Bangkok hemorrhagic A91
  - Barmah forest A92.8
  - Bartonella A44.Ø
  - bilious, hemoglobinuric B5Ø.8
  - blackwater B5Ø.8
  - blister BØØ.1
  - Bolivian hemorrhagic A96.1
  - Bonvale dam T73.3 ☑
  - boutonneuse A77.1
  - brain — *see* Encephalitis
  - Brazilian purpuric A48.4
  - breakbone A9Ø
  - Bullis A77.Ø
  - Bunyamwera A92.8
  - Burdwan B55.Ø
  - Bwamba A92.8
  - Cameroon — *see* Malaria
  - Canton A75.9
  - catarrhal (acute) JØØ
    - chronic J31.Ø
  - cat-scratch A28.1
  - Central Asian hemorrhagic A98.Ø
  - cerebral — *see* Encephalitis
  - cerebrospinal meningococcal A39.Ø
  - Chagres B5Ø.9
  - Chandipura A92.8
  - Changuinola A93.1
  - Charcot's (biliary) (hepatic) (intermittent) — *see* Calculus, bile duct
  - Chikungunya (viral) (hemorrhagic) A92.Ø
  - Chitral A93.1
  - Colombo — *see* Fever, paratyphoid
  - Colorado tick (virus) A93.2
  - congestive (remittent) — *see* Malaria
  - Congo virus A98.Ø
  - continued malarial B5Ø.9
  - Corsican — *see* Malaria
  - Crimean-Congo hemorrhagic A98.Ø
  - Cyprus — *see* Brucellosis
  - dandy A9Ø
  - deer fly — *see* Tularemia
  - dengue (virus) A9Ø
    - hemorrhagic A91
    - sandfly A93.1
  - desert B38.Ø
  - drug induced R5Ø.2
  - due to
    - conditions classified elsewhere R5Ø.81
    - heat T67.Ø ☑
  - enteric AØ1.ØØ
  - enteroviral exanthematous (Boston exanthem) A88.Ø
  - ephemeral (of unknown origin) R5Ø.9
  - epidemic hemorrhagic A98.5
  - erysipelatous — *see* Erysipelas
  - estivo-autumnal (malarial) B5Ø.9
  - famine A75.Ø
  - five day A79.Ø
  - following delivery O86.4
  - Fort Bragg A27.89
  - gastroenteric AØ1.ØØ
  - gastromalarial — *see* Malaria
  - Gibraltar — *see* Brucellosis
  - glandular — *see* Mononucleosis, infectious
  - Guama (viral) A92.8
  - Haverhill A25.1
  - hay (allergic) J3Ø.1
    - with asthma (bronchial) J45.9Ø9
      - with
        - exacerbation (acute) J45.9Ø1
        - status asthmaticus J45.9Ø2

Fever — *continued*
- Zika (viral) A92.8

Fibrillation
- atrial or auricular (established) I48.91
  - chronic I48.2
  - paroxysmal I48.Ø
  - permanent I48.2
  - persistent I48.1
- cardiac I49.8
- heart I49.8
- muscular M62.89
- ventricular I49.Ø1

Fibrin
- ball or bodies, pleural (sac) J94.1
- chamber, anterior (eye) (gelatinous exudate) — *see* Iridocyclitis, acute

Fibrinogenolysis — *see* Fibrinolysis

Fibrinogenopenia D68.8
- acquired D65
- congenital D68.2

Fibrinolysis (hemorrhagic) (acquired) D65
- antepartum hemorrhage — *see* Hemorrhage, antepartum, with coagulation defect
- following
  - abortion — *see* Abortion by type complicated by hemorrhage
  - ectopic or molar pregnancy OØ8.1
- intrapartum O67.Ø
- newborn, transient P6Ø
- postpartum O72.3

Fibrinopenia (hereditary) D68.2
- acquired D68.4

Fibrinopurulent — *see* condition

Fibrinous — *see* condition

Fibroadenoma
- cellular intracanalicular D24- ☑
- giant D24- ☑
- intracanalicular
  - cellular D24- ☑
  - giant D24- ☑
  - specified site — *see* Neoplasm, benign, by site
  - unspecified site D24- ☑
- juvenile D24- ☑
- pericanalicular
  - specified site — *see* Neoplasm, benign, by site
  - unspecified site D24- ☑
- phyllodes D24- ☑
- prostate D29.1
- specified site NEC — *see* Neoplasm, benign, by site
- unspecified site D24- ☑

Fibroadenosis, breast (chronic) (cystic) (diffuse) (periodic) (segmental) N6Ø.2- ☑

Fibroangioma (*see also* Neoplasm, benign, by site)
- juvenile
  - specified site — *see* Neoplasm, benign, by site
  - unspecified site D1Ø.6

Fibrochondrosarcoma — *see* Neoplasm, cartilage, malignant

Fibrocystic
- disease (*see also* Fibrosis, cystic)
  - breast — *see* Mastopathy, cystic
  - jaw M27.49
  - kidney (congenital) Q61.8
  - liver Q44.6
  - pancreas E84.9
- kidney (congenital) Q61.8

Fibrodysplasia ossificans progressiva — *see* Myositis, ossificans, progressiva

Fibroelastosis (cordis) (endocardial) (endomyocardial) I42.4

Fibroid (tumor) (*see also* Neoplasm, connective tissue, benign)
- disease, lung (chronic) — *see* Fibrosis, lung
- heart (disease) — *see* Myocarditis
- in pregnancy or childbirth O34.1- ☑
  - causing obstructed labor O65.5
- induration, lung (chronic) — *see* Fibrosis, lung
- lung — *see* Fibrosis, lung
- pneumonia (chronic) — *see* Fibrosis, lung
- uterus D25.9

Fibrolipoma — *see* Lipoma

Fibroliposarcoma — *see* Neoplasm, connective tissue, malignant

Fibroma (*see also* Neoplasm, connective tissue, benign)
- ameloblastic — *see* Cyst, calcifying odontogenic
- bone (nonossifying) — *see* Disorder, bone, specified type NEC

Fibroma — *continued*
- bone — *see* Disorder, bone, specified type — *continued*
  - ossifying — *see* Neoplasm, bone, benign
- cementifying — *see* Neoplasm, bone, benign
- chondromyxoid — *see* Neoplasm, bone, benign
- desmoplastic — *see* Neoplasm, connective tissue, uncertain behavior
- durum — *see* Neoplasm, connective tissue, benign
- fascial — *see* Neoplasm, connective tissue, benign
- invasive — *see* Neoplasm, connective tissue, uncertain behavior
- molle — *see* Lipoma
- myxoid — *see* Neoplasm, connective tissue, benign
- nasopharynx, nasopharyngeal (juvenile) D1Ø.6
- nonosteogenic (nonossifying) — *see* Dysplasia, fibrous
- odontogenic (central) — *see* Cyst, calcifying odontogenic
- ossifying — *see* Neoplasm, bone, benign
- periosteal — *see* Neoplasm, bone, benign
- soft — *see* Lipoma

Fibromatosis M72.9
- abdominal — *see* Neoplasm, connective tissue, uncertain behavior
- aggressive — *see* Neoplasm, connective tissue, uncertain behavior
- congenital generalized — *see* Neoplasm, connective tissue, uncertain behavior
- Dupuytren's M72.Ø
- gingival KØ6.1
- palmar (fascial) M72.Ø
- plantar (fascial) M72.2
- pseudosarcomatous (proliferative) (subcutaneous) M72.4
- retroperitoneal D48.3
- specified NEC M72.8

Fibromyalgia M79.7

Fibromyoma (*see also* Neoplasm, connective tissue, benign)
- uterus (corpus) (*see also* Leiomyoma, uterus)
  - in pregnancy or childbirth — *see* Fibroid, in pregnancy or childbirth
    - causing obstructed labor O65.5

Fibromyositis M79.7

Fibromyxolipoma D17.9

Fibromyxoma — *see* Neoplasm, connective tissue, benign

Fibromyxosarcoma — *see* Neoplasm, connective tissue, malignant

Fibro-odontoma, ameloblastic — *see* Cyst, calcifying odontogenic

Fibro-osteoma — *see* Neoplasm, bone, benign

Fibroplasia, retrolental H35.17- ☑

Fibropurulent — *see* condition

Fibrosarcoma (*see also* Neoplasm, connective tissue, malignant)
- ameloblastic C41.1
  - upper jaw (bone) C41.Ø
- congenital — *see* Neoplasm, connective tissue, malignant
- fascial — *see* Neoplasm, connective tissue, malignant
- infantile — *see* Neoplasm, connective tissue, malignant
- odontogenic C41.1
  - upper jaw (bone) C41.Ø
- periosteal — *see* Neoplasm, bone, malignant

Fibrosclerosis
- breast N6Ø.3- ☑
- multifocal M35.5
- penis (corpora cavernosa) N48.6

Fibrosis, fibrotic
- adrenal (gland) E27.8
- amnion O41.8X- ☑
- anal papillae K62.89
- arteriocapillary — *see* Arteriosclerosis
- bladder N32.89
  - interstitial — *see* Cystitis, chronic, interstitial
  - localized submucosal — *see* Cystitis, chronic, interstitial
  - panmural — *see* Cystitis, chronic, interstitial
- breast — *see* Fibrosclerosis, breast
- capillary (*see also* Arteriosclerosis) I7Ø.9Ø
  - lung (chronic) — *see* Fibrosis, lung
- cardiac — *see* Myocarditis
- cervix N88.8
- chorion O41.8X- ☑
- corpus cavernosum (sclerosing) N48.6

Fibrosis, fibrotic — *continued*
- cystic (of pancreas) E84.9
  - with
    - distal intestinal obstruction syndrome E84.19
    - fecal impaction E84.19
    - intestinal manifestations NEC E84.19
    - pulmonary manifestations E84.Ø
    - specified manifestations NEC E84.8
- due to device, implant or graft (*see also* Complications, by site and type, specified NEC) T85.82 ☑
  - arterial graft NEC T82.828 ☑
  - breast (implant) T85.82 ☑
  - catheter NEC T85.82 ☑
    - dialysis (renal) T82.828 ☑
      - intraperitoneal T85.82 ☑
    - infusion NEC T82.828 ☑
      - spinal (epidural) (subdural) T85.82 ☑
    - urinary (indwelling) T83.82 ☑
  - electronic (electrode) (pulse generator) (stimulator)
    - bone T84.82 ☑
    - cardiac T82.827 ☑
    - nervous system (brain) (peripheral nerve) (spinal) T85.82 ☑
    - urinary T83.82 ☑
  - fixation, internal (orthopedic) NEC T84.82 ☑
  - gastrointestinal (bile duct) (esophagus) T85.82 ☑
  - genital NEC T83.82 ☑
  - heart NEC T82.827 ☑
  - joint prosthesis T84.82 ☑
  - ocular (corneal graft) (orbital implant) NEC T85.82 ☑
  - orthopedic NEC T84.82 ☑
  - specified NEC T85.82 ☑
  - urinary NEC T83.82 ☑
  - vascular NEC T82.828 ☑
  - ventricular intracranial shunt T85.82 ☑
- ejaculatory duct N5Ø.8
- endocardium — *see* Endocarditis
- endomyocardial (tropical) I42.3
- epididymis N5Ø.8
- eye muscle — *see* Strabismus, mechanical
- heart — *see* Myocarditis
- hepatic — *see* Fibrosis, liver
- hepatolienal (portal hypertension) K76.6
- hepatosplenic (portal hypertension) K76.6
- infrapatellar fat pad M79.4
- intrascrotal N5Ø.8
- kidney N26.9
- liver K74.Ø
  - with sclerosis K74.2
  - alcoholic K7Ø.2
- lung (atrophic) (chronic) (confluent) (massive) (perialveolar) (peribronchial) J84.1Ø
  - with
    - anthracosilicosis J6Ø
    - anthracosis J6Ø
    - asbestosis J61
    - bagassosis J67.1
    - bauxite J63.1
    - berylliosis J63.2
    - byssinosis J66.Ø
    - calcicosis J62.8
    - chalicosis J62.8
    - dust reticulation J64
    - farmer's lung J67.Ø
    - ganister disease J62.8
    - graphite J63.3
    - pneumoconiosis NOS J64
    - siderosis J63.4
    - silicosis J62.8
  - capillary J84.1Ø
  - congenital P27.8
  - diffuse (idiopathic) J84.1Ø
    - chemicals, gases, fumes or vapors (inhalation) J68.4
    - interstitial J84.1Ø
      - acute J84.114
    - talc J62.Ø
  - following radiation J7Ø.1
  - idiopathic J84.112
  - postinflammatory J84.1Ø
  - silicotic J62.8
  - tuberculous — *see* Tuberculosis, pulmonary
- lymphatic gland I89.8
- median bar — *see* Hyperplasia, prostate
- mediastinum (idiopathic) J98.5
- meninges G96.19

- **Fibrosis, fibrotic** — *continued*
  - myocardium, myocardial — *see* Myocarditis
  - ovary N83.8
  - oviduct N83.8
  - pancreas K86.8
  - penis NEC N48.6
  - pericardium I31.Ø
  - perineum, in pregnancy or childbirth O34.7- ☑
    - causing obstructed labor O65.5
  - pleura J94.1
  - popliteal fat pad M79.4
  - prostate (chronic) — *see* Hyperplasia, prostate
  - pulmonary (*see also* Fibrosis, lung) J84.1Ø
    - congenital P27.8
    - idiopathic J84.112
  - rectal sphincter K62.89
  - retroperitoneal, idiopathic (with ureteral obstruction) N13.5
    - with infection N13.6
  - sclerosing mesenteric (idiopathic) K65.4
  - scrotum N5Ø.8
  - seminal vesicle N5Ø.8
  - senile R54
  - skin L9Ø.5
  - spermatic cord N5Ø.8
  - spleen D73.89
    - in schistosomiasis (bilharziasis) B65.9 [D77]
  - subepidermal nodular — *see* Neoplasm, skin, benign
  - submucous (oral) (tongue) K13.5
  - testis N44.8
    - chronic, due to syphilis A52.76
  - thymus (gland) E32.8
  - tongue, submucous K13.5
  - tunica vaginalis N5Ø.8
  - uterus (non-neoplastic) N85.8
  - vagina N89.8
  - valve, heart — *see* Endocarditis
  - vas deferens N5Ø.8
  - vein I87.8
- **Fibrositis** (periarticular) M79.7
  - nodular, chronic (Jaccoud's) (rheumatoid) — *see* Arthropathy, postrheumatic, chronic
- **Fibrothorax** J94.1
- **Fibrotic** — *see* Fibrosis
- **Fibrous** — *see* condition
- **Fibroxanthoma** (*see also* Neoplasm, connective tissue, benign)
  - atypical — *see* Neoplasm, connective tissue, uncertain behavior
  - malignant — *see* Neoplasm, connective tissue, malignant
- **Fibroxanthosarcoma** — *see* Neoplasm, connective tissue, malignant
- **Fiedler's**
  - disease (icterohemorrhagic leptospirosis) A27.Ø
  - myocarditis (acute) I4Ø.1
- **Fifth disease** BØ8.3
  - venereal A55
- **Filaria, filarial, filariasis** — *see* Infestation, filarial
- **Filatov's disease** — *see* Mononucleosis, infectious
- **File-cutter's disease** — *see* Poisoning, lead
- **Filling defect**
  - biliary tract R93.2
  - bladder R93.4
  - duodenum R93.3
  - gallbladder R93.2
  - gastrointestinal tract R93.3
  - intestine R93.3
  - kidney R93.4
  - stomach R93.3
  - ureter R93.4
- **Fimbrial cyst** Q5Ø.4
- **Financial problem affecting care NOS** Z59.9
  - bankruptcy Z59.8
  - foreclosure on loan Z59.8
- **Findings, abnormal, inconclusive, without diagnosis** (*see also* Abnormal)
  - 17-ketosteroids, elevated R82.5
  - acetonuria R82.4
  - alcohol in blood R78.Ø
  - anisocytosis R71.8
  - antenatal screening of mother O28.9
    - biochemical O28.1
    - chromosomal O28.5
    - cytological O28.2
    - genetic O28.5
    - hematological O28.Ø
    - radiological O28.4

Findings, abnormal, inconclusive, without diagnosis — *continued*

- antenatal screening of mother — *continued*
  - specified NEC O28.8
  - ultrasonic O28.3
- antibody titer, elevated R76.Ø
- anticardiolipin antibody R76.Ø
- antiphosphatidylglycerol antibody R76.Ø
- antiphosphatidylinositol antibody R76.Ø
- antiphosphatidylserine antibody R76.Ø
- antiphospholipid antibody R76.Ø
- bacteriuria N39.Ø
- bicarbonate E87.8
- bile in urine R82.2
- blood sugar R73.Ø9
  - high R73.9
  - low (transient) E16.2
- body fluid or substance, specified NEC R88.8
- casts, urine R82.99
- catecholamines R82.5
- cells, urine R82.99
- chloride E87.8
- cholesterol E78.9
  - high E78.Ø
    - with high triglycerides E78.2
- chyluria R82.Ø
- cloudy
  - dialysis effluent R88.Ø
  - urine R82.9Ø
- creatinine clearance R94.4
- crystals, urine R82.99
- culture
  - blood R78.81
  - positive — *see* Positive, culture
- echocardiogram R93.1
- electrolyte level, urinary R82.99
- function study NEC R94.8
  - bladder R94.8
  - endocrine NEC R94.7
    - thyroid R94.6
  - kidney R94.4
  - liver R94.5
  - pancreas R94.8
  - placenta R94.8
  - pulmonary R94.2
  - spleen R94.8
- gallbladder, nonvisualization R93.2
- glucose (tolerance test) (non-fasting) R73.Ø9
- glycosuria R81
- heart
  - shadow R93.1
  - sounds RØ1.2
- hematinuria R82.3
- hematocrit drop (precipitous) R71.Ø
- hemoglobinuria R82.3
- human papillomavirus (HPV) DNA test positive
  - cervix
    - high risk R87.81Ø
    - low risk R87.82Ø
  - vagina
    - high risk R87.811
    - low risk R87.821
- in blood (of substance not normally found in blood) R78.9
  - addictive drug NEC R78.4
  - alcohol (excessive level) R78.Ø
  - cocaine R78.2
  - hallucinogen R78.3
  - heavy metals (abnormal level) R78.79
  - lead R78.71
  - lithium (abnormal level) R78.89
  - opiate drug R78.1
  - psychotropic drug R78.5
  - specified substance NEC R78.89
  - steroid agent R78.6
- indoleacetic acid, elevated R82.5
- ketonuria R82.4
- lactic acid dehydrogenase (LDH) R74.Ø
- liver function test R79.89
- mammogram NEC R92.8
  - calcification (calculus) R92.1
  - inconclusive result (due to dense breasts) R92.2
  - microcalcification R92.Ø
- mediastinal shift R93.8
- melanin, urine R82.99
- myoglobinuria R82.1
- neonatal screening PØ9
- nonvisualization of gallbladder R93.2

Findings, abnormal, inconclusive, without diagnosis — *continued*

- odor of urine NOS R82.9Ø
- Papanicolaou cervix R87.619
  - non-atypical endometrial cells R87.618
- pneumoencephalogram R93.Ø
- poikilocytosis R71.8
- potassium (deficiency) E87.6
  - excess E87.5
- PPD R76.11
- radiologic (X-ray) R93.8
  - abdomen R93.5
  - biliary tract R93.2
  - breast R92.8
  - gastrointestinal tract R93.3
  - genitourinary organs R93.8
  - head R93.Ø
  - inconclusive due to excess body fat of patient R93.9
  - intrathoracic organs NEC R93.1
  - placenta R93.8
  - retroperitoneum R93.5
  - skin R93.8
  - skull R93.Ø
  - subcutaneous tissue R93.8
- red blood cell (count) (morphology) (sickling) (volume) R71.8
- scan NEC R94.8
  - bladder R94.8
  - bone R94.8
  - kidney R94.4
  - liver R93.2
  - lung R94.2
  - pancreas R94.8
  - placental R94.8
  - spleen R94.8
  - thyroid R94.6
- sedimentation rate, elevated R7Ø.Ø
- SGOT R74.Ø
- SGPT R74.Ø
- sodium (deficiency) E87.1
  - excess E87.Ø
- specified body fluid NEC R88.8
- stress test R94.39
- thyroid (function) (metabolic rate) (scan) (uptake) R94.6
- transaminase (level) R74.Ø
- triglycerides E78.9
  - high E78.1
    - with high cholesterol E78.2
- tuberculin skin test (without active tuberculosis) R76.11
- urine R82.9Ø
  - acetone R82.4
  - bacteria N39.Ø
  - bile R82.2
  - casts or cells R82.99
  - chyle R82.Ø
  - culture positive R82.7
  - glucose R81
  - hemoglobin R82.3
  - ketone R82.4
  - sugar R81
- vanillylmandelic acid (VMA), elevated R82.5
- vectorcardiogram (VCG) R94.39
- ventriculogram R93.Ø
- white blood cell (count) (differential) (morphology) D72.9
- xerography R92.8

- **Finger** — *see* condition
- **Fire, Saint Anthony's** — *see* Erysipelas
- **Fire-setting**
  - pathological (compulsive) F63.1
- **Fish hook stomach** K31.89
- **Fishmeal-worker's lung** J67.8
- **Fissure, fissured**
  - anus, anal K6Ø.2
    - acute K6Ø.Ø
    - chronic K6Ø.1
    - congenital Q43.8
  - ear, lobule, congenital Q17.8
  - epiglottis (congenital) Q31.8
  - larynx J38.7
    - congenital Q31.8
  - lip K13.Ø
    - congenital — *see* Cleft, lip
  - nipple N64.Ø
    - associated with
      - lactation O92.13

- **Fissure, fissured** — *continued*
  - nipple — *continued*
    - associated with — *continued*
      - pregnancy O92.11- ☑
      - puerperium O92.12
  - nose Q3Ø.2
  - palate (congenital) — *see* Cleft, palate
  - skin R23.4
  - spine (congenital) (*see also* Spina bifida)
    - with hydrocephalus — *see* Spina bifida, by site, with hydrocephalus
  - tongue (acquired) K14.5
    - congenital Q38.3
- **Fistula** (cutaneous) L98.8
  - abdomen (wall) K63.2
    - bladder N32.2
    - intestine NEC K63.2
    - ureter N28.89
    - uterus N82.5
  - abdominorectal K63.2
  - abdominosigmoidal K63.2
  - abdominothoracic J86.Ø
  - abdominouterine N82.5
    - congenital Q51.7
  - abdominovesical N32.2
  - accessory sinuses — *see* Sinusitis
  - actinomycotic — *see* Actinomycosis
  - alveolar antrum — *see* Sinusitis, maxillary
  - alveolar process KØ4.6
  - anorectal K6Ø.5
  - antrobuccal — *see* Sinusitis, maxillary
  - antrum — *see* Sinusitis, maxillary
  - anus, anal (recurrent) (infectional) K6Ø.3
    - congenital Q43.6
      - with absence, atresia and stenosis Q42.2
    - tuberculous A18.32
  - aorta-duodenal I77.2
  - appendix, appendicular K38.3
  - arteriovenous (acquired) (nonruptured) I77.Ø
    - brain I67.1
      - congenital Q28.2
        - ruptured I6Ø.8
      - ruptured I6Ø.8
    - cerebral — *see* Fistula, arteriovenous, brain
    - congenital (peripheral) (*see also* Malformation, arteriovenous)
      - brain Q28.2
        - ruptured I6Ø.8
      - coronary Q24.5
      - pulmonary Q25.72
    - coronary I25.41
      - congenital Q24.5
    - pulmonary I28.Ø
      - congenital Q25.72
    - surgically created (for dialysis) Z99.2
      - complication — *see* Complication, arteriovenous, fistula, surgically created
    - traumatic — *see* Injury, blood vessel
  - artery I77.2
  - aural (mastoid) — *see* Mastoiditis, chronic
  - auricle (*see also* Disorder, pinna, specified type NEC)
    - congenital Q18.1
  - Bartholin's gland N82.8
  - bile duct (common) (hepatic) K83.3
    - with calculus, stones — *see* Calculus, bile duct
  - biliary (tract) — *see* Fistula, bile duct
  - bladder (sphincter) NEC (*see also* Fistula, vesico-) N32.2
    - into seminal vesicle N32.2
  - bone (*see also* Disorder, bone, specified type NEC)
    - with osteomyelitis, chronic — *see* Osteomyelitis, chronic, with draining sinus
  - brain G93.89
    - arteriovenous (acquired) I67.1
      - congenital Q28.2
  - branchial (cleft) Q18.Ø
  - branchiogenous Q18.Ø
  - breast N61
    - puerperal, postpartum or gestational, due to mastitis (purulent) — *see* Mastitis, obstetric, purulent
  - bronchial J86.Ø
  - bronchocutaneous, bronchomediastinal, bronchopleural, bronchopleuromediastinal (infective) J86.Ø
    - tuberculous NEC A15.5
  - bronchoesophageal J86.Ø
    - congenital Q39.2
      - with atresia of esophagus Q39.1
  - bronchovisceral J86.Ø
- **Fistula** — *continued*
  - buccal cavity (infective) K12.2
  - cecosigmoidal K63.2
  - cecum K63.2
  - cerebrospinal (fluid) G96.Ø
  - cervical, lateral Q18.1
  - cervicoaural Q18.1
  - cervicosigmoidal N82.4
  - cervicovesical N82.1
  - cervix N82.8
  - chest (wall) J86.Ø
  - cholecystenteric — *see* Fistula, gallbladder
  - cholecystocolic — *see* Fistula, gallbladder
  - cholecystocolonic — *see* Fistula, gallbladder
  - cholecystoduodenal — *see* Fistula, gallbladder
  - cholecystogastric — *see* Fistula, gallbladder
  - cholecystointestinal — *see* Fistula, gallbladder
  - choledochoduodenal — *see* Fistula, bile duct
  - cholocolic K82.3
  - coccyx — *see* Sinus, pilonidal
  - colon K63.2
  - colostomy K94.Ø9
  - common duct — *see* Fistula, bile duct
  - congenital, site not listed — *see* Anomaly, by site
  - coronary, arteriovenous I25.41
    - congenital Q24.5
  - costal region J86.Ø
  - cul-de-sac, Douglas' N82.8
  - cystic duct (*see also* Fistula, gallbladder)
    - congenital Q44.5
  - dental KØ4.6
  - diaphragm J86.Ø
  - duodenum K31.6
  - ear (external) (canal) — *see* Disorder, ear, external, specified type NEC
  - enterocolic K63.2
  - enterocutaneous K63.2
  - enterouterine N82.4
    - congenital Q51.7
  - enterovaginal N82.4
    - congenital Q52.2
    - large intestine N82.3
    - small intestine N82.2
  - enterovesical N32.1
  - epididymis N5Ø.8
    - tuberculous A18.15
  - esophagobronchial J86.Ø
    - congenital Q39.2
      - with atresia of esophagus Q39.1
  - esophagocutaneous K22.8
  - esophagopleural-cutaneous J86.Ø
  - esophagotracheal J86.Ø
    - congenital Q39.2
      - with atresia of esophagus Q39.1
  - esophagus K22.8
    - congenital Q39.2
      - with atresia of esophagus Q39.1
  - ethmoid — *see* Sinusitis, ethmoidal
  - eyeball (cornea) (sclera) — *see* Disorder, globe, hypotony
  - eyelid HØ1.8
  - fallopian tube, external N82.5
  - fecal K63.2
    - congenital Q43.6
  - from periapical abscess KØ4.6
  - frontal sinus — *see* Sinusitis, frontal
  - gallbladder K82.3
    - with calculus, cholelithiasis, stones — *see* Calculus, gallbladder
  - gastric K31.6
  - gastrocolic K31.6
    - congenital Q4Ø.2
    - tuberculous A18.32
  - gastroenterocolic K31.6
  - gastroesophageal K31.6
  - gastrojejunal K31.6
  - gastrojejunocolic K31.6
  - genital tract (female) N82.9
    - specified NEC N82.8
    - to intestine NEC N82.4
    - to skin N82.5
  - hepatic artery-portal vein, congenital Q26.6
  - hepatopleural J86.Ø
  - hepatopulmonary J86.Ø
  - ileorectal or ileosigmoidal K63.2
  - ileovaginal N82.2
  - ileovesical N32.1
  - ileum K63.2
- **Fistula** — *continued*
  - in ano K6Ø.3
    - tuberculous A18.32
  - inner ear (labyrinth) — *see* subcategory H83.1 ☑
  - intestine NEC K63.2
  - intestinocolonic (abdominal) K63.2
  - intestinoureteral N28.89
  - intestinouterine N82.4
  - intestinovaginal N82.4
    - large intestine N82.3
    - small intestine N82.2
  - intestinovesical N32.1
  - ischiorectal (fossa) K61.3
  - jejunum K63.2
  - joint M25.1Ø
    - ankle M25.17- ☑
    - elbow M25.12- ☑
    - foot joint M25.17- ☑
    - hand joint M25.14- ☑
    - hip M25.15- ☑
    - knee M25.16- ☑
    - shoulder M25.11- ☑
    - specified joint NEC M25.18
    - tuberculous — *see* Tuberculosis, joint
    - vertebrae M25.18
    - wrist M25.13- ☑
  - kidney N28.89
  - labium (majus) (minus) N82.8
  - labyrinth — *see* subcategory H83.1 ☑
  - lacrimal (gland) (sac) HØ4.61- ☑
  - lacrimonasal duct — *see* Fistula, lacrimal
  - laryngotracheal, congenital Q34.8
  - larynx J38.7
  - lip K13.Ø
    - congenital Q38.Ø
  - lumbar, tuberculous A18.Ø1
  - lung J86.Ø
  - lymphatic I89.8
  - mammary (gland) N61
  - mastoid (process) (region) — *see* Mastoiditis, chronic
  - maxillary J32.Ø
  - medial, face and neck Q18.8
  - mediastinal J86.Ø
  - mediastinobronchial J86.Ø
  - mediastinocutaneous J86.Ø
  - middle ear — *see* subcategory H74.8 ☑
  - mouth K12.2
  - nasal J34.89
    - sinus — *see* Sinusitis
  - nasopharynx J39.2
  - nipple N64.Ø
  - nose J34.89
  - oral (cutaneous) K12.2
    - maxillary J32.Ø
    - nasal (with cleft palate) — *see* Cleft, palate
  - orbit, orbital — *see* Disorder, orbit, specified type NEC
  - oroantral J32.Ø
  - oviduct, external N82.5
  - palate (hard) M27.8
  - pancreatic K86.8
  - pancreaticoduodenal K86.8
  - parotid (gland) K11.4
    - region K12.2
  - penis N48.89
  - perianal K6Ø.3
  - pericardium (pleura) (sac) — *see* Pericarditis
  - pericecal K63.2
  - perineorectal K6Ø.4
  - perineosigmoidal K63.2
  - perineum, perineal (with urethral involvement) NEC N36.Ø
    - tuberculous A18.13
    - ureter N28.89
  - perirectal K6Ø.4
    - tuberculous A18.32
  - peritoneum K65.9
  - pharyngoesophageal J39.2
  - pharynx J39.2
    - branchial cleft (congenital) Q18.Ø
  - pilonidal (infected) (rectum) — *see* Sinus, pilonidal
  - pleura, pleural, pleurocutaneous, pleuroperitoneal J86.Ø
    - tuberculous NEC A15.6
  - pleuropericardial I31.8
  - portal vein-hepatic artery, congenital Q26.6
  - postauricular H7Ø.81- ☑
  - postoperative, persistent T81.83 ☑
    - specified site — *see* Fistula, by site

Fistula — *continued*
preauricular (congenital) Q18.1
prostate N42.89
pulmonary J86.Ø
arteriovenous I28.Ø
congenital Q25.72
tuberculous — *see* Tuberculosis, pulmonary
pulmonoperitoneal J86.Ø
rectolabial N82.4
rectosigmoid (intercommunicating) K63.2
rectoureteral N28.89
rectourethral N36.Ø
congenital Q64.73
rectouterine N82.4
congenital Q51.7
rectovaginal N82.3
congenital Q52.2
tuberculous A18.18
rectovesical N32.1
congenital Q64.79
rectovesicovaginal N82.3
rectovulval N82.4
congenital Q52.79
rectum (to skin) K6Ø.4
congenital Q43.6
with absence, atresia and stenosis Q42.Ø
tuberculous A18.32
renal N28.89
retroauricular — *see* Fistula, postauricular
salivary duct or gland (any) K11.4
congenital Q38.4
scrotum (urinary) N5Ø.8
tuberculous A18.15
semicircular canals — *see* subcategory H83.1 ☑
sigmoid K63.2
to bladder N32.1
sinus — *see* Sinusitis
skin L98.8
to genital tract (female) N82.5
splenocolic D73.89
stercoral K63.2
stomach K31.6
sublingual gland K11.4
submandibular gland K11.4
submaxillary (gland) K11.4
region K12.2
thoracic J86.Ø
duct I89.8
thoracoabdominal J86.Ø
thoracogastric J86.Ø
thoracointestinal J86.Ø
thorax J86.Ø
thyroglossal duct Q89.2
thyroid EØ7.89
trachea, congenital (external) (internal) Q32.1
tracheoesophageal J86.Ø
congenital Q39.2
with atresia of esophagus Q39.1
following tracheostomy J95.Ø4
traumatic arteriovenous — *see* Injury, blood vessel, by site
tuberculous — *code by* site under Tuberculosis
typhoid AØ1.Ø9
umbilicourinary Q64.8
urachus, congenital Q64.4
ureter (persistent) N28.89
ureteroabdominal N28.89
ureterorectal N28.89
ureterosigmoido-abdominal N28.89
ureterovaginal N82.1
ureterovesical N32.2
urethra N36.Ø
congenital Q64.79
tuberculous A18.13
urethroperineal N36.Ø
urethroperineovesical N32.2
urethrorectal N36.Ø
congenital Q64.73
urethroscrotal N5Ø.8
urethrovaginal N82.1
urethrovesical N32.2
urinary (tract) (persistent) (recurrent) N36.Ø
uteroabdominal N82.5
congenital Q51.7
uteroenteric, uterointestinal N82.4
congenital Q51.7
uterorectal N82.4
congenital Q51.7

Fistula — *continued*
uteroureteric N82.1
uterourethral Q51.7
uterovaginal N82.8
uterovesical N82.1
congenital Q51.7
uterus N82.8
vagina (postpartal) (wall) N82.8
vaginocutaneous (postpartal) N82.5
vaginointestinal NEC N82.4
large intestine N82.3
small intestine N82.2
vaginoperineal N82.5
vasocutaneous, congenital Q55.7
vesical NEC N32.2
vesicoabdominal N32.2
vesicocervicovaginal N82.1
vesicocolic N32.1
vesicocutaneous N32.2
vesicoenteric N32.1
vesicointestinal N32.1
vesicometrorectal N82.4
vesicoperineal N32.2
vesicorectal N32.1
congenital Q64.79
vesicosigmoidal N32.1
vesicosigmoidovaginal N82.3
vesicoureteral N32.2
vesicoureterovaginal N82.1
vesicourethral N32.2
vesicourethrorectal N32.1
vesicouterine N82.1
congenital Q51.7
vesicovaginal N82.Ø
vulvorectal N82.4
congenital Q52.79

Fit R56.9
epileptic — *see* Epilepsy
fainting R55
hysterical F44.5
newborn P9Ø

Fitting (and adjustment) (of)
artificial
arm — *see* Admission, adjustment, artificial, arm
breast Z44.3 ☑
eye Z44.2 ☑
leg — *see* Admission, adjustment, artificial, leg
automatic implantable cardiac defibrillator (with synchronous cardiac pacemaker) Z45.Ø2
brain neuropacemaker Z46.2
implanted Z45.42
cardiac defibrillator — *see* Fitting (and adjustment) (of), automatic implantable cardiac defibrillator
catheter, non-vascular Z46.82
colostomy belt Z46.89
contact lenses Z46.Ø
cystostomy device Z46.6
defibrillator, cardiac — *see* Fitting (and adjustment) (of), automatic implantable cardiac defibrillator
dentures Z46.3
device NOS Z46.9
abdominal Z46.89
gastrointestinal NEC Z46.59
implanted NEC Z45.89
nervous system Z46.2
implanted — *see* Admission, adjustment, device, implanted, nervous system
orthodontic Z46.4
orthoptic Z46.Ø
orthotic Z46.89
prosthetic (external) Z44.9
breast Z44.3 ☑
dental Z46.3
eye Z44.2 ☑
specified NEC Z44.8
specified NEC Z46.89
substitution
auditory Z46.2
implanted — *see* Admission, adjustment, device, implanted, hearing device
nervous system Z46.2
implanted — *see* Admission, adjustment, device, implanted, nervous system
visual Z46.2
implanted Z45.31
urinary Z46.6
gastric lap band Z46.51
gastrointestinal appliance NEC Z46.59

Fitting — *continued*
glasses (reading) Z46.Ø
hearing aid Z46.1
ileostomy device Z46.89
insulin pump Z46.81
intestinal appliance NEC Z46.89
myringotomy device (stent) (tube) Z45.82
neuropacemaker Z46.2
implanted Z45.42
non-vascular catheter Z46.82
orthodontic device Z46.4
orthopedic device (brace) (cast) (corset) (shoes) Z46.89
pacemaker (cardiac) Z45.Ø18
nervous system (brain) (peripheral nerve) (spinal cord) Z46.2
implanted Z45.42
pulse generator Z45.Ø1Ø
portacath (port-a-cath) Z45.2
prosthesis (external) Z44.9
arm — *see* Admission, adjustment, artificial, arm
breast Z44.3 ☑
dental Z46.3
eye Z44.2 ☑
leg — *see* Admission, adjustment, artificial, leg
specified NEC Z44.8
spectacles Z46.Ø
wheelchair Z46.89

Fitzhugh-Curtis syndrome
due to
Chlamydia trachomatis A74.81
Neisseria gonorrhorea (gonococcal peritonitis) A54.85

Fitz's syndrome (acute hemorrhagic pancreatitis) K85.8

Fixation
joint — *see* Ankylosis
larynx J38.7
stapes — *see* Ankylosis, ear ossicles
deafness — *see* Deafness, conductive
uterus (acquired) — *see* Malposition, uterus
vocal cord J38.3

Flabby ridge KØ6.8

Flaccid (*see also* condition)
palate, congenital Q38.5

Flail
chest S22.5 ☑
newborn (birth injury) P13.8
joint (paralytic) M25.2Ø
ankle M25.27- ☑
elbow M25.22- ☑
foot joint M25.27- ☑
hand joint M25.24- ☑
hip M25.25- ☑
knee M25.26- ☑
shoulder M25.21- ☑
specified joint NEC M25.28
wrist M25.23- ☑

Flajani's disease — *see* Hyperthyroidism, with, goiter (diffuse)

Flap, liver K71.3

Flashbacks (residual to hallucinogen use) F16.283

Flat
chamber (eye) — *see* Disorder, globe, hypotony, flat anterior chamber
chest, congenital Q67.8
foot (acquired) (fixed type) (painful) (postural) (*see also* Deformity, limb, flat foot)
congenital (rigid) (spastic (everted)) Q66.5- ☑
rachitic sequelae (late effect) E64.3
organ or site, congenital NEC — *see* Anomaly, by site
pelvis M95.5
with disproportion (fetopelvic) O33.Ø
causing obstructed labor O65.Ø
congenital Q74.2

Flatau-Schilder disease G37.Ø

Flatback syndrome M4Ø.3Ø
lumbar region M4Ø.36
lumbosacral region M4Ø.37
thoracolumbar region M4Ø.35

Flattening
head, femur M89.8X5
hip — *see* Coxa, plana
lip (congenital) Q18.8
nose (congenital) Q67.4
acquired M95.Ø

Flatulence R14.3
psychogenic F45.8

- **Flatus** R14.3
  - vaginalis N89.8
- **Flax-dresser's disease** J66.1
- **Flea bite** — *see* Injury, bite, by site, superficial, insect
- **Flecks, glaucomatous** (subcapsular) — *see* Cataract, complicated
- **Fleischer** (-Kayser) **ring** (cornea) H18.Ø4- ☑
- **Fleshy mole** OØ2.Ø
- **Flexibilitas cerea** — *see* Catalepsy
- **Flexion**
  - amputation stump (surgical) T87.89
  - cervix — *see* Malposition, uterus
  - contracture, joint — *see* Contraction, joint
  - deformity, joint (*see also* Deformity, limb, flexion) M21.2Ø
    - hip, congenital Q65.89
  - uterus (*see also* Malposition, uterus)
    - lateral — *see* Lateroversion, uterus
- **Flexner-Boyd dysentery** AØ3.2
- **Flexner's dysentery** AØ3.1
- **Flexure** — *see* Flexion
- **Flint murmur** (aortic insufficiency) I35.1
- **Floater, vitreous** — *see* Opacity, vitreous
- **Floating**
  - cartilage (joint) (*see also* Loose, body, joint)
    - knee — *see* Derangement, knee, loose body
  - gallbladder, congenital Q44.1
  - kidney N28.89
    - congenital Q63.8
  - spleen D73.89
- **Flooding** N92.Ø
- **Floor** — *see* condition
- **Floppy**
  - baby syndrome (nonspecific) P94.2
  - iris syndrome (intraoperative) (IFIS) H21.81
  - nonrheumatic mitral valve syndrome I34.1
- **Flu** (*see also* Influenza)
  - avian (*see also* Influenza, due to, identified novel influenza A virus) JØ9.X2
  - bird (*see also* Influenza, due to, identified novel influenza A virus) JØ9.X2
  - intestinal NEC AØ8.4
  - swine (viruses that normally cause infections in pigs) (*see also* Influenza, due to, identified novel influenza A virus) JØ9.X2
- **Fluctuating blood pressure** I99.8
- **Fluid**
  - abdomen R18.8
  - chest J94.8
  - heart — *see* Failure, heart, congestive
  - joint — *see* Effusion, joint
  - loss (acute) E86.9
    - with
      - hypernatremia E87.Ø
      - hyponatremia E87.1
  - lung — *see* Edema, lung
  - overload E87.7Ø
    - specified NEC E87.79
  - peritoneal cavity R18.8
  - pleural cavity J94.8
  - retention R6Ø.9
- **Flukes NEC** (*see also* Infestation, fluke)
  - blood NEC — *see* Schistosomiasis
  - liver B66.3
- **Fluor** (vaginalis) N89.8
  - trichomonal or due to Trichomonas (vaginalis) A59.ØØ
- **Fluorosis**
  - dental KØØ.3
  - skeletal M85.1Ø
    - ankle M85.17- ☑
    - foot M85.17- ☑
    - forearm M85.13- ☑
    - hand M85.14- ☑
    - lower leg M85.16- ☑
    - multiple site M85.19
    - neck M85.18
    - rib M85.18
    - shoulder M85.11- ☑
    - skull M85.18
    - specified site NEC M85.18
    - thigh M85.15- ☑
    - toe M85.17- ☑
    - upper arm M85.12- ☑
    - vertebra M85.18
- **Flush syndrome** E34.Ø
- **Flushing** R23.2
  - menopausal N95.1
- **Flutter**
  - atrial or auricular I48.92
    - atypical I48.4
    - type I I48.3
    - type II I48.4
    - typical I48.3
  - heart I49.8
    - atrial or auricular I48.92
      - atypical I48.4
      - type I I48.3
      - type II I48.4
      - typical I48.3
    - ventricular I49.Ø2
  - ventricular I49.Ø2
- **FNHTR** (febrile nonhemolytic transfusion reaction) R5Ø.84
- **Fochier's abscess** — *code by* site under Abscess
- **Focus, Assmann's** — *see* Tuberculosis, pulmonary
- **Fogo selvagem** L1Ø.3
- **Foix-Alajouanine syndrome** G95.19
- **Fold, folds** (anomalous) (*see also* Anomaly, by site)
  - Descemet's membrane — *see* Change, corneal membrane, Descemet's, fold
  - epicanthic Q1Ø.3
  - heart Q24.8
- **Folie à deux** F24
- **Follicle**
  - cervix (nabothian) (ruptured) N88.8
  - graafian, ruptured, with hemorrhage N83.Ø
  - nabothian N88.8
- **Follicular** — *see* condition
- **Folliculitis** (superficial) L73.9
  - abscedens et suffodiens L66.3
  - cyst N83.Ø
  - decalvans L66.2
  - deep — *see* Furuncle, by site
  - gonococcal (acute) (chronic) A54.Ø1
  - keloid, keloidalis L73.Ø
  - pustular LØ1.Ø2
  - ulerythematosa reticulata L66.4
- **Folliculome lipidique**
  - specified site — *see* Neoplasm, benign, by site
  - unspecified site
    - female D27.9
    - male D29.2Ø
- **Følling's disease** E7Ø.Ø
- **Follow-up** — *see* Examination, follow-up
- **Fong's syndrome** (hereditary osteo-onychodysplasia) Q78.5
- **Food**
  - allergy L27.2
  - asphyxia (from aspiration or inhalation) — *see* Foreign body, by site
  - choked on — *see* Foreign body, by site
  - deprivation T73.Ø ☑
    - specified kind of food NEC E63.8
  - intoxication — *see* Poisoning, food
  - lack of T73.Ø ☑
  - poisoning — *see* Poisoning, food
  - rejection NEC — *see* Disorder, eating
  - strangulation or suffocation — *see* Foreign body, by site
  - toxemia — *see* Poisoning, food
- **Foot** — *see* condition
- **Foramen ovale** (nonclosure) (patent) (persistent) Q21.1
- **Forbes' glycogen storage disease** E74.Ø3
- **Fordyce-Fox disease** L75.2
- **Fordyce's disease** (mouth) Q38.6
- **Forearm** — *see* condition
- **Foreign body**
  - with
    - laceration — *see* Laceration, by site, with foreign body
    - puncture wound — *see* Puncture, by site, with foreign body
  - accidentally left following a procedure T81.5Ø9 ☑
    - aspiration T81.5Ø6 ☑
      - resulting in
        - adhesions T81.516 ☑
        - obstruction T81.526 ☑
        - perforation T81.536 ☑
        - specified complication NEC T81.596 ☑
    - cardiac catheterization T81.5Ø5 ☑
      - resulting in
        - acute reaction T81.6Ø ☑
          - aseptic peritonitis T81.61 ☑
          - specified NEC T81.69 ☑
        - adhesions T81.515 ☑

- **Foreign body** — *continued*
  - accidentally left following a procedure — *continued*
    - cardiac catheterization — *continued*
      - resulting in — *continued*
        - obstruction T81.525 ☑
        - perforation T81.535 ☑
        - specified complication NEC T81.595 ☑
    - causing
      - acute reaction T81.6Ø ☑
        - aseptic peritonitis T81.61 ☑
        - specified complication NEC T81.69 ☑
      - adhesions T81.519 ☑
      - aseptic peritonitis T81.61 ☑
      - obstruction T81.529 ☑
      - perforation T81.539 ☑
      - specified complication NEC T81.599 ☑
    - endoscopy T81.5Ø4 ☑
      - resulting in
        - adhesions T81.514 ☑
        - obstruction T81.524 ☑
        - perforation T81.534 ☑
        - specified complication NEC T81.594 ☑
    - immunization T81.5Ø3 ☑
      - resulting in
        - adhesions T81.513 ☑
        - obstruction T81.523 ☑
        - perforation T81.533 ☑
        - specified complication NEC T81.593 ☑
    - infusion T81.5Ø1 ☑
      - resulting in
        - adhesions T81.511 ☑
        - obstruction T81.521 ☑
        - perforation T81.531 ☑
        - specified complication NEC T81.591 ☑
    - injection T81.5Ø3 ☑
      - resulting in
        - adhesions T81.513 ☑
        - obstruction T81.523 ☑
        - perforation T81.533 ☑
        - specified complication NEC T81.593 ☑
    - kidney dialysis T81.5Ø2 ☑
      - resulting in
        - adhesions T81.512 ☑
        - obstruction T81.522 ☑
        - perforation T81.532 ☑
        - specified complication NEC T81.592 ☑
    - packing removal T81.5Ø7 ☑
      - resulting in
        - acute reaction T81.6Ø ☑
          - aseptic peritonitis T81.61 ☑
          - specified NEC T81.69 ☑
        - adhesions T81.517 ☑
        - obstruction T81.527 ☑
        - perforation T81.537 ☑
        - specified complication NEC T81.597 ☑
    - puncture T81.5Ø6 ☑
      - resulting in
        - adhesions T81.516 ☑
        - obstruction T81.526 ☑
        - perforation T81.536 ☑
        - specified complication NEC T81.596 ☑
    - specified procedure NEC T81.5Ø8 ☑
      - resulting in
        - acute reaction T81.6Ø ☑
          - aseptic peritonitis T81.61 ☑
          - specified NEC T81.69 ☑
        - adhesions T81.518 ☑
        - obstruction T81.528 ☑
        - perforation T81.538 ☑
        - specified complication NEC T81.598 ☑
    - surgical operation T81.5ØØ ☑
      - resulting in
        - acute reaction T81.6Ø ☑
          - aseptic peritonitis T81.61 ☑
          - specified NEC T81.69 ☑
        - adhesions T81.51Ø ☑
        - obstruction T81.52Ø ☑
        - perforation T81.53Ø ☑
        - specified complication NEC T81.59Ø ☑
    - transfusion T81.5Ø1 ☑
      - resulting in
        - adhesions T81.511 ☑
        - obstruction T81.521 ☑
        - perforation T81.531 ☑
        - specified complication NEC T81.591 ☑

Foreign body — *continued*
- alimentary tract T18.9 ☑
  - anus T18.5 ☑
  - colon T18.4 ☑
  - esophagus — *see* Foreign body, esophagus
  - mouth T18.Ø ☑
  - multiple sites T18.8 ☑
  - rectosigmoid (junction) T18.5 ☑
  - rectum T18.5 ☑
  - small intestine T18.3 ☑
  - specified site NEC T18.8 ☑
  - stomach T18.2 ☑
- anterior chamber (eye) SØ5.5- ☑
- auditory canal — *see* Foreign body, entering through orifice, ear
- bronchus T17.5Ø8 ☑
  - causing
    - asphyxiation T17.5ØØ ☑
      - food (bone) (seed) T17.52Ø ☑
      - gastric contents (vomitus) T17.51Ø ☑
      - specified type NEC T17.59Ø ☑
    - injury NEC T17.5Ø8 ☑
      - food (bone) (seed) T17.528 ☑
      - gastric contents (vomitus) T17.518 ☑
      - specified type NEC T17.598 ☑
- canthus — *see* Foreign body, conjunctival sac
- ciliary body (eye) SØ5.5- ☑
- conjunctival sac T15.1- ☑
- cornea T15.Ø- ☑
- entering through orifice
  - accessory sinus T17.Ø ☑
  - alimentary canal T18.9 ☑
    - multiple parts T18.8 ☑
    - specified part NEC T18.8 ☑
  - alveolar process T18.Ø ☑
  - antrum (Highmore's) T17.Ø ☑
  - anus T18.5 ☑
  - appendix T18.4 ☑
  - auditory canal — *see* Foreign body, entering through orifice, ear
  - auricle — *see* Foreign body, entering through orifice, ear
  - bladder T19.1 ☑
  - bronchioles — *see* Foreign body, respiratory tract, specified site NEC
  - bronchus (main) — *see* Foreign body, bronchus
  - buccal cavity T18.Ø ☑
  - canthus (inner) — *see* Foreign body, conjunctival sac
  - cecum T18.4 ☑
  - cervix (canal) (uteri) T19.3 ☑
  - colon T18.4 ☑
  - conjunctival sac — *see* Foreign body, conjunctival sac
  - cornea — *see* Foreign body, cornea
  - digestive organ or tract NOS T18.9 ☑
    - multiple parts T18.8 ☑
    - specified part NEC T18.8 ☑
  - duodenum T18.3 ☑
  - ear (external) T16.- ☑
  - esophagus — *see* Foreign body, esophagus
  - eye (external) NOS T15.9- ☑
    - conjunctival sac — *see* Foreign body, conjunctival sac
    - cornea — *see* Foreign body, cornea
    - specified part NEC T15.8- ☑
  - eyeball (*see also* Foreign body, entering through orifice, eye, specified part NEC)
    - with penetrating wound — *see* Puncture, eyeball
  - eyelid (*see also* Foreign body, conjunctival sac)
    - with
      - laceration — *see* Laceration, eyelid, with foreign body
      - puncture — *see* Puncture, eyelid, with foreign body
      - superficial injury — *see* Foreign body, superficial, eyelid
  - gastrointestinal tract T18.9 ☑
    - multiple parts T18.8 ☑
    - specified part NEC T18.8 ☑
  - genitourinary tract T19.9 ☑
    - multiple parts T19.8 ☑
    - specified part NEC T19.8 ☑
  - globe — *see* Foreign body, entering through orifice, eyeball

Foreign body — *continued*
- entering through orifice — *continued*
  - gum T18.Ø ☑
  - Highmore's antrum T17.Ø ☑
  - hypopharynx — *see* Foreign body, pharynx
  - ileum T18.3 ☑
  - intestine (small) T18.3 ☑
    - large T18.4 ☑
  - lacrimal apparatus (punctum) — *see* Foreign body, entering through orifice, eye, specified part NEC
  - large intestine T18.4 ☑
  - larynx — *see* Foreign body, larynx
  - lung — *see* Foreign body, respiratory tract, specified site NEC
  - maxillary sinus T17.Ø ☑
  - mouth T18.Ø ☑
  - nasal sinus T17.Ø ☑
  - nasopharynx — *see* Foreign body, pharynx
  - nose (passage) T17.1 ☑
  - nostril T17.1 ☑
  - oral cavity T18.Ø ☑
  - palate T18.Ø ☑
  - penis T19.4 ☑
  - pharynx — *see* Foreign body, pharynx
  - piriform sinus — *see* Foreign body, pharynx
  - rectosigmoid (junction) T18.5 ☑
  - rectum T18.5 ☑
  - respiratory tract — *see* Foreign body, respiratory tract
  - sinus (accessory) (frontal) (maxillary) (nasal) T17.Ø ☑
    - piriform — *see* Foreign body, pharynx
  - small intestine T18.3 ☑
  - stomach T18.2 ☑
  - suffocation by — *see* Foreign body, by site
  - tear ducts or glands — *see* Foreign body, entering through orifice, eye, specified part NEC
  - throat — *see* Foreign body, pharynx
  - tongue T18.Ø ☑
  - tonsil, tonsillar (fossa) — *see* Foreign body, pharynx
  - trachea — *see* Foreign body, trachea
  - ureter T19.8 ☑
  - urethra T19.Ø ☑
  - uterus (any part) T19.3 ☑
  - vagina T19.2 ☑
  - vulva T19.2 ☑
- esophagus T18.1Ø8 ☑
  - causing
    - injury NEC T18.1Ø8 ☑
      - food (bone) (seed) T18.128 ☑
      - gastric contents (vomitus) T18.118 ☑
      - specified type NEC T18.198 ☑
    - tracheal compression T18.1ØØ ☑
      - food (bone) (seed) T18.12Ø ☑
      - gastric contents (vomitus) T18.11Ø ☑
      - specified type NEC T18.19Ø ☑
- felling of, in throat RØ9.89
- fragment — *see* Retained, foreign body fragments (type of)
- genitourinary tract T19.9 ☑
  - bladder T19.1 ☑
  - multiple parts T19.8 ☑
  - penis T19.4 ☑
  - specified site NEC T19.8 ☑
  - urethra T19.Ø ☑
  - uterus T19.3 ☑
    - IUD Z97.5
  - vagina T19.2 ☑
    - contraceptive device Z97.5
  - vulva T19.2 ☑
- granuloma (old) (soft tissue) (*see also* Granuloma, foreign body)
  - skin L92.3
- in
  - laceration — *see* Laceration, by site, with foreign body
  - puncture wound — *see* Puncture, by site, with foreign body
  - soft tissue (residual) M79.5
- inadvertently left in operation wound — *see* Foreign body, accidentally left during a procedure
- ingestion, ingested NOS T18.9 ☑
- inhalation or inspiration — *see* Foreign body, by site
- internal organ, not entering through a natural orifice — code as specific injury with foreign body

Foreign body — *continued*
- intraocular SØ5.5- ☑
  - old, retained (nonmagnetic) H44.7Ø- ☑
    - anterior chamber H44.71- ☑
    - ciliary body H44.72- ☑
    - iris H44.72- ☑
    - lens H44.73- ☑
    - magnetic H44.6Ø- ☑
      - anterior chamber H44.61- ☑
      - ciliary body H44.62- ☑
      - iris H44.62- ☑
      - lens H44.63- ☑
      - posterior wall H44.64- ☑
      - specified site NEC H44.69- ☑
      - vitreous body H44.65- ☑
    - posterior wall H44.74- ☑
    - specified site NEC H44.79- ☑
    - vitreous body H44.75- ☑
- iris — *see* Foreign body, intraocular
- lacrimal punctum — *see* Foreign body, entering through orifice, eye, specified part NEC
- larynx T17.3Ø8 ☑
  - causing
    - asphyxiation T17.3ØØ ☑
      - food (bone) (seed) T17.32Ø ☑
      - gastric contents (vomitus) T17.31Ø ☑
      - specified type NEC T17.39Ø ☑
    - injury NEC T17.3Ø8 ☑
      - food (bone) (seed) T17.328 ☑
      - gastric contents (vomitus) T17.318 ☑
      - specified type NEC T17.398 ☑
- lens — *see* Foreign body, intraocular
- ocular muscle SØ5.4- ☑
  - old, retained — *see* Foreign body, orbit, old
- old or residual
  - soft tissue (residual) M79.5
- operation wound, left accidentally — *see* Foreign body, accidentally left during a procedure
- orbit SØ5.4- ☑
  - old, retained HØ5.5- ☑
- pharynx T17.2Ø8 ☑
  - causing
    - asphyxiation T17.2ØØ ☑
      - food (bone) (seed) T17.22Ø ☑
      - gastric contents (vomitus) T17.21Ø ☑
      - specified type NEC T17.29Ø ☑
    - injury NEC T17.2Ø8 ☑
      - food (bone) (seed) T17.228 ☑
      - gastric contents (vomitus) T17.218 ☑
      - specified type NEC T17.298 ☑
- respiratory tract T17.9Ø8 ☑
  - bronchioles — *see* Foreign body, respiratory tract, specified site NEC
  - bronchus — *see* Foreign body, bronchus
  - causing
    - asphyxiation T17.9ØØ ☑
      - food (bone) (seed) T17.92Ø ☑
      - gastric contents (vomitus) T17.91Ø ☑
      - specified type NEC T17.99Ø ☑
    - injury NEC T17.9Ø8 ☑
      - food (bone) (seed) T17.928 ☑
      - gastric contents (vomitus) T17.918 ☑
      - specified type NEC T17.998 ☑
  - larynx — *see* Foreign body, larynx
  - lung — *see* Foreign body, respiratory tract, specified site NEC
  - multiple parts — *see* Foreign body, respiratory tract, specified site NEC
  - nasal sinus T17.Ø ☑
  - nasopharynx — *see* Foreign body, pharynx
  - nose T17.1 ☑
  - nostril T17.1 ☑
  - pharynx — *see* Foreign body, pharynx
  - specified site NEC T17.8Ø8 ☑
    - causing
      - asphyxiation T17.8ØØ ☑
        - food (bone) (seed) T17.82Ø ☑
        - gastric contents (vomitus) T17.81Ø ☑
        - specified type NEC T17.89Ø ☑
      - injury NEC T17.8Ø8 ☑
        - food (bone) (seed) T17.828 ☑
        - gastric contents (vomitus) T17.818 ☑
        - specified type NEC T17.898 ☑
  - throat — *see* Foreign body, pharynx
  - trachea — *see* Foreign body, trachea
- retained (old) (nonmagnetic) (in)

- **Foreign body** — *continued*
  - retained — *continued*
    - anterior chamber (eye) — *see* Foreign body, intraocular, old, retained, anterior chamber
      - magnetic — *see* Foreign body, intraocular, old, retained, magnetic, anterior chamber
    - ciliary body — *see* Foreign body, intraocular, old, retained, ciliary body
      - magnetic — *see* Foreign body, intraocular, old, retained, magnetic, ciliary body
    - eyelid HØ2.819
      - left HØ2.816
        - lower HØ2.815
        - upper HØ2.814
      - right HØ2.813
        - lower HØ2.812
        - upper HØ2.811
    - fragments — *see* Retained, foreign body fragments (type of)
    - globe — *see* Foreign body, intraocular, old, retained
      - magnetic — *see* Foreign body, intraocular, old, retained, magnetic
    - intraocular — *see* Foreign body, intraocular, old, retained
      - magnetic — *see* Foreign body, intraocular, old, retained, magnetic
    - iris — *see* Foreign body, intraocular, old, retained, iris
      - magnetic — *see* Foreign body, intraocular, old, retained, magnetic, iris
    - lens — *see* Foreign body, intraocular, old, retained, lens
      - magnetic — *see* Foreign body, intraocular, old, retained, magnetic, lens
    - muscle — *see* Foreign body, retained, soft tissue
    - orbit — *see* Foreign body, orbit, old
    - posterior wall of globe — *see* Foreign body, intraocular, old, retained, posterior wall
      - magnetic — *see* Foreign body, intraocular, old, retained, magnetic, posterior wall
    - retrobulbar — *see* Foreign body, orbit, old, retrobulbar
    - soft tissue M79.5
    - vitreous — *see* Foreign body, intraocular, old, retained, vitreous body
      - magnetic — *see* Foreign body, intraocular, old, retained, magnetic, vitreous body
  - retina SØ5.5- ☑
  - superficial, without open wound
    - abdomen, abdominal (wall) S3Ø.851 ☑
    - alveolar process SØØ.552 ☑
    - ankle S9Ø.55- ☑
    - antecubital space — *see* Foreign body, superficial, forearm
    - anus S3Ø.857 ☑
    - arm (upper) S4Ø.85- ☑
    - auditory canal — *see* Foreign body, superficial, ear
    - auricle — *see* Foreign body, superficial, ear
    - axilla — *see* Foreign body, superficial, arm
    - back, lower S3Ø.85Ø ☑
    - breast S2Ø.15- ☑
    - brow SØØ.85 ☑
    - buttock S3Ø.85Ø ☑
    - calf — *see* Foreign body, superficial, leg
    - canthus — *see* Foreign body, superficial, eyelid
    - cheek SØØ.85 ☑
      - internal SØØ.552 ☑
    - chest wall — *see* Foreign body, superficial, thorax
    - chin SØØ.85 ☑
    - clitoris S3Ø.854 ☑
    - costal region — *see* Foreign body, superficial, thorax
    - digit(s)
      - foot — *see* Foreign body, superficial, toe
      - hand — *see* Foreign body, superficial, finger
    - ear SØØ.45- ☑
    - elbow S5Ø.35- ☑
    - epididymis S3Ø.853 ☑
    - epigastric region S3Ø.851 ☑
    - epiglottis S1Ø.15 ☑
    - esophagus, cervical S1Ø.15 ☑
    - eyebrow — *see* Foreign body, superficial, eyelid
    - eyelid SØØ.25- ☑
    - face SØØ.85 ☑
    - finger(s) S6Ø.459 ☑
      - index S6Ø.45- ☑

- **Foreign body** — *continued*
  - superficial, without open wound — *continued*
    - finger(s) — *continued*
      - little S6Ø.45- ☑
      - middle S6Ø.45- ☑
      - ring S6Ø.45- ☑
    - flank S3Ø.851 ☑
    - foot (except toe(s) alone) S9Ø.85- ☑
      - toe — *see* Foreign body, superficial, toe
    - forearm S5Ø.85- ☑
      - elbow only — *see* Foreign body, superficial, elbow
    - forehead SØØ.85 ☑
    - genital organs, external
      - female S3Ø.856 ☑
      - male S3Ø.855 ☑
    - groin S3Ø.851 ☑
    - gum SØØ.552 ☑
    - hand S6Ø.55- ☑
    - head SØØ.95 ☑
      - ear — *see* Foreign body, superficial, ear
      - eyelid — *see* Foreign body, superficial, eyelid
      - lip SØØ.551 ☑
      - nose SØØ.35 ☑
      - oral cavity SØØ.552 ☑
      - scalp SØØ.Ø5 ☑
      - specified site NEC SØØ.85 ☑
    - heel — *see* Foreign body, superficial, foot
    - hip S7Ø.25- ☑
    - inguinal region S3Ø.851 ☑
    - interscapular region S2Ø.459 ☑
    - jaw SØØ.85 ☑
    - knee S8Ø.25- ☑
    - labium (majus) (minus) S3Ø.854 ☑
    - larynx S1Ø.15 ☑
    - leg (lower) S8Ø.85- ☑
      - knee — *see* Foreign body, superficial, knee
      - upper — *see* Foreign body, superficial, thigh
    - lip SØØ.551 ☑
    - lower back S3Ø.85Ø ☑
    - lumbar region S3Ø.85Ø ☑
    - malar region SØØ.85 ☑
    - mammary — *see* Foreign body, superficial, breast
    - mastoid region SØØ.85 ☑
    - mouth SØØ.552 ☑
    - nail
      - finger — *see* Foreign body, superficial, finger
      - toe — *see* Foreign body, superficial, toe
    - nape S1Ø.85 ☑
    - nasal SØØ.35 ☑
    - neck S1Ø.95 ☑
      - specified site NEC S1Ø.85 ☑
      - throat S1Ø.15 ☑
    - nose SØØ.35 ☑
    - occipital region SØØ.Ø5 ☑
    - oral cavity SØØ.552 ☑
    - orbital region — *see* Foreign body, superficial, eyelid
    - palate SØØ.552 ☑
    - palm — *see* Foreign body, superficial, hand
    - parietal region SØØ.Ø5 ☑
    - pelvis S3Ø.85Ø ☑
    - penis S3Ø.852 ☑
    - perineum
      - female S3Ø.854 ☑
      - male S3Ø.85Ø ☑
    - periocular area — *see* Foreign body, superficial, eyelid
    - phalanges
      - finger — *see* Foreign body, superficial, finger
      - toe — *see* Foreign body, superficial, toe
    - pharynx S1Ø.15 ☑
    - pinna — *see* Foreign body, superficial, ear
    - popliteal space — *see* Foreign body, superficial, knee
    - prepuce S3Ø.852 ☑
    - pubic region S3Ø.85Ø ☑
    - pudendum
      - female S3Ø.856 ☑
      - male S3Ø.855 ☑
    - sacral region S3Ø.85Ø ☑
    - scalp SØØ.Ø5 ☑
    - scapular region — *see* Foreign body, superficial, shoulder
    - scrotum S3Ø.853 ☑
    - shin — *see* Foreign body, superficial, leg

- **Foreign body** — *continued*
  - superficial, without open wound — *continued*
    - shoulder S4Ø.25- ☑
    - sternal region S2Ø.359 ☑
    - submaxillary region SØØ.85 ☑
    - submental region SØØ.85 ☑
    - subungual
      - finger(s) — *see* Foreign body, superficial, finger
      - toe(s) — *see* Foreign body, superficial, toe
    - supraclavicular fossa S1Ø.85 ☑
    - supraorbital SØØ.85 ☑
    - temple SØØ.85 ☑
    - temporal region SØØ.85 ☑
    - testis S3Ø.853 ☑
    - thigh S7Ø.35- ☑
    - thorax, thoracic (wall) S2Ø.95 ☑
      - back S2Ø.45- ☑
      - front S2Ø.35- ☑
    - throat S1Ø.15 ☑
    - thumb S6Ø.35- ☑
    - toe(s) (lesser) S9Ø.456 ☑
      - great S9Ø.45- ☑
    - tongue SØØ.552 ☑
    - trachea S1Ø.15 ☑
    - tunica vaginalis S3Ø.853 ☑
    - tympanum, tympanic membrane — *see* Foreign body, superficial, ear
    - uvula SØØ.552 ☑
    - vagina S3Ø.854 ☑
    - vocal cords S1Ø.15 ☑
    - vulva S3Ø.854 ☑
    - wrist S6Ø.85- ☑
  - swallowed T18.9 ☑
  - trachea T17.4Ø8 ☑
    - causing
      - asphyxiation T17.4ØØ ☑
        - food (bone) (seed) T17.42Ø ☑
        - gastric contents (vomitus) T17.41Ø ☑
        - specified type NEC T17.49Ø ☑
      - injury NEC T17.4Ø8 ☑
        - food (bone) (seed) T17.428 ☑
        - gastric contents (vomitus) T17.418 ☑
        - specified type NEC T17.498 ☑
  - type of fragment — *see* Retained, foreign body fragments (type of)
  - vitreous (humor) SØ5.5- ☑
- **Forestier's disease** (rhizomelic pseudopolyarthritis) M35.3
  - meaning ankylosing hyperostosis — *see* Hyperostosis, ankylosing
- **Formation**
  - hyalin in cornea — *see* Degeneration, cornea
  - sequestrum in bone (due to infection) — *see* Osteomyelitis, chronic
  - valve
    - colon, congenital Q43.8
    - ureter (congenital) Q62.39
- **Formication** R2Ø.2
- **Fort Bragg fever** A27.89
- **Fossa** (*see also* condition)
  - pyriform — *see* condition
- **Foster-Kennedy syndrome** H47.14- ☑
- **Fothergill's**
  - disease (trigeminal neuralgia) (*see also* Neuralgia, trigeminal)
  - scarlatina anginosa A38.9
- **Foul breath** R19.6
- **Foundling** Z76.1
- **Fournier disease or gangrene** N49.3
  - female N76.89
- **Fourth**
  - cranial nerve — *see* condition
  - molar KØØ.1
- **Foville's** (peduncular) **disease or syndrome** G46.3
- **Fox** (-Fordyce) disease (apocrine miliaria) L75.2
- **Fracture, burst** — *see* Fracture, traumatic, by site
- **Fracture, chronic** — *see* Fracture, pathological
- **Fracture, insufficiency** — *see* Fracture, pathologic, by site
- **Fracture, pathological** (pathologic) (*see also* Fracture, traumatic) M84.4Ø ☑
  - ankle M84.47- ☑
  - carpus M84.44- ☑
  - clavicle M84.41- ☑
  - dental implant M27.63
  - dental restorative material KØ8.539

- **Fracture, pathological** — *continued*
  - dental restorative material — *continued*
    - with loss of material KØ8.531
    - without loss of material KØ8.53Ø
  - due to
    - neoplastic disease NEC (*see also* Neoplasm) M84.5Ø
      - ankle M84.57- ☑
      - carpus M84.54- ☑
      - clavicle M84.51- ☑
      - femur M84.55- ☑
      - fibula M84.56- ☑
      - finger M84.54- ☑
      - hip M84.559 ☑
      - humerus M84.52- ☑
      - ilium M84.55Ø ☑
      - ischium M84.55Ø ☑
      - metacarpus M84.54- ☑
      - metatarsus M84.57- ☑
      - neck M84.58 ☑
      - pelvis M84.55Ø ☑
      - radius M84.53- ☑
      - rib M84.58 ☑
      - scapula M84.51- ☑
      - skull M84.58 ☑
      - specified site NEC M84.58 ☑
      - tarsus M84.57- ☑
      - tibia M84.56- ☑
      - toe M84.57- ☑
      - ulna M84.53- ☑
      - vertebra M84.58 ☑
    - osteoporosis M8Ø.8Ø ☑
      - disuse — *see* Osteoporosis, specified type NEC, with pathological fracture
      - drug-induced — *see* Osteoporosis, drug induced, with pathological fracture
      - idiopathic — *see* Osteoporosis, specified type NEC, with pathological fracture
      - postmenopausal — *see* Osteoporosis, postmenopausal, with pathological fracture
      - postoophorectomy — *see* Osteoporosis, postoophorectomy, with pathological fracture
      - postsurgical malabsorption — *see* Osteoporosis, specified type NEC, with pathological fracture
      - specified cause NEC — *see* Osteoporosis, specified type NEC, with pathological fracture
    - specified disease NEC M84.6Ø ☑
      - ankle M84.67- ☑
      - carpus M84.64- ☑
      - clavicle M84.61- ☑
      - femur M84.65- ☑
      - fibula M84.66- ☑
      - finger M84.64- ☑
      - hip M84.65- ☑
      - humerus M84.62- ☑
      - ilium M84.65Ø ☑
      - ischium M84.65Ø ☑
      - metacarpus M84.64- ☑
      - metatarsus M84.67- ☑
      - neck M84.68 ☑
      - radius M84.63- ☑
      - rib M84.68 ☑
      - scapula M84.61- ☑
      - skull M84.68 ☑
      - tarsus M84.67- ☑
      - tibia M84.66- ☑
      - toe M84.67- ☑
      - ulna M84.63- ☑
      - vertebra M84.68 ☑
  - femur M84.45- ☑
  - fibula M84.46- ☑
  - finger M84.44- ☑
  - hip M84.459 ☑
  - humerus M84.42- ☑
  - ilium M84.454 ☑
  - ischium M84.454 ☑
  - joint prosthesis — *see* Complications, joint prosthesis, mechanical, breakdown, by site
    - periprosthetic — *see* Complications, joint prosthesis, mechanical, periprosthesis, fracture, by site
  - metacarpus M84.44- ☑
  - metatarsus M84.47- ☑
  - neck M84.48 ☑

- **Fracture, pathological** — *continued*
  - pelvis M84.454 ☑
  - radius M84.43- ☑
  - restorative material (dental) KØ8.539
    - with loss of material KØ8.531
    - without loss of material KØ8.53Ø
  - rib M84.48 ☑
  - scapula M84.41- ☑
  - skull M84.48 ☑
  - tarsus M84.47- ☑
  - tibia M84.46- ☑
  - toe M84.47- ☑
  - ulna M84.43- ☑
  - vertebra M84.48 ☑
- **Fracture, traumatic** (abduction) (adduction) (separation) (*see also* Fracture, pathological) T14.8
  - acetabulum S32.4Ø- ☑
    - column
      - anterior (displaced) (iliopubic) S32.43- ☑
        - nondisplaced S32.436 ☑
      - posterior (displaced) (ilioischial) S32.443 ☑
        - nondisplaced S32.44- ☑
    - dome (displaced) S32.48- ☑
      - nondisplaced S32.48 ☑
    - specified NEC S32.49- ☑
    - transverse (displaced) S32.45- ☑
      - with associated posterior wall fracture (displaced) S32.46- ☑
        - nondisplaced S32.46- ☑
      - nondisplaced S32.45- ☑
    - wall
      - anterior (displaced) S32.41- ☑
        - nondisplaced S32.41- ☑
      - medial (displaced) S32.47- ☑
        - nondisplaced S32.47- ☑
      - posterior (displaced) S32.42- ☑
        - with associated transverse fracture (displaced) S32.46- ☑
          - nondisplaced S32.46- ☑
        - nondisplaced S32.42- ☑
  - acromion — *see* Fracture, scapula, acromial process
  - ankle S82.899 ☑
    - bimalleolar (displaced) S82.84- ☑
      - nondisplaced S82.84- ☑
    - lateral malleolus only (displaced) S82.6- ☑
      - nondisplaced S82.6- ☑
    - medial malleolus (displaced) S82.5- ☑
      - associated with Maisonneuve's fracture — *see* Fracture, Maisonneuve's
      - nondisplaced S82.5- ☑
    - talus — *see* Fracture, tarsal, talus
    - trimalleolar (displaced) S82.85- ☑
      - nondisplaced S82.85- ☑
  - arm (upper) (*see also* Fracture, humerus, shaft)
    - humerus — *see* Fracture, humerus
    - radius — *see* Fracture, radius
    - ulna — *see* Fracture, ulna
  - astragalus — *see* Fracture, tarsal, talus
  - atlas — *see* Fracture, neck, cervical vertebra, first
  - axis — *see* Fracture, neck, cervical vertebra, second
  - back — *see* Fracture, vertebra
  - Barton's — *see* Barton's fracture
  - base of skull — *see* Fracture, skull, base
  - basicervical (basal) (femoral) S72.Ø ☑
  - Bennett's — *see* Bennett's fracture
  - bimalleolar — *see* Fracture, ankle, bimalleolar
  - blow-out SØ2.3 ☑
  - bone NEC T14.8
    - birth injury P13.9
    - following insertion of orthopedic implant, joint prosthesis or bone plate — *see* Fracture, following insertion of orthopedic implant, joint prosthesis or bone plate
    - in (due to) neoplastic disease NEC — *see* Fracture, pathological, due to, neoplastic disease
    - pathological (cause unknown) — *see* Fracture, pathological
  - breast bone — *see* Fracture, sternum
  - bucket handle (semilunar cartilage) — *see* Tear, meniscus
  - burst — *see* Fracture, traumatic, by site
  - calcaneus — *see* Fracture, tarsal, calcaneus
  - carpal bone(s) S62.1Ø- ☑
    - capitate (displaced) S62.13- ☑
      - nondisplaced S62.13- ☑
    - cuneiform — *see* Fracture, carpal bone, triquetrum

- **Fracture, traumatic** — *continued*
  - carpal bone(s) — *continued*
    - hamate (body) (displaced) S62.143 ☑
      - hook process (displaced) S62.15- ☑
        - nondisplaced S62.15- ☑
      - nondisplaced S62.14- ☑
    - larger multangular — *see* Fracture, carpal bones, trapezium
    - lunate (displaced) S62.12- ☑
      - nondisplaced S62.12- ☑
    - navicular S62.ØØ- ☑
      - distal pole (displaced) S62.Ø1- ☑
        - nondisplaced S62.Ø1- ☑
      - middle third (displaced) S62.Ø2- ☑
        - nondisplaced S62.Ø2- ☑
      - proximal third (displaced) S62.Ø3- ☑
        - nondisplaced S62.Ø3- ☑
      - volar tuberosity — *see* Fracture, carpal bones, navicular, distal pole
    - os magnum — *see* Fracture, carpal bones, capitate
    - pisiform (displaced) S62.16- ☑
      - nondisplaced S62.16- ☑
    - semilunar — *see* Fracture, carpal bones, lunate
    - smaller multangular — *see* Fracture, carpal bones, trapezoid
    - trapezium (displaced) S62.17- ☑
      - nondisplaced S62.17- ☑
    - trapezoid (displaced) S62.18- ☑
      - nondisplaced S62.18- ☑
    - triquetrum (displaced) S62.11- ☑
      - nondisplaced S62.11- ☑
    - unciform — *see* Fracture, carpal bones, hamate
  - cervical — *see* Fracture, vertebra, cervical
  - clavicle S42.ØØ- ☑
    - acromial end (displaced) S42.Ø3- ☑
      - nondisplaced S42.Ø3- ☑
    - birth injury P13.4
    - lateral end — *see* Fracture, clavicle, acromial end
    - shaft (displaced) S42.Ø2- ☑
      - nondisplaced S42.Ø2- ☑
    - sternal end (anterior) (displaced) S42.Ø1- ☑
      - nondisplaced S42.Ø1- ☑
      - posterior S42.Ø1- ☑
  - coccyx S32.2 ☑
  - collapsed — *see* Collapse, vertebra
  - collar bone — *see* Fracture, clavicle
  - Colles' — *see* Colles' fracture
  - compression, not due to trauma — *see* Collapse, vertebra
  - coronoid process — *see* Fracture, ulna, upper end, coronoid process
  - corpus cavernosum penis S39.84Ø ☑
  - costochondral cartilage S23.41 ☑
  - costochondral, costosternal junction — *see* Fracture, rib
  - cranium — *see* Fracture, skull
  - cricoid cartilage S12.8 ☑
  - cuboid (ankle) — *see* Fracture, tarsal, cuboid
  - cuneiform
    - foot — *see* Fracture, tarsal, cuneiform
    - wrist — *see* Fracture, carpal, triquetrum
  - delayed union — *see* Delay, union, fracture
  - dental restorative material KØ8.539
    - with loss of material KØ8.531
    - without loss of material KØ8.53Ø
  - due to
    - birth injury — *see* Birth, injury, fracture
    - osteoporosis — *see* Osteoporosis, with fracture
  - Dupuytren's — *see* Fracture, ankle, lateral malleolus
  - elbow S42.4Ø- ☑
  - ethmoid (bone) (sinus) — *see* Fracture, skull, base
  - face bone SØ2.92 ☑
  - fatigue (*see also* Fracture, stress)
    - vertebra M48.4Ø ☑
      - cervical region M48.42 ☑
      - cervicothoracic region M48.43 ☑
      - lumbar region M48.46 ☑
      - lumbosacral region M48.47 ☑
      - occipito-atlanto-axial region M48.41 ☑
      - sacrococcygeal region M48.48 ☑
      - thoracic region M48.44 ☑
      - thoracolumbar region M48.45 ☑
  - femur, femoral S72.9- ☑
    - basicervical (basal) S72.Ø ☑
    - birth injury P13.2
    - capital epiphyseal S79.Ø1- ☑

Fracture, traumatic — *continued*
femur, femoral — *continued*
condyles, epicondyles — *see* Fracture, femur, lower end
distal end — *see* Fracture, femur, lower end
epiphysis
head — *see* Fracture, femur, upper end, epiphysis
lower — *see* Fracture, femur, lower end, epiphysis
upper — *see* Fracture, femur, upper end, epiphysis
following insertion of implant, prosthesis or plate M96.66- ☑
head — *see* Fracture, femur, upper end, head
intertrochanteric — *see* Fracture, femur, trochanteric
intratrochanteric — *see* Fracture, femur, trochanteric
lower end S72.4Ø- ☑
condyle (displaced) S72.41- ☑
lateral (displaced) S72.42- ☑
nondisplaced S72.42- ☑
medial (displaced) S72.43- ☑
nondisplaced S72.43- ☑
nondisplaced S72.41- ☑
epiphysis (displaced) S72.44- ☑
nondisplaced S72.44- ☑
physeal S79.1Ø- ☑
Salter-Harris
Type I S79.11- ☑
Type II S79.12- ☑
Type III S79.13- ☑
Type IV S79.14- ☑
specified NEC S79.19- ☑
specified NEC S72.49- ☑
supracondylar (displaced) S72.45- ☑
with intracondylar extension (displaced) S72.46- ☑
nondisplaced S72.46- ☑
nondisplaced S72.45- ☑
torus S72.47- ☑
neck — *see* Fracture, femur, upper end, neck
pertrochanteric — *see* Fracture, femur, trochanteric
shaft (lower third) (middle third) (upper third) S72.3Ø- ☑
comminuted (displaced) S72.35- ☑
nondisplaced S72.35- ☑
oblique (displaced) S72.33- ☑
nondisplaced S72.33- ☑
segmental (displaced) S72.36- ☑
nondisplaced S72.36- ☑
specified NEC S72.39- ☑
spiral (displaced) S72.34- ☑
nondisplaced S72.34- ☑
transverse (displaced) S72.32- ☑
nondisplaced S72.32- ☑
specified site NEC — *see* subcategory S72.8 ☑
subcapital (displaced) S72.Ø1- ☑
subtrochanteric (region) (section) (displaced) S72.2- ☑
nondisplaced S72.2- ☑
transcervical — *see* Fracture, femur, upper end, neck
transtrochanteric — *see* Fracture, femur, trochanteric
trochanteric S72.1Ø- ☑
apophyseal (displaced) S72.14- ☑
nondisplaced S72.14- ☑
greater trochanter (displaced) S72.11- ☑
nondisplaced S72.11- ☑
intertrochanteric (displaced) S72.13- ☑
nondisplaced S72.13- ☑
lesser trochanter (displaced) S72.12- ☑
nondisplaced S72.12- ☑
upper end S72.ØØ- ☑
apophyseal (displaced) S72.13- ☑
nondisplaced S72.13- ☑
cervicotrochanteric — *see* Fracture, femur, upper end, neck, base
epiphysis (displaced) S72.Ø2- ☑
nondisplaced S72.Ø2- ☑
head S72.Ø5- ☑
articular (displaced) S72.Ø6- ☑
nondisplaced S72.Ø6- ☑

Fracture, traumatic — *continued*
femur, femoral — *continued*
upper end — *continued*
head — *continued*
specified NEC S72.Ø9- ☑
intertrochanteric (displaced) S72.14- ☑
nondisplaced S72.14- ☑
intracapsular S72.Ø1- ☑
midcervical (displaced) S72.Ø3- ☑
nondisplaced S72.Ø3- ☑
neck S72.ØØ- ☑
base (displaced) S72.Ø4- ☑
nondisplaced S72.Ø4- ☑
specified NEC S72.Ø9- ☑
pertrochanteric — *see* Fracture, femur, upper end, trochanteric
physeal S79.ØØ- ☑
Salter-Harris type I S79.Ø1- ☑
specified NEC S79.Ø9- ☑
subcapital (displaced) S72.Ø1- ☑
subtrochanteric (displaced) S72.2- ☑
nondisplaced S72.2- ☑
transcervical — *see* Fracture, femur, upper end, midcervical
trochanteric S72.1Ø- ☑
greater (displaced) S72.11- ☑
nondisplaced S72.11- ☑
lesser (displaced) S72.12- ☑
nondisplaced S72.12- ☑
fibula (shaft) (styloid) S82.4Ø- ☑
comminuted (displaced) S82.45- ☑
nondisplaced S82.45- ☑
following insertion of implant, prosthesis or plate M96.67- ☑
involving ankle or malleolus — *see* Fracture, fibula, lateral malleolus
lateral malleolus (displaced) S82.6- ☑
nondisplaced S82.6- ☑
lower end
physeal S89.3Ø- ☑
Salter-Harris
Type I S89.31- ☑
Type II S89.32- ☑
specified NEC S89.39- ☑
specified NEC S82.83- ☑
torus S82.82- ☑
oblique (displaced) S82.43- ☑
nondisplaced S82.43- ☑
segmental (displaced) S82.46- ☑
nondisplaced S82.46- ☑
specified NEC S82.49- ☑
spiral (displaced) S82.44- ☑
nondisplaced S82.44- ☑
transverse (displaced) S82.42- ☑
nondisplaced S82.42- ☑
upper end
physeal S89.2Ø- ☑
Salter-Harris
Type I S89.21- ☑
Type II S89.22- ☑
specified NEC S89.29- ☑
specified NEC S82.83- ☑
torus S82.81- ☑
finger (except thumb) S62.6Ø- ☑
distal phalanx (displaced) S62.63- ☑
nondisplaced S62.66- ☑
index S62.6Ø- ☑
distal phalanx (displaced) S62.63- ☑
nondisplaced S62.66- ☑
medial phalanx (displaced) S62.62- ☑
nondisplaced S62.65- ☑
proximal phalanx (displaced) S62.61- ☑
nondisplaced S62.64- ☑
little S62.6Ø- ☑
distal phalanx (displaced) S62.63- ☑
nondisplaced S62.66- ☑
medial phalanx (displaced) S62.62- ☑
nondisplaced S62.65- ☑
proximal phalanx (displaced) S62.61- ☑
nondisplaced S62.64- ☑
medial phalanx (displaced) S62.62- ☑
nondisplaced S62.65- ☑
middle S62.6Ø- ☑
distal phalanx (displaced) S62.63- ☑
nondisplaced S62.66- ☑
medial phalanx (displaced) S62.62- ☑

Fracture, traumatic — *continued*
finger — *continued*
middle — *continued*
medial phalanx — *continued*
nondisplaced S62.65- ☑
proximal phalanx (displaced) S62.61- ☑
nondisplaced S62.64- ☑
proximal phalanx (displaced) S62.61- ☑
nondisplaced S62.64- ☑
ring S62.6Ø- ☑
distal phalanx (displaced) S62.63- ☑
nondisplaced S62.66- ☑
medial phalanx (displaced) S62.62- ☑
nondisplaced S62.65- ☑
proximal phalanx (displaced) S62.61- ☑
nondisplaced S62.64- ☑
thumb — *see* Fracture, thumb
following insertion (intraoperative) (postoperative) of orthopedic implant, joint prosthesis or bone plate M96.69
femur M96.66- ☑
fibula M96.67- ☑
humerus M96.62- ☑
pelvis M96.65
radius M96.63- ☑
specified bone NEC M96.69
tibia M96.67- ☑
ulna M96.63- ☑
foot S92.9Ø- ☑
astragalus — *see* Fracture, tarsal, talus
calcaneus — *see* Fracture, tarsal, calcaneus
cuboid — *see* Fracture, tarsal, cuboid
cuneiform — *see* Fracture, tarsal, cuneiform
metatarsal — *see* Fracture, metatarsal
navicular — *see* Fracture, tarsal, navicular
talus — *see* Fracture, tarsal, talus
tarsal — *see* Fracture, tarsal
toe — *see* Fracture, toe
forearm S52.9- ☑
radius — *see* Fracture, radius
ulna — *see* Fracture, ulna
fossa (anterior) (middle) (posterior) SØ2.19 ☑
frontal (bone) (skull) SØ2.Ø ☑
sinus SØ2.19 ☑
glenoid (cavity) (scapula) — *see* Fracture, scapula, glenoid cavity
greenstick — *see* Fracture, by site
hallux — *see* Fracture, toe, great
hand S62.9- ☑
carpal — *see* Fracture, carpal bone
finger (except thumb) — *see* Fracture, finger
metacarpal — *see* Fracture, metacarpal
navicular (scaphoid) (hand) — *see* Fracture, carpal bone, navicular
thumb — *see* Fracture, thumb
healed or old
with complications — *code by* Nature of the complication
heel bone — *see* Fracture, tarsal, calcaneus
Hill-Sachs S42.29- ☑
hip — *see* Fracture, femur, neck
humerus S42.3Ø- ☑
anatomical neck — *see* Fracture, humerus, upper end
articular process — *see* Fracture, humerus, lower end
capitellum — *see* Fracture, humerus, lower end, condyle, lateral
distal end — *see* Fracture, humerus, lower end
epiphysis
lower — *see* Fracture, humerus, lower end, physeal
upper — *see* Fracture, humerus, upper end, physeal
external condyle — *see* Fracture, humerus, lower end, condyle, lateral
following insertion of implant, prosthesis or plate M96.62- ☑
great tuberosity — *see* Fracture, humerus, upper end, greater tuberosity
intercondylar — *see* Fracture, humerus, lower end
internal epicondyle — *see* Fracture, humerus, lower end, epicondyle, medial
lesser tuberosity — *see* Fracture, humerus, upper end, lesser tuberosity
lower end S42.4Ø- ☑

Fracture, traumatic — *continued*
- neck — *continued*
  - hyoid bone S12.8 ☑
  - larynx S12.8 ☑
  - specified site NEC S12.8 ☑
  - thyroid cartilage S12.8 ☑
  - trachea S12.8 ☑
- neoplastic NEC — *see* Fracture, pathological, due to, neoplastic disease
- neural arch — *see* Fracture, vertebra
- newborn — *see* Birth, injury, fracture
- nontraumatic — *see* Fracture, pathological
- nonunion — *see* Nonunion, fracture
- nose, nasal (bone) (septum) SØ2.2 ☑
- occiput — *see* Fracture, skull, base, occiput
- odontoid process — *see* Fracture, neck, cervical vertebra, second
- olecranon (process) (ulna) — *see* Fracture, ulna, upper end, olecranon process
- orbit, orbital (bone) (region) SØ2.8 ☑
  - floor (blow-out) SØ2.3 ☑
  - roof SØ2.19 ☑
- os
  - calcis — *see* Fracture, tarsal, calcaneus
  - magnum — *see* Fracture, carpal, capitate
  - pubis — *see* Fracture, pubis
- palate SØ2.8 ☑
- parietal bone (skull) SØ2.Ø ☑
- patella S82.ØØ- ☑
  - comminuted (displaced) S82.Ø4- ☑
    - nondisplaced S82.Ø4- ☑
  - longitudinal (displaced) S82.Ø2- ☑
    - nondisplaced S82.Ø2- ☑
  - osteochondral (displaced) S82.Ø1- ☑
    - nondisplaced S82.Ø1- ☑
  - specified NEC S82.Ø9- ☑
  - transverse (displaced) S82.Ø3- ☑
    - nondisplaced S82.Ø3- ☑
- pedicle (of vertebral arch) — *see* Fracture, vertebra
- pelvis, pelvic (bone) S32.9 ☑
  - acetabulum — *see* Fracture, acetabulum
  - circle — *see* Disruption, pelvic ring
  - following insertion of implant, prosthesis or plate M96.65
  - ilium — *see* Fracture, ilium
  - ischium — *see* Fracture, ischium
  - multiple
    - with disruption of pelvic ring (circle) — *see* Disruption, pelvic ring
    - without disruption of pelvic ring (circle) S32.82 ☑
  - pubis — *see* Fracture, pubis
  - sacrum — *see* Fracture, sacrum
  - specified site NEC S32.89 ☑
- phalanx
  - foot — *see* Fracture, toe
  - hand — *see* Fracture, finger
- pisiform — *see* Fracture, carpal, pisiform
- pond — *see* Fracture, skull
- prosthetic device, internal — *see* Complications, prosthetic device, by site, mechanical
- pubis S32.5Ø- ☑
  - with disruption of pelvic ring — *see* Disruption, pelvic ring
  - specified site NEC S32.59- ☑
  - superior rim S32.51- ☑
- radius S52.9- ☑
  - distal end — *see* Fracture, radius, lower end
  - following insertion of implant, prosthesis or plate M96.63- ☑
  - head — *see* Fracture, radius, upper end, head
  - lower end S52.5Ø- ☑
    - Barton's — *see* Barton's fracture
    - Colles' — *see* Colles' fracture
    - extraarticular NEC S52.55- ☑
    - intraarticular NEC S52.57- ☑
    - physeal S59.2Ø- ☑
      - Salter-Harris
        - Type I S59.21- ☑
        - Type II S59.22- ☑
        - Type III S59.23- ☑
        - Type IV S59.24- ☑
      - specified NEC S59.29- ☑
    - Smith's — *see* Smith's fracture
    - specified NEC S52.59- ☑
    - styloid process (displaced) S52.51- ☑

Fracture, traumatic — *continued*
- radius — *continued*
  - lower end — *continued*
    - styloid process — *continued*
      - nondisplaced S52.51- ☑
    - torus S52.52- ☑
  - neck — *see* Fracture, radius, upper end
  - proximal end — *see* Fracture, radius, upper end
  - shaft S52.3Ø- ☑
    - bent bone S52.38- ☑
    - comminuted (displaced) S52.35- ☑
      - nondisplaced S52.35- ☑
    - Galeazzi's — *see* Galeazzi's fracture
    - greenstick S52.31- ☑
    - oblique (displaced) S52.33- ☑
      - nondisplaced S52.33- ☑
    - segmental (displaced) S52.36- ☑
      - nondisplaced S52.36- ☑
    - specified NEC S52.39- ☑
    - spiral (displaced) S52.34- ☑
      - nondisplaced S52.34- ☑
    - transverse (displaced) S52.32- ☑
      - nondisplaced S52.32- ☑
  - upper end S52.1Ø- ☑
    - head (displaced) S52.12- ☑
      - nondisplaced S52.12- ☑
    - neck (displaced) S52.13- ☑
      - nondisplaced S52.13- ☑
    - physeal S59.1Ø- ☑
      - Salter-Harris
        - Type I S59.11- ☑
        - Type II S59.12- ☑
        - Type III S59.13- ☑
        - Type IV S59.14- ☑
      - specified NEC S59.19- ☑
    - specified NEC S52.18- ☑
    - torus S52.11- ☑
- ramus
  - inferior or superior, pubis — *see* Fracture, pubis
  - mandible — *see* Fracture, mandible
- restorative material (dental) KØ8.539
  - with loss of material KØ8.531
  - without loss of material KØ8.53Ø
- rib S22.3- ☑
  - with flail chest — *see* Flail, chest
  - multiple S22.4- ☑
    - with flail chest — *see* Flail, chest
- root, tooth — *see* Fracture, tooth
- sacrum S32.1Ø ☑
  - specified NEC S32.19 ☑
  - Type
    - 1 S32.14 ☑
    - 2 S32.15 ☑
    - 3 S32.16 ☑
    - 4 S32.17 ☑
  - Zone
    - I S32.119 ☑
      - displaced (minimally) S32.111 ☑
        - severely S32.112 ☑
      - nondisplaced S32.11Ø ☑
    - II S32.129 ☑
      - displaced (minimally) S32.121 ☑
        - severely S32.122 ☑
      - nondisplaced S32.12Ø ☑
    - III S32.139 ☑
      - displaced (minimally) S32.131 ☑
        - severely S32.132 ☑
      - nondisplaced S32.13Ø ☑
- scaphoid (hand) (*see also* Fracture, carpal, navicular)
  - foot — *see* Fracture, tarsal, navicular
- scapula S42.1Ø- ☑
  - acromial process (displaced) S42.12- ☑
    - nondisplaced S42.12- ☑
  - body (displaced) S42.11- ☑
    - nondisplaced S42.11- ☑
  - coracoid process (displaced) S42.13- ☑
    - nondisplaced S42.13- ☑
  - glenoid cavity (displaced) S42.14- ☑
    - nondisplaced S42.14- ☑
  - neck (displaced) S42.15- ☑
    - nondisplaced S42.15- ☑
  - specified NEC S42.19- ☑
- semilunar bone, wrist — *see* Fracture, carpal, lunate
- sequelae — *see* Sequelae, fracture
- sesamoid bone
  - hand — *see* Fracture, carpal

Fracture, traumatic — *continued*
- sesamoid bone — *continued*
  - other — *code by* site under Fracture
- shepherd's — *see* Fracture, tarsal, talus
- shoulder (girdle) S42.9- ☑
  - blade — *see* Fracture, scapula
- sinus (ethmoid) (frontal) SØ2.19 ☑
- skull SØ2.91 ☑
  - base SØ2.1Ø ☑
    - occiput SØ2.119 ☑
      - condyle SØ2.113 ☑
        - type I SØ2.11Ø ☑
        - type II SØ2.111 ☑
        - type III SØ2.112 ☑
      - specified NEC SØ2.118 ☑
    - specified NEC SØ2.19 ☑
  - birth injury P13.Ø
  - frontal bone SØ2.Ø ☑
  - parietal bone SØ2.Ø ☑
  - specified site NEC SØ2.8 ☑
  - temporal bone SØ2.19 ☑
  - vault SØ2.Ø ☑
- Smith's — *see* Smith's fracture
- sphenoid (bone) (sinus) SØ2.19 ☑
- spine — *see* Fracture, vertebra
- spinous process — *see* Fracture, vertebra
- spontaneous (cause unknown) — *see* Fracture, pathological
- stave (of thumb) — *see* Fracture, metacarpal, first
- sternum S22.2Ø ☑
  - with flail chest — *see* Flail, chest
  - body S22.22 ☑
  - manubrium S22.21 ☑
  - xiphoid (process) S22.24 ☑
- stress M84.3Ø ☑
  - ankle M84.37- ☑
  - carpus M84.34- ☑
  - clavicle M84.31- ☑
  - femoral neck M84.359 ☑
  - femur M84.35- ☑
  - fibula M84.36- ☑
  - finger M84.34- ☑
  - hip M84.359 ☑
  - humerus M84.32- ☑
  - ilium M84.35Ø ☑
  - ischium M84.35Ø ☑
  - metacarpus M84.34- ☑
  - metatarsus M84.37- ☑
  - neck — *see* Fracture, fatigue, vertebra
  - pelvis M84.35Ø ☑
  - radius M84.33- ☑
  - rib M84.38 ☑
  - scapula M84.31- ☑
  - skull M84.38 ☑
  - tarsus M84.37- ☑
  - tibia M84.36- ☑
  - toe M84.37- ☑
  - ulna M84.33- ☑
  - vertebra — *see* Fracture, fatigue, vertebra
- supracondylar, elbow — *see* Fracture, humerus, lower end, supracondylar
- symphysis pubis — *see* Fracture, pubis
- talus (ankle bone) — *see* Fracture, tarsal, talus
- tarsal bone(s) S92.2Ø- ☑
  - astragalus — *see* Fracture, tarsal, talus
  - calcaneus S92.ØØ- ☑
    - anterior process (displaced) S92.Ø2- ☑
      - nondisplaced S92.Ø2- ☑
    - body (displaced) S92.Ø1- ☑
      - nondisplaced S92.Ø1- ☑
    - extraarticular NEC (displaced) S92.Ø5- ☑
      - nondisplaced S92.Ø5- ☑
    - intraarticular (displaced) S92.Ø6- ☑
      - nondisplaced S92.Ø6- ☑
    - tuberosity (displaced) S92.Ø4- ☑
      - avulsion (displaced) S92.Ø3- ☑
        - nondisplaced S92.Ø3- ☑
      - nondisplaced S92.Ø4- ☑
  - cuboid (displaced) S92.21- ☑
    - nondisplaced S92.21- ☑
  - cuneiform
    - intermediate (displaced) S92.23- ☑
      - nondisplaced S92.23- ☑
    - lateral (displaced) S92.22- ☑
      - nondisplaced S92.22- ☑
    - medial (displaced) S92.24- ☑

- **Fracture, traumatic** — *continued*
  - tarsal bone(s) — *continued*
    - cuneiform — *continued*
      - medial — *continued*
        - nondisplaced S92.24- ☑
    - navicular (displaced) S92.25- ☑
      - nondisplaced S92.25- ☑
    - scaphoid — *see* Fracture, tarsal, navicular
    - talus S92.10- ☑
      - avulsion (displaced) S92.15- ☑
        - nondisplaced S92.15- ☑
      - body (displaced) S92.12- ☑
        - nondisplaced S92.12- ☑
      - dome (displaced) S92.14- ☑
        - nondisplaced S92.14- ☑
      - head (displaced) S92.12- ☑
        - nondisplaced S92.12- ☑
      - lateral process (displaced) S92.14- ☑
        - nondisplaced S92.14- ☑
      - neck (displaced) S92.11- ☑
        - nondisplaced S92.11- ☑
      - posterior process (displaced) S92.13- ☑
        - nondisplaced S92.13- ☑
      - specified NEC S92.19- ☑
  - temporal bone (styloid) S02.19 ☑
  - thorax (bony) S22.9 ☑
    - with flail chest — *see* Flail, chest
    - rib S22.3- ☑
      - multiple S22.4- ☑
        - with flail chest — *see* Flail, chest
    - sternum S22.20 ☑
      - body S22.22 ☑
      - manubrium S22.21 ☑
      - xiphoid process S22.24 ☑
    - vertebra (displaced) S22.009 ☑
      - burst (stable) S22.001 ☑
        - unstable S22.002 ☑
      - eighth S22.069 ☑
        - burst (stable) S22.061 ☑
          - unstable S22.062 ☑
        - specified type NEC S22.068 ☑
        - wedge compression S22.060 ☑
      - eleventh S22.089 ☑
        - burst (stable) S22.081 ☑
          - unstable S22.082 ☑
        - specified type NEC S22.088 ☑
        - wedge compression S22.080 ☑
      - fifth S22.059 ☑
        - burst (stable) S22.051 ☑
          - unstable S22.052 ☑
        - specified type NEC S22.058 ☑
        - wedge compression S22.050 ☑
      - first S22.019 ☑
        - burst (stable) S22.011 ☑
          - unstable S22.012 ☑
        - specified type NEC S22.018 ☑
        - wedge compression S22.010 ☑
      - fourth S22.049 ☑
        - burst (stable) S22.041 ☑
          - unstable S22.042 ☑
        - specified type NEC S22.048 ☑
        - wedge compression S22.040 ☑
      - ninth S22.079 ☑
        - burst (stable) S22.071 ☑
          - unstable S22.072 ☑
        - specified type NEC S22.078 ☑
        - wedge compression S22.070 ☑
      - nondisplaced S22.001 ☑
      - second S22.029 ☑
        - burst (stable) S22.021 ☑
          - unstable S22.022 ☑
        - specified type NEC S22.028 ☑
        - wedge compression S22.020 ☑
      - seventh S22.069 ☑
        - burst (stable) S22.061 ☑
          - unstable S22.062 ☑
        - specified type NEC S22.068 ☑
        - wedge compression S22.060 ☑
      - sixth S22.059 ☑
        - burst (stable) S22.051 ☑
          - unstable S22.052 ☑
        - specified type NEC S22.058 ☑
        - wedge compression S22.050 ☑
      - specified type NEC S22.008 ☑
      - tenth S22.079 ☑

- **Fracture, traumatic** — *continued*
  - thorax — *continued*
    - vertebra — *continued*
      - tenth — *continued*
        - burst (stable) S22.071 ☑
          - unstable S22.072 ☑
        - specified type NEC S22.078 ☑
        - wedge compression S22.070 ☑
      - third S22.039 ☑
        - burst (stable) S22.031 ☑
          - unstable S22.032 ☑
        - specified type NEC S22.038 ☑
        - wedge compression S22.030 ☑
      - twelfth S22.089 ☑
        - burst (stable) S22.081 ☑
          - unstable S22.082 ☑
        - specified type NEC S22.088 ☑
        - wedge compression S22.080 ☑
      - wedge compression S22.000 ☑
  - thumb S62.50- ☑
    - distal phalanx (displaced) S62.52- ☑
      - nondisplaced S62.52- ☑
    - proximal phalanx (displaced) S62.51- ☑
      - nondisplaced S62.51- ☑
  - thyroid cartilage S12.8 ☑
  - tibia (shaft) S82.20- ☑
    - comminuted (displaced) S82.25- ☑
      - nondisplaced S82.25- ☑
    - condyles — *see* Fracture, tibia, upper end
    - distal end — *see* Fracture, tibia, lower end
    - epiphysis
      - lower — *see* Fracture, tibia, lower end
      - upper — *see* Fracture, tibia, upper end
    - following insertion of implant, prosthesis or plate M96.67- ☑
    - head (involving knee joint) — *see* Fracture, tibia, upper end
    - intercondyloid eminence — *see* Fracture, tibia, upper end
    - involving ankle or malleolus — *see* Fracture, ankle, medial malleolus
    - lower end S82.30- ☑
      - physeal S89.10- ☑
        - Salter-Harris
          - Type I S89.11- ☑
          - Type II S89.12- ☑
          - Type III S89.13- ☑
          - Type IV S89.14- ☑
        - specified NEC S89.19- ☑
      - pilon (displaced) S82.87- ☑
        - nondisplaced S82.87- ☑
      - specified NEC S82.39- ☑
      - torus S82.31- ☑
    - malleolus — *see* Fracture, ankle, medial malleolus
    - oblique (displaced) S82.23- ☑
      - nondisplaced S82.23- ☑
    - pilon — *see* Fracture, tibia, lower end, pilon
    - proximal end — *see* Fracture, tibia, upper end
    - segmental (displaced) S82.26- ☑
      - nondisplaced S82.26- ☑
    - specified NEC S82.29- ☑
    - spine — *see* Fracture, upper end, spine
    - spiral (displaced) S82.24- ☑
      - nondisplaced S82.24- ☑
    - transverse (displaced) S82.22- ☑
      - nondisplaced S82.22- ☑
    - tuberosity — *see* Fracture, tibia, upper end, tuberosity
    - upper end S82.10- ☑
      - bicondylar (displaced) S82.14- ☑
        - nondisplaced S82.14- ☑
      - lateral condyle (displaced) S82.12- ☑
        - nondisplaced S82.12- ☑
      - medial condyle (displaced) S82.13- ☑
        - nondisplaced S82.13- ☑
      - physeal S89.00- ☑
        - Salter-Harris
          - Type I S89.01- ☑
          - Type II S89.02- ☑
          - Type III S89.03- ☑
          - Type IV S89.04- ☑
        - specified NEC S89.09- ☑
      - plateau — *see* Fracture, tibia, upper end, bicondylar
      - specified NEC S82.19- ☑
      - spine (displaced) S82.11- ☑

- **Fracture, traumatic** — *continued*
  - tibia — *continued*
    - upper end — *continued*
      - spine — *continued*
        - nondisplaced S82.11- ☑
      - torus S82.16- ☑
      - tuberosity (displaced) S82.15- ☑
        - nondisplaced S82.15- ☑
  - toe S92.91- ☑
    - great (displaced) S92.40- ☑
      - distal phalanx (displaced) S92.42- ☑
        - nondisplaced S92.42- ☑
      - nondisplaced S92.40- ☑
      - proximal phalanx (displaced) S92.41- ☑
        - nondisplaced S92.41- ☑
      - specified NEC S92.49- ☑
    - lesser (displaced) S92.50- ☑
      - distal phalanx (displaced) S92.53- ☑
        - nondisplaced S92.53- ☑
      - medial phalanx (displaced) S92.52- ☑
        - nondisplaced S92.52- ☑
      - nondisplaced S92.50- ☑
      - proximal phalanx (displaced) S92.51- ☑
        - nondisplaced S92.51- ☑
      - specified NEC S92.59- ☑
  - tooth (root) S02.5 ☑
  - trachea (cartilage) S12.8 ☑
  - transverse process — *see* Fracture, vertebra
  - trapezium or trapezoid bone — *see* Fracture, carpal
  - trimalleolar — *see* Fracture, ankle, trimalleolar
  - triquetrum (cuneiform of carpus) — *see* Fracture, carpal, triquetrum
  - trochanter — *see* Fracture, femur, trochanteric
  - tuberosity (external) — *code by* site under Fracture
  - ulna (shaft) S52.20- ☑
    - bent bone S52.28- ☑
    - coronoid process — *see* Fracture, ulna, upper end, coronoid process
    - distal end — *see* Fracture, ulna, lower end
    - following insertion of implant, prosthesis or plate M96.63- ☑
    - head S52.00- ☑
    - lower end S52.60- ☑
      - physeal S59.00- ☑
        - Salter-Harris
          - Type I S59.01- ☑
          - Type II S59.02- ☑
          - Type III S59.03- ☑
          - Type IV S59.04- ☑
        - specified NEC S59.09- ☑
      - specified NEC S52.69- ☑
      - styloid process (displaced) S52.61- ☑
        - nondisplaced S52.61- ☑
      - torus S52.62- ☑
    - proximal end — *see* Fracture, ulna, upper end
    - shaft S52.20- ☑
      - comminuted (displaced) S52.25- ☑
        - nondisplaced S52.25- ☑
      - greenstick S52.21- ☑
      - Monteggia's — *see* Monteggia's fracture
      - oblique (displaced) S52.23- ☑
        - nondisplaced S52.23- ☑
      - segmental (displaced) S52.26- ☑
        - nondisplaced S52.26- ☑
      - specified NEC S52.29- ☑
      - spiral (displaced) S52.24- ☑
        - nondisplaced S52.24- ☑
      - transverse (displaced) S52.22- ☑
        - nondisplaced S52.22- ☑
    - upper end S52.00- ☑
      - coronoid process (displaced) S52.04- ☑
        - nondisplaced S52.04- ☑
      - olecranon process (displaced) S52.02- ☑
        - with intraarticular extension S52.03- ☑
        - nondisplaced S52.02- ☑
          - with intraarticular extension S52.03- ☑
      - specified NEC S52.09- ☑
      - torus S52.01- ☑
  - unciform — *see* Fracture, carpal, hamate
  - vault of skull S02.0 ☑
  - vertebra, vertebral (arch) (body) (column) (neural arch) (pedicle) (spinous process) (transverse process)
    - atlas — *see* Fracture, neck, cervical vertebra, first
    - axis — *see* Fracture, neck, cervical vertebra, second
    - cervical (teardrop) S12.9 ☑

Fracture, traumatic — *continued*
vertebra, vertebral — *continued*
cervical — *continued*
axis — *see* Fracture, neck, cervical vertebra, second
first (atlas) — *see* Fracture, neck, cervical vertebra, first
second (axis) — *see* Fracture, neck, cervical vertebra, second
chronic M84.48 ☑
coccyx S32.2 ☑
dorsal — *see* Fracture, thorax, vertebra
lumbar S32.ØØ9 ☑
burst (stable) S32.ØØ1 ☑
unstable S32.ØØ2 ☑
fifth S32.Ø59 ☑
burst (stable) S32.Ø51 ☑
unstable S32.Ø52 ☑
specified type NEC S32.Ø58 ☑
wedge compression S32.Ø5Ø ☑
first S32.Ø19 ☑
burst (stable) S32.Ø11 ☑
unstable S32.Ø12 ☑
specified type NEC S32.Ø18 ☑
wedge compression S32.Ø1Ø ☑
fourth S32.Ø49 ☑
burst (stable) S32.Ø41 ☑
unstable S32.Ø42 ☑
specified type NEC S32.Ø48 ☑
wedge compression S32.Ø4Ø ☑
second S32.Ø29 ☑
burst (stable) S32.Ø21 ☑
unstable S32.Ø22 ☑
specified type NEC S32.Ø28 ☑
wedge compression S32.Ø2Ø ☑
specified type NEC S32.ØØ8 ☑
third S32.Ø39 ☑
burst (stable) S32.Ø31 ☑
unstable S32.Ø32 ☑
specified type NEC S32.Ø38 ☑
wedge compression S32.Ø3Ø ☑
wedge compression S32.ØØØ ☑
metastatic — *see* Collapse, vertebra, in, specified disease NEC (*see also* Neoplasm)
newborn (birth injury) P11.5
sacrum S32.1Ø ☑
specified NEC S32.19 ☑
Type
1 S32.14 ☑
2 S32.15 ☑
3 S32.16 ☑
4 S32.17 ☑
Zone
I S32.119 ☑
displaced (minimally) S32.111 ☑
severely S32.112 ☑
nondisplaced S32.11Ø ☑
II S32.129 ☑
displaced (minimally) S32.121 ☑
severely S32.122 ☑
nondisplaced S32.12Ø ☑
III S32.139 ☑
displaced (minimally) S32.131 ☑
severely S32.132 ☑
nondisplaced S32.13Ø ☑
thoracic — *see* Fracture, thorax, vertebra
vertex SØ2.Ø ☑
vomer (bone) SØ2.2 ☑
wrist S62.1Ø- ☑
carpal — *see* Fracture, carpal bone
navicular (scaphoid) (hand) — *see* Fracture, carpal, navicular
xiphisternum, xiphoid (process) S22.24 ☑
zygoma SØ2.4Ø2 ☑
Fragile, fragility
autosomal site Q95.5
bone, congenital (with blue sclera) Q78.Ø
capillary (hereditary) D69.8
hair L67.8
nails L6Ø.3
non-sex chromosome site Q95.5
X chromosome Q99.2
Fragilitas
crinium L67.8
ossium (with blue sclerae) (hereditary) Q78.Ø
unguium L6Ø.3

Fragilitas — *continued*
unguium — *continued*
congenital Q84.6
Fragments, cataract (lens), **following cataract surgery** H59.Ø2- ☑
retained foreign body — *see* Retained, foreign body fragments (type of)
Frailty (frail) R54
mental R41.81
Frambesia, frambesial (tropica) (*see also* Yaws)
initial lesion or ulcer A66.Ø
primary A66.Ø
Frambeside
gummatous A66.4
of early yaws A66.2
Frambesioma A66.1
Franceschetti-Klein (-Wildervanck) **disease or syndrome** Q75.4
Francis' disease — *see* Tularemia
Franklin disease C88.2
Frank's essential thrombocytopenia D69.3
Fraser's syndrome Q87.Ø
Freckle(s) L81.2
malignant melanoma in — *see* Melanoma
melanotic (Hutchinson's) — *see* Melanoma, in situ
retinal D49.81
Frederickson's hyperlipoproteinemia, type
I and V E78.3
IIA E78.Ø
IIB and III E78.2
IV E78.1
Freeman Sheldon syndrome Q87.Ø
Freezing (*see also* Effect, adverse, cold) T69.9 ☑
Freiberg's disease (infraction of metatarsal head or osteochondrosis) — *see* Osteochondrosis, juvenile, metatarsus
Frei's disease A55
Fremitus, friction, cardiac RØ1.2
Frenum, frenulum
external os Q51.828
tongue (shortening) (congenital) Q38.1
Frequency micturition (nocturnal) R35.Ø
psychogenic F45.8
Frey's syndrome
auriculotemporal G5Ø.8
hyperhidrosis L74.52
Friction
burn — *see* Burn, by site
fremitus, cardiac RØ1.2
precordial RØ1.2
sounds, chest RØ9.89
Friderichsen-Waterhouse syndrome or disease A39.1
Friedländer's B (bacillus) **NEC** (*see also* condition) A49.8
Friedreich's
ataxia G11.1
combined systemic disease G11.1
facial hemihypertrophy Q67.4
sclerosis (cerebellum) (spinal cord) G11.1
Frigidity F52.22
Fröhlich's syndrome E23.6
Frontal (*see also* condition)
lobe syndrome FØ7.Ø
Frostbite (superficial) T33.9Ø ☑
with
partial thickness skin loss — *see* Frostbite (superficial), by site
tissue necrosis T34.9Ø ☑
abdominal wall T33.3 ☑
with tissue necrosis T34.3 ☑
ankle T33.81- ☑
with tissue necrosis T34.81- ☑
arm T33.4- ☑
with tissue necrosis T34.4- ☑
finger(s) — *see* Frostbite, finger
hand — *see* Frostbite, hand
wrist — *see* Frostbite, wrist
ear T33.Ø1- ☑
with tissue necrosis T34.Ø1- ☑
face T33.Ø9 ☑
with tissue necrosis T34.Ø9 ☑
finger T33.53- ☑
with tissue necrosis T34.53- ☑
foot T33.82- ☑
with tissue necrosis T34.82- ☑
hand T33.52- ☑
with tissue necrosis T34.52- ☑
head T33.Ø9 ☑

Frostbite — *continued*
head — *continued*
with tissue necrosis T34.Ø9 ☑
ear — *see* Frostbite, ear
nose — *see* Frostbite, nose
hip (and thigh) T33.6- ☑
with tissue necrosis T34.6- ☑
knee T33.7- ☑
with tissue necrosis T34.7- ☑
leg T33.9- ☑
with tissue necrosis T34.9- ☑
ankle — *see* Frostbite, ankle
foot — *see* Frostbite, foot
knee — *see* Frostbite, knee
lower T33.7- ☑
with tissue necrosis T34.7- ☑
thigh — *see* Frostbite, hip
toe — *see* Frostbite, toe
limb
lower T33.99 ☑
with tissue necrosis T34.99 ☑
upper — *see* Frostbite, arm
neck T33.1 ☑
with tissue necrosis T34.1 ☑
nose T33.Ø2 ☑
with tissue necrosis T34.Ø2 ☑
pelvis T33.3 ☑
with tissue necrosis T34.3 ☑
specified site NEC T33.99 ☑
with tissue necrosis T34.99 ☑
thigh — *see* Frostbite, hip
thorax T33.2 ☑
with tissue necrosis T34.2 ☑
toes T33.83- ☑
with tissue necrosis T34.83- ☑
trunk T33.99 ☑
with tissue necrosis T34.99 ☑
wrist T33.51- ☑
with tissue necrosis T34.51- ☑
Frotteurism F65.81
Frozen (*see also* Effect, adverse, cold) T69.9 ☑
pelvis (female) N94.89
male K66.8
shoulder — *see* Capsulitis, adhesive
Fructokinase deficiency E74.11
Fructose 1,6 diphosphatase deficiency E74.19
Fructosemia (benign) (essential) E74.12
Fructosuria (benign) (essential) E74.11
Fuchs'
black spot (myopic) H44.2- ☑
dystrophy (corneal endothelium) H18.51
heterochromic cyclitis — *see* Cyclitis, Fuchs' heterochromic
Fucosidosis E77.1
Fugue R68.89
dissociative F44.1
hysterical (dissociative) F44.1
postictal in epilepsy — *see* Epilepsy
reaction to exceptional stress (transient) F43.Ø
Fulminant, fulminating — *see* condition
Functional (*see also* condition)
bleeding (uterus) N93.8
Functioning, intellectual, borderline R41.83
Fundus — *see* condition
Fungemia NOS B49
Fungus, fungous
cerebral G93.89
disease NOS B49
infection — *see* Infection, fungus
Funiculitis (acute) (chronic) (endemic) N49.1
gonococcal (acute) (chronic) A54.23
tuberculous A18.15
Funnel
breast (acquired) M95.4
congenital Q67.6
sequelae (late effect) of rickets E64.3
chest (acquired) M95.4
congenital Q67.6
sequelae (late effect) of rickets E64.3
pelvis (acquired) M95.5
with disproportion (fetopelvic) O33.3 ☑
causing obstructed labor O65.3
congenital Q74.2
FUO (fever of unknown origin) R5Ø.9
Furfur L21.Ø
microsporon B36.Ø

G

- **Gain in weight** (abnormal) (excessive) (*see also* Weight, gain)
- **Gaisböck's disease** (polycythemia hypertonica) D75.1
- **Gait abnormality** R26.9
  - ataxic R26.Ø
  - falling R29.6
  - hysterical (ataxic) (staggering) F44.4
  - paralytic R26.1
  - spastic R26.1
  - specified type NEC R26.89
  - staggering R26.Ø
  - unsteadiness R26.81
  - walking difficulty NEC R26.2
- **Galactocele** (breast) N64.89
  - puerperal, postpartum O92.79
- **Galactokinase deficiency** E74.29
- **Galactophoritis** N61
  - gestational, puerperal, postpartum O91.2- ☑
- **Galactorrhea** O92.6
  - not associated with childbirth N64.3
- **Galactosemia** (classic) (congenital) E74.21
- **Galactosuria** E74.29
- **Galacturia** R82.Ø
  - schistosomiasis (bilharziasis) B65.Ø
- **Galeazzi's fracture** S52.37- ☑
- **Galen's vein** — *see* condition
- **Galeophobia** F4Ø.218
- **Gall duct** — *see* condition
- **Gallbladder** (*see also* condition)
  - acute K81.Ø
- **Gallop rhythm** RØØ.8
- **Gallstone** (colic) (cystic duct) (gallbladder) (impacted) (multiple) (*see also* Calculus, gallbladder)
  - with
    - cholecystitis — *see* Calculus, gallbladder, with cholecystitis
  - bile duct (common) (hepatic) — *see* Calculus, bile duct
  - causing intestinal obstruction K56.3
  - specified NEC K8Ø.8Ø
    - with obstruction K8Ø.81
- **Gambling** Z72.6
  - pathological (compulsive) F63.Ø
- **Gammopathy** (of undetermined significance [MGUS]) D47.2
  - associated with lymphoplasmacytic dyscrasia D47.2
  - monoclonal D47.2
  - polyclonal D89.Ø
- **Gamna's disease** (siderotic splenomegaly) D73.1
- **Gamophobia** F4Ø.298
- **Gampsodactylia** (congenital) Q66.7
- **Gamstorp's disease** (adynamia episodica hereditaria) G72.3
- **Gandy-Nanta disease** (siderotic splenomegaly) D73.1
- **Gang**
  - membership offenses Z72.81Ø
- **Gangliocytoma** D36.1Ø
- **Ganglioglioma** — *see* Neoplasm, uncertain behavior, by site
- **Ganglion** (compound) (diffuse) (joint) (tendon (sheath)) M67.4Ø
  - ankle M67.47- ☑
  - foot M67.47- ☑
  - forearm M67.43- ☑
  - hand M67.44- ☑
  - lower leg M67.46- ☑
  - multiple sites M67.49
  - of yaws (early) (late) A66.6
  - pelvic region M67.45- ☑
  - periosteal — *see* Periostitis
  - shoulder region M67.41- ☑
  - specified site NEC M67.48
  - thigh region M67.45- ☑
  - tuberculous A18.Ø9
  - upper arm M67.42- ☑
  - wrist M67.43- ☑
- **Ganglioneuroblastoma** — *see* Neoplasm, nerve, malignant
- **Ganglioneuroma** D36.1Ø
  - malignant — *see* Neoplasm, nerve, malignant
- **Ganglioneuromatosis** D36.1Ø
- **Ganglionitis**
  - fifth nerve — *see* Neuralgia, trigeminal
  - gasserian (postherpetic) (postzoster) BØ2.21
  - geniculate G51.1
    - newborn (birth injury) P11.3
    - postherpetic, postzoster BØ2.21
  - herpes zoster BØ2.21
  - postherpetic geniculate BØ2.21
- **Gangliosidosis** E75.1Ø
  - GM1 E75.19
  - GM2 E75.ØØ
    - other specified E75.Ø9
    - Sandhoff disease E75.Ø1
    - Tay-Sachs disease E75.Ø2
  - GM3 E75.19
  - mucolipidosis IV E75.11
- **Gangosa** A66.5
- **Gangrene, gangrenous** (connective tissue) (dropsical) (dry) (moist) (skin) (ulcer) (*see also* Necrosis) I96
  - with diabetes (mellitus) — *see* Diabetes, gangrene
  - abdomen (wall) I96
  - alveolar M27.3
  - appendix K35.8Ø
    - with
      - perforation or rupture K35.2
      - peritoneal abscess K35.3
      - peritonitis NEC K35.3
        - generalized (with perforation or rupture) K35.2
        - localized (with perforation or rupture) K35.3
  - arteriosclerotic (general) (senile) — *see* Arteriosclerosis, extremities, with, gangrene
  - auricle I96
  - Bacillus welchii A48.Ø
  - bladder (infectious) — *see* Cystitis, specified type NEC
  - bowel, cecum, or colon — *see* Gangrene, intestine
  - Clostridium perfringens or welchii A48.Ø
  - cornea H18.89- ☑
  - corpora cavernosa N48.29
    - noninfective N48.89
  - cutaneous, spreading I96
  - decubital — *see* Ulcer, pressure, by site
  - diabetic (any site) — *see* Diabetes, gangrene
  - emphysematous — *see* Gangrene, gas
  - epidemic — *see* Poisoning, food, noxious, plant
  - epididymis (infectional) N45.1
  - erysipelas — *see* Erysipelas
  - extremity (lower) (upper) I96
  - Fournier N49.3
    - female N76.89
  - fusospirochetal A69.Ø
  - gallbladder — *see* Cholecystitis, acute
  - gas (bacillus) A48.Ø
    - following
      - abortion — *see* Abortion by type complicated by infection
      - ectopic or molar pregnancy OØ8.Ø
  - glossitis K14.Ø
  - hernia — *see* Hernia, by site, with gangrene
  - intestine, intestinal (hemorrhagic) (massive) K55.Ø
    - with
      - mesenteric embolism K55.Ø
      - obstruction — *see* Obstruction, intestine
  - laryngitis JØ4.Ø
  - limb (lower) (upper) I96
  - lung J85.Ø
    - spirochetal A69.8
  - lymphangitis I89.1
  - Meleney's (synergistic) — *see* Ulcer, skin
  - mesentery K55.Ø
    - with
      - embolism K55.Ø
      - intestinal obstruction — *see* Obstruction, intestine
  - mouth A69.Ø
  - ovary — *see* Oophoritis
  - pancreas K85.9
  - penis N48.29
    - noninfective N48.89
  - perineum I96
  - pharynx (*see also* Pharyngitis)
    - Vincent's A69.1
  - presenile I73.1
  - progressive synergistic — *see* Ulcer, skin
  - pulmonary J85.Ø
  - pulpal (dental) KØ4.1
  - quinsy J36
  - Raynaud's (symmetric gangrene) I73.Ø1
  - retropharyngeal J39.2
  - scrotum N49.3
    - noninfective N5Ø.8
  - senile (atherosclerotic) — *see* Arteriosclerosis, extremities, with, gangrene
  - spermatic cord N49.1
    - noninfective N5Ø.8
  - spine I96
  - spirochetal NEC A69.8
  - spreading cutaneous I96
  - stomatitis A69.Ø
  - symmetrical I73.Ø1
  - testis (infectional) N45.2
    - noninfective N44.8
  - throat (*see also* Pharyngitis)
    - diphtheritic A36.Ø
    - Vincent's A69.1
  - thyroid (gland) EØ7.89
  - tooth (pulp) KØ4.1
  - tuberculous NEC — *see* Tuberculosis
  - tunica vaginalis N49.1
    - noninfective N5Ø.8
  - umbilicus I96
  - uterus — *see* Endometritis
  - uvulitis K12.2
  - vas deferens N49.1
    - noninfective N5Ø.8
  - vulva N76.89
- **Ganister disease** J62.8
- **Ganser's syndrome** (hysterical) F44.89
- **Gardner-Diamond syndrome** (autoerythrocyte sensitization) D69.2
- **Gargoylism** E76.Ø1
- **Garré's disease, osteitis** (sclerosing), osteomyelitis — *see* Osteomyelitis, specified type NEC
- **Garrod's pad, knuckle** M72.1
- **Gartner's duct**
  - cyst Q52.4
  - persistent Q5Ø.6
- **Gas** R14.3
  - asphyxiation, inhalation, poisoning, suffocation NEC — *see* Table of Drugs and Chemicals
  - excessive R14.Ø
  - gangrene A48.Ø
    - following
      - abortion — *see* Abortion by type complicated by infection
      - ectopic or molar pregnancy OØ8.Ø
  - on stomach R14.Ø
  - pains R14.1
- **Gastralgia** (*see also* Pain, abdominal)
- **Gastrectasis** K31.Ø
  - psychogenic F45.8
- **Gastric** — *see* condition
- **Gastrinoma**
  - malignant
    - pancreas C25.4
    - specified site NEC — *see* Neoplasm, malignant, by site
    - unspecified site C25.4
  - specified site — *see* Neoplasm, uncertain behavior
  - unspecified site D37.9
- **Gastritis** (simple) K29.7Ø
  - with bleeding K29.71
  - acute (erosive) K29.ØØ
    - with bleeding K29.Ø1
  - alcoholic K29.2Ø
    - with bleeding K29.21
  - allergic K29.6Ø
    - with bleeding K29.61
  - atrophic (chronic) K29.4Ø
    - with bleeding K29.41

- **Gastritis** — *continued*
  - chronic (antral) (fundal) K29.50
    - with bleeding K29.51
    - atrophic K29.40
      - with bleeding K29.41
    - superficial K29.30
      - with bleeding K29.31
  - dietary counseling and surveillance Z71.3
  - due to diet deficiency E63.9
  - eosinophilic K52.81
  - giant hypertrophic K29.60
    - with bleeding K29.61
  - granulomatous K29.60
    - with bleeding K29.61
  - hypertrophic (mucosa) K29.60
    - with bleeding K29.61
  - nervous F54
  - spastic K29.60
    - with bleeding K29.61
  - specified NEC K29.60
    - with bleeding K29.61
  - superficial chronic K29.30
    - with bleeding K29.31
  - tuberculous A18.83
  - viral NEC A08.4
- **Gastrocarcinoma** — *see* Neoplasm, malignant, stomach
- **Gastrocolic** — *see* condition
- **Gastrodisciasis, gastrodiscoidiasis** B66.8
- **Gastroduodenitis** K29.90
  - with bleeding K29.91
  - virus, viral A08.4
    - specified type NEC A08.39
- **Gastrodynia** — *see* Pain, abdominal
- **Gastroenteritis** (acute) (chronic) (noninfectious) (*see also* Enteritis) K52.9
  - allergic K52.2
  - dietetic K52.2
  - drug-induced K52.1
  - due to
    - Cryptosporidium A07.2
    - drugs K52.1
    - food poisoning — *see* intoxication, foodborne
    - radiation K52.0
  - eosinophilic K52.81
  - epidemic (infectious) A09
  - food hypersensitivity K52.2
  - infectious — *see* Enteritis, infectious
  - influenzal — *see* Influenza, with gastroenteritis
  - noninfectious K52.9
    - specified NEC K52.89
  - rotaviral A08.0
  - Salmonella A02.0
  - toxic K52.1
  - viral NEC A08.4
    - acute infectious A08.39
      - type Norwalk A08.11
    - infantile (acute) A08.39
    - Norwalk agent A08.11
    - rotaviral A08.0
    - severe of infants A08.39
    - specified type NEC A08.39
- **Gastroenteropathy** (*see also* Gastroenteritis) K52.9
  - acute, due to Norovirus A08.11
  - acute, due to Norwalk agent A08.11
  - infectious A09
- **Gastroenteroptosis** K63.4
- **Gastroesophageal laceration- hemorrhage syndrome** K22.6
- **Gastrointestinal** — *see* condition
- **Gastrojejunal** — *see* condition
- **Gastrojejunitis** (*see also* Enteritis) K52.9
- **Gastrojejunocolic** — *see* condition
- **Gastroliths** K31.89
- **Gastromalacia** K31.89
- **Gastroparalysis** K31.84
  - diabetic — *see* Diabetes, gastroparalysis
- **Gastroparesis** K31.84
  - diabetic — *see* Diabetes, by type, with gastroparesis
- **Gastropathy** K31.9
  - congestive portal K31.89
  - erythematous K29.70
  - exudative K90.89
  - portal hypertensive K31.89
- **Gastroptosis** K31.89
- **Gastrorrhagia** K92.2
  - psychogenic F45.8
- **Gastroschisis** (congenital) Q79.3
- **Gastrospasm** (neurogenic) (reflex) K31.89
- **Gastrospasm** — *continued*
  - neurotic F45.8
  - psychogenic F45.8
- **Gastrostaxis** — *see* Gastritis, with bleeding
- **Gastrostenosis** K31.89
- **Gastrostomy**
  - attention to Z43.1
  - status Z93.1
- **Gastrosuccorrhea** (continuous) (intermittent) K31.89
  - neurotic F45.8
  - psychogenic F45.8
- **Gatophobia** F40.218
- **Gaucher's disease or splenomegaly** (adult) (infantile) E75.22
- **Gee** (-Herter)(-Thaysen) **disease** (nontropical sprue) K90.0
- **Gélineau's syndrome** G47.419
  - with cataplexy G47.411
- **Gemination, tooth, teeth** K00.2
- **Gemistocytoma**
  - specified site — *see* Neoplasm, malignant, by site
  - unspecified site C71.9
- **General, generalized** — *see* condition
- **Genetic**
  - carrier (status)
    - cystic fibrosis Z14.1
    - hemophilia A (asymptomatic) Z14.01
      - symptomatic Z14.02
    - specified NEC Z14.8
  - susceptibility to disease NEC Z15.89
    - malignant neoplasm Z15.09
      - breast Z15.01
      - endometrium Z15.04
      - ovary Z15.02
      - prostate Z15.03
      - specified NEC Z15.09
    - multiple endocrine neoplasia Z15.81
- **Genital** — *see* condition
- **Genito-anorectal syndrome** A55
- **Genitourinary system** — *see* condition
- **Genu**
  - congenital Q74.1
  - extrorsum (acquired) (*see also* Deformity, varus, knee)
    - congenital Q74.1
    - sequelae (late effect) of rickets E64.3
  - introrsum (acquired) (*see also* Deformity, valgus, knee)
    - congenital Q74.1
    - sequelae (late effect) of rickets E64.3
  - rachitic (old) E64.3
  - recurvatum (acquired) (*see also* Deformity, limb, specified type NEC, lower leg)
    - congenital Q68.2
    - sequelae (late effect) of rickets E64.3
  - valgum (acquired) (knock-knee) M21.06- ☑
    - congenital Q74.1
    - sequelae (late effect) of rickets E64.3
  - varum (acquired) (bowleg) M21.16- ☑
    - congenital Q74.1
    - sequelae (late effect) of rickets E64.3
- **Geographic tongue** K14.1
- **Geophagia** — *see* Pica
- **Geotrichosis** B48.3
  - stomatitis B48.3
- **Gephyrophobia** F40.242
- **Gerbode defect** Q21.0
- **GERD** (gastroesophageal reflux disease) K21.9
- **Gerhardt's**
  - disease (erythromelalgia) I73.81
  - syndrome (vocal cord paralysis) J38.00
    - bilateral J38.02
    - unilateral J38.01
- **German measles** (*see also* Rubella)
  - exposure to Z20.4
- **Germinoblastoma** (diffuse) C85.9- ☑
  - follicular C82.9- ☑
- **Germinoma** — *see* Neoplasm, malignant, by site
- **Gerontoxon** — *see* Degeneration, cornea, senile
- **Gerstmann's syndrome** R48.8
  - developmental F81.2
- **Gerstmann-Sträussler-Scheinker syndrome** (GSS) A81.82
- **Gestation** (period) (*see also* Pregnancy)
  - ectopic — *see* Pregnancy, by site
  - multiple O30.9- ☑
    - greater than quadruplets — *see* Pregnancy, multiple (gestation), specified NEC
    - specified NEC — *see* Pregnancy, multiple (gestation), specified NEC
- **Gestational**
  - mammary abscess O91.11- ☑
  - purulent mastitis O91.11- ☑
  - subareolar abscess O91.11- ☑
- **Ghon tubercle, primary infection** A15.7
- **Ghost**
  - teeth K00.4
  - vessels (cornea) H16.41- ☑
- **Ghoul hand** A66.3
- **Gianotti-Crosti disease** L44.4
- **Giant**
  - cell
    - epulis K06.8
    - peripheral granuloma K06.8
  - esophagus, congenital Q39.5
  - kidney, congenital Q63.3
  - urticaria T78.3 ☑
    - hereditary D84.1
- **Giardiasis** A07.1
- **Gibert's disease or pityriasis** L42
- **Giddiness** R42
  - hysterical F44.89
  - psychogenic F45.8
- **Gierke's disease** (glycogenosis I) E74.01
- **Gigantism** (cerebral) (hypophyseal) (pituitary) E22.0
  - constitutional E34.4
- **Gilbert's disease or syndrome** E80.4
- **Gilchrist's disease** B40.9
- **Gilford-Hutchinson disease** E34.8
- **Gilles de la Tourette's disease or syndrome** (motor-verbal tic) F95.2
- **Gingivitis** K05.10
  - acute (catarrhal) K05.00
    - necrotizing A69.1
    - nonplaque induced K05.01
    - plaque induced K05.00
  - chronic (desquamative) (hyperplastic) (simple marginal) (ulcerative) K05.10
    - nonplaque induced K05.11
    - plaque induced K05.10
  - expulsiva — *see* Periodontitis
  - necrotizing ulcerative (acute) A69.1
  - pellagrous E52
    - acute necrotizing A69.1
  - Vincent's A69.1
- **Gingivoglossitis** K14.0
- **Gingivopericementitis** — *see* Periodontitis
- **Gingivosis** — *see* Gingivitis, chronic
- **Gingivostomatitis** K05.10
  - herpesviral B00.2
  - necrotizing ulcerative (acute) A69.1
- **Gland, glandular** — *see* condition
- **Glanders** A24.0
- **Glanzmann** (-Naegeli) **disease or thrombasthenia** D69.1
- **Glasgow coma scale**
  - total score
    - 3-8 R40.243
    - 9-12 R40.242
    - 13-15 R40.241
- **Glass-blower's disease** (cataract) — *see* Cataract, specified NEC
- **Glaucoma** H40.9
  - with
    - increased episcleral venous pressure H40.81- ☑
    - pseudoexfoliation of lens — *see* Glaucoma, open angle, primary, capsular
  - absolute H44.51- ☑
  - angle-closure (primary) H40.20- ☑
    - acute (attack) (crisis) H40.21- ☑
    - chronic H40.22- ☑
    - intermittent H40.23- ☑
    - residual stage H40.24- ☑
  - borderline H40.00- ☑
  - capsular (with pseudoexfoliation of lens) — *see* Glaucoma, open angle, primary, capsular
  - childhood Q15.0
  - closed angle — *see* Glaucoma, angle-closure
  - congenital Q15.0
  - corticosteroid-induced — *see* Glaucoma, secondary, drugs
  - hypersecretion H40.82- ☑
  - in (due to)
    - amyloidosis E85.4 [H42]
    - aniridia Q13.1 [H42]
    - concussion of globe — *see* Glaucoma, secondary, trauma

Glaucoma — *continued*
- in — *continued*
  - dislocation of lens — *see* Glaucoma, secondary
  - disorder of lens NEC — *see* Glaucoma, secondary
  - drugs — *see* Glaucoma, secondary, drugs
  - endocrine disease NOS E34.9 [H42]
  - eye
    - inflammation — *see* Glaucoma, secondary, inflammation
    - trauma — *see* Glaucoma, secondary, trauma
  - hypermature cataract — *see* Glaucoma, secondary
  - iridocyclitis — *see* Glaucoma, secondary, inflammation
  - lens disorder — *see* Glaucoma, secondary
  - Lowe's syndrome E72.03 [H42]
  - metabolic disease NOS E88.9 [H42]
  - ocular disorders NEC — *see* Glaucoma, secondary
  - onchocerciasis B73.02
  - pupillary block — *see* Glaucoma, secondary
  - retinal vein occlusion — *see* Glaucoma, secondary
  - Rieger's anomaly Q13.81 [H42]
  - rubeosis of iris — *see* Glaucoma, secondary
  - tumor of globe — *see* Glaucoma, secondary
- infantile Q15.0
- low tension — *see* Glaucoma, open angle, primary, low-tension
- malignant H40.83- ☑
- narrow angle — *see* Glaucoma, angle-closure
- newborn Q15.0
- noncongestive (chronic) — *see* Glaucoma, open angle
- nonobstructive — *see* Glaucoma, open angle
- obstructive (*see also* Glaucoma, angle-closure)
  - due to lens changes — *see* Glaucoma, secondary
- open angle H40.10- ☑
  - primary H40.11- ☑
    - capsular (with pseudoexfoliation of lens) H40.14- ☑
    - low-tension H40.12- ☑
    - pigmentary H40.13- ☑
    - residual stage H40.15- ☑
- phacolytic — *see* Glaucoma, secondary
- pigmentary — *see* Glaucoma, open angle, primary, pigmentary
- postinfectious — *see* Glaucoma, secondary, inflammation
- secondary (to) H40.5- ☑
  - drugs H40.6- ☑
  - inflammation H40.4- ☑
  - trauma H40.3- ☑
- simple (chronic) H40.11 ☑
- simplex H40.11 ☑
- specified type NEC H40.89
- suspect H40.00- ☑
- syphilitic A52.71
- traumatic (*see also* Glaucoma, secondary, trauma)
  - newborn (birth injury) P15.3
- tuberculous A18.59

Glaucomatous flecks (subcapsular) — *see* Cataract, complicated

Glazed tongue K14.4

Gleet (gonococcal) A54.01

Glénard's disease K63.4

Glioblastoma (multiforme)
- with sarcomatous component
  - specified site — *see* Neoplasm, malignant, by site
  - unspecified site C71.9
- giant cell
  - specified site — *see* Neoplasm, malignant, by site
  - unspecified site C71.9
- specified site — *see* Neoplasm, malignant, by site
- unspecified site C71.9

Glioma (malignant)
- astrocytic
  - specified site — *see* Neoplasm, malignant, by site
  - unspecified site C71.9
- mixed
  - specified site — *see* Neoplasm, malignant, by site
  - unspecified site C71.9
- nose Q30.8
- specified site NEC — *see* Neoplasm, malignant, by site
- subependymal D43.2
  - specified site — *see* Neoplasm, uncertain behavior, by site
  - unspecified site D43.2
- unspecified site C71.9

Gliomatosis cerebri C71.0

Glioneuroma — *see* Neoplasm, uncertain behavior, by site

Gliosarcoma
- specified site — *see* Neoplasm, malignant, by site
- unspecified site C71.9

Gliosis (cerebral) G93.89
- spinal G95.89

Glisson's disease — *see* Rickets

Globinuria R82.3

Globus (hystericus) F45.8

Glomangioma D18.00
- intra-abdominal D18.03
- intracranial D18.02
- skin D18.01
- specified site NEC D18.09

Glomangiomyoma D18.00
- intra-abdominal D18.03
- intracranial D18.02
- skin D18.01
- specified site NEC D18.09

Glomangiosarcoma — *see* Neoplasm, connective tissue, malignant

Glomerular
- disease in syphilis A52.75
- nephritis — *see* Glomerulonephritis

Glomerulitis — *see* Glomerulonephritis

Glomerulonephritis (*see also* Nephritis) N05.9
- with
  - edema — *see* Nephrosis
  - minimal change N05.0
  - minor glomerular abnormality N05.0
- acute N00.9
- chronic N03.9
- crescentic (diffuse) NEC (*see also* N00-N07 with fourth character .7) N05.7
- dense deposit (*see also* N00-N07 with fourth character .6) N05.6
- diffuse
  - crescentic (*see also* N00-N07 with fourth character .7) N05.7
  - endocapillary proliferative (*see also* N00-N07 with fourth character .4) N05.4
  - membranous (*see also* N00-N07 with fourth character .2) N05.2
  - mesangial proliferative (*see also* N00-N07 with fourth character .3) N05.3
  - mesangiocapillary (*see also* N00-N07 with fourth character .5) N05.5
  - sclerosing N05.8
- endocapillary proliferative (diffuse) NEC (*see also* N00-N07 with fourth character .4) N05.4
- extracapillary NEC (*see also* N00-N07 with fourth character .7) N05.7
- focal (and segmental) (*see also* N00-N07 with fourth character .1) N05.1
- hypocomplementemic — *see* Glomerulonephritis, membranoproliferative
- IgA — *see* Nephropathy, IgA
- immune complex (circulating) NEC N05.8
- in (due to)
  - amyloidosis E85.4 [N08]
  - bilharziasis B65.9 [N08]
  - cryoglobulinemia D89.1 [N08]
  - defibrination syndrome D65 [N08]
  - diabetes mellitus — *see* Diabetes, glomerulosclerosis
  - disseminated intravascular coagulation D65 [N08]
  - Fabry (-Anderson) disease E75.21 [N08]
  - Goodpasture's syndrome M31.0
  - hemolytic-uremic syndrome D59.3
  - Henoch (-Schönlein) purpura D69.0 [N08]
  - lecithin cholesterol acyltransferase deficiency E78.6 [N08]
  - microscopic polyangiitis M31.7 [N08]
  - multiple myeloma C90.0- ☑ [N08]
  - Plasmodium malariae B52.0
  - schistosomiasis B65.9 [N08]
  - sepsis A41.9 [N08]
    - streptococcal A40- ☑ [N08]
  - sickle-cell disorders D57.- ☑ [N08]
  - strongyloidiasis B78.9 [N08]
  - subacute bacterial endocarditis I33.0 [N08]
  - syphilis (late) congenital A50.59 [N08]
  - systemic lupus erythematosus M32.14
  - thrombotic thrombocytopenic purpura M31.1 [N08]
  - typhoid fever A01.09
  - Waldenström macroglobulinemia C88.0 [N08]

Glomerulonephritis — *continued*
- in — *continued*
  - Wegener's granulomatosis M31.31
- latent or quiescent N03.9
- lobular, lobulonodular — *see* Glomerulonephritis, membranoproliferative
- membranoproliferative (diffuse)(type 1 or 3) (*see also* N00-N07 with fourth character .5) N05.5
  - dense deposit (type 2) NEC (*see also* N00-N07 with fourth character .6) N05.6
- membranous (diffuse) NEC (*see also* N00-N07 with fourth character .2) N05.2
- mesangial
  - IgA/IgG — *see* Nephropathy, IgA
  - proliferative (diffuse) NEC (*see also* N00-N07 with fourth character .3) N05.3
- mesangiocapillary (diffuse) NEC (*see also* N00-N07 with fourth character .5) N05.5
- necrotic, necrotizing NEC (*see also* N00- N07 with fourth character .8) N05.8
- nodular — *see* Glomerulonephritis, membranoproliferative
- poststreptococcal NEC N05.9
  - acute N00.9
  - chronic N03.9
  - rapidly progressive N01.9
- proliferative NEC (*see also* N00-N07 with fourth character .8) N05.8
  - diffuse (lupus) M32.14
- rapidly progressive N01.9
- sclerosing, diffuse N05.8
- specified pathology NEC (*see also* N00- N07 with fourth character .8) N05.8
- subacute N01.9

Glomerulopathy — *see* Glomerulonephritis

Glomerulosclerosis (*see also* Sclerosis, renal)
- intercapillary (nodular) (with diabetes) — *see* Diabetes, glomerulosclerosis
- intracapillary — *see* Diabetes, glomerulosclerosis

Glossagra K14.6

Glossalgia K14.6

Glossitis (chronic superficial) (gangrenous) (Moeller's) K14.0
- areata exfoliativa K14.1
- atrophic K14.4
- benign migratory K14.1
- cortical superficial, sclerotic K14.0
- Hunter's D51.0
- interstitial, sclerous K14.0
- median rhomboid K14.2
- pellagrous E52
- superficial, chronic K14.0

Glossocele K14.8

Glossodynia K14.6
- exfoliativa K14.4

Glossoncus K14.8

Glossopathy K14.9

Glossophytia K14.3

Glossoplegia K14.8

Glossoptosis K14.8

Glossopyrosis K14.6

Glossotrichia K14.3

Glossy skin L90.8

Glottis — *see* condition

Glottitis (*see also* Laryngitis) J04.0

Glucagonoma
- pancreas
  - benign D13.7
  - malignant C25.4
  - uncertain behavior D37.8
- specified site NEC
  - benign — *see* Neoplasm, benign, by site
  - malignant — *see* Neoplasm, malignant, by site
  - uncertain behavior — *see* Neoplasm, uncertain behavior, by site
- unspecified site
  - benign D13.7
  - malignant C25.4
  - uncertain behavior D37.8

Glucoglycinuria E72.51

Glucose-galactose malabsorption E74.39

Glue
- ear — *see* Otitis, media, nonsuppurative, chronic, mucoid
- sniffing (airplane) — *see* Abuse, drug, inhalant
  - dependence — *see* Dependence, drug, inhalant

Glutaric aciduria E72.3

Glycinemia E72.51
Glycinuria (renal) (with ketosis) E72.Ø9
Glycogen
infiltration — *see* Disease, glycogen storage
storage disease — *see* Disease, glycogen storage
Glycogenosis (diffuse) (generalized) (*see also* Disease, glycogen storage)
cardiac E74.Ø2 [I43]
diabetic, secondary — *see* Diabetes, glycogenosis, secondary
pulmonary interstitial J84.842
Glycopenia E16.2
Glycosuria R81
renal E74.8
Gnathostoma spinigerum (infection) (infestation), **gnathostomiasis** (wandering swelling) B83.1
Goiter (plunging) (substernal) EØ4.9
with
hyperthyroidism (recurrent) — *see* Hyperthyroidism, with, goiter
thyrotoxicosis — *see* Hyperthyroidism, with, goiter
adenomatous — *see* Goiter, nodular
cancerous C73
congenital (nontoxic) EØ3.Ø
diffuse EØ3.Ø
parenchymatous EØ3.Ø
transitory, with normal functioning P72.Ø
cystic EØ4.2
due to iodine-deficiency EØ1.1
due to
enzyme defect in synthesis of thyroid hormone EØ7.1
iodine-deficiency (endemic) EØ1.2
dyshormonogenetic (familial) EØ7.1
endemic (iodine-deficiency) EØ1.2
diffuse EØ1.Ø
multinodular EØ1.1
exophthalmic — *see* Hyperthyroidism, with, goiter
iodine-deficiency (endemic) EØ1.2
diffuse EØ1.Ø
multinodular EØ1.1
nodular EØ1.1
lingual Q89.2
lymphadenoid EØ6.3
malignant C73
multinodular (cystic) (nontoxic) EØ4.2
toxic or with hyperthyroidism EØ5.2Ø
with thyroid storm EØ5.21
neonatal NEC P72.Ø
nodular (nontoxic) (due to) EØ4.9
with
hyperthyroidism EØ5.2Ø
with thyroid storm EØ5.21
thyrotoxicosis EØ5.2Ø
with thyroid storm EØ5.21
endemic EØ1.1
iodine-deficiency EØ1.1
sporadic EØ4.9
toxic EØ5.2Ø
with thyroid storm EØ5.21
nontoxic EØ4.9
diffuse (colloid) EØ4.Ø
multinodular EØ4.2
simple EØ4.Ø
specified NEC EØ4.8
uninodular EØ4.1
simple EØ4.Ø
toxic — *see* Hyperthyroidism, with, goiter
uninodular (nontoxic) EØ4.1
toxic or with hyperthyroidism EØ5.1Ø
with thyroid storm EØ5.11
Goiter-deafness syndrome EØ7.1
Goldberg syndrome Q89.8
Goldberg-Maxwell syndrome E34.51
Goldblatt's hypertension or kidney I7Ø.1
Goldenhar (-Gorlin) **syndrome** Q87.Ø
Goldflam-Erb disease or syndrome G7Ø.ØØ
with exacerbation (acute) G7Ø.Ø1
in crisis G7Ø.Ø1
Goldscheider's disease Q81.8
Goldstein's disease (familial hemorrhagic telangiectasia) I78.Ø
Golfer's elbow — *see* Epicondylitis, medial
Gonadoblastoma
specified site — *see* Neoplasm, uncertain behavior, by site
unspecified site
female D39.1Ø

Gonadoblastoma — *continued*
unspecified site — *continued*
male D4Ø.1Ø
Gonecystitis — *see* Vesiculitis
Gongylonemiasis B83.8
Goniosynechiae — *see* Adhesions, iris, goniosynechiae
Gonococcemia A54.86
Gonococcus, gonococcal (disease) (infection) (*see also* condition) A54.9
anus A54.6
bursa, bursitis A54.49
conjunctiva, conjunctivitis (neonatorum) A54.31
endocardium A54.83
eye A54.3Ø
conjunctivitis A54.31
iridocyclitis A54.32
keratitis A54.33
newborn A54.31
other specified A54.39
fallopian tubes (acute) (chronic) A54.24
genitourinary (organ) (system) (tract) (acute)
lower A54.ØØ
with abscess (accessory gland) (periurethral) A54.1
upper (*see also* condition) A54.29
heart A54.83
iridocyclitis A54.32
joint A54.42
lymphatic (gland) (node) A54.89
meninges, meningitis A54.81
musculoskeletal A54.4Ø
arthritis A54.42
osteomyelitis A54.43
other specified A54.49
spondylopathy A54.41
pelviperitonitis A54.24
pelvis (acute) (chronic) A54.24
pharynx A54.5
proctitis A54.6
pyosalpinx (acute) (chronic) A54.24
rectum A54.6
skin A54.89
specified site NEC A54.89
tendon sheath A54.49
throat A54.5
urethra (acute) (chronic) A54.Ø1
with abscess (accessory gland) (periurethral) A54.1
vulva (acute) (chronic) A54.Ø2
Gonocytoma
specified site — *see* Neoplasm, uncertain behavior, by site
unspecified site
female D39.1Ø
male D4Ø.1Ø
Gonorrhea (acute) (chronic) A54.9
Bartholin's gland (acute) (chronic) (purulent) A54.Ø2
with abscess (accessory gland) (periurethral) A54.1
bladder A54.Ø1
cervix A54.Ø3
conjunctiva, conjunctivitis (neonatorum) A54.31
contact Z2Ø.2
Cowper's gland (with abscess) A54.1
exposure to Z2Ø.2
fallopian tube (acute) (chronic) A54.24
kidney (acute) (chronic) A54.21
lower genitourinary tract A54.ØØ
with abscess (accessory gland) (periurethral) A54.1
ovary (acute) (chronic) A54.24
pelvis (acute) (chronic) A54.24
female pelvic inflammatory disease A54.24
penis A54.Ø9
prostate (acute) (chronic) A54.22
seminal vesicle (acute) (chronic) A54.23
specified site not listed (*see also* Gonococcus) A54.89
spermatic cord (acute) (chronic) A54.23
urethra A54.Ø1
with abscess (accessory gland) (periurethral) A54.1
vagina A54.Ø2
vas deferens (acute) (chronic) A54.23
vulva A54.Ø2
Goodall's disease AØ8.19
Goodpasture's syndrome M31.Ø
Gopalan's syndrome (burning feet) E53.Ø
Gorlin-Chaudry-Moss syndrome Q87.Ø
Gottron's papules L94.4
Gougerot-Blum syndrome (pigmented purpuric lichenoid dermatitis) L81.7

Gougerot-Carteaud disease or syndrome (confluent reticulate papillomatosis) L83
Gougerot's syndrome (trisymptomatic) L81.7
Gouley's syndrome (constrictive pericarditis) I31.1
Goundou A66.6
Gout, chronic (*see also* Gout, gouty) M1A.9 ☑ (*following* MØ8)
drug-induced M1A.2Ø ☑ (*following* MØ8)
ankle M1A.27- ☑ (*following* MØ8)
elbow M1A.22- ☑ (*following* MØ8)
foot joint M1A.27- ☑ (*following* MØ8)
hand joint M1A.24- ☑ (*following* MØ8)
hip M1A.25- ☑ (*following* MØ8)
knee M1A.26- ☑ (*following* MØ8)
multiple site M1A.29- ☑ (*following* MØ8)
shoulder M1A.21- ☑ (*following* MØ8)
vertebrae M1A.28 ☑ (*following* MØ8)
wrist M1A.23- ☑ (*following* MØ8)
idiopathic M1A.ØØ ☑ (*following* MØ8)
ankle M1A.Ø7- ☑ (*following* MØ8)
elbow M1A.Ø2- ☑ (*following* MØ8)
foot joint M1A.Ø7- ☑ (*following* MØ8)
hand joint M1A.Ø4- ☑ (*following* MØ8)
hip M1A.Ø5- ☑ (*following* MØ8)
knee M1A.Ø6- ☑ (*following* MØ8)
multiple site M1A.Ø9 ☑ (*following* MØ8)
shoulder M1A.Ø1- ☑ (*following* MØ8)
vertebrae M1A.Ø8 ☑ (*following* MØ8)
wrist M1A.Ø3- ☑ (*following* MØ8)
in (due to) renal impairment M1A.3Ø ☑ (*following* MØ8)
ankle M1A.37- ☑ (*following* MØ8)
elbow M1A.32- ☑ (*following* MØ8)
foot joint M1A.37- ☑ (*following* MØ8)
hand joint M1A.34- ☑ (*following* MØ8)
hip M1A.35- ☑ (*following* MØ8)
knee M1A.36- ☑ (*following* MØ8)
multiple site M1A.39 ☑ (*following* MØ8)
shoulder M1A.31- ☑ (*following* MØ8)
vertebrae M1A.38 ☑ (*following* MØ8)
wrist M1A.33- ☑ (*following* MØ8)
lead-induced M1A.1Ø ☑ (*following* MØ8)
ankle M1A.17- ☑ (*following* MØ8)
elbow M1A.12- ☑ (*following* MØ8)
foot joint M1A.17- ☑ (*following* MØ8)
hand joint M1A.14- ☑ (*following* MØ8)
hip M1A.15- ☑ (*following* MØ8)
knee M1A.16- ☑ (*following* MØ8)
multiple site M1A.19 ☑ (*following* MØ8)
shoulder M1A.11- ☑ (*following* MØ8)
vertebrae M1A.18 ☑ (*following* MØ8)
wrist M1A.13- ☑ (*following* MØ8)
primary — *see* Gout, chronic, idiopathic
saturnine — *see* Gout, chronic, lead-induced
secondary NEC M1A.4Ø ☑ (*following* MØ8)
ankle M1A.47- ☑ (*following* MØ8)
elbow M1A.42- ☑ (*following* MØ8)
foot joint M1A.47- ☑ (*following* MØ8)
hand joint M1A.44- ☑ (*following* MØ8)
hip M1A.45- ☑ (*following* MØ8)
knee M1A.46- ☑ (*following* MØ8)
multiple site M1A.49 ☑ (*following* MØ8)
shoulder M1A.41- ☑ (*following* MØ8)
vertebrae M1A.48 ☑ (*following* MØ8)
wrist M1A.43- ☑ (*following* MØ8)
syphilitic (*see also* subcategory M14.8-) A52.77
tophi M1A.9 ☑ (*following* MØ8)
Gout, gouty (acute) (attack) (flare) (*see also* Gout, chronic) M1Ø.9
drug-induced M1Ø.2Ø
ankle M1Ø.27- ☑
elbow M1Ø.22- ☑
foot joint M1Ø.27- ☑
hand joint M1Ø.24- ☑
hip M1Ø.25- ☑
knee M1Ø.26- ☑
multiple site M1Ø.29
shoulder M1Ø.21- ☑
vertebrae M1Ø.28
wrist M1Ø.23- ☑
idiopathic M1Ø.ØØ
ankle M1Ø.Ø7- ☑
elbow M1Ø.Ø2- ☑
foot joint M1Ø.Ø7- ☑
hand joint M1Ø.Ø4- ☑
hip M1Ø.Ø5- ☑

- **Growth** — *continued*
  - secondary — *see* Neoplasm, secondary, by site
- **Gruby's disease** B35.Ø
- **Gubler-Millard paralysis or syndrome** G46.3
- **Guerin-Stern syndrome** Q74.3
- **Guidance, insufficient anterior** (occlusal) M26.54
- **Guillain-Barré disease or syndrome** G61.Ø
  - sequelae G65.Ø
- **Guinea worms** (infection) (infestation) B72
- **Guinon's disease** (motor-verbal tic) F95.2
- **Gull's disease** EØ3.4
- **Gum** — *see* condition
- **Gumboil** KØ4.7
  - with sinus KØ4.6
- **Gumma** (syphilitic) A52.79
  - artery A52.Ø9
    - cerebral A52.Ø4
  - bone A52.77
    - of yaws (late) A66.6
  - brain A52.19
  - cauda equina A52.19
  - central nervous system A52.3
  - ciliary body A52.71
  - congenital A5Ø.59
  - eyelid A52.71
  - heart A52.Ø6
  - intracranial A52.19
  - iris A52.71
  - kidney A52.75
  - larynx A52.73
  - leptomeninges A52.19
  - liver A52.74
  - meninges A52.19
  - myocardium A52.Ø6
  - nasopharynx A52.73
  - neurosyphilitic A52.3
  - nose A52.73
  - orbit A52.71
  - palate (soft) A52.79
  - penis A52.76
  - pericardium A52.Ø6
  - pharynx A52.73
  - pituitary A52.79
  - scrofulous (tuberculous) A18.4
  - skin A52.79
  - specified site NEC A52.79
  - spinal cord A52.19
  - tongue A52.79
  - tonsil A52.73
  - trachea A52.73
  - tuberculous A18.4
  - ulcerative due to yaws A66.4
  - ureter A52.75
  - yaws A66.4
    - bone A66.6
- **Gunn's syndrome** QØ7.8
- **Gunshot wound** (*see also* Wound, open)
  - fracture — *code as* Fracture, by site
  - internal organs — *see* Injury, by site
- **Gynandrism** Q56.Ø
- **Gynandroblastoma**
  - specified site — *see* Neoplasm, uncertain behavior, by site
  - unspecified site
    - female D39.1Ø
    - male D4Ø.1Ø
- **Gynecological examination** (periodic) (routine) ZØ1.419
  - with abnormal findings ZØ1.411
- **Gynecomastia** N62
- **Gynephobia** F4Ø.291
- **Gyrate scalp** Q82.8

H

- **H** (Hartnup's) **disease** E72.Ø2
- **Haas' disease or osteochondrosis** (juvenile) (head of humerus) — *see* Osteochondrosis, juvenile, humerus
- **Habit, habituation**
  - bad sleep Z72.821
  - chorea F95.8
  - disturbance, child F98.9
  - drug — *see* Dependence, drug
  - irregular sleep Z72.821
  - laxative F55.2
  - spasm — *see* Tic
  - tic — *see* Tic
- **Haemophilus** (H.) **influenzae, as cause of disease classified elsewhere** B96.3
- **Haff disease** — *see* Poisoning, mercury
- **Hageman's factor defect, deficiency or disease** D68.2
- **Haglund's disease or osteochondrosis** (juvenile) (os tibiale externum) — *see* Osteochondrosis, juvenile, tarsus
- **Hailey-Hailey disease** Q82.8
- **Hair** (*see also* condition)
  - plucking F63.3
    - in stereotyped movement disorder F98.4
  - tourniquet syndrome (*see also* Constriction, external, by site)
    - finger S6Ø.44- ☑
    - penis S3Ø.842 ☑
    - thumb S6Ø.34- ☑
    - toe S9Ø.44- ☑
- **Hairball in stomach** T18.2 ☑
- **Hair-pulling, pathological** (compulsive) F63.3
- **Hairy black tongue** K14.3
- **Half vertebra** Q76.49
- **Halitosis** R19.6
- **Hallerman-Streiff syndrome** Q87.Ø
- **Hallervorden-Spatz disease** G23.Ø
- **Hallopeau's acrodermatitis or disease** L4Ø.2
- **Hallucination** R44.3
  - auditory R44.Ø
  - gustatory R44.2
  - olfactory R44.2
  - specified NEC R44.2
  - tactile R44.2
  - visual R44.1
- **Hallucinosis** (chronic) F28
  - alcoholic (acute) F1Ø.951
    - in
      - abuse F1Ø.151
      - dependence F1Ø.251
  - drug-induced F19.951
    - cannabis F12.951
    - cocaine F14.951
    - hallucinogen F16.151
    - in
      - abuse F19.151
        - cannabis F12.151
        - cocaine F14.151
        - hallucinogen F16.151
        - inhalant F18.151
        - opioid F11.151
        - sedative, anxiolytic or hypnotic F13.151
        - stimulant NEC F15.151
      - dependence F19.251
        - cannabis F12.251
        - cocaine F14.251
        - hallucinogen F16.251
        - inhalant F18.251
        - opioid F11.251
        - sedative, anxiolytic or hypnotic F13.251
        - stimulant NEC F15.251
    - inhalant F18.951
    - opioid F11.951
    - sedative, anxiolytic or hypnotic F13.951
    - stimulant NEC F15.951
  - organic FØ6.Ø
- **Hallux**
  - deformity (acquired) NEC M2Ø.5X- ☑
  - limitus M2Ø.5X- ☑
  - malleus (acquired) NEC M2Ø.3- ☑
  - rigidus (acquired) M2Ø.2- ☑
    - congenital Q74.2
    - sequelae (late effect) of rickets E64.3
  - valgus (acquired) M2Ø.1- ☑
    - congenital Q66.6
  - varus (acquired) M2Ø.3- ☑
    - congenital Q66.3
- **Halo, visual** H53.19
- **Hamartoma, hamartoblastoma** Q85.9
  - epithelial (gingival), odontogenic, central or peripheral — *see* Cyst, calcifying odontogenic
- **Hamartosis** Q85.9
- **Hamman-Rich syndrome** J84.114
- **Hammer toe** (acquired) NEC (*see also* Deformity, toe, hammer toe)
  - congenital Q66.89
  - sequelae (late effect) of rickets E64.3
- **Hand** — *see* condition
- **Hand-foot syndrome** L27.1
- **Handicap, handicapped**
  - educational Z55.9
    - specified NEC Z55.8
- **Hand-Schüller-Christian disease or syndrome** C96.5
- **Hanging** (asphyxia) (strangulation) (suffocation) — *see* Asphyxia, traumatic, due to mechanical threat
- **Hangnail** (*see also* Cellulitis, digit)
  - with lymphangitis — *see* Lymphangitis, acute, digit
- **Hangover** (alcohol) F1Ø.129
- **Hanhart's syndrome** Q87.Ø
- **Hanot-Chauffard** (-Troisier) **syndrome** E83.19
- **Hanot's cirrhosis or disease** K74.3
- **Hansen's disease** — *see* Leprosy
- **Hantaan virus disease** (Korean hemorrhagic fever) A98.5
- **Hantavirus disease** (with renal manifestations) (Dobrava) (Puumala) (Seoul) A98.5
  - with pulmonary manifestations (Andes) (Bayou) (Bermejo) (Black Creek Canal) (Choclo) (Juquitiba) (Laguna negra) (Lechiguanas) (New York) (Oran) (Sin nombre) B33.4
- **Happy puppet syndrome** Q93.5
- **Harada's disease or syndrome** H3Ø.81- ☑
- **Hardening**
  - artery — *see* Arteriosclerosis
  - brain G93.89
- **Harelip** (complete) (incomplete) — *see* Cleft, lip
- **Harlequin** (newborn) Q8Ø.4
- **Harley's disease** D59.6
- **Harmful use** (of)
  - alcohol F1Ø.1Ø
  - anxiolytics — *see* Abuse, drug, sedative
  - cannabinoids — *see* Abuse, drug, cannabis
  - cocaine — *see* Abuse, drug, cocaine
  - drug — *see* Abuse, drug
  - hallucinogens — *see* Abuse, drug, hallucinogen
  - hypnotics — *see* Abuse, drug, sedative
  - opioids — *see* Abuse, drug, opioid
  - PCP (phencyclidine) — *see* Abuse, drug, hallucinogen
  - sedatives — *see* Abuse, drug, sedative
  - stimulants NEC — *see* Abuse, drug, stimulant
- **Harris' lines** — *see* Arrest, epiphyseal
- **Hartnup's disease** E72.Ø2
- **Harvester's lung** J67.Ø
- **Harvesting ovum for in vitro fertilization** Z31.83
- **Hashimoto's disease or thyroiditis** EØ6.3
- **Hashitoxicosis** (transient) EØ6.3
- **Hassal-Henle bodies or warts** (cornea) H18.49
- **Haut mal** — *see* Epilepsy, generalized, specified NEC
- **Haverhill fever** A25.1
- **Hay fever** (*see also* Fever, hay) J3Ø.1
- **Hayem-Widal syndrome** D59.8
- **Haygarth's nodes** M15.8
- **Haymaker's lung** J67.Ø
- **Hb** (abnormal)
  - Bart's disease D56.Ø
  - disease — *see* Disease, hemoglobin
  - trait — *see* Trait
- **Head** — *see* condition
- **Headache** R51
  - allergic NEC G44.89
  - associated with sexual activity G44.82
  - chronic daily R51
  - cluster G44.ØØ9
    - chronic G44.Ø29
      - intractable G44.Ø21
      - not intractable G44.Ø29
    - episodic G44.Ø19
      - intractable G44.Ø11
      - not intractable G44.Ø19
    - intractable G44.ØØ1
    - not intractable G44.ØØ9
  - cough (primary) G44.83
  - daily chronic R51
  - drug-induced NEC G44.4Ø
    - intractable G44.41
    - not intractable G44.4Ø
  - exertional (primary) G44.84
  - histamine G44.ØØ9
    - intractable G44.ØØ1
    - not intractable G44.ØØ9
  - hypnic G44.81
  - lumbar puncture G97.1
  - medication overuse G44.4Ø
    - intractable G44.41
    - not intractable G44.4Ø
  - menstrual — *see* Migraine, menstrual
  - migraine (type) (*see also* Migraine) G43.9Ø9

- **Headache** — *continued*
  - nasal septum R51
  - neuralgiform, short lasting unilateral, with conjunctival injection and tearing (SUNCT) G44.059
    - intractable G44.051
    - not intractable G44.059
  - new daily persistent (NDPH) G44.52
  - orgasmic G44.82
  - periodic syndromes in adults and children G43.C0 (*following* G43.7)
    - with refractory migraine G43.C1 (*following* G43.7)
    - without refractory migraine G43.C0 (*following* G43.7)
    - intractable G43.C1 (*following* G43.7)
    - not intractable G43.C0 (*following* G43.7)
  - postspinal puncture G97.1
  - post-traumatic G44.309
    - acute G44.319
      - intractable G44.311
      - not intractable G44.319
    - chronic G44.329
      - intractable G44.321
      - not intractable G44.329
    - intractable G44.301
    - not intractable G44.309
  - pre-menstrual — *see* Migraine, menstrual
  - preorgasmic G44.82
  - primary
    - cough G44.83
    - exertional G44.84
    - stabbing G44.85
    - thunderclap G44.53
  - rebound G44.40
    - intractable G44.41
    - not intractable G44.40
  - short lasting unilateral neuralgiform, with conjunctival injection and tearing (SUNCT) G44.059
    - intractable G44.051
    - not intractable G44.059
  - specified syndrome NEC G44.89
  - spinal and epidural anesthesia - induced T88.59 ☑
    - in labor and delivery O74.5
    - in pregnancy O29.4- ☑
    - postpartum, puerperal O89.4
  - spinal fluid loss (from puncture) G97.1
  - stabbing (primary) G44.85
  - tension (-type) G44.209
    - chronic G44.229
      - intractable G44.221
      - not intractable G44.229
    - episodic G44.219
      - intractable G44.211
      - not intractable G44.219
    - intractable G44.201
    - not intractable G44.209
  - thunderclap (primary) G44.53
  - vascular NEC G44.1
- **Healthy**
  - infant
    - accompanying sick mother Z76.3
    - receiving care Z76.2
  - person accompanying sick person Z76.3
- **Hearing examination** Z01.10
  - with abnormal findings NEC Z01.118
  - following failed hearing screening Z01.110
  - for hearing conservation and treatment Z01.12
- **Heart** — *see* condition
- **Heart beat**
  - abnormality R00.9
    - specified NEC R00.8
  - awareness R00.2
  - rapid R00.0
  - slow R00.1
- **Heartburn** R12
  - psychogenic F45.8
- **Heat** (effects) T67.9 ☑
  - apoplexy T67.0 ☑
  - burn (*see also* Burn) L55.9
  - collapse T67.1 ☑
  - cramps T67.2 ☑
  - dermatitis or eczema L59.0
  - edema T67.7 ☑
  - erythema — *code by site under* Burn, first degree
  - excessive T67.9 ☑
    - specified effect NEC T67.8 ☑
  - exhaustion T67.5 ☑
    - anhydrotic T67.3 ☑
- **Heat** — *continued*
  - exhaustion — *continued*
    - due to
      - salt (and water) depletion T67.4 ☑
      - water depletion T67.3 ☑
        - with salt depletion T67.4 ☑
  - fatigue (transient) T67.6 ☑
  - fever T67.0 ☑
  - hyperpyrexia T67.0 ☑
  - prickly L74.0
  - prostration — *see* Heat, exhaustion
  - pyrexia T67.0 ☑
  - rash L74.0
  - specified effect NEC T67.8 ☑
  - stroke T67.0 ☑
  - sunburn — *see* Sunburn
  - syncope T67.1 ☑
- **Heavy-for-dates NEC** (infant) (4000g to 4499g) P08.1
  - exceptionally (4500g or more) P08.0
- **Hebephrenia, hebephrenic** (schizophrenia) F20.1
- **Heberden's disease or nodes** (with arthropathy) M15.1
- **Hebra's**
  - pityriasis L26
  - prurigo L28.2
- **Heel** — *see* condition
- **Heerfordt's disease** D86.89
- **Hegglin's anomaly or syndrome** D72.0
- **Heilmeyer-Schoner disease** D45
- **Heine-Medin disease** A80.9
- **Heinz body anemia, congenital** D58.2
- **Heliophobia** F40.228
- **Heller's disease or syndrome** F84.3
- **HELLP syndrome** (hemolysis, elevated liver enzymes and low platelet count) O14.2- ☑
- **Helminthiasis** (*see also* Infestation, helminth)
  - Ancylostoma B76.0
  - intestinal B82.0
    - mixed types (types classifiable to more than one of the titles B65.0-B81.3 and B81.8) B81.4
    - specified type NEC B81.8
  - mixed types (intestinal) (types classifiable to more than one of the titles B65.0-B81.3 and B81.8) B81.4
  - Necator (americanus) B76.1
  - specified type NEC B83.8
- **Heloma** L84
- **Hemangioblastoma** — *see* Neoplasm, connective tissue, uncertain behavior
  - malignant — *see* Neoplasm, connective tissue, malignant
- **Hemangioendothelioma** (*see also* Neoplasm, uncertain behavior, by site)
  - benign D18.00
    - intra-abdominal D18.03
    - intracranial D18.02
    - skin D18.01
    - specified site NEC D18.09
  - bone (diffuse) — *see* Neoplasm, bone, malignant
  - epithelioid (*see also* Neoplasm, uncertain behavior, by site)
    - malignant — *see* Neoplasm, malignant, by site
  - malignant — *see* Neoplasm, connective tissue, malignant
- **Hemangiofibroma** — *see* Neoplasm, benign, by site
- **Hemangiolipoma** — *see* Lipoma
- **Hemangioma** D18.00
  - arteriovenous D18.00
    - intra-abdominal D18.03
    - intracranial D18.02
    - skin D18.01
    - specified site NEC D18.09
  - capillary D18.00
    - intra-abdominal D18.03
    - intracranial D18.02
    - skin D18.01
    - specified site NEC D18.09
  - cavernous D18.00
    - intra-abdominal D18.03
    - intracranial D18.02
    - skin D18.01
    - specified site NEC D18.09
  - epithelioid D18.00
    - intra-abdominal D18.03
    - intracranial D18.02
    - skin D18.01
    - specified site NEC D18.09
  - histiocytoid D18.00
- **Hemangioma** — *continued*
  - histiocytoid — *continued*
    - intra-abdominal D18.03
    - intracranial D18.02
    - skin D18.01
    - specified site NEC D18.09
  - infantile D18.00
    - intra-abdominal D18.03
    - intracranial D18.02
    - skin D18.01
    - specified site NEC D18.09
  - intra-abdominal D18.03
  - intracranial D18.02
  - intramuscular D18.00
    - intra-abdominal D18.03
    - intracranial D18.02
    - skin D18.01
    - specified site NEC D18.09
  - juvenile D18.00
  - malignant — *see* Neoplasm,connective tissue, malignant
  - plexiform D18.00
    - intra-abdominal D18.03
    - intracranial D18.02
    - skin D18.01
    - specified site NEC D18.09
  - racemose D18.00
    - intra-abdominal D18.03
    - intracranial D18.02
    - skin D18.01
    - specified site NEC D18.09
  - sclerosing — *see* Neoplasm, skin, benign
  - simplex D18.00
    - intra-abdominal D18.03
    - intracranial D18.02
    - skin D18.01
    - specified site NEC D18.09
  - skin D18.01
  - specified site NEC D18.09
  - venous D18.00
    - intra-abdominal D18.03
    - intracranial D18.02
    - skin D18.01
    - specified site NEC D18.09
  - verrucous keratotic D18.00
    - intra-abdominal D18.03
    - intracranial D18.02
    - skin D18.01
    - specified site NEC D18.09
- **Hemangiomatosis** (systemic) I78.8
  - involving single site — *see* Hemangioma
- **Hemangiopericytoma** (*see also* Neoplasm, connective tissue, uncertain behavior)
  - benign — *see* Neoplasm, connective tissue, benign
  - malignant — *see* Neoplasm, connective tissue, malignant
- **Hemangiosarcoma** — *see* Neoplasm, connective tissue, malignant
- **Hemarthrosis** (nontraumatic) M25.00
  - ankle M25.07- ☑
  - elbow M25.02- ☑
  - foot joint M25.07- ☑
  - hand joint M25.04- ☑
  - hip M25.05- ☑
  - in hemophilic arthropathy — *see* Arthropathy, hemophilic
  - knee M25.06- ☑
  - shoulder M25.01- ☑
  - specified joint NEC M25.08
  - traumatic — *see* Sprain, by site
  - vertebrae M25.08
  - wrist M25.03- ☑
- **Hematemesis** K92.0
  - with ulcer — *code by site under* Ulcer, with hemorrhage K27.4
  - newborn, neonatal P54.0
    - due to swallowed maternal blood P78.2
- **Hematidrosis** L74.8
- **Hematinuria** (*see also* Hemoglobinuria)
  - malarial B50.8
- **Hematobilia** K83.8
- **Hematocele**
  - female NEC N94.89
    - with ectopic pregnancy O00.9
    - ovary N83.8
  - male N50.1
- **Hematochezia** (*see also* Melena) K92.1

Hematochyluria (*see also* Infestation, filarial)
  schistosomiasis (bilharziasis) B65.Ø
Hematocolpos (with hematometra or hematosalpinx) N89.7
Hematocornea — *see* Pigmentation, cornea, stromal
Hematogenous — *see* condition
Hematoma (traumatic) (skin surface intact) (*see also* Contusion)
  with
    injury of internal organs — *see* Injury, by site
    open wound — *see* Wound, open
  amputation stump (surgical) (late) T87.89
  aorta, dissecting I71.ØØ
    abdominal I71.Ø2
    thoracic I71.Ø1
    thoracoabdominal I71.Ø3
  aortic intramural — *see* Dissection, aorta
  arterial (complicating trauma) — *see* Injury, blood vessel, by site
  auricle — *see* Contusion, ear
    nontraumatic — *see* Disorder, pinna, hematoma
  birth injury NEC P15.8
  brain (traumatic)
    with
      cerebral laceration or contusion (diffuse) — *see* Injury, intracranial, diffuse
        focal — *see* Injury, intracranial, focal
    cerebellar, traumatic SØ6.37- ☑
    intracerebral, traumatic — *see* Injury, intracranial, intracerebral hemorrhage
    newborn NEC P52.4
      birth injury P1Ø.1
    nontraumatic — *see* Hemorrhage, intracranial
    subarachnoid, arachnoid, traumatic — *see* Injury, intracranial, subarachnoid hemorrhage
    subdural, traumatic — *see* Injury, intracranial, subdural hemorrhage
  breast (nontraumatic) N64.89
  broad ligament (nontraumatic) N83.7
    traumatic S37.892 ☑
  cerebellar, traumatic SØ6.37- ☑
  cerebral — *see* Hematoma, brain
  cerebrum SØ6.36- ☑
    left SØ6.35- ☑
    right SØ6.34- ☑
  cesarean delivery wound O9Ø.2
  complicating delivery (perineal) (pelvic) (vagina) (vulva) O71.7
  corpus cavernosum (nontraumatic) N48.89
  epididymis (nontraumatic) N5Ø.1
  epidural (traumatic) — *see* Injury, intracranial, epidural hemorrhage
    spinal — *see* Injury, spinal cord, by region
  episiotomy O9Ø.2
  face, birth injury P15.4
  genital organ NEC (nontraumatic)
    female (nonobstetric) N94.89
      traumatic S3Ø.2Ø2 ☑
    male N5Ø.1
      traumatic S3Ø.2Ø1 ☑
  internal organs — *see* Injury, by site
  intracerebral, traumatic — *see* Injury, intracranial, intracerebral hemorrhage
  intraoperative — *see* Complications, intraoperative, hemorrhage
  labia (nontraumatic) (nonobstetric) N9Ø.89
  liver (subcapsular) (nontraumatic) K76.89
    birth injury P15.Ø
  mediastinum — *see* Injury, intrathoracic
  mesosalpinx (nontraumatic) N83.7
    traumatic S37.898 ☑
  muscle — code by site under Contusion
  nontraumatic
    muscle M79.81
    soft tissue M79.81
  obstetrical surgical wound O9Ø.2
  orbit, orbital (nontraumatic) (*see also* Hemorrhage, orbit)
    traumatic — *see* Contusion, orbit
  pelvis (female) (nontraumatic) (nonobstetric) N94.89
    obstetric O71.7
    traumatic — *see* Injury, by site
  penis (nontraumatic) N48.89
    birth injury P15.5
  perianal (nontraumatic) K64.5
  perineal S3Ø.23 ☑
    complicating delivery O71.7
Hematoma — *continued*
  perirenal — *see* Injury, kidney
  pinna — *see* Contusion, ear
    nontraumatic — *see* Disorder, pinna, hematoma
  placenta O43.89- ☑
  postoperative (postprocedural) — *see* Complication, postprocedural, hemorrhage
  retroperitoneal (nontraumatic) K66.1
    traumatic S36.892 ☑
  scrotum, superficial S3Ø.22 ☑
    birth injury P15.5
  seminal vesicle (nontraumatic) N5Ø.1
    traumatic S37.892 ☑
  spermatic cord (traumatic) S37.892 ☑
    nontraumatic N5Ø.1
  spinal (cord) (meninges) (*see also* Injury, spinal cord, by region)
    newborn (birth injury) P11.5
  spleen D73.5
    intraoperative — *see* Complications, intraoperative, hemorrhage, spleen
    postprocedural (postoperative) — *see* Complications, postprocedural, hemorrhage, spleen
  sternocleidomastoid, birth injury P15.2
  sternomastoid, birth injury P15.2
  subarachnoid (traumatic) — *see* Injury, intracranial, subarachnoid hemorrhage
    newborn (nontraumatic) P52.5
      due to birth injury P1Ø.3
    nontraumatic — *see* Hemorrhage, intracranial, subarachnoid
  subdural (traumatic) — *see* Injury, intracranial, subdural hemorrhage
    newborn (localized) P52.8
      birth injury P1Ø.Ø
    nontraumatic — *see* Hemorrhage, intracranial, subdural
  superficial, newborn P54.5
  testis (nontraumatic) N5Ø.1
    birth injury P15.5
  tunica vaginalis (nontraumatic) N5Ø.1
  umbilical cord, complicating delivery O69.5 ☑
  uterine ligament (broad) (nontraumatic) N83.7
    traumatic S37.892 ☑
  vagina (ruptured) (nontraumatic) N89.8
    complicating delivery O71.7
  vas deferens (nontraumatic) N5Ø.1
    traumatic S37.892 ☑
  vitreous — *see* Hemorrhage, vitreous
  vulva (nontraumatic) (nonobstetric) N9Ø.89
    complicating delivery O71.7
    newborn (birth injury) P15.5
Hematometra N85.7
  with hematocolpos N89.7
Hematomyelia (central) G95.19
  newborn (birth injury) P11.5
  traumatic T14.8
Hematomyelitis GØ4.9Ø
Hematoperitoneum — *see* Hemoperitoneum
Hematophobia F4Ø.23Ø
Hematopneumothorax (see Hemothorax)
Hematopoiesis, cyclic D7Ø.4
Hematoporphyria — *see* Porphyria
Hematorachis, hematorrhachis G95.19
  newborn (birth injury) P11.5
Hematosalpinx N83.6
  with
    hematocolpos N89.7
    hematometra N85.7
      with hematocolpos N89.7
  infectional — *see* Salpingitis
Hematospermia R36.1
Hematothorax (see Hemothorax)
Hematuria R31.9
  benign (familial) (of childhood) (*see also* Hematuria, idiopathic)
    essential microscopic R31.1
  due to sulphonamide, sulfonamide — *see* Table of Drugs and Chemicals, by drug
  endemic (*see also* Schistosomiasis) B65.Ø
  gross R31.Ø
  idiopathic NØ2.9
    with glomerular lesion
      crescentic (diffuse) glomerulonephritis NØ2.7
      dense deposit disease NØ2.6
      endocapillary proliferative glomerulonephritis NØ2.4
Hematuria — *continued*
  idiopathic — *continued*
    with glomerular lesion — *continued*
      focal and segmental hyalinosis or sclerosis NØ2.1
      membranoproliferative (diffuse) NØ2.5
      membranous (diffuse) NØ2.2
      mesangial proliferative (diffuse) NØ2.3
      mesangiocapillary (diffuse) NØ2.5
      minor abnormality NØ2.Ø
      proliferative NEC NØ2.8
      specified pathology NEC NØ2.8
  intermittent — *see* Hematuria, idiopathic
  malarial B5Ø.8
  microscopic NEC R31.2
    benign essential R31.1
  paroxysmal (*see also* Hematuria, idiopathic)
    nocturnal D59.5
  persistent — *see* Hematuria, idiopathic
  recurrent — *see* Hematuria, idiopathic
  tropical (*see also* Schistosomiasis) B65.Ø
  tuberculous A18.13
Hemeralopia (day blindness) H53.11
  vitamin A deficiency E5Ø.5
Hemi-akinesia R41.4
Hemianalgesia R2Ø.Ø
Hemianencephaly QØØ.Ø
Hemianesthesia R2Ø.Ø
Hemianopia, hemianopsia (heteronymous) H53.47
  homonymous H53.46- ☑
  syphilitic A52.71
Hemiathetosis R25.8
Hemiatrophy R68.89
  cerebellar G31.9
  face, facial, progressive (Romberg) G51.8
  tongue K14.8
Hemiballism (us) G25.5
Hemicardia Q24.8
Hemicephalus, hemicephaly QØØ.Ø
Hemichorea G25.5
Hemicolitis, left — *see* Colitis, left sided
Hemicrania
  congenital malformation QØØ.Ø
  continua G44.51
  meaning migraine (*see also* Migraine) G43.9Ø9
  paroxysmal G44.Ø39
    chronic G44.Ø49
      intractable G44.Ø41
      not intractable G44.Ø49
    episodic G44.Ø39
      intractable G44.Ø31
      not intractable G44.Ø39
    intractable G44.Ø31
    not intractable G44.Ø39
Hemidystrophy — *see* Hemiatrophy
Hemiectromelia Q73.8
Hemihypalgesia R2Ø.8
Hemihypesthesia R2Ø.1
Hemi-inattention R41.4
Hemimelia Q73.8
  lower limb — *see* Defect, reduction, lower limb, specified type NEC
  upper limb — *see* Defect, reduction, upper limb, specified type NEC
Hemiparalysis — *see* Hemiplegia
Hemiparesis — *see* Hemiplegia
Hemiparesthesia R2Ø.2
Hemiparkinsonism G2Ø
Hemiplegia G81.9- ☑
  alternans facialis G83.89
  ascending NEC G81.9Ø
    spinal G95.89
  congenital (cerebral) G8Ø.8
    spastic G8Ø.2
  embolic (current episode) I63.4- ☑
  flaccid G81.Ø- ☑
  following
    cerebrovascular disease I69.959
      cerebral infarction I69.35- ☑
      intracerebral hemorrhage I69.15- ☑
      nontraumatic intracranial hemorrhage NEC I69.25- ☑
      specified disease NEC I69.85- ☑
      stroke NOS I69.35- ☑
      subarachnoid hemorrhage I69.Ø5- ☑
  hysterical F44.4
  newborn NEC P91.8

- **Hemiplegia** — *continued*
  - newborn — *continued*
    - birth injury P11.9
  - spastic G81.1- ☑
    - congenital G80.2
  - thrombotic (current episode) I63.3 ☑
- **Hemisection, spinal cord** — *see* Injury, spinal cord, by region
- **Hemispasm** (facial) R25.2
- **Hemisporosis** B48.8
- **Hemitremor** R25.1
- **Hemivertebra** Q76.49
  - failure of segmentation with scoliosis Q76.3
  - fusion with scoliosis Q76.3
- **Hemochromatosis** E83.119
  - with refractory anemia D46.1
  - due to repeated red blood cell transfusion E83.111
  - hereditary (primary) E83.110
  - primary E83.110
  - specified NEC E83.118
- **Hemoglobin** (*see also* condition)
  - abnormal (disease) — *see* Disease, hemoglobin
  - AS genotype D57.3
  - Constant Spring D58.2
  - E-beta thalassemia D56.5
  - fetal, hereditary persistence (HPFH) D56.4
  - H Constant Spring D56.0
  - low NOS D64.9
  - S (Hb S), heterozygous D57.3
- **Hemoglobinemia** D59.9
  - due to blood transfusion T80.89 ☑
  - paroxysmal D59.6
    - nocturnal D59.5
- **Hemoglobinopathy** (mixed) D58.2
  - with thalassemia D56.8
  - sickle-cell D57.1
    - with thalassemia D57.40
      - with crisis (vasoocclusive pain) D57.419
        - with
          - acute chest syndrome D57.411
          - splenic sequestration D57.412
      - without crisis D57.40
- **Hemoglobinuria** R82.3
  - with anemia, hemolytic, acquired (chronic) NEC D59.6
  - cold (agglutinin) (paroxysmal) (with Raynaud's syndrome) D59.6
  - due to exertion or hemolysis NEC D59.6
  - intermittent D59.6
  - malarial B50.8
  - march D59.6
  - nocturnal (paroxysmal) D59.5
  - paroxysmal (cold) D59.6
    - nocturnal D59.5
- **Hemolymphangioma** D18.1
- **Hemolysis**
  - intravascular
    - with
      - abortion — *see* Abortion, by type, complicated by, hemorrhage
      - ectopic or molar pregnancy O08.1
      - hemorrhage
        - antepartum — *see* Hemorrhage, antepartum, with coagulation defect
        - intrapartum (*see also* Hemorrhage, complicating, delivery) O67.0
    - postpartum O72.3
  - neonatal (excessive) P58.9
    - specified NEC P58.8
- **Hemolytic** — *see* condition
- **Hemopericardium** I31.2
  - following acute myocardial infarction (current complication) I23.0
  - newborn P54.8
  - traumatic — *see* Injury, heart, with hemopericardium
- **Hemoperitoneum** K66.1
  - infectional K65.9
  - traumatic S36.899 ☑
    - with open wound — *see* Wound, open, with penetration into peritoneal cavity
- **Hemophilia** (classical) (familial) (hereditary) D66
  - A D66
  - acquired D68.311
  - autoimmune D68.311
  - B D67
  - C D68.1
  - calcipriva (*see also* Defect, coagulation) D68.4
  - nonfamilial (*see also* Defect, coagulation) D68.4
  - secondary D68.311
- **Hemophilia** — *continued*
  - vascular D68.0
- **Hemophthalmos** H44.81- ☑
- **Hemopneumothorax** (*see also* Hemothorax)
  - traumatic S27.2 ☑
- **Hemoptysis** R04.2
  - newborn P26.9
  - tuberculous — *see* Tuberculosis, pulmonary
- **Hemorrhage, hemorrhagic** (concealed) R58
  - abdomen R58
  - accidental antepartum — *see* Hemorrhage, antepartum
  - acute idiopathic pulmonary, in infants R04.81
  - adenoid J35.8
  - adrenal (capsule) (gland) E27.49
    - medulla E27.8
    - newborn P54.4
  - after delivery — *see* Hemorrhage, postpartum
  - alveolar
    - lung, newborn P26.8
    - process K08.8
  - alveolus K08.8
  - amputation stump (surgical) T87.89
  - anemia (chronic) D50.0
    - acute D62
  - antepartum (with) O46.90
    - with coagulation defect O46.00- ☑
      - afibrinogenemia O46.01- ☑
      - disseminated intravascular coagulation O46.02- ☑
      - hypofibrinogenemia O46.01- ☑
      - specified defect NEC O46.09- ☑
    - before 20 weeks gestation O20.9
      - specified type NEC O20.8
      - threatened abortion O20.0
    - due to
      - abruptio placenta (*see also* Abruptio placentae) O45.9- ☑
      - leiomyoma, uterus — *see* Hemorrhage, antepartum, specified cause NEC
      - placenta previa O44.1- ☑
    - specified cause NEC — *see* subcategory O46.8X- ☑
  - anus (sphincter) K62.5
  - apoplexy (stroke) — *see* Hemorrhage, intracranial, intracerebral
  - arachnoid — *see* Hemorrhage, intracranial, subarachnoid
  - artery R58
    - brain — *see* Hemorrhage, intracranial, intracerebral
  - basilar (ganglion) I61.0
  - bladder N32.89
  - bowel K92.2
    - newborn P54.3
  - brain (miliary) (nontraumatic) — *see* Hemorrhage, intracranial, intracerebral
    - due to
      - birth injury P10.1
      - syphilis A52.05
    - epidural or extradural (traumatic) — *see* Injury, intracranial, epidural hemorrhage
    - newborn P52.4
      - birth injury P10.1
    - subarachnoid — *see* Hemorrhage, intracranial, subarachnoid
    - subdural — *see* Hemorrhage, intracranial, subdural
  - brainstem (nontraumatic) I61.3
    - traumatic S06.38- ☑
  - breast N64.59
  - bronchial tube — *see* Hemorrhage, lung
  - bronchopulmonary — *see* Hemorrhage, lung
  - bronchus — *see* Hemorrhage, lung
  - bulbar I61.5
  - capillary I78.8
    - primary D69.8
  - cecum K92.2
  - cerebellar, cerebellum (nontraumatic) I61.4
    - newborn P52.6
    - traumatic S06.37- ☑
  - cerebral, cerebrum (*see also* Hemorrhage, intracranial, intracerebral)
    - lobe I61.1
    - newborn (anoxic) P52.4
      - birth injury P10.1
  - cerebromeningeal I61.8
  - cerebrospinal — *see* Hemorrhage, intracranial, intracerebral
  - cervix (uteri) (stump) NEC N88.8
- **Hemorrhage, hemorrhagic** — *continued*
  - chamber, anterior (eye) — *see* Hyphema
  - childbirth — *see* Hemorrhage, complicating, delivery
  - choroid H31.30- ☑
    - expulsive H31.31- ☑
  - ciliary body — *see* Hyphema
  - cochlea — *see* subcategory H83.8 ☑
  - colon K92.2
  - complicating
    - abortion — *see* Abortion, by type, complicated by, hemorrhage
    - delivery O67.9
      - associated with coagulation defect (afibrinogenemia) (DIC) (hyperfibrinolysis) O67.0
      - specified cause NEC O67.8
    - surgical procedure — *see* Hemorrhage, intraoperative
  - conjunctiva H11.3- ☑
    - newborn P54.8
  - cord, newborn (stump) P51.9
  - corpus luteum (ruptured) cyst N83.1
  - cortical (brain) I61.1
  - cranial — *see* Hemorrhage, intracranial
  - cutaneous R23.3
    - due to autosensitivity, erythrocyte D69.2
    - newborn P54.5
  - delayed
    - following ectopic or molar pregnancy O08.1
    - postpartum O72.2
  - diathesis (familial) D69.9
  - disease D69.9
    - newborn P53
    - specified type NEC D69.8
  - due to or associated with
    - afibrinogenemia or other coagulation defect (conditions in categories D65- D69)
      - antepartum — *see* Hemorrhage, antepartum, with coagulation defect
      - intrapartum O67.0
    - dental implant M27.61
    - device, implant or graft (*see also* Complications, by site and type, specified NEC) T85.83 ☑
      - arterial graft NEC T82.838 ☑
      - breast T85.83 ☑
      - catheter NEC T85.83 ☑
        - dialysis (renal) T82.838 ☑
          - intraperitoneal T85.83 ☑
        - infusion NEC T82.838 ☑
          - spinal (epidural) (subdural) T85.83 ☑
        - urinary (indwelling) T83.83 ☑
      - electronic (electrode) (pulse generator) (stimulator)
        - bone T84.83 ☑
        - cardiac T82.837 ☑
        - nervous system (brain) (peripheral nerve) (spinal) T85.83 ☑
        - urinary T83.83 ☑
      - fixation, internal (orthopedic) NEC T84.83 ☑
      - gastrointestinal (bile duct) (esophagus) T85.83 ☑
      - genital NEC T83.83 ☑
      - heart NEC T82.837 ☑
      - joint prosthesis T84.83 ☑
      - ocular (corneal graft) (orbital implant) NEC T85.83 ☑
      - orthopedic NEC T84.83 ☑
        - bone graft T86.838
      - specified NEC T85.83 ☑
      - urinary NEC T83.83 ☑
      - vascular NEC T82.838 ☑
      - ventricular intracranial shunt T85.83 ☑
  - duodenum, duodenal K92.2
    - ulcer — *see* Ulcer, duodenum, with hemorrhage
  - dura mater — *see* Hemorrhage, intracranial, subdural
  - endotracheal — *see* Hemorrhage, lung
  - epicranial subaponeurotic (massive), birth injury P12.2
  - epidural (traumatic) (*see also* Injury, intracranial, epidural hemorrhage)
    - nontraumatic I62.1
  - esophagus K22.8
    - varix I85.01
      - secondary I85.11
  - excessive, following ectopic gestation (subsequent episode) O08.1
  - extradural (traumatic) — *see* Injury, intracranial, epidural hemorrhage
    - birth injury P10.8

- **Hemorrhage, hemorrhagic** — *continued*
  - extradural — *see* Injury, intracranial, epidural hemorrhage — *continued*
    - newborn (anoxic) (nontraumatic) P52.8
    - nontraumatic I62.1
  - eye NEC H57.8
    - fundus — *see* Hemorrhage, retina
    - lid — *see* Disorder, eyelid, specified type NEC
  - fallopian tube N83.6
  - fibrinogenolysis — *see* Fibrinolysis
  - fibrinolytic (acquired) — *see* Fibrinolysis
  - from
    - ear (nontraumatic) — *see* Otorrhagia
    - tracheostomy stoma J95.Ø1
  - fundus, eye — *see* Hemorrhage, retina
  - funis — *see* Hemorrhage, umbilicus, cord
  - gastric — *see* Hemorrhage, stomach
  - gastroenteric K92.2
    - newborn P54.3
  - gastrointestinal (tract) K92.2
    - newborn P54.3
  - genital organ, male N5Ø.1
  - genitourinary (tract) NOS R31.9
  - gingiva KØ6.8
  - globe (eye) — *see* Hemophthalmos
  - graafian follicle cyst (ruptured) N83.Ø
  - gum KØ6.8
  - heart I51.89
  - hypopharyngeal (throat) RØ4.1
  - intermenstrual (regular) N92.3
    - irregular N92.1
  - internal (organs) NEC R58
    - capsule I61.Ø
    - ear — *see* subcategory H83.8 ☑
    - newborn P54.8
  - intestine K92.2
    - newborn P54.3
  - intra-abdominal R58
  - intra-alveolar (lung), newborn P26.8
  - intracerebral (nontraumatic) — *see* Hemorrhage, intracranial, intracerebral
  - intracranial (nontraumatic) I62.9
    - birth injury P1Ø.9
    - epidural, nontraumatic I62.1
    - extradural, nontraumatic I62.1
    - intracerebral (nontraumatic) (in) I61.9
      - brain stem I61.3
      - cerebellum I61.4
      - hemisphere I61.2
        - cortical (superficial) I61.1
        - subcortical (deep) I61.Ø
      - intraoperative
        - during a nervous system procedure G97.31
        - during other procedure G97.32
      - intraventricular I61.5
      - multiple localized I61.6
      - newborn P52.4
        - birth injury P1Ø.1
      - postprocedural
        - following a nervous system procedure G97.51
        - following other procedure G97.52
      - specified NEC I61.8
      - superficial I61.1
      - traumatic (diffuse) — *see* Injury, intracranial, diffuse
        - focal — *see* Injury, intracranial, focal
    - newborn P52.9
      - specified NEC P52.8
    - subarachnoid (nontraumatic) (from) I6Ø.9
      - intracranial (cerebral) artery I6Ø.7
        - anterior communicating I6Ø.2- ☑
        - basilar I6Ø.4
        - carotid siphon and bifurcation I6Ø.Ø- ☑
        - communicating I6Ø.7
          - anterior I6Ø.2- ☑
          - posterior I6Ø.3- ☑
        - middle cerebral I6Ø.1- ☑
        - posterior communicating I6Ø.3- ☑
        - specified artery NEC I6Ø.6
        - vertebral I6Ø.5- ☑
      - newborn P52.5
        - birth injury P1Ø.3
      - specified NEC I6Ø.8
      - traumatic SØ6.6X- ☑
    - subdural (nontraumatic) I62.ØØ
      - acute I62.Ø1
      - birth injury P1Ø.Ø

- **Hemorrhage, hemorrhagic** — *continued*
  - intracranial — *continued*
    - subdural — *continued*
      - chronic I62.Ø3
      - newborn (anoxic) (hypoxic) P52.8
        - birth injury P1Ø.Ø
      - spinal G95.19
      - subacute I62.Ø2
      - traumatic — *see* Injury, intracranial, subdural hemorrhage
    - traumatic — *see* Injury, intracranial, focal brain injury
  - intramedullary NEC G95.19
  - intraocular — *see* Hemophthalmos
  - intraoperative, intraprocedural — *see* Complication, hemorrhage (hematoma), intraoperative (intraprocedural), by site
  - intrapartum — *see* Hemorrhage, complicating, delivery
  - intrapelvic
    - female N94.89
    - male K66.1
  - intraperitoneal K66.1
  - intrapontine I61.3
  - intraprocedural — *see* Complication, hemorrhage (hematoma), intraoperative (intraprocedural), by site
  - intrauterine N85.7
    - complicating delivery (*see also* Hemorrhage, complicating, delivery) O67.9
    - postpartum — *see* Hemorrhage, postpartum
  - intraventricular I61.5
    - newborn (nontraumatic) (*see also* Newborn, affected by, hemorrhage) P52.3
      - due to birth injury P1Ø.2
      - grade
        - 1 P52.Ø
        - 2 P52.1
        - 3 P52.21
        - 4 P52.22
  - intravesical N32.89
  - iris (postinfectional) (postinflammatory) (toxic) — *see* Hyphema
  - joint (nontraumatic) — *see* Hemarthrosis
  - kidney N28.89
  - knee (joint) (nontraumatic) — *see* Hemarthrosis, knee
  - labyrinth — *see* subcategory H83.8 ☑
  - lenticular striate artery I61.Ø
  - ligature, vessel — *see* Hemorrhage, postoperative
  - liver K76.89
  - lung RØ4.89
    - newborn P26.9
      - massive P26.1
      - specified NEC P26.8
    - tuberculous — *see* Tuberculosis, pulmonary
  - massive umbilical, newborn P51.Ø
  - mediastinum — *see* Hemorrhage, lung
  - medulla I61.3
  - membrane (brain) I6Ø.8
    - spinal cord — *see* Hemorrhage, spinal cord
  - meninges, meningeal (brain) (middle) I6Ø.8
    - spinal cord — *see* Hemorrhage, spinal cord
  - mesentery K66.1
  - metritis — *see* Endometritis
  - mouth K13.79
  - mucous membrane NEC R58
    - newborn P54.8
  - muscle M62.89
  - nail (subungual) L6Ø.8
  - nasal turbinate RØ4.Ø
    - newborn P54.8
  - navel, newborn P51.9
  - newborn P54.9
    - specified NEC P54.8
  - nipple N64.59
  - nose RØ4.Ø
    - newborn P54.8
  - omentum K66.1
  - optic nerve (sheath) H47.Ø2- ☑
  - orbit, orbital HØ5.23- ☑
  - ovary NEC N83.8
  - oviduct N83.6
  - pancreas K86.8
  - parathyroid (gland) (spontaneous) E21.4
  - parturition — *see* Hemorrhage, complicating, delivery
  - penis N48.89
  - pericardium, pericarditis I31.2
  - peritoneum, peritoneal K66.1

- **Hemorrhage, hemorrhagic** — *continued*
  - peritonsillar tissue J35.8
    - due to infection J36
  - petechial R23.3
    - due to autosensitivity, erythrocyte D69.2
  - pituitary (gland) E23.6
  - pleura — *see* Hemorrhage, lung
  - polioencephalitis, superior E51.2
  - polymyositis — *see* Polymyositis
  - pons, pontine I61.3
  - posterior fossa (nontraumatic) I61.8
    - newborn P52.6
  - postmenopausal N95.Ø
  - postnasal RØ4.Ø
  - postoperative — *see* Complications, postprocedural, hemorrhage, by site
  - postpartum NEC (following delivery of placenta) O72.1
    - delayed or secondary O72.2
    - retained placenta O72.Ø
    - third stage O72.Ø
  - pregnancy — *see* Hemorrhage, antepartum
  - preretinal — *see* Hemorrhage, retina
  - prostate N42.1
  - puerperal — *see* Hemorrhage, postpartum
    - delayed or secondary O72.2
  - pulmonary RØ4.89
    - newborn P26.9
      - massive P26.1
      - specified NEC P26.8
    - tuberculous — *see* Tuberculosis, pulmonary
  - purpura (primary) D69.3
  - rectum (sphincter) K62.5
    - newborn P54.2
  - recurring, following initial hemorrhage at time of injury T79.2 ☑
  - renal N28.89
  - respiratory passage or tract RØ4.9
    - specified NEC RØ4.89
  - retina, retinal (vessels) H35.6- ☑
    - diabetic — *see* Diabetes, retinal, hemorrhage
  - retroperitoneal R58
  - scalp R58
  - scrotum N5Ø.1
  - secondary (nontraumatic) R58
    - following initial hemorrhage at time of injury T79.2 ☑
  - seminal vesicle N5Ø.1
  - skin R23.3
    - newborn P54.5
  - slipped umbilical ligature P51.8
  - spermatic cord N5Ø.1
  - spinal (cord) G95.19
    - newborn (birth injury) P11.5
  - spleen D73.5
    - intraoperative — *see* Complications, intraoperative, hemorrhage, spleen
    - postprocedural — *see* Complications, postprocedural, hemorrhage, spleen
  - stomach K92.2
    - newborn P54.3
    - ulcer — *see* Ulcer, stomach, with hemorrhage
  - subarachnoid (nontraumatic) — *see* Hemorrhage, intracranial, subarachnoid
  - subconjunctival (*see also* Hemorrhage, conjunctiva)
    - birth injury P15.3
  - subcortical (brain) I61.Ø
  - subcutaneous R23.3
  - subdiaphragmatic R58
  - subdural (acute) (nontraumatic) — *see* Hemorrhage, intracranial, subdural
  - subependymal
    - newborn P52.Ø
      - with intraventricular extension P52.1
        - and intracerebral extension P52.22
  - subgaleal P12.1
  - subhyaloid — *see* Hemorrhage, retina
  - subperiosteal — *see* Disorder, bone, specified type NEC
  - subretinal — *see* Hemorrhage, retina
  - subtentorial — *see* Hemorrhage, intracranial, subdural
  - subungual L6Ø.8
  - suprarenal (capsule) (gland) E27.49
    - newborn P54.4
  - tentorium (traumatic) NEC — *see* Hemorrhage, brain
    - newborn (birth injury) P1Ø.4
  - testis N5Ø.1
  - third stage (postpartum) O72.Ø
  - thorax — *see* Hemorrhage, lung

- **Hemorrhage, hemorrhagic** — *continued*
  - throat RØ4.1
  - thymus (gland) E32.8
  - thyroid (cyst) (gland) EØ7.89
  - tongue K14.8
  - tonsil J35.8
  - trachea — *see* Hemorrhage, lung
  - tracheobronchial RØ4.89
    - newborn P26.Ø
  - traumatic — *code to* specific injury
    - cerebellar — *see* Hemorrhage, brain
    - intracranial — *see* Hemorrhage, brain
    - recurring or secondary (following initial hemorrhage at time of injury) T79.2 ☑
  - tuberculous NEC (*see also* Tuberculosis, pulmonary) A15.Ø
  - tunica vaginalis N5Ø.1
  - ulcer — *code by* site under Ulcer, with hemorrhage K27.4
  - umbilicus, umbilical
    - cord
      - after birth, newborn P51.9
      - complicating delivery O69.5 ☑
    - newborn P51.9
      - massive P51.Ø
      - slipped ligature P51.8
    - stump P51.9
  - urethra (idiopathic) N36.8
  - uterus, uterine (abnormal) N93.9
    - climacteric N92.4
    - complicating delivery — *see* Hemorrhage, complicating, delivery
    - dysfunctional or functional N93.8
    - intermenstrual (regular) N92.3
      - irregular N92.1
    - postmenopausal N95.Ø
    - postpartum — *see* Hemorrhage, postpartum
    - preclimacteric or premenopausal N92.4
    - prepubertal N93.8
    - pubertal N92.2
  - vagina (abnormal) N93.9
    - newborn P54.6
  - vas deferens N5Ø.1
  - vasa previa O69.4 ☑
  - ventricular I61.5
  - vesical N32.89
  - viscera NEC R58
    - newborn P54.8
  - vitreous (humor) (intraocular) H43.1- ☑
  - vulva N9Ø.89
- **Hemorrhoids** (bleeding) (without mention of degree) K64.9
  - 1st degree (grade/stage I) (without prolapse outside of anal canal) K64.Ø
  - 2nd degree (grade/stage II) (that prolapse with straining but retract spontaneously) K64.1
  - 3rd degree (grade/stage III) (that prolapse with straining and require manual replacement back inside anal canal) K64.2
  - 4th degree (grade/stage IV) (with prolapsed tissue that cannot be manually replaced) K64.3
  - complicating
    - pregnancy O22.4 ☑
    - puerperium O87.2
  - external K64.4
    - with
      - thrombosis K64.5
  - internal (without mention of degree) K64.8
  - prolapsed K64.8
  - skin tags
    - anus K64.4
    - residual K64.4
  - specified NEC K64.8
  - strangulated (*see also* Hemorrhoids, by degree) K64.8
  - thrombosed (*see also* Hemorrhoids, by degree) K64.5
  - ulcerated (*see also* Hemorrhoids, by degree) K64.8
- **Hemosalpinx** N83.6
  - with
    - hematocolpos N89.7
    - hematometra N85.7
      - with hematocolpos N89.7
- **Hemosiderosis** (dietary) E83.19
  - pulmonary, idiopathic E83.1- ☑ [J84.Ø3]
  - transfusion T8Ø.89 ☑
- **Hemothorax** (bacterial) (nontuberculous) J94.2
  - newborn P54.8
  - traumatic S27.1 ☑
    - with pneumothorax S27.2 ☑
- **Hemothorax** — *continued*
  - tuberculous NEC A15.6
- **Henoch** (-Schönlein) **disease or syndrome** (purpura) D69.Ø
- **Henpue, henpuye** A66.6
- **Hepar lobatum** (syphilitic) A52.74
- **Hepatalgia** K76.89
- **Hepatitis** K75.9
  - acute B17.9
    - with coma K72.Ø1
    - with hepatic failure — *see* Failure, hepatic
    - alcoholic — *see* Hepatitis, alcoholic
    - infectious B15.9
      - with hepatic coma B15.Ø
    - viral B17.9
  - alcoholic (acute) (chronic) K7Ø.1Ø
    - with ascites K7Ø.11
  - amebic — *see* Abscess, liver, amebic
  - anicteric, (viral) — *see* Hepatitis, viral
  - antigen-associated (HAA) — *see* Hepatitis, B
  - Australia-antigen (positive) — *see* Hepatitis, B
  - autoimmune K75.4
  - B B19.1Ø
    - with hepatic coma B19.11
    - acute B16.9
      - with
        - delta-agent (coinfection) (without hepatic coma) B16.1
          - with hepatic coma B16.Ø
        - hepatic coma (without delta-agent coinfection) B16.2
    - chronic B18.1
      - with delta-agent B18.Ø
  - bacterial NEC K75.89
  - C (viral) B19.2Ø
    - with hepatic coma B19.21
    - acute B17.1Ø
      - with hepatic coma B17.11
    - chronic B18.2
  - catarrhal (acute) B15.9
    - with hepatic coma B15.Ø
  - cholangiolitic K75.89
  - cholestatic K75.89
  - chronic K73.9
    - active NEC K73.2
    - lobular NEC K73.1
    - persistent NEC K73.Ø
    - specified NEC K73.8
  - cytomegaloviral B25.1
  - due to ethanol (acute) (chronic) — *see* Hepatitis, alcoholic
  - epidemic B15.9
    - with hepatic coma B15.Ø
  - fulminant NEC (viral) — *see* Hepatitis, viral
  - granulomatous NEC K75.3
  - herpesviral BØØ.81
  - history of
    - B Z86.19
    - C Z86.19
  - homologous serum — *see* Hepatitis, viral, type B
  - in (due to)
    - mumps B26.81
    - toxoplasmosis (acquired) B58.1
      - congenital (active) P37.1 [K77]
  - infectious, infective (acute) (chronic) (subacute) B15.9
    - with hepatic coma B15.Ø
  - inoculation — *see* Hepatitis, viral, type B
  - interstitial (chronic) K74.69
  - lupoid NEC K75.4
  - malignant NEC (with hepatic failure) K72.9Ø
    - with coma K72.91
  - neonatal (idiopathic) (toxic) P59.29
  - neonatal giant cell P59.29
  - newborn P59.29
  - postimmunization — *see* Hepatitis, viral, type B
  - post-transfusion — *see* Hepatitis, viral, type B
  - reactive, nonspecific K75.2
  - serum — *see* Hepatitis, viral, type B
  - specified type NEC
    - with hepatic failure — *see* Failure, hepatic
  - syphilitic (late) A52.74
    - congenital (early) A5Ø.Ø8 [K77]
      - late A5Ø.59 [K77]
    - secondary A51.45
  - toxic (*see also* Disease, liver, toxic) K71.6
  - tuberculous A18.83
  - viral, virus B19.9
    - with hepatic coma B19.Ø
- **Hepatitis** — *continued*
  - viral, virus — *continued*
    - acute B17.9
    - chronic B18.9
      - specified NEC B18.8
      - type
        - B B18.1
          - with delta-agent B18.Ø
        - C B18.2
    - congenital P35.3
    - coxsackie B33.8 [K77]
    - cytomegalic inclusion B25.1
    - in remission, any type — *code to* Hepatitis, chronic, by type
    - non-A, non-B B17.8
    - specified type NEC (with or without coma) B17.8
    - type
      - A B15.9
        - with hepatic coma B15.Ø
      - B B19.1Ø
        - with hepatic coma B19.11
        - acute B16.9
          - with
            - delta-agent (coinfection) (without hepatic coma) B16.1
              - with hepatic coma B16.Ø
            - hepatic coma (without delta-agent coinfection) B16.2
        - chronic B18.1
          - with delta-agent B18.Ø
      - C B19.2Ø
        - with hepatic coma B19.21
        - acute B17.1Ø
          - with hepatic coma B17.11
        - chronic B18.2
      - E B17.2
      - non-A, non-B B17.8
- **Hepatization lung** (acute) — *see* Pneumonia, lobar
- **Hepatoblastoma** C22.2
- **Hepatocarcinoma** C22.Ø
- **Hepatocholangiocarcinoma** C22.Ø
- **Hepatocholangioma, benign** D13.4
- **Hepatocholangitis** K75.89
- **Hepatolenticular degeneration** E83.Ø1
- **Hepatoma** (malignant) C22.Ø
  - benign D13.4
  - embryonal C22.Ø
- **Hepatomegaly** (*see also* Hypertrophy, liver)
  - with splenomegaly R16.2
  - congenital Q44.7
  - in mononucleosis
    - gammaherpesviral B27.Ø9
    - infectious specified NEC B27.89
- **Hepatoptosis** K76.89
- **Hepatorenal syndrome following labor and delivery** O9Ø.4
- **Hepatosis** K76.89
- **Hepatosplenomegaly** R16.2
  - hyperlipemic (Bürger-Grütz type) E78.3 [K77]
- **Hereditary** — *see* condition
- **Heredodegeneration, macular** — *see* Dystrophy, retina
- **Heredopathia atactica polyneuritiformis** G6Ø.1
- **Heredosyphilis** — *see* Syphilis, congenital
- **Herlitz' syndrome** Q81.1
- **Hermansky-Pudlak syndrome** E7Ø.331
- **Hermaphrodite, hermaphroditism** (true) Q56.Ø
  - 46,XX with streak gonads Q99.1
  - 46,XX/46,XY Q99.Ø
  - 46,XY with streak gonads Q99.1
  - chimera 46,XX/46,XY Q99.Ø
- **Hernia, hernial** (acquired) (recurrent) K46.9
  - with
    - gangrene — *see* Hernia, by site, with, gangrene
    - incarceration — *see* Hernia, by site, with, obstruction
    - irreducible — *see* Hernia, by site, with, obstruction
    - obstruction — *see* Hernia, by site, with, obstruction
    - strangulation — *see* Hernia, by site, with, obstruction
  - abdomen, abdominal K46.9
    - with
      - gangrene (and obstruction) K46.1
      - obstruction K46.Ø
    - femoral — *see* Hernia, femoral
    - incisional — *see* Hernia, incisional
    - inguinal — *see* Hernia, inguinal
    - specified site NEC K45.8

- **Hernia, hernial** — *continued*
  - abdomen, abdominal — *continued*
    - specified site — *continued*
      - with
        - gangrene (and obstruction) K45.1
        - obstruction K45.Ø
    - umbilical — *see* Hernia, umbilical
    - wall — *see* Hernia, ventral
  - appendix — *see* Hernia, abdomen
  - bladder (mucosa) (sphincter)
    - congenital (female) (male) Q79.51
    - female — *see* Cystocele
    - male N32.89
  - brain, congenital — *see* Encephalocele
  - cartilage, vertebra — *see* Displacement, intervertebral disc
  - cerebral, congenital (*see also* Encephalocele)
    - endaural QØ1.8
  - ciliary body (traumatic) SØ5.2- ☑
  - colon — *see* Hernia, abdomen
  - Cooper's — *see* Hernia, abdomen, specified site NEC
  - crural — *see* Hernia, femoral
  - diaphragm, diaphragmatic K44.9
    - with
      - gangrene (and obstruction) K44.1
      - obstruction K44.Ø
    - congenital Q79.Ø
  - direct (inguinal) — *see* Hernia, inguinal
  - diverticulum, intestine — *see* Hernia, abdomen
  - double (inguinal) — *see* Hernia, inguinal, bilateral
  - due to adhesions (with obstruction) K56.5
  - epigastric (*see also* Hernia, ventral) K43.9
  - esophageal hiatus — *see* Hernia, hiatal
  - external (inguinal) — *see* Hernia, inguinal
  - fallopian tube N83.4
  - fascia M62.89
  - femoral K41.9Ø
    - with
      - gangrene (and obstruction) K41.4Ø
        - not specified as recurrent K41.4Ø
        - recurrent K41.41
      - obstruction K41.3Ø
        - not specified as recurrent K41.3Ø
        - recurrent K41.31
    - bilateral K41.2Ø
      - with
        - gangrene (and obstruction) K41.1Ø
          - not specified as recurrent K41.1Ø
          - recurrent K41.11
        - obstruction K41.ØØ
          - not specified as recurrent K41.ØØ
          - recurrent K41.Ø1
      - not specified as recurrent K41.2Ø
      - recurrent K41.21
    - not specified as recurrent K41.9Ø
    - recurrent K41.91
    - unilateral K41.9Ø
      - with
        - gangrene (and obstruction) K41.4Ø
          - not specified as recurrent K41.4Ø
          - recurrent K41.41
        - obstruction K41.3Ø
          - not specified as recurrent K41.3Ø
          - recurrent K41.31
      - not specified as recurrent K41.9Ø
      - recurrent K41.91
  - foramen magnum G93.5
    - congenital QØ1.8
  - funicular (umbilical) (*see also* Hernia, umbilicus)
    - spermatic (cord) — *see* Hernia, inguinal
  - gastrointestinal tract — *see* Hernia, abdomen
  - Hesselbach's — *see* Hernia, femoral, specified site NEC
  - hiatal (esophageal) (sliding) K44.9
    - with
      - gangrene (and obstruction) K44.1
      - obstruction K44.Ø
    - congenital Q4Ø.1
  - hypogastric — *see* Hernia, ventral
  - incarcerated (*see also* Hernia, by site, with obstruction)
    - with gangrene — *see* Hernia, by site, with gangrene
  - incisional K43.2
    - with
      - gangrene (and obstruction) K43.1
      - obstruction K43.Ø
  - indirect (inguinal) — *see* Hernia, inguinal
  - inguinal (direct) (external) (funicular) (indirect) (internal) (oblique) (scrotal) (sliding) K4Ø.9Ø

- **Hernia, hernial** — *continued*
  - inguinal — *continued*
    - with
      - gangrene (and obstruction) K4Ø.4Ø
        - not specified as recurrent K4Ø.4Ø
        - recurrent K4Ø.41
      - obstruction K4Ø.3Ø
        - not specified as recurrent K4Ø.3Ø
        - recurrent K4Ø.31
    - bilateral K4Ø.2Ø
      - with
        - gangrene (and obstruction) K4Ø.1Ø
          - not specified as recurrent K4Ø.1Ø
          - recurrent K4Ø.11
        - obstruction K4Ø.ØØ
          - not specified as recurrent K4Ø.ØØ
          - recurrent K4Ø.Ø1
      - not specified as recurrent K4Ø.2Ø
      - recurrent K4Ø.21
    - not specified as recurrent K4Ø.9Ø
    - recurrent K4Ø.91
    - unilateral K4Ø.9Ø
      - with
        - gangrene (and obstruction) K4Ø.4Ø
          - not specified as recurrent K4Ø.4Ø
          - recurrent K4Ø.41
        - obstruction K4Ø.3Ø
          - not specified as recurrent K4Ø.3Ø
          - recurrent K4Ø.31
      - not specified as recurrent K4Ø.9Ø
      - recurrent K4Ø.91
  - internal (*see also* Hernia, abdomen)
    - inguinal — *see* Hernia, inguinal
  - interstitial — *see* Hernia, abdomen
  - intervertebral cartilage or disc — *see* Displacement, intervertebral disc
  - intestine, intestinal — *see* Hernia, by site
  - intra-abdominal — *see* Hernia, abdomen
  - iris (traumatic) SØ5.2- ☑
  - irreducible (*see also* Hernia, by site, with obstruction)
    - with gangrene — *see* Hernia, by site, with gangrene
  - ischiatic — *see* Hernia, abdomen, specified site NEC
  - ischiorectal — *see* Hernia, abdomen, specified site NEC
  - lens (traumatic) SØ5.2- ☑
  - linea (alba) (semilunaris) — *see* Hernia, ventral
  - Littre's — *see* Hernia, abdomen
  - lumbar — *see* Hernia, abdomen, specified site NEC
  - lung (subcutaneous) J98.4
  - mediastinum J98.5
  - mesenteric (internal) — *see* Hernia, abdomen
  - midline — *see* Hernia, ventral
  - muscle (sheath) M62.89
  - nucleus pulposus — *see* Displacement, intervertebral disc
  - oblique (inguinal) — *see* Hernia, inguinal
  - obstructive (*see also* Hernia, by site, with obstruction)
    - with gangrene — *see* Hernia, by site, with gangrene
  - obturator — *see* Hernia, abdomen, specified site NEC
  - omental — *see* Hernia, abdomen
  - ovary N83.4
  - oviduct N83.4
  - paraesophageal (*see also* Hernia, diaphragm)
    - congenital Q4Ø.1
  - parastomal K43.5
    - with
      - gangrene (and obstruction) K43.4
      - obstruction K43.3
  - paraumbilical — *see* Hernia, umbilicus
  - perineal — *see* Hernia, abdomen, specified site NEC
  - Petit's — *see* Hernia, abdomen, specified site NEC
  - postoperative — *see* Hernia, incisional
  - pregnant uterus — *see* Abnormal, uterus in pregnancy or childbirth
  - prevesical N32.89
  - properitoneal — *see* Hernia, abdomen, specified site NEC
  - pudendal — *see* Hernia, abdomen, specified site NEC
  - rectovaginal N81.6
  - retroperitoneal — *see* Hernia, abdomen, specified site NEC
  - Richter's — *see* Hernia, abdomen, with obstruction
  - Rieux's, Riex's — *see* Hernia, abdomen, specified site NEC

- **Hernia, hernial** — *continued*
  - sac condition (adhesion) (dropsy) (inflammation) (laceration) (suppuration) — *code by site under* Hernia
  - sciatic — *see* Hernia, abdomen, specified site NEC
  - scrotum, scrotal — *see* Hernia, inguinal
  - sliding (inguinal) (*see also* Hernia, inguinal)
    - hiatus — *see* Hernia, hiatal
  - spigelian — *see* Hernia, ventral
  - spinal — *see* Spina bifida
  - strangulated (*see also* Hernia, by site, with obstruction)
    - with gangrene — *see* Hernia, by site, with gangrene
  - subxiphoid — *see* Hernia, ventral
  - supra-umbilicus — *see* Hernia, ventral
  - tendon — *see* Disorder, tendon, specified type NEC
  - Treitz's (fossa) — *see* Hernia, abdomen, specified site NEC
  - tunica vaginalis Q55.29
  - umbilicus, umbilical K42.9
    - with
      - gangrene (and obstruction) K42.1
      - obstruction K42.Ø
  - ureter N28.89
  - urethra, congenital Q64.79
  - urinary meatus, congenital Q64.79
  - uterus N81.4
    - pregnant — *see* Abnormal, uterus in pregnancy or childbirth
  - vaginal (anterior) (wall) — *see* Cystocele
  - Velpeau's — *see* Hernia, femoral
  - ventral K43.9
    - with
      - gangrene (and obstruction) K43.7
      - obstruction K43.6
    - incisional K43.2
      - with
        - gangrene (and obstruction) K43.1
        - obstruction K43.Ø
    - recurrent — *see* Hernia, incisional
    - specified NEC K43.9
      - with
        - gangrene (and obstruction) K43.7
        - obstruction K43.6
  - vesical
    - congenital (female) (male) Q79.51
    - female — *see* Cystocele
    - male N32.89
  - vitreous (into wound) SØ5.2- ☑
    - into anterior chamber — *see* Prolapse, vitreous
- **Herniation** (*see also* Hernia)
  - brain (stem) G93.5
  - cerebral G93.5
  - mediastinum J98.5
  - nucleus pulposus — *see* Displacement, intervertebral disc
- **Herpangina** BØ8.5
- **Herpes, herpesvirus, herpetic** BØØ.9
  - anogenital A6Ø.9
    - perianal skin A6Ø.1
    - rectum A6Ø.1
    - urogenital tract A6Ø.ØØ
      - cervix A6Ø.Ø3
      - male genital organ NEC A6Ø.Ø2
      - penis A6Ø.Ø1
      - specified site NEC A6Ø.Ø9
      - vagina A6Ø.Ø4
      - vulva A6Ø.Ø4
  - blepharitis (zoster) BØ2.39
    - simplex BØØ.59
  - circinatus B35.4
    - bullosus L12.Ø
  - conjunctivitis (simplex) BØØ.53
    - zoster BØ2.31
  - cornea BØ2.33
  - encephalitis BØØ.4
    - due to herpesvirus 6 B1Ø.Ø1
    - due to herpesvirus 7 B1Ø.Ø9
    - specified NEC B1Ø.Ø9
  - eye (zoster) BØ2.3Ø
    - simplex BØØ.5Ø
  - eyelid (zoster) BØ2.39
    - simplex BØØ.59
  - facialis BØØ.1
  - febrilis BØØ.1
  - geniculate ganglionitis BØ2.21
  - genital, genitalis A6Ø.ØØ
    - female A6Ø.Ø9

Herpes, herpesvirus, herpetic — *continued*
- genital, genitalis — *continued*
  - male A6Ø.Ø2
- gestational, gestationis O26.4- ☑
- gingivostomatitis BØØ.2
- human BØØ.9
  - 1 — *see* Herpes, simplex
  - 2 — *see* Herpes, simplex
  - 3 — *see* Varicella
  - 4 — *see* Mononucleosis, Epstein-Barr (virus)
  - 5 — *see* Disease, cytomegalic inclusion (generalized)
  - 6
    - encephalitis B1Ø.Ø1
    - specified NEC B1Ø.81
  - 7
    - encephalitis B1Ø.Ø9
    - specified NEC B1Ø.82
  - 8 B1Ø.89
- infection NEC B1Ø.89
  - Kaposi's sarcoma associated B1Ø.89
- iridocyclitis (simplex) BØØ.51
  - zoster BØ2.32
- iris (vesicular erythema multiforme) L51.9
- iritis (simplex) BØØ.51
- Kaposi's sarcoma associated B1Ø.89
- keratitis (simplex) (dendritic) (disciform) (interstitial) BØØ.52
  - zoster (interstitial) BØ2.33
- keratoconjunctivitis (simplex) BØØ.52
  - zoster BØ2.33
- labialis BØØ.1
- lip BØØ.1
- meningitis (simplex) BØØ.3
  - zoster BØ2.1
- ophthalmicus (zoster) NEC BØ2.3Ø
  - simplex BØØ.5Ø
- penis A6Ø.Ø1
- perianal skin A6Ø.1
- pharyngitis, pharyngotonsillitis BØØ.2
- rectum A6Ø.1
- scrotum A6Ø.Ø2
- sepsis BØØ.7
- simplex BØØ.9
  - complicated NEC BØØ.89
  - congenital P35.2
  - conjunctivitis BØØ.53
  - external ear BØØ.1
  - eyelid BØØ.59
  - hepatitis BØØ.81
  - keratitis (interstitial) BØØ.52
  - myleitis BØØ.82
  - specified complication NEC BØØ.89
  - visceral BØØ.89
- stomatitis BØØ.2
- tonsurans B35.Ø
- visceral BØØ.89
- vulva A6Ø.Ø4
- whitlow BØØ.89
- zoster (*see also* condition) BØ2.9
  - auricularis BØ2.21
  - complicated NEC BØ2.8
  - conjunctivitis BØ2.31
  - disseminated BØ2.7
  - encephalitis BØ2.Ø
  - eye (lid) BØ2.39
  - geniculate ganglionitis BØ2.21
  - keratitis (interstitial) BØ2.33
  - meningitis BØ2.1
  - myelitis BØ2.24
  - neuritis, neuralgia BØ2.29
  - ophthalmicus NEC BØ2.3Ø
  - oticus BØ2.21
  - polyneuropathy BØ2.23
  - specified complication NEC BØ2.8
  - trigeminal neuralgia BØ2.22

Herpesvirus (human) — *see* Herpes

Herpetophobia F4Ø.218

Herrick's anemia — *see* Disease, sickle-cell

Hers' disease E74.Ø9

Herter-Gee syndrome K9Ø.Ø

Herxheimer's reaction R68.89

Hesitancy
- of micturition R39.11
- urinary R39.11

Hesselbach's hernia — *see* Hernia, femoral, specified site NEC

Heterochromia (congenital) Q13.2

Heterochromia — *continued*
- cataract — *see* Cataract, complicated
- cyclitis (Fuchs) — *see* Cyclitis, Fuchs' heterochromic
- hair L67.1
- iritis — *see* Cyclitis, Fuchs' heterochromic
- retained metallic foreign body (nonmagnetic) — *see* Foreign body, intraocular, old, retained
  - magnetic — *see* Foreign body, intraocular, old, retained, magnetic
- uveitis — *see* Cyclitis, Fuchs' heterochromic

Heterophoria — *see* Strabismus, heterophoria

Heterophyes, heterophyiasis (small intestine) B66.8

Heterotopia, heterotopic (*see also* Malposition, congenital)
- cerebralis QØ4.8

Heterotropia — *see* Strabismus

Heubner-Herter disease K9Ø.Ø

Hexadactylism Q69.9

HGSIL (cytology finding) (high grade squamous intraepithelial lesion on cytologic smear) (Pap smear finding)
- anus R85.613
- cervix R87.613
  - biopsy (histology) finding — *code to* CIN II or CIN III
- vagina R87.623
  - biopsy (histology) finding — *code to* VAIN II or VAIN III

Hibernoma — *see* Lipoma

Hiccup, hiccough RØ6.6
- epidemic B33.Ø
- psychogenic F45.8

Hidden penis (congenital) Q55.64
- acquired N48.83

Hidradenitis (axillaris) (suppurative) L73.2

Hidradenoma (nodular) (*see also* Neoplasm, skin, benign)
- clear cell — *see* Neoplasm, skin, benign
- papillary — *see* Neoplasm, skin, benign

Hidrocystoma — *see* Neoplasm, skin, benign

High
- altitude effects T7Ø.2Ø ☑
  - anoxia T7Ø.29 ☑
  - on
    - ears T7Ø.Ø ☑
    - sinuses T7Ø.1 ☑
  - polycythemia D75.1
- arch
  - foot Q66.7
  - palate, congenital Q38.5
- arterial tension — *see* Hypertension
- basal metabolic rate R94.8
- blood pressure (*see also* Hypertension)
  - borderline RØ3.Ø
  - reading (incidental) (isolated) (nonspecific), without diagnosis of hypertension RØ3.Ø
- cholesterol E78.Ø
  - with high triglycerides E78.2
- diaphragm (congenital) Q79.1
- expressed emotional level within family Z63.8
- head at term O32.4 ☑
- palate, congenital Q38.5
- risk
  - infant NEC Z76.2
  - sexual behavior (heterosexual) Z72.51
    - bisexual Z72.53
    - homosexual Z72.52
- temperature (of unknown origin) R5Ø.9
- thoracic rib Q76.6
- triglycerides E78.1
  - with high cholesterol E78.2

Hildenbrand's disease A75.Ø

Hilum — *see* condition

Hip — *see* condition

Hippel's disease Q85.8

Hippophobia F4Ø.218

Hippus H57.Ø9

Hirschsprung's disease or megacolon Q43.1

Hirsutism, hirsuties L68.Ø

Hirudiniasis
- external B88.3
- internal B83.4

Hiss-Russell dysentery AØ3.1

Histidinemia, histidinuria E7Ø.41

Histiocytoma (*see also* Neoplasm, skin, benign)
- fibrous (*see also* Neoplasm, skin, benign)
  - atypical — *see* Neoplasm, connective tissue, uncertain behavior

Histiocytoma — *continued*
- fibrous (*see also* Neoplasm, skin, benign) — *continued*
  - malignant — *see* Neoplasm, connective tissue, malignant

Histiocytosis D76.3
- acute differentiated progressive C96.Ø
- Langerhans' cell NEC C96.6
  - multifocal X
    - multisystemic (disseminated) C96.Ø
    - unisystemic C96.5
  - pulmonary, adult (adult PLCH) J84.82
  - unifocal (X) C96.6
- lipid, lipoid D76.3
  - essential E75.29
- malignant C96.A (*following* C96.6)
- mononuclear phagocytes NEC D76.1
  - Langerhans' cells C96.6
- non-Langerhans cell D76.3
- polyostotic sclerosing D76.3
- sinus, with massive lymphadenopathy D76.3
- syndrome NEC D76.3
- X NEC C96.6
  - acute (progressive) C96.Ø
  - chronic C96.6
  - multifocal C96.5
  - multisystemic C96.Ø
  - unifocal C96.6

Histoplasmosis B39.9
- with pneumonia NEC B39.2
- African B39.5
- American — *see* Histoplasmosis, capsulati
- capsulati B39.4
  - disseminated B39.3
  - generalized B39.3
  - pulmonary B39.2
    - acute B39.Ø
    - chronic B39.1
- Darling's B39.4
- duboisii B39.5
- lung NEC B39.2

History
- family (of) (*see also* History, personal (of))
  - alcohol abuse Z81.1
  - allergy NEC Z84.89
  - anemia Z83.2
  - arthritis Z82.61
  - asthma Z82.5
  - blindness Z82.1
  - cardiac death (sudden) Z82.41
  - carrier of genetic disease Z84.81
  - chromosomal anomaly Z82.79
  - chronic
    - disabling disease NEC Z82.8
    - lower respiratory disease Z82.5
  - colonic polyps Z83.71
  - congenital malformations and deformations Z82.79
    - polycystic kidney Z82.71
  - consanguinity Z84.3
  - deafness Z82.2
  - diabetes mellitus Z83.3
  - disability NEC Z82.8
  - disease or disorder (of)
    - allergic NEC Z84.89
    - behavioral NEC Z81.8
    - blood and blood-forming organs Z83.2
    - cardiovascular NEC Z82.49
    - chronic disabling NEC Z82.8
    - digestive Z83.79
    - ear NEC Z83.52
    - endocrine NEC Z83.49
    - eye NEC Z83.518
      - glaucoma Z83.511
    - genitourinary NEC Z84.2
    - glaucoma Z83.511
    - hematological Z83.2
    - immune mechanism Z83.2
    - infectious NEC Z83.1
    - ischemic heart Z82.49
    - kidney Z84.1
    - mental NEC Z81.8
    - metabolic Z83.49
    - musculoskeletal NEC Z82.69
    - neurological NEC Z82.Ø
    - nutritional Z83.49
    - parasitic NEC Z83.1
    - psychiatric NEC Z81.8
    - respiratory NEC Z83.6

- **History** — *continued*
  - family (*see also* History, personal) — *continued*
    - disease or disorder — *continued*
      - skin and subcutaneous tissue NEC Z84.Ø
      - specified NEC Z84.89
    - drug abuse NEC Z81.3
    - epilepsy Z82.Ø
    - genetic disease carrier Z84.81
    - glaucoma Z83.511
    - hearing loss Z82.2
    - human immunodeficiency virus (HIV) infection Z83.Ø
    - Huntington's chorea Z82.Ø
    - intellectual disability Z81.Ø
    - leukemia Z8Ø.6
    - malignant neoplasm (of) NOS Z8Ø.9
      - bladder Z8Ø.52
      - breast Z8Ø.3
      - bronchus Z8Ø.1
      - digestive organ Z8Ø.Ø
      - gastrointestinal tract Z8Ø.Ø
      - genital organ Z8Ø.49
        - ovary Z8Ø.41
        - prostate Z8Ø.42
        - specified organ NEC Z8Ø.49
        - testis Z8Ø.43
      - hematopoietic NEC Z8Ø.7
      - intrathoracic organ NEC Z8Ø.2
      - kidney Z8Ø.51
      - lung Z8Ø.1
      - lymphatic NEC Z8Ø.7
      - ovary Z8Ø.41
      - prostate Z8Ø.42
      - respiratory organ NEC Z8Ø.2
      - specified site NEC Z8Ø.8
      - testis Z8Ø.43
      - trachea Z8Ø.1
      - urinary organ or tract Z8Ø.59
        - bladder Z8Ø.52
        - kidney Z8Ø.51
    - mental
      - disorder NEC Z81.8
    - multiple endocrine neoplasia (MEN) syndrome Z83.41
    - osteoporosis Z82.62
    - polycystic kidney Z82.71
    - polyps (colon) Z83.71
    - psychiatric disorder Z81.8
    - psychoactive substance abuse NEC Z81.3
    - respiratory condition NEC Z83.6
      - asthma and other lower respiratory conditions Z82.5
    - self-harmful behavior Z81.8
    - skin condition Z84.Ø
    - specified condition NEC Z84.89
    - stroke (cerebrovascular) Z82.3
    - substance abuse NEC Z81.4
      - alcohol Z81.1
      - drug NEC Z81.3
      - psychoactive NEC Z81.3
      - tobacco Z81.2
    - sudden cardiac death Z82.41
    - tobacco abuse Z81.2
    - violence, violent behavior Z81.8
    - visual loss Z82.1
  - personal (of) (*see also* History, family (of))
    - abuse
      - adult Z91.419
        - physical and sexual Z91.41Ø
        - psychological Z91.411
      - childhood Z62.819
        - physical Z62.81Ø
        - psychological Z62.811
        - sexual Z62.81Ø
    - alcohol dependence F1Ø.21
    - allergy (to) Z88.9
      - analgesic agent NEC Z88.6
      - anesthetic Z88.4
      - antibiotic agent NEC Z88.1
      - anti-infective agent NEC Z88.3
      - contrast media Z91.Ø41
      - drugs, medicaments and biological substances Z88.9
        - specified NEC Z88.8
      - food Z91.Ø18
        - additives Z91.Ø2
        - eggs Z91.Ø12
        - milk products Z91.Ø11

- **History** — *continued*
  - personal (*see also* History, family) — *continued*
    - allergy — *continued*
      - food — *continued*
        - peanuts Z91.Ø1Ø
        - seafood Z91.Ø13
        - specified food NEC Z91.Ø18
      - insect Z91.Ø38
        - bee Z91.Ø3Ø
      - latex Z91.Ø4Ø
      - medicinal agents Z88.9
        - specified NEC Z88.8
      - narcotic agent NEC Z88.5
      - nonmedicinal agents Z91.Ø48
      - penicillin Z88.Ø
      - serum Z88.7
      - specified NEC Z91.Ø9
      - sulfonamides Z88.2
      - vaccine Z88.7
    - anaphylactic shock Z87.892
    - anaphylaxis Z87.892
    - behavioral disorders Z86.59
    - benign carcinoid tumor Z86.Ø12
    - benign neoplasm Z86.Ø18
      - brain Z86.Ø11
      - carcinoid Z86.Ø12
      - colonic polyps Z86.Ø1Ø
    - brain injury (traumatic) Z87.82Ø
    - breast implant removal Z98.86
    - calculi, renal Z87.442
    - cancer — *see* History, personal (of), malignant neoplasm (of)
    - cardiac arrest (death), successfully resuscitated Z86.74
    - cerebral infarction without residual deficit Z86.73
    - cervical dysplasia Z87.41Ø
    - chemotherapy for neoplastic condition Z92.21
    - childhood abuse — *see* History, personal (of), abuse
    - cleft lip (corrected) Z87.73Ø
    - cleft palate (corrected) Z87.73Ø
    - collapsed vertebra (healed) Z87.311
      - due to osteoporosis Z87.31Ø
    - combat and operational stress reaction Z86.51
    - congenital malformation (corrected) Z87.798
      - circulatory system (corrected) Z87.74
      - digestive system (corrected) NEC Z87.738
      - ear (corrected) Z87.72Ø
      - eye (corrected) Z87.721
      - face and neck (corrected) Z87.79Ø
      - genitourinary system (corrected) NEC Z87.718
      - heart (corrected) Z87.74
      - integument (corrected) Z87.76
      - limb(s) (corrected) Z87.76
      - musculoskeletal system (corrected) Z87.76
      - neck (corrected) Z87.79Ø
      - nervous system (corrected) NEC Z87.728
      - respiratory system (corrected) Z87.75
      - sense organs (corrected) NEC Z87.728
      - specified NEC Z87.798
    - contraception Z92.Ø
    - deployment (military) Z91.82
    - diabetic foot ulcer Z86.31
    - disease or disorder (of) Z87.898
      - anaphylaxis Z87.892
      - blood and blood-forming organs Z86.2
      - circulatory system Z86.79
        - specified condition NEC Z86.79
      - connective tissue Z87.39
      - digestive system Z87.19
        - colonic polyp Z86.Ø1Ø
        - peptic ulcer disease Z87.11
        - specified condition NEC Z87.19
      - ear Z86.69
      - endocrine Z86.39
        - diabetic foot ulcer Z86.31
        - gestational diabetes Z86.32
        - specified type NEC Z86.39
      - eye Z86.69
      - genital (track) system NEC
        - female Z87.42
        - male Z87.438
      - hematological Z86.2
      - Hodgkin Z85.71
      - immune mechanism Z86.2
      - infectious Z86.19
        - malaria Z86.13

- **History** — *continued*
  - personal (*see also* History, family) — *continued*
    - disease or disorder — *continued*
      - infectious — *continued*
        - Methicillin resistant Staphylococcus aureus (MRSA) Z86.14
        - poliomyelitis Z86.12
        - specified NEC Z86.19
        - tuberculosis Z86.11
      - mental NEC Z86.59
      - metabolic Z86.39
        - diabetic foot ulcer Z86.31
        - gestational diabetes Z86.32
        - specified type NEC Z86.39
      - musculoskeletal NEC Z87.39
      - nervous system Z86.69
      - nutritional Z86.39
      - parasitic Z86.19
      - respiratory system NEC Z87.Ø9
      - sense organs Z86.69
      - skin Z87.2
      - specified site or type NEC Z87.898
      - subcutaneous tissue Z87.2
      - trophoblastic Z87.59
      - urinary system NEC Z87.448
    - drug dependence — *see* Dependence, drug, by type, in remission
    - drug therapy
      - antineoplastic chemotherapy Z92.21
      - estrogen Z92.23
      - immunosupression Z92.25
      - inhaled steroids Z92.24Ø
      - monoclonal drug Z92.22
      - specified NEC Z92.29
      - steroid Z92.241
      - systemic steroids Z92.241
    - dysplasia
      - cervical Z87.41Ø
      - prostatic Z87.43Ø
      - vaginal Z87.411
      - vulvar Z87.412
    - embolism (venous) Z86.718
      - pulmonary Z86.711
    - encephalitis Z86.61
    - estrogen therapy Z92.23
    - extracorporeal membrane oxygenation (ECMO) Z92.81
    - failed conscious sedation Z92.83
    - failed moderate sedation Z92.83
    - fall, falling Z91.81
    - fracture (healed)
      - fatigue Z87.312
      - fragility Z87.31Ø
      - osteoporosis Z87.31Ø
      - pathological NEC Z87.311
      - stress Z87.312
      - traumatic Z87.81
    - gestational diabetes Z86.32
    - hepatitis
      - B Z86.19
      - C Z86.19
    - Hodgkin disease Z85.71
    - hyperthermia, malignant Z88.4
    - hypospadias (corrected) Z87.71Ø
    - hysterectomy Z9Ø.71Ø
    - immunosupression therapy Z92.25
    - in situ neoplasm
      - breast Z86.ØØØ
      - cervix uteri Z86.ØØ1
      - specified NEC Z86.ØØ8
    - in utero procedure during pregnancy Z98.87Ø
    - in utero procedure while a fetus Z98.871
    - infection NEC Z86.19
      - central nervous system Z86.61
      - Methicillin resistant Staphylococcus aureus (MRSA) Z86.14
      - urinary (recurrent) (tract) Z87.44Ø
    - injury NEC Z87.828
    - irradiation Z92.3
    - kidney stones Z87.442
    - leukemia Z85.6
    - lymphoma (non-Hodgkin) Z85.72
    - malignant melanoma (skin) Z85.82Ø
    - malignant neoplasm (of) Z85.9
      - accessory sinuses Z85.22
      - anus NEC Z85.Ø48
        - carcinoid Z85.Ø4Ø
      - bladder Z85.51

- **History** — *continued*
  - personal (*see also* History, family) — *continued*
    - malignant neoplasm — *continued*
      - bone Z85.83Ø
      - brain Z85.841
      - breast Z85.3
      - bronchus NEC Z85.118
        - carcinoid Z85.11Ø
      - carcinoid — *see* History, personal (of), malignant neoplasm, by site, carcinioid
      - cervix Z85.41
      - colon NEC Z85.Ø38
        - carcinoid Z85.Ø3Ø
      - digestive organ Z85.ØØ
        - specified NEC Z85.Ø9
      - endocrine gland NEC Z85.858
      - epididymis Z85.48
      - esophagus Z85.Ø1
      - eye Z85.84Ø
      - gastrointestinal tract — *see* History, malignant neoplasm, digestive organ
      - genital organ
        - female Z85.4Ø
          - specified NEC Z85.44
        - male Z85.45
          - specified NEC Z85.49
      - hematopoietic NEC Z85.79
      - intrathoracic organ Z85.2Ø
      - kidney NEC Z85.528
        - carcinoid Z85.52Ø
      - large intestine NEC Z85.Ø38
        - carcinoid Z85.Ø3Ø
      - larynx Z85.21
      - liver Z85.Ø5
      - lung NEC Z85.118
        - carcinoid Z85.11Ø
      - mediastinum Z85.29
      - Merkel cell Z85.821
      - middle ear Z85.22
      - nasal cavities Z85.22
      - nervous system NEC Z85.848
      - oral cavity Z85.819
        - specified site NEC Z85.818
      - ovary Z85.43
      - pancreas Z85.Ø7
      - pelvis Z85.53
      - pharynx Z85.819
        - specified site NEC Z85.818
      - pleura Z85.29
      - prostate Z85.46
      - rectosigmoid junction NEC Z85.Ø48
        - carcinoid Z85.Ø4Ø
      - rectum NEC Z85.Ø48
        - carcinoid Z85.Ø4Ø
      - respiratory organ Z85.2Ø
      - sinuses, accessory Z85.22
      - skin NEC Z85.828
        - melanoma Z85.82Ø
        - Merkel cell Z85.821
      - small intestine NEC Z85.Ø68
        - carcinoid Z85.Ø6Ø
      - soft tissue Z85.831
      - specified site NEC Z85.89
      - stomach NEC Z85.Ø28
        - carcinoid Z85.Ø2Ø
      - testis Z85.47
      - thymus NEC Z85.238
        - carcinoid Z85.23Ø
      - thyroid Z85.85Ø
      - tongue Z85.81Ø
      - trachea Z85.12
      - urinary organ or tract Z85.5Ø
        - specified NEC Z85.59
      - uterus Z85.42
    - maltreatment Z91.89
    - medical treatment NEC Z92.89
    - melanoma (malignant) (skin) Z85.82Ø
    - meningitis Z86.61
    - mental disorder Z86.59
    - Merkel cell carcinoma (skin) Z85.821
    - Methicillin resistant Staphylococcus aureus (MRSA) Z86.14
    - military deployment Z91.82
    - military war, peacekeeping and humanitarian deployment (current or past conflict) Z91.82
    - myocardial infarction (old) I25.2
    - neglect (in)
      - adult Z91.412

- **History** — *continued*
  - personal (*see also* History, family) — *continued*
    - neglect — *continued*
      - childhood Z62.812
    - neoplasm
      - benign Z86.Ø18
        - brain Z86.Ø11
        - colon polyp Z86.Ø1Ø
      - in situ
        - breast Z86.ØØØ
        - cervix uteri Z86.ØØ1
        - specified NEC Z86.ØØ8
      - malignant — *see* History of, malignant neoplasm
      - uncertain behavior Z86.Ø3
    - nephrotic syndrome Z87.441
    - nicotine dependence Z87.891
    - noncompliance with medical treatment or regimen — *see* Noncompliance
    - nutritional deficiency Z86.39
    - obstetric complications Z87.59
      - childbirth Z87.59
      - pregnancy Z87.59
      - pre-term labor Z87.51
      - puerperium Z87.59
    - osteoporosis fractures Z87.31 ☑
    - parasuicide (attempt) Z91.5
    - physical trauma NEC Z87.828
      - self-harm or suicide attempt Z91.5
    - pneumonia (recurrent) Z87.Ø1
    - poisoning NEC Z91.89
      - self-harm or suicide attempt Z91.5
    - poor personal hygiene Z91.89
    - preterm labor Z87.51
    - procedure during pregnancy Z98.87Ø
    - procedure while a fetus Z98.871
    - prolonged reversible ischemic neurologic deficit (PRIND) Z86.73
    - prostatic dysplasia Z87.43Ø
    - psychological
      - abuse
        - adult Z91.411
        - child Z62.811
      - trauma, specified NEC Z91.49
    - radiation therapy Z92.3
    - removal
      - implant
        - breast Z98.86
    - renal calculi Z87.442
    - respiratory condition NEC Z87.Ø9
    - retained foreign body fully removed Z87.821
    - risk factors NEC Z91.89
    - self-harm Z91.5
    - self-poisoning attempt Z91.5
    - sex reassignment Z87.89Ø
    - sleep-wake cycle problem Z72.821
    - specified NEC Z87.898
    - steroid therapy (systemic) Z92.241
      - inhaled Z92.24Ø
    - stroke without residual deficits Z86.73
    - substance abuse NEC F1Ø-F19 with fifth character 1
    - sudden cardiac arrest Z86.74
    - sudden cardiac death successfully resuscitated Z86.74
    - suicide attempt Z91.5
    - surgery NEC Z98.89
      - sex reassignment Z87.89Ø
      - transplant — *see* Transplant
    - thrombophlebitis Z86.72
    - thrombosis (venous) Z86.718
      - pulmonary Z86.711
    - tobacco dependence Z87.891
    - transient ischemic attack (TIA) without residual deficits Z86.73
    - trauma (physical) NEC Z87.828
      - psychological NEC Z91.49
      - self-harm Z91.5
    - traumatic brain injury Z87.82Ø
    - unhealthy sleep-wake cycle Z72.821
    - urinary calculi Z87.442
    - urinary (recurrent) (tract) infection(s) Z87.44Ø
    - vaginal dysplasia Z87.411
    - venous thrombosis or embolism Z86.718
      - pulmonary Z86.711
    - vulvar dysplasia Z87.412
- **His-Werner disease** A79.Ø
- **HIV** (*see also* Human, immunodeficiency virus) B2Ø

- **HIV** — *continued*
  - laboratory evidence (nonconclusive) R75
  - nonconclusive test (in infants) R75
  - positive, seropositive Z21
- **Hives** (bold) — *see* Urticaria
- **Hoarseness** R49.Ø
- **Hobo** Z59.Ø
- **Hodgkin disease** — *see* Lymphoma, Hodgkin
- **Hodgson's disease** I71.2
  - ruptured I71.1
- **Hoffa-Kastert disease** E88.89
- **Hoffa's disease** E88.89
- **Hoffmann-Bouveret syndrome** I47.9
- **Hoffmann's syndrome** EØ3.9 [G73.7]
- **Hole** (round)
  - macula H35.34- ☑
  - retina (without detachment) — *see* Break, retina, round hole
    - with detachment — *see* Detachment, retina, with retinal, break
- **Holiday relief care** Z75.5
- **Hollenhorst's plaque** — *see* Occlusion, artery, retina
- **Hollow foot** (congenital) Q66.7
  - acquired — *see* Deformity, limb, foot, specified NEC
- **Holoprosencephaly** QØ4.2
- **Holt-Oram syndrome** Q87.2
- **Homelessness** Z59.Ø
- **Homesickness** — *see* Disorder, adjustment
- **Homocystinemia, homocystinuria** E72.11
- **Homogentisate 1,2-dioxygenase deficiency** E7Ø.29
- **Homologous serum hepatitis** (prophylactic) (therapeutic) — *see* Hepatitis, viral, type B
- **Honeycomb lung** J98.4
  - congenital Q33.Ø
- **Hooded**
  - clitoris Q52.6
  - penis Q55.69
- **Hookworm** (anemia) (disease) (infection) (infestation) B76.9
  - specified NEC B76.8
- **Hordeolum** (eyelid) (externum) (recurrent) HØØ.Ø19
  - internum HØØ.Ø29
    - left HØØ.Ø26
      - lower HØØ.Ø25
      - upper HØØ.Ø24
    - right HØØ.Ø23
      - lower HØØ.Ø22
      - upper HØØ.Ø21
  - left HØØ.Ø16
    - lower HØØ.Ø15
    - upper HØØ.Ø14
  - right HØØ.Ø13
    - lower HØØ.Ø12
    - upper HØØ.Ø11
- **Horn**
  - cutaneous L85.8
  - nail L6Ø.2
    - congenital Q84.6
- **Horner** (-Claude Bernard) **syndrome** G9Ø.2
  - traumatic — *see* Injury, nerve, cervical sympathetic
- **Horseshoe kidney** (congenital) Q63.1
- **Horton's headache or neuralgia** G44.Ø99
  - intractable G44.Ø91
  - not intractable G44.Ø99
- **Hospital hopper syndrome** — *see* Disorder, factitious
- **Hospitalism in children** — *see* Disorder, adjustment
- **Hostility** R45.5
  - towards child Z62.3
- **Hot flashes**
  - menopausal N95.1
- **Hourglass** (contracture) (*see also* Contraction, hourglass)
  - stomach K31.89
    - congenital Q4Ø.2
    - stricture K31.2
- **Household, housing circumstance affecting care** Z59.9
  - specified NEC Z59.8
- **Housemaid's knee** — *see* Bursitis, prepatellar
- **Hudson** (-Stähli) **line** (cornea) — *see* Pigmentation, cornea, anterior
- **Human**
  - bite (open wound) (*see also* Bite)
    - intact skin surface — *see* Bite, superficial
  - herpesvirus — *see* Herpes
  - immunodeficiency virus (HIV) disease (infection) B2Ø
    - asymptomatic status Z21
    - contact Z2Ø.6

Human — *continued*
immunodeficiency virus disease — *continued*
counseling Z71.7
dementia B2Ø [FØ2.8Ø]
with behavioral disturbance B2Ø [FØ2.81]
exposure to Z2Ø.6
laboratory evidence R75
type-2 (HIV 2) as cause of disease classified elsewhere B97.35
papillomavirus (HPV)
DNA test positive
high risk
cervix R87.81Ø
vagina R87.811
low risk
cervix R87.82Ø
vagina R87.821
screening for Z11.51
T-cell lymphotropic virus
type-1 (HTLV-I) infection B33.3
as cause of disease classified elsewhere B97.33
carrier Z22.6
type-2 (HTLV-II) as cause of disease classified elsewhere B97.34
Humidifier lung or pneumonitis J67.7
Humiliation (experience) **in childhood** Z62.898
Humpback (acquired) — *see* Kyphosis
Hunchback (acquired) — *see* Kyphosis
Hunger T73.Ø ☑
air, psychogenic F45.8
Hungry bone syndrome E83.81
Hunner's ulcer — *see* Cystitis, chronic, interstitial
Hunter's
glossitis D51.Ø
syndrome E76.1
Huntington's disease or chorea G1Ø
with dementia G1Ø [FØ2.8Ø]
with behavioral disturbance G1Ø [FØ2.81]
Hunt's
disease or syndrome (herpetic geniculate ganglionitis) BØ2.21
dyssynergia cerebellaris myoclonica G11.1
neuralgia BØ2.21
Hurler (-Scheie) **disease or syndrome** E76.Ø2
Hurst's disease G36.1
Hurthle cell
adenocarcinoma C73
adenoma D34
carcinoma C73
tumor D34
Hutchinson-Boeck disease or syndrome — *see* Sarcoidosis
Hutchinson-Gilford disease or syndrome E34.8
Hutchinson's
disease, meaning
angioma serpiginosum L81.7
pompholyx (cheiropompholyx) L3Ø.1
prurigo estivalis L56.4
summer eruption or summer prurigo L56.4
melanotic freckle — *see* Melanoma, in situ
malignant melanoma in — *see* Melanoma
teeth or incisors (congenital syphilis) A5Ø.52
triad (congenital syphilis) A5Ø.53
Hyalin plaque, sclera, senile H15.89
Hyaline membrane (disease) (lung) (pulmonary) (newborn) P22.Ø
Hyalinosis
cutis (et mucosae) E78.89
focal and segmental (glomerular) (*see also* NØØ-NØ7 with fourth character .1) NØ5.1
Hyalitis, hyalosis, asteroid (*see also* Deposit, crystalline)
syphilitic (late) A52.71
Hydatid
cyst or tumor — *see* Echinococcus
mole — *see* Hydatidiform mole
Morgagni
female Q5Ø.5
male (epididymal) Q55.4
testicular Q55.29
Hydatidiform mole (benign) (complicating pregnancy) (delivered) (undelivered) OØ1.9
classical OØ1.Ø
complete OØ1.Ø
incomplete OØ1.1
invasive D39.2
malignant D39.2
partial OØ1.1
Hydatidosis — *see* Echinococcus
Hydradenitis (axillaris) (suppurative) L73.2
Hydradenoma — *see* Hidradenoma
Hydramnios O4Ø.- ☑
Hydrancephaly, hydranencephaly QØ4.3
with spina bifida — *see* Spina bifida, with hydrocephalus
Hydrargyrism NEC — *see* Poisoning, mercury
Hydrarthrosis (*see also* Effusion, joint)
gonococcal A54.42
intermittent M12.4Ø
ankle M12.47- ☑
elbow M12.42- ☑
foot joint M12.47- ☑
hand joint M12.44- ☑
hip M12.45- ☑
knee M12.46- ☑
multiple site M12.49
shoulder M12.41- ☑
specified joint NEC M12.48
wrist M12.43- ☑
of yaws (early) (late) (*see also* subcategory M14.8-) A66.6
syphilitic (late) A52.77
congenital A5Ø.55 [M12.8Ø]
Hydremia D64.89
Hydrencephalocele (congenital) — *see* Encephalocele
Hydrencephalomeningocele (congenital) — *see* Encephalocele
Hydroa R23.8
aestivale L56.4
vacciniforme L56.4
Hydroadenitis (axillaris) (suppurative) L73.2
Hydrocalycosis — *see* Hydronephrosis
Hydrocele (spermatic cord) (testis) (tunica vaginalis) N43.3
canal of Nuck N94.89
communicating N43.2
congenital P83.5
congenital P83.5
encysted N43.Ø
female NEC N94.89
infected N43.1
newborn P83.5
round ligament N94.89
specified NEC N43.2
spinalis — *see* Spina bifida
vulva N9Ø.89
Hydrocephalus (acquired) (external) (internal) (malignant) (recurrent) G91.9
aqueduct Sylvius stricture QØ3.Ø
causing disproportion O33.6 ☑
with obstructed labor O66.3
communicating G91.Ø
congenital (external) (internal) QØ3.9
with spina bifida QØ5.4
cervical QØ5.Ø
dorsal QØ5.1
lumbar QØ5.2
lumbosacral QØ5.2
sacral QØ5.3
thoracic QØ5.1
thoracolumbar QØ5.1
specified NEC QØ3.8
due to toxoplasmosis (congenital) P37.1
foramen Magendie block (acquired) G91.1
congenital (*see also* Hydrocephalus, congenital) QØ3.1
in (due to)
infectious disease NEC B89 [G91.4]
neoplastic disease NEC (*see also* Neoplasm) G91.4
parasitic disease B89 [G91.4]
newborn QØ3.9
with spina bifida — *see* Spina bifida, with hydrocephalus
noncommunicating G91.1
normal pressure G91.2
secondary G91.Ø
obstructive G91.1
otitic G93.2
post-traumatic NEC G91.3
secondary G91.4
post-traumatic G91.3
specified NEC G91.8
syphilitic, congenital A5Ø.49
Hydrocolpos (congenital) N89.8
Hydrocystoma — *see* Neoplasm, skin, benign
Hydroencephalocele (congenital) — *see* Encephalocele
Hydroencephalomeningocele (congenital) — *see* Encephalocele
Hydrohematopneumothorax — *see* Hemothorax
Hydromeningitis — *see* Meningitis
Hydromeningocele (spinal) (*see also* Spina bifida)
cranial — *see* Encephalocele
Hydrometra N85.8
Hydrometrocolpos N89.8
Hydromicrocephaly QØ2
Hydromphalos (since birth) Q45.8
Hydromyelia QØ6.4
Hydromyelocele — *see* Spina bifida
Hydronephrosis (atrophic) (early) (functionless) (intermittent) (primary) (secondary) NEC N13.3Ø
with
infection N13.6
obstruction (by) (of)
renal calculus N13.2
with infection N13.6
ureteral NEC N13.1
with infection N13.6
calculus N13.2
with infection N13.6
ureteropelvic junction (congenital) Q62.Ø
with infection N13.6
ureteral stricture NEC N13.1
with infection N13.6
congenital Q62.Ø
specified type NEC N13.39
tuberculous A18.11
Hydropericarditis — *see* Pericarditis
Hydropericardium — *see* Pericarditis
Hydroperitoneum R18.8
Hydrophobia — *see* Rabies
Hydrophthalmos Q15.Ø
Hydropneumohemothorax — *see* Hemothorax
Hydropneumopericarditis — *see* Pericarditis
Hydropneumopericardium — *see* Pericarditis
Hydropneumothorax J94.8
traumatic — *see* Injury, intrathoracic, lung
tuberculous NEC A15.6
Hydrops R6Ø.9
abdominis R18.8
articulorum intermittens — *see* Hydrarthrosis, intermittent
cardiac — *see* Failure, heart, congestive
causing obstructed labor (mother) O66.3
endolymphatic H81.Ø- ☑
fetal — *see* Pregnancy, complicated by, hydrops, fetalis
fetalis P83.2
due to
ABO isoimmunization P56.Ø
alpha thalassemia D56.Ø
hemolytic disease P56.9Ø
specified NEC P56.99
isoimmunization (ABO) (Rh) P56.Ø
other specified nonhemolytic disease NEC P83.2
Rh incompatibility P56.Ø
during pregnancy — *see* Pregnancy, complicated by, hydrops, fetalis
gallbladder K82.1
joint — *see* Effusion, joint
labyrinth H81.Ø- ☑
newborn (idiopathic) P83.2
due to
ABO isoimmunization P56.Ø
alpha thalassemia D56.Ø
hemolytic disease P56.9Ø
specified NEC P56.99
isoimmunization (ABO) (Rh) P56.Ø
Rh incompatibility P56.Ø
nutritional — *see* Malnutrition, severe
pericardium — *see* Pericarditis
pleura — *see* Hydrothorax
spermatic cord — *see* Hydrocele
Hydropyonephrosis N13.6
Hydrorachis QØ6.4
Hydrorrhea (nasal) J34.89
pregnancy — *see* Rupture, membranes, premature
Hydrosadenitis (axillaris) (suppurative) L73.2
Hydrosalpinx (fallopian tube) (follicularis) N7Ø.11
Hydrothorax (double) (pleura) J94.8
chylous (nonfilarial) I89.8
filarial (*see also* Infestation, filarial) B74.9 [J91.8]
traumatic — *see* Injury, intrathoracic
tuberculous NEC (non primary) A15.6
Hydroureter (*see also* Hydronephrosis) N13.4

- **Hydroureter** — *continued*
  - with infection N13.6
  - congenital Q62.39
- **Hydroureteronephrosis** — *see* Hydronephrosis
- **Hydrourethra** N36.8
- **Hydroxykynureninuria** E70.8
- **Hydroxylysinemia** E72.3
- **Hydroxyprolinemia** E72.59
- **Hygiene, sleep**
  - abuse Z72.821
  - inadequate Z72.821
  - poor Z72.821
- **Hygroma** (congenital) (cystic) D18.1
  - praepatellare, prepatellar — *see* Bursitis, prepatellar
- **Hymen** — *see* condition
- **Hymenolepis, hymenolepiasis** (diminuta) (infection) (infestation) (nana) B71.0
- **Hypalgesia** R20.8
- **Hyperacidity** (gastric) K31.89
  - psychogenic F45.8
- **Hyperactive, hyperactivity** F90.9
  - basal cell, uterine cervix — *see* Dysplasia, cervix
  - bowel sounds R19.12
  - cervix epithelial (basal) — *see* Dysplasia, cervix
  - child F90.9
    - attention deficit — *see* Disorder, attention-deficit hyperactivity
  - detrusor muscle N32.81
  - gastrointestinal K31.89
    - psychogenic F45.8
  - nasal mucous membrane J34.3
  - stomach K31.89
  - thyroid (gland) — *see* Hyperthyroidism
- **Hyperacusis** H93.23- ☑
- **Hyperadrenalism** E27.5
- **Hyperadrenocorticism** E24.9
  - congenital E25.0
  - iatrogenic E24.2
    - correct substance properly administered — *see* Table of Drugs and Chemicals, by drug, adverse effect
    - overdose or wrong substance given or taken — *see* Table of Drugs and Chemicals, by drug, poisoning
  - not associated with Cushing's syndrome E27.0
  - pituitary-dependent E24.0
- **Hyperaldosteronism** E26.9
  - familial (type I) E26.02
  - glucocorticoid-remediable E26.02
  - primary (due to (bilateral) adrenal hyperplasia) E26.09
  - primary NEC E26.09
  - secondary E26.1
  - specified NEC E26.89
- **Hyperalgesia** R20.8
- **Hyperalimentation** R63.2
  - carotene, carotin E67.1
  - specified NEC E67.8
  - vitamin
    - A E67.0
    - D E67.3
- **Hyperaminoaciduria**
  - arginine E72.21
  - cystine E72.01
  - lysine E72.3
  - ornithine E72.4
- **Hyperammonemia** (congenital) E72.20
- **Hyperazotemia** — *see* Uremia
- **Hyperbetalipoproteinemia** (familial) E78.0
  - with prebetalipoproteinemia E78.2
- **Hyperbilirubinemia**
  - constitutional E80.6
  - familial conjugated E80.6
  - neonatal (transient) — *see* Jaundice, newborn
- **Hypercalcemia, hypocalciuric, familial** E83.52
- **Hypercalciuria, idiopathic** E83.52
- **Hypercapnia** R06.89
  - newborn P84
- **Hypercarotenemia, hypercarotinemia** (dietary) E67.1
- **Hypercementosis** K03.4
- **Hyperchloremia** E87.8
- **Hyperchlorhydria** K31.89
  - neurotic F45.8
  - psychogenic F45.8
- **Hypercholesterinemia** — *see* Hypercholesterolemia
- **Hypercholesterolemia** (essential) (familial) (hereditary) (primary) (pure) E78.0
  - with hyperglyceridemia, endogenous E78.2
- **Hypercholesterolemia** — *continued*
  - dietary counseling and surveillance Z71.3
- **Hyperchylia gastrica, psychogenic** F45.8
- **Hyperchylomicronemia** (familial) (primary) E78.3
  - with hyperbetalipoproteinemia E78.3
- **Hypercoagulable** (state) D68.59
  - activated protein C resistance D68.51
  - antithrombin (III) deficiency D68.59
  - factor V Leiden mutation D68.51
  - primary NEC D68.59
  - protein C deficiency D68.59
  - protein S deficiency D68.59
  - prothrombin gene mutation D68.52
  - secondary D68.69
  - specified NEC D68.69
- **Hypercoagulation** (state) D68.59
- **Hypercorticalism, pituitary-dependent** E24.0
- **Hypercorticosolism** — *see* Cushing's, syndrome
- **Hypercorticosteronism** E24.2
  - correct substance properly administered — *see* Table of Drugs and Chemicals, by drug, adverse effect
  - overdose or wrong substance given or taken — *see* Table of Drugs and Chemicals, by drug, poisoning
- **Hypercortisonism** E24.2
  - correct substance properly administered — *see* Table of Drugs and Chemicals, by drug, adverse effect
  - overdose or wrong substance given or taken — *see* Table of Drugs and Chemicals, by drug, poisoning
- **Hyperekplexia** Q89.8
- **Hyperelectrolytemia** E87.8
- **Hyperemesis** R11.10
  - with nausea R11.2
  - gravidarum (mild) O21.0
    - with
      - carbohydrate depletion O21.1
      - dehydration O21.1
      - electrolyte imbalance O21.1
      - metabolic disturbance O21.1
    - severe (with metabolic disturbance) O21.1
  - projectile R11.12
  - psychogenic F45.8
- **Hyperemia** (acute) (passive) R68.89
  - anal mucosa K62.89
  - bladder N32.89
  - cerebral I67.89
  - conjunctiva H11.43- ☑
  - ear internal, acute — *see* subcategory H83.0 ☑
  - enteric K59.8
  - eye — *see* Hyperemia, conjunctiva
  - eyelid (active) (passive) — *see* Disorder, eyelid, specified type NEC
  - intestine K59.8
  - iris — *see* Disorder, iris, vascular
  - kidney N28.89
  - labyrinth — *see* subcategory H83.0 ☑
  - liver (active) K76.89
  - lung (passive) — *see* Edema, lung
  - pulmonary (passive) — *see* Edema, lung
  - renal N28.89
  - retina H35.89
  - stomach K31.89
- **Hyperesthesia** (body surface) R20.3
  - larynx (reflex) J38.7
    - hysterical F44.89
  - pharynx (reflex) J39.2
    - hysterical F44.89
- **Hyperestrogenism** (drug-induced) (iatrogenic) E28.0
- **Hyperexplexia** Q89.8
- **Hyperfibrinolysis** — *see* Fibrinolysis
- **Hyperfructosemia** E74.19
- **Hyperfunction**
  - adrenal cortex, not associated with Cushing's syndrome E27.0
    - medulla E27.5
      - adrenomedullary E27.5
    - virilism E25.9
      - congenital E25.0
  - ovarian E28.8
  - pancreas K86.8
  - parathyroid (gland) E21.3
  - pituitary (gland) (anterior) E22.9
    - specified NEC E22.8
  - polyglandular E31.1
  - testicular E29.0
- **Hypergammaglobulinemia** D89.2
  - polyclonal D89.0
  - Waldenström D89.0
- **Hypergastrinemia** E16.4
- **Hyperglobulinemia** R77.1
- **Hyperglycemia, hyperglycemic** (transient) R73.9
  - coma — *see* Diabetes, by type, with coma
  - postpancreatectomy E89.1
- **Hyperglyceridemia** (endogenous) (essential) (familial) (hereditary) (pure) E78.1
  - mixed E78.3
- **Hyperglycinemia** (non-ketotic) E72.51
- **Hypergonadism**
  - ovarian E28.8
  - testicular (primary) (infantile) E29.0
- **Hyperheparinemia** D68.32
- **Hyperhidrosis, hyperidrosis** R61
  - focal
    - primary L74.519
      - axilla L74.510
      - face L74.511
      - palms L74.512
      - soles L74.513
    - secondary L74.52
  - generalized R61
  - localized
    - primary L74.519
      - axilla L74.510
      - face L74.511
      - palms L74.512
      - soles L74.513
    - secondary L74.52
  - psychogenic F45.8
  - secondary R61
    - focal L74.52
- **Hyperhistidinemia** E70.41
- **Hyperhomocysteinemia** E72.11
- **Hyperhydroxyprolinemia** E72.59
- **Hyperinsulinism** (functional) E16.1
  - with
    - coma (hypoglycemic) E15
    - encephalopathy E16.1 [G94]
  - ectopic E16.1
  - therapeutic misadventure (from administration of insulin) — *see* subcategory T38.3 ☑
- **Hyperkalemia** E87.5
- **Hyperkeratosis** (*see also* Keratosis) L85.9
  - cervix N88.0
  - due to yaws (early) (late) (palmar or plantar) A66.3
  - follicularis Q82.8
    - penetrans (in cutem) L87.0
  - palmoplantaris climacterica L85.1
  - pinta A67.1
  - senile (with pruritus) L57.0
  - universalis congenita Q80.8
  - vocal cord J38.3
  - vulva N90.4
- **Hyperkinesia, hyperkinetic** (disease) (reaction) (syndrome) (childhood) (adolescence) (*see also* Disorder, attention-deficit hyperactivity)
  - heart I51.89
- **Hyperleucine-isoleucinemia** E71.19
- **Hyperlipemia, hyperlipidemia** E78.5
  - combined E78.2
    - familial E78.4
  - group
    - A E78.0
    - B E78.1
    - C E78.2
    - D E78.3
  - mixed E78.2
  - specified NEC E78.4
- **Hyperlipidosis** E75.6
  - hereditary NEC E75.5
- **Hyperlipoproteinemia** E78.5
  - Fredrickson's type
    - I E78.3
    - IIa E78.0
    - IIb E78.2
    - III E78.2
    - IV E78.1
    - V E78.3
  - low-density-lipoprotein-type (LDL) E78.0
  - very-low-density-lipoprotein-type (VLDL) E78.1
- **Hyperlucent lung, unilateral** J43.0
- **Hyperlysinemia** E72.3
- **Hypermagnesemia** E83.41
  - neonatal P71.8

- **Hypermenorrhea** N92.Ø
- **Hypermethioninemia** E72.19
- **Hypermetropia** (congenital) H52.Ø- ☑
- **Hypermobility, hypermotility**
  - cecum — *see* Syndrome, irritable bowel
  - coccyx — *see* subcategory M53.2 ☑
  - colon — *see* Syndrome, irritable bowel
    - psychogenic F45.8
  - ileum K58.9
  - intestine (*see also* Syndrome, irritable bowel) K58.9
    - psychogenic F45.8
  - meniscus (knee) — *see* Derangement, knee, meniscus
  - scapula — *see* Instability, joint, shoulder
  - stomach K31.89
    - psychogenic F45.8
  - syndrome M35.7
  - urethra N36.41
    - with intrinsic sphincter deficiency N36.43
- **Hypernasality** R49.21
- **Hypernatremia** E87.Ø
- **Hypernephroma** C64.- ☑
- **Hyperopia** — *see* Hypermetropia
- **Hyperorexia nervosa** F5Ø.2
- **Hyperornithinemia** E72.4
- **Hyperosmia** R43.1
- **Hyperosmolality** E87.Ø
- **Hyperostosis** (monomelic) (*see also* Disorder, bone, density and structure, specified NEC)
  - ankylosing (spine) M48.1Ø
    - cervical region M48.12
    - cervicothoracic region M48.13
    - lumbar region M48.16
    - lumbosacral region M48.17
    - multiple sites M48.19
    - occipito-atlanto-axial region M48.11
    - sacrococcygeal region M48.18
    - thoracic region M48.14
    - thoracolumbar region M48.15
  - cortical (skull) M85.2
    - infantile M89.8X- ☑
  - frontal, internal of skull M85.2
  - interna frontalis M85.2
  - skeletal, diffuse idiopathic — *see* Hyperostosis, ankylosing
  - skull M85.2
    - congenital Q75.8
  - vertebral, ankylosing — *see* Hyperostosis, ankylosing
- **Hyperovarism** E28.8
- **Hyperoxaluria** (primary) E72.53
- **Hyperparathyroidism** E21.3
  - primary E21.Ø
  - secondary (renal) N25.81
    - non-renal E21.1
  - specified NEC E21.2
  - tertiary E21.2
- **Hyperpathia** R2Ø.8
- **Hyperperistalsis** R19.2
  - psychogenic F45.8
- **Hyperpermeability, capillary** I78.8
- **Hyperphagia** R63.2
- **Hyperphenylalaninemia NEC** E7Ø.1
- **Hyperphoria** (alternating) H5Ø.53
- **Hyperphosphatemia** E83.39
- **Hyperpiesis, hyperpiesia** — *see* Hypertension
- **Hyperpigmentation** (*see also* Pigmentation)
  - melanin NEC L81.4
  - postinflammatory L81.Ø
- **Hyperpinealism** E34.8
- **Hyperpituitarism** E22.9
- **Hyperplasia, hyperplastic**
  - adenoids J35.2
  - adrenal (capsule) (cortex) (gland) E27.8
    - with
      - sexual precocity (male) E25.9
        - congenital E25.Ø
      - virilism, adrenal E25.9
        - congenital E25.Ø
      - virilization (female) E25.9
        - congenital E25.Ø
    - congenital E25.Ø
      - salt-losing E25.Ø
  - adrenomedullary E27.5
  - angiolymphoid, eosinophilia (ALHE) D18.Ø1
  - appendix (lymphoid) K38.Ø
  - artery, fibromuscular I77.3
  - bone (*see also* Hypertrophy, bone)
    - marrow D75.89

Hyperplasia, hyperplastic — *continued*

  - breast (*see also* Hypertrophy, breast)
    - ductal (atypical) N6Ø.9- ☑
  - C-cell, thyroid EØ7.Ø
  - cementation (tooth) (teeth) KØ3.4
  - cervical gland R59.Ø
  - cervix (uteri) (basal cell) (endometrium) (polypoid) (*see also* Dysplasia, cervix)
    - congenital Q51.828
  - clitoris, congenital Q52.6
  - denture KØ6.2
  - endocervicitis N72
  - endometrium, endometrial (adenomatous) (benign) (cystic) (glandular) (glandular-cystic) (polypoid) N85.ØØ
    - with atypia N85.Ø2
    - cervix — *see* Dysplasia, cervix
    - complex (without atypia) N85.Ø1
    - simple (without atypia) N85.Ø1
  - epithelial L85.9
    - focal, oral, including tongue K13.29
    - nipple N62
    - skin L85.9
    - tongue K13.29
    - vaginal wall N89.3
  - erythroid D75.89
  - fibromuscular of artery (carotid) (renal) I77.3
  - genital
    - female NEC N94.89
    - male N5Ø.8
  - gingiva KØ6.1
  - glandularis cystica uteri (interstitialis) (*see also* Hyperplasia, endometrial) N85.ØØ
  - gum KØ6.1
  - hymen, congenital Q52.4
  - irritative, edentulous (alveolar) KØ6.2
  - jaw M26.Ø9
    - alveolar M26.79
    - lower M26.Ø3
      - alveolar M26.72
    - upper M26.Ø1
      - alveolar M26.71
  - kidney (congenital) Q63.3
  - labia N9Ø.6
    - epithelial N9Ø.3
  - liver (congenital) Q44.7
    - nodular, focal K76.89
  - lymph gland or node R59.9
  - mandible, mandibular M26.Ø3
    - alveolar M26.72
    - unilateral condylar M27.8
  - maxilla, maxillary M26.Ø1
    - alveolar M26.71
  - myometrium, myometrial N85.2
  - neuroendocrine cell, of infancy J84.841
  - nose
    - lymphoid J34.89
    - polypoid J33.9
  - oral mucosa (irritative) K13.6
  - organ or site, congenital NEC — *see* Anomaly, by site
  - ovary N83.8
  - palate, papillary (irritative) K13.6
  - pancreatic islet cells E16.9
    - alpha E16.8
      - with excess
        - gastrin E16.4
        - glucagon E16.3
    - beta E16.1
  - parathyroid (gland) E21.Ø
  - pharynx (lymphoid) J39.2
  - prostate (adenofibromatous) (nodular) N4Ø.Ø
    - with lower urinary tract symptoms (LUTS) N4Ø.1
    - without lower urinary tract symtpoms (LUTS) N4Ø.Ø
  - renal artery I77.89
  - reticulo-endothelial (cell) D75.89
  - salivary gland (any) K11.1
  - Schimmelbusch's — *see* Mastopathy, cystic
  - suprarenal capsule (gland) E27.8
  - thymus (gland) (persistent) E32.Ø
  - thyroid (gland) — *see* Goiter
  - tonsils (faucial) (infective) (lingual) (lymphoid) J35.1
    - with adenoids J35.3
  - unilateral condylar M27.8
  - uterus, uterine N85.2
    - endometrium (glandular) (*see also* Hyperplasia, endometrial) N85.ØØ
  - vulva N9Ø.6
    - epithelial N9Ø.3
- **Hyperpnea** — *see* Hyperventilation
- **Hyperpotassemia** E87.5
- **Hyperprebetalipoproteinemia** (familial) E78.1
- **Hyperprolactinemia** E22.1
- **Hyperprolinemia** (type I) (type II) E72.59
- **Hyperproteinemia** E88.Ø9
- **Hyperprothrombinemia, causing coagulation factor deficiency** D68.4
- **Hyperpyrexia** R5Ø.9
  - heat (effects) T67.Ø ☑
  - malignant, due to anesthetic T88.3 ☑
  - rheumatic — *see* Fever, rheumatic
  - unknown origin R5Ø.9
- **Hyper-reflexia** R29.2
- **Hypersalivation** K11.7
- **Hypersecretion**
  - ACTH (not associated with Cushing's syndrome) E27.Ø
    - pituitary E24.Ø
  - adrenaline E27.5
  - adrenomedullary E27.5
  - androgen (testicular) E29.Ø
    - ovarian (drug-induced) (iatrogenic) E28.1
  - calcitonin EØ7.Ø
  - catecholamine E27.5
  - corticoadrenal E24.9
  - cortisol E24.9
  - epinephrine E27.5
  - estrogen E28.Ø
  - gastric K31.89
    - psychogenic F45.8
  - gastrin E16.4
  - glucagon E16.3
  - hormone(s)
    - ACTH (not associated with Cushing's syndrome) E27.Ø
      - pituitary E24.Ø
    - antidiuretic E22.2
    - growth E22.Ø
    - intestinal NEC E34.1
    - ovarian androgen E28.1
    - pituitary E22.9
    - testicular E29.Ø
    - thyroid stimulating EØ5.8Ø
      - with thyroid storm EØ5.81
  - insulin — *see* Hyperinsulinism
  - lacrimal glands — *see* Epiphora
  - medulloadrenal E27.5
  - milk O92.6
  - ovarian androgens E28.1
  - salivary gland (any) K11.7
  - thyrocalcitonin EØ7.Ø
  - upper respiratory J39.8
- **Hypersegmentation, leukocytic, hereditary** D72.Ø
- **Hypersensitive, hypersensitiveness, hypersensitivity** (*see also* Allergy)
  - carotid sinus G9Ø.Ø1
  - colon — *see* Irritable, colon
  - drug T88.7 ☑
  - gastrointestinal K52.2
    - psychogenic F45.8
  - labyrinth — *see* subcategory H83.2 ☑
  - pain R2Ø.8
  - pneumonitis — *see* Pneumonitis, allergic
  - reaction T78.4Ø ☑
    - upper respiratory tract NEC J39.3
- **Hypersomnia** (organic) G47.1Ø
  - due to
    - alcohol
      - abuse F1Ø.182
      - dependence F1Ø.282
      - use F1Ø.982
    - amphetamines
      - abuse F15.182
      - dependence F15.282
      - use F15.982
    - caffeine
      - abuse F15.182
      - dependence F15.282
      - use F15.982
    - cocaine
      - abuse F14.182
      - dependence F14.282
      - use F14.982
    - drug NEC
      - abuse F19.182
      - dependence F19.282
      - use F19.982
    - medical condition G47.14

- **Hypofunction** — *continued*
  - testicular E29.1
    - postprocedural (postsurgical) (postirradiation) (iatrogenic) E89.5
- **Hypogalactia** O92.4
- **Hypogammaglobulinemia** (*see also* Agammaglobulinemia) D8Ø.1
  - hereditary D8Ø.Ø
  - nonfamilial D8Ø.1
  - transient, of infancy D8Ø.7
- **Hypogenitalism** (congenital) — *see* Hypogonadism
- **Hypoglossia** Q38.3
- **Hypoglycemia** (spontaneous) E16.2
  - coma E15
    - diabetic — *see* Diabetes, coma
  - diabetic — *see* Diabetes, hypoglycemia
  - dietary counseling and surveillance Z71.3
  - drug-induced E16.Ø
    - with coma (nondiabetic) E15
  - due to insulin E16.Ø
    - with coma (nondiabetic) E15
    - therapeutic misadventure — *see* subcategory T38.3 ☑
  - functional, nonhyperinsulinemic E16.1
  - iatrogenic E16.Ø
    - with coma (nondiabetic) E15
  - in infant of diabetic mother P7Ø.1
    - gestational diabetes P7Ø.Ø
  - infantile E16.1
  - leucine-induced E71.19
  - neonatal (transitory) P7Ø.4
    - iatrogenic P7Ø.3
  - reactive (not drug-induced) E16.1
  - transitory neonatal P7Ø.4
- **Hypogonadism**
  - female E28.39
  - hypogonadotropic E23.Ø
  - male E29.1
  - ovarian (primary) E28.39
  - pituitary E23.Ø
  - testicular (primary) E29.1
- **Hypohidrosis, hypoidrosis** L74.4
- **Hypoinsulinemia, postprocedural** E89.1
- **Hypokalemia** E87.6
- **Hypoleukocytosis** — *see* Agranulocytosis
- **Hypolipoproteinemia** (alpha) (beta) E78.6
- **Hypomagnesemia** E83.42
  - neonatal P71.2
- **Hypomania, hypomanic reaction** F3Ø.8
- **Hypomenorrhea** — *see* Oligomenorrhea
- **Hypometabolism** R63.8
- **Hypomotility**
  - gastrointestinal (tract) K31.89
    - psychogenic F45.8
  - intestine K59.8
    - psychogenic F45.8
  - stomach K31.89
    - psychogenic F45.8
- **Hyponasality** R49.22
- **Hyponatremia** E87.1
- **Hypo-osmolality** E87.1
- **Hypo-ovarianism, hypo-ovarism** E28.39
- **Hypoparathyroidism** E2Ø.9
  - familial E2Ø.8
  - idiopathic E2Ø.Ø
  - neonatal, transitory P71.4
  - postprocedural E89.2
  - specified NEC E2Ø.8
- **Hypoperfusion** (in)
  - newborn P96.89
- **Hypopharyngitis** — *see* Laryngopharyngitis
- **Hypophoria** H5Ø.53
- **Hypophosphatemia, hypophosphatasia** (acquired) (congenital) (renal) E83.39
  - familial E83.31
- **Hypophyseal, hypophysis** (*see also* condition)
  - dwarfism E23.Ø
  - gigantism E22.Ø
- **Hypopiesis** — *see* Hypotension
- **Hypopinealism** E34.8
- **Hypopituitarism** (juvenile) E23.Ø
  - drug-induced E23.1
  - due to
    - hypophysectomy E89.3
    - radiotherapy E89.3
  - iatrogenic NEC E23.1
  - postirradiation E89.3
  - postpartum E23.Ø
  - postprocedural E89.3
- **Hypoplasia, hypoplastic**
  - adrenal (gland), congenital Q89.1
  - alimentary tract, congenital Q45.8
    - upper Q4Ø.8
  - anus, anal (canal) Q42.3
    - with fistula Q42.2
  - aorta, aortic Q25.4
    - ascending, in hypoplastic left heart syndrome Q23.4
    - valve Q23.1
      - in hypoplastic left heart syndrome Q23.4
  - areola, congenital Q83.8
  - arm (congenital) — *see* Defect, reduction, upper limb
  - artery (peripheral) Q27.8
    - brain (congenital) Q28.3
    - coronary Q24.5
    - digestive system Q27.8
    - lower limb Q27.8
    - pulmonary Q25.79
      - functional, unilateral J43.Ø
    - retinal (congenital) Q14.1
    - specified site NEC Q27.8
    - umbilical Q27.Ø
    - upper limb Q27.8
  - auditory canal Q17.8
    - causing impairment of hearing Q16.9
  - biliary duct or passage Q44.5
  - bone NOS Q79.9
    - face Q75.8
    - marrow D61.9
      - megakaryocytic D69.49
    - skull — *see* Hypoplasia, skull
  - brain QØ2
    - gyri QØ4.3
    - part of QØ4.3
  - breast (areola) N64.82
  - bronchus Q32.4
  - cardiac Q24.8
  - carpus — *see* Defect, reduction, upper limb, specified type NEC
  - cartilage hair Q78.5
  - cecum Q42.8
  - cementum KØØ.4
  - cephalic QØ2
  - cerebellum QØ4.3
  - cervix (uteri), congenital Q51.821
  - clavicle (congenital) Q74.Ø
  - coccyx Q76.49
  - colon Q42.9
    - specified NEC Q42.8
  - corpus callosum QØ4.Ø
  - cricoid cartilage Q31.2
  - digestive organ(s) or tract NEC Q45.8
    - upper (congenital) Q4Ø.8
  - ear (auricle) (lobe) Q17.2
    - middle Q16.4
  - enamel of teeth (neonatal) (postnatal) (prenatal) KØØ.4
  - endocrine (gland) NEC Q89.2
  - endometrium N85.8
  - epididymis (congenital) Q55.4
  - epiglottis Q31.2
  - erythroid, congenital D61.Ø1
  - esophagus (congenital) Q39.8
  - eustachian tube Q17.8
  - eye Q11.2
  - eyelid (congenital) Q1Ø.3
  - face Q18.8
    - bone(s) Q75.8
  - femur (congenital) — *see* Defect, reduction, lower limb, specified type NEC
  - fibula (congenital) — *see* Defect, reduction, lower limb, specified type NEC
  - finger (congenital) — *see* Defect, reduction, upper limb, specified type NEC
  - focal dermal Q82.8
  - foot — *see* Defect, reduction, lower limb, specified type NEC
  - gallbladder Q44.Ø
  - genitalia, genital organ(s)
    - female, congenital Q52.8
      - external Q52.79
      - internal NEC Q52.8
    - in adiposogenital dystrophy E23.6
  - glottis Q31.2
  - hair Q84.2
  - hand (congenital) — *see* Defect, reduction, upper limb, specified type NEC
  - heart Q24.8
  - humerus (congenital) — *see* Defect, reduction, upper limb, specified type NEC
  - intestine (small) Q41.9
    - large Q42.9
      - specified NEC Q42.8
  - jaw M26.Ø9
    - alveolar M26.79
    - lower M26.Ø4
      - alveolar M26.74
    - upper M26.Ø2
      - alveolar M26.73
  - kidney(s) Q6Ø.5
    - bilateral Q6Ø.4
    - unilateral Q6Ø.3
  - labium (majus) (minus), congenital Q52.79
  - larynx Q31.2
  - left heart syndrome Q23.4
  - leg (congenital) — *see* Defect, reduction, lower limb
  - limb Q73.8
    - lower (congenital) — *see* Defect, reduction, lower limb
    - upper (congenital) — *see* Defect, reduction, upper limb
  - liver Q44.7
  - lung (lobe) (not associated with short gestation) Q33.6
    - associated with immaturity, low birth weight, prematurity, or short gestation P28.Ø
  - mammary (areola), congenital Q83.8
  - mandible, mandibular M26.Ø4
    - alveolar M26.74
    - unilateral condylar M27.8
  - maxillary M26.Ø2
    - alveolar M26.73
  - medullary D61.9
  - megakaryocytic D69.49
  - metacarpus — *see* Defect, reduction, upper limb, specified type NEC
  - metatarsus — *see* Defect, reduction, lower limb, specified type NEC
  - muscle Q79.8
  - nail(s) Q84.6
  - nose, nasal Q3Ø.1
  - optic nerve H47.Ø3- ☑
  - osseous meatus (ear) Q17.8
  - ovary, congenital Q5Ø.39
  - pancreas Q45.Ø
  - parathyroid (gland) Q89.2
  - parotid gland Q38.4
  - patella Q74.1
  - pelvis, pelvic girdle Q74.2
  - penis (congenital) Q55.62
  - peripheral vascular system Q27.8
    - digestive system Q27.8
    - lower limb Q27.8
    - specified site NEC Q27.8
    - upper limb Q27.8
  - pituitary (gland) (congenital) Q89.2
  - pulmonary (not associated with short gestation) Q33.6
    - artery, functional J43.Ø
    - associated with short gestation P28.Ø
  - radioulnar — *see* Defect, reduction, upper limb, specified type NEC
  - radius — *see* Defect, reduction, upper limb
  - rectum Q42.1
    - with fistula Q42.Ø
  - respiratory system NEC Q34.8
  - rib Q76.6
  - right heart syndrome Q22.6
  - sacrum Q76.49
  - scapula Q74.Ø
  - scrotum Q55.1
  - shoulder girdle Q74.Ø
  - skin Q82.8
  - skull (bone) Q75.8
    - with
      - anencephaly QØØ.Ø
      - encephalocele — *see* Encephalocele
      - hydrocephalus QØ3.9
        - with spina bifida — *see* Spina bifida, by site, with hydrocephalus
      - microcephaly QØ2
  - spinal (cord) (ventral horn cell) QØ6.1
  - spine Q76.49
  - sternum Q76.7

- **Hypoplasia, hypoplastic** — *continued*
  - tarsus — *see* Defect, reduction, lower limb, specified type NEC
  - testis Q55.1
  - thymic, with immunodeficiency D82.1
  - thymus (gland) Q89.2
    - with immunodeficiency D82.1
  - thyroid (gland) EØ3.1
    - cartilage Q31.2
  - tibiofibular (congenital) — *see* Defect, reduction, lower limb, specified type NEC
  - toe — *see* Defect, reduction, lower limb, specified type NEC
  - tongue Q38.3
  - Turner's KØØ.4
  - ulna (congenital) — *see* Defect, reduction, upper limb
  - umbilical artery Q27.Ø
  - unilateral condylar M27.8
  - ureter Q62.8
  - uterus, congenital Q51.811
  - vagina Q52.4
  - vascular NEC peripheral Q27.8
    - brain Q28.3
    - digestive system Q27.8
    - lower limb Q27.8
    - specified site NEC Q27.8
    - upper limb Q27.8
  - vein(s) (peripheral) Q27.8
    - brain Q28.3
    - digestive system Q27.8
    - great Q26.8
    - lower limb Q27.8
    - specified site NEC Q27.8
    - upper limb Q27.8
  - vena cava (inferior) (superior) Q26.8
  - vertebra Q76.49
  - vulva, congenital Q52.79
  - zonule (ciliary) Q12.8
- **Hypopotassemia** E87.6
- **Hypoproconvertinemia, congenital** (hereditary) D68.2
- **Hypoproteinemia** E77.8
- **Hypoprothrombinemia** (congenital) (hereditary) (idiopathic) D68.2
  - acquired D68.4
  - newborn, transient P61.6
- **Hypoptyalism** K11.7
- **Hypopyon** (eye) (anterior chamber) — *see* Iridocyclitis, acute, hypopyon
- **Hypopyrexia** R68.Ø
- **Hyporeflexia** R29.2
- **Hyposecretion**
  - ACTH E23.Ø
  - antidiuretic hormone E23.2
  - ovary E28.39
  - salivary gland (any) K11.7
  - vasopressin E23.2
- **Hyposegmentation, leukocytic, hereditary** D72.Ø
- **Hyposiderinemia** D5Ø.9
- **Hypospadias** Q54.9
  - balanic Q54.Ø
  - coronal Q54.Ø
  - glandular Q54.Ø
  - penile Q54.1
  - penoscrotal Q54.2
  - perineal Q54.3
  - specified NEC Q54.8
- **Hypospermatogenesis** — *see* Oligospermia
- **Hyposplenism** D73.Ø
- **Hypostasis pulmonary, passive** — *see* Edema, lung
- **Hypostatic** — *see* condition
- **Hyposthenuria** N28.89
- **Hypotension** (arterial) (constitutional) I95.9
  - chronic I95.89
  - drug-induced I95.2
  - due to (of) hemodialysis I95.3
  - iatrogenic I95.89
  - idiopathic (permanent) I95.Ø
  - intracranial, following ventricular shunting (ventriculostomy) G97.2
  - intra-dialytic I95.3
  - maternal, syndrome (following labor and delivery) O26.5- ☑
  - neurogenic, orthostatic G9Ø.3
  - orthostatic (chronic) I95.1
    - due to drugs I95.2
    - neurogenic G9Ø.3
  - postoperative I95.81
  - postural I95.1
- **Hypotension** — *continued*
  - specified NEC I95.89
- **Hypothermia** (accidental) T68 ☑
  - due to anesthesia, anesthetic T88.51 ☑
  - low environmental temperature T68 ☑
  - neonatal P8Ø.9
    - environmental (mild) NEC P8Ø.8
    - mild P8Ø.8
    - severe (chronic) (cold injury syndrome) P8Ø.Ø
    - specified NEC P8Ø.8
  - not associated with low environmental temperature R68.Ø
- **Hypothyroidism** (acquired) EØ3.9
  - congenital (without goiter) EØ3.1
    - with goiter (diffuse) EØ3.Ø
  - due to
    - exogenous substance NEC EØ3.2
    - iodine-deficiency, acquired EØ1.8
      - subclinical EØ2
    - irradiation therapy E89.Ø
    - medicament NEC EØ3.2
    - P-aminosalicylic acid (PAS) EØ3.2
    - phenylbutazone EØ3.2
    - resorcinol EØ3.2
    - sulfonamide EØ3.2
    - surgery E89.Ø
    - thiourea group drugs EØ3.2
  - iatrogenic NEC EØ3.2
  - iodine-deficiency (acquired) EØ1.8
    - congenital — *see* Syndrome, iodine- deficiency, congenital
    - subclinical EØ2
  - neonatal, transitory P72.2
  - postinfectious EØ3.3
  - postirradiation E89.Ø
  - postprocedural E89.Ø
  - postsurgical E89.Ø
  - specified NEC EØ3.8
  - subclinical, iodine-deficiency related EØ2
- **Hypotonia, hypotonicity, hypotony**
  - bladder N31.2
  - congenital (benign) P94.2
  - eye — *see* Disorder, globe, hypotony
- **Hypotrichosis** — *see* Alopecia
- **Hypotropia** H5Ø.2- ☑
- **Hypoventilation** RØ6.89
  - congenital central alveolar G47.35
  - sleep related
    - idiopathic nonobstructive alveolar G47.34
    - in conditions classified elsewhere G47.36
- **Hypovitaminosis** — *see* Deficiency, vitamin
- **Hypovolemia** E86.1
  - surgical shock T81.19 ☑
  - traumatic (shock) T79.4 ☑
- **Hypoxemia** RØ9.Ø2
  - newborn P84
  - sleep related, in conditions classified elsewhere G47.36
- **Hypoxia** (*see also* Anoxia) RØ9.Ø2
  - cerebral, during a procedure NEC G97.81
    - postprocedural NEC G97.82
  - intrauterine P84
  - myocardial — *see* Insufficiency, coronary
  - newborn P84
  - sleep-related G47.34
- **Hypsarhythmia** — *see* Epilepsy, generalized, specified NEC
- **Hysteralgia, pregnant uterus** O26.89- ☑
- **Hysteria, hysterical** (conversion) (dissociative state) F44.9
  - anxiety F41.8
  - convulsions F44.5
  - psychosis, acute F44.9
- **Hysteroepilepsy** F44.5

I

- **Ichthyoparasitism due to Vandellia cirrhosa** B88.8
- **Ichthyosis** (congenital) Q8Ø.9
  - acquired L85.Ø
  - fetalis Q8Ø.4
  - hystrix Q8Ø.8
  - lamellar Q8Ø.2
  - lingual K13.29
  - palmaris and plantaris Q82.8
  - simplex Q8Ø.Ø
  - vera Q8Ø.8
  - vulgaris Q8Ø.Ø
- **Ichthyosis** — *continued*
  - X-linked Q8Ø.1
- **Ichthyotoxism** — *see* Poisoning, fish
  - bacterial — *see* Intoxication, foodborne
- **Icteroanemia, hemolytic** (acquired) D59.9
  - congenital — *see* Spherocytosis
- **Icterus** (*see also* Jaundice)
  - conjunctiva R17
  - gravis, newborn P55.Ø
  - hematogenous (acquired) D59.9
  - hemolytic (acquired) D59.9
    - congenital — *see* Spherocytosis
  - hemorrhagic (acute) (leptospiral) (spirochetal) A27.Ø
    - newborn P53
  - infectious B15.9
    - with hepatic coma B15.Ø
    - leptospiral A27.Ø
    - spirochetal A27.Ø
  - neonatorum — *see* Jaundice, newborn
  - newborn P59.9
  - spirochetal A27.Ø
- **Ictus solaris, solis** T67.Ø ☑
- **Id reaction** (due to bacteria) L3Ø.2
- **Ideation**
  - homicidal R45.85Ø
  - suicidal R45.851
- **Identity disorder** (child) F64.9
  - gender role F64.2
  - psychosexual F64.2
- **Idioglossia** F8Ø.Ø
- **Idiopathic** — *see* condition
- **Idiot, idiocy** (congenital) F73
  - amaurotic (Bielschowsky(-Jansky)) (family) (infantile (late)) (juvenile (late)) (Vogt-Spielmeyer) E75.4
  - microcephalic QØ2
- **IgE asthma** J45.9Ø9
- **IIAC** (idiopathic infantile arterial calcification) Q28.8
- **Ileitis** (chronic) (noninfectious) (*see also* Enteritis) K52.9
  - backwash — *see* Pancolitis, ulcerative (chronic)
  - infectious AØ9
  - regional (ulcerative) — *see* Enteritis, regional, small intestine
  - segmental — *see* Enteritis, regional
  - terminal (ulcerative) — *see* Enteritis, regional, small intestine
- **Ileocolitis** (*see also* Enteritis) K52.9
  - infectious AØ9
  - regional — *see* Enteritis, regional
- **Ileostomy**
  - attention to Z43.2
  - malfunctioning K94.13
  - status Z93.2
    - with complication — *see* Complications, enterostomy
- **Ileotyphus** — *see* Typhoid
- **Ileum** — *see* condition
- **Ileus** (bowel) (colon) (inhibitory) (intestine) K56.7
  - adynamic K56.Ø
  - due to gallstone (in intestine) K56.3
  - duodenal (chronic) K31.5
  - gallstone K56.3
  - mechanical NEC K56.69
  - meconium P76.Ø
    - in cystic fibrosis E84.11
    - meaning meconium plug (without cystic fibrosis) P76.Ø
  - myxedema K59.8
  - neurogenic K56.Ø
    - Hirschsprung's disease or megacolon Q43.1
  - newborn
    - due to meconium P76.Ø
      - in cystic fibrosis E84.11
      - meaning meconium plug (without cystic fibrosis) P76.Ø
    - transitory P76.1
  - obstructive K56.69
  - paralytic K56.Ø
- **Iliac** — *see* condition
- **Iliotibial band syndrome** M76.3- ☑
- **Illiteracy** Z55.Ø
- **Illness** (*see also* Disease) R69
  - manic-depressive — *see* Disorder, bipolar
- **Imbalance** R26.89
  - autonomic G9Ø.8
  - constituents of food intake E63.1
  - electrolyte E87.8

Imbalance — *continued*
- electrolyte — *continued*
  - with
    - abortion — *see* Abortion by type, complicated by, electrolyte imbalance
    - molar pregnancy O08.5
  - due to hyperemesis gravidarum O21.1
  - following ectopic or molar pregnancy O08.5
  - neonatal, transitory NEC P74.4
    - potassium P74.3
    - sodium P74.2
- endocrine E34.9
- eye muscle NOS H50.9
- hormone E34.9
- hysterical F44.4
- labyrinth — *see* subcategory H83.2 ☑
- posture R29.3
- protein-energy — *see* Malnutrition
- sympathetic G90.8

Imbecile, imbecility (I.Q. 35-49) F71

Imbedding, intrauterine device T83.39 ☑

Imbibition, cholesterol (gallbladder) K82.4

Imbrication, teeth,, fully erupted M26.30

Imerslund (-Gräsbeck) **syndrome** D51.1

Immature (*see also* Immaturity)
- birth (less than 37 completed weeks) — *see* Preterm, newborn
  - extremely (less than 28 completed weeks) — *see* Immaturity, extreme
- personality F60.89

Immaturity (less than 37 completed weeks) (*see also* Preterm, newborn)
- extreme of newborn (less than 28 completed weeks of gestation) (less than 196 completed days of gestation) (unspecified weeks of gestation) P07.20
  - gestational age
    - less than 23 completed weeks P07.21
    - 23 completed weeks (23 weeks, 0 days through 23 weeks, 6 days) P07.22
    - 24 completed weeks (24 weeks, 0 days through 24 weeks, 6 days) P07.23
    - 25 completed weeks (25 weeks, 0 days through 25 weeks, 6 days) P07.24
    - 26 completed weeks (26 weeks, 0 days through 26 weeks, 6 days) P07.25
    - 27 completed weeks (27 weeks, 0 days through 27 weeks, 6 days) P07.26
- fetus or infant light-for-dates — *see* Light-for-dates
- lung, newborn P28.0
- organ or site NEC — *see* Hypoplasia
- pulmonary, newborn P28.0
- reaction F60.89
- sexual (female) (male), after puberty E30.0

Immersion T75.1 ☑
- foot T69.02- ☑
- hand T69.01- ☑

Immobile, immobility
- complete, due to severe physical disability or frailty R53.2
- intestine K59.8
- syndrome (paraplegic) M62.3

Immune reconstitution (inflammatory) syndrome [IRIS] D89.3

Immunization (*see also* Vaccination)
- ABO — *see* Incompatibility, ABO
  - in newborn P55.1
- complication — *see* Complications, vaccination
- encounter for Z23
- not done (not carried out) Z28.9
  - because (of)
    - acute illness of patient Z28.01
    - allergy to vaccine (or component) Z28.04
    - caregiver refusal Z28.82
    - chronic illness of patient Z28.02
    - contraindication NEC Z28.09
    - group pressure Z28.1
    - guardian refusal Z28.82
    - immune compromised state of patient Z28.03
    - parent refusal Z28.82
    - patient had disease being vaccinated against Z28.81
    - patient refusal Z28.21
    - patient's belief Z28.1
    - religious beliefs of patient Z28.1
    - specified reason NEC Z28.89
      - of patient Z28.29
    - unspecified patient reason Z28.20

Immunization — *continued*
- Rh factor
  - affecting management of pregnancy NEC O36.09- ☑
    - anti-D antibody O36.01- ☑
  - from transfusion — *see* Complication(s), transfusion, incompatibility reaction, Rh (factor)

Immunocytoma C83.0- ☑

Immunodeficiency D84.9
- with
  - adenosine-deaminase deficiency D81.3
  - antibody defects D80.9
    - specified type NEC D80.8
  - hyperimmunoglobulinemia D80.6
  - increased immunoglobulin M (IgM) D80.5
  - major defect D82.9
    - specified type NEC D82.8
  - partial albinism D82.8
  - short-limbed stature D82.2
  - thrombocytopenia and eczema D82.0
- antibody with
  - hyperimmunoglobulinemia D80.6
  - near-normal immunoglobulins D80.6
- autosomal recessive, Swiss type D80.0
- combined D81.9
  - biotin-dependent carboxylase D81.819
    - biotinidase D81.810
    - holocarboxylase synthetase D81.818
    - specified type NEC D81.818
  - severe (SCID) D81.9
    - with
      - low or normal B-cell numbers D81.2
      - low T- and B-cell numbers D81.1
      - reticular dysgenesis D81.0
  - specified type NEC D81.89
- common variable D83.9
  - with
    - abnormalities of B-cell numbers and function D83.0
    - autoantibodies to B- or T-cells D83.2
    - immunoregulatory T-cell disorders D83.1
  - specified type NEC D83.8
- following hereditary defective response to Epstein-Barr virus (EBV) D82.3
- selective, immunoglobulin
  - A (IgA) D80.2
  - G (IgG) (subclasses) D80.3
  - M (IgM) D80.4
- severe combined (SCID) D81.9
- specified type NEC D84.8
- X-linked, with increased IgM D80.5

Immunotherapy (encounter for)
- antineoplastic Z51.12

Impaction, impacted
- bowel, colon, rectum (*see also* Impaction, fecal) K56.49
  - by gallstone K56.3
- calculus — *see* Calculus
- cerumen (ear) (external) H61.2- ☑
- cuspid — *see* Impaction, tooth
- dental (same or adjacent tooth) K01.1
- fecal, feces K56.41
- fracture — *see* Fracture, by site
- gallbladder — *see* Calculus, gallbladder
- gallstone(s) — *see* Calculus, gallbladder
  - bile duct (common) (hepatic) — *see* Calculus, bile duct
  - cystic duct — *see* Calculus, gallbladder
  - in intestine, with obstruction (any part) K56.3
- intestine (calculous) NEC (*see also* Impaction, fecal) K56.49
  - gallstone, with ileus K56.3
- intrauterine device (IUD) T83.39 ☑
- molar — *see* Impaction, tooth
- shoulder, causing obstructed labor O66.0
- tooth, teeth K01.1
- turbinate J34.89

Impaired, impairment (function)
- auditory discrimination — *see* Abnormal, auditory perception
- cognitive, mild, so stated G31.84
- dual sensory Z73.82
- fasting glucose R73.01
- glucose tolerance (oral) R73.02
- hearing — *see* Deafness
- heart — *see* Disease, heart
- kidney N28.9
  - disorder resulting from N25.9
    - specified NEC N25.89

Impaired, impairment — *continued*
- liver K72.90
  - with coma K72.91
- mastication K08.8
- mild cognitive, so stated G31.84
- mobility
  - ear ossicles — *see* Ankylosis, ear ossicles
  - requiring care provider Z74.09
- myocardium, myocardial — *see* Insufficiency, myocardial
- rectal sphincter R19.8
- renal (acute) (chronic) N28.9
  - disorder resulting from N25.9
    - specified NEC N25.89
- vision NEC H54.7
  - both eyes H54.3

Impediment, speech R47.9
- psychogenic (childhood) F98.8
- slurring R47.81
- specified NEC R47.89

Impending
- coronary syndrome I20.0
- delirium tremens F10.239
- myocardial infarction I20.0

Imperception auditory (acquired) (*see also* Deafness)
- congenital H93.25

Imperfect
- aeration, lung (newborn) NEC — *see* Atelectasis
- closure (congenital)
  - alimentary tract NEC Q45.8
    - lower Q43.8
    - upper Q40.8
  - atrioventricular ostium Q21.2
  - atrium (secundum) Q21.1
  - branchial cleft or sinus Q18.0
  - choroid Q14.3
  - cricoid cartilage Q31.8
  - cusps, heart valve NEC Q24.8
    - pulmonary Q22.3
  - ductus
    - arteriosus Q25.0
    - Botalli Q25.0
  - ear drum (causing impairment of hearing) Q16.4
  - esophagus with communication to bronchus or trachea Q39.1
  - eyelid Q10.3
  - foramen
    - botalli Q21.1
    - ovale Q21.1
  - genitalia, genital organ(s) or system
    - female Q52.8
      - external Q52.79
      - internal NEC Q52.8
    - male Q55.8
  - glottis Q31.8
  - interatrial ostium or septum Q21.1
  - interauricular ostium or septum Q21.1
  - interventricular ostium or septum Q21.0
  - larynx Q31.8
  - lip — *see* Cleft, lip
  - nasal septum Q30.3
  - nose Q30.2
  - omphalomesenteric duct Q43.0
  - optic nerve entry Q14.2
  - organ or site not listed — *see* Anomaly, by site
  - ostium
    - interatrial Q21.1
    - interauricular Q21.1
    - interventricular Q21.0
  - palate — *see* Cleft, palate
  - preauricular sinus Q18.1
  - retina Q14.1
  - roof of orbit Q75.8
  - sclera Q13.5
  - septum
    - aorticopulmonary Q21.4
    - atrial (secundum) Q21.1
    - between aorta and pulmonary artery Q21.4
    - heart Q21.9
    - interatrial (secundum) Q21.1
    - interauricular (secundum) Q21.1
    - interventricular Q21.0
      - in tetralogy of Fallot Q21.3
    - nasal Q30.3
    - ventricular Q21.0
      - with pulmonary stenosis or atresia, dextraposition of aorta, and hypertrophy of right ventricle Q21.3

- **Imperfect** — *continued*
  - closure — *continued*
    - septum — *continued*
      - ventricular — *continued*
        - in tetralogy of Fallot Q21.3
    - skull Q75.Ø
      - with
        - anencephaly QØØ.Ø
        - encephalocele — *see* Encephalocele
        - hydrocephalus QØ3.9
          - with spina bifida — *see* Spina bifida, by site, with hydrocephalus
        - microcephaly QØ2
    - spine (with meningocele) — *see* Spina bifida
    - trachea Q32.1
    - tympanic membrane (causing impairment of hearing) Q16.4
    - uterus Q51.818
    - vitelline duct Q43.Ø
  - erection — *see* Dysfunction, sexual, male, erectile
  - fusion — *see* Imperfect, closure
  - inflation, lung (newborn) — *see* Atelectasis
  - posture R29.3
  - rotation, intestine Q43.3
  - septum, ventricular Q21.Ø
- **Imperfectly descended testis** — *see* Cryptorchid
- **Imperforate** (congenital) (*see also* Atresia)
  - anus Q42.3
    - with fistula Q42.2
  - cervix (uteri) Q51.828
  - esophagus Q39.Ø
    - with tracheoesophageal fistula Q39.1
  - hymen Q52.3
  - jejunum Q41.1
  - pharynx Q38.8
  - rectum Q42.1
    - with fistula Q42.Ø
  - urethra Q64.39
  - vagina Q52.4
- **Impervious** (congenital) (*see also* Atresia)
  - anus Q42.3
    - with fistula Q42.2
  - bile duct Q44.2
  - esophagus Q39.Ø
    - with tracheoesophageal fistula Q39.1
  - intestine (small) Q41.9
    - large Q42.9
      - specified NEC Q42.8
  - rectum Q42.1
    - with fistula Q42.Ø
  - ureter — *see* Atresia, ureter
  - urethra Q64.39
- **Impetiginization of dermatoses** LØ1.1
- **Impetigo** (any organism) (any site) (circinate) (contagiosa) (simplex) (vulgaris) LØ1.ØØ
  - Bockhart's LØ1.Ø2
  - bullous, bullosa LØ1.Ø3
  - external ear LØ1.ØØ [H62.4Ø]
  - follicularis LØ1.Ø2
  - furfuracea L3Ø.5
  - herpetiformis L4Ø.1
    - nonobstetrical L4Ø.1
  - neonatorum LØ1.Ø3
  - nonbullous LØ1.Ø1
  - specified type NEC LØ1.Ø9
  - ulcerative LØ1.Ø9
- **Impingement** (on teeth)
  - soft tissue
    - anterior M26.81
    - posterior M26.82
- **Implant, endometrial** N8Ø.9
- **Implantation**
  - anomalous — *see* Anomaly, by site
    - ureter Q62.63
  - cyst
    - external area or site (skin) NEC L72.Ø
    - iris — *see* Cyst, iris, implantation
    - vagina N89.8
    - vulva N9Ø.7
  - dermoid (cyst) — *see* Implantation, cyst
- **Impotence** (sexual) N52.9
  - counseling Z7Ø.1
  - organic origin (*see also* Dysfunction, sexual, male, erectile) N52.9
  - psychogenic F52.21
- **Impression, basilar** Q75.8
- **Imprisonment, anxiety concerning** Z65.1
- **Improper care** (child) (newborn) — *see* Maltreatment
- **Improperly tied umbilical cord** (causing hemorrhage) P51.8
- **Impulsiveness** (impulsive) R45.87
- **Inability to swallow** — *see* Aphagia
- **Inaccessible, inaccessibility**
  - health care NEC Z75.3
    - due to
      - waiting period Z75.2
        - for admission to facility elsewhere Z75.1
  - other helping agencies Z75.4
- **Inactive** — *see* condition
- **Inadequate, inadequacy**
  - aesthetics of dental restoration KØ8.56
  - biologic, constitutional, functional, or social F6Ø.7
  - development
    - child R62.5Ø
    - genitalia
      - after puberty NEC E3Ø.Ø
      - congenital
        - female Q52.8
          - external Q52.79
          - internal Q52.8
        - male Q55.8
    - lungs Q33.6
      - associated with short gestation P28.Ø
    - organ or site not listed — *see* Anomaly, by site
  - diet (causing nutritional deficiency) E63.9
  - eating habits Z72.4
  - environment, household Z59.1
  - family support Z63.8
  - food (supply) NEC Z59.4
    - hunger effects T73.Ø ☑
  - functional F6Ø.7
  - household care, due to
    - family member
      - handicapped or ill Z74.2
      - on vacation Z75.5
      - temporarily away from home Z74.2
    - technical defects in home Z59.1
    - temporary absence from home of person rendering care Z74.2
  - housing (heating) (space) Z59.1
  - income (financial) Z59.6
  - intrafamilial communication Z63.8
  - material resources Z59.9
  - mental — *see* Disability, intellectual
  - parental supervision or control of child Z62.Ø
  - personality F6Ø.7
  - pulmonary
    - function RØ6.89
      - newborn P28.5
    - ventilation, newborn P28.5
  - sample of cytologic smear
    - anus R85.615
    - cervix R87.615
    - vagina R87.625
  - social F6Ø.7
    - insurance Z59.7
    - skills NEC Z73.4
  - supervision of child by parent Z62.Ø
  - teaching affecting education Z55.8
  - welfare support Z59.7
- **Inanition** R64
  - with edema — *see* Malnutrition, severe
  - due to
    - deprivation of food T73.Ø ☑
    - malnutrition — *see* Malnutrition
  - fever R5Ø.9
- **Inappropriate**
  - change in quantitative human chorionic gonadotropin (hCG) in early pregnancy OØ2.81
  - diet or eating habits Z72.4
  - level of quantitative human chorionic gonadotropin (hCG) for gestational age in early pregnancy OØ2.81
  - secretion
    - antidiuretic hormone (ADH) (excessive) E22.2
      - deficiency E23.2
    - pituitary (posterior) E22.2
- **Inattention at or after birth** — *see* Neglect
- **Incarceration, incarcerated**
  - enterocele K46.Ø
    - gangrenous K46.1
  - epiplocele K46.Ø
    - gangrenous K46.1
  - exophthalmos K42.Ø
    - gangrenous K42.1
  - hernia (*see also* Hernia, by site, with obstruction)
- **Incarceration, incarcerated** — *continued*
  - hernia (*see also* Hernia, by site, with obstruction) — *continued*
    - with gangrene — *see* Hernia, by site, with gangrene
  - iris, in wound — *see* Injury, eye, laceration, with prolapse
  - lens, in wound — *see* Injury, eye, laceration, with prolapse
  - omphalocele K42.Ø
  - prison, anxiety concerning Z65.1
  - rupture — *see* Hernia, by site
  - sarcoepiplocele K46.Ø
    - gangrenous K46.1
  - sarcoepiplomphalocele K42.Ø
    - with gangrene K42.1
  - uterus N85.8
    - gravid O34.51- ☑
      - causing obstructed labor O65.5
- **Incised wound**
  - external — *see* Laceration
  - internal organs — *see* Injury, by site
- **Incision, incisional**
  - hernia K43.2
    - with
      - gangrene (and obstruction) K43.1
      - obstruction K43.Ø
  - surgical, complication — *see* Complications, surgical procedure
  - traumatic
    - external — *see* Laceration
    - internal organs — *see* Injury, by site
- **Inclusion**
  - azurophilic leukocytic D72.Ø
  - blennorrhea (neonatal) (newborn) P39.1
  - gallbladder in liver (congenital) Q44.1
- **Incompatibility**
  - ABO
    - affecting management of pregnancy O36.11- ☑
      - anti-A sensitization O36.11- ☑
      - anti-B sensitization O36.19- ☑
      - specified NEC O36.19- ☑
    - infusion or transfusion reaction — *see* Complication(s), transfusion, incompatibility reaction, ABO
    - newborn P55.1
  - blood (group) (Duffy) (K(ell)) (Kidd) (Lewis) (M) (S) NEC
    - affecting management of pregnancy O36.11- ☑
      - anti-A sensitization O36.11- ☑
      - anti-B sensitization O36.19- ☑
    - infusion or transfusion reaction T8Ø.89 ☑
    - newborn P55.8
  - divorce or estrangement Z63.5
  - Rh (blood group) (factor) Z31.82
    - affecting management of pregnancy NEC O36.Ø9- ☑
      - anti-D antibody O36.Ø1- ☑
    - infusion or transfusion reaction — *see* Complication(s), transfusion, incompatibility reaction, Rh (factor)
    - newborn P55.Ø
  - rhesus — *see* Incompatibility, Rh
- **Incompetency, incompetent, incompetence**
  - annular
    - aortic (valve) — *see* Insufficiency, aortic
    - mitral (valve) I34.Ø
    - pulmonary valve (heart) I37.1
  - aortic (valve) — *see* Insufficiency, aortic
  - cardiac valve — *see* Endocarditis
  - cervix, cervical (os) N88.3
    - in pregnancy O34.3- ☑
  - chronotropic I45.89
    - with
      - autonomic dysfunction G9Ø.8
      - ischemic heart disease I25.89
      - left ventricular dysfunction I51.89
      - sinus node dysfunction I49.8
  - esophagogastric (junction) (sphincter) K22.Ø
  - mitral (valve) — *see* Insufficiency, mitral
  - pelvic fundus N81.89
  - pubocervical tissue N81.82
  - pulmonary valve (heart) I37.1
    - congenital Q22.3
  - rectovaginal tissue N81.83
  - tricuspid (annular) (valve) — *see* Insufficiency, tricuspid
  - valvular — *see* Endocarditis
    - congenital Q24.8

- **Incompetency, incompetent, incompetence** — *continued*
  - vein, venous (saphenous) (varicose) — *see* Varix, leg
- **Incomplete** (*see also* condition)
  - bladder, emptying R33.9
  - defecation R15.Ø
  - expansion lungs (newborn) NEC — *see* Atelectasis
  - rotation, intestine Q43.3
- **Inconclusive**
  - diagnostic imaging due to excess body fat of patient R93.9
  - findings on diagnostic imaging of breast NEC R92.8
  - mammogram (due to dense breasts) R92.2
- **Incontinence** R32
  - anal sphincter R15.9
  - feces R15.9
    - nonorganic origin F98.1
  - overflow N39.49Ø
  - psychogenic F45.8
  - rectal R15.9
  - reflex N39.498
  - stress (female) (male) N39.3
    - and urge N39.46
  - urethral sphincter R32
  - urge N39.41
    - and stress (female) (male) N39.46
  - urine (urinary) R32
    - continuous N39.45
    - due to cognitive impairment, or severe physical disability or immobility R39.81
    - functional R39.81
    - mixed (stress and urge) N39.46
    - nocturnal N39.44
    - nonorganic origin F98.Ø
    - overflow N39.49Ø
    - post dribbling N39.43
    - reflex N39.498
    - specified NEC N39.498
    - stress (female) (male) N39.3
      - and urge N39.46
    - total N39.498
    - unaware N39.42
    - urge N39.41
      - and stress (female) (male) N39.46
- **Incontinentia pigmenti** Q82.3
- **Incoordinate, incoordination**
  - esophageal-pharyngeal (newborn) — *see* Dysphagia
  - muscular R27.8
  - uterus (action) (contractions) (complicating delivery) O62.4
- **Increase, increased**
  - abnormal, in development R63.8
  - androgens (ovarian) E28.1
  - anticoagulants (antithrombin) (anti-VIIIa) (anti-IXa) (anti-Xa) (anti-XIa) — *see* Circulating anticoagulants
  - cold sense R2Ø.8
  - estrogen E28.Ø
  - function
    - adrenal
      - cortex — *see* Cushing's, syndrome
      - medulla E27.5
    - pituitary (gland) (anterior) (lobe) E22.9
      - posterior E22.2
  - heat sense R2Ø.8
  - intracranial pressure (benign) G93.2
  - permeability, capillaries I78.8
  - pressure, intracranial G93.2
  - secretion
    - gastrin E16.4
    - glucagon E16.3
    - pancreas, endocrine E16.9
      - growth hormone-releasing hormone E16.8
      - pancreatic polypeptide E16.8
      - somatostatin E16.8
      - vasoactive-intestinal polypeptide E16.8
  - sphericity, lens Q12.4
  - splenic activity D73.1
  - venous pressure I87.8
    - portal K76.6
- **Increta placenta** O43.22- ☑
- **Incrustation, cornea, foreign body** (lead)(zinc) — *see* Foreign body, cornea
- **Incyclophoria** H5Ø.54
- **Incyclotropia** — *see* Cyclotropia
- **Indeterminate sex** Q56.4
- **India rubber skin** Q82.8
- **Indigestion** (acid) (bilious) (functional) K3Ø
- **Indigestion** — *continued*
  - catarrhal K31.89
  - due to decomposed food NOS AØ5.9
  - nervous F45.8
  - psychogenic F45.8
- **Indirect** — *see* condition
- **Induratio penis plastica** N48.6
- **Induration, indurated**
  - brain G93.89
  - breast (fibrous) N64.51
    - puerperal, postpartum O92.29
  - broad ligament N83.8
  - chancre
    - anus A51.1
    - congenital A5Ø.Ø7
    - extragenital NEC A51.2
  - corpora cavernosa (penis) (plastic) N48.6
  - liver (chronic) K76.89
  - lung (black) (chronic) (fibroid) (*see also* Fibrosis, lung) J84.1Ø
    - essential brown J84.Ø3
  - penile (plastic) N48.6
  - phlebitic — *see* Phlebitis
  - skin R23.4
- **Inebriety** (without dependence) — *see* Alcohol, intoxication
- **Inefficiency, kidney** N28.9
- **Inelasticity, skin** R23.4
- **Inequality, leg** (length) (acquired) (*see also* Deformity, limb, unequal length)
  - congenital — *see* Defect, reduction, lower limb
  - lower leg — *see* Deformity, limb, unequal length
- **Inertia**
  - bladder (neurogenic) N31.2
  - stomach K31.89
    - psychogenic F45.8
  - uterus, uterine during labor O62.2
    - during latent phase of labor O62.Ø
    - primary O62.Ø
    - secondary O62.1
  - vesical (neurogenic) N31.2
- **Infancy, infantile, infantilism** (*see also* condition)
  - celiac K9Ø.Ø
  - genitalia, genitals (after puberty) E3Ø.Ø
  - Herter's (nontropical sprue) K9Ø.Ø
  - intestinal K9Ø.Ø
  - Lorain E23.Ø
  - pancreatic K86.8
  - pelvis M95.5
    - with disproportion (fetopelvic) O33.1
      - causing obstructed labor O65.1
  - pituitary E23.Ø
  - renal N25.Ø
  - uterus — *see* Infantile, genitalia
- **Infant(s)** (*see also* Infancy)
  - excessive crying R68.11
  - irritable child R68.12
  - lack of care — *see* Neglect
  - liveborn (singleton) Z38.2
    - born in hospital Z38.ØØ
      - by cesarean Z38.Ø1
    - born outside hospital Z38.1
    - multiple NEC Z38.8
      - born in hospital Z38.68
        - by cesarean Z38.69
      - born outside hospital Z38.7
    - quadruplet Z38.8
      - born in hospital Z38.63
        - by cesarean Z38.64
      - born outside hospital Z38.7
    - quintuplet Z38.8
      - born in hospital Z38.65
        - by cesarean Z38.66
      - born outside hospital Z38.7
    - triplet Z38.8
      - born in hospital Z38.61
        - by cesarean Z38.62
      - born outside hospital Z38.7
    - twin Z38.5
      - born in hospital Z38.3Ø
        - by cesarean Z38.31
      - born outside hospital Z38.4
  - of diabetic mother (syndrome of) P7Ø.1
    - gestational diabetes P7Ø.Ø
- **Infantile** (*see also* condition)
  - genitalia, genitals E3Ø.Ø
  - os, uterine E3Ø.Ø
  - penis E3Ø.Ø
- **Infantile** — *continued*
  - testis E29.1
  - uterus E3Ø.Ø
- **Infantilism** — *see* Infancy
- **Infarct, infarction**
  - adrenal (capsule) (gland) E27.49
  - appendices epiploicae K55.Ø
  - bowel K55.Ø
  - brain (stem) — *see* Infarct, cerebral
  - breast N64.89
  - brewer's (kidney) N28.Ø
  - cardiac — *see* Infarct, myocardium
  - cerebellar — *see* Infarct, cerebral
  - cerebral (*see also* Occlusion, artery cerebral or precerebral, with infarction) I63.9
    - aborted I63.9
    - cortical I63.9
    - due to
      - cerebral venous thrombosis, nonpyogenic I63.6
      - embolism
        - cerebral arteries I63.4- ☑
        - precerebral arteries I63.1- ☑
      - occlusion NEC
        - cerebral arteries I63.5- ☑
        - precerebral arteries I63.2- ☑
      - stenosis NEC
        - cerebral arteries I63.5- ☑
        - precerebral arteries I63.2- ☑
      - thrombosis
        - cerebral artery I63.3- ☑
        - precerebral artery I63.Ø- ☑
    - intraoperative
      - during cardiac surgery I97.81Ø
      - during other surgery I97.811
    - postprocedural
      - following cardiac surgery I97.82Ø
      - following other surgery I97.821
    - specified NEC I63.8
  - colon (acute) (agnogenic) (embolic) (hemorrhagic) (nonocclusive) (nonthrombotic) (occlusive) (segmental) (thrombotic) (with gangrene) K55.Ø
  - coronary artery — *see* Infarct, myocardium
  - embolic — *see* Embolism
  - fallopian tube N83.8
  - gallbladder K82.8
  - heart — *see* Infarct, myocardium
  - hepatic K76.3
  - hypophysis (anterior lobe) E23.6
  - impending (myocardium) I2Ø.Ø
  - intestine (acute) (agnogenic) (embolic) (hemorrhagic) (nonocclusive) (nonthrombotic) (occlusive) (thrombotic) (with gangrene) K55.Ø
  - kidney N28.Ø
  - liver K76.3
  - lung (embolic) (thrombotic) — *see* Embolism, pulmonary
  - lymph node I89.8
  - mesentery, mesenteric (embolic) (thrombotic) (with gangrene) K55.Ø
  - muscle (ischemic) M62.2Ø
    - ankle M62.27- ☑
    - foot M62.27- ☑
    - forearm M62.23- ☑
    - hand M62.24- ☑
    - lower leg M62.26- ☑
    - pelvic region M62.25- ☑
    - shoulder region M62.21- ☑
    - specified site NEC M62.28
    - thigh M62.25- ☑
    - upper arm M62.22- ☑
  - myocardium, myocardial (acute) (with stated duration of 4 weeks or less) I21.3
    - diagnosed on ECG, but presenting no symptoms I25.2
    - healed or old I25.2
    - intraoperative
      - during cardiac surgery I97.79Ø
      - during other surgery I97.791
    - non-Q wave I21.4
    - non-ST elevation (NSTEMI) I21.4
      - subsequent I22.2
    - nontransmural I21.4
    - past (diagnosed on ECG or other investigation, but currently presenting no symptoms) I25.2
    - postprocedural
      - following cardiac surgery I97.19Ø
      - following other surgery I97.191
    - Q wave (see also, Infarct, myocardium, by site) I21.3

Infarct, infarction — *continued*
- myocardium, myocardial — *continued*
  - ST elevation (STEMI) I21.3
    - anterior (anteroapical) (anterolateral) (anteroseptal) (Q wave) (wall) I21.Ø9
      - subsequent I22.Ø
    - inferior (diaphragmatic) (inferolateral) (inferoposterior) (wall) NEC I21.19
      - subsequent I22.1
    - inferoposterior transmural (Q wave) I21.11
    - involving
      - coronary artery of anterior wall NEC I21.Ø9
      - coronary artery of inferior wall NEC I21.19
      - diagonal coronary artery I21.Ø2
      - left anterior descending coronary artery I21.Ø2
      - left circumflex coronary artery I21.21
      - left main coronary artery I21.Ø1
      - oblique marginal coronary artery I21.21
      - right coronary artery I21.11
    - lateral (apical-lateral) (basal-lateral) (high) I21.29
      - subsequent I22.8
    - posterior (posterobasal) (posterolateral) (posteroseptal) (true) I21.29
      - subsequent I22.8
    - septal I21.29
      - subsequent I22.8
    - specified NEC I21.29
      - subsequent I22.8
    - subsequent I22.9
  - subsequent (recurrent) (reinfarction) I22.9
    - anterior (anteroapical) (anterolateral) (anteroseptal) (wall) I22.Ø
    - diaphragmatic (wall) I22.1
    - inferior (diaphragmatic) (inferolateral) (inferoposterior) (wall) I22.1
    - lateral (apical-lateral) (basal-lateral) (high) I22.8
    - non-ST elevation (NSTEMI) I22.2
    - posterior (posterobasal) (posterolateral) (posteroseptal) (true) I22.8
    - septal I22.8
    - specified NEC I22.8
    - ST elevation I22.9
      - anterior (anteroapical) (anterolateral) (anteroseptal) (wall) I22.Ø
      - inferior (diaphragmatic) (inferolateral) (inferoposterior) (wall) I22.1
      - specified NEC I22.8
    - subendocardial I22.2
    - transmural I22.9
      - anterior (anteroapical) (anterolateral) (anteroseptal) (wall) I22.Ø
      - diaphragmatic (wall) I22.1
      - inferior (diaphragmatic) (inferolateral) (inferoposterior) (wall) I22.1
      - lateral (apical-lateral) (basal-lateral) (high) I22.8
      - posterior (posterobasal) (posterolateral) (posteroseptal) (true) I22.8
      - specified NEC I22.8
  - syphilitic A52.Ø6
  - transmural I21.3
    - anterior (anteroapical) (anterolateral) (anteroseptal) (Q wave) (wall) NEC I21.Ø9
    - inferior (diaphragmatic) (inferolateral) (inferoposterior) (Q wave) (wall) NEC I21.19
    - inferoposterior (Q wave) I21.11
    - lateral (apical-lateral) (basal-lateral) (high) NEC I21.29
    - posterior (posterobasal) (posterolateral) (posteroseptal) (true) NEC I21.29
    - septal NEC I21.29
    - specified NEC I21.29
- nontransmural I21.4
- omentum K55.Ø
- ovary N83.8
- pancreas K86.8
- papillary muscle — *see* Infarct, myocardium
- parathyroid gland E21.4
- pituitary (gland) E23.6
- placenta O43.81- ☑
- prostate N42.89
- pulmonary (artery) (vein) (hemorrhagic) — *see* Embolism, pulmonary
- renal (embolic) (thrombotic) N28.Ø
- retina, retinal (artery) — *see* Occlusion, artery, retina
- spinal (cord) (acute) (embolic) (nonembolic) G95.11

Infarct, infarction — *continued*
- spleen D73.5
  - embolic or thrombotic I74.8
- subendocardial (acute) (nontransmural) I21.4
- suprarenal (capsule) (gland) E27.49
- testis N5Ø.1
- thrombotic (*see also* Thrombosis)
  - artery, arterial — *see* Embolism
- thyroid (gland) EØ7.89
- ventricle (heart) — *see* Infarct, myocardium

Infecting — *see* condition

Infection, infected, infective (opportunistic) B99.9
- with
  - drug resistant organism — *see* Resistance (to), drug (*see also* specific organism)
  - lymphangitis — *see* Lymphangitis
  - organ dysfunction (acute) R65.2Ø
    - with septic shock R65.21
- abscess (skin) — *code by* site under Abscess
- Absidia — *see* Mucormycosis
- Acanthamoeba — *see* Acanthamebiasis
- Acanthocheilonema (perstans) (streptocerca) B74.4
- accessory sinus (chronic) — *see* Sinusitis
- achorion — *see* Dermatophytosis
- Acremonium falciforme B47.Ø
- acromioclavicular MØØ.9
- Actinobacillus (actinomycetem-comitans) A28.8
  - mallei A24.Ø
  - muris A25.1
- Actinomadura B47.1
- Actinomyces (israelii) (*see also* Actinomycosis) A42.9
- Actinomycetales — *see* Actinomycosis
- actinomycotic NOS — *see* Actinomycosis
- adenoid (and tonsil) JØ3.9Ø
  - chronic J35.Ø2
- adenovirus NEC
  - as cause of disease classified elsewhere B97.Ø
  - unspecified nature or site B34.Ø
- aerogenes capsulatus A48.Ø
- aertrycke — *see* Infection, salmonella
- alimentary canal NOS — *see* Enteritis, infectious
- Allescheria boydii B48.2
- Alternaria B48.8
- alveolus, alveolar (process) KØ4.7
- Ameba, amebic (histolytica) — *see* Amebiasis
- amniotic fluid, sac or cavity O41.1Ø- ☑
  - chorioamnionitis O41.12- ☑
  - placentitis O41.14- ☑
- amputation stump (surgical) — *see* Complication, amputation stump, infection
- Ancylostoma (duodenalis) B76.Ø
- Anisakiasis, Anisakis larvae B81.Ø
- anthrax — *see* Anthrax
- antrum (chronic) — *see* Sinusitis, maxillary
- anus, anal (papillae) (sphincter) K62.89
- arbovirus (arbor virus) A94
  - specified type NEC A93.8
- artificial insemination N98.Ø
- Ascaris lumbricoides — *see* Ascariasis
- Ascomycetes B47.Ø
- Aspergillus (flavus) (fumigatus) (terreus) — *see* Aspergillosis
- atypical
  - acid-fast (bacilli) — *see* Mycobacterium, atypical
  - mycobacteria — *see* Mycobacterium, atypical
  - virus A81.9
    - specified type NEC A81.89
- auditory meatus (external) — *see* Otitis, externa, infective
- auricle (ear) — *see* Otitis, externa, infective
- axillary gland (lymph) LØ4.2
- Bacillus A49.9
  - abortus A23.1
  - anthracis — *see* Anthrax
  - Ducrey's (any location) A57
  - Flexner's AØ3.1
  - Friedländer's NEC A49.8
  - gas (gangrene) A48.Ø
  - mallei A24.Ø
  - melitensis A23.Ø
  - paratyphoid, paratyphosus AØ1.4
    - A AØ1.1
    - B AØ1.2
    - C AØ1.3
  - Shiga (-Kruse) AØ3.Ø
  - suipestifer — *see* Infection, salmonella
  - swimming pool A31.1

Infection, infected, infective — *continued*
- Bacillus — *continued*
  - typhosa AØ1.ØØ
  - welchii — *see* Gangrene, gas
- bacterial NOS A49.9
  - as cause of disease classified elsewhere B96.89
    - Bacteroides fragilis [B. fragilis] B96.6
    - Clostridium perfringens [C. perfringens] B96.7
    - Enterobacter sakazakii B96.89
    - Enterococcus B95.2
    - Escherichia coli [E. coli] (*see also* Escherichia coli) B96.2Ø
    - Helicobacter pylori [H.pylori] B96.81
    - Hemophilus influenzae [H. influenzae] B96.3
    - Klebsiella pneumoniae [K. pneumoniae] B96.1
    - Mycoplasma pneumoniae [M. pneumoniae] B96.Ø
    - Proteus (mirabilis) (morganii) B96.4
    - Pseudomonas (aeruginosa) (mallei) (pseudomallei) B96.5
    - Staphylococcus B95.8
      - aureus (methicillin susceptible) (MSSA) B95.61
        - methicillin resistant (MRSA) B95.62
      - specified NEC B95.7
    - Streptococcus B95.5
      - group A B95.Ø
      - group B B95.1
      - pneumoniae B95.3
      - specified NEC B95.4
    - Vibrio vulnificus B96.82
  - specified NEC A48.8
- Bacterium
  - paratyphosum AØ1.4
    - A AØ1.1
    - B AØ1.2
    - C AØ1.3
  - typhosum AØ1.ØØ
- Bacteroides NEC A49.8
  - fragilis, as cause of disease classified elsewhere B96.6
- Balantidium coli AØ7.Ø
- Bartholin's gland N75.8
- Basidiobolus B46.8
- bile duct (common) (hepatic) — *see* Cholangitis
- bladder — *see* Cystitis
- Blastomyces, blastomycotic (*see also* Blastomycosis)
  - brasiliensis — *see* Paracoccidioidomycosis
  - dermatitidis — *see* Blastomycosis
  - European — *see* Cryptococcosis
  - Loboi B48.Ø
  - North American B4Ø.9
  - South American — *see* Paracoccidioidomycosis
- bleb, postprocedure — *see* Blebitis
- bone — *see* Osteomyelitis
- Bordetella — *see* Whooping cough
- Borrelia bergdorfi A69.2Ø
- brain (*see also* Encephalitis) GØ4.9Ø
  - membranes — *see* Meningitis
  - septic GØ6.Ø
    - meninges — *see* Meningitis, bacterial
- branchial cyst Q18.Ø
- breast — *see* Mastitis
- bronchus — *see* Bronchitis
- Brucella A23.9
  - abortus A23.1
  - canis A23.3
  - melitensis A23.Ø
  - mixed A23.8
  - specified NEC A23.8
  - suis A23.2
- Brugia (malayi) B74.1
  - timori B74.2
- bursa — *see* Bursitis, infective
- buttocks (skin) LØ8.9
- Campylobacter, intestinal AØ4.5
  - as cause of disease classified elsewhere B96.81
- Candida (albicans) (tropicalis) — *see* Candidiasis
- candiru B88.8
- Capillaria (intestinal) B81.1
  - hepatica B83.8
  - philippinensis B81.1
- cartilage — *see* Disorder, cartilage, specified type NEC
- cat liver fluke B66.Ø
- catheter-related bloodstream (CRBSI) T8Ø.211 ☑
- cellulitis — *code by* site under Cellulitis
- central line-associated T8Ø.219 ☑
  - bloodstream (CLABSI) T8Ø.211 ☑

- **Infection, infected, infective** — *continued*
  - fungus — *continued*
    - hand B35.2
    - nail B35.1
    - pathogenic to compromised host only B48.8
    - perianal (area) B35.6
    - scalp B35.0
    - skin B36.9
      - foot B35.3
      - hand B35.2
      - toenails B35.1
  - Fusarium B48.8
  - gallbladder — *see* Cholecystitis
  - gas bacillus — *see* Gangrene, gas
  - gastrointestinal — *see* Enteritis, infectious
  - generalized NEC — *see* Sepsis
  - genital organ or tract
    - female — *see* Disease, pelvis, inflammatory
    - male N49.9
      - multiple sites N49.8
      - specified NEC N49.8
  - Ghon tubercle, primary A15.7
  - Giardia lamblia A07.1
  - gingiva (chronic) K05.10
    - acute K05.00
      - nonplaque induced K05.01
      - plaque induced K05.00
    - nonplaque induced K05.11
    - plaque induced K05.10
  - glanders A24.0
  - glenosporopsis B48.0
  - Gnathostoma (spinigerum) B83.1
  - Gongylonema B83.8
  - gonococcal — *see* Gonococcus
  - gram-negative bacilli NOS A49.9
  - guinea worm B72
  - gum (chronic) K05.10
    - acute K05.00
      - nonplaque induced K05.01
      - plaque induced K05.00
    - nonplaque induced K05.11
    - plaque induced K05.10
  - Haemophilus — *see* Infection, Hemophilus
  - heart — *see* Carditis
  - Helicobacter pylori A04.8
    - as cause of disease classified elsewhere B96.81
  - helminths B83.9
    - intestinal B82.0
      - mixed (types classifiable to more than one of the titles B65.0-B81.3 and B81.8) B81.4
      - specified type NEC B81.8
    - specified type NEC B83.8
  - Hemophilus
    - aegyptius, systemic A48.4
    - ducrey (any location) A57
    - generalized A41.3
    - influenzae NEC A49.2
      - as cause of disease classified elsewhere B96.3
  - herpes (simplex) (*see also* Herpes)
    - congenital P35.2
    - disseminated B00.7
    - zoster B02.9
  - herpesvirus, herpesviral — *see* Herpes
  - Heterophyes (heterophyes) B66.8
  - hip (joint) NEC M00.9
    - due to internal joint prosthesis
      - left T84.52 ☑
      - right T84.51 ☑
    - skin NEC L08.9
  - Histoplasma — *see* Histoplasmosis
    - American B39.4
    - capsulatum B39.4
  - hookworm B76.9
  - human
    - papilloma virus A63.0
    - T-cell lymphotropic virus type-1 (HTLV-1) B33.3
  - hydrocele N43.0
  - Hymenolepis B71.0
  - hypopharynx — *see* Pharyngitis
  - inguinal (lymph) glands L04.1
    - due to soft chancre A57
  - intervertebral disc, pyogenic M46.30
    - cervical region M46.32
    - cervicothoracic region M46.33
    - lumbar region M46.36
    - lumbosacral region M46.37
    - multiple sites M46.39
    - occipito-atlanto-axial region M46.31

- **Infection, infected, infective** — *continued*
  - intervertebral disc, pyogenic — *continued*
    - sacrococcygeal region M46.38
    - thoracic region M46.34
    - thoracolumbar region M46.35
  - intestine, intestinal — *see* Enteritis, infectious
    - specified NEC A08.8
  - intra-amniotic affecting newborn NEC P39.2
  - Isospora belli or hominis A07.3
  - Japanese B encephalitis A83.0
  - jaw (bone) (lower) (upper) M27.2
  - joint NEC M00.9
    - due to internal joint prosthesis T84.50 ☑
  - kidney (cortex) (hematogenous) N15.9
    - with calculus N20.0
      - with hydronephrosis N13.6
    - following ectopic gestation O08.83
    - pelvis and ureter (cystic) N28.85
    - puerperal (postpartum) O86.21
    - specified NEC N15.8
  - Klebsiella (K.) pneumoniae NEC A49.8
    - as cause of disease classified elsewhere B96.1
  - knee (joint) NEC M00.9
    - due to internal joint prosthesis
      - left T84.54 ☑
      - right T84.53 ☑
    - joint M00.9
    - skin L08.9
  - Koch's — *see* Tuberculosis
  - labia (majora) (minora) (acute) — *see* Vulvitis
  - lacrimal
    - gland — *see* Dacryoadenitis
    - passages (duct) (sac) — *see* Inflammation, lacrimal, passages
  - lancet fluke B66.2
  - larynx NEC J38.7
  - leg (skin) NOS L08.9
  - Legionella pneumophila A48.1
    - nonpneumonic A48.2
  - Leishmania (*see also* Leishmaniasis)
    - aethiopica B55.1
    - braziliensis B55.2
    - chagasi B55.0
    - donovani B55.0
    - infantum B55.0
    - major B55.1
    - mexicana B55.1
    - tropica B55.1
  - lentivirus, as cause of disease classified elsewhere B97.31
  - Leptosphaeria senegalensis B47.0
  - Leptospira interrogans A27.9
    - autumnalis A27.89
    - canicola A27.89
    - hebdomadis A27.89
    - icterohaemorrhagiae A27.0
    - pomona A27.89
    - specified type NEC A27.89
  - leptospirochetal NEC — *see* Leptospirosis
  - Listeria monocytogenes (*see also* Listeriosis)
    - congenital P37.2
  - Loa loa B74.3
    - with conjunctival infestation B74.3
    - eyelid B74.3
  - Loboa loboi B48.0
  - local, skin (staphylococcal) (streptococcal) L08.9
    - abscess — *code by* site under Abscess
    - cellulitis — *code by* site under Cellulitis
    - specified NEC L08.89
    - ulcer — *see* Ulcer, skin
  - Loefflerella mallei A24.0
  - lung (*see also* Pneumonia) J18.9
    - atypical Mycobacterium A31.0
    - spirochetal A69.8
    - tuberculous — *see* Tuberculosis, pulmonary
    - virus — *see* Pneumonia, viral
  - lymph gland (*see also* Lymphadenitis, acute)
    - mesenteric I88.0
  - lymphoid tissue, base of tongue or posterior pharynx, NEC (chronic) J35.03
  - Madurella (grisea) (mycetomii) B47.0
  - major
    - following ectopic or molar pregnancy O08.0
    - puerperal, postpartum, childbirth O85
  - Malassezia furfur B36.0
  - Malleomyces
    - mallei A24.0
    - pseudomallei (whitmori) — *see* Melioidosis

- **Infection, infected, infective** — *continued*
  - mammary gland N61
  - Mansonella (ozzardi) (perstans) (streptocerca) B74.4
  - mastoid — *see* Mastoiditis
  - maxilla, maxillary M27.2
    - sinus (chronic) — *see* Sinusitis, maxillary
  - mediastinum J98.5
  - Medina (worm) B72
  - meibomian cyst or gland — *see* Hordeolum
  - meninges — *see* Meningitis, bacterial
  - meningococcal (*see also* condition) A39.9
    - adrenals A39.1
    - brain A39.81
    - cerebrospinal A39.0
    - conjunctiva A39.89
    - endocardium A39.51
    - heart A39.50
      - endocardium A39.51
      - myocardium A39.52
      - pericardium A39.53
    - joint A39.83
    - meninges A39.0
    - meningococcemia A39.4
      - acute A39.2
      - chronic A39.3
    - myocardium A39.52
    - pericardium A39.53
    - retrobulbar neuritis A39.82
    - specified site NEC A39.89
  - mesenteric lymph nodes or glands NEC I88.0
  - Metagonimus B66.8
  - metatarsophalangeal M00.9
  - methicillin
    - resistant Staphylococcus aureus (MRSA) A49.02
    - susceptible Staphylococcus aureus (MSSA) A49.01
  - Microsporum, microsporic — *see* Dermatophytosis
  - mixed flora (bacterial) NEC A49.8
  - Monilia — *see* Candidiasis
  - Monosporium apiospermum B48.2
  - mouth, parasitic B37.0
  - Mucor — *see* Mucormycosis
  - muscle NEC — *see* Myositis, infective
  - mycelium NOS B49
  - mycetoma B47.9
    - actinomycotic NEC B47.1
    - mycotic NEC B47.0
  - Mycobacterium, mycobacterial — *see* Mycobacterium
  - Mycoplasma NEC A49.3
    - pneumoniae, as cause of disease classified elsewhere B96.0
  - mycotic NOS B49
    - pathogenic to compromised host only B48.8
    - skin NOS B36.9
  - myocardium NEC I40.0
  - nail (chronic)
    - with lymphangitis — *see* Lymphangitis, acute, digit
    - finger L03.01- ☑
      - fungus B35.1
    - ingrowing L60.0
    - toe L03.03- ☑
      - fungus B35.1
  - nasal sinus (chronic) — *see* Sinusitis
  - nasopharynx — *see* Nasopharyngitis
  - navel L08.82
  - Necator americanus B76.1
  - Neisseria — *see* Gonococcus
  - Neotestudina rosatii B47.0
  - newborn P39.9
    - intra-amniotic NEC P39.2
    - skin P39.4
    - specified type NEC P39.8
  - nipple N61
    - associated with
      - lactation O91.03
      - pregnancy O91.01- ☑
      - puerperium O91.02
  - Nocardia — *see* Nocardiosis
  - obstetrical surgical wound (puerperal) O86.0
  - Oesophagostomum (apiostomum) B81.8
  - Oestrus ovis — *see* Myiasis
  - Oidium albicans B37.9
  - Onchocerca (volvulus) — *see* Onchocerciasis
  - oncovirus, as cause of disease classified elsewhere B97.32
  - operation wound T81.4 ☑
  - Opisthorchis (felineus) (viverrini) B66.0
  - orbit, orbital — *see* Inflammation, orbit

Infection, infected, infective — *continued*
- orthopoxvirus NEC BØ8.Ø9
- ovary — *see* Salpingo-oophoritis
- Oxyuris vermicularis B8Ø
- pancreas (acute) K85.9
  - abscess — *see* Pancreatitis, acute
  - specified NEC K85.8
- papillomavirus, as cause of disease classified elsewhere B97.7
- papovavirus NEC B34.4
- Paracoccidioides brasiliensis — *see* Paracoccidioidomycosis
- Paragonimus (westermani) B66.4
- parainfluenza virus B34.8
- parameningococcus NOS A39.9
- parapoxvirus BØ8.6Ø
  - specified NEC BØ8.69
- parasitic B89
- Parastrongylus
  - cantonensis B83.2
  - costaricensis B81.3
  - paratyphoid AØ1.4
    - Type A AØ1.1
    - Type B AØ1.2
    - Type C AØ1.3
- paraurethral ducts N34.2
- parotid gland — *see* Sialoadenitis
- parvovirus NEC B34.3
  - as cause of disease classified elsewhere B97.6
- Pasteurella NEC A28.Ø
  - multocida A28.Ø
  - pestis — *see* Plague
  - pseudotuberculosis A28.Ø
  - septica (cat bite) (dog bite) A28.Ø
  - tularensis — *see* Tularemia
- pelvic, female — *see* Disease, pelvis, inflammatory
- Penicillium (marneffei) B48.4
- penis (glans) (retention) NEC N48.29
- periapical KØ4.5
- peridental, periodontal KØ5.2Ø
  - generalized KØ5.22
  - localized KØ5.21
- perinatal period P39.9
  - specified type NEC P39.8
- perineal repair (puerperal) O86.Ø
- periorbital — *see* Inflammation, orbit
- perirectal K62.89
- perirenal — *see* Infection, kidney
- peritoneal — *see* Peritonitis
- periureteral N28.89
- Petriellidium boydii B48.2
- pharynx (*see also* Pharyngitis)
  - coxsackievirus BØ8.5
  - posterior, lymphoid (chronic) J35.Ø3
- Phialophora
  - gougerotii (subcutaneous abscess or cyst) B43.2
  - jeanselmei (subcutaneous abscess or cyst) B43.2
  - verrucosa (skin) B43.Ø
- Piedraia hortae B36.3
- pinta A67.9
  - intermediate A67.1
  - late A67.2
  - mixed A67.3
  - primary A67.Ø
- pinworm B8Ø
- pityrosporum furfur B36.Ø
- pleuro-pneumonia-like organism (PPLO) NEC A49.3
  - as cause of disease classified elsewhere B96.Ø
- pneumococcus, pneumococcal NEC A49.1
  - as cause of disease classified elsewhere B95.3
  - generalized (purulent) A4Ø.3
    - with pneumonia J13
- Pneumocystis carinii (pneumonia) B59
- Pneumocystis jiroveci (pneumonia) B59
- port or reservoir T8Ø.212 ☑
- postoperative T81.4 ☑
- postoperative wound T81.4 ☑
- postprocedural T81.4 ☑
- postvaccinal T88.Ø ☑
- prepuce NEC N47.7
  - with penile inflammation N47.6
- prion — *see* Disease, prion, central nervous system
- prostate (capsule) — *see* Prostatitis
- Proteus (mirabilis) (morganii) (vulgaris) NEC A49.8
  - as cause of disease classified elsewhere B96.4
- protozoal NEC B64
  - intestinal AØ7.9
    - specified NEC AØ7.8

Infection, infected, infective — *continued*
- protozoal — *continued*
  - specified NEC B6Ø.8
- Pseudoallescheria boydii B48.2
- Pseudomonas NEC A49.8
  - as cause of disease classified elsewhere B96.5
  - mallei A24.Ø
  - pneumonia J15.1
  - pseudomallei — *see* Melioidosis
- puerperal O86.4
  - genitourinary tract NEC O86.89
  - major or generalized O85
  - minor O86.4
  - specified NEC O86.89
- pulmonary — *see* Infection, lung
- purulent — *see* Abscess
- Pyrenochaeta romeroi B47.Ø
- Q fever A78
- rectum (sphincter) K62.89
- renal (*see also* Infection, kidney)
  - pelvis and ureter (cystic) N28.85
- reovirus, as cause of disease classified elsewhere B97.5
- respiratory (tract) NEC J98.8
  - acute J22
  - chronic J98.8
  - influenzal (upper) (acute) — *see* Influenza, with, respiratory manifestations NEC
  - lower (acute) J22
    - chronic — *see* Bronchitis, chronic
  - rhinovirus JØØ
  - syncytial virus, as cause of disease classified elsewhere B97.4
  - upper (acute) NOS JØ6.9
    - chronic J39.8
    - streptococcal JØ6.9
    - viral NOS JØ6.9
- resulting from
  - presence of internal prosthesis, implant, graft — *see* Complications, by site and type, infection
- retortamoniasis AØ7.8
- retroperitoneal NEC K68.9
- retrovirus B33.3
  - as cause of disease classified elsewhere B97.3Ø
    - human
      - immunodeficiency, type 2 (HIV 2) B97.35
      - T-cell lymphotropic
        - type I (HTLV-I) B97.33
        - type II (HTLV-II) B97.34
    - lentivirus B97.31
    - oncovirus B97.32
    - specified NEC B97.39
- Rhinosporidium (seeberi) B48.1
- rhinovirus
  - as cause of disease classified elsewhere B97.89
  - unspecified nature or site B34.8
- Rhizopus — *see* Mucormycosis
- rickettsial NOS A79.9
- roundworm (large) NEC B82.Ø
  - Ascariasis (*see also* Ascariasis) B77.9
- rubella — *see* Rubella
- Saccharomyces — *see* Candidiasis
- salivary duct or gland (any) — *see* Sialoadenitis
- Salmonella (aertrycke) (arizonae) (callinarum) (cholerae-suis) (enteritidis) (suipestifer) (typhimurium) AØ2.9
  - with
    - (gastro)enteritis AØ2.Ø
    - sepsis AØ2.1
    - specified manifestation NEC AØ2.8
  - due to food (poisoning) AØ2.9
  - hirschfeldii AØ1.3
  - localized AØ2.2Ø
    - arthritis AØ2.23
    - meningitis AØ2.21
    - osteomyelitis AØ2.24
    - pneumonia AØ2.22
    - pyelonephritis AØ2.25
    - specified NEC AØ2.29
  - paratyphi AØ1.4
    - A AØ1.1
    - B AØ1.2
    - C AØ1.3
  - schottmuelleri AØ1.2
  - typhi, typhosa — *see* Typhoid
- Sarcocystis AØ7.8
- scabies B86
- Schistosoma — *see* Infestation, Schistosoma
- scrotum (acute) NEC N49.2

Infection, infected, infective — *continued*
- seminal vesicle — *see* Vesiculitis
- septic
  - localized, skin — *see* Abscess
- sheep liver fluke B66.3
- Shigella AØ3.9
  - boydii AØ3.2
  - dysenteriae AØ3.Ø
  - flexneri AØ3.1
  - group
    - A AØ3.Ø
    - B AØ3.1
    - C AØ3.2
    - D AØ3.3
  - Schmitz (-Stutzer) AØ3.Ø
  - schmitzii AØ3.Ø
  - shigae AØ3.Ø
  - sonnei AØ3.3
  - specified NEC AØ3.8
- shoulder (joint) NEC MØØ.9
  - due to internal joint prosthesis T84.59 ☑
  - skin NEC LØ8.9
- sinus (accessory) (chronic) (nasal) (*see also* Sinusitis)
  - pilonidal — *see* Sinus, pilonidal
  - skin NEC LØ8.89
- Skene's duct or gland — *see* Urethritis
- skin (local) (staphylococcal) (streptococcal) LØ8.9
  - abscess — *code by* site under Abscess
  - cellulitis — *code by* site under Cellulitis
  - due to fungus B36.9
    - specified type NEC B36.8
  - mycotic B36.9
    - specified type NEC B36.8
  - newborn P39.4
  - ulcer — *see* Ulcer, skin
- slow virus A81.9
  - specified NEC A81.89
- Sparganum (mansoni) (proliferum) (baxteri) B7Ø.1
- specific (*see also* Syphilis)
  - to perinatal period — *see* Infection, congenital
- specified NEC B99.8
- spermatic cord NEC N49.1
- sphenoidal (sinus) — *see* Sinusitis, sphenoidal
- spinal cord NOS (*see also* Myelitis) GØ4.91
  - abscess GØ6.1
  - meninges — *see* Meningitis
  - streptococcal GØ4.89
- Spirillum A25.Ø
- spirochetal NOS A69.9
  - lung A69.8
  - specified NEC A69.8
- Spirometra larvae B7Ø.1
- spleen D73.89
- Sporotrichum, Sporothrix (schenckii) — *see* Sporotrichosis
- staphylococcal, unspecified site
  - as cause of disease classified elsewhere B95.8
    - aureus (methicillin susceptible) (MSSA) B95.61
      - methicillin resistant (MRSA) B95.62
    - specified NEC B95.7
  - aureus (methicillin susceptible) (MSSA) A49.Ø1
    - methicillin resistant (MRSA) A49.Ø2
  - food poisoning AØ5.Ø
  - generalized (purulent) A41.2
  - pneumonia — *see* Pneumonia, staphylococcal
- Stellantchasmus falcatus B66.8
- streptobacillus moniliformis A25.1
- streptococcal NEC A49.1
  - as cause of disease classified elsewhere B95.5
  - B genitourinary complicating
    - childbirth O98.82
    - pregnancy O98.81- ☑
    - puerperium O98.83
  - congenital
    - sepsis P36.1Ø
      - group B P36.Ø
      - specified NEC P36.19
  - generalized (purulent) A4Ø.9
- Streptomyces B47.1
- Strongyloides (stercoralis) — *see* Strongyloidiasis
- stump (amputation) (surgical) — *see* Complication, amputation stump, infection
- subcutaneous tissue, local LØ8.9
- suipestifer — *see* Infection, salmonella
- swimming pool bacillus A31.1
- Taenia — *see* Infestation, Taenia
- Taeniarhynchus saginatus B68.1
- tapeworm — *see* Infestation, tapeworm

- **Infection, infected, infective** — *continued*
  - tendon (sheath) — *see* Tenosynovitis, infective NEC
  - Ternidens diminutus B81.8
  - testis — *see* Orchitis
  - threadworm B80
  - throat — *see* Pharyngitis
  - thyroglossal duct K14.8
  - toe (skin) L08.9
    - cellulitis L03.03- ☑
      - fungus B35.1
    - nail L03.03- ☑
      - fungus B35.1
  - tongue NEC K14.0
    - parasitic B37.0
  - tonsil (and adenoid) (faucial) (lingual) (pharyngeal) — *see* Tonsillitis
  - tooth, teeth K04.7
    - periapical K04.7
    - peridental, periodontal K05.20
      - generalized K05.22
      - localized K05.21
    - pulp K04.0
    - socket M27.3
  - TORCH — *see* Infection, congenital
    - without active infection P00.2
  - Torula histolytica — *see* Cryptococcosis
  - Toxocara (canis) (cati) (felis) B83.0
  - Toxoplasma gondii — *see* Toxoplasma
  - trachea, chronic J42
  - trematode NEC — *see* Infestation, fluke
  - trench fever A79.0
  - Treponèma pallidum — *see* Syphilis
  - Trichinella (spiralis) B75
  - Trichomonas A59.9
    - cervix A59.09
    - intestine A07.8
    - prostate A59.02
    - specified site NEC A59.8
    - urethra A59.03
    - urogenitalis A59.00
    - vagina A59.01
    - vulva A59.01
  - Trichophyton, trichophytic — *see* Dermatophytosis
  - Trichosporon (beigelii) cutaneum B36.2
  - Trichostrongylus B81.2
  - Trichuris (trichiura) B79
  - Trombicula (irritans) B88.0
  - Trypanosoma
    - brucei
      - gambiense B56.0
      - rhodesiense B56.1
    - cruzi — *see* Chagas' disease
  - tubal — *see* Salpingo-oophoritis
  - tuberculous NEC — *see* Tuberculosis
  - tubo-ovarian — *see* Salpingo-oophoritis
  - tunica vaginalis N49.1
  - tunnel T80.212 ☑
  - tympanic membrane NEC — *see* Myringitis
  - typhoid (abortive) (ambulant) (bacillus) — *see* Typhoid
  - typhus A75.9
    - flea-borne A75.2
    - mite-borne A75.3
    - recrudescent A75.1
    - tick-borne A77.9
      - African A77.1
      - North Asian A77.2
  - umbilicus L08.82
  - ureter N28.86
  - urethra — *see* Urethritis
  - urinary (tract) N39.0
    - bladder — *see* Cystitis
    - complicating
      - pregnancy O23.4- ☑
        - specified type NEC O23.3- ☑
    - kidney — *see* Infection, kidney
    - newborn P39.3
    - puerperal (postpartum) O86.20
    - tuberculous A18.13
    - urethra — *see* Urethritis
  - uterus, uterine — *see* Endometritis
  - vaccination T88.0 ☑
  - vaccinia not from vaccination B08.011
  - vagina (acute) — *see* Vaginitis
  - varicella B01.9
  - varicose veins — *see* Varix
  - vas deferens NEC N49.1
  - vesical — *see* Cystitis

- **Infection, infected, infective** — *continued*
  - Vibrio
    - cholerae A00.0
      - El Tor A00.1
    - parahaemolyticus (food poisoning) A05.3
    - vulnificus
      - as cause of disease classified elsewhere B96.82
      - foodborne intoxication A05.5
  - Vincent's (gum) (mouth) (tonsil) A69.1
  - virus, viral NOS B34.9
    - adenovirus
      - as cause of disease classified elsewhere B97.0
      - unspecified nature or site B34.0
    - arborvirus, arbovirus arthropod-borne A94
    - as cause of disease classified elsewhere B97.89
      - adenovirus B97.0
      - coronavirus B97.29
        - SARS-associated B97.21
      - coxsackievirus B97.11
      - echovirus B97.12
      - enterovirus B97.10
        - coxsackievirus B97.11
        - echovirus B97.12
        - specified NEC B97.19
      - human
        - immunodeficiency, type 2 (HIV 2) B97.35
        - metapneumovirus B97.81
        - T-cell lymphotropic,
          - type I (HTLV-I) B97.33
          - type II (HTLV-II) B97.34
      - papillomavirus B97.7
      - parvovirus B97.6
      - reovirus B97.5
      - respiratory syncytial B97.4
      - retrovirus B97.30
        - human
          - immunodeficiency, type 2 (HIV 2) B97.35
          - T-cell lymphotropic,
            - type I (HTLV-I) B97.33
            - type II (HTLV-II) B97.34
        - lentivirus B97.31
        - oncovirus B97.32
        - specified NEC B97.39
      - specified NEC B97.89
    - central nervous system A89
      - atypical A81.9
        - specified NEC A81.89
      - enterovirus NEC A88.8
        - meningitis A87.0
      - slow virus A81.9
        - specified NEC A81.89
      - specified NEC A88.8
    - chest J98.8
    - cotia B08.8
    - coxsackie (*see also* Infection, coxsackie) B34.1
      - as cause of disease classified elsewhere B97.11
    - ECHO
      - as cause of disease classified elsewhere B97.12
      - unspecified nature or site B34.1
    - encephalitis, tick-borne A84.9
    - enterovirus, as cause of disease classified elsewhere B97.10
      - coxsackievirus B97.11
      - echovirus B97.12
      - specified NEC B97.19
    - exanthem NOS B09
    - human metapneumovirus as cause of disease classified elsewhere B97.81
    - human papilloma as cause of disease classified elsewhere B97.7
    - intestine — *see* Enteritis, viral
    - respiratory syncytial
      - as cause of disease classified elsewhere B97.4
      - bronchopneumonia J12.1
      - common cold syndrome J00
      - nasopharyngitis (acute) J00
    - rhinovirus
      - as cause of disease classified elsewhere B97.89
      - unspecified nature or site B34.8
    - slow A81.9
      - specified NEC A81.89
    - specified type NEC B33.8
      - as cause of disease classified elsewhere B97.89
      - unspecified nature or site B34.8
    - unspecified nature or site B34.9
    - West Nile — *see* Virus, West Nile
  - vulva (acute) — *see* Vulvitis
  - West Nile — *see* Virus, West Nile

- **Infection, infected, infective** — *continued*
  - whipworm B79
  - worms B83.9
    - specified type NEC B83.8
  - Wuchereria (bancrofti) B74.0
    - malayi B74.1
  - yatapoxvirus B08.70
    - specified NEC B08.79
  - yeast (*see also* Candidiasis) B37.9
  - yellow fever — *see* Fever, yellow
  - Yersinia
    - enterocolitica (intestinal) A04.6
    - pestis — *see* Plague
    - pseudotuberculosis A28.2
  - Zeis' gland — *see* Hordeolum
  - zoonotic bacterial NOS A28.9
  - Zopfia senegalensis B47.0
- **Infective, infectious** — *see* condition
- **Infertility**
  - female N97.9
    - age-related N97.8
    - associated with
      - anovulation N97.0
      - cervical (mucus) disease or anomaly N88.3
      - congenital anomaly
        - cervix N88.3
        - fallopian tube N97.1
        - uterus N97.2
        - vagina N97.8
      - dysmucorrhea N88.3
      - fallopian tube disease or anomaly N97.1
      - pituitary-hypothalamic origin E23.0
      - specified origin NEC N97.8
      - Stein-Leventhal syndrome E28.2
      - uterine disease or anomaly N97.2
      - vaginal disease or anomaly N97.8
    - due to
      - cervical anomaly N88.3
      - fallopian tube anomaly N97.1
      - ovarian failure E28.39
      - Stein-Leventhal syndrome E28.2
      - uterine anomaly N97.2
      - vaginal anomaly N97.8
    - nonimplantation N97.2
    - origin
      - cervical N88.3
      - tubal (block) (occlusion) (stenosis) N97.1
      - uterine N97.2
      - vaginal N97.8
  - male N46.9
    - azoospermia N46.01
      - extratesticular cause N46.029
        - drug therapy N46.021
        - efferent duct obstruction N46.023
        - infection N46.022
        - radiation N46.024
        - specified cause NEC N46.029
        - systemic disease N46.025
    - oligospermia N46.11
      - extratesticular cause N46.129
        - drug therapy N46.121
        - efferent duct obstruction N46.123
        - infection N46.122
        - radiation N46.124
        - specified cause NEC N46.129
        - systemic disease N46.125
    - specified type NEC N46.8
- **Infestation** B88.9
  - Acanthocheilonema (perstans) (streptocerca) B74.4
  - Acariasis B88.0
    - demodex folliculorum B88.0
    - sarcoptes scabiei B86
    - trombiculae B88.0
  - Agamofilaria streptocerca B74.4
  - Ancylostoma, ankylostoma (braziliense) (caninum) (ceylanicum) (duodenale) B76.0
    - americanum B76.1
    - new world B76.1
  - Anisakis larvae, anisakiasis B81.0
  - arthropod NEC B88.2
  - Ascaris lumbricoides — *see* Ascariasis
  - Balantidium coli A07.0
  - beef tapeworm B68.1
  - Bothriocephalus (latus) B70.0
    - larval B70.1
  - broad tapeworm B70.0
    - larval B70.1
  - Brugia (malayi) B74.1

- **Infestation** — *continued*
  - Brugia — *continued*
    - timori B74.2
  - candiru B88.8
  - Capillaria
    - hepatica B83.8
    - philippinensis B81.1
  - cat liver fluke B66.Ø
  - cestodes B71.9
    - diphyllobothrium — *see* Infestation, diphyllobothrium
    - dipylidiasis B71.1
    - hymenolepiasis B71.Ø
    - specified type NEC B71.8
  - chigger B88.Ø
  - chigo, chigoe B88.1
  - Clonorchis (sinensis) (liver) B66.1
  - coccidial AØ7.3
  - crab-lice B85.3
  - Cysticercus cellulosae — *see* Cysticercosis
  - Demodex (folliculorum) B88.Ø
  - Dermanyssus gallinae B88.Ø
  - Dermatobia (hominis) — *see* Myiasis
  - Dibothriocephalus (latus) B7Ø.Ø
    - larval B7Ø.1
  - Dicrocoelium dendriticum B66.2
  - Diphyllobothrium (adult) (latum) (intestinal) (pacificum) B7Ø.Ø
    - larval B7Ø.1
  - Diplogonoporus (grandis) B71.8
  - Dipylidium caninum B67.4
  - Distoma hepaticum B66.3
  - dog tapeworm B67.4
  - Dracunculus medinensis B72
  - dragon worm B72
  - dwarf tapeworm B71.Ø
  - Echinococcus — *see* Echinococcus
  - Echinostomum ilocanum B66.8
  - Entamoeba (histolytica) — *see* Infection, Ameba
  - Enterobius vermicularis B8Ø
  - eyelid
    - in (due to)
      - leishmaniasis B55.1
      - loiasis B74.3
      - onchocerciasis B73.Ø9
      - phthiriasis B85.3
    - parasitic NOS B89
  - eyeworm B74.3
  - Fasciola (gigantica) (hepatica) (indica) B66.3
  - Fasciolopsis (buski) (intestine) B66.5
  - filarial B74.9
    - bancroftian B74.Ø
    - conjunctiva B74.9
    - due to
      - Acanthocheilonema (perstans) (streptocerca) B74.4
      - Brugia (malayi) B74.1
        - timori B74.2
      - Dracunculus medinensis B72
      - guinea worm B72
      - loa loa B74.3
      - Mansonella (ozzardi) (perstans) (streptocerca) B74.4
      - Onchocerca volvulus B73.ØØ
        - eye B73.ØØ
        - eyelid B73.Ø9
      - Wuchereria (bancrofti) B74.Ø
    - Malayan B74.1
    - ozzardi B74.4
    - specified type NEC B74.8
  - fish tapeworm B7Ø.Ø
    - larval B7Ø.1
  - fluke B66.9
    - blood NOS — *see* Schistosomiasis
    - cat liver B66.Ø
    - intestinal B66.5
    - lancet B66.2
    - liver (sheep) B66.3
      - cat B66.Ø
      - Chinese B66.1
      - due to clonorchiasis B66.1
      - oriental B66.1
    - lung (oriental) B66.4
    - sheep liver B66.3
    - specified type NEC B66.8
  - fly larvae — *see* Myiasis
  - Gasterophilus (intestinalis) — *see* Myiasis
  - Gastrodiscoides hominis B66.8

- **Infestation** — *continued*
  - Giardia lamblia AØ7.1
  - Gnathostoma (spinigerum) B83.1
  - Gongylonema B83.8
  - guinea worm B72
  - helminth B83.9
    - angiostrongyliasis B83.2
      - intestinal B81.3
    - gnathostomiasis B83.1
    - hirudiniasis, internal B83.4
    - intestinal B82.Ø
      - angiostrongyliasis B81.3
      - anisakiasis B81.Ø
      - ascariasis — *see* Ascariasis
      - capillariasis B81.1
      - cysticercosis — *see* Cysticercosis
      - diphyllobothriasis — *see* Infestation, diphyllobothriasis
      - dracunculiasis B72
      - echinococcus — *see* Echinococcosis
      - enterobiasis B8Ø
      - filariasis — *see* Infestation, filarial
      - fluke — *see* Infestation, fluke
      - hookworm — *see* Infestation, hookworm
      - mixed (types classifiable to more than one of the titles B65.Ø-B81.3 and B81.8) B81.4
      - onchocerciasis — *see* Onchocerciasis
      - schistosomiasis — *see* Infestation, schistosoma
      - specified
        - cestode NEC — *see* Infestation, cestode
        - type NEC B81.8
      - strongyloidiasis — *see* Strongyloidiasis
      - taenia — *see* Infestation, taenia
      - trichinellosis B75
      - trichostrongyliasis B81.2
      - trichuriasis B79
    - specified type NEC B83.8
    - syngamiasis B83.3
    - visceral larva migrans B83.Ø
  - Heterophyes (heterophyes) B66.8
  - hookworm B76.9
    - ancylostomiasis B76.Ø
    - necatoriasis B76.1
    - specified type NEC B76.8
  - Hymenolepis (diminuta) (nana) B71.Ø
  - intestinal NEC B82.9
  - leeches (aquatic) (land) — *see* Hirudiniasis
  - Leishmania — *see* Leishmaniasis
  - lice, louse — *see* Infestation, Pediculus
  - Linguatula B88.8
  - Liponyssoides sanguineus B88.Ø
  - Loa loa B74.3
    - conjunctival B74.3
    - eyelid B74.3
  - louse — *see* Infestation, Pediculus
  - maggots — *see* Myiasis
  - Mansonella (ozzardi) (perstans) (streptocerca) B74.4
  - Medina (worm) B72
  - Metagonimus (yokogawai) B66.8
  - microfilaria streptocerca — *see* Onchocerciasis
    - eye B73.ØØ
    - eyelid B73.Ø9
  - mites B88.9
    - scabic B86
  - Monilia (albicans) — *see* Candidiasis
  - mouth B37.Ø
  - Necator americanus B76.1
  - nematode NEC (intestinal) B82.Ø
    - Ancylostoma B76.Ø
    - conjunctiva NEC B83.9
    - Enterobius vermicularis B8Ø
    - Gnathostoma spinigerum B83.1
    - physaloptera B8Ø
    - specified NEC B81.8
    - trichostrongylus B81.2
    - trichuris (trichuria) B79
  - Oesophagostomum (apiostomum) B81.8
  - Oestrus ovis (*see also* Myiasis) B87.9
  - Onchocerca (volvulus) — *see* Onchocerciasis
  - Opisthorchis (felineus) (viverrini) B66.Ø
  - orbit, parasitic NOS B89
  - Oxyuris vermicularis B8Ø
  - Paragonimus (westermani) B66.4
  - parasite, parasitic B89
    - eyelid B89
    - intestinal NOS B82.9
    - mouth B37.Ø
    - skin B88.9

- **Infestation** — *continued*
  - parasite, parasitic — *continued*
    - tongue B37.Ø
  - Parastrongylus
    - cantonensis B83.2
    - costaricensis B81.3
  - Pediculus B85.2
    - body B85.1
    - capitis (humanus) (any site) B85.Ø
    - corporis (humanus) (any site) B85.1
    - head B85.Ø
    - mixed (classifiable to more than one of the titles B85.Ø - B85.3) B85.4
    - pubis (any site) B85.3
  - Pentastoma B88.8
  - Phthirus (pubis) (any site) B85.3
    - with any infestation classifiable to B85.Ø - B85.2 B85.4
  - pinworm B8Ø
  - pork tapeworm (adult) B68.Ø
  - protozoal NEC B64
    - intestinal AØ7.9
      - specified NEC AØ7.8
    - specified NEC B6Ø.8
  - pubic, louse B85.3
  - rat tapeworm B71.Ø
  - red bug B88.Ø
  - roundworm (large) NEC B82.Ø
    - Ascariasis (*see also* Ascariasis) B77.9
  - sandflea B88.1
  - Sarcoptes scabiei B86
  - scabies B86
  - Schistosoma B65.9
    - bovis B65.8
    - cercariae B65.3
    - haematobium B65.Ø
    - intercalatum B65.8
    - japonicum B65.2
    - mansoni B65.1
    - mattheei B65.8
    - mekongi B65.8
    - specified type NEC B65.8
    - spindale B65.8
  - screw worms — *see* Myiasis
  - skin NOS B88.9
  - Sparganum (mansoni) (proliferum) (baxteri) B7Ø.1
    - larval B7Ø.1
  - specified type NEC B88.8
  - Spirometra larvae B7Ø.1
  - Stellantchasmus falcatus B66.8
  - Strongyloides stercoralis — *see* Strongyloidiasis
  - Taenia B68.9
    - diminuta B71.Ø
    - echinococcus — *see* Echinococcus
    - mediocanellata B68.1
    - nana B71.Ø
    - saginata B68.1
    - solium (intestinal form) B68.Ø
      - larval form — *see* Cysticercosis
  - Taeniarhynchus saginatus B68.1
  - tapeworm B71.9
    - beef B68.1
    - broad B7Ø.Ø
      - larval B7Ø.1
    - dog B67.4
    - dwarf B71.Ø
    - fish B7Ø.Ø
      - larval B7Ø.1
    - pork B68.Ø
    - rat B71.Ø
  - Ternidens diminutus B81.8
  - Tetranychus molestissimus B88.Ø
  - threadworm B8Ø
  - tongue B37.Ø
  - Toxocara (canis) (cati) (felis) B83.Ø
  - trematode(s) NEC — *see* Infestation, fluke
  - Trichinella (spiralis) B75
  - Trichocephalus B79
  - Trichomonas — *see* Trichomoniasis
  - Trichostrongylus B81.2
  - Trichuris (trichiura) B79
  - Trombicula (irritans) B88.Ø
  - Tunga penetrans B88.1
  - Uncinaria americana B76.1
  - Vandellia cirrhosa B88.8
  - whipworm B79
  - worms B83.9
    - intestinal B82.Ø

Infestation — *continued*
- Wuchereria (bancrofti) B74.Ø

Infiltrate, infiltration
- amyloid (generalized) (localized) — *see* Amyloidosis
- calcareous NEC R89.7
  - localized — *see* Degeneration, by site
- calcium salt R89.7
- cardiac
  - fatty — *see* Degeneration, myocardial
  - glycogenic E74.Ø2 [I43]
- corneal — *see* Edema, cornea
- eyelid — *see* Inflammation, eyelid
- glycogen, glycogenic — *see* Disease, glycogen storage
- heart, cardiac
  - fatty — *see* Degeneration, myocardial
  - glycogenic E74.Ø2 [I43]
- inflammatory in vitreous H43.89
- kidney N28.89
- leukemic — *see* Leukemia
- liver K76.89
  - fatty — *see* Fatty, liver NEC
  - glycogen (*see also* Disease, glycogen storage) E74.Ø3 [K77]
- lung R91.8
  - eosinophilic J82
- lymphatic (*see also* Leukemia, lymphatic) C91.9- ☑
  - gland I88.9
- muscle, fatty M62.89
- myocardium, myocardial
  - fatty — *see* Degeneration, myocardial
  - glycogenic E74.Ø2 [I43]
- on chest x-ray R91.8
- pulmonary R91.8
  - with eosinophilia J82
- skin (lymphocytic) L98.6
- thymus (gland) (fatty) E32.8
- urine R39.Ø
- vesicant agent
  - antineoplastic chemotherapy T8Ø.81Ø ☑
  - other agent NEC T8Ø.818 ☑
- vitreous body H43.89

Infirmity R68.89
- senile R54

Inflammation, inflamed, inflammatory (with exudation)
- abducent (nerve) — *see* Strabismus, paralytic, sixth nerve
- accessory sinus (chronic) — *see* Sinusitis
- adrenal (gland) E27.8
- alveoli, teeth M27.3
  - scorbutic E54
- anal canal, anus K62.89
- antrum (chronic) — *see* Sinusitis, maxillary
- appendix — *see* Appendicitis
- arachnoid — *see* Meningitis
- areola N61
  - puerperal, postpartum or gestational — *see* Infection, nipple
- areolar tissue NOS LØ8.9
- artery — *see* Arteritis
- auditory meatus (external) — *see* Otitis, externa
- Bartholin's gland N75.8
- bile duct (common) (hepatic) or passage — *see* Cholangitis
- bladder — *see* Cystitis
- bone — *see* Osteomyelitis
- brain (*see also* Encephalitis)
  - membrane — *see* Meningitis
- breast N61
  - puerperal, postpartum, gestational — *see* Mastitis, obstetric
- broad ligament — *see* Disease, pelvis, inflammatory
- bronchi — *see* Bronchitis
- catarrhal JØØ
- cecum — *see* Appendicitis
- cerebral (*see also* Encephalitis)
  - membrane — *see* Meningitis
- cerebrospinal
  - meningococcal A39.Ø
- cervix (uteri) — *see* Cervicitis
- chest J98.8
- chorioretinal H3Ø.9- ☑
  - cyclitis — *see* Cyclitis
  - disseminated H3Ø.1Ø- ☑
    - generalized H3Ø.13- ☑
    - peripheral H3Ø.12- ☑
    - posterior pole H3Ø.11- ☑

Inflammation, inflamed, inflammatory — *continued*
- chorioretinal — *continued*
  - epitheliopathy — *see* Epitheliopathy
  - focal H3Ø.ØØ- ☑
    - juxtapapillary H3Ø.Ø1- ☑
    - macular H3Ø.Ø4- ☑
    - paramacular — *see* Inflammation, chorioretinal, focal, macular
    - peripheral H3Ø.Ø3- ☑
    - posterior pole H3Ø.Ø2- ☑
  - specified type NEC H3Ø.89- ☑
- choroid — *see* Inflammation, chorioretinal
- chronic, postmastoidectomy cavity — *see* Complications, postmastoidectomy, inflammation
- colon — *see* Enteritis
- connective tissue (diffuse) NEC — *see* Disorder, soft tissue, specified type NEC
- cornea — *see* Keratitis
- corpora cavernosa N48.29
- cranial nerve — *see* Disorder, nerve, cranial
- Douglas' cul-de-sac or pouch (chronic) N73.Ø
- due to device, implant or graft (*see also* Complications, by site and type, infection or inflammation)
  - arterial graft T82.7 ☑
  - breast (implant) T85.79 ☑
  - catheter T85.79 ☑
    - dialysis (renal) T82.7 ☑
      - intraperitoneal T85.71 ☑
    - infusion T82.7 ☑
      - spinal (epidural) (subdural) T85.79 ☑
    - urinary (indwelling) T83.51 ☑
  - electronic (electrode) (pulse generator) (stimulator)
    - bone T84.7 ☑
    - cardiac T82.7 ☑
    - nervous system (brain) (peripheral nerve) (spinal) T85.79 ☑
    - urinary T83.59 ☑
  - fixation, internal (orthopedic) NEC — *see* Complication, fixation device, infection
  - gastrointestinal (bile duct) (esophagus) T85.79 ☑
  - genital NEC T83.6 ☑
  - heart NEC T82.7 ☑
    - valve (prosthesis) T82.6 ☑
      - graft T82.7 ☑
  - joint prosthesis — *see* Complication, joint prosthesis, infection
  - ocular (corneal graft) (orbital implant) NEC T85.79 ☑
  - orthopedic NEC T84.7 ☑
  - specified NEC T85.79 ☑
  - urinary NEC T83.59 ☑
  - vascular NEC T82.7 ☑
  - ventricular intracranial shunt T85.79 ☑
- duodenum K29.8Ø
  - with bleeding K29.81
- dura mater — *see* Meningitis
- ear (middle) (*see also* Otitis, media)
  - external — *see* Otitis, externa
  - inner — *see* subcategory H83.Ø ☑
- epididymis — *see* Epididymitis
- esophagus K2Ø.9
- ethmoidal (sinus) (chronic) — *see* Sinusitis, ethmoidal
- eustachian tube (catarrhal) — *see* Salpingitis, eustachian
- eyelid HØ1.9
  - abscess — *see* Abscess, eyelid
  - blepharitis — *see* Blepharitis
  - chalazion — *see* Chalazion
  - dermatosis (noninfectious) — *see* Dermatosis, eyelid
  - hordeolum — *see* Hordeolum
  - specified NEC HØ1.8
- fallopian tube — *see* Salpingo-oophoritis
- fascia — *see* Myositis
- follicular, pharynx J31.2
- frontal (sinus) (chronic) — *see* Sinusitis, frontal
- gallbladder — *see* Cholecystitis
- gastric — *see* Gastritis
- gastrointestinal — *see* Enteritis
- genital organ (internal) (diffuse)
  - female — *see* Disease, pelvis, inflammatory
  - male N49.9
    - multiple sites N49.8
    - specified NEC N49.8
- gland (lymph) — *see* Lymphadenitis

Inflammation, inflamed, inflammatory — *continued*
- glottis — *see* Laryngitis
- granular, pharynx J31.2
- gum KØ5.1Ø
  - nonplaque induced KØ5.11
  - plaque induced KØ5.1Ø
- heart — *see* Carditis
- hepatic duct — *see* Cholangitis
- ileoanal (internal) pouch K91.85Ø
- ileum (*see also* Enteritis)
  - regional or terminal — *see* Enteritis, regional
- intestinal pouch K91.85Ø
- intestine (any part) — *see* Enteritis
- jaw (acute) (bone) (chronic) (lower) (suppurative) (upper) M27.2
- joint NEC — *see* Arthritis
  - sacroiliac M46.1
- kidney — *see* Nephritis
- knee (joint) M13.169
  - tuberculous A18.Ø2
- labium (majus) (minus) — *see* Vulvitis
- lacrimal
  - gland — *see* Dacryoadenitis
  - passages (duct) (sac) (*see also* Dacryocystitis)
    - canaliculitis — *see* Canaliculitis, lacrimal
- larynx — *see* Laryngitis
- leg NOS LØ8.9
- lip K13.Ø
- liver (capsule) (*see also* Hepatitis)
  - chronic K73.9
  - suppurative K75.Ø
- lung (acute) (*see also* Pneumonia)
  - chronic J98.4
- lymph gland or node — *see* Lymphadenitis
- lymphatic vessel — *see* Lymphangitis
- maxilla, maxillary M27.2
  - sinus (chronic) — *see* Sinusitis, maxillary
- membranes of brain or spinal cord — *see* Meningitis
- meninges — *see* Meningitis
- mouth K12.1
- muscle — *see* Myositis
- myocardium — *see* Myocarditis
- nasal sinus (chronic) — *see* Sinusitis
- nasopharynx — *see* Nasopharyngitis
- navel LØ8.82
- nerve NEC — *see* Neuralgia
- nipple N61
  - puerperal, postpartum or gestational — *see* Infection, nipple
- nose — *see* Rhinitis
- oculomotor (nerve) — *see* Strabismus, paralytic, third nerve
- optic nerve — *see* Neuritis, optic
- orbit (chronic) HØ5.1Ø
  - acute HØ5.ØØ
    - abscess — *see* Abscess, orbit
    - cellulitis — *see* Cellulitis, orbit
    - osteomyelitis — *see* Osteomyelitis, orbit
    - periostitis — *see* Periostitis, orbital
    - tenonitis — *see* Tenonitis, eye
  - granuloma — *see* Granuloma, orbit
  - myositis — *see* Myositis, orbital
- ovary — *see* Salpingo-oophoritis
- oviduct — *see* Salpingo-oophoritis
- pancreas (acute) — *see* Pancreatitis
- parametrium N73.Ø
- parotid region LØ8.9
- pelvis, female — *see* Disease, pelvis, inflammatory
- penis (corpora cavernosa) N48.29
- perianal K62.89
- pericardium — *see* Pericarditis
- perineum (female) (male) LØ8.9
- perirectal K62.89
- peritoneum — *see* Peritonitis
- periuterine — *see* Disease, pelvis, inflammatory
- perivesical — *see* Cystitis
- petrous bone (acute) (chronic) — *see* Petrositis
- pharynx (acute) — *see* Pharyngitis
- pia mater — *see* Meningitis
- pleura — *see* Pleurisy
- polyp, colon (*see also* Polyp, colon, inflammatory) K51.4Ø
- prostate (*see also* Prostatitis)
  - specified type NEC N41.8
- rectosigmoid — *see* Rectosigmoiditis
- rectum (*see also* Proctitis) K62.89

Inflammation, inflamed, inflammatory — *continued*
respiratory, upper (*see also* Infection, respiratory, upper) JØ6.9
acute, due to radiation J7Ø.Ø
chronic, due to external agent — *see* condition, respiratory, chronic, due to
due to
chemicals, gases, fumes or vapors (inhalation) J68.2
radiation J7Ø.1
retina — *see* Chorioretinitis
retrocecal — *see* Appendicitis
retroperitoneal — *see* Peritonitis
salivary duct or gland (any) (suppurative) — *see* Sialoadenitis
scorbutic, alveoli, teeth E54
scrotum N49.2
seminal vesicle — *see* Vesiculitis
sigmoid — *see* Enteritis
sinus — *see* Sinusitis
Skene's duct or gland — *see* Urethritis
skin LØ8.9
spermatic cord N49.1
sphenoidal (sinus) — *see* Sinusitis, sphenoidal
spinal
cord — *see* Encephalitis
membrane — *see* Meningitis
nerve — *see* Disorder, nerve
spine — *see* Spondylopathy, inflammatory
spleen (capsule) D73.89
stomach — *see* Gastritis
subcutaneous tissue LØ8.9
suprarenal (gland) E27.8
synovial — *see* Tenosynovitis
tendon (sheath) NEC — *see* Tenosynovitis
testis — *see* Orchitis
throat (acute) — *see* Pharyngitis
thymus (gland) E32.8
thyroid (gland) — *see* Thyroiditis
tongue K14.Ø
tonsil — *see* Tonsillitis
trachea — *see* Tracheitis
trochlear (nerve) — *see* Strabismus, paralytic, fourth nerve
tubal — *see* Salpingo-oophoritis
tuberculous NEC — *see* Tuberculosis
tubo-ovarian — *see* Salpingo-oophoritis
tunica vaginalis N49.1
tympanic membrane — *see* Tympanitis
umbilicus, umbilical LØ8.82
uterine ligament — *see* Disease, pelvis, inflammatory
uterus (catarrhal) — *see* Endometritis
uveal tract (anterior) NOS (*see also* Iridocyclitis)
posterior — *see* Chorioretinitis
vagina — *see* Vaginitis
vas deferens N49.1
vein (*see also* Phlebitis)
intracranial or intraspinal (septic) GØ8
thrombotic I8Ø.9
leg — *see* Phlebitis, leg
lower extremity — *see* Phlebitis, leg
vocal cord J38.3
vulva — *see* Vulvitis
Wharton's duct (suppurative) — *see* Sialoadenitis
Inflation, lung, imperfect (newborn) — *see* Atelectasis
Influenza (bronchial) (epidemic) (respiratory (upper)) (unidentified influenza virus) J11.1
with
digestive manifestations J11.2
encephalopathy J11.81
enteritis J11.2
gastroenteritis J11.2
gastrointestinal manifestations J11.2
laryngitis J11.1
myocarditis J11.82
otitis media J11.83
pharyngitis J11.1
pneumonia J11.ØØ
specified type J11.Ø8
respiratory manifestations NEC J11.1
specified manifestation NEC J11.89
A/H5N1 (*see also* Influenza, due to, identified novel influenza A virus) JØ9.X2
avian (*see also* Influenza, due to, identified novel influenza A virus) JØ9.X2

Influenza — *continued*
bird (*see also* Influenza, due to, identified novel influenza A virus) JØ9.X2
due to
avian (*see also* Influenza, due to, identified novel influenza A virus) JØ9.X2
identified influenza virus NEC J1Ø.1
with
digestive manifestations J1Ø.2
encephalopathy J1Ø.81
enteritis J1Ø.2
gastroenteritis J1Ø.2
gastrointestinal manifestations J1Ø.2
laryngitis J1Ø.1
myocarditis J1Ø.82
otitis media J1Ø.83
pharyngitis J1Ø.1
pneumonia (unspecified type) J1Ø.ØØ
with same identified influenza virus J1Ø.Ø1
specified type NEC J1Ø.Ø8
respiratory manifestations NEC J1Ø.1
specified manifestation NEC J1Ø.89
identified novel influenza A virus JØ9.X2
with
digestive manifestations JØ9.X3
encephalopathy JØ9.X9
enteritis JØ9.X3
gastroenteritis JØ9.X3
gastrointestinal manifestations JØ9.X3
laryngitis JØ9.X2
myocarditis JØ9.X9
otitis media JØ9.X9
pharyngitis JØ9.X2
pneumonia JØ9.X1
respiratory manifestations NEC JØ9.X2
specified manifestation NEC JØ9.X9
upper respiratory symptoms JØ9.X2
novel (2ØØ9) H1N1 influenza (*see also* Influenza, due to, identified influenza virus NEC) J1Ø.1
novel influenza A/H1N1 (*see also* Influenza, due to, identified influenza virus NEC) J1Ø.1
of other animal origin, not bird or swine (*see also* Influenza, due to, identified novel influenza A virus) JØ9.X2
swine (viruses that normally cause infections in pigs) (*see also* Influenza, due to, identified novel influenza A virus) JØ9.X2
Influenzal — *see* Influenza
Influenza-like disease — *see* Influenza
Infraction, Freiberg's (metatarsal head) — *see* Osteochondrosis, juvenile, metatarsus
Infraeruption of tooth (teeth) M26.34
Infusion complication, misadventure, or reaction — *see* Complications, infusion
Ingestion
chemical — *see* Table of Drugs and Chemicals, by substance, poisoning
drug or medicament
correct substance properly administered — *see* Table of Drugs and Chemicals, by drug, adverse effect
overdose or wrong substance given or taken — *see* Table of Drugs and Chemicals, by drug, poisoning
foreign body — *see* Foreign body, alimentary tract
tularemia A21.3
Ingrowing
hair (beard) L73.1
nail (finger) (toe) L6Ø.Ø
Inguinal (*see also* condition)
testicle Q53.9
bilateral Q53.21
unilateral Q53.11
Inhalation
anthrax A22.1
flame T27.3 ☑
food or foreign body — *see* Foreign body, by site
gases, fumes, or vapors NEC T59.9- ☑
specified agent — *see* Table of Drugs and Chemicals, by substance
liquid or vomitus — *see* Asphyxia
meconium (newborn) P24.ØØ
with
with respiratory symptoms P24.Ø1
pneumonia (pneumonitis) P24.Ø1
mucus — *see* Asphyxia, mucus

Inhalation — *continued*
oil or gasoline (causing suffocation) — *see* Foreign body, by site
smoke J7Ø.5
due to chemicals, gases, fumes and vapors J68.9
steam — *see* Toxicity, vapors
stomach contents or secretions — *see* Foreign body, by site
due to anesthesia (general) (local) or other sedation T88.59 ☑
in labor and delivery O74.Ø
in pregnancy O29.Ø1- ☑
postpartum, puerperal O89.Ø1
Inhibition, orgasm
female F52.31
male F52.32
Inhibitor, systemic lupus erythematosus (presence of) D68.62
Iniencephalus, iniencephaly QØØ.2
Injection, traumatic jet (air) (industrial) (water) (paint or dye) T7Ø.4 ☑
Injury (*see also* specified injury type) T14.9Ø
abdomen, abdominal S39.91 ☑
blood vessel — *see* Injury, blood vessel, abdomen
cavity — *see* Injury, intra-abdominal
contusion S3Ø.1 ☑
internal — *see* Injury, intra-abdominal
intra-abdominal organ — *see* Injury, intra-abdominal
nerve — *see* Injury, nerve, abdomen
open — *see* Wound, open, abdomen
specified NEC S39.81 ☑
superficial — *see* Injury, superficial, abdomen
Achilles tendon S86.ØØ- ☑
laceration S86.Ø2- ☑
specified type NEC S86.Ø9- ☑
strain S86.Ø1- ☑
acoustic, resulting in deafness — *see* Injury, nerve, acoustic
adrenal (gland) S37.819 ☑
contusion S37.812 ☑
laceration S37.813 ☑
specified type NEC S37.818 ☑
alveolar (process) SØ9.93 ☑
ankle S99.91- ☑
contusion — *see* Contusion, ankle
dislocation — *see* Dislocation, ankle
fracture — *see* Fracture, ankle
nerve — *see* Injury, nerve, ankle
open — *see* Wound, open, ankle
specified type NEC S99.81- ☑
sprain — *see* Sprain, ankle
superficial — *see* Injury, superficial, ankle
anterior chamber, eye — *see* Injury, eye, specified site NEC
anus — *see* Injury, abdomen
aorta (thoracic) S25.ØØ ☑
abdominal S35.ØØ ☑
laceration (minor) (superficial) S35.Ø1 ☑
major S35.Ø2 ☑
specified type NEC S35.Ø9 ☑
laceration (minor) (superficial) S25.Ø1 ☑
major S25.Ø2 ☑
specified type NEC S25.Ø9 ☑
arm (upper) S49.9- ☑
blood vessel — *see* Injury, blood vessel, arm
contusion — *see* Contusion, arm, upper
fracture — *see* Fracture, humerus
lower — *see* Injury, forearm
muscle — *see* Injury, muscle, shoulder
nerve — *see* Injury, nerve, arm
open — *see* Wound, open, arm
specified type NEC S49.8- ☑
superficial — *see* Injury, superficial, arm
artery (complicating trauma) (*see also* Injury, blood vessel, by site)
cerebral or meningeal — *see* Injury, intracranial
auditory canal (external) (meatus) SØ9.91 ☑
auricle, auris, ear SØ9.91 ☑
axilla — *see* Injury, shoulder
back — *see* Injury, back, lower
bile duct S36.13 ☑
birth (*see also* Birth, injury) P15.9
bladder (sphincter) S37.2Ø ☑
at delivery O71.5
contusion S37.22 ☑

- **Injury** — *continued*
  - bladder — *continued*
    - laceration S37.23 ☑
    - obstetrical trauma O71.5
    - specified type NEC S37.29 ☑
  - blast (air) (hydraulic) (immersion) (underwater) NEC T14.8
    - acoustic nerve trauma — *see* Injury, nerve, acoustic
    - bladder — *see* Injury, bladder
    - brain — *see* Concussion
    - colon — *see* Injury, intestine, large
    - ear (primary) S09.31- ☑
      - secondary S09.39- ☑
    - generalized T70.8 ☑
    - lung — *see* Injury, intrathoracic, lung
    - multiple body organs T70.8 ☑
    - peritoneum S36.81 ☑
    - rectum S36.61 ☑
    - retroperitoneum S36.898 ☑
    - small intestine S36.419 ☑
      - duodenum S36.410 ☑
      - specified site NEC S36.418 ☑
    - specified
      - intra-abdominal organ NEC S36.898 ☑
      - pelvic organ NEC S37.899 ☑
  - blood vessel NEC T14.8
    - abdomen S35.9 ☑
      - aorta — *see* Injury, aorta, abdominal
      - celiac artery — *see* Injury, blood vessel, celiac artery
      - iliac vessel — *see* Injury, blood vessel, iliac
      - laceration S35.91 ☑
      - mesenteric vessel — *see* Injury, mesenteric
      - portal vein — *see* Injury, blood vessel, portal vein
      - renal vessel — *see* Injury, blood vessel, renal
      - specified vessel NEC S35.8X- ☑
      - splenic vessel — *see* Injury, blood vessel, splenic
      - vena cava — *see* Injury, vena cava, inferior
    - ankle — *see* Injury, blood vessel, foot
    - aorta (abdominal) (thoracic) — *see* Injury, aorta
    - arm (upper) NEC S45.90- ☑
      - forearm — *see* Injury, blood vessel, forearm
      - laceration S45.91- ☑
      - specified
        - site NEC S45.80- ☑
          - laceration S45.81- ☑
          - specified type NEC S45.89- ☑
        - type NEC S45.99- ☑
      - superficial vein S45.30- ☑
        - laceration S45.31- ☑
        - specified type NEC S45.39- ☑
    - axillary
      - artery S45.00- ☑
        - laceration S45.01- ☑
        - specified type NEC S45.09- ☑
      - vein S45.20- ☑
        - laceration S45.21- ☑
        - specified type NEC S45.29- ☑
    - azygos vein — *see* Injury, blood vessel, thoracic, specified site NEC
    - brachial
      - artery S45.10- ☑
        - laceration S45.11- ☑
        - specified type NEC S45.19- ☑
      - vein S45.20- ☑
        - laceration S45.219 ☑
        - specified type NEC S45.29- ☑
    - carotid artery (common) (external) (internal, extracranial) S15.00- ☑
      - internal, intracranial S06.8- ☑
      - laceration (minor) (superficial) S15.01- ☑
        - major S15.02- ☑
      - specified type NEC S15.09- ☑
    - celiac artery S35.219 ☑
      - branch S35.299 ☑
        - laceration (minor) (superficial) S35.291 ☑
          - major S35.292 ☑
        - specified NEC S35.298 ☑
      - laceration (minor) (superficial) S35.211 ☑
        - major S35.212 ☑
      - specified type NEC S35.218 ☑
    - cerebral — *see* Injury, intracranial
    - deep plantar — *see* Injury, blood vessel, plantar artery

- **Injury** — *continued*
  - blood vessel — *continued*
    - digital (hand) — *see* Injury, blood vessel, finger
    - dorsal
      - artery (foot) S95.00- ☑
        - laceration S95.01- ☑
        - specified type NEC S95.09- ☑
      - vein (foot) S95.20- ☑
        - laceration S95.21- ☑
        - specified type NEC S95.29- ☑
    - due to accidental laceration during procedure — *see* Laceration, accidental complicating surgery
    - extremity — *see* Injury, blood vessel, limb
    - femoral
      - artery (common) (superficial) S75.00- ☑
        - laceration (minor) (superficial) S75.01- ☑
          - major S75.02- ☑
        - specified type NEC S75.09- ☑
      - vein (hip level) (thigh level) S75.10- ☑
        - laceration (minor) (superficial) S75.11- ☑
          - major S75.12- ☑
        - specified type NEC S75.19- ☑
    - finger S65.50- ☑
      - index S65.50- ☑
        - laceration S65.51- ☑
        - specified type NEC S65.59- ☑
      - laceration S65.51- ☑
      - little S65.50- ☑
        - laceration S65.51- ☑
        - specified type NEC S65.59- ☑
      - middle S65.50- ☑
        - laceration S65.51- ☑
        - specified type NEC S65.59- ☑
      - specified type NEC S65.59- ☑
      - thumb — *see* Injury, blood vessel, thumb
    - foot S95.90- ☑
      - dorsal
        - artery — *see* Injury, blood vessel, dorsal, artery
        - vein — *see* Injury, blood vessel, dorsal, vein
      - laceration S95.91- ☑
      - plantar artery — *see* Injury, blood vessel, plantar artery
      - specified
        - site NEC S95.80- ☑
          - laceration S95.81- ☑
          - specified type NEC S95.89- ☑
        - specified type NEC S95.99- ☑
    - forearm S55.90- ☑
      - laceration S55.91- ☑
      - radial artery — *see* Injury, blood vessel, radial artery
      - specified
        - site NEC S55.80- ☑
          - laceration S55.81- ☑
          - specified type NEC S55.89- ☑
        - type NEC S55.99- ☑
      - ulnar artery — *see* Injury, blood vessel, ulnar artery
      - vein S55.20- ☑
        - laceration S55.21- ☑
        - specified type NEC S55.29- ☑
    - gastric
      - artery — *see* Injury, mesenteric, artery, branch
      - vein — *see* Injury, blood vessel, abdomen
    - gastroduodenal artery — *see* Injury, mesenteric, artery, branch
    - greater saphenous vein (lower leg level) S85.30- ☑
      - hip (and thigh) level S75.20- ☑
        - laceration (minor) (superficial) S75.21- ☑
          - major S75.22- ☑
        - specified type NEC S75.29- ☑
      - laceration S85.31- ☑
      - specified type NEC S85.39- ☑
    - hand (level) S65.90- ☑
      - finger — *see* Injury, blood vessel, finger
      - laceration S65.91- ☑
      - palmar arch — *see* Injury, blood vessel, palmar arch
      - radial artery — *see* Injury, blood vessel, radial artery, hand
      - specified
        - site NEC S65.80- ☑
          - laceration S65.81- ☑
          - specified type NEC S65.89- ☑

- **Injury** — *continued*
  - blood vessel — *continued*
    - hand — *continued*
      - specified — *continued*
        - type NEC S65.99- ☑
      - thumb — *see* Injury, blood vessel, thumb
      - ulnar artery — *see* Injury, blood vessel, ulnar artery, hand
    - head S09.0 ☑
      - intracranial — *see* Injury, intracranial
      - multiple S09.0 ☑
    - hepatic
      - artery — *see* Injury, mesenteric, artery
      - vein — *see* Injury, vena cava, inferior
    - hip S75.90- ☑
      - femoral artery — *see* Injury, blood vessel, femoral, artery
      - femoral vein — *see* Injury, blood vessel, femoral, vein
      - greater saphenous vein — *see* Injury, blood vessel, greater saphenous, hip level
      - laceration S75.91- ☑
      - specified
        - site NEC S75.80- ☑
          - laceration S75.81- ☑
          - specified type NEC S75.89- ☑
        - type NEC S75.99- ☑
    - hypogastric (artery) (vein) — *see* Injury, blood vessel, iliac
    - iliac S35.5- ☑
      - artery S35.51- ☑
      - specified vessel NEC S35.5- ☑
      - uterine vessel — *see* Injury, blood vessel, uterine
      - vein S35.51- ☑
    - innominate — *see* Injury, blood vessel, thoracic, innominate
    - intercostal (artery) (vein) — *see* Injury, blood vessel, thoracic, intercostal
    - jugular vein (external) S15.20- ☑
      - internal S15.30- ☑
        - laceration (minor) (superficial) S15.31- ☑
          - major S15.32- ☑
        - specified type NEC S15.39- ☑
      - laceration (minor) (superficial) S15.21- ☑
        - major S15.22- ☑
      - specified type NEC S15.29- ☑
    - leg (level) (lower) S85.90- ☑
      - greater saphenous — *see* Injury, blood vessel, greater saphenous
      - laceration S85.91- ☑
      - lesser saphenous — *see* Injury, blood vessel, lesser saphenous
      - peroneal artery — *see* Injury, blood vessel, peroneal artery
      - popliteal
        - artery — *see* Injury, blood vessel, popliteal, artery
        - vein — *see* Injury, blood vessel, popliteal, vein
      - specified
        - site NEC S85.80- ☑
          - laceration S85.81- ☑
          - specified type NEC S85.89- ☑
        - type NEC S85.99- ☑
      - thigh — *see* Injury, blood vessel, hip
      - tibial artery — *see* Injury, blood vessel, tibial artery
    - lesser saphenous vein (lower leg level) S85.40- ☑
      - laceration S85.41- ☑
      - specified type NEC S85.49- ☑
    - limb
      - lower — *see* Injury, blood vessel, leg
      - upper — *see* Injury, blood vessel, arm
    - lower back — *see* Injury, blood vessel, abdomen
      - specified NEC — *see* Injury, blood vessel, abdomen, specified, site NEC
    - mammary (artery) (vein) — *see* Injury, blood vessel, thoracic, specified site NEC
    - mesenteric (inferior) (superior)
      - artery — *see* Injury, mesenteric, artery
      - vein — *see* Injury, blood vessel, mesenteric, vein
    - neck S15.9 ☑
      - specified site NEC S15.8 ☑
    - ovarian (artery) (vein) — *see* subcategory S35.8 ☑

Injury — *continued*
- blood vessel — *continued*
  - palmar arch (superficial) S65.2Ø- ☑
    - deep S65.3Ø- ☑
      - laceration S65.31- ☑
      - specified type NEC S65.39- ☑
    - laceration S65.21- ☑
    - specified type NEC S65.29- ☑
  - pelvis — *see* Injury, blood vessel, abdomen
    - specified NEC — *see* Injury, blood vessel, abdomen, specified, site NEC
  - peroneal artery S85.2Ø- ☑
    - laceration S85.21- ☑
    - specified type NEC S85.29- ☑
  - plantar artery (deep) (foot) S95.1Ø- ☑
    - laceration S95.11- ☑
    - specified type NEC S95.19- ☑
  - popliteal
    - artery S85.ØØ- ☑
      - laceration S85.Ø1- ☑
      - specified type NEC S85.Ø9- ☑
    - vein S85.5Ø- ☑
      - laceration S85.51- ☑
      - specified type NEC S85.59- ☑
  - portal vein S35.319 ☑
    - laceration S35.311 ☑
    - specified type NEC S35.318 ☑
  - precerebral — *see* Injury, blood vessel, neck
  - pulmonary (artery) (vein) — *see* Injury, blood vessel, thoracic, pulmonary
  - radial artery (forearm level) S55.1Ø- ☑
    - hand and wrist (level) S65.1Ø- ☑
      - laceration S65.11- ☑
      - specified type NEC S65.19- ☑
    - laceration S55.11- ☑
    - specified type NEC S55.19- ☑
  - renal
    - artery S35.4Ø- ☑
      - laceration S35.41- ☑
      - specified NEC S35.49- ☑
    - vein S35.4Ø- ☑
      - laceration S35.41- ☑
      - specified NEC S35.49- ☑
  - saphenous vein (greater) (lower leg level) — *see* Injury, blood vessel, greater saphenous
    - hip and thigh level — *see* Injury, blood vessel, greater saphenous, hip level
    - lesser — *see* Injury, blood vessel, lesser saphenous
  - shoulder
    - specified NEC — *see* Injury, blood vessel, arm, specified site NEC
    - superficial vein — *see* Injury, blood vessel, arm, superficial vein
  - specified NEC T14.8
  - splenic
    - artery — *see* Injury, blood vessel, celiac artery, branch
    - vein S35.329 ☑
      - laceration S35.321 ☑
      - specified NEC S35.328 ☑
  - subclavian — *see* Injury, blood vessel, thoracic, innominate
  - thigh — *see* Injury, blood vessel, hip
  - thoracic S25.9Ø ☑
    - aorta S25.ØØ ☑
      - laceration (minor) (superficial) S25.Ø1 ☑
        - major S25.Ø2 ☑
      - specified type NEC S25.Ø9 ☑
    - azygos vein — *see* Injury, blood vessel, thoracic, specified, site NEC
    - innominate
      - artery S25.1Ø- ☑
        - laceration (minor) (superficial) S25.11- ☑
          - major S25.12- ☑
        - specified type NEC S25.19- ☑
      - vein S25.3Ø- ☑
        - laceration (minor) (superficial) S25.31- ☑
          - major S25.32- ☑
        - specified type NEC S25.39- ☑
    - intercostal S25.5Ø- ☑
      - laceration S25.51- ☑
      - specified type NEC S25.59- ☑
    - laceration S25.91 ☑

Injury — *continued*
- blood vessel — *continued*
  - thoracic — *continued*
    - mammary vessel — *see* Injury, blood vessel, thoracic, specified, site NEC
    - pulmonary S25.4Ø- ☑
      - laceration (minor) (superficial) S25.41- ☑
        - major S25.42- ☑
      - specified type NEC S25.49- ☑
    - specified
      - site NEC S25.8Ø- ☑
        - laceration S25.81 ☑
        - specified type NEC S25.89 ☑
      - type NEC S25.99 ☑
    - subclavian — *see* Injury, blood vessel, thoracic, innominate
    - vena cava (superior) S25.2Ø ☑
      - laceration (minor) (superficial) S25.21 ☑
        - major S25.22 ☑
      - specified type NEC S25.29 ☑
  - thumb S65.4Ø- ☑
    - laceration S65.41- ☑
    - specified type NEC S65.49- ☑
  - tibial artery S85.1Ø- ☑
    - anterior S85.13- ☑
      - laceration S85.14- ☑
      - specified injury NEC S85.15- ☑
    - laceration S85.11- ☑
    - posterior S85.16- ☑
      - laceration S85.17- ☑
      - specified injury NEC S85.18- ☑
    - specified injury NEC S85.12- ☑
  - ulnar artery (forearm level) S55.ØØ- ☑
    - hand and wrist (level) S65.ØØ- ☑
      - laceration S65.Ø1- ☑
      - specified type NEC S65.Ø9- ☑
    - laceration S55.Ø1- ☑
    - specified type NEC S55.Ø9- ☑
  - upper arm (level) — *see* Injury, blood vessel, arm
    - superficial vein — *see* Injury, blood vessel, arm, superficial vein
  - uterine S35.5- ☑
    - artery S35.53- ☑
    - vein S35.53- ☑
  - vena cava — *see* Injury, vena cava
  - vertebral artery S15.1Ø- ☑
    - laceration (minor) (superficial) S15.11- ☑
      - major S15.12- ☑
    - specified type NEC S15.19- ☑
  - wrist (level) — *see* Injury, blood vessel, hand
- brachial plexus S14.3 ☑
  - newborn P14.3
- brain (traumatic) SØ6.9- ☑
  - diffuse (axonal) SØ6.2X- ☑
  - focal SØ6.3Ø- ☑
  - traumatic — *see* category SØ6 ☑
- brainstem SØ6.38- ☑
- breast NOS S29.9 ☑
- broad ligament — *see* Injury, pelvic organ, specified site NEC
- bronchus, bronchi — *see* Injury, intrathoracic, bronchus
- brow SØ9.9Ø ☑
- buttock S39.92 ☑
- canthus, eye SØ5.9Ø ☑
- cardiac plexus — *see* Injury, nerve, thorax, sympathetic
- cauda equina S34.3 ☑
- cavernous sinus — *see* Injury, intracranial
- cecum — *see* Injury, colon
- celiac ganglion or plexus — *see* Injury, nerve, lumbosacral, sympathetic
- cerebellum — *see* Injury, intracranial
- cerebral — *see* Injury, intracranial
- cervix (uteri) — *see* Injury, uterus
- cheek (wall) SØ9.93 ☑
- chest — *see* Injury, thorax
- childbirth (newborn) (*see also* Birth, injury)
  - maternal NEC O71.9
- chin SØ9.93 ☑
- choroid (eye) — *see* Injury, eye, specified site NEC
- clitoris S39.94 ☑
- coccyx (*see also* Injury, back, lower)
  - complicating delivery O71.6
- colon — *see* Injury, intestine, large
- common bile duct — *see* Injury, liver
- conjunctiva (superficial) — *see* Injury, eye, conjunctiva

Injury — *continued*
- conus medullaris — *see* Injury, spinal, sacral
- cord
  - spermatic (pelvic region) S37.898 ☑
    - scrotal region S39.848 ☑
  - spinal — *see* Injury, spinal cord, by region
- cornea — *see* Injury, eye, specified site NEC
  - abrasion — *see* Injury, eye, cornea, abrasion
- cortex (cerebral) (*see also* Injury, intracranial)
  - visual — *see* Injury, nerve, optic
- costal region NEC S29.9 ☑
- costochondral NEC S29.9 ☑
- cranial
  - cavity — *see* Injury, intracranial
  - nerve — *see* Injury, nerve, cranial
- crushing — *see* Crush
- cutaneous sensory nerve
- cystic duct — *see* Injury, liver
- deep tissue — *see* Contusion, by site
  - meaning pressure ulcer — *see* Ulcer, pressure, unstageable, by site
- delivery (newborn) P15.9
  - maternal NEC O71.9
- Descemet's membrane — *see* Injury, eyeball, penetrating
- diaphragm — *see* Injury, intrathoracic, diaphragm
- duodenum — *see* Injury, intestine, small, duodenum
- ear (auricle) (external) (canal) SØ9.91 ☑
  - abrasion — *see* Abrasion, ear
  - bite — *see* Bite, ear
  - blister — *see* Blister, ear
  - bruise — *see* Contusion, ear
  - contusion — *see* Contusion, ear
  - external constriction — *see* Constriction, external, ear
  - hematoma — *see* Hematoma, ear
  - inner — *see* Injury, ear, middle
  - laceration — *see* Laceration, ear
  - middle SØ9.3Ø- ☑
    - blast — *see* Injury, blast, ear
    - specified NEC SØ9.39- ☑
  - puncture — *see* Puncture, ear
  - superficial — *see* Injury, superficial, ear
- eighth cranial nerve (acoustic or auditory) — *see* Injury, nerve, acoustic
- elbow S59.9Ø- ☑
  - contusion — *see* Contusion, elbow
  - dislocation — *see* Dislocation, elbow
  - fracture — *see* Fracture, ulna, upper end
  - open — *see* Wound, open, elbow
  - specified NEC S59.8Ø- ☑
  - sprain — *see* Sprain, elbow
  - superficial — *see* Injury, superficial, elbow
- eleventh cranial nerve (accessory) — *see* Injury, nerve, accessory
- epididymis S39.94 ☑
- epigastric region S39.91 ☑
- epiglottis NEC S19.89 ☑
- esophageal plexus — *see* Injury, nerve, thorax, sympathetic
- esophagus (thoracic part) (*see also* Injury, intrathoracic, esophagus)
  - cervical NEC S19.85 ☑
- eustachian tube SØ9.3Ø ☑
- eye SØ5.9- ☑
  - avulsion SØ5.7- ☑
  - ball — *see* Injury, eyeball
  - conjunctiva SØ5.Ø- ☑
  - cornea
    - abrasion SØ5.Ø- ☑
  - laceration SØ5.3- ☑
    - with prolapse SØ5.2- ☑
  - lacrimal apparatus SØ5.8X- ☑
  - orbit penetration SØ5.4- ☑
  - specified site NEC SØ5.8X- ☑
- eyeball SØ5.8X- ☑
  - contusion SØ5.1- ☑
  - penetrating SØ5.6- ☑
    - with
      - foreign body SØ5.5- ☑
      - prolapse or loss of intraocular tissue SØ5.2- ☑
    - without prolapse or loss of intraocular tissue SØ5.3- ☑
  - specified type NEC SØ5.8- ☑
- eyebrow SØ9.93 ☑

- **Injury** — *continued*
  - eyelid S09.93 ☑
    - abrasion — *see* Abrasion, eyelid
    - contusion — *see* Contusion, eyelid
    - open — *see* Wound, open, eyelid
  - face S09.93 ☑
  - fallopian tube S37.509 ☑
    - bilateral S37.502 ☑
      - blast injury S37.512 ☑
      - contusion S37.522 ☑
      - laceration S37.532 ☑
      - specified type NEC S37.592 ☑
    - blast injury (primary) S37.519 ☑
      - bilateral S37.512 ☑
      - secondary — *see* Injury, fallopian tube, specified type NEC
      - unilateral S37.511 ☑
    - contusion S37.529 ☑
      - bilateral S37.522 ☑
      - unilateral S37.521 ☑
    - laceration S37.539 ☑
      - bilateral S37.532 ☑
      - unilateral S37.531 ☑
    - specified type NEC S37.599 ☑
      - bilateral S37.592 ☑
      - unilateral S37.591 ☑
    - unilateral S37.501 ☑
      - blast injury S37.511 ☑
      - contusion S37.521 ☑
      - laceration S37.531 ☑
      - specified type NEC S37.591 ☑
  - fascia — *see* Injury, muscle
  - fifth cranial nerve (trigeminal) — *see* Injury, nerve, trigeminal
  - finger (nail) S69.9- ☑
    - blood vessel — *see* Injury, blood vessel, finger
    - contusion — *see* Contusion, finger
    - dislocation — *see* Dislocation, finger
    - fracture — *see* Fracture, finger
    - muscle — *see* Injury, muscle, finger
    - nerve — *see* Injury, nerve, digital, finger
    - open — *see* Wound, open, finger
    - specified NEC S69.8- ☑
    - sprain — *see* Sprain, finger
    - superficial — *see* Injury, superficial, finger
  - first cranial nerve (olfactory) — *see* Injury, nerve, olfactory
  - flank — *see* Injury, abdomen
  - foot S99.92- ☑
    - blood vessel — *see* Injury, blood vessel, foot
    - contusion — *see* Contusion, foot
    - dislocation — *see* Dislocation, foot
    - fracture — *see* Fracture, foot
    - muscle — *see* Injury, muscle, foot
    - open — *see* Wound, open, foot
    - specified type NEC S99.82- ☑
    - sprain — *see* Sprain, foot
    - superficial — *see* Injury, superficial, foot
  - forceps NOS P15.9
  - forearm S59.91- ☑
    - blood vessel — *see* Injury, blood vessel, forearm
    - contusion — *see* Contusion, forearm
    - fracture — *see* Fracture, forearm
    - muscle — *see* Injury, muscle, forearm
    - nerve — *see* Injury, nerve, forearm
    - open — *see* Wound, open, forearm
    - specified NEC S59.81- ☑
    - superficial — *see* Injury, superficial, forearm
  - forehead S09.90 ☑
  - fourth cranial nerve (trochlear) — *see* Injury, nerve, trochlear
  - gallbladder S36.129 ☑
    - contusion S36.122 ☑
    - laceration S36.123 ☑
    - specified NEC S36.128 ☑
  - ganglion
    - celiac, coeliac — *see* Injury, nerve, lumbosacral, sympathetic
    - gasserian — *see* Injury, nerve, trigeminal
    - stellate — *see* Injury, nerve, thorax, sympathetic
    - thoracic sympathetic — *see* Injury, nerve, thorax, sympathetic
  - gasserian ganglion — *see* Injury, nerve, trigeminal
  - gastric artery — *see* Injury, blood vessel, celiac artery, branch

- **Injury** — *continued*
  - gastroduodenal artery — *see* Injury, blood vessel, celiac artery, branch
  - gastrointestinal tract — *see* Injury, intra-abdominal
    - with open wound into abdominal cavity — *see* Wound, open, with penetration into peritoneal cavity
    - colon — *see* Injury, intestine, large
    - rectum — *see* Injury, intestine, large, rectum
      - with open wound into abdominal cavity S36.61 ☑
    - small intestine — *see* Injury, intestine, small
    - specified site NEC — *see* Injury, intra-abdominal, specified, site NEC
    - stomach — *see* Injury, stomach
  - genital organ(s)
    - external S39.94 ☑
      - specified NEC S39.848 ☑
    - internal S37.90 ☑
      - fallopian tube — *see* Injury, fallopian tube
      - ovary — *see* Injury, ovary
      - prostate — *see* Injury, prostate
      - seminal vesicle — *see* Injury, pelvis, organ, specified site NEC
      - uterus — *see* Injury, uterus
      - vas deferens — *see* Injury, pelvis, organ, specified site NEC
    - obstetrical trauma O71.9
  - gland
    - lacrimal laceration — *see* Injury, eye, specified site NEC
    - salivary S09.90 ☑
    - thyroid NEC S19.84 ☑
  - globe (eye) S05.90 ☑
    - specified NEC S05.8X- ☑
  - groin — *see* Injury, abdomen
  - gum S09.90 ☑
  - hand S69.9- ☑
    - blood vessel — *see* Injury, blood vessel, hand
    - contusion — *see* Contusion, hand
    - fracture — *see* Fracture, hand
    - muscle — *see* Injury, muscle, hand
    - nerve — *see* Injury, nerve, hand
    - open — *see* Wound, open, hand
    - specified NEC S69.8- ☑
    - sprain — *see* Sprain, hand
    - superficial — *see* Injury, superficial, hand
  - head S09.90 ☑
    - with loss of consciousness S06.9- ☑
    - specified NEC S09.8 ☑
  - heart S26.90 ☑
    - with hemopericardium S26.00 ☑
      - contusion S26.01 ☑
      - laceration (mild) S26.020 ☑
        - major S26.022 ☑
        - moderate S26.021 ☑
      - specified type NEC S26.09 ☑
    - without hemopericardium S26.10 ☑
      - contusion S26.11 ☑
      - laceration S26.12 ☑
      - specified type NEC S26.19 ☑
    - contusion S26.91 ☑
    - laceration S26.92 ☑
    - specified type NEC S26.99 ☑
  - heel — *see* Injury, foot
  - hepatic
    - artery — *see* Injury, blood vessel, celiac artery, branch
    - duct — *see* Injury, liver
    - vein — *see* Injury, vena cava, inferior
  - hip S79.91- ☑
    - blood vessel — *see* Injury, blood vessel, hip
    - contusion — *see* Contusion, hip
    - dislocation — *see* Dislocation, hip
    - fracture — *see* Fracture, femur, neck
    - muscle — *see* Injury, muscle, hip
    - nerve — *see* Injury, nerve, hip
    - open — *see* Wound, open, hip
    - specified NEC S79.81- ☑
    - sprain — *see* Sprain, hip
    - superficial — *see* Injury, superficial, hip
  - hymen S39.94 ☑
  - hypogastric
    - blood vessel — *see* Injury, blood vessel, iliac
    - plexus — *see* Injury, nerve, lumbosacral, sympathetic

- **Injury** — *continued*
  - ileum — *see* Injury, intestine, small
  - iliac region S39.91 ☑
  - instrumental (during surgery) — *see* Laceration, accidental complicating surgery
    - birth injury — *see* Birth, injury
    - nonsurgical — *see* Injury, by site
    - obstetrical O71.9
      - bladder O71.5
      - cervix O71.3
      - high vaginal O71.4
      - perineal NOS O70.9
      - urethra O71.5
      - uterus O71.5
        - with rupture or perforation O71.1
  - internal T14.8
    - aorta — *see* Injury, aorta
    - bladder (sphincter) — *see* Injury, bladder
      - with
        - ectopic or molar pregnancy O08.6
      - following ectopic or molar pregnancy O08.6
      - obstetrical trauma O71.5
    - bronchus, bronchi — *see* Injury, intrathoracic, bronchus
    - cecum — *see* Injury, intestine, large
    - cervix (uteri) (*see also* Injury, uterus)
      - with ectopic or molar pregnancy O08.6
      - following ectopic or molar pregnancy O08.6
      - obstetrical trauma O71.3
    - chest — *see* Injury, intrathoracic
    - gastrointestinal tract — *see* Injury, intra-abdominal
    - heart — *see* Injury, heart
    - intestine NEC — *see* Injury, intestine
    - intrauterine — *see* Injury, uterus
    - mesentery — *see* Injury, intra-abdominal, specified, site NEC
    - pelvis, pelvic (organ) S37.90 ☑
      - following ectopic or molar pregnancy (subsequent episode) O08.6
      - obstetrical trauma NEC O71.5
        - rupture or perforation O71.1
      - specified NEC S39.83 ☑
    - rectum — *see* Injury, intestine, large, rectum
    - stomach — *see* Injury, stomach
    - ureter — *see* Injury, ureter
    - urethra (sphincter) following ectopic or molar pregnancy O08.6
    - uterus — *see* Injury, uterus
  - interscapular area — *see* Injury, thorax
  - intestine
    - large S36.509 ☑
      - ascending (right) S36.500 ☑
        - blast injury (primary) S36.510 ☑
          - secondary S36.590 ☑
        - contusion S36.520 ☑
        - laceration S36.530 ☑
        - specified type NEC S36.590 ☑
      - blast injury (primary) S36.519 ☑
        - ascending (right) S36.510 ☑
        - descending (left) S36.512 ☑
        - rectum S36.61 ☑
        - sigmoid S36.513 ☑
        - specified site NEC S36.518 ☑
        - transverse S36.511 ☑
      - contusion S36.529 ☑
        - ascending (right) S36.520 ☑
        - descending (left) S36.522 ☑
        - rectum S36.62 ☑
        - sigmoid S36.523 ☑
        - specified site NEC S36.528 ☑
        - transverse S36.521 ☑
      - descending (left) S36.502 ☑
        - blast injury (primary) S36.512 ☑
          - secondary S36.592 ☑
        - contusion S36.522 ☑
        - laceration S36.532 ☑
        - specified type NEC S36.592 ☑
      - laceration S36.539 ☑
        - ascending (right) S36.530 ☑
        - descending (left) S36.532 ☑
        - rectum S36.63 ☑
        - sigmoid S36.533 ☑
        - specified site NEC S36.538 ☑
        - transverse S36.531 ☑
      - rectum S36.60 ☑
        - blast injury (primary) S36.61 ☑

- **Injury** — *continued*
  - intestine — *continued*
    - large — *continued*
      - rectum — *continued*
        - blast injury — *continued*
          - secondary S36.69 ☑
        - contusion S36.62 ☑
        - laceration S36.63 ☑
        - specified type NEC S36.69 ☑
      - sigmoid S36.5Ø3 ☑
        - blast injury (primary) S36.513 ☑
          - secondary S36.593 ☑
        - contusion S36.523 ☑
        - laceration S36.533 ☑
        - specified type NEC S36.593 ☑
      - specified
        - site NEC S36.5Ø8 ☑
          - blast injury (primary) S36.518 ☑
            - secondary S36.598 ☑
          - contusion S36.528 ☑
          - laceration S36.538 ☑
          - specified type NEC S36.598 ☑
        - type NEC S36.599 ☑
          - ascending (right) S36.59Ø ☑
          - descending (left) S36.592 ☑
          - rectum S36.69 ☑
          - sigmoid S36.593 ☑
          - specified site NEC S36.598 ☑
          - transverse S36.591 ☑
      - transverse S36.5Ø1 ☑
        - blast injury (primary) S36.511 ☑
          - secondary S36.591 ☑
        - contusion S36.521 ☑
        - laceration S36.531 ☑
        - specified type NEC S36.591 ☑
    - small S36.4Ø9 ☑
      - blast injury (primary) S36.419 ☑
        - duodenum S36.41Ø ☑
        - secondary S36.499 ☑
          - duodenum S36.49Ø ☑
          - specified site NEC S36.498 ☑
        - specified site NEC S36.418 ☑
      - contusion S36.429 ☑
        - duodenum S36.42Ø ☑
        - specified site NEC S36.428 ☑
      - duodenum S36.4ØØ ☑
        - blast injury (primary) S36.41Ø ☑
          - secondary S36.49Ø ☑
        - contusion S36.42Ø ☑
        - laceration S36.43Ø ☑
        - specified NEC S36.49Ø ☑
      - laceration S36.439 ☑
        - duodenum S36.43Ø ☑
        - specified site NEC S36.438 ☑
      - specified
        - site NEC S36.4Ø8 ☑
        - type NEC S36.499 ☑
          - duodenum S36.49Ø ☑
          - specified site NEC S36.498 ☑
  - intra-abdominal S36.9Ø ☑
    - adrenal gland — *see* Injury, adrenal gland
    - bladder — *see* Injury, bladder
    - colon — *see* Injury, intestine, large
    - contusion S36.92 ☑
    - fallopian tube — *see* Injury, fallopian tube
    - gallbladder — *see* Injury, gallbladder
    - intestine — *see* Injury, intestine
    - kidney — *see* Injury, kidney
    - laceration S36.93 ☑
    - liver — *see* Injury, liver
    - ovary — *see* Injury, ovary
    - pancreas — *see* Injury, pancreas
    - pelvic NOS S37.9Ø ☑
    - peritoneum — *see* Injury, intra-abdominal, specified, site NEC
    - prostate — *see* Injury, prostate
    - rectum — *see* Injury, intestine, large, rectum
    - retroperitoneum — *see* Injury, intra-abdominal, specified, site NEC
    - seminal vesicle — *see* Injury, pelvis, organ, specified site NEC
    - small intestine — *see* Injury, intestine, small
    - specified
      - pelvic S37.9Ø ☑
        - specified
          - site NEC S37.899 ☑

- **Injury** — *continued*
  - intra-abdominal — *continued*
    - specified — *continued*
      - pelvic — *continued*
        - specified — *continued*
          - site — *continued*
            - specified type NEC S37.898 ☑
          - type NEC S37.99 ☑
      - site NEC S36.899 ☑
        - contusion S36.892 ☑
        - laceration S36.893 ☑
        - specified type NEC S36.898 ☑
      - type NEC S36.99 ☑
    - spleen — *see* Injury, spleen
    - stomach — *see* Injury, stomach
    - ureter — *see* Injury, ureter
    - urethra — *see* Injury, urethra
    - uterus — *see* Injury, uterus
    - vas deferens — *see* Injury, pelvis, organ, specified site NEC
  - intracranial (traumatic) SØ6.9- ☑
    - cerebellar hemorrhage, traumatic — *see* Injury, intracranial, focal
    - cerebral edema, traumatic SØ6.1X- ☑
      - diffuse SØ6.1X- ☑
      - focal SØ6.1X- ☑
    - diffuse (axonal) SØ6.2X- ☑
    - epidural hemorrhage (traumatic) SØ6.4X- ☑
    - focal brain injury SØ6.3Ø- ☑
      - contusion — *see* Contusion, cerebral
      - laceration — *see* Laceration, cerebral
    - intracerebral hemorrhage, traumatic SØ6.36- ☑
      - left side SØ6.35- ☑
      - right side SØ6.34- ☑
    - subarachnoid hemorrhage, traumatic SØ6.6X- ☑
    - subdural hemorrhage, traumatic SØ6.5X- ☑
  - intraocular — *see* Injury, eyeball, penetrating
  - intrathoracic S27.9 ☑
    - bronchus S27.4Ø9 ☑
      - bilateral S27.4Ø2 ☑
      - blast injury (primary) S27.419 ☑
        - bilateral S27.412 ☑
        - secondary — *see* Injury, intrathoracic, bronchus, specified type NEC
        - unilateral S27.411 ☑
      - contusion S27.429 ☑
        - bilateral S27.422 ☑
        - unilateral S27.421 ☑
      - laceration S27.439 ☑
        - bilateral S27.432 ☑
        - unilateral S27.431 ☑
      - specified type NEC S27.499 ☑
        - bilateral S27.492 ☑
        - unilateral S27.491 ☑
      - unilateral S27.4Ø1 ☑
    - diaphragm S27.8Ø9 ☑
      - contusion S27.8Ø2 ☑
      - laceration S27.8Ø3 ☑
      - specified type NEC S27.8Ø8 ☑
    - esophagus (thoracic) S27.819 ☑
      - contusion S27.812 ☑
      - laceration S27.813 ☑
      - specified type NEC S27.818 ☑
    - heart — *see* Injury, heart
    - hemopneumothorax S27.2 ☑
    - hemothorax S27.1 ☑
    - lung S27.3Ø9 ☑
      - aspiration J69.Ø
      - bilateral S27.3Ø2 ☑
      - blast injury (primary) S27.319 ☑
        - bilateral S27.312 ☑
        - secondary — *see* Injury, intrathoracic, lung, specified type NEC
        - unilateral S27.311 ☑
      - contusion S27.329 ☑
        - bilateral S27.322 ☑
        - unilateral S27.321 ☑
      - laceration S27.339 ☑
        - bilateral S27.332 ☑
        - unilateral S27.331 ☑
      - specified type NEC S27.399 ☑
        - bilateral S27.392 ☑
        - unilateral S27.391 ☑
      - unilateral S27.3Ø1 ☑
    - pleura S27.6Ø ☑
      - laceration S27.63 ☑

- **Injury** — *continued*
  - intrathoracic — *continued*
    - pleura — *continued*
      - specified type NEC S27.69 ☑
    - pneumothorax S27.Ø ☑
    - specified organ NEC S27.899 ☑
      - contusion S27.892 ☑
      - laceration S27.893 ☑
      - specified type NEC S27.898 ☑
    - thoracic duct — *see* Injury, intrathoracic, specified organ NEC
    - thymus gland — *see* Injury, intrathoracic, specified organ NEC
    - trachea, thoracic S27.5Ø ☑
      - blast (primary) S27.51 ☑
      - contusion S27.52 ☑
      - laceration S27.53 ☑
      - specified type NEC S27.59 ☑
  - iris — *see* Injury, eye, specified site NEC
    - penetrating — *see* Injury, eyeball, penetrating
  - jaw SØ9.93 ☑
  - jejunum — *see* Injury, intestine, small
  - joint NOS T14.8
    - old or residual — *see* Disorder, joint, specified type NEC
  - kidney S37.ØØ- ☑
    - acute (nontraumatic) N17.9
    - contusion — *see* Contusion, kidney
    - laceration — *see* Laceration, kidney
    - specified NEC S37.Ø9- ☑
  - knee S89.9- ☑
    - contusion — *see* Contusion, knee
    - dislocation — *see* Dislocation, knee
    - meniscus (lateral) (medial) — *see* Sprain, knee, specified site NEC
      - old injury or tear — *see* Derangement, knee, meniscus, due to old injury
    - open — *see* Wound, open, knee
    - specified NEC S89.8- ☑
    - sprain — *see* Sprain, knee
    - superficial — *see* Injury, superficial, knee
  - labium (majus) (minus) S39.94 ☑
  - labyrinth, ear SØ9.3Ø- ☑
  - lacrimal apparatus, duct, gland, or sac — *see* Injury, eye, specified site NEC
  - larynx NEC S19.81 ☑
  - leg (lower) S89.9- ☑
    - blood vessel — *see* Injury, blood vessel, leg
    - contusion — *see* Contusion, leg
    - fracture — *see* Fracture, leg
    - muscle — *see* Injury, muscle, leg
    - nerve — *see* Injury, nerve, leg
    - open — *see* Wound, open, leg
    - specified NEC S89.8- ☑
    - superficial — *see* Injury, superficial, leg
  - lens, eye — *see* Injury, eye, specified site NEC
    - penetrating — *see* Injury, eyeball, penetrating
  - limb NEC T14.8
  - lip SØ9.93 ☑
  - liver S36.119 ☑
    - contusion S36.112 ☑
    - laceration S36.113 ☑
      - major (stellate) S36.116 ☑
      - minor S36.114 ☑
      - moderate S36.115 ☑
    - specified NEC S36.118 ☑
  - lower back S39.92 ☑
    - specified NEC S39.82 ☑
  - lumbar, lumbosacral (region) S39.92 ☑
    - plexus — *see* Injury, lumbosacral plexus
  - lumbosacral plexus S34.4 ☑
  - lung (*see also* Injury, intrathoracic, lung)
    - aspiration J69.Ø
    - transfusion-related (TRALI) J95.84
  - lymphatic thoracic duct — *see* Injury, intrathoracic, specified organ NEC
  - malar region SØ9.93 ☑
  - mastoid region SØ9.9Ø ☑
  - maxilla SØ9.93 ☑
  - mediastinum — *see* Injury, intrathoracic, specified organ NEC
  - membrane, brain — *see* Injury, intracranial
  - meningeal artery — *see* Injury, intracranial, subdural hemorrhage
  - meninges (cerebral) — *see* Injury, intracranial

- **Injury** — *continued*
  - mesenteric
    - artery
      - branch S35.299 ☑
        - laceration (minor) (superficial) S35.291 ☑
          - major S35.292 ☑
        - specified NEC S35.298 ☑
      - inferior S35.239 ☑
        - laceration (minor) (superficial) S35.231 ☑
          - major S35.232 ☑
        - specified NEC S35.238 ☑
      - superior S35.229 ☑
        - laceration (minor) (superficial) S35.221 ☑
          - major S35.222 ☑
        - specified NEC S35.228 ☑
    - plexus (inferior) (superior) — *see* Injury, nerve, lumbosacral, sympathetic
    - vein
      - inferior S35.349 ☑
        - laceration S35.341 ☑
        - specified NEC S35.348 ☑
      - superior S35.339 ☑
        - laceration S35.331 ☑
        - specified NEC S35.338 ☑
  - mesentery — *see* Injury, intra-abdominal, specified site NEC
  - mesosalpinx — *see* Injury, pelvic organ, specified site NEC
  - middle ear S09.30- ☑
  - midthoracic region NOS S29.9 ☑
  - mouth S09.93 ☑
  - multiple NOS T07
  - muscle (and fascia) (and tendon)
    - abdomen S39.001 ☑
      - laceration S39.021 ☑
      - specified type NEC S39.091 ☑
      - strain S39.011 ☑
    - abductor
      - thumb, forearm level — *see* Injury, muscle, thumb, abductor
    - adductor
      - thigh S76.20- ☑
        - laceration S76.22- ☑
        - specified type NEC S76.29- ☑
        - strain S76.21- ☑
    - ankle — *see* Injury, muscle, foot
    - anterior muscle group, at leg level (lower) S86.20- ☑
      - laceration S86.22- ☑
      - specified type NEC S86.29- ☑
      - strain S86.21- ☑
    - arm (upper) — *see* Injury, muscle, shoulder
    - biceps (parts NEC) S46.20- ☑
      - laceration S46.22- ☑
      - long head S46.10- ☑
        - laceration S46.12- ☑
        - specified type NEC S46.19- ☑
        - strain S46.11- ☑
      - specified type NEC S46.29- ☑
      - strain S46.21- ☑
    - extensor
      - finger(s) (other than thumb) — *see* Injury, muscle, finger by site, extensor
      - forearm level, specified NEC — *see* Injury, muscle, forearm, extensor
      - thumb — *see* Injury, muscle, thumb, extensor
      - toe (large) (ankle level) (foot level) — *see* Injury, muscle, toe, extensor
    - finger
      - extensor (forearm level) S56.40- ☑
        - hand level S66.309 ☑
          - laceration S66.329 ☑
          - specified type NEC S66.399 ☑
          - strain S66.319 ☑
        - laceration S56.429 ☑
        - specified type NEC S56.499 ☑
        - strain S56.419 ☑
      - flexor (forearm level) S56.10- ☑
        - hand level S66.109 ☑
          - laceration S66.129 ☑
          - specified type NEC S66.199 ☑
          - strain S66.119 ☑
        - laceration S56.129 ☑
        - specified type NEC S56.199 ☑
        - strain S56.119 ☑
      - index

- **Injury** — *continued*
  - muscle — *continued*
    - finger — *continued*
      - index — *continued*
        - extensor (forearm level)
          - hand level S66.308 ☑
            - laceration S66.32- ☑
            - specified type NEC S66.39- ☑
            - strain S66.31- ☑
          - specified type NEC S56.492- ☑
        - flexor (forearm level)
          - hand level S66.108 ☑
            - laceration S66.12- ☑
            - specified type NEC S66.19- ☑
            - strain S66.11- ☑
          - specified type NEC S56.19- ☑
          - strain S56.11- ☑
        - intrinsic S66.50- ☑
          - laceration S66.52- ☑
          - specified type NEC S66.59- ☑
          - strain S66.51- ☑
      - intrinsic S66.509 ☑
        - laceration S66.529 ☑
        - specified type NEC S66.599 ☑
        - strain S66.519 ☑
      - little
        - extensor (forearm level)
          - hand level S66.30- ☑
            - laceration S66.32- ☑
            - specified type NEC S66.39- ☑
            - strain S66.31- ☑
          - laceration S56.42- ☑
          - specified type NEC S56.49- ☑
          - strain S56.41- ☑
        - flexor (forearm level)
          - hand level S66.10- ☑
            - laceration S66.12- ☑
            - specified type NEC S66.19- ☑
            - strain S66.11- ☑
          - laceration S56.12- ☑
          - specified type NEC S56.19- ☑
          - strain S56.11- ☑
        - intrinsic S66.50- ☑
          - laceration S66.52- ☑
          - specified type NEC S66.59- ☑
          - strain S66.51- ☑
      - middle
        - extensor (forearm level)
          - hand level S66.30- ☑
            - laceration S66.32- ☑
            - specified type NEC S66.39- ☑
            - strain S66.31- ☑
          - laceration S56.42- ☑
          - specified type NEC S56.49- ☑
          - strain S56.41- ☑
        - flexor (forearm level)
          - hand level S66.10- ☑
            - laceration S66.12- ☑
            - specified type NEC S66.19- ☑
            - strain S66.11- ☑
          - laceration S56.12- ☑
          - specified type NEC S56.19- ☑
          - strain S56.11- ☑
        - intrinsic S66.50- ☑
          - laceration S66.52- ☑
          - specified type NEC S66.59- ☑
          - strain S66.51- ☑
      - ring
        - extensor (forearm level)
          - hand level S66.30- ☑
            - laceration S66.32- ☑
            - specified type NEC S66.39- ☑
            - strain S66.31- ☑
          - laceration S56.42- ☑
          - specified type NEC S56.49- ☑
          - strain S56.41- ☑
        - flexor (forearm level)
          - hand level S66.10- ☑
            - laceration S66.12- ☑
            - specified type NEC S66.19- ☑
            - strain S66.11- ☑
          - laceration S56.12- ☑
          - specified type NEC S56.19- ☑
          - strain S56.11- ☑
        - intrinsic S66.50- ☑
          - laceration S66.52- ☑

- **Injury** — *continued*
  - muscle — *continued*
    - finger — *continued*
      - ring — *continued*
        - intrinsic — *continued*
          - specified type NEC S66.59- ☑
          - strain S66.51- ☑
    - flexor
      - finger(s) (other than thumb) — *see* Injury, muscle, finger
      - forearm level, specified NEC — *see* Injury, muscle, forearm, flexor
      - thumb — *see* Injury, muscle, thumb, flexor
      - toe (long) (ankle level) (foot level) — *see* Injury, muscle, toe, flexor
    - foot S96.90- ☑
      - intrinsic S96.20- ☑
        - laceration S96.22- ☑
        - specified type NEC S96.29- ☑
        - strain S96.21- ☑
      - laceration S96.92- ☑
      - long extensor, toe — *see* Injury, muscle, toe, extensor
      - long flexor, toe — *see* Injury, muscle, toe, flexor
      - specified
        - site NEC S96.80- ☑
          - laceration S96.82- ☑
          - specified type NEC S96.89- ☑
          - strain S96.81- ☑
        - type S96.99- ☑
      - strain S96.91- ☑
    - forearm (level) S56.90- ☑
      - extensor S56.50- ☑
        - laceration S56.52- ☑
        - specified type NEC S56.59- ☑
        - strain S56.51- ☑
      - flexor S56.20- ☑
        - laceration S56.22- ☑
        - specified type NEC S56.29- ☑
        - strain S56.21- ☑
      - laceration S56.92- ☑
      - specified S56.99- ☑
        - site NEC S56.80- ☑
          - laceration S56.82- ☑
          - strain S56.81- ☑
          - type NEC S56.89- ☑
      - strain S56.91- ☑
    - hand (level) S66.90- ☑
      - laceration S66.92- ☑
      - specified
        - site NEC S66.80- ☑
          - laceration S66.82- ☑
          - specified type NEC S66.89- ☑
          - strain S66.81- ☑
        - type NEC S66.99- ☑
      - strain S66.91- ☑
    - head S09.10 ☑
      - laceration S09.12 ☑
      - specified type NEC S09.19 ☑
      - strain S09.11 ☑
    - hip NEC S76.00- ☑
      - laceration S76.02- ☑
      - specified type NEC S76.09- ☑
      - strain S76.01- ☑
    - intrinsic
      - ankle and foot level — *see* Injury, muscle, foot, intrinsic
      - finger (other than thumb) — *see* Injury, muscle, finger by site, intrinsic
      - foot (level) — *see* Injury, muscle, foot, intrinsic
      - thumb — *see* Injury, muscle, thumb, intrinsic
    - leg (level) (lower) S86.90- ☑
      - Achilles tendon — *see* Injury, Achilles tendon
      - anterior muscle group — *see* Injury, muscle, anterior muscle group
      - laceration S86.92- ☑
      - peroneal muscle group — *see* Injury, muscle, peroneal muscle group
      - posterior muscle group — *see* Injury, muscle, posterior muscle group, leg level
      - specified
        - site NEC S86.80- ☑
          - laceration S86.82- ☑
          - specified type NEC S86.89- ☑
          - strain S86.81- ☑
        - type NEC S86.99- ☑

- **Injury** — *continued*
  - nerve — *continued*
    - hypoglossal — *continued*
      - specified type NEC S04.89- ☑
    - lateral plantar S94.0- ☑
    - leg (lower) S84.9- ☑
      - cutaneous sensory — *see* Injury, nerve, cutaneous sensory, leg
      - peroneal — *see* Injury, nerve, peroneal
      - specified site NEC — *see* subcategory S84.8 ☑
      - tibial — *see* Injury, nerve, tibial
      - upper — *see* Injury, nerve, thigh
    - lower
      - back — *see* Injury, nerve, abdomen, specified site NEC
        - peripheral — *see* Injury, nerve, abdomen, peripheral
      - limb — *see* Injury, nerve, leg
    - lumbar plexus — *see* Injury, nerve, lumbosacral, sympathetic
    - lumbar spinal — *see* Injury, nerve, spinal, lumbar
    - lumbosacral
      - plexus — *see* Injury, nerve, lumbosacral, sympathetic
      - sympathetic S34.5 ☑
    - medial plantar S94.1- ☑
    - median (forearm level) S54.1- ☑
      - hand (level) S64.1- ☑
      - upper arm (level) S44.1- ☑
      - wrist (level) — *see* Injury, nerve, median, hand
    - musculocutaneous S44.4- ☑
    - musculospiral (upper arm level) — *see* Injury, nerve, radial, upper arm
    - neck S14.9 ☑
      - peripheral S14.4 ☑
      - specified site NEC S14.8 ☑
      - sympathetic S14.5 ☑
    - ninth cranial (glossopharyngeal) — *see* Injury, nerve, glossopharyngeal
    - oculomotor S04.1- ☑
      - contusion S04.1- ☑
      - laceration S04.1- ☑
      - specified type NEC S04.1- ☑
    - olfactory S04.81- ☑
      - specified type NEC S04.81- ☑
    - optic S04.01- ☑
      - contusion S04.01- ☑
      - laceration S04.01- ☑
      - specified type NEC S04.01- ☑
    - pelvic girdle — *see* Injury, nerve, hip
    - pelvis — *see* Injury, nerve, abdomen, specified site NEC
      - peripheral — *see* Injury, nerve, abdomen, peripheral
    - peripheral NEC T14.8
      - abdomen — *see* Injury, nerve, abdomen, peripheral
      - lower back — *see* Injury, nerve, abdomen, peripheral
      - neck — *see* Injury, nerve, neck, peripheral
      - pelvis — *see* Injury, nerve, abdomen, peripheral
      - specified NEC T14.8
    - peroneal (lower leg level) S84.1- ☑
      - foot S94.2- ☑
    - plexus
      - brachial — *see* Injury, brachial plexus
      - celiac, coeliac — *see* Injury, nerve, lumbosacral, sympathetic
      - mesenteric, inferior — *see* Injury, nerve, lumbosacral, sympathetic
      - sacral — *see* Injury, lumbosacral plexus
      - spinal
        - brachial — *see* Injury, brachial plexus
        - lumbosacral — *see* Injury, lumbosacral plexus
    - pneumogastric — *see* Injury, nerve, vagus
    - radial (forearm level) S54.2- ☑
      - hand (level) S64.2- ☑
      - upper arm (level) S44.2- ☑
      - wrist (level) — *see* Injury, nerve, radial, hand
    - root — *see* Injury, nerve, spinal, root
    - sacral plexus — *see* Injury, lumbosacral plexus
    - sacral spinal — *see* Injury, nerve, spinal, sacral
    - sciatic (hip level) (thigh level) S74.0- ☑
    - second cranial (optic) — *see* Injury, nerve, optic
    - seventh cranial (facial) — *see* Injury, nerve, facial

- **Injury** — *continued*
  - nerve — *continued*
    - shoulder — *see* Injury, nerve, arm
    - sixth cranial (abducent) — *see* Injury, nerve, abducens
    - spinal
      - plexus — *see* Injury, nerve, plexus, spinal
      - root
        - cervical S14.2 ☑
        - dorsal S24.2 ☑
        - lumbar S34.21 ☑
        - sacral S34.22 ☑
        - thoracic — *see* Injury, nerve, spinal, root, dorsal
    - splanchnic — *see* Injury, nerve, lumbosacral, sympathetic
    - sympathetic NEC — *see* Injury, nerve, lumbosacral, sympathetic
      - cervical — *see* Injury, nerve, cervical sympathetic
    - tenth cranial (pneumogastric or vagus) — *see* Injury, nerve, vagus
    - thigh (level) — *see* Injury, nerve, hip
      - cutaneous sensory — *see* Injury, nerve, cutaneous sensory, hip
      - femoral — *see* Injury, nerve, femoral
      - sciatic — *see* Injury, nerve, sciatic
      - specified NEC — *see* Injury, nerve, hip
    - third cranial (oculomotor) — *see* Injury, nerve, oculomotor
    - thorax S24.9 ☑
      - peripheral S24.3 ☑
      - specified site NEC S24.8 ☑
      - sympathetic S24.4 ☑
    - thumb, digital — *see* Injury, nerve, digital, thumb
    - tibial (lower leg level) (posterior) S84.0- ☑
    - toe — *see* Injury, nerve, ankle
    - trigeminal S04.3- ☑
      - contusion S04.3- ☑
      - laceration S04.3- ☑
      - specified type NEC S04.3- ☑
    - trochlear S04.2- ☑
      - contusion S04.2- ☑
      - laceration S04.2- ☑
      - specified type NEC S04.2- ☑
    - twelfth cranial (hypoglossal) — *see* Injury, nerve, hypoglossal
    - ulnar (forearm level) S54.0- ☑
      - arm (upper) (level) S44.0- ☑
      - hand (level) S64.0- ☑
      - wrist (level) — *see* Injury, nerve, ulnar, hand
    - vagus S04.89- ☑
      - specified type NEC S04.89- ☑
    - wrist (level) — *see* Injury, nerve, hand
  - ninth cranial nerve (glossopharyngeal) — *see* Injury, nerve, glossopharyngeal
  - nose (septum) S09.92 ☑
  - obstetrical O71.9
    - specified NEC O71.89
  - occipital (region) (scalp) S09.90 ☑
    - lobe — *see* Injury, intracranial
  - optic chiasm S04.02 ☑
  - optic radiation S04.03- ☑
  - optic tract and pathways S04.03- ☑
  - orbit, orbital (region) — *see* Injury, eye
    - penetrating (with foreign body) — *see* Injury, eye, orbit, penetrating
    - specified NEC — *see* Injury, eye, specified site NEC
  - ovary, ovarian S37.409 ☑
    - bilateral S37.402 ☑
      - contusion S37.422 ☑
      - laceration S37.432 ☑
      - specified type NEC S37.492 ☑
    - blood vessel — *see* Injury, blood vessel, ovarian
    - contusion S37.429 ☑
      - bilateral S37.422 ☑
      - unilateral S37.421 ☑
    - laceration S37.439 ☑
      - bilateral S37.432 ☑
      - unilateral S37.431 ☑
    - specified type NEC S37.499 ☑
      - bilateral S37.492 ☑
      - unilateral S37.491 ☑
    - unilateral S37.401 ☑
      - contusion S37.421 ☑
      - laceration S37.431 ☑

- **Injury** — *continued*
  - ovary, ovarian — *continued*
    - unilateral — *continued*
      - specified type NEC S37.491 ☑
  - palate (hard) (soft) S09.93 ☑
  - pancreas S36.209 ☑
    - body S36.201 ☑
      - contusion S36.221 ☑
      - laceration S36.231 ☑
        - major S36.261 ☑
        - minor S36.241 ☑
        - moderate S36.251 ☑
      - specified type NEC S36.291 ☑
    - contusion S36.229 ☑
    - head S36.200 ☑
      - contusion S36.220 ☑
      - laceration S36.230 ☑
        - major S36.260 ☑
        - minor S36.240 ☑
        - moderate S36.250 ☑
      - specified type NEC S36.290 ☑
    - laceration S36.239 ☑
      - major S36.269 ☑
      - minor S36.249 ☑
      - moderate S36.259 ☑
    - specified type NEC S36.299 ☑
    - tail S36.202 ☑
      - contusion S36.222 ☑
      - laceration S36.232 ☑
        - major S36.262 ☑
        - minor S36.242 ☑
        - moderate S36.252 ☑
      - specified type NEC S36.292 ☑
  - parietal (region) (scalp) S09.90 ☑
    - lobe — *see* Injury, intracranial
  - patellar ligament (tendon) S76.10- ☑
    - laceration S76.12- ☑
    - specified NEC S76.19- ☑
    - strain S76.11- ☑
  - pelvis, pelvic (floor) S39.93 ☑
    - complicating delivery O70.1
    - joint or ligament, complicating delivery O71.6
    - organ S37.90 ☑
      - with ectopic or molar pregnancy O08.6
      - complication of abortion — *see* Abortion
      - contusion S37.92 ☑
      - following ectopic or molar pregnancy O08.6
      - laceration S37.93 ☑
      - obstetrical trauma NEC O71.5
      - specified
        - site NEC S37.899 ☑
          - contusion S37.892 ☑
          - laceration S37.893 ☑
          - specified type NEC S37.898 ☑
        - type NEC S37.99 ☑
    - specified NEC S39.83 ☑
  - penis S39.94 ☑
  - perineum S39.94 ☑
  - peritoneum S36.81 ☑
    - laceration S36.893 ☑
  - periurethral tissue — *see* Injury, urethra
    - complicating delivery O71.82
  - phalanges
    - foot — *see* Injury, foot
    - hand — *see* Injury, hand
  - pharynx NEC S19.85 ☑
  - pleura — *see* Injury, intrathoracic, pleura
  - plexus
    - brachial — *see* Injury, brachial plexus
    - cardiac — *see* Injury, nerve, thorax, sympathetic
    - celiac, coeliac — *see* Injury, nerve, lumbosacral, sympathetic
    - esophageal — *see* Injury, nerve, thorax, sympathetic
    - hypogastric — *see* Injury, nerve, lumbosacral, sympathetic
    - lumbar, lumbosacral — *see* Injury, lumbosacral plexus
    - mesenteric — *see* Injury, nerve, lumbosacral, sympathetic
    - pulmonary — *see* Injury, nerve, thorax, sympathetic
  - postcardiac surgery (syndrome) I97.0
  - prepuce S39.94 ☑
  - prostate S37.829 ☑
    - contusion S37.822 ☑

Injury — *continued*
- prostate — *continued*
  - laceration S37.823 ☑
  - specified type NEC S37.828 ☑
- pubic region S39.94 ☑
- pudendum S39.94 ☑
- pulmonary plexus — *see* Injury, nerve, thorax, sympathetic
- rectovaginal septum NEC S39.83 ☑
- rectum — *see* Injury, intestine, large, rectum
- retina — *see* Injury, eye, specified site NEC
  - penetrating — *see* Injury, eyeball, penetrating
- retroperitoneal — *see* Injury, intra-abdominal, specified site NEC
- rotator cuff (muscle(s)) (tendon(s)) S46.00- ☑
  - laceration S46.02- ☑
  - specified type NEC S46.09- ☑
  - strain S46.01- ☑
- round ligament — *see* Injury, pelvic organ, specified site NEC
- sacral plexus — *see* Injury, lumbosacral plexus
- salivary duct or gland S09.93 ☑
- scalp S09.90 ☑
  - newborn (birth injury) P12.9
    - due to monitoring (electrode) (sampling incision) P12.4
    - specified NEC P12.89
      - caput succedaneum P12.81
- scapular region — *see* Injury, shoulder
- sclera — *see* Injury, eye, specified site NEC
  - penetrating — *see* Injury, eyeball, penetrating
- scrotum S39.94 ☑
- second cranial nerve (optic) — *see* Injury, nerve, optic
- seminal vesicle — *see* Injury, pelvic organ, specified site NEC
- seventh cranial nerve (facial) — *see* Injury, nerve, facial
- shoulder S49.9- ☑
  - blood vessel — *see* Injury, blood vessel, arm
  - contusion — *see* Contusion, shoulder
  - dislocation — *see* Dislocation, shoulder
  - fracture — *see* Fracture, shoulder
  - muscle — *see* Injury, muscle, shoulder
  - nerve — *see* Injury, nerve, shoulder
  - open — *see* Wound, open, shoulder
  - specified type NEC S49.8- ☑
  - sprain — *see* Sprain, shoulder girdle
  - superficial — *see* Injury, superficial, shoulder
- sinus
  - cavernous — *see* Injury, intracranial
  - nasal S09.92 ☑
- sixth cranial nerve (abducent) — *see* Injury, nerve, abducens
- skeleton, birth injury P13.9
  - specified part NEC P13.8
- skin NEC T14.8
  - surface intact — *see* Injury, superficial
- skull NEC S09.90 ☑
- specified NEC T14.8
- spermatic cord (pelvic region) S37.898 ☑
  - scrotal region S39.848 ☑
- spinal (cord)
  - cervical (neck) S14.109 ☑
    - anterior cord syndrome S14.139 ☑
      - C1 level S14.131 ☑
      - C2 level S14.132 ☑
      - C3 level S14.133 ☑
      - C4 level S14.134 ☑
      - C5 level S14.135 ☑
      - C6 level S14.136 ☑
      - C7 level S14.137 ☑
      - C8 level S14.138 ☑
    - Brown-Séquard syndrome S14.149 ☑
      - C1 level S14.141 ☑
      - C2 level S14.142 ☑
      - C3 level S14.143 ☑
      - C4 level S14.144 ☑
      - C5 level S14.145 ☑
      - C6 level S14.146 ☑
      - C7 level S14.147 ☑
      - C8 level S14.148 ☑
    - C1 level S14.101 ☑
    - C2 level S14.102 ☑
    - C3 level S14.103 ☑
    - C4 level S14.104 ☑
    - C5 level S14.105 ☑
    - C6 level S14.106 ☑

Injury — *continued*
- spinal — *continued*
  - cervical — *continued*
    - C7 level S14.107 ☑
    - C8 level S14.108 ☑
    - central cord syndrome S14.129 ☑
      - C1 level S14.121 ☑
      - C2 level S14.122 ☑
      - C3 level S14.123 ☑
      - C4 level S14.124 ☑
      - C5 level S14.125 ☑
      - C6 level S14.126 ☑
      - C7 level S14.127 ☑
      - C8 level S14.128 ☑
    - complete lesion S14.119 ☑
      - C1 level S14.111 ☑
      - C2 level S14.112 ☑
      - C3 level S14.113 ☑
      - C4 level S14.114 ☑
      - C5 level S14.115 ☑
      - C6 level S14.116 ☑
      - C7 level S14.117 ☑
      - C8 level S14.118 ☑
    - concussion S14.0 ☑
    - edema S14.0 ☑
    - incomplete lesion specified NEC S14.159 ☑
      - C1 level S14.151 ☑
      - C2 level S14.152 ☑
      - C3 level S14.153 ☑
      - C4 level S14.154 ☑
      - C5 level S14.155 ☑
      - C6 level S14.156 ☑
      - C7 level S14.157 ☑
      - C8 level S14.158 ☑
    - posterior cord syndrome S14.159 ☑
      - C1 level S14.151 ☑
      - C2 level S14.152 ☑
      - C3 level S14.153 ☑
      - C4 level S14.154 ☑
      - C5 level S14.155 ☑
      - C6 level S14.156 ☑
      - C7 level S14.157 ☑
      - C8 level S14.158 ☑
  - dorsal — *see* Injury, spinal, thoracic
  - lumbar S34.109 ☑
    - complete lesion S34.119 ☑
      - L1 level S34.111 ☑
      - L2 level S34.112 ☑
      - L3 level S34.113 ☑
      - L4 level S34.114 ☑
      - L5 level S34.115 ☑
    - concussion S34.01 ☑
    - edema S34.01 ☑
    - incomplete lesion S34.129 ☑
      - L1 level S34.121 ☑
      - L2 level S34.122 ☑
      - L3 level S34.123 ☑
      - L4 level S34.124 ☑
      - L5 level S34.125 ☑
    - L1 level S34.101 ☑
    - L2 level S34.102 ☑
    - L3 level S34.103 ☑
    - L4 level S34.104 ☑
    - L5 level S34.105 ☑
  - nerve root NEC
    - cervical — *see* Injury, nerve, spinal, root, cervical
    - dorsal — *see* Injury, nerve, spinal, root, dorsal
    - lumbar S34.21 ☑
    - sacral S34.22 ☑
    - thoracic — *see* Injury, nerve, spinal, root, dorsal
  - plexus
    - brachial — *see* Injury, brachial plexus
    - lumbosacral — *see* Injury, lumbosacral plexus
  - sacral S34.139 ☑
    - complete lesion S34.131 ☑
    - incomplete lesion S34.132 ☑
  - thoracic S24.109 ☑
    - anterior cord syndrome S24.139 ☑
      - T1 level S24.131 ☑
      - T2-T6 level S24.132 ☑
      - T7-T10 level S24.133 ☑
      - T11-T12 level S24.134 ☑
    - Brown-Séquard syndrome S24.149 ☑
      - T1 level S24.141 ☑

Injury — *continued*
- spinal — *continued*
  - thoracic — *continued*
    - Brown-Séquard syndrome — *continued*
      - T2-T6 level S24.142 ☑
      - T7-T10 level S24.143 ☑
      - T11-T12 level S24.144 ☑
    - complete lesion S24.119 ☑
      - T1 level S24.111 ☑
      - T2-T6 level S24.112 ☑
      - T7-T10 level S24.113 ☑
      - T11-T12 level S24.114 ☑
    - concussion S24.0 ☑
    - edema S24.0 ☑
    - incomplete lesion specified NEC S24.159 ☑
      - T1 level S24.151 ☑
      - T2-T6 level S24.152 ☑
      - T7-T10 level S24.153 ☑
      - T11-T12 level S24.154 ☑
    - posterior cord syndrome S24.159 ☑
      - T1 level S24.151 ☑
      - T2-T6 level S24.152 ☑
      - T7-T10 level S24.153 ☑
      - T11-T12 level S24.154 ☑
    - T1 level S24.101 ☑
    - T2-T6 level S24.102 ☑
    - T7-T10 level S24.103 ☑
    - T11-T12 level S24.104 ☑
- splanchnic nerve — *see* Injury, nerve, lumbosacral, sympathetic
- spleen S36.00 ☑
  - contusion S36.029 ☑
    - major S36.021 ☑
    - minor S36.020 ☑
  - laceration S36.039 ☑
    - major (massive) (stellate) S36.032 ☑
    - moderate S36.031 ☑
    - superficial (capsular) (minor) S36.030 ☑
  - specified type NEC S36.09 ☑
- splenic artery — *see* Injury, blood vessel, celiac artery, branch
- stellate ganglion — *see* Injury, nerve, thorax, sympathetic
- sternal region S29.9 ☑
- stomach S36.30 ☑
  - contusion S36.32 ☑
  - laceration S36.33 ☑
  - specified type NEC S36.39 ☑
- subconjunctival — *see* Injury, eye, conjunctiva
- subcutaneous NEC T14.8
- submaxillary region S09.93 ☑
- submental region S09.93 ☑
- subungual
  - fingers — *see* Injury, hand
  - toes — *see* Injury, foot
- superficial NEC T14.8
  - abdomen, abdominal (wall) S30.92 ☑
    - abrasion S30.811 ☑
    - bite S30.871 ☑
      - insect S30.861 ☑
    - contusion S30.1 ☑
    - external constriction S30.841 ☑
    - foreign body S30.851 ☑
  - abrasion — *see* Abrasion, by site
  - adnexa, eye NEC — *see* Injury, eye, specified site NEC
  - alveolar process — *see* Injury, superficial, oral cavity
  - ankle S90.91- ☑
    - abrasion — *see* Abrasion, ankle
    - bite — *see* Bite, ankle
    - blister — *see* Blister, ankle
    - contusion — *see* Contusion, ankle
    - external constriction — *see* Constriction, external, ankle
    - foreign body — *see* Foreign body, superficial, ankle
  - anus S30.98 ☑
  - arm (upper) S40.92- ☑
    - abrasion — *see* Abrasion, arm
    - bite — *see* Bite, superficial, arm
    - blister — *see* Blister, arm (upper)
    - contusion — *see* Contusion, arm
    - external constriction — *see* Constriction, external, arm

- **Injury** — *continued*
  - superficial — *continued*
    - arm — *continued*
      - foreign body — *see* Foreign body, superficial, arm
    - auditory canal (external) (meatus) — *see* Injury, superficial, ear
    - auricle — *see* Injury, superficial, ear
    - axilla — *see* Injury, superficial, arm
    - back (*see also* Injury, superficial, thorax, back)
      - lower S30.91 ☑
        - abrasion S30.810 ☑
        - contusion S30.0 ☑
        - external constriction S30.840 ☑
        - superficial
          - bite NEC S30.870 ☑
            - insect S30.860 ☑
          - foreign body S30.850 ☑
    - bite NEC — *see* Bite, superficial NEC, by site
    - blister — *see* Blister, by site
    - breast S20.10- ☑
      - abrasion — *see* Abrasion, breast
      - bite — *see* Bite, superficial, breast
      - contusion — *see* Contusion, breast
      - external constriction — *see* Constriction, external, breast
      - foreign body — *see* Foreign body, superficial, breast
    - brow — *see* Injury, superficial, head, specified NEC
    - buttock S30.91 ☑
    - calf — *see* Injury, superficial, leg
    - canthus, eye — *see* Injury, superficial, periocular area
    - cheek (external) — *see* Injury, superficial, head, specified NEC
      - internal — *see* Injury, superficial, oral cavity
    - chest wall — *see* Injury, superficial, thorax
    - chin — *see* Injury, superficial, head NEC
    - clitoris S30.95 ☑
    - conjunctiva — *see* Injury, eye, conjunctiva
      - with foreign body (in conjunctival sac) — *see* Foreign body, conjunctival sac
    - contusion — *see* Contusion, by site
    - costal region — *see* Injury, superficial, thorax
    - digit(s)
      - hand — *see* Injury, superficial, finger
    - ear (auricle) (canal) (external) S00.40- ☑
      - abrasion — *see* Abrasion, ear
      - bite — *see* Bite, superficial, ear
      - contusion — *see* Contusion, ear
      - external constriction — *see* Constriction, external, ear
      - foreign body — *see* Foreign body, superficial, ear
    - elbow S50.90- ☑
      - abrasion — *see* Abrasion, elbow
      - bite — *see* Bite, superficial, elbow
      - blister — *see* Blister, elbow
      - contusion — *see* Contusion, elbow
      - external constriction — *see* Constriction, external, elbow
      - foreign body — *see* Foreign body, superficial, elbow
    - epididymis S30.94 ☑
    - epigastric region S30.92 ☑
    - epiglottis — *see* Injury, superficial, throat
    - esophagus
      - cervical — *see* Injury, superficial, throat
    - external constriction — *see* Constriction, external, by site
    - extremity NEC T14.8
    - eyeball NEC — *see* Injury, eye, specified site NEC
    - eyebrow — *see* Injury, superficial, periocular area
    - eyelid S00.20- ☑
      - abrasion — *see* Abrasion, eyelid
      - bite — *see* Bite, superficial, eyelid
      - contusion — *see* Contusion, eyelid
      - external constriction — *see* Constriction, external, eyelid
      - foreign body — *see* Foreign body, superficial, eyelid
    - face NEC — *see* Injury, superficial, head, specified NEC
    - finger(s) S60.949 ☑
      - abrasion — *see* Abrasion, finger
      - bite — *see* Bite, superficial, finger
      - blister — *see* Blister, finger
      - contusion — *see* Contusion, finger
      - external constriction — *see* Constriction, external, finger
      - foreign body — *see* Foreign body, superficial, finger
      - index S60.94- ☑
      - insect bite — *see* Bite, by site, superficial, insect
      - little S60.94- ☑
      - middle S60.94- ☑
      - ring S60.94- ☑
    - flank S30.92 ☑
    - foot S90.92- ☑
      - abrasion — *see* Abrasion, foot
      - bite — *see* Bite, foot
      - blister — *see* Blister, foot
      - contusion — *see* Contusion, foot
      - external constriction — *see* Constriction, external, foot
      - foreign body — *see* Foreign body, superficial, foot
    - forearm S50.91- ☑
      - abrasion — *see* Abrasion, forearm
      - bite — *see* Bite, forearm, superficial
      - blister — *see* Blister, forearm
      - contusion — *see* Contusion, forearm
      - elbow only — *see* Injury, superficial, elbow
      - external constriction — *see* Constriction, external, forearm
      - foreign body — *see* Foreign body, superficial, forearm
    - forehead — *see* Injury, superficial, head NEC
    - foreign body — *see* Foreign body, superficial
    - genital organs, external
      - female S30.97 ☑
      - male S30.96 ☑
    - globe (eye) — *see* Injury, eye, specified site NEC
    - groin S30.92 ☑
    - gum — *see* Injury, superficial, oral cavity
    - hand S60.92- ☑
      - abrasion — *see* Abrasion, hand
      - bite — *see* Bite, superficial, hand
      - contusion — *see* Contusion, hand
      - external constriction — *see* Constriction, external, hand
      - foreign body — *see* Foreign body, superficial, hand
    - head S00.90 ☑
      - ear — *see* Injury, superficial, ear
      - eyelid — *see* Injury, superficial, eyelid
      - nose S00.30 ☑
      - oral cavity S00.502 ☑
      - scalp S00.00 ☑
      - specified site NEC S00.80 ☑
    - heel — *see* Injury, superficial, foot
    - hip S70.91- ☑
      - abrasion — *see* Abrasion, hip
      - bite — *see* Bite, superficial, hip
      - blister — *see* Blister, hip
      - contusion — *see* Contusion, hip
      - external constriction — *see* Constriction, external, hip
      - foreign body — *see* Foreign body, superficial, hip
    - iliac region — *see* Injury, superficial, abdomen
    - inguinal region — *see* Injury, superficial, abdomen
    - insect bite — *see* Bite, by site, superficial, insect
    - interscapular region — *see* Injury, superficial, thorax, back
    - jaw — *see* Injury, superficial, head, specified NEC
    - knee S80.91- ☑
      - abrasion — *see* Abrasion, knee
      - bite — *see* Bite, superficial, knee
      - blister — *see* Blister, knee
      - contusion — *see* Contusion, knee
      - external constriction — *see* Constriction, external, knee
      - foreign body — *see* Foreign body, superficial, knee
    - labium (majus) (minus) S30.95 ☑
    - lacrimal (apparatus) (gland) (sac) — *see* Injury, eye, specified site NEC
    - larynx — *see* Injury, superficial, throat
    - leg (lower) S80.92- ☑
      - abrasion — *see* Abrasion, leg
      - bite — *see* Bite, superficial, leg
      - contusion — *see* Contusion, leg
      - external constriction — *see* Constriction, external, leg
      - foreign body — *see* Foreign body, superficial, leg
      - knee — *see* Injury, superficial, knee
    - limb NEC T14.8
    - lip S00.501 ☑
    - lower back S30.91 ☑
    - lumbar region S30.91 ☑
    - malar region — *see* Injury, superficial, head, specified NEC
    - mammary — *see* Injury, superficial, breast
    - mastoid region — *see* Injury, superficial, head, specified NEC
    - mouth — *see* Injury, superficial, oral cavity
    - muscle NEC T14.8
    - nail NEC T14.8
      - finger — *see* Injury, superficial, finger
      - toe — *see* Injury, superficial, toe
    - nasal (septum) — *see* Injury, superficial, nose
    - neck S10.90 ☑
      - specified site NEC S10.80 ☑
    - nose (septum) S00.30 ☑
    - occipital region — *see* Injury, superficial, scalp
    - oral cavity S00.502 ☑
    - orbital region — *see* Injury, superficial, periocular area
    - palate — *see* Injury, superficial, oral cavity
    - palm — *see* Injury, superficial, hand
    - parietal region — *see* Injury, superficial, scalp
    - pelvis S30.91 ☑
      - girdle — *see* Injury, superficial, hip
    - penis S30.93 ☑
    - perineum
      - female S30.95 ☑
      - male S30.91 ☑
    - periocular area S00.20- ☑
      - abrasion — *see* Abrasion, eyelid
      - bite — *see* Bite, superficial, eyelid
      - contusion — *see* Contusion, eyelid
      - external constriction — *see* Constriction, external, eyelid
      - foreign body — *see* Foreign body, superficial, eyelid
    - phalanges
      - finger — *see* Injury, superficial, finger
      - toe — *see* Injury, superficial, toe
    - pharynx — *see* Injury, superficial, throat
    - pinna — *see* Injury, superficial, ear
    - popliteal space — *see* Injury, superficial, knee
    - prepuce S30.93 ☑
    - pubic region S30.91 ☑
    - pudendum
      - female S30.97 ☑
      - male S30.96 ☑
    - sacral region S30.91 ☑
    - scalp S00.00 ☑
    - scapular region — *see* Injury, superficial, shoulder
    - sclera — *see* Injury, eye, specified site NEC
    - scrotum S30.94 ☑
    - shin — *see* Injury, superficial, leg
    - shoulder S40.91- ☑
      - abrasion — *see* Abrasion, shoulder
      - bite — *see* Bite, superficial, shoulder
      - blister — *see* Blister, shoulder
      - contusion — *see* Contusion, shoulder
      - external constriction — *see* Constriction, external, shoulder
      - foreign body — *see* Foreign body, superficial, shoulder
    - skin NEC T14.8
    - sternal region — *see* Injury, superficial, thorax, front
    - subconjunctival — *see* Injury, eye, specified site NEC
    - subcutaneous NEC T14.8
    - submaxillary region — *see* Injury, superficial, head, specified NEC
    - submental region — *see* Injury, superficial, head, specified NEC

- **Injury** — *continued*
  - superficial — *continued*
    - subungual
      - finger(s) — *see* Injury, superficial, finger
      - toe(s) — *see* Injury, superficial, toe
    - supraclavicular fossa — *see* Injury, superficial, neck
    - supraorbital — *see* Injury, superficial, head, specified NEC
    - temple — *see* Injury, superficial, head, specified NEC
    - temporal region — *see* Injury, superficial, head, specified NEC
    - testis S3Ø.94 ☑
    - thigh S7Ø.92- ☑
      - abrasion — *see* Abrasion, thigh
      - bite — *see* Bite, superficial, thigh
      - blister — *see* Blister, thigh
      - contusion — *see* Contusion, thigh
      - external constriction — *see* Constriction, external, thigh
      - foreign body — *see* Foreign body, superficial, thigh
    - thorax, thoracic (wall) S2Ø.9Ø ☑
      - abrasion — *see* Abrasion, thorax
      - back S2Ø.4Ø- ☑
      - bite — *see* Bite, thorax, superficial
      - blister — *see* Blister, thorax
      - contusion — *see* Contusion, thorax
      - external constriction — *see* Constriction, external, thorax
      - foreign body — *see* Foreign body, superficial, thorax
      - front S2Ø.3Ø- ☑
    - throat S1Ø.1Ø ☑
      - abrasion S1Ø.11 ☑
      - bite S1Ø.17 ☑
        - insect S1Ø.16 ☑
      - blister S1Ø.12 ☑
      - contusion S1Ø.Ø ☑
      - external constriction S1Ø.14 ☑
      - foreign body S1Ø.15 ☑
    - thumb S6Ø.93- ☑
      - abrasion — *see* Abrasion, thumb
      - bite — *see* Bite, superficial, thumb
      - blister — *see* Blister, thumb
      - contusion — *see* Contusion, thumb
      - external constriction — *see* Constriction, external, thumb
      - foreign body — *see* Foreign body, superficial, thumb
      - insect bite — *see* Bite, by site, superficial, insect
      - specified type NEC S6Ø.39 ☑
    - toe(s) S9Ø.93- ☑
      - abrasion — *see* Abrasion, toe
      - bite — *see* Bite, toe
      - blister — *see* Blister, toe
      - contusion — *see* Contusion, toe
      - external constriction — *see* Constriction, external, toe
      - foreign body — *see* Foreign body, superficial, toe
      - great S9Ø.93- ☑
    - tongue — *see* Injury, superficial, oral cavity
    - tooth, teeth — *see* Injury, superficial, oral cavity
    - trachea S1Ø.1Ø ☑
    - tunica vaginalis S3Ø.94 ☑
    - tympanum, tympanic membrane — *see* Injury, superficial, ear
    - uvula — *see* Injury, superficial, oral cavity
    - vagina S3Ø.95 ☑
    - vocal cords — *see* Injury, superficial, throat
    - vulva S3Ø.95 ☑
    - wrist S6Ø.91- ☑
  - supraclavicular region — *see* Injury, neck
  - supraorbital SØ9.93 ☑
  - suprarenal gland (multiple) — *see* Injury, adrenal
  - surgical complication (external or internal site) — *see* Laceration, accidental complicating surgery
  - temple SØ9.9Ø ☑
  - temporal region SØ9.9Ø ☑
  - tendon (*see also* Injury, muscle, by site)
    - abdomen — *see* Injury, muscle, abdomen
    - Achilles — *see* Injury, Achilles tendon
    - lower back — *see* Injury, muscle, lower back
    - pelvic organs — *see* Injury, muscle, pelvis

- **Injury** — *continued*
  - tenth cranial nerve (pneumogastric or vagus) — *see* Injury, nerve, vagus
  - testis S39.94 ☑
  - thigh S79.92- ☑
    - blood vessel — *see* Injury, blood vessel, hip
    - contusion — *see* Contusion, thigh
    - fracture — *see* Fracture, femur
    - muscle — *see* Injury, muscle, thigh
    - nerve — *see* Injury, nerve, thigh
    - open — *see* Wound, open, thigh
    - specified NEC S79.82- ☑
    - superficial — *see* Injury, superficial, thigh
  - third cranial nerve (oculomotor) — *see* Injury, nerve, oculomotor
  - thorax, thoracic S29.9 ☑
    - blood vessel — *see* Injury, blood vessel, thorax
    - cavity — *see* Injury, intrathoracic
    - dislocation — *see* Dislocation, thorax
    - external (wall) S29.9 ☑
      - contusion — *see* Contusion, thorax
      - nerve — *see* Injury, nerve, thorax
      - open — *see* Wound, open, thorax
      - specified NEC S29.8 ☑
      - sprain — *see* Sprain, thorax
      - superficial — *see* Injury, superficial, thorax
    - fracture — *see* Fracture, thorax
    - internal — *see* Injury, intrathoracic
    - intrathoracic organ — *see* Injury, intrathoracic
    - sympathetic ganglion — *see* Injury, nerve, thorax, sympathetic
  - throat (*see also* Injury, neck) S19.9 ☑
  - thumb S69.9- ☑
    - blood vessel — *see* Injury, blood vessel, thumb
    - contusion — *see* Contusion, thumb
    - dislocation — *see* Dislocation, thumb
    - fracture — *see* Fracture, thumb
    - muscle — *see* Injury, muscle, thumb
    - nerve — *see* Injury, nerve, digital, thumb
    - open — *see* Wound, open, thumb
    - specified NEC S69.8- ☑
    - sprain — *see* Sprain, thumb
    - superficial — *see* Injury, superficial, thumb
  - thymus (gland) — *see* Injury, intrathoracic, specified organ NEC
  - thyroid (gland) NEC S19.84 ☑
  - toe S99.92- ☑
    - contusion — *see* Contusion, toe
    - dislocation — *see* Dislocation, toe
    - fracture — *see* Fracture, toe
    - muscle — *see* Injury, muscle, toe
    - open — *see* Wound, open, toe
    - specified type NEC S99.82- ☑
    - sprain — *see* Sprain, toe
    - superficial — *see* Injury, superficial, toe
  - tongue SØ9.93 ☑
  - tonsil SØ9.93 ☑
  - tooth SØ9.93 ☑
  - trachea (cervical) NEC S19.82 ☑
    - thoracic — *see* Injury, intrathoracic, trachea, thoracic
  - transfusion-related acute lung (TRALI) J95.84
  - tunica vaginalis S39.94 ☑
  - twelfth cranial nerve (hypoglossal) — *see* Injury, nerve, hypoglossal
  - ureter S37.1Ø ☑
    - contusion S37.12 ☑
    - laceration S37.13 ☑
    - specified type NEC S37.19 ☑
  - urethra (sphincter) S37.3Ø ☑
    - at delivery O71.5
    - contusion S37.32 ☑
    - laceration S37.33 ☑
    - specified type NEC S37.39 ☑
  - urinary organ S37.9Ø ☑
    - contusion S37.92 ☑
    - laceration S37.93 ☑
    - specified
      - site NEC S37.899 ☑
        - contusion S37.892 ☑
        - laceration S37.893 ☑
        - specified type NEC S37.898 ☑
      - type NEC S37.99 ☑
  - uterus, uterine S37.6Ø ☑
    - with ectopic or molar pregnancy OØ8.6
    - blood vessel — *see* Injury, blood vessel, iliac

- **Injury** — *continued*
  - uterus, uterine — *continued*
    - contusion S37.62 ☑
    - laceration S37.63 ☑
      - cervix at delivery O71.3
    - rupture associated with obstetrics — *see* Rupture, uterus
    - specified type NEC S37.69 ☑
  - uvula SØ9.93 ☑
  - vagina S39.93 ☑
    - abrasion S3Ø.814 ☑
    - bite S31.45 ☑
      - insect S3Ø.864 ☑
      - superficial NEC S3Ø.874 ☑
    - contusion S3Ø.23 ☑
    - crush S38.Ø3 ☑
    - during delivery — *see* Laceration, vagina, during delivery
    - external constriction S3Ø.844 ☑
    - insect bite S3Ø.864 ☑
    - laceration S31.41 ☑
      - with foreign body S31.42 ☑
    - open wound S31.4Ø ☑
    - puncture S31.43 ☑
      - with foreign body S31.44 ☑
    - superficial S3Ø.95 ☑
      - foreign body S3Ø.854 ☑
  - vas deferens — *see* Injury, pelvic organ, specified site NEC
  - vascular NEC T14.8
  - vein — *see* Injury, blood vessel
  - vena cava (superior) S25.2Ø ☑
    - inferior S35.1Ø ☑
      - laceration (minor) (superficial) S35.11 ☑
        - major S35.12 ☑
      - specified type NEC S35.19 ☑
    - laceration (minor) (superficial) S25.21 ☑
      - major S25.22 ☑
    - specified type NEC S25.29 ☑
  - vesical (sphincter) — *see* Injury, bladder
  - visual cortex SØ4.Ø4- ☑
  - vitreous (humor) SØ5.9Ø ☑
    - specified NEC SØ5.8X- ☑
  - vocal cord NEC S19.83 ☑
  - vulva S39.94 ☑
    - abrasion S3Ø.814 ☑
    - bite S31.45 ☑
      - insect S3Ø.864 ☑
      - superficial NEC S3Ø.874 ☑
    - contusion S3Ø.23 ☑
    - crush S38.Ø3 ☑
    - during delivery — *see* Laceration, perineum, female, during delivery
    - external constriction S3Ø.844 ☑
    - insect bite S3Ø.864 ☑
    - laceration S31.41 ☑
      - with foreign body S31.42 ☑
    - open wound S31.4Ø ☑
    - puncture S31.43 ☑
      - with foreign body S31.44 ☑
    - superficial S3Ø.95 ☑
      - foreign body S3Ø.854 ☑
  - whiplash (cervical spine) S13.4 ☑
  - wrist S69.9- ☑
    - blood vessel — *see* Injury, blood vessel, hand
    - contusion — *see* Contusion, wrist
    - dislocation — *see* Dislocation, wrist
    - fracture — *see* Fracture, wrist
    - muscle — *see* Injury, muscle, hand
    - nerve — *see* Injury, nerve, hand
    - open — *see* Wound, open, wrist
    - specified NEC S69.8- ☑
    - sprain — *see* Sprain, wrist
    - superficial — *see* Injury, superficial, wrist
- **Inoculation** (*see also* Vaccination)
  - complication or reaction — *see* Complications, vaccination
- **Insanity, insane** (*see also* Psychosis)
  - adolescent — *see* Schizophrenia
  - confusional F28
    - acute or subacute FØ5
  - delusional F22
  - senile FØ3 ☑
- **Insect**
  - bite — *see* Bite, by site, superficial, insect

Insect — *continued*
- venomous, poisoning NEC (by) — *see* Venom, arthropod

Insensitivity
- adrenocorticotropin hormone (ACTH) E27.49
- androgen E34.5Ø
  - complete E34.51
  - partial E34.52

Insertion
- cord (umbilical) lateral or velamentous O43.12- ☑
- intrauterine contraceptive device (encounter for) — *see* Intrauterine contraceptive device

Insolation (sunstroke) T67.Ø ☑

Insomnia (organic) G47.ØØ
- without objective findings F51.Ø2
- adjustment F51.Ø2
- adjustment disorder F51.Ø2
- behavioral, of childhood Z73.819
  - combined type Z73.812
  - limit setting type Z73.811
  - sleep-onset association type Z73.81Ø
- childhood Z73.819
- chronic F51.Ø4
  - somatized tension F51.Ø4
- conditioned F51.Ø4
- due to
  - alcohol
    - abuse F1Ø.182
    - dependence F1Ø.282
    - use F1Ø.982
  - amphetamines
    - abuse F15.182
    - dependence F15.282
    - use F15.982
  - anxiety disorder F51.Ø5
  - caffeine
    - abuse F15.182
    - dependence F15.282
    - use F15.982
  - cocaine
    - abuse F14.182
    - dependence F14.282
    - use F14.982
  - depression F51.Ø5
  - drug NEC
    - abuse F19.182
    - dependence F19.282
    - use F19.982
  - medical condition G47.Ø1
  - mental disorder NEC F51.Ø5
  - opioid
    - abuse F11.182
    - dependence F11.282
    - use F11.982
  - psychoactive substance NEC
    - abuse F19.182
    - dependence F19.182
    - use F19.982
  - sedative, hypnotic, or anxiolytic
    - abuse F13.182
    - dependence F13.282
    - use F13.982
  - stimulant NEC
    - abuse F15.182
    - dependence F15.282
    - use F15.982
- fatal familial (FFI) A81.83
- idiopathic F51.Ø1
- learned F51.3
- nonorganic origin F51.Ø1
- not due to a substance or known physiological condition F51.Ø1
  - specified NEC F51.Ø9
- paradoxical F51.Ø3
- primary F51.Ø1
- psychiatric F51.Ø5
- psychophysiologic F51.Ø4
- related to psychopathology F51.Ø5
- short-term F51.Ø2
- specified NEC G47.Ø9
- stress-related F51.Ø2
- transient F51.Ø2

Inspiration
- food or foreign body — *see* Foreign body, by site
- mucus — *see* Asphyxia, mucus

Inspissated bile syndrome (newborn) P59.1

Instability
- emotional (excessive) F6Ø.3

Instability — *continued*
- joint (post-traumatic) M25.3Ø
  - ankle M25.37- ☑
  - due to old ligament injury — *see* Disorder, ligament
  - elbow M25.32- ☑
  - flail — *see* Flail, joint
  - foot M25.37- ☑
  - hand M25.34- ☑
  - hip M25.35- ☑
  - knee M25.36- ☑
  - lumbosacral — *see* subcategory M53.2 ☑
  - prosthesis — *see* Complications, joint prosthesis, mechanical, displacement, by site
  - sacroiliac — *see* subcategory M53.2 ☑
  - secondary to
    - old ligament injury — *see* Disorder, ligament
    - removal of joint prosthesis M96.89
  - shoulder (region) M25.31- ☑
  - spine — *see* subcategory M53.2 ☑
  - wrist M25.33- ☑
- knee (chronic) M23.5- ☑
- lumbosacral — *see* subcategory M53.2 ☑
- nervous F48.8
- personality (emotional) F6Ø.3
- spine — *see* Instability, joint, spine
- vasomotor R55

Institutional syndrome (childhood) F94.2

Institutionalization, affecting child Z62.22
- disinhibited attachment F94.2

Insufficiency, insufficient
- accommodation, old age H52.4
- adrenal (gland) E27.4Ø
  - primary E27.1
- adrenocortical E27.4Ø
  - drug-induced E27.3
  - iatrogenic E27.3
  - primary E27.1
- anterior (occlusal) guidance M26.54
- anus K62.89
- aortic (valve) I35.1
  - with
    - mitral (valve) disease IØ8.Ø
      - with tricuspid (valve) disease IØ8.3
    - stenosis I35.2
    - tricuspid (valve) disease IØ8.2
      - with mitral (valve) disease IØ8.3
  - congenital Q23.1
  - rheumatic IØ6.1
    - with
      - mitral (valve) disease IØ8.Ø
        - with tricuspid (valve) disease IØ8.3
      - stenosis IØ6.2
        - with mitral (valve) disease IØ8.Ø
          - with tricuspid (valve) disease IØ8.3
      - tricuspid (valve) disease IØ8.2
        - with mitral (valve) disease IØ8.3
  - specified cause NEC I35.1
  - syphilitic A52.Ø3
- arterial I77.1
  - basilar G45.Ø
  - carotid (hemispheric) G45.1
  - cerebral I67.81
  - coronary (acute or subacute) I24.8
  - mesenteric K55.1
  - peripheral I73.9
  - precerebral (multiple) (bilateral) G45.2
  - vertebral G45.Ø
- arteriovenous I99.8
- biliary K83.8
- cardiac (*see also* Insufficiency, myocardial)
  - due to presence of (cardiac) prosthesis I97.11- ☑
  - postprocedural I97.11- ☑
- cardiorenal, hypertensive I13.2
- cardiovascular — *see* Disease, cardiovascular
- cerebrovascular (acute) I67.81
  - with transient focal neurological signs and symptoms G45.8
- circulatory NEC I99.8
  - newborn P29.89
- convergence H51.11
- coronary (acute or subacute) I24.8
  - chronic or with a stated duration of over 4 weeks I25.89
- corticoadrenal E27.4Ø
  - primary E27.1
- dietary E63.9
- divergence H51.8

Insufficiency, insufficient — *continued*
- food T73.Ø ☑
- gastroesophageal K22.8
- gonadal
  - ovary E28.39
  - testis E29.1
- heart (*see also* Insufficiency, myocardial)
  - newborn P29.Ø
  - valve — *see* Endocarditis
- hepatic — *see* Failure, hepatic
- idiopathic autonomic G9Ø.Ø9
- interocclusal distance of fully erupted teeth (ridge) M26.36
- kidney N28.9
  - acute N28.9
  - chronic N18.9
- lacrimal (secretion) HØ4.12- ☑
  - passages — *see* Stenosis, lacrimal
- liver — *see* Failure, hepatic
- lung — *see* Insufficiency, pulmonary
- mental (congenital) — *see* Disability, intellectual
- mesenteric K55.1
- mitral (valve) I34.Ø
  - with
    - aortic valve disease IØ8.Ø
      - with tricuspid (valve) disease IØ8.3
    - obstruction or stenosis IØ5.2
      - with aortic valve disease IØ8.Ø
    - tricuspid (valve) disease IØ8.1
      - with aortic (valve) disease IØ8.3
  - congenital Q23.3
  - rheumatic IØ5.1
    - with
      - aortic valve disease IØ8.Ø
        - with tricuspid (valve) disease IØ8.3
      - obstruction or stenosis IØ5.2
        - with aortic valve disease IØ8.Ø
          - with tricuspid (valve) disease IØ8.3
      - tricuspid (valve) disease IØ8.1
        - with aortic (valve) disease IØ8.3
    - active or acute IØ1.1
      - with chorea, rheumatic (Sydenham's) IØ2.Ø
  - specified cause, except rheumatic I34.Ø
- muscle (*see also* Disease, muscle)
  - heart — *see* Insufficiency, myocardial
  - ocular NEC H5Ø.9
- myocardial, myocardium (with arteriosclerosis) I5Ø.9
  - with
    - rheumatic fever (conditions in IØØ) IØ9.Ø
      - active, acute or subacute IØ1.2
        - with chorea IØ2.Ø
      - inactive or quiescent (with chorea) IØ9.Ø
  - congenital Q24.8
  - hypertensive — *see* Hypertension, heart
  - newborn P29.Ø
  - rheumatic IØ9.Ø
    - active, acute, or subacute IØ1.2
  - syphilitic A52.Ø6
- nourishment T73.Ø ☑
- pancreatic K86.8
- parathyroid (gland) E2Ø.9
- peripheral vascular (arterial) I73.9
- pituitary E23.Ø
- placental (mother) O36.51- ☑
- platelets D69.6
- prenatal care affecting management of pregnancy OØ9.3- ☑
- progressive pluriglandular E31.Ø
- pulmonary J98.4
  - acute, following surgery (nonthoracic) J95.2
    - thoracic J95.1
  - chronic, following surgery J95.3
  - following
    - shock J98.4
    - trauma J98.4
  - newborn P28.5
  - valve I37.1
    - with stenosis I37.2
    - congenital Q22.2
    - rheumatic IØ9.89
      - with aortic, mitral or tricuspid (valve) disease IØ8.8
- pyloric K31.89
- renal (acute) N28.9
  - chronic N18.9
- respiratory RØ6.89
  - newborn P28.5
- rotation — *see* Malrotation

Insufficiency, insufficient — *continued*
- sleep syndrome F51.12
- social insurance Z59.7
- suprarenal E27.4Ø
  - primary E27.1
- tarso-orbital fascia, congenital Q1Ø.3
- testis E29.1
- thyroid (gland) (acquired) EØ3.9
  - congenital EØ3.1
- tricuspid (valve) (rheumatic) IØ7.1
  - with
    - aortic (valve) disease IØ8.2
      - with mitral (valve) disease IØ8.3
    - mitral (valve) disease IØ8.1
      - with aortic (valve) disease IØ8.3
    - obstruction or stenosis IØ7.2
      - with aortic (valve) disease IØ8.2
        - with mitral (valve) disease IØ8.3
  - congenital Q22.8
  - nonrheumatic I36.1
    - with stenosis I36.2
- urethral sphincter R32
- valve, valvular (heart) — *see* Endocarditis
  - congenital Q24.8
- vascular I99.8
  - intestine K55.9
    - acute K55.Ø
  - mesenteric K55.1
  - peripheral I73.9
  - renal — *see* Hypertension, kidney
- velopharyngeal
  - acquired K13.79
  - congenital Q38.8
- venous (chronic) (peripheral) I87.2
- ventricular — *see* Insufficiency, myocardial
- welfare support Z59.7

Insufflation, fallopian Z31.41

Insular — *see* condition

Insulinoma
- pancreas
  - benign D13.7
  - malignant C25.4
  - uncertain behavior D37.8
- specified site
  - benign — *see* Neoplasm, by site, benign
  - malignant — *see* Neoplasm, by site, malignant
  - uncertain behavior — *see* Neoplasm, by site, uncertain behavior
- unspecified site
  - benign D13.7
  - malignant C25.4
  - uncertain behavior D37.8

Insuloma — *see* Insulinoma

Interference
- balancing side M26.56
- non-working side M26.56

Intermenstrual — *see* condition

Intermittent — *see* condition

Internal — *see* condition

Interrogation
- cardiac defibrillator (automatic) (implantable) Z45.Ø2
- cardiac pacemaker Z45.Ø18
- cardiac (event) (loop) recorder Z45.Ø9
- infusion pump (implanted) (intrathecal) Z45.1
- neurostimulator Z46.2

Interruption
- bundle of His I44.3Ø
- phase-shift, sleep cycle — *see* Disorder, sleep, circadian rhythm
- sleep phase-shift, or 24 hour sleep-wake cycle — *see* Disorder, sleep, circadian rhythm

Interstitial — *see* condition

Intertrigo L3Ø.4
- labialis K13.Ø

Intervertebral disc — *see* condition

Intestine, intestinal — *see* condition

Intolerance
- carbohydrate K9Ø.4
- disaccharide, hereditary E73.Ø
- fat NEC K9Ø.4
  - pancreatic K9Ø.3
- food K9Ø.4
  - dietary counseling and surveillance Z71.3
- fructose E74.1Ø
  - hereditary E74.12
- glucose (-galactose) E74.39
- gluten K9Ø.Ø
- lactose E73.9

Intolerance — *continued*
- lactose — *continued*
  - specified NEC E73.8
- lysine E72.3
- milk NEC K9Ø.4
  - lactose E73.9
- protein K9Ø.4
- starch NEC K9Ø.4
- sucrose (-isomaltose) E74.31

Intoxicated NEC (without dependence) — *see* Alcohol, intoxication

Intoxication
- acid E87.2
- alcoholic (acute) (without dependence) — *see* Alcohol, intoxication
- alimentary canal K52.1
- amphetamine (without dependence) — *see* Abuse, drug, stimulant, with intoxication
  - with dependence — *see* Dependence, drug, stimulant, with intoxication
- anxiolytic (acute) (without dependence) — *see* Abuse, drug, sedative, with intoxication
  - with dependence — *see* Dependence, drug, sedative, with intoxication
- caffeine (acute) (without dependence) — *see* Abuse, drug, stimulant, with intoxication
  - with dependence — *see* Dependence, drug, stimulant, with intoxication
- cannabinoids (acute) (without dependence) — *see* Abuse, drug, cannabis, with intoxication
  - with dependence — *see* Dependence, drug, cannabis, with intoxication
- chemical — *see* Table of Drugs and Chemicals
  - via placenta or breast milk — *see* - Absorption, chemical, through placenta
- cocaine (acute) (without dependence) — *see* Abuse, drug, cocaine, with intoxication
  - with dependence — *see* Dependence, drug, cocaine, with intoxication
- drug
  - acute (without dependence) — *see* Abuse, drug, by type with intoxication
    - with dependence — *see* Dependence, drug, by type with intoxication
  - addictive
    - via placenta or breast milk — *see* Absorption, drug, addictive, through placenta
  - newborn P93.8
    - gray baby syndrome P93.Ø
  - overdose or wrong substance given or taken — *see* Table of Drugs and Chemicals, by drug, poisoning
- enteric K52.1
- foodborne AØ5.9
  - bacterial AØ5.9
  - classical (Clostridium botulinum) AØ5.1
  - due to
    - Bacillus cereus AØ5.4
    - bacterium AØ5.9
      - specified NEC AØ5.8
    - Clostridium
      - botulinum AØ5.1
      - perfringens AØ5.2
      - welchii AØ5.2
    - Salmonella AØ2.9
      - with
        - (gastro)enteritis AØ2.Ø
        - localized infection(s) AØ2.2Ø
          - arthritis AØ2.23
          - meningitis AØ2.21
          - osteomyelitis AØ2.24
          - pneumonia AØ2.22
          - pyelonephritis AØ2.25
          - specified NEC AØ2.29
        - sepsis AØ2.1
        - specified manifestation NEC AØ2.8
    - Staphylococcus AØ5.Ø
    - Vibrio
      - parahaemolyticus AØ5.3
      - vulnificus AØ5.5
  - enterotoxin, staphylococcal AØ5.Ø
  - noxious — *see* Poisoning, food, noxious
- gastrointestinal K52.1
- hallucinogenic (without dependence) — *see* Abuse, drug, hallucinogen, with intoxication
  - with dependence — *see* Dependence, drug, hallucinogen, with intoxication

Intoxication — *continued*
- hypnotic (acute) (without dependence) — *see* Abuse, drug, sedative, with intoxication
  - with dependence — *see* Dependence, drug, sedative, with intoxication
- inhalant (acute) (without dependence) — *see* Abuse, drug, inhalant, with intoxication
  - with dependence — *see* Dependence, drug, inhalant, with intoxication
- meaning
  - inebriation — *see* category F1Ø ☑
  - poisoning — *see* Table of Drugs and Chemicals
- methyl alcohol (acute) (without dependence) — *see* Alcohol, intoxication
- opioid (acute) (without dependence) — *see* Abuse, drug, opioid, with intoxication
  - with dependence — *see* Dependence, drug, opioid, with intoxication
- pathologic NEC (without dependence) — *see* Alcohol, intoxication
- phencyclidine (without dependence) — *see* Abuse, drug, psychoactive NEC, with intoxication
  - with dependence — *see* Dependence, drug, psychoactive NEC, with intoxication
- potassium (K) E87.5
- psychoactive substance NEC (without dependence) — *see* Abuse, drug, psychoactive NEC, with intoxication
  - with dependence — *see* Dependence, drug, psychoactive NEC, with intoxication
- sedative (acute) (without dependence) — *see* Abuse, drug, sedative, with intoxication
  - with dependence — *see* Dependence, drug, sedative, with intoxication
- serum (*see also* Reaction, serum) T8Ø.69 ☑
- uremic — *see* Uremia
- volatile solvents (acute) (without dependence) — *see* Abuse, drug, inhalant, with intoxication
  - with dependence — *see* Dependence, drug, inhalant, with intoxication
- water E87.79

Intracranial — *see* condition

Intrahepatic gallbladder Q44.1

Intraligamentous — *see* condition

Intrathoracic (*see also* condition)
- kidney Q63.2

Intrauterine contraceptive device
- checking Z3Ø.431
- in situ Z97.5
- insertion Z3Ø.43Ø
  - immediately following removal Z3Ø.433
- management Z3Ø.431
- reinsertion Z3Ø.433
- removal Z3Ø.432
- replacement Z3Ø.433
- retention in pregnancy O26.3- ☑

Intraventricular — *see* condition

Intrinsic deformity — *see* Deformity

Intubation, difficult or failed T88.4 ☑

Intumescence, lens (eye) (cataract) — *see* Cataract

Intussusception (bowel) (colon) (enteric) (ileocecal) (ileocolic) (intestine) (rectum) K56.1
- appendix K38.8
- congenital Q43.8
- ureter (with obstruction) N13.5

Invagination (bowel, colon, intestine or rectum) K56.1

Inversion
- albumin-globulin (A-G) ratio E88.Ø9
- bladder N32.89
- cecum — *see* Intussusception
- cervix N88.8
- chromosome in normal individual Q95.1
- circadian rhythm — *see* Disorder, sleep, circadian rhythm
- nipple N64.59
  - congenital Q83.8
  - gestational — *see* Retraction, nipple
  - puerperal, postpartum — *see* Retraction, nipple
- nyctohemeral rhythm — *see* Disorder, sleep, circadian rhythm
- optic papilla Q14.2
- organ or site, congenital NEC — *see* Anomaly, by site
- sleep rhythm — *see* Disorder, sleep, circadian rhythm
- testis (congenital) Q55.29
- uterus (chronic) (postinfectional) (postpartal, old) N85.5
  - postpartum O71.2

Inversion — *continued*
- vagina (posthysterectomy) N99.3
- ventricular Q2Ø.5

Investigation (*see also* Examination) ZØ4.9
- clinical research subject (control) (normal comparison) (participant) ZØØ.6

Involuntary movement, abnormal R25.9

Involution, involutional (*see also* condition)
- breast, cystic — *see* Dysplasia, mammary, specified type NEC
- depression (single episode) F32.8
  - recurrent episode F33.9
- melancholia (recurrent episode) (single episode) F32.8
- ovary, senile — *see* Atrophy, ovary
- thymus failure E32.8

I.Q.
- under 2Ø F73
- 2Ø-34 F72
- 35-49 F71
- 5Ø-69 F7Ø

IRDS (type I) P22.Ø
- type II P22.1

Irideremia Q13.1

Iridis rubeosis — *see* Disorder, iris, vascular

Iridochoroiditis (panuveitis) — *see* Panuveitis

Iridocyclitis H2Ø.9
- acute H2Ø.Ø- ☑
  - hypopyon H2Ø.Ø5- ☑
  - primary H2Ø.Ø1- ☑
  - recurrent H2Ø.Ø2- ☑
  - secondary (noninfectious) H2Ø.Ø4- ☑
    - infectious H2Ø.Ø3- ☑
- chronic H2Ø.1- ☑
- due to allergy — *see* Iridocyclitis, acute, secondary
- endogenous — *see* Iridocyclitis, acute, primary
- Fuchs' — *see* Cyclitis, Fuchs' heterochromic
- gonococcal A54.32
- granulomatous — *see* Iridocyclitis, chronic
- herpes, herpetic (simplex) BØØ.51
  - zoster BØ2.32
- hypopyon — *see* Iridocyclitis, acute, hypopyon
- in (due to)
  - ankylosing spondylitis M45.9
  - gonococcal infection A54.32
  - herpes (simplex) virus BØØ.51
    - zoster BØ2.32
  - infectious disease NOS B99 ☑
  - parasitic disease NOS B89 [H22]
  - sarcoidosis D86.83
  - syphilis A51.43
  - tuberculosis A18.54
  - zoster BØ2.32
- lens-induced H2Ø.2- ☑
- nongranulomatous — *see* Iridocyclitis, acute
- recurrent — *see* Iridocyclitis, acute, recurrent
- rheumatic — *see* Iridocyclitis, chronic
- subacute — *see* Iridocyclitis, acute
- sympathetic — *see* Uveitis, sympathetic
- syphilitic (secondary) A51.43
- tuberculous (chronic) A18.54
- Vogt-Koyanagi H2Ø.82- ☑

Iridocyclochoroiditis (panuveitis) — *see* Panuveitis

Iridodialysis H21.53- ☑

Iridodonesis H21.89

Iridoplegia (complete) (partial) (reflex) H57.Ø9

Iridoschisis H21.25- ☑

Iris (*see also* condition)
- bombé — *see* Membrane, pupillary

Iritis (*see also* Iridocyclitis)
- chronic — *see* Iridocyclitis, chronic
- diabetic — *see* EØ8-E13 with .39
- due to
  - herpes simplex BØØ.51
  - leprosy A3Ø.9 [H22]
- gonococcal A54.32
- gouty M1Ø.9
- granulomatous — *see* Iridocyclitis, chronic
- lens induced — *see* Iridocyclitis, lens-induced
- papulosa (syphilitic) A52.71
- rheumatic — *see* Iridocyclitis, chronic
- syphilitic (secondary) A51.43
  - congenital (early) A5Ø.Ø1
  - late A52.71
- tuberculous A18.54

Iron — *see* condition

Iron-miner's lung J63.4

Irradiated enamel (tooth, teeth) KØ3.89

Irradiation effects, adverse T66 ☑

Irreducible, irreducibility — *see* condition

Irregular, irregularity
- action, heart I49.9
- alveolar process KØ8.8
- bleeding N92.6
- breathing RØ6.89
- contour of cornea (acquired) — *see* Deformity, cornea
  - congenital Q13.4
- contour, reconstructed breast N65.Ø
- dentin (in pulp) KØ4.3
- eye movements H55.89
  - nystagmus — *see* Nystagmus
  - saccadic H55.81
- labor O62.2
- menstruation (cause unknown) N92.6
- periods N92.6
- prostate N42.9
- pupil — *see* Abnormality, pupillary
- reconstructed breast N65.Ø
- respiratory RØ6.89
- septum (nasal) J34.2
- shape, organ or site, congenital NEC — *see* Distortion
- sleep-wake pattern (rhythm) G47.23

Irritable, irritability R45.4
- bladder N32.89
- bowel (syndrome) K58.9
  - with diarrhea K58.Ø
  - psychogenic F45.8
- bronchial — *see* Bronchitis
- cerebral, in newborn P91.3
- colon K58.9
  - with diarrhea K58.Ø
  - psychogenic F45.8
- duodenum K59.8
- heart (psychogenic) F45.8
- hip — *see* Derangement, joint, specified type NEC, hip
- ileum K59.8
- infant R68.12
- jejunum K59.8
- rectum K59.8
- stomach K31.89
  - psychogenic F45.8
- sympathetic G9Ø.8
- urethra N36.8

Irritation
- anus K62.89
- axillary nerve G54.Ø
- bladder N32.89
- brachial plexus G54.Ø
- bronchial — *see* Bronchitis
- cervical plexus G54.2
- cervix — *see* Cervicitis
- choroid, sympathetic — *see* Endophthalmitis
- cranial nerve — *see* Disorder, nerve, cranial
- gastric K31.89
  - psychogenic F45.8
- globe, sympathetic — *see* Uveitis, sympathetic
- labyrinth — *see* subcategory H83.2 ☑
- lumbosacral plexus G54.1
- meninges (traumatic) — *see* Injury, intracranial
  - nontraumatic — *see* Meningismus
- nerve — *see* Disorder, nerve
- nervous R45.Ø
- penis N48.89
- perineum NEC L29.3
- peripheral autonomic nervous system G9Ø.8
- peritoneum — *see* Peritonitis
- pharynx J39.2
- plantar nerve — *see* Lesion, nerve, plantar
- spinal (cord) (traumatic) (*see also* Injury, spinal cord, by region)
  - nerve G58.9
    - root NEC — *see* Radiculopathy
  - nontraumatic — *see* Myelopathy
- stomach K31.89
  - psychogenic F45.8
- sympathetic nerve NEC G9Ø.8
- ulnar nerve — *see* Lesion, nerve, ulnar
- vagina N89.8

Ischemia, ischemic I99.8
- bowel (transient)
  - acute K55.Ø
  - chronic K55.1
  - due to mesenteric artery insufficiency K55.1
- brain — *see* Ischemia, cerebral
- cardiac (see Disease, heart, ischemic)
- cardiomyopathy I25.5

Ischemia, ischemic — *continued*
- cerebral (chronic) (generalized) I67.82
  - arteriosclerotic I67.2
  - intermittent G45.9
  - newborn P91.Ø
  - recurrent focal G45.8
  - transient G45.9
- colon chronic (due to mesenteric artery insufficiency) K55.1
- coronary — *see* Disease, heart, ischemic
- demand (coronary) (*see also* Angina) I24.8
- heart (chronic or with a stated duration of over 4 weeks) I25.9
  - acute or with a stated duration of 4 weeks or less I24.9
  - subacute I24.9
- infarction, muscle — *see* Infarct, muscle
- intestine (large) (small) (transient) K55.9
  - acute K55.Ø
  - chronic K55.1
  - due to mesenteric artery insufficiency K55.1
- kidney N28.Ø
- mesenteric, acute K55.Ø
- muscle, traumatic T79.6 ☑
- myocardium, myocardial (chronic or with a stated duration of over 4 weeks) I25.9
  - acute, without myocardial infarction I24.Ø
  - silent (asymptomatic) I25.6
  - transient of newborn P29.4
- renal N28.Ø
- retina, retinal — *see* Occlusion, artery, retina
- small bowel
  - acute K55.Ø
  - chronic K55.1
  - due to mesenteric artery insufficiency K55.1
- spinal cord G95.11
- subendocardial — *see* Insufficiency, coronary
- supply (coronary) (*see also* Angina) I25.9
  - due to vasospasm I2Ø.1

Ischial spine — *see* condition

Ischialgia — *see* Sciatica

Ischiopagus Q89.4

Ischium, ischial — *see* condition

Ischuria R34

Iselin's disease or osteochondrosis — *see* Osteochondrosis, juvenile, metatarsus

Islands of
- parotid tissue in
  - lymph nodes Q38.6
  - neck structures Q38.6
- submaxillary glands in
  - fascia Q38.6
  - lymph nodes Q38.6
  - neck muscles Q38.6

Islet cell tumor, pancreas D13.7

Isoimmunization NEC (*see also* Incompatibility)
- affecting management of pregnancy (ABO) (with hydrops fetalis) O36.11- ☑
  - anti-A sensitization O36.11- ☑
  - anti-B sensitization O36.19- ☑
  - anti-c sensitization O36.Ø9- ☑
  - anti-C sensitization O36.Ø9- ☑
  - anti-E sensitization O36.Ø9- ☑
  - anti-e sensitization O36.Ø9- ☑
  - Rh NEC O36.Ø9- ☑
    - anti-D antibody O36.Ø1- ☑
  - specified NEC O36.19- ☑
- newborn P55.9
  - with
    - hydrops fetalis P56.Ø
    - kernicterus P57.Ø
  - ABO (blood groups) P55.1
  - Rhesus (Rh) factor P55.Ø
  - specified type NEC P55.8

Isolation, isolated
- dwelling Z59.8
- family Z63.79
- social Z6Ø.4

Isoleucinosis E71.19

Isomerism atrial appendages (with asplenia or polysplenia) Q2Ø.6

Isosporiasis, isosporosis AØ7.3

Isovaleric acidemia E71.11Ø

Issue of
- medical certificate ZØ2.79
  - for disability determination ZØ2.71

- **Issue of** — *continued*
  - repeat prescription (appliance) (glasses) (medicinal substance, medicament, medicine) Z76.Ø
    - contraception — *see* Contraception
- **Itch, itching** (*see also* Pruritus)
  - baker's L23.6
  - barber's B35.Ø
  - bricklayer's L24.5
  - cheese B88.Ø
  - clam digger's B65.3
  - coolie B76.9
  - copra B88.Ø
  - dew B76.9
  - dhobi B35.6
  - filarial — *see* Infestation, filarial
  - grain B88.Ø
  - grocer's B88.Ø
  - ground B76.9
  - harvest B88.Ø
  - jock B35.6
  - Malabar B35.5
    - beard B35.Ø
    - foot B35.3
    - scalp B35.Ø
  - meaning scabies B86
  - Norwegian B86
  - perianal L29.Ø
  - poultrymen's B88.Ø
  - sarcoptic B86
  - scabies B86
  - scrub B88.Ø
  - straw B88.Ø
  - swimmer's B65.3
  - water B76.9
  - winter L29.8
- **Ivemark's syndrome** (asplenia with congenital heart disease) Q89.Ø1
- **Ivory bones** Q78.2
- **Ixodiasis NEC** B88.8

J

- **Jaccoud's syndrome** — *see* Arthropathy, postrheumatic, chronic
- **Jackson's**
  - membrane Q43.3
  - paralysis or syndrome G83.89
  - veil Q43.3
- **Jacquet's dermatitis** (diaper dermatitis) L22
- **Jadassohn-Pellizari's disease or anetoderma** L9Ø.2
- **Jadassohn's**
  - blue nevus — *see* Nevus
  - intraepidermal epithelioma — *see* Neoplasm, skin, benign
- **Jaffe-Lichtenstein** (-Uehlinger) **syndrome** — *see* Dysplasia, fibrous, bone NEC
- **Jakob-Creutzfeldt disease or syndrome** — *see* Creutzfeldt-Jakob disease or syndrome
- **Jaksch-Luzet disease** D64.89
- **Jamaican**
  - neuropathy G92
  - paraplegic tropical ataxic-spastic syndrome G92
- **Janet's disease** F48.8
- **Janiceps** Q89.4
- **Jansky-Bielschowsky amaurotic idiocy** E75.4
- **Japanese**
  - B-type encephalitis A83.Ø
  - river fever A75.3
- **Jaundice** (yellow) R17
  - acholuric (familial) (splenomegalic) (*see also* Spherocytosis)
    - acquired D59.8
  - breast-milk (inhibitor) P59.3
  - catarrhal (acute) B15.9
    - with hepatic coma B15.Ø
  - cholestatic (benign) R17
  - due to or associated with
    - delayed conjugation P59.8
      - associated with (due to) preterm delivery P59.Ø
    - preterm delivery P59.Ø
  - epidemic (catarrhal) B15.9
    - with hepatic coma B15.Ø
    - leptospiral A27.Ø
    - spirochetal A27.Ø
  - familial nonhemolytic (congenital) (Gilbert) E8Ø.4
    - Crigler-Najjar E8Ø.5
  - febrile (acute) B15.9
    - with hepatic coma B15.Ø
- **Jaundice** — *continued*
  - febrile — *continued*
    - leptospiral A27.Ø
    - spirochetal A27.Ø
  - hematogenous D59.9
  - hemolytic (acquired) D59.9
    - congenital — *see* Spherocytosis
  - hemorrhagic (acute) (leptospiral) (spirochetal) A27.Ø
  - infectious (acute) (subacute) B15.9
    - with hepatic coma B15.Ø
    - leptospiral A27.Ø
    - spirochetal A27.Ø
  - leptospiral (hemorrhagic) A27.Ø
  - malignant (without coma) K72.9Ø
    - with coma K72.91
  - neonatal — *see* Jaundice, newborn
  - newborn P59.9
    - due to or associated with
      - ABO
        - antibodies P55.1
        - incompatibility, maternal/fetal P55.1
        - isoimmunization P55.1
      - absence or deficiency of enzyme system for bilirubin conjugation (congenital) P59.8
      - bleeding P58.1
      - breast milk inhibitors to conjugation P59.3
        - associated with preterm delivery P59.Ø
      - bruising P58.Ø
      - Crigler-Najjar syndrome E8Ø.5
      - delayed conjugation P59.8
        - associated with preterm delivery P59.Ø
      - drugs or toxins
        - given to newborn P58.42
        - transmitted from mother P58.41
      - excessive hemolysis P58.9
        - due to
          - bleeding P58.1
          - bruising P58.Ø
          - drugs or toxins
            - given to newborn P58.42
            - transmitted from mother P58.41
          - infection P58.2
          - polycythemia P58.3
          - swallowed maternal blood P58.5
        - specified type NEC P58.8
      - galactosemia E74.21
      - Gilbert syndrome E8Ø.4
      - hemolytic disease P55.9
        - ABO isoimmunization P55.1
        - Rh isoimmunization P55.Ø
        - specified NEC P55.8
      - hepatocellular damage P59.2Ø
        - specified NEC P59.29
      - hereditary hemolytic anemia P58.8
      - hypothyroidism, congenital EØ3.1
      - incompatibility, maternal/fetal NOS P55.9
      - infection P58.2
      - inspissated bile syndrome P59.1
      - isoimmunization NOS P55.9
      - mucoviscidosis E84.9
      - polycythemia P58.3
      - preterm delivery P59.Ø
      - Rh
        - antibodies P55.Ø
        - incompatibility, maternal/fetal P55.Ø
        - isoimmunization P55.Ø
      - specified cause NEC P59.8
      - swallowed maternal blood P58.5
    - spherocytosis (congenital) D58.Ø
  - nonhemolytic congenital familial (Gilbert) E8Ø.4
  - nuclear, newborn (*see also* Kernicterus of newborn) P57.9
  - obstructive (*see also* Obstruction, bile duct) K83.1
  - post-immunization — *see* Hepatitis, viral, type, B
  - post-transfusion — *see* Hepatitis, viral, type, B
  - regurgitation (*see also* Obstruction, bile duct) K83.1
  - serum (homologous) (prophylactic) (therapeutic) — *see* Hepatitis, viral, type, B
  - spirochetal (hemorrhagic) A27.Ø
  - symptomatic R17
    - newborn P59.9
- **Jaw** — *see* condition
- **Jaw-winking phenomenon or syndrome** QØ7.8
- **Jealousy**
  - alcoholic F1Ø.988
  - childhood F93.8
  - sibling F93.8
- **Jejunitis** — *see* Enteritis
- **Jejunostomy status** Z93.4
- **Jejunum, jejunal** — *see* condition
- **Jensen's disease** — *see* Inflammation, chorioretinal, focal, juxtapapillary
- **Jerks, myoclonic** G25.3
- **Jervell-Lange-Nielsen syndrome** I45.81
- **Jeune's disease** Q77.2
- **Jigger disease** B88.1
- **Job's syndrome** (chronic granulomatous disease) D71
- **Joint** (*see also* condition)
  - mice — *see* Loose, body, joint
    - knee M23.4- ☑
- **Jordan's anomaly or syndrome** D72.Ø
- **Joseph-Diamond-Blackfan anemia** (congenital hypoplastic) D61.Ø1
- **Jungle yellow fever** A95.Ø
- **Jüngling's disease** — *see* Sarcoidosis
- **Juvenile** — *see* condition

K

- **Kahler's disease** C9Ø.Ø- ☑
- **Kakke** E51.11
- **Kala-azar** B55.Ø
- **Kallmann's syndrome** E23.Ø
- **Kanner's syndrome** (autism) — *see* Psychosis, childhood
- **Kaposi's**
  - dermatosis (xeroderma pigmentosum) Q82.1
  - lichen ruber L44.Ø
    - acuminatus L44.Ø
  - sarcoma
    - colon C46.4
    - connective tissue C46.1
    - gastrointestinal organ C46.4
    - lung C46.5- ☑
    - lymph node (multiple) C46.3
    - palate (hard) (soft) C46.2
    - rectum C46.4
    - skin (multiple sites) C46.Ø
    - specified site NEC C46.7
    - stomach C46.4
    - unspecified site C46.9
  - varicelliform eruption BØØ.Ø
    - vaccinia T88.1 ☑
- **Kartagener's syndrome or triad** (sinusitis, bronchiectasis, situs inversus) Q89.3
- **Karyotype**
  - with abnormality except iso (Xq) Q96.2
  - 45,X Q96.Ø
  - 46,X
    - iso (Xq) Q96.1
  - 46,XX Q98.3
    - with streak gonads Q5Ø.32
    - hermaphrodite (true) Q99.1
    - male Q98.3
  - 46,XY
    - with streak gonads Q56.1
    - female Q97.3
    - hermaphrodite (true) Q99.1
  - 47,XXX Q97.Ø
  - 47,XXY Q98.Ø
  - 47,XYY Q98.5
- **Kaschin-Beck disease** — *see* Disease, Kaschin-Beck
- **Katayama's disease or fever** B65.2
- **Kawasaki's syndrome** M3Ø.3
- **Kayser-Fleischer ring** (cornea) (pseudosclerosis) H18.Ø4- ☑
- **Kaznelson's syndrome** (congenital hypoplastic anemia) D61.Ø1
- **Kearns-Sayre syndrome** H49.81- ☑
- **Kedani fever** A75.3
- **Kelis** L91.Ø
- **Kelly** (-Patterson) **syndrome** (sideropenic dysphagia) D5Ø.1
- **Keloid, cheloid** L91.Ø
  - acne L73.Ø
  - Addison's L94.Ø
  - cornea — *see* Opacity, cornea
  - Hawkin's L91.Ø
  - scar L91.Ø
- **Keloma** L91.Ø
- **Kenya fever** A77.1
- **Keratectasia** (*see also* Ectasia, cornea)
  - congenital Q13.4
- **Keratinization of alveolar ridge mucosa**
  - excessive K13.23
  - minimal K13.22

- **Korsakow's disease, psychosis or syndrome** — *see* Korsakoff's disease
- **Kostmann's disease or syndrome** (infantile genetic agranulocytosis) — *see* Agranulocytosis
- **Kozhevnikof's epilepsy** G4Ø.1Ø9
  - intractable G4Ø.119
    - with status epilepticus G4Ø.111
    - without status epilepticus G4Ø.119
  - not intractable G4Ø.1Ø9
    - with status epilepticus G4Ø.1Ø1
    - without status epilepticus G4Ø.1Ø9
- **Krabbe's**
  - disease E75.23
  - syndrome, congenital muscle hypoplasia Q79.8
- **Kraepelin-Morel disease** — *see* Schizophrenia
- **Kraft-Weber-Dimitri disease** Q85.8
- **Kraurosis**
  - ani K62.89
  - penis N48.Ø
  - vagina N89.8
  - vulva N9Ø.4
- **Kreotoxism** AØ5.9
- **Krukenberg's**
  - spindle — *see* Pigmentation, cornea, posterior
  - tumor C79.6- ☑
- **Kufs' disease** E75.4
- **Kugelberg-Welander disease** G12.1
- **Kuhnt-Junius degeneration** (*see also* Degeneration, macula) H35.32
- **Kümmell's disease or spondylitis** — *see* Spondylopathy, traumatic
- **Kupffer cell sarcoma** C22.3
- **Kuru** A81.81
- **Kussmaul's**
  - disease M3Ø.Ø
  - respiration E87.2
    - in diabetic acidosis — *see* Diabetes, by type, with ketoacidosis
- **Kwashiorkor** E4Ø
  - marasmic, marasmus type E42
- **Kyasanur Forest disease** A98.2
- **Kyphoscoliosis, kyphoscoliotic** (acquired) (*see also* Scoliosis) M41.9
  - congenital Q67.5
  - heart (disease) I27.1
  - sequelae of rickets E64.3
  - tuberculous A18.Ø1
- **Kyphosis, kyphotic** (acquired) M4Ø.2Ø9
  - cervical region M4Ø.2Ø2
  - cervicothoracic region M4Ø.2Ø3
  - congenital Q76.419
    - cervical region Q76.412
    - cervicothoracic region Q76.413
    - occipito-atlanto-axial region Q76.411
    - thoracic region Q76.414
    - thoracolumbar region Q76.415
  - Morquio-Brailsford type (spinal) (*see also* subcategory M49.8) E76.219
  - postlaminectomy M96.3
  - postradiation therapy M96.2
  - postural (adolescent) M4Ø.ØØ
    - cervicothoracic region M4Ø.Ø3
    - thoracic region M4Ø.Ø4
    - thoracolumbar region M4Ø.Ø5
  - secondary NEC M4Ø.1Ø
    - cervical region M4Ø.12
    - cervicothoracic region M4Ø.13
    - thoracic region M4Ø.14
    - thoracolumbar region M4Ø.15
  - sequelae of rickets E64.3
  - specified type NEC M4Ø.299
    - cervical region M4Ø.292
    - cervicothoracic region M4Ø.293
    - thoracic region M4Ø.294
    - thoracolumbar region M4Ø.295
  - syphilitic, congenital A5Ø.56
  - thoracic region M4Ø.2Ø4
  - thoracolumbar region M4Ø.2Ø5
  - tuberculous A18.Ø1
- **Kyrle disease** L87.Ø

L

- **Labia, labium** — *see* condition
- **Labile**
  - blood pressure RØ9.89
  - vasomotor system I73.9
- **Labioglossal paralysis** G12.29
- **Labium leporinum** — *see* Cleft, lip
- **Labor** — *see* Delivery
- **Labored breathing** — *see* Hyperventilation
- **Labyrinthitis** (circumscribed) (destructive) (diffuse) (inner ear) (latent) (purulent) (suppurative) (*see also* subcategory) H83.Ø ☑
  - syphilitic A52.79
- **Laceration**
  - with abortion — *see* Abortion, by type, complicated by laceration of pelvic organs
  - abdomen, abdominal
    - wall S31.119 ☑
      - with
        - foreign body S31.129 ☑
        - penetration into peritoneal cavity S31.619 ☑
          - with foreign body S31.629 ☑
      - epigastric region S31.112 ☑
        - with
          - foreign body S31.122 ☑
          - penetration into peritoneal cavity S31.612 ☑
            - with foreign body S31.622 ☑
      - left
        - lower quadrant S31.114 ☑
          - with
            - foreign body S31.124 ☑
            - penetration into peritoneal cavity S31.614 ☑
              - with foreign body S31.624 ☑
        - upper quadrant S31.111 ☑
          - with
            - foreign body S31.121 ☑
            - penetration into peritoneal cavity S31.611 ☑
              - with foreign body S31.621 ☑
      - periumbilic region S31.115 ☑
        - with
          - foreign body S31.125 ☑
          - penetration into peritoneal cavity S31.615 ☑
            - with foreign body S31.625 ☑
      - right
        - lower quadrant S31.113 ☑
          - with
            - foreign body S31.123 ☑
            - penetration into peritoneal cavity S31.613 ☑
              - with foreign body S31.623 ☑
        - upper quadrant S31.11Ø ☑
          - with
            - foreign body S31.12Ø ☑
            - penetration into peritoneal cavity S31.61Ø ☑
              - with foreign body S31.62Ø ☑
  - accidental, complicating surgery — *see* Complications, surgical, accidental puncture or laceration
  - Achilles tendon S86.Ø2- ☑
  - adrenal gland S37.813 ☑
  - alveolar (process) — *see* Laceration, oral cavity
  - ankle S91.Ø1- ☑
    - with
      - foreign body S91.Ø2- ☑
  - antecubital space — *see* Laceration, elbow
  - anus (sphincter) S31.831 ☑
    - with
      - ectopic or molar pregnancy OØ8.6
      - foreign body S31.832 ☑
    - complicating delivery — *see* Delivery, complicated, by, laceration, anus (sphincter)
    - following ectopic or molar pregnancy OØ8.6
    - nontraumatic, nonpuerperal — *see* Fissure, anus
  - arm (upper) S41.11- ☑
    - with foreign body S41.12- ☑
    - lower — *see* Laceration, forearm
  - auditory canal (external) (meatus) — *see* Laceration, ear
  - auricle, ear — *see* Laceration, ear
  - axilla — *see* Laceration, arm
  - back (*see also* Laceration, thorax, back)
    - lower S31.Ø1Ø ☑
      - with
        - foreign body S31.Ø2Ø ☑
          - with penetration into retroperitoneal space S31.Ø21 ☑

Laceration — *continued*

  - back (*see also* Laceration, thorax, back) — *continued*
    - lower — *continued*
      - with — *continued*
        - penetration into retroperitoneal space S31.Ø11 ☑
  - bile duct S36.13 ☑
  - bladder S37.23 ☑
    - with ectopic or molar pregnancy OØ8.6
    - following ectopic or molar pregnancy OØ8.6
    - obstetrical trauma O71.5
  - blood vessel — *see* Injury, blood vessel
  - bowel (*see also* Laceration, intestine)
    - with ectopic or molar pregnancy OØ8.6
    - complicating abortion — *see* Abortion, by type, complicated by, specified condition NEC
    - following ectopic or molar pregnancy OØ8.6
    - obstetrical trauma O71.5
  - brain (any part) (cortex) (diffuse) (membrane) (*see also* Injury, intracranial, diffuse)
    - during birth P1Ø.8
      - with hemorrhage P1Ø.1
    - focal — *see* Injury, intracranial, focal brain injury
  - brainstem SØ6.38- ☑
  - breast S21.Ø1- ☑
    - with foreign body S21.Ø2- ☑
  - broad ligament S37.893 ☑
    - with ectopic or molar pregnancy OØ8.6
    - following ectopic or molar pregnancy OØ8.6
    - laceration syndrome N83.8
    - obstetrical trauma O71.6
    - syndrome (laceration) N83.8
  - buttock S31.8Ø1 ☑
    - with foreign body S31.8Ø2 ☑
    - left S31.821 ☑
      - with foreign body S31.822 ☑
    - right S31.811 ☑
      - with foreign body S31.812 ☑
  - calf — *see* Laceration, leg
  - canaliculus lacrimalis — *see* Laceration, eyelid
  - canthus, eye — *see* Laceration, eyelid
  - capsule, joint — *see* Sprain
  - causing eversion of cervix uteri (old) N86
  - central (perineal), complicating delivery O7Ø.9
  - cerebellum, traumatic SØ6.37- ☑
  - cerebral SØ6.33- ☑
    - during birth P1Ø.8
      - with hemorrhage P1Ø.1
    - left side SØ6.32- ☑
    - right side SØ6.31- ☑
  - cervix (uteri)
    - with ectopic or molar pregnancy OØ8.6
    - following ectopic or molar pregnancy OØ8.6
    - nonpuerperal, nontraumatic N88.1
    - obstetrical trauma (current) O71.3
    - old (postpartal) N88.1
    - traumatic S37.63 ☑
  - cheek (external) SØ1.41- ☑
    - with foreign body SØ1.42- ☑
    - internal — *see* Laceration, oral cavity
  - chest wall — *see* Laceration, thorax
  - chin — *see* Laceration, head, specified site NEC
  - chordae tendinae NEC I51.1
    - concurrent with acute myocardial infarction — *see* Infarct, myocardium
    - following acute myocardial infarction (current complication) I23.4
  - clitoris — *see* Laceration, vulva
  - colon — *see* Laceration, intestine, large, colon
  - common bile duct S36.13 ☑
  - cortex (cerebral) — *see* Injury, intracranial, diffuse
  - costal region — *see* Laceration, thorax
  - cystic duct S36.13 ☑
  - diaphragm S27.8Ø3 ☑
  - digit(s)
    - foot — *see* Laceration, toe
    - hand — *see* Laceration, finger
  - duodenum S36.43Ø ☑
  - ear (canal) (external) SØ1.31- ☑
    - with foreign body SØ1.32- ☑
    - drum SØ9.2- ☑
  - elbow S51.Ø1- ☑
    - with
      - foreign body S51.Ø2- ☑
  - epididymis — *see* Laceration, testis

Laceration — *continued*
- epigastric region — *see* Laceration, abdomen, wall, epigastric region
- esophagus K22.8
  - traumatic
    - cervical S11.21 ☑
      - with foreign body S11.22 ☑
    - thoracic S27.813 ☑
- eye (ball) S05.3- ☑
  - with prolapse or loss of intraocular tissue S05.2- ☑
  - penetrating S05.6- ☑
- eyebrow — *see* Laceration, eyelid
- eyelid S01.11- ☑
  - with foreign body S01.12- ☑
- face NEC — *see* Laceration, head, specified site NEC
- fallopian tube S37.539 ☑
  - bilateral S37.532 ☑
  - unilateral S37.531 ☑
- finger(s) S61.219 ☑
  - with
    - damage to nail S61.319 ☑
      - with
        - foreign body S61.329 ☑
    - foreign body S61.229 ☑
  - index S61.218 ☑
    - with
      - damage to nail S61.318 ☑
        - with
          - foreign body S61.328 ☑
      - foreign body S61.228 ☑
    - left S61.211 ☑
      - with
        - damage to nail S61.311 ☑
          - with
            - foreign body S61.321 ☑
        - foreign body S61.221 ☑
    - right S61.210 ☑
      - with
        - damage to nail S61.310 ☑
          - with
            - foreign body S61.320 ☑
        - foreign body S61.220 ☑
  - little S61.218 ☑
    - with
      - damage to nail S61.318 ☑
        - with
          - foreign body S61.328 ☑
      - foreign body S61.228 ☑
    - left S61.217 ☑
      - with
        - damage to nail S61.317 ☑
          - with
            - foreign body S61.327 ☑
        - foreign body S61.227 ☑
    - right S61.216 ☑
      - with
        - damage to nail S61.316 ☑
          - with
            - foreign body S61.326 ☑
        - foreign body S61.226 ☑
  - middle S61.218 ☑
    - with
      - damage to nail S61.318 ☑
        - with
          - foreign body S61.328 ☑
      - foreign body S61.228 ☑
    - left S61.213 ☑
      - with
        - damage to nail S61.313 ☑
          - with
            - foreign body S61.323 ☑
        - foreign body S61.223 ☑
    - right S61.212 ☑
      - with
        - damage to nail S61.312 ☑
          - with
            - foreign body S61.322 ☑
        - foreign body S61.222 ☑
  - ring S61.218 ☑
    - with
      - damage to nail S61.318 ☑
        - with
          - foreign body S61.328 ☑
      - foreign body S61.228 ☑
    - left S61.215 ☑

Laceration — *continued*
- finger(s) — *continued*
  - ring — *continued*
    - left — *continued*
      - with
        - damage to nail S61.315 ☑
          - with
            - foreign body S61.325 ☑
        - foreign body S61.225 ☑
    - right S61.214 ☑
      - with
        - damage to nail S61.314 ☑
          - with
            - foreign body S61.324 ☑
        - foreign body S61.224 ☑
- flank S31.119 ☑
  - with foreign body S31.129 ☑
- foot (except toe(s) alone) S91.319 ☑
  - with foreign body S91.329 ☑
  - left S91.312 ☑
    - with foreign body S91.322 ☑
  - right S91.311 ☑
    - with foreign body S91.321 ☑
  - toe — *see* Laceration, toe
- forearm S51.819 ☑
  - with
    - foreign body S51.829 ☑
  - elbow only — *see* Laceration, elbow
  - left S51.812 ☑
    - with
      - foreign body S51.822 ☑
  - right S51.811 ☑
    - with
      - foreign body S51.821 ☑
- forehead S01.81 ☑
  - with foreign body S01.82 ☑
- fourchette O70.0
  - with ectopic or molar pregnancy O08.6
  - complicating delivery O70.0
  - following ectopic or molar pregnancy O08.6
- gallbladder S36.123 ☑
- genital organs, external
  - female S31.512 ☑
    - with foreign body S31.522 ☑
    - vagina — *see* Laceration, vagina
    - vulva — *see* Laceration, vulva
  - male S31.511 ☑
    - with foreign body S31.521 ☑
    - penis — *see* Laceration, penis
    - scrotum — *see* Laceration, scrotum
    - testis — *see* Laceration, testis
- groin — *see* Laceration, abdomen, wall
- gum — *see* Laceration, oral cavity
- hand S61.419 ☑
  - with
    - foreign body S61.429 ☑
  - finger — *see* Laceration, finger
  - left S61.412 ☑
    - with
      - foreign body S61.422 ☑
  - right S61.411 ☑
    - with
      - foreign body S61.421 ☑
  - thumb — *see* Laceration, thumb
- head S01.91 ☑
  - with foreign body S01.92 ☑
  - cheek — *see* Laceration, cheek
  - ear — *see* Laceration, ear
  - eyelid — *see* Laceration, eyelid
  - lip — *see* Laceration, lip
  - nose — *see* Laceration, nose
  - oral cavity — *see* Laceration, oral cavity
  - scalp S01.01 ☑
    - with foreign body S01.02 ☑
  - specified site NEC S01.81 ☑
    - with foreign body S01.82 ☑
  - temporomandibular area — *see* Laceration, cheek
- heart — *see* Injury, heart, laceration
- heel — *see* Laceration, foot
- hepatic duct S36.13 ☑
- hip S71.019 ☑
  - with foreign body S71.029 ☑
  - left S71.012 ☑
    - with foreign body S71.022 ☑
  - right S71.011 ☑
    - with foreign body S71.021 ☑

Laceration — *continued*
- hymen — *see* Laceration, vagina
- hypochondrium — *see* Laceration, abdomen, wall
- hypogastric region — *see* Laceration, abdomen, wall
- ileum S36.438 ☑
- inguinal region — *see* Laceration, abdomen, wall
- instep — *see* Laceration, foot
- internal organ — *see* Injury, by site
- interscapular region — *see* Laceration, thorax, back
- intestine
  - large
    - colon S36.539 ☑
      - ascending S36.530 ☑
      - descending S36.532 ☑
      - sigmoid S36.533 ☑
      - specified site NEC S36.538 ☑
    - rectum S36.63 ☑
      - transverse S36.531 ☑
  - small S36.439 ☑
    - duodenum S36.430 ☑
    - specified site NEC S36.438 ☑
- intra-abdominal organ S36.93 ☑
  - intestine — *see* Laceration, intestine
  - liver — *see* Laceration, liver
  - pancreas — *see* Laceration, pancreas
  - peritoneum S36.81 ☑
  - specified site NEC S36.893 ☑
  - spleen — *see* Laceration, spleen
  - stomach — *see* Laceration, stomach
- intracranial NEC (*see also* Injury, intracranial, diffuse)
  - birth injury P10.9
- jaw — *see* Laceration, head, specified site NEC
- jejunum S36.438 ☑
- joint capsule — *see* Sprain, by site
- kidney S37.03- ☑
  - major (greater than 3 cm) (massive) (stellate) S37.06- ☑
  - minor (less than 1 cm) S37.04- ☑
  - moderate (1 to 3 cm) S37.05- ☑
    - multiple S37.06- ☑
- knee S81.01- ☑
  - with foreign body S81.02- ☑
- labium (majus) (minus) — *see* Laceration, vulva
- lacrimal duct — *see* Laceration, eyelid
- large intestine — *see* Laceration, intestine, large
- larynx S11.011 ☑
  - with foreign body S11.012 ☑
- leg (lower) S81.819 ☑
  - with foreign body S81.829 ☑
  - foot — *see* Laceration, foot
  - knee — *see* Laceration, knee
  - left S81.812 ☑
    - with foreign body S81.822 ☑
  - right S81.811 ☑
    - with foreign body S81.821 ☑
  - upper — *see* Laceration, thigh
- ligament — *see* Sprain
- lip S01.511 ☑
  - with foreign body S01.521 ☑
- liver S36.113 ☑
  - major (stellate) S36.116 ☑
  - minor S36.114 ☑
  - moderate S36.115 ☑
- loin — *see* Laceration, abdomen, wall
- lower back — *see* Laceration, back, lower
- lumbar region — *see* Laceration, back, lower
- lung S27.339 ☑
  - bilateral S27.332 ☑
  - unilateral S27.331 ☑
- malar region — *see* Laceration, head, specified site NEC
- mammary — *see* Laceration, breast
- mastoid region — *see* Laceration, head, specified site NEC
- meninges — *see* Injury, intracranial, diffuse
- meniscus — *see* Tear, meniscus
- mesentery S36.893 ☑
- mesosalpinx S37.893 ☑
- mouth — *see* Laceration, oral cavity
- muscle — *see* Injury, muscle, by site, laceration
- nail
  - finger — *see* Laceration, finger, with damage to nail
  - toe — *see* Laceration, toe, with damage to nail
- nasal (septum) (sinus) — *see* Laceration, nose

- **Laceration** — *continued*
  - nasopharynx — *see* Laceration, head, specified site NEC
  - neck S11.91 ☑
    - with foreign body S11.92 ☑
    - involving
      - cervical esophagus S11.21 ☑
        - with foreign body S11.22 ☑
      - larynx — *see* Laceration, larynx
      - pharynx — *see* Laceration, pharynx
      - thyroid gland — *see* Laceration, thyroid gland
      - trachea — *see* Laceration, trachea
    - specified site NEC S11.81 ☑
      - with foreign body S11.82 ☑
  - nerve — *see* Injury, nerve
  - nose (septum) (sinus) SØ1.21 ☑
    - with foreign body SØ1.22 ☑
  - ocular NOS SØ5.3- ☑
    - adnexa NOS SØ1.11- ☑
  - oral cavity SØ1.512 ☑
    - with foreign body SØ1.522 ☑
  - orbit (eye) — *see* Wound, open, ocular, orbit
  - ovary S37.439 ☑
    - bilateral S37.432 ☑
    - unilateral S37.431 ☑
  - palate — *see* Laceration, oral cavity
  - palm — *see* Laceration, hand
  - pancreas S36.239 ☑
  - pelvic S31.Ø1Ø ☑
    - with
      - foreign body S31.Ø2Ø ☑
        - penetration into retroperitoneal cavity S31.Ø21 ☑
      - penetration into retroperitoneal cavity S31.Ø11 ☑
    - floor (*see also* Laceration, back, lower)
      - with ectopic or molar pregnancy OØ8.6
      - complicating delivery O7Ø.1
      - following ectopic or molar pregnancy OØ8.6
      - old (postpartal) N81.89
    - organ S37.93 ☑
  - penis S31.21 ☑
    - with foreign body S31.22 ☑
  - perineum
    - female S31.41 ☑
      - with
        - ectopic or molar pregnancy OØ8.6
        - foreign body S31.42 ☑
      - during delivery O7Ø.9
        - first degree O7Ø.Ø
        - fourth degree O7Ø.3
        - second degree O7Ø.1
        - third degree O7Ø.2
      - old (postpartal) N81.89
      - postpartal N81.89
      - secondary (postpartal) O9Ø.1
    - male S31.119 ☑
      - with foreign body S31.129 ☑
  - periocular area (with or without lacrimal passages) — *see* Laceration, eyelid
  - peritoneum S36.893 ☑
  - periumbilic region — *see* Laceration, abdomen, wall, periumbilic
  - periurethral tissue — *see* Laceration, urethra
  - phalanges
    - finger — *see* Laceration, finger
    - toe — *see* Laceration, toe
  - pharynx S11.21 ☑
    - with foreign body S11.22 ☑
  - pinna — *see* Laceration, ear
  - popliteal space — *see* Laceration, knee
  - prepuce — *see* Laceration, penis
  - prostate S37.823 ☑
  - pubic region S31.119 ☑
    - with foreign body S31.129 ☑
  - pudendum — *see* Laceration, genital organs, external
  - rectovaginal septum — *see* Laceration, vagina
  - rectum S36.63 ☑
  - retroperitoneum S36.893 ☑
  - round ligament S37.893 ☑
  - sacral region — *see* Laceration, back, lower
  - sacroiliac region — *see* Laceration, back, lower
  - salivary gland — *see* Laceration, oral cavity
  - scalp SØ1.Ø1 ☑
    - with foreign body SØ1.Ø2 ☑
  - scapular region — *see* Laceration, shoulder

- **Laceration** — *continued*
  - scrotum S31.31 ☑
    - with foreign body S31.32 ☑
  - seminal vesicle S37.893 ☑
  - shin — *see* Laceration, leg
  - shoulder S41.Ø19 ☑
    - with foreign body S41.Ø29 ☑
    - left S41.Ø12 ☑
      - with foreign body S41.Ø22 ☑
    - right S41.Ø11 ☑
      - with foreign body S41.Ø21 ☑
  - small intestine — *see* Laceration, intestine, small
  - spermatic cord — *see* Laceration, testis
  - spinal cord (meninges) (*see also* Injury, spinal cord, by region)
    - due to injury at birth P11.5
    - newborn (birth injury) P11.5
  - spleen S36.Ø39 ☑
    - major (massive) (stellate) S36.Ø32 ☑
    - moderate S36.Ø31 ☑
    - superficial (minor) S36.Ø3Ø ☑
  - sternal region — *see* Laceration, thorax, front
  - stomach S36.33 ☑
  - submaxillary region — *see* Laceration, head, specified site NEC
  - submental region — *see* Laceration, head, specified site NEC
  - subungual
    - finger(s) — *see* Laceration, finger, with damage to nail
    - toe(s) — *see* Laceration, toe, with damage to nail
  - suprarenal gland — *see* Laceration, adrenal gland
  - temple, temporal region — *see* Laceration, head, specified site NEC
  - temporomandibular area — *see* Laceration, cheek
  - tendon — *see* Injury, muscle, by site, laceration
    - Achilles S86.Ø2- ☑
  - tentorium cerebelli — *see* Injury, intracranial, diffuse
  - testis S31.31 ☑
    - with foreign body S31.32 ☑
  - thigh S71.11- ☑
    - with foreign body S71.12- ☑
  - thorax, thoracic (wall) S21.91 ☑
    - with foreign body S21.92 ☑
      - back S21.22- ☑
        - with penetration into thoracic cavity S21.42- ☑
      - front S21.12- ☑
        - with penetration into thoracic cavity S21.32- ☑
    - back S21.21- ☑
      - with
        - foreign body S21.22- ☑
          - with penetration into thoracic cavity S21.42- ☑
        - penetration into thoracic cavity S21.41- ☑
    - breast — *see* Laceration, breast
    - front S21.11- ☑
      - with
        - foreign body S21.12- ☑
          - with penetration into thoracic cavity S21.32- ☑
        - penetration into thoracic cavity S21.31- ☑
  - thumb S61.Ø19 ☑
    - with
      - damage to nail S61.119 ☑
        - with
          - foreign body S61.129 ☑
      - foreign body S61.Ø29 ☑
    - left S61.Ø12 ☑
      - with
        - damage to nail S61.112 ☑
          - with
            - foreign body S61.122 ☑
        - foreign body S61.Ø22 ☑
    - right S61.Ø11 ☑
      - with
        - damage to nail S61.111 ☑
          - with
            - foreign body S61.121 ☑
        - foreign body S61.Ø21 ☑
  - thyroid gland S11.11 ☑
    - with foreign body S11.12 ☑
  - toe(s) S91.119 ☑
    - with
      - damage to nail S91.219 ☑

- **Laceration** — *continued*
  - toe(s) — *continued*
    - with — *continued*
      - damage to nail — *continued*
        - with
          - foreign body S91.229 ☑
      - foreign body S91.129 ☑
    - great S91.113 ☑
      - with
        - damage to nail S91.213 ☑
          - with
            - foreign body S91.223 ☑
        - foreign body S91.123 ☑
      - left S91.112 ☑
        - with
          - damage to nail S91.212 ☑
            - with
              - foreign body S91.222 ☑
          - foreign body S91.122 ☑
      - right S91.111 ☑
        - with
          - damage to nail S91.211 ☑
            - with
              - foreign body S91.221 ☑
          - foreign body S91.121 ☑
    - lesser S91.116 ☑
      - with
        - damage to nail S91.216 ☑
          - with
            - foreign body S91.226 ☑
        - foreign body S91.126 ☑
      - left S91.115 ☑
        - with
          - damage to nail S91.215 ☑
            - with
              - foreign body S91.225 ☑
          - foreign body S91.125 ☑
      - right S91.114 ☑
        - with
          - damage to nail S91.214 ☑
            - with
              - foreign body S91.224 ☑
          - foreign body S91.124 ☑
  - tongue — *see* Laceration, oral cavity
  - trachea S11.Ø21 ☑
    - with foreign body S11.Ø22 ☑
  - tunica vaginalis — *see* Laceration, testis
  - tympanum, tympanic membrane — *see* Laceration, ear, drum
  - umbilical region S31.115 ☑
    - with foreign body S31.125 ☑
  - ureter S37.13 ☑
  - urethra S37.33 ☑
    - with or following ectopic or molar pregnancy OØ8.6
    - obstetrical trauma O71.5
  - urinary organ NEC S37.893 ☑
  - uterus S37.63 ☑
    - with ectopic or molar pregnancy OØ8.6
    - following ectopic or molar pregnancy OØ8.6
    - nonpuerperal, nontraumatic N85.8
    - obstetrical trauma NEC O71.81
    - old (postpartal) N85.8
  - uvula — *see* Laceration, oral cavity
  - vagina S31.41 ☑
    - with
      - ectopic or molar pregnancy OØ8.6
      - foreign body S31.42 ☑
    - during delivery O71.4
      - with perineal laceration — *see* Laceration, perineum, female, during delivery
    - following ectopic or molar pregnancy OØ8.6
    - nonpuerperal, nontraumatic N89.8
    - old (postpartal) N89.8
  - vas deferens S37.893 ☑
  - vesical — *see* Laceration, bladder
  - vocal cords S11.Ø31 ☑
    - with foreign body S11.Ø32 ☑
  - vulva S31.41 ☑
    - with
      - ectopic or molar pregnancy OØ8.6
      - foreign body S31.42 ☑
    - complicating delivery O7Ø.Ø
    - following ectopic or molar pregnancy OØ8.6
    - nonpuerperal, nontraumatic N9Ø.89
    - old (postpartal) N9Ø.89
  - wrist S61.519 ☑

Laceration — *continued*
- wrist — *continued*
  - with
    - foreign body S61.529 ☑
  - left S61.512 ☑
    - with
      - foreign body S61.522 ☑
  - right S61.511 ☑
    - with
      - foreign body S61.521 ☑

Lack of
- achievement in school Z55.3
- adequate
  - food Z59.4
  - intermaxillary vertical dimension of fully erupted teeth M26.36
  - sleep Z72.82Ø
- appetite (see Anorexia) R63.Ø
- awareness R41.9
- care
  - in home Z74.2
  - of infant (at or after birth) T76.Ø2 ☑
    - confirmed T74.Ø2 ☑
- cognitive functions R41.9
- coordination R27.9
  - ataxia R27.Ø
  - specified type NEC R27.8
- development (physiological) R62.5Ø
  - failure to thrive (child over 28 days old) R62.51
    - adult R62.7
    - newborn P92.6
  - short stature R62.52
  - specified type NEC R62.59
- energy R53.83
- financial resources Z59.6
- food T73.Ø ☑
- growth R62.52
- heating Z59.1
- housing (permanent) (temporary) Z59.Ø
  - adequate Z59.1
- learning experiences in childhood Z62.898
- leisure time (affecting life-style) Z73.2
- material resources Z59.9
- memory (*see also* Amnesia)
  - mild, following organic brain damage FØ6.8
- ovulation N97.Ø
- parental supervision or control of child Z62.Ø
- person able to render necessary care Z74.2
- physical exercise Z72.3
- play experience in childhood Z62.898
- posterior occlusal support M26.57
- relaxation (affecting life-style) Z73.2
- sexual
  - desire F52.Ø
  - enjoyment F52.1
- shelter Z59.Ø
- sleep (adequate) Z72.82Ø
- supervision of child by parent Z62.Ø
- support, posterior occlusal M26.57
- water T73.1 ☑

Lacrimal — *see* condition

Lacrimation, abnormal — *see* Epiphora

Lacrimonasal duct — *see* condition

Lactation, lactating (breast) (puerperal, postpartum)
- associated
  - cracked nipple O92.13
  - retracted nipple O92.Ø3
- defective O92.4
- disorder NEC O92.79
- excessive O92.6
- failed (complete) O92.3
  - partial O92.4
- mastitis NEC — *see* Mastitis, obstetric
- mother (care and/or examination) Z39.1
- nonpuerperal N64.3

Lacticemia, excessive E87.2

Lacunar skull Q75.8

Laennec's cirrhosis K74.69
- alcoholic K7Ø.3Ø
  - with ascites K7Ø.31

Lafora's disease — *see* Epilepsy, generalized, idiopathic

Lag, lid (nervous) — *see* Retraction, lid

Lagophthalmos (eyelid) (nervous) HØ2.2Ø9
- cicatricial HØ2.219
  - left HØ2.216
    - lower HØ2.215
    - upper HØ2.214
  - right HØ2.213

Lagophthalmos — *continued*
- cicatricial — *continued*
  - right — *continued*
    - lower HØ2.212
    - upper HØ2.211
- keratoconjunctivitis — *see* Keratoconjunctivitis
- left HØ2.2Ø6
  - lower HØ2.2Ø5
  - upper HØ2.2Ø4
- mechanical HØ2.229
  - left HØ2.226
    - lower HØ2.225
    - upper HØ2.224
  - right HØ2.223
    - lower HØ2.222
    - upper HØ2.221
- paralytic HØ2.239
  - left HØ2.236
    - lower HØ2.235
    - upper HØ2.234
  - right HØ2.233
    - lower HØ2.232
    - upper HØ2.231
- right HØ2.2Ø3
  - lower HØ2.2Ø2
  - upper HØ2.2Ø1

Laki-Lorand factor deficiency — *see* Defect, coagulation, specified type NEC

Lalling F8Ø.Ø

Lambert-Eaton syndrome — *see* Syndrome, Lambert-Eaton

Lambliasis, lambliosis AØ7.1

Landau-Kleffner syndrome — *see* Epilepsy, specified NEC

Landouzy-Déjérine dystrophy or facioscapulohumeral atrophy G71.Ø

Landouzy's disease (icterohemorrhagic leptospirosis) A27.Ø

Landry-Guillain-Barré, syndrome or paralysis G61.Ø

Landry's disease or paralysis G61.Ø

Lane's
- band Q43.3
- kink — *see* Obstruction, intestine
- syndrome K9Ø.2

Langdon Down syndrome — *see* Trisomy, 21

Lapsed immunization schedule status Z28.3

Large
- baby (regardless of gestational age) (4ØØØg to 4499g) PØ8.1
- ear, congenital Q17.1
- physiological cup Q14.2
- stature R68.89

Large-for-dates NEC (infant) (4ØØØg to 4499g) PØ8.1
- affecting management of pregnancy O36.6- ☑
- exceptionally (45ØØg or more) PØ8.Ø

Larsen-Johansson disease orosteochondrosis — *see* Osteochondrosis, juvenile, patella

Larsen's syndrome (flattened facies and multiple congenital dislocations) Q74.8

Larva migrans
- cutaneous B76.9
  - Ancylostoma B76.Ø
- visceral B83.Ø

Laryngeal — *see* condition

Laryngismus (stridulus) J38.5
- congenital P28.89
- diphtheritic A36.2

Laryngitis (acute) (edematous) (fibrinous) (infective) (infiltrative) (malignant) (membranous) (phlegmonous) (pneumococcal) (pseudomembranous) (septic) (subglottic) (suppurative) (ulcerative) JØ4.Ø
- with
  - influenza, flu, or grippe — *see* Influenza, with, laryngitis
  - tracheitis (acute) — *see* Laryngotracheitis
- atrophic J37.Ø
- catarrhal J37.Ø
- chronic J37.Ø
  - with tracheitis (chronic) J37.1
- diphtheritic A36.2
- due to external agent — *see* Inflammation, respiratory, upper, due to
- H. influenzae JØ4.Ø
- Hemophilus influenzae JØ4.Ø
- hypertrophic J37.Ø
- influenzal — *see* Influenza, with, respiratory manifestations NEC
- obstructive JØ5.Ø

Laryngitis — *continued*
- sicca J37.Ø
- spasmodic JØ5.Ø
  - acute JØ4.Ø
- streptococcal JØ4.Ø
- stridulous JØ5.Ø
- syphilitic (late) A52.73
  - congenital A5Ø.59 [J99]
    - early A5Ø.Ø3 [J99]
- tuberculous A15.5
- Vincent's A69.1

Laryngocele (congenital) (ventricular) Q31.3

Laryngofissure J38.7
- congenital Q31.8

Laryngomalacia (congenital) Q31.5

Laryngopharyngitis (acute) JØ6.Ø
- chronic J37.Ø
- due to external agent — *see* Inflammation, respiratory, upper, due to

Laryngoplegia J38.ØØ
- bilateral J38.Ø2
- unilateral J38.Ø1

Laryngoptosis J38.7

Laryngospasm J38.5

Laryngostenosis J38.6

Laryngotracheitis (acute) (Infectional) (infective) (viral) JØ4.2
- atrophic J37.1
- catarrhal J37.1
- chronic J37.1
- diphtheritic A36.2
- due to external agent — *see* Inflammation, respiratory, upper, due to
- Hemophilus influenzae JØ4.2
- hypertrophic J37.1
- influenzal — *see* Influenza, with, respiratory manifestations NEC
- pachydermic J38.7
- sicca J37.1
- spasmodic J38.5
  - acute JØ5.Ø
- streptococcal JØ4.2
- stridulous J38.5
- syphilitic (late) A52.73
  - congenital A5Ø.59 [J99]
    - early A5Ø.Ø3 [J99]
- tuberculous A15.5
- Vincent's A69.1

Laryngotracheobronchitis — *see* Bronchitis

Larynx, laryngeal — *see* condition

Lassa fever A96.2

Lassitude — *see* Weakness

Late
- talker R62.Ø
- walker R62.Ø

Late effect(s) — *see* Sequelae

Latent — *see* condition

Laterocession — *see* Lateroversion

Lateroflexion — *see* Lateroversion

Lateroversion
- cervix — *see* Lateroversion, uterus
- uterus, uterine (cervix) (postinfectional) (postpartal, old) N85.4
  - congenital Q51.818
  - in pregnancy or childbirth O34.59- ☑

Lathyrism — *see* Poisoning, food, noxious, plant

Launois' syndrome (pituitary gigantism) E22.Ø

Launois-Bensaude adenolipomatosis E88.89

Laurence-Moon (-Bardet)-**Biedl syndrome** Q87.89

Lax, laxity (*see also* Relaxation)
- ligament (ous) (*see also* Disorder, ligament)
  - familial M35.7
  - knee — *see* Derangement, knee
- skin (acquired) L57.4
  - congenital Q82.8

Laxative habit F55.2

Lazy leukocyte syndrome D7Ø.8

Lead miner's lung J63.6

Leak, leakage
- air NEC J93.82
  - postprocedural J95.812
- amniotic fluid — *see* Rupture, membranes, premature
- blood (microscopic), fetal, into maternal circulation
  - affecting management of pregnancy — *see* Pregnancy, complicated by
- cerebrospinal fluid G96.Ø
  - from spinal (lumbar) puncture G97.Ø

Leak, leakage — *continued*
- device, implant or graft (*see also* Complications, by site and type, mechanical)
  - arterial graft NEC — *see* Complication, cardiovascular device, mechanical, vascular
  - breast (implant) T85.43 ☑
  - catheter NEC T85.638 ☑
    - dialysis (renal) T82.43 ☑
      - intraperitoneal T85.631 ☑
    - infusion NEC T82.534 ☑
      - spinal (epidural) (subdural) T85.63Ø ☑
    - urinary, indwelling T83.Ø38 ☑
      - cystostomy T83.Ø3Ø ☑
  - gastrointestinal — *see* Complications, prosthetic device, mechanical, gastrointestinal device
  - genital NEC T83.498 ☑
    - penile prosthesis T83.49Ø ☑
  - heart NEC — *see* Complication, cardiovascular device, mechanical
  - joint prosthesis — *see* Complications, joint prosthesis, mechanical, specified NEC, by site
  - ocular NEC — *see* Complications, prosthetic device, mechanical, ocular device
  - orthopedic NEC — *see* Complication, orthopedic, device, mechanical
  - persistent air J93.82
  - specified NEC T85.638 ☑
  - urinary NEC (*see also* Complication, genitourinary, device, urinary, mechanical)
    - graft T83.23 ☑
  - vascular NEC — *see* Complication, cardiovascular device, mechanical
  - ventricular intracranial shunt T85.Ø3 ☑
- urine — *see* Incontinence

Leaky heart — *see* Endocarditis
Learning defect (specific) F81.9
Leather bottle stomach C16.9
Leber's
- congenital amaurosis H35.5Ø
- optic atrophy (hereditary) H47.22

Lederer's anemia D59.1
Leeches (external) — *see* Hirudiniasis
Leg — *see* condition
Legg (-Calvé)-**Perthes disease, syndrome or osteochondrosis** M91.1- ☑
Legionellosis A48.1
- nonpneumonic A48.2

Legionnaires'
- disease A48.1
  - nonpneumonic A48.2
- pneumonia A48.1

Leigh's disease G31.82
Leiner's disease L21.1
Leiofibromyoma — *see* Leiomyoma
Leiomyoblastoma — *see* Neoplasm, connective tissue, benign
Leiomyofibroma (*see also* Neoplasm, connective tissue, benign)
- uterus (cervix) (corpus) D25.9

Leiomyoma (*see also* Neoplasm, connective tissue, benign)
- bizarre — *see* Neoplasm, connective tissue, benign
- cellular — *see* Neoplasm, connective tissue, benign
- epithelioid — *see* Neoplasm, connective tissue, benign
- uterus (cervix) (corpus) D25.9
  - intramural D25.1
  - submucous D25.Ø
  - subserosal D25.2
- vascular — *see* Neoplasm, connective tissue, benign

Leiomyoma, leiomyomatosis (intravascular) — *see* Neoplasm, connective tissue, uncertain behavior
Leiomyosarcoma (*see also* Neoplasm, connective tissue, malignant)
- epithelioid — *see* Neoplasm, connective tissue, malignant
- myxoid — *see* Neoplasm, connective tissue, malignant

Leishmaniasis B55.9
- American (mucocutaneous) B55.2
  - cutaneous B55.1
- Asian Desert B55.1
- Brazilian B55.2
- cutaneous (any type) B55.1
- dermal (*see also* Leishmaniasis, cutaneous)
  - post-kala-azar B55.Ø
- eyelid B55.1
- infantile B55.Ø
- Mediterranean B55.Ø

Leishmaniasis — *continued*
- mucocutaneous (American) (New World) B55.2
- naso-oral B55.2
- nasopharyngeal B55.2
- old world B55.1
- tegumentaria diffusa B55.1
- visceral B55.Ø

Leishmanoid, dermal (*see also* Leishmaniasis, cutaneous)
- post-kala-azar B55.Ø

Lenegre's disease I44.2
Lengthening, leg — *see* Deformity, limb, unequal length
Lennert's lymphoma — *see* Lymphoma, Lennert's
Lennox-Gastaut syndrome G4Ø.812
- intractable G4Ø.814
  - with status epilepticus G4Ø.813
  - without status epilepticus G4Ø.814
- not intractable G4Ø.812
  - with status epilepticus G4Ø.811
  - without status epilepticus G4Ø.812

Lens — *see* condition
Lenticonus (anterior) (posterior) (congenital) Q12.8
Lenticular degeneration, progressive E83.Ø1
Lentiglobus (posterior) (congenital) Q12.8
Lentigo (congenital) L81.4
- maligna (*see also* Melanoma, in situ)
  - melanoma — *see* Melanoma

Lentivirus, as cause of disease classified elsewhere B97.31
Leontiasis
- ossium M85.2
- syphilitic (late) A52.78
  - congenital A5Ø.59

Lepothrix A48.8
Lepra — *see* Leprosy
Leprechaunism E34.8
Leprosy A3Ø.- ☑
- with muscle disorder A3Ø.9 [M63.8Ø]
  - ankle A3Ø.9 [M63.87-] ☑
  - foot A3Ø.9 [M63.87-] ☑
  - forearm A3Ø.9 [M63.83-] ☑
  - hand A3Ø.9 [M63.84-] ☑
  - lower leg A3Ø.9 [M63.86-] ☑
  - multiple sites A3Ø.9 [M63.89]
  - pelvic region A3Ø.9 [M63.85-] ☑
  - shoulder region A3Ø.9 [M63.81-] ☑
  - specified site NEC A3Ø.9 [M63.88]
  - thigh A3Ø.9 [M63.85-] ☑
  - upper arm A3Ø.9 [M63.82-] ☑
- anesthetic A3Ø.9
- BB A3Ø.3
- BL A3Ø.4
- borderline (infiltrated) (neuritic) A3Ø.3
  - lepromatous A3Ø.4
  - tuberculoid A3Ø.2
- BT A3Ø.2
- dimorphous (infiltrated) (neuritic) A3Ø.3
- I A3Ø.Ø
- indeterminate (macular) (neuritic) A3Ø.Ø
- lepromatous (diffuse) (infiltrated) (macular) (neuritic) (nodular) A3Ø.5
- LL A3Ø.5
- macular (early) (neuritic) (simple) A3Ø.9
- maculoanesthetic A3Ø.9
- mixed A3Ø.3
- neural A3Ø.9
- nodular A3Ø.5
- primary neuritic A3Ø.3
- specified type NEC A3Ø.8
- TT A3Ø.1
- tuberculoid (major) (minor) A3Ø.1

Leptocytosis, hereditary D56.9
Leptomeningitis (chronic) (circumscribed) (hemorrhagic) (nonsuppurative) — *see* Meningitis
Leptomeningopathy G96.19
Leptospiral — *see* condition
Leptospirochetal — *see* condition
Leptospirosis A27.9
- canicola A27.89
- due to Leptospira interrogans serovar icterohaemorrhagiae A27.Ø
- icterohemorrhagica A27.Ø
- pomona A27.89
- Weil's disease A27.Ø

Leptus dermatitis B88.Ø
Leriche's syndrome (aortic bifurcation occlusion) I74.Ø9
Leri's pleonosteosis Q78.8
Leri-Weill syndrome Q77.8
Lermoyez' syndrome — *see* Vertigo, peripheral NEC
Lesch-Nyhan syndrome E79.1
Leser-Trélat disease L82.1
- inflamed L82.Ø

Lesion(s) (nontraumatic)
- abducens nerve — *see* Strabismus, paralytic, sixth nerve
- alveolar process KØ8.9
- angiocentric immunoproliferative D47.Z9 (*following* D47.4)
- anorectal K62.9
- aortic (valve) I35.9
- auditory nerve — *see* subcategory H93.3 ☑
- basal ganglion G25.9
- bile duct — *see* Disease, bile duct
- biomechanical M99.9
  - specified type NEC M99.89
    - abdomen M99.89
    - acromioclavicular M99.87
    - cervical region M99.81
    - cervicothoracic M99.81
    - costochondral M99.88
    - costovertebral M99.88
    - head region M99.8Ø
    - hip M99.85
    - lower extremity M99.86
    - lumbar region M99.83
    - lumbosacral M99.83
    - occipitocervical M99.8Ø
    - pelvic region M99.85
    - pubic M99.85
    - rib cage M99.88
    - sacral region M99.84
    - sacrococcygeal M99.84
    - sacroiliac M99.84
    - specified NEC M99.89
    - sternochondral M99.88
    - sternoclavicular M99.87
    - thoracic region M99.82
    - thoracolumbar M99.82
    - upper extremity M99.87
- bladder N32.9
- bone — *see* Disorder, bone
- brachial plexus G54.Ø
- brain G93.9
  - congenital QØ4.9
  - vascular I67.9
    - degenerative I67.9
    - hypertensive I67.4
- buccal cavity K13.79
- calcified — *see* Calcification
- canthus — *see* Disorder, eyelid
- carate — *see* Pinta, lesions
- cardia K22.9
- cardiac (*see also* Disease, heart) I51.9
  - congenital Q24.9
  - valvular — *see* Endocarditis
- cauda equina G83.4
- cecum K63.9
- cerebral — *see* Lesion, brain
- cerebrovascular I67.9
  - degenerative I67.9
  - hypertensive I67.4
- cervical (nerve) root NEC G54.2
- chiasmal — *see* Disorder, optic, chiasm
- chorda tympani G51.8
- coin, lung R91.1
- colon K63.9
- congenital — *see* Anomaly, by site
- conjunctiva H11.9
- conus medullaris — *see* Injury, conus medullaris
- coronary artery — *see* Ischemia, heart
- cranial nerve G52.9
  - eighth — *see* Disorder, ear
  - eleventh G52.9
  - fifth G5Ø.9
  - first G52.Ø
  - fourth — *see* Strabismus, paralytic, fourth nerve
  - seventh G51.9
  - sixth — *see* Strabismus, paralytic, sixth nerve
  - tenth G52.2
  - twelfth G52.3
- cystic — *see* Cyst
- degenerative — *see* Degeneration
- duodenum K31.9
- edentulous (alveolar) ridge, associated with trauma, due to traumatic occlusion KØ6.2

Index
Lesion — Leukopenia

Lesion(s) — *continued*
- en coup de sabre L94.1
- eyelid — *see* Disorder, eyelid
- gasserian ganglion G5Ø.8
- gastric K31.9
- gastroduodenal K31.9
- gastrointestinal K63.9
- gingiva, associated with trauma KØ6.2
- glomerular
  - focal and segmental (*see also* NØØ-NØ7 with fourth character .1) NØ5.1
  - minimal change (*see also* NØØ-NØ7 with fourth character .Ø) NØ5.Ø
- heart (organic) — *see* Disease, heart
- hyperchromic, due to pinta (carate) A67.1
- hyperkeratotic — *see* Hyperkeratosis
- hypothalamic E23.7
- ileocecal K63.9
- ileum K63.9
- iliohypogastric nerve G57.8- ☑
- inflammatory — *see* Inflammation
- intestine K63.9
- intracerebral — *see* Lesion, brain
- intrachiasmal (optic) — *see* Disorder, optic, chiasm
- intracranial, space-occupying R9Ø.Ø
- joint — *see* Disorder, joint
  - sacroiliac (old) M53.3
- keratotic — *see* Keratosis
- kidney — *see* Disease, renal
- laryngeal nerve (recurrent) G52.2
- lip K13.Ø
- liver K76.9
- lumbosacral
  - plexus G54.1
  - root (nerve) NEC G54.4
- lung (coin) R91.1
- maxillary sinus J32.Ø
- mitral IØ5.9
- Morel-Lavallée — *see* Hematoma, by site
- motor cortex NEC G93.89
- mouth K13.79
- nerve G58.9
  - femoral G57.2- ☑
  - median G56.1- ☑
    - carpal tunnel syndrome — *see* Syndrome, carpal tunnel
  - plantar G57.6- ☑
  - popliteal (lateral) G57.3- ☑
    - medial G57.4- ☑
  - radial G56.3- ☑
  - sciatic G57.Ø- ☑
  - spinal — *see* Injury, nerve, spinal
  - ulnar G56.2- ☑
- nervous system, congenital QØ7.9
- nonallopathic — *see* Lesion, biomechanical
- nose (internal) J34.89
- obstructive — *see* Obstruction
- obturator nerve G57.8- ☑
- oral mucosa K13.7Ø
- organ or site NEC — *see* Disease, by site
- osteolytic — *see* Osteolysis
- peptic K27.9
- periodontal, due to traumatic occlusion KØ5.5
- pharynx J39.2
- pigment, pigmented (skin) L81.9
- pinta — *see* Pinta, lesions
- polypoid — *see* Polyp
- prechiasmal (optic) — *see* Disorder, optic, chiasm
- primary (*see also* Syphilis, primary) A51.Ø
  - carate A67.Ø
  - pinta A67.Ø
  - yaws A66.Ø
- pulmonary J98.4
  - valve I37.9
- pylorus K31.9
- rectosigmoid K63.9
- retina, retinal H35.9
- sacroiliac (joint) (old) M53.3
- salivary gland K11.9
  - benign lymphoepithelial K11.8
- saphenous nerve G57.8- ☑
- sciatic nerve G57.Ø- ☑
- secondary — *see* Syphilis, secondary
- shoulder (region) M75.9- ☑
  - specified NEC M75.8- ☑
- sigmoid K63.9
- sinus (accessory) (nasal) J34.89

Lesion(s) — *continued*
- skin L98.9
  - suppurative LØ8.Ø
- SLAP S43.43- ☑
- spinal cord G95.9
  - congenital QØ6.9
- spleen D73.89
- stomach K31.9
- superior glenoid labrum S43.43- ☑
- syphilitic — *see* Syphilis
- tertiary — *see* Syphilis, tertiary
- thoracic root (nerve) NEC G54.3
- tonsillar fossa J35.9
- tooth, teeth KØ8.9
  - white spot
    - chewing surface KØ2.51
    - pit and fissure surface KØ2.51
    - smooth surface KØ2.61
- traumatic — *see* specific type of injury by site
- tricuspid (valve) IØ7.9
  - nonrheumatic I36.9
- trigeminal nerve G5Ø.9
- ulcerated or ulcerative — *see* Ulcer, skin
- uterus N85.9
- vagus nerve G52.2
- valvular — *see* Endocarditis
- vascular I99.9
  - affecting central nervous system I67.9
  - following trauma NEC T14.8
  - umbilical cord, complicating delivery O69.5 ☑
- warty — *see* Verruca
- white spot (tooth)
  - chewing surface KØ2.51
  - pit and fissure surface KØ2.51
  - smooth surface KØ2.61

Lethargic — *see* condition

Lethargy R53.83

Letterer-Siwe's disease C96.Ø

Leukemia, leukemic C95.9- ☑
- acute basophilic C94.8- ☑
- acute bilineal C95.Ø- ☑
- acute erythroid C94.Ø- ☑
- acute lymphoblastic C91.Ø- ☑
- acute megakaryoblastic C94.2- ☑
- acute megakaryocytic C94.2- ☑
- acute mixed lineage C95.Ø- ☑
- acute monoblastic (monoblastic/monocytic) C93.Ø- ☑
- acute monocytic (monoblastic/monocytic) C93.Ø- ☑
- acute myeloblastic (minimal differentiation) (with maturation) C92.Ø- ☑
- acute myeloid
  - with
    - 11q23-abnormality C92.6- ☑
    - dysplasia of remaining hematopoesis and/or myelodysplastic disease in its history C92.A- ☑ (*following* C92.6)
    - multilineage dysplasia C92.A- ☑ (*following* C92.6)
    - variation of MLL-gene C92.6- ☑
  - M6 (a)(b) C94.Ø- ☑
  - M7 C94.2- ☑
- acute myelomonocytic C92.5- ☑
- acute promyelocytic C92.4- ☑
- adult T-cell (HTLV-1-associated) (acute variant) (chronic variant) (lymphomatoid variant) (smouldering variant) C91.5- ☑
- aggressive NK-cell C94.8- ☑
- AML (1/ETO) (MØ) (M1) (M2) (without a FAB classification) C92.Ø- ☑
- AML M3 C92.4- ☑
- AML M4 (Eo with inv(16) or t(16;16)) C92.5- ☑
- AML M5 C93.Ø- ☑
- AML M5a C93.Ø- ☑
- AML M5b C93.Ø- ☑
- AML Me with t (15;17) and variants C92.4- ☑
- atypical chronic myeloid, BCR/ABL-negative C92.2- ☑
- biphenotypic acute C95.Ø- ☑
- blast cell C95.Ø- ☑
- Burkitt-type, mature B-cell C91.A- ☑ (*following* C91.6)
- chronic lymphocytic, of B-cell type C91.1- ☑
- chronic monocytic C93.1- ☑
- chronic myelogenous (Philadelphia chromosome (Ph1) positive) (t(9;22)) (q34;q11) (with crisis of blast cells) C92.1- ☑
- chronic myeloid, BCR/ABL-positive C92.1- ☑
  - atypical, BCR/ABL-negative C92.2- ☑
- chronic myelomonocytic C93.1- ☑

Leukemia, leukemic — *continued*
- chronic neutrophilic D47.1
- CMML (-1) (-2) (with eosinophilia) C93.1- ☑
- granulocytic (*see also* Category C92) C92.9- ☑
- hairy cell C91.4- ☑
- juvenile myelomonocytic C93.3- ☑
- lymphoid C91.9- ☑
  - specified NEC C91.Z- ☑ (*following* C91.6)
- mast cell C94.3- ☑
- mature B-cell, Burkitt-type C91.A- ☑ (*following* C91.6)
- monocytic (subacute) C93.9- ☑
  - specified NEC C93.Z- ☑ (*following* C93.3)
- myelogenous (*see also* Category C92) C92.9- ☑
- myeloid C92.9- ☑
  - specified NEC C92.Z- ☑ (*following* C92.6)
- plasma cell C9Ø.1- ☑
- plasmacytic C9Ø.1- ☑
- prolymphocytic
  - of B-cell type C91.3- ☑
  - of T-cell type C91.6- ☑
- specified NEC C94.8- ☑
- stem cell, of unclear lineage C95.Ø- ☑
- subacute lymphocytic C91.9- ☑
- T-cell large granular lymphocytic C91.Z- ☑ (*following* C91.6)
- unspecified cell type C95.9- ☑
  - acute C95.Ø- ☑
  - chronic C95.1- ☑

Leukemoid reaction (*see also* Reaction, leukemoid) D72.823

Leukoaraiosis (hypertensive) I67.81

Leukoariosis — *see* Leukoaraiosis

Leukocoria — *see* Disorder, globe, degenerated condition, leucocoria

Leukocytopenia D72.819

Leukocytosis D72.829
- eosinophilic D72.1

Leukoderma, leukodermia NEC L81.5
- syphilitic A51.39
  - late A52.79

Leukodystrophy E75.29

Leukoedema, oral epithelium K13.29

Leukoencephalitis GØ4.81
- acute (subacute) hemorrhagic G36.1
  - postimmunization or postvaccinal GØ4.Ø2
- postinfectious GØ4.Ø1
- subacute sclerosing A81.1
- van Bogaert's (sclerosing) A81.1

Leukoencephalopathy (*see also* Encephalopathy) G93.49
- Binswanger's I67.3
- heroin vapor G92
- metachromatic E75.25
- multifocal (progressive) A81.2
- postimmunization and postvaccinal GØ4.Ø2
- progressive multifocal A81.2
- reversible, posterior G93.6
- van Bogaert's (sclerosing) A81.1
- vascular, progressive I67.3

Leukoerythroblastosis D75.9

Leukokeratosis (*see also* Leukoplakia)
- mouth K13.21
- nicotina palati K13.24
- oral mucosa K13.21
- tongue K13.21
- vocal cord J38.3

Leukokraurosis vulva (e) N9Ø.4

Leukoma (cornea) (*see also* Opacity, cornea)
- adherent H17.Ø- ☑
- interfering with central vision — *see* Opacity, cornea, central

Leukomalacia, cerebral, newborn P91.2
- periventricular P91.2

Leukomelanopathy, hereditary D72.Ø

Leukonychia (punctata) (striata) L6Ø.8
- congenital Q84.4

Leukopathia unguium L6Ø.8
- congenital Q84.4

Leukopenia D72.819
- basophilic D72.818
- chemotherapy (cancer) induced D7Ø.1
- congenital D7Ø.Ø
- cyclic D7Ø.Ø
- drug induced NEC D7Ø.2
  - due to cytoreductive cancer chemotherapy D7Ø.1
- eosinophilic D72.818
- familial D7Ø.Ø

Leukopenia — *continued*
infantile genetic D70.0
malignant D70.9
periodic D70.0
transitory neonatal P61.5
Leukopenic — *see* condition
Leukoplakia
anus K62.89
bladder (postinfectional) N32.89
buccal K13.21
cervix (uteri) N88.0
esophagus K22.8
gingiva K13.21
hairy (oral mucosa) (tongue) K13.3
kidney (pelvis) N28.89
larynx J38.7
lip K13.21
mouth K13.21
oral epithelium, including tongue (mucosa) K13.21
palate K13.21
pelvis (kidney) N28.89
penis (infectional) N48.0
rectum K62.89
syphilitic (late) A52.79
tongue K13.21
ureter (postinfectional) N28.89
urethra (postinfectional) N36.8
uterus N85.8
vagina N89.4
vocal cord J38.3
vulva N90.4
Leukorrhea N89.8
due to Trichomonas (vaginalis) A59.00
trichomonal A59.00
Leukosarcoma C85.9- ☑
Levocardia (isolated) Q24.1
with situs inversus Q89.3
Levotransposition Q20.5
Lev's disease or syndrome (acquired complete heart block) I44.2
Levulosuria — *see* Fructosuria
Levurid L30.2
Lewy body (ies) (dementia) (disease) G31.83
Leyden-Moebius dystrophy G71.0
Leydig cell
carcinoma
specified site — *see* Neoplasm, malignant, by site
unspecified site
female C56.9
male C62.9- ☑
tumor
benign
specified site — *see* Neoplasm, benign, by site
unspecified site
female D27.- ☑
male D29.2- ☑
malignant
specified site — *see* Neoplasm, malignant, by site
unspecified site
female C56.- ☑
male C62.9- ☑
specified site — *see* Neoplasm, uncertain behavior, by site
unspecified site
female D39.1- ☑
male D40.1- ☑
Leydig-Sertoli cell tumor
specified site — *see* Neoplasm, benign, by site
unspecified site
female D27.- ☑
male D29.2- ☑
LGSIL (Low grade squamous intraepithelial lesion on cytologic smear of)
anus R85.612
cervix R87.612
vagina R87.622
Liar, pathologic F60.2
Libido
decreased R68.82
Libman-Sacks disease M32.11
Lice (infestation) B85.2
body (Pediculus corporis) B85.1
crab B85.3
head (Pediculus capitis) B85.0
mixed (classifiable to more than one of the titles B85.0-B85.3) B85.4

Lice — *continued*
pubic (Phthirus pubis) B85.3
Lichen L28.0
albus L90.0
penis N48.0
vulva N90.4
amyloidosis E85.4 [L99]
atrophicus L90.0
penis N48.0
vulva N90.4
congenital Q82.8
myxedematosus L98.5
nitidus L44.1
pilaris Q82.8
acquired L85.8
planopilaris L66.1
planus (chronicus) L43.9
annularis L43.8
bullous L43.1
follicular L66.1
hypertrophic L43.0
moniliformis L44.3
of Wilson L43.9
specified NEC L43.8
subacute (active) L43.3
tropicus L43.3
ruber
acuminatus L44.0
moniliformis L44.3
planus L43.9
sclerosus (et atrophicus) L90.0
penis N48.0
vulva N90.4
scrofulosus (primary) (tuberculous) A18.4
simplex (chronicus) (circumscriptus) L28.0
striatus L44.2
urticatus L28.2
Lichenification L28.0
Lichenoides tuberculosis (primary) A18.4
Lichtheim's disease or syndrome — *see* Degeneration, combined
Lien migrans D73.89
Ligament — *see* condition
Light
for gestational age — *see* Light for dates
headedness R42
Light-for-dates (infant) P05.00
with weight of
1000-1249 grams P05.04
1250-1499 grams P05.05
1500-1749 grams P05.06
1750-1999 grams P05.07
2000-2499 grams P05.08
499 grams or less P05.01
500-749 grams P05.02
750-999 grams P05.03
affecting management of pregnancy O36.59- ☑
and small-for-dates — *see* Small for dates
Lightning (effects) (stroke) (struck by) T75.00 ☑
burn — *see* Burn
foot E53.8
shock T75.01 ☑
specified effect NEC T75.09 ☑
Lightwood-Albright syndrome N25.89
Lightwood's disease or syndrome (renal tubular acidosis) N25.89
Lignac (-de Toni) (-Fanconi) (-Debré) **disease or syndrome** E72.09
with cystinosis E72.04
Ligneous thyroiditis E06.5
Likoff's syndrome I20.8
Limb — *see* condition
Limbic epilepsy personality syndrome F07.0
Limitation, limited
activities due to disability Z73.6
cardiac reserve — *see* Disease, heart
eye muscle duction, traumatic — *see* Strabismus, mechanical
mandibular range of motion M26.52
Lindau (-von Hippel) **disease** Q85.8
Line(s)
Beau's L60.4
Harris' — *see* Arrest, epiphyseal
Hudson's (cornea) — *see* Pigmentation, cornea, anterior
Stähli's (cornea) — *see* Pigmentation, cornea, anterior
Linea corneae senilis — *see* Change, cornea, senile

Lingua
geographica K14.1
nigra (villosa) K14.3
plicata K14.5
tylosis K13.29
Lingual — *see* condition
Linguatulosis B88.8
Linitis (gastric) **plastica** C16.9
Lip — *see* condition
Lipedema — *see* Edema
Lipemia (*see also* Hyperlipidemia)
retina, retinalis E78.3
Lipidosis E75.6
cerebral (infantile) (juvenile) (late) E75.4
cerebroretinal E75.4
cerebroside E75.22
cholesterol (cerebral) E75.5
glycolipid E75.21
hepatosplenomegalic E78.3
sphingomyelin — *see* Niemann-Pick disease or syndrome
sulfatide E75.29
Lipoadenoma — *see* Neoplasm, benign, by site
Lipoblastoma — *see* Lipoma
Lipoblastomatosis — *see* Lipoma
Lipochondrodystrophy E76.01
Lipochrome histiocytosis (familial) D71
Lipodermatosclerosis — *see* Varix, leg, with, inflammation
ulcerated — *see* Varix, leg, with, ulcer, with inflammation by site
Lipodystrophia progressiva E88.1
Lipodystrophy (progressive) E88.1
insulin E88.1
intestinal K90.81
mesenteric K65.4
Lipofibroma — *see* Lipoma
Lipofuscinosis, neuronal (with ceroidosis) E75.4
Lipogranuloma, sclerosing L92.8
Lipogranulomatosis E78.89
Lipoid (*see also* condition)
histiocytosis D76.3
essential E75.29
nephrosis N04.9
proteinosis of Urbach E78.89
Lipoidemia — *see* Hyperlipidemia
Lipoidosis — *see* Lipidosis
Lipoma D17.9
fetal D17.9
fat cell D17.9
infiltrating D17.9
intramuscular D17.9
pleomorphic D17.9
site classification
arms (skin) (subcutaneous) D17.2- ☑
connective tissue D17.30
intra-abdominal D17.5
intrathoracic D17.4
peritoneum D17.79
retroperitoneum D17.79
specified site NEC D17.39
spermatic cord D17.6
face (skin) (subcutaneous) D17.0
genitourinary organ NEC D17.72
head (skin) (subcutaneous) D17.0
intra-abdominal D17.5
intrathoracic D17.4
kidney D17.71
legs (skin) (subcutaneous) D17.2- ☑
neck (skin) (subcutaneous) D17.0
peritoneum D17.79
retroperitoneum D17.79
skin D17.30
specified site NEC D17.39
specified site NEC D17.79
spermatic cord D17.6
subcutaneous D17.30
specified site NEC D17.39
trunk (skin) (subcutaneous) D17.1
unspecified D17.9
spindle cell D17.9
Lipomatosis E88.2
dolorosa (Dercum) E88.2
fetal — *see* Lipoma
Launois-Bensaude E88.89
Lipomyoma — *see* Lipoma
Lipomyxoma — *see* Lipoma

Lipomyxosarcoma — *see* Neoplasm, connective tissue, malignant
Lipoprotein metabolism disorder E78.9
Lipoproteinemia E78.5
  broad-beta E78.2
  floating-beta E78.2
  hyper-pre-beta E78.1
Liposarcoma (*see also* Neoplasm, connective tissue, malignant)
  dedifferentiated — *see* Neoplasm, connective tissue, malignant
  differentiated type — *see* Neoplasm, connective tissue, malignant
  embryonal — *see* Neoplasm, connective tissue, malignant
  mixed type — *see* Neoplasm, connective tissue, malignant
  myxoid — *see* Neoplasm, connective tissue, malignant
  pleomorphic — *see* Neoplasm, connective tissue, malignant
  round cell — *see* Neoplasm, connective tissue, malignant
  well differentiated type — *see* Neoplasm, connective tissue, malignant
Liposynovitis prepatellaris E88.89
Lipping, cervix N86
Lipschütz disease or ulcer N76.6
Lipuria R82.Ø
  schistosomiasis (bilharziasis) B65.Ø
Lisping F8Ø.Ø
Lissauer's paralysis A52.17
Lissencephalia, lissencephaly QØ4.3
Listeriosis, listerellosis A32.9
  congenital (disseminated) P37.2
  cutaneous A32.Ø
  neonatal, newborn (disseminated) P37.2
  oculoglandular A32.81
  specified NEC A32.89
Lithemia E79.Ø
Lithiasis — *see* Calculus
Lithosis J62.8
Lithuria R82.99
Litigation, anxiety concerning Z65.3
Little leaguer's elbow — *see* Epicondylitis, medial
Little's disease G8Ø.9
Littre's
  gland — *see* condition
  hernia — *see* Hernia, abdomen
Littritis — *see* Urethritis
Livedo (annularis) (racemosa) (reticularis) R23.1
Liver — *see* condition
Living alone (problems with) Z6Ø.2
  with handicapped person Z74.2
Lloyd's syndrome — *see* Adenomatosis, endocrine
Loa loa, loaiasis, loasis B74.3
Lobar — *see* condition
Lobomycosis B48.Ø
Lobo's disease B48.Ø
Lobotomy syndrome FØ7.Ø
Lobstein (-Ekman) **disease or syndrome** Q78.Ø
Lobster-claw hand Q71.6- ☑
Lobulation (congenital) (*see also* Anomaly, by site)
  kidney, Q63.1
  liver, abnormal Q44.7
  spleen Q89.Ø9
Lobule, lobular — *see* condition
Local, localized — *see* condition
Locked twins causing obstructed labor O66.1
Locked-in state G83.5
Locking
  joint — *see* Derangement, joint, specified type NEC
    knee — *see* Derangement, knee
Lockjaw — *see* Tetanus
Löffler's
  endocarditis I42.3
  eosinophilia J82
  pneumonia J82
  syndrome (eosinophilic pneumonitis) J82
Loiasis (with conjunctival infestation) (eyelid) B74.3
Lone Star fever A77.Ø
Long
  labor O63.9
    first stage O63.Ø
    second stage O63.1
  QT syndrome I45.81
Longitudinal stripes or grooves, nails L6Ø.8
  congenital Q84.6
Long-term (current) (prophylactic) **drug therapy** (use of)
  agents affecting estrogen receptors and estrogen levels NEC Z79.818
  anastrozole (Arimidex) Z79.811
  antibiotics Z79.2
    short-term use — *omit code*
  anticoagulants Z79.Ø1
  anti-inflammatory, non-steroidal (NSAID) Z79.1
  antiplatelet Z79.Ø2
  antithrombotics Z79.Ø2
  aromatase inhibitors Z79.811
  aspirin Z79.82
  birth control pill or patch Z79.3
  bisphosphonates Z79.83
  contraceptive, oral Z79.3
  drug, specified NEC Z79.899
  estrogen receptor downregulators Z79.818
  Evista Z79.81Ø
  exemestane (Aromasin) Z79.811
  Fareston Z79.81Ø
  fulvestrant (Faslodex) Z79.818
  gonadotropin-releasing hormone (GnRH) agonist Z79.818
  goserelin acetate (Zoladex) Z79.818
  hormone replacement (postmenopausal) Z79.89Ø
  insulin Z79.4
  letrozole (Femara) Z79.811
  leuprolide acetate (leuprorelin) (Lupron) Z79.818
  megestrol acetate (Megace) Z79.818
  methadone for pain management Z79.891
  Nolvadex Z79.81Ø
  non-steroidal anti-inflammatories (NSAID) Z79.1
  opiate analgesic Z79.891
  oral contraceptive Z79.3
  raloxifene (Evista) Z79.81Ø
  selective estrogen receptor modulators (SERMs) Z79.81Ø
  steroids
    inhaled Z79.51
    systemic Z79.52
  tamoxifen (Nolvadex) Z79.81Ø
  toremifene (Fareston) Z79.81Ø
Loop
  intestine — *see* Volvulus
  vascular on papilla (optic) Q14.2
Loose (*see also* condition)
  body
    joint M24.ØØ
      ankle M24.Ø7- ☑
      elbow M24.Ø2- ☑
      hand M24.Ø4- ☑
      hip M24.Ø5- ☑
      knee M23.4- ☑
      shoulder (region) M24.Ø1- ☑
      specified site NEC M24.Ø8
      toe M24.Ø7- ☑
      vertebra M24.Ø8
      wrist M24.Ø3- ☑
    knee M23.4- ☑
    sheath, tendon — *see* Disorder, tendon, specified type NEC
  cartilage — *see* Loose, body, joint
  tooth, teeth KØ8.8
Loosening
  aseptic
    joint prosthesis — *see* Complications, joint prosthesis, mechanical, loosening, by site
  epiphysis — *see* Osteochondropathy
  mechanical
    joint prosthesis — *see* Complications, joint prosthesis, mechanical, loosening, by site
Looser-Milkman (-Debray) **syndrome** M83.8
Lop ear (deformity) Q17.3
Lorain (-Levi) **short stature syndrome** E23.Ø
Lordosis M4Ø.5Ø
  acquired — *see* Lordosis, specified type NEC
  congenital Q76.429
    lumbar region Q76.426
    lumbosacral region Q76.427
    sacral region Q76.428
    sacrococcygeal region Q76.428
    thoracolumbar region Q76.425
  lumbar region M4Ø.56
  lumbosacral region M4Ø.57
  postsurgical M96.4
  postural — *see* Lordosis, specified type NEC
  rachitic (late effect) (sequelae) E64.3
Lordosis — *continued*
  sequelae of rickets E64.3
  specified type NEC M4Ø.4Ø
    lumbar region M4Ø.46
    lumbosacral region M4Ø.47
    thoracolumbar region M4Ø.45
  thoracolumbar region M4Ø.55
  tuberculous A18.Ø1
Loss (of)
  appetite (see Anorexia) R63.Ø
    hysterical F5Ø.8
    nonorganic origin F5Ø.8
    psychogenic F5Ø.8
  blood — *see* Hemorrhage
  consciousness, transient R55
    traumatic — *see* Injury, intracranial
  control, sphincter, rectum R15.9
    nonorganic origin F98.1
  elasticity, skin R23.4
  family (member) in childhood Z62.898
  fluid (acute) E86.9
    with
      hypernatremia E87.Ø
      hyponatremia E87.1
  function of labyrinth — *see* subcategory H83.2 ☑
  hair, nonscarring — *see* Alopecia
  hearing (*see also* Deafness)
    central NOS H9Ø.5
    neural NOS H9Ø.5
    perceptive NOS H9Ø.5
    sensorineural NOS H9Ø.5
    sensory NOS H9Ø.5
  height R29.89Ø
  limb or member, traumatic, current — *see* Amputation, traumatic
  love relationship in childhood Z62.898
  memory (*see also* Amnesia)
    mild, following organic brain damage FØ6.8
  mind — *see* Psychosis
  occlusal vertical dimension of fully erupted teeth M26.37
  organ or part — *see* Absence, by site, acquired
  ossicles, ear (partial) H74.32- ☑
  parent in childhood Z63.4
  pregnancy, recurrent N96
    without current pregnancy N96
    care in current pregnancy O26.2- ☑
  recurrent pregnancy — *see* Loss, pregnancy, recurrent
  self-esteem, in childhood Z62.898
  sense of
    smell — *see* Disturbance, sensation, smell
    taste — *see* Disturbance, sensation, taste
    touch R2Ø.8
  sensory R44.9
    dissociative F44.6
  sexual desire F52.Ø
  sight (acquired) (complete) (congenital) — *see* Blindness
  substance of
    bone — *see* Disorder, bone, density and structure, specified NEC
    cartilage — *see* Disorder, cartilage, specified type NEC
      auricle (ear) — *see* Disorder, pinna, specified type NEC
    vitreous (humor) H15.89
  tooth, teeth — *see* Absence, teeth, acquired
  vision, visual H54.7
    both eyes H54.3
    one eye H54.6Ø
      left (normal vision on right) H54.62
      right (normal vision on left) H54.61
    specified as blindness — *see* Blindness
    subjective
      sudden H53.13- ☑
      transient H53.12- ☑
  vitreous — *see* Prolapse, vitreous
  voice — *see* Aphonia
  weight (abnormal) (cause unknown) R63.4
Louis-Bar syndrome (ataxia-telangiectasia) G11.3
Louping ill (encephalitis) A84.8
Louse, lousiness — *see* Lice
Low
  achiever, school Z55.3
  back syndrome M54.5
  basal metabolic rate R94.8
  birthweight (2499 grams or less) PØ7.1Ø

- **Low** — *continued*
  - birthweight — *continued*
    - with weight of
      - 1ØØØ-1249 grams PØ7.14
      - 125Ø-1499 grams PØ7.15
      - 15ØØ-1749 grams PØ7.16
      - 175Ø-1999 grams PØ7.17
      - 2ØØØ-2499 grams PØ7.18
    - extreme (999 grams or less) PØ7.ØØ
      - with weight of
        - 499 grams or less PØ7.Ø1
        - 5ØØ-749 grams PØ7.Ø2
        - 75Ø-999 grams PØ7.Ø3
    - for gestational age — *see* Light for dates
  - blood pressure (*see also* Hypotension)
    - reading (incidental) (isolated) (nonspecific) RØ3.1
  - cardiac reserve — *see* Disease, heart
  - function (*see also* Hypofunction)
    - kidney N28.9
  - hematocrit D64.9
  - hemoglobin D64.9
  - income Z59.6
  - level of literacy Z55.Ø
  - lying
    - kidney N28.89
    - organ or site, congenital — *see* Malposition, congenital
  - output syndrome (cardiac) — *see* Failure, heart
  - platelets (blood) — *see* Thrombocytopenia
  - reserve, kidney N28.89
  - salt syndrome E87.1
  - self esteem R45.81
  - set ears Q17.4
  - vision H54.2
    - one eye (other eye normal) H54.5Ø
      - left (normal vision on right) H54.52
      - other eye blind — *see* Blindness
      - right (normal vision on left) H54.51
- **Low-density-lipoprotein-type** (LDL) **hyperlipoproteinemia** E78.Ø
- **Lowe's syndrome** E72.Ø3
- **Lown-Ganong-Levine syndrome** I45.6
- **LSD reaction** (acute) (without dependence) F16.9Ø
  - with dependence F16.2Ø
- **L-shaped kidney** Q63.8
- **Ludwig's angina or disease** K12.2
- **Lues** (venerea), **luetic** — *see* Syphilis
- **Luetscher's syndrome** (dehydration) E86.Ø
- **Lumbago, lumbalgia** M54.5
  - with sciatica M54.4- ☑
    - due to intervertebral disc disorder M51.17
  - due to displacement, intervertebral disc M51.27
    - with sciatica M51.17
- **Lumbar** — *see* condition
- **Lumbarization, vertebra, congenital** Q76.49
- **Lumbermen's itch** B88.Ø
- **Lump** — *see* Mass
- **Lunacy** — *see* Psychosis
- **Lung** — *see* condition
- **Lupoid** (miliary) **of Boeck** D86.3
- **Lupus**
  - anticoagulant D68.62
    - with
      - hemorrhagic disorder D68.312
      - hypercoagulable state D68.62
    - finding without diagnosis R76.Ø
  - discoid (local) L93.Ø
  - erythematosus (discoid) (local) L93.Ø
    - disseminated — *see* Lupus, erythematosus, systemic
    - eyelid HØ1.129
      - left HØ1.126
        - lower HØ1.125
        - upper HØ1.124
      - right HØ1.123
        - lower HØ1.122
        - upper HØ1.121
    - profundus L93.2
    - specified NEC L93.2
    - subacute cutaneous L93.1
    - systemic M32.9
      - with organ or system involvement M32.1Ø
        - endocarditis M32.11
        - lung M32.13
        - pericarditis M32.12
        - renal (glomerular) M32.14
          - tubulo-interstitial M32.15
        - specified organ or system NEC M32.19
- **Lupus** — *continued*
  - erythematosus — *continued*
    - systemic — *continued*
      - drug-induced M32.Ø
      - inhibitor (presence of) D68.62
        - with
          - hemorrhagic disorder D68.312
          - hypercoagulable state D68.62
        - finding without diagnosis R76.Ø
      - specified NEC M32.8
  - exedens A18.4
  - hydralazine M32.Ø
    - correct substance properly administered — *see* Table of Drugs and Chemicals, by drug, adverse effect
    - overdose or wrong substance given or taken — *see* Table of Drugs and Chemicals, by drug, poisoning
  - nephritis (chronic) M32.14
  - nontuberculous, not disseminated L93.Ø
  - panniculitis L93.2
  - pernio (Besnier) D86.3
  - systemic — *see* Lupus, erythematosus, systemic
  - tuberculous A18.4
    - eyelid A18.4
  - vulgaris A18.4
    - eyelid A18.4
- **Luteinoma** D27.- ☑
- **Lutembacher's disease or syndrome** (atrial septal defect with mitral stenosis) Q21.1
- **Luteoma** D27.- ☑
- **Lutz** (-Splendore-de Almeida) **disease** — *see* Paracoccidioidomycosis
- **Luxation** (*see also* Dislocation)
  - eyeball (nontraumatic) — *see* Luxation, globe
    - birth injury P15.3
  - globe, nontraumatic H44.82- ☑
  - lacrimal gland — *see* Dislocation, lacrimal gland
  - lens (old) (partial) (spontaneous)
    - congenital Q12.1
      - syphilitic A5Ø.39
- **Lycanthropy** F22
- **Lyell's syndrome** L51.2
  - due to drug L51.2
    - correct substance properly administered — *see* Table of Drugs and Chemicals, by drug, adverse effect
    - overdose or wrong substance given or taken — *see* Table of Drugs and Chemicals, by drug, poisoning
- **Lyme disease** A69.2Ø
- **Lymph**
  - gland or node — *see* condition
  - scrotum — *see* Infestation, filarial
- **Lymphadenitis** I88.9
  - with ectopic or molar pregnancy OØ8.Ø
  - acute LØ4.9
    - axilla LØ4.2
    - face LØ4.Ø
    - head LØ4.Ø
    - hip LØ4.3
    - limb
      - lower LØ4.3
      - upper LØ4.2
    - neck LØ4.Ø
    - shoulder LØ4.2
    - specified site NEC LØ4.8
    - trunk LØ4.1
  - anthracosis (occupational) J6Ø
  - any site, except mesenteric I88.9
    - chronic I88.1
    - subacute I88.1
  - breast
    - gestational — *see* Mastitis, obstetric
    - puerperal, postpartum (nonpurulent) O91.22
  - chancroidal (congenital) A57
  - chronic I88.1
    - mesenteric I88.Ø
  - due to
    - Brugia (malayi) B74.1
      - timori B74.2
    - chlamydial lymphogranuloma A55
    - diphtheria (toxin) A36.89
    - lymphogranuloma venereum A55
    - Wuchereria bancrofti B74.Ø
  - following ectopic or molar pregnancy OØ8.Ø
  - gonorrheal A54.89
  - infective — *see* Lymphadenitis, acute
- **Lymphadenitis** — *continued*
  - mesenteric (acute) (chronic) (nonspecific) (subacute) I88.Ø
    - due to Salmonella typhi AØ1.Ø9
    - tuberculous A18.39
  - mycobacterial A31.8
  - purulent — *see* Lymphadenitis, acute
  - pyogenic — *see* Lymphadenitis, acute
  - regional, nonbacterial I88.8
  - septic — *see* Lymphadenitis, acute
  - subacute, unspecified site I88.1
  - suppurative — *see* Lymphadenitis, acute
  - syphilitic (early) (secondary) A51.49
    - late A52.79
  - tuberculous — *see* Tuberculosis, lymph gland
  - venereal (chlamydial) A55
- **Lymphadenoid goiter** EØ6.3
- **Lymphadenopathy** (generalized) R59.1
  - angioimmunoblastic, with dysproteinemia (AILD) C86.5
  - due to toxoplasmosis (acquired) B58.89
    - congenital (acute) (subacute) (chronic) P37.1
  - localized R59.Ø
  - syphilitic (early) (secondary) A51.49
- **Lymphadenosis** R59.1
- **Lymphangiectasis** I89.Ø
  - conjunctiva H11.89
  - postinfectional I89.Ø
  - scrotum I89.Ø
- **Lymphangiectatic elephantiasis, nonfilarial** I89.Ø
- **Lymphangioendothelioma** D18.1
  - malignant — *see* Neoplasm, connective tissue, malignant
- **Lymphangioleiomyomatosis** J84.81
- **Lymphangioma** D18.1
  - capillary D18.1
  - cavernous D18.1
  - cystic D18.1
  - malignant — *see* Neoplasm, connective tissue, malignant
- **Lymphangiomyoma** D18.1
- **Lymphangiomyomatosis** J84.81
- **Lymphangiosarcoma** — *see* Neoplasm, connective tissue, malignant
- **Lymphangitis** I89.1
  - with
    - abscess — *code by* site under Abscess
    - cellulitis — *code by* site under Cellulitis
    - ectopic or molar pregnancy OØ8.Ø
  - acute LØ3.91
    - abdominal wall LØ3.321
    - ankle — *see* Lymphangitis, acute, lower limb
    - arm — *see* Lymphangitis, acute, upper limb
    - auricle (ear) — *see* Lymphangitis, acute, ear
    - axilla LØ3.12- ☑
    - back (any part) LØ3.322
    - buttock LØ3.327
    - cervical (meaning neck) LØ3.222
    - cheek (external) LØ3.212
    - chest wall LØ3.323
    - digit
      - finger — *see* Lymphangitis, acute, finger
      - toe — *see* Lymphangitis, acute, toe
    - ear (external) H6Ø.1- ☑
    - external auditory canal — *see* Lymphangitis, acute, ear
    - eyelid — *see* Abscess, eyelid
    - face NEC LØ3.212
    - finger (intrathecal) (periosteal) (subcutaneous) (subcuticular) LØ3.Ø2- ☑
    - foot — *see* Lymphangitis, acute, lower limb
    - gluteal (region) LØ3.327
    - groin LØ3.324
    - hand — *see* Lymphangitis, acute, upper limb
    - head NEC LØ3.891
      - face (any part, except ear, eye and nose) LØ3.212
    - heel — *see* Lymphangitis, acute, lower limb
    - hip — *see* Lymphangitis, acute, lower limb
    - jaw (region) LØ3.212
    - knee — *see* Lymphangitis, acute, lower limb
    - leg — *see* Lymphangitis, acute, lower limb
    - lower limb LØ3.12- ☑
      - toe — *see* Lymphangitis, acute, toe
    - navel LØ3.326
    - neck (region) LØ3.222
    - orbit, orbital — *see* Cellulitis, orbit

- **Lymphangitis** — *continued*
  - acute — *continued*
    - pectoral (region) LØ3.323
    - perineal, perineum LØ3.325
    - scalp (any part) LØ3.891
    - shoulder — *see* Lymphangitis, acute, upper limb
    - specified site NEC LØ3.898
    - thigh — *see* Lymphangitis, acute, lower limb
    - thumb (intrathecal) (periosteal) (subcutaneous) (subcuticular) — *see* Lymphangitis, acute, finger
    - toe (intrathecal) (periosteal) (subcutaneous) (subcuticular) LØ3.Ø4- ☑
    - trunk LØ3.329
      - abdominal wall LØ3.321
      - back (any part) LØ3.322
      - buttock LØ3.327
      - chest wall LØ3.323
      - groin LØ3.324
      - perineal, perineum LØ3.325
      - umbilicus LØ3.326
    - umbilicus LØ3.326
    - upper limb LØ3.12- ☑
      - axilla — *see* Lymphangitis, acute, axilla
      - finger — *see* Lymphangitis, acute, finger
      - thumb — *see* Lymphangitis, acute, finger
    - wrist — *see* Lymphangitis, acute, upper limb
  - breast
    - gestational — *see* Mastitis, obstetric
  - chancroidal A57
  - chronic (any site) I89.1
  - due to
    - Brugia (malayi) B74.1
      - timori B74.2
    - Wuchereria bancrofti B74.Ø
  - following ectopic or molar pregnancy OØ8.89
  - penis
    - acute N48.29
    - gonococcal (acute) (chronic) A54.Ø9
  - puerperal, postpartum, childbirth O86.89
  - strumous, tuberculous A18.2
  - subacute (any site) I89.1
  - tuberculous — *see* Tuberculosis, lymph gland
- **Lymphatic** (vessel) — *see* condition
- **Lymphatism** E32.8
- **Lymphectasia** I89.Ø
- **Lymphedema** (acquired) (*see also* Elephantiasis)
  - congenital Q82.Ø
  - hereditary (chronic) (idiopathic) Q82.Ø
  - postmastectomy I97.2
  - praecox I89.Ø
  - secondary I89.Ø
  - surgical NEC I97.89
    - postmastectomy (syndrome) I97.2
- **Lymphoblastic** — *see* condition
- **Lymphoblastoma** (diffuse) — *see* Lymphoma, lymphoblastic (diffuse)
  - giant follicular — *see* Lymphoma, lymphoblastic (diffuse)
  - macrofollicular — *see* Lymphoma, lymphoblastic (diffuse)
- **Lymphocele** I89.8
- **Lymphocytic**
  - chorioencephalitis (acute) (serous) A87.2
  - choriomeningitis (acute) (serous) A87.2
  - meningoencephalitis A87.2
- **Lymphocytoma, benign cutis** L98.8
- **Lymphocytopenia** D72.81Ø
- **Lymphocytosis** (symptomatic) D72.82Ø
  - infectious (acute) B33.8
- **Lymphoepithelioma** — *see* Neoplasm, malignant, by site
- **Lymphogranuloma** (malignant) (*see also* Lymphoma, Hodgkin)
  - chlamydial A55
  - inguinale A55
  - venereum (any site) (chlamydial) (with stricture of rectum) A55
- **Lymphogranulomatosis** (malignant) (*see also* Lymphoma, Hodgkin)
  - benign (Boeck's sarcoid) (Schaumann's) D86.1
- **Lymphohistiocytosis, hemophagocytic** (familial) D76.1
- **Lymphoid** — *see* condition
- **Lymphoma** (of) (malignant) C85.9Ø
  - adult T-cell (HTLV-1-associated) (acute variant) (chronic variant) (lymphomatoid variant) (smouldering variant) C91.5- ☑
- **Lymphoma** — *continued*
  - anaplastic large cell
    - ALK-negative C84.7- ☑
    - ALK-positive C84.6- ☑
    - CD3Ø-positive C84.6- ☑
    - primary cutaneous C86.6
  - angioimmunoblastic T-cell C86.5
  - BALT C88.4
  - B-cell C85.1- ☑
  - blastic NK-cell C86.4
  - B-precursor C83.5- ☑
  - bronchial-associated lymphoid tissue [BALT-lymphoma] C88.4
  - Burkitt (atypical) C83.7- ☑
  - Burkitt-like C83.7- ☑
  - centrocytic C83.1- ☑
  - cutaneous follicle center C82.6- ☑
  - cutaneous T-cell C84.A- ☑ (*following* C84.7)
  - diffuse follicle center C82.5- ☑
  - diffuse large cell C83.3- ☑
    - anaplastic C83.3- ☑
    - B-cell C83.3- ☑
    - CD3Ø-positive C83.3- ☑
    - centroblastic C83.3- ☑
    - immunoblastic C83.3- ☑
    - plasmablastic C83.3- ☑
    - subtype not specified C83.3- ☑
    - T-cell rich C83.3- ☑
  - enteropathy-type (associated) (intestinal) T-cell C86.2
  - extranodal marginal zone B-cell lymphoma of mucosa-associated lymphoid tissue [MALT-lymphoma] C88.4
  - extranodal NK/T-cell, nasal type C86.Ø
  - follicular C82.9- ☑
    - grade
      - I C82.Ø- ☑
      - II C82.1- ☑
      - III C82.2- ☑
      - IIIa C82.3- ☑
      - IIIb C82.4- ☑
    - specified NEC C82.8- ☑
  - hepatosplenic T-cell (alpha-beta) (gamma-delta) C86.1
  - histiocytic C85.9- ☑
    - true C96.A (*following* C96.6)
  - Hodgkin C81.9 ☑
    - classical C81.7- ☑
      - lymphocyte depleted C81.3- ☑
      - lymphocyte-rich C81.4- ☑
      - mixed cellularity C81.2- ☑
      - nodular sclerosis C81.1- ☑
      - specified NEC C81.7- ☑
    - lymphocyte depleted classical C81.3- ☑
    - lymphocyte-rich classical C81.4- ☑
    - mixed cellularity classical C81.2- ☑
    - nodular
      - lymphocyte predominant C81.Ø- ☑
      - sclerosis classical C81.1- ☑
  - intravascular large B-cell C83.8- ☑
  - Lennert's C84.4- ☑
  - lymphoblastic (diffuse) C83.5- ☑
  - lymphoblastic B-cell C83.5- ☑
  - lymphoblastic T-cell C83.5- ☑
  - lymphoepithelioid C84.4- ☑
  - lymphoplasmacytic C83.Ø- ☑
    - with IgM-production C88.Ø
  - MALT C88.4
  - mantle cell C83.1- ☑
  - mature T-cell NEC C84.4- ☑
  - mature T/NK-cell C84.9- ☑
    - specified NEC C84.Z- ☑ (*following* C84.7)
  - mediastinal (thymic) large B-cell C85.2- ☑
  - Mediterranean C88.3
  - mucosa-associated lymphoid tissue [MALT-lymphoma] C88.4
  - NK/T cell C84.9- ☑
  - nodal marginal zone C83.Ø- ☑
  - non-follicular (diffuse) C83.9- ☑
    - specified NEC C83.8- ☑
  - non-Hodgkin (*see also* Lymphoma, by type) C85.9- ☑
    - specified NEC C85.8- ☑
  - non-leukemic variant of B-CLL C83.Ø- ☑
  - peripheral T-cell, not classified C84.4- ☑
  - primary cutaneous
    - anaplastic large cell C86.6
    - CD3Ø-positive large T-cell C86.6
  - primary effusion B-cell C83.8- ☑
- **Lymphoma** — *continued*
  - SALT C88.4
  - skin-associated lymphoid tissue [SALT-lymphoma] C88.4
  - small cell B-cell C83.Ø- ☑
  - splenic marginal zone C83.Ø- ☑
  - subcutaneous panniculitis-like T-cell C86.3
  - T-precursor C83.5- ☑
  - true histiocytic C96.A (*following* C96.6)
- **Lymphomatosis** — *see* Lymphoma
- **Lymphopathia venereum, veneris** A55
- **Lymphopenia** D72.81Ø
- **Lymphoplasmacytic leukemia** — *see* Leukemia, chronic lymphocytic, B-cell type
- **Lymphoproliferation, X-linked disease** D82.3
- **Lymphoreticulosis, benign** (of inoculation) A28.1
- **Lymphorrhea** I89.8
- **Lymphosarcoma** (diffuse) (*see also* Lymphoma) C85.9- ☑
- **Lymphostasis** I89.8
- **Lypemania** — *see* Melancholia
- **Lysine and hydroxylysine metabolism disorder** E72.3
- **Lyssa** — *see* Rabies

M

- **Macacus ear** Q17.3
- **Maceration, wet feet, tropical** (syndrome) T69.Ø2- ☑
- **MacLeod's syndrome** J43.Ø
- **Macrocephalia, macrocephaly** Q75.3
- **Macrocheilia, macrochilia** (congenital) Q18.6
- **Macrocolon** (*see also* Megacolon) Q43.1
- **Macrocornea** Q15.8
  - with glaucoma Q15.Ø
- **Macrocytic** — *see* condition
- **Macrocytosis** D75.89
- **Macrodactylia, macrodactylism** (fingers) (thumbs) Q74.Ø
  - toes Q74.2
- **Macrodontia** KØØ.2
- **Macrogenia** M26.Ø5
- **Macrogenitosomia** (adrenal) (male) (praecox) E25.9
  - congenital E25.Ø
- **Macroglobulinemia** (idiopathic) (primary) C88.Ø
  - monoclonal (essential) D47.2
  - Waldenström C88.Ø
- **Macroglossia** (congenital) Q38.2
  - acquired K14.8
- **Macrognathia, macrognathism** (congenital) (mandibular) (maxillary) M26.Ø9
- **Macrogyria** (congenital) QØ4.8
- **Macrohydrocephalus** — *see* Hydrocephalus
- **Macromastia** — *see* Hypertrophy, breast
- **Macrophthalmos** Q11.3
  - in congenital glaucoma Q15.Ø
- **Macropsia** H53.15
- **Macrosigmoid** K59.3
  - congenital Q43.2
- **Macrospondylitis , acromegalic** E22.Ø
- **Macrostomia** (congenital) Q18.4
- **Macrotia** (external ear) (congenital) Q17.1
- **Macula**
  - cornea, corneal — *see* Opacity, cornea
  - degeneration (atrophic) (exudative) (senile) (*see also* Degeneration, macula)
    - hereditary — *see* Dystrophy, retina
- **Maculae ceruleae** B85.1
- **Maculopathy, toxic** — *see* Degeneration, macula, toxic
- **Madarosis** (eyelid) HØ2.729
  - left HØ2.726
    - lower HØ2.725
    - upper HØ2.724
  - right HØ2.723
    - lower HØ2.722
    - upper HØ2.721
- **Madelung's**
  - deformity (radius) Q74.Ø
  - disease
    - radial deformity Q74.Ø
    - symmetrical lipomas, neck E88.89
- **Madness** — *see* Psychosis
- **Madura**
  - foot B47.9
    - actinomycotic B47.1
    - mycotic B47.Ø
- **Maduromycosis** B47.Ø
- **Maffucci's syndrome** Q78.4

- **Magnesium metabolism disorder** — *see* Disorder, metabolism, magnesium
- **Main en griffe** (acquired) (*see also* Deformity, limb, clawhand)
  - congenital Q74.Ø
- **Maintenance** (encounter for)
  - antineoplastic chemotherapy Z51.11
  - antineoplastic radiation therapy Z51.Ø
  - methadone F11.2Ø
- **Majocchi's**
  - disease L81.7
  - granuloma B35.8
- **Major** — *see* condition
- **Mal de los pintos** — *see* Pinta
- **Mal de mer** T75.3 ☑
- **Malabar itch** (any site) B35.5
- **Malabsorption** K9Ø.9
  - calcium K9Ø.89
  - carbohydrate K9Ø.4
  - disaccharide E73.9
  - fat K9Ø.4
  - galactose E74.2Ø
  - glucose (-galactose) E74.39
  - intestinal K9Ø.9
    - specified NEC K9Ø.89
  - isomaltose E74.31
  - lactose E73.9
  - methionine E72.19
  - monosaccharide E74.39
  - postgastrectomy K91.2
  - postsurgical K91.2
  - protein K9Ø.4
  - starch K9Ø.4
  - sucrose E74.39
  - syndrome K9Ø.9
    - postsurgical K91.2
- **Malacia, bone** (adult) M83.9
  - juvenile — *see* Rickets
- **Malacoplakia**
  - bladder N32.89
  - pelvis (kidney) N28.89
  - ureter N28.89
  - urethra N36.8
- **Malacosteon, juvenile** — *see* Rickets
- **Maladaptation** — *see* Maladjustment
- **Maladie de Roger** Q21.Ø
- **Maladjustment**
  - conjugal Z63.Ø
    - involving divorce or estrangement Z63.5
  - educational Z55.4
  - family Z63.9
  - marital Z63.Ø
    - involving divorce or estrangement Z63.5
  - occupational NEC Z56.89
  - simple, adult — *see* Disorder, adjustment
  - situational — *see* Disorder, adjustment
  - social Z6Ø.9
    - due to
      - acculturation difficulty Z6Ø.3
      - discrimination and persecution (perceived) Z6Ø.5
      - exclusion and isolation Z6Ø.4
      - life-cycle (phase of life) transition Z6Ø.Ø
      - rejection Z6Ø.4
      - specified reason NEC Z6Ø.8
- **Malaise** R53.81
- **Malakoplakia** — *see* Malacoplakia
- **Malaria, malarial** (fever) B54
  - with
    - blackwater fever B5Ø.8
      - hemoglobinuric (bilious) B5Ø.8
    - hemoglobinuria B5Ø.8
  - accidentally induced (therapeutically) — *code by* type under Malaria
  - algid B5Ø.9
  - cerebral B5Ø.Ø [G94]
  - clinically diagnosed (without parasitological confirmation) B54
  - congenital NEC P37.4
    - falciparum P37.3
  - congestion, congestive B54
  - continued (fever) B5Ø.9
  - estivo-autumnal B5Ø.9
  - falciparum B5Ø.9
    - with complications NEC B5Ø.8
      - cerebral B5Ø.Ø [G94]
    - severe B5Ø.8
  - hemorrhagic B54

- **Malaria, malarial** — *continued*
  - malariae B52.9
    - with
      - complications NEC B52.8
      - glomerular disorder B52.Ø
  - malignant (tertian) — *see* Malaria, falciparum
  - mixed infections — *code to* first listed type in B5Ø-B53
  - ovale B53.Ø
  - parasitologically confirmed NEC B53.8
  - pernicious, acute — *see* Malaria, falciparum
  - Plasmodium (P.)
    - falciparum NEC — *see* Malaria, falciparum
    - malariae NEC B52.9
      - with Plasmodium
        - falciparum (and or vivax) — *see* Malaria, falciparum
        - vivax (*see also* Malaria, vivax)
          - and falciparum — *see* Malaria, falciparum
    - ovale B53.Ø
      - with Plasmodium malariae (*see also* Malaria, malariae)
        - and vivax (*see also* Malaria, vivax)
          - and falciparum — *see* Malaria, falciparum
    - simian B53.1
      - with Plasmodium malariae (*see also* Malaria, malariae)
        - and vivax (*see also* Malaria, vivax)
          - and falciparum — *see* Malaria, falciparum
    - vivax NEC B51.9
      - with Plasmodium falciparum — *see* Malaria, falciparum
  - quartan — *see* Malaria, malariae
  - quotidian — *see* Malaria, falciparum
  - recurrent B54
  - remittent B54
  - specified type NEC (parasitologically confirmed) B53.8
  - spleen B54
  - subtertian (fever) — *see* Malaria, falciparum
  - tertian (benign) (*see also* Malaria, vivax)
    - malignant B5Ø.9
  - tropical B5Ø.9
  - typhoid B54
  - vivax B51.9
    - with
      - complications NEC B51.8
      - ruptured spleen B51.Ø
- **Malassez's disease** (cystic) N5Ø.8
- **Malassimilation** K9Ø.9
- **Maldescent, testis** Q53.9
  - bilateral Q53.2Ø
    - abdominal Q53.21
    - perineal Q53.22
  - unilateral Q53.1Ø
    - abdominal Q53.11
    - perineal Q53.12
- **Maldevelopment** (*see also* Anomaly)
  - brain Q07.9
  - colon Q43.9
  - hip Q74.2
    - congenital dislocation Q65.2
      - bilateral Q65.1
      - unilateral Q65.Ø- ☑
  - mastoid process Q75.8
  - middle ear Q16.4
    - except ossicles Q16.4
    - ossicles Q16.3
  - ossicles Q16.3
  - spine Q76.49
  - toe Q74.2
- **Male type pelvis** Q74.2
  - with disproportion (fetopelvic) O33.3 ☑
    - causing obstructed labor O65.3
- **Malformation** (congenital) (*see also* Anomaly)
  - adrenal gland Q89.1
  - affecting multiple systems with skeletal changes NEC Q87.5
  - alimentary tract Q45.9
    - specified type NEC Q45.8
    - upper Q4Ø.9
      - specified type NEC Q4Ø.8
  - aorta Q25.9
    - atresia Q25.2
    - coarctation (preductal) (postductal) Q25.1
    - patent ductus arteriosus Q25.Ø
    - specified type NEC Q25.4

- **Malformation** — *continued*
  - aorta — *continued*
    - stenosis (supravalvular) Q25.3
  - aortic valve Q23.9
    - specified NEC Q23.8
  - arteriovenous, aneurysmatic (congenital) Q27.3Ø
    - brain Q28.2
    - cerebral Q28.2
    - peripheral Q27.3Ø
      - digestive system Q27.33
      - lower limb Q27.32
      - other specified site Q27.39
      - renal vessel Q27.34
      - upper limb Q27.31
    - precerebral vessels (nonruptured) Q28.Ø
  - auricle
    - ear (congenital) Q17.3
      - acquired H61.119
        - left H61.112
          - with right H61.113
        - right H61.111
          - with left H61.113
  - bile duct Q44.5
  - bladder Q64.79
    - aplasia Q64.5
    - diverticulum Q64.6
    - exstrophy — *see* Exstrophy, bladder
    - neck obstruction Q64.31
  - bone Q79.9
    - face Q75.9
      - specified type NEC Q75.8
    - skull Q75.9
      - specified type NEC Q75.8
  - brain (multiple) QØ4.9
    - arteriovenous Q28.2
    - specified type NEC QØ4.8
  - branchial cleft Q18.2
  - breast Q83.9
    - specified type NEC Q83.8
  - broad ligament Q5Ø.6
  - bronchus Q32.4
  - bursa Q79.9
  - cardiac
    - chambers Q2Ø.9
      - specified type NEC Q2Ø.8
    - septum Q21.9
      - specified type NEC Q21.8
  - cerebral QØ4.9
    - vessels Q28.3
  - cervix uteri Q51.9
    - specified type NEC Q51.828
  - Chiari
    - Type I G93.5
    - Type II QØ7.Ø1
  - choroid (congenital) Q14.3
    - plexus QØ7.8
  - circulatory system Q28.9
  - cochlea Q16.5
  - cornea Q13.4
  - coronary vessels Q24.5
  - corpus callosum (congenital) QØ4.Ø
  - diaphragm Q79.1
  - digestive system NEC, specified type NEC Q45.8
  - dura QØ7.9
    - brain QØ4.9
    - spinal QØ6.9
  - ear Q17.9
    - causing impairment of hearing Q16.9
    - external Q17.9
      - accessory auricle Q17.Ø
      - causing impairment of hearing Q16.9
        - absence of
          - auditory canal Q16.1
          - auricle Q16.Ø
      - macrotia Q17.1
      - microtia Q17.2
      - misplacement Q17.4
      - misshapen NEC Q17.3
      - prominence Q17.5
      - specified type NEC Q17.8
    - inner Q16.5
    - middle Q16.4
      - absence of eustachian tube Q16.2
      - ossicles (fusion) Q16.3
    - ossicles Q16.3
    - specified type NEC Q17.8
  - epididymis Q55.4
  - esophagus Q39.9

- **Malformation** — *continued*
  - esophagus — *continued*
    - specified type NEC Q39.8
  - eye Q15.9
    - lid Q1Ø.3
    - specified NEC Q15.8
  - fallopian tube Q5Ø.6
  - genital organ — *see* Anomaly, genitalia
  - great
    - artery Q25.9
      - aorta — *see* Malformation, aorta
      - pulmonary artery — *see* Malformation, pulmonary, artery
      - specified type NEC Q25.8
    - vein Q26.9
      - anomalous
        - portal venous connection Q26.5
        - pulmonary venous connection Q26.4
          - partial Q26.3
          - total Q26.2
      - persistent left superior vena cava Q26.1
      - portal vein-hepatic artery fistula Q26.6
      - specified type NEC Q26.8
      - vena cava stenosis, congenital Q26.Ø
  - gum Q38.6
  - hair Q84.2
  - heart Q24.9
    - specified type NEC Q24.8
  - integument Q84.9
    - specified type NEC Q84.8
  - internal ear Q16.5
  - intestine Q43.9
    - specified type NEC Q43.8
  - iris Q13.2
  - joint Q74.9
    - ankle Q74.2
    - lumbosacral Q76.49
    - sacroiliac Q74.2
    - specified type NEC Q74.8
  - kidney Q63.9
    - accessory Q63.Ø
    - giant Q63.3
    - horseshoe Q63.1
    - hydronephrosis Q62.Ø
    - malposition Q63.2
    - specified type NEC Q63.8
  - lacrimal apparatus Q1Ø.6
  - lingual Q38.3
  - lip Q38.Ø
  - liver Q44.7
  - lung Q33.9
  - meninges or membrane (congenital) QØ7.9
    - cerebral QØ4.8
    - spinal (cord) QØ6.9
  - middle ear Q16.4
    - ossicles Q16.3
  - mitral valve Q23.9
    - specified NEC Q23.8
  - Mondini's (congenital) (malformation, cochlea) Q16.5
  - mouth (congenital) Q38.6
  - multiple types NEC Q89.7
  - musculoskeletal system Q79.9
  - myocardium Q24.8
  - nail Q84.6
  - nervous system (central) QØ7.9
  - nose Q3Ø.9
    - specified type NEC Q3Ø.8
  - optic disc Q14.2
  - orbit Q1Ø.7
  - ovary Q5Ø.39
  - palate Q38.5
  - parathyroid gland Q89.2
  - pelvic organs or tissues NEC
    - in pregnancy or childbirth O34.8- ☑
      - causing obstructed labor O65.5
  - penis Q55.69
    - aplasia Q55.5
    - curvature (lateral) Q55.61
    - hypoplasia Q55.62
  - pericardium Q24.8
  - peripheral vascular system Q27.9
    - specified type NEC Q27.8
  - pharynx Q38.8
  - precerebral vessels Q28.1
  - prostate Q55.4
  - pulmonary
    - arteriovenous Q25.72
    - artery Q25.9

- **Malformation** — *continued*
  - pulmonary — *continued*
    - artery — *continued*
      - atresia Q25.5
      - specified type NEC Q25.79
      - stenosis Q25.6
    - valve Q22.3
  - renal artery Q27.2
  - respiratory system Q34.9
  - retina Q14.1
  - scrotum — *see* Malformation, testis and scrotum
  - seminal vesicles Q55.4
  - sense organs NEC QØ7.9
  - skin Q82.9
  - specified NEC Q89.8
  - spinal
    - cord QØ6.9
    - nerve root QØ7.8
  - spine Q76.49
    - kyphosis — *see* Kyphosis, congenital
    - lordosis — *see* Lordosis, congenital
  - spleen Q89.Ø9
  - stomach Q4Ø.3
    - specified type NEC Q4Ø.2
  - teeth, tooth KØØ.9
  - tendon Q79.9
  - testis and scrotum Q55.2Ø
    - aplasia Q55.Ø
    - hypoplasia Q55.1
    - polyorchism Q55.21
    - retractile testis Q55.22
    - scrotal transposition Q55.23
    - specified NEC Q55.29
  - thorax, bony Q76.9
  - throat Q38.8
  - thyroid gland Q89.2
  - tongue (congenital) Q38.3
    - hypertrophy Q38.2
    - tie Q38.1
  - trachea Q32.1
  - tricuspid valve Q22.9
    - specified type NEC Q22.8
  - umbilical cord NEC (complicating delivery) O69.89 ☑
  - umbilicus Q89.9
  - ureter Q62.8
    - agenesis Q62.4
    - duplication Q62.5
    - malposition — *see* Malposition, congenital, ureter
    - obstructive defect — *see* Defect, obstructive, ureter
    - vesico-uretero-renal reflux Q62.7
  - urethra Q64.79
    - aplasia Q64.5
    - duplication Q64.74
    - posterior valves Q64.2
    - prolapse Q64.71
    - stricture Q64.32
  - urinary system Q64.9
  - uterus Q51.9
    - specified type NEC Q51.818
  - vagina Q52.4
  - vas deferens Q55.4
    - atresia Q55.3
  - vascular system, peripheral Q27.9
  - venous — *see* Anomaly, vein(s)
  - vulva Q52.7Ø
- **Malfunction** (*see also* Dysfunction)
  - cardiac electronic device T82.119 ☑
    - electrode T82.11Ø ☑
    - pulse generator T82.111 ☑
    - specified type NEC T82.118 ☑
  - catheter device NEC T85.618 ☑
    - cystostomy T83.Ø1Ø ☑
    - dialysis (renal) (vascular) T82.41 ☑
      - intraperitoneal T85.611 ☑
    - infusion NEC T82.514 ☑
      - spinal (epidural) (subdural) T85.61Ø ☑
    - urinary, indwelling T83.Ø18 ☑
  - colostomy K94.Ø3
    - valve K94.Ø3
  - cystostomy (stoma) N99.512
    - catheter T83.Ø1Ø ☑
  - enteric stoma K94.13
  - enterostomy K94.13
  - esophagostomy K94.33
  - gastroenteric K31.89
  - gastrostomy K94.23
  - ileostomy K94.13
    - valve K94.13

- **Malfunction** — *continued*
  - jejunostomy K94.13
  - pacemaker — *see* Malfunction, cardiac electronic device
  - prosthetic device, internal — *see* Complications, prosthetic device, by site, mechanical
  - tracheostomy J95.Ø3
  - urinary device NEC — *see* Complication, genitourinary, device, urinary, mechanical
  - valve
    - colostomy K94.Ø3
    - heart T82.Ø9 ☑
    - ileostomy K94.13
  - vascular graft or shunt NEC — *see* Complication, cardiovascular device, mechanical, vascular
  - ventricular (communicating shunt) T85.Ø1 ☑
- **Malherbe's tumor** — *see* Neoplasm, skin, benign
- **Malibu disease** L98.8
- **Malignancy** (*see also* Neoplasm, malignant, by site)
  - unspecified site (primary) C8Ø.1
- **Malignant** — *see* condition
- **Malingerer, malingering** Z76.5
- **Mallet finger** (acquired) — *see* Deformity, finger, mallet finger
  - congenital Q74.Ø
  - sequelae of rickets E64.3
- **Malleus** A24.Ø
- **Mallory's bodies** R89.7
- **Mallory-Weiss syndrome** K22.6
- **Malnutrition** E46
  - degree
    - first E44.1
    - mild (protein) E44.1
    - moderate (protein) E44.Ø
    - second E44.Ø
    - severe (protein-energy) E43
      - intermediate form E42
        - with
          - kwashiorkor (and marasmus) E42
          - marasmus E41
    - third E43
  - following gastrointestinal surgery K91.2
  - intrauterine
    - light-for-dates — *see* Light for dates
    - small-for-dates — *see* Small for dates
  - lack of care, or neglect (child) (infant) T76.Ø2 ☑
    - confirmed T74.Ø2 ☑
  - malignant E4Ø
  - protein E46
    - calorie E46
      - mild E44.1
      - moderate E44.Ø
      - severe E43
        - intermediate form E42
          - with
            - kwashiorkor (and marasmus) E42
            - marasmus E41
    - energy E46
      - mild E44.1
      - moderate E44.Ø
      - severe E43
        - intermediate form E42
          - with
            - kwashiorkor (and marasmus) E42
            - marasmus E41
  - severe (protein-energy) E43
    - with
      - kwashiorkor (and marasmus) E42
      - marasmus E41
- **Malocclusion** (teeth) M26.4
  - Angle's M26.219
    - class I M26.211
    - class II M26.212
    - class III M26.213
  - due to
    - abnormal swallowing M26.59
    - mouth breathing M26.59
    - tongue, lip or finger habits M26.59
  - temporomandibular (joint) M26.69
- **Malposition**
  - cervix — *see* Malposition, uterus
  - congenital
    - adrenal (gland) Q89.1
    - alimentary tract Q45.8
      - lower Q43.8
      - upper Q4Ø.8
    - aorta Q25.4
    - appendix Q43.8

- **Mania** — *continued*
  - recurrent F31.89
- **Manic-depressive insanity, psychosis, or syndrome** — *see* Disorder, bipolar
- **Mannosidosis** E77.1
- **Mansonelliasis, mansonellosis** B74.4
- **Manson's**
  - disease B65.1
  - schistosomiasis B65.1
- **Manual** — *see* condition
- **Maple-bark-stripper's lung** (disease) J67.6
- **Maple-syrup-urine disease** E71.Ø
- **Marable's syndrome** (celiac artery compression) I77.4
- **Marasmus** E41
  - due to malnutrition E41
  - intestinal E41
  - nutritional E41
  - senile R54
  - tuberculous NEC — *see* Tuberculosis
- **Marble**
  - bones Q78.2
  - skin R23.8
- **Marburg virus disease** A98.3
- **March**
  - fracture — *see* Fracture, traumatic, stress, by site
  - hemoglobinuria D59.6
- **Marchesani** (-Weill) **syndrome** Q87.Ø
- **Marchiafava** (-Bignami) **syndrome or disease** G37.1
- **Marchiafava-Micheli syndrome** D59.5
- **Marcus Gunn's syndrome** QØ7.8
- **Marfan's syndrome** — *see* Syndrome, Marfan's
- **Marie-Bamberger disease** — *see* Osteoarthropathy, hypertrophic, specified NEC
- **Marie-Charcot-Tooth neuropathic muscular atrophy** G6Ø.Ø
- **Marie's**
  - cerebellar ataxia (late-onset) G11.2
  - disease or syndrome (acromegaly) E22.Ø
- **Marie-Strümpell arthritis, disease or spondylitis** — *see* Spondylitis, ankylosing
- **Marion's disease** (bladder neck obstruction) N32.Ø
- **Marital conflict** Z63.Ø
- **Mark**
  - port wine Q82.5
  - raspberry Q82.5
  - strawberry Q82.5
  - stretch L9Ø.6
  - tattoo L81.8
- **Marker heterochromatin** — *see* Extra, marker chromosomes
- **Maroteaux-Lamy syndrome** (mild) (severe) E76.29
- **Marrow** (bone)
  - arrest D61.9
  - poor function D75.89
- **Marseilles fever** A77.1
- **Marsh fever** — *see* Malaria
- **Marshall's** (hidrotic) **ectodermal dysplasia** Q82.4
- **Marsh's disease** (exophthalmic goiter) EØ5.ØØ
  - with storm EØ5.Ø1
- **Masculinization** (female) **with adrenal hyperplasia** E25.9
  - congenital E25.Ø
- **Masculinovoblastoma** D27.- ☑
- **Masochism** (sexual) F65.51
- **Mason's lung** J62.8
- **Mass**
  - abdominal R19.ØØ
    - epigastric R19.Ø6
    - generalized R19.Ø7
    - left lower quadrant R19.Ø4
    - left upper quadrant R19.Ø2
    - periumbilic R19.Ø5
    - right lower quadrant R19.Ø3
    - right upper quadrant R19.Ø1
    - specified site NEC R19.Ø9
  - breast N63
  - chest R22.2
  - cystic — *see* Cyst
  - ear H93.8- ☑
  - head R22.Ø
  - intra-abdominal (diffuse) (generalized) — *see* Mass, abdominal
  - kidney N28.89
  - liver R16.Ø
  - localized (skin) R22.9
    - chest R22.2
    - head R22.Ø
- **Mass** — *continued*
  - localized — *continued*
    - limb
      - lower R22.4- ☑
      - upper R22.3- ☑
    - neck R22.1
    - trunk R22.2
  - lung R91.8
  - malignant — *see* Neoplasm, malignant, by site
  - neck R22.1
  - pelvic (diffuse) (generalized) — *see* Mass, abdominal
  - specified organ NEC — *see* Disease, by site
  - splenic R16.1
  - substernal thyroid — *see* Goiter
  - superficial (localized) R22.9
  - umbilical (diffuse) (generalized) R19.Ø9
- **Massive** — *see* condition
- **Mast cell**
  - disease, systemic tissue D47.Ø
  - leukemia C94.3- ☑
  - sarcoma C96.2
  - tumor D47.Ø
    - malignant C96.2
- **Mastalgia** N64.4
- **Masters-Allen syndrome** N83.8
- **Mastitis** (acute) (diffuse) (nonpuerperal) (subacute) N61
  - chronic (cystic) — *see* Mastopathy, cystic
  - cystic (Schimmelbusch's type) — *see* Mastopathy, cystic
  - fibrocystic — *see* Mastopathy, cystic
  - infective N61
    - newborn P39.Ø
  - interstitial, gestational or puerperal — *see* Mastitis, obstetric
  - neonatal (noninfective) P83.4
    - infective P39.Ø
  - obstetric (interstitial) (nonpurulent)
    - associated with
      - lactation O91.23
      - pregnancy O91.21- ☑
      - puerperium O91.22
    - purulent
      - associated with
        - lactation O91.13
        - pregnancy O91.11- ☑
        - puerperium O91.12
  - periductal — *see* Ectasia, mammary duct
  - phlegmonous — *see* Mastopathy, cystic
  - plasma cell — *see* Ectasia, mammary duct
- **Mastocytoma** D47.Ø
  - malignant C96.2
- **Mastocytosis** Q82.2
  - aggressive systemic C96.2
  - indolent systemic D47.Ø
  - malignant C96.2
  - systemic, associated with clonal hematopoetic non-mast-cell disease (SM-AHNMD) D47.Ø
- **Mastodynia** N64.4
- **Mastoid** — *see* condition
- **Mastoidalgia** — *see* subcategory H92.Ø ☑
- **Mastoiditis** (coalescent) (hemorrhagic) (suppurative) H7Ø.9- ☑
  - acute, subacute H7Ø.ØØ- ☑
    - complicated NEC H7Ø.Ø9- ☑
    - subperiosteal H7Ø.Ø1- ☑
  - chronic (necrotic) (recurrent) H7Ø.1- ☑
  - in (due to)
    - infectious disease NEC B99 ☑ [H75.Ø-] ☑
    - parasitic disease NEC B89 [H75.Ø-] ☑
    - tuberculosis A18.Ø3
  - petrositis — *see* Petrositis
  - postauricular fistula — *see* Fistula, postauricular
  - specified NEC H7Ø.89- ☑
  - tuberculous A18.Ø3
- **Mastopathy, mastopathia** N64.9
  - chronica cystica — *see* Mastopathy, cystic
  - cystic (chronic) (diffuse) N6Ø.1- ☑
    - with epithelial proliferation N6Ø.3- ☑
  - diffuse cystic — *see* Mastopathy, cystic
  - estrogenic, oestrogenica N64.89
  - ovarian origin N64.89
- **Mastoplasia, mastoplastia** N62
- **Masturbation** (excessive) F98.8
- **Maternal care** (for) — *see* Pregnancy (complicated by) (management affected by)
- **Matheiu's disease** (leptospiral jaundice) A27.Ø
- **Mauclaire's disease or osteochondrosis** — *see* Osteochondrosis, juvenile, hand, metacarpal
- **Maxcy's disease** A75.2
- **Maxilla, maxillary** — *see* condition
- **May** (-Hegglin) **anomaly or syndrome** D72.Ø
- **McArdle** (-Schmid)(-Pearson) **disease** (glycogen storage) E74.Ø4
- **McCune-Albright syndrome** Q78.1
- **McQuarrie's syndrome** (idiopathic familial hypoglycemia) E16.2
- **Meadow's syndrome** Q86.1
- **Measles** (black) (hemorrhagic) (suppressed) BØ5.9
  - with
    - complications NEC BØ5.89
    - encephalitis BØ5.Ø
    - intestinal complications BØ5.4
    - keratitis (keratoconjunctivitis) BØ5.81
    - meningitis BØ5.1
    - otitis media BØ5.3
    - pneumonia BØ5.2
  - French — *see* Rubella
  - German — *see* Rubella
  - Liberty — *see* Rubella
- **Meatitis, urethral** — *see* Urethritis
- **Meatus, meatal** — *see* condition
- **Meat-wrappers' asthma** J68.9
- **Meckel-Gruber syndrome** Q61.9
- **Meckel's diverticulitis, diverticulum** (displaced) (hypertrophic) Q43.Ø
  - malignant — *see* Table of Neoplasms, small intestine, malignant
- **Meconium**
  - ileus, newborn P76.Ø
    - in cystic fibrosis E84.11
    - meaning meconium plug (without cystic fibrosis) P76.Ø
  - obstruction, newborn P76.Ø
    - due to fecaliths P76.Ø
    - in mucoviscidosis E84.11
  - peritonitis P78.Ø
  - plug syndrome (newborn) NEC P76.Ø
- **Median** (*see also* condition)
  - arcuate ligament syndrome I77.4
  - bar (prostate) (vesical orifice) — *see* Hyperplasia, prostate
  - rhomboid glossitis K14.2
- **Mediastinal shift** R93.8
- **Mediastinitis** (acute) (chronic) J98.5
  - syphilitic A52.73
  - tuberculous A15.8
- **Mediastinopericarditis** (*see also* Pericarditis)
  - acute I3Ø.9
  - adhesive I31.Ø
  - chronic I31.8
    - rheumatic IØ9.2
- **Mediastinum, mediastinal** — *see* condition
- **Medicine poisoning** — *see* Table of Drugs and Chemicals, by drug, poisoning
- **Mediterranean**
  - fever — *see* Brucellosis
    - familial E85.Ø
    - tick A77.1
  - kala-azar B55.Ø
  - leishmaniasis B55.Ø
  - tick fever A77.1
- **Medulla** — *see* condition
- **Medullary cystic kidney** Q61.5
- **Medullated fibers**
  - optic (nerve) Q14.8
  - retina Q14.1
- **Medulloblastoma**
  - desmoplastic C71.6
  - specified site — *see* Neoplasm, malignant, by site
  - unspecified site C71.6
- **Medulloepithelioma** (*see also* Neoplasm, malignant, by site)
  - teratoid — *see* Neoplasm, malignant, by site
- **Medullomyoblastoma**
  - specified site — *see* Neoplasm, malignant, by site
  - unspecified site C71.6
- **Meekeren-Ehlers-Danlos syndrome** Q79.6
- **Megacolon** (acquired) (functional) (not Hirschsprung's disease) (in) K59.3
  - Chagas' disease B57.32
  - congenital, congenitum (aganglionic) Q43.1
  - Hirschsprung's (disease) Q43.1
  - toxic NEC K59.3

Index

Megacolon — Melanosarcoma

- **Melanosis** L81.4
  - addisonian E27.1
    - tuberculous A18.7
  - adrenal E27.1
  - colon K63.89
  - conjunctiva — *see* Pigmentation, conjunctiva
    - congenital Q13.89
  - cornea (presenile) (senile) (*see also* Pigmentation, cornea)
    - congenital Q13.4
  - eye NEC H57.8
    - congenital Q15.8
  - lenticularis progressiva Q82.1
  - liver K76.89
  - precancerous (*see also* Melanoma, in situ)
    - malignant melanoma in — *see* Melanoma
  - Riehl's L81.4
  - sclera H15.89
    - congenital Q13.89
  - suprarenal E27.1
  - tar L81.4
  - toxic L81.4
- **Melanuria** R82.99
- **MELAS syndrome** E88.41
- **Melasma** L81.1
  - adrenal (gland) E27.1
  - suprarenal (gland) E27.1
- **Melena** K92.1
  - with ulcer — *code by* site under Ulcer, with hemorrhage K27.4
  - due to swallowed maternal blood P78.2
  - newborn, neonatal P54.1
    - due to swallowed maternal blood P78.2
- **Meleney's**
  - gangrene (cutaneous) — *see* Ulcer, skin
  - ulcer (chronic undermining) — *see* Ulcer, skin
- **Melioidosis** A24.9
  - acute A24.1
  - chronic A24.2
  - fulminating A24.1
  - pneumonia A24.1
  - pulmonary (chronic) A24.2
    - acute A24.1
    - subacute A24.2
  - sepsis A24.1
  - specified NEC A24.3
  - subacute A24.2
- **Melitensis, febris** A23.Ø
- **Melkersson** (-Rosenthal) **syndrome** G51.2
- **Mellitus, diabetes** — *see* Diabetes
- **Melorheostosis** (bone) — *see* Disorder, bone, density and structure, specified NEC
- **Meloschisis** Q18.4
- **Melotia** Q17.4
- **Membrana**
  - capsularis lentis posterior Q13.89
  - epipapillaris Q14.2
- **Membranacea placenta** O43.19- ☑
- **Membranaceous uterus** N85.8
- **Membrane**(s), membranous (*see also* condition)
  - cyclitic — *see* Membrane, pupillary
  - folds, congenital — *see* Web
  - Jackson's Q43.3
  - over face of newborn P28.9
  - premature rupture — *see* Rupture, membranes, premature
  - pupillary H21.4- ☑
    - persistent Q13.89
  - retained (with hemorrhage) (complicating delivery) O72.2
    - without hemorrhage O73.1
  - secondary cataract — *see* Cataract, secondary
  - unruptured (causing asphyxia) — *see* Asphyxia, newborn
  - vitreous — *see* Opacity, vitreous, membranes and strands
- **Membranitis** — *see* Chorioamnionitis
- **Memory disturbance, lack or loss** (*see also* Amnesia)
  - mild, following organic brain damage FØ6.8
- **Menadione deficiency** E56.1
- **Menarche**
  - delayed E3Ø.Ø
  - precocious E3Ø.1
- **Mendacity, pathologic** F6Ø.2
- **Mendelson's syndrome** (due to anesthesia) J95.4
  - in labor and delivery O74.Ø
  - in pregnancy O29.Ø1- ☑

- **Mendelson's syndrome** — *continued*
  - obstetric O74.Ø
  - postpartum, puerperal O89.Ø1
- **Ménétrier's disease or syndrome** K29.6Ø
  - with bleeding K29.61
- **Ménière's disease, syndrome or vertigo** H81.Ø- ☑
- **Meninges, meningeal** — *see* condition
- **Meningioma** (*see also* Neoplasm, meninges, benign)
  - angioblastic — *see* Neoplasm, meninges, benign
  - angiomatous — *see* Neoplasm, meninges, benign
  - endotheliomatous — *see* Neoplasm, meninges, benign
  - fibroblastic — *see* Neoplasm, meninges, benign
  - fibrous — *see* Neoplasm, meninges, benign
  - hemangioblastic — *see* Neoplasm, meninges, benign
  - hemangiopericytic — *see* Neoplasm, meninges, benign
  - malignant — *see* Neoplasm, meninges, malignant
  - meningiothelial — *see* Neoplasm, meninges, benign
  - meningotheliomatous — *see* Neoplasm, meninges, benign
  - mixed — *see* Neoplasm, meninges, benign
  - multiple — *see* Neoplasm, meninges, uncertain behavior
  - papillary — *see* Neoplasm, meninges, uncertain behavior
  - psammomatous — *see* Neoplasm, meninges, benign
  - syncytial — *see* Neoplasm, meninges, benign
  - transitional — *see* Neoplasm, meninges, benign
- **Meningiomatosis** (diffuse) — *see* Neoplasm, meninges, uncertain behavior
- **Meningism** — *see* Meningismus
- **Meningismus** (infectional) (pneumococcal) R29.1
  - due to serum or vaccine R29.1
  - influenzal — *see* Influenza, with, manifestations NEC
- **Meningitis** (basal) (basic) (brain) (cerebral) (cervical) (congestive) (diffuse) (hemorrhagic) (infantile) (membranous) (metastatic) (nonspecific) (pontine) (progressive) (simple) (spinal) (subacute) (sympathetic) (toxic) GØ3.9
  - abacterial GØ3.Ø
  - actinomycotic A42.81
  - adenoviral A87.1
  - arbovirus A87.8
  - aseptic (acute) GØ3.Ø
  - bacterial GØØ.9
    - Escherichia coli (E. coli) GØØ.8
    - Friedländer (bacillus) GØØ.8
    - gram-negative GØØ.9
    - H. influenzae GØØ.Ø
    - Klebsiella GØØ.8
    - pneumococcal GØØ.1
    - specified organism NEC GØØ.8
    - staphylococcal GØØ.3
    - streptococcal (acute) GØØ.2
  - benign recurrent (Mollaret) GØ3.2
  - candidal B37.5
  - caseous (tuberculous) A17.Ø
  - cerebrospinal A39.Ø
  - chronic NEC GØ3.1
  - clear cerebrospinal fluid NEC GØ3.Ø
  - coxsackievirus A87.Ø
  - cryptococcal B45.1
  - diplococcal (gram positive) A39.Ø
  - echovirus A87.Ø
  - enteroviral A87.Ø
  - eosinophilic B83.2
  - epidemic NEC A39.Ø
  - Escherichia coli (E. coli) GØØ.8
  - fibrinopurulent GØØ.9
    - specified organism NEC GØØ.8
  - Friedländer (bacillus) GØØ.8
  - gonococcal A54.81
  - gram-negative cocci GØØ.9
  - gram-positive cocci GØØ.9
  - H. influenzae GØØ.Ø
  - Haemophilus (influenzae) GØØ.Ø
  - in (due to)
    - adenovirus A87.1
    - African trypanosomiasis B56.9 [GØ2]
    - anthrax A22.8
    - bacterial disease NEC A48.8 [GØ1]
    - Chagas' disease (chronic) B57.41
    - chickenpox BØ1.Ø
    - coccidioidomycosis B38.4
    - Diplococcus pneumoniae GØØ.1
    - enterovirus A87.Ø
    - herpes (simplex) virus BØØ.3
      - zoster BØ2.1

- **Meningitis** — *continued*
  - in — *continued*
    - infectious mononucleosis B27.92
    - leptospirosis A27.81
    - Listeria monocytogenes A32.11
    - Lyme disease A69.21
    - measles BØ5.1
    - mumps (virus) B26.1
    - neurosyphilis (late) A52.13
    - parasitic disease NEC B89 [GØ2]
    - poliovirus A8Ø.9 [GØ2]
    - preventive immunization, inoculation or vaccination GØ3.8
    - rubella BØ6.Ø2
    - Salmonella infection AØ2.21
    - specified cause NEC GØ3.8
    - typhoid fever AØ1.Ø1
    - varicella BØ1.Ø
    - viral disease NEC A87.8
    - whooping cough A37.9Ø
    - zoster BØ2.1
  - infectious GØØ.9
  - influenzal (H. influenzae) GØØ.Ø
  - Klebsiella GØØ.8
  - leptospiral (aseptic) A27.81
  - lymphocytic (acute) (benign) (serous) A87.2
  - meningococcal A39.Ø
  - Mima polymorpha GØØ.8
  - Mollaret (benign recurrent) GØ3.2
  - monilial B37.5
  - mycotic NEC B49 [GØ2]
  - Neisseria A39.Ø
  - nonbacterial GØ3.Ø
  - nonpyogenic NEC GØ3.Ø
  - ossificans G96.19
  - pneumococcal GØØ.1
  - poliovirus A8Ø.9 [GØ2]
  - postmeasles BØ5.1
  - purulent GØØ.9
    - specified organism NEC GØØ.8
  - pyogenic GØØ.9
    - specified organism NEC GØØ.8
  - Salmonella (arizonae) (Cholerae-Suis) (enteritidis) (typhimurium) AØ2.21
  - septic GØØ.9
    - specified organism NEC GØØ.8
  - serosa circumscripta NEC GØ3.Ø
  - serous NEC G93.2
  - specified organism NEC GØØ.8
  - sporotrichosis B42.81
  - staphylococcal GØØ.3
  - sterile GØ3.Ø
  - streptococcal (acute) GØØ.2
  - suppurative GØØ.9
    - specified organism NEC GØØ.8
  - syphilitic (late) (tertiary) A52.13
    - acute A51.41
    - congenital A5Ø.41
    - secondary A51.41
  - Torula histolytica (cryptococcal) B45.1
  - traumatic (complication of injury) T79.8 ☑
  - tuberculous A17.Ø
  - typhoid AØ1.Ø1
  - viral NEC A87.9
  - Yersinia pestis A2Ø.3
- **Meningocele** (spinal) (*see also* Spina bifida)
  - with hydrocephalus — *see* Spina bifida, by site, with hydrocephalus
  - acquired (traumatic) G96.19
  - cerebral — *see* Encephalocele
- **Meningocerebritis** — *see* Meningoencephalitis
- **Meningococcemia** A39.4
  - acute A39.2
  - chronic A39.3
- **Meningococcus, meningococcal** (*see also* condition) A39.9
  - adrenalitis, hemorrhagic A39.1
  - carrier (suspected) of Z22.31
  - meningitis (cerebrospinal) A39.Ø
- **Meningoencephalitis** (*see also* Encephalitis) GØ4.9Ø
  - acute NEC (*see also* Encephalitis, viral) A86
  - bacterial NEC GØ4.2
  - California A83.5
  - diphasic A84.1
  - eosinophilic B83.2
  - epidemic A39.81
  - herpesviral, herpetic BØØ.4
    - due to herpesvirus 6 B1Ø.Ø1

Meningoencephalitis — *continued*
herpesviral, herpetic — *continued*
due to herpesvirus 7 B10.Ø9
specified NEC B10.Ø9
in (due to)
blastomycosis NEC B4Ø.81
diseases classified elsewhere GØ5.3
free-living amebae B6Ø.2
H. influenzae GØØ.Ø
Hemophilus influenzae (H .influenzae) GØ4.2
herpes BØØ.4
due to herpesvirus 6 B10.Ø1
due to herpesvirus 7 B10.Ø9
specified NEC B10.Ø9
Lyme disease A69.22
mercury — *see* subcategory T56.1 ☑
mumps B26.2
Naegleria (amebae) (organisms) (fowleri) B6Ø.2
Parastrongylus cantonensis B83.2
toxoplasmosis (acquired) B58.2
congenital P37.1
infectious (acute) (viral) A86
influenzal (H. influenzae) GØ4.2
Listeria monocytogenes A32.12
lymphocytic (serous) A87.2
mumps B26.2
parasitic NEC B89 [GØ5.3]
pneumococcal GØØ.1
primary amebic B6Ø.2
specific (syphilitic) A52.14
specified organism NEC GØ4.81
staphylococcal GØ4.2
streptococcal GØ4.2
syphilitic A52.14
toxic NEC G92
due to mercury — *see* subcategory T56.1 ☑
tuberculous A17.82
virus NEC A86
Meningoencephalocele (*see also* Encephalocele)
syphilitic A52.19
congenital A5Ø.49
Meningoencephalomyelitis (*see also* Meningoencephalitis)
acute NEC (viral) A86
disseminated GØ4.ØØ
postimmunization or postvaccination GØ4.Ø2
postinfectious GØ4.Ø1
due to
actinomycosis A42.82
Torula B45.1
Toxoplasma or toxoplasmosis (acquired) B58.2
congenital P37.1
postimmunization or postvaccination GØ4.Ø2
Meningoencephalomyelopathy G96.9
Meningoencephalopathy G96.9
Meningomyelitis (*see also* Meningoencephalitis)
bacterial NEC GØ4.2
blastomycotic NEC B4Ø.81
cryptococcal B45.1
in diseases classified elsewhere GØ5.4
meningococcal A39.81
syphilitic A52.14
tuberculous A17.82
Meningomyelocele (*see also* Spina bifida)
syphilitic A52.19
Meningomyeloneuritis — *see* Meningoencephalitis
Meningoradiculitis — *see* Meningitis
Meningovascular — *see* condition
Menkes' disease or syndrome E83.Ø9
meaning maple-syrup-urine disease E71.Ø
Menometrorrhagia N92.1
Menopause, menopausal (asymptomatic) (state) Z78.Ø
arthritis (any site) NEC — *see* Arthritis, specified form NEC
bleeding N92.4
depression (single episode) F32.8
agitated (single episode) F32.2
recurrent episode F33.9
psychotic (single episode) F32.8
recurrent episode F33.9
recurrent episode F33.9
melancholia (single episode) F32.8
recurrent episode F33.9
paranoid state F22
premature E28.319
asymptomatic E28.319
postirradiation E89.4Ø
postsurgical E89.4Ø

Menopause, menopausal — *continued*
premature — *continued*
symptomatic E28.31Ø
postirradiation E89.41
postsurgical E89.41
psychosis NEC F28
symptomatic N95.1
toxic polyarthritis NEC — *see* Arthritis, specified form NEC
Menorrhagia (primary) N92.Ø
climacteric N92.4
menopausal N92.4
menopausal N92.4
postclimacteric N95.Ø
postmenopausal N95.Ø
preclimacteric or premenopausal N92.4
pubertal (menses retained) N92.2
Menostaxis N92.Ø
Menses, retention N94.89
Menstrual — *see* Menstruation
Menstruation
absent — *see* Amenorrhea
anovulatory N97.Ø
cycle, irregular N92.6
delayed N91.Ø
disorder N93.9
psychogenic F45.8
during pregnancy O2Ø.8
excessive (with regular cycle) N92.Ø
with irregular cycle N92.1
at puberty N92.2
frequent N92.Ø
infrequent — *see* Oligomenorrhea
irregular N92.6
specified NEC N92.5
latent N92.5
membranous N92.5
painful (*see also* Dysmenorrhea) N94.6
primary N94.4
psychogenic F45.8
secondary N94.5
passage of clots N92.Ø
precocious E3Ø.1
protracted N92.5
rare — *see* Oligomenorrhea
retained N94.89
retrograde N92.5
scanty — *see* Oligomenorrhea
suppression N94.89
vicarious (nasal) N94.89
Mental (*see also* condition)
deficiency — *see* Disability, intellectual
deterioration — *see* Psychosis
disorder — *see* Disorder, mental
exhaustion F48.8
insufficiency (congenital) — *see* Disability, intellectual
observation without need for further medical care Z03.89
retardation — *see* Disability, intellectual
subnormality — *see* Disability, intellectuall
upset — *see* Disorder, mental
Meralgia paresthetica G57.1- ☑
Mercurial — *see* condition
Mercurialism — *see* subcategory T56.1 ☑
Merkel cell tumor — *see* Carcinoma, Merkel cell
Merocele — *see* Hernia, femoral
Meromelia
lower limb — *see* Defect, reduction, lower limb
intercalary
femur — *see* Defect, reduction, lower limb, specified type NEC
tibiofibular (complete) (incomplete) — *see* Defect, reduction, lower limb
upper limb — *see* Defect, reduction, upper limb
intercalary, humeral, radioulnar — *see* Agenesis, arm, with hand present
MERRF syndrome (myoclonic epilepsy associated with ragged-red fiber) E88.42
Merzbacher-Pelizaeus disease E75.29
Mesaortitis — *see* Aortitis
Mesarteritis — *see* Arteritis
Mesencephalitis — *see* Encephalitis
Mesenchymoma (*see also* Neoplasm, connective tissue, uncertain behavior)
benign — *see* Neoplasm, connective tissue, benign
malignant — *see* Neoplasm, connective tissue, malignant

Mesenteritis
retractile K65.4
sclerosing K65.4
Mesentery, mesenteric — *see* condition
Mesiodens, mesiodentes KØØ.1
Mesio-occlusion M26.213
Mesocolon — *see* condition
Mesonephroma (malignant) — *see* Neoplasm, malignant, by site
benign — *see* Neoplasm, benign, by site
Mesophlebitis — *see* Phlebitis
Mesostromal dysgenesia Q13.89
Mesothelioma (malignant) C45.9
benign
mesentery D19.1
mesocolon D19.1
omentum D19.1
peritoneum D19.1
pleura D19.Ø
specified site NEC D19.7
unspecified site D19.9
biphasic C45.9
benign
mesentery D19.1
mesocolon D19.1
omentum D19.1
peritoneum D19.1
pleura D19.Ø
specified site NEC D19.7
unspecified site D19.9
cystic D48.4
epithelioid C45.9
benign
mesentery D19.1
mesocolon D19.1
omentum D19.1
peritoneum D19.1
pleura D19.Ø
specified site NEC D19.7
unspecified site D19.9
fibrous C45.9
benign
mesentery D19.1
mesocolon D19.1
omentum D19.1
peritoneum D19.1
pleura D19.Ø
specified site NEC D19.7
unspecified site D19.9
site classification
liver C45.7
lung C45.7
mediastinum C45.7
mesentery C45.1
mesocolon C45.1
omentum C45.1
pericardium C45.2
peritoneum C45.1
pleura C45.Ø
parietal C45.Ø
retroperitoneum C45.7
specified site NEC C45.7
unspecified C45.9
Metabolic syndrome E88.81
Metagonimiasis B66.8
Metagonimus infestation (intestine) B66.8
Metal
pigmentation L81.8
polisher's disease J62.8
Metamorphopsia H53.15
Metaplasia
apocrine (breast) — *see* Dysplasia, mammary, specified type NEC
cervix (squamous) — *see* Dysplasia, cervix
endometrium (squamous) (uterus) N85.8
esophagus
kidney (pelvis) (squamous) N28.89
myelogenous D73.1
myeloid (agnogenic) (megakaryocytic) D73.1
spleen D73.1
squamous cell, bladder N32.89
Metastasis, metastatic
abscess — *see* Abscess
calcification E83.59
cancer
from specified site — *see* Neoplasm, malignant, by site

Mononucleosis, infectious — *continued*
  gammaherpesviral B27.ØØ
    with
      complication NEC B27.Ø9
      meningitis B27.Ø2
      polyneuropathy B27.Ø1
  specified NEC B27.8Ø
    with
      complication NEC B27.89
      meningitis B27.82
      polyneuropathy B27.81
Monoplegia G83.3- ☑
  congenital (cerebral) G8Ø.8
    spastic G8Ø.1
  embolic (current episode) I63.4 ☑
  following
    cerebrovascular disease
      cerebral infarction
        lower limb I69.34- ☑
        upper limb I69.33- ☑
      intracerebral hemorrhage
        lower limb I69.14- ☑
        upper limb I69.13- ☑
      lower limb I69.94- ☑
      nontraumatic intracranial hemorrhage NEC
        lower limb I69.24- ☑
        upper limb I69.23- ☑
      specified disease NEC
        lower limb I69.84- ☑
        upper limb I69.83- ☑
      stroke NOS
        lower limb I69.34- ☑
        upper limb I69.33- ☑
      subarachnoid hemorrhage
        lower limb I69.Ø4- ☑
        upper limb I69.Ø3- ☑
      upper limb I69.93- ☑
  hysterical (transient) F44.4
  lower limb G83.1- ☑
  psychogenic (conversion reaction) F44.4
  thrombotic (current episode) I63.3 ☑
  transient R29.818
  upper limb G83.2- ☑
Monorchism, monorchidism Q55.Ø
Monosomy (*see also* Deletion, chromosome) Q93.9
  specified NEC Q93.89
  whole chromosome
    meiotic nondisjunction Q93.Ø
    mitotic nondisjunction Q93.1
    mosaicism Q93.1
  X Q96.9
Monster, monstrosity (single) Q89.7
  acephalic QØØ.Ø
  twin Q89.4
Monteggia's fracture (-dislocation) S52.27- ☑
Mooren's ulcer (cornea) — *see* Ulcer, cornea, Mooren's
Moore's syndrome — *see* Epilepsy, specified NEC
Mooser-Neill reaction A75.2
Mooser's bodies A75.2
Morbidity not stated or unknown R69
Morbilli — *see* Measles
Morbus (*see also* Disease)
  angelicus, anglorum E55.Ø
  Beigel B36.2
  caducus — *see* Epilepsy
  celiacus K9Ø.Ø
  comitialis — *see* Epilepsy
  cordis (*see also* Disease, heart) I51.9
    valvulorum — *see* Endocarditis
  coxae senilis M16.9
    tuberculous A18.Ø2
  hemorrhagicus neonatorum P53
  maculosus neonatorum P54.5
Morel (-Stewart)(-Morgagni) **syndrome** M85.2
Morel-Kraepelin disease — *see* Schizophrenia
Morel-Moore syndrome M85.2
Morgagni's
  cyst, organ, hydatid, or appendage
    female Q5Ø.5
    male (epididymal) Q55.4
      testicular Q55.29
  syndrome M85.2
Morgagni-Stewart-Morel syndrome M85.2
Morgagni-Stokes-Adams syndrome I45.9
Morgagni-Turner (-Albright) **syndrome** Q96.9
Moria FØ7.Ø
Moron (I.Q. 5Ø-69) F7Ø
Morphea L94.Ø
Morphinism (without remission) F11.2Ø
  with remission F11.21
Morphinomania (without remission) F11.2Ø
  with remission F11.21
Morquio (-Ullrich)(-Brailsford) **disease or syndrome** — *see* Mucopolysaccharidosis
Mortification (dry) (moist) — *see* Gangrene
Morton's metatarsalgia (neuralgia)(neuroma) (syndrome) G57.6- ☑
Morvan's disease or syndrome G6Ø.8
Mosaicism, mosaic (autosomal) (chromosomal)
  45,X/46,XX Q96.3
  45,X/other cell lines NEC with abnormal sex chromosome Q96.4
  sex chromosome
    female Q97.8
    lines with various numbers of X chromosomes Q97.2
    male Q98.7
  XY Q96.3
Moschowitz' disease M31.1
Mother yaw A66.Ø
Motion sickness (from travel, any vehicle) (from roundabouts or swings) T75.3 ☑
Mottled, mottling, teeth (enamel) (endemic) (nonendemic) KØØ.3
Mounier-Kuhn syndrome Q32.4
  with bronchiectasis J47.9
    exacerbation (acute) J47.1
    lower respiratory infection J47.Ø
  acquired J98.Ø9
    with bronchiectasis J47.9
      with
        exacerbation (acute) J47.1
        lower respiratory infection J47.Ø
Mountain
  sickness T7Ø.29 ☑
    with polycythemia , acquired (acute) D75.1
  tick fever A93.2
Mouse, joint — *see* Loose, body, joint
  knee M23.4- ☑
Mouth — *see* condition
Movable
  coccyx — *see* subcategory M53.2 ☑
  kidney N28.89
    congenital Q63.8
  spleen D73.89
Movements, dystonic R25.8
Moyamoya disease I67.5
MRSA (Methicillin resistant Staphylococcus aureus)
  infection A49.Ø2
    as the cause of diseases classified elsewhere B95.62
  sepsis A41.Ø2
MSSA (Methicillin susceptible Staphylococcus aureus)
  infection A49.Ø1
    as the cause of diseases classified elsewhere B95.61
  sepsis A41.Ø1
Mucha-Habermann disease L41.Ø
Mucinosis (cutaneous) (focal) (papular) (skin) L98.5
  oral K13.79
Mucocele
  appendix K38.8
  buccal cavity K13.79
  gallbladder K82.1
  lacrimal sac, chronic HØ4.43- ☑
  nasal sinus J34.1
  nose J34.1
  salivary gland (any) K11.6
  sinus (accessory) (nasal) J34.1
  turbinate (bone) (middle) (nasal) J34.1
  uterus N85.8
Mucolipidosis
  I E77.1
  II, III E77.Ø
  IV E75.11
Mucopolysaccharidosis E76.3
  beta-gluduronidase deficiency E76.29
  cardiopathy E76.3 [I52]
  Hunter's syndrome E76.1
  Hurler's syndrome E76.Ø1
  Hurler-Scheie syndrome E76.Ø2
  Maroteaux-Lamy syndrome E76.29
  Morquio syndrome E76.219
    A E76.21Ø
    B E76.211
    classic E76.21Ø
Mucopolysaccharidosis — *continued*
  Sanfilippo syndrome E76.22
  Scheie's syndrome E76.Ø3
  specified NEC E76.29
  type
    I
      Hurler's syndrome E76.Ø1
      Hurler-Scheie syndrome E76.Ø2
      Scheie's syndrome E76.Ø3
    II E76.1
    III E76.22
    IV E76.219
    IVA E76.21Ø
    IVB E76.211
    VI E76.29
    VII E76.29
Mucormycosis B46.5
  cutaneous B46.3
  disseminated B46.4
  gastrointestinal B46.2
  generalized B46.4
  pulmonary B46.Ø
  rhinocerebral B46.1
  skin B46.3
  subcutaneous B46.3
Mucositis (ulcerative) K12.3Ø
  due to drugs NEC K12.32
  gastrointestinal K92.81
  mouth (oral) (oropharyngeal) K12.3Ø
    due to antineoplastic therapy K12.31
    due to drugs NEC K12.32
    due to radiation K12.33
    specified NEC K12.39
    viral K12.39
  nasal J34.81
  oral cavity — *see* Mucositis, mouth
  oral soft tissues — *see* Mucositis, mouth
  vagina and vulva N76.81
Mucositis necroticans agranulocytica — *see* Agranulocytosis
Mucous (*see also* condition)
  patches (syphilitic) A51.39
    congenital A5Ø.Ø7
Mucoviscidosis E84.9
  with meconium obstruction E84.11
Mucus
  asphyxia or suffocation — *see* Asphyxia, mucus
  in stool R19.5
  plug — *see* Asphyxia, mucus
Muguet B37.Ø
Mulberry molars (congenital syphilis) A5Ø.52
Müllerian mixed tumor
  specified site — *see* Neoplasm, malignant, by site
  unspecified site C54.9
Multicystic kidney (development) Q61.4
Multiparity (grand) Z64.1
  affecting management of pregnancy, labor and delivery (supervision only) OØ9.4- ☑
  requiring contraceptive management — *see* Contraception
Multipartita placenta O43.19- ☑
Multiple, multiplex (*see also* condition)
  digits (congenital) Q69.9
  endocrine neoplasia — *see* Neoplasia, endocrine, multiple (MEN)
  personality F44.81
Mumps B26.9
  arthritis B26.85
  complication NEC B26.89
  encephalitis B26.2
  hepatitis B26.81
  meningitis (aseptic) B26.1
  meningoencephalitis B26.2
  myocarditis B26.82
  oophoritis B26.89
  orchitis B26.Ø
  pancreatitis B26.3
  polyneuropathy B26.84
Mumu (*see also* Infestation, filarial) B74.9 [N51]
Münchhausen's syndrome — *see* Disorder, factitious
Münchmeyer's syndrome — *see* Myositis, ossificans, progressiva
Mural — *see* condition
Murmur (cardiac) (heart) (organic) RØ1.1
  abdominal R19.15
  aortic (valve) — *see* Endocarditis, aortic
  benign RØ1.Ø
  diastolic — *see* Endocarditis

- **Murmur** — *continued*
  - Flint I35.1
  - functional RØ1.Ø
  - Graham Steell I37.1
  - innocent RØ1.Ø
  - mitral (valve) — *see* Insufficiency, mitral
  - nonorganic RØ1.Ø
  - presystolic, mitral — *see* Insufficiency, mitral
  - pulmonic (valve) I37.8
  - systolic (valvular) — *see* Endocarditis
  - tricuspid (valve) IØ7.9
  - valvular — *see* Endocarditis
- **Murri's disease** (intermittent hemoglobinuria) D59.6
- **Muscle, muscular** (*see also* condition)
  - carnitine (palmityltransferase) deficiency E71.314
- **Musculoneuralgia** — *see* Neuralgia
- **Mushrooming hip** — *see* Derangement, joint, specified NEC, hip
- **Mushroom-workers'** (pickers') **disease or lung** J67.5
- **Mutation**(s)
  - factor V Leiden D68.51
  - prothrombin gene D68.52
  - surfactant, of lung J84.83
- **Mutism** (*see also* Aphasia)
  - deaf (acquired) (congenital) NEC H91.3
  - elective (adjustment reaction) (childhood) F94.Ø
  - hysterical F44.4
  - selective (childhood) F94.Ø
- **MVD** (microvillus inclusion disease) Q43.8
- **MVID** (microvillus inclusion disease) Q43.8
- **Myalgia** M79.1
  - epidemic (cervical) B33.Ø
  - traumatic NEC T14.8
- **Myasthenia** G7Ø.9
  - congenital G7Ø.2
  - cordis — *see* Failure, heart
  - developmental G7Ø.2
  - gravis G7Ø.ØØ
    - with exacerbation (acute) G7Ø.Ø1
    - in crisis G7Ø.Ø1
    - neonatal, transient P94.Ø
    - pseudoparalytica G7Ø.ØØ
      - with exacerbation (acute) G7Ø.Ø1
      - in crisis G7Ø.Ø1
  - stomach, psychogenic F45.8
  - syndrome
    - in
      - diabetes mellitus — *see* EØ8-E13 with .44
      - neoplastic disease (*see also* Neoplasm) D49.9 [G73.3]
      - pernicious anemia D51.Ø [G73.3]
      - thyrotoxicosis EØ5.9Ø [G73.3]
        - with thyroid storm EØ5.91 [G73.3]
- **Myasthenic** M62.81
- **Mycelium infection** B49
- **Mycetismus** — *see* Poisoning, food, noxious, mushroom
- **Mycetoma** B47.9
  - actinomycotic B47.1
  - bone (mycotic) B47.9 [M9Ø.8Ø]
  - eumycotic B47.Ø
  - foot B47.9
    - actinomycotic B47.1
    - mycotic B47.Ø
  - madurae NEC B47.9
    - mycotic B47.Ø
  - maduromycotic B47.Ø
  - mycotic B47.Ø
  - nocardial B47.1
- **Mycobacteriosis** — *see* Mycobacterium
- **Mycobacterium, mycobacterial** (infection) A31.9
  - anonymous A31.9
  - atypical A31.9
    - cutaneous A31.1
    - pulmonary A31.Ø
      - tuberculous — *see* Tuberculosis, pulmonary
    - specified site NEC A31.8
  - avium (intracellulare complex) A31.Ø
  - balnei A31.1
  - Battey A31.Ø
  - chelonei A31.8
  - cutaneous A31.1
  - extrapulmonary systemic A31.8
  - fortuitum A31.8
  - intracellulare (Battey bacillus) A31.Ø
  - kakaferifu A31.8
  - kansasii (yellow bacillus) A31.Ø
  - kasongo A31.8
  - leprae (*see also* Leprosy) A3Ø.9
- **Mycobacterium, mycobacterial** — *continued*
  - luciflavum A31.1
  - marinum (M. balnei) A31.1
  - nonspecific — *see* Mycobacterium, atypical
  - pulmonary (atypical) A31.Ø
    - tuberculous — *see* Tuberculosis, pulmonary
  - scrofulaceum A31.8
  - simiae A31.8
  - systemic, extrapulmonary A31.8
  - szulgai A31.8
  - terrae A31.8
  - triviale A31.8
  - tuberculosis (human, bovine) — *see* Tuberculosis
  - ulcerans A31.1
  - xenopi A31.8
- **Mycoplasma** (M.) **pneumoniae, as cause of disease classified elsewhere** B96.Ø
- **Mycosis, mycotic** B49
  - cutaneous NEC B36.9
  - ear B36.8
  - fungoides (extranodal) (solid organ) C84.Ø- ☑
  - mouth B37.Ø
  - nails B35.1
  - opportunistic B48.8
  - skin NEC B36.9
  - specified NEC B48.8
  - stomatitis B37.Ø
  - vagina, vaginitis (candidal) B37.3
- **Mydriasis** (pupil) H57.Ø4
- **Myelatelia** QØ6.1
- **Myelinolysis, pontine, central** G37.2
- **Myelitis** (acute) (ascending) (childhood) (chronic) (descending) (diffuse) (disseminated) (idiopathic) (pressure) (progressive) (spinal cord) (subacute) (*see also* Encephalitis) GØ4.91
  - herpes simplex BØØ.82
  - herpes zoster BØ2.24
  - in diseases classified elsewhere GØ5.4
  - necrotizing, subacute G37.4
  - optic neuritis in G36.Ø
  - postchickenpox BØ1.12
  - postherpetic BØ2.24
  - postimmunization GØ4.Ø2
  - postinfectious NEC GØ4.89
  - postvaccinal GØ4.Ø2
  - specified NEC GØ4.89
  - syphilitic (transverse) A52.14
  - toxic G92
  - transverse (in demyelinating diseases of central nervous system) G37.3
  - tuberculous A17.82
  - varicella BØ1.12
- **Myeloblastic** — *see* condition
- **Myeloblastoma**
  - granular cell (*see also* Neoplasm, connective tissue)
    - malignant — *see* Neoplasm, connective tissue, malignant
  - tongue D1Ø.1
- **Myelocele** — *see* Spina bifida
- **Myelocystocele** — *see* Spina bifida
- **Myelocytic** — *see* condition
- **Myelodysplasia** D46.9
  - specified NEC D46.Z (*following* D46.4)
  - spinal cord (congenital) QØ6.1
- **Myelodysplastic syndrome** D46.9
  - with
    - 5q deletion D46.C (*following* D46.2)
    - isolated del (5q) chromosomal abnormality D46.C (*following* D46.2)
  - specified NEC D46.Z (*following* D46.4)
- **Myeloencephalitis** — *see* Encephalitis
- **Myelofibrosis** D75.81
  - with myeloid metaplasia D47.4
  - acute C94.4- ☑
  - idiopathic (chronic) D47.4
  - primary D47.1
  - secondary D75.81
    - in myeloproliferative disease D47.4
- **Myelogenous** — *see* condition
- **Myeloid** — *see* condition
- **Myelokathexis** D7Ø.9
- **Myeloleukodystrophy** E75.29
- **Myelolipoma** — *see* Lipoma
- **Myeloma** (multiple) C9Ø.Ø- ☑
  - monostotic C9Ø.3 ☑
    - plasma cell C9Ø.Ø- ☑
  - plasma cell C9Ø.Ø- ☑
- **Myeloma** — *continued*
  - solitary (*see also* Plasmacytoma, solitary) C9Ø.3- ☑
- **Myelomalacia** G95.89
- **Myelomatosis** C9Ø.Ø- ☑
- **Myelomeningitis** — *see* Meningoencephalitis
- **Myelomeningocele** (spinal cord) — *see* Spina bifida
- **Myelo-osteo-musculodysplasia hereditaria** Q79.8
- **Myelopathic**
  - anemia D64.89
  - muscle atrophy — *see* Atrophy, muscle, spinal
  - pain syndrome G89.Ø
- **Myelopathy** (spinal cord) G95.9
  - drug-induced G95.89
  - in (due to)
    - degeneration or displacement, intervertebral disc NEC — *see* Disorder, disc, with, myelopathy
    - infection — *see* Encephalitis
    - intervertebral disc disorder (*see also* Disorder, disc, with, myelopathy)
    - mercury — *see* subcategory T56.1 ☑
    - neoplastic disease (*see also* Neoplasm) D49.9 [G99.2]
    - pernicious anemia D51.Ø [G99.2]
    - spondylosis — *see* Spondylosis, with myelopathy NEC
  - necrotic (subacute) (vascular) G95.19
  - radiation-induced G95.89
  - spondylogenic NEC — *see* Spondylosis, with myelopathy NEC
  - toxic G95.89
  - transverse, acute G37.3
  - vascular G95.19
  - vitamin B12 E53.8 [G32.Ø]
- **Myelophthisis** D61.82
- **Myeloradiculitis** GØ4.91
- **Myeloradiculodysplasia** (spinal) QØ6.1
- **Myelosarcoma** C92.3- ☑
- **Myelosclerosis** D75.89
  - with myeloid metaplasia D47.4
  - disseminated, of nervous system G35
  - megakaryocytic D47.4
    - with myeloid metaplasia D47.4
- **Myelosis**
  - acute C92.Ø- ☑
  - aleukemic C92.9- ☑
  - chronic D47.1
  - erythremic (acute) C94.Ø- ☑
  - megakaryocytic C94.2- ☑
  - nonleukemic D72.828
  - subacute C92.9- ☑
- **Myiasis** (cavernous) B87.9
  - aural B87.4
  - creeping B87.Ø
  - cutaneous B87.Ø
  - dermal B87.Ø
  - ear (external) (middle) B87.4
  - eye B87.2
  - genitourinary B87.81
  - intestinal B87.82
  - laryngeal B87.3
  - nasopharyngeal B87.3
  - ocular B87.2
  - orbit B87.2
  - skin B87.Ø
  - specified site NEC B87.89
  - traumatic B87.1
  - wound B87.1
- **Myoadenoma, prostate** — *see* Hyperplasia, prostate
- **Myoblastoma**
  - granular cell (*see also* Neoplasm, connective tissue, benign)
    - malignant — *see* Neoplasm, connective tissue, malignant
  - tongue D1Ø.1
- **Myocardial** — *see* condition
- **Myocardiopathy** (congestive) (constrictive) (familial) (hypertrophic nonobstructive) (idiopathic) (infiltrative) (obstructive) (primary) (restrictive) (sporadic) (*see also* Cardiomyopathy) I42.9
  - alcoholic I42.6
  - cobalt-beer I42.6
  - glycogen storage E74.Ø2 [I43]
  - hypertrophic obstructive I42.1
  - in (due to)
    - beriberi E51.12
    - cardiac glycogenosis E74.Ø2 [I43]
    - Friedreich's ataxia G11.1 [I43]

N

- **Naegeli's**
  - disease Q82.8
  - leukemia, monocytic C93.1- ☑
- **Naegleriasis** (with meningoencephalitis) B6Ø.2
- **Naffziger's syndrome** G54.Ø
- **Naga sore** — *see* Ulcer, skin
- **Nägele's pelvis** M95.5
  - with disproportion (fetopelvic) O33.Ø
    - causing obstructed labor O65.Ø
- **Nail** (*see also* condition)
  - biting F98.8
  - patella syndrome Q87.2
- **Nanism, nanosomia** — *see* Dwarfism
- **Nanophyetiasis** B66.8
- **Nanukayami** A27.89
- **Napkin rash** L22
- **Narcolepsy** G47.419
  - with cataplexy G47.411
  - in conditions classified elsewhere G47.429
    - with cataplexy G47.421
- **Narcosis** RØ6.89
- **Narcotism** — *see* Dependence
- **NARP** (Neuropathy, Ataxia and Retinitis pigmentosa) syndrome E88.49
- **Narrow**
  - anterior chamber angle H4Ø.Ø3- ☑
  - pelvis — *see* Contraction, pelvis
- **Narrowing** (*see also* Stenosis)
  - artery I77.1
    - auditory, internal I65.8
    - basilar — *see* Occlusion, artery, basilar
    - carotid — *see* Occlusion, artery, carotid
    - cerebellar — *see* Occlusion, artery, cerebellar
    - cerebral — *see* Occlusion artery, cerebral
    - choroidal — *see* Occlusion, artery, cerebral, specified NEC
    - communicating posterior — *see* Occlusion, artery, cerebral, specified NEC
    - coronary (*see also* Disease, heart, ischemic, atherosclerotic)
      - congenital Q24.5
        - syphilitic A5Ø.54 [I52]
      - due to syphilis NEC A52.Ø6
    - hypophyseal — *see* Occlusion, artery, cerebral, specified NEC
    - pontine — *see* Occlusion, artery, cerebral, specified NEC
    - precerebral — *see* Occlusion, artery, precerebral
    - vertebral — *see* Occlusion, artery, vertebral
  - auditory canal (external) — *see* Stenosis, external ear canal
  - eustachian tube — *see* Obstruction, eustachian tube
  - eyelid — *see* Disorder, eyelid function
  - larynx J38.6
  - mesenteric artery K55.Ø
  - palate M26.89
  - palpebral fissure — *see* Disorder, eyelid function
  - ureter N13.5
    - with infection N13.6
  - urethra — *see* Stricture, urethra
- **Narrowness, abnormal, eyelid** Q1Ø.3
- **Nasal** — *see* condition
- **Nasolachrymal, nasolacrimal** — *see* condition
- **Nasopharyngeal** (*see also* condition)
  - pituitary gland Q89.2
  - torticollis M43.6
- **Nasopharyngitis** (acute) (infective) (streptococcal) (subacute) JØØ
  - chronic (suppurative) (ulcerative) J31.1
- **Nasopharynx, nasopharyngeal** — *see* condition
- **Natal tooth, teeth** KØØ.6
- **Nausea** (without vomiting) R11.Ø
  - with vomiting R11.2
  - gravidarum — *see* Hyperemesis, gravidarum
  - marina T75.3 ☑
  - navalis T75.3 ☑
- **Navel** — *see* condition
- **Neapolitan fever** — *see* Brucellosis
- **Near drowning** T75.1 ☑
- **Nearsightedness** — *see* Myopia
- **Near-syncope** R55
- **Nebula, cornea** — *see* Opacity, cornea
- **Necator americanus infestation** B76.1
- **Necatoriasis** B76.1
- **Neck** — *see* condition
- **Necrobiosis** R68.89
  - lipoidica NEC L92.1
    - with diabetes — *see* EØ8-E13 with .62Ø
- **Necrolysis, toxic epidermal** L51.2
  - due to drug
    - correct substance properly administered — *see* Table of Drugs and Chemicals, by drug, adverse effect
    - overdose or wrong substance given or taken — *see* Table of Drugs and Chemicals, by drug, poisoning
- **Necrophilia** F65.89
- **Necrosis, necrotic** (ischemic) (*see also* Gangrene)
  - adrenal (capsule) (gland) E27.49
  - amputation stump (surgical) (late) T87.5Ø
    - arm T87.5- ☑
    - leg T87.5- ☑
  - antrum J32.Ø
  - aorta (hyaline) (*see also* Aneurysm, aorta)
    - cystic medial — *see* Dissection, aorta
  - artery I77.5
  - bladder (aseptic) (sphincter) N32.89
  - bone (*see also* Osteonecrosis) M87.9
    - aseptic or avascular — *see* Osteonecrosis
      - idiopathic M87.ØØ
    - ethmoid J32.2
    - jaw M27.2
    - tuberculous — *see* Tuberculosis, bone
  - brain I67.89
  - breast (aseptic) (fat) (segmental) N64.1
  - bronchus J98.Ø9
  - central nervous system NEC I67.89
  - cerebellar I67.89
  - cerebral I67.89
  - colon K55.Ø
  - cornea H18.4Ø
  - cortical (acute) (renal) N17.1
  - cystic medial (aorta) — *see* Dissection, aorta
  - dental pulp KØ4.1
  - esophagus K22.8
  - ethmoid (bone) J32.2
  - eyelid — *see* Disorder, eyelid, degenerative
  - fat, fatty (generalized) (*see also* Disorder, soft tissue, specified type NEC)
    - abdominal wall K65.4
    - breast (aseptic) (segmental) N64.1
    - localized — *see* Degeneration, by site, fatty
    - mesentery K65.4
    - omentum K65.4
    - pancreas K86.8
    - peritoneum K65.4
    - skin (subcutaneous), newborn P83.Ø
    - subcutaneous, due to birth injury P15.6
  - gallbladder — *see* Cholecystitis, acute
  - heart — *see* Infarct, myocardium
  - hip, aseptic or avascular — *see* Osteonecrosis, by type, femur
  - intestine (acute) (hemorrhagic) (massive) K55.Ø
  - jaw M27.2
  - kidney (bilateral) N28.Ø
    - acute N17.9
    - cortical (acute) (bilateral) N17.1
      - with ectopic or molar pregnancy OØ8.4
    - medullary (bilateral) (in acute renal failure) (papillary) N17.2
    - papillary (bilateral) (in acute renal failure) N17.2
    - tubular N17.Ø
      - with ectopic or molar pregnancy OØ8.4
      - complicating
        - abortion — *see* Abortion, by type, complicated by, tubular necrosis
        - ectopic or molar pregnancy OØ8.4
        - pregnancy — *see* Pregnancy, complicated by, diseases of, specified type or system NEC

Necrosis, necrotic — *continued*

  - kidney — *continued*
    - tubular — *continued*
      - following ectopic or molar pregnancy OØ8.4
      - traumatic T79.5 ☑
  - larynx J38.7
  - liver (with hepatic failure) (cell) — *see* Failure, hepatic
    - hemorrhagic, central K76.2
  - lung J85.Ø
  - lymphatic gland — *see* Lymphadenitis, acute
  - mammary gland (fat) (segmental) N64.1
  - mastoid (chronic) — *see* Mastoiditis, chronic
  - medullary (acute) (renal) N17.2
  - mesentery K55.Ø
    - fat K65.4
  - mitral valve — *see* Insufficiency, mitral
  - myocardium, myocardial — *see* Infarct, myocardium
  - nose J34.Ø
  - omentum (with mesenteric infarction) K55.Ø
    - fat K65.4
  - orbit, orbital — *see* Osteomyelitis, orbit
  - ossicles, ear — *see* Abnormal, ear ossicles
  - ovary N7Ø.92
  - pancreas (aseptic) (duct) (fat) K86.8
    - acute (infective) — *see* Pancreatitis, acute
    - infective — *see* Pancreatitis, acute
  - papillary (acute) (renal) N17.2
  - perineum N9Ø.89
  - peritoneum (with mesenteric infarction) K55.Ø
    - fat K65.4
  - pharynx JØ2.9
    - in granulocytopenia — *see* Neutropenia
    - Vincent's A69.1
  - phosphorus — *see* subcategory T54.2 ☑
  - pituitary (gland) (postpartum) (Sheehan) E23.Ø
  - pressure — *see* Ulcer, pressure, by site
  - pulmonary J85.Ø
  - pulp (dental) KØ4.1
  - radiation — *see* Necrosis, by site
  - radium — *see* Necrosis, by site
  - renal — *see* Necrosis, kidney
  - sclera H15.89
  - scrotum N5Ø.8
  - skin or subcutaneous tissue NEC I96
  - spine, spinal (column) (*see also* Osteonecrosis, by type, vertebra)
    - cord G95.19
  - spleen D73.5
  - stomach K31.89
  - stomatitis (ulcerative) A69.Ø
  - subcutaneous fat, newborn P83.8
  - subendocardial (acute) I21.4
    - chronic I25.89
  - suprarenal (capsule) (gland) E27.49
  - testis N5Ø.8
  - thymus (gland) E32.8
  - tonsil J35.8
  - trachea J39.8
  - tuberculous NEC — *see* Tuberculosis
  - tubular (acute) (anoxic) (renal) (toxic) N17.Ø
    - postprocedural N99.Ø
  - vagina N89.8
  - vertebra (*see also* Osteonecrosis, by type, vertebra)
    - tuberculous A18.Ø1
  - vulva N9Ø.89
  - X-ray — *see* Necrosis, by site
- **Necrospermia** — *see* Infertility, male
- **Need** (for)
  - care provider because (of)
    - assistance with personal care Z74.1
    - continuous supervision required Z74.3
    - impaired mobility Z74.Ø9
    - no other household member able to render care Z74.2
    - specified reason NEC Z74.8
  - immunization — *see* Vaccination
  - vaccination — *see* Vaccination
- **Neglect**
  - adult
    - confirmed T74.Ø1 ☑
    - history of Z91.412
    - suspected T76.Ø1 ☑

- **Neglect** — *continued*
  - child (childhood)
    - confirmed T74.Ø2 ☑
    - history of Z62.812
    - suspected T76.Ø2 ☑
  - emotional, in childhood Z62.898
  - hemispatial R41.4
  - left-sided R41.4
  - sensory R41.4
  - visuospatial R41.4
- **Neisserian infection NEC** — *see* Gonococcus
- **Nelaton's syndrome** G6Ø.8
- **Nelson's syndrome** E24.1
- **Nematodiasis** (intestinal) B82.Ø
  - Ancylostoma B76.Ø
- **Neonatal** (*see also* Newborn)
  - acne L7Ø.4
  - bradycardia P29.12
  - screening, abnormal findings on PØ9
  - tachycardia P29.11
  - tooth, teeth KØØ.6
- **Neonatorum** — *see* condition
- **Neoplasia**
  - endocrine, multiple (MEN) E31.2Ø
    - type I E31.21
    - type IIA E31.22
    - type IIB E31.23
  - intraepithelial (histologically confirmed)
    - anal (AIN) (histologically confirmed) K62.82
      - grade I K62.82
      - grade II K62.82
      - severe DØ1.3
    - cervical glandular (histologically confirmed) DØ6.9
    - cervix (uteri) (CIN) (histologically confirmed) N87.9
      - glandular DØ6.9
      - grade I N87.Ø
      - grade II N87.1
      - grade III (severe dysplasia) (*see also* Carcinoma, cervix uteri, in situ) DØ6.9
    - prostate (histologically confirmed) (PIN I) (PIN II) N42.3
      - grade I N42.3
      - grade II N42.3
      - severe DØ7.5
    - vagina (histologically confirmed) (VAIN) N89.3
      - grade I N89.Ø
      - grade II N89.1
      - grade III (severe dysplasia) DØ7.2
    - vulva (histologically confirmed) (VIN) N9Ø.3
      - grade I N9Ø.Ø
      - grade II N9Ø.1
      - grade III (severe dysplasia) DØ7.1
- **Neoplasm, neoplastic** (*see also* Table of Neoplasms)
  - lipomatous, benign — *see* Lipoma
- **Neovascularization**
  - ciliary body — *see* Disorder, iris, vascular
  - cornea H16.4Ø- ☑
    - deep H16.44- ☑
    - ghost vessels — *see* Ghost, vessels
    - localized H16.43- ☑
    - pannus — *see* Pannus
  - iris — *see* Disorder, iris, vascular
  - retina H35.Ø5- ☑
- **Nephralgia** N23
- **Nephritis, nephritic** (albuminuric) (azotemic) (congenital) (disseminated) (epithelial) (familial) (focal) (granulomatous) (hemorrhagic) (infantile) (nonsuppurative, excretory) (uremic) NØ5.9
  - with
    - dense deposit disease NØ5.6
    - diffuse
      - crescentic glomerulonephritis NØ5.7
      - endocapillary proliferative glomerulonephritis NØ5.4
      - membranous glomerulonephritis NØ5.2
      - mesangial proliferative glomerulonephritis NØ5.3
      - mesangiocapillary glomerulonephritis NØ5.5
    - edema — *see* Nephrosis
    - focal and segmental glomerular lesions NØ5.1
    - foot process disease NØ4.9
    - glomerular lesion
      - diffuse sclerosing NØ5.8
      - hypocomplementemic — *see* Nephritis, membranoproliferative
      - IgA — *see* Nephropathy, IgA
      - lobular, lobulonodular — *see* Nephritis, membranoproliferative

- **Nephritis, nephritic** — *continued*
  - with — *continued*
    - glomerular lesion — *continued*
      - nodular — *see* Nephritis, membranoproliferative
    - lesion of
      - glomerulonephritis, proliferative NØ5.8
      - renal necrosis NØ5.9
    - minor glomerular abnormality NØ5.Ø
    - specified morphological changes NEC NØ5.8
  - acute NØØ.9
    - with
      - dense deposit disease NØØ.6
      - diffuse
        - crescentic glomerulonephritis NØØ.7
        - endocapillary proliferative glomerulonephritis NØØ.4
        - membranous glomerulonephritis NØØ.2
        - mesangial proliferative glomerulonephritis NØØ.3
        - mesangiocapillary glomerulonephritis NØØ.5
      - focal and segmental glomerular lesions NØØ.1
      - minor glomerular abnormality NØØ.Ø
      - specified morphological changes NEC NØØ.8
  - amyloid E85.4 [NØ8]
  - antiglomerular basement membrane (anti-GBM) antibody NEC
    - in Goodpasture's syndrome M31.Ø
  - antitubular basement membrane (tubulo-interstitial) NEC N12
    - toxic — *see* Nephropathy, toxic
  - arteriolar — *see* Hypertension, kidney
  - arteriosclerotic — *see* Hypertension, kidney
  - ascending — *see* Nephritis, tubulo-interstitial
  - atrophic NØ3.9
  - Balkan (endemic) N15.Ø
  - calculous, calculus — *see* Calculus, kidney
  - cardiac — *see* Hypertension, kidney
  - cardiovascular — *see* Hypertension, kidney
  - chronic NØ3.9
    - with
      - dense deposit disease NØ3.6
      - diffuse
        - crescentic glomerulonephritis NØ3.7
        - endocapillary proliferative glomerulonephritis NØ3.4
        - membranous glomerulonephritis NØ3.2
        - mesangial proliferative glomerulonephritis NØ3.3
        - mesangiocapillary glomerulonephritis NØ3.5
      - focal and segmental glomerular lesions NØ3.1
      - minor glomerular abnormality NØ3.Ø
      - specified morphological changes NEC NØ3.8
    - arteriosclerotic — *see* Hypertension, kidney
  - cirrhotic N26.9
  - complicating pregnancy O26.83- ☑
  - croupous NØØ.9
  - degenerative — *see* Nephrosis
  - diffuse sclerosing NØ5.8
  - due to
    - diabetes mellitus — *see* EØ8-E13 with .21
    - subacute bacterial endocarditis I33.Ø
    - systemic lupus erythematosus (chronic) M32.14
    - typhoid fever AØ1.Ø9
  - gonococcal (acute) (chronic) A54.21
  - hypocomplementemic — *see* Nephritis, membranoproliferative
  - IgA — *see* Nephropathy, IgA
  - immune complex (circulating) NEC NØ5.8
  - infective — *see* Nephritis, tubulo-interstitial
  - interstitial — *see* Nephritis, tubulo-interstitial
  - lead N14.3
  - membranoproliferative (diffuse) (type 1 or 3) (*see also* NØØ-NØ7 with fourth character .5) NØ5.5
    - type 2 (*see also* NØØ-NØ7 with fourth character .6) NØ5.6
  - minimal change NØ5.Ø
  - necrotic, necrotizing NEC (*see also* NØØ-NØ7 with fourth character .8) NØ5.8
  - nephrotic — *see* Nephrosis
  - nodular — *see* Nephritis, membranoproliferative
  - polycystic Q61.3
    - adult type Q61.2
    - autosomal
      - dominant Q61.2
      - recessive NEC Q61.19
    - childhood type NEC Q61.19
    - infantile type NEC Q61.19

- **Nephritis, nephritic** — *continued*
  - poststreptococcal NØ5.9
    - acute NØØ.9
    - chronic NØ3.9
    - rapidly progressive NØ1.9
  - proliferative NEC (*see also* NØØ-NØ7 with fourth character .8) NØ5.8
  - purulent — *see* Nephritis, tubulo-interstitial
  - rapidly progressive NØ1.9
    - with
      - dense deposit disease NØ1.6
      - diffuse
        - crescentic glomerulonephritis NØ1.7
        - endocapillary proliferative glomerulonephritis NØ1.4
        - membranous glomerulonephritis NØ1.2
        - mesangial proliferative glomerulonephritis NØ1.3
        - mesangiocapillary glomerulonephritis NØ1.5
      - focal and segmental glomerular lesions NØ1.1
      - minor glomerular abnormality NØ1.Ø
      - specified morphological changes NEC NØ1.8
  - salt losing or wasting NEC N28.89
  - saturnine N14.3
  - sclerosing, diffuse NØ5.8
  - septic — *see* Nephritis, tubulo-interstitial
  - specified pathology NEC (*see also* NØØ-NØ7 with fourth character .8) NØ5.8
  - subacute NØ1.9
  - suppurative — *see* Nephritis, tubulo-interstitial
  - syphilitic (late) A52.75
    - congenital A5Ø.59 [NØ8]
    - early (secondary) A51.44
  - toxic — *see* Nephropathy, toxic
  - tubal, tubular — *see* Nephritis, tubulo-interstitial
  - tuberculous A18.11
  - tubulo-interstitial (in) N12
    - acute (infectious) N1Ø
    - chronic (infectious) N11.9
      - nonobstructive N11.8
        - reflux-associated N11.Ø
      - obstructive N11.1
      - specified NEC N11.8
    - due to
      - brucellosis A23.9 [N16]
      - cryoglobulinemia D89.1 [N16]
      - glycogen storage disease E74.ØØ [N16]
    - Sjögren's syndrome M35.Ø4
  - vascular — *see* Hypertension, kidney
  - war NØØ.9
- **Nephroblastoma** (epithelial) (mesenchymal) C64- ☑
- **Nephrocalcinosis** E83.59 [N29]
- **Nephrocystitis, pustular** — *see* Nephritis, tubulo-interstitial
- **Nephrolithiasis** (congenital) (pelvis) (recurrent) (*see also* Calculus, kidney)
- **Nephroma** C64- ☑
  - mesoblastic D41.Ø- ☑
- **Nephronephritis** — *see* Nephrosis
- **Nephronophthisis** Q61.5
- **Nephropathia epidemica** A98.5
- **Nephropathy** (*see also* Nephritis) N28.9
  - with
    - edema — *see* Nephrosis
    - glomerular lesion — *see* Glomerulonephritis
  - amyloid, hereditary E85.Ø
  - analgesic N14.Ø
    - with medullary necrosis, acute N17.2
  - Balkan (endemic) N15.Ø
  - chemical — *see* Nephropathy, toxic
  - diabetic — *see* EØ8-E13 with .21
  - drug-induced N14.2
    - specified NEC N14.1
  - focal and segmental hyalinosis or sclerosis NØ2.1
  - heavy metal-induced N14.3
  - hereditary NEC NØ7.9
    - with
      - dense deposit disease NØ7.6
      - diffuse
        - crescentic glomerulonephritis NØ7.7
        - endocapillary proliferative glomerulonephritis NØ7.4
        - membranous glomerulonephritis NØ7.2
        - mesangial proliferative glomerulonephritis NØ7.3
        - mesangiocapillary glomerulonephritis NØ7.5
      - focal and segmental glomerular lesions NØ7.1
      - minor glomerular abnormality NØ7.Ø

- **Nephropathy** — *continued*
  - hereditary — *continued*
    - with — *continued*
      - specified morphological changes NEC NØ7.8
  - hypercalcemic N25.89
  - hypertensive — *see* Hypertension, kidney
  - hypokalemic (vacuolar) N25.89
  - IgA NØ2.8
    - with glomerular lesion NØ2.9
      - focal and segmental hyalinosis or sclerosis NØ2.1
      - membranoproliferative (diffuse) NØ2.5
      - membranous (diffuse) NØ2.2
      - mesangial proliferative (diffuse) NØ2.3
      - mesangiocapillary (diffuse) NØ2.5
      - proliferative NEC NØ2.8
      - specified pathology NEC NØ2.8
  - lead N14.3
  - membranoproliferative (diffuse) NØ2.5
  - membranous (diffuse) NØ2.2
  - mesangial (IgA/IgG) — *see* Nephropathy, IgA
    - proliferative (diffuse) NØ2.3
  - mesangiocapillary (diffuse) NØ2.5
  - obstructive N13.8
  - phenacetin N17.2
  - phosphate-losing N25.Ø
  - potassium depletion N25.89
  - pregnancy-related O26.83- ☑
  - proliferative NEC (*see also* NØØ-NØ7 with fourth character .8) NØ5.8
  - protein-losing N25.89
  - saturnine N14.3
  - sickle-cell D57.- ☑ [NØ8]
  - toxic NEC N14.4
    - due to
      - drugs N14.2
        - analgesic N14.Ø
        - specified NEC N14.1
      - heavy metals N14.3
  - vasomotor N17.Ø
  - water-losing N25.89
- **Nephroptosis** N28.83
- **Nephropyosis** — *see* Abscess, kidney
- **Nephrorrhagia** N28.89
- **Nephrosclerosis** (arteriolar)(arteriosclerotic) (chronic) (hyaline) (*see also* Hypertension, kidney)
  - hyperplastic — *see* Hypertension, kidney
  - senile N26.9
- **Nephrosis, nephrotic** (Epstein's) (syndrome) (congenital) NØ4.9
  - with
    - foot process disease NØ4.9
    - glomerular lesion NØ4.1
    - hypocomplementemic NØ4.5
  - acute NØ4.9
  - anoxic — *see* Nephrosis, tubular
  - chemical — *see* Nephrosis, tubular
  - cholemic K76.7
  - diabetic — *see* EØ8-E13 with .21
  - Finnish type (congenital) Q89.8
  - hemoglobin N1Ø
  - hemoglobinuric — *see* Nephrosis, tubular
  - in
    - amyloidosis E85.4 [NØ8]
    - diabetes mellitus — *see* EØ8-E13 with .21
    - epidemic hemorrhagic fever A98.5
    - malaria (malariae) B52.Ø
  - ischemic — *see* Nephrosis, tubular
  - lipoid NØ4.9
  - lower nephron — *see* Nephrosis, tubular
  - malarial (malariae) B52.Ø
  - minimal change NØ4.Ø
  - myoglobin N1Ø
  - necrotizing — *see* Nephrosis, tubular
  - osmotic (sucrose) N25.89
  - radiation NØ4.9
  - syphilitic (late) A52.75
  - toxic — *see* Nephrosis, tubular
  - tubular (acute) N17.Ø
    - postprocedural N99.Ø
    - radiation NØ4.9
- **Nephrosonephritis, hemorrhagic** (endemic) A98.5
- **Nephrostomy**
  - attention to Z43.6
  - status Z93.6
- **Nerve** (*see also* condition)
  - injury — *see* Injury, nerve, by body site
- **Nerves** R45.Ø
- **Nervous** (*see also* condition) R45.Ø
  - heart F45.8
  - stomach F45.8
  - tension R45.Ø
- **Nervousness** R45.Ø
- **Nesidioblastoma**
  - pancreas D13.7
  - specified site NEC — *see* Neoplasm, benign, by site
  - unspecified site D13.7
- **Nettleship's syndrome** Q82.2
- **Neumann's disease or syndrome** L1Ø.1
- **Neuralgia, neuralgic** (acute) M79.2
  - accessory (nerve) G52.8
  - acoustic (nerve) — *see* subcategory H93.3 ☑
  - auditory (nerve) — *see* subcategory H93.3 ☑
  - ciliary G44.ØØ9
    - intractable G44.ØØ1
    - not intractable G44.ØØ9
  - cranial
    - nerve (*see also* Disorder, nerve, cranial)
      - fifth or trigeminal — *see* Neuralgia, trigeminal
    - postherpetic, postzoster BØ2.29
  - ear — *see* subcategory H92.Ø ☑
  - facialis vera G51.1
  - Fothergill's — *see* Neuralgia, trigeminal
  - glossopharyngeal (nerve) G52.1
  - Horton's G44.Ø99
    - intractable G44.Ø91
    - not intractable G44.Ø99
  - Hunt's BØ2.21
  - hypoglossal (nerve) G52.3
  - infraorbital — *see* Neuralgia, trigeminal
  - malarial — *see* Malaria
  - migrainous G44.ØØ9
    - intractable G44.ØØ1
    - not intractable G44.ØØ9
  - Morton's G57.6- ☑
  - nerve, cranial — *see* Disorder, nerve, cranial
  - nose G52.Ø
  - occipital M54.81
  - olfactory G52.Ø
  - penis N48.9
  - perineum R1Ø.2
  - postherpetic NEC BØ2.29
    - trigeminal BØ2.22
  - pubic region R1Ø.2
  - scrotum R1Ø.2
  - Sluder's G44.89
  - specified nerve NEC G58.8
  - spermatic cord R1Ø.2
  - sphenopalatine (ganglion) G9Ø.Ø9
  - trifacial — *see* Neuralgia, trigeminal
  - trigeminal G5Ø.Ø
    - postherpetic, postzoster BØ2.22
  - vagus (nerve) G52.2
  - writer's F48.8
    - organic G25.89
- **Neurapraxia** — *see* Injury, nerve
- **Neurasthenia** F48.8
  - cardiac F45.8
  - gastric F45.8
  - heart F45.8
- **Neurilemmoma** (*see also* Neoplasm, nerve, benign)
  - acoustic (nerve) D33.3
  - malignant (*see also* Neoplasm, nerve, malignant)
    - acoustic (nerve) C72.4- ☑
- **Neurilemmosarcoma** — *see* Neoplasm, nerve, malignant
- **Neurinoma** — *see* Neoplasm, nerve, benign
- **Neurinomatosis** — *see* Neoplasm, nerve, uncertain behavior
- **Neuritis** (rheumatoid) M79.2
  - abducens (nerve) — *see* Strabismus, paralytic, sixth nerve
  - accessory (nerve) G52.8
  - acoustic (nerve) (*see also* subcategory) H93.3 ☑
    - in (due to)
      - infectious disease NEC B99 ☑ [H94.Ø-] ☑
      - parasitic disease NEC B89 [H94.Ø-] ☑
    - syphilitic A52.15
  - alcoholic G62.1
    - with psychosis — *see* Psychosis, alcoholic
  - amyloid, any site E85.4 [G63]
  - auditory (nerve) — *see* subcategory H93.3 ☑
  - brachial — *see* Radiculopathy
    - due to displacement, intervertebral disc — *see* Disorder, disc, cervical, with neuritis
- **Neuritis** — *continued*
  - cranial nerve
    - due to Lyme disease A69.22
    - eighth or acoustic or auditory — *see* subcategory H93.3 ☑
    - eleventh or accessory G52.8
    - fifth or trigeminal G51.Ø
    - first or olfactory G52.Ø
    - fourth or trochlear — *see* Strabismus, paralytic, fourth nerve
    - second or optic — *see* Neuritis, optic
    - seventh or facial G51.8
      - newborn (birth injury) P11.3
    - sixth or abducent — *see* Strabismus, paralytic, sixth nerve
    - tenth or vagus G52.2
    - third or oculomotor — *see* Strabismus, paralytic, third nerve
    - twelfth or hypoglossal G52.3
  - Déjérine-Sottas G6Ø.Ø
  - diabetic (mononeuropathy) — *see* EØ8-E13 with .41
    - polyneuropathy — *see* EØ8-E13 with .42
  - due to
    - beriberi E51.11
    - displacement, prolapse or rupture, intervertebral disc — *see* Disorder, disc, with, radiculopathy
    - herniation, nucleus pulposus M51.9 [G55]
  - endemic E51.11
  - facial G51.8
    - newborn (birth injury) P11.3
  - general — *see* Polyneuropathy
  - geniculate ganglion G51.1
    - due to herpes (zoster) BØ2.21
  - gouty M1Ø.ØØ [G63]
  - hypoglossal (nerve) G52.3
  - ilioinguinal (nerve) G57.9- ☑
  - infectious (multiple) NEC G61.Ø
  - interstitial hypertrophic progressive G6Ø.Ø
  - lumbar M54.16
  - lumbosacral M54.17
  - multiple (*see also* Polyneuropathy)
    - endemic E51.11
    - infective, acute G61.Ø
  - multiplex endemica E51.11
  - nerve root — *see* Radiculopathy
  - oculomotor (nerve) — *see* Strabismus, paralytic, third nerve
  - olfactory nerve G52.Ø
  - optic (nerve) (hereditary) (sympathetic) H46.9
    - with demyelination G36.Ø
    - in myelitis G36.Ø
    - nutritional H46.2
    - papillitis — *see* Papillitis, optic
    - retrobulbar H46.1- ☑
    - specified type NEC H46.8
    - toxic H46.3
  - peripheral (nerve) G62.9
    - multiple — *see* Polyneuropathy
    - single — *see* Mononeuritis
  - pneumogastric (nerve) G52.2
  - postherpetic, postzoster BØ2.29
  - progressive hypertrophic interstitial G6Ø.Ø
  - retrobulbar (*see also* Neuritis, optic, retrobulbar)
    - in (due to)
      - late syphilis A52.15
      - meningococcal infection A39.82
    - meningococcal A39.82
    - syphilitic A52.15
  - sciatic (nerve) (*see also* Sciatica)
    - due to displacement of intervertebral disc — *see* Disorder, disc, with, radiculopathy
  - serum (*see also* Reaction, serum) T8Ø.69 ☑
  - shoulder-girdle G54.5
  - specified nerve NEC G58.8
  - spinal (nerve) root — *see* Radiculopathy
  - syphilitic A52.15
  - thenar (median) G56.1- ☑
  - thoracic M54.14
  - toxic NEC G62.2
  - trochlear (nerve) — *see* Strabismus, paralytic, fourth nerve
  - vagus (nerve) G52.2
- **Neuroastrocytoma** — *see* Neoplasm, uncertain behavior, by site
- **Neuroavitaminosis** E56.9 [G99.8]
- **Neuroblastoma**
  - olfactory C3Ø.Ø
  - specified site — *see* Neoplasm, malignant, by site

- **Newborn** — *continued*
  - affected by — *continued*
    - intestinal perforation P78.0
    - intrauterine (fetal) blood loss P50.9
      - due to (from)
        - cut end of co-twin cord P50.5
        - hemorrhage into
          - co-twin P50.3
          - maternal circulation P50.4
        - placenta P50.2
        - ruptured cord blood P50.1
        - vasa previa P50.0
      - specified NEC P50.8
    - intrauterine (fetal) hemorrhage P50.9
    - intrauterine (in utero) procedure P96.5
    - malpresentation (malposition) NEC P03.1
    - maternal (complication of) (use of)
      - alcohol P04.3
      - analgesia (maternal) P04.0
      - anesthesia (maternal) P04.0
      - blood loss P02.1
      - circulatory disease P00.3
      - condition P00.9
        - specified NEC P00.89
      - delivery P03.9
        - Cesarean P03.4
        - forceps P03.2
        - vacuum extractor P03.3
      - diabetes mellitus (pre-existing) P70.1
      - disorder P00.9
        - specified NEC P00.89
      - drugs (addictive) (illegal) NEC P04.49
      - ectopic pregnancy P01.4
      - gestational diabetes P70.0
      - hemorrhage P02.1
      - hypertensive disorder P00.0
      - incompetent cervix P01.0
      - infectious disease P00.2
      - injury P00.5
      - labor and delivery P03.9
      - malpresentation before labor P01.7
      - maternal death P01.6
      - medical procedure P00.7
      - medication P04.1
      - multiple pregnancy P01.5
      - nutritional disorder P00.4
      - oligohydramnios P01.2
      - parasitic disease P00.2
      - periodontal disease P00.81
      - placenta previa P02.0
      - polyhydramnios P01.3
      - precipitate delivery P03.5
      - pregnancy P01.9
        - specified P01.8
      - premature rupture of membranes P01.1
      - renal disease P00.1
      - respiratory disease P00.3
      - surgical procedure P00.6
      - urinary tract disease P00.1
      - uterine contraction (abnormal) P03.6
    - meconium peritonitis P78.0
    - medication (legal) (maternal use) (prescribed) P04.1
    - membrane abnormalities P02.9
      - specified NEC P02.8
    - membranitis P02.7
    - methamphetamine(s) P04.49
    - mixed metabolic and respiratory acidosis P84
    - neonatal abstinence syndrome P96.1
    - noxious substances transmitted via placenta or breast milk P04.9
      - specified NEC P04.8
    - nutritional supplements P04.5
    - placenta previa P02.0
    - placental
      - abnormality (functional) (morphological) P02.20
        - specified NEC P02.29
      - dysfunction P02.29
      - infarction P02.29
      - insufficiency P02.29
      - separation NEC P02.1
      - transfusion syndromes P02.3
    - placentitis P02.7
    - precipitate delivery P03.5
    - prolapsed cord P02.4
    - respiratory arrest P28.81
    - slow intrauterine growth P05.9
    - tobacco P04.2

- **Newborn** — *continued*
  - affected by — *continued*
    - twin to twin transplacental transfusion P02.3
    - umbilical cord (tightly) around neck P02.5
    - umbilical cord condition P02.60
      - short cord P02.69
      - specified NEC P02.69
    - uterine contractions (abnormal) P03.6
    - vasa previa P02.69
      - from intrauterine blood loss P50.0
  - apnea P28.3
    - obstructive P28.4
    - primary P28.3
    - specified P28.4
  - born in hospital Z38.00
    - by cesarean Z38.01
  - born outside hospital Z38.1
  - breast buds P96.89
  - breast engorgement P83.4
  - check-up — *see* Newborn, examination
  - convulsion P90
  - dehydration P74.1
  - examination
    - 8 to 28 days old Z00.111
    - under 8 days old Z00.110
  - fever P81.9
    - environmentally-induced P81.0
  - hyperbilirubinemia P59.9
    - of prematurity P59.0
  - hypernatremia P74.2
  - hyponatremia P74.2
  - infection P39.9
    - candidal P37.5
    - specified NEC P39.8
    - urinary tract P39.3
  - jaundice P59.8
    - due to
      - breast milk inhibitor P59.3
      - hepatocellular damage P59.20
        - specified NEC P59.29
      - preterm delivery P59.0
    - of prematurity P59.0
    - specified NEC P59.8
  - late metabolic acidosis P74.0
  - mastitis P39.0
    - infective P39.0
    - noninfective P83.4
  - multiple born NEC Z38.8
    - born in hospital Z38.68
      - by cesarean Z38.69
    - born outside hospital Z38.7
  - omphalitis P38.9
    - with mild hemorrhage P38.1
    - without hemorrhage P38.9
  - post-term P08.21
  - prolonged gestation (over 42 completed weeks) P08.22
  - quadruplet Z38.8
    - born in hospital Z38.63
      - by cesarean Z38.64
    - born outside hospital Z38.7
  - quintuplet Z38.8
    - born in hospital Z38.65
      - by cesarean Z38.66
    - born outside hospital Z38.7
  - seizure P90
  - sepsis (congenital) P36.9
    - due to
      - anaerobes NEC P36.5
      - Escherichia coli P36.4
      - Staphylococcus P36.30
        - aureus P36.2
        - specified NEC P36.39
      - Streptococcus P36.10
        - group B P36.0
        - specified NEC P36.19
    - specified NEC P36.8
  - triplet Z38.8
    - born in hospital Z38.61
      - by cesarean Z38.62
    - born outside hospital Z38.7
  - twin Z38.5
    - born in hospital Z38.30
      - by cesarean Z38.31
    - born outside hospital Z38.4
  - vomiting P92.09
    - bilious P92.01
  - weight check Z00.111

- **Newcastle conjunctivitis or disease** B30.8
- **Nezelof's syndrome** (pure alymphocytosis) D81.4
- **Niacin** (amide) **deficiency** E52
- **Nicolas** (-Durand)-**Favre disease** A55
- **Nicotine** — *see* Tobacco
- **Nicotinic acid deficiency** E52
- **Niemann-Pick disease or syndrome** E75.249
  - specified NEC E75.248
  - type
    - A E75.240
    - B E75.241
    - C E75.242
    - D E75.243
- **Night**
  - blindness — *see* Blindness, night
  - sweats R61
  - terrors (child) F51.4
- **Nightmares** (REM sleep type) F51.5
- **Nipple** — *see* condition
- **Nisbet's chancre** A57
- **Nishimoto** (-Takeuchi) **disease** I67.5
- **Nitritoid crisis or reaction** — *see* Crisis, nitritoid
- **Nitrosohemoglobinemia** D74.8
- **Njovera** A65
- **Nocardiosis, nocardiasis** A43.9
  - cutaneous A43.1
  - lung A43.0
  - pneumonia A43.0
  - pulmonary A43.0
  - specified site NEC A43.8
- **Nocturia** R35.1
  - psychogenic F45.8
- **Nocturnal** — *see* condition
- **Nodal rhythm** I49.8
- **Node**(s) (*see also* Nodule)
  - Bouchard's (with arthropathy) M15.2
  - Haygarth's M15.8
  - Heberden's (with arthropathy) M15.1
  - larynx J38.7
  - lymph — *see* condition
  - milker's B08.03
  - Osler's I33.0
  - Schmorl's — *see* Schmorl's disease
  - singer's J38.2
  - teacher's J38.2
  - tuberculous — *see* Tuberculosis, lymph gland
  - vocal cord J38.2
- **Nodule**(s), **nodular**
  - actinomycotic — *see* Actinomycosis
  - breast NEC N63
  - colloid (cystic), thyroid E04.1
  - cutaneous — *see* Swelling, localized
  - endometrial (stromal) D26.1
  - Haygarth's M15.8
  - inflammatory — *see* Inflammation
  - juxta-articular
    - syphilitic A52.77
    - yaws A66.7
  - larynx J38.7
  - lung, solitary (subsegmental branch of the bronchial tree) R91.1
    - multiple R91.8
  - milker's B08.03
  - prostate N40.2
    - with lower urinary tract symptoms (LUTS) N40.3
    - without lower urinary tract symtpoms (LUTS) N40.2
  - pulmonary, solitary (subsegmental branch of the bronchial tree) R91.1
  - retrocardiac R09.89
  - rheumatoid M06.30
    - ankle M06.37- ☑
    - elbow M06.32- ☑
    - foot joint M06.37- ☑
    - hand joint M06.34- ☑
    - hip M06.35- ☑
    - knee M06.36- ☑
    - multiple site M06.39
    - shoulder M06.31- ☑
    - vertebra M06.38
    - wrist M06.33- ☑
  - scrotum (inflammatory) N49.2
  - singer's J38.2
  - solitary, lung (subsegmental branch of the bronchial tree) R91.1
    - multiple R91.8
  - subcutaneous — *see* Swelling, localized
  - teacher's J38.2

Nodule(s), **nodular** — *continued*
thyroid (cold) (gland) (nontoxic) EØ4.1
with thyrotoxicosis EØ5.2Ø
with thyroid storm EØ5.21
toxic or with hyperthyroidism EØ5.2Ø
with thyroid storm EØ5.21
vocal cord J38.2
Noma (gangrenous) (hospital) (infective) A69.Ø
auricle I96
mouth A69.Ø
pudendi N76.89
vulvae N76.89
Nomad, nomadism Z59.Ø
Nonautoimmune hemolytic anemia D59.4
drug-induced D59.2
Nonclosure (*see also* Imperfect, closure)
ductus arteriosus (Botallo's) Q25.Ø
foramen
botalli Q21.1
ovale Q21.1
Noncompliance Z91.19
with
dialysis Z91.15
dietary regimen Z91.11
medical treatment Z91.19
medication regimen NEC Z91.14
underdosing (*see also* Table of Drugs and Chemicals, categories T36-T5Ø, with final character 6) Z91.14
intentional NEC Z91.128
due to financial hardship of patient Z91.12Ø
unintentional NEC Z91.138
due to patient's age related debility Z91.13Ø
renal dialysis Z91.15
Nondescent (congenital) (*see also* Malposition, congenital)
cecum Q43.3
colon Q43.3
testicle Q53.9
bilateral Q53.2Ø
abdominal Q53.21
perineal Q53.22
unilateral Q53.1Ø
abdominal Q53.11
perineal Q53.12
Nondevelopment
brain QØ2
part of QØ4.3
heart Q24.8
organ or site, congenital NEC — *see* Hypoplasia
Nonengagement
head NEC O32.4 ☑
in labor, causing obstructed labor O64.8 ☑
Nonexanthematous tick fever A93.2
Nonexpansion, lung (newborn) P28.Ø
Nonfunctioning
cystic duct (*see also* Disease, gallbladder) K82.8
gallbladder (*see also* Disease, gallbladder) K82.8
kidney N28.9
labyrinth — *see* subcategory H83.2 ☑
Non-Hodgkin lymphoma NEC — *see* Lymphoma, non-Hodgkin
Nonimplantation, ovum N97.2
Noninsufflation, fallopian tube N97.1
Non-ketotic hyperglycinemia E72.51
Nonne-Milroy syndrome Q82.Ø
Nonovulation N97.Ø
Nonpatent fallopian tube N97.1
Nonpneumatization, lung NEC P28.Ø
Nonrotation — *see* Malrotation
Nonsecretion, urine — *see* Anuria
Nonunion
fracture — *see* Fracture, by site
organ or site, congenital NEC — *see* Imperfect, closure
symphysis pubis, congenital Q74.2
Nonvisualization, gallbladder R93.2
Nonvital, nonvitalized tooth KØ4.99
Non-working side interference M26.56
Noonan's syndrome Q87.1
Normocytic anemia (infectional) due to blood loss (chronic) D5Ø.Ø
acute D62
Norrie's disease (congenital) Q15.8
North American blastomycosis B4Ø.9
Norwegian itch B86
Nose, nasal — *see* condition
Nosebleed RØ4.Ø
Nose-picking F98.8
Nosomania F45.21
Nosophobia F45.22
Nostalgia F43.2Ø
Notch of iris Q13.2
Notching nose, congenital (tip) Q3Ø.2
Nothnagel's
syndrome — *see* Strabismus, paralytic, third nerve
vasomotor acroparesthesia I73.89
Novy's relapsing fever A68.9
louse-borne A68.Ø
tick-borne A68.1
Noxious
foodstuffs, poisoning by — *see* Poisoning, food, noxious, plant
substances transmitted through placenta or breast milk PØ4.9
Nucleus pulposus — *see* condition
Numbness R2Ø.Ø
Nuns' knee — *see* Bursitis, prepatellar
Nursemaid's elbow S53.Ø3- ☑
Nutcracker esophagus K22.4
Nutmeg liver K76.1
Nutrient element deficiency E61.9
specified NEC E61.8
Nutrition deficient or insufficient (*see also* Malnutrition) E46
due to
insufficient food T73.Ø ☑
lack of
care (child) T76.Ø2 ☑
adult T76.Ø1 ☑
food T73.Ø ☑
Nutritional stunting E45
Nyctalopia (night blindness) — *see* Blindness, night
Nycturia R35.1
psychogenic F45.8
Nymphomania F52.8
Nystagmus H55.ØØ
benign paroxysmal — *see* Vertigo, benign paroxysmal
central positional H81.4- ☑
congenital H55.Ø1
dissociated H55.Ø4
latent H55.Ø2
miners' H55.Ø9
positional
benign paroxysmal H81.4- ☑
central H81.4- ☑
specified form NEC H55.Ø9
visual deprivation H55.Ø3

O

Obermeyer's relapsing fever (European) A68.Ø
Obesity E66.9
with alveolar hyperventilation E66.2
adrenal E27.8
complicating
childbirth O99.214
pregnancy O99.21- ☑
puerperium O99.215
constitutional E66.8
dietary counseling and surveillance Z71.3
drug-induced E66.1
due to
drug E66.1
excess calories E66.Ø9
morbid E66.Ø1
severe E66.Ø1
endocrine E66.8
endogenous E66.8
familial E66.8
glandular E66.8
hypothyroid — *see* Hypothyroidism
morbid E66.Ø1
with alveolar hypoventilation E66.2
due to excess calories E66.Ø1
nutritional E66.Ø9
pituitary E23.6
severe E66.Ø1
specified type NEC E66.8
Oblique — *see* condition
Obliteration
appendix (lumen) K38.8
artery I77.1
Obliteration — *continued*
bile duct (noncalculous) K83.1
common duct (noncalculous) K83.1
cystic duct — *see* Obstruction, gallbladder
disease, arteriolar I77.1
endometrium N85.8
eye, anterior chamber — *see* Disorder, globe, hypotony
fallopian tube N97.1
lymphatic vessel I89.Ø
due to mastectomy I97.2
organ or site, congenital NEC — *see* Atresia, by site
ureter N13.5
with infection N13.6
urethra — *see* Stricture, urethra
vein I87.8
vestibule (oral) KØ8.8
Observation (following) (for) (without need for further medical care) ZØ4.9
accident NEC ZØ4.3
at work ZØ4.2
transport ZØ4.1
adverse effect of drug ZØ3.6
alleged rape or sexual assault (victim), ruled out
adult ZØ4.41
child ZØ4.42
criminal assault ZØ4.8
development state
adolescent ZØØ.3
period of rapid growth in childhood ZØØ.2
puberty ZØØ.3
disease, specified NEC ZØ3.89
following work accident ZØ4.2
growth and development state — *see* Observation, development state
injuries (accidental) NEC (*see also* Observation, accident)
newborn (for suspected condition, ruled out) — *see* Newborn, affected by (suspected to be), maternal (complication of) (use of)
postpartum
immediately after delivery Z39.Ø
routine follow-up Z39.2
pregnancy (normal) (without complication) Z34.9- ☑
high risk OØ9.9- ☑
suicide attempt, alleged NEC ZØ3.89
self-poisoning ZØ3.6
suspected, ruled out (*see also* Suspected condition, ruled out)
abuse, physical
adult ZØ4.71
child ZØ4.72
accident at work ZØ4.2
adult battering victim ZØ4.71
child battering victim ZØ4.72
condition NEC ZØ3.89
newborn — *see* Newborn, affected by (suspected to be), maternal (complication of) (use of)
drug poisoning or adverse effect ZØ3.6
exposure (to)
anthrax ZØ3.81Ø
biological agent NEC ZØ3.818
inflicted injury NEC ZØ4.8
suicide attempt, alleged ZØ3.89
self-poisoning ZØ3.6
toxic effects from ingested substance (drug) (poison) ZØ3.6
toxic effects from ingested substance (drug) (poison) ZØ3.6
Obsession, obsessional state F42
Obsessive-compulsive neurosis or reaction F42
Obstetric embolism, septic — *see* Embolism, obstetric, septic
Obstetrical trauma (complicating delivery) O71.9
with or following ectopic or molar pregnancy OØ8.6
specified type NEC O71.89
Obstipation — *see* Constipation
Obstruction, obstructed, obstructive
airway J98.8
with
allergic alveolitis J67.9
asthma J45.909
with
exacerbation (acute) J45.901
status asthmaticus J45.902
bronchiectasis J47.9

- **Occlusion, occluded** — *continued*
  - artery (*see also* Embolism, artery) — *continued*
    - brain or cerebral I66.9
      - with infarction (due to) I63.5 ☑
        - embolism I63.4 ☑
        - thrombosis I63.3 ☑
    - carotid I65.2- ☑
      - with
        - infarction I63.23- ☑
          - due to
            - embolism I63.13- ☑
            - thrombosis I63.Ø3- ☑
    - cerebellar (anterior inferior) (posterior inferior) (superior) I66.3
      - with infarction I63.54- ☑
        - due to
          - embolism I63.44- ☑
          - thrombosis I63.34- ☑
    - cerebral I66.9
      - with infarction I63.5Ø
        - due to
          - embolism I63.4Ø
            - specified NEC I63.49
          - thrombosis I63.3Ø
            - specified NEC I63.39
      - anterior I66.1- ☑
        - with infarction I63.52- ☑
          - due to
            - embolism I63.42- ☑
            - thrombosis I63.32- ☑
      - middle I66.Ø- ☑
        - with infarction I63.51- ☑
          - due to
            - embolism I63.41- ☑
            - thrombosis I63.31- ☑
      - posterior I66.2- ☑
        - with infarction I63.53- ☑
          - due to
            - embolism I63.43- ☑
            - thrombosis I63.33- ☑
      - specified NEC I66.8
        - with infarction I63.59
          - due to
            - embolism I63.4 ☑
            - thrombosis I63.3 ☑
    - choroidal (anterior) — *see* Occlusion, artery, precerebral, specified NEC
    - communicating posterior — *see* Occlusion, artery, cerebral, specified NEC
    - complete
      - coronary I25.82
      - extremities I7Ø.92
    - coronary (acute) (thrombotic) (without myocardial infarction) I24.Ø
      - with myocardial infarction — *see* Infarction, myocardium
      - chronic total I25.82
      - complete I25.82
      - healed or old I25.2
      - total (chronic) I25.82
    - hypophyseal — *see* Occlusion, artery, precerebral, specified NEC
    - iliac I74.5
    - lower extremities due to stenosis or stricture I77.1
    - mesenteric (embolic) (thrombotic) K55.Ø
    - perforating — *see* Occlusion, artery, cerebral, specified NEC
    - peripheral I77.9
      - thrombotic or embolic I74.4
    - pontine — *see* Occlusion, artery, cerebral, specified NEC
    - precerebral I65.9
      - with infarction I63.2Ø
        - due to
          - embolism I63.1Ø
            - specified NEC I63.19
          - thrombosis I63.ØØ
            - specified NEC I63.Ø9
        - specified NEC I63.29
      - basilar — *see* Occlusion, artery, basilar
      - carotid — *see* Occlusion, artery, carotid
      - puerperal O88.23
      - specified NEC I65.8
        - with infarction I63.29
          - due to
            - embolism I63.19
            - thrombosis I63.ØØ

- **Occlusion, occluded** — *continued*
  - artery (*see also* Embolism, artery) — *continued*
    - precerebral — *continued*
      - vertebral — *see* Occlusion, artery, vertebral
    - renal N28.Ø
    - retinal
      - branch H34.23- ☑
      - central H34.1- ☑
      - partial H34.21- ☑
      - transient H34.Ø- ☑
    - spinal — *see* Occlusion, artery, precerebral, vertebral
    - total (chronic)
      - coronary I25.82
      - extremities I7Ø.92
    - vertebral I65.Ø- ☑
      - with
        - infarction I63.21- ☑
          - due to
            - embolism I63.11- ☑
            - thrombosis I63.Ø1- ☑
  - basilar artery — *see* Occlusion, artery, basilar
  - bile duct (common) (hepatic) (noncalculous) K83.1
  - bowel — *see* Obstruction, intestine
  - carotid (artery) (common) (internal) — *see* Occlusion, artery, carotid
  - centric (of teeth) M26.59
    - maximum intercuspation discrepancy M26.55
  - cerebellar (artery) — *see* Occlusion, artery, cerebellar
  - cerebral (artery) — *see* Occlusion, artery, cerebral
  - cerebrovascular (*see also* Occlusion, artery, cerebral)
    - with infarction I63.5 ☑
  - cervical canal — *see* Stricture, cervix
  - cervix (uteri) — *see* Stricture, cervix
  - choanal Q3Ø.Ø
  - choroidal (artery) — *see* Occlusion, artery, precerebral, specified NEC
  - colon — *see* Obstruction, intestine
  - communicating posterior artery — *see* Occlusion, artery, precerebral, specified NEC
  - coronary (artery) (vein) (thrombotic) (*see also* Infarct, myocardium)
    - chronic total I25.82
    - healed or old I25.2
    - not resulting in infarction I24.Ø
    - total (chronic) I25.82
  - cystic duct — *see* Obstruction, gallbladder
  - embolic — *see* Embolism
  - fallopian tube N97.1
    - congenital Q5Ø.6
  - gallbladder (*see also* Obstruction, gallbladder)
    - congenital (causing jaundice) Q44.1
  - gingiva, traumatic KØ6.2
  - hymen N89.6
    - congenital Q52.3
  - hypophyseal (artery) — *see* Occlusion, artery, precerebral, specified NEC
  - iliac artery I74.5
  - intestine — *see* Obstruction, intestine
  - lacrimal passages — *see* Obstruction, lacrimal
  - lung J98.4
  - lymph or lymphatic channel I89.Ø
  - mammary duct N64.89
  - mesenteric artery (embolic) (thrombotic) K55.Ø
  - nose J34.89
    - congenital Q3Ø.Ø
  - organ or site, congenital NEC — *see* Atresia, by site
  - oviduct N97.1
    - congenital Q5Ø.6
  - peripheral arteries
    - due to stricture or stenosis I77.1
    - upper extremity I74.2
  - pontine (artery) — *see* Occlusion, artery, precerebral, specified NEC
  - posterior lingual, of mandibular teeth M26.29
  - precerebral artery — *see* Occlusion, artery, precerebral
  - punctum lacrimale — *see* Obstruction, lacrimal
  - pupil — *see* Membrane, pupillary
  - pylorus, adult (*see also* Stricture, pylorus) K31.1
  - renal artery N28.Ø
  - retina, retinal
    - artery — *see* Occlusion, artery, retinal
    - vein (central) H34.81- ☑
      - engorgement H34.82- ☑
      - tributary H34.83- ☑
    - vessels H34.9

- **Occlusion, occluded** — *continued*
  - spinal artery — *see* Occlusion, artery, precerebral, vertebral
  - teeth (mandibular) (posterior lingual) M26.29
  - thoracic duct I89.Ø
  - thrombotic — *see* Thrombosis, artery
  - traumatic
    - edentulous (alveolar) ridge KØ6.2
    - gingiva KØ6.2
    - periodontal KØ5.5
  - tubal N97.1
  - ureter (complete) (partial) N13.5
    - congenital Q62.1Ø
  - ureteropelvic junction N13.5
    - congenital Q62.11
  - ureterovesical orifice N13.5
    - congenital Q62.12
  - urethra — *see* Stricture, urethra
  - uterus N85.8
  - vagina N89.5
  - vascular NEC I99.8
  - vein — *see* Thrombosis
    - retinal — *see* Occlusion, retinal, vein
  - vena cava (inferior) (superior) — *see* Embolism, vena cava
  - ventricle (brain) NEC G91.1
  - vertebral (artery) — *see* Occlusion, artery, vertebral
  - vessel (blood) I99.8
  - vulva N9Ø.5
- **Occult**
  - blood in feces (stools) R19.5
- **Occupational**
  - problems NEC Z56.89
- **Ochlophobia** — *see* Agoraphobia
- **Ochronosis** (endogenous) E7Ø.29
- **Ocular muscle** — *see* condition
- **Oculogyric crisis or disturbance** H51.8
  - psychogenic F45.8
- **Oculomotor syndrome** H51.9
- **Oculopathy**
  - syphilitic NEC A52.71
    - congenital
      - early A5Ø.Ø1
      - late A5Ø.3Ø
    - early (secondary) A51.43
    - late A52.71
- **Oddi's sphincter spasm** K83.4
- **Odontalgia** KØ8.8
- **Odontoameloblastoma** — *see* Cyst, calcifying odontogenic
- **Odontoclasia** KØ3.89
- **Odontodysplasia, regional** KØØ.4
- **Odontogenesis imperfecta** KØØ.5
- **Odontoma** (ameloblastic) (complex) (compound) (fibroameloblastic) — *see* Cyst, calcifying odontogenic
- **Odontomyelitis** (closed) (open) KØ4.Ø
- **Odontorrhagia** KØ8.8
- **Odontosarcoma, ameloblastic** C41.1
  - upper jaw (bone) C41.Ø
- **Oestriasis** — *see* Myiasis
- **Oguchi's disease** H53.63
- **Ohara's disease** — *see* Tularemia
- **Oidiomycosis** — *see* Candidiasis
- **Oidium albicans infection** — *see* Candidiasis
- **Old age** (without mention of debility) R54
  - dementia FØ3 ☑
- **Old** (previous) **myocardial infarction** I25.2
- **Olfactory** — *see* condition
- **Oligemia** — *see* Anemia
- **Oligoastrocytoma**
  - specified site — *see* Neoplasm, malignant, by site
  - unspecified site C71.9
- **Oligocythemia** D64.9
- **Oligodendroblastoma**
  - specified site — *see* Neoplasm, malignant
  - unspecified site C71.9
- **Oligodendroglioma**
  - anaplastic type
    - specified site — *see* Neoplasm, malignant, by site
    - unspecified site C71.9
  - specified site — *see* Neoplasm, malignant, by site
  - unspecified site C71.9
- **Oligodontia** — *see* Anodontia
- **Oligoencephalon** QØ2
- **Oligohidrosis** L74.4
- **Oligohydramnios** O41.Ø- ☑
- **Oligohydrosis** L74.4

Oligomenorrhea N91.5
  primary N91.3
  secondary N91.4
Oligophrenia (*see also* Disability, intellectual)
  phenylpyruvic E7Ø.Ø
Oligospermia N46.11
  due to
    drug therapy N46.121
    efferent duct obstruction N46.123
    infection N46.122
    radiation N46.124
    specified cause NEC N46.129
    systemic disease N46.125
Oligotrichia — *see* Alopecia
Oliguria R34
  postprocedural N99.Ø
  with, complicating or following ectopic or molar pregnancy OØ8.4
Ollier's disease Q78.4
Omenotocele — *see* Hernia, abdomen, specified site NEC
Omentitis — *see* Peritonitis
Omentum, omental — *see* condition
Omphalitis (congenital) (newborn) P38.9
  with mild hemorrhage P38.1
  without hemorrhage P38.9
  not of newborn LØ8.82
  tetanus A33
Omphalocele Q79.2
Omphalomesenteric duct, persistent Q43.Ø
Omphalorrhagia, newborn P51.9
Omsk hemorrhagic fever A98.1
Onanism (excessive) F98.8
Onchocerciasis, onchocercosis B73.1
  with
    eye disease B73.ØØ
      endophthalmitis B73.Ø1
      eyelid B73.Ø9
      glaucoma B73.Ø2
      specified NEC B73.Ø9
  eyelid B73.Ø9
  eye NEC B73.ØØ
Oncocytoma — *see* Neoplasm, benign, by site
Oncovirus, as cause of disease classified elsewhere B97.32
Ondine's curse — *see* Apnea, sleep
Oneirophrenia F23
Onychauxis L6Ø.2
  congenital Q84.5
Onychia (*see also* Cellulitis, digit)
  with lymphangitis — *see* Lymphangitis, acute, digit
  candidal B37.2
  dermatophytic B35.1
Onychitis (*see also* Cellulitis, digit)
  with lymphangitis — *see* Lymphangitis, acute, digit
Onychocryptosis L6Ø.Ø
Onychodystrophy L6Ø.3
  congenital Q84.6
Onychogryphosis, onychogryposis L6Ø.2
Onycholysis L6Ø.1
Onychomadesis L6Ø.8
Onychomalacia L6Ø.3
Onychomycosis (finger) (toe) B35.1
Onycho-osteodysplasia Q79.8
Onychophagia F98.8
Onychophosis L6Ø.8
Onychoptosis L6Ø.8
Onychorrhexis L6Ø.3
  congenital Q84.6
Onychoschizia L6Ø.3
Onyxis (finger) (toe) L6Ø.Ø
Onyxitis (*see also* Cellulitis, digit)
  with lymphangitis — *see* Lymphangitis, acute, digit
Oophoritis (cystic) (infectional) (interstitial) N7Ø.92
  with salpingitis N7Ø.93
  acute N7Ø.Ø2
    with salpingitis N7Ø.Ø3
  chronic N7Ø.12
    with salpingitis N7Ø.13
  complicating abortion — *see* Abortion, by type, complicated by, oophoritis
Oophorocele N83.4
Opacity, opacities
  cornea H17.- ☑
    central H17.1- ☑
    congenital Q13.3
    degenerative — *see* Degeneration, cornea

Opacity, opacities — *continued*
  cornea — *continued*
    hereditary — *see* Dystrophy, cornea
    inflammatory — *see* Keratitis
    minor H17.81- ☑
    peripheral H17.82- ☑
    sequelae of trachoma (healed) B94.Ø
    specified NEC H17.89
  enamel (teeth) (fluoride) (nonfluoride) KØØ.3
  lens — *see* Cataract
  snowball — *see* Deposit, crystalline
  vitreous (humor) NEC H43.39- ☑
    congenital Q14.Ø
    membranes and strands H43.31- ☑
Opalescent dentin (hereditary) KØØ.5
Open, opening
  abnormal, organ or site, congenital — *see* Imperfect, closure
  angle with
    borderline
      findings
        high risk H4Ø.Ø2- ☑
        low risk H4Ø.Ø1- ☑
      intraocular pressure H4Ø.ØØ- ☑
    cupping of discs H4Ø.Ø1- ☑
    glaucoma (primary) — *see* Glaucoma, open angle
  bite
    anterior M26.22Ø
    posterior M26.221
  false — *see* Imperfect, closure
  margin on tooth restoration KØ8.51
  restoration margins of tooth KØ8.51
  wound — *see* Wound, open
Operational fatigue F48.8
Operative — *see* condition
Operculitis — *see* Periodontitis
Operculum — *see* Break, retina
Ophiasis L63.2
Ophthalmia (*see also* Conjunctivitis) H1Ø.9
  actinic rays — *see* Photokeratitis
  allergic (acute) — *see* Conjunctivitis, acute, atopic
  blennorrhagic (gonococcal) (neonatorum) A54.31
  diphtheritic A36.86
  Egyptian A71.1
  electrica — *see* Photokeratitis
  gonococcal (neonatorum) A54.31
  metastatic — *see* Endophthalmitis, purulent
  migraine — *see* Migraine, ophthalmoplegic
  neonatorum, newborn P39.1
    gonococcal A54.31
  nodosa H16.24- ☑
  purulent — *see* Conjunctivitis, acute, mucopurulent
  spring — *see* Conjunctivitis, acute, atopic
  sympathetic — *see* Uveitis, sympathetic
Ophthalmitis — *see* Ophthalmia
Ophthalmocele (congenital) Q15.8
Ophthalmoneuromyelitis G36.Ø
Ophthalmoplegia (*see also* Strabismus, paralytic)
  anterior internuclear — *see* Ophthalmoplegia, internuclear
  ataxia-areflexia G61.Ø
  diabetic — *see* EØ8-E13 with .39
  exophthalmic EØ5.ØØ
    with thyroid storm EØ5.Ø1
  external H49.88- ☑
    progressive H49.4- ☑
      with pigmentary retinopathy — *see* Kearns-Sayre syndrome
    total H49.3- ☑
  internal (complete) (total) H52.51- ☑
  internuclear H51.2- ☑
  migraine — *see* Migraine, ophthalmoplegic
  Parinaud's H49.88- ☑
  progressive external — *see* Ophthalmoplegia, external, progressive
  supranuclear, progressive G23.1
  total (external) — *see* Ophthalmoplegia, external, total
Opioid(s)
  abuse — *see* Abuse, drug, opioids
  dependence — *see* Dependence, drug, opioids
Opisthognathism M26.Ø9
Opisthorchiasis (felineus) (viverrini) B66.Ø
Opitz' disease D73.2
Opiumism — *see* Dependence, drug, opioid
Oppenheim's disease G7Ø.2
Oppenheim-Urbach disease (necrobiosis lipoidica diabeticorum) — *see* EØ8-E13 with .62Ø

Optic nerve — *see* condition
Orbit — *see* condition
Orchioblastoma C62.9- ☑
Orchitis (gangrenous) (nonspecific) (septic) (suppurative) N45.2
  blennorrhagic (gonococcal) (acute) (chronic) A54.23
  chlamydial A56.19
  filarial (*see also* Infestation, filarial) B74.9 [N51]
  gonococcal (acute) (chronic) A54.23
  mumps B26.Ø
  syphilitic A52.76
  tuberculous A18.15
Orf (virus disease) BØ8.Ø2
Organic (*see also* condition)
  brain syndrome FØ9
  heart — *see* Disease, heart
  mental disorder FØ9
  psychosis FØ9
Orgasm
  anejaculatory N53.13
Oriental
  bilharziasis B65.2
  schistosomiasis B65.2
Orifice — *see* condition
Origin of both great vessels from right ventricle Q2Ø.1
Ormond's disease (with ureteral obstruction) N13.5
  with infection N13.6
Ornithine metabolism disorder E72.4
Ornithinemia (Type I) (Type II) E72.4
Ornithosis A7Ø
Orotaciduria, oroticaciduria (congenital) (hereditary) (pyrimidine deficiency) E79.8
  anemia D53.Ø
Orthodontics
  adjustment Z46.4
  fitting Z46.4
Orthopnea RØ6.Ø1
Orthopoxvirus BØ8.Ø9
  specified NEC BØ8.Ø9
Os, uterus — *see* condition
Osgood-Schlatter disease or osteochondrosis — *see* Osteochondrosis, juvenile, tibia
Osler (-Weber)-**Rendu disease** I78.Ø
Osler's nodes I33.Ø
Osmidrosis L75.Ø
Osseous — *see* condition
Ossification
  artery — *see* Arteriosclerosis
  auricle (ear) — *see* Disorder, pinna, specified type NEC
  bronchial J98.Ø9
  cardiac — *see* Degeneration, myocardial
  cartilage (senile) — *see* Disorder, cartilage, specified type NEC
  coronary (artery) — *see* Disease, heart, ischemic, atherosclerotic
  diaphragm J98.6
  ear, middle — *see* Otosclerosis
  falx cerebri G96.19
  fontanel, premature Q75.Ø
  heart (*see also* Degeneration, myocardial)
    valve — *see* Endocarditis
  larynx J38.7
  ligament — *see* Disorder, tendon, specified type NEC
    posterior longitudinal — *see* Spondylopathy, specified NEC
  meninges (cerebral) (spinal) G96.19
  multiple, eccentric centers — *see* Disorder, bone, development or growth
  muscle (*see also* Calcification, muscle)
    due to burns — *see* Myositis, ossificans, in, burns
    paralytic — *see* Myositis, ossificans, in, quadriplegia
    progressive — *see* Myositis, ossificans, progressiva
    specified NEC M61.5Ø
      ankle M61.57- ☑
      foot M61.57- ☑
      forearm M61.53- ☑
      hand M61.54- ☑
      lower leg M61.56- ☑
      multiple sites M61.59
      pelvic region M61.55- ☑
      shoulder region M61.51- ☑
      specified site NEC M61.58
      thigh M61.55- ☑
      upper arm M61.52- ☑
    traumatic — *see* Myositis, ossificans, traumatica

Ossification — *continued*
- myocardium, myocardial — *see* Degeneration, myocardial
- penis N48.89
- periarticular — *see* Disorder, joint, specified type NEC
- pinna — *see* Disorder, pinna, specified type NEC
- rider's bone — *see* Ossification, muscle, specified NEC
- sclera H15.89
- subperiosteal, post-traumatic M89.8X- ☑
- tendon — *see* Disorder, tendon, specified type NEC
- trachea J39.8
- tympanic membrane — *see* Disorder, tympanic membrane, specified NEC
- vitreous (humor) — *see* Deposit, crystalline

Osteitis (*see also* Osteomyelitis)
- alveolar M27.3
- condensans M85.30
  - ankle M85.37- ☑
  - foot M85.37- ☑
  - forearm M85.33- ☑
  - hand M85.34- ☑
  - lower leg M85.36- ☑
  - multiple site M85.39
  - neck M85.38
  - rib M85.38
  - shoulder M85.31- ☑
  - skull M85.38
  - specified site NEC M85.38
  - thigh M85.35- ☑
  - toe M85.37- ☑
  - upper arm M85.32- ☑
  - vertebra M85.38
- deformans M88.9
  - in (due to)
    - malignant neoplasm of bone C41.9 [M90.60]
    - neoplastic disease (*see also* Neoplasm) D49.9 [M90.60]
      - carpus D49.9 [M90.64-] ☑
      - clavicle D49.9 [M90.61-] ☑
      - femur D49.9 [M90.65-] ☑
      - fibula D49.9 [M90.66-] ☑
      - finger D49.9 [M90.64-] ☑
      - humerus D49.9 [M90.62-] ☑
      - ilium D49.9 [M90.65-] ☑
      - ischium D49.9 [M90.65-] ☑
      - metacarpus D49.9 [M90.64-] ☑
      - metatarsus D49.9 [M90.67-] ☑
      - multiple sites D49.9 [M90.69]
      - neck D49.9 [M90.68]
      - radius D49.9 [M90.63-] ☑
      - rib D49.9 [M90.68]
      - scapula D49.9 [M90.61-] ☑
      - skull D49.9 [M90.68]
      - tarsus D49.9 [M90.67-] ☑
      - tibia D49.9 [M90.66-] ☑
      - toe D49.9 [M90.67-] ☑
      - ulna D49.9 [M90.63-] ☑
      - vertebra D49.9 [M90.68]
  - skull M88.0
  - specified NEC — *see* Paget's disease, bone, by site
  - vertebra M88.1
- due to yaws A66.6
- fibrosa NEC — *see* Cyst, bone, by site
  - circumscripta — *see* Dysplasia, fibrous, bone NEC
  - cystica (generalisata) E21.0
  - disseminata Q78.1
  - osteoplastica E21.0
- fragilitans Q78.0
- Garr's (sclerosing) — *see* Osteomyelitis, specified type NEC
- jaw (acute) (chronic) (lower) (suppurative) (upper) M27.2
- parathyroid E21.0
- petrous bone (acute) (chronic) — *see* Petrositis
- sclerotic, nonsuppurative — *see* Osteomyelitis, specified type NEC
- tuberculosa A18.09
  - cystica D86.89
  - multiplex cystoides D86.89

Osteoarthritis M19.90
- ankle M19.07- ☑
- elbow M19.02- ☑
- foot joint M19.07- ☑
- generalized M15.9
  - erosive M15.4
  - primary M15.0
  - specified NEC M15.8

Osteoarthritis — *continued*
- hand joint M19.04- ☑
  - first carpometacarpal joint M18.9
- hip M16.1- ☑
  - bilateral M16.0
  - due to hip dysplasia (unilateral) M16.3- ☑
    - bilateral M16.2
- interphalangeal
  - distal (Heberden) M15.1
  - proximal (Bouchard) M15.2
- knee M17.9
  - bilateral M17.0
- post-traumatic NEC M19.92
  - ankle M19.17- ☑
  - elbow M19.12- ☑
  - foot joint M19.17- ☑
  - hand joint M19.14- ☑
    - first carpometacarpal joint M18.3- ☑
      - bilateral M18.2
  - hip M16.5- ☑
    - bilateral M16.4
  - knee M17.3- ☑
    - bilateral M17.2
  - shoulder M19.11- ☑
  - wrist M19.13- ☑
- primary M19.91
  - ankle M19.07- ☑
  - elbow M19.02- ☑
  - foot joint M19.07- ☑
  - hand joint M19.04- ☑
    - first carpometacarpal joint M18.1- ☑
      - bilateral M18.0
  - hip M16.1- ☑
    - bilateral M16.0
  - knee M17.1- ☑
    - bilateral M17.0
  - shoulder M19.01- ☑
  - spine — *see* Spondylosis
  - wrist M19.03- ☑
- secondary M19.93
  - ankle M19.27- ☑
  - elbow M19.22- ☑
  - foot joint M19.27- ☑
  - hand joint M19.24- ☑
    - first carpometacarpal joint M18.5- ☑
      - bilateral M18.4
  - hip M16.7
    - bilateral M16.6
  - knee M17.5
    - bilateral M17.4
  - multiple M15.3
  - shoulder M19.21- ☑
  - spine — *see* Spondylosis
  - wrist M19.23- ☑
- shoulder M19.01- ☑
- spine — *see* Spondylosis
- wrist M19.03- ☑

Osteoarthropathy (hypertrophic) M19.90
- ankle — *see* Osteoarthritis, primary, ankle
- elbow — *see* Osteoarthritis, primary, elbow
- foot joint — *see* Osteoarthritis, primary, foot
- hand joint — *see* Osteoarthritis, primary, hand joint
- knee joint — *see* Osteoarthritis, primary, knee
- multiple site — *see* Osteoarthritis, primary, multiple joint
- pulmonary (*see also* Osteoarthropathy, specified type NEC)
  - hypertrophic — *see* Osteoarthropathy, hypertrophic, specified type NEC
- secondary — *see* Osteoarthropathy, specified type NEC
- secondary hypertrophic — *see* Osteoarthropathy, specified type NEC
- shoulder — *see* Osteoarthritis, primary, shoulder
- specified joint NEC — *see* Osteoarthritis, primary, specified joint NEC
- specified type NEC M89.40
  - carpus M89.44- ☑
  - clavicle M89.41- ☑
  - femur M89.45- ☑
  - fibula M89.46- ☑
  - finger M89.44- ☑
  - humerus M89.42- ☑
  - ilium M89.459
  - ischium M89.459
  - metacarpus M89.44- ☑

Osteoarthropathy — *continued*
- specified type — *continued*
  - metatarsus M89.47- ☑
  - multiple sites M89.49
  - neck M89.48
  - radius M89.43- ☑
  - rib M89.48
  - scapula M89.41- ☑
  - skull M89.48
  - tarsus M89.47- ☑
  - tibia M89.46- ☑
  - toe M89.47- ☑
  - ulna M89.43- ☑
  - vertebra M89.48
- spine — *see* Spondylosis
- wrist — *see* Osteoarthritis, primary, wrist

Osteoarthrosis (degenerative) (hypertrophic) (joint) (*see also* Osteoarthritis)
- deformans alkaptonurica E70.29 [M36.8]
- erosive M15.4
- generalized M15.9
  - primary M15.0
- polyarticular M15.9
- spine — *see* Spondylosis

Osteoblastoma — *see* Neoplasm, bone, benign
- aggressive — *see* Neoplasm, bone, uncertain behavior

Osteochondritis (*see also* Osteochondropathy, by site)
- Brailsford's — *see* Osteochondrosis, juvenile, radius
- dissecans M93.20
  - ankle M93.27- ☑
  - elbow M93.22- ☑
  - foot M93.27- ☑
  - hand M93.24- ☑
  - hip M93.25- ☑
  - knee M93.26- ☑
  - multiple sites M93.29
  - shoulder joint M93.21- ☑
  - specified site NEC M93.28
  - wrist M93.23- ☑
- juvenile M92.9
  - patellar — *see* Osteochondrosis, juvenile, patella
- syphilitic (congenital) (early) A50.02 [M90.80]
  - ankle A50.02 [M90.87-] ☑
  - elbow A50.02 [M90.82-] ☑
  - foot A50.02 [M90.87-] ☑
  - forearm A50.02 [M90.83-] ☑
  - hand A50.02 [M90.84-] ☑
  - hip A50.02 [M90.85-] ☑
  - knee A50.02 [M90.86-] ☑
  - multiple sites A50.02 [M90.89]
  - shoulder joint A50.02 [M90.81-] ☑
  - specified site NEC A50.02 [M90.88]

Osteochondroarthrosis deformans endemica — *see* Disease, Kaschin-Beck

Osteochondrodysplasia Q78.9
- with defects of growth of tubular bones and spine Q77.9
  - specified NEC Q77.8
- specified NEC Q78.8

Osteochondrodystrophy E78.9

Osteochondrolysis — *see* Osteochondritis, dissecans

Osteochondroma — *see* Neoplasm, bone, benign

Osteochondromatosis D48.0
- syndrome Q78.4

Osteochondromyxosarcoma — *see* Neoplasm, bone, malignant

Osteochondropathy M93.90
- ankle M93.97- ☑
- elbow M93.92- ☑
- foot M93.97- ☑
- hand M93.94- ☑
- hip M93.95- ☑
- Kienböck's disease of adults M93.1
- knee M93.96- ☑
- multiple joints M93.99
- osteochondritis dissecans — *see* Osteochondritis, dissecans
- osteochondrosis — *see* Osteochondrosis
- shoulder region M93.91- ☑
- slipped upper femoral epiphysis — *see* Slipped, epiphysis, upper femoral
- specified joint NEC M93.98
- specified type NEC M93.80
  - ankle M93.87- ☑
  - elbow M93.82- ☑
  - foot M93.87- ☑

- **Osteochondropathy** — *continued*
  - specified type — *continued*
    - hand M93.84- ☑
    - hip M93.85- ☑
    - knee M93.86- ☑
    - multiple joints M93.89
    - shoulder region M93.81- ☑
    - specified joint NEC M93.88
    - wrist M93.83- ☑
  - syphilitic, congenital
    - early A5Ø.Ø2 [M9Ø.8Ø]
    - late A5Ø.56 [M9Ø.8Ø]
  - wrist M93.93- ☑
- **Osteochondrosarcoma** — *see* Neoplasm, bone, malignant
- **Osteochondrosis** (*see also* Osteochondropathy, by site)
  - acetabulum (juvenile) M91.Ø
  - adult — *see* Osteochondropathy, specified type NEC, by site
  - astragalus (juvenile) — *see* Osteochondrosis, juvenile, tarsus
  - Blount's — *see* Osteochondrosis, juvenile, tibia
  - Buchanan's M91.Ø
  - Burns' — *see* Osteochondrosis, juvenile, ulna
  - calcaneus (juvenile) — *see* Osteochondrosis, juvenile, tarsus
  - capitular epiphysis (femur) (juvenile) — *see* Legg-Calvé-Perthes disease
  - carpal (juvenile) (lunate) (scaphoid) — *see* Osteochondrosis, juvenile, hand, carpal lunate
    - adult M93.1
  - coxae juvenilis — *see* Legg-Calvé-Perthes disease
  - deformans juvenilis, coxae — *see* Legg-Calvé-Perthes disease
  - Diaz's — *see* Osteochondrosis, juvenile, tarsus
  - dissecans (knee) (shoulder) — *see* Osteochondritis, dissecans
  - femoral capital epiphysis (juvenile) — *see* Legg-Calvé-Perthes disease
  - femur (head), juvenile — *see* Legg-Calvé-Perthes disease
  - fibula (juvenile) — *see* Osteochondrosis, juvenile, fibula
  - foot NEC (juvenile) M92.8
  - Freiberg's — *see* Osteochondrosis, juvenile, metatarsus
  - Haas' (juvenile) — *see* Osteochondrosis, juvenile, humerus
  - Haglund's — *see* Osteochondrosis, juvenile, tarsus
  - hip (juvenile) — *see* Legg-Calvé-Perthes disease
  - humerus (capitulum) (head) (juvenile) — *see* Osteochondrosis, juvenile, humerus
  - ilium, iliac crest (juvenile) M91.Ø
  - ischiopubic synchondrosis M91.Ø
  - Iselin's — *see* Osteochondrosis, juvenile, metatarsus
  - juvenile, juvenilis M92.9
    - after congenital dislocation of hip reduction — *see* Osteochondrosis, juvenile, hip, specified NEC
    - arm — *see* Osteochondrosis, juvenile, upper limb NEC
    - capitular epiphysis (femur) — *see* Legg-Calvé-Perthes disease
    - clavicle, sternal epiphysis — *see* Osteochondrosis, juvenile, upper limb NEC
    - coxae — *see* Legg-Calvé-Perthes disease
    - deformans M92.9
    - fibula M92.5- ☑
    - foot NEC M92.8
    - hand M92.2Ø- ☑
      - carpal lunate M92.21- ☑
      - metacarpal head M92.22- ☑
      - specified site NEC M92.29- ☑
    - head of femur — *see* Legg-Calvé-Perthes disease
    - hip and pelvis M91.9- ☑
      - coxa plana — *see* Coxa, plana
      - femoral head — *see* Legg-Calvé-Perthes disease
      - pelvis M91.Ø
      - pseudocoxalgia — *see* Pseudocoxalgia
      - specified NEC M91.8- ☑
    - humerus M92.Ø- ☑
    - limb
      - lower NEC M92.8
      - upper NEC — *see* Osteochondrosis, juvenile, upper limb NEC
    - medial cuneiform bone — *see* Osteochondrosis, juvenile, tarsus
    - metatarsus M92.7- ☑
    - patella M92.4- ☑

- **Osteochondrosis** — *continued*
  - juvenile, juvenilis — *continued*
    - radius M92.1- ☑
    - specified site NEC M92.8
    - spine M42.ØØ
      - cervical region M42.Ø2
      - cervicothoracic region M42.Ø3
      - lumbar region M42.Ø6
      - lumbosacral region M42.Ø7
      - multiple sites M42.Ø9
      - occipito-atlanto-axial region M42.Ø1
      - sacrococcygeal region M42.Ø8
      - thoracic region M42.Ø4
      - thoracolumbar region M42.Ø5
    - tarsus M92.6- ☑
    - tibia M92.5- ☑
    - ulna M92.1- ☑
    - upper limb NEC M92.3- ☑
    - vertebra (body) (epiphyseal plates) (Calvé's) (Scheuermann's) — *see* Osteochondrosis, juvenile, spine
  - Kienböck's — *see* Osteochondrosis, juvenile, hand, carpal lunate
    - adult M93.1
  - Köhler's
    - patellar — *see* Osteochondrosis, juvenile, patella
    - tarsal navicular — *see* Osteochondrosis, juvenile, tarsus
  - Legg-Perthes (-Calvé)(-Waldenström) — *see* Legg-Calvé-Perthes disease
  - limb
    - lower NEC (juvenile) M92.8
    - upper NEC (juvenile) — *see* Osteochondrosis, juvenile, upper limb NEC
  - lunate bone (carpal) (juvenile) (*see also* Osteochondrosis, juvenile, hand, carpal lunate)
    - adult M93.1
  - Mauclaire's — *see* Osteochondrosis, juvenile, hand, metacarpal
  - metacarpal (head) (juvenile) — *see* Osteochondrosis, juvenile, hand, metacarpal
  - metatarsus (fifth) (head) (juvenile) (second) — *see* Osteochondrosis, juvenile, metatarsus
  - navicular (juvenile) — *see* Osteochondrosis, juvenile, tarsus
  - os
    - calcis (juvenile) — *see* Osteochondrosis, juvenile, tarsus
    - tibiale externum (juvenile) — *see* Osteochondrosis, juvenile, tarsus
  - Osgood-Schlatter — *see* Osteochondrosis, juvenile, tibia
  - Panner's — *see* Osteochondrosis, juvenile, humerus
  - patellar center (juvenile) (primary) (secondary) — *see* Osteochondrosis, juvenile, patella
  - pelvis (juvenile) M91.Ø
  - Pierson's M91.Ø
  - radius (head) (juvenile) — *see* Osteochondrosis, juvenile, radius
  - Scheuermann's — *see* Osteochondrosis, juvenile, spine
  - Sever's — *see* Osteochondrosis, juvenile, tarsus
  - Sinding-Larsen — *see* Osteochondrosis, juvenile, patella
  - spine M42.9
    - adult M42.1Ø
      - cervical region M42.12
      - cervicothoracic region M42.13
      - lumbar region M42.16
      - lumbosacral region M42.17
      - multiple sites M42.19
      - occipito-atlanto-axial region M42.11
      - sacrococcygeal region M42.18
      - thoracic region M42.14
      - thoracolumbar region M42.15
    - juvenile — *see* Osteochondrosis, juvenile, spine
  - symphysis pubis (juvenile) M91.Ø
  - syphilitic (congenital) A5Ø.Ø2
  - talus (juvenile) — *see* Osteochondrosis, juvenile, tarsus
  - tarsus (navicular) (juvenile) — *see* Osteochondrosis, juvenile, tarsus
  - tibia (proximal) (tubercle) (juvenile) — *see* Osteochondrosis, juvenile, tibia
  - tuberculous — *see* Tuberculosis, bone
  - ulna (lower) (juvenile) — *see* Osteochondrosis, juvenile, ulna
  - van Neck's M91.Ø
  - vertebral — *see* Osteochondrosis, spine

- **Osteoclastoma** D48.Ø
  - malignant — *see* Neoplasm, bone, malignant
- **Osteodynia** — *see* Disorder, bone, specified type NEC
- **Osteodystrophy** Q78.9
  - azotemic N25.Ø
  - congenital Q78.9
  - parathyroid, secondary E21.1
  - renal N25.Ø
- **Osteofibroma** — *see* Neoplasm, bone, benign
- **Osteofibrosarcoma** — *see* Neoplasm, bone, malignant
- **Osteogenesis imperfecta** Q78.Ø
- **Osteogenic** — *see* condition
- **Osteolysis** M89.5Ø
  - carpus M89.54- ☑
  - clavicle M89.51- ☑
  - femur M89.55- ☑
  - fibula M89.56- ☑
  - finger M89.54- ☑
  - humerus M89.52- ☑
  - ilium M89.559
  - ischium M89.559
  - joint prosthesis (periprosthetic) — *see* Complications, joint prosthesis, mechanical, periprosthetic, osteolysis, by site
  - metacarpus M89.54- ☑
  - metatarsus M89.57- ☑
  - multiple sites M89.59
  - neck M89.58
  - periprosthetic — *see* Complications, joint prosthesis, mechanical, periprosthetic, osteolysis, by site
  - radius M89.53- ☑
  - rib M89.58
  - scapula M89.51- ☑
  - skull M89.58
  - tarsus M89.57- ☑
  - tibia M89.56- ☑
  - toe M89.57- ☑
  - ulna M89.53- ☑
  - vertebra M89.58
- **Osteoma** (*see also* Neoplasm, bone, benign)
  - osteoid (*see also* Neoplasm, bone, benign)
    - giant — *see* Neoplasm, bone, benign
- **Osteomalacia** M83.9
  - adult M83.9
    - drug-induced NEC M83.5
    - due to
      - malabsorption (postsurgical) M83.2
      - malnutrition M83.3
    - specified NEC M83.8
  - aluminium-induced M83.4
  - infantile — *see* Rickets
  - juvenile — *see* Rickets
  - oncogenic E83.89
  - pelvis M83.8
  - puerperal M83.Ø
  - senile M83.1
  - vitamin-D-resistant in adults E83.31 [M9Ø.8-] ☑
    - carpus E83.31 [M9Ø.84-] ☑
    - clavicle E83.31 [M9Ø.81-] ☑
    - femur E83.31 [M9Ø.85-] ☑
    - fibula E83.31 [M9Ø.86-] ☑
    - finger E83.31 [M9Ø.84-] ☑
    - humerus E83.31 [M9Ø.82-] ☑
    - ilium E83.31 [M9Ø.859]
    - ischium E83.31 [M9Ø.859]
    - metacarpus E83.31 [M9Ø.84-] ☑
    - metatarsus E83.31 [M9Ø.87-] ☑
    - multiple sites E83.31 [M9Ø.89]
    - neck E83.31 [M9Ø.88]
    - radius E83.31 [M9Ø.83-] ☑
    - rib E83.31 [M9Ø.88]
    - scapula E83.31 [M9Ø.819]
    - skull E83.31 [M9Ø.88]
    - tarsus E83.31 [M9Ø.879]
    - tibia E83.31 [M9Ø.869]
    - toe E83.31 [M9Ø.879]
    - ulna E83.31 [M9Ø.839]
    - vertebra E83.31 [M9Ø.88]
- **Osteomyelitis** (general) (infective) (localized) (neonatal) (purulent) (septic) (staphylococcal) (streptococcal) (suppurative) (with periostitis) M86.9
  - acute M86.1Ø
    - carpus M86.14- ☑
    - clavicle M86.11- ☑
    - femur M86.15- ☑
    - fibula M86.16- ☑
    - finger M86.14- ☑

- **Osteomyelitis** — *continued*
  - acute — *continued*
    - hematogenous M86.ØØ
      - carpus M86.Ø4- ☑
      - clavicle M86.Ø1- ☑
      - femur M86.Ø5- ☑
      - fibula M86.Ø6- ☑
      - finger M86.Ø4- ☑
      - humerus M86.Ø2- ☑
      - ilium M86.Ø59
      - ischium M86.Ø59
      - mandible M27.2
      - metacarpus M86.Ø4- ☑
      - metatarsus M86.Ø7- ☑
      - multiple sites M86.Ø9
      - neck M86.Ø8
      - orbit HØ5.Ø2- ☑
      - petrous bone — *see* Petrositis
      - radius M86.Ø3- ☑
      - rib M86.Ø8
      - scapula M86.Ø1- ☑
      - skull M86.Ø8
      - tarsus M86.Ø7- ☑
      - tibia M86.Ø6- ☑
      - toe M86.Ø7- ☑
      - ulna M86.Ø3- ☑
      - vertebra — *see* Osteomyelitis, vertebra
    - humerus M86.12- ☑
    - ilium M86.159
    - ischium M86.159
    - mandible M27.2
    - metacarpus M86.14- ☑
    - metatarsus M86.17- ☑
    - multiple sites M86.19
    - neck M86.18
    - orbit HØ5.Ø2- ☑
    - petrous bone — *see* Petrositis
    - radius M86.13- ☑
    - rib M86.18
    - scapula M86.11- ☑
    - skull M86.18
    - tarsus M86.17- ☑
    - tibia M86.16- ☑
    - toe M86.17- ☑
    - ulna M86.13- ☑
    - vertebra — *see* Osteomyelitis, vertebra
  - chronic (or old) M86.6Ø
    - with draining sinus M86.4Ø
      - carpus M86.44- ☑
      - clavicle M86.41- ☑
      - femur M86.45- ☑
      - fibula M86.46- ☑
      - finger M86.44- ☑
      - humerus M86.42- ☑
      - ilium M86.459
      - ischium M86.459
      - mandible M27.2
      - metacarpus M86.44- ☑
      - metatarsus M86.47- ☑
      - multiple sites M86.49
      - neck M86.48
      - orbit HØ5.Ø2- ☑
      - petrous bone — *see* Petrositis
      - radius M86.43- ☑
      - rib M86.48
      - scapula M86.41- ☑
      - skull M86.48
      - tarsus M86.47- ☑
      - tibia M86.46- ☑
      - toe M86.47- ☑
      - ulna M86.43- ☑
      - vertebra — *see* Osteomyelitis, vertebra
    - carpus M86.64- ☑
    - clavicle M86.61- ☑
    - femur M86.65- ☑
    - fibula M86.66- ☑
    - finger M86.64- ☑
    - hematogenous NEC M86.5Ø
      - carpus M86.54- ☑
      - clavicle M86.51- ☑
      - femur M86.55- ☑
      - fibula M86.56- ☑
      - finger M86.54- ☑
      - humerus M86.52- ☑
      - ilium M86.559
      - ischium M86.559

- **Osteomyelitis** — *continued*
  - chronic — *continued*
    - hematogenous — *continued*
      - mandible M27.2
      - metacarpus M86.54- ☑
      - metatarsus M86.57- ☑
      - multifocal M86.3Ø
        - carpus M86.34- ☑
        - clavicle M86.31- ☑
        - femur M86.35- ☑
        - fibula M86.36- ☑
        - finger M86.34- ☑
        - humerus M86.32- ☑
        - ilium M86.359
        - ischium M86.359
        - metacarpus M86.34- ☑
        - metatarsus M86.37- ☑
        - multiple sites M86.39
        - neck M86.38
        - radius M86.33- ☑
        - rib M86.38
        - scapula M86.31- ☑
        - skull M86.38
        - tarsus M86.37- ☑
        - tibia M86.36- ☑
        - toe M86.37- ☑
        - ulna M86.33- ☑
        - vertebra — *see* Osteomyelitis, vertebra
      - multiple sites M86.59
      - neck M86.58
      - orbit HØ5.Ø2- ☑
      - petrous bone — *see* Petrositis
      - radius M86.53- ☑
      - rib M86.58
      - scapula M86.51- ☑
      - skull M86.58
      - tarsus M86.57- ☑
      - tibia M86.56- ☑
      - toe M86.57- ☑
      - ulna M86.53- ☑
      - vertebra — *see* Osteomyelitis, vertebra
    - humerus M86.62- ☑
    - ilium M86.659
    - ischium M86.659
    - mandible M27.2
    - metacarpus M86.64- ☑
    - metatarsus M86.67- ☑
    - multifocal — *see* Osteomyelitis, chronic, hematogenous, multifocal
    - multiple sites M86.69
    - neck M86.68
    - orbit HØ5.Ø2- ☑
    - petrous bone — *see* Petrositis
    - radius M86.63- ☑
    - rib M86.68
    - scapula M86.61- ☑
    - skull M86.68
    - tarsus M86.67- ☑
    - tibia M86.66- ☑
    - toe M86.67- ☑
    - ulna M86.63- ☑
    - vertebra — *see* Osteomyelitis, vertebra
  - echinococcal B67.2
  - Garr's — *see* Osteomyelitis, specified type NEC
  - jaw (acute) (chronic) (lower) (neonatal) (suppurative) (upper) M27.2
  - nonsuppurating — *see* Osteomyelitis, specified type NEC
  - orbit HØ5.Ø2- ☑
  - petrous bone — *see* Petrositis
  - Salmonella (arizonae) (cholerae-suis) (enteritidis) (typhimurium) AØ2.24
  - sclerosing, nonsuppurative — *see* Osteomyelitis, specified type NEC
  - specified type NEC (*see also* subcategory) M86.8X- ☑
    - mandible M27.2
    - orbit HØ5.Ø2- ☑
    - petrous bone — *see* Petrositis
    - vertebra — *see* Osteomyelitis, vertebra
  - subacute M86.2Ø
    - carpus M86.24- ☑
    - clavicle M86.21- ☑
    - femur M86.25- ☑
    - fibula M86.26- ☑
    - finger M86.24- ☑
    - humerus M86.22- ☑

- **Osteomyelitis** — *continued*
  - subacute — *continued*
    - mandible M27.2
    - metacarpus M86.24- ☑
    - metatarsus M86.27- ☑
    - multiple sites M86.29
    - neck M86.28
    - orbit HØ5.Ø2- ☑
    - petrous bone — *see* Petrositis
    - radius M86.23- ☑
    - rib M86.28
    - scapula M86.21- ☑
    - skull M86.28
    - tarsus M86.27- ☑
    - tibia M86.26- ☑
    - toe M86.27- ☑
    - ulna M86.23- ☑
    - vertebra — *see* Osteomyelitis, vertebra
  - syphilitic A52.77
    - congenital (early) A5Ø.Ø2 [M9Ø.8Ø]
  - tuberculous — *see* Tuberculosis, bone
  - typhoid AØ1.Ø5
  - vertebra M46.2Ø
    - cervical region M46.22
    - cervicothoracic region M46.23
    - lumbar region M46.26
    - lumbosacral region M46.27
    - occipito-atlanto-axial region M46.21
    - sacrococcygeal region M46.28
    - thoracic region M46.24
    - thoracolumbar region M46.25
- **Osteomyelofibrosis** D75.89
- **Osteomyelosclerosis** D75.89
- **Osteonecrosis** M87.9
  - due to
    - drugs — *see* Osteonecrosis, secondary, due to, drugs
    - trauma — *see* Osteonecrosis, secondary, due to, trauma
  - idiopathic aseptic M87.ØØ
    - ankle M87.Ø7- ☑
    - carpus M87.Ø3- ☑
    - clavicle M87.Ø1- ☑
    - femur M87.Ø5- ☑
    - fibula M87.Ø6- ☑
    - finger M87.Ø4- ☑
    - humerus M87.Ø2- ☑
    - ilium M87.Ø5Ø
    - ischium M87.Ø5Ø
    - metacarpus M87.Ø4- ☑
    - metatarsus M87.Ø7- ☑
    - multiple sites M87.Ø9
    - neck M87.Ø8
    - pelvis M87.Ø5Ø
    - radius M87.Ø3- ☑
    - rib M87.Ø8
    - scapula M87.Ø1- ☑
    - skull M87.Ø8
    - tarsus M87.Ø7- ☑
    - tibia M87.Ø6- ☑
    - toe M87.Ø7- ☑
    - ulna M87.Ø3- ☑
    - vertebra M87.Ø8
  - secondary NEC M87.3Ø
    - carpus M87.33- ☑
    - clavicle M87.31- ☑
    - due to
      - drugs M87.1Ø
        - carpus M87.13- ☑
        - clavicle M87.11- ☑
        - femur M87.15- ☑
        - fibula M87.16- ☑
        - finger M87.14- ☑
        - humerus M87.12- ☑
        - ilium M87.159
        - ischium M87.159
        - jaw M87.18Ø
        - metacarpus M87.14- ☑
        - metatarsus M87.17- ☑
        - multiple sites M87.19
        - neck M87.18
        - radius M87.13- ☑
        - rib M87.18 ☑
        - scapula M87.11- ☑
        - skull M87.18 ☑
        - tarsus M87.17- ☑
        - tibia M87.16- ☑

- **Osteopsathyrosis** (idiopathica) Q78.0
- **Osteoradionecrosis, jaw** (acute) (chronic) (lower) (suppurative) (upper) M27.2
- **Osteosarcoma** (any form) — *see* Neoplasm, bone, malignant
- **Osteosclerosis** Q78.2
  - acquired M85.8- ☑
  - congenita Q77.4
  - fragilitas (generalisata) Q78.2
  - myelofibrosis D75.81
- **Osteosclerotic anemia** D64.89
- **Osteosis**
  - cutis L94.2
  - renal fibrocystic N25.0
- **Österreicher-Turner syndrome** Q87.2
- **Ostium**
  - atrioventriculare commune Q21.2
  - primum (arteriosum) (defect) (persistent) Q21.2
  - secundum (arteriosum) (defect) (patent) (persistent) Q21.1
- **Ostrum-Furst syndrome** Q75.8
- **Otalgia** H92.0 ☑
- **Otitis** (acute) H66.90
  - with effusion (*see also* Otitis, media, nonsuppurative)
    - purulent — *see* Otitis, media, suppurative
  - adhesive — *see* subcategory H74.1 ☑
  - chronic (*see also* Otitis, media, chronic)
    - with effusion (*see also* Otitis, media, nonsuppurative, chronic)
  - externa H60.9- ☑
    - abscess — *see* Abscess, ear, external
    - acute (noninfective) H60.50- ☑
      - actinic H60.51- ☑
      - chemical H60.52- ☑
      - contact H60.53- ☑
      - eczematoid H60.54- ☑
      - infective — *see* Otitis, externa, infective
      - reactive H60.55- ☑
      - specified NEC H60.59- ☑
    - cellulitis — *see* Cellulitis, ear
    - chronic H60.6- ☑
    - diffuse — *see* Otitis, externa, infective, diffuse
    - hemorrhagic — *see* Otitis, externa, infective, hemorrhagic
    - in (due to)
      - aspergillosis B44.89
      - candidiasis B37.84
      - erysipelas A46 [H62.40]
      - herpes (simplex) virus infection B00.1
        - zoster B02.8
      - impetigo L01.00 [H62.40]
      - infectious disease NEC B99 ☑ [H62.4-] ☑
      - mycosis NEC B36.9 [H62.40]
      - parasitic disease NEC B89 [H62.40]
      - viral disease NEC B34.9 [H62.40]
      - zoster B02.8
    - infective NEC H60.39- ☑
      - abscess — *see* Abscess, ear, external
      - cellulitis — *see* Cellulitis, ear
      - diffuse H60.31- ☑
      - hemorrhagic H60.32- ☑
      - swimmer's ear — *see* Swimmer's, ear
    - malignant H60.2- ☑
    - mycotic B36.9 [H62.40]
    - necrotizing — *see* Otitis, externa, malignant
    - Pseudomonas aeruginosa — *see* Otitis, externa, malignant
    - reactive — *see* Otitis, externa, acute, reactive
    - specified NEC — *see* subcategory H60.8 ☑
    - tropical B36.8
  - insidiosa — *see* Otosclerosis
  - interna H83.0 ☑
  - media (hemorrhagic) (staphylococcal) (streptococcal) H66.9- ☑
    - with effusion (nonpurulent) — *see* Otitis, media, nonsuppurative
    - acute, subacute H66.90
      - allergic — *see* Otitis, media, nonsuppurative, acute, allergic
      - exudative — *see* Otitis, media, nonsuppurative, acute
      - mucoid — *see* Otitis, media, nonsuppurative, acute
      - necrotizing (*see also* Otitis, media, suppurative, acute)
        - in
          - measles B05.3

Otitis — *continued*
- media — *continued*
  - acute, subacute — *continued*
    - necrotizing (*see also* Otitis, media, suppurative, acute) — *continued*
      - in — *continued*
        - scarlet fever A38.0
    - nonsuppurative NEC — *see* Otitis, media, nonsuppurative, acute
    - purulent — *see* Otitis, media, suppurative, acute
    - sanguinous — *see* Otitis, media, nonsuppurative, acute
    - secretory — *see* Otitis, media, nonsuppurative, acute, serous
    - seromucinous — *see* Otitis, media, nonsuppurative, acute
    - serous — *see* Otitis, media, nonsuppurative, acute, serous
    - suppurative — *see* Otitis, media, suppurative, acute
  - allergic — *see* Otitis, media, nonsuppurative
  - catarrhal — *see* Otitis, media, nonsuppurative
  - chronic H66.90
    - with effusion (nonpurulent) — *see* Otitis, media, nonsuppurative, chronic
    - allergic — *see* Otitis, media, nonsuppurative, chronic, allergic
    - benign suppurative — *see* Otitis, media, suppurative, chronic, tubotympanic
    - catarrhal — *see* Otitis, media, nonsuppurative, chronic, serous
    - exudative — *see* Otitis, media, nonsuppurative, chronic
    - mucinous — *see* Otitis, media, nonsuppurative, chronic, mucoid
    - mucoid — *see* Otitis, media, nonsuppurative, chronic, mucoid
    - nonsuppurative NEC — *see* Otitis, media, nonsuppurative, chronic
    - purulent — *see* Otitis, media, suppurative, chronic
    - secretory — *see* Otitis, media, nonsuppurative, chronic, mucoid
    - seromucinous — *see* Otitis, media, nonsuppurative, chronic
    - serous — *see* Otitis, media, nonsuppurative, chronic, serous
    - suppurative — *see* Otitis, media, suppurative, chronic
    - transudative — *see* Otitis, media, nonsuppurative, chronic, mucoid
  - exudative — *see* Otitis, media, nonsuppurative
  - in (due to) (with)
    - influenza — *see* Influenza, with, otitis media
    - measles B05.3
    - scarlet fever A38.0
    - tuberculosis A18.6
    - viral disease NEC B34.- ☑ [H67.-] ☑
  - mucoid — *see* Otitis, media, nonsuppurative
  - nonsuppurative H65.9- ☑
    - acute or subacute NEC H65.19- ☑
      - allergic H65.11- ☑
        - recurrent H65.11- ☑
      - recurrent H65.19- ☑
      - secretory — *see* Otitis, media, nonsuppurative, serous
      - serous H65.0- ☑
        - recurrent H65.0- ☑
    - chronic H65.49- ☑
      - allergic H65.41- ☑
      - mucoid H65.3- ☑
      - serous H65.2- ☑
  - postmeasles B05.3
  - purulent — *see* Otitis, media, suppurative
  - secretory — *see* Otitis, media, nonsuppurative
  - seromucinous — *see* Otitis, media, nonsuppurative
  - serous — *see* Otitis, media, nonsuppurative
  - suppurative H66.4- ☑
    - acute H66.00- ☑
      - with rupture of ear drum H66.01- ☑
      - recurrent H66.00- ☑
        - with rupture of ear drum H66.01- ☑
    - chronic (*see also* subcategory) H66.3 ☑
      - atticoantral H66.2- ☑
      - benign — *see* Otitis, media, suppurative, chronic, tubotympanic

Otitis — *continued*
- media — *continued*
  - suppurative — *continued*
    - chronic (*see also* subcategory) — *continued*
      - tubotympanic H66.1- ☑
  - transudative — *see* Otitis, media, nonsuppurative
  - tuberculous A18.6
- **Otocephaly** Q18.2
- **Otolith syndrome** — *see* subcategory H81.8 ☑
- **Otomycosis** (diffuse) **NEC** B36.9 [H62.40]
  - in
    - aspergillosis B44.89
    - candidiasis B37.84
    - moniliasis B37.84
- **Otoporosis** — *see* Otosclerosis
- **Otorrhagia** (nontraumatic) H92.2- ☑
  - traumatic — *code by* Type of injury
- **Otorrhea** H92.1- ☑
  - cerebrospinal G96.0
- **Otosclerosis** (general) H80.9- ☑
  - cochlear (endosteal) H80.2- ☑
  - involving
    - otic capsule — *see* Otosclerosis, cochlear
    - oval window
      - nonobliterative H80.0- ☑
      - obliterative H80.1- ☑
    - round window — *see* Otosclerosis, cochlear
  - nonobliterative — *see* Otosclerosis, involving, oval window, nonobliterative
  - obliterative — *see* Otosclerosis, involving, oval window, obliterative
  - specified NEC H80.8- ☑
- **Otospongiosis** — *see* Otosclerosis
- **Otto's disease or pelvis** M24.7
- **Outcome of delivery** Z37.9
  - multiple births Z37.9
    - all liveborn Z37.50
      - quadruplets Z37.52
      - quintuplets Z37.53
      - sextuplets Z37.54
      - specified number NEC Z37.59
      - triplets Z37.51
    - all stillborn Z37.7
    - some liveborn Z37.60
      - quadruplets Z37.62
      - quintuplets Z37.63
      - sextuplets Z37.64
      - specified number NEC Z37.69
      - triplets Z37.61
  - single NEC Z37.9
    - liveborn Z37.0
    - stillborn Z37.1
  - twins NEC Z37.9
    - both liveborn Z37.2
    - both stillborn Z37.4
    - one liveborn, one stillborn Z37.3
- **Outlet** — *see* condition
- **Ovalocytosis** (congenital) (hereditary) — *see* Elliptocytosis
- **Ovarian** — *see* Condition
- **Ovariocele** N83.4
- **Ovaritis** (cystic) — *see* Oophoritis
- **Ovary, ovarian** (*see also* condition)
  - resistant syndrome E28.39
  - vein syndrome N13.8
- **Overactive** (*see also* Hyperfunction)
  - adrenal cortex NEC E27.0
  - bladder N32.81
  - hypothalamus E23.3
  - thyroid — *see* Hyperthyroidism
- **Overactivity** R46.3
  - child — *see* Disorder, attention-deficit hyperactivity
- **Overbite** (deep) (excessive) (horizontal) (vertical) M26.29
- **Overbreathing** — *see* Hyperventilation
- **Overconscientious personality** F60.5
- **Overdevelopment** — *see* Hypertrophy
- **Overdistension** — *see* Distension
- **Overdose, overdosage** (drug) — *see* Table of Drugs and Chemicals, by drug, poisoning
- **Overeating** R63.2
  - nonorganic origin F50.8
  - psychogenic F50.8
- **Overexertion** (effects) (exhaustion) T73.3 ☑
- **Overexposure** (effects) T73.9 ☑
  - exhaustion T73.2 ☑
- **Overfeeding** — *see* Overeating
  - newborn P92.4

- **Overfill, endodontic** M27.52
- **Overgrowth, bone** — *see* Hypertrophy, bone
- **Overhanging of dental restorative material** (unrepairable) KØ8.52
- **Overheated** (places) (effects) — *see* Heat
- **Overjet** (excessive horizontal) M26.23
- **Overlaid, overlying** (suffocation) — *see* Asphyxia, traumatic, due to mechanical threat
- **Overlap, excessive horizontal** (teeth) M26.23
- **Overlapping toe** (acquired) (*see also* Deformity, toe, specified NEC)
  - congenital (fifth toe) Q66.89
- **Overload**
  - circulatory, due to transfusion (blood) (blood components) (TACO) E87.71
  - fluid E87.7Ø
    - due to transfusion (blood) (blood components) E87.71
    - specified NEC E87.79
  - iron, due to repeated red blood cell transfusions E83.111
  - potassium (K) E87.5
  - sodium (Na) E87.Ø
- **Overnutrition** — *see* Hyperalimentation
- **Overproduction** (*see also* Hypersecretion)
  - ACTH E27.Ø
  - catecholamine E27.5
  - growth hormone E22.Ø
- **Overprotection, child by parent** Z62.1
- **Overriding**
  - aorta Q25.4
  - finger (acquired) — *see* Deformity, finger
    - congenital Q68.1
  - toe (acquired) (*see also* Deformity, toe, specified NEC)
    - congenital Q66.89
- **Overstrained** R53.83
  - heart — *see* Hypertrophy, cardiac
- **Overuse, muscle NEC** M7Ø.8- ☑
- **Overweight** E66.3
- **Overworked** R53.83
- **Oviduct** — *see* condition
- **Ovotestis** Q56.Ø
- **Ovulation** (cycle)
  - failure or lack of N97.Ø
  - pain N94.Ø
- **Ovum** — *see* condition
- **Owren's disease or syndrome** (parahemophilia) D68.2
- **Ox heart** — *see* Hypertrophy, cardiac
- **Oxalosis** E72.53
- **Oxaluria** E72.53
- **Oxycephaly, oxycephalic** Q75.Ø
  - syphilitic, congenital A5Ø.Ø2
- **Oxyuriasis** B8Ø
- **Oxyuris vermicularis** (infestation) B8Ø
- **Ozena** J31.Ø

P

- **Pachyderma, pachydermia** L85.9
  - larynx (verrucosa) J38.7
- **Pachydermatocele** (congenital) Q82.8
- **Pachydermoperiostosis** (*see also* Osteoarthropathy, hypertrophic, specified type NEC)
  - clubbed nail M89.4Ø [L62]
- **Pachygyria** QØ4.3
- **Pachymeningitis** (adhesive) (basal) (brain) (cervical) (chronic)(circumscribed) (external) (fibrous) (hemorrhagic) (hypertrophic) (internal) (purulent) (spinal) (suppurative) — *see* Meningitis
- **Pachyonychia** (congenital) Q84.5
- **Pacinian tumor** — *see* Neoplasm, skin, benign
- **Pad, knuckle or Garrod's** M72.1
- **Paget's disease**
  - with infiltrating duct carcinoma — *see* Neoplasm, breast, malignant
  - bone M88.9
    - carpus M88.84- ☑
    - clavicle M88.81- ☑
    - femur M88.85- ☑
    - fibula M88.86- ☑
    - finger M88.84- ☑
    - humerus M88.82- ☑
    - ilium M88.85- ☑
    - in neoplastic disease — *see* Osteitis, deformans, in neoplastic disease
    - ischium M88.85- ☑
    - metacarpus M88.84- ☑

Paget's disease — *continued*
- bone — *continued*
  - metatarsus M88.87- ☑
  - multiple sites M88.89
  - neck M88.88
  - radius M88.83- ☑
  - rib M88.88
  - scapula M88.81- ☑
  - skull M88.Ø
  - tarsus M88.87- ☑
  - tibia M88.86- ☑
  - toe M88.87- ☑
  - ulna M88.83- ☑
  - vertebra M88.88
- breast (female) C5Ø.Ø1- ☑
  - male C5Ø.Ø2- ☑
- extramammary (*see also* Neoplasm, skin, malignant)
  - anus C21.Ø
    - margin C44.59Ø
    - skin C44.59Ø
- intraductal carcinoma — *see* Neoplasm, breast, malignant
- malignant — *see* Neoplasm, skin, malignant
  - breast (female) C5Ø.Ø1- ☑
    - male C5Ø.Ø2- ☑
  - unspecified site (female) C5Ø.Ø1- ☑
    - male C5Ø.Ø2- ☑
- mammary — *see* Paget's disease, breast
- nipple — *see* Paget's disease, breast
- osteitis deformans — *see* Paget's disease, bone

- **Paget-Schroetter syndrome** I82.89Ø
- **Pain**(s) (*see also* Painful) R52
  - abdominal R1Ø.9
    - colic R1Ø.83
    - generalized R1Ø.84
      - with acute abdomen R1Ø.Ø
    - lower R1Ø.3Ø
      - left quadrant R1Ø.32
      - pelvic or perineal R1Ø.2
      - periumbilical R1Ø.33
      - right quadrant R1Ø.31
    - rebound — *see* Tenderness, abdominal, rebound
    - severe with abdominal rigidity R1Ø.Ø
    - tenderness — *see* Tenderness, abdominal
    - upper R1Ø.1Ø
      - epigastric R1Ø.13
      - left quadrant R1Ø.12
      - right quadrant R1Ø.11
  - acute R52
    - due to trauma G89.11
    - neoplasm related G89.3
    - postprocedural NEC G89.18
    - post-thoracotomy G89.12
    - specified by site — *code to* Pain, by site
  - adnexa (uteri) R1Ø.2
  - anginoid — *see* Pain, precordial
  - anus K62.89
  - arm — *see* Pain, limb, upper
  - axillary (axilla) M79.62- ☑
  - back (postural) M54.9
  - bladder R39.89
    - associated with micturition — *see* Micturition, painful
  - bone — *see* Disorder, bone, specified type NEC
  - breast N64.4
  - broad ligament R1Ø.2
  - cancer associated (acute) (chronic) G89.3
  - cecum — *see* Pain, abdominal
  - cervicobrachial M53.1
  - chest (central) RØ7.9
    - anterior wall RØ7.89
    - atypical RØ7.89
    - ischemic I2Ø.9
    - musculoskeletal RØ7.89
    - non-cardiac RØ7.89
    - on breathing RØ7.1
    - pleurodynia RØ7.81
    - precordial RØ7.2
    - wall (anterior) RØ7.89
  - chronic G89.29
    - associated with significant psychosocial dysfunction G89.4
    - due to trauma G89.21
    - neoplasm related G89.3
    - postoperative NEC G89.28
    - postprocedural NEC G89.28
    - post-thoracotomy G89.22

Pain(s) — *continued*
- chronic — *continued*
  - specified NEC G89.29
- coccyx M53.3
- colon — *see* Pain, abdominal
- coronary — *see* Angina
- costochondral RØ7.1
- diaphragm RØ7.1
- due to cancer G89.3
- due to device, implant or graft (*see also* Complications, by site and type, specified NEC) T85.84 ☑
  - arterial graft NEC T82.848 ☑
  - breast (implant) T85.84 ☑
  - catheter NEC T85.84 ☑
    - dialysis (renal) T82.848 ☑
      - intraperitoneal T85.84 ☑
    - infusion NEC T82.848 ☑
      - spinal (epidural) (subdural) T85.84 ☑
    - urinary (indwelling) T83.84 ☑
  - electronic (electrode) (pulse generator) (stimulator)
    - bone T84.84 ☑
    - cardiac T82.847 ☑
    - nervous system (brain) (peripheral nerve) (spinal) T85.84 ☑
    - urinary T83.84 ☑
  - fixation, internal (orthopedic) NEC T84.84 ☑
  - gastrointestinal (bile duct) (esophagus) T85.84 ☑
  - genital NEC T83.84 ☑
  - heart NEC T82.847 ☑
  - infusion NEC T85.84 ☑
  - joint prosthesis T84.84 ☑
  - ocular (corneal graft) (orbital implant) NEC T85.84 ☑
  - orthopedic NEC T84.84 ☑
  - specified NEC T85.84 ☑
  - urinary NEC T83.84 ☑
  - vascular NEC T82.848 ☑
  - ventricular intracranial shunt T85.84 ☑
- due to malignancy (primary) (secondary) G89.3
- ear — *see* subcategory H92.Ø ☑
- epigastric, epigastrium R1Ø.13
- eye — *see* Pain, ocular
- face, facial R51
  - atypical G5Ø.1
- female genital organs NEC N94.89
- finger — *see* Pain, limb, upper
- flank — *see* Pain, abdominal
- foot — *see* Pain, limb, lower
- gallbladder K82.9
- gas (intestinal) R14.1
- gastric — *see* Pain, abdominal
- generalized NOS R52
- genital organ
  - female N94.89
  - male N5Ø.8
- groin — *see* Pain, abdominal, lower
- hand — *see* Pain, limb, upper
- head — *see* Headache
- heart — *see* Pain, precordial
- infra-orbital — *see* Neuralgia, trigeminal
- intercostal RØ7.82
- intermenstrual N94.Ø
- jaw R68.84
- joint M25.5Ø
  - ankle M25.57- ☑
  - elbow M25.52- ☑
  - finger M79.64- ☑
  - foot M25.57- ☑
  - hand M79.64- ☑
  - hip M25.55- ☑
  - knee M25.56- ☑
  - shoulder M25.51- ☑
  - toe M25.57- ☑
  - wrist M25.53- ☑
- kidney N23
- laryngeal RØ7.Ø
- leg — *see* Pain, limb, lower
- limb M79.6Ø9
  - lower M79.6Ø- ☑
    - foot M79.67- ☑
    - lower leg M79.66- ☑
    - thigh M79.65- ☑
    - toe M79.67- ☑
  - upper M79.6Ø- ☑
    - axilla M79.62- ☑
    - finger M79.64- ☑

- **Pain(s)** — *continued*
  - limb — *continued*
    - upper — *continued*
      - forearm M79.63- ☑
      - hand M79.64- ☑
      - upper arm M79.62- ☑
  - loin M54.5
  - low back M54.5
  - lumbar region M54.5
  - mandibular R68.84
  - mastoid — *see* subcategory H92.Ø ☑
  - maxilla R68.84
  - menstrual (*see also* Dysmenorrhea) N94.6
  - metacarpophalangeal (joint) — *see* Pain, joint, hand
  - metatarsophalangeal (joint) — *see* Pain, joint, foot
  - mouth K13.79
  - muscle — *see* Myalgia
  - musculoskeletal (*see also* Pain, by site) M79.1
  - myofascial M79.1
  - nasal J34.89
  - nasopharynx J39.2
  - neck NEC M54.2
  - nerve NEC — *see* Neuralgia
  - neuromuscular — *see* Neuralgia
  - nose J34.89
  - ocular H57.1- ☑
  - ophthalmic — *see* Pain, ocular
  - orbital region — *see* Pain, ocular
  - ovary N94.89
  - over heart — *see* Pain, precordial
  - ovulation N94.Ø
  - pelvic (female) R1Ø.2
  - penis N48.89
  - pericardial — *see* Pain, precordial
  - perineal, perineum R1Ø.2
  - pharynx J39.2
  - pleura, pleural, pleuritic RØ7.81
  - postoperative NOS G89.18
  - postprocedural NOS G89.18
  - post-thoracotomy G89.12
  - precordial (region) RØ7.2
  - premenstrual N94.3
  - psychogenic (persistent) (any site) F45.41
  - radicular (spinal) — *see* Radiculopathy
  - rectum K62.89
  - respiration RØ7.1
  - retrosternal RØ7.2
  - rheumatoid, muscular — *see* Myalgia
  - rib RØ7.81
  - root (spinal) — *see* Radiculopathy
  - round ligament (stretch) R1Ø.2
  - sacroiliac M53.3
  - sciatic — *see* Sciatica
  - scrotum N5Ø.8
  - seminal vesicle N5Ø.8
  - shoulder M25.51- ☑
  - spermatic cord N5Ø.8
  - spinal root — *see* Radiculopathy
  - spine M54.9
    - cervical M54.2
    - low back M54.5
      - with sciatica M54.4- ☑
    - thoracic M54.6
  - stomach — *see* Pain, abdominal
  - substernal RØ7.2
  - temporomandibular (joint) M26.62
  - testis N5Ø.8
  - thoracic spine M54.6
    - with radicular and visceral pain M54.14
  - throat RØ7.Ø
  - tibia — *see* Pain, limb, lower
  - toe — *see* Pain, limb, lower
  - tongue K14.6
  - tooth KØ8.8
  - trigeminal — *see* Neuralgia, trigeminal
  - tumor associated G89.3
  - ureter N23
  - urinary (organ) (system) N23
  - uterus NEC N94.89
  - vagina R1Ø.2
  - vertebrogenic (syndrome) M54.89
  - vesical R39.89
    - associated with micturition — *see* Micturition, painful
  - vulva R1Ø.2
- **Painful** (*see also* Pain)
  - coitus
    - female N94.1
    - male N53.12
    - psychogenic F52.6
  - ejaculation (semen) N53.12
    - psychogenic F52.6
  - erection — *see* Priapism
  - feet syndrome E53.8
  - joint replacement (hip) (knee) T84.84 ☑
  - menstruation — *see* Dysmenorrhea
    - psychogenic F45.8
  - micturition — *see* Micturition, painful
  - respiration RØ7.1
  - scar NEC L9Ø.5
  - wire sutures T81.89 ☑
- **Painter's colic** — *see* subcategory T56.Ø ☑
- **Palate** — *see* condition
- **Palatoplegia** K13.79
- **Palatoschisis** — *see* Cleft, palate
- **Palilalia** R48.8
- **Palliative care** Z51.5
- **Pallor** R23.1
  - optic disc, temporal — *see* Atrophy, optic
- **Palmar** (*see also* condition)
  - fascia — *see* condition
- **Palpable**
  - cecum K63.89
  - kidney N28.89
  - ovary N83.8
  - prostate N42.9
  - spleen — *see* Splenomegaly
- **Palpitations** (heart) RØØ.2
  - psychogenic F45.8
- **Palsy** (*see also* Paralysis) G83.9
  - atrophic diffuse (progressive) G12.22
  - Bell's (*see also* Palsy, facial)
    - newborn P11.3
  - brachial plexus NEC G54.Ø
    - newborn (birth injury) P14.3
  - brain — *see* Palsy, cerebral
  - bulbar (progressive) (chronic) G12.22
    - of childhood (Fazio-Londe) G12.1
    - pseudo NEC G12.29
    - supranuclear (progressive) G23.1
  - cerebral (congenital) G8Ø.9
    - ataxic G8Ø.4
    - athetoid G8Ø.3
    - choreathetoid G8Ø.3
    - dipiegic G8Ø.8
      - spastic G8Ø.1
    - dyskinetic G8Ø.3
      - athetoid G8Ø.3
      - choreathetoid G8Ø.3
      - distonic G8Ø.3
    - dystonic G8Ø.3
    - hemiplegic G8Ø.8
      - spastic G8Ø.2
    - mixed G8Ø.8
    - monoplegic G8Ø.8
      - spastic G8Ø.1
    - paraplegic G8Ø.8
      - spastic G8Ø.1
    - quadriplegic G8Ø.8
      - spastic G8Ø.Ø
    - spastic G8Ø.1
      - diplegic G8Ø.1
      - hemiplegic G8Ø.2
      - monoplegic G8Ø.1
      - quadriplegic G8Ø.Ø
      - specified NEC G8Ø.1
      - tetrapelgic G8Ø.Ø
    - specified NEC G8Ø.8
    - syphilitic A52.12
      - congenital A5Ø.49
    - tetraplegic G8Ø.8
      - spastic G8Ø.Ø
  - cranial nerve (*see also* Disorder, nerve, cranial)
    - multiple G52.7
      - in
        - infectious disease B99 ☑ [G53]
        - neoplastic disease (*see also* Neoplasm) D49.9 [G53]
        - parasitic disease B89 [G53]
        - sarcoidosis D86.82
  - creeping G12.22
  - diver's T7Ø.3 ☑
  - Erb's P14.Ø
  - facial G51.Ø
- **Palsy** — *continued*
  - facial — *continued*
    - newborn (birth injury) P11.3
  - glossopharyngeal G52.1
  - Klumpke (-Déjérine) P14.1
  - lead — *see* subcategory T56.Ø ☑
  - median nerve (tardy) G56.1- ☑
  - nerve G58.9
    - specified NEC G58.8
  - peroneal nerve (acute) (tardy) G57.3- ☑
  - progressive supranuclear G23.1
  - pseudobulbar NEC G12.29
  - radial nerve (acute) G56.3- ☑
  - seventh nerve (*see also* Palsy, facial)
    - newborn P11.3
  - shaking — *see* Parkinsonism
  - spastic (cerebral) (spinal) G8Ø.1
  - ulnar nerve (tardy) G56.2- ☑
  - wasting G12.29
- **Paludism** — *see* Malaria
- **Panangiitis** M3Ø.Ø
- **Panaris, panaritium** (*see also* Cellulitis, digit)
  - with lymphangitis — *see* Lymphangitis, acute, digit
- **Panarteritis nodosa** M3Ø.Ø
  - brain or cerebral I67.7
- **Pancake heart** R93.1
  - with cor pulmonale (chronic) I27.81
- **Pancarditis** (acute) (chronic) I51.89
  - rheumatic IØ9.89
    - active or acute IØ1.8
- **Pancoast's syndrome or tumor** C34.1- ☑
- **Pancolitis, ulcerative** (chronic) K51.ØØ
  - with
    - abscess K51.Ø14
    - complication K51.Ø19
    - fistula K51.Ø13
    - obstruction K51.Ø12
    - rectal bleeding K51.Ø11
    - specified complication NEC K51.Ø18
- **Pancreas, pancreatic** — *see* condition
- **Pancreatitis** (annular) (apoplectic) (calcareous) (edematous) (hemorrhagic) (malignant) (recurrent) (subacute) (suppurative) K85.9
  - acute K85.9
    - alcohol induced K85.2
    - biliary K85.1
    - drug induced K85.3
    - gallstone K85.1
    - idiopathic K85.Ø
    - specified NEC K85.8
  - chronic (infectious) K86.1
    - alcohol-induced K86.Ø
    - recurrent K86.1
    - relapsing K86.1
  - cystic (chronic) K86.1
  - cytomegaloviral B25.2
  - fibrous (chronic) K86.1
  - gallstone K85.1
  - gangrenous K85.8
  - interstitial (chronic) K86.1
    - acute K85.8
  - mumps B26.3
  - recurrent (chronic) K86.1
  - relapsing, chronic K86.1
  - syphilitic A52.74
- **Pancreatoblastoma** — *see* Neoplasm, pancreas, malignant
- **Pancreolithiasis** K86.8
- **Pancytolysis** D75.89
- **Pancytopenia** (acquired) D61.818
  - with
    - malformations D61.Ø9
    - myelodysplastic syndrome — *see* Syndrome, myelodysplastic
  - antineoplastic chemotherapy induced D61.81Ø
  - congenital D61.Ø9
  - drug-induced NEC D61.811
- **Panencephalitis, subacute, sclerosing** A81.1
- **Panhematopenia** D61.9
  - congenital D61.Ø9
  - constitutional D61.Ø9
  - splenic, primary D73.1
- **Panhemocytopenia** D61.9
  - congenital D61.Ø9
  - constitutional D61.Ø9
- **Panhypogonadism** E29.1
- **Panhypopituitarism** E23.Ø
  - prepubertal E23.Ø

Panic (attack) (state) F41.Ø
- reaction to exceptional stress (transient) F43.Ø

Panmyelopathy, familial, constitutional D61.Ø9
Panmyelophthisis D61.82
- congenital D61.Ø9

Panmyelosis (acute) (with myelofibrosis) C94.4- ☑
Panner's disease — *see* Osteochondrosis, juvenile, humerus
Panneuritis endemica E51.11
Panniculitis (nodular) (nonsuppurative) M79.3
- back M54.ØØ
  - cervical region M54.Ø2
  - cervicothoracic region M54.Ø3
  - lumbar region M54.Ø6
  - lumbosacral region M54.Ø7
  - multiple sites M54.Ø9
  - occipito-atlanto-axial region M54.Ø1
  - sacrococcygeal region M54.Ø8
  - thoracic region M54.Ø4
  - thoracolumbar region M54.Ø5
- lupus L93.2
- mesenteric K65.4
- neck M54.Ø2
  - cervicothoracic region M54.Ø3
  - occipito-atlanto-axial region M54.Ø1
- relapsing M35.6

Panniculus adiposus (abdominal) E65
Pannus (allergic) (cornea) (degenerativus) (keratic) H16.42- ☑
- abdominal (symptomatic) E65
- trachomatosus, trachomatous (active) A71.1

Panophthalmitis H44.Ø1- ☑
Pansinusitis (chronic) (hyperplastic) (nonpurulent) (purulent) J32.4
- acute JØ1.4Ø
  - recurrent JØ1.41
- tuberculous A15.8

Panuveitis (sympathetic) H44.11- ☑
Panvalvular disease IØ8.9
- specified NEC IØ8.8

Papanicolaou smear, cervix Z12.4
- as part of routine gynecological examination ZØ1.419
  - with abnormal findings ZØ1.411
- for suspected neoplasm Z12.4
- nonspecific abnormal finding R87.619
- routine ZØ1.419
  - with abnormal findings ZØ1.411

Papilledema (choked disc) H47.1Ø
- associated with
  - decreased ocular pressure H47.12
  - increased intracranial pressure H47.11
  - retinal disorder H47.13
- Foster-Kennedy syndrome H47.14- ☑

Papillitis H46.ØØ
- anus K62.89
- chronic lingual K14.4
- necrotizing, kidney N17.2
- optic H46.Ø- ☑
- rectum K62.89
- renal, necrotizing N17.2
- tongue K14.Ø

Papilloma (*see also* Neoplasm, benign, by site)
- acuminatum (female) (male) (anogenital) A63.Ø
- benign pinta (primary) A67.Ø
- bladder (urinary) (transitional cell) D41.4
- choroid plexus (lateral ventricle) (third ventricle) D33.Ø
  - anaplastic C71.5
  - fourth ventricle D33.1
  - malignant C71.5
- renal pelvis (transitional cell) D41.1- ☑
  - benign D3Ø.1- ☑
- Schneiderian
  - specified site — *see* Neoplasm, benign, by site
  - unspecified site D14.Ø
- serous surface
  - borderline malignancy
    - specified site — *see* Neoplasm, uncertain behavior, by site
    - unspecified site D39.1Ø
  - specified site — *see* Neoplasm, benign, by site
  - unspecified site D27.9
- transitional (cell)
  - bladder (urinary) D41.4
  - inverted type — *see* Neoplasm, uncertain behavior, by site
  - renal pelvis D41.1- ☑
  - ureter D41.2- ☑

Papilloma — *continued*
- ureter (transitional cell) D41.2- ☑
  - benign D3Ø.2- ☑
- urothelial — *see* Neoplasm, uncertain behavior, by site
- villous — *see* Neoplasm, uncertain behavior, by site
  - adenocarcinoma in — *see* Neoplasm, malignant, by site
  - in situ — *see* Neoplasm, in situ
- yaws, plantar or palmar A66.1

Papillomata, multiple, of yaws A66.1
Papillomatosis (*see also* Neoplasm, benign, by site)
- confluent and reticulated L83
- cystic, breast — *see* Mastopathy, cystic
- ductal, breast — *see* Mastopathy, cystic
- intraductal (diffuse) — *see* Neoplasm, benign, by site
- subareolar duct D24- ☑

Papillomavirus, as cause of disease classified elsewhere B97.7
Papillon-Léage and Psaume syndrome Q87.Ø
Papule(s) R23.8
- carate (primary) A67.Ø
- fibrous, of nose D22.39
- Gottron's L94.4
- pinta (primary) A67.Ø

Papulosis
- lymphomatoid C86.6
- malignant I77.89

Papyraceous fetus O31.Ø- ☑
Para-albuminemia E88.Ø9
Paracephalus Q89.7
Parachute mitral valve Q23.2
Paracoccidioidomycosis B41.9
- disseminated B41.7
- generalized B41.7
- mucocutaneous-lymphangitic B41.8
- pulmonary B41.Ø
- specified NEC B41.8
- visceral B41.8

Paradentosis KØ5.4
Paraffinoma T88.8 ☑
Paraganglioma D44.7
- adrenal D35.Ø- ☑
  - malignant C74.1- ☑
- aortic body D44.7
  - malignant C75.5
- carotid body D44.6
  - malignant C75.4
- chromaffin (*see also* Neoplasm, benign, by site)
  - malignant — *see* Neoplasm, malignant, by site
- extra-adrenal D44.7
  - malignant C75.5
    - specified site — *see* Neoplasm, malignant, by site
    - unspecified site C75.5
  - specified site — *see* Neoplasm, uncertain behavior, by site
  - unspecified site D44.7
- gangliocytic D13.2
  - specified site — *see* Neoplasm, benign, by site
  - unspecified site D13.2
- glomus jugulare D44.7
  - malignant C75.5
- jugular D44.7
- malignant C75.5
  - specified site — *see* Neoplasm, malignant, by site
  - unspecified site C75.5
- nonchromaffin D44.7
  - malignant C75.5
    - specified site — *see* Neoplasm, malignant, by site
    - unspecified site C75.5
  - specified site — *see* Neoplasm, uncertain behavior, by site
  - unspecified site D44.7
- parasympathetic D44.7
  - specified site — *see* Neoplasm, uncertain behavior, by site
  - unspecified site D44.7
- specified site — *see* Neoplasm, uncertain behavior, by site
- sympathetic D44.7
  - specified site — *see* Neoplasm, uncertain behavior, by site
  - unspecified site D44.7
- unspecified site D44.7

Parageusia R43.2

Parageusia — *continued*
- psychogenic F45.8

Paragonimiasis B66.4
Paragranuloma, Hodgkin — *see* Lymphoma, Hodgkin, classical, specified NEC
Parahemophilia (*see also* Defect, coagulation) D68.2
Parakeratosis R23.4
- variegata L41.Ø

Paralysis, paralytic (complete) (incomplete) G83.9
- with
  - syphilis A52.17
- abducens, abducent (nerve) — *see* Strabismus, paralytic, sixth nerve
- abductor, lower extremity G57.9- ☑
- accessory nerve G52.8
- accommodation (*see also* Paresis, of accommodation)
  - hysterical F44.89
- acoustic nerve (except Deafness) H93.3 ☑
- agitans (*see also* Parkinsonism) G2Ø
  - arteriosclerotic G21.4
- alternating (oculomotor) G83.89
- amyotrophic G12.21
- ankle G57.9- ☑
- anus (sphincter) K62.89
- arm — *see* Monoplegia, upper limb
- ascending (spinal), acute G61.Ø
- association G12.29
- asthenic bulbar G7Ø.ØØ
  - with exacerbation (acute) G7Ø.Ø1
  - in crisis G7Ø.Ø1
- ataxic (hereditary) G11.9
  - general (syphilitic) A52.17
- atrophic G58.9
  - infantile, acute — *see* Poliomyelitis, paralytic
  - progressive G12.22
  - spinal (acute) — *see* Poliomyelitis, paralytic
- axillary G54.Ø
- Babinski-Nageotte's G83.89
- Bell's G51.Ø
  - newborn P11.3
- Benedikt's G46.3
- birth injury P14.9
  - spinal cord P11.5
- bladder (neurogenic) (sphincter) N31.2
- bowel, colon or intestine K56.Ø
- brachial plexus G54.Ø
  - birth injury P14.3
  - newborn (birth injury) P14.3
- brain G83.9
  - diplegia G83.Ø
  - triplegia G83.89
- bronchial J98.Ø9
- Brown-Séquard G83.81
- bulbar (chronic) (progressive) G12.22
  - infantile — *see* Poliomyelitis, paralytic
  - poliomyelitic — *see* Poliomyelitis, paralytic
  - pseudo G12.29
- bulbospinal G7Ø.ØØ
  - with exacerbation (acute) G7Ø.Ø1
  - in crisis G7Ø.Ø1
- cardiac (*see also* Failure, heart) I5Ø.9
- cerebrocerebellar, diplegic G8Ø.1
- cervical
  - plexus G54.2
  - sympathetic G9Ø.Ø9
- Céstan-Chenais G46.3
- Charcot-Marie-Tooth type G6Ø.Ø
- Clark's G8Ø.9
- colon K56.Ø
- compressed air T7Ø.3 ☑
- compression
  - arm G56.9- ☑
  - leg G57.9- ☑
  - lower extremity G57.9- ☑
  - upper extremity G56.9- ☑
- congenital (cerebral) — *see* Palsy, cerebral
- conjugate movement (gaze) (of eye) H51.Ø
  - cortical (nuclear) (supranuclear) H51.Ø
- cordis — *see* Failure, heart
- cranial or cerebral nerve G52.9
- creeping G12.22
- crossed leg G83.89
- crutch — *see* Injury, brachial plexus
- deglutition R13.Ø
  - hysterical F44.4
- dementia A52.17
- descending (spinal) NEC G12.29
- diaphragm (flaccid) J98.6

Paralysis, paralytic — *continued*
- diaphragm — *continued*
  - due to accidental dissection of phrenic nerve during procedure — *see* Puncture, accidental complicating surgery
- digestive organs NEC K59.8
- diplegic — *see* Diplegia
- divergence (nuclear) H51.8
- diver's T7Ø.3 ☑
- Duchenne's
  - birth injury P14.Ø
  - due to or associated with
    - motor neuron disease G12.22
    - muscular dystrophy G71.Ø
- due to intracranial or spinal birth injury — *see* Palsy, cerebral
- embolic (current episode) I63.4 ☑
- Erb (-Duchenne) (birth) (newborn) P14.Ø
- Erb's syphilitic spastic spinal A52.17
- esophagus K22.8
- eye muscle (extrinsic) H49.9
  - intrinsic (*see also* Paresis, of accommodation)
- facial (nerve) G51.Ø
  - birth injury P11.3
  - congenital P11.3
  - following operation NEC — *see* Puncture, accidental complicating surgery
  - newborn (birth injury) P11.3
- familial (recurrent) (periodic) G72.3
  - spastic G11.4
- fauces J39.2
- finger G56.9- ☑
- gait R26.1
- gastric nerve (nondiabetic) G52.2
- gaze, conjugate H51.Ø
- general (progressive) (syphilitic) A52.17
  - juvenile A5Ø.45
- glottis J38.ØØ
  - bilateral J38.Ø2
  - unilateral J38.Ø1
- gluteal G54.1
- Gubler (-Millard) G46.3
- hand — *see* Monoplegia, upper limb
- heart — *see* Arrest, cardiac
- hemiplegic — *see* Hemiplegia
- hyperkalemic periodic (familial) G72.3
- hypoglossal (nerve) G52.3
- hypokalemic periodic G72.3
- hysterical F44.4
- ileus K56.Ø
- infantile (*see also* Poliomyelitis, paralytic) A8Ø.3Ø
  - bulbar — *see* Poliomyelitis, paralytic
  - cerebral — *see* Palsy, cerebral
  - spastic — *see* Palsy, cerebral, spastic
- infective — *see* Poliomyelitis, paralytic
- inferior nuclear G83.9
- internuclear — *see* Ophthalmoplegia, internuclear
- intestine K56.Ø
- iris H57.Ø9
  - due to diphtheria (toxin) A36.89
- ischemic, Volkmann's (complicating trauma) T79.6 ☑
- Jackson's G83.89
- jake — *see* Poisoning, food, noxious, plant
- Jamaica ginger (jake) G62.2
- juvenile general A5Ø.45
- Klumpke (-Déjérine) (birth) (newborn) P14.1
- labioglossal (laryngeal) (pharyngeal) G12.29
- Landry's G61.Ø
- laryngeal nerve (recurrent) (superior) (unilateral) J38.ØØ
  - bilateral J38.Ø2
  - unilateral J38.Ø1
- larynx J38.ØØ
  - bilateral J38.Ø2
  - due to diphtheria (toxin) A36.2
  - unilateral J38.Ø1
- lateral G12.21
- lead T56.Ø ☑
- left side — *see* Hemiplegia
- leg G83.1- ☑
  - both — *see* Paraplegia
  - crossed G83.89
  - hysterical F44.4
  - psychogenic F44.4
  - transient or transitory R29.818
    - traumatic NEC — *see* Injury, nerve, leg
- levator palpebrae superioris — *see* Blepharoptosis, paralytic
- limb — *see* Monoplegia

Paralysis, paralytic — *continued*
- lip K13.Ø
- Lissauer's A52.17
- lower limb — *see* Monoplegia, lower limb
  - both — *see* Paraplegia
- lung J98.4
- median nerve G56.1- ☑
- medullary (tegmental) G83.89
- mesencephalic NEC G83.89
  - tegmental G83.89
- middle alternating G83.89
- Millard-Gubler-Foville G46.3
- monoplegic — *see* Monoplegia
- motor G83.9
- muscle, muscular NEC G72.89
  - due to nerve lesion G58.9
  - eye (extrinsic) H49.9
    - intrinsic — *see* Paresis, of accommodation
    - oblique — *see* Strabismus, paralytic, fourth nerve
  - iris sphincter H21.9
  - ischemic (Volkmann's) (complicating trauma) T79.6 ☑
  - progressive G12.21
  - pseudohypertrophic G71.Ø
- musculocutaneous nerve G56.9- ☑
- musculospiral G56.9- ☑
- nerve (*see also* Disorder, nerve)
  - abducent — *see* Strabismus, paralytic, sixth nerve
  - accessory G52.8
  - auditory (except Deafness) H93.3 ☑
  - birth injury P14.9
  - cranial or cerebral G52.9
  - facial G51.Ø
    - birth injury P11.3
    - congenital P11.3
    - newborn (birth injury) P11.3
  - fourth or trochlear — *see* Strabismus, paralytic, fourth nerve
  - newborn (birth injury) P14.9
  - oculomotor — *see* Strabismus, paralytic, third nerve
  - phrenic (birth injury) P14.2
  - radial G56.3- ☑
  - seventh or facial G51.Ø
    - newborn (birth injury) P11.3
  - sixth or abducent — *see* Strabismus, paralytic, sixth nerve
  - syphilitic A52.15
  - third or oculomotor — *see* Strabismus, paralytic, third nerve
  - trigeminal G5Ø.9
  - trochlear — *see* Strabismus, paralytic, fourth nerve
  - ulnar G56.2- ☑
- normokalemic periodic G72.3
- ocular H49.9
  - alternating G83.89
- oculofacial, congenital (Moebius) Q87.Ø
- oculomotor (external bilateral) (nerve) — *see* Strabismus, paralytic, third nerve
- palate (soft) K13.79
- paratrigeminal G5Ø.9
- periodic (familial) (hyperkalemic) (hypokalemic) (myotonic) (normokalemic) (potassium sensitive) (secondary) G72.3
- peripheral autonomic nervous system — *see* Neuropathy, peripheral, autonomic
- peroneal (nerve) G57.3- ☑
- pharynx J39.2
- phrenic nerve G56.8- ☑
- plantar nerve(s) G57.6- ☑
- pneumogastric nerve G52.2
- poliomyelitis (current) — *see* Poliomyelitis, paralytic
- popliteal nerve G57.3- ☑
- postepileptic transitory G83.84
- progressive (atrophic) (bulbar) (spinal) G12.22
  - general A52.17
  - infantile acute — *see* Poliomyelitis, paralytic
  - supranuclear G23.1
- pseudobulbar G12.29
- pseudohypertrophic (muscle) G71.Ø
- psychogenic F44.4
- quadriceps G57.9- ☑
- quadriplegic — *see* Tetraplegia
- radial nerve G56.3- ☑
- rectus muscle (eye) H49.9
- recurrent isolated sleep G47.53

Paralysis, paralytic — *continued*
- respiratory (muscle) (system) (tract) RØ6.81
  - center NEC G93.89
  - congenital P28.89
  - newborn P28.89
- right side — *see* Hemiplegia
- saturnine T56.Ø ☑
- sciatic nerve G57.Ø- ☑
- senile G83.9
- shaking — *see* Parkinsonism
- shoulder G56.9- ☑
- sleep, recurrent isolated G47.53
- spastic G83.9
  - cerebral — *see* Palsy, cerebral, spastic
  - congenital (cerebral) — *see* Palsy, cerebral, spastic
  - familial G11.4
  - hereditary G11.4
  - quadriplegic G8Ø.Ø
  - syphilitic (spinal) A52.17
- sphincter, bladder — *see* Paralysis, bladder
- spinal (cord) G83.9
  - accessory nerve G52.8
  - acute — *see* Poliomyelitis, paralytic
  - ascending acute G61.Ø
  - atrophic (acute) (*see also* Poliomyelitis, paralytic)
    - spastic, syphilitic A52.17
  - congenital NEC — *see* Palsy, cerebral
  - hereditary G95.89
  - infantile — *see* Poliomyelitis, paralytic
  - progressive G12.21
  - sequelae NEC G83.89
- sternomastoid G52.8
- stomach K31.84
  - diabetic — *see* Diabetes, by type, with gastroparesis
  - nerve G52.2
    - diabetic — *see* Diabetes, by type, with gastroparesis
- stroke — *see* Infarct, brain
- subcapsularis G56.8- ☑
- supranuclear (progressive) G23.1
- sympathetic G9Ø.8
  - cervical G9Ø.Ø9
  - nervous system — *see* Neuropathy, peripheral, autonomic
- syndrome G83.9
  - specified NEC G83.89
- syphilitic spastic spinal (Erb's) A52.17
- thigh G57.9- ☑
- throat J39.2
  - diphtheritic A36.Ø
  - muscle J39.2
- thrombotic (current episode) I63.3 ☑
- thumb G56.9- ☑
- tick — *see* Toxicity, venom, arthropod, specified NEC
- Todd's (postepileptic transitory paralysis) G83.84
- toe G57.6- ☑
- tongue K14.8
- transient R29.5
  - arm or leg NEC R29.818
  - traumatic NEC — *see* Injury, nerve
- trapezius G52.8
- traumatic, transient NEC — *see* Injury, nerve
- trembling — *see* Parkinsonism
- triceps brachii G56.9- ☑
- trigeminal nerve G5Ø.9
- trochlear (nerve) — *see* Strabismus, paralytic, fourth nerve
- ulnar nerve G56.2- ☑
- upper limb — *see* Monoplegia, upper limb
- uremic N18.9 [G99.8]
- uveoparotitic D86.89
- uvula K13.79
  - postdiphtheritic A36.Ø
- vagus nerve G52.2
- vasomotor NEC G9Ø.8
- velum palati K13.79
- vesical — *see* Paralysis, bladder
- vestibular nerve (except Vertigo) H93.3 ☑
- vocal cords J38.ØØ
  - bilateral J38.Ø2
  - unilateral J38.Ø1
- Volkmann's (complicating trauma) T79.6 ☑
- wasting G12.29
- Weber's G46.3
- wrist G56.9- ☑

Paramedial urethrovesical orifice Q64.79

Paramenia N92.6
Parametritis (*see also* Disease, pelvis, inflammatory) N73.2
acute N73.Ø
complicating abortion — *see* Abortion, by type, complicated by, parametritis
Parametrium, parametric — *see* condition
Paramnesia — *see* Amnesia
Paramolar KØØ.1
Paramyloidosis E85.8
Paramyoclonus multiplex G25.3
Paramyotonia (congenita) G71.19
Parangi — *see* Yaws
Paranoia (querulans) F22
senile FØ3 ☑
Paranoid
dementia (senile) FØ3 ☑
praecox — *see* Schizophrenia
personality F6Ø.Ø
psychosis (climacteric) (involutional) (menopausal) F22
psychogenic (acute) F23
senile FØ3 ☑
reaction (acute) F23
chronic F22
schizophrenia F2Ø.Ø
state (climacteric) (involutional) (menopausal) (simple) F22
senile FØ3 ☑
tendencies F6Ø.Ø
traits F6Ø.Ø
trends F6Ø.Ø
type, psychopathic personality F6Ø.Ø
Paraparesis — *see* Paraplegia
Paraphasia R47.Ø2
Paraphilia F65.9
Paraphimosis (congenital) N47.2
chancroidal A57
Paraphrenia, paraphrenic (late) F22
schizophrenia F2Ø.Ø
Paraplegia (lower) G82.2Ø
ataxic — *see* Degeneration, combined, spinal cord
complete G82.21
congenital (cerebral) G8Ø.8
spastic G8Ø.1
familial spastic G11.4
functional (hysterical) F44.4
hereditary, spastic G11.4
hysterical F44.4
incomplete G82.22
Pott's A18.Ø1
psychogenic F44.4
spastic
Erb's spinal, syphilitic A52.17
hereditary G11.4
tropical GØ4.1
syphilitic (spastic) A52.17
tropical spastic GØ4.1
Parapoxvirus BØ8.6Ø
specified NEC BØ8.69
Paraproteinemia D89.2
benign (familial) D89.2
monoclonal D47.2
secondary to malignant disease D47.2
Parapsoriasis L41.9
en plaques L41.4
guttata L41.1
large plaque L41.4
retiform, retiformis L41.5
small plaque L41.3
specified NEC L41.8
varioliformis (acuta) L41.Ø
Parasitic (*see also* condition)
disease NEC B89
stomatitis B37.Ø
sycosis (beard) (scalp) B35.Ø
twin Q89.4
Parasitism B89
intestinal B82.9
skin B88.9
specified — *see* Infestation
Parasitophobia F4Ø.218
Parasomnia G47.5Ø
due to
alcohol
abuse F1Ø.182
dependence F1Ø.282
Parasomnia — *continued*
due to — *continued*
alcohol — *continued*
use F1Ø.982
amphetamines
abuse F15.182
dependence F15.282
use F15.982
caffeine
abuse F15.182
dependence F15.282
use F15.982
cocaine
abuse F14.182
dependence F14.282
use F14.982
drug NEC
abuse F19.182
dependence F19.282
use F19.982
opioid
abuse F11.182
dependence F11.282
use F11.982
psychoactive substance NEC
abuse F19.182
dependence F19.282
use F19.982
sedative, hypnotic, or anxiolytic
abuse F13.182
dependence F13.282
use F13.982
stimulant NEC
abuse F15.182
dependence F15.282
use F15.982
in conditions classified elsewhere G47.54
nonorganic origin F51.8
organic G47.5Ø
specified NEC G47.59
Paraspadias Q54.9
Paraspasmus facialis G51.8
Parasuicide (attempt)
history of (personal) Z91.5
in family Z81.8
Parathyroid gland — *see* condition
Parathyroid tetany E2Ø.9
Paratrachoma A74.Ø
Paratyphilitis — *see* Appendicitis
Paratyphoid (fever) — *see* Fever, paratyphoid
Paratyphus — *see* Fever, paratyphoid
Paraurethral duct Q64.79
nonorganic origin F51.5
Paraurethritis (*see also* Urethritis)
gonococcal (acute) (chronic) (with abscess) A54.1
Paravaccinia NEC BØ8.Ø4
Paravaginitis — *see* Vaginitis
Parencephalitis (*see also* Encephalitis)
sequelae GØ9
Parent-child conflict — *see* Conflict, parent-child
estrangement NEC Z62.89Ø
Paresis (*see also* Paralysis)
accommodation — *see* Paresis, of accommodation
Bernhardt's G57.1- ☑
bladder (sphincter) (*see also* Paralysis, bladder)
tabetic A52.17
bowel, colon or intestine K56.Ø
extrinsic muscle, eye H49.9
general (progressive) (syphilitic) A52.17
juvenile A5Ø.45
heart — *see* Failure, heart
insane (syphilitic) A52.17
juvenile (general) A5Ø.45
of accommodation H52.52- ☑
peripheral progressive (idiopathic) G6Ø.3
pseudohypertrophic G71.Ø
senile G83.9
syphilitic (general) A52.17
congenital A5Ø.45
vesical NEC N31.2
Paresthesia (*see also* Disturbance, sensation)
Bernhardt G57.1- ☑
Paretic — *see* condition
Parinaud's
conjunctivitis H1Ø.89
oculoglandular syndrome H1Ø.89
ophthalmoplegia H49.88- ☑
Parkinsonism (idiopathic) (primary) G2Ø
Parkinsonism — *continued*
with neurogenic orthostatic hypotension (symptomatic) G9Ø.3
arteriosclerotic G21.4
dementia G31.83 [FØ2.8Ø]
with behavioral disturbance G31.83 [FØ2.81]
due to
drugs NEC G21.19
neuroleptic G21.11
neuroleptic induced G21.11
postencephalitic G21.3
secondary G21.9
due to
arteriosclerosis G21.4
drugs NEC G21.19
neuroleptic G21.11
encephalitis G21.3
external agents NEC G21.2
syphilis A52.19
specified NEC G21.8
syphilitic A52.19
treatment-induced NEC G21.19
vascular G21.4
Parkinson's disease, syndrome or tremor — *see* Parkinsonism
Parodontitis — *see* Periodontitis
Parodontosis KØ5.4
Paronychia (*see also* Cellulitis, digit)
with lymphangitis — *see* Lymphangitis, acute, digit
candidal (chronic) B37.2
tuberculous (primary) A18.4
Parorexia (psychogenic) F5Ø.8
Parosmia R43.1
psychogenic F45.8
Parotid gland — *see* condition
Parotitis, parotiditis (allergic)(nonspecific toxic) (purulent) (septic) (suppurative) (*see also* Sialoadenitis)
epidemic — *see* Mumps
infectious — *see* Mumps
postoperative K91.89
surgical K91.89
Parrot fever A7Ø
Parrot's disease (early congenital syphilitic pseudoparalysis) A5Ø.Ø2
Parry-Romberg syndrome G51.8
Parry's disease or syndrome EØ5.ØØ
with thyroid storm EØ5.Ø1
Pars planitis — *see* Cyclitis
Parsonage (-Aldren)-**Turner syndrome** G54.5
Parson's disease (exophthalmic goiter) EØ5.ØØ
with thyroid storm EØ5.Ø1
Particolored infant Q82.8
Parturition — *see* Delivery
Parulis KØ4.7
with sinus KØ4.6
Parvovirus, as cause of disease classified elsewhere B97.6
Pasini and Pierini's atrophoderma L9Ø.3
Passage
false, urethra N36.5
meconium (newborn) during delivery PØ3.82
of sounds or bougies — *see* Attention to, artificial, opening
Passive — *see* condition
smoking Z77.22
Pasteurella septica A28.Ø
Pasteurellosis — *see* Infection, Pasteurella
PAT (paroxysmal atrial tachycardia) I47.1
Patau's syndrome — *see* Trisomy, 13
Patches
mucous (syphilitic) A51.39
congenital A5Ø.Ø7
smokers' (mouth) K13.24
Patellar — *see* condition
Patent (*see also* Imperfect, closure)
canal of Nuck Q52.4
cervix N88.3
ductus arteriosus or Botallo's Q25.Ø
foramen
botalli Q21.1
ovale Q21.1
interauricular septum Q21.1
interventricular septum Q21.Ø
omphalomesenteric duct Q43.Ø
os (uteri) — *see* Patent, cervix
ostium secundum Q21.1
urachus Q64.4

Patent — *continued*
- vitelline duct Q43.Ø

Paterson (-Brown)(-Kelly) **syndrome or web** D5Ø.1
Pathologic, pathological (*see also* condition)
- asphyxia RØ9.Ø1
- fire-setting F63.1
- gambling F63.Ø
- ovum OØ2.Ø
- resorption, tooth KØ3.3
- stealing F63.2

Pathology (of) — *see* Disease
- periradicular, associated with previous endodontic treatment NEC M27.59

Pattern, sleep-wake, irregular G47.23
Patulous (*see also* Imperfect, closure (congenital))
- alimentary tract Q45.8
  - lower Q43.8
  - upper Q4Ø.8
- eustachian tube H69.Ø- ☑

Pause, sinoatrial I49.5
Paxton's disease B36.2
Pearl(s)
- enamel KØØ.2
- Epstein's KØ9.8

Pearl-worker's disease — *see* Osteomyelitis, specified type NEC
Pectenosis K62.4
Pectoral — *see* condition
Pectus
- carinatum (congenital) Q67.7
  - acquired M95.4
  - rachitic sequelae (late effect) E64.3
- excavatum (congenital) Q67.6
  - acquired M95.4
  - rachitic sequelae (late effect) E64.3
- recurvatum (congenital) Q67.6

Pedatrophia E41
Pederosis F65.4
Pediculosis (infestation) B85.2
- capitis (head-louse) (any site) B85.Ø
- corporis (body-louse) (any site) B85.1
- eyelid B85.Ø
- mixed (classifiable to more than one of the titles B85.Ø-B85.3) B85.4
- pubis (pubic louse) (any site) B85.3
- vestimenti B85.1
- vulvae B85.3

Pediculus (infestation) — *see* Pediculosis
Pedophilia F65.4
Peg-shaped teeth KØØ.2
Pelade — *see* Alopecia, areata
Pelger-Huët anomaly or syndrome D72.Ø
Peliosis (rheumatica) D69.Ø
- hepatis K76.4
  - with toxic liver disease K71.8

Pelizaeus-Merzbacher disease E75.29
Pellagra (alcoholic) (with polyneuropathy) E52
Pellagra-cerebellar-ataxia-renal aminoaciduria syndrome E72.Ø2
Pellegrini (-Stieda) **disease or syndrome** — *see* Bursitis, tibial collateral
Pellizzi's syndrome E34.8
Pel's crisis A52.11
Pelvic (*see also* condition)
- examination (periodic) (routine) ZØ1.419
  - with abnormal findings ZØ1.411
- kidney, congenital Q63.2

Pelviolithiasis — *see* Calculus, kidney
Pelviperitonitis (*see also* Peritonitis, pelvic)
- gonococcal A54.24
- puerperal O85

Pelvis — *see* condition or type
Pemphigoid L12.9
- benign, mucous membrane L12.1
- bullous L12.Ø
- cicatricial L12.1
- juvenile L12.2
- ocular L12.1
- specified NEC L12.8

Pemphigus L1Ø.9
- benign familial (chronic) Q82.8
- Brazilian L1Ø.3
- circinatus L13.Ø
- conjunctiva L12.1
- drug-induced L1Ø.5
- erythematosus L1Ø.4
- foliaceous L1Ø.2

Pemphigus — *continued*
- gangrenous — *see* Gangrene
- neonatorum LØ1.Ø3
- ocular L12.1
- paraneoplastic L1Ø.81
- specified NEC L1Ø.89
- syphilitic (congenital) A5Ø.Ø6
- vegetans L1Ø.1
- vulgaris L1Ø.Ø
- wildfire L1Ø.3

Pendred's syndrome EØ7.1
Pendulous
- abdomen, in pregnancy — *see* Pregnancy, complicated by, abnormal, pelvic organs or tissues NEC
- breast N64.89

Penetrating wound (*see also* Puncture)
- with internal injury — *see* Injury, by site
- eyeball — *see* Puncture, eyeball
- orbit (with or without foreign body) — *see* Puncture, orbit
- uterus by instrument with or following ectopic or molar pregnancy OØ8.6

Penicillosis B48.4
Penis — *see* condition
Penitis N48.29
Pentalogy of Fallot Q21.8
Pentasomy X syndrome Q97.1
Pentosuria (essential) E74.8
Percreta placenta - O43.23 ☑
Peregrinating patient — *see* Disorder, factitious
Perforation, perforated (nontraumatic) (of)
- accidental during procedure (blood vessel) (nerve) (organ) — *see* Complication, accidental puncture or laceration
- antrum — *see* Sinusitis, maxillary
- appendix K35.2
- atrial septum, multiple Q21.1
- attic, ear — *see* Perforation, tympanum, attic
- bile duct (common) (hepatic) K83.2
  - cystic K82.2
- bladder (urinary)
  - with or following ectopic or molar pregnancy OØ8.6
  - obstetrical trauma O71.5
  - traumatic S37.29 ☑
    - at delivery O71.5
- bowel K63.1
  - with or following ectopic or molar pregnancy OØ8.6
  - newborn P78.Ø
  - obstetrical trauma O71.5
  - traumatic — *see* Laceration, intestine
- broad ligament N83.8
  - with or following ectopic or molar pregnancy OØ8.6
  - obstetrical trauma O71.6
- by
  - device, implant or graft (*see also* Complications, by site and type, mechanical) T85.628 ☑
    - arterial graft NEC — *see* Complication, cardiovascular device, mechanical, vascular
    - breast (implant) T85.49 ☑
    - catheter NEC T85.698 ☑
      - cystostomy T83.Ø9Ø ☑
      - dialysis (renal) T82.49 ☑
        - intraperitoneal T85.691 ☑
      - infusion NEC T82.594 ☑
        - spinal (epidural) (subdural) T85.69Ø ☑
    - electronic (electrode) (pulse generator) (stimulator)
      - bone T84.39Ø ☑
      - cardiac T82.199 ☑
        - electrode T82.19Ø ☑
        - pulse generator T82.191 ☑
        - specified type NEC T82.198 ☑
      - nervous system — *see* Complication, prosthetic device, mechanical, electronic nervous system stimulator
      - urinary — *see* Complication, genitourinary, device, urinary, mechanical
    - fixation, internal (orthopedic) NEC — *see* Complication, fixation device, mechanical
    - gastrointestinal — *see* Complications, prosthetic device, mechanical, gastrointestinal device
    - genital NEC T83.498 ☑
      - intrauterine contraceptive device T83.39 ☑
      - penile prosthesis T83.49Ø ☑
    - heart NEC — *see* Complication, cardiovascular device, mechanical

Perforation, perforated — *continued*
- by — *continued*
  - device, implant or graft (*see also* Complications, by site and type, mechanical) — *continued*
    - joint prosthesis — *see* Complications, joint prosthesis, mechanical, specified NEC, by site
    - ocular NEC — *see* Complications, prosthetic device, mechanical, ocular device
    - orthopedic NEC — *see* Complication, orthopedic, device, mechanical
    - specified NEC T85.628 ☑
    - urinary, indwelling T83.Ø98 ☑
    - urinary NEC (*see also* Complication, genitourinary, device, urinary, mechanical)
      - graft T83.29 ☑
    - vascular NEC — *see* Complication, cardiovascular device, mechanical
    - ventricular intracranial shunt T85.Ø9 ☑
  - foreign body left accidentally in operative wound T81.539 ☑
  - instrument (any) during a procedure, accidental — *see* Puncture, accidental complicating surgery
- cecum K35.2
- cervix (uteri) N88.8
  - with or following ectopic or molar pregnancy OØ8.6
  - obstetrical trauma O71.3
- colon K63.1
  - newborn P78.Ø
  - obstetrical trauma O71.5
  - traumatic — *see* Laceration, intestine, large
- common duct (bile) K83.2
- cornea (due to ulceration) — *see* Ulcer, cornea, perforated
- cystic duct K82.2
- diverticulum (intestine) K57.8Ø
  - with bleeding K57.81
  - large intestine K57.2Ø
    - with
      - bleeding K57.21
      - small intestine K57.4Ø
        - with bleeding K57.41
  - small intestine K57.ØØ
    - with
      - bleeding K57.Ø1
      - large intestine K57.4Ø
        - with bleeding K57.41
- ear drum — *see* Perforation, tympanum
- esophagus K22.3
- ethmoidal sinus — *see* Sinusitis, ethmoidal
- frontal sinus — *see* Sinusitis, frontal
- gallbladder K82.2
- heart valve — *see* Endocarditis
- ileum K63.1
  - newborn P78.Ø
  - obstetrical trauma O71.5
  - traumatic — *see* Laceration, intestine, small
- instrumental, surgical (accidental) (blood vessel) (nerve) (organ) — *see* Puncture, accidental complicating surgery
- intestine NEC K63.1
  - with ectopic or molar pregnancy OØ8.6
  - newborn P78.Ø
  - obstetrical trauma O71.5
  - traumatic — *see* Laceration, intestine
  - ulcerative NEC K63.1
    - newborn P78.Ø
- jejunum, jejunal K63.1
  - obstetrical trauma O71.5
  - traumatic — *see* Laceration, intestine, small
  - ulcer — *see* Ulcer, gastrojejunal, with perforation
- joint prosthesis — *see* Complications, joint prosthesis, mechanical, specified NEC, by site
- mastoid (antrum) (cell) — *see* Disorder, mastoid, specified NEC
- maxillary sinus — *see* Sinusitis, maxillary
- membrana tympani — *see* Perforation, tympanum
- nasal
  - septum J34.89
    - congenital Q3Ø.3
    - syphilitic A52.73
  - sinus J34.89
    - congenital Q3Ø.8
    - due to sinusitis — *see* Sinusitis
- palate (*see also* Cleft, palate) Q35.9
  - syphilitic A52.79

- **Perforation, perforated** — *continued*
  - palatine vault (*see also* Cleft, palate, hard) Q35.1
    - syphilitic A52.79
      - congenital A5Ø.59
  - pars flaccida (ear drum) — *see* Perforation, tympanum, attic
  - pelvic
    - floor S31.Ø3Ø ☑
      - with
        - ectopic or molar pregnancy OØ8.6
        - penetration into retroperitoneal space S31.Ø31 ☑
        - retained foreign body S31.Ø4Ø ☑
          - with penetration into retroperitoneal space S31.Ø41 ☑
      - following ectopic or molar pregnancy OØ8.6
      - obstetrical trauma O7Ø.1
    - organ S37.99 ☑
      - adrenal gland S37.818 ☑
      - bladder — *see* Perforation, bladder
      - fallopian tube S37.599 ☑
        - bilateral S37.592 ☑
        - unilateral S37.591 ☑
      - kidney S37.Ø9- ☑
      - obstetrical trauma O71.5
      - ovary S37.499 ☑
        - bilateral S37.492 ☑
        - unilateral S37.491 ☑
      - prostate S37.828 ☑
      - specified organ NEC S37.898 ☑
      - ureter — *see* Perforation, ureter
      - urethra — *see* Perforation, urethra
      - uterus — *see* Perforation, uterus
  - perineum — *see* Laceration, perineum
  - pharynx J39.2
  - rectum K63.1
    - newborn P78.Ø
    - obstetrical trauma O71.5
    - traumatic S36.63 ☑
  - root canal space due to endodontic treatment M27.51
  - sigmoid K63.1
    - newborn P78.Ø
    - obstetrical trauma O71.5
    - traumatic S36.533 ☑
  - sinus (accessory) (chronic) (nasal) J34.89
  - sphenoidal sinus — *see* Sinusitis, sphenoidal
  - surgical (accidental) (by instrument) (blood vessel) (nerve) (organ) — *see* Puncture, accidental complicating surgery
  - traumatic
    - external — *see* Puncture
    - eye — *see* Puncture, eyeball
    - internal organ — *see* Injury, by site
  - tympanum, tympanic (membrane) (persistent post-traumatic) (postinflammatory) H72.9- ☑
    - attic H72.1- ☑
      - multiple — *see* Perforation, tympanum, multiple
      - total — *see* Perforation, tympanum, total
    - central H72.Ø- ☑
      - multiple — *see* Perforation, tympanum, multiple
      - total — *see* Perforation, tympanum, total
    - marginal NEC — *see* subcategory H72.2 ☑
    - multiple H72.81- ☑
    - pars flaccida — *see* Perforation, tympanum, attic
    - total H72.82- ☑
    - traumatic, current episode SØ9.2- ☑
  - typhoid, gastrointestinal — *see* Typhoid
  - ulcer — *see* Ulcer, by site, with perforation
  - ureter N28.89
    - traumatic S37.19 ☑
  - urethra N36.8
    - with ectopic or molar pregnancy OØ8.6
    - following ectopic or molar pregnancy OØ8.6
    - obstetrical trauma O71.5
    - traumatic S37.39 ☑
      - at delivery O71.5
  - uterus
    - with ectopic or molar pregnancy OØ8.6
    - by intrauterine contraceptive device T83.39 ☑
    - following ectopic or molar pregnancy OØ8.6
    - obstetrical trauma O71.1
    - traumatic S37.69 ☑
      - obstetric O71.1
  - uvula K13.79
    - syphilitic A52.79

- **Perforation, perforated** — *continued*
  - vagina O71.4
    - obstetrical trauma O71.4
    - other trauma — *see* Puncture, vagina
- **Periadenitis mucosa necrotica recurrens** K12.Ø
- **Periappendicitis** (acute) — *see* Appendicitis
- **Periarteritis nodosa** (disseminated) (infectious) (necrotizing) M3Ø.Ø
- **Periarthritis** (joint) (*see also* Enthesopathy)
  - Duplay's M75.Ø- ☑
  - gonococcal A54.42
  - humeroscapularis — *see* Capsulitis, adhesive
  - scapulohumeral — *see* Capsulitis, adhesive
  - shoulder — *see* Capsulitis, adhesive
  - wrist M77.2- ☑
- **Periarthrosis** (angioneural) — *see* Enthesopathy
- **Pericapsulitis, adhesive** (shoulder) — *see* Capsulitis, adhesive
- **Pericarditis** (with decompensation) (with effusion) I31.9
  - with rheumatic fever (conditions in IØØ)
    - active — *see* Pericarditis, rheumatic
    - inactive or quiescent IØ9.2
  - acute (hemorrhagic) (nonrheumatic) (Sicca) I3Ø.9
    - with chorea (acute) (rheumatic) (Sydenham's) IØ2.Ø
    - benign I3Ø.8
    - nonspecific I3Ø.Ø
    - rheumatic IØ1.Ø
      - with chorea (acute) (Sydenham's) IØ2.Ø
  - adhesive or adherent (chronic) (external) (internal) I31.Ø
    - acute — *see* Pericarditis, acute
    - rheumatic IØ9.2
  - bacterial (acute) (subacute) (with serous or seropurulent effusion) I3Ø.1
  - calcareous I31.1
  - cholesterol (chronic) I31.8
    - acute I3Ø.9
  - chronic (nonrheumatic) I31.9
    - rheumatic IØ9.2
  - constrictive (chronic) I31.1
  - coxsackie B33.23
  - fibrinocaseous (tuberculous) A18.84
  - fibrinopurulent I3Ø.1
  - fibrinous I3Ø.8
  - fibrous I31.Ø
  - gonococcal A54.83
  - idiopathic I3Ø.Ø
  - in systemic lupus erythematosus M32.12
  - infective I3Ø.1
  - meningococcal A39.53
  - neoplastic (chronic) I31.8
    - acute I3Ø.9
  - obliterans, obliterating I31.Ø
  - plastic I31.Ø
  - pneumococcal I3Ø.1
  - postinfarction I24.1
  - purulent I3Ø.1
  - rheumatic (active) (acute) (with effusion) (with pneumonia) IØ1.Ø
    - with chorea (acute) (rheumatic) (Sydenham's) IØ2.Ø
    - chronic or inactive (with chorea) IØ9.2
  - rheumatoid — *see* Rheumatoid, carditis
  - septic I3Ø.1
  - serofibrinous I3Ø.8
  - staphylococcal I3Ø.1
  - streptococcal I3Ø.1
  - suppurative I3Ø.1
  - syphilitic A52.Ø6
  - tuberculous A18.84
  - uremic N18.9 [I32]
  - viral I3Ø.1
- **Pericardium, pericardial** — *see* condition
- **Pericellulitis** — *see* Cellulitis
- **Pericementitis** (chronic) (suppurative) (*see also* Periodontitis)
  - acute KØ5.2Ø
    - generalized KØ5.22
    - localized KØ5.21
- **Perichondritis**
  - auricle — *see* Perichondritis, ear
  - bronchus J98.Ø9
  - ear (external) H61.ØØ- ☑
    - acute H61.Ø1- ☑
    - chronic H61.Ø2- ☑
  - external auditory canal — *see* Perichondritis, ear
  - larynx J38.7
    - syphilitic A52.73
    - typhoid AØ1.Ø9

- **Perichondritis** — *continued*
  - nose J34.89
  - pinna — *see* Perichondritis, ear
  - trachea J39.8
- **Periclasia** KØ5.4
- **Pericoronitis** — *see* Periodontitis
- **Pericystitis** N3Ø.9Ø
  - with hematuria N3Ø.91
- **Peridiverticulitis** (intestine) K57.92
  - cecum — *see* Diverticulitis, intestine, large
  - colon — *see* Diverticulitis, intestine, large
  - duodenum — *see* Diverticulitis, intestine, small
  - intestine — *see* Diverticulitis, intestine
  - jejunum — *see* Diverticulitis, intestine, small
  - rectosigmoid — *see* Diverticulitis, intestine, large
  - rectum — *see* Diverticulitis, intestine, large
  - sigmoid — *see* Diverticulitis, intestine, large
- **Periendocarditis** — *see* Endocarditis
- **Periepididymitis** N45.1
- **Perifolliculitis** LØ1.Ø2
  - abscedens, caput, scalp L66.3
  - capitis, abscedens (et suffodiens) L66.3
  - superficial pustular LØ1.Ø2
- **Perihepatitis** K65.8
- **Perilabyrinthitis** (acute) — *see* subcategory H83.Ø ☑
- **Perimeningitis** — *see* Meningitis
- **Perimetritis** — *see* Endometritis
- **Perimetrosalpingitis** — *see* Salpingo-oophoritis
- **Perineocele** N81.81
- **Perinephric, perinephritic** — *see* condition
- **Perinephritis** (*see also* Infection, kidney)
  - purulent — *see* Abscess, kidney
- **Perineum, perineal** — *see* condition
- **Perineuritis NEC** — *see* Neuralgia
- **Periodic** — *see* condition
- **Periodontitis** (chronic) (complex) (compound) (local) (simplex) KØ5.3Ø
  - acute KØ5.2Ø
    - generalized KØ5.22
    - localized KØ5.21
  - apical KØ4.5
    - acute (pulpal origin) KØ4.4
  - generalized KØ5.32
  - localized KØ5.31
- **Periodontoclasia** KØ5.4
- **Periodontosis** (juvenile) KØ5.4
- **Periods** (*see also* Menstruation)
  - heavy N92.Ø
  - irregular N92.6
  - shortened intervals (irregular) N92.1
- **Perionychia** (*see also* Cellulitis, digit)
  - with lymphangitis — *see* Lymphangitis, acute, digit
- **Perioophoritis** — *see* Salpingo-oophoritis
- **Periorchitis** N45.2
- **Periosteum, periosteal** — *see* condition
- **Periostitis** (albuminosa) (circumscribed) (diffuse) (infective) (monomelic) (*see also* Osteomyelitis)
  - alveolar M27.3
  - alveolodental M27.3
  - dental M27.3
  - gonorrheal A54.43
  - jaw (lower) (upper) M27.2
  - orbit HØ5.Ø3- ☑
  - syphilitic A52.77
    - congenital (early) A5Ø.Ø2 [M9Ø.8Ø]
    - secondary A51.46
  - tuberculous — *see* Tuberculosis, bone
  - yaws (hypertrophic) (early) (late) A66.6 [M9Ø.8Ø]
- **Periostosis** (hyperplastic) (*see also* Disorder, bone, specified type NEC)
  - with osteomyelitis — *see* Osteomyelitis, specified type NEC
- **Peripartum**
  - cardiomyopathy O9Ø.3
- **Periphlebitis** — *see* Phlebitis
- **Periproctitis** K62.89
- **Periprostatitis** — *see* Prostatitis
- **Perirectal** — *see* condition
- **Perirenal** — *see* condition
- **Perisalpingitis** — *see* Salpingo-oophoritis
- **Perisplenitis** (infectional) D73.89
- **Peristalsis, visible or reversed** R19.2
- **Peritendinitis** — *see* Enthesopathy
- **Peritoneum, peritoneal** — *see* condition
- **Peritonitis** (adhesive) (bacterial) (fibrinous) (hemorrhagic) (idiopathic) (localized) (perforative) (primary) (with adhesions) (with effusion) K65.9

- **Perversion, perverted** — *continued*
  - sense of smell and taste R43.8
    - psychogenic F45.8
  - sexual — *see* Deviation, sexual
- **Pervious, congenital** (*see also* Imperfect, closure)
  - ductus arteriosus Q25.Ø
- **Pes** (congenital) (*see also* Talipes)
  - acquired (*see also* Deformity, limb, foot, specified NEC)
    - planus — *see* Deformity, limb, flat foot
  - adductus Q66.89
  - cavus Q66.7
  - deformity NEC, acquired — *see* Deformity, limb, foot, specified NEC
  - planus (acquired) (any degree) (*see also* Deformity, limb, flat foot)
    - rachitic sequelae (late effect) E64.3
  - valgus Q66.6
- **Pest, pestis** — *see* Plague
- **Petechia, petechiae** R23.3
  - newborn P54.5
- **Petechial typhus** A75.9
- **Peter's anomaly** Q13.4
- **Petit mal seizure** — *see* Epilepsy, generalized, specified NEC
- **Petit's hernia** — *see* Hernia, abdomen, specified site NEC
- **Petrellidosis** B48.2
- **Petrositis** H7Ø.2Ø- ☑
  - acute H7Ø.21- ☑
  - chronic H7Ø.22- ☑
- **Peutz-Jeghers disease or syndrome** Q85.8
- **Peyronie's disease** N48.6
- **Pfeiffer's disease** — *see* Mononucleosis, infectious
- **Phagedena** (dry) (moist) (sloughing) (*see also* Gangrene)
  - geometric L88
  - penis N48.29
  - tropical — *see* Ulcer, skin
  - vulva N76.6
- **Phagedenic** — *see* condition
- **Phakoma** H35.89
- **Phakomatosis** (*see also* specific eponymous syndromes) Q85.9
  - Bourneville's Q85.1
  - specified NEC Q85.8
- **Phantom limb syndrome** (without pain) G54.7
  - with pain G54.6
- **Pharyngeal pouch syndrome** D82.1
- **Pharyngitis** (acute) (catarrhal)(gangrenous) (infective) (malignant) (membranous) (phlegmonous) (pseudomembranous) (simple) (subacute) (suppurative) (ulcerative) (viral) JØ2.9
  - with influenza, flu, or grippe — *see* Influenza, with, pharyngitis
  - aphthous BØ8.5
  - atrophic J31.2
  - chlamydial A56.4
  - chronic (atrophic) (granular) (hypertrophic) J31.2
  - coxsackievirus BØ8.5
  - diphtheritic A36.Ø
  - enteroviral vesicular BØ8.5
  - follicular (chronic) J31.2
  - fusospirochetal A69.1
  - gonococcal A54.5
  - granular (chronic) J31.2
  - herpesviral BØØ.2
  - hypertrophic J31.2
  - infectional, chronic J31.2
  - influenzal — *see* Influenza, with, respiratory manifestations NEC
  - lymphonodular, acute (enteroviral) BØ8.8
  - pneumococcal JØ2.8
  - purulent JØ2.9
  - putrid JØ2.9
  - septic JØ2.Ø
  - sicca J31.2
  - specified organism NEC JØ2.8
  - staphylococcal JØ2.8
  - streptococcal JØ2.Ø
  - syphilitic, congenital (early) A5Ø.Ø3
  - tuberculous A15.8
  - vesicular, enteroviral BØ8.5
  - viral NEC JØ2.8
- **Pharyngoconjunctivitis, viral** B3Ø.2
- **Pharyngolaryngitis** (acute) JØ6.Ø
  - chronic J37.Ø
- **Pharyngoplegia** J39.2
- **Pharyngotonsillitis, herpesviral** BØØ.2
- **Pharyngotracheitis, chronic** J42
- **Pharynx, pharyngeal** — *see* condition
- **Phenomenon**
  - Arthus' — *see* Arthus' phenomenon
  - jaw-winking QØ7.8
  - lupus erythematosus (LE) cell M32.9
  - Raynaud's (secondary) I73.ØØ
    - with gangrene I73.Ø1
  - vasomotor R55
  - vasospastic I73.9
  - vasovagal R55
  - Wenckebach's I44.1
- **Phenylketonuria** E7Ø.1
  - classical E7Ø.Ø
  - maternal E7Ø.1
- **Pheochromoblastoma**
  - specified site — *see* Neoplasm, malignant, by site
  - unspecified site C74.1Ø
- **Pheochromocytoma**
  - malignant
    - specified site — *see* Neoplasm, malignant, by site
    - unspecified site C74.1Ø
  - specified site — *see* Neoplasm, benign, by site
  - unspecified site D35.ØØ
- **Pheohyphomycosis** — *see* Chromomycosis
- **Pheomycosis** — *see* Chromomycosis
- **Phimosis** (congenital) (due to infection) N47.1
  - chancroidal A57
- **Phlebectasia** (*see also* Varix)
  - congenital Q27.4
- **Phlebitis** (infective) (pyemic) (septic) (suppurative) I8Ø.9
  - antepartum — *see* Thrombophlebitis, antepartum
  - blue — *see* Phlebitis, leg, deep
  - breast, superficial I8Ø.8
  - cavernous (venous) sinus — *see* Phlebitis, intracranial (venous) sinus
  - cerebral (venous) sinus — *see* Phlebitis, intracranial (venous) sinus
  - chest wall, superficial I8Ø.8
  - cranial (venous) sinus — *see* Phlebitis, intracranial (venous) sinus
  - deep (vessels) — *see* Phlebitis, leg, deep
  - due to implanted device — *see* Complications, by site and type, specified NEC
  - during or resulting from a procedure T81.72 ☑
  - femoral vein (superficial) I8Ø.1- ☑
  - femoropopliteal vein I8Ø.Ø- ☑
  - gestational — *see* Phlebopathy, gestational
  - hepatic veins I8Ø.8
  - iliofemoral — *see* Phlebitis, femoral vein
  - intracranial (venous) sinus (any) GØ8
    - nonpyogenic I67.6
  - intraspinal venous sinuses and veins GØ8
    - nonpyogenic G95.19
  - lateral (venous) sinus — *see* Phlebitis, intracranial (venous) sinus
  - leg I8Ø.3
    - antepartum — *see* Thrombophlebitis, antepartum
    - deep (vessels) NEC I8Ø.2Ø- ☑
      - iliac I8Ø.21- ☑
      - popliteal vein I8Ø.22- ☑
      - specified vessel NEC I8Ø.29- ☑
      - tibial vein I8Ø.23- ☑
    - femoral vein (superficial) I8Ø.1- ☑
    - superficial (vessels) I8Ø.Ø- ☑
  - longitudinal sinus — *see* Phlebitis, intracranial (venous) sinus
  - lower limb — *see* Phlebitis, leg
  - migrans, migrating (superficial) I82.1
  - pelvic
    - with ectopic or molar pregnancy OØ8.Ø
    - following ectopic or molar pregnancy OØ8.Ø
    - puerperal, postpartum O87.1
  - popliteal vein — *see* Phlebitis, leg, deep, popliteal
  - portal (vein) K75.1
  - postoperative T81.72 ☑
  - pregnancy — *see* Thrombophlebitis, antepartum
  - puerperal, postpartum, childbirth O87.Ø
    - deep O87.1
    - pelvic O87.1
    - superficial O87.Ø
  - retina — *see* Vasculitis, retina
  - saphenous (accessory) (great) (long) (small) — *see* Phlebitis, leg, superficial
  - sinus (meninges) — *see* Phlebitis, intracranial (venous) sinus
  - specified site NEC I8Ø.8
- **Phlebitis** — *continued*
  - syphilitic A52.Ø9
  - tibial vein — *see* Phlebitis, leg, deep, tibial
  - ulcerative I8Ø.9
    - leg — *see* Phlebitis, leg
  - umbilicus I8Ø.8
  - uterus (septic) — *see* Endometritis
  - varicose (leg) (lower limb) — *see* Varix, leg, with, inflammation
- **Phlebofibrosis** I87.8
- **Phleboliths** I87.8
- **Phlebopathy,**
  - gestational O22.9- ☑
  - puerperal O87.9
- **Phlebosclerosis** I87.8
- **Phlebothrombosis** (*see also* Thrombosis)
  - antepartum — *see* Thrombophlebitis, antepartum
  - pregnancy — *see* Thrombophlebitis, antepartum
  - puerperal — *see* Thrombophlebitis, puerperal
- **Phlebotomus fever** A93.1
- **Phlegmasia**
  - alba dolens O87.1
    - nonpuerperal — *see* Phlebitis, femoral vein
  - cerulea dolens — *see* Phlebitis, leg, deep
- **Phlegmon** — *see* Abscess
- **Phlegmonous** — *see* condition
- **Phlyctenulosis** (allergic) (keratoconjunctivitis) (nontuberculous) (*see also* Keratoconjunctivitis)
  - cornea — *see* Keratoconjunctivitis
  - tuberculous A18.52
- **Phobia, phobic** F4Ø.9
  - animal F4Ø.218
    - spiders F4Ø.21Ø
  - examination F4Ø.298
  - reaction F4Ø.9
  - simple F4Ø.298
  - social F4Ø.1Ø
    - generalized F4Ø.11
  - specific (isolated) F4Ø.298
    - animal F4Ø.218
      - spiders F4Ø.21Ø
    - blood F4Ø.23Ø
    - injection F4Ø.231
    - injury F4Ø.233
    - men F4Ø.29Ø
    - natural environment F4Ø.228
      - thunderstorms F4Ø.22Ø
    - situational F4Ø.248
      - bridges F4Ø.242
      - closed in spaces F4Ø.24Ø
      - flying F4Ø.243
      - heights F4Ø.241
    - specified focus NEC F4Ø.298
    - transfusion F4Ø.231
    - women F4Ø.291
  - specified NEC F4Ø.8
    - medical care NEC F4Ø.232
  - state F4Ø.9
- **Phocas' disease** — *see* Mastopathy, cystic
- **Phocomelia** Q73.1
  - lower limb — *see* Agenesis, leg, with foot present
  - upper limb — *see* Agenesis, arm, with hand present
- **Phoria** H5Ø.5Ø
- **Phosphate-losing tubular disorder** N25.Ø
- **Phosphatemia** E83.39
- **Phosphaturia** E83.39
- **Photodermatitis** (sun) L56.8
  - chronic L57.8
  - due to drug L56.8
  - light other than sun L59.8
- **Photokeratitis** H16.13- ☑
- **Photophobia** H53.14- ☑
- **Photophthalmia** — *see* Photokeratitis
- **Photopsia** H53.19
- **Photoretinitis** — *see* Retinopathy, solar
- **Photosensitivity, photosensitization** (sun) skin L56.8
  - light other than sun L59.8
- **Phrenitis** — *see* Encephalitis
- **Phrynoderma** (vitamin A deficiency) E5Ø.8
- **Phthiriasis** (pubis) B85.3
  - with any infestation classifiable to B85.Ø-B85.2 B85.4
- **Phthirus infestation** — *see* Phthiriasis
- **Phthisis** (*see also* Tuberculosis)
  - bulbi (infectional) — *see* Disorder, globe, degenerated condition, atrophy
  - eyeball (due to infection) — *see* Disorder, globe, degenerated condition, atrophy

Phycomycosis — *see* Zygomycosis
Physalopteriasis B81.8
Physical restraint status Z78.1
Phytobezoar T18.9 ☑
- intestine T18.3 ☑
- stomach T18.2 ☑

Pian — *see* Yaws
Pianoma A66.1
Pica F5Ø.8
- in adults F5Ø.8
- infant or child F98.3

Picking, nose F98.8
Pick-Niemann disease — *see* Niemann-Pick disease or syndrome
Pick's
- cerebral atrophy G31.Ø1 [FØ2.8Ø]
  - with behavioral disturbance G31.Ø1 [FØ2.81]
- disease or syndrome (brain) G31.Ø1 [FØ2.8Ø]
  - with behavioral disturbance G31.Ø1 [FØ2.81]

Pickwickian syndrome E66.2
Piebaldism E7Ø.39
Piedra (beard) (scalp) B36.8
- black B36.3
- white B36.2

Pierre Robin deformity or syndrome Q87.Ø
Pierson's disease or osteochondrosis M91.Ø
Pig-bel AØ5.2
Pigeon
- breast or chest (acquired) M95.4
  - congenital Q67.7
  - rachitic sequelae (late effect) E64.3
- breeder's disease or lung J67.2
- fancier's disease or lung J67.2
- toe — *see* Deformity, toe, specified NEC

Pigmentation (abnormal) (anomaly) L81.9
- conjunctiva H11.13- ☑
- cornea (anterior) H18.Ø1- ☑
  - posterior H18.Ø5- ☑
  - stromal H18.Ø6- ☑
- diminished melanin formation NEC L81.6
- iron L81.8
- lids, congenital Q82.8
- limbus corneae — *see* Pigmentation, cornea
- metals L81.8
- optic papilla, congenital Q14.2
- retina, congenital (grouped) (nevoid) Q14.1
- scrotum, congenital Q82.8
- tattoo L81.8

Piles (*see also* Hemorrhoids) K64.9
Pili
- annulati or torti (congenital) Q84.1
- incarnati L73.1

Pill roller hand (intrinsic) — *see* Parkinsonism
Pilomatrixoma — *see* Neoplasm, skin, benign
- malignant — *see* Neoplasm, skin, malignant

Pilonidal — *see* condition
Pimple R23.8
Pinched nerve — *see* Neuropathy, entrapment
Pindborg tumor — *see* Cyst, calcifying odontogenic
Pineal body or gland — *see* condition
Pinealoblastoma C75.3
Pinealoma D44.5
- malignant C75.3

Pineoblastoma C75.3
Pineocytoma D44.5
Pinguecula H11.15- ☑
Pingueculitis H1Ø.81- ☑
Pinhole meatus (*see also* Stricture, urethra) N35.9
Pink
- disease — *see* subcategory T56.1 ☑
- eye — *see* Conjunctivitis, acute, mucopurulent

Pinkus' disease (lichen nitidus) L44.1
Pinpoint
- meatus — *see* Stricture, urethra
- os (uteri) — *see* Stricture, cervix

Pins and needles R2Ø.2
Pinta A67.9
- cardiovascular lesions A67.2
- chancre (primary) A67.Ø
- erythematous plaques A67.1
- hyperchromic lesions A67.1
- hyperkeratosis A67.1
- lesions A67.9
  - cardiovascular A67.2
  - hyperchromic A67.1
  - intermediate A67.1
  - late A67.2

Pinta — *continued*
- lesions — *continued*
  - mixed A67.3
  - primary A67.Ø
  - skin (achromic) (cicatricial) (dyschromic) A67.2
    - hyperchromic A67.1
    - mixed (achromic and hyperchromic) A67.3
- papule (primary) A67.Ø
- skin lesions (achromic) (cicatricial) (dyschromic) A67.2
  - hyperchromic A67.1
  - mixed (achromic and hyperchromic) A67.3
- vitiligo A67.2

Pintids A67.1
Pinworm (disease) (infection) (infestation) B8Ø
Piroplasmosis B6Ø.Ø
Pistol wound — *see* Gunshot wound
Pitchers' elbow — *see* Derangement, joint, specified type NEC, elbow
Pithecoid pelvis Q74.2
- with disproportion (fetopelvic) O33.Ø
  - causing obstructed labor O65.Ø

Pithiatism F48.8
Pitted — *see* Pitting
Pitting (*see also* Edema) R6Ø.9
- lip R6Ø.Ø
- nail L6Ø.8
- teeth KØØ.4

Pituitary gland — *see* condition
Pituitary-snuff-taker's disease J67.8
Pityriasis (capitis) L21.Ø
- alba L3Ø.5
- circinata (et maculata) L42
- furfuracea L21.Ø
- Hebra's L26
- lichenoides L41.Ø
  - chronica L41.1
  - et varioliformis (acuta) L41.Ø
- maculata (et circinata) L3Ø.5
- nigra B36.1
- pilaris, Hebra's L44.Ø
- rosea L42
- rotunda L44.8
- rubra (Hebra) pilaris L44.Ø
- simplex L3Ø.5
- specified type NEC L3Ø.5
- streptogenes L3Ø.5
- versicolor (scrotal) B36.Ø

Placenta, placental — *see* Pregnancy, complicated by (care of) (management affected by), specified condition
Placentitis O41.14- ☑
Plagiocephaly Q67.3
Plague A2Ø.9
- abortive A2Ø.8
- ambulatory A2Ø.8
- asymptomatic A2Ø.8
- bubonic A2Ø.Ø
- cellulocutaneous A2Ø.1
- cutaneobubonic A2Ø.1
- lymphatic gland A2Ø.Ø
- meningitis A2Ø.3
- pharyngeal A2Ø.8
- pneumonic (primary) (secondary) A2Ø.2
- pulmonary, pulmonic A2Ø.2
- septicemic A2Ø.7
- tonsillar A2Ø.8
  - septicemic A2Ø.7

Planning, family
- contraception Z3Ø.9
- procreation Z31.69

Plaque(s)
- artery, arterial — *see* Arteriosclerosis
- calcareous — *see* Calcification
- coronary, lipid rich I25.83
- epicardial I31.8
- erythematous, of pinta A67.1
- Hollenhorst's — *see* Occlusion, artery, retina
- lipid rich, coronary I25.83
- pleural (without asbestos) J92.9
  - with asbestos J92.Ø
- tongue K13.29

Plasmacytoma C9Ø.3- ☑
- extramedullary C9Ø.2- ☑
- medullary C9Ø.Ø- ☑
- solitary C9Ø.3- ☑

Plasmacytopenia D72.818
Plasmacytosis D72.822
Plaster ulcer — *see* Ulcer, pressure, by site
Plateau iris syndrome (post-iridectomy) (postprocedural) (without glaucoma) H21.82
- with glaucoma H4Ø.22- ☑

Platybasia Q75.8
Platyonychia (congenital) Q84.6
- acquired L6Ø.8

Platypelloid pelvis M95.5
- with disproportion (fetopelvic) O33.Ø
  - causing obstructed labor O65.Ø
- congenital Q74.2

Platyspondylisis Q76.49
Plaut (-Vincent) **disease** (*see also* Vincent's) A69.1
Plethora R23.2
- newborn P61.1

Pleura, pleural — *see* condition
Pleuralgia RØ7.81
Pleurisy (acute) (adhesive) (chronic) (costal) (diaphragmatic) (double) (dry) (fibrinous) (fibrous) (interlobar) (latent) (plastic) (primary) (residual) (sicca) (sterile) (subacute) (unresolved) RØ9.1
- with
  - adherent pleura J86.Ø
  - effusion J9Ø
    - chylous, chyliform J94.Ø
    - tuberculous (non primary) A15.6
      - primary (progressive) A15.7
  - tuberculosis — *see* Pleurisy, tuberculous (non primary)
- encysted — *see* Pleurisy, with effusion
- exudative — *see* Pleurisy, with effusion
- fibrinopurulent, fibropurulent — *see* Pyothorax
- hemorrhagic — *see* Hemothorax
- pneumococcal J9Ø
- purulent — *see* Pyothorax
- septic — *see* Pyothorax
- serofibrinous — *see* Pleurisy, with effusion
- seropurulent — *see* Pyothorax
- serous — *see* Pleurisy, with effusion
- staphylococcal J86.9
- streptococcal J9Ø
- suppurative — *see* Pyothorax
- traumatic (post) (current) — *see* Injury, intrathoracic, pleura
- tuberculous (with effusion) (non primary) A15.6
  - primary (progressive) A15.7

Pleuritis sicca — *see* Pleurisy
Pleurobronchopneumonia — *see* Pneumonia, broncho-
Pleurodynia RØ7.81
- epidemic B33.Ø
- viral B33.Ø

Pleuropericarditis (*see also* Pericarditis)
- acute I3Ø.9

Pleuropneumonia (acute) (bilateral) (double) (septic) (*see also* Pneumonia) J18.8
- chronic — *see* Fibrosis, lung

Pleuro-pneumonia-like-organism (PPLO), as cause of disease classified elsewhere B96.Ø
Pleurorrhea — *see* Pleurisy, with effusion
Plexitis, brachial G54.Ø
Plica
- polonica B85.Ø
- syndrome, knee M67.5- ☑
- tonsil J35.8

Plicated tongue K14.5
Plug
- bronchus NEC J98.Ø9
- meconium (newborn) NEC syndrome P76.Ø
- mucus — *see* Asphyxia, mucus

Plumbism — *see* subcategory T56.Ø ☑
Plummer's disease EØ5.2Ø
- with thyroid storm EØ5.21

Plummer-Vinson syndrome D5Ø.1
Pluricarential syndrome of infancy E4Ø
Plus (and minus) **hand** (intrinsic) — *see* Deformity, limb, specified type NEC, forearm
Pneumathemia — *see* Air, embolism
Pneumatic hammer (drill) syndrome T75.21 ☑
Pneumatocele (lung) J98.4
- intracranial G93.89
- tension J44.9

Pneumatosis
- cystoides intestinalis K63.89
- intestinalis K63.89
- peritonei K66.8

Pneumaturia R39.89
Pneumoblastoma — *see* Neoplasm, lung, malignant
Pneumocephalus G93.89

- **Pneumonia** — *continued*
  - interstitial — *continued*
    - lymphocytic (due to collagen vascular disease) (in diseases classified elsewhere) J84.17
    - lymphoid J84.2
    - non-specific J84.89
      - due to
        - collagen vascular disease J84.17
        - known underlying cause J84.17
      - idiopathic J84.113
      - in diseases classified elsewhere J84.17
    - plasma cell B59
    - pseudomonas J15.1
    - usual J84.112
      - due to collagen vascular disease J84.17
      - idiopathic J84.112
      - in diseases classified elsewhere J84.17
  - Klebsiella (pneumoniae) J15.Ø
  - lipid, lipoid (exogenous) J69.1
    - endogenous J84.89
  - lobar (disseminated) (double) (interstitial) J18.1
    - bacterial J15.9
      - specified NEC J15.8
    - chronic — *see* Fibrosis, lung
    - Escherichia coli (E. coli) J15.5
    - Friedländer's bacillus J15.Ø
    - Hemophilus influenzae J14
    - hypostatic J18.2
    - Klebsiella (pneumoniae) J15.Ø
    - pneumococcal J13
    - Proteus J15.6
    - Pseudomonas J15.1
    - specified organism NEC J16.8
    - staphylococcal — *see* Pneumonia, staphylococcal
    - streptococcal NEC J15.4
    - Streptococcus pneumoniae J13
    - viral, virus — *see* Pneumonia, viral
  - lobular — *see* Pneumonia, broncho
  - Löffler's J82
  - lymphoid interstitial J84.2
  - massive — *see* Pneumonia, lobar
  - meconium P24.Ø1
  - MSSA (methicillin susceptible Staphylococcus aureus) J15.211
  - multilobar — *see* Pneumonia, by type
  - Mycoplasma (pneumoniae) J15.7
  - necrotic J85.Ø
  - neonatal P23.9
    - aspiration — *see* Aspiration, by substance, with pneumonia
  - nitrogen dioxide J68.9
  - organizing J84.89
    - due to
      - collagen vascular disease J84.17
      - known underlying cause J84.17
    - in diseases classified elsewhere J84.17
  - orthostatic J18.2
  - parainfluenza virus J12.2
  - parenchymatous — *see* Fibrosis, lung
  - passive J18.2
  - patchy — *see* Pneumonia, broncho
  - Peptococcus J15.8
  - Peptostreptococcus J15.8
  - plasma cell (of infants) B59
  - pleurolobar — *see* Pneumonia, lobar
  - pleuro-pneumonia-like organism (PPLO) J15.7
  - pneumococcal (broncho) (lobar) J13
  - Pneumocystis (carinii) (jiroveci) B59
  - postinfectional NEC B99 ☑ [J17]
  - postmeasles BØ5.2
  - Proteus J15.6
  - Pseudomonas J15.1
  - psittacosis A7Ø
  - radiation J7Ø.Ø
  - respiratory syncytial virus J12.1
  - resulting from a procedure J95.89
  - rheumatic IØØ [J17]
  - Salmonella (arizonae) (cholerae-suis) (enteritidis) (typhimurium) AØ2.22
    - typhi AØ1.Ø3
    - typhoid fever AØ1.Ø3
  - SARS-associated coronavirus J12.81
  - segmented, segmental — *see* Pneumonia, broncho-
  - Serratia marcescens J15.6
  - specified NEC J18.8
    - bacterium NEC J15.8
    - organism NEC J16.8
    - virus NEC J12.89

- **Pneumonia** — *continued*
  - spirochetal NEC A69.8
  - staphylococcal (broncho) (lobar) J15.2Ø
    - aureus (methicillin susceptible) (MSSA) J15.211
      - methicillin resistant (MRSA) J15.212
    - specified NEC J15.29
  - static, stasis J18.2
  - streptococcal NEC (broncho) (lobar) J15.4
    - group
      - A J15.4
      - B J15.3
      - specified NEC J15.4
  - Streptococcus pneumoniae J13
  - syphilitic, congenital (early) A5Ø.Ø4
  - traumatic (complication) (early) (secondary) T79.8 ☑
  - tuberculous (any) — *see* Tuberculosis, pulmonary
  - tularemic A21.2
  - varicella BØ1.2
  - Veillonella J15.8
  - ventilator associated J95.851
  - viral, virus (broncho) (interstitial) (lobar) J12.9
    - adenoviral J12.Ø
    - congenital P23.Ø
    - human metapneumovirus J12.3
    - parainfluenza J12.2
    - respiratory syncytial J12.1
    - SARS-associated coronavirus J12.81
    - specified NEC J12.89
  - white (congenital) A5Ø.Ø4
- **Pneumonic** — *see* condition
- **Pneumonitis** (acute) (primary) (*see also* Pneumonia)
  - air-conditioner J67.7
  - allergic (due to) J67.9
    - organic dust NEC J67.8
    - red cedar dust J67.8
    - sequoiosis J67.8
    - wood dust J67.8
  - aspiration J69.Ø
    - due to
      - anesthesia J95.4
        - during
          - labor and delivery O74.Ø
          - pregnancy O29.Ø1- ☑
          - puerperium O89.Ø1
      - fumes or gases J68.Ø
    - obstetric O74.Ø
  - chemical (due to gases, fumes or vapors) (inhalation) J68.Ø
    - due to anesthesia J95.4
  - cholesterol J84.89
  - chronic — *see* Fibrosis, lung
  - congenital rubella P35.Ø
  - crack (cocaine) J68.Ø
  - due to
    - beryllium J68.Ø
    - cadmium J68.Ø
    - crack (cocaine) J68.Ø
    - detergent J69.8
    - fluorocarbon-polymer J68.Ø
    - food, vomit (aspiration) J69.Ø
    - fumes or vapors J68.Ø
    - gases, fumes or vapors (inhalation) J68.Ø
    - inhalation
      - blood J69.8
      - essences J69.1
      - food (regurgitated), milk, vomit J69.Ø
      - oils, essences J69.1
      - saliva J69.Ø
      - solids, liquids NEC J69.8
    - manganese J68.Ø
    - nitrogen dioxide J68.Ø
    - oils, essences J69.1
    - solids, liquids NEC J69.8
    - toxoplasmosis (acquired) B58.3
      - congenital P37.1
    - vanadium J68.Ø
    - ventilator J95.851
  - eosinophilic J82
  - hypersensitivity J67.9
    - air conditioner lung J67.7
    - bagassosis J67.1
    - bird fancier's lung J67.2
    - farmer's lung J67.Ø
    - maltworker's lung J67.4
    - maple bark-stripper's lung J67.6
    - mushroom worker's lung J67.5
    - specified organic dust NEC J67.8
    - suberosis J67.3

- **Pneumonitis** — *continued*
  - interstitial (chronic) J84.89
    - acute J84.114
    - lymphoid J84.2
    - non-specific J84.89
      - idiopathic J84.113
  - lymphoid, interstitial J84.2
  - meconium P24.Ø1
  - postanesthetic J95.4
    - correct substance properly administered — *see* Table of Drugs and Chemicals, by drug, adverse effect
    - in labor and delivery O74.Ø
    - in pregnancy O29.Ø1- ☑
    - obstetric O74.Ø
    - overdose or wrong substance given or taken (by accident) — *see* Table of Drugs and Chemicals, by drug, poisoning
    - postpartum, puerperal O89.Ø1
  - postoperative J95.4
    - obstetric O74.Ø
  - radiation J7Ø.Ø
  - rubella, congenital P35.Ø
  - ventilation (air-conditioning) J67.7
  - ventilator associated J95.851
  - wood-dust J67.8
- **Pneumonoconiosis** — *see* Pneumoconiosis
- **Pneumoparotid** K11.8
- **Pneumopathy NEC** J98.4
  - alveolar J84.Ø9
  - due to organic dust NEC J66.8
  - parietoalveolar J84.Ø9
- **Pneumopericarditis** (*see also* Pericarditis)
  - acute I3Ø.9
- **Pneumopericardium** (*see also* Pericarditis)
  - congenital P25.3
  - newborn P25.3
  - traumatic (post) — *see* Injury, heart
- **Pneumophagia** (psychogenic) F45.8
- **Pneumopleurisy, pneumopleuritis** (*see also* Pneumonia) J18.8
- **Pneumopyopericardium** I3Ø.1
- **Pneumopyothorax** — *see* Pyopneumothorax
  - with fistula J86.Ø
- **Pneumorrhagia** (*see also* Hemorrhage, lung)
  - tuberculous — *see* Tuberculosis, pulmonary
- **Pneumothorax NOS** J93.9
  - acute J93.83
  - chronic J93.81
  - congenital P25.1
  - perinatal period P25.1
  - postprocedural J95.811
  - specified NEC J93.83
  - spontaneous NOS J93.83
    - newborn P25.1
    - primary J93.11
    - secondary J93.12
    - tension J93.Ø
  - tense valvular, infectional J93.Ø
  - tension (spontaneous) J93.Ø
  - traumatic S27.Ø ☑
    - with hemothorax S27.2 ☑
  - tuberculous — *see* Tuberculosis, pulmonary
- **Podagra** (*see also* Gout) M1Ø.9
- **Podencephalus** QØ1.9
- **Poikilocytosis** R71.8
- **Poikiloderma** L81.6
  - Civatte's L57.3
  - congenital Q82.8
  - vasculare atrophicans L94.5
- **Poikilodermatomyositis** M33.1Ø
  - with
    - myopathy M33.12
    - respiratory involvement M33.11
    - specified organ involvement NEC M33.19
- **Pointed ear** (congenital) Q17.3
- **Poison ivy, oak, sumac or other plant dermatitis** (allergic) (contact) L23.7
- **Poisoning** (acute) (*see also* Table of Drugs and Chemicals)
  - algae and toxins T65.82- ☑
  - Bacillus B (aertrycke) (cholerae (suis)) (paratyphosus) (suipestifer) AØ2.9
    - botulinus AØ5.1
  - bacterial toxins AØ5.9
  - berries, noxious — *see* Poisoning, food, noxious, berries
  - botulism AØ5.1
  - ciguatera fish T61.Ø- ☑

Poisoning — *continued*
- Clostridium botulinum A05.1
- death-cap (Amanita phalloides) (Amanita verna) — *see* Poisoning, food, noxious, mushrooms
- drug — *see* Table of Drugs and Chemicals, by drug, poisoning
- epidemic, fish (noxious) — *see* Poisoning, seafood
  - bacterial A05.9
- fava bean D55.0
- fish (noxious) T61.9- ☑
  - bacterial — *see* Intoxication, foodborne, by agent
  - ciguatera fish — *see* Poisoning, ciguatera fish
  - scombroid fish — *see* Poisoning, scombroid fish
  - specified type NEC T61.77- ☑
- food (acute) (diseased) (infected) (noxious) NEC T62.9- ☑
  - bacterial — *see* Intoxication, foodborne, by agent
  - due to
    - Bacillus (aertrycke) (choleraesuis) (paratyphosus) (suipestifer) A02.9
      - botulinus A05.1
    - Clostridium (perfringens) (Welchii) A05.2
    - salmonella (aertrycke) (callinarum) (choleraesuis) (enteritidis) (paratyphi) (suipestifer) A02.9
      - with
        - gastroenteritis A02.0
        - sepsis A02.1
    - staphylococcus A05.0
    - Vibrio
      - parahaemolyticus A05.3
      - vulnificus A05.5
  - noxious or naturally toxic T62.9- ☑
    - berries — *see* subcategory T62.1 ☑
    - fish — *see* Poisoning, seafood
    - mushrooms — *see* subcategory T62.0X ☑
    - plants NEC — *see* subcategory T62.2X ☑
    - seafood — *see* Poisoning, seafood
    - specified NEC — *see* subcategory T62.8X ☑
- ichthyotoxism — *see* Poisoning, seafood
- kreotoxism, food A05.9
- latex T65.81- ☑
- lead T56.0- ☑
- mushroom — *see* Poisoning, food, noxious, mushroom
- mussels (*see also* Poisoning, shellfish)
  - bacterial — *see* Intoxication, foodborne, by agent
- nicotine (tobacco) T65.2- ☑
- noxious foodstuffs — *see* Poisoning, food, noxious
- plants, noxious — *see* Poisoning, food, noxious, plants NEC
- ptomaine — *see* Poisoning, food
- radiation J70.0
- Salmonella (arizonae) (cholerae-suis) (enteritidis) (typhimurium) A02.9
- scombroid fish T61.1- ☑
- seafood (noxious) T61.9- ☑
  - bacterial — *see* Intoxication, foodborne, by agent
  - fish — *see* Poisoning, fish
  - shellfish — *see* Poisoning, shellfish
  - specified NEC — *see* subcategory T61.8X ☑
- shellfish (amnesic) (azaspiracid) (diarrheic) (neurotoxic) (noxious) (paralytic) T61.78- ☑
  - bacterial — *see* Intoxication, foodborne, by agent
  - ciguatera mollusk — *see* Poisoning, ciguatera fish
- specified substance NEC T65.891 ☑
- Staphylococcus, food A05.0
- tobacco (nicotine) T65.2- ☑
- water E87.79

Poker spine — *see* Spondylitis, ankylosing

Poland syndrome Q79.8

Polioencephalitis (acute) (bulbar) A80.9
- inferior G12.22
- influenzal — *see* Influenza, with, encephalopathy
- superior hemorrhagic (acute) (Wernicke's) E51.2
- Wernicke's E51.2

Polioencephalomyelitis (acute) (anterior) A80.9
- with beriberi E51.2

Polioencephalopathy, superior hemorrhagic E51.2
- with
  - beriberi E51.11
  - pellagra E52

Poliomeningoencephalitis — *see* Meningoencephalitis

Poliomyelitis (acute) (anterior) (epidemic) A80.9
- with paralysis (bulbar) — *see* Poliomyelitis, paralytic
- abortive A80.4
- ascending (progressive) — *see* Poliomyelitis, paralytic
- bulbar (paralytic) — *see* Poliomyelitis, paralytic

Poliomyelitis — *continued*
- congenital P35.8
- nonepidemic A80.9
- nonparalytic A80.4
- paralytic A80.30
  - specified NEC A80.39
  - vaccine-associated A80.0
  - wild virus
    - imported A80.1
    - indigenous A80.2
- spinal, acute A80.9

Poliosis (eyebrow) (eyelashes) L67.1
- circumscripta, acquired L67.1

Pollakiuria R35.0
- psychogenic F45.8

Pollinosis J30.1

Pollitzer's disease L73.2

Polyadenitis (*see also* Lymphadenitis)
- malignant A20.0

Polyalgia M79.89

Polyangiitis M30.0
- microscopic M31.7
- overlap syndrome M30.8

Polyarteritis
- microscopic M31.7
- nodosa M30.0
  - with lung involvement M30.1
  - juvenile M30.2
  - related condition NEC M30.8

Polyarthralgia — *see* Pain, joint

Polyarthritis, polyarthropathy (*see also* Arthritis) M13.0
- due to or associated with other specified conditions — *see* Arthritis
- epidemic (Australian) (with exanthema) B33.1
- infective — *see* Arthritis, pyogenic or pyemic
- inflammatory M06.4
- juvenile (chronic) (seronegative) M08.3
- migratory — *see* Fever, rheumatic
- rheumatic, acute — *see* Fever, rheumatic

Polyarthrosis M15.9
- post-traumatic M15.3
- primary M15.0
- specified NEC M15.8

Polycarential syndrome of infancy E40

Polychondritis (atrophic) (chronic) (*see also* Disorder, cartilage, specified type NEC)
- relapsing M94.1

Polycoria Q13.2

Polycystic (disease)
- degeneration, kidney Q61.3
  - autosomal dominant (adult type) Q61.2
  - autosomal recessive (infantile type) NEC Q61.19
- kidney Q61.3
  - autosomal
    - dominant Q61.2
    - recessive NEC Q61.19
  - autosomal dominant (adult type) Q61.2
  - autosomal recessive (childhood type) NEC Q61.19
  - infantile type NEC Q61.19
- liver Q44.6
- lung J98.4
  - congenital Q33.0
- ovary, ovaries E28.2
- spleen Q89.09

Polycythemia (secondary) D75.1
- acquired D75.1
- benign (familial) D75.0
- due to
  - donor twin P61.1
  - erythropoietin D75.1
  - fall in plasma volume D75.1
  - high altitude D75.1
  - maternal-fetal transfusion P61.1
  - stress D75.1
- emotional D75.1
- erythropoietin D75.1
- familial (benign) D75.0
- Gaisböck's (hypertonica) D75.1
- high altitude D75.1
- hypertonica D75.1
- hypoxemic D75.1
- neonatorum P61.1
- nephrogenous D75.1
- relative D75.1
- secondary D75.1
- spurious D75.1
- stress D75.1
- vera D45

Polycytosis cryptogenica D75.1

Polydactylism, polydactyly Q69.9
- toes Q69.2

Polydipsia R63.1

Polydystrophy, pseudo-Hurler E77.0

Polyembryoma — *see* Neoplasm, malignant, by site

Polyglandular
- deficiency E31.0
- dyscrasia E31.9
- dysfunction E31.9
- syndrome E31.8

Polyhydramnios O40.- ☑

Polymastia Q83.1

Polymenorrhea N92.0

Polymyalgia M35.3
- arteritica, giant cell M31.5
- rheumatica M35.3
  - with giant cell arteritis M31.5

Polymyositis (acute) (chronic) (hemorrhagic) M33.20
- with
  - myopathy M33.22
  - respiratory involvement M33.21
  - skin involvement — *see* Dermatopolymyositis
  - specified organ involvement NEC M33.29
- ossificans (generalisata) (progressiva) — *see* Myositis, ossificans, progressiva

Polyneuritis, polyneuritic (*see also* Polyneuropathy)
- acute (post-)infective G61.0
- alcoholic G62.1
- cranialis G52.7
- demyelinating, chronic inflammatory (CIDP) G61.81
- diabetic — *see* Diabetes, polyneuropathy
- diphtheritic A36.83
- due to lack of vitamin NEC E56.9 [G63]
- endemic E51.11
- erythredema — *see* subcategory T56.1 ☑
- febrile, acute G61.0
- hereditary ataxic G60.1
- idiopathic, acute G61.0
- infective (acute) G61.0
- inflammatory, chronic demyelinating (CIDP) G61.81
- nutritional E63.9 [G63]
- postinfective (acute) G61.0
- specified NEC G62.89

Polyneuropathy (peripheral) G62.9
- alcoholic G62.1
- amyloid (Portuguese) E85.1 [G63]
- arsenical G62.2
- critical illness G62.81
- demyelinating, chronic inflammatory (CIDP) G61.81
- diabetic — *see* Diabetes, polyneuropathy
- drug-induced G62.0
- hereditary G60.9
  - specified NEC G60.8
- idiopathic G60.9
  - progressive G60.3
- in (due to)
  - alcohol G62.1
    - sequelae G65.2
  - amyloidosis, familial (Portuguese) E85.1 [G63]
  - antitetanus serum G61.1
  - arsenic G62.2
    - sequelae G65.2
  - avitaminosis NEC E56.9 [G63]
  - beriberi E51.11
  - collagen vascular disease NEC M35.9 [G63]
  - deficiency (of)
    - B (-complex) vitamins E53.9 [G63]
    - vitamin B6 E53.1 [G63]
  - diabetes — *see* Diabetes, polyneuropathy
  - diphtheria A36.83
  - drug or medicament G62.0
    - correct substance properly administered — *see* Table of Drugs and Chemicals, by drug, adverse effect
    - overdose or wrong substance given or taken — *see* Table of Drugs and Chemicals, by drug, poisoning
  - endocrine disease NEC E34.9 [G63]
  - herpes zoster B02.23
  - hypoglycemia E16.2 [G63]
  - infectious
    - disease NEC B99 ☑ [G63]
    - mononucleosis B27.91
  - lack of vitamin NEC E56.9 [G63]
  - lead G62.2
    - sequelae G65.2
  - leprosy A30.9 [G63]

Subterms under main terms may continue to next column or page

☑ Additional Character Required — Refer to the Tabular List for Character Selection

Polyneuropathy — *continued*
- in — *continued*
  - Lyme disease A69.22
  - metabolic disease NEC E88.9 [G63]
  - microscopic polyangiitis M31.7 [G63]
  - mumps B26.84
  - neoplastic disease (*see also* Neoplasm) D49.9 [G63]
  - nutritional deficiency NEC E63.9 [G63]
  - organophosphate compounds G62.2
    - sequelae G65.2
  - parasitic disease NEC B89 [G63]
  - pellagra E52 [G63]
  - polyarteritis nodosa M3Ø.Ø
  - porphyria E8Ø.2Ø [G63]
  - radiation G62.82
  - rheumatoid arthritis — *see* Rheumatoid, polyneuropathy
  - sarcoidosis D86.89
  - serum G61.1
  - syphilis (late) A52.15
    - congenital A5Ø.43
  - systemic
    - connective tissue disorder M35.9 [G63]
    - lupus erythematosus M32.19
  - toxic agent NEC G62.2
    - sequelae G65.2
  - triorthocresyl phosphate G62.2
    - sequelae G65.2
  - tuberculosis A17.89
  - uremia N18.9 [G63]
  - vitamin B12 deficiency E53.8 [G63]
    - with anemia (pernicious) D51.Ø [G63]
      - due to dietary deficiency D51.3 [G63]
  - zoster BØ2.23
- inflammatory G61.9
  - chronic demyelinating (CIDP) G61.81
  - sequelae G65.1
  - specified NEC G61.89
- lead G62.2
  - sequelae G65.2
- nutritional NEC E63.9 [G63]
- postherpetic (zoster) BØ2.23
- progressive G6Ø.3
- radiation-induced G62.82
- sensory (hereditary) (idiopathic) G6Ø.8
- specified NEC G62.89
- syphilitic (late) A52.15
  - congenital A5Ø.43

Polyopia H53.8

Polyorchism, polyorchidism Q55.21

Polyosteoarthritis (*see also* Osteoarthritis, generalized) M15.9
- post-traumatic M15.3
- specified NEC M15.8

Polyostotic fibrous dysplasia Q78.1

Polyotia Q17.Ø

Polyp, polypus
- accessory sinus J33.8
- adenocarcinoma in — *see* Neoplasm, malignant, by site
- adenocarcinoma in situ in — *see* Neoplasm, in situ, by site
- adenoid tissue J33.Ø
- adenomatous (*see also* Neoplasm, benign, by site)
  - adenocarcinoma in — *see* Neoplasm, malignant, by site
  - adenocarcinoma in situ in — *see* Neoplasm, in situ, by site
  - carcinoma in — *see* Neoplasm, malignant, by site
  - carcinoma in situ in — *see* Neoplasm, in situ, by site
  - multiple — *see* Neoplasm, benign
    - adenocarcinoma in — *see* Neoplasm, malignant, by site
    - adenocarcinoma in situ in — *see* Neoplasm, in situ, by site
- antrum J33.8
- anus, anal (canal) K62.Ø
- Bartholin's gland N84.3
- bladder D41.4
- carcinoma in — *see* Neoplasm, malignant, by site
- carcinoma in situ in — *see* Neoplasm, in situ, by site
- cecum D12.Ø
- cervix (uteri) N84.1
  - in pregnancy or childbirth — *see* Pregnancy, complicated by, abnormal, cervix
  - mucous N84.1
  - nonneoplastic N84.1

Polyp, polypus — *continued*
- choanal J33.Ø
- cholesterol K82.4
- clitoris N84.3
- colon K63.5
  - adenomatous D12.6
  - ascending D12.2
  - cecum D12.Ø
  - descending D12.4
  - inflammatory K51.4Ø
    - with
      - abscess K51.414
      - complication K51.419
        - specified NEC K51.418
      - fistula K51.413
      - intestinal obstruction K51.412
      - rectal bleeding K51.411
  - sigmoid D12.5
  - transverse D12.3
- corpus uteri N84.Ø
- dental KØ4.Ø
- duodenum K31.7
- ear (middle) H74.4- ☑
- endometrium N84.Ø
- ethmoidal (sinus) J33.8
- fallopian tube N84.8
- female genital tract N84.9
  - specified NEC N84.8
- frontal (sinus) J33.8
- gallbladder K82.4
- gingiva, gum KØ6.8
- labia, labium (majus) (minus) N84.3
- larynx (mucous) J38.1
  - adenomatous D14.1
- malignant — *see* Neoplasm, malignant, by site
- maxillary (sinus) J33.8
- middle ear — *see* Polyp, ear (middle)
- myometrium N84.Ø
- nares
  - anterior J33.9
  - posterior J33.Ø
- nasal (mucous) J33.9
  - cavity J33.Ø
  - septum J33.Ø
- nasopharyngeal J33.Ø
- nose (mucous) J33.9
- oviduct N84.8
- pharynx J39.2
- placenta O9Ø.89
- prostate — *see* Enlargement, enlarged, prostate
- pudenda, pudendum N84.3
- pulpal (dental) KØ4.Ø
- rectum (nonadenomatous) K62.1
  - adenomatous — *see* Polyp, adenomatous
- septum (nasal) J33.Ø
- sinus (accessory) (ethmoidal) (frontal) (maxillary) (sphenoidal) J33.8
- sphenoidal (sinus) J33.8
- stomach K31.7
  - adenomatous D13.1
- tube, fallopian N84.8
- turbinate, mucous membrane J33.8
- umbilical, newborn P83.6
- ureter N28.89
- urethra N36.2
- uterus (body) (corpus) (mucous) N84.Ø
  - cervix N84.1
  - in pregnancy or childbirth — *see* Pregnancy, complicated by, tumor, uterus
- vagina N84.2
- vocal cord (mucous) J38.1
- vulva N84.3

Polyphagia R63.2

Polyploidy Q92.7

Polypoid — *see* condition

Polyposis (*see also* Polyp)
- coli (adenomatous) D12.6
  - adenocarcinoma in C18.9
  - adenocarcinoma in situ in — *see* Neoplasm, in situ, by site
  - carcinoma in C18.9
- colon (adenomatous) D12.6
- familial D12.6
  - adenocarcinoma in situ in — *see* Neoplasm, in situ, by site
- intestinal (adenomatous) D12.6
- malignant lymphomatous C83.1- ☑

Polyposis — *continued*
- multiple, adenomatous (*see also* Neoplasm, benign) D36.9

Polyradiculitis — *see* Polyneuropathy

Polyradiculoneuropathy (acute) (postinfective) (segmentally demyelinating) G61.Ø

Polyserositis
- due to pericarditis I31.1
- pericardial I31.1
- periodic, familial E85.Ø
- tuberculous A19.9
  - acute A19.1
  - chronic A19.8

Polysplenia syndrome Q89.Ø9

Polysyndactyly (*see also* Syndactylism, syndactyly) Q7Ø.4

Polytrichia L68.3

Polyunguia Q84.6

Polyuria R35.8
- nocturnal R35.1
- psychogenic F45.8

Pompe's disease (glycogen storage) E74.Ø2

Pompholyx L3Ø.1

Poncet's disease (tuberculous rheumatism) A18.Ø9

Pond fracture — *see* Fracture, skull

Ponos B55.Ø

Pons, pontine — *see* condition

Poor
- aesthetic of existing restoration of tooth KØ8.56
- contractions, labor O62.2
- gingival margin to tooth restoration KØ8.51
- personal hygiene R46.Ø
- prenatal care, affecting management of pregnancy — *see* Pregnancy, complicated by, insufficient, prenatal care
- sucking reflex (newborn) R29.2
- urinary stream R39.12
- vision NEC H54.7

Poradenitis, nostras inguinalis or venerea A55

Porencephaly (congenital) (developmental) (true) QØ4.6
- acquired G93.Ø
- nondevelopmental G93.Ø
- traumatic (post) FØ7.89

Porocephaliasis B88.8

Porokeratosis Q82.8

Poroma, eccrine — *see* Neoplasm, skin, benign

Porphyria (South African) E8Ø.2Ø
- acquired E8Ø.2Ø
- acute intermittent (hepatic) (Swedish) E8Ø.21
- cutanea tarda (hereditary) (symptomatic) E8Ø.1
- due to drugs E8Ø.2Ø
  - correct substance properly administered — *see* Table of Drugs and Chemicals, by drug, adverse effect
  - overdose or wrong substance given or taken — *see* Table of Drugs and Chemicals, by drug, poisoning
- erythropoietic (congenital) (hereditary) E8Ø.Ø
- hepatocutaneous type E8Ø.1
- secondary E8Ø.2Ø
- toxic NEC E8Ø.2Ø
- variegata E8Ø.2Ø

Porphyrinuria — *see* Porphyria

Porphyruria — *see* Porphyria

Port wine nevus, mark, or stain Q82.5

Portal — *see* condition

Posadas-Wernicke disease B38.9

Positive
- culture (nonspecific)
  - blood R78.81
  - bronchial washings R84.5
  - cerebrospinal fluid R83.5
  - cervix uteri R87.5
  - nasal secretions R84.5
  - nipple discharge R89.5
  - nose R84.5
    - staphylococcus (Methicillin susceptible) Z22.321
      - Methicillin resistant Z22.322
  - peritoneal fluid R85.5
  - pleural fluid R84.5
  - prostatic secretions R86.5
  - saliva R85.5
  - seminal fluid R86.5
  - sputum R84.5
  - synovial fluid R89.5
  - throat scrapings R84.5
  - urine R82.7
  - vagina R87.5
  - vulva R87.5

Positive — *continued*
- culture — *continued*
  - wound secretions R89.5
- PPD (skin test) R76.11
- serology for syphilis A53.Ø
  - with signs or symptoms — *code as* Syphilis, by site and stage
  - false R76.8
- skin test, tuberculin (without active tuberculosis) R76.11
- test, human immunodeficiency virus (HIV) R75
- VDRL A53.Ø
  - with signs or symptoms — *code by* site and stage under Syphilis A53.9
- Wassermann reaction A53.Ø

Postcardiotomy syndrome I97.Ø
Postcaval ureter Q62.62
Postcholecystectomy syndrome K91.5
Postclimacteric bleeding N95.Ø
Postcommissurotomy syndrome I97.Ø
Postconcussional syndrome FØ7.81
Postcontusional syndrome FØ7.81
Postcricoid region — *see* condition
Post-dates (4Ø-42 weeks) (pregnancy) (mother) O48.Ø
- more than 42 weeks gestation O48.1

Postencephalitic syndrome FØ7.89
Posterior — *see* condition
Posterolateral sclerosis (spinal cord) — *see* Degeneration, combined
Postexanthematous — *see* condition
Postfebrile — *see* condition
Postgastrectomy dumping syndrome K91.1
Posthemiplegic chorea — *see* Monoplegia
Posthemorrhagic anemia (chronic) D5Ø.Ø
- acute D62
- newborn P61.3

Postherpetic neuralgia (zoster) BØ2.29
- trigeminal BØ2.22

Posthitis N47.7
Postimmunization complication or reaction — *see* Complications, vaccination
Postinfectious — *see* condition
Postlaminectomy syndrome NEC M96.1
Postleukotomy syndrome FØ7.Ø
Postmastectomy lymphedema (syndrome) I97.2
Postmaturity, postmature (over 42 weeks)
- maternal (over 42 weeks gestation) O48.1
- newborn PØ8.22

Postmeasles complication NEC (*see also* condition) BØ5.89
Postmenopausal
- endometrium (atrophic) N95.8
  - suppurative (*see also* Endometritis) N71.9
- osteoporosis — *see* Osteoporosis, postmenopausal

Postnasal drip RØ9.82
- due to
  - allergic rhinitis — *see* Rhinitis, allergic
  - common cold JØØ
  - gastroesophageal reflux — *see* Reflux, gastroesophageal
  - nasopharyngitis — *see* Nasopharyngitis
  - other known condition — *code to* condition
  - sinusitis — *see* Sinusitis

Postnatal — *see* condition
Postoperative (postprocedural) — *see* Complication, postoperative
- pneumothorax, therapeutic Z98.3
- state NEC Z98.89

Postpancreatectomy hyperglycemia E89.1
Postpartum — *see* Puerperal
Postphlebitic syndrome — *see* Syndrome, postthrombotic
Postpolio (myelitic) **syndrome** G14
Postpoliomyelitic (*see also* condition)
- osteopathy — *see* Osteopathy, after poliomyelitis

Postprocedural (*see also* Postoperative)
- hypoinsulinemia E89.1

Postschizophrenic depression F32.8
Postsurgery status (*see also* Status (post))
- pneumothorax, therapeutic Z98.3

Post-term (4Ø-42 weeks) (pregnancy) (mother) O48.Ø
- infant PØ8.21
- more than 42 weeks gestation (mother) O48.1

Post-traumatic brain syndrome, nonpsychotic FØ7.81
Post-typhoid abscess AØ1.Ø9
Postures, hysterical F44.2
Postvaccinal reaction or complication — *see* Complications, vaccination
Postvalvulotomy syndrome I97.Ø
Potain's
- disease (pulmonary edema) — *see* Edema, lung
- syndrome (gastrectasis with dyspepsia) K31.Ø

Potter's
- asthma J62.8
- facies Q6Ø.6
- lung J62.8
- syndrome (with renal agenesis) Q6Ø.6

Pott's
- curvature (spinal) A18.Ø1
- disease or paraplegia A18.Ø1
- spinal curvature A18.Ø1
- tumor, puffy — *see* Osteomyelitis, specified type NEC

Pouch
- bronchus Q32.4
- Douglas' — *see* condition
- esophagus, esophageal, congenital Q39.6
  - acquired K22.5
- gastric K31.4
- Hartmann's K82.8
- pharynx, pharyngeal (congenital) Q38.7

Pouchitis K91.85Ø
Poultrymen's itch B88.Ø
Poverty NEC Z59.6
- extreme Z59.5

Poxvirus NEC BØ8.8
Prader-Willi syndrome Q87.1
Preauricular appendage or tag Q17.Ø
Prebetalipoproteinemia (acquired) (essential) (familial) (hereditary) (primary) (secondary) E78.1
- with chylomicronemia E78.3

Precipitate labor or delivery O62.3
Preclimacteric bleeding (menorrhagia) N92.4
Precocious
- adrenarche E3Ø.1
- menarche E3Ø.1
- menstruation E3Ø.1
- pubarche E3Ø.1
- puberty E3Ø.1
  - central E22.8
- sexual development NEC E3Ø.1
- thelarche E3Ø.8

Precocity, sexual (constitutional) (cryptogenic) (female) (idiopathic) (male) E3Ø.1
- with adrenal hyperplasia E25.9
  - congenital E25.Ø

Precordial pain RØ7.2
Predeciduous teeth KØØ.2
Prediabetes, prediabetic R73.Ø9
- complicating
  - pregnancy — *see* Pregnancy, complicated by, diseases of, specified type or system NEC
  - puerperium O99.89

Predislocation status of hip at birth Q65.6
Pre-eclampsia O14.9- ☑
- with pre-existing hypertension — *see* Hypertension, complicating pregnancy, pre-existing, with, pre-eclampsia
- mild O14.Ø- ☑
- moderate O14.Ø- ☑
- severe O14.1- ☑
  - with hemolysis, elevated liver enzymes and low platelet count (HELLP) O14.2- ☑

Pre-eruptive color change, teeth, tooth KØØ.8
Pre-excitation atrioventricular conduction I45.6
Preglaucoma H4Ø.ØØ- ☑
Pregnancy (single) (uterine) (*see also* Delivery and Puerperal)

> *Note: The Tabular must be reviewed for assignment of appropriate seventh character for multiple gestation codes in Chapter 15*

> *Note: The Tabular must be reviewed for assignment of the appropriate character indicating the trimester of the pregnancy*

- abdominal (ectopic) OØØ.Ø
  - with viable fetus O36.7- ☑
- ampullar OØØ.1
- biochemical OØ2.81
- broad ligament OØØ.8
- cervical OØØ.8
- chemical OØ2.81

Pregnancy — *continued*
- complicated by (care of) (management affected by)
  - abnormal, abnormality
    - cervix O34.4- ☑
      - causing obstructed labor O65.5
    - cord (umbilical) O69.9 ☑
    - findings on antenatal screening of mother O28.9
      - biochemical O28.1
      - chromosomal O28.5
      - cytological O28.2
      - genetic O28.5
      - hematological O28.Ø
      - radiological O28.4
      - specified NEC O28.8
      - ultrasonic O28.3
    - glucose (tolerance) NEC O99.81Ø
    - pelvic organs O34.9- ☑
      - specified NEC O34.8- ☑
        - causing obstructed labor O65.5
    - pelvis (bony) (major) NEC O33.Ø
    - perineum O34.7- ☑
    - position
      - placenta O44.1- ☑
        - without hemorrhage O44.Ø- ☑
      - uterus O34.59- ☑
    - uterus O34.59- ☑
      - causing obstructed labor O65.5
      - congenital O34.Ø- ☑
    - vagina O34.6- ☑
      - causing obstructed labor O65.5
    - vulva O34.7- ☑
      - causing obstructed labor O65.5
  - abruptio placentae — *see* Abruptio placentae
  - abscess or cellulitis
    - bladder O23.1- ☑
    - breast O91.11- ☑
    - genital organ or tract O23.9- ☑
  - abuse
    - physical O9A.31 ☑ (*following* O99)
    - psychological O9A.51 ☑ (*following* O99)
    - sexual O9A.41 ☑ (*following* O99)
  - adverse effect anesthesia O29.9- ☑
    - aspiration pneumonitis O29.Ø1- ☑
    - cardiac arrest O29.11- ☑
    - cardiac complication NEC O29.19- ☑
    - cardiac failure O29.12- ☑
    - central nervous system complication NEC O29.29- ☑
    - cerebral anoxia O29.21- ☑
    - failed or difficult intubation O29.6- ☑
    - inhalation of stomach contents or secretions NOS O29.Ø1- ☑
    - local, toxic reaction O29.3X ☑
    - Mendelson's syndrome O29.Ø1- ☑
    - pressure collapse of lung O29.Ø2- ☑
    - pulmonary complications NEC O29.Ø9- ☑
    - specified NEC O29.8X- ☑
    - spinal and epidural type NEC O29.5X ☑
      - induced headache O29.4- ☑
  - albuminuria O12.1- ☑
  - alcohol use O99.31- ☑
  - amnionitis O41.12- ☑
  - anaphylactoid syndrome of pregnancy O88.Ø1- ☑
  - anemia (conditions in D5Ø-D64) (pre-existing) O99.Ø1- ☑
    - complicating the puerperium O99.Ø3
  - antepartum hemorrhage O46.9- ☑
    - with coagulation defect — *see* Hemorrhage, antepartum, with coagulation defect
    - specified NEC O46.8X- ☑
  - appendicitis O99.61- ☑
  - atrophy (yellow) (acute) liver (subacute) O26.61- ☑
  - bariatric surgery status O99.84- ☑
  - bicornis or bicornuate uterus O34.59- ☑
  - biliary tract problems O26.61- ☑
  - breech presentation O32.1 ☑
  - cardiovascular diseases (conditions in IØØ-IØ9, I2Ø-I52, I7Ø-I99) O99.41- ☑
  - cerebrovascular disorders (conditions in I6Ø-I69) O99.41- ☑
  - cervical shortening O26.87- ☑
  - cervicitis O23.51- ☑
  - chloasma (gravidarum) O26.89- ☑
  - cholecystitis O99.61- ☑
  - cholestasis (intrahepatic) O26.61- ☑

- **Pregnancy** — *continued*
  - complicated by — *continued*
    - chorioamnionitis O41.12- ☑
    - circulatory system disorder (conditions in IØØ-IØ9, I2Ø-I99, O99.41-)
    - compound presentation O32.6 ☑
    - conjoined twins O3Ø.Ø2- ☑
    - connective system disorders (conditions in MØØ-M99) O99.89
    - contracted pelvis (general) O33.1
      - inlet O33.2
      - outlet O33.3 ☑
    - convulsions (eclamptic) (uremic) (*see also* Eclampsia) O15.9
    - cracked nipple O92.11- ☑
    - cystitis O23.1- ☑
    - cystocele O34.8- ☑
    - death of fetus (near term) O36.4 ☑
      - early pregnancy OØ2.1
      - of one fetus or more in multiple gestation O31.2- ☑
    - deciduitis O41.14- ☑
    - decreased fetal movement O36.81- ☑
    - dental problems O99.61- ☑
    - diabetes (mellitus) O24.91- ☑
      - gestational (pregnancy induced) — *see* Diabetes, gestational
      - pre-existing O24.31- ☑
        - specified NEC O24.81- ☑
        - type 1 O24.Ø1- ☑
        - type 2 O24.11- ☑
    - digestive system disorders (conditions in KØØ-K93) O99.61- ☑
    - diseases of — *see* Pregnancy, complicated by, specified body system disease
      - biliary tract O26.61- ☑
      - blood NEC (conditions in D65-D77) O99.11- ☑
      - liver O26.61- ☑
      - specified NEC O99.89
    - disorders of — *see* Pregnancy, complicated by, specified body system disorder
      - amniotic fluid and membranes O41.9- ☑
        - specified NEC O41.8X- ☑
      - biliary tract O26.61- ☑
      - ear and mastoid process (conditions in H6Ø-H95) O99.89
      - eye and adnexa (conditions in HØØ-H59) O99.89
      - liver O26.61- ☑
      - skin (conditions in LØØ-L99) O99.71- ☑
      - specified NEC O99.89
    - displacement, uterus NEC O34.59- ☑
      - causing obstructed labor O65.5
    - disproportion (due to) O33.9
      - fetal deformities NEC O33.7
      - generally contracted pelvis O33.1
      - hydrocephalic fetus O33.6 ☑
      - inlet contraction of pelvis O33.2
      - mixed maternal and fetal origin O33.4 ☑
      - specified NEC O33.8
    - double uterus O34.59- ☑
      - causing obstructed labor O65.5
    - drug use (conditions in F11-F19) O99.32- ☑
    - eclampsia, eclamptic (coma) (convulsions) (delirium) (nephritis) (uremia) (*see also* Eclampsia) O15.- ☑
    - ectopic pregnancy — *see* Pregnancy, ectopic
    - edema O12.Ø- ☑
      - with
        - gestational hypertension, mild (*see also* Pre-eclampsia) O14.Ø- ☑
        - proteinuria O12.2- ☑
    - effusion, amniotic fluid — *see* Pregnancy, complicated by, premature rupture of membranes
    - elderly
      - multigravida OØ9.52- ☑
      - primigravida OØ9.51- ☑
    - embolism (*see also* Embolism, obstetric, pregnancy) O88.- ☑
    - endocrine diseases NEC O99.28- ☑
    - endometritis O86.12
    - excessive weight gain O26.Ø- ☑
    - exhaustion O26.81- ☑
      - during labor and delivery O75.81
    - face presentation O32.3 ☑
    - failed induction of labor O61.9
      - instrumental O61.1
      - mechanical O61.1

- **Pregnancy** — *continued*
  - complicated by — *continued*
    - failed induction of labor — *continued*
      - medical O61.Ø
      - specified NEC O61.8
      - surgical O61.1
    - failed or difficult intubation for anesthesia O29.6- ☑
    - false labor (pains) O47.9
      - at or after 37 completed weeks of pregnancy O47.1
      - before 37 completed weeks of pregnancy O47.Ø- ☑
    - fatigue O26.81- ☑
      - during labor and delivery O75.81
    - fatty metamorphosis of liver O26.61- ☑
    - female genital mutilation O34.8- ☑ [N9Ø.81-] ☑
    - fetal (maternal care for)
      - abnormality or damage O35.9 ☑
        - acid-base balance O68
        - specified type NEC O35.8 ☑
      - acidemia O68
      - acidosis O68
      - alkalosis O68
      - anemia and thrombocytopenia O36.82- ☑
      - anencephaly O35.Ø ☑
      - chromosomal abnormality (conditions in Q9Ø-Q99) O35.1 ☑
      - conjoined twins O3Ø.Ø2- ☑
      - damage from
        - amniocentesis O35.7 ☑
        - biopsy procedures O35.7 ☑
        - drug addiction O35.5 ☑
        - hematological investigation O35.7 ☑
        - intrauterine contraceptive device O35.7 ☑
        - maternal
          - alcohol addiction O35.4 ☑
          - cytomegalovirus infection O35.3 ☑
          - disease NEC O35.8 ☑
          - drug addiction O35.5 ☑
          - listeriosis O35.8 ☑
          - rubella O35.3 ☑
          - toxoplasmosis O35.8 ☑
          - viral infection O35.3 ☑
        - medical procedure NEC O35.7 ☑
        - radiation O35.6 ☑
      - death (near term) O36.4 ☑
        - early pregnancy OØ2.1
      - decreased movement O36.81- ☑
      - disproportion due to deformity (fetal) O33.7
      - excessive growth (large for dates) O36.6- ☑
      - growth retardation O36.59- ☑
        - light for dates O36.59- ☑
        - small for dates O36.59- ☑
      - heart rate irregularity (bradycardia) (decelerations) (tachycardia) O76
      - hereditary disease O35.2 ☑
      - hydrocephalus O35.Ø ☑
      - intrauterine death O36.4 ☑
      - poor growth O36.59- ☑
        - light for dates O36.59- ☑
        - small for dates O36.59- ☑
      - problem O36.9- ☑
        - specified NEC O36.89- ☑
      - reduction (elective) O31.3- ☑
      - selective termination O31.3- ☑
      - spina bifida O35.Ø ☑
      - thrombocytopenia O36.82- ☑
    - fibroid (tumor) (uterus) O34.1- ☑
    - fissure of nipple O92.11- ☑
    - gallstones O99.61- ☑
    - gastric banding status O99.84- ☑
    - gastric bypass status O99.84- ☑
    - genital herpes (asymptomatic) (history of) (inactive) O98.51- ☑
    - genital tract infection O23.9- ☑
    - glomerular diseases (conditions in NØØ-NØ7) O26.83- ☑
      - with hypertension, pre-existing — *see* Hypertension, complicating, pregnancy, pre-existing, with, renal disease
    - gonorrhea O98.21- ☑
    - grand multiparity OØ9.4 ☑
    - habitual aborter — *see* Pregnancy, complicated by, recurrent pregnancy loss

- **Pregnancy** — *continued*
  - complicated by — *continued*
    - HELLP syndrome (hemolysis, elevated liver enzymes and low platelet count) O14.2- ☑
    - hemorrhage
      - antepartum — *see* Hemorrhage, antepartum
      - before 2Ø completed weeks gestation O2Ø.9
        - specified NEC O2Ø.8
      - due to premature separation, placenta (*see also* Abruptio placentae) O45.9- ☑
      - early O2Ø.9
        - specified NEC O2Ø.8
      - threatened abortion O2Ø.Ø
    - hemorrhoids O22.4- ☑
    - hepatitis (viral) O98.41- ☑
    - herniation of uterus O34.59- ☑
    - high
      - head at term O32.4 ☑
      - risk — *see* Supervision (of) (for), high-risk
    - history of in utero procedure during previous pregnancy OØ9.82- ☑
    - HIV O98.71- ☑
    - human immunodeficiency virus (HIV) disease O98.71- ☑
    - hydatidiform mole (*see also* Mole, hydatidiform) OØ1.9
    - hydramnios O4Ø.- ☑
    - hydrocephalic fetus (disproportion) O33.6 ☑
    - hydrops
      - amnii O4Ø.- ☑
      - fetalis O36.2- ☑
        - associated with isoimmunization (*see also* Pregnancy, complicated by, isoimmunization) O36.11- ☑
    - hydrorrhea O42.9Ø
    - hyperemesis (gravidarum) (mild) (*see also* Hyperemesis, gravidarum) O21.Ø
    - hypertension — *see* Hypertension, complicating pregnancy
    - hypertensive
      - heart and renal disease, pre-existing — *see* Hypertension, complicating, pregnancy, pre-existing, with, heart disease, with renal disease
      - heart disease, pre-existing — *see* Hypertension, complicating, pregnancy, pre-existing, with, heart disease
      - renal disease, pre-existing — *see* Hypertension, complicating, pregnancy, pre-existing, with, renal disease
    - hypotension O26.5- ☑
    - immune disorders NEC (conditions in D8Ø-D89) O99.11- ☑
    - incarceration, uterus O34.51- ☑
    - incompetent cervix O34.3- ☑
    - inconclusive fetal viability O36.8Ø ☑
    - infection(s) O98.91- ☑
      - amniotic fluid or sac O41.1Ø- ☑
      - bladder O23.1- ☑
      - carrier state NEC O99.83Ø
        - streptococcus B O99.82Ø
      - genital organ or tract O23.9- ☑
        - specified NEC O23.59- ☑
      - genitourinary tract O23.9- ☑
      - gonorrhea O98.21- ☑
      - hepatitis (viral) O98.41- ☑
      - HIV O98.71- ☑
      - human immunodeficiency virus (HIV) O98.71- ☑
      - kidney O23.Ø- ☑
      - nipple O91.Ø1- ☑
      - parasitic disease O98.91- ☑
        - specified NEC O98.81- ☑
      - protozoal disease O98.61- ☑
      - sexually transmitted NEC O98.31- ☑
      - specified type NEC O98.81- ☑
      - syphilis O98.11- ☑
      - tuberculosis O98.Ø1- ☑
      - urethra O23.2- ☑
      - urinary (tract) O23.4- ☑
        - specified NEC O23.3- ☑
      - viral disease O98.51- ☑
    - injury or poisoning (conditions in SØØ-T88) O9A.21- ☑ (*following* O99)
      - due to abuse
        - physical O9A.31- ☑ (*following* O99)

- **Pregnancy** — *continued*
  - complicated by — *continued*
    - young mother — *continued*
      - primigravida OØ9.61- ☑
  - complicated NOS O26.9- ☑
  - concealed OØ9.3- ☑
  - continuing following
    - elective fetal reduction of one or more fetus O31.3- ☑
    - intrauterine death of one or more fetus O31.2- ☑
    - spontaneous abortion of one or more fetus O31.1- ☑
  - cornual OØØ.8
  - ectopic (ruptured) OØØ.9
    - abdominal OØØ.Ø
      - with viable fetus O36.7- ☑
    - cervical OØØ.8
    - complicated (by) OØ8.9
      - afibrinogenemia OØ8.1
      - cardiac arrest OØ8.81
      - chemical damage of pelvic organ(s) OØ8.6
      - circulatory collapse OØ8.3
      - defibrination syndrome OØ8.1
      - electrolyte imbalance OØ8.5
      - embolism (amniotic fluid) (blood clot) (pulmonary) (septic) OØ8.2
      - endometritis OØ8.Ø
      - genital tract and pelvic infection OØ8.Ø
      - hemorrhage (delayed) (excessive) OØ8.1
      - infection
        - genital tract or pelvic OØ8.Ø
        - kidney OØ8.83
        - urinary tract OØ8.3
      - intravascular coagulation OØ8.1
      - laceration of pelvic organ(s) OØ8.6
      - metabolic disorder OØ8.5
      - oliguria OØ8.4
      - oophoritis OØ8.Ø
      - parametritis OØ8.Ø
      - pelvic peritonitis OØ8.Ø
      - perforation of pelvic organ(s) OØ8.6
      - renal failure or shutdown OØ8.4
      - salpingitis or salpingo-oophoritis OØ8.Ø
      - sepsis OØ8.82
      - shock OØ8.83
        - septic OØ8.82
      - specified condition NEC OØ8.89
      - tubular necrosis (renal) OØ8.4
      - uremia OØ8.4
      - urinary infection OØ8.83
      - venous complication NEC OØ8.7
        - embolism OØ8.2
    - cornual OØØ.8
    - intraligamentous OØØ.8
    - mural OØØ.8
    - ovarian OØØ.2
    - specified site NEC OØØ.8
    - tubal (ruptured) OØØ.1
  - examination (normal) Z34.9- ☑
    - first Z34.Ø- ☑
    - high-risk — *see* Pregnancy, supervision of, high-risk
    - specified Z34.8- ☑
  - extrauterine — *see* Pregnancy, ectopic
  - fallopian OØØ.1
  - false F45.8
  - hidden OØ9.3- ☑
  - high-risk — *see* Pregnancy, supervision of, high-risk
  - incidental finding Z33.1
  - interstitial OØØ.8
  - intraligamentous OØØ.8
  - intramural OØØ.8
  - intraperitoneal OØØ.Ø
  - isthmian OØØ.1
  - mesometric (mural) OØØ.8
  - molar NEC OØ2.Ø
    - complicated (by) OØ8.9
      - afibrinogenemia OØ8.1
      - cardiac arrest OØ8.81
      - chemical damage of pelvic organ(s) OØ8.6
      - circulatory collapse OØ8.3
      - defibrination syndrome OØ8.1
      - electrolyte imbalance OØ8.5
      - embolism (amniotic fluid) (blood clot) (pulmonary) (septic) OØ8.2
      - endometritis OØ8.Ø
      - genital tract and pelvic infection OØ8.Ø
      - hemorrhage (delayed) (excessive) OØ8.1

- **Pregnancy** — *continued*
  - molar — *continued*
    - complicated — *continued*
      - infection
        - genital tract or pelvic OØ8.Ø
        - kidney OØ8.83
        - urinary tract OØ8.83
      - intravascular coagulation OØ8.1
      - laceration of pelvic organ(s) OØ8.6
      - metabolic disorder OØ8.5
      - oliguria OØ8.4
      - oophoritis OØ8.Ø
      - parametritis OØ8.Ø
      - pelvic peritonitis OØ8.Ø
      - perforation of pelvic organ(s) OØ8.6
      - renal failure or shutdown OØ8.4
      - salpingitis or salpingo-oophoritis OØ8.Ø
      - sepsis OØ8.82
      - shock OØ8.3
        - septic OØ8.82
      - specified condition NEC OØ8.89
      - tubular necrosis (renal) OØ8.4
      - uremia OØ8.4
      - urinary infection OØ8.83
      - venous complication NEC OØ8.7
        - embolism OØ8.2
    - hydatidiform (*see also* Mole, hydatidiform) OØ1.9
  - multiple (gestation) O3Ø.9- ☑
    - greater than quadruplets — *see* Pregnancy, multiple (gestation), specified NEC
    - specified NEC O3Ø.8Ø- ☑
      - with
        - two or more monoamniotic fetuses O3Ø.82- ☑
        - two or more monochorionic fetuses O3Ø.81- ☑
      - two or more monoamniotic fetuses O3Ø.82- ☑
      - two or more monochorionic fetuses O3Ø.81- ☑
      - unable to determine number of placenta and number of amniotic sacs O3Ø.89- ☑
      - unspecified number of placenta and unspecified number of amniotic sacs O3Ø.8Ø- ☑
  - mural OØØ.8
  - normal (supervision of) Z34.9- ☑
    - first Z34.Ø- ☑
    - high-risk — *see* Pregnancy, supervision of, high-risk
    - specified Z34.8- ☑
  - ovarian OØØ.2
  - postmature (4Ø to 42 weeks) O48.Ø
    - more than 42 weeks gestation O48.1
  - post-term (4Ø to 42 weeks) O48.Ø
  - prenatal care only Z34.9- ☑
    - first Z34.Ø- ☑
    - high-risk — *see* Pregnancy, supervision of, high-risk
    - specified Z34.8- ☑
  - prolonged (more than 42 weeks gestation) O48.1
  - quadruplet O3Ø.2Ø- ☑
    - with
      - two or more monoamniotic fetuses O3Ø.22- ☑
      - two or more monochorionic fetuses O3Ø.21- ☑
    - two or more monoamniotic fetuses O3Ø.22- ☑
    - two or more monochorionic fetuses O3Ø.21- ☑
    - unable to determine number of placenta and number of amniotic sacs O3Ø.29- ☑
    - unspecified number of placenta and unspecified number of amniotic sacs O3Ø.2Ø- ☑
  - quintuplet — *see* Pregnancy, multiple (gestation), specified NEC
  - sextuplet — *see* Pregnancy, multiple (gestation), specified NEC
  - supervision of
    - concealed pregnancy OØ9.3- ☑
    - elderly mother
      - multigravida OØ9.52- ☑
      - primigravida OØ9.51- ☑
    - hidden pregnancy OØ9.3- ☑
    - high-risk OØ9.9- ☑
      - due to (history of)
        - ectopic pregnancy OØ9.1- ☑
        - elderly — *see* Pregnancy, supervision, elderly mother
        - grand multiparity OØ9.4 ☑
        - in utero procedure during previous pregnancy OØ9.82- ☑
        - in vitro fertilization OØ9.81- ☑

- **Pregnancy** — *continued*
  - supervision of — *continued*
    - high-risk — *continued*
      - due to — *continued*
        - infertility OØ9.Ø- ☑
        - insufficient prenatal care OØ9.3- ☑
        - molar pregnancy OØ9.1- ☑
        - multiple previous pregnancies OØ9.4- ☑
        - older mother — *see* Pregnancy, supervision of, elderly mother
        - poor reproductive or obstetric history NEC OØ9.29- ☑
        - pre-term labor OØ9.21- ☑
        - previous
          - neonatal death OØ9.29- ☑
        - social problems OØ9.7- ☑
        - specified NEC OØ9.89- ☑
        - very young mother — *see* Pregnancy, supervision, young mother
      - resulting from in vitro fertilization OØ9.81- ☑
    - normal Z34.9- ☑
      - first Z34.Ø- ☑
      - specified NEC Z34.8- ☑
    - young mother
      - multigravida OØ9.62- ☑
      - primigravida OØ9.61- ☑
  - triplet O3Ø.1Ø- ☑
    - with
      - two or more monoamniotic fetuses O3Ø.12- ☑
      - two or more monochrorionic fetuses O3Ø.11- ☑
    - two or more monoamniotic fetuses O3Ø.12- ☑
    - two or more monochrorionic fetuses O3Ø.11- ☑
    - unable to determine number of placenta and number of amniotic sacs O3Ø.19- ☑
    - unspecified number of placenta and unspecified number of amniotic sacs O3Ø.1Ø- ☑
  - tubal (with abortion) (with rupture) OØØ.1
  - twin O3Ø.ØØ- ☑
    - conjoined O3Ø.Ø2- ☑
    - dichorionic/diamniotic (two placenta, two amniotic sacs) O3Ø.Ø4- ☑
    - monochorionic/diamniotic (one placenta, two amniotic sacs) O3Ø.Ø3- ☑
    - monochorionic/monoamniotic (one placenta, one amniotic sac) O3Ø.Ø1- ☑
    - unable to determine number of placenta and number of amniotic sacs O3Ø.Ø9- ☑
    - unspecified number of placenta and unspecified number of amniotic sacs O3Ø.ØØ- ☑
  - unwanted Z64.Ø
  - weeks of gestation
    - less than 8 weeks Z3A.Ø1 (*following* Z36)
    - 8 weeks Z3A.Ø8 (*following* Z36)
    - 9 weeks Z3A.Ø9 (*following* Z36)
    - 1Ø weeks Z3A.1Ø (*following* Z36)
    - 11 weeks Z3A.11 (*following* Z36)
    - 12 weeks Z3A.12 (*following* Z36)
    - 13 weeks Z3A.13 (*following* Z36)
    - 14 weeks Z3A.14 (*following* Z36)
    - 15 weeks Z3A.15 (*following* Z36)
    - 16 weeks Z3A.16 (*following* Z36)
    - 17 weeks Z3A.17 (*following* Z36)
    - 18 weeks Z3A.18 (*following* Z36)
    - 19 weeks Z3A.19 (*following* Z36)
    - 2Ø weeks Z3A.2Ø (*following* Z36)
    - 21 weeks Z3A.21 (*following* Z36)
    - 22 weeks Z3A.22 (*following* Z36)
    - 23 weeks Z3A.23 (*following* Z36)
    - 24 weeks Z3A.24 (*following* Z36)
    - 25 weeks Z3A.25 (*following* Z36)
    - 26 weeks Z3A.26 (*following* Z36)
    - 27 weeks Z3A.27 (*following* Z36)
    - 28 weeks Z3A.28 (*following* Z36)
    - 29 weeks Z3A.29 (*following* Z36)
    - 3Ø weeks Z3A.3Ø (*following* Z36)
    - 31 weeks Z3A.31 (*following* Z36)
    - 32 weeks Z3A.32 (*following* Z36)
    - 33 weeks Z3A.33 (*following* Z36)
    - 34 weeks Z3A.34 (*following* Z36)
    - 35 weeks Z3A.35 (*following* Z36)
    - 36 weeks Z3A.36 (*following* Z36)
    - 37 weeks Z3A.37 (*following* Z36)
    - 38 weeks Z3A.38 (*following* Z36)
    - 39 weeks Z3A.39 (*following* Z36)
    - 4Ø weeks Z3A.4Ø (*following* Z36)
    - 41 weeks Z3A.41 (*following* Z36)
    - 42 weeks Z3A.42 (*following* Z36)

- **Pregnancy** — *continued*
  - weeks of gestation — *continued*
    - greater than 42 weeks Z3A.49 (*following* Z36)
    - not specified Z3A.ØØ (*following* Z36)
- **Preiser's disease** — *see* Osteonecrosis, secondary, due to, trauma, metacarpus
- **Pre-kwashiorkor** — *see* Malnutrition, severe
- **Preleukemia** (syndrome) D46.9
- **Preluxation, hip, congenital** Q65.6
- **Premature** (*see also* condition)
  - adrenarche E27.Ø
  - aging E34.8
  - beats I49.4Ø
    - atrial I49.1
    - auricular I49.1
    - supraventricular I49.1
  - birth NEC — *see* Preterm, newborn
  - closure, foramen ovale Q21.8
  - contraction
    - atrial I49.1
    - atrioventricular I49.2
    - auricular I49.1
    - auriculoventricular I49.49
    - heart (extrasystole) I49.49
    - junctional I49.2
    - ventricular I49.3
  - delivery (*see also* Pregnancy, complicated by, preterm labor) O6Ø.1Ø ☑
  - ejaculation F52.4
  - infant NEC — *see* Preterm, newborn
    - light-for-dates — *see* Light for dates
  - labor — *see* Pregnancy, complicated by, preterm labor
  - lungs P28.Ø
  - menopause E28.319
    - asymptomatic E28.319
    - symptomatic E28.31Ø
  - newborn
    - less than 37 completed weeks — *see* Preterm, newborn
    - extreme (less than 28 completed weeks) — *see* Immaturity, extreme
  - puberty E3Ø.1
  - rupture membranes or amnion — *see* Pregnancy, complicated by, premature rupture of membranes
  - senility E34.8
  - thelarche E3Ø.8
  - ventricular systole I49.3
- **Prematurity NEC** (less than 37 completed weeks) — *see* Preterm, newborn
  - extreme (less than 28 completed weeks) — *see* Immaturity, extreme
- **Premenstrual**
  - dysphoric disorder (PMDD) N94.3
  - tension (syndrome) N94.3
- **Premolarization, cuspids** KØØ.2
- **Prenatal**
  - care, normal pregnancy — *see* Pregnancy, normal
  - screening of mother Z36
  - teeth KØØ.6
- **Preparatory care for subsequent treatment NEC**
  - for dialysis Z49.Ø1
    - peritoneal Z49.Ø2
- **Prepartum** — *see* condition
- **Preponderance, left or right ventricular** I51.7
- **Prepuce** — *see* condition
- **PRES** (posterior reversible encephalopathy syndrome) I67.83
- **Presbycardia** R54
- **Presbycusis, presbyacusia** H91.1- ☑
- **Presbyesophagus** K22.8
- **Presbyophrenia** FØ3 ☑
- **Presbyopia** H52.4
- **Prescription of contraceptives** (initial) Z3Ø.Ø19
  - emergency (postcoital) Z3Ø.Ø12
  - implantable subdermal Z3Ø.Ø19
  - injectable Z3Ø.Ø13
  - intrauterine contraceptive device Z3Ø.Ø14
  - pills Z3Ø.Ø11
  - postcoital (emergency) Z3Ø.Ø12
  - repeat Z3Ø.4Ø
    - implantable subdermal Z3Ø.49
    - injectable Z3Ø.42
    - pills Z3Ø.41
    - specified type NEC Z3Ø.49
  - specified type NEC Z3Ø.Ø18
- **Presence** (of)
  - ankle-joint implant (functional) (prosthesis) Z96.66- ☑
  - aortocoronary (bypass) graft Z95.1
  - arterial-venous shunt (dialysis) Z99.2
  - artificial
    - eye (globe) Z97.Ø
    - heart (fully implantable) (mechanical) Z95.812
      - valve Z95.2
    - larynx Z96.3
    - lens (intraocular) Z96.1
    - limb (complete) (partial) Z97.1- ☑
      - arm Z97.1- ☑
        - bilateral Z97.15
      - leg Z97.1- ☑
        - bilateral Z97.16
  - audiological implant (functional) Z96.29
  - bladder implant (functional) Z96.Ø
  - bone
    - conduction hearing device Z96.29
    - implant (functional) NEC Z96.7
    - joint (prosthesis) — *see* Presence, joint implant
  - cardiac
    - defibrillator (functional) (with synchronous cardiac pacemaker) Z95.81Ø
    - implant or graft Z95.9
      - specified type NEC Z95.818
    - pacemaker Z95.Ø
  - cerebrospinal fluid drainage device Z98.2
  - cochlear implant (functional) Z96.21
  - contact lens (es) Z97.3
  - coronary artery graft or prosthesis Z95.5
  - CSF shunt Z98.2
  - dental prosthesis device Z97.2
  - dentures Z97.2
  - device (external) NEC Z97.8
    - cardiac NEC Z95.818
    - heart assist Z95.811
    - implanted (functional) Z96.9
      - specified NEC Z96.89
    - prosthetic Z97.8
  - ear implant Z96.2Ø
    - cochlear implant Z96.21
    - myringotomy tube Z96.22
    - specified type NEC Z96.29
  - elbow-joint implant (functional) (prosthesis) Z96.62- ☑
  - endocrine implant (functional) NEC Z96.49
  - eustachian tube stent or device (functional) Z96.29
  - external hearing-aid or device Z97.4
  - finger-joint implant (functional) (prosthetic) Z96.69- ☑
  - functional implant Z96.9
    - specified NEC Z96.89
  - graft
    - cardiac NEC Z95.818
    - vascular NEC Z95.828
  - hearing-aid or device (external) Z97.4
    - implant (bone) (cochlear) (functional) Z96.21
  - heart assist device Z95.811
  - heart valve implant (functional) Z95.2
    - prosthetic Z95.2
    - specified type NEC Z95.4
    - xenogenic Z95.3
  - hip-joint implant (functional) (prosthesis) Z96.64- ☑
  - implanted device (artificial) (functional) (prosthetic) Z96.9
    - automatic cardiac defibrillator (with synchronous cardiac pacemaker) Z95.81Ø
    - cardiac pacemaker Z95.Ø
    - cochlear Z96.21
    - dental Z96.5
    - heart Z95.812
    - heart valve Z95.2
      - prosthetic Z95.2
      - specified NEC Z95.4
      - xenogenic Z95.3
    - insulin pump Z96.41
    - intraocular lens Z96.1
    - joint Z96.6Ø
      - ankle Z96.66- ☑
      - elbow Z96.62- ☑
      - finger Z96.69- ☑
      - hip Z96.64- ☑
      - knee Z96.65- ☑
      - shoulder Z96.61- ☑
      - specified NEC Z96.698
      - wrist Z96.63- ☑
    - larynx Z96.3
    - myringotomy tube Z96.22
- **Presence** — *continued*
  - implanted device — *continued*
    - otological Z96.2Ø
      - cochlear Z96.21
      - eustachian stent Z96.29
      - myringotomy Z96.22
      - specified NEC Z96.29
      - stapes Z96.29
    - skin Z96.81
    - skull plate Z96.7
    - specified NEC Z96.89
    - urogenital Z96.Ø
  - insulin pump (functional) Z96.41
  - intestinal bypass or anastomosis Z98.Ø
  - intraocular lens (functional) Z96.1
  - intrauterine contraceptive device (IUD) Z97.5
  - intravascular implant (functional) (prosthetic) NEC Z95.9
    - coronary artery Z95.5
    - defibrillator (with synchronous cardiac pacemaker) Z95.81Ø
    - peripheral vessel (with angioplasty) Z95.82Ø
  - joint implant (prosthetic) (any) Z96.6Ø
    - ankle — *see* Presence, ankle joint implant
    - elbow — *see* Presence, elbow joint implant
    - finger — *see* Presence, finger joint implant
    - hip — *see* Presence, hip joint implant
    - knee — *see* Presence, knee joint implant
    - shoulder — *see* Presence, shoulder joint implant
    - specified joint NEC Z96.698
    - wrist — *see* Presence, wrist joint implant
  - knee-joint implant (functional) (prosthesis) Z96.65- ☑
  - laryngeal implant (functional) Z96.3
  - mandibular implant (dental) Z96.5
  - myringotomy tube(s) Z96.22
  - orthopedic-joint implant (prosthetic) (any) — *see* Presence, joint implant
  - otological implant (functional) Z96.29
  - shoulder-joint implant (functional) (prosthesis) Z96.61- ☑
  - skull-plate implant Z96.7
  - spectacles Z97.3
  - stapes implant (functional) Z96.29
  - systemic lupus erythematosus [SLE] inhibitor D68.62
  - tendon implant (functional) (graft) Z96.7
  - tooth root(s) implant Z96.5
  - ureteral stent Z96.Ø
  - urethral stent Z96.Ø
  - urogenital implant (functional) Z96.Ø
  - vascular implant or device Z95.9
    - access port device Z95.828
    - specified type NEC Z95.828
  - wrist-joint implant (functional) (prosthesis) Z96.63- ☑
- **Presenile** (*see also* condition)
  - dementia FØ3 ☑
  - premature aging E34.8
- **Presentation, fetal** — *see* Delivery, complicated by, malposition
- **Prespondylolisthesis** (congenital) Q76.2
- **Pressure**
  - area, skin — *see* Ulcer, pressure, by site
  - brachial plexus G54.Ø
  - brain G93.5
    - injury at birth NEC P11.1
  - cerebral — *see* Pressure, brain
  - chest RØ7.89
  - cone, tentorial G93.5
  - hyposystolic (*see also* Hypotension)
    - incidental reading, without diagnosis of hypotension RØ3.1
  - increased
    - intracranial (benign) G93.2
      - injury at birth P11.Ø
    - intraocular H4Ø.Ø5- ☑
  - lumbosacral plexus G54.1
  - mediastinum J98.5
  - necrosis (chronic) — *see* Ulcer, pressure, by site
  - parental, inappropriate (excessive) Z62.6
  - sore (chronic) — *see* Ulcer, pressure, by site
  - spinal cord G95.2Ø
  - ulcer (chronic) — *see* Ulcer, pressure, by site
  - venous, increased I87.8
- **Pre-syncope** R55
- **Preterm**
  - delivery (*see also* Pregnancy, complicated by, preterm labor) O6Ø.1Ø ☑
  - labor — *see* Pregnancy, complicated by, preterm labor
  - newborn (infant) PØ7.3Ø

Problem — *continued*
work schedule (stressful) Z56.3
Procedure (surgical)
for purpose other than remedying health state Z41.9
specified NEC Z41.8
not done Z53.9
because of
administrative reasons Z53.8
contraindication Z53.Ø9
smoking Z53.Ø1
patient's decision Z53.2Ø
for reasons of belief or group pressure Z53.1
left against medical advice (AMA) Z53.21
specified reason NEC Z53.29
specified reason NEC Z53.8
Procidentia (uteri) N81.3
Proctalgia K62.89
fugax K59.4
spasmodic K59.4
Proctitis K62.89
amebic (acute) AØ6.Ø
chlamydial A56.3
gonococcal A54.6
granulomatous — *see* Enteritis, regional, large intestine
herpetic A6Ø.1
radiation K62.7
tuberculous A18.32
ulcerative (chronic) K51.2Ø
with
complication K51.219
abscess K51.214
fistula K51.213
obstruction K51.212
rectal bleeding K51.211
specified NEC K51.218
Proctocele
female (without uterine prolapse) N81.6
with uterine prolapse N81.2
complete N81.3
male K62.3
Proctocolitis, mucosal — *see* Rectosigmoiditis, ulcerative
Proctoptosis K62.3
Proctorrhagia K62.5
Proctosigmoiditis K63.89
ulcerative (chronic) — *see* Rectosigmoiditis, ulcerative
Proctospasm K59.4
psychogenic F45.8
Profichet's disease — *see* Disorder, soft tissue, specified type NEC
Progeria E34.8
Prognathism (mandibular) (maxillary) M26.19
Progonoma (melanotic) — *see* Neoplasm, benign, by site
Progressive — *see* condition
Prolactinoma
specified site — *see* Neoplasm, benign, by site
unspecified site D35.2
Prolapse, prolapsed
anus, anal (canal) (sphincter) K62.2
arm or hand O32.2 ☑
causing obstructed labor O64.4 ☑
bladder (mucosa) (sphincter) (acquired)
congenital Q79.4
female — *see* Cystocele
male N32.89
breast implant (prosthetic) T85.49 ☑
cecostomy K94.Ø9
cecum K63.4
cervix, cervical (hypertrophied) N81.2
anterior lip, obstructing labor O65.5
congenital Q51.828
postpartal, old N81.2
stump N81.85
ciliary body (traumatic) — *see* Laceration, eye(ball), with prolapse or loss of interocular tissue
colon (pedunculated) K63.4
colostomy K94.Ø9
disc (intervertebral) — *see* Displacement, intervertebral disc
eye implant (orbital) T85.398 ☑
lens (ocular) — *see* Complications, intraocular lens
fallopian tube N83.4
gastric (mucosa) K31.89
genital, female N81.9
specified NEC N81.89
globe, nontraumatic — *see* Luxation, globe

Prolapse, prolapsed — *continued*
ileostomy bud K94.19
intervertebral disc — *see* Displacement, intervertebral disc
intestine (small) K63.4
iris (traumatic) — *see* Laceration, eye(ball), with prolapse or loss of interocular tissue
nontraumatic H21.89
kidney N28.83
congenital Q63.2
laryngeal muscles or ventricle J38.7
liver K76.89
meatus urinarius N36.8
mitral (valve) I34.1
ocular lens implant — *see* Complications, intraocular lens
organ or site, congenital NEC — *see* Malposition, congenital
ovary N83.4
pelvic floor, female N81.89
perineum, female N81.89
rectum (mucosa) (sphincter) K62.3
due to trichuris trichuria B79
spleen D73.89
stomach K31.89
umbilical cord
complicating delivery O69.Ø ☑
urachus, congenital Q64.4
ureter N28.89
with obstruction N13.5
with infection N13.6
ureterovesical orifice N28.89
urethra (acquired) (infected) (mucosa) N36.8
congenital Q64.71
urinary meatus N36.8
congenital Q64.72
uterovaginal N81.4
complete N81.3
incomplete N81.2
uterus (with prolapse of vagina) N81.4
complete N81.3
congenital Q51.818
first degree N81.2
in pregnancy or childbirth — *see* Pregnancy, complicated by, abnormal, uterus
incomplete N81.2
postpartal (old) N81.4
second degree N81.2
third degree N81.3
uveal (traumatic) — *see* Laceration, eye(ball), with prolapse or loss of interocular tissue
vagina (anterior) (wall) — *see* Cystocele
with prolapse of uterus N81.4
complete N81.3
incomplete N81.2
posterior wall N81.6
posthysterectomy N99.3
vitreous (humor) H43.Ø- ☑
in wound — *see* Laceration, eye(ball), with prolapse or loss of interocular tissue
womb — *see* Prolapse, uterus
Prolapsus, female N81.9
specified NEC N81.89
Proliferation(s)
primary cutaneous CD3Ø-positive large T-cell C86.6
Proliferative — *see* condition
Prolonged, prolongation (of)
bleeding (time) (idiopathic) R79.1
coagulation (time) R79.1
gestation (over 42 completed weeks)
mother O48.1
newborn PØ8.22
interval I44.Ø
labor O63.9
first stage O63.Ø
second stage O63.1
partial thromboplastin time (PTT) R79.1
pregnancy (more than 42 weeks gestation) O48.1
prothrombin time R79.1
QT interval I45.81
uterine contractions in labor O62.4
Prominence, prominent
auricle (congenital) (ear) Q17.5
ischial spine or sacral promontory
with disproportion (fetopelvic) O33.Ø
causing obstructed labor O65.Ø
nose (congenital) acquired M95.Ø
Promiscuity — *see* High, risk, sexual behavior

Pronation
ankle — *see* Deformity, limb, foot, specified NEC
foot (*see also* Deformity, limb, foot, specified NEC)
congenital Q74.2
Prophylactic
administration of
antibiotics, long-term Z79.2
short-term use — *omit code*
drug (*see also* Long-term (current) drug therapy (use of)) Z79.899
medication Z79.899
organ removal (for neoplasia management) Z4Ø.ØØ
breast Z4Ø.Ø1
ovary Z4Ø.Ø2
specified site NEC Z4Ø.Ø9
surgery Z4Ø.9
for risk factors related to malignant neoplasm — *see* Prophylactic, organ removal
specified NEC Z4Ø.8
vaccination Z23
Propionic acidemia E71.121
Proptosis (ocular) (*see also* Exophthalmos)
thyroid — *see* Hyperthyroidism, with goiter
Prosecution, anxiety concerning Z65.3
Prosopagnosia R48.3
Prostadynia N42.81
Prostate, prostatic — *see* condition
Prostatism — *see* Hyperplasia, prostate
Prostatitis (congestive) (suppurative) (with cystitis) N41.9
acute N41.Ø
cavitary N41.8
chronic N41.1
diverticular N41.8
due to Trichomonas (vaginalis) A59.Ø2
fibrous N41.1
gonococcal (acute) (chronic) A54.22
granulomatous N41.4
hypertrophic N41.1
subacute N41.1
trichomonal A59.Ø2
tuberculous A18.14
Prostatocystitis N41.3
Prostatorrhea N42.89
Prostatosis N42.82
Prostration R53.83
heat (*see also* Heat, exhaustion)
anhydrotic T67.3 ☑
due to
salt (and water) depletion T67.4 ☑
water depletion T67.3 ☑
nervous F48.8
senile R54
Protanomaly (anomalous trichromat) H53.54
Protanopia (complete) (incomplete) H53.54
Protection (against) (from) — *see* Prophylactic
Protein
deficiency NEC — *see* Malnutrition
malnutrition — *see* Malnutrition
sickness (*see also* Reaction, serum) T8Ø.69 ☑
Proteinemia R77.9
Proteinosis
alveolar (pulmonary) J84.Ø1
lipid or lipoid (of Urbach) E78.89
Proteinuria R8Ø.9
Bence Jones R8Ø.3
complicating pregnancy — *see* Proteinuria, gestational
gestational O12.1- ☑
with edema O12.2- ☑
idiopathic R8Ø.Ø
isolated R8Ø.Ø
with glomerular lesion NØ6.9
dense deposit disease NØ6.6
diffuse
crescentic glomerulonephritis NØ6.7
endocapillary proliferative glomerulonephritis NØ6.4
mesangiocapillary glomerulonephritis NØ6.5
focal and segmental hyalinosis or sclerosis NØ6.1
membranous (diffuse) NØ6.2
mesangial proliferative (diffuse) NØ6.3
minimal change NØ6.Ø
specified pathology NEC NØ6.8
orthostatic R8Ø.2
with glomerular lesion — *see* Proteinuria, isolated, with glomerular lesion
persistent R8Ø.1

- **Proteinuria** — *continued*
  - persistent — *continued*
    - with glomerular lesion — *see* Proteinuria, isolated, with glomerular lesion
  - postural R8Ø.2
    - with glomerular lesion — *see* Proteinuria, isolated, with glomerular lesion
  - pre-eclamptic — *see* Pre-eclampsia
  - specified type NEC R8Ø.8
- **Proteolysis, pathologic** D65
- **Proteus** (mirabilis) (morganii), **as cause of disease classified elsewhere** B96.4
- **Prothrombin gene mutation** D68.52
- **Protoporphyria, erythropoietic** E8Ø.Ø
- **Protozoal** (*see also* condition)
  - disease B64
    - specified NEC B6Ø.8
- **Protrusion, protrusio**
  - acetabuli M24.7
  - acetabulum (into pelvis) M24.7
  - device, implant or graft (*see also* Complications, by site and type, mechanical) T85.698 ☑
    - arterial graft NEC — *see* Complication, cardiovascular device, mechanical, vascular
    - breast (implant) T85.49 ☑
    - catheter NEC T85.698 ☑
      - cystostomy T83.Ø9Ø ☑
      - dialysis (renal) T82.49 ☑
        - intraperitoneal T85.691 ☑
      - infusion NEC T82.594 ☑
        - spinal (epidural) (subdural) T85.69Ø ☑
      - urinary, indwelling T83.Ø98 ☑
    - electronic (electrode) (pulse generator) (stimulator)
      - bone T84.39Ø ☑
      - nervous system — *see* Complication, prosthetic device, mechanical, electronic nervous system stimulator
    - fixation, internal (orthopedic) NEC — *see* Complication, fixation device, mechanical
    - gastrointestinal — *see* Complications, prosthetic device, mechanical, gastrointestinal device
    - genital NEC T83.498 ☑
      - intrauterine contraceptive device T83.39 ☑
      - penile prosthesis T83.49Ø ☑
    - heart NEC — *see* Complication, cardiovascular device, mechanical
    - joint prosthesis — *see* Complications, joint prosthesis, mechanical, specified NEC, by site
    - ocular NEC — *see* Complications, prosthetic device, mechanical, ocular device
    - orthopedic NEC — *see* Complication, orthopedic, device, mechanical
    - specified NEC T85.628 ☑
    - urinary NEC (*see also* Complication, genitourinary, device, urinary, mechanical)
      - graft T83.29 ☑
    - vascular NEC — *see* Complication, cardiovascular device, mechanical
    - ventricular intracranial shunt T85.Ø9 ☑
  - intervertebral disc — *see* Displacement, intervertebral disc
  - joint prosthesis — *see* Complications, joint prosthesis, mechanical, specified NEC, by site
  - nucleus pulposus — *see* Displacement, intervertebral disc
- **Prune belly** (syndrome) Q79.4
- **Prurigo** (ferox) (gravis) (Hebrae) (Hebra's) (mitis) (simplex) L28.2
  - Besnier's L2Ø.Ø
  - estivalis L56.4
  - nodularis L28.1
  - psychogenic F45.8
- **Pruritus, pruritic** (essential) L29.9
  - ani, anus L29.Ø
    - psychogenic F45.8
  - anogenital L29.3
    - psychogenic F45.8
  - due to onchocerca volvulus B73.1
  - gravidarum — *see* Pregnancy, complicated by, specified pregnancy-related condition NEC
  - hiemalis L29.8
  - neurogenic (any site) F45.8
  - perianal L29.Ø
  - psychogenic (any site) F45.8
  - scroti, scrotum L29.1
    - psychogenic F45.8
  - senile, senilis L29.8
- **Pruritus, pruritic** — *continued*
  - specified NEC L29.8
    - psychogenic F45.8
  - Trichomonas A59.9
  - vulva, vulvae L29.2
    - psychogenic F45.8
- **Pseudarthrosis, pseudoarthrosis** (bone) — *see* Nonunion, fracture
  - clavicle, congenital Q74.Ø
  - joint, following fusion or arthrodesis M96.Ø
- **Pseudoaneurysm** — *see* Aneurysm
- **Pseudoangina** (pectoris) — *see* Angina
- **Pseudoangioma** I81
- **Pseudoarteriosus** Q28.8
- **Pseudoarthrosis** — *see* Pseudarthrosis
- **Pseudobulbar affect** (PBA) F48.8
- **Pseudochromhidrosis** L67.8
- **Pseudocirrhosis, liver, pericardial** I31.1
- **Pseudocowpox** BØ8.Ø3
- **Pseudocoxalgia** M91.3- ☑
- **Pseudocroup** J38.5
- **Pseudo-Cushing's syndrome, alcohol-induced** E24.4
- **Pseudocyesis** F45.8
- **Pseudocyst**
  - lung J98.4
  - pancreas K86.3
  - retina — *see* Cyst, retina
- **Pseudoelephantiasis neuroarthritica** Q82.Ø
- **Pseudoexfoliation, capsule** (lens) — *see* Cataract, specified NEC
- **Pseudofolliculitis barbae** L73.1
- **Pseudoglioma** H44.89
- **Pseudohemophilia** (Bernuth's) (hereditary) (type B) D68.Ø
  - Type A D69.8
  - vascular D69.8
- **Pseudohermaphroditism** Q56.3
  - adrenal E25.8
  - female Q56.2
    - with adrenocortical disorder E25.8
    - without adrenocortical disorder Q56.2
    - adrenal, congenital E25.Ø
  - male Q56.1
    - with
      - 5-alpha-reductase deficiency E29.1
      - adrenocortical disorder E25.8
      - androgen resistance E34.51
      - cleft scrotum Q56.1
      - feminizing testis E34.51
    - without gonadal disorder Q56.1
    - adrenal E25.8
- **Pseudo-Hurler's polydystrophy** E77.Ø
- **Pseudohydrocephalus** G93.2
- **Pseudohypertrophic muscular dystrophy** (Erb's) G71.Ø
- **Pseudohypertrophy, muscle** G71.Ø
- **Pseudohypoparathyroidism** E2Ø.1
- **Pseudoinsomnia** F51.Ø3
- **Pseudoleukemia, infantile** D64.89
- **Pseudomembranous** — *see* condition
- **Pseudomeningocele** (cerebral) (infective) (post-traumatic) G96.19
  - postprocedural (spinal) G97.82
- **Pseudomenses** (newborn) P54.6
- **Pseudomenstruation** (newborn) P54.6
- **Pseudomonas**
  - aeruginosa, as cause of disease classified elsewhere B96.5
  - mallei infection A24.Ø
    - as cause of disease classified elsewhere B96.5
  - pseudomallei, as cause of disease classified elsewhere B96.5
- **Pseudomyotonia** G71.19
- **Pseudomyxoma peritonei** C78.6
- **Pseudoneuritis, optic** (nerve) (disc) (papilla), **congenital** Q14.2
- **Pseudo-obstruction intestine** (acute) (chronic) (idiopathic) (intermittent secondary) (primary) K59.8
- **Pseudopapilledema** H47.33- ☑
  - congenital Q14.2
- **Pseudoparalysis**
  - arm or leg R29.818
  - atonic, congenital P94.2
- **Pseudopelade** L66.Ø
- **Pseudophakia** Z96.1
- **Pseudopolyarthritis, rhizomelic** M35.3
- **Pseudopolycythemia** D75.1
- **Pseudopseudohypoparathyroidism** E2Ø.1
- **Pseudopterygium** H11.81- ☑
- **Pseudoptosis** (eyelid) — *see* Blepharochalasis
- **Pseudopuberty, precocious**
  - female heterosexual E25.8
  - male isosexual E25.8
- **Pseudorickets** (renal) N25.Ø
- **Pseudorubella** BØ8.2Ø
- **Pseudosclerema, newborn** P83.8
- **Pseudosclerosis** (brain)
  - Jakob's — *see* Creutzfeldt-Jakob disease or syndrome
  - of Westphal (Strümpell) E83.Ø1
  - spastic — *see* Creutzfeldt-Jakob disease or syndrome
- **Pseudotetanus** — *see* Convulsions
- **Pseudotetany** R29.Ø
  - hysterical F44.5
- **Pseudotruncus arteriosus** Q25.4
- **Pseudotuberculosis** A28.2
  - enterocolitis AØ4.8
  - pasteurella (infection) A28.Ø
- **Pseudotumor**
  - cerebri G93.2
  - orbital HØ5.11 ☑
- **Pseudoxanthoma elasticum** Q82.8
- **Psilosis** (sprue) (tropical) K9Ø.1
  - nontropical K9Ø.Ø
- **Psittacosis** A7Ø
- **Psoitis** M6Ø.88
- **Psoriasis** L4Ø.9
  - arthropathic L4Ø.5Ø
    - arthritis mutilans L4Ø.52
    - distal interphalangeal L4Ø.51
    - juvenile L4Ø.54
    - other specified L4Ø.59
    - spondylitis L4Ø.53
  - buccal K13.29
  - flexural L4Ø.8
  - guttate L4Ø.4
  - mouth K13.29
  - nummular L4Ø.Ø
  - plaque L4Ø.Ø
  - psychogenic F54
  - pustular (generalized) L4Ø.1
    - palmaris et plantaris L4Ø.3
  - specified NEC L4Ø.8
  - vulgaris L4Ø.Ø
- **Psychasthenia** F48.8
- **Psychiatric disorder or problem** F99
- **Psychogenic** (*see also* condition)
  - factors associated with physical conditions F54
- **Psychological and behavioral factors affecting medical condition** F59
- **Psychoneurosis, psychoneurotic** (*see also* Neurosis)
  - anxiety (state) F41.1
  - depersonalization F48.1
  - hypochondriacal F45.21
  - hysteria F44.9
  - neurasthenic F48.8
  - personality NEC F6Ø.89
- **Psychopathy, psychopathic**
  - affectionless F94.2
  - autistic F84.5
  - constitution, post-traumatic FØ7.81
  - personality — *see* Disorder, personality
  - sexual — *see* Deviation, sexual
  - state F6Ø.2
- **Psychosexual identity disorder of childhood** F64.2
- **Psychosis, psychotic** F29
  - acute (transient) F23
    - hysterical F44.9
  - affective — *see* Disorder, mood
  - alcoholic F1Ø.959
    - with
      - abuse F1Ø.159
      - anxiety disorder F1Ø.98Ø
        - with
          - abuse F1Ø.18Ø
          - dependence F1Ø.28Ø
      - delirium tremens F1Ø.231
      - delusions F1Ø.95Ø
        - with
          - abuse F1Ø.15Ø
          - dependence F1Ø.25Ø
      - dementia F1Ø.97
        - with dependence F1Ø.27
      - dependence F1Ø.259
      - hallucinosis F1Ø.951

- **Psychosis, psychotic** — *continued*
  - alcoholic — *continued*
    - with
      - hallucinosis — *continued*
        - with
          - abuse F10.151
          - dependence F10.251
      - mood disorder F10.94
        - with
          - abuse F10.14
          - dependence F10.24
      - paranoia F10.950
        - with
          - abuse F10.150
          - dependence F10.250
      - persisting amnesia F10.96
        - with dependence F10.26
    - amnestic confabulatory F10.96
      - with dependence F10.26
    - delirium tremens F10.231
    - Korsakoff's, Korsakov's, Korsakow's F10.26
    - paranoid type F10.950
      - with
        - abuse F10.150
        - dependence F10.250
  - anergastic — *see* Psychosis, organic
  - arteriosclerotic (simple type) (uncomplicated) F01.50
    - with behavioral disturbance F01.51
  - childhood F84.0
    - atypical F84.8
  - climacteric — *see* Psychosis, involutional
  - confusional F29
    - acute or subacute F05
    - reactive F23
  - cycloid F23
  - depressive — *see* Disorder, depressive
  - disintegrative (childhood) F84.3
  - drug-induced — *see* F11-F19 with .X59
    - paranoid and hallucinatory states — *see* F11-F19 with .X50 or .X51
  - due to or associated with
    - addiction, drug — *see* F11-F19 with .X59
    - dependence
      - alcohol F10.259
      - drug — *see* F11-F19 with .X59
    - epilepsy F06.8
    - Huntington's chorea F06.8
    - ischemia, cerebrovascular (generalized) F06.8
    - multiple sclerosis F06.8
    - physical disease F06.8
    - presenile dementia F03 ☑
    - senile dementia F03 ☑
    - vascular disease (arteriosclerotic) (cerebral) F01.50
      - with behavioral disturbance F01.51
  - epileptic F06.8
  - episode F23
    - due to or associated with physical condition F06.8
  - exhaustive F43.0
  - hallucinatory, chronic F28
  - hypomanic F30.8
  - hysterical (acute) F44.9
  - induced F24
  - infantile F84.0
    - atypical F84.8
  - infective (acute) (subacute) F05
  - involutional F28
    - depressive — *see* Disorder, depressive
    - melancholic — *see* Disorder, depressive
    - paranoid (state) F22
  - Korsakoff's, Korsakov's, Korsakow's (nonalcoholic) F04
    - alcoholic F10.96
      - in dependence F10.26
    - induced by other psychoactive substance — *see* categories F11-F19 with .X5X
  - mania, manic (single episode) F30.2
    - recurrent type F31.89
  - manic-depressive — *see* Disorder, mood
  - menopausal — *see* Psychosis, involutional
  - mixed schizophrenic and affective F25.8
  - multi-infarct (cerebrovascular) F01.50
    - with behavioral disturbance F01.51
  - nonorganic F29
    - specified NEC F28
  - organic F09
    - due to or associated with
      - arteriosclerosis (cerebral) — *see* Psychosis, arteriosclerotic

- **Psychosis, psychotic** — *continued*
  - organic — *continued*
    - due to or associated with — *continued*
      - cerebrovascular disease, arteriosclerotic — *see* Psychosis, arteriosclerotic
      - childbirth — *see* Psychosis, puerperal
      - Creutzfeldt-Jakob disease or syndrome — *see* Creutzfeldt-Jakob disease or syndrome
      - dependence, alcohol F10.259
      - disease
        - alcoholic liver F10.259
        - brain, arteriosclerotic — *see* Psychosis, arteriosclerotic
        - cerebrovascular F01.50
          - with behavioral disturbance F01.51
        - Creutzfeldt-Jakob — *see* Creutzfeldt-Jakob disease or syndrome
        - endocrine or metabolic F06.8
          - acute or subacute F05
        - liver, alcoholic F10.259
      - epilepsy transient (acute) F05
      - infection
        - brain (intracranial) F06.8
          - acute or subacute F05
      - intoxication
        - alcoholic (acute) F10.259
        - drug F11-F19 with .X59
      - ischemia, cerebrovascular (generalized) — *see* Psychosis, arteriosclerotic
      - puerperium — *see* Psychosis, puerperal
      - trauma, brain (birth) (from electric current) (surgical) F06.8
        - acute or subacute F05
    - infective F06.8
      - acute or subacute F05
    - post-traumatic F06.8
      - acute or subacute F05
  - paranoiac F22
  - paranoid (climacteric) (involutional) (menopausal) F22
    - psychogenic (acute) F23
    - schizophrenic F20.0
    - senile F03 ☑
  - postpartum F53
  - presbyophrenic (type) F03 ☑
  - presenile F03 ☑
  - psychogenic (paranoid) F23
    - depressive F32.3
  - puerperal F53
    - specified type — *see* Psychosis, by type
  - reactive (brief) (transient) (emotional stress) (psychological trauma) F23
    - depressive F32.3
      - recurrent F33.3
    - excitative type F30.8
  - schizoaffective F25.9
    - depressive type F25.1
    - manic type F25.0
  - schizophrenia, schizophrenic — *see* Schizophrenia
  - schizophrenia-like, in epilepsy F06.2
  - schizophreniform F20.81
    - affective type F25.9
    - brief F23
    - confusional type F23
    - depressive type F25.1
    - manic type F25.0
    - mixed type F25.0
  - senile NEC F03 ☑
    - depressed or paranoid type F03 ☑
    - simple deterioration F03 ☑
    - specified type — *code to* condition
  - shared F24
  - situational (reactive) F23
  - symbiotic (childhood) F84.3
  - symptomatic F09
- **Psychosomatic** — *see* Disorder, psychosomatic
- **Psychosyndrome, organic** F07.9
- **Psychotic episode due to or associated with physical condition** F06.8
- **Pterygium** (eye) H11.00- ☑
  - amyloid H11.01- ☑
  - central H11.02- ☑
  - colli Q18.3
  - double H11.03- ☑
  - peripheral
    - progressive H11.05- ☑
    - stationary H11.04- ☑
  - recurrent H11.06- ☑
- **Ptilosis** (eyelid) — *see* Madarosis
- **Ptomaine** (poisoning) — *see* Poisoning, food
- **Ptosis** (*see also* Blepharoptosis)
  - adiposa (false) — *see* Blepharoptosis
  - breast N64.81
  - cecum K63.4
  - colon K63.4
  - congenital (eyelid) Q10.0
    - specified site NEC — *see* Anomaly, by site
  - eyelid — *see* Blepharoptosis
    - congenital Q10.0
  - gastric K31.89
  - intestine K63.4
  - kidney N28.83
  - liver K76.89
  - renal N28.83
  - splanchnic K63.4
  - spleen D73.89
  - stomach K31.89
  - viscera K63.4
- **PTP** D69.51
- **Ptyalism** (periodic) K11.7
  - hysterical F45.8
  - pregnancy — *see* Pregnancy, complicated by, specified pregnancy-related condition NEC
  - psychogenic F45.8
- **Ptyalolithiasis** K11.5
- **Pubarche, precocious** E30.1
- **Pubertas praecox** E30.1
- **Puberty** (development state) Z00.3
  - bleeding (excessive) N92.2
  - delayed E30.0
  - precocious (constitutional) (cryptogenic) (idiopathic) E30.1
    - central E22.8
    - due to
      - ovarian hyperfunction E28.1
        - estrogen E28.0
      - testicular hyperfunction E29.0
  - premature E30.1
    - due to
      - adrenal cortical hyperfunction E25.8
      - pineal tumor E34.8
      - pituitary (anterior) hyperfunction E22.8
- **Puckering, macula** — *see* Degeneration, macula, puckering
- **Pudenda, pudendum** — *see* condition
- **Puente's disease** (simple glandular cheilitis) K13.0
- **Puerperal, puerperium** (complicated by, complications)
  - abnormal glucose (tolerance test) O99.815
  - abscess
    - areola O91.02
      - associated with lactation O91.03
    - Bartholin's gland O86.19
    - breast O91.12
      - associated with lactation O91.13
    - cervix (uteri) O86.11
    - genital organ NEC O86.19
    - kidney O86.21
    - mammary O91.12
      - associated with lactation O91.13
    - nipple O91.02
      - associated with lactation O91.03
    - peritoneum O85
    - subareolar O91.12
      - associated with lactation O91.13
    - urinary tract — *see* Puerperal, infection, urinary
    - uterus O86.12
    - vagina (wall) O86.13
    - vaginorectal O86.13
    - vulvovaginal gland O86.13
  - adnexitis O86.19
  - afibrinogenemia, or other coagulation defect O72.3
  - albuminuria (acute) (subacute) — *see* Proteinuria, gestational
  - alcohol use O99.315
  - anemia O90.81
    - pre-existing (pre-pregnancy) O99.03
  - anesthetic death O89.8
  - apoplexy O99.43
  - bariatric surgery status O99.845
  - blood disorder NEC O99.13
  - blood dyscrasia O72.3
  - cardiomyopathy O90.3
  - cerebrovascular disorder (conditions in I60-I69) O99.43
  - cervicitis O86.11
  - circulatory system disorder O99.43
  - coagulopathy (any) O72.3

Puerperal, puerperium — *continued*
- complications O90.9
  - specified NEC O90.89
- convulsions — *see* Eclampsia
- cystitis O86.22
- cystopyelitis O86.29
- delirium NEC F05
- diabetes O24.93
  - gestational — *see* Puerperal, gestational diabetes
  - pre-existing O24.33
    - specified NEC O24.83
    - type 1 O24.03
    - type 2 O24.13
- digestive system disorder O99.63
- disease O90.9
  - breast NEC O92.29
  - cerebrovascular (acute) O99.43
  - nonobstetric NEC O99.89
  - tubo-ovarian O86.19
  - Valsuani's O99.03
- disorder O90.9
  - biliary tract O26.63
  - lactation O92.70
  - liver O26.63
  - nonobstetric NEC O99.89
- disruption
  - cesarean wound O90.0
  - episiotomy wound O90.1
  - perineal laceration wound O90.1
- drug use O99.325
- eclampsia (with pre-existing hypertension) O15.2
- embolism (pulmonary) (blood clot) — *see* Embolism, obstetric, puerperal
- endocrine, nutritional or metabolic disease NEC O99.285
- endophlebitis — *see* Puerperal, phlebitis
- endotrachelitis O86.11
- failure
  - lactation (complete) O92.3
    - partial O92.4
  - renal, acute O90.4
- fever (of unknown origin) O86.4
  - septic O85
- fissure, nipple O92.12
  - associated with lactation O92.13
- fistula
  - breast (due to mastitis) O91.12
    - associated with lactation O91.13
  - nipple O91.02
    - associated with lactation O91.03
- galactophoritis O91.22
  - associated with lactation O91.23
- galactorrhea O92.6
- gastric banding status O99.845
- gastric bypass status O99.845
- gastrointestinal disease NEC O99.63
- gestational diabetes O24.439
  - diet controlled O24.430
  - insulin (and diet) controlled O24.434
- gonorrhea O98.23
- hematoma, subdural O99.43
- hemiplegia, cerebral O99.355
  - due to cerbrovascular disorder O99.43
- hemorrhage O72.1
  - brain O99.43
  - bulbar O99.43
  - cerebellar O99.43
  - cerebral O99.43
  - cortical O99.43
  - delayed or secondary O72.2
  - extradural O99.43
  - internal capsule O99.43
  - intracranial O99.43
  - intrapontine O99.43
  - meningeal O99.43
  - pontine O99.43
  - retained placenta O72.0
  - subarachnoid O99.43
  - subcortical O99.43
  - subdural O99.43
  - third stage O72.0
  - uterine, delayed O72.2
  - ventricular O99.43
- hemorrhoids O87.2
- hepatorenal syndrome O90.4
- hypertension — *see* Hypertension, complicating, puerperium
- hypertrophy, breast O92.29

Puerperal, puerperium — *continued*
- induration breast (fibrous) O92.29
- infection O86.4
  - cervix O86.11
  - generalized O85
  - genital tract NEC O86.19
    - obstetric surgical wound O86.0
  - kidney (bacillus coli) O86.21
  - maternal O98.93
    - carrier state NEC O99.835
    - gonorrhea O98.23
    - human immunodeficiency virus (HIV) O98.73
    - protozoal O98.63
    - sexually transmitted NEC O98.33
    - specified NEC O98.83
    - streptococcus B carrier state O99.825
    - syphilis O98.13
    - tuberculosis O98.03
    - viral hepatitis O98.43
    - viral NEC O98.53
  - nipple O91.02
    - associated with lactation O91.03
  - peritoneum O85
  - renal O86.21
  - specified NEC O86.89
  - urinary (asymptomatic) (tract) NEC O86.20
    - bladder O86.22
    - kidney O86.21
    - specified site NEC O86.29
    - urethra O86.22
  - vagina O86.13
  - vein — *see* Puerperal, phlebitis
- ischemia, cerebral O99.43
- lymphangitis O86.89
  - breast O91.22
    - associated with lactation O91.23
- malignancy O9A.13 (*following* O99)
- malnutrition O25.3
- mammillitis O91.02
  - associated with lactation O91.03
- mammitis O91.22
  - associated with lactation O91.23
- mania F30.8
- mastitis O91.22
  - associated with lactation O91.23
  - purulent O91.12
    - associated with lactation O91.13
- melancholia — *see* Disorder, depressive
- mental disorder NEC O99.345
- metroperitonitis O85
- metrorrhagia — *see* Hemorrhage, postpartum
- metrosalpingitis O86.19
- metrovaginitis O86.13
- milk leg O87.1
- monoplegia, cerebral O99.43
- mood disturbance O90.6
- necrosis, liver (acute) (subacute) (conditions in subcategory K72.0) O26.63
  - with renal failure O90.4
- nervous system disorder O99.355
- obesity (pre-existing prior to pregnancy) O99.215
- obesity surgery status O99.845
- occlusion, precerebral artery O99.43
- paralysis
  - bladder (sphincter) O90.89
  - cerebral O99.43
- paralytic stroke O99.43
- parametritis O85
- paravaginitis O86.13
- pelviperitonitis O85
- perimetritis O86.12
- perimetrosalpingitis O86.19
- perinephritis O86.21
- periphlebitis — *see* Puerperal phlebitis
- peritoneal infection O85
- peritonitis (pelvic) O85
- perivaginitis O86.13
- phlebitis O87.0
  - deep O87.1
  - pelvic O87.1
  - superficial O87.0
- phlebothrombosis, deep O87.1
- phlegmasia alba dolens O87.1
- placental polyp O90.89
- pneumonia, embolic — *see* Embolism, obstetric, puerperal
- pre-eclampsia — *see* Pre-eclampsia
- psychosis F53

Puerperal, puerperium — *continued*
- pyelitis O86.21
- pyelocystitis O86.29
- pyelonephritis O86.21
- pyelonephrosis O86.21
- pyemia O85
- pyocystitis O86.29
- pyohemia O85
- pyometra O86.12
- pyonephritis O86.21
- pyosalpingitis O86.19
- pyrexia (of unknown origin) O86.4
- renal
  - disease NEC O90.89
  - failure O90.4
- respiratory disease NEC O99.53
- retention
  - decidua — *see* Retention, decidua
  - placenta O72.0
  - secundines — *see* Retention, secundines
- retrated nipple O92.02
- salpingo-ovaritis O86.19
- salpingoperitonitis O85
- secondary perineal tear O90.1
- sepsis (pelvic) O85
- sepsis O85
- septic thrombophlebitis O86.81
- skin disorder NEC O99.73
- specified condition NEC O99.89
- stroke O99.43
- subinvolution (uterus) O90.89
- subluxation of symphysis (pubis) O26.73
- suppuration — *see* Puerperal, abscess
- tetanus A34
- thelitis O91.02
  - associated with lactation O91.03
- thrombocytopenia O72.3
- thrombophlebitis (superficial) O87.0
  - deep O87.1
  - pelvic O87.1
  - septic O86.81
- thrombosis (venous) — *see* Thrombosis, puerperal
- thyroiditis O90.5
- toxemia (eclamptic) (pre-eclamptic) (with convulsions) O15.2
- trauma, non-obstetric O9A.23 (*following* O99)
  - caused by abuse (physical) (suspected) O9A.33 (*following* O99)
    - confirmed O9A.33 (*following* O99)
    - psychological (suspected) O9A.53 (*following* O99)
      - confirmed O9A.53 (*following* O99)
    - sexual (suspected) O9A.43 (*following* O99)
      - confirmed O9A.43 (*following* O99)
- uremia (due to renal failure) O90.4
- urethritis O86.22
- vaginitis O86.13
- varicose veins (legs) O87.4
  - vulva or perineum O87.8
- venous O87.9
- vulvitis O86.19
- vulvovaginitis O86.13
- white leg O87.1

Puerperium — *see* Puerperal
Pulmolithiasis J98.4
Pulmonary — *see* condition
Pulpitis (acute) (anachoretic) (chronic) (hyperplastic) (irreversible) (putrescent) (reversible) (suppurative) (ulcerative) K04.0
Pulpless tooth K04.99
Pulse
- alternating R00.8
- bigeminal R00.8
- fast R00.0
- feeble, rapid due to shock following injury T79.4 ☑
- rapid R00.0
- weak R09.89

Pulsus alternans or trigeminus R00.8
Punch drunk F07.81
Punctum lacrimale occlusion — *see* Obstruction, lacrimal
Puncture
- abdomen, abdominal
  - wall S31.139 ☑
    - with
      - foreign body S31.149 ☑
      - penetration into peritoneal cavity S31.639 ☑

- **Puncture** — *continued*
  - abdomen, abdominal — *continued*
    - wall — *continued*
      - with — *continued*
        - penetration into peritoneal cavity — *continued*
          - with foreign body S31.649 ☑
      - epigastric region S31.132 ☑
        - with
          - foreign body S31.142 ☑
          - penetration into peritoneal cavity S31.632 ☑
            - with foreign body S31.642 ☑
      - left
        - lower quadrant S31.134 ☑
          - with
            - foreign body S31.144 ☑
            - penetration into peritoneal cavity S31.634 ☑
              - with foreign body S31.644 ☑
        - upper quadrant S31.131 ☑
          - with
            - foreign body S31.141 ☑
            - penetration into peritoneal cavity S31.631 ☑
              - with foreign body S31.641 ☑
      - periumbilic region S31.135 ☑
        - with
          - foreign body S31.145 ☑
          - penetration into peritoneal cavity S31.635 ☑
            - with foreign body S31.645 ☑
      - right
        - lower quadrant S31.133 ☑
          - with
            - foreign body S31.143 ☑
            - penetration into peritoneal cavity S31.633 ☑
              - with foreign body S31.643 ☑
        - upper quadrant S31.13Ø ☑
          - with
            - foreign body S31.14Ø ☑
            - penetration into peritoneal cavity S31.63Ø ☑
              - with foreign body S31.64Ø ☑
  - accidental, complicating surgery — *see* Complication, accidental puncture or laceration
  - alveolar (process) — *see* Puncture, oral cavity
  - ankle S91.Ø39 ☑
    - with
      - foreign body S91.Ø49 ☑
    - left S91.Ø32 ☑
      - with
        - foreign body S91.Ø42 ☑
    - right S91.Ø31 ☑
      - with
        - foreign body S91.Ø41 ☑
  - anus S31.833 ☑
    - with foreign body S31.834 ☑
  - arm (upper) S41.139 ☑
    - with foreign body S41.149 ☑
    - left S41.132 ☑
      - with foreign body S41.142 ☑
    - lower — *see* Puncture, forearm
    - right S41.131 ☑
      - with foreign body S41.141 ☑
  - auditory canal (external) (meatus) — *see* Puncture, ear
  - auricle, ear — *see* Puncture, ear
  - axilla — *see* Puncture, arm
  - back (*see also* Puncture, thorax, back)
    - lower S31.Ø3Ø ☑
      - with
        - foreign body S31.Ø4Ø ☑
          - with penetration into retroperitoneal space S31.Ø41 ☑
        - penetration into retroperitoneal space S31.Ø31 ☑
  - bladder (traumatic) S37.29 ☑
    - nontraumatic N32.89
  - breast S21.Ø39 ☑
    - with foreign body S21.Ø49 ☑
    - left S21.Ø32 ☑
      - with foreign body S21.Ø42 ☑
    - right S21.Ø31 ☑
      - with foreign body S21.Ø41 ☑

- **Puncture** — *continued*
  - buttock S31.8Ø3 ☑
    - with foreign body S31.8Ø4 ☑
    - left S31.823 ☑
      - with foreign body S31.824 ☑
    - right S31.813 ☑
      - with foreign body S31.814 ☑
  - by
    - device, implant or graft — *see* Complications, by site and type, mechanical
    - foreign body left accidentally in operative wound T81.539 ☑
    - instrument (any) during a procedure, accidental — *see* Puncture, accidental complicating surgery
  - calf — *see* Puncture, leg
  - canaliculus lacrimalis — *see* Puncture, eyelid
  - canthus, eye — *see* Puncture, eyelid
  - cervical esophagus S11.23 ☑
    - with foreign body S11.24 ☑
  - cheek (external) SØ1.439 ☑
    - with foreign body SØ1.449 ☑
    - internal — *see* Puncture, oral cavity
    - left SØ1.432 ☑
      - with foreign body SØ1.442 ☑
    - right SØ1.431 ☑
      - with foreign body SØ1.441 ☑
  - chest wall — *see* Puncture, thorax
  - chin — *see* Puncture, head, specified site NEC
  - clitoris — *see* Puncture, vulva
  - costal region — *see* Puncture, thorax
  - digit(s)
    - foot — *see* Puncture, toe
    - hand — *see* Puncture, finger
  - ear (canal) (external) SØ1.339 ☑
    - with foreign body SØ1.349 ☑
    - drum SØ9.2- ☑
    - left SØ1.332 ☑
      - with foreign body SØ1.342 ☑
    - right SØ1.331 ☑
      - with foreign body SØ1.341 ☑
  - elbow S51.Ø39 ☑
    - with
      - foreign body S51.Ø49 ☑
    - left S51.Ø32 ☑
      - with
        - foreign body S51.Ø42 ☑
    - right S51.Ø31 ☑
      - with
        - foreign body S51.Ø41 ☑
  - epididymis — *see* Puncture, testis
  - epigastric region — *see* Puncture, abdomen, wall, epigastric
  - epiglottis S11.83 ☑
    - with foreign body S11.84 ☑
  - esophagus
    - cervical S11.23 ☑
      - with foreign body S11.24 ☑
    - thoracic S27.818 ☑
  - eyeball SØ5.6- ☑
    - with foreign body SØ5.5- ☑
  - eyebrow — *see* Puncture, eyelid
  - eyelid SØ1.13- ☑
    - with foreign body SØ1.14- ☑
    - left SØ1.132 ☑
      - with foreign body SØ1.142 ☑
    - right SØ1.131 ☑
      - with foreign body SØ1.141 ☑
  - face NEC — *see* Puncture, head, specified site NEC
  - finger(s) S61.239 ☑
    - with
      - damage to nail S61.339 ☑
        - with
          - foreign body S61.349 ☑
      - foreign body S61.249 ☑
    - index S61.238 ☑
      - with
        - damage to nail S61.338 ☑
          - with
            - foreign body S61.348 ☑
        - foreign body S61.248 ☑
      - left S61.231 ☑
        - with
          - damage to nail S61.331 ☑
            - with
              - foreign body S61.341 ☑

- **Puncture** -- *continued*
  - finger(s) — *continued*
    - index — *continued*
      - left — *continued*
        - with — *continued*
          - foreign body S61.241 ☑
      - right S61.23Ø ☑
        - with
          - damage to nail S61.33Ø ☑
            - with
              - foreign body S61.34Ø ☑
          - foreign body S61.24Ø ☑
    - little S61.238 ☑
      - with
        - damage to nail S61.338 ☑
          - with
            - foreign body S61.348 ☑
        - foreign body S61.248 ☑
      - left S61.237 ☑
        - with
          - damage to nail S61.337 ☑
            - with
              - foreign body S61.347 ☑
          - foreign body S61.247 ☑
      - right S61.236 ☑
        - with
          - damage to nail S61.336 ☑
            - with
              - foreign body S61.346 ☑
          - foreign body S61.246 ☑
    - middle S61.238 ☑
      - with
        - damage to nail S61.338 ☑
          - with
            - foreign body S61.348 ☑
        - foreign body S61.248 ☑
      - left S61.233 ☑
        - with
          - damage to nail S61.333 ☑
            - with
              - foreign body S61.343 ☑
          - foreign body S61.243 ☑
      - right S61.232 ☑
        - with
          - damage to nail S61.332 ☑
            - with
              - foreign body S61.342 ☑
          - foreign body S61.242 ☑
    - ring S61.238 ☑
      - with
        - damage to nail S61.338 ☑
          - with
            - foreign body S61.348 ☑
        - foreign body S61.248 ☑
      - left S61.235 ☑
        - with
          - damage to nail S61.335 ☑
            - with
              - foreign body S61.345 ☑
          - foreign body S61.245 ☑
      - right S61.234 ☑
        - with
          - damage to nail S61.334 ☑
            - with
              - foreign body S61.344 ☑
          - foreign body S61.244 ☑
  - flank S31.139 ☑
    - with foreign body S31.149 ☑
  - foot (except toe(s) alone) S91.339 ☑
    - with foreign body S91.349 ☑
    - left S91.332 ☑
      - with foreign body S91.342 ☑
    - right S91.331 ☑
      - with foreign body S91.341 ☑
    - toe — *see* Puncture, toe
  - forearm S51.839 ☑
    - with
      - foreign body S51.849 ☑
    - elbow only — *see* Puncture, elbow
    - left S51.832 ☑
      - with
        - foreign body S51.842 ☑
    - right S51.831 ☑
      - with
        - foreign body S51.841 ☑
  - forehead — *see* Puncture, head, specified site NEC

DRAFT

Puncture — *continued*
- genital organs, external
  - female S31.532 ☑
    - with foreign body S31.542 ☑
    - vagina — *see* Puncture, vagina
    - vulva — *see* Puncture, vulva
  - male S31.531 ☑
    - with foreign body S31.541 ☑
    - penis — *see* Puncture, penis
    - scrotum — *see* Puncture, scrotum
    - testis — *see* Puncture, testis
- groin — *see* Puncture, abdomen, wall
- gum — *see* Puncture, oral cavity
- hand S61.439 ☑
  - with
    - foreign body S61.449 ☑
  - finger — *see* Puncture, finger
  - left S61.432 ☑
    - with
      - foreign body S61.442 ☑
  - right S61.431 ☑
    - with
      - foreign body S61.441 ☑
  - thumb — *see* Puncture, thumb
- head S01.93 ☑
  - with foreign body S01.94 ☑
  - cheek — *see* Puncture, cheek
  - ear — *see* Puncture, ear
  - eyelid — *see* Puncture, eyelid
  - lip — *see* Puncture, oral cavity
  - nose — *see* Puncture, nose
  - oral cavity — *see* Puncture, oral cavity
  - scalp S01.03 ☑
    - with foreign body S01.04 ☑
  - specified site NEC S01.83 ☑
    - with foreign body S01.84 ☑
  - temporomandibular area — *see* Puncture, cheek
- heart S26.99 ☑
  - with hemopericardium S26.09 ☑
  - without hemopericardium S26.19 ☑
- heel — *see* Puncture, foot
- hip S71.039 ☑
  - with foreign body S71.049 ☑
  - left S71.032 ☑
    - with foreign body S71.042 ☑
  - right S71.031 ☑
    - with foreign body S71.041 ☑
- hymen — *see* Puncture, vagina
- hypochondrium — *see* Puncture, abdomen, wall
- hypogastric region — *see* Puncture, abdomen, wall
- inguinal region — *see* Puncture, abdomen, wall
- instep — *see* Puncture, foot
- internal organs — *see* Injury, by site
- interscapular region — *see* Puncture, thorax, back
- intestine
  - large
    - colon S36.599 ☑
      - ascending S36.590 ☑
      - descending S36.592 ☑
      - sigmoid S36.593 ☑
      - specified site NEC S36.598 ☑
      - transverse S36.591 ☑
    - rectum S36.69 ☑
  - small S36.499 ☑
    - duodenum S36.490 ☑
    - specified site NEC S36.498 ☑
- intra-abdominal organ S36.99 ☑
  - gallbladder S36.128 ☑
  - intestine — *see* Puncture, intestine
  - liver S36.118 ☑
  - pancreas — *see* Puncture, pancreas
  - peritoneum S36.81 ☑
  - specified site NEC S36.898 ☑
  - spleen S36.09 ☑
  - stomach S36.39 ☑
- jaw — *see* Puncture, head, specified site NEC
- knee S81.039 ☑
  - with foreign body S81.049 ☑
  - left S81.032 ☑
    - with foreign body S81.042 ☑
  - right S81.031 ☑
    - with foreign body S81.041 ☑
- labium (majus) (minus) — *see* Puncture, vulva
- lacrimal duct — *see* Puncture, eyelid
- larynx S11.013 ☑
  - with foreign body S11.014 ☑

Puncture — *continued*
- leg (lower) S81.839 ☑
  - with foreign body S81.849 ☑
  - foot — *see* Puncture, foot
  - knee — *see* Puncture, knee
  - left S81.832 ☑
    - with foreign body S81.842 ☑
  - right S81.831 ☑
    - with foreign body S81.841 ☑
  - upper — *see* Puncture, thigh
- lip S01.531 ☑
  - with foreign body S01.541 ☑
- loin — *see* Puncture, abdomen, wall
- lower back — *see* Puncture, back, lower
- lumbar region — *see* Puncture, back, lower
- malar region — *see* Puncture, head, specified site NEC
- mammary — *see* Puncture, breast
- mastoid region — *see* Puncture, head, specified site NEC
- mouth — *see* Puncture, oral cavity
- nail
  - finger — *see* Puncture, finger, with damage to nail
  - toe — *see* Puncture, toe, with damage to nail
- nasal (septum) (sinus) — *see* Puncture, nose
- nasopharynx — *see* Puncture, head, specified site NEC
- neck S11.93 ☑
  - with foreign body S11.94 ☑
  - involving
    - cervical esophagus — *see* Puncture, cervical esophagus
    - larynx — *see* Puncture, larynx
    - pharynx — *see* Puncture, pharynx
    - thyroid gland — *see* Puncture, thyroid gland
    - trachea — *see* Puncture, trachea
  - specified site NEC S11.83 ☑
    - with foreign body S11.84 ☑
- nose (septum) (sinus) S01.23 ☑
  - with foreign body S01.24 ☑
- ocular — *see* Puncture, eyeball
- oral cavity S01.532 ☑
  - with foreign body S01.542 ☑
- orbit S05.4- ☑
- palate — *see* Puncture, oral cavity
- palm — *see* Puncture, hand
- pancreas S36.299 ☑
  - body S36.291 ☑
  - head S36.290 ☑
  - tail S36.292 ☑
- pelvis — *see* Puncture, back, lower
- penis S31.23 ☑
  - with foreign body S31.24 ☑
- perineum
  - female S31.43 ☑
    - with foreign body S31.44 ☑
  - male S31.139 ☑
    - with foreign body S31.149 ☑
- periocular area (with or without lacrimal passages) — *see* Puncture, eyelid
- phalanges
  - finger — *see* Puncture, finger
  - toe — *see* Puncture, toe
- pharynx S11.23 ☑
  - with foreign body S11.24 ☑
- pinna — *see* Puncture, ear
- popliteal space — *see* Puncture, knee
- prepuce — *see* Puncture, penis
- pubic region S31.139 ☑
  - with foreign body S31.149 ☑
- pudendum — *see* Puncture, genital organs, external
- rectovaginal septum — *see* Puncture, vagina
- sacral region — *see* Puncture, back, lower
- sacroiliac region — *see* Puncture, back, lower
- salivary gland — *see* Puncture, oral cavity
- scalp S01.03 ☑
  - with foreign body S01.04 ☑
- scapular region — *see* Puncture, shoulder
- scrotum S31.33 ☑
  - with foreign body S31.34 ☑
- shin — *see* Puncture, leg
- shoulder S41.039 ☑
  - with foreign body S41.049 ☑
  - left S41.032 ☑
    - with foreign body S41.042 ☑
  - right S41.031 ☑
    - with foreign body S41.041 ☑
- spermatic cord — *see* Puncture, testis

Puncture — *continued*
- sternal region — *see* Puncture, thorax, front
- submaxillary region — *see* Puncture, head, specified site NEC
- submental region — *see* Puncture, head, specified site NEC
- subungual
  - finger(s) — *see* Puncture, finger, with damage to nail
  - toe — *see* Puncture, toe, with damage to nail
- supraclavicular fossa — *see* Puncture, neck, specified site NEC
- temple, temporal region — *see* Puncture, head, specified site NEC
- temporomandibular area — *see* Puncture, cheek
- testis S31.33 ☑
  - with foreign body S31.34 ☑
- thigh S71.139 ☑
  - with foreign body S71.149 ☑
  - left S71.132 ☑
    - with foreign body S71.142 ☑
  - right S71.131 ☑
    - with foreign body S71.141 ☑
- thorax, thoracic (wall) S21.93 ☑
  - with foreign body S21.94 ☑
  - back S21.23- ☑
    - with
      - foreign body S21.24- ☑
        - with penetration S21.44 ☑
      - penetration S21.43 ☑
  - breast — *see* Puncture, breast
  - front S21.13- ☑
    - with
      - foreign body S21.14- ☑
        - with penetration S21.34 ☑
      - penetration S21.33 ☑
- throat — *see* Puncture, neck
- thumb S61.039 ☑
  - with
    - damage to nail S61.139 ☑
      - with
        - foreign body S61.149 ☑
    - foreign body S61.049 ☑
  - left S61.032 ☑
    - with
      - damage to nail S61.132 ☑
        - with
          - foreign body S61.142 ☑
      - foreign body S61.042 ☑
  - right S61.031 ☑
    - with
      - damage to nail S61.131 ☑
        - with
          - foreign body S61.141 ☑
      - foreign body S61.041 ☑
- thyroid gland S11.13 ☑
  - with foreign body S11.14 ☑
- toe(s) S91.139 ☑
  - with
    - damage to nail S91.239 ☑
      - with
        - foreign body S91.249 ☑
    - foreign body S91.149 ☑
  - great S91.133 ☑
    - with
      - damage to nail S91.233 ☑
        - with
          - foreign body S91.243 ☑
      - foreign body S91.143 ☑
    - left S91.132 ☑
      - with
        - damage to nail S91.232 ☑
          - with
            - foreign body S91.242 ☑
        - foreign body S91.142 ☑
    - right S91.131 ☑
      - with
        - damage to nail S91.231 ☑
          - with
            - foreign body S91.241 ☑
        - foreign body S91.141 ☑
  - lesser S91.136 ☑
    - with
      - damage to nail S91.236 ☑
        - with
          - foreign body S91.246 ☑

- **Puncture** — *continued*
  - toe(s) — *continued*
    - lesser — *continued*
      - with — *continued*
        - foreign body S91.146 ☑
    - left S91.135 ☑
      - with
        - damage to nail S91.235 ☑
          - with
            - foreign body S91.245 ☑
        - foreign body S91.145 ☑
    - right S91.134 ☑
      - with
        - damage to nail S91.234 ☑
          - with
            - foreign body S91.244 ☑
        - foreign body S91.144 ☑
  - tongue — *see* Puncture, oral cavity
  - trachea S11.Ø23 ☑
    - with foreign body S11.Ø24 ☑
  - tunica vaginalis — *see* Puncture, testis
  - tympanum, tympanic membrane SØ9.2- ☑
  - umbilical region S31.135 ☑
    - with foreign body S31.145 ☑
  - uvula — *see* Puncture, oral cavity
  - vagina S31.43 ☑
    - with foreign body S31.44 ☑
  - vocal cords S11.Ø33 ☑
    - with foreign body S11.Ø34 ☑
  - vulva S31.43 ☑
    - with foreign body S31.44 ☑
  - wrist S61.539 ☑
    - with
      - foreign body S61.549 ☑
    - left S61.532 ☑
      - with
        - foreign body S61.542 ☑
    - right S61.531 ☑
      - with
        - foreign body S61.541 ☑
- **PUO** (pyrexia of unknown origin) R5Ø.9
- **Pupillary membrane** (persistent) Q13.89
- **Pupillotonia** — *see* Anomaly, pupil, function, tonic pupil
- **Purpura** D69.2
  - abdominal D69.Ø
  - allergic D69.Ø
  - anaphylactoid D69.Ø
  - annularis telangiectodes L81.7
  - arthritic D69.Ø
  - autoerythrocyte sensitization D69.2
  - autoimmune D69.Ø
  - bacterial D69.Ø
  - Bateman's (senile) D69.2
  - capillary fragility (hereditary) (idiopathic) D69.8
  - cryoglobulinemic D89.1
  - Devil's pinches D69.2
  - fibrinolytic — *see* Fibrinolysis
  - fulminans, fulminous D65
  - gangrenous D65
  - hemorrhagic, hemorrhagica D69.3
    - not due to thrombocytopenia D69.Ø
  - Henoch (-Schönlein) (allergic) D69.Ø
  - hypergammaglobulinemic (benign) (Waldenström) D89.Ø
  - idiopathic (thrombocytopenic) D69.3
    - nonthrombocytopenic D69.Ø
  - immune thrombocytopenic D69.3
  - infectious D69.Ø
  - malignant D69.Ø
  - neonatorum P54.5
  - nervosa D69.Ø
  - newborn P54.5
  - nonthrombocytopenic D69.2
    - hemorrhagic D69.Ø
    - idiopathic D69.Ø
  - nonthrombopenic D69.2
  - peliosis rheumatica D69.Ø
  - posttransfusion (post-transfusion) (from (fresh) whole blood or blood products) D69.51
  - primary D69.49
  - red cell membrane sensitivity D69.2
  - rheumatica D69.Ø
  - Schönlein (-Henoch) (allergic) D69.Ø
  - scorbutic E54 [D77]
  - senile D69.2
  - simplex D69.2
  - symptomatica D69.Ø

- **Purpura** — *continued*
  - telangiectasia annularis L81.7
  - thrombocytopenic D69.49
    - congenital D69.42
    - hemorrhagic D69.3
    - hereditary D69.42
    - idiopathic D69.3
    - immune D69.3
    - neonatal, transitory P61.Ø
    - thrombotic M31.1
  - thrombohemolytic — *see* Fibrinolysis
  - thrombolytic — *see* Fibrinolysis
  - thrombopenic D69.49
  - thrombotic, thrombocytopenic M31.1
  - toxic D69.Ø
  - vascular D69.Ø
  - visceral symptoms D69.Ø
- **Purpuric spots** R23.3
- **Purulent** — *see* condition
- **Pus**
  - in
    - stool R19.5
    - urine N39.Ø
  - tube (rupture) — *see* Salpingo-oophoritis
- **Pustular rash** LØ8.Ø
- **Pustule** (nonmalignant) LØ8.9
  - malignant A22.Ø
- **Pustulosis palmaris et plantaris** L4Ø.3
- **Putnam** (-Dana) **disease or syndrome** — *see* Degeneration, combined
- **Putrescent pulp** (dental) KØ4.1
- **Pyarthritis, pyarthrosis** — *see* Arthritis, pyogenic or pyemic
  - tuberculous — *see* Tuberculosis, joint
- **Pyelectasis** — *see* Hydronephrosis
- **Pyelitis** (congenital) (uremic) (*see also* Pyelonephritis)
  - with
    - calculus — *see* category N2Ø ☑
      - with hydronephrosis N13.2
    - contracted kidney N11.9
  - acute N1Ø
  - chronic N11.9
    - with calculus — *see* category N2Ø ☑
      - with hydronephrosis N13.2
  - cystica N28.84
  - puerperal (postpartum) O86.21
  - tuberculous A18.11
- **Pyelocystitis** — *see* Pyelonephritis
- **Pyelonephritis** (*see also* Nephritis, tubulo-interstitial)
  - with
    - calculus — *see* category N2Ø ☑
      - with hydronephrosis N13.2
    - contracted kidney N11.9
  - acute N1Ø
  - calculous — *see* category N2Ø ☑
    - with hydronephrosis N13.2
  - chronic N11.9
    - with calculus — *see* category N2Ø ☑
      - with hydronephrosis N13.2
    - associated with ureteral obstruction or stricture N11.1
    - nonobstructive N11.8
      - with reflux (vesicoureteral) N11.Ø
    - obstructive N11.1
    - specified NEC N11.8
  - in (due to)
    - brucellosis A23.9 [N16]
    - cryoglobulinemia (mixed) D89.1 [N16]
    - cystinosis E72.Ø4
    - diphtheria A36.84
    - glycogen storage disease E74.Ø9 [N16]
    - leukemia NEC C95.9- ☑ [N16]
    - lymphoma NEC C85.9Ø [N16]
    - multiple myeloma C9Ø.Ø- ☑ [N16]
    - obstruction N11.1
    - Salmonella infection AØ2.25
    - sarcoidosis D86.84
    - sepsis A41.9 [N16]
    - Sjögren's disease M35.Ø4
    - toxoplasmosis B58.83
    - transplant rejection T86.91 [N16]
    - Wilson's disease E83.Ø1 [N16]
  - nonobstructive N12
    - with reflux (vesicoureteral) N11.Ø
    - chronic N11.8
  - syphilitic A52.75
- **Pyelonephrosis** (obstructive) N11.1
  - chronic N11.9

- **Pyelophlebitis** I8Ø.8
- **Pyeloureteritis cystica** N28.85
- **Pyemia, pyemic** (fever) (infection) (purulent) (*see also* Sepsis)
  - joint — *see* Arthritis, pyogenic or pyemic
  - liver K75.1
  - pneumococcal A4Ø.3
  - portal K75.1
  - postvaccinal T88.Ø ☑
  - puerperal, postpartum, childbirth O85
  - specified organism NEC A41.89
  - tuberculous — *see* Tuberculosis, miliary
- **Pygopagus** Q89.4
- **Pyknoepilepsy** (idiopathic) — *see* Pyknolepsy
- **Pyknolepsy** G4Ø.AØ9 (*following* G4Ø.3)
  - intractable G4Ø.A19 (*following* G4Ø.3)
    - with status epilepticus G4Ø.A11 (*following* G4Ø.3)
    - without status epilepticus G4Ø.A19 (*following* G4Ø.3)
  - not intractable G4Ø.AØ9 (*following* G4Ø.3)
    - with status epilepticus G4Ø.AØ1 (*following* G4Ø.3)
    - without status epilepticus G4Ø.AØ9 (*following* G4Ø.3)
- **Pylephlebitis** K75.1
- **Pyle's syndrome** Q78.5
- **Pylethrombophlebitis** K75.1
- **Pylethrombosis** K75.1
- **Pyloritis** K29.9Ø
  - with bleeding K29.91
- **Pylorospasm** (reflex) **NEC** K31.3
  - congenital or infantile Q4Ø.Ø
  - neurotic F45.8
  - newborn Q4Ø.Ø
  - psychogenic F45.8
- **Pylorus, pyloric** — *see* condition
- **Pyoarthrosis** — *see* Arthritis, pyogenic or pyemic
- **Pyocele**
  - mastoid — *see* Mastoiditis, acute
  - sinus (accessory) — *see* Sinusitis
  - turbinate (bone) J32.9
  - urethra (*see also* Urethritis) N34.Ø
- **Pyocolpos** — *see* Vaginitis
- **Pyocystitis** N3Ø.8Ø
  - with hematuria N3Ø.81
- **Pyoderma, pyodermia** LØ8.Ø
  - gangrenosum L88
  - newborn P39.4
  - phagedenic L88
  - vegetans LØ8.81
- **Pyodermatitis** LØ8.Ø
  - vegetans LØ8.81
- **Pyogenic** — *see* condition
- **Pyohydronephrosis** N13.6
- **Pyometra, pyometrium, pyometritis** — *see* Endometritis
- **Pyomyositis** (tropical) — *see* Myositis, infective
- **Pyonephritis** N12
- **Pyonephrosis** N13.6
  - tuberculous A18.11
- **Pyo-oophoritis** — *see* Salpingo-oophoritis
- **Pyo-ovarium** — *see* Salpingo-oophoritis
- **Pyopericarditis, pyopericardium** I3Ø.1
- **Pyophlebitis** — *see* Phlebitis
- **Pyopneumopericardium** I3Ø.1
- **Pyopneumothorax** (infective) J86.9
  - with fistula J86.Ø
  - tuberculous NEC A15.6
- **Pyosalpinx, pyosalpingitis** (*see also* Salpingo-oophoritis)
- **Pyothorax** J86.9
  - with fistula J86.Ø
  - tuberculous NEC A15.6
- **Pyoureter** N28.89
  - tuberculous A18.11
- **Pyramidopallidonigral syndrome** G2Ø
- **Pyrexia** (of unknown origin) R5Ø.9
  - atmospheric T67.Ø ☑
  - during labor NEC O75.2
  - heat T67.Ø ☑
  - newborn P81.9
    - environmentally-induced P81.Ø
  - persistent R5Ø.9
  - puerperal O86.4
- **Pyroglobulinemia NEC** E88.Ø9
- **Pyromania** F63.1
- **Pyrosis** R12
- **Pyuria** (bacterial) N39.Ø

Q

- **Q fever** A78
  - with pneumonia A78
- **Quadricuspid aortic valve** Q23.8
- **Quadrilateral fever** A78
- **Quadriparesis** — *see* Quadriplegia
  - meaning muscle weakness M62.81
- **Quadriplegia** G82.5Ø
  - complete
    - C1-C4 level G82.51
    - C5-C7 level G82.53
  - congenital (cerebral) (spinal) G8Ø.8
    - spastic G8Ø.Ø
  - embolic (current episode) I63.4 ☑
  - functional R53.2
  - incomplete
    - C1-C4 level G82.52
    - C5-C7 level G82.54
  - thrombotic (current episode) I63.3 ☑
  - traumatic — *code to* injury with seventh character S
    - current episode — *see* Injury, spinal (cord), cervical
- **Quadruplet, pregnancy** — *see* Pregnancy, quadruplet
- **Quarrelsomeness** F6Ø.3
- **Queensland fever** A77.3
- **Quervain's disease** M65.4
  - thyroid EØ6.1
- **Queyrat's erythroplasia** DØ7.4
  - penis DØ7.4
  - specified site — *see* Neoplasm, skin, in situ
  - unspecified site DØ7.4
- **Quincke's disease or edema** T78.3 ☑
  - hereditary D84.1
- **Quinsy** (gangrenous) J36
- **Quintan fever** A79.Ø
- **Quintuplet, pregnancy** — *see* Pregnancy, quintuplet

R

- **Rabbit fever** — *see* Tularemia
- **Rabies** A82.9
  - contact Z2Ø.3
  - exposure to Z2Ø.3
  - inoculation reaction — *see* Complications, vaccination
  - sylvatic A82.Ø
  - urban A82.1
- **Rachischisis** — *see* Spina bifida
- **Rachitic** (*see also* condition)
  - deformities of spine (late effect) (sequelae) E64.3
  - pelvis (late effect) (sequelae) E64.3
    - with disproportion (fetopelvic) O33.Ø
      - causing obstructed labor O65.Ø
- **Rachitis, rachitism** (acute) (tarda) (*see also* Rickets)
  - renalis N25.Ø
  - sequelae E64.3
- **Radial nerve** — *see* condition
- **Radiation**
  - burn — *see* Burn
  - effects NOS T66 ☑
  - sickness NOS T66 ☑
  - therapy, encounter for Z51.Ø
- **Radiculitis** (pressure) (vertebrogenic) — *see* Radiculopathy
- **Radiculomyelitis** (*see also* Encephalitis)
  - toxic, due to
    - Clostridium tetani A35
    - Corynebacterium diphtheriae A36.82
- **Radiculopathy** M54.1Ø
  - cervical region M54.12
  - cervicothoracic region M54.13
  - due to
    - disc disorder
      - C3 M5Ø.11
      - C4 M5Ø.11
      - C5 M5Ø.12
      - C6 M5Ø.12
      - C7 M5Ø.12
      - C8 M5Ø.13
    - displacement of intervertebral disc — *see* Disorder, disc, with, radiculopathy
  - leg M54.1- ☑
  - lumbar region M54.16
  - lumbosacral region M54.17
  - occipito-atlanto-axial region M54.11
  - postherpetic BØ2.29
  - sacrococcygeal region M54.18

Radiculopathy — *continued*

  - syphilitic A52.11
  - thoracic region (with visceral pain) M54.14
  - thoracolumbar region M54.15
- **Radiodermal burns** (acute, chronic, or occupational) — *see* Burn
- **Radiodermatitis** L58.9
  - acute L58.Ø
  - chronic L58.1
- **Radiotherapy session** Z51.Ø
- **Rage, meaning rabies** — *see* Rabies
- **Ragpicker's disease** A22.1
- **Ragsorter's disease** A22.1
- **Raillietiniasis** B71.8
- **Railroad neurosis** F48.8
- **Railway spine** F48.8
- **Raised** (*see also* Elevated)
  - antibody titer R76.Ø
- **Rake teeth, tooth** M26.39
- **Rales** RØ9.89
- **Ramifying renal pelvis** Q63.8
- **Ramsay-Hunt disease or syndrome** (*see also* Hunt's disease) BØ2.21
  - meaning dyssynergia cerebellaris myoclonica G11.1
- **Ranula** K11.6
  - congenital Q38.4
- **Rape**
  - adult
    - confirmed T74.21 ☑
    - suspected T76.21 ☑
  - alleged, observation or examination, ruled out
    - adult ZØ4.41
    - child ZØ4.42
  - child
    - confirmed T74.22 ☑
    - suspected T76.22 ☑
- **Rapid**
  - feeble pulse, due to shock, following injury T79.4 ☑
  - heart (beat) RØØ.Ø
    - psychogenic F45.8
  - second stage (delivery) O62.3
  - time-zone change syndrome — *see* Disorder, sleep, circadian rhythm, psychogenic
- **Rarefaction, bone** — *see* Disorder, bone, density and structure, specified NEC
- **Rash** (toxic) R21
  - canker A38.9
  - diaper L22
  - drug (internal use) L27.Ø
    - contact (*see also* Dermatitis, due to, drugs, external) L25.1
  - following immunization T88.1 ☑
  - food — *see* Dermatitis, due to, food
  - heat L74.Ø
  - napkin (psoriasiform) L22
  - nettle — *see* Urticaria
  - pustular LØ8.Ø
  - rose R21
    - epidemic BØ6.9
  - scarlet A38.9
  - serum (*see also* Reaction, serum) T8Ø.69 ☑
  - wandering tongue K14.1
- **Rasmussen aneurysm** — *see* Tuberculosis, pulmonary
- **Rasmussen encephalitis** GØ4.81
- **Rat-bite fever** A25.9
  - due to Streptobacillus moniliformis A25.1
  - spirochetal (morsus muris) A25.Ø
- **Rathke's pouch tumor** D44.3
- **Raymond** (-Céstan) **syndrome** I65.8
- **Raynaud's disease, phenomenon or syndrome** (secondary) I73.ØØ
  - with gangrene (symmetric) I73.Ø1
- **RDS** (newborn) (type I) P22.Ø
  - type II P22.1
- **Reaction** (*see also* Disorder)
  - adaptation — *see* Disorder, adjustment
  - adjustment (anxiety) (conduct disorder) (depressiveness) (distress) — *see* Disorder, adjustment
    - with
      - mutism, elective (child) (adolescent) F94.Ø
  - adverse
    - food (any) (ingested) NEC T78.1 ☑
      - anaphylactic — *see* Shock, anaphylactic, due to food
  - affective — *see* Disorder, mood
  - allergic — *see* Allergy
  - anaphylactic — *see* Shock, anaphylactic

Reaction — *continued*

  - anaphylactoid — *see* Shock, anaphylactic
  - anesthesia — *see* Anesthesia, complication
  - antitoxin (prophylactic) (therapeutic) — *see* Complications, vaccination
  - anxiety F41.1
  - Arthus — *see* Arthus' phenomenon
  - asthenic F48.8
  - combat and operational stress F43.Ø
  - compulsive F42
  - conversion F44.9
  - crisis, acute F43.Ø
  - deoxyribonuclease (DNA) (DNase) hypersensitivity D69.2
  - depressive (single episode) F32.9
    - affective (single episode) F31.4
      - recurrent episode F33.9
    - neurotic F34.1
    - psychoneurotic F34.1
    - psychotic F32.3
    - recurrent — *see* Disorder, depressive, recurrent
  - dissociative F44.9
  - drug NEC T88.7 ☑
    - addictive — *see* Dependence, drug
      - transmitted via placenta or breast milk — *see* Absorption, drug, addictive, through placenta
    - allergic — *see* Allergy, drug
    - lichenoid L43.2
    - newborn P93.8
      - gray baby syndrome P93.Ø
    - overdose or poisoning (by accident) — *see* Table of Drugs and Chemicals, by drug, poisoning
    - photoallergic L56.1
    - phototoxic L56.Ø
    - withdrawal — *see* Dependence, by drug, with, withdrawal
      - infant of dependent mother P96.1
      - newborn P96.1
    - wrong substance given or taken (by accident) — *see* Table of Drugs and Chemicals, by drug, poisoning
  - fear F4Ø.9
    - child (abnormal) F93.8
  - febrile nonhemolytic transfusion (FNHTR) R5Ø.84
  - fluid loss, cerebrospinal G97.1
  - foreign
    - body NEC — *see* Granuloma, foreign body
      - in operative wound (inadvertently left) — *see* Foreign body, accidentally left during a procedure
    - substance accidentally left during a procedure (chemical) (powder) (talc) T81.6Ø ☑
      - aseptic peritonitis T81.61 ☑
      - body or object (instrument) (sponge) (swab) — *see* Foreign body, accidentally left during a procedure
      - specified reaction NEC T81.69 ☑
  - grief — *see* Disorder, adjustment
  - Herxheimer's R68.89
  - hyperkinetic — *see* Hyperkinesia
  - hypochondriacal F45.2Ø
  - hypoglycemic, due to insulin E16.Ø
    - with coma (diabetic) — *see* Diabetes, coma
      - nondiabetic E15
    - therapeutic misadventure — *see* subcategory T38.3 ☑
  - hypomanic F3Ø.8
  - hysterical F44.9
  - immunization — *see* Complications, vaccination
  - incompatibility
    - ABO blood group (infusion) (transfusion) — *see* Complication(s), transfusion, incompatibility reaction, ABO
      - delayed serologic T8Ø.39 ☑
    - minor blood group (Duffy) (E) (K(ell)) (Kidd) (Lewis) (M) (N) (P) (S) T8Ø.89 ☑
    - Rh (factor) (infusion) (transfusion) — *see* Complication(s), transfusion, incompatibility reaction, Rh (factor)
  - inflammatory — *see* Infection
  - infusion — *see* Complications, infusion
  - inoculation (immune serum) — *see* Complications, vaccination
  - insulin T38.3- ☑
  - involutional psychotic — *see* Disorder, depressive
  - leukemoid D72.823

- **Reaction** — *continued*
  - leukemoid — *continued*
    - basophilic D72.823
    - lymphocytic D72.823
    - monocytic D72.823
    - myelocytic D72.823
    - neutrophilic D72.823
  - LSD (acute)
    - due to drug abuse — *see* Abuse, drug, hallucinogen
    - due to drug dependence — *see* Dependence, drug, hallucinogen
  - lumbar puncture G97.1
  - manic-depressive — *see* Disorder, bipolar
  - neurasthenic F48.8
  - neurogenic — *see* Neurosis
  - neurotic F48.9
  - neurotic-depressive F34.1
  - nitritoid — *see* Crisis, nitritoid
  - nonspecific
    - to
      - cell mediated immunity measurement of gamma interferon antigen response without active tuberculosis R76.12
      - QuantiFERON-TB test (QFT) without active tuberculosis R76.12
      - tuberculin test (*see also* Reaction, tuberculin skin test) R76.11
  - obsessive-compulsive F42
  - organic, acute or subacute — *see* Delirium
  - paranoid (acute) F23
    - chronic F22
    - senile FØ3 ☑
  - passive dependency F6Ø.7
  - phobic F4Ø.9
  - post-traumatic stress, uncomplicated Z73.3
  - psychogenic F99
  - psychoneurotic (*see also* Neurosis)
    - compulsive F42
    - depersonalization F48.1
    - depressive F34.1
    - hypochondriacal F45.2Ø
    - neurasthenic F48.8
    - obsessive F42
  - psychophysiologic — *see* Disorder, somatoform
  - psychosomatic — *see* Disorder, somatoform
  - psychotic — *see* Psychosis
  - scarlet fever toxin — *see* Complications, vaccination
  - schizophrenic F23
    - acute (brief) (undifferentiated) F23
    - latent F21
    - undifferentiated (acute) (brief) F23
  - serological for syphilis — *see* Serology for syphilis
  - serum T8Ø.69 ☑
    - anaphylactic (immediate) (*see also* Shock, anaphylactic) T8Ø.59 ☑
    - specified reaction NEC
      - due to
        - administration of blood and blood products T8Ø.61 ☑
        - immunization T8Ø.62 ☑
        - serum specified NEC T8Ø.69 ☑
        - vaccination T8Ø.62 ☑
  - situational — *see* Disorder, adjustment
  - somatization — *see* Disorder, somatoform
  - spinal puncture G97.1
  - stress (severe) F43.9
    - acute (agitation) ("daze") (disorientation) (disturbance of consciousness) (flight reaction) (fugue) F43.Ø
    - specified NEC F43.8
  - surgical procedure — *see* Complications, surgical procedure
  - tetanus antitoxin — *see* Complications, vaccination
  - toxic, to local anesthesia T81.89 ☑
    - in labor and delivery O74.4
    - in pregnancy O29.3X- ☑
    - postpartum, puerperal O89.3
  - toxin-antitoxin — *see* Complications, vaccination
  - transfusion (blood) (bone marrow) (lymphocytes) (allergic) — *see* Complications, transfusion
  - tuberculin skin test, abnormal R76.11
  - vaccination (any) — *see* Complications, vaccination
  - withdrawing, child or adolescent F93.8
- **Reactive airway disease** — *see* Asthma
- **Reactive depression** — *see* Reaction, depressive
- **Rearrangement**
  - chromosomal
    - balanced (in) Q95.9
      - abnormal individual (autosomal) Q95.2
        - non-sex (autosomal) chromosomes Q95.2
        - sex/non-sex chromosomes Q95.3
      - specified NEC Q95.8
- **Recalcitrant patient** — *see* Noncompliance
- **Recanalization, thrombus** — *see* Thrombosis
- **Recession, receding**
  - chamber angle (eye) H21.55- ☑
  - chin M26.Ø9
  - gingival (generalized) (localized) (postinfective) (postoperative) KØ6.Ø
- **Recklinghausen disease** Q85.Ø1
  - bones E21.Ø
- **Reclus' disease** (cystic) — *see* Mastopathy, cystic
- **Recrudescent typhus** (fever) A75.1
- **Recruitment, auditory** H93.21- ☑
- **Rectalgia** K62.89
- **Rectitis** K62.89
- **Rectocele**
  - female (without uterine prolapse) N81.6
    - with uterine prolapse N81.4
      - incomplete N81.2
  - in pregnancy — *see* Pregnancy, complicated by, abnormal, pelvic organs or tissues NEC
  - male K62.3
- **Rectosigmoid junction** — *see* condition
- **Rectosigmoiditis** K63.89
  - ulcerative (chronic) K51.3Ø
    - with
      - complication K51.319
        - abscess K51.314
        - fistula K51.313
        - obstruction K51.312
        - rectal bleeding K51.311
        - specified NEC K51.318
- **Rectourethral** — *see* condition
- **Rectovaginal** — *see* condition
- **Rectovesical** — *see* condition
- **Rectum, rectal** — *see* condition
- **Recurrent** — *see* condition
  - pregnancy loss — *see* Loss (of), pregnancy, recurrent
- **Red bugs** B88.Ø
- **Red tide** (*see also* Table of Drugs and Chemicals) T65.82- ☑
- **Red-cedar lung or pneumonitis** J67.8
- **Reduced**
  - mobility Z74.Ø9
  - ventilatory or vital capacity R94.2
- **Redundant, redundancy**
  - anus (congenital) Q43.8
  - clitoris N9Ø.89
  - colon (congenital) Q43.8
  - foreskin (congenital) N47.8
  - intestine (congenital) Q43.8
  - labia N9Ø.6
  - organ or site, congenital NEC — *see* Accessory
  - panniculus (abdominal) E65
  - prepuce (congenital) N47.8
  - pylorus K31.89
  - rectum (congenital) Q43.8
  - scrotum N5Ø.8
  - sigmoid (congenital) Q43.8
  - skin (of face) L57.4
    - eyelids — *see* Blepharochalasis
  - stomach K31.89
- **Reduplication** — *see* Duplication
- **Reflex** R29.2
  - hyperactive gag J39.2
  - pupillary, abnormal — *see* Anomaly, pupil, function
  - vasoconstriction I73.9
  - vasovagal R55
- **Reflux** K21.9
  - acid K21.9
  - esophageal K21.9
    - with esophagitis K21.Ø
    - newborn P78.83
  - gastroesophageal K21.9
    - with esophagitis K21.Ø
  - mitral — *see* Insufficiency, mitral
  - ureteral — *see* Reflux, vesicoureteral
  - vesicoureteral (with scarring) N13.7Ø
    - with
      - nephropathy N13.729
        - with hydroureter N13.739
- **Reflux** — *continued*
  - vesicoureteral — *continued*
    - with — *continued*
      - nephropathy — *continued*
        - with hydroureter — *continued*
          - bilateral N13.732
          - unilateral N13.731
        - without hydroureter N13.729
          - bilateral N13.722
          - unilateral N13.721
        - bilateral N13.722
        - unilateral N13.721
      - pyelonephritis (chronic) N11.Ø
    - without nephropathy N13.71
  - congenital Q62.7
- **Reforming, artificial openings** — *see* Attention to, artificial, opening
- **Refractive error** — *see* Disorder, refraction
- **Refsum's disease or syndrome** G6Ø.1
- **Refusal of**
  - food, psychogenic F5Ø.8
  - treatment (because of) Z53.2Ø
    - left against medical advice (AMA) Z53.21
    - patient's decision NEC Z53.29
    - reasons of belief or group pressure Z53.1
- **Regional** — *see* condition
- **Regurgitation** R11.1Ø
  - aortic (valve) — *see* Insufficiency, aortic
  - food (*see also* Vomiting)
    - with reswallowing — *see* Rumination
    - newborn P92.1
  - gastric contents — *see* Vomiting
  - heart — *see* Endocarditis
  - mitral (valve) — *see* Insufficiency, mitral
    - congenital Q23.3
  - myocardial — *see* Endocarditis
  - pulmonary (valve) (heart) I37.1
    - congenital Q22.2
    - syphilitic A52.Ø3
  - tricuspid — *see* Insufficiency, tricuspid
  - valve, valvular — *see* Endocarditis
    - congenital Q24.8
  - vesicoureteral — *see* Reflux, vesicoureteral
- **Reichmann's disease or syndrome** K31.89
- **Reifenstein syndrome** E34.52
- **Reinsertion, contraceptive device** Z3Ø.433
- **Reiter's disease, syndrome, or urethritis** MØ2.3Ø
  - ankle MØ2.37- ☑
  - elbow MØ2.32- ☑
  - foot joint MØ2.37- ☑
  - hand joint MØ2.34- ☑
  - hip MØ2.35- ☑
  - knee MØ2.36- ☑
  - multiple site MØ2.39
  - shoulder MØ2.31- ☑
  - vertebra MØ2.38
  - wrist MØ2.33- ☑
- **Rejection**
  - food, psychogenic F5Ø.8
  - transplant T86.91
    - bone T86.83Ø
      - marrow T86.Ø1
    - cornea T86.84Ø
    - heart T86.21
      - with lung(s) T86.31
    - intestine T86.85Ø
    - kidney T86.11
    - liver T86.41
    - lung(s) T86.81Ø
      - with heart T86.31
    - organ (immune or nonimmune cause) T86.91
    - pancreas T86.89Ø
    - skin (allograft) (autograft) T86.82Ø
    - specified NEC T86.89Ø
    - stem cell (peripheral blood) (umbilical cord) T86.5
- **Relapsing fever** A68.9
  - Carter's (Asiatic) A68.1
  - Dutton's (West African) A68.1
  - Koch's A68.9
  - louse-borne (epidemic) A68.Ø
  - Novy's (American) A68.1
  - Obermeyers's (European) A68.Ø
  - Spirillum A68.9
  - tick-borne (endemic) A68.1
- **Relationship**
  - occlusal
    - open anterior M26.22Ø

DRAFT

- **Retained** — *continued*
  - fragments (type of) Z18.9
    - acrylics Z18.2
    - animal quill(s) or spines Z18.31
    - cement Z18.83
    - concrete Z18.83
    - crystalline Z18.83
    - depleted isotope Z18.09
    - depleted uranium Z18.01
    - diethylhexylphthalates Z18.2
    - glass Z18.81
    - isocyanate Z18.2
    - magnetic metal Z18.11
    - metal Z18.10
    - nonmagnectic metal Z18.12
    - nontherapeutic radioactive Z18.09
    - organic NEC Z18.39
    - plastic Z18.2
    - quill(s) (animal) Z18.31
    - radioactive (nontherapeutic) NEC Z18.09
    - specified NEC Z18.89
    - spine(s) (animal) Z18.31
    - stone Z18.83
    - tooth (teeth) Z18.32
    - wood Z18.33
  - gallstones, following cholecystectomy K91.86
- **Retardation**
  - development, developmental, specific — *see* Disorder, developmental
  - endochondral bone growth — *see* Disorder, bone, development or growth
  - growth R62.50
    - due to malnutrition E45
  - mental — *see* Disability, intellectual
  - motor function, specific F82
  - physical (child) R62.52
    - due to malnutrition E45
  - reading (specific) F81.0
  - spelling (specific) (without reading disorder) F81.81
- **Retching** — *see* Vomiting
- **Retention** (*see also* Retained)
  - bladder — *see* Retention, urine
  - carbon dioxide E87.2
  - cholelithiasis following cholecystectomy K91.86
  - cyst — *see* Cyst
  - dead
    - fetus (at or near term) (mother) O36.4 ☑
      - early fetal death O02.1
    - ovum O02.0
  - decidua (fragments) (following delivery) (with hemorrhage) O72.2
    - without hemorrhage O73.1
  - deciduous tooth K00.6
  - dental root K08.3
  - fecal — *see* Constipation
  - fetus
    - dead O36.4 ☑
      - early O02.1
  - fluid R60.9
  - foreign body (*see also* Foreign body, retained)
    - current trauma — *code as* Foreign body, by site or type
  - gallstones, following cholecystectomy K91.86
  - gastric K31.89
  - intrauterine contraceptive device, in pregnancy — *see* Pregnancy, complicated by, retention, intrauterine device
  - membranes (complicating delivery) (with hemorrhage) O72.2
    - with abortion — *see* Abortion, by type
    - without hemorrhage O73.1
  - meniscus — *see* Derangement, meniscus
  - menses N94.89
  - milk (puerperal, postpartum) O92.79
  - nitrogen, extrarenal R39.2
  - ovary syndrome N99.83
  - placenta (total) (with hemorrhage) O72.0
    - without hemorrhage O73.0
    - portions or fragments (with hemorrhage) O72.2
      - without hemorrhage O73.1
  - products of conception
    - early pregnancy (dead fetus) O02.1
    - following
      - delivery (with hemorrhage) O72.2
        - without hemorrhage O73.1
  - secundines (following delivery) (with hemorrhage) O72.0
    - without hemorrhage O73.0
- **Retention** — *continued*
  - secundines — *continued*
    - complicating puerperium (delayed hemorrhage) O72.2
    - partial O72.2
      - without hemorrhage O73.1
  - smegma, clitoris N90.89
  - urine R33.9
    - drug-induced R33.0
    - due to hyperplasia (hypertrophy) of prostate — *see* Hyperplasia, prostate
    - organic R33.8
      - drug-induced R33.0
    - psychogenic F45.8
    - specified NEC R33.8
  - water (in tissues) — *see* Edema
- **Reticulation, dust** — *see* Pneumoconiosis
- **Reticulocytosis** R70.1
- **Reticuloendotheliosis**
  - acute infantile C96.0
  - leukemic C91.4- ☑
  - malignant C96.9
  - nonlipid C96.0
- **Reticulohistiocytoma** (giant-cell) D76.3
- **Reticuloid, actinic** L57.1
- **Reticulosis** (skin)
  - acute of infancy C96.0
  - hemophagocytic, familial D76.1
  - histiocytic medullary C96.9
  - lipomelanotic I89.8
  - malignant (midline) C86.0
  - nonlipid C96.0
  - polymorphic C83.8- ☑
  - Sézary — *see* Sézary disease
- **Retina, retinal** (*see also* condition)
  - dark area D49.81
- **Retinitis** (*see also* Inflammation, chorioretinal)
  - albuminurica N18.9 [H32]
  - diabetic — *see* Diabetes, retinitis
  - disciformis — *see* Degeneration, macula
  - focal — *see* Inflammation, chorioretinal, focal
  - gravidarum — *see* Pregnancy, complicated by, specified pregnancy-related condition NEC
  - juxtapapillaris — *see* Inflammation, chorioretinal, focal, juxtapapillary
  - luetic — *see* Retinitis, syphilitic
  - pigmentosa H35.52
  - proliferans — *see* Disorder, globe, degenerative, specified type NEC
  - proliferating — *see* Disorder, globe, degenerative, specified type NEC
  - renal N18.9 [H32]
  - syphilitic (early) (secondary) A51.43
    - central, recurrent A52.71
    - congenital (early) A50.01 [H32]
    - late A52.71
  - tuberculous A18.53
- **Retinoblastoma** C69.2- ☑
  - differentiated C69.2- ☑
  - undifferentiated C69.2- ☑
- **Retinochoroiditis** (*see also* Inflammation, chorioretinal)
  - disseminated — *see* Inflammation, chorioretinal, disseminated
    - syphilitic A52.71
  - focal — *see* Inflammation, chorioretinal
  - juxtapapillaris — *see* Inflammation, chorioretinal, focal, juxtapapillary
- **Retinopathy** (background) H35.00
  - arteriosclerotic I70.8 [H35.0-] ☑
  - atherosclerotic I70.8 [H35.0-] ☑
  - central serous — *see* Chorioretinopathy, central serous
  - Coats H35.02- ☑
  - diabetic — *see* Diabetes, retinopathy
  - exudative H35.02- ☑
  - hypertensive H35.03- ☑
  - in (due to)
    - diabetes — *see* Diabetes, retinopathy
    - sickle-cell disorders D57.- ☑ [H36]
  - of prematurity H35.10- ☑
    - stage 0 H35.11- ☑
    - stage 1 H35.12- ☑
    - stage 2 H35.13- ☑
    - stage 3 H35.14- ☑
    - stage 4 H35.15- ☑
    - stage 5 H35.16- ☑
  - pigmentary, congenital — *see* Dystrophy, retina
  - proliferative NEC H35.2- ☑
- **Retinopathy** — *continued*
  - proliferative — *continued*
    - diabetic — *see* Diabetes, retinopathy, proliferative
    - sickle-cell D57.- ☑ [H36]
  - solar H31.02- ☑
- **Retinoschisis** H33.10- ☑
  - congenital Q14.1
  - specified type NEC H33.19- ☑
- **Retortamoniasis** A07.8
- **Retractile testis** Q55.22
- **Retraction**
  - cervix — *see* Retroversion, uterus
  - drum (membrane) — *see* Disorder, tympanic membrane, specified NEC
  - finger — *see* Deformity, finger
  - lid H02.539
    - left H02.536
      - lower H02.535
      - upper H02.534
    - right H02.533
      - lower H02.532
      - upper H02.531
  - lung J98.4
  - mediastinum J98.5
  - nipple N64.53
    - associated with
      - lactation O92.03
      - pregnancy O92.01- ☑
      - puerperium O92.02
    - congenital Q83.8
  - palmar fascia M72.0
  - pleura — *see* Pleurisy
  - ring, uterus (Bandl's) (pathological) O62.4
  - sternum (congenital) Q76.7
    - acquired M95.4
  - uterus — *see* Retroversion, uterus
  - valve (heart) — *see* Endocarditis
- **Retrobulbar** — *see* condition
- **Retrocecal** — *see* condition
- **Retrocession** — *see* Retroversion
- **Retrodisplacement** — *see* Retroversion
- **Retroflection, retroflexion** — *see* Retroversion
- **Retrognathia, retrognathism** (mandibular) (maxillary) M26.19
- **Retrograde menstruation** N92.5
- **Retroperineal** — *see* condition
- **Retroperitoneal** — *see* condition
- **Retroperitonitis** K68.9
- **Retropharyngeal** — *see* condition
- **Retroplacental** — *see* condition
- **Retroposition** — *see* Retroversion
- **Retroprosthetic membrane** T85.398 ☑
- **Retrosternal thyroid** (congenital) Q89.2
- **Retroversion, retroverted**
  - cervix — *see* Retroversion, uterus
  - female NEC — *see* Retroversion, uterus
  - iris H21.89
  - testis (congenital) Q55.29
  - uterus (acquired) (acute) (any degree) (asymptomatic) (cervix) (postinfectional) (postpartal, old) N85.4
    - congenital Q51.818
    - in pregnancy O34.53- ☑
- **Retrovirus, as cause of disease classified elsewhere** B97.30
  - human
    - immunodeficiency, type 2 (HIV 2) B97.35
    - T-cell lymphotropic
      - type I (HTLV-I) B97.33
      - type II (HTLV-II) B97.34
  - lentivirus B97.31
  - oncovirus B97.32
  - specified NEC B97.39
- **Retrusion, premaxilla** (developmental) M26.09
- **Rett's disease or syndrome** F84.2
- **Reverse peristalsis** R19.2
- **Reye's syndrome** G93.7
- **Rh** (factor)
  - hemolytic disease (newborn) P55.0
  - incompatibility, immunization or sensitization
    - affecting management of pregnancy NEC O36.09- ☑
      - anti-D antibody O36.01- ☑
    - newborn P55.0
    - transfusion reaction — *see* Complication(s), transfusion, incompatibility reaction, Rh (factor)
  - negative mother affecting newborn P55.0

- **Rh** — *continued*
  - titer elevated — *see* Complication(s), transfusion, incompatibility reaction, Rh (factor)
  - transfusion reaction — *see* Complication(s), transfusion, incompatibility reaction, Rh (factor)
- **Rhabdomyolysis** (idiopathic) NEC M62.82
  - traumatic T79.6 ☑
- **Rhabdomyoma** (*see also* Neoplasm, connective tissue, benign)
  - adult — *see* Neoplasm, connective tissue, benign
  - fetal — *see* Neoplasm, connective tissue, benign
  - glycogenic — *see* Neoplasm, connective tissue, benign
- **Rhabdomyosarcoma** (any type) — *see* Neoplasm, connective tissue, malignant
- **Rhabdosarcoma** — *see* Rhabdomyosarcoma
- **Rhesus** (factor) **incompatibility** — *see* Rh, incompatibility
- **Rheumatic** (acute) (subacute) (chronic)
  - adherent pericardium I09.2
  - coronary arteritis I01.9
  - degeneration, myocardium I09.Ø
  - fever (acute) — *see* Fever, rheumatic
  - heart — *see* Disease, heart, rheumatic
  - myocardial degeneration — *see* Degeneration, myocardium
  - myocarditis (chronic) (inactive) (with chorea) I09.Ø
    - with chorea (acute) (rheumatic) (Sydenham's) I02.Ø
    - active or acute I01.2
  - pancarditis, acute I01.8
    - with chorea (acute (rheumatic) Sydenham's) I02.Ø
  - pericarditis (active) (acute) (with effusion) (with pneumonia) I01.Ø
    - with chorea (acute) (rheumatic) (Sydenham's) I02.Ø
    - chronic or inactive I09.2
  - pneumonia I00 [J17]
  - torticollis M43.6
  - typhoid fever A01.09
- **Rheumatism** (articular) (neuralgic) (nonarticular) M79.Ø
  - gout — *see* Arthritis, rheumatoid
  - intercostal, meaning Tietze's disease M94.Ø
  - palindromic (any site) M12.30
    - ankle M12.37- ☑
    - elbow M12.32- ☑
    - foot joint M12.37- ☑
    - hand joint M12.34- ☑
    - hip M12.35- ☑
    - knee M12.36- ☑
    - multiple site M12.39
    - shoulder M12.31- ☑
    - specified joint NEC M12.38
    - vertebrae M12.38
    - wrist M12.33- ☑
  - sciatic M54.4- ☑
- **Rheumatoid** (*see also* condition)
  - arthritis (*see also* Arthritis, rheumatoid)
    - with involvement of organs NEC MØ5.6Ø
      - ankle MØ5.67- ☑
      - elbow MØ5.62- ☑
      - foot joint MØ5.67- ☑
      - hand joint MØ5.64- ☑
      - hip MØ5.65- ☑
      - knee MØ5.66- ☑
      - multiple site MØ5.69
      - shoulder MØ5.61- ☑
      - vertebra — *see* Spondylitis, ankylosing
      - wrist MØ5.63- ☑
    - seronegative — *see* Arthritis, rheumatoid, seronegative
    - seropositive — *see* Arthritis, rheumatoid, seropositive
  - carditis MØ5.3Ø
    - ankle MØ5.37- ☑
    - elbow MØ5.32- ☑
    - foot joint MØ5.37- ☑
    - hand joint MØ5.34- ☑
    - hip MØ5.35- ☑
    - knee MØ5.36- ☑
    - multiple site MØ5.39
    - shoulder MØ5.31- ☑
    - vertebra — *see* Spondylitis, ankylosing
    - wrist MØ5.33- ☑
  - endocarditis — *see* Rheumatoid, carditis
  - lung (disease) MØ5.1Ø
    - ankle MØ5.17- ☑
    - elbow MØ5.12- ☑
    - foot joint MØ5.17- ☑
    - hand joint MØ5.14- ☑
- **Rheumatoid** — *continued*
  - lung — *continued*
    - hip MØ5.15- ☑
    - knee MØ5.16- ☑
    - multiple site MØ5.19
    - shoulder MØ5.11- ☑
    - vertebra — *see* Spondylitis, ankylosing
    - wrist MØ5.13- ☑
  - myocarditis — *see* Rheumatoid, carditis
  - myopathy MØ5.4Ø
    - ankle MØ5.47- ☑
    - elbow MØ5.42- ☑
    - foot joint MØ5.47- ☑
    - hand joint MØ5.44- ☑
    - hip MØ5.45- ☑
    - knee MØ5.46- ☑
    - multiple site MØ5.49
    - shoulder MØ5.41- ☑
    - vertebra — *see* Spondylitis, ankylosing
    - wrist MØ5.43- ☑
  - pericarditis — *see* Rheumatoid, carditis
  - polyarthritis — *see* Arthritis, rheumatoid
  - polyneuropathy MØ5.5Ø
    - ankle MØ5.57- ☑
    - elbow MØ5.52- ☑
    - foot joint MØ5.57- ☑
    - hand joint MØ5.54- ☑
    - hip MØ5.55- ☑
    - knee MØ5.56- ☑
    - multiple site MØ5.59
    - shoulder MØ5.51- ☑
    - vertebra — *see* Spondylitis, ankylosing
    - wrist MØ5.53- ☑
  - vasculitis MØ5.2Ø
    - ankle MØ5.27- ☑
    - elbow MØ5.22- ☑
    - foot joint MØ5.27- ☑
    - hand joint MØ5.24- ☑
    - hip MØ5.25- ☑
    - knee MØ5.26- ☑
    - multiple site MØ5.29
    - shoulder MØ5.21- ☑
    - vertebra — *see* Spondylitis, ankylosing
    - wrist MØ5.23- ☑
- **Rhinitis** (atrophic) (catarrhal) (chronic) (croupous) (fibrinous) (granulomatous) (hyperplastic) (hypertrophic) (membranous) (obstructive) (purulent) (suppurative) (ulcerative) J31.Ø
  - with
    - sore throat — *see* Nasopharyngitis
  - acute JØØ
  - allergic J3Ø.9
    - with asthma J45.9Ø9
      - with
        - exacerbation (acute) J45.9Ø1
        - status asthmaticus J45.9Ø2
    - due to
      - food J3Ø.5
      - pollen J3Ø.1
    - nonseasonal J3Ø.89
    - perennial J3Ø.89
    - seasonal NEC J3Ø.2
    - specified NEC J3Ø.89
  - infective JØØ
  - pneumococcal JØØ
  - syphilitic A52.73
    - congenital A5Ø.Ø5 [J99]
  - tuberculous A15.8
  - vasomotor J3Ø.Ø
- **Rhinoantritis** (chronic) — *see* Sinusitis, maxillary
- **Rhinodacryolith** — *see* Dacryolith
- **Rhinolith** (nasal sinus) J34.89
- **Rhinomegaly** J34.89
- **Rhinopharyngitis** (acute) (subacute) (*see also* Nasopharyngitis)
  - chronic J31.1
  - destructive ulcerating A66.5
  - mutilans A66.5
- **Rhinophyma** L71.1
- **Rhinorrhea** J34.89
  - cerebrospinal (fluid) G96.Ø
  - paroxysmal — *see* Rhinitis, allergic
  - spasmodic — *see* Rhinitis, allergic
- **Rhinosalpingitis** — *see* Salpingitis, eustachian
- **Rhinoscleroma** A48.8
- **Rhinosporidiosis** B48.1
- **Rhinovirus infection NEC** B34.8
- **Rhizomelic chondrodysplasia punctata** E71.54Ø
- **Rhythm**
  - atrioventricular nodal I49.8
  - disorder I49.9
    - coronary sinus I49.8
    - ectopic I49.8
    - nodal I49.8
  - escape I49.9
  - heart, abnormal I49.9
  - idioventricular I44.2
  - nodal I49.8
  - sleep, inversion G47.2- ☑
    - nonorganic origin — *see* Disorder, sleep, circadian rhythm, psychogenic
- **Rhytidosis facialis** L98.8
- **Rib** (*see also* condition)
  - cervical Q76.5
- **Riboflavin deficiency** E53.Ø
- **Rice bodies** (*see also* Loose, body, joint)
  - knee M23.4- ☑
- **Richter syndrome** — *see* Leukemia, chronic lymphocytic, B-cell type
- **Richter's hernia** — *see* Hernia, abdomen, with obstruction
- **Ricinism** — *see* Poisoning, food, noxious, plant
- **Rickets** (active) (acute) (adolescent) (chest wall) (congenital) (current) (infantile) (intestinal) E55.Ø
  - adult — *see* Osteomalacia
  - celiac K9Ø.Ø
  - hypophosphatemic with nephrotic-glycosuric dwarfism E72.Ø9
  - inactive E64.3
  - kidney N25.Ø
  - renal N25.Ø
  - sequelae, any E64.3
  - vitamin-D-resistant E83.31 [M9Ø.8Ø]
- **Rickettsial disease** A79.9
  - specified type NEC A79.89
- **Rickettsialpox** (Rickettsia akari) A79.1
- **Rickettsiosis** A79.9
  - due to
    - Ehrlichia sennetsu A79.81
    - Rickettsia akari (rickettsialpox) A79.1
  - specified type NEC A79.89
  - tick-borne A77.9
  - vesicular A79.1
- **Rider's bone** — *see* Ossification, muscle, specified NEC
- **Ridge, alveolus** (*see also* condition)
  - flabby KØ6.8
- **Ridged ear, congenital** Q17.3
- **Riedel's**
  - lobe, liver Q44.7
  - struma, thyroiditis or disease EØ6.5
- **Rieger's anomaly or syndrome** Q13.81
- **Riehl's melanosis** L81.4
- **Rietti-Greppi-Micheli anemia** D56.9
- **Rieux's hernia** — *see* Hernia, abdomen, specified site NEC
- **Riga** (-Fede) **disease** K14.Ø
- **Riggs' disease** — *see* Periodontitis
- **Right middle lobe syndrome** J98.11
- **Rigid, rigidity** (*see also* condition)
  - abdominal R19.3Ø
    - with severe abdominal pain R1Ø.Ø
    - epigastric R19.36
    - generalized R19.37
    - left lower quadrant R19.34
    - left upper quadrant R19.32
    - periumbilic R19.35
    - right lower quadrant R19.33
    - right upper quadrant R19.31
  - articular, multiple, congenital Q68.8
  - cervix (uteri) in pregnancy — *see* Pregnancy, complicated by, abnormal, cervix
  - hymen (acquired) (congenital) N89.6
  - nuchal R29.1
  - pelvic floor in pregnancy — *see* Pregnancy, complicated by, abnormal, pelvic organs or tissues NEC
  - perineum or vulva in pregnancy — *see* Pregnancy, complicated by, abnormal, vulva
  - spine — *see* Dorsopathy, specified NEC
  - vagina in pregnancy — *see* Pregnancy, complicated by, abnormal, vagina
- **Rigors** R68.89
  - with fever R5Ø.9
- **Riley-Day syndrome** G9Ø.1
- **RIND** (reversible ischemic neurologic deficit) I63.9

Ring(s)
- aorta (vascular) Q25.4
- Bandl's O62.4
- contraction, complicating delivery O62.4
- esophageal, lower (muscular) K22.2
- Fleischer's (cornea) H18.Ø4- ☑
- hymenal, tight (acquired) (congenital) N89.6
- Kayser-Fleischer (cornea) H18.Ø4- ☑
- retraction, uterus, pathological O62.4
- Schatzki's (esophagus) (lower) K22.2
  - congenital Q39.3
- Soemmerring's — *see* Cataract, secondary
- vascular (congenital) Q25.8
  - aorta Q25.4

Ringed hair (congenital) Q84.1

Ringworm B35.9
- beard B35.Ø
- black dot B35.Ø
- body B35.4
- Burmese B35.5
- corporeal B35.4
- foot B35.3
- groin B35.6
- hand B35.2
- honeycomb B35.Ø
- nails B35.1
- perianal (area) B35.6
- scalp B35.Ø
- specified NEC B35.8
- Tokelau B35.5

Rise, venous pressure I87.8

Risk, suicidal
- meaning personal history of attempted suicide Z91.5
- meaning suicidal ideation — *see* Ideation, suicidal

Ritter's disease LØØ

Rivalry, sibling Z62.891

Rivalta's disease A42.2

River blindness B73.Ø1

Robert's pelvis Q74.2
- with disproportion (fetopelvic) O33.Ø
  - causing obstructed labor O65.Ø

Robin (-Pierre) **syndrome** Q87.Ø

Robinow-Silvermann-Smith syndrome Q87.1

Robinson's (hidrotic) **ectodermal dysplasia or syndrome** Q82.4

Robles' disease B73.Ø1

Rocky Mountain (spotted) **fever** A77.Ø

Roetheln — *see* Rubella

Roger's disease Q21.Ø

Rokitansky-Aschoff sinuses (gallbladder) K82.8

Rolando's fracture (displaced) S62.22- ☑
- nondisplaced S62.22- ☑

Romano-Ward (prolonged QT interval) **syndrome** I45.81

Romberg's disease or syndrome G51.8

Roof, mouth — *see* condition

Rosacea L71.9
- acne L71.9
- keratitis L71.8
- specified NEC L71.8

Rosary, rachitic E55.Ø

Rose
- cold J3Ø.1
- fever J3Ø.1
- rash R21
  - epidemic BØ6.9

Rosenbach's erysipeloid A26.Ø

Rosenthal's disease or syndrome D68.1

Roseola BØ9
- infantum BØ8.2Ø
  - due to human herpesvirus 6 BØ8.21
  - due to human herpesvirus 7 BØ8.22

Ross River disease or fever B33.1

Rossbach's disease K31.89
- psychogenic F45.8

Rostan's asthma (cardiac) — *see* Failure, ventricular, left

Rotation
- anomalous, incomplete or insufficient, intestine Q43.3
- cecum (congenital) Q43.3
- colon (congenital) Q43.3
- spine, incomplete or insufficient — *see* Dorsopathy, deforming, specified NEC
- tooth, teeth, fully erupted M26.35
- vertebra, incomplete or insufficient — *see* Dorsopathy, deforming, specified NEC

Rotes Quérol disease or syndrome — *see* Hyperostosis, ankylosing

Roth (-Bernhardt) **disease or syndrome** — *see* Meralgia paraesthetica

Rothmund (-Thomson) **syndrome** Q82.8

Rotor's disease or syndrome E8Ø.6

Round
- back (with wedging of vertebrae) — *see* Kyphosis
  - sequelae (late effect) of rickets E64.3
- worms (large) (infestation) NEC B82.Ø
  - Ascariasis (*see also* Ascariasis) B77.9

Roussy-Lévy syndrome G6Ø.Ø

Rubella (German measles) BØ6.9
- complication NEC BØ6.Ø9
  - neurological BØ6.ØØ
- congenital P35.Ø
- contact Z2Ø.4
- exposure to Z2Ø.4
- maternal
  - care for (suspected) damage to fetus O35.3 ☑
  - manifest rubella in infant P35.Ø
  - suspected damage to fetus affecting management of pregnancy O35.3 ☑
- specified complications NEC BØ6.89

Rubeola (meaning measles) — *see* Measles
- meaning rubella — *see* Rubella

Rubeosis, iris — *see* Disorder, iris, vascular

Rubinstein-Taybi syndrome Q87.2

Rudimentary (congenital) (*see also* Agenesis)
- arm — *see* Defect, reduction, upper limb
- bone Q79.9
- cervix uteri Q51.828
- eye Q11.2
- lobule of ear Q17.3
- patella Q74.1
- respiratory organs in thoracopagus Q89.4
- tracheal bronchus Q32.4
- uterus Q51.818
  - in male Q56.1
- vagina Q52.Ø

Ruled out condition — *see* Observation, suspected

Rumination R11.1Ø
- with nausea R11.2
- disorder of infancy F98.21
- neurotic F42
- newborn P92.1
- obsessional F42
- psychogenic F42

Runeberg's disease D51.Ø

Runny nose RØ9.89

Rupia (syphilitic) A51.39
- congenital A5Ø.Ø6
- tertiary A52.79

Rupture, ruptured
- abscess (spontaneous) — *code by* site under Abscess
- aneurysm — *see* Aneurysm
- anus (sphincter) — *see* Laceration, anus
- aorta, aortic I71.8
  - abdominal I71.3
  - arch I71.1
  - ascending I71.1
  - descending I71.8
    - abdominal I71.3
    - thoracic I71.1
  - syphilitic A52.Ø1
  - thoracoabdominal I71.5
  - thorax, thoracic I71.1
  - transverse I71.1
  - traumatic — *see* Injury, aorta, laceration, major
  - valve or cusp (*see also* Endocarditis, aortic) I35.8
- appendix (with peritonitis) K35.2
- arteriovenous fistula, brain I6Ø.8
- artery I77.2
  - brain — *see* Hemorrhage, intracranial, intracerebral
  - coronary — *see* Infarct, myocardium
  - heart — *see* Infarct, myocardium
  - pulmonary I28.8
  - traumatic (complication) — *see* Injury, blood vessel
- bile duct (common) (hepatic) K83.2
  - cystic K82.2
- bladder (sphincter) (nontraumatic) (spontaneous) N32.89
  - following ectopic or molar pregnancy OØ8.6
  - obstetrical trauma O71.5
  - traumatic S37.29 ☑
- blood vessel (*see also* Hemorrhage)
  - brain — *see* Hemorrhage, intracranial, intracerebral
  - heart — *see* Infarct, myocardium

Rupture, ruptured — *continued*
- blood vessel (*see also* Hemorrhage) — *continued*
  - traumatic (complication) — *see* Injury, blood vessel, laceration, major, by site
- bone — *see* Fracture
- bowel (nontraumatic) K63.1
- brain
  - aneurysm (congenital) (*see also* Hemorrhage, intracranial, subarachnoid)
    - syphilitic A52.Ø5
  - hemorrhagic — *see* Hemorrhage, intracranial, intracerebral
- capillaries I78.8
- cardiac (auricle) (ventricle) (wall) I23.3
  - with hemopericardium I23.Ø
  - infectional I4Ø.9
  - traumatic — *see* Injury, heart
- cartilage (articular) (current) (*see also* Sprain)
  - knee S83.3- ☑
  - semilunar — *see* Tear, meniscus
- cecum (with peritonitis) K65.Ø
  - with peritoneal abscess K35.3
  - traumatic S36.598 ☑
- celiac artery, traumatic — *see* Injury, blood vessel, celiac artery, laceration, major
- cerebral aneurysm (congenital) (see Hemorrhage, intracranial, subarachnoid)
- cervix (uteri)
  - with ectopic or molar pregnancy OØ8.6
  - following ectopic or molar pregnancy OØ8.6
  - obstetrical trauma O71.3
  - traumatic S37.69 ☑
- chordae tendineae NEC I51.1
  - concurrent with acute myocardial infarction — *see* Infarct, myocardium
  - following acute myocardial infarction (current complication) I23.4
- choroid (direct) (indirect) (traumatic) H31.32- ☑
- circle of Willis I6Ø.6
- colon (nontraumatic) K63.1
  - traumatic — *see* Injury, intestine, large
- cornea (traumatic) — *see* Injury, eye, laceration
- coronary (artery) (thrombotic) — *see* Infarct, myocardium
- corpus luteum (infected) (ovary) N83.1
- cyst — *see* Cyst
- cystic duct K82.2
- Descemet's membrane — *see* Change, corneal membrane, Descemet's, rupture
  - traumatic — *see* Injury, eye, laceration
- diaphragm, traumatic — *see* Injury, intrathoracic, diaphragm
- disc — *see* Rupture, intervertebral disc
- diverticulum (intestine) K57.8Ø
  - with bleeding K57.81
  - bladder N32.3
  - large intestine K57.2Ø
    - with
      - bleeding K57.21
      - small intestine K57.4Ø
        - with bleeding K57.41
  - small intestine K57.ØØ
    - with
      - bleeding K57.Ø1
      - large intestine K57.4Ø
        - with bleeding K57.41
- duodenal stump K31.89
- ear drum (nontraumatic) (*see also* Perforation, tympanum)
  - traumatic SØ9.2- ☑
    - due to blast injury — *see* Injury, blast, ear
- esophagus K22.3
- eye (without prolapse or loss of intraocular tissue) — *see* Injury, eye, laceration
- fallopian tube NEC (nonobstetric) (nontraumatic) N83.8
  - due to pregnancy OØØ.1
- fontanel P13.1
- gallbladder K82.2
  - traumatic S36.128 ☑
- gastric (*see also* Rupture, stomach)
  - vessel K92.2
- globe (eye) (traumatic) — *see* Injury, eye, laceration
- graafian follicle (hematoma) N83.Ø
- heart — *see* Rupture, cardiac
- hymen (nontraumatic) (nonintentional) N89.8
- internal organ, traumatic — *see* Injury, by site

Rupture, ruptured — *continued*
tympanum, tympanic (membrane) (nontraumatic) (*see also* Perforation, tympanic membrane) H72.9- ☑
traumatic — *see* Rupture, ear drum, traumatic
umbilical cord, complicating delivery O69.89 ☑
ureter (traumatic) S37.19 ☑
nontraumatic N28.89
urethra (nontraumatic) N36.8
with ectopic or molar pregnancy O08.6
following ectopic or molar pregnancy O08.6
obstetrical trauma O71.5
traumatic S37.39 ☑
uterosacral ligament (nonobstetric) (nontraumatic) N83.8
uterus (traumatic) S37.69 ☑
before labor O71.Ø- ☑
during or after labor O71.1
nonpuerperal, nontraumatic N85.8
pregnant (during labor) O71.1
before labor O71.Ø- ☑
vagina — *see* Injury, vagina
valve, valvular (heart) — *see* Endocarditis
varicose vein — *see* Varix
varix — *see* Varix
vena cava R58
traumatic — *see* Injury, vena cava, laceration, major
vesical (urinary) N32.89
vessel (blood) R58
pulmonary I28.8
traumatic — *see* Injury, blood vessel
viscus R19.8
vulva complicating delivery O7Ø.Ø
Russell-Silver syndrome Q87.1
Russian spring-summer type encephalitis A84.Ø
Rust's disease (tuberculous cervical spondylitis) A18.Ø1
Ruvalcaba-Myhre-Smith syndrome E71.44Ø
Rytand-Lipsitch syndrome I44.2

S

Saber, sabre shin or tibia (syphilitic) A5Ø.56 [M9Ø.8-] ☑
Sac lacrimal — *see* condition
Saccharomyces infection B37.9
Saccharopinuria E72.3
Saccular — *see* condition
Sacculation
aorta (nonsyphilitic) — *see* Aneurysm, aorta
bladder N32.3
intralaryngeal (congenital) (ventricular) Q31.3
larynx (congenital) (ventricular) Q31.3
organ or site, congenital — *see* Distortion
pregnant uterus — *see* Pregnancy, complicated by, abnormal, uterus
ureter N28.89
urethra N36.1
vesical N32.3
Sachs' amaurotic familial idiocy or disease E75.Ø2
Sachs-Tay disease E75.Ø2
Sacks-Libman disease M32.11
Sacralgia M53.3
Sacralization Q76.49
Sacrodynia M53.3
Sacroiliac joint — *see* condition
Sacroiliitis NEC M46.1
Sacrum — *see* condition
Saddle
back — *see* Lordosis
embolus
abdominal aorta I74.Ø1
pulmonary artery I26.92
with acute cor pulmonale I26.Ø2
injury — *code to* condition
nose M95.Ø
due to syphilis A5Ø.57
Sadism (sexual) F65.52
Sadness, postpartal O9Ø.6
Sadomasochism F65.5Ø
Saemisch's ulcer (cornea) — *see* Ulcer, cornea, central
Sahib disease B55.Ø
Sailors' skin L57.8
Saint
Anthony's fire — *see* Erysipelas
triad — *see* Hernia, diaphragm
Vitus' dance — *see* Chorea, Sydenham's
Salaam
attack(s) — *see* Epilepsy, spasms

Salaam — *continued*
tic R25.8
Salicylism
abuse F55.8
overdose or wrong substance given — *see* Table of Drugs and Chemicals, by drug, poisoning
Salivary duct or gland — *see* condition
Salivation, excessive K11.7
Salmonella — *see* Infection, Salmonella
Salmonellosis AØ2.Ø
Salpingitis (catarrhal) (fallopian tube) (nodular) (pseudofollicular) (purulent) (septic) N7Ø.91
with oophoritis N7Ø.93
acute N7Ø.Ø1
with oophoritis N7Ø.Ø3
chlamydial A56.11
chronic N7Ø.11
with oophoritis N7Ø.13
complicating abortion — *see* Abortion, by type, complicated by, salpingitis
ear — *see* Salpingitis, eustachian
eustachian (tube) H68.ØØ- ☑
acute H68.Ø1- ☑
chronic H68.Ø2- ☑
follicularis N7Ø.11
with oophoritis N7Ø.13
gonococcal (acute) (chronic) A54.24
interstitial, chronic N7Ø.11
with oophoritis N7Ø.13
isthmica nodosa N7Ø.11
with oophoritis N7Ø.13
specific (gonococcal) (acute) (chronic) A54.24
tuberculous (acute) (chronic) A18.17
venereal (gonococcal) (acute) (chronic) A54.24
Salpingocele N83.4
Salpingo-oophoritis (catarrhal) (purulent) (ruptured) (septic) (suppurative) N7Ø.93
acute N7Ø.Ø3
with ectopic or molar pregnancy OØ8.Ø
following ectopic or molar pregnancy OØ8.Ø
gonococcal A54.24
chronic N7Ø.13
following ectopic or molar pregnancy OØ8.Ø
gonococcal (acute) (chronic) A54.24
puerperal O86.19
specific (gonococcal) (acute) (chronic) A54.24
subacute N7Ø.Ø3
tuberculous (acute) (chronic) A18.17
venereal (gonococcal) (acute) (chronic) A54.24
Salpingo-ovaritis — *see* Salpingo-oophoritis
Salpingoperitonitis — *see* Salpingo-oophoritis
Salzmann's nodular dystrophy — *see* Degeneration, cornea, nodular
Sampson's cyst or tumor N8Ø.1
San Joaquin (Valley) **fever** B38.Ø
Sandblaster's asthma, lung or pneumoconiosis J62.8
Sander's disease (paranoia) F22
Sandfly fever A93.1
Sandhoff's disease E75.Ø1
Sanfilippo (Type B) (Type C) (Type D) **syndrome** E76.22
Sanger-Brown ataxia G11.2
Sao Paulo fever or typhus A77.Ø
Saponification, mesenteric K65.8
Sarcocele (benign)
syphilitic A52.76
congenital A5Ø.59
Sarcocystosis AØ7.8
Sarcoepiplocele — *see* Hernia
Sarcoepiplomphalocele Q79.2
Sarcoid (*see also* Sarcoidosis)
arthropathy D86.86
Boeck's D86.9
Darier-Roussy D86.3
iridocyclitis D86.83
meningitis D86.81
myocarditis D86.85
myositis D86.87
pyelonephritis D86.84
Spiegler-Fendt LØ8.89
Sarcoidosis D86.9
with
cranial nerve palsies D86.82
hepatic granuloma D86.89
polyarthritis D86.86
tubulo-interstitial nephropathy D86.84
combined sites NEC D86.89
lung D86.Ø

Sarcoidosis — *continued*
lung — *continued*
and lymph nodes D86.2
lymph nodes D86.1
and lung D86.2
meninges D86.81
skin D86.3
specified type NEC D86.89
Sarcoma (of) (*see also* Neoplasm, connective tissue, malignant)
alveolar soft part — *see* Neoplasm, connective tissue, malignant
ameloblastic C41.1
upper jaw (bone) C41.Ø
botryoid — *see* Neoplasm, connective tissue, malignant
botryoides — *see* Neoplasm, connective tissue, malignant
cerebellar C71.6
circumscribed (arachnoidal) C71.6
circumscribed (arachnoidal) cerebellar C71.6
clear cell (*see also* Neoplasm, connective tissue, malignant)
kidney C64.- ☑
dendritic cells (accessory cells) C96.4
embryonal — *see* Neoplasm, connective tissue, malignant
endometrial (stromal) C54.1
isthmus C54.Ø
epithelioid (cell) — *see* Neoplasm, connective tissue, malignant
Ewing's — *see* Neoplasm, bone, malignant
follicular dendritic cell C96.4
germinoblastic (diffuse) — *see* Lymphoma, diffuse large cell
follicular — *see* Lymphoma, follicular, specified NEC
giant cell (except of bone) (*see also* Neoplasm, connective tissue, malignant)
bone — *see* Neoplasm, bone, malignant
glomoid — *see* Neoplasm, connective tissue, malignant
granulocytic C92.3- ☑
hemangioendothelial — *see* Neoplasm, connective tissue, malignant
hemorrhagic, multiple — *see* Sarcoma, Kaposi's
histiocytic C96.A (*following* C96.6)
Hodgkin — *see* Lymphoma, Hodgkin
immunoblastic (diffuse) — *see* Lymphoma, diffuse large cell
interdigitating dendritic cell C96.4
Kaposi's
colon C46.4
connective tissue C46.1
gastrointestinal organ C46.4
lung C46.5- ☑
lymph node(s) C46.3
palate (hard) (soft) C46.2
rectum C46.4
skin C46.Ø
specified site NEC C46.7
stomach C46.4
unspecified site C46.9
Kupffer cell C22.3
Langerhans cell C96.4
leptomeningeal — *see* Neoplasm, meninges, malignant
liver NEC C22.4
lymphangioendothelial — *see* Neoplasm, connective tissue, malignant
lymphoblastic — *see* Lymphoma, lymphoblastic (diffuse)
lymphocytic — *see* Lymphoma, small cell B-cell
mast cell C96.2
melanotic — *see* Melanoma
meningeal — *see* Neoplasm, meninges, malignant
meningothelial — *see* Neoplasm, meninges, malignant
mesenchymal (*see also* Neoplasm, connective tissue, malignant)
mixed — *see* Neoplasm, connective tissue, malignant
mesothelial — *see* Mesothelioma
monstrocellular
specified site — *see* Neoplasm, malignant, by site
unspecified site C71.9
myeloid C92.3- ☑
neurogenic — *see* Neoplasm, nerve, malignant

Index
Rupture, ruptured — Sarcoma

Sarcoma — *continued*
- odontogenic C41.1
  - upper jaw (bone) C41.Ø
- osteoblastic — *see* Neoplasm, bone, malignant
- osteogenic (*see also* Neoplasm, bone, malignant)
  - juxtacortical — *see* Neoplasm, bone, malignant
  - periosteal — *see* Neoplasm, bone, malignant
- periosteal (*see also* Neoplasm, bone, malignant)
  - osteogenic — *see* Neoplasm, bone, malignant
- pleomorphic cell — *see* Neoplasm, connective tissue, malignant
- reticulum cell (diffuse) — *see* Lymphoma, diffuse large cell
  - nodular — *see* Lymphoma, follicular
  - pleomorphic cell type — *see* Lymphoma, diffuse large cell
- rhabdoid — *see* Neoplasm, malignant, by site
- round cell — *see* Neoplasm, connective tissue, malignant
- small cell — *see* Neoplasm, connective tissue, malignant
- soft tissue — *see* Neoplasm, connective tissue, malignant
- spindle cell — *see* Neoplasm, connective tissue, malignant
- stromal (endometrial) C54.1
  - isthmus C54.Ø
- synovial (*see also* Neoplasm, connective tissue, malignant)
  - biphasic — *see* Neoplasm, connective tissue, malignant
  - epithelioid cell — *see* Neoplasm, connective tissue, malignant
  - spindle cell — *see* Neoplasm, connective tissue, malignant

Sarcomatosis
- meningeal — *see* Neoplasm, meninges, malignant
- specified site NEC — *see* Neoplasm, connective tissue, malignant
- unspecified site C8Ø.1

Sarcosinemia E72.59
Sarcosporidiosis (intestinal) AØ7.8
Satiety, early R68.81
Saturnine — *see* condition
Saturnism
- overdose or wrong substance given or taken — *see* Table of Drugs and Chemicals, by drug, poisoning

Satyriasis F52.8
Sauriasis — *see* Ichthyosis
SBE (subacute bacterial endocarditis) I33.Ø
Scabies (any site) B86
Scabs R23.4
Scaglietti-Dagnini syndrome E22.Ø
Scald — *see* Burn
Scalenus anticus (anterior) **syndrome** G54.Ø
Scales R23.4
Scaling, skin R23.4
Scalp — *see* condition
Scapegoating affecting child Z62.3
Scaphocephaly Q75.Ø
Scapulalgia M89.8X1
Scapulohumeral myopathy G71.Ø
Scar, scarring (*see also* Cicatrix) L9Ø.5
- adherent L9Ø.5
- atrophic L9Ø.5
- cervix
  - in pregnancy or childbirth — *see* Pregnancy, complicated by, abnormal cervix
- cheloid L91.Ø
- chorioretinal H31.ØØ- ☑
  - posterior pole macula H31.Ø1- ☑
  - postsurgical H59.81- ☑
  - solar retinopathy H31.Ø2- ☑
  - specified type NEC H31.Ø9- ☑
- choroid — *see* Scar, chorioretinal
- conjunctiva H11.24- ☑
- cornea H17.9
  - xerophthalmic (*see also* Opacity, cornea)
    - vitamin A deficiency E5Ø.6
- duodenum, obstructive K31.5
- hypertrophic L91.Ø
- keloid L91.Ø
- labia N9Ø.89
- lung (base) J98.4
- macula — *see* Scar, chorioretinal, posterior pole
- muscle M62.89

Scar, scarring — *continued*
- myocardium, myocardial I25.2
- painful L9Ø.5
- posterior pole (eye) — *see* Scar, chorioretinal, posterior pole
- retina — *see* Scar, chorioretinal
- trachea J39.8
- uterus N85.8
  - in pregnancy O34.29
- vagina N89.8
  - postoperative N99.2
- vulva N9Ø.89

Scarabiasis B88.2
Scarlatina (anginosa) (maligna) (ulcerosa) A38.9
- myocarditis (acute) A38.1
  - old — *see* Myocarditis
- otitis media A38.Ø

Scarlet fever (albuminuria) (angina) A38.9
Schamberg's disease (progressive pigmentary dermatosis) L81.7
Schatzki's ring (acquired) (esophagus) (lower) K22.2
- congenital Q39.3

Schaufenster krankheit I2Ø.8
Schaumann's
- benign lymphogranulomatosis D86.1
- disease or syndrome — *see* Sarcoidosis

Scheie's syndrome E76.Ø3
Schenck's disease B42.1
Scheuermann's disease or osteochondrosis — *see* Osteochondrosis, juvenile, spine
Schilder (-Flatau) **disease** G37.Ø
Schilling-type monocytic leukemia C93.Ø- ☑
Schimmelbusch's disease, cystic mastitis, or hyperplasia — *see* Mastopathy, cystic
Schistosoma infestation — *see* Infestation, Schistosoma
Schistosomiasis B65.9
- with muscle disorder B65.9 [M63.8Ø]
  - ankle B65.9 [M63.87-] ☑
  - foot B65.9 [M63.87-] ☑
  - forearm B65.9 [M63.83-] ☑
  - hand B65.9 [M63.84-] ☑
  - lower leg B65.9 [M63.86-] ☑
  - multiple sites B65.9 [M63.89]
  - pelvic region B65.9 [M63.85-] ☑
  - shoulder region B65.9 [M63.81-] ☑
  - specified site NEC B65.9 [M63.88]
  - thigh B65.9 [M63.85-] ☑
  - upper arm B65.9 [M63.82-] ☑
- Asiatic B65.2
- bladder B65.Ø
- chestermani B65.8
- colon B65.1
- cutaneous B65.3
- due to
  - S. haematobium B65.Ø
  - S. japonicum B65.2
  - S. mansoni B65.1
  - S. mattheii B65.8
- Eastern B65.2
- genitourinary tract B65.Ø
- intestinal B65.1
- lung NEC B65.9 [J99]
  - pneumonia B65.9 [J17]
- Manson's (intestinal) B65.1
- oriental B65.2
- pulmonary NEC B65.9 [J99]
  - pneumonia B65.9
- Schistosoma
  - haematobium B65.Ø
  - japonicum B65.2
  - mansoni B65.1
- specified type NEC B65.8
- urinary B65.Ø
- vesical B65.Ø

Schizencephaly QØ4.6
Schizoaffective psychosis F25.9
Schizodontia KØØ.2
Schizoid personality F6Ø.1
Schizophrenia, schizophrenic F2Ø.9
- acute (brief) (undifferentiated) F23
- atypical (form) F2Ø.3
- borderline F21
- catalepsy F2Ø.2
- catatonic (type) (excited) (withdrawn) F2Ø.2
- cenesthopathic, cenesthesiopathic F2Ø.89
- childhood type F84.5
- chronic undifferentiated F2Ø.5

Schizophrenia, schizophrenic — *continued*
- cyclic F25.Ø
- disorganized (type) F2Ø.1
- flexibilitas cerea F2Ø.2
- hebephrenic (type) F2Ø.1
- incipient F21
- latent F21
- negative type F2Ø.5
- paranoid (type) F2Ø.Ø
- paraphrenic F2Ø.Ø
- post-psychotic depression F32.8
- prepsychotic F21
- prodromal F21
- pseudoneurotic F21
- pseudopsychopathic F21
- reaction F23
- residual (state) (type) F2Ø.5
- restzustand F2Ø.5
- schizoaffective (type) — *see* Psychosis, schizoaffective
- simple (type) F2Ø.89
- simplex F2Ø.89
- specified type NEC F2Ø.89
- stupor F2Ø.2
- syndrome of childhood F84.5
- undifferentiated (type) F2Ø.3
  - chronic F2Ø.5

Schizothymia (persistent) F6Ø.1
Schlatter-Osgood disease or osteochondrosis — *see* Osteochondrosis, juvenile, tibia
Schlatter's tibia — *see* Osteochondrosis, juvenile, tibia
Schmidt's syndrome (polyglandular, autoimmune) E31.Ø
Schmincke's carcinoma or tumor — *see* Neoplasm, nasopharynx, malignant
Schmitz (-Stutzer) **dysentery** AØ3.Ø
Schmorl's disease or nodes
- lumbar region M51.46
- lumbosacral region M51.47
- sacrococcygeal region M53.3
- thoracic region M51.44
- thoracolumbar region M51.45

Schneiderian
- papilloma — *see* Neoplasm, nasopharynx, benign
  - specified site — *see* Neoplasm, benign, by site
  - unspecified site D14.Ø
- specified site — *see* Neoplasm, malignant, by site
  - unspecified site C3Ø.Ø

Scholte's syndrome (malignant carcinoid) E34.Ø
Scholz (-Bielchowsky-Henneberg) **disease or syndrome** E75.25
Schönlein (-Henoch) disease or purpura (primary) (rheumatic) D69.Ø
Schottmuller's disease AØ1.4
Schroeder's syndrome (endocrine hypertensive) E27.Ø
Schüller-Christian disease or syndrome C96.5
Schultze's type acroparesthesia, simple I73.89
Schultz's disease or syndrome — *see* Agranulocytosis
Schwalbe-Ziehen-Oppenheim disease G24.1
Schwannoma (*see also* Neoplasm, nerve, benign)
- malignant (*see also* Neoplasm, nerve, malignant)
  - with rhabdomyoblastic differentiation — *see* Neoplasm, nerve, malignant
- melanocytic — *see* Neoplasm, nerve, benign
- pigmented — *see* Neoplasm, nerve, benign

Schwannomatosis Q85.Ø3
Schwartz (-Jampel) **syndrome** G71.13
Schwartz-Bartter syndrome E22.2
Schweniger-Buzzi anetoderma L9Ø.1
Sciatic — *see* condition
Sciatica (infective)
- with lumbago M54.4- ☑
  - due to intervertebral disc disorder — *see* Disorder, disc, with, radiculopathy
- due to displacement of intervertebral disc (with lumbago) — *see* Disorder, disc, with, radiculopathy
- wallet M54.3- ☑

Scimitar syndrome Q26.8
Sclera — *see* condition
Sclerectasia H15.84- ☑
Scleredema
- adultorum — *see* Sclerosis, systemic
- Buschke's — *see* Sclerosis, systemic
- newborn P83.Ø

Sclerema (adiposum) (edematosum) (neonatorum) (newborn) P83.Ø
- adultorum — *see* Sclerosis, systemic

Scleriasis — *see* Scleroderma
Scleritis H15.ØØ- ☑

☑ **Additional Character Required — Refer to the Tabular List for Character Selection**
Subterms under main terms may continue to next column or page

- **Scleritis** — *continued*
  - with corneal involvement H15.Ø4- ☑
  - anterior H15.Ø1- ☑
  - brawny H15.Ø2- ☑
  - in (due to) zoster BØ2.34
  - posterior H15.Ø3- ☑
  - specified type NEC H15.Ø9- ☑
  - syphilitic A52.71
  - tuberculous (nodular) A18.51
- **Sclerochoroiditis** H31.8
- **Scleroconjunctivitis** — *see* Scleritis
- **Sclerocystic ovary syndrome** E28.2
- **Sclerodactyly, sclerodactylia** L94.3
- **Scleroderma, sclerodermia** (acrosclerotic) (diffuse) (generalized) (progressive) (pulmonary) (*see also* Sclerosis, systemic) M34.9
  - circumscribed L94.Ø
  - linear L94.1
  - localized L94.Ø
  - newborn P83.8
  - systemic M34.9
- **Sclerokeratitis** H16.8
  - tuberculous A18.52
- **Scleroma nasi** A48.8
- **Scleromalacia** (perforans) H15.Ø5- ☑
- **Scleromyxedema** L98.5
- **Sclérose en plaques** G35
- **Sclerosis, sclerotic**
  - adrenal (gland) E27.8
  - Alzheimer's — *see* Disease, Alzheimer's
  - amyotrophic (lateral) G12.21
  - aorta, aortic I7Ø.Ø
    - valve — *see* Endocarditis, aortic
  - artery, arterial, arteriolar, arteriovascular — *see* Arteriosclerosis
  - ascending multiple G35
  - brain (generalized) (lobular) G37.9
    - artery, arterial I67.2
    - diffuse G37.Ø
    - disseminated G35
    - insular G35
    - Krabbe's E75.23
    - miliary G35
    - multiple G35
    - presenile (Alzheimer's) — *see* Disease, Alzheimer's, early onset
    - senile (arteriosclerotic) I67.2
    - stem, multiple G35
    - tuberous Q85.1
  - bulbar, multiple G35
  - bundle of His I44.39
  - cardiac — *see* Disease, heart, ischemic, atherosclerotic
  - cardiorenal — *see* Hypertension, cardiorenal
  - cardiovascular (*see also* Disease, cardiovascular)
    - renal — *see* Hypertension, cardiorenal
  - cerebellar — *see* Sclerosis, brain
  - cerebral — *see* Sclerosis, brain
  - cerebrospinal (disseminated) (multiple) G35
  - cerebrovascular I67.2
  - choroid — *see* Degeneration, choroid
  - combined (spinal cord) (*see also* Degeneration, combined)
    - multiple G35
  - concentric (Balo) G37.5
  - cornea — *see* Opacity, cornea
  - coronary (artery) I25.1Ø
    - with angina pectoris — *see* Arteriosclerosis, coronary (artery),
  - corpus cavernosum
    - female N9Ø.89
    - male N48.6
  - diffuse (brain) (spinal cord) G37.Ø
  - disseminated G35
  - dorsal G35
  - dorsolateral (spinal cord) — *see* Degeneration, combined
  - endometrium N85.5
  - extrapyramidal G25.9
  - eye, nuclear (senile) — *see* Cataract, senile, nuclear
  - focal and segmental (glomerular) (*see also* NØØ-NØ7 with fourth character .1) NØ5.1
  - Friedreich's (spinal cord) G11.1
  - funicular (spermatic cord) N5Ø.8
  - general (vascular) — *see* Arteriosclerosis
  - gland (lymphatic) I89.8
  - hepatic K74.1
    - alcoholic K7Ø.2
- **Sclerosis, sclerotic** — *continued*
  - hereditary
    - cerebellar G11.9
    - spinal (Friedreich's ataxia) G11.1
  - hippocampal G93.81
  - insular G35
  - kidney — *see* Sclerosis, renal
  - larynx J38.7
  - lateral (amyotrophic) (descending) (primary) (spinal) G12.21
  - lens, senile nuclear — *see* Cataract, senile, nuclear
  - liver K74.1
    - with fibrosis K74.2
      - alcoholic K7Ø.2
    - alcoholic K7Ø.2
    - cardiac K76.1
  - lung — *see* Fibrosis, lung
  - mastoid — *see* Mastoiditis, chronic
  - mesial temporal G93.81
  - mitral IØ5.8
  - Mönckeberg's (medial) — *see* Arteriosclerosis, extremities
  - multiple (brain stem) (cerebral) (generalized) (spinal cord) G35
  - myocardium, myocardial — *see* Disease, heart, ischemic, atherosclerotic
  - nuclear (senile), eye — *see* Cataract, senile, nuclear
  - ovary N83.8
  - pancreas K86.8
  - penis N48.6
  - peripheral arteries — *see* Arteriosclerosis, extremities
  - plaques G35
  - pluriglandular E31.8
  - polyglandular E31.8
  - posterolateral (spinal cord) — *see* Degeneration, combined
  - presenile (Alzheimer's) — *see* Disease, Alzheimer's, early onset
  - primary, lateral G12.29
  - progressive, systemic M34.Ø
  - pulmonary — *see* Fibrosis, lung
    - artery I27.Ø
    - valve (heart) — *see* Endocarditis, pulmonary
  - renal N26.9
    - with
      - cystine storage disease E72.Ø9
      - hypertensive heart disease (conditions in I11) — *see* Hypertension, cardiorenal
    - arteriolar (hyaline) (hyperplastic) — *see* Hypertension, kidney
  - retina (senile) (vascular) H35.ØØ
  - senile (vascular) — *see* Arteriosclerosis
  - spinal (cord) (progressive) G95.89
    - ascending G61.Ø
    - combined (*see also* Degeneration, combined)
      - multiple G35
      - syphilitic A52.11
    - disseminated G35
    - dorsolateral — *see* Degeneration, combined
    - hereditary (Friedreich's) (mixed form) G11.1
    - lateral (amyotrophic) G12.21
    - multiple G35
    - posterior (syphilitic) A52.11
  - stomach K31.89
  - subendocardial, congenital I42.4
  - systemic M34.9
    - with
      - lung involvement M34.81
      - myopathy M34.82
      - polyneuropathy M34.83
    - drug-induced M34.2
    - due to chemicals NEC M34.2
    - progressive M34.Ø
    - specified NEC M34.89
  - temporal (mesial) G93.81
  - tricuspid (heart) (valve) IØ7.8
  - tuberous (brain) Q85.1
  - tympanic membrane — *see* Disorder, tympanic membrane, specified NEC
  - valve, valvular (heart) — *see* Endocarditis
  - vascular — *see* Arteriosclerosis
  - vein I87.8
- **Scoliosis** (acquired) (postural) M41.9
  - adolescent (idiopathic) — *see* Scoliosis, idiopathic, juvenile
  - congenital Q67.5
    - due to bony malformation Q76.3
    - failure of segmentation (hemivertebra) Q76.3
- **Scoliosis** — *continued*
  - congenital — *continued*
    - hemivertebra fusion Q76.3
    - postural Q67.5
  - idiopathic M41.2Ø
    - adolescent M41.129
      - cervical region M41.122
      - cervicothoracic region M41.123
      - lumbar region M41.126
      - lumbosacral region M41.127
      - thoracic region M41.124
      - thoracolumbar region M41.125
    - cervical region M41.22
    - cervicothoracic region M41.23
    - infantile M41.ØØ
      - cervical region M41.Ø2
      - cervicothoracic region M41.Ø3
      - lumbar region M41.Ø6
      - lumbosacral region M41.Ø7
      - sacrococcygeal region M41.Ø8
      - thoracic region M41.Ø4
      - thoracolumbar region M41.Ø5
    - juvenile M41.119
      - cervical region M41.112
      - cervicothoracic region M41.113
      - lumbar region M41.116
      - lumbosacral region M41.117
      - thoracic region M41.114
      - thoracolumbar region M41.115
    - lumbar region M41.26
    - lumbosacral region M41.27
    - thoracic region M41.24
    - thoracolumbar region M41.25
  - neuromuscular M41.4Ø
    - cervical region M41.42
    - cervicothoracic region M41.43
    - lumbar region M41.46
    - lumbosacral region M41.47
    - occipito-atlanto-axial region M41.41
    - thoracic region M41.44
    - thoracolumbar region M41.45
  - paralytic — *see* Scoliosis, neuromuscular
  - postradiation therapy M96.5
  - rachitic (late effect or sequelae) E64.3 [M49.8Ø]
    - cervical region E64.3 [M49.82]
    - cervicothoracic region E64.3 [M49.83]
    - lumbar region E64.3 [M49.86]
    - lumbosacral region E64.3 [M49.87]
    - multiple sites E64.3 [M49.89]
    - occipito-atlanto-axial region E64.3 [M49.81]
    - sacrococcygeal region E64.3 [M49.88]
    - thoracic region E64.3 [M49.84]
    - thoracolumbar region E64.3 [M49.85]
  - sciatic M54.4- ☑
  - secondary (to) NEC M41.5Ø
    - cerebral palsy, Friedreich's ataxia, poliomyelitis, neuromuscular disorders — *see* Scoliosis, neuromuscular
    - cervical region M41.52
    - cervicothoracic region M41.53
    - lumbar region M41.56
    - lumbosacral region M41.57
    - thoracic region M41.54
    - thoracolumbar region M41.55
  - specified form NEC M41.8Ø
    - cervical region M41.82
    - cervicothoracic region M41.83
    - lumbar region M41.86
    - lumbosacral region M41.87
    - thoracic region M41.84
    - thoracolumbar region M41.85
  - thoracogenic M41.3Ø
    - thoracic region M41.34
    - thoracolumbar region M41.35
  - tuberculous A18.Ø1
- **Scoliotic pelvis**
  - with disproportion (fetopelvic) O33.Ø
    - causing obstructed labor O65.Ø
- **Scorbutus, scorbutic** (*see also* Scurvy)
  - anemia D53.2
- **Scotoma** (arcuate) (Bjerrum) (central) (ring) (*see also* Defect, visual field, localized, scotoma)
  - scintillating H53.19
- **Scratch** — *see* Abrasion
- **Scratchy throat** RØ9.89
- **Screening** (for) Z13.9
  - alcoholism Z13.89
  - anemia Z13.Ø

- **Screening** — *continued*
  - anomaly, congenital Z13.89
  - antenatal, of mother Z36
  - arterial hypertension Z13.6
  - arthropod-borne viral disease NEC Z11.59
  - bacteriuria, asymptomatic Z13.89
  - behavioral disorder Z13.89
  - brain injury, traumatic Z13.85Ø
  - bronchitis, chronic Z13.83
  - brucellosis Z11.2
  - cardiovascular disorder Z13.6
  - cataract Z13.5
  - chlamydial diseases Z11.8
  - cholera Z11.Ø
  - chromosomal abnormalities (nonprocreative) NEC Z13.79
  - colonoscopy Z12.11
  - congenital
    - dislocation of hip Z13.89
    - eye disorder Z13.5
    - malformation or deformation Z13.89
  - contamination NEC Z13.88
  - cystic fibrosis Z13.228
  - dengue fever Z11.59
  - dental disorder Z13.84
  - depression Z13.89
  - developmental handicap Z13.4
    - in early childhood Z13.4
  - diabetes mellitus Z13.1
  - diphtheria Z11.2
  - disability, intellectual Z13.4
  - disease or disorder Z13.9
    - bacterial NEC Z11.2
      - intestinal infectious Z11.Ø
      - respiratory tuberculosis Z11.1
    - blood or blood-forming organ Z13.Ø
    - cardiovascular Z13.6
    - Chagas' Z11.6
    - chlamydial Z11.8
    - dental Z13.89
    - developmental Z13.4
    - digestive tract NEC Z13.818
      - lower GI Z13.811
      - upper GI Z13.81Ø
    - ear Z13.5
    - endocrine Z13.29
    - eye Z13.5
    - genitourinary Z13.89
    - heart Z13.6
    - human immunodeficiency virus (HIV) infection Z11.4
    - immunity Z13.Ø
    - infection
      - intestinal Z11.Ø
        - specified NEC Z11.6
    - infectious Z11.9
    - mental Z13.89
    - metabolic Z13.228
    - neurological Z13.89
    - nutritional Z13.21
      - metabolic Z13.228
        - lipoid disorders Z13.22Ø
    - protozoal Z11.6
      - intestinal Z11.Ø
    - respiratory Z13.83
    - rheumatic Z13.828
    - rickettsial Z11.8
    - sexually-transmitted NEC Z11.3
      - human immunodeficiency virus (HIV) Z11.4
    - sickle-cell (trait) Z13.Ø
    - skin Z13.89
    - specified NEC Z13.89
    - spirochetal Z11.8
    - thyroid Z13.29
    - vascular Z13.6
    - venereal Z11.3
    - viral NEC Z11.59
      - human immunodeficiency virus (HIV) Z11.4
      - intestinal Z11.Ø
  - elevated titer Z13.89
  - emphysema Z13.83
  - encephalitis, viral (mosquito- or tick-borne) Z11.59
  - exposure to contaminants (toxic) Z13.88
  - fever
    - dengue Z11.59
    - hemorrhagic Z11.59
    - yellow Z11.59
  - filariasis Z11.6

- **Screening** — *continued*
  - galactosemia Z13.228
  - gastrointestinal condition Z13.818
  - genetic (nonprocreative) - for procreative management — *see* Testing, genetic, for procreative management
    - disease carrier status (nonprocreative) Z13.71
    - specified NEC (nonprocreative) Z13.79
  - genitourinary condition Z13.89
  - glaucoma Z13.5
  - gonorrhea Z11.3
  - gout Z13.89
  - helminthiasis (intestinal) Z11.6
  - hematopoietic malignancy Z12.89
  - hemoglobinopathies NEC Z13.Ø
  - hemorrhagic fever Z11.59
  - Hodgkin disease Z12.89
  - human immunodeficiency virus (HIV) Z11.4
  - human papillomavirus Z11.51
  - hypertension Z13.6
  - immunity disorders Z13.Ø
  - infection
    - mycotic Z11.8
    - parasitic Z11.8
  - ingestion of radioactive substance Z13.88
  - intellectual disability Z13.4
  - intestinal
    - helminthiasis Z11.6
    - infectious disease Z11.Ø
  - leishmaniasis Z11.6
  - leprosy Z11.2
  - leptospirosis Z11.8
  - leukemia Z12.89
  - lymphoma Z12.89
  - malaria Z11.6
  - malnutrition Z13.29
    - metabolic Z13.228
    - nutritional Z13.21
  - measles Z11.59
  - mental disorder Z13.89
  - metabolic errors, inborn Z13.228
  - multiphasic Z13.89
  - musculoskeletal disorder Z13.828
    - osteoporosis Z13.82Ø
  - mycoses Z11.8
  - myocardial infarction (acute) Z13.6
  - neoplasm (malignant) (of) Z12.9
    - bladder Z12.6
    - blood Z12.89
    - breast Z12.39
      - routine mammogram Z12.31
    - cervix Z12.4
    - colon Z12.11
    - genitourinary organs NEC Z12.79
      - bladder Z12.6
      - cervix Z12.4
      - ovary Z12.73
      - prostate Z12.5
      - testis Z12.71
      - vagina Z12.72
    - hematopoietic system Z12.89
    - intestinal tract Z12.1Ø
      - colon Z12.11
      - rectum Z12.12
      - small intestine Z12.13
    - lung Z12.2
    - lymph (glands) Z12.89
    - nervous system Z12.82
    - oral cavity Z12.81
    - prostate Z12.5
    - rectum Z12.12
    - respiratory organs Z12.2
    - skin Z12.83
    - small intestine Z12.13
    - specified site NEC Z12.89
    - stomach Z12.Ø
  - nephropathy Z13.89
  - nervous system disorders NEC Z13.858
  - neurological condition Z13.89
  - osteoporosis Z13.82Ø
  - parasitic infestation Z11.9
    - specified NEC Z11.8
  - phenylketonuria Z13.228
  - plague Z11.2
  - poisoning (chemical) (heavy metal) Z13.88
  - poliomyelitis Z11.59
  - postnatal, chromosomal abnormalities Z13.89
  - prenatal, of mother Z36

- **Screening** — *continued*
  - protozoal disease Z11.6
    - intestinal Z11.Ø
  - pulmonary tuberculosis Z11.1
  - radiation exposure Z13.88
  - respiratory condition Z13.83
  - respiratory tuberculosis Z11.1
  - rheumatoid arthritis Z13.828
  - rubella Z11.59
  - schistosomiasis Z11.6
  - sexually-transmitted disease NEC Z11.3
    - human immunodeficiency virus (HIV) Z11.4
  - sickle-cell disease or trait Z13.Ø
  - skin condition Z13.89
  - sleeping sickness Z11.6
  - special Z13.9
    - specified NEC Z13.89
  - syphilis Z11.3
  - tetanus Z11.2
  - trachoma Z11.8
  - traumatic brain injury Z13.85Ø
  - trypanosomiasis Z11.6
  - tuberculosis, respiratory Z11.1
  - venereal disease Z11.3
  - viral encephalitis (mosquito- or tick-borne) Z11.59
  - whooping cough Z11.2
  - worms, intestinal Z11.6
  - yaws Z11.8
  - yellow fever Z11.59
- **Scrofula, scrofulosis** (tuberculosis of cervical lymph glands) A18.2
- **Scrofulide** (primary) (tuberculous) A18.4
- **Scrofuloderma, scrofulodermia** (any site) (primary) A18.4
- **Scrofulosus lichen** (primary) (tuberculous) A18.4
- **Scrofulous** — *see* condition
- **Scrotal tongue** K14.5
- **Scrotum** — *see* condition
- **Scurvy, scorbutic** E54
  - anemia D53.2
  - gum E54
  - infantile E54
  - rickets E55.Ø [M9Ø.8Ø]
- **Sealpox** BØ8.62
- **Seasickness** T75.3 ☑
- **Seatworm** (infection) (infestation) B8Ø
- **Sebaceous** (*see also* condition)
  - cyst — *see* Cyst, sebaceous
- **Seborrhea, seborrheic** L21.9
  - capillitii R23.8
  - capitis L21.Ø
  - dermatitis L21.9
    - infantile L21.1
  - eczema L21.9
    - infantile L21.1
  - sicca L21.Ø
- **Seckel's syndrome** Q87.1
- **Seclusion, pupil** — *see* Membrane, pupillary
- **Second hand tobacco smoke exposure** (acute) (chronic) Z77.22
  - in the perinatal period P96.81
- **Secondary**
  - dentin (in pulp) KØ4.3
  - neoplasm, secondaries — *see* Table of Neoplasms, secondary
- **Secretion**
  - antidiuretic hormone, inappropriate E22.2
  - catecholamine, by pheochromocytoma E27.5
  - hormone
    - antidiuretic, inappropriate (syndrome) E22.2
    - by
      - carcinoid tumor E34.Ø
      - pheochromocytoma E27.5
    - ectopic NEC E34.2
  - urinary
    - excessive R35.8
    - suppression R34
- **Section**
  - nerve, traumatic — *see* Injury, nerve
- **Segmentation, incomplete** (congenital) (*see also* Fusion)
  - bone NEC Q78.8
  - lumbosacral (joint) (vertebra) Q76.49
- **Seitelberger's syndrome** (infantile neuraxonal dystrophy) G31.89
- **Seizure(s)** (*see also* Convulsions) R56.9
  - akinetic — *see* Epilepsy, generalized, specified NEC
  - atonic — *see* Epilepsy, generalized, specified NEC

Seizure(s) — *continued*
- autonomic (hysterical) F44.5
- convulsive — *see* Convulsions
- cortical (focal) (motor) — *see* Epilepsy, localization-related, symptomatic, with simple partial seizures
- disorder (*see also* Epilepsy) G4Ø.9Ø9
- due to stroke — *see* Sequelae (of), disease, cerebrovascular, by type, specified NEC
- epileptic — *see* Epilepsy
- febrile (simple) R56.ØØ
  - with status epilepticus G4Ø.9Ø1
  - complex (atypical) (complicated) R56.Ø1
    - with status epilepticus G4Ø.9Ø1
- grand mal G4Ø.4Ø9
  - intractable G4Ø.419
    - with status epilepticus G4Ø.411
    - without status epilepticus G4Ø.419
  - not intractable G4Ø.4Ø9
    - with status epilepticus G4Ø.4Ø1
    - without status epilepticus G4Ø.4Ø9
- heart — *see* Disease, heart
- hysterical F44.5
- intractable G4Ø.919
  - with status epilepticus G4Ø.911
- Jacksonian (focal) (motor type) (sensory type) — *see* Epilepsy, localization-related, symptomatic, with simple partial seizures
- newborn P9Ø
- nonspecific epileptic
  - atonic — *see* Epilepsy, generalized, specified NEC
  - clonic — *see* Epilepsy, generalized, specified NEC
  - myoclonic — *see* Epilepsy, generalized, specified NEC
  - tonic — *see* Epilepsy, generalized, specified NEC
  - tonic-clonic — *see* Epilepsy, generalized, specified NEC
- partial, developing into secondarily generalized seizures
  - complex — *see* Epilepsy, localization-related, symptomatic, with complex partial seizures
  - simple — *see* Epilepsy, localization-related, symptomatic, with simple partial seizures
- petit mal G4Ø.4Ø9
  - intractable G4Ø.419
    - with status epilepticus G4Ø.411
    - without status epilepticus G4Ø.419
  - not intractable G4Ø.4Ø9
    - with status epilepticus G4Ø.4Ø1
    - without status epilepticus G4Ø.4Ø9
- post traumatic R56.1
- recurrent G4Ø.9Ø9
- specified NEC G4Ø.89
- uncinate — *see* Epilepsy, localization-related, symptomatic, with complex partial seizures

Selenium deficiency, dietary E59

Self-damaging behavior (life-style) Z72.89

Self-harm (attempted)
- history (personal) Z91.5
  - in family Z81.8

Self-mutilation (attempted)
- history (personal) Z91.5
  - in family Z81.8

Self-poisoning
- history (personal) Z91.5
  - in family Z81.8
- observation following (alleged) attempt ZØ3.6

Semicoma R4Ø.1

Seminal vesiculitis N49.Ø

Seminoma C62.9- ☑
- specified site — *see* Neoplasm, malignant, by site

Senear-Usher disease or syndrome L1Ø.4

Senectus R54

Senescence (without mention of psychosis) R54

Senile, senility (*see also* condition) R41.81
- with
  - acute confusional state FØ5
  - mental changes NOS FØ3 ☑
  - psychosis NEC — *see* Psychosis, senile
- asthenia R54
- cervix (atrophic) N88.8
- debility R54
- endometrium (atrophic) N85.8
- fallopian tube (atrophic) — *see* Atrophy, fallopian tube
- heart (failure) R54
- ovary (atrophic) — *see* Atrophy, ovary
- premature E34.8

Senile, senility — *continued*
- vagina, vaginitis (atrophic) N95.2
- wart L82.1

Sensation
- burning (skin) R2Ø.8
  - tongue K14.6
- loss of R2Ø.8
- prickling (skin) R2Ø.2
- tingling (skin) R2Ø.2

Sense loss
- smell — *see* Disturbance, sensation, smell
- taste — *see* Disturbance, sensation, taste
- touch R2Ø.8

Sensibility disturbance (cortical) (deep) (vibratory) R2Ø.9

Sensitive, sensitivity (*see also* Allergy)
- carotid sinus G9Ø.Ø1
- child (excessive) F93.8
- cold, autoimmune D59.1
- dentin KØ3.89
- latex Z91.Ø4Ø
- methemoglobin D74.8
- tuberculin, without clinical or radiological symptoms R76.11
- visual
  - glare H53.71
  - impaired contrast H53.72

Sensitiver Beziehungswahn F22

Sensitization, auto-erythrocytic D69.2

Separation
- anxiety, abnormal (of childhood) F93.Ø
- apophysis, traumatic — *code as* Fracture, by site
- choroid — *see* Detachment, choroid
- epiphysis, epiphyseal
  - nontraumatic (*see also* Osteochondropathy, specified type NEC)
    - upper femoral — *see* Slipped, epiphysis, upper femoral
  - traumatic — *code as* Fracture, by site
- fracture — *see* Fracture
- infundibulum cardiac from right ventricle by a partition Q24.3
- joint (traumatic) (current) — *code by* site under Dislocation
- pubic bone, obstetrical trauma O71.6
- retina, retinal — *see* Detachment, retina
- symphysis pubis, obstetrical trauma O71.6
- tracheal ring, incomplete, congenital Q32.1

Sepsis (generalized) (unspecified organism) A41.9
- with
  - organ dysfunction (acute) (multiple) R65.2Ø
    - with septic shock R65.21
- actinomycotic A42.7
- adrenal hemorrhage syndrome (meningococcal) A39.1
- anaerobic A41.4
- Bacillus anthracis A22.7
- Brucella (*see also* Brucellosis) A23.9
- candidal B37.7
- cryptogenic A41.9
- due to device, implant or graft T85.79 ☑
  - arterial graft NEC T82.7 ☑
  - breast (implant) T85.79 ☑
  - catheter NEC T85.79 ☑
    - dialysis (renal) T82.7 ☑
      - intraperitoneal T85.71 ☑
    - infusion NEC T82.7 ☑
      - spinal (epidural) (subdural) T85.79 ☑
    - urinary (indwelling) T83.51 ☑
  - ectopic or molar pregnancy OØ8.82
  - electronic (electrode) (pulse generator) (stimulator)
    - bone T84.7 ☑
    - cardiac T82.7 ☑
    - nervous system (brain) (peripheral nerve) (spinal) T85.79 ☑
    - urinary T83.59 ☑
  - fixation, internal (orthopedic) — *see* Complication, fixation device, infection
  - gastrointestinal (bile duct) (esophagus) T85.79 ☑
  - genital T83.6 ☑
  - heart NEC T82.7 ☑
    - valve (prosthesis) T82.6 ☑
      - graft T82.7 ☑
  - joint prosthesis — *see* Complication, joint prosthesis, infection
  - ocular (corneal graft) (orbital implant) T85.79 ☑
  - orthopedic NEC T84.7 ☑

Sepsis — *continued*
- due to device, implant or graft — *continued*
  - orthopedic — *continued*
    - fixation device, internal — *see* Complication, fixation device, infection
    - specified NEC T85.79 ☑
  - vascular T82.7 ☑
  - ventricular intracranial shunt T85.79 ☑
- during labor O75.3
- Enterococcus A41.81
- Erysipelothrix (rhusiopathiae) (erysipeloid) A26.7
- Escherichia coli (E. coli) A41.5 ☑
- extraintestinal yersiniosis A28.2
- following
  - abortion (subsequent episode) OØ8.Ø
    - current episode — *see* Abortion
  - ectopic or molar pregnancy OØ8.82
  - immunization T88.Ø ☑
  - infusion, therapeutic injection or transfusion NEC T8Ø.29 ☑
- gangrenous A41.9
- gonococcal A54.86
- Gram-negative (organism) A41.5 ☑
  - anaerobic A41.4
- Haemophilus influenzae A41.3
- herpesviral BØØ.7
- intra-abdominal K65.1
- intraocular — *see* Endophthalmitis, purulent
- Listeria monocytogenes A32.7
- localized — *code to* specific localized infection
  - in operation wound T81.4 ☑
  - skin — *see* Abscess
- malleus A24.Ø
- melioidosis A24.1
- meningeal — *see* Meningitis
- meningococcal A39.4
  - acute A39.2
  - chronic A39.3
- MSSA (Methicillin susceptible Staphylococcus aureus) A41.Ø1
- newborn P36.9
  - due to
    - anaerobes NEC P36.5
    - Escherichia coli P36.4
    - Staphylococcus P36.3Ø
      - aureus P36.2
      - specified NEC P36.39
    - Streptococcus P36.1Ø
      - group B P36.Ø
      - specified NEC P36.19
  - specified NEC P36.8
- Pasteurella multocida A28.Ø
- pelvic, puerperal, postpartum, childbirth O85
- pneumococcal A4Ø.3
- postprocedural T81.4 ☑
- puerperal, postpartum, childbirth (pelvic) O85
- Salmonella (arizonae) (cholerae-suis) (enteritidis) (typhimurium) AØ2.1
- severe R65.2Ø
  - with septic shock R65.21
- Shigella (*see also* Dysentery, bacillary) AØ3.9
- skin, localized — *see* Abscess
- specified organism NEC A41.89
- Staphylococcus, staphylococcal A41.2
  - aureus (methicillin susceptible) (MSSA) A41.Ø1
    - methicillin resistant (MRSA) A41.Ø2
  - coagulase-negative A41.1
  - specified NEC A41.1
- Streptococcus, streptococcal A4Ø.9
  - agalactiae A4Ø.1
  - group
    - A A4Ø.Ø
    - B A4Ø.1
    - D A41.81
  - neonatal P36.1Ø
    - group B P36.Ø
    - specified NEC P36.19
  - pneumoniae A4Ø.3
  - pyogenes A4Ø.Ø
  - specified NEC A4Ø.8
- tracheostomy stoma J95.Ø2
- tularemic A21.7
- umbilical, umbilical cord (newborn) — *see* Sepsis, newborn
- Yersinia pestis A2Ø.7

Septate — *see* Septum

Septic — *see* condition
- arm — *see* Cellulitis, upper limb

- **Septic** — *continued*
  - arm — *see* Cellulitis, upper limb — *continued*
    - with lymphangitis — *see* Lymphangitis, acute, upper limb
  - embolus — *see* Embolism
  - finger — *see* Cellulitis, digit
    - with lymphangitis — *see* Lymphangitis, acute, digit
  - foot — *see* Cellulitis, lower limb
    - with lymphangitis — *see* Lymphangitis, acute, lower limb
  - gallbladder (acute) K81.Ø
  - hand — *see* Cellulitis, upper limb
    - with lymphangitis — *see* Lymphangitis, acute, upper limb
  - joint — *see* Arthritis, pyogenic or pyemic
  - leg — *see* Cellulitis, lower limb
    - with lymphangitis — *see* Lymphangitis, acute, lower limb
  - nail (*see also* Cellulitis, digit)
    - with lymphangitis — *see* Lymphangitis, acute, digit
  - sore (*see also* Abscess)
    - throat JØ2.Ø
      - streptococcal JØ2.Ø
  - spleen (acute) D73.89
  - teeth, tooth (pulpal origin) KØ4.4
  - throat — *see* Pharyngitis
  - thrombus — *see* Thrombosis
  - toe — *see* Cellulitis, digit
    - with lymphangitis — *see* Lymphangitis, acute, digit
  - tonsils, chronic J35.Ø1
    - with adenoiditis J35.Ø3
  - uterus — *see* Endometritis
- **Septicemia** A41.9
  - meaning sepsis — *see* Sepsis
- **Septum, septate** (congenital) (*see also* Anomaly, by site)
  - anal Q42.3
    - with fistula Q42.2
  - aqueduct of Sylvius QØ3.Ø
    - with spina bifida — *see* Spina bifida, by site, with hydrocephalus
  - uterus (complete) (partial) Q51.2
  - vagina Q52.1Ø
    - in pregnancy — *see* Pregnancy, complicated by, abnormal vagina
      - causing obstructed labor O65.5
    - longitudinal (with or without obstruction) Q52.12
    - transverse Q52.11
- **Sequelae** (of) (*see also* condition)
  - abscess, intracranial or intraspinal (conditions in GØ6) GØ9
  - amputation — *code to* injury with seventh character S
  - burn and corrosion — *code to* injury with seventh character S
  - calcium deficiency E64.8
  - cerebrovascular disease — *see* Sequelae, disease, cerebrovascular
  - childbirth O94
  - contusion — *code to* injury with seventh character S
  - corrosion — *see* Sequelae, burn and corrosion
  - crushing injury — *code to* injury with seventh character S
  - disease
    - cerebrovascular I69.9Ø
      - alteration of sensation I69.998
      - aphasia I69.92Ø
      - apraxia I69.99Ø
      - ataxia I69.993
      - cognitive deficits I69.91
      - disturbance of vision I69.998
      - dysarthria I69.922
      - dysphagia I69.991
      - dysphasia I69.921
      - facial droop I69.992
      - facial weakness I69.992
      - fluency disorder I69.923
      - hemiplegia I69.95- ☑
      - hemorrhage
        - intracerebral — *see* Sequelae, hemorrhage, intracerebral
        - intracranial, nontraumatic NEC — *see* Sequelae, hemorrhage, intracranial, nontraumatic

- **Sequelae** — *continued*
  - disease — *continued*
    - cerebrovascular — *continued*
      - hemorrhage — *continued*
        - subarachnoid — *see* Sequelae, hemorrhage, subarachnoid
      - language deficit I69.928
      - monoplegia
        - lower limb I69.84- ☑
        - upper limb I69.93- ☑
      - paralytic syndrome I69.96- ☑
      - specified effect NEC I69.998
      - specified type NEC I69.8Ø
        - alteration of sensation I69.898
        - aphasia I69.82Ø
        - apraxia I69.89Ø
        - ataxia I69.893
        - cognitive deficits I69.81
        - disturbance of vision I69.898
        - dysarthria I69.822
        - dysphagia I69.891
        - dysphasia I69.821
        - facial droop I69.892
        - facial weakness I69.892
        - fluency disorder I69.823
        - hemiplegia I69.85- ☑
        - language deficit I69.828
        - monoplegia
          - lower limb I69.84- ☑
          - upper limb I69.83- ☑
        - paralytic syndrome I69.86- ☑
        - specified effect NEC I69.898
      - speech deficit I69.928
        - speech deficit I69.828
      - stroke NOS — *see* Sequelae, stroke NOS
  - dislocation — *code to* injury with seventh character S
  - encephalitis or encephalomyelitis (conditions in GØ4) GØ9
    - in infectious disease NEC B94.8
    - viral B94.1
  - external cause — *code to* injury with seventh character S
  - foreign body entering natural orifice — *code to* injury with seventh character S
  - fracture — *code to* injury with seventh character S
  - frostbite — *code to* injury with seventh character S
  - Hansen's disease B92
  - hemorrhage
    - intracerebral I69.1Ø
      - alteration of sensation I69.198
      - aphasia I69.12Ø
      - apraxia I69.19Ø
      - ataxia I69.193
      - cognitive deficits I69.11
      - disturbance of vision I69.198
      - dysarthria I69.122
      - dysphagia I69.191
      - dysphasia I69.121
      - facial droop I69.192
      - facial weakness I69.192
      - fluency disorder I69.123
      - hemiplegia I69.15- ☑
      - language deficit NEC I69.128
      - monoplegia
        - lower limb I69.14- ☑
        - upper limb I69.13- ☑
      - paralytic syndrome I69.16- ☑
      - specified effect NEC I69.198
      - speech deficit NEC I69.128
    - intracranial, nontraumatic NEC I69.2Ø
      - alteration of sensation I69.298
      - aphasia I69.22Ø
      - apraxia I69.29Ø
      - ataxia I69.293
      - cognitive deficits I69.21
      - disturbance of vision I69.298
      - dysarthria I69.222
      - dysphagia I69.291
      - dysphasia I69.221
      - facial droop I69.292
      - facial weakness I69.292
      - fluency disorder I69.223
      - hemiplegia I69.25- ☑
      - language deficit NEC I69.228
      - monoplegia
        - lower limb I69.24- ☑
        - upper limb I69.23- ☑
      - paralytic syndrome I69.26- ☑

- **Sequelae** — *continued*
  - hemorrhage — *continued*
    - intracranial, nontraumatic — *continued*
      - specified effect NEC I69.298
      - speech deficit NEC I69.228
    - subarachnoid I69.ØØ
      - alteration of sensation I69.Ø98
      - aphasia I69.Ø2Ø
      - apraxia I69.Ø9Ø
      - ataxia I69.Ø93
      - cognitive deficits I69.Ø1
      - disturbance of vision I69.Ø98
      - dysarthria I69.Ø22
      - dysphagia I69.Ø91
      - dysphasia I69.Ø21
      - facial droop I69.Ø92
      - facial weakness I69.Ø92
      - fluency disorder I69.Ø23
      - hemiplegia I69.Ø5- ☑
      - language deficit NEC I69.Ø28
      - monoplegia
        - lower limb I69.Ø4- ☑
        - upper limb I69.Ø3- ☑
      - paralytic syndrome I69.Ø6- ☑
      - specified effect NEC I69.Ø98
      - speech deficit NEC I69.Ø28
  - hepatitis, viral B94.2
  - hyperalimentation E68
  - infarction
    - cerebral I69.3Ø
      - alteration of sensation I69.398
      - aphasia I69.32Ø
      - apraxia I69.39Ø
      - ataxia I69.393
      - cognitive deficits I69.31
      - disturbance of vision I69.398
      - dysarthria I69.322
      - dysphagia I69.391
      - dysphasia I69.321
      - facial droop I69.392
      - facial weakness I69.392
      - fluency disorder I69.323
      - hemiplegia I69.35- ☑
      - language deficit NEC I69.328
      - monoplegia
        - lower limb I69.34- ☑
        - upper limb I69.33- ☑
      - paralytic syndrome I69.36- ☑
      - specified effect NEC I69.398
      - speech deficit NEC I69.328
  - infection, pyogenic, intracranial or intraspinal GØ9
  - infectious disease B94.9
    - specified NEC B94.8
  - injury — *code to* injury with seventh character S
  - leprosy B92
  - meningitis
    - bacterial (conditions in GØØ) GØ9
    - other or unspecified cause (conditions in GØ3) GØ9
  - muscle (and tendon) injury — *code to* injury with seventh character S
  - myelitis — *see* Sequelae, encephalitis
  - niacin deficiency E64.8
  - nutritional deficiency E64.9
    - specified NEC E64.8
  - obstetrical condition O94
  - parasitic disease B94.9
  - phlebitis or thrombophlebitis of intracranial or intraspinal venous sinuses and veins (conditions in GØ8) GØ9
  - poisoning — *code to* poisoning with seventh character S
    - nonmedicinal substance — *see* Sequelae, toxic effect, nonmedicinal substance
  - poliomyelitis (acute) B91
  - pregnancy O94
  - protein-energy malnutrition E64.Ø
  - puerperium O94
  - rickets E64.3
  - selenium deficiency E64.8
  - sprain and strain — *code to* injury with seventh character S
  - stroke NOS I69.3Ø
    - alteration in sensation I69.398
    - aphasia I69.32Ø
    - apraxia I69.39Ø
    - ataxia I69.393
    - cognitive deficits I69.31
    - disturbance of vision I69.398

- **Sequelae** — *continued*
  - stroke — *continued*
    - dysarthria I69.322
    - dysphagia I69.391
    - dysphasia I69.321
    - facial droop I69.392
    - facial weakness I69.392
    - hemiplegia I69.35- ☑
    - language deficit NEC I69.328
    - monoplegia
      - lower limb I69.34- ☑
      - upper limb I69.33- ☑
    - paralytic syndrome I69.36- ☑
    - specified effect NEC I69.398
    - speech deficit NEC I69.328
  - tendon and muscle injury — *code to* injury with seventh character S
  - thiamine deficiency E64.8
  - trachoma B94.Ø
  - tuberculosis B9Ø.9
    - bones and joints B9Ø.2
    - central nervous system B9Ø.Ø
    - genitourinary B9Ø.1
    - pulmonary (respiratory) B9Ø.9
    - specified organs NEC B9Ø.8
  - viral
    - encephalitis B94.1
    - hepatitis B94.2
  - vitamin deficiency NEC E64.8
    - A E64.1
    - B E64.8
    - C E64.2
  - wound, open — *code to* injury with seventh character S
- **Sequestration** (*see also* Sequestrum)
  - lung, congenital Q33.2
- **Sequestrum**
  - bone — *see* Osteomyelitis, chronic
  - dental M27.2
  - jaw bone M27.2
  - orbit — *see* Osteomyelitis, orbit
  - sinus (accessory) (nasal) — *see* Sinusitis
- **Sequoiosis lung or pneumonitis** J67.8
- **Serology for syphilis**
  - doubtful
    - with signs or symptoms — *code by* site and stage under Syphilis
    - follow-up of latent syphilis — *see* Syphilis, latent
  - negative, with signs or symptoms — *code by* site and stage under Syphilis
  - positive A53.Ø
    - with signs or symptoms — *code by* site and stage under Syphilis
  - reactivated A53.Ø
- **Seroma** (*see also* Hematoma)
  - traumatic, secondary and recurrent T79.2 ☑
- **Seropurulent** — *see* condition
- **Serositis, multiple** K65.8
  - pericardial I31.1
  - peritoneal K65.8
- **Serous** — *see* condition
- **Sertoli cell**
  - adenoma
    - specified site — *see* Neoplasm, benign, by site
    - unspecified site
      - female D27.9
      - male D29.2Ø
  - carcinoma
    - specified site — *see* Neoplasm, malignant, by site
    - unspecified site (male) C62.9- ☑
      - female C56.9
  - tumor
    - with lipid storage
      - specified site — *see* Neoplasm, benign, by site
      - unspecified site
        - female D27.9
        - male D29.2Ø
    - specified site — *see* Neoplasm, benign, by site
    - unspecified site
      - female D27.9
      - male D29.2Ø
- **Sertoli-Leydig cell tumor** — *see* Neoplasm, benign, by site
  - specified site — *see* Neoplasm, benign, by site
  - unspecified site
    - female D27.9
    - male D29.2Ø
- **Serum**
  - allergy, allergic reaction (*see also* Reaction, serum) T8Ø.69 ☑
    - shock (*see also* Shock, anaphylactic) T8Ø.59 ☑
  - arthritis (*see also* Reaction, serum) T8Ø.69 ☑
  - complication or reaction NEC (*see also* Reaction, serum) T8Ø.69 ☑
  - disease NEC (*see also* Reaction, serum) T8Ø.69 ☑
  - hepatitis (*see also* Hepatitis, viral, type B)
    - carrier (suspected) of Z22.51
  - intoxication (*see also* Reaction, serum) T8Ø.69 ☑
  - neuritis (*see also* Reaction, serum) T8Ø.69 ☑
  - neuropathy G61.1
  - poisoning NEC (*see also* Reaction, serum) T8Ø.69 ☑
  - rash NEC (*see also* Reaction, serum) T8Ø.69 ☑
  - reaction NEC (*see also* Reaction, serum) T8Ø.69 ☑
  - sickness NEC (*see also* Reaction, serum) T8Ø.69 ☑
  - urticaria (*see also* Reaction, serum) T8Ø.69 ☑
- **Sesamoiditis** M25.8- ☑
- **Severe sepsis** R65.2Ø
  - with septic shock R65.21
- **Sever's disease or osteochondrosis** — *see* Osteochondrosis, juvenile, tarsus
- **Sex**
  - chromosome mosaics Q97.8
    - lines with various numbers of X chromosomes Q97.2
  - education Z7Ø.8
  - reassignment surgery status Z87.89Ø
- **Sextuplet pregnancy** — *see* Pregnancy, sextuplet
- **Sexual**
  - function, disorder of (psychogenic) F52.9
  - immaturity (female) (male) E3Ø.Ø
  - impotence (psychogenic) organic origin NEC — *see* Dysfunction, sexual, male
  - precocity (constitutional) (cryptogenic)(female) (idiopathic) (male) E3Ø.1
- **Sexuality, pathologic** — *see* Deviation, sexual
- **Sézary disease** C84.1- ☑
- **Shadow, lung** R91.8
- **Shaking palsy or paralysis** — *see* Parkinsonism
- **Shallowness, acetabulum** — *see* Derangement, joint, specified type NEC, hip
- **Shaver's disease** J63.1
- **Sheath** (tendon) — *see* condition
- **Sheathing, retinal vessels** H35.Ø1- ☑
- **Shedding**
  - nail L6Ø.8
  - premature, primary (deciduous) teeth KØØ.6
- **Sheehan's disease or syndrome** E23.Ø
- **Shelf, rectal** K62.89
- **Shell teeth** KØØ.5
- **Shellshock** (current) F43.Ø
  - lasting state — *see* Disorder, post-traumatic stress
- **Shield kidney** Q63.1
- **Shift**
  - auditory threshold (temporary) H93.24- ☑
  - mediastinal R93.8
- **Shifting sleep-work schedule** (affecting sleep) G47.26
- **Shiga** (-Kruse) **dysentery** AØ3.Ø
- **Shiga's bacillus** AØ3.Ø
- **Shigella** (dysentery) — *see* Dysentery, bacillary
- **Shigellosis** AØ3.9
  - Group A AØ3.Ø
  - Group B AØ3.1
  - Group C AØ3.2
  - Group D AØ3.3
- **Shin splints** S86.89- ☑
- **Shingles** — *see* Herpes, zoster
- **Shipyard disease or eye** B3Ø.Ø
- **Shirodkar suture, in pregnancy** — *see* Pregnancy, complicated by, incompetent cervix
- **Shock** R57.9
  - with ectopic or molar pregnancy OØ8.3
  - adrenal (cortical) (Addisonian) E27.2
  - adverse food reaction (anaphylactic) — *see* Shock, anaphylactic, due to food
  - allergic — *see* Shock, anaphylactic
  - anaphylactic T78.2 ☑
    - chemical — *see* Table of Drugs and Chemicals
    - due to drug or medicinal substance
      - correct substance properly administered T88.6 ☑
      - overdose or wrong substance given or taken (by accident) — *see* Table of Drugs and Chemicals, by drug, poisoning
- **Shock** — *continued*
  - anaphylactic — *continued*
    - due to food (nonpoisonous) T78.ØØ ☑
      - additives T78.Ø6 ☑
      - dairy products T78.Ø7 ☑
      - eggs T78.Ø8 ☑
      - fish T78.Ø3 ☑
        - shellfish T78.Ø2 ☑
      - fruit T78.Ø4 ☑
      - milk T78.Ø7 ☑
      - nuts T78.Ø5 ☑
        - peanuts T78.Ø1 ☑
      - peanuts T78.Ø1 ☑
      - seeds T78.Ø5 ☑
      - specified type NEC T78.Ø9 ☑
      - vegetable T78.Ø4 ☑
    - following sting(s) — *see* Venom
    - immunization T8Ø.52 ☑
    - serum T8Ø.59 ☑
      - blood and blood products T8Ø.51 ☑
      - immunization T8Ø.52 ☑
      - specified NEC T8Ø.59 ☑
      - vaccination T8Ø.52 ☑
  - anaphylactoid — *see* Shock, anaphylactic
  - anesthetic
    - correct substance properly administered T88.2 ☑
    - overdose or wrong substance given or taken — *see* Table of Drugs and Chemicals, by drug, poisoning
    - specified anesthetic — *see* Table of Drugs and Chemicals, by drug, poisoning
  - cardiogenic R57.Ø
  - chemical substance — *see* Table of Drugs and Chemicals
  - complicating ectopic or molar pregnancy OØ8.3
  - culture — *see* Disorder, adjustment
  - drug
    - due to correct substance properly administered T88.6 ☑
    - overdose or wrong substance given or taken (by accident) — *see* Table of Drugs and Chemicals, by drug, poisoning
  - during or after labor and delivery O75.1
  - electric T75.4 ☑
    - (taser) T75.4 ☑
  - endotoxic R65.21
    - postprocedural (during or resulting from a procedure, not elsewhere classified) T81.12 ☑
  - following
    - ectopic or molar pregnancy OØ8.3
    - injury (immediate) (delayed) T79.4 ☑
    - labor and delivery O75.1
  - food (anaphylactic) — *see* Shock, anaphylactic, due to food
  - from electroshock gun (taser) T75.4 ☑
  - gram-negative R65.21
    - postprocedural (during or resulting from a procedure, not elsewhere classified) T81.12 ☑
  - hematologic R57.8
  - hemorrhagic
    - surgery (intraoperative) (postoperative) T81.19 ☑
    - trauma T79.4 ☑
  - hypovolemic R57.1
    - surgical T81.19 ☑
    - traumatic T79.4 ☑
  - insulin E15
    - therapeutic misadventure — *see* subcategory T38.3 ☑
  - kidney N17.Ø
    - traumatic (following crushing) T79.5 ☑
  - lightning T75.Ø1 ☑
  - lung J8Ø
  - obstetric O75.1
    - with ectopic or molar pregnancy OØ8.3
    - following ectopic or molar pregnancy OØ8.3
  - pleural (surgical) T81.19 ☑
    - due to trauma T79.4 ☑
  - postprocedural (postoperative) T81.1Ø ☑
    - with ectopic or molar pregnancy OØ8.3
    - cardiogenic T81.11 ☑
    - endotoxic T81.12 ☑
    - following ectopic or molar pregnancy OØ8.3
    - gram-negative T81.12 ☑
    - hypovolemic T81.19 ☑
    - septic T81.12 ☑
    - specified type NEC T81.19 ☑

Sinusitis — *continued*
- involving more than one sinus but not pansinusitis J32.8
  - acute J01.80
    - recurrent J01.81
- maxillary J32.0
  - acute J01.00
    - recurrent J01.01
- sphenoidal J32.3
  - acute J01.30
    - recurrent J01.31
- tuberculous, any sinus A15.8

Sinusitis-bronchiectasis-situs inversus (syndrome) (triad) Q89.3
Sipple's syndrome E31.22
Sirenomelia (syndrome) Q87.2
Siriasis T67.0 ☑
Sirkari's disease B55.0
Siti A65
Situation, psychiatric F99
Situational
- disturbance (transient) — *see* Disorder, adjustment
  - acute F43.0
- maladjustment — *see* Disorder, adjustment
- reaction — *see* Disorder, adjustment
  - acute F43.0

Situs inversus or transversus (abdominalis) (thoracis) Q89.3
Sixth disease B08.20
- due to human herpesvirus 6 B08.21
- due to human herpesvirus 7 B08.22

Sjögren-Larsson syndrome Q87.1
Sjögren's syndrome or disease — *see* Sicca syndrome
Skeletal — *see* condition
Skene's gland — *see* condition
Skenitis — *see* Urethritis
Skerljevo A65
Skevas-Zerfus disease — *see* Toxicity, venom, marine animal, sea anemone
Skin (*see also* condition)
- clammy R23.1
- donor — *see* Donor, skin
- hidebound M35.9

Slate-dressers' or slate-miners' lung J62.8
Sleep
- apnea — *see* Apnea, sleep
- deprivation Z72.820
- disorder or disturbance G47.9
  - child F51.9
  - nonorganic origin F51.9
  - specified NEC G47.8
- disturbance G47.9
  - nonorganic origin F51.9
- drunkenness F51.9
- rhythm inversion G47.2- ☑
- terrors F51.4
- walking F51.3
  - hysterical F44.89

Sleep hygiene
- abuse Z72.821
- inadequate Z72.821
- poor Z72.821

Sleeping sickness — *see* Sickness, sleeping
Sleeplessness — *see* Insomnia
- menopausal N95.1

Sleep-wake schedule disorder G47.20
Slim disease (in HIV infection) B20
Slipped, slipping
- epiphysis (traumatic) (*see also* Osteochondropathy, specified type NEC)
  - capital femoral (traumatic)
    - acute (on chronic) S79.01- ☑
  - current traumatic — *code as* Fracture, by site
  - upper femoral (nontraumatic) M93.00- ☑
    - acute M93.01- ☑
      - on chronic M93.03- ☑
    - chronic M93.02- ☑
- intervertebral disc — *see* Displacement, intervertebral disc
- ligature, umbilical P51.8
- patella — *see* Disorder, patella, derangement NEC
- rib M89.8X8
- sacroiliac joint — *see* subcategory M53.2 ☑
- tendon — *see* Disorder, tendon
- ulnar nerve, nontraumatic — *see* Lesion, nerve, ulnar
- vertebra NEC — *see* Spondylolisthesis

Slocumb's syndrome E27.0
Sloughing (multiple) (phagedena) (skin) (*see also* Gangrene)
- abscess — *see* Abscess
- appendix K38.8
- fascia — *see* Disorder, soft tissue, specified type NEC
- scrotum N50.8
- tendon — *see* Disorder, tendon
- transplanted organ — *see* Rejection, transplant
- ulcer — *see* Ulcer, skin

Slow
- feeding, newborn P92.2
- flow syndrome, coronary I20.8
- heart (beat) R00.1

Slowing, urinary stream R39.19
Sluder's neuralgia (syndrome) G44.89
Slurred, slurring speech R47.81
Small (ness)
- for gestational age — *see* Small for dates
- introitus, vagina N89.6
- kidney (unknown cause) N27.9
  - bilateral N27.1
  - unilateral N27.0
- ovary (congenital) Q50.39
- pelvis
  - with disproportion (fetopelvic) O33.1
    - causing obstructed labor O65.1
- uterus N85.8
- white kidney N03.9

Small-and-light-for-dates — *see* Small for dates
Small-for-dates (infant) P05.10
- with weight of
  - 1000-1249 grams P05.14
  - 1250-1499 grams P05.15
  - 1500-1749 grams P05.16
  - 1750-1999 grams P05.17
  - 2000-2499 grams P05.18
  - 499 grams or less P05.11
  - 500-749 grams P05.12
  - 750-999 grams P05.13

Smallpox B03
Smearing, fecal R15.1
Smith-Lemli-Opitz syndrome E78.72
Smith's fracture S52.54- ☑
Smoker — *see* Dependence, drug, nicotine
Smoker's
- bronchitis J41.0
- cough J41.0
- palate K13.24
- throat J31.2
- tongue K13.24

Smoking
- passive Z77.22

Smothering spells R06.81
Snaggle teeth, tooth M26.39
Snapping
- finger — *see* Trigger finger
- hip — *see* Derangement, joint, specified type NEC, hip
  - involving the iliotiblial band M76.3- ☑
- knee — *see* Derangement, knee
  - involving the iliotiblial band M76.3- ☑

Sneddon-Wilkinson disease or syndrome (sub-corneal pustular dermatosis) L13.1
Sneezing (intractable) R06.7
Sniffing
- cocaine
  - abuse — *see* Abuse, drug, cocaine
  - dependence — *see* Dependence, drug, cocaine
- gasoline
  - abuse — *see* Abuse, drug, inhalant
  - dependence — *see* Dependence, drug, inhalant
- glue (airplane)
  - abuse — *see* Abuse, drug, inhalant
  - drug dependence — *see* Dependence, drug, inhalant

Sniffles
- newborn P28.89

Snoring R06.83
Snow blindness — *see* Photokeratitis
Snuffles (non-syphilitic) R06.5
- newborn P28.89
- syphilitic (infant) A50.05 [J99]

Social
- exclusion Z60.4
  - due to discrimination or persecution (perceived) Z60.5
- migrant Z59.0
  - acculturation difficulty Z60.3

Social — *continued*
- rejection Z60.4
  - due to discrimination or persecution Z60.5
- role conflict NEC Z73.5
- skills inadequacy NEC Z73.4
- transplantation Z60.3

Sodoku A25.0
Soemmerring's ring — *see* Cataract, secondary
Soft (*see also* condition)
- nails L60.3

Softening
- bone — *see* Osteomalacia
- brain (necrotic) (progressive) G93.89
  - congenital Q04.8
  - embolic I63.4 ☑
  - hemorrhagic — *see* Hemorrhage, intracranial, intracerebral
  - occlusive I63.5 ☑
  - thrombotic I63.3 ☑
- cartilage M94.2- ☑
  - patella M22.4- ☑
- cerebellar — *see* Softening, brain
- cerebral — *see* Softening, brain
- cerebrospinal — *see* Softening, brain
- myocardial, heart — *see* Degeneration, myocardial
- spinal cord G95.89
- stomach K31.89

Soldier's
- heart F45.8
- patches I31.0

Solitary
- cyst, kidney N28.1
- kidney, congenital Q60.0

Solvent abuse — *see* Abuse, drug, inhalant
- dependence — *see* Dependence, drug, inhalant

Somatization reaction, somatic reaction — *see* Disorder, somatoform
Somnambulism F51.3
- hysterical F44.89

Somnolence R40.0
- nonorganic origin F51.11

Sonne dysentery A03.3
Soor B37.0
Sore
- bed — *see* Ulcer, pressure, by site
- chiclero B55.1
- Delhi B55.1
- desert — *see* Ulcer, skin
- eye H57.1- ☑
- Lahore B55.1
- mouth K13.79
  - canker K12.0
- muscle M79.1
- Naga — *see* Ulcer, skin
- of skin — *see* Ulcer, skin
- oriental B55.1
- pressure — *see* Ulcer, pressure, by site
- skin L98.9
- soft A57
- throat (acute) (*see also* Pharyngitis)
  - with influenza, flu, or grippe — *see* Influenza, with, respiratory manifestations NEC
  - chronic J31.2
  - coxsackie (virus) B08.5
  - diphtheritic A36.0
  - herpesviral B00.2
  - influenzal — *see* Influenza, with, respiratory manifestations NEC
  - septic J02.0
  - streptococcal (ulcerative) J02.0
  - viral NEC J02.8
    - coxsackie B08.5
- tropical — *see* Ulcer, skin
- veldt — *see* Ulcer, skin

Soto's syndrome (cerebral gigantism) Q87.3
South African cardiomyopathy syndrome I42.8
Southeast Asian hemorrhagic fever A91
Spacing
- abnormal, tooth, teeth, fully erupted M26.30
- excessive, tooth, fully erupted M26.32

Spade-like hand (congenital) Q68.1
Spading nail L60.8
- congenital Q84.6

Spanish collar N47.1
Sparganosis B70.1
Spasm(s), spastic, spasticity (*see also* condition) R25.2
- accommodation — *see* Spasm, of accommodation

Spasm(s), spastic, spasticity — *continued*
- ampulla of Vater K83.4
- anus, ani (sphincter) (reflex) K59.4
  - psychogenic F45.8
- artery I73.9
  - cerebral G45.9
- Bell's G51.3
- bladder (sphincter, external or internal) N32.89
  - psychogenic F45.8
- bronchus, bronchiole J98.Ø1
- cardia K22.Ø
- cardiac I2Ø.1
- carpopedal — *see* Tetany
- cerebral (arteries) (vascular) G45.9
- cervix, complicating delivery O62.4
- ciliary body (of accommodation) — *see* Spasm, of accommodation
- colon K58.9
  - with diarrhea K58.Ø
  - psychogenic F45.8
- common duct K83.8
- compulsive — *see* Tic
- conjugate H51.8
- coronary (artery) I2Ø.1
- diaphragm (reflex) RØ6.6
  - epidemic B33.Ø
  - psychogenic F45.8
- duodenum K59.8
- epidemic diaphragmatic (transient) B33.Ø
- esophagus (diffuse) K22.4
  - psychogenic F45.8
- facial G51.3
- fallopian tube N83.8
- gastrointestinal (tract) K31.89
  - psychogenic F45.8
- glottis J38.5
  - hysterical F44.4
  - psychogenic F45.8
    - conversion reaction F44.4
  - reflex through recurrent laryngeal nerve J38.5
- habit — *see* Tic
- heart I2Ø.1
- hemifacial (clonic) G51.3
- hourglass — *see* Contraction, hourglass
- hysterical F44.4
- infantile — *see* Epilepsy, spasms
- inferior oblique, eye H51.8
- intestinal (*see also* Syndrome, irritable bowel) K58.9
  - psychogenic F45.8
- larynx, laryngeal J38.5
  - hysterical F44.4
  - psychogenic F45.8
    - conversion reaction F44.4
- levator palpebrae superioris — *see* Disorder, eyelid function
- muscle NEC M62.838
  - back M62.83Ø
- nerve, trigeminal G51.Ø
- nervous F45.8
- nodding F98.4
- occupational F48.8
- oculogyric H51.8
  - psychogenic F45.8
- of accommodation H52.53- ☑
- ophthalmic artery — *see* Occlusion, artery, retina
- perineal, female N94.89
- peroneo-extensor (*see also* Deformity, limb, flat foot)
- pharynx (reflex) J39.2
  - hysterical F45.8
  - psychogenic F45.8
- psychogenic F45.8
- pylorus NEC K31.3
  - adult hypertrophic K31.89
  - congenital or infantile Q4Ø.Ø
  - psychogenic F45.8
- rectum (sphincter) K59.4
  - psychogenic F45.8
- retinal (artery) — *see* Occlusion, artery, retina
- sigmoid (*see also* Syndrome, irritable bowel) K58.9
  - psychogenic F45.8
- sphincter of Oddi K83.4
- stomach K31.89
  - neurotic F45.8
- throat J39.2
  - hysterical F45.8
  - psychogenic F45.8
- tic F95.9
  - chronic F95.1

Spasm(s), spastic, spasticity — *continued*
- tic — *continued*
  - transient of childhood F95.Ø
- tongue K14.8
- torsion (progressive) G24.1
- trigeminal nerve — *see* Neuralgia, trigeminal
- ureter N13.5
- urethra (sphincter) N35.9
- uterus N85.8
  - complicating labor O62.4
- vagina N94.2
  - psychogenic F52.5
- vascular I73.9
- vasomotor I73.9
- vein NEC I87.8
- viscera — *see* Pain, abdominal

Spasmodic — *see* condition

Spasmophilia — *see* Tetany

Spasmus nutans F98.4

Spastic, spasticity (*see also* Spasm)
- child (cerebral) (congenital) (paralysis) G8Ø.1

Speaker's throat R49.8

Specific, specified — *see* condition

Speech
- defect, disorder, disturbance, impediment R47.9
  - psychogenic, in childhood and adolescence F98.8
  - slurring R47.81
  - specified NEC R47.89

Spencer's disease AØ8.19

Spens' syndrome (syncope with heart block) I45.9

Sperm counts (fertility testing) Z31.41
- postvasectomy Z3Ø.8
  - reversal Z31.42

Spermatic cord — *see* condition

Spermatocele N43.4Ø
- congenital Q55.4
- multiple N43.42
- single N43.41

Spermatocystitis N49.Ø

Spermatocytoma C62.9- ☑
- specified site — *see* Neoplasm, malignant, by site

Spermatorrhea N5Ø.8

Sphacelus — *see* Gangrene

Sphenoidal — *see* condition

Sphenoiditis (chronic) — *see* Sinusitis, sphenoidal

Sphenopalatine ganglion neuralgia G9Ø.Ø9

Sphericity, increased, lens (congenital) Q12.4

Spherocytosis (congenital) (familial) (hereditary) D58.Ø
- hemoglobin disease D58.Ø
- sickle-cell (disease) D57.8- ☑

Spherophakia Q12.4

Sphincter — *see* condition

Sphincteritis, sphincter of Oddi — *see* Cholangitis

Sphingolipidosis E75.3
- specified NEC E75.29

Sphingomyelinosis E75.3

Spicule tooth KØØ.2

Spider
- bite — *see* Toxicity, venom, spider
- fingers — *see* Syndrome, Marfan's
- nevus I78.1
- toes — *see* Syndrome, Marfan's
- vascular I78.1

Spiegler-Fendt
- benign lymphocytoma L98.8
- sarcoid LØ8.89

Spielmeyer-Vogt disease E75.4

Spina bifida (aperta) QØ5.9
- with hydrocephalus NEC QØ5.4
- cervical QØ5.5
  - with hydrocephalus QØ5.Ø
- dorsal QØ5.6
  - with hydrocephalus QØ5.1
- lumbar QØ5.7
  - with hydrocephalus QØ5.2
- lumbosacral QØ5.7
  - with hydrocephalus QØ5.2
- occulta Q76.Ø
- sacral QØ5.8
  - with hydrocephalus QØ5.3
- thoracic QØ5.6
  - with hydrocephalus QØ5.1
- thoracolumbar QØ5.6
  - with hydrocephalus QØ5.1

Spindle, Krukenberg's — *see* Pigmentation, cornea, posterior

Spine, spinal — *see* condition

Spiradenoma (eccrine) — *see* Neoplasm, skin, benign

Spirillosis A25.Ø

Spirillum
- minus A25.Ø
- obermeieri infection A68.Ø

Spirochetal — *see* condition

Spirochetosis A69.9
- arthritic, arthritica A69.9
- bronchopulmonary A69.8
- icterohemorrhagic A27.Ø
- lung A69.8

Spirometrosis B7Ø.1

Spitting blood — *see* Hemoptysis

Splanchnoptosis K63.4

Spleen, splenic — *see* condition

Splenectasis — *see* Splenomegaly

Splenitis (interstitial) (malignant) (nonspecific) D73.89
- malarial (*see also* Malaria) B54 [D77]
- tuberculous A18.85

Splenocele D73.89

Splenomegaly, splenomegalia (Bengal) (cryptogenic) (idiopathic) (tropical) R16.1
- with hepatomegaly R16.2
- cirrhotic D73.2
- congenital Q89.Ø9
- congestive, chronic D73.2
- Egyptian B65.1
- Gaucher's E75.22
- malarial (*see also* Malaria) B54 [D77]
- neutropenic D73.81
- Niemann-Pick — *see* Niemann-Pick disease or syndrome
- siderotic D73.2
- syphilitic A52.79
  - congenital (early) A5Ø.Ø8 [D77]

Splenopathy D73.9

Splenoptosis D73.89

Splenosis D73.89

Splinter — *see* Foreign body, superficial, by site

Split, splitting
- foot Q72.7- ☑
- heart sounds RØ1.2
- lip, congenital — *see* Cleft, lip
- nails L6Ø.3
- urinary stream R39.13

Spondylarthrosis — *see* Spondylosis

Spondylitis (chronic) (*see also* Spondylopathy, inflammatory)
- ankylopoietica — *see* Spondylitis, ankylosing
- ankylosing (chronic) M45.9
  - with lung involvement M45.9 [J99]
  - cervical region M45.2
  - cervicothoracic region M45.3
  - juvenile MØ8.1
  - lumbar region M45.6
  - lumbosacral region M45.7
  - multiple sites M45.Ø
  - occipito-atlanto-axial region M45.1
  - sacrococcygeal region M45.8
  - thoracic region M45.4
  - thoracolumbar region M45.5
- atrophic (ligamentous) — *see* Spondylitis, ankylosing
- deformans (chronic) — *see* Spondylosis
- gonococcal A54.41
- gouty M1Ø.Ø8
- in (due to)
  - brucellosis A23.9 [M49.8Ø]
    - cervical region A23.9 [M49.82]
    - cervicothoracic region A23.9 [M49.83]
    - lumbar region A23.9 [M49.86]
    - lumbosacral region A23.9 [M49.87]
    - multiple sites A23.9 [M49.89]
    - occipito-atlanto-axial region A23.9 [M49.81]
    - sacrococcygeal region A23.9 [M49.88]
    - thoracic region A23.9 [M49.84]
    - thoracolumbar region A23.9 [M49.85]
  - enterobacteria (*see also* subcategory M49.8) AØ4.9
  - tuberculosis A18.Ø1
- infectious NEC — *see* Spondylopathy, infective
- juvenile ankylosing (chronic) MØ8.1
- Kümmell's — *see* Spondylopathy, traumatic
- Marie-Strümpell — *see* Spondylitis, ankylosing
- muscularis — *see* Spondylopathy, specified NEC
- psoriatic L4Ø.53
- rheumatoid — *see* Spondylitis, ankylosing
- rhizomelica — *see* Spondylitis, ankylosing
- sacroiliac NEC M46.1

Sprain — *continued*
- foot — *continued*
  - tarsometatarsal ligament S93.62- ☑
  - toe — *see* Sprain, toe
- hand S63.9- ☑
  - finger — *see* Sprain, finger
  - specified site NEC — *see* subcategory S63.8 ☑
  - thumb — *see* Sprain, thumb
- head S03.9 ☑
- hip S73.10- ☑
  - iliofemoral ligament S73.11- ☑
  - ischiocapsular (ligament) S73.12- ☑
  - specified NEC S73.19- ☑
- iliofemoral — *see* Sprain, hip
- innominate
  - acetabulum — *see* Sprain, hip
  - sacral junction S33.6 ☑
- internal
  - collateral, ankle — *see* Sprain, ankle
  - semilunar cartilage — *see* Sprain, knee, specified site NEC
- interphalangeal
  - finger — *see* Sprain, finger, interphalangeal (joint)
  - toe — *see* Sprain, toe, interphalangeal joint
- ischiocapsular — *see* Sprain, hip
- ischiofemoral — *see* Sprain, hip
- jaw (articular disc) (cartilage) (meniscus) S03.4 ☑
  - old M26.69
- knee S83.9- ☑
  - collateral ligament S83.40- ☑
    - lateral (fibular) S83.42- ☑
    - medial (tibial) S83.41- ☑
  - cruciate ligament S83.50- ☑
    - anterior S83.51- ☑
    - posterior S83.52- ☑
  - lateral (fibular) collateral ligament S83.42- ☑
  - medial (tibial) collateral ligament S83.41- ☑
  - patellar ligament S76.11- ☑
  - specified site NEC S83.8X- ☑
  - superior tibiofibular joint (ligament) S83.6- ☑
- lateral collateral, knee — *see* Sprain, knee, collateral
- lumbar (spine) S33.5 ☑
- lumbosacral S33.9 ☑
- mandible (articular disc) S03.4 ☑
  - old M26.69
- medial collateral, knee — *see* Sprain, knee, collateral
- meniscus
  - jaw S03.4 ☑
    - old M26.69
  - knee — *see* Sprain, knee, specified site NEC
    - with current tear — *see* Tear, meniscus
      - old — *see* Derangement, knee, meniscus, due to old tear
  - mandible S03.4 ☑
    - old M26.69
- metacarpal (distal) (proximal) — *see* Sprain, hand, specified site NEC
- metacarpophalangeal — *see* Sprain, finger, metacarpophalangeal (joint)
- metatarsophalangeal — *see* Sprain, toe, metatarsophalangeal joint
- midcarpal — *see* Sprain, hand, specified site NEC
- midtarsal — *see* Sprain, foot, specified site NEC
- neck S13.9 ☑
  - anterior longitudinal cervical ligament S13.4 ☑
  - atlanto-axial joint S13.4 ☑
  - atlanto-occipital joint S13.4 ☑
  - cervical spine S13.4 ☑
  - cricoarytenoid ligament S13.5 ☑
  - cricothyroid ligament S13.5 ☑
  - specified site NEC S13.8 ☑
  - thyroid region (cartilage) S13.5 ☑
- nose S03.8 ☑
- orbicular, hip — *see* Sprain, hip
- patella — *see* Sprain, knee, specified site NEC
- patellar ligament S76.11- ☑
- pelvis NEC S33.8 ☑
- phalanx
  - finger — *see* Sprain, finger
  - toe — *see* Sprain, toe
- pubofemoral — *see* Sprain, hip
- radiocarpal — *see* Sprain, wrist
- radiohumeral — *see* Sprain, elbow
- radius, collateral — *see* Rupture, traumatic, ligament, radial collateral
- rib (cage) S23.41 ☑

Sprain — *continued*
- rotator cuff (capsule) S43.42- ☑
- sacroiliac (region)
  - chronic or old — *see* subcategory M53.2 ☑
  - joint S33.6 ☑
- scaphoid (hand) — *see* Sprain, hand, specified site NEC
- scapula (r) — *see* Sprain, shoulder girdle, specified site NEC
- semilunar cartilage (knee) — *see* Sprain, knee, specified site NEC
  - with current tear — *see* Tear, meniscus
    - old — *see* Derangement, knee, meniscus, due to old tear
- shoulder joint S43.40- ☑
  - acromioclavicular joint (ligament) — *see* Sprain, acromioclavicular joint
  - blade — *see* Sprain, shoulder, girdle, specified site NEC
  - coracoclavicular joint (ligament) — *see* Sprain, coracoclavicular joint
  - coracohumeral ligament — *see* Sprain, coracohumeral joint
  - girdle S43.9- ☑
    - specified site NEC S43.8- ☑
  - rotator cuff — *see* Sprain, rotator cuff
  - specified site NEC S43.49- ☑
  - sternoclavicular joint (ligament) — *see* Sprain, sternoclavicular joint
- spine
  - cervical S13.4 ☑
  - lumbar S33.5 ☑
  - thoracic S23.3 ☑
- sternoclavicular joint S43.6- ☑
- sternum S23.429 ☑
  - chondrosternal joint S23.421 ☑
  - specified site NEC S23.428 ☑
  - sternoclavicular (joint) (ligament) S23.420 ☑
- symphysis
  - jaw S03.4 ☑
    - old M26.69
  - mandibular S03.4 ☑
    - old M26.69
- talofibular — *see* Sprain, ankle
- tarsal — *see* Sprain, foot, specified site NEC
- tarsometatarsal — *see* Sprain, foot, specified site NEC
- temporomandibular S03.4 ☑
  - old M26.69
- thorax S23.9 ☑
  - ribs S23.41 ☑
  - specified site NEC S23.8 ☑
  - spine S23.3 ☑
  - sternum — *see* Sprain, sternum
- thumb S63.60- ☑
  - interphalangeal (joint) S63.62- ☑
  - metacarpophalangeal (joint) S63.64- ☑
  - specified site NEC S63.68- ☑
- thyroid cartilage or region S13.5 ☑
- tibia (proximal end) — *see* Sprain, knee, specified site NEC
- tibial collateral, knee — *see* Sprain, knee, collateral
- tibiofibular
  - distal — *see* Sprain, ankle
  - superior — *see* Sprain, knee, specified site NEC
- toe(s) S93.50- ☑
  - great S93.50- ☑
  - interphalangeal joint S93.51- ☑
    - great S93.51- ☑
    - lesser S93.51- ☑
  - lesser S93.50- ☑
  - metatarsophalangeal joint S93.52- ☑
    - great S93.52- ☑
    - lesser S93.52- ☑
- ulna, collateral — *see* Rupture, traumatic, ligament, ulnar collateral
- ulnohumeral — *see* Sprain, elbow
- wrist S63.50- ☑
  - carpal S63.51- ☑
  - radiocarpal S63.52- ☑
  - specified site NEC S63.59- ☑
- xiphoid cartilage — *see* Sprain, sternum

Sprengel's deformity (congenital) Q74.0

Sprue (tropical) K90.1
- celiac K90.0
- idiopathic K90.0
- meaning thrush B37.0

Sprue — *continued*
- nontropical K90.0

Spur, bone (*see also* Enthesopathy)
- calcaneal M77.3- ☑
- iliac crest M76.2- ☑
- nose (septum) J34.89

Spurway's syndrome Q78.0

Sputum
- abnormal (amount) (color) (odor) (purulent) R09.3
- blood-stained R04.2
- excessive (cause unknown) R09.3

Squamous (*see also* condition)
- epithelium in
  - cervical canal (congenital) Q51.828
  - uterine mucosa (congenital) Q51.818

Squashed nose M95.0
- congenital Q67.4

Squeeze, diver's T70.3 ☑

Squint (*see also* Strabismus)
- accommodative — *see* Strabismus, convergent concomitant

St. Hubert's disease A82.9

Stab (*see also* Laceration)
- internal organs — *see* Injury, by site

Stafne's cyst or cavity M27.0

Staggering gait R26.0
- hysterical F44.4

Staghorn calculus — *see* Calculus, kidney

Stähli's line (cornea) (pigment) — *see* Pigmentation, cornea, anterior

Stain, staining
- meconium (newborn) P96.83
- port wine Q82.5
- tooth, teeth (hard tissues) (extrinsic) K03.6
  - due to
    - accretions K03.6
    - deposits (betel) (black) (green) (materia alba) (orange) (soft) (tobacco) K03.6
    - metals (copper) (silver) K03.7
    - nicotine K03.6
    - pulpal bleeding K03.7
    - tobacco K03.6
  - intrinsic K00.8

Stammering (*see also* Disorder, fluency) F80.81

Standstill
- auricular I45.5
- cardiac — *see* Arrest, cardiac
- sinoatrial I45.5
- ventricular — *see* Arrest, cardiac

Stannosis J63.5

Stanton's disease — *see* Melioidosis

Staphylitis (acute) (catarrhal) (chronic) (gangrenous) (membranous) (suppurative) (ulcerative) K12.2

Staphylococcal scalded skin syndrome L00

Staphylococcemia A41.2

Staphylococcus, staphylococcal (*see also* condition)
- as cause of disease classified elsewhere B95.8
  - aureus (methicillin susceptible) (MSSA) B95.61
    - methicillin resistant (MRSA) B95.62
- specified NEC, as cause of disease classified elsewhere B95.7

Staphyloma (sclera)
- cornea H18.72- ☑
- equatorial H15.81- ☑
- localized (anterior) H15.82- ☑
- posticum H15.83- ☑
- ring H15.85- ☑

Stargardt's disease — *see* Dystrophy, retina

Starvation (inanition) (due to lack of food) T73.0 ☑
- edema — *see* Malnutrition, severe

Stasis
- bile (noncalculous) K83.1
- bronchus J98.09
  - with infection — *see* Bronchitis
- cardiac — *see* Failure, heart, congestive
- cecum K59.8
- colon K59.8
- dermatitis — *see* Varix, leg, with, inflammation
- duodenal K31.5
- eczema — *see* Varix, leg, with, inflammation
- edema — *see* Hypertension, venous (chronic), idiopathic
- foot T69.0- ☑
- ileocecal coil K59.8
- ileum K59.8
- intestinal K59.8
- jejunum K59.8

- **Stasis**— *continued*
  - kidney N19
  - liver (cirrhotic) K76.1
  - lymphatic I89.8
  - pneumonia J18.2
  - pulmonary — *see* Edema, lung
  - rectal K59.8
  - renal N19
    - tubular N17.0
  - ulcer — *see* Varix, leg, with, ulcer
    - without varicose veins I87.2
  - urine — *see* Retention, urine
  - venous I87.8
- **State** (of)
  - affective and paranoid, mixed, organic psychotic F06.8
  - agitated R45.1
    - acute reaction to stress F43.0
  - anxiety (neurotic) F41.1
  - apprehension F41.1
  - burn-out Z73.0
  - climacteric, female Z78.0
    - symptomatic N95.1
  - compulsive F42
    - mixed with obsessional thoughts F42
  - confusional (psychogenic) F44.89
    - acute (*see also* Delirium)
      - with
        - arteriosclerotic dementia F01.50
          - with behavioral disturbance F01.51
        - senility or dementia F05
      - alcoholic F10.231
    - epileptic F05
    - reactive (from emotional stress, psychological trauma) F44.89
    - subacute — *see* Delirium
  - convulsive — *see* Convulsions
  - crisis F43.0
  - depressive F32.9
    - neurotic F34.1
  - dissociative F44.9
  - emotional shock (stress) R45.7
  - hypercoagulation — *see* Hypercoagulable
  - locked-in G83.5
  - menopausal Z78.0
    - symptomatic N95.1
  - neurotic F48.9
    - with depersonalization F48.1
  - obsessional F42
  - oneiroid (schizophrenia-like) F23
  - organic
    - hallucinatory (nonalcoholic) F06.0
    - paranoid (hallucinatory) F06.2
  - panic F41.0
  - paranoid F22
    - climacteric F22
    - involutional F22
    - menopausal F22
    - organic F06.2
    - senile F03 ☑
    - simple F22
  - persistent vegetative R40.3
  - phobic F40.9
  - postleukotomy F07.0
  - pregnant, incidental Z33.1
  - psychogenic, twilight F44.89
  - psychopathic (constitutional) F60.2
  - psychotic, organic (*see also* Psychosis, organic)
    - mixed paranoid and affective F06.8
    - senile or presenile F03 ☑
    - transient NEC F06.8
      - with
        - depression F06.31
        - hallucinations F06.0
  - residual schizophrenic F20.5
  - restlessness R45.1
  - stress (emotional) R45.7
  - tension (mental) F48.9
    - specified NEC F48.8
  - transient organic psychotic NEC F06.8
    - depressive type F06.31
    - hallucinatory type F06.30
  - twilight
    - epileptic F05
    - psychogenic F44.89
  - vegetative, persistent R40.3
  - vital exhaustion Z73.0
  - withdrawal, — *see* Withdrawal, state
- **Status** (post) (*see also* Presence (of))
  - absence, epileptic — *see* Epilepsy, by type, with status epilepticus
  - administration of tPA (rtPA) in a different facility within the last 24 hours prior to admission to current facility Z92.82
  - adrenalectomy (unilateral) (bilateral) E89.6
  - anastomosis Z98.0
  - anginosus I20.9
  - angioplasty (peripheral) Z98.62
    - with implant Z95.820
    - coronary artery Z98.61
      - with implant Z95.5
  - aortocoronary bypass Z95.1
  - arthrodesis Z98.1
  - artificial opening (of) Z93.9
    - gastrointestinal tract Z93.4
    - specified NEC Z93.8
    - urinary tract Z93.6
    - vagina Z93.8
  - asthmaticus — *see* Asthma, by type, with status asthmaticus
  - awaiting organ transplant Z76.82
  - bariatric surgery Z98.84
  - bed confinement Z74.01
  - bleb, filtering (vitreous), after glaucoma surgery Z98.83
  - breast implant Z98.82
    - removal Z98.86
  - cataract extraction Z98.4- ☑
  - cholecystectomy Z90.49
  - clitorectomy N90.811
    - with excision of labia minora N90.812
  - colectomy (complete) (partial) Z90.49
  - colonization — *see* Carrier (suspected) of
  - colostomy Z93.3
  - convulsivus idiopathicus — *see* Epilepsy, by type, with status epilepticus
  - coronary artery angioplasty — *see* Status, angioplasty, coronary artery
  - cystectomy (urinary bladder) Z90.6
  - cystostomy Z93.50
    - appendico-vesicostomy Z93.52
    - cutaneous Z93.51
    - specified NEC Z93.59
  - delinquent immunization Z28.3
  - dental Z98.818
    - crown Z98.811
    - fillings Z98.811
    - restoration Z98.811
    - sealant Z98.810
    - specified NEC Z98.818
  - deployment (current) (military) Z56.82
  - dialysis (hemodialysis) (peritoneal) Z99.2
  - do not resuscitate (DNR) Z66
  - donor — *see* Donor
  - embedded fragments — *see* Retained, foreign body fragments (type of)
  - embedded splinter — *see* Retained, foreign body fragments (type of)
  - enterostomy Z93.4
  - epileptic, epilepticus (*see also* Epilepsy, by type, with status epilepticus) G40.901
  - estrogen receptor
    - negative Z17.1
    - positive Z17.0
  - female genital cutting — *see* Female genital mutilation status
  - female genital mutilation — *see* Female genital mutilation status
  - filtering (vitreous) bleb after glaucoma surgery Z98.83
  - gastrectomy (complete) (partial) Z90.3
  - gastric banding Z98.84
  - gastric bypass for obesity Z98.84
  - gastrostomy Z93.1
  - human immunodeficiency virus (HIV) infection, asymptomatic Z21
  - hysterectomy (complete) (total) Z90.710
    - partial (with remaining cervial stump) Z90.711
  - ileostomy Z93.2
  - implant
    - breast Z98.82
  - infibulation N90.813
  - intestinal bypass Z98.0
  - jejunostomy Z93.4
  - lapsed immunization schedule Z28.3
  - laryngectomy Z90.02
  - lymphaticus E32.8
  - marmoratus G80.3
- **Status** — *continued*
  - mastectomy (unilateral) (bilateral) Z90.1- ☑
  - military deployment status (current) Z56.82
    - in theater or in support of military war, peacekeeping and humanitarian operations Z56.82
  - nephrectomy (unilateral) (bilateral) Z90.5
  - nephrostomy Z93.6
  - obesity surgery Z98.84
  - oophorectomy
    - bilateral Z90.722
    - unilateral Z90.721
  - organ replacement
    - by artificial or mechanical device or prosthesis of
      - artery Z95.828
      - bladder Z96.0
      - blood vessel Z95.828
      - breast Z97.8
      - eye globe Z97.0
      - heart Z95.812
        - valve Z95.2
      - intestine Z97.8
      - joint Z96.60
        - hip — *see* Presence, hip joint implant
        - knee — *see* Presence, knee joint implant
        - specified site NEC Z96.698
      - kidney Z97.8
      - larynx Z96.3
      - lens Z96.1
      - limbs — *see* Presence, artificial, limb
      - liver Z97.8
      - lung Z97.8
      - pancreas Z97.8
    - by organ transplant (heterologous)(homologous) — *see* Transplant
  - pacemaker
    - brain Z96.89
    - cardiac Z95.0
    - specified NEC Z96.89
  - pancreatectomy Z90.410
    - complete Z90.410
    - partial Z90.411
    - total Z90.410
  - physical restraint Z78.1
  - pneumonectomy (complete) (partial) Z90.2
  - pneumothorax, therapeutic Z98.3
  - postcommotio cerebri F07.81
  - postoperative (postprocedural) NEC Z98.89
    - breast implant Z98.82
    - dental Z98.818
      - crown Z98.811
      - fillings Z98.811
      - restoration Z98.811
      - sealant Z98.810
      - specified NEC Z98.818
    - pneumothorax, therapeutic Z98.3
  - postpartum (routine follow-up) Z39.2
    - care immediately after delivery Z39.0
  - postsurgical (postprocedural) NEC Z98.89
    - pneumothorax, therapeutic Z98.3
  - pregnancy, incidental Z33.1
  - prosthesis coronary angioplasty Z95.5
  - pseudophakia Z96.1
  - renal dialysis (hemodialysis) (peritoneal) Z99.2
  - retained foreign body — *see* Retained, foreign body fragments (type of)
  - reversed jejunal transposition (for bypass) Z98.0
  - salpingo-oophorectomy
    - bilateral Z90.722
    - unilateral Z90.721
  - sex reassignment surgery status Z87.890
  - shunt
    - arteriovenous (for dialysis) Z99.2
    - cerebrospinal fluid Z98.2
    - ventricular (communicating) (for drainage) Z98.2
  - splenectomy Z90.81
  - thymicolymphaticus E32.8
  - thymicus E32.8
  - thymolymphaticus E32.8
  - thyroidectomy (hypothyroidism) E89.0
  - tooth (teeth) extraction (*see also* Absence, teeth, acquired) K08.409
  - tPA (rtPA) administration in a different facility within the last 24 hours prior to admission to current facility Z92.82
  - tracheostomy Z93.0
  - transplant — *see* Transplant
    - organ removed Z98.85
  - tubal ligation Z98.51

Status — *continued*
- underimmunization Z28.3
- ureterostomy Z93.6
- urethrostomy Z93.6
- vagina, artificial Z93.8
- vasectomy Z98.52
- wheelchair confinement Z99.3

Stealing
- child problem F91.8
  - in company with others Z72.81Ø
- pathological (compulsive) F63.2

Steam burn — *see* Burn
Steatocystoma multiplex L72.2
Steatohepatitis (nonalcoholic) (NASH) K75.81
Steatoma L72.3
- eyelid (cystic) — *see* Dermatosis, eyelid
  - infected — *see* Hordeolum

Steatorrhea (chronic) K9Ø.4
- with lacteal obstruction K9Ø.2
- idiopathic (adult) (infantile) K9Ø.Ø
- pancreatic K9Ø.3
- primary K9Ø.Ø
- tropical K9Ø.1

Steatosis E88.89
- heart — *see* Degeneration, myocardial
- kidney N28.89
- liver NEC K76.Ø

Steele-Richardson-Olszewski disease or syndrome G23.1
Steinbrocker's syndrome G9Ø.8
Steinert's disease G71.11
Stein-Leventhal syndrome E28.2
Stein's syndrome E28.2
STEMI (*see also* Infarct, myocardium, ST elevation) I21.3
Stenocardia I2Ø.8
Stenocephaly Q75.8
Stenosis, stenotic (cicatricial) (*see also* Stricture)
- ampulla of Vater K83.1
- anus, anal (canal) (sphincter) K62.4
  - and rectum K62.4
  - congenital Q42.3
    - with fistula Q42.2
- aorta (ascending) (supraventricular) (congenital) Q25.3
  - arteriosclerotic I7Ø.Ø
  - calcified I7Ø.Ø
- aortic (valve) I35.Ø
  - with insufficiency I35.2
  - congenital Q23.Ø
  - rheumatic IØ6.Ø
    - with
      - incompetency, insufficiency or regurgitation IØ6.2
        - with mitral (valve) disease IØ8.Ø
          - with tricuspid (valve) disease IØ8.3
      - mitral (valve) disease IØ8.Ø
        - with tricuspid (valve) disease IØ8.3
      - tricuspid (valve) disease IØ8.2
        - with mitral (valve) disease IØ8.3
  - specified cause NEC I35.Ø
  - syphilitic A52.Ø3
- aqueduct of Sylvius (congenital) QØ3.Ø
  - with spina bifida — *see* Spina bifida, by site, with hydrocephalus
  - acquired G91.1
- artery NEC (*see also* Arteriosclerosis) I77.1
  - celiac I77.4
  - cerebral — *see* Occlusion, artery, cerebral
  - extremities — *see* Arteriosclerosis, extremities
  - precerebral — *see* Occlusion, artery, precerebral
  - pulmonary (congenital) Q25.6
    - acquired I28.8
  - renal I7Ø.1
- bile duct (common) (hepatic) K83.1
  - congenital Q44.3
- bladder-neck (acquired) N32.Ø
  - congenital Q64.31
- brain G93.89
- bronchus J98.Ø9
  - congenital Q32.3
  - syphilitic A52.72
- cardia (stomach) K22.2
  - congenital Q39.3
- cardiovascular — *see* Disease, cardiovascular
- caudal M48.Ø8
- cervix, cervical (canal) N88.2
  - congenital Q51.828
  - in pregnancy or childbirth — *see* Pregnancy, complicated by, abnormal cervix

Stenosis, stenotic — *continued*
- colon (*see also* Obstruction, intestine)
  - congenital Q42.9
    - specified NEC Q42.8
- colostomy K94.Ø3
- common (bile) duct K83.1
  - congenital Q44.3
- coronary (artery) — *see* Disease, heart, ischemic, atherosclerotic
- cystic duct — *see* Obstruction, gallbladder
- due to presence of device, implant or graft (*see also* Complications, by site and type, specified NEC) T85.85 ☑
  - arterial graft NEC T82.858 ☑
  - breast (implant) T85.85 ☑
  - catheter T85.85 ☑
    - dialysis (renal) T82.858 ☑
      - intraperitoneal T85.85 ☑
    - infusion NEC T82.858 ☑
      - spinal (epidural) (subdural) T85.85 ☑
    - urinary (indwelling) T83.85 ☑
  - fixation, internal (orthopedic) NEC T84.85 ☑
  - gastrointestinal (bile duct) (esophagus) T85.85 ☑
  - genital NEC T83.85 ☑
  - heart NEC T82.857 ☑
  - joint prosthesis T84.85 ☑
  - ocular (corneal graft) (orbital implant) NEC T85.85 ☑
  - orthopedic NEC T84.85 ☑
  - specified NEC T85.85 ☑
  - urinary NEC T83.85 ☑
  - vascular NEC T82.858 ☑
  - ventricular intracranial shunt T85.85 ☑
- duodenum K31.5
  - congenital Q41.Ø
- ejaculatory duct NEC N5Ø.8
- endocervical os — *see* Stenosis, cervix
- enterostomy K94.13
- esophagus K22.2
  - congenital Q39.3
  - syphilitic A52.79
    - congenital A5Ø.59 [K23]
- eustachian tube — *see* Obstruction, eustachian tube
- external ear canal (acquired) H61.3Ø- ☑
  - congenital Q16.1
  - due to
    - inflammation H61.32- ☑
    - trauma H61.31- ☑
  - postprocedural H95.81- ☑
  - specified cause NEC H61.39- ☑
- gallbladder — *see* Obstruction, gallbladder
- glottis J38.6
- heart valve (congenital) Q24.8
  - aortic Q23.Ø
  - mitral Q23.2
  - pulmonary Q22.1
  - tricuspid Q22.4
- hepatic duct K83.1
- hymen N89.6
- hypertrophic subaortic (idiopathic) I42.1
- ileum K56.69
  - congenital Q41.2
- infundibulum cardia Q24.3
- intervertebral foramina (*see also* Lesion, biomechanical, specified NEC)
  - connective tissue M99.79
    - abdomen M99.79
    - cervical region M99.71
    - cervicothoracic M99.71
    - head region M99.7Ø
    - lumbar region M99.73
    - lumbosacral M99.73
    - occipitocervical M99.7Ø
    - sacral region M99.74
    - sacrococcygeal M99.74
    - sacroiliac M99.74
    - specified NEC M99.79
    - thoracic region M99.72
    - thoracolumbar M99.72
  - disc M99.79
    - abdomen M99.79
    - cervical region M99.71
    - cervicothoracic M99.71
    - head region M99.7Ø
    - lower extremity M99.76
    - lumbar region M99.73
    - lumbosacral M99.73

Stenosis, stenotic — *continued*
- intervertebral foramina (*see also* Lesion, biomechanical, specified) — *continued*
  - disc — *continued*
    - occipitocervical M99.7Ø
    - pelvic M99.75
    - rib cage M99.78
    - sacral region M99.74
    - sacrococcygeal M99.74
    - sacroiliac M99.74
    - specified NEC M99.79
    - thoracic region M99.72
    - thoracolumbar M99.72
    - upper extremity M99.77
  - osseous M99.69
    - abdomen M99.69
    - cervical region M99.61
    - cervicothoracic M99.61
    - head region M99.6Ø
    - lower extremity M99.66
    - lumbar region M99.63
    - lumbosacral M99.63
    - occipitocervical M99.6Ø
    - pelvic M99.65
    - rib cage M99.68
    - sacral region M99.64
    - sacrococcygeal M99.64
    - sacroiliac M99.64
    - specified NEC M99.69
    - thoracic region M99.62
    - thoracolumbar M99.62
    - upper extremity M99.67
  - subluxation — *see* Stenosis, intervertebral foramina, osseous
- intestine (*see also* Obstruction, intestine)
  - congenital (small) Q41.9
    - large Q42.9
      - specified NEC Q42.8
    - specified NEC Q41.8
- jejunum K56.69
  - congenital Q41.1
- lacrimal (passage)
  - canaliculi HØ4.54- ☑
  - congenital Q1Ø.5
  - duct HØ4.55- ☑
  - punctum HØ4.56- ☑
  - sac HØ4.57- ☑
- lacrimonasal duct — *see* Stenosis, lacrimal, duct
  - congenital Q1Ø.5
- larynx J38.6
  - congenital NEC Q31.8
    - subglottic Q31.1
  - syphilitic A52.73
    - congenital A5Ø.59 [J99]
- mitral (chronic) (inactive) (valve) IØ5.Ø
  - with
    - aortic valve disease IØ8.Ø
    - incompetency, insufficiency or regurgitation IØ5.2
  - active or acute IØ1.1
    - with rheumatic or Sydenham's chorea IØ2.Ø
  - congenital Q23.2
  - specified cause, except rheumatic I34.2
  - syphilitic A52.Ø3
- myocardium, myocardial (*see also* Degeneration, myocardial)
  - hypertrophic subaortic (idiopathic) I42.1
- nares (anterior) (posterior) J34.89
  - congenital Q3Ø.Ø
- nasal duct (*see also* Stenosis, lacrimal, duct)
  - congenital Q1Ø.5
- nasolacrimal duct (*see also* Stenosis, lacrimal, duct)
  - congenital Q1Ø.5
- neural canal (*see also* Lesion, biomechanical, specified NEC)
  - connective tissue M99.49
    - abdomen M99.49
    - cervical region M99.41
    - cervicothoracic M99.41
    - head region M99.4Ø
    - lower extremity M99.46
    - lumbar region M99.43
    - lumbosacral M99.43
    - occipitocervical M99.4Ø
    - pelvic M99.45
    - rib cage M99.48
    - sacral region M99.44
    - sacrococcygeal M99.44

Stomatitis — *continued*
  monilial B37.Ø
  mycotic B37.Ø
  necrotizing ulcerative A69.Ø
  parasitic B37.Ø
  septic K12.1
  spirochetal A69.1
  suppurative (acute) K12.2
  ulceromembranous A69.1
  vesicular K12.1
    with exanthem (enteroviral) BØ8.4
    virus disease A93.8
  Vincent's A69.1
Stomatocytosis D58.8
Stomatomycosis B37.Ø
Stomatorrhagia K13.79
Stone(s) (*see also* Calculus)
  bladder (diverticulum) N21.Ø
  cystine E72.Ø9
  heart syndrome I5Ø.1
  kidney N2Ø.Ø
  prostate N42.Ø
  pulpal (dental) KØ4.2
  renal N2Ø.Ø
  salivary gland or duct (any) K11.5
  urethra (impacted) N21.1
  urinary (duct) (impacted) (passage) N2Ø.9
    bladder (diverticulum) N21.Ø
    lower tract N21.9
    specified NEC N21.8
  xanthine E79.8 [N22]
Stonecutter's lung J62.8
Stonemason's asthma, disease, lung or pneumoconiosis J62.8
Stoppage
  heart — *see* Arrest, cardiac
  urine — *see* Retention, urine
Storm, thyroid — *see* Thyrotoxicosis
Strabismus (congenital) (nonparalytic) H5Ø.9
  concomitant H5Ø.4Ø
    convergent — *see* Strabismus, convergent concomitant
    divergent — *see* Strabismus, divergent concomitant
  convergent concomitant H5Ø.ØØ
    accommodative component H5Ø.43
    alternating H5Ø.Ø5
      with
        A pattern H5Ø.Ø6
        specified nonconcomitances NEC H5Ø.Ø8
        V pattern H5Ø.Ø7
    monocular H5Ø.Ø1- ☑
      with
        A pattern H5Ø.Ø2- ☑
        specified nonconcomitances NEC H5Ø.Ø4- ☑
        V pattern H5Ø.Ø3- ☑
      intermittent H5Ø.31- ☑
        alternating H5Ø.32
  cyclotropia H5Ø.1- ☑
  divergent concomitant H5Ø.1Ø
    alternating H5Ø.15
      with
        A pattern H5Ø.16
        specified noncomitances NEC H5Ø.18
        V pattern H5Ø.17
    monocular H5Ø.11- ☑
      with
        A pattern H5Ø.12- ☑
        specified noncomitances NEC H5Ø.14- ☑
        V pattern H5Ø.13- ☑
      intermittent H5Ø.33 ☑
        alternating H5Ø.34
  Duane's syndrome H5Ø.81- ☑
  due to adhesions, scars H5Ø.69
  heterophoria H5Ø.5Ø
    alternating H5Ø.55
    cyclophoria H5Ø.54
    esophoria H5Ø.51
    exophoria H5Ø.52
    vertical H5Ø.53
  heterotropia H5Ø.4Ø
    intermittent H5Ø.3Ø
  hypertropia H5Ø.2- ☑
  hypotropia — *see* Hypertropia
  latent H5Ø.5Ø
  mechanical H5Ø.6Ø
    Brown's sheath syndrome H5Ø.61- ☑
Strabismus — *continued*
  mechanical — *continued*
    specified type NEC H5Ø.69
  monofixation syndrome H5Ø.42
  paralytic H49.9
    abducens nerve H49.2- ☑
    fourth nerve H49.1- ☑
    Kearns-Sayre syndrome H49.81- ☑
    ophthalmoplegia (external)
      progressive H49.4- ☑
        with pigmentary retinopathy H49.81- ☑
      total H49.3- ☑
    sixth nerve H49.2- ☑
    specified type NEC H49.88- ☑
    third nerve H49.Ø- ☑
    trochlear nerve H49.1- ☑
  specified type NEC H5Ø.89
  vertical H5Ø.2- ☑
Strain
  back S39.Ø12 ☑
  cervical S16.1 ☑
  eye NEC — *see* Disturbance, vision, subjective
  heart — *see* Disease, heart
  low back S39.Ø12 ☑
  mental NOS Z73.3
    work-related Z56.6
  muscle (tendon) — *see* Injury, muscle, by site, strain
  neck S16.1 ☑
  physical NOS Z73.3
    work-related Z56.6
  postural (*see also* Disorder, soft tissue, due to use)
  psychological NEC Z73.3
  tendon — *see* Injury, muscle, by site, strain
Straining, on urination R39.16
Strand, vitreous — *see* Opacity, vitreous, membranes and strands
Strangulation, strangulated (*see also* Asphyxia, traumatic)
  appendix K38.8
  bladder-neck N32.Ø
  bowel or colon K56.2
  food or foreign body — *see* Foreign body, by site
  hemorrhoids — *see* Hemorrhoids, with complication
  hernia (*see also* Hernia, by site, with obstruction)
    with gangrene — *see* Hernia, by site, with gangrene
  intestine (large) (small) K56.2
    with hernia (*see also* Hernia, by site, with obstruction)
      with gangrene — *see* Hernia, by site, with gangrene
  mesentery K56.2
  mucus — *see* Asphyxia, mucus
  omentum K56.2
  organ or site, congenital NEC — *see* Atresia, by site
  ovary — *see* Torsion, ovary
  penis N48.89
    foreign body T19.4 ☑
  rupture — *see* Hernia, by site, with obstruction
  stomach due to hernia (*see also* Hernia, by site, with obstruction)
    with gangrene — *see* Hernia, by site, with gangrene
  vesicourethral orifice N32.Ø
Strangury R3Ø.Ø
Straw itch B88.Ø
Strawberry
  gallbladder K82.4
  mark Q82.5
  tongue (red) (white) K14.3
Streak(s)
  macula, angioid H35.33
  ovarian Q5Ø.32
Strephosymbolia F81.Ø
  secondary to organic lesion R48.8
Streptobacillary fever A25.1
Streptobacillosis A25.1
Streptobacillus moniliformis A25.1
Streptococcus, streptococcal (*see also* condition)
  as cause of disease classified elsewhere B95.5
  group
    A, as cause of disease classified elsewhere B95.Ø
    B, as cause of disease classified elsewhere B95.1
    D, as cause of disease classified elsewhere B95.2
  pneumoniae, as cause of disease classified elsewhere B95.3
Streptococcus, streptococcal — *continued*
  specified NEC, as cause of disease classified elsewhere B95.4
Streptomycosis B47.1
Streptotrichosis A48.8
Stress F43.9
  family — *see* Disruption, family
  fetal P84
    complicating pregnancy O77.9
      due to drug administration O77.1
  mental NEC Z73.3
    work-related Z56.6
  physical NEC Z73.3
    work-related Z56.6
  polycythemia D75.1
  reaction (*see also* Reaction, stress) F43.9
  work schedule Z56.3
Stretching, nerve — *see* Injury, nerve
Striae albicantes, atrophicae or distensae (cutis) L9Ø.6
Stricture (*see also* Stenosis)
  ampulla of Vater K83.1
  anus (sphincter) K62.4
    congenital Q42.3
      with fistula Q42.2
    infantile Q42.3
      with fistula Q42.2
  aorta (ascending) (congenital) Q25.3
    arteriosclerotic I7Ø.Ø
    calcified I7Ø.Ø
    supravalvular, congenital Q25.3
  aortic (valve) — *see* Stenosis, aortic
  aqueduct of Sylvius (congenital) QØ3.Ø
    with spina bifida — *see* Spina bifida, by site, with hydrocephalus
    acquired G91.1
  artery I77.1
    basilar — *see* Occlusion, artery, basilar
    carotid — *see* Occlusion, artery, carotid
    celiac I77.4
    congenital (peripheral) Q27.8
      cerebral Q28.3
      coronary Q24.5
      digestive system Q27.8
      lower limb Q27.8
      retinal Q14.1
      specified site NEC Q27.8
      umbilical Q27.Ø
      upper limb Q27.8
    coronary — *see* Disease, heart, ischemic, atherosclerotic
      congenital Q24.5
    precerebral — *see* Occlusion, artery, precerebral
    pulmonary (congenital) Q25.6
      acquired I28.8
    renal I7Ø.1
    vertebral — *see* Occlusion, artery, vertebral
  auditory canal (external) (congenital)
    acquired — *see* Stenosis, external ear canal
  bile duct (common) (hepatic) K83.1
    congenital Q44.3
    postoperative K91.89
  bladder N32.89
    neck N32.Ø
  bowel — *see* Obstruction, intestine
  brain G93.89
  bronchus J98.Ø9
    congenital Q32.3
    syphilitic A52.72
  cardia (stomach) K22.2
    congenital Q39.3
  cardiac (*see also* Disease, heart)
    orifice (stomach) K22.2
  cecum — *see* Obstruction, intestine
  cervix, cervical (canal) N88.2
    congenital Q51.828
    in pregnancy — *see* Pregnancy, complicated by, abnormal cervix
      causing obstructed labor O65.5
  colon (*see also* Obstruction, intestine)
    congenital Q42.9
      specified NEC Q42.8
  colostomy K94.Ø3
  common (bile) duct K83.1
  coronary (artery) — *see* Disease, heart, ischemic, atherosclerotic
  cystic duct — *see* Obstruction, gallbladder
  digestive organs NEC, congenital Q45.8
  duodenum K31.5

- **Stricture** — *continued*
  - duodenum — *continued*
    - congenital Q41.Ø
  - ear canal (external) (congenital) Q16.1
    - acquired — *see* Stricture, auditory canal, acquired
  - ejaculatory duct N5Ø.8
  - enterostomy K94.13
  - esophagus K22.2
    - congenital Q39.3
    - syphilitic A52.79
      - congenital A5Ø.59 [K23]
  - eustachian tube (*see also* Obstruction, eustachian tube)
    - congenital Q17.8
  - fallopian tube N97.1
    - gonococcal A54.24
    - tuberculous A18.17
  - gallbladder — *see* Obstruction, gallbladder
  - glottis J38.6
  - heart (*see also* Disease, heart)
    - valve (*see also* Endocarditis) I38
      - aortic Q23.Ø
      - mitral Q23.4
      - pulmonary Q22.1
      - tricuspid Q22.4
  - hepatic duct K83.1
  - hourglass, of stomach K31.2
  - hymen N89.6
  - hypopharynx J39.2
  - ileum K56.69
    - congenital Q41.2
  - intestine (*see also* Obstruction, intestine)
    - congenital (small) Q41.9
      - large Q42.9
        - specified NEC Q42.8
      - specified NEC Q41.8
    - ischemic K55.1
  - jejunum K56.69
    - congenital Q41.1
  - lacrimal passages (*see also* Stenosis, lacrimal)
    - congenital Q1Ø.5
  - larynx J38.6
    - congenital NEC Q31.8
      - subglottic Q31.1
    - syphilitic A52.73
      - congenital A5Ø.59 [J99]
  - meatus
    - ear (congenital) Q16.1
      - acquired — *see* Stricture, auditory canal, acquired
    - osseous (ear) (congenital) Q16.1
      - acquired — *see* Stricture, auditory canal, acquired
    - urinarius (*see also* Stricture, urethra)
      - congenital Q64.33
  - mitral (valve) — *see* Stenosis, mitral
  - myocardium, myocardial I51.5
    - hypertrophic subaortic (idiopathic) I42.1
  - nares (anterior) (posterior) J34.89
    - congenital Q3Ø.Ø
  - nasal duct (*see also* Stenosis, lacrimal, duct)
    - congenital Q1Ø.5
  - nasolacrimal duct (*see also* Stenosis, lacrimal, duct)
    - congenital Q1Ø.5
  - nasopharynx J39.2
    - syphilitic A52.73
  - nose J34.89
    - congenital Q3Ø.Ø
  - nostril (anterior) (posterior) J34.89
    - congenital Q3Ø.Ø
    - syphilitic A52.73
      - congenital A5Ø.59 [J99]
  - organ or site, congenital NEC — *see* Atresia, by site
  - os uteri — *see* Stricture, cervix
  - osseous meatus (ear) (congenital) Q16.1
    - acquired — *see* Stricture, auditory canal, acquired
  - oviduct — *see* Stricture, fallopian tube
  - pelviureteric junction (congenital) Q62.11
  - penis, by foreign body T19.4 ☑
  - pharynx J39.2
  - prostate N42.89
  - pulmonary, pulmonic
    - artery (congenital) Q25.6
      - acquired I28.8
      - noncongenital I28.8
    - infundibulum (congenital) Q24.3
    - valve I37.Ø
      - congenital Q22.1
    - vein, acquired I28.8

- **Stricture** — *continued*
  - pulmonary, pulmonic — *continued*
    - vessel NEC I28.8
  - punctum lacrimale (*see also* Stenosis, lacrimal, punctum)
    - congenital Q1Ø.5
  - pylorus (hypertrophic) K31.1
    - adult K31.1
    - congenital Q4Ø.Ø
    - infantile Q4Ø.Ø
  - rectosigmoid K56.69
  - rectum (sphincter) K62.4
    - congenital Q42.1
      - with fistula Q42.Ø
    - due to
      - chlamydial lymphogranuloma A55
      - irradiation K91.89
      - lymphogranuloma venereum A55
    - gonococcal A54.6
    - inflammatory (chlamydial) A55
    - syphilitic A52.74
    - tuberculous A18.32
  - renal artery I7Ø.1
    - congenital Q27.1
  - salivary duct or gland (any) K11.8
  - sigmoid (flexure) — *see* Obstruction, intestine
  - spermatic cord N5Ø.8
  - stoma (following) (of)
    - colostomy K94.Ø3
    - enterostomy K94.13
    - gastrostomy K94.23
    - ileostomy K94.13
    - tracheostomy J95.Ø3
  - stomach K31.89
    - congenital Q4Ø.2
    - hourglass K31.2
  - subaortic Q24.4
    - hypertrophic (acquired) (idiopathic) I42.1
  - subglottic J38.6
  - syphilitic NEC A52.79
  - trachea J39.8
    - congenital Q32.1
    - syphilitic A52.73
    - tuberculous NEC A15.5
  - tracheostomy J95.Ø3
  - tricuspid (valve) — *see* Stenosis, tricuspid
  - tunica vaginalis N5Ø.8
  - ureter (postoperative) N13.5
    - with
      - hydronephrosis N13.1
        - with infection N13.6
      - pyelonephritis (chronic) N11.1
    - congenital — *see* Atresia, ureter
    - tuberculous A18.11
  - ureteropelvic junction (congenital) Q62.11
  - ureterovesical orifice N13.5
    - with infection N13.6
  - urethra (organic) (spasmodic) N35.9
    - associated with schistosomiasis B65.Ø [N37]
    - congenital Q64.39
      - valvular (posterior) Q64.2
    - due to
      - infection — *see* Stricture, urethra, postinfective
      - trauma — *see* Stricture, urethra, post-traumatic
    - gonococcal, gonorrheal A54.Ø1
    - infective NEC — *see* Stricture, urethra, postinfective
    - late effect (sequelae) of injury — *see* Stricture, urethra, post-traumatic
    - postcatheterization — *see* Stricture, urethra, postprocedural
    - postinfective NEC
      - female N35.12
      - male N35.119
        - anterior urethra N35.114
        - bulbous urethra N35.112
        - meatal N35.111
        - membranous urethra N35.113
    - postobstetric N35.Ø21
    - postoperative — *see* Stricture, urethra, postprocedural
    - postprocedural
      - female N99.12
      - male N99.114
        - anterior urethra N99.113
        - bulbous urethra N99.111
        - meatal N99.11Ø
        - membranous urethra N99.112

- **Stricture** — *continued*
  - urethra — *continued*
    - post-traumatic
      - female N35.Ø28
        - due to childbirth N35.Ø21
      - male N35.Ø14
        - anterior urethra N35.Ø13
        - bulbous urethra N35.Ø11
        - meatal N35.Ø1Ø
        - membranous urethra N35.Ø12
    - sequela (late effect) of
      - childbirth N35.Ø21
      - injury — *see* Stricture, urethra, post-traumatic
    - specified cause NEC N35.8
    - syphilitic A52.76
    - traumatic — *see* Stricture, urethra, post-traumatic
    - valvular (posterior), congenital Q64.2
  - urinary meatus — *see* Stricture, urethra
  - uterus, uterine (synechiae) N85.6
    - os (external) (internal) — *see* Stricture, cervix
  - vagina (outlet) — *see* Stenosis, vagina
  - valve (cardiac) (heart) (*see also* Endocarditis)
    - congenital
      - aortic Q23.Ø
      - mitral Q23.2
      - pulmonary Q22.1
      - tricuspid Q22.4
  - vas deferens N5Ø.8
    - congenital Q55.4
  - vein I87.1
  - vena cava (inferior) (superior) NEC I87.1
    - congenital Q26.Ø
  - vesicourethral orifice N32.Ø
    - congenital Q64.31
  - vulva (acquired) N9Ø.5
- **Stridor** RØ6.1
  - congenital (larynx) P28.89
- **Stridulous** — *see* condition
- **Stroke** (apoplectic) (brain) (embolic) (ischemic) (paralytic) (thrombotic) I63.9
  - epileptic — *see* Epilepsy
  - heat T67.Ø ☑
  - in evolution I63.9
  - intraoperative
    - during cardiac surgery I97.81Ø
    - during other surgery I97.811
  - lightning — *see* Lightning
  - meaning
    - cerebral hemorrhage — *code to* Hemorrhage, intracranial
    - cerebral infarction — *code to* Infarction, cerebral
  - postprocedural
    - following cardiac surgery I97.82Ø
    - following other surgery I97.821
  - unspecified (NOS) I63.9
- **Stromatosis, endometrial** D39.Ø
- **Strongyloidiasis, strongyloidosis** B78.9
  - cutaneous B78.1
  - disseminated B78.7
  - intestinal B78.Ø
- **Strophulus pruriginosus** L28.2
- **Struck by lightning** — *see* Lightning
- **Struma** (*see also* Goiter)
  - Hashimoto EØ6.3
  - lymphomatosa EØ6.3
  - nodosa (simplex) EØ4.9
    - endemic EØ1.2
      - multinodular EØ1.1
    - multinodular EØ4.2
      - iodine-deficiency related EØ1.1
    - toxic or with hyperthyroidism EØ5.2Ø
      - with thyroid storm EØ5.21
      - multinodular EØ5.2Ø
        - with thyroid storm EØ5.21
      - uninodular EØ5.1Ø
        - with thyroid storm EØ5.11
    - toxicosa EØ5.2Ø
      - with thyroid storm EØ5.21
      - multinodular EØ5.2Ø
        - with thyroid storm EØ5.21
      - uninodular EØ5.1Ø
        - with thyroid storm EØ5.11
    - uninodular EØ4.1
  - ovarii D27.- ☑
  - Riedel's EØ6.5
- **Strumipriva cachexia** EØ3.4
- **Strümpell-Marie spine** — *see* Spondylitis, ankylosing
- **Strümpell-Westphal pseudosclerosis** E83.Ø1

- **Stuart deficiency disease** (factor X) D68.2
- **Stuart-Prower factor deficiency** (factor X) D68.2
- **Student's elbow** — *see* Bursitis, elbow, olecranon
- **Stump** — *see* Amputation
- **Stunting, nutritional** E45
- **Stupor** (catatonic) R40.1
  - depressive F32.8
  - dissociative F44.2
  - manic F30.2
  - manic-depressive F31.89
  - psychogenic (anergic) F44.2
  - reaction to exceptional stress (transient) F43.0
- **Sturge** (-Weber) (-Dimitri) (-Kalischer) **disease or syndrome** Q85.8
- **Stuttering** F80.81
  - adult onset F98.5
  - childhood onset F80.81
  - following cerebrovascular disease — *see* Disorder, fluency. following cerebrovascular disease
  - in conditions classified elsewhere R47.82
- **Sty, stye** (external) (internal) (meibomian) (zeisian) — *see* Hordeolum
- **Subacidity, gastric** K31.89
  - psychogenic F45.8
- **Subacute** — *see* condition
- **Subarachnoid** — *see* condition
- **Subcortical** — *see* condition
- **Subcostal syndrome, nerve compression** — *see* Mononeuropathy, upper limb, specified site NEC
- **Subcutaneous, subcuticular** — *see* condition
- **Subdural** — *see* condition
- **Subendocardium** — *see* condition
- **Subependymoma**
  - specified site — *see* Neoplasm, uncertain behavior, by site
  - unspecified site D43.2
- **Suberosis** J67.3
- **Subglossitis** — *see* Glossitis
- **Subhemophilia** D66
- **Subinvolution**
  - breast (postlactational) (postpuerperal) N64.89
  - puerperal O90.89
  - uterus (chronic) (nonpuerperal) N85.3
    - puerperal O90.89
- **Sublingual** — *see* condition
- **Sublinguitis** — *see* Sialoadenitis
- **Subluxatable hip** Q65.6
- **Subluxation** (*see also* Dislocation)
  - acromioclavicular S43.11- ☑
  - ankle S93.0- ☑
  - atlantoaxial, recurrent M43.4
    - with myelopathy M43.3
  - carpometacarpal (joint) NEC S63.05- ☑
    - thumb S63.04- ☑
  - complex, vertebral — *see* Complex, subluxation
  - congenital (*see also* Malposition, congenital)
    - hip — *see* Dislocation, hip, congenital, partial
    - joint (excluding hip)
      - lower limb Q68.8
      - shoulder Q68.8
      - upper limb Q68.8
  - elbow (traumatic) S53.10- ☑
    - anterior S53.11- ☑
    - lateral S53.14- ☑
    - medial S53.13- ☑
    - posterior S53.12- ☑
    - specified type NEC S53.19- ☑
  - finger S63.20- ☑
    - index S63.20- ☑
    - interphalangeal S63.22- ☑
      - distal S63.24- ☑
        - index S63.24- ☑
        - little S63.24- ☑
        - middle S63.24- ☑
        - ring S63.24- ☑
      - index S63.22- ☑
      - little S63.22- ☑
      - middle S63.22- ☑
      - proximal S63.23- ☑
        - index S63.23- ☑
        - little S63.23- ☑
        - middle S63.23- ☑
        - ring S63.23- ☑
      - ring S63.22- ☑
    - little S63.20- ☑
    - metacarpophalangeal S63.21- ☑

- **Subluxation** — *continued*
  - finger — *continued*
    - metacarpophalangeal — *continued*
      - index S63.21- ☑
      - little S63.21- ☑
      - middle S63.21- ☑
      - ring S63.21- ☑
    - middle S63.20- ☑
    - ring S63.20- ☑
  - foot S93.30- ☑
    - specified site NEC S93.33- ☑
    - tarsal joint S93.31- ☑
    - tarsometatarsal joint S93.32- ☑
    - toe — *see* Subluxation, toe
  - hip S73.00- ☑
    - anterior S73.03- ☑
      - obturator S73.02- ☑
    - central S73.04- ☑
    - posterior S73.01- ☑
  - interphalangeal (joint)
    - finger S63.22- ☑
      - distal joint S63.24- ☑
        - index S63.24- ☑
        - little S63.24- ☑
        - middle S63.24- ☑
        - ring S63.24- ☑
      - index S63.22- ☑
      - little S63.22- ☑
      - middle S63.22- ☑
      - proximal joint S63.23- ☑
        - index S63.23- ☑
        - little S63.23- ☑
        - middle S63.23- ☑
        - ring S63.23- ☑
      - ring S63.22- ☑
    - thumb S63.12- ☑
      - distal joint S63.14- ☑
      - proximal joint S63.13- ☑
    - toe S93.13- ☑
      - great S93.13- ☑
      - lesser S93.13- ☑
  - joint prosthesis — *see* Complications, joint prosthesis, mechanical, displacement, by site
  - knee S83.10- ☑
    - cap — *see* Subluxation, patella
    - patella — *see* Subluxation, patella
    - proximal tibia
      - anteriorly S83.11- ☑
      - laterally S83.14- ☑
      - medially S83.13- ☑
      - posteriorly S83.12- ☑
    - specified type NEC S83.19- ☑
  - lens — *see* Dislocation, lens, partial
  - ligament, traumatic — *see* Sprain, by site
  - metacarpal (bone)
    - proximal end S63.06- ☑
  - metacarpophalangeal (joint)
    - finger S63.21- ☑
      - index S63.21- ☑
      - little S63.21- ☑
      - middle S63.21- ☑
      - ring S63.21- ☑
    - thumb S63.11- ☑
  - metatarsophalangeal joint S93.14- ☑
    - great toe S93.14- ☑
    - lesser toe S93.14- ☑
  - midcarpal (joint) S63.03- ☑
  - patella S83.00- ☑
    - lateral S83.01- ☑
    - recurrent (nontraumatic) — *see* Dislocation, patella, recurrent, incomplete
    - specified type NEC S83.09- ☑
  - pathological — *see* Dislocation, pathological
  - radial head S53.00- ☑
    - anterior S53.01- ☑
    - nursemaid's elbow S53.03- ☑
    - posterior S53.02- ☑
    - specified type NEC S53.09- ☑
  - radiocarpal (joint) S63.02- ☑
  - radioulnar (joint)
    - distal S63.01- ☑
    - proximal — *see* Subluxation, elbow
  - shoulder
    - congenital Q68.8
    - girdle S43.30- ☑
      - scapula S43.31- ☑

- **Subluxation** — *continued*
  - shoulder — *continued*
    - girdle — *continued*
      - specified site NEC S43.39- ☑
    - traumatic S43.00- ☑
      - anterior S43.01- ☑
      - inferior S43.03- ☑
      - posterior S43.02- ☑
      - specified type NEC S43.08- ☑
  - sternoclavicular (joint) S43.20- ☑
    - anterior S43.21- ☑
    - posterior S43.22- ☑
  - symphysis (pubis)
  - thumb S63.103 ☑
    - interphalangeal joint — *see* Subluxation, interphalangeal (joint), thumb
    - metacarpophalangeal joint — *see* Subluxation, metacarpophalangeal (joint), thumb
  - toe(s) S93.10- ☑
    - great S93.10- ☑
      - interphalangeal joint S93.13- ☑
      - metatarsophalangeal joint S93.14- ☑
    - interphalangeal joint S93.13- ☑
    - lesser S93.10- ☑
      - interphalangeal joint S93.13- ☑
      - metatarsophalangeal joint S93.14- ☑
    - metatarsophalangeal joint S93.149 ☑
  - ulna
    - distal end S63.07- ☑
    - proximal end — *see* Subluxation, elbow
  - ulnohumeral joint — *see* Subluxation, elbow
  - vertebral
    - recurrent NEC — *see* subcategory M43.5 ☑
    - traumatic
      - cervical S13.100 ☑
        - atlantoaxial joint S13.120 ☑
        - atlantooccipital joint S13.110 ☑
        - atloidooccipital joint S13.110 ☑
        - joint between
          - C0 and C1 S13.110 ☑
          - C1 and C2 S13.120 ☑
          - C2 and C3 S13.130 ☑
          - C3 and C4 S13.140 ☑
          - C4 and C5 S13.150 ☑
          - C5 and C6 S13.160 ☑
          - C6 and C7 S13.170 ☑
          - C7 and T1 S13.180 ☑
        - occipitoatloid joint S13.110 ☑
      - lumbar S33.100 ☑
        - joint between
          - L1 and L2 S33.110 ☑
          - L2 and L3 S33.120 ☑
          - L3 and L4 S33.130 ☑
          - L4 and L5 S33.140 ☑
      - thoracic S23.100 ☑
        - joint between
          - T1 and T2 S23.110 ☑
          - T2 and T3 S23.120 ☑
          - T3 and T4 S23.122 ☑
          - T4 and T5 S23.130 ☑
          - T5 and T6 S23.132 ☑
          - T6 and T7 S23.140 ☑
          - T7 and T8 S23.142 ☑
          - T8 and T9 S23.150 ☑
          - T9 and T10 S23.152 ☑
          - T10 and T11 S23.160 ☑
          - T11 and T12 S23.162 ☑
          - T12 and L1 S23.170 ☑
  - wrist (carpal bone) S63.00- ☑
    - carpometacarpal joint — *see* Subluxation, carpometacarpal (joint)
    - distal radioulnar joint — *see* Subluxation, radioulnar (joint), distal
    - metacarpal bone, proximal — *see* Subluxation, metacarpal (bone), proximal end
    - midcarpal — *see* Subluxation, midcarpal (joint)
    - radiocarpal joint — *see* Subluxation, radiocarpal (joint)
    - recurrent — *see* Dislocation, recurrent, wrist
    - specified site NEC S63.09- ☑
    - ulna — *see* Subluxation, ulna, distal end
- **Submaxillary** — *see* condition
- **Submersion** (fatal) (nonfatal) T75.1 ☑
- **Submucous** — *see* condition
- **Subnormal, subnormality**
  - accommodation (old age) H52.4

Subnormal, subnormality — *continued*
- mental — *see* Disability, intellectual
- temperature (accidental) T68 ☑

Subphrenic — *see* condition
Subscapular nerve — *see* condition
Subseptus uterus Q51.2
Subsiding appendicitis K36
Substernal thyroid EØ4.9
- congenital Q89.2

Substitution disorder F44.9
Subtentorial — *see* condition
Subthyroidism (acquired) (*see also* Hypothyroidism)
- congenital EØ3.1

Succenturiate placenta O43.19- ☑
Sucking thumb, child (excessive) F98.8
Sudamen, sudamina L74.1
Sudanese kala-azar B55.Ø
Sudden
- hearing loss — *see* Deafness, sudden
- heart failure — *see* Failure, heart

Sudeck's atrophy, disease, or syndrome — *see* Algoneurodystrophy
Suffocation — *see* Asphyxia, traumatic
Sugar
- blood
  - high (transient) R73.9
  - low (transient) E16.2
- in urine R81

Suicide, suicidal (attempted) T14.91
- by poisoning — *see* Table of Drugs and Chemicals
- history of (personal) Z91.5
  - in family Z81.8
- ideation — *see* Ideation, suicidal
- risk
  - meaning personal history of attempted suicide Z91.5
  - meaning suicidal ideation — *see* Ideation, suicidal
- tendencies
  - meaning personal history of attempted suicide Z91.5
  - meaning suicidal ideation — *see* Ideation, suicidal
- trauma — *see* nature of injury by site

Suipestifer infection — *see* Infection, salmonella
Sulfhemoglobinemia, sulphemoglobinemia (acquired) (with methemoglobinemia) D74.8
Sumatran mite fever A75.3
Summer — *see* condition
Sunburn L55.9
- first degree L55.Ø
- second degree L55.1
- third degree L55.2

SUNCT (short lasting unilateral neuralgiform headache with conjunctival injection and tearing) G44.Ø59
- intractable G44.Ø51
- not intractable G44.Ø59

Sunken acetabulum — *see* Derangement, joint, specified type NEC, hip
Sunstroke T67.Ø ☑
Superfecundation — *see* Pregnancy, multiple
Superfetation — *see* Pregnancy, multiple
Superinvolution (uterus) N85.8
Supernumerary (congenital)
- aortic cusps Q23.8
- auditory ossicles Q16.3
- bone Q79.8
- breast Q83.1
- carpal bones Q74.Ø
- cusps, heart valve NEC Q24.8
  - aortic Q23.8
  - mitral Q23.2
  - pulmonary Q22.3
- digit(s) Q69.9
- ear (lobule) Q17.Ø
- fallopian tube Q5Ø.6
- finger Q69.Ø
- hymen Q52.4
- kidney Q63.Ø
- lacrimonasal duct Q1Ø.6
- lobule (ear) Q17.Ø
- mitral cusps Q23.2
- muscle Q79.8
- nipple(s) Q83.3
- organ or site not listed — *see* Accessory
- ossicles, auditory Q16.3
- ovary Q5Ø.31
- oviduct Q5Ø.6
- pulmonary, pulmonic cusps Q22.3

Supernumerary — *continued*
- rib Q76.6
  - cervical or first (syndrome) Q76.5
- roots (of teeth) KØØ.2
- spleen Q89.Ø9
- tarsal bones Q74.2
- teeth KØØ.1
- testis Q55.29
- thumb Q69.1
- toe Q69.2
- uterus Q51.2
- vagina Q52.1 ☑
- vertebra Q76.49

Supervision (of)
- contraceptive — *see* Prescription, contraceptives
- dietary (for) Z71.3
  - allergy (food) Z71.3
  - colitis Z71.3
  - diabetes mellitus Z71.3
  - food allergy or intolerance Z71.3
  - gastritis Z71.3
  - hypercholesterolemia Z71.3
  - hypoglycemia Z71.3
  - intolerance (food) Z71.3
  - obesity Z71.3
  - specified NEC Z71.3
- healthy infant or child Z76.2
  - foundling Z76.1
- high-risk pregnancy — *see* Pregnancy, complicated by, high, risk
- lactation Z39.1
- pregnancy — *see* Pregnancy, supervision of

Supplemental teeth KØØ.1
Suppression
- binocular vision H53.34
- lactation O92.5
- menstruation N94.89
- ovarian secretion E28.39
- renal N28.9
- urine, urinary secretion R34

Suppuration, suppurative (*see also* condition)
- accessory sinus (chronic) — *see* Sinusitis
- adrenal gland
- antrum (chronic) — *see* Sinusitis, maxillary
- bladder — *see* Cystitis
- brain GØ6.Ø
  - sequelae GØ9
- breast N61
  - puerperal, postpartum or gestational — *see* Mastitis, obstetric, purulent
- dental periosteum M27.3
- ear (middle) (*see also* Otitis, media)
  - external NEC — *see* Otitis, externa, infective
  - internal — *see* subcategory H83.Ø ☑
- ethmoidal (chronic) (sinus) — *see* Sinusitis, ethmoidal
- fallopian tube — *see* Salpingo-oophoritis
- frontal (chronic) (sinus) — *see* Sinusitis, frontal
- gallbladder (acute) K81.Ø
- gum KØ5.2Ø
  - generalized KØ5.22
  - localized KØ5.21
- intracranial GØ6.Ø
- joint — *see* Arthritis, pyogenic or pyemic
- labyrinthine — *see* subcategory H83.Ø ☑
- lung — *see* Abscess, lung
- mammary gland N61
  - puerperal, postpartum O91.12
    - associated with lactation O91.13
- maxilla, maxillary M27.2
  - sinus (chronic) — *see* Sinusitis, maxillary
- muscle — *see* Myositis, infective
- nasal sinus (chronic) — *see* Sinusitis
- pancreas, acute K85.8
- parotid gland — *see* Sialoadenitis
- pelvis, pelvic
  - female — *see* Disease, pelvis, inflammatory
  - male K65.Ø
- pericranial — *see* Osteomyelitis
- salivary duct or gland (any) — *see* Sialoadenitis
- sinus (accessory) (chronic) (nasal) — *see* Sinusitis
- sphenoidal sinus (chronic) — *see* Sinusitis, sphenoidal
- thymus (gland) E32.1
- thyroid (gland) EØ6.Ø
- tonsil — *see* Tonsillitis
- uterus — *see* Endometritis

Supraeruption of tooth (teeth) M26.34
Supraglottitis JØ4.3Ø

Supraglottitis — *continued*
- with obstruction JØ4.31

Suprarenal (gland) — *see* condition
Suprascapular nerve — *see* condition
Suprasellar — *see* condition
Surfer's knots or nodules S89.8- ☑
Surgical
- emphysema T81.82 ☑
- procedures, complication or misadventure — *see* Complications, surgical procedures
- shock T81.1Ø ☑

Surveillance (of) (for) (*see also* Observation)
- alcohol abuse Z71.41
- contraceptive — *see* Prescription, contraceptives
- dietary Z71.3
- drug abuse Z71.51

Susceptibility to disease, genetic Z15.89
- malignant neoplasm Z15.Ø9
  - breast Z15.Ø1
  - endometrium Z15.Ø4
  - ovary Z15.Ø2
  - prostate Z15.Ø3
  - specified NEC Z15.Ø9
- multiple endocrine neoplasia Z15.81

Suspected condition, ruled out (*see also* Observation, suspected)
- amniotic cavity and membrane ZØ3.71
- cervical shortening ZØ3.75
- fetal anomaly ZØ3.73
- fetal growth ZØ3.74
- maternal and fetal conditions NEC ZØ3.79
- oligohydramnios ZØ3.71
- placental problem ZØ3.72
- polyhydramnios ZØ3.71

Suspended uterus
- in pregnancy or childbirth — *see* Pregnancy, complicated by, abnormal uterus

Sutton's nevus D22.9
Suture
- burst (in operation wound) T81.31 ☑
  - external operation wound T81.31 ☑
  - internal operation wound T81.32 ☑
- inadvertently left in operation wound — *see* Foreign body, accidentally left during a procedure
- removal Z48.Ø2

Swab inadvertently left in operation wound — *see* Foreign body, accidentally left during a procedure
Swallowed, swallowing
- difficulty — *see* Dysphagia
- foreign body — *see* Foreign body, alimentary tract

Swan-neck deformity (finger) — *see* Deformity, finger, swan-neck
Swearing, compulsive F42
- in Gilles de la Tourette's syndrome F95.2

Sweat, sweats
- fetid L75.Ø
- night R61

Sweating, excessive R61
Sweeley-Klionsky disease E75.21
Sweet's disease or dermatosis L98.2
Swelling (of) R6Ø.9
- abdomen, abdominal (not referable to any particular organ) — *see* Mass, abdominal
- ankle — *see* Effusion, joint, ankle
- arm M79.89
  - forearm M79.89
- breast N63
- Calabar B74.3
- cervical gland R59.Ø
- chest, localized R22.2
- ear H93.8- ☑
- extremity (lower) (upper) — *see* Disorder, soft tissue, specified type NEC
- finger M79.89
- foot M79.89
- glands R59.9
  - generalized R59.1
  - localized R59.Ø
- hand M79.89
- head (localized) R22.Ø
- inflammatory — *see* Inflammation
- intra-abdominal — *see* Mass, abdominal
- joint — *see* Effusion, joint
- leg M79.89
  - lower M79.89
- limb — *see* Disorder, soft tissue, specified type NEC

- **Swelling** — *continued*
  - localized (skin) R22.9
    - chest R22.2
    - head R22.Ø
    - limb
      - lower — *see* Mass, localized, limb, lower
      - upper — *see* Mass, localized, limb, upper
    - neck R22.1
    - trunk R22.2
  - neck (localized) R22.1
  - pelvic — *see* Mass, abdominal
  - scrotum N5Ø.8
  - splenic — *see* Splenomegaly
  - testis N5Ø.8
  - toe M79.89
  - umbilical R19.Ø9
  - wandering, due to Gnathostoma (spinigerum) B83.1
  - white — *see* Tuberculosis, arthritis
- **Swift** (-Feer) **disease**
  - overdose or wrong substance given or taken — *see* Table of Drugs and Chemicals, by drug, poisoning
- **Swimmer's**
  - cramp T75.1 ☑
  - ear H6Ø.33- ☑
  - itch B65.3
- **Swimming in the head** R42
- **Swollen** — *see* Swelling
- **Swyer syndrome** Q99.1
- **Sycosis** L73.8
  - barbae (not parasitic) L73.8
  - contagiosa (mycotic) B35.Ø
  - lupoides L73.8
  - mycotic B35.Ø
  - parasitic B35.Ø
  - vulgaris L73.8
- **Sydenham's chorea** — *see* Chorea, Sydenham's
- **Sylvatic yellow fever** A95.Ø
- **Sylvest's disease** B33.Ø
- **Symblepharon** H11.23- ☑
  - congenital Q1Ø.3
- **Symond's syndrome** G93.2
- **Sympathetic** — *see* condition
- **Sympatheticotonia** G9Ø.8
- **Sympathicoblastoma**
  - specified site — *see* Neoplasm, malignant, by site
  - unspecified site C74.9Ø
- **Sympathogonioma** — *see* Sympathicoblastoma
- **Symphalangy** (fingers) (toes) Q7Ø.9
- **Symptoms NEC** R68.89
  - breast NEC N64.59
  - development NEC R63.8
  - factitious, self-induced — *see* Disorder, factitious
  - genital organs, female R1Ø.2
  - involving
    - abdomen NEC R19.8
    - appearance NEC R46.89
    - awareness R41.9
      - altered mental status R41.82
      - amnesia — *see* Amnesia
      - borderline intellectual functioning R41.83
      - coma — *see* Coma
      - disorientation R41.Ø
      - neurologic neglect syndrome R41.4
      - senile cognitive decline R41.81
      - specified symptom NEC R41.89
    - behavior NEC R46.89
    - cardiovascular system NEC RØ9.89
    - chest NEC RØ9.89
    - circulatory system NEC RØ9.89
    - cognitive functions R41.9
      - altered mental status R41.82
      - amnesia — *see* Amnesia
      - borderline intellectual functioning R41.83
      - coma — *see* Coma
      - disorientation R41.Ø
      - neurologic neglect syndrome R41.4
      - senile cognitive decline R41.81
      - specified symptom NEC R41.89
    - development NEC R62.5Ø
    - digestive system NEC R19.8
    - emotional state NEC R45.89
      - emotional lability R45.86
    - food and fluid intake R63.8
    - general perceptions and sensations R44.9
      - specified NEC R44.8
    - musculoskeletal system R29.91

- **Symptoms** — *continued*
  - involving — *continued*
    - musculoskeletal system — *continued*
      - specified NEC R29.898
    - nervous system R29.9Ø
      - specified NEC R29.818
    - pelvis NEC R19.8
    - respiratory system NEC RØ9.89
    - skin and integument R23.9
    - urinary system R39.9
  - menopausal N95.1
  - metabolism NEC R63.8
  - neurotic F48.8
  - of infancy R68.19
  - pelvis NEC, female R1Ø.2
  - skin and integument NEC R23.9
  - subcutaneous tissue NEC R23.9
- **Sympus** Q74.2
- **Syncephalus** Q89.4
- **Synchondrosis**
  - abnormal (congenital) Q78.8
  - ischiopubic M91.Ø
- **Synchysis** (scintillans) (senile) (vitreous body) H43.89
- **Syncope** (near) (pre-) R55
  - anginosa I2Ø.8
  - bradycardia RØØ.1
  - cardiac R55
  - carotid sinus G9Ø.Ø1
  - due to spinal (lumbar) puncture G97.1
  - heart R55
  - heat T67.1 ☑
  - laryngeal RØ5
  - psychogenic F48.8
  - tussive RØ5
  - vasoconstriction R55
  - vasodepressor R55
  - vasomotor R55
  - vasovagal R55
- **Syndactylism, syndactyly** Q7Ø.9
  - complex (with synostosis)
    - fingers Q7Ø.Ø- ☑
    - toes Q7Ø.2- ☑
  - simple (without synostosis)
    - fingers Q7Ø.1- ☑
    - toes Q7Ø.3- ☑
- **Syndrome** (*see also* Disease)
  - 48,XXXX Q97.1
  - 49,XXXXX Q97.1
  - 5q minus NOS D46.C (*following* D46.2)
  - abdominal
    - acute R1Ø.Ø
    - muscle deficiency Q79.4
  - abnormal innervation HØ2.519
    - left HØ2.516
      - lower HØ2.515
      - upper HØ2.514
    - right HØ2.513
      - lower HØ2.512
      - upper HØ2.511
  - abstinence, neonatal P96.1
  - acid pulmonary aspiration, obstetric O74.Ø
  - acquired immunodeficiency — *see* Human, immunodeficiency virus (HIV) disease
  - acute abdominal R1Ø.Ø
  - acute respiratory distress (adult) (child) J8Ø
  - Adair-Dighton Q78.Ø
  - Adams-Stokes (-Morgagni) I45.9
  - adiposogenital E23.6
  - adrenal
    - hemorrhage (meningococcal) A39.1
    - meningococcic A39.1
  - adrenocortical — *see* Cushing's, syndrome
  - adrenogenital E25.9
    - congenital, associated with enzyme deficiency E25.Ø
  - afferent loop NEC K91.89
  - Alagille's Q44.7
  - alcohol withdrawal (without convulsions) — *see* Dependence, alcohol, with, withdrawal
  - Alder's D72.Ø
  - Aldrich (-Wiskott) D82.Ø
  - alien hand R41.4
  - Alport Q87.81
  - alveolar hypoventilation E66.2
  - alveolocapillary block J84.1Ø
  - amnesic, amnestic (confabulatory) (due to) — *see* Disorder, amnesic
  - amyostatic (Wilson's disease) E83.Ø1

- **Syndrome** — *continued*
  - androgen insensitivity E34.5Ø
    - complete E34.51
    - partial E34.52
  - androgen resistance (*see also* Syndrome, androgen insensitivity) E34.5Ø
  - Angelman Q93.5
  - anginal — *see* Angina
  - ankyloglossia superior Q38.1
  - anterior
    - chest wall RØ7.89
    - cord G83.82
    - spinal artery G95.19
      - compression M47.Ø19
        - cervical region M47.Ø12
        - cervicothoracic region M47.Ø13
        - lumbar region M47.Ø16
        - occipito-atlanto-axial region M47.Ø11
        - thoracic region M47.Ø14
        - thoracolumbar region M47.Ø15
    - tibial M76.81- ☑
  - antibody deficiency D8Ø.9
    - agammaglobulinemic D8Ø.1
      - hereditary D8Ø.Ø
    - congenital D8Ø.Ø
    - hypogammaglobulinemic D8Ø.1
      - hereditary D8Ø.Ø
  - anticardiolipin (-antibody) D68.61
  - antiphospholipid (-antibody) D68.61
  - aortic
    - arch M31.4
    - bifurcation I74.Ø9
  - aortomesenteric duodenum occlusion K31.5
  - apical ballooning (transient left ventricular) I51.81
  - arcuate ligament I77.4
  - argentaffin, argintaffinoma E34.Ø
  - Arnold-Chiari — *see* Arnold-Chiari disease
  - Arrillaga-Ayerza I27.Ø
  - Asherman's N85.6
  - aspiration, of newborn — *see* Aspiration, by substance, with pneumonia
    - meconium P24.Ø1
  - ataxia-telangiectasia G11.3
  - auriculotemporal G5Ø.8
  - autoerythrocyte sensitization (Gardner-Diamond) D69.2
  - autoimmune lymphoproliferative [ALPS] D89.82
  - autoimmune polyglandular E31.Ø
  - autosomal — *see* Abnormal, autosomes
  - Avellis' G46.8
  - Ayerza (-Arrillaga) I27.Ø
  - Babinski-Nageotte G83.89
  - Bakwin-Krida Q79.8
  - bare lymphocyte D81.6
  - Barré-Guillain G61.Ø
  - Barré-Liéou M53.Ø
  - Barrett's — *see* Barrett's, esophagus
  - Barsony-Polgar K22.4
  - Bársony-Teschendorf K22.4
  - Barth E78.71
  - Bartter's E26.81
  - basal cell nevus Q87.89
  - Basedow's EØ5.ØØ
    - with thyroid storm EØ5.Ø1
  - basilar artery G45.Ø
  - Batten-Steinert G71.11
  - battered
    - baby or child — *see* Maltreatment, child, physical abuse
    - spouse — *see* Maltreatment, adult, physical abuse
  - Beals Q87.4Ø
  - Beau's I51.5
  - Beck's I65.8
  - Benedikt's G46.3
  - Béquez César (-Steinbrinck-Chédiak-Higashi) E7Ø.33Ø
  - Bernhardt-Roth — *see* Meralgia paresthetica
  - Bernheim's I5Ø.9
  - big spleen D73.1
  - bilateral polycystic ovarian E28.2
  - Bing-Horton's — *see* Horton's headache
  - Birt-Hogg-Dube syndrome Q87.89
  - Björck (-Thorsen) E34.Ø
  - black
    - lung J6Ø
    - widow spider bite — *see* Toxicity, venom, spider, black widow
  - Blackfan-Diamond D61.Ø1

Syndrome — *continued*
- endocrine-hypertensive E27.Ø
- entrapment — *see* Neuropathy, entrapment
- eosinophilia-myalgia M35.8
- epileptic (*see also* Epilepsy, by type)
  - absence G40.AØ9 (*following* G40.3)
    - intractable G40.A19 (*following* G40.3)
      - with status epilepticus G40.A11 (*following* G40.3)
      - without status epilepticus G40.A19 (*following* G40.3)
    - not intractable G40.AØ9 (*following* G40.3)
      - with status epilepticus G40.AØ1 (*following* G40.3)
      - without status epilepticus G40.AØ9 (*following* G40.3)
- Erdheim-Chester (ECD) E88.89
- Erdheim's E22.Ø
- erythrocyte fragmentation D59.4
- Evans D69.41
- exhaustion F48.8
- extrapyramidal G25.9
  - specified NEC G25.89
- eye retraction — *see* Strabismus
- eyelid-malar-mandible Q87.Ø
- Faber's D5Ø.9
- facial pain, paroxysmal G5Ø.Ø
- Fallot's Q21.3
- familial eczema-thrombocytopenia (Wiskott-Aldrich) D82.Ø
- Fanconi (-de Toni) (-Debré) E72.Ø9
  - with cystinosis E72.Ø4
- Fanconi's (anemia) (congenital pancytopenia) D61.Ø9
- fatigue
  - chronic R53.82
  - psychogenic F48.8
- faulty bowel habit K59.3
- Feil-Klippel (brevicollis) Q76.1
- Felty's — *see* Felty's syndrome
- fertile eunuch E23.Ø
- fetal
  - alcohol (dysmorphic) Q86.Ø
  - hydantoin Q86.1
- Fiedler's I4Ø.1
- first arch Q87.Ø
- fish odor E72.8
- Fisher's G61.Ø
- Fitzhugh-Curtis
  - due to
    - Chlamydia trachomatis A74.81
    - Neisseria gonorrhorea (gonococcal peritonitis) A54.85
- Fitz's K85.8
- Flajani (-Basedow) EØ5.ØØ
  - with thyroid storm EØ5.Ø1
- flatback — *see* Flatback syndrome
- floppy
  - baby P94.2
  - iris (intraoeprative) (IFIS) H21.81
  - mitral valve I34.1
- flush E34.Ø
- Foix-Alajouanine G95.19
- Fong's Q79.8
- foramen magnum G93.5
- Foster-Kennedy H47.14- ☑
- Foville's (peduncular) G46.3
- fragile X Q99.2
- Franceschetti Q75.4
- Frey's
  - auriculotemporal G5Ø.8
  - hyperhidrosis L74.52
- Friderichsen-Waterhouse A39.1
- Froin's G95.89
- frontal lobe FØ7.Ø
- Fukuhara E88.49
- functional
  - bowel K59.9
  - prepubertal castrate E29.1
- Gaisböck's D75.1
- ganglion (basal ganglia brain) G25.9
  - geniculi G51.1
- Gardner-Diamond D69.2
- gastroesophageal
  - junction K22.Ø
  - laceration-hemorrhage K22.6
- gastrojejunal loop obstruction K91.89
- Gee-Herter-Heubner K9Ø.Ø
- Gelineau's G47.419

Syndrome — *continued*
- Gelineau's — *continued*
  - with cataplexy G47.411
- genito-anorectal A55
- Gerstmann-Sträussler-Scheinker (GSS) A81.82
- Gianotti-Crosti L44.4
- giant platelet (Bernard-Soulier) D69.1
- Gilles de la Tourette's F95.2
- goiter-deafness EØ7.1
- Goldberg Q89.8
- Goldberg-Maxwell E34.51
- Good's D83.8
- Gopalan' (burning feet) E53.8
- Gorlin's Q87.89
- Gougerot-Blum L81.7
- Gouley's I31.1
- Gower's R55
- gray or grey (newborn) P93.Ø
  - platelet D69.1
- Gubler-Millard G46.3
- Guillain-Barré (-Strohl) G61.Ø
- gustatory sweating G5Ø.8
- Hadfield-Clarke K86.8
- hair tourniquet — *see* Constriction, external, by site
- Hamman's J98.19
- hand-foot L27.1
- hand-shoulder G9Ø.8
- hantavirus (cardio)-pulmonary (HPS) (HCPS) B33.4
- happy puppet Q93.5
- Harada's H3Ø.81- ☑
- Hayem-Faber D5Ø.9
- headache NEC G44.89
  - complicated NEC G44.59
- Heberden's I2Ø.8
- Hedinger's E34.Ø
- Hegglin's D72.Ø
- HELLP (hemolysis, elevated liver enzymes and low platelet count) O14.2- ☑
- hemolytic-uremic D59.3
- hemophagocytic, infection-associated D76.2
- Henoch-Schönlein D69.Ø
- hepatic flexure K59.8
- hepatopulmonary K76.81
- hepatorenal K76.7
  - following delivery O9Ø.4
  - postoperative or postprocedural K91.83
  - postpartum, puerperal O9Ø.4
- hepatourologic K76.7
- Herter (-Gee) (nontropical sprue) K9Ø.Ø
- Heubner-Herter K9Ø.Ø
- Heyd's K76.7
- Hilger's G9Ø.Ø9
- histamine-like (fish poisoning) — *see* Poisoning, fish
- histiocytic D76.3
- histiocytosis NEC D76.3
- HIV infection, acute B2Ø
- Hoffmann-Werdnig G12.Ø
- Hollander-Simons E88.1
- Hoppe-Goldflam G7Ø.ØØ
  - with exacerbation (acute) G7Ø.Ø1
  - in crisis G7Ø.Ø1
- Horner's G9Ø.2
- hungry bone E83.81
- hunterian glossitis D51.Ø
- Hutchinson's triad A5Ø.53
- hyperabduction G54.Ø
- hyperammonemia-hyperornithinemia-homocitrullinemia E72.4
- hypereosinophilic (idiopathic) D72.1
- hyperimmunoglobulin E (IgE) D82.4
- hyperkalemic E87.5
- hyperkinetic — *see* Hyperkinesia
- hypermobility M35.7
- hypernatremia E87.Ø
- hyperosmolarity E87.Ø
- hyperperfusion G97.82
- hypersplenic D73.1
- hypertransfusion, newborn P61.1
- hyperventilation F45.8
- hyperviscosity (of serum)
  - polycythemic D75.1
  - sclerothymic D58.8
- hypoglycemic (familial) (neonatal) E16.2
- hypokalemic E87.6
- hyponatremic E87.1
- hypopituitarism E23.Ø
- hypoplastic left-heart Q23.4
- hypopotassemia E87.6

Syndrome — *continued*
- hyposmolality E87.1
- hypotension, maternal O26.5- ☑
- hypothenar hammer I73.89
- ICF (intravascular coagulation-fibrinolysis) D65
- idiopathic
  - cardiorespiratory distress, newborn P22.Ø
  - nephrotic (infantile) NØ4.9
- iliotibial band M76.3- ☑
- immobility, immobilization (paraplegic) M62.3
- immune reconstitution D89.3
- immune reconstitution inflammatory [IRIS] D89.3
- immunity deficiency, combined D81.9
- immunodeficiency
  - acquired — *see* Human, immunodeficiency virus (HIV) disease
  - combined D81.9
- impending coronary I2Ø.Ø
- impingement, shoulder M75.4- ☑
- inappropriate secretion of antidiuretic hormone E22.2
- infant
  - gestational diabetes P7Ø.Ø
  - of diabetic mother P7Ø.1
- infantilism (pituitary) E23.Ø
- inferior vena cava I87.1
- inspissated bile (newborn) P59.1
- institutional (childhood) F94.2
- insufficient sleep F51.12
- intermediate coronary (artery) I2Ø.Ø
- interspinous ligament — *see* Spondylopathy, specified NEC
- intestinal
  - carcinoid E34.Ø
  - knot K56.2
- intravascular coagulation-fibrinolysis (ICF) D65
- iodine-deficiency, congenital EØØ.9
  - type
    - mixed EØØ.2
    - myxedematous EØØ.1
    - neurological EØØ.Ø
- IRDS (idiopathic respiratory distress, newborn) P22.Ø
- irritable
  - bowel K58.9
    - with diarrhea K58.Ø
    - psychogenic F45.8
  - heart (psychogenic) F45.8
  - weakness F48.8
- ischemic bowel (transient) K55.9
  - chronic K55.1
  - due to mesenteric artery insufficiency K55.1
- IVC (intravascular coagulopathy) D65
- Ivemark's Q89.Ø1
- Jaccoud's — *see* Arthropathy, postrheumatic, chronic
- Jackson's G83.89
- Jakob-Creutzfeldt — *see* Creutzfeldt-Jakob disease or syndrome
- jaw-winking QØ7.8
- Jervell-Lange-Nielsen I45.81
- jet lag G47.25
- Job's D71
- Joseph-Diamond-Blackfan D61.Ø1
- jugular foramen G52.7
- Kabuki Q89.8
- Kanner's (autism) F84.Ø
- Kartagener's Q89.3
- Kelly's D5Ø.1
- Kimmelsteil-Wilson — *see* Diabetes, specified type, with Kimmelsteil-Wilson disease
- Klein (e)-Levine G47.13
- Klippel-Feil (brevicollis) Q76.1
- Köhler-Pellegrini-Steida — *see* Bursitis, tibial collateral
- König's K59.8
- Korsakoff (-Wernicke) (nonalcoholic) FØ4
  - alcoholic F1Ø.26
- Kostmann's D7Ø.Ø
- Krabbe's congenital muscle hypoplasia Q79.8
- labyrinthine — *see* subcategory H83.2 ☑
- lacunar NEC G46.7
- Lambert-Eaton G7Ø.8Ø
  - in
    - neoplastic disease G73.1
    - specified disease NEC G7Ø.81
- Landau-Kleffner — *see* Epilepsy, specified NEC
- Larsen's Q74.8
- lateral
  - cutaneous nerve of thigh G57.1- ☑
  - medullary G46.4
- Launois' E22.Ø

Syndrome — *continued*
- lazy
  - leukocyte D7Ø.8
  - posture M62.3
- Lemiere I8Ø.8
- Lennox-Gastaut G4Ø.812
  - intractable G4Ø.814
    - with status epilepticus G4Ø.813
    - without status epilepticus G4Ø.814
  - not intractable G4Ø.812
    - with status epilepticus G4Ø.811
    - without status epilepticus G4Ø.812
- lenticular, progressive E83.Ø1
- Leopold-Levi's EØ5.9Ø
- Lev's I44.2
- Lichtheim's D51.Ø
- Li-Fraumeni Z15.Ø1
- Lightwood's N25.89
- Lignac (de Toni) (-Fanconi) (-Debré) E72.Ø9
  - with cystinosis E72.Ø4
- Likoff's I2Ø.8
- limbic epilepsy personality FØ7.Ø
- liver-kidney K76.7
- lobotomy FØ7.Ø
- Loffler's J82
- long arm 18 or 21 deletion Q93.89
- long QT I45.81
- Louis-Barré G11.3
- low
  - atmospheric pressure T7Ø.29 ☑
  - back M54.5
  - output (cardiac) I5Ø.9
- lower radicular, newborn (birth injury) P14.8
- Luetscher's (dehydration) E86.Ø
- Lupus anticoagulant D68.62
- Lutembacher's Q21.1
- macrophage activation D76.1
  - due to infection D76.2
- magnesium-deficiency R29.Ø
- Mal de Debarquement R42
- malabsorption K9Ø.9
  - postsurgical K91.2
- malformation, congenital, due to
  - alcohol Q86.Ø
  - exogenous cause NEC Q86.8
  - hydantoin Q86.1
  - warfarin Q86.2
- malignant
  - carcinoid E34.Ø
  - neuroleptic G21.Ø
- Mallory-Weiss K22.6
- mandibulofacial dysostosis Q75.4
- manic-depressive — *see* Disorder, bipolar, affective
- maple-syrup-urine E71.Ø
- Marable's I77.4
- Marfan's Q87.4Ø
  - with
    - cardiovascular manifestations Q87.418
      - aortic dilation Q87.41Ø
    - ocular manifestations Q87.42
    - skeletal manifestations Q87.43
- Marie's (acromegaly) E22.Ø
- maternal hypotension — *see* Syndrome, hypotension, maternal
- May (-Hegglin) D72.Ø
- McArdle (-Schmidt) (-Pearson) E74.Ø4
- McQuarrie's E16.2
- meconium plug (newborn) P76.Ø
- median arcuate ligament I77.4
- Meekeren-Ehlers-Danlos Q79.6
- megavitamin-B6 E67.2
- Meige G24.4
- MELAS E88.41
- Mendelson's O74.Ø
- MERRF (myoclonic epilepsy associated with ragged-red fibers) E88.42
- mesenteric
  - artery (superior) K55.1
  - vascular insufficiency K55.1
- metabolic E88.81
- metastatic carcinoid E34.Ø
- micrognathia-glossoptosis Q87.Ø
- midbrain NEC G93.89
- middle lobe (lung) J98.19
- middle radicular G54.Ø
- migraine (*see also* Migraine) G43.9Ø9
- Mikulicz' K11.8
- milk-alkali E83.52

Syndrome — *continued*
- Millard-Gubler G46.3
- Miller-Dieker Q93.88
- Miller-Fisher G61.Ø
- Minkowski-Chauffard D58.Ø
- Mirizzi's K83.1
- MNGIE (Mitochondrial Neurogastrointestinal Encephalopathy) E88.49
- Möbius, ophthalmoplegic migraine — *see* Migraine, ophthalmoplegic
- monofixation H5Ø.42
- Morel-Moore M85.2
- Morel-Morgagni M85.2
- Morgagni (-Morel) (-Stewart) M85.2
- Morgagni-Adams-Stokes I45.9
- Mounier-Kuhn Q32.4
  - with bronchiectasis J47.9
    - with
      - exacerbation (acute) J47.1
      - lower respiratory infection J47.Ø
  - acquired J98.Ø9
    - with bronchiectasis J47.9
      - with
        - exacerbation (acute) J47.1
        - lower respiratory infection J47.Ø
- mucocutaneous lymph node (acute febrile) (MCLS) M3Ø.3
- multiple endocrine neoplasia (MEN) — *see* Neoplasia, endocrine, multiple (MEN)
- multiple operations — *see* Disorder, factitious
- myasthenic G7Ø.9
  - in
    - diabetes mellitus — *see* Diabetes, amyotrophy
    - endocrine disease NEC E34.9 [G73.3]
    - neoplastic disease (*see also* Neoplasm) D49.9 [G73.3]
    - thyrotoxicosis (hyperthyroidism) EØ5.9Ø [G73.3]
      - with thyroid storm EØ5.91 [G73.3]
- myelodysplastic D46.9
  - with
    - 5q deletion D46.C (*following* D46.2)
    - isolated del (5q) chromosomal abnormality D46.C (*following* D46.2)
  - lesions, low grade D46.2Ø
  - specified NEC D46.Z (*following* D46.4)
- myelopathic pain G89.Ø
- myeloproliferative (chronic) D47.1
- myofascial pain M79.1
- Naffziger's G54.Ø
- nail patella Q87.2
- NARP (Neuropathy, Ataxia and Retinitis pigmentosa) E88.49
- neonatal abstinence P96.1
- nephritic (*see also* Nephritis)
  - with edema — *see* Nephrosis
  - acute NØØ.9
  - chronic NØ3.9
  - rapidly progressive NØ1.9
- nephrotic (congenital) (*see also* Nephrosis) NØ4.9
  - with
    - dense deposit disease NØ4.6
    - diffuse
      - crescentic glomerulonephritis NØ4.7
      - endocapillary proliferative glomerulonephritis NØ4.4
      - membranous glomerulonephritis NØ4.2
      - mesangial proliferative glomerulonephritis NØ4.3
      - mesangiocapillary glomerulonephritis NØ4.5
    - focal and segmental glomerular lesions NØ4.1
    - minor glomerular abnormality NØ4.Ø
    - specified morphological changes NEC NØ4.8
  - diabetic — *see* Diabetes, nephrosis
- neurologic neglect R41.4
- Nezelof's D81.4
- Nonne-Milroy-Meige Q82.Ø
- Nothnagel's vasomotor acroparesthesia I73.89
- oculomotor H51.9
- ophthalmoplegia-cerebellar ataxia — *see* Strabismus, paralytic, third nerve
- oral-facial-digital Q87.Ø
- organic
  - affective FØ6.3Ø
  - amnesic (not alcohol- or drug-induced) FØ4
  - brain FØ9
  - depressive FØ6.31
  - hallucinosis FØ6.Ø
  - personality FØ7.Ø

Syndrome — *continued*
- Ormond's N13.5
- oro-facial-digital Q87.Ø
- os trigonum Q68.8
- Osler-Weber-Rendu I78.Ø
- osteoporosis-osteomalacia M83.8
- Osterreicher-Turner Q79.8
- otolith — *see* subcategory H81.8 ☑
- oto-palatal-digital Q87.Ø
- outlet (thoracic) G54.Ø
- ovary
  - polycystic E28.2
  - resistant E28.39
  - sclerocystic E28.2
- Owren's D68.2
- Paget-Schroetter I82.89Ø
- pain (*see also* Pain)
  - complex regional I G9Ø.5Ø
    - lower limb G9Ø.52- ☑
    - specified site NEC G9Ø.59
    - upper limb G9Ø.51- ☑
  - complex regional II — *see* Causalgia
- painful
  - bruising D69.2
  - feet E53.8
  - prostate N42.81
- paralysis agitans — *see* Parkinsonism
- paralytic G83.9
  - specified NEC G83.89
- Parinaud's H51.Ø
- parkinsonian — *see* Parkinsonism
- Parkinson's — *see* Parkinsonism
- paroxysmal facial pain G5Ø.Ø
- Parry's EØ5.ØØ
  - with thyroid storm EØ5.Ø1
- Parsonage (-Aldren)-Turner G54.5
- patella clunk M25.86- ☑
- Paterson (-Brown) (-Kelly) D5Ø.1
- pectoral girdle I77.89
- pectoralis minor I77.89
- Pelger-Huet D72.Ø
- pellagra-cerebellar ataxia-renal aminoaciduria E72.Ø2
- pellagroid E52
- Pellegrini-Stieda — *see* Bursitis, tibial collateral
- pelvic congestion-fibrosis, female N94.89
- penta X Q97.1
- peptic ulcer — *see* Ulcer, peptic
- perabduction I77.89
- periodic headache, in adults and children — *see* Headache, periodic syndromes in adults and children
- periurethral fibrosis N13.5
- phantom limb (without pain) G54.7
  - with pain G54.6
- pharyngeal pouch D82.1
- Pick's (heart) (liver) I31.1
- Pickwickian E66.2
- PIE (pulmonary infiltration with eosinophilia) J82
- pigmentary pallidal degeneration (progressive) G23.Ø
- pineal E34.8
- pituitary E22.Ø
- placental transfusion — *see* Pregnancy, complicated by, placental transfusion syndromes
- plantar fascia M72.2
- plateau iris (post-iridectomy) (postprocedural) H21.82
- Plummer-Vinson D5Ø.1
- pluricarential of infancy E4Ø
- plurideficiency E4Ø
- pluriglandular (compensatory) E31.8
  - autoimmune E31.Ø
- pneumatic hammer T75.21 ☑
- polyangiitis overlap M3Ø.8
- polycarential of infancy E4Ø
- polyglandular E31.8
  - autoimmune E31.Ø
- polysplenia Q89.Ø9
- pontine NEC G93.89
- popliteal
  - artery entrapment I77.89
  - web Q87.89
- post chemoembolization — *code to* associated conditions
- postcardiac injury
  - postcardiotomy I97.Ø
  - postmyocardial infarction I24.1
- postcardiotomy I97.Ø
- postcholecystectomy K91.5
- postcommissurotomy I97.Ø

Syndrome — *continued*
- postconcussional FØ7.81
- postcontusional FØ7.81
- postencephalitic FØ7.89
- posterior
  - cervical sympathetic M53.Ø
  - cord G83.83
  - fossa compression G93.5
  - reversible encephalopathy (PRES) I67.83
- postgastrectomy (dumping) K91.1
- postgastric surgery K91.1
- postinfarction I24.1
- postlaminectomy NEC M96.1
- postleukotomy FØ7.Ø
- postmastectomy lymphedema I97.2
- postmyocardial infarction I24.1
- postoperative NEC T81.9 ☑
  - blind loop K9Ø.2
- postpartum panhypopituitary (Sheehan) E23.Ø
- postpolio (myelitic) G14
- postthrombotic I87.ØØ9
  - with
    - inflammation I87.Ø2- ☑
      - with ulcer I87.Ø3- ☑
    - specified complication NEC I87.Ø9- ☑
    - ulcer I87.Ø1- ☑
      - with inflammation I87.Ø3- ☑
  - asymptomatic I87.ØØ- ☑
- postvagotomy K91.1
- postvalvulotomy I97.Ø
- postviral NEC G93.3
  - fatigue G93.3
- Potain's K31.Ø
- potassium intoxication E87.5
- precerebral artery (multiple) (bilateral) G45.2
- preinfarction I2Ø.Ø
- preleukemic D46.9
- premature senility E34.8
- premenstrual dysphoric N94.3
- premenstrual tension N94.3
- Prinzmetal-Massumi RØ7.1
- prune belly Q79.4
- pseudo -Turner's Q87.1
- pseudocarpal tunnel (sublimis) — *see* Syndrome, carpal tunnel
- pseudoparalytica G7Ø.ØØ
  - with exacerbation (acute) G7Ø.Ø1
  - in crisis G7Ø.Ø1
- psycho-organic (nonpsychotic severity) FØ7.9
  - acute or subacute FØ5
  - depressive type FØ6.31
  - hallucinatory type FØ6.Ø
  - nonpsychotic severity FØ7.Ø
  - specified NEC FØ7.89
- pulmonary
  - arteriosclerosis I27.Ø
  - dysmaturity (Wilson-Mikity) P27.Ø
  - hypoperfusion (idiopathic) P22.Ø
  - renal (hemorrhagic) (Goodpasture's) M31.Ø
- pure
  - motor lacunar G46.5
  - sensory lacunar G46.6
- Putnam-Dana D51.Ø
- pyramidopallidonigral G2Ø
- pyriformis — *see* Lesion, nerve, sciatic
- QT interval prolongation I45.81
- radicular NEC — *see* Radiculopathy
  - upper limbs, newborn (birth injury) P14.3
- rapid time-zone change G47.25
- Rasmussen GØ4.81
- Raymond (-Céstan) I65.8
- Raynaud's I73.ØØ
  - with gangrene I73.Ø1
- RDS (respiratory distress syndrome, newborn) P22.Ø
- reactive airways dysfunction J68.3
- Refsum's G6Ø.1
- Reifenstein E34.52
- renal glomerulohyalinosis-diabetic — *see* Diabetes, nephrosis
- Rendu-Osler-Weber I78.Ø
- residual ovary N99.83
- resistant ovary E28.39
- respiratory
  - distress
    - acute J8Ø
      - adult J8Ø
      - child J8Ø
    - newborn (idiopathic) (type I) P22.Ø

Syndrome — *continued*
- respiratory — *continued*
  - distress — *continued*
    - newborn — *continued*
      - type II P22.1
- restless legs G25.81
- retinoblastoma (familial) C69.2 ☑
- retroperitoneal fibrosis N13.5
- retroviral seroconversion (acute) Z21
- Reye's G93.7
- Richter — *see* Leukemia, chronic lymphocytic, B-cell type
- Ridley's I5Ø.1
- right
  - heart, hypoplastic Q22.6
  - ventricular obstruction — *see* Failure, heart, congestive
- Romano-Ward (prolonged QT interval) I45.81
- rotator cuff, shoulder (*see also* Tear, rotator cuff) M75.1Ø- ☑
- Rotes Quérol — *see* Hyperostosis, ankylosing
- Roth — *see* Meralgia paresthetica
- rubella (congenital) P35.Ø
- Ruvalcaba-Myhre-Smith E71.44Ø
- Rytand-Lipsitch I44.2
- salt
  - depletion E87.1
    - due to heat NEC T67.8 ☑
      - causing heat exhaustion or prostration T67.4 ☑
  - low E87.1
- salt-losing N28.89
- Scaglietti-Dagnini E22.Ø
- scalenus anticus (anterior) G54.Ø
- scapulocostal — *see* Mononeuropathy, upper limb, specified site NEC
- scapuloperoneal G71.Ø
- schizophrenic, of childhood NEC F84.5
- Schnitzler D47.2
- Scholte's E34.Ø
- Schroeder's E27.Ø
- Schüller-Christian C96.5
- Schwachman's — *see* Syndrome, Shwachman's
- Schwartz (-Jampel) G71.13
- Schwartz-Bartter E22.2
- scimitar Q26.8
- sclerocystic ovary E28.2
- Seitelberger's G31.89
- septicemic adrenal hemorrhage A39.1
- seroconversion, retroviral (acute) Z21
- serous meningitis G93.2
- severe acute respiratory (SARS) J12.81
- shaken infant T74.4 ☑
- shock (traumatic) T79.4 ☑
  - kidney N17.Ø
    - following crush injury T79.5 ☑
  - toxic A48.3
- shock-lung J8Ø
- Shone's — *code to* specific anomalies
- short
  - bowel K91.2
  - rib Q77.2
- shoulder-hand — *see* Algoneurodystrophy
- Shwachman's D7Ø.4
- sicca — *see* Sicca syndrome
- sick
  - cell E87.1
  - sinus I49.5
- sick-euthyroid EØ7.81
- sideropenic D5Ø.1
- Siemens' ectodermal dysplasia Q82.4
- Silfverskiöld's Q78.9
- Simons' E88.1
- sinus tarsi M25.57- ☑
- sinusitis-bronchiectasis-situs inversus Q89.3
- Sipple's E31.22
- sirenomelia Q87.2
- Slocumb's E27.Ø
- slow flow, coronary I2Ø.8
- Sluder's G44.89
- Smith-Magenis Q93.88
- Sneddon-Wilkinson L13.1
- Sotos' E22.Ø
- South African cardiomyopathy I42.8
- spasmodic
  - upward movement, eyes H51.8
  - winking F95.8
- Spen's I45.9

Syndrome — *continued*
- splenic
  - agenesis Q89.Ø1
  - flexure K59.8
  - neutropenia D73.81
- Spurway's Q78.Ø
- staphylococcal scalded skin LØØ
- Stein-Leventhal E28.2
- Stein's E28.2
- Stevens-Johnson syndrome L51.1
  - toxic epidermal necrolysis overlap L51.3
- Stewart-Morel M85.2
- Stickler Q89.8
- stiff baby Q89.8
- stiff man G25.82
- Still-Felty — *see* Felty's syndrome
- Stokes (-Adams) I45.9
- stone heart I5Ø.1
- straight back, congenital Q76.49
- subclavian steal G45.8
- subcoracoid-pectoralis minor G54.Ø
- subcostal nerve compression I77.89
- subphrenic interposition Q43.3
- superior
  - cerebellar artery I63.8
  - mesenteric artery K55.1
  - semi-circular canal dehiscence H83.8X- ☑
  - vena cava I87.1
- supine hypotensive (maternal) — *see* Syndrome, hypotension, maternal
- suprarenal cortical E27.Ø
- supraspinatus (*see also* Tear, rotator cuff) M75.1Ø- ☑
- Susac G93.49
- swallowed blood P78.2
- sweat retention L74.Ø
- Swyer Q99.1
- Symond's G93.2
- sympathetic
  - cervical paralysis G9Ø.2
  - pelvic, female N94.89
- systemic inflammatory response (SIRS), of non-infectious origin (without organ dysfunction) R65.1Ø
  - with acute organ dysfunction R65.11
- tachycardia-bradycardia I49.5
- takotsubo I51.81
- TAR (thrombocytopenia with absent radius) Q87.2
- tarsal tunnel G57.5- ☑
- teething KØØ.7
- tegmental G93.89
- telangiectasic-pigmentation-cataract Q82.8
- temporal pyramidal apex — *see* Otitis, media, suppurative, acute
- temporomandibular joint-pain-dysfunction M26.62
- Terry's H44.2- ☑
- testicular feminization (*see also* Syndrome, androgen insensitivity) E34.51
- thalamic pain (hyperesthetic) G89.Ø
- thoracic outlet (compression) G54.Ø
- Thorson-Björck E34.Ø
- thrombocytopenia with absent radius (TAR) Q87.2
- thyroid-adrenocortical insufficiency E31.Ø
- tibial
  - anterior M76.81- ☑
  - posterior M76.82- ☑
- Tietze's M94.Ø
- time-zone (rapid) G47.25
- Toni-Fanconi E72.Ø9
  - with cystinosis E72.Ø4
- Touraine's Q79.8
- tourniquet — *see* Constriction, external, by site
- toxic shock A48.3
- transient left ventricular apical ballooning I51.81
- traumatic vasospastic T75.22 ☑
- Treacher Collins Q75.4
- triple X, female Q97.Ø
- trisomy Q92.9
  - 13 Q91.7
    - meiotic nondisjunction Q91.4
    - mitotic nondisjunction Q91.5
    - mosaicism Q91.5
    - translocation Q91.6
  - 18 Q91.3
    - meiotic nondisjunction Q91.Ø
    - mitotic nondisjunction Q91.1
    - mosaicism Q91.1
    - translocation Q91.2
  - 2Ø (q)(p) Q92.8
  - 21 Q9Ø.9

Syphilis, syphilitic — *continued*
- congenital — *continued*
  - early, or less than 2 years after birth — *continued*
    - symptomatic — *continued*
      - visceral A5Ø.Ø8
  - chorioretinitis, choroiditis A5Ø.Ø1 [H32]
  - interstitial keratitis A5Ø.31
  - juvenile neurosyphilis A5Ø.45
  - late, or 2 years or more after birth NEC A5Ø.7
    - chorioretinitis, choroiditis A5Ø.32
    - interstitial keratitis A5Ø.31
    - juvenile neurosyphilis A5Ø.45
    - latent (without manifestations) A5Ø.6
      - negative spinal fluid test A5Ø.6
      - serology positive A5Ø.6
    - symptomatic or with manifestations NEC A5Ø.59
      - arthropathy A5Ø.55
      - cardiovascular A5Ø.54
      - Clutton's joints A5Ø.51
      - Hutchinson's teeth A5Ø.52
      - Hutchinson's triad A5Ø.53
      - osteochondropathy A5Ø.56
      - saddle nose A5Ø.57
- conjugal A53.9
  - tabes A52.11
- conjunctiva (late) A52.71
- contact Z2Ø.2
- cord bladder A52.19
- cornea, late A52.71
- coronary (artery) (sclerosis) A52.Ø6
- coryza, congenital A5Ø.Ø5
- cranial nerve A52.15
  - multiple palsies A52.15
- cutaneous — *see* Syphilis, skin
- dacryocystitis (late) A52.71
- degeneration, spinal cord A52.12
- dementia paralytica A52.17
  - juvenilis A5Ø.45
- destruction of bone A52.77
- dilatation, aorta A52.Ø1
- due to blood transfusion A53.9
- dura mater A52.13
- ear A52.79
  - inner A52.79
    - nerve (eighth) A52.15
    - neurorecurrence A52.15
- early A51.9
  - cardiovascular A52.ØØ
  - central nervous system A52.3
  - latent (without manifestations) (less than 2 years after infection) A51.5
    - negative spinal fluid test A51.5
    - serological relapse after treatment A51.5
    - serology positive A51.5
  - relapse (treated, untreated) A51.9
  - skin A51.39
  - symptomatic A51.9
    - extragenital chancre A51.2
    - primary, except extragenital chancre A51.Ø
    - secondary (*see also* Syphilis, secondary) A51.39
      - relapse (treated, untreated) A51.49
  - ulcer A51.39
- eighth nerve (neuritis) A52.15
- endemic A65
- endocarditis A52.Ø3
  - aortic A52.Ø3
  - pulmonary A52.Ø3
- epididymis (late) A52.76
- epiglottis (late) A52.73
- epiphysitis (congenital) (early) A5Ø.Ø2
- episcleritis (late) A52.71
- esophagus A52.79
- eustachian tube A52.73
- exposure to Z2Ø.2
- eye A52.71
- eyelid (late) (with gumma) A52.71
- fallopian tube (late) A52.76
- fracture A52.77
- gallbladder (late) A52.74
- gastric (polyposis) (late) A52.74
- general A53.9
  - paralysis A52.17
    - juvenile A5Ø.45
- genital (primary) A51.Ø
- glaucoma A52.71
- gumma NEC A52.79

Syphilis, syphilitic — *continued*
- gumma — *continued*
  - cardiovascular system A52.ØØ
  - central nervous system A52.3
  - congenital A5Ø.59
- heart (block) (decompensation) (disease) (failure) A52.Ø6 [I52]
  - valve NEC A52.Ø3
- hemianesthesia A52.19
- hemianopsia A52.71
- hemiparesis A52.17
- hemiplegia A52.17
- hepatic artery A52.Ø9
- hepatis A52.74
- hepatomegaly, congenital A5Ø.Ø8
- hereditaria tarda — *see* Syphilis, congenital, late
- hereditary — *see* Syphilis, congenital
- Hutchinson's teeth A5Ø.52
- hyalitis A52.71
- inactive — *see* Syphilis, latent
- infantum — *see* Syphilis, congenital
- inherited — *see* Syphilis, congenital
- internal ear A52.79
- intestine (late) A52.74
- iris, iritis (secondary) A51.43
  - late A52.71
- joint (late) A52.77
- keratitis (congenital) (interstitial) (late) A5Ø.31
- kidney (late) A52.75
- lacrimal passages (late) A52.71
- larynx (late) A52.73
- late A52.9
  - cardiovascular A52.ØØ
  - central nervous system A52.3
  - kidney A52.75
  - latent or 2 years or more after infection (without manifestations) A52.8
    - negative spinal fluid test A52.8
    - serology positive A52.8
  - paresis A52.17
  - specified site NEC A52.79
  - symptomatic or with manifestations A52.79
  - tabes A52.11
- latent A53.Ø
  - with signs or symptoms — *code by* site and stage under Syphilis
  - early, or less than 2 years after infection A51.5
  - central nervous system A52.2
  - date of infection unspecified A53.Ø
  - follow-up of latent syphilis A53.Ø
    - date of infection unspecified A53.Ø
    - late, or 2 years or more after infection A52.8
  - late, or 2 years or more after infection A52.8
  - positive serology (only finding) A53.Ø
    - early, or less than 2 years after infection A51.5
    - date of infection unspecified A53.Ø
    - late, or 2 years or more after infection A52.8
- lens (late) A52.71
- leukoderma A51.39
  - late A52.79
- lienitis A52.79
- lip A51.39
  - chancre (primary) A51.2
  - late A52.79
- Lissauer's paralysis A52.17
- liver A52.74
- locomotor ataxia A52.11
- lung A52.72
- lymph gland (early) (secondary) A51.49
  - late A52.79
- lymphadenitis (secondary) A51.49
- macular atrophy of skin A51.39
  - striated A52.79
- mediastinum (late) A52.73
- meninges (adhesive) (brain) (spinal cord) A52.13
- meningitis A52.13
  - acute (secondary) A51.41
  - congenital A5Ø.41
- meningoencephalitis A52.14
- meningovascular A52.13
  - congenital A5Ø.41
- mesarteritis A52.Ø9
  - brain A52.Ø4
- middle ear A52.77
- mitral stenosis A52.Ø3
- monoplegia A52.17
- mouth (secondary) A51.39
  - late A52.79

Syphilis, syphilitic — *continued*
- mucocutaneous (secondary) A51.39
  - late A52.79
- mucous
  - membrane (secondary) A51.39
    - late A52.79
  - patches A51.39
    - congenital A5Ø.Ø7
- mulberry molars A5Ø.52
- muscle A52.78
- myocardium A52.Ø6
- nasal sinus (late) A52.73
- neonatorum — *see* Syphilis, congenital
- nephrotic syndrome (secondary) A51.44
- nerve palsy (any cranial nerve) A52.15
  - multiple A52.15
- nervous system, central A52.3
- neuritis A52.15
  - acoustic A52.15
- neurorecidive of retina A52.19
- neuroretinitis A52.19
- newborn — *see* Syphilis, congenital
- nodular superficial (late) A52.79
- nonvenereal A65
- nose (late) A52.73
  - saddle back deformity A5Ø.57
- occlusive arterial disease A52.Ø9
- oculopathy A52.71
- ophthalmic (late) A52.71
- optic nerve (atrophy) (neuritis) (papilla) A52.15
- orbit (late) A52.71
- organic A53.9
- osseous (late) A52.77
- osteochondritis (congenital) (early) A5Ø.Ø2 [M9Ø.8Ø]
- osteoporosis A52.77
- ovary (late) A52.76
- oviduct (late) A52.76
- palate (late) A52.79
- pancreas (late) A52.74
- paralysis A52.17
  - general A52.17
    - juvenile A5Ø.45
- paresis (general) A52.17
  - juvenile A5Ø.45
- paresthesia A52.19
- Parkinson's disease or syndrome A52.19
- paroxysmal tachycardia A52.Ø6
- pemphigus (congenital) A5Ø.Ø6
- penis (chancre) A51.Ø
  - late A52.76
- pericardium A52.Ø6
- perichondritis, larynx (late) A52.73
- periosteum (late) A52.77
  - congenital (early) A5Ø.Ø2 [M9Ø.8Ø]
  - early (secondary) A51.46
- peripheral nerve A52.79
- petrous bone (late) A52.77
- pharynx (late) A52.73
  - secondary A51.39
- pituitary (gland) A52.79
- pleura (late) A52.73
- pneumonia, white A5Ø.Ø4
- pontine lesion A52.17
- portal vein A52.Ø9
- primary A51.Ø
  - anal A51.1
  - and secondary — *see* Syphilis, secondary
  - central nervous system A52.3
  - extragenital chancre NEC A51.2
  - fingers A51.2
  - genital A51.Ø
  - lip A51.2
  - specified site NEC A51.2
  - tonsils A51.2
- prostate (late) A52.76
- ptosis (eyelid) A52.71
- pulmonary (late) A52.72
  - artery A52.Ø9
- pyelonephritis (late) A52.75
- recently acquired, symptomatic A51.9
- rectum (late) A52.74
- respiratory tract (late) A52.73
- retina, late A52.71
- retrobulbar neuritis A52.15
- salpingitis A52.76
- sclera (late) A52.71
- sclerosis
  - cerebral A52.17

T

Tabacism, tabacosis, tabagism (*see also* Poisoning, tobacco)
- meaning dependence (without remission) F17.2ØØ
  - with
    - disorder F17.299
      - remission F17.211
      - specified disorder NEC F17.298
      - withdrawal F17.2Ø3

Tabardillo A75.9
- flea-borne A75.2
- louse-borne A75.Ø

Tabes, tabetic A52.1Ø
- with
  - central nervous system syphilis A52.1Ø
  - Charcot's joint A52.16
  - cord bladder A52.19
  - crisis, viscera (any) A52.19
  - paralysis, general A52.17
  - paresis (general) A52.17
  - perforating ulcer (foot) A52.19
- arthropathy (Charcot) A52.16
- bladder A52.19
- bone A52.11
- cerebrospinal A52.12
- congenital A5Ø.45
- conjugal A52.1Ø
- dorsalis A52.11
  - juvenile A5Ø.49
- juvenile A5Ø.49
- latent A52.19
- mesenterica A18.39
- paralysis, insane, general A52.17
- spasmodic A52.17
- syphilis (cerebrospinal) A52.12

Taboparalysis A52.17

Taboparesis (remission) A52.17
- juvenile A5Ø.45

TAC (trigeminal autonomic cephalgia) **NEC** G44.Ø99
- intractable G44.Ø91
- not intractable G44.Ø99

Tache noir S6Ø.22- ☑

Tachyalimentation K91.2

Tachyarrhythmia, tachyrhythmia — *see* Tachycardia

Tachycardia RØØ.Ø
- atrial (paroxysmal) I47.1
- auricular I47.1
- AV nodal re-entry (re-entrant) I47.1
- junctional (paroxysmal) I47.1
- newborn P29.11
- nodal (paroxysmal) I47.1
- non-paroxysmal AV nodal I45.89
- paroxysmal (sustained) (nonsustained) I47.9
  - with sinus bradycardia I49.5
  - atrial (PAT) I47.1
  - atrioventricular (AV) (re-entrant) I47.1
    - psychogenic F54
  - junctional I47.1
    - ectopic I47.1
  - nodal I47.1
  - psychogenic (atrial) (supraventricular) (ventricular) F54
  - supraventricular (sustained) I47.1
    - psychogenic F54
  - ventricular I47.2
    - psychogenic F54
- psychogenic F45.8
- sick sinus I49.5
- sinoauricular NOS RØØ.Ø
  - paroxysmal I47.1
- sinus [sinusal] NOS RØØ.Ø
  - paroxysmal I47.1
- supraventricular I47.1
- ventricular (paroxysmal) (sustained) I47.2
  - psychogenic F54

Tachygastria K31.89

Tachypnea RØ6.82
- hysterical F45.8
- newborn (idiopathic) (transitory) P22.1
- psychogenic F45.8
- transitory, of newborn P22.1

TACO (transfusion associated circulatory overload) E87.71

Taenia (infection) (infestation) B68.9
- diminuta B71.Ø
- echinococcal infestation B67.9Ø
- mediocanellata B68.1
- nana B71.Ø
- saginata B68.1
- solium (intestinal form) B68.Ø
  - larval form — *see* Cysticercosis

Taeniasis (intestine) — *see* Taenia

Tag (hypertrophied skin) (infected) L91.8
- adenoid J35.8
- anus K64.4
- hemorrhoidal K64.4
- hymen N89.8
- perineal N9Ø.89
- preauricular Q17.Ø
- sentinel K64.4
- skin L91.8
  - accessory (congenital) Q82.8
  - anus K64.4
  - congenital Q82.8
  - preauricular Q17.Ø
- tonsil J35.8
- urethra, urethral N36.8
- vulva N9Ø.89

Tahyna fever B33.8

Takahara's disease E8Ø.3

Takayasu's disease or syndrome M31.4

Talcosis (pulmonary) J62.Ø

Talipes (congenital) Q66.89
- acquired, planus — *see* Deformity, limb, flat foot
- asymmetric Q66.89
- calcaneovalgus Q66.4
- calcaneovarus Q66.1
- calcaneus Q66.89
- cavus Q66.7
- equinovalgus Q66.6
- equinovarus Q66.Ø
- equinus Q66.89
- percavus Q66.7
- planovalgus Q66.6
- planus (acquired) (any degree) (*see also* Deformity, limb, flat foot)
  - congenital Q66.5- ☑
  - due to rickets (sequelae) E64.3
- valgus Q66.6
- varus Q66.3

Tall stature, constitutional E34.4

Talma's disease M62.89

Talon noir S9Ø.3- ☑
- hand S6Ø.22- ☑
- heel S9Ø.3- ☑
- toe S9Ø.1- ☑

Tamponade, heart I31.4

Tanapox (virus disease) BØ8.71

Tangier disease E78.6

Tantrum, child problem F91.8

Tapeworm (infection) (infestation) — *see* Infestation, tapeworm

Tapia's syndrome G52.7

TAR (thrombocytopenia with absent radius) **syndrome** Q87.2

Tarral-Besnier disease L44.Ø

Tarsal tunnel syndrome — *see* Syndrome, tarsal tunnel

Tarsalgia — *see* Pain, limb, lower

Tarsitis (eyelid) HØ1.8
- syphilitic A52.71
- tuberculous A18.4

Tartar (teeth) (dental calculus) KØ3.6

Tattoo (mark) L81.8

Tauri's disease E74.Ø9

Taurodontism KØØ.2

Taussig-Bing syndrome Q2Ø.1

Taybi's syndrome Q87.2

Tay-Sachs amaurotic familial idiocy or disease E75.Ø2

TBI (traumatic brain injury) — *see* category SØ6 ☑

Teacher's node or nodule J38.2

Tear, torn (traumatic) (*see also* Laceration)
- with abortion — *see* Abortion
- annular fibrosis M51.35
- anus, anal (sphincter) S31.831 ☑

Tear, torn — *continued*
- anus, anal — *continued*
  - complicating delivery
    - with third degree perineal laceration O7Ø.2
      - with mucosa O7Ø.3
    - without third degree perineal laceration O7Ø.4
  - nontraumatic (healed) (old) K62.81
- articular cartilage, old — *see* Derangement, joint, articular cartilage, by site
- bladder
  - with ectopic or molar pregnancy OØ8.6
  - following ectopic or molar pregnancy OØ8.6
  - obstetrical O71.5
  - traumatic — *see* Injury, bladder
- bowel
  - with ectopic or molar pregnancy OØ8.6
  - following ectopic or molar pregnancy OØ8.6
  - obstetrical trauma O71.5
- broad ligament
  - with ectopic or molar pregnancy OØ8.6
  - following ectopic or molar pregnancy OØ8.6
  - obstetrical trauma O71.6
- bucket handle (knee) (meniscus) — *see* Tear, meniscus
- capsule, joint — *see* Sprain
- cartilage (*see also* Sprain)
  - articular, old — *see* Derangement, joint, articular cartilage, by site
- cervix
  - with ectopic or molar pregnancy OØ8.6
  - following ectopic or molar pregnancy OØ8.6
  - obstetrical trauma (current) O71.3
  - old N88.1
  - traumatic — *see* Injury, uterus
- dural G97.41
  - nontraumatic G96.11
- internal organ — *see* Injury, by site
- knee cartilage
  - articular (current) S83.3- ☑
  - old — *see* Derangement, knee, meniscus, due to old tear
- ligament — *see* Sprain
- meniscus (knee) (current injury) S83.2Ø9 ☑
  - bucket-handle S83.2Ø- ☑
  - lateral
    - bucket-handle S83.25- ☑
    - complex S83.27- ☑
    - peripheral S83.26- ☑
    - specified type NEC S83.28- ☑
  - medial
    - bucket-handle S83.21- ☑
    - complex S83.23- ☑
    - peripheral S83.22- ☑
    - specified type NEC S83.24- ☑
  - old — *see* Derangement, knee, meniscus, due to old tear
  - site other than knee — *code as* Sprain
  - specified type NEC S83.2Ø- ☑
- muscle — *see* Strain
- pelvic
  - floor, complicating delivery O7Ø.1
  - organ NEC, obstetrical trauma O71.5
    - with ectopic or molar pregnancy OØ8.6
    - following ectopic or molar pregnancy OØ8.6
- perineal, secondary O9Ø.1
- periurethral tissue, obstetrical trauma O71.82
  - with ectopic or molar pregnancy OØ8.6
  - following ectopic or molar pregnancy OØ8.6
- rectovaginal septum — *see* Laceration, vagina
- retina, retinal (without detachment) (horseshoe) (*see also* Break, retina, horseshoe)
  - with detachment — *see* Detachment, retina, with retinal, break
- rotator cuff (nontraumatic) M75.1Ø- ☑
  - complete M75.12- ☑
  - incomplete M75.11- ☑
  - traumatic S46.Ø1- ☑
    - capsule S43.42- ☑
- semilunar cartilage, knee — *see* Tear, meniscus
- supraspinatus (complete) (incomplete) (nontraumatic) (*see also* Tear, rotator cuff) M75.1Ø- ☑
- tendon — *see* Strain
- tentorial, at birth P1Ø.4

- **Test, tests, testing** — *continued*
  - skin, diagnostic — *continued*
    - Mantoux Z11.1
    - tuberculin Z11.1
  - specified NEC ZØ1.89
  - tuberculin Z11.1
    - abnormal result R76.11
  - vision ZØ1.ØØ
    - with abnormal findings ZØ1.Ø1
  - Wassermann Z11.3
    - positive — *see* Serology for syphilis, positive
- **Testicle, testicular, testis** (*see also* condition)
  - feminization syndrome (*see also* Syndrome, androgen insensitivity) E34.51
  - migrans Q55.29
- **Tetanus, tetanic** (cephalic) (convulsions) A35
  - with
    - abortion A34
    - ectopic or molar pregnancy OØ8.Ø
  - following ectopic or molar pregnancy OØ8.Ø
  - inoculation reaction (due to serum) — *see* Complications, vaccination
  - neonatorum A33
  - obstetrical A34
  - puerperal, postpartum, childbirth A34
- **Tetany** (due to) R29.Ø
  - alkalosis E87.3
  - associated with rickets E55.Ø
  - convulsions R29.Ø
    - hysterical F44.5
  - functional (hysterical) F44.5
  - hyperkinetic R29.Ø
    - hysterical F44.5
  - hyperpnea RØ6.4
    - hysterical F44.5
    - psychogenic F45.8
  - hyperventilation (*see also* Hyperventilation) RØ6.4
    - hysterical F44.5
  - neonatal (without calcium or magnesium deficiency) P71.3
  - parathyroid (gland) E2Ø.9
  - parathyroprival E89.2
  - post- (para)thyroidectomy E89.2
  - postoperative E89.2
  - pseudotetany R29.Ø
  - psychogenic (conversion reaction) F44.5
- **Tetralogy of Fallot** Q21.3
- **Tetraplegia** (chronic) (*see also* Quadriplegia) G82.5Ø
- **Thailand hemorrhagic fever** A91
- **Thalassanemia** — *see* Thalassemia
- **Thalassemia** (anemia) (disease) D56.9
  - with other hemoglobinopathy D56.8
  - alpha (major) (severe) (triple gene defect) D56.Ø
    - minor D56.3
    - silent carrier D56.3
    - trait D56.3
  - beta (severe) D56.1
    - homozygous D56.1
    - major D56.1
    - minor D56.3
    - trait D56.3
  - delta-beta (homozygous) D56.2
    - minor D56.3
    - trait D56.3
  - dominant D56.8
  - hemoglobin
    - C D56.8
    - E-beta D56.5
  - intermedia D56.1
  - major D56.1
  - minor D56.3
  - mixed D56.8
  - sickle-cell — *see* Disease, sickle-cell, thalassemia
  - specified type NEC D56.8
  - trait D56.3
  - variants D56.8
- **Thanatophoric dwarfism or short stature** Q77.1
- **Thaysen-Gee disease** (nontropical sprue) K9Ø.Ø
- **Thaysen's disease** K9Ø.Ø
- **Thecoma** D27- ☑
  - luteinized D27- ☑
  - malignant C56- ☑
- **Thelarche, premature** E3Ø.8
- **Thelaziasis** B83.8
- **Thelitis** N61
  - puerperal, postpartum or gestational — *see* Infection, nipple
- **Therapeutic** — *see* condition
- **Therapy**
  - drug, long-term (current) (prophylactic)
    - agents affecting estrogen receptors and estrogen levels NEC Z79.818
    - anastrozole (Arimidex) Z79.811
    - antibiotics Z79.2
      - short-term use — *omit code*
    - anticoagulants Z79.Ø1
    - anti-inflammatory Z79.1
    - antiplatelet Z79.Ø2
    - antithrombotics Z79.Ø2
    - aromatase inhibitors Z79.811
    - aspirin Z79.82
    - birth control pill or patch Z79.3
    - bisphosphonates Z79.83
    - contraceptive, oral Z79.3
    - drug, specified NEC Z79.899
    - estrogen receptor downregulators Z79.818
    - Evista Z79.81Ø
    - exemestane (Aromasin) Z79.811
    - Fareston Z79.81Ø
    - fulvestrant (Faslodex) Z79.818
    - gonadotropin-releasing hormone (GnRH) agonist Z79.818
    - goserelin acetate (Zoladex) Z79.818
    - hormone replacement (postmenopausal) Z79.89Ø
    - insulin Z79.4
    - letrozole (Femara) Z79.811
    - leuprolide acetate (leuprorelin) (Lupron) Z79.818
    - megestrol acetate (Megace) Z79.818
    - methadone
      - for pain management Z79.891
      - maintenance therapy F11.2Ø
    - Nolvadex Z79.81Ø
    - opiate analgesic Z79.891
    - oral contraceptive Z79.3
    - raloxifene (Evista) Z79.81Ø
    - selective estrogen receptor modulators (SERMs) Z79.81Ø
    - short term — *omit code*
    - steroids
      - inhaled Z79.51
      - systemic Z79.52
    - tamoxifen (Nolvadex) Z79.81Ø
    - toremifene (Fareston) Z79.81Ø
- **Thermic** — *see* condition
- **Thermography** (abnormal) (*see also* Abnormal, diagnostic imaging) R93.8
  - breast R92.8
- **Thermoplegia** T67.Ø ☑
- **Thesaurismosis, glycogen** — *see* Disease, glycogen storage
- **Thiamin deficiency** E51.9
  - specified NEC E51.8
- **Thiaminic deficiency with beriberi** E51.11
- **Thibierge-Weissenbach syndrome** — *see* Sclerosis, systemic
- **Thickening**
  - bone — *see* Hypertrophy, bone
  - breast N64.59
  - endometrium R93.8
  - epidermal L85.9
    - specified NEC L85.8
  - hymen N89.6
  - larynx J38.7
  - nail L6Ø.2
    - congenital Q84.5
  - periosteal — *see* Hypertrophy, bone
  - pleura J92.9
    - with asbestos J92.Ø
  - skin R23.4
  - subepiglottic J38.7
  - tongue K14.8
  - valve, heart — *see* Endocarditis
- **Thigh** — *see* condition
- **Thinning vertebra** — *see* Spondylopathy, specified NEC
- **Thirst, excessive** R63.1
  - due to deprivation of water T73.1 ☑
- **Thomsen disease** G71.12
- **Thoracic** (*see also* condition)
  - kidney Q63.2
  - outlet syndrome G54.Ø
- **Thoracogastroschisis** (congenital) Q79.8
- **Thoracopagus** Q89.4
- **Thorax** — *see* condition
- **Thorn's syndrome** N28.89
- **Thorson-Björck syndrome** E34.Ø
- **Threadworm** (infection) (infestation) B8Ø
- **Threatened**
  - abortion O2Ø.Ø
    - with subsequent abortion OØ3.9
  - job loss, anxiety concerning Z56.2
  - labor (without delivery) O47.9
    - after 37 completed weeks of gestation O47.1
    - before 37 completed weeks of gestation O47.Ø- ☑
  - loss of job, anxiety concerning Z56.2
  - miscarriage O2Ø.Ø
  - unemployment, anxiety concerning Z56.2
- **Three-day fever** A93.1
- **Threshers' lung** J67.Ø
- **Thrix annulata** (congenital) Q84.1
- **Throat** — *see* condition
- **Thrombasthenia** (Glanzmann) (hemorrhagic) (hereditary) D69.1
- **Thromboangiitis** I73.1
  - obliterans (general) I73.1
    - cerebral I67.89
    - vessels
      - brain I67.89
      - spinal cord I67.89
- **Thromboarteritis** — *see* Arteritis
- **Thromboasthenia** (Glanzmann) (hemorrhagic) (hereditary) D69.1
- **Thrombocytasthenia** (Glanzmann) D69.1
- **Thrombocythemia** (essential) (hemorrhagic) (idiopathic) (primary) D47.3
- **Thrombocytopathy** (dystrophic) (granulopenic) D69.1
- **Thrombocytopenia, thrombocytopenic** D69.6
  - with absent radius (TAR) Q87.2
  - congenital D69.42
  - dilutional D69.59
  - due to
    - (massive) blood transfusion D69.59
    - drugs D69.59
    - extracorporeal circulation of blood D69.59
    - platelet alloimmunization D69.59
  - essential D69.3
  - heparin induced (HIT) D75.82
  - hereditary D69.42
  - idiopathic D69.3
  - neonatal, transitory P61.Ø
    - due to
      - exchange transfusion P61.Ø
      - idiopathic maternal thrombocytopenia P61.Ø
      - isoimmunization P61.Ø
  - primary NEC D69.49
    - idiopathic D69.3
  - puerperal, postpartum O72.3
  - secondary D69.59
  - transient neonatal P61.Ø
- **Thrombocytosis, essential** D47.3
  - primary D47.3
- **Thromboembolism** — *see* Embolism
- **Thrombopathy** (Bernard-Soulier) D69.1
  - constitutional D68.Ø
  - Willebrand-Jurgens D68.Ø
- **Thrombopenia** — *see* Thrombocytopenia
- **Thrombophilia** D68.59
  - primary NEC D68.59
  - secondary NEC D68.69
  - specified NEC D68.69
- **Thrombophlebitis** I8Ø.9
  - antepartum O22.2- ☑
    - deep O22.3- ☑
    - superficial O22.2- ☑
  - cavernous (venous) sinus GØ8
    - complicating pregnancy O22.5- ☑
    - nonpyogenic I67.6
  - cerebral (sinus) (vein) GØ8
    - nonpyogenic I67.6
    - sequelae GØ9
  - due to implanted device — *see* Complications, by site and type, specified NEC
  - during or resulting from a procedure NEC T81.72 ☑
  - femoral vein (superficial) I8Ø.1- ☑
  - femoropopliteal vein I8Ø.Ø- ☑
  - hepatic (vein) I8Ø.8
  - idiopathic, recurrent I82.1
  - iliofemoral I8Ø.1- ☑
  - intracranial venous sinus (any) GØ8
    - nonpyogenic I67.6
    - sequelae GØ9
  - intraspinal venous sinuses and veins GØ8
    - nonpyogenic G95.19
  - lateral (venous) sinus GØ8
    - nonpyogenic I67.6

- **Thrombophlebitis** — *continued*
  - leg I80.299
    - superficial I80.0- ☑
  - longitudinal (venous) sinus G08
    - nonpyogenic I67.6
  - lower extremity I80.299
  - migrans, migrating I82.1
  - pelvic
    - with ectopic or molar pregnancy O08.0
    - following ectopic or molar pregnancy O08.0
    - puerperal O87.1
  - popliteal vein — *see* Phlebitis, leg, deep, popliteal
  - portal (vein) K75.1
  - postoperative T81.72 ☑
  - pregnancy — *see* Thrombophlebitis, antepartum
  - puerperal, postpartum, childbirth O87.0
    - deep O87.1
    - pelvic O87.1
    - septic O86.81
    - superficial O87.0
  - saphenous (greater) (lesser) I80.0- ☑
  - sinus (intracranial) G08
    - nonpyogenic I67.6
  - specified site NEC I80.8
  - tibial vein I80.23- ☑
- **Thrombosis, thrombotic** (bland) (multiple) (progressive) (silent) (vessel) I82.90
  - anal K64.5
  - antepartum — *see* Thrombophlebitis, antepartum
  - aorta, aortic I74.10
    - abdominal I74.09
      - saddle I74.01
    - bifurcation I74.09
    - saddle I74.01
    - specified site NEC I74.19
    - terminal I74.09
    - thoracic I74.11
    - valve — *see* Endocarditis, aortic
  - apoplexy I63.3 ☑
  - artery, arteries (postinfectional) I74.9
    - auditory, internal — *see* Occlusion, artery, precerebral, specified NEC
    - basilar — *see* Occlusion, artery, basilar
    - carotid (common) (internal) — *see* Occlusion, artery, carotid
    - cerebellar (anterior inferior) (posterior inferior) (superior) — *see* Occlusion, artery, cerebellar
    - cerebral — *see* Occlusion, artery, cerebral
    - choroidal (anterior) — *see* Occlusion, artery, cerebral, specified NEC
    - communicating, posterior — *see* Occlusion, artery, cerebral, specified NEC
    - coronary (*see also* Infarct, myocardium)
      - not resulting in infarction I24.0
    - hepatic I74.8
    - hypophyseal — *see* Occlusion, artery, cerebral, specified NEC
    - iliac I74.5
    - limb I74.4
      - lower I74.3
      - upper I74.2
    - meningeal, anterior or posterior — *see* Occlusion, artery, cerebral, specified NEC
    - mesenteric (with gangrene) K55.0
    - ophthalmic — *see* Occlusion, artery, retina
    - pontine — *see* Occlusion, artery, cerebral, specified NEC
    - precerebral — *see* Occlusion, artery, precerebral
    - pulmonary (iatrogenic) — *see* Embolism, pulmonary
    - renal N28.0
    - retinal — *see* Occlusion, artery, retina
    - spinal, anterior or posterior G95.11
    - traumatic NEC T14.8
    - vertebral — *see* Occlusion, artery, vertebral
  - atrium, auricular (*see also* Infarct, myocardium)
    - following acute myocardial infarction (current complication) I23.6
    - not resulting in infarction I24.0
  - basilar (artery) — *see* Occlusion, artery, basilar
  - brain (artery) (stem) (*see also* Occlusion, artery, cerebral)
    - due to syphilis A52.05
    - puerperal O99.43
    - sinus — *see* Thrombosis, intracranial venous sinus
  - capillary I78.8
  - cardiac (*see also* Infarct, myocardium)
    - not resulting in infarction I24.0
    - valve — *see* Endocarditis
  - carotid (artery) (common) (internal) — *see* Occlusion, artery, carotid
  - cavernous (venous) sinus — *see* Thrombosis, intracranial venous sinus
  - cerebellar artery (anterior inferior) (posterior inferior) (superior) I66.3
  - cerebral (artery) — *see* Occlusion, artery, cerebral
  - cerebrovenous sinus (*see also* Thrombosis, intracranial venous sinus)
    - puerperium O87.3
  - chronic I82.91
  - coronary (artery) (vein) (*see also* Infarct, myocardium)
    - not resulting in infarction I24.0
  - corpus cavernosum N48.89
  - cortical I66.9
  - deep — *see* Embolism, vein, lower extremity
  - due to device, implant or graft (*see also* Complications, by site and type, specified NEC) T85.86 ☑
    - arterial graft NEC T82.868 ☑
    - breast (implant) T85.86 ☑
    - catheter NEC T85.86 ☑
      - dialysis (renal) T82.868 ☑
        - intraperitoneal T85.86 ☑
      - infusion NEC T82.868 ☑
        - spinal (epidural) (subdural) T85.86 ☑
      - urinary (indwelling) T83.86 ☑
    - electronic (electrode) (pulse generator) (stimulator)
      - bone T84.86 ☑
      - cardiac T82.867 ☑
      - nervous system (brain) (peripheral nerve) (spinal) T85.86 ☑
      - urinary T83.86 ☑
    - fixation, internal (orthopedic) NEC T84.86 ☑
    - gastrointestinal (bile duct) (esophagus) T85.86 ☑
    - genital NEC T83.86 ☑
    - heart T82.867 ☑
    - joint prosthesis T84.86 ☑
    - ocular (corneal graft) (orbital implant) NEC T85.86 ☑
    - orthopedic NEC T84.86 ☑
    - specified NEC T85.86 ☑
    - urinary NEC T83.86 ☑
    - vascular NEC T82.868 ☑
    - ventricular intracranial shunt T85.86 ☑
  - during the puerperium — *see* Thrombosis, puerperal
  - endocardial (*see also* Infarct, myocardium)
    - not resulting in infarction I24.0
  - eye — *see* Occlusion, retina
  - genital organ
    - female NEC N94.89
      - pregnancy — *see* Thrombophlebitis, antepartum
    - male N50.1
  - gestational — *see* Phlebopathy, gestational
  - heart (chamber) (*see also* Infarct, myocardium)
    - not resulting in infarction I24.0
  - hepatic (vein) I82.0
    - artery I74.8
  - history (of) Z86.718
  - intestine (with gangrene) K55.0
  - intracardiac NEC (apical) (atrial) (auricular) (ventricular) (old) I51.3
  - intracranial (arterial) I66.9
    - venous sinus (any) G08
      - nonpyogenic origin I67.6
      - puerperium O87.3
  - intramural (*see also* Infarct, myocardium)
    - not resulting in infarction I24.0
  - intraspinal venous sinuses and veins G08
    - nonpyogenic G95.19
  - kidney (artery) N28.0
  - lateral (venous) sinus — *see* Thrombosis, intracranial venous sinus
  - leg — *see* Thrombosis, vein, lower extremity
    - arterial I74.3
  - liver (venous) I82.0
    - artery I74.8
    - portal vein I81
  - longitudinal (venous) sinus — *see* Thrombosis, intracranial venous sinus
  - lower limb — *see* Thrombosis, vein, lower extremity
  - lung (iatrogenic) (postoperative) — *see* Embolism, pulmonary
  - meninges (brain) (arterial) I66.8
  - mesenteric (artery) (with gangrene) K55.0
    - vein (inferior) (superior) I81
  - mitral I34.8
  - mural (*see also* Infarct, myocardium)
    - due to syphilis A52.06
    - not resulting in infarction I24.0
  - omentum (with gangrene) K55.0
  - ophthalmic — *see* Occlusion, retina
  - pampiniform plexus (male) N50.1
  - parietal (*see also* Infarct, myocardium)
    - not resulting in infarction I24.0
  - penis, superficial vein N48.81
  - perianal venous K64.5
  - peripheral arteries I74.4
    - upper I74.2
  - personal history (of) Z86.718
  - portal I81
    - due to syphilis A52.09
  - precerebral artery — *see* Occlusion, artery, precerebral
  - puerperal, postpartum O87.0
    - brain (artery) O99.43
      - venous (sinus) O87.3
    - cardiac O99.43
    - cerebral (artery) O99.43
      - venous (sinus) O87.3
    - superficial O87.0
  - pulmonary (artery) (iatrogenic) (postoperative) (vein) — *see* Embolism, pulmonary
  - renal (artery) N28.0
    - vein I82.3
  - resulting from presence of device, implant or graft — *see* Complications, by site and type, specified NEC
  - retina, retinal — *see* Occlusion, retina
  - scrotum N50.1
  - seminal vesicle N50.1
  - sigmoid (venous) sinus — *see* Thrombosis, intracranial venous sinus
  - sinus, intracranial (any) — *see* Thrombosis, intracranial venous sinus
  - specified site NEC I82.890
    - chronic I82.891
  - spermatic cord N50.1
  - spinal cord (arterial) G95.11
    - due to syphilis A52.09
    - pyogenic origin G06.1
  - spleen, splenic D73.5
    - artery I74.8
  - testis N50.1
  - traumatic NEC T14.8
  - tricuspid I07.8
  - tumor — *see* Neoplasm, unspecified behavior, by site
  - tunica vaginalis N50.1
  - umbilical cord (vessels), complicating delivery O69.5 ☑
  - vas deferens N50.1
  - vein (acute) I82.90
    - antecubital I82.61- ☑
      - chronic I82.71- ☑
    - axillary I82.A1- ☑ (*following* I82.7)
      - chronic I82.A2- ☑ (*following* I82.7)
    - basilic I82.61- ☑
      - chronic I82.71- ☑
    - brachial I82.62- ☑
      - chronic I82.72- ☑
    - brachiocephalic (innominate) I82.290
      - chronic I82.291
    - cephalic I82.61- ☑
      - chronic I82.71- ☑
    - cerebral, nonpyogenic I67.6
    - chronic I82.91
    - deep (DVT) I82.40- ☑
      - calf I82.4Z- ☑
        - chronic I82.5Z- ☑
      - lower leg I82.4Z- ☑
        - chronic I82.5Z- ☑
      - thigh I82.4Y- ☑
        - chronic I82.5Y- ☑
      - upper leg I82.4Y ☑
        - chronic I82.5y-
    - femoral I82.41- ☑
      - chronic I82.51- ☑
    - iliac (iliofemoral) I82.42- ☑
      - chronic I82.52- ☑
    - innominate I82.290
      - chronic I82.291

- **Thrombosis, thrombotic** — *continued*
  - vein — *continued*
    - internal jugular I82.C1- ☑ (*following* I82.7)
      - chronic I82.C2- ☑ (*following* I82.7)
    - lower extremity
      - deep I82.40- ☑
        - chronic I82.50- ☑
        - specified NEC I82.49- ☑
          - chronic NEC I82.59- ☑
      - distal
        - deep I82.4Z- ☑
      - proximal
        - deep I82.4Y- ☑
          - chronic I82.5Y- ☑
      - superficial I82.81- ☑
    - perianal K64.5
    - popliteal I82.43- ☑
      - chronic I82.53- ☑
    - radial I82.62- ☑
      - chronic I82.72- ☑
    - renal I82.3
    - saphenous (greater) (lesser) I82.81- ☑
    - specified NEC I82.890
      - chronic NEC I82.891
    - subclavian I82.B1- ☑ (*following* I82.7)
      - chronic I82.B2- ☑ (*following* I82.7)
    - thoracic NEC I82.290
      - chronic I82.291
    - tibial I82.44- ☑
      - chronic I82.54- ☑
    - ulnar I82.62- ☑
      - chronic I82.72- ☑
    - upper extremity I82.60- ☑
      - chronic I82.70- ☑
      - deep I82.62- ☑
        - chronic I82.72- ☑
      - superficial I82.61- ☑
        - chronic I82.71- ☑
  - vena cava
    - inferior I82.220
      - chronic I82.221
    - superior I82.210
      - chronic I82.211
  - venous, perianal K64.5
  - ventricle (*see also* Infarct, myocardium)
    - following acute myocardial infarction (current complication) I23.6
      - not resulting in infarction I24.0
- **Thrombus** — *see* Thrombosis
- **Thrush** (*see also* Candidiasis)
  - newborn P37.5
  - oral B37.0
  - vaginal B37.3
- **Thumb** (*see also* condition)
  - sucking (child problem) F98.8
- **Thymitis** E32.8
- **Thymoma** (benign) D15.0
  - malignant C37
- **Thymus, thymic** (gland) — *see* condition
- **Thyrocele** — *see* Goiter
- **Thyroglossal** (*see also* condition)
  - cyst Q89.2
  - duct, persistent Q89.2
- **Thyroid** (gland) (body) (*see also* condition)
  - hormone resistance E07.89
  - lingual Q89.2
  - nodule (cystic) (nontoxic) (single) E04.1
- **Thyroiditis** E06.9
  - acute (nonsuppurative) (pyogenic) (suppurative) E06.0
  - autoimmune E06.3
  - chronic (nonspecific) (sclerosing) E06.5
    - with thyrotoxicosis, transient E06.2
    - fibrous E06.5
    - lymphadenoid E06.3
    - lymphocytic E06.3
    - lymphoid E06.3
  - de Quervain's E06.1
  - drug-induced E06.4
  - fibrous (chronic) E06.5
  - giant-cell (follicular) E06.1
  - granulomatous (de Quervain) (subacute) E06.1
  - Hashimoto's (struma lymphomatosa) E06.3
  - iatrogenic E06.4
  - ligneous E06.5
  - lymphocytic (chronic) E06.3
  - lymphoid E06.3
  - lymphomatous E06.3
- **Thyroiditis** — *continued*
  - nonsuppurative E06.1
  - postpartum, puerperal O90.5
  - pseudotuberculous E06.1
  - pyogenic E06.0
  - radiation E06.4
  - Riedel's E06.5
  - subacute (granulomatous) E06.1
  - suppurative E06.0
  - tuberculous A18.81
  - viral E06.1
  - woody E06.5
- **Thyrolingual duct, persistent** Q89.2
- **Thyromegaly** E01.0
- **Thyrotoxic**
  - crisis — *see* Thyrotoxicosis
  - heart disease or failure (*see also* Thyrotoxicosis) E05.90 [I43]
    - with thyroid storm E05.91 [I43]
  - storm — *see* Thyrotoxicosis
- **Thyrotoxicosis** (recurrent) E05.90
  - with
    - goiter (diffuse) E05.00
      - with thyroid storm E05.01
      - adenomatous uninodular E05.10
        - with thyroid storm E05.11
      - multinodular E05.20
        - with thyroid storm E05.21
      - nodular E05.20
        - with thyroid storm E05.21
      - uninodular E05.10
        - with thyroid storm E05.11
    - infiltrative
      - dermopathy E05.00
        - with thyroid storm E05.01
      - ophthalmopathy E05.00
        - with thyroid storm E05.01
    - single thyroid nodule E05.10
      - with thyroid storm E05.11
    - thyroid storm E05.91
  - due to
    - ectopic thyroid nodule or tissue E05.30
      - with thyroid storm E05.31
    - ingestion of (excessive) thyroid material E05.40
      - with thyroid storm E05.41
    - overproduction of thyroid-stimulating hormone E05.80
      - with thyroid storm E05.81
    - specified cause NEC E05.80
      - with thyroid storm E05.81
  - factitia E05.40
    - with thyroid storm E05.41
  - heart E05.90 [I43]
    - with thyroid storm E05.91 [I43]
    - failure E05.90 [I43]
  - neonatal (transient) P72.1
  - transient with chronic thyroiditis E06.2
- **Tibia vara** — *see* Osteochondrosis, juvenile, tibia
- **Tic** (disorder) F95.9
  - breathing F95.8
  - child problem F95.0
  - compulsive F95.1
  - de la Tourette F95.2
  - degenerative (generalized) (localized) G25.69
    - facial G25.69
  - disorder
    - chronic
      - motor F95.1
      - vocal F95.1
    - combined vocal and multiple motor F95.2
    - transient F95.0
  - douloureux G50.0
    - atypical G50.1
    - postherpetic, postzoster B02.22
  - drug-induced G25.61
  - eyelid F95.8
  - habit F95.9
    - chronic F95.1
    - transient of childhood F95.0
  - lid, transient of childhood F95.0
  - motor-verbal F95.2
  - occupational F48.8
  - orbicularis F95.8
    - transient of childhood F95.0
  - organic origin G25.69
  - postchoreic G25.69
  - psychogenic, compulsive F95.1
  - salaam R25.8
- **Tic** — *continued*
  - spasm (motor or vocal) F95.9
    - chronic F95.1
    - transient of childhood F95.0
  - specified NEC F95.8
- **Tick-borne** — *see* condition
- **Tietze's disease or syndrome** M94.0
- **Tight, tightness**
  - anus K62.89
  - chest R07.89
  - fascia (lata) M62.89
  - foreskin (congenital) N47.1
  - hymen, hymenal ring N89.6
  - introitus (acquired) (congenital) N89.6
  - rectal sphincter K62.89
  - tendon — *see* Short, tendon
  - urethral sphincter N35.9
- **Tilting vertebra** — *see* Dorsopathy, deforming, specified NEC
- **Timidity, child** F93.8
- **Tinea** (intersecta) (tarsi) B35.9
  - amiantacea L44.8
  - asbestina B35.0
  - barbae B35.0
  - beard B35.0
  - black dot B35.0
  - blanca B36.2
  - capitis B35.0
  - corporis B35.4
  - cruris B35.6
  - flava B36.0
  - foot B35.3
  - furfuracea B36.0
  - imbricata (Tokelau) B35.5
  - kerion B35.0
  - manuum B35.2
  - microsporic — *see* Dermatophytosis
  - nigra B36.1
  - nodosa — *see* Piedra
  - pedis B35.3
  - scalp B35.0
  - specified site NEC B35.8
  - sycosis B35.0
  - tonsurans B35.0
  - trichophytic — *see* Dermatophytosis
  - unguium B35.1
  - versicolor B36.0
- **Tingling sensation** (skin) R20.2
- **Tin-miner's lung** J63.5
- **Tinnitus** (audible) (aurium) (subjective) — *see* subcategory H93.1 ☑
- **Tipped tooth** (teeth) M26.33
- **Tipping**
  - pelvis M95.5
    - with disproportion (fetopelvic) O33.0
      - causing obstructed labor O65.0
  - tooth (teeth), fully erupted M26.33
- **Tiredness** R53.83
- **Tissue** — *see* condition
- **Tobacco** (nicotine)
  - dependence — *see* Dependence, drug, nicotine
  - harmful use Z72.0
  - heart — *see* Tobacco, toxic effect
  - maternal use, affecting newborn P04.2
  - toxic effect — *see* Table of Drugs and Chemicals, by substance, poisoning
    - chewing tobacco — *see* Table of Drugs and Chemicals, by substance, poisoning
    - cigarettes — *see* Table of Drugs and Chemicals, by substance, poisoning
  - use Z72.0
    - complicating
      - childbirth O99.334
      - pregnancy O99.33- ☑
      - puerperium O99.335
    - counseling and surveillance Z71.6
  - withdrawal state — *see* Dependence, drug, nicotine
- **Tocopherol deficiency** E56.0
- **Todd's**
  - cirrhosis K74.3
  - paralysis (postepileptic) (transitory) G83.84
- **Toe** — *see* condition
- **Toilet, artificial opening** — *see* Attention to, artificial, opening
- **Tokelau** (ringworm) B35.5
- **Tollwut** — *see* Rabies

Tommaselli's disease R31.9
- correct substance properly administered — *see* Table of Drugs and Chemicals, by drug, adverse effect
- overdose or wrong substance given or taken — *see* Table of Drugs and Chemicals, by drug, poisoning

Tongue (*see also* condition)
- tie Q38.1

Tonic pupil — *see* Anomaly, pupil, function, tonic pupil
Toni-Fanconi syndrome (cystinosis) E72.Ø9
- with cystinosis E72.Ø4

Tonsil — *see* condition
Tonsillitis (acute) (catarrhal) (croupous) (follicular) (gangrenous) (infective) (lacunar) (lingual) (malignant) (membranous) (parenchymatous) (phlegmonous) (pseudomembranous) (purulent) (septic) (subacute) (suppurative) (toxic) (ulcerative) (vesicular) (viral) JØ3.9Ø
- chronic J35.Ø1
  - with adenoiditis J35.Ø3
- diphtheritic A36.Ø
- hypertrophic J35.Ø1
  - with adenoiditis J35.Ø3
- recurrent JØ3.91
- specified organism NEC JØ3.8Ø
  - recurrent JØ3.81
- staphylococcal JØ3.8Ø
  - recurrent JØ3.81
- streptococcal JØ3.ØØ
  - recurrent JØ3.Ø1
- tuberculous A15.8
- Vincent's A69.1

Tooth, teeth — *see* condition
Toothache KØ8.8
Topagnosis R2Ø.8
Tophi — *see* Gout, chronic
TORCH infection — *see* Infection, congenital
- without active infection PØØ.2

Torn — *see* Tear
Tornwaldt's cyst or disease J39.2
Torsion
- accessory tube — *see* Torsion, fallopian tube
- adnexa (female) — *see* Torsion, fallopian tube
- aorta, acquired I77.1
- appendix epididymis N44.Ø4
- appendix testis N44.Ø3
- bile duct (common) (hepatic) K83.8
  - congenital Q44.5
- bowel, colon or intestine K56.2
- cervix — *see* Malposition, uterus
- cystic duct K82.8
- dystonia — *see* Dystonia, torsion
- epididymis (appendix) N44.Ø4
- fallopian tube N83.52
  - with ovary N83.53
- gallbladder K82.8
  - congenital Q44.1
- hydatid of Morgagni
  - female N83.52
  - male N44.Ø3
- kidney (pedicle) (leading to infarction) N28.Ø
- Meckel's diverticulum (congenital) Q43.Ø
  - malignant — *see* Table of Neoplasms, small intestine, malignant
- mesentery K56.2
- omentum K56.2
- organ or site, congenital NEC — *see* Anomaly, by site
- ovary (pedicle) N83.51
  - with fallopian tube N83.53
  - congenital Q5Ø.2
- oviduct — *see* Torsion, fallopian tube
- penis (acquired) N48.82
  - congenital Q55.63
- spasm — *see* Dystonia, torsion
- spermatic cord N44.Ø2
  - extravaginal N44.Ø1
  - intravaginal N44.Ø2
- spleen D73.5
- testis, testicle N44.ØØ
  - appendix N44.Ø3
- tibia — *see* Deformity, limb, specified type NEC, lower leg
- uterus — *see* Malposition, uterus

Torticollis (intermittent) (spastic) M43.6
- congenital (sternomastoid) Q68.Ø
- due to birth injury P15.8
- hysterical F44.4
- ocular R29.891
- psychogenic F45.8
  - conversion reaction F44.4
- rheumatic M43.6
- rheumatoid MØ6.88
- spasmodic G24.3
- traumatic, current S13.4 ☑

Tortipelvis G24.1
Tortuous
- artery I77.1
- organ or site, congenital NEC — *see* Distortion
- retinal vessel, congenital Q14.1
- ureter N13.8
- urethra N36.8
- vein — *see* Varix

Torture, victim of Z65.4
Torula, torular (histolytica) (infection) — *see* Cryptococcosis
Torulosis — *see* Cryptococcosis
Torus (mandibularis) (palatinus) M27.Ø
- fracture — *see* Fracture, by site, torus

Touraine's syndrome Q79.8
Tourette's syndrome F95.2
Tourniquet syndrome — *see* Constriction, external, by site
Tower skull Q75.Ø
- with exophthalmos Q87.Ø

Toxemia R68.89
- bacterial — *see* Sepsis
- burn — *see* Burn
- eclamptic (with pre-existing hypertension) — *see* Eclampsia
- erysipelatous — *see* Erysipelas
- fatigue R68.89
- food — *see* Poisoning, food
- gastrointestinal K52.1
- intestinal K52.1
- kidney — *see* Uremia
- malarial — *see* Malaria
- myocardial — *see* Myocarditis, toxic
- of pregnancy — *see* Pre-eclampsia
- pre-eclamptic — *see* Pre-eclampsia
- small intestine K52.1
- staphylococcal, due to food AØ5.Ø
- stasis R68.89
- uremic — *see* Uremia
- urinary — *see* Uremia

Toxemica cerebropathia psychica (nonalcoholic) FØ4
- alcoholic — *see* Alcohol, amnestic disorder

Toxic (poisoning) (*see also* condition) T65.91 ☑
- effect — *see* Table of Drugs and Chemicals, by substance, poisoning
- shock syndrome A48.3
- thyroid (gland) — *see* Thyrotoxicosis

Toxicemia — *see* Toxemia
Toxicity — *see* Table of Drugs and Chemicals, by substance, poisoning
- fava bean D55.Ø
- food, noxious — *see* Poisoning, food
- from drug or nonmedicinal substance — *see* Table of Drugs and Chemicals, by drug

Toxicosis (*see also* Toxemia)
- capillary, hemorrhagic D69.Ø

Toxinfection, gastrointestinal K52.1
Toxocariasis B83.Ø
Toxoplasma, toxoplasmosis (acquired) B58.9
- with
  - hepatitis B58.1
  - meningoencephalitis B58.2
  - ocular involvement B58.ØØ
  - other organ involvement B58.89
  - pneumonia, pneumonitis B58.3
- congenital (acute) (subacute) (chronic) P37.1
- maternal, manifest toxoplasmosis in infant (acute) (subacute) (chronic) P37.1

tPA (rtPA) **administation in a different facility within the last 24 hours prior to admission to current facility** Z92.82
Trabeculation, bladder N32.89
Trachea — *see* condition
Tracheitis (catarrhal) (infantile) (membranous) (plastic) (septal) (suppurative) (viral) JØ4.1Ø
- with
  - bronchitis (15 years of age and above) J4Ø
    - acute or subacute — *see* Bronchitis, acute
    - chronic J42
    - tuberculous NEC A15.5
    - under 15 years of age J2Ø.9
  - laryngitis (acute) JØ4.2
    - chronic J37.1
    - tuberculous NEC A15.5
- acute JØ4.1Ø
  - with obstruction JØ4.11
- chronic J42
  - with
    - bronchitis (chronic) J42
    - laryngitis (chronic) J37.1
- diphtheritic (membranous) A36.89
- due to external agent — *see* Inflammation, respiratory, upper, due to
- syphilitic A52.73
- tuberculous A15.5

Trachelitis (nonvenereal) — *see* Cervicitis
Tracheobronchial — *see* condition
Tracheobronchitis (15 years of age and above) (*see also* Bronchitis)
- due to
  - Bordetella bronchiseptica A37.8Ø
    - with pneumonia A37.81
  - Francisella tularensis A21.8

Tracheobronchomegaly Q32.4
- with bronchiectasis J47.9
  - with
    - exacerbation (acute) J47.1
    - lower respiratory infection J47.Ø
- acquired J98.Ø9
  - with bronchiectasis J47.9
    - with
      - exacerbation (acute) J47.1
      - lower respiratory infection J47.Ø

Tracheobronchopneumonitis — *see* Pneumonia, broncho-
Tracheocele (external) (internal) J39.8
- congenital Q32.1

Tracheomalacia J39.8
- congenital Q32.Ø

Tracheopharyngitis (acute) JØ6.9
- chronic J42
- due to external agent — *see* Inflammation, respiratory, upper, due to

Tracheostenosis J39.8
Tracheostomy
- complication — *see* Complication, tracheostomy
- status Z93.Ø
  - attention to Z43.Ø
  - malfunctioning J95.Ø3

Trachoma, trachomatous A71.9
- active (stage) A71.1
- contraction of conjunctiva A71.1
- dubium A71.Ø
- healed or sequelae B94.Ø
- initial (stage) A71.Ø
- pannus A71.1
- Türck's J37.Ø

Traction, vitreomacular H43.82- ☑
Train sickness T75.3 ☑
Trait(s)
- Hb-S D57.3
- hemoglobin
  - abnormal NEC D58.2
    - with thalassemia D56.3
  - C — *see* Disease, hemoglobin C
  - S (Hb-S) D57.3
- Lepore D56.3
- personality, accentuated Z73.1
- sickle-cell D57.3
  - with elliptocytosis or spherocytosis D57.3
- type A personality Z73.1

Tramp Z59.Ø
Trance R41.89
- hysterical F44.89

Transaminasemia R74.Ø
Transection
- abdomen (partial) S38.3 ☑
- aorta (incomplete) (*see also* Injury, aorta)
  - complete — *see* Injury, aorta, laceration, major
- carotid artery (incomplete) (*see also* Injury, blood vessel, carotid, laceration)
  - complete — *see* Injury, blood vessel, carotid, laceration, major
- celiac artery (incomplete) S35.211 ☑
  - branch (incomplete) S35.291 ☑

Index

Tommaselli's disease — Transection

Transection — *continued*
- celiac artery — *continued*
  - branch — *continued*
    - complete S35.292 ☑
  - complete S35.212 ☑
- innominate
  - artery (incomplete) (*see also* Injury, blood vessel, thoracic, innominate, artery, laceration)
    - complete — *see* Injury, blood vessel, thoracic, innominate, artery, laceration, major
  - vein (incomplete) (*see also* Injury, blood vessel, thoracic, innominate, vein, laceration)
    - complete — *see* Injury, blood vessel, thoracic, innominate, vein, laceration, major
- jugular vein (external) (incomplete) (*see also* Injury, blood vessel, jugular vein, laceration)
  - complete — *see* Injury, blood vessel, jugular vein, laceration, major
  - internal (incomplete) (*see also* Injury, blood vessel, jugular vein, internal, laceration)
    - complete — *see* Injury, blood vessel, jugular vein, internal, laceration, major
- mesenteric artery (incomplete) (*see also* Injury, mesenteric, artery, laceration)
  - complete — *see* Injury, mesenteric artery, laceration, major
- pulmonary vessel (incomplete) (*see also* Injury, blood vessel, thoracic, pulmonary, laceration)
  - complete — *see* Injury, blood vessel, thoracic, pulmonary, laceration, major
- subclavian — *see* Transection, innominate
- vena cava (incomplete) (*see also* Injury, vena cava)
  - complete — *see* Injury, vena cava, laceration, major
- vertebral artery (incomplete) (*see also* Injury, blood vessel, vertebral, laceration)
  - complete — *see* Injury, blood vessel, vertebral, laceration, major

Transfusion
- associated (red blood cell) hemochromatosis E83.111
- blood
  - ABO incompatible — *see* Complication(s), transfusion, incompatibility reaction, ABO
  - minor blood group (Duffy) (E) (K(ell)) (Kidd) (Lewis) (M) (N) (P) (S) T8Ø.89 ☑
  - reaction or complication — *see* Complications, transfusion
- fetomaternal (mother) — *see* Pregnancy, complicated by, placenta, transfusion syndrome
- maternofetal (mother) — *see* Pregnancy, complicated by, placenta, transfusion syndrome
- placental (syndrome) (mother) — *see* Pregnancy, complicated by, placenta, transfusion syndrome
- reaction (adverse) — *see* Complications, transfusion
- related acute lung injury (TRALI) J95.84
- twin-to-twin — *see* Pregnancy, complicated by, placenta, transfusion syndrome, fetus to fetus

Transient (meaning homeless) (*see also* condition) Z59.Ø

Translocation
- balanced autosomal Q95.9
  - in normal individual Q95.Ø
- chromosomes NEC Q99.8
  - balanced and insertion in normal individual Q95.Ø
- Down syndrome Q9Ø.2
- trisomy
  - 13 Q91.6
  - 18 Q91.2
  - 21 Q9Ø.2

Translucency, iris — *see* Degeneration, iris

Transmission of chemical substances through the placenta — *see* Absorption, chemical, through placenta

Transparency, lung, unilateral J43.Ø

Transplant (ed) (status) Z94.9
- awaiting organ Z76.82
- bone Z94.6
  - marrow Z94.81
- candidate Z76.82
- complication — *see* Complication, transplant
- cornea Z94.7
- heart Z94.1
  - and lung(s) Z94.3
  - valve Z95.2
    - prosthetic Z95.2
    - specified NEC Z95.4
    - xenogenic Z95.3
- intestine Z94.82
- kidney Z94.Ø

Transplant — *continued*
- liver Z94.4
- lung(s) Z94.2
  - and heart Z94.3
- organ (failure) (infection) (rejection) Z94.9
  - removal status Z98.85
- pancreas Z94.83
- skin Z94.5
- social Z6Ø.3
- specified organ or tissue NEC Z94.89
- stem cells Z94.84
- tissue Z94.9

Transplants, ovarian, endometrial N8Ø.1

Transposed — *see* Transposition

Transposition (congenital) (*see also* Malposition, congenital)
- abdominal viscera Q89.3
- aorta (dextra) Q2Ø.3
- appendix Q43.8
- colon Q43.8
- corrected Q2Ø.5
- great vessels (complete) (partial) Q2Ø.3
- heart Q24.Ø
  - with complete transposition of viscera Q89.3
- intestine (large) (small) Q43.8
- reversed jejunal (for bypass) (status) Z98.Ø
- scrotum Q55.23
- stomach Q4Ø.2
  - with general transposition of viscera Q89.3
- tooth, teeth, fully erupted M26.3Ø
- vessels, great (complete) (partial) Q2Ø.3
- viscera (abdominal) (thoracic) Q89.3

Transsexualism F64.1

Transverse (*see also* condition)
- arrest (deep), in labor O64.Ø ☑
- lie (mother) O32.2 ☑
  - causing obstructed labor O64.8 ☑

Transvestism, transvestitism (dual-role) F64.1
- fetishistic F65.1

Trapped placenta (with hemorrhage) O72.Ø
- without hemorrhage O73.Ø

Trauma, traumatism (*see also* Injury)
- acoustic — *see* subcategory H83.3 ☑
- birth — *see* Birth, injury
- complicating ectopic or molar pregnancy OØ8.6
- during delivery O71.9
- following ectopic or molar pregnancy OØ8.6
- obstetric O71.9
  - specified NEC O71.89

Traumatic (*see also* condition)
- brain injury — *see* category SØ6 ☑

Treacher Collins syndrome Q75.4

Treitz's hernia — *see* Hernia, abdomen, specified site NEC

Trematode infestation — *see* Infestation, fluke

Trematodiasis — *see* Infestation, fluke

Trembling paralysis — *see* Parkinsonism

Tremor(s) R25.1
- drug induced G25.1
- essential (benign) G25.Ø
- familial G25.Ø
- hereditary G25.Ø
- hysterical F44.4
- intention G25.2
- medication induced postural G25.1
- mercurial — *see* subcategory T56.1 ☑
- Parkinson's — *see* Parkinsonism
- psychogenic (conversion reaction) F44.4
- senilis R54
- specified type NEC G25.2

Trench
- fever A79.Ø
- foot — *see* Immersion, foot
- mouth A69.1

Treponema pallidum infection — *see* Syphilis

Treponematosis
- due to
  - T. pallidum — *see* Syphilis
  - T. pertenue — *see* Yaws

Triad
- Hutchinson's (congenital syphilis) A5Ø.53
- Kartagener's Q89.3
- Saint's — *see* Hernia, diaphragm

Trichiasis (eyelid) HØ2.Ø59
- with entropion — *see* Entropion
- left HØ2.Ø56
  - lower HØ2.Ø55

Trichiasis — *continued*
- left — *continued*
  - upper HØ2.Ø54
- right HØ2.Ø53
  - lower HØ2.Ø52
  - upper HØ2.Ø51

Trichinella spiralis (infection) (infestation) B75

Trichinellosis, trichiniasis, trichinelliasis, trichinosis B75
- with muscle disorder B75 [M63.8Ø]
  - ankle B75 [M63.87-] ☑
  - foot B75 [M63.87-] ☑
  - forearm B75 [M63.83-] ☑
  - hand B75 [M63.84-] ☑
  - lower leg B75 [M63.86-] ☑
  - multiple sites B75 [M63.89]
  - pelvic region B75 [M63.85-] ☑
  - shoulder region B75 [M63.81-] ☑
  - specified site NEC B75 [M63.88]
  - thigh B75 [M63.85-] ☑
  - upper arm B75 [M63.82-] ☑

Trichobezoar T18.9 ☑
- intestine T18.3 ☑
- stomach T18.2 ☑

Trichocephaliasis, trichocephalosis B79

Trichocephalus infestation B79

Trichoclasis L67.8

Trichoepithelioma (*see also* Neoplasm, skin, benign)
- malignant — *see* Neoplasm, skin, malignant

Trichofolliculoma — *see* Neoplasm, skin, benign

Tricholemmoma — *see* Neoplasm, skin, benign

Trichomoniasis A59.9
- bladder A59.Ø3
- cervix A59.Ø9
- intestinal AØ7.8
- prostate A59.Ø2
- seminal vesicles A59.Ø9
- specified site NEC A59.8
- urethra A59.Ø3
- urogenitalis A59.ØØ
- vagina A59.Ø1
- vulva A59.Ø1

Trichomycosis
- axillaris A48.8
- nodosa, nodularis B36.8

Trichonodosis L67.8

Trichophytid, trichophyton infection — *see* Dermatophytosis

Trichophytobezoar T18.9 ☑
- intestine T18.3 ☑
- stomach T18.2 ☑

Trichophytosis — *see* Dermatophytosis

Trichoptilosis L67.8

Trichorrhexis (nodosa) (invaginata) L67.Ø

Trichosis axillaris A48.8

Trichosporosis nodosa B36.2

Trichostasis spinulosa (congenital) Q84.1

Trichostrongyliasis, trichostrongylosis (small intestine) B81.2

Trichostrongylus infection B81.2

Trichotillomania F63.3

Trichromat, trichromatopsia, anomalous (congenital) H53.55

Trichuriasis B79

Trichuris trichiura (infection) (infestation) (any site) B79

Tricuspid (valve) — *see* condition

Trifid (*see also* Accessory)
- kidney (pelvis) Q63.8
- tongue Q38.3

Trigeminal neuralgia — *see* Neuralgia, trigeminal

Trigeminy RØØ.8

Trigger finger (acquired) M65.3Ø
- congenital Q74.Ø
- index finger M65.32- ☑
- little finger M65.35- ☑
- middle finger M65.33- ☑
- ring finger M65.34- ☑
- thumb M65.31- ☑

Trigonitis (bladder) (chronic) (pseudomembranous) N3Ø.3Ø
- with hematuria N3Ø.31

Trigonocephaly Q75.Ø

Trilocular heart — *see* Cor triloculare

Trimethylaminuria E72.52

Tripartite placenta O43.19- ☑

Triphalangeal thumb Q74.Ø

- **Triple** (*see also* Accessory)
  - kidneys Q63.Ø
  - uteri Q51.818
  - X, female Q97.Ø
- **Triplegia** G83.89
  - congenital G8Ø.8
- **Triplet** (newborn) (*see also* Newborn, triplet)
  - complicating pregnancy — *see* Pregnancy, triplet
- **Triplication** — *see* Accessory
- **Triploidy** Q92.7
- **Trismus** R25.2
  - neonatorum A33
  - newborn A33
- **Trisomy** (syndrome) Q92.9
  - 13 (partial) Q91.7
    - meiotic nondisjunction Q91.4
    - mitotic nondisjunction Q91.5
    - mosaicism Q91.5
    - translocation Q91.6
  - 18 (partial) Q91.3
    - meiotic nondisjunction Q91.Ø
    - mitotic nondisjunction Q91.1
    - mosaicism Q91.1
    - translocation Q91.2
  - 2Ø Q92.8
  - 21 (partial) Q9Ø.9
    - meiotic nondisjunction Q9Ø.Ø
    - mitotic nondisjunction Q9Ø.1
    - mosaicism Q9Ø.1
    - translocation Q9Ø.2
  - 22 Q92.8
  - autosomes Q92.9
  - chromosome specified NEC Q92.8
    - partial Q92.2
      - due to unbalanced translocation Q92.5
    - specified NEC Q92.8
    - whole (nonsex chromosome)
      - meiotic nondisjunction Q92.Ø
      - mitotic nondisjunction Q92.1
      - mosaicism Q92.1
  - due to
    - dicentrics — *see* Extra, marker chromosomes
    - extra rings — *see* Extra, marker chromosomes
    - isochromosomes — *see* Extra, marker chromosomes
  - specified NEC Q92.8
  - whole chromosome Q92.9
    - meiotic nondisjunction Q92.Ø
    - mitotic nondisjunction Q92.1
    - mosaicism Q92.1
    - partial Q92.9
    - specified NEC Q92.8
- **Tritanomaly, tritanopia** H53.55
- **Trombiculosis, trombiculiasis, trombidiosis** B88.Ø
- **Trophedema** (congenital) (hereditary) Q82.Ø
- **Trophoblastic disease** (*see also* Mole, hydatidiform) OØ1.9
- **Tropholymphedema** Q82.Ø
- **Trophoneurosis NEC** G96.8
  - disseminated M34.9
- **Tropical** — *see* condition
- **Trouble** (*see also* Disease)
  - heart — *see* Disease, heart
  - kidney — *see* Disease, renal
  - nervous R45.Ø
  - sinus — *see* Sinusitis
- **Trousseau's syndrome** (thrombophlebitis migrans) I82.1
- **Truancy, childhood**
  - from school Z72.81Ø
- **Truncus**
  - arteriosus (persistent) Q2Ø.Ø
  - communis Q2Ø.Ø
- **Trunk** — *see* condition
- **Trypanosomiasis**
  - African B56.9
    - by Trypanosoma brucei
      - gambiense B56.Ø
      - rhodesiense B56.1
  - American — *see* Chagas' disease
  - Brazilian — *see* Chagas' disease
  - by Trypanosoma
    - brucei gambiense B56.Ø
    - brucei rhodesiense B56.1
    - cruzi — *see* Chagas' disease
  - gambiensis, Gambian B56.Ø
  - rhodesiensis, Rhodesian B56.1
  - South American — *see* Chagas' disease

- **Trypanosomiasis** — *continued*
  - where
    - African trypanosomiasis is prevalent B56.9
    - Chagas' disease is prevalent B57.2
- **T-shaped incisors** KØØ.2
- **Tsutsugamushi** (disease) (fever) A75.3
- **Tube, tubal, tubular** — *see* condition
- **Tubercle** (*see also* Tuberculosis)
  - brain, solitary A17.81
  - Darwin's Q17.8
  - Ghon, primary infection A15.7
- **Tuberculid, tuberculide** (indurating, subcutaneous) (lichenoid) (miliary) (papulonecrotic) (primary) (skin) A18.4
- **Tuberculoma** (*see also* Tuberculosis)
  - brain A17.81
  - meninges (cerebral) (spinal) A17.1
  - spinal cord A17.81
- **Tuberculosis, tubercular, tuberculous** (calcification) (calcified) (caseous) (chromogenic acid-fast bacilli) (degeneration) (fibrocaseous) (fistula) (interstitial) (isolated circumscribed lesions) (necrosis) (parenchymatous) (ulcerative) A15.9
  - with pneumoconiosis (any condition in J6Ø-J64) J65
  - abdomen (lymph gland) A18.39
  - abscess (respiratory) A15.9
    - bone A18.Ø3
      - hip A18.Ø2
      - knee A18.Ø2
      - sacrum A18.Ø1
      - specified site NEC A18.Ø3
      - spinal A18.Ø1
      - vertebra A18.Ø1
    - brain A17.81
    - breast A18.89
    - Cowper's gland A18.15
    - dura (mater) (cerebral) (spinal) A17.81
    - epidural (cerebral) (spinal) A17.81
    - female pelvis A18.17
    - frontal sinus A15.8
    - genital organs NEC A18.1Ø
    - genitourinary A18.1Ø
    - gland (lymphatic) — *see* Tuberculosis, lymph gland
    - hip A18.Ø2
    - intestine A18.32
    - ischiorectal A18.32
    - joint NEC A18.Ø2
      - hip A18.Ø2
      - knee A18.Ø2
      - specified NEC A18.Ø2
      - vertebral A18.Ø1
    - kidney A18.11
    - knee A18.Ø2
    - latent R76.11
    - lumbar (spine) A18.Ø1
    - lung — *see* Tuberculosis, pulmonary
    - meninges (cerebral) (spinal) A17.Ø
    - muscle A18.Ø9
    - perianal (fistula) A18.32
    - perinephritic A18.11
    - perirectal A18.32
    - rectum A18.32
    - retropharyngeal A15.8
    - sacrum A18.Ø1
    - scrofulous A18.2
    - scrotum A18.15
    - skin (primary) A18.4
    - spinal cord A17.81
    - spine or vertebra (column) A18.Ø1
    - subdiaphragmatic A18.31
    - testis A18.15
    - urinary A18.13
    - uterus A18.17
  - accessory sinus — *see* Tuberculosis, sinus
  - Addison's disease A18.7
  - adenitis — *see* Tuberculosis, lymph gland
  - adenoids A15.8
  - adenopathy — *see* Tuberculosis, lymph gland
  - adherent pericardium A18.84
  - adnexa (uteri) A18.17
  - adrenal (capsule) (gland) A18.7
  - alimentary canal A18.32
  - anemia A18.89
  - ankle (joint) (bone) A18.Ø2
  - anus A18.32
  - apex, apical — *see* Tuberculosis, pulmonary
  - appendicitis, appendix A18.32
  - arachnoid A17.Ø

- **Tuberculosis, tubercular, tuberculous** — *continued*
  - artery, arteritis A18.89
    - cerebral A18.89
  - arthritis (chronic) (synovial) A18.Ø2
    - spine or vertebra (column) A18.Ø1
  - articular — *see* Tuberculosis, joint
  - ascites A18.31
  - asthma — *see* Tuberculosis, pulmonary
  - axilla, axillary (gland) A18.2
  - bladder A18.12
  - bone A18.Ø3
    - hip A18.Ø2
    - knee A18.Ø2
    - limb NEC A18.Ø3
    - sacrum A18.Ø1
    - spine or vertebral column A18.Ø1
  - bowel (miliary) A18.32
  - brain A17.81
  - breast A18.89
  - broad ligament A18.17
  - bronchi, bronchial, bronchus A15.5
    - ectasia, ectasis (bronchiectasis) — *see* Tuberculosis, pulmonary
    - fistula A15.5
      - primary (progressive) A15.7
    - gland or node A15.4
      - primary (progressive) A15.7
    - lymph gland or node A15.4
      - primary (progressive) A15.7
  - bronchiectasis — *see* Tuberculosis, pulmonary
  - bronchitis A15.5
  - bronchopleural A15.6
  - bronchopneumonia, bronchopneumonic — *see* Tuberculosis, pulmonary
  - bronchorrhagia A15.5
  - bronchotracheal A15.5
  - bronze disease A18.7
  - buccal cavity A18.83
  - bulbourethral gland A18.15
  - bursa A18.Ø9
  - cachexia A15.9
  - cardiomyopathy A18.84
  - caries — *see* Tuberculosis, bone
  - cartilage A18.Ø2
    - intervertebral A18.Ø1
  - catarrhal — *see* Tuberculosis, respiratory
  - cecum A18.32
  - cellulitis (primary) A18.4
  - cerebellum A17.81
  - cerebral, cerebrum A17.81
  - cerebrospinal A17.81
    - meninges A17.Ø
  - cervical (lymph gland or node) A18.2
  - cervicitis, cervix (uteri) A18.16
  - chest — *see* Tuberculosis, respiratory
  - chorioretinitis A18.53
  - choroid, choroiditis A18.53
  - ciliary body A18.54
  - colitis A18.32
  - collier's J65
  - colliquativa (primary) A18.4
  - colon A18.32
  - complex, primary A15.7
  - congenital P37.Ø
  - conjunctiva A18.59
  - connective tissue (systemic) A18.89
  - contact Z2Ø.1
  - cornea (ulcer) A18.52
  - Cowper's gland A18.15
  - coxae A18.Ø2
  - coxalgia A18.Ø2
  - cul-de-sac of Douglas A18.17
  - curvature, spine A18.Ø1
  - cutis (colliquativa) (primary) A18.4
  - cyst, ovary A18.18
  - cystitis A18.12
  - dactylitis A18.Ø3
  - diarrhea A18.32
  - diffuse — *see* Tuberculosis, miliary
  - digestive tract A18.32
  - disseminated — *see* Tuberculosis, miliary
  - duodenum A18.32
  - dura (mater) (cerebral) (spinal) A17.Ø
    - abscess (cerebral) (spinal) A17.81
  - dysentery A18.32
  - ear (inner) (middle) A18.6
    - bone A18.Ø3
    - external (primary) A18.4

Tuberculosis, tubercular, tuberculous — *continued*
  subcutis (primary) A18.4
  subdeltoid bursa A18.83
  submaxillary (region) A18.83
  supraclavicular gland A18.2
  suprarenal (capsule) (gland) A18.7
  swelling, joint (*see also* category MØ1) (*see also* Tuberculosis, joint) A18.Ø2
  symphysis pubis A18.Ø2
  synovitis A18.Ø9
    articular A18.Ø2
    spine or vertebra A18.Ø1
  systemic — *see* Tuberculosis, miliary
  tarsitis A18.4
  tendon (sheath) — *see* Tuberculosis, tenosynovitis
  tenosynovitis A18.Ø9
    spine or vertebra A18.Ø1
  testis A18.15
  throat A15.8
  thymus gland A18.82
  thyroid gland A18.81
  tongue A18.83
  tonsil, tonsillitis A15.8
  trachea, tracheal A15.5
    lymph gland or node A15.4
      primary (progressive) A15.7
  tracheobronchial A15.5
    lymph gland or node A15.4
      primary (progressive) A15.7
  tubal (acute) (chronic) A18.17
  tunica vaginalis A18.15
  ulcer (skin) (primary) A18.4
    bowel or intestine A18.32
    specified NEC — *see* Tuberculosis, by site
  unspecified site A15.9
  ureter A18.11
  urethra, urethral (gland) A18.13
  urinary organ or tract A18.13
  uterus A18.17
  uveal tract A18.54
  uvula A18.83
  vagina A18.18
  vas deferens A18.15
  verruca, verrucosa (cutis) (primary) A18.4
  vertebra (column) A18.Ø1
  vesiculitis A18.15
  vulva A18.18
  wrist (joint) A18.Ø2
Tuberculum
  Carabelli — *see* Excludes Note at KØØ.2
  occlusal — *see* Excludes Note at KØØ.2
  paramolare KØØ.2
Tuberosity, enitre maxillary M26.Ø7
Tuberous sclerosis (brain) Q85.1
Tubo-ovarian — *see* condition
Tuboplasty, after previous sterilization Z31.Ø
  aftercare Z31.42
Tubotympanitis, catarrhal (chronic) — *see* Otitis, media, nonsuppurative, chronic, serous
Tularemia A21.9
  with
    conjunctivitis A21.1
    pneumonia A21.2
  abdominal A21.3
  bronchopneumonic A21.2
  conjunctivitis A21.1
  cryptogenic A21.3
  enteric A21.3
  gastrointestinal A21.3
  generalized A21.7
  ingestion A21.3
  intestinal A21.3
  oculoglandular A21.1
  ophthalmic A21.1
  pneumonia (any), pneumonic A21.2
  pulmonary A21.2
  sepsis A21.7
  specified NEC A21.8
  typhoidal A21.7
  ulceroglandular A21.Ø
Tularensis conjunctivitis A21.1
Tumefaction (*see also* Swelling)
  liver — *see* Hypertrophy, liver
Tumor (*see also* Neoplasm, unspecified behavior, by site)
  acinar cell — *see* Neoplasm, uncertain behavior, by site
  acinic cell — *see* Neoplasm, uncertain behavior, by site

Tumor — *continued*
  adenocarcinoid — *see* Neoplasm, malignant, by site
  adenomatoid (*see also* Neoplasm, benign, by site)
    odontogenic — *see* Cyst, calcifying odontogenic
  adnexal (skin) — *see* Neoplasm, skin, benign, by site
  adrenal
    cortical (benign) D35.Ø- ☑
      malignant C74.Ø- ☑
    rest — *see* Neoplasm, benign, by site
  alpha-cell
    malignant
      pancreas C25.4
      specified site NEC — *see* Neoplasm, malignant, by site
      unspecified site C25.4
    pancreas D13.7
    specified site NEC — *see* Neoplasm, benign, by site
    unspecified site D13.7
  aneurysmal — *see* Aneurysm
  aortic body D44.7
    malignant C75.5
  Askin's — *see* Neoplasm, connective tissue, malignant
  basal cell (*see also* Neoplasm, skin, uncertain behavior) D48.5
  Bednar — *see* Neoplasm, skin, malignant
  benign (unclassified) — *see* Neoplasm, benign, by site
  beta-cell
    malignant
      pancreas C25.4
      specified site NEC — *see* Neoplasm, malignant, by site
      unspecified site C25.4
    pancreas D13.7
    specified site NEC — *see* Neoplasm, benign, by site
    unspecified site D13.7
  Brenner D27.9
    borderline malignancy D39.1- ☑
    malignant C56- ☑
    proliferating D39.1- ☑
  bronchial alveolar, intravascular D38.1
  Brooke's — *see* Neoplasm, skin, benign
  brown fat — *see* Lipoma
  Burkitt — *see* Lymphoma, Burkitt
  calcifying epithelial odontogenic — *see* Cyst, calcifying odontogenic
  carcinoid
    benign D3A.ØØ (*following* D36)
      appendix D3A.Ø2Ø (*following* D36)
      ascending colon D3A.Ø22 (*following* D36)
      bronchus (lung) D3A.Ø9Ø (*following* D36)
      cecum D3A.Ø21 (*following* D36)
      colon D3A.Ø29 (*following* D36)
      descending colon D3A.Ø24 (*following* D36)
      duodenum D3A.Ø1Ø (*following* D36)
      foregut NOS D3A.Ø94 (*following* D36)
      hindgut NOS D3A.Ø96 (*following* D36)
      ileum D3A.Ø12 (*following* D36)
      jejunum D3A.Ø11 (*following* D36)
      kidney D3A.Ø93 (*following* D36)
      large intestine D3A.Ø29 (*following* D36)
      lung (bronchus) D3A.Ø9Ø (*following* D36)
      midgut NOS D3A.Ø95 (*following* D36)
      rectum D3A.Ø26 (*following* D36)
      sigmoid colon D3A.Ø25 (*following* D36)
      small intestine D3A.Ø19 (*following* D36)
      specified NEC D3A.Ø98 (*following* D36)
      stomach D3A.Ø92 (*following* D36)
      thymus D3A.Ø91 (*following* D36)
      transverse colon D3A.Ø23 (*following* D36)
    malignant C7A.ØØ (*following* C75)
      appendix C7A.Ø2Ø (*following* C75)
      ascending colon C7A.Ø22 (*following* C75)
      bronchus (lung) C7A.Ø9Ø (*following* C75)
      cecum C7A.Ø21 (*following* C75)
      colon C7A.Ø29 (*following* C75)
      descending colon C7A.Ø24 (*following* C75)
      duodenum C7A.Ø1Ø (*following* C75)
      foregut NOS C7A.Ø94 (*following* C75)
      hindgut NOS C7A.Ø96 (*following* C75)
      ileum C7A.Ø12 (*following* C75)
      jejunum C7A.Ø11 (*following* C75)
      kidney C7A.Ø93 (*following* C75)
      large intestine C7A.Ø29 (*following* C75)
      lung (bronchus) C7A.Ø9Ø (*following* C75)
      midgut NOS C7A.Ø95 (*following* C75)
      rectum C7A.Ø26 (*following* C75)
      sigmoid colon C7A.Ø25 (*following* C75)
      small intestine C7A.Ø19 (*following* C75)

Tumor — *continued*
  carcinoid — *continued*
    malignant — *continued*
      specified NEC C7A.Ø98 (*following* C75)
      stomach C7A.Ø92 (*following* C75)
      thymus C7A.Ø91 (*following* C75)
      transverse colon C7A.Ø23 (*following* C75)
    mesentary metastasis C7B.Ø4 (*following* C75)
    secondary C7B.ØØ (*following* C75)
      bone C7B.Ø3 (*following* C75)
      distant lymph nodes C7B.Ø1 (*following* C75)
      liver C7B.Ø2 (*following* C75)
      peritoneum C7B.Ø4 (*following* C75)
      specified NEC C7B.Ø9 (*following* C75)
  carotid body D44.6
    malignant C75.4
  cells (*see also* Neoplasm, unspecified behavior, by site)
    benign — *see* Neoplasm, benign, by site
    malignant — *see* Neoplasm, malignant, by site
    uncertain whether benign or malignant — *see* Neoplasm, uncertain behavior, by site
  cervix, in pregnancy or childbirth — *see* Pregnancy, complicated by, tumor, cervix
  chondromatous giant cell — *see* Neoplasm, bone, benign
  chromaffin (*see also* Neoplasm, benign, by site)
    malignant — *see* Neoplasm, malignant, by site
  Cock's peculiar L72.3
  Codman's — *see* Neoplasm, bone, benign
  dentigerous, mixed — *see* Cyst, calcifying odontogenic
  dermoid — *see* Neoplasm, benign, by site
    with malignant transformation C56- ☑
  desmoid (extra-abdominal) (*see also* Neoplasm, connective tissue, uncertain behavior)
    abdominal — *see* Neoplasm, connective tissue, uncertain behavior
  embolus — *see* Neoplasm, secondary, by site
  embryonal (mixed) (*see also* Neoplasm, uncertain behavior, by site)
    liver C22.7
  endodermal sinus
    specified site — *see* Neoplasm, malignant, by site
    unspecified site
      female C56.- ☑
      male C62.9Ø
  epithelial
    benign — *see* Neoplasm, benign, by site
    malignant — *see* Neoplasm, malignant, by site
  Ewing's — *see* Neoplasm, bone, malignant, by site
  fatty — *see* Lipoma
  fibroid — *see* Leiomyoma
  G cell
    malignant
      pancreas C25.4
      specified site NEC — *see* Neoplasm, malignant, by site
      unspecified site C25.4
    specified site — *see* Neoplasm, uncertain behavior, by site
    unspecified site D37.8
  germ cell (*see also* Neoplasm, malignant, by site)
    mixed — *see* Neoplasm, malignant, by site
  ghost cell, odontogenic — *see* Cyst, calcifying odontogenic
  giant cell (*see also* Neoplasm, uncertain behavior, by site)
    bone D48.Ø
      malignant — *see* Neoplasm, bone, malignant
    chondromatous — *see* Neoplasm, bone, benign
    malignant — *see* Neoplasm, malignant, by site
    soft parts — *see* Neoplasm, connective tissue, uncertain behavior
      malignant — *see* Neoplasm, connective tissue, malignant
  glomus D18.ØØ
    intra-abdominal D18.Ø3
    intracranial D18.Ø2
    jugulare D44.7
      malignant C75.5
    skin D18.Ø1
    specified site NEC D18.Ø9
  gonadal stromal — *see* Neoplasm, uncertain behavior, by site
  granular cell (*see also* Neoplasm, connective tissue, benign)
    malignant — *see* Neoplasm, connective tissue, malignant

- **Turner's** — *continued*
  - tooth KØØ.4
- **Turner-Ullrich syndrome** Q96.9
- **Tussis convulsiva** — *see* Whooping cough
- **Twiddler's syndrome** (due to)
  - automatic implantable defibrillatorT82.198
  - cardiac pacemaker T82.198 ☑
- **Twilight state**
  - epileptic FØ5
  - psychogenic F44.89
- **Twin** (newborn) (*see also* Newborn, twin)
  - conjoined Q89.4
  - pregnancy — *see* Pregnancy, twin, conjoined
- **Twinning, teeth** KØØ.2
- **Twist, twisted**
  - bowel, colon or intestine K56.2
  - hair (congenital) Q84.1
  - mesentery K56.2
  - omentum K56.2
  - organ or site, congenital NEC — *see* Anomaly, by site
  - ovarian pedicle — *see* Torsion, ovary
- **Twitching** R25.3
- **Tylosis** (acquired) L84
  - buccalis K13.29
  - linguae K13.29
  - palmaris et plantaris (congenital) (inherited) Q82.8
    - acquired L85.1
- **Tympanism** R14.Ø
- **Tympanites** (abdominal) (intestinal) R14.Ø
- **Tympanitis** — *see* Myringitis
- **Tympanosclerosis** H74.Ø ☑
- **Tympanum** — *see* condition
- **Tympany**
  - abdomen R14.Ø
  - chest RØ9.89
- **Type A behavior pattern** Z73.1
- **Typhlitis** — *see* Appendicitis
- **Typhoenteritis** — *see* Typhoid
- **Typhoid** (abortive) (ambulant) (any site) (clinical) (fever) (hemorrhagic) (infection) (intermittent) (malignant) (rheumatic) (Widal negative) AØ1.ØØ
  - with pneumonia AØ1.Ø3
  - abdominal AØ1.Ø9
  - arthritis AØ1.Ø4
  - carrier (suspected) of Z22.Ø
  - cholecystitis (current) AØ1.Ø9
  - endocarditis AØ1.Ø2
  - heart involvement AØ1.Ø2
  - inoculation reaction — *see* Complications, vaccination
  - meningitis AØ1.Ø1
  - mesenteric lymph nodes AØ1.Ø9
  - myocarditis AØ1.Ø2
  - osteomyelitis AØ1.Ø5
  - perichondritis, larynx AØ1.Ø9
  - pneumonia AØ1.Ø3
  - specified NEC AØ1.Ø9
  - spine AØ1.Ø5
  - ulcer (perforating) AØ1.Ø9
- **Typhomalaria** (fever) — *see* Malaria
- **Typhomania** AØ1.ØØ
- **Typhoperitonitis** AØ1.Ø9
- **Typhus** (fever) A75.9
  - abdominal, abdominalis — *see* Typhoid
  - African tick A77.1
  - amarillic A95.9
  - brain A75.9 [G94]
  - cerebral A75.9 [G94]
  - classical A75.Ø
  - due to Rickettsia
    - prowazekii A75.Ø
      - recrudescent A75.1
    - tsutsugamushi A75.3
    - typhi A75.2
  - endemic (flea-borne) A75.2
  - epidemic (louse-borne) A75.Ø
  - exanthematicus SAI A75.Ø
    - brillii SAI A75.1
    - mexicanus SAI A75.2
    - typhus murinus A75.2
  - exanthematic NEC A75.Ø
  - flea-borne A75.2
  - India tick A77.1
  - Kenya (tick) A77.1
  - louse-borne A75.Ø
  - Mexican A75.2
  - mite-borne A75.3
  - murine A75.2
  - North Asian tick-borne A77.2
- **Typhus** — *continued*
  - petechial A75.9
  - Queensland tick A77.3
  - rat A75.2
  - recrudescent A75.1
  - recurrens — *see* Fever, relapsing
  - Sao Paulo A77.Ø
  - scrub (China) (India) (Malaysia) (New Guinea) A75.3
  - shop (of Malaysia) A75.2
  - Siberian tick A77.2
  - tick-borne A77.9
  - tropical (mite-borne) A75.3
- **Tyrosinemia** E7Ø.21
  - newborn, transitory P74.5
- **Tyrosinosis** E7Ø.21
- **Tyrosinuria** E7Ø.29

U

- **Uhl's anomaly or disease** Q24.8
- **Ulcer, ulcerated, ulcerating, ulceration, ulcerative**
  - alveolar process M27.3
  - amebic (intestine) AØ6.1
    - skin AØ6.7
  - anastomotic — *see* Ulcer, gastrojejunal
  - anorectal K62.6
  - antral — *see* Ulcer, stomach
  - anus (sphincter) (solitary) K62.6
  - aorta — *see* Aneurysm
  - aphthous (oral) (recurrent) K12.Ø
    - genital organ(s)
      - female N76.6
      - male N5Ø.8
  - artery I77.2
  - atrophic — *see* Ulcer, skin
    - decubitus — *see* Ulcer, pressure, by site
  - back L98.429
    - with
      - bone necrosis L98.424
      - exposed fat layer L98.422
      - muscle necrosis L98.423
      - skin breakdown only L98.421
  - Barrett's (esophagus) K22.1Ø
    - with bleeding K22.11
  - bile duct (common) (hepatic) K83.8
  - bladder (solitary) (sphincter) NEC N32.89
    - bilharzial B65.9 [N33]
    - in schistosomiasis (bilharzial) B65.9 [N33]
    - submucosal — *see* Cystitis, interstitial
    - tuberculous A18.12
  - bleeding K27.4
  - bone — *see* Osteomyelitis, specified type NEC
  - bowel — *see* Ulcer, intestine
  - breast N61
  - bronchus J98.Ø9
  - buccal (cavity) (traumatic) K12.1
  - Buruli A31.1
  - buttock L98.419
    - with
      - bone necrosis L98.414
      - exposed fat layer L98.412
      - muscle necrosis L98.413
      - skin breakdown only L98.411
  - cancerous — *see* Neoplasm, malignant, by site
  - cardia K22.1Ø
    - with bleeding K22.11
  - cardioesophageal (peptic) K22.1Ø
    - with bleeding K22.11
  - cecum — *see* Ulcer, intestine
  - cervix (uteri) (decubitus) (trophic) N86
    - with cervicitis N72
  - chancroidal A57
  - chiclero B55.1
  - chronic (cause unknown) — *see* Ulcer, skin
  - Cochin-China B55.1
  - colon — *see* Ulcer, intestine
  - conjunctiva H1Ø.89
  - cornea H16.ØØ- ☑
    - with hypopyon H16.Ø3- ☑
    - central H16.Ø1- ☑
    - dendritic (herpes simplex) BØØ.52
    - marginal H16.Ø4- ☑
    - Mooren's H16.Ø5- ☑
    - mycotic H16.Ø6- ☑
    - perforated H16.Ø7- ☑
    - ring H16.Ø2- ☑
    - tuberculous (phlyctenular) A18.52
- **Ulcer, ulcerated, ulcerating, ulceration, ulcerative** — *continued*
  - corpus cavernosum (chronic) N48.5
  - crural — *see* Ulcer, lower limb
  - Curling's — *see* Ulcer, peptic, acute
  - Cushing's — *see* Ulcer, peptic, acute
  - cystic duct K82.8
  - cystitis (interstitial) — *see* Cystitis, interstitial
  - decubitus — *see* Ulcer, pressure, by site
  - dendritic, cornea (herpes simplex) BØØ.52
  - diabetes, diabetic — *see* Diabetes, ulcer
  - Dieulafoy's K25.Ø
  - due to
    - infection NEC — *see* Ulcer, skin
    - radiation NEC L59.8
    - trophic disturbance (any region) — *see* Ulcer, skin
    - X-ray L58.1
  - duodenum, duodenal (eroded) (peptic) K26.9
    - with
      - hemorrhage K26.4
        - and perforation K26.6
      - perforation K26.5
    - acute K26.3
      - with
        - hemorrhage K26.Ø
          - and perforation K26.2
        - perforation K26.1
    - chronic K26.7
      - with
        - hemorrhage K26.4
          - and perforation K26.6
        - perforation K26.5
  - dysenteric AØ9
  - elusive — *see* Cystitis, interstitial
  - endocarditis (acute) (chronic) (subacute) I28.8
  - epiglottis J38.7
  - esophagus (peptic) K22.1Ø
    - with bleeding K22.11
    - due to
      - aspirin K22.1Ø
        - with bleeding K22.11
      - gastrointestinal reflux disease K21.Ø
      - ingestion of chemical or medicament K22.1Ø
        - with bleeding K22.11
    - fungal K22.1Ø
      - with bleeding K22.11
    - infective K22.1Ø
      - with bleeding K22.11
    - varicose — *see* Varix, esophagus
  - eyelid (region) HØ1.8
  - fauces J39.2
  - Fenwick (-Hunner) (solitary) — *see* Cystitis, interstitial
  - fistulous — *see* Ulcer, skin
  - foot (indolent) (trophic) — *see* Ulcer, lower limb
  - frambesial, initial A66.Ø
  - frenum (tongue) K14.Ø
  - gallbladder or duct K82.8
  - gangrenous — *see* Gangrene
  - gastric — *see* Ulcer, stomach
  - gastrocolic — *see* Ulcer, gastrojejunal
  - gastroduodenal — *see* Ulcer, peptic
  - gastroesophageal — *see* Ulcer, stomach
  - gastrointestinal — *see* Ulcer, gastrojejunal
  - gastrojejunal (peptic) K28.9
    - with
      - hemorrhage K28.4
        - and perforation K28.6
      - perforation K28.5
    - acute K28.3
      - with
        - hemorrhage K28.Ø
          - and perforation K28.2
        - perforation K28.1
    - chronic K28.7
      - with
        - hemorrhage K28.4
          - and perforation K28.6
        - perforation K28.5
  - gastrojejunocolic — *see* Ulcer, gastrojejunal
  - gingiva KØ6.8
  - gingivitis KØ5.1Ø
    - nonplaque induced KØ5.11
    - plaque induced KØ5.1Ø
  - glottis J38.7
  - granuloma of pudenda A58
  - gum KØ6.8
  - gumma, due to yaws A66.4
  - heel — *see* Ulcer, lower limb

Ulcer, ulcerated, ulcerating, ulceration, ulcerative *— continued*
- hemorrhoid (*see also* Hemorrhoids, by degree) K64.8
- Hunner's — *see* Cystitis, interstitial
- hypopharynx J39.2
- hypopyon (chronic) (subacute) — *see* Ulcer, cornea, with hypopyon
- hypostaticum — *see* Ulcer, varicose
- ileum — *see* Ulcer, intestine
- intestine, intestinal K63.3
  - with perforation K63.1
  - amebic A06.1
  - duodenal — *see* Ulcer, duodenum
  - granulocytopenic (with hemorrhage) — *see* Neutropenia
  - marginal — *see* Ulcer, gastrojejunal
  - perforating K63.1
    - newborn P78.0
  - primary, small intestine K63.3
  - rectum K62.6
  - stercoraceous, stercoral K63.3
  - tuberculous A18.32
  - typhoid (fever) — *see* Typhoid
  - varicose I86.8
- jejunum, jejunal — *see* Ulcer, gastrojejunal
- keratitis — *see* Ulcer, cornea
- knee — *see* Ulcer, lower limb
- labium (majus) (minus) N76.6
- laryngitis — *see* Laryngitis
- larynx (aphthous) (contact) J38.7
  - diphtheritic A36.2
- leg — *see* Ulcer, lower limb
- lip K13.0
- Lipschütz's N76.6
- lower limb (atrophic) (chronic) (neurogenic) (perforating) (pyogenic) (trophic) (tropical) L97.909
  - with
    - bone necrosis L97.904
    - exposed fat layer L97.902
    - muscle necrosis L97.903
    - skin breakdown only L97.901
  - ankle L97.309
    - with
      - bone necrosis L97.304
      - exposed fat layer L97.302
      - muscle necrosis L97.303
      - skin breakdown only L97.301
    - left L97.329
      - with
        - bone necrosis L97.324
        - exposed fat layer L97.322
        - muscle necrosis L97.323
        - skin breakdown only L97.321
    - right L97.319
      - with
        - bone necrosis L97.314
        - exposed fat layer L97.312
        - muscle necrosis L97.313
        - skin breakdown only L97.311
  - calf L97.209
    - with
      - bone necrosis L97.204
      - exposed fat layer L97.202
      - muscle necrosis L97.203
      - skin breakdown only L97.201
    - left L97.229
      - with
        - bone necrosis L97.224
        - exposed fat layer L97.222
        - muscle necrosis L97.223
        - skin breakdown only L97.221
    - right L97.219
      - with
        - bone necrosis L97.214
        - exposed fat layer L97.212
        - muscle necrosis L97.213
        - skin breakdown only L97.211
  - decubitus — *see* Ulcer, pressure, by site
  - foot specified NEC L97.509
    - with
      - bone necrosis L97.504
      - exposed fat layer L97.502
      - muscle necrosis L97.503
      - skin breakdown only L97.501
    - left L97.529
      - with
        - bone necrosis L97.524
        - exposed fat layer L97.522

Ulcer, ulcerated, ulcerating, ulceration, ulcerative *— continued*
- lower limb *— continued*
  - foot specified *— continued*
    - left *— continued*
      - with *— continued*
        - muscle necrosis L97.523
        - skin breakdown only L97.521
    - right L97.519
      - with
        - bone necrosis L97.514
        - exposed fat layer L97.512
        - muscle necrosis L97.513
        - skin breakdown only L97.511
  - heel L97.409
    - with
      - bone necrosis L97.404
      - exposed fat layer L97.402
      - muscle necrosis L97.403
      - skin breakdown only L97.401
    - left L97.429
      - with
        - bone necrosis L97.424
        - exposed fat layer L97.422
        - muscle necrosis L97.423
        - skin breakdown only L97.421
    - right L97.419
      - with
        - bone necrosis L97.414
        - exposed fat layer L97.412
        - muscle necrosis L97.413
        - skin breakdown only L97.411
  - left L97.929
    - with
      - bone necrosis L97.924
      - exposed fat layer L97.922
      - muscle necrosis L97.923
      - skin breakdown only L97.921
  - leprous A30.1
  - lower leg NOS L97.909
    - with
      - bone necrosis L97.904
      - exposed fat layer L97.902
      - muscle necrosis L97.903
      - skin breakdown only L97.901
    - left L97.929
      - with
        - bone necrosis L97.924
        - exposed fat layer L97.922
        - muscle necrosis L97.923
        - skin breakdown only L97.921
    - right L97.919
      - with
        - bone necrosis L97.914
        - exposed fat layer L97.912
        - muscle necrosis L97.913
        - skin breakdown only L97.911
    - specified site NEC L97.809
      - with
        - bone necrosis L97.804
        - exposed fat layer L97.802
        - muscle necrosis L97.803
        - skin breakdown only L97.801
      - left L97.829
        - with
          - bone necrosis L97.824
          - exposed fat layer L97.822
          - muscle necrosis L97.823
          - skin breakdown only L97.821
      - right L97.819
        - with
          - bone necrosis L97.814
          - exposed fat layer L97.812
          - muscle necrosis L97.813
          - skin breakdown only L97.811
  - midfoot L97.409
    - with
      - bone necrosis L97.404
      - exposed fat layer L97.402
      - muscle necrosis L97.403
      - skin breakdown only L97.401
    - left L97.429
      - with
        - bone necrosis L97.424
        - exposed fat layer L97.422
        - muscle necrosis L97.423
        - skin breakdown only L97.421

Ulcer, ulcerated, ulcerating, ulceration, ulcerative *— continued*
- lower limb *— continued*
  - midfoot *— continued*
    - right L97.419
      - with
        - bone necrosis L97.414
        - exposed fat layer L97.412
        - muscle necrosis L97.413
        - skin breakdown only L97.411
  - right L97.919
    - with
      - bone necrosis L97.914
      - exposed fat layer L97.912
      - muscle necrosis L97.913
      - skin breakdown only L97.911
  - syphilitic A52.19
  - thigh L97.109
    - with
      - bone necrosis L97.104
      - exposed fat layer L97.102
      - muscle necrosis L97.103
      - skin breakdown only L97.101
    - left L97.129
      - with
        - bone necrosis L97.124
        - exposed fat layer L97.122
        - muscle necrosis L97.123
        - skin breakdown only L97.121
    - right L97.119
      - with
        - bone necrosis L97.114
        - exposed fat layer L97.112
        - muscle necrosis L97.113
        - skin breakdown only L97.111
  - toe L97.509
    - with
      - bone necrosis L97.504
      - exposed fat layer L97.502
      - muscle necrosis L97.503
      - skin breakdown only L97.501
    - left L97.529
      - with
        - bone necrosis L97.524
        - exposed fat layer L97.522
        - muscle necrosis L97.523
        - skin breakdown only L97.521
    - right L97.519
      - with
        - bone necrosis L97.514
        - exposed fat layer L97.512
        - muscle necrosis L97.513
        - skin breakdown only L97.511
  - varicose — *see* Varix, leg, with, ulcer
- luetic — *see* Ulcer, syphilitic
- lung J98.4
  - tuberculous — *see* Tuberculosis, pulmonary
- malignant — *see* Neoplasm, malignant, by site
- marginal NEC — *see* Ulcer, gastrojejunal
- meatus (urinarius) N34.2
- Meckel's diverticulum Q43.0
  - malignant — *see* Table of Neoplasms, small intestine, malignant
- Meleney's (chronic undermining) — *see* Ulcer, skin
- Mooren's (cornea) — *see* Ulcer, cornea, Mooren's
- mycobacterial (skin) A31.1
- nasopharynx J39.2
- neck, uterus N86
- neurogenic NEC — *see* Ulcer, skin
- nose, nasal (passage) (infective) (septum) J34.0
  - skin — *see* Ulcer, skin
  - spirochetal A69.8
  - varicose (bleeding) I86.8
- oral mucosa (traumatic) K12.1
- palate (soft) K12.1
- penis (chronic) N48.5
- peptic (site unspecified) K27.9
  - with
    - hemorrhage K27.4
      - and perforation K27.6
    - perforation K27.5
  - acute K27.3
    - with
      - hemorrhage K27.0
        - and perforation K27.2
      - perforation K27.1
  - chronic K27.7

Ulcer, ulcerated, ulcerating, ulceration, ulcerative — *continued*
- peptic — *continued*
  - chronic — *continued*
    - with
      - hemorrhage K27.4
        - and perforation K27.6
      - perforation K27.5
  - esophagus K22.1Ø
    - with bleeding K22.11
  - newborn P78.82
- perforating K27.5
  - skin — *see* Ulcer, skin
- peritonsillar J35.8
- phagedenic (tropical) — *see* Ulcer, skin
- pharynx J39.2
- phlebitis — *see* Phlebitis
- plaster — *see* Ulcer, pressure, by site
- popliteal space — *see* Ulcer, lower limb
- postpyloric — *see* Ulcer, duodenum
- prepuce N47.7
- prepyloric — *see* Ulcer, stomach
- pressure (pressure area) L89.9- ☑
  - ankle L89.5- ☑
  - back L89.1- ☑
  - buttock L89.3- ☑
  - coccyx L89.15- ☑
  - contiguous site of back, buttock, hip L89.4- ☑
  - elbow L89.Ø- ☑
  - face L89.81- ☑
  - head L89.81- ☑
  - heel L89.6- ☑
  - hip L89.2- ☑
  - sacral region (tailbone) L89.15- ☑
  - specified site NEC L89.89- ☑
  - stage 1 (healing) (pre-ulcer skin changes limited to persistent focal edema)
    - ankle L89.5- ☑
    - back L89.1- ☑
    - buttock L89.3- ☑
    - coccyx L89.15- ☑
    - contiguous site of back, buttock, hip L89.4- ☑
    - elbow L89.Ø- ☑
    - face L89.81- ☑
    - head L89.81- ☑
    - heel L89.6- ☑
    - hip L89.2- ☑
    - sacral region (tailbone) L89.15- ☑
    - specified site NEC L89.89- ☑
  - stage 2 (healing) (abrasion, blister, partial thickness skin loss involving epidermis and/or dermis)
    - ankle L89.5- ☑
    - back L89.1- ☑
    - buttock L89.3- ☑
    - coccyx L89.15- ☑
    - contiguous site of back, buttock, hip L89.4- ☑
    - elbow L89.Ø- ☑
    - face L89.81- ☑
    - head L89.81- ☑
    - heel L89.6- ☑
    - hip L89.2- ☑
    - sacral region (tailbone) L89.15- ☑
    - specified site NEC L89.89- ☑
  - stage 3 (healing) (full thickness skin loss involving damage or necrosis of subcutaneous tissue)
    - ankle L89.5- ☑
    - back L89.1- ☑
    - buttock L89.3- ☑
    - coccyx L89.15- ☑
    - contiguous site of back, buttock, hip L89.4- ☑
    - elbow L89.Ø- ☑
    - face L89.81- ☑
    - head L89.81- ☑
    - heel L89.6- ☑
    - hip L89.2- ☑
    - sacral region (tailbone) L89.15- ☑
    - specified site NEC L89.89- ☑
  - stage 4 (healing) (necrosis of soft tissues through to underlying muscle, tendon, or bone)
    - ankle L89.5- ☑
    - back L89.1- ☑
    - buttock L89.3- ☑
    - coccyx L89.15- ☑
    - contiguous site of back, buttock, hip L89.4- ☑
    - elbow L89.Ø- ☑
    - face L89.81- ☑

Ulcer, ulcerated, ulcerating, ulceration, ulcerative — *continued*
- pressure — *continued*
  - stage 4 — *continued*
    - head L89.81- ☑
    - heel L89.6- ☑
    - hip L89.2- ☑
    - sacral region (tailbone) L89.15- ☑
    - specified site NEC L89.89- ☑
  - unspecified stage
    - ankle L89.5- ☑
    - back L89.1- ☑
    - buttock L89.3- ☑
    - coccyx L89.15- ☑
    - contiguous site of back, buttock, hip L89.4- ☑
    - elbow L89.Ø- ☑
    - face L89.81- ☑
    - head L89.81- ☑
    - heel L89.6- ☑
    - hip L89.2- ☑
    - sacral region (tailbone) L89.15- ☑
    - specified site NEC L89.89- ☑
  - unstageable
    - ankle L89.5- ☑
    - back L89.1- ☑
    - buttock L89.3- ☑
    - coccyx L89.15- ☑
    - contiguous site of back, buttock, hip L89.4- ☑
    - elbow L89.Ø- ☑
    - face L89.81- ☑
    - head L89.81- ☑
    - heel L89.6- ☑
    - hip L89.2- ☑
    - sacral region (tailbone) L89.15- ☑
    - specified site NEC L89.89- ☑
- primary of intestine K63.3
  - with perforation K63.1
- prostate N41.9
- pyloric — *see* Ulcer, stomach
- rectosigmoid K63.3
  - with perforation K63.1
- rectum (sphincter) (solitary) K62.6
  - stercoraceous, stercoral K62.6
- retina — *see* Inflammation, chorioretinal
- rodent (*see also* Neoplasm, skin, malignant)
- sclera — *see* Scleritis
- scrofulous (tuberculous) A18.2
- scrotum N5Ø.8
  - tuberculous A18.15
  - varicose I86.1
- seminal vesicle N5Ø.8
- sigmoid — *see* Ulcer, intestine
- skin (atrophic) (chronic) (neurogenic) (non-healing) (perforating) (pyogenic) (trophic) (tropical) L98.499
  - with gangrene — *see* Gangrene
  - amebic AØ6.7
  - back — *see* Ulcer, back
  - buttock — *see* Ulcer, buttock
  - decubitus — *see* Ulcer, pressure
  - lower limb — *see* Ulcer, lower limb
  - mycobacterial A31.1
  - specified site NEC L98.499
    - with
      - bone necrosis L98.494
      - exposed fat layer L98.492
      - muscle necrosis L98.493
      - skin breakdown only L98.491
  - tuberculous (primary) A18.4
  - varicose — *see* Ulcer, varicose
- sloughing — *see* Ulcer, skin
- solitary, anus or rectum (sphincter) K62.6
- sore throat JØ2.9
  - streptococcal JØ2.Ø
- spermatic cord N5Ø.8
- spine (tuberculous) A18.Ø1
- stasis (venous) — *see* Varix, leg, with, ulcer
  - without varicose veins I87.2
- stercoraceous, stercoral K63.3
  - with perforation K63.1
  - anus or rectum K62.6
- stoma, stomal — *see* Ulcer, gastrojejunal
- stomach (eroded) (peptic) (round) K25.9
  - with
    - hemorrhage K25.4
      - and perforation K25.6
    - perforation K25.5

Ulcer, ulcerated, ulcerating, ulceration, ulcerative — *continued*
- stomach — *continued*
  - acute K25.3
    - with
      - hemorrhage K25.Ø
        - and perforation K25.2
      - perforation K25.1
  - chronic K25.7
    - with
      - hemorrhage K25.4
        - and perforation K25.6
      - perforation K25.5
- stomal — *see* Ulcer, gastrojejunal
- stomatitis K12.1
- stress — *see* Ulcer, peptic
- strumous (tuberculous) A18.2
- submucosal, bladder — *see* Cystitis, interstitial
- syphilitic (any site) (early) (secondary) A51.39
  - late A52.79
  - perforating A52.79
    - foot A52.11
- testis N5Ø.8
- thigh — *see* Ulcer, lower limb
- throat J39.2
  - diphtheritic A36.Ø
- toe — *see* Ulcer, lower limb
- tongue (traumatic) K14.Ø
- tonsil J35.8
  - diphtheritic A36.Ø
- trachea J39.8
- trophic — *see* Ulcer, skin
- tropical — *see* Ulcer, skin
- tuberculous — *see* Tuberculosis, ulcer
- tunica vaginalis N5Ø.8
- turbinate J34.89
- typhoid (perforating) — *see* Typhoid
- unspecified site — *see* Ulcer, skin
- urethra (meatus) — *see* Urethritis
- uterus N85.8
  - cervix N86
    - with cervicitis N72
  - neck N86
    - with cervicitis N72
- vagina N76.5
  - in Behçet's disease M35.2 [N77.Ø]
  - pessary N89.8
- valve, heart I33.Ø
- varicose (lower limb, any part) (*see also* Varix, leg, with, ulcer)
  - broad ligament I86.2
  - esophagus — *see* Varix, esophagus
  - inflamed or infected — *see* Varix, leg, with ulcer, with inflammation
  - nasal septum I86.8
  - perineum I86.3
  - scrotum I86.1
  - specified site NEC I86.8
  - sublingual I86.Ø
  - vulva I86.3
- vas deferens N5Ø.8
- vulva (acute) (infectional) N76.6
  - in (due to)
    - Behçet's disease M35.2 [N77.Ø]
    - herpesviral (herpes simplex) infection A6Ø.Ø4
    - tuberculosis A18.18
- vulvobuccal, recurring N76.6
- X-ray L58.1
- yaws A66.4

Ulcerosa scarlatina A38.8

Ulcus (*see also* Ulcer)
- cutis tuberculosum A18.4
- duodeni — *see* Ulcer, duodenum
- durum (syphilitic) A51.Ø
  - extragenital A51.2
- gastrojejunale — *see* Ulcer, gastrojejunal
- hypostaticum — *see* Ulcer, varicose
- molle (cutis) (skin) A57
- serpens corneae — *see* Ulcer, cornea, central
- ventriculi — *see* Ulcer, stomach

Ulegyria QØ4.8

Ulerythema
- ophryogenes, congenital Q84.2
- sycosiforme L73.8

Ullrich (-Bonnevie)(-Turner) **syndrome** Q87.1

Ullrich-Feichtiger syndrome Q87.Ø

Ulnar — *see* condition

Ulorrhagia, ulorrhea KØ6.8

- **Umbilicus, umbilical** — *see* condition
- **Unacceptable**
  - contours of tooth K08.54
  - morphology of tooth K08.54
- **Unavailability** (of)
  - bed at medical facility Z75.1
  - health service-related agencies Z75.4
  - medical facilities (at) Z75.3
    - due to
      - investigation by social service agency Z75.2
      - lack of services at home Z75.0
      - remoteness from facility Z75.3
      - waiting list Z75.1
    - home Z75.0
    - outpatient clinic Z75.3
  - schooling Z55.1
  - social service agencies Z75.4
- **Uncinaria americana infestation** B76.1
- **Uncinariasis** B76.9
- **Uncongenial work** Z56.5
- **Unconscious** (ness) — *see* Coma
- **Under observation** — *see* Observation
- **Underachievement in school** Z55.3
- **Underdevelopment** (*see also* Undeveloped)
  - nose Q30.1
  - sexual E30.0
- **Underdosing** (*see also* Table of Drugs and Chemicals, categories T36-T50, with final character 6) Z91.14
  - intentional NEC Z91.128
    - due to financial hardship of patient Z91.120
  - unintentional NEC Z91.138
    - due to patient's age related debility Z91.130
- **Underfeeding, newborn** P92.3
- **Underfill, endodontic** M27.53
- **Underimmunization status** Z28.3
- **Undernourishment** — *see* Malnutrition
- **Undernutrition** — *see* Malnutrition
- **Underweight** R63.6
  - for gestational age — *see* Light for dates
- **Underwood's disease** P83.0
- **Undescended** (*see also* Malposition, congenital)
  - cecum Q43.3
  - colon Q43.3
  - testicle — *see* Cryptorchid
- **Undeveloped, undevelopment** (*see also* Hypoplasia)
  - brain (congenital) Q02
  - cerebral (congenital) Q02
  - heart Q24.8
  - lung Q33.6
  - testis E29.1
  - uterus E30.0
- **Undiagnosed** (disease) R69
- **Undulant fever** — *see* Brucellosis
- **Unemployment, anxiety concerning** Z56.0
  - threatened Z56.2
- **Unequal length** (acquired) (limb) (*see also* Deformity, limb, unequal length)
  - leg (*see also* Deformity, limb, unequal length)
    - congenital Q72.9- ☑
- **Unextracted dental root** K08.3
- **Unguis incarnatus** L60.0
- **Unhappiness** R45.2
- **Unicornate uterus** Q51.4
- **Unilateral** (*see also* condition)
  - development, breast N64.89
  - organ or site, congenital NEC — *see* Agenesis, by site
- **Unilocular heart** Q20.8
- **Union, abnormal** (*see also* Fusion)
  - larynx and trachea Q34.8
- **Universal mesentery** Q43.3
- **Unrepairable overhanging of dental restorative materials** K08.52
- **Unsatisfactory**
  - restoration of tooth K08.50
    - specified NEC K08.59
  - sample of cytologic smear
    - anus R85.615
    - cervix R87.615
    - vagina R87.625
  - surroundings Z59.1
    - work Z56.5
- **Unsoundness of mind** — *see* Psychosis
- **Unstable**
  - back NEC — *see* Instability, joint, spine
  - hip (congenital) Q65.6
    - acquired — *see* Derangement, joint, specified type NEC, hip
- **Unstable** — *continued*
  - joint — *see* Instability, joint
    - secondary to removal of joint prosthesis M96.89
  - lie (mother) O32.0 ☑
  - lumbosacral joint (congenital)
    - acquired — *see* subcategory M53.2 ☑
  - sacroiliac — *see* subcategory M53.2 ☑
  - spine NEC — *see* Instability, joint, spine
- **Unsteadiness on feet** R26.81
- **Untruthfulness, child problem** F91.8
- **Unverricht** (-Lundborg) **disease or epilepsy** — *see* Epilepsy, generalized, idiopathic
- **Unwanted pregnancy** Z64.0
- **Upbringing, institutional** Z62.22
  - away from parents NEC Z62.29
  - in care of non-parental family member Z62.21
  - in foster care Z62.21
  - in orphanage or group home Z62.22
  - in welfare custody Z62.21
- **Upper respiratory** — *see* condition
- **Upset**
  - gastric K30
  - gastrointestinal K30
    - psychogenic F45.8
  - intestinal (large) (small) K59.9
    - psychogenic F45.8
  - menstruation N93.9
  - mental F48.9
  - stomach K30
    - psychogenic F45.8
- **Urachus** (*see also* condition)
  - patent or persistent Q64.4
- **Urbach-Oppenheim disease** (necrobiosis lipoidica diabeticorum) — *see* E08-E13 with .620
- **Urbach's lipoid proteinosis** E78.89
- **Urbach-Wiethe disease** E78.89
- **Urban yellow fever** A95.1
- **Urea**
  - blood, high — *see* Uremia
  - cycle metabolism disorder — *see* Disorder, urea cycle metabolism
- **Uremia, uremic** N19
  - with
    - ectopic or molar pregnancy O08.4
    - polyneuropathy N18.9 [G63]
  - chronic (*see also* Disease, kidney, chronic) N18.9
    - due to hypertension — *see* Hypertensive, kidney
  - complicating
    - ectopic or molar pregnancy O08.4
  - congenital P96.0
  - extrarenal R39.2
  - following ectopic or molar pregnancy O08.4
  - newborn P96.0
  - prerenal R39.2
- **Ureter, ureteral** — *see* condition
- **Ureteralgia** N23
- **Ureterectasis** — *see* Hydroureter
- **Ureteritis** N28.89
  - cystica N28.86
  - due to calculus N20.1
    - with calculus, kidney N20.2
      - with hydronephrosis N13.2
  - gonococcal (acute) (chronic) A54.21
  - nonspecific N28.89
- **Ureterocele** N28.89
  - congenital (orthotopic) Q62.31
    - ectopic Q62.32
- **Ureterolith, ureterolithiasis** — *see* Calculus, ureter
- **Ureterostomy**
  - attention to Z43.6
  - status Z93.6
- **Urethra, urethral** — *see* condition
- **Urethralgia** R39.89
- **Urethritis** (anterior) (posterior) N34.2
  - calculous N21.1
  - candidal B37.41
  - chlamydial A56.01
  - diplococcal (gonococcal) A54.01
    - with abscess (accessory gland) (periurethral) A54.1
  - gonococcal A54.01
    - with abscess (accessory gland) (periurethral) A54.1
  - nongonococcal N34.1
    - Reiter's — *see* Reiter's disease
  - nonspecific N34.1
  - nonvenereal N34.1
  - postmenopausal N34.2
  - puerperal O86.22
- **Urethritis** — *continued*
  - Reiter's — *see* Reiter's disease
  - specified NEC N34.2
  - trichomonal or due to Trichomonas (vaginalis) A59.03
- **Urethrocele** N81.0
  - with
    - cystocele — *see* Cystocele
    - prolapse of uterus — *see* Prolapse, uterus
- **Urethrolithiasis** (with colic or infection) N21.1
- **Urethrorectal** — *see* condition
- **Urethrorrhagia** N36.8
- **Urethrorrhea** R36.9
- **Urethrostomy**
  - attention to Z43.6
  - status Z93.6
- **Urethrotrigonitis** — *see* Trigonitis
- **Urethrovaginal** — *see* condition
- **Urgency**
  - fecal R15.2
  - hypertensive — *see* Hypertension
  - urinary N39.41
- **Urhidrosis, uridrosis** L74.8
- **Uric acid in blood** (increased) E79.0
- **Uricacidemia** (asymptomatic) E79.0
- **Uricemia** (asymptomatic) E79.0
- **Uricosuria** R82.99
- **Urinary** — *see* condition
- **Urination**
  - frequent R35.0
  - painful R30.9
- **Urine**
  - blood in — *see* Hematuria
  - discharge, excessive R35.8
  - enuresis, nonorganic origin F98.0
  - extravasation R39.0
  - frequency R35.0
  - incontinence R32
    - nonorganic origin F98.0
  - intermittent stream R39.19
  - pus in N39.0
  - retention or stasis R33.9
    - organic R33.8
      - drug-induced R33.0
    - psychogenic F45.8
  - secretion
    - deficient R34
    - excessive R35.8
    - frequency R35.0
  - stream
    - intermittent R39.19
    - slowing R39.19
    - splitting R39.13
    - weak R39.12
- **Urinemia** — *see* Uremia
- **Urinoma, urethra** N36.8
- **Uroarthritis, infectious** (Reiter's) — *see* Reiter's disease
- **Urodialysis** R34
- **Urolithiasis** — *see* Calculus, urinary
- **Uronephrosis** — *see* Hydronephrosis
- **Uropathy** N39.9
  - obstructive N13.9
    - specified NEC N13.8
  - reflux N13.9
    - specified NEC N13.8
  - vesicoureteral reflux-associated — *see* Reflux, vesicoureteral
- **Urosepsis** — *code to* condition
- **Urticaria** L50.9
  - with angioneurotic edema T78.3 ☑
    - hereditary D84.1
  - allergic L50.0
  - cholinergic L50.5
  - chronic L50.8
  - cold, familial L50.2
  - contact L50.6
  - dermatographic L50.3
  - due to
    - cold or heat L50.2
    - drugs L50.0
    - food L50.0
    - inhalants L50.0
    - plants L50.6
    - serum (*see also* Reaction, serum) T80.69 ☑
  - factitial L50.3
  - giant T78.3 ☑
    - hereditary D84.1
  - gigantea T78.3 ☑

- **Urticaria** — *continued*
  - idiopathic L5Ø.1
  - larynx T78.3 ☑
    - hereditary D84.1
  - neonatorum P83.8
  - nonallergic L5Ø.1
  - papulosa (Hebra) L28.2
  - pigmentosa Q82.2
  - recurrent periodic L5Ø.8
  - serum (*see also* Reaction, serum) T8Ø.69 ☑
  - solar L56.3
  - specified type NEC L5Ø.8
  - thermal (cold) (heat) L5Ø.2
  - vibratory L5Ø.4
  - xanthelasmoidea Q82.2
- **Use** (of)
  - alcohol F1Ø.99
    - with sleep disorder F1Ø.982
    - harmful — *see* Abuse, alcohol
  - amphetamines — *see* Use, stimulant NEC
  - caffeine — *see* Use, stimulant NEC
  - cannabis F12.9Ø
    - with
      - anxiety disorder F12.98Ø
      - intoxication F12.929
        - with
          - delirium F12.921
          - perceptual disturbance F12.922
        - uncomplicated F12.92Ø
      - other specified disorder F12.988
      - psychosis F12.959
        - delusions F12.95Ø
        - hallucinations F12.951
      - unspecified disorder F12.99
  - cocaine F14.9Ø
    - with
      - anxiety disorder F14.98Ø
      - intoxication F14.929
        - with
          - delirium F14.921
          - perceptual disturbance F14.922
        - uncomplicated F14.92Ø
      - other specified disorder F14.988
      - psychosis F14.959
        - delusions F14.95Ø
        - hallucinations F14.951
      - sexual dysfunction F14.981
      - sleep disorder F14.982
      - unspecified disorder F14.99
    - harmful — *see* Abuse, drug, cocaine
  - drug(s) NEC F19.9Ø
    - with sleep disorder F19.982
    - harmful — *see* Abuse, drug, by type
  - hallucinogen NEC F16.9Ø
    - with
      - anxiety disorder F16.98Ø
      - intoxication F16.929
        - with
          - delirium F16.921
        - uncomplicated F16.92Ø
      - mood disorder F16.94
      - other specified disorder F16.988
      - perception disorder (flashbacks) F16.983
      - psychosis F16.959
        - delusions F16.95Ø
        - hallucinations F16.951
      - unspecified disorder F16.99
    - harmful — *see* Abuse, drug, hallucinogen NEC
  - inhalants F18.9Ø
    - with
      - anxiety disorder F18.98Ø
      - intoxication F18.929
        - with delirium F18.921
        - uncomplicated F18.92Ø
      - mood disorder F18.94
      - other specified disorder F18.988
      - persisting dementia F18.97
      - psychosis F18.959
        - delusions F18.95Ø
        - hallucinations F18.951
      - unspecified disorder F18.99
    - harmful — *see* Abuse, drug, inhalant
  - methadone F11.2Ø
  - nonprescribed drugs F19.9Ø
    - harmful — *see* Abuse, non-psychoactive substance
  - opioid F11.9Ø
- **Use** — *continued*
  - opioid — *continued*
    - with
      - disorder F11.99
        - mood F11.94
        - sleep F11.982
        - specified type NEC F11.988
      - intoxication F11.929
        - with
          - delirium F11.921
          - perceptual disturbance F11.922
        - uncomplicated F11.92Ø
      - withdrawal F11.93
    - harmful — *see* Abuse, drug, opioid
  - patent medicines F19.9Ø
    - harmful — *see* Abuse, non-psychoactive substance
  - psychoactive drug NEC F19.9Ø
    - with
      - anxiety disorder F19.98Ø
      - intoxication F19.929
        - with
          - delirium F19.921
          - perceptual disturbance F19.922
        - uncomplicated F19.92Ø
      - mood disorder F19.94
      - other specified disorder F19.988
      - persisting
        - amnestic disorder F19.96
        - dementia F19.97
      - psychosis F19.959
        - delusions F19.95Ø
        - hallucinations F19.951
      - sexual dysfunction F19.981
      - sleep disorder F19.982
      - unspecified disorder F19.99
      - withdrawal F19.939
        - with
          - delirium F19.931
          - perceptual disturbance F19.932
        - uncomplicated F19.93Ø
    - harmful — *see* Abuse, drug NEC, psychoactive NEC
  - sedative, hypnotic, or anxiolytic F13.9Ø
    - with
      - anxiety disorder F13.98Ø
      - intoxication F13.929
        - with
          - delirium F13.921
        - uncomplicated F13.92Ø
      - other specified disorder F13.988
      - persisting
        - amnestic disorder F13.96
        - dementia F13.97
      - psychosis F13.959
        - delusions F13.95Ø
        - hallucinations F13.951
      - sexual dysfunction F13.981
      - sleep disorder F13.982
      - unspecified disorder F13.99
    - harmful — *see* Abuse, drug, sedative, hypnotic, or anxiolytic
  - stimulant NEC F15.9Ø
    - with
      - anxiety disorder F15.98Ø
      - intoxication F15.929
        - with
          - delirium F15.921
          - perceptual disturbance F15.922
        - uncomplicated F15.92Ø
      - mood disorder F15.94
      - other specified disorder F15.988
      - psychosis F15.959
        - delusions F15.95Ø
        - hallucinations F15.951
      - sexual dysfunction F15.981
      - sleep disorder F15.982
      - unspecified disorder F15.99
      - withdrawal F15.93
    - harmful — *see* Abuse, drug, stimulant NEC
  - tobacco Z72.Ø
    - with dependence — *see* Dependence, drug, nicotine
  - volatile solvents (*see also* Use, inhalant) F18.9Ø
    - harmful — *see* Abuse, drug, inhalant
- **Usher-Senear disease or syndrome** L1Ø.4
- **Uta** B55.1
- **Uteromegaly** N85.2
- **Uterovaginal** — *see* condition
- **Uterovesical** — *see* condition
- **Uveal** — *see* condition
- **Uveitis** (anterior) (*see also* Iridocyclitis)
  - acute — *see* Iridocyclitis, acute
  - chronic — *see* Iridocyclitis, chronic
  - due to toxoplasmosis (acquired) B58.Ø9
    - congenital P37.1
  - granulomatous — *see* Iridocyclitis, chronic
  - heterochromic — *see* Cyclitis, Fuchs' heterochromic
  - lens-induced — *see* Iridocyclitis, lens-induced
  - posterior — *see* Chorioretinitis
  - sympathetic H44.13- ☑
  - syphilitic (secondary) A51.43
    - congenital (early) A5Ø.Ø1
    - late A52.71
  - tuberculous A18.54
- **Uveoencephalitis** — *see* Inflammation, chorioretinal
- **Uveokeratitis** — *see* Iridocyclitis
- **Uveoparotitis** D86.89
- **Uvula** — *see* condition
- **Uvulitis** (acute) (catarrhal) (chronic) (membranous) (suppurative) (ulcerative) K12.2

V

- **Vaccination** (prophylactic)
  - complication or reaction — *see* Complications, vaccination
  - delayed Z28.9
  - encounter for Z23
  - not done — *see* Immunization, not done, because (of)
- **Vaccinia** (generalized) (localized) T88.1 ☑
  - without vaccination BØ8.Ø11
  - congenital P35.8
- **Vacuum, in sinus** (accessory) (nasal) J34.89
- **Vagabond, vagabondage** Z59.Ø
- **Vagabond's disease** B85.1
- **Vagina, vaginal** — *see* condition
- **Vaginalitis** (tunica) (testis) N49.1
- **Vaginismus** (reflex) N94.2
  - functional F52.5
  - nonorganic F52.5
  - psychogenic F52.5
  - secondary N94.2
- **Vaginitis** (acute) (circumscribed) (diffuse) (emphysematous) (nonvenereal) (ulcerative) N76.Ø
  - with ectopic or molar pregnancy OØ8.Ø
  - amebic AØ6.82
  - atrophic, postmenopausal N95.2
  - bacterial N76.Ø
  - blennorrhagic (gonococcal) A54.Ø2
  - candidal B37.3
  - chlamydial A56.Ø2
  - chronic N76.1
  - due to Trichomonas (vaginalis) A59.Ø1
  - following ectopic or molar pregnancy OØ8.Ø
  - gonococcal A54.Ø2
    - with abscess (accessory gland) (periurethral) A54.1
  - granuloma A58
  - in (due to)
    - candidiasis B37.3
    - herpesviral (herpes simplex) infection A6Ø.Ø4
    - pinworm infection B8Ø [N77.1]
  - monilial B37.3
  - mycotic (candidal) B37.3
  - postmenopausal atrophic N95.2
  - puerperal (postpartum) O86.13
  - senile (atrophic) N95.2
  - subacute or chronic N76.1
  - syphilitic (early) A51.Ø
    - late A52.76
  - trichomonal A59.Ø1
  - tuberculous A18.18
- **Vaginosis** — *see* Vaginitis
- **Vagotonia** G52.2
- **Vagrancy** Z59.Ø
- **VAIN** — *see* Neoplasia, intraepithelial, vagina
- **Vallecula** — *see* condition
- **Valley fever** B38.Ø
- **Valsuani's disease** — *see* Anemia, obstetric
- **Valve, valvular** (formation) (*see also* condition)
  - cerebral ventricle (communicating) in situ Z98.2
  - cervix, internal os Q51.828
  - congenital NEC — *see* Atresia, by site
  - ureter (pelvic junction) (vesical orifice) Q62.39
  - urethra (congenital) (posterior) Q64.2
- **Valvulitis** (chronic) — *see* Endocarditis
- **Valvulopathy** — *see* Endocarditis

- **Van Bogaert's leukoencephalopathy** (sclerosing) (subacute) A81.1
- **Van Bogaert-Scherer-Epstein disease or syndrome** E75.5
- **Van Buchem's syndrome** M85.2
- **Van Creveld-von Gierke disease** E74.Ø1
- **Van der Hoeve** (-de Kleyn) **syndrome** Q78.Ø
- **Van der Woude's syndrome** Q38.Ø
- **Van Neck's disease or osteochondrosis** M91.Ø
- **Vanishing lung** J44.9
- **Vapor asphyxia or suffocation** T59.9 ☑
  - specified agent — *see* Table of Drugs and Chemicals
- **Variance, lethal ball, prosthetic heart valve** T82.Ø9 ☑
- **Variants, thalassemic** D56.8
- **Variations in hair color** L67.1
- **Varicella** BØ1.9
  - with
    - complications NEC BØ1.89
    - encephalitis BØ1.11
    - encephalomyelitis BØ1.11
    - meningitis BØ1.Ø
    - myelitis BØ1.12
    - pneumonia BØ1.2
  - congenital P35.8
- **Varices** — *see* Varix
- **Varicocele** (scrotum) (thrombosed) I86.1
  - ovary I86.2
  - perineum I86.3
  - spermatic cord (ulcerated) I86.1
- **Varicose**
  - aneurysm (ruptured) I77.Ø
  - dermatitis — *see* Varix, leg, with, inflammation
  - eczema — *see* Varix, leg, with, inflammation
  - phlebitis — *see* Varix, with, inflammation
  - tumor — *see* Varix
  - ulcer (lower limb, any part) (*see also* Varix, leg, with, ulcer)
    - anus (*see also* Hemorrhoids) K64.8
    - esophagus — *see* Varix, esophagus
    - inflamed or infected — *see* Varix, leg, with ulcer, with inflammation
    - nasal septum I86.8
    - perineum I86.3
    - scrotum I86.1
    - specified site NEC I86.8
  - vein — *see* Varix
  - vessel — *see* Varix, leg
- **Varicosis, varicosities, varicosity** — *see* Varix
- **Variola** (major) (minor) BØ3
- **Varioloid** BØ3
- **Varix** (lower limb) (ruptured) I83.9Ø
  - with
    - edema I83.899
    - inflammation I83.1Ø
      - with ulcer (venous) I83.2Ø9
    - pain I83.819
    - specified complication NEC I83.899
    - stasis dermatitis I83.1Ø
      - with ulcer (venous) I83.2Ø9
    - swelling I83.899
    - ulcer I83.ØØ9
      - with inflammation I83.2Ø9
  - aneurysmal I77.Ø
  - asymptomatic I83.9- ☑
  - bladder I86.2
  - broad ligament I86.2
  - complicating
    - childbirth (lower extremity) O87.4
      - anus or rectum O87.2
      - genital (vagina, vulva or perineum) O87.8
    - pregnancy (lower extremity) O22.Ø- ☑
      - anus or rectum O22.4- ☑
      - genital (vagina, vulva or perineum) O22.1- ☑
    - puerperium (lower extremity) O87.4
      - anus or rectum O87.2
      - genital (vagina, vulva, perineum) O87.8
  - congenital (any site) Q27.8
  - esophagus (idiopathic) (primary) (ulcerated) I85.ØØ
    - bleeding I85.Ø1
    - congenital Q27.8
    - in (due to)
      - alcoholic liver disease I85.1Ø
        - bleeding I85.11
      - cirrhosis of liver I85.1Ø
        - bleeding I85.11
      - portal hypertension I85.1Ø
        - bleeding I85.11

Varix — *continued*

  - esophagus — *continued*
    - in — *continued*
      - schistosomiasis I85.1Ø
        - bleeding I85.11
      - toxic liver disease I85.1Ø
        - bleeding I85.11
    - secondary I85.1Ø
      - bleeding I85.11
  - gastric I86.4
  - inflamed or infected I83.1Ø
    - ulcerated I83.2Ø9
  - labia (majora) I86.3
  - leg (asymptomatic) I83.9Ø
    - with
      - edema I83.899
      - inflammation I83.1Ø
        - with ulcer — *see* Varix, leg, with, ulcer, with inflammation by site
      - pain I83.819
      - specified complication NEC I83.899
      - swelling I83.899
      - ulcer I83.ØØ9
        - with inflammation I83.2Ø9
        - ankle I83.ØØ3
          - with inflammation I83.2Ø3
        - calf I83.ØØ2
          - with inflammation I83.2Ø2
        - foot NEC I83.ØØ5
          - with inflammation I83.2Ø5
        - heel I83.ØØ4
          - with inflammation I83.2Ø4
        - lower leg NEC I83.ØØ8
          - with inflammation I83.2Ø8
        - midfoot I83.ØØ4
          - with inflammation I83.2Ø4
        - thigh I83.ØØ1
          - with inflammation I83.2Ø1
    - bilateral (asymptomatic) I83.93
      - with
        - edema I83.893
        - pain I83.813
        - specified complication NEC I83.893
        - swelling I83.893
        - ulcer I83.ØØ9
          - with inflammation I83.2Ø9
    - left (asymptomatic) I83.92
      - with
        - edema I83.892
        - inflammation I83.12
          - with ulcer — *see* Varix, leg, with, ulcer, with inflammation by site
        - pain I83.812
        - specified complication NEC I83.892
        - swelling I83.892
        - ulcer I83.Ø29
          - with inflammation I83.229
          - ankle I83.Ø23
            - with inflammation I83.223
          - calf I83.Ø22
            - with inflammation I83.222
          - foot NEC I83.Ø25
            - with inflammation I83.225
          - heel I83.Ø24
            - with inflammation I83.224
          - lower leg NEC I83.Ø28
            - with inflammation I83.228
          - midfoot I83.Ø24
            - with inflammation I83.224
          - thigh I83.Ø21
            - with inflammation I83.221
    - right (asymptomatic) I83.91
      - with
        - edema I83.891
        - inflammation I83.11
          - with ulcer — *see* Varix, leg, with, ulcer, with inflammation by site
        - pain I83.811
        - specified complication NEC I83.891
        - swelling I83.891
        - ulcer I83.Ø19
          - with inflammation I83.219
          - ankle I83.Ø13
            - with inflammation I83.213
          - calf I83.Ø12
            - with inflammation I83.212
          - foot NEC I83.Ø15
            - with inflammation I83.215

Varix — *continued*

  - leg — *continued*
    - right — *continued*
      - with — *continued*
        - ulcer — *continued*
          - heel I83.Ø14
            - with inflammation I83.214
          - lower leg NEC I83.Ø18
            - with inflammation I83.218
          - midfoot I83.Ø14
            - with inflammation I83.214
          - thigh I83.Ø11
            - with inflammation I83.211
  - nasal septum I86.8
  - orbit I86.8
    - congenital Q27.8
  - ovary I86.2
  - papillary I78.1
  - pelvis I86.2
  - perineum I86.3
  - pharynx I86.8
  - placenta O43.89- ☑
  - renal papilla I86.8
  - retina H35.Ø9
  - scrotum (ulcerated) I86.1
  - sigmoid colon I86.8
  - specified site NEC I86.8
  - spinal (cord) (vessels) I86.8
  - spleen, splenic (vein) (with phlebolith) I86.8
  - stomach I86.4
  - sublingual I86.Ø
  - ulcerated I83.ØØ9
    - inflamed or infected I83.2Ø9
  - uterine ligament I86.2
  - vagina I86.8
  - vocal cord I86.8
  - vulva I86.3
- **Vas deferens** — *see* condition
- **Vas deferentitis** N49.1
- **Vasa previa** O69.4 ☑
  - hemorrhage from, affecting newborn P5Ø.Ø
- **Vascular** (*see also* condition)
  - loop on optic papilla Q14.2
  - spasm I73.9
  - spider I78.1
- **Vascularization, cornea** — *see* Neovascularization, cornea
- **Vasculitis** I77.6
  - allergic D69.Ø
  - cryoglobulinemic D89.1
  - disseminated I77.6
  - hypocomplementemic M31.8
  - kidney I77.89
  - livedoid L95.Ø
  - nodular L95.8
  - retina H35.Ø6- ☑
  - rheumatic — *see* Fever, rheumatic
  - rheumatoid — *see* Rheumatoid, vasculitis
  - skin (limited to) L95.9
    - specified NEC L95.8
- **Vasculopathy, necrotizing** M31.9
  - cardiac allograft T86.29Ø
  - specified NEC M31.8
- **Vasitis** (nodosa) N49.1
  - tuberculous A18.15
- **Vasodilation** I73.9
- **Vasomotor** — *see* condition
- **Vasoplasty, after previous sterilization** Z31.Ø
  - aftercare Z31.42
- **Vasospasm** (vasoconstriction) I73.9
  - cerebral (cerebrovascular) (artery) I67.848
    - reversible I67.841
  - coronary I2Ø.1
  - nerve
    - arm — *see* Mononeuropathy, upper limb
    - brachial plexus G54.Ø
    - cervical plexus G54.2
    - leg — *see* Mononeuropathy, lower limb
  - peripheral NOS I73.9
  - retina (artery) — *see* Occlusion, artery, retina
- **Vasospastic** — *see* condition
- **Vasovagal attack** (paroxysmal) R55
  - psychogenic F45.8
- **VATER syndrome** Q87.2
- **Vater's ampulla** — *see* condition
- **Vegetation, vegetative**
  - adenoid (nasal fossa) J35.8
  - endocarditis (acute) (any valve) (subacute) I33.Ø

Vegetation, vegetative — *continued*
  heart (mycotic) (valve) I33.Ø
Veil
  Jackson's Q43.3
Vein, venous — *see* condition
Veldt sore — *see* Ulcer, skin
Velpeau's hernia — *see* Hernia, femoral
Venereal
  bubo A55
  disease A64
  granuloma inguinale A58
  lymphogranuloma (Durand-Nicolas-Favre) A55
Venofibrosis I87.8
Venom, venomous — *see* Table of Drugs and Chemicals, by animal or substance, poisoning
Venous — *see* condition
Ventilator lung, newborn P27.8
Ventral — *see* condition
Ventricle, ventricular (*see also* condition)
  escape I49.3
  inversion Q2Ø.5
Ventriculitis (cerebral) (*see also* Encephalitis) GØ4.9Ø
Ventriculostomy status Z98.2
Vernet's syndrome G52.7
Verneuil's disease (syphilitic bursitis) A52.78
Verruca (due to HPV) (filiformis) (simplex) (viral) (vulgaris) BØ7.9
  acuminata A63.Ø
  necrogenica (primary) (tuberculosa) A18.4
  plana BØ7.8
  plantaris BØ7.Ø
  seborrheica L82.1
    inflamed L82.Ø
  senile (seborrheic) L82.1
    inflamed L82.Ø
  tuberculosa (primary) A18.4
  venereal A63.Ø
Verrucosities — *see* Verruca
Verruga peruana, peruviana A44.1
Version
  with extraction
  cervix — *see* Malposition, uterus
  uterus (postinfectional) (postpartal, old) — *see* Malposition, uterus
Vertebra, vertebral — *see* condition
Vertical talus (congenital) Q66.8Ø
  left foot Q66.82
  right foot Q66.81
Vertigo R42
  auditory — *see* Vertigo, aural
  aural H81.31- ☑
  benign paroxysmal (positional) H81.1- ☑
  central (origin) H81.4- ☑
  cerebral H81.4- ☑
  Dix and Hallpike (epidemic) — *see* Neuronitis, vestibular
  due to infrasound T75.23 ☑
  epidemic A88.1
    Dix and Hallpike — *see* Neuronitis, vestibular
    Pedersen's — *see* Neuronitis, vestibular
    vestibular neuronitis — *see* Neuronitis, vestibular
  hysterical F44.89
  infrasound T75.23 ☑
  labyrinthine — *see* subcategory H81.Ø ☑
  laryngeal RØ5
  malignant positional H81.4- ☑
  Ménière's — *see* subcategory H81.Ø ☑
  menopausal N95.1
  otogenic — *see* Vertigo, aural
  paroxysmal positional, benign — *see* Vertigo, benign paroxysmal
  Pedersen's (epidemic) — *see* Neuronitis, vestibular
  peripheral NEC H81.39- ☑
  positional
    benign paroxysmal — *see* Vertigo, benign paroxysmal
    malignant H81.4- ☑
Very-low-density-lipoprotein-type (VLDL) **hyperlipoproteinemia** E78.1
Vesania — *see* Psychosis
Vesical — *see* condition
Vesicle
  cutaneous R23.8
  seminal — *see* condition
  skin R23.8
Vesicocolic — *see* condition
Vesicoperineal — *see* condition
Vesicorectal — *see* condition
Vesicourethrorectal — *see* condition
Vesicovaginal — *see* condition
Vesicular — *see* condition
Vesiculitis (seminal) N49.Ø
  amebic AØ6.82
  gonorrheal (acute) (chronic) A54.23
  trichomonal A59.Ø9
  tuberculous A18.15
Vestibulitis (ear) (*see also* subcategory) H83.Ø ☑
  nose (external) J34.89
  vulvar N94.81Ø
Vestibulopathy , acute peripheral (recurrent) — *see* Neuronitis, vestibular
Vestige, vestigial (*see also* Persistence)
  branchial Q18.Ø
  structures in vitreous Q14.Ø
Vibration
  adverse effects T75.2Ø ☑
    pneumatic hammer syndrome T75.21 ☑
    specified effect NEC T75.29 ☑
    vasospastic syndrome T75.22 ☑
    vertigo from infrasound T75.23 ☑
  exposure (occupational) Z57.7
  vertigo T75.23 ☑
Vibriosis A28.9
Victim (of)
  crime Z65.4
  disaster Z65.5
  terrorism Z65.4
  torture Z65.4
  war Z65.5
Vidal's disease L28.Ø
Villaret's syndrome G52.7
Villous — *see* condition
VIN — *see* Neoplasia, intraepithelial, vulva
Vincent's infection (angina) (gingivitis) A69.1
  stomatitis NEC A69.1
Vinson-Plummer syndrome D5Ø.1
Violence, physical R45.6
Viosterol deficiency — *see* Deficiency, calciferol
Vipoma — *see* Neoplasm, malignant, by site
Viremia B34.9
Virilism (adrenal) E25.9
  congenital E25.Ø
Virilization (female) (suprarenal) E25.9
  congenital E25.Ø
  isosexual E28.2
Virulent bubo A57
Virus, viral (*see also* condition)
  as cause of disease classified elsewhere B97.89
  cytomegalovirus B25.9
  human immunodeficiency (HIV) — *see* Human, immunodeficiency virus (HIV) disease
  infection — *see* Infection, virus
  specified NEC B34.8
  swine influneza (viruses that normally cause infections in pigs) (*see also* Influenza, due to, identified novel influenza A virus) JØ9.X2
  West Nile (fever) A92.3Ø
    with
      complications NEC A92.39
      cranial nerve disorders A92.32
      encephalitis A92.31
      encephalomyelitis A92.31
      neurologic manifestation NEC A92.32
      optic neuritis A92.32
      polyradiculitis A92.32
Viscera, visceral — *see* condition
Visceroptosis K63.4
Visible peristalsis R19.2
Vision, visual
  binocular, suppression H53.34
  blurred, blurring H53.8
    hysterical F44.6
  defect, defective NEC H54.7
  disorientation (syndrome) H53.8
  disturbance H53.9
    hysterical F44.6
  double H53.2
  examination ZØ1.ØØ
    with abnormal findings ZØ1.Ø1
  field, limitation (defect) — *see* Defect, visual field
  hallucinations R44.1
  halos H53.19
  loss — *see* Loss, vision
Vision, visual — *continued*
  loss — *see* Loss, vision — *continued*
    sudden — *see* Disturbance, vision, subjective, loss, sudden
  low (both eyes) — *see* Low, vision
  perception, simultaneous without fusion H53.33
Vitality, lack or want of R53.83
  newborn P96.89
Vitamin deficiency — *see* Deficiency, vitamin
Vitelline duct, persistent Q43.Ø
Vitiligo L8Ø
  eyelid HØ2.739
    left HØ2.736
      lower HØ2.735
      upper HØ2.734
    right HØ2.733
      lower HØ2.732
      upper HØ2.731
  pinta A67.2
  vulva N9Ø.89
Vitreal corneal syndrome H59.Ø1- ☑
Vitreoretinopathy, proliferative (*see also* Retinopathy, proliferative)
  with retinal detachment — *see* Detachment, retina, traction
Vitreous (*see also* condition)
  touch syndrome — *see* Complication, postprocedural, following cataract surgery
Vocal cord — *see* condition
Vogt-Koyanagi syndrome H2Ø.82- ☑
Vogt's disease or syndrome G8Ø.3
Vogt-Spieimeyer amaurotic idiocy or disease E75.4
Voice
  change R49.9
    specified NEC R49.8
  loss — *see* Aphonia
Volhynian fever A79.Ø
Volkmann's ischemic contracture or paralysis (complicating trauma) T79.6 ☑
Volvulus (bowel) (colon) (duodenum) (intestine) K56.2
  with perforation K56.2
  congenital Q43.8
  fallopian tube — *see* Torsion, fallopian tube
  oviduct — *see* Torsion, fallopian tube
  stomach (due to absence of gastrocolic ligament) K31.89
Vomiting R11.1Ø
  with nausea R11.2
  without nausea R11.11
  asphyxia — *see* Foreign body, by site, causing asphyxia, gastric contents
  bilious (cause unknown) R11.14
    following gastro-intestinal surgery K91.Ø
    in newborn P92.Ø1
  blood — *see* Hematemesis
  causing asphyxia, choking, or suffocation — *see* Foreign body, by site
  cyclical G43.AØ (*following* G43.7)
    with refractory migraine G43.A1 (*following* G43.7)
    without refractory migraine G43.AØ (*following* G43.7)
    intractable G43.A1 (*following* G43.7)
    not intractable G43.AØ (*following* G43.7)
    psychogenic F5Ø.8
  fecal mater R11.13
  following gastrointestinal surgery K91.Ø
    psychogenic F5Ø.8
  functional K31.89
  hysterical F5Ø.8
  nervous F5Ø.8
  neurotic F5Ø.8
  newborn NEC P92.Ø9
    bilious P92.Ø1
  periodic R11.1Ø
    psychogenic F5Ø.8
  projectile R11.12
  psychogenic F5Ø.8
  uremic — *see* Uremia
Vomito negro — *see* Fever, yellow
Von Bezold's abscess — *see* Mastoiditis, acute
Von Economo-Cruchet disease A85.8
Von Eulenburg's disease G71.19
Von Gierke's disease E74.Ø1
Von Hippel (-Lindau) **disease or syndrome** Q85.8
Von Jaksch's anemia or disease D64.89
Von Recklinghausen
  disease (neurofibromatosis) Q85.Ø1

Von Recklinghausen — *continued*
- disease — *continued*
  - bones E21.Ø

Von Schroetter's syndrome I82.89Ø
Von Willebrand (-Jurgens)(-Minot) **disease or syndrome** D68.Ø
Von Zumbusch's disease L4Ø.1
Voyeurism F65.3
Vrolik's disease Q78.Ø
Vulva — *see* condition
Vulvismus N94.2
Vulvitis (acute) (allergic) (atrophic) (hypertrophic) (intertriginous) (senile) N76.2
- with ectopic or molar pregnancy OØ8.Ø
- adhesive, congenital Q52.79
- blennorrhagic (gonococcal) A54.Ø2
- candidal B37.3
- chlamydial A56.Ø2
- due to Haemophilus ducreyi A57
- following ectopic or molar pregnancy OØ8.Ø
- gonococcal A54.Ø2
  - with abscess (accessory gland) (periurethral) A54.1
- herpesviral A6Ø.Ø4
- leukoplakic N9Ø.4
- monilial B37.3
- puerperal (postpartum) O86.19
- subacute or chronic N76.3
- syphilitic (early) A51.Ø
  - late A52.76
- trichomonal A59.Ø1
- tuberculous A18.18

Vulvodynia N94.819
- specified NEC N94.818

Vulvorectal — *see* condition
Vulvovaginitis (acute) — *see* Vaginitis

W

Waiting list, person on Z75.1
- for organ transplant Z76.82
- undergoing social agency investigation Z75.2

Waldenström
- hypergammaglobulinemia D89.Ø
- syndrome or macroglobulinemia C88.Ø

Waldenström-Kjellberg syndrome D5Ø.1
Walking
- difficulty R26.2
  - psychogenic F44.4
- sleep F51.3
  - hysterical F44.89

Wall, abdominal — *see* condition
Wallenberg's disease or syndrome G46.3
Wallgren's disease I87.8
Wandering
- gallbladder, congenital Q44.1
- in diseases classified elsewhere Z91.83
- kidney, congenital Q63.8
- organ or site, congenital NEC — *see* Malposition, congenital, by site
- pacemaker (heart) I49.8
- spleen D73.89

War neurosis F48.8
Wart (due to HPV) (filiform) (infectious) (viral) BØ7.9
- anogenital region (venereal) A63.Ø
- common BØ7.8
- external genital organs (venereal) A63.Ø
- flat BØ7.8
- Hassal-Henle's (of cornea) H18.49
- Peruvian A44.1
- plantar BØ7.Ø
- prosector (tuberculous) A18.4
- seborrheic L82.1
  - inflamed L82.Ø
- senile (seborrheic) L82.1
  - inflamed L82.Ø
- tuberculous A18.4
- venereal A63.Ø

Warthin's tumor — *see* Neoplasm, salivary gland, benign
Wassilieff's disease A27.Ø
Wasting
- disease R64
  - due to malnutrition E41
- extreme (due to malnutrition) E41
- muscle NEC — *see* Atrophy, muscle

Water
- clefts (senile cataract) — *see* Cataract, senile, incipient
- deprivation of T73.1 ☑

Water — *continued*
- intoxication E87.79
- itch B76.9
- lack of T73.1 ☑
- loading E87.7Ø
- on
  - brain — *see* Hydrocephalus
  - chest J94.8
- poisoning E87.79

Waterbrash R12
Waterhouse (-Friderichsen) **syndrome or disease** (meningococcal) A39.1
Water-losing nephritis N25.89
Watermelon stomach K31.819
- with hemorrhage K31.811
- without hemorrhage K31.819

Watsoniasis B66.8
Wax in ear — *see* Impaction, cerumen
Weak, weakening, weakness (generalized) R53.1
- arches (acquired) (*see also* Deformity, limb, flat foot)
- bladder (sphincter) R32
- facial R29.81Ø
  - following
    - cerebrovascular disease I69.992
      - cerebral infarction I69.392
      - intracerebral hemorrhage I69.192
      - nontraumatic intracranial hemorrhage NEC I69.292
      - specified disease NEC I69.892
      - stroke I69.392
      - subarachnoid hemorrhage I69.Ø92
- foot (double) — *see* Weak, arches
- heart, cardiac — *see* Failure, heart
- mind F7Ø
- muscle M62.81
- myocardium — *see* Failure, heart
- newborn P96.89
- pelvic fundus N81.89
- pubocervical tissue N81.82
- rectovaginal tissue N81.83
- senile R54
- urinary stream R39.12
- valvular — *see* Endocarditis

Wear, worn (with normal or routine use)
- articular bearing surface of internal joint prosthesis — *see* Complications, joint prosthesis, mechanical, wear of articular bearing surfaces, by site
- device, implant or graft — *see* Complications, by site, mechanical complication
- tooth, teeth (approximal) (hard tissues) (interproximal) (occlusal) KØ3.Ø

Weather, weathered
- effects of
  - cold T69.9 ☑
    - specified effect NEC T69.8 ☑
  - hot — *see* Heat
- skin L57.8

Weaver's syndrome Q87.3
Web, webbed (congenital)
- duodenal Q43.8
- esophagus Q39.4
- fingers Q7Ø.1- ☑
- larynx (glottic) (subglottic) Q31.Ø
- neck (pterygium colli) Q18.3
- Paterson-Kelly D5Ø.1
- popliteal syndrome Q87.89
- toes Q7Ø.3- ☑

Weber-Christian disease M35.6
Weber-Cockayne syndrome (epidermolysis bullosa) Q81.8
Weber-Gubler syndrome G46.3
Weber-Leyden syndrome G46.3
Weber-Osler syndrome I78.Ø
Weber's paralysis or syndrome G46.3
Wedge-shaped or wedging vertebra — *see* Collapse, vertebra NEC
Wegener's granulomatosis or syndrome M31.3Ø
- with
  - kidney involvement M31.31
  - lung involvement M31.3Ø
    - with kidney involvement M31.31

Wegner's disease A5Ø.Ø2
Weight
- 1ØØØ-2499 grams at birth (low) — *see* Low, birthweight
- 999 grams or less at birth (extremely low) — *see* Low, birthweight, extreme

Weight — *continued*
- gain (abnormal) (excessive) R63.5
  - in pregnancy — *see* Pregnancy, complicated by, excessive weight gain
    - low — *see* Pregnancy, complicated by, insufficient, weight gain
- loss (abnormal) (cause unknown) R63.4

Weightlessness (effect of) T75.82 ☑
Weil (l)-Marchesani syndrome Q87.1
Weil's disease A27.Ø
Weingarten's syndrome J82
Weir Mitchell's disease I73.81
Weiss-Baker syndrome G9Ø.Ø9
Wells' disease L98.3
Wen — *see* Cyst, sebaceous
Wenckebach's block or phenomenon I44.1
Werdnig-Hoffmann syndrome (muscular atrophy) G12.Ø
Werlhof's disease D69.3
Wermer's disease or syndrome E31.21
Werner-His disease A79.Ø
Werner's disease or syndrome E34.8
Wernicke-Korsakoff's syndrome or psychosis (alcoholic) F1Ø.96
- with dependence F1Ø.26
- drug-induced
  - due to drug abuse — *see* Abuse, drug, by type, with amnestic disorder
  - due to drug dependence — *see* Dependence, drug, by type, with amnestic disorder
- nonalcoholic FØ4

Wernicke-Posadas disease B38.9
Wernicke's
- developmental aphasia F8Ø.2
- disease or syndrome E51.2
- encephalopathy E51.2
- polioencephalitis, superior E51.2

West African fever B5Ø.8
Westphal-Strümpell syndrome E83.Ø1
West's syndrome — *see* Epilepsy, spasms
Wet
- feet, tropical (maceration) (syndrome) — *see* Immersion, foot
- lung (syndrome), newborn P22.1

Wharton's duct — *see* condition
Wheal — *see* Urticaria
Wheezing RØ6.2
Whiplash injury S13.4 ☑
Whipple's disease (*see also* subcategory M14.8-) K9Ø.81
Whipworm (disease) (infection) (infestation) B79
Whistling face Q87.Ø
White (*see also* condition)
- kidney, small NØ3.9
- leg, puerperal, postpartum, childbirth O87.1
- mouth B37.Ø
- patches of mouth K13.29
- spot lesions, teeth
  - chewing surface KØ2.51
  - pit and fissure surface KØ2.51
  - smooth surface KØ2.61

Whitehead L7Ø.Ø
Whitlow (*see also* Cellulitis, digit)
- with lymphangitis — *see* Lymphangitis, acute, digit
- herpesviral BØØ.89

Whitmore's disease or fever — *see* Melioidosis
Whooping cough A37.9Ø
- with pneumonia A37.91
  - due to Bordetella
    - bronchiseptica A37.81
    - parapertussis A37.11
    - pertussis A37.Ø1
  - specified organism NEC A37.81
- due to
  - Bordetella
    - bronchiseptica A37.8Ø
      - with pneumonia A37.81
    - parapertussis A37.1Ø
      - with pneumonia A37.11
    - pertussis A37.ØØ
      - with pneumonia A37.Ø1
    - specified NEC A37.8Ø
      - with pneumonia A37.81

Wichman's asthma J38.5
Wide cranial sutures, newborn P96.3
Widening aorta — *see* Ectasia, aorta
- with aneurysm — *see* Aneurysm, aorta

Wilkie's disease or syndrome K55.1

Wound, open — *continued*
finger(s) — *continued*
ring — *continued*
left — *continued*
with damage to nail S61.3Ø5 ☑
right S61.2Ø4 ☑
with damage to nail S61.3Ø4 ☑
flank — *see* Wound, open, abdomen, wall
foot (except toe(s) alone) S91.3Ø- ☑
with amputation — *see* Amputation, traumatic, foot
bite — *see* Bite, foot
laceration — *see* Laceration, foot
puncture — *see* Puncture, foot
toe — *see* Wound, open, toe
forearm S51.8Ø- ☑
with
amputation — *see* Amputation, traumatic, forearm
bite — *see* Bite, forearm
elbow only — *see* Wound, open, elbow
laceration — *see* Laceration, forearm
puncture — *see* Puncture, forearm
forehead — *see* Wound, open, head, specified site NEC
genital organs, external
with amputation — *see* Amputation, traumatic, genital organs
bite — *see* Bite, genital organ
female S31.5Ø2 ☑
vagina S31.4Ø ☑
vulva S31.4Ø ☑
laceration — *see* Laceration, genital organ
male S31.5Ø1 ☑
penis S31.2Ø ☑
scrotum S31.3Ø ☑
testes S31.3Ø ☑
puncture — *see* Puncture, genital organ
globe (eye) — *see* Wound, open, ocular
groin — *see* Wound, open, abdomen, wall
gum — *see* Wound, open, oral cavity
hand S61.4Ø- ☑
with
amputation — *see* Amputation, traumatic, hand
bite — *see* Bite, hand
finger(s) — *see* Wound, open, finger
laceration — *see* Laceration, hand
puncture — *see* Puncture, hand
thumb — *see* Wound, open, thumb
head SØ1.9Ø ☑
bite — *see* Bite, head
cheek — *see* Wound, open, cheek
ear — *see* Wound, open, ear
eyelid — *see* Wound, open, eyelid
laceration — *see* Laceration, head
lip — *see* Wound, open, lip
nose SØ1.2Ø ☑
oral cavity — *see* Wound, open, oral cavity
puncture — *see* Puncture, head
scalp — *see* Wound, open, scalp
specified site NEC SØ1.8Ø ☑
temporomandibular area — *see* Wound, open, cheek
heel — *see* Wound, open, foot
hip S71.ØØ- ☑
with amputation — *see* Amputation, traumatic, hip
bite — *see* Bite, hip
laceration — *see* Laceration, hip
puncture — *see* Puncture, hip
hymen S31.4Ø ☑
bite — *see* Bite, vulva
laceration — *see* Laceration, vagina
puncture — *see* Puncture, vagina
hypochondrium S31.1Ø9 ☑
bite — *see* Bite, hypochondrium
laceration — *see* Laceration, hypochondrium
puncture — *see* Puncture, hypochondrium
hypogastric region S31.1Ø9 ☑
bite — *see* Bite, hypogastric region
laceration — *see* Laceration, hypogastric region
puncture — *see* Puncture, hypogastric region
iliac (region) — *see* Wound, open, inguinal region
inguinal region S31.1Ø9 ☑
bite — *see* Bite, abdomen, wall, lower quadrant
laceration — *see* Laceration, inguinal region

Wound, open — *continued*
inguinal region — *continued*
puncture — *see* Puncture, inguinal region
instep — *see* Wound, open, foot
interscapular region — *see* Wound, open, thorax, back
intraocular — *see* Wound, open, ocular
iris — *see* Wound, open, ocular
jaw — *see* Wound, open, head, specified site NEC
knee S81.ØØ- ☑
bite — *see* Bite, knee
laceration — *see* Laceration, knee
puncture — *see* Puncture, knee
labium (majus) (minus) — *see* Wound, open, vulva
laceration — *see* Laceration, by site
lacrimal duct — *see* Wound, open, eyelid
larynx S11.Ø19 ☑
bite — *see* Bite, larynx
laceration — *see* Laceration, larynx
puncture — *see* Puncture, larynx
left
lower quadrant S31.1Ø4 ☑
with penetration into peritoneal cavity S31.6Ø4 ☑
bite — *see* Bite, abdomen, wall, left, lower quadrant
laceration — *see* Laceration, abdomen, wall, left, lower quadrant
puncture — *see* Puncture, abdomen, wall, left, lower quadrant
upper quadrant S31.1Ø1 ☑
with penetration into peritoneal cavity S31.6Ø1 ☑
bite — *see* Bite, abdomen, wall, left, upper quadrant
laceration — *see* Laceration, abdomen, wall, left, upper quadrant
puncture — *see* Puncture, abdomen, wall, left, upper quadrant
leg (lower) S81.8Ø- ☑
with amputation — *see* Amputation, traumatic, leg
ankle — *see* Wound, open, ankle
bite — *see* Bite, leg
foot — *see* Wound, open, foot
knee — *see* Wound, open, knee
laceration — *see* Laceration, leg
puncture — *see* Puncture, leg
toe — *see* Wound, open, toe
upper — *see* Wound, open, thigh
lip SØ1.5Ø1 ☑
bite — *see* Bite, lip
laceration — *see* Laceration, lip
puncture — *see* Puncture, lip
loin S31.1Ø9 ☑
bite — *see* Bite, abdomen, wall
laceration — *see* Laceration, loin
puncture — *see* Puncture, loin
lower back — *see* Wound, open, back, lower
lumbar region — *see* Wound, open, back, lower
malar region — *see* Wound, open, head, specified site NEC
mammary — *see* Wound, open, breast
mastoid region — *see* Wound, open, head, specified site NEC
mouth — *see* Wound, open, oral cavity
nail
finger — *see* Wound, open, finger, with damage to nail
toe — *see* Wound, open, toe, with damage to nail
nape (neck) — *see* Wound, open, neck
nasal (septum) (sinus) — *see* Wound, open, nose
nasopharynx — *see* Wound, open, head, specified site NEC
neck S11.9Ø ☑
bite — *see* Bite, neck
involving
cervical esophagus S11.2Ø ☑
larynx — *see* Wound, open, larynx
pharynx S11.2Ø ☑
thyroid S11.1Ø ☑
trachea (cervical) S11.Ø29 ☑
bite — *see* Bite, trachea
laceration S11.Ø21 ☑
with foreign body S11.Ø22 ☑
puncture S11.Ø23 ☑
with foreign body S11.Ø24 ☑

Wound, open — *continued*
neck — *continued*
laceration — *see* Laceration, neck
puncture — *see* Puncture, neck
specified site NEC S11.8Ø ☑
specified type NEC S11.89 ☑
nose (septum) (sinus) SØ1.2Ø ☑
with amputation — *see* Amputation, traumatic, nose
bite — *see* Bite, nose
laceration — *see* Laceration, nose
puncture — *see* Puncture, nose
ocular SØ5.9Ø ☑
avulsion (traumatic enucleation) SØ5.7- ☑
eyeball SØ5.6- ☑
with foreign body SØ5.5- ☑
eyelid — *see* Wound, open, eyelid
laceration and rupture SØ5.3- ☑
with prolapse or loss of intraocular tissue SØ5.2- ☑
orbit (penetrating) (with or without foreign body) SØ5.4- ☑
periocular area — *see* Wound, open, eyelid
specified NEC SØ5.8X- ☑
oral cavity SØ1.5Ø2 ☑
bite SØ1.552 ☑
laceration — *see* Laceration, oral cavity
puncture — *see* Puncture, oral cavity
orbit — *see* Wound, open, ocular, orbit
palate — *see* Wound, open, oral cavity
palm — *see* Wound, open, hand
pelvis, pelvic (*see also* Wound, open, back, lower)
girdle — *see* Wound, open, hip
penetrating — *see* Puncture, by site
penis S31.2Ø ☑
with amputation — *see* Amputation, traumatic, penis
bite S31.25 ☑
laceration — *see* Laceration, penis
puncture — *see* Puncture, penis
perineum
bite — *see* Bite, perineum
female S31.5Ø2 ☑
laceration — *see* Laceration, perineum
male S31.5Ø1 ☑
puncture — *see* Puncture, perineum
periocular area (with or without lacrimal passages) — *see* Wound, open, eyelid
periumbilic region S31.1Ø5 ☑
with penetration into peritoneal cavity S31.6Ø5 ☑
bite — *see* Bite, abdomen, wall, periumbilic region
laceration — *see* Laceration, abdomen, wall, periumbilic region
puncture — *see* Puncture, abdomen, wall, periumbilic region
phalanges
finger — *see* Wound, open, finger
toe — *see* Wound, open, toe
pharynx S11.2Ø ☑
pinna — *see* Wound, open, ear
popliteal space — *see* Wound, open, knee
prepuce — *see* Wound, open, penis
pubic region — *see* Wound, open, back, lower
pudendum — *see* Wound, open, genital organs, external
puncture wound — *see* Puncture
rectovaginal septum — *see* Wound, open, vagina
right
lower quadrant S31.1Ø3 ☑
with penetration into peritoneal cavity S31.6Ø3 ☑
bite — *see* Bite, abdomen, wall, right, lower quadrant
laceration — *see* Laceration, abdomen, wall, right, lower quadrant
puncture — *see* Puncture, abdomen, wall, right, lower quadrant
upper quadrant S31.1ØØ ☑
with penetration into peritoneal cavity S31.6ØØ ☑
bite — *see* Bite, abdomen, wall, right, upper quadrant
laceration — *see* Laceration, abdomen, wall, right, upper quadrant
puncture — *see* Puncture, abdomen, wall, right, upper quadrant

- **Wound, open** — *continued*
  - sacral region — *see* Wound, open, back, lower
  - sacroiliac region — *see* Wound, open, back, lower
  - salivary gland — *see* Wound, open, oral cavity
  - scalp S01.00 ☑
    - bite S01.05 ☑
    - laceration — *see* Laceration, scalp
    - puncture — *see* Puncture, scalp
  - scalpel, newborn (birth injury) P15.8
  - scapular region — *see* Wound, open, shoulder
  - sclera — *see* Wound, open, ocular
  - scrotum S31.30 ☑
    - with amputation — *see* Amputation, traumatic, scrotum
    - bite S31.35 ☑
    - laceration — *see* Laceration, scrotum
    - puncture — *see* Puncture, scrotum
  - shin — *see* Wound, open, leg
  - shoulder S41.00- ☑
    - with amputation — *see* Amputation, traumatic, arm
    - bite — *see* Bite, shoulder
    - laceration — *see* Laceration, shoulder
    - puncture — *see* Puncture, shoulder
  - skin NOS T14.8
  - spermatic cord — *see* Wound, open, testis
  - sternal region — *see* Wound, open, thorax, front wall
  - submaxillary region — *see* Wound, open, head, specified site NEC
  - submental region — *see* Wound, open, head, specified site NEC
  - subungual
    - finger(s) — *see* Wound, open, finger
    - toe(s) — *see* Wound, open, toe
  - supraclavicular region — *see* Wound, open, neck, specified site NEC
  - temple, temporal region — *see* Wound, open, head, specified site NEC
  - temporomandibular area — *see* Wound, open, cheek
  - testis S31.30 ☑
    - with amputation — *see* Amputation, traumatic, testes
    - bite S31.35 ☑
    - laceration — *see* Laceration, testis
    - puncture — *see* Puncture, testis
  - thigh S71.10- ☑
    - with amputation — *see* Amputation, traumatic, hip
    - bite — *see* Bite, thigh
    - laceration — *see* Laceration, thigh
    - puncture — *see* Puncture, thigh
  - thorax, thoracic (wall) S21.90 ☑
    - back S21.20- ☑
      - with penetration S21.40 ☑
    - bite — *see* Bite, thorax
    - breast — *see* Wound, open, breast
    - front S21.10- ☑
      - with penetration S21.30 ☑
    - laceration — *see* Laceration, thorax
    - puncture — *see* Puncture, thorax
  - throat — *see* Wound, open, neck
  - thumb S61.009 ☑
    - with
      - amputation — *see* Amputation, traumatic, thumb
      - damage to nail S61.109 ☑
    - bite — *see* Bite, thumb
    - laceration — *see* Laceration, thumb
    - left S61.002 ☑
      - with
        - damage to nail S61.102 ☑
    - puncture — *see* Puncture, thumb
    - right S61.001 ☑
      - with
        - damage to nail S61.101 ☑
  - thyroid (gland) — *see* Wound, open, neck, thyroid
  - toe(s) S91.109 ☑
    - with
      - amputation — *see* Amputation, traumatic, toe
      - damage to nail S91.209 ☑
    - bite — *see* Bite, toe
    - great S91.103 ☑
      - with
        - damage to nail S91.203 ☑
      - left S91.102 ☑

- **Wound, open** — *continued*
  - toe(s) — *continued*
    - great — *continued*
      - left — *continued*
        - with
          - damage to nail S91.202 ☑
      - right S91.101 ☑
        - with
          - damage to nail S91.201 ☑
    - laceration — *see* Laceration, toe
    - lesser S91.106 ☑
      - with
        - damage to nail S91.206 ☑
      - left S91.105 ☑
        - with
          - damage to nail S91.205 ☑
      - right S91.104 ☑
        - with
          - damage to nail S91.204 ☑
    - puncture — *see* Puncture, toe
  - tongue — *see* Wound, open, oral cavity
  - trachea (cervical region) — *see* Wound, open, neck, trachea
  - tunica vaginalis — *see* Wound, open, testis
  - tympanum, tympanic membrane S09.2- ☑
    - laceration — *see* Laceration, ear, drum
    - puncture — *see* Puncture, tympanum
  - umbilical region — *see* Wound, open, abdomen, wall, periumbilic region
  - uvula — *see* Wound, open, oral cavity
  - vagina S31.40 ☑
    - bite S31.45 ☑
    - laceration — *see* Laceration, vagina
    - puncture — *see* Puncture, vagina
  - vitreous (humor) — *see* Wound, open, ocular
  - vocal cord S11.039 ☑
    - bite — *see* Bite, vocal cord
    - laceration S11.031 ☑
      - with foreign body S11.032 ☑
    - puncture S11.033 ☑
      - with foreign body S11.034 ☑
  - vulva S31.40 ☑
    - with amputation — *see* Amputation, traumatic, vulva
    - bite S31.45 ☑
    - laceration — *see* Laceration, vulva
    - puncture — *see* Puncture, vulva
  - wrist S61.50- ☑
    - bite — *see* Bite, wrist
    - laceration — *see* Laceration, wrist
    - puncture — *see* Puncture, wrist
- **Wound, superficial** — *see* Injury (*see also* specified injury type)
- **Wright's syndrome** G54.0
- **Wrist** — *see* condition
- **Wrong drug** (by accident) (given in error) — *see* Table of Drugs and Chemicals, by drug, poisoning
- **Wry neck** — *see* Torticollis
- **Wuchereria** (bancrofti) **infestation** B74.0
- **Wuchereriasis** B74.0
- **Wuchernde Struma Langhans** C73

X

- **Xanthelasma** (eyelid) (palpebrarum) H02.60
  - left H02.66
    - lower H02.65
    - upper H02.64
  - right H02.63
    - lower H02.62
    - upper H02.61
- **Xanthelasmatosis** (essential) E78.2
- **Xanthinuria, hereditary** E79.8
- **Xanthoastrocytoma**
  - specified site — *see* Neoplasm, malignant, by site
  - unspecified site C71.9
- **Xanthofibroma** — *see* Neoplasm, connective tissue, benign
- **Xanthogranuloma** D76.3
- **Xanthoma(s), xanthomatosis** (primary) (familial) (hereditary) E75.5
  - with
    - hyperlipoproteinemia
      - Type I E78.3
      - Type III E78.2
      - Type IV E78.1

- **Xanthoma(s), xanthomatosis** — *continued*
  - with — *continued*
    - hyperlipoproteinemia — *continued*
      - Type V E78.3
  - cerebrotendinous E75.5
  - cutaneotendinous E75.5
  - disseminatum (skin) E78.2
  - eruptive E78.2
  - hypercholesterinemic E78.0
  - hypercholesterolemic E78.0
  - hyperlipidemic E78.5
  - joint E75.5
  - multiple (skin) E78.2
  - tendon (sheath) E75.5
  - tuberosum E78.2
  - tuberous E78.2
  - tubo-eruptive E78.2
  - verrucous, oral mucosa K13.4
- **Xanthosis** R23.8
- **Xenophobia** F40.10
- **Xeroderma** (*see also* Ichthyosis)
  - acquired L85.0
    - eyelid H01.149
      - left H01.146
        - lower H01.145
        - upper H01.144
      - right H01.143
        - lower H01.142
        - upper H01.141
  - pigmentosum Q82.1
  - vitamin A deficiency E50.8
- **Xerophthalmia** (vitamin A deficiency) E50.7
  - unrelated to vitamin A deficiency — *see* Keratoconjunctivitis
- **Xerosis**
  - conjunctiva H11.14- ☑
    - with Bitot's spots (*see also* Pigmentation, conjunctiva)
      - vitamin A deficiency E50.1
    - vitamin A deficiency E50.0
  - cornea H18.89- ☑
    - with ulceration — *see* Ulcer, cornea
      - vitamin A deficiency E50.3
    - vitamin A deficiency E50.2
  - cutis L85.3
  - skin L85.3
- **Xerostomia** K11.7
- **Xiphopagus** Q89.4
- **XO syndrome** Q96.9
- **X-ray** (of)
  - abnormal findings — *see* Abnormal, diagnostic imaging
  - breast (mammogram) (routine) Z12.31
  - chest
    - routine (as part of a general medical examination) Z00.00
      - with abnormal findings Z00.01
  - routine (as part of a general medical examination) Z00.00
    - with abnormal findings Z00.01
- **XXXXY syndrome** Q98.1
- **XXY syndrome** Q98.0

Y

- **Yaba pox** (virus disease) B08.72
- **Yatapoxvirus** B08.70
  - specified NEC B08.79
- **Yawning** R06.89
  - psychogenic F45.8
- **Yaws** A66.9
  - cutaneous, less than five years after infection A66.2
  - bone lesions A66.6
  - butter A66.1
  - chancre A66.0
  - early (cutaneous) (macular) (maculopapular) (micropapular) (papular) A66.2
    - frambeside A66.2
    - skin lesions NEC A66.2
  - eyelid A66.2
  - ganglion A66.6
  - gangosis, gangosa A66.5
  - gumma, gummata A66.4
    - bone A66.6
  - gummatous
    - frambeside A66.4
    - osteitis A66.6
    - periostitis A66.6

Z

ICD-1Ø-CM Neoplasm Table

Note: The list below gives the code number for neoplasms by anatomical site. For each site there are six possible code numbers according to whether the neoplasm in question is malignant, benign, in situ, of uncertain behavior, or of unspecified nature. The description of the neoplasm will often indicate which of the six columns is appropriate; e.g., malignant melanoma of skin, benign fibroadenoma of breast, carcinoma in situ of cervix uteri. Where such descriptors are not present, the remainder of the Index should be consulted where guidance is given to the appropriate column for each morphological (histological) variety listed; e.g., Mesonephroma – see Neoplasm, malignant; Embryoma (see also Neoplasm, uncertain behavior); Disease, Bowen's – see Neoplasm, skin, in situ. However, the guidance in the Index can be overridden if one of the descriptors mentioned above is present; e.g., malignant adenoma of colon is coded to C18.9 and not to D12.6 as the adjective "malignant" overrides the Index entry "Adenoma (see also Neoplasm, benign)." Codes listed with a dash -, following the code have a required 5th character for laterality. The tabular list must be reviewed for the complete code.

	Malignant Primary	Malignant Secondary	Ca in situ	Benign	Uncertain	Unspecified Behavior
Neoplasm, neoplastic	C8Ø.1	C79.9	DØ9.9	D36.9	D48.9	D49.9
abdomen, abdominal	C76.2	C79.8-☑	DØ9.8	D36.7	D48.7	D49.89
cavity	C76.2	C79.8-☑	DØ9.8	D36.7	D48.7	D49.89
organ	C76.2	C79.8-☑	DØ9.8	D36.7	D48.7	D49.89
viscera	C76.2	C79.8-☑	DØ9.8	D36.7	D48.7	D49.89
wall — *see also* Neoplasm, abdomen, wall, skin	C44.5Ø9	C79.2	DØ4.5	D23.5	D48.5	D49.2
connective tissue	C49.4	C79.8-☑	—	D21.4	D48.1	D49.2
skin	C44.5Ø9	—	—	—	—	—
basal cell carcinoma	C44.519	—	—	—	—	—
specified type NEC	C44.599	—	—	—	—	—
squamous cell carcinoma	C44.529	—	—	—	—	—
abdominopelvic	C76.8	C79.8-☑	—	D36.7	D48.7	D49.89
accessory sinus — *see* Neoplasm, sinus						
acoustic nerve	C72.4-☑	C79.49	—	D33.3	D43.3	D49.7
adenoid (pharynx) (tissue)	C11.1	C79.89	DØØ.Ø8	D1Ø.6	D37.Ø5	D49.Ø
adipose tissue — *see also* Neoplasm, connective tissue	C49.4	C79.89	—	D21.9	D48.1	D49.2
adnexa (uterine)	C57.4	C79.89	DØ7.39	D28.7	D39.8	D49.5
adrenal	C74.9-☑	C79.7-☑	DØ9.3	D35.Ø-☑	D44.1-☑	D49.7
capsule	C74.9-☑	C79.7-☑	DØ9.3	D35.Ø-☑	D44.1-☑	D49.7
cortex	C74.Ø-☑	C79.7-☑	DØ9.3	D35.Ø-☑	D44.1-☑	D49.7
gland	C74.9-☑	C79.7-☑	DØ9.3	D35.Ø-☑	D44.1-☑	D49.7
medulla	C74.1-☑	C79.7-☑	DØ9.3	D35.Ø-☑	D44.1-☑	D49.7
ala nasi (external) — *see also* Neoplasm, skin, nose	C44.3Ø1	C79.2	DØ4.39	D23.39	D48.5	D49.2
alimentary canal or tract NEC	C26.9	C78.8Ø	DØ1.9	D13.9	D37.9	D49.Ø
alveolar	CØ3.9	C79.89	DØØ.Ø3	D1Ø.39	D37.Ø9	D49.Ø
mucosa	CØ3.9	C79.89	DØØ.Ø3	D1Ø.39	D37.Ø9	D49.Ø
lower	CØ3.1	C79.89	DØØ.Ø3	D1Ø.39	D37.Ø9	D49.Ø
upper	CØ3.Ø	C79.89	DØØ.Ø3	D1Ø.39	D37.Ø9	D49.Ø
ridge or process	C41.1	C79.51	—	D16.5	D48.Ø	D49.2
carcinoma	CØ3.9	C79.8-☑	—	—	—	—
lower	CØ3.1	C79.8-☑	—	—	—	—
upper	CØ3.Ø	C79.8-☑	—	—	—	—
lower	C41.1	C79.51	—	D16.5	D48.Ø	D49.2
mucosa	CØ3.9	C79.89	DØØ.Ø3	D1Ø.39	D37.Ø9	D49.Ø
lower	CØ3.1	C79.89	DØØ.Ø3	D1Ø.39	D37.Ø9	D49.Ø
upper	CØ3.Ø	C79.89	DØØ.Ø3	D1Ø.39	D37.Ø9	D49.Ø
upper	C41.Ø	C79.51	—	D16.4	D48.Ø	D49.2
sulcus	CØ6.1	C79.89	DØØ.Ø2	D1Ø.39	D37.Ø9	D49.Ø
alveolus	CØ3.9	C79.89	DØØ.Ø3	D1Ø.39	D37.Ø9	D49.Ø
lower	CØ3.1	C79.89	DØØ.Ø3	D1Ø.39	D37.Ø9	D49.Ø
upper	CØ3.Ø	C79.89	DØØ.Ø3	D1Ø.39	D37.Ø9	D49.Ø
ampulla of Vater	C24.1	C78.89	DØ1.5	D13.5	D37.6	D49.Ø
ankle NEC	C76.5-☑	C79.89	DØ4.7-☑	D36.7	D48.7	D49.89

	Malignant Primary	Malignant Secondary	Ca in situ	Benign	Uncertain	Unspecified Behavior
Neoplasm, neoplastic — *continued*						
anorectum, anorectal (junction)	C21.8	C78.5	DØ1.3	D12.9	D37.8	D49.Ø
antecubital fossa or space	C76.4-☑	C79.89	DØ4.6-☑	D36.7	D48.7	D49.89
antrum (Highmore) (maxillary)	C31.Ø	C78.39	DØ2.3	D14.Ø	D38.5	D49.1
pyloric	C16.3	C78.89	DØØ.2	D13.1	D37.1	D49.Ø
tympanicum	C3Ø.1	C78.39	DØ2.3	D14.Ø	D38.5	D49.1
anus, anal	C21.Ø	C78.5	DØ1.3	D12.9	D37.8	D49.Ø
canal	C21.1	C78.5	DØ1.3	D12.9	D37.8	D49.Ø
cloacogenic zone	C21.2	C78.5	DØ1.3	D12.9	D37.8	D49.Ø
margin — *see also* Neoplasm, anus, skin	C44.5ØØ	C79.2	DØ4.5	D23.5	D48.5	D49.2
overlapping lesion with rectosigmoid junction or rectum	C21.8	—	—	—	—	—
skin	C44.5ØØ	C79.2	DØ4.5	D23.5	D48.5	D49.2
basal cell carcinoma	C44.51Ø	—	—	—	—	—
specified type NEC	C44.59Ø	—	—	—	—	—
squamous cell carcinoma	C44.52Ø	—	—	—	—	—
sphincter	C21.1	C78.5	DØ1.3	D12.9	D37.8	D49.Ø
aorta (thoracic)	C49.3	C79.89	—	D21.3	D48.1	D49.2
abdominal	C49.4	C79.89	—	D21.4	D48.1	D49.2
aortic body	C75.5	C79.89	—	D35.6	D44.7	D49.7
aponeurosis	C49.9	C79.89	—	D21.9	D48.1	D49.2
palmar	C49.1-☑	C79.89	—	D21.1-☑	D48.1	D49.2
plantar	C49.2-☑	C79.89	—	D21.2-☑	D48.1	D49.2
appendix	C18.1	C78.5	DØ1.Ø	D12.1	D37.3	D49.Ø
arachnoid	C7Ø.9	C79.49	—	D32.9	D42.9	D49.7
cerebral	C7Ø.Ø	C79.32	—	D32.Ø	D42.Ø	D49.7
spinal	C7Ø.1	C79.49	—	D32.1	D42.1	D49.7
areola	C5Ø.Ø-☑	C79.81	DØ5-☑	D24-☑	D48.6-☑	D49.3
arm NEC	C76.4-☑	C79.89	DØ4.6-☑	D36.7	D48.7	D49.89
artery — *see* Neoplasm, connective tissue						
aryepiglottic fold	C13.1	C79.89	DØØ.Ø8	D1Ø.7	D37.Ø5	D49.Ø
hypopharyngeal aspect	C13.1	C79.89	DØØ.Ø8	D1Ø.7	D37.Ø5	D49.Ø
laryngeal aspect	C32.1	C78.39	DØ2.Ø	D14.1	D38.Ø	D49.1
marginal zone	C13.1	C79.89	DØØ.Ø8	D1Ø.7	D37.Ø5	D49.Ø
arytenoid (cartilage)	C32.3	C78.39	DØ2.Ø	D14.1	D38.Ø	D49.1
fold — *see* Neoplasm, aryepiglottic						
associated with transplanted organ	C8Ø.2	—	—	—	—	—
atlas	C41.2	C79.51	—	D16.6	D48.Ø	D49.2
atrium, cardiac	C38.Ø	C79.89	—	D15.1	D48.7	D49.89
auditory						
canal (external) (skin) A81	C44.2Ø-☑	C79.2	DØ4.2-☑	D23.2-☑	D48.5	D49.2
internal	C3Ø.1	C78.39	DØ2.3	D14.Ø	D38.5	D49.1
nerve	C72.4-☑	C79.49	—	D33.3	D43.3	D49.7
tube	C3Ø.1	C78.39	DØ2.3	D14.Ø	D38.5	D49.1
opening	C11.2	C79.89	DØØ.Ø8	D1Ø.6	D37.Ø5	D49.Ø
auricle, ear — *see also* Neoplasm, skin, ear	C44.2Ø-☑	C79.2	DØ4.2-☑	D23.2-☑	D48.5	D49.2
auricular canal (external) — *see also* Neoplasm, skin, ear	C44.2Ø-☑	C79.2	DØ4.2-☑	D23.2-☑	D48.5	D49.2
internal	C3Ø.1	C78.39	DØ2.3	D14.Ø	D38.5	D49.2
autonomic nerve or nervous system NEC (*see* Neoplasm, nerve, peripheral)						
axilla, axillary	C76.1	C79.89	DØ9.8	D36.7	D48.7	D49.89
fold — *see also* Neoplasm, skin, trunk	C44.5Ø9	C79.2	DØ4.5	D23.5	D48.5	D49.2
back NEC	C76.8	C79.89	DØ4.5	D36.7	D48.7	D49.89

	Malignant Primary	Malignant Secondary	Ca in situ	Benign	Uncertain	Unspecified Behavior
Neoplasm, neoplastic — *continued*						
Bartholin's gland	C51.Ø	C79.82	DØ7.1	D28.Ø	D39.8	D49.5
basal ganglia	C71.Ø	C79.31	—	D33.Ø	D43.Ø	D49.6
basis pedunculi	C71.7	C79.31	—	D33.1	D43.1	D49.6
bile or biliary (tract)	C24.9	C78.89	DØ1.5	D13.5	D37.6	D49.Ø
canaliculi (biliferi) (intrahepatic)	C22.1	C78.7	DØ1.5	D13.4	D37.6	D49.Ø
canals, interlobular	C22.1	C78.89	DØ1.5	D13.4	D37.6	D49.Ø
duct or passage (common) (cystic) (extrahepatic)	C24.Ø	C78.89	DØ1.5	D13.5	D37.6	D49.Ø
interlobular	C22.1	C78.89	DØ1.5	D13.4	D37.6	D49.Ø
intrahepatic	C22.1	C78.7	DØ1.5	D13.4	D37.6	D49.Ø
and extrahepatic	C24.8	C78.89	DØ1.5	D13.5	D37.6	D49.Ø
bladder (urinary)	C67.9	C79.11	DØ9.Ø	D3Ø.3	D41.4	D49.4
dome	C67.1	C79.11	DØ9.Ø	D3Ø.3	D41.4	D49.4
neck	C67.5	C79.11	DØ9.Ø	D3Ø.3	D41.4	D49.4
orifice	C67.9	C79.11	DØ9.Ø	D3Ø.3	D41.4	D49.4
ureteric	C67.6	C79.11	DØ9.Ø	D3Ø.3	D41.4	D49.4
urethral	C67.5	C79.11	DØ9.Ø	D3Ø.3	D41.4	D49.4
overlapping lesion	C67.8	—	—	—	—	—
sphincter	C67.8	C79.11	DØ9.Ø	D3Ø.3	D41.4	D49.4
trigone	C67.Ø	C79.11	DØ9.Ø	D3Ø.3	D41.4	D49.4
urachus	C67.7	C79.11	DØ9.Ø	D3Ø.3	D41.4	D49.4
wall	C67.9	C79.11	DØ9.Ø	D3Ø.3	D41.4	D49.4
anterior	C67.3	C79.11	DØ9.Ø	D3Ø.3	D41.4	D49.4
lateral	C67.2	C79.11	DØ9.Ø	D3Ø.3	D41.4	D49.4
posterior	C67.4	C79.11	DØ9.Ø	D3Ø.3	D41.4	D49.4
blood vessel — *see* Neoplasm, connective tissue						
bone (periosteum)	C41.9	C79.51	—	D16.9	D48.Ø	D49.2
acetabulum	C41.4	C79.51	—	D16.8	D48.Ø	D49.2
ankle	C4Ø.3-☑	C79.51	—	D16.3-☑	—	—
arm NEC	C4Ø.Ø-☑	C79.51	—	D16.Ø-☑	—	—
astragalus	C4Ø.3-☑	C79.51	—	D16.3-☑	—	—
atlas	C41.2	C79.51	—	D16.6	D48.Ø	D49.2
axis	C41.2	C79.51	—	D16.6	D48.Ø	D49.2
back NEC	C41.2	C79.51	—	D16.6	D48.Ø	D49.2
calcaneus	C4Ø.3-☑	C79.51	—	D16.3-☑	—	—
calvarium	C41.Ø	C79.51	—	D16.4	D48.Ø	D49.2
carpus (any)	C4Ø.1-☑	C79.51	—	D16.1-☑	—	—
cartilage NEC	C41.9	C79.51	—	D16.9	D48.Ø	D49.2
clavicle	C41.3	C79.51	—	D16.7	D48.Ø	D49.2
clivus	C41.Ø	C79.51	—	D16.4	D48.Ø	D49.2
coccygeal vertebra	C41.4	C79.51	—	D16.8	D48.Ø	D49.2
coccyx	C41.4	C79.51	—	D16.8	D48.Ø	D49.2
costal cartilage	C41.3	C79.51	—	D16.7	D48.Ø	D49.2
costovertebral joint	C41.3	C79.51	—	D16.7	D48.Ø	D49.2
cranial	C41.Ø	C79.51	—	D16.4	D48.Ø	D49.2
cuboid	C4Ø.3-☑	C79.51	—	D16.3-☑	—	—
cuneiform	C41.9	C79.51	—	D16.9	D48.Ø	D49.2
elbow	C4Ø.Ø-☑	C79.51	—	D16.Ø-☑	—	—
ethmoid (labyrinth)	C41.Ø	C79.51	—	D16.4	D48.Ø	D49.2
face	C41.Ø	C79.51	—	D16.4	D48.Ø	D49.2
femur (any part)	C4Ø.2-☑	C79.51	—	D16.2-☑	—	—
fibula (any part)	C4Ø.2-☑	C79.51	—	D16.2-☑	—	—
finger (any)	C4Ø.1-☑	C79.51	—	D16.1-☑	—	—
foot	C4Ø.3-☑	C79.51	—	D16.3-☑	—	—
forearm	C4Ø.Ø-☑	C79.51	—	D16.Ø-☑	—	—
frontal	C41.Ø	C79.51	—	D16.4	D48.Ø	D49.2
hand	C4Ø.1-☑	C79.51	—	D16.1-☑	—	—
heel	C4Ø.3-☑	C79.51	—	D16.3-☑	—	—
hip	C41.4	C79.51	—	D16.8	D48.Ø	D49.2
humerus (any part)	C4Ø.Ø-☑	C79.51	—	D16.Ø-☑	—	—
hyoid	C41.Ø	C79.51	—	D16.4	D48.Ø	D49.2
ilium	C41.4	C79.51	—	D16.8	D48.Ø	D49.2
innominate	C41.4	C79.51	—	D16.8	D48.Ø	D49.2
intervertebral cartilage or disc	C41.2	C79.51	—	D16.6	D48.Ø	D49.2
ischium	C41.4	C79.51	—	D16.8	D48.Ø	D49.2
jaw (lower)	C41.1	C79.51	—	D16.5	D48.Ø	D49.2
knee	C4Ø.2-☑	C79.51	—	D16.2-☑	—	—
leg NEC	C4Ø.2-☑	C79.51	—	D16.2-☑	—	—
limb NEC	C4Ø.9-☑	C79.51	—	D16.9	—	—
Neoplasm, neoplastic — *continued*						
bone — *continued*						
limb — *continued*						
lower (long bones)	C4Ø.2-☑	C79.51	—	D16.2-☑	—	—
short bones	C4Ø.3-☑	C79.51	—	D16.3-☑	—	—
upper (long bones)	C4Ø.Ø-☑	C79.51	—	D16.Ø-☑	—	—
short bones	C4Ø.1-☑	C79.51	—	D16.1-☑	—	—
malar	C41.Ø	C79.51	—	D16.4	D48.Ø	D49.2
mandible	C41.1	C79.51	—	D16.5	D48.Ø	D49.2
marrow NEC (any bone)	C96.9	C79.52	—	—	D47.9	D49.89
mastoid	C41.Ø	C79.51	—	D16.4	D48.Ø	D49.2
maxilla, maxillary (superior)	C41.Ø	C79.51	—	D16.4	D48.Ø	D49.2
inferior	C41.1	C79.51	—	D16.5	D48.Ø	D49.2
metacarpus (any)	C4Ø.1-☑	C79.51	—	D16.1-☑	—	—
metatarsus (any)	C4Ø.3-☑	C79.51	—	D16.3-☑	—	—
navicular						
ankle	C4Ø.3-☑	C79.51	—	—	—	—
hand	C4Ø.1-☑	C79.51	—	—	—	—
nose, nasal	C41.Ø	C79.51	—	D16.4	D48.Ø	D49.2
occipital	C41.Ø	C79.51	—	D16.4	D48.Ø	D49.2
orbit	C41.Ø	C79.51	—	D16.4	D48.Ø	D49.2
overlapping sites	C4Ø.8-☑	—	—	—	—	—
parietal	C41.Ø	C79.51	—	D16.4	D48.Ø	D49.2
patella	C4Ø.2-☑	C79.51	—	—	—	—
pelvic	C41.4	C79.51	—	D16.8	D48.Ø	D49.2
phalanges						
foot	C4Ø.3-☑	C79.51	—	—	—	—
hand	C4Ø.1-☑	C79.51	—	—	—	—
pubic	C41.4	C79.51	—	D16.8	D48.Ø	D49.2
radius (any part)	C4Ø.Ø-☑	C79.51	—	D16.Ø-☑	—	—
rib	C41.3	C79.51	—	D16.7	D48.Ø	D49.2
sacral vertebra	C41.4	C79.51	—	D16.8	D48.Ø	D49.2
sacrum	C41.4	C79.51	—	D16.8	D48.Ø	D49.2
scaphoid						
of ankle	C4Ø.3-☑	C79.51	—	—	—	—
of hand	C4Ø.1-☑	C79.51	—	—	—	—
scapula (any part)	C4Ø.Ø-☑	C79.51	—	D16.Ø-☑	—	—
sella turcica	C41.Ø	C79.51	—	D16.4	D48.Ø	D49.2
shoulder	C4Ø.Ø-☑	C79.51	—	D16.Ø-☑	—	—
skull	C41.Ø	C79.51	—	D16.4	D48.Ø	D49.2
sphenoid	C41.Ø	C79.51	—	D16.4	D48.Ø	D49.2
spine, spinal (column)	C41.2	C79.51	—	D16.6	D48.Ø	D49.2
coccyx	C41.4	C79.51	—	D16.8	D48.Ø	D49.2
sacrum	C41.4	C79.51	—	D16.8	D48.Ø	D49.2
sternum	C41.3	C79.51	—	D16.7	D48.Ø	D49.2
tarsus (any)	C4Ø.3-☑	C79.51	—	—	—	—
temporal	C41.Ø	C79.51	—	D16.4	D48.Ø	D49.2
thumb	C4Ø.1-☑	C79.51	—	—	—	—
tibia (any part)	C4Ø.2-☑	C79.51	—	—	—	—
toe (any)	C4Ø.3-☑	C79.51	—	—	—	—
trapezium	C4Ø.1-☑	C79.51	—	—	—	—
trapezoid	C4Ø.1-☑	C79.51	—	—	—	—
turbinate	C41.Ø	C79.51	—	D16.4	D48.Ø	D49.2
ulna (any part)	C4Ø.Ø-☑	C79.51	—	D16.Ø-☑	—	—
unciform	C4Ø.1-☑	C79.51	—	—	—	—
vertebra (column)	C41.2	C79.51	—	D16.6	D48.Ø	D49.2
coccyx	C41.4	C79.51	—	D16.8	D48.Ø	D49.2
sacrum	C41.4	C79.51	—	D16.8	D48.Ø	D49.2
vomer	C41.Ø	C79.51	—	D16.4	D48.Ø	D49.2
wrist	C4Ø.1-☑	C79.51	—	—	—	—
xiphoid process	C41.3	C79.51	—	D16.7	D48.Ø	D49.2
zygomatic	C41.Ø	C79.51	—	D16.4	D48.Ø	D49.2
book-leaf (mouth) — *ventral surface of tongue and floor of mouth*	CØ6.89	C79.89	DØØ.ØØ	D1Ø.39	D37.Ø9	D49.Ø
bowel — *see* Neoplasm, intestine						
brachial plexus	C47.1-☑	C79.89	—	D36.12	D48.2	D49.2
brain NEC	C71.9	C79.31	—	D33.2	D43.2	D49.6
basal ganglia	C71.Ø	C79.31	—	D33.Ø	D43.Ø	D49.6
cerebellopontine angle	C71.6	C79.31	—	D33.1	D43.1	D49.6
cerebellum NOS	C71.6	C79.31	—	D33.1	D43.1	D49.6
cerebrum	C71.Ø	C79.31	—	D33.Ø	D43.Ø	D49.6

	Malignant Primary	Malignant Secondary	Ca in situ	Benign	Uncertain	Unspecified Behavior
Neoplasm, neoplastic — *continued*						
brain — *continued*						
choroid plexus	C71.7	C79.31	—	D33.1	D43.1	D49.6
corpus callosum	C71.8	C79.31	—	D33.2	D43.2	D49.6
corpus striatum	C71.Ø	C79.31	—	D33.Ø	D43.Ø	D49.6
cortex (cerebral)	C71.Ø	C79.31	—	D33.Ø	D43.Ø	D49.6
frontal lobe	C71.1	C79.31	—	D33.Ø	D43.Ø	D49.6
globus pallidus	C71.Ø	C79.31	—	D33.Ø	D43.Ø	D49.6
hippocampus	C71.2	C79.31	—	D33.Ø	D43.Ø	D49.6
hypothalamus	C71.Ø	C79.31	—	D33.Ø	D43.Ø	D49.6
internal capsule	C71.Ø	C79.31	—	D33.Ø	D43.Ø	D49.6
medulla oblongata	C71.7	C79.31	—	D33.1	D43.1	D49.6
meninges	C70.Ø	C79.32	—	D32.Ø	D42.Ø	D49.7
midbrain	C71.7	C79.31	—	D33.1	D43.1	D49.6
occipital lobe	C71.4	C79.31	—	D33.Ø	D43.Ø	D49.6
overlapping lesion	C71.8	C79.31	—	—	—	—
parietal lobe	C71.3	C79.31	—	D33.Ø	D43.Ø	D49.6
peduncle	C71.7	C79.31	—	D33.1	D43.1	D49.6
pons	C71.7	C79.31	—	D33.1	D43.1	D49.6
stem	C71.7	C79.31	—	D33.1	D43.1	D49.6
tapetum	C71.8	C79.31	—	D33.2	D43.2	D49.6
temporal lobe	C71.2	C79.31	—	D33.Ø	D43.Ø	D49.6
thalamus	C71.Ø	C79.31	—	D33.Ø	D43.Ø	D49.6
uncus	C71.2	C79.31	—	D33.Ø	D43.Ø	D49.6
ventricle (floor)	C71.5	C79.31	—	D33.Ø	D43.Ø	D49.6
fourth	C71.7	C79.31	—	D33.1	D43.1	D49.6
branchial (cleft) (cyst) (vestiges)	C1Ø.4	C79.89	DØØ.Ø8	D1Ø.5	D37.Ø5	D49.Ø
breast (connective tissue) (glandular tissue) (soft parts)	C5Ø.9-☑	C79.81	DØ5.-☑	D24.-☑	D48.6-☑	D49.3
areola	C5Ø.Ø-☑	C79.81	DØ5.-☑	D24.-☑	D48.6-☑	D49.3
axillary tail	C5Ø.6-☑	C79.81	DØ5.-☑	D24.-☑	D48.6-☑	D49.3
central portion	C5Ø.1-☑	C79.81	DØ5.-☑	D24.-☑	D48.6-☑	D49.3
inner	C5Ø.8-☑	C79.81	DØ5.-☑	D24.-☑	D48.6-☑	D49.3
lower	C5Ø.8-☑	C79.81	DØ5.-☑	D24.-☑	D48.6-☑	D49.3
lower-inner quadrant	C5Ø.3-☑	C79.81	DØ5.-☑	D24.-☑	D48.6-☑	D49.3
lower-outer quadrant	C5Ø.5-☑	C79.81	DØ5.-☑	D24.-☑	D48.6-☑	D49.3
mastectomy site (skin) — *see also* Neoplasm, breast, skin	C44.5Ø1	C79.2	—	—	—	—
specified as breast tissue	C5Ø.8-☑	C79.81	—	—	—	—
midline	C5Ø.8-☑	C79.81	DØ5.-☑	D24.-☑	D48.6-☑	D49.3
nipple	C5Ø.Ø-☑	C79.81	DØ5.-☑	D24.-☑	D48.6-☑	D49.3
outer	C5Ø.8-☑	C79.81	DØ5.-☑	D24.-☑	D48.6-☑	D49.3
overlapping lesion	C5Ø.8-☑	—	—	—	—	—
skin	C44.5Ø1	C79.2	DØ4.5	D23.5	D48.5	D49.2
basal cell carcinoma	C44.511	—	—	—	—	—
specified type NEC	C44.591	—	—	—	—	—
squamous cell carcinoma	C44.521	—	—	—	—	—
tail (axillary)	C5Ø.6-☑	C79.81	DØ5.-☑	D24.-☑	D48.6-☑	D49.3
upper	C5Ø.8-☑	C79.81	DØ5.-☑	D24.-☑	D48.6-☑	D49.3
upper-inner quadrant	C5Ø.2-☑	C79.81	DØ5.-☑	D24.-☑	D48.6-☑	D49.3
upper-outer quadrant	C5Ø.4-☑	C79.81	DØ5.-☑	D24.-☑	D48.6-☑	D49.3
broad ligament	C57.1-☑	C79.82	DØ7.39	D28.2	D39.8	D49.5
bronchiogenic, bronchogenic (lung)	C34.9-☑	C78.Ø-☑	DØ2.2-☑	D14.3-☑	D38.1	D49.1
bronchiole	C34.9-☑	C78.Ø-☑	DØ2.2-☑	D14.3-☑	D38.1	D49.1
bronchus	C34.9-☑	C78.Ø-☑	DØ2.2-☑	D14.3-☑	D38.1	D49.1
carina	C34.Ø-☑	C78.Ø-☑	DØ2.2-☑	D14.3-☑	D38.1	D49.1
lower lobe of lung	C34.3-☑	C78.Ø-☑	DØ2.2-☑	D14.3-☑	D38.1	D49.1
main	C34.Ø-☑	C78.Ø-☑	DØ2.2-☑	D14.3-☑	D38.1	D49.1
middle lobe of lung	C34.2	C78.Ø-☑	DØ2.21	D14.31	D38.1	D49.1
overlapping lesion	C34.8-☑	—	—	—	—	—
upper lobe of lung	C34.1-☑	C78.Ø-☑	DØ2.2-☑	D14.3-☑	D38.1	D49.1
brow	C44.3Ø9	C79.2	DØ4.39	D23.39	D48.5	D49.2
basal cell carcinoma	C44.319	—	—	—	—	—
specified type NEC	C44.399	—	—	—	—	—

	Malignant Primary	Malignant Secondary	Ca in situ	Benign	Uncertain	Unspecified Behavior
Neoplasm, neoplastic — *continued*						
brow — *continued*						
squamous cell carcinoma	C44.329	—	—	—	—	—
buccal (cavity)	CØ6.9	C79.89	DØØ.ØØ	D1Ø.39	D37.Ø9	D49.Ø
commissure	CØ6.Ø	C79.89	DØØ.Ø2	D1Ø.39	D37.Ø9	D49.Ø
groove (lower) (upper)	CØ6.1	C79.89	DØØ.Ø2	D1Ø.39	D37.Ø9	D49.Ø
mucosa	CØ6.Ø	C79.89	DØØ.Ø2	D1Ø.39	D37.Ø9	D49.Ø
sulcus (lower) (upper)	CØ6.1	C79.89	DØØ.Ø2	D1Ø.39	D37.Ø9	D49.Ø
bulbourethral gland	C68.Ø	C79.19	DØ9.19	D3Ø.4	D41.3	D49.5
bursa — *see* Neoplasm, connective tissue						
buttock NEC	C76.3	C79.89	DØ4.5	D36.7	D48.7	D49.89
calf	C76.5-☑	C79.89	DØ4.7-☑	D36.7	D48.7	D49.89
calvarium	C41.Ø	C79.51	—	D16.4	D48.Ø	D49.2
calyx, renal	C65.-☑	C79.Ø-☑	DØ9.19	D3Ø.1-☑	D41.1-☑	D49.5
canal						
anal	C21.1	C78.5	DØ1.3	D12.9	D37.8	D49.Ø
auditory (external) — *see also* Neoplasm, skin, ear	C44.2Ø-☑	C79.2	DØ4.2-☑	D23.2-☑	D48.5	D49.2
auricular (external) — *see also* Neoplasm, skin, ear	C44.2Ø-☑	C79.2	DØ4.2-☑	D23.2-☑	D48.5	D49.2
canaliculi, biliary (biliferi) (intrahepatic)	C22.1	C78.7	DØ1.5	D13.4	D37.6	D49.Ø
canthus (eye) (inner) (outer)	C44.1Ø-☑	C79.2	DØ4.1-☑	D23.1-☑	D48.5	D49.2
basal cell carcinoma	C44.11-☑	—	—	—	—	—
specified type NEC	C44.19-☑	—	—	—	—	—
squamous cell carcinoma	C44.12-☑	—	—	—	—	—
capillary — *see* Neoplasm, connective tissue						
caput coli	C18.Ø	C78.5	DØ1.Ø	D12.Ø	D37.4	D49.Ø
carcinoid — *see* Tumor, carcinoid						
cardia (gastric)	C16.Ø	C78.89	DØØ.2	D13.1	D37.1	D49.Ø
cardiac orifice (stomach)	C16.Ø	C78.89	DØØ.2	D13.1	D37.1	D49.Ø
cardio-esophageal junction	C16.Ø	C78.89	DØØ.2	D13.1	D37.1	D49.Ø
cardio-esophagus	C16.Ø	C78.89	DØØ.2	D13.1	D37.1	D49.Ø
carina (bronchus)	C34.Ø-☑	C78.Ø-☑	DØ2.2-☑	D14.3-☑	D38.1	D49.1
carotid (artery)	C49.Ø	C79.89	—	D21.Ø	D48.1	D49.2
body	C75.4	C79.89	—	D35.5	D44.6	D49.7
carpus (any bone)	C4Ø.1-☑	C79.51	—	D16.1-☑	—	—
cartilage (articular) (joint) NEC — *see also* Neoplasm, bone	C41.9	C79.51	—	D16.9	D48.Ø	D49.2
arytenoid	C32.3	C78.39	DØ2.Ø	D14.1	D38.Ø	D49.1
auricular	C49.Ø	C79.89	—	D21.Ø	D48.1	D49.2
bronchi	C34.Ø-☑	C78.39	—	D14.3-☑	D38.1	D49.1
costal	C41.3	C79.51	—	D16.7	D48.Ø	D49.2
cricoid	C32.3	C78.39	DØ2.Ø	D14.1	D38.Ø	D49.1
cuneiform	C32.3	C78.39	DØ2.Ø	D14.1	D38.Ø	D49.1
ear (external)	C49.Ø	C79.89	—	D21.Ø	D48.1	D49.2
ensiform	C41.3	C79.51	—	D16.7	D48.Ø	D49.2
epiglottis	C32.1	C78.39	DØ2.Ø	D14.1	D38.Ø	D49.1
anterior surface	C1Ø.1	C79.89	DØØ.Ø8	D1Ø.5	D37.Ø5	D49.Ø
eyelid	C49.Ø	C79.89	—	D21.Ø	D48.1	D49.2
intervertebral	C41.2	C79.51	—	D16.6	D48.Ø	D49.2
larynx, laryngeal	C32.3	C78.39	DØ2.Ø	D14.1	D38.Ø	D49.1
nose, nasal	C3Ø.Ø	C78.39	DØ2.3	D14.Ø	D38.5	D49.1
pinna	C49.Ø	C79.89	—	D21.Ø	D48.1	D49.2
rib	C41.3	C79.51	—	D16.7	D48.Ø	D49.2
semilunar (knee)	C4Ø.2-☑	C79.51	—	D16.2-☑	D48.Ø	D49.2
thyroid	C32.3	C78.39	DØ2.Ø	D14.1	D38.Ø	D49.1
trachea	C33	C78.39	DØ2.1	D14.2	D38.1	D49.1
cauda equina	C72.1	C79.49	—	D33.4	D43.4	D49.7
cavity						
buccal	CØ6.9	C79.89	DØØ.ØØ	D1Ø.3Ø	D37.Ø9	D49.Ø
nasal	C3Ø.Ø	C78.39	DØ2.3	D14.Ø	D38.5	D49.1
oral	CØ6.9	C79.89	DØØ.ØØ	D1Ø.3Ø	D37.Ø9	D49.Ø
peritoneal	C48.2	C78.6	—	D2Ø.1	D48.4	D49.Ø
tympanic	C3Ø.1	C78.39	DØ2.3	D14.Ø	D38.5	D49.1
cecum	C18.Ø	C78.5	DØ1.Ø	D12.Ø	D37.4	D49.Ø

	Malignant Primary	Malignant Secondary	Ca in situ	Benign	Uncertain	Unspecified Behavior
Neoplasm, neoplastic — *continued*						
central nervous system	C72.9	C79.4Ø	—	—	—	—
cerebellopontine (angle)	C71.6	C79.31	—	D33.1	D43.1	D49.6
cerebellum, cerebellar	C71.6	C79.31	—	D33.1	D43.1	D49.6
cerebrum, cerebral (cortex) (hemisphere) (white matter)	C71.Ø	C79.31	—	D33.Ø	D43.Ø	D49.6
meninges	C7Ø.Ø	C79.32	—	D32.Ø	D42.Ø	D49.7
peduncle	C71.7	C79.31	—	D33.1	D43.1	D49.6
ventricle	C71.5	C79.31	—	D33.Ø	D43.Ø	D49.6
fourth	C71.7	C79.31	—	D33.1	D43.1	D49.6
cervical region	C76.Ø	C79.89	DØ9.8	D36.7	D48.7	D49.89
cervix (cervical) (uteri) (uterus)	C53.9	C79.82	DØ6.9	D26.Ø	D39.Ø	D49.5
canal	C53.Ø	C79.82	DØ6.Ø	D26.Ø	D39.Ø	D49.5
endocervix (canal) (gland)	C53.Ø	C79.82	DØ6.Ø	D26.Ø	D39.Ø	D49.5
exocervix	C53.1	C79.82	DØ6.1	D26.Ø	D39.Ø	D49.5
external os	C53.1	C79.82	DØ6.1	D26.Ø	D39.Ø	D49.5
internal os	C53.Ø	C79.82	DØ6.Ø	D26.Ø	D39.Ø	D49.5
nabothian gland	C53.Ø	C79.82	DØ6.Ø	D26.Ø	D39.Ø	D49.5
overlapping lesion	C53.8	—	—	—	—	—
squamocolumnar junction	C53.8	C79.82	DØ6.7	D26.Ø	D39.Ø	D49.5
stump	C53.8	C79.82	DØ6.7	D26.Ø	D39.Ø	D49.5
cheek	C76.Ø	C79.89	DØ9.8	D36.7	D48.7	D49.89
external	C44.3Ø9	C79.2	DØ4.39	D23.39	D48.5	D49.2
basal cell carcinoma	C44.319	—	—	—	—	—
specified type NEC	C44.399	—	—	—	—	—
squamous cell carcinoma	C44.329	—	—	—	—	—
inner aspect	CØ6.Ø	C79.89	DØØ.Ø2	D1Ø.39	D37.Ø9	D49.Ø
internal	CØ6.Ø	C79.89	DØØ.Ø2	D1Ø.39	D37.Ø9	D49.Ø
mucosa	CØ6.Ø	C79.89	DØØ.Ø2	D1Ø.39	D37.Ø9	D49.Ø
chest (wall) NEC	C76.1	C79.89	DØ9.8	D36.7	D48.7	D49.89
chiasma opticum	C72.3-☑	C79.49	—	D33.3	D43.3	D49.7
chin	C44.3Ø9	C79.2	DØ4.39	D23.39	D48.5	D49.2
basal cell carcinoma	C44.319	—	—	—	—	—
specified type NEC	C44.399	—	—	—	—	—
squamous cell carcinoma	C44.329	—	—	—	—	—
choana	C11.3	C79.89	DØØ.Ø8	D1Ø.6	D37.Ø5	D49.Ø
cholangiole	C22.1	C78.89	DØ1.5	D13.4	D37.6	D49.Ø
choledochal duct	C24.Ø	C78.89	DØ1.5	D13.5	D37.6	D49.Ø
choroid	C69.3-☑	C79.49	DØ9.2-☑	D31.3-☑	D48.7	D49.81
plexus	C71.5	C79.31	—	D33.Ø	D43.Ø	D49.6
ciliary body	C69.4-☑	C79.49	DØ9.2-☑	D31.4-☑	D48.7	D49.89
clavicle	C41.3	C79.51	—	D16.7	D48.Ø	D49.2
clitoris	C51.2	C79.82	DØ7.1	D28.Ø	D39.8	D49.5
clivus	C41.Ø	C79.51	—	D16.4	D48.Ø	D49.2
cloacogenic zone	C21.2	C78.5	DØ1.3	D12.9	D37.8	D49.Ø
coccygeal						
body or glomus	C49.5	C79.89	—	D21.5	D48.1	D49.2
vertebra	C41.4	C79.51	—	D16.8	D48.Ø	D49.2
coccyx	C41.4	C79.51	—	D16.8	D48.Ø	D49.2
colon — *see also* Neoplasm, intestine, large	C18.9	C78.5	—	—	—	—
with rectum	C19	C78.5	DØ1.1	D12.7	D37.5	D49.Ø
columnella — *see also* Neoplasm, skin, face	C44.39Ø	C79.2	DØ4.39	D23.39	D48.5	D49.2
column, spinal — *see* Neoplasm, spine						
commissure						
labial, lip	CØØ.6	C79.89	DØØ.Ø1	D1Ø.39	D37.Ø1	D49.Ø
laryngeal	C32.Ø	C78.39	DØ2.Ø	D14.1	D38.Ø	D49.1
common (bile) duct	C24.Ø	C78.89	DØ1.5	D13.5	D37.6	D49.Ø
concha — *see also* Neoplasm, skin, ear	C44.2Ø-☑	C79.2	DØ4.2-☑	D23.2-☑	D48.5	D49.2
nose	C3Ø.Ø	C78.39	DØ2.3	D14.Ø	D38.5	D49.1
conjunctiva	C69.Ø-☑	C79.49	DØ9.2-☑	D31.Ø-☑	D48.7	D49.89

	Malignant Primary	Malignant Secondary	Ca in situ	Benign	Uncertain	Unspecified Behavior
Neoplasm, neoplastic — *continued*						
connective tissue NEC	C49.9	C79.89	—	D21.9	D48.1	D49.2

Note: For neoplasms of connective tissue (blood vessel, bursa, fascia, ligament, muscle, peripheral nerves, sympathetic and parasympathetic nerves and ganglia, synovia, tendon, etc.) or of morphological types that indicate connective tissue, code according to the list under "Neoplasm, connective tissue". For sites that do not appear in this list, code to neoplasm of that site; e.g., fibrosarcoma, pancreas (C25.9)

Note: Morphological types that indicate connective tissue appear in their proper place in the alphabetic index with the instruction "see Neoplasm, connective tissue ...."

	Malignant Primary	Malignant Secondary	Ca in situ	Benign	Uncertain	Unspecified Behavior
abdomen	C49.4	C79.89	—	D21.4	D48.1	D49.2
abdominal wall	C49.4	C79.89	—	D21.4	D48.1	D49.2
ankle	C49.2-☑	C79.89	—	D21.2-☑	D48.1	D49.2
antecubital fossa or space	C49.1-☑	C79.89	—	D21.1-☑	D48.1	D49.2
arm	C49.1-☑	C79.89	—	D21.1-☑	D48.1	D49.2
auricle (ear)	C49.Ø	C79.89	—	D21.Ø	D48.1	D49.2
axilla	C49.3	C79.89	—	D21.3	D48.1	D49.2
back	C49.6	C79.89	—	D21.6	D48.1	D49.2
breast — *see* Neoplasm, breast						
buttock	C49.5	C79.89	—	D21.5	D48.1	D49.2
calf	C49.2-☑	C79.89	—	D21.2-☑	D48.1	D49.2
cervical region	C49.Ø	C79.89	—	D21.Ø	D48.1	D49.2
cheek	C49.Ø	C79.89	—	D21.Ø	D48.1	D49.2
chest (wall)	C49.3	C79.89	—	D21.3	D48.1	D49.2
chin	C49.Ø	C79.89	—	D21.Ø	D48.1	D49.2
diaphragm	C49.3	C79.89	—	D21.3	D48.1	D49.2
ear (external)	C49.Ø	C79.89	—	D21.Ø	D48.1	D49.2
elbow	C49.1-☑	C79.89	—	D21.1-☑	D48.1	D49.2
extrarectal	C49.5	C79.89	—	D21.5	D48.1	D49.2
extremity	C49.9	C79.89	—	D21.9	D48.1	D49.2
lower	C49.2-☑	C79.89	—	D21.2-☑	D48.1	D49.2
upper	C49.1-☑	C79.89	—	D21.1-☑	D48.1	D49.2
eyelid	C49.Ø	C79.89	—	D21.Ø	D48.1	D49.2
face	C49.Ø	C79.89	—	D21.Ø	D48.1	D49.2
finger	C49.1-☑	C79.89	—	D21.1-☑	D48.1	D49.2
flank	C49.6	C79.89	—	D21.6	D48.1	D49.2
foot	C49.2-☑	C79.89	—	D21.2-☑	D48.1	D49.2
forearm	C49.1-☑	C79.89	—	D21.1-☑	D48.1	D49.2
forehead	C49.Ø	C79.89	—	D21.Ø	D48.1	D49.2
gastric	C49.4	C79.89	—	D21.4	D48.1	D49.2
gastrointestinal	C49.4	C79.89	—	D21.4	D48.1	D49.2
gluteal region	C49.5	C79.89	—	D21.5	D48.1	D49.2
great vessels NEC	C49.3	C79.89	—	D21.3	D48.1	D49.2
groin	C49.5	C79.89	—	D21.5	D48.1	D49.2
hand	C49.1-☑	C79.89	—	D21.1-☑	D48.1	D49.2
head	C49.Ø	C79.89	—	D21.Ø	D48.1	D49.2
heel	C49.2-☑	C79.89	—	D21.2-☑	D48.1	D49.2
hip	C49.2-☑	C79.89	—	D21.2-☑	D48.1	D49.2
hypochondrium	C49.4	C79.89	—	D21.4	D48.1	D49.2
iliopsoas muscle	C49.5	C79.89	—	D21.5	D48.1	D49.2
infraclavicular region	C49.3	C79.89	—	D21.3	D48.1	D49.2
inguinal (canal) (region)	C49.5	C79.89	—	D21.5	D48.1	D49.2
intestinal	C49.4	C79.89	—	D21.4	D48.1	D49.2
intrathoracic	C49.3	C79.89	—	D21.3	D48.1	D49.2
ischiorectal fossa	C49.5	C79.89	—	D21.5	D48.1	D49.2
jaw	CØ3.9	C79.89	DØØ.Ø3	D1Ø.39	D48.1	D49.Ø
knee	C49.2-☑	C79.89	—	D21.2-☑	D48.1	D49.2
leg	C49.2-☑	C79.89	—	D21.2-☑	D48.1	D49.2
limb NEC	C49.9	C79.89	—	D21.9	D48.1	D49.2
lower	C49.2-☑	C79.89	—	D21.2-☑	D48.1	D49.2
upper	C49.1-☑	C79.89	—	D21.1-☑	D48.1	D49.2
nates	C49.5	C79.89	—	D21.5	D48.1	D49.2
neck	C49.Ø	C79.89	—	D21.Ø	D48.1	D49.2
orbit	C69.6-☑	C79.49	DØ9.2-☑	D31.6-☑	D48.1	D49.89
overlapping lesion	C49.8	—	—	—	—	—
pararectal	C49.5	C79.89	—	D21.5	D48.1	D49.2
para-urethral	C49.5	C79.89	—	D21.5	D48.1	D49.2
paravaginal	C49.5	C79.89	—	D21.5	D48.1	D49.2
pelvis (floor)	C49.5	C79.89	—	D21.5	D48.1	D49.2
pelvo-abdominal	C49.8	C79.89	—	D21.6	D48.1	D49.2
perineum	C49.5	C79.89	—	D21.5	D48.1	D49.2
perirectal (tissue)	C49.5	C79.89	—	D21.5	D48.1	D49.2

	Malignant Primary	Malignant Secondary	Ca in situ	Benign	Uncertain	Unspecified Behavior
Neoplasm, neoplastic — *continued*						
connective tissue — *continued*						
periurethral (tissue)	C49.5	C79.89	—	D21.5	D48.1	D49.2
popliteal fossa or space	C49.2-☑	C79.89	—	D21.2-☑	D48.1	D49.2
presacral	C49.5	C79.89	—	D21.5	D48.1	D49.2
psoas muscle	C49.4	C79.89	—	D21.4	D48.1	D49.2
pterygoid fossa	C49.Ø	C79.89	—	D21.Ø	D48.1	D49.2
rectovaginal septum or wall	C49.5	C79.89	—	D21.5	D48.1	D49.2
rectovesical	C49.5	C79.89	—	D21.5	D48.1	D49.2
retroperitoneum	C48.Ø	C78.6	—	D2Ø.Ø	D48.3	D49.Ø
sacrococcygeal region	C49.5	C79.89	—	D21.5	D48.1	D49.2
scalp	C49.Ø	C79.89	—	D21.Ø	D48.1	D49.2
scapular region	C49.3	C79.89	—	D21.3	D48.1	D49.2
shoulder	C49.1-☑	C79.89	—	D21.1-☑	D48.1	D49.2
skin (dermis) NEC — *see also* Neoplasm, skin, by site	C44.9Ø	C79.2	DØ4.9	D23.9	D48.5	D49.2
stomach	C49.4	C79.89	—	D21.4	D48.1	D49.2
submental	C49.Ø	C79.89	—	D21.Ø	D48.1	D49.2
supraclavicular region	C49.Ø	C79.89	—	D21.Ø	D48.1	D49.2
temple	C49.Ø	C79.89	—	D21.Ø	D48.1	D49.2
temporal region	C49.Ø	C79.89	—	D21.Ø	D48.1	D49.2
thigh	C49.2-☑	C79.89	—	D21.2-☑	D48.1	D49.2
thoracic (duct) (wall)	C49.3	C79.89	—	D21.3	D48.1	D49.2
thorax	C49.3	C79.89	—	D21.3	D48.1	D49.2
thumb	C49.1-☑	C79.89	—	D21.1-☑	D48.1	D49.2
toe	C49.2-☑	C79.89	—	D21.2-☑	D48.1	D49.2
trunk	C49.6	C79.89	—	D21.6	D48.1	D49.2
umbilicus	C49.4	C79.89	—	D21.4	D48.1	D49.2
vesicorectal	C49.5	C79.89	—	D21.5	D48.1	D49.2
wrist	C49.1-☑	C79.89	—	D21.1-☑	D48.1	D49.2
conus medullaris	C72.Ø	C79.49	—	D33.4	D43.4	D49.7
cord (true) (vocal)	C32.Ø	C78.39	DØ2.Ø	D14.1	D38.Ø	D49.1
false	C32.1	C78.39	DØ2.Ø	D14.1	D38.Ø	D49.1
spermatic	C63.1-☑	C79.82	DØ7.69	D29.8	D4Ø.8	D49.5
spinal (cervical) (lumbar) (thoracic)	C72.Ø	C79.49	—	D33.4	D43.4	D49.7
cornea (limbus)	C69.1-☑	C79.49	DØ9.2-☑	D31.1-☑	D48.7	D49.89
corpus						
albicans	C56.-☑	C79.6-☑	DØ7.39	D27.-☑	D39.1-☑	D49.5
callosum, brain	C71.Ø	C79.31	—	D33.2	D43.2	D49.6
cavernosum	C6Ø.2	C79.82	DØ7.4	D29.Ø	D4Ø.8	D49.5
gastric	C16.2	C78.89	DØØ.2	D13.1	D37.1	D49.Ø
overlapping sites	C54.8	—	—	—	—	—
penis	C6Ø.2	C79.82	DØ7.4	D29.Ø	D4Ø.8	D49.5
striatum, cerebrum	C71.Ø	C79.31	—	D33.Ø	D43.Ø	D49.6
uteri	C54.9	C79.82	DØ7.Ø	D26.1	D39.Ø	D49.5
isthmus	C54.Ø	C79.82	DØ7.Ø	D26.1	D39.Ø	D49.5
cortex						
adrenal	C74.Ø-☑	C79.7-☑	DØ9.3	D35.Ø-☑	D44.1-☑	D49.7
cerebral	C71.Ø	C79.31	—	D33.Ø	D43.Ø	D49.6
costal cartilage	C41.3	C79.51	—	D16.7	D48.Ø	D49.2
costovertebral joint	C41.3	C79.51	—	D16.7	D48.Ø	D49.2
Cowper's gland	C68.Ø	C79.19	DØ9.19	D3Ø.4	D41.3	D49.5
cranial (fossa, any)	C71.9	C79.31	—	D33.2	D43.2	D49.6
meninges	C7Ø.Ø	C79.32	—	D32.Ø	D42.Ø	D49.7
nerve	C72.5Ø	C79.49	—	D33.3	D43.3	D49.7
specified NEC	C72.59	C79.49	—	D33.3	D43.3	D49.7
craniobuccal pouch	C75.2	C79.89	DØ9.3	D35.2	D44.3	D49.7
craniopharyngeal (duct) (pouch)	C75.2	C79.89	DØ9.3	D35.3	D44.4	D49.7
cricoid	C13.Ø	C79.89	DØØ.Ø8	D1Ø.7	D37.Ø5	D49.Ø
cartilage	C32.3	C78.39	DØ2.Ø	D14.1	D38.Ø	D49.1
cricopharynx	C13.Ø	C79.89	DØØ.Ø8	D1Ø.7	D37.Ø5	D49.Ø
crypt of Morgagni	C21.8	C78.5	DØ1.3	D12.9	D37.8	D49.Ø
crystalline lens	C69.4-☑	C79.49	DØ9.2-☑	D31.4-☑	D48.7	D49.89
cul-de-sac (Douglas')	C48.1	C78.6	—	D2Ø.1	D48.4	D49.Ø
cuneiform cartilage	C32.3	C78.39	DØ2.Ø	D14.1	D38.Ø	D49.1
cutaneous — *see* Neoplasm, skin						
cutis — *see* Neoplasm, skin						
Neoplasm, neoplastic — *continued*						
cystic (bile) duct (common)	C24.Ø	C78.89	DØ1.5	D13.5	D37.6	D49.Ø
dermis — *see* Neoplasm, skin						
diaphragm	C49.3	C79.89	—	D21.3	D48.1	D49.2
digestive organs, system, tube, or tract NEC	C26.9	C78.89	DØ1.9	D13.9	D37.9	D49.Ø
disc, intervertebral	C41.2	C79.51	—	D16.6	D48.Ø	D49.2
disease, generalized	C8Ø.Ø	—	—	—	—	—
disseminated	C8Ø.Ø	—	—	—	—	—
Douglas' cul-de-sac or pouch	C48.1	C78.6	—	D2Ø.1	D48.4	D49.Ø
duodenojejunal junction	C17.8	C78.4	DØ1.49	D13.39	D37.2	D49.Ø
duodenum	C17.Ø	C78.4	DØ1.49	D13.2	D37.2	D49.Ø
dura (cranial) (mater)	C7Ø.9	C79.49	—	D32.9	D42.9	D49.7
cerebral	C7Ø.Ø	C79.32	—	D32.Ø	D42.Ø	D49.7
spinal	C7Ø.1	C79.49	—	D32.1	D42.1	D49.7
ear (external) — *see also* Neoplasm, skin, ear	C44.2Ø-☑	C79.2	DØ4.2-☑	D23.2-☑	D48.5	D49.2
auricle or auris — *see also* Neoplasm, skin, ear	C44.2Ø-☑	C79.2	DØ4.2-☑	D23.2-☑	D48.5	D49.2
canal, external — *see also* Neoplasm, skin, ear	C44.2Ø-☑	C79.2	DØ4.2-☑	D23.2-☑	D48.5	D49.2
cartilage	C49.Ø	C79.89	—	D21.Ø	D48.1	D49.2
external meatus — *see also* Neoplasm, skin, ear	C44.2Ø-☑	C79.2	DØ4.2-☑	D23.2-☑	D48.5	D49.2
inner	C3Ø.1	C78.39	DØ2.3	D14.Ø	D38.5	D49.1
lobule — *see also* Neoplasm, skin, ear	C44.2Ø-☑	C79.2	DØ4.2-☑	D23.2-☑	D48.5	D49.2
middle	C3Ø.1	C78.39	DØ2.3	D14.Ø	D38.5	D49.1
overlapping lesion with accessory sinuses	C31.8	—	—	—	—	—
skin	C44.2Ø-☑	C79.2	DØ4.2-☑	D23.2-☑	D48.5	D49.2
basal cell carcinoma	C44.21-☑	—	—	—	—	—
specified type NEC	C44.29-☑	—	—	—	—	—
squamous cell carcinoma	C44.22-☑	—	—	—	—	—
earlobe	C44.2Ø-☑	C79.2	DØ4.2-☑	D23.2-☑	D48.5	D49.2
basal cell carcinoma	C44.21-☑	—	—	—	—	—
specified type NEC	C44.29-☑	—	—	—	—	—
squamous cell carcinoma	C44.22-☑	—	—	—	—	—
ejaculatory duct	C63.7	C79.82	DØ7.69	D29.8	D4Ø.8	D49.5
elbow NEC	C76.4-☑	C79.89	DØ4.6-☑	D36.7	D48.7	D49.89
endocardium	C38.Ø	C79.89	—	D15.1	D48.7	D49.89
endocervix (canal) (gland)	C53.Ø	C79.82	DØ6.Ø	D26.Ø	D39.Ø	D49.5
endocrine gland NEC	C75.9	C79.89	DØ9.3	D35.9	D44.9	D49.7
pluriglandular	C75.8	C79.89	DØ9.3	D35.7	D44.9	D49.7
endometrium (gland) (stroma)	C54.1	C79.82	DØ7.Ø	D26.1	D39.Ø	D49.5
ensiform cartilage	C41.3	C79.51	—	D16.7	D48.Ø	D49.2
enteric — *see* Neoplasm, intestine						
ependyma (brain)	C71.5	C79.31	—	D33.Ø	D43.Ø	D49.6
fourth ventricle	C71.7	C79.31	—	D33.1	D43.1	D49.6
epicardium	C38.Ø	C79.89	—	D15.1	D48.7	D49.89
epididymis	C63.Ø-☑	C79.82	DØ7.69	D29.3-☑	D4Ø.8	D49.5
epidural	C72.9	C79.49	—	D33.9	D43.9	D49.7
epiglottis	C32.1	C78.39	DØ2.Ø	D14.1	D38.Ø	D49.1
anterior aspect or surface	C1Ø.1	C79.89	DØØ.Ø8	D1Ø.5	D37.Ø5	D49.Ø
cartilage	C32.3	C78.39	DØ2.Ø	D14.1	D38.Ø	D49.1
free border (margin)	C1Ø.1	C79.89	DØØ.Ø8	D1Ø.5	D37.Ø5	D49.Ø
junctional region	C1Ø.8	C79.89	DØØ.Ø8	D1Ø.5	D37.Ø5	D49.Ø
posterior (laryngeal) surface	C32.1	C78.39	DØ2.Ø	D14.1	D38.Ø	D49.1

	Malignant Primary	Malignant Secondary	Ca in situ	Benign	Uncertain	Unspecified Behavior
Neoplasm, neoplastic — *continued*						
epiglottis — *continued*						
suprahyoid portion	C32.1	C78.39	DØ2.Ø	D14.1	D38.Ø	D49.1
esophagogastric junction	C16.Ø	C78.89	DØØ.2	D13.1	D37.1	D49.Ø
esophagus	C15.9	C78.89	DØØ.1	D13.Ø	D37.8	D49.Ø
abdominal	C15.5	C78.89	DØØ.1	D13.Ø	D37.8	D49.Ø
cervical	C15.3	C78.89	DØØ.1	D13.Ø	D37.8	D49.Ø
distal (third)	C15.5	C78.89	DØØ.1	D13.Ø	D37.8	D49.Ø
lower (third)	C15.5	C78.89	DØØ.1	D13.Ø	D37.8	D49.Ø
middle (third)	C15.4	C78.89	DØØ.1	D13.Ø	D37.8	D49.Ø
overlapping lesion	C15.8	—	—	—	—	—
proximal (third)	C15.3	C78.89	DØØ.1	D13.Ø	D37.8	D49.Ø
thoracic	C15.4	C78.89	DØØ.1	D13.Ø	D37.8	D49.Ø
upper (third)	C15.3	C78.89	DØØ.1	D13.Ø	D37.8	D49.Ø
ethmoid (sinus)	C31.1	C78.39	DØ2.3	D14.Ø	D38.5	D49.1
bone or labyrinth	C41.Ø	C79.51	—	D16.4	D48.Ø	D49.2
eustachian tube	C3Ø.1	C78.39	DØ2.3	D14.Ø	D38.5	D49.1
exocervix	C53.1	C79.82	DØ6.1	D26.Ø	D39.Ø	D49.5
external						
meatus (ear) — *see also* Neoplasm, skin, ear	C44.2Ø-☑	C79.2	DØ4.2-☑	D23.2-☑	D48.5	D49.2
os, cervix uteri	C53.1	C79.82	DØ6.1	D26.Ø	D39.Ø	D49.5
extradural	C72.9	C79.49	—	D33.9	D43.9	D49.7
extrahepatic (bile) duct	C24.Ø	C78.89	DØ1.5	D13.5	D37.6	D49.Ø
overlapping lesion with gallbladder	C24.8	—	—	—	—	—
extraocular muscle	C69.6-☑	C79.49	DØ9.2-☑	D31.6-☑	D48.7	D49.89
extrarectal	C76.3	C79.89	DØ9.8	D36.7	D48.7	D49.89
extremity	C76.8	C79.89	DØ4.8	D36.7	D48.7	D49.89
lower	C76.5-☑	C79.89	DØ4.7-☑	D36.7	D48.7	D49.89
upper	C76.4-☑	C79.89	DØ4.6-☑	D36.7	D48.7	D49.89
eyeball	C69.9-☑	C79.49	DØ9.2-☑	D31.9-☑	D48.7	D49.89
eyebrow	C44.3Ø9	C79.2	DØ4.39	D23.39	D48.5	D49.2
basal cell carcinoma	C44.319	—	—	—	—	—
specified type NEC	C44.399	—	—	—	—	—
squamous cell carcinoma	C44.329	—	—	—	—	—
eyelid (lower) (skin) (upper)	C44.1Ø-☑	—	—	—	—	—
basal cell carcinoma	C44.11-☑	—	—	—	—	—
cartilage	C49.Ø	C79.89	—	D21.Ø	D48.1	D49.2
specified type NEC	C44.19-☑	—	—	—	—	—
squamous cell carcinoma	C44.12-☑	—	—	—	—	—
eye NEC	C69.9-☑	C79.49	DØ9.2-☑	D31.9-☑	D48.7	D49.89
overlapping sites	C69.8-☑	—	—	—	—	—
face NEC	C76.Ø	C79.89	DØ4.39	D36.7	D48.7	D49.89
fallopian tube (accessory)	C57.Ø-☑	C79.82	DØ7.39	D28.2	D39.8	D49.5
falx (cerebella) (cerebri)	C7Ø.Ø	C79.32	—	D32.Ø	D42.Ø	D49.7
fascia — *see also* Neoplasm, connective tissue						
palmar	C49.1-☑	C79.89	—	D21.1-☑	D48.1	D49.2
plantar	C49.2-☑	C79.89	—	D21.2-☑	D48.1	D49.2
fatty tissue — *see* Neoplasm, connective tissue						
fauces, faucial NEC	C1Ø.9	C79.89	DØØ.Ø8	D1Ø.5	D37.Ø5	D49.Ø
pillars	CØ9.1	C79.89	DØØ.Ø8	D1Ø.5	D37.Ø5	D49.Ø
tonsil	CØ9.9	C79.89	DØØ.Ø8	D1Ø.4	D37.Ø5	D49.Ø
femur (any part)	C4Ø.2-☑	—	—	D16.2-☑	—	—
fetal membrane	C58	C79.82	DØ7.Ø	D26.7	D39.2	D49.5
fibrous tissue — *see* Neoplasm, connective tissue						
fibula (any part)	C4Ø.2-☑	C79.51	—	D16.2-☑	—	—
filum terminale	C72.Ø	C79.49	—	D33.4	D43.4	D49.7
finger NEC	C76.4-☑	C79.89	DØ4.6-☑	D36.7	D48.7	D49.89
flank NEC	C76.8	C79.89	DØ4.5	D36.7	D48.7	D49.89
follicle, nabothian	C53.Ø	C79.82	DØ6.Ø	D26.Ø	D39.Ø	D49.5
foot NEC	C76.5-☑	C79.89	DØ4.7-☑	D36.7	D48.7	D49.89
forearm NEC	C76.4-☑	C79.89	DØ4.6-☑	D36.7	D48.7	D49.89
forehead (skin)	C44.3Ø9	C79.2	DØ4.39	D23.39	D48.5	D49.2

	Malignant Primary	Malignant Secondary	Ca in situ	Benign	Uncertain	Unspecified Behavior
Neoplasm, neoplastic — *continued*						
forehead — *continued*						
basal cell carcinoma	C44.319	—	—	—	—	—
specified type NEC	C44.399	—	—	—	—	—
squamous cell carcinoma	C44.329	—	—	—	—	—
foreskin	C6Ø.Ø	C79.82	DØ7.4	D29.Ø	D4Ø.8	D49.5
fornix						
pharyngeal	C11.3	C79.89	DØØ.Ø8	D1Ø.6	D37.Ø5	D49.Ø
vagina	C52	C79.82	DØ7.2	D28.1	D39.8	D49.5
fossa (of)						
anterior (cranial)	C71.9	C79.31	—	D33.2	D43.2	D49.6
cranial	C71.9	C79.31	—	D33.2	D43.2	D49.6
ischiorectal	C76.3	C79.89	DØ9.8	D36.7	D48.7	D49.89
middle (cranial)	C71.9	C79.31	—	D33.2	D43.2	D49.6
piriform	C12	C79.89	DØØ.Ø8	D1Ø.7	D37.Ø5	D49.Ø
pituitary	C75.1	C79.89	DØ9.3	D35.2	D44.3	D49.7
posterior (cranial)	C71.9	C79.31	—	D33.2	D43.2	D49.6
pterygoid	C49.Ø	C79.89	—	D21.Ø	D48.1	D49.2
pyriform	C12	C79.89	DØØ.Ø8	D1Ø.7	D37.Ø5	D49.Ø
Rosenmuller	C11.2	C79.89	DØØ.Ø8	D1Ø.6	D37.Ø5	D49.Ø
tonsillar	CØ9.Ø	C79.89	DØØ.Ø8	D1Ø.5	D37.Ø5	D49.Ø
fourchette	C51.9	C79.82	DØ7.1	D28.Ø	D39.8	D49.5
frenulum						
labii — *see* Neoplasm, lip, internal						
linguae	CØ2.2	C79.89	DØØ.Ø7	D1Ø.1	D37.Ø2	D49.Ø
frontal						
bone	C41.Ø	C79.51	—	D16.4	D48.Ø	D49.2
lobe, brain	C71.1	C79.31	—	D33.Ø	D43.Ø	D49.6
pole	C71.1	C79.31	—	D33.Ø	D43.Ø	D49.6
sinus	C31.2	C78.39	DØ2.3	D14.Ø	D38.5	D49.1
fundus						
stomach	C16.1	C78.89	DØØ.2	D13.1	D37.1	D49.Ø
uterus	C54.3	C79.82	DØ7.Ø	D26.1	D39.Ø	D49.5
gallbladder	C23	C78.89	DØ1.5	D13.5	D37.6	D49.Ø
overlapping lesion with extrahepatic bile ducts	C24.8	—	—	—	—	—
gall duct (extrahepatic)	C24.Ø	C78.89	DØ1.5	D13.5	D37.6	D49.Ø
intrahepatic	C22.1	C78.7	DØ1.5	D13.4	D37.6	D49.Ø
ganglia — *see also* Neoplasm, nerve, peripheral	C47.9	C79.89	—	D36.1Ø	D48.2	D49.2
basal	C71.Ø	C79.31	—	D33.Ø	D43.Ø	D49.6
cranial nerve	C72.5Ø	C79.49	—	D33.3	D43.3	D49.7
Gartner's duct	C52	C79.82	DØ7.2	D28.1	D39.8	D49.5
gastric — *see* Neoplasm, stomach						
gastrocolic	C26.9	C78.89	DØ1.9	D13.9	D37.9	D49.Ø
gastroesophageal junction	C16.Ø	C78.89	DØØ.2	D13.1	D37.1	D49.Ø
gastrointestinal (tract) NEC	C26.9	C78.89	DØ1.9	D13.9	D37.9	D49.Ø
generalized	C8Ø.Ø	—	—	—	—	—
genital organ or tract						
female NEC	C57.9	C79.82	DØ7.3Ø	D28.9	D39.9	D49.5
overlapping lesion	C57.8	—	—	—	—	—
specified site NEC	C57.7	C79.82	DØ7.39	D28.7	D39.8	D49.5
male NEC	C63.9	C79.82	DØ7.6Ø	D29.9	D4Ø.9	D49.5
overlapping lesion	C63.8	—	—	—	—	—
specified site NEC	C63.7	C79.82	DØ7.69	D29.8	D4Ø.8	D49.5
genitourinary tract						
female	C57.9	C79.82	DØ7.3Ø	D28.9	D39.9	D49.5
male	C63.9	C79.82	DØ7.6Ø	D29.9	D4Ø.9	D49.5
gingiva (alveolar) (marginal)	CØ3.9	C79.89	DØØ.Ø3	D1Ø.39	D37.Ø9	D49.Ø
lower	CØ3.1	C79.89	DØØ.Ø3	D1Ø.39	D37.Ø9	D49.Ø
mandibular	CØ3.1	C79.89	DØØ.Ø3	D1Ø.39	D37.Ø9	D49.Ø
maxillary	CØ3.Ø	C79.89	DØØ.Ø3	D1Ø.39	D37.Ø9	D49.Ø
upper	CØ3.Ø	C79.89	DØØ.Ø3	D1Ø.39	D37.Ø9	D49.Ø
gland, glandular (lymphatic) (system) — *see also* Neoplasm, lymph gland						
endocrine NEC	C75.9	C79.89	DØ9.3	D35.9	D44.9	D49.7

	Malignant Primary	Malignant Secondary	Ca in situ	Benign	Uncertain	Unspecified Behavior
Neoplasm, neoplastic — *continued*						
gland, glandular — *see also* Neoplasm, lymph gland — *continued*						
salivary — *see* Neoplasm, salivary gland						
glans penis	C60.1	C79.82	D07.4	D29.0	D40.8	D49.5
globus pallidus	C71.0	C79.31	—	D33.0	D43.0	D49.6
glomus						
coccygeal	C49.5	C79.89	—	D21.5	D48.1	D49.2
jugularis	C75.5	C79.89	—	D35.6	D44.7	D49.7
glosso-epiglottic fold(s)	C10.1	C79.89	D00.08	D10.5	D37.05	D49.0
glossopalatine fold	C09.1	C79.89	D00.08	D10.5	D37.05	D49.0
glossopharyngeal sulcus	C09.0	C79.89	D00.08	D10.5	D37.05	D49.0
glottis	C32.0	C78.39	D02.0	D14.1	D38.0	D49.1
gluteal region	C76.3	C79.89	D04.5	D36.7	D48.7	D49.89
great vessels NEC	C49.3	C79.89	—	D21.3	D48.1	D49.2
groin NEC	C76.3	C79.89	D04.5	D36.7	D48.7	D49.89
gum	C03.9	C79.89	D00.03	D10.39	D37.09	D49.0
lower	C03.1	C79.89	D00.03	D10.39	D37.09	D49.0
upper	C03.0	C79.89	D00.03	D10.39	D37.09	D49.0
hand NEC	C76.4-☑	C79.89	D04.6-☑	D36.7	D48.7	D49.89
head NEC	C76.0	C79.89	D04.4	D36.7	D48.7	D49.89
heart	C38.0	C79.89	—	D15.1	D48.7	D49.89
heel NEC	C76.5-☑	C79.89	D04.7-☑	D36.7	D48.7	D49.89
helix — *see also* Neoplasm, skin, ear	C44.20-☑	C79.2	D04.2-☑	D23.2-☑	D48.5	D49.2
hematopoietic, hemopoietic tissue NEC	C96.9	—	—	—	—	—
specified NEC	C96.Z	—	—	—	—	—
hemisphere, cerebral	C71.0	C79.31	—	D33.0	D43.0	D49.6
hemorrhoidal zone	C21.1	C78.5	D01.3	D12.9	D37.8	D49.0
hepatic — *see also* Index to disease, by histology	C22.9	C78.7	D01.5	D13.4	D37.6	D49.0
duct (bile)	C24.0	C78.89	D01.5	D13.5	D37.6	D49.0
flexure (colon)	C18.3	C78.5	D01.0	D12.3	D37.4	D49.0
primary	C22.8	C78.7	D01.5	D13.4	D37.6	D49.0
hepatobiliary	C24.9	C78.89	D01.5	D13.5	D37.6	D49.0
hepatoblastoma	C22.2	C78.7	D01.5	D13.4	D37.6	D49.0
hepatoma	C22.0	C78.7	D01.5	D13.4	D37.6	D49.0
hilus of lung	C34.0-☑	C78.0-☑	D02.2-☑	D14.3-☑	D38.1	D49.1
hippocampus, brain	C71.2	C79.31	—	D33.0	D43.0	D49.6
hip NEC	C76.5-☑	C79.89	D04.7-☑	D36.7	D48.7	D49.89
humerus (any part)	C40.0-☑	C79.51	—	D16.0-☑	—	—
hymen	C52	C79.82	D07.2	D28.1	D39.8	D49.5
hypopharynx, hypopharyngeal NEC	C13.9	C79.89	D00.08	D10.7	D37.05	D49.0
overlapping lesion	C13.8	—	—	—	—	—
postcricoid region	C13.0	C79.89	D00.08	D10.7	D37.05	D49.0
posterior wall	C13.2	C79.89	D00.08	D10.7	D37.05	D49.0
pyriform fossa (sinus)	C12	C79.89	D00.08	D10.7	D37.05	D49.0
hypophysis	C75.1	C79.89	D09.3	D35.2	D44.3	D49.7
hypothalamus	C71.0	C79.31	—	D33.0	D43.0	D49.6
ileocecum, ileocecal (coil) (junction) (valve)	C18.0	C78.5	D01.0	D12.0	D37.4	D49.0
ileum	C17.2	C78.4	D01.49	D13.39	D37.2	D49.0
ilium	C41.4	C79.51	—	D16.8	D48.0	D49.2
immunoproliferative NEC	C88.9	—	—	—	—	—
infraclavicular (region)	C76.1	C79.89	D04.5	D36.7	D48.7	D49.89
inguinal (region)	C76.3	C79.89	D04.5	D36.7	D48.7	D49.89
insula	C71.0	C79.31	—	D33.0	D43.0	D49.6
insular tissue (pancreas)	C25.4	C78.89	D01.7	D13.7	D37.8	D49.0
brain	C71.0	C79.31	—	D33.0	D43.0	D49.6
interarytenoid fold	C13.1	C78.39	D00.08	D10.7	D37.05	D49.0
hypopharyngeal aspect	C13.1	C79.89	D00.08	D10.7	D37.05	D49.0
laryngeal aspect	C32.1	C78.39	D02.0	D14.1	D38.0	D49.1
marginal zone	C13.1	C79.89	D00.08	D10.7	D37.05	D49.0
interdental papillae	C03.9	C79.89	D00.03	D10.39	D37.09	D49.0

	Malignant Primary	Malignant Secondary	Ca in situ	Benign	Uncertain	Unspecified Behavior
Neoplasm, neoplastic — *continued*						
interdental papillae — *continued*						
lower	C03.1	C79.89	D00.03	D10.39	D37.09	D49.0
upper	C03.0	C79.89	D00.03	D10.39	D37.09	D49.0
internal						
capsule	C71.0	C79.31	—	D33.0	D43.0	D49.6
os (cervix)	C53.0	C79.82	D06.0	D26.0	D39.0	D49.5
intervertebral cartilage or disc	C41.2	C79.51	—	D16.6	D48.0	D49.2
intestine, intestinal	C26.0	C78.80	D01.40	D13.9	D37.8	D49.0
large	C18.9	C78.5	D01.0	D12.6	D37.4	D49.0
appendix	C18.1	C78.5	D01.0	D12.1	D37.3	D49.0
caput coli	C18.0	C78.5	D01.0	D12.0	D37.4	D49.0
cecum	C18.0	C78.5	D01.0	D12.0	D37.4	D49.0
colon	C18.9	C78.5	D01.0	D12.6	D37.4	D49.0
and rectum	C19	C78.5	D01.1	D12.7	D37.5	D49.0
ascending	C18.2	C78.5	D01.0	D12.2	D37.4	D49.0
caput	C18.0	C78.5	D01.0	D12.0	D37.4	D49.0
descending	C18.6	C78.5	D01.0	D12.4	D37.4	D49.0
distal	C18.6	C78.5	D01.0	D12.4	D37.4	D49.0
left	C18.6	C78.5	D01.0	D12.4	D37.4	D49.0
overlapping lesion	C18.8	—	—	—	—	—
pelvic	C18.7	C78.5	D01.0	D12.5	D37.4	D49.0
right	C18.2	C78.5	D01.0	D12.2	D37.4	D49.0
sigmoid (flexure)	C18.7	C78.5	D01.0	D12.5	D37.4	D49.0
transverse	C18.4	C78.5	D01.0	D12.3	D37.4	D49.0
hepatic flexure	C18.3	C78.5	D01.0	D12.3	D37.4	D49.0
ileocecum, ileocecal (coil) (valve)	C18.0	C78.5	D01.0	D12.0	D37.4	D49.0
overlapping lesion	C18.8	—	—	—	—	—
sigmoid flexure (lower) (upper)	C18.7	C78.5	D01.0	D12.5	D37.4	D49.0
splenic flexure	C18.5	C78.5	D01.0	D12.3	D37.4	D49.0
small	C17.9	C78.4	D01.40	D13.30	D37.2	D49.0
duodenum	C17.0	C78.4	D01.49	D13.2	D37.2	D49.0
ileum	C17.2	C78.4	D01.49	D13.39	D37.2	D49.0
jejunum	C17.1	C78.4	D01.49	D13.39	D37.2	D49.0
overlapping lesion	C17.8	—	—	—	—	—
tract NEC	C26.0	C78.89	D01.40	D13.9	D37.8	D49.0
intra-abdominal	C76.2	C79.89	D09.8	D36.7	D48.7	D49.89
intracranial NEC	C71.9	C79.31	—	D33.2	D43.2	D49.6
intrahepatic (bile) duct	C22.1	C78.7	D01.5	D13.4	D37.6	D49.0
intraocular	C69.9-☑	C79.49	D09.2-☑	D31.9-☑	D48.7	D49.89
intraorbital	C69.6-☑	C79.49	D09.2-☑	D31.6-☑	D48.7	D49.89
intrasellar	C75.1	C79.89	D09.3	D35.2	D44.3	D49.7
intrathoracic (cavity) (organs)	C76.1	C79.89	D09.8	D15.9	D48.7	D49.89
specified NEC	C76.1	C79.89	D09.8	D15.7	—	—
iris	C69.4-☑	C79.49	D09.2-☑	D31.4-☑	D48.7	D49.89
ischiorectal (fossa)	C76.3	C79.89	D09.8	D36.7	D48.7	D49.89
ischium	C41.4	C79.51	—	D16.8	D48.0	D49.2
island of Reil	C71.0	C79.31	—	D33.0	D43.0	D49.6
islands or islets of Langerhans	C25.4	C78.89	D01.7	D13.7	D37.8	D49.0
isthmus uteri	C54.0	C79.82	D07.0	D26.1	D39.0	D49.5
jaw	C76.0	C79.89	D09.8	D36.7	D48.7	D49.89
bone	C41.1	C79.51	—	D16.5	D48.0	D49.2
lower	C41.1	C79.51	—	D16.5	—	—
upper	C41.0	C79.51	—	D16.4	—	—
carcinoma (any type) (lower) (upper)	C76.0	C79.89	—	—	—	—
skin — *see also* Neoplasm, skin, face	C44.309	C79.2	D04.39	D23.39	D48.5	D49.2
soft tissues	C03.9	C79.89	D00.03	D10.39	D37.09	D49.0
lower	C03.1	C79.89	D00.03	D10.39	D37.09	D49.0
upper	C03.0	C79.89	D00.03	D10.39	D37.09	D49.0
jejunum	C17.1	C78.4	D01.49	D13.39	D37.2	D49.0
joint NEC — *see also* Neoplasm, bone	C41.9	C79.51	—	D16.9	D48.0	D49.2
acromioclavicular	C40.0-☑	C79.51	—	D16.0-☑	—	—
bursa or synovial membrane — *see*						

	Malignant Primary	Malignant Secondary	Ca in situ	Benign	Uncertain	Unspecified Behavior
Neoplasm, neoplastic — *continued*						
joint — *see also* Neoplasm, bone — *continued*						
bursa or synovial membrane — *see* Neoplasm, connective tissue — *continued* Neoplasm, connective tissue						
costovertebral	C41.3	C79.51	—	D16.7	D48.Ø	D49.2
sternocostal	C41.3	C79.51	—	D16.7	D48.Ø	D49.2
temporomandibular	C41.1	C79.51	—	D16.5	D48.Ø	D49.2
junction						
anorectal	C21.8	C78.5	DØ1.3	D12.9	D37.8	D49.Ø
cardioesophageal	C16.Ø	C78.89	DØØ.2	D13.1	D37.1	D49.Ø
esophagogastric	C16.Ø	C78.89	DØØ.2	D13.1	D37.1	D49.Ø
gastroesophageal	C16.Ø	C78.89	DØØ.2	D13.1	D37.1	D49.Ø
hard and soft palate	CØ5.9	C79.89	DØØ.ØØ	D1Ø.39	D37.Ø9	D49.Ø
ileocecal	C18.Ø	C78.5	DØ1.Ø	D12.Ø	D37.4	D49.Ø
pelvirectal	C19	C78.5	DØ1.1	D12.7	D37.5	D49.Ø
pelviureteric	C65.-☑	C79.Ø-☑	DØ9.19	D3Ø.1-☑	D41.1-☑	D49.5
rectosigmoid	C19	C78.5	DØ1.1	D12.7	D37.5	D49.Ø
squamocolumnar, of cervix	C53.8	C79.82	DØ6.7	D26.Ø	D39.Ø	D49.5
Kaposi's sarcoma — *see* Kaposi's, sarcoma						
kidney (parenchymal)	C64.-☑	C79.Ø-☑	DØ9.19	D3Ø.Ø-☑	D41.Ø-☑	D49.5
calyx	C65.-☑	C79.Ø-☑	DØ9.19	D3Ø.1-☑	D41.1-☑	D49.5
hilus	C65.-☑	C79.Ø-☑	DØ9.19	D3Ø.1-☑	D41.1-☑	D49.5
pelvis	C65.-☑	C79.Ø-☑	DØ9.19	D3Ø.1-☑	D41.1-☑	D49.5
knee NEC	C76.5-☑	C79.89	DØ4.7-☑	D36.7	D48.7	D49.89
labia (skin)	C51.9	C79.82	DØ7.1	D28.Ø	D39.8	D49.5
majora	C51.Ø	C79.82	DØ7.1	D28.Ø	D39.8	D49.5
minora	C51.1	C79.82	DØ7.1	D28.Ø	D39.8	D49.5
labial — *see also* Neoplasm, lip	CØØ.9	C79.89	DØØ.Ø1	D1Ø.Ø	D37.Ø1	D49.Ø
sulcus (lower) (upper)	CØ6.1	C79.89	DØØ.Ø2	D1Ø.39	D37.Ø9	D49.Ø
labium (skin)	C51.9	C79.82	DØ7.1	D28.Ø	D39.8	D49.5
majus	C51.Ø	C79.82	DØ7.1	D28.Ø	D39.8	D49.5
minus	C51.1	C79.82	DØ7.1	D28.Ø	D39.8	D49.5
lacrimal						
canaliculi	C69.5-☑	C79.49	DØ9.2-☑	D31.5-☑	D48.7	D49.89
duct (nasal)	C69.5-☑	C79.49	DØ9.2-☑	D31.5-☑	D48.7	D49.89
gland	C69.5-☑	C79.49	DØ9.2-☑	D31.5-☑	D48.7	D49.89
punctum	C69.5-☑	C79.49	DØ9.2-☑	D31.5-☑	D48.7	D49.89
sac	C69.5-☑	C79.49	DØ9.2-☑	D31.5-☑	D48.7	D49.89
Langerhans, islands or islets	C25.4	C78.89	DØ1.7	D13.7	D37.8	D49.Ø
laryngopharynx	C13.9	C79.89	DØØ.Ø8	D1Ø.7	D37.Ø5	D49.Ø
larynx, laryngeal NEC	C32.9	C78.39	DØ2.Ø	D14.1	D38.Ø	D49.1
aryepiglottic fold	C32.1	C78.39	DØ2.Ø	D14.1	D38.Ø	D49.1
cartilage (arytenoid) (cricoid) (cuneiform) (thyroid)	C32.3	C78.39	DØ2.Ø	D14.1	D38.Ø	D49.1
commissure (anterior) (posterior)	C32.Ø	C78.39	DØ2.Ø	D14.1	D38.Ø	D49.1
extrinsic NEC	C32.1	C78.39	DØ2.Ø	D14.1	D38.Ø	D49.1
meaning hypopharynx	C13.9	C79.89	DØØ.Ø8	D1Ø.7	D37.Ø5	D49.Ø
interarytenoid fold	C32.1	C78.39	DØ2.Ø	D14.1	D38.Ø	D49.1
intrinsic	C32.Ø	C78.39	DØ2.Ø	D14.1	D38.Ø	D49.1
overlapping lesion	C32.8	—	—	—	—	—
ventricular band	C32.1	C78.39	DØ2.Ø	D14.1	D38.Ø	D49.1
leg NEC	C76.5-☑	C79.89	DØ4.7-☑	D36.7	D48.7	D49.89
lens, crystalline	C69.4-☑	C79.49	DØ9.2-☑	D31.4-☑	D48.7	D49.89
lid (lower) (upper)	C44.1Ø-☑	C79.2	DØ4.1-☑	D23.1-☑	D48.5	D49.2
basal cell carcinoma	C44.11-☑	—	—	—	—	—
specified type NEC	C44.19-☑	—	—	—	—	—
squamous cell carcinoma	C44.12-☑	—	—	—	—	—
ligament — *see also* Neoplasm, connective tissue						

	Malignant Primary	Malignant Secondary	Ca in situ	Benign	Uncertain	Unspecified Behavior
Neoplasm, neoplastic — *continued*						
ligament — *see also* Neoplasm, connective tissue — *continued*						
broad	C57.1-☑	C79.82	DØ7.39	D28.2	D39.8	D49.5
Mackenrodt's	C57.7	C79.82	DØ7.39	D28.7	D39.8	D49.5
non-uterine — *see* Neoplasm, connective tissue						
round	C57.2-☑	C79.82	—	D28.2	D39.8	D49.5
sacro-uterine	C57.3	C79.82	—	D28.2	D39.8	D49.5
uterine	C57.3	C79.82	—	D28.2	D39.8	D49.5
utero-ovarian	C57.7	C79.82	DØ7.39	D28.2	D39.8	D49.5
uterosacral	C57.3	C79.82	—	D28.2	D39.8	D49.5
limb	C76.8	C79.89	DØ4.8	D36.7	D48.7	D49.89
lower	C76.5-☑	C79.89	DØ4.7-☑	D36.7	D48.7	D49.89
upper	C76.4-☑	C79.89	DØ4.6-☑	D36.7	D48.7	D49.89
limbus of cornea	C69.1-☑	C79.49	DØ9.2-☑	D31.1-☑	D48.7	D49.89
lingual NEC — *see also* Neoplasm, tongue	CØ2.9	C79.89	DØØ.Ø7	D1Ø.1	D37.Ø2	D49.Ø
lingula, lung	C34.1-☑	C78.Ø-☑	DØ2.2-☑	D14.3-☑	D38.1	D49.1
lip	CØØ.9	C79.89	DØØ.Ø1	D1Ø.Ø	D37.Ø1	D49.Ø
buccal aspect — *see* Neoplasm, lip, internal						
commissure	CØØ.6	C79.89	DØØ.Ø1	D1Ø.Ø	D37.Ø1	D49.Ø
external	CØØ.2	C79.89	DØØ.Ø1	D1Ø.Ø	D37.Ø1	D49.Ø
lower	CØØ.1	C79.89	DØØ.Ø1	D1Ø.Ø	D37.Ø1	D49.Ø
upper	CØØ.Ø	C79.89	DØØ.Ø1	D1Ø.Ø	D37.Ø1	D49.Ø
frenulum — *see* Neoplasm, lip, internal						
inner aspect — *see* Neoplasm, lip, internal						
internal	CØØ.5	C79.89	DØØ.Ø1	D1Ø.Ø	D37.Ø1	D49.Ø
lower	CØØ.4	C79.89	DØØ.Ø1	D1Ø.Ø	D37.Ø1	D49.Ø
upper	CØØ.3	C79.89	DØØ.Ø1	D1Ø.Ø	D37.Ø1	D49.Ø
lipstick area	CØØ.2	C79.89	DØØ.Ø1	D1Ø.Ø	D37.Ø1	D49.Ø
lower	CØØ.1	C79.89	DØØ.Ø1	D1Ø.Ø	D37.Ø1	D49.Ø
upper	CØØ.Ø	C79.89	DØØ.Ø1	D1Ø.Ø	D37.Ø1	D49.Ø
lower	CØØ.1	C79.89	DØØ.Ø1	D1Ø.Ø	D37.Ø1	D49.Ø
internal	CØØ.4	C79.89	DØØ.Ø1	D1Ø.Ø	D37.Ø1	D49.Ø
mucosa — *see* Neoplasm, lip, internal						
oral aspect — *see* Neoplasm, lip, internal						
overlapping lesion	CØØ.8	—	—	—	—	—
with oral cavity or pharynx	C14.8	—	—	—	—	—
skin (commissure) (lower) (upper)	C44.ØØ	C79.2	DØ4.Ø	D23.Ø	D48.5	D49.2
basal cell carcinoma	C44.Ø1	—	—	—	—	—
specified type NEC	C44.Ø9	—	—	—	—	—
squamous cell carcinoma	C44.Ø2	—	—	—	—	—
upper	CØØ.Ø	C79.89	DØØ.Ø1	D1Ø.Ø	D37.Ø1	D49.Ø
internal	CØØ.3	C79.89	DØØ.Ø1	D1Ø.Ø	D37.Ø1	D49.Ø
vermilion border	CØØ.2	C79.89	DØØ.Ø1	D1Ø.Ø	D37.Ø1	D49.Ø
lower	CØØ.1	C79.89	DØØ.Ø1	D1Ø.Ø	D37.Ø1	D49.Ø
upper	CØØ.Ø	C79.89	DØØ.Ø1	D1Ø.Ø	D37.Ø1	D49.Ø
lipomatous — *see* Lipoma, by site						
liver — *see also* Index to disease, by histology	C22.9	C78.7	DØ1.5	D13.4	D37.6	D49.Ø
primary	C22.8	C78.7	DØ1.5	D13.4	D37.6	D49.Ø
lumbosacral plexus	C47.5	C79.89	—	D36.16	D48.2	D49.2
lung	C34.9-☑	C78.Ø-☑	DØ2.2-☑	D14.3-☑	D38.1	D49.1
azygos lobe	C34.1-☑	C78.Ø-☑	DØ2.2-☑	D14.3-☑	D38.1	D49.1
carina	C34.Ø-☑	C78.Ø-☑	DØ2.2-☑	D14.3-☑	D38.1	D49.1
hilus	C34.Ø-☑	C78.Ø-☑	DØ2.2-☑	D14.3-☑	D38.1	D49.1
lingula	C34.1-☑	C78.Ø-☑	DØ2.2-☑	D14.3-☑	D38.1	D49.1
lobe NEC	C34.9-☑	C78.Ø-☑	DØ2.2-☑	D14.3-☑	D38.1	D49.1
lower lobe	C34.3-☑	C78.Ø-☑	DØ2.2-☑	D14.3-☑	D38.1	D49.1

	Malignant Primary	Malignant Secondary	Ca in situ	Benign	Uncertain	Unspecified Behavior
Neoplasm, neoplastic — *continued*						
lung — *continued*						
main bronchus	C34.Ø-☑	C78.Ø-☑	DØ2.2-☑	D14.3-☑	D38.1	D49.1
mesothelioma — *see* Mesothelioma						
middle lobe	C34.2	C78.Ø-☑	DØ2.21	D14.31	D38.1	D49.1
overlapping lesion	C34.8-☑	—	—	—	—	—
upper lobe	C34.1-☑	C78.Ø-☑	DØ2.2-☑	D14.3-☑	D38.1	D49.1
lymph, lymphatic channel NEC	C49.9	C79.89	—	D21.9	D48.1	D49.2
gland (secondary)	—	C77.9	—	D36.Ø	D48.7	D49.89
abdominal	—	C77.2	—	D36.Ø	D48.7	D49.89
aortic	—	C77.2	—	D36.Ø	D48.7	D49.89
arm	—	C77.3	—	D36.Ø	D48.7	D49.89
auricular (anterior) (posterior)	—	C77.Ø	—	D36.Ø	D48.7	D49.89
axilla, axillary	—	C77.3	—	D36.Ø	D48.7	D49.89
brachial	—	C77.3	—	D36.Ø	D48.7	D49.89
bronchial	—	C77.1	—	D36.Ø	D48.7	D49.89
bronchopulmonary	—	C77.1	—	D36.Ø	D48.7	D49.89
celiac	—	C77.2	—	D36.Ø	D48.7	D49.89
cervical	—	C77.Ø	—	D36.Ø	D48.7	D49.89
cervicofacial	—	C77.Ø	—	D36.Ø	D48.7	D49.89
Cloquet	—	C77.4	—	D36.Ø	D48.7	D49.89
colic	—	C77.2	—	D36.Ø	D48.7	D49.89
common duct	—	C77.2	—	D36.Ø	D48.7	D49.89
cubital	—	C77.3	—	D36.Ø	D48.7	D49.89
diaphragmatic	—	C77.1	—	D36.Ø	D48.7	D49.89
epigastric, inferior	—	C77.1	—	D36.Ø	D48.7	D49.89
epitrochlear	—	C77.3	—	D36.Ø	D48.7	D49.89
esophageal	—	C77.1	—	D36.Ø	D48.7	D49.89
face	—	C77.Ø	—	D36.Ø	D48.7	D49.89
femoral	—	C77.4	—	D36.Ø	D48.7	D49.89
gastric	—	C77.2	—	D36.Ø	D48.7	D49.89
groin	—	C77.4	—	D36.Ø	D48.7	D49.89
head	—	C77.Ø	—	D36.Ø	D48.7	D49.89
hepatic	—	C77.2	—	D36.Ø	D48.7	D49.89
hilar (pulmonary)	—	C77.1	—	D36.Ø	D48.7	D49.89
splenic	—	C77.2	—	D36.Ø	D48.7	D49.89
hypogastric	—	C77.5	—	D36.Ø	D48.7	D49.89
ileocolic	—	C77.2	—	D36.Ø	D48.7	D49.89
iliac	—	C77.5	—	D36.Ø	D48.7	D49.89
infraclavicular	—	C77.3	—	D36.Ø	D48.7	D49.89
inguina, inguinal	—	C77.4	—	D36.Ø	D48.7	D49.89
innominate	—	C77.1	—	D36.Ø	D48.7	D49.89
intercostal	—	C77.1	—	D36.Ø	D48.7	D49.89
intestinal	—	C77.2	—	D36.Ø	D48.7	D49.89
intrabdominal	—	C77.2	—	D36.Ø	D48.7	D49.89
intrapelvic	—	C77.5	—	D36.Ø	D48.7	D49.89
intrathoracic	—	C77.1	—	D36.Ø	D48.7	D49.89
jugular	—	C77.Ø	—	D36.Ø	D48.7	D49.89
leg	—	C77.4	—	D36.Ø	D48.7	D49.89
limb						
lower	—	C77.4	—	D36.Ø	D48.7	D49.89
upper	—	C77.3	—	D36.Ø	D48.7	D49.89
lower limb	—	C77.4	—	D36.Ø	D48.7	D49.89
lumbar	—	C77.2	—	D36.Ø	D48.7	D49.89
mandibular	—	C77.Ø	—	D36.Ø	D48.7	D49.89
mediastinal	—	C77.1	—	D36.Ø	D48.7	D49.89
mesenteric (inferior) (superior)	—	C77.2	—	D36.Ø	D48.7	D49.89
midcolic	—	C77.2	—	D36.Ø	D48.7	D49.89
multiple sites in categories C77.Ø - C77.5	—	C77.8	—	D36.Ø	D48.7	D49.89
neck	—	C77.Ø	—	D36.Ø	D48.7	D49.89
obturator	—	C77.5	—	D36.Ø	D48.7	D49.89
occipital	—	C77.Ø	—	D36.Ø	D48.7	D49.89
pancreatic	—	C77.2	—	D36.Ø	D48.7	D49.89
para-aortic	—	C77.2	—	D36.Ø	D48.7	D49.89
paracervical	—	C77.5	—	D36.Ø	D48.7	D49.89
parametrial	—	C77.5	—	D36.Ø	D48.7	D49.89
parasternal	—	C77.1	—	D36.Ø	D48.7	D49.89
parotid	—	C77.Ø	—	D36.Ø	D48.7	D49.89
pectoral	—	C77.3	—	D36.Ø	D48.7	D49.89
pelvic	—	C77.5	—	D36.Ø	D48.7	D49.89
peri-aortic	—	C77.2	—	D36.Ø	D48.7	D49.89
peripancreatic	—	C77.2	—	D36.Ø	D48.7	D49.89
popliteal	—	C77.4	—	D36.Ø	D48.7	D49.89
porta hepatis	—	C77.2	—	D36.Ø	D48.7	D49.89

	Malignant Primary	Malignant Secondary	Ca in situ	Benign	Uncertain	Unspecified Behavior
Neoplasm, neoplastic — *continued*						
lymph, lymphatic channel — *continued*						
gland — *continued*						
portal	—	C77.2	—	D36.Ø	D48.7	D49.89
preauricular	—	C77.Ø	—	D36.Ø	D48.7	D49.89
prelaryngeal	—	C77.Ø	—	D36.Ø	D48.7	D49.89
presymphysial	—	C77.5	—	D36.Ø	D48.7	D49.89
pretracheal	—	C77.Ø	—	D36.Ø	D48.7	D49.89
primary (any site) NEC	C96.9	—	—	—	—	—
pulmonary (hiler)	—	C77.1	—	D36.Ø	D48.7	D49.89
pyloric	—	C77.2	—	D36.Ø	D48.7	D49.89
retroperitoneal	—	C77.2	—	D36.Ø	D48.7	D49.89
retropharyngeal	—	C77.Ø	—	D36.Ø	D48.7	D49.89
Rosenmuller's	—	C77.4	—	D36.Ø	D48.7	D49.89
sacral	—	C77.5	—	D36.Ø	D48.7	D49.89
scalene	—	C77.Ø	—	D36.Ø	D48.7	D49.89
site NEC	—	C77.9	—	D36.Ø	D48.7	D49.89
splenic (hilar)	—	C77.2	—	D36.Ø	D48.7	D49.89
subclavicular	—	C77.3	—	D36.Ø	D48.7	D49.89
subinguinal	—	C77.4	—	D36.Ø	D48.7	D49.89
sublingual	—	C77.Ø	—	D36.Ø	D48.7	D49.89
submandibular	—	C77.Ø	—	D36.Ø	D48.7	D49.89
submaxillary	—	C77.Ø	—	D36.Ø	D48.7	D49.89
submental	—	C77.Ø	—	D36.Ø	D48.7	D49.89
subscapular	—	C77.3	—	D36.Ø	D48.7	D49.89
supraclavicular	—	C77.Ø	—	D36.Ø	D48.7	D49.89
thoracic	—	C77.1	—	D36.Ø	D48.7	D49.89
tibial	—	C77.4	—	D36.Ø	D48.7	D49.89
tracheal	—	C77.1	—	D36.Ø	D48.7	D49.89
tracheobronchial	—	C77.1	—	D36.Ø	D48.7	D49.89
upper limb	—	C77.3	—	D36.Ø	D48.7	D49.89
Virchow's	—	C77.Ø	—	D36.Ø	D48.7	D49.89
node — *see also* Neoplasm, lymph gland						
primary NEC	C96.9	—	—	—	—	—
vessel — *see also* Neoplasm, connective tissue	C49.9	C79.89	—	D21.9	D48.1	D49.2
Mackenrodt's ligament	C57.7	C79.82	DØ7.39	D28.7	D39.8	D49.5
malar	C41.Ø	C79.51	—	D16.4	D48.Ø	D49.2
region — *see* Neoplasm, cheek						
mammary gland — *see* Neoplasm, breast						
mandible	C41.1	C79.51	—	D16.5	D48.Ø	D49.2
alveolar						
mucosa (carcinoma)	CØ3.1	C79.89	DØØ.Ø3	D1Ø.39	D37.Ø9	D49.Ø
ridge or process	C41.1	C79.51	—	D16.5	D48.Ø	D49.2
marrow (bone) NEC	C96.9	C79.52	—	—	D47.9	D49.89
mastectomy site (skin) — *see also* Neoplasm, breast, skin	C44.5Ø1	C79.2	—	—	—	—
specified as breast tissue	C5Ø.8-☑	C79.81	—	—	—	—
mastoid (air cells) (antrum) (cavity)	C3Ø.1	C78.39	DØ2.3	D14.Ø	D38.5	D49.1
bone or process	C41.Ø	C79.51	—	D16.4	D48.Ø	D49.2
maxilla, maxillary (superior)	C41.Ø	C79.51	—	D16.4	D48.Ø	D49.2
alveolar						
mucosa	CØ3.Ø	C79.89	DØØ.Ø3	D1Ø.39	D37.Ø9	D49.Ø
ridge or process (carcinoma)	C41.Ø	C79.51	—	D16.4	D48.Ø	D49.2
antrum	C31.Ø	C78.39	DØ2.3	D14.Ø	D38.5	D49.1
carcinoma	CØ3.Ø	C79.51	—	—	—	—
inferior — *see* Neoplasm, mandible						
sinus	C31.Ø	C78.39	DØ2.3	D14.Ø	D38.5	D49.1
meatus external (ear) — *see also* Neoplasm, skin, ear	C44.2Ø-☑	C79.2	DØ4.2-☑	D23.2-☑	D48.5	D49.2
Meckel diverticulum, malignant	C17.3	C78.4	DØ1.49	D13.39	D37.2	D49.Ø

	Malignant Primary	Malignant Secondary	Ca in situ	Benign	Uncertain	Unspecified Behavior
Neoplasm, neoplastic — *continued*						
mediastinum, mediastinal	C38.3	C78.1	—	D15.2	D38.3	D49.89
anterior	C38.1	C78.1	—	D15.2	D38.3	D49.89
posterior	C38.2	C78.1	—	D15.2	D38.3	D49.89
medulla						
adrenal	C74.1-☑	C79.7-☑	D09.3	D35.Ø-☑	D44.1-☑	D49.7
oblongata	C71.7	C79.31	—	D33.1	D43.1	D49.6
meibomian gland	C44.1Ø-☑	C79.2	DØ4.1-☑	D23.1-☑	D48.5	D49.2
basal cell carcinoma	C44.11-☑	—	—	—	—	—
specified type NEC	C44.19-☑	—	—	—	—	—
squamous cell carcinoma	C44.12-☑	—	—	—	—	—
melanoma — *see* Melanoma						
meninges	C7Ø.9	C79.49	—	D32.9	D42.9	D49.7
brain	C7Ø.Ø	C79.32	—	D32.Ø	D42.Ø	D49.7
cerebral	C7Ø.Ø	C79.32	—	D32.Ø	D42.Ø	D49.7
crainial	C7Ø.Ø	C79.32	—	D32.Ø	D42.Ø	D49.7
intracranial	C7Ø.Ø	C79.32	—	D32.Ø	D42.Ø	D49.7
spinal (cord)	C7Ø.1	C79.49	—	D32.1	D42.1	D49.7
meniscus, knee joint (lateral) (medial)	C4Ø.2-☑	C79.51	—	D16.2-☑	D48.Ø	D49.2
Merkel cell — *see* Carcinoma, Merkel cell						
mesentery, mesenteric	C48.1	C78.6	—	D2Ø.1	D48.4	D49.Ø
mesoappendix	C48.1	C78.6	—	D2Ø.1	D48.4	D49.Ø
mesocolon	C48.1	C78.6	—	D2Ø.1	D48.4	D49.Ø
mesopharynx — *see* Neoplasm, oropharynx						
mesosalpinx	C57.1-☑	C79.82	DØ7.39	D28.2	D39.8	D49.5
mesothelial tissue — *see* Mesothelioma						
mesothelioma — *see* Mesothelioma						
mesovarium	C57.1-☑	C79.82	DØ7.39	D28.2	D39.8	D49.5
metacarpus (any bone)	C4Ø.1-☑	C79.51	—	D16.1-☑	—	—
metastatic NEC — *see also* Neoplasm, by site, secondary	—	C79.9	—	—	—	—
metatarsus (any bone)	C4Ø.3-☑	C79.51	—	D16.3-☑	—	—
midbrain	C71.7	C79.31	—	D33.1	D43.1	D49.6
milk duct — *see* Neoplasm, breast						
mons						
pubis	C51.9	C79.82	DØ7.1	D28.Ø	D39.8	D49.5
veneris	C51.9	C79.82	DØ7.1	D28.Ø	D39.8	D49.5
motor tract	C72.9	C79.49	—	D33.9	D43.9	D49.7
brain	C71.9	C79.31	—	D33.2	D43.2	D49.6
cauda equina	C72.1	C79.49	—	D33.4	D43.4	D49.7
spinal	C72.Ø	C79.49	—	D33.4	D43.4	D49.7
mouth	CØ6.9	C79.89	DØØ.ØØ	D1Ø.3Ø	D37.Ø9	D49.Ø
book-leaf	CØ6.89	C79.89	—	—	—	—
floor	CØ4.9	C79.89	DØØ.Ø6	D1Ø.2	D37.Ø9	D49.Ø
anterior portion	CØ4.Ø	C79.89	DØØ.Ø6	D1Ø.2	D37.Ø9	D49.Ø
lateral portion	CØ4.1	C79.89	DØØ.Ø6	D1Ø.2	D37.Ø9	D49.Ø
overlapping lesion	CØ4.8	—	—	—	—	—
overlapping NEC	CØ6.8Ø	—	—	—	—	—
roof	CØ5.9	C79.89	DØØ.ØØ	D1Ø.39	D37.Ø9	D49.Ø
specified part NEC	CØ6.89	C79.89	DØØ.ØØ	D1Ø.39	D37.Ø9	D49.Ø
vestibule	CØ6.1	C79.89	DØØ.ØØ	D1Ø.39	D37.Ø9	D49.Ø
mucosa						
alveolar (ridge or process)	CØ3.9	C79.89	DØØ.Ø3	D1Ø.39	D37.Ø9	D49.Ø
lower	CØ3.1	C79.89	DØØ.Ø3	D1Ø.39	D37.Ø9	D49.Ø
upper	CØ3.Ø	C79.89	DØØ.Ø3	D1Ø.39	D37.Ø9	D49.Ø
buccal	CØ6.Ø	C79.89	DØØ.Ø2	D1Ø.39	D37.Ø9	D49.Ø
cheek	CØ6.Ø	C79.89	DØØ.Ø2	D1Ø.39	D37.Ø9	D49.Ø
lip — *see* Neoplasm, lip, internal						
nasal	C3Ø.Ø	C78.39	DØ2.3	D14.Ø	D38.5	D49.1
oral	CØ6.Ø	C79.89	DØØ.Ø2	D1Ø.39	D37.Ø9	D49.Ø
Mullerian duct						
female	C57.7	C79.82	DØ7.39	D28.7	D39.8	D49.5
male	C63.7	C79.82	DØ7.69	D29.8	D4Ø.8	D49.5

	Malignant Primary	Malignant Secondary	Ca in situ	Benign	Uncertain	Unspecified Behavior
Neoplasm, neoplastic — *continued*						
muscle — *see also* Neoplasm, connective tissue						
extraocular	C69.6-☑	C79.49	DØ9.2-☑	D31.6-☑	D48.7	D49.89
myocardium	C38.Ø	C79.89	—	D15.1	D48.7	D49.89
myometrium	C54.2	C79.82	DØ7.Ø	D26.1	D39.Ø	D49.5
myopericardium	C38.Ø	C79.89	—	D15.1	D48.7	D49.89
nabothian gland (follicle)	C53.Ø	C79.82	DØ6.Ø	D26.Ø	D39.Ø	D49.5
nail — *see also* Neoplasm, skin, limb	C44.9Ø	C79.2	DØ4.9	D23.9	D48.5	D49.2
finger — *see also* Neoplasm, skin, limb, upper	C44.6Ø-☑	C79.2	DØ4.6-☑	D23.6-☑	D48.5	D49.2
toe — *see also* Neoplasm, skin, limb, lower	C44.7Ø-☑	C79.2	DØ4.7-☑	D23.7-☑	D48.5	D49.2
nares, naris (anterior) (posterior)	C3Ø.Ø	C78.39	DØ2.3	D14.Ø	D38.5	D49.1
nasal — *see* Neoplasm, nose						
nasolabial groove — *see also* Neoplasm, skin, face	C44.3Ø9	C79.2	DØ4.39	D23.39	D48.5	D49.2
nasolacrimal duct	C69.5-☑	C79.49	DØ9.2-☑	D31.5-☑	D48.7	D49.89
nasopharynx, nasopharyngeal	C11.9	C79.89	DØØ.Ø8	D1Ø.6	D37.Ø5	D49.Ø
floor	C11.3	C79.89	DØØ.Ø8	D1Ø.6	D37.Ø5	D49.Ø
overlapping lesion	C11.8	—	—	—	—	—
roof	C11.Ø	C79.89	DØØ.Ø8	D1Ø.6	D37.Ø5	D49.Ø
wall	C11.9	C79.89	DØØ.Ø8	D1Ø.6	D37.Ø5	D49.Ø
anterior	C11.3	C79.89	DØØ.Ø8	D1Ø.6	D37.Ø5	D49.Ø
lateral	C11.2	C79.89	DØØ.Ø8	D1Ø.6	D37.Ø5	D49.Ø
posterior	C11.1	C79.89	DØØ.Ø8	D1Ø.6	D37.Ø5	D49.Ø
superior	C11.Ø	C79.89	DØØ.Ø8	D1Ø.6	D37.Ø5	D49.Ø
nates — *see also* Neoplasm, skin, trunk	C44.5Ø9	C79.2	DØ4.5	D23.5	D48.5	D49.2
neck NEC	C76.Ø	C79.89	DØ9.8	D36.7	D48.7	D49.89
skin	C44.4Ø	—	—	—	—	—
basal cell carcinoma	C44.41	—	—	—	—	—
specified type NEC	C44.49	—	—	—	—	—
squamous cell carcinoma	C44.42	—	—	—	—	—
nerve (ganglion)	C47.9	C79.89	—	D36.1Ø	D48.2	D49.2
abducens	C72.59	C79.49	—	D33.3	D43.3	D49.7
accessory (spinal)	C72.59	C79.49	—	D33.3	D43.3	D49.7
acoustic	C72.4-☑	C79.49	—	D33.3	D43.3	D49.7
auditory	C72.4-☑	C79.49	—	D33.3	D43.3	D49.7
autonomic NEC — *see also* Neoplasm, nerve, peripheral	C47.9	C79.89	—	D36.1Ø	D48.2	D49.2
brachial	C47.1-☑	C79.89	—	D36.12	D48.2	D49.2
cranial	C72.5Ø	C79.49	—	D33.3	D43.3	D49.7
specified NEC	C72.59	C79.49	—	D33.3	D43.3	D49.7
facial	C72.59	C79.49	—	D33.3	D43.3	D49.7
femoral	C47.2-☑	C79.89	—	D36.13	D48.2	D49.2
ganglion NEC — *see also* Neoplasm, nerve, peripheral	C47.9	C79.89	—	D36.1Ø	D48.2	D49.2
glossopharyngeal	C72.59	C79.49	—	D33.3	D43.3	D49.7
hypoglossal	C72.59	C79.49	—	D33.3	D43.3	D49.7
intercostal	C47.3	C79.89	—	D36.14	D48.2	D49.2
lumbar	C47.6	C79.89	—	D36.17	D48.2	D49.2
median	C47.1-☑	C79.89	—	D36.12	D48.2	D49.2
obturator	C47.2-☑	C79.89	—	D36.13	D48.2	D49.2
oculomotor	C72.59	C79.49	—	D33.3	D43.3	D49.7
olfactory	C47.2-☑	C79.49	—	D33.3	D43.3	D49.7
optic	C72.3-☑	C79.49	—	D33.3	D43.3	D49.7
parasympathetic NEC	C47.9	C79.89	—	D36.1Ø	D48.2	D49.2
peripheral NEC	C47.9	C79.89	—	D36.1Ø	D48.2	D49.2
abdomen	C47.4	C79.89	—	D36.15	D48.2	D49.2
abdominal wall	C47.4	C79.89	—	D36.15	D48.2	D49.2
ankle	C47.2-☑	C79.89	—	D36.13	D48.2	D49.2

	Malignant Primary	Malignant Secondary	Ca in situ	Benign	Uncertain	Unspecified Behavior
Neoplasm, neoplastic — *continued*						
nerve — *continued*						
peripheral — *continued*						
antecubital fossa or space	C47.1-☑	C79.89	—	D36.12	D48.2	D49.2
arm	C47.1-☑	C79.89	—	D36.12	D48.2	D49.2
auricle (ear)	C47.Ø	C79.89	—	D36.11	D48.2	D49.2
axilla	C47.3	C79.89	—	D36.12	D48.2	D49.2
back	C47.6	C79.89	—	D36.17	D48.2	D49.2
buttock	C47.5	C79.89	—	D36.16	D48.2	D49.2
calf	C47.2-☑	C79.89	—	D36.13	D48.2	D49.2
cervical region	C47.Ø	C79.89	—	D36.11	D48.2	D49.2
cheek	C47.Ø	C79.89	—	D36.11	D48.2	D49.2
chest (wall)	C47.3	C79.89	—	D36.14	D48.2	D49.2
chin	C47.Ø	C79.89	—	D36.11	D48.2	D49.2
ear (external)	C47.Ø	C79.89	—	D36.11	D48.2	D49.2
elbow	C47.1-☑	C79.89	—	D36.12	D48.2	D49.2
extrarectal	C47.5	C79.89	—	D36.16	D48.2	D49.2
extremity	C47.9	C79.89	—	D36.1Ø	D48.2	D49.2
lower	C47.2-☑	C79.89	—	D36.13	D48.2	D49.2
upper	C47.1-☑	C79.89	—	D36.12	D48.2	D49.2
eyelid	C47.Ø	C79.89	—	D36.11	D48.2	D49.2
face	C47.Ø	C79.89	—	D36.11	D48.2	D49.2
finger	C47.1-☑	C79.89	—	D36.12	D48.2	D49.2
flank	C47.6	C79.89	—	D36.17	D48.2	D49.2
foot	C47.2-☑	C79.89	—	D36.13	D48.2	D49.2
forearm	C47.1-☑	C79.89	—	D36.12	D48.2	D49.2
forehead	C47.Ø	C79.89	—	D36.11	D48.2	D49.2
gluteal region	C47.5	C79.89	—	D36.16	D48.2	D49.2
groin	C47.5	C79.89	—	D36.16	D48.2	D49.2
hand	C47.1-☑	C79.89	—	D36.12	D48.2	D49.2
head	C47.Ø	C79.89	—	D36.11	D48.2	D49.2
heel	C47.2-☑	C79.89	—	D36.13	D48.2	D49.2
hip	C47.2-☑	C79.89	—	D36.13	D48.2	D49.2
infraclavicular region	C47.3	C79.89	—	D36.14	D48.2	D49.2
inguinal (canal) (region)	C47.5	C79.89	—	D36.16	D48.2	D49.2
intrathoracic	C47.3	C79.89	—	D36.14	D48.2	D49.2
ischiorectal fossa	C47.5	C79.89	—	D36.16	D48.2	D49.2
knee	C47.2-☑	C79.89	—	D36.13	D48.2	D49.2
leg	C47.2-☑	C79.89	—	D36.13	D48.2	D49.2
limb NEC	C47.9	C79.89	—	D36.1Ø	D48.2	D49.2
lower	C47.2-☑	C79.89	—	D36.13	D48.2	D49.2
upper	C47.1-☑	C79.89	—	D36.12	D48.2	D49.2
nates	C47.5	C79.89	—	D36.16	D48.2	D49.2
neck	C47.Ø	C79.89	—	D36.11	D48.2	D49.2
orbit	C69.6-☑	C79.49	—	D31.6-☑	D48.7	D49.2
pararectal	C47.5	C79.89	—	D36.16	D48.2	D49.2
paraurethral	C47.5	C79.89	—	D36.16	D48.2	D49.2
paravaginal	C47.5	C79.89	—	D36.16	D48.2	D49.2
pelvis (floor)	C47.5	C79.89	—	D36.16	D48.2	D49.2
pelvoabdominal	C47.8	C79.89	—	D36.17	D48.2	D49.2
perineum	C47.5	C79.89	—	D36.16	D48.2	D49.2
perirectal (tissue)	C47.5	C79.89	—	D36.16	D48.2	D49.2
periurethral (tissue)	C47.5	C79.89	—	D36.16	D48.2	D49.2
popliteal fossa or space	C47.2-☑	C79.89	—	D36.13	D48.2	D49.2
presacral	C47.5	C79.89	—	D36.16	D48.2	D49.2
pterygoid fossa	C47.Ø	C79.89	—	D36.11	D48.2	D49.2
rectovaginal septum or wall	C47.5	C79.89	—	D36.16	D48.2	D49.2
rectovesical	C47.5	C79.89	—	D36.16	D48.2	D49.2
sacrococcygeal region	C47.5	C79.89	—	D36.16	D48.2	D49.2
scalp	C47.Ø	C79.89	—	D36.11	D48.2	D49.2
scapular region	C47.3	C79.89	—	D36.14	D48.2	D49.2
shoulder	C47.1-☑	C79.89	—	D36.12	D48.2	D49.2
submental	C47.Ø	C79.89	—	D36.11	D48.2	D49.2
supraclavicular region	C47.Ø	C79.89	—	D36.11	D48.2	D49.2
temple	C47.Ø	C79.89	—	D36.11	D48.2	D49.2
temporal region	C47.Ø	C79.89	—	D36.11	D48.2	D49.2
thigh	C47.2-☑	C79.89	—	D36.13	D48.2	D49.2
thoracic (duct) (wall)	C47.3	C79.89	—	D36.14	D48.2	D49.2
thorax	C47.3	C79.89	—	D36.14	D48.2	D49.2
thumb	C47.1-☑	C79.89	—	D36.12	D48.2	D49.2
Neoplasm, neoplastic — *continued*						
nerve — *continued*						
peripheral — *continued*						
toe	C47.2-☑	C79.89	—	D36.13	D48.2	D49.2
trunk	C47.6	C79.89	—	D36.17	D48.2	D49.2
umbilicus	C47.4	C79.89	—	D36.15	D48.2	D49.2
vesicorectal	C47.5	C79.89	—	D36.16	D48.2	D49.2
wrist	C47.1-☑	C79.89	—	D36.12	D48.2	D49.2
radial	C47.1-☑	C79.89	—	D36.12	D48.2	D49.2
sacral	C47.5	C79.89	—	D36.16	D48.2	D49.2
sciatic	C47.2-☑	C79.89	—	D36.13	D48.2	D49.2
spinal NEC	C47.9	C79.89	—	D36.1Ø	D48.2	D49.2
accessory	C72.59	C79.49	—	D33.3	D43.3	D49.7
sympathetic NEC — *see also* Neoplasm, nerve, peripheral	C47.9	C79.89	—	D36.1Ø	D48.2	D49.2
trigeminal	C72.59	C79.49	—	D33.3	D43.3	D49.7
trochlear	C72.59	C79.49	—	D33.3	D43.3	D49.7
ulnar	C47.1-☑	C79.89	—	D36.12	D48.2	D49.2
vagus	C72.59	C79.49	—	D33.3	D43.3	D49.7
nervous system (central)	C72.9	C79.4Ø	—	D33.9	D43.9	D49.7
autonomic — *see* Neoplasm, nerve, peripheral						
parasympathetic — *see* Neoplasm, nerve, peripheral						
specified site NEC	—	C79.49	—	D33.7	D43.8	—
sympathetic — *see* Neoplasm, nerve, peripheral						
nevus — *see* Nevus						
nipple	C5Ø.Ø-☑	C79.81	DØ5.-☑	D24.-☑	—	—
nose, nasal	C76.Ø	C79.89	DØ9.8	D36.7	D48.7	D49.89
ala (external) (nasi) — *see also* Neoplasm, nose, skin	C44.3Ø1	C79.2	DØ4.39	D23.39	D48.5	D49.2
bone	C41.Ø	C79.51	—	D16.4	D48.Ø	D49.2
cartilage	C3Ø.Ø	C78.39	DØ2.3	D14.Ø	D38.5	D49.1
cavity	C3Ø.Ø	C78.39	DØ2.3	D14.Ø	D38.5	D49.1
choana	C11.3	C79.89	DØØ.Ø8	D1Ø.6	D37.Ø5	D49.Ø
external (skin) — *see also* Neoplasm, nose, skin	C44.3Ø1	C79.2	DØ4.39	D23.39	D48.5	D49.2
fossa	C3Ø.Ø	C78.39	DØ2.3	D14.Ø	D38.5	D49.1
internal	C3Ø.Ø	C78.39	DØ2.3	D14.Ø	D38.5	D49.1
mucosa	C3Ø.Ø	C78.39	DØ2.3	D14.Ø	D38.5	D49.1
septum	C3Ø.Ø	C78.39	DØ2.3	D14.Ø	D38.5	D49.1
posterior margin	C11.3	C79.89	DØØ.Ø8	D1Ø.6	D37.Ø5	D49.Ø
sinus — *see* Neoplasm, sinus						
skin	C44.3Ø1	C79.2	DØ4.39	D23.39	D48.5	D49.2
basal cell carcinoma	C44.311	—	—	—	—	—
specified type NEC	C44.391	—	—	—	—	—
squamous cell carcinoma	C44.321	—	—	—	—	—
turbinate (mucosa)	C3Ø.Ø	C78.39	DØ2.3	D14.Ø	D38.5	D49.1
bone	C41.Ø	C79.51	—	D16.4	D48.Ø	D49.2
vestibule	C3Ø.Ø	C78.39	DØ2.3	D14.Ø	D38.5	D49.1
nostril	C3Ø.Ø	C78.39	DØ2.3	D14.Ø	D38.5	D49.1
nucleus pulposus	C41.2	C79.51	—	D16.6	D48.Ø	D49.2
occipital						
bone	C41.Ø	C79.51	—	D16.4	D48.Ø	D49.2
lobe or pole, brain	C71.4	C79.31	—	D33.Ø	D43.Ø	D49.6
odontogenic — *see* Neoplasm, jaw bone						
olfactory nerve or bulb	C72.2-☑	C79.49	—	D33.3	D43.3	D49.7
olive (brain)	C71.7	C79.31	—	D33.1	D43.1	D49.6
omentum	C48.1	C78.6	—	D2Ø.1	D48.4	D49.Ø
operculum (brain)	C71.Ø	C79.31	—	D33.Ø	D43.Ø	D49.6
optic nerve, chiasm, or tract	C72.3-☑	C79.49	—	D33.3	D43.3	D49.7
oral (cavity)	CØ6.9	C79.89	DØØ.ØØ	D1Ø.3Ø	D37.Ø9	D49.Ø
ill-defined	C14.8	C79.89	DØØ.ØØ	D1Ø.3Ø	D37.Ø9	D49.Ø
mucosa	CØ6.Ø	C79.89	DØØ.Ø2	D1Ø.39	D37.Ø9	D49.Ø
orbit	C69.6-☑	C79.49	DØ9.2-☑	D31.6-☑	D48.7	D49.89

	Malignant Primary	Malignant Secondary	Ca in situ	Benign	Uncertain	Unspecified Behavior
Neoplasm, neoplastic — *continued*						
orbit — *continued*						
autonomic nerve	C69.6-☑	C79.49	—	D31.6-☑	D48.7	D49.2
bone	C41.0	C79.51	—	D16.4	D48.0	D49.2
eye	C69.6-☑	C79.49	D09.2-☑	D31.6-☑	D48.7	D49.89
peripheral nerves	C69.6-☑	C79.49	—	D31.6-☑	D48.7	D49.2
soft parts	C69.6-☑	C79.49	D09.2-☑	D31.6-☑	D48.7	D49.89
organ of Zuckerkandl	C75.5	C79.89	—	D35.6	D44.7	D49.7
oropharynx	C10.9	C79.89	D00.08	D10.5	D37.05	D49.0
branchial cleft (vestige)	C10.4	C79.89	D00.08	D10.5	D37.05	D49.0
junctional region	C10.8	C79.89	D00.08	D10.5	D37.05	D49.0
lateral wall	C10.2	C79.89	D00.08	D10.5	D37.05	D49.0
overlapping lesion	C10.8	—	—	—	—	—
pillars or fauces	C09.1	C79.89	D00.08	D10.5	D37.05	D49.0
posterior wall	C10.3	C79.89	D00.08	D10.5	D37.05	D49.0
vallecula	C10.0	C79.89	D00.08	D10.5	D37.05	D49.0
os						
external	C53.1	C79.82	D06.1	D26.0	D39.0	D49.5
internal	C53.0	C79.82	D06.0	D26.0	D39.0	D49.5
ovary	C56.-☑	C79.6-☑	D07.39	D27.-☑	D39.1-☑	D49.5
oviduct	C57.0-☑	C79.82	D07.39	D28.2	D39.8	D49.5
palate	C05.9	C79.89	D00.00	D10.39	D37.09	D49.0
hard	C05.0	C79.89	D00.05	D10.39	D37.09	D49.0
junction of hard and soft palate	C05.9	C79.89	D00.00	D10.39	D37.09	D49.0
overlapping lesions	C05.8	—	—	—	—	—
soft	C05.1	C79.89	D00.04	D10.39	D37.09	D49.0
nasopharyngeal surface	C11.3	C79.89	D00.08	D10.6	D37.05	D49.0
posterior surface	C11.3	C79.89	D00.08	D10.6	D37.05	D49.0
superior surface	C11.3	C79.89	D00.08	D10.6	D37.05	D49.0
palatoglossal arch	C09.1	C79.89	D00.00	D10.5	D37.09	D49.0
palatopharyngeal arch	C09.1	C79.89	D00.00	D10.5	D37.09	D49.0
pallium	C71.0	C79.31	—	D33.0	D43.0	D49.6
palpebra	C44.10-☑	C79.2	D04.1-☑	D23.1-☑	D48.5	D49.2
basal cell carcinoma	C44.11-☑	—	—	—	—	—
specified type NEC	C44.19-☑	—	—	—	—	—
squamous cell carcinoma	C44.12-☑	—	—	—	—	—
pancreas	C25.9	C78.89	D01.7	D13.6	D37.8	D49.0
body	C25.1	C78.89	D01.7	D13.6	D37.8	D49.0
duct (of Santorini) (of Wirsung)	C25.3	C78.89	D01.7	D13.6	D37.8	D49.0
ectopic tissue	C25.7	C78.89	—	D13.6	D37.8	D49.0
head	C25.0	C78.89	D01.7	D13.6	D37.8	D49.0
islet cells	C25.4	C78.89	D01.7	D13.7	D37.8	D49.0
neck	C25.7	C78.89	D01.7	D13.6	D37.8	D49.0
overlapping lesion	C25.8	—	—	—	—	—
tail	C25.2	C78.89	D01.7	D13.6	D37.8	D49.0
para-aortic body	C75.5	C79.89	—	D35.6	D44.7	D49.7
paraganglion NEC	C75.5	C79.89	—	D35.6	D44.7	D49.7
parametrium	C57.3	C79.82	—	D28.2	D39.8	D49.5
paranephric	C48.0	C78.6	—	D20.0	D48.3	D49.0
pararectal	C76.3	C79.89	—	D36.7	D48.7	D49.89
parasagittal (region)	C76.0	C79.89	D09.8	D36.7	D48.7	D49.89
parasellar	C72.9	C79.49	—	D33.9	D43.8	D49.7
parathyroid (gland)	C75.0	C79.89	D09.3	D35.1	D44.2	D49.7
paraurethral	C76.3	C79.89	—	D36.7	D48.7	D49.89
gland	C68.1	C79.19	D09.19	D30.8	D41.8	D49.5
paravaginal	C76.3	C79.89	—	D36.7	D48.7	D49.89
parenchyma, kidney	C64.-☑	C79.0-☑	D09.19	D30.0-☑	D41.0-☑	D49.5
parietal						
bone	C41.0	C79.51	—	D16.4	D48.0	D49.2
lobe, brain	C71.3	C79.31	—	D33.0	D43.0	D49.6
paroophoron	C57.1-☑	C79.82	D07.39	D28.2	D39.8	D49.5
parotid (duct) (gland)	C07	C79.89	D00.00	D11.0	D37.030	D49.0
parovarium	C57.1-☑	C79.82	D07.39	D28.2	D39.8	D49.5
patella	C40.20	C79.51	—	—	—	—
peduncle, cerebral	C71.7	C79.31	—	D33.1	D43.1	D49.6
pelvirectal junction	C19	C78.5	D01.1	D12.7	D37.5	D49.0
pelvis, pelvic	C76.3	C79.89	D09.8	D36.7	D48.7	D49.89
bone	C41.4	C79.51	—	D16.8	D48.0	D49.2
floor	C76.3	C79.89	D09.8	D36.7	D48.7	D49.89
renal	C65.-☑	C79.0-☑	D09.19	D30.1-☑	D41.1-☑	D49.5
viscera	C76.3	C79.89	D09.8	D36.7	D48.7	D49.89
Neoplasm, neoplastic — *continued*						
pelvis, pelvic — *continued*						
wall	C76.3	C79.89	D09.8	D36.7	D48.7	D49.89
pelvo-abdominal	C76.8	C79.89	D09.8	D36.7	D48.7	D49.89
penis	C60.9	C79.82	D07.4	D29.0	D40.8	D49.5
body	C60.2	C79.82	D07.4	D29.0	D40.8	D49.5
corpus (cavernosum)	C60.2	C79.82	D07.4	D29.0	D40.8	D49.5
glans	C60.1	C79.82	D07.4	D29.0	D40.8	D49.5
overlapping sites	C60.8	—	—	—	—	—
skin NEC	C60.9	C79.82	D07.4	D29.0	D40.8	D49.5
periadrenal (tissue)	C48.0	C78.6	—	D20.0	D48.3	D49.0
perianal (skin) — *see also* Neoplasm, anus, skin	C44.500	C79.2	D04.5	D23.5	D48.5	D49.2
pericardium	C38.0	C79.89	—	D15.1	D48.7	D49.89
perinephric	C48.0	C78.6	—	D20.0	D48.3	D49.0
perineum	C76.3	C79.89	D09.8	D36.7	D48.7	D49.89
periodontal tissue NEC	C03.9	C79.89	D00.03	D10.39	D37.09	D49.0
periosteum — *see* Neoplasm, bone						
peripancreatic	C48.0	C78.6	—	D20.0	D48.3	D49.0
peripheral nerve NEC	C47.9	C79.89	—	D36.10	D48.2	D49.2
perirectal (tissue)	C76.3	C79.89	—	D36.7	D48.7	D49.89
perirenal (tissue)	C48.0	C78.6	—	D20.0	D48.3	D49.0
peritoneum, peritoneal (cavity)	C48.2	C78.6	—	D20.1	D48.4	D49.0
benign mesothelial tissue — *see* Mesothelioma, benign						
overlapping lesion	C48.8	—	—	—	—	—
with digestive organs	C26.9	—	—	—	—	—
parietal	C48.1	C78.6	—	D20.1	D48.4	D49.0
pelvic	C48.1	C78.6	—	D20.1	D48.4	D49.0
specified part NEC	C48.1	C78.6	—	D20.1	D48.4	D49.0
peritonsillar (tissue)	C76.0	C79.89	D09.8	D36.7	D48.7	D49.89
periurethral tissue	C76.3	C79.89	—	D36.7	D48.7	D49.89
phalanges						
foot	C40.3-☑	C79.51	—	D16.3-☑	—	—
hand	C40.1-☑	C79.51	—	D16.1-☑	—	—
pharynx, pharyngeal	C14.0	C79.89	D00.08	D10.9	D37.05	D49.0
bursa	C11.1	C79.89	D00.08	D10.6	D37.05	D49.0
fornix	C11.3	C79.89	D00.08	D10.6	D37.05	D49.0
recess	C11.2	C79.89	D00.08	D10.6	D37.05	D49.0
region	C14.0	C79.89	D00.08	D10.9	D37.05	D49.0
tonsil	C11.1	C79.89	D00.08	D10.6	D37.05	D49.0
wall (lateral) (posterior)	C14.0	C79.89	D00.08	D10.9	D37.05	D49.0
pia mater	C70.9	C79.40	—	D32.9	D42.9	D49.7
cerebral	C70.0	C79.32	—	D32.0	D42.0	D49.7
cranial	C70.0	C79.32	—	D32.0	D42.0	D49.7
spinal	C70.1	C79.49	—	D32.1	D42.1	D49.7
pillars of fauces	C09.1	C79.89	D00.08	D10.5	D37.05	D49.0
pineal (body) (gland)	C75.3	C79.89	D09.3	D35.4	D44.5	D49.7
pinna (ear) NEC — *see also* Neoplasm, skin, ear	C44.20-☑	C79.2	D04.2-☑	D23.2-☑	D48.5	D49.2
piriform fossa or sinus	C12	C79.89	D00.08	D10.7	D37.05	D49.0
pituitary (body) (fossa) (gland) (lobe)	C75.1	C79.89	D09.3	D35.2	D44.3	D49.7
placenta	C58	C79.82	D07.0	D26.7	D39.2	D49.5
pleura, pleural (cavity)	C38.4	C78.2	—	D19.0	D38.2	D49.1
overlapping lesion with heart or mediastinum	C38.8	—	—	—	—	—
parietal	C38.4	C78.2	—	D19.0	D38.2	D49.1
visceral	C38.4	C78.2	—	D19.0	D38.2	D49.1
plexus						
brachial	C47.1-☑	C79.89	—	D36.12	D48.2	D49.2
cervical	C47.0	C79.89	—	D36.11	D48.2	D49.2
choroid	C71.5	C79.31	—	D33.0	D43.0	D49.6
lumbosacral	C47.5	C79.89	—	D36.16	D48.2	D49.2
sacral	C47.5	C79.89	—	D36.16	D48.2	D49.2
pluriendocrine	C75.8	C79.89	D09.3	D35.7	D44.9	D49.7
pole						

	Malignant Primary	Malignant Secondary	Ca in situ	Benign	Uncertain	Unspecified Behavior
Neoplasm, neoplastic — *continued*						
pole — *continued*						
frontal	C71.1	C79.31	—	D33.0	D43.0	D49.6
occipital	C71.4	C79.31	—	D33.0	D43.0	D49.6
pons (varolii)	C71.7	C79.31	—	D33.1	D43.1	D49.6
popliteal fossa or space	C76.5-☑	C79.89	D04.7-☑	D36.7	D48.7	D49.89
postcricoid (region)	C13.0	C79.89	D00.08	D10.7	D37.05	D49.0
posterior fossa (cranial)	C71.9	C79.31	—	D33.2	D43.2	D49.6
postnasal space	C11.9	C79.89	D00.08	D10.6	D37.05	D49.0
prepuce	C60.0	C79.82	D07.4	D29.0	D40.8	D49.5
prepylorus	C16.4	C78.89	D00.2	D13.1	D37.1	D49.0
presacral (region)	C76.3	C79.89	—	D36.7	D48.7	D49.89
prostate (gland)	C61	C79.82	D07.5	D29.1	D40.0	D49.59
utricle	C68.0	C79.19	D09.19	D30.4	D41.3	D49.5
pterygoid fossa	C49.0	C79.89	—	D21.0	D48.1	D49.2
pubic bone	C41.4	C79.51	—	D16.8	D48.0	D49.2
pudenda, pudendum (femaie)	C51.9	C79.82	D07.1	D28.0	D39.8	D49.5
pulmonary — *see also* Neoplasm, lung	C34.9-☑	C78.0-☑	D02.2-☑	D14.3-☑	D38.1	D49.1
putamen	C71.0	C79.31	—	D33.0	D43.0	D49.6
pyloric						
antrum	C16.3	C78.89	D00.2	D13.1	D37.1	D49.0
canal	C16.4	C78.89	D00.2	D13.1	D37.1	D49.0
pylorus	C16.4	C78.89	D00.2	D13.1	D37.1	D49.0
pyramid (brain)	C71.7	C79.31	—	D33.1	D43.1	D49.6
pyriform fossa or sinus	C12	C79.89	D00.08	D10.7	D37.05	D49.0
radius (any part)	C40.0-☑	C79.51	—	D16.0-☑	—	—
Rathke's pouch	C75.1	C79.89	D09.3	D35.2	D44.3	D49.7
rectosigmoid (junction)	C19	C78.5	D01.1	D12.7	D37.5	D49.0
overlapping lesion with anus or rectum	C21.8	—	—	—	—	—
rectouterine pouch	C48.1	C78.6	—	D20.1	D48.4	D49.0
rectovaginal septum or wall	C76.3	C79.89	D09.8	D36.7	D48.7	D49.89
rectovesical septum	C76.3	C79.89	D09.8	D36.7	D48.7	D49.89
rectum (ampulla)	C20	C78.5	D01.2	D12.8	D37.5	D49.0
and colon	C19	C78.5	D01.1	D12.7	D37.5	D49.0
overlapping lesion with anus or rectosigmoid junction	C21.8	—	—	—	—	—
renal	C64.-☑	C79.0-☑	D09.19	D30.0-☑	D41.0-☑	D49.5
calyx	C65.-☑	C79.0-☑	D09.19	D30.1-☑	D41.1-☑	D49.5
hilus	C65.-☑	C79.0-☑	D09.19	D30.1-☑	D41.1-☑	D49.5
parenchyma	C64.-☑	C79.0-☑	D09.19	D30.0-☑	D41.0-☑	D49.5
pelvis	C65.-☑	C79.0-☑	D09.19	D30.1-☑	D41.1-☑	D49.5
respiratory						
organs or system NEC	C39.9	C78.30	D02.4	D14.4	D38.6	D49.1
tract NEC	C39.9	C78.30	D02.4	D14.4	D38.5	D49.1
upper	C39.0	C78.30	D02.4	D14.4	D38.5	D49.1
retina	C69.2-☑	C79.49	D09.2-☑	D31.2-☑	D48.7	D49.81
retrobulbar	C69.6-☑	C79.49	—	D31.6-☑	D48.7	D49.89
retrocecal	C48.0	C78.6	—	D20.0	D48.3	D49.0
retromolar (area) (triangle) (trigone)	C06.2	C79.89	D00.00	D10.39	D37.09	D49.0
retro-orbital	C76.0	C79.89	D09.8	D36.7	D48.7	D49.89
retroperitoneal (space) (tissue)	C48.0	C78.6	—	D20.0	D48.3	D49.0
retroperitoneum	C48.0	C78.6	—	D20.0	D48.3	D49.0
retropharyngeal	C14.0	C79.89	D00.08	D10.9	D37.05	D49.0
retrovesical (septum)	C76.3	C79.89	D09.8	D36.7	D48.7	D49.89
rhinencephalon	C71.0	C79.31	—	D33.0	D43.0	D49.6
rib	C41.3	C79.51	—	D16.7	D48.0	D49.2
Rosenmuller's fossa	C11.2	C79.89	D00.08	D10.6	D37.05	D49.0
round ligament	C57.2☑	C79.82	—	D28.2	D39.8	D49.5
sacrococcyx, sacrococcygeal	C41.4	C79.51	—	D16.8	D48.0	D49.2
region	C76.3	C79.89	D09.8	D36.7	D48.7	D49.89
sacrouterine ligament	C57.3	C79.82	—	D28.2	D39.8	D49.5
sacrum, sacral (vertebra)	C41.4	C79.51	—	D16.8	D48.0	D49.2
Neoplasm, neoplastic — *continued*						
salivary gland or duct (major)	C08.9	C79.89	D00.00	D11.9	D37.039	D49.0
minor NEC	C06.9	C79.89	D00.00	D10.39	D37.04	D49.0
overlapping lesion	C08.9	—	—	—	—	—
parotid	C07	C79.89	D00.00	D11.0	D37.030	D49.0
pluriglandular	C08.9	C79.89	D00.00	D11.9	D37.039	D49.0
sublingual	C08.1	C79.89	D00.00	D11.7	D37.031	D49.0
submandibular	C08.0	C79.89	D00.00	D11.7	D37.032	D49.0
submaxillary	C08.0	C79.89	D00.00	D11.7	D37.032	D49.0
salpinx (uterine)	C57.0-☑	C79.82	D07.39	D28.2	D39.8	D49.5
Santorini's duct	C25.3	C78.89	D01.7	D13.6	D37.8	D49.0
scalp	C44.40	C79.2	D04.4	D23.4	D48.5	D49.2
basal cell carcinoma	C44.41	—	—	—	—	—
specified type NEC	C44.49	—	—	—	—	—
squamous cell carcinoma	C44.42	—	—	—	—	—
scapula (any part)	C40.0-☑	C79.51	—	D16.0-☑	—	—
scapular region	C76.1	C79.89	D09.8	D36.7	D48.7	D49.89
scar NEC — *see also* Neoplasm, skin, by site	C44.90	C79.2	D04.9	D23.9	D48.5	D49.2
sciatic nerve	C47.2-☑	C79.89	—	D36.13	D48.2	D49.2
sclera	C69.4-☑	C79.49	D09.2-☑	D31.4-☑	D48.7	D49.89
scrotum (skin)	C63.2	C79.82	D07.61	D29.4	D40.8	D49.5
sebaceous gland — *see* Neoplasm, skin						
sella turcica	C75.1	C79.89	D09.3	D35.2	D44.3	D49.7
bone	C41.0	C79.51	—	D16.4	D48.0	D49.2
semilunar cartilage (knee)	C40.2-☑	C79.51	—	D16.2-☑	D48.0	D49.2
seminal vesicle	C63.7	C79.82	D07.69	D29.8	D40.8	D49.5
septum						
nasal	C30.0	C78.39	D02.3	D14.0	D38.5	D49.1
posterior margin	C11.3	C79.89	D00.08	D10.6	D37.05	D49.0
rectovaginal	C76.3	C79.89	D09.8	D36.7	D48.7	D49.89
rectovesical	C76.3	C79.89	D09.8	D36.7	D48.7	D49.89
urethrovaginal	C57.9	C79.82	D07.30	D28.9	D39.9	D49.5
vesicovaginal	C57.9	C79.82	D07.30	D28.9	D39.9	D49.5
shoulder NEC	C76.4-☑	C79.89	D04.6-☑	D36.7	D48.7	D49.89
sigmoid flexure (lower) (upper)	C18.7	C78.5	D01.0	D12.5	D37.4	D49.0
sinus (accessory)	C31.9	C78.39	D02.3	D14.0	D38.5	D49.1
bone (any)	C41.0	C79.51	—	D16.4	D48.0	D49.2
ethmoidal	C31.1	C78.39	D02.3	D14.0	D38.5	D49.1
frontal	C31.2	C78.39	D02.3	D14.0	D38.5	D49.1
maxillary	C31.0	C78.39	D02.3	D14.0	D38.5	D49.1
nasal, paranasal NEC	C31.9	C78.39	D02.3	D14.0	D38.5	D49.1
overlapping lesion	C31.8	—	—	—	—	—
pyriform	C12	C79.89	D00.08	D10.7	D37.05	D49.0
sphenoid	C31.3	C78.39	D02.3	D14.0	D38.5	D49.1
skeleton, skeletal NEC	C41.9	C79.51	—	D16.9	D48.0	D49.2
Skene's gland	C68.1	C79.19	D09.19	D30.8	D41.8	D49.5
skin NOS	C44.90	C79.2	D04.9	D23.9	D48.5	D49.2
abdominal wall	C44.509	C79.2	D04.5	D23.5	D48.5	D49.2
basal cell carcinoma	C44.519	—	—	—	—	—
specified type NEC	C44.599	—	—	—	—	—
squamous cell carcinoma	C44.529	—	—	—	—	—
ala nasi — *see also* Neoplasm, nose, skin	C44.301	C79.2	D04.39	D23.39	D48.5	D49.2
ankle — *see also* Neoplasm, skin, limb, lower	C44.70-☑	C79.2	D04.7-☑	D23.7-☑	D48.5	D49.2
antecubital space — *see also* Neoplasm, skin, limb, upper	C44.60-☑	C79.2	D04.6-☑	D23.6-☑	D48.5	D49.2
anus	C44.500	C79.2	D04.5	D23.5	D48.5	D49.2
basal cell carcinoma	C44.510	—	—	—	—	—
specified type NEC	C44.590	—	—	—	—	—
squamous cell carcinoma	C44.520	—	—	—	—	—

	Malignant Primary	Malignant Secondary	Ca in situ	Benign	Uncertain	Unspecified Behavior
Neoplasm, neoplastic — *continued*						
skin — *continued*						
arm — *see also* Neoplasm, skin, limb, upper	C44.60-☑	C79.2	D04.6-☑	D23.6-☑	D48.5	D49.2
auditory canal (external) — *see also* Neoplasm, skin, ear	C44.20-☑	C79.2	D04.2-☑	D23.2-☑	D48.5	D49.2
auricle (ear) — *see also* Neoplasm, skin, ear	C44.20-☑	C79.2	D04.2-☑	D23.2-☑	D48.5	D49.2
auricular canal (external) — *see also* Neoplasm, skin, ear	C44.20-☑	C79.2	D04.2-☑	D23.2-☑	D48.5	D49.2
axilla, axillary fold — *see also* Neoplasm, skin, trunk	C44.509	C79.2	D04.5	D23.5	D48.5	D49.2
back — *see also* Neoplasm, skin, trunk	C44.509	C79.2	D04.5	D23.5	D48.5	D49.2
basal cell carcinoma	C44.91	—	—	—	—	—
breast	C44.501	C79.2	D04.5	D23.5	D48.5	D49.2
basal cell carcinoma	C44.511	—	—	—	—	—
specified type NEC	C44.591	—	—	—	—	—
squamous cell carcinoma	C44.521	—	—	—	—	—
brow — *see also* Neoplasm, skin, face	C44.309	C79.2	D04.39	D23.39	D48.5	D49.2
buttock — *see also* Neoplasm, skin, trunk	C44.509	C79.2	D04.5	D23.5	D48.5	D49.2
calf — *see also* Neoplasm, skin, limb, lower	C44.70-☑	C79.2	D04.7-☑	D23.7-☑	D48.5	D49.2
canthus (eye) (inner) (outer)	C44.10-☑	C79.2	D04.1-☑	D23.1-☑	D48.5	D49.2
basal cell carcinoma	C44.11-☑	—	—	—	—	—
specified type NEC	C44.19-☑	—	—	—	—	—
squamous cell carcinoma	C44.12-☑	—	—	—	—	—
cervical region — *see also* Neoplasm, skin, neck	C44.40	C79.2	D04.4	D23.4	D48.5	D49.2
cheek (external) — *see also* Neoplasm, skin, face	C44.309	C79.2	D04.39	D23.39	D48.5	D49.2
chest (wall) — *see also* Neoplasm, skin, trunk	C44.509	C79.2	D04.5	D23.5	D48.5	D49.2
chin — *see also* Neoplasm, skin, face	C44.309	C79.2	D04.39	D23.39	D48.5	D49.2
clavicular area — *see also* Neoplasm, skin, trunk	C44.509	C79.2	D04.5	D23.5	D48.5	D49.2
clitoris	C51.2	C79.82	D07.1	D28.0	D39.8	D49.5
columnella — *see also* Neoplasm, skin, face	C44.309	C79.2	D04.39	D23.39	D48.5	D49.2
concha — *see also* Neoplasm, skin, ear	C44.20-☑	C79.2	D04.2-☑	D23.2-☑	D48.5	D49.2
ear (external)	C44.20-☑	C79.2	D04.2-☑	D23.2-☑	D48.5	D49.2
basal cell carcinoma	C44.21-☑	—	—	—	—	—
specified type NEC	C44.29-☑	—	—	—	—	—
squamous cell carcinoma	C44.22-☑	—	—	—	—	—
elbow — *see also* Neoplasm, skin, limb, upper	C44.60-☑	C79.2	D04.6-☑	D23.6-☑	D48.5	D49.2
Neoplasm, neoplastic — *continued*						
skin — *continued*						
eyebrow — *see also* Neoplasm, skin, face	C44.309	C79.2	D04.39	D23.39	D48.5	D49.2
eyelid	C44.10-☑	C79.2	D04.1-☑	D23.1-☑	D48.5	D49.2
basal cell carcinoma	C44.11-☑	—	—	—	—	—
specified type NEC	C44.19-☑	—	—	—	—	—
squamous cell carcinoma	C44.12-☑	—	—	—	—	—
face NOS	C44.300	C79.2	D04.30	D23.30	D48.5	D49.2
basal cell carcinoma	C44.310	—	—	—	—	—
specified type NEC	C44.390	—	—	—	—	—
squamous cell carcinoma	C44.320	—	—	—	—	—
female genital organs (external)	C51.9	C79.82	D07.1	D28.0	D39.8	D49.5
clitoris	C51.2	C79.82	D07.1	D28.0	D39.8	D49.5
labium NEC	C51.9	C79.82	D07.1	D28.0	D39.8	D49.5
majus	C51.0	C79.82	D07.1	D28.0	D39.8	D49.5
minus	C51.1	C79.82	D07.1	D28.0	D39.8	D49.5
pudendum	C51.9	C79.82	D07.1	D28.0	D39.8	D49.5
vulva	C51.9	C79.82	D07.1	D28.0	D39.8	D49.5
finger — *see also* Neoplasm, skin, limb, upper	C44.60-☑	C79.2	D04.6-☑	D23.6-☑	D48.5	D49.2
flank — *see also* Neoplasm, skin, trunk	C44.509	C79.2	D04.5	D23.5	D48.5	D49.2
foot — *see also* Neoplasm, skin, limb, lower	C44.70-☑	C79.2	D04.7-☑	D23.7-☑	D48.5	D49.2
forearm — *see also* Neoplasm, skin, limb, upper	C44.60-☑	C79.2	D04.6-☑	D23.6-☑	D48.5	D49.2
forehead — *see also* Neoplasm, skin, face	C44.309	C79.2	D04.39	D23.39	D48.5	D49.2
glabella — *see also* Neoplasm, skin, face	C44.309	C79.2	D04.39	D23.39	D48.5	D49.2
gluteal region — *see also* Neoplasm, skin, trunk	C44.509	C79.2	D04.5	D23.5	D48.5	D49.2
groin — *see also* Neoplasm, skin, trunk	C44.509	C79.2	D04.5	D23.5	D48.5	D49.2
hand — *see also* Neoplasm, skin, limb, upper	C44.60-☑	C79.2	D04.6-☑	D23.6-☑	D48.5	D49.2
head NEC — *see also* Neoplasm, skin, scalp	C44.40	C79.2	D04.4	D23.4	D48.5	D49.2
heel — *see also* Neoplasm, skin, limb, lower	C44.70-☑	C79.2	D04.7-☑	D23.7-☑	D48.5	D49.2
helix — *see also* Neoplasm, skin, ear	C44.20-☑	C79.2	D04.2-☑	D23.2-☑	D48.5	D49.2
hip — *see also* Neoplasm, skin, limb, lower	C44.70-☑	C79.2	D04.7-☑	D23.7-☑	D48.5	D49.2
infraclavicular region — *see also* Neoplasm, skin, trunk	C44.509	C79.2	D04.5	D23.5	D48.5	D49.2
inguinal region — *see also* Neoplasm, skin, trunk	C44.509	C79.2	D04.5	D23.5	D48.5	D49.2
jaw — *see also* Neoplasm, skin, face	C44.309	C79.2	D04.39	D23.39	D48.5	D49.2
Kaposi's sarcoma — *see* Kaposi's, sarcoma, skin						
knee — *see also* Neoplasm, skin, limb, lower	C44.70-☑	C79.2	D04.7-☑	D23.7-☑	D48.5	D49.2
labia						

	Malignant Primary	Malignant Secondary	Ca in situ	Benign	Uncertain	Unspecified Behavior
Neoplasm, neoplastic — *continued*						
skin — *continued*						
labia — *continued*						
majora	C51.Ø	C79.82	DØ7.1	D28.Ø	D39.8	D49.5
minora	C51.1	C79.82	DØ7.1	D28.Ø	D39.8	D49.5
leg — *see also* Neoplasm, skin, limb, lower	C44.7Ø-☑	C79.2	DØ4.7-☑	D23.7-☑	D48.5	D49.2
lid (lower) (upper)	C44.1Ø-☑	C79.2	DØ4.1-☑	D23.1-☑	D48.5	D49.2
basal cell carcinoma	C44.11-☑	—	—	—	—	—
specified type NEC	C44.19-☑	—	—	—	—	—
squamous cell carcinoma	C44.12-☑	—	—	—	—	—
limb NEC	C44.9Ø	C79.2	DØ4.9	D23.9	D48.5	D49.2
basal cell carcinoma	C44.91	—	—	—	—	—
lower	C44.7Ø-☑	C79.2	DØ4.7-☑	D23.7-☑	D48.5	D49.2
basal cell carcinoma	C44.71-☑	—	—	—	—	—
specified type NEC	C44.79-☑	—	—	—	—	—
squamous cell carcinoma	C44.72-☑	—	—	—	—	—
upper	C44.6Ø-☑	C79.2	DØ4.6-☑	D23.6-☑	D48.5	D49.2
basal cell carcinoma	C44.61-☑	—	—	—	—	—
specified type NEC	C44.69-☑	—	—	—	—	—
squamous cell carcinoma	C44.62-☑	—	—	—	—	—
lip (lower) (upper)	C44.ØØ	C79.2	DØ4.Ø	D23.Ø	D48.5	D49.2
basal cell carcinoma	C44.Ø1	—	—	—	—	—
specified type NEC	C44.Ø9	—	—	—	—	—
squamous cell carcinoma	C44.Ø2	—	—	—	—	—
male genital organs	C63.9	C79.82	DØ7.6Ø	D29.9	D4Ø.8	D49.5
penis	C6Ø.9	C79.82	DØ7.4	D29.Ø	D4Ø.8	D49.5
prepuce	C6Ø.Ø	C79.82	DØ7.4	D29.Ø	D4Ø.8	D49.5
scrotum	C63.2	C79.82	DØ7.61	D29.4	D4Ø.8	D49.5
mastectomy site (skin) — *see also* Neoplasm, skin, breast	C44.5Ø1	C79.2	—	—	—	—
specified as breast tissue	C5Ø.8-☑	C79.81	—	—	—	—
meatus, acoustic (external) — *see also* Neoplasm, skin, ear	C44.2Ø-☑	C79.2	DØ4.2-☑	D23.2-☑	D48.5	D49.2
melanotic — *see* Melanoma						
Merkel cell — *see* Carcinoma, Merkel cell						
nates — *see also* Neoplasm, skin, trunk	C44.5Ø9	C79.2	DØ4.5	D23.5	D48.5	D49.2
neck	C44.4Ø	C79.2	DØ4.4	D23.4	D48.5	D49.2
basal cell carcinoma	C44.41	—	—	—	—	—
specified type NEC	C44.49	—	—	—	—	—
squamous cell carcinoma	C44.42	—	—	—	—	—
nevus — *see* Nevus, skin						
nose (external) — *see also* Neoplasm, nose, skin	C44.3Ø1	C79.2	DØ4.39	D23.39	D48.5	D49.2
overlapping lesion	C44.8Ø	—	—	—	—	—
basal cell carcinoma	C44.81	—	—	—	—	—
specified type NEC	C44.89	—	—	—	—	—
squamous cell carcinoma	C44.82	—	—	—	—	—
Neoplasm, neoplastic — *continued*						
skin — *continued*						
palm — *see also* Neoplasm, skin, limb, upper	C44.6Ø-☑	C79.2	DØ4.6-☑	D23.6-☑	D48.5	D49.2
palpebra	C44.1Ø-☑	C79.2	DØ4.1-☑	D23.1-☑	D48.5	D49.2
basal cell carcinoma	C44.11-☑	—	—	—	—	—
specified type NEC	C44.19-☑	—	—	—	—	—
squamous cell carcinoma	C44.12-☑	—	—	—	—	—
penis NEC	C6Ø.9	C79.82	DØ7.4	D29.Ø	D4Ø.8	D49.5
perianal — *see also* Neoplasm, skin, anus	C44.5ØØ	C79.2	DØ4.5	D23.5	D48.5	D49.2
perineum — *see also* Neoplasm, skin, anus	C44.5ØØ	C79.2	DØ4.5	D23.5	D48.5	D49.2
pinna — *see also* Neoplasm, skin, ear	C44.2Ø-☑	C79.2	DØ4.2-☑	D23.2-☑	D48.5	D49.2
plantar — *see also* Neoplasm, skin, limb, lower	C44.7Ø-☑	C79.2	DØ4.7-☑	D23.7-☑	D48.5	D49.2
popliteal fossa or space — *see also* Neoplasm, skin, limb, lower	C44.7Ø-☑	C79.2	DØ4.7-☑	D23.7-☑	D48.5	D49.2
prepuce	C6Ø.Ø	C79.82	DØ7.4	D29.Ø	D4Ø.8	D49.5
pubes — *see also* Neoplasm, skin, trunk	C44.5Ø9	C79.2	DØ4.5	D23.5	D48.5	D49.2
sacrococcygeal region — *see also* Neoplasm, skin, trunk	C44.5Ø9	C79.2	DØ4.5	D23.5	D48.5	D49.2
scalp	C44.4Ø	C79.2	DØ4.4	D23.4	D48.5	D49.2
basal cell carcinoma	C44.41	—	—	—	—	—
specified type NEC	C44.49	—	—	—	—	—
squamous cell carcinoma	C44.42	—	—	—	—	—
scapular region — *see also* Neoplasm, skin, trunk	C44.5Ø9	C79.2	DØ4.5	D23.5	D48.5	D49.2
scrotum	C63.2	C79.82	DØ7.61	D29.4	D4Ø.8	D49.5
shoulder — *see also* Neoplasm, skin, limb, upper	C44.6Ø-☑	C79.2	DØ4.6-☑	D23.6-☑	D48.5	D49.2
sole (foot) — *see also* Neoplasm, skin, limb, lower	C44.7Ø-☑	C79.2	DØ4.7-☑	D23.7-☑	D48.5	D49.2
specified sites NEC	C44.8Ø	C79.2	DØ4.8	D23.9	D48.5	D49.2
basal cell carcinoma	C44.81	—	—	—	—	—
specified type NEC	C44.89	—	—	—	—	—
squamous cell carcinoma	C44.82	—	—	—	—	—
specified type NEC	C44.99	—	—	—	—	—
squamous cell carcinoma	C44.92	—	—	—	—	—
submammary fold — *see also* Neoplasm, skin, trunk	C44.5Ø9	C79.2	DØ4.5	D23.5	D48.5	D49.2
supraclavicular region — *see also* Neoplasm, skin, neck	C44.4Ø	C79.2	DØ4.4	D23.4	D48.5	D49.2
temple — *see also* Neoplasm, skin, face	C44.3Ø9	C79.2	DØ4.39	D23.39	D48.5	D49.2
thigh — *see also* Neoplasm, skin, limb, lower	C44.7Ø-☑	C79.2	DØ4.7-☑	D23.7-☑	D48.5	D49.2
thoracic wall — *see also* Neoplasm, skin, trunk	C44.5Ø9	C79.2	DØ4.5	D23.5	D48.5	D49.2

	Malignant Primary	Malignant Secondary	Ca in situ	Benign	Uncertain	Unspecified Behavior
Neoplasm, neoplastic — *continued*						
skin — *continued*						
thumb — *see also* Neoplasm, skin, limb, upper	C44.60-☑	C79.2	D04.6-☑	D23.6-☑	D48.5	D49.2
toe — *see also* Neoplasm, skin, limb, lower	C44.70-☑	C79.2	D04.7-☑	D23.7-☑	D48.5	D49.2
tragus — *see also* Neoplasm, skin, ear	C44.20-☑	C79.2	D04.2-☑	D23.2-☑	D48.5	D49.2
trunk	C44.509	C79.2	D04.5	D23.5	D48.5	D49.2
basal cell carcinoma	C44.519	—	—	—	—	—
specified type NEC	C44.599	—	—	—	—	—
squamous cell carcinoma	C44.529	—	—	—	—	—
umbilicus — *see also* Neoplasm, skin, trunk	C44.509	C79.2	D04.5	D23.5	D48.5	D49.2
vulva	C51.9	C79.82	D07.1	D28.0	D39.8	D49.5
overlapping lesion	C51.8	—	—	—	—	—
wrist — *see also* Neoplasm, skin, limb, upper	C44.60-☑	C79.2	D04.6-☑	D23.6-☑	D48.5	D49.2
skull	C41.0	C79.51	—	D16.4	D48.0	D49.2
soft parts or tissues — *see* Neoplasm, connective tissue						
specified site NEC	C76.8	C79.89	D09.8	D36.7	D48.7	D49.89
spermatic cord	C63.1-☑	C79.82	D07.69	D29.8	D40.8	D49.5
sphenoid	C31.3	C78.39	D02.3	D14.0	D38.5	D49.1
bone	C41.0	C79.51	—	D16.4	D48.0	D49.2
sinus	C31.3	C78.39	D02.3	D14.0	D38.5	D49.1
sphincter						
anal	C21.1	C78.5	D01.3	D12.9	D37.8	D49.0
of Oddi	C24.0	C78.89	D01.5	D13.5	D37.6	D49.0
spine, spinal (column)	C41.2	C79.51	—	D16.6	D48.0	D49.2
bulb	C71.7	C79.31	—	D33.1	D43.1	D49.6
coccyx	C41.4	C79.51	—	D16.8	D48.0	D49.2
cord (cervical) (lumbar) (sacral) (thoracic)	C72.0	C79.49	—	D33.4	D43.4	D49.7
dura mater	C70.1	C79.49	—	D32.1	D42.1	D49.7
lumbosacral	C41.2	C79.51	—	D16.6	D48.0	D49.2
marrow NEC	C96.9	C79.52	—	—	D47.9	D49.89
membrane	C70.1	C79.49	—	D32.1	D42.1	D49.7
meninges	C70.1	C79.49	—	D32.1	D42.1	D49.7
nerve (root)	C47.9	C79.89	—	D36.10	D48.2	D49.2
pia mater	C70.1	C79.49	—	D32.1	D42.1	D49.7
root	C47.9	C79.89	—	D36.10	D48.2	D49.2
sacrum	C41.4	C79.51	—	D16.8	D48.0	D49.2
spleen, splenic NEC	C26.1	C78.89	D01.7	D13.9	D37.8	D49.0
flexure (colon)	C18.5	C78.5	D01.0	D12.3	D37.4	D49.0
stem, brain	C71.7	C79.31	—	D33.1	D43.1	D49.6
Stensen's duct	C07	C79.89	D00.00	D11.0	D37.030	D49.0
sternum	C41.3	C79.51	—	D16.7	D48.0	D49.2
stomach	C16.9	C78.89	D00.2	D13.1	D37.1	D49.0
antrum (pyloric)	C16.3	C78.89	D00.2	D13.1	D37.1	D49.0
body	C16.2	C78.89	D00.2	D13.1	D37.1	D49.0
cardia	C16.0	C78.89	D00.2	D13.1	D37.1	D49.0
cardiac orifice	C16.0	C78.89	D00.2	D13.1	D37.1	D49.0
corpus	C16.2	C78.89	D00.2	D13.1	D37.1	D49.0
fundus	C16.1	C78.89	D00.2	D13.1	D37.1	D49.0
greater curvature NEC	C16.6	C78.89	D00.2	D13.1	D37.1	D49.0
lesser curvature NEC	C16.5	C78.89	D00.2	D13.1	D37.1	D49.0
overlapping lesion	C16.8	—	—	—	—	—
prepylorus	C16.4	C78.89	D00.2	D13.1	D37.1	D49.0
pylorus	C16.4	C78.89	D00.2	D13.1	D37.1	D49.0
wall NEC	C16.9	C78.89	D00.2	D13.1	D37.1	D49.0
anterior NEC	C16.8	C78.89	D00.2	D13.1	D37.1	D49.0
posterior NEC	C16.8	C78.89	D00.2	D13.1	D37.1	D49.0
stroma, endometrial	C54.1	C79.82	D07.0	D26.1	D39.0	D49.5
stump, cervical	C53.8	C79.82	D06.7	D26.0	D39.0	D49.5
subcutaneous (nodule) (tissue) NEC — *see* Neoplasm, connective tissue						
Neoplasm, neoplastic — *continued*						
subcutaneous — *see* Neoplasm, connective tissue — *continued* Neoplasm, connective tissue						
subdural	C70.9	C79.32	—	D32.9	D42.9	D49.7
subglottis, subglottic	C32.2	C78.39	D02.0	D14.1	D38.0	D49.1
sublingual	C04.9	C79.89	D00.06	D10.2	D37.09	D49.0
gland or duct	C08.1	C79.89	D00.00	D11.7	D37.031	D49.0
submandibular gland	C08.0	C79.89	D00.00	D11.7	D37.032	D49.0
submaxillary gland or duct	C08.0	C79.89	D00.00	D11.7	D37.032	D49.0
submental	C76.0	C79.89	D09.8	D36.7	D48.7	D49.89
subpleural	C34.9-☑	C78.0-☑	D02.2-☑	D14.3-☑	D38.1	D49.1
substernal	C38.1	C78.1	—	D15.2	D38.3	D49.89
sudoriferous, sudoriparous gland, site unspecified	C44.90	C79.2	D04.9	D23.9	D48.5	D49.2
specified site — *see* Neoplasm, skin						
supraclavicular region	C76.0	C79.89	D09.8	D36.7	D48.7	D49.89
supraglottis	C32.1	C78.39	D02.0	D14.1	D38.0	D49.1
suprarenal	C74.9-☑	C79.7-☑	D09.3	D35.0-☑	D44.1-☑	D49.7
capsule	C74.9-☑	C79.7-☑	D09.3	D35.0-☑	D44.1-☑	D49.7
cortex	C74.0-☑	C79.7-☑	D09.3	D35.0-☑	D44.1-☑	D49.7
gland	C74.9-☑	C79.7-☑	D09.3	D35.0-☑	D44.1-☑	D49.7
medulla	C74.1-☑	C79.7-☑	D09.3	D35.0-☑	D44.1-☑	D49.7
suprasellar (region)	C71.9	C79.31	—	D33.2	D43.2	D49.6
supratentorial (brain) NEC	C71.0	C79.31	—	D33.0	D43.0	D49.6
sweat gland (apocrine) (eccrine), site unspecified	C44.90	C79.2	D04.9	D23.9	D48.5	D49.2
specified site — *see* Neoplasm, skin						
sympathetic nerve or nervous system NEC	C47.9	C79.89	—	D36.10	D48.2	D49.2
symphysis pubis	C41.4	C79.51	—	D16.8	D48.0	D49.2
synovial membrane — *see* Neoplasm, connective tissue						
tapetum, brain	C71.8	C79.31	—	D33.2	D43.2	D49.6
tarsus (any bone)	C40.3-☑	C79.51	—	D16.3-☑	—	—
temple (skin) — *see also* Neoplasm, skin, face	C44.309	C79.2	D04.39	D23.39	D48.5	D49.2
temporal						
bone	C41.0	C79.51	—	D16.4	D48.0	D49.2
lobe or pole	C71.2	C79.31	—	D33.0	D43.0	D49.6
region	C76.0	C79.89	D09.8	D36.7	D48.7	D49.89
skin — *see also* Neoplasm, skin, face	C44.309	C79.2	D04.39	D23.39	D48.5	D49.2
tendon (sheath) — *see* Neoplasm, connective tissue						
tentorium (cerebelli)	C70.0	C79.32	—	D32.0	D42.0	D49.7
testis, testes	C62.9-☑	C79.82	D07.69	D29.2-☑	D40.1-☑	D49.5
descended	C62.1-☑	C79.82	D07.69	D29.2-☑	D40.1-☑	D49.5
ectopic	C62.0-☑	C79.82	D07.69	D29.2-☑	D40.1-☑	D49.5
retained	C62.0-☑	C79.82	D07.69	D29.2-☑	D40.1-☑	D49.5
scrotal	C62.1-☑	C79.82	D07.69	D29.2-☑	D40.1-☑	D49.5
undescended	C62.0-☑	C79.82	D07.69	D29.2-☑	D40.1-☑	D49.5
unspecified whether descended or undescended	C62.9-☑	C79.82	D07.69	D29.2-☑	D40.1-☑	D49.5
thalamus	C71.0	C79.31	—	D33.0	D43.0	D49.6
thigh NEC	C76.5-☑	C79.89	D04.7-☑	D36.7	D48.7	D49.89
thorax, thoracic (cavity) (organs NEC)	C76.1	C79.89	D09.8	D36.7	D48.7	D49.89
duct	C49.3	C79.89	—	D21.3	D48.1	D49.2
wall NEC	C76.1	C79.89	D09.8	D36.7	D48.7	D49.89
throat	C14.0	C79.89	D00.08	D10.9	D37.05	D49.0
thumb NEC	C76.4-☑	C79.89	D04.6-☑	D36.7	D48.7	D49.89
thymus (gland)	C37	C79.89	D09.3	D15.0	D38.4	D49.89
thyroglossal duct	C73	C79.89	D09.3	D34	D44.0	D49.7

	Malignant Primary	Malignant Secondary	Ca in situ	Benign	Uncertain	Unspecified Behavior
Neoplasm, neoplastic — *continued*						
thyroid (gland)	C73	C79.89	D09.3	D34	D44.0	D49.7
cartilage	C32.3	C78.39	D02.0	D14.1	D38.0	D49.1
tibia (any part)	C40.2-☑	C79.51	—	D16.2-☑	—	—
toe NEC	C76.5-☑	C79.89	D04.7-☑	D36.7	D48.7	D49.89
tongue	C02.9	C79.89	D00.07	D10.1	D37.02	D49.0
anterior (two-thirds) NEC	C02.3	C79.89	D00.07	D10.1	D37.02	D49.0
dorsal surface	C02.0	C79.89	D00.07	D10.1	D37.02	D49.0
ventral surface	C02.2	C79.89	D00.07	D10.1	D37.02	D49.0
base (dorsal surface)	C01	C79.89	D00.07	D10.1	D37.02	D49.0
border (lateral)	C02.1	C79.89	D00.07	D10.1	D37.02	D49.0
dorsal surface NEC	C02.0	C79.89	D00.07	D10.1	D37.02	D49.0
fixed part NEC	C01	C79.89	D00.07	D10.1	D37.02	D49.0
foreamen cecum	C02.0	C79.89	D00.07	D10.1	D37.02	D49.0
frenulum linguae	C02.2	C79.89	D00.07	D10.1	D37.02	D49.0
junctional zone	C02.8	C79.89	D00.07	D10.1	D37.02	D49.0
margin (lateral)	C02.1	C79.89	D00.07	D10.1	D37.02	D49.0
midline NEC	C02.0	C79.89	D00.07	D10.1	D37.02	D49.0
mobile part NEC	C02.3	C79.89	D00.07	D10.1	D37.02	D49.0
overlapping lesion	C02.8	—	—	—	—	—
posterior (third)	C01	C79.89	D00.07	D10.1	D37.02	D49.0
root	C01	C79.89	D00.07	D10.1	D37.02	D49.0
surface (dorsal)	C02.0	C79.89	D00.07	D10.1	D37.02	D49.0
base	C01	C79.89	D00.07	D10.1	D37.02	D49.0
ventral	C02.2	C79.89	D00.07	D10.1	D37.02	D49.0
tip	C02.1	C79.89	D00.07	D10.1	D37.02	D49.0
tonsil	C02.4	C79.89	D00.07	D10.1	D37.02	D49.0
tonsil	C09.9	C79.89	D00.08	D10.4	D37.05	D49.0
fauces, faucial	C09.9	C79.89	D00.08	D10.4	D37.05	D49.0
lingual	C02.4	C79.89	D00.07	D10.1	D37.02	D49.0
overlapping sites	C09.8	—	—	—	—	—
palatine	C09.9	C79.89	D00.08	D10.4	D37.05	D49.0
pharyngeal	C11.1	C79.89	D00.08	D10.6	D37.05	D49.0
pillar (anterior) (posterior)	C09.1	C79.89	D00.08	D10.5	D37.05	D49.0
tonsillar fossa	C09.0	C79.89	D00.08	D10.5	D37.05	D49.0
tooth socket NEC	C03.9	C79.89	D00.03	D10.39	D37.09	D49.0
trachea (cartilage) (mucosa)	C33	C78.39	D02.1	D14.2	D38.1	D49.1
overlapping lesion with bronchus or lung	C34.8-☑	—	—	—	—	—
tracheobronchial	C34.8-☑	C78.39	D02.1	D14.2	D38.1	D49.1
overlapping lesion with lung	C34.8-☑	—	—	—	—	—
tragus — *see also* Neoplasm, skin, ear	C44.20-☑	C79.2	D04.2-☑	D23.2-☑	D48.5	D49.2
trunk NEC	C76.8	C79.89	D04.5	D36.7	D48.7	D49.89
tubo-ovarian	C57.8	C79.82	D07.39	D28.7	D39.8	D49.5
tunica vaginalis	C63.7	C79.82	D07.69	D29.8	D40.8	D49.5
turbinate (bone)	C41.0	C79.51	—	D16.4	D48.0	D49.2
nasal	C30.0	C78.39	D02.3	D14.0	D38.5	D49.1
tympanic cavity	C30.1	C78.39	D02.3	D14.0	D38.5	D49.1
ulna (any part)	C40.0-☑	C79.51	—	D16.0-☑	—	—
umbilicus, umbilical — *see also* Neoplasm, skin, trunk	C44.509	C79.2	D04.5	D23.5	D48.5	D49.2
uncus, brain	C71.2	C79.31	—	D33.0	D43.0	D49.6
unknown site or unspecified	C80.1	C79.9	D09.9	D36.9	D48.9	D49.9
urachus	C67.7	C79.11	D09.0	D30.3	D41.4	D49.4
ureter-bladder (junction)	C67.6	C79.11	D09.0	D30.3	D41.4	D49.4
ureter, ureteral	C66.-☑	C79.19	D09.19	D30.2-☑	D41.2-☑	D49.5
orifice (bladder)	C67.6	C79.11	D09.0	D30.3	D41.4	D49.4
urethra, urethral (gland)	C68.0	C79.19	D09.19	D30.4	D41.3	D49.5
orifice, internal	C67.5	C79.11	D09.0	D30.3	D41.4	D49.4
urethrovaginal (septum)	C57.9	C79.82	D07.30	D28.9	D39.8	D49.5
urinary organ or system	C68.9	C79.10	D09.10	D30.9	D41.9	D49.5
bladder — *see* Neoplasm, bladder						
overlapping lesion	C68.8	—	—	—	—	—
specified sites NEC	C68.8	C79.19	D09.19	D30.8	D41.8	D49.5
utero-ovarian	C57.8	C79.82	D07.39	D28.7	D39.8	D49.5
ligament	C57.1-☑	C79.82	D07.39	D28.2	D39.8	D49.5
uterosacral ligament	C57.3	C79.82	—	D28.2	D39.8	D49.5
uterus, uteri, uterine	C55	C79.82	D07.0	D26.9	D39.0	D49.5
adnexa NEC	C57.4	C79.82	D07.39	D28.7	D39.8	D49.5
body	C54.9	C79.82	D07.0	D26.1	D39.0	D49.5
cervix	C53.9	C79.82	D06.9	D26.0	D39.0	D49.5
cornu	C54.9	C79.82	D07.0	D26.1	D39.0	D49.5
corpus	C54.9	C79.82	D07.0	D26.1	D39.0	D49.5
endocervix (canal) (gland)	C53.0	C79.82	D06.0	D26.0	D39.0	D49.5
endometrium	C54.1	C79.82	D07.0	D26.1	D39.0	D49.5
exocervix	C53.1	C79.82	D06.1	D26.0	D39.0	D49.5
external os	C53.1	C79.82	D06.1	D26.0	D39.0	D49.5
fundus	C54.3	C79.82	D07.0	D26.1	D39.0	D49.5
internal os	C53.0	C79.82	D06.0	D26.0	D39.0	D49.5
isthmus	C54.0	C79.82	D07.0	D26.1	D39.0	D49.5
ligament	C57.3	C79.82	—	D28.2	D39.8	D49.5
broad	C57.1-☑	C79.82	D07.39	D28.2	D39.8	D49.5
round	C57.2-☑	C79.82	—	D28.2	D39.8	D49.5
lower segment	C54.0	C79.82	D07.0	D26.1	D39.0	D49.5
myometrium	C54.2	C79.82	D07.0	D26.1	D39.0	D49.5
overlapping sites	C54.8	—	—	—	—	—
squamocolumnar junction	C53.8	C79.82	D06.7	D26.0	D39.0	D49.5
tube	C57.0-☑	C79.82	D07.39	D28.2	D39.8	D49.5
utricle, prostatic	C68.0	C79.19	D09.19	D30.4	D41.3	D49.5
uveal tract	C69.4-☑	C79.49	D09.2-☑	D31.4-☑	D48.7	D49.89
uvula	C05.2	C79.89	D00.04	D10.39	D37.09	D49.0
vagina, vaginal (fornix) (vault) (wall)	C52	C79.82	D07.2	D28.1	D39.8	D49.5
vaginovesical	C57.9	C79.82	D07.30	D28.9	D39.9	D49.5
septum	C57.9	C79.82	D07.30	D28.9	D39.9	D49.5
vallecula (epigiottis)	C10.0	C79.89	D00.08	D10.5	D37.05	D49.0
vascular — *see* Neoplasm, connective tissue						
vas deferens	C63.1-☑	C79.82	D07.69	D29.8	D40.8	D49.5
Vater's ampulla	C24.1	C78.89	D01.5	D13.5	D37.6	D49.0
vein, venous — *see* Neoplasm, connective tissue						
vena cava (abdominal) (inferior)	C49.4	C79.89	—	D21.4	D48.1	D49.2
superior	C49.3	C79.89	—	D21.3	D48.1	D49.2
ventricle (cerebral) (floor) (lateral) (third)	C71.5	C79.31	—	D33.0	D43.0	D49.6
cardiac (left) (right)	C38.0	C79.89	—	D15.1	D48.7	D49.89
fourth	C71.7	C79.31	—	D33.1	D43.1	D49.6
ventricular band of larynx	C32.1	C78.39	D02.0	D14.1	D38.0	D49.1
ventriculus — *see* Neoplasm, stomach						
vermillion border — *see* Neoplasm, lip						
vermis, cerebellum	C71.6	C79.31	—	D33.1	D43.1	D49.6
vertebra (column)	C41.2	C79.51	—	D16.6	D48.0	D49.2
coccyx	C41.4	C79.51	—	D16.8	D48.0	D49.2
marrow NEC	C96.9	C79.52	—	—	D47.9	D49.89
sacrum	C41.4	C79.51	—	D16.8	D48.0	D49.2
vesical — *see* Neoplasm, bladder						
vesicle, seminal	C63.7	C79.82	D07.69	D29.8	D40.8	D49.5
vesicocervical tissue	C57.9	C79.82	D07.30	D28.9	D39.9	D49.5
vesicorectal	C76.3	C79.82	D09.8	D36.7	D48.7	D49.89
vesicovaginal	C57.9	C79.82	D07.30	D28.9	D39.9	D49.5
septum	C57.9	C79.82	D07.30	D28.9	D39.8	D49.5
vessel (blood) — *see* Neoplasm, connective tissue						
vestibular gland, greater	C51.0	C79.82	D07.1	D28.0	D39.8	D49.5
vestibule						
mouth	C06.1	C79.89	D00.00	D10.39	D37.09	D49.0
nose	C30.0	C78.39	D02.3	D14.0	D38.5	D49.1
Virchow's gland	C77.0	C77.0	—	D36.0	D48.7	D49.89
viscera NEC	C76.8	C79.89	D09.8	D36.7	D48.7	D49.89
vocal cords (true)	C32.0	C78.39	D02.0	D14.1	D38.0	D49.1
false	C32.1	C78.39	D02.0	D14.1	D38.0	D49.1
vomer	C41.0	C79.51	—	D16.4	D48.0	D49.2
vulva	C51.9	C79.82	D07.1	D28.0	D39.8	D49.5
vulvovaginal gland	C51.0	C79.82	D07.1	D28.0	D39.8	D49.5
Waldeyer's ring	C14.2	C79.89	D00.08	D10.9	D37.05	D49.0
Wharton's duct	C08.0	C79.89	D00.00	D11.7	D37.032	D49.0

	Malignant Primary	Malignant Secondary	Ca in situ	Benign	Uncertain	Unspecified Behavior
Neoplasm, neoplastic — *continued*						
white matter (central) (cerebral)	C71.Ø	C79.31	—	D33.Ø	D43.Ø	D49.6
windpipe	C33	C78.39	DØ2.1	D14.2	D38.1	D49.1
Wirsung's duct	C25.3	C78.89	DØ1.7	D13.6	D37.8	D49.Ø
wolffian (body) (duct)						
female	C57.7	C79.82	DØ7.39	D28.7	D39.8	D49.5
male	C63.7	C79.82	DØ7.69	D29.8	D4Ø.8	D49.5
womb — *see* Neoplasm, uterus						
wrist NEC	C76.4-☑	C79.89	DØ4.6-☑	D36.7	D48.7	D49.89
xiphoid process	C41.3	C79.51	—	D16.7	D48.Ø	D49.2
Zuckerkandl organ	C75.5	C79.89	—	D35.6	D44.7	D49.7

ICD-1Ø-CM Table of Drugs and Chemicals

Substance	Poisoning, Accidental (unintentional)	Poisoning, Intentional Self-harm	Poisoning, Assault	Poisoning, Undetermined	Adverse Effect	Under-dosing
14-Hydroxydihydromorphinone	T4Ø.2X1	T4Ø.2X2	T4Ø.2X3	T4Ø.2X4	T4Ø.2X5	T4Ø.2X6
1-Propanol	T51.3X1	T51.3X2	T51.3X3	T51.3X4	—	—
2,3,7,8-Tetrachlorodibenzo-p-dioxin	T53.7X1	T53.7X2	T53.7X3	T53.7X4	—	—
2,4,5-T (trichlorophenoxyacetic acid)	T6Ø.1X1	T6Ø.1X2	T6Ø.1X3	T6Ø.1X4	—	—
2,4,5-Trichlorophenoxyacetic acid	T6Ø.3X1	T6Ø.3X2	T6Ø.3X3	T6Ø.3X4	—	—
2,4-D (dichlorophenoxyacetic acid)	T6Ø.3X1	T6Ø.3X2	T6Ø.3X3	T6Ø.3X4	—	—
2,4-Toluene diisocyanate	T65.ØX1	T65.ØX2	T65.ØX3	T65.ØX4	—	—
2-Deoxy-5-fluorouridine	T45.1X1	T45.1X2	T45.1X3	T45.1X4	T45.1X5	T45.1X6
2-Ethoxyethanol	T52.3X1	T52.3X2	T52.3X3	T52.3X4	—	—
2-Methoxyethanol	T52.3X1	T52.3X2	T52.3X3	T52.3X4	—	—
2-Propanol	T51.2X1	T51.2X2	T51.2X3	T51.2X4	—	—
4-Aminobutyric acid	T43.8X1	T43.8X2	T43.8X3	T43.8X4	T43.8X5	T43.8X6
4-Aminophenol derivatives	T39.1X1	T39.1X2	T39.1X3	T39.1X4	T39.1X5	T39.1X6
5-Deoxy-5-fluorouridine	T45.1X1	T45.1X2	T45.1X3	T45.1X4	T45.1X5	T45.1X6
5-Methoxypsoralen (5-MOP)	T5Ø.991	T5Ø.992	T5Ø.993	T5Ø.994	T5Ø.995	T5Ø.996
8-Aminoquinoline drugs	T37.2X1	T37.2X2	T37.2X3	T37.2X4	T37.2X5	T37.2X6
8-Methoxypsoralen (8-MOP)	T5Ø.991	T5Ø.992	T5Ø.993	T5Ø.994	T5Ø.995	T5Ø.996
ABOB	T37.5X1	T37.5X2	T37.5X3	T37.5X4	T37.5X5	T37.5X6
Abrine	T62.2X1	T62.2X2	T62.2X3	T62.2X4	—	—
Abrus (seed)	T62.2X1	T62.2X2	T62.2X3	T62.2X4	—	—
Absinthe	T51.ØX1	T51.ØX2	T51.ØX3	T51.ØX4	—	—
beverage	T51.ØX1	T51.ØX2	T51.ØX3	T51.ØX4	—	—
Acaricide	T6Ø.8X1	T6Ø.8X2	T6Ø.8X3	T6Ø.8X4	—	—
Acebutolol	T44.7X1	T44.7X2	T44.7X3	T44.7X4	T44.7X5	T44.7X6
Acecarbromal	T42.6X1	T42.6X2	T42.6X3	T42.6X4	T42.6X5	T42.6X6
Aceclidine	T44.1X1	T44.1X2	T44.1X3	T44.1X4	T44.1X5	T44.1X6
Acedapsone	T37.ØX1	T37.ØX2	T37.ØX3	T37.ØX4	T37.ØX5	T37.ØX6
Acefylline piperazine	T48.6X1	T48.6X2	T48.6X3	T48.6X4	T48.6X5	T48.6X6
Acemorphan	T4Ø.2X1	T4Ø.2X2	T4Ø.2X3	T4Ø.2X4	T4Ø.2X5	T4Ø.2X6
Acenocoumarin	T45.511	T45.512	T45.513	T45.514	T45.515	T45.516
Acenocoumarol	T45.511	T45.512	T45.513	T45.514	T45.515	T45.516
Acepifylline	T48.6X1	T48.6X2	T48.6X3	T48.6X4	T48.6X5	T48.6X6
Acepromazine	T43.3X1	T43.3X2	T43.3X3	T43.3X4	T43.3X5	T43.3X6
Acesulfamethoxypyridazine	T37.ØX1	T37.ØX2	T37.ØX3	T37.ØX4	T37.ØX5	T37.ØX6
Acetal	T52.8X1	T52.8X2	T52.8X3	T52.8X4	—	—
Acetaldehyde (vapor)	T52.8X1	T52.8X2	T52.8X3	T52.8X4	—	—
liquid	T65.891	T65.892	T65.893	T65.894	—	—
Acetaminophen	T39.1X1	T39.1X2	T39.1X3	T39.1X4	T39.1X5	T39.1X6
Acetaminosalol	T39.1X1	T39.1X2	T39.1X3	T39.1X4	T39.1X5	T39.1X6
Acetanilide	T39.1X1	T39.1X2	T39.1X3	T39.1X4	T39.1X5	T39.1X6
Acetarsol	T37.3X1	T37.3X2	T37.3X3	T37.3X4	T37.3X5	T37.3X6
Acetazolamide	T5Ø.2X1	T5Ø.2X2	T5Ø.2X3	T5Ø.2X4	T5Ø.2X5	T5Ø.2X6
Acetiamine	T45.2X1	T45.2X2	T45.2X3	T45.2X4	T45.2X5	T45.2X6
Acetic						
acid	T54.2X1	T54.2X2	T54.2X3	T54.2X4	—	—
with sodium acetate (ointment)	T49.3X1	T49.3X2	T49.3X3	T49.3X4	T49.3X5	T49.3X6
ester (solvent)(vapor)	T52.8X1	T52.8X2	T52.8X3	T52.8X4	—	—
irrigating solution	T5Ø.3X1	T5Ø.3X2	T5Ø.3X3	T5Ø.3X4	T5Ø.3X5	T5Ø.3X6
medicinal (lotion)	T49.2X1	T49.2X2	T49.2X3	T49.2X4	T49.2X5	T49.2X6
anhydride	T65.891	T65.892	T65.893	T65.894	—	—
ether (vapor)	T52.8X1	T52.8X2	T52.8X3	T52.8X4	—	—
Acetohexamide	T38.3X1	T38.3X2	T38.3X3	T38.3X4	T38.3X5	T38.3X6
Acetohydroxamic acid	T5Ø.991	T5Ø.992	T5Ø.993	T5Ø.994	T5Ø.995	T5Ø.996
Acetomenaphthone	T45.7X1	T45.7X2	T45.7X3	T45.7X4	T45.7X5	T45.7X6
Acetomorphine	T4Ø.1X1	T4Ø.1X2	T4Ø.1X3	T4Ø.1X4	—	—
Acetone (oils)	T52.4X1	T52.4X2	T52.4X3	T52.4X4	—	—
chlorinated	T52.4X1	T52.4X2	T52.4X3	T52.4X4	—	—
vapor	T52.4X1	T52.4X2	T52.4X3	T52.4X4	—	—
Acetonitrile	T52.8X1	T52.8X2	T52.8X3	T52.8X4	—	—
Acetophenazine	T43.3X1	T43.3X2	T43.3X3	T43.3X4	T43.3X5	T43.3X6
Acetophenetedin	T39.1X1	T39.1X2	T39.1X3	T39.1X4	T39.1X5	T39.1X6
Acetophenone	T52.4X1	T52.4X2	T52.4X3	T52.4X4	—	—
Acetorphine	T4Ø.2X1	T4Ø.2X2	T4Ø.2X3	T4Ø.2X4	—	—
Acetosulfone (sodium)	T37.1X1	T37.1X2	T37.1X3	T37.1X4	T37.1X5	T37.1X6
Acetrizoate (sodium)	T5Ø.8X1	T5Ø.8X2	T5Ø.8X3	T5Ø.8X4	T5Ø.8X5	T5Ø.8X6
Acetrizoic acid	T5Ø.8X1	T5Ø.8X2	T5Ø.8X3	T5Ø.8X4	T5Ø.8X5	T5Ø.8X6
Acetyl						
bromide	T53.6X1	T53.6X2	T53.6X3	T53.6X4	—	—
chloride	T53.6X1	T53.6X2	T53.6X3	T53.6X4	—	—
Acetylcarbromal	T42.6X1	T42.6X2	T42.6X3	T42.6X4	T42.6X5	T42.6X6
Acetylcholine						
chloride	T44.1X1	T44.1X2	T44.1X3	T44.1X4	T44.1X5	T44.1X6
derivative	T44.1X1	T44.1X2	T44.1X3	T44.1X4	T44.1X5	T44.1X6
Acetylcysteine	T48.4X1	T48.4X2	T48.4X3	T48.4X4	T48.4X5	T48.4X6
Acetyldigitoxin	T46.ØX1	T46.ØX2	T46.ØX3	T46.ØX4	T46.ØX5	T46.ØX6
Acetyldigoxin	T46.ØX1	T46.ØX2	T46.ØX3	T46.ØX4	T46.ØX5	T46.ØX6
Acetyldihydrocodeine	T4Ø.2X1	T4Ø.2X2	T4Ø.2X3	T4Ø.2X4	—	—
Acetyldihydrocodeinone	T4Ø.2X1	T4Ø.2X2	T4Ø.2X3	T4Ø.2X4	—	—
Acetylene (gas)	T59.891	T59.892	T59.893	T59.894	—	—
dichloride	T53.6X1	T53.6X2	T53.6X3	T53.6X4	—	—
incomplete combustion of	T58.11	T58.12	T58.13	T58.14	—	—
industrial	T59.891	T59.892	T59.893	T59.894	—	—
tetrachloride	T53.6X1	T53.6X2	T53.6X3	T53.6X4	—	—
vapor	T53.6X1	T53.6X2	T53.6X3	T53.6X4	—	—
Acetylpheneturide	T42.6X1	T42.6X2	T42.6X3	T42.6X4	T42.6X5	T42.6X6
Acetylphenylhydrazine	T39.8X1	T39.8X2	T39.8X3	T39.8X4	T39.8X5	T39.8X6
Acetylsalicylic acid (salts)	T39.Ø11	T39.Ø12	T39.Ø13	T39.Ø14	T39.Ø15	T39.Ø16
enteric coated	T39.Ø11	T39.Ø12	T39.Ø13	T39.Ø14	T39.Ø15	T39.Ø16
Acetylsulfamethoxypyridazine	T37.ØX1	T37.ØX2	T37.ØX3	T37.ØX4	T37.ØX5	T37.ØX6
Achromycin	T36.4X1	T36.4X2	T36.4X3	T36.4X4	T36.4X5	T36.4X6
ophthalmic preparation	T49.5X1	T49.5X2	T49.5X3	T49.5X4	T49.5X5	T49.5X6
topical NEC	T49.ØX1	T49.ØX2	T49.ØX3	T49.ØX4	T49.ØX5	T49.ØX6
Aciclovir	T37.5X1	T37.5X2	T37.5X3	T37.5X4	T37.5X5	T37.5X6
Acidifying agent NEC	T5Ø.9Ø1	T5Ø.9Ø2	T5Ø.9Ø3	T5Ø.9Ø4	T5Ø.9Ø5	T5Ø.9Ø6
Acid (corrosive) **NEC**	T54.2X1	T54.2X2	T54.2X3	T54.2X4	—	—
Acipimox	T46.6X1	T46.6X2	T46.6X3	T46.6X4	T46.6X5	T46.6X6
Acitretin	T5Ø.991	T5Ø.992	T5Ø.993	T5Ø.994	T5Ø.995	T5Ø.996
Aclarubicin	T45.1X1	T45.1X2	T45.1X3	T45.1X4	T45.1X5	T45.1X6
Aclatonium napadisilate	T48.1X1	T48.1X2	T48.1X3	T48.1X4	T48.1X5	T48.1X6
Aconite (wild)	T46.991	T46.992	T46.993	T46.994	T46.995	T46.996
Aconitine	T46.991	T46.992	T46.993	T46.994	T46.995	T46.996
Aconitum ferox	T46.991	T46.992	T46.993	T46.994	T46.995	T46.996
Acridine	T65.6X1	T65.6X2	T65.6X3	T65.6X4	—	—
vapor	T59.891	T59.892	T59.893	T59.894	—	—
Acriflavine	T37.91	T37.92	T37.93	T37.94	T37.95	T37.96
Acriflavinium chloride	T49.ØX1	T49.ØX2	T49.ØX3	T49.ØX4	T49.ØX5	T49.ØX6
Acrinol	T49.ØX1	T49.ØX2	T49.ØX3	T49.ØX4	T49.ØX5	T49.ØX6
Acrisorcin	T49.ØX1	T49.ØX2	T49.ØX3	T49.ØX4	T49.ØX5	T49.ØX6
Acrivastine	T45.ØX1	T45.ØX2	T45.ØX3	T45.ØX4	T45.ØX5	T45.ØX6
Acrolein (gas)	T59.891	T59.892	T59.893	T59.894	—	—
liquid	T54.1X1	T54.1X2	T54.1X3	T54.1X4	—	—
Acrylamide	T65.891	T65.892	T65.893	T65.894	—	—
Acrylic resin	T49.3X1	T49.3X2	T49.3X3	T49.3X4	T49.3X5	T49.3X6
Acrylonitrile	T65.891	T65.892	T65.893	T65.894	—	—
Actaea spicata	T62.2X1	T62.2X2	T62.2X3	T62.2X4	—	—
berry	T62.1X1	T62.1X2	T62.1X3	T62.1X4	—	—
Acterol	T37.3X1	T37.3X2	T37.3X3	T37.3X4	T37.3X5	T37.3X6
ACTH	T38.811	T38.812	T38.813	T38.814	T38.815	T38.816
Actinomycin C	T45.1X1	T45.1X2	T45.1X3	T45.1X4	T45.1X5	T45.1X6
Actinomycin D	T45.1X1	T45.1X2	T45.1X3	T45.1X4	T45.1X5	T45.1X6
Activated charcoal — *see also* Charcoal, medicinal	T47.6X1	T47.6X2	T47.6X3	T47.6X4	T47.6X5	T47.6X6
Acyclovir	T37.5X1	T37.5X2	T37.5X3	T37.5X4	T37.5X5	T37.5X6
Adenine	T45.2X1	T45.2X2	T45.2X3	T45.2X4	T45.2X5	T45.2X6
arabinoside	T37.5X1	T37.5X2	T37.5X3	T37.5X4	T37.5X5	T37.5X6
Adenosine (phosphate)	T46.2X1	T46.2X2	T46.2X3	T46.2X4	T46.2X5	T46.2X6
ADH	T38.891	T38.892	T38.893	T38.894	T38.895	T38.896
Adhesive NEC	T65.891	T65.892	T65.893	T65.894	—	—
Adicillin	T36.ØX1	T36.ØX2	T36.ØX3	T36.ØX4	T36.ØX5	T36.ØX6
Adiphenine	T44.3X1	T44.3X2	T44.3X3	T44.3X4	T44.3X5	T44.3X6
Adipiodone	T5Ø.8X1	T5Ø.8X2	T5Ø.8X3	T5Ø.8X4	T5Ø.8X5	T5Ø.8X6
Adjunct, pharmaceutical	T5Ø.9Ø1	T5Ø.9Ø2	T5Ø.9Ø3	T5Ø.9Ø4	T5Ø.9Ø5	T5Ø.9Ø6
Adrenal (extract, cortex or medulla) (glucocorticoids) (hormones) (mineralocorticoids)	T38.ØX1	T38.ØX2	T38.ØX3	T38.ØX4	T38.ØX5	T38.ØX6
ENT agent	T49.6X1	T49.6X2	T49.6X3	T49.6X4	T49.6X5	T49.6X6
ophthalmic preparation	T49.5X1	T49.5X2	T49.5X3	T49.5X4	T49.5X5	T49.5X6
topical NEC	T49.ØX1	T49.ØX2	T49.ØX3	T49.ØX4	T49.ØX5	T49.ØX6
Adrenalin — *see* Adrenaline						
Adrenaline	T44.5X1	T44.5X2	T44.5X3	T44.5X4	T44.5X5	T44.5X6
Adrenergic NEC	T44.9Ø1	T44.9Ø2	T44.9Ø3	T44.9Ø4	T44.9Ø5	T44.9Ø6
blocking agent NEC	T44.8X1	T44.8X2	T44.8X3	T44.8X4	T44.8X5	T44.8X6
beta, heart	T44.7X1	T44.7X2	T44.7X3	T44.7X4	T44.7X5	T44.7X6
specified NEC	T44.991	T44.992	T44.993	T44.994	T44.995	T44.996
Adrenochrome						
derivative	T46.991	T46.992	T46.993	T46.994	T46.995	T46.996

Substance	Poisoning, Accidental (unintentional)	Poisoning, Intentional Self-harm	Poisoning, Assault	Poisoning, Undetermined	Adverse Effect	Under-dosing
Adrenochrome — *continued*						
(mono) semicarbazone	T46.991	T46.992	T46.993	T46.994	T46.995	T46.996
Adrenocorticotrophic hormone	T38.811	T38.812	T38.813	T38.814	T38.815	T38.816
Adrenocorticotrophin	T38.811	T38.812	T38.813	T38.814	T38.815	T38.816
Adriamycin	T45.1X1	T45.1X2	T45.1X3	T45.1X4	T45.1X5	T45.1X6
Aerosol spray NEC	T65.91	T65.92	T65.93	T65.94	—	—
Aerosporin	T36.8X1	T36.8X2	T36.8X3	T36.8X4	T36.8X5	T36.8X6
ENT agent	T49.6X1	T49.6X2	T49.6X3	T49.6X4	T49.6X5	T49.6X6
ophthalmic preparation	T49.5X1	T49.5X2	T49.5X3	T49.5X4	T49.5X5	T49.5X6
topical NEC	T49.ØX1	T49.ØX2	T49.ØX3	T49.ØX4	T49.ØX5	T49.ØX6
Aethusa cynapium	T62.2X1	T62.2X2	T62.2X3	T62.2X4	—	—
Afghanistan black	T4Ø.7X1	T4Ø.7X2	T4Ø.7X3	T4Ø.7X4	T4Ø.7X5	T4Ø.7X6
Aflatoxin	T64.Ø1	T64.Ø2	T64.Ø3	T64.Ø4	—	—
Afloqualone	T42.8X1	T42.8X2	T42.8X3	T42.8X4	T42.8X5	T42.8X6
African boxwood	T62.2X1	T62.2X2	T62.2X3	T62.2X4	—	—
Agar	T47.4X1	T47.4X2	T47.4X3	T47.4X4	T47.4X5	T47.4X6
Agonist						
predominantly						
alpha-adrenoreceptor	T44.4X1	T44.4X2	T44.4X3	T44.4X4	T44.4X5	T44.4X6
beta-adrenoreceptor	T44.5X1	T44.5X2	T44.5X3	T44.5X4	T44.5X5	T44.5X6
Agricultural agent NEC	T65.91	T65.92	T65.93	T65.94	—	—
Agrypnal	T42.3X1	T42.3X2	T42.3X3	T42.3X4	T42.3X5	T42.3X6
AHLG	T5Ø.Z11	T5Ø.Z12	T5Ø.Z13	T5Ø.Z14	T5Ø.Z15	T5Ø.Z16
Air contaminant(s), **source/type NOS**	T65.91	T65.92	T65.93	T65.94	—	—
Ajmaline	T46.2X1	T46.2X2	T46.2X3	T46.2X4	T46.2X5	T46.2X6
Akee	T62.1X1	T62.1X2	T62.1X3	T62.1X4	—	—
Akrinol	T49.ØX1	T49.ØX2	T49.ØX3	T49.ØX4	T49.ØX5	T49.ØX6
Akritoin	T37.8X1	T37.8X2	T37.8X3	T37.8X4	T37.8X5	T37.8X6
Alacepril	T46.4X1	T46.4X2	T46.4X3	T46.4X4	T46.4X5	T46.4X6
Alantolactone	T37.4X1	T37.4X2	T37.4X3	T37.4X4	T37.4X5	T37.4X6
Albamycin	T36.8X1	T36.8X2	T36.8X3	T36.8X4	T36.8X5	T36.8X6
Albendazole	T37.4X1	T37.4X2	T37.4X3	T37.4X4	T37.4X5	T37.4X6
Albumin						
bovine	T45.8X1	T45.8X2	T45.8X3	T45.8X4	T45.8X5	T45.8X6
human serum	T45.8X1	T45.8X2	T45.8X3	T45.8X4	T45.8X5	T45.8X6
salt-poor	T45.8X1	T45.8X2	T45.8X3	T45.8X4	T45.8X5	T45.8X6
normal human serum	T45.8X1	T45.8X2	T45.8X3	T45.8X4	T45.8X5	T45.8X6
Albuterol	T48.6X1	T48.6X2	T48.6X3	T48.6X4	T48.6X5	T48.6X6
Albutoin	T42.ØX1	T42.ØX2	T42.ØX3	T42.ØX4	T42.ØX5	T42.ØX6
Alclometasone	T49.ØX1	T49.ØX2	T49.ØX3	T49.ØX4	T49.ØX5	T49.ØX6
Alcohol	T51.91	T51.92	T51.93	T51.94	—	—
absolute	T51.ØX1	T51.ØX2	T51.ØX3	T51.ØX4	—	—
beverage	T51.ØX1	T51.ØX2	T51.ØX3	T51.ØX4	—	—
allyl	T51.8X1	T51.8X2	T51.8X3	T51.8X4	—	—
amyl	T51.3X1	T51.3X2	T51.3X3	T51.3X4	—	—
antifreeze	T51.1X1	T51.1X2	T51.1X3	T51.1X4	—	—
beverage	T51.ØX1	T51.ØX2	T51.ØX3	T51.ØX4	—	—
butyl	T51.3X1	T51.3X2	T51.3X3	T51.3X4	—	—
dehydrated	T51.ØX1	T51.ØX2	T51.ØX3	T51.ØX4	—	—
beverage	T51.ØX1	T51.ØX2	T51.ØX3	T51.ØX4	—	—
denatured	T51.ØX1	T51.ØX2	T51.ØX3	T51.ØX4	—	—
deterrent NEC	T5Ø.6X1	T5Ø.6X2	T5Ø.6X3	T5Ø.6X4	T5Ø.6X5	T5Ø.6X6
diagnostic (gastric function)	T5Ø.8X1	T5Ø.8X2	T5Ø.8X3	T5Ø.8X4	T5Ø.8X5	T5Ø.8X6
ethyl	T51.ØX1	T51.ØX2	T51.ØX3	T51.ØX4	—	—
beverage	T51.ØX1	T51.ØX2	T51.ØX3	T51.ØX4	—	—
grain	T51.ØX1	T51.ØX2	T51.ØX3	T51.ØX4	—	—
beverage	T51.ØX1	T51.ØX2	T51.ØX3	T51.ØX4	—	—
industrial	T51.ØX1	T51.ØX2	T51.ØX3	T51.ØX4	—	—
isopropyl	T51.2X1	T51.2X2	T51.2X3	T51.2X4	—	—
methyl	T51.1X1	T51.1X2	T51.1X3	T51.1X4	—	—
preparation for consumption	T51.ØX1	T51.ØX2	T51.ØX3	T51.ØX4	—	—
propyl	T51.3X1	T51.3X2	T51.3X3	T51.3X4	—	—
secondary	T51.2X1	T51.2X2	T51.2X3	T51.2X4	—	—
radiator	T51.1X1	T51.1X2	T51.1X3	T51.1X4	—	—
rubbing	T51.2X1	T51.2X2	T51.2X3	T51.2X4	—	—
specified type NEC	T51.8X1	T51.8X2	T51.8X3	T51.8X4	—	—
surgical	T51.ØX1	T51.ØX2	T51.ØX3	T51.ØX4	—	—
vapor (from any type of Alcohol)	T59.891	T59.892	T59.893	T59.894	—	—
wood	T51.1X1	T51.1X2	T51.1X3	T51.1X4	—	—
Alcuronium (chloride)	T48.1X1	T48.1X2	T48.1X3	T48.1X4	T48.1X5	T48.1X6
Aldactone	T5Ø.ØX1	T5Ø.ØX2	T5Ø.ØX3	T5Ø.ØX4	T5Ø.ØX5	T5Ø.ØX6
Aldesulfone sodium	T37.1X1	T37.1X2	T37.1X3	T37.1X4	T37.1X5	T37.1X6
Aldicarb	T6Ø.ØX1	T6Ø.ØX2	T6Ø.ØX3	T6Ø.ØX4	—	—
Aldomet	T46.5X1	T46.5X2	T46.5X3	T46.5X4	T46.5X5	T46.5X6
Aldosterone	T5Ø.ØX1	T5Ø.ØX2	T5Ø.ØX3	T5Ø.ØX4	T5Ø.ØX5	T5Ø.ØX6
Aldrin (dust)	T6Ø.1X1	T6Ø.1X2	T6Ø.1X3	T6Ø.1X4	—	—
Aleve — *see* Naproxen						
Alexitol sodium	T47.1X1	T47.1X2	T47.1X3	T47.1X4	T47.1X5	T47.1X6

Substance	Poisoning, Accidental (unintentional)	Poisoning, Intentional Self-harm	Poisoning, Assault	Poisoning, Undetermined	Adverse Effect	Under-dosing
Alfacalcidol	T45.2X1	T45.2X2	T45.2X3	T45.2X4	T45.2X5	T45.2X6
Alfadolone	T41.1X1	T41.1X2	T41.1X3	T41.1X4	T41.1X5	T41.1X6
Alfaxalone	T41.1X1	T41.1X2	T41.1X3	T41.1X4	T41.1X5	T41.1X6
Alfentanil	T4Ø.4X1	T4Ø.4X2	T4Ø.4X3	T4Ø.4X4	T4Ø.4X5	T4Ø.4X6
Alfuzosin (hydrochloride)	T44.8X1	T44.8X2	T44.8X3	T44.8X4	T44.8X5	T44.8X6
Algae (harmful) (toxin)	T65.821	T65.822	T65.823	T65.824	—	—
Algeldrate	T47.1X1	T47.1X2	T47.1X3	T47.1X4	T47.1X5	T47.1X6
Algin	T47.8X1	T47.8X2	T47.8X3	T47.8X4	T47.8X5	T47.8X6
Alglucerase	T45.3X1	T45.3X2	T45.3X3	T45.3X4	T45.3X5	T45.3X6
Alidase	T45.3X1	T45.3X2	T45.3X3	T45.3X4	T45.3X5	T45.3X6
Alimemazine	T43.3X1	T43.3X2	T43.3X3	T43.3X4	T43.3X5	T43.3X6
Aliphatic thiocyanates	T65.ØX1	T65.ØX2	T65.ØX3	T65.ØX4	—	—
Alizapride	T45.ØX1	T45.ØX2	T45.ØX3	T45.ØX4	T45.ØX5	T45.ØX6
Alkali (caustic)	T54.3X1	T54.3X2	T54.3X3	T54.3X4	—	—
Alkaline antiseptic solution (aromatic)	T49.6X1	T49.6X2	T49.6X3	T49.6X4	T49.6X5	T49.6X6
Alkalinizing agents (medicinal)	T5Ø.9Ø1	T5Ø.9Ø2	T5Ø.9Ø3	T5Ø.9Ø4	T5Ø.9Ø5	T5Ø.9Ø6
Alkalizing agent NEC	T5Ø.9Ø1	T5Ø.9Ø2	T5Ø.9Ø3	T5Ø.9Ø4	T5Ø.9Ø5	T5Ø.9Ø6
Alka-seltzer	T39.Ø11	T39.Ø12	T39.Ø13	T39.Ø14	T39.Ø15	T39.Ø16
Alkavervir	T46.5X1	T46.5X2	T46.5X3	T46.5X4	T46.5X5	T46.5X6
Alkonium (bromide)	T49.ØX1	T49.ØX2	T49.ØX3	T49.ØX4	T49.ØX5	T49.ØX6
Alkylating drug NEC	T45.1X1	T45.1X2	T45.1X3	T45.1X4	T45.1X5	T45.1X6
antimyeloproliferative	T45.1X1	T45.1X2	T45.1X3	T45.1X4	T45.1X5	T45.1X6
lymphatic	T45.1X1	T45.1X2	T45.1X3	T45.1X4	T45.1X5	T45.1X6
Alkylisocyanate	T65.ØX1	T65.ØX2	T65.ØX3	T65.ØX4	—	—
Allantoin	T49.4X1	T49.4X2	T49.4X3	T49.4X4	T49.4X5	T49.4X6
Allegron	T43.Ø11	T43.Ø12	T43.Ø13	T43.Ø14	T43.Ø15	T43.Ø16
Allethrin	T49.ØX1	T49.ØX2	T49.ØX3	T49.ØX4	T49.ØX5	T49.ØX6
Allobarbital	T42.3X1	T42.3X2	T42.3X3	T42.3X4	T42.3X5	T42.3X6
Allopurinol	T5Ø.4X1	T5Ø.4X2	T5Ø.4X3	T5Ø.4X4	T5Ø.4X5	T5Ø.4X6
Allyl						
alcohol	T51.8X1	T51.8X2	T51.8X3	T51.8X4	—	—
disulfide	T46.6X1	T46.6X2	T46.6X3	T46.6X4	T46.6X5	T46.6X6
Allylestrenol	T38.5X1	T38.5X2	T38.5X3	T38.5X4	T38.5X5	T38.5X6
Allylisopropylacetylurea	T42.6X1	T42.6X2	T42.6X3	T42.6X4	T42.6X5	T42.6X6
Allylisopropylmalonylurea	T42.3X1	T42.3X2	T42.3X3	T42.3X4	T42.3X5	T42.3X6
Allylthiourea	T49.3X1	T49.3X2	T49.3X3	T49.3X4	T49.3X5	T49.3X6
Allyltribromide	T42.6X1	T42.6X2	T42.6X3	T42.6X4	T42.6X5	T42.6X6
Allypropymal	T42.3X1	T42.3X2	T42.3X3	T42.3X4	T42.3X5	T42.3X6
Almagate	T47.1X1	T47.1X2	T47.1X3	T47.1X4	T47.1X5	T47.1X6
Almasilate	T47.1X1	T47.1X2	T47.1X3	T47.1X4	T47.1X5	T47.1X6
Almitrine	T5Ø.7X1	T5Ø.7X2	T5Ø.7X3	T5Ø.7X4	T5Ø.7X5	T5Ø.7X6
Aloes	T47.2X1	T47.2X2	T47.2X3	T47.2X4	T47.2X5	T47.2X6
Aloglutamol	T47.1X1	T47.1X2	T47.1X3	T47.1X4	T47.1X5	T47.1X6
Aloin	T47.2X1	T47.2X2	T47.2X3	T47.2X4	T47.2X5	T47.2X6
Aloxidone	T42.2X1	T42.2X2	T42.2X3	T42.2X4	T42.2X5	T42.2X6
Alpha						
acetyldigoxin	T46.ØX1	T46.ØX2	T46.ØX3	T46.ØX4	T46.ØX5	T46.ØX6
adrenergic blocking drug	T44.6X1	T44.6X2	T44.6X3	T44.6X4	T44.6X5	T44.6X6
amylase	T45.3X1	T45.3X2	T45.3X3	T45.3X4	T45.3X5	T45.3X6
tocoferol (acetate)	T45.2X1	T45.2X2	T45.2X3	T45.2X4	T45.2X5	T45.2X6
tocopherol	T45.2X1	T45.2X2	T45.2X3	T45.2X4	T45.2X5	T45.2X6
Alphadolone	T41.1X1	T41.1X2	T41.1X3	T41.1X4	T41.1X5	T41.1X6
Alphaprodine	T4Ø.4X1	T4Ø.4X2	T4Ø.4X3	T4Ø.4X4	T4Ø.4X5	T4Ø.4X6
Alphaxalone	T41.1X1	T41.1X2	T41.1X3	T41.1X4	T41.1X5	T41.1X6
Alprazolam	T42.4X1	T42.4X2	T42.4X3	T42.4X4	T42.4X5	T42.4X6
Alprenolol	T44.7X1	T44.7X2	T44.7X3	T44.7X4	T44.7X5	T44.7X6
Alprostadil	T46.7X1	T46.7X2	T46.7X3	T46.7X4	T46.7X5	T46.7X6
Alsactide	T38.811	T38.812	T38.813	T38.814	T38.815	T38.816
Alseroxylon	T46.5X1	T46.5X2	T46.5X3	T46.5X4	T46.5X5	T46.5X6
Alteplase	T45.611	T45.612	T45.613	T45.614	T45.615	T45.616
Altizide	T5Ø.2X1	T5Ø.2X2	T5Ø.2X3	T5Ø.2X4	T5Ø.2X5	T5Ø.2X6
Altretamine	T45.1X1	T45.1X2	T45.1X3	T45.1X4	T45.1X5	T45.1X6
Alum (medicinal)	T49.4X1	T49.4X2	T49.4X3	T49.4X4	T49.4X5	T49.4X6
nonmedicinal (ammonium) (potassium)	T56.891	T56.892	T56.893	T56.894	—	—
Aluminium, aluminum						
acetate	T49.2X1	T49.2X2	T49.2X3	T49.2X4	T49.2X5	T49.2X6
solution	T49.ØX1	T49.ØX2	T49.ØX3	T49.ØX4	T49.ØX5	T49.ØX6
aspirin	T39.Ø11	T39.Ø12	T39.Ø13	T39.Ø14	T39.Ø15	T39.Ø16
bis (acetylsalicylate)	T39.Ø11	T39.Ø12	T39.Ø13	T39.Ø14	T39.Ø15	T39.Ø16
carbonate (gel, basic)	T47.1X1	T47.1X2	T47.1X3	T47.1X4	T47.1X5	T47.1X6
chlorhydroxide-complex	T47.1X1	T47.1X2	T47.1X3	T47.1X4	T47.1X5	T47.1X6
chloride	T49.2X1	T49.2X2	T49.2X3	T49.2X4	T49.2X5	T49.2X6
clofibrate	T46.6X1	T46.6X2	T46.6X3	T46.6X4	T46.6X5	T46.6X6
diacetate	T49.2X1	T49.2X2	T49.2X3	T49.2X4	T49.2X5	T49.2X6
glycinate	T47.1X1	T47.1X2	T47.1X3	T47.1X4	T47.1X5	T47.1X6
hydroxide (gel)	T47.1X1	T47.1X2	T47.1X3	T47.1X4	T47.1X5	T47.1X6
hydroxide-magnesium carb. gel	T47.1X1	T47.1X2	T47.1X3	T47.1X4	T47.1X5	T47.1X6
magnesium silicate	T47.1X1	T47.1X2	T47.1X3	T47.1X4	T47.1X5	T47.1X6
nicotinate	T46.7X1	T46.7X2	T46.7X3	T46.7X4	T46.7X5	T46.7X6

Substance	Poisoning, Accidental (unintentional)	Poisoning, Intentional Self-harm	Poisoning, Assault	Poisoning, Undetermined	Adverse Effect	Under-dosing
Aluminium, aluminum — *continued*						
ointment (surgical) (topical)	T49.3X1	T49.3X2	T49.3X3	T49.3X4	T49.3X5	T49.3X6
phosphate	T47.1X1	T47.1X2	T47.1X3	T47.1X4	T47.1X5	T47.1X6
salicylate	T39.Ø91	T39.Ø92	T39.Ø93	T39.Ø94	T39.Ø95	T39.Ø96
silicate	T47.1X1	T47.1X2	T47.1X3	T47.1X4	T47.1X5	T47.1X6
sodium silicate	T47.1X1	T47.1X2	T47.1X3	T47.1X4	T47.1X5	T47.1X6
subacetate	T49.2X1	T49.2X2	T49.2X3	T49.2X4	T49.2X5	T49.2X6
sulfate	T49.ØX1	T49.ØX2	T49.ØX3	T49.ØX4	T49.ØX5	T49.ØX6
tannate	T47.6X1	T47.6X2	T47.6X3	T47.6X4	T47.6X5	T47.6X6
topical NEC	T49.3X1	T49.3X2	T49.3X3	T49.3X4	T49.3X5	T49.3X6
Alurate	T42.3X1	T42.3X2	T42.3X3	T42.3X4	T42.3X5	T42.3X6
Alverine	T44.3X1	T44.3X2	T44.3X3	T44.3X4	T44.3X5	T44.3X6
Alvodine	T4Ø.2X1	T4Ø.2X2	T4Ø.2X3	T4Ø.2X4	T4Ø.2X5	T4Ø.2X6
Amanita phalloides	T62.ØX1	T62.ØX2	T62.ØX3	T62.ØX4	—	—
Amanitine	T62.ØX1	T62.ØX2	T62.ØX3	T62.ØX4	—	—
Amantadine	T42.8X1	T42.8X2	T42.8X3	T42.8X4	T42.8X5	T42.8X6
Ambazone	T49.6X1	T49.6X2	T49.6X3	T49.6X4	T49.6X5	T49.6X6
Ambenonium (chloride)	T44.ØX1	T44.ØX2	T44.ØX3	T44.ØX4	T44.ØX5	T44.ØX6
Ambroxol	T48.4X1	T48.4X2	T48.4X3	T48.4X4	T48.4X5	T48.4X6
Ambuphylline	T48.6X1	T48.6X2	T48.6X3	T48.6X4	T48.6X5	T48.6X6
Ambutonium bromide	T44.3X1	T44.3X2	T44.3X3	T44.3X4	T44.3X5	T44.3X6
Amcinonide	T49.ØX1	T49.ØX2	T49.ØX3	T49.ØX4	T49.ØX5	T49.ØX6
Amdinocilline	T36.ØX1	T36.ØX2	T36.ØX3	T36.ØX4	T36.ØX5	T36.ØX6
Ametazole	T5Ø.8X1	T5Ø.8X2	T5Ø.8X3	T5Ø.8X4	T5Ø.8X5	T5Ø.8X6
Amethocaine	T41.3X1	T41.3X2	T41.3X3	T41.3X4	T41.3X5	T41.3X6
regional	T41.3X1	T41.3X2	T41.3X3	T41.3X4	T41.3X5	T41.3X6
spinal	T41.3X1	T41.3X2	T41.3X3	T41.3X4	T41.3X5	T41.3X6
Amethopterin	T45.1X1	T45.1X2	T45.1X3	T45.1X4	T45.1X5	T45.1X6
Amezinium metilsulfate	T44.991	T44.992	T44.993	T44.994	T44.995	T44.996
Amfebutamone	T43.291	T43.292	T43.293	T43.294	T43.295	T43.296
Amfepramone	T5Ø.5X1	T5Ø.5X2	T5Ø.5X3	T5Ø.5X4	T5Ø.5X5	T5Ø.5X6
Amfetamine	T43.621	T43.622	T43.623	T43.624	T43.625	T43.626
Amfetaminil	T43.621	T43.622	T43.623	T43.624	T43.625	T43.626
Amfomycin	T36.8X1	T36.8X2	T36.8X3	T36.8X4	T36.8X5	T36.8X6
Amidefrine mesilate	T48.5X1	T48.5X2	T48.5X3	T48.5X4	T48.5X5	T48.5X6
Amidone	T4Ø.3X1	T4Ø.3X2	T4Ø.3X3	T4Ø.3X4	T4Ø.3X5	T4Ø.3X6
Amidopyrine	T39.2X1	T39.2X2	T39.2X3	T39.2X4	T39.2X5	T39.2X6
Amidotrizoate	T5Ø.8X1	T5Ø.8X2	T5Ø.8X3	T5Ø.8X4	T5Ø.8X5	T5Ø.8X6
Amiflamine	T43.1X1	T43.1X2	T43.1X3	T43.1X4	T43.1X5	T43.1X6
Amikacin	T36.5X1	T36.5X2	T36.5X3	T36.5X4	T36.5X5	T36.5X6
Amikhelline	T46.3X1	T46.3X2	T46.3X3	T46.3X4	T46.3X5	T46.3X6
Amiloride	T5Ø.2X1	T5Ø.2X2	T5Ø.2X3	T5Ø.2X4	T5Ø.2X5	T5Ø.2X6
Aminacrine	T49.ØX1	T49.ØX2	T49.ØX3	T49.ØX4	T49.ØX5	T49.ØX6
Amineptine	T43.Ø11	T43.Ø12	T43.Ø13	T43.Ø14	T43.Ø15	T43.Ø16
Aminitrozole	T37.3X1	T37.3X2	T37.3X3	T37.3X4	T37.3X5	T37.3X6
Aminoacetic acid (derivatives)	T5Ø.3X1	T5Ø.3X2	T5Ø.3X3	T5Ø.3X4	T5Ø.3X5	T5Ø.3X6
Amino acids	T5Ø.3X1	T5Ø.3X2	T5Ø.3X3	T5Ø.3X4	T5Ø.3X5	T5Ø.3X6
Aminoacridine	T49.ØX1	T49.ØX2	T49.ØX3	T49.ØX4	T49.ØX5	T49.ØX6
Aminobenzoic acid (-p)	T49.3X1	T49.3X2	T49.3X3	T49.3X4	T49.3X5	T49.3X6
Aminocaproic acid	T45.621	T45.622	T45.623	T45.624	T45.625	T45.626
Aminoethylisothiourium	T45.8X1	T45.8X2	T45.8X3	T45.8X4	T45.8X5	T45.8X6
Aminofenazone	T39.2X1	T39.2X2	T39.2X3	T39.2X4	T39.2X5	T39.2X6
Aminoglutethimide	T45.1X1	T45.1X2	T45.1X3	T45.1X4	T45.1X5	T45.1X6
Aminohippuric acid	T5Ø.8X1	T5Ø.8X2	T5Ø.8X3	T5Ø.8X4	T5Ø.8X5	T5Ø.8X6
Aminomethylbenzoic acid	T45.691	T45.692	T45.693	T45.694	T45.695	T45.696
Aminometradine	T5Ø.2X1	T5Ø.2X2	T5Ø.2X3	T5Ø.2X4	T5Ø.2X5	T5Ø.2X6
Aminopentamide	T44.3X1	T44.3X2	T44.3X3	T44.3X4	T44.3X5	T44.3X6
Aminophenazone	T39.2X1	T39.2X2	T39.2X3	T39.2X4	T39.2X5	T39.2X6
Aminophenol	T54.ØX1	T54.ØX2	T54.ØX3	T54.ØX4	—	—
Aminophenylpyridone	T43.591	T43.592	T43.593	T43.594	T43.595	T43.596
Aminophylline	T48.6X1	T48.6X2	T48.6X3	T48.6X4	T48.6X5	T48.6X6
Aminopterin sodium	T45.1X1	T45.1X2	T45.1X3	T45.1X4	T45.1X5	T45.1X6
Aminopyrine	T39.2X1	T39.2X2	T39.2X3	T39.2X4	T39.2X5	T39.2X6
Aminorex	T5Ø.5X1	T5Ø.5X2	T5Ø.5X3	T5Ø.5X4	T5Ø.5X5	T5Ø.5X6
Aminosalicylic acid	T37.1X1	T37.1X2	T37.1X3	T37.1X4	T37.1X5	T37.1X6
Aminosalylum	T37.1X1	T37.1X2	T37.1X3	T37.1X4	T37.1X5	T37.1X6
Amiodarone	T46.2X1	T46.2X2	T46.2X3	T46.2X4	T46.2X5	T46.2X6
Amiphenazole	T5Ø.7X1	T5Ø.7X2	T5Ø.7X3	T5Ø.7X4	T5Ø.7X5	T5Ø.7X6
Amiquinsin	T46.5X1	T46.5X2	T46.5X3	T46.5X4	T46.5X5	T46.5X6
Amisometradine	T5Ø.2X1	T5Ø.2X2	T5Ø.2X3	T5Ø.2X4	T5Ø.2X5	T5Ø.2X6
Amisulpride	T43.591	T43.592	T43.593	T43.594	T43.595	T43.596
Amitriptyline	T43.Ø11	T43.Ø12	T43.Ø13	T43.Ø14	T43.Ø15	T43.Ø16
Amitriptylinoxide	T43.Ø11	T43.Ø12	T43.Ø13	T43.Ø14	T43.Ø15	T43.Ø16
Amlexanox	T48.6X1	T48.6X2	T48.6X3	T48.6X4	T48.6X5	T48.6X6
Ammonia (fumes) (gas) (vapor)	T59.891	T59.892	T59.893	T59.894	—	—
aromatic spirit	T48.991	T48.992	T48.993	T48.994	T48.995	T48.996
liquid (household)	T54.3X1	T54.3X2	T54.3X3	T54.3X4	—	—
Ammoniated mercury	T49.ØX1	T49.ØX2	T49.ØX3	T49.ØX4	T49.ØX5	T49.ØX6
Ammonium						
acid tartrate	T49.5X1	T49.5X2	T49.5X3	T49.5X4	T49.5X5	T49.5X6

Substance	Poisoning, Accidental (unintentional)	Poisoning, Intentional Self-harm	Poisoning, Assault	Poisoning, Undetermined	Adverse Effect	Under-dosing
Ammonium — *continued*						
bromide	T42.6X1	T42.6X2	T42.6X3	T42.6X4	T42.6X5	T42.6X6
carbonate	T54.3X1	T54.3X2	T54.3X3	T54.3X4	—	—
chloride	T5Ø.991	T5Ø.992	T5Ø.993	T5Ø.994	T5Ø.995	T5Ø.996
expectorant	T48.4X1	T48.4X2	T48.4X3	T48.4X4	T48.4X5	T48.4X6
compounds (household) NEC	T54.3X1	T54.3X2	T54.3X3	T54.3X4	—	—
fumes (any usage)	T59.891	T59.892	T59.893	T59.894	—	—
industrial	T54.3X1	T54.3X2	T54.3X3	T54.3X4	—	—
ichthyosulronate	T49.4X1	T49.4X2	T49.4X3	T49.4X4	T49.4X5	T49.4X6
mandelate	T37.91	T37.92	T37.93	T37.94	T37.95	T37.96
sulfamate	T6Ø.3X1	T6Ø.3X2	T6Ø.3X3	T6Ø.3X4	—	—
sulfonate resin	T47.8X1	T47.8X2	T47.8X3	T47.8X4	T47.8X5	T47.8X6
Amobarbital (sodium)	T42.3X1	T42.3X2	T42.3X3	T42.3X4	T42.3X5	T42.3X6
Amodiaquine	T37.2X1	T37.2X2	T37.2X3	T37.2X4	T37.2X5	T37.2X6
Amopyroquin (e)	T37.2X1	T37.2X2	T37.2X3	T37.2X4	T37.2X5	T37.2X6
Amoxapine	T43.Ø11	T43.Ø12	T43.Ø13	T43.Ø14	T43.Ø15	T43.Ø16
Amoxicillin	T36.ØX1	T36.ØX2	T36.ØX3	T36.ØX4	T36.ØX5	T36.ØX6
Amperozide	T43.591	T43.592	T43.593	T43.594	T43.595	T43.596
Amphenidone	T43.591	T43.592	T43.593	T43.594	T43.595	T43.596
Amphetamine NEC	T43.621	T43.622	T43.623	T43.624	T43.625	T43.626
Amphomycin	T36.8X1	T36.8X2	T36.8X3	T36.8X4	T36.8X5	T36.8X6
Amphotalide	T37.4X1	T37.4X2	T37.4X3	T37.4X4	T37.4X5	T37.4X6
Amphotericin B	T36.7X1	T36.7X2	T36.7X3	T36.7X4	T36.7X5	T36.7X6
topical	T49.ØX1	T49.ØX2	T49.ØX3	T49.ØX4	T49.ØX5	T49.ØX6
Ampicillin	T36.ØX1	T36.ØX2	T36.ØX3	T36.ØX4	T36.ØX5	T36.ØX6
Amprotropine	T44.3X1	T44.3X2	T44.3X3	T44.3X4	T44.3X5	T44.3X6
Amsacrine	T45.1X1	T45.1X2	T45.1X3	T45.1X4	T45.1X5	T45.1X6
Amygdaline	T62.2X1	T62.2X2	T62.2X3	T62.2X4	—	—
Amyl						
acetate	T52.8X1	T52.8X2	T52.8X3	T52.8X4	—	—
vapor	T59.891	T59.892	T59.893	T59.894	—	—
alcohol	T51.3X1	T51.3X2	T51.3X3	T51.3X4	—	—
chloride	T53.6X1	T53.6X2	T53.6X3	T53.6X4	—	—
formate	T52.8X1	T52.8X2	T52.8X3	T52.8X4	—	—
nitrite	T46.3X1	T46.3X2	T46.3X3	T46.3X4	T46.3X5	T46.3X6
propionate	T65.891	T65.892	T65.893	T65.894	—	—
Amylase	T47.5X1	T47.5X2	T47.5X3	T47.5X4	T47.5X5	T47.5X6
Amyleine, regional	T41.3X1	T41.3X2	T41.3X3	T41.3X4	T41.3X5	T41.3X6
Amylene						
dichloride	T53.6X1	T53.6X2	T53.6X3	T53.6X4	—	—
hydrate	T51.3X1	T51.3X2	T51.3X3	T51.3X4	—	—
Amylmetacresol	T49.6X1	T49.6X2	T49.6X3	T49.6X4	T49.6X5	T49.6X6
Amylobarbitone	T42.3X1	T42.3X2	T42.3X3	T42.3X4	T42.3X5	T42.3X6
Amylocaine, regional	T41.3X1	T41.3X2	T41.3X3	T41.3X4	T41.3X5	T41.3X6
infiltration (subcutaneous)	T41.3X1	T41.3X2	T41.3X3	T41.3X4	T41.3X5	T41.3X6
nerve block (peripheral) (plexus)	T41.3X1	T41.3X2	T41.3X3	T41.3X4	T41.3X5	T41.3X6
spinal	T41.3X1	T41.3X2	T41.3X3	T41.3X4	T41.3X5	T41.3X6
topical (surface)	T41.3X1	T41.3X2	T41.3X3	T41.3X4	T41.3X5	T41.3X6
Amylopectin	T47.6X1	T47.6X2	T47.6X3	T47.6X4	T47.6X5	T47.6X6
Amytal (sodium)	T42.3X1	T42.3X2	T42.3X3	T42.3X4	T42.3X5	T42.3X6
Anabolic steroid	T38.7X1	T38.7X2	T38.7X3	T38.7X4	T38.7X5	T38.7X6
Analeptic NEC	T5Ø.7X1	T5Ø.7X2	T5Ø.7X3	T5Ø.7X4	T5Ø.7X5	T5Ø.7X6
Analgesic	T39.91	T39.92	T39.93	T39.94	T39.95	T39.96
anti-inflammatory NEC	T39.91	T39.92	T39.93	T39.94	T39.95	T39.96
propionic acid derivative	T39.311	T39.312	T39.313	T39.314	T39.315	T39.316
antirheumatic NEC	T39.4X1	T39.4X2	T39.4X3	T39.4X4	T39.4X5	T39.4X6
aromatic NEC	T39.1X1	T39.1X2	T39.1X3	T39.1X4	T39.1X5	T39.1X6
narcotic NEC	T4Ø.6Ø1	T4Ø.6Ø2	T4Ø.6Ø3	T4Ø.6Ø4	T4Ø.6Ø5	T4Ø.6Ø6
combination	T4Ø.6Ø1	T4Ø.6Ø2	T4Ø.6Ø3	T4Ø.6Ø4	T4Ø.6Ø5	T4Ø.6Ø6
obstetric	T4Ø.6Ø1	T4Ø.6Ø2	T4Ø.6Ø3	T4Ø.6Ø4	T4Ø.6Ø5	T4Ø.6Ø6
non-narcotic NEC	T39.91	T39.92	T39.93	T39.94	T39.95	T39.96
combination	T39.91	T39.92	T39.93	T39.94	T39.95	T39.96
pyrazole	T39.2X1	T39.2X2	T39.2X3	T39.2X4	T39.2X5	T39.2X6
specified NEC	T39.8X1	T39.8X2	T39.8X3	T39.8X4	T39.8X5	T39.8X6
Analgin	T39.2X1	T39.2X2	T39.2X3	T39.2X4	T39.2X5	T39.2X6
Anamirta cocculus	T62.1X1	T62.1X2	T62.1X3	T62.1X4	—	—
Ancillin	T36.ØX1	T36.ØX2	T36.ØX3	T36.ØX4	T36.ØX5	T36.ØX6
Ancrod	T45.691	T45.692	T45.693	T45.694	T45.695	T45.696
Androgen	T38.7X1	T38.7X2	T38.7X3	T38.7X4	T38.7X5	T38.7X6
Androgen-estrogen mixture	T38.7X1	T38.7X2	T38.7X3	T38.7X4	T38.7X5	T38.7X6
Androstalone	T38.7X1	T38.7X2	T38.7X3	T38.7X4	T38.7X5	T38.7X6
Androstanolone	T38.7X1	T38.7X2	T38.7X3	T38.7X4	T38.7X5	T38.7X6
Androsterone	T38.7X1	T38.7X2	T38.7X3	T38.7X4	T38.7X5	T38.7X6
Anemone pulsatilla	T62.2X1	T62.2X2	T62.2X3	T62.2X4	—	—
Anesthesia						
caudal	T41.3X1	T41.3X2	T41.3X3	T41.3X4	T41.3X5	T41.3X6
endotracheal	T41.ØX1	T41.ØX2	T41.ØX3	T41.ØX4	T41.ØX5	T41.ØX6
epidural	T41.3X1	T41.3X2	T41.3X3	T41.3X4	T41.3X5	T41.3X6
inhalation	T41.ØX1	T41.ØX2	T41.ØX3	T41.ØX4	T41.ØX5	T41.ØX6
local	T41.3X1	T41.3X2	T41.3X3	T41.3X4	T41.3X5	T41.3X6

Substance	Poisoning, Accidental (unintentional)	Poisoning, Intentional Self-harm	Poisoning, Assault	Poisoning, Undetermined	Adverse Effect	Under-dosing
Anesthesia — *continued*						
mucosal	T41.3X1	T41.3X2	T41.3X3	T41.3X4	T41.3X5	T41.3X6
muscle relaxation	T48.1X1	T48.1X2	T48.1X3	T48.1X4	T48.1X5	T48.1X6
nerve blocking	T41.3X1	T41.3X2	T41.3X3	T41.3X4	T41.3X5	T41.3X6
plexus blocking	T41.3X1	T41.3X2	T41.3X3	T41.3X4	T41.3X5	T41.3X6
potentiated	T41.2Ø1	T41.2Ø2	T41.2Ø3	T41.2Ø4	T41.2Ø5	T41.2Ø6
rectal	T41.2Ø1	T41.2Ø2	T41.2Ø3	T41.2Ø4	T41.2Ø5	T41.2Ø6
general	T41.2Ø1	T41.2Ø2	T41.2Ø3	T41.2Ø4	T41.2Ø5	T41.2Ø6
local	T41.3X1	T41.3X2	T41.3X3	T41.3X4	T41.3X5	T41.3X6
regional	T41.3X1	T41.3X2	T41.3X3	T41.3X4	T41.3X5	T41.3X6
surface	T41.3X1	T41.3X2	T41.3X3	T41.3X4	T41.3X5	T41.3X6
Anesthetic NEC — *see also* Anesthesia	T41.41	T41.42	T41.43	T41.44	T41.45	T41.46
with muscle relaxant	T41.2Ø1	T41.2Ø2	T41.2Ø3	T41.2Ø4	T41.2Ø5	T41.2Ø6
general	T41.2Ø1	T41.2Ø2	T41.2Ø3	T41.2Ø4	T41.2Ø5	T41.2Ø6
local	T41.3X1	T41.3X2	T41.3X3	T41.3X4	T41.3X5	T41.3X6
gaseous NEC	T41.ØX1	T41.ØX2	T41.ØX3	T41.ØX4	T41.ØX5	T41.ØX6
general NEC	T41.2Ø1	T41.2Ø2	T41.2Ø3	T41.2Ø4	T41.2Ø5	T41.2Ø6
halogenated hydrocarbon derivatives NEC	T41.ØX1	T41.ØX2	T41.ØX3	T41.ØX4	T41.ØX5	T41.ØX6
infiltration NEC	T41.3X1	T41.3X2	T41.3X3	T41.3X4	T41.3X5	T41.3X6
intravenous NEC	T41.1X1	T41.1X2	T41.1X3	T41.1X4	T41.1X5	T41.1X6
local NEC	T41.3X1	T41.3X2	T41.3X3	T41.3X4	T41.3X5	T41.3X6
rectal	T41.2Ø1	T41.2Ø2	T41.2Ø3	T41.2Ø4	T41.2Ø5	T41.2Ø6
general	T41.2Ø1	T41.2Ø2	T41.2Ø3	T41.2Ø4	T41.2Ø5	T41.2Ø6
local	T41.3X1	T41.3X2	T41.3X3	T41.3X4	T41.3X5	T41.3X6
regional NEC	T41.3X1	T41.3X2	T41.3X3	T41.3X4	T41.3X5	T41.3X6
spinal NEC	T41.3X1	T41.3X2	T41.3X3	T41.3X4	T41.3X5	T41.3X6
thiobarbiturate	T41.1X1	T41.1X2	T41.1X3	T41.1X4	T41.1X5	T41.1X6
topical	T41.3X1	T41.3X2	T41.3X3	T41.3X4	T41.3X5	T41.3X6
Aneurine	T45.2X1	T45.2X2	T45.2X3	T45.2X4	T45.2X5	T45.2X6
Angio-Conray	T5Ø.8X1	T5Ø.8X2	T5Ø.8X3	T5Ø.8X4	T5Ø.8X5	T5Ø.8X6
Angiotensin	T44.5X1	T44.5X2	T44.5X3	T44.5X4	T44.5X5	T44.5X6
Angiotensinamide	T44.991	T44.992	T44.993	T44.994	T44.995	T44.996
Anhydrohydroxy-progesterone	T38.5X1	T38.5X2	T38.5X3	T38.5X4	T38.5X5	T38.5X6
Anhydron	T5Ø.2X1	T5Ø.2X2	T5Ø.2X3	T5Ø.2X4	T5Ø.2X5	T5Ø.2X6
Anileridine	T4Ø.4X1	T4Ø.4X2	T4Ø.4X3	T4Ø.4X4	T4Ø.4X5	T4Ø.4X6
Aniline (dye) (liquid)	T65.3X1	T65.3X2	T65.3X3	T65.3X4	—	—
analgesic	T39.1X1	T39.1X2	T39.1X3	T39.1X4	T39.1X5	T39.1X6
derivatives, therapeutic NEC	T39.1X1	T39.1X2	T39.1X3	T39.1X4	T39.1X5	T39.1X6
vapor	T65.3X1	T65.3X2	T65.3X3	T65.3X4	—	—
Aniscoropine	T44.3X1	T44.3X2	T44.3X3	T44.3X4	T44.3X5	T44.3X6
Anise oil	T47.5X1	T47.5X2	T47.5X3	T47.5X4	T47.5X5	T47.5X6
Anisidine	T65.3X1	T65.3X2	T65.3X3	T65.3X4	—	—
Anisindione	T45.511	T45.512	T45.513	T45.514	T45.515	T45.516
Anisotropine methyl-bromide	T44.3X1	T44.3X2	T44.3X3	T44.3X4	T44.3X5	T44.3X6
Anistreplase	T45.611	T45.612	T45.613	T45.614	T45.615	T45.616
Anorexiant (central)	T5Ø.5X1	T5Ø.5X2	T5Ø.5X3	T5Ø.5X4	T5Ø.5X5	T5Ø.5X6
Anorexic agents	T5Ø.5X1	T5Ø.5X2	T5Ø.5X3	T5Ø.5X4	T5Ø.5X5	T5Ø.5X6
Ansamycin	T36.6X1	T36.6X2	T36.6X3	T36.6X4	T36.6X5	T36.6X6
Ant (bite) (sting)	T63.421	T63.422	T63.423	T63.424	—	—
Antabuse	T5Ø.6X1	T5Ø.6X2	T5Ø.6X3	T5Ø.6X4	T5Ø.6X5	T5Ø.6X6
Antacid NEC	T47.1X1	T47.1X2	T47.1X3	T47.1X4	T47.1X5	T47.1X6
Antagonist						
Aldosterone	T5Ø.ØX1	T5Ø.ØX2	T5Ø.ØX3	T5Ø.ØX4	T5Ø.ØX5	T5Ø.ØX6
alpha-adrenoreceptor	T44.6X1	T44.6X2	T44.6X3	T44.6X4	T44.6X5	T44.6X6
anticoagulant	T45.7X1	T45.7X2	T45.7X3	T45.7X4	T45.7X5	T45.7X6
beta-adrenoreceptor	T44.7X1	T44.7X2	T44.7X3	T44.7X4	T44.7X5	T44.7X6
extrapyramidal NEC	T44.3X1	T44.3X2	T44.3X3	T44.3X4	T44.3X5	T44.3X6
folic acid	T45.1X1	T45.1X2	T45.1X3	T45.1X4	T45.1X5	T45.1X6
H2 receptor	T47.ØX1	T47.ØX2	T47.ØX3	T47.ØX4	T47.ØX5	T47.ØX6
heavy metal	T45.8X1	T45.8X2	T45.8X3	T45.8X4	T45.8X5	T45.8X6
narcotic analgesic	T5Ø.7X1	T5Ø.7X2	T5Ø.7X3	T5Ø.7X4	T5Ø.7X5	T5Ø.7X6
opiate	T5Ø.7X1	T5Ø.7X2	T5Ø.7X3	T5Ø.7X4	T5Ø.7X5	T5Ø.7X6
pyrimidine	T45.1X1	T45.1X2	T45.1X3	T45.1X4	T45.1X5	T45.1X6
serotonin	T46.5X1	T46.5X2	T46.5X3	T46.5X4	T46.5X5	T46.5X6
Antazolin (e)	T45.ØX1	T45.ØX2	T45.ØX3	T45.ØX4	T45.ØX5	T45.ØX6
Anterior pituitary hormone NEC	T38.811	T38.812	T38.813	T38.814	T38.815	T38.816
Anthelmintic NEC	T37.4X1	T37.4X2	T37.4X3	T37.4X4	T37.4X5	T37.4X6
Anthiolimine	T37.4X1	T37.4X2	T37.4X3	T37.4X4	T37.4X5	T37.4X6
Anthralin	T49.4X1	T49.4X2	T49.4X3	T49.4X4	T49.4X5	T49.4X6
Anthramycin	T45.1X1	T45.1X2	T45.1X3	T45.1X4	T45.1X5	T45.1X6
Antiadrenergic NEC	T44.8X1	T44.8X2	T44.8X3	T44.8X4	T44.8X5	T44.8X6
Antiallergic NEC	T45.ØX1	T45.ØX2	T45.ØX3	T45.ØX4	T45.ØX5	T45.ØX6
Antiandrogen NEC	T38.6X1	T38.6X2	T38.6X3	T38.6X4	T38.6X5	T38.6X6
Anti-anemic (drug) (preparation)	T45.8X1	T45.8X2	T45.8X3	T45.8X4	T45.8X5	T45.8X6
Antianxiety drug NEC	T43.5Ø1	T43.5Ø2	T43.5Ø3	T43.5Ø4	T43.5Ø5	T43.5Ø6
Antiaris toxicaria	T65.891	T65.892	T65.893	T65.894	—	—
Antiarteriosclerotic drug	T46.6X1	T46.6X2	T46.6X3	T46.6X4	T46.6X5	T46.6X6

Substance	Poisoning, Accidental (unintentional)	Poisoning, Intentional Self-harm	Poisoning, Assault	Poisoning, Undetermined	Adverse Effect	Under-dosing
Antiasthmatic drug NEC	T48.6X1	T48.6X2	T48.6X3	T48.6X4	T48.6X5	T48.6X6
Antibiotic NEC	T36.91	T36.92	T36.93	T36.94	T36.95	T36.96
aminoglycoside	T36.5X1	T36.5X2	T36.5X3	T36.5X4	T36.5X5	T36.5X6
anticancer	T45.1X1	T45.1X2	T45.1X3	T45.1X4	T45.1X5	T45.1X6
antifungal	T36.7X1	T36.7X2	T36.7X3	T36.7X4	T36.7X5	T36.7X6
antimycobacterial	T36.5X1	T36.5X2	T36.5X3	T36.5X4	T36.5X5	T36.5X6
antineoplastic	T45.1X1	T45.1X2	T45.1X3	T45.1X4	T45.1X5	T45.1X6
b-lactam NEC	T36.1X1	T36.1X2	T36.1X3	T36.1X4	T36.1X5	T36.1X6
cephalosporin (group)	T36.1X1	T36.1X2	T36.1X3	T36.1X4	T36.1X5	T36.1X6
chloramphenicol (group)	T36.2X1	T36.2X2	T36.2X3	T36.2X4	T36.2X5	T36.2X6
ENT	T49.6X1	T49.6X2	T49.6X3	T49.6X4	T49.6X5	T49.6X6
eye	T49.5X1	T49.5X2	T49.5X3	T49.5X4	T49.5X5	T49.5X6
fungicidal (local)	T49.ØX1	T49.ØX2	T49.ØX3	T49.ØX4	T49.ØX5	T49.ØX6
intestinal	T36.8X1	T36.8X2	T36.8X3	T36.8X4	T36.8X5	T36.8X6
local	T49.ØX1	T49.ØX2	T49.ØX3	T49.ØX4	T49.ØX5	T49.ØX6
macrolides	T36.3X1	T36.3X2	T36.3X3	T36.3X4	T36.3X5	T36.3X6
polypeptide	T36.8X1	T36.8X2	T36.8X3	T36.8X4	T36.8X5	T36.8X6
specified NEC	T36.8X1	T36.8X2	T36.8X3	T36.8X4	T36.8X5	T36.8X6
tetracycline (group)	T36.4X1	T36.4X2	T36.4X3	T36.4X4	T36.4X5	T36.4X6
throat	T49.6X1	T49.6X2	T49.6X3	T49.6X4	T49.6X5	T49.6X6
Anticancer agents NEC	T45.1X1	T45.1X2	T45.1X3	T45.1X4	T45.1X5	T45.1X6
Anticholesterolemic drug NEC	T46.6X1	T46.6X2	T46.6X3	T46.6X4	T46.6X5	T46.6X6
Anticholinergic NEC	T44.3X1	T44.3X2	T44.3X3	T44.3X4	T44.3X5	T44.3X6
Anticholinesterase	T44.ØX1	T44.ØX2	T44.ØX3	T44.ØX4	T44.ØX5	T44.ØX6
organophosphorus	T44.ØX1	T44.ØX2	T44.ØX3	T44.ØX4	T44.ØX5	T44.ØX6
insecticide	T6Ø.ØX1	T6Ø.ØX2	T6Ø.ØX3	T6Ø.ØX4	—	—
nerve gas	T59.891	T59.892	T59.893	T59.894	—	—
reversible	T44.ØX1	T44.ØX2	T44.ØX3	T44.ØX4	T44.ØX5	T44.ØX6
ophthalmological	T49.5X1	T49.5X2	T49.5X3	T49.5X4	T49.5X5	T49.5X6
Anticoagulant NEC	T45.511	T45.512	T45.513	T45.514	T45.515	T45.516
Antagonist	T45.7X1	T45.7X2	T45.7X3	T45.7X4	T45.7X5	T45.7X6
Anti-common-cold drug NEC	T48.5X1	T48.5X2	T48.5X3	T48.5X4	T48.5X5	T48.5X6
Anticonvulsant	T42.71	T42.72	T42.73	T42.74	T42.75	T42.76
barbiturate	T42.3X1	T42.3X2	T42.3X3	T42.3X4	T42.3X5	T42.3X6
combination (with barbiturate)	T42.3X1	T42.3X2	T42.3X3	T42.3X4	T42.3X5	T42.3X6
hydantoin	T42.ØX1	T42.ØX2	T42.ØX3	T42.ØX4	T42.ØX5	T42.ØX6
hypnotic NEC	T42.6X1	T42.6X2	T42.6X3	T42.6X4	T42.6X5	T42.6X6
oxazolidinedione	T42.2X1	T42.2X2	T42.2X3	T42.2X4	T42.2X5	T42.2X6
pyrimidinedione	T42.6X1	T42.6X2	T42.6X3	T42.6X4	T42.6X5	T42.6X6
specified NEC	T42.6X1	T42.6X2	T42.6X3	T42.6X4	T42.6X5	T42.6X6
succinimide	T42.2X1	T42.2X2	T42.2X3	T42.2X4	T42.2X5	T42.2X6
Antidepressant	T43.2Ø1	T43.2Ø2	T43.2Ø3	T43.2Ø4	T43.2Ø5	T43.2Ø6
monoamine oxidase inhibitor	T43.1X1	T43.1X2	T43.1X3	T43.1X4	T43.1X5	T43.1X6
selective serotonin norepinephrine reuptake inhibitor	T43.211	T43.212	T43.213	T43.214	T43.215	T43.216
selective serotonin reuptake inhibitor	T43.221	T43.222	T43.223	T43.224	T43.225	T43.226
specified NEC	T43.291	T43.292	T43.293	T43.294	T43.295	T43.296
tetracyclic	T43.Ø21	T43.Ø22	T43.Ø23	T43.Ø24	T43.Ø25	T43.Ø26
triazolopyridine	T43.211	T43.212	T43.213	T43.214	T43.215	T43.216
tricyclic	T43.Ø11	T43.Ø12	T43.Ø13	T43.Ø14	T43.Ø15	T43.Ø16
Antidiabetic NEC	T38.3X1	T38.3X2	T38.3X3	T38.3X4	T38.3X5	T38.3X6
biguanide	T38.3X1	T38.3X2	T38.3X3	T38.3X4	T38.3X5	T38.3X6
and sulfonyl combined	T38.3X1	T38.3X2	T38.3X3	T38.3X4	T38.3X5	T38.3X6
combined	T38.3X1	T38.3X2	T38.3X3	T38.3X4	T38.3X5	T38.3X6
sulfonylurea	T38.3X1	T38.3X2	T38.3X3	T38.3X4	T38.3X5	T38.3X6
Antidiarrheal drug NEC	T47.6X1	T47.6X2	T47.6X3	T47.6X4	T47.6X5	T47.6X6
absorbent	T47.6X1	T47.6X2	T47.6X3	T47.6X4	T47.6X5	T47.6X6
Anti-D immunoglobulin (human)	T5Ø.Z11	T5Ø.Z12	T5Ø.Z13	T5Ø.Z14	T5Ø.Z15	T5Ø.Z16
Antidiphtheria serum	T5Ø.Z11	T5Ø.Z12	T5Ø.Z13	T5Ø.Z14	T5Ø.Z15	T5Ø.Z16
Antidiuretic hormone	T38.891	T38.892	T38.893	T38.894	T38.895	T38.896
Antidote NEC	T5Ø.6X1	T5Ø.6X2	T5Ø.6X3	T5Ø.6X4	T5Ø.6X5	T5Ø.6X6
heavy metal	T45.8X1	T45.8X2	T45.8X3	T45.8X4	T45.8X5	T45.8X6
Antidysrhythmic NEC	T46.2X1	T46.2X2	T46.2X3	T46.2X4	T46.2X5	T46.2X6
Antiemetic drug	T45.ØX1	T45.ØX2	T45.ØX3	T45.ØX4	T45.ØX5	T45.ØX6
Antiepilepsy agent	T42.71	T42.72	T42.73	T42.74	T42.75	T42.76
combination	T42.5X1	T42.5X2	T42.5X3	T42.5X4	T42.5X5	T42.5X6
mixed	T42.5X1	T42.5X2	T42.5X3	T42.5X4	T42.5X5	T42.5X6
specified, NEC	T42.6X1	T42.6X2	T42.6X3	T42.6X4	T42.6X5	T42.6X6
Antiestrogen NEC	T38.6X1	T38.6X2	T38.6X3	T38.6X4	T38.6X5	T38.6X6
Antifertility pill	T38.4X1	T38.4X2	T38.4X3	T38.4X4	T38.4X5	T38.4X6
Antifibrinolytic drug	T45.621	T45.622	T45.623	T45.624	T45.625	T45.626
Antifilarial drug	T37.4X1	T37.4X2	T37.4X3	T37.4X4	T37.4X5	T37.4X6
Antiflatulent	T47.5X1	T47.5X2	T47.5X3	T47.5X4	T47.5X5	T47.5X6
Antifreeze	T65.91	T65.92	T65.93	T65.94	—	—
alcohol	T51.1X1	T51.1X2	T51.1X3	T51.1X4	—	—
ethylene glycol	T51.8X1	T51.8X2	T51.8X3	T51.8X4	—	—

Substance	Poisoning, Accidental (unintentional)	Poisoning, Intentional Self-harm	Poisoning, Assault	Poisoning, Undetermined	Adverse Effect	Under-dosing
Antifungal						
antibiotic (systemic)	T36.7X1	T36.7X2	T36.7X3	T36.7X4	T36.7X5	T36.7X6
anti-infective NEC	T37.91	T37.92	T37.93	T37.94	T37.95	T37.96
disinfectant, local	T49.ØX1	T49.ØX2	T49.ØX3	T49.ØX4	T49.ØX5	T49.ØX6
nonmedicinal (spray)	T6Ø.3X1	T6Ø.3X2	T6Ø.3X3	T6Ø.3X4	—	—
topical	T49.ØX1	T49.ØX2	T49.ØX3	T49.ØX4	T49.ØX5	T49.ØX6
Anti-gastric-secretion drug NEC	T47.1X1	T47.1X2	T47.1X3	T47.1X4	T47.1X5	T47.1X6
Antigonadotrophin NEC	T38.6X1	T38.6X2	T38.6X3	T38.6X4	T38.6X5	T38.6X6
Antihallucinogen	T43.5Ø1	T43.5Ø2	T43.5Ø3	T43.5Ø4	T43.5Ø5	T43.5Ø6
Antihelmintics	T37.4X1	T37.4X2	T37.4X3	T37.4X4	T37.4X5	T37.4X6
Antihemophilic						
factor	T45.8X1	T45.8X2	T45.8X3	T45.8X4	T45.8X5	T45.8X6
fraction	T45.8X1	T45.8X2	T45.8X3	T45.8X4	T45.8X5	T45.8X6
globulin concentrate	T45.7X1	T45.7X2	T45.7X3	T45.7X4	T45.7X5	T45.7X6
human plasma	T45.8X1	T45.8X2	T45.8X3	T45.8X4	T45.8X5	T45.8X6
plasma, dried	T45.7X1	T45.7X2	T45.7X3	T45.7X4	T45.7X5	T45.7X6
Antihemorrhoidal preparation	T49.2X1	T49.2X2	T49.2X3	T49.2X4	T49.2X5	T49.2X6
Antiheparin drug	T45.7X1	T45.7X2	T45.7X3	T45.7X4	T45.7X5	T45.7X6
Antihistamine	T45.ØX1	T45.ØX2	T45.ØX3	T45.ØX4	T45.ØX5	T45.ØX6
Antihookworm drug	T37.4X1	T37.4X2	T37.4X3	T37.4X4	T37.4X5	T37.4X6
Anti-human lymphocytic globulin	T5Ø.Z11	T5Ø.Z12	T5Ø.Z13	T5Ø.Z14	T5Ø.Z15	T5Ø.Z16
Antihyperlipidemic drug	T46.6X1	T46.6X2	T46.6X3	T46.6X4	T46.6X5	T46.6X6
Antihypertensive drug NEC	T46.5X1	T46.5X2	T46.5X3	T46.5X4	T46.5X5	T46.5X6
Anti-infective NEC	T37.91	T37.92	T37.93	T37.94	T37.95	T37.96
anthelmintic	T37.4X1	T37.4X2	T37.4X3	T37.4X4	T37.4X5	T37.4X6
antibiotics	T36.91	T36.92	T36.93	T36.94	T36.95	T36.96
specified NEC	T36.8X1	T36.8X2	T36.8X3	T36.8X4	T36.8X5	T36.8X6
antimalarial	T37.2X1	T37.2X2	T37.2X3	T37.2X4	T37.2X5	T37.2X6
antimycobacterial NEC	T37.1X1	T37.1X2	T37.1X3	T37.1X4	T37.1X5	T37.1X6
antibiotics	T36.5X1	T36.5X2	T36.5X3	T36.5X4	T36.5X5	T36.5X6
antiprotozoal NEC	T37.3X1	T37.3X2	T37.3X3	T37.3X4	T37.3X5	T37.3X6
blood	T37.2X1	T37.2X2	T37.2X3	T37.2X4	T37.2X5	T37.2X6
antiviral	T37.5X1	T37.5X2	T37.5X3	T37.5X4	T37.5X5	T37.5X6
arsenical	T37.8X1	T37.8X2	T37.8X3	T37.8X4	T37.8X5	T37.8X6
bismuth, local	T49.ØX1	T49.ØX2	T49.ØX3	T49.ØX4	T49.ØX5	T49.ØX6
ENT	T49.6X1	T49.6X2	T49.6X3	T49.6X4	T49.6X5	T49.6X6
eye NEC	T49.5X1	T49.5X2	T49.5X3	T49.5X4	T49.5X5	T49.5X6
heavy metals NEC	T37.8X1	T37.8X2	T37.8X3	T37.8X4	T37.8X5	T37.8X6
local NEC	T49.ØX1	T49.ØX2	T49.ØX3	T49.ØX4	T49.ØX5	T49.ØX6
specified NEC	T49.ØX1	T49.ØX2	T49.ØX3	T49.ØX4	T49.ØX5	T49.ØX6
mixed	T37.91	T37.92	T37.93	T37.94	T37.95	T37.96
ophthalmic preparation	T49.5X1	T49.5X2	T49.5X3	T49.5X4	T49.5X5	T49.5X6
topical NEC	T49.ØX1	T49.ØX2	T49.ØX3	T49.ØX4	T49.ØX5	T49.ØX6
Anti-inflammatory drug NEC	T39.391	T39.392	T39.393	T39.394	T39.395	T39.396
local	T49.ØX1	T49.ØX2	T49.ØX3	T49.ØX4	T49.ØX5	T49.ØX6
nonsteroidal NEC	T39.391	T39.392	T39.393	T39.394	T39.395	T39.396
propionic acid derivative	T39.311	T39.312	T39.313	T39.314	T39.315	T39.316
specified NEC	T39.391	T39.392	T39.393	T39.394	T39.395	T39.396
Antikaluretic	T5Ø.3X1	T5Ø.3X2	T5Ø.3X3	T5Ø.3X4	T5Ø.3X5	T5Ø.3X6
Antiknock (tetraethyl lead)	T56.ØX1	T56.ØX2	T56.ØX3	T56.ØX4	—	—
Antilipemic drug NEC	T46.6X1	T46.6X2	T46.6X3	T46.6X4	T46.6X5	T46.6X6
Antimalarial	T37.2X1	T37.2X2	T37.2X3	T37.2X4	T37.2X5	T37.2X6
prophylactic NEC	T37.2X1	T37.2X2	T37.2X3	T37.2X4	T37.2X5	T37.2X6
pyrimidine derivative	T37.2X1	T37.2X2	T37.2X3	T37.2X4	T37.2X5	T37.2X6
Antimetabolite	T45.1X1	T45.1X2	T45.1X3	T45.1X4	T45.1X5	T45.1X6
Antimitotic agent	T45.1X1	T45.1X2	T45.1X3	T45.1X4	T45.1X5	T45.1X6
Antimony (compounds) (vapor) **NEC**	T56.891	T56.892	T56.893	T56.894	—	—
anti-infectives	T37.8X1	T37.8X2	T37.8X3	T37.8X4	T37.8X5	T37.8X6
dimercaptosuccinate	T37.3X1	T37.3X2	T37.3X3	T37.3X4	T37.3X5	T37.3X6
hydride	T56.891	T56.892	T56.893	T56.894	—	—
pesticide (vapor)	T6Ø.8X1	T6Ø.8X2	T6Ø.8X3	T6Ø.8X4	—	—
potassium (sodium) tartrate	T37.8X1	T37.8X2	T37.8X3	T37.8X4	T37.8X5	T37.8X6
sodium dimercaptosuccinate	T37.3X1	T37.3X2	T37.3X3	T37.3X4	T37.3X5	T37.3X6
tartrated	T37.8X1	T37.8X2	T37.8X3	T37.8X4	T37.8X5	T37.8X6
Antimuscarinic NEC	T44.3X1	T44.3X2	T44.3X3	T44.3X4	T44.3X5	T44.3X6
Antimycobacterial drug NEC	T37.1X1	T37.1X2	T37.1X3	T37.1X4	T37.1X5	T37.1X6
antibiotics	T36.5X1	T36.5X2	T36.5X3	T36.5X4	T36.5X5	T36.5X6
combination	T37.1X1	T37.1X2	T37.1X3	T37.1X4	T37.1X5	T37.1X6
Antinausea drug	T45.ØX1	T45.ØX2	T45.ØX3	T45.ØX4	T45.ØX5	T45.ØX6
Antinematode drug	T37.4X1	T37.4X2	T37.4X3	T37.4X4	T37.4X5	T37.4X6
Antineoplastic NEC	T45.1X1	T45.1X2	T45.1X3	T45.1X4	T45.1X5	T45.1X6
alkaloidal	T45.1X1	T45.1X2	T45.1X3	T45.1X4	T45.1X5	T45.1X6
antibiotics	T45.1X1	T45.1X2	T45.1X3	T45.1X4	T45.1X5	T45.1X6
combination	T45.1X1	T45.1X2	T45.1X3	T45.1X4	T45.1X5	T45.1X6
estrogen	T38.5X1	T38.5X2	T38.5X3	T38.5X4	T38.5X5	T38.5X6
Antineoplastic — *continued*						
steroid	T38.7X1	T38.7X2	T38.7X3	T38.7X4	T38.7X5	T38.7X6
Antiparasitic drug (systemic)	T37.91	T37.92	T37.93	T37.94	T37.95	T37.96
local	T49.ØX1	T49.ØX2	T49.ØX3	T49.ØX4	T49.ØX5	T49.ØX6
specified NEC	T37.8X1	T37.8X2	T37.8X3	T37.8X4	T37.8X5	T37.8X6
Antiparkinsonism drug NEC	T42.8X1	T42.8X2	T42.8X3	T42.8X4	T42.8X5	T42.8X6
Antiperspirant NEC	T49.2X1	T49.2X2	T49.2X3	T49.2X4	T49.2X5	T49.2X6
Antiphlogistic NEC	T39.4X1	T39.4X2	T39.4X3	T39.4X4	T39.4X5	T39.4X6
Antiplatyhelmintic drug	T37.4X1	T37.4X2	T37.4X3	T37.4X4	T37.4X5	T37.4X6
Antiprotozoal drug NEC	T37.3X1	T37.3X2	T37.3X3	T37.3X4	T37.3X5	T37.3X6
blood	T37.2X1	T37.2X2	T37.2X3	T37.2X4	T37.2X5	T37.2X6
local	T49.ØX1	T49.ØX2	T49.ØX3	T49.ØX4	T49.ØX5	T49.ØX6
Antipruritic drug NEC	T49.1X1	T49.1X2	T49.1X3	T49.1X4	T49.1X5	T49.1X6
Antipsychotic drug	T43.5Ø1	T43.5Ø2	T43.5Ø3	T43.5Ø4	T43.5Ø5	T43.5Ø6
specified NEC	T43.591	T43.592	T43.593	T43.594	T43.595	T43.596
Antipyretic	T39.91	T39.92	T39.93	T39.94	T39.95	T39.96
specified NEC	T39.8X1	T39.8X2	T39.8X3	T39.8X4	T39.8X5	T39.8X6
Antipyrine	T39.2X1	T39.2X2	T39.2X3	T39.2X4	T39.2X5	T39.2X6
Antirabies hyperimmune serum	T5Ø.Z11	T5Ø.Z12	T5Ø.Z13	T5Ø.Z14	T5Ø.Z15	T5Ø.Z16
Antirheumatic NEC	T39.4X1	T39.4X2	T39.4X3	T39.4X4	T39.4X5	T39.4X6
Antirigidity drug NEC	T42.8X1	T42.8X2	T42.8X3	T42.8X4	T42.8X5	T42.8X6
Antischistosomal drug	T37.4X1	T37.4X2	T37.4X3	T37.4X4	T37.4X5	T37.4X6
Antiscorpion sera	T5Ø.Z11	T5Ø.Z12	T5Ø.Z13	T5Ø.Z14	T5Ø.Z15	T5Ø.Z16
Antiseborrheics	T49.4X1	T49.4X2	T49.4X3	T49.4X4	T49.4X5	T49.4X6
Antiseptics (external) (medicinal)	T49.ØX1	T49.ØX2	T49.ØX3	T49.ØX4	T49.ØX5	T49.ØX6
Antistine	T45.ØX1	T45.ØX2	T45.ØX3	T45.ØX4	T45.ØX5	T45.ØX6
Antitapeworm drug	T37.4X1	T37.4X2	T37.4X3	T37.4X4	T37.4X5	T37.4X6
Antitetanus immunoglobulin	T5Ø.Z11	T5Ø.Z12	T5Ø.Z13	T5Ø.Z14	T5Ø.Z15	T5Ø.Z16
Antithyroid drug NEC	T38.2X1	T38.2X2	T38.2X3	T38.2X4	T38.2X5	T38.2X6
Antitoxin	T5Ø.Z11	T5Ø.Z12	T5Ø.Z13	T5Ø.Z14	T5Ø.Z15	T5Ø.Z16
diphtheria	T5Ø.Z11	T5Ø.Z12	T5Ø.Z13	T5Ø.Z14	T5Ø.Z15	T5Ø.Z16
gas gangrene	T5Ø.Z11	T5Ø.Z12	T5Ø.Z13	T5Ø.Z14	T5Ø.Z15	T5Ø.Z16
tetanus	T5Ø.Z11	T5Ø.Z12	T5Ø.Z13	T5Ø.Z14	T5Ø.Z15	T5Ø.Z16
Antitrichomonal drug	T37.3X1	T37.3X2	T37.3X3	T37.3X4	T37.3X5	T37.3X6
Antituberculars	T37.1X1	T37.1X2	T37.1X3	T37.1X4	T37.1X5	T37.1X6
antibiotics	T36.5X1	T36.5X2	T36.5X3	T36.5X4	T36.5X5	T36.5X6
Antitussive NEC	T48.3X1	T48.3X2	T48.3X3	T48.3X4	T48.3X5	T48.3X6
codeine mixture	T4Ø.2X1	T4Ø.2X2	T4Ø.2X3	T4Ø.2X4	T4Ø.2X5	T4Ø.2X6
opiate	T4Ø.2X1	T4Ø.2X2	T4Ø.2X3	T4Ø.2X4	T4Ø.2X5	T4Ø.2X6
Antivaricose drug	T46.8X1	T46.8X2	T46.8X3	T46.8X4	T46.8X5	T46.8X6
Antivenin, antivenom (sera)	T5Ø.Z11	T5Ø.Z12	T5Ø.Z13	T5Ø.Z14	T5Ø.Z15	T5Ø.Z16
crotaline	T5Ø.Z11	T5Ø.Z12	T5Ø.Z13	T5Ø.Z14	T5Ø.Z15	T5Ø.Z16
spider bite	T5Ø.Z11	T5Ø.Z12	T5Ø.Z13	T5Ø.Z14	T5Ø.Z15	T5Ø.Z16
Antivertigo drug	T45.ØX1	T45.ØX2	T45.ØX3	T45.ØX4	T45.ØX5	T45.ØX6
Antiviral drug NEC	T37.5X1	T37.5X2	T37.5X3	T37.5X4	T37.5X5	T37.5X6
eye	T49.5X1	T49.5X2	T49.5X3	T49.5X4	T49.5X5	T49.5X6
Antiwhipworm drug	T37.4X1	T37.4X2	T37.4X3	T37.4X4	T37.4X5	T37.4X6
Ant poison — *see* Insecticide						
Antrol — *see also* by specific chemical substance	T6Ø.91	T6Ø.92	T6Ø.93	T6Ø.94	—	—
fungicide	T6Ø.91	T6Ø.92	T6Ø.93	T6Ø.94	—	—
ANTU (alpha naphthylthiourea)	T6Ø.4X1	T6Ø.4X2	T6Ø.4X3	T6Ø.4X4	—	—
Apalcillin	T36.ØX1	T36.ØX2	T36.ØX3	T36.ØX4	T36.ØX5	T36.ØX6
APC	T48.5X1	T48.5X2	T48.5X3	T48.5X4	T48.5X5	T48.5X6
Aplonidine	T44.4X1	T44.4X2	T44.4X3	T44.4X4	T44.4X5	T44.4X6
Apomorphine	T47.7X1	T47.7X2	T47.7X3	T47.7X4	T47.7X5	T47.7X6
Appetite depressants, central	T5Ø.5X1	T5Ø.5X2	T5Ø.5X3	T5Ø.5X4	T5Ø.5X5	T5Ø.5X6
Apraclonidine (hydrochloride)	T44.4X1	T44.4X2	T44.4X3	T44.4X4	T44.4X5	T44.4X6
Apresoline	T46.5X1	T46.5X2	T46.5X3	T46.5X4	T46.5X5	T46.5X6
Aprindine	T46.2X1	T46.2X2	T46.2X3	T46.2X4	T46.2X5	T46.2X6
Aprobarbital	T42.3X1	T42.3X2	T42.3X3	T42.3X4	T42.3X5	T42.3X6
Apronalide	T42.6X1	T42.6X2	T42.6X3	T42.6X4	T42.6X5	T42.6X6
Aprotinin	T45.621	T45.622	T45.623	T45.624	T45.625	T45.626
Aptocaine	T41.3X1	T41.3X2	T41.3X3	T41.3X4	T41.3X5	T41.3X6
Aqua fortis	T54.2X1	T54.2X2	T54.2X3	T54.2X4	—	—
Ara-A	T37.5X1	T37.5X2	T37.5X3	T37.5X4	T37.5X5	T37.5X6
Ara-C	T45.1X1	T45.1X2	T45.1X3	T45.1X4	T45.1X5	T45.1X6
Arachis oil	T49.3X1	T49.3X2	T49.3X3	T49.3X4	T49.3X5	T49.3X6
cathartic	T47.4X1	T47.4X2	T47.4X3	T47.4X4	T47.4X5	T47.4X6
Aralen	T37.2X1	T37.2X2	T37.2X3	T37.2X4	T37.2X5	T37.2X6
Arecoline	T44.1X1	T44.1X2	T44.1X3	T44.1X4	T44.1X5	T44.1X6
Arginine	T5Ø.991	T5Ø.992	T5Ø.993	T5Ø.994	T5Ø.995	T5Ø.996
glutamate	T5Ø.991	T5Ø.992	T5Ø.993	T5Ø.994	T5Ø.995	T5Ø.996
Argyrol	T49.ØX1	T49.ØX2	T49.ØX3	T49.ØX4	T49.ØX5	T49.ØX6
ENT agent	T49.6X1	T49.6X2	T49.6X3	T49.6X4	T49.6X5	T49.6X6

Substance	Poisoning, Accidental (unintentional)	Poisoning, Intentional Self-harm	Poisoning, Assault	Poisoning, Undetermined	Adverse Effect	Under-dosing
Argyrol — *continued*						
ophthalmic preparation	T49.5X1	T49.5X2	T49.5X3	T49.5X4	T49.5X5	T49.5X6
Aristocort	T38.ØX1	T38.ØX2	T38.ØX3	T38.ØX4	T38.ØX5	T38.ØX6
ENT agent	T49.6X1	T49.6X2	T49.6X3	T49.6X4	T49.6X5	T49.6X6
ophthalmic preparation	T49.5X1	T49.5X2	T49.5X3	T49.5X4	T49.5X5	T49.5X6
topical NEC	T49.ØX1	T49.ØX2	T49.ØX3	T49.ØX4	T49.ØX5	T49.ØX6
Aromatics, corrosive	T54.1X1	T54.1X2	T54.1X3	T54.1X4	—	—
disinfectants	T54.1X1	T54.1X2	T54.1X3	T54.1X4	—	—
Arsenate of lead	T57.ØX1	T57.ØX2	T57.ØX3	T57.ØX4	—	—
herbicide	T57.ØX1	T57.ØX2	T57.ØX3	T57.ØX4	—	—
Arsenic, arsenicals (compounds) (dust) (vapor) **NEC**	T57.ØX1	T57.ØX2	T57.ØX3	T57.ØX4	—	—
anti-infectives	T37.8X1	T37.8X2	T37.8X3	T37.8X4	T37.8X5	T37.8X6
pesticide (dust) (fumes)	T57.ØX1	T57.ØX2	T57.ØX3	T57.ØX4	—	—
Arsine (gas)	T57.ØX1	T57.ØX2	T57.ØX3	T57.ØX4	—	—
Arsphenamine (silver)	T37.8X1	T37.8X2	T37.8X3	T37.8X4	T37.8X5	T37.8X6
Arsthinol	T37.3X1	T37.3X2	T37.3X3	T37.3X4	T37.3X5	T37.3X6
Artane	T44.3X1	T44.3X2	T44.3X3	T44.3X4	T44.3X5	T44.3X6
Arthropod (venomous) **NEC**	T63.481	T63.482	T63.483	T63.484	—	—
Articaine	T41.3X1	T41.3X2	T41.3X3	T41.3X4	T41.3X5	T41.3X6
Asbestos	T57.8X1	T57.8X2	T57.8X3	T57.8X4	—	—
Ascaridole	T37.4X1	T37.4X2	T37.4X3	T37.4X4	T37.4X5	T37.4X6
Ascorbic acid	T45.2X1	T45.2X2	T45.2X3	T45.2X4	T45.2X5	T45.2X6
Asiaticoside	T49.ØX1	T49.ØX2	T49.ØX3	T49.ØX4	T49.ØX5	T49.ØX6
Asparaginase	T45.1X1	T45.1X2	T45.1X3	T45.1X4	T45.1X5	T45.1X6
Aspidium (oleoresin)	T37.4X1	T37.4X2	T37.4X3	T37.4X4	T37.4X5	T37.4X6
Aspirin (aluminum) (soluble)	T39.Ø11	T39.Ø12	T39.Ø13	T39.Ø14	T39.Ø15	T39.Ø16
Aspoxicillin	T36.ØX1	T36.ØX2	T36.ØX3	T36.ØX4	T36.ØX5	T36.ØX6
Astemizole	T45.ØX1	T45.ØX2	T45.ØX3	T45.ØX4	T45.ØX5	T45.ØX6
Astringent (local)	T49.2X1	T49.2X2	T49.2X3	T49.2X4	T49.2X5	T49.2X6
specified NEC	T49.2X1	T49.2X2	T49.2X3	T49.2X4	T49.2X5	T49.2X6
Astromicin	T36.5X1	T36.5X2	T36.5X3	T36.5X4	T36.5X5	T36.5X6
Ataractic drug NEC	T43.5Ø1	T43.5Ø2	T43.5Ø3	T43.5Ø4	T43.5Ø5	T43.5Ø6
Atenolol	T44.7X1	T44.7X2	T44.7X3	T44.7X4	T44.7X5	T44.7X6
Atonia drug, intestinal	T47.4X1	T47.4X2	T47.4X3	T47.4X4	T47.4X5	T47.4X6
Atophan	T5Ø.4X1	T5Ø.4X2	T5Ø.4X3	T5Ø.4X4	T5Ø.4X5	T5Ø.4X6
Atracurium besilate	T48.1X1	T48.1X2	T48.1X3	T48.1X4	T48.1X5	T48.1X6
Atropine	T44.3X1	T44.3X2	T44.3X3	T44.3X4	T44.3X5	T44.3X6
derivative	T44.3X1	T44.3X2	T44.3X3	T44.3X4	T44.3X5	T44.3X6
methonitrate	T44.3X1	T44.3X2	T44.3X3	T44.3X4	T44.3X5	T44.3X6
Attapulgite	T47.6X1	T47.6X2	T47.6X3	T47.6X4	T47.6X5	T47.6X6
Auramine	T65.891	T65.892	T65.893	T65.894	—	—
dye	T65.6X1	T65.6X2	T65.6X3	T65.6X4	—	—
fungicide	T6Ø.3X1	T6Ø.3X2	T6Ø.3X3	T6Ø.3X4	—	—
Auranofin	T39.4X1	T39.4X2	T39.4X3	T39.4X4	T39.4X5	T39.4X6
Aurantiin	T46.991	T46.992	T46.993	T46.994	T46.995	T46.996
Aureomycin	T36.4X1	T36.4X2	T36.4X3	T36.4X4	T36.4X5	T36.4X6
ophthalmic preparation	T49.5X1	T49.5X2	T49.5X3	T49.5X4	T49.5X5	T49.5X6
topical NEC	T49.ØX1	T49.ØX2	T49.ØX3	T49.ØX4	T49.ØX5	T49.ØX6
Aurothioglucose	T39.4X1	T39.4X2	T39.4X3	T39.4X4	T39.4X5	T39.4X6
Aurothioglycanide	T39.4X1	T39.4X2	T39.4X3	T39.4X4	T39.4X5	T39.4X6
Aurothiomalate sodium	T39.4X1	T39.4X2	T39.4X3	T39.4X4	T39.4X5	T39.4X6
Aurotioprol	T39.4X1	T39.4X2	T39.4X3	T39.4X4	T39.4X5	T39.4X6
Automobile fuel	T52.ØX1	T52.ØX2	T52.ØX3	T52.ØX4	—	—
Autonomic nervous system agent NEC	T44.9Ø1	T44.9Ø2	T44.9Ø3	T44.9Ø4	T44.9Ø5	T44.9Ø6
Avlosulfon	T37.1X1	T37.1X2	T37.1X3	T37.1X4	T37.1X5	T37.1X6
Avomine	T42.6X1	T42.6X2	T42.6X3	T42.6X4	T42.6X5	T42.6X6
Axerophthol	T45.2X1	T45.2X2	T45.2X3	T45.2X4	T45.2X5	T45.2X6
Azacitidine	T45.1X1	T45.1X2	T45.1X3	T45.1X4	T45.1X5	T45.1X6
Azacyclonol	T43.591	T43.592	T43.593	T43.594	T43.595	T43.596
Azadirachta	T6Ø.2X1	T6Ø.2X2	T6Ø.2X3	T6Ø.2X4	—	—
Azanidazole	T37.3X1	T37.3X2	T37.3X3	T37.3X4	T37.3X5	T37.3X6
Azapetine	T46.7X1	T46.7X2	T46.7X3	T46.7X4	T46.7X5	T46.7X6
Azapropazone	T39.2X1	T39.2X2	T39.2X3	T39.2X4	T39.2X5	T39.2X6
Azaribine	T45.1X1	T45.1X2	T45.1X3	T45.1X4	T45.1X5	T45.1X6
Azaserine	T45.1X1	T45.1X2	T45.1X3	T45.1X4	T45.1X5	T45.1X6
Azatadine	T45.ØX1	T45.ØX2	T45.ØX3	T45.ØX4	T45.ØX5	T45.ØX6
Azatepa	T45.1X1	T45.1X2	T45.1X3	T45.1X4	T45.1X5	T45.1X6
Azathioprine	T45.1X1	T45.1X2	T45.1X3	T45.1X4	T45.1X5	T45.1X6
Azelaic acid	T49.ØX1	T49.ØX2	T49.ØX3	T49.ØX4	T49.ØX5	T49.ØX6
Azelastine	T45.ØX1	T45.ØX2	T45.ØX3	T45.ØX4	T45.ØX5	T45.ØX6
Azidocillin	T36.ØX1	T36.ØX2	T36.ØX3	T36.ØX4	T36.ØX5	T36.ØX6
Azidothymidine	T37.5X1	T37.5X2	T37.5X3	T37.5X4	T37.5X5	T37.5X6
Azinphos (ethyl) (methyl)	T6Ø.ØX1	T6Ø.ØX2	T6Ø.ØX3	T6Ø.ØX4	—	—
Aziridine (chelating)	T54.1X1	T54.1X2	T54.1X3	T54.1X4	—	—
Azithromycin	T36.3X1	T36.3X2	T36.3X3	T36.3X4	T36.3X5	T36.3X6
Azlocillin	T36.ØX1	T36.ØX2	T36.ØX3	T36.ØX4	T36.ØX5	T36.ØX6
Azobenzene smoke	T65.3X1	T65.3X2	T65.3X3	T65.3X4	—	—
acaricide	T6Ø.8X1	T6Ø.8X2	T6Ø.8X3	T6Ø.8X4	—	—
Azosulfamide	T37.ØX1	T37.ØX2	T37.ØX3	T37.ØX4	T37.ØX5	T37.ØX6
AZT	T37.5X1	T37.5X2	T37.5X3	T37.5X4	T37.5X5	T37.5X6
Aztreonam	T36.1X1	T36.1X2	T36.1X3	T36.1X4	T36.1X5	T36.1X6

Substance	Poisoning, Accidental (unintentional)	Poisoning, Intentional Self-harm	Poisoning, Assault	Poisoning, Undetermined	Adverse Effect	Under-dosing
Azulfidine	T37.ØX1	T37.ØX2	T37.ØX3	T37.ØX4	T37.ØX5	T37.ØX6
Azuresin	T5Ø.8X1	T5Ø.8X2	T5Ø.8X3	T5Ø.8X4	T5Ø.8X5	T5Ø.8X6
b-acetyldigoxin	T46.ØX1	T46.ØX2	T46.ØX3	T46.ØX4	T46.ØX5	T46.ØX6
P-Acetamidophenol	T39.1X1	T39.1X2	T39.1X3	T39.1X4	T39.1X5	T39.1X6
Bacampicillin	T36.ØX1	T36.ØX2	T36.ØX3	T36.ØX4	T36.ØX5	T36.ØX6
Bacillus						
lactobacillus	T47.8X1	T47.8X2	T47.8X3	T47.8X4	T47.8X5	T47.8X6
subtilis	T47.6X1	T47.6X2	T47.6X3	T47.6X4	T47.6X5	T47.6X6
Bacimycin	T49.ØX1	T49.ØX2	T49.ØX3	T49.ØX4	T49.ØX5	T49.ØX6
ophthalmic preparation	T49.5X1	T49.5X2	T49.5X3	T49.5X4	T49.5X5	T49.5X6
Bacitracin zinc	T49.ØX1	T49.ØX2	T49.ØX3	T49.ØX4	T49.ØX5	T49.ØX6
with neomycin	T49.ØX1	T49.ØX2	T49.ØX3	T49.ØX4	T49.ØX5	T49.ØX6
ENT agent	T49.6X1	T49.6X2	T49.6X3	T49.6X4	T49.6X5	T49.6X6
ophthalmic preparation	T49.5X1	T49.5X2	T49.5X3	T49.5X4	T49.5X5	T49.5X6
topical NEC	T49.ØX1	T49.ØX2	T49.ØX3	T49.ØX4	T49.ØX5	T49.ØX6
Baclofen	T42.8X1	T42.8X2	T42.8X3	T42.8X4	T42.8X5	T42.8X6
Baking soda	T5Ø.991	T5Ø.992	T5Ø.993	T5Ø.994	T5Ø.995	T5Ø.996
BAL	T45.8X1	T45.8X2	T45.8X3	T45.8X4	T45.8X5	T45.8X6
Bambuterol	T48.6X1	T48.6X2	T48.6X3	T48.6X4	T48.6X5	T48.6X6
Bamethan (sulfate)	T46.7X1	T46.7X2	T46.7X3	T46.7X4	T46.7X5	T46.7X6
Bamifylline	T48.6X1	T48.6X2	T48.6X3	T48.6X4	T48.6X5	T48.6X6
Bamipine	T45.ØX1	T45.ØX2	T45.ØX3	T45.ØX4	T45.ØX5	T45.ØX6
Baneberry — *see* Actaea spicata						
Banewort — *see* Belladonna						
Barbenyl	T42.3X1	T42.3X2	T42.3X3	T42.3X4	T42.3X5	T42.3X6
Barbexaclone	T42.6X1	T42.6X2	T42.6X3	T42.6X4	T42.6X5	T42.6X6
Barbital	T42.3X1	T42.3X2	T42.3X3	T42.3X4	T42.3X5	T42.3X6
sodium	T42.3X1	T42.3X2	T42.3X3	T42.3X4	T42.3X5	T42.3X6
Barbitone	T42.3X1	T42.3X2	T42.3X3	T42.3X4	T42.3X5	T42.3X6
Barbiturate NEC	T42.3X1	T42.3X2	T42.3X3	T42.3X4	T42.3X5	T42.3X6
with tranquilizer	T42.3X1	T42.3X2	T42.3X3	T42.3X4	T42.3X5	T42.3X6
anesthetic (intravenous)	T41.1X1	T41.1X2	T41.1X3	T41.1X4	T41.1X5	T41.1X6
Barium (carbonate) (chloride) (sulfite)	T57.8X1	T57.8X2	T57.8X3	T57.8X4	—	—
diagnostic agent	T5Ø.8X1	T5Ø.8X2	T5Ø.8X3	T5Ø.8X4	T5Ø.8X5	T5Ø.8X6
pesticide	T6Ø.4X1	T6Ø.4X2	T6Ø.4X3	T6Ø.4X4	—	—
rodenticide	T6Ø.4X1	T6Ø.4X2	T6Ø.4X3	T6Ø.4X4	—	—
sulfate (medicinal)	T5Ø.8X1	T5Ø.8X2	T5Ø.8X3	T5Ø.8X4	T5Ø.8X5	T5Ø.8X6
Barrier cream	T49.3X1	T49.3X2	T49.3X3	T49.3X4	T49.3X5	T49.3X6
Basic fuchsin	T49.ØX1	T49.ØX2	T49.ØX3	T49.ØX4	T49.ØX5	T49.ØX6
Battery acid or fluid	T54.2X1	T54.2X2	T54.2X3	T54.2X4	—	—
Bay rum	T51.8X1	T51.8X2	T51.8X3	T51.8X4	—	—
b-benzalbutyramide	T46.6X1	T46.6X2	T46.6X3	T46.6X4	T46.6X5	T46.6X6
BCG (vaccine)	T5Ø.A91	T5Ø.A92	T5Ø.A93	T5Ø.A94	T5Ø.A95	T5Ø.A96
BCNU	T45.1X1	T45.1X2	T45.1X3	T45.1X4	T45.1X5	T45.1X6
Bearsfoot	T62.2X1	T62.2X2	T62.2X3	T62.2X4	—	—
Beclamide	T42.6X1	T42.6X2	T42.6X3	T42.6X4	T42.6X5	T42.6X6
Beclomethasone	T44.5X1	T44.5X2	T44.5X3	T44.5X4	T44.5X5	T44.5X6
Bee (sting) (venom)	T63.441	T63.442	T63.443	T63.444	—	—
Befunolol	T49.5X1	T49.5X2	T49.5X3	T49.5X4	T49.5X5	T49.5X6
Bekanamycin	T36.5X1	T36.5X2	T36.5X3	T36.5X4	T36.5X5	T36.5X6
Belladonna — *see also* Nightshade						
alkaloids	T44.3X1	T44.3X2	T44.3X3	T44.3X4	T44.3X5	T44.3X6
extract	T44.3X1	T44.3X2	T44.3X3	T44.3X4	T44.3X5	T44.3X6
herb	T44.3X1	T44.3X2	T44.3X3	T44.3X4	T44.3X5	T44.3X6
Bemegride	T5Ø.7X1	T5Ø.7X2	T5Ø.7X3	T5Ø.7X4	T5Ø.7X5	T5Ø.7X6
Benactyzine	T44.3X1	T44.3X2	T44.3X3	T44.3X4	T44.3X5	T44.3X6
Benadryl	T45.ØX1	T45.ØX2	T45.ØX3	T45.ØX4	T45.ØX5	T45.ØX6
Benaprizine	T44.3X1	T44.3X2	T44.3X3	T44.3X4	T44.3X5	T44.3X6
Benazepril	T46.4X1	T46.4X2	T46.4X3	T46.4X4	T46.4X5	T46.4X6
Bencyclane	T46.7X1	T46.7X2	T46.7X3	T46.7X4	T46.7X5	T46.7X6
Bendazol	T46.3X1	T46.3X2	T46.3X3	T46.3X4	T46.3X5	T46.3X6
Bendrofluazide	T5Ø.2X1	T5Ø.2X2	T5Ø.2X3	T5Ø.2X4	T5Ø.2X5	T5Ø.2X6
Bendroflumethiazide	T5Ø.2X1	T5Ø.2X2	T5Ø.2X3	T5Ø.2X4	T5Ø.2X5	T5Ø.2X6
Benemid	T5Ø.4X1	T5Ø.4X2	T5Ø.4X3	T5Ø.4X4	T5Ø.4X5	T5Ø.4X6
Benethamine penicillin	T36.ØX1	T36.ØX2	T36.ØX3	T36.ØX4	T36.ØX5	T36.ØX6
Benexate	T47.1X1	T47.1X2	T47.1X3	T47.1X4	T47.1X5	T47.1X6
Benfluorex	T46.6X1	T46.6X2	T46.6X3	T46.6X4	T46.6X5	T46.6X6
Benfotiamine	T45.2X1	T45.2X2	T45.2X3	T45.2X4	T45.2X5	T45.2X6
Benisone	T49.ØX1	T49.ØX2	T49.ØX3	T49.ØX4	T49.ØX5	T49.ØX6
Benomyl	T6Ø.ØX1	T6Ø.ØX2	T6Ø.ØX3	T6Ø.ØX4	—	—
Benoquin	T49.8X1	T49.8X2	T49.8X3	T49.8X4	T49.8X5	T49.8X6
Benoxinate	T41.3X1	T41.3X2	T41.3X3	T41.3X4	T41.3X5	T41.3X6
Benperidol	T43.4X1	T43.4X2	T43.4X3	T43.4X4	T43.4X5	T43.4X6
Benproperine	T48.3X1	T48.3X2	T48.3X3	T48.3X4	T48.3X5	T48.3X6
Benserazide	T42.8X1	T42.8X2	T42.8X3	T42.8X4	T42.8X5	T42.8X6
Bentazepam	T42.4X1	T42.4X2	T42.4X3	T42.4X4	T42.4X5	T42.4X6
Bentiromide	T5Ø.8X1	T5Ø.8X2	T5Ø.8X3	T5Ø.8X4	T5Ø.8X5	T5Ø.8X6
Bentonite	T49.3X1	T49.3X2	T49.3X3	T49.3X4	T49.3X5	T49.3X6
Benzalbutyramide	T46.6X1	T46.6X2	T46.6X3	T46.6X4	T46.6X5	T46.6X6
Benzalkonium (chloride)	T49.ØX1	T49.ØX2	T49.ØX3	T49.ØX4	T49.ØX5	T49.ØX6
ophthalmic preparation	T49.5X1	T49.5X2	T49.5X3	T49.5X4	T49.5X5	T49.5X6

Substance	Poisoning, Accidental (unintentional)	Poisoning, Intentional Self-harm	Poisoning, Assault	Poisoning, Undetermined	Adverse Effect	Under-dosing
Benzamidosalicylate (calcium)	T37.1X1	T37.1X2	T37.1X3	T37.1X4	T37.1X5	T37.1X6
Benzamine	T41.3X1	T41.3X2	T41.3X3	T41.3X4	T41.3X5	T41.3X6
lactate	T49.1X1	T49.1X2	T49.1X3	T49.1X4	T49.1X5	T49.1X6
Benzamphetamine	T5Ø.5X1	T5Ø.5X2	T5Ø.5X3	T5Ø.5X4	T5Ø.5X5	T5Ø.5X6
Benzapril hydrochloride	T46.5X1	T46.5X2	T46.5X3	T46.5X4	T46.5X5	T46.5X6
Benzathine benzylpenicillin	T36.ØX1	T36.ØX2	T36.ØX3	T36.ØX4	T36.ØX5	T36.ØX6
Benzathine penicillin	T36.ØX1	T36.ØX2	T36.ØX3	T36.ØX4	T36.ØX5	T36.ØX6
Benzatropine	T42.8X1	T42.8X2	T42.8X3	T42.8X4	T42.8X5	T42.8X6
Benzbromarone	T5Ø.4X1	T5Ø.4X2	T5Ø.4X3	T5Ø.4X4	T5Ø.4X5	T5Ø.4X6
Benzcarbimine	T45.1X1	T45.1X2	T45.1X3	T45.1X4	T45.1X5	T45.1X6
Benzedrex	T44.991	T44.992	T44.993	T44.994	T44.995	T44.996
Benzedrine (amphetamine)	T43.621	T43.622	T43.623	T43.624	T43.625	T43.626
Benzenamine	T65.3X1	T65.3X2	T65.3X3	T65.3X4	—	—
Benzene	T52.1X1	T52.1X2	T52.1X3	T52.1X4	—	—
homologues (acetyl) (dimethyl) (methyl) (solvent)	T52.2X1	T52.2X2	T52.2X3	T52.2X4	—	—
Benzethonium (chloride)	T49.ØX1	T49.ØX2	T49.ØX3	T49.ØX4	T49.ØX5	T49.ØX6
Benzfetamine	T5Ø.5X1	T5Ø.5X2	T5Ø.5X3	T5Ø.5X4	T5Ø.5X5	T5Ø.5X6
Benzhexol	T44.3X1	T44.3X2	T44.3X3	T44.3X4	T44.3X5	T44.3X6
Benzhydramine (chloride)	T45.ØX1	T45.ØX2	T45.ØX3	T45.ØX4	T45.ØX5	T45.ØX6
Benzidine	T65.891	T65.892	T65.893	T65.894	—	—
Benzilonium bromide	T44.3X1	T44.3X2	T44.3X3	T44.3X4	T44.3X5	T44.3X6
Benzimidazole	T6Ø.3X1	T6Ø.3X2	T6Ø.3X3	T6Ø.3X4	—	—
Benzin (e) — *see* Ligroin						
Benziodarone	T46.3X1	T46.3X2	T46.3X3	T46.3X4	T46.3X5	T46.3X6
Benznidazole	T37.3X1	T37.3X2	T37.3X3	T37.3X4	T37.3X5	T37.3X6
Benzocaine	T41.3X1	T41.3X2	T41.3X3	T41.3X4	T41.3X5	T41.3X6
Benzodiapin	T42.4X1	T42.4X2	T42.4X3	T42.4X4	T42.4X5	T42.4X6
Benzodiazepine NEC	T42.4X1	T42.4X2	T42.4X3	T42.4X4	T42.4X5	T42.4X6
Benzoic acid	T49.ØX1	T49.ØX2	T49.ØX3	T49.ØX4	T49.ØX5	T49.ØX6
with salicylic acid	T49.ØX1	T49.ØX2	T49.ØX3	T49.ØX4	T49.ØX5	T49.ØX6
Benzoin (tincture)	T48.5X1	T48.5X2	T48.5X3	T48.5X4	T48.5X5	T48.5X6
Benzol (benzene)	T52.1X1	T52.1X2	T52.1X3	T52.1X4	—	—
vapor	T52.ØX1	T52.ØX2	T52.ØX3	T52.ØX4	—	—
Benzomorphan	T4Ø.2X1	T4Ø.2X2	T4Ø.2X3	T4Ø.2X4	T4Ø.2X5	T4Ø.2X6
Benzonatate	T48.3X1	T48.3X2	T48.3X3	T48.3X4	T48.3X5	T48.3X6
Benzophenones	T49.3X1	T49.3X2	T49.3X3	T49.3X4	T49.3X5	T49.3X6
Benzopyrone	T46.991	T46.992	T46.993	T46.994	T46.995	T46.996
Benzothiadiazides	T5Ø.2X1	T5Ø.2X2	T5Ø.2X3	T5Ø.2X4	T5Ø.2X5	T5Ø.2X6
Benzoxonium chloride	T49.ØX1	T49.ØX2	T49.ØX3	T49.ØX4	T49.ØX5	T49.ØX6
Benzoylpas calcium	T37.1X1	T37.1X2	T37.1X3	T37.1X4	T37.1X5	T37.1X6
Benzoyl peroxide	T49.ØX1	T49.ØX2	T49.ØX3	T49.ØX4	T49.ØX5	T49.ØX6
Benzperidin	T43.591	T43.592	T43.593	T43.594	T43.595	T43.596
Benzperidol	T43.591	T43.592	T43.593	T43.594	T43.595	T43.596
Benzphetamine	T5Ø.5X1	T5Ø.5X2	T5Ø.5X3	T5Ø.5X4	T5Ø.5X5	T5Ø.5X6
Benzpyrinium bromide	T44.1X1	T44.1X2	T44.1X3	T44.1X4	T44.1X5	T44.1X6
Benzquinamide	T45.ØX1	T45.ØX2	T45.ØX3	T45.ØX4	T45.ØX5	T45.ØX6
Benzthiazide	T5Ø.2X1	T5Ø.2X2	T5Ø.2X3	T5Ø.2X4	T5Ø.2X5	T5Ø.2X6
Benztropine						
anticholinergic	T44.3X1	T44.3X2	T44.3X3	T44.3X4	T44.3X5	T44.3X6
antiparkinson	T42.8X1	T42.8X2	T42.8X3	T42.8X4	T42.8X5	T42.8X6
Benzydamine	T49.ØX1	T49.ØX2	T49.ØX3	T49.ØX4	T49.ØX5	T49.ØX6
Benzyl						
acetate	T52.8X1	T52.8X2	T52.8X3	T52.8X4	—	—
alcohol	T49.ØX1	T49.ØX2	T49.ØX3	T49.ØX4	T49.ØX5	T49.ØX6
benzoate	T49.ØX1	T49.ØX2	T49.ØX3	T49.ØX4	T49.ØX5	T49.ØX6
Benzoic acid	T49.ØX1	T49.ØX2	T49.ØX3	T49.ØX4	T49.ØX5	T49.ØX6
morphine	T4Ø.2X1	T4Ø.2X2	T4Ø.2X3	T4Ø.2X4	—	—
nicotinate	T46.6X1	T46.6X2	T46.6X3	T46.6X4	T46.6X5	T46.6X6
penicillin	T36.ØX1	T36.ØX2	T36.ØX3	T36.ØX4	T36.ØX5	T36.ØX6
Benzylhydrochlorthiazide	T5Ø.2X1	T5Ø.2X2	T5Ø.2X3	T5Ø.2X4	T5Ø.2X5	T5Ø.2X6
Benzylpenicillin	T36.ØX1	T36.ØX2	T36.ØX3	T36.ØX4	T36.ØX5	T36.ØX6
Benzylthiouracil	T38.2X1	T38.2X2	T38.2X3	T38.2X4	T38.2X5	T38.2X6
Bephenium hydroxynaphthoate	T37.4X1	T37.4X2	T37.4X3	T37.4X4	T37.4X5	T37.4X6
Bepridil	T46.1X1	T46.1X2	T46.1X3	T46.1X4	T46.1X5	T46.1X6
Bergamot oil	T65.891	T65.892	T65.893	T65.894	—	—
Bergapten	T5Ø.991	T5Ø.992	T5Ø.993	T5Ø.994	T5Ø.995	T5Ø.996
Berries, poisonous	T62.1X1	T62.1X2	T62.1X3	T62.1X4	—	—
Beryllium (compounds)	T56.7X1	T56.7X2	T56.7X3	T56.7X4	—	—
beta adrenergic blocking agent, heart	T44.7X1	T44.7X2	T44.7X3	T44.7X4	T44.7X5	T44.7X6
Betacarotene	T45.2X1	T45.2X2	T45.2X3	T45.2X4	T45.2X5	T45.2X6
Beta-Chlor	T42.6X1	T42.6X2	T42.6X3	T42.6X4	T42.6X5	T42.6X6
Betahistine	T46.7X1	T46.7X2	T46.7X3	T46.7X4	T46.7X5	T46.7X6
Betaine	T47.5X1	T47.5X2	T47.5X3	T47.5X4	T47.5X5	T47.5X6
Betamethasone	T49.ØX1	T49.ØX2	T49.ØX3	T49.ØX4	T49.ØX5	T49.ØX6
topical	T49.ØX1	T49.ØX2	T49.ØX3	T49.ØX4	T49.ØX5	T49.ØX6
Betamicin	T36.8X1	T36.8X2	T36.8X3	T36.8X4	T36.8X5	T36.8X6
Betanidine	T46.5X1	T46.5X2	T46.5X3	T46.5X4	T46.5X5	T46.5X6
Betaxolol	T44.7X1	T44.7X2	T44.7X3	T44.7X4	T44.7X5	T44.7X6

Substance	Poisoning, Accidental (unintentional)	Poisoning, Intentional Self-harm	Poisoning, Assault	Poisoning, Undetermined	Adverse Effect	Under-dosing
Betazole	T5Ø.8X1	T5Ø.8X2	T5Ø.8X3	T5Ø.8X4	T5Ø.8X5	T5Ø.8X6
Bethanechol	T44.1X1	T44.1X2	T44.1X3	T44.1X4	T44.1X5	T44.1X6
chloride	T44.1X1	T44.1X2	T44.1X3	T44.1X4	T44.1X5	T44.1X6
Bethanidine	T46.5X1	T46.5X2	T46.5X3	T46.5X4	T46.5X5	T46.5X6
Betoxycaine	T41.3X1	T41.3X2	T41.3X3	T41.3X4	T41.3X5	T41.3X6
Betula oil	T49.3X1	T49.3X2	T49.3X3	T49.3X4	T49.3X5	T49.3X6
Bevantolol	T44.7X1	T44.7X2	T44.7X3	T44.7X4	T44.7X5	T44.7X6
Bevonium metilsulfate	T44.3X1	T44.3X2	T44.3X3	T44.3X4	T44.3X5	T44.3X6
Bezafibrate	T46.6X1	T46.6X2	T46.6X3	T46.6X4	T46.6X5	T46.6X6
Bezitramide	T4Ø.4X1	T4Ø.4X2	T4Ø.4X3	T4Ø.4X4	T4Ø.4X5	T4Ø.4X6
BHA	T5Ø.991	T5Ø.992	T5Ø.993	T5Ø.994	T5Ø.995	T5Ø.996
Bhang	T4Ø.7X1	T4Ø.7X2	T4Ø.7X3	T4Ø.7X4	T4Ø.7X5	T4Ø.7X6
BHC (medicinal)	T49.ØX1	T49.ØX2	T49.ØX3	T49.ØX4	T49.ØX5	T49.ØX6
nonmedicinal (vapor)	T53.6X1	T53.6X2	T53.6X3	T53.6X4	—	—
Bialamicol	T37.3X1	T37.3X2	T37.3X3	T37.3X4	T37.3X5	T37.3X6
Bibenzonium bromide	T48.3X1	T48.3X2	T48.3X3	T48.3X4	T48.3X5	T48.3X6
Bibrocathol	T49.5X1	T49.5X2	T49.5X3	T49.5X4	T49.5X5	T49.5X6
Bichloride of mercury — *see* Mercury, chloride						
Bichromates (calcium) (potassium)(sodium) (crystals)	T57.8X1	T57.8X2	T57.8X3	T57.8X4	—	—
fumes	T56.2X1	T56.2X2	T56.2X3	T56.2X4	—	—
Biclotymol	T49.6X1	T49.6X2	T49.6X3	T49.6X4	T49.6X5	T49.6X6
Bicucculine	T5Ø.7X1	T5Ø.7X2	T5Ø.7X3	T5Ø.7X4	T5Ø.7X5	T5Ø.7X6
Bifemelane	T43.291	T43.292	T43.293	T43.294	T43.295	T43.296
Biguanide derivatives, oral	T38.3X1	T38.3X2	T38.3X3	T38.3X4	T38.3X5	T38.3X6
Bile salts	T47.5X1	T47.5X2	T47.5X3	T47.5X4	T47.5X5	T47.5X6
Biligrafin	T5Ø.8X1	T5Ø.8X2	T5Ø.8X3	T5Ø.8X4	T5Ø.8X5	T5Ø.8X6
Bilopaque	T5Ø.8X1	T5Ø.8X2	T5Ø.8X3	T5Ø.8X4	T5Ø.8X5	T5Ø.8X6
Binifibrate	T46.6X1	T46.6X2	T46.6X3	T46.6X4	T46.6X5	T46.6X6
Binitrobenzol	T65.3X1	T65.3X2	T65.3X3	T65.3X4	—	—
Bioflavonoid(s)	T46.991	T46.992	T46.993	T46.994	T46.995	T46.996
Biological substance NEC	T5Ø.901	T5Ø.902	T5Ø.903	T5Ø.904	T5Ø.905	T5Ø.906
Biotin	T45.2X1	T45.2X2	T45.2X3	T45.2X4	T45.2X5	T45.2X6
Biperiden	T44.3X1	T44.3X2	T44.3X3	T44.3X4	T44.3X5	T44.3X6
Bisacodyl	T47.2X1	T47.2X2	T47.2X3	T47.2X4	T47.2X5	T47.2X6
Bisbentiamine	T45.2X1	T45.2X2	T45.2X3	T45.2X4	T45.2X5	T45.2X6
Bisbutiamine	T45.2X1	T45.2X2	T45.2X3	T45.2X4	T45.2X5	T45.2X6
Bisdequalinium (salts) (diacetate)	T49.6X1	T49.6X2	T49.6X3	T49.6X4	T49.6X5	T49.6X6
Bishydroxycoumarin	T45.511	T45.512	T45.513	T45.514	T45.515	T45.516
Bismarsen	T37.8X1	T37.8X2	T37.8X3	T37.8X4	T37.8X5	T37.8X6
Bismuth salts	T47.6X1	T47.6X2	T47.6X3	T47.6X4	T47.6X5	T47.6X6
aluminate	T47.1X1	T47.1X2	T47.1X3	T47.1X4	T47.1X5	T47.1X6
anti-infectives	T37.8X1	T37.8X2	T37.8X3	T37.8X4	T37.8X5	T37.8X6
formic iodide	T49.ØX1	T49.ØX2	T49.ØX3	T49.ØX4	T49.ØX5	T49.ØX6
glycolylarsenate	T49.ØX1	T49.ØX2	T49.ØX3	T49.ØX4	T49.ØX5	T49.ØX6
nonmedicinal (compounds) NEC	T65.91	T65.92	T65.93	T65.94	—	—
subcarbonate	T47.6X1	T47.6X2	T47.6X3	T47.6X4	T47.6X5	T47.6X6
subsalicylate	T37.8X1	T37.8X2	T37.8X3	T37.8X4	T37.8X5	T37.8X6
sulfarsphenamine	T37.8X1	T37.8X2	T37.8X3	T37.8X4	T37.8X5	T37.8X6
Bisoprolol	T44.7X1	T44.7X2	T44.7X3	T44.7X4	T44.7X5	T44.7X6
Bisoxatin	T47.2X1	T47.2X2	T47.2X3	T47.2X4	T47.2X5	T47.2X6
Bisulepin (hydrochloride)	T45.ØX1	T45.ØX2	T45.ØX3	T45.ØX4	T45.ØX5	T45.ØX6
Bithionol	T37.8X1	T37.8X2	T37.8X3	T37.8X4	T37.8X5	T37.8X6
anthelminthic	T37.4X1	T37.4X2	T37.4X3	T37.4X4	T37.4X5	T37.4X6
Bitolterol	T48.6X1	T48.6X2	T48.6X3	T48.6X4	T48.6X5	T48.6X6
Bitoscanate	T37.4X1	T37.4X2	T37.4X3	T37.4X4	T37.4X5	T37.4X6
Bitter almond oil	T62.8X1	T62.8X2	T62.8X3	T62.8X4	—	—
Bittersweet	T62.2X1	T62.2X2	T62.2X3	T62.2X4	—	—
Black						
flag	T6Ø.91	T6Ø.92	T6Ø.93	T6Ø.94	—	—
henbane	T62.2X1	T62.2X2	T62.2X3	T62.2X4	—	—
leaf (40)	T6Ø.91	T6Ø.92	T6Ø.93	T6Ø.94	—	—
widow spider (bite)	T63.311	T63.312	T63.313	T63.314	—	—
antivenin	T5Ø.Z11	T5Ø.Z12	T5Ø.Z13	T5Ø.Z14	T5Ø.Z15	T5Ø.Z16
Blast furnace gas (carbon monoxide from)	T58.8X1	T58.8X2	T58.8X3	T58.8X4	—	—
Bleach	T54.91	T54.92	T54.93	T54.94	—	—
Bleaching agent (medicinal)	T49.4X1	T49.4X2	T49.4X3	T49.4X4	T49.4X5	T49.4X6
Bleomycin	T45.1X1	T45.1X2	T45.1X3	T45.1X4	T45.1X5	T45.1X6
Blockain	T41.3X1	T41.3X2	T41.3X3	T41.3X4	T41.3X5	T41.3X6
infiltration (subcutaneous)	T41.3X1	T41.3X2	T41.3X3	T41.3X4	T41.3X5	T41.3X6
nerve block (peripheral) (plexus)	T41.3X1	T41.3X2	T41.3X3	T41.3X4	T41.3X5	T41.3X6
topical (surface)	T41.3X1	T41.3X2	T41.3X3	T41.3X4	T41.3X5	T41.3X6
Blockers, calcium channel	T46.1X1	T46.1X2	T46.1X3	T46.1X4	T46.1X5	T46.1X6
Blood (derivatives) (natural) (plasma) (whole)	T45.8X1	T45.8X2	T45.8X3	T45.8X4	T45.8X5	T45.8X6
dried	T45.8X1	T45.8X2	T45.8X3	T45.8X4	T45.8X5	T45.8X6
drug affecting NEC	T45.91	T45.92	T45.93	T45.94	T45.95	T45.96

Substance	Poisoning, Accidental (unintentional)	Poisoning, Intentional Self-harm	Poisoning, Assault	Poisoning, Undetermined	Adverse Effect	Under-dosing
Blood — *continued*						
expander NEC	T45.8X1	T45.8X2	T45.8X3	T45.8X4	T45.8X5	T45.8X6
fraction NEC	T45.8X1	T45.8X2	T45.8X3	T45.8X4	T45.8X5	T45.8X6
substitute (macromolecular)	T45.8X1	T45.8X2	T45.8X3	T45.8X4	T45.8X5	T45.8X6
Blue velvet	T4Ø.2X1	T4Ø.2X2	T4Ø.2X3	T4Ø.2X4	—	—
Bone meal	T62.8X1	T62.8X2	T62.8X3	T62.8X4	—	—
Bonine	T45.ØX1	T45.ØX2	T45.ØX3	T45.ØX4	T45.ØX5	T45.ØX6
Bopindolol	T44.7X1	T44.7X2	T44.7X3	T44.7X4	T44.7X5	T44.7X6
Boracic acid	T49.ØX1	T49.ØX2	T49.ØX3	T49.ØX4	T49.ØX5	T49.ØX6
ENT agent	T49.6X1	T49.6X2	T49.6X3	T49.6X4	T49.6X5	T49.6X6
ophthalmic preparation	T49.5X1	T49.5X2	T49.5X3	T49.5X4	T49.5X5	T49.5X6
Borane complex	T57.8X1	T57.8X2	T57.8X3	T57.8X4	—	—
Borate(s)	T57.8X1	T57.8X2	T57.8X3	T57.8X4	—	—
buffer	T5Ø.991	T5Ø.992	T5Ø.993	T5Ø.994	T5Ø.995	T5Ø.996
cleanser	T54.91	T54.92	T54.93	T54.94	—	—
sodium	T57.8X1	T57.8X2	T57.8X3	T57.8X4	—	—
Borax (cleanser)	T54.91	T54.92	T54.93	T54.94	—	—
Bordeaux mixture	T6Ø.3X1	T6Ø.3X2	T6Ø.3X3	T6Ø.3X4	—	—
Boric acid	T49.ØX1	T49.ØX2	T49.ØX3	T49.ØX4	T49.ØX5	T49.ØX6
ENT agent	T49.6X1	T49.6X2	T49.6X3	T49.6X4	T49.6X5	T49.6X6
ophthalmic preparation	T49.5X1	T49.5X2	T49.5X3	T49.5X4	T49.5X5	T49.5X6
Bornaprine	T44.3X1	T44.3X2	T44.3X3	T44.3X4	T44.3X5	T44.3X6
Boron	T57.8X1	T57.8X2	T57.8X3	T57.8X4	—	—
hydride NEC	T57.8X1	T57.8X2	T57.8X3	T57.8X4	—	—
fumes or gas	T57.8X1	T57.8X2	T57.8X3	T57.8X4	—	—
trifluoride	T59.891	T59.892	T59.893	T59.894	—	—
Botox	T48.291	T48.292	T48.293	T48.294	T48.295	T48.296
Botulinus anti-toxin (type A, B)	T5Ø.Z11	T5Ø.Z12	T5Ø.Z13	T5Ø.Z14	T5Ø.Z15	T5Ø.Z16
Brake fluid vapor	T59.891	T59.892	T59.893	T59.894	—	—
Brallobarbital	T42.3X1	T42.3X2	T42.3X3	T42.3X4	T42.3X5	T42.3X6
Bran (wheat)	T47.4X1	T47.4X2	T47.4X3	T47.4X4	T47.4X5	T47.4X6
Brass (fumes)	T56.891	T56.892	T56.893	T56.894	—	—
Brasso	T52.ØX1	T52.ØX2	T52.ØX3	T52.ØX4	—	—
Bretylium tosilate	T46.2X1	T46.2X2	T46.2X3	T46.2X4	T46.2X5	T46.2X6
Brevital (sodium)	T41.1X1	T41.1X2	T41.1X3	T41.1X4	T41.1X5	T41.1X6
Brinase	T45.3X1	T45.3X2	T45.3X3	T45.3X4	T45.3X5	T45.3X6
British antilewisite	T45.8X1	T45.8X2	T45.8X3	T45.8X4	T45.8X5	T45.8X6
Brodifacoum	T6Ø.4X1	T6Ø.4X2	T6Ø.4X3	T6Ø.4X4	—	—
Bromal (hydrate)	T42.6X1	T42.6X2	T42.6X3	T42.6X4	T42.6X5	T42.6X6
Bromazepam	T42.4X1	T42.4X2	T42.4X3	T42.4X4	T42.4X5	T42.4X6
Bromazine	T45.ØX1	T45.ØX2	T45.ØX3	T45.ØX4	T45.ØX5	T45.ØX6
Brombenzylcyanide	T59.3X1	T59.3X2	T59.3X3	T59.3X4	—	—
Bromelains	T45.3X1	T45.3X2	T45.3X3	T45.3X4	T45.3X5	T45.3X6
Bromethalin	T6Ø.4X1	T6Ø.4X2	T6Ø.4X3	T6Ø.4X4	—	—
Bromhexine	T48.4X1	T48.4X2	T48.4X3	T48.4X4	T48.4X5	T48.4X6
Bromide salts	T42.6X1	T42.6X2	T42.6X3	T42.6X4	T42.6X5	T42.6X6
Bromindione	T45.511	T45.512	T45.513	T45.514	T45.515	T45.516
Bromine						
compounds (medicinal)	T42.6X1	T42.6X2	T42.6X3	T42.6X4	T42.6X5	T42.6X6
sedative	T42.6X1	T42.6X2	T42.6X3	T42.6X4	T42.6X5	T42.6X6
vapor	T59.891	T59.892	T59.893	T59.894	—	—
Bromisoval	T42.6X1	T42.6X2	T42.6X3	T42.6X4	T42.6X5	T42.6X6
Bromisovalum	T42.6X1	T42.6X2	T42.6X3	T42.6X4	T42.6X5	T42.6X6
Bromobenzylcyanide	T59.3X1	T59.3X2	T59.3X3	T59.3X4	—	—
Bromochlorosalicylani-lide	T49.ØX1	T49.ØX2	T49.ØX3	T49.ØX4	T49.ØX5	T49.ØX6
Bromocriptine	T42.8X1	T42.8X2	T42.8X3	T42.8X4	T42.8X5	T42.8X6
Bromodiphenhydramine	T45.ØX1	T45.ØX2	T45.ØX3	T45.ØX4	T45.ØX5	T45.ØX6
Bromoform	T42.6X1	T42.6X2	T42.6X3	T42.6X4	T42.6X5	T42.6X6
Bromophenol blue reagent	T5Ø.991	T5Ø.992	T5Ø.993	T5Ø.994	T5Ø.995	T5Ø.996
Bromopride	T47.8X1	T47.8X2	T47.8X3	T47.8X4	T47.8X5	T47.8X6
Bromosalicylchloranitide	T49.ØX1	T49.ØX2	T49.ØX3	T49.ØX4	T49.ØX5	T49.ØX6
Bromosalicylhydroxamic acid	T37.1X1	T37.1X2	T37.1X3	T37.1X4	T37.1X5	T37.1X6
Bromo-seltzer	T39.1X1	T39.1X2	T39.1X3	T39.1X4	T39.1X5	T39.1X6
Bromoxynil	T6Ø.3X1	T6Ø.3X2	T6Ø.3X3	T6Ø.3X4	—	—
Bromperidol	T43.4X1	T43.4X2	T43.4X3	T43.4X4	T43.4X5	T43.4X6
Brompheniramine	T45.ØX1	T45.ØX2	T45.ØX3	T45.ØX4	T45.ØX5	T45.ØX6
Bromsulfophthalein	T5Ø.8X1	T5Ø.8X2	T5Ø.8X3	T5Ø.8X4	T5Ø.8X5	T5Ø.8X6
Bromural	T42.6X1	T42.6X2	T42.6X3	T42.6X4	T42.6X5	T42.6X6
Bromvaletone	T42.6X1	T42.6X2	T42.6X3	T42.6X4	T42.6X5	T42.6X6
Bronchodilator NEC	T48.6X1	T48.6X2	T48.6X3	T48.6X4	T48.6X5	T48.6X6
Brotizolam	T42.4X1	T42.4X2	T42.4X3	T42.4X4	T42.4X5	T42.4X6
Brovincamine	T46.7X1	T46.7X2	T46.7X3	T46.7X4	T46.7X5	T46.7X6
Brown recluse spider (bite) (venom)	T63.331	T63.332	T63.333	T63.334	—	—
Brown spider (bite) (venom)	T63.391	T63.392	T63.393	T63.394	—	—
Broxaterol	T48.6X1	T48.6X2	T48.6X3	T48.6X4	T48.6X5	T48.6X6
Broxuridine	T45.1X1	T45.1X2	T45.1X3	T45.1X4	T45.1X5	T45.1X6
Broxyquinoline	T37.8X1	T37.8X2	T37.8X3	T37.8X4	T37.8X5	T37.8X6
Bruceine	T48.291	T48.292	T48.293	T48.294	T48.295	T48.296
Brucia	T62.2X1	T62.2X2	T62.2X3	T62.2X4	—	—

Substance	Poisoning, Accidental (unintentional)	Poisoning, Intentional Self-harm	Poisoning, Assault	Poisoning, Undetermined	Adverse Effect	Under-dosing
Brucine	T65.1X1	T65.1X2	T65.1X3	T65.1X4	—	—
Brunswick green — *see* Copper						
Bruten — *see* Ibuprofen						
Bryonia	T47.2X1	T47.2X2	T47.2X3	T47.2X4	T47.2X5	T47.2X6
Buclizine	T45.ØX1	T45.ØX2	T45.ØX3	T45.ØX4	T45.ØX5	T45.ØX6
Buclosamide	T49.ØX1	T49.ØX2	T49.ØX3	T49.ØX4	T49.ØX5	T49.ØX6
Budesonide	T44.5X1	T44.5X2	T44.5X3	T44.5X4	T44.5X5	T44.5X6
Budralazine	T46.5X1	T46.5X2	T46.5X3	T46.5X4	T46.5X5	T46.5X6
Bufferin	T39.Ø11	T39.Ø12	T39.Ø13	T39.Ø14	T39.Ø15	T39.Ø16
Buflomedil	T46.7X1	T46.7X2	T46.7X3	T46.7X4	T46.7X5	T46.7X6
Buformin	T38.3X1	T38.3X2	T38.3X3	T38.3X4	T38.3X5	T38.3X6
Bufotenine	T4Ø.991	T4Ø.992	T4Ø.993	T4Ø.994	—	—
Bufrolin	T48.6X1	T48.6X2	T48.6X3	T48.6X4	T48.6X5	T48.6X6
Bufylline	T48.6X1	T48.6X2	T48.6X3	T48.6X4	T48.6X5	T48.6X6
Bulk filler	T5Ø.5X1	T5Ø.5X2	T5Ø.5X3	T5Ø.5X4	T5Ø.5X5	T5Ø.5X6
cathartic	T47.4X1	T47.4X2	T47.4X3	T47.4X4	T47.4X5	T47.4X6
Bumetanide	T5Ø.1X1	T5Ø.1X2	T5Ø.1X3	T5Ø.1X4	T5Ø.1X5	T5Ø.1X6
Bunaftine	T46.2X1	T46.2X2	T46.2X3	T46.2X4	T46.2X5	T46.2X6
Bunamiodyl	T5Ø.8X1	T5Ø.8X2	T5Ø.8X3	T5Ø.8X4	T5Ø.8X5	T5Ø.8X6
Bunazosin	T44.6X1	T44.6X2	T44.6X3	T44.6X4	T44.6X5	T44.6X6
Bunitrolol	T44.7X1	T44.7X2	T44.7X3	T44.7X4	T44.7X5	T44.7X6
Buphenine	T46.7X1	T46.7X2	T46.7X3	T46.7X4	T46.7X5	T46.7X6
Bupivacaine	T41.3X1	T41.3X2	T41.3X3	T41.3X4	T41.3X5	T41.3X6
infiltration (subcutaneous)	T41.3X1	T41.3X2	T41.3X3	T41.3X4	T41.3X5	T41.3X6
nerve block (peripheral) (plexus)	T41.3X1	T41.3X2	T41.3X3	T41.3X4	T41.3X5	T41.3X6
spinal	T41.3X1	T41.3X2	T41.3X3	T41.3X4	T41.3X5	T41.3X6
Bupranolol	T44.7X1	T44.7X2	T44.7X3	T44.7X4	T44.7X5	T44.7X6
Buprenorphine	T4Ø.4X1	T4Ø.4X2	T4Ø.4X3	T4Ø.4X4	T4Ø.4X5	T4Ø.4X6
Bupropion	T43.291	T43.292	T43.293	T43.294	T43.295	T43.296
Burimamide	T47.1X1	T47.1X2	T47.1X3	T47.1X4	T47.1X5	T47.1X6
Buserelin	T38.891	T38.892	T38.893	T38.894	T38.895	T38.896
Buspirone	T43.591	T43.592	T43.593	T43.594	T43.595	T43.596
Busulfan, busulphan	T45.1X1	T45.1X2	T45.1X3	T45.1X4	T45.1X5	T45.1X6
Butabarbital (sodium)	T42.3X1	T42.3X2	T42.3X3	T42.3X4	T42.3X5	T42.3X6
Butabarbitone	T42.3X1	T42.3X2	T42.3X3	T42.3X4	T42.3X5	T42.3X6
Butabarpal	T42.3X1	T42.3X2	T42.3X3	T42.3X4	T42.3X5	T42.3X6
Butacaine	T41.3X1	T41.3X2	T41.3X3	T41.3X4	T41.3X5	T41.3X6
Butalamine	T46.7X1	T46.7X2	T46.7X3	T46.7X4	T46.7X5	T46.7X6
Butalbital	T42.3X1	T42.3X2	T42.3X3	T42.3X4	T42.3X5	T42.3X6
Butallylonal	T42.3X1	T42.3X2	T42.3X3	T42.3X4	T42.3X5	T42.3X6
Butamben	T41.3X1	T41.3X2	T41.3X3	T41.3X4	T41.3X5	T41.3X6
Butamirate	T48.3X1	T48.3X2	T48.3X3	T48.3X4	T48.3X5	T48.3X6
Butane (distributed in mobile container)	T59.891	T59.892	T59.893	T59.894	—	—
distributed through pipes	T59.891	T59.892	T59.893	T59.894	—	—
incomplete combustion	T58.11	T58.12	T58.13	T58.14	—	—
Butanilicaine	T41.3X1	T41.3X2	T41.3X3	T41.3X4	T41.3X5	T41.3X6
Butanol	T51.3X1	T51.3X2	T51.3X3	T51.3X4	—	—
Butanone, 2-butanone	T52.4X1	T52.4X2	T52.4X3	T52.4X4	—	—
Butantrone	T49.4X1	T49.4X2	T49.4X3	T49.4X4	T49.4X5	T49.4X6
Butaperazine	T43.3X1	T43.3X2	T43.3X3	T43.3X4	T43.3X5	T43.3X6
Butazolidin	T39.2X1	T39.2X2	T39.2X3	T39.2X4	T39.2X5	T39.2X6
Butetamate	T48.6X1	T48.6X2	T48.6X3	T48.6X4	T48.6X5	T48.6X6
Butethal	T42.3X1	T42.3X2	T42.3X3	T42.3X4	T42.3X5	T42.3X6
Butethamate	T44.3X1	T44.3X2	T44.3X3	T44.3X4	T44.3X5	T44.3X6
Buthalitone (sodium)	T41.1X1	T41.1X2	T41.1X3	T41.1X4	T41.1X5	T41.1X6
Butisol (sodium)	T42.3X1	T42.3X2	T42.3X3	T42.3X4	T42.3X5	T42.3X6
Butizide	T5Ø.2X1	T5Ø.2X2	T5Ø.2X3	T5Ø.2X4	T5Ø.2X5	T5Ø.2X6
Butobarbital	T42.3X1	T42.3X2	T42.3X3	T42.3X4	T42.3X5	T42.3X6
sodium	T42.3X1	T42.3X2	T42.3X3	T42.3X4	T42.3X5	T42.3X6
Butobarbitone	T42.3X1	T42.3X2	T42.3X3	T42.3X4	T42.3X5	T42.3X6
Butoconazole (nitrate)	T49.ØX1	T49.ØX2	T49.ØX3	T49.ØX4	T49.ØX5	T49.ØX6
Butorphanol	T4Ø.4X1	T4Ø.4X2	T4Ø.4X3	T4Ø.4X4	T4Ø.4X5	T4Ø.4X6
Butriptyline	T43.Ø11	T43.Ø12	T43.Ø13	T43.Ø14	T43.Ø15	T43.Ø16
Butropium bromide	T44.3X1	T44.3X2	T44.3X3	T44.3X4	T44.3X5	T44.3X6
Buttercups	T62.2X1	T62.2X2	T62.2X3	T62.2X4	—	—
Butter of antimony — *see* Antimony						
Butyl						
acetate (secondary)	T52.8X1	T52.8X2	T52.8X3	T52.8X4	—	—
alcohol	T51.3X1	T51.3X2	T51.3X3	T51.3X4	—	—
aminobenzoate	T41.3X1	T41.3X2	T41.3X3	T41.3X4	T41.3X5	T41.3X6
butyrate	T52.8X1	T52.8X2	T52.8X3	T52.8X4	—	—
carbinol	T51.3X1	T51.3X2	T51.3X3	T51.3X4	—	—
carbitol	T52.3X1	T52.3X2	T52.3X3	T52.3X4	—	—
cellosolve	T52.3X1	T52.3X2	T52.3X3	T52.3X4	—	—
chloral (hydrate)	T42.6X1	T42.6X2	T42.6X3	T42.6X4	T42.6X5	T42.6X6
formate	T52.8X1	T52.8X2	T52.8X3	T52.8X4	—	—
lactate	T52.8X1	T52.8X2	T52.8X3	T52.8X4	—	—
propionate	T52.8X1	T52.8X2	T52.8X3	T52.8X4	—	—
scopolamine bromide	T44.3X1	T44.3X2	T44.3X3	T44.3X4	T44.3X5	T44.3X6
thiobarbital sodium	T41.1X1	T41.1X2	T41.1X3	T41.1X4	T41.1X5	T41.1X6

Substance	Poisoning, Accidental (unintentional)	Poisoning, Intentional Self-harm	Poisoning, Assault	Poisoning, Undetermined	Adverse Effect	Under-dosing
Butylated hydroxyanisole	T50.991	T50.992	T50.993	T50.994	T50.995	T50.996
Butylchloral hydrate	T42.6X1	T42.6X2	T42.6X3	T42.6X4	T42.6X5	T42.6X6
Butyltoluene	T52.2X1	T52.2X2	T52.2X3	T52.2X4	—	—
Butyn	T41.3X1	T41.3X2	T41.3X3	T41.3X4	T41.3X5	T41.3X6
Butyrophenone (-based tranquilizers)	T43.4X1	T43.4X2	T43.4X3	T43.4X4	T43.4X5	T43.4X6
Cabergoline	T42.8X1	T42.8X2	T42.8X3	T42.8X4	T42.8X5	T42.8X6
Cacodyl, cacodylic acid	T57.0X1	T57.0X2	T57.0X3	T57.0X4	—	—
Cactinomycin	T45.1X1	T45.1X2	T45.1X3	T45.1X4	T45.1X5	T45.1X6
Cade oil	T49.4X1	T49.4X2	T49.4X3	T49.4X4	T49.4X5	T49.4X6
Cadexomer iodine	T49.0X1	T49.0X2	T49.0X3	T49.0X4	T49.0X5	T49.0X6
Cadmium (chloride) (fumes) (oxide)	T56.3X1	T56.3X2	T56.3X3	T56.3X4	—	—
sulfide (medicinal) NEC	T49.4X1	T49.4X2	T49.4X3	T49.4X4	T49.4X5	T49.4X6
Cadralazine	T46.5X1	T46.5X2	T46.5X3	T46.5X4	T46.5X5	T46.5X6
Caffeine	T43.611	T43.612	T43.613	T43.614	T43.615	T43.616
Calabar bean	T62.2X1	T62.2X2	T62.2X3	T62.2X4	—	—
Caladium seguinum	T62.2X1	T62.2X2	T62.2X3	T62.2X4	—	—
Calamine (lotion)	T49.3X1	T49.3X2	T49.3X3	T49.3X4	T49.3X5	T49.3X6
Calcifediol	T45.2X1	T45.2X2	T45.2X3	T45.2X4	T45.2X5	T45.2X6
Calciferol	T45.2X1	T45.2X2	T45.2X3	T45.2X4	T45.2X5	T45.2X6
Calcitonin	T50.991	T50.992	T50.993	T50.994	T50.995	T50.996
Calcitriol	T45.2X1	T45.2X2	T45.2X3	T45.2X4	T45.2X5	T45.2X6
Calcium	T50.3X1	T50.3X2	T50.3X3	T50.3X4	T50.3X5	T50.3X6
actylsalicylate	T39.011	T39.012	T39.013	T39.014	T39.015	T39.016
benzamidosalicylate	T37.1X1	T37.1X2	T37.1X3	T37.1X4	T37.1X5	T37.1X6
bromide	T42.6X1	T42.6X2	T42.6X3	T42.6X4	T42.6X5	T42.6X6
bromolactobionate	T42.6X1	T42.6X2	T42.6X3	T42.6X4	T42.6X5	T42.6X6
carbaspirin	T39.011	T39.012	T39.013	T39.014	T39.015	T39.016
carbimide	T50.6X1	T50.6X2	T50.6X3	T50.6X4	T50.6X5	T50.6X6
carbonate	T47.1X1	T47.1X2	T47.1X3	T47.1X4	T47.1X5	T47.1X6
chloride	T50.991	T50.992	T50.993	T50.994	T50.995	T50.996
anhydrous	T50.991	T50.992	T50.993	T50.994	T50.995	T50.996
cyanide	T57.8X1	T57.8X2	T57.8X3	T57.8X4	—	—
dioctyl sulfosuccinate	T47.4X1	T47.4X2	T47.4X3	T47.4X4	T47.4X5	T47.4X6
disodium edathamil	T45.8X1	T45.8X2	T45.8X3	T45.8X4	T45.8X5	T45.8X6
disodium edetate	T45.8X1	T45.8X2	T45.8X3	T45.8X4	T45.8X5	T45.8X6
dobesilate	T46.991	T46.992	T46.993	T46.994	T46.995	T46.996
EDTA	T45.8X1	T45.8X2	T45.8X3	T45.8X4	T45.8X5	T45.8X6
ferrous citrate	T45.4X1	T45.4X2	T45.4X3	T45.4X4	T45.4X5	T45.4X6
folinate	T45.8X1	T45.8X2	T45.8X3	T45.8X4	T45.8X5	T45.8X6
glubionate	T50.3X1	T50.3X2	T50.3X3	T50.3X4	T50.3X5	T50.3X6
gluconate	T50.3X1	T50.3X2	T50.3X3	T50.3X4	T50.3X5	T50.3X6
gluconogalactogluconate	T50.3X1	T50.3X2	T50.3X3	T50.3X4	T50.3X5	T50.3X6
hydrate, hydroxide	T54.3X1	T54.3X2	T54.3X3	T54.3X4	—	—
hypochlorite	T54.3X1	T54.3X2	T54.3X3	T54.3X4	—	—
iodide	T48.4X1	T48.4X2	T48.4X3	T48.4X4	T48.4X5	T48.4X6
ipodate	T50.8X1	T50.8X2	T50.8X3	T50.8X4	T50.8X5	T50.8X6
lactate	T50.3X1	T50.3X2	T50.3X3	T50.3X4	T50.3X5	T50.3X6
leucovorin	T45.8X1	T45.8X2	T45.8X3	T45.8X4	T45.8X5	T45.8X6
mandelate	T37.91	T37.92	T37.93	T37.94	T37.95	T37.96
oxide	T54.3X1	T54.3X2	T54.3X3	T54.3X4	—	—
pantothenate	T45.2X1	T45.2X2	T45.2X3	T45.2X4	T45.2X5	T45.2X6
phosphate	T50.3X1	T50.3X2	T50.3X3	T50.3X4	T50.3X5	T50.3X6
salicylate	T39.091	T39.092	T39.093	T39.094	T39.095	T39.096
salts	T50.3X1	T50.3X2	T50.3X3	T50.3X4	T50.3X5	T50.3X6
Calculus-dissolving drug	T50.991	T50.992	T50.993	T50.994	T50.995	T50.996
Calomel	T49.0X1	T49.0X2	T49.0X3	T49.0X4	T49.0X5	T49.0X6
Caloric agent	T50.3X1	T50.3X2	T50.3X3	T50.3X4	T50.3X5	T50.3X6
Calusterone	T38.7X1	T38.7X2	T38.7X3	T38.7X4	T38.7X5	T38.7X6
Camazepam	T42.4X1	T42.4X2	T42.4X3	T42.4X4	T42.4X5	T42.4X6
Camomile	T49.0X1	T49.0X2	T49.0X3	T49.0X4	T49.0X5	T49.0X6
Camoquin	T37.2X1	T37.2X2	T37.2X3	T37.2X4	T37.2X5	T37.2X6
Camphor						
insecticide	T60.2X1	T60.2X2	T60.2X3	T60.2X4	—	—
medicinal	T49.8X1	T49.8X2	T49.8X3	T49.8X4	T49.8X5	T49.8X6
Camylofin	T44.3X1	T44.3X2	T44.3X3	T44.3X4	T44.3X5	T44.3X6
Cancer chemotherapy drug regimen	T45.1X1	T45.1X2	T45.1X3	T45.1X4	T45.1X5	T45.1X6
Candeptin	T49.0X1	T49.0X2	T49.0X3	T49.0X4	T49.0X5	T49.0X6
Candicidin	T49.0X1	T49.0X2	T49.0X3	T49.0X4	T49.0X5	T49.0X6
Cannabinol	T40.7X1	T40.7X2	T40.7X3	T40.7X4	T40.7X5	T40.7X6
Cannabis (derivatives)	T40.7X1	T40.7X2	T40.7X3	T40.7X4	T40.7X5	T40.7X6
Canned heat	T51.1X1	T51.1X2	T51.1X3	T51.1X4	—	—
Canrenoic acid	T50.0X1	T50.0X2	T50.0X3	T50.0X4	T50.0X5	T50.0X6
Canrenone	T50.0X1	T50.0X2	T50.0X3	T50.0X4	T50.0X5	T50.0X6
Cantharides, cantharidin, cantharis	T49.8X1	T49.8X2	T49.8X3	T49.8X4	T49.8X5	T49.8X6
Canthaxanthin	T50.991	T50.992	T50.993	T50.994	T50.995	T50.996
Capillary-active drug NEC	T46.901	T46.902	T46.903	T46.904	T46.905	T46.906
Capreomycin	T36.8X1	T36.8X2	T36.8X3	T36.8X4	T36.8X5	T36.8X6
Capsicum	T49.4X1	T49.4X2	T49.4X3	T49.4X4	T49.4X5	T49.4X6
Captafol	T60.3X1	T60.3X2	T60.3X3	T60.3X4	—	—

Substance	Poisoning, Accidental (unintentional)	Poisoning, Intentional Self-harm	Poisoning, Assault	Poisoning, Undetermined	Adverse Effect	Under-dosing
Captan	T60.3X1	T60.3X2	T60.3X3	T60.3X4	—	—
Captodiame, captodiamine	T43.591	T43.592	T43.593	T43.594	T43.595	T43.596
Captopril	T46.4X1	T46.4X2	T46.4X3	T46.4X4	T46.4X5	T46.4X6
Caramiphen	T44.3X1	T44.3X2	T44.3X3	T44.3X4	T44.3X5	T44.3X6
Carazolol	T44.7X1	T44.7X2	T44.7X3	T44.7X4	T44.7X5	T44.7X6
Carbachol	T44.1X1	T44.1X2	T44.1X3	T44.1X4	T44.1X5	T44.1X6
Carbacrylamine (resin)	T50.3X1	T50.3X2	T50.3X3	T50.3X4	T50.3X5	T50.3X6
Carbamate (insecticide)	T60.0X1	T60.0X2	T60.0X3	T60.0X4	—	—
Carbamate (sedative)	T42.6X1	T42.6X2	T42.6X3	T42.6X4	T42.6X5	T42.6X6
herbicide	T60.0X1	T60.0X2	T60.0X3	T60.0X4	—	—
insecticide	T60.0X1	T60.0X2	T60.0X3	T60.0X4	—	—
Carbamazepine	T42.1X1	T42.1X2	T42.1X3	T42.1X4	T42.1X5	T42.1X6
Carbamide	T47.3X1	T47.3X2	T47.3X3	T47.3X4	T47.3X5	T47.3X6
peroxide	T49.0X1	T49.0X2	T49.0X3	T49.0X4	T49.0X5	T49.0X6
topical	T49.8X1	T49.8X2	T49.8X3	T49.8X4	T49.8X5	T49.8X6
Carbamylcholine chloride	T44.1X1	T44.1X2	T44.1X3	T44.1X4	T44.1X5	T44.1X6
Carbaril	T60.0X1	T60.0X2	T60.0X3	T60.0X4	—	—
Carbarsone	T37.3X1	T37.3X2	T37.3X3	T37.3X4	T37.3X5	T37.3X6
Carbaryl	T60.0X1	T60.0X2	T60.0X3	T60.0X4	—	—
Carbaspirin	T39.011	T39.012	T39.013	T39.014	T39.015	T39.016
Carbazochrome (salicylate) (sodium sulfonate)	T49.4X1	T49.4X2	T49.4X3	T49.4X4	T49.4X5	T49.4X6
Carbenicillin	T36.0X1	T36.0X2	T36.0X3	T36.0X4	T36.0X5	T36.0X6
Carbenoxolone	T47.1X1	T47.1X2	T47.1X3	T47.1X4	T47.1X5	T47.1X6
Carbetapentane	T48.3X1	T48.3X2	T48.3X3	T48.3X4	T48.3X5	T48.3X6
Carbethyl salicylate	T39.091	T39.092	T39.093	T39.094	T39.095	T39.096
Carbidopa (with levodopa)	T42.8X1	T42.8X2	T42.8X3	T42.8X4	T42.8X5	T42.8X6
Carbimazole	T38.2X1	T38.2X2	T38.2X3	T38.2X4	T38.2X5	T38.2X6
Carbinol	T51.1X1	T51.1X2	T51.1X3	T51.1X4	—	—
Carbinoxamine	T45.0X1	T45.0X2	T45.0X3	T45.0X4	T45.0X5	T45.0X6
Carbiphene	T39.8X1	T39.8X2	T39.8X3	T39.8X4	T39.8X5	T39.8X6
Carbitol	T52.3X1	T52.3X2	T52.3X3	T52.3X4	—	—
Carbocaine	T41.3X1	T41.3X2	T41.3X3	T41.3X4	T41.3X5	T41.3X6
infiltration (subcutaneous)	T41.3X1	T41.3X2	T41.3X3	T41.3X4	T41.3X5	T41.3X6
nerve block (peripheral) (plexus)	T41.3X1	T41.3X2	T41.3X3	T41.3X4	T41.3X5	T41.3X6
topical (surface)	T41.3X1	T41.3X2	T41.3X3	T41.3X4	T41.3X5	T41.3X6
Carbocisteine	T48.4X1	T48.4X2	T48.4X3	T48.4X4	T48.4X5	T48.4X6
Carbocromen	T46.3X1	T46.3X2	T46.3X3	T46.3X4	T46.3X5	T46.3X6
Carbol fuchsin	T49.0X1	T49.0X2	T49.0X3	T49.0X4	T49.0X5	T49.0X6
Carbolic acid — *see also* Phenol	T54.0X1	T54.0X2	T54.0X3	T54.0X4	—	—
Carbolonium (bromide)	T48.1X1	T48.1X2	T48.1X3	T48.1X4	T48.1X5	T48.1X6
Carbo medicinalis	T47.6X1	T47.6X2	T47.6X3	T47.6X4	T47.6X5	T47.6X6
Carbomycin	T36.8X1	T36.8X2	T36.8X3	T36.8X4	T36.8X5	T36.8X6
Carbon						
bisulfide (liquid)	T65.4X1	T65.4X2	T65.4X3	T65.4X4	—	—
vapor	T65.4X1	T65.4X2	T65.4X3	T65.4X4	—	—
dioxide (gas)	T59.7X1	T59.7X2	T59.7X3	T59.7X4	—	—
medicinal	T41.5X1	T41.5X2	T41.5X3	T41.5X4	T41.5X5	T41.5X6
nonmedicinal	T59.7X1	T59.7X2	T59.7X3	T59.7X4	—	—
snow	T49.4X1	T49.4X2	T49.4X3	T49.4X4	T49.4X5	T49.4X6
disulfide (liquid)	T65.4X1	T65.4X2	T65.4X3	T65.4X4	—	—
vapor	T65.4X1	T65.4X2	T65.4X3	T65.4X4	—	—
monoxide (from incomplete combustion)	T58.91	T58.92	T58.93	T58.94	—	—
blast furnace gas	T58.8X1	T58.8X2	T58.8X3	T58.8X4	—	—
butane (distributed in mobile container)	T58.11	T58.12	T58.13	T58.14	—	—
distributed through pipes	T58.11	T58.12	T58.13	T58.14	—	—
charcoal fumes	T58.2X1	T58.2X2	T58.2X3	T58.2X4	—	—
coal	T58.2X1	T58.2X2	T58.2X3	T58.2X4	—	—
coke (in domestic stoves, fireplaces)	T58.2X1	T58.2X2	T58.2X3	T58.2X4	—	—
exhaust gas (motor) not in transit	T58.01	T58.02	T58.03	T58.04	—	—
combustion engine, any not in watercraft	T58.01	T58.02	T58.03	T58.04	—	—
farm tractor, not in transit	T58.01	T58.02	T58.03	T58.04	—	—
gas engine	T58.01	T58.02	T58.03	T58.04	—	—
motor pump	T58.01	T58.02	T58.03	T58.04	—	—
motor vehicle, not in transit	T58.01	T58.02	T58.03	T58.04	—	—
fuel (in domestic use)	T58.2X1	T58.2X2	T58.2X3	T58.2X4	—	—
gas (piped)	T58.11	T58.12	T58.13	T58.14	—	—
in mobile container	T58.11	T58.12	T58.13	T58.14	—	—
piped (natural)	T58.11	T58.12	T58.13	T58.14	—	—
utility	T58.11	T58.12	T58.13	T58.14	—	—
in mobile container	T58.11	T58.12	T58.13	T58.14	—	—
gas (piped)	T58.11	T58.12	T58.13	T58.14	—	—
illuminating gas	T58.11	T58.12	T58.13	T58.14	—	—

Substance	Poisoning, Accidental (unintentional)	Poisoning, Intentional Self-harm	Poisoning, Assault	Poisoning, Undetermined	Adverse Effect	Under-dosing
Carbon — *continued*						
monoxide — *continued*						
industrial fuels or gases, any	T58.8X1	T58.8X2	T58.8X3	T58.8X4	—	—
kerosene (in domestic stoves, fireplaces)	T58.2X1	T58.2X2	T58.2X3	T58.2X4	—	—
kiln gas or vapor	T58.8X1	T58.8X2	T58.8X3	T58.8X4	—	—
motor exhaust gas, not in transit	T58.Ø1	T58.Ø2	T58.Ø3	T58.Ø4	—	—
piped gas (manufactured) (natural)	T58.11	T58.12	T58.13	T58.14	—	—
producer gas	T58.8X1	T58.8X2	T58.8X3	T58.8X4	—	—
propane (distributed in mobile container)	T58.11	T58.12	T58.13	T58.14	—	—
distributed through pipes	T58.11	T58.12	T58.13	T58.14	—	—
solid (in domestic stoves, fireplaces)	T58.2X1	T58.2X2	T58.2X3	T58.2X4	—	—
specified source NEC	T58.8X1	T58.8X2	T58.8X3	T58.8X4	—	—
stove gas	T58.11	T58.12	T58.13	T58.14	—	—
piped	T58.11	T58.12	T58.13	T58.14	—	—
utility gas	T58.11	T58.12	T58.13	T58.14	—	—
piped	T58.11	T58.12	T58.13	T58.14	—	—
water gas	T58.11	T58.12	T58.13	T58.14	—	—
wood (in domestic stoves, fireplaces)	T58.2X1	T58.2X2	T58.2X3	T58.2X4	—	—
tetrachloride (vapor) NEC	T53.ØX1	T53.ØX2	T53.ØX3	T53.ØX4	—	—
liquid (cleansing agent) NEC	T53.ØX1	T53.ØX2	T53.ØX3	T53.ØX4	—	—
solvent	T53.ØX1	T53.ØX2	T53.ØX3	T53.ØX4	—	—
Carbonic acid gas	T59.7X1	T59.7X2	T59.7X3	T59.7X4	—	—
anhydrase inhibitor NEC	T5Ø.2X1	T5Ø.2X2	T5Ø.2X3	T5Ø.2X4	T5Ø.2X5	T5Ø.2X6
Carbophenothion	T6Ø.ØX1	T6Ø.ØX2	T6Ø.ØX3	T6Ø.ØX4	—	—
Carboplatin	T45.1X1	T45.1X2	T45.1X3	T45.1X4	T45.1X5	T45.1X6
Carboprost	T48.ØX1	T48.ØX2	T48.ØX3	T48.ØX4	T48.ØX5	T48.ØX6
Carboquone	T45.1X1	T45.1X2	T45.1X3	T45.1X4	T45.1X5	T45.1X6
Carbowax	T49.3X1	T49.3X2	T49.3X3	T49.3X4	T49.3X5	T49.3X6
Carboxymethylcellulose	T47.4X1	T47.4X2	T47.4X3	T47.4X4	T47.4X5	T47.4X6
Carbrital	T42.3X1	T42.3X2	T42.3X3	T42.3X4	T42.3X5	T42.3X6
Carbromal	T42.6X1	T42.6X2	T42.6X3	T42.6X4	T42.6X5	T42.6X6
Carbutamide	T38.3X1	T38.3X2	T38.3X3	T38.3X4	T38.3X5	T38.3X6
Carbuterol	T48.6X1	T48.6X2	T48.6X3	T48.6X4	T48.6X5	T48.6X6
Cardiac						
depressants	T46.2X1	T46.2X2	T46.2X3	T46.2X4	T46.2X5	T46.2X6
rhythm regulator	T46.2X1	T46.2X2	T46.2X3	T46.2X4	T46.2X5	T46.2X6
specified NEC	T46.2X1	T46.2X2	T46.2X3	T46.2X4	T46.2X5	T46.2X6
Cardiografin	T5Ø.8X1	T5Ø.8X2	T5Ø.8X3	T5Ø.8X4	T5Ø.8X5	T5Ø.8X6
Cardiogreen	T5Ø.8X1	T5Ø.8X2	T5Ø.8X3	T5Ø.8X4	T5Ø.8X5	T5Ø.8X6
Cardiotonic (glycoside) **NEC**	T46.ØX1	T46.ØX2	T46.ØX3	T46.ØX4	T46.ØX5	T46.ØX6
Cardiovascular drug NEC	T46.9Ø1	T46.9Ø2	T46.9Ø3	T46.9Ø4	T46.9Ø5	T46.9Ø6
Cardrase	T5Ø.2X1	T5Ø.2X2	T5Ø.2X3	T5Ø.2X4	T5Ø.2X5	T5Ø.2X6
Carfecillin	T36.ØX1	T36.ØX2	T36.ØX3	T36.ØX4	T36.ØX5	T36.ØX6
Carfenazine	T43.3X1	T43.3X2	T43.3X3	T43.3X4	T43.3X5	T43.3X6
Carfusin	T49.ØX1	T49.ØX2	T49.ØX3	T49.ØX4	T49.ØX5	T49.ØX6
Carindacillin	T36.ØX1	T36.ØX2	T36.ØX3	T36.ØX4	T36.ØX5	T36.ØX6
Carisoprodol	T42.8X1	T42.8X2	T42.8X3	T42.8X4	T42.8X5	T42.8X6
Carmellose	T47.4X1	T47.4X2	T47.4X3	T47.4X4	T47.4X5	T47.4X6
Carminative	T47.5X1	T47.5X2	T47.5X3	T47.5X4	T47.5X5	T47.5X6
Carmofur	T45.1X1	T45.1X2	T45.1X3	T45.1X4	T45.1X5	T45.1X6
Carmustine	T45.1X1	T45.1X2	T45.1X3	T45.1X4	T45.1X5	T45.1X6
Carotene	T45.2X1	T45.2X2	T45.2X3	T45.2X4	T45.2X5	T45.2X6
Carphenazine	T43.3X1	T43.3X2	T43.3X3	T43.3X4	T43.3X5	T43.3X6
Carpipramine	T42.4X1	T42.4X2	T42.4X3	T42.4X4	T42.4X5	T42.4X6
Carprofen	T39.311	T39.312	T39.313	T39.314	T39.315	T39.316
Carpronium chloride	T44.3X1	T44.3X2	T44.3X3	T44.3X4	T44.3X5	T44.3X6
Carrageenan	T47.8X1	T47.8X2	T47.8X3	T47.8X4	T47.8X5	T47.8X6
Carteolol	T44.7X1	T44.7X2	T44.7X3	T44.7X4	T44.7X5	T44.7X6
Carter's Little Pills	T47.2X1	T47.2X2	T47.2X3	T47.2X4	T47.2X5	T47.2X6
Cascara (sagrada)	T47.2X1	T47.2X2	T47.2X3	T47.2X4	T47.2X5	T47.2X6
Cassava	T62.2X1	T62.2X2	T62.2X3	T62.2X4	—	—
Castellani's paint	T49.ØX1	T49.ØX2	T49.ØX3	T49.ØX4	T49.ØX5	T49.ØX6
Castor						
bean	T62.2X1	T62.2X2	T62.2X3	T62.2X4	—	—
oil	T47.2X1	T47.2X2	T47.2X3	T47.2X4	T47.2X5	T47.2X6
Catalase	T45.3X1	T45.3X2	T45.3X3	T45.3X4	T45.3X5	T45.3X6
Caterpillar (sting)	T63.431	T63.432	T63.433	T63.434	—	—
Catha (edulis) (tea)	T43.691	T43.692	T43.693	T43.694	—	—
Cathartic NEC	T47.4X1	T47.4X2	T47.4X3	T47.4X4	T47.4X5	T47.4X6
anthacene derivative	T47.2X1	T47.2X2	T47.2X3	T47.2X4	T47.2X5	T47.2X6
bulk	T47.4X1	T47.4X2	T47.4X3	T47.4X4	T47.4X5	T47.4X6
contact	T47.2X1	T47.2X2	T47.2X3	T47.2X4	T47.2X5	T47.2X6
emollient NEC	T47.4X1	T47.4X2	T47.4X3	T47.4X4	T47.4X5	T47.4X6
irritant NEC	T47.2X1	T47.2X2	T47.2X3	T47.2X4	T47.2X5	T47.2X6
Cathartic — *continued*						
mucilage	T47.4X1	T47.4X2	T47.4X3	T47.4X4	T47.4X5	T47.4X6
saline	T47.3X1	T47.3X2	T47.3X3	T47.3X4	T47.3X5	T47.3X6
vegetable	T47.2X1	T47.2X2	T47.2X3	T47.2X4	T47.2X5	T47.2X6
Cathine	T5Ø.5X1	T5Ø.5X2	T5Ø.5X3	T5Ø.5X4	T5Ø.5X5	T5Ø.5X6
Cathomycin	T36.8X1	T36.8X2	T36.8X3	T36.8X4	T36.8X5	T36.8X6
Cation exchange resin	T5Ø.3X1	T5Ø.3X2	T5Ø.3X3	T5Ø.3X4	T5Ø.3X5	T5Ø.3X6
Caustic(s) **NEC**	T54.91	T54.92	T54.93	T54.94	—	—
alkali	T54.3X1	T54.3X2	T54.3X3	T54.3X4	—	—
hydroxide	T54.3X1	T54.3X2	T54.3X3	T54.3X4	—	—
potash	T54.3X1	T54.3X2	T54.3X3	T54.3X4	—	—
soda	T54.3X1	T54.3X2	T54.3X3	T54.3X4	—	—
specified NEC	T54.91	T54.92	T54.93	T54.94	—	—
Ceepryn	T49.ØX1	T49.ØX2	T49.ØX3	T49.ØX4	T49.ØX5	T49.ØX6
ENT agent	T49.6X1	T49.6X2	T49.6X3	T49.6X4	T49.6X5	T49.6X6
lozenges	T49.6X1	T49.6X2	T49.6X3	T49.6X4	T49.6X5	T49.6X6
Cefacetrile	T36.1X1	T36.1X2	T36.1X3	T36.1X4	T36.1X5	T36.1X6
Cefaclor	T36.1X1	T36.1X2	T36.1X3	T36.1X4	T36.1X5	T36.1X6
Cefadroxil	T36.1X1	T36.1X2	T36.1X3	T36.1X4	T36.1X5	T36.1X6
Cefalexin	T36.1X1	T36.1X2	T36.1X3	T36.1X4	T36.1X5	T36.1X6
Cefaloglycin	T36.1X1	T36.1X2	T36.1X3	T36.1X4	T36.1X5	T36.1X6
Cefaloridine	T36.1X1	T36.1X2	T36.1X3	T36.1X4	T36.1X5	T36.1X6
Cefalosporins	T36.1X1	T36.1X2	T36.1X3	T36.1X4	T36.1X5	T36.1X6
Cefalotin	T36.1X1	T36.1X2	T36.1X3	T36.1X4	T36.1X5	T36.1X6
Cefamandole	T36.1X1	T36.1X2	T36.1X3	T36.1X4	T36.1X5	T36.1X6
Cefamycin antibiotic	T36.1X1	T36.1X2	T36.1X3	T36.1X4	T36.1X5	T36.1X6
Cefapirin	T36.1X1	T36.1X2	T36.1X3	T36.1X4	T36.1X5	T36.1X6
Cefatrizine	T36.1X1	T36.1X2	T36.1X3	T36.1X4	T36.1X5	T36.1X6
Cefazedone	T36.1X1	T36.1X2	T36.1X3	T36.1X4	T36.1X5	T36.1X6
Cefazolin	T36.1X1	T36.1X2	T36.1X3	T36.1X4	T36.1X5	T36.1X6
Cefbuperazone	T36.1X1	T36.1X2	T36.1X3	T36.1X4	T36.1X5	T36.1X6
Cefetamet	T36.1X1	T36.1X2	T36.1X3	T36.1X4	T36.1X5	T36.1X6
Cefixime	T36.1X1	T36.1X2	T36.1X3	T36.1X4	T36.1X5	T36.1X6
Cefmenoxime	T36.1X1	T36.1X2	T36.1X3	T36.1X4	T36.1X5	T36.1X6
Cefmetazole	T36.1X1	T36.1X2	T36.1X3	T36.1X4	T36.1X5	T36.1X6
Cefminox	T36.1X1	T36.1X2	T36.1X3	T36.1X4	T36.1X5	T36.1X6
Cefonicid	T36.1X1	T36.1X2	T36.1X3	T36.1X4	T36.1X5	T36.1X6
Cefoperazone	T36.1X1	T36.1X2	T36.1X3	T36.1X4	T36.1X5	T36.1X6
Ceforanide	T36.1X1	T36.1X2	T36.1X3	T36.1X4	T36.1X5	T36.1X6
Cefotaxime	T36.1X1	T36.1X2	T36.1X3	T36.1X4	T36.1X5	T36.1X6
Cefotetan	T36.1X1	T36.1X2	T36.1X3	T36.1X4	T36.1X5	T36.1X6
Cefotiam	T36.1X1	T36.1X2	T36.1X3	T36.1X4	T36.1X5	T36.1X6
Cefoxitin	T36.1X1	T36.1X2	T36.1X3	T36.1X4	T36.1X5	T36.1X6
Cefpimizole	T36.1X1	T36.1X2	T36.1X3	T36.1X4	T36.1X5	T36.1X6
Cefpiramide	T36.1X1	T36.1X2	T36.1X3	T36.1X4	T36.1X5	T36.1X6
Cefradine	T36.1X1	T36.1X2	T36.1X3	T36.1X4	T36.1X5	T36.1X6
Cefroxadine	T36.1X1	T36.1X2	T36.1X3	T36.1X4	T36.1X5	T36.1X6
Cefsulodin	T36.1X1	T36.1X2	T36.1X3	T36.1X4	T36.1X5	T36.1X6
Ceftazidime	T36.1X1	T36.1X2	T36.1X3	T36.1X4	T36.1X5	T36.1X6
Cefteram	T36.1X1	T36.1X2	T36.1X3	T36.1X4	T36.1X5	T36.1X6
Ceftezole	T36.1X1	T36.1X2	T36.1X3	T36.1X4	T36.1X5	T36.1X6
Ceftizoxime	T36.1X1	T36.1X2	T36.1X3	T36.1X4	T36.1X5	T36.1X6
Ceftriaxone	T36.1X1	T36.1X2	T36.1X3	T36.1X4	T36.1X5	T36.1X6
Cefuroxime	T36.1X1	T36.1X2	T36.1X3	T36.1X4	T36.1X5	T36.1X6
Cefuzonam	T36.1X1	T36.1X2	T36.1X3	T36.1X4	T36.1X5	T36.1X6
Celestone	T38.ØX1	T38.ØX2	T38.ØX3	T38.ØX4	T38.ØX5	T38.ØX6
topical	T49.ØX1	T49.ØX2	T49.ØX3	T49.ØX4	T49.ØX5	T49.ØX6
Celiprolol	T44.7X1	T44.7X2	T44.7X3	T44.7X4	T44.7X5	T44.7X6
Cell stimulants and proliferants	T49.8X1	T49.8X2	T49.8X3	T49.8X4	T49.8X5	T49.8X6
Cellosolve	T52.91	T52.92	T52.93	T52.94	—	—
Cellulose						
cathartic	T47.4X1	T47.4X2	T47.4X3	T47.4X4	T47.4X5	T47.4X6
hydroxyethyl	T47.4X1	T47.4X2	T47.4X3	T47.4X4	T47.4X5	T47.4X6
nitrates (topical)	T49.3X1	T49.3X2	T49.3X3	T49.3X4	T49.3X5	T49.3X6
oxidized	T49.4X1	T49.4X2	T49.4X3	T49.4X4	T49.4X5	T49.4X6
Centipede (bite)	T63.411	T63.412	T63.413	T63.414	—	—
Central nervous system						
depressants	T42.71	T42.72	T42.73	T42.74	T42.75	T42.76
anesthetic (general) NEC	T41.2Ø1	T41.2Ø2	T41.2Ø3	T41.2Ø4	T41.2Ø5	T41.2Ø6
gases NEC	T41.ØX1	T41.ØX2	T41.ØX3	T41.ØX4	T41.ØX5	T41.ØX6
intravenous	T41.1X1	T41.1X2	T41.1X3	T41.1X4	T41.1X5	T41.1X6
barbiturates	T42.3X1	T42.3X2	T42.3X3	T42.3X4	T42.3X5	T42.3X6
benzodiazepines	T42.4X1	T42.4X2	T42.4X3	T42.4X4	T42.4X5	T42.4X6
bromides	T42.6X1	T42.6X2	T42.6X3	T42.6X4	T42.6X5	T42.6X6
cannabis sativa	T4Ø.7X1	T4Ø.7X2	T4Ø.7X3	T4Ø.7X4	T4Ø.7X5	T4Ø.7X6
chloral hydrate	T42.6X1	T42.6X2	T42.6X3	T42.6X4	T42.6X5	T42.6X6
ethanol	T51.ØX1	T51.ØX2	T51.ØX3	T51.ØX4	—	—
hallucinogenics	T4Ø.9Ø1	T4Ø.9Ø2	T4Ø.9Ø3	T4Ø.9Ø4	T4Ø.9Ø5	T4Ø.9Ø6
hypnotics	T42.71	T42.72	T42.73	T42.74	T42.75	T42.76
specified NEC	T42.6X1	T42.6X2	T42.6X3	T42.6X4	T42.6X5	T42.6X6
muscle relaxants	T42.8X1	T42.8X2	T42.8X3	T42.8X4	T42.8X5	T42.8X6
paraldehyde	T42.6X1	T42.6X2	T42.6X3	T42.6X4	T42.6X5	T42.6X6

Substance	Poisoning, Accidental (unintentional)	Poisoning, Intentional Self-harm	Poisoning, Assault	Poisoning, Undetermined	Adverse Effect	Under-dosing
Central nervous system — *continued*						
depressants — *continued*						
sedatives; sedative-hypnotics	T42.71	T42.72	T42.73	T42.74	T42.75	T42.76
mixed NEC	T42.6X1	T42.6X2	T42.6X3	T42.6X4	T42.6X5	T42.6X6
specified NEC	T42.6X1	T42.6X2	T42.6X3	T42.6X4	T42.6X5	T42.6X6
muscle-tone depressants	T42.8X1	T42.8X2	T42.8X3	T42.8X4	T42.8X5	T42.8X6
stimulants	T43.6Ø1	T43.6Ø2	T43.6Ø3	T43.6Ø4	T43.6Ø5	T43.6Ø6
amphetamines	T43.621	T43.622	T43.623	T43.624	T43.625	T43.626
analeptics	T5Ø.7X1	T5Ø.7X2	T5Ø.7X3	T5Ø.7X4	T5Ø.7X5	T5Ø.7X6
antidepressants	T43.2Ø1	T43.2Ø2	T43.2Ø3	T43.2Ø4	T43.2Ø5	T43.2Ø6
opiate antagonists	T5Ø.7X1	T5Ø.7X2	T5Ø.7X3	T5Ø.7X4	T5Ø.7X5	T5Ø.7X6
specified NEC	T43.691	T43.692	T43.693	T43.694	T43.695	T43.696
Cephalexin	T36.1X1	T36.1X2	T36.1X3	T36.1X4	T36.1X5	T36.1X6
Cephaloglycin	T36.1X1	T36.1X2	T36.1X3	T36.1X4	T36.1X5	T36.1X6
Cephaloridine	T36.1X1	T36.1X2	T36.1X3	T36.1X4	T36.1X5	T36.1X6
Cephalosporins	T36.1X1	T36.1X2	T36.1X3	T36.1X4	T36.1X5	T36.1X6
N (adicillin)	T36.ØX1	T36.ØX2	T36.ØX3	T36.ØX4	T36.ØX5	T36.ØX6
Cephalothin	T36.1X1	T36.1X2	T36.1X3	T36.1X4	T36.1X5	T36.1X6
Cephalotin	T36.1X1	T36.1X2	T36.1X3	T36.1X4	T36.1X5	T36.1X6
Cephradine	T36.1X1	T36.1X2	T36.1X3	T36.1X4	T36.1X5	T36.1X6
Cerbera (odallam)	T62.2X1	T62.2X2	T62.2X3	T62.2X4	—	—
Cerberin	T46.ØX1	T46.ØX2	T46.ØX3	T46.ØX4	T46.ØX5	T46.ØX6
Cerebral stimulants	T43.6Ø1	T43.6Ø2	T43.6Ø3	T43.6Ø4	T43.6Ø5	T43.6Ø6
psychotherapeutic	T43.6Ø1	T43.6Ø2	T43.6Ø3	T43.6Ø4	T43.6Ø5	T43.6Ø6
specified NEC	T43.691	T43.692	T43.693	T43.694	T43.695	T43.696
Cerium oxalate	T45.ØX1	T45.ØX2	T45.ØX3	T45.ØX4	T45.ØX5	T45.ØX6
Cerous oxalate	T45.ØX1	T45.ØX2	T45.ØX3	T45.ØX4	T45.ØX5	T45.ØX6
Ceruletide	T5Ø.8X1	T5Ø.8X2	T5Ø.8X3	T5Ø.8X4	T5Ø.8X5	T5Ø.8X6
Cetalkonium (chloride)	T49.ØX1	T49.ØX2	T49.ØX3	T49.ØX4	T49.ØX5	T49.ØX6
Cethexonium chloride	T49.ØX1	T49.ØX2	T49.ØX3	T49.ØX4	T49.ØX5	T49.ØX6
Cetiedil	T46.7X1	T46.7X2	T46.7X3	T46.7X4	T46.7X5	T46.7X6
Cetirizine	T45.ØX1	T45.ØX2	T45.ØX3	T45.ØX4	T45.ØX5	T45.ØX6
Cetomacrogol	T5Ø.991	T5Ø.992	T5Ø.993	T5Ø.994	T5Ø.995	T5Ø.996
Cetotiamine	T45.2X1	T45.2X2	T45.2X3	T45.2X4	T45.2X5	T45.2X6
Cetoxime	T45.ØX1	T45.ØX2	T45.ØX3	T45.ØX4	T45.ØX5	T45.ØX6
Cetraxate	T47.1X1	T47.1X2	T47.1X3	T47.1X4	T47.1X5	T47.1X6
Cetrimide	T49.ØX1	T49.ØX2	T49.ØX3	T49.ØX4	T49.ØX5	T49.ØX6
Cetrimonium (bromide)	T49.ØX1	T49.ØX2	T49.ØX3	T49.ØX4	T49.ØX5	T49.ØX6
Cetylpyridinium chloride	T49.ØX1	T49.ØX2	T49.ØX3	T49.ØX4	T49.ØX5	T49.ØX6
ENT agent	T49.6X1	T49.6X2	T49.6X3	T49.6X4	T49.6X5	T49.6X6
lozenges	T49.6X1	T49.6X2	T49.6X3	T49.6X4	T49.6X5	T49.6X6
Cevadilla — *see* Sabadilla						
Cevitamic acid	T45.2X1	T45.2X2	T45.2X3	T45.2X4	T45.2X5	T45.2X6
Chalk, precipitated	T47.1X1	T47.1X2	T47.1X3	T47.1X4	T47.1X5	T47.1X6
Chamomile	T49.ØX1	T49.ØX2	T49.ØX3	T49.ØX4	T49.ØX5	T49.ØX6
Ch'an su	T46.ØX1	T46.ØX2	T46.ØX3	T46.ØX4	T46.ØX5	T46.ØX6
Charcoal	T47.6X1	T47.6X2	T47.6X3	T47.6X4	T47.6X5	T47.6X6
activated — *see also* Charcoal, medicinal	T47.6X1	T47.6X2	T47.6X3	T47.6X4	T47.6X5	T47.6X6
fumes (Carbon monoxide)	T58.2X1	T58.2X2	T58.2X3	T58.2X4	—	—
industrial	T58.8X1	T58.8X2	T58.8X3	T58.8X4	—	—
medicinal (activated)	T47.6X1	T47.6X2	T47.6X3	T47.6X4	T47.6X5	T47.6X6
antidiarrheal	T47.6X1	T47.6X2	T47.6X3	T47.6X4	T47.6X5	T47.6X6
poison control	T47.8X1	T47.8X2	T47.8X3	T47.8X4	T47.8X5	T47.8X6
specified use other than for diarrhea	T47.8X1	T47.8X2	T47.8X3	T47.8X4	T47.8X5	T47.8X6
topical	T49.8X1	T49.8X2	T49.8X3	T49.8X4	T49.8X5	T49.8X6
Chaulmosulfone	T37.1X1	T37.1X2	T37.1X3	T37.1X4	T37.1X5	T37.1X6
Chelating agent NEC	T5Ø.6X1	T5Ø.6X2	T5Ø.6X3	T5Ø.6X4	T5Ø.6X5	T5Ø.6X6
Chelidonium majus	T62.2X1	T62.2X2	T62.2X3	T62.2X4	—	—
Chemical substance NEC	T65.91	T65.92	T65.93	T65.94	—	—
Chenodeoxycholic acid	T47.5X1	T47.5X2	T47.5X3	T47.5X4	T47.5X5	T47.5X6
Chenodiol	T47.5X1	T47.5X2	T47.5X3	T47.5X4	T47.5X5	T47.5X6
Chenopodium	T37.4X1	T37.4X2	T37.4X3	T37.4X4	T37.4X5	T37.4X6
Cherry laurel	T62.2X1	T62.2X2	T62.2X3	T62.2X4	—	—
Chinidin (e)	T46.2X1	T46.2X2	T46.2X3	T46.2X4	T46.2X5	T46.2X6
Chiniofon	T37.8X1	T37.8X2	T37.8X3	T37.8X4	T37.8X5	T37.8X6
Chlophedianol	T48.3X1	T48.3X2	T48.3X3	T48.3X4	T48.3X5	T48.3X6
Chloral	T42.6X1	T42.6X2	T42.6X3	T42.6X4	T42.6X5	T42.6X6
derivative	T42.6X1	T42.6X2	T42.6X3	T42.6X4	T42.6X5	T42.6X6
hydrate	T42.6X1	T42.6X2	T42.6X3	T42.6X4	T42.6X5	T42.6X6
Chloralamide	T42.6X1	T42.6X2	T42.6X3	T42.6X4	T42.6X5	T42.6X6
Chloralodol	T42.6X1	T42.6X2	T42.6X3	T42.6X4	T42.6X5	T42.6X6
Chloralose	T6Ø.4X1	T6Ø.4X2	T6Ø.4X3	T6Ø.4X4	—	—
Chlorambucil	T45.1X1	T45.1X2	T45.1X3	T45.1X4	T45.1X5	T45.1X6
Chloramine	T57.8X1	T57.8X2	T57.8X3	T57.8X4	—	—
T	T49.ØX1	T49.ØX2	T49.ØX3	T49.ØX4	T49.ØX5	T49.ØX6
topical	T49.ØX1	T49.ØX2	T49.ØX3	T49.ØX4	T49.ØX5	T49.ØX6
Chloramphenicol	T36.2X1	T36.2X2	T36.2X3	T36.2X4	T36.2X5	T36.2X6
ENT agent	T49.6X1	T49.6X2	T49.6X3	T49.6X4	T49.6X5	T49.6X6
ophthalmic preparation	T49.5X1	T49.5X2	T49.5X3	T49.5X4	T49.5X5	T49.5X6
Chloramphenicol — *continued*						
topical NEC	T49.ØX1	T49.ØX2	T49.ØX3	T49.ØX4	T49.ØX5	T49.ØX6
Chlorate (potassium) (sodium) **NEC**	T6Ø.3X1	T6Ø.3X2	T6Ø.3X3	T6Ø.3X4	—	—
herbicide	T6Ø.3X1	T6Ø.3X2	T6Ø.3X3	T6Ø.3X4	—	—
Chlorazanil	T5Ø.2X1	T5Ø.2X2	T5Ø.2X3	T5Ø.2X4	T5Ø.2X5	T5Ø.2X6
Chlorbenzene, chlorbenzol	T53.7X1	T53.7X2	T53.7X3	T53.7X4	—	—
Chlorbenzoxamine	T44.3X1	T44.3X2	T44.3X3	T44.3X4	T44.3X5	T44.3X6
Chlorbutol	T42.6X1	T42.6X2	T42.6X3	T42.6X4	T42.6X5	T42.6X6
Chlorcyclizine	T45.ØX1	T45.ØX2	T45.ØX3	T45.ØX4	T45.ØX5	T45.ØX6
Chlordan (e) (dust)	T6Ø.1X1	T6Ø.1X2	T6Ø.1X3	T6Ø.1X4	—	—
Chlordantoin	T49.ØX1	T49.ØX2	T49.ØX3	T49.ØX4	T49.ØX5	T49.ØX6
Chlordiazepoxide	T42.4X1	T42.4X2	T42.4X3	T42.4X4	T42.4X5	T42.4X6
Chlordiethyl benzamide	T49.3X1	T49.3X2	T49.3X3	T49.3X4	T49.3X5	T49.3X6
Chloresium	T49.8X1	T49.8X2	T49.8X3	T49.8X4	T49.8X5	T49.8X6
Chlorethiazol	T42.6X1	T42.6X2	T42.6X3	T42.6X4	T42.6X5	T42.6X6
Chlorethyl — *see* Ethyl chloride						
Chloretone	T42.6X1	T42.6X2	T42.6X3	T42.6X4	T42.6X5	T42.6X6
Chlorex	T53.6X1	T53.6X2	T53.6X3	T53.6X4	—	—
insecticide	T6Ø.1X1	T6Ø.1X2	T6Ø.1X3	T6Ø.1X4	—	—
Chlorfenvinphos	T6Ø.ØX1	T6Ø.ØX2	T6Ø.ØX3	T6Ø.ØX4	—	—
Chlorhexadol	T42.6X1	T42.6X2	T42.6X3	T42.6X4	T42.6X5	T42.6X6
Chlorhexamide	T45.1X1	T45.1X2	T45.1X3	T45.1X4	T45.1X5	T45.1X6
Chlorhexidine	T49.ØX1	T49.ØX2	T49.ØX3	T49.ØX4	T49.ØX5	T49.ØX6
Chlorhydroxyquinolin	T49.ØX1	T49.ØX2	T49.ØX3	T49.ØX4	T49.ØX5	T49.ØX6
Chloride of lime (bleach)	T54.3X1	T54.3X2	T54.3X3	T54.3X4	—	—
Chlorimipramine	T43.Ø11	T43.Ø12	T43.Ø13	T43.Ø14	T43.Ø15	T43.Ø16
Chlorinated						
camphene	T53.6X1	T53.6X2	T53.6X3	T53.6X4	—	—
diphenyl	T53.7X1	T53.7X2	T53.7X3	T53.7X4	—	—
hydrocarbons NEC	T53.91	T53.92	T53.93	T53.94	—	—
solvents	T53.91	T53.92	T53.93	T53.94	—	—
lime (bleach)	T54.3X1	T54.3X2	T54.3X3	T54.3X4	—	—
and boric acid solution	T49.ØX1	T49.ØX2	T49.ØX3	T49.ØX4	T49.ØX5	T49.ØX6
naphthalene (insecticide)	T6Ø.1X1	T6Ø.1X2	T6Ø.1X3	T6Ø.1X4	—	—
industrial (non-pesticide)	T53.7X1	T53.7X2	T53.7X3	T53.7X4	—	—
pesticide NEC	T6Ø.8X1	T6Ø.8X2	T6Ø.8X3	T6Ø.8X4	—	—
soda — *see also* sodium hypochlorite						
solution	T49.ØX1	T49.ØX2	T49.ØX3	T49.ØX4	T49.ØX5	T49.ØX6
Chlorine (fumes) (gas)	T59.4X1	T59.4X2	T59.4X3	T59.4X4	—	—
bleach	T54.3X1	T54.3X2	T54.3X3	T54.3X4	—	—
compound gas NEC	T59.4X1	T59.4X2	T59.4X3	T59.4X4	—	—
disinfectant	T59.4X1	T59.4X2	T59.4X3	T59.4X4	—	—
releasing agents NEC	T59.4X1	T59.4X2	T59.4X3	T59.4X4	—	—
Chlorisondamine chloride	T46.991	T46.992	T46.993	T46.994	T46.995	T46.996
Chlormadinone	T38.5X1	T38.5X2	T38.5X3	T38.5X4	T38.5X5	T38.5X6
Chlormephos	T6Ø.ØX1	T6Ø.ØX2	T6Ø.ØX3	T6Ø.ØX4	—	—
Chlormerodrin	T5Ø.2X1	T5Ø.2X2	T5Ø.2X3	T5Ø.2X4	T5Ø.2X5	T5Ø.2X6
Chlormethiazole	T42.6X1	T42.6X2	T42.6X3	T42.6X4	T42.6X5	T42.6X6
Chlormethine	T45.1X1	T45.1X2	T45.1X3	T45.1X4	T45.1X5	T45.1X6
Chlormethylenecycline	T36.4X1	T36.4X2	T36.4X3	T36.4X4	T36.4X5	T36.4X6
Chlormezanone	T42.6X1	T42.6X2	T42.6X3	T42.6X4	T42.6X5	T42.6X6
Chloroacetic acid	T6Ø.3X1	T6Ø.3X2	T6Ø.3X3	T6Ø.3X4	—	—
Chloroacetone	T59.3X1	T59.3X2	T59.3X3	T59.3X4	—	—
Chloroacetophenone	T59.3X1	T59.3X2	T59.3X3	T59.3X4	—	—
Chloroaniline	T53.7X1	T53.7X2	T53.7X3	T53.7X4	—	—
Chlorobenzene, chlorobenzol	T53.7X1	T53.7X2	T53.7X3	T53.7X4	—	—
Chlorobromomethane (fire extinguisher)	T53.6X1	T53.6X2	T53.6X3	T53.6X4	—	—
Chlorobutanol	T49.ØX1	T49.ØX2	T49.ØX3	T49.ØX4	T49.ØX5	T49.ØX6
Chlorocresol	T49.ØX1	T49.ØX2	T49.ØX3	T49.ØX4	T49.ØX5	T49.ØX6
Chlorodehydromethyltestosterone	T38.7X1	T38.7X2	T38.7X3	T38.7X4	T38.7X5	T38.7X6
Chlorodinitrobenzene	T53.7X1	T53.7X2	T53.7X3	T53.7X4	—	—
dust or vapor	T53.7X1	T53.7X2	T53.7X3	T53.7X4	—	—
Chlorodiphenyl	T53.7X1	T53.7X2	T53.7X3	T53.7X4	—	—
Chloroethane — *see* Ethyl chloride						
Chloroethylene	T53.6X1	T53.6X2	T53.6X3	T53.6X4	—	—
Chlorofluorocarbons	T53.5X1	T53.5X2	T53.5X3	T53.5X4	—	—
Chloroform (fumes) (vapor)	T53.1X1	T53.1X2	T53.1X3	T53.1X4	—	—
anesthetic	T41.ØX1	T41.ØX2	T41.ØX3	T41.ØX4	T41.ØX5	T41.ØX6
solvent	T53.1X1	T53.1X2	T53.1X3	T53.1X4	—	—
water, concentrated	T41.ØX1	T41.ØX2	T41.ØX3	T41.ØX4	T41.ØX5	T41.ØX6
Chloroguanide	T37.2X1	T37.2X2	T37.2X3	T37.2X4	T37.2X5	T37.2X6
Chloromycetin	T36.2X1	T36.2X2	T36.2X3	T36.2X4	T36.2X5	T36.2X6
ENT agent	T49.6X1	T49.6X2	T49.6X3	T49.6X4	T49.6X5	T49.6X6
ophthalmic preparation	T49.5X1	T49.5X2	T49.5X3	T49.5X4	T49.5X5	T49.5X6
otic solution	T49.6X1	T49.6X2	T49.6X3	T49.6X4	T49.6X5	T49.6X6
topical NEC	T49.ØX1	T49.ØX2	T49.ØX3	T49.ØX4	T49.ØX5	T49.ØX6
Chloronitrobenzene	T53.7X1	T53.7X2	T53.7X3	T53.7X4	—	—
dust or vapor	T53.7X1	T53.7X2	T53.7X3	T53.7X4	—	—

Substance	Poisoning, Accidental (unintentional)	Poisoning, Intentional Self-harm	Poisoning, Assault	Poisoning, Undetermined	Adverse Effect	Under-dosing
Chlorophacinone	T6Ø.4X1	T6Ø.4X2	T6Ø.4X3	T6Ø.4X4	—	—
Chlorophenol	T53.7X1	T53.7X2	T53.7X3	T53.7X4	—	—
Chlorophenothane	T6Ø.1X1	T6Ø.1X2	T6Ø.1X3	T6Ø.1X4	—	—
Chlorophyll	T5Ø.991	T5Ø.992	T5Ø.993	T5Ø.994	T5Ø.995	T5Ø.996
Chloropicrin (fumes)	T53.6X1	T53.6X2	T53.6X3	T53.6X4	—	—
fumigant	T6Ø.8X1	T6Ø.8X2	T6Ø.8X3	T6Ø.8X4	—	—
fungicide	T6Ø.3X1	T6Ø.3X2	T6Ø.3X3	T6Ø.3X4	—	—
pesticide	T6Ø.8X1	T6Ø.8X2	T6Ø.8X3	T6Ø.8X4	—	—
Chloroprocaine	T41.3X1	T41.3X2	T41.3X3	T41.3X4	T41.3X5	T41.3X6
infiltration (subcutaneous)	T41.3X1	T41.3X2	T41.3X3	T41.3X4	T41.3X5	T41.3X6
nerve block (peripheral) (plexus)	T41.3X1	T41.3X2	T41.3X3	T41.3X4	T41.3X5	T41.3X6
spinal	T41.3X1	T41.3X2	T41.3X3	T41.3X4	T41.3X5	T41.3X6
Chloroptic	T49.5X1	T49.5X2	T49.5X3	T49.5X4	T49.5X5	T49.5X6
Chloropurine	T45.1X1	T45.1X2	T45.1X3	T45.1X4	T45.1X5	T45.1X6
Chloropyramine	T45.ØX1	T45.ØX2	T45.ØX3	T45.ØX4	T45.ØX5	T45.ØX6
Chloropyrifos	T6Ø.ØX1	T6Ø.ØX2	T6Ø.ØX3	T6Ø.ØX4	—	—
Chloropyrilene	T45.ØX1	T45.ØX2	T45.ØX3	T45.ØX4	T45.ØX5	T45.ØX6
Chloroquine	T37.2X1	T37.2X2	T37.2X3	T37.2X4	T37.2X5	T37.2X6
Chlorothalonil	T6Ø.3X1	T6Ø.3X2	T6Ø.3X3	T6Ø.3X4	—	—
Chlorothen	T45.ØX1	T45.ØX2	T45.ØX3	T45.ØX4	T45.ØX5	T45.ØX6
Chlorothiazide	T5Ø.2X1	T5Ø.2X2	T5Ø.2X3	T5Ø.2X4	T5Ø.2X5	T5Ø.2X6
Chlorothymol	T49.4X1	T49.4X2	T49.4X3	T49.4X4	T49.4X5	T49.4X6
Chlorotrianisene	T38.5X1	T38.5X2	T38.5X3	T38.5X4	T38.5X5	T38.5X6
Chlorovinyldichloroarsine, not in war	T57.ØX1	T57.ØX2	T57.ØX3	T57.ØX4	—	—
Chloroxine	T49.4X1	T49.4X2	T49.4X3	T49.4X4	T49.4X5	T49.4X6
Chloroxylenol	T49.ØX1	T49.ØX2	T49.ØX3	T49.ØX4	T49.ØX5	T49.ØX6
Chlorphenamine	T45.ØX1	T45.ØX2	T45.ØX3	T45.ØX4	T45.ØX5	T45.ØX6
Chlorphenesin	T42.8X1	T42.8X2	T42.8X3	T42.8X4	T42.8X5	T42.8X6
topical (antifungal)	T49.ØX1	T49.ØX2	T49.ØX3	T49.ØX4	T49.ØX5	T49.ØX6
Chlorpheniramine	T45.ØX1	T45.ØX2	T45.ØX3	T45.ØX4	T45.ØX5	T45.ØX6
Chlorphenoxamine	T45.ØX1	T45.ØX2	T45.ØX3	T45.ØX4	T45.ØX5	T45.ØX6
Chlorphentermine	T5Ø.5X1	T5Ø.5X2	T5Ø.5X3	T5Ø.5X4	T5Ø.5X5	T5Ø.5X6
Chlorprocaine — *see* Chloroprocaine						
Chlorproguanil	T37.2X1	T37.2X2	T37.2X3	T37.2X4	T37.2X5	T37.2X6
Chlorpromazine	T43.3X1	T43.3X2	T43.3X3	T43.3X4	T43.3X5	T43.3X6
Chlorpropamide	T38.3X1	T38.3X2	T38.3X3	T38.3X4	T38.3X5	T38.3X6
Chlorprothixene	T43.4X1	T43.4X2	T43.4X3	T43.4X4	T43.4X5	T43.4X6
Chlorquinaldol	T49.ØX1	T49.ØX2	T49.ØX3	T49.ØX4	T49.ØX5	T49.ØX6
Chlorquinol	T49.ØX1	T49.ØX2	T49.ØX3	T49.ØX4	T49.ØX5	T49.ØX6
Chlortalidone	T5Ø.2X1	T5Ø.2X2	T5Ø.2X3	T5Ø.2X4	T5Ø.2X5	T5Ø.2X6
Chlortetracycline	T36.4X1	T36.4X2	T36.4X3	T36.4X4	T36.4X5	T36.4X6
Chlorthalidone	T5Ø.2X1	T5Ø.2X2	T5Ø.2X3	T5Ø.2X4	T5Ø.2X5	T5Ø.2X6
Chlorthion	T6Ø.ØX1	T6Ø.ØX2	T6Ø.ØX3	T6Ø.ØX4	—	—
Chlorthiophos	T6Ø.ØX1	T6Ø.ØX2	T6Ø.ØX3	T6Ø.ØX4	—	—
Chlortrianisene	T38.5X1	T38.5X2	T38.5X3	T38.5X4	T38.5X5	T38.5X6
Chlor-Trimeton	T45.ØX1	T45.ØX2	T45.ØX3	T45.ØX4	T45.ØX5	T45.ØX6
Chlorzoxazone	T42.8X1	T42.8X2	T42.8X3	T42.8X4	T42.8X5	T42.8X6
Choke damp	T59.7X1	T59.7X2	T59.7X3	T59.7X4	—	—
Cholagogues	T47.5X1	T47.5X2	T47.5X3	T47.5X4	T47.5X5	T47.5X6
Cholebrine	T5Ø.8X1	T5Ø.8X2	T5Ø.8X3	T5Ø.8X4	T5Ø.8X5	T5Ø.8X6
Cholecalciferol	T45.2X1	T45.2X2	T45.2X3	T45.2X4	T45.2X5	T45.2X6
Cholecystokinin	T5Ø.8X1	T5Ø.8X2	T5Ø.8X3	T5Ø.8X4	T5Ø.8X5	T5Ø.8X6
Cholera vaccine	T5Ø.A91	T5Ø.A92	T5Ø.A93	T5Ø.A94	T5Ø.A95	T5Ø.A96
Choleretic	T47.5X1	T47.5X2	T47.5X3	T47.5X4	T47.5X5	T47.5X6
Cholesterol-lowering agents	T46.6X1	T46.6X2	T46.6X3	T46.6X4	T46.6X5	T46.6X6
Cholestyramine (resin)	T46.6X1	T46.6X2	T46.6X3	T46.6X4	T46.6X5	T46.6X6
Cholic acid	T47.5X1	T47.5X2	T47.5X3	T47.5X4	T47.5X5	T47.5X6
Choline	T48.6X1	T48.6X2	T48.6X3	T48.6X4	T48.6X5	T48.6X6
chloride	T5Ø.991	T5Ø.992	T5Ø.993	T5Ø.994	T5Ø.995	T5Ø.996
dihydrogen citrate	T5Ø.991	T5Ø.992	T5Ø.993	T5Ø.994	T5Ø.995	T5Ø.996
salicylate	T39.Ø91	T39.Ø92	T39.Ø93	T39.Ø94	T39.Ø95	T39.Ø96
theophyllinate	T48.6X1	T48.6X2	T48.6X3	T48.6X4	T48.6X5	T48.6X6
Cholinergic (drug) **NEC**	T44.1X1	T44.1X2	T44.1X3	T44.1X4	T44.1X5	T44.1X6
muscle tone enhancer	T44.1X1	T44.1X2	T44.1X3	T44.1X4	T44.1X5	T44.1X6
organophosphorus	T44.ØX1	T44.ØX2	T44.ØX3	T44.ØX4	T44.ØX5	T44.ØX6
insecticide	T6Ø.ØX1	T6Ø.ØX2	T6Ø.ØX3	T6Ø.ØX4	—	—
nerve gas	T59.891	T59.892	T59.893	T59.894	—	—
trimethyl ammonium propanediol	T44.1X1	T44.1X2	T44.1X3	T44.1X4	T44.1X5	T44.1X6
Cholinesterase reactivator	T5Ø.6X1	T5Ø.6X2	T5Ø.6X3	T5Ø.6X4	T5Ø.6X5	T5Ø.6X6
Cholografin	T5Ø.8X1	T5Ø.8X2	T5Ø.8X3	T5Ø.8X4	T5Ø.8X5	T5Ø.8X6
Chorionic gonadotropin	T38.891	T38.892	T38.893	T38.894	T38.895	T38.896
Chromate	T56.2X1	T56.2X2	T56.2X3	T56.2X4	—	—
dust or mist	T56.2X1	T56.2X2	T56.2X3	T56.2X4	—	—
lead — *see also* lead	T56.ØX1	T56.ØX2	T56.ØX3	T56.ØX4	—	—
paint	T56.ØX1	T56.ØX2	T56.ØX3	T56.ØX4	—	—
Chromic						
acid	T56.2X1	T56.2X2	T56.2X3	T56.2X4	—	—
dust or mist	T56.2X1	T56.2X2	T56.2X3	T56.2X4	—	—

Substance	Poisoning, Accidental (unintentional)	Poisoning, Intentional Self-harm	Poisoning, Assault	Poisoning, Undetermined	Adverse Effect	Under-dosing
Chromic — *continued*						
phosphate 32P	T45.1X1	T45.1X2	T45.1X3	T45.1X4	T45.1X5	T45.1X6
Chromium	T56.2X1	T56.2X2	T56.2X3	T56.2X4	—	—
compounds — *see* Chromate						
sesquioxide	T5Ø.8X1	T5Ø.8X2	T5Ø.8X3	T5Ø.8X4	T5Ø.8X5	T5Ø.8X6
Chromomycin A3	T45.1X1	T45.1X2	T45.1X3	T45.1X4	T45.1X5	T45.1X6
Chromonar	T46.3X1	T46.3X2	T46.3X3	T46.3X4	T46.3X5	T46.3X6
Chromyl chloride	T56.2X1	T56.2X2	T56.2X3	T56.2X4	—	—
Chrysarobin	T49.4X1	T49.4X2	T49.4X3	T49.4X4	T49.4X5	T49.4X6
Chrysazin	T47.2X1	T47.2X2	T47.2X3	T47.2X4	T47.2X5	T47.2X6
Chymar	T45.3X1	T45.3X2	T45.3X3	T45.3X4	T45.3X5	T45.3X6
ophthalmic preparation	T49.5X1	T49.5X2	T49.5X3	T49.5X4	T49.5X5	T49.5X6
Chymopapain	T45.3X1	T45.3X2	T45.3X3	T45.3X4	T45.3X5	T45.3X6
Chymotrypsin	T45.3X1	T45.3X2	T45.3X3	T45.3X4	T45.3X5	T45.3X6
ophthalmic preparation	T49.5X1	T49.5X2	T49.5X3	T49.5X4	T49.5X5	T49.5X6
Cianidanol	T5Ø.991	T5Ø.992	T5Ø.993	T5Ø.994	T5Ø.995	T5Ø.996
Cianopramine	T43.Ø11	T43.Ø12	T43.Ø13	T43.Ø14	T43.Ø15	T43.Ø16
Cibenzoline	T46.2X1	T46.2X2	T46.2X3	T46.2X4	T46.2X5	T46.2X6
Ciclacillin	T36.ØX1	T36.ØX2	T36.ØX3	T36.ØX4	T36.ØX5	T36.ØX6
Ciclobarbital — *see* Hexobarbital						
Ciclonicate	T46.7X1	T46.7X2	T46.7X3	T46.7X4	T46.7X5	T46.7X6
Ciclopirox (olamine)	T49.ØX1	T49.ØX2	T49.ØX3	T49.ØX4	T49.ØX5	T49.ØX6
Ciclosporin	T45.1X1	T45.1X2	T45.1X3	T45.1X4	T45.1X5	T45.1X6
Cicuta maculata or virosa	T62.2X1	T62.2X2	T62.2X3	T62.2X4	—	—
Cicutoxin	T62.2X1	T62.2X2	T62.2X3	T62.2X4	—	—
Cigarette lighter fluid	T52.ØX1	T52.ØX2	T52.ØX3	T52.ØX4	—	—
Cigarettes (tobacco)	T65.221	T65.222	T65.223	T65.224	—	—
Ciguatoxin	T61.Ø1	T61.Ø2	T61.Ø3	T61.Ø4	—	—
Cilazapril	T46.4X1	T46.4X2	T46.4X3	T46.4X4	T46.4X5	T46.4X6
Cimetidine	T47.ØX1	T47.ØX2	T47.ØX3	T47.ØX4	T47.ØX5	T47.ØX6
Cimetropium bromide	T44.3X1	T44.3X2	T44.3X3	T44.3X4	T44.3X5	T44.3X6
Cinchocaine	T41.3X1	T41.3X2	T41.3X3	T41.3X4	T41.3X5	T41.3X6
topical (surface)	T41.3X1	T41.3X2	T41.3X3	T41.3X4	T41.3X5	T41.3X6
Cinchona	T37.2X1	T37.2X2	T37.2X3	T37.2X4	T37.2X5	T37.2X6
Cinchonine alkaloids	T37.2X1	T37.2X2	T37.2X3	T37.2X4	T37.2X5	T37.2X6
Cinchophen	T5Ø.4X1	T5Ø.4X2	T5Ø.4X3	T5Ø.4X4	T5Ø.4X5	T5Ø.4X6
Cinepazide	T46.7X1	T46.7X2	T46.7X3	T46.7X4	T46.7X5	T46.7X6
Cinnamedrine	T48.5X1	T48.5X2	T48.5X3	T48.5X4	T48.5X5	T48.5X6
Cinnarizine	T45.ØX1	T45.ØX2	T45.ØX3	T45.ØX4	T45.ØX5	T45.ØX6
Cinoxacin	T37.8X1	T37.8X2	T37.8X3	T37.8X4	T37.8X5	T37.8X6
Ciprofibrate	T46.6X1	T46.6X2	T46.6X3	T46.6X4	T46.6X5	T46.6X6
Ciprofloxacin	T36.8X1	T36.8X2	T36.8X3	T36.8X4	T36.8X5	T36.8X6
Cisapride	T47.8X1	T47.8X2	T47.8X3	T47.8X4	T47.8X5	T47.8X6
Cisplatin	T45.1X1	T45.1X2	T45.1X3	T45.1X4	T45.1X5	T45.1X6
Citalopram	T43.221	T43.222	T43.223	T43.224	T43.225	T43.226
Citanest	T41.3X1	T41.3X2	T41.3X3	T41.3X4	T41.3X5	T41.3X6
infiltration (subcutaneous)	T41.3X1	T41.3X2	T41.3X3	T41.3X4	T41.3X5	T41.3X6
nerve block (peripheral) (plexus)	T41.3X1	T41.3X2	T41.3X3	T41.3X4	T41.3X5	T41.3X6
Citric acid	T47.5X1	T47.5X2	T47.5X3	T47.5X4	T47.5X5	T47.5X6
Citrovorum (factor)	T45.8X1	T45.8X2	T45.8X3	T45.8X4	T45.8X5	T45.8X6
Claviceps purpurea	T62.2X1	T62.2X2	T62.2X3	T62.2X4	—	—
Clavulanic acid	T36.1X1	T36.1X2	T36.1X3	T36.1X4	T36.1X5	T36.1X6
Cleaner, cleansing agent, type not specified	T65.891	T65.892	T65.893	T65.894	—	—
of paint or varnish	T52.91	T52.92	T52.93	T52.94	—	—
specified type NEC	T65.891	T65.892	T65.893	T65.894	—	—
Clebopride	T47.8X1	T47.8X2	T47.8X3	T47.8X4	T47.8X5	T47.8X6
Clefamide	T37.3X1	T37.3X2	T37.3X3	T37.3X4	T37.3X5	T37.3X6
Clemastine	T45.ØX1	T45.ØX2	T45.ØX3	T45.ØX4	T45.ØX5	T45.ØX6
Clematis vitalba	T62.2X1	T62.2X2	T62.2X3	T62.2X4	—	—
Clemizole	T45.ØX1	T45.ØX2	T45.ØX3	T45.ØX4	T45.ØX5	T45.ØX6
penicillin	T36.ØX1	T36.ØX2	T36.ØX3	T36.ØX4	T36.ØX5	T36.ØX6
Clenbuterol	T48.6X1	T48.6X2	T48.6X3	T48.6X4	T48.6X5	T48.6X6
Clidinium bromide	T44.3X1	T44.3X2	T44.3X3	T44.3X4	T44.3X5	T44.3X6
Clindamycin	T36.8X1	T36.8X2	T36.8X3	T36.8X4	T36.8X5	T36.8X6
Clinofibrate	T46.6X1	T46.6X2	T46.6X3	T46.6X4	T46.6X5	T46.6X6
Clioquinol	T37.8X1	T37.8X2	T37.8X3	T37.8X4	T37.8X5	T37.8X6
Cliradon	T4Ø.2X1	T4Ø.2X2	T4Ø.2X3	T4Ø.2X4	—	—
Clobazam	T42.4X1	T42.4X2	T42.4X3	T42.4X4	T42.4X5	T42.4X6
Clobenzorex	T5Ø.5X1	T5Ø.5X2	T5Ø.5X3	T5Ø.5X4	T5Ø.5X5	T5Ø.5X6
Clobetasol	T49.ØX1	T49.ØX2	T49.ØX3	T49.ØX4	T49.ØX5	T49.ØX6
Clobetasone	T49.ØX1	T49.ØX2	T49.ØX3	T49.ØX4	T49.ØX5	T49.ØX6
Clobutinol	T48.3X1	T48.3X2	T48.3X3	T48.3X4	T48.3X5	T48.3X6
Clocortolone	T38.ØX1	T38.ØX2	T38.ØX3	T38.ØX4	T38.ØX5	T38.ØX6
Clodantoin	T49.ØX1	T49.ØX2	T49.ØX3	T49.ØX4	T49.ØX5	T49.ØX6
Clodronic acid	T5Ø.991	T5Ø.992	T5Ø.993	T5Ø.994	T5Ø.995	T5Ø.996
Clofazimine	T37.1X1	T37.1X2	T37.1X3	T37.1X4	T37.1X5	T37.1X6
Clofedanol	T48.3X1	T48.3X2	T48.3X3	T48.3X4	T48.3X5	T48.3X6
Clofenamide	T5Ø.2X1	T5Ø.2X2	T5Ø.2X3	T5Ø.2X4	T5Ø.2X5	T5Ø.2X6
Clofenotane	T49.ØX1	T49.ØX2	T49.ØX3	T49.ØX4	T49.ØX5	T49.ØX6
Clofezone	T39.2X1	T39.2X2	T39.2X3	T39.2X4	T39.2X5	T39.2X6
Clofibrate	T46.6X1	T46.6X2	T46.6X3	T46.6X4	T46.6X5	T46.6X6

Substance	Poisoning, Accidental (unintentional)	Poisoning, Intentional Self-harm	Poisoning, Assault	Poisoning, Undetermined	Adverse Effect	Under-dosing
Clofibride	T46.6X1	T46.6X2	T46.6X3	T46.6X4	T46.6X5	T46.6X6
Cloforex	T5Ø.5X1	T5Ø.5X2	T5Ø.5X3	T5Ø.5X4	T5Ø.5X5	T5Ø.5X6
Clomethiazole	T42.6X1	T42.6X2	T42.6X3	T42.6X4	T42.6X5	T42.6X6
Clometocillin	T36.ØX1	T36.ØX2	T36.ØX3	T36.ØX4	T36.ØX5	T36.ØX6
Clomifene	T38.5X1	T38.5X2	T38.5X3	T38.5X4	T38.5X5	T38.5X6
Clomiphene	T38.5X1	T38.5X2	T38.5X3	T38.5X4	T38.5X5	T38.5X6
Clomipramine	T43.Ø11	T43.Ø12	T43.Ø13	T43.Ø14	T43.Ø15	T43.Ø16
Clomocycline	T36.4X1	T36.4X2	T36.4X3	T36.4X4	T36.4X5	T36.4X6
Clonazepam	T42.4X1	T42.4X2	T42.4X3	T42.4X4	T42.4X5	T42.4X6
Clonidine	T46.5X1	T46.5X2	T46.5X3	T46.5X4	T46.5X5	T46.5X6
Clonixin	T39.8X1	T39.8X2	T39.8X3	T39.8X4	T39.8X5	T39.8X6
Clopamide	T5Ø.2X1	T5Ø.2X2	T5Ø.2X3	T5Ø.2X4	T5Ø.2X5	T5Ø.2X6
Clopenthixol	T43.4X1	T43.4X2	T43.4X3	T43.4X4	T43.4X5	T43.4X6
Cloperastine	T48.3X1	T48.3X2	T48.3X3	T48.3X4	T48.3X5	T48.3X6
Clophedianol	T48.3X1	T48.3X2	T48.3X3	T48.3X4	T48.3X5	T48.3X6
Cloponone	T36.2X1	T36.2X2	T36.2X3	T36.2X4	T36.2X5	T36.2X6
Cloprednol	T38.ØX1	T38.ØX2	T38.ØX3	T38.ØX4	T38.ØX5	T38.ØX6
Cloral betaine	T42.6X1	T42.6X2	T42.6X3	T42.6X4	T42.6X5	T42.6X6
Cloramfenicol	T36.2X1	T36.2X2	T36.2X3	T36.2X4	T36.2X5	T36.2X6
Clorazepate (dipotassium)	T42.4X1	T42.4X2	T42.4X3	T42.4X4	T42.4X5	T42.4X6
Clorexolone	T5Ø.2X1	T5Ø.2X2	T5Ø.2X3	T5Ø.2X4	T5Ø.2X5	T5Ø.2X6
Clorfenamine	T45.ØX1	T45.ØX2	T45.ØX3	T45.ØX4	T45.ØX5	T45.ØX6
Clorgiline	T43.1X1	T43.1X2	T43.1X3	T43.1X4	T43.1X5	T43.1X6
Clorotepine	T44.3X1	T44.3X2	T44.3X3	T44.3X4	T44.3X5	T44.3X6
Clorox (bleach)	T54.91	T54.92	T54.93	T54.94	—	—
Clorprenaline	T48.6X1	T48.6X2	T48.6X3	T48.6X4	T48.6X5	T48.6X6
Clortermine	T5Ø.5X1	T5Ø.5X2	T5Ø.5X3	T5Ø.5X4	T5Ø.5X5	T5Ø.5X6
Clotiapine	T43.591	T43.592	T43.593	T43.594	T43.595	T43.596
Clotiazepam	T42.4X1	T42.4X2	T42.4X3	T42.4X4	T42.4X5	T42.4X6
Clotibric acid	T46.6X1	T46.6X2	T46.6X3	T46.6X4	T46.6X5	T46.6X6
Clotrimazole	T49.ØX1	T49.ØX2	T49.ØX3	T49.ØX4	T49.ØX5	T49.ØX6
Cloxacillin	T36.ØX1	T36.ØX2	T36.ØX3	T36.ØX4	T36.ØX5	T36.ØX6
Cloxazolam	T42.4X1	T42.4X2	T42.4X3	T42.4X4	T42.4X5	T42.4X6
Cloxiquine	T49.ØX1	T49.ØX2	T49.ØX3	T49.ØX4	T49.ØX5	T49.ØX6
Clozapine	T42.4X1	T42.4X2	T42.4X3	T42.4X4	T42.4X5	T42.4X6
Coagulant NEC	T45.7X1	T45.7X2	T45.7X3	T45.7X4	T45.7X5	T45.7X6
Coal (carbon monoxide from) — *see also* Carbon, monoxide, coal	T58.2X1	T58.2X2	T58.2X3	T58.2X4	—	—
oil — *see* Kerosene						
tar	T49.1X1	T49.1X2	T49.1X3	T49.1X4	T49.1X5	T49.1X6
fumes	T59.891	T59.892	T59.893	T59.894	—	—
medicinal (ointment)	T49.4X1	T49.4X2	T49.4X3	T49.4X4	T49.4X5	T49.4X6
analgesics NEC	T39.2X1	T39.2X2	T39.2X3	T39.2X4	T39.2X5	T39.2X6
naphtha (solvent)	T52.ØX1	T52.ØX2	T52.ØX3	T52.ØX4	—	—
Cobalamine	T45.2X1	T45.2X2	T45.2X3	T45.2X4	T45.2X5	T45.2X6
Cobalt (nonmedicinal) (fumes) (industrial)	T56.891	T56.892	T56.893	T56.894	—	—
medicinal (trace) (chloride)	T45.8X1	T45.8X2	T45.8X3	T45.8X4	T45.8X5	T45.8X6
Cobra (venom)	T63.Ø41	T63.Ø42	T63.Ø43	T63.Ø44	—	—
Coca (leaf)	T4Ø.5X1	T4Ø.5X2	T4Ø.5X3	T4Ø.5X4	T4Ø.5X5	T4Ø.5X6
Cocaine	T4Ø.5X1	T4Ø.5X2	T4Ø.5X3	T4Ø.5X4	T4Ø.5X5	T4Ø.5X6
topical anesthetic	T41.3X1	T41.3X2	T41.3X3	T41.3X4	T41.3X5	T41.3X6
Cocarboxylase	T45.3X1	T45.3X2	T45.3X3	T45.3X4	T45.3X5	T45.3X6
Coccidioidin	T5Ø.8X1	T5Ø.8X2	T5Ø.8X3	T5Ø.8X4	T5Ø.8X5	T5Ø.8X6
Cocculus indicus	T62.1X1	T62.1X2	T62.1X3	T62.1X4	—	—
Cochineal	T65.6X1	T65.6X2	T65.6X3	T65.6X4	—	—
medicinal products	T5Ø.991	T5Ø.992	T5Ø.993	T5Ø.994	T5Ø.995	T5Ø.996
Codeine	T4Ø.2X1	T4Ø.2X2	T4Ø.2X3	T4Ø.2X4	T4Ø.2X5	T4Ø.2X6
Cod-liver oil	T45.2X1	T45.2X2	T45.2X3	T45.2X4	T45.2X5	T45.2X6
Coenzyme A	T5Ø.991	T5Ø.992	T5Ø.993	T5Ø.994	T5Ø.995	T5Ø.996
Coffee	T62.8X1	T62.8X2	T62.8X3	T62.8X4	—	—
Cogalactoisomerase	T5Ø.991	T5Ø.992	T5Ø.993	T5Ø.994	T5Ø.995	T5Ø.996
Cogentin	T44.3X1	T44.3X2	T44.3X3	T44.3X4	T44.3X5	T44.3X6
Coke fumes or gas (carbon monoxide)	T58.2X1	T58.2X2	T58.2X3	T58.2X4	—	—
industrial use	T58.8X1	T58.8X2	T58.8X3	T58.8X4	—	—
Colace	T47.4X1	T47.4X2	T47.4X3	T47.4X4	T47.4X5	T47.4X6
Colaspase	T45.1X1	T45.1X2	T45.1X3	T45.1X4	T45.1X5	T45.1X6
Colchicine	T5Ø.4X1	T5Ø.4X2	T5Ø.4X3	T5Ø.4X4	T5Ø.4X5	T5Ø.4X6
Colchicum	T62.2X1	T62.2X2	T62.2X3	T62.2X4	—	—
Cold cream	T49.3X1	T49.3X2	T49.3X3	T49.3X4	T49.3X5	T49.3X6
Colecalciferol	T45.2X1	T45.2X2	T45.2X3	T45.2X4	T45.2X5	T45.2X6
Colestipol	T46.6X1	T46.6X2	T46.6X3	T46.6X4	T46.6X5	T46.6X6
Colestyramine	T46.6X1	T46.6X2	T46.6X3	T46.6X4	T46.6X5	T46.6X6
Colimycin	T36.8X1	T36.8X2	T36.8X3	T36.8X4	T36.8X5	T36.8X6
Colistimethate	T36.8X1	T36.8X2	T36.8X3	T36.8X4	T36.8X5	T36.8X6
Colistin	T36.8X1	T36.8X2	T36.8X3	T36.8X4	T36.8X5	T36.8X6
sulfate (eye preparation)	T49.5X1	T49.5X2	T49.5X3	T49.5X4	T49.5X5	T49.5X6
Collagen	T5Ø.991	T5Ø.992	T5Ø.993	T5Ø.994	T5Ø.995	T5Ø.996
Collagenase	T49.4X1	T49.4X2	T49.4X3	T49.4X4	T49.4X5	T49.4X6
Collodion	T49.3X1	T49.3X2	T49.3X3	T49.3X4	T49.3X5	T49.3X6
Colocynth	T47.2X1	T47.2X2	T47.2X3	T47.2X4	T47.2X5	T47.2X6
Colophony adhesive	T49.3X1	T49.3X2	T49.3X3	T49.3X4	T49.3X5	T49.3X6
Colorant — *see also* Dye	T5Ø.991	T5Ø.992	T5Ø.993	T5Ø.994	T5Ø.995	T5Ø.996
Coloring matter — *see* Dye(s)						
Combustion gas (after combustion) — *see* Carbon, monoxide						
prior to combustion	T59.891	T59.892	T59.893	T59.894	—	—
Compazine	T43.3X1	T43.3X2	T43.3X3	T43.3X4	T43.3X5	T43.3X6
Compound						
42 (warfarin)	T6Ø.4X1	T6Ø.4X2	T6Ø.4X3	T6Ø.4X4	—	—
269 (endrin)	T6Ø.1X1	T6Ø.1X2	T6Ø.1X3	T6Ø.1X4	—	—
497 (dieldrin)	T6Ø.1X1	T6Ø.1X2	T6Ø.1X3	T6Ø.1X4	—	—
1080 (sodium fluoroacetate)	T6Ø.4X1	T6Ø.4X2	T6Ø.4X3	T6Ø.4X4	—	—
3422 (parathion)	T6Ø.ØX1	T6Ø.ØX2	T6Ø.ØX3	T6Ø.ØX4	—	—
3911 (phorate)	T6Ø.ØX1	T6Ø.ØX2	T6Ø.ØX3	T6Ø.ØX4	—	—
3956 (toxaphene)	T6Ø.1X1	T6Ø.1X2	T6Ø.1X3	T6Ø.1X4	—	—
4049 (malathion)	T6Ø.ØX1	T6Ø.ØX2	T6Ø.ØX3	T6Ø.ØX4	—	—
4069 (malathion)	T6Ø.ØX1	T6Ø.ØX2	T6Ø.ØX3	T6Ø.ØX4	—	—
4124 (dicapthon)	T6Ø.ØX1	T6Ø.ØX2	T6Ø.ØX3	T6Ø.ØX4	—	—
E (cortisone)	T38.ØX1	T38.ØX2	T38.ØX3	T38.ØX4	T38.ØX5	T38.ØX6
F (hydrocortisone)	T38.ØX1	T38.ØX2	T38.ØX3	T38.ØX4	T38.ØX5	T38.ØX6
Congener, anabolic	T38.7X1	T38.7X2	T38.7X3	T38.7X4	T38.7X5	T38.7X6
Congo red	T5Ø.8X1	T5Ø.8X2	T5Ø.8X3	T5Ø.8X4	T5Ø.8X5	T5Ø.8X6
Coniine, conine	T62.2X1	T62.2X2	T62.2X3	T62.2X4	—	—
Conium (maculatum)	T62.2X1	T62.2X2	T62.2X3	T62.2X4	—	—
Conjugated estrogenic substances	T38.5X1	T38.5X2	T38.5X3	T38.5X4	T38.5X5	T38.5X6
Contac	T48.5X1	T48.5X2	T48.5X3	T48.5X4	T48.5X5	T48.5X6
Contact lens solution	T49.5X1	T49.5X2	T49.5X3	T49.5X4	T49.5X5	T49.5X6
Contraceptive (oral)	T38.4X1	T38.4X2	T38.4X3	T38.4X4	T38.4X5	T38.4X6
vaginal	T49.8X1	T49.8X2	T49.8X3	T49.8X4	T49.8X5	T49.8X6
Contrast medium, radiography	T5Ø.8X1	T5Ø.8X2	T5Ø.8X3	T5Ø.8X4	T5Ø.8X5	T5Ø.8X6
Convallaria glycosides	T46.ØX1	T46.ØX2	T46.ØX3	T46.ØX4	T46.ØX5	T46.ØX6
Convallaria majalis	T62.2X1	T62.2X2	T62.2X3	T62.2X4	—	—
berry	T62.1X1	T62.1X2	T62.1X3	T62.1X4	—	—
Copperhead snake (bite) (venom)	T63.Ø61	T63.Ø62	T63.Ø63	T63.Ø64	—	—
Copper (dust) (fumes) (nonmedicinal) **NEC**	T56.4X1	T56.4X2	T56.4X3	T56.4X4	—	—
arsenate, arsenite	T57.ØX1	T57.ØX2	T57.ØX3	T57.ØX4	—	—
insecticide	T6Ø.2X1	T6Ø.2X2	T6Ø.2X3	T6Ø.2X4	—	—
emetic	T47.7X1	T47.7X2	T47.7X3	T47.7X4	T47.7X5	T47.7X6
fungicide	T6Ø.3X1	T6Ø.3X2	T6Ø.3X3	T6Ø.3X4	—	—
gluconate	T49.ØX1	T49.ØX2	T49.ØX3	T49.ØX4	T49.ØX5	T49.ØX6
insecticide	T6Ø.2X1	T6Ø.2X2	T6Ø.2X3	T6Ø.2X4	—	—
medicinal (trace)	T45.8X1	T45.8X2	T45.8X3	T45.8X4	T45.8X5	T45.8X6
oleate	T49.ØX1	T49.ØX2	T49.ØX3	T49.ØX4	T49.ØX5	T49.ØX6
sulfate	T56.4X1	T56.4X2	T56.4X3	T56.4X4	—	—
cupric	T56.4X1	T56.4X2	T56.4X3	T56.4X4	—	—
fungicide	T6Ø.3X1	T6Ø.3X2	T6Ø.3X3	T6Ø.3X4	—	—
medicinal						
ear	T49.6X1	T49.6X2	T49.6X3	T49.6X4	T49.6X5	T49.6X6
emetic	T47.7X1	T47.7X2	T47.7X3	T47.7X4	T47.7X5	T47.7X6
eye	T49.5X1	T49.5X2	T49.5X3	T49.5X4	T49.5X5	T49.5X6
cuprous	T56.4X1	T56.4X2	T56.4X3	T56.4X4	—	—
fungicide	T6Ø.3X1	T6Ø.3X2	T6Ø.3X3	T6Ø.3X4	—	—
medicinal						
ear	T49.6X1	T49.6X2	T49.6X3	T49.6X4	T49.6X5	T49.6X6
emetic	T47.7X1	T47.7X2	T47.7X3	T47.7X4	T47.7X5	T47.7X6
eye	T49.5X1	T49.5X2	T49.5X3	T49.5X4	T49.5X5	T49.5X6
Coral (sting)	T63.691	T63.692	T63.693	T63.694	—	—
snake (bite) (venom)	T63.Ø21	T63.Ø22	T63.Ø23	T63.Ø24	—	—
Corbadrine	T49.6X1	T49.6X2	T49.6X3	T49.6X4	T49.6X5	T49.6X6
Cordite	T65.891	T65.892	T65.893	T65.894	—	—
vapor	T59.891	T59.892	T59.893	T59.894	—	—
Cordran	T49.ØX1	T49.ØX2	T49.ØX3	T49.ØX4	T49.ØX5	T49.ØX6
Corn cures	T49.4X1	T49.4X2	T49.4X3	T49.4X4	T49.4X5	T49.4X6
Cornhusker's lotion	T49.3X1	T49.3X2	T49.3X3	T49.3X4	T49.3X5	T49.3X6
Corn starch	T49.3X1	T49.3X2	T49.3X3	T49.3X4	T49.3X5	T49.3X6
Coronary vasodilator NEC	T46.3X1	T46.3X2	T46.3X3	T46.3X4	T46.3X5	T46.3X6
Corrosive NEC	T54.91	T54.92	T54.93	T54.94	—	—
acid NEC	T54.2X1	T54.2X2	T54.2X3	T54.2X4	—	—
aromatics	T54.1X1	T54.1X2	T54.1X3	T54.1X4	—	—
disinfectant	T54.1X1	T54.1X2	T54.1X3	T54.1X4	—	—
fumes NEC	T54.91	T54.92	T54.93	T54.94	—	—
specified NEC	T54.91	T54.92	T54.93	T54.94	—	—
sublimate	T56.1X1	T56.1X2	T56.1X3	T56.1X4	—	—
Cortate	T38.ØX1	T38.ØX2	T38.ØX3	T38.ØX4	T38.ØX5	T38.ØX6
Cort-Dome	T38.ØX1	T38.ØX2	T38.ØX3	T38.ØX4	T38.ØX5	T38.ØX6
ENT agent	T49.6X1	T49.6X2	T49.6X3	T49.6X4	T49.6X5	T49.6X6
ophthalmic preparation	T49.5X1	T49.5X2	T49.5X3	T49.5X4	T49.5X5	T49.5X6

Substance	Poisoning, Accidental (unintentional)	Poisoning, Intentional Self-harm	Poisoning, Assault	Poisoning, Undetermined	Adverse Effect	Under-dosing
Cort-Dome — *continued*						
topical NEC	T49.ØX1	T49.ØX2	T49.ØX3	T49.ØX4	T49.ØX5	T49.ØX6
Cortef	T38.ØX1	T38.ØX2	T38.ØX3	T38.ØX4	T38.ØX5	T38.ØX6
ENT agent	T49.6X1	T49.6X2	T49.6X3	T49.6X4	T49.6X5	T49.6X6
ophthalmic preparation	T49.5X1	T49.5X2	T49.5X3	T49.5X4	T49.5X5	T49.5X6
topical NEC	T49.ØX1	T49.ØX2	T49.ØX3	T49.ØX4	T49.ØX5	T49.ØX6
Corticosteroid	T38.ØX1	T38.ØX2	T38.ØX3	T38.ØX4	T38.ØX5	T38.ØX6
ENT agent	T49.6X1	T49.6X2	T49.6X3	T49.6X4	T49.6X5	T49.6X6
mineral	T5Ø.ØX1	T5Ø.ØX2	T5Ø.ØX3	T5Ø.ØX4	T5Ø.ØX5	T5Ø.ØX6
ophthalmic	T49.5X1	T49.5X2	T49.5X3	T49.5X4	T49.5X5	T49.5X6
topical NEC	T49.ØX1	T49.ØX2	T49.ØX3	T49.ØX4	T49.ØX5	T49.ØX6
Corticotropin	T38.811	T38.812	T38.813	T38.814	T38.815	T38.816
Cortisol	T49.ØX1	T49.ØX2	T49.ØX3	T49.ØX4	T49.ØX5	T49.ØX6
ENT agent	T49.6X1	T49.6X2	T49.6X3	T49.6X4	T49.6X5	T49.6X6
ophthalmic preparation	T49.5X1	T49.5X2	T49.5X3	T49.5X4	T49.5X5	T49.5X6
topical NEC	T49.ØX1	T49.ØX2	T49.ØX3	T49.ØX4	T49.ØX5	T49.ØX6
Cortisone (acetate)	T38.ØX1	T38.ØX2	T38.ØX3	T38.ØX4	T38.ØX5	T38.ØX6
ENT agent	T49.6X1	T49.6X2	T49.6X3	T49.6X4	T49.6X5	T49.6X6
ophthalmic preparation	T49.5X1	T49.5X2	T49.5X3	T49.5X4	T49.5X5	T49.5X6
topical NEC	T49.ØX1	T49.ØX2	T49.ØX3	T49.ØX4	T49.ØX5	T49.ØX6
Cortivazol	T38.ØX1	T38.ØX2	T38.ØX3	T38.ØX4	T38.ØX5	T38.ØX6
Cortogen	T38.ØX1	T38.ØX2	T38.ØX3	T38.ØX4	T38.ØX5	T38.ØX6
ENT agent	T49.6X1	T49.6X2	T49.6X3	T49.6X4	T49.6X5	T49.6X6
ophthalmic preparation	T49.5X1	T49.5X2	T49.5X3	T49.5X4	T49.5X5	T49.5X6
Cortone	T38.ØX1	T38.ØX2	T38.ØX3	T38.ØX4	T38.ØX5	T38.ØX6
ENT agent	T49.6X1	T49.6X2	T49.6X3	T49.6X4	T49.6X5	T49.6X6
ophthalmic preparation	T49.5X1	T49.5X2	T49.5X3	T49.5X4	T49.5X5	T49.5X6
Cortril	T38.ØX1	T38.ØX2	T38.ØX3	T38.ØX4	T38.ØX5	T38.ØX6
ENT agent	T49.6X1	T49.6X2	T49.6X3	T49.6X4	T49.6X5	T49.6X6
ophthalmic preparation	T49.5X1	T49.5X2	T49.5X3	T49.5X4	T49.5X5	T49.5X6
topical NEC	T49.ØX1	T49.ØX2	T49.ØX3	T49.ØX4	T49.ØX5	T49.ØX6
Corynebacterium parvum	T45.1X1	T45.1X2	T45.1X3	T45.1X4	T45.1X5	T45.1X6
Cosmetic preparation	T49.8X1	T49.8X2	T49.8X3	T49.8X4	T49.8X5	T49.8X6
Cosmetics	T49.8X1	T49.8X2	T49.8X3	T49.8X4	T49.8X5	T49.8X6
Cosyntropin	T38.811	T38.812	T38.813	T38.814	T38.815	T38.816
Cotarnine	T45.7X1	T45.7X2	T45.7X3	T45.7X4	T45.7X5	T45.7X6
Co-trimoxazole	T36.8X1	T36.8X2	T36.8X3	T36.8X4	T36.8X5	T36.8X6
Cottonseed oil	T49.3X1	T49.3X2	T49.3X3	T49.3X4	T49.3X5	T49.3X6
Cough mixture (syrup)	T48.4X1	T48.4X2	T48.4X3	T48.4X4	T48.4X5	T48.4X6
containing opiates	T4Ø.2X1	T4Ø.2X2	T4Ø.2X3	T4Ø.2X4	T4Ø.2X5	T4Ø.2X6
expectorants	T48.4X1	T48.4X2	T48.4X3	T48.4X4	T48.4X5	T48.4X6
Coumadin	T45.511	T45.512	T45.513	T45.514	T45.515	T45.516
rodenticide	T6Ø.4X1	T6Ø.4X2	T6Ø.4X3	T6Ø.4X4	—	—
Coumaphos	T6Ø.ØX1	T6Ø.ØX2	T6Ø.ØX3	T6Ø.ØX4	—	—
Coumarin	T45.511	T45.512	T45.513	T45.514	T45.515	T45.516
Coumetarol	T45.511	T45.512	T45.513	T45.514	T45.515	T45.516
Cowbane	T62.2X1	T62.2X2	T62.2X3	T62.2X4	—	—
Cozyme	T45.2X1	T45.2X2	T45.2X3	T45.2X4	T45.2X5	T45.2X6
Crack	T4Ø.5X1	T4Ø.5X2	T4Ø.5X3	T4Ø.5X4	—	—
Crataegus extract	T46.ØX1	T46.ØX2	T46.ØX3	T46.ØX4	T46.ØX5	T46.ØX6
Creolin	T54.1X1	T54.1X2	T54.1X3	T54.1X4	—	—
disinfectant	T54.1X1	T54.1X2	T54.1X3	T54.1X4	—	—
Creosol (compound)	T49.ØX1	T49.ØX2	T49.ØX3	T49.ØX4	T49.ØX5	T49.ØX6
Creosote (coal tar) (beechwood)	T49.ØX1	T49.ØX2	T49.ØX3	T49.ØX4	T49.ØX5	T49.ØX6
medicinal (expectorant)	T48.4X1	T48.4X2	T48.4X3	T48.4X4	T48.4X5	T48.4X6
syrup	T48.4X1	T48.4X2	T48.4X3	T48.4X4	T48.4X5	T48.4X6
Cresol(s)	T49.ØX1	T49.ØX2	T49.ØX3	T49.ØX4	T49.ØX5	T49.ØX6
and soap solution	T49.ØX1	T49.ØX2	T49.ØX3	T49.ØX4	T49.ØX5	T49.ØX6
Cresyl acetate	T49.ØX1	T49.ØX2	T49.ØX3	T49.ØX4	T49.ØX5	T49.ØX6
Cresylic acid	T49.ØX1	T49.ØX2	T49.ØX3	T49.ØX4	T49.ØX5	T49.ØX6
Crimidine	T6Ø.4X1	T6Ø.4X2	T6Ø.4X3	T6Ø.4X4	—	—
Croconazole	T37.8X1	T37.8X2	T37.8X3	T37.8X4	T37.8X5	T37.8X6
Cromoglicic acid	T48.6X1	T48.6X2	T48.6X3	T48.6X4	T48.6X5	T48.6X6
Cromolyn	T48.6X1	T48.6X2	T48.6X3	T48.6X4	T48.6X5	T48.6X6
Cromonar	T46.3X1	T46.3X2	T46.3X3	T46.3X4	T46.3X5	T46.3X6
Cropropamide	T39.8X1	T39.8X2	T39.8X3	T39.8X4	T39.8X5	T39.8X6
with crotethamide	T5Ø.7X1	T5Ø.7X2	T5Ø.7X3	T5Ø.7X4	T5Ø.7X5	T5Ø.7X6
Crotamiton	T49.ØX1	T49.ØX2	T49.ØX3	T49.ØX4	T49.ØX5	T49.ØX6
Crotethamide	T39.8X1	T39.8X2	T39.8X3	T39.8X4	T39.8X5	T39.8X6
with cropropamide	T5Ø.7X1	T5Ø.7X2	T5Ø.7X3	T5Ø.7X4	T5Ø.7X5	T5Ø.7X6
Croton (oil)	T47.2X1	T47.2X2	T47.2X3	T47.2X4	T47.2X5	T47.2X6
chloral	T42.6X1	T42.6X2	T42.6X3	T42.6X4	T42.6X5	T42.6X6
Crude oil	T52.ØX1	T52.ØX2	T52.ØX3	T52.ØX4	—	—
Cryogenine	T39.8X1	T39.8X2	T39.8X3	T39.8X4	T39.8X5	T39.8X6
Cryolite (vapor)	T6Ø.1X1	T6Ø.1X2	T6Ø.1X3	T6Ø.1X4	—	—
insecticide	T6Ø.1X1	T6Ø.1X2	T6Ø.1X3	T6Ø.1X4	—	—
Cryptenamine (tannates)	T46.5X1	T46.5X2	T46.5X3	T46.5X4	T46.5X5	T46.5X6
Crystal violet	T49.ØX1	T49.ØX2	T49.ØX3	T49.ØX4	T49.ØX5	T49.ØX6
Cuckoopint	T62.2X1	T62.2X2	T62.2X3	T62.2X4	—	—
Cumetharol	T45.511	T45.512	T45.513	T45.514	T45.515	T45.516
Cupric						
acetate	T6Ø.3X1	T6Ø.3X2	T6Ø.3X3	T6Ø.3X4	—	—

Substance	Poisoning, Accidental (unintentional)	Poisoning, Intentional Self-harm	Poisoning, Assault	Poisoning, Undetermined	Adverse Effect	Under-dosing
Cupric — *continued*						
acetoarsenite	T57.ØX1	T57.ØX2	T57.ØX3	T57.ØX4	—	—
arsenate	T57.ØX1	T57.ØX2	T57.ØX3	T57.ØX4	—	—
gluconate	T49.ØX1	T49.ØX2	T49.ØX3	T49.ØX4	T49.ØX5	T49.ØX6
oleate	T49.ØX1	T49.ØX2	T49.ØX3	T49.ØX4	T49.ØX5	T49.ØX6
sulfate	T56.4X1	T56.4X2	T56.4X3	T56.4X4	—	—
Cuprous sulfate — *see also* Copper sulfate	T56.4X1	T56.4X2	T56.4X3	T56.4X4	—	—
Curare, curarine	T48.1X1	T48.1X2	T48.1X3	T48.1X4	T48.1X5	T48.1X6
Cyamemazine	T43.3X1	T43.3X2	T43.3X3	T43.3X4	T43.3X5	T43.3X6
Cyamopsis tetragonoloba	T46.6X1	T46.6X2	T46.6X3	T46.6X4	T46.6X5	T46.6X6
Cyanacetyl hydrazide	T37.1X1	T37.1X2	T37.1X3	T37.1X4	T37.1X5	T37.1X6
Cyanic acid (gas)	T59.891	T59.892	T59.893	T59.894	—	—
Cyanide(s) (compounds) (potassium) (sodium) **NEC**	T65.ØX1	T65.ØX2	T65.ØX3	T65.ØX4	—	—
dust or gas (inhalation) NEC	T57.3X1	T57.3X2	T57.3X3	T57.3X4	—	—
fumigant	T65.ØX1	T65.ØX2	T65.ØX3	T65.ØX4	—	—
hydrogen	T57.3X1	T57.3X2	T57.3X3	T57.3X4	—	—
mercuric — *see* Mercury						
pesticide (dust) (fumes)	T65.ØX1	T65.ØX2	T65.ØX3	T65.ØX4	—	—
Cyanoacrylate adhesive	T49.3X1	T49.3X2	T49.3X3	T49.3X4	T49.3X5	T49.3X6
Cyanocobalamin	T45.8X1	T45.8X2	T45.8X3	T45.8X4	T45.8X5	T45.8X6
Cyanogen (chloride) (gas) **NEC**	T59.891	T59.892	T59.893	T59.894	—	—
Cyclacillin	T36.ØX1	T36.ØX2	T36.ØX3	T36.ØX4	T36.ØX5	T36.ØX6
Cyclaine	T41.3X1	T41.3X2	T41.3X3	T41.3X4	T41.3X5	T41.3X6
Cyclamate	T5Ø.991	T5Ø.992	T5Ø.993	T5Ø.994	T5Ø.995	T5Ø.996
Cyclamen europaeum	T62.2X1	T62.2X2	T62.2X3	T62.2X4	—	—
Cyclandelate	T46.7X1	T46.7X2	T46.7X3	T46.7X4	T46.7X5	T46.7X6
Cyclazocine	T5Ø.7X1	T5Ø.7X2	T5Ø.7X3	T5Ø.7X4	T5Ø.7X5	T5Ø.7X6
Cyclizine	T45.ØX1	T45.ØX2	T45.ØX3	T45.ØX4	T45.ØX5	T45.ØX6
Cyclobarbital	T42.3X1	T42.3X2	T42.3X3	T42.3X4	T42.3X5	T42.3X6
Cyclobarbitone	T42.3X1	T42.3X2	T42.3X3	T42.3X4	T42.3X5	T42.3X6
Cyclobenzaprine	T48.1X1	T48.1X2	T48.1X3	T48.1X4	T48.1X5	T48.1X6
Cyclodrine	T44.3X1	T44.3X2	T44.3X3	T44.3X4	T44.3X5	T44.3X6
Cycloguanil embonate	T37.2X1	T37.2X2	T37.2X3	T37.2X4	T37.2X5	T37.2X6
Cyclohexane	T52.8X1	T52.8X2	T52.8X3	T52.8X4	—	—
Cyclohexanol	T51.8X1	T51.8X2	T51.8X3	T51.8X4	—	—
Cyclohexanone	T52.4X1	T52.4X2	T52.4X3	T52.4X4	—	—
Cycloheximide	T6Ø.3X1	T6Ø.3X2	T6Ø.3X3	T6Ø.3X4	—	—
Cyclohexyl acetate	T52.8X1	T52.8X2	T52.8X3	T52.8X4	—	—
Cycloleucin	T45.1X1	T45.1X2	T45.1X3	T45.1X4	T45.1X5	T45.1X6
Cyclomethycaine	T41.3X1	T41.3X2	T41.3X3	T41.3X4	T41.3X5	T41.3X6
Cyclopentamine	T44.4X1	T44.4X2	T44.4X3	T44.4X4	T44.4X5	T44.4X6
Cyclopenthiazide	T5Ø.2X1	T5Ø.2X2	T5Ø.2X3	T5Ø.2X4	T5Ø.2X5	T5Ø.2X6
Cyclopentolate	T44.3X1	T44.3X2	T44.3X3	T44.3X4	T44.3X5	T44.3X6
Cyclophosphamide	T45.1X1	T45.1X2	T45.1X3	T45.1X4	T45.1X5	T45.1X6
Cycloplegic drug	T49.5X1	T49.5X2	T49.5X3	T49.5X4	T49.5X5	T49.5X6
Cyclopropane	T41.291	T41.292	T41.293	T41.294	T41.295	T41.296
Cyclopyrabital	T39.8X1	T39.8X2	T39.8X3	T39.8X4	T39.8X5	T39.8X6
Cycloserine	T37.1X1	T37.1X2	T37.1X3	T37.1X4	T37.1X5	T37.1X6
Cyclosporin	T45.1X1	T45.1X2	T45.1X3	T45.1X4	T45.1X5	T45.1X6
Cyclothiazide	T5Ø.2X1	T5Ø.2X2	T5Ø.2X3	T5Ø.2X4	T5Ø.2X5	T5Ø.2X6
Cycrimine	T44.3X1	T44.3X2	T44.3X3	T44.3X4	T44.3X5	T44.3X6
Cyhalothrin	T6Ø.1X1	T6Ø.1X2	T6Ø.1X3	T6Ø.1X4	—	—
Cymarin	T46.ØX1	T46.ØX2	T46.ØX3	T46.ØX4	T46.ØX5	T46.ØX6
Cypermethrin	T6Ø.1X1	T6Ø.1X2	T6Ø.1X3	T6Ø.1X4	—	—
Cyphenothrin	T6Ø.2X1	T6Ø.2X2	T6Ø.2X3	T6Ø.2X4	—	—
Cyproheptadine	T45.ØX1	T45.ØX2	T45.ØX3	T45.ØX4	T45.ØX5	T45.ØX6
Cyproterone	T38.6X1	T38.6X2	T38.6X3	T38.6X4	T38.6X5	T38.6X6
Cysteamine	T5Ø.6X1	T5Ø.6X2	T5Ø.6X3	T5Ø.6X4	T5Ø.6X5	T5Ø.6X6
Cytarabine	T45.1X1	T45.1X2	T45.1X3	T45.1X4	T45.1X5	T45.1X6
Cytisus						
laburnum	T62.2X1	T62.2X2	T62.2X3	T62.2X4	—	—
scoparius	T62.2X1	T62.2X2	T62.2X3	T62.2X4	—	—
Cytochrome C	T47.5X1	T47.5X2	T47.5X3	T47.5X4	T47.5X5	T47.5X6
Cytomel	T38.1X1	T38.1X2	T38.1X3	T38.1X4	T38.1X5	T38.1X6
Cytosine arabinoside	T45.1X1	T45.1X2	T45.1X3	T45.1X4	T45.1X5	T45.1X6
Cytoxan	T45.1X1	T45.1X2	T45.1X3	T45.1X4	T45.1X5	T45.1X6
Cytozyme	T45.7X1	T45.7X2	T45.7X3	T45.7X4	T45.7X5	T45.7X6
S-Carboxymethylcysteine	T48.4X1	T48.4X2	T48.4X3	T48.4X4	T48.4X5	T48.4X6
Dacarbazine	T45.1X1	T45.1X2	T45.1X3	T45.1X4	T45.1X5	T45.1X6
Dactinomycin	T45.1X1	T45.1X2	T45.1X3	T45.1X4	T45.1X5	T45.1X6
DADPS	T37.1X1	T37.1X2	T37.1X3	T37.1X4	T37.1X5	T37.1X6
Dakin's solution	T49.ØX1	T49.ØX2	T49.ØX3	T49.ØX4	T49.ØX5	T49.ØX6
Dalapon (sodium)	T6Ø.3X1	T6Ø.3X2	T6Ø.3X3	T6Ø.3X4	—	—
Dalmane	T42.4X1	T42.4X2	T42.4X3	T42.4X4	T42.4X5	T42.4X6
Danazol	T38.6X1	T38.6X2	T38.6X3	T38.6X4	T38.6X5	T38.6X6
Danilone	T45.511	T45.512	T45.513	T45.514	T45.515	T45.516
Danthron	T47.2X1	T47.2X2	T47.2X3	T47.2X4	T47.2X5	T47.2X6
Dantrolene	T42.8X1	T42.8X2	T42.8X3	T42.8X4	T42.8X5	T42.8X6
Dantron	T47.2X1	T47.2X2	T47.2X3	T47.2X4	T47.2X5	T47.2X6

Substance	Poisoning, Accidental (unintentional)	Poisoning, Intentional Self-harm	Poisoning, Assault	Poisoning, Undetermined	Adverse Effect	Under-dosing
Daphne (gnidium) (mezereum)	T62.2X1	T62.2X2	T62.2X3	T62.2X4	—	—
berry	T62.1X1	T62.1X2	T62.1X3	T62.1X4	—	—
Dapsone	T37.1X1	T37.1X2	T37.1X3	T37.1X4	T37.1X5	T37.1X6
Daraprim	T37.2X1	T37.2X2	T37.2X3	T37.2X4	T37.2X5	T37.2X6
Darnel	T62.2X1	T62.2X2	T62.2X3	T62.2X4	—	—
Darvon	T39.8X1	T39.8X2	T39.8X3	T39.8X4	T39.8X5	T39.8X6
Daunomycin	T45.1X1	T45.1X2	T45.1X3	T45.1X4	T45.1X5	T45.1X6
Daunorubicin	T45.1X1	T45.1X2	T45.1X3	T45.1X4	T45.1X5	T45.1X6
DBI	T38.3X1	T38.3X2	T38.3X3	T38.3X4	T38.3X5	T38.3X6
D-Con	T6Ø.91	T6Ø.92	T6Ø.93	T6Ø.94	—	—
insecticide	T6Ø.2X1	T6Ø.2X2	T6Ø.2X3	T6Ø.2X4	—	—
rodenticide	T6Ø.4X1	T6Ø.4X2	T6Ø.4X3	T6Ø.4X4	—	—
DDAVP	T38.891	T38.892	T38.893	T38.894	T38.895	T38.896
DDE (bis(chlorophenyl)-dichloroethylene)	T6Ø.2X1	T6Ø.2X2	T6Ø.2X3	T6Ø.2X4	—	—
DDS	T37.1X1	T37.1X2	T37.1X3	T37.1X4	T37.1X5	T37.1X6
DDT (dust)	T6Ø.1X1	T6Ø.1X2	T6Ø.1X3	T6Ø.1X4	—	—
Deadly nightshade — *see also* Belladonna	T62.2X1	T62.2X2	T62.2X3	T62.2X4	—	—
berry	T62.1X1	T62.1X2	T62.1X3	T62.1X4	—	—
Deamino-D-arginine vasopressin	T38.891	T38.892	T38.893	T38.894	T38.895	T38.896
Deanol (aceglumate)	T5Ø.991	T5Ø.992	T5Ø.993	T5Ø.994	T5Ø.995	T5Ø.996
Debrisoquine	T46.5X1	T46.5X2	T46.5X3	T46.5X4	T46.5X5	T46.5X6
Decaborane	T57.8X1	T57.8X2	T57.8X3	T57.8X4	—	—
fumes	T59.891	T59.892	T59.893	T59.894	—	—
Decadron	T38.ØX1	T38.ØX2	T38.ØX3	T38.ØX4	T38.ØX5	T38.ØX6
ENT agent	T49.6X1	T49.6X2	T49.6X3	T49.6X4	T49.6X5	T49.6X6
ophthalmic preparation	T49.5X1	T49.5X2	T49.5X3	T49.5X4	T49.5X5	T49.5X6
topical NEC	T49.ØX1	T49.ØX2	T49.ØX3	T49.ØX4	T49.ØX5	T49.ØX6
Decahydronaphthalene	T52.8X1	T52.8X2	T52.8X3	T52.8X4	—	—
Decalin	T52.8X1	T52.8X2	T52.8X3	T52.8X4	—	—
Decamethonium (bromide)	T48.1X1	T48.1X2	T48.1X3	T48.1X4	T48.1X5	T48.1X6
Decholin	T47.5X1	T47.5X2	T47.5X3	T47.5X4	T47.5X5	T47.5X6
Declomycin	T36.4X1	T36.4X2	T36.4X3	T36.4X4	T36.4X5	T36.4X6
Decongestant, nasal (mucosa)	T48.5X1	T48.5X2	T48.5X3	T48.5X4	T48.5X5	T48.5X6
combination	T48.5X1	T48.5X2	T48.5X3	T48.5X4	T48.5X5	T48.5X6
Deet	T6Ø.8X1	T6Ø.8X2	T6Ø.8X3	T6Ø.8X4	—	—
Deferoxamine	T45.8X1	T45.8X2	T45.8X3	T45.8X4	T45.8X5	T45.8X6
Deflazacort	T38.ØX1	T38.ØX2	T38.ØX3	T38.ØX4	T38.ØX5	T38.ØX6
Deglycyrrhizinized extract of licorice	T48.4X1	T48.4X2	T48.4X3	T48.4X4	T48.4X5	T48.4X6
Dehydrocholic acid	T47.5X1	T47.5X2	T47.5X3	T47.5X4	T47.5X5	T47.5X6
Dehydroemetine	T37.3X1	T37.3X2	T37.3X3	T37.3X4	T37.3X5	T37.3X6
Dekalin	T52.8X1	T52.8X2	T52.8X3	T52.8X4	—	—
Delalutin	T38.5X1	T38.5X2	T38.5X3	T38.5X4	T38.5X5	T38.5X6
Delorazepam	T42.4X1	T42.4X2	T42.4X3	T42.4X4	T42.4X5	T42.4X6
Delphinium	T62.2X1	T62.2X2	T62.2X3	T62.2X4	—	—
Deltamethrin	T6Ø.1X1	T6Ø.1X2	T6Ø.1X3	T6Ø.1X4	—	—
Deltasone	T38.ØX1	T38.ØX2	T38.ØX3	T38.ØX4	T38.ØX5	T38.ØX6
Deltra	T38.ØX1	T38.ØX2	T38.ØX3	T38.ØX4	T38.ØX5	T38.ØX6
Delvinal	T42.3X1	T42.3X2	T42.3X3	T42.3X4	T42.3X5	T42.3X6
Demecarium (bromide)	T49.5X1	T49.5X2	T49.5X3	T49.5X4	T49.5X5	T49.5X6
Demeclocycline	T36.4X1	T36.4X2	T36.4X3	T36.4X4	T36.4X5	T36.4X6
Demecolcine	T45.1X1	T45.1X2	T45.1X3	T45.1X4	T45.1X5	T45.1X6
Demegestone	T38.5X1	T38.5X2	T38.5X3	T38.5X4	T38.5X5	T38.5X6
Demelanizing agents	T49.8X1	T49.8X2	T49.8X3	T49.8X4	T49.8X5	T49.8X6
Demephion -O and -S	T6Ø.ØX1	T6Ø.ØX2	T6Ø.ØX3	T6Ø.ØX4	—	—
Demerol	T4Ø.2X1	T4Ø.2X2	T4Ø.2X3	T4Ø.2X4	T4Ø.2X5	T4Ø.2X6
Demethylchlortetracycline	T36.4X1	T36.4X2	T36.4X3	T36.4X4	T36.4X5	T36.4X6
Demethyltetracycline	T36.4X1	T36.4X2	T36.4X3	T36.4X4	T36.4X5	T36.4X6
Demeton -O and -S	T6Ø.ØX1	T6Ø.ØX2	T6Ø.ØX3	T6Ø.ØX4	—	—
Demulcent (external)	T49.3X1	T49.3X2	T49.3X3	T49.3X4	T49.3X5	T49.3X6
specified NEC	T49.3X1	T49.3X2	T49.3X3	T49.3X4	T49.3X5	T49.3X6
Demulen	T38.4X1	T38.4X2	T38.4X3	T38.4X4	T38.4X5	T38.4X6
Denatured alcohol	T51.ØX1	T51.ØX2	T51.ØX3	T51.ØX4	—	—
Dendrid	T49.5X1	T49.5X2	T49.5X3	T49.5X4	T49.5X5	T49.5X6
Dental drug, topical application NEC	T49.7X1	T49.7X2	T49.7X3	T49.7X4	T49.7X5	T49.7X6
Dentifrice	T49.7X1	T49.7X2	T49.7X3	T49.7X4	T49.7X5	T49.7X6
Deodorant spray (feminine hygiene)	T49.8X1	T49.8X2	T49.8X3	T49.8X4	T49.8X5	T49.8X6
Deoxycortone	T5Ø.ØX1	T5Ø.ØX2	T5Ø.ØX3	T5Ø.ØX4	T5Ø.ØX5	T5Ø.ØX6
Deoxyribonuclease (pancreatic)	T45.3X1	T45.3X2	T45.3X3	T45.3X4	T45.3X5	T45.3X6
Depilatory	T49.4X1	T49.4X2	T49.4X3	T49.4X4	T49.4X5	T49.4X6
Deprenalin	T42.8X1	T42.8X2	T42.8X3	T42.8X4	T42.8X5	T42.8X6
Deprenyl	T42.8X1	T42.8X2	T42.8X3	T42.8X4	T42.8X5	T42.8X6
Depressant						
appetite (central)	T5Ø.5X1	T5Ø.5X2	T5Ø.5X3	T5Ø.5X4	T5Ø.5X5	T5Ø.5X6
cardiac	T46.2X1	T46.2X2	T46.2X3	T46.2X4	T46.2X5	T46.2X6
Depressant — *continued*						
central nervous system (anesthetic) — *see also* Central nervous system, depressants	T42.71	T42.72	T42.73	T42.74	T42.75	T42.76
general anesthetic	T41.2Ø1	T41.2Ø2	T41.2Ø3	T41.2Ø4	T41.2Ø5	T41.2Ø6
muscle tone	T42.8X1	T42.8X2	T42.8X3	T42.8X4	T42.8X5	T42.8X6
muscle tone, central	T42.8X1	T42.8X2	T42.8X3	T42.8X4	T42.8X5	T42.8X6
psychotherapeutic	T43.5Ø1	T43.5Ø2	T43.5Ø3	T43.5Ø4	T43.5Ø5	T43.5Ø6
Depressant, appetite	T5Ø.5X1	T5Ø.5X2	T5Ø.5X3	T5Ø.5X4	T5Ø.5X5	T5Ø.5X6
Deptropine	T45.ØX1	T45.ØX2	T45.ØX3	T45.ØX4	T45.ØX5	T45.ØX6
Dequalinium (chloride)	T49.ØX1	T49.ØX2	T49.ØX3	T49.ØX4	T49.ØX5	T49.ØX6
Derris root	T6Ø.2X1	T6Ø.2X2	T6Ø.2X3	T6Ø.2X4	—	—
Deserpidine	T46.5X1	T46.5X2	T46.5X3	T46.5X4	T46.5X5	T46.5X6
Desferrioxamine	T45.8X1	T45.8X2	T45.8X3	T45.8X4	T45.8X5	T45.8X6
Desipramine	T43.Ø11	T43.Ø12	T43.Ø13	T43.Ø14	T43.Ø15	T43.Ø16
Deslanoside	T46.ØX1	T46.ØX2	T46.ØX3	T46.ØX4	T46.ØX5	T46.ØX6
Desloughing agent	T49.4X1	T49.4X2	T49.4X3	T49.4X4	T49.4X5	T49.4X6
Desmethylimipramine	T43.Ø11	T43.Ø12	T43.Ø13	T43.Ø14	T43.Ø15	T43.Ø16
Desmopressin	T38.891	T38.892	T38.893	T38.894	T38.895	T38.896
Desocodeine	T4Ø.2X1	T4Ø.2X2	T4Ø.2X3	T4Ø.2X4	T4Ø.2X5	T4Ø.2X6
Desogestrel	T38.5X1	T38.5X2	T38.5X3	T38.5X4	T38.5X5	T38.5X6
Desomorphine	T4Ø.2X1	T4Ø.2X2	T4Ø.2X3	T4Ø.2X4	—	—
Desonide	T49.ØX1	T49.ØX2	T49.ØX3	T49.ØX4	T49.ØX5	T49.ØX6
Desoximetasone	T49.ØX1	T49.ØX2	T49.ØX3	T49.ØX4	T49.ØX5	T49.ØX6
Desoxycorticosteroid	T5Ø.ØX1	T5Ø.ØX2	T5Ø.ØX3	T5Ø.ØX4	T5Ø.ØX5	T5Ø.ØX6
Desoxycortone	T5Ø.ØX1	T5Ø.ØX2	T5Ø.ØX3	T5Ø.ØX4	T5Ø.ØX5	T5Ø.ØX6
Desoxyephedrine	T43.621	T43.622	T43.623	T43.624	T43.625	T43.626
Detaxtran	T46.6X1	T46.6X2	T46.6X3	T46.6X4	T46.6X5	T46.6X6
Detergent	T49.2X1	T49.2X2	T49.2X3	T49.2X4	T49.2X5	T49.2X6
external medication	T49.2X1	T49.2X2	T49.2X3	T49.2X4	T49.2X5	T49.2X6
local	T49.2X1	T49.2X2	T49.2X3	T49.2X4	T49.2X5	T49.2X6
medicinal	T49.2X1	T49.2X2	T49.2X3	T49.2X4	T49.2X5	T49.2X6
nonmedicinal	T55.1X1	T55.1X2	T55.1X3	T55.1X4	—	—
specified NEC	T55.1X1	T55.1X2	T55.1X3	T55.1X4	—	—
Deterrent, alcohol	T5Ø.6X1	T5Ø.6X2	T5Ø.6X3	T5Ø.6X4	T5Ø.6X5	T5Ø.6X6
Detoxifying agent	T5Ø.6X1	T5Ø.6X2	T5Ø.6X3	T5Ø.6X4	T5Ø.6X5	T5Ø.6X6
Detrothyronine	T38.1X1	T38.1X2	T38.1X3	T38.1X4	T38.1X5	T38.1X6
Dettol (external medication)	T49.ØX1	T49.ØX2	T49.ØX3	T49.ØX4	T49.ØX5	T49.ØX6
Dexamethasone	T38.ØX1	T38.ØX2	T38.ØX3	T38.ØX4	T38.ØX5	T38.ØX6
ENT agent	T49.6X1	T49.6X2	T49.6X3	T49.6X4	T49.6X5	T49.6X6
ophthalmic preparation	T49.5X1	T49.5X2	T49.5X3	T49.5X4	T49.5X5	T49.5X6
topical NEC	T49.ØX1	T49.ØX2	T49.ØX3	T49.ØX4	T49.ØX5	T49.ØX6
Dexamfetamine	T43.621	T43.622	T43.623	T43.624	T43.625	T43.626
Dexamphetamine	T43.621	T43.622	T43.623	T43.624	T43.625	T43.626
Dexbrompheniramine	T45.ØX1	T45.ØX2	T45.ØX3	T45.ØX4	T45.ØX5	T45.ØX6
Dexchlorpheniramine	T45.ØX1	T45.ØX2	T45.ØX3	T45.ØX4	T45.ØX5	T45.ØX6
Dexedrine	T43.621	T43.622	T43.623	T43.624	T43.625	T43.626
Dexetimide	T44.3X1	T44.3X2	T44.3X3	T44.3X4	T44.3X5	T44.3X6
Dexfenfluramine	T5Ø.5X1	T5Ø.5X2	T5Ø.5X3	T5Ø.5X4	T5Ø.5X5	T5Ø.5X6
Dexpanthenol	T45.2X1	T45.2X2	T45.2X3	T45.2X4	T45.2X5	T45.2X6
Dextran (40) (70) (150)	T45.8X1	T45.8X2	T45.8X3	T45.8X4	T45.8X5	T45.8X6
Dextriferron	T45.4X1	T45.4X2	T45.4X3	T45.4X4	T45.4X5	T45.4X6
Dextroamphetamine	T43.621	T43.622	T43.623	T43.624	T43.625	T43.626
Dextro calcium pantothenate	T45.2X1	T45.2X2	T45.2X3	T45.2X4	T45.2X5	T45.2X6
Dextromethorphan	T48.3X1	T48.3X2	T48.3X3	T48.3X4	T48.3X5	T48.3X6
Dextromoramide	T4Ø.4X1	T4Ø.4X2	T4Ø.4X3	T4Ø.4X4	—	—
topical	T49.8X1	T49.8X2	T49.8X3	T49.8X4	T49.8X5	T49.8X6
Dextro pantothenyl alcohol	T45.2X1	T45.2X2	T45.2X3	T45.2X4	T45.2X5	T45.2X6
Dextropropoxyphene	T4Ø.4X1	T4Ø.4X2	T4Ø.4X3	T4Ø.4X4	T4Ø.4X5	T4Ø.4X6
Dextrorphan	T4Ø.2X1	T4Ø.2X2	T4Ø.2X3	T4Ø.2X4	T4Ø.2X5	T4Ø.2X6
Dextrose	T5Ø.3X1	T5Ø.3X2	T5Ø.3X3	T5Ø.3X4	T5Ø.3X5	T5Ø.3X6
concentrated solution, intravenous	T46.8X1	T46.8X2	T46.8X3	T46.8X4	T46.8X5	T46.8X6
Dextrothyroxin	T38.1X1	T38.1X2	T38.1X3	T38.1X4	T38.1X5	T38.1X6
Dextrothyroxine sodium	T38.1X1	T38.1X2	T38.1X3	T38.1X4	T38.1X5	T38.1X6
DFP	T44.ØX1	T44.ØX2	T44.ØX3	T44.ØX4	T44.ØX5	T44.ØX6
DHE	T37.3X1	T37.3X2	T37.3X3	T37.3X4	T37.3X5	T37.3X6
45	T46.5X1	T46.5X2	T46.5X3	T46.5X4	T46.5X5	T46.5X6
Diabinese	T38.3X1	T38.3X2	T38.3X3	T38.3X4	T38.3X5	T38.3X6
Diacetone alcohol	T52.4X1	T52.4X2	T52.4X3	T52.4X4	—	—
Diacetyl monoxime	T5Ø.991	T5Ø.992	T5Ø.993	T5Ø.994	—	—
Diacetylmorphine	T4Ø.1X1	T4Ø.1X2	T4Ø.1X3	T4Ø.1X4	—	—
Diachylon plaster	T49.4X1	T49.4X2	T49.4X3	T49.4X4	T49.4X5	T49.4X6
Diaethylstilboestrolum	T38.5X1	T38.5X2	T38.5X3	T38.5X4	T38.5X5	T38.5X6
Diagnostic agent NEC	T5Ø.8X1	T5Ø.8X2	T5Ø.8X3	T5Ø.8X4	T5Ø.8X5	T5Ø.8X6
Dial (soap)	T49.2X1	T49.2X2	T49.2X3	T49.2X4	T49.2X5	T49.2X6
sedative	T42.3X1	T42.3X2	T42.3X3	T42.3X4	T42.3X5	T42.3X6
Dialkyl carbonate	T52.91	T52.92	T52.93	T52.94	—	—
Diallylbarbituric acid	T42.3X1	T42.3X2	T42.3X3	T42.3X4	T42.3X5	T42.3X6
Diallymal	T42.3X1	T42.3X2	T42.3X3	T42.3X4	T42.3X5	T42.3X6

Substance	Poisoning, Accidental (unintentional)	Poisoning, Intentional Self-harm	Poisoning, Assault	Poisoning, Undetermined	Adverse Effect	Under-dosing
Dialysis solution (intraperitoneal)	T5Ø.3X1	T5Ø.3X2	T5Ø.3X3	T5Ø.3X4	T5Ø.3X5	T5Ø.3X6
Diaminodiphenylsulfone	T37.1X1	T37.1X2	T37.1X3	T37.1X4	T37.1X5	T37.1X6
Diamorphine	T4Ø.1X1	T4Ø.1X2	T4Ø.1X3	T4Ø.1X4	—	—
Diamox	T5Ø.2X1	T5Ø.2X2	T5Ø.2X3	T5Ø.2X4	T5Ø.2X5	T5Ø.2X6
Diamthazole	T49.ØX1	T49.ØX2	T49.ØX3	T49.ØX4	T49.ØX5	T49.ØX6
Dianthone	T47.2X1	T47.2X2	T47.2X3	T47.2X4	T47.2X5	T47.2X6
Diaphenylsulfone	T37.ØX1	T37.ØX2	T37.ØX3	T37.ØX4	T37.ØX5	T37.ØX6
Diasone (sodium)	T37.1X1	T37.1X2	T37.1X3	T37.1X4	T37.1X5	T37.1X6
Diastase	T47.5X1	T47.5X2	T47.5X3	T47.5X4	T47.5X5	T47.5X6
Diatrizoate	T5Ø.8X1	T5Ø.8X2	T5Ø.8X3	T5Ø.8X4	T5Ø.8X5	T5Ø.8X6
Diazepam	T42.4X1	T42.4X2	T42.4X3	T42.4X4	T42.4X5	T42.4X6
Diazinon	T6Ø.ØX1	T6Ø.ØX2	T6Ø.ØX3	T6Ø.ØX4	—	—
Diazomethane (gas)	T59.891	T59.892	T59.893	T59.894	—	—
Diazoxide	T46.5X1	T46.5X2	T46.5X3	T46.5X4	T46.5X5	T46.5X6
Dibekacin	T36.5X1	T36.5X2	T36.5X3	T36.5X4	T36.5X5	T36.5X6
Dibenamine	T44.6X1	T44.6X2	T44.6X3	T44.6X4	T44.6X5	T44.6X6
Dibenzepin	T43.Ø11	T43.Ø12	T43.Ø13	T43.Ø14	T43.Ø15	T43.Ø16
Dibenzheptropine	T45.ØX1	T45.ØX2	T45.ØX3	T45.ØX4	T45.ØX5	T45.ØX6
Dibenzyline	T44.6X1	T44.6X2	T44.6X3	T44.6X4	T44.6X5	T44.6X6
Diborane (gas)	T59.891	T59.892	T59.893	T59.894	—	—
Dibromochloropropane	T6Ø.8X1	T6Ø.8X2	T6Ø.8X3	T6Ø.8X4	—	—
Dibromodulcitol	T45.1X1	T45.1X2	T45.1X3	T45.1X4	T45.1X5	T45.1X6
Dibromoethane	T53.6X1	T53.6X2	T53.6X3	T53.6X4	—	—
Dibromomannitol	T45.1X1	T45.1X2	T45.1X3	T45.1X4	T45.1X5	T45.1X6
Dibromopropamidine isethionate	T49.ØX1	T49.ØX2	T49.ØX3	T49.ØX4	T49.ØX5	T49.ØX6
Dibrompropamidine	T49.ØX1	T49.ØX2	T49.ØX3	T49.ØX4	T49.ØX5	T49.ØX6
Dibucaine	T41.3X1	T41.3X2	T41.3X3	T41.3X4	T41.3X5	T41.3X6
topical (surface)	T41.3X1	T41.3X2	T41.3X3	T41.3X4	T41.3X5	T41.3X6
Dibunate sodium	T48.3X1	T48.3X2	T48.3X3	T48.3X4	T48.3X5	T48.3X6
Dibutoline sulfate	T44.3X1	T44.3X2	T44.3X3	T44.3X4	T44.3X5	T44.3X6
Dicamba	T6Ø.3X1	T6Ø.3X2	T6Ø.3X3	T6Ø.3X4	—	—
Dicapthon	T6Ø.ØX1	T6Ø.ØX2	T6Ø.ØX3	T6Ø.ØX4	—	—
Dichlobenil	T6Ø.3X1	T6Ø.3X2	T6Ø.3X3	T6Ø.3X4	—	—
Dichlone	T6Ø.3X1	T6Ø.3X2	T6Ø.3X3	T6Ø.3X4	—	—
Dichloralphenozone	T42.6X1	T42.6X2	T42.6X3	T42.6X4	T42.6X5	T42.6X6
Dichlorbenzidine	T65.3X1	T65.3X2	T65.3X3	T65.3X4	—	—
Dichlorhydrin	T52.8X1	T52.8X2	T52.8X3	T52.8X4	—	—
Dichlorhydroxyquinoline	T37.8X1	T37.8X2	T37.8X3	T37.8X4	T37.8X5	T37.8X6
Dichlorobenzene	T53.7X1	T53.7X2	T53.7X3	T53.7X4	—	—
Dichlorobenzyl alcohol	T49.6X1	T49.6X2	T49.6X3	T49.6X4	T49.6X5	T49.6X6
Dichlorodifluoromethane	T53.5X1	T53.5X2	T53.5X3	T53.5X4	—	—
Dichloroethane	T52.8X1	T52.8X2	T52.8X3	T52.8X4	—	—
Dichloroethylene	T53.6X1	T53.6X2	T53.6X3	T53.6X4	—	—
Dichloroethyl sulfide, not in war	T59.891	T59.892	T59.893	T59.894	—	—
Dichloroformoxine, not in war	T59.891	T59.892	T59.893	T59.894	—	—
Dichlorohydrin, alpha-dichlorohydrin	T52.8X1	T52.8X2	T52.8X3	T52.8X4	—	—
Dichloromethane (solvent)	T53.4X1	T53.4X2	T53.4X3	T53.4X4	—	—
vapor	T53.4X1	T53.4X2	T53.4X3	T53.4X4	—	—
Dichloronaphthoquinone	T6Ø.3X1	T6Ø.3X2	T6Ø.3X3	T6Ø.3X4	—	—
Dichlorophen	T37.4X1	T37.4X2	T37.4X3	T37.4X4	T37.4X5	T37.4X6
Dichloropropene	T6Ø.3X1	T6Ø.3X2	T6Ø.3X3	T6Ø.3X4	—	—
Dichloropropionic acid	T6Ø.3X1	T6Ø.3X2	T6Ø.3X3	T6Ø.3X4	—	—
Dichlorphenamide	T5Ø.2X1	T5Ø.2X2	T5Ø.2X3	T5Ø.2X4	T5Ø.2X5	T5Ø.2X6
Dichlorvos	T6Ø.ØX1	T6Ø.ØX2	T6Ø.ØX3	T6Ø.ØX4	—	—
Diclofenac	T39.391	T39.392	T39.393	T39.394	T39.395	T39.396
Diclofenamide	T5Ø.2X1	T5Ø.2X2	T5Ø.2X3	T5Ø.2X4	T5Ø.2X5	T5Ø.2X6
Diclofensine	T43.291	T43.292	T43.293	T43.294	T43.295	T43.296
Diclonixine	T39.8X1	T39.8X2	T39.8X3	T39.8X4	T39.8X5	T39.8X6
Dicloxacillin	T36.ØX1	T36.ØX2	T36.ØX3	T36.ØX4	T36.ØX5	T36.ØX6
Dicophane	T49.ØX1	T49.ØX2	T49.ØX3	T49.ØX4	T49.ØX5	T49.ØX6
Dicoumarol, dicoumarin, dicumarol	T45.511	T45.512	T45.513	T45.514	T45.515	T45.516
Dicrotophos	T6Ø.ØX1	T6Ø.ØX2	T6Ø.ØX3	T6Ø.ØX4	—	—
Dicyanogen (gas)	T65.ØX1	T65.ØX2	T65.ØX3	T65.ØX4	—	—
Dicyclomine	T44.3X1	T44.3X2	T44.3X3	T44.3X4	T44.3X5	T44.3X6
Dicycloverine	T44.3X1	T44.3X2	T44.3X3	T44.3X4	T44.3X5	T44.3X6
Dideoxycytidine	T37.5X1	T37.5X2	T37.5X3	T37.5X4	T37.5X5	T37.5X6
Dideoxyinosine	T37.5X1	T37.5X2	T37.5X3	T37.5X4	T37.5X5	T37.5X6
Dieldrin (vapor)	T6Ø.1X1	T6Ø.1X2	T6Ø.1X3	T6Ø.1X4	—	—
Diemal	T42.3X1	T42.3X2	T42.3X3	T42.3X4	T42.3X5	T42.3X6
Dienestrol	T38.5X1	T38.5X2	T38.5X3	T38.5X4	T38.5X5	T38.5X6
Dienoestrol	T38.5X1	T38.5X2	T38.5X3	T38.5X4	T38.5X5	T38.5X6
Dietetic drug NEC	T5Ø.9Ø1	T5Ø.9Ø2	T5Ø.9Ø3	T5Ø.9Ø4	T5Ø.9Ø5	T5Ø.9Ø6
Diethazine	T42.8X1	T42.8X2	T42.8X3	T42.8X4	T42.8X5	T42.8X6
Diethyl						
barbituric acid	T42.3X1	T42.3X2	T42.3X3	T42.3X4	T42.3X5	T42.3X6
carbamazine	T37.4X1	T37.4X2	T37.4X3	T37.4X4	T37.4X5	T37.4X6
carbinol	T51.3X1	T51.3X2	T51.3X3	T51.3X4	—	—
Diethyl — *continued*						
carbonate	T52.8X1	T52.8X2	T52.8X3	T52.8X4	—	—
ether (vapor) — *see also* ether	T41.ØX1	T41.ØX2	T41.ØX3	T41.ØX4	T41.ØX5	T41.ØX6
oxide	T52.8X1	T52.8X2	T52.8X3	T52.8X4	—	—
propion	T5Ø.5X1	T5Ø.5X2	T5Ø.5X3	T5Ø.5X4	T5Ø.5X5	T5Ø.5X6
stilbestrol	T38.5X1	T38.5X2	T38.5X3	T38.5X4	T38.5X5	T38.5X6
toluamide (nonmedicinal)	T6Ø.8X1	T6Ø.8X2	T6Ø.8X3	T6Ø.8X4	—	—
medicinal	T49.3X1	T49.3X2	T49.3X3	T49.3X4	T49.3X5	T49.3X6
Diethylcarbamazine	T37.4X1	T37.4X2	T37.4X3	T37.4X4	T37.4X5	T37.4X6
Diethylene						
dioxide	T52.8X1	T52.8X2	T52.8X3	T52.8X4	—	—
glycol (monoacetate) (monobutyl ether) (monoethyl ether)	T52.3X1	T52.3X2	T52.3X3	T52.3X4	—	—
Diethylhexylphthalate	T65.891	T65.892	T65.893	T65.894	—	—
Diethylpropion	T5Ø.5X1	T5Ø.5X2	T5Ø.5X3	T5Ø.5X4	T5Ø.5X5	T5Ø.5X6
Diethylstilbestrol	T38.5X1	T38.5X2	T38.5X3	T38.5X4	T38.5X5	T38.5X6
Diethylstilboestrol	T38.5X1	T38.5X2	T38.5X3	T38.5X4	T38.5X5	T38.5X6
Diethylsulfone-diethylmethane	T42.6X1	T42.6X2	T42.6X3	T42.6X4	T42.6X5	T42.6X6
Diethyltoluamide	T49.ØX1	T49.ØX2	T49.ØX3	T49.ØX4	T49.ØX5	T49.ØX6
Diethyltryptamine (DET)	T4Ø.991	T4Ø.992	T4Ø.993	T4Ø.994	—	—
Difebarbamate	T42.3X1	T42.3X2	T42.3X3	T42.3X4	T42.3X5	T42.3X6
Difencloxazine	T4Ø.2X1	T4Ø.2X2	T4Ø.2X3	T4Ø.2X4	T4Ø.2X5	T4Ø.2X6
Difenidol	T45.ØX1	T45.ØX2	T45.ØX3	T45.ØX4	T45.ØX5	T45.ØX6
Difenoxin	T47.6X1	T47.6X2	T47.6X3	T47.6X4	T47.6X5	T47.6X6
Difetarsone	T37.3X1	T37.3X2	T37.3X3	T37.3X4	T37.3X5	T37.3X6
Diffusin	T45.3X1	T45.3X2	T45.3X3	T45.3X4	T45.3X5	T45.3X6
Diflorasone	T49.ØX1	T49.ØX2	T49.ØX3	T49.ØX4	T49.ØX5	T49.ØX6
Diflos	T44.ØX1	T44.ØX2	T44.ØX3	T44.ØX4	T44.ØX5	T44.ØX6
Diflubenzuron	T6Ø.1X1	T6Ø.1X2	T6Ø.1X3	T6Ø.1X4	—	—
Diflucortolone	T49.ØX1	T49.ØX2	T49.ØX3	T49.ØX4	T49.ØX5	T49.ØX6
Diflunisal	T39.Ø91	T39.Ø92	T39.Ø93	T39.Ø94	T39.Ø95	T39.Ø96
Difluoromethyldopa	T42.8X1	T42.8X2	T42.8X3	T42.8X4	T42.8X5	T42.8X6
Difluorophate	T44.ØX1	T44.ØX2	T44.ØX3	T44.ØX4	T44.ØX5	T44.ØX6
Digestant NEC	T47.5X1	T47.5X2	T47.5X3	T47.5X4	T47.5X5	T47.5X6
Digitalin (e)	T46.ØX1	T46.ØX2	T46.ØX3	T46.ØX4	T46.ØX5	T46.ØX6
Digitalis (leaf)(glycoside)	T46.ØX1	T46.ØX2	T46.ØX3	T46.ØX4	T46.ØX5	T46.ØX6
lanata	T46.ØX1	T46.ØX2	T46.ØX3	T46.ØX4	T46.ØX5	T46.ØX6
purpurea	T46.ØX1	T46.ØX2	T46.ØX3	T46.ØX4	T46.ØX5	T46.ØX6
Digitoxin	T46.ØX1	T46.ØX2	T46.ØX3	T46.ØX4	T46.ØX5	T46.ØX6
Digitoxose	T46.ØX1	T46.ØX2	T46.ØX3	T46.ØX4	T46.ØX5	T46.ØX6
Digoxin	T46.ØX1	T46.ØX2	T46.ØX3	T46.ØX4	T46.ØX5	T46.ØX6
Digoxine	T46.ØX1	T46.ØX2	T46.ØX3	T46.ØX4	T46.ØX5	T46.ØX6
Dihydralazine	T46.5X1	T46.5X2	T46.5X3	T46.5X4	T46.5X5	T46.5X6
Dihydrazine	T46.5X1	T46.5X2	T46.5X3	T46.5X4	T46.5X5	T46.5X6
Dihydrocodeine	T4Ø.2X1	T4Ø.2X2	T4Ø.2X3	T4Ø.2X4	T4Ø.2X5	T4Ø.2X6
Dihydrocodeinone	T4Ø.2X1	T4Ø.2X2	T4Ø.2X3	T4Ø.2X4	T4Ø.2X5	T4Ø.2X6
Dihydroergocornine	T46.7X1	T46.7X2	T46.7X3	T46.7X4	T46.7X5	T46.7X6
Dihydroergocristine (mesilate)	T46.7X1	T46.7X2	T46.7X3	T46.7X4	T46.7X5	T46.7X6
Dihydroergokryptine	T46.7X1	T46.7X2	T46.7X3	T46.7X4	T46.7X5	T46.7X6
Dihydroergotamine	T46.5X1	T46.5X2	T46.5X3	T46.5X4	T46.5X5	T46.5X6
Dihydroergotoxine	T46.7X1	T46.7X2	T46.7X3	T46.7X4	T46.7X5	T46.7X6
mesilate	T46.7X1	T46.7X2	T46.7X3	T46.7X4	T46.7X5	T46.7X6
Dihydrohydroxycodeinone	T4Ø.2X1	T4Ø.2X2	T4Ø.2X3	T4Ø.2X4	T4Ø.2X5	T4Ø.2X6
Dihydrohydroxymorphinone	T4Ø.2X1	T4Ø.2X2	T4Ø.2X3	T4Ø.2X4	T4Ø.2X5	T4Ø.2X6
Dihydroisocodeine	T4Ø.2X1	T4Ø.2X2	T4Ø.2X3	T4Ø.2X4	T4Ø.2X5	T4Ø.2X6
Dihydromorphine	T4Ø.2X1	T4Ø.2X2	T4Ø.2X3	T4Ø.2X4	—	—
Dihydromorphinone	T4Ø.2X1	T4Ø.2X2	T4Ø.2X3	T4Ø.2X4	T4Ø.2X5	T4Ø.2X6
Dihydrostreptomycin	T36.5X1	T36.5X2	T36.5X3	T36.5X4	T36.5X5	T36.5X6
Dihydrotachysterol	T45.2X1	T45.2X2	T45.2X3	T45.2X4	T45.2X5	T45.2X6
Dihydroxyaluminum aminoacetate	T47.1X1	T47.1X2	T47.1X3	T47.1X4	T47.1X5	T47.1X6
Dihydroxyaluminum sodium carbonate	T47.1X1	T47.1X2	T47.1X3	T47.1X4	T47.1X5	T47.1X6
Dihydroxyanthraquinone	T47.2X1	T47.2X2	T47.2X3	T47.2X4	T47.2X5	T47.2X6
Dihydroxycodeinone	T4Ø.2X1	T4Ø.2X2	T4Ø.2X3	T4Ø.2X4	T4Ø.2X5	T4Ø.2X6
Dihydroxypropyl theophylline	T5Ø.2X1	T5Ø.2X2	T5Ø.2X3	T5Ø.2X4	T5Ø.2X5	T5Ø.2X6
Diiodohydroxyquin	T37.8X1	T37.8X2	T37.8X3	T37.8X4	T37.8X5	T37.8X6
topical	T49.ØX1	T49.ØX2	T49.ØX3	T49.ØX4	T49.ØX5	T49.ØX6
Diiodohydroxyquinoline	T37.8X1	T37.8X2	T37.8X3	T37.8X4	T37.8X5	T37.8X6
Diiodotyrosine	T38.2X1	T38.2X2	T38.2X3	T38.2X4	T38.2X5	T38.2X6
Diisopromine	T44.3X1	T44.3X2	T44.3X3	T44.3X4	T44.3X5	T44.3X6
Diisopropylamine	T46.3X1	T46.3X2	T46.3X3	T46.3X4	T46.3X5	T46.3X6
Diisopropylfluorophosphonate	T44.ØX1	T44.ØX2	T44.ØX3	T44.ØX4	T44.ØX5	T44.ØX6
Dilantin	T42.ØX1	T42.ØX2	T42.ØX3	T42.ØX4	T42.ØX5	T42.ØX6
Dilaudid	T4Ø.2X1	T4Ø.2X2	T4Ø.2X3	T4Ø.2X4	T4Ø.2X5	T4Ø.2X6
Dilazep	T46.3X1	T46.3X2	T46.3X3	T46.3X4	T46.3X5	T46.3X6
Dill	T47.5X1	T47.5X2	T47.5X3	T47.5X4	T47.5X5	T47.5X6
Diloxanide	T37.3X1	T37.3X2	T37.3X3	T37.3X4	T37.3X5	T37.3X6
Diltiazem	T46.1X1	T46.1X2	T46.1X3	T46.1X4	T46.1X5	T46.1X6

Substance	Poisoning, Accidental (unintentional)	Poisoning, Intentional Self-harm	Poisoning, Assault	Poisoning, Undetermined	Adverse Effect	Under-dosing
Dimazole	T49.ØX1	T49.ØX2	T49.ØX3	T49.ØX4	T49.ØX5	T49.ØX6
Dimefline	T5Ø.7X1	T5Ø.7X2	T5Ø.7X3	T5Ø.7X4	T5Ø.7X5	T5Ø.7X6
Dimefox	T6Ø.ØX1	T6Ø.ØX2	T6Ø.ØX3	T6Ø.ØX4	—	—
Dimemorfan	T48.3X1	T48.3X2	T48.3X3	T48.3X4	T48.3X5	T48.3X6
Dimenhydrinate	T45.ØX1	T45.ØX2	T45.ØX3	T45.ØX4	T45.ØX5	T45.ØX6
Dimercaprol (British anti-lewisite)	T45.8X1	T45.8X2	T45.8X3	T45.8X4	T45.8X5	T45.8X6
Dimercaptopropanol	T45.8X1	T45.8X2	T45.8X3	T45.8X4	T45.8X5	T45.8X6
Dimestrol	T38.5X1	T38.5X2	T38.5X3	T38.5X4	T38.5X5	T38.5X6
Dimetane	T45.ØX1	T45.ØX2	T45.ØX3	T45.ØX4	T45.ØX5	T45.ØX6
Dimethicone	T47.1X1	T47.1X2	T47.1X3	T47.1X4	T47.1X5	T47.1X6
Dimethindene	T45.ØX1	T45.ØX2	T45.ØX3	T45.ØX4	T45.ØX5	T45.ØX6
Dimethisoquin	T49.1X1	T49.1X2	T49.1X3	T49.1X4	T49.1X5	T49.1X6
Dimethisterone	T38.5X1	T38.5X2	T38.5X3	T38.5X4	T38.5X5	T38.5X6
Dimethoate	T6Ø.ØX1	T6Ø.ØX2	T6Ø.ØX3	T6Ø.ØX4	—	—
Dimethocaine	T41.3X1	T41.3X2	T41.3X3	T41.3X4	T41.3X5	T41.3X6
Dimethoxanate	T48.3X1	T48.3X2	T48.3X3	T48.3X4	T48.3X5	T48.3X6
Dimethyl						
arsine, arsinic acid	T57.ØX1	T57.ØX2	T57.ØX3	T57.ØX4	—	—
carbinol	T51.2X1	T51.2X2	T51.2X3	T51.2X4	—	—
carbonate	T52.8X1	T52.8X2	T52.8X3	T52.8X4	—	—
diguanide	T38.3X1	T38.3X2	T38.3X3	T38.3X4	T38.3X5	T38.3X6
ketone	T52.4X1	T52.4X2	T52.4X3	T52.4X4	—	—
vapor	T52.4X1	T52.4X2	T52.4X3	T52.4X4	—	—
meperidine	T4Ø.2X1	T4Ø.2X2	T4Ø.2X3	T4Ø.2X4	T4Ø.2X5	T4Ø.2X6
parathion	T6Ø.ØX1	T6Ø.ØX2	T6Ø.ØX3	T6Ø.ØX4	—	—
phthlate	T49.3X1	T49.3X2	T49.3X3	T49.3X4	T49.3X5	T49.3X6
polysiloxane	T47.8X1	T47.8X2	T47.8X3	T47.8X4	T47.8X5	T47.8X6
sulfate (fumes)	T59.891	T59.892	T59.893	T59.894	—	—
liquid	T65.891	T65.892	T65.893	T65.894	—	—
sulfoxide (nonmedicinal)	T52.8X1	T52.8X2	T52.8X3	T52.8X4	—	—
medicinal	T49.4X1	T49.4X2	T49.4X3	T49.4X4	T49.4X5	T49.4X6
tryptamine	T4Ø.991	T4Ø.992	T4Ø.993	T4Ø.994	—	—
tubocurarine	T48.1X1	T48.1X2	T48.1X3	T48.1X4	T48.1X5	T48.1X6
Dimethylamine sulfate	T49.4X1	T49.4X2	T49.4X3	T49.4X4	T49.4X5	T49.4X6
Dimethylformamide	T52.8X1	T52.8X2	T52.8X3	T52.8X4	—	—
Dimethyltubocurarinium chloride	T48.1X1	T48.1X2	T48.1X3	T48.1X4	T48.1X5	T48.1X6
Dimeticone	T47.1X1	T47.1X2	T47.1X3	T47.1X4	T47.1X5	T47.1X6
Dimetilan	T6Ø.ØX1	T6Ø.ØX2	T6Ø.ØX3	T6Ø.ØX4	—	—
Dimetindene	T45.ØX1	T45.ØX2	T45.ØX3	T45.ØX4	T45.ØX5	T45.ØX6
Dimetotiazine	T43.3X1	T43.3X2	T43.3X3	T43.3X4	T43.3X5	T43.3X6
Dimorpholamine	T5Ø.7X1	T5Ø.7X2	T5Ø.7X3	T5Ø.7X4	T5Ø.7X5	T5Ø.7X6
Dimoxyline	T46.3X1	T46.3X2	T46.3X3	T46.3X4	T46.3X5	T46.3X6
Dinitrobenzene	T65.3X1	T65.3X2	T65.3X3	T65.3X4	—	—
vapor	T59.891	T59.892	T59.893	T59.894	—	—
Dinitrobenzol	T65.3X1	T65.3X2	T65.3X3	T65.3X4	—	—
vapor	T59.891	T59.892	T59.893	T59.894	—	—
Dinitrobutylphenol	T65.3X1	T65.3X2	T65.3X3	T65.3X4	—	—
Dinitro (-ortho-)cresol (pesticide) (spray)	T65.3X1	T65.3X2	T65.3X3	T65.3X4	—	—
Dinitrocyclohexylphenol	T65.3X1	T65.3X2	T65.3X3	T65.3X4	—	—
Dinitrophenol	T65.3X1	T65.3X2	T65.3X3	T65.3X4	—	—
Dinoprost	T48.ØX1	T48.ØX2	T48.ØX3	T48.ØX4	T48.ØX5	T48.ØX6
Dinoprostone	T48.ØX1	T48.ØX2	T48.ØX3	T48.ØX4	T48.ØX5	T48.ØX6
Dinoseb	T6Ø.3X1	T6Ø.3X2	T6Ø.3X3	T6Ø.3X4	—	—
Dioctyl sulfosuccinate (calcium) (sodium)	T47.4X1	T47.4X2	T47.4X3	T47.4X4	T47.4X5	T47.4X6
Diodone	T5Ø.8X1	T5Ø.8X2	T5Ø.8X3	T5Ø.8X4	T5Ø.8X5	T5Ø.8X6
Diodoquin	T37.8X1	T37.8X2	T37.8X3	T37.8X4	T37.8X5	T37.8X6
Dionin	T4Ø.2X1	T4Ø.2X2	T4Ø.2X3	T4Ø.2X4	T4Ø.2X5	T4Ø.2X6
Diosmin	T46.991	T46.992	T46.993	T46.994	T46.995	T46.996
Dioxane	T52.8X1	T52.8X2	T52.8X3	T52.8X4	—	—
Dioxathion	T6Ø.ØX1	T6Ø.ØX2	T6Ø.ØX3	T6Ø.ØX4	—	—
Dioxin	T53.7X1	T53.7X2	T53.7X3	T53.7X4	—	—
Dioxopromethazine	T43.3X1	T43.3X2	T43.3X3	T43.3X4	T43.3X5	T43.3X6
Dioxyline	T46.3X1	T46.3X2	T46.3X3	T46.3X4	T46.3X5	T46.3X6
Dipentene	T52.8X1	T52.8X2	T52.8X3	T52.8X4	—	—
Diperodon	T41.3X1	T41.3X2	T41.3X3	T41.3X4	T41.3X5	T41.3X6
Diphacinone	T6Ø.4X1	T6Ø.4X2	T6Ø.4X3	T6Ø.4X4	—	—
Diphemanil	T44.3X1	T44.3X2	T44.3X3	T44.3X4	T44.3X5	T44.3X6
metilsulfate	T44.3X1	T44.3X2	T44.3X3	T44.3X4	T44.3X5	T44.3X6
Diphenadione	T45.511	T45.512	T45.513	T45.514	T45.515	T45.516
rodenticide	T6Ø.4X1	T6Ø.4X2	T6Ø.4X3	T6Ø.4X4	—	—
Diphenhydramine	T45.ØX1	T45.ØX2	T45.ØX3	T45.ØX4	T45.ØX5	T45.ØX6
Diphenidol	T45.ØX1	T45.ØX2	T45.ØX3	T45.ØX4	T45.ØX5	T45.ØX6
Diphenoxylate	T47.6X1	T47.6X2	T47.6X3	T47.6X4	T47.6X5	T47.6X6
Diphenylamine	T65.3X1	T65.3X2	T65.3X3	T65.3X4	—	—
Diphenylbutazone	T39.2X1	T39.2X2	T39.2X3	T39.2X4	T39.2X5	T39.2X6
Diphenylchloroarsine, not in war	T57.ØX1	T57.ØX2	T57.ØX3	T57.ØX4	—	—
Diphenylhydantoin	T42.ØX1	T42.ØX2	T42.ØX3	T42.ØX4	T42.ØX5	T42.ØX6
Diphenylmethane dye	T52.1X1	T52.1X2	T52.1X3	T52.1X4	—	—

Substance	Poisoning, Accidental (unintentional)	Poisoning, Intentional Self-harm	Poisoning, Assault	Poisoning, Undetermined	Adverse Effect	Under-dosing
Diphenylpyraline	T45.ØX1	T45.ØX2	T45.ØX3	T45.ØX4	T45.ØX5	T45.ØX6
Diphtheria						
antitoxin	T5Ø.Z11	T5Ø.Z12	T5Ø.Z13	T5Ø.Z14	T5Ø.Z15	T5Ø.Z16
toxoid	T5Ø.A91	T5Ø.A92	T5Ø.A93	T5Ø.A94	T5Ø.A95	T5Ø.A96
with tetanus toxoid	T5Ø.A21	T5Ø.A22	T5Ø.A23	T5Ø.A24	T5Ø.A25	T5Ø.A26
with pertussis component	T5Ø.A11	T5Ø.A12	T5Ø.A13	T5Ø.A14	T5Ø.A15	T5Ø.A16
vaccine	T5Ø.A91	T5Ø.A92	T5Ø.A93	T5Ø.A94	T5Ø.A95	T5Ø.A96
combination						
without pertussis	T5Ø.A21	T5Ø.A22	T5Ø.A23	T5Ø.A24	T5Ø.A25	T5Ø.A26
including pertussis	T5Ø.A11	T5Ø.A12	T5Ø.A13	T5Ø.A14	T5Ø.A15	T5Ø.A16
Diphylline	T5Ø.2X1	T5Ø.2X2	T5Ø.2X3	T5Ø.2X4	T5Ø.2X5	T5Ø.2X6
Dipipanone	T4Ø.4X1	T4Ø.4X2	T4Ø.4X3	T4Ø.4X4	—	—
Dipivefrine	T49.5X1	T49.5X2	T49.5X3	T49.5X4	T49.5X5	T49.5X6
Diplovax	T5Ø.B91	T5Ø.B92	T5Ø.B93	T5Ø.B94	T5Ø.B95	T5Ø.B96
Diprophylline	T5Ø.2X1	T5Ø.2X2	T5Ø.2X3	T5Ø.2X4	T5Ø.2X5	T5Ø.2X6
Dipropyline	T48.291	T48.292	T48.293	T48.294	T48.295	T48.296
Dipyridamole	T46.3X1	T46.3X2	T46.3X3	T46.3X4	T46.3X5	T46.3X6
Dipyrone	T39.2X1	T39.2X2	T39.2X3	T39.2X4	T39.2X5	T39.2X6
Diquat (dibromide)	T6Ø.3X1	T6Ø.3X2	T6Ø.3X3	T6Ø.3X4	—	—
Disinfectant	T65.891	T65.892	T65.893	T65.894	—	—
alkaline	T54.3X1	T54.3X2	T54.3X3	T54.3X4	—	—
aromatic	T54.1X1	T54.1X2	T54.1X3	T54.1X4	—	—
intestinal	T37.8X1	T37.8X2	T37.8X3	T37.8X4	T37.8X5	T37.8X6
Disipal	T42.8X1	T42.8X2	T42.8X3	T42.8X4	T42.8X5	T42.8X6
Disodium edetate	T5Ø.6X1	T5Ø.6X2	T5Ø.6X3	T5Ø.6X4	T5Ø.6X5	T5Ø.6X6
Disoprofol	T41.291	T41.292	T41.293	T41.294	T41.295	T41.296
Disopyramide	T46.2X1	T46.2X2	T46.2X3	T46.2X4	T46.2X5	T46.2X6
Distigmine (bromide)	T44.ØX1	T44.ØX2	T44.ØX3	T44.ØX4	T44.ØX5	T44.ØX6
Disulfamide	T5Ø.2X1	T5Ø.2X2	T5Ø.2X3	T5Ø.2X4	T5Ø.2X5	T5Ø.2X6
Disulfanilamide	T37.ØX1	T37.ØX2	T37.ØX3	T37.ØX4	T37.ØX5	T37.ØX6
Disulfiram	T5Ø.6X1	T5Ø.6X2	T5Ø.6X3	T5Ø.6X4	T5Ø.6X5	T5Ø.6X6
Disulfoton	T6Ø.ØX1	T6Ø.ØX2	T6Ø.ØX3	T6Ø.ØX4	—	—
Dithiazanine iodide	T37.4X1	T37.4X2	T37.4X3	T37.4X4	T37.4X5	T37.4X6
Dithiocarbamate	T6Ø.ØX1	T6Ø.ØX2	T6Ø.ØX3	T6Ø.ØX4	—	—
Dithranol	T49.4X1	T49.4X2	T49.4X3	T49.4X4	T49.4X5	T49.4X6
Diucardin	T5Ø.2X1	T5Ø.2X2	T5Ø.2X3	T5Ø.2X4	T5Ø.2X5	T5Ø.2X6
Diupres	T5Ø.2X1	T5Ø.2X2	T5Ø.2X3	T5Ø.2X4	T5Ø.2X5	T5Ø.2X6
Diuretic NEC	T5Ø.2X1	T5Ø.2X2	T5Ø.2X3	T5Ø.2X4	T5Ø.2X5	T5Ø.2X6
benzothiadiazine	T5Ø.2X1	T5Ø.2X2	T5Ø.2X3	T5Ø.2X4	T5Ø.2X5	T5Ø.2X6
carbonic acid anhydrase inhibitors	T5Ø.2X1	T5Ø.2X2	T5Ø.2X3	T5Ø.2X4	T5Ø.2X5	T5Ø.2X6
furfuryl NEC	T5Ø.2X1	T5Ø.2X2	T5Ø.2X3	T5Ø.2X4	T5Ø.2X5	T5Ø.2X6
loop (high-ceiling)	T5Ø.1X1	T5Ø.1X2	T5Ø.1X3	T5Ø.1X4	T5Ø.1X5	T5Ø.1X6
mercurial NEC	T5Ø.2X1	T5Ø.2X2	T5Ø.2X3	T5Ø.2X4	T5Ø.2X5	T5Ø.2X6
osmotic	T5Ø.2X1	T5Ø.2X2	T5Ø.2X3	T5Ø.2X4	T5Ø.2X5	T5Ø.2X6
purine NEC	T5Ø.2X1	T5Ø.2X2	T5Ø.2X3	T5Ø.2X4	T5Ø.2X5	T5Ø.2X6
saluretic NEC	T5Ø.2X1	T5Ø.2X2	T5Ø.2X3	T5Ø.2X4	T5Ø.2X5	T5Ø.2X6
sulfonamide	T5Ø.2X1	T5Ø.2X2	T5Ø.2X3	T5Ø.2X4	T5Ø.2X5	T5Ø.2X6
thiazide NEC	T5Ø.2X1	T5Ø.2X2	T5Ø.2X3	T5Ø.2X4	T5Ø.2X5	T5Ø.2X6
xanthine	T5Ø.2X1	T5Ø.2X2	T5Ø.2X3	T5Ø.2X4	T5Ø.2X5	T5Ø.2X6
Diurgin	T5Ø.2X1	T5Ø.2X2	T5Ø.2X3	T5Ø.2X4	T5Ø.2X5	T5Ø.2X6
Diuril	T5Ø.2X1	T5Ø.2X2	T5Ø.2X3	T5Ø.2X4	T5Ø.2X5	T5Ø.2X6
Diuron	T6Ø.3X1	T6Ø.3X2	T6Ø.3X3	T6Ø.3X4	—	—
Divalproex	T42.6X1	T42.6X2	T42.6X3	T42.6X4	T42.6X5	T42.6X6
Divinyl ether	T41.ØX1	T41.ØX2	T41.ØX3	T41.ØX4	T41.ØX5	T41.ØX6
Dixanthogen	T49.ØX1	T49.ØX2	T49.ØX3	T49.ØX4	T49.ØX5	T49.ØX6
Dixyrazine	T43.3X1	T43.3X2	T43.3X3	T43.3X4	T43.3X5	T43.3X6
D-lysergic acid diethylamide	T4Ø.8X1	T4Ø.8X2	T4Ø.8X3	T4Ø.8X4	—	—
DMCT	T36.4X1	T36.4X2	T36.4X3	T36.4X4	T36.4X5	T36.4X6
DMSO — *see* Dimethyl sulfoxide						
DNBP	T6Ø.3X1	T6Ø.3X2	T6Ø.3X3	T6Ø.3X4	—	—
DNOC	T65.3X1	T65.3X2	T65.3X3	T65.3X4	—	—
Dobutamine	T44.5X1	T44.5X2	T44.5X3	T44.5X4	T44.5X5	T44.5X6
DOCA	T38.ØX1	T38.ØX2	T38.ØX3	T38.ØX4	T38.ØX5	T38.ØX6
Docusate sodium	T47.4X1	T47.4X2	T47.4X3	T47.4X4	T47.4X5	T47.4X6
Dodicin	T49.ØX1	T49.ØX2	T49.ØX3	T49.ØX4	T49.ØX5	T49.ØX6
Dofamium chloride	T49.ØX1	T49.ØX2	T49.ØX3	T49.ØX4	T49.ØX5	T49.ØX6
Dolophine	T4Ø.3X1	T4Ø.3X2	T4Ø.3X3	T4Ø.3X4	T4Ø.3X5	T4Ø.3X6
Doloxene	T39.8X1	T39.8X2	T39.8X3	T39.8X4	T39.8X5	T39.8X6
Domestic gas (after combustion) — *see* Gas, utility						
prior to combustion	T59.891	T59.892	T59.893	T59.894	—	—
Domiodol	T48.4X1	T48.4X2	T48.4X3	T48.4X4	T48.4X5	T48.4X6
Domiphen (bromide)	T49.ØX1	T49.ØX2	T49.ØX3	T49.ØX4	T49.ØX5	T49.ØX6
Domperidone	T45.ØX1	T45.ØX2	T45.ØX3	T45.ØX4	T45.ØX5	T45.ØX6
Dopa	T42.8X1	T42.8X2	T42.8X3	T42.8X4	T42.8X5	T42.8X6
Dopamine	T44.991	T44.992	T44.993	T44.994	T44.995	T44.996
Doriden	T42.6X1	T42.6X2	T42.6X3	T42.6X4	T42.6X5	T42.6X6
Dormiral	T42.3X1	T42.3X2	T42.3X3	T42.3X4	T42.3X5	T42.3X6
Dormison	T42.6X1	T42.6X2	T42.6X3	T42.6X4	T42.6X5	T42.6X6
Dornase	T48.4X1	T48.4X2	T48.4X3	T48.4X4	T48.4X5	T48.4X6

Substance	Poisoning, Accidental (unintentional)	Poisoning, Intentional Self-harm	Poisoning, Assault	Poisoning, Undetermined	Adverse Effect	Under-dosing
Dorsacaine	T41.3X1	T41.3X2	T41.3X3	T41.3X4	T41.3X5	T41.3X6
Dosulepin	T43.011	T43.012	T43.013	T43.014	T43.015	T43.016
Dothiepin	T43.011	T43.012	T43.013	T43.014	T43.015	T43.016
Doxantrazole	T48.6X1	T48.6X2	T48.6X3	T48.6X4	T48.6X5	T48.6X6
Doxapram	T50.7X1	T50.7X2	T50.7X3	T50.7X4	T50.7X5	T50.7X6
Doxazosin	T44.6X1	T44.6X2	T44.6X3	T44.6X4	T44.6X5	T44.6X6
Doxepin	T43.011	T43.012	T43.013	T43.014	T43.015	T43.016
Doxifluridine	T45.1X1	T45.1X2	T45.1X3	T45.1X4	T45.1X5	T45.1X6
Doxorubicin	T45.1X1	T45.1X2	T45.1X3	T45.1X4	T45.1X5	T45.1X6
Doxycycline	T36.4X1	T36.4X2	T36.4X3	T36.4X4	T36.4X5	T36.4X6
Doxylamine	T45.0X1	T45.0X2	T45.0X3	T45.0X4	T45.0X5	T45.0X6
Dramamine	T45.0X1	T45.0X2	T45.0X3	T45.0X4	T45.0X5	T45.0X6
Drano (drain cleaner)	T54.3X1	T54.3X2	T54.3X3	T54.3X4	—	—
Dressing, live pulp	T49.7X1	T49.7X2	T49.7X3	T49.7X4	T49.7X5	T49.7X6
Drocode	T40.2X1	T40.2X2	T40.2X3	T40.2X4	T40.2X5	T40.2X6
Dromoran	T40.2X1	T40.2X2	T40.2X3	T40.2X4	T40.2X5	T40.2X6
Dromostanolone	T38.7X1	T38.7X2	T38.7X3	T38.7X4	T38.7X5	T38.7X6
Dronabinol	T40.7X1	T40.7X2	T40.7X3	T40.7X4	T40.7X5	T40.7X6
Droperidol	T43.591	T43.592	T43.593	T43.594	T43.595	T43.596
Dropropizine	T48.3X1	T48.3X2	T48.3X3	T48.3X4	T48.3X5	T48.3X6
Drostanolone	T38.7X1	T38.7X2	T38.7X3	T38.7X4	T38.7X5	T38.7X6
Drotaverine	T44.3X1	T44.3X2	T44.3X3	T44.3X4	T44.3X5	T44.3X6
Drotrecogin alfa	T45.511	T45.512	T45.513	T45.514	T45.515	T45.516
Drug NEC	T50.901	T50.902	T50.903	T50.904	T50.905	T50.906
specified NEC	T50.991	T50.992	T50.993	T50.994	T50.995	T50.996
DTIC	T45.1X1	T45.1X2	T45.1X3	T45.1X4	T45.1X5	T45.1X6
Duboisine	T44.3X1	T44.3X2	T44.3X3	T44.3X4	T44.3X5	T44.3X6
Dulcolax	T47.2X1	T47.2X2	T47.2X3	T47.2X4	T47.2X5	T47.2X6
Duponol (C) (EP)	T49.2X1	T49.2X2	T49.2X3	T49.2X4	T49.2X5	T49.2X6
Durabolin	T38.7X1	T38.7X2	T38.7X3	T38.7X4	T38.7X5	T38.7X6
Dyclone	T41.3X1	T41.3X2	T41.3X3	T41.3X4	T41.3X5	T41.3X6
Dyclonine	T41.3X1	T41.3X2	T41.3X3	T41.3X4	T41.3X5	T41.3X6
Dydrogesterone	T38.5X1	T38.5X2	T38.5X3	T38.5X4	T38.5X5	T38.5X6
Dye NEC	T65.6X1	T65.6X2	T65.6X3	T65.6X4	—	—
antiseptic	T49.0X1	T49.0X2	T49.0X3	T49.0X4	T49.0X5	T49.0X6
diagnostic agents	T50.8X1	T50.8X2	T50.8X3	T50.8X4	T50.8X5	T50.8X6
pharmaceutical NEC	T50.901	T50.902	T50.903	T50.904	T50.905	T50.906
Dyflos	T44.0X1	T44.0X2	T44.0X3	T44.0X4	T44.0X5	T44.0X6
Dymelor	T38.3X1	T38.3X2	T38.3X3	T38.3X4	T38.3X5	T38.3X6
Dynamite	T65.3X1	T65.3X2	T65.3X3	T65.3X4	—	—
fumes	T59.891	T59.892	T59.893	T59.894	—	—
Dyphylline	T44.3X1	T44.3X2	T44.3X3	T44.3X4	T44.3X5	T44.3X6
b-eucaine	T49.1X1	T49.1X2	T49.1X3	T49.1X4	T49.1X5	T49.1X6
Ear drug NEC	T49.6X1	T49.6X2	T49.6X3	T49.6X4	T49.6X5	T49.6X6
Ear preparations	T49.6X1	T49.6X2	T49.6X3	T49.6X4	T49.6X5	T49.6X6
Echothiophate, echothiopate, ecothiopate	T49.5X1	T49.5X2	T49.5X3	T49.5X4	T49.5X5	T49.5X6
Econazole	T49.0X1	T49.0X2	T49.0X3	T49.0X4	T49.0X5	T49.0X6
Ecothiopate iodide	T49.5X1	T49.5X2	T49.5X3	T49.5X4	T49.5X5	T49.5X6
Ecstasy	T43.621	T43.622	T43.623	T43.624	T43.625	T43.626
Ectylurea	T42.6X1	T42.6X2	T42.6X3	T42.6X4	T42.6X5	T42.6X6
Edathamil disodium	T45.8X1	T45.8X2	T45.8X3	T45.8X4	T45.8X5	T45.8X6
Edecrin	T50.1X1	T50.1X2	T50.1X3	T50.1X4	T50.1X5	T50.1X6
Edetate, disodium (calcium)	T45.8X1	T45.8X2	T45.8X3	T45.8X4	T45.8X5	T45.8X6
Edoxudine	T49.5X1	T49.5X2	T49.5X3	T49.5X4	T49.5X5	T49.5X6
Edrophonium	T44.0X1	T44.0X2	T44.0X3	T44.0X4	T44.0X5	T44.0X6
chloride	T44.0X1	T44.0X2	T44.0X3	T44.0X4	T44.0X5	T44.0X6
EDTA	T50.6X1	T50.6X2	T50.6X3	T50.6X4	T50.6X5	T50.6X6
Eflornithine	T37.2X1	T37.2X2	T37.2X3	T37.2X4	T37.2X5	T37.2X6
Efloxate	T46.3X1	T46.3X2	T46.3X3	T46.3X4	T46.3X5	T46.3X6
Elase	T49.8X1	T49.8X2	T49.8X3	T49.8X4	T49.8X5	T49.8X6
Elastase	T47.5X1	T47.5X2	T47.5X3	T47.5X4	T47.5X5	T47.5X6
Elaterium	T47.2X1	T47.2X2	T47.2X3	T47.2X4	T47.2X5	T47.2X6
Elcatonin	T50.991	T50.992	T50.993	T50.994	T50.995	T50.996
Elder	T62.2X1	T62.2X2	T62.2X3	T62.2X4	—	—
berry, (unripe)	T62.1X1	T62.1X2	T62.1X3	T62.1X4	—	—
Electrolyte balance drug	T50.3X1	T50.3X2	T50.3X3	T50.3X4	T50.3X5	T50.3X6
Electrolytes NEC	T50.3X1	T50.3X2	T50.3X3	T50.3X4	T50.3X5	T50.3X6
Electrolytic agent NEC	T50.3X1	T50.3X2	T50.3X3	T50.3X4	T50.3X5	T50.3X6
Elemental diet	T50.901	T50.902	T50.903	T50.904	T50.905	T50.906
Elliptinium acetate	T45.1X1	T45.1X2	T45.1X3	T45.1X4	T45.1X5	T45.1X6
Embramine	T45.0X1	T45.0X2	T45.0X3	T45.0X4	T45.0X5	T45.0X6
Emepronium (salts)	T44.3X1	T44.3X2	T44.3X3	T44.3X4	T44.3X5	T44.3X6
bromide	T44.3X1	T44.3X2	T44.3X3	T44.3X4	T44.3X5	T44.3X6
Emetic NEC	T47.7X1	T47.7X2	T47.7X3	T47.7X4	T47.7X5	T47.7X6
Emetine	T37.3X1	T37.3X2	T37.3X3	T37.3X4	T37.3X5	T37.3X6
Emollient NEC	T49.3X1	T49.3X2	T49.3X3	T49.3X4	T49.3X5	T49.3X6
Emorfazone	T39.8X1	T39.8X2	T39.8X3	T39.8X4	T39.8X5	T39.8X6
Emylcamate	T43.591	T43.592	T43.593	T43.594	T43.595	T43.596
Enalapril	T46.4X1	T46.4X2	T46.4X3	T46.4X4	T46.4X5	T46.4X6
Enalaprilat	T46.4X1	T46.4X2	T46.4X3	T46.4X4	T46.4X5	T46.4X6
Encainide	T46.2X1	T46.2X2	T46.2X3	T46.2X4	T46.2X5	T46.2X6
Endocaine	T41.3X1	T41.3X2	T41.3X3	T41.3X4	T41.3X5	T41.3X6

Substance	Poisoning, Accidental (unintentional)	Poisoning, Intentional Self-harm	Poisoning, Assault	Poisoning, Undetermined	Adverse Effect	Under-dosing
Endosulfan	T60.2X1	T60.2X2	T60.2X3	T60.2X4	—	—
Endothall	T60.3X1	T60.3X2	T60.3X3	T60.3X4	—	—
Endralazine	T46.5X1	T46.5X2	T46.5X3	T46.5X4	T46.5X5	T46.5X6
Endrin	T60.1X1	T60.1X2	T60.1X3	T60.1X4	—	—
Enflurane	T41.0X1	T41.0X2	T41.0X3	T41.0X4	T41.0X5	T41.0X6
Enhexymal	T42.3X1	T42.3X2	T42.3X3	T42.3X4	T42.3X5	T42.3X6
Enocitabine	T45.1X1	T45.1X2	T45.1X3	T45.1X4	T45.1X5	T45.1X6
Enovid	T38.4X1	T38.4X2	T38.4X3	T38.4X4	T38.4X5	T38.4X6
Enoxacin	T36.8X1	T36.8X2	T36.8X3	T36.8X4	T36.8X5	T36.8X6
Enoxaparin (sodium)	T45.511	T45.512	T45.513	T45.514	T45.515	T45.516
Enpiprazole	T43.591	T43.592	T43.593	T43.594	T43.595	T43.596
Enprofylline	T48.6X1	T48.6X2	T48.6X3	T48.6X4	T48.6X5	T48.6X6
Enprostil	T47.1X1	T47.1X2	T47.1X3	T47.1X4	T47.1X5	T47.1X6
Enterogastrone	T38.891	T38.892	T38.893	T38.894	T38.895	T38.896
ENT preparations (anti-infectives)	T49.6X1	T49.6X2	T49.6X3	T49.6X4	T49.6X5	T49.6X6
Enviomycin	T36.8X1	T36.8X2	T36.8X3	T36.8X4	T36.8X5	T36.8X6
Enzodase	T45.3X1	T45.3X2	T45.3X3	T45.3X4	T45.3X5	T45.3X6
Enzyme NEC	T45.3X1	T45.3X2	T45.3X3	T45.3X4	T45.3X5	T45.3X6
depolymerizing	T49.8X1	T49.8X2	T49.8X3	T49.8X4	T49.8X5	T49.8X6
fibrolytic	T45.3X1	T45.3X2	T45.3X3	T45.3X4	T45.3X5	T45.3X6
gastric	T47.5X1	T47.5X2	T47.5X3	T47.5X4	T47.5X5	T47.5X6
intestinal	T47.5X1	T47.5X2	T47.5X3	T47.5X4	T47.5X5	T47.5X6
local action	T49.4X1	T49.4X2	T49.4X3	T49.4X4	T49.4X5	T49.4X6
proteolytic	T49.4X1	T49.4X2	T49.4X3	T49.4X4	T49.4X5	T49.4X6
thrombolytic	T45.3X1	T45.3X2	T45.3X3	T45.3X4	T45.3X5	T45.3X6
EPAB	T41.3X1	T41.3X2	T41.3X3	T41.3X4	T41.3X5	T41.3X6
Epanutin	T42.0X1	T42.0X2	T42.0X3	T42.0X4	T42.0X5	T42.0X6
Ephedra	T44.991	T44.992	T44.993	T44.994	T44.995	T44.996
Ephedrine	T44.991	T44.992	T44.993	T44.994	T44.995	T44.996
Epichlorhydrin, epichlorohydrin	T52.8X1	T52.8X2	T52.8X3	T52.8X4	—	—
Epicillin	T36.0X1	T36.0X2	T36.0X3	T36.0X4	T36.0X5	T36.0X6
Epiestriol	T38.5X1	T38.5X2	T38.5X3	T38.5X4	T38.5X5	T38.5X6
Epilim — *see* Sodium valproate						
Epimestrol	T38.5X1	T38.5X2	T38.5X3	T38.5X4	T38.5X5	T38.5X6
Epinephrine	T44.5X1	T44.5X2	T44.5X3	T44.5X4	T44.5X5	T44.5X6
Epirubicin	T45.1X1	T45.1X2	T45.1X3	T45.1X4	T45.1X5	T45.1X6
Epitiostanol	T38.7X1	T38.7X2	T38.7X3	T38.7X4	T38.7X5	T38.7X6
Epitizide	T50.2X1	T50.2X2	T50.2X3	T50.2X4	T50.2X5	T50.2X6
EPN	T60.0X1	T60.0X2	T60.0X3	T60.0X4	—	—
EPO	T45.8X1	T45.8X2	T45.8X3	T45.8X4	T45.8X5	T45.8X6
Epoetin alpha	T45.8X1	T45.8X2	T45.8X3	T45.8X4	T45.8X5	T45.8X6
Epomediol	T50.991	T50.992	T50.993	T50.994	T50.995	T50.996
Epoprostenol	T45.521	T45.522	T45.523	T45.524	T45.525	T45.526
Epoxy resin	T65.891	T65.892	T65.893	T65.894	—	—
Eprazinone	T48.4X1	T48.4X2	T48.4X3	T48.4X4	T48.4X5	T48.4X6
Epsilon aminocaproic acid	T45.621	T45.622	T45.623	T45.624	T45.625	T45.626
Epsom salt	T47.3X1	T47.3X2	T47.3X3	T47.3X4	T47.3X5	T47.3X6
Eptazocine	T40.4X1	T40.4X2	T40.4X3	T40.4X4	T40.4X5	T40.4X6
Equanil	T43.591	T43.592	T43.593	T43.594	T43.595	T43.596
Equisetum	T62.2X1	T62.2X2	T62.2X3	T62.2X4	—	—
diuretic	T50.2X1	T50.2X2	T50.2X3	T50.2X4	T50.2X5	T50.2X6
Ergobasine	T48.0X1	T48.0X2	T48.0X3	T48.0X4	T48.0X5	T48.0X6
Ergocalciferol	T45.2X1	T45.2X2	T45.2X3	T45.2X4	T45.2X5	T45.2X6
Ergoloid mesylates	T46.7X1	T46.7X2	T46.7X3	T46.7X4	T46.7X5	T46.7X6
Ergometrine	T48.0X1	T48.0X2	T48.0X3	T48.0X4	T48.0X5	T48.0X6
Ergonovine	T48.0X1	T48.0X2	T48.0X3	T48.0X4	T48.0X5	T48.0X6
Ergotamine	T46.5X1	T46.5X2	T46.5X3	T46.5X4	T46.5X5	T46.5X6
Ergotocine	T48.0X1	T48.0X2	T48.0X3	T48.0X4	T48.0X5	T48.0X6
Ergotrate	T48.0X1	T48.0X2	T48.0X3	T48.0X4	T48.0X5	T48.0X6
Ergot NEC	T64.81	T64.82	T64.83	T64.84	—	—
derivative	T48.0X1	T48.0X2	T48.0X3	T48.0X4	T48.0X5	T48.0X6
medicinal (alkaloids)	T48.0X1	T48.0X2	T48.0X3	T48.0X4	T48.0X5	T48.0X6
prepared	T48.0X1	T48.0X2	T48.0X3	T48.0X4	T48.0X5	T48.0X6
Eritrityl tetranitrate	T46.3X1	T46.3X2	T46.3X3	T46.3X4	T46.3X5	T46.3X6
Erythrityl tetranitrate	T46.3X1	T46.3X2	T46.3X3	T46.3X4	T46.3X5	T46.3X6
Erythrol tetranitrate	T46.3X1	T46.3X2	T46.3X3	T46.3X4	T46.3X5	T46.3X6
Erythromycin (salts)	T36.3X1	T36.3X2	T36.3X3	T36.3X4	T36.3X5	T36.3X6
ophthalmic preparation	T49.5X1	T49.5X2	T49.5X3	T49.5X4	T49.5X5	T49.5X6
topical NEC	T49.0X1	T49.0X2	T49.0X3	T49.0X4	T49.0X5	T49.0X6
Erythropoietin	T45.8X1	T45.8X2	T45.8X3	T45.8X4	T45.8X5	T45.8X6
human	T45.8X1	T45.8X2	T45.8X3	T45.8X4	T45.8X5	T45.8X6
Escin	T46.991	T46.992	T46.993	T46.994	T46.995	T46.996
Esculin	T45.2X1	T45.2X2	T45.2X3	T45.2X4	T45.2X5	T45.2X6
Esculoside	T45.2X1	T45.2X2	T45.2X3	T45.2X4	T45.2X5	T45.2X6
ESDT (ether-soluble tar distillate)	T49.1X1	T49.1X2	T49.1X3	T49.1X4	T49.1X5	T49.1X6
Eserine	T49.5X1	T49.5X2	T49.5X3	T49.5X4	T49.5X5	T49.5X6
Esflurbiprofen	T39.311	T39.312	T39.313	T39.314	T39.315	T39.316
Eskabarb	T42.3X1	T42.3X2	T42.3X3	T42.3X4	T42.3X5	T42.3X6
Eskalith	T43.8X1	T43.8X2	T43.8X3	T43.8X4	T43.8X5	T43.8X6
Esmolol	T44.7X1	T44.7X2	T44.7X3	T44.7X4	T44.7X5	T44.7X6

Substance	Poisoning, Accidental (unintentional)	Poisoning, Intentional Self-harm	Poisoning, Assault	Poisoning, Undetermined	Adverse Effect	Under-dosing
Estanozolol	T38.7X1	T38.7X2	T38.7X3	T38.7X4	T38.7X5	T38.7X6
Estazolam	T42.4X1	T42.4X2	T42.4X3	T42.4X4	T42.4X5	T42.4X6
Estradiol	T38.5X1	T38.5X2	T38.5X3	T38.5X4	T38.5X5	T38.5X6
with testosterone	T38.7X1	T38.7X2	T38.7X3	T38.7X4	T38.7X5	T38.7X6
benzoate	T38.5X1	T38.5X2	T38.5X3	T38.5X4	T38.5X5	T38.5X6
Estramustine	T45.1X1	T45.1X2	T45.1X3	T45.1X4	T45.1X5	T45.1X6
Estriol	T38.5X1	T38.5X2	T38.5X3	T38.5X4	T38.5X5	T38.5X6
Estrogen	T38.5X1	T38.5X2	T38.5X3	T38.5X4	T38.5X5	T38.5X6
with progesterone	T38.5X1	T38.5X2	T38.5X3	T38.5X4	T38.5X5	T38.5X6
conjugated	T38.5X1	T38.5X2	T38.5X3	T38.5X4	T38.5X5	T38.5X6
Estrone	T38.5X1	T38.5X2	T38.5X3	T38.5X4	T38.5X5	T38.5X6
Estropipate	T38.5X1	T38.5X2	T38.5X3	T38.5X4	T38.5X5	T38.5X6
Etacrynate sodium	T5Ø.1X1	T5Ø.1X2	T5Ø.1X3	T5Ø.1X4	T5Ø.1X5	T5Ø.1X6
Etacrynic acid	T5Ø.1X1	T5Ø.1X2	T5Ø.1X3	T5Ø.1X4	T5Ø.1X5	T5Ø.1X6
Etafedrine	T48.6X1	T48.6X2	T48.6X3	T48.6X4	T48.6X5	T48.6X6
Etafenone	T46.3X1	T46.3X2	T46.3X3	T46.3X4	T46.3X5	T46.3X6
Etambutol	T37.1X1	T37.1X2	T37.1X3	T37.1X4	T37.1X5	T37.1X6
Etamiphyllin	T48.6X1	T48.6X2	T48.6X3	T48.6X4	T48.6X5	T48.6X6
Etamivan	T5Ø.7X1	T5Ø.7X2	T5Ø.7X3	T5Ø.7X4	T5Ø.7X5	T5Ø.7X6
Etamsylate	T45.7X1	T45.7X2	T45.7X3	T45.7X4	T45.7X5	T45.7X6
Etebenecid	T5Ø.4X1	T5Ø.4X2	T5Ø.4X3	T5Ø.4X4	T5Ø.4X5	T5Ø.4X6
Ethacridine	T49.ØX1	T49.ØX2	T49.ØX3	T49.ØX4	T49.ØX5	T49.ØX6
Ethacrynic acid	T5Ø.1X1	T5Ø.1X2	T5Ø.1X3	T5Ø.1X4	T5Ø.1X5	T5Ø.1X6
Ethadione	T42.2X1	T42.2X2	T42.2X3	T42.2X4	T42.2X5	T42.2X6
Ethambutol	T37.1X1	T37.1X2	T37.1X3	T37.1X4	T37.1X5	T37.1X6
Ethamide	T5Ø.2X1	T5Ø.2X2	T5Ø.2X3	T5Ø.2X4	T5Ø.2X5	T5Ø.2X6
Ethamivan	T5Ø.7X1	T5Ø.7X2	T5Ø.7X3	T5Ø.7X4	T5Ø.7X5	T5Ø.7X6
Ethamsylate	T45.7X1	T45.7X2	T45.7X3	T45.7X4	T45.7X5	T45.7X6
Ethanol	T51.ØX1	T51.ØX2	T51.ØX3	T51.ØX4	—	—
beverage	T51.ØX1	T51.ØX2	T51.ØX3	T51.ØX4	—	—
Ethanolamine oleate	T46.8X1	T46.8X2	T46.8X3	T46.8X4	T46.8X5	T46.8X6
Ethaverine	T44.3X1	T44.3X2	T44.3X3	T44.3X4	T44.3X5	T44.3X6
Ethchlorvynol	T42.6X1	T42.6X2	T42.6X3	T42.6X4	T42.6X5	T42.6X6
Ethebenecid	T5Ø.4X1	T5Ø.4X2	T5Ø.4X3	T5Ø.4X4	T5Ø.4X5	T5Ø.4X6
Ether (vapor)	T41.ØX1	T41.ØX2	T41.ØX3	T41.ØX4	T41.ØX5	T41.ØX6
anesthetic	T41.ØX1	T41.ØX2	T41.ØX3	T41.ØX4	T41.ØX5	T41.ØX6
divinyl	T41.ØX1	T41.ØX2	T41.ØX3	T41.ØX4	T41.ØX5	T41.ØX6
ethyl (medicinal)	T41.ØX1	T41.ØX2	T41.ØX3	T41.ØX4	T41.ØX5	T41.ØX6
nonmedicinal	T52.8X1	T52.8X2	T52.8X3	T52.8X4	—	—
petroleum — *see* Ligroin						
solvent	T52.8X1	T52.8X2	T52.8X3	T52.8X4	—	—
Ethiazide	T5Ø.2X1	T5Ø.2X2	T5Ø.2X3	T5Ø.2X4	T5Ø.2X5	T5Ø.2X6
Ethidium chloride (vapor)	T59.891	T59.892	T59.893	T59.894	—	—
Ethinamate	T42.6X1	T42.6X2	T42.6X3	T42.6X4	T42.6X5	T42.6X6
Ethinylestradiol, ethinyloestradiol	T38.5X1	T38.5X2	T38.5X3	T38.5X4	T38.5X5	T38.5X6
with						
levonorgestrel	T38.4X1	T38.4X2	T38.4X3	T38.4X4	T38.4X5	T38.4X6
norethisterone	T38.4X1	T38.4X2	T38.4X3	T38.4X4	T38.4X5	T38.4X6
Ethiodized oil (131 I)	T5Ø.8X1	T5Ø.8X2	T5Ø.8X3	T5Ø.8X4	T5Ø.8X5	T5Ø.8X6
Ethion	T6Ø.ØX1	T6Ø.ØX2	T6Ø.ØX3	T6Ø.ØX4	—	—
Ethionamide	T37.1X1	T37.1X2	T37.1X3	T37.1X4	T37.1X5	T37.1X6
Ethioniamide	T37.1X1	T37.1X2	T37.1X3	T37.1X4	T37.1X5	T37.1X6
Ethisterone	T38.5X1	T38.5X2	T38.5X3	T38.5X4	T38.5X5	T38.5X6
Ethobral	T42.3X1	T42.3X2	T42.3X3	T42.3X4	T42.3X5	T42.3X6
Ethocaine (infiltration) (topical)	T41.3X1	T41.3X2	T41.3X3	T41.3X4	T41.3X5	T41.3X6
nerve block (peripheral) (plexus)	T41.3X1	T41.3X2	T41.3X3	T41.3X4	T41.3X5	T41.3X6
spinal	T41.3X1	T41.3X2	T41.3X3	T41.3X4	T41.3X5	T41.3X6
Ethoheptazine	T4Ø.4X1	T4Ø.4X2	T4Ø.4X3	T4Ø.4X4	T4Ø.4X5	T4Ø.4X6
Ethopropazine	T44.3X1	T44.3X2	T44.3X3	T44.3X4	T44.3X5	T44.3X6
Ethosuximide	T42.2X1	T42.2X2	T42.2X3	T42.2X4	T42.2X5	T42.2X6
Ethotoin	T42.ØX1	T42.ØX2	T42.ØX3	T42.ØX4	T42.ØX5	T42.ØX6
Ethoxazene	T37.91	T37.92	T37.93	T37.94	T37.95	T37.96
Ethoxazorutoside	T46.991	T46.992	T46.993	T46.994	T46.995	T46.996
Ethoxzolamide	T5Ø.2X1	T5Ø.2X2	T5Ø.2X3	T5Ø.2X4	T5Ø.2X5	T5Ø.2X6
Ethyl						
acetate	T52.8X1	T52.8X2	T52.8X3	T52.8X4	—	—
alcohol	T51.ØX1	T51.ØX2	T51.ØX3	T51.ØX4	—	—
beverage	T51.ØX1	T51.ØX2	T51.ØX3	T51.ØX4	—	—
aldehyde (vapor)	T59.891	T59.892	T59.893	T59.894	—	—
liquid	T52.8X1	T52.8X2	T52.8X3	T52.8X4	—	—
aminobenzoate	T41.3X1	T41.3X2	T41.3X3	T41.3X4	T41.3X5	T41.3X6
aminophenothiazine	T43.3X1	T43.3X2	T43.3X3	T43.3X4	T43.3X5	T43.3X6
benzoate	T52.8X1	T52.8X2	T52.8X3	T52.8X4	—	—
biscoumacetate	T45.511	T45.512	T45.513	T45.514	T45.515	T45.516
bromide (anesthetic)	T41.ØX1	T41.ØX2	T41.ØX3	T41.ØX4	T41.ØX5	T41.ØX6
carbamate	T45.1X1	T45.1X2	T45.1X3	T45.1X4	T45.1X5	T45.1X6
carbinol	T51.3X1	T51.3X2	T51.3X3	T51.3X4	—	—
carbonate	T52.8X1	T52.8X2	T52.8X3	T52.8X4	—	—
chaulmoograte	T37.1X1	T37.1X2	T37.1X3	T37.1X4	T37.1X5	T37.1X6
chloride (anesthetic)	T41.ØX1	T41.ØX2	T41.ØX3	T41.ØX4	T41.ØX5	T41.ØX6

Substance	Poisoning, Accidental (unintentional)	Poisoning, Intentional Self-harm	Poisoning, Assault	Poisoning, Undetermined	Adverse Effect	Under-dosing
Ethyl — *continued*						
chloride — *continued*						
anesthetic (local)	T41.3X1	T41.3X2	T41.3X3	T41.3X4	T41.3X5	T41.3X6
inhaled	T41.ØX1	T41.ØX2	T41.ØX3	T41.ØX4	T41.ØX5	T41.ØX6
local	T49.4X1	T49.4X2	T49.4X3	T49.4X4	T49.4X5	T49.4X6
solvent	T53.6X1	T53.6X2	T53.6X3	T53.6X4	—	—
dibunate	T48.3X1	T48.3X2	T48.3X3	T48.3X4	T48.3X5	T48.3X6
dichloroarsine (vapor)	T57.ØX1	T57.ØX2	T57.ØX3	T57.ØX4	—	—
estranol	T38.7X1	T38.7X2	T38.7X3	T38.7X4	T38.7X5	T38.7X6
ether — *see also* ether	T52.8X1	T52.8X2	T52.8X3	T52.8X4	—	—
formate NEC (solvent)	T52.ØX1	T52.ØX2	T52.ØX3	T52.ØX4	—	—
fumarate	T49.4X1	T49.4X2	T49.4X3	T49.4X4	T49.4X5	T49.4X6
hydroxyisobutyrate NEC (solvent)	T52.8X1	T52.8X2	T52.8X3	T52.8X4	—	—
iodoacetate	T59.3X1	T59.3X2	T59.3X3	T59.3X4	—	—
lactate NEC (solvent)	T52.8X1	T52.8X2	T52.8X3	T52.8X4	—	—
loflazepate	T42.4X1	T42.4X2	T42.4X3	T42.4X4	T42.4X5	T42.4X6
mercuric chloride	T56.1X1	T56.1X2	T56.1X3	T56.1X4	—	—
methylcarbinol	T51.8X1	T51.8X2	T51.8X3	T51.8X4	—	—
morphine	T4Ø.2X1	T4Ø.2X2	T4Ø.2X3	T4Ø.2X4	T4Ø.2X5	T4Ø.2X6
noradrenaline	T48.6X1	T48.6X2	T48.6X3	T48.6X4	T48.6X5	T48.6X6
oxybutyrate NEC (solvent)	T52.8X1	T52.8X2	T52.8X3	T52.8X4	—	—
Ethylene (gas)	T59.891	T59.892	T59.893	T59.894	—	—
anesthetic (general)	T41.ØX1	T41.ØX2	T41.ØX3	T41.ØX4	T41.ØX5	T41.ØX6
chlorohydrin	T52.8X1	T52.8X2	T52.8X3	T52.8X4	—	—
vapor	T53.6X1	T53.6X2	T53.6X3	T53.6X4	—	—
dichloride	T52.8X1	T52.8X2	T52.8X3	T52.8X4	—	—
vapor	T53.6X1	T53.6X2	T53.6X3	T53.6X4	—	—
dinitrate	T52.3X1	T52.3X2	T52.3X3	T52.3X4	—	—
glycol(s)	T52.8X1	T52.8X2	T52.8X3	T52.8X4	—	—
dinitrate	T52.3X1	T52.3X2	T52.3X3	T52.3X4	—	—
monobutyl ether	T52.3X1	T52.3X2	T52.3X3	T52.3X4	—	—
imine	T54.1X1	T54.1X2	T54.1X3	T54.1X4	—	—
oxide (fumigant) (nonmedicinal)	T59.891	T59.892	T59.893	T59.894	—	—
medicinal	T49.ØX1	T49.ØX2	T49.ØX3	T49.ØX4	T49.ØX5	T49.ØX6
Ethylenediaminetetra-acetic acid	T5Ø.6X1	T5Ø.6X2	T5Ø.6X3	T5Ø.6X4	T5Ø.6X5	T5Ø.6X6
Ethylenediamine theophylline	T48.6X1	T48.6X2	T48.6X3	T48.6X4	T48.6X5	T48.6X6
Ethylenedinitrilotetra-acetate	T5Ø.6X1	T5Ø.6X2	T5Ø.6X3	T5Ø.6X4	T5Ø.6X5	T5Ø.6X6
Ethylestrenol	T38.7X1	T38.7X2	T38.7X3	T38.7X4	T38.7X5	T38.7X6
Ethylhydroxycellulose	T47.4X1	T47.4X2	T47.4X3	T47.4X4	T47.4X5	T47.4X6
Ethylidene						
chloride NEC	T53.6X1	T53.6X2	T53.6X3	T53.6X4	—	—
diacetate	T6Ø.3X1	T6Ø.3X2	T6Ø.3X3	T6Ø.3X4	—	—
dicoumarin	T45.511	T45.512	T45.513	T45.514	T45.515	T45.516
dicoumarol	T45.511	T45.512	T45.513	T45.514	T45.515	T45.516
diethyl ether	T52.ØX1	T52.ØX2	T52.ØX3	T52.ØX4	—	—
Ethylmorphine	T4Ø.2X1	T4Ø.2X2	T4Ø.2X3	T4Ø.2X4	T4Ø.2X5	T4Ø.2X6
Ethylnorepinephrine	T48.6X1	T48.6X2	T48.6X3	T48.6X4	T48.6X5	T48.6X6
Ethylparachlorophen-oxyisobutyrate	T46.6X1	T46.6X2	T46.6X3	T46.6X4	T46.6X5	T46.6X6
Ethynodiol	T38.4X1	T38.4X2	T38.4X3	T38.4X4	T38.4X5	T38.4X6
with mestranol diacetate	T38.4X1	T38.4X2	T38.4X3	T38.4X4	T38.4X5	T38.4X6
Etidocaine	T41.3X1	T41.3X2	T41.3X3	T41.3X4	T41.3X5	T41.3X6
infiltration (subcutaneous)	T41.3X1	T41.3X2	T41.3X3	T41.3X4	T41.3X5	T41.3X6
nerve (peripheral) (plexus)	T41.3X1	T41.3X2	T41.3X3	T41.3X4	T41.3X5	T41.3X6
Etidronate	T5Ø.991	T5Ø.992	T5Ø.993	T5Ø.994	T5Ø.995	T5Ø.996
Etidronic acid (disodium salt)	T5Ø.991	T5Ø.992	T5Ø.993	T5Ø.994	T5Ø.995	T5Ø.996
Etifoxine	T42.6X1	T42.6X2	T42.6X3	T42.6X4	T42.6X5	T42.6X6
Etilefrine	T44.4X1	T44.4X2	T44.4X3	T44.4X4	T44.4X5	T44.4X6
Etilfen	T42.3X1	T42.3X2	T42.3X3	T42.3X4	T42.3X5	T42.3X6
Etinodiol	T38.4X1	T38.4X2	T38.4X3	T38.4X4	T38.4X5	T38.4X6
Etiroxate	T46.6X1	T46.6X2	T46.6X3	T46.6X4	T46.6X5	T46.6X6
Etizolam	T42.4X1	T42.4X2	T42.4X3	T42.4X4	T42.4X5	T42.4X6
Etodolac	T39.391	T39.392	T39.393	T39.394	T39.395	T39.396
Etofamide	T37.3X1	T37.3X2	T37.3X3	T37.3X4	T37.3X5	T37.3X6
Etofibrate	T46.6X1	T46.6X2	T46.6X3	T46.6X4	T46.6X5	T46.6X6
Etofylline	T46.7X1	T46.7X2	T46.7X3	T46.7X4	T46.7X5	T46.7X6
clofibrate	T46.6X1	T46.6X2	T46.6X3	T46.6X4	T46.6X5	T46.6X6
Etoglucid	T45.1X1	T45.1X2	T45.1X3	T45.1X4	T45.1X5	T45.1X6
Etomidate	T41.1X1	T41.1X2	T41.1X3	T41.1X4	T41.1X5	T41.1X6
Etomide	T39.8X1	T39.8X2	T39.8X3	T39.8X4	T39.8X5	T39.8X6
Etomidoline	T44.3X1	T44.3X2	T44.3X3	T44.3X4	T44.3X5	T44.3X6
Etoposide	T45.1X1	T45.1X2	T45.1X3	T45.1X4	T45.1X5	T45.1X6
Etorphine	T4Ø.2X1	T4Ø.2X2	T4Ø.2X3	T4Ø.2X4	T4Ø.2X5	T4Ø.2X6
Etoval	T42.3X1	T42.3X2	T42.3X3	T42.3X4	T42.3X5	T42.3X6
Etozolin	T5Ø.1X1	T5Ø.1X2	T5Ø.1X3	T5Ø.1X4	T5Ø.1X5	T5Ø.1X6
Etretinate	T5Ø.991	T5Ø.992	T5Ø.993	T5Ø.994	T5Ø.995	T5Ø.996
Etryptamine	T43.691	T43.692	T43.693	T43.694	T43.695	T43.696
Etybenzatropine	T44.3X1	T44.3X2	T44.3X3	T44.3X4	T44.3X5	T44.3X6

Substance	Poisoning, Accidental (unintentional)	Poisoning, Intentional Self-harm	Poisoning, Assault	Poisoning, Undetermined	Adverse Effect	Under-dosing
Etynodiol	T38.4X1	T38.4X2	T38.4X3	T38.4X4	T38.4X5	T38.4X6
Eucaine	T41.3X1	T41.3X2	T41.3X3	T41.3X4	T41.3X5	T41.3X6
Eucalyptus oil	T49.7X1	T49.7X2	T49.7X3	T49.7X4	T49.7X5	T49.7X6
Eucatropine	T49.5X1	T49.5X2	T49.5X3	T49.5X4	T49.5X5	T49.5X6
Eucodal	T40.2X1	T40.2X2	T40.2X3	T40.2X4	T40.2X5	T40.2X6
Euneryl	T42.3X1	T42.3X2	T42.3X3	T42.3X4	T42.3X5	T42.3X6
Euphthalmine	T44.3X1	T44.3X2	T44.3X3	T44.3X4	T44.3X5	T44.3X6
Eurax	T49.0X1	T49.0X2	T49.0X3	T49.0X4	T49.0X5	T49.0X6
Euresol	T49.4X1	T49.4X2	T49.4X3	T49.4X4	T49.4X5	T49.4X6
Euthroid	T38.1X1	T38.1X2	T38.1X3	T38.1X4	T38.1X5	T38.1X6
Evans blue	T50.8X1	T50.8X2	T50.8X3	T50.8X4	T50.8X5	T50.8X6
Evipal	T42.3X1	T42.3X2	T42.3X3	T42.3X4	T42.3X5	T42.3X6
sodium	T41.1X1	T41.1X2	T41.1X3	T41.1X4	T41.1X5	T41.1X6
Evipan	T42.3X1	T42.3X2	T42.3X3	T42.3X4	T42.3X5	T42.3X6
sodium	T41.1X1	T41.1X2	T41.1X3	T41.1X4	T41.1X5	T41.1X6
Exalamide	T49.0X1	T49.0X2	T49.0X3	T49.0X4	T49.0X5	T49.0X6
Exalgin	T39.1X1	T39.1X2	T39.1X3	T39.1X4	T39.1X5	T39.1X6
Excipients, pharmaceutical	T50.901	T50.902	T50.903	T50.904	T50.905	T50.906
Exhaust gas (engine) (motor vehicle)	T58.01	T58.02	T58.03	T58.04	—	—
Ex-Lax (phenolphthalein)	T47.2X1	T47.2X2	T47.2X3	T47.2X4	T47.2X5	T47.2X6
Expectorant NEC	T48.4X1	T48.4X2	T48.4X3	T48.4X4	T48.4X5	T48.4X6
Extended insulin zinc suspension	T38.3X1	T38.3X2	T38.3X3	T38.3X4	T38.3X5	T38.3X6
External medications (skin) (mucous membrane)	T49.91	T49.92	T49.93	T49.94	T49.95	T49.96
dental agent	T49.7X1	T49.7X2	T49.7X3	T49.7X4	T49.7X5	T49.7X6
ENT agent	T49.6X1	T49.6X2	T49.6X3	T49.6X4	T49.6X5	T49.6X6
ophthalmic preparation	T49.5X1	T49.5X2	T49.5X3	T49.5X4	T49.5X5	T49.5X6
specified NEC	T49.8X1	T49.8X2	T49.8X3	T49.8X4	T49.8X5	T49.8X6
Extrapyramidal antagonist NEC	T44.3X1	T44.3X2	T44.3X3	T44.3X4	T44.3X5	T44.3X6
Eye agents (anti-infective)	T49.5X1	T49.5X2	T49.5X3	T49.5X4	T49.5X5	T49.5X6
Eye drug NEC	T49.5X1	T49.5X2	T49.5X3	T49.5X4	T49.5X5	T49.5X6
FAC (fluorouracil + doxorubicin + cyclophosphamide)	T45.1X1	T45.1X2	T45.1X3	T45.1X4	T45.1X5	T45.1X6
Factor						
I (fibrinogen)	T45.8X1	T45.8X2	T45.8X3	T45.8X4	T45.8X5	T45.8X6
III (thromboplastin)	T45.8X1	T45.8X2	T45.8X3	T45.8X4	T45.8X5	T45.8X6
IX complex	T45.7X1	T45.7X2	T45.7X3	T45.7X4	T45.7X5	T45.7X6
human	T45.8X1	T45.8X2	T45.8X3	T45.8X4	T45.8X5	T45.8X6
VIII (antihemophilic Factor) (concentrate)	T45.8X1	T45.8X2	T45.8X3	T45.8X4	T45.8X5	T45.8X6
Famotidine	T47.0X1	T47.0X2	T47.0X3	T47.0X4	T47.0X5	T47.0X6
Fat suspension, intravenous	T50.991	T50.992	T50.993	T50.994	T50.995	T50.996
Fazadinium bromide	T48.1X1	T48.1X2	T48.1X3	T48.1X4	T48.1X5	T48.1X6
Febarbamate	T42.3X1	T42.3X2	T42.3X3	T42.3X4	T42.3X5	T42.3X6
Fecal softener	T47.4X1	T47.4X2	T47.4X3	T47.4X4	T47.4X5	T47.4X6
Fedrilate	T48.3X1	T48.3X2	T48.3X3	T48.3X4	T48.3X5	T48.3X6
Felodipine	T46.1X1	T46.1X2	T46.1X3	T46.1X4	T46.1X5	T46.1X6
Felypressin	T38.891	T38.892	T38.893	T38.894	T38.895	T38.896
Femoxetine	T43.221	T43.222	T43.223	T43.224	T43.225	T43.226
Fenalcomine	T46.3X1	T46.3X2	T46.3X3	T46.3X4	T46.3X5	T46.3X6
Fenamisal	T37.1X1	T37.1X2	T37.1X3	T37.1X4	T37.1X5	T37.1X6
Fenazone	T39.2X1	T39.2X2	T39.2X3	T39.2X4	T39.2X5	T39.2X6
Fenbendazole	T37.4X1	T37.4X2	T37.4X3	T37.4X4	T37.4X5	T37.4X6
Fenbutrazate	T50.5X1	T50.5X2	T50.5X3	T50.5X4	T50.5X5	T50.5X6
Fencamfamine	T43.691	T43.692	T43.693	T43.694	T43.695	T43.696
Fendiline	T46.1X1	T46.1X2	T46.1X3	T46.1X4	T46.1X5	T46.1X6
Fenetylline	T43.691	T43.692	T43.693	T43.694	T43.695	T43.696
Fenflumizole	T39.391	T39.392	T39.393	T39.394	T39.395	T39.396
Fenfluramine	T50.5X1	T50.5X2	T50.5X3	T50.5X4	T50.5X5	T50.5X6
Fenobarbital	T42.3X1	T42.3X2	T42.3X3	T42.3X4	T42.3X5	T42.3X6
Fenofibrate	T46.6X1	T46.6X2	T46.6X3	T46.6X4	T46.6X5	T46.6X6
Fenoprofen	T39.311	T39.312	T39.313	T39.314	T39.315	T39.316
Fenoterol	T48.6X1	T48.6X2	T48.6X3	T48.6X4	T48.6X5	T48.6X6
Fenoverine	T44.3X1	T44.3X2	T44.3X3	T44.3X4	T44.3X5	T44.3X6
Fenoxazoline	T48.5X1	T48.5X2	T48.5X3	T48.5X4	T48.5X5	T48.5X6
Fenproporex	T50.5X1	T50.5X2	T50.5X3	T50.5X4	T50.5X5	T50.5X6
Fenquizone	T50.2X1	T50.2X2	T50.2X3	T50.2X4	T50.2X5	T50.2X6
Fentanyl	T40.4X1	T40.4X2	T40.4X3	T40.4X4	T40.4X5	T40.4X6
Fentazin	T43.3X1	T43.3X2	T43.3X3	T43.3X4	T43.3X5	T43.3X6
Fenthion	T60.0X1	T60.0X2	T60.0X3	T60.0X4	—	—
Fenticlor	T49.0X1	T49.0X2	T49.0X3	T49.0X4	T49.0X5	T49.0X6
Fenylbutazone	T39.2X1	T39.2X2	T39.2X3	T39.2X4	T39.2X5	T39.2X6
Feprazone	T39.2X1	T39.2X2	T39.2X3	T39.2X4	T39.2X5	T39.2X6
Fer de lance (bite) (venom)	T63.061	T63.062	T63.063	T63.064	—	—
Ferric — *see also* Iron						
chloride	T45.4X1	T45.4X2	T45.4X3	T45.4X4	T45.4X5	T45.4X6
citrate	T45.4X1	T45.4X2	T45.4X3	T45.4X4	T45.4X5	T45.4X6
hydroxide						
colloidal	T45.4X1	T45.4X2	T45.4X3	T45.4X4	T45.4X5	T45.4X6
Ferric — *see also* Iron — *continued*						
hydroxide — *continued*						
polymaltose	T45.4X1	T45.4X2	T45.4X3	T45.4X4	T45.4X5	T45.4X6
pyrophosphate	T45.4X1	T45.4X2	T45.4X3	T45.4X4	T45.4X5	T45.4X6
Ferritin	T45.4X1	T45.4X2	T45.4X3	T45.4X4	T45.4X5	T45.4X6
Ferrocholinate	T45.4X1	T45.4X2	T45.4X3	T45.4X4	T45.4X5	T45.4X6
Ferrodextrane	T45.4X1	T45.4X2	T45.4X3	T45.4X4	T45.4X5	T45.4X6
Ferropolimaler	T45.4X1	T45.4X2	T45.4X3	T45.4X4	T45.4X5	T45.4X6
Ferrous — *see also* Iron						
phosphate	T45.4X1	T45.4X2	T45.4X3	T45.4X4	T45.4X5	T45.4X6
salt	T45.4X1	T45.4X2	T45.4X3	T45.4X4	T45.4X5	T45.4X6
with folic acid	T45.4X1	T45.4X2	T45.4X3	T45.4X4	T45.4X5	T45.4X6
Ferrous fumerate, gluconate, lactate, salt NEC, sulfate (medicinal)	T45.4X1	T45.4X2	T45.4X3	T45.4X4	T45.4X5	T45.4X6
Ferrovanadium (fumes)	T59.891	T59.892	T59.893	T59.894	—	—
Ferrum — *see* Iron						
Fertilizers NEC	T65.891	T65.892	T65.893	T65.894	—	—
with herbicide mixture	T60.3X1	T60.3X2	T60.3X3	T60.3X4	—	—
Fetoxilate	T47.6X1	T47.6X2	T47.6X3	T47.6X4	T47.6X5	T47.6X6
Fiber, dietary	T47.4X1	T47.4X2	T47.4X3	T47.4X4	T47.4X5	T47.4X6
Fiberglass	T65.831	T65.832	T65.833	T65.834	—	—
Fibrinogen (human)	T45.8X1	T45.8X2	T45.8X3	T45.8X4	T45.8X5	T45.8X6
Fibrinolysin (human)	T45.691	T45.692	T45.693	T45.694	T45.695	T45.696
Fibrinolysis						
affecting drug	T45.601	T45.602	T45.603	T45.604	T45.605	T45.606
inhibitor NEC	T45.621	T45.622	T45.623	T45.624	T45.625	T45.626
Fibrinolytic drug	T45.611	T45.612	T45.613	T45.614	T45.615	T45.616
Filix mas	T37.4X1	T37.4X2	T37.4X3	T37.4X4	T37.4X5	T37.4X6
Filtering cream	T49.3X1	T49.3X2	T49.3X3	T49.3X4	T49.3X5	T49.3X6
Fiorinal	T39.011	T39.012	T39.013	T39.014	T39.015	T39.016
Firedamp	T59.891	T59.892	T59.893	T59.894	—	—
Fish, noxious, nonbacterial	T61.91	T61.92	T61.93	T61.94	—	—
ciguatera	T61.01	T61.02	T61.03	T61.04	—	—
scombroid	T61.11	T61.12	T61.13	T61.14	—	—
shell	T61.781	T61.782	T61.783	T61.784	—	—
specified NEC	T61.771	T61.772	T61.773	T61.774	—	—
Flagyl	T37.3X1	T37.3X2	T37.3X3	T37.3X4	T37.3X5	T37.3X6
Flavine adenine dinucleotide	T45.2X1	T45.2X2	T45.2X3	T45.2X4	T45.2X5	T45.2X6
Flavodic acid	T46.991	T46.992	T46.993	T46.994	T46.995	T46.996
Flavoxate	T44.3X1	T44.3X2	T44.3X3	T44.3X4	T44.3X5	T44.3X6
Flaxedil	T48.1X1	T48.1X2	T48.1X3	T48.1X4	T48.1X5	T48.1X6
Flaxseed (medicinal)	T49.3X1	T49.3X2	T49.3X3	T49.3X4	T49.3X5	T49.3X6
Flecainide	T46.2X1	T46.2X2	T46.2X3	T46.2X4	T46.2X5	T46.2X6
Fleroxacin	T36.8X1	T36.8X2	T36.8X3	T36.8X4	T36.8X5	T36.8X6
Floctafenine	T39.8X1	T39.8X2	T39.8X3	T39.8X4	T39.8X5	T39.8X6
Flomax	T44.6X1	T44.6X2	T44.6X3	T44.6X4	T44.6X5	T44.6X6
Flomoxef	T36.1X1	T36.1X2	T36.1X3	T36.1X4	T36.1X5	T36.1X6
Flopropione	T44.3X1	T44.3X2	T44.3X3	T44.3X4	T44.3X5	T44.3X6
Florantyrone	T47.5X1	T47.5X2	T47.5X3	T47.5X4	T47.5X5	T47.5X6
Floraquin	T37.8X1	T37.8X2	T37.8X3	T37.8X4	T37.8X5	T37.8X6
Florinef	T38.0X1	T38.0X2	T38.0X3	T38.0X4	T38.0X5	T38.0X6
ENT agent	T49.6X1	T49.6X2	T49.6X3	T49.6X4	T49.6X5	T49.6X6
ophthalmic preparation	T49.5X1	T49.5X2	T49.5X3	T49.5X4	T49.5X5	T49.5X6
topical NEC	T49.0X1	T49.0X2	T49.0X3	T49.0X4	T49.0X5	T49.0X6
Flowers of sulfur	T49.4X1	T49.4X2	T49.4X3	T49.4X4	T49.4X5	T49.4X6
Floxuridine	T45.1X1	T45.1X2	T45.1X3	T45.1X4	T45.1X5	T45.1X6
Fluanisone	T43.4X1	T43.4X2	T43.4X3	T43.4X4	T43.4X5	T43.4X6
Flubendazole	T37.4X1	T37.4X2	T37.4X3	T37.4X4	T37.4X5	T37.4X6
Fluclorolone acetonide	T49.0X1	T49.0X2	T49.0X3	T49.0X4	T49.0X5	T49.0X6
Flucloxacillin	T36.0X1	T36.0X2	T36.0X3	T36.0X4	T36.0X5	T36.0X6
Fluconazole	T37.8X1	T37.8X2	T37.8X3	T37.8X4	T37.8X5	T37.8X6
Flucytosine	T37.8X1	T37.8X2	T37.8X3	T37.8X4	T37.8X5	T37.8X6
Fludeoxyglucose (18F)	T50.8X1	T50.8X2	T50.8X3	T50.8X4	T50.8X5	T50.8X6
Fludiazepam	T42.4X1	T42.4X2	T42.4X3	T42.4X4	T42.4X5	T42.4X6
Fludrocortisone	T50.0X1	T50.0X2	T50.0X3	T50.0X4	T50.0X5	T50.0X6
ENT agent	T49.6X1	T49.6X2	T49.6X3	T49.6X4	T49.6X5	T49.6X6
ophthalmic preparation	T49.5X1	T49.5X2	T49.5X3	T49.5X4	T49.5X5	T49.5X6
topical NEC	T49.0X1	T49.0X2	T49.0X3	T49.0X4	T49.0X5	T49.0X6
Fludroxycortide	T49.0X1	T49.0X2	T49.0X3	T49.0X4	T49.0X5	T49.0X6
Flufenamic acid	T39.391	T39.392	T39.393	T39.394	T39.395	T39.396
Fluindione	T45.511	T45.512	T45.513	T45.514	T45.515	T45.516
Flumequine	T37.8X1	T37.8X2	T37.8X3	T37.8X4	T37.8X5	T37.8X6
Flumethasone	T49.0X1	T49.0X2	T49.0X3	T49.0X4	T49.0X5	T49.0X6
Flumethiazide	T50.2X1	T50.2X2	T50.2X3	T50.2X4	T50.2X5	T50.2X6
Flumidin	T37.5X1	T37.5X2	T37.5X3	T37.5X4	T37.5X5	T37.5X6
Flunarizine	T46.7X1	T46.7X2	T46.7X3	T46.7X4	T46.7X5	T46.7X6
Flunidazole	T37.8X1	T37.8X2	T37.8X3	T37.8X4	T37.8X5	T37.8X6
Flunisolide	T48.6X1	T48.6X2	T48.6X3	T48.6X4	T48.6X5	T48.6X6
Flunitrazepam	T42.4X1	T42.4X2	T42.4X3	T42.4X4	T42.4X5	T42.4X6
Fluocinolone (acetonide)	T49.0X1	T49.0X2	T49.0X3	T49.0X4	T49.0X5	T49.0X6
Fluocinonide	T49.0X1	T49.0X2	T49.0X3	T49.0X4	T49.0X5	T49.0X6

Substance	Poisoning, Accidental (unintentional)	Poisoning, Intentional Self-harm	Poisoning, Assault	Poisoning, Undetermined	Adverse Effect	Under-dosing
Fluocortin (butyl)	T49.0X1	T49.0X2	T49.0X3	T49.0X4	T49.0X5	T49.0X6
Fluocortolone	T49.0X1	T49.0X2	T49.0X3	T49.0X4	T49.0X5	T49.0X6
Fluohydrocortisone	T38.0X1	T38.0X2	T38.0X3	T38.0X4	T38.0X5	T38.0X6
ENT agent	T49.6X1	T49.6X2	T49.6X3	T49.6X4	T49.6X5	T49.6X6
ophthalmic preparation	T49.5X1	T49.5X2	T49.5X3	T49.5X4	T49.5X5	T49.5X6
topical NEC	T49.0X1	T49.0X2	T49.0X3	T49.0X4	T49.0X5	T49.0X6
Fluonid	T49.0X1	T49.0X2	T49.0X3	T49.0X4	T49.0X5	T49.0X6
Fluopromazine	T43.3X1	T43.3X2	T43.3X3	T43.3X4	T43.3X5	T43.3X6
Fluoracetate	T60.8X1	T60.8X2	T60.8X3	T60.8X4	—	—
Fluorescein	T50.8X1	T50.8X2	T50.8X3	T50.8X4	T50.8X5	T50.8X6
Fluorhydrocortisone	T50.0X1	T50.0X2	T50.0X3	T50.0X4	T50.0X5	T50.0X6
Fluoride (nonmedicinal) (pesticide) (sodium) **NEC**	T60.8X1	T60.8X2	T60.8X3	T60.8X4	—	—
hydrogen — *see* Hydrofluoric acid						
medicinal NEC	T50.991	T50.992	T50.993	T50.994	T50.995	T50.996
dental use	T49.7X1	T49.7X2	T49.7X3	T49.7X4	T49.7X5	T49.7X6
not pesticide NEC	T54.91	T54.92	T54.93	T54.94	—	—
stannous	T49.7X1	T49.7X2	T49.7X3	T49.7X4	T49.7X5	T49.7X6
Fluorinated corticosteroids	T38.0X1	T38.0X2	T38.0X3	T38.0X4	T38.0X5	T38.0X6
Fluorine (gas)	T59.5X1	T59.5X2	T59.5X3	T59.5X4	—	—
salt — *see* Fluoride(s)						
Fluoristan	T49.7X1	T49.7X2	T49.7X3	T49.7X4	T49.7X5	T49.7X6
Fluormetholone	T49.0X1	T49.0X2	T49.0X3	T49.0X4	T49.0X5	T49.0X6
Fluoroacetate	T60.8X1	T60.8X2	T60.8X3	T60.8X4	—	—
Fluorocarbon monomer	T53.6X1	T53.6X2	T53.6X3	T53.6X4	—	—
Fluorocytosine	T37.8X1	T37.8X2	T37.8X3	T37.8X4	T37.8X5	T37.8X6
Fluorodeoxyuridine	T45.1X1	T45.1X2	T45.1X3	T45.1X4	T45.1X5	T45.1X6
Fluorometholone	T49.0X1	T49.0X2	T49.0X3	T49.0X4	T49.0X5	T49.0X6
ophthalmic preparation	T49.5X1	T49.5X2	T49.5X3	T49.5X4	T49.5X5	T49.5X6
Fluorophosphate insecticide	T60.0X1	T60.0X2	T60.0X3	T60.0X4	—	—
Fluorosol	T46.3X1	T46.3X2	T46.3X3	T46.3X4	T46.3X5	T46.3X6
Fluorouracil	T45.1X1	T45.1X2	T45.1X3	T45.1X4	T45.1X5	T45.1X6
Fluorphenylalanine	T49.5X1	T49.5X2	T49.5X3	T49.5X4	T49.5X5	T49.5X6
Fluothane	T41.0X1	T41.0X2	T41.0X3	T41.0X4	T41.0X5	T41.0X6
Fluoxetine	T43.221	T43.222	T43.223	T43.224	T43.225	T43.226
Fluoxymesterone	T38.7X1	T38.7X2	T38.7X3	T38.7X4	T38.7X5	T38.7X6
Flupenthixol	T43.4X1	T43.4X2	T43.4X3	T43.4X4	T43.4X5	T43.4X6
Flupentixol	T43.4X1	T43.4X2	T43.4X3	T43.4X4	T43.4X5	T43.4X6
Fluphenazine	T43.3X1	T43.3X2	T43.3X3	T43.3X4	T43.3X5	T43.3X6
Fluprednidene	T49.0X1	T49.0X2	T49.0X3	T49.0X4	T49.0X5	T49.0X6
Fluprednisolone	T38.0X1	T38.0X2	T38.0X3	T38.0X4	T38.0X5	T38.0X6
Fluradoline	T39.8X1	T39.8X2	T39.8X3	T39.8X4	T39.8X5	T39.8X6
Flurandrenolide	T49.0X1	T49.0X2	T49.0X3	T49.0X4	T49.0X5	T49.0X6
Flurandrenolone	T49.0X1	T49.0X2	T49.0X3	T49.0X4	T49.0X5	T49.0X6
Flurazepam	T42.4X1	T42.4X2	T42.4X3	T42.4X4	T42.4X5	T42.4X6
Flurbiprofen	T39.311	T39.312	T39.313	T39.314	T39.315	T39.316
Flurobate	T49.0X1	T49.0X2	T49.0X3	T49.0X4	T49.0X5	T49.0X6
Fluroxene	T41.0X1	T41.0X2	T41.0X3	T41.0X4	T41.0X5	T41.0X6
Fluspirilene	T43.591	T43.592	T43.593	T43.594	T43.595	T43.596
Flutamide	T38.6X1	T38.6X2	T38.6X3	T38.6X4	T38.6X5	T38.6X6
Flutazolam	T42.4X1	T42.4X2	T42.4X3	T42.4X4	T42.4X5	T42.4X6
Fluticasone propionate	T49.1X1	T49.1X2	T49.1X3	T49.1X4	T49.1X5	T49.1X6
Flutoprazepam	T42.4X1	T42.4X2	T42.4X3	T42.4X4	T42.4X5	T42.4X6
Flutropium bromide	T48.6X1	T48.6X2	T48.6X3	T48.6X4	T48.6X5	T48.6X6
Fluvoxamine	T43.221	T43.222	T43.223	T43.224	T43.225	T43.226
Folacin	T45.8X1	T45.8X2	T45.8X3	T45.8X4	T45.8X5	T45.8X6
Folic acid	T45.8X1	T45.8X2	T45.8X3	T45.8X4	T45.8X5	T45.8X6
with ferrous salt	T45.2X1	T45.2X2	T45.2X3	T45.2X4	T45.2X5	T45.2X6
antagonist	T45.1X1	T45.1X2	T45.1X3	T45.1X4	T45.1X5	T45.1X6
Folinic acid	T45.8X1	T45.8X2	T45.8X3	T45.8X4	T45.8X5	T45.8X6
Folium stramoniae	T48.6X1	T48.6X2	T48.6X3	T48.6X4	T48.6X5	T48.6X6
Follicle-stimulating hormone, human	T38.811	T38.812	T38.813	T38.814	T38.815	T38.816
Folpet	T60.3X1	T60.3X2	T60.3X3	T60.3X4	—	—
Fominoben	T48.3X1	T48.3X2	T48.3X3	T48.3X4	T48.3X5	T48.3X6
Food, foodstuffs, noxious, nonbacterial, NEC	T62.91	T62.92	T62.93	T62.94	—	—
berries	T62.1X1	T62.1X2	T62.1X3	T62.1X4	—	—
fish — *see also* Fish	T61.91	T61.92	T61.93	T61.94	—	—
mushrooms	T62.0X1	T62.0X2	T62.0X3	T62.0X4	—	—
plants	T62.2X1	T62.2X2	T62.2X3	T62.2X4	—	—
seafood	T61.91	T61.92	T61.93	T61.94	—	—
specified NEC	T61.8X1	T61.8X2	T61.8X3	T61.8X4	—	—
seeds	T62.2X1	T62.2X2	T62.2X3	T62.2X4	—	—
shellfish	T61.781	T61.782	T61.783	T61.784	—	—
specified NEC	T62.8X1	T62.8X2	T62.8X3	T62.8X4	—	—
Fool's parsley	T62.2X1	T62.2X2	T62.2X3	T62.2X4	—	—
Formaldehyde (solution), gas or vapor	T59.2X1	T59.2X2	T59.2X3	T59.2X4	—	—
fungicide	T60.3X1	T60.3X2	T60.3X3	T60.3X4	—	—
Formalin	T59.2X1	T59.2X2	T59.2X3	T59.2X4	—	—
Formalin — *continued*						
fungicide	T60.3X1	T60.3X2	T60.3X3	T60.3X4	—	—
vapor	T59.2X1	T59.2X2	T59.2X3	T59.2X4	—	—
Formic acid	T54.2X1	T54.2X2	T54.2X3	T54.2X4	—	—
vapor	T59.891	T59.892	T59.893	T59.894	—	—
Foscarnet sodium	T37.5X1	T37.5X2	T37.5X3	T37.5X4	T37.5X5	T37.5X6
Fosfestrol	T38.5X1	T38.5X2	T38.5X3	T38.5X4	T38.5X5	T38.5X6
Fosfomycin	T36.8X1	T36.8X2	T36.8X3	T36.8X4	T36.8X5	T36.8X6
Fosfonet sodium	T37.5X1	T37.5X2	T37.5X3	T37.5X4	T37.5X5	T37.5X6
Fosinopril	T46.4X1	T46.4X2	T46.4X3	T46.4X4	T46.4X5	T46.4X6
sodium	T46.4X1	T46.4X2	T46.4X3	T46.4X4	T46.4X5	T46.4X6
Fowler's solution	T57.0X1	T57.0X2	T57.0X3	T57.0X4	—	—
Foxglove	T62.2X1	T62.2X2	T62.2X3	T62.2X4	—	—
Framycetin	T36.5X1	T36.5X2	T36.5X3	T36.5X4	T36.5X5	T36.5X6
Frangula	T47.2X1	T47.2X2	T47.2X3	T47.2X4	T47.2X5	T47.2X6
extract	T47.2X1	T47.2X2	T47.2X3	T47.2X4	T47.2X5	T47.2X6
Frei antigen	T50.8X1	T50.8X2	T50.8X3	T50.8X4	T50.8X5	T50.8X6
Freon	T53.5X1	T53.5X2	T53.5X3	T53.5X4	—	—
Fructose	T50.3X1	T50.3X2	T50.3X3	T50.3X4	T50.3X5	T50.3X6
Frusemide	T50.1X1	T50.1X2	T50.1X3	T50.1X4	T50.1X5	T50.1X6
FSH	T38.811	T38.812	T38.813	T38.814	T38.815	T38.816
Ftorafur	T45.1X1	T45.1X2	T45.1X3	T45.1X4	T45.1X5	T45.1X6
Fuel						
automobile	T52.0X1	T52.0X2	T52.0X3	T52.0X4	—	—
exhaust gas, not in transit	T58.01	T58.02	T58.03	T58.04	—	—
vapor NEC	T52.0X1	T52.0X2	T52.0X3	T52.0X4	—	—
gas (domestic use) — *see also* Carbon, monoxide, fuel, utility	T59.891	T59.892	T59.893	T59.894	—	—
utility	T59.891	T59.892	T59.893	T59.894	—	—
incomplete combustion of — *see* Carbon, monoxide, fuel, utility						
in mobile container	T59.891	T59.892	T59.893	T59.894	—	—
piped (natural)	T59.891	T59.892	T59.893	T59.894	—	—
industrial, incomplete combustion	T58.8X1	T58.8X2	T58.8X3	T58.8X4	—	—
Fugillin	T36.8X1	T36.8X2	T36.8X3	T36.8X4	T36.8X5	T36.8X6
Fulminate of mercury	T56.1X1	T56.1X2	T56.1X3	T56.1X4	—	—
Fulvicin	T36.7X1	T36.7X2	T36.7X3	T36.7X4	T36.7X5	T36.7X6
Fumadil	T36.8X1	T36.8X2	T36.8X3	T36.8X4	T36.8X5	T36.8X6
Fumagillin	T36.8X1	T36.8X2	T36.8X3	T36.8X4	T36.8X5	T36.8X6
Fumaric acid	T49.4X1	T49.4X2	T49.4X3	T49.4X4	T49.4X5	T49.4X6
Fumes (from)	T59.91	T59.92	T59.93	T59.94	—	—
carbon monoxide — *see* Carbon, monoxide						
charcoal (domestic use) — *see* Charcoal, fumes						
chloroform — *see* Chloroform						
coke (in domestic stoves, fireplaces) — *see* Coke fumes						
corrosive NEC	T54.91	T54.92	T54.93	T54.94	—	—
ether — *see* ether						
freons	T53.5X1	T53.5X2	T53.5X3	T53.5X4	—	—
hydrocarbons	T59.891	T59.892	T59.893	T59.894	—	—
petroleum (liquefied)	T59.891	T59.892	T59.893	T59.894	—	—
distributed through pipes (pure or mixed with air)	T59.891	T59.892	T59.893	T59.894	—	—
lead — *see* lead						
metal — *see* Metals, or the specified metal						
nitrogen dioxide	T59.0X1	T59.0X2	T59.0X3	T59.0X4	—	—
pesticides — *see* Pesticides						
petroleum (liquefied)	T59.891	T59.892	T59.893	T59.894	—	—
distributed through pipes (pure or mixed with air)	T59.891	T59.892	T59.893	T59.894	—	—
polyester	T59.891	T59.892	T59.893	T59.894	—	—
specified source NEC — *see also* substance specified	T59.891	T59.892	T59.893	T59.894	—	—
sulfur dioxide	T59.1X1	T59.1X2	T59.1X3	T59.1X4	—	—
Fumigant NEC	T60.91	T60.92	T60.93	T60.94	—	—
Fungicide NEC (nonmedicinal)	T60.3X1	T60.3X2	T60.3X3	T60.3X4	—	—
Fungi, noxious, used as food	T62.0X1	T62.0X2	T62.0X3	T62.0X4	—	—
Fungizone	T36.7X1	T36.7X2	T36.7X3	T36.7X4	T36.7X5	T36.7X6
topical	T49.0X1	T49.0X2	T49.0X3	T49.0X4	T49.0X5	T49.0X6
Furacin	T49.0X1	T49.0X2	T49.0X3	T49.0X4	T49.0X5	T49.0X6
Furadantin	T37.91	T37.92	T37.93	T37.94	T37.95	T37.96
Furazolidone	T37.8X1	T37.8X2	T37.8X3	T37.8X4	T37.8X5	T37.8X6

Substance	Poisoning, Accidental (unintentional)	Poisoning, Intentional Self-harm	Poisoning, Assault	Poisoning, Undetermined	Adverse Effect	Under-dosing
Furazolium chloride	T49.ØX1	T49.ØX2	T49.ØX3	T49.ØX4	T49.ØX5	T49.ØX6
Furfural	T52.8X1	T52.8X2	T52.8X3	T52.8X4	—	—
Furnace (coal burning) (domestic), gas from	T58.2X1	T58.2X2	T58.2X3	T58.2X4	—	—
industrial	T58.8X1	T58.8X2	T58.8X3	T58.8X4	—	—
Furniture polish	T65.891	T65.892	T65.893	T65.894	—	—
Furosemide	T5Ø.1X1	T5Ø.1X2	T5Ø.1X3	T5Ø.1X4	T5Ø.1X5	T5Ø.1X6
Furoxone	T37.91	T37.92	T37.93	T37.94	T37.95	T37.96
Fursultiamine	T45.2X1	T45.2X2	T45.2X3	T45.2X4	T45.2X5	T45.2X6
Fusafungine	T36.8X1	T36.8X2	T36.8X3	T36.8X4	T36.8X5	T36.8X6
Fusel oil (any) (amyl) (butyl) (propyl), vapor	T51.3X1	T51.3X2	T51.3X3	T51.3X4	—	—
Fusidate (ethanolamine) (sodium)	T36.8X1	T36.8X2	T36.8X3	T36.8X4	T36.8X5	T36.8X6
Fusidic acid	T36.8X1	T36.8X2	T36.8X3	T36.8X4	T36.8X5	T36.8X6
Fytic acid, nonasodium	T5Ø.6X1	T5Ø.6X2	T5Ø.6X3	T5Ø.6X4	T5Ø.6X5	T5Ø.6X6
b-Galactosidase	T47.5X1	T47.5X2	T47.5X3	T47.5X4	T47.5X5	T47.5X6
GABA	T43.8X1	T43.8X2	T43.8X3	T43.8X4	T43.8X5	T43.8X6
Gadopentetic acid	T5Ø.8X1	T5Ø.8X2	T5Ø.8X3	T5Ø.8X4	T5Ø.8X5	T5Ø.8X6
Galactose	T5Ø.3X1	T5Ø.3X2	T5Ø.3X3	T5Ø.3X4	T5Ø.3X5	T5Ø.3X6
Galantamine	T44.ØX1	T44.ØX2	T44.ØX3	T44.ØX4	T44.ØX5	T44.ØX6
Gallamine (triethiodide)	T48.1X1	T48.1X2	T48.1X3	T48.1X4	T48.1X5	T48.1X6
Gallium citrate	T5Ø.991	T5Ø.992	T5Ø.993	T5Ø.994	T5Ø.995	T5Ø.996
Gallopamil	T46.1X1	T46.1X2	T46.1X3	T46.1X4	T46.1X5	T46.1X6
Gamboge	T47.2X1	T47.2X2	T47.2X3	T47.2X4	T47.2X5	T47.2X6
Gamimune	T5Ø.Z11	T5Ø.Z12	T5Ø.Z13	T5Ø.Z14	T5Ø.Z15	T5Ø.Z16
Gamma-aminobutyric acid	T43.8X1	T43.8X2	T43.8X3	T43.8X4	T43.8X5	T43.8X6
Gamma-benzene hexachloride (medicinal)	T49.ØX1	T49.ØX2	T49.ØX3	T49.ØX4	T49.ØX5	T49.ØX6
nonmedicinal, vapor	T53.6X1	T53.6X2	T53.6X3	T53.6X4	—	—
Gamma-BHC (medicinal) — *see also* Gamma-benzene hexachloride	T49.ØX1	T49.ØX2	T49.ØX3	T49.ØX4	T49.ØX5	T49.ØX6
Gamma globulin	T5Ø.Z11	T5Ø.Z12	T5Ø.Z13	T5Ø.Z14	T5Ø.Z15	T5Ø.Z16
Gamulin	T5Ø.Z11	T5Ø.Z12	T5Ø.Z13	T5Ø.Z14	T5Ø.Z15	T5Ø.Z16
Ganciclovir (sodium)	T37.5X1	T37.5X2	T37.5X3	T37.5X4	T37.5X5	T37.5X6
Ganglionic blocking drug NEC	T44.2X1	T44.2X2	T44.2X3	T44.2X4	T44.2X5	T44.2X6
specified NEC	T44.2X1	T44.2X2	T44.2X3	T44.2X4	T44.2X5	T44.2X6
Ganja	T4Ø.7X1	T4Ø.7X2	T4Ø.7X3	T4Ø.7X4	T4Ø.7X5	T4Ø.7X6
Garamycin	T36.5X1	T36.5X2	T36.5X3	T36.5X4	T36.5X5	T36.5X6
ophthalmic preparation	T49.5X1	T49.5X2	T49.5X3	T49.5X4	T49.5X5	T49.5X6
topical NEC	T49.ØX1	T49.ØX2	T49.ØX3	T49.ØX4	T49.ØX5	T49.ØX6
Gardenal	T42.3X1	T42.3X2	T42.3X3	T42.3X4	T42.3X5	T42.3X6
Gardepanyl	T42.3X1	T42.3X2	T42.3X3	T42.3X4	T42.3X5	T42.3X6
Gas	T59.91	T59.92	T59.93	T59.94	—	—
acetylene	T59.891	T59.892	T59.893	T59.894	—	—
incomplete combustion of	T58.11	T58.12	T58.13	T58.14	—	—
air contaminants, source or type not specified	T59.91	T59.92	T59.93	T59.94	—	—
anesthetic	T41.ØX1	T41.ØX2	T41.ØX3	T41.ØX4	T41.ØX5	T41.ØX6
blast furnace	T58.8X1	T58.8X2	T58.8X3	T58.8X4	—	—
butane — *see* butane						
carbon monoxide — *see* Carbon, monoxide						
chlorine	T59.4X1	T59.4X2	T59.4X3	T59.4X4	—	—
coal	T58.2X1	T58.2X2	T58.2X3	T58.2X4	—	—
cyanide	T57.3X1	T57.3X2	T57.3X3	T57.3X4	—	—
dicyanogen	T65.ØX1	T65.ØX2	T65.ØX3	T65.ØX4	—	—
domestic — *see* Domestic gas						
exhaust	T58.Ø1	T58.Ø2	T58.Ø3	T58.Ø4	—	—
from utility (for cooking, heating, or lighting) (after combustion) — *see* Carbon, monoxide, fuel, utility						
prior to combustion	T59.891	T59.892	T59.893	T59.894	—	—
from wood- or coal-burning stove or fireplace	T58.2X1	T58.2X2	T58.2X3	T58.2X4	—	—
fuel (domestic use) (after combustion) — *see also* Carbon, monoxide, fuel						
industrial use	T58.8X1	T58.8X2	T58.8X3	T58.8X4	—	—
prior to combustion	T59.891	T59.892	T59.893	T59.894	—	—
utility	T59.891	T59.892	T59.893	T59.894	—	—
incomplete combustion of — *see* Carbon, monoxide, fuel, utility						
in mobile container	T59.891	T59.892	T59.893	T59.894	—	—
piped (natural)	T59.891	T59.892	T59.893	T59.894	—	—
garage	T58.Ø1	T58.Ø2	T58.Ø3	T58.Ø4	—	—
hydrocarbon NEC	T59.891	T59.892	T59.893	T59.894	—	—
Gas — *continued*						
hydrocarbon — *continued*						
incomplete combustion of — *see* Carbon, monoxide, fuel, utility						
liquefied — *see* butane						
piped	T59.891	T59.892	T59.893	T59.894	—	—
hydrocyanic acid	T65.ØX1	T65.ØX2	T65.ØX3	T65.ØX4	—	—
illuminating (after combustion)	T58.11	T58.12	T58.13	T58.14	—	—
prior to combustion	T59.891	T59.892	T59.893	T59.894	—	—
incomplete combustion, any — *see* Carbon, monoxide						
kiln	T58.8X1	T58.8X2	T58.8X3	T58.8X4	—	—
lacrimogenic	T59.3X1	T59.3X2	T59.3X3	T59.3X4	—	—
liquefied petroleum — *see* butane						
marsh	T59.891	T59.892	T59.893	T59.894	—	—
motor exhaust, not in transit	T58.Ø1	T58.Ø2	T58.Ø3	T58.Ø4	—	—
mustard, not in war	T59.891	T59.892	T59.893	T59.894	—	—
natural	T59.891	T59.892	T59.893	T59.894	—	—
nerve, not in war	T59.91	T59.92	T59.93	T59.94	—	—
oil	T52.ØX1	T52.ØX2	T52.ØX3	T52.ØX4	—	—
petroleum (liquefied) (distributed in mobile containers)	T59.891	T59.892	T59.893	T59.894	—	—
piped (pure or mixed with air)	T59.891	T59.892	T59.893	T59.894	—	—
piped (manufactured) (natural) NEC	T59.891	T59.892	T59.893	T59.894	—	—
producer	T58.8X1	T58.8X2	T58.8X3	T58.8X4	—	—
propane — *see* propane						
refrigerant (chlorofluoro-carbon)	T53.5X1	T53.5X2	T53.5X3	T53.5X4	—	—
not chlorofluoro-carbon	T59.891	T59.892	T59.893	T59.894	—	—
sewer	T59.91	T59.92	T59.93	T59.94	—	—
specified source NEC	T59.91	T59.92	T59.93	T59.94	—	—
stove (after combustion)	T58.11	T58.12	T58.13	T58.14	—	—
prior to combustion	T59.891	T59.892	T59.893	T59.894	—	—
tear	T59.3X1	T59.3X2	T59.3X3	T59.3X4	—	—
therapeutic	T41.5X1	T41.5X2	T41.5X3	T41.5X4	T41.5X5	T41.5X6
utility (for cooking, heating, or lighting) (piped) NEC	T59.891	T59.892	T59.893	T59.894	—	—
incomplete combustion of — *see* Carbon, monoxide, fuel, utilty						
in mobile container	T59.891	T59.892	T59.893	T59.894	—	—
piped (natural)	T59.891	T59.892	T59.893	T59.894	—	—
water	T58.11	T58.12	T58.13	T58.14	—	—
incomplete combustion of — *see* Carbon, monoxide, fuel, utility						
Gaseous substance — *see* Gas						
Gasoline	T52.ØX1	T52.ØX2	T52.ØX3	T52.ØX4	—	—
vapor	T52.ØX1	T52.ØX2	T52.ØX3	T52.ØX4	—	—
Gastric enzymes	T47.5X1	T47.5X2	T47.5X3	T47.5X4	T47.5X5	T47.5X6
Gastrografin	T5Ø.8X1	T5Ø.8X2	T5Ø.8X3	T5Ø.8X4	T5Ø.8X5	T5Ø.8X6
Gastrointestinal drug	T47.91	T47.92	T47.93	T47.94	T47.95	T47.96
biological	T47.8X1	T47.8X2	T47.8X3	T47.8X4	T47.8X5	T47.8X6
specified NEC	T47.8X1	T47.8X2	T47.8X3	T47.8X4	T47.8X5	T47.8X6
Gaultheria procumbens	T62.2X1	T62.2X2	T62.2X3	T62.2X4	—	—
Gefarnate	T44.3X1	T44.3X2	T44.3X3	T44.3X4	T44.3X5	T44.3X6
Gelatin (intravenous)	T45.8X1	T45.8X2	T45.8X3	T45.8X4	T45.8X5	T45.8X6
absorbable (sponge)	T45.7X1	T45.7X2	T45.7X3	T45.7X4	T45.7X5	T45.7X6
Gelfilm	T49.8X1	T49.8X2	T49.8X3	T49.8X4	T49.8X5	T49.8X6
Gelfoam	T45.7X1	T45.7X2	T45.7X3	T45.7X4	T45.7X5	T45.7X6
Gelsemine	T5Ø.991	T5Ø.992	T5Ø.993	T5Ø.994	T5Ø.995	T5Ø.996
Gelsemium (sempervirens)	T62.2X1	T62.2X2	T62.2X3	T62.2X4	—	—
Gemeprost	T48.ØX1	T48.ØX2	T48.ØX3	T48.ØX4	T48.ØX5	T48.ØX6
Gemfibrozil	T46.6X1	T46.6X2	T46.6X3	T46.6X4	T46.6X5	T46.6X6
Gemonil	T42.3X1	T42.3X2	T42.3X3	T42.3X4	T42.3X5	T42.3X6
Gentamicin	T36.5X1	T36.5X2	T36.5X3	T36.5X4	T36.5X5	T36.5X6
ophthalmic preparation	T49.5X1	T49.5X2	T49.5X3	T49.5X4	T49.5X5	T49.5X6
topical NEC	T49.ØX1	T49.ØX2	T49.ØX3	T49.ØX4	T49.ØX5	T49.ØX6
Gentian	T47.5X1	T47.5X2	T47.5X3	T47.5X4	T47.5X5	T47.5X6
violet	T49.ØX1	T49.ØX2	T49.ØX3	T49.ØX4	T49.ØX5	T49.ØX6
Gepefrine	T44.4X1	T44.4X2	T44.4X3	T44.4X4	T44.4X5	T44.4X6
Gestonorone caproate	T38.5X1	T38.5X2	T38.5X3	T38.5X4	T38.5X5	T38.5X6
Gexane	T49.ØX1	T49.ØX2	T49.ØX3	T49.ØX4	T49.ØX5	T49.ØX6
Gila monster (venom)	T63.111	T63.112	T63.113	T63.114	—	—
Ginger	T47.5X1	T47.5X2	T47.5X3	T47.5X4	T47.5X5	T47.5X6
Jamaica — *see* Jamaica, ginger						

Substance	Poisoning, Accidental (unintentional)	Poisoning, Intentional Self-harm	Poisoning, Assault	Poisoning, Undetermined	Adverse Effect	Under-dosing
Gitalin	T46.ØX1	T46.ØX2	T46.ØX3	T46.ØX4	T46.ØX5	T46.ØX6
amorphous	T46.ØX1	T46.ØX2	T46.ØX3	T46.ØX4	T46.ØX5	T46.ØX6
Gitaloxin	T46.ØX1	T46.ØX2	T46.ØX3	T46.ØX4	T46.ØX5	T46.ØX6
Gitoxin	T46.ØX1	T46.ØX2	T46.ØX3	T46.ØX4	T46.ØX5	T46.ØX6
Glafenine	T39.8X1	T39.8X2	T39.8X3	T39.8X4	T39.8X5	T39.8X6
Glandular extract (medicinal) **NEC**	T5Ø.Z91	T5Ø.Z92	T5Ø.Z93	T5Ø.Z94	T5Ø.Z95	T5Ø.Z96
Glaucarubin	T37.3X1	T37.3X2	T37.3X3	T37.3X4	T37.3X5	T37.3X6
Glibenclamide	T38.3X1	T38.3X2	T38.3X3	T38.3X4	T38.3X5	T38.3X6
Glibornuride	T38.3X1	T38.3X2	T38.3X3	T38.3X4	T38.3X5	T38.3X6
Gliclazide	T38.3X1	T38.3X2	T38.3X3	T38.3X4	T38.3X5	T38.3X6
Glimidine	T38.3X1	T38.3X2	T38.3X3	T38.3X4	T38.3X5	T38.3X6
Glipizide	T38.3X1	T38.3X2	T38.3X3	T38.3X4	T38.3X5	T38.3X6
Gliquidone	T38.3X1	T38.3X2	T38.3X3	T38.3X4	T38.3X5	T38.3X6
Glisolamide	T38.3X1	T38.3X2	T38.3X3	T38.3X4	T38.3X5	T38.3X6
Glisoxepide	T38.3X1	T38.3X2	T38.3X3	T38.3X4	T38.3X5	T38.3X6
Globin zinc insulin	T38.3X1	T38.3X2	T38.3X3	T38.3X4	T38.3X5	T38.3X6
Globulin						
antilymphocytic	T5Ø.Z11	T5Ø.Z12	T5Ø.Z13	T5Ø.Z14	T5Ø.Z15	T5Ø.Z16
antirhesus	T5Ø.Z11	T5Ø.Z12	T5Ø.Z13	T5Ø.Z14	T5Ø.Z15	T5Ø.Z16
antivenin	T5Ø.Z11	T5Ø.Z12	T5Ø.Z13	T5Ø.Z14	T5Ø.Z15	T5Ø.Z16
antiviral	T5Ø.Z11	T5Ø.Z12	T5Ø.Z13	T5Ø.Z14	T5Ø.Z15	T5Ø.Z16
Glucagon	T38.3X1	T38.3X2	T38.3X3	T38.3X4	T38.3X5	T38.3X6
Glucocorticoids	T38.ØX1	T38.ØX2	T38.ØX3	T38.ØX4	T38.ØX5	T38.ØX6
Glucocorticosteroid	T38.ØX1	T38.ØX2	T38.ØX3	T38.ØX4	T38.ØX5	T38.ØX6
Gluconic acid	T5Ø.991	T5Ø.992	T5Ø.993	T5Ø.994	T5Ø.995	T5Ø.996
Glucosamine sulfate	T39.4X1	T39.4X2	T39.4X3	T39.4X4	T39.4X5	T39.4X6
Glucose	T5Ø.3X1	T5Ø.3X2	T5Ø.3X3	T5Ø.3X4	T5Ø.3X5	T5Ø.3X6
with sodium chloride	T5Ø.3X1	T5Ø.3X2	T5Ø.3X3	T5Ø.3X4	T5Ø.3X5	T5Ø.3X6
Glucosulfone sodium	T37.1X1	T37.1X2	T37.1X3	T37.1X4	T37.1X5	T37.1X6
Glucurolactone	T47.8X1	T47.8X2	T47.8X3	T47.8X4	T47.8X5	T47.8X6
Glue NEC	T52.8X1	T52.8X2	T52.8X3	T52.8X4	—	—
Glutamic acid	T47.5X1	T47.5X2	T47.5X3	T47.5X4	T47.5X5	T47.5X6
Glutaral (medicinal)	T49.ØX1	T49.ØX2	T49.ØX3	T49.ØX4	T49.ØX5	T49.ØX6
nonmedicinal	T65.891	T65.892	T65.893	T65.894	—	—
Glutaraldehyde (nonmedicinal)	T65.891	T65.892	T65.893	T65.894	—	—
medicinal	T49.ØX1	T49.ØX2	T49.ØX3	T49.ØX4	T49.ØX5	T49.ØX6
Glutathione	T5Ø.6X1	T5Ø.6X2	T5Ø.6X3	T5Ø.6X4	T5Ø.6X5	T5Ø.6X6
Glutethimide	T42.6X1	T42.6X2	T42.6X3	T42.6X4	T42.6X5	T42.6X6
Glyburide	T38.3X1	T38.3X2	T38.3X3	T38.3X4	T38.3X5	T38.3X6
Glycerin	T47.4X1	T47.4X2	T47.4X3	T47.4X4	T47.4X5	T47.4X6
Glycerol	T47.4X1	T47.4X2	T47.4X3	T47.4X4	T47.4X5	T47.4X6
borax	T49.6X1	T49.6X2	T49.6X3	T49.6X4	T49.6X5	T49.6X6
intravenous	T5Ø.3X1	T5Ø.3X2	T5Ø.3X3	T5Ø.3X4	T5Ø.3X5	T5Ø.3X6
iodinated	T48.4X1	T48.4X2	T48.4X3	T48.4X4	T48.4X5	T48.4X6
Glycerophosphate	T5Ø.991	T5Ø.992	T5Ø.993	T5Ø.994	T5Ø.995	T5Ø.996
Glyceryl						
gualacolate	T48.4X1	T48.4X2	T48.4X3	T48.4X4	T48.4X5	T48.4X6
nitrate	T46.3X1	T46.3X2	T46.3X3	T46.3X4	T46.3X5	T46.3X6
triacetate (topical)	T49.ØX1	T49.ØX2	T49.ØX3	T49.ØX4	T49.ØX5	T49.ØX6
trinitrate	T46.3X1	T46.3X2	T46.3X3	T46.3X4	T46.3X5	T46.3X6
Glycine	T5Ø.3X1	T5Ø.3X2	T5Ø.3X3	T5Ø.3X4	T5Ø.3X5	T5Ø.3X6
Glyclopyramide	T38.3X1	T38.3X2	T38.3X3	T38.3X4	T38.3X5	T38.3X6
Glycobiarsol	T37.3X1	T37.3X2	T37.3X3	T37.3X4	T37.3X5	T37.3X6
Glycols (ether)	T52.3X1	T52.3X2	T52.3X3	T52.3X4	—	—
Glyconiazide	T37.1X1	T37.1X2	T37.1X3	T37.1X4	T37.1X5	T37.1X6
Glycopyrrolate	T44.3X1	T44.3X2	T44.3X3	T44.3X4	T44.3X5	T44.3X6
Glycopyrronium	T44.3X1	T44.3X2	T44.3X3	T44.3X4	T44.3X5	T44.3X6
bromide	T44.3X1	T44.3X2	T44.3X3	T44.3X4	T44.3X5	T44.3X6
Glycoside, cardiac (stimulant)	T46.ØX1	T46.ØX2	T46.ØX3	T46.ØX4	T46.ØX5	T46.ØX6
Glycyclamide	T38.3X1	T38.3X2	T38.3X3	T38.3X4	T38.3X5	T38.3X6
Glycyrrhiza extract	T48.4X1	T48.4X2	T48.4X3	T48.4X4	T48.4X5	T48.4X6
Glycyrrhizic acid	T48.4X1	T48.4X2	T48.4X3	T48.4X4	T48.4X5	T48.4X6
Glycyrrhizinate potassium	T48.4X1	T48.4X2	T48.4X3	T48.4X4	T48.4X5	T48.4X6
Glymidine sodium	T38.3X1	T38.3X2	T38.3X3	T38.3X4	T38.3X5	T38.3X6
Glyphosate	T6Ø.3X1	T6Ø.3X2	T6Ø.3X3	T6Ø.3X4	—	—
Glyphylline	T48.6X1	T48.6X2	T48.6X3	T48.6X4	T48.6X5	T48.6X6
Gold						
colloidal (I98Au)	T45.1X1	T45.1X2	T45.1X3	T45.1X4	T45.1X5	T45.1X6
salts	T39.4X1	T39.4X2	T39.4X3	T39.4X4	T39.4X5	T39.4X6
Golden sulfide of antimony	T56.891	T56.892	T56.893	T56.894	—	—
Goldylocks	T62.2X1	T62.2X2	T62.2X3	T62.2X4	—	—
Gonadal tissue extract	T38.9Ø1	T38.9Ø2	T38.9Ø3	T38.9Ø4	T38.9Ø5	T38.9Ø6
female	T38.5X1	T38.5X2	T38.5X3	T38.5X4	T38.5X5	T38.5X6
male	T38.7X1	T38.7X2	T38.7X3	T38.7X4	T38.7X5	T38.7X6
Gonadorelin	T38.891	T38.892	T38.893	T38.894	T38.895	T38.896
Gonadotropin	T38.891	T38.892	T38.893	T38.894	T38.895	T38.896
chorionic	T38.891	T38.892	T38.893	T38.894	T38.895	T38.896
pituitary	T38.811	T38.812	T38.813	T38.814	T38.815	T38.816
Goserelin	T45.1X1	T45.1X2	T45.1X3	T45.1X4	T45.1X5	T45.1X6
Grain alcohol	T51.ØX1	T51.ØX2	T51.ØX3	T51.ØX4	—	—
Gramicidin	T49.ØX1	T49.ØX2	T49.ØX3	T49.ØX4	T49.ØX5	T49.ØX6
Granisetron	T45.ØX1	T45.ØX2	T45.ØX3	T45.ØX4	T45.ØX5	T45.ØX6
Gratiola officinalis	T62.2X1	T62.2X2	T62.2X3	T62.2X4	—	—
Grease	T65.891	T65.892	T65.893	T65.894	—	—
Green hellebore	T62.2X1	T62.2X2	T62.2X3	T62.2X4	—	—
Green soap	T49.2X1	T49.2X2	T49.2X3	T49.2X4	T49.2X5	T49.2X6
Grifulvin	T36.7X1	T36.7X2	T36.7X3	T36.7X4	T36.7X5	T36.7X6
Griseofulvin	T36.7X1	T36.7X2	T36.7X3	T36.7X4	T36.7X5	T36.7X6
Growth hormone	T38.811	T38.812	T38.813	T38.814	T38.815	T38.816
Guaiacol derivatives	T48.4X1	T48.4X2	T48.4X3	T48.4X4	T48.4X5	T48.4X6
Guaiac reagent	T5Ø.991	T5Ø.992	T5Ø.993	T5Ø.994	T5Ø.995	T5Ø.996
Guaifenesin	T48.4X1	T48.4X2	T48.4X3	T48.4X4	T48.4X5	T48.4X6
Guaimesal	T48.4X1	T48.4X2	T48.4X3	T48.4X4	T48.4X5	T48.4X6
Guaiphenesin	T48.4X1	T48.4X2	T48.4X3	T48.4X4	T48.4X5	T48.4X6
Guamecycline	T36.4X1	T36.4X2	T36.4X3	T36.4X4	T36.4X5	T36.4X6
Guanabenz	T46.5X1	T46.5X2	T46.5X3	T46.5X4	T46.5X5	T46.5X6
Guanacline	T46.5X1	T46.5X2	T46.5X3	T46.5X4	T46.5X5	T46.5X6
Guanadrel	T46.5X1	T46.5X2	T46.5X3	T46.5X4	T46.5X5	T46.5X6
Guanatol	T37.2X1	T37.2X2	T37.2X3	T37.2X4	T37.2X5	T37.2X6
Guanethidine	T46.5X1	T46.5X2	T46.5X3	T46.5X4	T46.5X5	T46.5X6
Guanfacine	T46.5X1	T46.5X2	T46.5X3	T46.5X4	T46.5X5	T46.5X6
Guano	T65.891	T65.892	T65.893	T65.894	—	—
Guanochlor	T46.5X1	T46.5X2	T46.5X3	T46.5X4	T46.5X5	T46.5X6
Guanoclor	T46.5X1	T46.5X2	T46.5X3	T46.5X4	T46.5X5	T46.5X6
Guanoctine	T46.5X1	T46.5X2	T46.5X3	T46.5X4	T46.5X5	T46.5X6
Guanoxabenz	T46.5X1	T46.5X2	T46.5X3	T46.5X4	T46.5X5	T46.5X6
Guanoxan	T46.5X1	T46.5X2	T46.5X3	T46.5X4	T46.5X5	T46.5X6
Guar gum (medicinal)	T46.6X1	T46.6X2	T46.6X3	T46.6X4	T46.6X5	T46.6X6
Hachimycin	T36.7X1	T36.7X2	T36.7X3	T36.7X4	T36.7X5	T36.7X6
Hair						
dye	T49.4X1	T49.4X2	T49.4X3	T49.4X4	T49.4X5	T49.4X6
preparation NEC	T49.4X1	T49.4X2	T49.4X3	T49.4X4	T49.4X5	T49.4X6
Halazepam	T42.4X1	T42.4X2	T42.4X3	T42.4X4	T42.4X5	T42.4X6
Halcinolone	T49.ØX1	T49.ØX2	T49.ØX3	T49.ØX4	T49.ØX5	T49.ØX6
Halcinonide	T49.ØX1	T49.ØX2	T49.ØX3	T49.ØX4	T49.ØX5	T49.ØX6
Halethazole	T49.ØX1	T49.ØX2	T49.ØX3	T49.ØX4	T49.ØX5	T49.ØX6
Hallucinogen NEC	T4Ø.9Ø1	T4Ø.9Ø2	T4Ø.9Ø3	T4Ø.9Ø4	T4Ø.9Ø5	T4Ø.9Ø6
Halofantrine	T37.2X1	T37.2X2	T37.2X3	T37.2X4	T37.2X5	T37.2X6
Halofenate	T46.6X1	T46.6X2	T46.6X3	T46.6X4	T46.6X5	T46.6X6
Halometasone	T49.ØX1	T49.ØX2	T49.ØX3	T49.ØX4	T49.ØX5	T49.ØX6
Haloperidol	T43.4X1	T43.4X2	T43.4X3	T43.4X4	T43.4X5	T43.4X6
Haloprogin	T49.ØX1	T49.ØX2	T49.ØX3	T49.ØX4	T49.ØX5	T49.ØX6
Halotex	T49.ØX1	T49.ØX2	T49.ØX3	T49.ØX4	T49.ØX5	T49.ØX6
Halothane	T41.ØX1	T41.ØX2	T41.ØX3	T41.ØX4	T41.ØX5	T41.ØX6
Haloxazolam	T42.4X1	T42.4X2	T42.4X3	T42.4X4	T42.4X5	T42.4X6
Halquinols	T49.ØX1	T49.ØX2	T49.ØX3	T49.ØX4	T49.ØX5	T49.ØX6
Hamamelis	T49.2X1	T49.2X2	T49.2X3	T49.2X4	T49.2X5	T49.2X6
Haptendextran	T45.8X1	T45.8X2	T45.8X3	T45.8X4	T45.8X5	T45.8X6
Harmonyl	T46.5X1	T46.5X2	T46.5X3	T46.5X4	T46.5X5	T46.5X6
Hartmann's solution	T5Ø.3X1	T5Ø.3X2	T5Ø.3X3	T5Ø.3X4	T5Ø.3X5	T5Ø.3X6
Hashish	T4Ø.7X1	T4Ø.7X2	T4Ø.7X3	T4Ø.7X4	T4Ø.7X5	T4Ø.7X6
Hawaiian Woodrose seeds	T4Ø.991	T4Ø.992	T4Ø.993	T4Ø.994	—	—
HCB	T6Ø.3X1	T6Ø.3X2	T6Ø.3X3	T6Ø.3X4	—	—
HCH	T53.6X1	T53.6X2	T53.6X3	T53.6X4	—	—
medicinal	T49.ØX1	T49.ØX2	T49.ØX3	T49.ØX4	T49.ØX5	T49.ØX6
HCN	T57.3X1	T57.3X2	T57.3X3	T57.3X4	—	—
Headache cures, drugs, powders NEC	T5Ø.9Ø1	T5Ø.9Ø2	T5Ø.9Ø3	T5Ø.9Ø4	T5Ø.9Ø5	T5Ø.9Ø6
Heavenly Blue (morning glory)	T4Ø.991	T4Ø.992	T4Ø.993	T4Ø.994	—	—
Heavy metal antidote	T45.8X1	T45.8X2	T45.8X3	T45.8X4	T45.8X5	T45.8X6
Hedaquinium	T49.ØX1	T49.ØX2	T49.ØX3	T49.ØX4	T49.ØX5	T49.ØX6
Hedge hyssop	T62.2X1	T62.2X2	T62.2X3	T62.2X4	—	—
Heet	T49.8X1	T49.8X2	T49.8X3	T49.8X4	T49.8X5	T49.8X6
Helenin	T37.4X1	T37.4X2	T37.4X3	T37.4X4	T37.4X5	T37.4X6
Helium (nonmedicinal) **NEC**	T59.891	T59.892	T59.893	T59.894	—	—
medicinal	T48.991	T48.992	T48.993	T48.994	T48.995	T48.996
Hellebore (black) (green) (white)	T62.2X1	T62.2X2	T62.2X3	T62.2X4	—	—
Hematin	T45.8X1	T45.8X2	T45.8X3	T45.8X4	T45.8X5	T45.8X6
Hematinic preparation	T45.8X1	T45.8X2	T45.8X3	T45.8X4	T45.8X5	T45.8X6
Hematological agent	T45.91	T45.92	T45.93	T45.94	T45.95	T45.96
specified NEC	T45.8X1	T45.8X2	T45.8X3	T45.8X4	T45.8X5	T45.8X6
Hemlock	T62.2X1	T62.2X2	T62.2X3	T62.2X4	—	—
Hemostatic	T45.621	T45.622	T45.623	T45.624	T45.625	T45.626
drug, systemic	T45.621	T45.622	T45.623	T45.624	T45.625	T45.626
Hemostyptic	T49.4X1	T49.4X2	T49.4X3	T49.4X4	T49.4X5	T49.4X6
Henbane	T62.2X1	T62.2X2	T62.2X3	T62.2X4	—	—
Heparin (sodium)	T45.511	T45.512	T45.513	T45.514	T45.515	T45.516
action reverser	T45.7X1	T45.7X2	T45.7X3	T45.7X4	T45.7X5	T45.7X6
Heparin-fraction	T45.511	T45.512	T45.513	T45.514	T45.515	T45.516
Heparinoid (systemic)	T45.511	T45.512	T45.513	T45.514	T45.515	T45.516

Substance	Poisoning, Accidental (unintentional)	Poisoning, Intentional Self-harm	Poisoning, Assault	Poisoning, Undetermined	Adverse Effect	Under-dosing
Hepatic secretion stimulant	T47.8X1	T47.8X2	T47.8X3	T47.8X4	T47.8X5	T47.8X6
Hepatitis B						
immune globulin	T5Ø.Z11	T5Ø.Z12	T5Ø.Z13	T5Ø.Z14	T5Ø.Z15	T5Ø.Z16
vaccine	T5Ø.B91	T5Ø.B92	T5Ø.B93	T5Ø.B94	T5Ø.B95	T5Ø.B96
Hepronicate	T46.7X1	T46.7X2	T46.7X3	T46.7X4	T46.7X5	T46.7X6
Heptabarb	T42.3X1	T42.3X2	T42.3X3	T42.3X4	T42.3X5	T42.3X6
Heptabarbital	T42.3X1	T42.3X2	T42.3X3	T42.3X4	T42.3X5	T42.3X6
Heptabarbitone	T42.3X1	T42.3X2	T42.3X3	T42.3X4	T42.3X5	T42.3X6
Heptachlor	T6Ø.1X1	T6Ø.1X2	T6Ø.1X3	T6Ø.1X4	—	—
Heptalgin	T4Ø.2X1	T4Ø.2X2	T4Ø.2X3	T4Ø.2X4	T4Ø.2X5	T4Ø.2X6
Heptaminol	T46.3X1	T46.3X2	T46.3X3	T46.3X4	T46.3X5	T46.3X6
Herbicide NEC	T6Ø.3X1	T6Ø.3X2	T6Ø.3X3	T6Ø.3X4	—	—
Heroin	T4Ø.1X1	T4Ø.1X2	T4Ø.1X3	T4Ø.1X4	—	—
Herplex	T49.5X1	T49.5X2	T49.5X3	T49.5X4	T49.5X5	T49.5X6
HES	T45.8X1	T45.8X2	T45.8X3	T45.8X4	T45.8X5	T45.8X6
Hesperidin	T46.991	T46.992	T46.993	T46.994	T46.995	T46.996
Hetacillin	T36.ØX1	T36.ØX2	T36.ØX3	T36.ØX4	T36.ØX5	T36.ØX6
Hetastarch	T45.8X1	T45.8X2	T45.8X3	T45.8X4	T45.8X5	T45.8X6
HETP	T6Ø.ØX1	T6Ø.ØX2	T6Ø.ØX3	T6Ø.ØX4	—	—
Hexachlorobenzene (vapor)	T6Ø.3X1	T6Ø.3X2	T6Ø.3X3	T6Ø.3X4	—	—
Hexachlorocyclohexane	T53.6X1	T53.6X2	T53.6X3	T53.6X4	—	—
Hexachlorophene	T49.ØX1	T49.ØX2	T49.ØX3	T49.ØX4	T49.ØX5	T49.ØX6
Hexadiline	T46.3X1	T46.3X2	T46.3X3	T46.3X4	T46.3X5	T46.3X6
Hexadimethrine (bromide)	T45.7X1	T45.7X2	T45.7X3	T45.7X4	T45.7X5	T45.7X6
Hexadylamine	T46.3X1	T46.3X2	T46.3X3	T46.3X4	T46.3X5	T46.3X6
Hexaethyl tetraphosphate	T6Ø.ØX1	T6Ø.ØX2	T6Ø.ØX3	T6Ø.ØX4	—	—
Hexafluorenium bromide	T48.1X1	T48.1X2	T48.1X3	T48.1X4	T48.1X5	T48.1X6
Hexafluronium (bromide)	T48.1X1	T48.1X2	T48.1X3	T48.1X4	T48.1X5	T48.1X6
Hexa-germ	T49.2X1	T49.2X2	T49.2X3	T49.2X4	T49.2X5	T49.2X6
Hexahydrobenzol	T52.8X1	T52.8X2	T52.8X3	T52.8X4	—	—
Hexahydrocresol(s)	T51.8X1	T51.8X2	T51.8X3	T51.8X4	—	—
arsenide	T57.ØX1	T57.ØX2	T57.ØX3	T57.ØX4	—	—
arseniurated	T57.ØX1	T57.ØX2	T57.ØX3	T57.ØX4	—	—
cyanide	T57.3X1	T57.3X2	T57.3X3	T57.3X4	—	—
gas	T59.891	T59.892	T59.893	T59.894	—	—
Fluoride (liquid)	T57.8X1	T57.8X2	T57.8X3	T57.8X4	—	—
vapor	T59.891	T59.892	T59.893	T59.894	—	—
phophorated	T6Ø.ØX1	T6Ø.ØX2	T6Ø.ØX3	T6Ø.ØX4	—	—
sulfate	T57.8X1	T57.8X2	T57.8X3	T57.8X4	—	—
sulfide (gas)	T59.6X1	T59.6X2	T59.6X3	T59.6X4	—	—
arseniurated	T57.ØX1	T57.ØX2	T57.ØX3	T57.ØX4	—	—
sulfurated	T57.8X1	T57.8X2	T57.8X3	T57.8X4	—	—
Hexahydrophenol	T51.8X1	T51.8X2	T51.8X3	T51.8X4	—	—
Hexalen	T51.8X1	T51.8X2	T51.8X3	T51.8X4	—	—
Hexamethonium bromide	T44.2X1	T44.2X2	T44.2X3	T44.2X4	T44.2X5	T44.2X6
Hexamethylene	T52.8X1	T52.8X2	T52.8X3	T52.8X4	—	—
Hexamethylmelamine	T45.1X1	T45.1X2	T45.1X3	T45.1X4	T45.1X5	T45.1X6
Hexamidine	T49.ØX1	T49.ØX2	T49.ØX3	T49.ØX4	T49.ØX5	T49.ØX6
Hexamine (mandelate)	T37.8X1	T37.8X2	T37.8X3	T37.8X4	T37.8X5	T37.8X6
Hexanone, 2-hexanone	T52.4X1	T52.4X2	T52.4X3	T52.4X4	—	—
Hexanuorenium	T48.1X1	T48.1X2	T48.1X3	T48.1X4	T48.1X5	T48.1X6
Hexapropymate	T42.6X1	T42.6X2	T42.6X3	T42.6X4	T42.6X5	T42.6X6
Hexasonium iodide	T44.3X1	T44.3X2	T44.3X3	T44.3X4	T44.3X5	T44.3X6
Hexcarbacholine bromide	T48.1X1	T48.1X2	T48.1X3	T48.1X4	T48.1X5	T48.1X6
Hexemal	T42.3X1	T42.3X2	T42.3X3	T42.3X4	T42.3X5	T42.3X6
Hexestrol	T38.5X1	T38.5X2	T38.5X3	T38.5X4	T38.5X5	T38.5X6
Hexethal (sodium)	T42.3X1	T42.3X2	T42.3X3	T42.3X4	T42.3X5	T42.3X6
Hexetidine	T37.8X1	T37.8X2	T37.8X3	T37.8X4	T37.8X5	T37.8X6
Hexobarbital	T42.3X1	T42.3X2	T42.3X3	T42.3X4	T42.3X5	T42.3X6
rectal	T41.291	T41.292	T41.293	T41.294	T41.295	T41.296
sodium	T41.1X1	T41.1X2	T41.1X3	T41.1X4	T41.1X5	T41.1X6
Hexobendine	T46.3X1	T46.3X2	T46.3X3	T46.3X4	T46.3X5	T46.3X6
Hexocyclium	T44.3X1	T44.3X2	T44.3X3	T44.3X4	T44.3X5	T44.3X6
metilsulfate	T44.3X1	T44.3X2	T44.3X3	T44.3X4	T44.3X5	T44.3X6
Hexoestrol	T38.5X1	T38.5X2	T38.5X3	T38.5X4	T38.5X5	T38.5X6
Hexone	T52.4X1	T52.4X2	T52.4X3	T52.4X4	—	—
Hexoprenaline	T48.6X1	T48.6X2	T48.6X3	T48.6X4	T48.6X5	T48.6X6
Hexylcaine	T41.3X1	T41.3X2	T41.3X3	T41.3X4	T41.3X5	T41.3X6
Hexylresorcinol	T52.2X1	T52.2X2	T52.2X3	T52.2X4	—	—
HGH (human growth hormone)	T38.811	T38.812	T38.813	T38.814	T38.815	T38.816
Hinkle's pills	T47.2X1	T47.2X2	T47.2X3	T47.2X4	T47.2X5	T47.2X6
Histalog	T5Ø.8X1	T5Ø.8X2	T5Ø.8X3	T5Ø.8X4	T5Ø.8X5	T5Ø.8X6
Histamine (phosphate)	T5Ø.8X1	T5Ø.8X2	T5Ø.8X3	T5Ø.8X4	T5Ø.8X5	T5Ø.8X6
Histoplasmin	T5Ø.8X1	T5Ø.8X2	T5Ø.8X3	T5Ø.8X4	T5Ø.8X5	T5Ø.8X6
Holly berries	T62.2X1	T62.2X2	T62.2X3	T62.2X4	—	—
Homatropine	T44.3X1	T44.3X2	T44.3X3	T44.3X4	T44.3X5	T44.3X6
methylbromide	T44.3X1	T44.3X2	T44.3X3	T44.3X4	T44.3X5	T44.3X6
Homochlorcyclizine	T45.ØX1	T45.ØX2	T45.ØX3	T45.ØX4	T45.ØX5	T45.ØX6
Homosalate	T49.3X1	T49.3X2	T49.3X3	T49.3X4	T49.3X5	T49.3X6
Homo-tet	T5Ø.Z11	T5Ø.Z12	T5Ø.Z13	T5Ø.Z14	T5Ø.Z15	T5Ø.Z16
Hormone	T38.8Ø1	T38.8Ø2	T38.8Ø3	T38.8Ø4	T38.8Ø5	T38.8Ø6
Hormone — *continued*						
adrenal cortical steroids	T38.ØX1	T38.ØX2	T38.ØX3	T38.ØX4	T38.ØX5	T38.ØX6
androgenic	T38.7X1	T38.7X2	T38.7X3	T38.7X4	T38.7X5	T38.7X6
anterior pituitary NEC	T38.811	T38.812	T38.813	T38.814	T38.815	T38.816
antidiabetic agents	T38.3X1	T38.3X2	T38.3X3	T38.3X4	T38.3X5	T38.3X6
antidiuretic	T38.891	T38.892	T38.893	T38.894	T38.895	T38.896
cancer therapy	T45.1X1	T45.1X2	T45.1X3	T45.1X4	T45.1X5	T45.1X6
follicle stimulating	T38.811	T38.812	T38.813	T38.814	T38.815	T38.816
gonadotropic	T38.891	T38.892	T38.893	T38.894	T38.895	T38.896
pituitary	T38.811	T38.812	T38.813	T38.814	T38.815	T38.816
growth	T38.811	T38.812	T38.813	T38.814	T38.815	T38.816
luteinizing	T38.811	T38.812	T38.813	T38.814	T38.815	T38.816
ovarian	T38.5X1	T38.5X2	T38.5X3	T38.5X4	T38.5X5	T38.5X6
oxytocic	T48.ØX1	T48.ØX2	T48.ØX3	T48.ØX4	T48.ØX5	T48.ØX6
parathyroid (derivatives)	T5Ø.991	T5Ø.992	T5Ø.993	T5Ø.994	T5Ø.995	T5Ø.996
pituitary (posterior) NEC	T38.891	T38.892	T38.893	T38.894	T38.895	T38.896
anterior	T38.811	T38.812	T38.813	T38.814	T38.815	T38.816
specified, NEC	T38.891	T38.892	T38.893	T38.894	T38.895	T38.896
thyroid	T38.1X1	T38.1X2	T38.1X3	T38.1X4	T38.1X5	T38.1X6
Hornet (sting)	T63.451	T63.452	T63.453	T63.454	—	—
Horse anti-human lymphocytic serum	T5Ø.Z11	T5Ø.Z12	T5Ø.Z13	T5Ø.Z14	T5Ø.Z15	T5Ø.Z16
Horticulture agent NEC	T65.91	T65.92	T65.93	T65.94	—	—
with pesticide	T6Ø.91	T6Ø.92	T6Ø.93	T6Ø.94	—	—
Human						
albumin	T45.8X1	T45.8X2	T45.8X3	T45.8X4	T45.8X5	T45.8X6
growth hormone (HGH)	T38.811	T38.812	T38.813	T38.814	T38.815	T38.816
immune serum	T5Ø.Z11	T5Ø.Z12	T5Ø.Z13	T5Ø.Z14	T5Ø.Z15	T5Ø.Z16
Hyaluronidase	T45.3X1	T45.3X2	T45.3X3	T45.3X4	T45.3X5	T45.3X6
Hyazyme	T45.3X1	T45.3X2	T45.3X3	T45.3X4	T45.3X5	T45.3X6
Hycodan	T4Ø.2X1	T4Ø.2X2	T4Ø.2X3	T4Ø.2X4	T4Ø.2X5	T4Ø.2X6
Hydantoin derivative NEC	T42.ØX1	T42.ØX2	T42.ØX3	T42.ØX4	T42.ØX5	T42.ØX6
Hydeltra	T38.ØX1	T38.ØX2	T38.ØX3	T38.ØX4	T38.ØX5	T38.ØX6
Hydergine	T44.6X1	T44.6X2	T44.6X3	T44.6X4	T44.6X5	T44.6X6
Hydrabamine penicillin	T36.ØX1	T36.ØX2	T36.ØX3	T36.ØX4	T36.ØX5	T36.ØX6
Hydralazine	T46.5X1	T46.5X2	T46.5X3	T46.5X4	T46.5X5	T46.5X6
Hydrargaphen	T49.ØX1	T49.ØX2	T49.ØX3	T49.ØX4	T49.ØX5	T49.ØX6
Hydrargyri aminochloridum	T49.ØX1	T49.ØX2	T49.ØX3	T49.ØX4	T49.ØX5	T49.ØX6
Hydrastine	T48.291	T48.292	T48.293	T48.294	T48.295	T48.296
Hydrazine	T54.1X1	T54.1X2	T54.1X3	T54.1X4	—	—
monoamine oxidase inhibitors	T43.1X1	T43.1X2	T43.1X3	T43.1X4	T43.1X5	T43.1X6
Hydrazoic acid, azides	T54.2X1	T54.2X2	T54.2X3	T54.2X4	—	—
Hydriodic acid	T48.4X1	T48.4X2	T48.4X3	T48.4X4	T48.4X5	T48.4X6
Hydrocarbon gas	T59.891	T59.892	T59.893	T59.894	—	—
incomplete combustion of — *see* Carbon, monoxide, fuel, utility						
liquefied (mobile container)	T59.891	T59.892	T59.893	T59.894	—	—
piped (natural)	T59.891	T59.892	T59.893	T59.894	—	—
Hydrochloric acid (liquid)	T54.2X1	T54.2X2	T54.2X3	T54.2X4	—	—
medicinal (digestant)	T47.5X1	T47.5X2	T47.5X3	T47.5X4	T47.5X5	T47.5X6
vapor	T59.891	T59.892	T59.893	T59.894	—	—
Hydrochlorothiazide	T5Ø.2X1	T5Ø.2X2	T5Ø.2X3	T5Ø.2X4	T5Ø.2X5	T5Ø.2X6
Hydrocodone	T4Ø.2X1	T4Ø.2X2	T4Ø.2X3	T4Ø.2X4	T4Ø.2X5	T4Ø.2X6
Hydrocortisone (derivatives)	T49.ØX1	T49.ØX2	T49.ØX3	T49.ØX4	T49.ØX5	T49.ØX6
aceponate	T49.ØX1	T49.ØX2	T49.ØX3	T49.ØX4	T49.ØX5	T49.ØX6
ENT agent	T49.6X1	T49.6X2	T49.6X3	T49.6X4	T49.6X5	T49.6X6
ophthalmic preparation	T49.5X1	T49.5X2	T49.5X3	T49.5X4	T49.5X5	T49.5X6
topical NEC	T49.ØX1	T49.ØX2	T49.ØX3	T49.ØX4	T49.ØX5	T49.ØX6
Hydrocortone	T38.ØX1	T38.ØX2	T38.ØX3	T38.ØX4	T38.ØX5	T38.ØX6
ENT agent	T49.6X1	T49.6X2	T49.6X3	T49.6X4	T49.6X5	T49.6X6
ophthalmic preparation	T49.5X1	T49.5X2	T49.5X3	T49.5X4	T49.5X5	T49.5X6
topical NEC	T49.ØX1	T49.ØX2	T49.ØX3	T49.ØX4	T49.ØX5	T49.ØX6
Hydrocyanic acid (liquid)	T57.3X1	T57.3X2	T57.3X3	T57.3X4	—	—
gas	T65.ØX1	T65.ØX2	T65.ØX3	T65.ØX4	—	—
Hydroflumethiazide	T5Ø.2X1	T5Ø.2X2	T5Ø.2X3	T5Ø.2X4	T5Ø.2X5	T5Ø.2X6
Hydrofluoric acid (liquid)	T54.2X1	T54.2X2	T54.2X3	T54.2X4	—	—
vapor	T59.891	T59.892	T59.893	T59.894	—	—
Hydrogen	T59.891	T59.892	T59.893	T59.894	—	—
arsenide	T57.ØX1	T57.ØX2	T57.ØX3	T57.ØX4	—	—
arseniureted	T57.ØX1	T57.ØX2	T57.ØX3	T57.ØX4	—	—
chloride	T57.8X1	T57.8X2	T57.8X3	T57.8X4	—	—
cyanide (salts)	T57.3X1	T57.3X2	T57.3X3	T57.3X4	—	—
gas	T57.3X1	T57.3X2	T57.3X3	T57.3X4	—	—
Fluoride	T59.5X1	T59.5X2	T59.5X3	T59.5X4	—	—
vapor	T59.5X1	T59.5X2	T59.5X3	T59.5X4	—	—
peroxide	T49.ØX1	T49.ØX2	T49.ØX3	T49.ØX4	T49.ØX5	T49.ØX6
phosphureted	T57.1X1	T57.1X2	T57.1X3	T57.1X4	—	—
sulfide	T59.6X1	T59.6X2	T59.6X3	T59.6X4	—	—
arseniureted	T57.ØX1	T57.ØX2	T57.ØX3	T57.ØX4	—	—
sulfureted	T59.6X1	T59.6X2	T59.6X3	T59.6X4	—	—

Substance	Poisoning, Accidental (unintentional)	Poisoning, Intentional Self-harm	Poisoning, Assault	Poisoning, Undetermined	Adverse Effect	Under-dosing
Hydromethylpyridine	T46.7X1	T46.7X2	T46.7X3	T46.7X4	T46.7X5	T46.7X6
Hydromorphinol	T4Ø.2X1	T4Ø.2X2	T4Ø.2X3	T4Ø.2X4	—	—
Hydromorphinone	T4Ø.2X1	T4Ø.2X2	T4Ø.2X3	T4Ø.2X4	T4Ø.2X5	T4Ø.2X6
Hydromorphone	T4Ø.2X1	T4Ø.2X2	T4Ø.2X3	T4Ø.2X4	T4Ø.2X5	T4Ø.2X6
Hydromox	T5Ø.2X1	T5Ø.2X2	T5Ø.2X3	T5Ø.2X4	T5Ø.2X5	T5Ø.2X6
Hydrophilic lotion	T49.3X1	T49.3X2	T49.3X3	T49.3X4	T49.3X5	T49.3X6
Hydroquinidine	T46.2X1	T46.2X2	T46.2X3	T46.2X4	T46.2X5	T46.2X6
Hydroquinone	T52.2X1	T52.2X2	T52.2X3	T52.2X4	—	—
vapor	T59.891	T59.892	T59.893	T59.894	—	—
Hydrosulfuric acid (gas)	T59.6X1	T59.6X2	T59.6X3	T59.6X4	—	—
Hydrotalcite	T47.1X1	T47.1X2	T47.1X3	T47.1X4	T47.1X5	T47.1X6
Hydrous wool fat	T49.3X1	T49.3X2	T49.3X3	T49.3X4	T49.3X5	T49.3X6
Hydroxide, caustic	T54.3X1	T54.3X2	T54.3X3	T54.3X4	—	—
Hydroxocobalamin	T45.8X1	T45.8X2	T45.8X3	T45.8X4	T45.8X5	T45.8X6
Hydroxyamphetamine	T49.5X1	T49.5X2	T49.5X3	T49.5X4	T49.5X5	T49.5X6
Hydroxycarbamide	T45.1X1	T45.1X2	T45.1X3	T45.1X4	T45.1X5	T45.1X6
Hydroxychloroquine	T37.8X1	T37.8X2	T37.8X3	T37.8X4	T37.8X5	T37.8X6
Hydroxydihydrocodeinone	T4Ø.2X1	T4Ø.2X2	T4Ø.2X3	T4Ø.2X4	T4Ø.2X5	T4Ø.2X6
Hydroxyestrone	T38.5X1	T38.5X2	T38.5X3	T38.5X4	T38.5X5	T38.5X6
Hydroxyethyl starch	T45.8X1	T45.8X2	T45.8X3	T45.8X4	T45.8X5	T45.8X6
Hydroxymethylpentanone	T52.4X1	T52.4X2	T52.4X3	T52.4X4	—	—
Hydroxyphenamate	T43.591	T43.592	T43.593	T43.594	T43.595	T43.596
Hydroxyphenylbutazone	T39.2X1	T39.2X2	T39.2X3	T39.2X4	T39.2X5	T39.2X6
Hydroxyprogesterone	T38.5X1	T38.5X2	T38.5X3	T38.5X4	T38.5X5	T38.5X6
caproate	T38.5X1	T38.5X2	T38.5X3	T38.5X4	T38.5X5	T38.5X6
Hydroxyquinoline (derivatives) **NEC**	T37.8X1	T37.8X2	T37.8X3	T37.8X4	T37.8X5	T37.8X6
Hydroxystilbamidine	T37.3X1	T37.3X2	T37.3X3	T37.3X4	T37.3X5	T37.3X6
Hydroxytoluene (nonmedicinal)	T54.ØX1	T54.ØX2	T54.ØX3	T54.ØX4	—	—
medicinal	T49.ØX1	T49.ØX2	T49.ØX3	T49.ØX4	T49.ØX5	T49.ØX6
Hydroxyurea	T45.1X1	T45.1X2	T45.1X3	T45.1X4	T45.1X5	T45.1X6
Hydroxyzine	T43.591	T43.592	T43.593	T43.594	T43.595	T43.596
Hyoscine	T44.3X1	T44.3X2	T44.3X3	T44.3X4	T44.3X5	T44.3X6
Hyoscyamine	T44.3X1	T44.3X2	T44.3X3	T44.3X4	T44.3X5	T44.3X6
Hyoscyamus	T44.3X1	T44.3X2	T44.3X3	T44.3X4	T44.3X5	T44.3X6
dry extract	T44.3X1	T44.3X2	T44.3X3	T44.3X4	T44.3X5	T44.3X6
Hypaque	T5Ø.8X1	T5Ø.8X2	T5Ø.8X3	T5Ø.8X4	T5Ø.8X5	T5Ø.8X6
Hypertussis	T5Ø.Z11	T5Ø.Z12	T5Ø.Z13	T5Ø.Z14	T5Ø.Z15	T5Ø.Z16
Hypnotic	T42.71	T42.72	T42.73	T42.74	T42.75	T42.76
anticonvulsant	T42.71	T42.72	T42.73	T42.74	T42.75	T42.76
specified NEC	T42.6X1	T42.6X2	T42.6X3	T42.6X4	T42.6X5	T42.6X6
Hypochlorite	T49.ØX1	T49.ØX2	T49.ØX3	T49.ØX4	T49.ØX5	T49.ØX6
Hypophysis, posterior	T38.891	T38.892	T38.893	T38.894	T38.895	T38.896
Hypotensive NEC	T46.5X1	T46.5X2	T46.5X3	T46.5X4	T46.5X5	T46.5X6
Hypromellose	T49.5X1	T49.5X2	T49.5X3	T49.5X4	T49.5X5	T49.5X6
Ibacitabine	T37.5X1	T37.5X2	T37.5X3	T37.5X4	T37.5X5	T37.5X6
Ibopamine	T44.991	T44.992	T44.993	T44.994	T44.995	T44.996
Ibufenac	T39.311	T39.312	T39.313	T39.314	T39.315	T39.316
Ibuprofen	T39.311	T39.312	T39.313	T39.314	T39.315	T39.316
Ibuproxam	T39.311	T39.312	T39.313	T39.314	T39.315	T39.316
Ibuterol	T48.6X1	T48.6X2	T48.6X3	T48.6X4	T48.6X5	T48.6X6
Ichthammol	T49.ØX1	T49.ØX2	T49.ØX3	T49.ØX4	T49.ØX5	T49.ØX6
Ichthyol	T49.4X1	T49.4X2	T49.4X3	T49.4X4	T49.4X5	T49.4X6
Idarubicin	T45.1X1	T45.1X2	T45.1X3	T45.1X4	T45.1X5	T45.1X6
Idrocilamide	T42.8X1	T42.8X2	T42.8X3	T42.8X4	T42.8X5	T42.8X6
Ifenprodil	T46.7X1	T46.7X2	T46.7X3	T46.7X4	T46.7X5	T46.7X6
Ifosfamide	T45.1X1	T45.1X2	T45.1X3	T45.1X4	T45.1X5	T45.1X6
Iletin	T38.3X1	T38.3X2	T38.3X3	T38.3X4	T38.3X5	T38.3X6
Ilex	T62.2X1	T62.2X2	T62.2X3	T62.2X4	—	—
Illuminating gas (after combustion)	T58.11	T58.12	T58.13	T58.14	—	—
prior to combustion	T59.891	T59.892	T59.893	T59.894	—	—
Ilopan	T45.2X1	T45.2X2	T45.2X3	T45.2X4	T45.2X5	T45.2X6
Iloprost	T46.7X1	T46.7X2	T46.7X3	T46.7X4	T46.7X5	T46.7X6
Ilotycin	T36.3X1	T36.3X2	T36.3X3	T36.3X4	T36.3X5	T36.3X6
ophthalmic preparation	T49.5X1	T49.5X2	T49.5X3	T49.5X4	T49.5X5	T49.5X6
topical NEC	T49.ØX1	T49.ØX2	T49.ØX3	T49.ØX4	T49.ØX5	T49.ØX6
Imidazole-4-carboxamide	T45.1X1	T45.1X2	T45.1X3	T45.1X4	T45.1X5	T45.1X6
Iminostilbene	T42.1X1	T42.1X2	T42.1X3	T42.1X4	T42.1X5	T42.1X6
Imipenem	T36.ØX1	T36.ØX2	T36.ØX3	T36.ØX4	T36.ØX5	T36.ØX6
Imipramine	T43.Ø11	T43.Ø12	T43.Ø13	T43.Ø14	T43.Ø15	T43.Ø16
Immu-G	T5Ø.Z11	T5Ø.Z12	T5Ø.Z13	T5Ø.Z14	T5Ø.Z15	T5Ø.Z16
Immuglobin	T5Ø.Z11	T5Ø.Z12	T5Ø.Z13	T5Ø.Z14	T5Ø.Z15	T5Ø.Z16
Immune						
globulin	T5Ø.Z11	T5Ø.Z12	T5Ø.Z13	T5Ø.Z14	T5Ø.Z15	T5Ø.Z16
serum globulin	T5Ø.Z11	T5Ø.Z12	T5Ø.Z13	T5Ø.Z14	T5Ø.Z15	T5Ø.Z16
Immunoglobin human (intravenous) (normal)	T5Ø.Z11	T5Ø.Z12	T5Ø.Z13	T5Ø.Z14	T5Ø.Z15	T5Ø.Z16
unmodified	T5Ø.Z11	T5Ø.Z12	T5Ø.Z13	T5Ø.Z14	T5Ø.Z15	T5Ø.Z16
Immunosuppressive drug	T45.1X1	T45.1X2	T45.1X3	T45.1X4	T45.1X5	T45.1X6
Immu-tetanus	T5Ø.Z11	T5Ø.Z12	T5Ø.Z13	T5Ø.Z14	T5Ø.Z15	T5Ø.Z16
Indalpine	T43.221	T43.222	T43.223	T43.224	T43.225	T43.226
Indanazoline	T48.5X1	T48.5X2	T48.5X3	T48.5X4	T48.5X5	T48.5X6
Indandione (derivatives)	T45.511	T45.512	T45.513	T45.514	T45.515	T45.516
Indapamide	T46.5X1	T46.5X2	T46.5X3	T46.5X4	T46.5X5	T46.5X6
Indendione (derivatives)	T45.511	T45.512	T45.513	T45.514	T45.515	T45.516
Indenolol	T44.7X1	T44.7X2	T44.7X3	T44.7X4	T44.7X5	T44.7X6
Inderal	T44.7X1	T44.7X2	T44.7X3	T44.7X4	T44.7X5	T44.7X6
Indian						
hemp	T4Ø.7X1	T4Ø.7X2	T4Ø.7X3	T4Ø.7X4	T4Ø.7X5	T4Ø.7X6
tobacco	T62.2X1	T62.2X2	T62.2X3	T62.2X4	—	—
Indigo carmine	T5Ø.8X1	T5Ø.8X2	T5Ø.8X3	T5Ø.8X4	T5Ø.8X5	T5Ø.8X6
Indobufen	T45.521	T45.522	T45.523	T45.524	T45.525	T45.526
Indocin	T39.2X1	T39.2X2	T39.2X3	T39.2X4	T39.2X5	T39.2X6
Indocyanine green	T5Ø.8X1	T5Ø.8X2	T5Ø.8X3	T5Ø.8X4	T5Ø.8X5	T5Ø.8X6
Indometacin	T39.391	T39.392	T39.393	T39.394	T39.395	T39.396
Indomethacin	T39.391	T39.392	T39.393	T39.394	T39.395	T39.396
farnesil	T39.4X1	T39.4X2	T39.4X3	T39.4X4	T39.4X5	T39.4X6
Indoramin	T44.6X1	T44.6X2	T44.6X3	T44.6X4	T44.6X5	T44.6X6
Industrial						
alcohol	T51.ØX1	T51.ØX2	T51.ØX3	T51.ØX4	—	—
fumes	T59.891	T59.892	T59.893	T59.894	—	—
solvents (fumes) (vapors)	T52.91	T52.92	T52.93	T52.94	—	—
Influenza vaccine	T5Ø.B91	T5Ø.B92	T5Ø.B93	T5Ø.B94	T5Ø.B95	T5Ø.B96
Ingested substance NEC	T65.91	T65.92	T65.93	T65.94	—	—
INH	T37.1X1	T37.1X2	T37.1X3	T37.1X4	T37.1X5	T37.1X6
Inhalation, gas (noxious) — *see* Gas						
Inhibitor						
angiotensin-converting enzyme	T46.4X1	T46.4X2	T46.4X3	T46.4X4	T46.4X5	T46.4X6
carbonic anhydrase	T5Ø.2X1	T5Ø.2X2	T5Ø.2X3	T5Ø.2X4	T5Ø.2X5	T5Ø.2X6
fibrinolysis	T45.621	T45.622	T45.623	T45.624	T45.625	T45.626
monoamine oxidase NEC	T43.1X1	T43.1X2	T43.1X3	T43.1X4	T43.1X5	T43.1X6
hydrazine	T43.1X1	T43.1X2	T43.1X3	T43.1X4	T43.1X5	T43.1X6
postsynaptic	T43.8X1	T43.8X2	T43.8X3	T43.8X4	T43.8X5	T43.8X6
prothrombin synthesis	T45.511	T45.512	T45.513	T45.514	T45.515	T45.516
Ink	T65.891	T65.892	T65.893	T65.894	—	—
Inorganic substance NEC	T57.91	T57.92	T57.93	T57.94	—	—
Inosine pranobex	T37.5X1	T37.5X2	T37.5X3	T37.5X4	T37.5X5	T37.5X6
Inositol	T5Ø.991	T5Ø.992	T5Ø.993	T5Ø.994	T5Ø.995	T5Ø.996
nicotinate	T46.7X1	T46.7X2	T46.7X3	T46.7X4	T46.7X5	T46.7X6
Inproquone	T45.1X1	T45.1X2	T45.1X3	T45.1X4	T45.1X5	T45.1X6
Insecticide NEC	T6Ø.91	T6Ø.92	T6Ø.93	T6Ø.94	—	—
carbamate	T6Ø.ØX1	T6Ø.ØX2	T6Ø.ØX3	T6Ø.ØX4	—	—
chlorinated	T6Ø.1X1	T6Ø.1X2	T6Ø.1X3	T6Ø.1X4	—	—
mixed	T6Ø.91	T6Ø.92	T6Ø.93	T6Ø.94	—	—
organochlorine	T6Ø.1X1	T6Ø.1X2	T6Ø.1X3	T6Ø.1X4	—	—
organophosphorus	T6Ø.ØX1	T6Ø.ØX2	T6Ø.ØX3	T6Ø.ØX4	—	—
Insect (sting), venomous	T63.481	T63.482	T63.483	T63.484	—	—
ant	T63.421	T63.422	T63.423	T63.424	—	—
bee	T63.441	T63.442	T63.443	T63.444	—	—
caterpillar	T63.431	T63.432	T63.433	T63.434	—	—
hornet	T63.451	T63.452	T63.453	T63.454	—	—
wasp	T63.461	T63.462	T63.463	T63.464	—	—
Insular tissue extract	T38.3X1	T38.3X2	T38.3X3	T38.3X4	T38.3X5	T38.3X6
Insulin (amorphous) (globin) (isophane) (Lente) (NPH) (Semilente) (Ultralente)	T38.3X1	T38.3X2	T38.3X3	T38.3X4	T38.3X5	T38.3X6
defalan	T38.3X1	T38.3X2	T38.3X3	T38.3X4	T38.3X5	T38.3X6
human	T38.3X1	T38.3X2	T38.3X3	T38.3X4	T38.3X5	T38.3X6
injection, soluble	T38.3X1	T38.3X2	T38.3X3	T38.3X4	T38.3X5	T38.3X6
biphasic	T38.3X1	T38.3X2	T38.3X3	T38.3X4	T38.3X5	T38.3X6
intermediate acting	T38.3X1	T38.3X2	T38.3X3	T38.3X4	T38.3X5	T38.3X6
protamine zinc	T38.3X1	T38.3X2	T38.3X3	T38.3X4	T38.3X5	T38.3X6
slow acting	T38.3X1	T38.3X2	T38.3X3	T38.3X4	T38.3X5	T38.3X6
zinc						
protamine injection	T38.3X1	T38.3X2	T38.3X3	T38.3X4	T38.3X5	T38.3X6
suspension (amorphous) (crystalline)	T38.3X1	T38.3X2	T38.3X3	T38.3X4	T38.3X5	T38.3X6
Interferon (alpha) (beta) (gamma)	T37.5X1	T37.5X2	T37.5X3	T37.5X4	T37.5X5	T37.5X6
Intestinal motility control drug	T47.6X1	T47.6X2	T47.6X3	T47.6X4	T47.6X5	T47.6X6
biological	T47.8X1	T47.8X2	T47.8X3	T47.8X4	T47.8X5	T47.8X6
Intranarcon	T41.1X1	T41.1X2	T41.1X3	T41.1X4	T41.1X5	T41.1X6
Intravenous						
amino acids	T5Ø.991	T5Ø.992	T5Ø.993	T5Ø.994	T5Ø.995	T5Ø.996
fat suspension	T5Ø.991	T5Ø.992	T5Ø.993	T5Ø.994	T5Ø.995	T5Ø.996
Inulin	T5Ø.8X1	T5Ø.8X2	T5Ø.8X3	T5Ø.8X4	T5Ø.8X5	T5Ø.8X6
Invert sugar	T5Ø.3X1	T5Ø.3X2	T5Ø.3X3	T5Ø.3X4	T5Ø.3X5	T5Ø.3X6
Inza — *see* Naproxen						
Iobenzamic acid	T5Ø.8X1	T5Ø.8X2	T5Ø.8X3	T5Ø.8X4	T5Ø.8X5	T5Ø.8X6
Iocarmic acid	T5Ø.8X1	T5Ø.8X2	T5Ø.8X3	T5Ø.8X4	T5Ø.8X5	T5Ø.8X6
Iocetamic acid	T5Ø.8X1	T5Ø.8X2	T5Ø.8X3	T5Ø.8X4	T5Ø.8X5	T5Ø.8X6

Substance	Poisoning, Accidental (unintentional)	Poisoning, Intentional Self-harm	Poisoning, Assault	Poisoning, Undetermined	Adverse Effect	Under-dosing
Iodamide	T5Ø.8X1	T5Ø.8X2	T5Ø.8X3	T5Ø.8X4	T5Ø.8X5	T5Ø.8X6
Iodide NEC — *see also* Iodine	T49.ØX1	T49.ØX2	T49.ØX3	T49.ØX4	T49.ØX5	T49.ØX6
mercury (ointment)	T49.ØX1	T49.ØX2	T49.ØX3	T49.ØX4	T49.ØX5	T49.ØX6
methylate	T49.ØX1	T49.ØX2	T49.ØX3	T49.ØX4	T49.ØX5	T49.ØX6
potassium (expectorant) NEC	T48.4X1	T48.4X2	T48.4X3	T48.4X4	T48.4X5	T48.4X6
Iodinated						
contrast medium	T5Ø.8X1	T5Ø.8X2	T5Ø.8X3	T5Ø.8X4	T5Ø.8X5	T5Ø.8X6
glycerol	T48.4X1	T48.4X2	T48.4X3	T48.4X4	T48.4X5	T48.4X6
human serum albumin (131I)	T5Ø.8X1	T5Ø.8X2	T5Ø.8X3	T5Ø.8X4	T5Ø.8X5	T5Ø.8X6
Iodine (antiseptic, external) (tincture) **NEC**	T49.ØX1	T49.ØX2	T49.ØX3	T49.ØX4	T49.ØX5	T49.ØX6
125 — *see also* Radiation sickness, and Exposure to radioactivce isotopes	T5Ø.8X1	T5Ø.8X2	T5Ø.8X3	T5Ø.8X4	T5Ø.8X5	T5Ø.8X6
therapeutic	T5Ø.991	T5Ø.992	T5Ø.993	T5Ø.994	T5Ø.995	T5Ø.996
131 — *see also* Radiation sickness, and Exposure to radioactivce isotopes	T5Ø.8X1	T5Ø.8X2	T5Ø.8X3	T5Ø.8X4	T5Ø.8X5	T5Ø.8X6
therapeutic	T38.2X1	T38.2X2	T38.2X3	T38.2X4	T38.2X5	T38.2X6
diagnostic	T5Ø.8X1	T5Ø.8X2	T5Ø.8X3	T5Ø.8X4	T5Ø.8X5	T5Ø.8X6
for thyroid conditions (antithyroid)	T38.2X1	T38.2X2	T38.2X3	T38.2X4	T38.2X5	T38.2X6
solution	T49.ØX1	T49.ØX2	T49.ØX3	T49.ØX4	T49.ØX5	T49.ØX6
vapor	T59.891	T59.892	T59.893	T59.894	—	—
Iodipamide	T5Ø.8X1	T5Ø.8X2	T5Ø.8X3	T5Ø.8X4	T5Ø.8X5	T5Ø.8X6
Iodized (poppy seed) oil	T5Ø.8X1	T5Ø.8X2	T5Ø.8X3	T5Ø.8X4	T5Ø.8X5	T5Ø.8X6
Iodobismitol	T37.8X1	T37.8X2	T37.8X3	T37.8X4	T37.8X5	T37.8X6
Iodochlorhydroxyquin	T37.8X1	T37.8X2	T37.8X3	T37.8X4	T37.8X5	T37.8X6
topical	T49.ØX1	T49.ØX2	T49.ØX3	T49.ØX4	T49.ØX5	T49.ØX6
Iodochlorhydroxyquinoline	T37.8X1	T37.8X2	T37.8X3	T37.8X4	T37.8X5	T37.8X6
Iodocholesterol (131I)	T5Ø.8X1	T5Ø.8X2	T5Ø.8X3	T5Ø.8X4	T5Ø.8X5	T5Ø.8X6
Iodoform	T49.ØX1	T49.ØX2	T49.ØX3	T49.ØX4	T49.ØX5	T49.ØX6
Iodohippuric acid	T5Ø.8X1	T5Ø.8X2	T5Ø.8X3	T5Ø.8X4	T5Ø.8X5	T5Ø.8X6
Iodopanoic acid	T5Ø.8X1	T5Ø.8X2	T5Ø.8X3	T5Ø.8X4	T5Ø.8X5	T5Ø.8X6
Iodophthalein (sodium)	T5Ø.8X1	T5Ø.8X2	T5Ø.8X3	T5Ø.8X4	T5Ø.8X5	T5Ø.8X6
Iodopyracet	T5Ø.8X1	T5Ø.8X2	T5Ø.8X3	T5Ø.8X4	T5Ø.8X5	T5Ø.8X6
Iodoquinol	T37.8X1	T37.8X2	T37.8X3	T37.8X4	T37.8X5	T37.8X6
Iodoxamic acid	T5Ø.8X1	T5Ø.8X2	T5Ø.8X3	T5Ø.8X4	T5Ø.8X5	T5Ø.8X6
Iofendylate	T5Ø.8X1	T5Ø.8X2	T5Ø.8X3	T5Ø.8X4	T5Ø.8X5	T5Ø.8X6
Ioglycamic acid	T5Ø.8X1	T5Ø.8X2	T5Ø.8X3	T5Ø.8X4	T5Ø.8X5	T5Ø.8X6
Iohexol	T5Ø.8X1	T5Ø.8X2	T5Ø.8X3	T5Ø.8X4	T5Ø.8X5	T5Ø.8X6
Ion exchange resin						
anion	T47.8X1	T47.8X2	T47.8X3	T47.8X4	T47.8X5	T47.8X6
cation	T5Ø.3X1	T5Ø.3X2	T5Ø.3X3	T5Ø.3X4	T5Ø.3X5	T5Ø.3X6
cholestyramine	T46.6X1	T46.6X2	T46.6X3	T46.6X4	T46.6X5	T46.6X6
intestinal	T47.8X1	T47.8X2	T47.8X3	T47.8X4	T47.8X5	T47.8X6
Iopamidol	T5Ø.8X1	T5Ø.8X2	T5Ø.8X3	T5Ø.8X4	T5Ø.8X5	T5Ø.8X6
Iopanoic acid	T5Ø.8X1	T5Ø.8X2	T5Ø.8X3	T5Ø.8X4	T5Ø.8X5	T5Ø.8X6
Iophenoic acid	T5Ø.8X1	T5Ø.8X2	T5Ø.8X3	T5Ø.8X4	T5Ø.8X5	T5Ø.8X6
Iopodate, sodium	T5Ø.8X1	T5Ø.8X2	T5Ø.8X3	T5Ø.8X4	T5Ø.8X5	T5Ø.8X6
Iopodic acid	T5Ø.8X1	T5Ø.8X2	T5Ø.8X3	T5Ø.8X4	T5Ø.8X5	T5Ø.8X6
Iopromide	T5Ø.8X1	T5Ø.8X2	T5Ø.8X3	T5Ø.8X4	T5Ø.8X5	T5Ø.8X6
Iopydol	T5Ø.8X1	T5Ø.8X2	T5Ø.8X3	T5Ø.8X4	T5Ø.8X5	T5Ø.8X6
Iotalamic acid	T5Ø.8X1	T5Ø.8X2	T5Ø.8X3	T5Ø.8X4	T5Ø.8X5	T5Ø.8X6
Iothalamate	T5Ø.8X1	T5Ø.8X2	T5Ø.8X3	T5Ø.8X4	T5Ø.8X5	T5Ø.8X6
Iothiouracil	T38.2X1	T38.2X2	T38.2X3	T38.2X4	T38.2X5	T38.2X6
Iotrol	T5Ø.8X1	T5Ø.8X2	T5Ø.8X3	T5Ø.8X4	T5Ø.8X5	T5Ø.8X6
Iotrolan	T5Ø.8X1	T5Ø.8X2	T5Ø.8X3	T5Ø.8X4	T5Ø.8X5	T5Ø.8X6
Iotroxate	T5Ø.8X1	T5Ø.8X2	T5Ø.8X3	T5Ø.8X4	T5Ø.8X5	T5Ø.8X6
Iotroxic acid	T5Ø.8X1	T5Ø.8X2	T5Ø.8X3	T5Ø.8X4	T5Ø.8X5	T5Ø.8X6
Ioversol	T5Ø.8X1	T5Ø.8X2	T5Ø.8X3	T5Ø.8X4	T5Ø.8X5	T5Ø.8X6
Ioxaglate	T5Ø.8X1	T5Ø.8X2	T5Ø.8X3	T5Ø.8X4	T5Ø.8X5	T5Ø.8X6
Ioxaglic acid	T5Ø.8X1	T5Ø.8X2	T5Ø.8X3	T5Ø.8X4	T5Ø.8X5	T5Ø.8X6
Ioxitalamic acid	T5Ø.8X1	T5Ø.8X2	T5Ø.8X3	T5Ø.8X4	T5Ø.8X5	T5Ø.8X6
Ipecac	T47.7X1	T47.7X2	T47.7X3	T47.7X4	T47.7X5	T47.7X6
Ipecacuanha	T48.4X1	T48.4X2	T48.4X3	T48.4X4	T48.4X5	T48.4X6
Ipodate, calcium	T5Ø.8X1	T5Ø.8X2	T5Ø.8X3	T5Ø.8X4	T5Ø.8X5	T5Ø.8X6
Ipral	T42.3X1	T42.3X2	T42.3X3	T42.3X4	T42.3X5	T42.3X6
Ipratropium (bromide)	T48.6X1	T48.6X2	T48.6X3	T48.6X4	T48.6X5	T48.6X6
Ipriflavone	T46.3X1	T46.3X2	T46.3X3	T46.3X4	T46.3X5	T46.3X6
Iprindole	T43.Ø11	T43.Ø12	T43.Ø13	T43.Ø14	T43.Ø15	T43.Ø16
Iproclozide	T43.1X1	T43.1X2	T43.1X3	T43.1X4	T43.1X5	T43.1X6
Iprofenin	T5Ø.8X1	T5Ø.8X2	T5Ø.8X3	T5Ø.8X4	T5Ø.8X5	T5Ø.8X6
Iproheptine	T49.2X1	T49.2X2	T49.2X3	T49.2X4	T49.2X5	T49.2X6
Iproniazid	T43.1X1	T43.1X2	T43.1X3	T43.1X4	T43.1X5	T43.1X6
Iproplatin	T45.1X1	T45.1X2	T45.1X3	T45.1X4	T45.1X5	T45.1X6
Iproveratril	T46.1X1	T46.1X2	T46.1X3	T46.1X4	T46.1X5	T46.1X6
Iron (compounds) (medicinal) **NEC**	T45.4X1	T45.4X2	T45.4X3	T45.4X4	T45.4X5	T45.4X6
ammonium	T45.4X1	T45.4X2	T45.4X3	T45.4X4	T45.4X5	T45.4X6
dextran injection	T45.4X1	T45.4X2	T45.4X3	T45.4X4	T45.4X5	T45.4X6

Substance	Poisoning, Accidental (unintentional)	Poisoning, Intentional Self-harm	Poisoning, Assault	Poisoning, Undetermined	Adverse Effect	Under-dosing
Iron (compounds) (medicinal) **NEC** — *continued*						
nonmedicinal	T56.891	T56.892	T56.893	T56.894	—	—
salts	T45.4X1	T45.4X2	T45.4X3	T45.4X4	T45.4X5	T45.4X6
sorbitex	T45.4X1	T45.4X2	T45.4X3	T45.4X4	T45.4X5	T45.4X6
sorbitol citric acid complex	T45.4X1	T45.4X2	T45.4X3	T45.4X4	T45.4X5	T45.4X6
Irrigating fluid (vaginal)	T49.8X1	T49.8X2	T49.8X3	T49.8X4	T49.8X5	T49.8X6
eye	T49.5X1	T49.5X2	T49.5X3	T49.5X4	T49.5X5	T49.5X6
Isepamicin	T36.5X1	T36.5X2	T36.5X3	T36.5X4	T36.5X5	T36.5X6
Isoaminile (citrate)	T48.3X1	T48.3X2	T48.3X3	T48.3X4	T48.3X5	T48.3X6
Isoamyl nitrite	T46.3X1	T46.3X2	T46.3X3	T46.3X4	T46.3X5	T46.3X6
Isobenzan	T6Ø.1X1	T6Ø.1X2	T6Ø.1X3	T6Ø.1X4	—	—
Isobutyl acetate	T52.8X1	T52.8X2	T52.8X3	T52.8X4	—	—
Isocarboxazid	T43.1X1	T43.1X2	T43.1X3	T43.1X4	T43.1X5	T43.1X6
Isoconazole	T49.ØX1	T49.ØX2	T49.ØX3	T49.ØX4	T49.ØX5	T49.ØX6
Isocyanate	T65.ØX1	T65.ØX2	T65.ØX3	T65.ØX4	—	—
Isoephedrine	T44.991	T44.992	T44.993	T44.994	T44.995	T44.996
Isoetarine	T48.6X1	T48.6X2	T48.6X3	T48.6X4	T48.6X5	T48.6X6
Isoethadione	T42.2X1	T42.2X2	T42.2X3	T42.2X4	T42.2X5	T42.2X6
Isoetharine	T44.5X1	T44.5X2	T44.5X3	T44.5X4	T44.5X5	T44.5X6
Isoflurane	T41.ØX1	T41.ØX2	T41.ØX3	T41.ØX4	T41.ØX5	T41.ØX6
Isoflurophate	T44.ØX1	T44.ØX2	T44.ØX3	T44.ØX4	T44.ØX5	T44.ØX6
Isomaltose, ferric complex	T45.4X1	T45.4X2	T45.4X3	T45.4X4	T45.4X5	T45.4X6
Isometheptene	T44.3X1	T44.3X2	T44.3X3	T44.3X4	T44.3X5	T44.3X6
Isoniazid	T37.1X1	T37.1X2	T37.1X3	T37.1X4	T37.1X5	T37.1X6
with						
rifampicin	T36.6X1	T36.6X2	T36.6X3	T36.6X4	T36.6X5	T36.6X6
thioacetazone	T37.1X1	T37.1X2	T37.1X3	T37.1X4	T37.1X5	T37.1X6
Isonicotinic acid hydrazide	T37.1X1	T37.1X2	T37.1X3	T37.1X4	T37.1X5	T37.1X6
Isonipecaine	T4Ø.4X1	T4Ø.4X2	T4Ø.4X3	T4Ø.4X4	T4Ø.4X5	T4Ø.4X6
Isopentaquine	T37.2X1	T37.2X2	T37.2X3	T37.2X4	T37.2X5	T37.2X6
Isophane insulin	T38.3X1	T38.3X2	T38.3X3	T38.3X4	T38.3X5	T38.3X6
Isophorone	T65.891	T65.892	T65.893	T65.894	—	—
Isophosphamide	T45.1X1	T45.1X2	T45.1X3	T45.1X4	T45.1X5	T45.1X6
Isopregnenone	T38.5X1	T38.5X2	T38.5X3	T38.5X4	T38.5X5	T38.5X6
Isoprenaline	T48.6X1	T48.6X2	T48.6X3	T48.6X4	T48.6X5	T48.6X6
Isopromethazine	T43.3X1	T43.3X2	T43.3X3	T43.3X4	T43.3X5	T43.3X6
Isopropamide	T44.3X1	T44.3X2	T44.3X3	T44.3X4	T44.3X5	T44.3X6
iodide	T44.3X1	T44.3X2	T44.3X3	T44.3X4	T44.3X5	T44.3X6
Isopropanol	T51.2X1	T51.2X2	T51.2X3	T51.2X4	—	—
Isopropyl						
acetate	T52.8X1	T52.8X2	T52.8X3	T52.8X4	—	—
alcohol	T51.2X1	T51.2X2	T51.2X3	T51.2X4	—	—
medicinal	T49.4X1	T49.4X2	T49.4X3	T49.4X4	T49.4X5	T49.4X6
ether	T52.8X1	T52.8X2	T52.8X3	T52.8X4	—	—
Isopropylaminophenazone	T39.2X1	T39.2X2	T39.2X3	T39.2X4	T39.2X5	T39.2X6
Isoproterenol	T48.6X1	T48.6X2	T48.6X3	T48.6X4	T48.6X5	T48.6X6
Isosorbide dinitrate	T46.3X1	T46.3X2	T46.3X3	T46.3X4	T46.3X5	T46.3X6
Isothipendyl	T45.ØX1	T45.ØX2	T45.ØX3	T45.ØX4	T45.ØX5	T45.ØX6
Isotretinoin	T5Ø.991	T5Ø.992	T5Ø.993	T5Ø.994	T5Ø.995	T5Ø.996
Isoxazolyl penicillin	T36.ØX1	T36.ØX2	T36.ØX3	T36.ØX4	T36.ØX5	T36.ØX6
Isoxicam	T39.391	T39.392	T39.393	T39.394	T39.395	T39.396
Isoxsuprine	T46.7X1	T46.7X2	T46.7X3	T46.7X4	T46.7X5	T46.7X6
Ispagula	T47.4X1	T47.4X2	T47.4X3	T47.4X4	T47.4X5	T47.4X6
husk	T47.4X1	T47.4X2	T47.4X3	T47.4X4	T47.4X5	T47.4X6
Isradipine	T46.1X1	T46.1X2	T46.1X3	T46.1X4	T46.1X5	T46.1X6
l-thyroxine sodium	T38.1X1	T38.1X2	T38.1X3	T38.1X4	T38.1X5	T38.1X6
Itraconazole	T37.8X1	T37.8X2	T37.8X3	T37.8X4	T37.8X5	T37.8X6
Itramin tosilate	T46.3X1	T46.3X2	T46.3X3	T46.3X4	T46.3X5	T46.3X6
Ivermectin	T37.4X1	T37.4X2	T37.4X3	T37.4X4	T37.4X5	T37.4X6
Izoniazid	T37.1X1	T37.1X2	T37.1X3	T37.1X4	T37.1X5	T37.1X6
with thioacetazone	T37.1X1	T37.1X2	T37.1X3	T37.1X4	T37.1X5	T37.1X6
Jalap	T47.2X1	T47.2X2	T47.2X3	T47.2X4	T47.2X5	T47.2X6
Jamaica						
dogwood (bark)	T39.8X1	T39.8X2	T39.8X3	T39.8X4	T39.8X5	T39.8X6
ginger	T65.891	T65.892	T65.893	T65.894	—	—
root	T62.2X1	T62.2X2	T62.2X3	T62.2X4	—	—
Jatropha	T62.2X1	T62.2X2	T62.2X3	T62.2X4	—	—
curcas	T62.2X1	T62.2X2	T62.2X3	T62.2X4	—	—
Jectofer	T45.4X1	T45.4X2	T45.4X3	T45.4X4	T45.4X5	T45.4X6
Jellyfish (sting)	T63.621	T63.622	T63.623	T63.624	—	—
Jequirity (bean)	T62.2X1	T62.2X2	T62.2X3	T62.2X4	—	—
Jimson weed (stramonium)	T62.2X1	T62.2X2	T62.2X3	T62.2X4	—	—
seeds	T62.2X1	T62.2X2	T62.2X3	T62.2X4	—	—
Josamycin	T36.3X1	T36.3X2	T36.3X3	T36.3X4	T36.3X5	T36.3X6
Juniper tar	T49.1X1	T49.1X2	T49.1X3	T49.1X4	T49.1X5	T49.1X6
Kallidinogenase	T46.7X1	T46.7X2	T46.7X3	T46.7X4	T46.7X5	T46.7X6
Kallikrein	T46.7X1	T46.7X2	T46.7X3	T46.7X4	T46.7X5	T46.7X6
Kanamycin	T36.5X1	T36.5X2	T36.5X3	T36.5X4	T36.5X5	T36.5X6
Kantrex	T36.5X1	T36.5X2	T36.5X3	T36.5X4	T36.5X5	T36.5X6
Kaolin	T47.6X1	T47.6X2	T47.6X3	T47.6X4	T47.6X5	T47.6X6
light	T47.6X1	T47.6X2	T47.6X3	T47.6X4	T47.6X5	T47.6X6
Karaya (gum)	T47.4X1	T47.4X2	T47.4X3	T47.4X4	T47.4X5	T47.4X6

Substance	Poisoning, Accidental (unintentional)	Poisoning, Intentional Self-harm	Poisoning, Assault	Poisoning, Undetermined	Adverse Effect	Under-dosing
Kebuzone	T39.2X1	T39.2X2	T39.2X3	T39.2X4	T39.2X5	T39.2X6
Kelevan	T6Ø.1X1	T6Ø.1X2	T6Ø.1X3	T6Ø.1X4	—	—
Kemithal	T41.1X1	T41.1X2	T41.1X3	T41.1X4	T41.1X5	T41.1X6
Kenacort	T38.ØX1	T38.ØX2	T38.ØX3	T38.ØX4	T38.ØX5	T38.ØX6
Keratolytic drug NEC	T49.4X1	T49.4X2	T49.4X3	T49.4X4	T49.4X5	T49.4X6
anthracene	T49.4X1	T49.4X2	T49.4X3	T49.4X4	T49.4X5	T49.4X6
Keratoplastic NEC	T49.4X1	T49.4X2	T49.4X3	T49.4X4	T49.4X5	T49.4X6
Kerosene, kerosine (fuel) (solvent) **NEC**	T52.ØX1	T52.ØX2	T52.ØX3	T52.ØX4	—	—
insecticide	T52.ØX1	T52.ØX2	T52.ØX3	T52.ØX4	—	—
vapor	T52.ØX1	T52.ØX2	T52.ØX3	T52.ØX4	—	—
Ketamine	T41.291	T41.292	T41.293	T41.294	T41.295	T41.296
Ketazolam	T42.4X1	T42.4X2	T42.4X3	T42.4X4	T42.4X5	T42.4X6
Ketazon	T39.2X1	T39.2X2	T39.2X3	T39.2X4	T39.2X5	T39.2X6
Ketobemidone	T4Ø.4X1	T4Ø.4X2	T4Ø.4X3	T4Ø.4X4	—	—
Ketoconazole	T49.ØX1	T49.ØX2	T49.ØX3	T49.ØX4	T49.ØX5	T49.ØX6
Ketols	T52.4X1	T52.4X2	T52.4X3	T52.4X4	—	—
Ketone oils	T52.4X1	T52.4X2	T52.4X3	T52.4X4	—	—
Ketoprofen	T39.311	T39.312	T39.313	T39.314	T39.315	T39.316
Ketorolac	T39.8X1	T39.8X2	T39.8X3	T39.8X4	T39.8X5	T39.8X6
Ketotifen	T45.ØX1	T45.ØX2	T45.ØX3	T45.ØX4	T45.ØX5	T45.ØX6
Khat	T43.691	T43.692	T43.693	T43.694	—	—
Khellin	T46.3X1	T46.3X2	T46.3X3	T46.3X4	T46.3X5	T46.3X6
Khelloside	T46.3X1	T46.3X2	T46.3X3	T46.3X4	T46.3X5	T46.3X6
Kiln gas or vapor (carbon monoxide)	T58.8X1	T58.8X2	T58.8X3	T58.8X4	—	—
Kitasamycin	T36.3X1	T36.3X2	T36.3X3	T36.3X4	T36.3X5	T36.3X6
Konsyl	T47.4X1	T47.4X2	T47.4X3	T47.4X4	T47.4X5	T47.4X6
Kosam seed	T62.2X1	T62.2X2	T62.2X3	T62.2X4	—	—
Krait (venom)	T63.Ø91	T63.Ø92	T63.Ø93	T63.Ø94	—	—
Kwell (insecticide)	T6Ø.1X1	T6Ø.1X2	T6Ø.1X3	T6Ø.1X4	—	—
anti-infective (topical)	T49.ØX1	T49.ØX2	T49.ØX3	T49.ØX4	T49.ØX5	T49.ØX6
Labetalol	T44.8X1	T44.8X2	T44.8X3	T44.8X4	T44.8X5	T44.8X6
Laburnum (seeds)	T62.2X1	T62.2X2	T62.2X3	T62.2X4	—	—
leaves	T62.2X1	T62.2X2	T62.2X3	T62.2X4	—	—
Lachesine	T49.5X1	T49.5X2	T49.5X3	T49.5X4	T49.5X5	T49.5X6
Lacidipine	T46.5X1	T46.5X2	T46.5X3	T46.5X4	T46.5X5	T46.5X6
Lacquer	T65.6X1	T65.6X2	T65.6X3	T65.6X4	—	—
Lacrimogenic gas	T59.3X1	T59.3X2	T59.3X3	T59.3X4	—	—
Lactated potassic saline	T5Ø.3X1	T5Ø.3X2	T5Ø.3X3	T5Ø.3X4	T5Ø.3X5	T5Ø.3X6
Lactic acid	T49.8X1	T49.8X2	T49.8X3	T49.8X4	T49.8X5	T49.8X6
Lactobacillus						
acidophilus	T47.6X1	T47.6X2	T47.6X3	T47.6X4	T47.6X5	T47.6X6
compound	T47.6X1	T47.6X2	T47.6X3	T47.6X4	T47.6X5	T47.6X6
bifidus, lyophilized	T47.6X1	T47.6X2	T47.6X3	T47.6X4	T47.6X5	T47.6X6
bulgaricus	T47.6X1	T47.6X2	T47.6X3	T47.6X4	T47.6X5	T47.6X6
sporogenes	T47.6X1	T47.6X2	T47.6X3	T47.6X4	T47.6X5	T47.6X6
Lactoflavin	T45.2X1	T45.2X2	T45.2X3	T45.2X4	T45.2X5	T45.2X6
Lactose (as excipient)	T5Ø.9Ø1	T5Ø.9Ø2	T5Ø.9Ø3	T5Ø.9Ø4	T5Ø.9Ø5	T5Ø.9Ø6
Lactuca (virosa) (extract)	T42.6X1	T42.6X2	T42.6X3	T42.6X4	T42.6X5	T42.6X6
Lactucarium	T42.6X1	T42.6X2	T42.6X3	T42.6X4	T42.6X5	T42.6X6
Lactulose	T47.3X1	T47.3X2	T47.3X3	T47.3X4	T47.3X5	T47.3X6
Laevo — *see* Levo-						
Lanatosides	T46.ØX1	T46.ØX2	T46.ØX3	T46.ØX4	T46.ØX5	T46.ØX6
Lanolin	T49.3X1	T49.3X2	T49.3X3	T49.3X4	T49.3X5	T49.3X6
Largactil	T43.3X1	T43.3X2	T43.3X3	T43.3X4	T43.3X5	T43.3X6
Larkspur	T62.2X1	T62.2X2	T62.2X3	T62.2X4	—	—
Laroxyl	T43.Ø11	T43.Ø12	T43.Ø13	T43.Ø14	T43.Ø15	T43.Ø16
Lasix	T5Ø.1X1	T5Ø.1X2	T5Ø.1X3	T5Ø.1X4	T5Ø.1X5	T5Ø.1X6
Lassar's paste	T49.4X1	T49.4X2	T49.4X3	T49.4X4	T49.4X5	T49.4X6
Latamoxef	T36.1X1	T36.1X2	T36.1X3	T36.1X4	T36.1X5	T36.1X6
Latex	T65.811	T65.812	T65.813	T65.814	—	—
Lathyrus (seed)	T62.2X1	T62.2X2	T62.2X3	T62.2X4	—	—
Laudanum	T4Ø.ØX1	T4Ø.ØX2	T4Ø.ØX3	T4Ø.ØX4	T4Ø.ØX5	T4Ø.ØX6
Laudexium	T48.1X1	T48.1X2	T48.1X3	T48.1X4	T48.1X5	T48.1X6
Laughing gas	T41.ØX1	T41.ØX2	T41.ØX3	T41.ØX4	T41.ØX5	T41.ØX6
Laurel, black or cherry	T62.2X1	T62.2X2	T62.2X3	T62.2X4	—	—
Laurolinium	T49.ØX1	T49.ØX2	T49.ØX3	T49.ØX4	T49.ØX5	T49.ØX6
Lauryl sulfoacetate	T49.2X1	T49.2X2	T49.2X3	T49.2X4	T49.2X5	T49.2X6
Laxative NEC	T47.4X1	T47.4X2	T47.4X3	T47.4X4	T47.4X5	T47.4X6
osmotic	T47.3X1	T47.3X2	T47.3X3	T47.3X4	T47.3X5	T47.3X6
saline	T47.3X1	T47.3X2	T47.3X3	T47.3X4	T47.3X5	T47.3X6
stimulant	T47.2X1	T47.2X2	T47.2X3	T47.2X4	T47.2X5	T47.2X6
L-dopa	T42.8X1	T42.8X2	T42.8X3	T42.8X4	T42.8X5	T42.8X6
Lead (dust) (fumes) (vapor) **NEC**	T56.ØX1	T56.ØX2	T56.ØX3	T56.ØX4	—	—
acetate	T49.2X1	T49.2X2	T49.2X3	T49.2X4	T49.2X5	T49.2X6
alkyl (fuel additive)	T56.ØX1	T56.ØX2	T56.ØX3	T56.ØX4	—	—
anti-infectives	T37.8X1	T37.8X2	T37.8X3	T37.8X4	T37.8X5	T37.8X6
antiknock compound (tetraethyl)	T56.ØX1	T56.ØX2	T56.ØX3	T56.ØX4	—	—
Lead (dust) (fumes) (vapor) **NEC** — *continued*						
arsenate, arsenite (dust)(herbicide) (insecticide) (vapor)	T57.ØX1	T57.ØX2	T57.ØX3	T57.ØX4	—	—
carbonate	T56.ØX1	T56.ØX2	T56.ØX3	T56.ØX4	—	—
paint	T56.ØX1	T56.ØX2	T56.ØX3	T56.ØX4	—	—
chromate	T56.ØX1	T56.ØX2	T56.ØX3	T56.ØX4	—	—
paint	T56.ØX1	T56.ØX2	T56.ØX3	T56.ØX4	—	—
dioxide	T56.ØX1	T56.ØX2	T56.ØX3	T56.ØX4	—	—
inorganic	T56.ØX1	T56.ØX2	T56.ØX3	T56.ØX4	—	—
iodide	T56.ØX1	T56.ØX2	T56.ØX3	T56.ØX4	—	—
pigment (paint)	T56.ØX1	T56.ØX2	T56.ØX3	T56.ØX4	—	—
monoxide (dust)	T56.ØX1	T56.ØX2	T56.ØX3	T56.ØX4	—	—
paint	T56.ØX1	T56.ØX2	T56.ØX3	T56.ØX4	—	—
organic	T56.ØX1	T56.ØX2	T56.ØX3	T56.ØX4	—	—
oxide	T56.ØX1	T56.ØX2	T56.ØX3	T56.ØX4	—	—
paint	T56.ØX1	T56.ØX2	T56.ØX3	T56.ØX4	—	—
paint	T56.ØX1	T56.ØX2	T56.ØX3	T56.ØX4	—	—
salts	T56.ØX1	T56.ØX2	T56.ØX3	T56.ØX4	—	—
specified compound NEC	T56.ØX1	T56.ØX2	T56.ØX3	T56.ØX4	—	—
tetra-ethyl	T56.ØX1	T56.ØX2	T56.ØX3	T56.ØX4	—	—
Lebanese red	T4Ø.7X1	T4Ø.7X2	T4Ø.7X3	T4Ø.7X4	T4Ø.7X5	T4Ø.7X6
Lefetamine	T39.8X1	T39.8X2	T39.8X3	T39.8X4	T39.8X5	T39.8X6
Lenperone	T43.4X1	T43.4X2	T43.4X3	T43.4X4	T43.4X5	T43.4X6
Lente lietin (insulin)	T38.3X1	T38.3X2	T38.3X3	T38.3X4	T38.3X5	T38.3X6
Leptazol	T5Ø.7X1	T5Ø.7X2	T5Ø.7X3	T5Ø.7X4	T5Ø.7X5	T5Ø.7X6
Leptophos	T6Ø.ØX1	T6Ø.ØX2	T6Ø.ØX3	T6Ø.ØX4	—	—
Leritine	T4Ø.2X1	T4Ø.2X2	T4Ø.2X3	T4Ø.2X4	T4Ø.2X5	T4Ø.2X6
Letosteine	T48.4X1	T48.4X2	T48.4X3	T48.4X4	T48.4X5	T48.4X6
Letter	T38.1X1	T38.1X2	T38.1X3	T38.1X4	T38.1X5	T38.1X6
Lettuce opium	T42.6X1	T42.6X2	T42.6X3	T42.6X4	T42.6X5	T42.6X6
Leucinocaine	T41.3X1	T41.3X2	T41.3X3	T41.3X4	T41.3X5	T41.3X6
Leucocianidol	T46.991	T46.992	T46.993	T46.994	T46.995	T46.996
Leucovorin (factor)	T45.8X1	T45.8X2	T45.8X3	T45.8X4	T45.8X5	T45.8X6
Leukeran	T45.1X1	T45.1X2	T45.1X3	T45.1X4	T45.1X5	T45.1X6
Leuprolide	T38.891	T38.892	T38.893	T38.894	T38.895	T38.896
Levalbuterol	T48.6X1	T48.6X2	T48.6X3	T48.6X4	T48.6X5	T48.6X6
Levallorphan	T5Ø.7X1	T5Ø.7X2	T5Ø.7X3	T5Ø.7X4	T5Ø.7X5	T5Ø.7X6
Levamisole	T37.4X1	T37.4X2	T37.4X3	T37.4X4	T37.4X5	T37.4X6
Levanil	T42.6X1	T42.6X2	T42.6X3	T42.6X4	T42.6X5	T42.6X6
Levarterenol	T44.4X1	T44.4X2	T44.4X3	T44.4X4	T44.4X5	T44.4X6
Levdropropizine	T48.3X1	T48.3X2	T48.3X3	T48.3X4	T48.3X5	T48.3X6
Levobunolol	T49.5X1	T49.5X2	T49.5X3	T49.5X4	T49.5X5	T49.5X6
Levocabastine (hydrochloride)	T45.ØX1	T45.ØX2	T45.ØX3	T45.ØX4	T45.ØX5	T45.ØX6
Levocarnitine	T5Ø.991	T5Ø.992	T5Ø.993	T5Ø.994	T5Ø.995	T5Ø.996
Levodopa	T42.8X1	T42.8X2	T42.8X3	T42.8X4	T42.8X5	T42.8X6
with carbidopa	T42.8X1	T42.8X2	T42.8X3	T42.8X4	T42.8X5	T42.8X6
Levo-dromoran	T4Ø.2X1	T4Ø.2X2	T4Ø.2X3	T4Ø.2X4	T4Ø.2X5	T4Ø.2X6
Levoglutamide	T5Ø.991	T5Ø.992	T5Ø.993	T5Ø.994	T5Ø.995	T5Ø.996
Levoid	T38.1X1	T38.1X2	T38.1X3	T38.1X4	T38.1X5	T38.1X6
Levo-isomethadone	T4Ø.3X1	T4Ø.3X2	T4Ø.3X3	T4Ø.3X4	T4Ø.3X5	T4Ø.3X6
Levomepromazine	T43.3X1	T43.3X2	T43.3X3	T43.3X4	T43.3X5	T43.3X6
Levonordefrin	T49.6X1	T49.6X2	T49.6X3	T49.6X4	T49.6X5	T49.6X6
Levonorgestrel	T38.4X1	T38.4X2	T38.4X3	T38.4X4	T38.4X5	T38.4X6
with ethinylestradiol	T38.5X1	T38.5X2	T38.5X3	T38.5X4	T38.5X5	T38.5X6
Levopromazine	T43.3X1	T43.3X2	T43.3X3	T43.3X4	T43.3X5	T43.3X6
Levoprome	T42.6X1	T42.6X2	T42.6X3	T42.6X4	T42.6X5	T42.6X6
Levopropoxyphene	T4Ø.4X1	T4Ø.4X2	T4Ø.4X3	T4Ø.4X4	T4Ø.4X5	T4Ø.4X6
Levopropylhexedrine	T5Ø.5X1	T5Ø.5X2	T5Ø.5X3	T5Ø.5X4	T5Ø.5X5	T5Ø.5X6
Levoproxyphylline	T48.6X1	T48.6X2	T48.6X3	T48.6X4	T48.6X5	T48.6X6
Levorphanol	T4Ø.4X1	T4Ø.4X2	T4Ø.4X3	T4Ø.4X4	T4Ø.4X5	T4Ø.4X6
Levothyroxine	T38.1X1	T38.1X2	T38.1X3	T38.1X4	T38.1X5	T38.1X6
sodium	T38.1X1	T38.1X2	T38.1X3	T38.1X4	T38.1X5	T38.1X6
Levsin	T44.3X1	T44.3X2	T44.3X3	T44.3X4	T44.3X5	T44.3X6
Levulose	T5Ø.3X1	T5Ø.3X2	T5Ø.3X3	T5Ø.3X4	T5Ø.3X5	T5Ø.3X6
Lewisite (gas), not in war	T57.ØX1	T57.ØX2	T57.ØX3	T57.ØX4	—	—
Librium	T42.4X1	T42.4X2	T42.4X3	T42.4X4	T42.4X5	T42.4X6
Lidex	T49.ØX1	T49.ØX2	T49.ØX3	T49.ØX4	T49.ØX5	T49.ØX6
Lidocaine	T41.3X1	T41.3X2	T41.3X3	T41.3X4	T41.3X5	T41.3X6
regional	T41.3X1	T41.3X2	T41.3X3	T41.3X4	T41.3X5	T41.3X6
spinal	T41.3X1	T41.3X2	T41.3X3	T41.3X4	T41.3X5	T41.3X6
Lidofenin	T5Ø.8X1	T5Ø.8X2	T5Ø.8X3	T5Ø.8X4	T5Ø.8X5	T5Ø.8X6
Lidoflazine	T46.1X1	T46.1X2	T46.1X3	T46.1X4	T46.1X5	T46.1X6
Lighter fluid	T52.ØX1	T52.ØX2	T52.ØX3	T52.ØX4	—	—
Lignin hemicellulose	T47.6X1	T47.6X2	T47.6X3	T47.6X4	T47.6X5	T47.6X6
Lignocaine	T41.3X1	T41.3X2	T41.3X3	T41.3X4	T41.3X5	T41.3X6
regional	T41.3X1	T41.3X2	T41.3X3	T41.3X4	T41.3X5	T41.3X6
spinal	T41.3X1	T41.3X2	T41.3X3	T41.3X4	T41.3X5	T41.3X6
Ligroin (e) (solvent)	T52.ØX1	T52.ØX2	T52.ØX3	T52.ØX4	—	—
vapor	T59.891	T59.892	T59.893	T59.894	—	—
Ligustrum vulgare	T62.2X1	T62.2X2	T62.2X3	T62.2X4	—	—

Substance	Poisoning, Accidental (unintentional)	Poisoning, Intentional Self-harm	Poisoning, Assault	Poisoning, Undetermined	Adverse Effect	Under-dosing
Lily of the valley	T62.2X1	T62.2X2	T62.2X3	T62.2X4	—	—
Lime (chloride)	T54.3X1	T54.3X2	T54.3X3	T54.3X4	—	—
Limonene	T52.8X1	T52.8X2	T52.8X3	T52.8X4	—	—
Lincomycin	T36.8X1	T36.8X2	T36.8X3	T36.8X4	T36.8X5	T36.8X6
Lindane (insecticide) (nonmedicinal) (vapor)	T53.6X1	T53.6X2	T53.6X3	T53.6X4	—	—
medicinal	T49.ØX1	T49.ØX2	T49.ØX3	T49.ØX4	T49.ØX5	T49.ØX6
Liniments NEC	T49.91	T49.92	T49.93	T49.94	T49.95	T49.96
Linoleic acid	T46.6X1	T46.6X2	T46.6X3	T46.6X4	T46.6X5	T46.6X6
Linolenic acid	T46.6X1	T46.6X2	T46.6X3	T46.6X4	T46.6X5	T46.6X6
Linseed	T47.4X1	T47.4X2	T47.4X3	T47.4X4	T47.4X5	T47.4X6
Liothyronine	T38.1X1	T38.1X2	T38.1X3	T38.1X4	T38.1X5	T38.1X6
Liotrix	T38.1X1	T38.1X2	T38.1X3	T38.1X4	T38.1X5	T38.1X6
Lipancreatin	T47.5X1	T47.5X2	T47.5X3	T47.5X4	T47.5X5	T47.5X6
Lipo-alprostadil	T46.7X1	T46.7X2	T46.7X3	T46.7X4	T46.7X5	T46.7X6
Lipo-Lutin	T38.5X1	T38.5X2	T38.5X3	T38.5X4	T38.5X5	T38.5X6
Lipotropic drug NEC	T5Ø.9Ø1	T5Ø.9Ø2	T5Ø.9Ø3	T5Ø.9Ø4	T5Ø.9Ø5	T5Ø.9Ø6
Liquefied petroleum gases	T59.891	T59.892	T59.893	T59.894	—	—
piped (pure or mixed with air)	T59.891	T59.892	T59.893	T59.894	—	—
Liquid						
paraffin	T47.4X1	T47.4X2	T47.4X3	T47.4X4	T47.4X5	T47.4X6
petrolatum	T47.4X1	T47.4X2	T47.4X3	T47.4X4	T47.4X5	T47.4X6
topical	T49.3X1	T49.3X2	T49.3X3	T49.3X4	T49.3X5	T49.3X6
specified NEC	T65.891	T65.892	T65.893	T65.894	—	—
substance	T65.91	T65.92	T65.93	T65.94	—	—
Liquor creosolis compositus	T65.891	T65.892	T65.893	T65.894	—	—
Liquorice	T48.4X1	T48.4X2	T48.4X3	T48.4X4	T48.4X5	T48.4X6
extract	T47.8X1	T47.8X2	T47.8X3	T47.8X4	T47.8X5	T47.8X6
Lisinopril	T46.4X1	T46.4X2	T46.4X3	T46.4X4	T46.4X5	T46.4X6
Lisuride	T42.8X1	T42.8X2	T42.8X3	T42.8X4	T42.8X5	T42.8X6
Lithane	T43.8X1	T43.8X2	T43.8X3	T43.8X4	T43.8X5	T43.8X6
Lithium	T56.891	T56.892	T56.893	T56.894	—	—
gluconate	T43.591	T43.592	T43.593	T43.594	T43.595	T43.596
salts (carbonate)	T43.591	T43.592	T43.593	T43.594	T43.595	T43.596
Lithonate	T43.8X1	T43.8X2	T43.8X3	T43.8X4	T43.8X5	T43.8X6
Liver						
extract	T45.8X1	T45.8X2	T45.8X3	T45.8X4	T45.8X5	T45.8X6
for parenteral use	T45.8X1	T45.8X2	T45.8X3	T45.8X4	T45.8X5	T45.8X6
fraction 1	T45.8X1	T45.8X2	T45.8X3	T45.8X4	T45.8X5	T45.8X6
hydrolysate	T45.8X1	T45.8X2	T45.8X3	T45.8X4	T45.8X5	T45.8X6
Lizard (bite) (venom)	T63.121	T63.122	T63.123	T63.124	—	—
LMD	T45.8X1	T45.8X2	T45.8X3	T45.8X4	T45.8X5	T45.8X6
Lobelia	T62.2X1	T62.2X2	T62.2X3	T62.2X4	—	—
Lobeline	T5Ø.7X1	T5Ø.7X2	T5Ø.7X3	T5Ø.7X4	T5Ø.7X5	T5Ø.7X6
Local action drug NEC	T49.8X1	T49.8X2	T49.8X3	T49.8X4	T49.8X5	T49.8X6
Locorten	T49.ØX1	T49.ØX2	T49.ØX3	T49.ØX4	T49.ØX5	T49.ØX6
Lofepramine	T43.Ø11	T43.Ø12	T43.Ø13	T43.Ø14	T43.Ø15	T43.Ø16
Lolium temulentum	T62.2X1	T62.2X2	T62.2X3	T62.2X4	—	—
Lomotil	T47.6X1	T47.6X2	T47.6X3	T47.6X4	T47.6X5	T47.6X6
Lomustine	T45.1X1	T45.1X2	T45.1X3	T45.1X4	T45.1X5	T45.1X6
Lonidamine	T45.1X1	T45.1X2	T45.1X3	T45.1X4	T45.1X5	T45.1X6
Loperamide	T47.6X1	T47.6X2	T47.6X3	T47.6X4	T47.6X5	T47.6X6
Loprazolam	T42.4X1	T42.4X2	T42.4X3	T42.4X4	T42.4X5	T42.4X6
Lorajmine	T46.2X1	T46.2X2	T46.2X3	T46.2X4	T46.2X5	T46.2X6
Loratidine	T45.ØX1	T45.ØX2	T45.ØX3	T45.ØX4	T45.ØX5	T45.ØX6
Lorazepam	T42.4X1	T42.4X2	T42.4X3	T42.4X4	T42.4X5	T42.4X6
Lorcainide	T46.2X1	T46.2X2	T46.2X3	T46.2X4	T46.2X5	T46.2X6
Lormetazepam	T42.4X1	T42.4X2	T42.4X3	T42.4X4	T42.4X5	T42.4X6
Lotions NEC	T49.91	T49.92	T49.93	T49.94	T49.95	T49.96
Lotusate	T42.3X1	T42.3X2	T42.3X3	T42.3X4	T42.3X5	T42.3X6
Lovastatin	T46.6X1	T46.6X2	T46.6X3	T46.6X4	T46.6X5	T46.6X6
Lowila	T49.2X1	T49.2X2	T49.2X3	T49.2X4	T49.2X5	T49.2X6
Loxapine	T43.591	T43.592	T43.593	T43.594	T43.595	T43.596
Lozenges (throat)	T49.6X1	T49.6X2	T49.6X3	T49.6X4	T49.6X5	T49.6X6
LSD	T4Ø.8X1	T4Ø.8X2	T4Ø.8X3	T4Ø.8X4	—	—
L-Tryptophan — *see* amino acid						
Lubricant, eye	T49.5X1	T49.5X2	T49.5X3	T49.5X4	T49.5X5	T49.5X6
Lubricating oil NEC	T52.ØX1	T52.ØX2	T52.ØX3	T52.ØX4	—	—
Lucanthone	T37.4X1	T37.4X2	T37.4X3	T37.4X4	T37.4X5	T37.4X6
Luminal	T42.3X1	T42.3X2	T42.3X3	T42.3X4	T42.3X5	T42.3X6
Lung irritant (gas) **NEC**	T59.91	T59.92	T59.93	T59.94	—	—
Luteinizing hormone	T38.811	T38.812	T38.813	T38.814	T38.815	T38.816
Lutocylol	T38.5X1	T38.5X2	T38.5X3	T38.5X4	T38.5X5	T38.5X6
Lutromone	T38.5X1	T38.5X2	T38.5X3	T38.5X4	T38.5X5	T38.5X6
Lututrin	T48.291	T48.292	T48.293	T48.294	T48.295	T48.296
Lye (concentrated)	T54.3X1	T54.3X2	T54.3X3	T54.3X4	—	—
Lygranum (skin test)	T5Ø.8X1	T5Ø.8X2	T5Ø.8X3	T5Ø.8X4	T5Ø.8X5	T5Ø.8X6
Lymecycline	T36.4X1	T36.4X2	T36.4X3	T36.4X4	T36.4X5	T36.4X6
Lymphogranuloma venereum antigen	T5Ø.8X1	T5Ø.8X2	T5Ø.8X3	T5Ø.8X4	T5Ø.8X5	T5Ø.8X6
Lynestrenol	T38.4X1	T38.4X2	T38.4X3	T38.4X4	T38.4X5	T38.4X6
Lyovac Sodium Edecrin	T5Ø.1X1	T5Ø.1X2	T5Ø.1X3	T5Ø.1X4	T5Ø.1X5	T5Ø.1X6
Lypressin	T38.891	T38.892	T38.893	T38.894	T38.895	T38.896
Lysergic acid diethylamide	T4Ø.8X1	T4Ø.8X2	T4Ø.8X3	T4Ø.8X4	—	—
Lysergide	T4Ø.8X1	T4Ø.8X2	T4Ø.8X3	T4Ø.8X4	—	—
Lysine vasopressin	T38.891	T38.892	T38.893	T38.894	T38.895	T38.896
Lysol	T54.1X1	T54.1X2	T54.1X3	T54.1X4	—	—
Lysozyme	T49.ØX1	T49.ØX2	T49.ØX3	T49.ØX4	T49.ØX5	T49.ØX6
Lytta (vitatta)	T49.8X1	T49.8X2	T49.8X3	T49.8X4	T49.8X5	T49.8X6
Mace	T59.3X1	T59.3X2	T59.3X3	T59.3X4	—	—
Macrogol	T5Ø.991	T5Ø.992	T5Ø.993	T5Ø.994	T5Ø.995	T5Ø.996
Macrolide						
anabolic drug	T38.7X1	T38.7X2	T38.7X3	T38.7X4	T38.7X5	T38.7X6
antibiotic	T36.3X1	T36.3X2	T36.3X3	T36.3X4	T36.3X5	T36.3X6
Mafenide	T49.ØX1	T49.ØX2	T49.ØX3	T49.ØX4	T49.ØX5	T49.ØX6
Magaldrate	T47.1X1	T47.1X2	T47.1X3	T47.1X4	T47.1X5	T47.1X6
Magic mushroom	T4Ø.991	T4Ø.992	T4Ø.993	T4Ø.994	—	—
Magnamycin	T36.8X1	T36.8X2	T36.8X3	T36.8X4	T36.8X5	T36.8X6
Magnesia magma	T47.1X1	T47.1X2	T47.1X3	T47.1X4	T47.1X5	T47.1X6
Magnesium NEC	T56.891	T56.892	T56.893	T56.894	—	—
carbonate	T47.1X1	T47.1X2	T47.1X3	T47.1X4	T47.1X5	T47.1X6
citrate	T47.4X1	T47.4X2	T47.4X3	T47.4X4	T47.4X5	T47.4X6
hydroxide	T47.1X1	T47.1X2	T47.1X3	T47.1X4	T47.1X5	T47.1X6
oxide	T47.1X1	T47.1X2	T47.1X3	T47.1X4	T47.1X5	T47.1X6
peroxide	T49.ØX1	T49.ØX2	T49.ØX3	T49.ØX4	T49.ØX5	T49.ØX6
salicylate	T39.Ø91	T39.Ø92	T39.Ø93	T39.Ø94	T39.Ø95	T39.Ø96
silicofluoride	T5Ø.3X1	T5Ø.3X2	T5Ø.3X3	T5Ø.3X4	T5Ø.3X5	T5Ø.3X6
sulfate	T47.4X1	T47.4X2	T47.4X3	T47.4X4	T47.4X5	T47.4X6
thiosulfate	T45.ØX1	T45.ØX2	T45.ØX3	T45.ØX4	T45.ØX5	T45.ØX6
trisilicate	T47.1X1	T47.1X2	T47.1X3	T47.1X4	T47.1X5	T47.1X6
Malathion (medicinal)	T49.ØX1	T49.ØX2	T49.ØX3	T49.ØX4	T49.ØX5	T49.ØX6
insecticide	T6Ø.ØX1	T6Ø.ØX2	T6Ø.ØX3	T6Ø.ØX4	—	—
Male fern extract	T37.4X1	T37.4X2	T37.4X3	T37.4X4	T37.4X5	T37.4X6
M-AMSA	T45.1X1	T45.1X2	T45.1X3	T45.1X4	T45.1X5	T45.1X6
Mandelic acid	T37.8X1	T37.8X2	T37.8X3	T37.8X4	T37.8X5	T37.8X6
Manganese (dioxide) (salts)	T57.2X1	T57.2X2	T57.2X3	T57.2X4	—	—
medicinal	T5Ø.991	T5Ø.992	T5Ø.993	T5Ø.994	T5Ø.995	T5Ø.996
Mannitol	T47.3X1	T47.3X2	T47.3X3	T47.3X4	T47.3X5	T47.3X6
hexanitrate	T46.3X1	T46.3X2	T46.3X3	T46.3X4	T46.3X5	T46.3X6
Mannomustine	T45.1X1	T45.1X2	T45.1X3	T45.1X4	T45.1X5	T45.1X6
MAO inhibitors	T43.1X1	T43.1X2	T43.1X3	T43.1X4	T43.1X5	T43.1X6
Mapharsen	T37.8X1	T37.8X2	T37.8X3	T37.8X4	T37.8X5	T37.8X6
Maphenide	T49.ØX1	T49.ØX2	T49.ØX3	T49.ØX4	T49.ØX5	T49.ØX6
Maprotiline	T43.Ø21	T43.Ø22	T43.Ø23	T43.Ø24	T43.Ø25	T43.Ø26
Marcaine	T41.3X1	T41.3X2	T41.3X3	T41.3X4	T41.3X5	T41.3X6
infiltration (subcutaneous)	T41.3X1	T41.3X2	T41.3X3	T41.3X4	T41.3X5	T41.3X6
nerve block (peripheral) (plexus)	T41.3X1	T41.3X2	T41.3X3	T41.3X4	T41.3X5	T41.3X6
Marezine	T45.ØX1	T45.ØX2	T45.ØX3	T45.ØX4	T45.ØX5	T45.ØX6
Marihuana	T4Ø.7X1	T4Ø.7X2	T4Ø.7X3	T4Ø.7X4	T4Ø.7X5	T4Ø.7X6
Marijuana	T4Ø.7X1	T4Ø.7X2	T4Ø.7X3	T4Ø.7X4	T4Ø.7X5	T4Ø.7X6
Marine (sting)	T63.691	T63.692	T63.693	T63.694	—	—
animals (sting)	T63.691	T63.692	T63.693	T63.694	—	—
plants (sting)	T63.711	T63.712	T63.713	T63.714	—	—
Marplan	T43.1X1	T43.1X2	T43.1X3	T43.1X4	T43.1X5	T43.1X6
Marsh gas	T59.891	T59.892	T59.893	T59.894	—	—
Marsilid	T43.1X1	T43.1X2	T43.1X3	T43.1X4	T43.1X5	T43.1X6
Matulane	T45.1X1	T45.1X2	T45.1X3	T45.1X4	T45.1X5	T45.1X6
Mazindol	T5Ø.5X1	T5Ø.5X2	T5Ø.5X3	T5Ø.5X4	T5Ø.5X5	T5Ø.5X6
MCPA	T6Ø.3X1	T6Ø.3X2	T6Ø.3X3	T6Ø.3X4	—	—
MDMA	T43.621	T43.622	T43.623	T43.624	T43.625	T43.626
Meadow saffron	T62.2X1	T62.2X2	T62.2X3	T62.2X4	—	—
Measles virus vaccine (attenuated)	T5Ø.B91	T5Ø.B92	T5Ø.B93	T5Ø.B94	T5Ø.B95	T5Ø.B96
Meat, noxious	T62.8X1	T62.8X2	T62.8X3	T62.8X4	—	—
Meballymal	T42.3X1	T42.3X2	T42.3X3	T42.3X4	T42.3X5	T42.3X6
Mebanazine	T43.1X1	T43.1X2	T43.1X3	T43.1X4	T43.1X5	T43.1X6
Mebaral	T42.3X1	T42.3X2	T42.3X3	T42.3X4	T42.3X5	T42.3X6
Mebendazole	T37.4X1	T37.4X2	T37.4X3	T37.4X4	T37.4X5	T37.4X6
Mebeverine	T44.3X1	T44.3X2	T44.3X3	T44.3X4	T44.3X5	T44.3X6
Mebhydrolin	T45.ØX1	T45.ØX2	T45.ØX3	T45.ØX4	T45.ØX5	T45.ØX6
Mebumal	T42.3X1	T42.3X2	T42.3X3	T42.3X4	T42.3X5	T42.3X6
Mebutamate	T43.591	T43.592	T43.593	T43.594	T43.595	T43.596
Mecamylamine	T44.2X1	T44.2X2	T44.2X3	T44.2X4	T44.2X5	T44.2X6
Mechlorethamine	T45.1X1	T45.1X2	T45.1X3	T45.1X4	T45.1X5	T45.1X6
Mecillinam	T36.ØX1	T36.ØX2	T36.ØX3	T36.ØX4	T36.ØX5	T36.ØX6
Meclizine (hydrochloride)	T45.ØX1	T45.ØX2	T45.ØX3	T45.ØX4	T45.ØX5	T45.ØX6
Meclocycline	T36.4X1	T36.4X2	T36.4X3	T36.4X4	T36.4X5	T36.4X6
Meclofenamate	T39.391	T39.392	T39.393	T39.394	T39.395	T39.396
Meclofenamic acid	T39.391	T39.392	T39.393	T39.394	T39.395	T39.396
Meclofenoxate	T43.691	T43.692	T43.693	T43.694	T43.695	T43.696
Meclozine	T45.ØX1	T45.ØX2	T45.ØX3	T45.ØX4	T45.ØX5	T45.ØX6
Mecobalamin	T45.8X1	T45.8X2	T45.8X3	T45.8X4	T45.8X5	T45.8X6
Mecoprop	T6Ø.3X1	T6Ø.3X2	T6Ø.3X3	T6Ø.3X4	—	—

Substance	Poisoning, Accidental (unintentional)	Poisoning, Intentional Self-harm	Poisoning, Assault	Poisoning, Undetermined	Adverse Effect	Under-dosing
Mecrilate	T49.3X1	T49.3X2	T49.3X3	T49.3X4	T49.3X5	T49.3X6
Mecysteine	T48.4X1	T48.4X2	T48.4X3	T48.4X4	T48.4X5	T48.4X6
Medazepam	T42.4X1	T42.4X2	T42.4X3	T42.4X4	T42.4X5	T42.4X6
Medicament NEC	T5Ø.9Ø1	T5Ø.9Ø2	T5Ø.9Ø3	T5Ø.9Ø4	T5Ø.9Ø5	T5Ø.9Ø6
Medinal	T42.3X1	T42.3X2	T42.3X3	T42.3X4	T42.3X5	T42.3X6
Medomin	T42.3X1	T42.3X2	T42.3X3	T42.3X4	T42.3X5	T42.3X6
Medrogestone	T38.5X1	T38.5X2	T38.5X3	T38.5X4	T38.5X5	T38.5X6
Medroxalol	T44.8X1	T44.8X2	T44.8X3	T44.8X4	T44.8X5	T44.8X6
Medroxyprogesterone acetate (depot)	T38.5X1	T38.5X2	T38.5X3	T38.5X4	T38.5X5	T38.5X6
Medrysone	T49.ØX1	T49.ØX2	T49.ØX3	T49.ØX4	T49.ØX5	T49.ØX6
Mefenamic acid	T39.391	T39.392	T39.393	T39.394	T39.395	T39.396
Mefenorex	T5Ø.5X1	T5Ø.5X2	T5Ø.5X3	T5Ø.5X4	T5Ø.5X5	T5Ø.5X6
Mefloquine	T37.2X1	T37.2X2	T37.2X3	T37.2X4	T37.2X5	T37.2X6
Mefruside	T5Ø.2X1	T5Ø.2X2	T5Ø.2X3	T5Ø.2X4	T5Ø.2X5	T5Ø.2X6
Megahallucinogen	T4Ø.9Ø1	T4Ø.9Ø2	T4Ø.9Ø3	T4Ø.9Ø4	T4Ø.9Ø5	T4Ø.9Ø6
Megestrol	T38.5X1	T38.5X2	T38.5X3	T38.5X4	T38.5X5	T38.5X6
Meglumine						
antimoniate	T37.8X1	T37.8X2	T37.8X3	T37.8X4	T37.8X5	T37.8X6
diatrizoate	T5Ø.8X1	T5Ø.8X2	T5Ø.8X3	T5Ø.8X4	T5Ø.8X5	T5Ø.8X6
iodipamide	T5Ø.8X1	T5Ø.8X2	T5Ø.8X3	T5Ø.8X4	T5Ø.8X5	T5Ø.8X6
iotroxate	T5Ø.8X1	T5Ø.8X2	T5Ø.8X3	T5Ø.8X4	T5Ø.8X5	T5Ø.8X6
MEK (methyl ethyl ketone)	T52.4X1	T52.4X2	T52.4X3	T52.4X4	—	—
Meladinin	T49.3X1	T49.3X2	T49.3X3	T49.3X4	T49.3X5	T49.3X6
Meladrazine	T44.3X1	T44.3X2	T44.3X3	T44.3X4	T44.3X5	T44.3X6
Melaleuca alternifolia oil	T49.ØX1	T49.ØX2	T49.ØX3	T49.ØX4	T49.ØX5	T49.ØX6
Melanizing agents	T49.3X1	T49.3X2	T49.3X3	T49.3X4	T49.3X5	T49.3X6
Melanocyte-stimulating hormone	T38.891	T38.892	T38.893	T38.894	T38.895	T38.896
Melarsonyl potassium	T37.3X1	T37.3X2	T37.3X3	T37.3X4	T37.3X5	T37.3X6
Melarsoprol	T37.3X1	T37.3X2	T37.3X3	T37.3X4	T37.3X5	T37.3X6
Melia azedarach	T62.2X1	T62.2X2	T62.2X3	T62.2X4	—	—
Melitracen	T43.Ø11	T43.Ø12	T43.Ø13	T43.Ø14	T43.Ø15	T43.Ø16
Mellaril	T43.3X1	T43.3X2	T43.3X3	T43.3X4	T43.3X5	T43.3X6
Meloxine	T49.3X1	T49.3X2	T49.3X3	T49.3X4	T49.3X5	T49.3X6
Melperone	T43.4X1	T43.4X2	T43.4X3	T43.4X4	T43.4X5	T43.4X6
Melphalan	T45.1X1	T45.1X2	T45.1X3	T45.1X4	T45.1X5	T45.1X6
Memantine	T43.8X1	T43.8X2	T43.8X3	T43.8X4	T43.8X5	T43.8X6
Menadiol	T45.7X1	T45.7X2	T45.7X3	T45.7X4	T45.7X5	T45.7X6
sodium sulfate	T45.7X1	T45.7X2	T45.7X3	T45.7X4	T45.7X5	T45.7X6
Menadione	T45.7X1	T45.7X2	T45.7X3	T45.7X4	T45.7X5	T45.7X6
sodium bisulfite	T45.7X1	T45.7X2	T45.7X3	T45.7X4	T45.7X5	T45.7X6
Menaphthone	T45.7X1	T45.7X2	T45.7X3	T45.7X4	T45.7X5	T45.7X6
Menaquinone	T45.7X1	T45.7X2	T45.7X3	T45.7X4	T45.7X5	T45.7X6
Menatetrenone	T45.7X1	T45.7X2	T45.7X3	T45.7X4	T45.7X5	T45.7X6
Meningococcal vaccine	T5Ø.A91	T5Ø.A92	T5Ø.A93	T5Ø.A94	T5Ø.A95	T5Ø.A96
Menningovax (-AC) (-C)	T5Ø.A91	T5Ø.A92	T5Ø.A93	T5Ø.A94	T5Ø.A95	T5Ø.A96
Menotropins	T38.811	T38.812	T38.813	T38.814	T38.815	T38.816
Menthol	T48.5X1	T48.5X2	T48.5X3	T48.5X4	T48.5X5	T48.5X6
Mepacrine	T37.2X1	T37.2X2	T37.2X3	T37.2X4	T37.2X5	T37.2X6
Meparfynol	T42.6X1	T42.6X2	T42.6X3	T42.6X4	T42.6X5	T42.6X6
Mepartricin	T36.7X1	T36.7X2	T36.7X3	T36.7X4	T36.7X5	T36.7X6
Mepazine	T43.3X1	T43.3X2	T43.3X3	T43.3X4	T43.3X5	T43.3X6
Mepenzolate	T44.3X1	T44.3X2	T44.3X3	T44.3X4	T44.3X5	T44.3X6
bromide	T44.3X1	T44.3X2	T44.3X3	T44.3X4	T44.3X5	T44.3X6
Meperidine	T4Ø.4X1	T4Ø.4X2	T4Ø.4X3	T4Ø.4X4	T4Ø.4X5	T4Ø.4X6
Mephebarbital	T42.3X1	T42.3X2	T42.3X3	T42.3X4	T42.3X5	T42.3X6
Mephenamin (e)	T42.8X1	T42.8X2	T42.8X3	T42.8X4	T42.8X5	T42.8X6
Mephenesin	T42.8X1	T42.8X2	T42.8X3	T42.8X4	T42.8X5	T42.8X6
Mephenhydramine	T45.ØX1	T45.ØX2	T45.ØX3	T45.ØX4	T45.ØX5	T45.ØX6
Mephenoxalone	T42.8X1	T42.8X2	T42.8X3	T42.8X4	T42.8X5	T42.8X6
Mephentermine	T44.991	T44.992	T44.993	T44.994	T44.995	T44.996
Mephenytoin	T42.ØX1	T42.ØX2	T42.ØX3	T42.ØX4	T42.ØX5	T42.ØX6
with phenobarbital	T42.3X1	T42.3X2	T42.3X3	T42.3X4	T42.3X5	T42.3X6
Mephobarbital	T42.3X1	T42.3X2	T42.3X3	T42.3X4	T42.3X5	T42.3X6
Mephosfolan	T6Ø.ØX1	T6Ø.ØX2	T6Ø.ØX3	T6Ø.ØX4	—	—
Mepindolol	T44.7X1	T44.7X2	T44.7X3	T44.7X4	T44.7X5	T44.7X6
Mepiperphenidol	T44.3X1	T44.3X2	T44.3X3	T44.3X4	T44.3X5	T44.3X6
Mepitiostane	T38.7X1	T38.7X2	T38.7X3	T38.7X4	T38.7X5	T38.7X6
Mepivacaine	T41.3X1	T41.3X2	T41.3X3	T41.3X4	T41.3X5	T41.3X6
epidural	T41.3X1	T41.3X2	T41.3X3	T41.3X4	T41.3X5	T41.3X6
Meprednisone	T38.ØX1	T38.ØX2	T38.ØX3	T38.ØX4	T38.ØX5	T38.ØX6
Meprobam	T43.591	T43.592	T43.593	T43.594	T43.595	T43.596
Meprobamate	T43.591	T43.592	T43.593	T43.594	T43.595	T43.596
Meproscillarin	T46.ØX1	T46.ØX2	T46.ØX3	T46.ØX4	T46.ØX5	T46.ØX6
Meprylcaine	T41.3X1	T41.3X2	T41.3X3	T41.3X4	T41.3X5	T41.3X6
Meptazinol	T39.8X1	T39.8X2	T39.8X3	T39.8X4	T39.8X5	T39.8X6
Mepyramine	T45.ØX1	T45.ØX2	T45.ØX3	T45.ØX4	T45.ØX5	T45.ØX6
Mequitazine	T43.3X1	T43.3X2	T43.3X3	T43.3X4	T43.3X5	T43.3X6
Meralluride	T5Ø.2X1	T5Ø.2X2	T5Ø.2X3	T5Ø.2X4	T5Ø.2X5	T5Ø.2X6
Merbaphen	T5Ø.2X1	T5Ø.2X2	T5Ø.2X3	T5Ø.2X4	T5Ø.2X5	T5Ø.2X6
Merbromin	T49.ØX1	T49.ØX2	T49.ØX3	T49.ØX4	T49.ØX5	T49.ØX6

Substance	Poisoning, Accidental (unintentional)	Poisoning, Intentional Self-harm	Poisoning, Assault	Poisoning, Undetermined	Adverse Effect	Under-dosing
Mercaptobenzothiazole salts	T49.ØX1	T49.ØX2	T49.ØX3	T49.ØX4	T49.ØX5	T49.ØX6
Mercaptomerin	T5Ø.2X1	T5Ø.2X2	T5Ø.2X3	T5Ø.2X4	T5Ø.2X5	T5Ø.2X6
Mercaptopurine	T45.1X1	T45.1X2	T45.1X3	T45.1X4	T45.1X5	T45.1X6
Mercumatilin	T5Ø.2X1	T5Ø.2X2	T5Ø.2X3	T5Ø.2X4	T5Ø.2X5	T5Ø.2X6
Mercuramide	T5Ø.2X1	T5Ø.2X2	T5Ø.2X3	T5Ø.2X4	T5Ø.2X5	T5Ø.2X6
Mercurochrome	T49.ØX1	T49.ØX2	T49.ØX3	T49.ØX4	T49.ØX5	T49.ØX6
Mercurophylline	T5Ø.2X1	T5Ø.2X2	T5Ø.2X3	T5Ø.2X4	T5Ø.2X5	T5Ø.2X6
Mercury, mercurial, mercuric, mercurous (compounds) (cyanide) (fumes) (nonmedicinal) (vapor) **NEC**	T56.1X1	T56.1X2	T56.1X3	T56.1X4	—	—
ammoniated	T49.ØX1	T49.ØX2	T49.ØX3	T49.ØX4	T49.ØX5	T49.ØX6
anti-infective						
local	T49.ØX1	T49.ØX2	T49.ØX3	T49.ØX4	T49.ØX5	T49.ØX6
systemic	T37.8X1	T37.8X2	T37.8X3	T37.8X4	T37.8X5	T37.8X6
topical	T49.ØX1	T49.ØX2	T49.ØX3	T49.ØX4	T49.ØX5	T49.ØX6
chloride (ammoniated)	T49.ØX1	T49.ØX2	T49.ØX3	T49.ØX4	T49.ØX5	T49.ØX6
fungicide	T56.1X1	T56.1X2	T56.1X3	T56.1X4	—	—
diuretic NEC	T5Ø.2X1	T5Ø.2X2	T5Ø.2X3	T5Ø.2X4	T5Ø.2X5	T5Ø.2X6
fungicide	T56.1X1	T56.1X2	T56.1X3	T56.1X4	—	—
organic (fungicide)	T56.1X1	T56.1X2	T56.1X3	T56.1X4	—	—
oxide, yellow	T49.ØX1	T49.ØX2	T49.ØX3	T49.ØX4	T49.ØX5	T49.ØX6
Mersalyl	T5Ø.2X1	T5Ø.2X2	T5Ø.2X3	T5Ø.2X4	T5Ø.2X5	T5Ø.2X6
Merthiolate	T49.ØX1	T49.ØX2	T49.ØX3	T49.ØX4	T49.ØX5	T49.ØX6
ophthalmic preparation	T49.5X1	T49.5X2	T49.5X3	T49.5X4	T49.5X5	T49.5X6
Meruvax	T5Ø.B91	T5Ø.B92	T5Ø.B93	T5Ø.B94	T5Ø.B95	T5Ø.B96
Mesalazine	T47.8X1	T47.8X2	T47.8X3	T47.8X4	T47.8X5	T47.8X6
Mescal buttons	T4Ø.991	T4Ø.992	T4Ø.993	T4Ø.994	—	—
Mescaline	T4Ø.991	T4Ø.992	T4Ø.993	T4Ø.994	—	—
Mesna	T48.4X1	T48.4X2	T48.4X3	T48.4X4	T48.4X5	T48.4X6
Mesoglycan	T46.6X1	T46.6X2	T46.6X3	T46.6X4	T46.6X5	T46.6X6
Mesoridazine	T43.3X1	T43.3X2	T43.3X3	T43.3X4	T43.3X5	T43.3X6
Mestanolone	T38.7X1	T38.7X2	T38.7X3	T38.7X4	T38.7X5	T38.7X6
Mesterolone	T38.7X1	T38.7X2	T38.7X3	T38.7X4	T38.7X5	T38.7X6
Mestranol	T38.5X1	T38.5X2	T38.5X3	T38.5X4	T38.5X5	T38.5X6
Mesulergine	T42.8X1	T42.8X2	T42.8X3	T42.8X4	T42.8X5	T42.8X6
Mesulfen	T49.ØX1	T49.ØX2	T49.ØX3	T49.ØX4	T49.ØX5	T49.ØX6
Mesuximide	T42.2X1	T42.2X2	T42.2X3	T42.2X4	T42.2X5	T42.2X6
Metabutethamine	T41.3X1	T41.3X2	T41.3X3	T41.3X4	T41.3X5	T41.3X6
Metactesylacetate	T49.ØX1	T49.ØX2	T49.ØX3	T49.ØX4	T49.ØX5	T49.ØX6
Metacycline	T36.4X1	T36.4X2	T36.4X3	T36.4X4	T36.4X5	T36.4X6
Metaldehyde (snail killer) **NEC**	T6Ø.8X1	T6Ø.8X2	T6Ø.8X3	T6Ø.8X4	—	—
Metals (heavy) (nonmedicinal)	T56.91	T56.92	T56.93	T56.94	—	—
dust, fumes, or vapor NEC	T56.91	T56.92	T56.93	T56.94	—	—
light NEC	T56.91	T56.92	T56.93	T56.94	—	—
dust, fumes, or vapor NEC	T56.91	T56.92	T56.93	T56.94	—	—
specified NEC	T56.891	T56.892	T56.893	T56.894	—	—
thallium	T56.811	T56.812	T56.813	T56.814	—	—
Metamfetamine	T43.621	T43.622	T43.623	T43.624	T43.625	T43.626
Metamizole sodium	T39.2X1	T39.2X2	T39.2X3	T39.2X4	T39.2X5	T39.2X6
Metampicillin	T36.ØX1	T36.ØX2	T36.ØX3	T36.ØX4	T36.ØX5	T36.ØX6
Metamucil	T47.4X1	T47.4X2	T47.4X3	T47.4X4	T47.4X5	T47.4X6
Metandienone	T38.7X1	T38.7X2	T38.7X3	T38.7X4	T38.7X5	T38.7X6
Metandrostenolone	T38.7X1	T38.7X2	T38.7X3	T38.7X4	T38.7X5	T38.7X6
Metaphen	T49.ØX1	T49.ØX2	T49.ØX3	T49.ØX4	T49.ØX5	T49.ØX6
Metaphos	T6Ø.ØX1	T6Ø.ØX2	T6Ø.ØX3	T6Ø.ØX4	—	—
Metapramine	T43.Ø11	T43.Ø12	T43.Ø13	T43.Ø14	T43.Ø15	T43.Ø16
Metaproterenol	T48.291	T48.292	T48.293	T48.294	T48.295	T48.296
Metaraminol	T44.4X1	T44.4X2	T44.4X3	T44.4X4	T44.4X5	T44.4X6
Metaxalone	T42.8X1	T42.8X2	T42.8X3	T42.8X4	T42.8X5	T42.8X6
Metenolone	T38.7X1	T38.7X2	T38.7X3	T38.7X4	T38.7X5	T38.7X6
Metergoline	T42.8X1	T42.8X2	T42.8X3	T42.8X4	T42.8X5	T42.8X6
Metescufylline	T46.991	T46.992	T46.993	T46.994	T46.995	T46.996
Metetoin	T42.ØX1	T42.ØX2	T42.ØX3	T42.ØX4	T42.ØX5	T42.ØX6
Metformin	T38.3X1	T38.3X2	T38.3X3	T38.3X4	T38.3X5	T38.3X6
Methacholine	T44.1X1	T44.1X2	T44.1X3	T44.1X4	T44.1X5	T44.1X6
Methacycline	T36.4X1	T36.4X2	T36.4X3	T36.4X4	T36.4X5	T36.4X6
Methadone	T4Ø.3X1	T4Ø.3X2	T4Ø.3X3	T4Ø.3X4	T4Ø.3X5	T4Ø.3X6
Methallenestril	T38.5X1	T38.5X2	T38.5X3	T38.5X4	T38.5X5	T38.5X6
Methallenoestril	T38.5X1	T38.5X2	T38.5X3	T38.5X4	T38.5X5	T38.5X6
Methamphetamine	T43.621	T43.622	T43.623	T43.624	T43.625	T43.626
Methampyrone	T39.2X1	T39.2X2	T39.2X3	T39.2X4	T39.2X5	T39.2X6
Methandienone	T38.7X1	T38.7X2	T38.7X3	T38.7X4	T38.7X5	T38.7X6
Methandriol	T38.7X1	T38.7X2	T38.7X3	T38.7X4	T38.7X5	T38.7X6
Methandrostenolone	T38.7X1	T38.7X2	T38.7X3	T38.7X4	T38.7X5	T38.7X6
Methane	T59.891	T59.892	T59.893	T59.894	—	—
Methanethiol	T59.891	T59.892	T59.893	T59.894	—	—
Methaniazide	T37.1X1	T37.1X2	T37.1X3	T37.1X4	T37.1X5	T37.1X6
Methanol (vapor)	T51.1X1	T51.1X2	T51.1X3	T51.1X4	—	—

Table of Drugs and Chemicals

Mecrilate — Methanol

Substance	Poisoning, Accidental (unintentional)	Poisoning, Intentional Self-harm	Poisoning, Assault	Poisoning, Undetermined	Adverse Effect	Under-dosing
Methantheline	T44.3X1	T44.3X2	T44.3X3	T44.3X4	T44.3X5	T44.3X6
Methanthelinium bromide	T44.3X1	T44.3X2	T44.3X3	T44.3X4	T44.3X5	T44.3X6
Methaphenilene	T45.ØX1	T45.ØX2	T45.ØX3	T45.ØX4	T45.ØX5	T45.ØX6
Methapyrilene	T45.ØX1	T45.ØX2	T45.ØX3	T45.ØX4	T45.ØX5	T45.ØX6
Methaqualone (compound)	T42.6X1	T42.6X2	T42.6X3	T42.6X4	T42.6X5	T42.6X6
Metharbital	T42.3X1	T42.3X2	T42.3X3	T42.3X4	T42.3X5	T42.3X6
Methazolamide	T5Ø.2X1	T5Ø.2X2	T5Ø.2X3	T5Ø.2X4	T5Ø.2X5	T5Ø.2X6
Methdilazine	T43.3X1	T43.3X2	T43.3X3	T43.3X4	T43.3X5	T43.3X6
Methedrine	T43.621	T43.622	T43.623	T43.624	T43.625	T43.626
Methenamine (mandelate)	T37.8X1	T37.8X2	T37.8X3	T37.8X4	T37.8X5	T37.8X6
Methenolone	T38.7X1	T38.7X2	T38.7X3	T38.7X4	T38.7X5	T38.7X6
Methergine	T48.ØX1	T48.ØX2	T48.ØX3	T48.ØX4	T48.ØX5	T48.ØX6
Methetoin	T42.ØX1	T42.ØX2	T42.ØX3	T42.ØX4	T42.ØX5	T42.ØX6
Methiacil	T38.2X1	T38.2X2	T38.2X3	T38.2X4	T38.2X5	T38.2X6
Methicillin	T36.ØX1	T36.ØX2	T36.ØX3	T36.ØX4	T36.ØX5	T36.ØX6
Methimazole	T38.2X1	T38.2X2	T38.2X3	T38.2X4	T38.2X5	T38.2X6
Methiodal sodium	T5Ø.8X1	T5Ø.8X2	T5Ø.8X3	T5Ø.8X4	T5Ø.8X5	T5Ø.8X6
Methionine	T5Ø.991	T5Ø.992	T5Ø.993	T5Ø.994	T5Ø.995	T5Ø.996
Methisazone	T37.5X1	T37.5X2	T37.5X3	T37.5X4	T37.5X5	T37.5X6
Methisoprinol	T37.5X1	T37.5X2	T37.5X3	T37.5X4	T37.5X5	T37.5X6
Methitural	T42.3X1	T42.3X2	T42.3X3	T42.3X4	T42.3X5	T42.3X6
Methixene	T44.3X1	T44.3X2	T44.3X3	T44.3X4	T44.3X5	T44.3X6
Methobarbital, methobarbitone	T42.3X1	T42.3X2	T42.3X3	T42.3X4	T42.3X5	T42.3X6
Methocarbamol	T42.8X1	T42.8X2	T42.8X3	T42.8X4	T42.8X5	T42.8X6
skeletal muscle relaxant	T48.1X1	T48.1X2	T48.1X3	T48.1X4	T48.1X5	T48.1X6
Methohexital	T41.1X1	T41.1X2	T41.1X3	T41.1X4	T41.1X5	T41.1X6
Methohexitone	T41.1X1	T41.1X2	T41.1X3	T41.1X4	T41.1X5	T41.1X6
Methoin	T42.ØX1	T42.ØX2	T42.ØX3	T42.ØX4	T42.ØX5	T42.ØX6
Methopholine	T39.8X1	T39.8X2	T39.8X3	T39.8X4	T39.8X5	T39.8X6
Methopromazine	T43.3X1	T43.3X2	T43.3X3	T43.3X4	T43.3X5	T43.3X6
Methorate	T48.3X1	T48.3X2	T48.3X3	T48.3X4	T48.3X5	T48.3X6
Methoserpidine	T46.5X1	T46.5X2	T46.5X3	T46.5X4	T46.5X5	T46.5X6
Methotrexate	T45.1X1	T45.1X2	T45.1X3	T45.1X4	T45.1X5	T45.1X6
Methotrimeprazine	T43.3X1	T43.3X2	T43.3X3	T43.3X4	T43.3X5	T43.3X6
Methoxa-Dome	T49.3X1	T49.3X2	T49.3X3	T49.3X4	T49.3X5	T49.3X6
Methoxamine	T44.4X1	T44.4X2	T44.4X3	T44.4X4	T44.4X5	T44.4X6
Methoxsalen	T5Ø.991	T5Ø.992	T5Ø.993	T5Ø.994	T5Ø.995	T5Ø.996
Methoxyaniline	T65.3X1	T65.3X2	T65.3X3	T65.3X4	—	—
Methoxybenzyl penicillin	T36.ØX1	T36.ØX2	T36.ØX3	T36.ØX4	T36.ØX5	T36.ØX6
Methoxychlor	T53.7X1	T53.7X2	T53.7X3	T53.7X4	—	—
Methoxy-DDT	T53.7X1	T53.7X2	T53.7X3	T53.7X4	—	—
Methoxyflurane	T41.ØX1	T41.ØX2	T41.ØX3	T41.ØX4	T41.ØX5	T41.ØX6
Methoxyphenamine	T48.6X1	T48.6X2	T48.6X3	T48.6X4	T48.6X5	T48.6X6
Methoxypromazine	T43.3X1	T43.3X2	T43.3X3	T43.3X4	T43.3X5	T43.3X6
Methscopolamine bromide	T44.3X1	T44.3X2	T44.3X3	T44.3X4	T44.3X5	T44.3X6
Methsuximide	T42.2X1	T42.2X2	T42.2X3	T42.2X4	T42.2X5	T42.2X6
Methyclothiazide	T5Ø.2X1	T5Ø.2X2	T5Ø.2X3	T5Ø.2X4	T5Ø.2X5	T5Ø.2X6
Methyl						
acetate	T52.4X1	T52.4X2	T52.4X3	T52.4X4	—	—
acetone	T52.4X1	T52.4X2	T52.4X3	T52.4X4	—	—
acrylate	T65.891	T65.892	T65.893	T65.894	—	—
alcohol	T51.1X1	T51.1X2	T51.1X3	T51.1X4	—	—
aminophenol	T65.3X1	T65.3X2	T65.3X3	T65.3X4	—	—
amphetamine	T43.621	T43.622	T43.623	T43.624	T43.625	T43.626
androstanolone	T38.7X1	T38.7X2	T38.7X3	T38.7X4	T38.7X5	T38.7X6
atropine	T44.3X1	T44.3X2	T44.3X3	T44.3X4	T44.3X5	T44.3X6
benzene	T52.2X1	T52.2X2	T52.2X3	T52.2X4	—	—
benzoate	T52.8X1	T52.8X2	T52.8X3	T52.8X4	—	—
benzol	T52.2X1	T52.2X2	T52.2X3	T52.2X4	—	—
bromide (gas)	T59.891	T59.892	T59.893	T59.894	—	—
fumigant	T6Ø.8X1	T6Ø.8X2	T6Ø.8X3	T6Ø.8X4	—	—
butanol	T51.3X1	T51.3X2	T51.3X3	T51.3X4	—	—
carbinol	T51.1X1	T51.1X2	T51.1X3	T51.1X4	—	—
carbonate	T52.8X1	T52.8X2	T52.8X3	T52.8X4	—	—
CCNU	T45.1X1	T45.1X2	T45.1X3	T45.1X4	T45.1X5	T45.1X6
cellosolve	T52.91	T52.92	T52.93	T52.94	—	—
cellulose	T47.4X1	T47.4X2	T47.4X3	T47.4X4	T47.4X5	T47.4X6
chloride (gas)	T59.891	T59.892	T59.893	T59.894	—	—
chloroformate	T59.3X1	T59.3X2	T59.3X3	T59.3X4	—	—
cyclohexane	T52.8X1	T52.8X2	T52.8X3	T52.8X4	—	—
cyclohexanol	T51.8X1	T51.8X2	T51.8X3	T51.8X4	—	—
cyclohexanone	T52.8X1	T52.8X2	T52.8X3	T52.8X4	—	—
cyclohexyl acetate	T52.8X1	T52.8X2	T52.8X3	T52.8X4	—	—
demeton	T6Ø.ØX1	T6Ø.ØX2	T6Ø.ØX3	T6Ø.ØX4	—	—
dihydromorphinone	T4Ø.2X1	T4Ø.2X2	T4Ø.2X3	T4Ø.2X4	T4Ø.2X5	T4Ø.2X6
ergometrine	T48.ØX1	T48.ØX2	T48.ØX3	T48.ØX4	T48.ØX5	T48.ØX6
ergonovine	T48.ØX1	T48.ØX2	T48.ØX3	T48.ØX4	T48.ØX5	T48.ØX6
ethyl ketone	T52.4X1	T52.4X2	T52.4X3	T52.4X4	—	—
glucamine antimonate	T37.8X1	T37.8X2	T37.8X3	T37.8X4	T37.8X5	T37.8X6
hydrazine	T65.891	T65.892	T65.893	T65.894	—	—
iodide	T65.891	T65.892	T65.893	T65.894	—	—
isobutyl ketone	T52.4X1	T52.4X2	T52.4X3	T52.4X4	—	—

Substance	Poisoning, Accidental (unintentional)	Poisoning, Intentional Self-harm	Poisoning, Assault	Poisoning, Undetermined	Adverse Effect	Under-dosing
Methyl — *continued*						
isothiocyanate	T6Ø.3X1	T6Ø.3X2	T6Ø.3X3	T6Ø.3X4	—	—
mercaptan	T59.891	T59.892	T59.893	T59.894	—	—
morphine NEC	T4Ø.2X1	T4Ø.2X2	T4Ø.2X3	T4Ø.2X4	T4Ø.2X5	T4Ø.2X6
nicotinate	T49.4X1	T49.4X2	T49.4X3	T49.4X4	T49.4X5	T49.4X6
paraben	T49.ØX1	T49.ØX2	T49.ØX3	T49.ØX4	T49.ØX5	T49.ØX6
parafynol	T42.6X1	T42.6X2	T42.6X3	T42.6X4	T42.6X5	T42.6X6
parathion	T6Ø.ØX1	T6Ø.ØX2	T6Ø.ØX3	T6Ø.ØX4	—	—
peridol	T43.4X1	T43.4X2	T43.4X3	T43.4X4	T43.4X5	T43.4X6
phenidate	T43.631	T43.632	T43.633	T43.634	T43.635	T43.636
prednisolone	T38.ØX1	T38.ØX2	T38.ØX3	T38.ØX4	T38.ØX5	T38.ØX6
ENT agent	T49.6X1	T49.6X2	T49.6X3	T49.6X4	T49.6X5	T49.6X6
ophthalmic preparation	T49.5X1	T49.5X2	T49.5X3	T49.5X4	T49.5X5	T49.5X6
topical NEC	T49.ØX1	T49.ØX2	T49.ØX3	T49.ØX4	T49.ØX5	T49.ØX6
propylcarbinol	T51.3X1	T51.3X2	T51.3X3	T51.3X4	—	—
rosaniline NEC	T49.ØX1	T49.ØX2	T49.ØX3	T49.ØX4	T49.ØX5	T49.ØX6
salicylate	T49.2X1	T49.2X2	T49.2X3	T49.2X4	T49.2X5	T49.2X6
sulfate (fumes)	T59.891	T59.892	T59.893	T59.894	—	—
liquid	T52.8X1	T52.8X2	T52.8X3	T52.8X4	—	—
sulfonal	T42.6X1	T42.6X2	T42.6X3	T42.6X4	T42.6X5	T42.6X6
testosterone	T38.7X1	T38.7X2	T38.7X3	T38.7X4	T38.7X5	T38.7X6
thiouracil	T38.2X1	T38.2X2	T38.2X3	T38.2X4	T38.2X5	T38.2X6
Methylamphetamine	T43.621	T43.622	T43.623	T43.624	T43.625	T43.626
Methylated spirit	T51.1X1	T51.1X2	T51.1X3	T51.1X4	—	—
Methylatropine nitrate	T44.3X1	T44.3X2	T44.3X3	T44.3X4	T44.3X5	T44.3X6
Methylbenactyzium bromide	T44.3X1	T44.3X2	T44.3X3	T44.3X4	T44.3X5	T44.3X6
Methylbenzethonium chloride	T49.ØX1	T49.ØX2	T49.ØX3	T49.ØX4	T49.ØX5	T49.ØX6
Methylcellulose	T47.4X1	T47.4X2	T47.4X3	T47.4X4	T47.4X5	T47.4X6
laxative	T47.4X1	T47.4X2	T47.4X3	T47.4X4	T47.4X5	T47.4X6
Methylchlorophenoxyacetic acid	T6Ø.3X1	T6Ø.3X2	T6Ø.3X3	T6Ø.3X4	—	—
Methyldopa	T46.5X1	T46.5X2	T46.5X3	T46.5X4	T46.5X5	T46.5X6
Methyldopate	T46.5X1	T46.5X2	T46.5X3	T46.5X4	T46.5X5	T46.5X6
Methylene						
blue	T5Ø.6X1	T5Ø.6X2	T5Ø.6X3	T5Ø.6X4	T5Ø.6X5	T5Ø.6X6
chloride or dichloride (solvent) NEC	T53.4X1	T53.4X2	T53.4X3	T53.4X4	—	—
Methylenedioxyamphetamine	T43.621	T43.622	T43.623	T43.624	T43.625	T43.626
Methylenedioxymethamphetamine	T43.621	T43.622	T43.623	T43.624	T43.625	T43.626
Methylergometrine	T48.ØX1	T48.ØX2	T48.ØX3	T48.ØX4	T48.ØX5	T48.ØX6
Methylergonovine	T48.ØX1	T48.ØX2	T48.ØX3	T48.ØX4	T48.ØX5	T48.ØX6
Methylestrenolone	T38.5X1	T38.5X2	T38.5X3	T38.5X4	T38.5X5	T38.5X6
Methylethyl cellulose	T5Ø.991	T5Ø.992	T5Ø.993	T5Ø.994	T5Ø.995	T5Ø.996
Methylhexabital	T42.3X1	T42.3X2	T42.3X3	T42.3X4	T42.3X5	T42.3X6
Methylmorphine	T4Ø.2X1	T4Ø.2X2	T4Ø.2X3	T4Ø.2X4	T4Ø.2X5	T4Ø.2X6
Methylparaben (ophthalmic)	T49.5X1	T49.5X2	T49.5X3	T49.5X4	T49.5X5	T49.5X6
Methylparafynol	T42.6X1	T42.6X2	T42.6X3	T42.6X4	T42.6X5	T42.6X6
Methylpentynol, methylpenthynol	T42.6X1	T42.6X2	T42.6X3	T42.6X4	T42.6X5	T42.6X6
Methylphenidate	T43.631	T43.632	T43.633	T43.634	T43.635	T43.636
Methylphenobarbital	T42.3X1	T42.3X2	T42.3X3	T42.3X4	T42.3X5	T42.3X6
Methylpolysiloxane	T47.1X1	T47.1X2	T47.1X3	T47.1X4	T47.1X5	T47.1X6
Methylprednisolone — *see* Methyl, prednisolone						
Methylrosaniline	T49.ØX1	T49.ØX2	T49.ØX3	T49.ØX4	T49.ØX5	T49.ØX6
Methylrosanilinium chloride	T49.ØX1	T49.ØX2	T49.ØX3	T49.ØX4	T49.ØX5	T49.ØX6
Methyltestosterone	T38.7X1	T38.7X2	T38.7X3	T38.7X4	T38.7X5	T38.7X6
Methylthionine chloride	T5Ø.6X1	T5Ø.6X2	T5Ø.6X3	T5Ø.6X4	T5Ø.6X5	T5Ø.6X6
Methylthioninium chloride	T5Ø.6X1	T5Ø.6X2	T5Ø.6X3	T5Ø.6X4	T5Ø.6X5	T5Ø.6X6
Methylthiouracil	T38.2X1	T38.2X2	T38.2X3	T38.2X4	T38.2X5	T38.2X6
Methyprylon	T42.6X1	T42.6X2	T42.6X3	T42.6X4	T42.6X5	T42.6X6
Methysergide	T46.5X1	T46.5X2	T46.5X3	T46.5X4	T46.5X5	T46.5X6
Metiamide	T47.1X1	T47.1X2	T47.1X3	T47.1X4	T47.1X5	T47.1X6
Meticillin	T36.ØX1	T36.ØX2	T36.ØX3	T36.ØX4	T36.ØX5	T36.ØX6
Meticrane	T5Ø.2X1	T5Ø.2X2	T5Ø.2X3	T5Ø.2X4	T5Ø.2X5	T5Ø.2X6
Metildigoxin	T46.ØX1	T46.ØX2	T46.ØX3	T46.ØX4	T46.ØX5	T46.ØX6
Metipranolol	T49.5X1	T49.5X2	T49.5X3	T49.5X4	T49.5X5	T49.5X6
Metirosine	T46.5X1	T46.5X2	T46.5X3	T46.5X4	T46.5X5	T46.5X6
Metisazone	T37.5X1	T37.5X2	T37.5X3	T37.5X4	T37.5X5	T37.5X6
Metixene	T44.3X1	T44.3X2	T44.3X3	T44.3X4	T44.3X5	T44.3X6
Metizoline	T48.5X1	T48.5X2	T48.5X3	T48.5X4	T48.5X5	T48.5X6
Metoclopramide	T45.ØX1	T45.ØX2	T45.ØX3	T45.ØX4	T45.ØX5	T45.ØX6
Metofenazate	T43.3X1	T43.3X2	T43.3X3	T43.3X4	T43.3X5	T43.3X6
Metofoline	T39.8X1	T39.8X2	T39.8X3	T39.8X4	T39.8X5	T39.8X6
Metolazone	T5Ø.2X1	T5Ø.2X2	T5Ø.2X3	T5Ø.2X4	T5Ø.2X5	T5Ø.2X6
Metopon	T4Ø.2X1	T4Ø.2X2	T4Ø.2X3	T4Ø.2X4	T4Ø.2X5	T4Ø.2X6
Metoprine	T45.1X1	T45.1X2	T45.1X3	T45.1X4	T45.1X5	T45.1X6
Metoprolol	T44.7X1	T44.7X2	T44.7X3	T44.7X4	T44.7X5	T44.7X6
Metrifonate	T6Ø.ØX1	T6Ø.ØX2	T6Ø.ØX3	T6Ø.ØX4	—	—

Substance	Poisoning, Accidental (unintentional)	Poisoning, Intentional Self-harm	Poisoning, Assault	Poisoning, Undetermined	Adverse Effect	Under-dosing
Metrizamide	T5Ø.8X1	T5Ø.8X2	T5Ø.8X3	T5Ø.8X4	T5Ø.8X5	T5Ø.8X6
Metrizoic acid	T5Ø.8X1	T5Ø.8X2	T5Ø.8X3	T5Ø.8X4	T5Ø.8X5	T5Ø.8X6
Metronidazole	T37.8X1	T37.8X2	T37.8X3	T37.8X4	T37.8X5	T37.8X6
Metycaine	T41.3X1	T41.3X2	T41.3X3	T41.3X4	T41.3X5	T41.3X6
infiltration (subcutaneous)	T41.3X1	T41.3X2	T41.3X3	T41.3X4	T41.3X5	T41.3X6
nerve block (peripheral) (plexus)	T41.3X1	T41.3X2	T41.3X3	T41.3X4	T41.3X5	T41.3X6
topical (surface)	T41.3X1	T41.3X2	T41.3X3	T41.3X4	T41.3X5	T41.3X6
Metyrapone	T5Ø.8X1	T5Ø.8X2	T5Ø.8X3	T5Ø.8X4	T5Ø.8X5	T5Ø.8X6
Mevinphos	T6Ø.ØX1	T6Ø.ØX2	T6Ø.ØX3	T6Ø.ØX4	—	—
Mexazolam	T42.4X1	T42.4X2	T42.4X3	T42.4X4	T42.4X5	T42.4X6
Mexenone	T49.3X1	T49.3X2	T49.3X3	T49.3X4	T49.3X5	T49.3X6
Mexiletine	T46.2X1	T46.2X2	T46.2X3	T46.2X4	T46.2X5	T46.2X6
Mezereon	T62.2X1	T62.2X2	T62.2X3	T62.2X4	—	—
berries	T62.1X1	T62.1X2	T62.1X3	T62.1X4	—	—
Mezlocillin	T36.ØX1	T36.ØX2	T36.ØX3	T36.ØX4	T36.ØX5	T36.ØX6
Mianserin	T43.Ø21	T43.Ø22	T43.Ø23	T43.Ø24	T43.Ø25	T43.Ø26
Micatin	T49.ØX1	T49.ØX2	T49.ØX3	T49.ØX4	T49.ØX5	T49.ØX6
Miconazole	T49.ØX1	T49.ØX2	T49.ØX3	T49.ØX4	T49.ØX5	T49.ØX6
Micronomicin	T36.5X1	T36.5X2	T36.5X3	T36.5X4	T36.5X5	T36.5X6
Midazolam	T42.4X1	T42.4X2	T42.4X3	T42.4X4	T42.4X5	T42.4X6
Midecamycin	T36.3X1	T36.3X2	T36.3X3	T36.3X4	T36.3X5	T36.3X6
Mifepristone	T38.6X1	T38.6X2	T38.6X3	T38.6X4	T38.6X5	T38.6X6
Milk of magnesia	T47.1X1	T47.1X2	T47.1X3	T47.1X4	T47.1X5	T47.1X6
Millipede (tropical) (venomous)	T63.411	T63.412	T63.413	T63.414	—	—
Miltown	T43.591	T43.592	T43.593	T43.594	T43.595	T43.596
Milverine	T44.3X1	T44.3X2	T44.3X3	T44.3X4	T44.3X5	T44.3X6
Minaprine	T43.291	T43.292	T43.293	T43.294	T43.295	T43.296
Minaxolone	T41.291	T41.292	T41.293	T41.294	T41.295	T41.296
Mineral						
acids	T54.2X1	T54.2X2	T54.2X3	T54.2X4	—	—
oil (laxative)(medicinal)	T47.4X1	T47.4X2	T47.4X3	T47.4X4	T47.4X5	T47.4X6
emulsion	T47.2X1	T47.2X2	T47.2X3	T47.2X4	T47.2X5	T47.2X6
nonmedicinal	T52.ØX1	T52.ØX2	T52.ØX3	T52.ØX4	—	—
topical	T49.3X1	T49.3X2	T49.3X3	T49.3X4	T49.3X5	T49.3X6
salt NEC	T5Ø.3X1	T5Ø.3X2	T5Ø.3X3	T5Ø.3X4	T5Ø.3X5	T5Ø.3X6
spirits	T52.ØX1	T52.ØX2	T52.ØX3	T52.ØX4	—	—
Mineralocorticosteroid	T5Ø.ØX1	T5Ø.ØX2	T5Ø.ØX3	T5Ø.ØX4	T5Ø.ØX5	T5Ø.ØX6
Minocycline	T36.4X1	T36.4X2	T36.4X3	T36.4X4	T36.4X5	T36.4X6
Minoxidil	T46.7X1	T46.7X2	T46.7X3	T46.7X4	T46.7X5	T46.7X6
Miokamycin	T36.3X1	T36.3X2	T36.3X3	T36.3X4	T36.3X5	T36.3X6
Miotic drug	T49.5X1	T49.5X2	T49.5X3	T49.5X4	T49.5X5	T49.5X6
Mipafox	T6Ø.ØX1	T6Ø.ØX2	T6Ø.ØX3	T6Ø.ØX4	—	—
Mirex	T6Ø.1X1	T6Ø.1X2	T6Ø.1X3	T6Ø.1X4	—	—
Mirtazapine	T43.Ø21	T43.Ø22	T43.Ø23	T43.Ø24	T43.Ø25	T43.Ø26
Misonidazole	T37.3X1	T37.3X2	T37.3X3	T37.3X4	T37.3X5	T37.3X6
Misoprostol	T47.1X1	T47.1X2	T47.1X3	T47.1X4	T47.1X5	T47.1X6
Mithramycin	T45.1X1	T45.1X2	T45.1X3	T45.1X4	T45.1X5	T45.1X6
Mitobronitol	T45.1X1	T45.1X2	T45.1X3	T45.1X4	T45.1X5	T45.1X6
Mitoguazone	T45.1X1	T45.1X2	T45.1X3	T45.1X4	T45.1X5	T45.1X6
Mitolactol	T45.1X1	T45.1X2	T45.1X3	T45.1X4	T45.1X5	T45.1X6
Mitomycin	T45.1X1	T45.1X2	T45.1X3	T45.1X4	T45.1X5	T45.1X6
Mitopodozide	T45.1X1	T45.1X2	T45.1X3	T45.1X4	T45.1X5	T45.1X6
Mitotane	T45.1X1	T45.1X2	T45.1X3	T45.1X4	T45.1X5	T45.1X6
Mitoxantrone	T45.1X1	T45.1X2	T45.1X3	T45.1X4	T45.1X5	T45.1X6
Mivacurium chloride	T48.1X1	T48.1X2	T48.1X3	T48.1X4	T48.1X5	T48.1X6
Miyari bacteria	T47.6X1	T47.6X2	T47.6X3	T47.6X4	T47.6X5	T47.6X6
Moclobemide	T43.1X1	T43.1X2	T43.1X3	T43.1X4	T43.1X5	T43.1X6
Moderil	T46.5X1	T46.5X2	T46.5X3	T46.5X4	T46.5X5	T46.5X6
Mofebutazone	T39.2X1	T39.2X2	T39.2X3	T39.2X4	T39.2X5	T39.2X6
Mogadon — *see* Nitrazepam						
Molindone	T43.591	T43.592	T43.593	T43.594	T43.595	T43.596
Molsidomine	T46.3X1	T46.3X2	T46.3X3	T46.3X4	T46.3X5	T46.3X6
Mometasone	T49.ØX1	T49.ØX2	T49.ØX3	T49.ØX4	T49.ØX5	T49.ØX6
Monistat	T49.ØX1	T49.ØX2	T49.ØX3	T49.ØX4	T49.ØX5	T49.ØX6
Monkshood	T62.2X1	T62.2X2	T62.2X3	T62.2X4	—	—
Monoamine oxidase inhibitor NEC	T43.1X1	T43.1X2	T43.1X3	T43.1X4	T43.1X5	T43.1X6
hydrazine	T43.1X1	T43.1X2	T43.1X3	T43.1X4	T43.1X5	T43.1X6
Monobenzone	T49.4X1	T49.4X2	T49.4X3	T49.4X4	T49.4X5	T49.4X6
Monochloroacetic acid	T6Ø.3X1	T6Ø.3X2	T6Ø.3X3	T6Ø.3X4	—	—
Monochlorobenzene	T53.7X1	T53.7X2	T53.7X3	T53.7X4	—	—
Monoethanolamine	T46.8X1	T46.8X2	T46.8X3	T46.8X4	T46.8X5	T46.8X6
oleate	T46.8X1	T46.8X2	T46.8X3	T46.8X4	T46.8X5	T46.8X6
Monooctanoin	T5Ø.991	T5Ø.992	T5Ø.993	T5Ø.994	T5Ø.995	T5Ø.996
Monophenylbutazone	T39.2X1	T39.2X2	T39.2X3	T39.2X4	T39.2X5	T39.2X6
Monosodium glutamate	T65.891	T65.892	T65.893	T65.894	—	—
Monosulfiram	T49.ØX1	T49.ØX2	T49.ØX3	T49.ØX4	T49.ØX5	T49.ØX6
Monoxide, carbon — *see* Carbon, monoxide						
Monoxidine hydrochloride	T46.1X1	T46.1X2	T46.1X3	T46.1X4	T46.1X5	T46.1X6
Monuron	T6Ø.3X1	T6Ø.3X2	T6Ø.3X3	T6Ø.3X4	—	—
Moperone	T43.4X1	T43.4X2	T43.4X3	T43.4X4	T43.4X5	T43.4X6
Mopidamol	T45.1X1	T45.1X2	T45.1X3	T45.1X4	T45.1X5	T45.1X6
MOPP (mechloreth-amine + vincristine + prednisone + procarba-zine)	T45.1X1	T45.1X2	T45.1X3	T45.1X4	T45.1X5	T45.1X6
Morfin	T4Ø.2X1	T4Ø.2X2	T4Ø.2X3	T4Ø.2X4	T4Ø.2X5	T4Ø.2X6
Morinamide	T37.1X1	T37.1X2	T37.1X3	T37.1X4	T37.1X5	T37.1X6
Morning glory seeds	T4Ø.991	T4Ø.992	T4Ø.993	T4Ø.994	—	—
Moroxydine	T37.5X1	T37.5X2	T37.5X3	T37.5X4	T37.5X5	T37.5X6
Morphazinamide	T37.1X1	T37.1X2	T37.1X3	T37.1X4	T37.1X5	T37.1X6
Morphine	T4Ø.2X1	T4Ø.2X2	T4Ø.2X3	T4Ø.2X4	T4Ø.2X5	T4Ø.2X6
antagonist	T5Ø.7X1	T5Ø.7X2	T5Ø.7X3	T5Ø.7X4	T5Ø.7X5	T5Ø.7X6
Morpholinylethylmorphine	T4Ø.2X1	T4Ø.2X2	T4Ø.2X3	T4Ø.2X4	—	—
Morsuximide	T42.2X1	T42.2X2	T42.2X3	T42.2X4	T42.2X5	T42.2X6
Mosapramine	T43.591	T43.592	T43.593	T43.594	T43.595	T43.596
Moth balls — *see also* Pesticides	T6Ø.2X1	T6Ø.2X2	T6Ø.2X3	T6Ø.2X4	—	—
naphthalene	T6Ø.2X1	T6Ø.2X2	T6Ø.2X3	T6Ø.2X4	—	—
paradichlorobenzene	T6Ø.1X1	T6Ø.1X2	T6Ø.1X3	T6Ø.1X4	—	—
Motor exhaust gas	T58.Ø1	T58.Ø2	T58.Ø3	T58.Ø4	—	—
Mouthwash (antiseptic) (zinc chloride)	T49.6X1	T49.6X2	T49.6X3	T49.6X4	T49.6X5	T49.6X6
Moxastine	T45.ØX1	T45.ØX2	T45.ØX3	T45.ØX4	T45.ØX5	T45.ØX6
Moxaverine	T44.3X1	T44.3X2	T44.3X3	T44.3X4	T44.3X5	T44.3X6
Moxisylyte	T46.7X1	T46.7X2	T46.7X3	T46.7X4	T46.7X5	T46.7X6
Mucilage, plant	T47.4X1	T47.4X2	T47.4X3	T47.4X4	T47.4X5	T47.4X6
Mucolytic drug	T48.4X1	T48.4X2	T48.4X3	T48.4X4	T48.4X5	T48.4X6
Mucomyst	T48.4X1	T48.4X2	T48.4X3	T48.4X4	T48.4X5	T48.4X6
Mucous membrane agents (external)	T49.91	T49.92	T49.93	T49.94	T49.95	T49.96
specified NEC	T49.8X1	T49.8X2	T49.8X3	T49.8X4	T49.8X5	T49.8X6
Mumps						
immune globulin (human)	T5Ø.Z11	T5Ø.Z12	T5Ø.Z13	T5Ø.Z14	T5Ø.Z15	T5Ø.Z16
skin test antigen	T5Ø.8X1	T5Ø.8X2	T5Ø.8X3	T5Ø.8X4	T5Ø.8X5	T5Ø.8X6
vaccine	T5Ø.B91	T5Ø.B92	T5Ø.B93	T5Ø.B94	T5Ø.B95	T5Ø.B96
Mumpsvax	T5Ø.B91	T5Ø.B92	T5Ø.B93	T5Ø.B94	T5Ø.B95	T5Ø.B96
Mupirocin	T49.ØX1	T49.ØX2	T49.ØX3	T49.ØX4	T49.ØX5	T49.ØX6
Muriatic acid — *see* Hydrochloric acid						
Muromonab-CD3	T45.1X1	T45.1X2	T45.1X3	T45.1X4	T45.1X5	T45.1X6
Muscle-action drug NEC	T48.2Ø1	T48.2Ø2	T48.2Ø3	T48.2Ø4	T48.2Ø5	T48.2Ø6
Muscle affecting agents NEC	T48.2Ø1	T48.2Ø2	T48.2Ø3	T48.2Ø4	T48.2Ø5	T48.2Ø6
oxytocic	T48.ØX1	T48.ØX2	T48.ØX3	T48.ØX4	T48.ØX5	T48.ØX6
relaxants	T48.2Ø1	T48.2Ø2	T48.2Ø3	T48.2Ø4	T48.2Ø5	T48.2Ø6
central nervous system	T42.8X1	T42.8X2	T42.8X3	T42.8X4	T42.8X5	T42.8X6
skeletal	T48.1X1	T48.1X2	T48.1X3	T48.1X4	T48.1X5	T48.1X6
smooth	T44.3X1	T44.3X2	T44.3X3	T44.3X4	T44.3X5	T44.3X6
Muscle relaxant — *see* Relaxant, muscle						
Muscle-tone depressant, central NEC	T42.8X1	T42.8X2	T42.8X3	T42.8X4	T42.8X5	T42.8X6
specified NEC	T42.8X1	T42.8X2	T42.8X3	T42.8X4	T42.8X5	T42.8X6
Mushroom, noxious	T62.ØX1	T62.ØX2	T62.ØX3	T62.ØX4	—	—
Mussel, noxious	T61.781	T61.782	T61.783	T61.784	—	—
Mustard (emetic)	T47.7X1	T47.7X2	T47.7X3	T47.7X4	T47.7X5	T47.7X6
black	T47.7X1	T47.7X2	T47.7X3	T47.7X4	T47.7X5	T47.7X6
gas, not in war	T59.91	T59.92	T59.93	T59.94	—	—
nitrogen	T45.1X1	T45.1X2	T45.1X3	T45.1X4	T45.1X5	T45.1X6
Mustine	T45.1X1	T45.1X2	T45.1X3	T45.1X4	T45.1X5	T45.1X6
M-vac	T45.1X1	T45.1X2	T45.1X3	T45.1X4	T45.1X5	T45.1X6
Mycifradin	T36.5X1	T36.5X2	T36.5X3	T36.5X4	T36.5X5	T36.5X6
topical	T49.ØX1	T49.ØX2	T49.ØX3	T49.ØX4	T49.ØX5	T49.ØX6
Mycitracin	T36.8X1	T36.8X2	T36.8X3	T36.8X4	T36.8X5	T36.8X6
ophthalmic preparation	T49.5X1	T49.5X2	T49.5X3	T49.5X4	T49.5X5	T49.5X6
Mycostatin	T36.7X1	T36.7X2	T36.7X3	T36.7X4	T36.7X5	T36.7X6
topical	T49.ØX1	T49.ØX2	T49.ØX3	T49.ØX4	T49.ØX5	T49.ØX6
Mycotoxins	T64.81	T64.82	T64.83	T64.84	—	—
aflatoxin	T64.Ø1	T64.Ø2	T64.Ø3	T64.Ø4	—	—
specified NEC	T64.81	T64.82	T64.83	T64.84	—	—
Mydriacyl	T44.3X1	T44.3X2	T44.3X3	T44.3X4	T44.3X5	T44.3X6
Mydriatic drug	T49.5X1	T49.5X2	T49.5X3	T49.5X4	T49.5X5	T49.5X6
Myelobromal	T45.1X1	T45.1X2	T45.1X3	T45.1X4	T45.1X5	T45.1X6
Myleran	T45.1X1	T45.1X2	T45.1X3	T45.1X4	T45.1X5	T45.1X6
Myochrysin (e)	T39.2X1	T39.2X2	T39.2X3	T39.2X4	T39.2X5	T39.2X6
Myoneural blocking agents	T48.1X1	T48.1X2	T48.1X3	T48.1X4	T48.1X5	T48.1X6
Myralact	T49.ØX1	T49.ØX2	T49.ØX3	T49.ØX4	T49.ØX5	T49.ØX6
Myristica fragrans	T62.2X1	T62.2X2	T62.2X3	T62.2X4	—	—
Myristicin	T65.891	T65.892	T65.893	T65.894	—	—
Mysoline	T42.3X1	T42.3X2	T42.3X3	T42.3X4	T42.3X5	T42.3X6
Nabilone	T4Ø.7X1	T4Ø.7X2	T4Ø.7X3	T4Ø.7X4	T4Ø.7X5	T4Ø.7X6
Nabumetone	T39.391	T39.392	T39.393	T39.394	T39.395	T39.396
Nadolol	T44.7X1	T44.7X2	T44.7X3	T44.7X4	T44.7X5	T44.7X6

Substance	Poisoning, Accidental (unintentional)	Poisoning, Intentional Self-harm	Poisoning, Assault	Poisoning, Undetermined	Adverse Effect	Under-dosing
Nafcillin	T36.ØX1	T36.ØX2	T36.ØX3	T36.ØX4	T36.ØX5	T36.ØX6
Nafoxidine	T38.6X1	T38.6X2	T38.6X3	T38.6X4	T38.6X5	T38.6X6
Naftazone	T46.991	T46.992	T46.993	T46.994	T46.995	T46.996
Naftidrofuryl (oxalate)	T46.7X1	T46.7X2	T46.7X3	T46.7X4	T46.7X5	T46.7X6
Naftifine	T49.ØX1	T49.ØX2	T49.ØX3	T49.ØX4	T49.ØX5	T49.ØX6
Nail polish remover	T52.91	T52.92	T52.93	T52.94	—	—
Nalbuphine	T4Ø.4X1	T4Ø.4X2	T4Ø.4X3	T4Ø.4X4	T4Ø.4X5	T4Ø.4X6
Naled	T6Ø.ØX1	T6Ø.ØX2	T6Ø.ØX3	T6Ø.ØX4	—	—
Nalidixic acid	T37.8X1	T37.8X2	T37.8X3	T37.8X4	T37.8X5	T37.8X6
Nalorphine	T5Ø.7X1	T5Ø.7X2	T5Ø.7X3	T5Ø.7X4	T5Ø.7X5	T5Ø.7X6
Naloxone	T5Ø.7X1	T5Ø.7X2	T5Ø.7X3	T5Ø.7X4	T5Ø.7X5	T5Ø.7X6
Naltrexone	T5Ø.7X1	T5Ø.7X2	T5Ø.7X3	T5Ø.7X4	T5Ø.7X5	T5Ø.7X6
Namenda	T43.8X1	T43.8X2	T43.8X3	T43.8X4	T43.8X5	T43.8X6
Nandrolone	T38.7X1	T38.7X2	T38.7X3	T38.7X4	T38.7X5	T38.7X6
Naphazoline	T48.5X1	T48.5X2	T48.5X3	T48.5X4	T48.5X5	T48.5X6
Naphtha (painters') (petroleum)	T52.ØX1	T52.ØX2	T52.ØX3	T52.ØX4	—	—
solvent	T52.ØX1	T52.ØX2	T52.ØX3	T52.ØX4	—	—
vapor	T52.ØX1	T52.ØX2	T52.ØX3	T52.ØX4	—	—
Naphthalene (non-chlorinated)	T6Ø.2X1	T6Ø.2X2	T6Ø.2X3	T6Ø.2X4	—	—
chlorinated	T6Ø.1X1	T6Ø.1X2	T6Ø.1X3	T6Ø.1X4	—	—
vapor	T6Ø.1X1	T6Ø.1X2	T6Ø.1X3	T6Ø.1X4	—	—
insecticide or moth repellent	T6Ø.2X1	T6Ø.2X2	T6Ø.2X3	T6Ø.2X4	—	—
chlorinated	T6Ø.1X1	T6Ø.1X2	T6Ø.1X3	T6Ø.1X4	—	—
vapor	T6Ø.2X1	T6Ø.2X2	T6Ø.2X3	T6Ø.2X4	—	—
chlorinated	T6Ø.1X1	T6Ø.1X2	T6Ø.1X3	T6Ø.1X4	—	—
Naphthol	T65.891	T65.892	T65.893	T65.894	—	—
Naphthylamine	T65.891	T65.892	T65.893	T65.894	—	—
Naphthylthiourea (ANTU)	T6Ø.4X1	T6Ø.4X2	T6Ø.4X3	T6Ø.4X4	—	—
Naprosyn — *see* Naproxen						
Naproxen	T39.311	T39.312	T39.313	T39.314	T39.315	T39.316
Narcotic (drug)	T4Ø.6Ø1	T4Ø.6Ø2	T4Ø.6Ø3	T4Ø.6Ø4	T4Ø.6Ø5	T4Ø.6Ø6
analgesic NEC	T4Ø.6Ø1	T4Ø.6Ø2	T4Ø.6Ø3	T4Ø.6Ø4	T4Ø.6Ø5	T4Ø.6Ø6
antagonist	T5Ø.7X1	T5Ø.7X2	T5Ø.7X3	T5Ø.7X4	T5Ø.7X5	T5Ø.7X6
specified NEC	T4Ø.691	T4Ø.692	T4Ø.693	T4Ø.694	T4Ø.695	T4Ø.696
synthetic	T4Ø.4X1	T4Ø.4X2	T4Ø.4X3	T4Ø.4X4	T4Ø.4X5	T4Ø.4X6
Narcotine	T48.3X1	T48.3X2	T48.3X3	T48.3X4	T48.3X5	T48.3X6
Nardil	T43.1X1	T43.1X2	T43.1X3	T43.1X4	T43.1X5	T43.1X6
Nasal drug NEC	T49.6X1	T49.6X2	T49.6X3	T49.6X4	T49.6X5	T49.6X6
Natamycin	T49.ØX1	T49.ØX2	T49.ØX3	T49.ØX4	T49.ØX5	T49.ØX6
Natrium cyanide — *see* Cyanide(s)						
Natural						
blood (product)	T45.8X1	T45.8X2	T45.8X3	T45.8X4	T45.8X5	T45.8X6
gas (piped)	T59.891	T59.892	T59.893	T59.894	—	—
incomplete combustion	T58.11	T58.12	T58.13	T58.14	—	—
Nealbarbital	T42.3X1	T42.3X2	T42.3X3	T42.3X4	T42.3X5	T42.3X6
Nectadon	T48.3X1	T48.3X2	T48.3X3	T48.3X4	T48.3X5	T48.3X6
Nedocromil	T48.6X1	T48.6X2	T48.6X3	T48.6X4	T48.6X5	T48.6X6
Nefopam	T39.8X1	T39.8X2	T39.8X3	T39.8X4	T39.8X5	T39.8X6
Nematocyst (sting)	T63.691	T63.692	T63.693	T63.694	—	—
Nembutal	T42.3X1	T42.3X2	T42.3X3	T42.3X4	T42.3X5	T42.3X6
Nemonapride	T43.591	T43.592	T43.593	T43.594	T43.595	T43.596
Neoarsphenamine	T37.8X1	T37.8X2	T37.8X3	T37.8X4	T37.8X5	T37.8X6
Neocinchophen	T5Ø.4X1	T5Ø.4X2	T5Ø.4X3	T5Ø.4X4	T5Ø.4X5	T5Ø.4X6
Neomycin (derivatives)	T36.5X1	T36.5X2	T36.5X3	T36.5X4	T36.5X5	T36.5X6
with						
bacitracin	T49.ØX1	T49.ØX2	T49.ØX3	T49.ØX4	T49.ØX5	T49.ØX6
neostigmine	T44.ØX1	T44.ØX2	T44.ØX3	T44.ØX4	T44.ØX5	T44.ØX6
ENT agent	T49.6X1	T49.6X2	T49.6X3	T49.6X4	T49.6X5	T49.6X6
ophthalmic preparation	T49.5X1	T49.5X2	T49.5X3	T49.5X4	T49.5X5	T49.5X6
topical NEC	T49.ØX1	T49.ØX2	T49.ØX3	T49.ØX4	T49.ØX5	T49.ØX6
Neonal	T42.3X1	T42.3X2	T42.3X3	T42.3X4	T42.3X5	T42.3X6
Neoprontosil	T37.ØX1	T37.ØX2	T37.ØX3	T37.ØX4	T37.ØX5	T37.ØX6
Neosalvarsan	T37.8X1	T37.8X2	T37.8X3	T37.8X4	T37.8X5	T37.8X6
Neosilversalvarsan	T37.8X1	T37.8X2	T37.8X3	T37.8X4	T37.8X5	T37.8X6
Neosporin	T36.8X1	T36.8X2	T36.8X3	T36.8X4	T36.8X5	T36.8X6
ENT agent	T49.6X1	T49.6X2	T49.6X3	T49.6X4	T49.6X5	T49.6X6
opthalmic preparation	T49.5X1	T49.5X2	T49.5X3	T49.5X4	T49.5X5	T49.5X6
topical NEC	T49.ØX1	T49.ØX2	T49.ØX3	T49.ØX4	T49.ØX5	T49.ØX6
Neostigmine bromide	T44.ØX1	T44.ØX2	T44.ØX3	T44.ØX4	T44.ØX5	T44.ØX6
Neraval	T42.3X1	T42.3X2	T42.3X3	T42.3X4	T42.3X5	T42.3X6
Neravan	T42.3X1	T42.3X2	T42.3X3	T42.3X4	T42.3X5	T42.3X6
Nerium oleander	T62.2X1	T62.2X2	T62.2X3	T62.2X4	—	—
Nerve gas, not in war	T59.91	T59.92	T59.93	T59.94	—	—
Nesacaine	T41.3X1	T41.3X2	T41.3X3	T41.3X4	T41.3X5	T41.3X6
infiltration (subcutaneous)	T41.3X1	T41.3X2	T41.3X3	T41.3X4	T41.3X5	T41.3X6
nerve block (peripheral) (plexus)	T41.3X1	T41.3X2	T41.3X3	T41.3X4	T41.3X5	T41.3X6
Netilmicin	T36.5X1	T36.5X2	T36.5X3	T36.5X4	T36.5X5	T36.5X6
Neurobarb	T42.3X1	T42.3X2	T42.3X3	T42.3X4	T42.3X5	T42.3X6

Substance	Poisoning, Accidental (unintentional)	Poisoning, Intentional Self-harm	Poisoning, Assault	Poisoning, Undetermined	Adverse Effect	Under-dosing
Neuroleptic drug NEC	T43.5Ø1	T43.5Ø2	T43.5Ø3	T43.5Ø4	T43.5Ø5	T43.5Ø6
Neuromuscular blocking drug	T48.1X1	T48.1X2	T48.1X3	T48.1X4	T48.1X5	T48.1X6
Neutral insulin injection	T38.3X1	T38.3X2	T38.3X3	T38.3X4	T38.3X5	T38.3X6
Neutral spirits	T51.ØX1	T51.ØX2	T51.ØX3	T51.ØX4	—	—
beverage	T51.ØX1	T51.ØX2	T51.ØX3	T51.ØX4	—	—
Niacin	T46.7X1	T46.7X2	T46.7X3	T46.7X4	T46.7X5	T46.7X6
Niacinamide	T45.2X1	T45.2X2	T45.2X3	T45.2X4	T45.2X5	T45.2X6
Nialamide	T43.1X1	T43.1X2	T43.1X3	T43.1X4	T43.1X5	T43.1X6
Niaprazine	T42.6X1	T42.6X2	T42.6X3	T42.6X4	T42.6X5	T42.6X6
Nicametate	T46.7X1	T46.7X2	T46.7X3	T46.7X4	T46.7X5	T46.7X6
Nicardipine	T46.1X1	T46.1X2	T46.1X3	T46.1X4	T46.1X5	T46.1X6
Nicergoline	T46.7X1	T46.7X2	T46.7X3	T46.7X4	T46.7X5	T46.7X6
Nickel (carbonyl) (tetra-carbonyl)(fumes) (vapor)	T56.891	T56.892	T56.893	T56.894	—	—
Nickelocene	T56.891	T56.892	T56.893	T56.894	—	—
Niclosamide	T37.4X1	T37.4X2	T37.4X3	T37.4X4	T37.4X5	T37.4X6
Nicofuranose	T46.7X1	T46.7X2	T46.7X3	T46.7X4	T46.7X5	T46.7X6
Nicomorphine	T4Ø.2X1	T4Ø.2X2	T4Ø.2X3	T4Ø.2X4	—	—
Nicorandil	T46.3X1	T46.3X2	T46.3X3	T46.3X4	T46.3X5	T46.3X6
Nicotiana (plant)	T62.2X1	T62.2X2	T62.2X3	T62.2X4	—	—
Nicotinamide	T45.2X1	T45.2X2	T45.2X3	T45.2X4	T45.2X5	T45.2X6
Nicotine (insecticide) (spray) (sulfate) **NEC**	T6Ø.2X1	T6Ø.2X2	T6Ø.2X3	T6Ø.2X4	—	—
from tobacco	T65.291	T65.292	T65.293	T65.294	—	—
cigarettes	T65.221	T65.222	T65.223	T65.224	—	—
not insecticide	T65.291	T65.292	T65.293	T65.294	—	—
Nicotinic acid	T46.7X1	T46.7X2	T46.7X3	T46.7X4	T46.7X5	T46.7X6
Nicotinyl alcohol	T46.7X1	T46.7X2	T46.7X3	T46.7X4	T46.7X5	T46.7X6
Nicoumalone	T45.511	T45.512	T45.513	T45.514	T45.515	T45.516
Nifedipine	T46.1X1	T46.1X2	T46.1X3	T46.1X4	T46.1X5	T46.1X6
Nifenazone	T39.2X1	T39.2X2	T39.2X3	T39.2X4	T39.2X5	T39.2X6
Nifuraldezone	T37.91	T37.92	T37.93	T37.94	T37.95	T37.96
Nifuratel	T37.8X1	T37.8X2	T37.8X3	T37.8X4	T37.8X5	T37.8X6
Nifurtimox	T37.3X1	T37.3X2	T37.3X3	T37.3X4	T37.3X5	T37.3X6
Nifurtoinol	T37.8X1	T37.8X2	T37.8X3	T37.8X4	T37.8X5	T37.8X6
Nightshade, deadly (solanum) — *see also* Belladonna	T62.2X1	T62.2X2	T62.2X3	T62.2X4	—	—
berry	T62.1X1	T62.1X2	T62.1X3	T62.1X4	—	—
Nikethamide	T5Ø.7X1	T5Ø.7X2	T5Ø.7X3	T5Ø.7X4	T5Ø.7X5	T5Ø.7X6
Nilstat	T36.7X1	T36.7X2	T36.7X3	T36.7X4	T36.7X5	T36.7X6
topical	T49.ØX1	T49.ØX2	T49.ØX3	T49.ØX4	T49.ØX5	T49.ØX6
Nilutamide	T38.6X1	T38.6X2	T38.6X3	T38.6X4	T38.6X5	T38.6X6
Nimesulide	T39.391	T39.392	T39.393	T39.394	T39.395	T39.396
Nimetazepam	T42.4X1	T42.4X2	T42.4X3	T42.4X4	T42.4X5	T42.4X6
Nimodipine	T46.1X1	T46.1X2	T46.1X3	T46.1X4	T46.1X5	T46.1X6
Nimorazole	T37.3X1	T37.3X2	T37.3X3	T37.3X4	T37.3X5	T37.3X6
Nimustine	T45.1X1	T45.1X2	T45.1X3	T45.1X4	T45.1X5	T45.1X6
Niridazole	T37.4X1	T37.4X2	T37.4X3	T37.4X4	T37.4X5	T37.4X6
Nisentil	T4Ø.2X1	T4Ø.2X2	T4Ø.2X3	T4Ø.2X4	T4Ø.2X5	T4Ø.2X6
Nisoldipine	T46.1X1	T46.1X2	T46.1X3	T46.1X4	T46.1X5	T46.1X6
Nitramine	T65.3X1	T65.3X2	T65.3X3	T65.3X4	—	—
Nitrate, organic	T46.3X1	T46.3X2	T46.3X3	T46.3X4	T46.3X5	T46.3X6
Nitrazepam	T42.4X1	T42.4X2	T42.4X3	T42.4X4	T42.4X5	T42.4X6
Nitrefazole	T5Ø.6X1	T5Ø.6X2	T5Ø.6X3	T5Ø.6X4	T5Ø.6X5	T5Ø.6X6
Nitrendipine	T46.1X1	T46.1X2	T46.1X3	T46.1X4	T46.1X5	T46.1X6
Nitric						
acid (liquid)	T54.2X1	T54.2X2	T54.2X3	T54.2X4	—	—
vapor	T59.891	T59.892	T59.893	T59.894	—	—
oxide (gas)	T59.ØX1	T59.ØX2	T59.ØX3	T59.ØX4	—	—
Nitrimidazine	T37.3X1	T37.3X2	T37.3X3	T37.3X4	T37.3X5	T37.3X6
Nitrite, amyl (medicinal) (vapor)	T46.3X1	T46.3X2	T46.3X3	T46.3X4	T46.3X5	T46.3X6
Nitroaniline	T65.3X1	T65.3X2	T65.3X3	T65.3X4	—	—
vapor	T59.891	T59.892	T59.893	T59.894	—	—
Nitrobenzene, nitrobenzol	T65.3X1	T65.3X2	T65.3X3	T65.3X4	—	—
vapor	T65.3X1	T65.3X2	T65.3X3	T65.3X4	—	—
Nitrocellulose	T65.891	T65.892	T65.893	T65.894	—	—
lacquer	T65.891	T65.892	T65.893	T65.894	—	—
Nitrodiphenyl	T65.3X1	T65.3X2	T65.3X3	T65.3X4	—	—
Nitrofural	T49.ØX1	T49.ØX2	T49.ØX3	T49.ØX4	T49.ØX5	T49.ØX6
Nitrofurantoin	T37.8X1	T37.8X2	T37.8X3	T37.8X4	T37.8X5	T37.8X6
Nitrofurazone	T49.ØX1	T49.ØX2	T49.ØX3	T49.ØX4	T49.ØX5	T49.ØX6
Nitrogen	T59.ØX1	T59.ØX2	T59.ØX3	T59.ØX4	—	—
mustard	T45.1X1	T45.1X2	T45.1X3	T45.1X4	T45.1X5	T45.1X6
Nitroglycerin, nitroglycerol (medicinal)	T46.3X1	T46.3X2	T46.3X3	T46.3X4	T46.3X5	T46.3X6
nonmedicinal	T65.5X1	T65.5X2	T65.5X3	T65.5X4	—	—
fumes	T65.5X1	T65.5X2	T65.5X3	T65.5X4	—	—
Nitroglycol	T52.3X1	T52.3X2	T52.3X3	T52.3X4	—	—
Nitrohydrochloric acid	T54.2X1	T54.2X2	T54.2X3	T54.2X4	—	—
Nitromersol	T49.ØX1	T49.ØX2	T49.ØX3	T49.ØX4	T49.ØX5	T49.ØX6

Substance	Poisoning, Accidental (unintentional)	Poisoning, Intentional Self-harm	Poisoning, Assault	Poisoning, Undetermined	Adverse Effect	Under-dosing
Nitronaphthalene	T65.891	T65.892	T65.893	T65.894	—	—
Nitrophenol	T54.ØX1	T54.ØX2	T54.ØX3	T54.ØX4	—	—
Nitropropane	T52.8X1	T52.8X2	T52.8X3	T52.8X4	—	—
Nitroprusside	T46.5X1	T46.5X2	T46.5X3	T46.5X4	T46.5X5	T46.5X6
Nitrosodimethylamine	T65.3X1	T65.3X2	T65.3X3	T65.3X4	—	—
Nitrothiazol	T37.4X1	T37.4X2	T37.4X3	T37.4X4	T37.4X5	T37.4X6
Nitrotoluene, nitrotoluol	T65.3X1	T65.3X2	T65.3X3	T65.3X4	—	—
vapor	T65.3X1	T65.3X2	T65.3X3	T65.3X4	—	—
Nitrous						
acid (liquid)	T54.2X1	T54.2X2	T54.2X3	T54.2X4	—	—
fumes	T59.891	T59.892	T59.893	T59.894	—	—
ether spirit	T46.3X1	T46.3X2	T46.3X3	T46.3X4	T46.3X5	T46.3X6
oxide	T41.ØX1	T41.ØX2	T41.ØX3	T41.ØX4	T41.ØX5	T41.ØX6
Nitroxoline	T37.8X1	T37.8X2	T37.8X3	T37.8X4	T37.8X5	T37.8X6
Nitrozone	T49.ØX1	T49.ØX2	T49.ØX3	T49.ØX4	T49.ØX5	T49.ØX6
Nizatidine	T47.ØX1	T47.ØX2	T47.ØX3	T47.ØX4	T47.ØX5	T47.ØX6
Nizofenone	T43.8X1	T43.8X2	T43.8X3	T43.8X4	T43.8X5	T43.8X6
Noctec	T42.6X1	T42.6X2	T42.6X3	T42.6X4	T42.6X5	T42.6X6
Noludar	T42.6X1	T42.6X2	T42.6X3	T42.6X4	T42.6X5	T42.6X6
Nomegestrol	T38.5X1	T38.5X2	T38.5X3	T38.5X4	T38.5X5	T38.5X6
Nomifensine	T43.291	T43.292	T43.293	T43.294	T43.295	T43.296
Nonoxinol	T49.8X1	T49.8X2	T49.8X3	T49.8X4	T49.8X5	T49.8X6
Nonylphenoxy (polyethoxyethanol)	T49.8X1	T49.8X2	T49.8X3	T49.8X4	T49.8X5	T49.8X6
Noptil	T42.3X1	T42.3X2	T42.3X3	T42.3X4	T42.3X5	T42.3X6
Noradrenaline	T44.4X1	T44.4X2	T44.4X3	T44.4X4	T44.4X5	T44.4X6
Noramidopyrine	T39.2X1	T39.2X2	T39.2X3	T39.2X4	T39.2X5	T39.2X6
methanesulfonate sodium	T39.2X1	T39.2X2	T39.2X3	T39.2X4	T39.2X5	T39.2X6
Norbormide	T6Ø.4X1	T6Ø.4X2	T6Ø.4X3	T6Ø.4X4	—	—
Nordazepam	T42.4X1	T42.4X2	T42.4X3	T42.4X4	T42.4X5	T42.4X6
Norepinephrine	T44.4X1	T44.4X2	T44.4X3	T44.4X4	T44.4X5	T44.4X6
Norethandrolone	T38.7X1	T38.7X2	T38.7X3	T38.7X4	T38.7X5	T38.7X6
Norethindrone	T38.4X1	T38.4X2	T38.4X3	T38.4X4	T38.4X5	T38.4X6
Norethisterone (acetate) (enantate)	T38.4X1	T38.4X2	T38.4X3	T38.4X4	T38.4X5	T38.4X6
with ethinylestradiol	T38.5X1	T38.5X2	T38.5X3	T38.5X4	T38.5X5	T38.5X6
Noretynodrel	T38.5X1	T38.5X2	T38.5X3	T38.5X4	T38.5X5	T38.5X6
Norfenefrine	T44.4X1	T44.4X2	T44.4X3	T44.4X4	T44.4X5	T44.4X6
Norfloxacin	T36.8X1	T36.8X2	T36.8X3	T36.8X4	T36.8X5	T36.8X6
Norgestrel	T38.4X1	T38.4X2	T38.4X3	T38.4X4	T38.4X5	T38.4X6
Norgestrienone	T38.4X1	T38.4X2	T38.4X3	T38.4X4	T38.4X5	T38.4X6
Norlestrin	T38.4X1	T38.4X2	T38.4X3	T38.4X4	T38.4X5	T38.4X6
Norlutin	T38.4X1	T38.4X2	T38.4X3	T38.4X4	T38.4X5	T38.4X6
Normal serum albumin (human), salt-poor	T45.8X1	T45.8X2	T45.8X3	T45.8X4	T45.8X5	T45.8X6
Normethandrone	T38.5X1	T38.5X2	T38.5X3	T38.5X4	T38.5X5	T38.5X6
Normison — *see* Benzodiazepines						
Normorphine	T4Ø.2X1	T4Ø.2X2	T4Ø.2X3	T4Ø.2X4	—	—
Norpseudoephedrine	T5Ø.5X1	T5Ø.5X2	T5Ø.5X3	T5Ø.5X4	T5Ø.5X5	T5Ø.5X6
Nortestosterone (furanpropionate)	T38.7X1	T38.7X2	T38.7X3	T38.7X4	T38.7X5	T38.7X6
Nortriptyline	T43.Ø11	T43.Ø12	T43.Ø13	T43.Ø14	T43.Ø15	T43.Ø16
Noscapine	T48.3X1	T48.3X2	T48.3X3	T48.3X4	T48.3X5	T48.3X6
Nose preparations	T49.6X1	T49.6X2	T49.6X3	T49.6X4	T49.6X5	T49.6X6
Novobiocin	T36.5X1	T36.5X2	T36.5X3	T36.5X4	T36.5X5	T36.5X6
Novocain (infiltration) (topical)	T41.3X1	T41.3X2	T41.3X3	T41.3X4	T41.3X5	T41.3X6
nerve block (peripheral) (plexus)	T41.3X1	T41.3X2	T41.3X3	T41.3X4	T41.3X5	T41.3X6
spinal	T41.3X1	T41.3X2	T41.3X3	T41.3X4	T41.3X5	T41.3X6
Noxious foodstuff	T62.91	T62.92	T62.93	T62.94	—	—
specified NEC	T62.8X1	T62.8X2	T62.8X3	T62.8X4	—	—
Noxiptiline	T43.Ø11	T43.Ø12	T43.Ø13	T43.Ø14	T43.Ø15	T43.Ø16
Noxytiolin	T49.ØX1	T49.ØX2	T49.ØX3	T49.ØX4	T49.ØX5	T49.ØX6
NPH Iletin (insulin)	T38.3X1	T38.3X2	T38.3X3	T38.3X4	T38.3X5	T38.3X6
Numorphan	T4Ø.2X1	T4Ø.2X2	T4Ø.2X3	T4Ø.2X4	T4Ø.2X5	T4Ø.2X6
Nunol	T42.3X1	T42.3X2	T42.3X3	T42.3X4	T42.3X5	T42.3X6
Nupercaine (spinal anesthetic)	T41.3X1	T41.3X2	T41.3X3	T41.3X4	T41.3X5	T41.3X6
topical (surface)	T41.3X1	T41.3X2	T41.3X3	T41.3X4	T41.3X5	T41.3X6
Nutmeg oil (liniment)	T49.3X1	T49.3X2	T49.3X3	T49.3X4	T49.3X5	T49.3X6
Nutritional supplement	T5Ø.9Ø1	T5Ø.9Ø2	T5Ø.9Ø3	T5Ø.9Ø4	T5Ø.9Ø5	T5Ø.9Ø6
Nux vomica	T65.1X1	T65.1X2	T65.1X3	T65.1X4	—	—
Nydrazid	T37.1X1	T37.1X2	T37.1X3	T37.1X4	T37.1X5	T37.1X6
Nylidrin	T46.7X1	T46.7X2	T46.7X3	T46.7X4	T46.7X5	T46.7X6
Nystatin	T36.7X1	T36.7X2	T36.7X3	T36.7X4	T36.7X5	T36.7X6
topical	T49.ØX1	T49.ØX2	T49.ØX3	T49.ØX4	T49.ØX5	T49.ØX6
Nytol	T45.ØX1	T45.ØX2	T45.ØX3	T45.ØX4	T45.ØX5	T45.ØX6
Obidoxime chloride	T5Ø.6X1	T5Ø.6X2	T5Ø.6X3	T5Ø.6X4	T5Ø.6X5	T5Ø.6X6
Octafonium (chloride)	T49.3X1	T49.3X2	T49.3X3	T49.3X4	T49.3X5	T49.3X6
Octamethyl pyrophosphoramide	T6Ø.ØX1	T6Ø.ØX2	T6Ø.ØX3	T6Ø.ØX4	—	—
Octanoin	T5Ø.991	T5Ø.992	T5Ø.993	T5Ø.994	T5Ø.995	T5Ø.996
Octatropine methylbromide	T44.3X1	T44.3X2	T44.3X3	T44.3X4	T44.3X5	T44.3X6
Octotiamine	T45.2X1	T45.2X2	T45.2X3	T45.2X4	T45.2X5	T45.2X6
Octoxinol (9)	T49.8X1	T49.8X2	T49.8X3	T49.8X4	T49.8X5	T49.8X6
Octreotide	T38.991	T38.992	T38.993	T38.994	T38.995	T38.996
Octyl nitrite	T46.3X1	T46.3X2	T46.3X3	T46.3X4	T46.3X5	T46.3X6
Oestradiol	T38.5X1	T38.5X2	T38.5X3	T38.5X4	T38.5X5	T38.5X6
Oestriol	T38.5X1	T38.5X2	T38.5X3	T38.5X4	T38.5X5	T38.5X6
Oestrogen	T38.5X1	T38.5X2	T38.5X3	T38.5X4	T38.5X5	T38.5X6
Oestrone	T38.5X1	T38.5X2	T38.5X3	T38.5X4	T38.5X5	T38.5X6
Ofloxacin	T36.8X1	T36.8X2	T36.8X3	T36.8X4	T36.8X5	T36.8X6
Oil (of)	T65.891	T65.892	T65.893	T65.894	—	—
bitter almond	T62.8X1	T62.8X2	T62.8X3	T62.8X4	—	—
cloves	T49.7X1	T49.7X2	T49.7X3	T49.7X4	T49.7X5	T49.7X6
colors	T65.6X1	T65.6X2	T65.6X3	T65.6X4	—	—
fumes	T59.891	T59.892	T59.893	T59.894	—	—
lubricating	T52.ØX1	T52.ØX2	T52.ØX3	T52.ØX4	—	—
Niobe	T52.8X1	T52.8X2	T52.8X3	T52.8X4	—	—
vitriol (liquid)	T54.2X1	T54.2X2	T54.2X3	T54.2X4	—	—
fumes	T54.2X1	T54.2X2	T54.2X3	T54.2X4	—	—
wintergreen (bitter) NEC	T49.3X1	T49.3X2	T49.3X3	T49.3X4	T49.3X5	T49.3X6
Oily preparation (for skin)	T49.3X1	T49.3X2	T49.3X3	T49.3X4	T49.3X5	T49.3X6
Ointment NEC	T49.3X1	T49.3X2	T49.3X3	T49.3X4	T49.3X5	T49.3X6
Olanzapine	T43.591	T43.592	T43.593	T43.594	T43.595	T43.596
Oleander	T62.2X1	T62.2X2	T62.2X3	T62.2X4	—	—
Oleandomycin	T36.3X1	T36.3X2	T36.3X3	T36.3X4	T36.3X5	T36.3X6
Oleandrin	T46.ØX1	T46.ØX2	T46.ØX3	T46.ØX4	T46.ØX5	T46.ØX6
Oleic acid	T46.6X1	T46.6X2	T46.6X3	T46.6X4	T46.6X5	T46.6X6
Oleovitamin A	T45.2X1	T45.2X2	T45.2X3	T45.2X4	T45.2X5	T45.2X6
Oleum ricini	T47.2X1	T47.2X2	T47.2X3	T47.2X4	T47.2X5	T47.2X6
Olive oil (medicinal) **NEC**	T47.4X1	T47.4X2	T47.4X3	T47.4X4	T47.4X5	T47.4X6
Olivomycin	T45.1X1	T45.1X2	T45.1X3	T45.1X4	T45.1X5	T45.1X6
Olsalazine	T47.8X1	T47.8X2	T47.8X3	T47.8X4	T47.8X5	T47.8X6
Omeprazole	T47.1X1	T47.1X2	T47.1X3	T47.1X4	T47.1X5	T47.1X6
OMPA	T6Ø.ØX1	T6Ø.ØX2	T6Ø.ØX3	T6Ø.ØX4	—	—
Oncovin	T45.1X1	T45.1X2	T45.1X3	T45.1X4	T45.1X5	T45.1X6
Ondansetron	T45.ØX1	T45.ØX2	T45.ØX3	T45.ØX4	T45.ØX5	T45.ØX6
Ophthaine	T41.3X1	T41.3X2	T41.3X3	T41.3X4	T41.3X5	T41.3X6
Ophthetic	T41.3X1	T41.3X2	T41.3X3	T41.3X4	T41.3X5	T41.3X6
Opiate NEC	T4Ø.6Ø1	T4Ø.6Ø2	T4Ø.6Ø3	T4Ø.6Ø4	T4Ø.6Ø5	T4Ø.6Ø6
antagonists	T5Ø.7X1	T5Ø.7X2	T5Ø.7X3	T5Ø.7X4	T5Ø.7X5	T5Ø.7X6
Opioid NEC	T4Ø.2X1	T4Ø.2X2	T4Ø.2X3	T4Ø.2X4	T4Ø.2X5	T4Ø.2X6
Opipramol	T43.Ø11	T43.Ø12	T43.Ø13	T43.Ø14	T43.Ø15	T43.Ø16
Opium alkaloids (total)	T4Ø.ØX1	T4Ø.ØX2	T4Ø.ØX3	T4Ø.ØX4	T4Ø.ØX5	T4Ø.ØX6
standardized powdered	T4Ø.ØX1	T4Ø.ØX2	T4Ø.ØX3	T4Ø.ØX4	T4Ø.ØX5	T4Ø.ØX6
tincture (camphorated)	T4Ø.ØX1	T4Ø.ØX2	T4Ø.ØX3	T4Ø.ØX4	T4Ø.ØX5	T4Ø.ØX6
Oracon	T38.4X1	T38.4X2	T38.4X3	T38.4X4	T38.4X5	T38.4X6
Oragrafin	T5Ø.8X1	T5Ø.8X2	T5Ø.8X3	T5Ø.8X4	T5Ø.8X5	T5Ø.8X6
Oral contraceptives	T38.4X1	T38.4X2	T38.4X3	T38.4X4	T38.4X5	T38.4X6
Oral rehydration salts	T5Ø.3X1	T5Ø.3X2	T5Ø.3X3	T5Ø.3X4	T5Ø.3X5	T5Ø.3X6
Orazamide	T5Ø.991	T5Ø.992	T5Ø.993	T5Ø.994	T5Ø.995	T5Ø.996
Orciprenaline	T48.291	T48.292	T48.293	T48.294	T48.295	T48.296
Organidin	T48.4X1	T48.4X2	T48.4X3	T48.4X4	T48.4X5	T48.4X6
Organonitrate NEC	T46.3X1	T46.3X2	T46.3X3	T46.3X4	T46.3X5	T46.3X6
Organophosphates	T6Ø.ØX1	T6Ø.ØX2	T6Ø.ØX3	T6Ø.ØX4	—	—
Orimune	T5Ø.B91	T5Ø.B92	T5Ø.B93	T5Ø.B94	T5Ø.B95	T5Ø.B96
Orinase	T38.3X1	T38.3X2	T38.3X3	T38.3X4	T38.3X5	T38.3X6
Ormeloxifene	T38.6X1	T38.6X2	T38.6X3	T38.6X4	T38.6X5	T38.6X6
Ornidazole	T37.3X1	T37.3X2	T37.3X3	T37.3X4	T37.3X5	T37.3X6
Ornithine aspartate	T5Ø.991	T5Ø.992	T5Ø.993	T5Ø.994	T5Ø.995	T5Ø.996
Ornoprostil	T47.1X1	T47.1X2	T47.1X3	T47.1X4	T47.1X5	T47.1X6
Orphenadrine (hydrochloride)	T42.8X1	T42.8X2	T42.8X3	T42.8X4	T42.8X5	T42.8X6
Ortal (sodium)	T42.3X1	T42.3X2	T42.3X3	T42.3X4	T42.3X5	T42.3X6
Orthoboric acid	T49.ØX1	T49.ØX2	T49.ØX3	T49.ØX4	T49.ØX5	T49.ØX6
ENT agent	T49.6X1	T49.6X2	T49.6X3	T49.6X4	T49.6X5	T49.6X6
ophthalmic preparation	T49.5X1	T49.5X2	T49.5X3	T49.5X4	T49.5X5	T49.5X6
Orthocaine	T41.3X1	T41.3X2	T41.3X3	T41.3X4	T41.3X5	T41.3X6
Orthodichlorobenzene	T53.7X1	T53.7X2	T53.7X3	T53.7X4	—	—
Ortho-Novum	T38.4X1	T38.4X2	T38.4X3	T38.4X4	T38.4X5	T38.4X6
Orthotolidine (reagent)	T54.2X1	T54.2X2	T54.2X3	T54.2X4	—	—
Osmic acid (liquid)	T54.2X1	T54.2X2	T54.2X3	T54.2X4	—	—
fumes	T54.2X1	T54.2X2	T54.2X3	T54.2X4	—	—
Osmotic diuretics	T5Ø.2X1	T5Ø.2X2	T5Ø.2X3	T5Ø.2X4	T5Ø.2X5	T5Ø.2X6
Otilonium bromide	T44.3X1	T44.3X2	T44.3X3	T44.3X4	T44.3X5	T44.3X6
Otorhinolaryngological drug NEC	T49.6X1	T49.6X2	T49.6X3	T49.6X4	T49.6X5	T49.6X6
Ouabain (e)	T46.ØX1	T46.ØX2	T46.ØX3	T46.ØX4	T46.ØX5	T46.ØX6
Ovarian						
hormone	T38.5X1	T38.5X2	T38.5X3	T38.5X4	T38.5X5	T38.5X6
stimulant	T38.5X1	T38.5X2	T38.5X3	T38.5X4	T38.5X5	T38.5X6
Ovral	T38.4X1	T38.4X2	T38.4X3	T38.4X4	T38.4X5	T38.4X6

Substance	Poisoning, Accidental (unintentional)	Poisoning, Intentional Self-harm	Poisoning, Assault	Poisoning, Undetermined	Adverse Effect	Under-dosing
Ovulen	T38.4X1	T38.4X2	T38.4X3	T38.4X4	T38.4X5	T38.4X6
Oxacillin	T36.ØX1	T36.ØX2	T36.ØX3	T36.ØX4	T36.ØX5	T36.ØX6
Oxalic acid	T54.2X1	T54.2X2	T54.2X3	T54.2X4	—	—
ammonium salt	T5Ø.991	T5Ø.992	T5Ø.993	T5Ø.994	T5Ø.995	T5Ø.996
Oxamniquine	T37.4X1	T37.4X2	T37.4X3	T37.4X4	T37.4X5	T37.4X6
Oxanamide	T43.591	T43.592	T43.593	T43.594	T43.595	T43.596
Oxandrolone	T38.7X1	T38.7X2	T38.7X3	T38.7X4	T38.7X5	T38.7X6
Oxantel	T37.4X1	T37.4X2	T37.4X3	T37.4X4	T37.4X5	T37.4X6
Oxapium iodide	T44.3X1	T44.3X2	T44.3X3	T44.3X4	T44.3X5	T44.3X6
Oxaprotiline	T43.Ø21	T43.Ø22	T43.Ø23	T43.Ø24	T43.Ø25	T43.Ø26
Oxaprozin	T39.311	T39.312	T39.313	T39.314	T39.315	T39.316
Oxatomide	T45.ØX1	T45.ØX2	T45.ØX3	T45.ØX4	T45.ØX5	T45.ØX6
Oxazepam	T42.4X1	T42.4X2	T42.4X3	T42.4X4	T42.4X5	T42.4X6
Oxazimedrine	T5Ø.5X1	T5Ø.5X2	T5Ø.5X3	T5Ø.5X4	T5Ø.5X5	T5Ø.5X6
Oxazolam	T42.4X1	T42.4X2	T42.4X3	T42.4X4	T42.4X5	T42.4X6
Oxazolidine derivatives	T42.2X1	T42.2X2	T42.2X3	T42.2X4	T42.2X5	T42.2X6
Oxazolidinedione (derivative)	T42.2X1	T42.2X2	T42.2X3	T42.2X4	T42.2X5	T42.2X6
Ox bile extract	T47.5X1	T47.5X2	T47.5X3	T47.5X4	T47.5X5	T47.5X6
Oxcarbazepine	T42.1X1	T42.1X2	T42.1X3	T42.1X4	T42.1X5	T42.1X6
Oxedrine	T44.4X1	T44.4X2	T44.4X3	T44.4X4	T44.4X5	T44.4X6
Oxeladin (citrate)	T48.3X1	T48.3X2	T48.3X3	T48.3X4	T48.3X5	T48.3X6
Oxendolone	T38.5X1	T38.5X2	T38.5X3	T38.5X4	T38.5X5	T38.5X6
Oxetacaine	T41.3X1	T41.3X2	T41.3X3	T41.3X4	T41.3X5	T41.3X6
Oxethazine	T41.3X1	T41.3X2	T41.3X3	T41.3X4	T41.3X5	T41.3X6
Oxetorone	T39.8X1	T39.8X2	T39.8X3	T39.8X4	T39.8X5	T39.8X6
Oxiconazole	T49.ØX1	T49.ØX2	T49.ØX3	T49.ØX4	T49.ØX5	T49.ØX6
Oxidizing agent NEC	T54.91	T54.92	T54.93	T54.94	—	—
Oxipurinol	T5Ø.4X1	T5Ø.4X2	T5Ø.4X3	T5Ø.4X4	T5Ø.4X5	T5Ø.4X6
Oxitriptan	T43.291	T43.292	T43.293	T43.294	T43.295	T43.296
Oxitropium bromide	T48.6X1	T48.6X2	T48.6X3	T48.6X4	T48.6X5	T48.6X6
Oxodipine	T46.1X1	T46.1X2	T46.1X3	T46.1X4	T46.1X5	T46.1X6
Oxolamine	T48.3X1	T48.3X2	T48.3X3	T48.3X4	T48.3X5	T48.3X6
Oxolinic acid	T37.8X1	T37.8X2	T37.8X3	T37.8X4	T37.8X5	T37.8X6
Oxomemazine	T43.3X1	T43.3X2	T43.3X3	T43.3X4	T43.3X5	T43.3X6
Oxophenarsine	T37.3X1	T37.3X2	T37.3X3	T37.3X4	T37.3X5	T37.3X6
Oxprenolol	T44.7X1	T44.7X2	T44.7X3	T44.7X4	T44.7X5	T44.7X6
Oxsoralen	T49.3X1	T49.3X2	T49.3X3	T49.3X4	T49.3X5	T49.3X6
Oxtriphylline	T48.6X1	T48.6X2	T48.6X3	T48.6X4	T48.6X5	T48.6X6
Oxybate sodium	T41.291	T41.292	T41.293	T41.294	T41.295	T41.296
Oxybuprocaine	T41.3X1	T41.3X2	T41.3X3	T41.3X4	T41.3X5	T41.3X6
Oxybutynin	T44.3X1	T44.3X2	T44.3X3	T44.3X4	T44.3X5	T44.3X6
Oxychlorosene	T49.ØX1	T49.ØX2	T49.ØX3	T49.ØX4	T49.ØX5	T49.ØX6
Oxycodone	T4Ø.2X1	T4Ø.2X2	T4Ø.2X3	T4Ø.2X4	T4Ø.2X5	T4Ø.2X6
Oxyfedrine	T46.3X1	T46.3X2	T46.3X3	T46.3X4	T46.3X5	T46.3X6
Oxygen	T41.5X1	T41.5X2	T41.5X3	T41.5X4	T41.5X5	T41.5X6
Oxylone	T49.ØX1	T49.ØX2	T49.ØX3	T49.ØX4	T49.ØX5	T49.ØX6
ophthalmic preparation	T49.5X1	T49.5X2	T49.5X3	T49.5X4	T49.5X5	T49.5X6
Oxymesterone	T38.7X1	T38.7X2	T38.7X3	T38.7X4	T38.7X5	T38.7X6
Oxymetazoline	T48.5X1	T48.5X2	T48.5X3	T48.5X4	T48.5X5	T48.5X6
Oxymetholone	T38.7X1	T38.7X2	T38.7X3	T38.7X4	T38.7X5	T38.7X6
Oxymorphone	T4Ø.2X1	T4Ø.2X2	T4Ø.2X3	T4Ø.2X4	T4Ø.2X5	T4Ø.2X6
Oxypertine	T43.591	T43.592	T43.593	T43.594	T43.595	T43.596
Oxyphenbutazone	T39.2X1	T39.2X2	T39.2X3	T39.2X4	T39.2X5	T39.2X6
Oxyphencyclimine	T44.3X1	T44.3X2	T44.3X3	T44.3X4	T44.3X5	T44.3X6
Oxyphenisatine	T47.2X1	T47.2X2	T47.2X3	T47.2X4	T47.2X5	T47.2X6
Oxyphenonium bromide	T44.3X1	T44.3X2	T44.3X3	T44.3X4	T44.3X5	T44.3X6
Oxypolygelatin	T45.8X1	T45.8X2	T45.8X3	T45.8X4	T45.8X5	T45.8X6
Oxyquinoline (derivatives)	T37.8X1	T37.8X2	T37.8X3	T37.8X4	T37.8X5	T37.8X6
Oxytetracycline	T36.4X1	T36.4X2	T36.4X3	T36.4X4	T36.4X5	T36.4X6
Oxytocic drug NEC	T48.ØX1	T48.ØX2	T48.ØX3	T48.ØX4	T48.ØX5	T48.ØX6
Oxytocin (synthetic)	T48.ØX1	T48.ØX2	T48.ØX3	T48.ØX4	T48.ØX5	T48.ØX6
Ozone	T59.891	T59.892	T59.893	T59.894	—	—
PABA	T49.3X1	T49.3X2	T49.3X3	T49.3X4	T49.3X5	T49.3X6
Packed red cells	T45.8X1	T45.8X2	T45.8X3	T45.8X4	T45.8X5	T45.8X6
Padimate	T49.3X1	T49.3X2	T49.3X3	T49.3X4	T49.3X5	T49.3X6
Paint NEC	T65.6X1	T65.6X2	T65.6X3	T65.6X4	—	—
cleaner	T52.91	T52.92	T52.93	T52.94	—	—
fumes NEC	T59.891	T59.892	T59.893	T59.894	—	—
lead (fumes)	T56.ØX1	T56.ØX2	T56.ØX3	T56.ØX4	—	—
solvent NEC	T52.8X1	T52.8X2	T52.8X3	T52.8X4	—	—
stripper	T52.8X1	T52.8X2	T52.8X3	T52.8X4	—	—
Palfium	T4Ø.2X1	T4Ø.2X2	T4Ø.2X3	T4Ø.2X4	—	—
Palm kernel oil	T5Ø.991	T5Ø.992	T5Ø.993	T5Ø.994	T5Ø.995	T5Ø.996
Paludrine	T37.2X1	T37.2X2	T37.2X3	T37.2X4	T37.2X5	T37.2X6
PAM (pralidoxime)	T5Ø.6X1	T5Ø.6X2	T5Ø.6X3	T5Ø.6X4	T5Ø.6X5	T5Ø.6X6
Pamaquine (naphthoute)	T37.2X1	T37.2X2	T37.2X3	T37.2X4	T37.2X5	T37.2X6
Panadol	T39.1X1	T39.1X2	T39.1X3	T39.1X4	T39.1X5	T39.1X6
Pancreatic						
digestive secretion stimulant	T47.8X1	T47.8X2	T47.8X3	T47.8X4	T47.8X5	T47.8X6
dornase	T45.3X1	T45.3X2	T45.3X3	T45.3X4	T45.3X5	T45.3X6
Pancreatin	T47.5X1	T47.5X2	T47.5X3	T47.5X4	T47.5X5	T47.5X6

Substance	Poisoning, Accidental (unintentional)	Poisoning, Intentional Self-harm	Poisoning, Assault	Poisoning, Undetermined	Adverse Effect	Under-dosing
Pancrelipase	T47.5X1	T47.5X2	T47.5X3	T47.5X4	T47.5X5	T47.5X6
Pancuronium (bromide)	T48.1X1	T48.1X2	T48.1X3	T48.1X4	T48.1X5	T48.1X6
Pangamic acid	T45.2X1	T45.2X2	T45.2X3	T45.2X4	T45.2X5	T45.2X6
Panthenol	T45.2X1	T45.2X2	T45.2X3	T45.2X4	T45.2X5	T45.2X6
topical	T49.8X1	T49.8X2	T49.8X3	T49.8X4	T49.8X5	T49.8X6
Pantopon	T4Ø.ØX1	T4Ø.ØX2	T4Ø.ØX3	T4Ø.ØX4	T4Ø.ØX5	T4Ø.ØX6
Pantothenic acid	T45.2X1	T45.2X2	T45.2X3	T45.2X4	T45.2X5	T45.2X6
Panwarfin	T45.511	T45.512	T45.513	T45.514	T45.515	T45.516
Papain	T47.5X1	T47.5X2	T47.5X3	T47.5X4	T47.5X5	T47.5X6
digestant	T47.5X1	T47.5X2	T47.5X3	T47.5X4	T47.5X5	T47.5X6
Papaveretum	T4Ø.ØX1	T4Ø.ØX2	T4Ø.ØX3	T4Ø.ØX4	T4Ø.ØX5	T4Ø.ØX6
Papaverine	T44.3X1	T44.3X2	T44.3X3	T44.3X4	T44.3X5	T44.3X6
Para-acetamidophenol	T39.1X1	T39.1X2	T39.1X3	T39.1X4	T39.1X5	T39.1X6
Para-aminobenzoic acid	T49.3X1	T49.3X2	T49.3X3	T49.3X4	T49.3X5	T49.3X6
Para-aminophenol derivatives	T39.1X1	T39.1X2	T39.1X3	T39.1X4	T39.1X5	T39.1X6
Para-aminosalicylic acid	T37.1X1	T37.1X2	T37.1X3	T37.1X4	T37.1X5	T37.1X6
Paracetaldehyde	T42.6X1	T42.6X2	T42.6X3	T42.6X4	T42.6X5	T42.6X6
Paracetamol	T39.1X1	T39.1X2	T39.1X3	T39.1X4	T39.1X5	T39.1X6
Parachlorophenol (camphorated)	T49.ØX1	T49.ØX2	T49.ØX3	T49.ØX4	T49.ØX5	T49.ØX6
Paracodin	T4Ø.2X1	T4Ø.2X2	T4Ø.2X3	T4Ø.2X4	T4Ø.2X5	T4Ø.2X6
Paradione	T42.2X1	T42.2X2	T42.2X3	T42.2X4	T42.2X5	T42.2X6
Paraffin(s) (wax)	T52.ØX1	T52.ØX2	T52.ØX3	T52.ØX4	—	—
liquid (medicinal)	T47.4X1	T47.4X2	T47.4X3	T47.4X4	T47.4X5	T47.4X6
nonmedicinal	T52.ØX1	T52.ØX2	T52.ØX3	T52.ØX4	—	—
Paraformaldehyde	T6Ø.3X1	T6Ø.3X2	T6Ø.3X3	T6Ø.3X4	—	—
Paraldehyde	T42.6X1	T42.6X2	T42.6X3	T42.6X4	T42.6X5	T42.6X6
Paramethadione	T42.2X1	T42.2X2	T42.2X3	T42.2X4	T42.2X5	T42.2X6
Paramethasone	T38.ØX1	T38.ØX2	T38.ØX3	T38.ØX4	T38.ØX5	T38.ØX6
acetate	T49.ØX1	T49.ØX2	T49.ØX3	T49.ØX4	T49.ØX5	T49.ØX6
Paraoxon	T6Ø.ØX1	T6Ø.ØX2	T6Ø.ØX3	T6Ø.ØX4	—	—
Paraquat	T6Ø.3X1	T6Ø.3X2	T6Ø.3X3	T6Ø.3X4	—	—
Parasympatholytic NEC	T44.3X1	T44.3X2	T44.3X3	T44.3X4	T44.3X5	T44.3X6
Parasympathomimetic drug NEC	T44.1X1	T44.1X2	T44.1X3	T44.1X4	T44.1X5	T44.1X6
Parathion	T6Ø.ØX1	T6Ø.ØX2	T6Ø.ØX3	T6Ø.ØX4	—	—
Parathormone	T5Ø.991	T5Ø.992	T5Ø.993	T5Ø.994	T5Ø.995	T5Ø.996
Parathyroid extract	T5Ø.991	T5Ø.992	T5Ø.993	T5Ø.994	T5Ø.995	T5Ø.996
Paratyphoid vaccine	T5Ø.A91	T5Ø.A92	T5Ø.A93	T5Ø.A94	T5Ø.A95	T5Ø.A96
Paredrine	T44.4X1	T44.4X2	T44.4X3	T44.4X4	T44.4X5	T44.4X6
Paregoric	T4Ø.ØX1	T4Ø.ØX2	T4Ø.ØX3	T4Ø.ØX4	T4Ø.ØX5	T4Ø.ØX6
Pargyline	T46.5X1	T46.5X2	T46.5X3	T46.5X4	T46.5X5	T46.5X6
Paris green	T57.ØX1	T57.ØX2	T57.ØX3	T57.ØX4	—	—
insecticide	T57.ØX1	T57.ØX2	T57.ØX3	T57.ØX4	—	—
Parnate	T43.1X1	T43.1X2	T43.1X3	T43.1X4	T43.1X5	T43.1X6
Paromomycin	T36.5X1	T36.5X2	T36.5X3	T36.5X4	T36.5X5	T36.5X6
Paroxypropione	T45.1X1	T45.1X2	T45.1X3	T45.1X4	T45.1X5	T45.1X6
Parzone	T4Ø.2X1	T4Ø.2X2	T4Ø.2X3	T4Ø.2X4	T4Ø.2X5	T4Ø.2X6
PAS	T37.1X1	T37.1X2	T37.1X3	T37.1X4	T37.1X5	T37.1X6
Pasiniazid	T37.1X1	T37.1X2	T37.1X3	T37.1X4	T37.1X5	T37.1X6
PBB (polybrominated biphenyls)	T65.891	T65.892	T65.893	T65.894	—	—
PCB	T65.891	T65.892	T65.893	T65.894	—	—
PCP						
meaning pentachlorophenol	T6Ø.1X1	T6Ø.1X2	T6Ø.1X3	T6Ø.1X4	—	—
fungicide	T6Ø.3X1	T6Ø.3X2	T6Ø.3X3	T6Ø.3X4	—	—
herbicide	T6Ø.3X1	T6Ø.3X2	T6Ø.3X3	T6Ø.3X4	—	—
insecticide	T6Ø.1X1	T6Ø.1X2	T6Ø.1X3	T6Ø.1X4	—	—
meaning phencyclidine	T4Ø.991	T4Ø.992	T4Ø.993	T4Ø.994	—	—
Peach kernel oil (emulsion)	T47.4X1	T47.4X2	T47.4X3	T47.4X4	T47.4X5	T47.4X6
Peanut oil (emulsion) **NEC**	T47.4X1	T47.4X2	T47.4X3	T47.4X4	T47.4X5	T47.4X6
topical	T49.3X1	T49.3X2	T49.3X3	T49.3X4	T49.3X5	T49.3X6
Pearly Gates (morning glory seeds)	T4Ø.991	T4Ø.992	T4Ø.993	T4Ø.994	—	—
Pecazine	T43.3X1	T43.3X2	T43.3X3	T43.3X4	T43.3X5	T43.3X6
Pectin	T47.6X1	T47.6X2	T47.6X3	T47.6X4	T47.6X5	T47.6X6
Pefloxacin	T37.8X1	T37.8X2	T37.8X3	T37.8X4	T37.8X5	T37.8X6
Pegademase, bovine	T5Ø.Z91	T5Ø.Z92	T5Ø.Z93	T5Ø.Z94	T5Ø.Z95	T5Ø.Z96
Pelletierine tannate	T37.4X1	T37.4X2	T37.4X3	T37.4X4	T37.4X5	T37.4X6
Pemirolast (potassium)	T48.6X1	T48.6X2	T48.6X3	T48.6X4	T48.6X5	T48.6X6
Pemoline	T5Ø.7X1	T5Ø.7X2	T5Ø.7X3	T5Ø.7X4	T5Ø.7X5	T5Ø.7X6
Pempidine	T44.2X1	T44.2X2	T44.2X3	T44.2X4	T44.2X5	T44.2X6
Penamecillin	T36.ØX1	T36.ØX2	T36.ØX3	T36.ØX4	T36.ØX5	T36.ØX6
Penbutolol	T44.7X1	T44.7X2	T44.7X3	T44.7X4	T44.7X5	T44.7X6
Penethamate	T36.ØX1	T36.ØX2	T36.ØX3	T36.ØX4	T36.ØX5	T36.ØX6
Penfluridol	T43.591	T43.592	T43.593	T43.594	T43.595	T43.596
Penflutizide	T5Ø.2X1	T5Ø.2X2	T5Ø.2X3	T5Ø.2X4	T5Ø.2X5	T5Ø.2X6
Pengitoxin	T46.ØX1	T46.ØX2	T46.ØX3	T46.ØX4	T46.ØX5	T46.ØX6
Penicillamine	T5Ø.6X1	T5Ø.6X2	T5Ø.6X3	T5Ø.6X4	T5Ø.6X5	T5Ø.6X6
Penicillin (any)	T36.ØX1	T36.ØX2	T36.ØX3	T36.ØX4	T36.ØX5	T36.ØX6
Penicillinase	T45.3X1	T45.3X2	T45.3X3	T45.3X4	T45.3X5	T45.3X6

Substance	Poisoning, Accidental (unintentional)	Poisoning, Intentional Self-harm	Poisoning, Assault	Poisoning, Undetermined	Adverse Effect	Under-dosing
Penicilloyl polylysine	T5Ø.8X1	T5Ø.8X2	T5Ø.8X3	T5Ø.8X4	T5Ø.8X5	T5Ø.8X6
Penimepicycline	T36.4X1	T36.4X2	T36.4X3	T36.4X4	T36.4X5	T36.4X6
Pentachloroethane	T53.6X1	T53.6X2	T53.6X3	T53.6X4	—	—
Pentachloronaphthalene	T53.7X1	T53.7X2	T53.7X3	T53.7X4	—	—
Pentachlorophenol (pesticide)	T6Ø.1X1	T6Ø.1X2	T6Ø.1X3	T6Ø.1X4	—	—
fungicide	T6Ø.3X1	T6Ø.3X2	T6Ø.3X3	T6Ø.3X4	—	—
herbicide	T6Ø.3X1	T6Ø.3X2	T6Ø.3X3	T6Ø.3X4	—	—
insecticide	T6Ø.1X1	T6Ø.1X2	T6Ø.1X3	T6Ø.1X4	—	—
Pentaerythritol	T46.3X1	T46.3X2	T46.3X3	T46.3X4	T46.3X5	T46.3X6
chloral	T42.6X1	T42.6X2	T42.6X3	T42.6X4	T42.6X5	T42.6X6
tetranitrate NEC	T46.3X1	T46.3X2	T46.3X3	T46.3X4	T46.3X5	T46.3X6
Pentaerythrityl tetranitrate	T46.3X1	T46.3X2	T46.3X3	T46.3X4	T46.3X5	T46.3X6
Pentagastrin	T5Ø.8X1	T5Ø.8X2	T5Ø.8X3	T5Ø.8X4	T5Ø.8X5	T5Ø.8X6
Pentalin	T53.6X1	T53.6X2	T53.6X3	T53.6X4	—	—
Pentamethonium bromide	T44.2X1	T44.2X2	T44.2X3	T44.2X4	T44.2X5	T44.2X6
Pentamidine	T37.3X1	T37.3X2	T37.3X3	T37.3X4	T37.3X5	T37.3X6
Pentanol	T51.3X1	T51.3X2	T51.3X3	T51.3X4	—	—
Pentapyrrolinium (bitartrate)	T44.2X1	T44.2X2	T44.2X3	T44.2X4	T44.2X5	T44.2X6
Pentaquine	T37.2X1	T37.2X2	T37.2X3	T37.2X4	T37.2X5	T37.2X6
Pentazocine	T4Ø.4X1	T4Ø.4X2	T4Ø.4X3	T4Ø.4X4	T4Ø.4X5	T4Ø.4X6
Pentetrazole	T5Ø.7X1	T5Ø.7X2	T5Ø.7X3	T5Ø.7X4	T5Ø.7X5	T5Ø.7X6
Penthienate bromide	T44.3X1	T44.3X2	T44.3X3	T44.3X4	T44.3X5	T44.3X6
Pentifylline	T46.7X1	T46.7X2	T46.7X3	T46.7X4	T46.7X5	T46.7X6
Pentobarbital	T42.3X1	T42.3X2	T42.3X3	T42.3X4	T42.3X5	T42.3X6
sodium	T42.3X1	T42.3X2	T42.3X3	T42.3X4	T42.3X5	T42.3X6
Pentobarbitone	T42.3X1	T42.3X2	T42.3X3	T42.3X4	T42.3X5	T42.3X6
Pentolonium tartrate	T44.2X1	T44.2X2	T44.2X3	T44.2X4	T44.2X5	T44.2X6
Pentosan polysulfate (sodium)	T39.8X1	T39.8X2	T39.8X3	T39.8X4	T39.8X5	T39.8X6
Pentostatin	T45.1X1	T45.1X2	T45.1X3	T45.1X4	T45.1X5	T45.1X6
Pentothal	T41.1X1	T41.1X2	T41.1X3	T41.1X4	T41.1X5	T41.1X6
Pentoxifylline	T46.7X1	T46.7X2	T46.7X3	T46.7X4	T46.7X5	T46.7X6
Pentoxyverine	T48.3X1	T48.3X2	T48.3X3	T48.3X4	T48.3X5	T48.3X6
Pentrinat	T46.3X1	T46.3X2	T46.3X3	T46.3X4	T46.3X5	T46.3X6
Pentylenetetrazole	T5Ø.7X1	T5Ø.7X2	T5Ø.7X3	T5Ø.7X4	T5Ø.7X5	T5Ø.7X6
Pentylsalicylamide	T37.1X1	T37.1X2	T37.1X3	T37.1X4	T37.1X5	T37.1X6
Pentymal	T42.3X1	T42.3X2	T42.3X3	T42.3X4	T42.3X5	T42.3X6
Peplomycin	T45.1X1	T45.1X2	T45.1X3	T45.1X4	T45.1X5	T45.1X6
Peppermint (oil)	T47.5X1	T47.5X2	T47.5X3	T47.5X4	T47.5X5	T47.5X6
Pepsin	T47.5X1	T47.5X2	T47.5X3	T47.5X4	T47.5X5	T47.5X6
digestant	T47.5X1	T47.5X2	T47.5X3	T47.5X4	T47.5X5	T47.5X6
Pepstatin	T47.1X1	T47.1X2	T47.1X3	T47.1X4	T47.1X5	T47.1X6
Peptavlon	T5Ø.8X1	T5Ø.8X2	T5Ø.8X3	T5Ø.8X4	T5Ø.8X5	T5Ø.8X6
Perazine	T43.3X1	T43.3X2	T43.3X3	T43.3X4	T43.3X5	T43.3X6
Percaine (spinal)	T41.3X1	T41.3X2	T41.3X3	T41.3X4	T41.3X5	T41.3X6
topical (surface)	T41.3X1	T41.3X2	T41.3X3	T41.3X4	T41.3X5	T41.3X6
Perchloroethylene	T53.3X1	T53.3X2	T53.3X3	T53.3X4	—	—
medicinal	T37.4X1	T37.4X2	T37.4X3	T37.4X4	T37.4X5	T37.4X6
vapor	T53.3X1	T53.3X2	T53.3X3	T53.3X4	—	—
Percodan	T4Ø.2X1	T4Ø.2X2	T4Ø.2X3	T4Ø.2X4	T4Ø.2X5	T4Ø.2X6
Percogesic — *see also* acetaminophen	T45.ØX1	T45.ØX2	T45.ØX3	T45.ØX4	T45.ØX5	T45.ØX6
Percorten	T38.ØX1	T38.ØX2	T38.ØX3	T38.ØX4	T38.ØX5	T38.ØX6
Pergolide	T42.8X1	T42.8X2	T42.8X3	T42.8X4	T42.8X5	T42.8X6
Pergonal	T38.811	T38.812	T38.813	T38.814	T38.815	T38.816
Perhexilene	T46.3X1	T46.3X2	T46.3X3	T46.3X4	T46.3X5	T46.3X6
Perhexiline (maleate)	T46.3X1	T46.3X2	T46.3X3	T46.3X4	T46.3X5	T46.3X6
Periactin	T45.ØX1	T45.ØX2	T45.ØX3	T45.ØX4	T45.ØX5	T45.ØX6
Periciazine	T43.3X1	T43.3X2	T43.3X3	T43.3X4	T43.3X5	T43.3X6
Periclor	T42.6X1	T42.6X2	T42.6X3	T42.6X4	T42.6X5	T42.6X6
Perindopril	T46.4X1	T46.4X2	T46.4X3	T46.4X4	T46.4X5	T46.4X6
Perisoxal	T39.8X1	T39.8X2	T39.8X3	T39.8X4	T39.8X5	T39.8X6
Peritoneal dialysis solution	T5Ø.3X1	T5Ø.3X2	T5Ø.3X3	T5Ø.3X4	T5Ø.3X5	T5Ø.3X6
Peritrate	T46.3X1	T46.3X2	T46.3X3	T46.3X4	T46.3X5	T46.3X6
Perlapine	T42.4X1	T42.4X2	T42.4X3	T42.4X4	T42.4X5	T42.4X6
Permanganate	T65.891	T65.892	T65.893	T65.894	—	—
Permethrin	T6Ø.1X1	T6Ø.1X2	T6Ø.1X3	T6Ø.1X4	—	—
Pernocton	T42.3X1	T42.3X2	T42.3X3	T42.3X4	T42.3X5	T42.3X6
Pernoston	T42.3X1	T42.3X2	T42.3X3	T42.3X4	T42.3X5	T42.3X6
Peronine	T4Ø.2X1	T4Ø.2X2	T4Ø.2X3	T4Ø.2X4	—	—
Perphenazine	T43.3X1	T43.3X2	T43.3X3	T43.3X4	T43.3X5	T43.3X6
Pertofrane	T43.Ø11	T43.Ø12	T43.Ø13	T43.Ø14	T43.Ø15	T43.Ø16
Pertussis						
immune serum (human)	T5Ø.Z11	T5Ø.Z12	T5Ø.Z13	T5Ø.Z14	T5Ø.Z15	T5Ø.Z16
vaccine (with diphtheria toxoid) (with tetanus toxoid)	T5Ø.A11	T5Ø.A12	T5Ø.A13	T5Ø.A14	T5Ø.A15	T5Ø.A16
Peruvian balsam	T49.ØX1	T49.ØX2	T49.ØX3	T49.ØX4	T49.ØX5	T49.ØX6
Peruvoside	T46.ØX1	T46.ØX2	T46.ØX3	T46.ØX4	T46.ØX5	T46.ØX6
Pesticide (dust) (fumes) (vapor) **NEC**	T6Ø.91	T6Ø.92	T6Ø.93	T6Ø.94	—	—
Pesticide (dust) (fumes) (vapor) **NEC** — *continued*						
arsenic	T57.ØX1	T57.ØX2	T57.ØX3	T57.ØX4	—	—
chlorinated	T6Ø.1X1	T6Ø.1X2	T6Ø.1X3	T6Ø.1X4	—	—
cyanide	T65.ØX1	T65.ØX2	T65.ØX3	T65.ØX4	—	—
kerosene	T52.ØX1	T52.ØX2	T52.ØX3	T52.ØX4	—	—
mixture (of compounds)	T6Ø.91	T6Ø.92	T6Ø.93	T6Ø.94	—	—
naphthalene	T6Ø.2X1	T6Ø.2X2	T6Ø.2X3	T6Ø.2X4	—	—
organochlorine (compounds)	T6Ø.1X1	T6Ø.1X2	T6Ø.1X3	T6Ø.1X4	—	—
petroleum (distillate) (products) NEC	T6Ø.8X1	T6Ø.8X2	T6Ø.8X3	T6Ø.8X4	—	—
specified ingredient NEC	T6Ø.8X1	T6Ø.8X2	T6Ø.8X3	T6Ø.8X4	—	—
strychnine	T65.1X1	T65.1X2	T65.1X3	T65.1X4	—	—
thallium	T6Ø.4X1	T6Ø.4X2	T6Ø.4X3	T6Ø.4X4	—	—
Pethidine	T4Ø.4X1	T4Ø.4X2	T4Ø.4X3	T4Ø.4X4	T4Ø.4X5	T4Ø.4X6
Petrichloral	T42.6X1	T42.6X2	T42.6X3	T42.6X4	T42.6X5	T42.6X6
Petrol	T52.ØX1	T52.ØX2	T52.ØX3	T52.ØX4	—	—
vapor	T52.ØX1	T52.ØX2	T52.ØX3	T52.ØX4	—	—
Petrolatum	T49.3X1	T49.3X2	T49.3X3	T49.3X4	T49.3X5	T49.3X6
hydrophilic	T49.3X1	T49.3X2	T49.3X3	T49.3X4	T49.3X5	T49.3X6
liquid	T47.4X1	T47.4X2	T47.4X3	T47.4X4	T47.4X5	T47.4X6
topical	T49.3X1	T49.3X2	T49.3X3	T49.3X4	T49.3X5	T49.3X6
nonmedicinal	T52.ØX1	T52.ØX2	T52.ØX3	T52.ØX4	—	—
red veterinary	T49.3X1	T49.3X2	T49.3X3	T49.3X4	T49.3X5	T49.3X6
white	T49.3X1	T49.3X2	T49.3X3	T49.3X4	T49.3X5	T49.3X6
Petroleum (products) **NEC**	T52.ØX1	T52.ØX2	T52.ØX3	T52.ØX4	—	—
benzine(s) — *see* Ligroin						
ether — *see* Ligroin						
jelly — *see* Petrolatum						
naphtha — *see* Ligroin						
pesticide	T6Ø.8X1	T6Ø.8X2	T6Ø.8X3	T6Ø.8X4	—	—
solids	T52.ØX1	T52.ØX2	T52.ØX3	T52.ØX4	—	—
solvents	T52.ØX1	T52.ØX2	T52.ØX3	T52.ØX4	—	—
vapor	T52.ØX1	T52.ØX2	T52.ØX3	T52.ØX4	—	—
Peyote	T4Ø.991	T4Ø.992	T4Ø.993	T4Ø.994	—	—
Phanodorm, phanodorn	T42.3X1	T42.3X2	T42.3X3	T42.3X4	T42.3X5	T42.3X6
Phanquinone	T37.3X1	T37.3X2	T37.3X3	T37.3X4	T37.3X5	T37.3X6
Phanquone	T37.3X1	T37.3X2	T37.3X3	T37.3X4	T37.3X5	T37.3X6
Pharmaceutical						
adjunct NEC	T5Ø.9Ø1	T5Ø.9Ø2	T5Ø.9Ø3	T5Ø.9Ø4	T5Ø.9Ø5	T5Ø.9Ø6
excipient NEC	T5Ø.9Ø1	T5Ø.9Ø2	T5Ø.9Ø3	T5Ø.9Ø4	T5Ø.9Ø5	T5Ø.9Ø6
sweetener	T5Ø.9Ø1	T5Ø.9Ø2	T5Ø.9Ø3	T5Ø.9Ø4	T5Ø.9Ø5	T5Ø.9Ø6
viscous agent	T5Ø.9Ø1	T5Ø.9Ø2	T5Ø.9Ø3	T5Ø.9Ø4	T5Ø.9Ø5	T5Ø.9Ø6
Phemitone	T42.3X1	T42.3X2	T42.3X3	T42.3X4	T42.3X5	T42.3X6
Phenacaine	T41.3X1	T41.3X2	T41.3X3	T41.3X4	T41.3X5	T41.3X6
Phenacemide	T42.6X1	T42.6X2	T42.6X3	T42.6X4	T42.6X5	T42.6X6
Phenacetin	T39.1X1	T39.1X2	T39.1X3	T39.1X4	T39.1X5	T39.1X6
Phenadoxone	T4Ø.2X1	T4Ø.2X2	T4Ø.2X3	T4Ø.2X4	—	—
Phenaglycodol	T43.591	T43.592	T43.593	T43.594	T43.595	T43.596
Phenantoin	T42.ØX1	T42.ØX2	T42.ØX3	T42.ØX4	T42.ØX5	T42.ØX6
Phenaphthazine reagent	T5Ø.991	T5Ø.992	T5Ø.993	T5Ø.994	T5Ø.995	T5Ø.996
Phenazocine	T4Ø.4X1	T4Ø.4X2	T4Ø.4X3	T4Ø.4X4	T4Ø.4X5	T4Ø.4X6
Phenazone	T39.2X1	T39.2X2	T39.2X3	T39.2X4	T39.2X5	T39.2X6
Phenazopyridine	T39.8X1	T39.8X2	T39.8X3	T39.8X4	T39.8X5	T39.8X6
Phenbenicillin	T36.ØX1	T36.ØX2	T36.ØX3	T36.ØX4	T36.ØX5	T36.ØX6
Phenbutrazate	T5Ø.5X1	T5Ø.5X2	T5Ø.5X3	T5Ø.5X4	T5Ø.5X5	T5Ø.5X6
Phencyclidine	T4Ø.991	T4Ø.992	T4Ø.993	T4Ø.994	T4Ø.995	T4Ø.996
Phendimetrazine	T5Ø.5X1	T5Ø.5X2	T5Ø.5X3	T5Ø.5X4	T5Ø.5X5	T5Ø.5X6
Phenelzine	T43.1X1	T43.1X2	T43.1X3	T43.1X4	T43.1X5	T43.1X6
Phenemal	T42.3X1	T42.3X2	T42.3X3	T42.3X4	T42.3X5	T42.3X6
Phenergan	T42.6X1	T42.6X2	T42.6X3	T42.6X4	T42.6X5	T42.6X6
Pheneticillin	T36.ØX1	T36.ØX2	T36.ØX3	T36.ØX4	T36.ØX5	T36.ØX6
Pheneturide	T42.6X1	T42.6X2	T42.6X3	T42.6X4	T42.6X5	T42.6X6
Phenformin	T38.3X1	T38.3X2	T38.3X3	T38.3X4	T38.3X5	T38.3X6
Phenglutarimide	T44.3X1	T44.3X2	T44.3X3	T44.3X4	T44.3X5	T44.3X6
Phenicarbazide	T39.8X1	T39.8X2	T39.8X3	T39.8X4	T39.8X5	T39.8X6
Phenindamine	T45.ØX1	T45.ØX2	T45.ØX3	T45.ØX4	T45.ØX5	T45.ØX6
Phenindione	T45.511	T45.512	T45.513	T45.514	T45.515	T45.516
Pheniprazine	T43.1X1	T43.1X2	T43.1X3	T43.1X4	T43.1X5	T43.1X6
Pheniramine	T45.ØX1	T45.ØX2	T45.ØX3	T45.ØX4	T45.ØX5	T45.ØX6
Phenisatin	T47.2X1	T47.2X2	T47.2X3	T47.2X4	T47.2X5	T47.2X6
Phenmetrazine	T5Ø.5X1	T5Ø.5X2	T5Ø.5X3	T5Ø.5X4	T5Ø.5X5	T5Ø.5X6
Phenobal	T42.3X1	T42.3X2	T42.3X3	T42.3X4	T42.3X5	T42.3X6
Phenobarbital	T42.3X1	T42.3X2	T42.3X3	T42.3X4	T42.3X5	T42.3X6
with						
mephenytoin	T42.3X1	T42.3X2	T42.3X3	T42.3X4	T42.3X5	T42.3X6
phenytoin	T42.3X1	T42.3X2	T42.3X3	T42.3X4	T42.3X5	T42.3X6
sodium	T42.3X1	T42.3X2	T42.3X3	T42.3X4	T42.3X5	T42.3X6
Phenobarbitone	T42.3X1	T42.3X2	T42.3X3	T42.3X4	T42.3X5	T42.3X6
Phenobutiodil	T5Ø.8X1	T5Ø.8X2	T5Ø.8X3	T5Ø.8X4	T5Ø.8X5	T5Ø.8X6
Phenoctide	T49.ØX1	T49.ØX2	T49.ØX3	T49.ØX4	T49.ØX5	T49.ØX6
Phenol	T49.ØX1	T49.ØX2	T49.ØX3	T49.ØX4	T49.ØX5	T49.ØX6

Substance	Poisoning, Accidental (unintentional)	Poisoning, Intentional Self-harm	Poisoning, Assault	Poisoning, Undetermined	Adverse Effect	Under-dosing
Phenol — *continued*						
disinfectant	T54.ØX1	T54.ØX2	T54.ØX3	T54.ØX4	—	—
in oil injection	T46.8X1	T46.8X2	T46.8X3	T46.8X4	T46.8X5	T46.8X6
medicinal	T49.1X1	T49.1X2	T49.1X3	T49.1X4	T49.1X5	T49.1X6
nonmedicinal NEC	T54.ØX1	T54.ØX2	T54.ØX3	T54.ØX4	—	—
pesticide	T6Ø.8X1	T6Ø.8X2	T6Ø.8X3	T6Ø.8X4	—	—
red	T5Ø.8X1	T5Ø.8X2	T5Ø.8X3	T5Ø.8X4	T5Ø.8X5	T5Ø.8X6
Phenolic preparation	T49.1X1	T49.1X2	T49.1X3	T49.1X4	T49.1X5	T49.1X6
Phenolphthalein	T47.2X1	T47.2X2	T47.2X3	T47.2X4	T47.2X5	T47.2X6
Phenolsulfonphthalein	T5Ø.8X1	T5Ø.8X2	T5Ø.8X3	T5Ø.8X4	T5Ø.8X5	T5Ø.8X6
Phenomorphan	T4Ø.2X1	T4Ø.2X2	T4Ø.2X3	T4Ø.2X4	—	—
Phenonyl	T42.3X1	T42.3X2	T42.3X3	T42.3X4	T42.3X5	T42.3X6
Phenoperidine	T4Ø.4X1	T4Ø.4X2	T4Ø.4X3	T4Ø.4X4	—	—
Phenopyrazone	T46.991	T46.992	T46.993	T46.994	T46.995	T46.996
Phenoquin	T5Ø.4X1	T5Ø.4X2	T5Ø.4X3	T5Ø.4X4	T5Ø.4X5	T5Ø.4X6
Phenothiazine (psychotropic) **NEC**	T43.3X1	T43.3X2	T43.3X3	T43.3X4	T43.3X5	T43.3X6
insecticide	T6Ø.2X1	T6Ø.2X2	T6Ø.2X3	T6Ø.2X4	—	—
Phenothrin	T49.ØX1	T49.ØX2	T49.ØX3	T49.ØX4	T49.ØX5	T49.ØX6
Phenoxybenzamine	T46.7X1	T46.7X2	T46.7X3	T46.7X4	T46.7X5	T46.7X6
Phenoxyethanol	T49.ØX1	T49.ØX2	T49.ØX3	T49.ØX4	T49.ØX5	T49.ØX6
Phenoxymethyl penicillin	T36.ØX1	T36.ØX2	T36.ØX3	T36.ØX4	T36.ØX5	T36.ØX6
Phenprobamate	T42.8X1	T42.8X2	T42.8X3	T42.8X4	T42.8X5	T42.8X6
Phenprocoumon	T45.511	T45.512	T45.513	T45.514	T45.515	T45.516
Phensuximide	T42.2X1	T42.2X2	T42.2X3	T42.2X4	T42.2X5	T42.2X6
Phentermine	T5Ø.5X1	T5Ø.5X2	T5Ø.5X3	T5Ø.5X4	T5Ø.5X5	T5Ø.5X6
Phenthicillin	T36.ØX1	T36.ØX2	T36.ØX3	T36.ØX4	T36.ØX5	T36.ØX6
Phentolamine	T46.7X1	T46.7X2	T46.7X3	T46.7X4	T46.7X5	T46.7X6
Phenyl						
butazone	T39.2X1	T39.2X2	T39.2X3	T39.2X4	T39.2X5	T39.2X6
enediamine	T65.3X1	T65.3X2	T65.3X3	T65.3X4	—	—
hydrazine	T65.3X1	T65.3X2	T65.3X3	T65.3X4	—	—
antineoplastic	T45.1X1	T45.1X2	T45.1X3	T45.1X4	T45.1X5	T45.1X6
mercuric compounds — *see* Mercury						
salicylate	T49.3X1	T49.3X2	T49.3X3	T49.3X4	T49.3X5	T49.3X6
Phenylalanine mustard	T45.1X1	T45.1X2	T45.1X3	T45.1X4	T45.1X5	T45.1X6
Phenylbutazone	T39.2X1	T39.2X2	T39.2X3	T39.2X4	T39.2X5	T39.2X6
Phenylenediamine	T65.3X1	T65.3X2	T65.3X3	T65.3X4	—	—
Phenylephrine	T44.4X1	T44.4X2	T44.4X3	T44.4X4	T44.4X5	T44.4X6
Phenylethylbiguanide	T38.3X1	T38.3X2	T38.3X3	T38.3X4	T38.3X5	T38.3X6
Phenylmercuric						
acetate	T49.ØX1	T49.ØX2	T49.ØX3	T49.ØX4	T49.ØX5	T49.ØX6
borate	T49.ØX1	T49.ØX2	T49.ØX3	T49.ØX4	T49.ØX5	T49.ØX6
nitrate	T49.ØX1	T49.ØX2	T49.ØX3	T49.ØX4	T49.ØX5	T49.ØX6
Phenylmethylbarbitone	T42.3X1	T42.3X2	T42.3X3	T42.3X4	T42.3X5	T42.3X6
Phenylpropanol	T47.5X1	T47.5X2	T47.5X3	T47.5X4	T47.5X5	T47.5X6
Phenylpropanolamine	T44.991	T44.992	T44.993	T44.994	T44.995	T44.996
Phenylsulfthion	T6Ø.ØX1	T6Ø.ØX2	T6Ø.ØX3	T6Ø.ØX4	—	—
Phenyltoloxamine	T45.ØX1	T45.ØX2	T45.ØX3	T45.ØX4	T45.ØX5	T45.ØX6
Phenyramidol, phenyramidon	T39.8X1	T39.8X2	T39.8X3	T39.8X4	T39.8X5	T39.8X6
Phenytoin	T42.ØX1	T42.ØX2	T42.ØX3	T42.ØX4	T42.ØX5	T42.ØX6
with Phenobarbital	T42.3X1	T42.3X2	T42.3X3	T42.3X4	T42.3X5	T42.3X6
pHisoHex	T49.2X1	T49.2X2	T49.2X3	T49.2X4	T49.2X5	T49.2X6
Pholcodine	T48.3X1	T48.3X2	T48.3X3	T48.3X4	T48.3X5	T48.3X6
Pholedrine	T46.991	T46.992	T46.993	T46.994	T46.995	T46.996
Phorate	T6Ø.ØX1	T6Ø.ØX2	T6Ø.ØX3	T6Ø.ØX4	—	—
Phosdrin	T6Ø.ØX1	T6Ø.ØX2	T6Ø.ØX3	T6Ø.ØX4	—	—
Phosfolan	T6Ø.ØX1	T6Ø.ØX2	T6Ø.ØX3	T6Ø.ØX4	—	—
Phosgene (gas)	T59.891	T59.892	T59.893	T59.894	—	—
Phosphamidon	T6Ø.ØX1	T6Ø.ØX2	T6Ø.ØX3	T6Ø.ØX4	—	—
Phosphate	T65.891	T65.892	T65.893	T65.894	—	—
laxative	T47.4X1	T47.4X2	T47.4X3	T47.4X4	T47.4X5	T47.4X6
organic	T6Ø.ØX1	T6Ø.ØX2	T6Ø.ØX3	T6Ø.ØX4	—	—
solvent	T52.91	T52.92	T52.93	T52.94	—	—
tricresyl	T65.891	T65.892	T65.893	T65.894	—	—
Phosphine	T57.1X1	T57.1X2	T57.1X3	T57.1X4	—	—
fumigant	T57.1X1	T57.1X2	T57.1X3	T57.1X4	—	—
Phospholine	T49.5X1	T49.5X2	T49.5X3	T49.5X4	T49.5X5	T49.5X6
Phosphoric acid	T54.2X1	T54.2X2	T54.2X3	T54.2X4	—	—
Phosphorus (compound) **NEC**	T57.1X1	T57.1X2	T57.1X3	T57.1X4	—	—
pesticide	T6Ø.ØX1	T6Ø.ØX2	T6Ø.ØX3	T6Ø.ØX4	—	—
Phthalates	T65.891	T65.892	T65.893	T65.894	—	—
Phthalic anhydride	T65.891	T65.892	T65.893	T65.894	—	—
Phthalimidoglutarimide	T42.6X1	T42.6X2	T42.6X3	T42.6X4	T42.6X5	T42.6X6
Phthalylsulfathiazole	T37.ØX1	T37.ØX2	T37.ØX3	T37.ØX4	T37.ØX5	T37.ØX6
Phylloquinone	T45.7X1	T45.7X2	T45.7X3	T45.7X4	T45.7X5	T45.7X6
Physeptone	T4Ø.3X1	T4Ø.3X2	T4Ø.3X3	T4Ø.3X4	T4Ø.3X5	T4Ø.3X6
Physostigma venenosum	T62.2X1	T62.2X2	T62.2X3	T62.2X4	—	—
Physostigmine	T49.5X1	T49.5X2	T49.5X3	T49.5X4	T49.5X5	T49.5X6
Phytolacca decandra	T62.2X1	T62.2X2	T62.2X3	T62.2X4	—	—
Phytolacca decandra — *continued*						
berries	T62.1X1	T62.1X2	T62.1X3	T62.1X4	—	—
Phytomenadione	T45.7X1	T45.7X2	T45.7X3	T45.7X4	T45.7X5	T45.7X6
Phytonadione	T45.7X1	T45.7X2	T45.7X3	T45.7X4	T45.7X5	T45.7X6
Picoperine	T48.3X1	T48.3X2	T48.3X3	T48.3X4	T48.3X5	T48.3X6
Picosulfate (sodium)	T47.2X1	T47.2X2	T47.2X3	T47.2X4	T47.2X5	T47.2X6
Picric (acid)	T54.2X1	T54.2X2	T54.2X3	T54.2X4	—	—
Picrotoxin	T5Ø.7X1	T5Ø.7X2	T5Ø.7X3	T5Ø.7X4	T5Ø.7X5	T5Ø.7X6
Piketoprofen	T49.ØX1	T49.ØX2	T49.ØX3	T49.ØX4	T49.ØX5	T49.ØX6
Pilocarpine	T44.1X1	T44.1X2	T44.1X3	T44.1X4	T44.1X5	T44.1X6
Pilocarpus (jaborandi) extract	T44.1X1	T44.1X2	T44.1X3	T44.1X4	T44.1X5	T44.1X6
Pilsicainide (hydrochloride)	T46.2X1	T46.2X2	T46.2X3	T46.2X4	T46.2X5	T46.2X6
Pimaricin	T36.7X1	T36.7X2	T36.7X3	T36.7X4	T36.7X5	T36.7X6
Pimeclone	T5Ø.7X1	T5Ø.7X2	T5Ø.7X3	T5Ø.7X4	T5Ø.7X5	T5Ø.7X6
Pimelic ketone	T52.8X1	T52.8X2	T52.8X3	T52.8X4	—	—
Pimethixene	T45.ØX1	T45.ØX2	T45.ØX3	T45.ØX4	T45.ØX5	T45.ØX6
Piminodine	T4Ø.2X1	T4Ø.2X2	T4Ø.2X3	T4Ø.2X4	T4Ø.2X5	T4Ø.2X6
Pimozide	T43.591	T43.592	T43.593	T43.594	T43.595	T43.596
Pinacidil	T46.5X1	T46.5X2	T46.5X3	T46.5X4	T46.5X5	T46.5X6
Pinaverium bromide	T44.3X1	T44.3X2	T44.3X3	T44.3X4	T44.3X5	T44.3X6
Pinazepam	T42.4X1	T42.4X2	T42.4X3	T42.4X4	T42.4X5	T42.4X6
Pindolol	T44.7X1	T44.7X2	T44.7X3	T44.7X4	T44.7X5	T44.7X6
Pindone	T6Ø.4X1	T6Ø.4X2	T6Ø.4X3	T6Ø.4X4	—	—
Pine oil (disinfectant)	T65.891	T65.892	T65.893	T65.894	—	—
Pinkroot	T37.4X1	T37.4X2	T37.4X3	T37.4X4	T37.4X5	T37.4X6
Pipadone	T4Ø.2X1	T4Ø.2X2	T4Ø.2X3	T4Ø.2X4	—	—
Pipamazine	T45.ØX1	T45.ØX2	T45.ØX3	T45.ØX4	T45.ØX5	T45.ØX6
Pipamperone	T43.4X1	T43.4X2	T43.4X3	T43.4X4	T43.4X5	T43.4X6
Pipazetate	T48.3X1	T48.3X2	T48.3X3	T48.3X4	T48.3X5	T48.3X6
Pipemidic acid	T37.8X1	T37.8X2	T37.8X3	T37.8X4	T37.8X5	T37.8X6
Pipenzolate bromide	T44.3X1	T44.3X2	T44.3X3	T44.3X4	T44.3X5	T44.3X6
Piperacetazine	T43.3X1	T43.3X2	T43.3X3	T43.3X4	T43.3X5	T43.3X6
Piperacillin	T36.ØX1	T36.ØX2	T36.ØX3	T36.ØX4	T36.ØX5	T36.ØX6
Piperazine	T37.4X1	T37.4X2	T37.4X3	T37.4X4	T37.4X5	T37.4X6
estrone sulfate	T38.5X1	T38.5X2	T38.5X3	T38.5X4	T38.5X5	T38.5X6
Piper cubeba	T62.2X1	T62.2X2	T62.2X3	T62.2X4	—	—
Piperidione	T48.3X1	T48.3X2	T48.3X3	T48.3X4	T48.3X5	T48.3X6
Piperidolate	T44.3X1	T44.3X2	T44.3X3	T44.3X4	T44.3X5	T44.3X6
Piperocaine	T41.3X1	T41.3X2	T41.3X3	T41.3X4	T41.3X5	T41.3X6
infiltration (subcutaneous)	T41.3X1	T41.3X2	T41.3X3	T41.3X4	T41.3X5	T41.3X6
nerve block (peripheral) (plexus)	T41.3X1	T41.3X2	T41.3X3	T41.3X4	T41.3X5	T41.3X6
topical (surface)	T41.3X1	T41.3X2	T41.3X3	T41.3X4	T41.3X5	T41.3X6
Piperonyl butoxide	T6Ø.8X1	T6Ø.8X2	T6Ø.8X3	T6Ø.8X4	—	—
Pipethanate	T44.3X1	T44.3X2	T44.3X3	T44.3X4	T44.3X5	T44.3X6
Pipobroman	T45.1X1	T45.1X2	T45.1X3	T45.1X4	T45.1X5	T45.1X6
Pipotiazine	T43.3X1	T43.3X2	T43.3X3	T43.3X4	T43.3X5	T43.3X6
Pipoxizine	T45.ØX1	T45.ØX2	T45.ØX3	T45.ØX4	T45.ØX5	T45.ØX6
Pipradrol	T43.691	T43.692	T43.693	T43.694	T43.695	T43.696
Piprinhydrinate	T45.ØX1	T45.ØX2	T45.ØX3	T45.ØX4	T45.ØX5	T45.ØX6
Pirarubicin	T45.1X1	T45.1X2	T45.1X3	T45.1X4	T45.1X5	T45.1X6
Pirazinamide	T37.1X1	T37.1X2	T37.1X3	T37.1X4	T37.1X5	T37.1X6
Pirbuterol	T48.6X1	T48.6X2	T48.6X3	T48.6X4	T48.6X5	T48.6X6
Pirenzepine	T47.1X1	T47.1X2	T47.1X3	T47.1X4	T47.1X5	T47.1X6
Piretanide	T5Ø.1X1	T5Ø.1X2	T5Ø.1X3	T5Ø.1X4	T5Ø.1X5	T5Ø.1X6
Piribedil	T42.8X1	T42.8X2	T42.8X3	T42.8X4	T42.8X5	T42.8X6
Piridoxilate	T46.3X1	T46.3X2	T46.3X3	T46.3X4	T46.3X5	T46.3X6
Piritramide	T4Ø.4X1	T4Ø.4X2	T4Ø.4X3	T4Ø.4X4	—	—
Piromidic acid	T37.8X1	T37.8X2	T37.8X3	T37.8X4	T37.8X5	T37.8X6
Piroxicam	T39.391	T39.392	T39.393	T39.394	T39.395	T39.396
beta-cyclodextrin complex	T39.8X1	T39.8X2	T39.8X3	T39.8X4	T39.8X5	T39.8X6
Pirozadil	T46.6X1	T46.6X2	T46.6X3	T46.6X4	T46.6X5	T46.6X6
Piscidia (bark) (erythrina)	T39.8X1	T39.8X2	T39.8X3	T39.8X4	T39.8X5	T39.8X6
Pitch	T65.891	T65.892	T65.893	T65.894	—	—
Pitkin's solution	T41.3X1	T41.3X2	T41.3X3	T41.3X4	T41.3X5	T41.3X6
Pitocin	T48.ØX1	T48.ØX2	T48.ØX3	T48.ØX4	T48.ØX5	T48.ØX6
Pitressin (tannate)	T38.891	T38.892	T38.893	T38.894	T38.895	T38.896
Pituitary extracts (posterior)	T38.891	T38.892	T38.893	T38.894	T38.895	T38.896
anterior	T38.811	T38.812	T38.813	T38.814	T38.815	T38.816
Pituitrin	T38.891	T38.892	T38.893	T38.894	T38.895	T38.896
Pivampicillin	T36.ØX1	T36.ØX2	T36.ØX3	T36.ØX4	T36.ØX5	T36.ØX6
Pivmecillinam	T36.ØX1	T36.ØX2	T36.ØX3	T36.ØX4	T36.ØX5	T36.ØX6
Placental hormone	T38.891	T38.892	T38.893	T38.894	T38.895	T38.896
Placidyl	T42.6X1	T42.6X2	T42.6X3	T42.6X4	T42.6X5	T42.6X6
Plague vaccine	T5Ø.A91	T5Ø.A92	T5Ø.A93	T5Ø.A94	T5Ø.A95	T5Ø.A96
Plant						
food or fertilizer NEC	T65.891	T65.892	T65.893	T65.894	—	—
containing herbicide	T6Ø.3X1	T6Ø.3X2	T6Ø.3X3	T6Ø.3X4	—	—
noxious, used as food	T62.2X1	T62.2X2	T62.2X3	T62.2X4	—	—
berries	T62.1X1	T62.1X2	T62.1X3	T62.1X4	—	—
seeds	T62.2X1	T62.2X2	T62.2X3	T62.2X4	—	—

Substance	Poisoning, Accidental (unintentional)	Poisoning, Intentional Self-harm	Poisoning, Assault	Poisoning, Undetermined	Adverse Effect	Under-dosing
Plant — *continued*						
noxious, used as food — *continued*						
specified type NEC	T62.2X1	T62.2X2	T62.2X3	T62.2X4	—	—
Plasma	T45.8X1	T45.8X2	T45.8X3	T45.8X4	T45.8X5	T45.8X6
expander NEC	T45.8X1	T45.8X2	T45.8X3	T45.8X4	T45.8X5	T45.8X6
protein fraction (human)	T45.8X1	T45.8X2	T45.8X3	T45.8X4	T45.8X5	T45.8X6
Plasmanate	T45.8X1	T45.8X2	T45.8X3	T45.8X4	T45.8X5	T45.8X6
Plasminogen (tissue) activator	T45.611	T45.612	T45.613	T45.614	T45.615	T45.616
Plaster dressing	T49.3X1	T49.3X2	T49.3X3	T49.3X4	T49.3X5	T49.3X6
Plastic dressing	T49.3X1	T49.3X2	T49.3X3	T49.3X4	T49.3X5	T49.3X6
Plegicil	T43.3X1	T43.3X2	T43.3X3	T43.3X4	T43.3X5	T43.3X6
Plicamycin	T45.1X1	T45.1X2	T45.1X3	T45.1X4	T45.1X5	T45.1X6
Podophyllotoxin	T49.8X1	T49.8X2	T49.8X3	T49.8X4	T49.8X5	T49.8X6
Podophyllum (resin)	T49.4X1	T49.4X2	T49.4X3	T49.4X4	T49.4X5	T49.4X6
Poisonous berries	T62.1X1	T62.1X2	T62.1X3	T62.1X4	—	—
Poison NEC	T65.91	T65.92	T65.93	T65.94	—	—
Pokeweed (any part)	T62.2X1	T62.2X2	T62.2X3	T62.2X4	—	—
Poldine metilsulfate	T44.3X1	T44.3X2	T44.3X3	T44.3X4	T44.3X5	T44.3X6
Polidexide (sulfate)	T46.6X1	T46.6X2	T46.6X3	T46.6X4	T46.6X5	T46.6X6
Polidocanol	T46.8X1	T46.8X2	T46.8X3	T46.8X4	T46.8X5	T46.8X6
Poliomyelitis vaccine	T5Ø.B91	T5Ø.B92	T5Ø.B93	T5Ø.B94	T5Ø.B95	T5Ø.B96
Polish (car) (floor) (furni-ture) (metal) (porcelain) (silver)	T65.891	T65.892	T65.893	T65.894	—	—
abrasive	T65.891	T65.892	T65.893	T65.894	—	—
porcelain	T65.891	T65.892	T65.893	T65.894	—	—
Poloxalkol	T47.4X1	T47.4X2	T47.4X3	T47.4X4	T47.4X5	T47.4X6
Poloxamer	T47.4X1	T47.4X2	T47.4X3	T47.4X4	T47.4X5	T47.4X6
Polyaminostyrene resins	T5Ø.3X1	T5Ø.3X2	T5Ø.3X3	T5Ø.3X4	T5Ø.3X5	T5Ø.3X6
Polycarbophil	T47.4X1	T47.4X2	T47.4X3	T47.4X4	T47.4X5	T47.4X6
Polychlorinated biphenyl	T65.891	T65.892	T65.893	T65.894	—	—
Polycycline	T36.4X1	T36.4X2	T36.4X3	T36.4X4	T36.4X5	T36.4X6
Polyester fumes	T59.891	T59.892	T59.893	T59.894	—	—
Polyester resin hardener	T52.91	T52.92	T52.93	T52.94	—	—
fumes	T59.891	T59.892	T59.893	T59.894	—	—
Polyestradiol phosphate	T38.5X1	T38.5X2	T38.5X3	T38.5X4	T38.5X5	T38.5X6
Polyethanolamine alkyl sulfate	T49.2X1	T49.2X2	T49.2X3	T49.2X4	T49.2X5	T49.2X6
Polyethylene adhesive	T49.3X1	T49.3X2	T49.3X3	T49.3X4	T49.3X5	T49.3X6
Polyferose	T45.4X1	T45.4X2	T45.4X3	T45.4X4	T45.4X5	T45.4X6
Polygeline	T45.8X1	T45.8X2	T45.8X3	T45.8X4	T45.8X5	T45.8X6
Polymyxin	T36.8X1	T36.8X2	T36.8X3	T36.8X4	T36.8X5	T36.8X6
B	T36.8X1	T36.8X2	T36.8X3	T36.8X4	T36.8X5	T36.8X6
ENT agent	T49.6X1	T49.6X2	T49.6X3	T49.6X4	T49.6X5	T49.6X6
ophthalmic preparation	T49.5X1	T49.5X2	T49.5X3	T49.5X4	T49.5X5	T49.5X6
topical NEC	T49.ØX1	T49.ØX2	T49.ØX3	T49.ØX4	T49.ØX5	T49.ØX6
E sulfate (eye preparation)	T49.5X1	T49.5X2	T49.5X3	T49.5X4	T49.5X5	T49.5X6
Polynoxylin	T49.ØX1	T49.ØX2	T49.ØX3	T49.ØX4	T49.ØX5	T49.ØX6
Polyoestradiol phosphate	T38.5X1	T38.5X2	T38.5X3	T38.5X4	T38.5X5	T38.5X6
Polyoxymethyleneurea	T49.ØX1	T49.ØX2	T49.ØX3	T49.ØX4	T49.ØX5	T49.ØX6
Polysilane	T47.8X1	T47.8X2	T47.8X3	T47.8X4	T47.8X5	T47.8X6
Polytetrafluoroethylene (inhaled)	T59.891	T59.892	T59.893	T59.894	—	—
Polythiazide	T5Ø.2X1	T5Ø.2X2	T5Ø.2X3	T5Ø.2X4	T5Ø.2X5	T5Ø.2X6
Polyvidone	T45.8X1	T45.8X2	T45.8X3	T45.8X4	T45.8X5	T45.8X6
Polyvinylpyrrolidone	T45.8X1	T45.8X2	T45.8X3	T45.8X4	T45.8X5	T45.8X6
Pontocaine (hydrochloride) (infiltration) (topical)	T41.3X1	T41.3X2	T41.3X3	T41.3X4	T41.3X5	T41.3X6
nerve block (peripheral) (plexus)	T41.3X1	T41.3X2	T41.3X3	T41.3X4	T41.3X5	T41.3X6
spinal	T41.3X1	T41.3X2	T41.3X3	T41.3X4	T41.3X5	T41.3X6
Porfiromycin	T45.1X1	T45.1X2	T45.1X3	T45.1X4	T45.1X5	T45.1X6
Posterior pituitary hormone NEC	T38.891	T38.892	T38.893	T38.894	T38.895	T38.896
Pot	T4Ø.7X1	T4Ø.7X2	T4Ø.7X3	T4Ø.7X4	T4Ø.7X5	T4Ø.7X6
Potash (caustic)	T54.3X1	T54.3X2	T54.3X3	T54.3X4	—	—
Potassic saline injection (lactated)	T5Ø.3X1	T5Ø.3X2	T5Ø.3X3	T5Ø.3X4	T5Ø.3X5	T5Ø.3X6
Potassium-removing resin	T5Ø.3X1	T5Ø.3X2	T5Ø.3X3	T5Ø.3X4	T5Ø.3X5	T5Ø.3X6
Potassium-retaining drug	T5Ø.3X1	T5Ø.3X2	T5Ø.3X3	T5Ø.3X4	T5Ø.3X5	T5Ø.3X6
Potassium (salts) **NEC**	T5Ø.3X1	T5Ø.3X2	T5Ø.3X3	T5Ø.3X4	T5Ø.3X5	T5Ø.3X6
aminobenzoate	T45.8X1	T45.8X2	T45.8X3	T45.8X4	T45.8X5	T45.8X6
aminosalicylate	T37.1X1	T37.1X2	T37.1X3	T37.1X4	T37.1X5	T37.1X6
antimony ' tartrate'	T37.8X1	T37.8X2	T37.8X3	T37.8X4	T37.8X5	T37.8X6
arsenite (solution)	T57.ØX1	T57.ØX2	T57.ØX3	T57.ØX4	—	—
bichromate	T56.2X1	T56.2X2	T56.2X3	T56.2X4	—	—
bisulfate	T47.3X1	T47.3X2	T47.3X3	T47.3X4	T47.3X5	T47.3X6
bromide	T42.6X1	T42.6X2	T42.6X3	T42.6X4	T42.6X5	T42.6X6
canrenoate	T5Ø.ØX1	T5Ø.ØX2	T5Ø.ØX3	T5Ø.ØX4	T5Ø.ØX5	T5Ø.ØX6
carbonate	T54.3X1	T54.3X2	T54.3X3	T54.3X4	—	—
chlorate NEC	T65.891	T65.892	T65.893	T65.894	—	—
chloride	T5Ø.3X1	T5Ø.3X2	T5Ø.3X3	T5Ø.3X4	T5Ø.3X5	T5Ø.3X6

Substance	Poisoning, Accidental (unintentional)	Poisoning, Intentional Self-harm	Poisoning, Assault	Poisoning, Undetermined	Adverse Effect	Under-dosing
Potassium (salts) **NEC** — *continued*						
citrate	T5Ø.991	T5Ø.992	T5Ø.993	T5Ø.994	T5Ø.995	T5Ø.996
cyanide	T65.ØX1	T65.ØX2	T65.ØX3	T65.ØX4	—	—
ferric hexacyanoferrate (medicinal)	T5Ø.6X1	T5Ø.6X2	T5Ø.6X3	T5Ø.6X4	T5Ø.6X5	T5Ø.6X6
nonmedicinal	T65.891	T65.892	T65.893	T65.894	—	—
Fluoride	T57.8X1	T57.8X2	T57.8X3	T57.8X4	—	—
glucaldrate	T47.1X1	T47.1X2	T47.1X3	T47.1X4	T47.1X5	T47.1X6
hydroxide	T54.3X1	T54.3X2	T54.3X3	T54.3X4	—	—
iodate	T49.ØX1	T49.ØX2	T49.ØX3	T49.ØX4	T49.ØX5	T49.ØX6
iodide	T48.4X1	T48.4X2	T48.4X3	T48.4X4	T48.4X5	T48.4X6
nitrate	T57.8X1	T57.8X2	T57.8X3	T57.8X4	—	—
oxalate	T65.891	T65.892	T65.893	T65.894	—	—
perchlorate (nonmedicinal) NEC	T65.891	T65.892	T65.893	T65.894	—	—
antithyroid	T38.2X1	T38.2X2	T38.2X3	T38.2X4	T38.2X5	T38.2X6
medicinal	T38.2X1	T38.2X2	T38.2X3	T38.2X4	T38.2X5	T38.2X6
Permanganate (nonmedicinal)	T65.891	T65.892	T65.893	T65.894	—	—
medicinal	T49.ØX1	T49.ØX2	T49.ØX3	T49.ØX4	T49.ØX5	T49.ØX6
sulfate	T47.2X1	T47.2X2	T47.2X3	T47.2X4	T47.2X5	T47.2X6
Povidone	T45.8X1	T45.8X2	T45.8X3	T45.8X4	T45.8X5	T45.8X6
iodine	T49.ØX1	T49.ØX2	T49.ØX3	T49.ØX4	T49.ØX5	T49.ØX6
Practolol	T44.7X1	T44.7X2	T44.7X3	T44.7X4	T44.7X5	T44.7X6
Prajmalium bitartrate	T46.2X1	T46.2X2	T46.2X3	T46.2X4	T46.2X5	T46.2X6
Pralidoxime (iodide)	T5Ø.6X1	T5Ø.6X2	T5Ø.6X3	T5Ø.6X4	T5Ø.6X5	T5Ø.6X6
chloride	T5Ø.6X1	T5Ø.6X2	T5Ø.6X3	T5Ø.6X4	T5Ø.6X5	T5Ø.6X6
Pramiverine	T44.3X1	T44.3X2	T44.3X3	T44.3X4	T44.3X5	T44.3X6
Pramocaine	T49.1X1	T49.1X2	T49.1X3	T49.1X4	T49.1X5	T49.1X6
Pramoxine	T49.1X1	T49.1X2	T49.1X3	T49.1X4	T49.1X5	T49.1X6
Prasterone	T38.7X1	T38.7X2	T38.7X3	T38.7X4	T38.7X5	T38.7X6
Pravastatin	T46.6X1	T46.6X2	T46.6X3	T46.6X4	T46.6X5	T46.6X6
Prazepam	T42.4X1	T42.4X2	T42.4X3	T42.4X4	T42.4X5	T42.4X6
Praziquantel	T37.4X1	T37.4X2	T37.4X3	T37.4X4	T37.4X5	T37.4X6
Prazitone	T43.291	T43.292	T43.293	T43.294	T43.295	T43.296
Prazosin	T44.6X1	T44.6X2	T44.6X3	T44.6X4	T44.6X5	T44.6X6
Prednicarbate	T49.ØX1	T49.ØX2	T49.ØX3	T49.ØX4	T49.ØX5	T49.ØX6
Prednimustine	T45.1X1	T45.1X2	T45.1X3	T45.1X4	T45.1X5	T45.1X6
Prednisolone	T38.ØX1	T38.ØX2	T38.ØX3	T38.ØX4	T38.ØX5	T38.ØX6
ENT agent	T49.6X1	T49.6X2	T49.6X3	T49.6X4	T49.6X5	T49.6X6
ophthalmic preparation	T49.5X1	T49.5X2	T49.5X3	T49.5X4	T49.5X5	T49.5X6
steaglate	T49.ØX1	T49.ØX2	T49.ØX3	T49.ØX4	T49.ØX5	T49.ØX6
topical NEC	T49.ØX1	T49.ØX2	T49.ØX3	T49.ØX4	T49.ØX5	T49.ØX6
Prednisone	T38.ØX1	T38.ØX2	T38.ØX3	T38.ØX4	T38.ØX5	T38.ØX6
Prednylidene	T38.ØX1	T38.ØX2	T38.ØX3	T38.ØX4	T38.ØX5	T38.ØX6
Pregnandiol	T38.5X1	T38.5X2	T38.5X3	T38.5X4	T38.5X5	T38.5X6
Pregneninolone	T38.5X1	T38.5X2	T38.5X3	T38.5X4	T38.5X5	T38.5X6
Preludin	T43.691	T43.692	T43.693	T43.694	T43.695	T43.696
Premarin	T38.5X1	T38.5X2	T38.5X3	T38.5X4	T38.5X5	T38.5X6
Premedication anesthetic	T41.2Ø1	T41.2Ø2	T41.2Ø3	T41.2Ø4	T41.2Ø5	T41.2Ø6
Prenalterol	T44.5X1	T44.5X2	T44.5X3	T44.5X4	T44.5X5	T44.5X6
Prenoxdiazine	T48.3X1	T48.3X2	T48.3X3	T48.3X4	T48.3X5	T48.3X6
Prenylamine	T46.3X1	T46.3X2	T46.3X3	T46.3X4	T46.3X5	T46.3X6
Preparation H	T49.8X1	T49.8X2	T49.8X3	T49.8X4	T49.8X5	T49.8X6
Preparation, local	T49.4X1	T49.4X2	T49.4X3	T49.4X4	T49.4X5	T49.4X6
Preservative (nonmedicinal)	T65.891	T65.892	T65.893	T65.894	—	—
medicinal	T5Ø.9Ø1	T5Ø.9Ø2	T5Ø.9Ø3	T5Ø.9Ø4	T5Ø.9Ø5	T5Ø.9Ø6
wood	T6Ø.91	T6Ø.92	T6Ø.93	T6Ø.94	—	—
Prethcamide	T5Ø.7X1	T5Ø.7X2	T5Ø.7X3	T5Ø.7X4	T5Ø.7X5	T5Ø.7X6
Pride of China	T62.2X1	T62.2X2	T62.2X3	T62.2X4	—	—
Pridinol	T44.3X1	T44.3X2	T44.3X3	T44.3X4	T44.3X5	T44.3X6
Prifinium bromide	T44.3X1	T44.3X2	T44.3X3	T44.3X4	T44.3X5	T44.3X6
Prilocaine	T41.3X1	T41.3X2	T41.3X3	T41.3X4	T41.3X5	T41.3X6
infiltration (subcutaneous)	T41.3X1	T41.3X2	T41.3X3	T41.3X4	T41.3X5	T41.3X6
nerve block (peripheral) (plexus)	T41.3X1	T41.3X2	T41.3X3	T41.3X4	T41.3X5	T41.3X6
regional	T41.3X1	T41.3X2	T41.3X3	T41.3X4	T41.3X5	T41.3X6
Primaquine	T37.2X1	T37.2X2	T37.2X3	T37.2X4	T37.2X5	T37.2X6
Primidone	T42.6X1	T42.6X2	T42.6X3	T42.6X4	T42.6X5	T42.6X6
Primula (veris)	T62.2X1	T62.2X2	T62.2X3	T62.2X4	—	—
Prinadol	T4Ø.2X1	T4Ø.2X2	T4Ø.2X3	T4Ø.2X4	T4Ø.2X5	T4Ø.2X6
Priscol, Priscoline	T44.6X1	T44.6X2	T44.6X3	T44.6X4	T44.6X5	T44.6X6
Pristinamycin	T36.3X1	T36.3X2	T36.3X3	T36.3X4	T36.3X5	T36.3X6
Privet	T62.2X1	T62.2X2	T62.2X3	T62.2X4	—	—
berries	T62.1X1	T62.1X2	T62.1X3	T62.1X4	—	—
Privine	T44.4X1	T44.4X2	T44.4X3	T44.4X4	T44.4X5	T44.4X6
Pro-Banthine	T44.3X1	T44.3X2	T44.3X3	T44.3X4	T44.3X5	T44.3X6
Probarbital	T42.3X1	T42.3X2	T42.3X3	T42.3X4	T42.3X5	T42.3X6
Probenecid	T5Ø.4X1	T5Ø.4X2	T5Ø.4X3	T5Ø.4X4	T5Ø.4X5	T5Ø.4X6
Probucol	T46.6X1	T46.6X2	T46.6X3	T46.6X4	T46.6X5	T46.6X6
Procainamide	T46.2X1	T46.2X2	T46.2X3	T46.2X4	T46.2X5	T46.2X6
Procaine	T41.3X1	T41.3X2	T41.3X3	T41.3X4	T41.3X5	T41.3X6

Substance	Poisoning, Accidental (unintentional)	Poisoning, Intentional Self-harm	Poisoning, Assault	Poisoning, Undetermined	Adverse Effect	Under-dosing
Procaine — *continued*						
benzylpenicillin	T36.ØX1	T36.ØX2	T36.ØX3	T36.ØX4	T36.ØX5	T36.ØX6
nerve block (periphreal) (plexus)	T41.3X1	T41.3X2	T41.3X3	T41.3X4	T41.3X5	T41.3X6
penicillin G	T36.ØX1	T36.ØX2	T36.ØX3	T36.ØX4	T36.ØX5	T36.ØX6
regional	T41.3X1	T41.3X2	T41.3X3	T41.3X4	T41.3X5	T41.3X6
spinal	T41.3X1	T41.3X2	T41.3X3	T41.3X4	T41.3X5	T41.3X6
Procalmidol	T43.591	T43.592	T43.593	T43.594	T43.595	T43.596
Procarbazine	T45.1X1	T45.1X2	T45.1X3	T45.1X4	T45.1X5	T45.1X6
Procaterol	T44.5X1	T44.5X2	T44.5X3	T44.5X4	T44.5X5	T44.5X6
Prochlorperazine	T43.3X1	T43.3X2	T43.3X3	T43.3X4	T43.3X5	T43.3X6
Procyclidine	T44.3X1	T44.3X2	T44.3X3	T44.3X4	T44.3X5	T44.3X6
Producer gas	T58.8X1	T58.8X2	T58.8X3	T58.8X4	—	—
Profadol	T4Ø.4X1	T4Ø.4X2	T4Ø.4X3	T4Ø.4X4	T4Ø.4X5	T4Ø.4X6
Profenamine	T44.3X1	T44.3X2	T44.3X3	T44.3X4	T44.3X5	T44.3X6
Profenil	T44.3X1	T44.3X2	T44.3X3	T44.3X4	T44.3X5	T44.3X6
Proflavine	T49.ØX1	T49.ØX2	T49.ØX3	T49.ØX4	T49.ØX5	T49.ØX6
Progabide	T42.6X1	T42.6X2	T42.6X3	T42.6X4	T42.6X5	T42.6X6
Progesterone	T38.5X1	T38.5X2	T38.5X3	T38.5X4	T38.5X5	T38.5X6
Progestin	T38.5X1	T38.5X2	T38.5X3	T38.5X4	T38.5X5	T38.5X6
oral contraceptive	T38.4X1	T38.4X2	T38.4X3	T38.4X4	T38.4X5	T38.4X6
Progestogen NEC	T38.5X1	T38.5X2	T38.5X3	T38.5X4	T38.5X5	T38.5X6
Progestone	T38.5X1	T38.5X2	T38.5X3	T38.5X4	T38.5X5	T38.5X6
Proglumide	T47.1X1	T47.1X2	T47.1X3	T47.1X4	T47.1X5	T47.1X6
Proguanil	T37.2X1	T37.2X2	T37.2X3	T37.2X4	T37.2X5	T37.2X6
Prolactin	T38.811	T38.812	T38.813	T38.814	T38.815	T38.816
Prolintane	T43.691	T43.692	T43.693	T43.694	T43.695	T43.696
Proloid	T38.1X1	T38.1X2	T38.1X3	T38.1X4	T38.1X5	T38.1X6
Proluton	T38.5X1	T38.5X2	T38.5X3	T38.5X4	T38.5X5	T38.5X6
Promacetin	T37.1X1	T37.1X2	T37.1X3	T37.1X4	T37.1X5	T37.1X6
Promazine	T43.3X1	T43.3X2	T43.3X3	T43.3X4	T43.3X5	T43.3X6
Promedol	T4Ø.2X1	T4Ø.2X2	T4Ø.2X3	T4Ø.2X4	—	—
Promegestone	T38.5X1	T38.5X2	T38.5X3	T38.5X4	T38.5X5	T38.5X6
Promethazine (teoclate)	T43.3X1	T43.3X2	T43.3X3	T43.3X4	T43.3X5	T43.3X6
Promin	T37.1X1	T37.1X2	T37.1X3	T37.1X4	T37.1X5	T37.1X6
Pronase	T45.3X1	T45.3X2	T45.3X3	T45.3X4	T45.3X5	T45.3X6
Pronestyl (hydrochloride)	T46.2X1	T46.2X2	T46.2X3	T46.2X4	T46.2X5	T46.2X6
Pronetalol	T44.7X1	T44.7X2	T44.7X3	T44.7X4	T44.7X5	T44.7X6
Prontosil	T37.ØX1	T37.ØX2	T37.ØX3	T37.ØX4	T37.ØX5	T37.ØX6
Propachlor	T6Ø.3X1	T6Ø.3X2	T6Ø.3X3	T6Ø.3X4	—	—
Propafenone	T46.2X1	T46.2X2	T46.2X3	T46.2X4	T46.2X5	T46.2X6
Propallylonal	T42.3X1	T42.3X2	T42.3X3	T42.3X4	T42.3X5	T42.3X6
Propamidine	T49.ØX1	T49.ØX2	T49.ØX3	T49.ØX4	T49.ØX5	T49.ØX6
Propane (distributed in mobile container)	T59.891	T59.892	T59.893	T59.894	—	—
distributed through pipes	T59.891	T59.892	T59.893	T59.894	—	—
incomplete combustion	T58.11	T58.12	T58.13	T58.14	—	—
Propanidid	T41.291	T41.292	T41.293	T41.294	T41.295	T41.296
Propanil	T6Ø.3X1	T6Ø.3X2	T6Ø.3X3	T6Ø.3X4	—	—
Propantheline	T44.3X1	T44.3X2	T44.3X3	T44.3X4	T44.3X5	T44.3X6
bromide	T44.3X1	T44.3X2	T44.3X3	T44.3X4	T44.3X5	T44.3X6
Proparacaine	T41.3X1	T41.3X2	T41.3X3	T41.3X4	T41.3X5	T41.3X6
Propatylnitrate	T46.3X1	T46.3X2	T46.3X3	T46.3X4	T46.3X5	T46.3X6
Propicillin	T36.ØX1	T36.ØX2	T36.ØX3	T36.ØX4	T36.ØX5	T36.ØX6
Propiolactone	T49.ØX1	T49.ØX2	T49.ØX3	T49.ØX4	T49.ØX5	T49.ØX6
Propiomazine	T45.ØX1	T45.ØX2	T45.ØX3	T45.ØX4	T45.ØX5	T45.ØX6
Propionaidehyde (medicinal)	T42.6X1	T42.6X2	T42.6X3	T42.6X4	T42.6X5	T42.6X6
Propionate (calcium) (sodium)	T49.ØX1	T49.ØX2	T49.ØX3	T49.ØX4	T49.ØX5	T49.ØX6
Propion gel	T49.ØX1	T49.ØX2	T49.ØX3	T49.ØX4	T49.ØX5	T49.ØX6
Propitocaine	T41.3X1	T41.3X2	T41.3X3	T41.3X4	T41.3X5	T41.3X6
infiltration (subcutaneous)	T41.3X1	T41.3X2	T41.3X3	T41.3X4	T41.3X5	T41.3X6
nerve block (peripheral) (plexus)	T41.3X1	T41.3X2	T41.3X3	T41.3X4	T41.3X5	T41.3X6
Propofol	T41.291	T41.292	T41.293	T41.294	T41.295	T41.296
Propoxur	T6Ø.ØX1	T6Ø.ØX2	T6Ø.ØX3	T6Ø.ØX4	—	—
Propoxycaine	T41.3X1	T41.3X2	T41.3X3	T41.3X4	T41.3X5	T41.3X6
infiltration (subcutaneous)	T41.3X1	T41.3X2	T41.3X3	T41.3X4	T41.3X5	T41.3X6
nerve block (peripheral) (plexus)	T41.3X1	T41.3X2	T41.3X3	T41.3X4	T41.3X5	T41.3X6
topical (surface)	T41.3X1	T41.3X2	T41.3X3	T41.3X4	T41.3X5	T41.3X6
Propoxyphene	T4Ø.4X1	T4Ø.4X2	T4Ø.4X3	T4Ø.4X4	T4Ø.4X5	T4Ø.4X6
Propranolol	T44.7X1	T44.7X2	T44.7X3	T44.7X4	T44.7X5	T44.7X6
Propyl						
alcohol	T51.3X1	T51.3X2	T51.3X3	T51.3X4	—	—
carbinol	T51.3X1	T51.3X2	T51.3X3	T51.3X4	—	—
hexadrine	T44.4X1	T44.4X2	T44.4X3	T44.4X4	T44.4X5	T44.4X6
iodone	T5Ø.8X1	T5Ø.8X2	T5Ø.8X3	T5Ø.8X4	T5Ø.8X5	T5Ø.8X6
thiouracil	T38.2X1	T38.2X2	T38.2X3	T38.2X4	T38.2X5	T38.2X6
Propylaminophenothiazine	T43.3X1	T43.3X2	T43.3X3	T43.3X4	T43.3X5	T43.3X6
Propylene	T59.891	T59.892	T59.893	T59.894	—	—
Propylhexedrine	T48.5X1	T48.5X2	T48.5X3	T48.5X4	T48.5X5	T48.5X6

Substance	Poisoning, Accidental (unintentional)	Poisoning, Intentional Self-harm	Poisoning, Assault	Poisoning, Undetermined	Adverse Effect	Under-dosing
Propyliodone	T5Ø.8X1	T5Ø.8X2	T5Ø.8X3	T5Ø.8X4	T5Ø.8X5	T5Ø.8X6
Propylparaben (ophthalmic)	T49.5X1	T49.5X2	T49.5X3	T49.5X4	T49.5X5	T49.5X6
Propylthiouracil	T38.2X1	T38.2X2	T38.2X3	T38.2X4	T38.2X5	T38.2X6
Propyphenazone	T39.2X1	T39.2X2	T39.2X3	T39.2X4	T39.2X5	T39.2X6
Proquazone	T39.391	T39.392	T39.393	T39.394	T39.395	T39.396
Proscillaridin	T46.ØX1	T46.ØX2	T46.ØX3	T46.ØX4	T46.ØX5	T46.ØX6
Prostacyclin	T45.521	T45.522	T45.523	T45.524	T45.525	T45.526
Prostaglandin (I2)	T45.521	T45.522	T45.523	T45.524	T45.525	T45.526
E1	T46.7X1	T46.7X2	T46.7X3	T46.7X4	T46.7X5	T46.7X6
E2	T48.ØX1	T48.ØX2	T48.ØX3	T48.ØX4	T48.ØX5	T48.ØX6
F2 alpha	T48.ØX1	T48.ØX2	T48.ØX3	T48.ØX4	T48.ØX5	T48.ØX6
Prostigmin	T44.ØX1	T44.ØX2	T44.ØX3	T44.ØX4	T44.ØX5	T44.ØX6
Prosultiamine	T45.2X1	T45.2X2	T45.2X3	T45.2X4	T45.2X5	T45.2X6
Protamine sulfate	T45.7X1	T45.7X2	T45.7X3	T45.7X4	T45.7X5	T45.7X6
zinc insulin	T38.3X1	T38.3X2	T38.3X3	T38.3X4	T38.3X5	T38.3X6
Protease	T47.5X1	T47.5X2	T47.5X3	T47.5X4	T47.5X5	T47.5X6
Protectant, skin NEC	T49.3X1	T49.3X2	T49.3X3	T49.3X4	T49.3X5	T49.3X6
Protein hydrolysate	T5Ø.991	T5Ø.992	T5Ø.993	T5Ø.994	T5Ø.995	T5Ø.996
Prothiaden — *see* Dothiepin hydrochloride						
Prothionamide	T37.1X1	T37.1X2	T37.1X3	T37.1X4	T37.1X5	T37.1X6
Prothipendyl	T43.591	T43.592	T43.593	T43.594	T43.595	T43.596
Prothoate	T6Ø.ØX1	T6Ø.ØX2	T6Ø.ØX3	T6Ø.ØX4	—	—
Prothrombin						
activator	T45.7X1	T45.7X2	T45.7X3	T45.7X4	T45.7X5	T45.7X6
synthesis inhibitor	T45.511	T45.512	T45.513	T45.514	T45.515	T45.516
Protionamide	T37.1X1	T37.1X2	T37.1X3	T37.1X4	T37.1X5	T37.1X6
Protirelin	T38.891	T38.892	T38.893	T38.894	T38.895	T38.896
Protokylol	T48.6X1	T48.6X2	T48.6X3	T48.6X4	T48.6X5	T48.6X6
Protopam	T5Ø.6X1	T5Ø.6X2	T5Ø.6X3	T5Ø.6X4	T5Ø.6X5	T5Ø.6X6
Protoveratrine(s) (A) (B)	T46.5X1	T46.5X2	T46.5X3	T46.5X4	T46.5X5	T46.5X6
Protriptyline	T43.Ø11	T43.Ø12	T43.Ø13	T43.Ø14	T43.Ø15	T43.Ø16
Provera	T38.5X1	T38.5X2	T38.5X3	T38.5X4	T38.5X5	T38.5X6
Provitamin A	T45.2X1	T45.2X2	T45.2X3	T45.2X4	T45.2X5	T45.2X6
Proxibarbal	T42.3X1	T42.3X2	T42.3X3	T42.3X4	T42.3X5	T42.3X6
Proxymetacaine	T41.3X1	T41.3X2	T41.3X3	T41.3X4	T41.3X5	T41.3X6
Proxyphylline	T48.6X1	T48.6X2	T48.6X3	T48.6X4	T48.6X5	T48.6X6
Prozac — *see* Fluoxetine hydrochloride						
Prunus						
laurocerasus	T62.2X1	T62.2X2	T62.2X3	T62.2X4	—	—
virginiana	T62.2X1	T62.2X2	T62.2X3	T62.2X4	—	—
Prussian blue						
commercial	T65.891	T65.892	T65.893	T65.894	—	—
therapeutic	T5Ø.6X1	T5Ø.6X2	T5Ø.6X3	T5Ø.6X4	T5Ø.6X5	T5Ø.6X6
Prussic acid	T65.ØX1	T65.ØX2	T65.ØX3	T65.ØX4	—	—
vapor	T57.3X1	T57.3X2	T57.3X3	T57.3X4	—	—
Pseudoephedrine	T44.991	T44.992	T44.993	T44.994	T44.995	T44.996
Psilocin	T4Ø.991	T4Ø.992	T4Ø.993	T4Ø.994	—	—
Psilocybin	T4Ø.991	T4Ø.992	T4Ø.993	T4Ø.994	—	—
Psilocybine	T4Ø.991	T4Ø.992	T4Ø.993	T4Ø.994	—	—
Psoralene (nonmedicinal)	T65.891	T65.892	T65.893	T65.894	—	—
Psoralens (medicinal)	T5Ø.991	T5Ø.992	T5Ø.993	T5Ø.994	T5Ø.995	T5Ø.996
PSP (phenolsulfonphthalein)	T5Ø.8X1	T5Ø.8X2	T5Ø.8X3	T5Ø.8X4	T5Ø.8X5	T5Ø.8X6
Psychodysleptic drug NEC	T4Ø.9Ø1	T4Ø.9Ø2	T4Ø.9Ø3	T4Ø.9Ø4	T4Ø.9Ø5	T4Ø.9Ø6
Psychostimulant	T43.6Ø1	T43.6Ø2	T43.6Ø3	T43.6Ø4	T43.6Ø5	T43.6Ø6
amphetamine	T43.621	T43.622	T43.623	T43.624	T43.625	T43.626
caffeine	T43.611	T43.612	T43.613	T43.614	T43.615	T43.616
methylphenidate	T43.631	T43.632	T43.633	T43.634	T43.635	T43.636
specified NEC	T43.691	T43.692	T43.693	T43.694	T43.695	T43.696
Psychotherapeutic drug NEC	T43.91	T43.92	T43.93	T43.94	T43.95	T43.96
antidepressants — *see also* Antidepressant	T43.2Ø1	T43.2Ø2	T43.2Ø3	T43.2Ø4	T43.2Ø5	T43.2Ø6
specified NEC	T43.8X1	T43.8X2	T43.8X3	T43.8X4	T43.8X5	T43.8X6
tranquilizers NEC	T43.5Ø1	T43.5Ø2	T43.5Ø3	T43.5Ø4	T43.5Ø5	T43.5Ø6
Psychotomimetic agents	T4Ø.9Ø1	T4Ø.9Ø2	T4Ø.9Ø3	T4Ø.9Ø4	T4Ø.9Ø5	T4Ø.9Ø6
Psychotropic drug NEC	T43.91	T43.92	T43.93	T43.94	T43.95	T43.96
specified NEC	T43.8X1	T43.8X2	T43.8X3	T43.8X4	T43.8X5	T43.8X6
Psyllium hydrophilic mucilloid	T47.4X1	T47.4X2	T47.4X3	T47.4X4	T47.4X5	T47.4X6
Pteroylglutamic acid	T45.8X1	T45.8X2	T45.8X3	T45.8X4	T45.8X5	T45.8X6
Pteroyltriglutamate	T45.1X1	T45.1X2	T45.1X3	T45.1X4	T45.1X5	T45.1X6
PTFE — *see* Polytetrafluoroethylene						
Pulp						
devitalizing paste	T49.7X1	T49.7X2	T49.7X3	T49.7X4	T49.7X5	T49.7X6
dressing	T49.7X1	T49.7X2	T49.7X3	T49.7X4	T49.7X5	T49.7X6
Pulsatilla	T62.2X1	T62.2X2	T62.2X3	T62.2X4	—	—
Pumpkin seed extract	T37.4X1	T37.4X2	T37.4X3	T37.4X4	T37.4X5	T37.4X6
Purex (bleach)	T54.91	T54.92	T54.93	T54.94	—	—
Purgative NEC — *see also* Cathartic	T47.4X1	T47.4X2	T47.4X3	T47.4X4	T47.4X5	T47.4X6

Substance	Poisoning, Accidental (unintentional)	Poisoning, Intentional Self-harm	Poisoning, Assault	Poisoning, Undetermined	Adverse Effect	Under-dosing
Purine analogue (antineoplastic)	T45.1X1	T45.1X2	T45.1X3	T45.1X4	T45.1X5	T45.1X6
Purine diuretics	T5Ø.2X1	T5Ø.2X2	T5Ø.2X3	T5Ø.2X4	T5Ø.2X5	T5Ø.2X6
Purinethol	T45.1X1	T45.1X2	T45.1X3	T45.1X4	T45.1X5	T45.1X6
PVP	T45.8X1	T45.8X2	T45.8X3	T45.8X4	T45.8X5	T45.8X6
Pyrabital	T39.8X1	T39.8X2	T39.8X3	T39.8X4	T39.8X5	T39.8X6
Pyramidon	T39.2X1	T39.2X2	T39.2X3	T39.2X4	T39.2X5	T39.2X6
Pyrantel	T37.4X1	T37.4X2	T37.4X3	T37.4X4	T37.4X5	T37.4X6
Pyrathiazine	T45.ØX1	T45.ØX2	T45.ØX3	T45.ØX4	T45.ØX5	T45.ØX6
Pyrazinamide	T37.1X1	T37.1X2	T37.1X3	T37.1X4	T37.1X5	T37.1X6
Pyrazinoic acid (amide)	T37.1X1	T37.1X2	T37.1X3	T37.1X4	T37.1X5	T37.1X6
Pyrazole (derivatives)	T39.2X1	T39.2X2	T39.2X3	T39.2X4	T39.2X5	T39.2X6
Pyrazolone analgesic NEC	T39.2X1	T39.2X2	T39.2X3	T39.2X4	T39.2X5	T39.2X6
Pyrethrin, pyrethrum (nonmedicinal)	T6Ø.2X1	T6Ø.2X2	T6Ø.2X3	T6Ø.2X4	—	—
Pyrethrum extract	T49.ØX1	T49.ØX2	T49.ØX3	T49.ØX4	T49.ØX5	T49.ØX6
Pyribenzamine	T45.ØX1	T45.ØX2	T45.ØX3	T45.ØX4	T45.ØX5	T45.ØX6
Pyridine	T52.8X1	T52.8X2	T52.8X3	T52.8X4	—	—
aldoxime methiodide	T5Ø.6X1	T5Ø.6X2	T5Ø.6X3	T5Ø.6X4	T5Ø.6X5	T5Ø.6X6
aldoxime methyl chloride	T5Ø.6X1	T5Ø.6X2	T5Ø.6X3	T5Ø.6X4	T5Ø.6X5	T5Ø.6X6
vapor	T59.891	T59.892	T59.893	T59.894	—	—
Pyridium	T39.8X1	T39.8X2	T39.8X3	T39.8X4	T39.8X5	T39.8X6
Pyridostigmine bromide	T44.ØX1	T44.ØX2	T44.ØX3	T44.ØX4	T44.ØX5	T44.ØX6
Pyridoxal phosphate	T45.2X1	T45.2X2	T45.2X3	T45.2X4	T45.2X5	T45.2X6
Pyridoxine	T45.2X1	T45.2X2	T45.2X3	T45.2X4	T45.2X5	T45.2X6
Pyrilamine	T45.ØX1	T45.ØX2	T45.ØX3	T45.ØX4	T45.ØX5	T45.ØX6
Pyrimethamine	T37.2X1	T37.2X2	T37.2X3	T37.2X4	T37.2X5	T37.2X6
with sulfadoxine	T37.2X1	T37.2X2	T37.2X3	T37.2X4	T37.2X5	T37.2X6
Pyrimidine antagonist	T45.1X1	T45.1X2	T45.1X3	T45.1X4	T45.1X5	T45.1X6
Pyriminil	T6Ø.4X1	T6Ø.4X2	T6Ø.4X3	T6Ø.4X4	—	—
Pyrithione zinc	T49.4X1	T49.4X2	T49.4X3	T49.4X4	T49.4X5	T49.4X6
Pyrithyldione	T42.6X1	T42.6X2	T42.6X3	T42.6X4	T42.6X5	T42.6X6
Pyrogallic acid	T49.ØX1	T49.ØX2	T49.ØX3	T49.ØX4	T49.ØX5	T49.ØX6
Pyrogallol	T49.ØX1	T49.ØX2	T49.ØX3	T49.ØX4	T49.ØX5	T49.ØX6
Pyroxylin	T49.3X1	T49.3X2	T49.3X3	T49.3X4	T49.3X5	T49.3X6
Pyrrobutamine	T45.ØX1	T45.ØX2	T45.ØX3	T45.ØX4	T45.ØX5	T45.ØX6
Pyrrolizidine alkaloids	T62.8X1	T62.8X2	T62.8X3	T62.8X4	—	—
Pyrvinium chloride	T37.4X1	T37.4X2	T37.4X3	T37.4X4	T37.4X5	T37.4X6
PZI	T38.3X1	T38.3X2	T38.3X3	T38.3X4	T38.3X5	T38.3X6
Quaalude	T42.6X1	T42.6X2	T42.6X3	T42.6X4	T42.6X5	T42.6X6
Quarternary ammonium						
anti-infective	T49.ØX1	T49.ØX2	T49.ØX3	T49.ØX4	T49.ØX5	T49.ØX6
ganglion blocking	T44.2X1	T44.2X2	T44.2X3	T44.2X4	T44.2X5	T44.2X6
parasympatholytic	T44.3X1	T44.3X2	T44.3X3	T44.3X4	T44.3X5	T44.3X6
Quazepam	T42.4X1	T42.4X2	T42.4X3	T42.4X4	T42.4X5	T42.4X6
Quicklime	T54.3X1	T54.3X2	T54.3X3	T54.3X4	—	—
Quillaja extract	T48.4X1	T48.4X2	T48.4X3	T48.4X4	T48.4X5	T48.4X6
Quinacrine	T37.2X1	T37.2X2	T37.2X3	T37.2X4	T37.2X5	T37.2X6
Quinaglute	T46.2X1	T46.2X2	T46.2X3	T46.2X4	T46.2X5	T46.2X6
Quinalbarbital	T42.3X1	T42.3X2	T42.3X3	T42.3X4	T42.3X5	T42.3X6
Quinalbarbitone sodium	T42.3X1	T42.3X2	T42.3X3	T42.3X4	T42.3X5	T42.3X6
Quinalphos	T6Ø.ØX1	T6Ø.ØX2	T6Ø.ØX3	T6Ø.ØX4	—	—
Quinapril	T46.4X1	T46.4X2	T46.4X3	T46.4X4	T46.4X5	T46.4X6
Quinestradiol	T38.5X1	T38.5X2	T38.5X3	T38.5X4	T38.5X5	T38.5X6
Quinestradol	T38.5X1	T38.5X2	T38.5X3	T38.5X4	T38.5X5	T38.5X6
Quinestrol	T38.5X1	T38.5X2	T38.5X3	T38.5X4	T38.5X5	T38.5X6
Quinethazone	T5Ø.2X1	T5Ø.2X2	T5Ø.2X3	T5Ø.2X4	T5Ø.2X5	T5Ø.2X6
Quingestanol	T38.4X1	T38.4X2	T38.4X3	T38.4X4	T38.4X5	T38.4X6
Quinidine	T46.2X1	T46.2X2	T46.2X3	T46.2X4	T46.2X5	T46.2X6
Quinine	T37.2X1	T37.2X2	T37.2X3	T37.2X4	T37.2X5	T37.2X6
Quiniobine	T37.8X1	T37.8X2	T37.8X3	T37.8X4	T37.8X5	T37.8X6
Quinisocaine	T49.1X1	T49.1X2	T49.1X3	T49.1X4	T49.1X5	T49.1X6
Quinocide	T37.2X1	T37.2X2	T37.2X3	T37.2X4	T37.2X5	T37.2X6
Quinoline (derivatives) **NEC**	T37.8X1	T37.8X2	T37.8X3	T37.8X4	T37.8X5	T37.8X6
Quinupramine	T43.Ø11	T43.Ø12	T43.Ø13	T43.Ø14	T43.Ø15	T43.Ø16
Quotane	T41.3X1	T41.3X2	T41.3X3	T41.3X4	T41.3X5	T41.3X6
Rabies						
immune globulin (human)	T5Ø.Z11	T5Ø.Z12	T5Ø.Z13	T5Ø.Z14	T5Ø.Z15	T5Ø.Z16
vaccine	T5Ø.B91	T5Ø.B92	T5Ø.B93	T5Ø.B94	T5Ø.B95	T5Ø.B96
Racemoramide	T4Ø.2X1	T4Ø.2X2	T4Ø.2X3	T4Ø.2X4	—	—
Racemorphan	T4Ø.2X1	T4Ø.2X2	T4Ø.2X3	T4Ø.2X4	T4Ø.2X5	T4Ø.2X6
Racepinefrin	T44.5X1	T44.5X2	T44.5X3	T44.5X4	T44.5X5	T44.5X6
Raclopride	T43.591	T43.592	T43.593	T43.594	T43.595	T43.596
Radiator alcohol	T51.1X1	T51.1X2	T51.1X3	T51.1X4	—	—
Radioactive drug NEC	T5Ø.8X1	T5Ø.8X2	T5Ø.8X3	T5Ø.8X4	T5Ø.8X5	T5Ø.8X6
Radio-opaque (drugs) (materials)	T5Ø.8X1	T5Ø.8X2	T5Ø.8X3	T5Ø.8X4	T5Ø.8X5	T5Ø.8X6
Ramifenazone	T39.2X1	T39.2X2	T39.2X3	T39.2X4	T39.2X5	T39.2X6
Ramipril	T46.4X1	T46.4X2	T46.4X3	T46.4X4	T46.4X5	T46.4X6
Ranitidine	T47.ØX1	T47.ØX2	T47.ØX3	T47.ØX4	T47.ØX5	T47.ØX6
Ranunculus	T62.2X1	T62.2X2	T62.2X3	T62.2X4	—	—
Rat poison NEC	T6Ø.4X1	T6Ø.4X2	T6Ø.4X3	T6Ø.4X4	—	—
Rattlesnake (venom)	T63.Ø11	T63.Ø12	T63.Ø13	T63.Ø14	—	—
Raubasine	T46.7X1	T46.7X2	T46.7X3	T46.7X4	T46.7X5	T46.7X6
Raudixin	T46.5X1	T46.5X2	T46.5X3	T46.5X4	T46.5X5	T46.5X6
Rautensin	T46.5X1	T46.5X2	T46.5X3	T46.5X4	T46.5X5	T46.5X6
Rautina	T46.5X1	T46.5X2	T46.5X3	T46.5X4	T46.5X5	T46.5X6
Rautotal	T46.5X1	T46.5X2	T46.5X3	T46.5X4	T46.5X5	T46.5X6
Rauwiloid	T46.5X1	T46.5X2	T46.5X3	T46.5X4	T46.5X5	T46.5X6
Rauwoldin	T46.5X1	T46.5X2	T46.5X3	T46.5X4	T46.5X5	T46.5X6
Rauwolfia (alkaloids)	T46.5X1	T46.5X2	T46.5X3	T46.5X4	T46.5X5	T46.5X6
Razoxane	T45.1X1	T45.1X2	T45.1X3	T45.1X4	T45.1X5	T45.1X6
Realgar	T57.ØX1	T57.ØX2	T57.ØX3	T57.ØX4	—	—
Recombinant (R) — *see* specific protein						
Red blood cells, packed	T45.8X1	T45.8X2	T45.8X3	T45.8X4	T45.8X5	T45.8X6
Red squill (scilliroside)	T6Ø.4X1	T6Ø.4X2	T6Ø.4X3	T6Ø.4X4	—	—
Reducing agent, industrial NEC	T65.891	T65.892	T65.893	T65.894	—	—
Refrigerant gas (chlorofluorocarbon)	T53.5X1	T53.5X2	T53.5X3	T53.5X4	—	—
not chlorofluorocarbon	T59.891	T59.892	T59.893	T59.894	—	—
Regroton	T5Ø.2X1	T5Ø.2X2	T5Ø.2X3	T5Ø.2X4	T5Ø.2X5	T5Ø.2X6
Rehydration salts (oral)	T5Ø.3X1	T5Ø.3X2	T5Ø.3X3	T5Ø.3X4	T5Ø.3X5	T5Ø.3X6
Rela	T42.8X1	T42.8X2	T42.8X3	T42.8X4	T42.8X5	T42.8X6
Relaxant, muscle						
anesthetic	T48.1X1	T48.1X2	T48.1X3	T48.1X4	T48.1X5	T48.1X6
central nervous system	T42.8X1	T42.8X2	T42.8X3	T42.8X4	T42.8X5	T42.8X6
skeletal NEC	T48.1X1	T48.1X2	T48.1X3	T48.1X4	T48.1X5	T48.1X6
smooth NEC	T44.3X1	T44.3X2	T44.3X3	T44.3X4	T44.3X5	T44.3X6
Remoxipride	T43.591	T43.592	T43.593	T43.594	T43.595	T43.596
Renese	T5Ø.2X1	T5Ø.2X2	T5Ø.2X3	T5Ø.2X4	T5Ø.2X5	T5Ø.2X6
Renografin	T5Ø.8X1	T5Ø.8X2	T5Ø.8X3	T5Ø.8X4	T5Ø.8X5	T5Ø.8X6
Replacement solution	T5Ø.3X1	T5Ø.3X2	T5Ø.3X3	T5Ø.3X4	T5Ø.3X5	T5Ø.3X6
Reproterol	T48.6X1	T48.6X2	T48.6X3	T48.6X4	T48.6X5	T48.6X6
Rescinnamine	T46.5X1	T46.5X2	T46.5X3	T46.5X4	T46.5X5	T46.5X6
Reserpin (e)	T46.5X1	T46.5X2	T46.5X3	T46.5X4	T46.5X5	T46.5X6
Resorcin, resorcinol (nonmedicinal)	T65.891	T65.892	T65.893	T65.894	—	—
medicinal	T49.4X1	T49.4X2	T49.4X3	T49.4X4	T49.4X5	T49.4X6
Respaire	T48.4X1	T48.4X2	T48.4X3	T48.4X4	T48.4X5	T48.4X6
Respiratory drug NEC	T48.9Ø1	T48.9Ø2	T48.9Ø3	T48.9Ø4	T48.9Ø5	T48.9Ø6
antiasthmatic NEC	T48.6X1	T48.6X2	T48.6X3	T48.6X4	T48.6X5	T48.6X6
anti-common-cold NEC	T48.5X1	T48.5X2	T48.5X3	T48.5X4	T48.5X5	T48.5X6
expectorant NEC	T48.4X1	T48.4X2	T48.4X3	T48.4X4	T48.4X5	T48.4X6
stimulant	T48.9Ø1	T48.9Ø2	T48.9Ø3	T48.9Ø4	T48.9Ø5	T48.9Ø6
Retinoic acid	T49.ØX1	T49.ØX2	T49.ØX3	T49.ØX4	T49.ØX5	T49.ØX6
Retinol	T45.2X1	T45.2X2	T45.2X3	T45.2X4	T45.2X5	T45.2X6
Rh (D) **immune globulin** (human)	T5Ø.Z11	T5Ø.Z12	T5Ø.Z13	T5Ø.Z14	T5Ø.Z15	T5Ø.Z16
Rhodine	T39.Ø11	T39.Ø12	T39.Ø13	T39.Ø14	T39.Ø15	T39.Ø16
RhoGAM	T5Ø.Z11	T5Ø.Z12	T5Ø.Z13	T5Ø.Z14	T5Ø.Z15	T5Ø.Z16
Rhubarb						
dry extract	T47.2X1	T47.2X2	T47.2X3	T47.2X4	T47.2X5	T47.2X6
tincture, compound	T47.2X1	T47.2X2	T47.2X3	T47.2X4	T47.2X5	T47.2X6
Ribavirin	T37.5X1	T37.5X2	T37.5X3	T37.5X4	T37.5X5	T37.5X6
Riboflavin	T45.2X1	T45.2X2	T45.2X3	T45.2X4	T45.2X5	T45.2X6
Ribostamycin	T36.5X1	T36.5X2	T36.5X3	T36.5X4	T36.5X5	T36.5X6
Ricin	T62.2X1	T62.2X2	T62.2X3	T62.2X4	—	—
Ricinus communis	T62.2X1	T62.2X2	T62.2X3	T62.2X4	—	—
Rickettsial vaccine NEC	T5Ø.A91	T5Ø.A92	T5Ø.A93	T5Ø.A94	T5Ø.A95	T5Ø.A96
Rifabutin	T36.6X1	T36.6X2	T36.6X3	T36.6X4	T36.6X5	T36.6X6
Rifamide	T36.6X1	T36.6X2	T36.6X3	T36.6X4	T36.6X5	T36.6X6
Rifampicin	T36.6X1	T36.6X2	T36.6X3	T36.6X4	T36.6X5	T36.6X6
with isoniazid	T37.1X1	T37.1X2	T37.1X3	T37.1X4	T37.1X5	T37.1X6
Rifampin	T36.6X1	T36.6X2	T36.6X3	T36.6X4	T36.6X5	T36.6X6
Rifamycin	T36.6X1	T36.6X2	T36.6X3	T36.6X4	T36.6X5	T36.6X6
Rifaximin	T36.6X1	T36.6X2	T36.6X3	T36.6X4	T36.6X5	T36.6X6
Rimantadine	T37.5X1	T37.5X2	T37.5X3	T37.5X4	T37.5X5	T37.5X6
Rimazolium metilsulfate	T39.8X1	T39.8X2	T39.8X3	T39.8X4	T39.8X5	T39.8X6
Rimifon	T37.1X1	T37.1X2	T37.1X3	T37.1X4	T37.1X5	T37.1X6
Rimiterol	T48.6X1	T48.6X2	T48.6X3	T48.6X4	T48.6X5	T48.6X6
Ringer (lactate) **solution**	T5Ø.3X1	T5Ø.3X2	T5Ø.3X3	T5Ø.3X4	T5Ø.3X5	T5Ø.3X6
Ristocetin	T36.8X1	T36.8X2	T36.8X3	T36.8X4	T36.8X5	T36.8X6
Ritalin	T43.631	T43.632	T43.633	T43.634	T43.635	T43.636
Ritodrine	T44.5X1	T44.5X2	T44.5X3	T44.5X4	T44.5X5	T44.5X6
Roach killer — *see* Insecticide						
Rociverine	T44.3X1	T44.3X2	T44.3X3	T44.3X4	T44.3X5	T44.3X6
Rocky Mountain spotted fever vaccine	T5Ø.A91	T5Ø.A92	T5Ø.A93	T5Ø.A94	T5Ø.A95	T5Ø.A96
Rodenticide NEC	T6Ø.4X1	T6Ø.4X2	T6Ø.4X3	T6Ø.4X4	—	—
Rohypnol	T42.4X1	T42.4X2	T42.4X3	T42.4X4	T42.4X5	T42.4X6
Rokitamycin	T36.3X1	T36.3X2	T36.3X3	T36.3X4	T36.3X5	T36.3X6
Rolaids	T47.1X1	T47.1X2	T47.1X3	T47.1X4	T47.1X5	T47.1X6
Rolitetracycline	T36.4X1	T36.4X2	T36.4X3	T36.4X4	T36.4X5	T36.4X6
Romilar	T48.3X1	T48.3X2	T48.3X3	T48.3X4	T48.3X5	T48.3X6

Substance	Poisoning, Accidental (unintentional)	Poisoning, Intentional Self-harm	Poisoning, Assault	Poisoning, Undetermined	Adverse Effect	Under-dosing
Ronifibrate	T46.6X1	T46.6X2	T46.6X3	T46.6X4	T46.6X5	T46.6X6
Rosaprostol	T47.1X1	T47.1X2	T47.1X3	T47.1X4	T47.1X5	T47.1X6
Rose bengal sodium (131I)	T5Ø.8X1	T5Ø.8X2	T5Ø.8X3	T5Ø.8X4	T5Ø.8X5	T5Ø.8X6
Rose water ointment	T49.3X1	T49.3X2	T49.3X3	T49.3X4	T49.3X5	T49.3X6
Rosoxacin	T37.8X1	T37.8X2	T37.8X3	T37.8X4	T37.8X5	T37.8X6
Rotenone	T6Ø.2X1	T6Ø.2X2	T6Ø.2X3	T6Ø.2X4	—	—
Rotoxamine	T45.ØX1	T45.ØX2	T45.ØX3	T45.ØX4	T45.ØX5	T45.ØX6
Rough-on-rats	T6Ø.4X1	T6Ø.4X2	T6Ø.4X3	T6Ø.4X4	—	—
Roxatidine	T47.ØX1	T47.ØX2	T47.ØX3	T47.ØX4	T47.ØX5	T47.ØX6
Roxithromycin	T36.3X1	T36.3X2	T36.3X3	T36.3X4	T36.3X5	T36.3X6
Rt-PA	T45.611	T45.612	T45.613	T45.614	T45.615	T45.616
Rubbing alcohol	T51.2X1	T51.2X2	T51.2X3	T51.2X4	—	—
Rubefacient	T49.4X1	T49.4X2	T49.4X3	T49.4X4	T49.4X5	T49.4X6
Rubella vaccine	T5Ø.B91	T5Ø.B92	T5Ø.B93	T5Ø.B94	T5Ø.B95	T5Ø.B96
Rubeola vaccine	T5Ø.B91	T5Ø.B92	T5Ø.B93	T5Ø.B94	T5Ø.B95	T5Ø.B96
Rubidium chloride Rb82	T5Ø.8X1	T5Ø.8X2	T5Ø.8X3	T5Ø.8X4	T5Ø.8X5	T5Ø.8X6
Rubidomycin	T45.1X1	T45.1X2	T45.1X3	T45.1X4	T45.1X5	T45.1X6
Rue	T62.2X1	T62.2X2	T62.2X3	T62.2X4	—	—
Rufocromomycin	T45.1X1	T45.1X2	T45.1X3	T45.1X4	T45.1X5	T45.1X6
Russel's viper venin	T45.7X1	T45.7X2	T45.7X3	T45.7X4	T45.7X5	T45.7X6
Ruta (graveolens)	T62.2X1	T62.2X2	T62.2X3	T62.2X4	—	—
Rutinum	T46.991	T46.992	T46.993	T46.994	T46.995	T46.996
Rutoside	T46.991	T46.992	T46.993	T46.994	T46.995	T46.996
b-sitosterol(s)	T46.6X1	T46.6X2	T46.6X3	T46.6X4	T46.6X5	T46.6X6
Sabadilla (plant)	T62.2X1	T62.2X2	T62.2X3	T62.2X4	—	—
pesticide	T6Ø.2X1	T6Ø.2X2	T6Ø.2X3	T6Ø.2X4	—	—
Saccharated iron oxide	T45.8X1	T45.8X2	T45.8X3	T45.8X4	T45.8X5	T45.8X6
Saccharin	T5Ø.9Ø1	T5Ø.9Ø2	T5Ø.9Ø3	T5Ø.9Ø4	T5Ø.9Ø5	T5Ø.9Ø6
Saccharomyces boulardii	T47.6X1	T47.6X2	T47.6X3	T47.6X4	T47.6X5	T47.6X6
Safflower oil	T46.6X1	T46.6X2	T46.6X3	T46.6X4	T46.6X5	T46.6X6
Safrazine	T43.1X1	T43.1X2	T43.1X3	T43.1X4	T43.1X5	T43.1X6
Salazosulfapyridine	T37.ØX1	T37.ØX2	T37.ØX3	T37.ØX4	T37.ØX5	T37.ØX6
Salbutamol	T48.6X1	T48.6X2	T48.6X3	T48.6X4	T48.6X5	T48.6X6
Salicylamide	T39.Ø91	T39.Ø92	T39.Ø93	T39.Ø94	T39.Ø95	T39.Ø96
Salicylate NEC	T39.Ø91	T39.Ø92	T39.Ø93	T39.Ø94	T39.Ø95	T39.Ø96
methyl	T49.3X1	T49.3X2	T49.3X3	T49.3X4	T49.3X5	T49.3X6
theobromine calcium	T5Ø.2X1	T5Ø.2X2	T5Ø.2X3	T5Ø.2X4	T5Ø.2X5	T5Ø.2X6
Salicylazosulfapyridine	T37.ØX1	T37.ØX2	T37.ØX3	T37.ØX4	T37.ØX5	T37.ØX6
Salicylhydroxamic acid	T49.ØX1	T49.ØX2	T49.ØX3	T49.ØX4	T49.ØX5	T49.ØX6
Salicylic acid	T49.4X1	T49.4X2	T49.4X3	T49.4X4	T49.4X5	T49.4X6
with benzoic acid	T49.4X1	T49.4X2	T49.4X3	T49.4X4	T49.4X5	T49.4X6
congeners	T39.Ø91	T39.Ø92	T39.Ø93	T39.Ø94	T39.Ø95	T39.Ø96
derivative	T39.Ø91	T39.Ø92	T39.Ø93	T39.Ø94	T39.Ø95	T39.Ø96
salts	T39.Ø91	T39.Ø92	T39.Ø93	T39.Ø94	T39.Ø95	T39.Ø96
Salinazid	T37.1X1	T37.1X2	T37.1X3	T37.1X4	T37.1X5	T37.1X6
Salmeterol	T48.6X1	T48.6X2	T48.6X3	T48.6X4	T48.6X5	T48.6X6
Salol	T49.3X1	T49.3X2	T49.3X3	T49.3X4	T49.3X5	T49.3X6
Salsalate	T39.Ø91	T39.Ø92	T39.Ø93	T39.Ø94	T39.Ø95	T39.Ø96
Salt-replacing drug	T5Ø.9Ø1	T5Ø.9Ø2	T5Ø.9Ø3	T5Ø.9Ø4	T5Ø.9Ø5	T5Ø.9Ø6
Salt-retaining mineralocorticoid	T5Ø.ØX1	T5Ø.ØX2	T5Ø.ØX3	T5Ø.ØX4	T5Ø.ØX5	T5Ø.ØX6
Salt substitute	T5Ø.9Ø1	T5Ø.9Ø2	T5Ø.9Ø3	T5Ø.9Ø4	T5Ø.9Ø5	T5Ø.9Ø6
Saluretic NEC	T5Ø.2X1	T5Ø.2X2	T5Ø.2X3	T5Ø.2X4	T5Ø.2X5	T5Ø.2X6
Saluron	T5Ø.2X1	T5Ø.2X2	T5Ø.2X3	T5Ø.2X4	T5Ø.2X5	T5Ø.2X6
Salvarsan 606 (neosilver) (silver)	T37.8X1	T37.8X2	T37.8X3	T37.8X4	T37.8X5	T37.8X6
Sambucus canadensis	T62.2X1	T62.2X2	T62.2X3	T62.2X4	—	—
berry	T62.1X1	T62.1X2	T62.1X3	T62.1X4	—	—
Sandril	T46.5X1	T46.5X2	T46.5X3	T46.5X4	T46.5X5	T46.5X6
Sanguinaria canadensis	T62.2X1	T62.2X2	T62.2X3	T62.2X4	—	—
Saniflush (cleaner)	T54.2X1	T54.2X2	T54.2X3	T54.2X4	—	—
Santonin	T37.4X1	T37.4X2	T37.4X3	T37.4X4	T37.4X5	T37.4X6
Santyl	T49.8X1	T49.8X2	T49.8X3	T49.8X4	T49.8X5	T49.8X6
Saralasin	T46.5X1	T46.5X2	T46.5X3	T46.5X4	T46.5X5	T46.5X6
Sarcolysin	T45.1X1	T45.1X2	T45.1X3	T45.1X4	T45.1X5	T45.1X6
Sarkomycin	T45.1X1	T45.1X2	T45.1X3	T45.1X4	T45.1X5	T45.1X6
Saroten	T43.Ø11	T43.Ø12	T43.Ø13	T43.Ø14	T43.Ø15	T43.Ø16
Saturnine — *see* Lead						
Savin (oil)	T49.4X1	T49.4X2	T49.4X3	T49.4X4	T49.4X5	T49.4X6
Scammony	T47.2X1	T47.2X2	T47.2X3	T47.2X4	T47.2X5	T47.2X6
Scarlet red	T49.8X1	T49.8X2	T49.8X3	T49.8X4	T49.8X5	T49.8X6
Scheele's green	T57.ØX1	T57.ØX2	T57.ØX3	T57.ØX4	—	—
insecticide	T57.ØX1	T57.ØX2	T57.ØX3	T57.ØX4	—	—
Schizontozide (blood) (tissue)	T37.2X1	T37.2X2	T37.2X3	T37.2X4	T37.2X5	T37.2X6
Schradan	T6Ø.ØX1	T6Ø.ØX2	T6Ø.ØX3	T6Ø.ØX4	—	—
Schweinfurth green	T57.ØX1	T57.ØX2	T57.ØX3	T57.ØX4	—	—
insecticide	T57.ØX1	T57.ØX2	T57.ØX3	T57.ØX4	—	—
Scilla, rat poison	T6Ø.4X1	T6Ø.4X2	T6Ø.4X3	T6Ø.4X4	—	—
Scillaren	T6Ø.4X1	T6Ø.4X2	T6Ø.4X3	T6Ø.4X4	—	—
Sclerosing agent	T46.8X1	T46.8X2	T46.8X3	T46.8X4	T46.8X5	T46.8X6
Scombrotoxin	T61.11	T61.12	T61.13	T61.14	—	—
Scopolamine	T44.3X1	T44.3X2	T44.3X3	T44.3X4	T44.3X5	T44.3X6

Substance	Poisoning, Accidental (unintentional)	Poisoning, Intentional Self-harm	Poisoning, Assault	Poisoning, Undetermined	Adverse Effect	Under-dosing
Scopolia extract	T44.3X1	T44.3X2	T44.3X3	T44.3X4	T44.3X5	T44.3X6
Scouring powder	T65.891	T65.892	T65.893	T65.894	—	—
Sea						
anemone (sting)	T63.631	T63.632	T63.633	T63.634	—	—
cucumber (sting)	T63.691	T63.692	T63.693	T63.694	—	—
snake (bite) (venom)	T63.Ø91	T63.Ø92	T63.Ø93	T63.Ø94	—	—
urchin spine (puncture)	T63.691	T63.692	T63.693	T63.694	—	—
Seafood	T61.91	T61.92	T61.93	T61.94	—	—
specified NEC	T61.8X1	T61.8X2	T61.8X3	T61.8X4	—	—
Secbutabarbital	T42.3X1	T42.3X2	T42.3X3	T42.3X4	T42.3X5	T42.3X6
Secbutabarbitone	T42.3X1	T42.3X2	T42.3X3	T42.3X4	T42.3X5	T42.3X6
Secnidazole	T37.3X1	T37.3X2	T37.3X3	T37.3X4	T37.3X5	T37.3X6
Secobarbital	T42.3X1	T42.3X2	T42.3X3	T42.3X4	T42.3X5	T42.3X6
Seconal	T42.3X1	T42.3X2	T42.3X3	T42.3X4	T42.3X5	T42.3X6
Secretin	T5Ø.8X1	T5Ø.8X2	T5Ø.8X3	T5Ø.8X4	T5Ø.8X5	T5Ø.8X6
Sedative NEC	T42.71	T42.72	T42.73	T42.74	T42.75	T42.76
mixed NEC	T42.6X1	T42.6X2	T42.6X3	T42.6X4	T42.6X5	T42.6X6
Sedormid	T42.6X1	T42.6X2	T42.6X3	T42.6X4	T42.6X5	T42.6X6
Seed disinfectant or dressing	T6Ø.8X1	T6Ø.8X2	T6Ø.8X3	T6Ø.8X4	—	—
Seeds (poisonous)	T62.2X1	T62.2X2	T62.2X3	T62.2X4	—	—
Selegiline	T42.8X1	T42.8X2	T42.8X3	T42.8X4	T42.8X5	T42.8X6
Selenium NEC	T56.891	T56.892	T56.893	T56.894	—	—
disulfide or sulfide	T49.4X1	T49.4X2	T49.4X3	T49.4X4	T49.4X5	T49.4X6
fumes	T59.891	T59.892	T59.893	T59.894	—	—
sulfide	T49.4X1	T49.4X2	T49.4X3	T49.4X4	T49.4X5	T49.4X6
Selenomethionine (75Se)	T5Ø.8X1	T5Ø.8X2	T5Ø.8X3	T5Ø.8X4	T5Ø.8X5	T5Ø.8X6
Selsun	T49.4X1	T49.4X2	T49.4X3	T49.4X4	T49.4X5	T49.4X6
Semustine	T45.1X1	T45.1X2	T45.1X3	T45.1X4	T45.1X5	T45.1X6
Senega syrup	T48.4X1	T48.4X2	T48.4X3	T48.4X4	T48.4X5	T48.4X6
Senna	T47.2X1	T47.2X2	T47.2X3	T47.2X4	T47.2X5	T47.2X6
Sennoside A+B	T47.2X1	T47.2X2	T47.2X3	T47.2X4	T47.2X5	T47.2X6
Septisol	T49.2X1	T49.2X2	T49.2X3	T49.2X4	T49.2X5	T49.2X6
Seractide	T38.811	T38.812	T38.813	T38.814	T38.815	T38.816
Serax	T42.4X1	T42.4X2	T42.4X3	T42.4X4	T42.4X5	T42.4X6
Serenesil	T42.6X1	T42.6X2	T42.6X3	T42.6X4	T42.6X5	T42.6X6
Serenium (hydrochloride)	T37.91	T37.92	T37.93	T37.94	T37.95	T37.96
Serepax — *see* Oxazepam						
Sermorelin	T38.891	T38.892	T38.893	T38.894	T38.895	T38.896
Sernyl	T41.1X1	T41.1X2	T41.1X3	T41.1X4	T41.1X5	T41.1X6
Serotonin	T5Ø.991	T5Ø.992	T5Ø.993	T5Ø.994	T5Ø.995	T5Ø.996
Serpasil	T46.5X1	T46.5X2	T46.5X3	T46.5X4	T46.5X5	T46.5X6
Serrapeptase	T45.3X1	T45.3X2	T45.3X3	T45.3X4	T45.3X5	T45.3X6
Serum						
antibotulinus	T5Ø.Z11	T5Ø.Z12	T5Ø.Z13	T5Ø.Z14	T5Ø.Z15	T5Ø.Z16
anticytotoxic	T5Ø.Z11	T5Ø.Z12	T5Ø.Z13	T5Ø.Z14	T5Ø.Z15	T5Ø.Z16
antidiphtheria	T5Ø.Z11	T5Ø.Z12	T5Ø.Z13	T5Ø.Z14	T5Ø.Z15	T5Ø.Z16
antimeningococcus	T5Ø.Z11	T5Ø.Z12	T5Ø.Z13	T5Ø.Z14	T5Ø.Z15	T5Ø.Z16
anti-Rh	T5Ø.Z11	T5Ø.Z12	T5Ø.Z13	T5Ø.Z14	T5Ø.Z15	T5Ø.Z16
anti-snake-bite	T5Ø.Z11	T5Ø.Z12	T5Ø.Z13	T5Ø.Z14	T5Ø.Z15	T5Ø.Z16
antitetanic	T5Ø.Z11	T5Ø.Z12	T5Ø.Z13	T5Ø.Z14	T5Ø.Z15	T5Ø.Z16
antitoxic	T5Ø.Z11	T5Ø.Z12	T5Ø.Z13	T5Ø.Z14	T5Ø.Z15	T5Ø.Z16
complement (inhibitor)	T45.8X1	T45.8X2	T45.8X3	T45.8X4	T45.8X5	T45.8X6
convalescent	T5Ø.Z11	T5Ø.Z12	T5Ø.Z13	T5Ø.Z14	T5Ø.Z15	T5Ø.Z16
hemolytic complement	T45.8X1	T45.8X2	T45.8X3	T45.8X4	T45.8X5	T45.8X6
immune (human)	T5Ø.Z11	T5Ø.Z12	T5Ø.Z13	T5Ø.Z14	T5Ø.Z15	T5Ø.Z16
protective NEC	T5Ø.Z11	T5Ø.Z12	T5Ø.Z13	T5Ø.Z14	T5Ø.Z15	T5Ø.Z16
Setastine	T45.ØX1	T45.ØX2	T45.ØX3	T45.ØX4	T45.ØX5	T45.ØX6
Setoperone	T43.591	T43.592	T43.593	T43.594	T43.595	T43.596
Sewer gas	T59.91	T59.92	T59.93	T59.94	—	—
Shampoo	T55.ØX1	T55.ØX2	T55.ØX3	T55.ØX4	—	—
Shellfish, noxious, nonbacterial	T61.781	T61.782	T61.783	T61.784	—	—
Sildenafil	T46.7X1	T46.7X2	T46.7X3	T46.7X4	T46.7X5	T46.7X6
Silibinin	T5Ø.991	T5Ø.992	T5Ø.993	T5Ø.994	T5Ø.995	T5Ø.996
Silicone NEC	T65.891	T65.892	T65.893	T65.894	—	—
medicinal	T49.3X1	T49.3X2	T49.3X3	T49.3X4	T49.3X5	T49.3X6
Silvadene	T49.ØX1	T49.ØX2	T49.ØX3	T49.ØX4	T49.ØX5	T49.ØX6
Silver	T49.ØX1	T49.ØX2	T49.ØX3	T49.ØX4	T49.ØX5	T49.ØX6
anti-infectives	T49.ØX1	T49.ØX2	T49.ØX3	T49.ØX4	T49.ØX5	T49.ØX6
arsphenamine	T37.8X1	T37.8X2	T37.8X3	T37.8X4	T37.8X5	T37.8X6
colloidal	T49.ØX1	T49.ØX2	T49.ØX3	T49.ØX4	T49.ØX5	T49.ØX6
nitrate	T49.ØX1	T49.ØX2	T49.ØX3	T49.ØX4	T49.ØX5	T49.ØX6
ophthalmic preparation	T49.5X1	T49.5X2	T49.5X3	T49.5X4	T49.5X5	T49.5X6
toughened (keratolytic)	T49.4X1	T49.4X2	T49.4X3	T49.4X4	T49.4X5	T49.4X6
nonmedicinal (dust)	T56.891	T56.892	T56.893	T56.894	—	—
protein	T49.5X1	T49.5X2	T49.5X3	T49.5X4	T49.5X5	T49.5X6
salvarsan	T37.8X1	T37.8X2	T37.8X3	T37.8X4	T37.8X5	T37.8X6
sulfadiazine	T49.4X1	T49.4X2	T49.4X3	T49.4X4	T49.4X5	T49.4X6
Silymarin	T5Ø.991	T5Ø.992	T5Ø.993	T5Ø.994	T5Ø.995	T5Ø.996
Simaldrate	T47.1X1	T47.1X2	T47.1X3	T47.1X4	T47.1X5	T47.1X6
Simazine	T6Ø.3X1	T6Ø.3X2	T6Ø.3X3	T6Ø.3X4	—	—
Simethicone	T47.1X1	T47.1X2	T47.1X3	T47.1X4	T47.1X5	T47.1X6

Substance	Poisoning, Accidental (unintentional)	Poisoning, Intentional Self-harm	Poisoning, Assault	Poisoning, Undetermined	Adverse Effect	Under-dosing
Simfibrate	T46.6X1	T46.6X2	T46.6X3	T46.6X4	T46.6X5	T46.6X6
Simvastatin	T46.6X1	T46.6X2	T46.6X3	T46.6X4	T46.6X5	T46.6X6
Sincalide	T5Ø.8X1	T5Ø.8X2	T5Ø.8X3	T5Ø.8X4	T5Ø.8X5	T5Ø.8X6
Sinequan	T43.Ø11	T43.Ø12	T43.Ø13	T43.Ø14	T43.Ø15	T43.Ø16
Singoserp	T46.5X1	T46.5X2	T46.5X3	T46.5X4	T46.5X5	T46.5X6
Sintrom	T45.511	T45.512	T45.513	T45.514	T45.515	T45.516
Sisomicin	T36.5X1	T36.5X2	T36.5X3	T36.5X4	T36.5X5	T36.5X6
Sitosterols	T46.6X1	T46.6X2	T46.6X3	T46.6X4	T46.6X5	T46.6X6
Skeletal muscle relaxants	T48.1X1	T48.1X2	T48.1X3	T48.1X4	T48.1X5	T48.1X6
Skin						
agents (external)	T49.91	T49.92	T49.93	T49.94	T49.95	T49.96
specified NEC	T49.8X1	T49.8X2	T49.8X3	T49.8X4	T49.8X5	T49.8X6
test antigen	T5Ø.8X1	T5Ø.8X2	T5Ø.8X3	T5Ø.8X4	T5Ø.8X5	T5Ø.8X6
Sleep-eze	T45.ØX1	T45.ØX2	T45.ØX3	T45.ØX4	T45.ØX5	T45.ØX6
Sleeping draught, pill	T42.71	T42.72	T42.73	T42.74	T42.75	T42.76
Smallpox vaccine	T5Ø.B11	T5Ø.B12	T5Ø.B13	T5Ø.B14	T5Ø.B15	T5Ø.B16
Smelter fumes NEC	T56.91	T56.92	T56.93	T56.94	—	—
Smog	T59.1X1	T59.1X2	T59.1X3	T59.1X4	—	—
Smoke NEC	T59.811	T59.812	T59.813	T59.814	—	—
Smooth muscle relaxant	T44.3X1	T44.3X2	T44.3X3	T44.3X4	T44.3X5	T44.3X6
Snail killer NEC	T6Ø.8X1	T6Ø.8X2	T6Ø.8X3	T6Ø.8X4	—	—
Snake venom or bite	T63.ØØ1	T63.ØØ2	T63.ØØ3	T63.ØØ4	—	—
hemocoagulase	T45.7X1	T45.7X2	T45.7X3	T45.7X4	T45.7X5	T45.7X6
Snuff	T65.211	T65.212	T65.213	T65.214	—	—
Soap (powder) (product)	T55.ØX1	T55.ØX2	T55.ØX3	T55.ØX4	—	—
enema	T47.4X1	T47.4X2	T47.4X3	T47.4X4	T47.4X5	T47.4X6
medicinal, soft	T49.2X1	T49.2X2	T49.2X3	T49.2X4	T49.2X5	T49.2X6
superfatted	T49.2X1	T49.2X2	T49.2X3	T49.2X4	T49.2X5	T49.2X6
Sobrerol	T48.4X1	T48.4X2	T48.4X3	T48.4X4	T48.4X5	T48.4X6
Soda (caustic)	T54.3X1	T54.3X2	T54.3X3	T54.3X4	—	—
bicarb	T47.1X1	T47.1X2	T47.1X3	T47.1X4	T47.1X5	T47.1X6
chlorinated — *see* Sodium, hypochlorite						
Sodium						
acetosulfone	T37.1X1	T37.1X2	T37.1X3	T37.1X4	T37.1X5	T37.1X6
acetrizoate	T5Ø.8X1	T5Ø.8X2	T5Ø.8X3	T5Ø.8X4	T5Ø.8X5	T5Ø.8X6
acid phosphate	T5Ø.3X1	T5Ø.3X2	T5Ø.3X3	T5Ø.3X4	T5Ø.3X5	T5Ø.3X6
alginate	T47.8X1	T47.8X2	T47.8X3	T47.8X4	T47.8X5	T47.8X6
amidotrizoate	T5Ø.8X1	T5Ø.8X2	T5Ø.8X3	T5Ø.8X4	T5Ø.8X5	T5Ø.8X6
aminopterin	T45.1X1	T45.1X2	T45.1X3	T45.1X4	T45.1X5	T45.1X6
amylosulfate	T47.8X1	T47.8X2	T47.8X3	T47.8X4	T47.8X5	T47.8X6
amytal	T42.3X1	T42.3X2	T42.3X3	T42.3X4	T42.3X5	T42.3X6
antimony gluconate	T37.3X1	T37.3X2	T37.3X3	T37.3X4	T37.3X5	T37.3X6
arsenate	T57.ØX1	T57.ØX2	T57.ØX3	T57.ØX4	—	—
aurothiomalate	T39.4X1	T39.4X2	T39.4X3	T39.4X4	T39.4X5	T39.4X6
aurothiosulfate	T39.4X1	T39.4X2	T39.4X3	T39.4X4	T39.4X5	T39.4X6
barbiturate	T42.3X1	T42.3X2	T42.3X3	T42.3X4	T42.3X5	T42.3X6
basic phosphate	T47.4X1	T47.4X2	T47.4X3	T47.4X4	T47.4X5	T47.4X6
bicarbonate	T47.1X1	T47.1X2	T47.1X3	T47.1X4	T47.1X5	T47.1X6
bichromate	T57.8X1	T57.8X2	T57.8X3	T57.8X4	—	—
biphosphate	T5Ø.3X1	T5Ø.3X2	T5Ø.3X3	T5Ø.3X4	T5Ø.3X5	T5Ø.3X6
bisulfate	T65.891	T65.892	T65.893	T65.894	—	—
borate						
cleanser	T57.8X1	T57.8X2	T57.8X3	T57.8X4	—	—
eye	T49.5X1	T49.5X2	T49.5X3	T49.5X4	T49.5X5	T49.5X6
therapeutic	T49.8X1	T49.8X2	T49.8X3	T49.8X4	T49.8X5	T49.8X6
bromide	T42.6X1	T42.6X2	T42.6X3	T42.6X4	T42.6X5	T42.6X6
cacodylate (nonmedicinal) NEC	T5Ø.8X1	T5Ø.8X2	T5Ø.8X3	T5Ø.8X4	T5Ø.8X5	T5Ø.8X6
anti-infective	T37.8X1	T37.8X2	T37.8X3	T37.8X4	T37.8X5	T37.8X6
herbicide	T6Ø.3X1	T6Ø.3X2	T6Ø.3X3	T6Ø.3X4	—	—
calcium edetate	T45.8X1	T45.8X2	T45.8X3	T45.8X4	T45.8X5	T45.8X6
carbonate NEC	T54.3X1	T54.3X2	T54.3X3	T54.3X4	—	—
chlorate NEC	T65.891	T65.892	T65.893	T65.894	—	—
herbicide	T54.91	T54.92	T54.93	T54.94	—	—
chloride	T5Ø.3X1	T5Ø.3X2	T5Ø.3X3	T5Ø.3X4	T5Ø.3X5	T5Ø.3X6
with glucose	T5Ø.3X1	T5Ø.3X2	T5Ø.3X3	T5Ø.3X4	T5Ø.3X5	T5Ø.3X6
chromate	T65.891	T65.892	T65.893	T65.894	—	—
citrate	T5Ø.991	T5Ø.992	T5Ø.993	T5Ø.994	T5Ø.995	T5Ø.996
cromoglicate	T48.6X1	T48.6X2	T48.6X3	T48.6X4	T48.6X5	T48.6X6
cyanide	T65.ØX1	T65.ØX2	T65.ØX3	T65.ØX4	—	—
cyclamate	T5Ø.3X1	T5Ø.3X2	T5Ø.3X3	T5Ø.3X4	T5Ø.3X5	T5Ø.3X6
dehydrocholate	T45.8X1	T45.8X2	T45.8X3	T45.8X4	T45.8X5	T45.8X6
diatrizoate	T5Ø.8X1	T5Ø.8X2	T5Ø.8X3	T5Ø.8X4	T5Ø.8X5	T5Ø.8X6
dibunate	T48.4X1	T48.4X2	T48.4X3	T48.4X4	T48.4X5	T48.4X6
dioctyl sulfosuccinate	T47.4X1	T47.4X2	T47.4X3	T47.4X4	T47.4X5	T47.4X6
dipantoyl ferrate	T45.8X1	T45.8X2	T45.8X3	T45.8X4	T45.8X5	T45.8X6
edetate	T45.8X1	T45.8X2	T45.8X3	T45.8X4	T45.8X5	T45.8X6
ethacrynate	T5Ø.1X1	T5Ø.1X2	T5Ø.1X3	T5Ø.1X4	T5Ø.1X5	T5Ø.1X6
feredetate	T45.8X1	T45.8X2	T45.8X3	T45.8X4	T45.8X5	T45.8X6
Fluoride — *see* Fluoride						
fluoroacetate (dust) (pesticide)	T6Ø.4X1	T6Ø.4X2	T6Ø.4X3	T6Ø.4X4	—	—
Sodium — *continued*						
free salt	T5Ø.3X1	T5Ø.3X2	T5Ø.3X3	T5Ø.3X4	T5Ø.3X5	T5Ø.3X6
fusidate	T36.8X1	T36.8X2	T36.8X3	T36.8X4	T36.8X5	T36.8X6
glucaldrate	T47.1X1	T47.1X2	T47.1X3	T47.1X4	T47.1X5	T47.1X6
glucosulfone	T37.1X1	T37.1X2	T37.1X3	T37.1X4	T37.1X5	T37.1X6
glutamate	T45.8X1	T45.8X2	T45.8X3	T45.8X4	T45.8X5	T45.8X6
hydrogen carbonate	T5Ø.3X1	T5Ø.3X2	T5Ø.3X3	T5Ø.3X4	T5Ø.3X5	T5Ø.3X6
hydroxide	T54.3X1	T54.3X2	T54.3X3	T54.3X4	—	—
hypochlorite (bleach) NEC	T54.3X1	T54.3X2	T54.3X3	T54.3X4	—	—
disinfectant	T54.3X1	T54.3X2	T54.3X3	T54.3X4	—	—
medicinal (anti-infective) (external)	T49.ØX1	T49.ØX2	T49.ØX3	T49.ØX4	T49.ØX5	T49.ØX6
vapor	T54.3X1	T54.3X2	T54.3X3	T54.3X4	—	—
hyposulfite	T49.ØX1	T49.ØX2	T49.ØX3	T49.ØX4	T49.ØX5	T49.ØX6
indigotin disulfonate	T5Ø.8X1	T5Ø.8X2	T5Ø.8X3	T5Ø.8X4	T5Ø.8X5	T5Ø.8X6
iodide	T5Ø.991	T5Ø.992	T5Ø.993	T5Ø.994	T5Ø.995	T5Ø.996
I-131	T5Ø.8X1	T5Ø.8X2	T5Ø.8X3	T5Ø.8X4	T5Ø.8X5	T5Ø.8X6
therapeutic	T38.2X1	T38.2X2	T38.2X3	T38.2X4	T38.2X5	T38.2X6
iodohippurate (131I)	T5Ø.8X1	T5Ø.8X2	T5Ø.8X3	T5Ø.8X4	T5Ø.8X5	T5Ø.8X6
iopodate	T5Ø.8X1	T5Ø.8X2	T5Ø.8X3	T5Ø.8X4	T5Ø.8X5	T5Ø.8X6
iothalamate	T5Ø.8X1	T5Ø.8X2	T5Ø.8X3	T5Ø.8X4	T5Ø.8X5	T5Ø.8X6
iron edetate	T45.4X1	T45.4X2	T45.4X3	T45.4X4	T45.4X5	T45.4X6
lactate (compound solution)	T45.8X1	T45.8X2	T45.8X3	T45.8X4	T45.8X5	T45.8X6
lauryl (sulfate)	T49.2X1	T49.2X2	T49.2X3	T49.2X4	T49.2X5	T49.2X6
L-triiodothyronine	T38.1X1	T38.1X2	T38.1X3	T38.1X4	T38.1X5	T38.1X6
magnesium citrate	T5Ø.991	T5Ø.992	T5Ø.993	T5Ø.994	T5Ø.995	T5Ø.996
mersalate	T5Ø.2X1	T5Ø.2X2	T5Ø.2X3	T5Ø.2X4	T5Ø.2X5	T5Ø.2X6
metasilicate	T65.891	T65.892	T65.893	T65.894	—	—
metrizoate	T5Ø.8X1	T5Ø.8X2	T5Ø.8X3	T5Ø.8X4	T5Ø.8X5	T5Ø.8X6
monofluoroacetate (pesticide)	T6Ø.1X1	T6Ø.1X2	T6Ø.1X3	T6Ø.1X4	—	—
morrhuate	T46.8X1	T46.8X2	T46.8X3	T46.8X4	T46.8X5	T46.8X6
nafcillin	T36.ØX1	T36.ØX2	T36.ØX3	T36.ØX4	T36.ØX5	T36.ØX6
nitrate (oxidizing agent)	T65.891	T65.892	T65.893	T65.894	—	—
nitrite	T5Ø.6X1	T5Ø.6X2	T5Ø.6X3	T5Ø.6X4	T5Ø.6X5	T5Ø.6X6
nitroferricyanide	T46.5X1	T46.5X2	T46.5X3	T46.5X4	T46.5X5	T46.5X6
nitroprusside	T46.5X1	T46.5X2	T46.5X3	T46.5X4	T46.5X5	T46.5X6
oxalate	T65.891	T65.892	T65.893	T65.894	—	—
oxide/peroxide	T65.891	T65.892	T65.893	T65.894	—	—
oxybate	T41.291	T41.292	T41.293	T41.294	T41.295	T41.296
para-aminohippurate	T5Ø.8X1	T5Ø.8X2	T5Ø.8X3	T5Ø.8X4	T5Ø.8X5	T5Ø.8X6
perborate (nonmedicinal) NEC	T65.891	T65.892	T65.893	T65.894	—	—
medicinal	T49.ØX1	T49.ØX2	T49.ØX3	T49.ØX4	T49.ØX5	T49.ØX6
soap	T55.ØX1	T55.ØX2	T55.ØX3	T55.ØX4	—	—
percarbonate — *see* Sodium, perborate						
pertechnetate Tc99m	T5Ø.8X1	T5Ø.8X2	T5Ø.8X3	T5Ø.8X4	T5Ø.8X5	T5Ø.8X6
phosphate						
cellulose	T45.8X1	T45.8X2	T45.8X3	T45.8X4	T45.8X5	T45.8X6
dibasic	T47.2X1	T47.2X2	T47.2X3	T47.2X4	T47.2X5	T47.2X6
monobasic	T47.2X1	T47.2X2	T47.2X3	T47.2X4	T47.2X5	T47.2X6
phytate	T5Ø.6X1	T5Ø.6X2	T5Ø.6X3	T5Ø.6X4	T5Ø.6X5	T5Ø.6X6
picosulfate	T47.2X1	T47.2X2	T47.2X3	T47.2X4	T47.2X5	T47.2X6
polyhydroxyaluminium monocarbonate	T47.1X1	T47.1X2	T47.1X3	T47.1X4	T47.1X5	T47.1X6
polystyrene sulfonate	T5Ø.3X1	T5Ø.3X2	T5Ø.3X3	T5Ø.3X4	T5Ø.3X5	T5Ø.3X6
propionate	T49.ØX1	T49.ØX2	T49.ØX3	T49.ØX4	T49.ØX5	T49.ØX6
propyl hydroxybenzoate	T5Ø.991	T5Ø.992	T5Ø.993	T5Ø.994	T5Ø.995	T5Ø.996
psylliate	T46.8X1	T46.8X2	T46.8X3	T46.8X4	T46.8X5	T46.8X6
removing resins	T5Ø.3X1	T5Ø.3X2	T5Ø.3X3	T5Ø.3X4	T5Ø.3X5	T5Ø.3X6
salicylate	T39.Ø91	T39.Ø92	T39.Ø93	T39.Ø94	T39.Ø95	T39.Ø96
salt NEC	T5Ø.3X1	T5Ø.3X2	T5Ø.3X3	T5Ø.3X4	T5Ø.3X5	T5Ø.3X6
selenate	T6Ø.2X1	T6Ø.2X2	T6Ø.2X3	T6Ø.2X4	—	—
stibogluconate	T37.3X1	T37.3X2	T37.3X3	T37.3X4	T37.3X5	T37.3X6
sulfate	T47.4X1	T47.4X2	T47.4X3	T47.4X4	T47.4X5	T47.4X6
sulfoxone	T37.1X1	T37.1X2	T37.1X3	T37.1X4	T37.1X5	T37.1X6
tetradecyl sulfate	T46.8X1	T46.8X2	T46.8X3	T46.8X4	T46.8X5	T46.8X6
thiopental	T41.1X1	T41.1X2	T41.1X3	T41.1X4	T41.1X5	T41.1X6
thiosalicylate	T39.Ø91	T39.Ø92	T39.Ø93	T39.Ø94	T39.Ø95	T39.Ø96
thiosulfate	T5Ø.6X1	T5Ø.6X2	T5Ø.6X3	T5Ø.6X4	T5Ø.6X5	T5Ø.6X6
tolbutamide	T38.3X1	T38.3X2	T38.3X3	T38.3X4	T38.3X5	T38.3X6
(L)-triiodothyronine	T38.1X1	T38.1X2	T38.1X3	T38.1X4	T38.1X5	T38.1X6
tyropanoate	T5Ø.8X1	T5Ø.8X2	T5Ø.8X3	T5Ø.8X4	T5Ø.8X5	T5Ø.8X6
valproate	T42.6X1	T42.6X2	T42.6X3	T42.6X4	T42.6X5	T42.6X6
versenate	T5Ø.6X1	T5Ø.6X2	T5Ø.6X3	T5Ø.6X4	T5Ø.6X5	T5Ø.6X6
Sodium-free salt	T5Ø.9Ø1	T5Ø.9Ø2	T5Ø.9Ø3	T5Ø.9Ø4	T5Ø.9Ø5	T5Ø.9Ø6
Sodium-removing resin	T5Ø.3X1	T5Ø.3X2	T5Ø.3X3	T5Ø.3X4	T5Ø.3X5	T5Ø.3X6
Soft soap	T55.ØX1	T55.ØX2	T55.ØX3	T55.ØX4	—	—
Solanine	T62.2X1	T62.2X2	T62.2X3	T62.2X4	—	—
berries	T62.1X1	T62.1X2	T62.1X3	T62.1X4	—	—
Solanum dulcamara	T62.2X1	T62.2X2	T62.2X3	T62.2X4	—	—

Substance	Poisoning, Accidental (unintentional)	Poisoning, Intentional Self-harm	Poisoning, Assault	Poisoning, Undetermined	Adverse Effect	Under-dosing
Solanum dulcamara — *continued*						
berries	T62.1X1	T62.1X2	T62.1X3	T62.1X4	—	—
Solapsone	T37.1X1	T37.1X2	T37.1X3	T37.1X4	T37.1X5	T37.1X6
Solar lotion	T49.3X1	T49.3X2	T49.3X3	T49.3X4	T49.3X5	T49.3X6
Solasulfone	T37.1X1	T37.1X2	T37.1X3	T37.1X4	T37.1X5	T37.1X6
Soldering fluid	T65.891	T65.892	T65.893	T65.894	—	—
Solid substance	T65.91	T65.92	T65.93	T65.94	—	—
specified NEC	T65.891	T65.892	T65.893	T65.894	—	—
Solvent, industrial NEC	T52.91	T52.92	T52.93	T52.94	—	—
naphtha	T52.ØX1	T52.ØX2	T52.ØX3	T52.ØX4	—	—
petroleum	T52.ØX1	T52.ØX2	T52.ØX3	T52.ØX4	—	—
specified NEC	T52.8X1	T52.8X2	T52.8X3	T52.8X4	—	—
Soma	T42.8X1	T42.8X2	T42.8X3	T42.8X4	T42.8X5	T42.8X6
Somatorelin	T38.891	T38.892	T38.893	T38.894	T38.895	T38.896
Somatostatin	T38.991	T38.992	T38.993	T38.994	T38.995	T38.996
Somatotropin	T38.811	T38.812	T38.813	T38.814	T38.815	T38.816
Somatrem	T38.811	T38.812	T38.813	T38.814	T38.815	T38.816
Somatropin	T38.811	T38.812	T38.813	T38.814	T38.815	T38.816
Sominex	T45.ØX1	T45.ØX2	T45.ØX3	T45.ØX4	T45.ØX5	T45.ØX6
Somnos	T42.6X1	T42.6X2	T42.6X3	T42.6X4	T42.6X5	T42.6X6
Somonal	T42.3X1	T42.3X2	T42.3X3	T42.3X4	T42.3X5	T42.3X6
Soneryl	T42.3X1	T42.3X2	T42.3X3	T42.3X4	T42.3X5	T42.3X6
Soothing syrup	T5Ø.9Ø1	T5Ø.9Ø2	T5Ø.9Ø3	T5Ø.9Ø4	T5Ø.9Ø5	T5Ø.9Ø6
Sopor	T42.6X1	T42.6X2	T42.6X3	T42.6X4	T42.6X5	T42.6X6
Soporific	T42.71	T42.72	T42.73	T42.74	T42.75	T42.76
Soporific drug	T42.71	T42.72	T42.73	T42.74	T42.75	T42.76
specified type NEC	T42.6X1	T42.6X2	T42.6X3	T42.6X4	T42.6X5	T42.6X6
Sorbide nitrate	T46.3X1	T46.3X2	T46.3X3	T46.3X4	T46.3X5	T46.3X6
Sorbitol	T47.4X1	T47.4X2	T47.4X3	T47.4X4	T47.4X5	T47.4X6
Sotalol	T44.7X1	T44.7X2	T44.7X3	T44.7X4	T44.7X5	T44.7X6
Sotradecol	T46.8X1	T46.8X2	T46.8X3	T46.8X4	T46.8X5	T46.8X6
Soysterol	T46.6X1	T46.6X2	T46.6X3	T46.6X4	T46.6X5	T46.6X6
Spacoline	T44.3X1	T44.3X2	T44.3X3	T44.3X4	T44.3X5	T44.3X6
Spanish fly	T49.8X1	T49.8X2	T49.8X3	T49.8X4	T49.8X5	T49.8X6
Sparine	T43.3X1	T43.3X2	T43.3X3	T43.3X4	T43.3X5	T43.3X6
Sparteine	T48.ØX1	T48.ØX2	T48.ØX3	T48.ØX4	T48.ØX5	T48.ØX6
Spasmolytic						
anticholinergics	T44.3X1	T44.3X2	T44.3X3	T44.3X4	T44.3X5	T44.3X6
autonomic	T44.3X1	T44.3X2	T44.3X3	T44.3X4	T44.3X5	T44.3X6
bronchial NEC	T48.6X1	T48.6X2	T48.6X3	T48.6X4	T48.6X5	T48.6X6
quaternary ammonium	T44.3X1	T44.3X2	T44.3X3	T44.3X4	T44.3X5	T44.3X6
skeletal muscle NEC	T48.1X1	T48.1X2	T48.1X3	T48.1X4	T48.1X5	T48.1X6
Spectinomycin	T36.5X1	T36.5X2	T36.5X3	T36.5X4	T36.5X5	T36.5X6
Speed	T43.621	T43.622	T43.623	T43.624	T43.625	T43.626
Spermicide	T49.8X1	T49.8X2	T49.8X3	T49.8X4	T49.8X5	T49.8X6
Spider (bite) (venom)	T63.391	T63.392	T63.393	T63.394	—	—
antivenin	T5Ø.Z11	T5Ø.Z12	T5Ø.Z13	T5Ø.Z14	T5Ø.Z15	T5Ø.Z16
Spigelia (root)	T37.4X1	T37.4X2	T37.4X3	T37.4X4	T37.4X5	T37.4X6
Spindle inactivator	T5Ø.4X1	T5Ø.4X2	T5Ø.4X3	T5Ø.4X4	T5Ø.4X5	T5Ø.4X6
Spiperone	T43.4X1	T43.4X2	T43.4X3	T43.4X4	T43.4X5	T43.4X6
Spiramycin	T36.3X1	T36.3X2	T36.3X3	T36.3X4	T36.3X5	T36.3X6
Spirapril	T46.4X1	T46.4X2	T46.4X3	T46.4X4	T46.4X5	T46.4X6
Spirilene	T43.591	T43.592	T43.593	T43.594	T43.595	T43.596
Spirit(s) (neutral) **NEC**	T51.ØX1	T51.ØX2	T51.ØX3	T51.ØX4	—	—
beverage	T51.ØX1	T51.ØX2	T51.ØX3	T51.ØX4	—	—
industrial	T51.ØX1	T51.ØX2	T51.ØX3	T51.ØX4	—	—
mineral	T52.ØX1	T52.ØX2	T52.ØX3	T52.ØX4	—	—
of salt — *see* Hydrochloric acid						
surgical	T51.ØX1	T51.ØX2	T51.ØX3	T51.ØX4	—	—
Spironolactone	T5Ø.ØX1	T5Ø.ØX2	T5Ø.ØX3	T5Ø.ØX4	T5Ø.ØX5	T5Ø.ØX6
Spiroperidol	T43.4X1	T43.4X2	T43.4X3	T43.4X4	T43.4X5	T43.4X6
Sponge, absorbable (gelatin)	T45.7X1	T45.7X2	T45.7X3	T45.7X4	T45.7X5	T45.7X6
Sporostacin	T49.ØX1	T49.ØX2	T49.ØX3	T49.ØX4	T49.ØX5	T49.ØX6
Spray (aerosol)	T65.91	T65.92	T65.93	T65.94	—	—
cosmetic	T65.891	T65.892	T65.893	T65.894	—	—
medicinal NEC	T5Ø.9Ø1	T5Ø.9Ø2	T5Ø.9Ø3	T5Ø.9Ø4	T5Ø.9Ø5	T5Ø.9Ø6
pesticides — *see* Pesticides						
specified content — *see* specific substance						
Spurge flax	T62.2X1	T62.2X2	T62.2X3	T62.2X4	—	—
Spurges	T62.2X1	T62.2X2	T62.2X3	T62.2X4	—	—
Sputum viscosity-lowering drug	T48.4X1	T48.4X2	T48.4X3	T48.4X4	T48.4X5	T48.4X6
Squill	T46.ØX1	T46.ØX2	T46.ØX3	T46.ØX4	T46.ØX5	T46.ØX6
rat poison	T6Ø.4X1	T6Ø.4X2	T6Ø.4X3	T6Ø.4X4	—	—
Squirting cucumber (cathartic)	T47.2X1	T47.2X2	T47.2X3	T47.2X4	T47.2X5	T47.2X6
Stains	T65.6X1	T65.6X2	T65.6X3	T65.6X4	—	—
Stannous fluoride	T49.7X1	T49.7X2	T49.7X3	T49.7X4	T49.7X5	T49.7X6
Stanolone	T38.7X1	T38.7X2	T38.7X3	T38.7X4	T38.7X5	T38.7X6
Stanozolol	T38.7X1	T38.7X2	T38.7X3	T38.7X4	T38.7X5	T38.7X6

Substance	Poisoning, Accidental (unintentional)	Poisoning, Intentional Self-harm	Poisoning, Assault	Poisoning, Undetermined	Adverse Effect	Under-dosing
Staphisagria or stavesacre (pediculicide)	T49.ØX1	T49.ØX2	T49.ØX3	T49.ØX4	T49.ØX5	T49.ØX6
Starch	T5Ø.9Ø1	T5Ø.9Ø2	T5Ø.9Ø3	T5Ø.9Ø4	T5Ø.9Ø5	T5Ø.9Ø6
Stelazine	T43.3X1	T43.3X2	T43.3X3	T43.3X4	T43.3X5	T43.3X6
Stemetil	T43.3X1	T43.3X2	T43.3X3	T43.3X4	T43.3X5	T43.3X6
Stepronin	T48.4X1	T48.4X2	T48.4X3	T48.4X4	T48.4X5	T48.4X6
Sterculia	T47.4X1	T47.4X2	T47.4X3	T47.4X4	T47.4X5	T47.4X6
Sternutator gas	T59.891	T59.892	T59.893	T59.894	—	—
Steroid	T38.ØX1	T38.ØX2	T38.ØX3	T38.ØX4	T38.ØX5	T38.ØX6
anabolic	T38.7X1	T38.7X2	T38.7X3	T38.7X4	T38.7X5	T38.7X6
androgenic	T38.7X1	T38.7X2	T38.7X3	T38.7X4	T38.7X5	T38.7X6
antineoplastic, hormone	T38.7X1	T38.7X2	T38.7X3	T38.7X4	T38.7X5	T38.7X6
estrogen	T38.5X1	T38.5X2	T38.5X3	T38.5X4	T38.5X5	T38.5X6
ENT agent	T49.6X1	T49.6X2	T49.6X3	T49.6X4	T49.6X5	T49.6X6
ophthalmic preparation	T49.5X1	T49.5X2	T49.5X3	T49.5X4	T49.5X5	T49.5X6
topical NEC	T49.ØX1	T49.ØX2	T49.ØX3	T49.ØX4	T49.ØX5	T49.ØX6
Stibine	T56.891	T56.892	T56.893	T56.894	—	—
Stibogluconate	T37.3X1	T37.3X2	T37.3X3	T37.3X4	T37.3X5	T37.3X6
Stibophen	T37.4X1	T37.4X2	T37.4X3	T37.4X4	T37.4X5	T37.4X6
Stilbamidine (isetionate)	T37.3X1	T37.3X2	T37.3X3	T37.3X4	T37.3X5	T37.3X6
Stilbestrol	T38.5X1	T38.5X2	T38.5X3	T38.5X4	T38.5X5	T38.5X6
Stilboestrol	T38.5X1	T38.5X2	T38.5X3	T38.5X4	T38.5X5	T38.5X6
Stimulant						
central nervous system — *see also* Psychostimulant	T43.6Ø1	T43.6Ø2	T43.6Ø3	T43.6Ø4	T43.6Ø5	T43.6Ø6
analeptics	T5Ø.7X1	T5Ø.7X2	T5Ø.7X3	T5Ø.7X4	T5Ø.7X5	T5Ø.7X6
opiate antagonist	T5Ø.7X1	T5Ø.7X2	T5Ø.7X3	T5Ø.7X4	T5Ø.7X5	T5Ø.7X6
psychotherapeutic NEC — *see also* Psychotherapeutic drug	T43.6Ø1	T43.6Ø2	T43.6Ø3	T43.6Ø4	T43.6Ø5	T43.6Ø6
specified NEC	T43.691	T43.692	T43.693	T43.694	T43.695	T43.696
respiratory	T48.9Ø1	T48.9Ø2	T48.9Ø3	T48.9Ø4	T48.9Ø5	T48.9Ø6
Stone-dissolving drug	T5Ø.9Ø1	T5Ø.9Ø2	T5Ø.9Ø3	T5Ø.9Ø4	T5Ø.9Ø5	T5Ø.9Ø6
Storage battery (cells) (acid)	T54.2X1	T54.2X2	T54.2X3	T54.2X4	—	—
Stovaine	T41.3X1	T41.3X2	T41.3X3	T41.3X4	T41.3X5	T41.3X6
infiltration (subcutaneous)	T41.3X1	T41.3X2	T41.3X3	T41.3X4	T41.3X5	T41.3X6
nerve block (peripheral) (plexus)	T41.3X1	T41.3X2	T41.3X3	T41.3X4	T41.3X5	T41.3X6
spinal	T41.3X1	T41.3X2	T41.3X3	T41.3X4	T41.3X5	T41.3X6
topical (surface)	T41.3X1	T41.3X2	T41.3X3	T41.3X4	T41.3X5	T41.3X6
Stovarsal	T37.8X1	T37.8X2	T37.8X3	T37.8X4	T37.8X5	T37.8X6
Stove gas — *see* Gas, stove						
Stoxil	T49.5X1	T49.5X2	T49.5X3	T49.5X4	T49.5X5	T49.5X6
Stramonium	T48.6X1	T48.6X2	T48.6X3	T48.6X4	T48.6X5	T48.6X6
natural state	T62.2X1	T62.2X2	T62.2X3	T62.2X4	—	—
Streptodornase	T45.3X1	T45.3X2	T45.3X3	T45.3X4	T45.3X5	T45.3X6
Streptoduocin	T36.5X1	T36.5X2	T36.5X3	T36.5X4	T36.5X5	T36.5X6
Streptokinase	T45.611	T45.612	T45.613	T45.614	T45.615	T45.616
Streptomycin (derivative)	T36.5X1	T36.5X2	T36.5X3	T36.5X4	T36.5X5	T36.5X6
Streptonivicin	T36.5X1	T36.5X2	T36.5X3	T36.5X4	T36.5X5	T36.5X6
Streptovarycin	T36.5X1	T36.5X2	T36.5X3	T36.5X4	T36.5X5	T36.5X6
Streptozocin	T45.1X1	T45.1X2	T45.1X3	T45.1X4	T45.1X5	T45.1X6
Streptozotocin	T45.1X1	T45.1X2	T45.1X3	T45.1X4	T45.1X5	T45.1X6
Stripper (paint) (solvent)	T52.8X1	T52.8X2	T52.8X3	T52.8X4	—	—
Strobane	T6Ø.1X1	T6Ø.1X2	T6Ø.1X3	T6Ø.1X4	—	—
Strofantina	T46.ØX1	T46.ØX2	T46.ØX3	T46.ØX4	T46.ØX5	T46.ØX6
Strophanthin (g) (k)	T46.ØX1	T46.ØX2	T46.ØX3	T46.ØX4	T46.ØX5	T46.ØX6
Strophanthus	T46.ØX1	T46.ØX2	T46.ØX3	T46.ØX4	T46.ØX5	T46.ØX6
Strophantin	T46.ØX1	T46.ØX2	T46.ØX3	T46.ØX4	T46.ØX5	T46.ØX6
Strophantin-g	T46.ØX1	T46.ØX2	T46.ØX3	T46.ØX4	T46.ØX5	T46.ØX6
Strychnine (nonmedicinal) (pesticide) (salts)	T65.1X1	T65.1X2	T65.1X3	T65.1X4	—	—
medicinal	T48.291	T48.292	T48.293	T48.294	T48.295	T48.296
Strychnos (ignatii) — *see* Strychnine						
Styramate	T42.8X1	T42.8X2	T42.8X3	T42.8X4	T42.8X5	T42.8X6
Styrene	T65.891	T65.892	T65.893	T65.894	—	—
Succinimide, antiepileptic or anticonvulsant	T42.2X1	T42.2X2	T42.2X3	T42.2X4	T42.2X5	T42.2X6
mercuric — *see* Mercury						
Succinylcholine	T48.1X1	T48.1X2	T48.1X3	T48.1X4	T48.1X5	T48.1X6
Succinylsulfathiazole	T37.ØX1	T37.ØX2	T37.ØX3	T37.ØX4	T37.ØX5	T37.ØX6
Sucralfate	T47.1X1	T47.1X2	T47.1X3	T47.1X4	T47.1X5	T47.1X6
Sucrose	T5Ø.3X1	T5Ø.3X2	T5Ø.3X3	T5Ø.3X4	T5Ø.3X5	T5Ø.3X6
Sufentanil	T4Ø.4X1	T4Ø.4X2	T4Ø.4X3	T4Ø.4X4	T4Ø.4X5	T4Ø.4X6
Sulbactam	T36.ØX1	T36.ØX2	T36.ØX3	T36.ØX4	T36.ØX5	T36.ØX6
Sulbenicillin	T36.ØX1	T36.ØX2	T36.ØX3	T36.ØX4	T36.ØX5	T36.ØX6
Sulbentine	T49.ØX1	T49.ØX2	T49.ØX3	T49.ØX4	T49.ØX5	T49.ØX6
Sulfacetamide	T49.ØX1	T49.ØX2	T49.ØX3	T49.ØX4	T49.ØX5	T49.ØX6
ophthalmic preparation	T49.5X1	T49.5X2	T49.5X3	T49.5X4	T49.5X5	T49.5X6
Sulfachlorpyridazine	T37.ØX1	T37.ØX2	T37.ØX3	T37.ØX4	T37.ØX5	T37.ØX6
Sulfacitine	T37.ØX1	T37.ØX2	T37.ØX3	T37.ØX4	T37.ØX5	T37.ØX6
Sulfadiasulfone sodium	T37.ØX1	T37.ØX2	T37.ØX3	T37.ØX4	T37.ØX5	T37.ØX6

Substance	Poisoning, Accidental (unintentional)	Poisoning, Intentional Self-harm	Poisoning, Assault	Poisoning, Undetermined	Adverse Effect	Under-dosing
Sulfadiazine	T37.ØX1	T37.ØX2	T37.ØX3	T37.ØX4	T37.ØX5	T37.ØX6
silver (topical)	T49.ØX1	T49.ØX2	T49.ØX3	T49.ØX4	T49.ØX5	T49.ØX6
Sulfadimethoxine	T37.ØX1	T37.ØX2	T37.ØX3	T37.ØX4	T37.ØX5	T37.ØX6
Sulfadimidine	T37.ØX1	T37.ØX2	T37.ØX3	T37.ØX4	T37.ØX5	T37.ØX6
Sulfadoxine	T37.ØX1	T37.ØX2	T37.ØX3	T37.ØX4	T37.ØX5	T37.ØX6
with pyrimethamine	T37.2X1	T37.2X2	T37.2X3	T37.2X4	T37.2X5	T37.2X6
Sulfaethidole	T37.ØX1	T37.ØX2	T37.ØX3	T37.ØX4	T37.ØX5	T37.ØX6
Sulfafurazole	T37.ØX1	T37.ØX2	T37.ØX3	T37.ØX4	T37.ØX5	T37.ØX6
Sulfaguanidine	T37.ØX1	T37.ØX2	T37.ØX3	T37.ØX4	T37.ØX5	T37.ØX6
Sulfalene	T37.ØX1	T37.ØX2	T37.ØX3	T37.ØX4	T37.ØX5	T37.ØX6
Sulfaloxate	T37.ØX1	T37.ØX2	T37.ØX3	T37.ØX4	T37.ØX5	T37.ØX6
Sulfaloxic acid	T37.ØX1	T37.ØX2	T37.ØX3	T37.ØX4	T37.ØX5	T37.ØX6
Sulfamazone	T39.2X1	T39.2X2	T39.2X3	T39.2X4	T39.2X5	T39.2X6
Sulfamerazine	T37.ØX1	T37.ØX2	T37.ØX3	T37.ØX4	T37.ØX5	T37.ØX6
Sulfameter	T37.ØX1	T37.ØX2	T37.ØX3	T37.ØX4	T37.ØX5	T37.ØX6
Sulfamethazine	T37.ØX1	T37.ØX2	T37.ØX3	T37.ØX4	T37.ØX5	T37.ØX6
Sulfamethizole	T37.ØX1	T37.ØX2	T37.ØX3	T37.ØX4	T37.ØX5	T37.ØX6
Sulfamethoxazole	T37.ØX1	T37.ØX2	T37.ØX3	T37.ØX4	T37.ØX5	T37.ØX6
with trimethoprim	T36.8X1	T36.8X2	T36.8X3	T36.8X4	T36.8X5	T36.8X6
Sulfamethoxydiazine	T37.ØX1	T37.ØX2	T37.ØX3	T37.ØX4	T37.ØX5	T37.ØX6
Sulfamethoxypyridazine	T37.ØX1	T37.ØX2	T37.ØX3	T37.ØX4	T37.ØX5	T37.ØX6
Sulfamethylthiazole	T37.ØX1	T37.ØX2	T37.ØX3	T37.ØX4	T37.ØX5	T37.ØX6
Sulfametoxydiazine	T37.ØX1	T37.ØX2	T37.ØX3	T37.ØX4	T37.ØX5	T37.ØX6
Sulfamidopyrine	T39.2X1	T39.2X2	T39.2X3	T39.2X4	T39.2X5	T39.2X6
Sulfamonomethoxine	T37.ØX1	T37.ØX2	T37.ØX3	T37.ØX4	T37.ØX5	T37.ØX6
Sulfamoxole	T37.ØX1	T37.ØX2	T37.ØX3	T37.ØX4	T37.ØX5	T37.ØX6
Sulfamylon	T49.ØX1	T49.ØX2	T49.ØX3	T49.ØX4	T49.ØX5	T49.ØX6
Sulfan blue (diagnostic dye)	T5Ø.8X1	T5Ø.8X2	T5Ø.8X3	T5Ø.8X4	T5Ø.8X5	T5Ø.8X6
Sulfanilamide	T37.ØX1	T37.ØX2	T37.ØX3	T37.ØX4	T37.ØX5	T37.ØX6
Sulfanilylguanidine	T37.ØX1	T37.ØX2	T37.ØX3	T37.ØX4	T37.ØX5	T37.ØX6
Sulfaperin	T37.ØX1	T37.ØX2	T37.ØX3	T37.ØX4	T37.ØX5	T37.ØX6
Sulfaphenazole	T37.ØX1	T37.ØX2	T37.ØX3	T37.ØX4	T37.ØX5	T37.ØX6
Sulfaphenylthiazole	T37.ØX1	T37.ØX2	T37.ØX3	T37.ØX4	T37.ØX5	T37.ØX6
Sulfaproxyline	T37.ØX1	T37.ØX2	T37.ØX3	T37.ØX4	T37.ØX5	T37.ØX6
Sulfapyridine	T37.ØX1	T37.ØX2	T37.ØX3	T37.ØX4	T37.ØX5	T37.ØX6
Sulfapyrimidine	T37.ØX1	T37.ØX2	T37.ØX3	T37.ØX4	T37.ØX5	T37.ØX6
Sulfarsphenamine	T37.8X1	T37.8X2	T37.8X3	T37.8X4	T37.8X5	T37.8X6
Sulfasalazine	T37.ØX1	T37.ØX2	T37.ØX3	T37.ØX4	T37.ØX5	T37.ØX6
Sulfasuxidine	T37.ØX1	T37.ØX2	T37.ØX3	T37.ØX4	T37.ØX5	T37.ØX6
Sulfasymazine	T37.ØX1	T37.ØX2	T37.ØX3	T37.ØX4	T37.ØX5	T37.ØX6
Sulfated amylopectin	T47.8X1	T47.8X2	T47.8X3	T47.8X4	T47.8X5	T47.8X6
Sulfathiazole	T37.ØX1	T37.ØX2	T37.ØX3	T37.ØX4	T37.ØX5	T37.ØX6
Sulfatostearate	T49.2X1	T49.2X2	T49.2X3	T49.2X4	T49.2X5	T49.2X6
Sulfinpyrazone	T5Ø.4X1	T5Ø.4X2	T5Ø.4X3	T5Ø.4X4	T5Ø.4X5	T5Ø.4X6
Sulfiram	T49.ØX1	T49.ØX2	T49.ØX3	T49.ØX4	T49.ØX5	T49.ØX6
Sulfisomidine	T37.ØX1	T37.ØX2	T37.ØX3	T37.ØX4	T37.ØX5	T37.ØX6
Sulfisoxazole	T37.ØX1	T37.ØX2	T37.ØX3	T37.ØX4	T37.ØX5	T37.ØX6
ophthalmic preparation	T49.5X1	T49.5X2	T49.5X3	T49.5X4	T49.5X5	T49.5X6
Sulfobromophthalein (sodium)	T5Ø.8X1	T5Ø.8X2	T5Ø.8X3	T5Ø.8X4	T5Ø.8X5	T5Ø.8X6
Sulfobromphthalein	T5Ø.8X1	T5Ø.8X2	T5Ø.8X3	T5Ø.8X4	T5Ø.8X5	T5Ø.8X6
Sulfogaiacol	T48.4X1	T48.4X2	T48.4X3	T48.4X4	T48.4X5	T48.4X6
Sulfomyxin	T36.8X1	T36.8X2	T36.8X3	T36.8X4	T36.8X5	T36.8X6
Sulfonal	T42.6X1	T42.6X2	T42.6X3	T42.6X4	T42.6X5	T42.6X6
Sulfonamide NEC	T37.ØX1	T37.ØX2	T37.ØX3	T37.ØX4	T37.ØX5	T37.ØX6
eye	T49.5X1	T49.5X2	T49.5X3	T49.5X4	T49.5X5	T49.5X6
Sulfonazide	T37.1X1	T37.1X2	T37.1X3	T37.1X4	T37.1X5	T37.1X6
Sulfones	T37.1X1	T37.1X2	T37.1X3	T37.1X4	T37.1X5	T37.1X6
Sulfonethylmethane	T42.6X1	T42.6X2	T42.6X3	T42.6X4	T42.6X5	T42.6X6
Sulfonmethane	T42.6X1	T42.6X2	T42.6X3	T42.6X4	T42.6X5	T42.6X6
Sulfonphthal, sulfonphthol	T5Ø.8X1	T5Ø.8X2	T5Ø.8X3	T5Ø.8X4	T5Ø.8X5	T5Ø.8X6
Sulfonylurea derivatives, oral	T38.3X1	T38.3X2	T38.3X3	T38.3X4	T38.3X5	T38.3X6
Sulforidazine	T43.3X1	T43.3X2	T43.3X3	T43.3X4	T43.3X5	T43.3X6
Sulfoxone	T37.1X1	T37.1X2	T37.1X3	T37.1X4	T37.1X5	T37.1X6
Sulfuric acid	T54.2X1	T54.2X2	T54.2X3	T54.2X4	—	—
Sulfur, sulfurated, sulfuric, sulfurous, sulfuryl (compounds NEC) (medicinal)	T49.4X1	T49.4X2	T49.4X3	T49.4X4	T49.4X5	T49.4X6
acid	T54.2X1	T54.2X2	T54.2X3	T54.2X4	—	—
dioxide (gas)	T59.1X1	T59.1X2	T59.1X3	T59.1X4	—	—
ether — *see* Ether(s)						
hydrogen	T59.6X1	T59.6X2	T59.6X3	T59.6X4	—	—
medicinal (keratolytic) (ointment) NEC	T49.4X1	T49.4X2	T49.4X3	T49.4X4	T49.4X5	T49.4X6
ointment	T49.ØX1	T49.ØX2	T49.ØX3	T49.ØX4	T49.ØX5	T49.ØX6
pesticide (vapor)	T6Ø.91	T6Ø.92	T6Ø.93	T6Ø.94	—	—
vapor NEC	T59.891	T59.892	T59.893	T59.894	—	—
Sulglicotide	T47.1X1	T47.1X2	T47.1X3	T47.1X4	T47.1X5	T47.1X6
Sulindac	T39.391	T39.392	T39.393	T39.394	T39.395	T39.396
Sulisatin	T47.2X1	T47.2X2	T47.2X3	T47.2X4	T47.2X5	T47.2X6
Sulisobenzone	T49.3X1	T49.3X2	T49.3X3	T49.3X4	T49.3X5	T49.3X6

Substance	Poisoning, Accidental (unintentional)	Poisoning, Intentional Self-harm	Poisoning, Assault	Poisoning, Undetermined	Adverse Effect	Under-dosing
Sulkowitch's reagent	T5Ø.8X1	T5Ø.8X2	T5Ø.8X3	T5Ø.8X4	T5Ø.8X5	T5Ø.8X6
Sulmetozine	T44.3X1	T44.3X2	T44.3X3	T44.3X4	T44.3X5	T44.3X6
Suloctidil	T46.7X1	T46.7X2	T46.7X3	T46.7X4	T46.7X5	T46.7X6
Sulph- — *see also* Sulf-						
Sulphadiazine	T37.ØX1	T37.ØX2	T37.ØX3	T37.ØX4	T37.ØX5	T37.ØX6
Sulphadimethoxine	T37.ØX1	T37.ØX2	T37.ØX3	T37.ØX4	T37.ØX5	T37.ØX6
Sulphadimidine	T37.ØX1	T37.ØX2	T37.ØX3	T37.ØX4	T37.ØX5	T37.ØX6
Sulphadione	T37.1X1	T37.1X2	T37.1X3	T37.1X4	T37.1X5	T37.1X6
Sulphafurazole	T37.ØX1	T37.ØX2	T37.ØX3	T37.ØX4	T37.ØX5	T37.ØX6
Sulphamethizole	T37.ØX1	T37.ØX2	T37.ØX3	T37.ØX4	T37.ØX5	T37.ØX6
Sulphamethoxazole	T37.ØX1	T37.ØX2	T37.ØX3	T37.ØX4	T37.ØX5	T37.ØX6
Sulphan blue	T5Ø.8X1	T5Ø.8X2	T5Ø.8X3	T5Ø.8X4	T5Ø.8X5	T5Ø.8X6
Sulphaphenazole	T37.ØX1	T37.ØX2	T37.ØX3	T37.ØX4	T37.ØX5	T37.ØX6
Sulphapyridine	T37.ØX1	T37.ØX2	T37.ØX3	T37.ØX4	T37.ØX5	T37.ØX6
Sulphasalazine	T37.ØX1	T37.ØX2	T37.ØX3	T37.ØX4	T37.ØX5	T37.ØX6
Sulphinpyrazone	T5Ø.4X1	T5Ø.4X2	T5Ø.4X3	T5Ø.4X4	T5Ø.4X5	T5Ø.4X6
Sulpiride	T43.591	T43.592	T43.593	T43.594	T43.595	T43.596
Sulprostone	T48.ØX1	T48.ØX2	T48.ØX3	T48.ØX4	T48.ØX5	T48.ØX6
Sulpyrine	T39.2X1	T39.2X2	T39.2X3	T39.2X4	T39.2X5	T39.2X6
Sultamicillin	T36.ØX1	T36.ØX2	T36.ØX3	T36.ØX4	T36.ØX5	T36.ØX6
Sulthiame	T42.6X1	T42.6X2	T42.6X3	T42.6X4	T42.6X5	T42.6X6
Sultiame	T42.6X1	T42.6X2	T42.6X3	T42.6X4	T42.6X5	T42.6X6
Sultopride	T43.591	T43.592	T43.593	T43.594	T43.595	T43.596
Sumatriptan	T39.8X1	T39.8X2	T39.8X3	T39.8X4	T39.8X5	T39.8X6
Sunflower seed oil	T46.6X1	T46.6X2	T46.6X3	T46.6X4	T46.6X5	T46.6X6
Superinone	T48.4X1	T48.4X2	T48.4X3	T48.4X4	T48.4X5	T48.4X6
Suprofen	T39.311	T39.312	T39.313	T39.314	T39.315	T39.316
Suramin (sodium)	T37.4X1	T37.4X2	T37.4X3	T37.4X4	T37.4X5	T37.4X6
Surfacaine	T41.3X1	T41.3X2	T41.3X3	T41.3X4	T41.3X5	T41.3X6
Surital	T41.1X1	T41.1X2	T41.1X3	T41.1X4	T41.1X5	T41.1X6
Sutilains	T45.3X1	T45.3X2	T45.3X3	T45.3X4	T45.3X5	T45.3X6
Suxamethonium (chloride)	T48.1X1	T48.1X2	T48.1X3	T48.1X4	T48.1X5	T48.1X6
Suxethonium (chloride)	T48.1X1	T48.1X2	T48.1X3	T48.1X4	T48.1X5	T48.1X6
Suxibuzone	T39.2X1	T39.2X2	T39.2X3	T39.2X4	T39.2X5	T39.2X6
Sweetener	T5Ø.9Ø1	T5Ø.9Ø2	T5Ø.9Ø3	T5Ø.9Ø4	T5Ø.9Ø5	T5Ø.9Ø6
Sweet niter spirit	T46.3X1	T46.3X2	T46.3X3	T46.3X4	T46.3X5	T46.3X6
Sweet oil (birch)	T49.3X1	T49.3X2	T49.3X3	T49.3X4	T49.3X5	T49.3X6
Sym-dichloroethyl ether	T53.6X1	T53.6X2	T53.6X3	T53.6X4	—	—
Sympatholytic NEC	T44.8X1	T44.8X2	T44.8X3	T44.8X4	T44.8X5	T44.8X6
haloalkylamine	T44.8X1	T44.8X2	T44.8X3	T44.8X4	T44.8X5	T44.8X6
Sympathomimetic NEC	T44.9Ø1	T44.9Ø2	T44.9Ø3	T44.9Ø4	T44.9Ø5	T44.9Ø6
anti-common-cold	T48.5X1	T48.5X2	T48.5X3	T48.5X4	T48.5X5	T48.5X6
bronchodilator	T48.6X1	T48.6X2	T48.6X3	T48.6X4	T48.6X5	T48.6X6
specified NEC	T44.991	T44.992	T44.993	T44.994	T44.995	T44.996
Synagis	T5Ø.B91	T5Ø.B92	T5Ø.B93	T5Ø.B94	T5Ø.B95	T5Ø.B96
Synalar	T49.ØX1	T49.ØX2	T49.ØX3	T49.ØX4	T49.ØX5	T49.ØX6
Synthroid	T38.1X1	T38.1X2	T38.1X3	T38.1X4	T38.1X5	T38.1X6
Syntocinon	T48.ØX1	T48.ØX2	T48.ØX3	T48.ØX4	T48.ØX5	T48.ØX6
Syrosingopine	T46.5X1	T46.5X2	T46.5X3	T46.5X4	T46.5X5	T46.5X6
Systemic drug	T45.91	T45.92	T45.93	T45.94	T45.95	T45.96
specified NEC	T45.8X1	T45.8X2	T45.8X3	T45.8X4	T45.8X5	T45.8X6
Tablets — *see also* specified substance	T5Ø.9Ø1	T5Ø.9Ø2	T5Ø.9Ø3	T5Ø.9Ø4	T5Ø.9Ø5	T5Ø.9Ø6
Tace	T38.5X1	T38.5X2	T38.5X3	T38.5X4	T38.5X5	T38.5X6
Tacrine	T44.ØX1	T44.ØX2	T44.ØX3	T44.ØX4	T44.ØX5	T44.ØX6
Tadalafil	T46.7X1	T46.7X2	T46.7X3	T46.7X4	T46.7X5	T46.7X6
Talampicillin	T36.ØX1	T36.ØX2	T36.ØX3	T36.ØX4	T36.ØX5	T36.ØX6
Talbutal	T42.3X1	T42.3X2	T42.3X3	T42.3X4	T42.3X5	T42.3X6
Talc powder	T49.3X1	T49.3X2	T49.3X3	T49.3X4	T49.3X5	T49.3X6
Talcum	T49.3X1	T49.3X2	T49.3X3	T49.3X4	T49.3X5	T49.3X6
Taleranol	T38.6X1	T38.6X2	T38.6X3	T38.6X4	T38.6X5	T38.6X6
Tamoxifen	T38.6X1	T38.6X2	T38.6X3	T38.6X4	T38.6X5	T38.6X6
Tamsulosin	T44.6X1	T44.6X2	T44.6X3	T44.6X4	T44.6X5	T44.6X6
Tandearil, tanderil	T39.2X1	T39.2X2	T39.2X3	T39.2X4	T39.2X5	T39.2X6
Tannic acid	T49.2X1	T49.2X2	T49.2X3	T49.2X4	T49.2X5	T49.2X6
medicinal (astringent)	T49.2X1	T49.2X2	T49.2X3	T49.2X4	T49.2X5	T49.2X6
Tannin — *see* Tannic acid						
Tansy	T62.2X1	T62.2X2	T62.2X3	T62.2X4	—	—
TAO	T36.3X1	T36.3X2	T36.3X3	T36.3X4	T36.3X5	T36.3X6
Tapazole	T38.2X1	T38.2X2	T38.2X3	T38.2X4	T38.2X5	T38.2X6
Taractan	T43.591	T43.592	T43.593	T43.594	T43.595	T43.596
Tarantula (venomous)	T63.321	T63.322	T63.323	T63.324	—	—
Tartar emetic	T37.8X1	T37.8X2	T37.8X3	T37.8X4	T37.8X5	T37.8X6
Tartaric acid	T65.891	T65.892	T65.893	T65.894	—	—
Tartrated antimony (anti-infective)	T37.8X1	T37.8X2	T37.8X3	T37.8X4	T37.8X5	T37.8X6
Tartrate, laxative	T47.4X1	T47.4X2	T47.4X3	T47.4X4	T47.4X5	T47.4X6
Tar NEC	T52.ØX1	T52.ØX2	T52.ØX3	T52.ØX4	—	—
camphor	T6Ø.1X1	T6Ø.1X2	T6Ø.1X3	T6Ø.1X4	—	—
distillate	T49.1X1	T49.1X2	T49.1X3	T49.1X4	T49.1X5	T49.1X6
fumes	T59.891	T59.892	T59.893	T59.894	—	—
medicinal	T49.1X1	T49.1X2	T49.1X3	T49.1X4	T49.1X5	T49.1X6
ointment	T49.1X1	T49.1X2	T49.1X3	T49.1X4	T49.1X5	T49.1X6

Substance	Poisoning, Accidental (unintentional)	Poisoning, Intentional Self-harm	Poisoning, Assault	Poisoning, Undetermined	Adverse Effect	Under-dosing
Tauromustine	T45.1X1	T45.1X2	T45.1X3	T45.1X4	T45.1X5	T45.1X6
TCA — *see* Trichloroacetic acid						
TCDD	T53.7X1	T53.7X2	T53.7X3	T53.7X4	—	—
TDI (vapor)	T65.ØX1	T65.ØX2	T65.ØX3	T65.ØX4	—	—
Tear						
gas	T59.3X1	T59.3X2	T59.3X3	T59.3X4	—	—
solution	T49.5X1	T49.5X2	T49.5X3	T49.5X4	T49.5X5	T49.5X6
Teclothiazide	T5Ø.2X1	T5Ø.2X2	T5Ø.2X3	T5Ø.2X4	T5Ø.2X5	T5Ø.2X6
Teclozan	T37.3X1	T37.3X2	T37.3X3	T37.3X4	T37.3X5	T37.3X6
Tegafur	T45.1X1	T45.1X2	T45.1X3	T45.1X4	T45.1X5	T45.1X6
Tegretol	T42.1X1	T42.1X2	T42.1X3	T42.1X4	T42.1X5	T42.1X6
Teicoplanin	T36.8X1	T36.8X2	T36.8X3	T36.8X4	T36.8X5	T36.8X6
Telepaque	T5Ø.8X1	T5Ø.8X2	T5Ø.8X3	T5Ø.8X4	T5Ø.8X5	T5Ø.8X6
Tellurium	T56.891	T56.892	T56.893	T56.894	—	—
fumes	T56.891	T56.892	T56.893	T56.894	—	—
TEM	T45.1X1	T45.1X2	T45.1X3	T45.1X4	T45.1X5	T45.1X6
Temazepam	T42.4X1	T42.4X2	T42.4X3	T42.4X4	T42.4X5	T42.4X6
Temocillin	T36.ØX1	T36.ØX2	T36.ØX3	T36.ØX4	T36.ØX5	T36.ØX6
Tenamfetamine	T43.621	T43.622	T43.623	T43.624	T43.625	T43.626
Teniposide	T45.1X1	T45.1X2	T45.1X3	T45.1X4	T45.1X5	T45.1X6
Tenitramine	T46.3X1	T46.3X2	T46.3X3	T46.3X4	T46.3X5	T46.3X6
Tenoglicin	T48.4X1	T48.4X2	T48.4X3	T48.4X4	T48.4X5	T48.4X6
Tenonitrozole	T37.3X1	T37.3X2	T37.3X3	T37.3X4	T37.3X5	T37.3X6
Tenoxicam	T39.391	T39.392	T39.393	T39.394	T39.395	T39.396
TEPA	T45.1X1	T45.1X2	T45.1X3	T45.1X4	T45.1X5	T45.1X6
TEPP	T6Ø.ØX1	T6Ø.ØX2	T6Ø.ØX3	T6Ø.ØX4	—	—
Teprotide	T46.5X1	T46.5X2	T46.5X3	T46.5X4	T46.5X5	T46.5X6
Terazosin	T44.6X1	T44.6X2	T44.6X3	T44.6X4	T44.6X5	T44.6X6
Terbufos	T6Ø.ØX1	T6Ø.ØX2	T6Ø.ØX3	T6Ø.ØX4	—	—
Terbutaline	T48.6X1	T48.6X2	T48.6X3	T48.6X4	T48.6X5	T48.6X6
Terconazole	T49.ØX1	T49.ØX2	T49.ØX3	T49.ØX4	T49.ØX5	T49.ØX6
Terfenadine	T45.ØX1	T45.ØX2	T45.ØX3	T45.ØX4	T45.ØX5	T45.ØX6
Teriparatide (acetate)	T5Ø.991	T5Ø.992	T5Ø.993	T5Ø.994	T5Ø.995	T5Ø.996
Terizidone	T37.1X1	T37.1X2	T37.1X3	T37.1X4	T37.1X5	T37.1X6
Terlipressin	T38.891	T38.892	T38.893	T38.894	T38.895	T38.896
Terodiline	T46.3X1	T46.3X2	T46.3X3	T46.3X4	T46.3X5	T46.3X6
Teroxalene	T37.4X1	T37.4X2	T37.4X3	T37.4X4	T37.4X5	T37.4X6
Terpin (cis) **hydrate**	T48.4X1	T48.4X2	T48.4X3	T48.4X4	T48.4X5	T48.4X6
Terramycin	T36.4X1	T36.4X2	T36.4X3	T36.4X4	T36.4X5	T36.4X6
Tertatolol	T44.7X1	T44.7X2	T44.7X3	T44.7X4	T44.7X5	T44.7X6
Tessalon	T48.3X1	T48.3X2	T48.3X3	T48.3X4	T48.3X5	T48.3X6
Testolactone	T38.7X1	T38.7X2	T38.7X3	T38.7X4	T38.7X5	T38.7X6
Testosterone	T38.7X1	T38.7X2	T38.7X3	T38.7X4	T38.7X5	T38.7X6
Tetanus toxoid or vaccine	T5Ø.A91	T5Ø.A92	T5Ø.A93	T5Ø.A94	T5Ø.A95	T5Ø.A96
antitoxin	T5Ø.Z11	T5Ø.Z12	T5Ø.Z13	T5Ø.Z14	T5Ø.Z15	T5Ø.Z16
immune globulin (human)	T5Ø.Z11	T5Ø.Z12	T5Ø.Z13	T5Ø.Z14	T5Ø.Z15	T5Ø.Z16
toxoid	T5Ø.A91	T5Ø.A92	T5Ø.A93	T5Ø.A94	T5Ø.A95	T5Ø.A96
with diphtheria toxoid	T5Ø.A21	T5Ø.A22	T5Ø.A23	T5Ø.A24	T5Ø.A25	T5Ø.A26
with pertussis	T5Ø.A11	T5Ø.A12	T5Ø.A13	T5Ø.A14	T5Ø.A15	T5Ø.A16
Tetrabenazine	T43.591	T43.592	T43.593	T43.594	T43.595	T43.596
Tetracaine	T41.3X1	T41.3X2	T41.3X3	T41.3X4	T41.3X5	T41.3X6
nerve block (peripheral) (plexus)	T41.3X1	T41.3X2	T41.3X3	T41.3X4	T41.3X5	T41.3X6
regional	T41.3X1	T41.3X2	T41.3X3	T41.3X4	T41.3X5	T41.3X6
spinal	T41.3X1	T41.3X2	T41.3X3	T41.3X4	T41.3X5	T41.3X6
Tetrachlorethylene — *see* Tetrachloroethylene						
Tetrachlormethiazide	T5Ø.2X1	T5Ø.2X2	T5Ø.2X3	T5Ø.2X4	T5Ø.2X5	T5Ø.2X6
Tetrachloroethane	T53.6X1	T53.6X2	T53.6X3	T53.6X4	—	—
vapor	T53.6X1	T53.6X2	T53.6X3	T53.6X4	—	—
paint or varnish	T53.6X1	T53.6X2	T53.6X3	T53.6X4	—	—
Tetrachloroethylene (liquid)	T53.3X1	T53.3X2	T53.3X3	T53.3X4	—	—
medicinal	T37.4X1	T37.4X2	T37.4X3	T37.4X4	T37.4X5	T37.4X6
vapor	T53.3X1	T53.3X2	T53.3X3	T53.3X4	—	—
Tetrachloromethane — *see* Carbon tetrachloride						
Tetracosactide	T38.811	T38.812	T38.813	T38.814	T38.815	T38.816
Tetracosactrin	T38.811	T38.812	T38.813	T38.814	T38.815	T38.816
Tetracycline	T36.4X1	T36.4X2	T36.4X3	T36.4X4	T36.4X5	T36.4X6
ophthalmic preparation	T49.5X1	T49.5X2	T49.5X3	T49.5X4	T49.5X5	T49.5X6
topical NEC	T49.ØX1	T49.ØX2	T49.ØX3	T49.ØX4	T49.ØX5	T49.ØX6
Tetradifon	T6Ø.8X1	T6Ø.8X2	T6Ø.8X3	T6Ø.8X4	—	—
Tetradotoxin	T61.771	T61.772	T61.773	T61.774	—	—
Tetraethyl						
lead	T56.ØX1	T56.ØX2	T56.ØX3	T56.ØX4	—	—
pyrophosphate	T6Ø.ØX1	T6Ø.ØX2	T6Ø.ØX3	T6Ø.ØX4	—	—
Tetraethylammonium chloride	T44.2X1	T44.2X2	T44.2X3	T44.2X4	T44.2X5	T44.2X6
Tetraethylthiuram disulfide	T5Ø.6X1	T5Ø.6X2	T5Ø.6X3	T5Ø.6X4	T5Ø.6X5	T5Ø.6X6
Tetrahydroaminoacridine	T44.ØX1	T44.ØX2	T44.ØX3	T44.ØX4	T44.ØX5	T44.ØX6
Tetrahydrocannabinol	T4Ø.7X1	T4Ø.7X2	T4Ø.7X3	T4Ø.7X4	T4Ø.7X5	T4Ø.7X6
Tetrahydrofuran	T52.8X1	T52.8X2	T52.8X3	T52.8X4	—	—
Tetrahydronaphthalene	T52.8X1	T52.8X2	T52.8X3	T52.8X4	—	—
Tetrahydrozoline	T49.5X1	T49.5X2	T49.5X3	T49.5X4	T49.5X5	T49.5X6
Tetralin	T52.8X1	T52.8X2	T52.8X3	T52.8X4	—	—
Tetramethrin	T6Ø.2X1	T6Ø.2X2	T6Ø.2X3	T6Ø.2X4	—	—
Tetramethylthiuram (disulfide) **NEC**	T6Ø.3X1	T6Ø.3X2	T6Ø.3X3	T6Ø.3X4	—	—
medicinal	T49.ØX1	T49.ØX2	T49.ØX3	T49.ØX4	T49.ØX5	T49.ØX6
Tetramisole	T37.4X1	T37.4X2	T37.4X3	T37.4X4	T37.4X5	T37.4X6
Tetranicotinoyl fructose	T46.7X1	T46.7X2	T46.7X3	T46.7X4	T46.7X5	T46.7X6
Tetrazepam	T42.4X1	T42.4X2	T42.4X3	T42.4X4	T42.4X5	T42.4X6
Tetronal	T42.6X1	T42.6X2	T42.6X3	T42.6X4	T42.6X5	T42.6X6
Tetryl	T65.3X1	T65.3X2	T65.3X3	T65.3X4	—	—
Tetrylammonium chloride	T44.2X1	T44.2X2	T44.2X3	T44.2X4	T44.2X5	T44.2X6
Tetryzoline	T49.5X1	T49.5X2	T49.5X3	T49.5X4	T49.5X5	T49.5X6
Thalidomide	T45.1X1	T45.1X2	T45.1X3	T45.1X4	T45.1X5	T45.1X6
Thallium (compounds) (dust) **NEC**	T56.811	T56.812	T56.813	T56.814	—	—
pesticide	T6Ø.4X1	T6Ø.4X2	T6Ø.4X3	T6Ø.4X4	—	—
THC	T4Ø.7X1	T4Ø.7X2	T4Ø.7X3	T4Ø.7X4	T4Ø.7X5	T4Ø.7X6
Thebacon	T48.3X1	T48.3X2	T48.3X3	T48.3X4	T48.3X5	T48.3X6
Thebaine	T4Ø.2X1	T4Ø.2X2	T4Ø.2X3	T4Ø.2X4	T4Ø.2X5	T4Ø.2X6
Thenoic acid	T49.6X1	T49.6X2	T49.6X3	T49.6X4	T49.6X5	T49.6X6
Thenyldiamine	T45.ØX1	T45.ØX2	T45.ØX3	T45.ØX4	T45.ØX5	T45.ØX6
Theobromine (calcium salicylate)	T48.6X1	T48.6X2	T48.6X3	T48.6X4	T48.6X5	T48.6X6
sodium salicylate	T48.6X1	T48.6X2	T48.6X3	T48.6X4	T48.6X5	T48.6X6
Theophyllamine	T48.6X1	T48.6X2	T48.6X3	T48.6X4	T48.6X5	T48.6X6
Theophylline	T48.6X1	T48.6X2	T48.6X3	T48.6X4	T48.6X5	T48.6X6
aminobenzoic acid	T48.6X1	T48.6X2	T48.6X3	T48.6X4	T48.6X5	T48.6X6
ethylenediamine	T48.6X1	T48.6X2	T48.6X3	T48.6X4	T48.6X5	T48.6X6
piperazine p-amino-benzoate	T48.6X1	T48.6X2	T48.6X3	T48.6X4	T48.6X5	T48.6X6
Thiabendazole	T37.4X1	T37.4X2	T37.4X3	T37.4X4	T37.4X5	T37.4X6
Thialbarbital	T41.1X1	T41.1X2	T41.1X3	T41.1X4	T41.1X5	T41.1X6
Thiamazole	T38.2X1	T38.2X2	T38.2X3	T38.2X4	T38.2X5	T38.2X6
Thiambutosine	T37.1X1	T37.1X2	T37.1X3	T37.1X4	T37.1X5	T37.1X6
Thiamine	T45.2X1	T45.2X2	T45.2X3	T45.2X4	T45.2X5	T45.2X6
Thiamphenicol	T36.2X1	T36.2X2	T36.2X3	T36.2X4	T36.2X5	T36.2X6
Thiamylal	T41.1X1	T41.1X2	T41.1X3	T41.1X4	T41.1X5	T41.1X6
sodium	T41.1X1	T41.1X2	T41.1X3	T41.1X4	T41.1X5	T41.1X6
Thiazesim	T43.291	T43.292	T43.293	T43.294	T43.295	T43.296
Thiazides (diuretics)	T5Ø.2X1	T5Ø.2X2	T5Ø.2X3	T5Ø.2X4	T5Ø.2X5	T5Ø.2X6
Thiazinamium metilsulfate	T43.3X1	T43.3X2	T43.3X3	T43.3X4	T43.3X5	T43.3X6
Thiethylperazine	T43.3X1	T43.3X2	T43.3X3	T43.3X4	T43.3X5	T43.3X6
Thimerosal	T49.ØX1	T49.ØX2	T49.ØX3	T49.ØX4	T49.ØX5	T49.ØX6
ophthalmic preparation	T49.5X1	T49.5X2	T49.5X3	T49.5X4	T49.5X5	T49.5X6
Thioacetazone	T37.1X1	T37.1X2	T37.1X3	T37.1X4	T37.1X5	T37.1X6
with isoniazid	T37.1X1	T37.1X2	T37.1X3	T37.1X4	T37.1X5	T37.1X6
Thiobarbital sodium	T41.1X1	T41.1X2	T41.1X3	T41.1X4	T41.1X5	T41.1X6
Thiobarbiturate anesthetic	T41.1X1	T41.1X2	T41.1X3	T41.1X4	T41.1X5	T41.1X6
Thiobismol	T37.8X1	T37.8X2	T37.8X3	T37.8X4	T37.8X5	T37.8X6
Thiobutabarbital sodium	T41.1X1	T41.1X2	T41.1X3	T41.1X4	T41.1X5	T41.1X6
Thiocarbamate (insecticide)	T6Ø.ØX1	T6Ø.ØX2	T6Ø.ØX3	T6Ø.ØX4	—	—
Thiocarbamide	T38.2X1	T38.2X2	T38.2X3	T38.2X4	T38.2X5	T38.2X6
Thiocarbarsone	T37.8X1	T37.8X2	T37.8X3	T37.8X4	T37.8X5	T37.8X6
Thiocarlide	T37.1X1	T37.1X2	T37.1X3	T37.1X4	T37.1X5	T37.1X6
Thioctamide	T5Ø.991	T5Ø.992	T5Ø.993	T5Ø.994	T5Ø.995	T5Ø.996
Thioctic acid	T5Ø.991	T5Ø.992	T5Ø.993	T5Ø.994	T5Ø.995	T5Ø.996
Thiofos	T6Ø.ØX1	T6Ø.ØX2	T6Ø.ØX3	T6Ø.ØX4	—	—
Thioglycolate	T49.4X1	T49.4X2	T49.4X3	T49.4X4	T49.4X5	T49.4X6
Thioglycolic acid	T65.891	T65.892	T65.893	T65.894	—	—
Thioguanine	T45.1X1	T45.1X2	T45.1X3	T45.1X4	T45.1X5	T45.1X6
Thiomercaptomerin	T5Ø.2X1	T5Ø.2X2	T5Ø.2X3	T5Ø.2X4	T5Ø.2X5	T5Ø.2X6
Thiomerin	T5Ø.2X1	T5Ø.2X2	T5Ø.2X3	T5Ø.2X4	T5Ø.2X5	T5Ø.2X6
Thiomersal	T49.ØX1	T49.ØX2	T49.ØX3	T49.ØX4	T49.ØX5	T49.ØX6
Thionazin	T6Ø.ØX1	T6Ø.ØX2	T6Ø.ØX3	T6Ø.ØX4	—	—
Thiopental (sodium)	T41.1X1	T41.1X2	T41.1X3	T41.1X4	T41.1X5	T41.1X6
Thiopentone (sodium)	T41.1X1	T41.1X2	T41.1X3	T41.1X4	T41.1X5	T41.1X6
Thiopropazate	T43.3X1	T43.3X2	T43.3X3	T43.3X4	T43.3X5	T43.3X6
Thioproperazine	T43.3X1	T43.3X2	T43.3X3	T43.3X4	T43.3X5	T43.3X6
Thioridazine	T43.3X1	T43.3X2	T43.3X3	T43.3X4	T43.3X5	T43.3X6
Thiosinamine	T49.3X1	T49.3X2	T49.3X3	T49.3X4	T49.3X5	T49.3X6
Thiotepa	T45.1X1	T45.1X2	T45.1X3	T45.1X4	T45.1X5	T45.1X6
Thiothixene	T43.4X1	T43.4X2	T43.4X3	T43.4X4	T43.4X5	T43.4X6
Thiouracil (benzyl) (methyl) (propyl)	T38.2X1	T38.2X2	T38.2X3	T38.2X4	T38.2X5	T38.2X6
Thiourea	T38.2X1	T38.2X2	T38.2X3	T38.2X4	T38.2X5	T38.2X6
Thiphenamil	T44.3X1	T44.3X2	T44.3X3	T44.3X4	T44.3X5	T44.3X6
Thiram	T6Ø.3X1	T6Ø.3X2	T6Ø.3X3	T6Ø.3X4	—	—
medicinal	T49.2X1	T49.2X2	T49.2X3	T49.2X4	T49.2X5	T49.2X6
Thonzylamine (systemic)	T45.ØX1	T45.ØX2	T45.ØX3	T45.ØX4	T45.ØX5	T45.ØX6
mucosal decongestant	T48.5X1	T48.5X2	T48.5X3	T48.5X4	T48.5X5	T48.5X6

Substance	Poisoning, Accidental (unintentional)	Poisoning, Intentional Self-harm	Poisoning, Assault	Poisoning, Undetermined	Adverse Effect	Under-dosing
Thorazine	T43.3X1	T43.3X2	T43.3X3	T43.3X4	T43.3X5	T43.3X6
Thorium dioxide suspension	T50.8X1	T50.8X2	T50.8X3	T50.8X4	T50.8X5	T50.8X6
Thornapple	T62.2X1	T62.2X2	T62.2X3	T62.2X4	—	—
Throat drug NEC	T49.6X1	T49.6X2	T49.6X3	T49.6X4	T49.6X5	T49.6X6
Thrombin	T45.7X1	T45.7X2	T45.7X3	T45.7X4	T45.7X5	T45.7X6
Thrombolysin	T45.611	T45.612	T45.613	T45.614	T45.615	T45.616
Thromboplastin	T45.7X1	T45.7X2	T45.7X3	T45.7X4	T45.7X5	T45.7X6
Thurfyl nicotinate	T46.7X1	T46.7X2	T46.7X3	T46.7X4	T46.7X5	T46.7X6
Thymol	T49.0X1	T49.0X2	T49.0X3	T49.0X4	T49.0X5	T49.0X6
Thymopentin	T37.5X1	T37.5X2	T37.5X3	T37.5X4	T37.5X5	T37.5X6
Thymoxamine	T46.7X1	T46.7X2	T46.7X3	T46.7X4	T46.7X5	T46.7X6
Thymus extract	T38.891	T38.892	T38.893	T38.894	T38.895	T38.896
Thyreotrophic hormone	T38.811	T38.812	T38.813	T38.814	T38.815	T38.816
Thyroglobulin	T38.1X1	T38.1X2	T38.1X3	T38.1X4	T38.1X5	T38.1X6
Thyroid (hormone)	T38.1X1	T38.1X2	T38.1X3	T38.1X4	T38.1X5	T38.1X6
Thyrolar	T38.1X1	T38.1X2	T38.1X3	T38.1X4	T38.1X5	T38.1X6
Thyrotrophin	T38.811	T38.812	T38.813	T38.814	T38.815	T38.816
Thyrotropic hormone	T38.811	T38.812	T38.813	T38.814	T38.815	T38.816
Thyroxine	T38.1X1	T38.1X2	T38.1X3	T38.1X4	T38.1X5	T38.1X6
Tiabendazole	T37.4X1	T37.4X2	T37.4X3	T37.4X4	T37.4X5	T37.4X6
Tiamizide	T50.2X1	T50.2X2	T50.2X3	T50.2X4	T50.2X5	T50.2X6
Tianeptine	T43.291	T43.292	T43.293	T43.294	T43.295	T43.296
Tiapamil	T46.1X1	T46.1X2	T46.1X3	T46.1X4	T46.1X5	T46.1X6
Tiapride	T43.591	T43.592	T43.593	T43.594	T43.595	T43.596
Tiaprofenic acid	T39.311	T39.312	T39.313	T39.314	T39.315	T39.316
Tiaramide	T39.8X1	T39.8X2	T39.8X3	T39.8X4	T39.8X5	T39.8X6
Ticarcillin	T36.0X1	T36.0X2	T36.0X3	T36.0X4	T36.0X5	T36.0X6
Ticlatone	T49.0X1	T49.0X2	T49.0X3	T49.0X4	T49.0X5	T49.0X6
Ticlopidine	T45.521	T45.522	T45.523	T45.524	T45.525	T45.526
Ticrynafen	T50.1X1	T50.1X2	T50.1X3	T50.1X4	T50.1X5	T50.1X6
Tidiacic	T50.991	T50.992	T50.993	T50.994	T50.995	T50.996
Tiemonium	T44.3X1	T44.3X2	T44.3X3	T44.3X4	T44.3X5	T44.3X6
iodide	T44.3X1	T44.3X2	T44.3X3	T44.3X4	T44.3X5	T44.3X6
Tienilic acid	T50.1X1	T50.1X2	T50.1X3	T50.1X4	T50.1X5	T50.1X6
Tifenamil	T44.3X1	T44.3X2	T44.3X3	T44.3X4	T44.3X5	T44.3X6
Tigan	T45.0X1	T45.0X2	T45.0X3	T45.0X4	T45.0X5	T45.0X6
Tigloidine	T44.3X1	T44.3X2	T44.3X3	T44.3X4	T44.3X5	T44.3X6
Tilactase	T47.5X1	T47.5X2	T47.5X3	T47.5X4	T47.5X5	T47.5X6
Tiletamine	T41.291	T41.292	T41.293	T41.294	T41.295	T41.296
Tilidine	T40.4X1	T40.4X2	T40.4X3	T40.4X4	—	—
Timepidium bromide	T44.3X1	T44.3X2	T44.3X3	T44.3X4	T44.3X5	T44.3X6
Timiperone	T43.4X1	T43.4X2	T43.4X3	T43.4X4	T43.4X5	T43.4X6
Timolol	T44.7X1	T44.7X2	T44.7X3	T44.7X4	T44.7X5	T44.7X6
Tincture, iodine — *see* Iodine						
Tindal	T43.3X1	T43.3X2	T43.3X3	T43.3X4	T43.3X5	T43.3X6
Tinidazole	T37.3X1	T37.3X2	T37.3X3	T37.3X4	T37.3X5	T37.3X6
Tinoridine	T39.8X1	T39.8X2	T39.8X3	T39.8X4	T39.8X5	T39.8X6
Tin (chloride) (dust) (oxide) **NEC**	T56.6X1	T56.6X2	T56.6X3	T56.6X4	—	—
anti-infectives	T37.8X1	T37.8X2	T37.8X3	T37.8X4	T37.8X5	T37.8X6
Tiocarlide	T37.1X1	T37.1X2	T37.1X3	T37.1X4	T37.1X5	T37.1X6
Tioclomarol	T45.511	T45.512	T45.513	T45.514	T45.515	T45.516
Tioconazole	T49.0X1	T49.0X2	T49.0X3	T49.0X4	T49.0X5	T49.0X6
Tioguanine	T45.1X1	T45.1X2	T45.1X3	T45.1X4	T45.1X5	T45.1X6
Tiopronin	T50.991	T50.992	T50.993	T50.994	T50.995	T50.996
Tiotixene	T43.4X1	T43.4X2	T43.4X3	T43.4X4	T43.4X5	T43.4X6
Tioxolone	T49.4X1	T49.4X2	T49.4X3	T49.4X4	T49.4X5	T49.4X6
Tipepidine	T48.3X1	T48.3X2	T48.3X3	T48.3X4	T48.3X5	T48.3X6
Tiquizium bromide	T44.3X1	T44.3X2	T44.3X3	T44.3X4	T44.3X5	T44.3X6
Tiratricol	T38.1X1	T38.1X2	T38.1X3	T38.1X4	T38.1X5	T38.1X6
Tisopurine	T50.4X1	T50.4X2	T50.4X3	T50.4X4	T50.4X5	T50.4X6
Titanium (compounds) (vapor)	T56.891	T56.892	T56.893	T56.894	—	—
dioxide	T49.3X1	T49.3X2	T49.3X3	T49.3X4	T49.3X5	T49.3X6
ointment	T49.3X1	T49.3X2	T49.3X3	T49.3X4	T49.3X5	T49.3X6
oxide	T49.3X1	T49.3X2	T49.3X3	T49.3X4	T49.3X5	T49.3X6
tetrachloride	T56.891	T56.892	T56.893	T56.894	—	—
Titanocene	T56.891	T56.892	T56.893	T56.894	—	—
Titroid	T38.1X1	T38.1X2	T38.1X3	T38.1X4	T38.1X5	T38.1X6
Tizanidine	T42.8X1	T42.8X2	T42.8X3	T42.8X4	T42.8X5	T42.8X6
TMTD	T60.3X1	T60.3X2	T60.3X3	T60.3X4	—	—
TNT (fumes)	T65.3X1	T65.3X2	T65.3X3	T65.3X4	—	—
Toadstool	T62.0X1	T62.0X2	T62.0X3	T62.0X4	—	—
Tobacco NEC	T65.291	T65.292	T65.293	T65.294	—	—
cigarettes	T65.221	T65.222	T65.223	T65.224	—	—
Indian	T62.2X1	T62.2X2	T62.2X3	T62.2X4	—	—
smoke, second-hand	T65.221	T65.222	T65.223	T65.224	—	—
Tobramycin	T36.5X1	T36.5X2	T36.5X3	T36.5X4	T36.5X5	T36.5X6
Tocainide	T46.2X1	T46.2X2	T46.2X3	T46.2X4	T46.2X5	T46.2X6
Tocoferol	T45.2X1	T45.2X2	T45.2X3	T45.2X4	T45.2X5	T45.2X6
Tocopherol	T45.2X1	T45.2X2	T45.2X3	T45.2X4	T45.2X5	T45.2X6
acetate	T45.2X1	T45.2X2	T45.2X3	T45.2X4	T45.2X5	T45.2X6
Tocosamine	T48.0X1	T48.0X2	T48.0X3	T48.0X4	T48.0X5	T48.0X6
Todralazine	T46.5X1	T46.5X2	T46.5X3	T46.5X4	T46.5X5	T46.5X6
Tofisopam	T42.4X1	T42.4X2	T42.4X3	T42.4X4	T42.4X5	T42.4X6
Tofranil	T43.011	T43.012	T43.013	T43.014	T43.015	T43.016
Toilet deodorizer	T65.891	T65.892	T65.893	T65.894	—	—
Tolamolol	T44.7X1	T44.7X2	T44.7X3	T44.7X4	T44.7X5	T44.7X6
Tolazamide	T38.3X1	T38.3X2	T38.3X3	T38.3X4	T38.3X5	T38.3X6
Tolazoline	T46.7X1	T46.7X2	T46.7X3	T46.7X4	T46.7X5	T46.7X6
Tolbutamide (sodium)	T38.3X1	T38.3X2	T38.3X3	T38.3X4	T38.3X5	T38.3X6
Tolciclate	T49.0X1	T49.0X2	T49.0X3	T49.0X4	T49.0X5	T49.0X6
Tolmetin	T39.391	T39.392	T39.393	T39.394	T39.395	T39.396
Tolnaftate	T49.0X1	T49.0X2	T49.0X3	T49.0X4	T49.0X5	T49.0X6
Tolonidine	T46.5X1	T46.5X2	T46.5X3	T46.5X4	T46.5X5	T46.5X6
Toloxatone	T42.6X1	T42.6X2	T42.6X3	T42.6X4	T42.6X5	T42.6X6
Tolperisone	T44.3X1	T44.3X2	T44.3X3	T44.3X4	T44.3X5	T44.3X6
Tolserol	T42.8X1	T42.8X2	T42.8X3	T42.8X4	T42.8X5	T42.8X6
Toluene (liquid)	T52.2X1	T52.2X2	T52.2X3	T52.2X4	—	—
diisocyanate	T65.0X1	T65.0X2	T65.0X3	T65.0X4	—	—
Toluidine	T65.891	T65.892	T65.893	T65.894	—	—
vapor	T59.891	T59.892	T59.893	T59.894	—	—
Toluol (liquid)	T52.2X1	T52.2X2	T52.2X3	T52.2X4	—	—
vapor	T52.2X1	T52.2X2	T52.2X3	T52.2X4	—	—
Toluylenediamine	T65.3X1	T65.3X2	T65.3X3	T65.3X4	—	—
Tolylene-2,4-diisocyanate	T65.0X1	T65.0X2	T65.0X3	T65.0X4	—	—
Tonic NEC	T50.901	T50.902	T50.903	T50.904	T50.905	T50.906
Topical action drug NEC	T49.91	T49.92	T49.93	T49.94	T49.95	T49.96
ear, nose or throat	T49.6X1	T49.6X2	T49.6X3	T49.6X4	T49.6X5	T49.6X6
eye	T49.5X1	T49.5X2	T49.5X3	T49.5X4	T49.5X5	T49.5X6
skin	T49.91	T49.92	T49.93	T49.94	T49.95	T49.96
specified NEC	T49.8X1	T49.8X2	T49.8X3	T49.8X4	T49.8X5	T49.8X6
Toquizine	T44.3X1	T44.3X2	T44.3X3	T44.3X4	T44.3X5	T44.3X6
Toremifene	T38.6X1	T38.6X2	T38.6X3	T38.6X4	T38.6X5	T38.6X6
Tosylchloramide sodium	T49.8X1	T49.8X2	T49.8X3	T49.8X4	T49.8X5	T49.8X6
Toxaphene (dust) (spray)	T60.1X1	T60.1X2	T60.1X3	T60.1X4	—	—
Toxin, diphtheria (Schick Test)	T50.8X1	T50.8X2	T50.8X3	T50.8X4	T50.8X5	T50.8X6
Toxoid						
combined	T50.A21	T50.A22	T50.A23	T50.A24	T50.A25	T50.A26
diphtheria	T50.A91	T50.A92	T50.A93	T50.A94	T50.A95	T50.A96
tetanus	T50.A91	T50.A92	T50.A93	T50.A94	T50.A95	T50.A96
Trace element NEC	T45.8X1	T45.8X2	T45.8X3	T45.8X4	T45.8X5	T45.8X6
Tractor fuel NEC	T52.0X1	T52.0X2	T52.0X3	T52.0X4	—	—
Tragacanth	T50.991	T50.992	T50.993	T50.994	T50.995	T50.996
Tramadol	T40.4X1	T40.4X2	T40.4X3	T40.4X4	T40.4X5	T40.4X6
Tramazoline	T48.5X1	T48.5X2	T48.5X3	T48.5X4	T48.5X5	T48.5X6
Tranexamic acid	T45.621	T45.622	T45.623	T45.624	T45.625	T45.626
Tranilast	T45.0X1	T45.0X2	T45.0X3	T45.0X4	T45.0X5	T45.0X6
Tranquilizer NEC	T43.501	T43.502	T43.503	T43.504	T43.505	T43.506
with hypnotic or sedative	T42.6X1	T42.6X2	T42.6X3	T42.6X4	T42.6X5	T42.6X6
benzodiazepine NEC	T42.4X1	T42.4X2	T42.4X3	T42.4X4	T42.4X5	T42.4X6
butyrophenone NEC	T43.4X1	T43.4X2	T43.4X3	T43.4X4	T43.4X5	T43.4X6
carbamate	T43.591	T43.592	T43.593	T43.594	T43.595	T43.596
dimethylamine	T43.3X1	T43.3X2	T43.3X3	T43.3X4	T43.3X5	T43.3X6
ethylamine	T43.3X1	T43.3X2	T43.3X3	T43.3X4	T43.3X5	T43.3X6
hydroxyzine	T43.591	T43.592	T43.593	T43.594	T43.595	T43.596
major NEC	T43.501	T43.502	T43.503	T43.504	T43.505	T43.506
penothiazine NEC	T43.3X1	T43.3X2	T43.3X3	T43.3X4	T43.3X5	T43.3X6
phenothiazine-based	T43.3X1	T43.3X2	T43.3X3	T43.3X4	T43.3X5	T43.3X6
piperazine NEC	T43.3X1	T43.3X2	T43.3X3	T43.3X4	T43.3X5	T43.3X6
piperidine	T43.3X1	T43.3X2	T43.3X3	T43.3X4	T43.3X5	T43.3X6
propylamine	T43.3X1	T43.3X2	T43.3X3	T43.3X4	T43.3X5	T43.3X6
specified NEC	T43.591	T43.592	T43.593	T43.594	T43.595	T43.596
thioxanthene NEC	T43.591	T43.592	T43.593	T43.594	T43.595	T43.596
Tranxene	T42.4X1	T42.4X2	T42.4X3	T42.4X4	T42.4X5	T42.4X6
Tranylcypromine	T43.1X1	T43.1X2	T43.1X3	T43.1X4	T43.1X5	T43.1X6
Trapidil	T46.3X1	T46.3X2	T46.3X3	T46.3X4	T46.3X5	T46.3X6
Trasentine	T44.3X1	T44.3X2	T44.3X3	T44.3X4	T44.3X5	T44.3X6
Travert	T50.3X1	T50.3X2	T50.3X3	T50.3X4	T50.3X5	T50.3X6
Trazodone	T43.211	T43.212	T43.213	T43.214	T43.215	T43.216
Trecator	T37.1X1	T37.1X2	T37.1X3	T37.1X4	T37.1X5	T37.1X6
Treosulfan	T45.1X1	T45.1X2	T45.1X3	T45.1X4	T45.1X5	T45.1X6
Tretamine	T45.1X1	T45.1X2	T45.1X3	T45.1X4	T45.1X5	T45.1X6
Tretinoin	T49.0X1	T49.0X2	T49.0X3	T49.0X4	T49.0X5	T49.0X6
Tretoquinol	T48.6X1	T48.6X2	T48.6X3	T48.6X4	T48.6X5	T48.6X6
Triacetin	T49.0X1	T49.0X2	T49.0X3	T49.0X4	T49.0X5	T49.0X6
Triacetoxyanthracene	T49.4X1	T49.4X2	T49.4X3	T49.4X4	T49.4X5	T49.4X6
Triacetyloleandomycin	T36.3X1	T36.3X2	T36.3X3	T36.3X4	T36.3X5	T36.3X6
Triamcinolone	T49.0X1	T49.0X2	T49.0X3	T49.0X4	T49.0X5	T49.0X6
ENT agent	T49.6X1	T49.6X2	T49.6X3	T49.6X4	T49.6X5	T49.6X6
hexacetonide	T49.0X1	T49.0X2	T49.0X3	T49.0X4	T49.0X5	T49.0X6
ophthalmic preparation	T49.5X1	T49.5X2	T49.5X3	T49.5X4	T49.5X5	T49.5X6
topical NEC	T49.0X1	T49.0X2	T49.0X3	T49.0X4	T49.0X5	T49.0X6
Triampyzine	T44.3X1	T44.3X2	T44.3X3	T44.3X4	T44.3X5	T44.3X6

Substance	Poisoning, Accidental (unintentional)	Poisoning, Intentional Self-harm	Poisoning, Assault	Poisoning, Undetermined	Adverse Effect	Under-dosing
Triamterene	T5Ø.2X1	T5Ø.2X2	T5Ø.2X3	T5Ø.2X4	T5Ø.2X5	T5Ø.2X6
Triazine (herbicide)	T6Ø.3X1	T6Ø.3X2	T6Ø.3X3	T6Ø.3X4	—	—
Triaziquone	T45.1X1	T45.1X2	T45.1X3	T45.1X4	T45.1X5	T45.1X6
Triazolam	T42.4X1	T42.4X2	T42.4X3	T42.4X4	T42.4X5	T42.4X6
Triazole (herbicide)	T6Ø.3X1	T6Ø.3X2	T6Ø.3X3	T6Ø.3X4	—	—
Tribenoside	T46.991	T46.992	T46.993	T46.994	T46.995	T46.996
Tribromacetaldehyde	T42.6X1	T42.6X2	T42.6X3	T42.6X4	T42.6X5	T42.6X6
Tribromoethanol, rectal	T41.291	T41.292	T41.293	T41.294	T41.295	T41.296
Tribromomethane	T42.6X1	T42.6X2	T42.6X3	T42.6X4	T42.6X5	T42.6X6
Trichlorethane	T53.2X1	T53.2X2	T53.2X3	T53.2X4	—	—
Trichlorethylene	T53.2X1	T53.2X2	T53.2X3	T53.2X4	—	—
Trichlorfon	T6Ø.ØX1	T6Ø.ØX2	T6Ø.ØX3	T6Ø.ØX4	—	—
Trichlormethiazide	T5Ø.2X1	T5Ø.2X2	T5Ø.2X3	T5Ø.2X4	T5Ø.2X5	T5Ø.2X6
Trichlormethine	T45.1X1	T45.1X2	T45.1X3	T45.1X4	T45.1X5	T45.1X6
Trichloroacetic acid, Trichloracetic acid	T54.2X1	T54.2X2	T54.2X3	T54.2X4	—	—
medicinal	T49.4X1	T49.4X2	T49.4X3	T49.4X4	T49.4X5	T49.4X6
Trichloroethane	T53.2X1	T53.2X2	T53.2X3	T53.2X4	—	—
Trichloroethanol	T42.6X1	T42.6X2	T42.6X3	T42.6X4	T42.6X5	T42.6X6
Trichloroethylene (liquid) (vapor)	T53.2X1	T53.2X2	T53.2X3	T53.2X4	—	—
anesthetic (gas)	T41.ØX1	T41.ØX2	T41.ØX3	T41.ØX4	T41.ØX5	T41.ØX6
vapor NEC	T53.2X1	T53.2X2	T53.2X3	T53.2X4	—	—
Trichloroethyl phosphate	T42.6X1	T42.6X2	T42.6X3	T42.6X4	T42.6X5	T42.6X6
Trichlorofluoromethane NEC	T53.5X1	T53.5X2	T53.5X3	T53.5X4	—	—
Trichloronate	T6Ø.ØX1	T6Ø.ØX2	T6Ø.ØX3	T6Ø.ØX4	—	—
Trichloropropane	T53.6X1	T53.6X2	T53.6X3	T53.6X4	—	—
Trichlorotriethylamine	T45.1X1	T45.1X2	T45.1X3	T45.1X4	T45.1X5	T45.1X6
Trichomonacides NEC	T37.3X1	T37.3X2	T37.3X3	T37.3X4	T37.3X5	T37.3X6
Trichomycin	T36.7X1	T36.7X2	T36.7X3	T36.7X4	T36.7X5	T36.7X6
Triclobisonium chloride	T49.ØX1	T49.ØX2	T49.ØX3	T49.ØX4	T49.ØX5	T49.ØX6
Triclocarban	T49.ØX1	T49.ØX2	T49.ØX3	T49.ØX4	T49.ØX5	T49.ØX6
Triclofos	T42.6X1	T42.6X2	T42.6X3	T42.6X4	T42.6X5	T42.6X6
Triclosan	T49.ØX1	T49.ØX2	T49.ØX3	T49.ØX4	T49.ØX5	T49.ØX6
Tricresyl phosphate	T65.891	T65.892	T65.893	T65.894	—	—
solvent	T52.91	T52.92	T52.93	T52.94	—	—
Tricyclamol chloride	T44.3X1	T44.3X2	T44.3X3	T44.3X4	T44.3X5	T44.3X6
Tridesilon	T49.ØX1	T49.ØX2	T49.ØX3	T49.ØX4	T49.ØX5	T49.ØX6
Tridihexethyl iodide	T44.3X1	T44.3X2	T44.3X3	T44.3X4	T44.3X5	T44.3X6
Tridione	T42.2X1	T42.2X2	T42.2X3	T42.2X4	T42.2X5	T42.2X6
Trientine	T45.8X1	T45.8X2	T45.8X3	T45.8X4	T45.8X5	T45.8X6
Triethanolamine NEC	T54.3X1	T54.3X2	T54.3X3	T54.3X4	—	—
detergent	T54.3X1	T54.3X2	T54.3X3	T54.3X4	—	—
trinitrate (biphosphate)	T46.3X1	T46.3X2	T46.3X3	T46.3X4	T46.3X5	T46.3X6
Triethanomelamine	T45.1X1	T45.1X2	T45.1X3	T45.1X4	T45.1X5	T45.1X6
Triethylenemelamine	T45.1X1	T45.1X2	T45.1X3	T45.1X4	T45.1X5	T45.1X6
Triethylenephosphoramide	T45.1X1	T45.1X2	T45.1X3	T45.1X4	T45.1X5	T45.1X6
Triethylenethiophosphoramide	T45.1X1	T45.1X2	T45.1X3	T45.1X4	T45.1X5	T45.1X6
Trifluoperazine	T43.3X1	T43.3X2	T43.3X3	T43.3X4	T43.3X5	T43.3X6
Trifluoroethyl vinyl ether	T41.ØX1	T41.ØX2	T41.ØX3	T41.ØX4	T41.ØX5	T41.ØX6
Trifluperidol	T43.4X1	T43.4X2	T43.4X3	T43.4X4	T43.4X5	T43.4X6
Triflupromazine	T43.3X1	T43.3X2	T43.3X3	T43.3X4	T43.3X5	T43.3X6
Trifluridine	T37.5X1	T37.5X2	T37.5X3	T37.5X4	T37.5X5	T37.5X6
Triflusal	T45.521	T45.522	T45.523	T45.524	T45.525	T45.526
Trihexyphenidyl	T44.3X1	T44.3X2	T44.3X3	T44.3X4	T44.3X5	T44.3X6
Triiodothyronine	T38.1X1	T38.1X2	T38.1X3	T38.1X4	T38.1X5	T38.1X6
Trilene	T41.ØX1	T41.ØX2	T41.ØX3	T41.ØX4	T41.ØX5	T41.ØX6
Trilostane	T38.991	T38.992	T38.993	T38.994	T38.995	T38.996
Trimebutine	T44.3X1	T44.3X2	T44.3X3	T44.3X4	T44.3X5	T44.3X6
Trimecaine	T41.3X1	T41.3X2	T41.3X3	T41.3X4	T41.3X5	T41.3X6
Trimeprazine (tartrate)	T44.3X1	T44.3X2	T44.3X3	T44.3X4	T44.3X5	T44.3X6
Trimetaphan camsilate	T44.2X1	T44.2X2	T44.2X3	T44.2X4	T44.2X5	T44.2X6
Trimetazidine	T46.7X1	T46.7X2	T46.7X3	T46.7X4	T46.7X5	T46.7X6
Trimethadione	T42.2X1	T42.2X2	T42.2X3	T42.2X4	T42.2X5	T42.2X6
Trimethaphan	T44.2X1	T44.2X2	T44.2X3	T44.2X4	T44.2X5	T44.2X6
Trimethidinium	T44.2X1	T44.2X2	T44.2X3	T44.2X4	T44.2X5	T44.2X6
Trimethobenzamide	T45.ØX1	T45.ØX2	T45.ØX3	T45.ØX4	T45.ØX5	T45.ØX6
Trimethoprim	T37.8X1	T37.8X2	T37.8X3	T37.8X4	T37.8X5	T37.8X6
with sulfamethoxazole	T36.8X1	T36.8X2	T36.8X3	T36.8X4	T36.8X5	T36.8X6
Trimethylcarbinol	T51.3X1	T51.3X2	T51.3X3	T51.3X4	—	—
Trimethylpsoralen	T49.3X1	T49.3X2	T49.3X3	T49.3X4	T49.3X5	T49.3X6
Trimeton	T45.ØX1	T45.ØX2	T45.ØX3	T45.ØX4	T45.ØX5	T45.ØX6
Trimetrexate	T45.1X1	T45.1X2	T45.1X3	T45.1X4	T45.1X5	T45.1X6
Trimipramine	T43.Ø11	T43.Ø12	T43.Ø13	T43.Ø14	T43.Ø15	T43.Ø16
Trimustine	T45.1X1	T45.1X2	T45.1X3	T45.1X4	T45.1X5	T45.1X6
Trinitrine	T46.3X1	T46.3X2	T46.3X3	T46.3X4	T46.3X5	T46.3X6
Trinitrobenzol	T65.3X1	T65.3X2	T65.3X3	T65.3X4	—	—
Trinitrophenol	T65.3X1	T65.3X2	T65.3X3	T65.3X4	—	—
Trinitrotoluene (fumes)	T65.3X1	T65.3X2	T65.3X3	T65.3X4	—	—
Trional	T42.6X1	T42.6X2	T42.6X3	T42.6X4	T42.6X5	T42.6X6
Triorthocresyl phosphate	T65.891	T65.892	T65.893	T65.894	—	—
Trioxide of arsenic	T57.ØX1	T57.ØX2	T57.ØX3	T57.ØX4	—	—
Trioxysalen	T49.4X1	T49.4X2	T49.4X3	T49.4X4	T49.4X5	T49.4X6
Tripamide	T5Ø.2X1	T5Ø.2X2	T5Ø.2X3	T5Ø.2X4	T5Ø.2X5	T5Ø.2X6
Triparanol	T46.6X1	T46.6X2	T46.6X3	T46.6X4	T46.6X5	T46.6X6
Tripelennamine	T45.ØX1	T45.ØX2	T45.ØX3	T45.ØX4	T45.ØX5	T45.ØX6
Triperiden	T44.3X1	T44.3X2	T44.3X3	T44.3X4	T44.3X5	T44.3X6
Triperidol	T43.4X1	T43.4X2	T43.4X3	T43.4X4	T43.4X5	T43.4X6
Triphenylphosphate	T65.891	T65.892	T65.893	T65.894	—	—
Triple						
bromides	T42.6X1	T42.6X2	T42.6X3	T42.6X4	T42.6X5	T42.6X6
carbonate	T47.1X1	T47.1X2	T47.1X3	T47.1X4	T47.1X5	T47.1X6
vaccine						
DPT	T5Ø.A11	T5Ø.A12	T5Ø.A13	T5Ø.A14	T5Ø.A15	T5Ø.A16
including pertussis	T5Ø.A11	T5Ø.A12	T5Ø.A13	T5Ø.A14	T5Ø.A15	T5Ø.A16
MMR	T5Ø.B91	T5Ø.B92	T5Ø.B93	T5Ø.B94	T5Ø.B95	T5Ø.B96
Triprolidine	T45.ØX1	T45.ØX2	T45.ØX3	T45.ØX4	T45.ØX5	T45.ØX6
Trisodium hydrogen edetate	T5Ø.6X1	T5Ø.6X2	T5Ø.6X3	T5Ø.6X4	T5Ø.6X5	T5Ø.6X6
Trisoralen	T49.3X1	T49.3X2	T49.3X3	T49.3X4	T49.3X5	T49.3X6
Trisulfapyrimidines	T37.ØX1	T37.ØX2	T37.ØX3	T37.ØX4	T37.ØX5	T37.ØX6
Trithiozine	T44.3X1	T44.3X2	T44.3X3	T44.3X4	T44.3X5	T44.3X6
Tritiozine	T44.3X1	T44.3X2	T44.3X3	T44.3X4	T44.3X5	T44.3X6
Tritoqualine	T45.ØX1	T45.ØX2	T45.ØX3	T45.ØX4	T45.ØX5	T45.ØX6
Trofosfamide	T45.1X1	T45.1X2	T45.1X3	T45.1X4	T45.1X5	T45.1X6
Troleandomycin	T36.3X1	T36.3X2	T36.3X3	T36.3X4	T36.3X5	T36.3X6
Trolnitrate (phosphate)	T46.3X1	T46.3X2	T46.3X3	T46.3X4	T46.3X5	T46.3X6
Tromantadine	T37.5X1	T37.5X2	T37.5X3	T37.5X4	T37.5X5	T37.5X6
Trometamol	T5Ø.2X1	T5Ø.2X2	T5Ø.2X3	T5Ø.2X4	T5Ø.2X5	T5Ø.2X6
Tromethamine	T5Ø.2X1	T5Ø.2X2	T5Ø.2X3	T5Ø.2X4	T5Ø.2X5	T5Ø.2X6
Tronothane	T41.3X1	T41.3X2	T41.3X3	T41.3X4	T41.3X5	T41.3X6
Tropacine	T44.3X1	T44.3X2	T44.3X3	T44.3X4	T44.3X5	T44.3X6
Tropatepine	T44.3X1	T44.3X2	T44.3X3	T44.3X4	T44.3X5	T44.3X6
Tropicamide	T44.3X1	T44.3X2	T44.3X3	T44.3X4	T44.3X5	T44.3X6
Trospium chloride	T44.3X1	T44.3X2	T44.3X3	T44.3X4	T44.3X5	T44.3X6
Troxerutin	T46.991	T46.992	T46.993	T46.994	T46.995	T46.996
Troxidone	T42.2X1	T42.2X2	T42.2X3	T42.2X4	T42.2X5	T42.2X6
Tryparsamide	T37.3X1	T37.3X2	T37.3X3	T37.3X4	T37.3X5	T37.3X6
Trypsin	T45.3X1	T45.3X2	T45.3X3	T45.3X4	T45.3X5	T45.3X6
Tryptizol	T43.Ø11	T43.Ø12	T43.Ø13	T43.Ø14	T43.Ø15	T43.Ø16
TSH	T38.811	T38.812	T38.813	T38.814	T38.815	T38.816
Tuaminoheptane	T48.5X1	T48.5X2	T48.5X3	T48.5X4	T48.5X5	T48.5X6
Tuberculin, purified protein derivative (PPD)	T5Ø.8X1	T5Ø.8X2	T5Ø.8X3	T5Ø.8X4	T5Ø.8X5	T5Ø.8X6
Tubocurare	T48.1X1	T48.1X2	T48.1X3	T48.1X4	T48.1X5	T48.1X6
Tubocurarine (chloride)	T48.1X1	T48.1X2	T48.1X3	T48.1X4	T48.1X5	T48.1X6
Tulobuterol	T48.6X1	T48.6X2	T48.6X3	T48.6X4	T48.6X5	T48.6X6
Turpentine (spirits of)	T52.8X1	T52.8X2	T52.8X3	T52.8X4	—	—
vapor	T52.8X1	T52.8X2	T52.8X3	T52.8X4	—	—
Tybamate	T43.591	T43.592	T43.593	T43.594	T43.595	T43.596
Tyloxapol	T48.4X1	T48.4X2	T48.4X3	T48.4X4	T48.4X5	T48.4X6
Tymazoline	T48.5X1	T48.5X2	T48.5X3	T48.5X4	T48.5X5	T48.5X6
Typhoid-paratyphoid vaccine	T5Ø.A91	T5Ø.A92	T5Ø.A93	T5Ø.A94	T5Ø.A95	T5Ø.A96
Typhus vaccine	T5Ø.A91	T5Ø.A92	T5Ø.A93	T5Ø.A94	T5Ø.A95	T5Ø.A96
Tyropanoate	T5Ø.8X1	T5Ø.8X2	T5Ø.8X3	T5Ø.8X4	T5Ø.8X5	T5Ø.8X6
Tyrothricin	T49.6X1	T49.6X2	T49.6X3	T49.6X4	T49.6X5	T49.6X6
ENT agent	T49.6X1	T49.6X2	T49.6X3	T49.6X4	T49.6X5	T49.6X6
ophthalmic preparation	T49.5X1	T49.5X2	T49.5X3	T49.5X4	T49.5X5	T49.5X6
Ufenamate	T39.391	T39.392	T39.393	T39.394	T39.395	T39.396
Ultraviolet light protectant	T49.3X1	T49.3X2	T49.3X3	T49.3X4	T49.3X5	T49.3X6
Undecenoic acid	T49.ØX1	T49.ØX2	T49.ØX3	T49.ØX4	T49.ØX5	T49.ØX6
Undecoylium	T49.ØX1	T49.ØX2	T49.ØX3	T49.ØX4	T49.ØX5	T49.ØX6
Undecylenic acid (derivatives)	T49.ØX1	T49.ØX2	T49.ØX3	T49.ØX4	T49.ØX5	T49.ØX6
Unna's boot	T49.3X1	T49.3X2	T49.3X3	T49.3X4	T49.3X5	T49.3X6
Unsaturated fatty acid	T46.6X1	T46.6X2	T46.6X3	T46.6X4	T46.6X5	T46.6X6
Uracil mustard	T45.1X1	T45.1X2	T45.1X3	T45.1X4	T45.1X5	T45.1X6
Uramustine	T45.1X1	T45.1X2	T45.1X3	T45.1X4	T45.1X5	T45.1X6
Urapidil	T46.5X1	T46.5X2	T46.5X3	T46.5X4	T46.5X5	T46.5X6
Urari	T48.1X1	T48.1X2	T48.1X3	T48.1X4	T48.1X5	T48.1X6
Urate oxidase	T5Ø.4X1	T5Ø.4X2	T5Ø.4X3	T5Ø.4X4	T5Ø.4X5	T5Ø.4X6
Urea	T47.3X1	T47.3X2	T47.3X3	T47.3X4	T47.3X5	T47.3X6
peroxide	T49.ØX1	T49.ØX2	T49.ØX3	T49.ØX4	T49.ØX5	T49.ØX6
stibamine	T37.4X1	T37.4X2	T37.4X3	T37.4X4	T37.4X5	T37.4X6
topical	T49.8X1	T49.8X2	T49.8X3	T49.8X4	T49.8X5	T49.8X6
Urethane	T45.1X1	T45.1X2	T45.1X3	T45.1X4	T45.1X5	T45.1X6
Urginea (maritima) (scilla) — *see* Squill						
Uric acid metabolism drug NEC	T5Ø.4X1	T5Ø.4X2	T5Ø.4X3	T5Ø.4X4	T5Ø.4X5	T5Ø.4X6
Uricosuric agent	T5Ø.4X1	T5Ø.4X2	T5Ø.4X3	T5Ø.4X4	T5Ø.4X5	T5Ø.4X6
Urinary anti-infective	T37.8X1	T37.8X2	T37.8X3	T37.8X4	T37.8X5	T37.8X6
Urofollitropin	T38.811	T38.812	T38.813	T38.814	T38.815	T38.816
Urokinase	T45.611	T45.612	T45.613	T45.614	T45.615	T45.616

Substance	Poisoning, Accidental (unintentional)	Poisoning, Intentional Self-harm	Poisoning, Assault	Poisoning, Undetermined	Adverse Effect	Under-dosing
Urokon	T5Ø.8X1	T5Ø.8X2	T5Ø.8X3	T5Ø.8X4	T5Ø.8X5	T5Ø.8X6
Ursodeoxycholic acid	T5Ø.991	T5Ø.992	T5Ø.993	T5Ø.994	T5Ø.995	T5Ø.996
Ursodiol	T5Ø.991	T5Ø.992	T5Ø.993	T5Ø.994	T5Ø.995	T5Ø.996
Urtica	T62.2X1	T62.2X2	T62.2X3	T62.2X4	—	—
Utility gas — *see* Gas, utility						
Vaccine NEC	T5Ø.Z91	T5Ø.Z92	T5Ø.Z93	T5Ø.Z94	T5Ø.Z95	T5Ø.Z96
antineoplastic	T5Ø.Z91	T5Ø.Z92	T5Ø.Z93	T5Ø.Z94	T5Ø.Z95	T5Ø.Z96
bacterial NEC	T5Ø.A91	T5Ø.A92	T5Ø.A93	T5Ø.A94	T5Ø.A95	T5Ø.A96
with						
other bacterial component	T5Ø.A21	T5Ø.A22	T5Ø.A23	T5Ø.A24	T5Ø.A25	T5Ø.A26
pertussis component	T5Ø.A11	T5Ø.A12	T5Ø.A13	T5Ø.A14	T5Ø.A15	T5Ø.A16
viral-rickettsial component	T5Ø.A21	T5Ø.A22	T5Ø.A23	T5Ø.A24	T5Ø.A25	T5Ø.A26
mixed NEC	T5Ø.A21	T5Ø.A22	T5Ø.A23	T5Ø.A24	T5Ø.A25	T5Ø.A26
BCG	T5Ø.A91	T5Ø.A92	T5Ø.A93	T5Ø.A94	T5Ø.A95	T5Ø.A96
cholera	T5Ø.A91	T5Ø.A92	T5Ø.A93	T5Ø.A94	T5Ø.A95	T5Ø.A96
diphtheria	T5Ø.A91	T5Ø.A92	T5Ø.A93	T5Ø.A94	T5Ø.A95	T5Ø.A96
with tetanus	T5Ø.A21	T5Ø.A22	T5Ø.A23	T5Ø.A24	T5Ø.A25	T5Ø.A26
and pertussis	T5Ø.A11	T5Ø.A12	T5Ø.A13	T5Ø.A14	T5Ø.A15	T5Ø.A16
influenza	T5Ø.B91	T5Ø.B92	T5Ø.B93	T5Ø.B94	T5Ø.B95	T5Ø.B96
measles	T5Ø.B91	T5Ø.B92	T5Ø.B93	T5Ø.B94	T5Ø.B95	T5Ø.B96
with mumps and rubella	T5Ø.B91	T5Ø.B92	T5Ø.B93	T5Ø.B94	T5Ø.B95	T5Ø.B96
meningococcal	T5Ø.A91	T5Ø.A92	T5Ø.A93	T5Ø.A94	T5Ø.A95	T5Ø.A96
mumps	T5Ø.B91	T5Ø.B92	T5Ø.B93	T5Ø.B94	T5Ø.B95	T5Ø.B96
paratyphoid	T5Ø.A91	T5Ø.A92	T5Ø.A93	T5Ø.A94	T5Ø.A95	T5Ø.A96
pertussis	T5Ø.A11	T5Ø.A12	T5Ø.A13	T5Ø.A14	T5Ø.A15	T5Ø.A16
with diphtheria	T5Ø.A11	T5Ø.A12	T5Ø.A13	T5Ø.A14	T5Ø.A15	T5Ø.A16
and tetanus	T5Ø.A11	T5Ø.A12	T5Ø.A13	T5Ø.A14	T5Ø.A15	T5Ø.A16
with other component	T5Ø.A11	T5Ø.A12	T5Ø.A13	T5Ø.A14	T5Ø.A15	T5Ø.A16
plague	T5Ø.A91	T5Ø.A92	T5Ø.A93	T5Ø.A94	T5Ø.A95	T5Ø.A96
poliomyelitis	T5Ø.B91	T5Ø.B92	T5Ø.B93	T5Ø.B94	T5Ø.B95	T5Ø.B96
poliovirus	T5Ø.B91	T5Ø.B92	T5Ø.B93	T5Ø.B94	T5Ø.B95	T5Ø.B96
rabies	T5Ø.B91	T5Ø.B92	T5Ø.B93	T5Ø.B94	T5Ø.B95	T5Ø.B96
respiratory syncytial virus	T5Ø.B91	T5Ø.B92	T5Ø.B93	T5Ø.B94	T5Ø.B95	T5Ø.B96
rickettsial NEC	T5Ø.A91	T5Ø.A92	T5Ø.A93	T5Ø.A94	T5Ø.A95	T5Ø.A96
with						
bacterial component	T5Ø.A21	T5Ø.A22	T5Ø.A23	T5Ø.A24	T5Ø.A25	T5Ø.A26
Rocky Mountain spotted fever	T5Ø.A91	T5Ø.A92	T5Ø.A93	T5Ø.A94	T5Ø.A95	T5Ø.A96
rubella	T5Ø.B91	T5Ø.B92	T5Ø.B93	T5Ø.B94	T5Ø.B95	T5Ø.B96
sabin oral	T5Ø.B91	T5Ø.B92	T5Ø.B93	T5Ø.B94	T5Ø.B95	T5Ø.B96
smallpox	T5Ø.B11	T5Ø.B12	T5Ø.B13	T5Ø.B14	T5Ø.B15	T5Ø.B16
TAB	T5Ø.A91	T5Ø.A92	T5Ø.A93	T5Ø.A94	T5Ø.A95	T5Ø.A96
tetanus	T5Ø.A91	T5Ø.A92	T5Ø.A93	T5Ø.A94	T5Ø.A95	T5Ø.A96
typhoid	T5Ø.A91	T5Ø.A92	T5Ø.A93	T5Ø.A94	T5Ø.A95	T5Ø.A96
typhus	T5Ø.A91	T5Ø.A92	T5Ø.A93	T5Ø.A94	T5Ø.A95	T5Ø.A96
viral NEC	T5Ø.B91	T5Ø.B92	T5Ø.B93	T5Ø.B94	T5Ø.B95	T5Ø.B96
yellow fever	T5Ø.B91	T5Ø.B92	T5Ø.B93	T5Ø.B94	T5Ø.B95	T5Ø.B96
Vaccinia immune globulin	T5Ø.Z11	T5Ø.Z12	T5Ø.Z13	T5Ø.Z14	T5Ø.Z15	T5Ø.Z16
Vaginal contraceptives	T49.8X1	T49.8X2	T49.8X3	T49.8X4	T49.8X5	T49.8X6
Valerian						
root	T42.6X1	T42.6X2	T42.6X3	T42.6X4	T42.6X5	T42.6X6
tincture	T42.6X1	T42.6X2	T42.6X3	T42.6X4	T42.6X5	T42.6X6
Valethamate bromide	T44.3X1	T44.3X2	T44.3X3	T44.3X4	T44.3X5	T44.3X6
Valisone	T49.ØX1	T49.ØX2	T49.ØX3	T49.ØX4	T49.ØX5	T49.ØX6
Valium	T42.4X1	T42.4X2	T42.4X3	T42.4X4	T42.4X5	T42.4X6
Valmid	T42.6X1	T42.6X2	T42.6X3	T42.6X4	T42.6X5	T42.6X6
Valnoctamide	T42.6X1	T42.6X2	T42.6X3	T42.6X4	T42.6X5	T42.6X6
Valproate (sodium)	T42.6X1	T42.6X2	T42.6X3	T42.6X4	T42.6X5	T42.6X6
Valproic acid	T42.6X1	T42.6X2	T42.6X3	T42.6X4	T42.6X5	T42.6X6
Valpromide	T42.6X1	T42.6X2	T42.6X3	T42.6X4	T42.6X5	T42.6X6
Vanadium	T56.891	T56.892	T56.893	T56.894	—	—
Vancomycin	T36.8X1	T36.8X2	T36.8X3	T36.8X4	T36.8X5	T36.8X6
Vapor — *see also* Gas	T59.91	T59.92	T59.93	T59.94	—	—
kiln (carbon monoxide)	T58.8X1	T58.8X2	T58.8X3	T58.8X4	—	—
lead — *see* lead						
specified source NEC	T59.891	T59.892	T59.893	T59.894	—	—
Vardenafil	T46.7X1	T46.7X2	T46.7X3	T46.7X4	T46.7X5	T46.7X6
Varicose reduction drug	T46.8X1	T46.8X2	T46.8X3	T46.8X4	T46.8X5	T46.8X6
Varnish	T65.4X1	T65.4X2	T65.4X3	T65.4X4	—	—
cleaner	T52.91	T52.92	T52.93	T52.94	—	—
Vaseline	T49.3X1	T49.3X2	T49.3X3	T49.3X4	T49.3X5	T49.3X6
Vasodilan	T46.7X1	T46.7X2	T46.7X3	T46.7X4	T46.7X5	T46.7X6
Vasodilator						
coronary NEC	T46.3X1	T46.3X2	T46.3X3	T46.3X4	T46.3X5	T46.3X6
peripheral NEC	T46.7X1	T46.7X2	T46.7X3	T46.7X4	T46.7X5	T46.7X6
Vasopressin	T38.891	T38.892	T38.893	T38.894	T38.895	T38.896
Vasopressor drugs	T38.891	T38.892	T38.893	T38.894	T38.895	T38.896
Vecuronium bromide	T48.1X1	T48.1X2	T48.1X3	T48.1X4	T48.1X5	T48.1X6
Vegetable extract, astringent	T49.2X1	T49.2X2	T49.2X3	T49.2X4	T49.2X5	T49.2X6
Venlafaxine	T43.211	T43.212	T43.213	T43.214	T43.215	T43.216

Substance	Poisoning, Accidental (unintentional)	Poisoning, Intentional Self-harm	Poisoning, Assault	Poisoning, Undetermined	Adverse Effect	Under-dosing
Venom, venomous (bite) (sting)	T63.91	T63.92	T63.93	T63.94	—	—
amphibian NEC	T63.831	T63.832	T63.833	T63.834	—	—
animal NEC	T63.891	T63.892	T63.893	T63.894	—	—
ant	T63.421	T63.422	T63.423	T63.424	—	—
arthropod NEC	T63.481	T63.482	T63.483	T63.484	—	—
bee	T63.441	T63.442	T63.443	T63.444	—	—
centipede	T63.411	T63.412	T63.413	T63.414	—	—
fish	T63.591	T63.592	T63.593	T63.594	—	—
frog	T63.811	T63.812	T63.813	T63.814	—	—
hornet	T63.451	T63.452	T63.453	T63.454	—	—
insect NEC	T63.481	T63.482	T63.483	T63.484	—	—
lizard	T63.121	T63.122	T63.123	T63.124	—	—
marine						
animals	T63.691	T63.692	T63.693	T63.694	—	—
bluebottle	T63.611	T63.612	T63.613	T63.614	—	—
jellyfish NEC	T63.621	T63.622	T63.623	T63.624	—	—
Portugese Man-o-war	T63.611	T63.612	T63.613	T63.614	—	—
sea anemone	T63.631	T63.632	T63.633	T63.634	—	—
specified NEC	T63.691	T63.692	T63.693	T63.694	—	—
fish	T63.591	T63.592	T63.593	T63.594	—	—
plants	T63.711	T63.712	T63.713	T63.714	—	—
sting ray	T63.511	T63.512	T63.513	T63.514	—	—
millipede (tropical)	T63.411	T63.412	T63.413	T63.414	—	—
plant NEC	T63.791	T63.792	T63.793	T63.794	—	—
marine	T63.711	T63.712	T63.713	T63.714	—	—
reptile	T63.191	T63.192	T63.193	T63.194	—	—
gila monster	T63.111	T63.112	T63.113	T63.114	—	—
lizard NEC	T63.121	T63.122	T63.123	T63.124	—	—
scorpion	T63.2X1	T63.2X2	T63.2X3	T63.2X4	—	—
snake	T63.ØØ1	T63.ØØ2	T63.ØØ3	T63.ØØ4	—	—
African NEC	T63.Ø81	T63.Ø82	T63.Ø83	T63.Ø84	—	—
American (North) (South) NEC	T63.Ø61	T63.Ø62	T63.Ø63	T63.Ø64	—	—
Asian	T63.Ø81	T63.Ø82	T63.Ø83	T63.Ø84	—	—
Australian	T63.Ø71	T63.Ø72	T63.Ø73	T63.Ø74	—	—
cobra	T63.Ø41	T63.Ø42	T63.Ø43	T63.Ø44	—	—
coral snake	T63.Ø21	T63.Ø22	T63.Ø23	T63.Ø24	—	—
rattlesnake	T63.Ø11	T63.Ø12	T63.Ø13	T63.Ø14	—	—
specified NEC	T63.Ø91	T63.Ø92	T63.Ø93	T63.Ø94	—	—
taipan	T63.Ø31	T63.Ø32	T63.Ø33	T63.Ø34	—	—
specified NEC	T63.891	T63.892	T63.893	T63.894	—	—
spider	T63.3Ø1	T63.3Ø2	T63.3Ø3	T63.3Ø4	—	—
black widow	T63.311	T63.312	T63.313	T63.314	—	—
brown recluse	T63.331	T63.332	T63.333	T63.334	—	—
specified NEC	T63.391	T63.392	T63.393	T63.394	—	—
tarantula	T63.321	T63.322	T63.323	T63.324	—	—
sting ray	T63.511	T63.512	T63.513	T63.514	—	—
toad	T63.821	T63.822	T63.823	T63.824	—	—
wasp	T63.461	T63.462	T63.463	T63.464	—	—
Venous sclerosing drug NEC	T46.8X1	T46.8X2	T46.8X3	T46.8X4	T46.8X5	T46.8X6
Ventolin — *see* Albuterol						
Veramon	T42.3X1	T42.3X2	T42.3X3	T42.3X4	T42.3X5	T42.3X6
Verapamil	T46.1X1	T46.1X2	T46.1X3	T46.1X4	T46.1X5	T46.1X6
Veratrine	T46.5X1	T46.5X2	T46.5X3	T46.5X4	T46.5X5	T46.5X6
Veratrum						
album	T62.2X1	T62.2X2	T62.2X3	T62.2X4	—	—
alkaloids	T46.5X1	T46.5X2	T46.5X3	T46.5X4	T46.5X5	T46.5X6
viride	T62.2X1	T62.2X2	T62.2X3	T62.2X4	—	—
Verdigris	T6Ø.3X1	T6Ø.3X2	T6Ø.3X3	T6Ø.3X4	—	—
Veronal	T42.3X1	T42.3X2	T42.3X3	T42.3X4	T42.3X5	T42.3X6
Veroxil	T37.4X1	T37.4X2	T37.4X3	T37.4X4	T37.4X5	T37.4X6
Versenate	T5Ø.6X1	T5Ø.6X2	T5Ø.6X3	T5Ø.6X4	T5Ø.6X5	T5Ø.6X6
Versidyne	T39.8X1	T39.8X2	T39.8X3	T39.8X4	T39.8X5	T39.8X6
Vetrabutine	T48.ØX1	T48.ØX2	T48.ØX3	T48.ØX4	T48.ØX5	T48.ØX6
Vidarabine	T37.5X1	T37.5X2	T37.5X3	T37.5X4	T37.5X5	T37.5X6
Vienna						
green	T57.ØX1	T57.ØX2	T57.ØX3	T57.ØX4	—	—
insecticide	T6Ø.2X1	T6Ø.2X2	T6Ø.2X3	T6Ø.2X4	—	—
red	T57.ØX1	T57.ØX2	T57.ØX3	T57.ØX4	—	—
pharmaceutical dye	T5Ø.991	T5Ø.992	T5Ø.993	T5Ø.994	T5Ø.995	T5Ø.996
Vigabatrin	T42.6X1	T42.6X2	T42.6X3	T42.6X4	T42.6X5	T42.6X6
Viloxazine	T43.291	T43.292	T43.293	T43.294	T43.295	T43.296
Viminol	T39.8X1	T39.8X2	T39.8X3	T39.8X4	T39.8X5	T39.8X6
Vinbarbital, vinbarbitone	T42.3X1	T42.3X2	T42.3X3	T42.3X4	T42.3X5	T42.3X6
Vinblastine	T45.1X1	T45.1X2	T45.1X3	T45.1X4	T45.1X5	T45.1X6
Vinburnine	T46.7X1	T46.7X2	T46.7X3	T46.7X4	T46.7X5	T46.7X6
Vincamine	T45.1X1	T45.1X2	T45.1X3	T45.1X4	T45.1X5	T45.1X6
Vincristine	T45.1X1	T45.1X2	T45.1X3	T45.1X4	T45.1X5	T45.1X6
Vindesine	T45.1X1	T45.1X2	T45.1X3	T45.1X4	T45.1X5	T45.1X6
Vinesthene, vinethene	T41.ØX1	T41.ØX2	T41.ØX3	T41.ØX4	T41.ØX5	T41.ØX6
Vinorelbine tartrate	T45.1X1	T45.1X2	T45.1X3	T45.1X4	T45.1X5	T45.1X6

Substance	Poisoning, Accidental (unintentional)	Poisoning, Intentional Self-harm	Poisoning, Assault	Poisoning, Undetermined	Adverse Effect	Under-dosing
Vinpocetine	T46.7X1	T46.7X2	T46.7X3	T46.7X4	T46.7X5	T46.7X6
Vinyl						
acetate	T65.891	T65.892	T65.893	T65.894	—	—
bital	T42.3X1	T42.3X2	T42.3X3	T42.3X4	T42.3X5	T42.3X6
bromide	T65.891	T65.892	T65.893	T65.894	—	—
chloride	T59.891	T59.892	T59.893	T59.894	—	—
ether	T41.ØX1	T41.ØX2	T41.ØX3	T41.ØX4	T41.ØX5	T41.ØX6
Vinylbital	T42.3X1	T42.3X2	T42.3X3	T42.3X4	T42.3X5	T42.3X6
Vinylidene chloride	T65.891	T65.892	T65.893	T65.894	—	—
Vioform	T37.8X1	T37.8X2	T37.8X3	T37.8X4	T37.8X5	T37.8X6
topical	T49.ØX1	T49.ØX2	T49.ØX3	T49.ØX4	T49.ØX5	T49.ØX6
Viomycin	T36.8X1	T36.8X2	T36.8X3	T36.8X4	T36.8X5	T36.8X6
Viosterol	T45.2X1	T45.2X2	T45.2X3	T45.2X4	T45.2X5	T45.2X6
Viper (venom)	T63.Ø91	T63.Ø92	T63.Ø93	T63.Ø94	—	—
Viprynium	T37.4X1	T37.4X2	T37.4X3	T37.4X4	T37.4X5	T37.4X6
Viquidil	T46.7X1	T46.7X2	T46.7X3	T46.7X4	T46.7X5	T46.7X6
Viral vaccine NEC	T5Ø.B91	T5Ø.B92	T5Ø.B93	T5Ø.B94	T5Ø.B95	T5Ø.B96
Virginiamycin	T36.8X1	T36.8X2	T36.8X3	T36.8X4	T36.8X5	T36.8X6
Virugon	T37.5X1	T37.5X2	T37.5X3	T37.5X4	T37.5X5	T37.5X6
Viscous agent	T5Ø.9Ø1	T5Ø.9Ø2	T5Ø.9Ø3	T5Ø.9Ø4	T5Ø.9Ø5	T5Ø.9Ø6
Visine	T49.5X1	T49.5X2	T49.5X3	T49.5X4	T49.5X5	T49.5X6
Visnadine	T46.3X1	T46.3X2	T46.3X3	T46.3X4	T46.3X5	T46.3X6
Vitamin NEC	T45.2X1	T45.2X2	T45.2X3	T45.2X4	T45.2X5	T45.2X6
A	T45.2X1	T45.2X2	T45.2X3	T45.2X4	T45.2X5	T45.2X6
B1	T45.2X1	T45.2X2	T45.2X3	T45.2X4	T45.2X5	T45.2X6
B2	T45.2X1	T45.2X2	T45.2X3	T45.2X4	T45.2X5	T45.2X6
B6	T45.2X1	T45.2X2	T45.2X3	T45.2X4	T45.2X5	T45.2X6
B12	T45.2X1	T45.2X2	T45.2X3	T45.2X4	T45.2X5	T45.2X6
B15	T45.2X1	T45.2X2	T45.2X3	T45.2X4	T45.2X5	T45.2X6
B NEC	T45.2X1	T45.2X2	T45.2X3	T45.2X4	T45.2X5	T45.2X6
nicotinic acid	T46.7X1	T46.7X2	T46.7X3	T46.7X4	T46.7X5	T46.7X6
C	T45.2X1	T45.2X2	T45.2X3	T45.2X4	T45.2X5	T45.2X6
D	T45.2X1	T45.2X2	T45.2X3	T45.2X4	T45.2X5	T45.2X6
D2	T45.2X1	T45.2X2	T45.2X3	T45.2X4	T45.2X5	T45.2X6
D3	T45.2X1	T45.2X2	T45.2X3	T45.2X4	T45.2X5	T45.2X6
E	T45.2X1	T45.2X2	T45.2X3	T45.2X4	T45.2X5	T45.2X6
E acetate	T45.2X1	T45.2X2	T45.2X3	T45.2X4	T45.2X5	T45.2X6
hematopoietic	T45.8X1	T45.8X2	T45.8X3	T45.8X4	T45.8X5	T45.8X6
K1	T45.7X1	T45.7X2	T45.7X3	T45.7X4	T45.7X5	T45.7X6
K2	T45.7X1	T45.7X2	T45.7X3	T45.7X4	T45.7X5	T45.7X6
K NEC	T45.7X1	T45.7X2	T45.7X3	T45.7X4	T45.7X5	T45.7X6
PP	T45.2X1	T45.2X2	T45.2X3	T45.2X4	T45.2X5	T45.2X6
ulceroprotectant	T47.1X1	T47.1X2	T47.1X3	T47.1X4	T47.1X5	T47.1X6
Vleminckx's solution	T49.4X1	T49.4X2	T49.4X3	T49.4X4	T49.4X5	T49.4X6
Voltaren — *see* Diclofenac sodium						
Warfarin	T45.511	T45.512	T45.513	T45.514	T45.515	T45.516
rodenticide	T6Ø.4X1	T6Ø.4X2	T6Ø.4X3	T6Ø.4X4	—	—
sodium	T6Ø.4X1	T6Ø.4X2	T6Ø.4X3	T6Ø.4X4	—	—
Wasp (sting)	T63.461	T63.462	T63.463	T63.464		
Water						
balance drug	T5Ø.3X1	T5Ø.3X2	T5Ø.3X3	T5Ø.3X4	T5Ø.3X5	T5Ø.3X6
distilled	T5Ø.3X1	T5Ø.3X2	T5Ø.3X3	T5Ø.3X4	T5Ø.3X5	T5Ø.3X6
gas — *see* Gas, water						
incomplete combustion of — *see* Carbon, monoxide, fuel, utility						
hemlock	T62.2X1	T62.2X2	T62.2X3	T62.2X4	—	—
moccasin (venom)	T63.Ø61	T63.Ø62	T63.Ø63	T63.Ø64	—	—
purified	T5Ø.3X1	T5Ø.3X2	T5Ø.3X3	T5Ø.3X4	T5Ø.3X5	T5Ø.3X6
Wax (paraffin) (petroleum)	T52.ØX1	T52.ØX2	T52.ØX3	T52.ØX4	—	—
automobile	T65.891	T65.892	T65.893	T65.894	—	—
floor	T52.ØX1	T52.ØX2	T52.ØX3	T52.ØX4	—	—
Weed killers NEC	T6Ø.3X1	T6Ø.3X2	T6Ø.3X3	T6Ø.3X4	—	—
Welldorm	T42.6X1	T42.6X2	T42.6X3	T42.6X4	T42.6X5	T42.6X6
White						
arsenic	T57.ØX1	T57.ØX2	T57.ØX3	T57.ØX4	—	—
hellebore	T62.2X1	T62.2X2	T62.2X3	T62.2X4	—	—
lotion (keratolytic)	T49.4X1	T49.4X2	T49.4X3	T49.4X4	T49.4X5	T49.4X6
spirit	T52.ØX1	T52.ØX2	T52.ØX3	T52.ØX4	—	—
Whitewash	T65.891	T65.892	T65.893	T65.894	—	—
Whole blood (human)	T45.8X1	T45.8X2	T45.8X3	T45.8X4	T45.8X5	T45.8X6
Wild						
black cherry	T62.2X1	T62.2X2	T62.2X3	T62.2X4	—	—
poisonous plants NEC	T62.2X1	T62.2X2	T62.2X3	T62.2X4	—	—
Window cleaning fluid	T65.891	T65.892	T65.893	T65.894	—	—
Wintergreen (oil)	T49.3X1	T49.3X2	T49.3X3	T49.3X4	T49.3X5	T49.3X6
Wisterine	T62.2X1	T62.2X2	T62.2X3	T62.2X4	—	—
Witch hazel	T49.2X1	T49.2X2	T49.2X3	T49.2X4	T49.2X5	T49.2X6
Wood alcohol or spirit	T51.1X1	T51.1X2	T51.1X3	T51.1X4	—	—
Wool fat (hydrous)	T49.3X1	T49.3X2	T49.3X3	T49.3X4	T49.3X5	T49.3X6
Woorali	T48.1X1	T48.1X2	T48.1X3	T48.1X4	T48.1X5	T48.1X6
Wormseed, American	T37.4X1	T37.4X2	T37.4X3	T37.4X4	T37.4X5	T37.4X6

Substance	Poisoning, Accidental (unintentional)	Poisoning, Intentional Self-harm	Poisoning, Assault	Poisoning, Undetermined	Adverse Effect	Under-dosing
Xamoterol	T44.5X1	T44.5X2	T44.5X3	T44.5X4	T44.5X5	T44.5X6
Xanthine diuretics	T5Ø.2X1	T5Ø.2X2	T5Ø.2X3	T5Ø.2X4	T5Ø.2X5	T5Ø.2X6
Xanthinol nicotinate	T46.7X1	T46.7X2	T46.7X3	T46.7X4	T46.7X5	T46.7X6
Xanthotoxin	T49.3X1	T49.3X2	T49.3X3	T49.3X4	T49.3X5	T49.3X6
Xantinol nicotinate	T46.7X1	T46.7X2	T46.7X3	T46.7X4	T46.7X5	T46.7X6
Xantocillin	T36.ØX1	T36.ØX2	T36.ØX3	T36.ØX4	T36.ØX5	T36.ØX6
Xenon (127Xe) (133Xe)	T5Ø.8X1	T5Ø.8X2	T5Ø.8X3	T5Ø.8X4	T5Ø.8X5	T5Ø.8X6
Xenysalate	T49.4X1	T49.4X2	T49.4X3	T49.4X4	T49.4X5	T49.4X6
Xibornol	T37.8X1	T37.8X2	T37.8X3	T37.8X4	T37.8X5	T37.8X6
Xigris	T45.511	T45.512	T45.513	T45.514	T45.515	T45.516
Xipamide	T5Ø.2X1	T5Ø.2X2	T5Ø.2X3	T5Ø.2X4	T5Ø.2X5	T5Ø.2X6
Xylene (vapor)	T52.2X1	T52.2X2	T52.2X3	T52.2X4	—	—
Xylocaine (infiltration) (topical)	T41.3X1	T41.3X2	T41.3X3	T41.3X4	T41.3X5	T41.3X6
nerve block (peripheral) (plexus)	T41.3X1	T41.3X2	T41.3X3	T41.3X4	T41.3X5	T41.3X6
spinal	T41.3X1	T41.3X2	T41.3X3	T41.3X4	T41.3X5	T41.3X6
Xylol (vapor)	T52.2X1	T52.2X2	T52.2X3	T52.2X4	—	—
Xylometazoline	T48.5X1	T48.5X2	T48.5X3	T48.5X4	T48.5X5	T48.5X6
Yeast	T45.2X1	T45.2X2	T45.2X3	T45.2X4	T45.2X5	T45.2X6
dried	T45.2X1	T45.2X2	T45.2X3	T45.2X4	T45.2X5	T45.2X6
Yellow						
fever vaccine	T5Ø.B91	T5Ø.B92	T5Ø.B93	T5Ø.B94	T5Ø.B95	T5Ø.B96
jasmine	T62.2X1	T62.2X2	T62.2X3	T62.2X4	—	—
phenolphthalein	T47.2X1	T47.2X2	T47.2X3	T47.2X4	T47.2X5	T47.2X6
Yew	T62.2X1	T62.2X2	T62.2X3	T62.2X4	—	—
Yohimbic acid	T4Ø.991	T4Ø.992	T4Ø.993	T4Ø.994	T4Ø.995	T4Ø.996
Zactane	T39.8X1	T39.8X2	T39.8X3	T39.8X4	T39.8X5	T39.8X6
Zalcitabine	T37.5X1	T37.5X2	T37.5X3	T37.5X4	T37.5X5	T37.5X6
Zaroxolyn	T5Ø.2X1	T5Ø.2X2	T5Ø.2X3	T5Ø.2X4	T5Ø.2X5	T5Ø.2X6
Zephiran (topical)	T49.ØX1	T49.ØX2	T49.ØX3	T49.ØX4	T49.ØX5	T49.ØX6
ophthalmic preparation	T49.5X1	T49.5X2	T49.5X3	T49.5X4	T49.5X5	T49.5X6
Zeranol	T38.7X1	T38.7X2	T38.7X3	T38.7X4	T38.7X5	T38.7X6
Zerone	T51.1X1	T51.1X2	T51.1X3	T51.1X4	—	—
Zidovudine	T37.5X1	T37.5X2	T37.5X3	T37.5X4	T37.5X5	T37.5X6
Zimeldine	T43.221	T43.222	T43.223	T43.224	T43.225	T43.226
Zinc (compounds) (fumes) (vapor) **NEC**	T56.5X1	T56.5X2	T56.5X3	T56.5X4	—	—
anti-infectives	T49.ØX1	T49.ØX2	T49.ØX3	T49.ØX4	T49.ØX5	T49.ØX6
antivaricose	T46.8X1	T46.8X2	T46.8X3	T46.8X4	T46.8X5	T46.8X6
bacitracin	T49.ØX1	T49.ØX2	T49.ØX3	T49.ØX4	T49.ØX5	T49.ØX6
chloride (mouthwash)	T49.6X1	T49.6X2	T49.6X3	T49.6X4	T49.6X5	T49.6X6
chromate	T56.5X1	T56.5X2	T56.5X3	T56.5X4	—	—
gelatin	T49.3X1	T49.3X2	T49.3X3	T49.3X4	T49.3X5	T49.3X6
oxide	T49.3X1	T49.3X2	T49.3X3	T49.3X4	T49.3X5	T49.3X6
plaster	T49.3X1	T49.3X2	T49.3X3	T49.3X4	T49.3X5	T49.3X6
peroxide	T49.ØX1	T49.ØX2	T49.ØX3	T49.ØX4	T49.ØX5	T49.ØX6
pesticides	T56.5X1	T56.5X2	T56.5X3	T56.5X4	—	—
phosphide	T6Ø.4X1	T6Ø.4X2	T6Ø.4X3	T6Ø.4X4	—	—
pyrithionate	T49.4X1	T49.4X2	T49.4X3	T49.4X4	T49.4X5	T49.4X6
stearate	T49.3X1	T49.3X2	T49.3X3	T49.3X4	T49.3X5	T49.3X6
sulfate	T49.5X1	T49.5X2	T49.5X3	T49.5X4	T49.5X5	T49.5X6
ENT agent	T49.6X1	T49.6X2	T49.6X3	T49.6X4	T49.6X5	T49.6X6
ophthalmic solution	T49.5X1	T49.5X2	T49.5X3	T49.5X4	T49.5X5	T49.5X6
topical NEC	T49.ØX1	T49.ØX2	T49.ØX3	T49.ØX4	T49.ØX5	T49.ØX6
undecylenate	T49.ØX1	T49.ØX2	T49.ØX3	T49.ØX4	T49.ØX5	T49.ØX6
Zineb	T6Ø.ØX1	T6Ø.ØX2	T6Ø.ØX3	T6Ø.ØX4	—	—
Zinostatin	T45.1X1	T45.1X2	T45.1X3	T45.1X4	T45.1X5	T45.1X6
Zipeprol	T48.3X1	T48.3X2	T48.3X3	T48.3X4	T48.3X5	T48.3X6
Zofenopril	T46.4X1	T46.4X2	T46.4X3	T46.4X4	T46.4X5	T46.4X6
Zolpidem	T42.6X1	T42.6X2	T42.6X3	T42.6X4	T42.6X5	T42.6X6
Zomepirac	T39.391	T39.392	T39.393	T39.394	T39.395	T39.396
Zopiclone	T42.6X1	T42.6X2	T42.6X3	T42.6X4	T42.6X5	T42.6X6
Zorubicin	T45.1X1	T45.1X2	T45.1X3	T45.1X4	T45.1X5	T45.1X6
Zotepine	T43.591	T43.592	T43.593	T43.594	T43.595	T43.596
Zovant	T45.511	T45.512	T45.513	T45.514	T45.515	T45.516
Zoxazolamine	T42.8X1	T42.8X2	T42.8X3	T42.8X4	T42.8X5	T42.8X6
Zuclopenthixol	T43.4X1	T43.4X2	T43.4X3	T43.4X4	T43.4X5	T43.4X6
Zygadenus (venenosus)	T62.2X1	T62.2X2	T62.2X3	T62.2X4	—	—
Zyprexa	T43.591	T43.592	T43.593	T43.594	T43.595	T43.596

A

- **Abandonment** (causing exposure to weather conditions) (with intent to injure or kill) NEC X58 ☑
- **Abuse** (adult) (child) (mental) (physical) (sexual) X58 ☑
- **Accident** (to) X58 ☑
  - aircraft (in transit) (powered) (*see also* Accident, transport, aircraft)
    - due to, caused by cataclysm — *see* Forces of nature, by type
  - animal-drawn vehicle — *see* Accident, transport, animal-drawn vehicle occupant
  - animal-rider — *see* Accident, transport, animal-rider
  - automobile — *see* Accident, transport, car occupant
  - bare foot water skier V94.4 ☑
  - boat, boating (*see also* Accident, watercraft)
    - striking swimmer
      - powered V94.11 ☑
      - unpowered V94.12 ☑
  - bus — *see* Accident, transport, bus occupant
  - <Insert new term here>
  - cable car, not on rails V98.Ø ☑
    - on rails — *see* Accident, transport, streetcar occupant
  - car — *see* Accident, transport, car occupant
  - caused by, due to
    - animal NEC W64 ☑
    - chain hoist W24.Ø ☑
    - cold (excessive) — *see* Exposure, cold
    - corrosive liquid, substance — *see* Table of Drugs and Chemicals
    - cutting or piercing instrument — *see* Contact, with, by type of instrument
    - drive belt W24.Ø ☑
    - electric
      - current — *see* Exposure, electric current
      - motor (*see also* Contact, with, by type of machine) W31.3 ☑
        - current (of) W86.8 ☑
    - environmental factor NEC X58 ☑
    - explosive material — *see* Explosion
    - fire, flames — *see* Exposure, fire
    - firearm missile — *see* Discharge, firearm by type
    - heat (excessive) — *see* Heat
    - hot — *see* Contact, with, hot
    - ignition — *see* Ignition
    - lifting device W24.Ø ☑
    - lightning — *see* subcategory T75.Ø ☑
      - causing fire — *see* Exposure, fire
    - machine, machinery — *see* Contact, with, by type of machine
    - natural factor NEC X58 ☑
    - pulley (block) W24.Ø ☑
    - radiation — *see* Radiation
    - steam X13.1 ☑
      - inhalation X13.Ø ☑
      - pipe X16 ☑
    - thunderbolt — *see* subcategory T75.Ø ☑
      - causing fire — *see* Exposure, fire
    - transmission device W24.1 ☑
  - coach — *see* Accident, transport, bus occupant
  - coal car — *see* Accident, transport, industrial vehicle occupant
  - diving (*see also* Fall, into, water)
    - with
      - drowning or submersion — *see* Drowning
  - forklift — *see* Accident, transport, industrial vehicle occupant
  - heavy transport vehicle NOS — *see* Accident, transport, truck occupant
  - ice yacht V98.2 ☑
  - in
    - medical, surgical procedure
      - as, or due to misadventure — *see* Misadventure
      - causing an abnormal reaction or later complication without mention of misadventure (*see also* Complication of or following, by type of procedure) Y84.9
  - land yacht V98.1 ☑
  - late effect of — *see* WØØ-X58 with 7th character S

Accident — *continued*

  - logging car — *see* Accident, transport, industrial vehicle occupant
  - machine, machinery (*see also* Contact, with, by type of machine)
    - on board watercraft V93.69 ☑
      - explosion — *see* Explosion, in, watercraft
      - fire — *see* Burn, on board watercraft
      - powered craft V93.63 ☑
        - ferry boat V93.61 ☑
        - fishing boat V93.62 ☑
        - jetskis V93.63 ☑
        - liner V93.61 ☑
        - merchant ship V93.6Ø ☑
        - passenger ship V93.61 ☑
        - sailboat V93.64 ☑
  - mine tram — *see* Accident, transport, industrial vehicle occupant
  - mobility scooter (motorized) — *see* Accident, transport, pedestrian, conveyance, specified type NEC
  - motor scooter — *see* Accident, transport, motorcyclist
  - motor vehicle NOS (traffic) (*see also* Accident, transport) V89.2 ☑
    - nontraffic V89.Ø ☑
    - three-wheeled NOS — *see* Accident, transport, three-wheeled motor vehicle occupant
  - motorcycle NOS — *see* Accident, transport, motorcyclist
  - nonmotor vehicle NOS (nontraffic) (*see also* Accident, transport) V89.1 ☑
    - traffic NOS V89.3 ☑
  - nontraffic (victim's mode of transport NOS) V88.9 ☑
    - collision (between) V88.7 ☑
      - bus and truck V88.5 ☑
      - car and:
        - bus V88.3 ☑
        - pickup V88.2 ☑
        - three-wheeled motor vehicle V88.Ø ☑
        - train V88.6 ☑
        - truck V88.4 ☑
        - two-wheeled motor vehicle V88.Ø ☑
        - van V88.2 ☑
      - specified vehicle NEC and:
        - three-wheeled motor vehicle V88.1 ☑
        - two-wheeled motor vehicle V88.1 ☑
    - known mode of transport — *see* Accident, transport, by type of vehicle
    - noncollision V88.8 ☑
  - on board watercraft V93.89 ☑
    - powered craft V93.83 ☑
      - ferry boat V93.81 ☑
      - fishing boat V93.82 ☑
      - jetskis V93.83 ☑
      - liner V93.81 ☑
      - merchant ship V93.8Ø ☑
      - passenger ship V93.81 ☑
    - unpowered craft V93.88 ☑
      - canoe V93.85 ☑
      - inflatable V93.86 ☑
        - in tow
          - recreational V94.31 ☑
          - specified NEC V94.32 ☑
      - kayak V93.85 ☑
      - sailboat V93.84 ☑
      - surf-board V93.88 ☑
      - water skis V93.87 ☑
      - windsurfer V93.88 ☑
  - parachutist V97.29 ☑
    - entangled in object V97.21 ☑
    - injured on landing V97.22 ☑
  - pedal cycle — *see* Accident, transport, pedal cyclist
  - pedestrian (on foot)
    - with
      - another pedestrian W51 ☑
        - with fall WØ3 ☑
          - due to ice or snow WØØ.Ø ☑
        - on pedestrian conveyance NEC VØØ.Ø9 ☑
      - roller skater (in-line) VØØ.Ø1 ☑
      - skate boarder VØØ.Ø2 ☑
      - transport vehicle — *see* Accident, transport

Accident — *continued*

  - pedestrian — *continued*
    - on pedestrian conveyance — *see* Accident, transport, pedestrian, conveyance
  - pick-up truck or van — *see* Accident, transport, pickup truck occupant
  - quarry truck — *see* Accident, transport, industrial vehicle occupant
  - railway vehicle (any) (in motion) — *see* Accident, transport, railway vehicle occupant
    - due to cataclysm — *see* Forces of nature, by type
  - scooter (non-motorized) — *see* Accident, transport, pedestrian, conveyance, scooter
  - sequelae of — *see* categories WØØ-X58 with 7th character S
  - skateboard — *see* Accident, transport, pedestrian, conveyance, skateboard
  - ski(ing) — *see* Accident, transport, pedestrian, conveyance
    - lift V98.3 ☑
  - specified cause NEC X58 ☑
  - streetcar — *see* Accident, transport, streetcar occupant
  - traffic (victim's mode of transport NOS) V87.9 ☑
    - collision (between) V87.7 ☑
      - bus and truck V87.5 ☑
      - car and:
        - bus V87.3 ☑
        - pickup V87.2 ☑
        - three-wheeled motor vehicle V87.Ø ☑
        - train V87.6 ☑
        - truck V87.4 ☑
        - two-wheeled motor vehicle V87.Ø ☑
        - van V87.2 ☑
      - specified vehicle NEC and:
        - three-wheeled motor vehicle V87.1 ☑
        - two-wheeled motor vehicle V87.1 ☑
    - known mode of transport — *see* Accident, transport, by type of vehicle
    - noncollision V87.8 ☑
  - transport (involving injury to) V99 ☑
    - 18 wheeler — *see* Accident, transport, truck occupant
    - agricultural vehicle occupant (nontraffic) V84.9 ☑
      - driver V84.5 ☑
      - hanger-on V84.7 ☑
      - passenger V84.6 ☑
      - traffic V84.3 ☑
        - driver V84.Ø ☑
        - hanger-on V84.2 ☑
        - passenger V84.1 ☑
      - while boarding or alighting V84.4 ☑
    - aircraft NEC V97.89 ☑
      - military NEC V97.818 ☑
        - with civlian aircraft V97.81Ø ☑
        - civilian injured by V97.811 ☑
      - occupant injured (in)
        - nonpowered craft accident V96.9 ☑
          - balloon V96.ØØ ☑
            - collision V96.Ø3 ☑
            - crash V96.Ø1 ☑
            - explosion V96.Ø5 ☑
            - fire V96.Ø4 ☑
            - forced landing V96.Ø2 ☑
            - specified type NEC V96.Ø9 ☑
          - glider V96.2Ø ☑
            - collision V96.23 ☑
            - crash V96.21 ☑
            - explosion V96.25 ☑
            - fire V96.24 ☑
            - forced landing V96.22 ☑
            - specified type NEC V96.29 ☑
          - hang glider V96.1Ø ☑
            - collision V96.13 ☑
            - crash V96.11 ☑
            - explosion V96.15 ☑
            - fire V96.14 ☑
            - forced landing V96.12 ☑
            - specified type NEC V96.19 ☑
          - specified craft NEC V96.8 ☑
        - powered craft accident V95.9 ☑

- **Accident** — *continued*
  - transport — *continued*
    - aircraft — *continued*
      - occupant injured — *continued*
        - powered craft accident — *continued*
          - fixed wing
            - commercial V95.3Ø ☑
              - collision V95.33 ☑
              - crash V95.31 ☑
              - explosion V95.35 ☑
              - fire V95.34 ☑
              - forced landing V95.32 ☑
              - specified type NEC V95.39 ☑
            - private V95.2Ø ☑
              - collision V95.23 ☑
              - crash V95.21 ☑
              - explosion V95.25 ☑
              - fire V95.24 ☑
              - forced landing V95.22 ☑
              - specified type NEC V95.29 ☑
          - glider V95.1Ø ☑
            - collision V95.13 ☑
            - crash V95.11 ☑
            - explosion V95.15 ☑
            - fire V95.14 ☑
            - forced landing V95.12 ☑
            - specified type NEC V95.19 ☑
          - helicopter V95.ØØ ☑
            - collision V95.Ø3 ☑
            - crash V95.Ø1 ☑
            - explosion V95.Ø5 ☑
            - fire V95.Ø4 ☑
            - forced landing V95.Ø2 ☑
            - specified type NEC V95.Ø9 ☑
          - spacecraft V95.4Ø ☑
            - collision V95.43 ☑
            - crash V95.41 ☑
            - explosion V95.45 ☑
            - fire V95.44 ☑
            - forced landing V95.42 ☑
            - specified type NEC V95.49 ☑
          - specified craft NEC V95.8 ☑
          - ultralight V95.1Ø ☑
            - collision V95.13 ☑
            - crash V95.11 ☑
            - explosion V95.15 ☑
            - fire V95.14 ☑
            - forced landing V95.12 ☑
            - specified type NEC V95.19 ☑
        - specified accident NEC V97.Ø ☑
        - while boarding or alighting V97.1 ☑
      - person (injured by)
        - falling from, in or on aircraft V97.Ø ☑
        - machinery on aircraft V97.89 ☑
        - on ground with aircraft involvement V97.39 ☑
        - rotating propeller V97.32 ☑
        - struck by object falling from aircraft V97.31 ☑
        - sucked into aircraft jet V97.33 ☑
        - while boarding or alighting aircraft V97.1 ☑
    - airport (battery-powered) passenger vehicle — *see* Accident, transport, industrial vehicle occupant
    - all-terrain vehicle occupant (nontraffic) V86.99 ☑
      - driver V86.59 ☑
      - dune buggy — *see* Accident, transport, dune buggy occupant
      - hanger-on V86.79 ☑
      - passenger V86.69 ☑
      - snowmobile — *see* Accident, transport, snowmobile occupant
      - traffic V86.39 ☑
        - driver V86.Ø9 ☑
        - hanger-on V86.29 ☑
        - passenger V86.19 ☑
      - while boarding or alighting V86.49 ☑
    - ambulance occupant (traffic) V86.31 ☑
      - driver V86.Ø1 ☑
      - hanger-on V86.21 ☑
      - nontraffic V86.91 ☑
        - driver V86.51 ☑
        - hanger-on V86.71 ☑
        - passenger V86.61 ☑
      - passenger V86.11 ☑
      - while boarding or alighting V86.41 ☑

- **Accident** — *continued*
  - transport — *continued*
    - animal-drawn vehicle occupant (in) V8Ø.929 ☑
      - collision (with)
        - animal V8Ø.12 ☑
          - being ridden V8Ø.711 ☑
        - animal-drawn vehicle V8Ø.721 ☑
        - bus V8Ø.42 ☑
        - car V8Ø.42 ☑
        - fixed or stationary object V8Ø.82 ☑
        - military vehicle V8Ø.92Ø ☑
        - nonmotor vehicle V8Ø.791 ☑
        - pedal cycle V8Ø.22 ☑
        - pedestrian V8Ø.12 ☑
        - pickup V8Ø.42 ☑
        - railway train or vehicle V8Ø.62 ☑
        - specified motor vehicle NEC V8Ø.52 ☑
        - streetcar V8Ø.731 ☑
        - truck V8Ø.42 ☑
        - two- or three-wheeled motor vehicle V8Ø.32 ☑
        - van V8Ø.42 ☑
      - noncollision V8Ø.Ø2 ☑
      - specified circumstance NEC V8Ø.928 ☑
    - animal-rider V8Ø.919 ☑
      - collision (with)
        - animal V8Ø.11 ☑
          - being ridden V8Ø.71Ø ☑
        - animal-drawn vehicle V8Ø.72Ø ☑
        - bus V8Ø.41 ☑
        - car V8Ø.41 ☑
        - fixed or stationary object V8Ø.81 ☑
        - military vehicle V8Ø.91Ø ☑
        - nonmotor vehicle V8Ø.79Ø ☑
        - pedal cycle V8Ø.21 ☑
        - pedestrian V8Ø.11 ☑
        - pickup V8Ø.41 ☑
        - railway train or vehicle V8Ø.61 ☑
        - specified motor vehicle NEC V8Ø.51 ☑
        - streetcar V8Ø.73Ø ☑
        - truck V8Ø.41 ☑
        - two- or three-wheeled motor vehicle V8Ø.31 ☑
        - van V8Ø.41 ☑
      - noncollision V8Ø.Ø18 ☑
        - specified as horse rider V8Ø.Ø1Ø ☑
      - specified circumstance NEC V8Ø.918 ☑
    - armored car — *see* Accident, transport, truck occupant
    - battery-powered truck (baggage) (mail) — *see* Accident, transport, industrial vehicle occupant
    - bus occupant V79.9 ☑
      - collision (with)
        - animal (traffic) V7Ø.9 ☑
          - being ridden (traffic) V76.9 ☑
            - nontraffic V76.3 ☑
            - while boarding or alighting V76.4 ☑
          - nontraffic V7Ø.3 ☑
          - while boarding or alighting V7Ø.4 ☑
        - animal-drawn vehicle (traffic) V76.9 ☑
          - nontraffic V76.3 ☑
          - while boarding or alighting V76.4 ☑
        - bus (traffic) V74.9 ☑
          - nontraffic V74.3 ☑
          - while boarding or alighting V74.4 ☑
        - car (traffic) V73.9 ☑
          - nontraffic V73.3 ☑
          - while boarding or alighting V73.4 ☑
        - motor vehicle NOS (traffic) V79.6Ø ☑
          - nontraffic V79.2Ø ☑
          - specified type NEC (traffic) V79.69 ☑
            - nontraffic V79.29 ☑
        - pedal cycle (traffic) V71.9 ☑
          - nontraffic V71.3 ☑
          - while boarding or alighting V71.4 ☑
        - pickup truck (traffic) V73.9 ☑
          - nontraffic V73.3 ☑
          - while boarding or alighting V73.4 ☑
        - railway vehicle (traffic) V75.9 ☑
          - nontraffic V75.3 ☑
          - while boarding or alighting V75.4 ☑
        - specified vehicle NEC (traffic) V76.9 ☑
          - nontraffic V76.3 ☑
          - while boarding or alighting V76.4 ☑
        - stationary object (traffic) V77.9 ☑

- **Accident** — *continued*
  - transport — *continued*
    - bus occupant — *continued*
      - collision — *continued*
        - stationary object — *continued*
          - nontraffic V77.3 ☑
          - while boarding or alighting V77.4 ☑
        - streetcar (traffic) V76.9 ☑
          - nontraffic V76.3 ☑
          - while boarding or alighting V76.4 ☑
        - three wheeled motor vehicle (traffic) V72.9 ☑
          - nontraffic V72.3 ☑
          - while boarding or alighting V72.4 ☑
        - truck (traffic) V74.9 ☑
          - nontraffic V74.3 ☑
          - while boarding or alighting V74.4 ☑
        - two wheeled motor vehicle (traffic) V72.9 ☑
          - nontraffic V72.3 ☑
          - while boarding or alighting V72.4 ☑
        - van (traffic) V73.9 ☑
          - nontraffic V73.3 ☑
          - while boarding or alighting V73.4 ☑
      - driver
        - collision (with)
          - animal (traffic) V7Ø.5 ☑
            - being ridden (traffic) V76.5 ☑
              - nontraffic V76.Ø ☑
            - nontraffic V7Ø.Ø ☑
          - animal-drawn vehicle (traffic) V76.5 ☑
            - nontraffic V76.Ø ☑
          - bus (traffic) V74.5 ☑
            - nontraffic V74.Ø ☑
          - car (traffic) V73.5 ☑
            - nontraffic V73.Ø ☑
          - motor vehicle NOS (traffic) V79.4Ø ☑
            - nontraffic V79.ØØ ☑
            - specified type NEC (traffic) V79.49 ☑
              - nontraffic V79.Ø9 ☑
          - pedal cycle (traffic) V71.5 ☑
            - nontraffic V71.Ø ☑
          - pickup truck (traffic) V73.5 ☑
            - nontraffic V73.Ø ☑
          - railway vehicle (traffic) V75.5 ☑
            - nontraffic V75.Ø ☑
          - specified vehicle NEC (traffic) V76.5 ☑
            - nontraffic V76.Ø ☑
          - stationary object (traffic) V77.5 ☑
            - nontraffic V77.Ø ☑
          - streetcar (traffic) V76.5 ☑
            - nontraffic V76.Ø ☑
          - three wheeled motor vehicle (traffic) V72.5 ☑
            - nontraffic V72.Ø ☑
          - truck (traffic) V74.5 ☑
            - nontraffic V74.Ø ☑
          - two wheeled motor vehicle (traffic) V72.5 ☑
            - nontraffic V72.Ø ☑
          - van (traffic) V73.5 ☑
            - nontraffic V73.Ø ☑
        - noncollision accident (traffic) V78.5 ☑
          - nontraffic V78.Ø ☑
      - hanger-on
        - collision (with)
          - animal (traffic) V7Ø.7 ☑
            - being ridden (traffic) V76.7 ☑
              - nontraffic V76.2 ☑
            - nontraffic V7Ø.2 ☑
          - animal-drawn vehicle (traffic) V76.7 ☑
            - nontraffic V76.2 ☑
          - bus (traffic) V74.7 ☑
            - nontraffic V74.2 ☑
          - car (traffic) V73.7 ☑
            - nontraffic V73.2 ☑
          - pedal cycle (traffic) V71.7 ☑
            - nontraffic V71.2 ☑
          - pickup truck (traffic) V73.7 ☑
            - nontraffic V73.2 ☑
          - railway vehicle (traffic) V75.7 ☑
            - nontraffic V75.2 ☑
          - specified vehicle NEC (traffic) V76.7 ☑
            - nontraffic V76.2 ☑
          - stationary object (traffic) V77.7 ☑
            - nontraffic V77.2 ☑
          - streetcar (traffic) V76.7 ☑

- **Accident** — *continued*
  - transport — *continued*
    - bus occupant — *continued*
      - hanger-on — *continued*
        - collision — *continued*
          - streetcar — *continued*
            - nontraffic V76.2 ☑
          - three wheeled motor vehicle (traffic) V72.7 ☑
            - nontraffic V72.2 ☑
          - truck (traffic) V74.7 ☑
            - nontraffic V74.2 ☑
          - two wheeled motor vehicle (traffic) V72.7 ☑
            - nontraffic V72.2 ☑
          - van (traffic) V73.7 ☑
            - nontraffic V73.2 ☑
        - noncollision accident (traffic) V78.7 ☑
          - nontraffic V78.2 ☑
      - noncollision accident (traffic) V78.9 ☑
        - nontraffic V78.3 ☑
        - while boarding or alighting V78.4 ☑
      - nontraffic V79.3 ☑
      - passenger
        - collision (with)
          - animal (traffic) V70.6 ☑
            - being ridden (traffic) V76.6 ☑
              - nontraffic V76.1 ☑
            - nontraffic V70.1 ☑
          - animal-drawn vehicle (traffic) V76.6 ☑
            - nontraffic V76.1 ☑
          - bus (traffic) V74.6 ☑
            - nontraffic V74.1 ☑
          - car (traffic) V73.6 ☑
            - nontraffic V73.1 ☑
          - motor vehicle NOS (traffic) V79.50 ☑
            - nontraffic V79.10 ☑
            - specified type NEC (traffic) V79.59 ☑
              - nontraffic V79.19 ☑
          - pedal cycle (traffic) V71.6 ☑
            - nontraffic V71.1 ☑
          - pickup truck (traffic) V73.6 ☑
            - nontraffic V73.1 ☑
          - railway vehicle (traffic) V75.6 ☑
            - nontraffic V75.1 ☑
          - specified vehicle NEC (traffic) V76.6 ☑
            - nontraffic V76.1 ☑
          - stationary object (traffic) V77.6 ☑
            - nontraffic V77.1 ☑
          - streetcar (traffic) V76.6 ☑
            - nontraffic V76.1 ☑
          - three wheeled motor vehicle (traffic) V72.6 ☑
            - nontraffic V72.1 ☑
          - truck (traffic) V74.6 ☑
            - nontraffic V74.1 ☑
          - two wheeled motor vehicle (traffic) V72.6 ☑
            - nontraffic V72.1 ☑
          - van (traffic) V73.6 ☑
            - nontraffic V73.1 ☑
        - noncollision accident (traffic) V78.6 ☑
          - nontraffic V78.1 ☑
    - specified type NEC V79.88 ☑
      - military vehicle V79.81 ☑
  - cable car, not on rails V98.0 ☑
    - on rails — *see* Accident, transport, streetcar occupant
  - car occupant V49.9 ☑
    - ambulance occupant — *see* Accident, transport, ambulance occupant
    - collision (with)
      - animal (traffic) V40.9 ☑
        - being ridden (traffic) V46.9 ☑
          - nontraffic V46.3 ☑
          - while boarding or alighting V46.4 ☑
        - nontraffic V40.3 ☑
        - while boarding or alighting V40.4 ☑
      - animal-drawn vehicle (traffic) V46.9 ☑
        - nontraffic V46.3 ☑
        - while boarding or alighting V46.4 ☑
      - bus (traffic) V44.9 ☑
        - nontraffic V44.3 ☑
        - while boarding or alighting V44.4 ☑
      - car (traffic) V43.92 ☑
        - nontraffic V43.32 ☑

- **Accident** — *continued*
  - transport — *continued*
    - car occupant — *continued*
      - collision — *continued*
        - car — *continued*
          - while boarding or alighting V43.42 ☑
        - motor vehicle NOS (traffic) V49.60 ☑
          - nontraffic V49.20 ☑
          - specified type NEC (traffic) V49.69 ☑
            - nontraffic V49.29 ☑
        - pedal cycle (traffic) V41.9 ☑
          - nontraffic V41.3 ☑
          - while boarding or alighting V41.4 ☑
        - pickup truck (traffic) V43.93 ☑
          - nontraffic V43.33 ☑
          - while boarding or alighting V43.43 ☑
        - railway vehicle (traffic) V45.9 ☑
          - nontraffic V45.3 ☑
          - while boarding or alighting V45.4 ☑
        - specified vehicle NEC (traffic) V46.9 ☑
          - nontraffic V46.3 ☑
          - while boarding or alighting V46.4 ☑
        - sport utility vehicle (traffic) V43.91 ☑
          - nontraffic V43.31 ☑
          - while boarding or alighting V43.41 ☑
        - stationary object (traffic) V47.92 ☑
          - nontraffic V47.32 ☑
          - while boarding or alighting V47.4 ☑
        - streetcar (traffic) V46.9 ☑
          - nontraffic V46.3 ☑
          - while boarding or alighting V46.4 ☑
        - three wheeled motor vehicle (traffic) V42.9 ☑
          - nontraffic V42.3 ☑
          - while boarding or alighting V42.4 ☑
        - truck (traffic) V44.9 ☑
          - nontraffic V44.3 ☑
          - while boarding or alighting V44.4 ☑
        - two wheeled motor vehicle (traffic) V42.9 ☑
          - nontraffic V42.3 ☑
          - while boarding or alighting V42.4 ☑
        - van (traffic) V43.94 ☑
          - nontraffic V43.34 ☑
          - while boarding or alighting V43.44 ☑
      - driver
        - collision (with)
          - animal (traffic) V40.5 ☑
            - being ridden (traffic) V46.5 ☑
              - nontraffic V46.0 ☑
            - nontraffic V40.0 ☑
          - animal-drawn vehicle (traffic) V46.5 ☑
            - nontraffic V46.0 ☑
          - bus (traffic) V44.5 ☑
            - nontraffic V44.0 ☑
          - car (traffic) V43.52 ☑
            - nontraffic V43.02 ☑
          - motor vehicle NOS (traffic) V49.40 ☑
            - nontraffic V49.00 ☑
            - specified type NEC (traffic) V49.49 ☑
              - nontraffic V49.09 ☑
          - pedal cycle (traffic) V41.5 ☑
            - nontraffic V41.0 ☑
          - pickup truck (traffic) V43.53 ☑
            - nontraffic V43.03 ☑
          - railway vehicle (traffic) V45.5 ☑
            - nontraffic V45.0 ☑
          - specified vehicle NEC (traffic) V46.5 ☑
            - nontraffic V46.0 ☑
          - sport utility vehicle (traffic) V43.51 ☑
            - nontraffic V43.01 ☑
          - stationary object (traffic) V47.52 ☑
            - nontraffic V47.02 ☑
          - streetcar (traffic) V46.5 ☑
            - nontraffic V46.0 ☑
          - three wheeled motor vehicle (traffic) V42.5 ☑
            - nontraffic V42.0 ☑
          - truck (traffic) V44.5 ☑
            - nontraffic V44.0 ☑
          - two wheeled motor vehicle (traffic) V42.5 ☑
            - nontraffic V42.0 ☑
          - van (traffic) V43.54 ☑
            - nontraffic V43.04 ☑
        - noncollision accident (traffic) V48.5 ☑
          - nontraffic V48.0 ☑

- **Accident** — *continued*
  - transport — *continued*
    - car occupant — *continued*
      - hanger-on
        - collision (with)
          - animal (traffic) V40.7 ☑
            - being ridden (traffic) V46.7 ☑
              - nontraffic V46.2 ☑
            - nontraffic V40.2 ☑
          - animal-drawn vehicle (traffic) V46.7 ☑
            - nontraffic V46.2 ☑
          - bus (traffic) V44.7 ☑
            - nontraffic V44.2 ☑
          - car (traffic) V43.72 ☑
            - nontraffic V43.22 ☑
          - pedal cycle (traffic) V41.7 ☑
            - nontraffic V41.2 ☑
          - pickup truck (traffic) V43.73 ☑
            - nontraffic V43.23 ☑
          - railway vehicle (traffic) V45.7 ☑
            - nontraffic V45.2 ☑
          - specified vehicle NEC (traffic) V46.7 ☑
            - nontraffic V46.2 ☑
          - sport utility vehicle (traffic) V43.71 ☑
            - nontraffic V43.21 ☑
          - stationary object (traffic) V47.7 ☑
            - nontraffic V47.2 ☑
          - streetcar (traffic) V46.7 ☑
            - nontraffic V46.2 ☑
          - three wheeled motor vehicle (traffic) V42.7 ☑
            - nontraffic V42.2 ☑
          - truck (traffic) V44.7 ☑
            - nontraffic V44.2 ☑
          - two wheeled motor vehicle (traffic) V42.7 ☑
            - nontraffic V42.2 ☑
          - van (traffic) V43.74 ☑
            - nontraffic V43.24 ☑
        - noncollision accident (traffic) V48.7 ☑
          - nontraffic V48.2 ☑
      - noncollision accident (traffic) V48.9 ☑
        - nontraffic V48.3 ☑
        - while boarding or alighting V48.4 ☑
      - nontraffic V49.3 ☑
      - passenger
        - collision (with)
          - animal (traffic) V40.6 ☑
            - being ridden (traffic) V46.6 ☑
              - nontraffic V46.1 ☑
            - nontraffic V40.1 ☑
          - animal-drawn vehicle (traffic) V46.6 ☑
            - nontraffic V46.1 ☑
          - bus (traffic) V44.6 ☑
            - nontraffic V44.1 ☑
          - car (traffic) V43.62 ☑
            - nontraffic V43.12 ☑
          - motor vehicle NOS (traffic) V49.50 ☑
            - nontraffic V49.10 ☑
            - specified type NEC (traffic) V49.59 ☑
              - nontraffic V49.19 ☑
          - pedal cycle (traffic) V41.6 ☑
            - nontraffic V41.1 ☑
          - pickup truck (traffic) V43.63 ☑
            - nontraffic V43.13 ☑
          - railway vehicle (traffic) V45.6 ☑
            - nontraffic V45.1 ☑
          - specified vehicle NEC (traffic) V46.6 ☑
            - nontraffic V46.1 ☑
          - sport utility vehicle (traffic) V43.61 ☑
            - nontraffic V43.11 ☑
          - stationary object (traffic) V47.62 ☑
            - nontraffic V47.12 ☑
          - streetcar (traffic) V46.6 ☑
            - nontraffic V46.1 ☑
          - three wheeled motor vehicle (traffic) V42.6 ☑
            - nontraffic V42.1 ☑
          - truck (traffic) V44.6 ☑
            - nontraffic V44.1 ☑
          - two wheeled motor vehicle (traffic) V42.6 ☑
            - nontraffic V42.1 ☑
          - van (traffic) V43.64 ☑
            - nontraffic V43.14 ☑
        - noncollision accident (traffic) V48.6 ☑

- **Accident** — *continued*
  - transport — *continued*
    - car occupant — *continued*
      - passenger — *continued*
        - noncollision accident — *continued*
          - nontraffic V48.1 ☑
      - specified type NEC V49.88 ☑
        - military vehicle V49.81 ☑
    - coal car — *see* Accident, transport, industrial vehicle occupant
    - construction vehicle occupant (nontraffic) V85.9 ☑
      - driver V85.5 ☑
      - hanger-on V85.7 ☑
      - passenger V85.6 ☑
      - traffic V85.3 ☑
        - driver V85.0 ☑
        - hanger-on V85.2 ☑
        - passenger V85.1 ☑
      - while boarding or alighting V85.4 ☑
    - dirt bike rider — *see* Accident, transport, all-terrain vehicle occupant
    - due to cataclysm — *see* Forces of nature, by type
    - dune buggy occupant (nontraffic) V86.93 ☑
      - driver V86.53 ☑
      - hanger-on V86.73 ☑
      - passenger V86.63 ☑
      - traffic V86.33 ☑
        - driver V86.03 ☑
        - hanger-on V86.23 ☑
        - passenger V86.13 ☑
      - while boarding or alighting V86.43 ☑
    - forklift — *see* Accident, transport, industrial vehicle occupant
    - go cart — *see* Accident, transport, all-terrain vehicle occupant
    - golf cart — *see* Accident, transport, all-terrain vehicle occupant
    - heavy transport vehicle occupant — *see* Accident, transport, truck occupant
    - ice yacht V98.2 ☑
    - industrial vehicle occupant (nontraffic) V83.9 ☑
      - driver V83.5 ☑
      - hanger-on V83.7 ☑
      - passenger V83.6 ☑
      - traffic V83.3 ☑
        - driver V83.0 ☑
        - hanger-on V83.2 ☑
        - passenger V83.1 ☑
      - while boarding or alighting V83.4 ☑
    - interurban electric car — *see* Accident, transport, streetcar
    - land yacht V98.1 ☑
    - logging car — *see* Accident, transport, industrial vehicle occupant
    - military vehicle occupant (traffic) V86.34 ☑
      - driver V86.04 ☑
      - hanger-on V86.24 ☑
      - nontraffic V86.94 ☑
        - driver V86.54 ☑
        - hanger-on V86.74 ☑
        - passenger V86.64 ☑
      - passenger V86.14 ☑
      - while boarding or alighting V86.44 ☑
    - mine tram — *see* Accident, transport, industrial vehicle occupant
    - motor vehicle NEC occupant (traffic) V86.39 ☑
      - driver V86.09 ☑
      - hanger-on V86.29 ☑
      - nontraffic V86.99 ☑
        - driver V86.59 ☑
        - hanger-on V86.79 ☑
        - passenger V86.69 ☑
      - passenger V86.19 ☑
      - while boarding or alighting V86.49 ☑
    - motorcoach — *see* Accident, transport, bus occupant
    - motorcyclist V29.9 ☑
      - collision (with)
        - animal (traffic) V20.9 ☑
          - being ridden (traffic) V26.9 ☑
            - nontraffic V26.2 ☑
            - while boarding or alighting V26.3 ☑
          - nontraffic V20.2 ☑
          - while boarding or alighting V20.3 ☑
        - animal-drawn vehicle (traffic) V26.9 ☑
          - nontraffic V26.2 ☑

- **Accident** — *continued*
  - transport — *continued*
    - motorcyclist — *continued*
      - collision — *continued*
        - animal-drawn vehicle — *continued*
          - while boarding or alighting V26.3 ☑
        - bus (traffic) V24.9 ☑
          - nontraffic V24.2 ☑
          - while boarding or alighting V24.3 ☑
        - car (traffic) V23.9 ☑
          - nontraffic V23.2 ☑
          - while boarding or alighting V23.3 ☑
        - motor vehicle NOS (traffic) V29.60 ☑
          - nontraffic V29.20 ☑
          - specified type NEC (traffic) V29.69 ☑
            - nontraffic V29.29 ☑
        - pedal cycle (traffic) V21.9 ☑
          - nontraffic V21.2 ☑
          - while boarding or alighting V21.3 ☑
        - pickup truck (traffic) V23.9 ☑
          - nontraffic V23.2 ☑
          - while boarding or alighting V23.3 ☑
        - railway vehicle (traffic) V25.9 ☑
          - nontraffic V25.2 ☑
          - while boarding or alighting V25.3 ☑
        - specified vehicle NEC (traffic) V26.9 ☑
          - nontraffic V26.2 ☑
          - while boarding or alighting V26.3 ☑
        - stationary object (traffic) V27.9 ☑
          - nontraffic V27.2 ☑
          - while boarding or alighting V27.3 ☑
        - streetcar (traffic) V26.9 ☑
          - nontraffic V26.2 ☑
          - while boarding or alighting V26.3 ☑
        - three wheeled motor vehicle (traffic) V22.9 ☑
          - nontraffic V22.2 ☑
          - while boarding or alighting V22.3 ☑
        - truck (traffic) V24.9 ☑
          - nontraffic V24.2 ☑
          - while boarding or alighting V24.3 ☑
        - two wheeled motor vehicle (traffic) V22.9 ☑
          - nontraffic V22.2 ☑
          - while boarding or alighting V22.3 ☑
        - van (traffic) V23.9 ☑
          - nontraffic V23.2 ☑
          - while boarding or alighting V23.3 ☑
      - driver
        - collision (with)
          - animal (traffic) V20.4 ☑
            - being ridden (traffic) V26.4 ☑
              - nontraffic V26.0 ☑
            - nontraffic V20.0 ☑
          - animal-drawn vehicle (traffic) V26.4 ☑
            - nontraffic V26.0 ☑
          - bus (traffic) V24.4 ☑
            - nontraffic V24.0 ☑
          - car (traffic) V23.4 ☑
            - nontraffic V23.0 ☑
          - motor vehicle NOS (traffic) V29.40 ☑
            - nontraffic V29.00 ☑
            - specified type NEC (traffic) V29.49 ☑
              - nontraffic V29.09 ☑
          - pedal cycle (traffic) V21.4 ☑
            - nontraffic V21.0 ☑
          - pickup truck (traffic) V23.4 ☑
            - nontraffic V23.0 ☑
          - railway vehicle (traffic) V25.4 ☑
            - nontraffic V25.0 ☑
          - specified vehicle NEC (traffic) V26.4 ☑
            - nontraffic V26.0 ☑
          - stationary object (traffic) V27.4 ☑
            - nontraffic V27.0 ☑
          - streetcar (traffic) V26.4 ☑
            - nontraffic V26.0 ☑
          - three wheeled motor vehicle (traffic) V22.4 ☑
            - nontraffic V22.0 ☑
          - truck (traffic) V24.4 ☑
            - nontraffic V24.0 ☑
          - two wheeled motor vehicle (traffic) V22.4 ☑
            - nontraffic V22.0 ☑
          - van (traffic) V23.4 ☑
            - nontraffic V23.0 ☑
        - noncollision accident (traffic) V28.4 ☑

- **Accident** — *continued*
  - transport — *continued*
    - motorcyclist — *continued*
      - driver — *continued*
        - noncollision accident — *continued*
          - nontraffic V28.0 ☑
        - noncollision accident (traffic) V28.9 ☑
          - nontraffic V28.2 ☑
          - while boarding or alighting V28.3 ☑
        - nontraffic V29.3 ☑
      - passenger
        - collision (with)
          - animal (traffic) V20.5 ☑
            - being ridden (traffic) V26.5 ☑
              - nontraffic V26.1 ☑
            - nontraffic V20.1 ☑
          - animal-drawn vehicle (traffic) V26.5 ☑
            - nontraffic V26.1 ☑
          - bus (traffic) V24.5 ☑
            - nontraffic V24.1 ☑
          - car (traffic) V23.5 ☑
            - nontraffic V23.1 ☑
          - motor vehicle NOS (traffic) V29.50 ☑
            - nontraffic V29.10 ☑
            - specified type NEC (traffic) V29.59 ☑
              - nontraffic V29.19 ☑
          - pedal cycle (traffic) V21.5 ☑
            - nontraffic V21.1 ☑
          - pickup truck (traffic) V23.5 ☑
            - nontraffic V23.1 ☑
          - railway vehicle (traffic) V25.5 ☑
            - nontraffic V25.1 ☑
          - specified vehicle NEC (traffic) V26.5 ☑
            - nontraffic V26.1 ☑
          - stationary object (traffic) V27.5 ☑
            - nontraffic V27.1 ☑
          - streetcar (traffic) V26.5 ☑
            - nontraffic V26.1 ☑
          - three wheeled motor vehicle (traffic) V22.5 ☑
            - nontraffic V22.1 ☑
          - truck (traffic) V24.5 ☑
            - nontraffic V24.1 ☑
          - two wheeled motor vehicle (traffic) V22.5 ☑
            - nontraffic V22.1 ☑
          - van (traffic) V23.5 ☑
            - nontraffic V23.1 ☑
        - noncollision accident (traffic) V28.5 ☑
          - nontraffic V28.1 ☑
      - specified type NEC V29.88 ☑
        - military vehicle V29.81 ☑
    - occupant (of)
      - aircraft (powered) V95.9 ☑
        - fixed wing
          - commercial — *see* Accident, transport, aircraft, occupant, powered, fixed wing, commercial
          - private — *see* Accident, transport, aircraft, occupant, powered, fixed wing, private
        - nonpowered V96.9 ☑
        - specified NEC V95.8 ☑
      - airport battery-powered vehicle — *see* Accident, transport, industrial vehicle occupant
      - all-terrain vehicle (ATV) — *see* Accident, transport, all-terrain vehicle occupant
      - animal-drawn vehicle — *see* Accident, transport, animal-drawn vehicle occupant
      - automobile — *see* Accident, transport, car occupant
      - balloon V96.00 ☑
      - battery-powered vehicle — *see* Accident, transport, industrial vehicle occupant
      - bicycle — *see* Accident, transport, pedal cyclist
        - motorized — *see* Accident, transport, motorcycle rider
      - boat NEC — *see* Accident, watercraft
      - bulldozer — *see* Accident, transport, construction vehicle occupant
      - bus — *see* Accident, transport, bus occupant
      - cable car (on rails) (*see also* Accident, transport, streetcar occupant)
        - not on rails V98.0 ☑
      - car (*see also* Accident, transport, car occupant)

- **Accident** — *continued*
  - transport — *continued*
    - pedal cyclist — *continued*
      - passenger — *continued*
        - noncollision accident — *continued*
          - nontraffic V18.1 ☑
      - specified type NEC V19.88 ☑
        - military vehicle V19.81 ☑
    - pedestrian
      - conveyance (occupant) VØ9.9 ☑
        - babystroller VØØ.828 ☑
          - collision (with) VØ9.9 ☑
            - animal being ridden or animal drawn vehicle VØ6.99 ☑
              - nontraffic VØ6.Ø9 ☑
              - traffic VØ6.19 ☑
            - bus or heavy transport VØ4.99 ☑
              - nontraffic VØ4.Ø9 ☑
              - traffic VØ4.19 ☑
            - car VØ3.99 ☑
              - nontraffic VØ3.Ø9 ☑
              - traffic VØ3.19 ☑
            - pedal cycle VØ1.99 ☑
              - nontraffic VØ1.Ø9 ☑
              - traffic VØ1.19 ☑
            - pick-up truck or van VØ3.99 ☑
              - nontraffic VØ3.Ø9 ☑
              - traffic VØ3.19 ☑
            - railway (train) (vehicle) VØ5.99 ☑
              - nontraffic VØ5.Ø9 ☑
              - traffic VØ5.19 ☑
            - stationary object VØØ.822 ☑
            - streetcar VØ6.99 ☑
              - nontraffic VØ6.Ø9 ☑
              - traffic VØ6.19 ☑
            - two- or three-wheeled motor vehicle VØ2.99 ☑
              - nontraffic VØ2.Ø9 ☑
              - traffic VØ2.19 ☑
            - vehicle VØ9.9 ☑
              - animal-drawn VØ6.99 ☑
                - nontraffic VØ6.Ø9 ☑
                - traffic VØ6.19 ☑
              - motor
                - nontraffic VØ9.ØØ ☑
                - traffic VØ9.2Ø ☑
          - fall VØØ.821 ☑
          - nontraffic VØ9.1 ☑
            - involving motor vehicle NEC VØ9.ØØ ☑
          - traffic VØ9.3 ☑
            - involving motor vehicle NEC VØ9.2Ø ☑
        - flat-bottomed NEC VØØ.388 ☑
          - collision (with) VØ9.9 ☑
            - animal being ridden or animal drawn vehicle VØ6.99 ☑
              - nontraffic VØ6.Ø9 ☑
              - traffic VØ6.19 ☑
            - bus or heavy transport VØ4.99 ☑
              - nontraffic VØ4.Ø9 ☑
              - traffic VØ4.19 ☑
            - car VØ3.99 ☑
              - nontraffic VØ3.Ø9 ☑
              - traffic VØ3.19 ☑
            - pedal cycle VØ1.99 ☑
              - nontraffic VØ1.Ø9 ☑
              - traffic VØ1.19 ☑
            - pick-up truck or van VØ3.99 ☑
              - nontraffic VØ3.Ø9 ☑
              - traffic VØ3.19 ☑
            - railway (train) (vehicle) VØ5.99 ☑
              - nontraffic VØ5.Ø9 ☑
              - traffic VØ5.19 ☑
            - stationary object VØØ.382 ☑
            - streetcar VØ6.99 ☑
              - nontraffic VØ6.Ø9 ☑
              - traffic VØ6.19 ☑
            - two- or three-wheeled motor vehicle VØ2.99 ☑
              - nontraffic VØ2.Ø9 ☑
              - traffic VØ2.19 ☑
            - vehicle VØ9.9 ☑
              - animal-drawn VØ6.99 ☑
                - nontraffic VØ6.Ø9 ☑
                - traffic VØ6.19 ☑

- **Accident** — *continued*
  - transport — *continued*
    - pedestrian — *continued*
      - conveyance — *continued*
        - flat-bottomed — *continued*
          - collision — *continued*
            - vehicle — *continued*
              - motor
                - nontraffic VØ9.ØØ ☑
                - traffic VØ9.2Ø ☑
          - fall VØØ.381 ☑
          - nontraffic VØ9.1 ☑
            - involving motor vehicle NEC VØ9.ØØ ☑
          - snow
            - board — *see* Accident, transport, pedestrian, conveyance, snow board
            - ski — *see* Accident, transport, pedestrian, conveyance, skis (snow)
          - traffic VØ9.3 ☑
            - involving motor vehicle NEC VØ9.2Ø ☑
        - gliding type NEC VØØ.288 ☑
          - collision (with) VØ9.9 ☑
            - animal being ridden or animal drawn vehicle VØ6.99 ☑
              - nontraffic VØ6.Ø9 ☑
              - traffic VØ6.19 ☑
            - bus or heavy transport VØ4.99 ☑
              - nontraffic VØ4.Ø9 ☑
              - traffic VØ4.19 ☑
            - car VØ3.99 ☑
              - nontraffic VØ3.Ø9 ☑
              - traffic VØ3.19 ☑
            - pedal cycle VØ1.99 ☑
              - nontraffic VØ1.Ø9 ☑
              - traffic VØ1.19 ☑
            - pick-up truck or van VØ3.99 ☑
              - nontraffic VØ3.Ø9 ☑
              - traffic VØ3.19 ☑
            - railway (train) (vehicle) VØ5.99 ☑
              - nontraffic VØ5.Ø9 ☑
              - traffic VØ5.19 ☑
            - stationary object VØØ.282 ☑
            - streetcar VØ6.99 ☑
              - nontraffic VØ6.Ø9 ☑
              - traffic VØ6.19- ☑
            - two- or three-wheeled motor vehicle VØ2.99 ☑
              - nontraffic VØ2.Ø9 ☑
              - traffic VØ2.19 ☑
            - vehicle VØ9.9 ☑
              - animal-drawn VØ6.99 ☑
                - nontraffic VØ6.Ø9 ☑
                - traffic VØ6.19 ☑
              - motor
                - nontraffic VØ9.ØØ ☑
                - traffic VØ9.2Ø ☑
          - fall VØØ.281 ☑
          - heelies — *see* Accident, transport, pedestrian, conveyance, heelies
          - ice skate — *see* Accident, transport, pedestrian, conveyance, ice skate
          - nontraffic VØ9.1 ☑
            - involving motor vehicle NEC VØ9.ØØ ☑
          - sled — *see* Accident, transport, pedestrian, conveyance, sled
          - traffic VØ9.3 ☑
            - involving motor vehicle NEC VØ9.2Ø ☑
          - wheelies — *see* Accident, transport, pedestrian, conveyance, heelies
        - heelies VØØ.158 ☑
          - colliding with stationary object VØØ.152 ☑
          - fall VØØ.151 ☑
        - ice skates VØØ.218 ☑
          - collision (with) VØ9.9 ☑
            - animal being ridden or animal drawn vehicle VØ6.99 ☑
              - nontraffic VØ6.Ø9 ☑
              - traffic VØ6.19 ☑

- **Accident** — *continued*
  - transport — *continued*
    - pedestrian — *continued*
      - conveyance — *continued*
        - ice skates — *continued*
          - collision — *continued*
            - bus or heavy transport VØ4.99 ☑
              - nontraffic VØ4.Ø9 ☑
              - traffic VØ4.19 ☑
            - car VØ3.99 ☑
              - nontraffic VØ3.Ø9 ☑
              - traffic VØ3.19 ☑
            - pedal cycle VØ1.99 ☑
              - nontraffic VØ1.Ø9 ☑
              - traffic VØ1.19 ☑
            - pick-up truck or van VØ3.99 ☑
              - nontraffic VØ3.Ø9 ☑
              - traffic VØ3.19 ☑
            - railway (train) (vehicle) VØ5.99 ☑
              - nontraffic VØ5.Ø9 ☑
              - traffic VØ5.19 ☑
            - stationary object VØØ.212 ☑
            - streetcar VØ6.99 ☑
              - nontraffic VØ6.Ø9 ☑
              - traffic VØ6.19 ☑
            - two- or three-wheeled motor vehicle VØ2.99 ☑
              - nontraffic VØ2.Ø9 ☑
              - traffic VØ2.19 ☑
            - vehicle VØ9.9 ☑
              - animal-drawn VØ6.99 ☑
                - nontraffic VØ6.Ø9 ☑
                - traffic VØ6.19 ☑
              - motor
                - nontraffic VØ9.ØØ ☑
                - traffic VØ9.2Ø ☑
          - fall VØØ.211 ☑
          - nontraffic VØ9.1 ☑
            - involving motor vehicle NEC VØ9.ØØ ☑
          - traffic VØ9.3 ☑
            - involving motor vehicle NEC VØ9.2Ø ☑
        - motorized mobility scooter VØØ.838 ☑
          - collision with stationary object VØØ.832 ☑
          - fall from VØØ.831 ☑
          - nontraffic VØ9.1 ☑
            - involving motor vehicle VØ9.ØØ ☑
            - military VØ9.Ø1 ☑
            - specified type NEC VØ9.Ø9 ☑
        - roller skates (non in-line) VØØ.128 ☑
          - collision (with) VØ9.9 ☑
            - animal being ridden or animal drawn vehicle VØ6.91 ☑
              - nontraffic VØ6.Ø1 ☑
              - traffic VØ6.11 ☑
            - bus or heavy transport VØ4.91 ☑
              - nontraffic VØ4.Ø1 ☑
              - traffic VØ4.11 ☑
            - car VØ3.91 ☑
              - nontraffic VØ3.Ø1 ☑
              - traffic VØ3.11 ☑
            - pedal cycle VØ1.91 ☑
              - nontraffic VØ1.Ø1 ☑
              - traffic VØ1.11 ☑
            - pick-up truck or van VØ3.91 ☑
              - nontraffic VØ3.Ø1 ☑
              - traffic VØ3.11 ☑
            - railway (train) (vehicle) VØ5.91 ☑
              - nontraffic VØ5.Ø1 ☑
              - traffic VØ5.11 ☑
            - stationary object VØØ.122 ☑
            - streetcar VØ6.91 ☑
              - nontraffic VØ6.Ø1 ☑
              - traffic VØ6.11 ☑
            - two- or three-wheeled motor vehicle VØ2.91 ☑
              - nontraffic VØ2.Ø1 ☑
              - traffic VØ2.11 ☑
            - vehicle VØ9.9 ☑
              - animal-drawn VØ6.91 ☑
                - nontraffic VØ6.Ø1 ☑
                - traffic VØ6.11 ☑
              - motor
                - nontraffic VØ9.ØØ ☑

- **Accident** — *continued*
  - transport — *continued*
    - pedestrian — *continued*
      - conveyance — *continued*
        - sled — *continued*
          - collision — *continued*
            - vehicle — *continued*
              - animal-drawn — *continued*
                - traffic V06.19 ☑
              - motor
                - nontraffic V09.00 ☑
                - traffic V09.20 ☑
          - fall V00.221 ☑
          - nontraffic V09.1 ☑
            - involving motor vehicle NEC V09.00 ☑
          - traffic V09.3 ☑
            - involving motor vehicle NEC V09.20 ☑
        - snow board V00.318 ☑
          - collision (with) V09.9 ☑
            - animal being ridden or animal drawn vehicle V06.99 ☑
              - nontraffic V06.09 ☑
              - traffic V06.19 ☑
            - bus or heavy transport V04.99 ☑
              - nontraffic V04.09 ☑
              - traffic V04.19 ☑
            - car V03.99 ☑
              - nontraffic V03.09 ☑
              - traffic V03.19 ☑
            - pedal cycle V01.99 ☑
              - nontraffic V01.09 ☑
              - traffic V01.19 ☑
            - pick-up truck or van V03.99 ☑
              - nontraffic V03.09 ☑
              - traffic V03.19 ☑
            - railway (train) (vehicle) V05.99 ☑
              - nontraffic V05.09 ☑
              - traffic V05.19 ☑
            - stationary object V00.312 ☑
            - streetcar V06.99 ☑
              - nontraffic V06.09 ☑
              - traffic V06.19 ☑
            - two- or three-wheeled motor vehicle V02.99 ☑
              - nontraffic V02.09 ☑
              - traffic V02.19 ☑
            - vehicle V09.9 ☑
              - animal-drawn V06.99 ☑
                - nontraffic V06.09 ☑
                - traffic V06.19 ☑
              - motor
                - nontraffic V09.00 ☑
                - traffic V09.20 ☑
          - fall V00.311 ☑
          - nontraffic V09.1 ☑
            - involving motor vehicle NEC V09.00 ☑
          - traffic V09.3 ☑
            - involving motor vehicle NEC V09.20 ☑
        - specified type NEC V00.898 ☑
          - collision (with) V09.9 ☑
            - animal being ridden or animal drawn vehicle V06.99 ☑
              - nontraffic V06.09 ☑
              - traffic V06.19 ☑
            - bus or heavy transport V04.99 ☑
              - nontraffic V04.09 ☑
              - traffic V04.19 ☑
            - car V03.99 ☑
              - nontraffic V03.09 ☑
              - traffic V03.19 ☑
            - pedal cycle V01.99 ☑
              - nontraffic V01.09 ☑
              - traffic V01.19 ☑
            - pick-up truck or van V03.99 ☑
              - nontraffic V03.09 ☑
              - traffic V03.19 ☑
            - railway (train) (vehicle) V05.99 ☑
              - nontraffic V05.09 ☑
              - traffic V05.19 ☑
            - stationary object V00.892 ☑
            - streetcar V06.99 ☑
              - nontraffic V06.09 ☑

- **Accident** — *continued*
  - transport — *continued*
    - pedestrian — *continued*
      - conveyance — *continued*
        - specified type — *continued*
          - collision — *continued*
            - streetcar — *continued*
              - traffic V06.19 ☑
            - two- or three-wheeled motor vehicle V02.99 ☑
              - nontraffic V02.09 ☑
              - traffic V02.19 ☑
            - vehicle V09.9 ☑
              - animal-drawn V06.99 ☑
                - nontraffic V06.09 ☑
                - traffic V06.19 ☑
              - motor
                - nontraffic V09.00 ☑
                - traffic V09.20 ☑
          - fall V00.891 ☑
          - nontraffic V09.1 ☑
            - involving motor vehicle NEC V09.00 ☑
          - traffic V09.3 ☑
            - involving motor vehicle NEC V09.20 ☑
        - traffic V09.3 ☑
          - involving motor vehicle V09.20 ☑
            - military V09.21 ☑
            - specified type NEC V09.29 ☑
        - wheelchair (powered) V00.818 ☑
          - collision (with) V09.9 ☑
            - animal being ridden or animal drawn vehicle V06.99 ☑
              - nontraffic V06.09 ☑
              - traffic V06.19 ☑
            - bus or heavy transport V04.99 ☑
              - nontraffic V04.09 ☑
              - traffic V04.19 ☑
            - car V03.99 ☑
              - nontraffic V03.09 ☑
              - traffic V03.19 ☑
            - pedal cycle V01.99 ☑
              - nontraffic V01.09 ☑
              - traffic V01.19 ☑
            - pick-up truck or van V03.99 ☑
              - nontraffic V03.09 ☑
              - traffic V03.19 ☑
            - railway (train) (vehicle) V05.99 ☑
              - nontraffic V05.09 ☑
              - traffic V05.19 ☑
            - stationary object V00.812 ☑
            - streetcar V06.99 ☑
              - nontraffic V06.09 ☑
              - traffic V06.19 ☑
            - two- or three-wheeled motor vehicle V02.99 ☑
              - nontraffic V02.09 ☑
              - traffic V02.19 ☑
            - vehicle V09.9 ☑
              - animal-drawn V06.99 ☑
                - nontraffic V06.09 ☑
                - traffic V06.19 ☑
              - motor
                - nontraffic V09.00 ☑
                - traffic V09.20 ☑
          - fall V00.811 ☑
          - nontraffic V09.1 ☑
            - involving motor vehicle NEC V09.00 ☑
          - traffic V09.3 ☑
            - involving motor vehicle NEC V09.20 ☑
        - wheeled shoe V00.158 ☑
          - colliding with stationary object V00.152 ☑
          - fall V00.151 ☑
      - on foot (*see also* Accident, pedestrian)
        - collision (with)
          - animal being ridden or animal drawn vehicle V06.90 ☑
            - nontraffic V06.00 ☑
            - traffic V06.10 ☑
          - bus or heavy transport V04.90 ☑
            - nontraffic V04.00 ☑
            - traffic V04.10 ☑

- **Accident** — *continued*
  - transport — *continued*
    - pedestrian — *continued*
      - on foot (*see also* Accident, pedestrian) — *continued*
        - collision — *continued*
          - car V03.90 ☑
            - nontraffic V03.00 ☑
            - traffic V03.10 ☑
          - pedal cycle V01.90 ☑
            - nontraffic V01.00 ☑
            - traffic V01.10 ☑
          - pick-up truck or van V03.90 ☑
            - nontraffic V03.00 ☑
            - traffic V03.10 ☑
          - railway (train) (vehicle) V05.90 ☑
            - nontraffic V05.00 ☑
            - traffic V05.10 ☑
          - streetcar V06.90 ☑
            - nontraffic V06.00 ☑
            - traffic V06.10 ☑
          - two- or three-wheeled motor vehicle V02.90 ☑
            - nontraffic V02.00 ☑
            - traffic V02.10 ☑
          - vehicle V09.9 ☑
            - animal-drawn V06.90 ☑
              - nontraffic V06.00 ☑
              - traffic V06.10 ☑
            - motor
        - nontraffic V09.1 ☑
          - involving motor vehicle V09.00 ☑
            - military V09.01 ☑
            - specified type NEC V09.09 ☑
        - traffic V09.3 ☑
          - involving motor vehicle V09.20 ☑
            - military V09.21 ☑
            - specified type NEC V09.29 ☑
    - person NEC (unknown way or transportation) V99 ☑
      - collision (between)
        - bus (with)
          - heavy transport vehicle (traffic) V87.5 ☑
            - nontraffic V88.5 ☑
        - car (with)
          - bus (traffic) V87.3 ☑
            - nontraffic V88.3 ☑
          - heavy transport vehicle (traffic) V87.4 ☑
            - nontraffic V88.4 ☑
          - nontraffic V88.5 ☑
          - pick-up truck or van (traffic) V87.2 ☑
            - nontraffic V88.2 ☑
          - train or railway vehicle (traffic) V87.6 ☑
            - nontraffic V88.6 ☑
          - two-or three-wheeled motor vehicle (traffic) V87.0 ☑
            - nontraffic V88.0 ☑
        - motor vehicle (traffic) NEC V87.7 ☑
          - nontraffic V88.7 ☑
        - two-or three-wheeled vehicle (with) (traffic) motor vehicle NEC V87.1 ☑
          - nontraffic V88.1 ☑
      - nonmotor vehicle (collision) (noncollision) (traffic) V87.9 ☑
        - nontraffic V88.9 ☑
    - pickup truck occupant V59.9 ☑
      - collision (with)
        - animal (traffic) V50.9 ☑
          - being ridden (traffic) V56.9 ☑
            - nontraffic V56.3 ☑
            - while boarding or alighting V56.4 ☑
          - nontraffic V50.3 ☑
          - while boarding or alighting V50.4 ☑
        - animal-drawn vehicle (traffic) V56.9 ☑
          - nontraffic V56.3 ☑
          - while boarding or alighting V56.4 ☑
        - bus (traffic) V54.9 ☑
          - nontraffic V54.3 ☑
          - while boarding or alighting V54.4 ☑
        - car (traffic) V53.9 ☑
          - nontraffic V53.3 ☑
          - while boarding or alighting V53.4 ☑
        - motor vehicle NOS (traffic) V59.60 ☑
          - nontraffic V59.20 ☑
          - specified type NEC (traffic) V59.69 ☑
            - nontraffic V59.29 ☑

- **Accident** — *continued*
  - transport — *continued*
    - pickup truck occupant — *continued*
      - collision — *continued*
        - pedal cycle (traffic) V51.9 ☑
          - nontraffic V51.3 ☑
          - while boarding or alighting V51.4 ☑
        - pickup truck (traffic) V53.9 ☑
          - nontraffic V53.3 ☑
          - while boarding or alighting V53.4 ☑
        - railway vehicle (traffic) V55.9 ☑
          - nontraffic V55.3 ☑
          - while boarding or alighting V55.4 ☑
        - specified vehicle NEC (traffic) V56.9 ☑
          - nontraffic V56.3 ☑
          - while boarding or alighting V56.4 ☑
        - stationary object (traffic) V57.9 ☑
          - nontraffic V57.3 ☑
          - while boarding or alighting V57.4 ☑
        - streetcar (traffic) V56.9 ☑
          - nontraffic V56.3 ☑
          - while boarding or alighting V56.4 ☑
        - three wheeled motor vehicle (traffic) V52.9 ☑
          - nontraffic V52.3 ☑
          - while boarding or alighting V52.4 ☑
        - truck (traffic) V54.9 ☑
          - nontraffic V54.3 ☑
          - while boarding or alighting V54.4 ☑
        - two wheeled motor vehicle (traffic) V52.9 ☑
          - nontraffic V52.3 ☑
          - while boarding or alighting V52.4 ☑
        - van (traffic) V53.9 ☑
          - nontraffic V53.3 ☑
          - while boarding or alighting V53.4 ☑
      - driver
        - collision (with)
          - animal (traffic) V5Ø.5 ☑
            - being ridden (traffic) V56.5 ☑
              - nontraffic V56.Ø ☑
            - nontraffic V5Ø.Ø ☑
          - animal-drawn vehicle (traffic) V56.5 ☑
            - nontraffic V56.Ø ☑
          - bus (traffic) V54.5 ☑
            - nontraffic V54.Ø ☑
          - car (traffic) V53.5 ☑
            - nontraffic V53.Ø ☑
          - motor vehicle NOS (traffic) V59.4Ø ☑
            - nontraffic V59.ØØ ☑
            - specified type NEC (traffic) V59.49 ☑
              - nontraffic V59.Ø9 ☑
          - pedal cycle (traffic) V51.5 ☑
            - nontraffic V51.Ø ☑
          - pickup truck (traffic) V53.5 ☑
            - nontraffic V53.Ø ☑
          - railway vehicle (traffic) V55.5 ☑
            - nontraffic V55.Ø ☑
          - specified vehicle NEC (traffic) V56.5 ☑
            - nontraffic V56.Ø ☑
          - stationary object (traffic) V57.5 ☑
            - nontraffic V57.Ø ☑
          - streetcar (traffic) V56.5 ☑
            - nontraffic V56.Ø ☑
          - three wheeled motor vehicle (traffic) V52.5 ☑
            - nontraffic V52.Ø ☑
          - truck (traffic) V54.5 ☑
            - nontraffic V54.Ø ☑
          - two wheeled motor vehicle (traffic) V52.5 ☑
            - nontraffic V52.Ø ☑
          - van (traffic) V53.5 ☑
            - nontraffic V53.Ø ☑
        - noncollision accident (traffic) V58.5 ☑
          - nontraffic V58.Ø ☑
      - hanger-on
        - collision (with)
          - animal (traffic) V5Ø.7 ☑
            - being ridden (traffic) V56.7 ☑
              - nontraffic V56.2 ☑
            - nontraffic V5Ø.2 ☑
          - animal-drawn vehicle (traffic) V56.7 ☑
            - nontraffic V56.2 ☑
          - bus (traffic) V54.7 ☑
            - nontraffic V54.2 ☑
          - car (traffic) V53.7 ☑

- **Accident** — *continued*
  - transport — *continued*
    - pickup truck occupant — *continued*
      - hanger-on — *continued*
        - collision — *continued*
          - car — *continued*
            - nontraffic V53.2 ☑
          - pedal cycle (traffic) V51.7 ☑
            - nontraffic V51.2 ☑
          - pickup truck (traffic) V53.7 ☑
            - nontraffic V53.2 ☑
          - railway vehicle (traffic) V55.7 ☑
            - nontraffic V55.2 ☑
          - specified vehicle NEC (traffic) V56.7 ☑
            - nontraffic V56.2 ☑
          - stationary object (traffic) V57.7 ☑
            - nontraffic V57.2 ☑
          - streetcar (traffic) V56.7 ☑
            - nontraffic V56.2 ☑
          - three wheeled motor vehicle (traffic) V52.7 ☑
            - nontraffic V52.2 ☑
          - truck (traffic) V54.7 ☑
            - nontraffic V54.2 ☑
          - two wheeled motor vehicle (traffic) V52.7 ☑
            - nontraffic V52.2 ☑
          - van (traffic) V53.7 ☑
            - nontraffic V53.2 ☑
        - noncollision accident (traffic) V58.7 ☑
          - nontraffic V58.2 ☑
      - noncollision accident (traffic) V58.9 ☑
        - nontraffic V58.3 ☑
        - while boarding or alighting V58.4 ☑
      - nontraffic V59.3 ☑
      - passenger
        - collision (with)
          - animal (traffic) V5Ø.6 ☑
            - being ridden (traffic) V56.6 ☑
              - nontraffic V56.1 ☑
            - nontraffic V5Ø.1 ☑
          - animal-drawn vehicle (traffic) V56.6 ☑
            - nontraffic V56.1 ☑
          - bus (traffic) V54.6 ☑
            - nontraffic V54.1 ☑
          - car (traffic) V53.6 ☑
            - nontraffic V53.1 ☑
          - motor vehicle NOS (traffic) V59.5Ø ☑
            - nontraffic V59.1Ø ☑
            - specified type NEC (traffic) V59.59 ☑
              - nontraffic V59.19 ☑
          - pedal cycle (traffic) V51.6 ☑
            - nontraffic V51.1 ☑
          - pickup truck (traffic) V53.6 ☑
            - nontraffic V53.1 ☑
          - railway vehicle (traffic) V55.6 ☑
            - nontraffic V55.1 ☑
          - specified vehicle NEC (traffic) V56.6 ☑
            - nontraffic V56.1 ☑
          - stationary object (traffic) V57.6 ☑
            - nontraffic V57.1 ☑
          - streetcar (traffic) V56.6 ☑
            - nontraffic V56.1 ☑
          - three wheeled motor vehicle (traffic) V52.6 ☑
            - nontraffic V52.1 ☑
          - truck (traffic) V54.6 ☑
            - nontraffic V54.1 ☑
          - two wheeled motor vehicle (traffic) V52.6 ☑
            - nontraffic V52.1 ☑
          - van (traffic) V53.6 ☑
            - nontraffic V53.1 ☑
        - noncollision accident (traffic) V58.6 ☑
          - nontraffic V58.1 ☑
      - specified type NEC V59.88 ☑
        - military vehicle V59.81 ☑
    - quarry truck — *see* Accident, transport, industrial vehicle occupant
    - race car — *see* Accident, transport, motor vehicle NEC occupant
    - railway vehicle occupant V81.9 ☑
      - collision (with) V81.3 ☑
        - motor vehicle (non-military) (traffic) V81.1 ☑
          - military V81.83 ☑

- **Accident** — *continued*
  - transport — *continued*
    - railway vehicle occupant — *continued*
      - collision — *continued*
        - motor vehicle — *continued*
          - nontraffic V81.Ø ☑
        - rolling stock V81.2 ☑
        - specified object NEC V81.3 ☑
      - during derailment V81.7 ☑
        - with antecedent collision B — *see* Accident, transport, railway vehicle occupant, collision
      - explosion V81.81 ☑
      - fall (in railway vehicle) V81.5 ☑
        - during derailment V81.7 ☑
          - with antecedent collision B — *see* Accident, transport, railway vehicle occupant, collision
        - from railway vehicle V81.6 ☑
          - during derailment V81.7 ☑
            - with antecedent collision B — *see* Accident, transport, railway vehicle occupant, collision
        - while boarding or alighting V81.4 ☑
      - fire V81.81 ☑
      - object falling onto train V81.82 ☑
      - specified type NEC V81.89 ☑
      - while boarding or alighting V81.4 ☑
    - ski lift V98.3 ☑
    - snowmobile occupant (nontraffic) V86.92 ☑
      - driver V86.52 ☑
      - hanger-on V86.72 ☑
      - passenger V86.62 ☑
      - traffic V86.32 ☑
        - driver V86.Ø2 ☑
        - hanger-on V86.22 ☑
        - passenger V86.12 ☑
      - while boarding or alighting V86.42 ☑
    - specified NEC V98.8 ☑
    - sport utility vehicle occupant (*see also* Accident, transport, car occupant)
      - collision (with)
        - stationary object (traffic) V47.91 ☑
          - nontraffic V47.31 ☑
      - driver
        - collision (with)
          - stationary object (traffic) V47.51 ☑
            - nontraffic V47.Ø1 ☑
      - passenger
        - collision (with)
          - stationary object (traffic) V47.61 ☑
            - nontraffic V47.11 ☑
    - streetcar occupant V82.9 ☑
      - collision (with) V82.3 ☑
        - motor vehicle (traffic) V82.1 ☑
          - nontraffic V82.Ø ☑
        - rolling stock V82.2 ☑
      - during derailment V82.7 ☑
        - with antecedent collision B — *see* Accident, transport, streetcar occupant, collision
      - fall (in streetcar) V82.5 ☑
        - during derailment V82.7 ☑
          - with antecedent collision B — *see* Accident, transport, streetcar occupant, collision
        - from streetcar V82.6 ☑
          - during derailment V82.7 ☑
            - with antecedent collision B — *see* Accident, transport, streetcar occupant, collision
          - while boarding or alighting V82.4 ☑
        - while boarding or alighting V82.4 ☑
      - specified type NEC V82.8 ☑
      - while boarding or alighting V82.4 ☑
    - three-wheeled motor vehicle occupant V39.9 ☑
      - collision (with)
        - animal (traffic) V3Ø.9 ☑
          - being ridden (traffic) V36.9 ☑
            - nontraffic V36.3 ☑
            - while boarding or alighting V36.4 ☑
          - nontraffic V3Ø.3 ☑
          - while boarding or alighting V3Ø.4 ☑
        - animal-drawn vehicle (traffic) V36.9 ☑
          - nontraffic V36.3 ☑
          - while boarding or alighting V36.4 ☑
        - bus (traffic) V34.9 ☑

- **Accident** — *continued*
  - transport — *continued*
    - truck occupant — *continued*
      - driver — *continued*
        - collision — *continued*
          - stationary object (traffic) V67.5 ☑
            - nontraffic V67.0 ☑
          - streetcar (traffic) V66.5 ☑
            - nontraffic V66.0 ☑
          - three wheeled motor vehicle (traffic) V62.5 ☑
            - nontraffic V62.0 ☑
          - truck (traffic) V64.5 ☑
            - nontraffic V64.0 ☑
          - two wheeled motor vehicle (traffic) V62.5 ☑
            - nontraffic V62.0 ☑
          - van (traffic) V63.5 ☑
            - nontraffic V63.0 ☑
        - noncollision accident (traffic) V68.5 ☑
          - nontraffic V68.0 ☑
      - dump — *see* Accident, transport, construction vehicle occupant
      - hanger-on
        - collision (with)
          - animal (traffic) V60.7 ☑
            - being ridden (traffic) V66.7 ☑
              - nontraffic V66.2 ☑
            - nontraffic V60.2 ☑
          - animal-drawn vehicle (traffic) V66.7 ☑
            - nontraffic V66.2 ☑
          - bus (traffic) V64.7 ☑
            - nontraffic V64.2 ☑
          - car (traffic) V63.7 ☑
            - nontraffic V63.2 ☑
          - pedal cycle (traffic) V61.7 ☑
            - nontraffic V61.2 ☑
          - pickup truck (traffic) V63.7 ☑
            - nontraffic V63.2 ☑
          - railway vehicle (traffic) V65.7 ☑
            - nontraffic V65.2 ☑
          - specified vehicle NEC (traffic) V66.7 ☑
            - nontraffic V66.2 ☑
          - stationary object (traffic) V67.7 ☑
            - nontraffic V67.2 ☑
          - streetcar (traffic) V66.7 ☑
            - nontraffic V66.2 ☑
          - three wheeled motor vehicle (traffic) V62.7 ☑
            - nontraffic V62.2 ☑
          - truck (traffic) V64.7 ☑
            - nontraffic V64.2 ☑
          - two wheeled motor vehicle (traffic) V62.7 ☑
            - nontraffic V62.2 ☑
          - van (traffic) V63.7 ☑
            - nontraffic V63.2 ☑
        - noncollision accident (traffic) V68.7 ☑
          - nontraffic V68.2 ☑
      - noncollision accident (traffic) V68.9 ☑
        - nontraffic V68.3 ☑
        - while boarding or alighting V68.4 ☑
      - nontraffic V69.3 ☑
      - passenger
        - collision (with)
          - animal (traffic) V60.6 ☑
            - being ridden (traffic) V66.6 ☑
              - nontraffic V66.1- ☑
            - nontraffic V60.1 ☑
          - animal-drawn vehicle (traffic) V66.6 ☑
            - nontraffic V66.1 ☑
          - bus (traffic) V64.6 ☑
            - nontraffic V64.1 ☑
          - car (traffic) V63.6 ☑
            - nontraffic V63.1 ☑
          - motor vehicle NOS (traffic) V69.50 ☑
            - nontraffic V69.10 ☑
            - specified type NEC (traffic) V69.59 ☑
              - nontraffic V69.19 ☑
          - pedal cycle (traffic) V61.6 ☑
            - nontraffic V61.1 ☑
          - pickup truck (traffic) V63.6 ☑
            - nontraffic V63.1 ☑
          - railway vehicle (traffic) V65.6 ☑
            - nontraffic V65.1 ☑
          - specified vehicle NEC (traffic) V66.6 ☑

- **Accident** — *continued*
  - transport — *continued*
    - truck occupant — *continued*
      - passenger — *continued*
        - collision — *continued*
          - specified vehicle — *continued*
            - nontraffic V66.1 ☑
          - stationary object (traffic) V67.6 ☑
            - nontraffic V67.1 ☑
          - streetcar (traffic) V66.6 ☑
            - nontraffic V66.1 ☑
          - three wheeled motor vehicle (traffic) V62.6 ☑
            - nontraffic V62.1 ☑
          - truck (traffic) V64.6 ☑
            - nontraffic V64.1 ☑
          - two wheeled motor vehicle (traffic) V62.6 ☑
            - nontraffic V62.1 ☑
          - van (traffic) V63.6 ☑
            - nontraffic V63.1 ☑
        - noncollision accident (traffic) V68.6 ☑
          - nontraffic V68.1 ☑
      - pickup — *see* Accident, transport, pickup truck occupant
      - specified type NEC V69.88 ☑
        - military vehicle V69.81 ☑
    - van occupant V59.9 ☑
      - collision (with)
        - animal (traffic) V50.9 ☑
          - being ridden (traffic) V56.9 ☑
            - nontraffic V56.3 ☑
            - while boarding or alighting V56.4 ☑
          - nontraffic V50.3 ☑
          - while boarding or alighting V50.4 ☑
        - animal-drawn vehicle (traffic) V56.9 ☑
          - nontraffic V56.3 ☑
          - while boarding or alighting V56.4 ☑
        - bus (traffic) V54.9 ☑
          - nontraffic V54.3 ☑
          - while boarding or alighting V54.4 ☑
        - car (traffic) V53.9 ☑
          - nontraffic V53.3 ☑
          - while boarding or alighting V53.4 ☑
        - motor vehicle NOS (traffic) V59.60 ☑
          - nontraffic V59.20 ☑
          - specified type NEC (traffic) V59.69 ☑
            - nontraffic V59.29 ☑
        - pedal cycle (traffic) V51.9 ☑
          - nontraffic V51.3 ☑
          - while boarding or alighting V51.4 ☑
        - pickup truck (traffic) V53.9 ☑
          - nontraffic V53.3 ☑
          - while boarding or alighting V53.4 ☑
        - railway vehicle (traffic) V55.9 ☑
          - nontraffic V55.3 ☑
          - while boarding or alighting V55.4 ☑
        - specified vehicle NEC (traffic) V56.9 ☑
          - nontraffic V56.3 ☑
          - while boarding or alighting V56.4 ☑
        - stationary object (traffic) V57.9 ☑
          - nontraffic V57.3 ☑
          - while boarding or alighting V57.4 ☑
        - streetcar (traffic) V56.9 ☑
          - nontraffic V56.3 ☑
          - while boarding or alighting V56.4 ☑
        - three wheeled motor vehicle (traffic) V52.9 ☑
          - nontraffic V52.3 ☑
          - while boarding or alighting V52.4 ☑
        - truck (traffic) V54.9 ☑
          - nontraffic V54.3 ☑
          - while boarding or alighting V54.4 ☑
        - two wheeled motor vehicle (traffic) V52.9 ☑
          - nontraffic V52.3 ☑
          - while boarding or alighting V52.4 ☑
        - van (traffic) V53.9 ☑
          - nontraffic V53.3 ☑
          - while boarding or alighting V53.4 ☑
      - driver
        - collision (with)
          - animal (traffic) V50.5 ☑
            - being ridden (traffic) V56.5 ☑
              - nontraffic V56.0 ☑
            - nontraffic V50.0 ☑
          - animal-drawn vehicle (traffic) V56.5 ☑

- **Accident** — *continued*
  - transport — *continued*
    - van occupant — *continued*
      - driver — *continued*
        - collision — *continued*
          - animal-drawn vehicle — *continued*
            - nontraffic V56.0 ☑
          - bus (traffic) V54.5 ☑
            - nontraffic V54.0 ☑
          - car (traffic) V53.5 ☑
            - nontraffic V53.0 ☑
          - motor vehicle NOS (traffic) V59.40 ☑
            - nontraffic V59.00 ☑
            - specified type NEC (traffic) V59.49 ☑
              - nontraffic V59.09 ☑
          - pedal cycle (traffic) V51.5 ☑
            - nontraffic V51.0 ☑
          - pickup truck (traffic) V53.5 ☑
            - nontraffic V53.0 ☑
          - railway vehicle (traffic) V55.5 ☑
            - nontraffic V55.0 ☑
          - specified vehicle NEC (traffic) V56.5 ☑
            - nontraffic V56.0 ☑
          - stationary object (traffic) V57.5 ☑
            - nontraffic V57.0 ☑
          - streetcar (traffic) V56.5 ☑
            - nontraffic V56.0 ☑
          - three wheeled motor vehicle (traffic) V52.5 ☑
            - nontraffic V52.0 ☑
          - truck (traffic) V54.5 ☑
            - nontraffic V54.0 ☑
          - two wheeled motor vehicle (traffic) V52.5 ☑
            - nontraffic V52.0 ☑
          - van (traffic) V53.5 ☑
            - nontraffic V53.0 ☑
        - noncollision accident (traffic) V58.5 ☑
          - nontraffic V58.0 ☑
      - hanger-on
        - collision (with)
          - animal (traffic) V50.7 ☑
            - being ridden (traffic) V56.7 ☑
              - nontraffic V56.2 ☑
            - nontraffic V50.2 ☑
          - animal-drawn vehicle (traffic) V56.7 ☑
            - nontraffic V56.2 ☑
          - bus (traffic) V54.7 ☑
            - nontraffic V54.2 ☑
          - car (traffic) V53.7 ☑
            - nontraffic V53.2 ☑
          - pedal cycle (traffic) V51.7 ☑
            - nontraffic V51.2 ☑
          - pickup truck (traffic) V53.7 ☑
            - nontraffic V53.2 ☑
          - railway vehicle (traffic) V55.7 ☑
            - nontraffic V55.2 ☑
          - specified vehicle NEC (traffic) V56.7 ☑
            - nontraffic V56.2 ☑
          - stationary object (traffic) V57.7 ☑
            - nontraffic V57.2 ☑
          - streetcar (traffic) V56.7 ☑
            - nontraffic V56.2 ☑
          - three wheeled motor vehicle (traffic) V52.7 ☑
            - nontraffic V52.2 ☑
          - truck (traffic) V54.7 ☑
            - nontraffic V54.2 ☑
          - two wheeled motor vehicle (traffic) V52.7 ☑
            - nontraffic V52.2 ☑
          - van (traffic) V53.7 ☑
            - nontraffic V53.2 ☑
        - noncollision accident (traffic) V58.7 ☑
          - nontraffic V58.2 ☑
      - noncollision accident (traffic) V58.9 ☑
        - nontraffic V58.3 ☑
        - while boarding or alighting V58.4 ☑
      - nontraffic V59.3 ☑
      - passenger
        - collision (with)
          - animal (traffic) V50.6 ☑
            - being ridden (traffic) V56.6 ☑
              - nontraffic V56.1 ☑
            - nontraffic V50.1 ☑
          - animal-drawn vehicle (traffic) V56.6 ☑

- **Accident** — *continued*
  - transport — *continued*
    - van occupant — *continued*
      - passenger — *continued*
        - collision — *continued*
          - animal-drawn vehicle — *continued*
            - nontraffic V56.1 ☑
          - bus (traffic) V54.6 ☑
            - nontraffic V54.1 ☑
          - car (traffic) V53.6 ☑
            - nontraffic V53.1 ☑
          - motor vehicle NOS (traffic) V59.5Ø ☑
            - nontraffic V59.1Ø ☑
            - specified type NEC (traffic) V59.59 ☑
              - nontraffic V59.19 ☑
          - pedal cycle (traffic) V51.6 ☑
            - nontraffic V51.1 ☑
          - pickup truck (traffic) V53.6 ☑
            - nontraffic V53.1 ☑
          - railway vehicle (traffic) V55.6 ☑
            - nontraffic V55.1 ☑
          - specified vehicle NEC (traffic) V56.6 ☑
            - nontraffic V56.1 ☑
          - stationary object (traffic) V57.6 ☑
            - nontraffic V57.1 ☑
          - streetcar (traffic) V56.6 ☑
            - nontraffic V56.1 ☑
          - three wheeled motor vehicle (traffic) V52.6 ☑
            - nontraffic V52.1 ☑
          - truck (traffic) V54.6 ☑
            - nontraffic V54.1 ☑
          - two wheeled motor vehicle (traffic) V52.6 ☑
            - nontraffic V52.1 ☑
          - van (traffic) V53.6 ☑
            - nontraffic V53.1 ☑
        - noncollision accident (traffic) V58.6 ☑
          - nontraffic V58.1 ☑
      - specified type NEC V59.88 ☑
        - military vehicle V59.81 ☑
    - watercraft occupant — *see* Accident, watercraft
  - vehicle NEC V89.9 ☑
    - animal-drawn NEC — *see* Accident, transport, animal-drawn vehicle occupant
    - special
      - agricultural — *see* Accident, transport, agricultural vehicle occupant
      - construction — *see* Accident, transport, construction vehicle occupant
      - industrial — *see* Accident, transport, industrial vehicle occupant
    - three-wheeled NEC (motorized) — *see* Accident, transport, three-wheeled motor vehicle occupant
  - watercraft V94.9 ☑
    - causing
      - drowning B — *see* Drowning, due to, accident to, watercraft
      - injury NEC V91.89 ☑
        - crushed between craft and object V91.19 ☑
          - powered craft V91.13 ☑
            - ferry boat V91.11 ☑
            - fishing boat V91.12 ☑
            - jetskis V91.13 ☑
            - liner V91.11 ☑
            - merchant ship V91.1Ø ☑
            - passenger ship V91.11 ☑
          - unpowered craft V91.18 ☑
            - canoe V91.15 ☑
            - inflatable V91.16 ☑
            - kayak V91.15 ☑
            - sailboat V91.14 ☑
            - surf-board V91.18 ☑
            - windsurfer V91.18 ☑
        - fall on board V91.29 ☑
          - powered craft V91.23 ☑
            - ferry boat V91.21 ☑
            - fishing boat V91.22 ☑
            - jetskis V91.23 ☑
            - liner V91.21 ☑
            - merchant ship V91.2Ø ☑
            - passenger ship V91.21 ☑
          - unpowered craft
            - canoe V91.25 ☑
            - inflatable V91.26 ☑

- **Accident** — *continued*
  - watercraft — *continued*
    - causing — *continued*
      - injury — *continued*
        - fall on board — *continued*
          - unpowered craft — *continued*
            - kayak V91.25 ☑
            - sailboat V91.24 ☑
        - fire on board causing burn V91.Ø9 ☑
          - powered craft V91.Ø3 ☑
            - ferry boat V91.Ø1 ☑
            - fishing boat V91.Ø2 ☑
            - jetskis V91.Ø3 ☑
            - liner V91.Ø1 ☑
            - merchant ship V91.ØØ ☑
            - passenger ship V91.Ø1 ☑
          - unpowered craft V91.Ø8 ☑
            - canoe V91.Ø5 ☑
            - inflatable V91.Ø6 ☑
            - kayak V91.Ø5 ☑
            - sailboat V91.Ø4 ☑
            - surf-board V91.Ø8 ☑
            - water skis V91.Ø7 ☑
            - windsurfer V91.Ø8 ☑
        - hit by falling object V91.39 ☑
          - powered craft V91.33 ☑
            - ferry boat V91.31 ☑
            - fishing boat V91.32 ☑
            - jetskis V91.33 ☑
            - liner V91.31 ☑
            - merchant ship V91.3Ø ☑
            - passenger ship V91.31 ☑
          - unpowered craft V91.38 ☑
            - canoe V91.35 ☑
            - inflatable V91.36 ☑
            - kayak V91.35 ☑
            - sailboat V91.34 ☑
            - surf-board V91.38 ☑
            - water skis V91.37 ☑
            - windsurfer V91.38 ☑
        - specified type NEC V91.89 ☑
          - powered craft V91.83 ☑
            - ferry boat V91.81 ☑
            - fishing boat V91.82 ☑
            - jetskis V91.83 ☑
            - liner V91.81 ☑
            - merchant ship V91.8Ø ☑
            - passenger ship V91.81 ☑
          - unpowered craft V91.88 ☑
            - canoe V91.85 ☑
            - inflatable V91.86 ☑
            - kayak V91.85 ☑
            - sailboat V91.84 ☑
            - surf-board V91.88 ☑
            - water skis V91.87 ☑
            - windsurfer V91.88 ☑
    - due to, caused by cataclysm — *see* Forces of nature, by type
    - military NEC V94.818 ☑
      - with civilian watercraft V94.81Ø ☑
      - civilian in water injured by V94.811 ☑
    - nonpowered, struck by
      - nonpowered vessel V94.22 ☑
      - powered vessel V94.21 ☑
    - specified type NEC V94.89 ☑
    - striking swimmer
      - powered V94.11 ☑
      - unpowered V94.12 ☑
- **Acid throwing** (assault) YØ8.89 ☑
- **Activity** (involving) (of victim at time of event) Y93.9
  - aerobic and step exercise (class) Y93.A3 (*following* Y93.7)
  - alpine skiing Y93.23
  - animal care NEC Y93.K9 (*following* Y93.7)
  - arts and handcrafts NEC Y93.D9 (*following* Y93.7)
  - athletics played as a team or group NEC Y93.69
  - athletics played individually NEC Y93.59
  - athletics NEC Y93.79
  - baking Y93.G3 (*following* Y93.7)
  - ballet Y93.41
  - barbells Y93.B3 (*following* Y93.7)
  - BASE (Building, Antenna, Span, Earth) jumping Y93.33
  - baseball Y93.64
  - basketball Y93.67
  - bathing (personal) Y93.E1 (*following* Y93.7)
  - beach volleyball Y93.68

- **Activity** — *continued*
  - bike riding Y93.55
  - boogie boarding Y93.18
  - bowling Y93.54
  - boxing Y93.71
  - brass instrument playing Y93.J4 (*following* Y93.7)
  - building construction Y93.H3 (*following* Y93.7)
  - bungee jumping Y93.34
  - calisthenics Y93.A2 (*following* Y93.7)
  - canoeing (in calm and turbulent water) Y93.16
  - capture the flag Y93.6A
  - cardiorespiratory exercise NEC Y93.A9 (*following* Y93.7)
  - caregiving (providing) NEC Y93.F9 (*following* Y93.7)
    - bathing Y93.F1 (*following* Y93.7)
    - lifting Y93.F2 (*following* Y93.7)
  - cellular
    - communication device Y93.C2 (*following* Y93.7)
    - telephone Y93.C2 (*following* Y93.7)
  - challenge course Y93.A5 (*following* Y93.7)
  - cheerleading Y93.45
  - circuit training Y93.A4 (*following* Y93.7)
  - cleaning
    - floor Y93.E5 (*following* Y93.7)
  - climbing NEC Y93.39
    - mountain Y93.31
    - rock Y93.31
    - wall Y93.31
  - clothing care and maintenance NEC Y93.E9 (*following* Y93.7)
  - combatives Y93.75
  - computer
    - keyboarding Y93.C1 (*following* Y93.7)
    - technology NEC Y93.C9 (*following* Y93.7)
  - confidence course Y93.A5 (*following* Y93.7)
  - construction (building) Y93.H3 (*following* Y93.7)
  - cooking and baking Y93.G3 (*following* Y93.7)
  - cool down exercises Y93.A2 (*following* Y93.7)
  - cricket Y93.69
  - crocheting Y93.D1 (*following* Y93.7)
  - cross country skiing Y93.24
  - dancing (all types) Y93.41
  - digging
    - dirt Y93.H1 (*following* Y93.7)
  - dirt digging Y93.H1 (*following* Y93.7)
  - dishwashing Y93.G1 (*following* Y93.7)
  - diving (platform) (springboard) Y93.12
    - underwater Y93.15
  - dodge ball Y93.6A
  - downhill skiing Y93.23
  - drum playing Y93.J2 (*following* Y93.7)
  - dumbbells Y93.B3 (*following* Y93.7)
  - electronic
    - devices NEC Y93.C9 (*following* Y93.7)
      - hand held interactive Y93.C2 (*following* Y93.7)
    - game playing (using) (with)
      - interactive device Y93.C2 (*following* Y93.7)
      - keyboard or other stationary device Y93.C1 (*following* Y93.7)
  - elliptical machine Y93.A1 (*following* Y93.7)
  - exercise(s)
    - machines ((primarily) for)
      - cardiorespiratory conditioning Y93.A1 (*following* Y93.7)
      - muscle strengthening Y93.B1 (*following* Y93.7)
    - muscle strengthening (non-machine) NEC Y93.B9 (*following* Y93.7)
  - external motion NEC Y93.I9 (*following* Y93.7)
    - rollercoaster Y93.I1 (*following* Y93.7)
  - field hockey Y93.65
  - figure skating (pairs) (singles) Y93.21
  - flag football Y93.62
  - floor mopping and cleaning Y93.E5 (*following* Y93.7)
  - food preparation and clean up Y93.G1 (*following* Y93.7)
  - football (American) NOS Y93.61
    - flag Y93.62
    - tackle Y93.61
    - touch Y93.62
  - four square Y93.6A
  - free weights Y93.B3 (*following* Y93.7)
  - frisbee (ultimate) Y93.74
  - furniture
    - building Y93.D3 (*following* Y93.7)
    - finishing Y93.D3 (*following* Y93.7)
    - repair Y93.D3 (*following* Y93.7)
  - game playing (electronic)
    - using interactive device Y93.C2 (*following* Y93.7)
    - using keyboard or other stationary device Y93.C1 (*following* Y93.7)

Activity — *continued*
- gardening Y93.H2 (*following* Y93.7)
- golf Y93.53
- grass drills Y93.A6 (*following* Y93.7)
- grilling and smoking food Y93.G2 (*following* Y93.7)
- grooming and shearing an animal Y93.K3 (*following* Y93.7)
- guerilla drills Y93.A6 (*following* Y93.7)
- gymnastics (rhythmic) Y93.43
- hand held interactive electronic device Y93.C2 (*following* Y93.7)
- handball Y93.73
- handcrafts NEC Y93.D9 (*following* Y93.7)
- hang gliding Y93.35
- hiking (on level or elevated terrain) Y93.Ø1
- hockey (ice) Y93.22
  - field Y93.65
- horseback riding Y93.52
- household (interior) maintenance NEC Y93.E9 (*following* Y93.7)
- ice NEC Y93.29
  - dancing Y93.21
  - hockey Y93.22
  - skating Y93.21
- inline roller skating Y93.51
- ironing Y93.E4 (*following* Y93.7)
- judo Y93.75
- jumping jacks Y93.A2 (*following* Y93.7)
- jumping rope Y93.56
- jumping (off) NEC Y93.39
  - BASE (Building, Antenna, Span, Earth) Y93.33
  - bungee Y93.34
  - jacks Y93.A2 (*following* Y93.7)
  - rope Y93.56
- karate Y93.75
- kayaking (in calm and turbulent water) Y93.16
- keyboarding (computer) Y93.C1 (*following* Y93.7)
- kickball Y93.6A
- knitting Y93.D1 (*following* Y93.7)
- lacrosse Y93.65
- land maintenance NEC Y93.H9 (*following* Y93.7)
- landscaping Y93.H2 (*following* Y93.7)
- laundry Y93.E2 (*following* Y93.7)
- machines (exercise)
  - primarily for cardiorespiratory conditioning Y93.A1 (*following* Y93.7)
  - primarily for muscle strengthening Y93.B1 (*following* Y93.7)
- maintenance
  - exterior building NEC Y93.H9 (*following* Y93.7)
  - household (interior) NEC Y93.E9 (*following* Y93.7)
  - land Y93.H9 (*following* Y93.7)
  - property Y93.H9 (*following* Y93.7)
- marching (on level or elevated terrain) Y93.Ø1
- martial arts Y93.75
- microwave oven Y93.G3 (*following* Y93.7)
- milking an animal Y93.K2 (*following* Y93.7)
- mopping (floor) Y93.E5 (*following* Y93.7)
- mountain climbing Y93.31
- muscle strengthening
  - exercises (non-machine) NEC Y93.B9 (*following* Y93.7)
  - machines Y93.B1 (*following* Y93.7)
- musical keyboard (electronic) playing Y93.J1 (*following* Y93.7)
- nordic skiing Y93.24
- obstacle course Y93.A5 (*following* Y93.7)
- oven (microwave) Y93.G3 (*following* Y93.7)
- packing up and unpacking in moving to a new residence Y93.E6 (*following* Y93.7)
- parasailing Y93.19
- percussion instrument playing NEC Y93.J2 (*following* Y93.7)
- personal
  - bathing and showering Y93.E1 (*following* Y93.7)
  - hygiene NEC Y93.E8 (*following* Y93.7)
  - showering Y93.E1 (*following* Y93.7)
- physical games generally associated with school recess, summer camp and children Y93.6A
- physical training NEC Y93.A9 (*following* Y93.7)
- piano playing Y93.J1 (*following* Y93.7)
- pilates Y93.B4 (*following* Y93.7)
- platform diving Y93.12
- playing musical instrument
  - brass instrument Y93.J4 (*following* Y93.7)
  - drum Y93.J2 (*following* Y93.7)
  - musical keyboard (electronic) Y93.J1 (*following* Y93.7)

Activity — *continued*
- playing musical instrument — *continued*
  - percussion instrument NEC Y93.J2 (*following* Y93.7)
  - piano Y93.J1 (*following* Y93.7)
  - string instrument Y93.J3 (*following* Y93.7)
  - winds instrument Y93.J4 (*following* Y93.7)
- property maintenance
  - exterior NEC Y93.H9 (*following* Y93.7)
  - interior NEC Y93.E9 (*following* Y93.7)
- pruning (garden and lawn) Y93.H2 (*following* Y93.7)
- pull-ups Y93.B2 (*following* Y93.7)
- push-ups Y93.B2 (*following* Y93.7)
- racquetball Y93.73
- rafting (in calm and turbulent water) Y93.16
- raking (leaves) Y93.H1 (*following* Y93.7)
- rappelling Y93.32
- refereeing a sports activity Y93.81
- residential relocation Y93.E6 (*following* Y93.7)
- rhythmic gymnastics Y93.43
- rhythmic movement NEC Y93.49
- riding
  - horseback Y93.52
  - rollercoaster Y93.I1 (*following* Y93.7)
- rock climbing Y93.31
- roller skating (inline) Y93.51
- rollercoaster riding Y93.I1 (*following* Y93.7)
- rough housing and horseplay Y93.83
- rowing (in calm and turbulent water) Y93.16
- rugby Y93.63
- running Y93.Ø2
- SCUBA diving Y93.15
- sewing Y93.D2 (*following* Y93.7)
- shoveling Y93.H1 (*following* Y93.7)
  - dirt Y93.H1 (*following* Y93.7)
  - snow Y93.H1 (*following* Y93.7)
- showering (personal) Y93.E1 (*following* Y93.7)
- sit-ups Y93.B2 (*following* Y93.7)
- skateboarding Y93.51
- skating (ice) Y93.21
  - roller Y93.51
- skiing (alpine) (downhill) Y93.23
  - cross country Y93.24
  - nordic Y93.24
  - water Y93.17
- sledding (snow) Y93.23
- sleeping (sleep) Y93.84
- smoking and grilling food Y93.G2 (*following* Y93.7)
- snorkeling Y93.15
- snow NEC Y93.29
  - boarding Y93.23
  - shoveling Y93.H1 (*following* Y93.7)
  - sledding Y93.23
  - tubing Y93.23
- soccer Y93.66
- softball Y93.64
- specified NEC Y93.89
- spectator at an event Y93.82
- sports NEC Y93.79
  - sports played as a team or group NEC Y93.69
  - sports played individually NEC Y93.59
- springboard diving Y93.12
- squash Y93.73
- stationary bike Y93.A1 (*following* Y93.7)
- step (stepping) exercise (class) Y93.A3 (*following* Y93.7)
- stepper machine Y93.A1 (*following* Y93.7)
- stove Y93.G3 (*following* Y93.7)
- string instrument playing Y93.J3 (*following* Y93.7)
- surfing Y93.18
  - wind Y93.18
- swimming Y93.11
- tackle football Y93.61
- tap dancing Y93.41
- tennis Y93.73
- tobogganing Y93.23
- touch football Y93.62
- track and field events (non-running) Y93.57
  - running Y93.Ø2
- trampoline Y93.44
- treadmill Y93.A1 (*following* Y93.7)
- trimming shrubs Y93.H2 (*following* Y93.7)
- tubing (in calm and turbulent water) Y93.16
  - snow Y93.23
- ultimate frisbee Y93.74
- underwater diving Y93.15
- unpacking in moving to a new residence Y93.E6 (*following* Y93.7)
- use of stove, oven and microwave oven Y93.G3 (*following* Y93.7)

Activity — *continued*
- vacuuming Y93.E3 (*following* Y93.7)
- volleyball (beach) (court) Y93.68
- wake boarding Y93.17
- walking (on level or elevated terrain) Y93.Ø1
  - an animal Y93.K1 (*following* Y93.7)
- walking an animal Y93.K1 (*following* Y93.7)
- wall climbing Y93.31
- warm up and cool down exercises Y93.A2 (*following* Y93.7)
- water NEC Y93.19
  - aerobics Y93.14
  - craft NEC Y93.19
  - exercise Y93.14
  - polo Y93.13
  - skiing Y93.17
  - sliding Y93.18
  - survival training and testing Y93.19
- weeding (garden and lawn) Y93.H2 (*following* Y93.7)
- wind instrument playing Y93.J4 (*following* Y93.7)
- windsurfing Y93.18
- wrestling Y93.72
- yoga Y93.42

Adverse effect of drugs — *see* Table of Drugs and Chemicals

Aerosinusitis — *see* Air, pressure

After-effect, late — *see* Sequelae

Air
- blast in war operations — *see* War operations, air blast
- pressure
  - change, rapid
    - during
      - ascent W94.29 ☑
        - while (in) (surfacing from)
          - aircraft W94.23 ☑
          - deep water diving W94.21 ☑
          - underground W94.22 ☑
      - descent W94.39 ☑
        - in
          - aircraft W94.31 ☑
          - water W94.32 ☑
  - high, prolonged W94.Ø ☑
  - low, prolonged W94.12 ☑
    - due to residence or long visit at high altitude W94.11 ☑

Alpine sickness W94.11 ☑

Altitude sickness W94.11 ☑

Anaphylactic shock, anaphylaxis — *see* Table of Drugs and Chemicals

Andes disease W94.11 ☑

Arachnidism, arachnoidism X58 ☑

Arson (with intent to injure or kill) X97 ☑

Asphyxia, asphyxiation
- by
  - food (bone) (seed) — *see* categories T17 and T18 ☑
  - gas (*see also* Table of Drugs and Chemicals)
    - legal
      - execution — *see* Legal, intervention, gas
      - intervention — *see* Legal, intervention, gas
- from
  - fire (*see also* Exposure, fire)
    - in war operations — *see* War operations, fire
  - ignition — *see* Ignition
  - vomitus T17.81 ☑
- in war operations — *see* War operations, restriction of airway

Aspiration
- food (any type) (into respiratory tract) (with asphyxia, obstruction respiratory tract, suffocation) — *see* categories T17 and T18 ☑
- foreign body — *see* Foreign body, aspiration
- vomitus (with asphyxia, obstruction respiratory tract, suffocation) T17.81 ☑

Assassination (attempt) — *see* Assault

Assault (homicidal) (by) (in) YØ9
- arson X97 ☑
- bite (of human being) YØ4.1 ☑
- bodily force YØ4.8 ☑
  - bite YØ4.1 ☑
  - bumping into YØ4.2 ☑
  - sexual — *see* subcategories T74.Ø, T76.Ø ☑
  - unarmed fight YØ4.Ø ☑
- bomb X96.9 ☑
  - antipersonnel X96.Ø ☑
  - fertilizer X96.3 ☑
  - gasoline X96.1 ☑

- **Assault** — *continued*
  - bomb — *continued*
    - letter X96.2 ☑
    - petrol X96.1 ☑
    - pipe X96.3 ☑
    - specified NEC X96.8 ☑
  - brawl (hand) (fists) (foot) (unarmed) Y04.0 ☑
  - burning, burns (by fire) NEC X97 ☑
    - acid Y08.89 ☑
    - caustic, corrosive substance Y08.89 ☑
    - chemical from swallowing caustic, corrosive substance — *see* Table of Drugs and Chemicals
    - cigarette(s) X97 ☑
    - hot object X98.9 ☑
      - fluid NEC X98.2 ☑
      - household appliance X98.3 ☑
      - specified NEC X98.8 ☑
      - steam X98.0 ☑
      - tap water X98.1 ☑
      - vapors X98.0 ☑
    - scalding — *see* Assault, burning
    - steam X98.0 ☑
    - vitriol Y08.89 ☑
  - caustic, corrosive substance (gas) Y08.89 ☑
  - crashing of
    - aircraft Y08.81 ☑
    - motor vehicle Y03.8 ☑
      - pushed in front of Y02.0 ☑
      - run over Y03.0 ☑
      - specified NEC Y03.8 ☑
  - cutting or piercing instrument X99.9 ☑
    - dagger X99.2 ☑
    - glass X99.0 ☑
    - knife X99.1 ☑
    - specified NEC X99.8 ☑
    - sword X99.2 ☑
  - dagger X99.2 ☑
  - drowning (in) X92.9 ☑
    - bathtub X92.0 ☑
    - natural water X92.3 ☑
    - specified NEC X92.8 ☑
    - swimming pool X92.1 ☑
      - following fall X92.2 ☑
  - dynamite X96.8 ☑
  - explosive(s) (material) X96.9 ☑
  - fight (hand) (fists) (foot) (unarmed) Y04.0 ☑
    - with weapon — *see* Assault, by type of weapon
  - fire X97 ☑
  - firearm X95.9 ☑
    - airgun X95.01 ☑
    - handgun X93 ☑
    - hunting rifle X94.1 ☑
    - larger X94.9 ☑
      - specified NEC X94.8 ☑
    - machine gun X94.2 ☑
    - shotgun X94.0 ☑
    - specified NEC X95.8 ☑
  - from high place Y01 ☑
  - gunshot (wound) NEC — *see* Assault, firearm, by type
  - incendiary device X97 ☑
  - injury Y09
    - to child due to criminal abortion attempt NEC Y08.89 ☑
  - knife X99.1 ☑
  - late effect of — *see* categories X92-Y08 with 7th character S
  - placing before moving object NEC Y02.8 ☑
    - motor vehicle Y02.0 ☑
  - poisoning — *see* categories T36-T65 with 7th character S
  - puncture, any part of body — *see* Assault, cutting or piercing instrument
  - pushing
    - before moving object NEC Y02.8 ☑
      - motor vehicle Y02.0 ☑
      - subway train Y02.1 ☑
      - train Y02.1 ☑
    - from high place Y01 ☑
  - rape T74.2- ☑
  - scalding — *see* Assault, burning
  - sequelae of — *see* categories X92-Y08 with 7th character S
  - sexual (by bodily force) T74.2- ☑
  - shooting — *see* Assault, firearm
  - specified means NEC Y08.89 ☑
- **Assault** — *continued*
  - stab, any part of body — *see* Assault, cutting or piercing instrument
  - steam X98.0 ☑
  - striking against
    - other person Y04.2 ☑
    - sports equipment Y08.09 ☑
      - baseball bat Y08.02 ☑
      - hockey stick Y08.01 ☑
  - struck by
    - sports equipment Y08.09 ☑
      - baseball bat Y08.02 ☑
      - hockey stick Y08.01 ☑
  - submersion — *see* Assault, drowning
  - violence Y09
  - weapon Y09
    - blunt Y00 ☑
    - cutting or piercing — *see* Assault, cutting or piercing instrument
    - firearm — *see* Assault, firearm
  - wound Y09
    - cutting — *see* Assault, cutting or piercing instrument
    - gunshot — *see* Assault, firearm
    - knife X99.1 ☑
    - piercing — *see* Assault, cutting or piercing instrument
    - puncture — *see* Assault, cutting or piercing instrument
    - stab — *see* Assault, cutting or piercing instrument
- **Attack by mammals NEC** W55.89 ☑
- **Avalanche** — *see* Landslide
- **Aviator's disease** — *see* Air, pressure

B

- **Barotitis, barodontalgia, barosinusitis, barotrauma** (otitic) (sinus) — *see* Air, pressure
- **Battered** (baby) (child) (person) (syndrome) X58 ☑
- **Bayonet wound** W26.1 ☑
  - in
    - legal intervention — *see* Legal, intervention, sharp object, bayonet
    - war operations — *see* War operations, combat
  - stated as undetermined whether accidental or intentional Y28.8 ☑
  - suicide (attempt) X78.2 ☑
- **Bean in nose** — *see* categories T17 and T18 ☑
- **Bed set on fire NEC** — *see* Exposure, fire, uncontrolled, building, bed
- **Beheading** (by guillotine)
  - homicide X99.9 ☑
  - legal execution — *see* Legal, intervention
- **Bending, injury in** — *see* category Y93 ☑
- **Bends** — *see* Air, pressure, change
- **Bite, bitten by**
  - alligator W58.01 ☑
  - arthropod (nonvenomous) NEC W57 ☑
  - bull W55.21 ☑
  - cat W55.01 ☑
  - cow W55.21 ☑
  - crocodile W58.11 ☑
  - dog W54.0 ☑
  - goat W55.31 ☑
  - hoof stock NEC W55.31 ☑
  - horse W55.11 ☑
  - human being (accidentally) W50.3 ☑
    - with intent to injure or kill Y04.1 ☑
    - as, or caused by, a crowd or human stampede (with fall) W52 ☑
    - assault Y04.1 ☑
    - homicide (attempt) Y04.1 ☑
    - in
      - fight Y04.1 ☑
  - insect (nonvenomous) W57 ☑
  - lizard (nonvenomous) W59.01 ☑
  - mammal NEC W55.81 ☑
  - mammal NEC W55.81 ☑
    - marine W56.31 ☑
  - marine animal (nonvenomous) W56.81 ☑
  - millipede W57 ☑
  - moray eel W56.51 ☑
  - mouse W53.01 ☑
  - person(s) (accidentally) W50.3 ☑
    - with intent to injure or kill Y04.1 ☑
- **Bite, bitten by** — *continued*
  - person(s) — *continued*
    - as, or caused by, a crowd or human stampede (with fall) W52 ☑
    - assault Y04.1 ☑
    - homicide (attempt) Y04.1 ☑
    - in
      - fight Y04.1 ☑
  - pig W55.41 ☑
  - raccoon W55.51 ☑
  - rat W53.11 ☑
  - reptile W59.81 ☑
    - lizard W59.01 ☑
    - snake W59.11 ☑
    - turtle W59.21 ☑
      - terrestrial W59.81 ☑
  - rodent W53.81 ☑
    - mouse W53.01 ☑
    - rat W53.11 ☑
    - specified NEC W53.81 ☑
    - squirrel W53.21 ☑
  - shark W56.41 ☑
  - sheep W55.31 ☑
  - snake (nonvenomous) W59.11 ☑
  - spider (nonvenomous) W57 ☑
  - squirrel W53.21 ☑
- **Blast** (air) in war operations — *see* War operations, blast
- **Blizzard** X37.2 ☑
- **Blood alcohol level** Y90.9
  - less than 20mg/100ml Y90.0
  - 20-39mg/100ml Y90.1
  - 40-59mg/100ml Y90.2
  - 60-79mg/100ml Y90.3
  - 80-99mg/100ml Y90.4
  - 100-119mg/100ml Y90.5
  - 120-199mg/100ml Y90.6
  - 200-239mg/100ml Y90.7
  - presence in blood, level not specified Y90.9
- **Blow** X58 ☑
  - by law-enforcing agent, police (on duty) — *see* Legal, intervention, manhandling
    - blunt object — *see* Legal, intervention, blunt object
- **Blowing up** — *see* Explosion
- **Brawl** (hand) (fists) (foot) Y04.0 ☑
- **Breakage** (accidental) (part of)
  - ladder (causing fall) W11 ☑
  - scaffolding (causing fall) W12 ☑
- **Broken**
  - glass, contact with — *see* Contact, with, glass
  - power line (causing electric shock) W85 ☑
- **Bumping against, into** (accidentally)
  - object NEC W22.8 ☑
    - with fall — *see* Fall, due to, bumping against, object
    - caused by crowd or human stampede (with fall) W52 ☑
    - sports equipment W21.9 ☑
  - person(s) W51 ☑
    - with fall W03 ☑
      - due to ice or snow W00.0 ☑
    - assault Y04.2 ☑
    - caused by, a crowd or human stampede (with fall) W52 ☑
    - homicide (attempt) Y04.2 ☑
  - sports equipment W21.9 ☑
- **Burn, burned, burning** (accidental) (by) (from) (on)
  - acid NEC — *see* Table of Drugs and Chemicals
  - bed linen — *see* Exposure, fire, uncontrolled, in building, bed
  - blowtorch X08.8 ☑
    - with ignition of clothing NEC X06.2 ☑
      - nightwear X05 ☑
  - bonfire, campfire (controlled) (*see also* Exposure, fire, controlled, not in building)
    - uncontrolled — *see* Exposure, fire, uncontrolled, not in building
  - candle X08.8 ☑
    - with ignition of clothing NEC X06.2 ☑
      - nightwear X05 ☑
  - caustic liquid, substance (external) (internal) NEC — *see* Table of Drugs and Chemicals
  - chemical (external) (internal) (*see also* Table of Drugs and Chemicals)
    - in war operations — *see* War operations. fire
  - cigar(s) or cigarette(s) X08.8 ☑
    - with ignition of clothing NEC X06.2 ☑

- **Burn, burned, burning** — *continued*
  - cigar(s) or cigarette(s) — *continued*
    - with ignition of clothing — *continued*
      - nightwear XØ5 ☑
  - clothes, clothing NEC (from controlled fire) XØ6.2 ☑
    - with conflagration — *see* Exposure, fire, uncontrolled, building
      - not in building or structure — *see* Exposure, fire, uncontrolled, not in building
  - cooker (hot) X15.8 ☑
    - stated as undetermined whether accidental or intentional Y27.3 ☑
    - suicide (attempt) X77.3 ☑
  - electric blanket X16 ☑
  - engine (hot) X17 ☑
  - fire, flames — *see* Exposure, fire
  - flare, Very pistol — *see* Discharge, firearm NEC
  - heat
    - from appliance (electrical) (household) X15.8 ☑
      - cooker X15.8 ☑
      - hotplate X15.2 ☑
      - kettle X15.8 ☑
      - light bulb X15.8 ☑
      - saucepan X15.3 ☑
      - skillet X15.3 ☑
      - stated as undetermined whether accidental or intentional Y27.3 ☑
      - stove X15.Ø ☑
      - suicide (attempt) X77.3 ☑
      - toaster X15.1 ☑
    - in local application or packing during medical or surgical procedure Y63.5
  - heating
    - appliance, radiator or pipe X16 ☑
  - homicide (attempt) — *see* Assault, burning
  - hot
    - air X14.1 ☑
    - cooker X15.8 ☑
    - drink X1Ø.Ø ☑
    - engine X17 ☑
    - fat X1Ø.2 ☑
    - fluid NEC X12 ☑
    - food X1Ø.1 ☑
    - gases X14.1 ☑
    - heating appliance X16 ☑
    - household appliance NEC X15.8 ☑
    - kettle X15.8 ☑
    - liquid NEC X12 ☑
    - machinery X17 ☑
    - metal (molten) (liquid) NEC X18 ☑
    - object (not producing fire or flames) NEC X19 ☑
    - oil (cooking) X1Ø.2 ☑
    - pipe(s) X16 ☑
    - radiator X16 ☑
    - saucepan (glass) (metal) X15.3 ☑
    - stove (kitchen) X15.Ø ☑
    - substance NEC X19 ☑
      - caustic or corrosive NEC — *see* Table of Drugs and Chemicals
    - toaster X15.1 ☑
    - tool X17 ☑
    - vapor X13.1 ☑
    - water (tap) — *see* Contact, with, hot, tap water
  - hotplate X15.2 ☑
    - suicide (attempt) X77.3 ☑
  - ignition — *see* Ignition
  - in war operations — *see* War operations, fire
  - inflicted by other person X97 ☑
    - by hot objects, hot vapor, and steam — *see* Assault, burning, hot object
  - internal, from swallowed caustic, corrosive liquid, substance — *see* Table of Drugs and Chemicals
  - iron (hot) X15.8 ☑
    - stated as undetermined whether accidental or intentional Y27.3 ☑
    - suicide (attempt) X77.3 ☑
  - kettle (hot) X15.8 ☑
    - stated as undetermined whether accidental or intentional Y27.3 ☑
    - suicide (attempt) X77.3 ☑
  - lamp (flame) XØ8.8 ☑
    - with ignition of clothing NEC XØ6.2 ☑
      - nightwear XØ5 ☑
  - lighter (cigar) (cigarette) XØ8.8 ☑
    - with ignition of clothing NEC XØ6.2 ☑
      - nightwear XØ5 ☑

- **Burn, burned, burning** — *continued*
  - lightning — *see* subcategory T75.Ø ☑
    - causing fire — *see* Exposure, fire
  - liquid (boiling) (hot) NEC X12 ☑
    - stated as undetermined whether accidental or intentional Y27.2 ☑
    - suicide (attempt) X77.2 ☑
  - local application of externally applied substance in medical or surgical care Y63.5
  - machinery (hot) X17 ☑
  - matches XØ8.8 ☑
    - with ignition of clothing NEC XØ6.2 ☑
      - nightwear XØ5 ☑
  - mattress — *see* Exposure, fire, uncontrolled, building, bed
  - medicament, externally applied Y63.5
  - metal (hot) (liquid) (molten) NEC X18 ☑
  - nightwear (nightclothes, nightdress, gown, pajamas, robe) XØ5 ☑
  - object (hot) NEC X19 ☑
  - on board watercraft
    - due to
      - accident to watercraft V91.Ø9 ☑
        - powered craft V91.Ø3 ☑
          - ferry boat V91.Ø1 ☑
          - fishing boat V91.Ø2 ☑
          - jetskis V91.Ø3 ☑
          - liner V91.Ø1 ☑
          - merchant ship V91.ØØ ☑
          - passenger ship V91.Ø1 ☑
        - unpowered craft V91.Ø8 ☑
          - canoe V91.Ø5 ☑
          - inflatable V91.Ø6 ☑
          - kayak V91.Ø5 ☑
          - sailboat V91.Ø4 ☑
          - surf-board V91.Ø8 ☑
          - water skis V91.Ø7 ☑
          - windsurfer V91.Ø8 ☑
      - fire on board V93.Ø9 ☑
        - ferry boat V93.Ø1 ☑
        - fishing boat V93.Ø2 ☑
        - jetskis V93.Ø3 ☑
        - liner V93.Ø1 ☑
        - merchant ship V93.ØØ ☑
        - passenger ship V93.Ø1 ☑
        - powered craft NEC V93.Ø3 ☑
        - sailboat V93.Ø4 ☑
      - specified heat source NEC on board V93.19 ☑
        - ferry boat V93.11 ☑
        - fishing boat V93.12 ☑
        - jetskis V93.13 ☑
        - liner V93.11 ☑
        - merchant ship V93.1Ø ☑
        - passenger ship V93.11 ☑
        - powered craft NEC V93.13 ☑
        - sailboat V93.14 ☑
  - pipe (hot) X16 ☑
    - smoking XØ8.8 ☑
      - with ignition of clothing NEC XØ6.2 ☑
        - nightwear XØ5 ☑
  - powder — *see* Powder burn
  - radiator (hot) X16 ☑
  - saucepan (hot) (glass) (metal) X15.3 ☑
    - stated as undetermined whether accidental or intentional Y27.3 ☑
    - suicide (attempt) X77.3 ☑
  - self-inflicted X76 ☑
    - stated as undetermined whether accidental or intentional Y26 ☑
  - stated as undetermined whether accidental or intentional Y27.Ø ☑
  - steam X13.1 ☑
    - pipe X16 ☑
      - stated as undetermined whether accidental or intentional Y27.8 ☑
    - stated as undetermined whether accidental or intentional Y27.Ø ☑
    - suicide (attempt) X77.Ø ☑
  - stove (hot) (kitchen) X15.Ø ☑
    - stated as undetermined whether accidental or intentional Y27.3 ☑
    - suicide (attempt) X77.3 ☑
  - substance (hot) NEC X19 ☑
    - boiling X12 ☑
      - stated as undetermined whether accidental or intentional Y27.2 ☑

- **Burn, burned, burning** — *continued*
  - substance — *continued*
    - boiling — *continued*
      - suicide (attempt) X77.2 ☑
    - molten (metal) X18 ☑
  - suicide (attempt) NEC X76 ☑
    - hot
      - household appliance X77.3 ☑
      - object X77.9 ☑
  - therapeutic misadventure
    - heat in local application or packing during medical or surgical procedure Y63.5
    - overdose of radiation Y63.2
  - toaster (hot) X15.1 ☑
    - stated as undetermined whether accidental or intentional Y27.3 ☑
    - suicide (attempt) X77.3 ☑
  - tool (hot) X17 ☑
  - torch, welding XØ8.8 ☑
    - with ignition of clothing NEC XØ6.2 ☑
      - nightwear XØ5 ☑
  - trash fire (controlled) — *see* Exposure, fire, controlled, not in building
    - uncontrolled — *see* Exposure, fire, uncontrolled, not in building
  - vapor (hot) X13.1 ☑
    - stated as undetermined whether accidental or intentional Y27.Ø ☑
    - suicide (attempt) X77.Ø ☑
  - Very pistol — *see* Discharge, firearm NEC
- **Butted by animal** W55.82 ☑
  - bull W55.22 ☑
  - cow W55.22 ☑
  - goat W55.32 ☑
  - horse W55.12 ☑
  - pig W55.42 ☑
  - sheep W55.32 ☑

C

- **Caisson disease** — *see* Air, pressure, change
- **Campfire** (exposure to) (controlled) (*see also* Exposure, fire, controlled, not in building)
  - uncontrolled — *see* Exposure, fire, uncontrolled, not in building
- **Capital punishment** (any means) — *see* Legal, intervention
- **Car sickness** T75.3 ☑
- **Casualty** (not due to war) NEC X58 ☑
  - war — *see* War operations
- **Cat**
  - bite W55.Ø1 ☑
  - scratch W55.Ø3 ☑
- **Cataclysm, cataclysmic** (any injury) NEC — *see* Forces of nature
- **Catching fire** — *see* Exposure, fire
- **Caught**
  - between
    - folding object W23.Ø ☑
    - objects (moving) (stationary and moving) W23.Ø ☑
      - and machinery — *see* Contact, with, by type of machine
      - stationary W23.1 ☑
    - sliding door and door frame W23.Ø ☑
  - by, in
    - machinery (moving parts of) — *see* Contact, with, by type of machine
    - washing-machine wringer W23.Ø ☑
  - under packing crate (due to losing grip) W23.1 ☑
- **Cave-in caused by cataclysmic earth surface movement or eruption** — *see* Landslide
- **Change**(s) in air pressure — *see* Air, pressure, change
- **Choked, choking** (on) (any object except food or vomitus)
  - food (bone) (seed) — *see* categories T17 and T18 ☑
  - vomitus T17.81- ☑
- **Civil insurrection** — *see* War operations
- **Cloudburst** (any injury) X37.8 ☑
- **Cold, exposure to** (accidental) (excessive) (extreme) (natural) (place) NEC — *see* Exposure, cold
- **Collapse**
  - building W2Ø.1 ☑
    - burning (uncontrolled fire) XØØ.2 ☑
  - dam or man-made structure (causing earth movement) X36.Ø ☑
  - machinery — *see* Contact, with, by type of machine

- **Collapse** — *continued*
  - structure W20.1 ☑
    - burning (uncontrolled fire) X00.2 ☑
- **Collision** (accidental) NEC (*see also* Accident, transport) V89.9 ☑
  - pedestrian W51 ☑
    - with fall W03 ☑
      - due to ice or snow W00.0 ☑
      - involving pedestrian conveyance — *see* Accident, transport, pedestrian, conveyance
    - and
      - crowd or human stampede (with fall) W52 ☑
      - object W22.8 ☑
        - with fall — *see* Fall, due to, bumping against, object
  - person(s) — *see* Collision, pedestrian
  - transport vehicle NEC V89.9 ☑
    - and
      - avalanche, fallen or not moving — *see* Accident, transport
        - falling or moving — *see* Landslide
      - landslide, fallen or not moving — *see* Accident, transport
        - falling or moving — *see* Landslide
    - due to cataclysm — *see* Forces of nature, by type
    - intentional, purposeful suicide (attempt) — *see* Suicide, collision
- **Combustion, spontaneous** — *see* Ignition
- **Complication** (delayed) **of or following** (medical or surgical procedure) Y84.9
  - with misadventure — *see* Misadventure
  - amputation of limb(s) Y83.5
  - anastomosis (arteriovenous) (blood vessel) (gastrojejunal) (tendon) (natural or artificial material) Y83.2
  - aspiration (of fluid) Y84.4
    - tissue Y84.8
  - biopsy Y84.8
  - blood
    - sampling Y84.7
    - transfusion
      - procedure Y84.8
  - bypass Y83.2
  - catheterization (urinary) Y84.6
    - cardiac Y84.0
  - colostomy Y83.3
  - cystostomy Y83.3
  - dialysis (kidney) Y84.1
  - drug — *see* Table of Drugs and Chemicals
  - due to misadventure — *see* Misadventure
  - duodenostomy Y83.3
  - electroshock therapy Y84.3
  - external stoma, creation of Y83.3
  - formation of external stoma Y83.3
  - gastrostomy Y83.3
  - graft Y83.2
  - hypothermia (medically-induced) Y84.8
  - implant, implantation (of)
    - artificial
      - internal device (cardiac pacemaker) (electrodes in brain) (heart valve prosthesis) (orthopedic) Y83.1
      - material or tissue (for anastomosis or bypass) Y83.2
        - with creation of external stoma Y83.3
    - natural tissues (for anastomosis or bypass) Y83.2
      - with creation of external stoma Y83.3
  - infusion
    - procedure Y84.8
  - injection — *see* Table of Drugs and Chemicals
    - procedure Y84.8
  - insertion of gastric or duodenal sound Y84.5
  - insulin-shock therapy Y84.3
  - paracentesis (abdominal) (thoracic) (aspirative) Y84.4
  - procedures other than surgical operation — *see* Complication of or following, by type of procedure
  - radiological procedure or therapy Y84.2
  - removal of organ (partial) (total) NEC Y83.6
  - sampling
    - blood Y84.7
    - fluid NEC Y84.4
    - tissue Y84.8
  - shock therapy Y84.3
  - surgical operation NEC (*see also* Complication of or following, by type of operation) Y83.9
    - reconstructive NEC Y83.4

- **Complication** (delayed) **of or following** — *continued*
  - surgical operation (*see also* Complication of or following, by type of operation) — *continued*
    - reconstructive — *continued*
      - with
        - anastomosis, bypass or graft Y83.2
        - formation of external stoma Y83.3
    - specified NEC Y83.8
  - transfusion (*see also* Table of Drugs and Chemicals)
    - procedure Y84.8
  - transplant, transplantation (heart) (kidney) (liver) (whole organ, any) Y83.0
    - partial organ Y83.4
  - ureterostomy Y83.3
  - vaccination (*see also* Table of Drugs and Chemicals)
    - procedure Y84.8
- **Compression**
  - divers' squeeze — *see* Air, pressure, change
  - trachea by
    - food (lodged in esophagus) — *see* categories T17 and T18 ☑
    - vomitus (lodged in esophagus) T17.81- ☑
- **Conflagration** — *see* Exposure, fire, uncontrolled
- **Constriction** (external)
  - hair W49.01 ☑
  - jewelry W49.04 ☑
  - ring W49.04 ☑
  - rubber band W49.03 ☑
  - specified item NEC W49.09 ☑
  - string W49.02 ☑
  - thread W49.02 ☑
- **Contact** (accidental)
  - with
    - abrasive wheel (metalworking) W31.1 ☑
    - alligator W58.09 ☑
      - bite W58.01 ☑
      - crushing W58.03 ☑
      - strike W58.02 ☑
    - amphibian W62.9 ☑
      - frog W62.0 ☑
      - toad W62.1 ☑
    - animal (nonvenomous) NEC W64 ☑
      - marine W56.89 ☑
        - bite W56.81 ☑
        - dolphin — *see* Contact, with, dolphin
        - fish NEC — *see* Contact, with, fish
        - mammal — *see* Contact, with, mammal, marine
        - orca — *see* Contact, with, orca
        - sea lion — *see* Contact, with, sea lion
        - shark — *see* Contact, with, shark
        - strike W56.82 ☑
    - animate mechanical force NEC W64 ☑
    - arrow W21.89 ☑
      - not thrown, projected or falling W45.8 ☑
    - arthropods (nonvenomous) W57 ☑
    - axe W27.0 ☑
    - band-saw (industrial) W31.2 ☑
    - bayonet — *see* Bayonet wound
    - bee(s) X58 ☑
    - bench-saw (industrial) W31.2 ☑
    - bird W61.99 ☑
      - bite W61.91 ☑
      - chicken — *see* Contact, with, chicken
      - duck — *see* Contact, with, duck
      - goose — *see* Contact, with, goose
      - macaw — *see* Contact, with, macaw
      - parrot — *see* Contact, with, parrot
      - psittacine — *see* Contact, with, psittacine
      - strike W61.92 ☑
      - turkey — *see* Contact, with, turkey
    - blender W29.0 ☑
    - boiling water X12 ☑
      - stated as undetermined whether accidental or intentional Y27.2 ☑
      - suicide (attempt) X77.2 ☑
    - bore, earth-drilling or mining (land) (seabed) W31.0 ☑
    - buffalo — *see* Contact, with, hoof stock NEC
    - bull W55.29 ☑
      - bite W55.21 ☑
      - gored W55.22 ☑
      - strike W55.22 ☑
    - bumper cars W31.81 ☑
    - camel — *see* Contact, with, hoof stock NEC

- **Contact** — *continued*
  - with — *continued*
    - can
      - lid W45.2 ☑
      - opener W27.4 ☑
        - powered W29.0 ☑
    - cat W55.09 ☑
      - bite W55.01 ☑
      - scratch W55.03 ☑
    - caterpillar (venomous) X58 ☑
    - centipede (venomous) X58 ☑
    - chain
      - hoist W24.0 ☑
        - agricultural operations W30.89 ☑
      - saw W29.3 ☑
    - chicken W61.39 ☑
      - peck W61.33 ☑
      - strike W61.32 ☑
    - chisel W27.0 ☑
    - circular saw W31.2 ☑
    - cobra X58 ☑
    - combine (harvester) W30.0 ☑
    - conveyer belt W24.1 ☑
    - cooker (hot) X15.8 ☑
      - stated as undetermined whether accidental or intentional Y27.3 ☑
      - suicide (attempt) X77.3 ☑
    - coral X58 ☑
    - cotton gin W31.82 ☑
    - cow W55.29 ☑
      - bite W55.21 ☑
      - strike W55.22 ☑
    - crane W24.0 ☑
      - agricultural operations W30.89 ☑
    - crocodile W58.19 ☑
      - bite W58.11 ☑
      - crushing W58.13 ☑
      - strike W58.12 ☑
    - dagger W26.1 ☑
      - stated as undetermined whether accidental or intentional Y28.2 ☑
      - suicide (attempt) X78.2 ☑
    - dairy equipment W31.82 ☑
    - dart W21.89 ☑
      - not thrown, projected or falling W45.8 ☑
    - deer — *see* Contact, with, hoof stock NEC
    - derrick W24.0 ☑
      - agricultural operations W30.89 ☑
        - hay W30.2 ☑
    - dog W54.8 ☑
      - bite W54.0 ☑
      - strike W54.1 ☑
    - dolphin W56.09 ☑
      - bite W56.01 ☑
      - strike W56.02 ☑
    - donkey — *see* Contact, with, hoof stock NEC
    - drill (powered) W29.8 ☑
      - earth (land) (seabed) W31.0 ☑
      - nonpowered W27.8 ☑
    - drive belt W24.0 ☑
      - agricultural operations W30.89 ☑
    - dry ice — *see* Exposure, cold, man-made
    - dryer (clothes) (powered) (spin) W29.2 ☑
    - duck W61.69 ☑
      - bite W61.61 ☑
      - strike W61.62 ☑
    - earth (-)
      - drilling machine (industrial) W31.0 ☑
      - scraping machine in stationary use W31.83 ☑
    - edge of stiff paper W45.1 ☑
    - electric
      - beater W29.0 ☑
      - blanket X16 ☑
      - fan W29.2 ☑
        - commercial W31.82 ☑
      - knife W29.1 ☑
      - mixer W29.0 ☑
    - elevator (building) W24.0 ☑
      - agricultural operations W30.89 ☑
        - grain W30.3 ☑
    - engine(s), hot NEC X17 ☑
    - excavating machine W31.0 ☑
    - farm machine W30.9 ☑
    - feces — *see* Contact, with, by type of animal
    - fer de lance X58 ☑

- **Contact** — *continued*
  - with — *continued*
    - fish W56.59 ☑
      - bite W56.51 ☑
      - shark — *see* Contact, with, shark
      - strike W56.52 ☑
    - flying horses W31.81 ☑
    - forging (metalworking) machine W31.1 ☑
    - fork W27.4 ☑
    - forklift (truck) W24.Ø ☑
      - agricultural operations W3Ø.89 ☑
    - frog W62.Ø ☑
    - garden
      - cultivator (powered) W29.3 ☑
        - riding W3Ø.89 ☑
      - fork W27.1 ☑
    - gas turbine W31.3 ☑
    - Gila monster X58 ☑
    - giraffe — *see* Contact, with, hoof stock NEC
    - glass (sharp) (broken) W25 ☑
      - with subsequent fall W18.Ø2 ☑
      - assault X99.Ø ☑
      - due to fall — *see* Fall, by type
      - stated as undetermined whether accidental or intentional Y28.Ø ☑
      - suicide (attempt) X78.Ø ☑
    - goat W55.39 ☑
      - bite W55.31 ☑
      - strike W55.32 ☑
    - goose W61.59 ☑
      - bite W61.51 ☑
      - strike W61.52 ☑
    - hand
      - saw W27.Ø ☑
      - tool (not powered) NEC W27.8 ☑
        - powered W29.8 ☑
    - harvester W3Ø.Ø ☑
    - hay-derrick W3Ø.2 ☑
    - heating
      - appliance (hot) X16 ☑
      - pad (electric) X16 ☑
    - heat NEC X19 ☑
      - from appliance (electrical) (household) — *see* Contact, with, hot, household appliance heating appliance X16 ☑
    - hedge-trimmer (powered) W29.3 ☑
    - hoe W27.1 ☑
    - hoist (chain) (shaft) NEC W24.Ø ☑
      - agricultural W3Ø.89 ☑
    - hoof stock NEC W55.39 ☑
      - bite W55.31 ☑
      - strike W55.32 ☑
    - hornet(s) X58 ☑
    - horse W55.19 ☑
      - bite W55.11 ☑
      - strike W55.12 ☑
    - hot
      - air X14.1 ☑
        - inhalation X14.Ø ☑
      - cooker X15.8 ☑
      - drinks X1Ø.Ø ☑
      - engine X17 ☑
      - fats X1Ø.2 ☑
      - fluids NEC X12 ☑
        - assault X98.2 ☑
        - suicide (attempt) X77.2 ☑
        - undetermined whether accidental or intentional Y27.2 ☑
      - food X1Ø.1 ☑
      - gases X14.1 ☑
        - inhalation X14.Ø ☑
      - heating appliance X16 ☑
      - household appliance X15.8 ☑
        - assault X98.3 ☑
        - cooker X15.8 ☑
        - hotplate X15.2 ☑
        - kettle X15.8 ☑
        - light bulb X15.8 ☑
        - object NEC X19 ☑
          - assault X98.8 ☑
          - stated as undetermined whether accidental or intentional Y27.9 ☑
          - suicide (attempt) X77.8 ☑
        - saucepan X15.3 ☑
        - skillet X15.3 ☑

- **Contact** — *continued*
  - with — *continued*
    - hot — *continued*
      - household appliance — *continued*
        - stated as undetermined whether accidental or intentional Y27.3 ☑
        - stove X15.Ø ☑
        - suicide (attempt) X77.3 ☑
        - toaster X15.1 ☑
      - kettle X15.8 ☑
      - light bulb X15.8 ☑
      - liquid NEC (*see also* Burn) X12 ☑
        - drinks X1Ø.Ø ☑
        - stated as undetermined whether accidental or intentional Y27.2 ☑
        - suicide (attempt) X77.2 ☑
        - tap water X11.8 ☑
          - stated as undetermined whether accidental or intentional Y27.1 ☑
          - suicide (attempt) X77.1 ☑
      - machinery X17 ☑
      - metal (molten) (liquid) NEC X18 ☑
      - object (not producing fire or flames) NEC X19 ☑
      - oil (cooking) X1Ø.2 ☑
      - pipe X16 ☑
      - plate X15.2 ☑
      - radiator X16 ☑
      - saucepan (glass) (metal) X15.3 ☑
      - skillet X15.3 ☑
      - stove (kitchen) X15.Ø ☑
      - substance NEC X19 ☑
      - tap-water X11.8 ☑
        - assault X98.1 ☑
        - heated on stove X12 ☑
          - stated as undetermined whether accidental or intentional Y27.2 ☑
          - suicide (attempt) X77.2 ☑
        - in bathtub X11.Ø ☑
        - running X11.1 ☑
        - stated as undetermined whether accidental or intentional Y27.1 ☑
        - suicide (attempt) X77.1 ☑
      - toaster X15.1 ☑
      - tool X17 ☑
      - vapors X13.1 ☑
        - inhalation X13.Ø ☑
      - water (tap) X11.8 ☑
        - boiling X12 ☑
          - stated as undetermined whether accidental or intentional Y27.2 ☑
          - suicide (attempt) X77.2 ☑
        - heated on stove X12 ☑
          - stated as undetermined whether accidental or intentional Y27.2 ☑
          - suicide (attempt) X77.2 ☑
        - in bathtub X11.Ø ☑
        - running X11.1 ☑
        - stated as undetermined whether accidental or intentional Y27.1 ☑
        - suicide (attempt) X77.1 ☑
    - hotplate X15.2 ☑
    - ice-pick W27.4 ☑
    - insect (nonvenomous) NEC W57 ☑
    - kettle (hot) X15.8 ☑
    - knife W26.Ø ☑
      - assault X99.1 ☑
      - electric W29.1 ☑
      - stated as undetermined whether accidental or intentional Y28.1 ☑
      - suicide (attempt) X78.1 ☑
    - lathe (metalworking) W31.1 ☑
      - turnings W45.8 ☑
      - woodworking W31.2 ☑
    - lawnmower (powered) (ridden) W28 ☑
      - causing electrocution W86.8 ☑
        - suicide (attempt) X83.1 ☑
      - unpowered W27.1 ☑
    - lift, lifting (devices) W24.Ø ☑
      - agricultural operations W3Ø.89 ☑
      - shaft W24.Ø ☑
    - liquefied gas — *see* Exposure, cold, man-made
    - liquid air, hydrogen, nitrogen — *see* Exposure, cold, man-made
    - lizard (nonvenomous) W59.Ø9 ☑
      - bite W59.Ø1 ☑
      - strike W59.Ø2 ☑

- **Contact** — *continued*
  - with — *continued*
    - llama — *see* Contact, with, hoof stock NEC
    - macaw W61.19 ☑
      - bite W61.11 ☑
      - strike W61.12 ☑
    - machine, machinery W31.9 ☑
      - abrasive wheel W31.1 ☑
      - agricultural including animal-powered W3Ø.9 ☑
        - combine harvester W3Ø.Ø ☑
        - grain storage elevator W3Ø.3 ☑
        - hay derrick W3Ø.2 ☑
        - power take-off device W3Ø.1 ☑
        - reaper W3Ø.Ø ☑
        - specified NEC W3Ø.89 ☑
        - thresher W3Ø.Ø ☑
        - transport vehicle, stationary W3Ø.81 ☑
      - band saw W31.2 ☑
      - bench saw W31.2 ☑
      - circular saw W31.2 ☑
      - commercial NEC W31.82 ☑
      - drilling, metal (industrial) W31.1 ☑
      - earth-drilling W31.Ø ☑
      - earthmoving or scraping W31.89 ☑
      - excavating W31.89 ☑
      - forging machine W31.1 ☑
      - gas turbine W31.3 ☑
      - hot X17 ☑
      - internal combustion engine W31.3 ☑
      - land drill W31.Ø ☑
      - lathe W31.1 ☑
      - lifting (devices) W24.Ø ☑
      - metal drill W31.1 ☑
      - metalworking (industrial) W31.1 ☑
      - milling, metal W31.1 ☑
      - mining W31.Ø ☑
      - molding W31.2 ☑
      - overhead plane W31.2 ☑
      - power press, metal W31.1 ☑
      - prime mover W31.3 ☑
      - printing W31.89 ☑
      - radial saw W31.2 ☑
      - recreational W31.81 ☑
      - roller-coaster W31.81 ☑
      - rolling mill, metal W31.1 ☑
      - sander W31.2 ☑
      - seabed drill W31.Ø ☑
      - shaft
        - hoist W31.Ø ☑
        - lift W31.Ø ☑
      - specified NEC W31.89 ☑
      - spinning W31.89 ☑
      - steam engine W31.3 ☑
      - transmission W24.1 ☑
      - undercutter W31.Ø ☑
      - water driven turbine W31.3 ☑
      - weaving W31.89 ☑
      - woodworking or forming (industrial) W31.2 ☑
    - mammal (feces) (urine) W55.89 ☑
      - bull — *see* Contact, with, bull
      - cat — *see* Contact, with, cat
      - cow — *see* Contact, with, cow
      - goat — *see* Contact, with, goat
      - hoof stock — *see* Contact, with, hoof stock
      - horse — *see* Contact, with, horse
      - marine W56.39 ☑
        - dolphin — *see* Contact, with, dolphin
        - orca — *see* Contact, with, orca
        - sea lion — *see* Contact, with, sea lion
        - specified NEC W56.39 ☑
          - bite W56.31 ☑
          - strike W56.32 ☑
      - pig — *see* Contact, with, pig
      - raccoon — *see* Contact, with, raccoon
      - rodent — *see* Contact, with, rodent
      - sheep — *see* Contact, with, sheep
      - specified NEC W55.89 ☑
        - bite W55.81 ☑
        - strike W55.82 ☑
    - marine
      - animal W56.89 ☑
        - bite W56.81 ☑
        - dolphin — *see* Contact, with, dolphin
        - fish NEC — *see* Contact, with, fish

External Causes Index

Contact — Contact

- **Contact** — *continued*
  - with — *continued*
    - marine — *continued*
      - animal — *continued*
        - mammal — *see* Contact, with, mammal, marine
        - orca — *see* Contact, with, orca
        - sea lion — *see* Contact, with, sea lion
        - shark — *see* Contact, with, shark
        - strike W56.82 ☑
    - meat
      - grinder (domestic) W29.Ø ☑
        - industrial W31.82 ☑
        - nonpowered W27.4 ☑
      - slicer (domestic) W29.Ø ☑
        - industrial W31.82 ☑
    - merry go round W31.81 ☑
    - metal, hot (liquid) (molten) NEC X18 ☑
    - millipede W57 ☑
    - nail W45.Ø ☑
      - gun W29.4 ☑
    - needle (sewing) W27.3 ☑
      - hypodermic W46.Ø ☑
        - contaminated W46.1 ☑
    - object (blunt) NEC
      - hot NEC X19 ☑
      - legal intervention — *see* Legal, intervention, blunt object
      - sharp NEC W45.8 ☑
        - inflicted by other person NEC W45.8 ☑
          - stated as
            - intentional homicide (attempt) — *see* Assault, cutting or piercing instrument
          - legal intervention — *see* Legal, intervention, sharp object
        - self-inflicted X78.9 ☑
    - orca W56.29 ☑
      - bite W56.21 ☑
      - strike W56.22 ☑
    - overhead plane W31.2 ☑
    - paper (as sharp object) W45.1 ☑
    - paper-cutter W27.5 ☑
    - parrot W61.Ø9 ☑
      - bite W61.Ø1 ☑
      - strike W61.Ø2 ☑
    - pig W55.49 ☑
      - bite W55.41 ☑
      - strike W55.42 ☑
    - pipe, hot X16 ☑
    - pitchfork W27.1 ☑
    - plane (metal) (wood) W27.Ø ☑
      - overhead W31.2 ☑
    - plant thorns, spines, sharp leaves or other mechanisms W6Ø ☑
    - powered
      - garden cultivator W29.3 ☑
      - household appliance, implement, or machine W29.8 ☑
      - saw (industrial) W31.2 ☑
        - hand W29.8 ☑
    - printing machine W31.89 ☑
    - psittacine bird W61.29 ☑
      - bite W61.21 ☑
      - macaw — *see* Contact, with, macaw
      - parrot — *see* Contact, with, parrot
      - strike W61.22 ☑
    - pulley (block) (transmission) W24.Ø ☑
      - agricultural operations W3Ø.89 ☑
    - raccoon W55.59 ☑
      - bite W55.51 ☑
      - strike W55.52 ☑
    - radial-saw (industrial) W31.2 ☑
    - radiator (hot) X16 ☑
    - rake W27.1 ☑
    - rattlesnake X58 ☑
    - reaper W3Ø.Ø ☑
    - reptile W59.89 ☑
      - lizard — *see* Contact, with, lizard
      - snake — *see* Contact, with, snake
      - specified NEC W59.89 ☑
        - bite W59.81 ☑
        - crushing W59.83 ☑
        - strike W59.82 ☑
      - turtle — *see* Contact, with, turtle
    - rivet gun (powered) W29.4 ☑

- **Contact** — *continued*
  - with — *continued*
    - road scraper — *see* Accident, transport, construction vehicle
    - rodent (feces) (urine) W53.89 ☑
      - bite W53.81 ☑
      - mouse W53.Ø9 ☑
        - bite W53.Ø1 ☑
      - rat W53.19 ☑
        - bite W53.11 ☑
      - specified NEC W53.89 ☑
        - bite W53.81 ☑
      - squirrel W53.29 ☑
        - bite W53.21 ☑
    - roller coaster W31.81 ☑
    - rope NEC W24.Ø ☑
      - agricultural operations W3Ø.89 ☑
    - saliva — *see* Contact, with, by type of animal
    - sander W29.8 ☑
      - industrial W31.2 ☑
    - saucepan (hot) (glass) (metal) X15.3 ☑
    - saw W27.Ø ☑
      - band (industrial) W31.2 ☑
      - bench (industrial) W31.2 ☑
      - chain W29.3 ☑
      - hand W27.Ø ☑
    - sawing machine, metal W31.1 ☑
    - scissors W27.2 ☑
    - scorpion X58 ☑
    - screwdriver W27.Ø ☑
      - powered W29.8 ☑
    - sea
      - anemone, cucumber or urchin (spine) X58 ☑
      - lion W56.19 ☑
        - bite W56.11 ☑
        - strike W56.12 ☑
    - serpent — *see* Contact, with, snake, by type
    - sewing-machine (electric) (powered) W29.2 ☑
      - not powered W27.8 ☑
    - shaft (hoist) (lift) (transmission) NEC W24.Ø ☑
      - agricultural W3Ø.89 ☑
    - shark W56.49 ☑
      - bite W56.41 ☑
      - strike W56.42 ☑
    - shears (hand) W27.2 ☑
      - powered (industrial) W31.1 ☑
        - domestic W29.2 ☑
    - sheep W55.39 ☑
      - bite W55.31 ☑
      - strike W55.32 ☑
    - shovel W27.8 ☑
      - steam — *see* Accident, transport, construction vehicle
    - snake (nonvenomous) W59.19 ☑
      - bite W59.11 ☑
      - crushing W59.13 ☑
      - strike W59.12 ☑
    - spade W27.1 ☑
    - spider (venomous) X58 ☑
    - spin-drier W29.2 ☑
    - spinning machine W31.89 ☑
    - splinter W45.8 ☑
    - sports equipment W21.9 ☑
    - staple gun (powered) W29.8 ☑
    - steam X13.1 ☑
      - engine W31.3 ☑
      - inhalation X13.Ø ☑
      - pipe X16 ☑
      - shovel W31.89 ☑
    - stove (hot) (kitchen) X15.Ø ☑
    - substance, hot NEC X19 ☑
      - molten (metal) X18 ☑
    - sword W26.1 ☑
      - assault X99.2 ☑
      - stated as undetermined whether accidental or intentional Y28.2 ☑
      - suicide (attempt) X78.2 ☑
    - tarantula X58 ☑
    - thresher W3Ø.Ø ☑
    - tin can lid W45.2 ☑
    - toad W62.1 ☑
    - toaster (hot) X15.1 ☑
    - tool W27.8 ☑
      - hand (not powered) W27.8 ☑
        - auger W27.Ø ☑

- **Contact** — *continued*
  - with — *continued*
    - tool — *continued*
      - hand — *continued*
        - axe W27.Ø ☑
        - can opener W27.4 ☑
        - chisel W27.Ø ☑
        - fork W27.4 ☑
        - garden W27.1 ☑
        - handsaw W27.Ø ☑
        - hoe W27.1 ☑
        - ice-pick W27.4 ☑
        - kitchen utensil W27.4 ☑
        - manual
          - lawn mower W27.1 ☑
          - sewing machine W27.8 ☑
        - meat grinder W27.4 ☑
        - needle (sewing) W27.3 ☑
          - hypodermic W46.Ø ☑
            - contaminated W46.1 ☑
        - paper cutter W27.5 ☑
        - pitchfork W27.1 ☑
        - rake W27.1 ☑
        - scissors W27.2 ☑
        - screwdriver W27.Ø ☑
        - specified NEC W27.8 ☑
        - workbench W27.Ø ☑
      - hot X17 ☑
      - powered W29.8 ☑
        - blender W29.Ø ☑
          - commercial W31.82 ☑
        - can opener W29.Ø ☑
          - commercial W31.82 ☑
        - chainsaw W29.3 ☑
        - clothes dryer W29.2 ☑
          - commercial W31.82 ☑
        - dishwasher W29.2 ☑
          - commercial W31.82 ☑
        - edger W29.3 ☑
        - electric fan W29.2 ☑
          - commercial W31.82 ☑
        - electric knife W29.1 ☑
        - food processor W29.Ø ☑
          - commercial W31.82 ☑
        - garbage disposal W29.Ø ☑
          - commercial W31.82 ☑
        - garden tool W29.3 ☑
        - hedge trimmer W29.3 ☑
        - ice maker W29.Ø ☑
          - commercial W31.82 ☑
        - kitchen appliance W29.Ø ☑
          - commercial W31.82 ☑
        - lawn mower W28 ☑
        - meat grinder W29.Ø ☑
          - commercial W31.82 ☑
        - mixer W29.Ø ☑
          - commercial W31.82 ☑
        - rototiller W29.3 ☑
        - sewing machine W29.2 ☑
          - commercial W31.82 ☑
        - washing machine W29.2 ☑
          - commercial W31.82 ☑
    - transmission device (belt, cable, chain, gear, pinion, shaft) W24.1 ☑
      - agricultural operations W3Ø.89 ☑
    - turbine (gas) (water-driven) W31.3 ☑
    - turkey W61.49 ☑
      - peck W61.43 ☑
      - strike W61.42 ☑
    - turtle (nonvenomous) W59.29 ☑
      - bite W59.21 ☑
      - strike W59.22 ☑
      - terrestrial W59.89 ☑
        - bite W59.81 ☑
        - crushing W59.83 ☑
        - strike W59.82 ☑
    - under-cutter W31.Ø ☑
    - urine — *see* Contact, with, by type of animal
    - vehicle
      - agricultural use (transport) — *see* Accident, transport, agricultural vehicle
        - not on public highway W3Ø.81 ☑
      - industrial use (transport) — *see* Accident, transport, industrial vehicle
        - not on public highway W31.83 ☑

- **Drowning** — *continued*
  - in — *continued*
    - river — *see* Drowning, in, natural water
    - sea — *see* Drowning, in, natural water
    - specified place NEC W73 ☑
      - assault X92.8 ☑
      - following
        - dive or jump W16.811 ☑
          - striking
            - bottom W16.821 ☑
            - wall W16.831 ☑
        - fall W16.311 ☑
          - striking
            - bottom W16.321 ☑
            - wall W16.331 ☑
      - stated as undetermined whether accidental or intentional Y21.8 ☑
      - suicide (attempt) X71.8 ☑
    - stream — *see* Drowning, in, natural water
    - swimming-pool W67 ☑
      - assault X92.1 ☑
        - following fall X92.2 ☑
      - following
        - dive or jump W16.511 ☑
          - striking
            - bottom W16.521 ☑
            - wall W16.531 ☑
        - fall W16.Ø11 ☑
          - striking
            - bottom W16.Ø21 ☑
            - wall W16.Ø31 ☑
      - stated as undetermined whether accidental or intentional Y21.2 ☑
        - following fall Y21.3 ☑
      - suicide (attempt) X71.1 ☑
        - following fall X71.2 ☑
    - war operations — *see* War operations, restriction of airway
  - resulting from accident to watercraft — *see* Drowning, due to, accident, watercraft
  - self-inflicted X71.9 ☑
  - stated as undetermined whether accidental or intentional Y21.9 ☑
  - suicide (attempt) X71.9 ☑

E

- **Earth falling** (on) W2Ø.Ø ☑
  - caused by cataclysmic earth surface movement or eruption — *see* Landslide
- **Earth** (surface) movement NEC — *see* Forces of nature, earth movement
- **Earthquake** (any injury) X34 ☑
- **Effect**(s) (adverse) **of**
  - air pressure (any) — *see* Air, pressure
  - cold, excessive (exposure to) — *see* Exposure, cold
  - heat (excessive) — *see* Heat
  - hot place (weather) B — *see* Heat
  - insolation X3Ø ☑
  - late — *see* Sequelae
  - motion — *see* Motion
  - nuclear explosion or weapon in war operations — *see* War operations, nuclear weapon
  - radiation — *see* Radiation
  - travel — *see* Travel
- **Electric shock** (accidental) (by) (in) — *see* Exposure, electric current
- **Electrocution** (accidental) — *see* Exposure, electric current
- **Endotracheal tube wrongly placed during anesthetic procedure**
- **Entanglement**
  - in
    - bed linen, causing suffocation T71 ☑
    - wheel of pedal cycle V19.88 ☑
- **Entry of foreign body or material** — *see* Foreign body
- **Environmental pollution related condition** — *see* category Z57 ☑
- **Execution, legal** (any method) — *see* Legal, intervention
- **Exhaustion**
  - cold — *see* Exposure, cold
  - due to excessive exertion — *see* category Y93 ☑
  - heat — *see* Heat
- **Explosion** (accidental) (of) (with secondary fire) W4Ø.9 ☑
  - acetylene W4Ø.1 ☑
  - aerosol can W36.1 ☑
  - air tank (compressed) (in machinery) W36.2 ☑
  - aircraft (in transit) (powered) NEC V95.9 ☑
    - balloon V96.Ø5 ☑
    - fixed wing NEC (private) V95.25 ☑
      - commercial V95.35 ☑
    - glider V96.25 ☑
      - hang V96.15 ☑
      - powered V95.15 ☑
    - helicopter V95.Ø5 ☑
    - in war operations — *see* War operations, destruction of aircraft
    - microlight V95.15 ☑
    - nonpowered V96.9 ☑
      - specified NEC V96.8 ☑
    - powered NEC V95.8 ☑
    - stated as
      - homicide (attempt) YØ3.8 ☑
      - suicide (attempt) X83.Ø ☑
    - ultralight V95.15 ☑
  - anesthetic gas in operating room W4Ø.1 ☑
  - antipersonnel bomb W4Ø.8 ☑
    - assault X96.Ø ☑
    - homicide (attempt) X96.Ø ☑
    - suicide (attempt) X75 ☑
  - assault X96.9 ☑
  - bicycle tire W37.Ø ☑
  - blasting (cap) (materials) W4Ø.Ø ☑
  - boiler (machinery), not on transport vehicle W35 ☑
    - on watercraft — *see* Explosion, in, watercraft
  - butane W4Ø.1 ☑
  - caused by other person X96.9 ☑
  - coal gas W4Ø.1 ☑
  - detonator W4Ø.Ø ☑
  - dump (munitions) W4Ø.8 ☑
  - dynamite W4Ø.Ø ☑
    - in
      - assault X96.8 ☑
      - homicide (attempt) X96.8 ☑
      - legal intervention
        - injuring
          - bystander Y35.112 ☑
          - law enforcement personnel Y35.111 ☑
          - suspect Y35.113 ☑
      - suicide (attempt) X75 ☑
  - explosive (material) W4Ø.9 ☑
    - gas W4Ø.1 ☑
    - in blasting operation W4Ø.Ø ☑
    - specified NEC W4Ø.8 ☑
      - in
        - assault X96.8 ☑
        - homicide (attempt) X96.8 ☑
        - legal intervention
          - injuring
            - bystander Y35.192 ☑
            - law enforcement personnel Y35.191 ☑
            - suspect Y35.193 ☑
        - suicide (attempt) X75 ☑
  - factory (munitions) W4Ø.8 ☑
  - fertilizer bomb W4Ø.8 ☑
    - assault X96.3 ☑
    - homicide (attempt) X96.3 ☑
    - suicide (attempt) X75 ☑
  - firearm (parts) NEC W34.19 ☑
    - airgun W34.11Ø ☑
    - BB gun W34.11Ø ☑
    - gas, air or spring-operated gun NEC W34.118 ☑
    - hangun W32.1 ☑
    - hunting rifle W33.12 ☑
    - larger firearm W33.1Ø ☑
      - specified NEC W33.19 ☑
    - machine gun W33.13 ☑
    - paintball gun W34.111 ☑
    - pellet gun W34.11Ø ☑
    - shotgun W33.11 ☑
    - Very pistol [flare] W34.19 ☑
  - fire-damp W4Ø.1 ☑
  - fireworks W39 ☑
  - gas (coal) (explosive) W4Ø.1 ☑
    - cylinder W36.9 ☑
      - aerosol can W36.1 ☑
      - air tank W36.2 ☑
      - pressurized W36.3 ☑
      - specified NEC W36.8 ☑
  - gasoline (fumes) (tank) not in moving motor vehicle W4Ø.1 ☑
    - bomb W4Ø.8 ☑
      - assault X96.1 ☑
      - homicide (attempt) X96.1 ☑
      - suicide (attempt) X75 ☑
    - in motor vehicle — *see* Accident, transport, by type of vehicle
  - grain store W4Ø.8 ☑
  - grenade W4Ø.8 ☑
    - in
      - assault X96.8 ☑
      - homicide (attempt) X96.8 ☑
      - legal intervention
        - injuring
          - bystander Y35.192 ☑
          - law enforcement personnel Y35.191 ☑
          - suspect Y35.193 ☑
      - suicide (attempt) X75 ☑
  - handgun (parts) — *see* Explosion, firearm, hangun (parts)
  - homicide (attempt) X96.9 ☑
    - antipersonnel bomb — *see* Explosion, antipersonnel bomb
    - fertilizer bomb — *see* Explosion, fertilizer bomb
    - gasoline bomb — *see* Explosion, gasoline bomb
    - letter bomb — *see* Explosion, letter bomb
    - pipe bomb — *see* Explosion, pipe bomb
    - specified NEC X96.8 ☑
  - hose, pressurized W37.8 ☑
  - hot water heater, tank (in machinery) W35 ☑
    - on watercraft — *see* Explosion, in, watercraft
  - in, on
    - dump W4Ø.8 ☑
    - factory W4Ø.8 ☑
    - mine (of explosive gases) NEC W4Ø.1 ☑
    - watercraft V93.59 ☑
      - powered craft V93.53 ☑
        - ferry boat V93.51 ☑
        - fishing boat V93.52 ☑
        - jetskis V93.53 ☑
        - liner V93.51 ☑
        - merchant ship V93.5Ø ☑
        - passenger ship V93.51 ☑
        - sailboat V93.54 ☑
  - letter bomb W4Ø.8 ☑
    - assault X96.2 ☑
    - homicide (attempt) X96.2 ☑
    - suicide (attempt) X75 ☑
  - machinery (*see also* Contact, with, by type of machine)
    - on board watercraft — *see* Explosion, in, watercraft
    - pressure vessel — *see* Explosion, by type of vessel
  - methane W4Ø.1 ☑
  - mine W4Ø.1 ☑
  - missile NEC W4Ø.8 ☑
  - mortar bomb W4Ø.8 ☑
    - in
      - assault X96.8 ☑
      - homicide (attempt) X96.8 ☑
      - legal intervention
        - injuring
          - bystander Y35.192 ☑
          - law enforcement personnel Y35.191 ☑
          - suspect Y35.193 ☑
      - suicide (attempt) X75 ☑
  - munitions (dump) (factory) W4Ø.8 ☑
  - pipe, pressurized W37.8 ☑
    - bomb W4Ø.8 ☑
      - assault X96.4 ☑
      - homicide (attempt) X96.4 ☑
      - suicide (attempt) X75 ☑
  - pressure, pressurized
    - cooker W38 ☑
    - gas tank (in machinery) W36.3 ☑
    - hose W37.8 ☑
    - pipe W37.8 ☑
    - specified device NEC W38 ☑
    - tire W37.8 ☑
      - bicycle W37.Ø ☑
    - vessel (in machinery) W38 ☑
  - propane W4Ø.1 ☑
  - self-inflicted X75 ☑
  - shell (artillery) NEC W4Ø.8 ☑
    - during war operations — *see* War operations, explosion

External cause status — *continued*
- hobby not done for income Y99.8
- leisure activity Y99.8
- military activity Y99.1
- off-duty activity of military personnel Y99.8
- recreation or sport not for income or while a student Y99.8
- specified NEC Y99.8
- student activity Y99.8
- volunteer activity Y99.2

F

Factors, supplemental
- alcohol
  - blood level
    - less than 2Ømg/1ØØml Y9Ø.Ø
    - 2Ø-39mg/1ØØml Y9Ø.1
    - 4Ø-59mg/1ØØml Y9Ø.2
    - 6Ø-79mg/1ØØml Y9Ø.3
    - 8Ø-99mg/1ØØml Y9Ø.4
    - 1ØØ-119mg/1ØØml Y9Ø.5
    - 12Ø-199mg/1ØØml Y9Ø.6
    - 2ØØ-239mg/1ØØml Y9Ø.7
    - 24Ømg/1ØØml or more Y9Ø.8
    - presence in blood, level not specified Y9Ø.9
  - presence in blood, but level not specified Y9Ø.9
- environmental-pollution-related condition- see Z57 ☑
- nosocomial condition Y95
- work-related condition Y99.Ø

Failure
- in suture or ligature during surgical procedure Y65.2
- mechanical, of instrument or apparatus (any) (during any medical or surgical procedure) Y65.8
- sterile precautions (during medical and surgical care) — *see* Misadventure, failure, sterile precautions, by type of procedure
- to
  - introduce tube or instrument Y65.4
    - endotracheal tube during anesthesia Y65.3
  - make curve (transport vehicle) NEC — *see* Accident, transport
  - remove tube or instrument Y65.4

Fall, falling (accidental) W19 ☑
- building W2Ø.1 ☑
  - burning (uncontrolled fire) XØØ.3 ☑
- down
  - embankment W17.81 ☑
  - escalator W1Ø.Ø ☑
  - hill W17.81 ☑
  - ladder W11 ☑
  - ramp W1Ø.2 ☑
  - stairs, steps W1Ø.9 ☑
- due to
  - bumping against
    - object W18.ØØ ☑
      - sharp glass W18.Ø2 ☑
      - specified NEC W18.Ø9 ☑
      - sports equipment W18.Ø1 ☑
    - person WØ3 ☑
      - due to ice or snow WØØ.Ø ☑
      - on pedestrian conveyance — *see* Accident, transport, pedestrian, conveyance
  - collision with another person WØ3 ☑
    - due to ice or snow WØØ.Ø ☑
    - involving pedestrian conveyance — *see* Accident, transport, pedestrian, conveyance
  - grocery cart tipping over W17.82 ☑
  - ice or snow WØØ.9 ☑
    - from one level to another WØØ.2 ☑
      - on stairs or steps WØØ.1 ☑
    - involving pedestrian conveyance — *see* Accident, transport, pedestrian, conveyance
    - on same level WØØ.Ø ☑
  - slipping (on moving sidewalk) WØ1.Ø ☑
    - with subsequent striking against object WØ1.1Ø ☑
      - furniture WØ1.19Ø ☑
      - sharp object WØ1.119 ☑
        - glass WØ1.11Ø ☑
        - power tool or machine WØ1.111 ☑
        - specified NEC WØ1.118 ☑
      - specified NEC WØ1.198 ☑
  - striking against
    - object W18.ØØ ☑
      - sharp glass W18.Ø2 ☑
      - specified NEC W18.Ø9 ☑

Fall, falling — *continued*
- due to — *continued*
  - striking against — *continued*
    - object — *continued*
      - sports equipment W18.Ø1 ☑
    - person WØ3 ☑
      - due to ice or snow WØØ.Ø ☑
      - on pedestrian conveyance — *see* Accident, transport, pedestrian, conveyance
- earth (with asphyxia or suffocation (by pressure)) — *see* Earth, falling
- from, off, out of
  - aircraft NEC (with accident to aircraft NEC) V97.Ø ☑
    - while boarding or alighting V97.1 ☑
  - balcony W13.Ø ☑
  - bed WØ6 ☑
  - boat, ship, watercraft NEC (with drowning or submersion) — *see* Drowning, due to, fall overboard
    - with hitting bottom or object V94.Ø ☑
  - bridge W13.1 ☑
  - building W13.9 ☑
    - burning (uncontrolled fire) XØØ.3 ☑
  - cavity W17.2 ☑
  - chair WØ7 ☑
  - cherry picker W17.89 ☑
  - cliff W15 ☑
  - dock W17.4 ☑
  - embankment W17.81 ☑
  - escalator W1Ø.Ø ☑
  - flagpole W13.8 ☑
  - furniture NEC WØ8 ☑
  - grocery cart W17.82 ☑
  - haystack W17.89 ☑
  - high place NEC W17.89 ☑
    - stated as undetermined whether accidental or intentional Y3Ø ☑
  - hole W17.2 ☑
  - incline W1Ø.2 ☑
  - ladder W11 ☑
  - lifting device W17.89 ☑
  - machine, machinery (*see also* Contact, with, by type of machine)
    - not in operation W17.89 ☑
  - manhole W17.1 ☑
  - mobile elevated work platform [MEWP] W17.89 ☑
  - motorized mobility scooter WØ5.2 ☑
  - one level to another NEC W17.89 ☑
    - intentional, purposeful, suicide (attempt) X8Ø ☑
    - stated as undetermined whether accidental or intentional Y3Ø ☑
  - pit W17.2 ☑
  - playground equipment WØ9.8 ☑
    - jungle gym WØ9.2 ☑
    - slide WØ9.Ø ☑
    - swing WØ9.1 ☑
  - quarry W17.89 ☑
  - railing W13.9 ☑
  - ramp W1Ø.2 ☑
  - roof W13.2 ☑
  - scaffolding W12 ☑
  - scooter (nonmotorized) WØ5.1 ☑
    - motorized mobility WØ5.2 ☑
  - sky lift W17.89 ☑
  - stairs, steps W1Ø.9 ☑
    - curb W1Ø.1 ☑
    - due to ice or snow WØØ.1 ☑
    - escalator W1Ø.Ø ☑
    - incline W1Ø.2 ☑
    - ramp W1Ø.2 ☑
    - sidewalk curb W1Ø.1 ☑
    - specified NEC W1Ø.8 ☑
  - stepladder W11 ☑
  - storm drain W17.1 ☑
  - streetcar NEC V82.6 ☑
    - with antecedent collision — *see* Accident, transport, streetcar occupant
    - while boarding or alighting V82.4 ☑
  - structure NEC W13.8 ☑
    - burning (uncontrolled fire) XØØ.3 ☑
  - table WØ8 ☑
  - toilet W18.11 ☑
    - with subsequent striking against object W18.12 ☑
  - train NEC V81.6 ☑

Fall, falling — *continued*
- from, off, out of — *continued*
  - train — *continued*
    - during derailment (without antecedent collision) V81.7 ☑
      - with antecedent collision — *see* Accident, transport, railway vehicle occupant
    - while boarding or alighting V81.4 ☑
  - transport vehicle after collision — *see* Accident, transport, by type of vehicle, collision
  - tree W14 ☑
  - vehicle (in motion) NEC (*see also* Accident, transport) V89.9 ☑
    - motor NEC (*see also* Accident, transport, occupant, by type of vehicle) V87.8 ☑
    - stationary W17.89 ☑
      - while boarding or alighting B — *see* Accident, transport, by type of vehicle, while boarding or alighting
  - viaduct W13.8 ☑
  - wall W13.8 ☑
  - watercraft (*see also* Drowning, due to, fall overboard)
    - with hitting bottom or object V94.Ø ☑
  - well W17.Ø ☑
  - wheelchair, non-moving WØ5.Ø ☑
    - powered — *see* Accident, transport, pedestrian, conveyance occupant, specified type NEC
  - window W13.4 ☑
- in, on
  - aircraft NEC V97.Ø ☑
    - with accident to aircraft V97.Ø ☑
    - while boarding or alighting V97.1 ☑
  - bathtub (empty) W18.2 ☑
    - filled W16.212 ☑
      - causing drowning W16.211 ☑
  - escalator W1Ø.Ø ☑
  - incline W1Ø.2 ☑
  - ladder W11 ☑
  - machine, machinery — *see* Contact, with, by type of machine
  - object, edged, pointed or sharp (with cut) — *see* Fall, by type
  - playground equipment WØ9.8 ☑
    - jungle gym WØ9.2 ☑
    - slide WØ9.Ø ☑
    - swing WØ9.1 ☑
  - ramp W1Ø.2 ☑
  - scaffolding W12 ☑
  - shower W18.2 ☑
    - causing drowning W16.211 ☑
  - staircase, stairs, steps W1Ø.9 ☑
    - curb W1Ø.1 ☑
    - due to ice or snow WØØ.1 ☑
    - escalator W1Ø.Ø ☑
    - incline W1Ø.2 ☑
    - specified NEC W1Ø.8 ☑
  - streetcar (without antecedent collision) V82.5 ☑
    - with antecedent collision — *see* Accident, transport, streetcar occupant
    - while boarding or alighting V82.4 ☑
  - train (without antecedent collision) V81.5 ☑
    - with antecedent collision — *see* Accident, transport, railway vehicle occupant
    - during derailment (without antecedent collision) V81.7 ☑
      - with antecedent collision — *see* Accident, transport, railway vehicle occupant
    - while boarding or alighting V81.4 ☑
  - transport vehicle after collision — *see* Accident, transport, by type of vehicle, collision
  - watercraft V93.39 ☑
    - due to
      - accident to craft V91.29 ☑
        - powered craft V91.23 ☑
          - ferry boat V91.21 ☑
          - fishing boat V91.22 ☑
          - jetskis V91.23 ☑
          - liner V91.21 ☑
          - merchant ship V91.2Ø ☑
          - passenger ship V91.21 ☑
        - unpowered craft
          - canoe V91.25 ☑
          - inflatable V91.26 ☑
          - kayak V91.25 ☑
          - sailboat V91.24 ☑

- **Fall, falling** — *continued*
  - in, on — *continued*
    - watercraft — *continued*
      - powered craft V93.33 ☑
        - ferry boat V93.31 ☑
        - fishing boat V93.32 ☑
        - jetskis V93.33 ☑
        - liner V93.31 ☑
        - merchant ship V93.30 ☑
        - passenger ship V93.31 ☑
      - unpowered craft V93.38 ☑
        - canoe V93.35 ☑
        - inflatable V93.36 ☑
        - kayak V93.35 ☑
        - sailboat V93.34 ☑
        - surf-board V93.38 ☑
        - windsurfer V93.38 ☑
  - into
    - cavity W17.2 ☑
    - dock W17.4 ☑
    - fire — *see* Exposure, fire, by type
    - haystack W17.89 ☑
    - hole W17.2 ☑
    - lake — *see* Fall, into, water
    - lake — *see* Fall, into, water
    - manhole W17.1 ☑
    - moving part of machinery — *see* Contact, with, by type of machine
    - ocean — *see* Fall, into, water
    - opening in surface NEC W17.89 ☑
    - pit W17.2 ☑
    - pond — *see* Fall, into, water
    - quarry W17.89 ☑
    - river — *see* Fall, into, water
    - shaft W17.89 ☑
    - storm drain W17.1 ☑
    - stream — *see* Fall, into, water
    - swimming pool (*see also* Fall, into, water, in, swimming pool)
      - empty W17.3 ☑
    - tank W17.89 ☑
    - water W16.42 ☑
      - causing drowning W16.41 ☑
      - from watercraft — *see* Drowning, due to, fall overboard
      - hitting diving board W21.4 ☑
      - in
        - bathtub W16.212 ☑
          - causing drowning W16.211 ☑
        - bucket W16.222 ☑
          - causing drowning W16.221 ☑
        - natural body of water W16.112 ☑
          - causing drowning W16.111 ☑
          - striking
            - bottom W16.122 ☑
              - causing drowning W16.121 ☑
            - side W16.132 ☑
              - causing drowning W16.131 ☑
        - specified water NEC W16.312 ☑
          - causing drowning W16.311 ☑
          - striking
            - bottom W16.322 ☑
              - causing drowning W16.321 ☑
            - wall W16.332 ☑
              - causing drowning W16.331 ☑
        - swimming pool W16.012 ☑
          - causing drowning W16.011 ☑
          - striking
            - bottom W16.022 ☑
              - causing drowning W16.031 ☑
            - wall W16.032 ☑
              - causing drowning W16.021 ☑
        - utility bucket W16.222 ☑
          - causing drowning W16.221 ☑
    - well W17.0 ☑
  - involving
    - bed W06 ☑
    - chair W07 ☑
    - furniture NEC W08 ☑
    - glass — *see* Fall, by type
    - playground equipment W09.8 ☑
      - jungle gym W09.2 ☑
      - slide W09.0 ☑
      - swing W09.1 ☑
    - roller blades — *see* Accident, transport, pedestrian, conveyance

- **Fall, falling** — *continued*
  - involving — *continued*
    - skateboard(s) — *see* Accident, transport, pedestrian, conveyance
    - skates (ice) (in line) (roller) — *see* Accident, transport, pedestrian, conveyance
    - skis — *see* Accident, transport, pedestrian, conveyance
    - table W08 ☑
    - wheelchair, non-moving W05.0 ☑
      - powered — *see* Accident, transport, pedestrian, conveyance, specified type NEC
  - object — *see* Struck by, object, falling
  - off
    - toilet W18.11 ☑
      - with subsequent striking against object W18.12 ☑
  - on same level W18.30 ☑
    - due to
      - specified NEC W18.39 ☑
      - stepping on an object W18.31 ☑
  - out of
    - bed W06 ☑
    - building NEC W13.8 ☑
    - chair W07 ☑
    - furniture NEC W08 ☑
    - wheelchair, non-moving W05.0 ☑
      - powered — *see* Accident, transport, pedestrian, conveyance, specified type NEC
    - window W13.4 ☑
  - over
    - animal W01.0 ☑
    - cliff W15 ☑
    - embankment W17.81 ☑
    - small object W01.0 ☑
  - rock W20.8 ☑
  - same level W18.30 ☑
    - from
      - being crushed, pushed, or stepped on by a crowd or human stampede W52 ☑
      - collision, pushing, shoving, by or with other person W03 ☑
      - slipping, stumbling, tripping W01.0 ☑
    - involving ice or snow W00.0 ☑
      - involving skates (ice) (roller), skateboard, skis — *see* Accident, transport, pedestrian, conveyance
  - snowslide (avalanche) — *see* Landslide
  - stone W20.8 ☑
  - structure W20.1 ☑
    - burning (uncontrolled fire) X00.3 ☑
  - through
    - bridge W13.1 ☑
    - floor W13.3 ☑
    - roof W13.2 ☑
    - wall W13.8 ☑
    - window W13.4 ☑
  - timber W20.8 ☑
  - tree (caused by lightning) W20.8 ☑
  - while being carried or supported by other person(s) W04 ☑
- **Fallen on by**
  - animal (not being ridden) NEC W55.89 ☑
- **Felo-de-se** — *see* Suicide
- **Fight** (hand) (fists) (foot) — *see* Assault, fight
- **Fire** (accidental) — *see* Exposure, fire
- **Firearm discharge** — *see* Discharge, firearm
- **Fireball effects from nuclear explosion in war operations** — *see* War operations, nuclear weapons
- **Fireworks** (explosion) W39 ☑
- **Flash burns from explosion** — *see* Explosion
- **Flood** (any injury) (caused by) X38 ☑
  - collapse of man-made structure causing earth movement X36.0 ☑
  - tidal wave — *see* Forces of nature, tidal wave
- **Food** (any type) **in**
  - air passages (with asphyxia, obstruction, or suffocation) — *see* categories T17 and T18 ☑
  - alimentary tract causing asphyxia (due to compression of trachea) — *see* categories T17 and T18 ☑
- **Forces of nature** X39.8 ☑
  - avalanche X36.1 ☑
    - causing transport accident — *see* Accident, transport, by type of vehicle
  - blizzard X37.2 ☑
  - cataclysmic storm X37.9 ☑

- **Forces of nature** — *continued*
  - cataclysmic storm — *continued*
    - with flood X38 ☑
    - blizzard X37.2 ☑
    - cloudburst X37.8 ☑
    - cyclone X37.1 ☑
    - dust storm X37.3 ☑
    - hurricane X37.0 ☑
    - specified storm NEC X37.8 ☑
    - storm surge X37.0 ☑
    - tornado X37.1 ☑
    - twister X37.1 ☑
    - typhoon X37.0 ☑
  - cloudburst X37.8 ☑
  - cold (natural) X31 ☑
  - cyclone X37.1 ☑
  - dam collapse causing earth movement X36.0 ☑
  - dust storm X37.3 ☑
  - earth movement X36.1 ☑
    - caused by dam or structure collapse X36.0 ☑
    - earthquake X34 ☑
  - earthquake X34 ☑
  - flood (caused by) X38 ☑
    - dam collapse X36.0 ☑
    - tidal wave B — *see* Forces of nature, tidal wave
  - heat (natural) X30 ☑
  - hurricane X37.0 ☑
  - landslide X36.1 ☑
    - causing transport accident — *see* Accident, transport, by type of vehicle
  - lightning — *see* subcategory T75.0 ☑
    - causing fire — *see* Exposure, fire
  - mudslide X36.1 ☑
    - causing transport accident — *see* Accident, transport, by type of vehicle
  - radiation (natural) X39.08 ☑
    - radon X39.01 ☑
  - radon X39.01 ☑
  - specified force NEC X39.8 ☑
  - storm surge X37.0 ☑
  - structure collapse causing earth movement X36.0 ☑
  - sunlight X32 ☑
  - tidal wave X37.41 ☑
    - due to
      - earthquake X37.41 ☑
      - landslide X37.43 ☑
      - storm X37.42 ☑
      - volcanic eruption X37.41 ☑
  - tornado X37.1 ☑
  - tsunami X37.41 ☑
  - twister X37.1 ☑
  - typhoon X37.0 ☑
  - volcanic eruption X35 ☑
- **Foreign body**
  - aspiration — *see* Index to Diseases and Injuries, Foreign body, respiratory tract
  - entering through skin W45.8 ☑
    - can lid W45.2 ☑
    - nail W45.0 ☑
    - paper W45.1 ☑
    - specified NEC W45.8 ☑
    - splinter W45.8 ☑
- **Forest fire** (exposure to) — *see* Exposure, fire, uncontrolled, not in building
- **Found injured** X58 ☑
  - from exposure (to) — *see* Exposure
  - on
    - highway, road(way), street V89.9 ☑
    - railway right of way V81.9 ☑
- **Fracture** (circumstances unknown or unspecified) X58 ☑
  - due to specified cause NEC X58 ☑
- **Freezing** — *see* Exposure, cold
- **Frostbite** X31 ☑
  - due to man-made conditions — *see* Exposure, cold, man-made
- **Frozen** — *see* Exposure, cold

G

- **Gored by bull** W55.22 ☑
- **Gunshot wound** W34.00 ☑

H

- **Hailstones, injured by** X39.8 ☑

- **Hanged herself or himself** — *see* Hanging, self-inflicted
- **Hanging** (accidental) (*see also* category) T71 ☑
  - legal execution — *see* Legal, intervention, specified means NEC
- **Heat** (effects of) (excessive) X30 ☑
  - due to
    - man-made conditions W92 ☑
      - on board watercraft V93.29 ☑
        - fishing boat V93.22 ☑
        - merchant ship V93.20 ☑
        - passenger ship V93.21 ☑
        - sailboat V93.24 ☑
        - specified powered craft NEC V93.23 ☑
    - weather (conditions) X30 ☑
  - from
    - electric heating apparatus causing burning X16 ☑
    - nuclear explosion in war operations — *see* War operations, nuclear weapons
  - inappropriate in local application or packing in medical or surgical procedure Y63.5
- **Hemorrhage**
  - delayed following medical or surgical treatment without mention of misadventure — *see* Index to Diseases and Injuries, Complication(s)
  - during medical or surgical treatment as misadventure — *see* Index to Diseases and Injuries, Complication(s)
- **High**
  - altitude (effects) — *see* Air, pressure, low
  - level of radioactivity, effects — *see* Radiation
  - pressure (effects) — *see* Air, pressure, high
  - temperature, effects — *see* Heat
- **Hit, hitting** (accidental) by — *see* Struck by
- **Hitting against** — *see* Striking against
- **Homicide** (attempt) (justifiable) — *see* Assault
- **Hot**
  - place, effects (*see also* Heat)
  - weather, effects X30 ☑
- **House fire** (uncontrolled) — *see* Exposure, fire, uncontrolled, building
- **Humidity, causing problem** X39.8 ☑
- **Hunger** X58 ☑
- **Hurricane** (any injury) X37.0 ☑
- **Hypobarism, hypobaropathy** — *see* Air, pressure, low

I

- **Ictus**
  - caloris (*see also* Heat)
  - solaris X30 ☑
- **Ignition** (accidental) (*see also* Exposure, fire) X08.8 ☑
  - anesthetic gas in operating room W40.1 ☑
  - apparel X06.2 ☑
    - from highly flammable material X04 ☑
    - nightwear X05 ☑
  - bed linen (sheets) (spreads) (pillows) (mattress) — *see* Exposure, fire, uncontrolled, building, bed
  - benzine X04 ☑
  - clothes, clothing NEC (from controlled fire) X06.2 ☑
    - from
      - highly flammable material X04 ☑
  - ether X04 ☑
    - in operating room W40.1 ☑
  - explosive material — *see* Explosion
  - gasoline X04 ☑
  - jewelry (plastic) (any) X06.0 ☑
  - kerosene X04 ☑
  - material
    - explosive — *see* Explosion
    - highly flammable with secondary explosion X04 ☑
  - nightwear X05 ☑
  - paraffin X04 ☑
  - petrol X04 ☑
- **Immersion** (accidental) (*see also* Drowning)
  - hand or foot due to cold (excessive) X31 ☑
- **Implantation of quills of porcupine** W55.89 ☑
- **Inanition** (from) (hunger) X58 ☑
  - thirst X58 ☑
- **Inappropriate operation performed**
  - correct operation on wrong side or body part (wrong side) (wrong site) Y65.53
  - operation intended for another patient done on wrong patient Y65.52
  - wrong operation performed on correct patient Y65.51
- **Inattention after, at birth** (homicidal intent) (infanticidal intent) X58 ☑
- **Incident, adverse**
  - device
    - anesthesiology Y70.8
      - accessory Y70.2
      - diagnostic Y70.0
      - miscellaneous Y70.8
      - monitoring Y70.0
      - prosthetic Y70.2
      - rehabilitative Y70.1
      - surgical Y70.3
      - therapeutic Y70.1
    - cardiovascular Y71.8
      - accessory Y71.2
      - diagnostic Y71.0
      - miscellaneous Y71.8
      - monitoring Y71.0
      - prosthetic Y71.2
      - rehabilitative Y71.1
      - surgical Y71.3
      - therapeutic Y71.1
    - gastroenterology Y73.8
      - accessory Y73.2
      - diagnostic Y73.0
      - miscellaneous Y73.8
      - monitoring Y73.0
      - prosthetic Y73.2
      - rehabilitative Y73.1
      - surgical Y73.3
      - therapeutic Y73.1
    - general
      - hospital Y74.8
        - accessory Y74.2
        - diagnostic Y74.0
        - miscellaneous Y74.8
        - monitoring Y74.0
        - prosthetic Y74.2
        - rehabilitative Y74.1
        - surgical Y74.3
        - therapeutic Y74.1
      - surgical Y81.8
        - accessory Y81.2
        - diagnostic Y81.0
        - miscellaneous Y81.8
        - monitoring Y81.0
        - prosthetic Y81.2
        - rehabilitative Y81.1
        - surgical Y81.3
        - therapeutic Y81.1
    - gynecological Y76.8
      - accessory Y76.2
      - diagnostic Y76.0
      - miscellaneous Y76.8
      - monitoring Y76.0
      - prosthetic Y76.2
      - rehabilitative Y76.1
      - surgical Y76.3
      - therapeutic Y76.1
    - medical Y82.9
      - specified type NEC Y82.8
    - neurological Y75.8
      - accessory Y75.2
      - diagnostic Y75.0
      - miscellaneous Y75.8
      - monitoring Y75.0
      - prosthetic Y75.2
      - rehabilitative Y75.1
      - surgical Y75.3
      - therapeutic Y75.1
    - obstetrical Y76.8
      - accessory Y76.2
      - diagnostic Y76.0
      - miscellaneous Y76.8
      - monitoring Y76.0
      - prosthetic Y76.2
      - rehabilitative Y76.1
      - surgical Y76.3
      - therapeutic Y76.1
    - ophthalmic Y77.8
      - accessory Y77.2
      - diagnostic Y77.0
      - miscellaneous Y77.8
      - monitoring Y77.0
      - prosthetic Y77.2
      - rehabilitative Y77.1
      - surgical Y77.3
      - therapeutic Y77.1
    - orthopedic Y79.8
      - accessory Y79.2

Incident, adverse — *continued*

- device — *continued*
  - orthopedic — *continued*
    - diagnostic Y79.0
    - miscellaneous Y79.8
    - monitoring Y79.0
    - prosthetic Y79.2
    - rehabilitative Y79.1
    - surgical Y79.3
    - therapeutic Y79.1
  - otorhinolaryngological Y72.8
    - accessory Y72.2
    - diagnostic Y72.0
    - miscellaneous Y72.8
    - monitoring Y72.0
    - prosthetic Y72.2
    - rehabilitative Y72.1
    - surgical Y72.3
    - therapeutic Y72.1
  - personal use Y74.8
    - accessory Y74.2
    - diagnostic Y74.0
    - miscellaneous Y74.8
    - monitoring Y74.0
    - prosthetic Y74.2
    - rehabilitative Y74.1
    - surgical Y74.3
    - therapeutic Y74.1
  - physical medicine Y80.8
    - accessory Y80.2
    - diagnostic Y80.0
    - miscellaneous Y80.8
    - monitoring Y80.0
    - prosthetic Y80.2
    - rehabilitative Y80.1
    - surgical Y80.3
    - therapeutic Y80.1
  - plastic surgical Y81.8
    - accessory Y81.2
    - diagnostic Y81.0
    - miscellaneous Y81.8
    - monitoring Y81.0
    - prosthetic Y81.2
    - rehabilitative Y81.1
    - surgical Y81.3
    - therapeutic Y81.1
  - radiological Y78.8
    - accessory Y78.2
    - diagnostic Y78.0
    - miscellaneous Y78.8
    - monitoring Y78.0
    - prosthetic Y78.2
    - rehabilitative Y78.1
    - surgical Y78.3
    - therapeutic Y78.1
  - urology Y73.8
    - accessory Y73.2
    - diagnostic Y73.0
    - miscellaneous Y73.8
    - monitoring Y73.0
    - prosthetic Y73.2
    - rehabilitative Y73.1
    - surgical Y73.3
    - therapeutic Y73.1

- **Incineration** (accidental) — *see* Exposure, fire
- **Infanticide** — *see* Assault
- **Infrasound waves** (causing injury) W49.9 ☑
- **Ingestion**
  - foreign body (causing injury) (with obstruction) — *see* Foreign body, alimentary canal
  - poisonous
    - plant(s) X58 ☑
    - substance NEC — *see* Table of Drugs and Chemicals
- **Inhalation**
  - excessively cold substance, man-made — *see* Exposure, cold, man-made
  - food (any type) (into respiratory tract) (with asphyxia, obstruction respiratory tract, suffocation) — *see* categories T17 and T18 ☑
  - foreign body — *see* Foreign body, aspiration
  - gastric contents (with asphyxia, obstruction respiratory passage, suffocation) T17.81- ☑
  - hot air or gases X14.0 ☑
  - liquid air, hydrogen, nitrogen W93.12 ☑
    - suicide (attempt) X83.2 ☑
  - steam X13.0 ☑
    - assault X98.0 ☑

Inhalation — *continued*
steam — *continued*
stated as undetermined whether accidental or intentional Y27.Ø ☑
suicide (attempt) X77.Ø ☑
toxic gas — *see* Table of Drugs and Chemicals
vomitus (with asphyxia, obstruction respiratory passage, suffocation) T17.81- ☑
Injury, injured (accidental(ly)) NOS X58 ☑
by, caused by, from
assault — *see* Assault
law-enforcing agent, police, in course of legal intervention — *see* Legal intervention
suicide (attempt) X83.8 ☑
due to, in
civil insurrection — *see* War operations
fight (*see also* Assault, fight) YØ4.Ø ☑
war operations — *see* War operations
homicide (*see also* Assault) YØ9
inflicted (by)
in course of arrest (attempted), suppression of disturbance, maintenance of order, by law-enforcing agents — *see* Legal intervention
other person
stated as
accidental X58 ☑
intentional, homicide (attempt) — *see* Assault
undetermined whether accidental or intentional Y33 ☑
purposely (inflicted) by other person(s) — *see* Assault
self-inflicted X83.8 ☑
stated as accidental X58 ☑
specified cause NEC X58 ☑
undetermined whether accidental or intentional Y33 ☑
Insolation, effects X3Ø ☑
Insufficient nourishment X58 ☑
Interruption of respiration (by)
food (lodged in esophagus) — *see* categories T17 and T18 ☑
vomitus (lodged in esophagus) T17.81- ☑
Intervention, legal — *see* Legal intervention
Intoxication
drug — *see* Table of Drugs and Chemicals
poison — *see* Table of Drugs and Chemicals

J

Jammed (accidentally)
between objects (moving) (stationary and moving) W23.Ø ☑
stationary W23.1 ☑
Jumped, jumping
before moving object NEC X81.8 ☑
motor vehicle X81.Ø ☑
subway train X81.1 ☑
train X81.1 ☑
undetermined whether accidental or intentional Y31 ☑
from
boat (into water) voluntarily, without accident (to or on boat) W16.712 ☑
with
accident to or on boat — *see* Accident, watercraft
drowning or submersion W16.711 ☑
suicide (attempt) X71.3 ☑
striking bottom W16.722 ☑
causing drowning W16.721 ☑
building (*see also* Jumped, from, high place) W13.9 ☑
burning (uncontrolled fire) XØØ.5 ☑
high place NEC W17.89 ☑
suicide (attempt) X8Ø ☑
undetermined whether accidental or intentional Y3Ø ☑
structure (*see also* Jumped, from, high place) W13.9 ☑
burning (uncontrolled fire) XØØ.5 ☑
into water W16.92 ☑
causing drowning W16.91 ☑
from, off watercraft — *see* Jumped, from, boat
in
natural body W16.612 ☑
causing drowning W16.611 ☑

Jumped, jumping — *continued*
into water — *continued*
in — *continued*
natural body — *continued*
striking bottom W16.622 ☑
causing drowning W16.621 ☑
specified place NEC W16.812 ☑
causing drowning W16.811 ☑
striking
bottom W16.822 ☑
causing drowning W16.821 ☑
wall W16.832 ☑
causing drowning W16.831 ☑
swimming pool W16.512 ☑
causing drowning W16.511 ☑
striking
bottom W16.522 ☑
causing drowning W16.521 ☑
wall W16.532 ☑
causing drowning W16.531 ☑
suicide (attempt) X71.3 ☑

K

Kicked by
animal NEC W55.82 ☑
person(s) (accidentally) W5Ø.1 ☑
with intent to injure or kill YØ4.Ø ☑
as, or caused by, a crowd or human stampede (with fall) W52 ☑
assault YØ4.Ø ☑
homicide (attempt) YØ4.Ø ☑
in
fight YØ4.Ø ☑
legal intervention
injuring
bystander Y35.812 ☑
law enforcement personnel Y35.811 ☑
suspect Y35.813 ☑
Kicking against
object W22.8 ☑
sports equipment W21.9 ☑
stationary wW22.Ø9
sports equipment W21.89 ☑
person — *see* Striking against, person
sports equipment W21.9 ☑
Killed, killing (accidentally) NOS (*see also* Injury) X58 ☑
in
action — *see* War operations
brawl, fight (hand) (fists) (foot) YØ4.Ø ☑
by weapon (*see also* Assault)
cutting, piercing — *see* Assault, cutting or piercing instrument
firearm — *see* Discharge, firearm, by type, homicide
self
stated as
accident NOS X58 ☑
suicide — *see* Suicide
undetermined whether accidental or intentional Y33 ☑
Knocked down (accidentally) (by) NOS X58 ☑
animal (not being ridden) NEC (*see also* Struck by, by type of animal)
crowd or human stampede W52 ☑
person W51 ☑
in brawl, fight YØ4.Ø ☑
transport vehicle NEC (*see also* Accident, transport) VØ9.9 ☑

L

Laceration NEC — *see* Injury
Lack of
care (helpless person) (infant) (newborn) X58 ☑
food except as result of abandonment or neglect X58 ☑
due to abandonment or neglect X58 ☑
water except as result of transport accident X58 ☑
due to transport accident B — *see* Accident, transport, by type
helpless person, infant, newborn X58 ☑
Landslide (falling on transport vehicle) X36.1 ☑
caused by collapse of man-made structure X36.Ø ☑
Late effect — *see* Sequelae

Legal
execution (any method) — *see* Legal, intervention
intervention (by)
baton — *see* Legal, intervention, blunt object, baton
bayonet — *see* Legal, intervention, sharp object, bayonet
blow — *see* Legal, intervention, manhandling
blunt object
baton
injuring
bystander Y35.312 ☑
law enforcement personnel Y35.311 ☑
suspect Y35.313 ☑
injuring
bystander Y35.3Ø2 ☑
law enforcement personnel Y35.3Ø1 ☑
suspect Y35.3Ø3 ☑
specified NEC
injuring
bystander Y35.392 ☑
law enforcement personnel Y35.391 ☑
suspect Y35.393 ☑
stave
injuring
bystander Y35.392 ☑
law enforcement personnel Y35.391 ☑
suspect Y35.393 ☑
bomb — *see* Legal, intervention, explosive
cutting or piercing instrument — *see* Legal, intervention, sharp object
dynamite — *see* Legal, intervention, explosive, dynamite
explosive(s)
dynamite
injuring
bystander Y35.112 ☑
law enforcement personnel Y35.111 ☑
suspect Y35.113 ☑
grenade
injuring
bystander Y35.192 ☑
law enforcement personnel Y35.191 ☑
suspect Y35.193 ☑
injuring
bystander Y35.1Ø2 ☑
law enforcement personnel Y35.1Ø1 ☑
suspect Y35.1Ø3 ☑
mortar bomb
injuring
bystander Y35.192 ☑
law enforcement personnel Y35.191 ☑
suspect Y35.193 ☑
shell
injuring
bystander Y35.122 ☑
law enforcement personnel Y35.121 ☑
suspect Y35.123 ☑
specified NEC
injuring
bystander Y35.192 ☑
law enforcement personnel Y35.191 ☑
suspect Y35.193 ☑
firearm(s) (discharge)
handgun
injuring
bystander Y35.Ø22 ☑
law enforcement personnel Y35.Ø21 ☑
suspect Y35.Ø23 ☑
injuring
bystander Y35.ØØ2 ☑
law enforcement personnel Y35.ØØ1 ☑
suspect Y35.ØØ3 ☑
machine gun
injuring
bystander Y35.Ø12 ☑
law enforcement personnel Y35.Ø11 ☑
suspect Y35.Ø13 ☑
rifle pellet
injuring
bystander Y35.Ø32 ☑
law enforcement personnel Y35.Ø31 ☑
suspect Y35.Ø33 ☑
rubber bullet
injuring
bystander Y35.Ø42 ☑
law enforcement personnel Y35.Ø41 ☑

- **Legal** — *continued*
  - intervention — *continued*
    - firearm(s) — *continued*
      - rubber bullet — *continued*
        - injuring — *continued*
          - suspect Y35.Ø43 ☑
      - shotgun — *see* Legal, intervention, firearm, specified NEC
      - specified NEC
        - injuring
          - bystander Y35.Ø92 ☑
          - law enforcement personnel Y35.Ø91 ☑
          - suspect Y35.Ø93 ☑
    - gas (asphyxiation) (poisoning)
      - injuring
        - bystander Y35.2Ø2 ☑
        - law enforcement personnel Y35.2Ø1 ☑
        - suspect Y35.2Ø3 ☑
      - specified NEC
        - injuring
          - bystander Y35.292 ☑
          - law enforcement personnel Y35.291 ☑
          - suspect Y35.293 ☑
      - tear gas
        - injuring
          - bystander Y35.212 ☑
          - law enforcement personnel Y35.211 ☑
          - suspect Y35.213 ☑
    - grenade — *see* Legal, intervention, explosive, grenade
    - injuring
      - bystander Y35.92 ☑
      - law enforcement personnel Y35.91 ☑
      - suspect Y35.93 ☑
    - late effect (of) — *see* with 7th character S Y35 ☑
    - manhandling
      - injuring
        - bystander Y35.812 ☑
        - law enforcement personnel Y35.811 ☑
        - suspect Y35.813 ☑
    - sequelae (of) — *see* with 7th character S Y35 ☑
    - sharp objects
      - bayonet
        - injuring
          - bystander Y35.412 ☑
          - law enforcement personnel Y35.411 ☑
          - suspect Y35.413 ☑
      - injuring
        - bystander Y35.4Ø2 ☑
        - law enforcement personnel Y35.4Ø1 ☑
        - suspect Y35.4Ø3 ☑
      - specified NEC
        - injuring
          - bystander Y35.492 ☑
          - law enforcement personnel Y35.491 ☑
          - suspect Y35.493 ☑
    - specified means NEC
      - injuring
        - bystander Y35.892 ☑
        - law enforcement personnel Y35.891 ☑
        - suspect Y35.893 ☑
    - stabbing — *see* Legal, intervention, sharp object
    - stave — *see* Legal, intervention, blunt object, stave
    - tear gas — *see* Legal, intervention, gas, tear gas
    - truncheon — *see* Legal, intervention, blunt object, stave
- **Lightning** (shock) (stroke) (struck by) — *see* subcategory T75.Ø ☑
  - causing fire — *see* Exposure, fire
- **Loss of control** (transport vehicle) NEC — *see* Accident, transport
- **Lost at sea NOS** — *see* Drowning, due to, fall overboard
- **Low**
  - pressure (effects) — *see* Air, pressure, low
  - temperature (effects) — *see* Exposure, cold
- **Lying before train, vehicle or other moving object** X81.8 ☑
  - subway train X81.1 ☑
  - train X81.1 ☑
  - undetermined whether accidental or intentional Y31 ☑
- **Lynching** — *see* Assault

M

- **Malfunction** (mechanism or component) (of)
- **Malfunction** — *continued*
  - firearm W34.1Ø ☑
    - airgun W34.11Ø ☑
    - BB gun W34.11Ø ☑
    - gas, air or spring-operated gun NEC W34.118 ☑
    - handgun W32.1 ☑
    - hunting rifle W33.12 ☑
    - larger firearm W33.1Ø ☑
      - specified NEC W33.19 ☑
    - machine gun W33.13 ☑
    - paintball gun W34.111 ☑
    - pellet gun W34.11Ø ☑
    - shotgun W33.11 ☑
    - specified NEC W34.19 ☑
    - Very pistol [flare] W34.19 ☑
  - handgun — *see* Malfunction, firearm, handgun
- **Maltreatment** — *see* Perpetrator
- **Mangled** (accidentally) NOS X58 ☑
- **Manhandling** (in brawl, fight) YØ4.Ø ☑
  - legal intervention — *see* Legal, intervention, manhandling
- **Manslaughter** (nonaccidental) — *see* Assault
- **Mauled by animal NEC** W55.89 ☑
- **Medical procedure, complication of** (delayed or as an abnormal reaction without mention of misadventure) — *see* Complication of or following, by specified type of procedure
  - due to or as a result of misadventure — *see* Misadventure
- **Melting** (due to fire) (*see also* Exposure, fire)
  - apparel NEC XØ6.3 ☑
  - clothes, clothing NEC XØ6.3 ☑
    - nightwear XØ5 ☑
  - fittings or furniture (burning building) (uncontrolled fire) XØØ.8 ☑
  - nightwear XØ5 ☑
  - plastic jewelry XØ6.1 ☑
- **Mental cruelty** X58 ☑
- **Military operations** (injuries to military and civilians occuring during peacetime on military property and during routine military exercises and operations) (by) (from) (involving) Y37.9Ø- ☑
  - air blast Y37.2Ø- ☑
  - aircraft
    - destruction — *see* Military operations, destruction of aircraft
  - airway restriction — *see* Military operations, restriction of airways
  - asphyxiation — *see* Military operations, restriction of airways
  - biological weapons Y37.6X- ☑
  - blast Y37.2Ø- ☑
  - blast fragments Y37.2Ø- ☑
  - blast wave Y37.2Ø- ☑
  - blast wind Y37.2Ø- ☑
  - bomb Y37.2Ø- ☑
    - dirty Y37.5Ø- ☑
    - gasoline Y37.31- ☑
    - incendiary Y37.31- ☑
    - petrol Y37.31- ☑
  - bullet Y37.43- ☑
    - incendiary Y37.32- ☑
    - rubber Y37.41- ☑
  - chemical weapons Y37.7X- ☑
  - combat
    - hand to hand (unarmed) combat Y37.44- ☑
    - using blunt or piercing object Y37.45- ☑
  - conflagration — *see* Military operations, fire
  - conventional warfare NEC Y37.49- ☑
  - depth-charge Y37.Ø1- ☑
  - destruction of aircraft Y37.1Ø- ☑
    - due to
      - air to air missile Y37.11- ☑
      - collision with other aircraft Y37.12- ☑
      - detonation (accidental) of onboard munitions and explosives Y37.14- ☑
      - enemy fire or explosives Y37.11- ☑
      - explosive placed on aircraft Y37.11- ☑
      - onboard fire Y37.13- ☑
      - rocket propelled grenade [RPG] Y37.11- ☑
      - small arms fire Y37.11- ☑
      - surface to air missile Y37.11- ☑
    - specified NEC Y37.19- ☑
  - detonation (accidental) of
    - onboard marine weapons Y37.Ø5- ☑
- **Military operations** — *continued*
  - detonation of — *continued*
    - own munitions or munitions launch device Y37.24- ☑
  - dirty bomb Y37.5Ø- ☑
  - explosion (of) Y37.2Ø- ☑
    - aerial bomb Y37.21- ☑
    - bomb NOS (*see also* Military operations, bomb(s)) Y37.2Ø- ☑
    - fragments Y37.2Ø- ☑
    - grenade Y37.29- ☑
    - guided missile Y37.22- ☑
    - improvised explosive device [IED] (person-borne) (roadside) (vehicle-borne) Y37.23- ☑
    - land mine Y37.29- ☑
    - marine mine (at sea) (in harbor) Y37.Ø2- ☑
    - marine weapon Y37.ØØ- ☑
      - specified NEC Y37.Ø9- ☑
    - own munitions or munitions launch device (accidental) Y37.24- ☑
    - sea-based artillery shell Y37.Ø3- ☑
    - specified NEC Y37.29- ☑
    - torpedo Y37.Ø4- ☑
  - fire Y37.3Ø- ☑
    - specified NEC Y37.39- ☑
  - firearms
    - discharge Y37.43- ☑
    - pellets Y37.42- ☑
  - flamethrower Y37.33- ☑
  - fragments (from) (of)
    - improvised explosive device [IED] (person-borne) (roadside) (vehicle-borne) Y37.26- ☑
    - munitions Y37.25- ☑
    - specified NEC Y37.29- ☑
    - weapons Y37.27- ☑
  - friendly fire Y37.92- ☑
  - hand to hand (unarmed) combat Y37.44- ☑
  - hot substances — *see* Military operations, fire
  - incendiary bullet Y37.32- ☑
  - nuclear weapon (effects of) Y37.5Ø- ☑
    - acute radiation exposure Y37.54- ☑
    - blast pressure Y37.51- ☑
    - direct blast Y37.51- ☑
    - direct heat Y37.53- ☑
    - fallout exposure Y37.54- ☑
    - fireball Y37.53- ☑
    - indirect blast (struck or crushed by blast debris) (being thrown by blast) Y37.52- ☑
    - ionizing radiation (immediate exposure) Y37.54- ☑
    - nuclear radiation Y37.54- ☑
    - radiation
      - ionizing (immediate exposure) Y37.54- ☑
      - nuclear Y37.54- ☑
      - thermal Y37.53- ☑
    - secondary effects Y37.54- ☑
    - specified NEC Y37.59- ☑
    - thermal radiation Y37.53- ☑
  - restriction of air (airway)
    - intentional Y37.46- ☑
    - unintentional Y37.47- ☑
  - rubber bullets Y37.41- ☑
  - shrapnel NOS Y37.29- ☑
  - suffocation — *see* Military operations, restriction of airways
  - unconventional warfare NEC Y37.7X- ☑
  - underwater blast NOS Y37.ØØ- ☑
  - warfare
    - conventional NEC Y37.49- ☑
    - unconventional NEC Y37.7X- ☑
  - weapon of mass destruction [WMD] Y37.91- ☑
  - weapons
    - biological weapons Y37.6X- ☑
    - chemical Y37.7X- ☑
    - nuclear (effects of) Y37.5Ø- ☑
      - acute radiation exposure Y37.54- ☑
      - blast pressure Y37.51- ☑
      - direct blast Y37.51- ☑
      - direct heat Y37.53- ☑
      - fallout exposure Y37.54- ☑
      - fireball Y37.53- ☑
      - indirect blast (struck or crushed by blast debris) (being thrown by blast) Y37.52- ☑
      - radiation
        - ionizing (immediate exposure) Y37.54- ☑
        - nuclear Y37.54- ☑
        - thermal Y37.53- ☑

- **Military operations** — *continued*
  - weapons — *continued*
    - nuclear — *continued*
      - secondary effects Y37.54- ☑
      - specified NEC Y37.59- ☑
    - of mass destruction [WMD] Y37.91- ☑
- **Misadventure**(s) **to patient**(s) **during surgical or medical care** Y69
  - contaminated medical or biological substance (blood, drug, fluid) Y64.9
    - administered (by) NEC Y64.9
      - immunization Y64.1
      - infusion Y64.Ø
      - injection Y64.1
      - specified means NEC Y64.8
      - transfusion Y64.Ø
      - vaccination Y64.1
  - excessive amount of blood or other fluid during transfusion or infusion Y63.Ø
  - failure
    - in dosage Y63.9
      - electroshock therapy Y63.4
      - inappropriate temperature (too hot or too cold) in local application and packing Y63.5
      - infusion
        - excessive amount of fluid Y63.Ø
        - incorrect dilution of fluid Y63.1
      - insulin-shock therapy Y63.4
      - nonadministration of necessary drug or biological substance Y63.6
      - overdose — *see* Table of Drugs and Chemicals
        - radiation, in therapy Y63.2
      - radiation
        - overdose Y63.2
      - specified procedure NEC Y63.8
      - transfusion
        - excessive amount of blood Y63.Ø
    - mechanical, of instrument or apparatus (any) (during any procedure) Y65.8
    - sterile precautions (during procedure) Y62.9
      - aspiration of fluid or tissue (by puncture or catheterization, except heart) Y62.6
      - biopsy (except needle aspiration) Y62.8
        - needle (aspirating) Y62.6
      - blood sampling Y62.6
      - catheterization Y62.6
        - heart Y62.5
      - dialysis (kidney) Y62.2
      - endoscopic examination Y62.4
      - enema Y62.8
      - immunization Y62.3
      - infusion Y62.1
      - injection Y62.3
      - needle biopsy Y62.6
      - paracentesis (abdominal) (thoracic) Y62.6
      - perfusion Y62.2
      - puncture (lumbar) Y62.6
      - removal of catheter or packing Y62.8
      - specified procedure NEC Y62.8
      - surgical operation Y62.Ø
      - transfusion Y62.1
      - vaccination Y62.3
    - suture or ligature during surgical procedure Y65.2
    - to introduce or to remove tube or instrument B — *see* Failure, to
  - hemorrhage — *see* Index to Diseases and Injuries, Complication(s)
  - inadvertent exposure of patient to radiation Y63.3
  - inappropriate
    - operation performed — *see* Inappropriate operation performed
    - temperature (too hot or too cold) in local application or packing Y63.5
  - infusion (*see also* Misadventure, by type, infusion) Y69
    - excessive amount of fluid Y63.Ø
    - incorrect dilution of fluid Y63.1
    - wrong fluid Y65.1
  - mismatched blood in transfusion Y65.Ø
  - nonadministration of necessary drug or biological substance
  - overdose — *see* Table of Drugs and Chemicals
    - radiation (in therapy) Y63.2
  - perforation — *see* Index to Diseases and Injuries, Complication(s)
  - performance of inappropriate operation — *see* Inappropriate operation performed
  - puncture — *see* Index to Diseases and Injuries, Complication(s)
  - specified type NEC Y65.8
    - failure
      - suture or ligature during surgical operation Y65.2
      - to introduce or to remove tube or instrument B — *see* Failure, to
    - infusion of wrong fluid Y65.1
    - performance of inappropriate operation — *see* Inappropriate operation performed
    - transfusion of mismatched blood Y65.Ø
    - wrong
      - fluid in infusion Y65.1
      - placement of endotracheal tube during anesthetic procedure Y65.3
  - transfusion — *see* Misadventure, by type, transfusion
    - excessive amount of blood Y63.Ø
    - mismatched blood Y65.Ø
  - wrong
    - drug given in error — *see* Table of Drugs and Chemicals
    - fluid in infusion Y65.1
    - placement of endotracheal tube during anesthetic procedure Y65.3
- **Mismatched blood in transfusion** Y65.Ø
- **Motion sickness** T75.3 ☑
- **Mountain sickness** W94.11 ☑
- **Mudslide** (of cataclysmic nature) — *see* Landslide
- **Murder** (attempt) — *see* Assault

N

- **Nail, contact with** W45.Ø ☑
  - gun W29.4 ☑
- **Neglect** (criminal) (homicidal intent) X58 ☑
- **Noise** (causing injury) (pollution) W42.9 ☑
  - supersonic W42.Ø ☑
- **Nonadministration** (of)
  - drug or biological substance (necessary) Y63.6
  - surgical and medical care Y66
- **Nosocomial condition** Y95

O

- **Object**
  - falling
    - from, in, on, hitting
      - machinery — *see* Contact, with, by type of machine
  - set in motion by
    - accidental explosion or rupture of pressure vessel W38 ☑
    - firearm — *see* Discharge, firearm, by type
    - machine(ry) — *see* Contact, with, by type of machine
- **Overdose** (drug) — *see* Table of Drugs and Chemicals
  - radiation Y63.2
- **Overexertion** — *see* category Y93 ☑
- **Overexposure** (accidental) (to)
  - cold (*see also* Exposure, cold) X31 ☑
    - due to man-made conditions — *see* Exposure, cold, man-made
  - heat (*see also* Heat) X3Ø ☑
  - radiation — *see* Radiation
  - radioactivity W88.Ø ☑
  - sun (sunburn) X32 ☑
  - weather NEC — *see* Forces of nature
  - wind NEC — *see* Forces of nature
- **Overheated** — *see* Heat
- **Overturning** (accidental)
  - machinery — *see* Contact, with, by type of machine
  - transport vehicle NEC (*see also* Accident, transport) V89.9 ☑
  - watercraft (causing drowning, submersion) (*see also* Drowning, due to, accident to, watercraft, overturning)
    - causing injury except drowning or submersion B — *see* Accident, watercraft, causing, injury NEC

P

- **Parachute descent** (voluntary) (without accident to aircraft) V97.29 ☑
  - due to accident to aircraft — *see* Accident, transport, aircraft
- **Pecked by bird** W61.99 ☑
- **Perforation during medical or surgical treatment as misadventure** — *see* Index to Diseases and Injuries, Complication(s)
- **Perpetrator, perpetration, of assault, maltreatment and neglect** (by) YØ7.9
  - boyfriend YØ7.Ø3
  - brother YØ7.41Ø
    - stepbrother YØ7.435
  - coach YØ7.53
  - cousin
    - female YØ7.491
    - male YØ7.49Ø
  - daycare provider YØ7.519
    - at-home
      - adult care YØ7.512
      - childcare YØ7.51Ø
    - care center
      - adult care YØ7.513
      - childcare YØ7.511
  - family member NEC YØ7.499
  - father YØ7.11
    - adoptive YØ7.13
    - foster YØ7.42Ø
    - stepfather YØ7.43Ø
  - foster father YØ7.42Ø
  - foster mother YØ7.421
  - girl friend YØ7.Ø4
  - healthcare provider YØ7.529
    - mental health YØ7.521
    - specified NEC YØ7.528
  - husband YØ7.Ø1
  - instructor YØ7.53
  - mother YØ7.12
    - adoptive YØ7.14
    - foster YØ7.421
    - stepmother YØ7.433
  - nonfamily member YØ7.5Ø
    - specified NEC YØ7.59
  - nurse YØ7.528
  - occupational therapist YØ7.528
  - partner of parent
    - female YØ7.434
    - male YØ7.432
  - physical therapist YØ7.528
  - sister YØ7.411
  - speech therapist YØ7.528
  - stepbrother YØ7.435
  - stepfather YØ7.43Ø
  - stepmother YØ7.433
  - stepsister YØ7.436
  - teacher YØ7.53
  - wife YØ7.Ø2
- **Piercing** — *see* Contact, with, by type of object or machine
- **Pinched**
  - between objects (moving) (stationary and moving) W23.Ø ☑
    - stationary W23.1 ☑
- **Pinned under machine**(ry) — *see* Contact, with, by type of machine
- **Place of occurrence** Y92.9
  - abandoned house Y92.89
  - airplane Y92.813
  - airport Y92.52Ø
  - ambulatory health services establishment NEC Y92.538
  - ambulatory surgery center Y92.53Ø
  - amusement park Y92.831
  - apartment (co-op) — *see* Place of occurrence, residence, apartment
  - assembly hall Y92.29
  - bank Y92.51Ø
  - barn Y92.71
  - baseball field Y92.32Ø
  - basketball court Y92.31Ø
  - beach Y92.832
  - boarding house — *see* Place of occurrence, residence, boarding house
  - boat Y92.814
  - bowling alley Y92.39
  - bridge Y92.89
  - building under construction Y92.61
  - bus Y92.811
    - station Y92.521
  - cafe Y92.511

Place of occurrence — *continued*
- campsite Y92.833
- campus — *see* Place of occurrence, school
- canal Y92.89
- car Y92.810
- casino Y92.59
- children's home — *see* Place of occurrence, residence, institutional, orphanage
- church Y92.22
- cinema Y92.26
- clubhouse Y92.29
- coal pit Y92.64
- college (community) Y92.214
- condominium — *see* Place of occurrence, residence, apartment
- construction area — *see* Place of occurrence, industrial and construction area
- convalescent home — *see* Place of occurrence, residence, institutional, nursing home
- court-house Y92.240
- cricket ground Y92.328
- cultural building Y92.258
  - art gallery Y92.250
  - museum Y92.251
  - music hall Y92.252
  - opera house Y92.253
  - specified NEC Y92.258
  - theater Y92.254
- dancehall Y92.252
- day nursery Y92.210
- dentist office Y92.531
- derelict house Y92.89
- desert Y92.820
- dockyard Y92.62
- dock NOS Y92.89
- doctor's office Y92.531
- dormitory — *see* Place of occurrence, residence, institutional, school dormitory
- dry dock Y92.62
- factory (building) (premises) Y92.63
- farm (land under cultivation) (outbuildings) Y92.79
  - barn Y92.71
  - chicken coop Y92.72
  - field Y92.73
  - hen house Y92.72
  - house — *see* Place of occurrence, residence, house
  - orchard Y92.74
  - specified NEC Y92.79
- football field Y92.321
- forest Y92.821
- freeway Y92.411
- gallery Y92.250
- garage (commercial) Y92.59
  - boarding house Y92.044
  - military base Y92.135
  - mobile home Y92.025
  - nursing home Y92.124
  - orphanage Y92.114
  - private house Y92.015
  - reform school Y92.155
- gas station Y92.524
- gasworks Y92.69
- golf course Y92.39
- gravel pit Y92.64
- grocery Y92.512
- gymnasium Y92.39
- handball court Y92.318
- harbor Y92.89
- harness racing course Y92.39
- healthcare provider office Y92.531
- highway (interstate) Y92.411
- hill Y92.828
- hockey rink Y92.330
- home — *see* Place of occurrence, residence
- hospice — *see* Place of occurrence, residence, institutional, nursing home
- hospital Y92.239
  - cafeteria Y92.233
  - corridor Y92.232
  - operating room Y92.234
  - patient
    - bathroom Y92.231
    - room Y92.230
  - specified NEC Y92.238
- hotel Y92.59
- house (*see also* Place of occurrence, residence)
  - abandoned Y92.89
  - under construction Y92.61

Place of occurrence — *continued*
- industrial and construction area (yard) Y92.69
  - building under construction Y92.61
  - dock Y92.62
  - dry dock Y92.62
  - factory Y92.63
  - gasworks Y92.69
  - mine Y92.64
  - oil rig Y92.65
  - pit Y92.64
  - power station Y92.69
  - shipyard Y92.62
  - specified NEC Y92.69
  - tunnel under construction Y92.69
  - workshop Y92.69
- kindergarten Y92.211
- lacrosse field Y92.328
- lake Y92.828
- library Y92.241
- mall Y92.59
- market Y92.512
- marsh Y92.828
- military
  - base — *see* Place of occurrence, residence, institutional, military base
  - training ground Y92.84
- mine Y92.64
- mosque Y92.22
- motel Y92.59
- motorway (interstate) Y92.411
- mountain Y92.828
- movie-house Y92.26
- museum Y92.251
- music-hall Y92.252
- not applicable Y92.9
- nuclear power station Y92.69
- nursing home — *see* Place of occurrence, residence, institutional, nursing home
- office building Y92.59
- offshore installation Y92.65
- oil rig Y92.65
- old people's home — *see* Place of occurrence, residence, institutional, specified NEC
- opera-house Y92.253
- orphanage — *see* Place of occurrence, residence, institutional, orphanage
- outpatient surgery center Y92.530
- park (public) Y92.830
  - amusement Y92.831
- parking garage Y92.89
  - lot Y92.481
- pavement Y92.480
- physician office Y92.531
- polo field Y92.328
- pond Y92.828
- post office Y92.242
- power station Y92.69
- prairie Y92.828
- prison — *see* Place of occurrence, residence, institutional, prison
- public
  - administration building Y92.248
    - city hall Y92.243
    - courthouse Y92.240
    - library Y92.241
    - post office Y92.242
    - specified NEC Y92.248
  - building NEC Y92.29
  - hall Y92.29
  - place NOS Y92.89
- race course Y92.39
- radio station Y92.59
- railway line (bridge) Y92.85
- ranch (outbuildings) — *see* Place of occurrence, farm
- recreation area Y92.838
  - amusement park Y92.831
  - beach Y92.832
  - campsite Y92.833
  - park (public) Y92.830
  - seashore Y92.832
  - specified NEC Y92.838
- reform school - — *see* Place of occurrence, residence, institutional, reform school
- religious institution Y92.22
- residence (non-institutional) (private) Y92.009
  - apartment Y92.039
    - bathroom Y92.031
    - bedroom Y92.032

Place of occurrence — *continued*
- residence — *continued*
  - apartment — *continued*
    - kitchen Y92.030
    - specified NEC Y92.038
  - bathroom Y92.002
  - bedroom Y92.003
  - boarding house Y92.049
    - bathroom Y92.041
    - bedroom Y92.042
    - driveway Y92.043
    - garage Y92.044
    - garden Y92.046
    - kitchen Y92.040
    - specified NEC Y92.048
    - swimming pool Y92.045
    - yard Y92.046
  - dining room Y92.001
  - garden Y92.007
  - home Y92.009
  - house, single family Y92.019
    - bathroom Y92.012
    - bedroom Y92.013
    - dining room Y92.011
    - driveway Y92.014
    - garage Y92.015
    - garden Y92.017
    - kitchen Y92.010
    - specified NEC Y92.018
    - swimming pool Y92.016
    - yard Y92.017
  - institutional Y92.10
    - children's home — *see* Place of occurrence, residence, institutional, orphanage
    - hospice — *see* Place of occurrence, residence, institutional, nursing home
    - military base Y92.139
      - barracks Y92.133
      - garage Y92.135
      - garden Y92.137
      - kitchen Y92.130
      - mess hall Y92.131
      - specified NEC Y92.138
      - swimming pool Y92.136
      - yard Y92.137
    - nursing home Y92.129
      - bathroom Y92.121
      - bedroom Y92.122
      - driveway Y92.123
      - garage Y92.124
      - garden Y92.126
      - kitchen Y92.120
      - specified NEC Y92.128
      - swimming pool Y92.125
      - yard Y92.126
    - orphanage Y92.119
      - bathroom Y92.111
      - bedroom Y92.112
      - driveway Y92.113
      - garage Y92.114
      - garden Y92.116
      - kitchen Y92.110
      - specified NEC Y92.118
      - swimming pool Y92.115
      - yard Y92.116
    - prison Y92.149
      - bathroom Y92.142
      - cell Y92.143
      - courtyard Y92.147
      - dining room Y92.141
      - kitchen Y92.140
      - specified NEC Y92.148
      - swimming pool Y92.146
    - reform school Y92.159
      - bathroom Y92.152
      - bedroom Y92.153
      - dining room Y92.151
      - driveway Y92.154
      - garage Y92.155
      - garden Y92.157
      - kitchen Y92.150
      - specified NEC Y92.158
      - swimming pool Y92.156
      - yard Y92.157
    - school dormitory Y92.169
      - bathroom Y92.162
      - bedroom Y92.163
      - dining room Y92.161

- **Place of occurrence** — *continued*
  - residence — *continued*
    - institutional — *continued*
      - school dormitory — *continued*
        - kitchen Y92.160
        - specified NEC Y92.168
      - specified NEC Y92.199
        - bathroom Y92.192
        - bedroom Y92.193
        - dining room Y92.191
        - driveway Y92.194
        - garage Y92.195
        - garden Y92.197
        - kitchen Y92.190
        - specified NEC Y92.198
        - swimming pool Y92.196
        - yard Y92.197
    - kitchen Y92.000
    - mobile home Y92.029
      - bathroom Y92.022
      - bedroom Y92.023
      - dining room Y92.021
      - driveway Y92.024
      - garage Y92.025
      - garden Y92.027
      - kitchen Y92.020
      - specified NEC Y92.028
      - swimming pool Y92.026
      - yard Y92.027
    - specified place in residence NEC Y92.009
    - specified residence type NEC Y92.099
      - bathroom Y92.091
      - bedroom Y92.092
      - driveway Y92.093
      - garage Y92.094
      - garden Y92.096
      - kitchen Y92.090
      - specified NEC Y92.098
      - swimming pool Y92.095
      - yard Y92.096
  - restaurant Y92.511
  - riding school Y92.39
  - river Y92.828
  - road Y92.488
  - rodeo ring Y92.39
  - rugby field Y92.328
  - same day surgery center Y92.530
  - sand pit Y92.64
  - school (private) (public) (state) Y92.219
    - college Y92.214
    - daycare center Y92.210
    - elementary school Y92.211
    - high school Y92.213
    - kindergarten Y92.211
    - middle school Y92.212
    - specified NEC Y92.218
    - trace school Y92.215
    - university Y92.214
    - vocational school Y92.215
  - sea (shore) Y92.832
  - senior citizen center Y92.29
  - service area
    - airport Y92.520
    - bus station Y92.521
    - gas station Y92.524
    - highway rest stop Y92.523
    - railway station Y92.522
  - shipyard Y92.62
  - shop (commercial) Y92.513
  - sidewalk Y92.480
  - silo Y92.79
  - skating rink (roller) Y92.331
    - ice Y92.330
  - slaughter house Y92.86
  - soccer field Y92.322
  - specified place NEC Y92.89
  - sports area Y92.39
    - athletic
      - court Y92.318
        - basketball Y92.310
        - specified NEC Y92.318
        - squash Y92.311
        - tennis Y92.312
      - field Y92.328
        - baseball Y92.320
        - cricket ground Y92.328
        - football Y92.321
        - hockey Y92.328

- **Place of occurrence** — *continued*
  - sports area — *continued*
    - athletic — *continued*
      - field — *continued*
        - soccer Y92.322
        - specified NEC Y92.328
    - golf course Y92.39
    - gymnasium Y92.39
    - riding school Y92.39
    - skating rink (roller) Y92.331
      - ice Y92.330
    - stadium Y92.39
    - swimming pool Y92.34
  - squash court Y92.311
  - stadium Y92.39
  - steeplechasing course Y92.39
  - store Y92.512
  - stream Y92.828
  - street and highway Y92.410
    - bike path Y92.482
    - freeway Y92.411
    - highway ramp Y92.415
    - interstate highway Y92.411
    - local residential or business street Y92.414
    - motorway Y92.411
    - parking lot Y92.481
    - parkway Y92.412
    - sidewalk Y92.480
    - specified NEC Y92.488
    - state road Y92.413
  - subway car Y92.816
  - supermarket Y92.512
  - swamp Y92.828
  - swimming pool (public) Y92.34
    - private (at) Y92.095
      - boarding house Y92.045
      - military base Y92.136
      - mobile home Y92.026
      - nursing home Y92.125
      - orphanage Y92.115
      - prison Y92.146
      - reform school Y92.156
      - single family residence Y92.016
  - synagogue Y92.22
  - television station Y92.59
  - tennis court Y92.312
  - theater Y92.254
  - trade area Y92.59
    - bank Y92.510
    - cafe Y92.511
    - casino Y92.59
    - garage Y92.59
    - hotel Y92.59
    - market Y92.512
    - office building Y92.59
    - radio station Y92.59
    - restaurant Y92.511
    - shop Y92.513
    - shopping mall Y92.59
    - store Y92.512
    - supermarket Y92.512
    - television station Y92.59
    - warehouse Y92.59
  - trailer park, residential — *see* Place of occurrence, residence, mobile home
  - trailer site NOS Y92.89
  - train Y92.815
    - station Y92.522
  - truck Y92.812
  - tunnel under construction Y92.69
  - university Y92.214
  - urgent (health) care center Y92.532
  - vehicle (transport) Y92.818
    - airplane Y92.813
    - boat Y92.814
    - bus Y92.811
    - car Y92.810
    - specified NEC Y92.818
    - subway car Y92.816
    - train Y92.815
    - truck Y92.812
  - warehouse Y92.59
  - water reservoir Y92.89
  - wilderness area Y92.828
    - desert Y92.820
    - forest Y92.821
    - marsh Y92.828
    - mountain Y92.828

- **Place of occurrence** — *continued*
  - wilderness area — *continued*
    - prairie Y92.828
    - specified NEC Y92.828
    - swamp Y92.828
  - workshop Y92.69
  - yard, private Y92.096
    - boarding house Y92.046
    - mobile home Y92.027
    - single family house Y92.017
  - youth center Y92.29
  - zoo (zoological garden) Y92.834
- **Plumbism** — *see* Table of Drugs and Chemicals, lead
- **Poisoning** (accidental) (by) (*see also* Table of Drugs and Chemicals)
  - by plant, thorns, spines, sharp leaves or other mechanisms NEC X58 ☑
  - carbon monoxide
    - generated by
      - motor vehicle — *see* Accident, transport
      - watercraft (in transit) (not in transit) V93.89 ☑
        - ferry boat V93.81 ☑
        - fishing boat V93.82 ☑
        - jet skis V93.83 ☑
        - liner V93.81 ☑
        - merchant ship V93.80 ☑
        - passenger ship V93.81 ☑
        - powered craft NEC V93.83 ☑
  - caused by injection of poisons into skin by plant thorns, spines, sharp leaves X58 ☑
    - marine or sea plants (venomous) X58 ☑
  - execution — *see* Legal, intervention, gas
    - intervention
      - by gas — *see* Legal, intervention, gas
      - other specified means — *see* Legal, intervention, specified means NEC
  - exhaust gas
    - generated by
      - motor vehicle — *see* Accident, transport
      - watercraft (in transit) (not in transit) V93.89 ☑
        - ferry boat V93.81 ☑
        - fishing boat V93.82 ☑
        - jet skis V93.83 ☑
        - liner V93.81 ☑
        - merchant ship V93.80 ☑
        - passenger ship V93.81 ☑
        - powered craft NEC V93.83 ☑
  - fumes or smoke due to
    - explosion (*see also* Explosion) W40.9 ☑
    - fire — *see* Exposure, fire
    - ignition — *see* Ignition
  - gas
    - in legal intervention — *see* Legal, intervention, gas
    - legal execution — *see* Legal, intervention, gas
  - in war operations — *see* War operations
  - legal
- **Powder burn** (by) (from)
  - airgun W34.110 ☑
  - BB gun W34.110 ☑
  - firearn NEC W34.19 ☑
  - gas, air or spring-operated gun NEC W34.118 ☑
  - handgun W32.1 ☑
  - hunting rifle W33.12 ☑
  - larger firearm W33.10 ☑
    - specified NEC W33.19 ☑
  - machine gun W33.13 ☑
  - paintball gun W34.111 ☑
  - pellet gun W34.110 ☑
  - shotgun W33.11 ☑
  - Very pistol [flare] W34.19 ☑
- **Premature cessation** (of) **surgical and medical care** Y66
- **Privation** (food) (water) X58 ☑
- **Procedure** (operation)
  - correct, on wrong side or body part (wrong side) (wrong site) Y65.53
  - intended for another patient done on wrong patient Y65.52
  - performed on patient not scheduled for surgery Y65.52
  - performed on wrong patient Y65.52
  - wrong, performed on correct patient Y65.51
- **Prolonged**
  - sitting in transport vehicle — *see* Travel, by type of vehicle
  - stay in
    - high altitude as cause of anoxia, barodontalgia, barotitis or hypoxia W94.11 ☑

Prolonged — *continued*
- stay in — *continued*
  - weightless environment X52 ☑

Pulling, excessive — *see* category Y93 ☑

Puncture, puncturing (*see also* Contact, with, by type of object or machine)
- by
  - plant thorns, spines, sharp leaves or other mechanisms NEC W6Ø ☑
- during medical or surgical treatment as misadventure — *see* Index to Diseases and Injuries, Complication(s)

Pushed, pushing (accidental) (injury in) (overexertion) *see* category Y93 ☑
- by other person(s) (accidental) W51 ☑
  - with fall WØ3 ☑
    - due to ice or snow WØØ.Ø ☑
  - as, or caused by, a crowd or human stampede (with fall) W52 ☑
  - before moving object NEC YØ2.8 ☑
    - motor vehicle YØ2.Ø ☑
    - subway train YØ2.1 ☑
    - train YØ2.1 ☑
  - from
    - high place NEC
      - in accidental circumstances W17.89 ☑
      - stated as
        - intentional, homicide (attempt) YØ1 ☑
        - undetermined whether accidental or intentional Y3Ø ☑
    - transport vehicle NEC (*see also* Accident, transport) V89.9 ☑
      - stated as
        - intentional, homicide (attempt) YØ8.89 ☑

R

Radiation (exposure to)
- arc lamps W89.Ø ☑
- atomic power plant (malfunction) NEC W88.1 ☑
- complication of or abnormal reaction to medical radiotherapy Y84.2
- electromagnetic, ionizing W88.Ø ☑
- gamma rays W88.1 ☑
- in
  - war operations (from or following nuclear explosion) — *see* War operations
- inadvertent exposure of patient (receiving test or therapy) Y63.3
- infrared (heaters and lamps) W9Ø.1 ☑
  - excessive heat from W92 ☑
- ionized, ionizing (particles, artificially accelerated)
  - radioisotopes W88.1 ☑
  - specified NEC W88.8 ☑
  - x-rays W88.Ø ☑
- isotopes, radioactive — *see* Radiation, radioactive isotopes
- laser(s) W9Ø.2 ☑
  - in war operations — *see* War operations
  - misadventure in medical care Y63.2
- light sources (man-made visible and ultraviolet) W89.9 ☑
  - natural X32 ☑
  - specified NEC W89.8 ☑
  - tanning bed W89.1 ☑
  - welding light W89.Ø ☑
- man-made visible light W89.9 ☑
  - specified NEC W89.8 ☑
  - tanning bed W89.1 ☑
  - welding light W89.Ø ☑
- microwave W9Ø.8 ☑
- misadventure in medical or surgical procedure Y63.2
- natural NEC X39.Ø8 ☑
  - radon X39.Ø1 ☑
- overdose (in medical or surgical procedure) Y63.2
- radar W9Ø.Ø ☑
- radioactive isotopes (any) W88.1 ☑
  - atomic power plant malfunction W88.1 ☑
  - misadventure in medical or surgical treatment Y63.2
- radiofrequency W9Ø.Ø ☑
- radium NEC W88.1 ☑
- sun X32 ☑
- ultraviolet (light) (man-made) W89.9 ☑
  - natural X32 ☑

Radiation — *continued*
- ultraviolet — *continued*
  - specified NEC W89.8 ☑
  - tanning bed W89.1 ☑
  - welding light W89.Ø ☑
- welding arc, torch, or light W89.Ø ☑
  - excessive heat from W92 ☑
- x-rays (hard) (soft) W88.Ø ☑

Range disease W94.11 ☑

Rape (attempted) T74.2- ☑

Rat bite W53.11 ☑

Reaction, abnormal to medical procedure (*see also* Complication of or following, by type of procedure) Y84.9
- with misadventure — *see* Misadventure
- biologicals — *see* Table of Drugs and Chemicals
- drugs — *see* Table of Drugs and Chemicals
- vaccine — *see* Table of Drugs and Chemicals

Recoil
- airgun W34.11Ø ☑
- BB gun W34.11Ø ☑
- firearn NEC W34.19 ☑
- gas, air or spring-operated gun NEC W34.118 ☑
- handgun W32.1 ☑
- hunting rifle W33.12 ☑
- larger firearm W33.1Ø ☑
  - specified NEC W33.19 ☑
- machine gun W33.13 ☑
- paintball gun W34.111 ☑
- pellet W34.11Ø ☑
- shotgun W33.11 ☑
- Very pistol [flare] W34.19 ☑

Reduction in
- atmospheric pressure — *see* Air, pressure, change

Rock falling on or hitting (accidentally) (person) W2Ø.8 ☑
- in cave-in W2Ø.Ø ☑

Run over (accidentally) (by)
- animal (not being ridden) NEC W55.89 ☑
- machinery — *see* Contact, with, by specified type of machine
- transport vehicle NEC (*see also* Accident, transport) VØ9.9 ☑
  - intentional homicide (attempt) YØ3.Ø ☑
  - motor NEC VØ9.2Ø ☑
    - intentional homicide (attempt) YØ3.Ø ☑

Running
- before moving object X81.8 ☑
  - motor vehicle X81.Ø ☑

Running off, away
- animal (being ridden) (*see also* Accident, transport) V8Ø.918 ☑
  - not being ridden W55.89 ☑
- animal-drawn vehicle NEC (*see also* Accident, transport) V8Ø.928 ☑
- highway, road(way), street
  - transport vehicle NEC (*see also* Accident, transport) V89.9 ☑

Rupture pressurized devices — *see* Explosion, by type of device

S

Saturnism — *see* Table of Drugs and Chemicals, lead

Scald, scalding (accidental) (by) (from) (in) X19 ☑
- air (hot) X14.1 ☑
- gases (hot) X14.1 ☑
- homicide (attempt) — *see* Assault, burning, hot object
- inflicted by other person
  - stated as intentional, homicide (attempt) — *see* Assault, burning, hot object
- liquid (boiling) (hot) NEC X12 ☑
  - stated as undetermined whether accidental or intentional Y27.2 ☑
  - suicide (attempt) X77.2 ☑
- local application of externally applied substance in medical or surgical care Y63.5
- metal (molten) (liquid) (hot) NEC X18 ☑
- self-inflicted X77.9 ☑
- stated as undetermined whether accidental or intentional Y27.8 ☑
- steam X13.1 ☑
  - assault X98.Ø ☑
  - stated as undetermined whether accidental or intentional Y27.Ø ☑
  - suicide (attempt) X77.Ø ☑

Scald, scalding — *continued*
- suicide (attempt) X77.9 ☑
- vapor (hot) X13.1 ☑
  - assault X98.Ø ☑
  - stated as undetermined whether accidental or intentional Y27.Ø ☑
  - suicide (attempt) X77.Ø ☑

Scratched by
- cat W55.Ø3 ☑
- person(s) (accidentally) W5Ø.4 ☑
  - with intent to injure or kill YØ4.Ø ☑
  - as, or caused by, a crowd or human stampede (with fall) W52 ☑
  - assault YØ4.Ø ☑
  - homicide (attempt) YØ4.Ø ☑
  - in
    - fight YØ4.Ø ☑
    - legal intervention
      - injuring
        - bystander Y35.892 ☑
        - law enforcement personnel Y35.891 ☑
        - suspect Y35.893 ☑

Seasickness T75.3 ☑

Self-harm NEC (*see also* External cause by type, undetermined whether accidental or intentional)
- intentional — *see* Suicide
- poisoning NEC — *see* Table of Drugs and Chemicals, poisoning, accidental

Self-inflicted (injury) **NEC** (*see also* External cause by type, undetermined whether accidental or intentional)
- intentional — *see* Suicide
- poisoning NEC — *see* Table of Drugs and Chemicals, poisoning, accidental

Sequelae (of)
- accident NEC — *see* WØØ-X58 with 7th character S
- assault (homicidal) (any means) — *see* X92-YØ8 with 7th character S
- homicide, attempt (any means) — *see* X92-YØ8 with 7th character S
- injury undetermined whether accidentally or purposely inflicted — *see* Y21-Y33 with 7th character S
- intentional self-harm (classifiable to X71-X83) — *see* X71-X83 with 7th character S
- legal intervention — *see* with 7th character S Y35 ☑
- motor vehicle accident — *see* VØØ-V99 with 7th character S
- suicide, attempt (any means) — *see* X71-X83 with 7th character S
- transport accident — *see* VØØ-V99 with 7th character S
- war operations — *see* War operations

Shock
- electric — *see* Exposure, electric current
- from electric appliance (any) (faulty) W86.8 ☑
  - domestic W86.Ø ☑
  - suicide (attempt) X83.1 ☑

Shooting, shot (accidental(ly)) (*see also* Discharge, firearm, by type)
- herself or himself — *see* Discharge, firearm by type, self-inflicted
- homicide (attempt) — *see* Discharge, firearm by type, homicide
- in war operations — *see* War operations
- inflicted by other person — *see* Discharge, firearm by type, homicide
  - accidental — *see* Discharge, firearm, by type of firearm
- legal
  - execution — *see* Legal, intervention, firearm
  - intervention — *see* Legal, intervention, firearm
- self-inflicted — *see* Discharge, firearm by type, suicide
  - accidental — *see* Discharge, firearm, by type of firearm
- suicide (attempt) — *see* Discharge, firearm by type, suicide

Shoving (accidentally) **by other person** — *see* Pushed, by other person

Sickness
- alpine W94.11 ☑
- motion — *see* Motion
- mountain W94.11 ☑

Sinking (accidental)
- watercraft (causing drowning, submersion) (*see also* Drowning, due to, accident to, watercraft, sinking)

Sinking — *continued*
- watercraft (*see also* Drowning, due to, accident to, watercraft, sinking) — *continued*
  - causing injury except drowning or submersion B — *see* Accident, watercraft, causing, injury NEC

Siriasis X32 ☑

Slashed wrists — *see* Cut, self-inflicted

Slipping (accidental) (on same level) (with fall) WØ1.Ø ☑
- without fall W18.4Ø ☑
  - due to
    - specified NEC W18.49 ☑
    - stepping from one level to another W18.43 ☑
    - stepping into hole or opening W18.42 ☑
    - stepping on object W18.41 ☑
- on
  - ice WØØ.Ø ☑
    - with skates — *see* Accident, transport, pedestrian, conveyance
  - mud WØ1.Ø ☑
  - oil WØ1.Ø ☑
  - snow WØØ.Ø ☑
    - with skis — *see* Accident, transport, pedestrian, conveyance
  - surface (slippery) (wet) NEC WØ1.Ø ☑

Sliver, wood, contact with W45.8 ☑

Smoldering (due to fire) — *see* Exposure, fire

Sodomy (attempted) **by force** T74.2 ☑

Sound waves (causing injury) W42.9 ☑
- supersonic W42.Ø ☑

Splinter, contact with W45.8 ☑

Stab, stabbing B — *see* Cut

Starvation X58 ☑

Status of external cause Y99.9
- child assisting in compensated work for family Y99.8
- civilian activity done for financial or other compensation Y99.Ø
- civilian activity done for income or pay Y99.Ø
- family member assisting in compensated work for other family member Y99.8
- hobby not done for income Y99.8
- leisure activity Y99.8
- military activity Y99.1
- off-duty activity of military personnel Y99.8
- recreation or sport not for income or while a student Y99.8
- specified NEC Y99.8
- student activity Y99.8
- volunteer activity Y99.2

Stepped on
- by
  - animal (not being ridden) NEC W55.89 ☑
  - crowd or human stampede W52 ☑
  - person W5Ø.Ø ☑

Stepping on
- object W22.8 ☑
  - with fall W18.31 ☑
  - sports equipment W21.9 ☑
  - stationary W22.Ø9 ☑
    - sports equipment W21.89 ☑
- person W51 ☑
  - by crowd or human stampede W52 ☑
- sports equipment W21.9 ☑

Sting
- arthropod, nonvenomous W57 ☑
- insect, nonvenomous W57 ☑

Storm (cataclysmic) — *see* Forces of nature, cataclysmic storm

Straining, excessive — *see* category Y93 ☑

Strangling — *see* Strangulation

Strangulation (accidental) T71 ☑

Strenuous movements — *see* category Y93 ☑

Striking against
- airbag (automobile) W22.1Ø ☑
  - driver side W22.11 ☑
  - front passenger side W22.12 ☑
  - specified NEC W22.19 ☑
- bottom when
  - diving or jumping into water (in) W16.822 ☑
    - causing drowning W16.821 ☑
    - from boat W16.722 ☑
      - causing drowning W16.721 ☑
    - natural body W16.622 ☑
      - causing drowning W16.821 ☑
    - swimming pool W16.522 ☑
      - causing drowning W16.521 ☑

Striking against — *continued*
- bottom when — *continued*
  - falling into water (in) W16.322 ☑
    - causing drowning W16.321 ☑
    - fountain — *see* Striking against, bottom when, falling into water, specified NEC
    - natural body W16.122 ☑
      - causing drowning W16.121 ☑
    - reservoir — *see* Striking against, bottom when, falling into water, specified NEC
    - specified NEC W16.322 ☑
      - causing drowning W16.321 ☑
    - swimming pool W16.Ø22 ☑
      - causing drowning W16.Ø21 ☑
- diving board (swimming-pool) W21.4 ☑
- object W22.8 ☑
  - with
    - drowning or submersion — *see* Drowning
    - fall — *see* Fall, due to, bumping against, object
  - caused by crowd or human stampede (with fall) W52 ☑
  - furniture W22.Ø3 ☑
  - lamppost W22.Ø2 ☑
  - sports equipment W21.9 ☑
  - stationary W22.Ø9 ☑
    - sports equipment W21.89 ☑
  - wall W22.Ø1 ☑
- person(s) W51 ☑
  - with fall WØ3 ☑
    - due to ice or snow WØØ.Ø ☑
  - as, or caused by, a crowd or human stampede (with fall) W52 ☑
  - assault YØ4.2 ☑
  - homicide (attempt) YØ4.2 ☑
- sports equipment W21.9 ☑
- wall (when) W22.Ø1 ☑
  - diving or jumping into water (in) W16.832 ☑
    - causing drowning W16.831 ☑
    - swimming pool W16.532 ☑
      - causing drowning W16.531 ☑
  - falling into water (in) W16.332 ☑
    - causing drowning W16.331 ☑
    - fountain — *see* Striking against, wall when, falling into water, specified NEC
    - natural body W16.132 ☑
      - causing drowning W16.131 ☑
    - reservoir — *see* Striking against, wall when, falling into water, specified NEC
    - specified NEC W16.332 ☑
      - causing drowning W16.331 ☑
    - swimming pool W16.Ø32 ☑
      - causing drowning W16.Ø31 ☑
  - swimming pool (when) W22.Ø42 ☑
    - causing drowning W22.Ø41 ☑
    - diving or jumping into water W16.532 ☑
      - causing drowning W16.531 ☑
    - falling into water W16.Ø32 ☑
      - causing drowning W16.Ø31 ☑

Struck (accidentally) **by**
- airbag (automobile) W22.1Ø ☑
  - driver side W22.11 ☑
  - front passenger side W22.12 ☑
  - specified NEC W22.19 ☑
- alligator W58.Ø2 ☑
- animal (not being ridden) NEC W55.89 ☑
- avalanche — *see* Landslide
- ball (hit) (thrown) W21.ØØ ☑
  - assault YØ8.Ø9 ☑
  - baseball W21.Ø3 ☑
  - basketball W21.Ø5 ☑
  - football W21.Ø1 ☑
  - golf ball W21.Ø4 ☑
  - soccer W21.Ø2 ☑
  - softball W21.Ø7 ☑
  - specified NEC W21.Ø9 ☑
  - volleyball W21.Ø6 ☑
- bat or racquet
  - baseball bat W21.11 ☑
    - assault YØ8.Ø2 ☑
  - golf club W21.13 ☑
    - assault YØ8.Ø9 ☑
  - specified NEC W21.19 ☑
    - assault YØ8.Ø9 ☑
  - tennis racquet W21.12 ☑
    - assault YØ8.Ø9 ☑
- bullet (*see also* Discharge, firearm by type)

Struck (accidentally) **by** — *continued*
- bullet (*see also* Discharge, firearm by type) — *continued*
  - in war operations — *see* War operations
- crocodile W58.12 ☑
- dog W54.1 ☑
- flare, Very pistol — *see* Discharge, firearm NEC
- hailstones X39.8 ☑
- hockey (ice)
  - field
    - puck W21.221 ☑
    - stick W21.211 ☑
  - puck W21.22Ø ☑
  - stick W21.21Ø ☑
    - assault YØ8.Ø1 ☑
- landslide — *see* Landslide
- law-enforcement agent (on duty) — *see* Legal, intervention, manhandling
  - with blunt object — *see* Legal, intervention, blunt object
- lightning T75.Ø ☑
  - causing fire — *see* Exposure, fire
- machine — *see* Contact, with, by type of machine
- mammal NEC W55.89 ☑
  - marine W56.32 ☑
- marine animal W56.82 ☑
- missile
  - firearm — *see* Discharge, firearm by type
  - in war operations — *see* War operations, missile
- object W22.8 ☑
  - blunt W22.8 ☑
    - assault YØØ ☑
    - suicide (attempt) X79 ☑
    - undetermined whether accidental or intentional Y29 ☑
  - falling W2Ø.8 ☑
    - from, in, on
      - building W2Ø.1 ☑
        - burning (uncontrolled fire) XØØ.4 ☑
      - cataclysmic
        - earth surface movement NEC — *see* Landslide
        - storm — *see* Forces of nature, cataclysmic storm
      - cave-in W2Ø.Ø ☑
      - earthquake X34 ☑
      - machine (in operation) — *see* Contact, with, by type of machine
      - structure W2Ø.1 ☑
        - burning XØØ.4 ☑
      - transport vehicle (in motion) — *see* Accident, transport, by type of vehicle
      - watercraft V93.49 ☑
        - due to
          - accident to craft V91.39 ☑
            - powered craft V91.33 ☑
              - ferry boat V91.31 ☑
              - fishing boat V91.32 ☑
              - jetskis V91.33 ☑
              - liner V91.31 ☑
              - merchant ship V91.3Ø ☑
              - passenger ship V91.31 ☑
            - unpowered craft V91.38 ☑
              - canoe V91.35 ☑
              - inflatable V91.36 ☑
              - kayak V91.35 ☑
              - sailboat V91.34 ☑
              - surf-board V91.38 ☑
              - windsurfer V91.38 ☑
        - powered craft V93.43 ☑
          - ferry boat V93.41 ☑
          - fishing boat V93.42 ☑
          - jetskis V93.43 ☑
          - liner V93.41 ☑
          - merchant ship V93.4Ø ☑
          - passenger ship V93.41 ☑
        - unpowered craft V93.48 ☑
          - sailboat V93.44 ☑
          - surf-board V93.48 ☑
          - windsurfer V93.48 ☑
  - moving NEC W2Ø.8 ☑
  - projected W2Ø.8 ☑
    - assault YØØ ☑
    - in sports W21.9 ☑
      - assault YØ8.Ø9 ☑
      - ball W21.ØØ ☑

T

Terrorism — *continued*
- fire Y38.3X- ☑
- firearms Y38.4X- ☑
- hot substances Y38.5X- ☑
- nuclear weapons Y38.5X- ☑
- specified method NEC Y38.89- ☑

Thirst X58 ☑

Threat to breathing
- aspiration — *see* Aspiration
- due to cave-in, falling earth or substance NEC T71 ☑

Thrown (accidentally)
- against part (any) of or object in transport vehicle (in motion) NEC (*see also* Accident, transport)
- from
  - high place, homicide (attempt) YØ1 ☑
  - machinery — *see* Contact, with, by type of machine
  - transport vehicle NEC (*see also* Accident, transport) V89.9 ☑
- off — *see* Thrown, from

Thunderbolt — *see* subcategory T75.Ø ☑
- causing fire — *see* Exposure, fire

Tidal wave (any injury) NEC — *see* Forces of nature, tidal wave

Took
- overdose (drug) — *see* Table of Drugs and Chemicals
- poison — *see* Table of Drugs and Chemicals

Tornado (any injury) X37.1 ☑

Torrential rain (any injury) X37.8 ☑

Torture X58 ☑

Trampled by animal NEC W55.89 ☑

Trapped (accidentally)
- between objects (moving) (stationary and moving) — *see* Caught
- by part (any) of
  - motorcycle V29.88 ☑
  - pedal cycle V19.88 ☑
  - transport vehicle NEC (*see also* Accident, transport) V89.9 ☑

Travel (effects) (sickness) T75.3 ☑

Tree falling on or hitting (accidentally) (person) W2Ø.8 ☑

Tripping
- without fall W18.4Ø ☑
  - due to
    - specified NEC W18.49 ☑
    - stepping from one level to another W18.43 ☑
    - stepping into hole or opening W18.42 ☑
    - stepping on object W18.41 ☑
- over
  - animal WØ1.Ø ☑
    - with fall WØ1.Ø ☑
  - carpet, rug or (small) object W22.8 ☑
    - with fall W18.Ø9 ☑
  - person W51 ☑
    - with fall WØ3 ☑
      - due to ice or snow WØØ.Ø ☑

Twisted by person(s) (accidentally) W5Ø.2 ☑
- with intent to injure or kill YØ4.Ø ☑
- as, or caused by, a crowd or human stampede (with fall) W52 ☑
- assault YØ4.Ø ☑
- homicide (attempt) YØ4.Ø ☑
- in
  - fight YØ4.Ø ☑
  - legal intervention — *see* Legal, intervention, manhandling

Twisting, excessive — *see* category Y93 ☑

U

Underdosing of necessary drugs, medicaments or biological substances Y63.6

Undetermined intent (contact) (exposure)
- automobile collision Y32 ☑
- blunt object Y29 ☑
- drowning (submersion) (in) Y21.9 ☑
  - bathtub Y21.Ø ☑
    - after fall Y21.1 ☑
  - natural water (lake) (ocean) (pond) (river) (stream) Y21.4 ☑
  - specified place NEC Y21.8 ☑
  - swimming pool Y21.2 ☑
    - after fall Y21.3 ☑
- explosive material Y25 ☑
- fall, jump or push from high place Y3Ø ☑
- falling, lying or running before moving object Y31 ☑

Undetermined intent — *continued*
- fire Y26 ☑
- firearm discharge Y24.9 ☑
  - airgun (BB) (pellet) Y24.Ø ☑
  - handgun (pistol) (revolver) Y22 ☑
  - hunting rifle Y23.1 ☑
  - larger Y23.9 ☑
    - hunting rifle Y23.1 ☑
    - machine gun Y23.3 ☑
    - military Y23.2 ☑
    - shotgun Y23.Ø ☑
    - specified type NEC Y23.8 ☑
  - machine gun Y23.3 ☑
  - military Y23.2 ☑
  - shotgun Y23.Ø ☑
  - specified type NEC Y24.8 ☑
  - Very pistol Y24.8 ☑
- hot object Y27.9 ☑
  - fluid NEC Y27.2 ☑
  - household appliance Y27.3 ☑
  - specified object NEC Y27.8 ☑
  - steam Y27.Ø ☑
  - tap water Y27.1 ☑
  - vapor Y27.Ø ☑
- jump, fall or push from high place Y3Ø ☑
- lying, falling or running before moving object Y31 ☑
- motor vehicle crash Y32 ☑
- push, fall or jump from high place Y3Ø ☑
- running, falling or lying before moving object Y31 ☑
- sharp object Y28.9 ☑
  - dagger Y28.2 ☑
  - glass Y28.Ø ☑
  - knife Y28.1 ☑
  - specified object NEC Y28.8 ☑
  - sword Y28.2 ☑
- smoke Y26 ☑
- specified event NEC Y33 ☑

V

Vibration (causing injury) W49.9 ☑

Victim (of)
- avalanche — *see* Landslide
- earth movements NEC — *see* Forces of nature, earth movement
- earthquake X34 ☑
- flood — *see* Flood
- landslide — *see* Landslide
- lightning — *see* subcategory T75.Ø ☑
  - causing fire — *see* Exposure, fire
- storm (cataclysmic) NEC — *see* Forces of nature, cataclysmic storm
- volcanic eruption X35 ☑

Volcanic eruption (any injury) X35 ☑

Vomitus, gastric contents in air passages (with asphyxia, obstruction or suffocation) T17.81- ☑

W

Walked into stationary object (any) W22.Ø9 ☑
- furniture W22.Ø3 ☑
- lamppost W22.Ø2 ☑
- wall W22.Ø1 ☑

War operations (injuries to military personnel and civilians during war, civil insurrection and peacekeeping missions) (by) (from) (involving) Y36.9Ø ☑
- after cessation of hostilities Y36.89- ☑
  - explosion (of)
    - bomb placed during war operations Y36.82- ☑
    - mine placed during war operations Y36.81- ☑
  - specified NEC Y36.88- ☑
- air blast Y36.2Ø- ☑
- aircraft
  - destruction — *see* War operations, destruction of aircraft
- airway restriction — *see* War operations, restriction of airways
- asphyxiation — *see* War operations, restriction of airways
- biological weapons Y36.6X- ☑
- blast Y36.2Ø- ☑
- blast fragments Y36.2Ø- ☑
- blast wave Y36.2Ø- ☑
- blast wind Y36.2Ø- ☑
- bomb Y36.2Ø- ☑

War operations — *continued*
- bomb — *continued*
  - dirty Y36.5Ø- ☑
  - gasoline Y36.31- ☑
  - incendiary Y36.31- ☑
  - petrol Y36.31- ☑
- bullet Y36.43- ☑
  - incendiary Y36.32- ☑
  - rubber Y36.41- ☑
- chemical weapons Y36.7X- ☑
- combat
  - hand to hand (unarmed) combat Y36.44- ☑
  - using blunt or piercing object Y36.45- ☑
- conflagration — *see* War operations, fire
- conventional warfare NEC Y36.49- ☑
- depth-charge Y36.Ø1- ☑
- destruction of aircraft Y36.1Ø- ☑
  - due to
    - air to air missile Y36.11- ☑
    - collision with other aircraft Y36.12- ☑
    - detonation (accidental) of onboard munitions and explosives Y36.14- ☑
    - enemy fire or explosives Y36.11- ☑
    - explosive placed on aircraft Y36.11- ☑
    - onboard fire Y36.13- ☑
    - rocket propelled grenade [RPG] Y36.11- ☑
    - small arms fire Y36.11- ☑
    - surface to air missile Y36.11- ☑
  - specified NEC Y36.19- ☑
- detonation (accidental) of
  - onboard marine weapons Y36.Ø5- ☑
  - own munitions or munitions launch device Y36.24- ☑
- dirty bomb Y36.5Ø- ☑
- explosion (of) Y36.2Ø- ☑
  - aerial bomb Y36.21- ☑
  - after cessation of hostilities
    - bomb placed during war operations Y36.82- ☑
    - mine placed during war operations Y36.81- ☑
  - bomb NOS (*see also* War operations, bomb(s)) Y36.2Ø- ☑
  - fragments Y36.2Ø- ☑
  - grenade Y36.29- ☑
  - guided missile Y36.22- ☑
  - improvised explosive device [IED] (person-borne) (roadside) (vehicle-borne) Y36.23- ☑
  - land mine Y36.29- ☑
  - marine mine (at sea) (in harbor) Y36.Ø2- ☑
  - marine weapon Y36.ØØ- ☑
    - specified NEC Y36.Ø9- ☑
  - own munitions or munitions launch device (accidental) Y36.24- ☑
  - sea-based artillery shell Y36.Ø3- ☑
  - specified NEC Y36.29- ☑
  - torpedo Y36.Ø4- ☑
- fire Y36.3Ø- ☑
  - specified NEC Y36.39- ☑
- firearms
  - discharge Y36.43- ☑
  - pellets Y36.42- ☑
- flamethrower Y36.33- ☑
- fragments (from) (of)
  - improvised explosive device [IED] (person-borne) (roadside) (vehicle-borne) Y36.26- ☑
  - munitions Y36.25- ☑
  - specified NEC Y36.29- ☑
  - weapons Y36.27- ☑
- friendly fire Y36.92 ☑
- hand to hand (unarmed) combat Y36.44- ☑
- hot substances — *see* War operations, fire
- incendiary bullet Y36.32- ☑
- nuclear weapon (effects of) Y36.5Ø- ☑
  - acute radiation exposure Y36.54- ☑
  - blast pressure Y36.51- ☑
  - direct blast Y36.51- ☑
  - direct heat Y36.53- ☑
  - fallout exposure Y36.54- ☑
  - fireball Y36.53- ☑
  - indirect blast (struck or crushed by blast debris) (being thrown by blast) Y36.52- ☑
  - ionizing radiation (immediate exposure) Y36.54- ☑
  - nuclear radiation Y36.54- ☑
  - radiation
    - ionizing (immediate exposure) Y36.54- ☑
    - nuclear Y36.54- ☑
    - thermal Y36.53- ☑

ICD-1Ø-CM Tabular List of Diseases and Injuries

Chapter 1. Certain Infectious and Parasitic Diseases (AØØ-B99)

INCLUDES diseases generally recognized as communicable or transmissible

Use additional code to identify resistance to antimicrobial drugs (Z16.-)

EXCLUDES 1 *certain localized infections—see body system-related chapters*

EXCLUDES 2 *carrier or suspected carrier of infectious disease (Z22.-)*
infectious and parasitic diseases complicating pregnancy, childbirth and the puerperium (O98.-)
infectious and parasitic diseases specific to the perinatal period (P35-P39)
influenza and other acute respiratory infections (JØØ-J22)

This chapter contains the following blocks:

AØØ-AØ9	Intestinal infectious diseases
A15-A19	Tuberculosis
A2Ø-A28	Certain zoonotic bacterial diseases
A3Ø-A49	Other bacterial diseases
A5Ø-A64	Infections with a predominantly sexual mode of transmission
A65-A69	Other spirochetal diseases
A7Ø-A74	Other diseases caused by chlamydiae
A75-A79	Rickettsioses
A8Ø-A89	Viral infections of the central nervous system
A9Ø-A99	Arthropod-borne viral fevers and viral hemorrhagic fevers
BØØ-BØ9	Viral infections characterized by skin and mucous membrane lesions
B1Ø	Other human herpesviruses
B15-B19	Viral hepatitis
B2Ø	Human immunodeficiency virus [HIV] disease
B25-B34	Other viral diseases
B35-B49	Mycoses
B5Ø-B64	Protozoal diseases
B65-B83	Helminthiases
B85-B89	Pediculosis, acariasis and other infestations
B9Ø-B94	Sequelae of infectious and parasitic diseases
B95-B97	Bacterial and viral infectious agents
B99	Other infectious diseases

Intestinal Infectious Diseases (AØØ-AØ9)

✓4th **AØØ Cholera**

CC Excl: For CC codes in category AØØ, unless otherwise noted: AØØ.Ø-AØØ.9

AØØ.Ø Cholera due to Vibrio cholerae Ø1, biovar cholerae CC
Classical cholera

AØØ.1 Cholera due to Vibrio cholerae Ø1, biovar eltor CC
Cholera eltor

AØØ.9 Cholera, unspecified CC

✓4th **AØ1 Typhoid and paratyphoid fevers**

CC Excl: For CC codes in category AØ1, unless otherwise noted: AØ1.ØØ-AØ1.4

✓5th **AØ1.Ø Typhoid fever**
Infection due to Salmonella typhi

AØ1.ØØ Typhoid fever, unspecified CC

AØ1.Ø1 Typhoid meningitis CC

AØ1.Ø2 Typhoid fever with heart involvement CC
Typhoid endocarditis Typhoid myocarditis

AØ1.Ø3 Typhoid pneumonia CC

AØ1.Ø4 Typhoid arthritis CC

AØ1.Ø5 Typhoid osteomyelitis CC

AØ1.Ø9 Typhoid fever with other complications CC

AØ1.1 Paratyphoid fever A CC

AØ1.2 Paratyphoid fever B CC

AØ1.3 Paratyphoid fever C CC

AØ1.4 Paratyphoid fever, unspecified CC
Infection due to Salmonella paratyphi NOS

✓4th **AØ2 Other salmonella infections**

INCLUDES infection or foodborne intoxication due to any Salmonella species other than S. typhi and S. paratyphi

AØ2.Ø Salmonella enteritis CC
Salmonellosis
CC Excl: AØ1.ØØ-AØ1.Ø9, AØ1.4-AØ2.Ø, AØ3.9-AØ5.2, AØ7.4, AØ8.Ø-AØ9, A48.51-A48.52, K3Ø, K52.1-K52.2, K52.82-K52.9, K58.Ø-K58.9, K65.Ø, K65.2, K65.8, K68.12-K68.9, P76.8-P77.9, P78.1, P78.3-P78.89

AØ2.1 Salmonella sepsis HIV MCC
CC Excl: AØ2.1, A2Ø.7, A22.7, A26.7, A32.7, A39.2-A39.4, A4Ø.Ø-A4Ø.1, A4Ø.8-A41.9, A42.7, A48.2-A48.4, A48.8-A49.9, A54.86, BØØ.7, B37.7, B92, B94.2-B96.89, MØØ.Ø11-MØØ.Ø12, MØØ.Ø21-MØØ.Ø22, MØØ.Ø31- MØØ.Ø32, MØØ.Ø41-MØØ.Ø42, MØØ.Ø51-MØØ.Ø52, MØØ.Ø61-MØØ.Ø62, MØØ.Ø71-MØØ.Ø72, P36.Ø-P36.9, P39.2, P39.4-P39.9, R65.1Ø-R65.2Ø, Z16.1Ø-Z16.39

✓5th **AØ2.2 Localized salmonella infections**

AØ2.2Ø Localized salmonella infection, unspecified HIV

AØ2.21 Salmonella meningitis HIV MCC
CC Excl: AØ2.21, A17.Ø-A17.1, A27.81, A39.Ø, A5Ø.41, A51.41, A52.13, A54.82, A54.84, A54.89-A54.9, A74.81-A74.9, A87.Ø-A87.9, A96.2, A98.3-A98.4, B26.1, B33.24, B33.4-B33.8, B34.1-B34.2, B34.4-B34.8, B37.5, B38.4, B45.1, B58.2, B92, B94.2-B94.9, B97.1Ø, B97.19, B97.29, B97.5-B97.6, B97.81-B97.89, GØØ.Ø-GØ3.9, GØ4.2, G32.89, G96.8-G96.9, G98.Ø-G98.8, G99.8

AØ2.22 Salmonella pneumonia HIV MCC
CC Excl: AØ2.22, A15.Ø-A15.6, A15.8-A15.9, A17.9, A18.82, A18.84, A18.89, A2Ø.2, A21.1, A22.1, A31.Ø, A37.Ø1, A37.11, A37.81, A37.91, A42.Ø, A43.Ø, A48.1, B25.Ø, B39.Ø-B39.2, B44.Ø, B58.3, B59, B67.1, JØ9.X1-JØ9.X2, J1Ø.ØØ-J1Ø.1, J11.ØØ-J11.1, J12.Ø-J12.3, J12.89-J18.1, J18.8-J18.9, J22, J6Ø, J62.Ø-J67.7, J68.Ø-J7Ø.4, J7Ø.8-J7Ø.9, J98.4, J98.8-J99, R91.1

AØ2.23 Salmonella arthritis HIV CC
CC Excl: AØ2.23, A18.Ø2, A18.Ø9, A39.83-A39.84, A54.4Ø, A54.42-A54.43, A54.82, A54.84, A54.89-A54.9, BØ6.82, MØØ.ØØ, MØØ.19, MØØ.29, MØØ.39, MØØ.49, MØØ.59, MØØ.69, MØØ.79, MØØ.Ø8-MØ2.9, MØ5.4Ø-MØ5.59, MØ5.7Ø-MØ6.Ø9, MØ6.2Ø-MØ6.39, MØ6.8Ø-MØ7.69, M11.ØØ-M11.9, M12.1Ø-M15.Ø, M15.3-M15.9, M16.2-M16.9, M17.2-M17.9, M18.2-M18.9, M19.111-M19.93, M24.1Ø-M24.176, M25.ØØ, M25.Ø8-M25.18, M25.4Ø-M25.676, M25.8Ø-M25.9, M35.2, M36.1-M36.4, R29.4

AØ2.24 Salmonella osteomyelitis HIV CC
CC Excl: AØ2.24, A18.Ø3-A18.Ø9, M46.2Ø-M46.39, M86.ØØ-M86.9

AØ2.25 Salmonella pyelonephritis HIV CC
Salmonella tubulo-interstitial nephropathy
CC Excl: AØ2.25-AØ2.29

AØ2.29 Salmonella with other localized infection HIV CC
CC Excl: See code: AØ2.25

AØ2.8 Other specified salmonella infections HIV CC
CC Excl:AØ2.8

AØ2.9 Salmonella infection, unspecified HIV CC
CC Excl: AØ2.9

✓4th **AØ3 Shigellosis**

AØ3.Ø Shigellosis due to Shigella dysenteriae CC
Group A shigellosis [Shiga-Kruse dysentery]
CC Excl: AØØ.1, AØ1.ØØ-AØ1.Ø9, AØ1.4-AØ2.Ø, AØ3.Ø, AØ3.9, AØ4.9-AØ5.2, AØ6.Ø-AØ6.2, AØ6.9, AØ7.1-AØ7.9, AØ8.4-AØ9, A18.32-A18.39, A18.83, A48.51-A48.52, B37.82, B82.9, JØ9.X3-JØ9.X9, J1Ø.2-J1Ø.89, J11.2-J11.89, K3Ø, K31.84, K5Ø.ØØ-K51.919, K52.1-K52.2, K52.82-K55.1, K55.8-K55.9, K58.Ø-K58.9, P7Ø.Ø-P7Ø.4, P7Ø.9-P71.9, P72.1, P72.9-P74.4, P74.9, P76.8-P77.9, P78.1, P78.3-P78.89, P94.Ø

AØ3.1 Shigellosis due to Shigella flexneri
Group B shigellosis

AØ3.2 Shigellosis due to Shigella boydii
Group C shigellosis

AØ3.3 Shigellosis due to Shigella sonnei
Group D shigellosis

AØ3.8 Other shigellosis

AØ3.9 Shigellosis, unspecified
Bacillary dysentery NOS

✓4th **AØ4 Other bacterial intestinal infections**

EXCLUDES 1 *bacterial foodborne intoxications, NEC (AØ5.-)*
tuberculous enteritis (A18.32)

CC Excl: For CC codes in category AØ4, unless otherwise noted: For codes AØ4.Ø-AØ4.4: AØ2.Ø, AØ3.9-AØ5.Ø, AØ5.2, AØ7.4, AØ8.Ø-AØ9, JØ9.X3-JØ9.X9, J1Ø.2-J1Ø.89, J11.2-J11.89, K3Ø, K31.84, K52.1-K52.2, K52.82-K52.9, K58.Ø-K58.9, K65.Ø, K65.2, K65.8, K68.12-K68.9, P76.8-P77.9, P78.1, P78.3-P78.89 **For codes AØ4.5-AØ4.8:** AØØ.1, AØ1.ØØ-AØ1.Ø9, AØ1.4-AØ2.Ø, AØ3.9-AØ5.2, AØ6.Ø-AØ6.2, AØ6.9, AØ7.1-AØ9, A18.32-A18.39, A18.83, A48.51-A48.52, B37.82, B82.9, JØ9.X3-JØ9.X9, J1Ø.2-J1Ø.89, J11.2-J11.89, K3Ø, K31.84, K5Ø.ØØ-K51.919, K52.1-K52.2, K52.82-K55.1, K55.8-K55.9, K58.Ø-K58.9, P7Ø.Ø-P7Ø.4, P7Ø.9-P71.9, P72.1, P72.9-P74.4, P74.9, P76.8-P77.9, P78.1, P78.3-P78.89, P94.Ø

AØ4.Ø Enteropathogenic Escherichia coli infection CC

A04.1 Enterotoxigenic Escherichia coli infection CC

A04.2 Enteroinvasive Escherichia coli infection CC

A04.3 Enterohemorrhagic Escherichia coli infection CC

A04.4 Other intestinal Escherichia coli infections CC
Escherichia coli enteritis NOS

A04.5 Campylobacter enteritis CC

A04.6 Enteritis due to Yersinia enterocolitica CC
EXCLUDES 1 *extraintestinal yersiniosis (A28.2)*

A04.7 Enterocolitis due to Clostridium difficile CC
Foodborne intoxication by Clostridium difficile
Pseudomembraneous colitis

A04.8 Other specified bacterial intestinal infections CC

A04.9 Bacterial intestinal infection, unspecified CC
Bacterial enteritis NOS
CC Excl: A00.1, A01.00-A01.09, A01.4-A02.0, A03.9-A05.0, A05.2, A06.0-A06.2, A06.9, A07.1-A09, A18.32-A18.39, A18.83, B37.82, B82.9, J09.X3-J09.X9, J10.2-J10.89, J11.2-J11.89, K30, K31.84, K52.1-K52.2, K52.82-K52.9, K58.0-K58.9, K65.0, K65.2, K65.8, K68.12-K68.9, P76.8-P77.9, P78.1, P78.3-P78.89

✓4th A05 Other bacterial foodborne intoxications, not elsewhere classified

EXCLUDES 1 *Clostridium difficile foodborne intoxication and infection (A04.7)*
Escherichia coli infection (A04.0-A04.4)
listeriosis (A32.-)
salmonella foodborne intoxication and infection (A02.-)
toxic effect of noxious foodstuffs (T61-T62)

A05.0 Foodborne staphylococcal intoxication CC
CC Excl: A00.0-A09, A48.51-A48.52

A05.1 Botulism food poisoning CC
Botulism NOS
Classical foodborne intoxication due to Clostridium botulinum
EXCLUDES 1 *infant botulism (A48.51)*
wound botulism (A48.52)
CC Excl: A04.7-A05.2, A48.51-A48.52

A05.2 Foodborne Clostridium perfringens [Clostridium welchii] intoxication CC
Enteritis necroticans
Pig-bel
CC Excl: A02.0, A03.9-A05.2, A07.4, A08.0-A09, A48.51-A48.52, J09.X3-J09.X9, J10.2-J10.89, J11.2-J11.89, K30, K31.84, K52.1-K52.2, K52.82-K52.9, K58.0-K58.9, K65.0, K65.2, K65.8, K68.12-K68.9, P76.8-P77.9, P78.1, P78.3-P78.89

A05.3 Foodborne Vibrio parahaemolyticus intoxication CC
CC Excl: See code: A05.0

A05.4 Foodborne Bacillus cereus intoxication CC
CC Excl: See code: A05.0

A05.5 Foodborne Vibrio vulnificus intoxication CC
CC Excl: See code: A05.0

A05.8 Other specified bacterial foodborne intoxications CC
CC Excl: See code: A05.0

A05.9 Bacterial foodborne intoxication, unspecified

✓4th A06 Amebiasis

INCLUDES infection due to Entamoeba histolytica
EXCLUDES 1 *other protozoal intestinal diseases (A07.-)*
EXCLUDES 2 *acanthamebiasis (B60.1-)*
Naegleriasis (B60.2)

A06.0 Acute amebic dysentery CC
Acute amebiasis
Intestinal amebiasis NOS
CC Excl: A06.0-A06.1, A07.4

A06.1 Chronic intestinal amebiasis CC
CC Excl: See code: A06.0

A06.2 Amebic nondysenteric colitis CC
CC Excl: A02.0, A03.9-A05.0, A05.2, A06.0-A06.2, A06.9, A07.1-A09, B82.9, J09.X3-J09.X9, J10.2-J10.89, J11.2-J11.89, K30, K31.84, K50.00-K51.919, K52.1-K52.2, K52.82-K55.1, K55.8-K55.9, K58.0-K58.9, P76.8-P77.9, P78.1, P78.3-P78.89

A06.3 Ameboma of intestine CC
Ameboma NOS
CC Excl: A06.0-A06.6, A06.81-A06.89

A06.4 Amebic liver abscess MCC
Hepatic amebiasis
CC Excl: A06.4, K75.0

A06.5 Amebic lung abscess MCC
Amebic abscess of lung (and liver)
CC Excl: A06.5, J85.0-J85.2

A06.6 Amebic brain abscess MCC
Amebic abscess of brain (and liver) (and lung)
CC Excl: A06.6, G06.0

A06.7 Cutaneous amebiasis

✓5th A06.8 Amebic infection of other sites

A06.81 Amebic cystitis CC
CC Excl: A06.0-A06.6, A06.81-A06.89

A06.82 Other amebic genitourinary infections CC
Amebic balanitis
Amebic vesiculitis
Amebic vulvovaginitis
CC Excl: See code: A06.3

A06.89 Other amebic infections CC
Amebic appendicitis
Amebic splenic abscess
CC Excl: See code: A06.3

A06.9 Amebiasis, unspecified

✓4th A07 Other protozoal intestinal diseases

CC Excl: For CC codes in category A07, unless otherwise noted: A02.0, A03.9-A05.0, A05.2, A06.0-A06.2, A06.9, A07.1-A09, B82.9, J09.X3-J09.X9, J10.2-J10.89, J11.2-J11.89, K30, K31.84, K52.1-K52.2, K52.82-K52.9, K58.0-K58.9

A07.0 Balantidiasis
Balantidial dysentery

A07.1 Giardiasis [lambliasis] CC

A07.2 Cryptosporidiosis CC

A07.3 Isosporiasis HIV CC
Infection due to Isospora belli and Isospora hominis
Intestinal coccidiosis
Isosporosis

A07.4 Cyclosporiasis CC
CC Excl: A02.0, A03.9-A05.0, A05.2, A06.0-A06.2, A06.9, A07.1-A09, B82.9, J09.X3-J09.X9, J10.2-J10.89, J11.2-J11.89, K30, K31.84, K52.1-K52.2, K52.82-K52.9, K58.0-K58.9, K65.0, K65.2, K65.8, K68.12-K68.9

A07.8 Other specified protozoal intestinal diseases CC
Intestinal microsporidiosis
Intestinal trichomoniasis
Sarcocystosis
Sarcosporidiosis

A07.9 Protozoal intestinal disease, unspecified CC
Flagellate diarrhea
Protozoal colitis
Protozoal diarrhea
Protozoal dysentery

✓4th A08 Viral and other specified intestinal infections

EXCLUDES 1 *influenza with involvement of gastrointestinal tract (J09.X3, J10.2, J11.2)*

CC Excl: For CC codes in category A08, unless otherwise noted: A02.0, A03.9-A05.0, A05.2, A06.0-A06.2, A06.9, A07.1-A09, A18.32-A18.39, A18.83, B37.82, B82.9, J09.X3-J09.X9, J10.2-J10.89, J11.2-J11.89, K30, K31.84, K52.1-K52.2, K52.82-K52.9, K58.0-K58.9, K65.0, K65.2, K65.8, K68.12-K68.9, P76.8-P77.9, P78.1, P78.3-P78.89

A08.0 Rotaviral enteritis CC

✓5th A08.1 Acute gastroenteropathy due to Norwalk agent and other small round viruses

A08.11 Acute gastroenteropathy due to Norwalk agent CC
Acute gastroenteropathy due to Norovirus
Acute gastroenteropathy due to Norwalk-like agent

A08.19 Acute gastroenteropathy due to other small round viruses CC
Acute gastroenteropathy due to small round virus [SRV] NOS

A08.2 Adenoviral enteritis CC

✓5th A08.3 Other viral enteritis

A08.31 Calicivirus enteritis CC

A08.32 Astrovirus enteritis CC

A08.39 Other viral enteritis CC
Coxsackie virus enteritis
Echovirus enteritis
Enterovirus enteritis NEC
Torovirus enteritis

A08.4 Viral intestinal infection, unspecified
Viral enteritis NOS
Viral gastroenteritis NOS
Viral gastroenteropathy NOS

A08.8 Other specified intestinal infections

A09 Infectious gastroenteritis and colitis, unspecified CC

Infectious colitis NOS
Infectious enteritis NOS
Infectious gastroenteritis NOS
EXCLUDES 1 *colitis NOS (K52.9)*
diarrhea NOS (R19.7)
enteritis NOS (K52.9)
gastroenteritis NOS (K52.9)
noninfective gastroenteritis and colitis, unspecified (K52.9)
CC Excl: A00.0-A09, A48.51-A48.52

Tuberculosis (A15-A19)

INCLUDES infections due to Mycobacterium tuberculosis and Mycobacterium bovis

EXCLUDES 1 *congenital tuberculosis (P37.Ø)*
nonspecific reaction to test for tuberculosis without active tuberculosis (R76.1-)
pneumoconiosis associated with tuberculosis, any type in A15 (J65)
positive PPD (R76.11)
positive tuberculin skin test without active tuberculosis (R76.11)
sequelae of tuberculosis (B9Ø.-)
silicotuberculosis (J65)

✓4th A15 Respiratory tuberculosis

A15.Ø Tuberculosis of lung HIV CC
Tuberculous bronchiectasis
Tuberculous fibrosis of lung
Tuberculous pneumonia
Tuberculous pneumothorax
CC Excl: A15.Ø-A15.6, A15.8-A15.9, A17.9, A18.82, A18.84, A18.89-A19.9, A22.1, A31.Ø, A31.2-A31.9, A37.Ø1, A37.11, A37.81, A37.91, A48.1, A49.3-A49.9, B25.Ø, B44.Ø, B9Ø.9, B92, B94.2-B94.9, B96.Ø, B96.6-B96.89, JØ9.X1-JØ9.X2, J1Ø.ØØ-J1Ø.1, J11.ØØ-J11.1, J12.Ø-J12.3, J12.89-J18.1, J18.8-J18.9, J44.9, J47.Ø-J7Ø.4, J7Ø.8-J7Ø.9, J98.4, R91.1

A15.4 Tuberculosis of intrathoracic lymph nodes HIV CC
Tuberculosis of hilar lymph nodes
Tuberculosis of mediastinal lymph nodes
Tuberculosis of tracheobronchial lymph nodes
EXCLUDES 1 *tuberculosis specified as primary (A15.7)*
CC Excl: See code: A15.Ø

A15.5 Tuberculosis of larynx, trachea and bronchus HIV CC
Tuberculosis of bronchus
Tuberculosis of glottis
Tuberculosis of larynx
Tuberculosis of trachea
CC Excl: See code: A15.Ø

A15.6 Tuberculous pleurisy HIV CC
Tuberculosis of pleura Tuberculous empyema
EXCLUDES 1 *primary respiratory tuberculosis (A15.7)*
CC Excl: See code: A15.Ø

A15.7 Primary respiratory tuberculosis HIV CC
CC Excl: A15.Ø-A17.82, A17.89-A19.9

A15.8 Other respiratory tuberculosis HIV CC
Mediastinal tuberculosis
Nasopharyngeal tuberculosis
Tuberculosis of nose
Tuberculosis of sinus [any nasal]
CC Excl: A15.Ø-A17.82, A17.89, A18.31-A18.39, A18.83, A19.Ø-A19.9

A15.9 Respiratory tuberculosis unspecified HIV CC
CC Excl: See code: A15.8

✓4th A17 Tuberculosis of nervous system

A17.Ø Tuberculous meningitis HIV MCC
Tuberculosis of meninges (cerebral)(spinal)
Tuberculous leptomeningitis
EXCLUDES 1 *tuberculous meningoencephalitis (A17.82)*
CC Excl: AØ2.21, A17.Ø-A17.1, A17.89-A17.9, A18.82, A18.84, A18.89, A27.81, A31.2-A31.9, A39.Ø, A49.3-A49.9, A5Ø.41, A51.41, A52.13, A54.82, A54.84, A54.89-A54.9, A87.Ø-A87.9, BØØ.3, BØ2.1, B26.1, B37.5, B38.4, B45.1, B58.2, B9Ø.Ø, B92, B94.2-B94.9, B96.Ø, B96.6-B96.89, GØØ.Ø-GØ3.9, GØ4.2, G32.89, G61.Ø, G96.8-G96.9, G98.Ø-G98.8, G99.8

A17.1 Meningeal tuberculoma HIV MCC
Tuberculoma of meninges (cerebral) (spinal)
EXCLUDES 2 *tuberculoma of brain and spinal cord (A17.81)*
CC Excl: See code: A17.Ø

✓5th A17.8 Other tuberculosis of nervous system

A17.81 Tuberculoma of brain and spinal cord HIV MCC
Tuberculous abscess of brain and spinal cord
CC Excl: A17.81-A17.82, A17.89-A17.9, A18.82, A18.84, A18.89, A31.2-A31.9, A49.3-A49.9, B9Ø.Ø, B92, B94.2-B94.9, B96.Ø, B96.6-B96.89

A17.82 Tuberculous meningoencephalitis HIV MCC
Tuberculous myelitis
CC Excl: See code: A17.81

A17.83 Tuberculous neuritis HIV MCC
Tuberculous mononeuropathy
CC Excl: No Excl

A17.89 Other tuberculosis of nervous system HIV MCC
Tuberculous polyneuropathy
CC Excl: A17.89-A17.9, A18.82, A18.84, A18.89, A31.2-A31.9, A49.3-A49.9, B9Ø.Ø, B92, B94.2-B94.9, B96.Ø, B96.6-B96.89

A17.9 Tuberculosis of nervous system, unspecified HIV CC
CC Excl: A17.9, A18.82, A18.84, A18.89, A31.2-A31.9, A49.3-A49.9, B92, B94.2-B94.9, B96.Ø, B96.6-B96.89

✓4th A18 Tuberculosis of other organs

✓5th A18.Ø Tuberculosis of bones and joints

A18.Ø1 Tuberculosis of spine HIV CC
Pott's disease or curvature of spine
Tuberculous arthritis
Tuberculous osteomyelitis of spine
Tuberculous spondylitis
CC Excl: A18.Ø1

A18.Ø2 Tuberculous arthritis of other joints HIV CC
Tuberculosis of hip (joint)
Tuberculosis of knee (joint)
CC Excl: A18.Ø2

A18.Ø3 Tuberculosis of other bones HIV CC
Tuberculous mastoiditis
Tuberculous osteomyelitis
CC Excl: A18.Ø1-A18.Ø3

A18.Ø9 Other musculoskeletal tuberculosis HIV CC
Tuberculous myositis
Tuberculous synovitis
Tuberculous tenosynovitis
CC Excl: A18.Ø1-A18.Ø2, A18.Ø9

✓5th A18.1 Tuberculosis of genitourinary system

A18.1Ø Tuberculosis of genitourinary system, unspecified HIV CC
CC Excl: A17.9, A18.1Ø, A18.82, A18.84, A18.89, A31.2-A31.9, A49.3-A49.9, B9Ø.1, B92, B94.2-B94.9, B96.Ø, B96.6-B96.89

A18.11 Tuberculosis of kidney and ureter HIV CC
CC Excl: A17.9-A18.13, A18.82, A18.84, A18.89, A31.2-A31.9, A49.3-A49.9, B9Ø.1, B92, B94.2-B94.9, B96.Ø, B96.6-B96.89

A18.12 Tuberculosis of bladder HIV CC
CC Excl: See code: A18.11

A18.13 Tuberculosis of other urinary organs HIV CC
Tuberculous urethritis
CC Excl: See code: A18.11

A18.14 Tuberculosis of prostate HIV CC A ♂
CC Excl: A17.9, A18.1Ø, A18.14-A18.15, A18.82, A18.84, A18.89, A31.2-A31.9, A49.3-A49.9, B9Ø.1, B92, B94.2-B94.9, B96.Ø, B96.6-B96.89

A18.15 Tuberculosis of other male genital organs HIV CC ♂
CC Excl: See code: A18.14

A18.16 Tuberculosis of cervix HIV CC ♀
CC Excl: A17.9, A18.1Ø, A18.16-A18.18, A18.82, A18.84, A18.89, A31.2-A31.9, A49.3-A49.9, B9Ø.1, B92, B94.2-B94.9, B96.Ø, B96.6-B96.89

A18.17 Tuberculous female pelvic inflammatory disease HIV CC ♀
Tuberculous endometritis
Tuberculous oophoritis and salpingitis
CC Excl: See code: A18.16

A18.18 Tuberculosis of other female genital organs HIV CC ♀
Tuberculous ulceration of vulva
CC Excl: See code: A18.16

A18.2 Tuberculous peripheral lymphadenopathy HIV CC
Tuberculous adenitis
EXCLUDES 2 *tuberculosis of bronchial and mediastinal lymph nodes (A15.4)*
tuberculosis of mesenteric and retroperitoneal lymph nodes (A18.39)
tuberculous tracheobronchial adenopathy (A15.4)
CC Excl: A17.9, A18.2, A18.82, A18.84, A18.89, A31.2-A31.9, A49.3-A49.9, B92, B94.2-B94.9, B96.Ø, B96.6-B96.89

✓5th A18.3 Tuberculosis of intestines, peritoneum and mesenteric glands

CC Excl: For CC/MCC codes in subcategory A18.3, unless otherwise noted: A17.9, A18.31-A18.39, A18.82-A18.84, A18.89, A31.2-A31.9, A49.3-A49.9, B92, B94.2-B94.9, B96.Ø, B96.6-B96.89

A18.31 Tuberculous peritonitis HIV MCC
Tuberculous ascites

A18.32 Tuberculous enteritis HIV CC
Tuberculosis of anus and rectum
Tuberculosis of intestine (large) (small)

A18.39 Retroperitoneal tuberculosis HIV CC
Tuberculosis of mesenteric glands
Tuberculosis of retroperitoneal (lymph glands)

A18.4 Tuberculosis of skin and subcutaneous tissue HIV CC
Erythema induratum, tuberculous
Lupus excedens
Lupus vulgaris NOS
Lupus vulgaris of eyelid
Scrofuloderma
Tuberculosis of external ear
EXCLUDES 2 *lupus erythematosus (L93.-)*
lupus NOS (M32.9)
systemic (M32.-)
CC Excl: A15.Ø-A17.82, A17.89-A19.9

✓5th **A18.5 Tuberculosis of eye**
EXCLUDES 2 *lupus vulgaris of eyelid (A18.4)*

CC Excl: For CC codes in subcategory A18.5, unless otherwise noted: A17.9, A18.5Ø-A18.59, A18.82, A18.84, A18.89, A31.2-A31.9, A49.3-A49.9, B92, B94.2-B94.9, B96.Ø, B96.6-B96.89

A18.5Ø Tuberculosis of eye, unspecified HIV CC
A18.51 Tuberculous episcleritis HIV CC
A18.52 Tuberculous keratitis HIV CC
Tuberculous interstitial keratitis
Tuberculous keratoconjunctivitis (interstitial) (phlyctenular)
A18.53 Tuberculous chorioretinitis HIV CC
A18.54 Tuberculous iridocyclitis HIV CC
A18.59 Other tuberculosis of eye HIV CC
Tuberculous conjunctivitis

A18.6 Tuberculosis of (inner) (middle) ear HIV CC
Tuberculous otitis media
EXCLUDES 2 *tuberculosis of external ear (A18.4)*
tuberculous mastoiditis (A18.Ø3)
CC Excl: A17.9, A18.6, A18.82, A18.84, A18.89, A31.2-A31.9, A49.3-A49.9, B92, B94.2-B94.9, B96.Ø, B96.6-B96.89

A18.7 Tuberculosis of adrenal glands HIV CC
Tuberculous Addison's disease
CC Excl: A17.9, A18.7, A18.82, A18.84, A18.89, A31.2-A31.9, A49.3-A49.9, B92, B94.2-B94.9, B96.Ø, B96.6-B96.89

✓5th **A18.8 Tuberculosis of other specified organs**
A18.81 Tuberculosis of thyroid gland HIV CC
CC Excl: A17.9, A18.81-A18.82, A18.84, A18.89, A31.2-A31.9, A49.3-A49.9, B92, B94.2-B94.9, B96.Ø, B96.6-B96.89
A18.82 Tuberculosis of other endocrine glands HIV CC
Tuberculosis of pituitary gland
Tuberculosis of thymus gland
CC Excl: A17.9, A18.82, A18.84, A18.89, A31.2-A31.9, A49.3-A49.9, B92, B94.2-B94.9, B96.Ø, B96.6-B96.89
A18.83 Tuberculosis of digestive tract organs, not elsewhere classified HIV CC
EXCLUDES 1 *tuberculosis of intestine (A18.32)*
CC Excl: A17.9, A18.31-A18.39, A18.82-A18.84, A18.89, A31.2-A31.9, A49.3-A49.9, B92, B94.2-B94.9, B96.Ø, B96.6-B96.89
A18.84 Tuberculosis of heart HIV CC
Tuberculous cardiomyopathy
Tuberculous endocarditis
Tuberculous myocarditis
Tuberculous pericarditis
CC Excl: See code: A18.82
A18.85 Tuberculosis of spleen HIV CC
CC Excl: A17.9-A18.82, A18.84-A18.89, A31.2-A31.9, A49.3-A49.9, B92, B94.2-B94.9, B96.Ø, B96.6-B96.89
A18.89 Tuberculosis of other sites HIV CC
Tuberculosis of muscle
Tuberculous cerebral arteritis
CC Excl: See code: A18.82

✓4th **A19 Miliary tuberculosis**
INCLUDES disseminated tuberculosis
generalized tuberculosis
tuberculous polyserositis

CC Excl: For MCC codes in category A19, unless otherwise noted: A17.9, A18.82, A18.84, A18.89-A19.9, A31.2-A31.9, A49.3-A49.9, B92, B94.2-B94.9, B96.Ø, B96.6-B96.89

A19.Ø Acute miliary tuberculosis of a single specified site HIV MCC
A19.1 Acute miliary tuberculosis of multiple sites HIV MCC
A19.2 Acute miliary tuberculosis, unspecified HIV MCC
A19.8 Other miliary tuberculosis HIV MCC
A19.9 Miliary tuberculosis, unspecified HIV MCC

Certain zoonotic bacterial diseases (A2Ø-A28)

✓4th **A2Ø Plague**
INCLUDES infection due to Yersinia pestis

A2Ø.Ø Bubonic plague MCC
CC Excl: A2Ø.Ø-A2Ø.9
A2Ø.1 Cellulocutaneous plague MCC
CC Excl: See code: A2Ø.Ø
A2Ø.2 Pneumonic plague MCC
CC Excl: A2Ø.2-J12.81
A2Ø.3 Plague meningitis MCC
CC Excl: A2Ø.3-A2Ø.8
A2Ø.7 Septicemic plague MCC
CC Excl: AØ2.1, A2Ø.Ø-A2Ø.9, A22.7, A26.7, A32.7, A4Ø.Ø-A4Ø.1, A4Ø.8-A41.9, A42.7, A54.86, B37.7, P36.Ø-P36.9, P39.2, P39.4-P39.9, R65.1Ø-R65.2Ø
A2Ø.8 Other forms of plague MCC
Abortive plague
Asymptomatic plague
Pestis minor
CC Excl: See code: A2Ø.3
A2Ø.9 Plague, unspecified MCC
CC Excl: A2Ø.9

✓4th **A21 Tularemia**
INCLUDES deer-fly fever
infection due to Francisella tularensis
rabbit fever

A21.Ø Ulceroglandular tularemia CC
CC Excl: A21.Ø
A21.1 Oculoglandular tularemia CC
Ophthalmic tularemia
CC Excl: A21.1-J12.81
A21.2 Pulmonary tularemia CC
CC Excl: A22.1-A37.Ø1, A37.11, A37.81, A37.91, A48.1, B25.Ø, B44.Ø, JØ9.X1-JØ9.X2, J1Ø.ØØ-J1Ø.1, J11.ØØ-J11.1, J15.29, J15.5-J18.Ø, J18.8-J18.9, J22, J6Ø-J7Ø.4, J7Ø.8-J7Ø.9, J98.4, J98.8-J99, R91.1
A21.3 Gastrointestinal tularemia CC
Abdominal tularemia
CC Excl: A21.3
A21.7 Generalized tularemia CC
CC Excl: A21.Ø-A21.9
A21.8 Other forms of tularemia CC
CC Excl: See code: A21.7
A21.9 Tulamirea, unspecified CC
CC Excl: See code: A21.7

✓4th **A22 Anthrax**
INCLUDES infection due to Bacillus anthracis

A22.Ø Cutaneous anthrax CC
Malignant carbuncle
Malignant pustule
CC Excl: A22.Ø
A22.1 Pulmonary anthrax MCC
Inhalation anthrax
Woolsorter's disease
Ragpicker's disease
CC Excl: A15.Ø-A15.6, A15.8-A15.9, A17.9, A18.82, A18.84, A18.89, A2Ø.2, A21.1-A21.2, A22.1, A31.Ø, A37.Ø1, A37.11, A37.81,A37.91, A42.Ø, A43.Ø, A48.1, B25.Ø, B39.Ø-B39.2, B44.Ø, B58.3, B59, B67.1, JØ9.X1-JØ9.X2, J1Ø.ØØ-J1Ø.1, J11.ØØ-J11.1, J12.Ø-J18.1, J18.8-J18.9, J22, J44.9, J47.Ø-J7Ø.4, J7Ø.8-J7Ø.9, J98.4, J98.8-J99, Q33.4, R91.1
A22.2 Gastrointestinal anthrax CC
CC Excl: A22.2
A22.7 Anthrax sepsis PDx MCC MCC
CC Excl: AØ2.1-A2Ø.7, A22.7, A26.7, A32.7, A39.2-A39.4, A4Ø.Ø-A4Ø.1, A4Ø.8-A41.9, A42.7, A48.2-A48.4, A48.8-A49.9, A54.86, BØØ.7, B37.7, B92, B94.2-B96.89, MØØ.Ø11-MØØ.Ø12, MØØ.Ø21-MØØ.Ø22, MØØ.Ø31- MØØ.Ø32, MØØ.Ø41-MØØ.Ø42, MØØ.Ø51-MØØ.Ø52, MØØ.Ø61-MØØ.Ø62, MØØ.Ø71-MØØ.Ø72, P36.Ø-P36.9, P39.2, P39.4-P39.9, R65.1Ø-R65.2Ø, Z16.1Ø-Z16.39
A22.8 Other forms of anthrax CC
Anthrax meningitis
CC Excl: A22.8
A22.9 Anthrax, unspecified CC
CC Excl: A22.Ø-A22.9

✓4th **A23 Brucellosis**
Malta fever
Undulant fever
Mediterranean fever

A23.Ø Brucellosis due to Brucella melitensis
A23.1 Brucellosis due to Brucella abortus
A23.2 Brucellosis due to Brucella suis
A23.3 Brucellosis due to Brucella canis

A23.8 Other brucellosis CC
CC Excl: A23.0-A23.9

A23.9 Brucellosis, unspecified CC
CC Excl: See code: A23.8

✓4th A24 Glanders and melioidosis

A24.0 Glanders CC
Infection due to Pseudomonas mallei
Malleus
CC Excl: A24.0

A24.1 Acute and fulminating melioidosis CC
Melioidosis pneumonia
Melioidosis sepsis
CC Excl: A24.1-A24.9

A24.2 Subacute and chronic melioidosis CC
CC Excl: See code: A24.1

A24.3 Other melioidosis CC
CC Excl: See code: A24.1

A24.9 Melioidosis, unspecified CC
Infection due to Pseudomonas pseudomallei NOS
Whitmore's disease
CC Excl: See code: A24.1

✓4th A25 Rat-bite fevers

CC Excl: For CC codes in category A25, unless otherwise noted: A25.0-A25.9

A25.0 Spirillosis CC
Sodoku

A25.1 Streptobacillosis CC
Epidemic arthritic erythema
Streptobacillary rat-bite fever
Haverhill fever

A25.9 Rat-bite fever, unspecified CC

✓4th A26 Erysipeloid

A26.0 Cutaneous erysipeloid
Erythema migrans

A26.7 Erysipelothrix sepsis PDx MCC MCC
CC Excl: A02.1, A20.7, A22.7, A26.7, A32.7, A39.2-A39.4, A40.0-A40.1, A40.8-A41.9, A42.7, A48.2-A48.4, A48.8-A49.9, A54.86, B00.7, B37.7, B92, B94.2-B96.89, M00.011-M00.012, M00.021-M00.022, M00.031- M00.032, M00.041-M00.042, M00.051-M00.052, M00.061-M00.062, M00.071-M00.072, R65.10-R65.20, Z16.10-Z16.39

A26.8 Other forms of erysipeloid

A26.9 Erysipeloid, unspecified

✓4th A27 Leptospirosis

CC Excl: For CC/MCC codes in category A27, unless otherwise noted: A27.0-A27.9

A27.0 Leptospirosis icterohemorrhagica CC
Leptospiral or spirochetal jaundice (hemorrhagic)
Weil's disease

✓5th A27.8 Other forms of leptospirosis

A27.81 Aseptic meningitis in leptospirosis MCC
CC Excl: A02.21, A17.0-A17.1, A27.0-A27.9, A39.0, A50.41, A51.41, A52.13, A54.82, A54.84, A54.89-A54.9, A74.81-A74.9, A87.0-A87.9, A96.2, A98.3-A98.4, B26.1, B33.24, B33.4-B33.8, B34.1-B34.2, B34.4-B34.8, B37.5, B38.4, B45.1, B58.2, B92, B94.2-B94.9, B97.10, B97.19, B97.29, B97.5-B97.6, B97.81-B97.89, G00.0-G03.9, G04.2, G32.89, G61.0, G96.8-G96.9, G98.0-G98.8, G99.8

A27.89 Other forms of leptospirosis CC

A27.9 Leptospirosis, unspecified CC

✓4th A28 Other zoonotic bacterial diseases, not elsewhere classified

CC Excl: For CC codes in category A28, unless otherwise noted: :A26.0, A26.8-A26.9, A28.0, A28.2-A28.9, A32.0-A32.12, A32.81-A32.9

A28.0 Pasteurellosis CC

A28.1 Cat-scratch disease CC
Cat-scratch fever
CC Excl: A28.1-B97.21

A28.2 Extraintestinal yersiniosis CC
EXCLUDES 1 *enteritis due to Yersinia enterocolitica (A04.6)*
plague (A20.-)

A28.8 Other specified zoonotic bacterial diseases, not elsewhere classified CC

A28.9 Zoonotic bacterial disease, unspecified CC

Other bacterial diseases (A30-A49)

✓4th A30 Leprosy [Hansen's disease]
INCLUDES infection due to Mycobacterium leprae
EXCLUDES 1 *sequelae of leprosy (B92)*

A30.0 Indeterminate leprosy CC
I leprosy
CC Excl: A30.0

A30.1 Tuberculoid leprosy CC
TT leprosy
CC Excl: A30.1

A30.2 Borderline tuberculoid leprosy CC
BT leprosy
CC Excl: A30.2-A30.4

A30.3 Borderline leprosy CC
BB leprosy
CC Excl: See code: A30.2

A30.4 Borderline lepromatous leprosy CC
BL leprosy
CC Excl: See code: A30.2

A30.5 Lepromatous leprosy CC
LL leprosy
CC Excl: A30.5

A30.8 Other forms of leprosy CC
CC Excl: A30.8

A30.9 Leprosy, unspecified CC
CC Excl: A30.9

✓4th A31 Infection due to other mycobacteria

CC Excl: For CC codes in category A31, unless otherwise noted: A31.0-A31.9

EXCLUDES 2 *leprosy (A30.-)*
tuberculosis (A15-A19)

A31.0 Pulmonary mycobacterial infection CC
Infection due to Mycobacterium avium
Infection due to Mycobacterium intracellulare [Battey bacillus]
Infection due to Mycobacterium kansasii
CC Excl: A15.0-A15.6, A15.8-A15.9, A17.9, A18.82, A18.84, A18.89, A22.1, A31.0, A31.2-A31.9, A37.01, A37.11, A37.81, A37.91, A48.1, A49.3-A49.9, B25.0, B44.0, B90.9, B92, B94.2-B94.9, B96.0, B96.6-B96.89, J09.X1-J09.X2, J10.00-J10.1, J11.00-J11.1, J12.0-J12.3, J12.89-J18.1, J18.8-J18.9, J44.9, J47.0-J70.4, J70.8-J70.9, J98.4, R91.1

A31.1 Cutaneous mycobacterial infection CC
Buruli ulcer
Infection due to Mycobacterium marinum
Infection due to Mycobacterium ulcerans

A31.2 Disseminated mycobacterium avium-intracellulare complex (DMAC) HIV CC
MAC sepsis

A31.8 Other mycobacterial infections HIV CC

A31.9 Mycobacterial infection, unspecified HIV CC
Atypical mycobacterial infection NOS
Mycobacteriosis NOS

✓4th A32 Listeriosis
INCLUDES listerial foodborne infection
EXCLUDES 1 *neonatal (disseminated) listeriosis (P37.2)*

CC Excl: For CC/MCC codes in category A32, unless otherwise noted: A26.0, A26.8-A26.9, A28.0, A28.2-A28.9, A32.0-A32.12, A32.81-A32.9

A32.0 Cutaneous listeriosis CC

✓5th A32.1 Listerial meningitis and meningoencephalitis

A32.11 Listerial meningitis CC

A32.12 Listerial meningoencephalitis CC

A32.7 Listerial sepsis PDx MCC MCC
CC Excl: A02.1, A20.7, A22.7, A26.7, A32.7, A39.2-A39.4, A40.0-A40.1, A40.8-A41.9, A42.7, A48.2-A48.4, A48.8-A49.9, A54.86, B00.7, B37.7, B92, B94.2-B96.89, M00.011-M00.012, M00.021-M00.022, M00.031- M00.032, M00.041-M00.042, M00.051-M00.052, M00.061-M00.062, M00.071-M00.072, R65.10-R65.20, Z16.10-Z16.39

✓5th A32.8 Other forms of listeriosis

A32.81 Oculoglandular listeriosis CC

A32.82 Listerial endocarditis CC

A32.89 Other forms of listeriosis CC
Listerial cerebral arteritis

A32.9 Listeriosis, unspecified CC

A33 Tetanus neonatorum MCC N
CC Excl: A33-P29.2, P29.4, P29.89-P29.9, P94.1-P94.9, P96.0, P96.3-P96.5, P96.82-P96.89

A34 Obstetrical tetanus CC M ♀
CC Excl: A34, O08.0, O08.2-O08.9, O20.0-O20.9, O25.10-O25.3, O26.10-O26.13, O26.30-O26.43, O26.63-O26.819, O26.841-O26.86, O26.891-O26.93, O29.011-O29.93, O35.7X-O35.7X, O44.00-O44.13, O45.8X1-O45.93, O75.4, O75.81, O75.89-O75.9, O80, O90.89, O99.111-O99.285, O99.330-O99.335, O99.350-O99.355, O99.511-O99.73, O99.820-O99.825, O99.840-O9A.53

A35 Other tetanus MCC
Tetanus NOS
EXCLUDES 1 *obstetrical tetanus (A34)*
tetanus neonatorum (A33)
CC Excl: A35, B92, B94.2-B94.9

A36 Diphtheria (4th)

CC Excl: For CC codes in category A36, unless otherwise noted: A36.0-A36.9

A36.0 Pharyngeal diphtheria CC
Diphtheritic membranous angina
Tonsillar diphtheria

A36.1 Nasopharyngeal diphtheria CC

A36.2 Laryngeal diphtheria CC
Diphtheritic laryngotracheitis

A36.3 Cutaneous diphtheria CC
EXCLUDES 2 *erythrasma (L08.1)*

A36.8 Other diphtheria (5th)

A36.81 Diphtheritic cardiomyopathy CC
Diphtheritic myocarditis
CC Excl: A36.81, A52.06, B33.20-B33.22, I00, I01.2-I01.9, I09.0, I09.9, I23.0-I23.3, I23.6-I23.8, I40.0-I41, I51.0, I51.4, I87.8, I99.8-I99.9

A36.82 Diphtheritic radiculomyelitis CC

A36.83 Diphtheritic polyneuritis CC

A36.84 Diphtheritic tubulo-interstitial nephropathy CC

A36.85 Diphtheritic cystitis CC

A36.86 Diphtheritic conjunctivitis CC

A36.89 Other diphtheritic complications CC
Diphtheritic peritonitis

A36.9 Diphtheria, unspecified CC

A37 Whooping cough (4th)

CC Excl: For CC/MCC codes in category A37, unless otherwise noted: For codes A37.00, A37.10, A37.80 and A37.90: A37.00-A37.91 **For codes A37.01, A37.11, A37.81 and A37.91:** A15.0-A15.6, A15.8-A15.9, A17.9, A18.82, A18.84, A18.89, A21.2, A22.1, A31.0, A37.00-A37.91, A42.0, A43.0, A48.1, B25.0, B39.0-B39.2, B44.0, B58.3, B59, B67.1, J09.X1-J09.X2, J10.00-J10.1, J11.00-J11.1, J12.0-J12.3, J12.89-J18.1, J18.8-J18.9, J22, J44.9, J47.0-J70.4, J70.8-J70.9, J98.4, J98.8-J99, Q33.4, R91.1

A37.0 Whooping cough due to Bordetella pertussis (5th)

A37.00 Whooping cough due to Bordetella pertussis without pneumonia CC

A37.01 Whooping cough due to Bordetella pertussis with pneumonia PDx MCC MCC

A37.1 Whooping cough due to Bordetella parapertussis (5th)

A37.10 Whooping cough due to Bordetella parapertussis without pneumonia CC

A37.11 Whooping cough due to Bordetella with parapertussispneumonia PDx MCC MCC

A37.8 Whooping cough due to other Bordetella species (5th)

A37.80 Whooping cough due to other Bordetella species without pneumonia CC

A37.81 Whooping cough due to other Bordetella species with pneumonia PDx MCC MCC

A37.9 Whooping cough, unspecified species (5th)

A37.90 Whooping cough, unspecified species without pneumonia CC

A37.91 Whooping cough, unspecified species with pneumonia PDx MCC MCC

A38 Scarlet fever (4th)
INCLUDES scarlatina
EXCLUDES 2 *streptococcal sore throat (J02.0)*

CC Excl: For MCC codes in category A38, unless otherwise noted: A38.0-A38.9, A46, J02.0, J03.00-J03.01

A38.0 Scarlet fever with otitis media CC

A38.1 Scarlet fever with myocarditis CC

A38.8 Scarlet fever with other complications CC

A38.9 Scarlet fever, uncomplicated CC
Scarlet fever, NOS

A39 Meningococcal infection (4th)

A39.0 Meningococcal meningitis MCC
CC Excl: A02.21, A17.0-A17.1, A27.81, A39.0, A39.89-A39.9, A49.3-A49.9, A50.41, A51.41, A52.13, A54.82, A54.84, A54.89-A54.9, A87.0-A87.9, B00.3, B02.1, B26.1, B37.5, B38.4, B45.1, B58.2, B92, B94.2-B94.9, B96.0, B96.6-B96.89, G00.0-G03.9, G04.2, G32.89, G61.0, G96.8-G96.9, G98.0-G98.8, G99.8

A39.1 Waterhouse-Friderichsen syndrome MCC
Meningococcal hemorrhagic adrenalitis
Meningococcic adrenal syndrome
CC Excl: A39.1, A39.89-A39.9, A49.3-A49.9, B92, B94.2-B94.9, B96.0, B96.6-B96.89

A39.2 Acute meningococcemia MCC
CC Excl: A02.1, A20.7, A22.7, A26.7, A32.7, A39.2-A39.4, A39.89-A40.1, A40.8-A41.9, A42.7, A49.3-A49.9, A54.86, B00.7, B37.7, B92, B94.2-B94.9, B96.0, B96.6-B96.89, R65.10-R65.20

A39.3 Chronic meningococcemia MCC
CC Excl: See code: A39.2

A39.4 Meningococcemia, unspecified MCC
CC Excl: See code: A39.2

A39.5 Meningococcal heart disease (5th)

A39.50 Meningococcal carditis, unspecified MCC
CC Excl: A39.50, A39.89-A39.9, A49.3-A49.9, B92, B94.2-B94.9, B96.0, B96.6-B96.89

A39.51 Meningococcal endocarditis MCC
CC Excl: A39.51, A39.89-A39.9, A49.3-A49.9, B92, B94.2-B94.9, B96.0, B96.6-B96.89

A39.52 Meningococcal myocarditis MCC
CC Excl:A39.52, A49.3-A49.9, B92, B94.2-B94.9, B96.0, B96.6-B96.89

A39.53 Meningococcal pericarditis MCC
CC Excl: A39.53, A39.89-A39.9, A49.3-A49.9, B92, B94.2-B94.9, B96.0, B96.6-B96.89

A39.8 Other meningococcal infections (5th)

A39.81 Meningococcal encephalitis MCC
CC Excl: A39.81, A39.89-A39.9, A49.3-A49.9, B92, B94.2-B94.9, B96.0, B96.6-B96.89

A39.82 Meningococcal retrobulbar neuritis CC
CC Excl: A39.82, A39.89-A39.9, A49.3-A49.9, B92, B94.2-B94.9, B96.0, B96.6-B96.89

A39.83 Meningococcal arthritis CC
CC Excl: A39.83-A39.9, A49.3-A49.9, B92, B94.2-B94.9, B96.0, B96.6-B96.89

A39.84 Postmeningococcal arthritis CC
CC Excl: See code: A39.83

A39.89 Other meningococcal infections CC
Meningococcal conjunctivitis
CC Excl: A39.89-A39.9, A49.3-A49.9, B92, B94.2-B94.9, B96.0, B96.6-B96.89

A39.9 Meningococcal infection, unspecified CC
Meningococcal disease NOS
CC Excl: See code: A39.89

A40 Streptococcal sepsis (4th)
Code first: postprocedural streptococcal sepsis (T81.4)
streptococcal sepsis during labor (O75.3)
streptococcal sepsis following abortion or ectopic or molar pregnancy (O03-O07, O08.0)
streptococcal sepsis following immunization (T88.0)
streptococcal sepsis following infusion, transfusion or therapeutic injection (T80.2-)
EXCLUDES 1 *neonatal (P36.0-P36.1)*
puerperal sepsis (O85)
sepsis due to Streptococcus, group D (A41.81)

CC Excl: For MCC codes in category A40, unless otherwise noted: A02.1, A20.7, A22.7, A26.7, A32.7, A39.2-A39.4, A40.0-A40.1, A40.8-A41.9, A42.7, A48.2-A48.4, A48.8-A49.9, A54.86, B00.7, B37.7, B92, B94.2-B96.89, M00.011-M00.012, M00.021-M00.022, M00.031-M00.032, M00.041-M00.042, M00.051- M00.052, M00.061-M00.062, M00.071-M00.072, R65.10-R65.20, Z16.10-Z16.39

A40.0 Sepsis due to streptococcus, group A MCC

A40.1 Sepsis due to streptococcus, group B MCC

A40.3 Sepsis due to Streptococcus pneumoniae MCC
Pneumococcal sepsis
CC Excl: No Excl

A40.8 Other streptococcal sepsis MCC

A40.9 Streptococcal sepsis, unspecified HIV MCC

4th A41 Other sepsis

Code first: postprocedural sepsis (T81.4)
sepsis during labor (O75.3)
sepsis following abortion, ectopic or molar pregnancy (OØ3-OØ7, OØ8.Ø)
sepsis following immunization (T88.Ø)
sepsis following infusion, transfusion or therapeutic injection (T8Ø.2-)

EXCLUDES 1 *bacteremia NOS (R78.81)*
neonatal (P36.-)
puerperal sepsis (O85)
sepsis NOS (A41.9)
streptococcal sepsis (A4Ø.-)

EXCLUDES 2 *sepsis (due to) (in) actinomycotic (A42.7)*
sepsis (due to) (in) anthrax (A22.7)
sepsis (due to) (in) candidal (B37.7)
sepsis (due to) (in) Erysipelothrix (A26.7)
sepsis (due to) (in) extraintestinal yersiniosis (A28.2)
sepsis (due to) (in) gonococcal (A54.86)
sepsis (due to) (in) herpesviral (BØØ.7)
sepsis (due to) (in) listerial (A32.7)
sepsis (due to) (in) melioidosis (A24.1)
sepsis (due to) (in) meningococcal (A39.2-A39.4)
sepsis (due to) (in) plague (A2Ø.7)
sepsis (due to) (in) tularemia (A21.7)
toxic shock syndrome (A48.3)

AHA: 2Ø14, 2Q, 13

CC Excl: For MCC codes in category A41, unless otherwise noted: AØ2.1, A2Ø.7, A22.7, A26.7, A32.7, A39.2-A39.4, A4Ø.Ø-A4Ø.1, A4Ø.8-A41.9, A42.7, A48.2-A48.4, A48.8-A49.9, A54.86, BØØ.7, B37.7, B92, B94.2-B96.89, MØØ.Ø11-MØØ.Ø12, MØØ.Ø21-MØØ.Ø22, MØØ.Ø31-MØØ.Ø32, MØØ.Ø41-MØØ.Ø42, MØØ.Ø51- MØØ.Ø52, MØØ.Ø61-MØØ.Ø62, MØØ.Ø71-MØØ.Ø72, R65.1Ø-R65.2Ø, Z16.1Ø-Z16.39

5th A41.Ø Sepsis due to Staphylococcus aureus

A41.Ø1 Sepsis due to methicillin susceptible Staphylococcus aureus HIV MCC
MSSA sepsis
Staphylococcus aureus sepsis NOS

A41.Ø2 Sepsis due to methicillin resistant Staphylococcus aureus HIV MCC

A41.1 Sepsis due to other specified staphylococcus HIV MCC
Coagulase negative staphylococcus sepsis

A41.2 Sepsis due to unspecified staphylococcus HIV MCC

A41.3 Sepsis due to Hemophilus influenzae HIV MCC

A41.4 Sepsis due to anaerobes HIV MCC
EXCLUDES 1 *gas gangrene (A48.Ø)*

5th A41.5 Sepsis due to other Gram-negative organisms

A41.5Ø Gram-negative sepsis, unspecified HIV MCC
Gram-negative sepsis NOS

A41.51 Sepsis due to Escherichia coli [E. coli] HIV MCC

A41.52 Sepsis due to Pseudomonas HIV MCC
Pseudomonas aeroginosa

A41.53 Sepsis due to Serratia HIV MCC

A41.59 Other Gram-negative sepsis HIV MCC

5th A41.8 Other specified sepsis

A41.81 Sepsis due to Enterococcus HIV MCC

A41.89 Other specified sepsis HIV MCC

A41.9 Sepsis, unspecified organism HIV MCC
Septicemia NOS

4th A42 Actinomycosis

EXCLUDES 1 *actinomycetoma (B47.1)*

A42.Ø Pulmonary actinomycosis HIV CC
CC Excl: A42.Ø, A42.81-A43.Ø, A43.8-A43.9, B47.1, J12.81

A42.1 Abdominal actinomycosis HIV CC
CC Excl: A42.1, A42.81-A42.9, A43.8-A43.9, B47.1

A42.2 Cervicofacial actinomycosis HIV CC
CC Excl: A42.2, A42.81-A42.9, A43.8-A43.9, B47.1

A42.7 Actinomycotic sepsis HIV MCC
CC Excl: AØ2.1, A2Ø.7, A22.7, A26.7, A32.7, A39.2-A39.4, A4Ø.Ø-A4Ø.1, A4Ø.8-A41.9, A42.7, A48.2-A48.4, A48.8-A49.9, A54.86, BØØ.7, B37.7, B92, B94.2-B96.89, MØØ.Ø11-MØØ.Ø12, MØØ.Ø21-MØØ.Ø22, MØØ.Ø31- MØØ.Ø32, MØØ.Ø41-MØØ.Ø42, MØØ.Ø51-MØØ.Ø52, MØØ.Ø61-MØØ.Ø62, MØØ.Ø71-MØØ.Ø72, R65.1Ø-R65.2Ø, Z16.1Ø-Z16.39

5th A42.8 Other forms of actinomycosis

CC Excl: For CC codes in subcategory A42.8, unless otherwise noted: A42.Ø-A42.2, A42.81-A43.9, B47.1-B47.9, LØ8.1

A42.81 Actinomycotic meningitis HIV CC

A42.82 Actinomycotic encephalitis HIV CC

A42.89 Other forms of actinomycosis HIV CC

A42.9 Actinomycosis, unspecified HIV CC
CC Excl: See code: A42.8

4th A43 Nocardiosis

A43.Ø Pulmonary nocardiosis HIV CC
CC Excl: A42.Ø, A42.81-A43.Ø, A43.8-A43.9, B47.1, J12.81

A43.1 Cutaneous nocardiosis HIV CC
CC Excl: A42.81-A42.9, A43.1-A43.9, B47.1, LØ8.1

A43.8 Other forms of nocardiosis HIV CC
CC Excl: A42.Ø-A42.2, A42.81-A43.9, B47.1-B47.9, LØ8.1

A43.9 Nocardiosis, unspecified HIV CC
CC Excl: See code: A43.8

4th A44 Bartonellosis

CC Excl: For CC codes in category A44, unless otherwise noted: A44.Ø-A44.9, A68.Ø-A68.9, A69.2Ø-A69.29, A75.Ø-A79.9, B55.Ø-B57.5, B6Ø.Ø

A44.Ø Systemic bartonellosis CC
Oroya fever

A44.1 Cutaneous and mucocutaneous bartonellosis CC
Verruga peruana

A44.8 Other forms of bartonellosis CC

A44.9 Bartonellosis, unspecified CC

A46 Erysipelas

EXCLUDES 1 *postpartum or puerperal erysipelas (O86.89)*

4th A48 Other bacterial diseases, not elsewhere classified

EXCLUDES 1 *actinomycetoma (B47.1)*

A48.Ø Gas gangrene MCC
Clostridial cellulitis
Clostridial myonecrosis
CC Excl: A48.Ø, B92, B94.2-B94.9

A48.1 Legionnaires' disease HIV MCC
CC Excl: A15.Ø-A15.6, A15.8-A15.9, A17.9, A18.82, A18.84, A18.89, A21.2, A22.1, A31.Ø, A37.Ø1, A37.11, A37.81, A37.91, A42.Ø, A43.Ø, A48.1, B25.Ø, B39.Ø-B39.2, B44.Ø, B58.3, B59, B67.1, JØ9.X1-JØ9.X2, J1Ø.ØØ-J1Ø.1, J11.ØØ-J11.1, J12.Ø-J12.3, J12.89-J18.1, J18.8-J18.9, J22, J44.9, J47.Ø-J7Ø.4, J7Ø.8-J7Ø.9, J98.4, J98.8-J99, Q33.4, R91.1

A48.2 Nonpneumonic Legionnaires' disease [Pontiac fever]

A48.3 Toxic shock syndrome MCC
Use additional code to identify the organism (B95, B96)
EXCLUDES 1 *endotoxic shock NOS (R57.8)*
sepsis NOS (A41.9)
CC Excl: A48.3, G89.Ø-G89.4, RØ9.89, R41.Ø-R41.3, R41.82, R41.9, R44.8-R44.9, R45.83-R45.84, R46.Ø-R46.89, R52, R57.Ø-R57.9, R65.21-R68.19, R68.81-R68.83, R68.89-R69

A48.4 Brazilian purpuric fever
Systemic Hemophilus aegyptius infection

5th A48.5 Other specified botulism
Non-foodborne intoxication due to toxins of Clostridium botulinum [C. botulinum]
EXCLUDES 1 *food poisoning due to toxins of Clostridium botulinum (AØ5.1)*

CC Excl: For CC codes in subcategory A48.5, unless otherwise noted: AØ4.7, AØ5.Ø-AØ5.2, A48.51-A48.52

A48.51 Infant botulism CC P

A48.52 Wound botulism CC
Non-foodborne botulism NOS
Use additional code for associated wound

A48.8 Other specified bacterial diseases

4th A49 Bacterial infection of unspecified site

EXCLUDES 1 *bacterial agents as the cause of diseases classified elsewhere (B95-B96)*
chlamydial infection NOS (A74.9)
meningococcal infection NOS (A39.9)
rickettsial infection NOS (A79.9)
spirochetal infection NOS (A69.9)

5th A49.Ø Staphylococcal infection, unspecified site

A49.Ø1 Methicillin susceptible Staphylococcus aureus infection, unspecified site
Methicillin susceptible Staphylococcus aureus (MSSA) infection
Staphylococcus aureus infection NOS

A49.02 Methicillin resistant Staphylococcus aureus infection, unspecified site
Methicillin resistant Staphylococcus aureus (MRSA) infection

A49.1 Streptococcal infection, unspecified site

A49.2 Hemophilus influenzae infection, unspecified site

A49.3 Mycoplasma infection, unspecified site

A49.8 Other bacterial infections of unspecified site

A49.9 Bacterial infection, unspecified
EXCLUDES 1 *bacteremia NOS (R78.81)*

Infections with a predominantly sexual mode of transmission (A50-A64)

EXCLUDES 1 *human immunodeficiency virus [HIV] disease (B20)*
nonspecific and nongonococcal urethritis (N34.1)
Reiter's disease (M02.3-)

✓4th A50 Congenital syphilis

✓5th A50.0 Early congenital syphilis, symptomatic
Any congenital syphilitic condition specified as early or manifest less than two years after birth.)

CC Excl: For CC codes in subcategory A50.0, unless otherwise noted: A50.01-A51.46, A51.5-A53.9

A50.01 Early congenital syphilitic oculopathy CC

A50.02 Early congenital syphilitic osteochondropathy CC

A50.03 Early congenital syphilitic pharyngitis CC
Early congenital syphilitic laryngitis

A50.04 Early congenital syphilitic pneumonia CC

A50.05 Early congenital syphilitic rhinitis CC

A50.06 Early cutaneous congenital syphilis CC

A50.07 Early mucocutaneous congenital syphilis CC

A50.08 Early visceral congenital syphilis CC

A50.09 Other early congenital syphilis, symptomatic CC

A50.1 Early congenital syphilis, latent
Congenital syphilis without clinical manifestations, with positive serological reaction and negative spinal fluid test, less than two years after birth.

A50.2 Early congenital syphilis, unspecified CC
Congenital syphilis NOS less than two years after birth.
CC Excl: A50.01-A51.46, A51.5-A54.85, A54.89-A58, A63.8-A64, B92, B94.2-B94.9, M02.30-M02.342

✓5th A50.3 Late congenital syphilitic oculopathy
EXCLUDES 1 *Hutchinson's triad (A50.53)*

CC Excl: For CC/MCC codes in subcategory A50.3, unless otherwise noted: A50.01-A51.46, A51.5-A53.9

A50.30 Late congenital syphilitic oculopathy, unspecified CC

A50.31 Late congenital syphilitic interstitial keratitis CC

A50.32 Late congenital syphilitic chorioretinitis CC

A50.39 Other late congenital syphilitic oculopathy CC

✓5th A50.4 Late congenital neurosyphilis [juvenile neurosyphilis]
Use additional code to identify any associated mental disorder
EXCLUDES 1 *Hutchinson's triad (A50.53)*

A50.40 Late congenital neurosyphilis, unspecified CC
Juvenile neurosyphilis NOS
CC Excl: A50.01-A51.46, A51.5-A53.9, A56.00-A56.8, A63.8-A64, B92, B94.2-B94.9, N34.1

A50.41 Late congenital syphilitic meningitis MCC
CC Excl: A02.21, A17.0-A17.1, A27.81, A39.0, A50.01-A51.46, A51.5-A53.9, A54.82, A54.84, A54.89-A54.9, A56.00-A56.8, A63.8-A64, A87.0-A87.9, B00.3, B02.1, B26.1, B37.5, B38.4, B45.1, B58.2, B92, B94.2-B94.9, G00.0-G03.9, G04.2, G32.89, G61.0, G96.8-G96.9, G98.0-G98.8, G99.8, N34.1

A50.42 Late congenital syphilitic encephalitis MCC
CC Excl: A50.01-A51.46, A51.5-A53.9, A56.00-A56.8, A63.8-A64, B92, B94.2-B94.9, N34.1

A50.43 Late congenital syphilitic polyneuropathy CC
CC Excl: See code: A50.42

A50.44 Late congenital syphilitic optic nerve atrophy CC
CC Excl: A50.01-A51.46, A51.5-A53.9

A50.45 Juvenile general paresis CC
Dementia paralytica juvenilis
Juvenile tabetoparetic neurosyphilis
CC Excl: See code: A50.40

A50.49 Other late congenital neurosyphilis CC
Juvenile tabes dorsalis
CC Excl: See code: A50.40

✓5th A50.5 Other late congenital syphilis, symptomatic
Any congenital syphilitic condition specified as late or manifest two years or more after birth.

CC Excl: For CC codes in subcategory A50.5, unless otherwise noted: A50.01-A51.46, A51.5-A53.9

A50.51 Clutton's joints CC

A50.52 Hutchinson's teeth CC

A50.53 Hutchinson's triad CC

A50.54 Late congenital cardiovascular syphilis CC

A50.55 Late congenital syphilitic arthropathy CC

A50.56 Late congenital syphilitic osteochondropathy CC

A50.57 Syphilitic saddle nose CC

A50.59 Other late congenital syphilis, symptomatic CC

A50.6 Late congenital syphilis, latent
Congenital syphilis without clinical manifestations, with positive serological reaction and negative spinal fluid test, two years or more after birth.

A50.7 Late congenital syphilis, unspecified
Congenital syphilis NOS two years or more after birth.

A50.9 Congenital syphilis, unspecified

✓4th A51 Early syphilis

A51.0 Primary genital syphilis
Syphilitic chancre NOS

A51.1 Primary anal syphilis

A51.2 Primary syphilis of other sites

✓5th A51.3 Secondary syphilis of skin and mucous membranes

A51.31 Condyloma latum CC
CC Excl: A50.01-A51.46, A51.5-A53.9

A51.32 Syphilitic alopecia CC
CC Excl: A50.01-A51.46, A51.5-A54.85, A54.89-A58, A63.8-A64, M02.30-M02.39, N34.1

A51.39 Other secondary syphilis of skin CC
Syphilitic leukoderma Syphilitic mucous patch
EXCLUDES 1 *late syphilitic leukoderma (A52.79)*
CC Excl: See code: A51.31

✓5th A51.4 Other secondary syphilis

A51.41 Secondary syphilitic meningitis MCC
CC Excl: A02.21, A17.0-A17.1, A27.81, A39.0, A50.01-A51.46, A51.5-A54.85, A54.89-A58, A63.8-A64, A74.81-A74.9, A87.0-A87.9, A96.2, A98.3-A98.4, B26.1, B33.24, B33.4-B33.8, B34.1-B34.2, B34.4-B34.8, B37.5, B38.4, B45.1, B58.2, B92, B94.2-B94.9, B97.10, B97.19, B97.29, B97.5-B97.6, B97.81-B97.89, G00.0-G03.9, G04.2, G32.89, G61.0, G96.8-G96.9, G98.0-G98.8, G99.8, M02.30-M02.39, N34.1

A51.42 Secondary syphilitic female pelvic disease CC ♀
CC Excl: A50.01-A51.46, A51.5-A54.85, A54.89-A58, A63.8-A64, B92, B94.2-B94.9, M02.30-M02.39, N34.1

A51.43 Secondary syphilitic oculopathy CC
Secondary syphilitic chorioretinitis
Secondary syphilitic iridocyclitis, iritis
Secondary syphilitic uveitis
CC Excl: A50.01-A51.46, A51.5-A53.9

A51.44 Secondary syphilitic nephritis CC
CC Excl: A50.01-A51.46, A51.5-A54.85, A54.89-A58, A63.8-A64, B92, B94.2-B94.9, M02.30-M02.39, N34.1

A51.45 Secondary syphilitic hepatitis CC
CC Excl: A50.01-A51.46, A51.5-A54.85, A54.89-A58, A63.8-A64, K71.0-K71.9, K73.1-K73.8, K74.0-K74.69, K75.2-K76.0, K76.4-K76.5, K76.89-K76.9, M02.30-M02.39, N34.1

A51.46 Secondary syphilitic osteopathy CC
CC Excl: A18.09, A50.01-A51.46, A51.5-A54.85, A54.89-A58, A63.8-A64, A66.6, M02.30-M02.39, M84.80-M84.9, M85.10-M85.19, M85.80-M85.89, M86.30-M86.8X9, M89.20-M89.39, M89.50-M89.59, M89.8X0-M89.8X9, M94.1, M94.351-M94.8X9, N34.1

A51.49 Other secondary syphilitic conditions CC
Secondary syphilitic lymphadenopathy
Secondary syphilitic myositis
CC Excl: No Excl

A51.5 Early syphilis, latent
Syphilis (acquired) without clinical manifestations, with positive serological reaction and negative spinal fluid test, less than two years after infection.

A51.9 Early syphilis, unspecified

A52 Late syphilis

A52.0 Cardiovascular and cerebrovascular syphilis

CC Excl: For CC codes in subcategory A52.0, unless otherwise noted: A50.01-A51.46, A51.5-A53.9, A56.00-A56.8, A63.8-A64, B92, B94.2-B94.9, N34.1

A52.00 Cardiovascular syphilis, unspecified CC

A52.01 Syphilitic aneurysm of aorta CC

A52.02 Syphilitic aortitis CC

A52.03 Syphilitic endocarditis CC
Syphilitic aortic valve incompetence or stenosis
Syphilitic mitral valve stenosis
Syphilitic pulmonary valve regurgitation

A52.04 Syphilitic cerebral arteritis CC

A52.05 Other cerebrovascular syphilis CC
Syphilitic cerebral aneurysm (ruptured) (non-ruptured)
Syphilitic cerebral thrombosis

A52.06 Other syphilitic heart involvement CC
Syphilitic coronary artery disease
Syphilitic myocarditis
Syphilitic pericarditis

A52.09 Other cardiovascular syphilis CC

A52.1 Symptomatic neurosyphilis

CC Excl: For CC/MCC codes in subcategory A52.1, unless otherwise noted: A50.01-A51.46, A51.5-A53.9, A56.00-A56.8, A63.8-A64, B92, B94.2-B94.9, N34.1

A52.10 Symptomatic neurosyphilis, unspecified CC

A52.11 Tabes dorsalis CC
Locomotor ataxia (progressive)
Tabetic neurosyphilis

A52.12 Other cerebrospinal syphilis CC

A52.13 Late syphilitic meningitis MCC
CC Excl: A02.21, A17.0-A17.1, A27.81, A39.0, A50.01-A51.46, A51.5-A53.9, A54.82, A54.84, A54.89-A54.9, A56.00-A56.8, A63.8-A64, A87.0-A87.9, B00.3, B02.1, B26.1, B37.5, B38.4, B45.1, B58.2, B92, B94.2-B94.9, G00.0-G03.9, G04.2, G32.89, G61.0, G96.8-G96.9, G98.0-G98.8, G99.8, N34.1

A52.14 Late syphilitic encephalitis MCC

A52.15 Late syphilitic neuropathy CC
Late syphilitic acoustic neuritis
Late syphilitic optic (nerve) atrophy
Late syphilitic polyneuropathy
Late syphilitic retrobulbar neuritis

A52.16 Charcôt's arthropathy (tabetic) CC

A52.17 General paresis CC
Dementia paralytica

A52.19 Other symptomatic neurosyphilis CC
Syphilitic parkinsonism

A52.2 Asymptomatic neurosyphilis CC
CC Excl: See code: A52.1

A52.3 Neurosyphilis, unspecified CC
Gumma (syphilitic) Syphiloma
Syphilis (late)
CC Excl: See code: A52.1

A52.7 Other symptomatic late syphilis

CC Excl: For CC codes in subcategory A52.7, unless otherwise noted: A50.01-A51.46, A51.5-A54.85, A54.89-A58, A63.8-A64, M02.30-M02.39, N34.1

A52.71 Late syphilitic oculopathy CC
Late syphilitic chorioretinitis
Late syphilitic episcleritis
CC Excl: A18.50-A18.59, A50.01-A51.46, A51.5-A54.85, A54.89-A58, A63.8-A64, H15.001-H15.009, H15.091-H15.129, M02.30-M02.39, N34.1

A52.72 Syphilis of lung and bronchus CC

A52.73 Symptomatic late syphilis of other respiratory organs CC

A52.74 Syphilis of liver and other viscera CC
Late syphilitic peritonitis

A52.75 Syphilis of kidney and ureter CC
Syphilitic glomerular disease

A52.76 Other genitourinary symptomatic late syphilis CC
Late syphilitic female pelvic inflammatory disease

A52.77 Syphilis of bone and joint CC

A52.78 Syphilis of other musculoskeletal tissue CC
Late syphilitic bursitis
Syphilis [stage unspecified] of bursa
Syphilis [stage unspecified] of muscle
Syphilis [stage unspecified] of synovium
Syphilis [stage unspecified] of tendon

A52.79 Other symptomatic late syphilis CC
Late syphilitic leukoderma
Syphilis of adrenal gland
Syphilis of pituitary gland
Syphilis of thyroid gland
Syphilitic splenomegaly
EXCLUDES 1 *syphilitic leukoderma (secondary) (A51.39)*

A52.8 Late syphilis, latent
Syphilis (acquired) without clinical manifestations, with positive serological reaction and negative spinal fluid test, two years or more after infection

A52.9 Late syphilis, unspecified

A53 Other and unspecified syphilis

A53.0 Latent syphilis, unspecified as early or late
Latent syphilis NOS Positive serological reaction for syphilis

A53.9 Syphilis, unspecified
Infection due to Treponema pallidum NOS
Syphilis (acquired) NOS
EXCLUDES 1 *syphilis NOS under two years of age (A50.2)*

A54 Gonococcal infection

A54.0 Gonococcal infection of lower genitourinary tract without periurethral or accessory gland abscess

CC Excl: For CC codes in subcategory A54.0, unless otherwise noted: A54.00-A54.29, A54.82, A54.84, A54.89-A54.9, A56.00-A56.8, A63.8-A64, B92, B94.2-B94.9, N34.1

EXCLUDES 1 *gonococcal infection with genitourinary gland abscess (A54.1)*
gonococcal infection with periurethral abscess (A54.1)

A54.00 Gonococcal infection of lower genitourinary tract, unspecified CC

A54.01 Gonococcal cystitis and urethritis, unspecified CC

A54.02 Gonococcal vulvovaginitis, unspecified CC ♀

A54.03 Gonococcal cervicitis, unspecified CC ♀

A54.09 Other gonococcal infection of lower genitourinary tract CC

A54.1 Gonococcal infection of lower genitourinary tract with periurethral and accessory gland abscess CC
Gonococcal Bartholin's gland abscess
CC Excl: See code: A54.0

A54.2 Gonococcal pelviperitonitis and other gonococcal genitourinary infection

CC Excl: For CC codes in subcategory A54.2, unless otherwise noted: A54.00-A54.29, A54.82, A54.84, A54.89-A54.9, A56.00-A56.8, A63.8-A64, B92, B94.2-B94.9, N34.1

A54.21 Gonococcal infection of kidney and ureter CC

A54.22 Gonococcal prostatitis CC ♂

A54.23 Gonococcal infection of other male genital organs CC ♂
Gonococcal epididymitis Gonococcal orchitis

A54.24 Gonococcal female pelvic inflammatory disease CC ♀
Gonococcal pelviperitonitis
EXCLUDES 1 *gonococcal peritonitis (A54.85)*

A54.29 Other gonococcal genitourinary infections CC

A54.3 Gonococcal infection of eye

CC Excl: For CC codes in subcategory A54.3, unless otherwise noted: A50.01-A51.46, A51.5-A54.85, A54.89-A58, A63.8-A64, M02.30-M02.39, N34.1

A54.30 Gonococcal infection of eye, unspecified CC

A54.31 Gonococcal conjunctivitis CC
Ophthalmia neonatorum due to gonococcus

A54.32 Gonococcal iridocyclitis CC

A54.33 Gonococcal keratitis CC

A54.39 Other gonococcal eye infection CC
Gonococcal endophthalmia

A54.4 Gonococcal infection of musculoskeletal system

CC Excl: For CC codes in subcategory A54.4, unless otherwise noted: A02.23, A17.9, A18.02, A18.09, A18.82, A18.84, A18.89, A39.83-A39.84, A50.01-A51.46, A51.5-A54.85, A54.89-A58, A63.8-A64, B06.82, M00.00, M00.19, M00.29, M00.39, M00.49, M00.59, M00.69, M00.79, M00.08-M02.9, M05.40-M05.59, M05.70-M06.09, M06.20-M06.39, M06.80-M07.69, M11.00-M11.9, M12.10-M15.0, M15.3-M15.9, M16.2-M16.9, M17.2-M17.9, M18.2-M18.9, M19.111-M19.93, M24.10-M24.176, M25.00, M25.08-M25.18, M25.40-M25.676, M25.80-M25.9, M35.2, M36.1-M36.4, N34.1, R29.4

A54.40 Gonococcal infection of musculoskeletal system, unspecified CC

A54.41 Gonococcal spondylopathy CC

A54.42 Gonococcal arthritis CC
EXCLUDES 2 *gonococcal infection of spine (A54.41)*

A54.43 Gonococcal osteomyelitis CC
EXCLUDES 2 *gonococcal infection of spine (A54.41)*

A54.49 Gonococcal infection of other musculoskeletal tissue CC
Gonococcal bursitis
Gonococcal myositis
Gonococcal synovitis
Gonococcal tenosynovitis

A54.5 Gonococcal pharyngitis

A54.6 Gonococcal infection of anus and rectum

A54.8 Other gonococcal infections

A54.81 Gonococcal meningitis MCC
CC Excl: A02.21, A17.0-A17.1, A27.81, A39.0, A50.01-A51.46, A51.5-A54.85, A54.89-A58, A63.8-A64, A74.81-A74.9, A87.0-A87.9, A96.2, A98.3-A98.4, B26.1, B33.24, B33.4-B33.8, B34.1-B34.2, B34.4-B34.8, B37.5, B38.4, B45.1, B58.2, B92, B94.2-B94.9, B97.10, B97.19, B97.29, B97.5-B97.6, B97.81-B97.89, G00.0-G03.9, G04.2, G32.89, G61.0, G96.8-G96.9, G98.0-G98.8, G99.8, M02.30-M02.39, N34.1

A54.82 Gonococcal brain abscess CC
CC Excl: A50.01-A51.46, A51.5-A54.85, A54.89-A58, A63.8-A64, M02.30-M02.39, N25.81-N25.89, N34.1

A54.83 Gonococcal heart infection CC
Gonococcal endocarditis
Gonococcal myocarditis
Gonococcal pericarditis
CC Excl: A01.00-A01.09, A39.51, A50.01-A51.46, A51.5-A54.85, A54.89-A58, A63.8-A64, A78, B33.20-B33.22, B37.6, B40.0-B40.9, I00, I01.1-I02.0, I05.0-I07.9, I08.1-I08.3, I08.9-I09.1, I09.89-I09.9, I23.0-I23.3, I23.6-I23.8, I33.0-I41, I42.4, I51.0, I51.4, I87.8, I99.8-I99.9, M00.00, M00.08-M00.10, M00.18-M00.20, M00.28-M00.80, M00.88-M00.9, M02.30-M02.39, N34.1, Q22.2, Q23.8-Q23.9, Q24.8, T82.6XXA

A54.84 Gonococcal pneumonia CC
CC Excl: See code: A54.82

A54.85 Gonococcal peritonitis CC
EXCLUDES 1 *gonococcal pelviperitonitis (A54.24)*
CC Excl: A18.31-A34, A50.01-A51.46, A51.5-A54.85, A54.89-A58, A63.8-A64, K35.2-K35.3, K63.4, K63.89-K63.9, K65.1, K65.3, K65.9, K67, K86.8, K92.89-K92.9, M02.30-M02.39, N34.1, N73.3-N73.4, N73.6, O08.0, O08.82, O85, O86.12, O86.81-O86.89, P78.0, R11.13, T81.60XA, T81.61XA, T81.69XA

A54.86 Gonococcal sepsis PDx MCC MCC
CC Excl: A02.1, A20.7, A22.7, A26.7, A32.7, A39.2-A39.4, A40.0-A40.1, A40.8-A41.9, A42.7, A48.2-A48.4, A48.8-A49.9, A54.86, B00.7, B37.7, B92, B94.2-B96.89, M00.011-M00.012, M00.021-M00.022, M00.031- M00.032, M00.041-M00.042, M00.051- M00.052, M00.061-M00.062, M00.071-M00.072, R65.10-R65.20, Z16.10-Z16.39

A54.89 Other gonococcal infections CC
Gonococcal keratoderma
Gonococcal lymphadenitis
CC Excl: See code: A54.82

A54.9 Gonococcal infection, unspecified CC
CC Excl: See code: A54.82

A55 Chlamydial lymphogranuloma (venereum)
Climatic or tropical bubo
Durand-Nicolas-Favre disease
Esthiomene
Lymphogranuloma inguinale

A56 Other sexually transmitted chlamydial diseases
INCLUDES sexually transmitted diseases due to Chlamydia trachomatis
EXCLUDES 1 *neonatal chlamydial conjunctivitis (P39.1)*
neonatal chlamydial pneumonia (P23.1)
EXCLUDES 2 *chlamydial lymphogranuloma (A55)*
conditions classified to A74-

A56.0 Chlamydial infection of lower genitourinary tract

A56.00 Chlamydial infection of lower genitourinary tract, unspecified

A56.01 Chlamydial cystitis and urethritis

A56.02 Chlamydial vulvovaginitis ♀

A56.09 Other chlamydial infection of lower genitourinary tract
Chlamydial cervicitis

A56.1 Chlamydial infection of pelviperitoneum and other genitourinary organs

A56.11 Chlamydial female pelvic inflammatory disease ♀

A56.19 Other chlamydial genitourinary infection
Chlamydial epididymitis
Chlamydial orchitis

A56.2 Chlamydial infection of genitourinary tract, unspecified

A56.3 Chlamydial infection of anus and rectum

A56.4 Chlamydial infection of pharynx

A56.8 Sexually transmitted chlamydial infection of other sites

A57 Chancroid
Ulcus molle

A58 Granuloma inguinale
Donovanosis

A59 Trichomoniasis
EXCLUDES 2 *intestinal trichomoniasis (A07.8)*

A59.0 Urogenital trichomoniasis

A59.00 Urogenital trichomoniasis, unspecified
Fluor (vaginalis) due to Trichomonas
Leukorrhea (vaginalis) due to Trichomonas

A59.01 Trichomonal vulvovaginitis ♀

A59.02 Trichomonal prostatitis ♂

A59.03 Trichomonal cystitis and urethritis

A59.09 Other urogenital trichomoniasis
Trichomonas cervicitis

A59.8 Trichomoniasis of other sites

A59.9 Trichomoniasis, unspecified

A60 Anogenital herpesviral [herpes simplex] infections

A60.0 Herpesviral infection of genitalia and urogenital tract

A60.00 Herpesviral infection of urogenital system, unspecified HIV

A60.01 Herpesviral infection of penis HIV ♂

A60.02 Herpesviral infection of other male genital organs ♂

A60.03 Herpesviral cervicitis ♀

A60.04 Herpesviral vulvovaginitis HIV ♀
Herpesviral [herpes simplex] ulceration
Herpesviral [herpes simplex] vaginitis
Herpesviral [herpes simplex] vulvitis

A60.09 Herpesviral infection of other urogenital tract HIV

A60.1 Herpesviral infection of perianal skin and rectum HIV

A60.9 Anogenital herpesviral infection, unspecified HIV

A63 Other predominantly sexually transmitted diseases, not elsewhere classified
EXCLUDES 2 *molluscum contagiosum (B08.1)*
papilloma of cervix (D26.0)

A63.0 Anogenital (venereal) warts
Anogenital warts due to (human) papillomavirus [HPV]
Condyloma acuminatum

A63.8 Other specified predominantly sexually transmitted diseases

A64 Unspecified sexually transmitted disease

Other spirochetal diseases (A65-A69)

EXCLUDES 2 *leptospirosis (A27.-)*
syphilis (A50-A53)

A65 Nonvenereal syphilis
Bejel
Endemic syphilis
Njovera

✓4th **A66 Yaws**
INCLUDES bouba
frambesia (tropica)
pian

A66.0 Initial lesions of yaws
Chancre of yaws
Frambesia, initial or primary
Initial frambesial ulcer
Mother yaw

A66.1 Multiple papillomata and wet crab yaws
Frambesioma
Pianoma
Plantar or palmar papilloma of yaws

A66.2 Other early skin lesions of yaws
Cutaneous yaws, less than five years after infection
Early yaws (cutaneous) (macular) (maculopapular) (micropapular) (papular)
Frambeside of early yaws

A66.3 Hyperkeratosis of yaws
Ghoul hand
Hyperkeratosis, palmar or plantar (early) (late) due to yaws
Worm-eaten soles

A66.4 Gummata and ulcers of yaws
Gummatous frambeside
Nodular late yaws (ulcerated)

A66.5 Gangosa
Rhinopharyngitis mutilans

A66.6 Bone and joint lesions of yaws
Yaws ganglion
Yaws goundou
Yaws gumma, bone
Yaws gummatous osteitis or periostitis
Yaws hydrarthrosis
Yaws osteitis
Yaws periostitis (hypertrophic)

A66.7 Other manifestations of yaws
Juxta-articular nodules of yaws
Mucosal yaws

A66.8 Latent yaws
Yaws without clinical manifestations, with positive serology

A66.9 Yaws, unspecified

✓4th **A67 Pinta [carate]**

A67.0 Primary lesions of pinta
Chancre (primary) of pinta
Papule (primary) of pinta

A67.1 Intermediate lesions of pinta
Erythematous plaques of pinta
Hyperchromic lesions of pinta
Hyperkeratosis of pinta
Pintids

A67.2 Late lesions of pinta
Achromic skin lesions of pinta
Cicatricial skin lesions of pinta
Dyschromic skin lesions of pinta

A67.3 Mixed lesions of pinta
Achromic with hyperchromic skin lesions of pinta [carate]

A67.9 Pinta, unspecified

✓4th **A68 Relapsing fevers**
INCLUDES recurrent fever
EXCLUDES 2 *Lyme disease (A69.2-)*

CC Excl: For CC codes in category A68, unless otherwise noted: A44.0-A44.9, A68.0-A68.9, A69.20-A69.29, A75.0-A79.9, B55.0-B57.5, B60.0

A68.0 Louse-borne relapsing fever CC
Relapsing fever due to Borrelia recurrentis

A68.1 Tick-borne relapsing fever CC
Relapsing fever due to any Borrelia species other than Borrelia recurrentis

A68.9 Relapsing fever, unspecified CC

✓4th **A69 Other spirochetal infections**

A69.0 Necrotizing ulcerative stomatitis
Cancrum oris
Fusospirochetal gangrene
Noma
Stomatitis gangrenosa

A69.1 Other Vincent's infections CC
Fusospirochetal pharyngitis
Necrotizing ulcerative (acute) gingivitis
Necrotizing ulcerative (acute) gingivostomatitis
Spirochetal stomatitis
Trench mouth
Vincent's angina
Vincent's gingivitis
CC Excl: A69.1

✓5th **A69.2 Lyme disease**
Erythema chronicum migrans due to Borrelia burgdorferi

CC Excl: For CC codes in subcategory A69.2, unless otherwise noted: A44.0-A44.9, A68.0-A68.9, A69.20-A69.29, A75.0-A79.9, B55.0-B57.5, B60.0

A69.20 Lyme disease, unspecified CC
A69.21 Meningitis due to Lyme disease CC
A69.22 Other neurologic disorders in Lyme disease CC
Cranial neuritis
Meningoencephalitis
Polyneuropathy
A69.23 Arthritis due to Lyme disease CC
A69.29 Other conditions associated with Lyme disease CC
Myopericarditis due to Lyme disease

A69.8 Other specified spirochetal infections
A69.9 Spirochetal infection, unspecified

Other diseases caused by chlamydiae (A70-A74)

EXCLUDES 1 *sexually transmitted chlamydial diseases (A55-A56)*

A70 Chlamydia psittaci infections CC
Ornithosis
Parrot fever
Psittacosis
CC Excl: A70

✓4th **A71 Trachoma**
EXCLUDES 1 *sequelae of trachoma (B94.0)*

A71.0 Initial stage of trachoma
Trachoma dubium

A71.1 Active stage of trachoma
Granular conjunctivitis (trachomatous)
Trachomatous follicular conjunctivitis
Trachomatous pannus

A71.9 Trachoma, unspecified

✓4th **A74 Other diseases caused by chlamydiae**
EXCLUDES 1 *neonatal chlamydial conjunctivitis (P39.1)*
neonatal chlamydial pneumonia (P23.1)
Reiter's disease (M02.3-)
sexually transmitted chlamydial diseases (A55-A56)
EXCLUDES 2 *chlamydial pneumonia (J16.0)*

A74.0 Chlamydial conjunctivitis
Paratrachoma

✓5th **A74.8 Other chlamydial diseases**
A74.81 Chlamydial peritonitis
A74.89 Other chlamydial diseases

A74.9 Chlamydial infection, unspecified
Chlamydiosis NOS

Rickettsioses (A75-A79)

✓4th **A75 Typhus fever**
EXCLUDES 1 *rickettsiosis due to Ehrlichia sennetsu (A79.81)*

CC Excl: For CC codes in category A75, unless otherwise noted: A44.0-A44.9, A68.0-A68.9, A69.20-A69.29, A75.0-A79.9, B55.0-B57.5, B60.0

A75.0 Epidemic louse-borne typhus fever due to Rickettsia prowazekii CC
Classical typhus (fever)
Epidemic (louse-borne) typhus

A75.1 Recrudescent typhus [Brill's disease] CC
Brill-Zinsser disease

A75.2 Typhus fever due to Rickettsia typhi CC
Murine (flea-borne) typhus

A75.3 Typhus fever due to Rickettsia tsutsugamushi CC
Scrub (mite-borne) typhus
Tsutsugamushi fever

A75.9 Typhus fever, unspecified CC
Typhus (fever) NOS
CC Excl: A17.82, A44.Ø-A44.9, A5Ø.42, A52.14, A68.Ø-A68.9, A69.2Ø-A69.29, A75.Ø-A79.9, A81.1, A81.82-A81.89, A83.Ø-A85.8, A87.2, A88.Ø, A88.8, A92.1-A92.8, A93.Ø, BØØ.4, BØØ.82, BØ1.11-BØ1.12, BØ4, BØ6.Ø1, BØ8.Ø9, BØ8.2Ø-BØ8.22, BØ8.6Ø-BØ8.79, BØ9-B1Ø.Ø9, B26.2, B33.1, B45.Ø, B45.2-B45.9, B5Ø.9, B55.Ø-B57.5, B58.2, B6Ø.Ø, B75, B97.1Ø, B97.21, GØ4.ØØ-GØ4.Ø1, GØ4.31, GØ4.81-GØ5.4, G37.Ø, G37.4-G37.5, JØ9.X3-JØ9.X9, J1Ø.2-J1Ø.89, J11.2-J11.89, L44.4, M1A.1Ø-M1A.19, P35.2-P35.9, P37.Ø-P37.4, P37.8-P37.9, T56.ØX1-T56.ØX4 with 7th character A

✓4th **A77 Spotted fever [tick-borne rickettsioses]**

CC Excl: For CC codes in category A77, unless otherwise noted: A44.Ø-A44.9, A68.Ø-A68.9, A69.2Ø-A69.29, A75.Ø-A79.9, B55.Ø-B57.5, B6Ø.Ø

A77.Ø Spotted fever due to Rickettsia rickettsii CC
Rocky Mountain spotted fever
Sao Paulo fever

A77.1 Spotted fever due to Rickettsia conorii CC
African tick typhus
Boutonneuse fever
India tick typhus
Kenya tick typhus
Marseilles fever
Mediterranean tick fever

A77.2 Spotted fever due to Rickettsia siberica CC
North Asian tick fever
Siberian tick typhus

A77.3 Spotted fever due to Rickettsia australis CC
Queensland tick typhus

✓5th **A77.4 Ehrlichiosis**
EXCLUDES1 *Rickettsiosis due to Ehrlichia sennetsu (A79.81)*

A77.4Ø Ehrlichiosis, unspecified CC
A77.41 Ehrlichiosis chafeensis [E. chafeensis] CC
A77.49 Other ehrlichiosis CC

A77.8 Other spotted fevers CC
A77.9 Spotted fever, unspecified CC
Tick-borne typhus NOS

A78 Q fever CC
Infection due to Coxiella burnetii
Nine Mile fever
Quadrilateral fever
CC Excl: See code: A77

✓4th **A79 Other rickettsioses**

A79.Ø Trench fever CC
Quintan fever Wolhynian fever
CC Excl: See code: A77

A79.1 Rickettsialpox due to Rickettsia akari CC
Kew Garden fever Vesicular rickettsiosis
CC Excl: A77.Ø-A79.9

✓5th **A79.8 Other specified rickettsioses**

A79.81 Rickettsiosis due to Ehrlichia sennetsu CC
CC Excl: See code: A79.1

A79.89 Other specified rickettsioses CC
CC Excl: See code: A79.1

A79.9 Rickettsiosis, unspecified CC
Rickettsial infection NOS
CC Excl: See code: A79.1

Viral and prion infections of the central nervous system (A8Ø-A89)

EXCLUDES1 *postpolio syndrome (G14)*
sequelae of poliomyelitis (B91)
sequelae of viral encephalitis (B94.1)

✓4th **A8Ø Acute poliomyelitis**

CC Excl: For MCC codes in category A8Ø, unless otherwise noted: A8Ø.Ø-A8Ø.39

A8Ø.Ø Acute paralytic poliomyelitis, vaccine-associated MCC
A8Ø.1 Acute paralytic poliomyelitis, wild virus, imported MCC
A8Ø.2 Acute paralytic poliomyelitis, wild virus, indigenous MCC

✓5th **A8Ø.3 Acute paralytic poliomyelitis, other and unspecified**

A8Ø.3Ø Acute paralytic poliomyelitis, unspecified MCC
A8Ø.39 Other acute paralytic poliomyelitis MCC

A8Ø.4 Acute nonparalytic poliomyelitis
A8Ø.9 Acute poliomyelitis, unspecified

✓4th **A81 Atypical virus infections of central nervous system**
INCLUDES diseases of the central nervous system caused by prions
Use additional code to identify:
dementia with behavioral disturbance (FØ2.81)
dementia without behavioral disturbance (FØ2.8Ø)

✓5th **A81.Ø Creutzfeldt-Jakob disease**

A81.ØØ Creutzfeldt-Jakob disease, unspecified CC
Jakob-Creutzfeldt disease, unspecified
CC Excl: A17.82, A5Ø.42, A52.14, A75.9, A79.9, A81.ØØ-A81.9, A83.Ø-A85.8, A87.2, A88.Ø, A88.8, A92.1-A92.2, A92.4-A92.8, A93.Ø, BØØ.4, BØØ.82, BØ1.11-BØ1.12, BØ4, BØ6.Ø1, BØ8.Ø9, BØ8.2Ø-BØ8.22, BØ8.6Ø-BØ8.79, BØ9-B1Ø.Ø9, B26.2, B33.1, B45.Ø, B45.2-B45.9, B58.2, B75, B97.1Ø, GØ4.ØØ-GØ4.Ø1, GØ4.31, GØ4.81-GØ5.4, G37.Ø, G37.4-G37.5, I67.3, JØ9.X3-JØ9.X9, J1Ø.2-J1Ø.89, J11.2-J11.89, L44.4, M1A.1Ø-M1A.19, P35.2-P35.9, P37.Ø-P37.4, P37.8-P37.9, T56.ØX1-T56.ØX4A

A81.Ø1 Variant Creutzfeldt-Jakob disease CC
vCJD
CC Excl: See code: A81.ØØ

A81.Ø9 Other Creutzfeldt-Jakob disease CC
CJD
Familial Creutzfeldt-Jakob disease
Iatrogenic Creutzfeldt-Jakob disease
Sporadic Creutzfeldt-Jakob disease
Subacute spongiform encephalopathy (with dementia)
CC Excl: See code: A81.ØØ

A81.1 Subacute sclerosing panencephalitis CC
Dawson's inclusion body encephalitis
Van Bogaert's sclerosing leukoencephalopathy
CC Excl: A81.1, B92, B94.2-B94.9

A81.2 Progressive multifocal leukoencephalopathy HIV CC
Multifocal leukoencephalopathy NOS
CC Excl: A17.82, A5Ø.42, A52.14, A75.9, A79.9, A81.ØØ-A81.9, A83.Ø-A85.8, A87.2, A88.Ø, A88.8, A92.1-A92.2, A92.4-A92.8, A93.Ø, BØØ.4, BØØ.82, BØ1.11-BØ1.12, BØ4, BØ6.Ø1, BØ8.Ø9, BØ8.2Ø-BØ8.22, BØ8.6Ø-BØ8.79, BØ9-B1Ø.Ø9, B26.2, B27.ØØ-B27.99, B33.1, B45.Ø, B45.2-B45.9, B58.2, B75, GØ4.ØØ-GØ4.Ø1, GØ4.31, GØ4.81-GØ5.4, G37.Ø, G37.4-G37.5, I67.3, JØ9.X3-JØ9.X9, J1Ø.2-J1Ø.89, J11.2-J11.89, L44.4, M1A.1ØXØ-M1A.19X1, P35.2-P35.9, P37.Ø-P37.4, P37.8-P37.9, T56.ØX1A, T56.ØX2A, T56.ØX3A, T56.ØX4A

✓5th **A81.8 Other atypical virus infections of central nervous system**

A81.81 Kuru CC
CC Excl: A81.ØØ-A81.9, I67.3

A81.82 Gerstmann-Sträussler-Scheinker syndrome HIV CC
GSS syndrome
CC Excl: A81.ØØ-A81.9, A92.3Ø-A92.39, B97.21, I67.3

A81.83 Fatal familial insomnia HIV CC
FFI
CC Excl: See code: A81.82

A81.89 Other atypical virus infections of central nervous system HIV CC
CC Excl: See code: A81.82

A81.9 Atypical virus infection of central nervous system, unspecified HIV CC
Prion diseases of the central nervous system NOS
CC Excl: See code: A81.81

✓4th **A82 Rabies**

CC Excl: For CC codes in category A82, unless otherwise noted: A82.Ø-A82.9

A82.Ø Sylvatic rabies CC
A82.1 Urban rabies CC
A82.9 Rabies, unspecified CC

✓4th **A83 Mosquito-borne viral encephalitis**
INCLUDES mosquito-borne viral meningoencephalitis
EXCLUDES2 *Venezuelan equine encephalitis (A92.2)*
West Nile fever (A92.3-)
West Nile virus (A92.3-)

CC Excl: For MCC codes in category A83, unless otherwise noted: A17.82, A5Ø.42, A52.14, A75.9, A79.9, A81.1, A81.82-A81.89, A83.Ø-A85.8, A87.2, A88.Ø, A88.8, A92.1-A92.8, A93.Ø, BØØ.4, BØØ.82, BØ1.11-BØ1.12, BØ4, BØ6.Ø1, BØ8.Ø9, BØ8.2Ø-BØ8.22, BØ8.6Ø-BØ8.79, BØ9-B1Ø.Ø9, B26.2, B27.ØØ-B27.99, B33.1, B45.Ø, B45.2-B45.9, B58.2, B75, B97.1Ø, B97.21, GØ4.ØØ-GØ4.Ø1, GØ4.31, GØ4.81-GØ5.4, G37.Ø, G37.4-G37.5, JØ9.X3-JØ9.X9, J1Ø.2-J1Ø.89, J11.2-J11.89, L44.4, M1A.1ØXØ-M1A.19X1, P35.2-P35.9, P37.Ø-P37.4, P37.8-P37.9, T56.ØX1A, T56.ØX2A, T56.ØX3A, T56.ØX4A

A83.Ø Japanese encephalitis MCC
A83.1 Western equine encephalitis MCC

A83.2 Eastern equine encephalitis MCC

A83.3 St Louis encephalitis MCC

A83.4 Australian encephalitis MCC
Kunjin virus disease

A83.5 California encephalitis MCC
California meningoencephalitis
La Crosse encephalitis

A83.6 Rocio virus disease MCC

A83.8 Other mosquito-borne viral encephalitis MCC

A83.9 Mosquito-borne viral encephalitis, unspecified MCC

✓4th **A84 Tick-borne viral encephalitis**
INCLUDES tick-borne viral meningoencephalitis

CC Excl: For MCC codes in category A84, unless otherwise noted: A17.82, A5Ø.42, A52.14, A75.9, A79.9, A81.1, A81.82-A81.89, A83.Ø-A85.8, A87.2, A88.Ø, A88.8, A92.1-A92.8, A93.Ø, BØØ.4, BØØ.82, BØ1.11-BØ1.12, BØ4, BØ6.Ø1, BØ8.Ø9, BØ8.2Ø-BØ8.22, BØ8.6Ø-BØ8.79, BØ9-B1Ø.Ø9, B26.2, B27.ØØ-B27.99, B33.1, B45.Ø, B45.2-B45.9, B58.2, B75, B97.1Ø, B97.21, GØ4.ØØ-GØ4.Ø1, GØ4.31, GØ4.81-GØ5.4, G37.Ø, G37.4-G37.5, JØ9.X3-JØ9.X9, J1Ø.2-J1Ø.89, J11.2-J11.89, L44.4, M1A.1ØXØ-M1A.19X1, P35.2-P35.9, P37.Ø-P37.4, P37.8-P37.9, T56.ØX1A, T56.ØX2A, T56.ØX3A, T56.ØX4A

A84.Ø Far Eastern tick-borne encephalitis [Russian spring-summer encephalitis] MCC

A84.1 Central European tick-borne encephalitis MCC

A84.8 Other tick-borne viral encephalitis MCC
Louping ill
Powassan virus disease

A84.9 Tick-borne viral encephalitis, unspecified MCC

✓4th **A85 Other viral encephalitis, not elsewhere classified**
INCLUDES specified viral encephalomyelitis NEC
specified viral meningoencephalitis NEC
EXCLUDES 1 *benign myalgic encephalomyelitis (G93.3)*
encephalitis due to cytomegalovirus (B25.8)
encephalitis due to herpesvirus NEC (B1Ø.Ø-)
encephalitis due to herpesvirus [herpes simplex] (BØØ.4)
encephalitis due to measles virus (BØ5.Ø)
encephalitis due to mumps virus (B26.2)
encephalitis due to poliomyelitis virus (A8Ø.-)
encephalitis due to zoster (BØ2.Ø)
lymphocytic choriomeningitis (A87.2)

CC Excl: For CC/MCC codes in category A85, unless otherwise noted: A17.82, A5Ø.42, A52.14, A75.9, A79.9, A81.1, A81.82-A81.89, A83.Ø-A85.8, A87.2, A88.Ø, A88.8, A92.1-A92.8, A93.Ø, BØØ.4, BØØ.82, BØ1.11-BØ1.12, BØ4, BØ6.Ø1, BØ8.Ø9, BØ8.2Ø-BØ8.22, BØ8.6Ø-BØ8.79, BØ9-B1Ø.Ø9, B26.2, B27.ØØ-B27.99, B33.1, B45.Ø, B45.2-B45.9, B58.2, B75, B97.1Ø, B97.21, GØ4.ØØ-GØ4.Ø1, GØ4.31, GØ4.81-GØ5.4, G37.Ø, G37.4-G37.5, H66.4Ø-H66.43, JØ9.X3-JØ9.X9, J1Ø.2-J1Ø.89, J11.2-J11.89, L44.4, M1A.1ØXØ-M1A.19X1, M32.Ø-M32.9, P35.2-P35.9, P37.Ø-P37.4, P37.8-P37.9, T56.ØX1A, T56.ØX2A, T56.ØX3A, T56.ØX4A

A85.Ø Enteroviral encephalitis HIV CC
Enteroviral encephalomyelitis

A85.1 Adenoviral encephalitis HIV CC
Adenoviral meningoencephalitis

A85.2 Arthropod-borne viral encephalitis, unspecified MCC
EXCLUDES 1 *West nile virus with encephalitis (A92.31)*

A85.8 Other specified viral encephalitis HIV CC
Encephalitis lethargica
Von Economo-Cruchet disease

A86 Unspecified viral encephalitis HIV CC
Viral encephalomyelitis NOS
Viral meningoencephalitis NOS
CC Excl: A17.82, A5Ø.42, A52.14, A75.9, A79.9, A81.1, A81.82-A81.89, A83.Ø-A86, A87.2, A88.Ø, A88.8-A89, A92.1-A92.2, A92.4-A92.8, A93.Ø, BØØ.4, BØØ.82, BØ1.11-BØ1.12, BØ4, BØ6.Ø1, BØ8.Ø9, BØ8.2Ø-BØ8.22, BØ8.6Ø-BØ8.79, BØ9-B1Ø.Ø9, B26.2, B27.ØØ-B27.99, B33.1, B45.Ø, B45.2-B45.9, B58.2, B75, B97.1Ø, GØ4.ØØ-GØ4.Ø1, GØ4.31, GØ4.81-GØ5.4, G37.Ø, G37.4-G37.5, H66.4Ø-H66.43, JØ9.X3-JØ9.X9, J1Ø.2-J1Ø.89, J11.2-J11.89, L44.4, M1A.1ØXØ-M1A.19X1, M32.Ø-M32.9, P35.2-P35.9, P37.Ø-P37.4, P37.8-P37.9, T56.ØX1A, T56.ØX2A, T56.ØX3A, T56.ØX4A

✓4th **A87 Viral meningitis**
EXCLUDES 1 *meningitis due to herpesvirus [herpes simplex] (BØØ.3)*
meningitis due to measles virus (BØ5.1)
meningitis due to mumps virus (B26.1)
meningitis due to poliomyelitis virus (A8Ø.-)
meningitis due to zoster (BØ2.1)

CC Excl: For CC/MCC codes in category A87, unless otherwise noted: AØ2.21, A17.Ø-A17.1, A27.81, A39.Ø, A5Ø.41, A51.41, A52.13, A54.82, A54.84, A54.89-A54.9, A74.81-A74.9, A87.Ø-A87.9, A96.2, A98.3-A98.4, B26.1, B33.24, B33.4-B33.8, B34.1-B34.2, B34.4-B34.8, B37.5, B38.4, B45.1, B58.2, B92, B94.2-B94.9, B97.1Ø, B97.19, B97.29, B97.5-B97.6, B97.81-B97.89, GØØ.Ø-GØ3.9, GØ4.2, G32.89, G61.Ø, G96.8-G96.9, G98.Ø-G98.8, G99.8

A87.Ø Enteroviral meningitis CC
Coxsackievirus meningitis
Echovirus meningitis

A87.1 Adenoviral meningitis CC

A87.2 Lymphocytic choriomeningitis CC
Lymphocytic meningoencephalitis
CC Excl: AØ2.21, A17.Ø-A17.1, A27.81, A39.Ø, A5Ø.41, A51.41, A52.13, A54.82, A54.84, A54.89-A54.9, A74.81-A74.9, A87.Ø-A87.9, A92.3Ø-A92.39, A96.2, A98.3-A98.4, B26.1, B33.24, B33.4-B33.8, B34.1-B34.2, B34.4-B34.8, B37.5, B38.4, B45.1, B58.2, B92, B94.2-B94.9, B97.1Ø, B97.19-B97.29, B97.5-B97.6, B97.81-B97.89, GØØ.Ø-GØ3.9, GØ4.2, G32.89, G61.Ø, G96.8-G96.9, G98.Ø-G98.8, G99.8

A87.8 Other viral meningitis CC

A87.9 Viral meningitis, unspecified CC

✓4th **A88 Other viral infections of central nervous system, not elsewhere classified**
EXCLUDES 1 *viral encephalitis NOS (A86)*
viral meningitis NOS (A87.9)

A88.Ø Enteroviral exanthematous fever [Boston exanthem] CC
CC Excl: A17.82, A5Ø.42, A52.14, A75.9, A79.9, A81.1, A81.82-A81.89, A83.Ø-A85.8, A87.2, A88.Ø, A88.8, A92.1-A92.8, A93.Ø, BØØ.4, BØØ.82, BØ1.11-BØ1.12, BØ4, BØ6.Ø1, BØ8.Ø9, BØ8.2Ø-BØ8.22, BØ8.6Ø-BØ8.79, BØ9-B1Ø.Ø9, B26.2, B27.ØØ-B27.99, B33.1, B45.Ø, B45.2-B45.9, B58.2, B75, B97.1Ø, B97.21, GØ4.ØØ-GØ4.Ø1, GØ4.31, GØ4.81-GØ5.4, G37.Ø, G37.4-G37.5, JØ9.X3-JØ9.X9, J1Ø.2-J1Ø.89, J11.2-J11.89, L44.4, M1A.1ØXØ-M1A.19X1, P35.2-P35.9, P37.Ø-P37.4, P37.8-P37.9, T56.ØX1A, T56.ØX2A, T56.ØX3A, T56.ØX4A

A88.1 Epidemic vertigo

A88.8 Other specified viral infections of central nervous system HIV CC
CC Excl: See code: A85

A89 Unspecified viral infection of central nervous system HIV CC
CC Excl: See code: A86

Arthropod-borne viral fevers and viral hemorrhagic fevers (A9Ø-A99)

A9Ø Dengue fever [classical dengue] CC
EXCLUDES 1 *dengue hemorrhagic fever (A91)*
CC Excl: A9Ø

A91 Dengue hemorrhagic fever CC
CC Excl: A91-A94, A98.Ø-A98.2, A98.8-A99, B33.1

✓4th **A92 Other mosquito-borne viral fevers**
EXCLUDES 1 *Ross River disease (B33.1)*

A92.Ø Chikungunya virus disease CC
Chikungunya (hemorrhagic) fever
CC Excl: See code: A91

A92.1 O'nyong-nyong fever CC
CC Excl: A17.82, A5Ø.42, A52.14, A75.9, A79.9, A81.1, A81.82-A81.89, A83.Ø-A85.8, A87.2, A88.Ø, A88.8, A91-A94, A98.Ø-A98.2, A98.8-A99, BØØ.4, BØØ.82, BØ1.11-BØ1.12, BØ4, BØ6.Ø1, BØ8.Ø9, BØ8.2Ø-BØ8.22, BØ8.6Ø-BØ8.79, BØ9-B1Ø.Ø9, B26.2, B27.ØØ-B27.99, B33.1, B45.Ø, B45.2-B45.9, B58.2, B75, B97.1Ø, B97.21, GØ4.ØØ-GØ4.Ø1, GØ4.31, GØ4.81-GØ5.4, G37.Ø, G37.4-G37.5, JØ9.X3-JØ9.X9, J1Ø.2-J1Ø.89, J11.2-J11.89, L44.4, M1A.1ØXØ-M1A.19X1, P35.2-P35.9, P37.Ø-P37.4, P37.8-P37.9, T56.ØX1A, T56.ØX2A, T56.ØX3A, T56.ØX4A

A92.2 Venezuelan equine fever CC
Venezuelan equine encephalitis
Venezuelan equine encephalomyelitis virus disease
CC Excl: See code: A92.1

5th A92.3 West Nile virus infection
West Nile fever

CC Excl: For MCC codes in subcategory A92.3, unless otherwise noted: A17.82, A50.42, A52.14, A75.9, A79.9, A81.1, A81.82-A81.89, A83.0-A85.8, A87.2, A88.0, A88.8, A91-A92.2, A92.4-A94, A98.0-A98.2, A98.8-A99, B00.4, B00.82, B01.11-B01.12, B04, B06.01, B08.09, B08.20-B08.22, B08.60-B08.79, B09-B10.09, B26.2, B27.00-B27.99, B33.1, B45.0, B45.2-B45.9, B58.2, B75, B97.10, G04.00-G04.01, G04.31, G04.81-G05.4, G37.0, G37.4-G37.5, J09.X3-J09.X9, J10.2-J10.89, J11.2-J11.89, L44.4, P35.2-P35.9, P37.0-P37.4, P37.8-P37.9

A92.30 West Nile virus infection, unspecified MCC
West Nile fever NOS
West Nile fever without complications
West Nile virus NOS

A92.31 West Nile virus infection with encephalitis MCC
West Nile encephalitis
West Nile encephalomyelitis

A92.32 West Nile virus infection with other neurologic manifestation MCC
Use additional code to specify the neurologic manifestation

A92.39 West Nile virus infection with other complications MCC
Use additional code to specify the other conditions

A92.4 Rift Valley fever CC
CC Excl: See code: A92.1

A92.8 Other specified mosquito-borne viral fevers CC
CC Excl: See code: A92.1

A92.9 Mosquito-borne viral fever, unspecified CC
CC Excl: See code: A91

4th A93 Other arthropod-borne viral fevers, not elsewhere classified

A93.0 Oropouche virus disease CC
Oropouche fever
CC Excl: A17.82, A50.42, A52.14, A75.9, A79.9, A81.1, A81.82-A81.89, A83.0-A85.8, A87.2, A88.0, A88.8, A91-A94, A98.0-A98.2, A98.8-A99, B00.4, B00.82, B01.11-B01.12, B04, B06.01, B08.09, B08.20-B08.22, B08.60-B08.79, B09-B10.09, B26.2, B27.00-B27.99, B33.1, B45.0, B45.2-B45.9, B58.2, B75, B97.10, B97.21, G04.00-G04.01, G04.31, G04.81-G05.4, G37.0, G37.4-G37.5, J09.X3-J09.X9, J10.2-J10.89, J11.2-J11.89, L44.4, M1A.10-M1A.19, P35.2-P35.9, P37.0-P37.4, P37.8-P37.9, T56.0X1-T56.0X4 with 7th A

A93.1 Sandfly fever CC
Pappataci fever
Phlebotomus fever
CC Excl: A91-A94, A98.0-A98.2, A98.8-A99, B33.1

A93.2 Colorado tick fever CC
CC Excl: See code: A93.1

A93.8 Other specified arthropod-borne viral fevers CC
Piry virus disease
Vesicular stomatitis virus disease [Indiana fever]
CC Excl: See code: A91

A94 Unspecified arthropod-borne viral fever CC
Arboviral fever NOS
Arbovirus infection NOS
CC Excl: A91-A94, A98.0-A98.2, A98.8-A99, B33.1

4th A95 Yellow fever

CC Excl: For CC codes in category A95, unless otherwise noted: A95.0-A95.9

A95.0 Sylvatic yellow fever CC
Jungle yellow fever

A95.1 Urban yellow fever CC

A95.9 Yellow fever, unspecified CC

4th A96 Arenaviral hemorrhagic feverr

CC Excl: For CC codes in category A96, unless otherwise noted: A74.81-A74.9, A88.1, A96.0-A96.9, A98.3-A98.5, B25.8-B25.9, B33.24-B34.2, B34.4-B34.8, B97.0-B97.89

A96.0 Junin hemorrhagic fever CC
Argentinian hemorrhagic fever

A96.1 Machupo hemorrhagic fever CC
Bolivian hemorrhagic fever

A96.2 Lassa fever

A96.8 Other arenaviral hemorrhagic fevers CC

A96.9 Arenaviral hemorrhagic fever, unspecified CC

4th A98 Other viral hemorrhagic fevers, not elsewhere classified
EXCLUDES 1 *chikungunya hemorrhagic fever (A92.0)*
dengue hemorrhagic fever (A91)

CC Excl: For CC codes in category A98, unless otherwise noted: A91-A94, A98.0-A98.2, A98.8-A99, B33.1

A98.0 Crimean-Congo hemorrhagic fever CC
Central Asian hemorrhagic fever

A98.1 Omsk hemorrhagic fever CC

A98.2 Kyasanur Forest disease CC

A98.3 Marburg virus disease

A98.4 Ebola virus disease

A98.5 Hemorrhagic fever with renal syndrome CC
Epidemic hemorrhagic fever
Korean hemorrhagic fever
Russian hemorrhagic fever
Hantaan virus disease
Hantavirus disease with renal manifestations
Nephropathia epidemica
Songo fever
EXCLUDES 1 *hantavirus (cardio)-pulmonary syndrome (B33.4)*
CC Excl: A17.9, A18.10-A18.11, A18.13, A18.82, A18.84, A18.89, A54.21, A54.29, A54.82, A54.84, A54.89-A54.9, A59.00, A59.8-A59.9, A98.5, B37.41-B37.49, B97.21, E08.21-E08.29, E08.618-E08.638, E08.649-E08.8, E09.21-E09.29, E09.618-E09.638, E09.649-E09.8, E10.21-E10.29, E10.618-E10.638, E10.649, E10.69-E10.8, E11.21-E11.29, E11.618-E11.638, E11.649, E11.69-E11.8, E13.21-E13.29, E13.618-E13.638, E13.649-E13.8, M10.30-M10.39, N00.0-N11.0, N11.8-N13.39, N13.6, N14.0-N17.9, N19, N25.0-N26.1, N26.9-N27.9, N28.1-N29, N36.41-N36.43, N36.8-N36.9, N39.8-N39.9, R31.0-R31.9

A98.8 Other specified viral hemorrhagic fevers CC

A99 Unspecified viral hemorrhagic fever CC
CC Excl: See code: A98

Viral infections characterized by skin and mucous membrane lesions (B00-B09)

4th B00 Herpesviral [herpes simplex] infections
EXCLUDES 1 *congenital herpesviral infections (P35.2)*
EXCLUDES 2 *anogenital herpesviral infection (A60.-)*
gammaherpesviral mononucleosis (B27.0-)
herpangina (B08.5)

B00.0 Eczema herpeticum HIV
Kaposi's varicelliform eruption

B00.1 Herpesviral vesicular dermatitis HIV
Herpes simplex facialis
Herpes simplex labialis
Herpes simplex otitis externa
Vesicular dermatitis of ear
Vesicular dermatitis of lip

B00.2 Herpesviral gingivostomatitis and pharyngotonsillitis HIV CC
Herpesviral pharyngitis
CC Excl: B00.2

B00.3 Herpesviral meningitis HIV MCC
CC Excl: A02.21, A17.0-A17.1, A27.81, A39.0, A50.41, A51.41, A52.13, A54.82, A54.84, A54.89-A54.9, A87.0-A87.9, B00.3, B00.82-B00.9, B02.1, B10.81-B10.89, B26.1, B37.5, B38.4, B45.1, B58.2, B92, B94.2-B94.9, G00.0-G03.9, G04.2, G32.89, G61.0, G96.8-G96.9, G98.0-G98.8, G99.8

B00.4 Herpesviral encephalitis HIV MCC
Herpesviral meningoencephalitis
Simian B disease
EXCLUDES 1 *herpesviral encephalitis due to herpesvirus 6 and 7 (B10.01, B10.09)*
non-simplex herpesviral encephalitis (B10.0-)
CC Excl: B00.4-B00.9, B10.01-B10.89, B92, B94.2-B94.9

5th B00.5 Herpesviral ocular disease

CC Excl: For CC codes in subcategory B00.5, unless otherwise noted: B00.50-B00.59, B00.89-B00.9, B10.81-B10.89

B00.50 Herpesviral ocular disease, unspecified HIV CC

B00.51 Herpesviral iridocyclitis HIV CC
Herpesviral iritis
Herpesviral uveitis, anterior

B00.52 Herpesviral keratitis HIV CC
Herpesviral keratoconjunctivitis

B00.53 Herpesviral conjunctivitis HIV CC

B00.59 Other herpesviral disease of eye HIV CC
Herpesviral dermatitis of eyelid

B00.7 Disseminated herpesviral disease HIV MCC
Herpesviral sepsis
CC Excl: A02.1, A20.7, A22.7, A26.7, A32.7, A39.2-A39.4, A40.0-A40.1, A40.8-A41.9, A42.7, A54.86, B00.7, B00.82-B00.9, B10.81-B10.89, B37.7, B92, B94.2-B94.9, R65.10-R65.20

✓5th **B00.8 Other forms of herpesviral infections**

B00.81 Herpesviral hepatitis HIV CC
CC Excl: B00.3, B00.81-B00.9, B10.81-B10.89, B92, B94.2-B94.9

B00.82 Herpes simplex myelitis MCC
CC Excl: A74.81-A74.9, A96.2, A98.3-A98.4, B00.82-B00.9, B01.12, B02.24, B10.81-B10.89, B33.24, B33.4-B33.8, B34.1-B34.2, B34.4-B34.8, B92, B94.2-B94.9, B97.10, B97.19, B97.29, B97.5-B97.6, B97.81-B97.89, G04.00-G04.01, G04.31, G04.81-G04.89, G05.3-G05.4, G37.3

B00.89 Other herpesviral infection HIV CC
Herpesviral whitlow
CC Excl: A74.81-A74.9, A96.2, A98.3-A98.4, B00.82-B00.9, B10.81-B10.89, B33.24, B33.4-B33.8, B34.1-B34.2, B34.4-B34.8, B92, B94.2-B94.9, B97.10, B97.19, B97.29, B97.5-B97.6, B97.81-B97.89

B00.9 Herpesviral infection, unspecified HIV
Herpes simplex infection NOS

✓4th **B01 Varicella [chickenpox]**

B01.0 Varicella meningitis CC
CC Excl: A74.81-A74.9, A96.2, A98.3-A98.4, B01.0, B01.12, B01.81-B01.9, B08.04, B33.24, B33.4-B33.8, B34.1-B34.2, B34.4-B34.8, B92, B94.2-B94.9, B97.10, B97.19, B97.29, B97.5-B97.6, B97.81-B97.89

✓5th **B01.1 Varicella encephalitis, myelitis and encephalomyelitis**
Postchickenpox encephalitis, myelitis and encephalomyelitis

B01.11 Varicella encephalitis and encephalomyelitis MCC
Postchickenpox encephalitis and encephalomyelitis
CC Excl: A74.81-A74.9, A96.2, A98.3-A98.4, B01.0-B01.12, B01.81-B01.9, B08.04, B33.24, B33.4-B33.8, B34.1-B34.2, B34.4-B34.8, B92, B94.2-B94.9, B97.10, B97.19, B97.29, B97.5-B97.6, B97.81-B97.89

B01.12 Varicella myelitis MCC
Postchickenpox myelitis
CC Excl: A74.81-A74.9, A96.2, A98.3-A98.4, B00.82, B01.0, B01.12, B01.81-B01.9, B02.24, B08.04, B33.24, B33.4-B33.8, B34.1-B34.2, B34.4-B34.8, B92, B94.2-B94.9, B97.10, B97.19, B97.29, B97.5-B97.6, B97.81-B97.89, G04.00-G04.01, G04.31, G04.81-G04.89, G05.3-G05.4, G37.3

B01.2 Varicella pneumonia MCC
CC Excl: A74.81-A74.9, A96.2, A98.3-A98.4, B01.0, B01.12-B01.9, B08.04, B33.24, B33.4-B33.8, B34.1-B34.2, B34.4-B34.8, B92, B94.2-B94.9, B97.10, B97.19, B97.29, B97.5-B97.6, B97.81-B97.89

✓5th **B01.8 Varicella with other complications**

B01.81 Varicella keratitis CC
CC Excl: See code: B01.0

B01.89 Other varicella complications CC
CC Excl: See code: B01.0

B01.9 Varicella without complication CC
Varicella NOS
CC Excl: See code: B01.0

✓4th **B02 Zoster [herpes zoster]**
INCLUDES shingles
zona

B02.0 Zoster encephalitis HIV CC
Zoster meningoencephalitis
CC Excl: A74.81-A74.9, A96.2, A98.3-A98.4, B00.3, B00.82-B00.9, B02.0-B02.29, B02.7-B02.9, B10.81-B10.89, B33.24, B33.4-B33.8, B34.1-B34.2, B34.4-B34.8, B92, B94.2-B94.9, B97.10, B97.19, B97.29, B97.5-B97.6, B97.81-B97.89

B02.1 Zoster meningitis HIV MCC
CC Excl: A02.21, A17.0-A17.1, A27.81, A39.0, A50.41, A51.41, A52.13, A54.82, A54.84, A54.89-A54.9, A74.81-A74.9, A87.0-A87.9, A96.2, A98.3-A98.4, B00.3, B00.82-B00.9, B02.0-B02.29, B02.7-B02.9, B10.81-B10.89, B26.1, B33.24, B33.4-B33.8, B34.1-B34.2, B34.4-B34.8, B37.5, B38.4, B45.1, B58.2, B92, B94.2-B94.9, B97.10, B97.19, B97.29, B97.5-B97.6, B97.81-B97.89, G00.0-G03.9, G04.2, G32.89, G61.0, G96.8-G96.9, G98.0-G98.8, G99.8

✓5th **B02.2 Zoster with other nervous system involvement**

CC Excl: For CC/MCC codes in subcategory B02.2, unless otherwise noted: A74.81-A74.9, A96.2, A98.3-A98.4, B00.3, B00.82-B00.9, B02.0-B02.29, B02.7-B02.9, B10.81-B10.89, B33.24, B33.4-B33.8, B34.1-B34.2, B34.4-B34.8, B92, B94.2-B94.9, B97.10, B97.19, B97.29, B97.5-B97.6, B97.81-B97.89

B02.21 Postherpetic geniculate ganglionitis HIV CC

B02.22 Postherpetic trigeminal neuralgia HIV CC

B02.23 Postherpetic polyneuropathy HIV CC

B02.24 Postherpetic myelitis MCC
Herpes zoster myelitis
CC Excl: A74.81-A74.9, A96.2, A98.3-A98.4, B00.3, B00.82-B00.9, B01.12, B02.0-B02.29, B02.7-B02.9, B10.81-B10.89, B33.24, B33.4-B33.8, B34.1-B34.2, B34.4-B34.8, B92, B94.2-B94.9, B97.10, B97.19, B97.29, B97.5-B97.6, B97.81-B97.89, G04.00-G04.01, G04.31, G04.81-G04.89, G05.3-G05.4, G37.3

B02.29 Other postherpetic nervous system involvement HIV CC
Postherpetic radiculopathy

✓5th **B02.3 Zoster ocular disease**

CC Excl: For CC codes in subcategory B02.3, unless otherwise noted: B02.30-B02.39

B02.30 Zoster ocular disease, unspecified HIV CC

B02.31 Zoster conjunctivitis HIV CC

B02.32 Zoster iridocyclitis HIV CC

B02.33 Zoster keratitis HIV CC
Herpes zoster keratoconjunctivitis

B02.34 Zoster scleritis HIV CC

B02.39 Other herpes zoster eye disease HIV CC
Zoster blepharitis

B02.7 Disseminated zoster HIV CC
CC Excl: A60.00-A60.9, A74.81-A74.9, A96.2, A98.3-A98.4, B00.0-B00.2, B00.4-B00.9, B02.0-B02.9, B10.01-B10.89, B33.24, B33.4-B33.8, B34.1-B34.2, B34.4-B34.8, B92, B94.2-B94.9, B97.10, B97.19, B97.29, B97.5-B97.6, B97.81-B97.89

B02.8 Zoster with other complications HIV CC
Herpes zoster otitis externa
CC Excl: See code: B02.7

B02.9 Zoster without complications HIV
Zoster NOS

B03 Smallpox CC
NOTE In 1980 the 33rd World Health Assembly declared that smallpox had been eradicated.
The classification is maintained for surveillance purposes.
CC Excl: B01.0-B01.9, B03, B08.010-B08.04

B04 Monkeypox CC
CC Excl: B04-B08.011, B08.09, B08.3, B08.60-B08.79, B09, L44.4

✓4th **B05 Measles**
INCLUDES morbilli
EXCLUDES 1 *subacute sclerosing panencephalitis (A81.1)*

B05.0 Measles complicated by encephalitis MCC
Postmeasles encephalitis
CC Excl: A74.81-A74.9, A96.2, A98.3-A98.4, B05.0-B05.1, B05.4, B05.89-B05.9, B33.24, B33.4-B33.8, B34.1-B34.2, B34.4-B34.8, B92, B94.2-B94.9, B97.10, B97.19, B97.29, B97.5-B97.6, B97.81-B97.89

B05.1 Measles complicated by meningitis CC
Postmeasles meningitis
CC Excl: A74.81-A74.9, A96.2, A98.3-A98.4, B05.1, B05.4, B05.89-B05.9, B33.24, B33.4-B33.8, B34.1-B34.2, B34.4-B34.8, B92, B94.2-B94.9, B97.10, B97.19, B97.29, B97.5-B97.6, B97.81-B97.89

B05.2 Measles complicated by pneumonia MCC
Postmeasles pneumonia
CC Excl: A74.81-A74.9, A96.2, A98.3-A98.4, B05.1-B05.2, B05.4, B05.89-B05.9, B33.24, B33.4-B33.8, B34.1-B34.2, B34.4-B34.8, B92, B94.2-B94.9, B97.10, B97.19, B97.29, B97.5-B97.6, B97.81-B97.89

B05.3 Measles complicated by otitis media
Postmeasles otitis media

B05.4 Measles with intestinal complications CC
CC Excl: See code: B05.1

✓5th **B05.8 Measles with other complications**

B05.81 Measles keratitis and keratoconjunctivitis CC
CC Excl: A74.81-A74.9, A96.2, A98.3-A98.4, B05.1, B05.4-B05.9, B33.24, B33.4-B33.8, B34.1-B34.2, B34.4-B34.8, B92, B94.2-B94.9, B97.10, B97.19, B97.29, B97.5-B97.6, B97.81-B97.89

B05.89 Other measles complications CC
CC Excl: See code: B05.1

B05.9 Measles without complication
Measles NOS

4th B06 Rubella [German measles]
EXCLUDES 1 *congenital rubella (P35.0)c*

5th B06.0 Rubella with neurological complications

CC Excl: For CC/MCC codes in subcategory B06.0, unless otherwise noted: A74.81-A74.9, A96.2, A98.3-A98.4, B06.00-B06.81, B06.89-B06.9, B33.24, B33.4-B33.8, B34.1-B34.2, B34.4-B34.8, B92, B94.2-B94.9, B97.10, B97.19, B97.29, B97.5-B97.6, B97.81-B97.89

B06.00 Rubella with neurological complication, unspecified CC
B06.01 Rubella encephalitis MCC
Rubella meningoencephalitis
B06.02 Rubella meningitis CC
B06.09 Other neurological complications of rubella CC

5th B06.8 Rubella with other complications
B06.81 Rubella pneumonia CC
CC Excl: See code: B06.00
B06.82 Rubella arthritis CC
CC Excl: A74.81-A74.9, A96.2, A98.3-A98.4, B06.81-B06.9, B33.24, B33.4-B33.8, B34.1-B34.2, B34.4-B34.8, B92, B94.2-B94.9, B97.10, B97.19, B97.29, B97.5-B97.6, B97.81-B97.89
B06.89 Other rubella complications CC
CC Excl: See code: B06.0

B06.9 Rubella without complication
Rubella NOS

4th B07 Viral warts
INCLUDES verruca simplex
verruca vulgaris
viral warts due to human papillomavirus
EXCLUDES 2 *anogenital (venereal) warts (A63.0)*
papilloma of bladder (D41.4)
papilloma of cervix (D26.0)
papilloma larynx (D14.1)

B07.0 Plantar wart
Verruca plantaris
B07.8 Other viral warts
Common wart
Flat wart
Verruca plana
B07.9 Viral wart, unspecified

4th B08 Other viral infections characterized by skin and mucous membrane lesions, not elsewhere classified
EXCLUDES 1 *vesicular stomatitis virus disease (A93.8)*

5th B08.0 Other orthopoxvirus infections
EXCLUDES 2 *monkeypox (B04)*
6th B08.01 Cowpox and vaccinia not from vaccine
B08.010 Cowpox
B08.011 Vaccinia not from vaccine
EXCLUDES 1 *vaccinia (from vaccination) (generalized) (T88.1)*
B08.02 Orf virus disease
Contagious pustular dermatitis
Ecthyma contagiosum
B08.03 Pseudocowpox [milker's node]
B08.04 Paravaccinia, unspecified
B08.09 Other orthopoxvirus infections
Orthopoxvirus infection NOS

B08.1 Molluscum contagiosum

5th B08.2 Exanthema subitum [sixth disease]
Roseola infantum
B08.20 Exanthema subitum [sixth disease], unspecified P
Roseola infantum, unspecified
B08.21 Exanthema subitum [sixth disease] due to human herpesvirus 6 P
Roseola infantum due to human herpesvirus 6
B08.22 Exanthema subitum [sixth disease] due to human herpesvirus 7 P
Roseola infantum due to human herpesvirus 7

B08.3 Erythema infectiosum [fifth disease] CC
CC Excl: B08.3-B34.3

B08.4 Enteroviral vesicular stomatitis with exanthem
Hand, foot and mouth disease

B08.5 Enteroviral vesicular pharyngitis
Herpangina

5th B08.6 Parapoxvirus infections
B08.60 Parapoxvirus infection, unspecified
B08.61 Bovine stomatitis
B08.62 Sealpox
B08.69 Other parapoxvirus infections

5th B08.7 Yatapoxvirus infections
B08.70 Yatapoxvirus infection, unspecified
B08.71 Tanapox virus disease CC
CC Excl: B04, B08.010-B08.011, B08.09, B08.3, B08.60-B08.79, B09, L44.4
B08.72 Yaba pox virus disease
Yaba monkey tumor disease
B08.79 Other yatapoxvirus infections

B08.8 Other specified viral infections characterized by skin and mucous membrane lesions
Enteroviral lymphonodular pharyngitis
Foot-and-mouth disease
Poxvirus NEC

B09 Unspecified viral infection characterized by skin and mucous membrane lesions
Viral enanthema NOS
Viral exanthema NOS

Other human herpesviruses (B10)

4th B10 Other human herpesviruses
EXCLUDES 2 *cytomegalovirus (B25.9)*
Epstein-Barr virus (B27.0-)
herpes NOS (B00.9)
herpes simplex (B00.-)
herpes zoster (B02.-)
human herpesvirus NOS (B00.-)
human herpesvirus 1 and 2 (B00.-)
human herpesvirus 3 (B01.-, B02.-)
human herpesvirus 4 (B27.0-)
human herpesvirus 5 (B25.-)
varicella (B01.-)
zoster (B02.-)

5th B10.0 Other human herpesvirus encephalitis
EXCLUDES 2 *herpes encephalitis NOS (B00.4)*
herpes simplex encephalitis (B00.4)
human herpesvirus encephalitis (B00.4)
simian B herpes virus encephalitis (B00.4)
B10.01 Human herpesvirus 6 encephalitis HIV MCC
CC Excl: B00.4, B00.82-B00.9, B10.01-B10.89, B92, B94.2-B94.9
B10.09 Other human herpesvirus encephalitis HIV MCC
Human herpesvirus 7 encephalitis
CC Excl: See code: B10.01

5th B10.8 Other human herpesvirus infection
B10.81 Human herpesvirus 6 infection
B10.82 Human herpesvirus 7 infection
B10.89 Other human herpesvirus infection
Human herpesvirus 8 infection
Kaposi's sarcoma-associated herpesvirus infection

Viral hepatitis (B15-B19)

EXCLUDES 1 *sequelae of viral hepatitis (B94.2)*
EXCLUDES 2 *cytomegaloviral hepatitis (B25.1)*
herpesviral [herpes simplex] hepatitis (B00.81)

4th B15 Acute hepatitis A
B15.0 Hepatitis A with hepatic coma MCC
CC Excl: A74.81-A74.9, A96.2, A98.3-A98.4, B15.0-B19.9, B33.24, B33.4-B33.8, B34.1-B34.2, B34.4-B34.8, B92, B94.2-B94.9, B97.10, B97.19, B97.29, B97.5-B97.6, B97.81-B97.89
B15.9 Hepatitis A without hepatic coma CC
Hepatitis A (acute)(viral) NOS
CC Excl: See code: B15.0

4th B16 Acute hepatitis B

CC Excl: For CC/MCC codes in category B16, unless otherwise noted: A74.81-A74.9, A96.2, A98.3-A98.4, B15.0-B19.9, B33.24, B33.4-B33.8, B34.1-B34.2, B34.4-B34.8, B92, B94.2-B94.9, B97.10, B97.19, B97.29, B97.5-B97.6, B97.81-B97.89

B16.0 Acute hepatitis B with delta-agent with hepatic coma MCC
B16.1 Acute hepatitis B with delta-agent without hepatic coma CC
B16.2 Acute hepatitis B without delta-agent with hepatic coma MCC

B16.9 **Acute hepatitis B** without delta-agent and without hepatic coma CC
Hepatitis B (acute) (viral) NOS

✓4th **B17** Other acute **viral hepatitis**

CC Excl: For CC/MCC codes in category B17, unless otherwise noted: A74.81-A74.9, A96.2, A98.3-A98.4, B15.Ø-B19.9, B33.24, B33.4-B33.8, B34.1-B34.2, B34.4-B34.8, B92, B94.2-B94.9, B97.1Ø, B97.19, B97.29, B97.5-B97.6, B97.81-B97.89

B17.Ø **Acute** delta-(super) infection **of hepatitis B carrier** CC

✓5th **B17.1** **Acute** hepatitis C

B17.1Ø **Acute hepatitis C** without hepatic coma CC
Acute hepatitis C NOS

B17.11 **Acute hepatitis C** with hepatic coma MCC

B17.2 **Acute** hepatitis E CC

B17.8 Other **specified acute viral hepatitis** CC
Hepatitis non-A non-B (acute) (viral) NEC

B17.9 **Acute viral hepatitis,** unspecified CC
Acute hepatitis NOS

✓4th **B18** Chronic **viral hepatitis**

CC Excl: For CC codes in category B18, unless otherwise noted: A74.81-A74.9, A96.2, A98.3-A98.4, B15.Ø-B19.9, B33.24, B33.4-B33.8, B34.1-B34.2, B34.4-B34.8, B92, B94.2-B94.9, B97.1Ø, B97.19, B97.29, B97.5-B97.6, B97.81-B97.89

B18.Ø **Chronic viral hepatitis B** with delta-agent CC

B18.1 **Chronic viral hepatitis B** without delta-agent CC
Chronic (viral) hepatitis B

B18.2 **Chronic viral** hepatitis C

B18.8 Other **chronic viral hepatitis** CC

B18.9 **Chronic viral hepatitis,** unspecified CC

✓4th **B19** Unspecified **viral hepatitis**

CC Excl: For CC/MCC codes in category B19, unless otherwise noted: A74.81-A74.9, A96.2, A98.3-A98.4, B15.Ø-B19.9, B33.24, B33.4-B33.8, B34.1-B34.2, B34.4-B34.8, B92, B94.2-B94.9, B97.1Ø, B97.19, B97.29, B97.5-B97.6, B97.81-B97.89

B19.Ø **Unspecified viral hepatitis** with hepatic coma MCC

✓5th **B19.1** **Unspecified viral** hepatitis B

B19.1Ø **Unspecified viral hepatitis B** without hepatic coma CC
Unspecified viral hepatitis B NOS

B19.11 **Unspecified viral hepatitis B** with hepatic coma MCC

✓5th **B19.2** **Unspecified viral** hepatitis C

B19.2Ø **Unspecified viral hepatitis C** without hepatic coma
Viral hepatitis C NOS

B19.21 **Unspecified viral hepatitis C** with hepatic coma MCC

B19.9 Unspecified **viral hepatitis** without hepatic coma CC
Viral hepatitis NOS

Human immunodeficiency virus [HIV] disease (B2Ø)

B2Ø **Human immunodeficiency virus [HIV] disease** MCC

INCLUDES acquired immune deficiency syndrome [AIDS]
AIDS-related complex [ARC]
HIV infection, symptomatic

Code first human immunodeficiency virus [HIV] disease complicating pregnancy, childbirth and the puerperium, if applicable (O98.7-)

Use additional code(s) to identify all manifestations of HIV infection

EXCLUDES 1 *asymptomatic human immunodeficiency virus [HIV] infection status (Z21)*
exposure to HIV virus (Z2Ø.6)
inconclusive serologic evidence of HIV (R75)

CC Excl: B2Ø, B92, B94.2-B94.9

Other viral diseases (B25-B34)

✓4th **B25** **Cytomegaloviral disease**

EXCLUDES 1 *congenital cytomegalovirus infection (P35.1)*
cytomegaloviral mononucleosis (B27.1-)

B25.Ø **Cytomegaloviral** pneumonitis PDx MCC MCC
CC Excl: A15.Ø-A15.6, A15.8-A15.9, A17.9, A18.82, A18.84, A18.89, A21.2, A22.1, A31.Ø, A37.Ø1, A37.11, A37.81, A37.91, A42.Ø, A43.Ø, A48.1, B25.Ø, B39.Ø-B39.2, B44.Ø, B58.3, B59, B67.1, JØ9.X1-JØ9.X2, J1Ø.ØØ-J1Ø.1, J11.ØØ-J11.1, J12.Ø-J12.3, J12.89-J18.1, J18.8-J18.9, J22, J44.9, J47.Ø-J7Ø.4, J7Ø.8-J7Ø.9, J98.4, J98.8-J99, Q33.4, R91.1

B25.1 **Cytomegaloviral** hepatitis PDx CC CC
CC Excl: No Excl

B25.2 **Cytomegaloviral** pancreatitis PDx MCC MCC
CC Excl: B25.2, K85.Ø-K86.1, K86.8-K86.9

B25.8 Other **cytomegaloviral diseases** HIV CC
Cytomegaloviral encephalitis
CC Excl: A96.Ø-A96.9, A98.3-A98.5, B25.8-B25.9, B33.24-B34.2, B34.4-B34.8, B97.Ø-B97.32, B97.39, B97.5-B97.89

B25.9 **Cytomegaloviral disease,** unspecified HIV CC
CC Excl: See code: B25.8

✓4th **B26** **Mumps**

INCLUDES epidemic parotitis
infectious parotitis

B26.Ø **Mumps** orchitis CC ♂
CC Excl: A74.81-A74.9, A96.2, A98.3-A98.4, B26.Ø, B26.82-B26.83, B26.85-B26.9, B33.24, B33.4-B33.8, B34.1-B34.2, B34.4-B34.8, B92, B94.2-B94.9, B97.1Ø, B97.19, B97.29, B97.5-B97.6, B97.81-B97.89

B26.1 **Mumps** meningitis MCC
CC Excl: AØ2.21-A17.1, A27.81, A39.Ø, A5Ø.41, A51.41, A52.13, A54.82, A54.84, A54.89-A54.9, A74.81-A74.9, A87.Ø-A87.9, A96.2, A98.3-A98.4, BØØ.3, BØ2.1, B26.1, B26.82-B26.83, B26.85-B26.9, B33.24, B33.4-B33.8, B34.1-B34.2, B34.4-B34.8, B37.5, B38.4, B45.1, B58.2, B92, B94.2-B94.9, B97.1Ø, B97.19, B97.29, B97.5-B97.6, B97.81-B97.89, GØØ.Ø-GØ3.9, GØ4.2, G32.89, G61.Ø, G96.8-G96.9, G98.Ø-G98.8, G99.8

B26.2 **Mumps** encephalitis MCC
CC Excl: A74.81-A74.9, A96.2, A98.3-A98.4, B26.2, B26.82-B26.83, B26.85-B26.9, B33.24, B33.4-B33.8, B34.1-B34.2, B34.4-B34.8, B92, B94.2-B94.9, B97.1Ø, B97.19, B97.29, B97.5-B97.6, B97.81-B97.89

B26.3 **Mumps** pancreatitis CC
CC Excl: A74.81-A74.9, A96.2, A98.3-A98.4, B26.3, B26.82-B26.83, B26.85-B26.9, B33.24, B33.4-B33.8, B34.1-B34.2, B34.4-B34.8, B92, B94.2-B94.9, B97.1Ø, B97.19, B97.29, B97.5-B97.6, B97.81-B97.89

✓5th **B26.8** **Mumps with** other complications

B26.81 **Mumps** hepatitis CC
CC Excl: A74.81-A74.9, A96.2, A98.3-A98.4, B26.81-B26.83, B26.85-B26.9, B33.24, B33.4-B33.8, B34.1-B34.2, B34.4-B34.8, B92, B94.2-B94.9, B97.1Ø, B97.19, B97.29, B97.5-B97.6, B97.81-B97.89

B26.82 **Mumps** myocarditis CC
CC Excl: A74.81-A74.9, A96.2, A98.3-A98.4, B26.82-B26.83, B26.85-B26.9, B33.24, B33.4-B33.8, B34.1-B34.2, B34.4-B34.8, B92, B94.2-B94.9, B97.1Ø, B97.19, B97.29, B97.5-B97.6, B97.81-B97.89

B26.83 **Mumps** nephritis CC
CC Excl: See code: B26.82

B26.84 **Mumps** polyneuropathy CC
CC Excl: A74.81-A74.9, A96.2, A98.3-A98.4, B26.82-B26.9, B33.24, B33.4-B33.8, B34.1-B34.2, B34.4-B34.8, B92, B94.2-B94.9, B97.1Ø, B97.19, B97.29, B97.5-B97.6, B97.81-B97.89

B26.85 **Mumps** arthritis CC
CC Excl: See code: B26.82

B26.89 Other **mumps complications** CC
CC Excl: See code: B26.82

B26.9 **Mumps** without complication
Mumps NOS
Mumps parotitis NOS

✓4th **B27** **Infectious mononucleosis**

INCLUDES glandular fever
monocytic angina
Pfeiffer's disease

✓5th **B27.Ø** Gammaherpesviral **mononucleosis**
Mononucleosis due to Epstein-Barr virus

B27.ØØ **Gammaherpesviral mononucleosis** without complication

B27.Ø1 **Gammaherpesviral mononucleosis** with polyneuropathy

B27.Ø2 **Gammaherpesviral mononucleosis** with meningitis

B27.Ø9 **Gammaherpesviral mononucleosis** with other complications
Hepatomegaly in gammaherpesviral mononucleosis

✓5th **B27.1** Cytomegaloviral **mononucleosis**

B27.1Ø **Cytomegaloviral mononucleosis** without complications

B27.11 **Cytomegaloviral mononucleosis** with polyneuropathy

B27.12 **Cytomegaloviral mononucleosis** with meningitis

B27.19 **Cytomegaloviral mononucleosis** with other complication
Hepatomegaly in cytomegaloviral mononucleosis

✓5th **B27.8 Other infectious mononucleosis**

B27.80 Other infectious mononucleosis without complication

B27.81 Other infectious mononucleosis with polyneuropathy

B27.82 Other infectious mononucleosis with meningitis

B27.89 Other infectious mononucleosis with other complication
Hepatomegaly in other infectious mononucleosis

✓5th **B27.9 Infectious mononucleosis, unspecified**

B27.90 Infectious mononucleosis, unspecified without complication

B27.91 Infectious mononucleosis, unspecified with polyneuropathy

B27.92 Infectious mononucleosis, unspecified with meningitis

B27.99 Infectious mononucleosis, unspecified with other complication
Hepatomegaly in unspecified infectious mononucleosis

✓4th **B30 Viral conjunctivitis**

EXCLUDES 1 *herpesviral [herpes simplex] ocular disease (B00.5)*
ocular zoster (B02.3)

B30.0 Keratoconjunctivitis due to adenovirus
Epidemic keratoconjunctivitis
Shipyard eye

B30.1 Conjunctivitis due to adenovirus
Acute adenoviral follicular conjunctivitis
Swimming-pool conjunctivitis

B30.2 Viral pharyngoconjunctivitis

B30.3 Acute epidemic hemorrhagic conjunctivitis (enteroviral)
Conjunctivitis due to coxsackievirus 24
Conjunctivitis due to enterovirus 70
Hemorrhagic conjunctivitis (acute)(epidemic)

B30.8 Other viral conjunctivitis
Newcastle conjunctivitis

B30.9 Viral conjunctivitis, unspecified

✓4th **B33 Other viral diseases, not elsewhere classified**

B33.0 Epidemic myalgia
Bornholm disease

B33.1 Ross River disease CC
Epidemic polyarthritis and exanthema
Ross River fever
CC Excl: A17.82, A50.42, A52.14, A75.9, A79.9, A81.1, A81.82-A81.89, A83.0-A85.8, A87.2, A88.0, A88.8, A91-A94, A98.0-A98.2, A98.8-A99, B00.4, B00.82, B01.11-B01.12, B04, B06.01, B08.09, B08.20-B08.22, B08.60-B08.79, B09-B10.09, B26.2, B27.00-B27.99, B33.1, B45.0, B45.2-B45.9, B58.2, B75, B97.10, B97.21, G04.00-G04.01, G04.31, G04.81-G05.4, G37.0, G37.4-G37.5, J09.X3-J09.X9, J10.2-J10.89, J11.2-J11.89, L44.4, M1A.10X0-M1A.19X1, P35.2-P35.9, P37.0-P37.4, P37.8-P37.9, T56.0X1A, T56.0X2A, T56.0X3A, T56.0X4A

✓5th **B33.2 Viral carditis**
Coxsackie (virus) carditis

B33.20 Viral carditis, unspecified CC
CC Excl: A52.06, B33.20-B33.22, I00, I01.2-I01.9, I09.0, I09.9, I23.0-I23.3, I23.6-I23.8, I40.0-I41, I51.0, I51.4, I87.8, I99.8-I99.9

B33.21 Viral endocarditis CC
CC Excl: A01.00-A01.09, A39.51, A52.03, A78, B33.21, B37.6, B40.0-B40.9, I00, I01.1, I01.8-I02.0, I05.0-I07.9, I08.1-I08.3, I08.9, I09.1, I09.89-I09.9, I33.0-I39, I42.4, I87.8, I99.8-I99.9, Q22.2, Q23.8-Q23.9, Q24.8, T82.6XXA

B33.22 Viral myocarditis CC
CC Excl: See code: B33.20

B33.23 Viral pericarditis CC
CC Excl: B33.23, I01.0, I09.2, I30.0-I30.9, I31.3-I32, I87.8, I99.8-I99.9

B33.24 Viral cardiomyopathy

B33.3 Retrovirus infections, not elsewhere classified
Retrovirus infection NOS

B33.4 Hantavirus (cardio)-pulmonary syndrome [HPS] [HCPS] CC
Hantavirus disease with pulmonary manifestations
Sin nombre virus disease
Use additional code to identify any associated acute kidney failure (N17.9)
EXCLUDES 1 *hantavirus disease with renal manifestations (A98.5)*
hemorrhagic fever with renal manifestations (A98.5)
CC Excl: A74.81-A74.9, A88.1, A96.0-A96.9, A98.3-A98.5, B19.20-B19.21, B25.8-B25.9, B33.24-B34.2, B34.4-B34.8, B97.0-B97.89

B33.8 Other specified viral diseases
EXCLUDES 1 *anogenital human papillomavirus infection (A63.0)*
viral warts due to human papillomavirus infection (B07)

✓4th **B34 Viral infection of unspecified site**

EXCLUDES 1 *anogenital human papillomavirus infection (A63.0)*
cytomegaloviral disease NOS (B25.9)
herpesvirus [herpes simplex] infection NOS (B00.9)
retrovirus infection NOS (B33.3)
viral agents as the cause of diseases classified elsewhere (B97.-)
viral warts due to human papillomavirus infection (B07)

B34.0 Adenovirus infection, unspecified

B34.1 Enterovirus infection, unspecified
Coxsackievirus infection NOS
Echovirus infection NOS

B34.2 Coronavirus infection, unspecified
EXCLUDES 1 *pneumonia due to SARS-associated coronavirus (J12.81)*

B34.3 Parvovirus infection, unspecified CC
CC Excl: B08.3, B34.3

B34.4 Papovavirus infection, unspecified

B34.8 Other viral infections of unspecified site

B34.9 Viral infection, unspecified
Viremia NOS

Mycoses (B35-B49)

EXCLUDES 2 *hypersensitivity pneumonitis due to organic dust (J67.-)*
mycosis fungoides (C84.0-)

✓4th **B35 Dermatophytosis**

INCLUDES favus
infections due to species of Epidermophyton, Micro-sporum and Trichophyton
tinea, any type except those in B36-

B35.0 Tinea barbae and tinea capitis
Beard ringworm
Kerion
Scalp ringworm
Sycosis, mycotic

B35.1 Tinea unguium
Dermatophytic onychia
Dermatophytosis of nail
Onychomycosis
Ringworm of nails

B35.2 Tinea manuum
Dermatophytosis of hand
Hand ringworm

B35.3 Tinea pedis
Athlete's foot
Dermatophytosis of foot
Foot ringworm

B35.4 Tinea corporis
Ringworm of the body

B35.5 Tinea imbricata
Tokelau

B35.6 Tinea cruris
Dhobi itch
Groin ringworm
Jock itch

B35.8 Other dermatophytoses
Disseminated dermatophytosis
Granulomatous dermatophytosis

B35.9 Dermatophytosis, unspecified
Ringworm NOS

✓4th **B36 Other superficial mycoses**

B36.0 Pityriasis versicolor
Tinea flava
Tinea versicolor

B36.1 Tinea nigra
Keratomycosis nigricans palmaris
Microsporosis nigra
Pityriasis nigra

B36.2 White piedra
Tinea blanca

B36.3 Black piedra

B36.8 Other specified superficial mycoses

B36.9 Superficial mycosis, unspecified

B37 Candidiasis
INCLUDES candidosis
moniliasis
EXCLUDES 1 *neonatal candidiasis (P37.5)*

B37.0 Candidal stomatitis HIV CC
Oral thrush
CC Excl: B37.0-B37.9, B48.3, B49, B92, B94.2-B94.9

B37.1 Pulmonary candidiasis HIV MCC
Candidal bronchitis
Candidal pneumonia
CC Excl: See code: B37.0

B37.2 Candidiasis of skin and nail HIV
Candidal onychia
Candidal paronychia
EXCLUDES 2 *diaper dermatitis (L22)*

B37.3 Candidiasis of vulva and vagina ♀
Candidal vulvovaginitis
Monilial vulvovaginitis
Vaginal thrush

B37.4 Candidiasis of other urogenital sites

1 **B37.41 Candidal cystitis and urethritis** CC
CC Excl: B37.1, B37.41-B37.82, B37.84-B37.9, N25.81-N25.89

B37.42 Candidal balanitis

1 **B37.49 Other urogenital candidiasis** CC
Candidal pyelonephritis
CC Excl: See code: B37.41

B37.5 Candidal meningitis HIV MCC
CC Excl: A02.21, A17.0-A17.1, A27.81, A39.0, A50.41, A51.41, A52.13, A54.82, A54.84, A54.89-A54.9, A87.0-A87.9, B00.3, B02.1, B26.1, B37.0-B37.9, B38.4, B45.1, B48.3, B49, B58.2, B92, B94.2-B94.9, G00.0-G03.9, G04.2, G32.89, G61.0, G96.8-G96.9, G98.0-G98.8, G99.8

B37.6 Candidal endocarditis HIV MCC
CC Excl: B37.0-B37.9, B48.3, B49, B92, B94.2-B94.9

B37.7 Candidal sepsis PDx MCC MCC
Disseminated candidiasis
Systemic candidiasis
CC Excl: A02.1, A20.7, A22.7, A26.7, A32.7, A39.2-A39.4, A40.0-A40.1, A40.8-A41.9, A42.7, A48.2-A48.4, A48.8-A49.9, A54.86, B00.7, B37.0-B37.9, B48.3, B49, B92, B94.2-B96.89, M00.011-M00.012, M00.021-M00.022, M00.031- M00.032, M00.041-M00.042, M00.051- M00.052, M00.061-M00.062, M00.071-M00.072, R65.10-R65.20, Z16.10-Z16.39

B37.8 Candidiasis of other sites

CC Excl: For CC codes in subcategory B37.8, unless otherwise noted: B37.0-B37.9, B48.3, B49, B92, B94.2-B94.9

B37.81 Candidal esophagitis HIV CC

B37.82 Candidal enteritis HIV CC
Candidal proctitis

B37.83 Candidal cheilitis HIV CC

B37.84 Candidal otitis externa HIV CC

B37.89 Other sites of candidiasis HIV CC
Candidal osteomyelitis
CC Excl: B37.1, B37.5-B37.82, B37.84-B37.9

B37.9 Candidiasis, unspecified HIV
Thrush NOS

B38 Coccidioidomycosis

B38.0 Acute pulmonary coccidioidomycosis HIV CC
CC Excl: B38.0-B38.2, B38.7, B38.89-B38.9, B48.3, B49, B92, B94.2-B94.9

B38.1 Chronic pulmonary coccidioidomycosis HIV CC
CC Excl: B38.0-B39.9

B38.2 Pulmonary coccidioidomycosis, unspecified HIV CC
CC Excl: See code: B38.1

B38.3 Cutaneous coccidioidomycosis HIV CC
CC Excl: B38.0-B38.9

B38.4 Coccidioidomycosis meningitis HIV MCC
CC Excl: A02.21, A17.0-A17.1, A27.81, A39.0, A50.41, A51.41, A52.13, A54.82, A54.84, A54.89-A54.9, A87.0-A87.9, B00.3, B02.1, B26.1, B37.5, B38.4-B38.7, B38.89-B38.9, B45.1, B48.3, B49, B58.2, B92, B94.2-B94.9, G00.0-G03.9, G04.2, G32.89, G61.0, G96.8-G96.9, G98.0-G98.8, G99

B38.7 Disseminated coccidioidomycosis HIV CC
Generalized coccidioidomycosis
CC Excl: B38.7, B38.89-B38.9, B48.3, B49, B92, B94.2-B94.9

B38.8 Other forms of coccidioidomycosis

B38.81 Prostatic coccidioidomycosis HIV CC ♂
CC Excl: See code: B38.3

B38.89 Other forms of coccidioidomycosis HIV CC
CC Excl: See code: B38.7

B38.9 Coccidioidomycosis, unspecified HIV
CC Excl: See code: B38.7

B39 Histoplasmosis
Code first associated AIDS (B20)
Use additional code for any associated manifestations, such as:
endocarditis (I39)
meningitis (G02)
pericarditis (I32)
retinitits (H32)

B39.0 Acute pulmonary histoplasmosis capsulati HIV MCC
CC Excl: A22.1, A37.01, A37.11, A37.81, A37.91, A48.1, B25.0, B39.0-B39.4, B39.9, B44.0, B48.3, B49, B92, B94.2-B94.9, J09.X1-J09.X2, J10.00-J10.1, J11.00-J11.1, J12.0-J12.3, J12.89-J18.1, J18.8-J18.9, J44.9, J47.0-J70.4, J70.8-J70.9, J98.4, R91.1

B39.1 Chronic pulmonary histoplasmosis capsulati HIV MCC
CC Excl: See code: B39.0

B39.2 Pulmonary histoplasmosis capsulati, unspecified HIV MCC
CC Excl: See code: B39.0

B39.3 Disseminated histoplasmosis capsulati HIV CC
Generalized histoplasmosis capsulati
CC Excl: B38.0-B39.4

B39.4 Histoplasmosis capsulati, unspecified HIV
American histoplasmosis

B39.5 Histoplasmosis duboisii HIV
African histoplasmosis

B39.9 Histoplasmosis, unspecified HIV

B40 Blastomycosis
EXCLUDES 1 *Brazilian blastomycosis (B41.-)*
keloidal blastomycosis (B48.0)

CC Excl: For CC codes in category B40, unless otherwise noted: B40.0-B40.9, B48.3, B49, B92, B94.2-B94.9

B40.0 Acute pulmonary blastomycosis CC
B40.1 Chronic pulmonary blastomycosis CC
B40.2 Pulmonary blastomycosis, unspecified CC
B40.3 Cutaneous blastomycosis CC
B40.7 Disseminated blastomycosis CC
Generalized blastomycosis

B40.8 Other forms of blastomycosis

B40.81 Blastomycotic meningoencephalitis CC
Meningomyelitis due to blastomycosis

B40.89 Other forms of blastomycosis CC

B40.9 Blastomycosis, unspecified CC

B41 Paracoccidioidomycosis
INCLUDES Brazilian blastomycosis
Lutz' disease

CC Excl: For CC codes in category B41, unless otherwise noted: B41.0-B41.9, B48.3, B49, B92, B94.2-B94.9

B41.0 Pulmonary paracoccidioidomycosis CC
B41.7 Disseminated paracoccidioidomycosis CC
Generalized paracoccidioidomycosis
B41.8 Other forms of paracoccidioidomycosis CC
B41.9 Paracoccidioidomycosis, unspecified CC

B42 Sporotrichosis

B42.0 Pulmonary sporotrichosis
B42.1 Lymphocutaneous sporotrichosis
B42.7 Disseminated sporotrichosis
Generalized sporotrichosis

B42.8 Other forms of sporotrichosis

B42.81 Cerebral sporotrichosis
Meningitis due to sporotrichosis
B42.82 Sporotrichosis arthritis
B42.89 Other forms of sporotrichosis

B42.9 Sporotrichosis, unspecified

B43 Chromomycosis and pheomycotic abscess

B43.0 Cutaneous chromomycosis
Dermatitis verrucosa

1 HAC = as SDx not POA, in combination with SDx code T83.51XA also not POA.

B43.1 Pheomycotic brain abscess
Cerebral chromomycosis

B43.2 Subcutaneous pheomycotic abscess and cyst

B43.8 Other forms of chromomycosis

B43.9 Chromomycosis, unspecified

4th B44 Aspergillosis
INCLUDES aspergilloma

CC Excl: For CC/MCC codes in category B44, unless otherwise noted: B44.1-B44.7, B44.89-B44.9, B48.3-B48.4, B49, B92, B94.2-B94.9

B44.0 Invasive pulmonary aspergillosis PDx MCC MCC
CC Excl: A15.0-A15.6, A15.8-A15.9, A17.9, A18.82, A18.84, A18.89, A21.2, A22.1, A31.0, A37.01, A37.11, A37.81, A37.91, A42.0, A43.0, A48.1, B25.0, B39.0-B39.2, B44.0, B58.3, B59, B67.1, J09.X1-J09.X2, J10.00-J10.1, J11.00-J11.1, J12.0-J12.3, J12.89-J18.1, J18.8-J18.9, J22, J44.9, J47.0-J70.4, J70.8-J70.9, J98.4, J98.8-J99, Q33.4, R91.1

B44.1 Other pulmonary aspergillosis CC

B44.2 Tonsillar aspergillosis CC

B44.7 Disseminated aspergillosis CC
Generalized aspergillosis

5th B44.8 Other forms of aspergillosis

B44.81 Allergic bronchopulmonary aspergillosis CC
CC Excl: B44.81, J22, J98.8-J98.9

B44.89 Other forms of aspergillosis CC

B44.9 Aspergillosis, unspecified CC

4th B45 Cryptococcosis

CC Excl: For CC/MCC codes in category B45, unless otherwise noted: B45.0-B45.9, B48.3, B49, B92, B94.2-B94.9

B45.0 Pulmonary cryptococcosis HIV CC
CC Excl: B45.0, B45.2-B45.9, B48.3, B49, B92, B94.2-B94.9

B45.1 Cerebral cryptococcosis PDx MCC MCC
Cryptococcal meningitis
Cryptococcosis meningocerebralis
CC Excl: A02.21, A17.0-A17.1, A27.81, A39.0, A50.41, A51.41, A52.13, A54.82, A54.84, A54.89-A54.9, A87.0-A87.9, B00.3, B02.1, B26.1, B37.5, B38.4, B45.1, B58.2, E08.40-E08.49, E08.618-E08.638, E08.649-E08.8, E09.40-E09.49, E09.618-E09.638, E09.649-E09.8, E10.40-E10.49, E10.618-E10.638, E10.649, E10.69-E10.8, E11.40-E11.49, E11.618-E11.638, E11.649, E11.69-E11.8, E13.40-E13.49, E13.618-E13.638, E13.649-E13.8, G00.0-G03.9, G04.2, G32.89, G61.0, G96.8-G96.9, G98.0-G98.8, G99.8

B45.2 Cutaneous cryptococcosis HIV CC

B45.3 Osseous cryptococcosis HIV CC

B45.7 Disseminated cryptococcosis HIV CC
Generalized cryptococcosis

B45.8 Other forms of cryptococcosis HIV CC

B45.9 Cryptococcosis, unspecified HIV CC

4th B46 Zygomycosis

CC Excl: For MCC codes in category B46, unless otherwise noted: B46.0-B46.9, B48.3, B49, B92, B94.2-B94.9

B46.0 Pulmonary mucormycosis MCC

B46.1 Rhinocerebral mucormycosis MCC

B46.2 Gastrointestinal mucormycosis MCC

B46.3 Cutaneous mucormycosis MCC
Subcutaneous mucormycosis

B46.4 Disseminated mucormycosis MCC
Generalized mucormycosis

B46.5 Mucormycosis, unspecified MCC

B46.8 Other zygomycoses MCC
Entomophthoromycosis

B46.9 Zygomycosis, unspecified MCC
Phycomycosis NOS

4th B47 Mycetoma

B47.0 Eumycetoma CC
Madura foot, mycotic
Maduromycosis
CC Excl: B47.0, B48.3, B49, B92, B94.2-B94.9

B47.1 Actinomycetoma HIV CC
CC Excl: A42.0-A42.2, A42.81-A43.9, B47.1-B47.9, L08.1

B47.9 Mycetoma, unspecified HIV CC
Madura foot NOS
CC Excl: A42.81-A42.9, A43.8-A43.9, B47.1-B47.9

4th B48 Other mycoses, not elsewhere classified

B48.0 Lobomycosis
Keloidal blastomycosis
Lobo's disease

B48.1 Rhinosporidiosis

B48.2 Allescheriasis CC
Infection due to Pseudallescheria boydii
EXCLUDES 1 *eumycetoma (B47.0)*
CC Excl: B48.2-B48.3, B49, B92, B94.2-B94.9

B48.3 Geotrichosis CC
Geotrichum stomatitis
CC Excl: B48.3-B49

B48.4 Penicillosis CC
CC Excl: B44.1-B44.7, B44.89-B44.9, B48.3-B48.4, B49, B92, B94.2-B94.9

B48.8 Other specified mycoses HIV CC
Adiaspiromycosis
Infection of tissue and organs by Alternaria
Infection of tissue and organs by Drechslera
Infection of tissue and organs by Fusarium
Infection of tissue and organs by saprophytic fungi NEC
AHA: 2014, 2Q, 13
CC Excl: B48.3, B48.8-B49, B92, B94.2-B94.9

B49 Unspecified mycosis CC
Fungemia NOS
CC Excl: See code: B48.3

Protozoal diseases (B50-B64)

EXCLUDES 1 *amebiasis (A06.-)*
other protozoal intestinal diseases (A07.-)

4th B50 Plasmodium falciparum malaria
INCLUDES mixed infections of Plasmodium falciparum with any other Plasmodium species

CC Excl: For CC/MCC codes in category B50, unless otherwise noted: B50.0-B57.5

B50.0 Plasmodium falciparum malaria with cerebral complications CC
Cerebral malaria NOS

B50.8 Other severe and complicated Plasmodium falciparum malaria CC
Severe or complicated Plasmodium falciparum malaria NOS

B50.9 Plasmodium falciparum malaria, unspecified MCC

4th B51 Plasmodium vivax malaria
INCLUDES mixed infections of Plasmodium vivax with other Plasmodium species, except Plasmodium falciparum
EXCLUDES 1 *plasmodium vivax with Plasmodium falciparum (B50.-)*

CC Excl: For CC codes in category B51, unless otherwise noted: B50.0-B57.5

B51.0 Plasmodium vivax malaria with rupture of spleen CC

B51.8 Plasmodium vivax malaria with other complications CC

B51.9 Plasmodium vivax malaria without complication CC
Plasmodium vivax malaria NOS
CC Excl: A44.0-A44.9, A68.0-A68.9, A69.20-A69.29, B50.0-B57.5, B60.0

4th B52 Plasmodium malariae malaria
INCLUDES mixed infections of Plasmodium malariae with other Plasmodium species, except Plasmodium falciparum and Plasmodium vivax
EXCLUDES 1 *Plasmodium falciparum (B50.-)*
Plasmodium vivax (B51.-)

CC Excl: For CC codes in category B52, unless otherwise noted: B50.0-B57.5

B52.0 Plasmodium malariae malaria with nephropathy PDx CC CC
CC Excl: A17.9, A18.10-A18.11, A18.13, A18.82, A18.84, A18.89, A54.21, A54.29, A54.82, A54.84, A54.89-A54.9, A59.00, A59.8-A59.9, B37.41-B37.49, B50.0-B57.5, E08.21-E08.29, E08.618-E08.638, E08.649-E08.8, E09.21-E09.29, E09.618-E09.638, E09.649-E09.8, E10.21-E10.29, E10.618-E10.638, E10.649, E10.69-E10.8, E11.21-E11.29, E11.618-E11.638, E11.649, E11.69-E11.8, E13.21-E13.29, E13.618-E13.638, E13.649-E13.8, E88.3, M10.30-M10.39, N00.0-N11.0, N11.8-N13.39, N13.6, N14.0-N19, N25.0-N26.1, N26.9-N27.9, N28.1-N29, N36.41-N36.43, N36.8-N36.9, N39.8-N39.9, R31.0-R31.9

B52.8 Plasmodium malariae malaria with other complications CC

B52.9 Plasmodium malariae malaria without complication CC
Plasmodium malariae malaria NOS

B53 Other specified malaria

CC Excl: For CC codes in subcategory B53, unless otherwise noted: B50.0-B57.5

B53.0 Plasmodium ovale malaria CC

EXCLUDES 1 *Plasmodium ovale with Plasmodium falciparum (B50.-)*
Plasmodium ovale with Plasmodium malariae (B52.-)
Plasmodium ovale with Plasmodium vivax (B51.-)

B53.1 Malaria due to simian plasmodia CC

EXCLUDES 1 *Malaria due to simian plasmodia with Plasmodium falciparum (B50.-)*
Malaria due to simian plasmodia with Plasmodium malariae (B52.-)
Malaria due to simian plasmodia with Plasmodium ovale (B53.0)
Malaria due to simian plasmodia with Plasmodium vivax (B51.-)

B53.8 Other malaria, not elsewhere classified CC

B54 Unspecified malaria CC
CC Excl: B50.0-B57.5, B97.21

B55 Leishmaniasis

CC Excl: For CC codes in category B55, unless otherwise noted: A44.0-A44.9, A68.0-A68.9, A69.20-A69.29, A75.0-A79.9, B50.0-B57.5, B60.0

B55.0 Visceral leishmaniasis CC
Kala-azar
Post-kala-azar dermal leishmaniasis

B55.1 Cutaneous leishmaniasis CC

B55.2 Mucocutaneous leishmaniasis CC

B55.9 Leishmaniasis, unspecified CC

B56 African trypanosomiasis

CC Excl: For CC codes in category B56, unless otherwise noted: A44.0-A44.9, A68.0-A68.9, A69.20-A69.29, A75.0-A79.9, B50.0-B57.5, B60.0

B56.0 Gambiense trypanosomiasis CC
Infection due to Trypanosoma brucei gambiense
West African sleeping sickness

B56.1 Rhodesiense trypanosomiasis CC
East African sleeping sickness
Infection due to Trypanosoma brucei rhodesiense

B56.9 African trypanosomiasis, unspecified CC
Sleeping sickness NOS

B57 Chagas' disease

INCLUDES American trypanosomiasis
infection due to Trypanosoma cruzi

CC Excl: For CC codes in category B57, unless otherwise noted: A44.0-A44.9, A68.0-A68.9, A69.20-A69.29, A75.0-A79.9, B50.0-B57.5, B60.0

B57.0 Acute Chagas' disease with heart involvement CC
Acute Chagas' disease with myocarditis
CC Excl: B57.0-B57.2, B92, B94.2-B94.9

B57.1 Acute Chagas' disease without heart involvement CC
Acute Chagas' disease NOS

B57.2 Chagas' disease (chronic) with heart involvement CC
American trypanosomiasis NOS
Chagas' disease (chronic) NOS
Chagas' disease (chronic) with myocarditis
Trypanosomiasis NOS
CC Excl: See code: B57.0

B57.3 Chagas' disease (chronic) with digestive system involvement

B57.30 Chagas' disease with digestive system involvement, unspecified CC

B57.31 Megaesophagus in Chagas' disease CC

B57.32 Megacolon in Chagas' disease CC

B57.39 Other digestive system involvement in Chagas' disease CC

B57.4 Chagas' disease (chronic) with nervous system involvement

B57.40 Chagas' disease with nervous system involvement, unspecified CC

B57.41 Meningitis in Chagas' disease CC

B57.42 Meningoencephalitis in Chagas' disease CC

B57.49 Other nervous system involvement in Chagas' disease CC

B57.5 Chagas' disease (chronic) with other organ involvement CC

B58 Toxoplasmosis

INCLUDES infection due to Toxoplasma gondii

EXCLUDES 1 *congenital toxoplasmosis (P37.1)*

B58.0 Toxoplasma oculopathy

B58.00 Toxoplasma oculopathy, unspecified HIV CC
CC Excl: B58.00-B58.9, B92, B94.2-B94.9

B58.01 Toxoplasma chorioretinitis HIV CC
CC Excl: B58.00-B58.01, B58.82-B58.9, B92, B94.2-B94.9

B58.09 Other toxoplasma oculopathy HIV CC
Toxoplasma uveitis
CC Excl: B58.00-B58.09, B58.82-B58.9, B92, B94.2-B94.9

B58.1 Toxoplasma hepatitis HIV CC
CC Excl: B58.00-B58.1, B58.82-B58.9, B92, B94.2-B94.9

B58.2 Toxoplasma meningoencephalitis HIV MCC
CC Excl: B58.00-B58.2, B58.82-B58.9, B92, B94.2-B94.9

B58.3 Pulmonary toxoplasmosis HIV MCC
CC Excl: A22.1, A37.01, A37.11, A37.81, A37.91, A48.1, B25.0, B44.0, B58.00, B58.3, B58.82-B58.9, B92, B94.2-B94.9, J09.X1-J09.X2, J10.00-J10.1, J11.00-J11.1, J12.0-J12.3, J12.89-J18.1, J18.8-J18.9, J44.9, J47.0-J70.4, J70.8-J70.9, J98.4, R91.1

B58.8 Toxoplasmosis with other organ involvement

CC Excl: For CC/MCC codes in subcategory B58.8, unless otherwise noted: B58.00, B58.81-B58.9, B92, B94.2-B94.9

B58.81 Toxoplasma myocarditis HIV MCC

B58.82 Toxoplasma myositis HIV CC
CC Excl: B58.00, B58.82-B58.9, B92, B94.2-B94.9

B58.83 Toxoplasma tubulo-interstitial nephropathy HIV CC
Toxoplasma pyelonephritis

B58.89 Toxoplasmosis with other organ involvement HIV CC

B58.9 Toxoplasmosis, unspecified HIV CC
CC Excl: B58.9

B59 Pneumocystosis HIV MCC
Pneumonia due to Pneumocystis carinii
Pneumonia due to Pneumocystis jiroveci
CC Excl: A22.1, A37.01, A37.11, A37.81, A37.91, A48.1, B25.0, B44.0, B59, B92, B94.2-B94.9, J09.X1-J09.X2, J10.00-J10.1, J11.00-J11.1, J12.0-J12.3, J12.89-J18.1, J18.8-J18.9, J44.9, J47.0-J70.4, J70.8-J70.9, J98.4, R91.1

B60 Other protozoal diseases, not elsewhere classified

EXCLUDES 1 *cryptosporidiosis (A07.2)*
intestinal microsporidiosis (A07.8)
isosporiasis (A07.3)

B60.0 Babesiosis CC
Piroplasmosis
CC Excl: A44.0-A44.9, A68.0-A68.9, A69.20-A69.29, A75.0-A79.9, B50.0-B57.5, B60.0

B60.1 Acanthamebiasis

B60.10 Acanthamebiasis, unspecified CC
CC Excl: B59, B60.11, B60.19-B64, B89, B99.8-B99.9, L94.6, M35.2

B60.11 Meningoencephalitis due to Acanthamoeba (culbertsoni)

B60.12 Conjunctivitis due to Acanthamoeba

B60.13 Keratoconjunctivitis due to Acanthamoeba

B60.19 Other acanthamebic disease CC
CC Excl: See code: B60.10

B60.2 Naegleriasis CC
Primary amebic meningoencephalitis
CC Excl: See code: B60.10

B60.8 Other specified protozoal diseases HIV
Microsporidiosis

B64 Unspecified protozoal disease

Helminthiases (B65-B83)

B65 Schistosomiasis [bilharziasis]

INCLUDES snail fever

CC Excl: For CC codes in category B65, unless otherwise noted: B65.0-B65.9

B65.0 Schistosomiasis due to Schistosoma haematobium [urinary schistosomiasis] CC

B65.1 Schistosomiasis due to Schistosoma mansoni [intestinal schistosomiasis] CC

B65.2 Schistosomiasis due to Schistosoma japonicum CC
Asiatic schistosomiasis

B65.3 Cercarial dermatitis CC
Swimmer's itch

B65.8 Other schistosomiasis CC
Infection due to Schistosoma intercalatum
Infection due to Schistosoma mattheei
Infection due to Schistosoma mekongi

B65.9 Schistosomiasis, unspecified CC

4th B66 Other fluke infections

CC Excl: For CC codes in category B66, unless otherwise noted: B66.0-B66.9

B66.0 Opisthorchiasis CC
Infection due to cat liver fluke
Infection due to Opisthorchis (felineus)(viverrini)

B66.1 Clonorchiasis CC
Chinese liver fluke disease
Infection due to Clonorchis sinensis
Oriental liver fluke disease

B66.2 Dicroceliasis CC
Infection due to Dicrocoelium dendriticum
Lancet fluke infection

B66.3 Fascioliasis CC
Infection due to Fasciola gigantica
Infection due to Fasciola hepatica
Infection due to Fasciola indica
Sheep liver fluke disease

B66.4 Paragonimiasis CC
Infection due to Paragonimus species
Lung fluke disease
Pulmonary distomiasis

B66.5 Fasciolopsiasis CC
Infection due to Fasciolopsis buski
Intestinal distomiasis

B66.8 Other specified fluke infections CC
Echinostomiasis
Heterophyiasis
Metagonimiasis
Nanophyetiasis
Watsoniasis

B66.9 Fluke infection, unspecified CC

4th B67 Echinococcosis
INCLUDES hydatidosis

B67.0 Echinococcus granulosus infection of liver CC
CC Excl: B67.0, B67.8-B67.99

B67.1 Echinococcus granulosus infection of lung CC
CC Excl: B67.1, B67.8-B67.99, J12.81

B67.2 Echinococcus granulosus infection of bone CC
CC Excl: B67.2, B67.32-B67.39, B67.8-B67.99

5th B67.3 Echinococcus granulosus infection, other and multiple sites

B67.31 Echinococcus granulosus infection, thyroid gland CC
CC Excl: B67.31, B67.8-B67.99

B67.32 Echinococcus granulosus infection, multiple sites CC
CC Excl: B67.2, B67.32-B67.39, B67.8-B67.99

B67.39 Echinococcus granulosus infection, other sites CC
CC Excl: See code: B67.32

B67.4 Echinococcus granulosus infection, unspecified CC
Dog tapeworm (infection)
CC Excl: B67.4, B67.8-B67.99

B67.5 Echinococcus multilocularis infection of liver CC
CC Excl: B67.5, B67.8-B67.99

5th B67.6 Echinococcus multilocularis infection, other and multiple sites

B67.61 Echinococcus multilocularis infection, multiple sites CC
CC Excl: B67.61-B67.69, B67.8-B67.99

B67.69 Echinococcus multilocularis infection, other sites CC
CC Excl: See code: B67.61

B67.7 Echinococcus multilocularis infection, unspecified CC
CC Excl: B67.7-B67.99

B67.8 Echinococcosis, unspecified, of liver CC
CC Excl: B67.8-B67.99

5th B67.9 Echinococcosis, other and unspecified

B67.90 Echinococcosis, unspecified CC
Echinococcosis NOS
CC Excl: See code: B67.8

B67.99 Other echinococcosis CC
CC Excl: See code: B67.8

4th B68 Taeniasis
EXCLUDES 1 *cysticercosis (B69.-)*

B68.0 Taenia solium taeniasis CC
Pork tapeworm (infection)
CC Excl: A00.1, A01.00-A01.09, A01.4-A02.0, A03.9-A05.2, A06.0-A06.2, A06.9, A07.1-A09, A18.32-A18.39, A18.83, A48.51-A48.52, B37.82, B68.0-B71.9, B82.9, J09.X3-J09.X9, J10.2-J10.89, J11.2-J11.89, K30, K31.84, K52.1-K52.2, K52.82-K52.9, K58.0-K58.9, P76.8-P77.9, P78.1, P78.3-P78.89

B68.1 Taenia saginata taeniasis CC
Beef tapeworm (infection)
Infection due to adult tapeworm Taenia saginata
CC Excl: B68.0-B71.9

B68.9 Taeniasis, unspecified CC
CC Excl: See code: B68.1

4th B69 Cysticercosis
INCLUDES cysticerciasis infection due to larval form of Taenia solium

CC Excl: For CC codes in category B69, unless otherwise noted: B68.0-B71.9

B69.0 Cysticercosis of central nervous system CC

B69.1 Cysticercosis of eye CC

5th B69.8 Cysticercosis of other sites

B69.81 Myositis in cysticercosis CC

B69.89 Cysticercosis of other sites CC

B69.9 Cysticercosis, unspecified CC

4th B70 Diphyllobothriasis and sparganosis

CC Excl: For CC codes in category B70, unless otherwise noted: B68.0-B71.9

B70.0 Diphyllobothriasis CC
Diphyllobothrium (adult) (latum) (pacificum) infection
Fish tapeworm (infection)
EXCLUDES 2 *larval diphyllobothriasis (B70.1)*

B70.1 Sparganosis CC
Infection due to Sparganum (mansoni) (proliferum)
Infection due to Spirometra larva
Larval diphyllobothriasis
Spirometrosis

4th B71 Other cestode infections

CC Excl: For CC codes in category B71, unless otherwise noted: B68.0-B71.9

B71.0 Hymenolepiasis CC
Dwarf tapeworm infection
Rat tapeworm (infection)

B71.1 Dipylidiasis CC

B71.8 Other specified cestode infections CC
Coenurosis

B71.9 Cestode infection, unspecified
Tapeworm (infection) NOS

B72 Dracunculiasis CC
INCLUDES guinea worm infection
infection due to Dracunculus medinensis
CC Excl: B72-B74.9

4th B73 Onchocerciasis
INCLUDES onchocerca volvulus infection
onchocercosis
river blindness

CC Excl: For CC codes in category B73, unless otherwise noted: B72-B74.9

5th B73.0 Onchocerciasis with eye disease

B73.00 Onchocerciasis with eye involvement, unspecified CC

B73.01 Onchocerciasis with endophthalmitis CC

B73.02 Onchocerciasis with glaucoma CC

B73.09 Onchocerciasis with other eye involvement CC
Infestation of eyelid due to onchocerciasis

B73.1 Onchocerciasis without eye disease CC

B74 Filariasis
EXCLUDES 2 *onchocerciasis (B73)*
tropical (pulmonary) eosinophilia NOS (J82)

CC Excl: For CC codes in category B74, unless otherwise noted: B72-B74.9

B74.0 Filariasis due to Wuchereria bancrofti CC
Bancroftian elephantiasis
Bancroftian filariasis

B74.1 Filariasis due to Brugia malayi CC

B74.2 Filariasis due to Brugia timori CC

B74.3 Loiasis CC
Calabar swelling
Eyeworm disease of Africa
Loa loa infection

B74.4 Mansonelliasis CC
Infection due to Mansonella ozzardi
Infection due to Mansonella perstans
Infection due to Mansonella streptocerca

B74.8 Other filariases CC
Dirofilariasis

B74.9 Filariasis, unspecified CC

B75 Trichinellosis CC
INCLUDES infection due to Trichinella species
trichiniasis
CC Excl: A17.82- A50.42, A52.14, A75.9, A79.9, A81.1, A81.82-A81.89, A83.0-A85.8, A87.2, A88.0, A88.8, A92.1-A92.8, A93.0, B00.4, B00.82, B01.11-B01.12, B04, B06.01, B08.09, B08.20-B08.22, B08.60-B08.79, B09-B10.09, B26.2, B33.1, B45.0, B45.2-B45.9, B58.2, B75, B97.10, B97.21, G04.00-G04.01, G04.31, G04.81-G05.4, G37.0, G37.4-G37.5, J09.X3-J09.X9, J10.2-J10.89, J11.2-J11.89, L44.4, M1A.10X0-M1A.19X1, P35.2-P35.9, P37.0-P37.4, P37.8-P37.9, T56.0X1A, T56.0X2A, T56.0X3A, T56.0X4A

B76 Hookworm diseases
INCLUDES uncinariasis

CC Excl: For CC codes in category B76, unless otherwise noted: B76.0-B76.9

B76.0 Ancylostomiasis CC
Infection due to Ancylostoma species

B76.1 Necatoriasis CC
Infection due to Necator americanus

B76.8 Other hookworm diseases CC

B76.9 Hookworm disease, unspecified CC
Cutaneous larva migrans NOS

B77 Ascariasis
INCLUDES ascaridiasis
roundworm infection

B77.0 Ascariasis with intestinal complications CC
CC Excl: B77.0-B78.0, B78.7-B82.0

B77.8 Ascariasis with other complications

B77.81 Ascariasis pneumonia PDx MCC MCC
CC Excl: A15.0-A15.6, A15.8-A15.9, A17.9, A18.82, A18.84, A18.89, A21.2, A22.1, A31.0, A37.01, A37.11, A37.81, A37.91, A42.0, A43.0, A48.1, B25.0, B39.0-B39.2, B44.0, B58.3, B59, B67.1, B77.0-B78.0, B78.7-B82.0, J09.X1-J09.X2, J10.00-J10.1, J11.00-J11.1, J12.0-J12.3, J12.89-J18.1, J18.8-J18.9, J22, J44.9, J47.0-J70.4, J70.8-J70.9, J98.4, J98.8-J99, Q33.4, R91.1

B77.89 Ascariasis with other complications CC
CC Excl: B77.0-B78.0, B78.7-B82.0

B77.9 Ascariasis, unspecified CC
CC Excl: See code B77.0

B78 Strongyloidiasis
EXCLUDES 1 *trichostrongyliasis (B81.2)*

CC Excl: For CC codes in category B78, unless otherwise noted: B77.0-B78.0, B78.7-B82.0

B78.0 Intestinal strongyloidiasis HIV CC

B78.1 Cutaneous strongyloidiasis

B78.7 Disseminated strongyloidiasis HIV CC

B78.9 Strongyloidiasis, unspecified HIV CC

B79 Trichuriasis CC
INCLUDES trichocephaliasis
whipworm (disease)(infection)
CC Excl: See code: B77.89

B80 Enterobiasis CC
INCLUDES oxyuriasis
pinworm infection
threadworm infection
CC Excl: See code: B77.89

B81 Other intestinal helminthiases, not elsewhere classified
EXCLUDES 1 *angiostrongyliasis due to Parastrongylus cantonensis (B83.2)*

CC Excl: For CC codes in subcategories B81.0-B81.2, unless otherwise noted: B77.0-B78.0, B78.7-B82.0 **For CC codes in subcategories B81.3-B81.8:** B77.0-B78.0, B78.7-B83.3, B83.8-B83.9

B81.0 Anisakiasis CC
Infection due to Anisakis larva

B81.1 Intestinal capillariasis CC
Capillariasis NOS
Infection due to Capillaria philippinensis
EXCLUDES 2 *hepatic capillariasis (B83.8)*

B81.2 Trichostrongyliasis CC

B81.3 Intestinal angiostrongyliasis CC
Angiostrongyliasis due to Parastrongylus costaricensis

B81.4 Mixed intestinal helminthiases CC
Infection due to intestinal helminths classified to more than one of the categories B65.0-B81.3 and B81.8
Mixed helminthiasis NOS

B81.8 Other specified intestinal helminthiases CC
Infection due to Oesophagostomum species [esophagostomiasis]
Infection due to Ternidens diminutus [ternidensiasis]

B82 Unspecified intestinal parasitism

B82.0 Intestinal helminthiasis, unspecified CC
CC Excl: See code: B81.3

B82.9 Intestinal parasitism, unspecified

B83 Other helminthiases
EXCLUDES 1 *capillariasis NOS (B81.1)*
EXCLUDES 2 *intestinal capillariasis (B81.1)*

B83.0 Visceral larva migrans
Toxocariasis

B83.1 Gnathostomiasis
Wandering swelling

B83.2 Angiostrongyliasis due to Parastrongylus cantonensis
Eosinophilic meningoencephalitis due to Parastrongylus cantonensis
EXCLUDES 2 *intestinal angiostrongyliasis (B81.3)*

B83.3 Syngamiasis
Syngamosis

B83.4 Internal hirudiniasis
EXCLUDES 2 *external hirudiniasis (B88.3)*

B83.8 Other specified helminthiases
Acanthocephaliasis
Gongylonemiasis
Hepatic capillariasis
Metastrongyliasis
Thelaziasis

B83.9 Helminthiasis, unspecified
Worms NOS
EXCLUDES 1 *intestinal helminthiasis NOS (B82.0)*

Pediculosis, acariasis and other infestations (B85-B89)

B85 Pediculosis and phthiriasis

B85.0 Pediculosis due to Pediculus humanus capitis
Head-louse infestation

B85.1 Pediculosis due to Pediculus humanus corporis
Body-louse infestation

B85.2 Pediculosis, unspecified

B85.3 Phthiriasis
Infestation by crab-louse
Infestation by Phthirus pubis

B85.4 Mixed pediculosis and phthiriasis
Infestation classifiable to more than one of the categories B85.0-B85.3

B86 Scabies
Sarcoptic itch

B87 Myiasis
INCLUDES infestation by larva of flies

B87.0 Cutaneous myiasis
Creeping myiasis

B87.1 Wound myiasis
Traumatic myiasis

B87.2 Ocular **myiasis**

B87.3 Nasopharyngeal **myiasis**
Laryngeal myiasis

B87.4 Aural **myiasis**

✓5th **B87.8 Myiasis of** other sites

B87.81 Genitourinary **myiasis**

B87.82 Intestinal **myiasis**

B87.89 Myiasis of other sites

B87.9 Myiasis, unspecified

✓4th **B88 Other infestations**

B88.0 Other acariasis
Acarine dermatitis
Dermatitis due to Demodex species
Dermatitis due to Dermanyssus gallinae
Dermatitis due to Liponyssoides sanguineus
Trombiculosis
EXCLUDES 2 *scabies (B86)*

B88.1 Tungiasis [sandflea infestation]

B88.2 Other arthropod infestations
Scarabiasis

B88.3 External hirudiniasis
Leech infestation NOS
EXCLUDES 2 *internal hirudiniasis (B83.4)*

B88.8 Other specified infestations
Ichthyoparasitism due to Vandellia cirrhosa
Linguatulosis
Porocephaliasis

B88.9 Infestation, unspecified
Infestation (skin) NOS
Skin parasites NOS
Infestation by mites NOS

B89 Unspecified parasitic disease

Sequelae of infectious and parasitic diseases (B90-B94)

NOTE Categories B90-B94 are to be used to indicate conditions in categories A00-B89 as the cause of sequelae, which are themselves classified elsewhere. The "sequelae" include conditions specified as such; they also include residuals of diseases classifiable to the above categories if there is evidence that the disease itself is no longer present. Codes from these categories are not to be used for chronic infections. Code chronic current infections to active infectious disease as appropriate.

Code first condition resulting from (sequela) the infectious or parasitic disease

✓4th **B90 Sequelae of** tuberculosis

B90.0 Sequelae of central nervous system **tuberculosis**

B90.1 Sequelae of genitourinary **tuberculosis**

B90.2 Sequelae of tuberculosis of bones and joints

B90.8 Sequelae of tuberculosis of other **organs**
EXCLUDES 2 *sequelae of respiratory tuberculosis (B90.9)*

B90.9 Sequelae of respiratory and unspecified **tuberculosis**
Sequelae of tuberculosis NOS

B91 Sequelae of poliomyelitis
EXCLUDES 1 *postpolio syndrome (G14)*

B92 Sequelae of leprosy

✓4th **B94 Sequelae of** other and unspecified **infectious and parasitic diseases**

B94.0 Sequelae of trachoma

B94.1 Sequelae of viral encephalitis

B94.2 Sequelae of viral hepatitis

B94.8 Sequelae of other **specified infectious and parasitic diseases**

B94.9 Sequelae of unspecified **infectious and parasitic disease**

Bacterial and viral infectious agents (B95-B97)

NOTE These categories are provided for use as supplementary or additional codes to identify the infectious agent(s) in diseases classified elsewhere.

✓4th **B95 Streptococcus, Staphylococcus, and Enterococcus as the cause of diseases classified elsewhere**

B95.0 Streptococcus, group A, **as the cause of diseases classified elsewhere**

B95.1 Streptococcus, group B, **as the cause of diseases classified elsewhere**

B95.2 Enterococcus **as the cause of diseases classified elsewhere**

B95.3 Streptococcus pneumoniae **as the cause of diseases classified elsewhere**

B95.4 Other streptococcus **as the cause of diseases classified elsewhere**

B95.5 Unspecified streptococcus **as the cause of diseases classified elsewhere**

✓5th **B95.6** Staphylococcus aureus **as the cause of diseases classified elsewhere**

B95.61 Methicillin susceptible **Staphylococcus aureus infection as the cause of diseases classified elsewhere**
Methicillin susceptible Staphylococcus aureus (MSSA) infection as the cause of diseases classified elsewhere
Staphylococcus aureus infection NOS as the cause of diseases classified elsewhere

B95.62 Methicillin resistant **Staphylococcus aureus infection as the cause of diseases classified elsewhere**
Methicillin resistant Staphylococcus aureus (MRSA) infection as the cause of diseases classified elsewhere

B95.7 Other **staphylococcus as the cause of diseases classified elsewhere**

B95.8 Unspecified **staphylococcus as the cause of diseases classified elsewhere**

✓4th **B96 Other bacterial agents as the cause of diseases classified elsewhere**

B96.0 Mycoplasma pneumoniae **[M. pneumoniae] as the cause of diseases classified elsewhere**
Pleuro-pneumonia-like-organism [PPLO]

B96.1 Klebsiella pneumoniae **[K. pneumoniae] as the cause of diseases classified elsewhere**

✓5th **B96.2** Escherichia coli **[E. coli] as the cause of diseases classified elsewhere**

B96.20 Unspecified **Escherichia coli [E. coli] as the cause of diseases classified elsewhere**
Escherichia coli [E. coli] NOS

B96.21 Shiga toxin-producing **Escherichia coli [E. coli] (STEC)** O157 **as the cause of diseases classified elsewhere**
E. coli O157:H- (nonmotile) with confirmation of Shiga toxin
E. coli O157 with confirmation of Shiga toxin when H antigen is unknown, or is not H7
O157:H7 Escherichia coli [E.coli] with or without confirmation of Shiga toxin-production
Shiga toxin-producing Escherichia coli [E.coli] O157:H7 with or without confirmation of Shiga toxin-production
STEC O157:H7 with or without confirmation of Shiga toxin-production

B96.22 Other specified Shiga toxin-producing **Escherichia coli [E. coli] (STEC) as the cause of diseases classified elsewhere**
Non-O157 Shiga toxin-producing Escherichia coli [E.coli]
Non-O157 Shiga toxin-producing Escherichia coli [E.coli] with known O group

B96.23 Unspecified Shiga toxin-producing **Escherichia coli [E. coli] (STEC) as the cause of diseases classified elsewhere**
Shiga toxin-producing Escherichia coli [E. coli] with unspecified O group
STEC NOS

B96.29 Other **Escherichia coli [E. coli] as the cause of diseases classified elsewhere**
Non-Shiga toxin-producing E. coli

B96.3 Hemophilus influenzae **[H. influenzae] as the cause of diseases classified elsewhere**

B96.4 Proteus **(mirabilis) (morganii) as the cause of diseases classified elsewhere**

B96.5 Pseudomonas **(aeruginosa) (mallei) (pseudomallei) as the cause of diseases classified elsewhere**

B96.6 Bacteroides fragilis **[B. fragilis] as the cause of diseases classified elsewhere**

B96.7 Clostridium perfringens **[C. perfringens] as the cause of diseases classified elsewhere**

✓5th **B96.8 Other specified bacterial agents as the cause of diseases classified elsewhere**

B96.81 Helicobacter pylori **[H. pylori] as the cause of diseases classified elsewhere**

B96.82 **Vibrio vulnificus as the cause of diseases classified elsewhere**

B96.89 **Other specified bacterial agents as the cause of diseases classified elsewhere**

✓4th **B97 Viral agents as the cause of diseases classified elsewhere**

B97.0 **Adenovirus as the cause of diseases classified elsewhere**

✓5th **B97.1 Enterovirus as the cause of diseases classified elsewhere**

B97.10 **Unspecified enterovirus as the cause of diseases classified elsewhere**

B97.11 **Coxsackievirus as the cause of diseases classified elsewhere**

B97.12 **Echovirus as the cause of diseases classified elsewhere**

B97.19 **Other enterovirus as the cause of diseases classified elsewhere**

✓5th **B97.2 Coronavirus as the cause of diseases classified elsewhere**

B97.21 **SARS-associated coronavirus as the cause of diseases classified elsewhere** CC

EXCLUDES 1 *pneumonia due to SARS-associated coronavirus (J12.81)*

CC Excl: A15.0-A15.6, A15.8-A15.9, A17.9, A18.82, A18.84, A18.89, A21.2, A22.1, A31.0, A37.01, A37.11, A37.81, A37.91, A42.0, A43.0, A48.1, B25.0, B34.1-B34.2, B34.4-B34.8, B39.0-B39.2, B44.0, B58.3, B59, B67.1, B97.19-B97.29, B97.5-B97.6, B97.81-B97.89, J09.X1-J09.X2, J10.00-J10.1, J11.00-J11.1, J12.0-J12.3, J12.89-J18.1, J18.8-J18.9, J22, J44.9, J47.0-J70.4, J70.8-J70.9, J98.4, J98.8-J99, Q33.4, R91.1

B97.29 **Other coronavirus as the cause of diseases classified elsewhere**

✓5th **B97.3 Retrovirus as the cause of diseases classified elsewhere**

EXCLUDES 1 *human immunodeficiency virus [HIV] disease (B20)*

B97.30 **Unspecified retrovirus as the cause of diseases classified elsewhere**

B97.31 **Lentivirus as the cause of diseases classified elsewhere**

B97.32 **Oncovirus as the cause of diseases classified elsewhere**

B97.33 **Human T-cell lymphotrophic virus, type I [HTLV-I] as the cause of diseases classified elsewhere** CC

CC Excl: A74.81, A74.9, B33.3-B33.4, B34.1-B34.2, B34.4-B34.8, B97.10, B97.19-B97.29, B97.31-B97.39, B97.5-B97.6, B97.81-B97.89

B97.34 **Human T-cell lymphotrophic virus, type II [HTLV-II] as the cause of diseases classified elsewhere** CC

CC Excl: A74.81, A74.9, B33.3-B33.4, B34.1-B34.2, B34.4-B34.8, B97.10, B97.19-B97.39, B97.5-B97.6, B97.81-B97.89

B97.35 **Human immunodeficiency virus, type 2 [HIV 2] as the cause of diseases classified elsewhere** CC

CC Excl: A74.81, A74.9, B20, B33.3-B33.4, B34.1-B34.2, B34.4-B34.8, B97.10, B97.19-B97.39, B97.5-B97.6, B97.81-B97.89

B97.39 **Other retrovirus as the cause of diseases classified elsewhere**

B97.4 **Respiratory syncytial virus as the cause of diseases classified elsewhere**

B97.5 **Reovirus as the cause of diseases classified elsewhere**

B97.6 **Parvovirus as the cause of diseases classified elsewhere**

B97.7 **Papillomavirus as the cause of diseases classified elsewhere**

✓5th **B97.8 Other viral agents as the cause of diseases classified elsewhere**

B97.81 **Human metapneumovirus as the cause of diseases classified elsewhere**

B97.89 **Other viral agents as the cause of diseases classified elsewhere**

Other infectious diseases (B99)

✓4th **B99 Other and unspecified infectious diseases**

B99.8 **Other infectious disease** HIV

B99.9 **Unspecified infectious disease**

Chapter 2. Neoplasms (C00-D49)

NOTE

Functional activity
All neoplasms are classified in this chapter, whether they are functionally active or not. An additional code from Chapter 4 may be used, to identify functional activity associated with any neoplasm.

Morphology [Histology]
Chapter 2 classifies neoplasms primarily by site (topography), with broad groupings for behavior, malignant, in situ, benign, etc. The Table of Neoplasms should be used to identify the correct topography code. In a few cases, such as for malignant melanoma and certain neuroendocrine tumors, the morphology (histologic type) is included in the category and codes.

Primary malignant neoplasms overlapping site boundaries
A primary malignant neoplasm that overlaps two or more contiguous (next to each other) sites should be classified to the subcategory/code 8 ("overlapping lesion"), unless the combination is specifically indexed elsewhere. For multiple neoplasms of the same site that are not contiguous, such as tumors in different quadrants of the same breast, codes for each site should be assigned.

Malignant neoplasm of ectopic tissue
Malignant neoplasms of ectopic tissue are to be coded to the site mentioned, e.g., ectopic pancreatic malignant neoplasms are coded to pancreas, unspecified (C25.9).

This chapter contains the following blocks:

C00-C14	Malignant neoplasms of lip, oral cavity and pharynx
C15-C26	Malignant neoplasms of digestive organs
C30-C39	Malignant neoplasms of respiratory and intrathoracic organs
C40-C41	Malignant neoplasms of bone and articular cartilage
C43-C44	Melanoma and other malignant neoplasms of skin
C45-C49	Malignant neoplasms of mesothelial and soft tissue
C50	Malignant neoplasms of breast
C51-C58	Malignant neoplasms of female genital organs
C60-C63	Malignant neoplasms of male genital organs
C64-C68	Malignant neoplasms of urinary tract
C69-C72	Malignant neoplasms of eye, brain and other parts of central nervous system
C73-C75	Malignant neoplasms of thyroid and other endocrine glands
C7A	Malignant neuroendocrine tumors
C7B	Secondary neuroendocrine tumors
C76-C80	Malignant neoplasms of ill-defined, other secondary and unspecified sites
C81-C96	Malignant neoplasms of lymphoid, hematopoietic and related tissue
D00-D09	In situ neoplasms
D10-D36	Benign neoplasms, except benign neuroendocrine tumors
D3A	Benign neuroendocrine tumors
D37-D48	Neoplasms of uncertain behavior, polycythemia vera and myelodysplastic syndromes
D49	Neoplasms of unspecified behavior

MALIGNANT NEOPLASMS (C00-C96)

NOTE Malignant neoplasms, stated or presumed to be primary (of specified sites), and certain specified histologies, except neuroendocrine, and of lymphoid, hematopoietic and related tissue (C00-C75)

Malignant neoplasms of lip, oral cavity and pharynx (C00-C14)

✓4th **C00 Malignant neoplasm of lip**
Use additional code to identify:
- alcohol abuse and dependence (F10.-)
- history of tobacco use (Z87.891)
- tobacco dependence (F17.-)
- tobacco use (Z72.0)

EXCLUDES 1 *malignant melanoma of lip (C43.0)*
Merkel cell carcinoma of lip (C4A.0)
other and unspecified malignant neoplasm of skin of lip (C44.0-)

C00.0 Malignant neoplasm of external upper lip
Malignant neoplasm of lipstick area of upper lip
Malignant neoplasm of upper lip NOS
Malignant neoplasm of vermilion border of upper lip

C00.1 Malignant neoplasm of external lower lip
Malignant neoplasm of lower lip NOS
Malignant neoplasm of lipstick area of lower lip
Malignant neoplasm of vermilion border of lower lip

C00.2 Malignant neoplasm of external lip, unspecified
Malignant neoplasm of vermilion border of lip NOS

C00.3 Malignant neoplasm of upper lip, inner aspect
Malignant neoplasm of buccal aspect of upper lip
Malignant neoplasm of frenulum of upper lip
Malignant neoplasm of mucosa of upper lip
Malignant neoplasm of oral aspect of upper lip

C00.4 Malignant neoplasm of lower lip, inner aspect
Malignant neoplasm of buccal aspect of lower lip
Malignant neoplasm of frenulum of lower lip
Malignant neoplasm of mucosa of lower lip
Malignant neoplasm of oral aspect of lower lip

C00.5 Malignant neoplasm of lip, unspecified, inner aspect
Malignant neoplasm of buccal aspect of lip, unspecified
Malignant neoplasm of frenulum of lip, unspecified
Malignant neoplasm of mucosa of lip, unspecified
Malignant neoplasm of oral aspect of lip, unspecified

C00.6 Malignant neoplasm of commissure of lip, unspecified

C00.8 Malignant neoplasm of overlapping sites of lip

C00.9 Malignant neoplasm of lip, unspecified

C01 Malignant neoplasm of base of tongue
Malignant neoplasm of dorsal surface of base of tongue
Malignant neoplasm of fixed part of tongue NOS
Malignant neoplasm of posterior third of tongue
Use additional code to identify:
- alcohol abuse and dependence (F10.-)
- history of tobacco use (Z87.891)
- tobacco dependence (F17.-)
- tobacco use (Z72.0)

✓4th **C02 Malignant neoplasm of other and unspecified parts of tongue**
Use additional code to identify:
- alcohol abuse and dependence (F10.-)
- history of tobacco use (Z87.891)
- tobacco dependence (F17.-)
- tobacco use (Z72.0)

C02.0 Malignant neoplasm of dorsal surface of tongue
Malignant neoplasm of anterior two-thirds of tongue, dorsal surface
EXCLUDES 2 *malignant neoplasm of dorsal surface of base of tongue (C01)*

C02.1 Malignant neoplasm of border of tongue
Malignant neoplasm of tip of tongue

C02.2 Malignant neoplasm of ventral surface of tongue
Malignant neoplasm of anterior two-thirds of tongue, ventral surface
Malignant neoplasm of frenulum linguae

C02.3 Malignant neoplasm of anterior two-thirds of tongue, part unspecified
Malignant neoplasm of middle third of tongue NOS
Malignant neoplasm of mobile part of tongue NOS

C02.4 Malignant neoplasm of lingual tonsil
EXCLUDES 2 *malignant neoplasm of tonsil NOS (C09.9)*

C02.8 Malignant neoplasm of overlapping sites of tongue
Malignant neoplasm of two or more contiguous sites of tongue

C02.9 Malignant neoplasm of tongue, unspecified

✓4th **C03 Malignant neoplasm of gum**
INCLUDES malignant neoplasm of alveolar (ridge) mucosa
malignant neoplasm of gingiva
Use additional code to identify:
- alcohol abuse and dependence (F10.-)
- history of tobacco use (Z87.891)
- tobacco dependence (F17.-)
- tobacco use (Z72.0)

EXCLUDES 2 *malignant odontogenic neoplasms (C41.0-C41.1)*

C03.0 Malignant neoplasm of upper gum

C03.1 Malignant neoplasm of lower gum

C03.9 Malignant neoplasm of gum, unspecified

✓4th **C04 Malignant neoplasm of floor of mouth**
Use additional code to identify:
- alcohol abuse and dependence (F10.-)
- history of tobacco use (Z87.891)
- tobacco dependence (F17.-)
- tobacco use (Z72.0)

C04.0 Malignant neoplasm of anterior floor of mouth
Malignant neoplasm of anterior to the premolar-canine junction

C04.1 Malignant neoplasm of lateral floor of mouth

C04.8 Malignant neoplasm of overlapping sites of floor of mouth

C04.9 Malignant neoplasm of floor of mouth, unspecified

C05 Malignant neoplasm of palate
Use additional code to identify:
alcohol abuse and dependence (F10.-)
history of tobacco use (Z87.891)
tobacco dependence (F17.-)
tobacco use (Z72.0)
EXCLUDES 1 *Kaposi's sarcoma of palate (C46.2)*

C05.0 Malignant neoplasm of hard palate

C05.1 Malignant neoplasm of soft palate
EXCLUDES 2 *malignant neoplasm of nasopharyngeal surface of soft palate (C11.3)*

C05.2 Malignant neoplasm of uvula

C05.8 Malignant neoplasm of overlapping sites of palate

C05.9 Malignant neoplasm of palate, unspecified
Malignant neoplasm of roof of mouth

C06 Malignant neoplasm of other and unspecified parts of mouth
Use additional code to identify:
alcohol abuse and dependence (F10.-)
history of tobacco use (Z87.891)
tobacco dependence (F17.-)
tobacco use (Z72.0)

C06.0 Malignant neoplasm of cheek mucosa
Malignant neoplasm of buccal mucosa NOS
Malignant neoplasm of internal cheek

C06.1 Malignant neoplasm of vestibule of mouth
Malignant neoplasm of buccal sulcus (upper) (lower)
Malignant neoplasm of labial sulcus (upper) (lower)

C06.2 Malignant neoplasm of retromolar area

C06.8 Malignant neoplasm of overlapping sites of other and unspecified parts of mouth

C06.80 Malignant neoplasm of overlapping sites of unspecified parts of mouth

C06.89 Malignant neoplasm of overlapping sites of other parts of mouth
"book leaf" neoplasm [ventral surface of tongue and floor of mouth]

C06.9 Malignant neoplasm of mouth, unspecified
Malignant neoplasm of minor salivary gland, unspecified site
Malignant neoplasm of oral cavity NOS

C07 Malignant neoplasm of parotid gland
Use additional code to identify:
alcohol abuse and dependence (F10.-)
exposure to environmental tobacco smoke (Z77.22)
exposure to tobacco smoke in the perinatal period (P96.81)
history of tobacco use (Z87.891)
occupational exposure to environmental tobacco smoke (Z57.31)
tobacco dependence (F17.-)
tobacco use (Z72.0)

C08 Malignant neoplasm of other and unspecified major salivary glands
INCLUDES malignant neoplasm of salivary ducts
Use additional code to identify:
alcohol abuse and dependence (F10.-)
exposure to environmental tobacco smoke (Z77.22)
exposure to tobacco smoke in the perinatal period (P96.81)
history of tobacco use (Z87.891)
occupational exposure to environmental tobacco smoke (Z57.31)
tobacco dependence (F17.-)
tobacco use (Z72.0)
EXCLUDES 1 *malignant neoplasms of specified minor salivary glands which are classified according to their anatomical location*
EXCLUDES 2 *malignant neoplasms of minor salivary glands NOS (C06.9)*
malignant neoplasm of parotid gland (C07)

C08.0 Malignant neoplasm of submandibular gland
Malignant neoplasm of submaxillary gland

C08.1 Malignant neoplasm of sublingual gland

C08.9 Malignant neoplasm of major salivary gland, unspecified
Malignant neoplasm of salivary gland (major) NOS

C09 Malignant neoplasm of tonsil
Use additional code to identify:
alcohol abuse and dependence (F10.-)
exposure to environmental tobacco smoke (Z77.22)
exposure to tobacco smoke in the perinatal period (P96.81)
history of tobacco use (Z87.891)
occupational exposure to environmental tobacco smoke (Z57.31)
tobacco dependence (F17.-)
tobacco use (Z72.0)
EXCLUDES 2 *malignant neoplasm of lingual tonsil (C02.4)*
malignant neoplasm of pharyngeal tonsil (C11.1)

C09.0 Malignant neoplasm of tonsillar fossa

C09.1 Malignant neoplasm of tonsillar pillar (anterior) (posterior)

C09.8 Malignant neoplasm of overlapping sites of tonsil

C09.9 Malignant neoplasm of tonsil, unspecified
Malignant neoplasm of tonsil NOS
Malignant neoplasm of faucial tonsils
Malignant neoplasm of palatine tonsils

C10 Malignant neoplasm of oropharynx
Use additional code to identify:
alcohol abuse and dependence (F10.-)
exposure to environmental tobacco smoke (Z77.22)
exposure to tobacco smoke in the perinatal period (P96.81)
history of tobacco use (Z87.891)
occupational exposure to environmental tobacco smoke (Z57.31)
tobacco dependence (F17.-)
tobacco use (Z72.0)
EXCLUDES 2 *malignant neoplasm of tonsil (C09.-)*

C10.0 Malignant neoplasm of vallecula

C10.1 Malignant neoplasm of anterior surface of epiglottis
Malignant neoplasm of epiglottis, free border [margin]
Malignant neoplasm of glossoepiglottic fold(s)
EXCLUDES 2 *malignant neoplasm of epiglottis (suprahyoid portion) NOS (C32.1)*

C10.2 Malignant neoplasm of lateral wall of oropharynx

C10.3 Malignant neoplasm of posterior wall of oropharynx

C10.4 Malignant neoplasm of branchial cleft
Malignant neoplasm of branchial cyst [site of neoplasm]

C10.8 Malignant neoplasm of overlapping sites of oropharynx
Malignant neoplasm of junctional region of oropharynx

C10.9 Malignant neoplasm of oropharynx, unspecified

C11 Malignant neoplasm of nasopharynx
Use additional code to identify:
exposure to environmental tobacco smoke (Z77.22)
exposure to tobacco smoke in the perinatal period (P96.81)
history of tobacco use (Z87.891)
occupational exposure to environmental tobacco smoke (Z57.31)
tobacco dependence (F17.-)
tobacco use (Z72.0)

C11.0 Malignant neoplasm of superior wall of nasopharynx
Malignant neoplasm of roof of nasopharynx

C11.1 Malignant neoplasm of posterior wall of nasopharynx
Malignant neoplasm of adenoid
Malignant neoplasm of pharyngeal tonsil

C11.2 Malignant neoplasm of lateral wall of nasopharynx
Malignant neoplasm of fossa of Rosenmüller
Malignant neoplasm of opening of auditory tube
Malignant neoplasm of pharyngeal recess

C11.3 Malignant neoplasm of anterior wall of nasopharynx
Malignant neoplasm of floor of nasopharynx
Malignant neoplasm of nasopharyngeal (anterior) (posterior) surface of soft palate
Malignant neoplasm of posterior margin of nasal choana
Malignant neoplasm of posterior margin of nasal septum

C11.8 Malignant neoplasm of overlapping sites of nasopharynx

C11.9 Malignant neoplasm of nasopharynx, unspecified
Malignant neoplasm of nasopharyngeal wall NOS

C12 Malignant neoplasm of pyriform sinus
Malignant neoplasm of pyriform fossa
Use additional code to identify:
exposure to environmental tobacco smoke (Z77.22)
exposure to tobacco smoke in the perinatal period (P96.81)
history of tobacco use (Z87.891)
occupational exposure to environmental tobacco smoke (Z57.31)
tobacco dependence (F17.-)
tobacco use (Z72.0)

✓4th C13 Malignant neoplasm of hypopharynx
Use additional code to identify:
exposure to environmental tobacco smoke (Z77.22)
exposure to tobacco smoke in the perinatal period (P96.81)
history of tobacco use (Z87.891)
occupational exposure to environmental tobacco smoke (Z57.31)
tobacco dependence (F17.-)
tobacco use (Z72.Ø)
EXCLUDES 2 *malignant neoplasm of pyriform sinus (C12)*

C13.Ø Malignant neoplasm of postcricoid region

C13.1 Malignant neoplasm of aryepiglottic fold, hypopharyngeal aspect
Malignant neoplasm of aryepiglottic fold, marginal zone
Malignant neoplasm of aryepiglottic fold NOS
Malignant neoplasm of interarytenoid fold, marginal zone
Malignant neoplasm of interarytenoid fold NOS
EXCLUDES 2 *malignant neoplasm of aryepiglottic fold or interarytenoid fold, laryngeal aspect (C32.1)*

C13.2 Malignant neoplasm of posterior wall of hypopharynx

C13.8 Malignant neoplasm of overlapping sites of hypopharynx

C13.9 Malignant neoplasm of hypopharynx, unspecified
Malignant neoplasm of hypopharyngeal wall NOS

✓4th C14 Malignant neoplasm of other and ill-defined sites in the lip, oral cavity and pharynx
Use additional code to identify:
alcohol abuse and dependence (F1Ø.-)
exposure to environmental tobacco smoke (Z77.22)
exposure to tobacco smoke in the perinatal period (P96.81)
history of tobacco use (Z87.891)
occupational exposure to environmental tobacco smoke (Z57.31)
tobacco dependence (F17.-)
tobacco use (Z72.Ø)
EXCLUDES 1 *malignant neoplasm of oral cavity NOS (CØ6.9)*

C14.Ø Malignant neoplasm of pharynx, unspecified

C14.2 Malignant neoplasm of Waldeyer's ring

C14.8 Malignant neoplasm of overlapping sites of lip, oral cavity and pharynx
Primary malignant neoplasm of two or more contiguous sites of lip, oral cavity and pharynx
EXCLUDES 1 *"book leaf" neoplasm [ventral surface of tongue and floor of mouth] (CØ6.89)*

Malignant neoplasms of digestive organs (C15-C26)

EXCLUDES 1 *Kaposi's sarcoma of gastrointestinal sites (C46.4)*

✓4th C15 Malignant neoplasm of esophagus
Use additional code to identify:
alcohol abuse and dependence (F1Ø.-)

CC Excl: For CC codes in category C15, unless otherwise noted: C15.3-C15.9, C26.Ø, C26.9, C45.7-C45.9, C46.4, C76.8, C7A.ØØ, C7A.Ø98-C7B.ØØ, C7B.1, C8Ø.Ø-C8Ø.2, D49.Ø, D49.81-D49.9

C15.3 Malignant neoplasm of upper third of esophagus CC

C15.4 Malignant neoplasm of middle third of esophagus CC

C15.5 Malignant neoplasm of lower third of esophagus CC
EXCLUDES 1 *malignant neoplasm of cardio-esophageal junction (C16.Ø)*

C15.8 Malignant neoplasm of overlapping sites of esophagus CC

C15.9 Malignant neoplasm of esophagus, unspecified CC

✓4th C16 Malignant neoplasm of stomach
Use additional code to identify:
alcohol abuse and dependence (F1Ø.-)
EXCLUDES 2 *malignant carcinoid tumor of the stomach (C7A.Ø92)*

CC Excl: For CC codes in category C16, unless otherwise noted: C16.Ø-C16.9, C26.Ø, C26.9, C45.7-C45.9, C46.4, C76.8, C7A.ØØ, C7A.Ø92, C7A.Ø94-C7B.ØØ, C7B.1, C8Ø.Ø-C8Ø.2, D49.Ø, D49.81-D49.9

C16.Ø Malignant neoplasm of cardia CC
Malignant neoplasm of cardiac orifice
Malignant neoplasm of cardio-esophageal junction
Malignant neoplasm of esophagus and stomach
Malignant neoplasm of gastro-esophageal junction

C16.1 Malignant neoplasm of fundus of stomach CC

C16.2 Malignant neoplasm of body of stomach CC

C16.3 Malignant neoplasm of pyloric antrum CC
Malignant neoplasm of gastric antrum

C16.4 Malignant neoplasm of pylorus CC
Malignant neoplasm of prepylorus
Malignant neoplasm of pyloric canal

C16.5 Malignant neoplasm of lesser curvature of stomach, unspecified CC
Malignant neoplasm of lesser curvature of stomach, not classifiable to C16.1-C16.4

C16.6 Malignant neoplasm of greater curvature of stomach, unspecified CC
Malignant neoplasm of greater curvature of stomach, not classifiable to C16.Ø-C16.4

C16.8 Malignant neoplasm of overlapping sites of stomach CC

C16.9 Malignant neoplasm of stomach, unspecified CC
Gastric cancer NOS

✓4th C17 Malignant neoplasm of small intestine
EXCLUDES 1 *malignant carcinoid tumors of the small intestine (C7A.Ø1)*

C17.Ø Malignant neoplasm of duodenum CC
CC Excl: C17.Ø, C17.8-C17.9, C26.Ø, C26.9, C45.7-C45.9, C46.4, C7A.ØØ-C7A.Ø1Ø, C7A.Ø19, C7A.Ø98-C7B.ØØ, C7B.1, C76.8, C8Ø.Ø-C8Ø.2, D49.Ø, D49.81-D49.9

C17.1 Malignant neoplasm of jejunum CC
CC Excl: C17.Ø, C17.8-C17.9, C26.Ø, C26.9, C45.7-C45.9, C46.4, C7A.ØØ-C7A.Ø1Ø, C7A.Ø19, C7A.Ø98-C7B.ØØ, C7B.1, C76.8, C8Ø.Ø-C8Ø.2, D49.Ø, D49.81-D49.9

C17.2 Malignant neoplasm of ileum CC
EXCLUDES 1 *malignant neoplasm of ileocecal valve (C18.Ø)*
CC Excl: C17.Ø, C17.8-C17.9, C26.Ø, C26.9, C45.7-C45.9, C46.4, C7A.ØØ-C7A.Ø1Ø, C7A.Ø19, C7A.Ø98-C7B.ØØ, C7B.1, C76.8, C8Ø.Ø-C8Ø.2, D49.Ø, D49.81-D49.9

C17.3 Meckel's diverticulum, malignant CC
EXCLUDES 1 *Meckel's diverticulum, congenital (Q43.Ø)*
CC Excl: C17.Ø, C17.8-C17.9, C26.Ø, C26.9, C45.7-C45.9, C46.4, C7A.ØØ-C7A.Ø1Ø, C7A.Ø19, C7A.Ø98-C7B.ØØ, C7B.1, C76.8, C8Ø.Ø-C8Ø.2, D49.Ø, D49.81-D49.9

C17.8 Malignant neoplasm of overlapping sites of small intestine CC
CC Excl: C17.Ø, C17.8-C17.9, C26.Ø, C26.9, C45.7-C45.9, C46.4, C7A.ØØ-C7A.Ø1Ø, C7A.Ø19, C7A.Ø98-C7B.ØØ, C7B.1, C76.8, C8Ø.Ø-C8Ø.2, D49.Ø, D49.81-D49.9

C17.9 Malignant neoplasm of small intestine, unspecified CC
CC Excl: See code: C17.8

✓4th C18 Malignant neoplasm of colon
EXCLUDES 1 *malignant carcinoid tumors of the colon (C7A.Ø2-)*

C18.Ø Malignant neoplasm of cecum CC
Malignant neoplasm of ileocecal valve
CC Excl: C18.Ø, C18.8-C18.9, C26.Ø, C26.9, C45.7-C45.9, C46.4, C7A.ØØ, C7A.Ø21, C7A.Ø29, C7A.Ø98-C7B.ØØ, C7B.1, C76.8, C8Ø.Ø-C8Ø.2, D49.Ø, D49.81-D49.9

C18.1 Malignant neoplasm of appendix CC
CC Excl: C18.Ø, C18.8-C18.9, C26.Ø, C26.9, C45.7-C45.9, C46.4, C7A.ØØ, C7A.Ø21, C7A.Ø29, C7A.Ø98-C7B.ØØ, C7B.1, C76.8, C8Ø.Ø-C8Ø.2, D49.Ø, D49.81-D49.9

C18.2 Malignant neoplasm of ascending colon CC
CC Excl: C18.Ø, C18.8-C18.9, C26.Ø, C26.9, C45.7-C45.9, C46.4, C7A.ØØ, C7A.Ø21, C7A.Ø29, C7A.Ø98-C7B.ØØ, C7B.1, C76.8, C8Ø.Ø-C8Ø.2, D49.Ø, D49.81-D49.9

C18.3 Malignant neoplasm of hepatic flexure CC
CC Excl: C18.3, C18.8-C18.9, C26.Ø, C26.9, C45.7-C45.9, C46.4, C7A.ØØ, C7A.Ø29, C7A.Ø98-C7B.ØØ, C7B.1, C76.8, C8Ø.Ø-C8Ø.2, D49.Ø, D49.81-D49.9

C18.4 Malignant neoplasm of transverse colon CC
CC Excl: C18.4, C18.8-C18.9, C26.Ø, C26.9, C45.7-C45.9, C46.4, C7A.ØØ, C7A.Ø23, C7A.Ø29, C7A.Ø98-C7B.ØØ, C7B.1, C76.8, C8Ø.Ø-C8Ø.2, D49.Ø, D49.81-D49.9

C18.5 Malignant neoplasm of splenic flexure CC
CC Excl: C18.5, C18.8-C18.9, C26.Ø, C26.9, C45.7-C45.9, C46.4, C7A.ØØ, C7A.Ø29, C7A.Ø98-C7B.ØØ, C7B.1, C76.8, C8Ø.Ø-C8Ø.2, D49.Ø, D49.81-D49.9

C18.6 Malignant neoplasm of descending colon CC
CC Excl: C18.6, C18.8-C18.9, C26.Ø, C26.9, C45.7-C45.9, C46.4, C7A.ØØ, C7A.Ø24, C7A.Ø29, C7A.Ø98-C7B.ØØ, C7B.1, C76.8, C8Ø.Ø-C8Ø.2, D49.Ø, D49.81-D49.9

C18.7 Malignant neoplasm of sigmoid colon CC
Malignant neoplasm of sigmoid (flexure)
EXCLUDES 1 *malignant neoplasm of rectosigmoid junction (C19)*
CC Excl: C18.7-C18.9, C26.Ø, C26.9, C45.7-C45.9, C46.4, C7A.ØØ, C7A.Ø25, C7A.Ø29, C7A.Ø98-C7B.ØØ, C7B.1, C76.8, C8Ø.Ø-C8Ø.2, D49.Ø, D49.81-D49.9

C18.8 Malignant neoplasm of overlapping sites of colon CC
CC Excl: C18.8-C18.9, C26.Ø, C26.9, C45.7-C45.9, C46.4, C7A.ØØ, C7A.Ø29, C7A.Ø98-C7B.ØØ, C7B.1, C76.8, C8Ø.Ø-C8Ø.2, D49.Ø, D49.81-D49.9

C18.9 Malignant neoplasm of colon, unspecified CC
Malignant neoplasm of large intestine NOS
CC Excl: See code: C18.8

C19 Malignant neoplasm of rectosigmoid junction CC
Malignant neoplasm of colon with rectum
Malignant neoplasm of rectosigmoid (colon)
EXCLUDES 1 *malignant carcinoid tumors of the colon (C7A.02-)*
CC Excl: C19, C21.2-C21.8, C26.0, C26.9, C45.7-C45.9, C46.4, C7A.00, C7A.098-C7B.00, C7B.1, C76.8, C80.0-C80.2, D49.0, D49.81-D49.9

C20 Malignant neoplasm of rectum CC
Malignant neoplasm of rectal ampulla
EXCLUDES 1 *malignant carcinoid tumor of the rectum (C7A.026)*
CC Excl: C20, C21.2-C21.8, C26.0, C26.9, C45.7-C45.9, C46.4, C7A.00, C7A.026, C7A.098-C7B.00, C7B.1, C76.8, C80.0-C80.2, D49.0, D49.81-D49.9

✓4th **C21 Malignant neoplasm of anus and anal canal**
EXCLUDES 2 *malignant carcinoid tumors of the colon (C7A.02-)*
malignant melanoma of anal margin (C43.51)
malignant melanoma of anal skin (C43.51)
malignant melanoma of perianal skin (C43.51)
other and unspecified malignant neoplasm of anal margin (C44.500, C44.510, C44.520, C44.590)
other and unspecified malignant neoplasm of anal skin (C44.500, C44.510, C44.520, C44.590)
other and unspecified malignant neoplasm of perianal skin (C44.500, C44.510, C44.520, C44.590)

C21.0 Malignant neoplasm of anus, unspecified CC
CC Excl: C21.0-C21.8, C26.0, C26.9, C45.7-C45.9, C46.4, C76.8, C7A.00, C7A.098-C7B.00, C7B.1, C80.0-C80.2, D49.0, D49.81-D49.9

C21.1 Malignant neoplasm of anal canal CC
Malignant neoplasm of anal sphincter
CC Excl: See code: C21.0

C21.2 Malignant neoplasm of cloacogenic zone CC
CC Excl: C21.2-C21.8, C26.0, C26.9, C45.7-C45.9, C46.4, C76.8, C7A.00, C7A.098-C7B.00, C7B.1, C80.0-C80.2, D49.0, D49.81-D49.9

C21.8 Malignant neoplasm of overlapping sites of rectum, anus and anal canal CC
Malignant neoplasm of anorectal junction
Malignant neoplasm of anorectum
Primary malignant neoplasm of two or more contiguous sites of rectum, anus and anal canal
CC Excl: See code: C21.2

✓4th **C22 Malignant neoplasm of liver and intrahepatic bile ducts**
Use additional code to identify:
alcohol abuse and dependence (F10.-)
hepatitis B (B16.-, B18.0-B18.1)
hepatitis C (B17.1-, B18.2)
EXCLUDES 1 *malignant neoplasm of biliary tract NOS (C24.9)*
secondary malignant neoplasm of liver and intrahepatic bile duct (C78.7)

CC Excl: For CC codes in category C22, unless otherwise noted: C22.0-C22.9, C26.0, C26.9, C45.7-C45.9, C46.4, C76.8, C7A.00, C7A.098-C7B.00, C7B.1, C80.0-C80.2, D49.0, D49.81-D49.9

C22.0 Liver cell carcinoma CC
Hepatocellular carcinoma
Hepatoma

C22.1 Intrahepatic bile duct carcinoma CC
Cholangiocarcinoma
EXCLUDES 1 *malignant neoplasm of hepatic duct (C24.0)*

C22.2 Hepatoblastoma CC

C22.3 Angiosarcoma of liver CC
Kupffer cell sarcoma

C22.4 Other sarcomas of liver CC

C22.7 Other specified carcinomas of liver CC

C22.8 Malignant neoplasm of liver, primary, unspecified as to type CC

C22.9 Malignant neoplasm of liver, not specified as primary or secondary CC

C23 Malignant neoplasm of gallbladder CC
CC Excl: C23, C24.8-C24.9, C26.0, C26.9, C45.7-C45.9, C46.4, C7A.00, C7A.098-C7B.00, C7B.1, C76.8, C80.0-C80.2, D49.0, D49.81-D49.9

✓4th **C24 Malignant neoplasm of other and unspecified parts of biliary tract**
EXCLUDES 1 *malignant neoplasm of intrahepatic bile duct (C22.1)*

C24.0 Malignant neoplasm of extrahepatic bile duct CC
Malignant neoplasm of biliary duct or passage NOS
Malignant neoplasm of common bile duct
Malignant neoplasm of cystic duct
Malignant neoplasm of hepatic duct
CC Excl: C24.0, C24.8-C24.9, C26.0, C26.9, C45.7-C45.9, C46.4, C7A.00, C7A.098-C7B.00, C7B.1, C76.8, C80.0-C80.2, D49.0, D49.81-D49.9

C24.1 Malignant neoplasm of ampulla of Vater CC
CC Excl: C24.1-C24.9, C26.0, C26.9, C45.7-C45.9, C46.4, C76.8, C7A.00, C7A.098-C7B.00, C7B.1, C80.0-C80.2, D49.0, D49.81-D49.9

C24.8 Malignant neoplasm of overlapping sites of biliary tract CC
Malignant neoplasm involving both intrahepatic and extrahepatic bile ducts
Primary malignant neoplasm of two or more contiguous sites of biliary tract
CC Excl: C24.8-C24.9, C26.0, C26.9, C45.7-C45.9, C46.4, C76.8, C7A.00, C7A.098-C7B.00, C7B.1, C80.0-C80.2, D49.0, D49.81-D49.9

C24.9 Malignant neoplasm of biliary tract, unspecified CC
CC Excl: See code: C24.8

✓4th **C25 Malignant neoplasm of pancreas**
Use additional code to identify:
alcohol abuse and dependence (F10.-)

CC Excl: For CC codes in category C25, unless otherwise noted: C25.0-C26.0, C26.9, C45.7-C45.9, C46.4, C76.8, C7A.00, C7A.098-C7B.00, C7B.1, C80.0-C80.2, D49.0, D49.81-D49.9

C25.0 Malignant neoplasm of head of pancreas CC

C25.1 Malignant neoplasm of body of pancreas CC

C25.2 Malignant neoplasm of tail of pancreas CC

C25.3 Malignant neoplasm of pancreatic duct CC

C25.4 Malignant neoplasm of endocrine pancreas CC
Malignant neoplasm of islets of Langerhans
Use additional code to identify any functional activity

C25.7 Malignant neoplasm of other parts of pancreas CC
Malignant neoplasm of neck of pancreas

C25.8 Malignant neoplasm of overlapping sites of pancreas CC

C25.9 Malignant neoplasm of pancreas, unspecified CC

✓4th **C26 Malignant neoplasm of other and ill-defined digestive organs**
EXCLUDES 1 *malignant neoplasm of peritoneum and retroperitoneum (C48.-)*

C26.0 Malignant neoplasm of intestinal tract, part unspecified
Malignant neoplasm of intestine NOS

C26.1 Malignant neoplasm of spleen
EXCLUDES 1 *Hodgkin lymphoma (C81.-)*
non-Hodgkin lymphoma (C82-C85)

C26.9 Malignant neoplasm of ill-defined sites within the digestive system
Malignant neoplasm of alimentary canal or tract NOS
Malignant neoplasm of gastrointestinal tract NOS
EXCLUDES 1 *malignant neoplasm of abdominal NOS (C76.2)*
malignant neoplasm of intra-abdominal NOS (C76.2)

Malignant neoplasms of respiratory and intrathoracic organs (C30-C39)

INCLUDES malignant neoplasm of middle ear
EXCLUDES 1 *mesothelioma (C45.-)*

✓4th **C30 Malignant neoplasm of nasal cavity and middle ear**

C30.0 Malignant neoplasm of nasal cavity
Malignant neoplasm of cartilage of nose
Malignant neoplasm of nasal concha
Malignant neoplasm of internal nose
Malignant neoplasm of septum of nose
Malignant neoplasm of vestibule of nose
EXCLUDES 1 *malignant melanoma of skin of nose (C43.31)*
malignant neoplasm of nasal bone (C41.0)
malignant neoplasm of nose NOS (C76.0)
malignant neoplasm of olfactory bulb (C72.2-)
malignant neoplasm of posterior margin of nasal septum and choana (C11.3)
malignant neoplasm of turbinates (C41.0)
other and unspecified malignant neoplasm of skin of nose (C44.301, C44.311, C44.321, C44.391)

C30.1 Malignant neoplasm of middle ear
Malignant neoplasm of antrum tympanicum
Malignant neoplasm of auditory tube
Malignant neoplasm of eustachian tube
Malignant neoplasm of inner ear
Malignant neoplasm of mastoid air cells
Malignant neoplasm of tympanic cavity
EXCLUDES 1 *malignant melanoma of skin of (external) ear (C43.2-)*
malignant neoplasm of auricular canal (external) (C43.2-, C44.2-)
malignant neoplasm of bone of ear (meatus) (C41.0)
malignant neoplasm of cartilage of ear (C49.0)
other and unspecified malignant neoplasm of skin of (external) ear (C44.2-)

✓4th **C31 Malignant neoplasm of accessory sinuses**

C31.0 Malignant neoplasm of maxillary sinus
Malignant neoplasm of antrum (Highmore) (maxillary)

C31.1 Malignant neoplasm of ethmoidal sinus

C31.2 Malignant neoplasm of frontal sinus

C31.3 Malignant neoplasm of sphenoid sinus

C31.8 Malignant neoplasm of overlapping sites of accessory sinuses

C31.9 Malignant neoplasm of accessory sinus, unspecified

✓4th **C32 Malignant neoplasm of larynx**
Use additional code to identify:
alcohol abuse and dependence (F10.-)
exposure to environmental tobacco smoke (Z77.22)
exposure to tobacco smoke in the perinatal period (P96.81)
history of tobacco use (Z87.891)
occupational exposure to environmental tobacco smoke (Z57.31)
tobacco dependence (F17.-)
tobacco use (Z72.0)

C32.0 Malignant neoplasm of glottis
Malignant neoplasm of intrinsic larynx
Malignant neoplasm of laryngeal commissure (anterior)(posterior)
Malignant neoplasm of vocal cord (true) NOS

C32.1 Malignant neoplasm of supraglottis
Malignant neoplasm of aryepiglottic fold or interarytenoid fold, laryngeal aspect
Malignant neoplasm of epiglottis (suprahyoid portion) NOS
Malignant neoplasm of extrinsic larynx
Malignant neoplasm of false vocal cord
Malignant neoplasm of posterior (laryngeal) surface of epiglottis
Malignant neoplasm of ventricular bands
EXCLUDES 2 *malignant neoplasm of anterior surface of epiglottis (C10.1)*
malignant neoplasm of aryepiglottic fold or interarytenoid fold, hypopharyngeal aspect (C13.1)
malignant neoplasm of aryepiglottic fold or interarytenoid fold, marginal zone (C13.1)
malignant neoplasm of aryepiglottic fold or interarytenoid fold NOS (C13.1)

C32.2 Malignant neoplasm of subglottis

C32.3 Malignant neoplasm of laryngeal cartilage

C32.8 Malignant neoplasm of overlapping sites of larynx

C32.9 Malignant neoplasm of larynx, unspecified

C33 Malignant neoplasm of trachea CC
Use additional code to identify:
exposure to environmental tobacco smoke (Z77.22)
exposure to tobacco smoke in the perinatal period (P96.81)
history of tobacco use (Z87.891)
occupational exposure to environmental tobacco smoke (Z57.31)
tobacco dependence (F17.-)
tobacco use (Z72.0)
CC Excl: C33-C34.92, C39.9, C45.7-C45.9, C46.50-C46.52, C76.1, C76.8, C78.00-C78.1, C78.30-C78.39, C7A.00, C7A.090, C7A.098-C7B.00, C7B.1, C80.0-C80.2, D49.1, D49.81-D49.9

✓4th **C34 Malignant neoplasm of bronchus and lung**
Use additional code to identify:
exposure to environmental tobacco smoke (Z77.22)
exposure to tobacco smoke in the perinatal period (P96.81)
history of tobacco use (Z87.891)
occupational exposure to environmental tobacco smoke (Z57.31)
tobacco dependence (F17.-)
tobacco use (Z72.0)
EXCLUDES 1 *Kaposi's sarcoma of lung (C46.5-)*
malignant carcinoid tumor of the bronchus and lung (C7A.090)

✓5th **C34.0 Malignant neoplasm of main bronchus**
Malignant neoplasm of carina
Malignant neoplasm of hilus (of lung)

CC Excl: For CC codes in subcategory C34.0, unless otherwise noted: C34.00-C34.02, C34.80-C34.92, C39.9, C45.7-C45.9, C46.50-C46.52, C76.8, C7A.00, C7A.090, C7A.098-C7B.00, C7B.1, C80.0-C80.2, D49.1, D49.81-D49.9

C34.00 Malignant neoplasm of unspecified main bronchus CC

C34.01 Malignant neoplasm of right main bronchus CC

C34.02 Malignant neoplasm of left main bronchus CC

✓5th **C34.1 Malignant neoplasm of upper lobe, bronchus or lung**

CC Excl: For CC codes in subcategory C34.1, unless otherwise noted: C34.10-C34.12, C34.80-C34.92, C39.9, C45.7-C45.9, C46.50-C46.52, C76.8, C7A.00, C7A.090, C7A.098-C7B.00, C7B.1, C80.0-C80.2, D49.1, D49.81-D49.9

C34.10 Malignant neoplasm of upper lobe, unspecified bronchus or lung CC

C34.11 Malignant neoplasm of upper lobe, right bronchus or lung CC

C34.12 Malignant neoplasm of upper lobe, left bronchus or lung CC

C34.2 Malignant neoplasm of middle lobe, bronchus or lung CC
CC Excl: C34.2, C34.80-C34.92, C39.9, C45.7-C45.9, C46.50-C46.52, C7A.00, C7A.090, C7A.098-C7B.00, C7B.1, C76.8, C80.0-C80.2, D49.1, D49.81-D49.9

✓5th **C34.3 Malignant neoplasm of lower lobe, bronchus or lung**

CC Excl: For CC codes in subcategory C34.3, unless otherwise noted: C34.30-C34.92, C39.9, C45.7-C45.9, C46.50-C46.52, C76.8, C7A.00, C7A.090, C7A.098-C7B.00, C7B.1, C80.0-C80.2, D49.1, D49.81-D49.9

C34.30 Malignant neoplasm of lower lobe, unspecified bronchus or lung CC

C34.31 Malignant neoplasm of lower lobe, right bronchus or lung CC

C34.32 Malignant neoplasm of lower lobe, left bronchus or lung CC

✓5th **C34.8 Malignant neoplasm of overlapping sites of bronchus and lung**

CC Excl: For CC codes in subcategory C34.8, unless otherwise noted: C34.80-C34.92, C39.9, C45.7-C45.9, C46.50-C46.52, C76.8, C7A.00, C7A.090, C7A.098-C7B.00, C7B.1, C80.0-C80.2, D49.1, D49.81-D49.9

C34.80 Malignant neoplasm of overlapping sites of unspecified bronchus and lung CC

C34.81 Malignant neoplasm of overlapping sites of right bronchus and lung CC

C34.82 Malignant neoplasm of overlapping sites of left bronchus and lung CC

✓5th **C34.9 Malignant neoplasm of unspecified part of bronchus or lung**

CC Excl: For CC codes in subcategory C34.9, unless otherwise noted: C34.80-C34.92, C39.9, C45.7-C45.9, C46.50-C46.52, C76.8, C7A.00, C7A.090, C7A.098-C7B.00, C7B.1, C80.0-C80.2, D49.1, D49.81-D49.9

C34.90 Malignant neoplasm of unspecified part of unspecified bronchus or lung CC
Lung cancer NOS

C34.91 Malignant neoplasm of unspecified part of right bronchus or lung CC

C34.92 Malignant neoplasm of unspecified part of left bronchus or lung CC

C37 Malignant neoplasm of thymus CC
EXCLUDES 1 *malignant carcinoid tumor of the thymus (C7A.091)*
CC Excl: C37, C7A.091

✓4th **C38 Malignant neoplasm of heart, mediastinum and pleura**
EXCLUDES 1 *mesothelioma (C45.-)*

C38.0 Malignant neoplasm of heart CC
Malignant neoplasm of pericardium
EXCLUDES 1 *malignant neoplasm of great vessels (C49.3)*
CC Excl: C38.0, C45.2

C38.1 Malignant neoplasm of anterior mediastinum CC
CC Excl: C38.1-C38.3, C38.8, C39.9, C45.7-C45.9, C76.8, C7A.00, C7A.098-C7B.00, C7B.1, C80.0-C80.2, D49.1, D49.81-D49.9

C38.2 Malignant neoplasm of posterior mediastinum CC
CC Excl: See code: C38.1

C38.3 Malignant neoplasm of mediastinum, part unspecified CC
CC Excl: See code: C38.1

C38.4 Malignant neoplasm of pleura CC
CC Excl: C38.4-C39.9, C45.0, C45.7-C45.9, C76.8, C7A.00, C7A.098-C7B.00, C7B.1, C80.0-C80.2, D49.1, D49.81-D49.9

C38.8 Malignant neoplasm of overlapping sites of heart, mediastinum and pleura CC
CC Excl: See code: C38.1

C39 Malignant neoplasm of other and ill-defined sites in the respiratory system and intrathoracic organs
Use additional code to identify:
exposure to environmental tobacco smoke (Z77.22)
exposure to tobacco smoke in the perinatal period (P96.81)
history of tobacco use (Z87.891)
occupational exposure to environmental tobacco smoke (Z57.31)
tobacco dependence (F17.-)
tobacco use (Z72.0)
EXCLUDES 1 *intrathoracic malignant neoplasm NOS (C76.1)*
thoracic malignant neoplasm NOS (C76.1)

C39.0 Malignant neoplasm of upper respiratory tract, part unspecified

C39.9 Malignant neoplasm of lower respiratory tract, part unspecified
Malignant neoplasm of respiratory tract NOS

Malignant neoplasms of bone and articular cartilage (C40-C41)

INCLUDES malignant neoplasm of cartilage (articular) (joint)
malignant neoplasm of periosteum
EXCLUDES 1 *malignant neoplasm of bone marrow NOS (C96.9)*
malignant neoplasm of synovia (C49.-)

C40 Malignant neoplasm of bone and articular cartilage of limbs
Use additional code to identify major osseous defect, if applicable (M89.7-)

C40.0 Malignant neoplasm of scapula and long bones of upper limb
CC Excl: For CC codes in subcategory C40.0, unless otherwise noted: C40.00-C40.02, C40.80, C40.92, C41.9, Z51.0

C40.00 Malignant neoplasm of scapula and long bones of unspecified upper limb CC
C40.01 Malignant neoplasm of scapula and long bones of right upper limb CC
C40.02 Malignant neoplasm of scapula and long bones of left upper limb CC

C40.1 Malignant neoplasm of short bones of upper limb
CC Excl: For CC codes in subcategory C40.1, unless otherwise noted: C40.10-C40.12, C40.80-C40.92, C41.9, Z51.0

C40.10 Malignant neoplasm of short bones of unspecified upper limb CC
C40.11 Malignant neoplasm of short bones of right upper limb CC
C40.12 Malignant neoplasm of short bones of left upper limb CC

C40.2 Malignant neoplasm of long bones of lower limb
CC Excl: For CC codes in subcategory C40.2, unless otherwise noted: C40.20-C40.22, C40.80-C40.92, C41.9, Z51.0

C40.20 Malignant neoplasm of long bones of unspecified lower limb CC
C40.21 Malignant neoplasm of long bones of right lower limb CC
C40.22 Malignant neoplasm of long bones of left lower limb CC

C40.3 Malignant neoplasm of short bones of lower limb
CC Excl: For CC codes in subcategory C40.3, unless otherwise noted: C40.30-C40.92, C41.9, Z51.0

C40.30 Malignant neoplasm of short bones of unspecified lower limb CC
C40.31 Malignant neoplasm of short bones of right lower limb CC
C40.32 Malignant neoplasm of short bones of left lower limb CC

C40.8 Malignant neoplasm of overlapping sites of bone and articular cartilage of limb
CC Excl: For CC codes in subcategory C40.8, unless otherwise noted: C40.00-C41.9, Z51.0

C40.80 Malignant neoplasm of overlapping sites of bone and articular cartilage of unspecified limb CC
C40.81 Malignant neoplasm of overlapping sites of bone and articular cartilage of right limb CC
C40.82 Malignant neoplasm of overlapping sites of bone and articular cartilage of left limb CC

C40.9 Malignant neoplasm of unspecified bones and articular cartilage of limb
CC Excl: For CC codes in subcategory C40.9, ulless otherwise noted: C40.00-C41.9, Z51.0

C40.90 Malignant neoplasm of unspecified bones and articular cartilage of unspecified limb CC
C40.91 Malignant neoplasm of unspecified bones and articular cartilage of right limb CC
C40.92 Malignant neoplasm of unspecified bones and articular cartilage of left limb CC

C41 Malignant neoplasm of bone and articular cartilage of other and unspecified sites
EXCLUDES 1 *malignant neoplasm of bones of limbs (C40.-)*
malignant neoplasm of cartilage of ear (C49.0)
malignant neoplasm of cartilage of eyelid (C49.0)
malignant neoplasm of cartilage of larynx (C32.3)
malignant neoplasm of cartilage of limbs (C40.-)
malignant neoplasm of cartilage of nose (C30.0)

C41.0 Malignant neoplasm of bones of skull and face CC
Malignant neoplasm of maxilla (superior)
Malignant neoplasm of orbital bone
EXCLUDES 2 *carcinoma, any type except intraosseous or odontogenic of:*
maxillary sinus (C31.0)
upper jaw (C03.0)
malignant neoplasm of jaw bone (lower) (C41.1)
CC Excl: C40.80-C41.0, C41.9, Z51.0

C41.1 Malignant neoplasm of mandible CC
Malignant neoplasm of inferior maxilla
Malignant neoplasm of lower jaw bone
EXCLUDES 2 *carcinoma, any type except intraosseous or odontogenic of:*
jaw NOS (C03.9)
lower (C03.1)
malignant neoplasm of upper jaw bone (C41.0)
CC Excl: C40.80-C40.92, C41.1, C41.9, Z51.0

C41.2 Malignant neoplasm of vertebral column CC
EXCLUDES 1 *malignant neoplasm of sacrum and coccyx (C41.4)*
CC Excl: C40.80-C40.92, C41.2, C41.9, Z51.0

C41.3 Malignant neoplasm of ribs, sternum and clavicle CC
CC Excl: C40.80-C40.92, C41.3, C41.9, Z51.0

C41.4 Malignant neoplasm of pelvic bones, sacrum and coccyx CC
CC Excl: C40.80-C40.92, C41.4-C41.9, Z51.0

C41.9 Malignant neoplasm of bone and articular cartilage, unspecified CC
CC Excl: C40.00-C41.9, Z51.0

Melanoma and other malignant neoplasms of skin (C43-C44)

C43 Malignant melanoma of skin
EXCLUDES 1 *melanoma in situ (D03.-)*
EXCLUDES 2 *malignant melanoma of skin of genital organs (C51-C52, C60.-, C63.-)*
Merkel cell carcinoma (C4A.-)
sites other than skin—code to malignant neoplasm of the site

C43.0 Malignant melanoma of lip
EXCLUDES 1 *malignant neoplasm of vermilion border of lip (C00.0-C00.2)*

C43.1 Malignant melanoma of eyelid, including canthus
C43.10 Malignant melanoma of unspecified eyelid, including canthus
C43.11 Malignant melanoma of right eyelid, including canthus
C43.12 Malignant melanoma of left eyelid, including canthus

C43.2 Malignant melanoma of ear and external auricular canal
C43.20 Malignant melanoma of unspecified ear and external auricular canal
C43.21 Malignant melanoma of right ear and external auricular canal
C43.22 Malignant melanoma of left ear and external auricular canal

C43.3 Malignant melanoma of other and unspecified parts of face
C43.30 Malignant melanoma of unspecified part of face
C43.31 Malignant melanoma of nose
C43.39 Malignant melanoma of other parts of face

C43.4 Malignant melanoma of scalp and neck

✓5th **C43.5 Malignant melanoma of trunk**

EXCLUDES 2 *malignant neoplasm of anus NOS (C21.0)*
malignant neoplasm of scrotum (C63.2)

C43.51 Malignant melanoma of anal skin
Malignant melanoma of anal margin
Malignant melanoma of perianal skin

C43.52 Malignant melanoma of skin of breast

C43.59 Malignant melanoma of other part of trunk

✓5th **C43.6 Malignant melanoma of upper limb, including shoulder**

C43.60 Malignant melanoma of unspecified upper limb, including shoulder

C43.61 Malignant melanoma of right upper limb, including shoulder

C43.62 Malignant melanoma of left upper limb, including shoulder

✓5th **C43.7 Malignant melanoma of lower limb, including hip**

C43.70 Malignant melanoma of unspecified lower limb, including hip

C43.71 Malignant melanoma of right lower limb, including hip

C43.72 Malignant melanoma of left lower limb, including hip

C43.8 Malignant melanoma of overlapping sites of skin

C43.9 Malignant melanoma of skin, unspecified
Malignant melanoma of unspecified site of skin

✓4th **C4A Merkel cell carcinoma**

C4A.0 Merkel cell carcinoma of lip

EXCLUDES 1 *malignant neoplasm of vermilion border of lip (C00.0-C00.2)*

✓5th **C4A.1 Merkel cell carcinoma of eyelid, including canthus**

C4A.10 Merkel cell carcinoma of unspecified eyelid, including canthus

C4A.11 Merkel cell carcinoma of right eyelid, including canthus

C4A.12 Merkel cell carcinoma of left eyelid, including canthus

✓5th **C4A.2 Merkel cell carcinoma of ear and external auricular canal**

C4A.20 Merkel cell carcinoma of unspecified ear and external auricular canal

C4A.21 Merkel cell carcinoma of right ear and external auricular canal

C4A.22 Merkel cell carcinoma of left ear and external auricular canal

✓5th **C4A.3 Merkel cell carcinoma of other and unspecified parts of face**

C4A.30 Merkel cell carcinoma of unspecified part of face

C4A.31 Merkel cell carcinoma of nose

C4A.39 Merkel cell carcinoma of other parts of face

C4A.4 Merkel cell carcinoma of scalp and neck

✓5th **C4A.5 Merkel cell carcinoma of trunk**

EXCLUDES 2 *malignant neoplasm of anus NOS (C21.0)*
malignant neoplasm of scrotum (C63.2)

C4A.51 Merkel cell carcinoma of anal skin
Merkel cell carcinoma of anal margin
Merkel cell carcinoma of perianal skin

C4A.52 Merkel cell carcinoma of skin of breast

C4A.59 Merkel cell carcinoma of other part of trunk

✓5th **C4A.6 Merkel cell carcinoma of upper limb, including shoulder**

C4A.60 Merkel cell carcinoma of unspecified upper limb, including shoulder

C4A.61 Merkel cell carcinoma of right upper limb, including shoulder

C4A.62 Merkel cell carcinoma of left upper limb, including shoulder

✓5th **C4A.7 Merkel cell carcinoma of lower limb, including hip**

C4A.70 Merkel cell carcinoma of unspecified lower limb, including hip

C4A.71 Merkel cell carcinoma of right lower limb, including hip

C4A.72 Merkel cell carcinoma of left lower limb, including hip

C4A.8 Merkel cell carcinoma of overlapping sites

C4A.9 Merkel cell carcinoma, unspecified
Merkel cell carcinoma of unspecified site

✓4th **C44 Other and unspecified malignant neoplasm of skin**

INCLUDES malignant neoplasm of sebaceous glands
malignant neoplasm of sweat glands

EXCLUDES 1 *Kaposi's sarcoma of skin (C46.0)*
malignant melanoma of skin (C43.-)
malignant neoplasm of skin of genital organs (C51-C52, C60-, C63.2)
Merkel cell carcinoma (C4A.-)

✓5th **C44.0 Other and unspecified malignant neoplasm of skin of lip**

EXCLUDES 1 *malignant neoplasm of lip (C00.-)*

C44.00 Unspecified malignant neoplasm of skin of lip

C44.01 Basal cell carcinoma of skin of lip

C44.02 Squamous cell carcinoma of skin of lip

C44.09 Other specified malignant neoplasm of skin of lip

✓5th **C44.1 Other and unspecified malignant neoplasm of skin of eyelid, including canthus**

EXCLUDES 1 *connective tissue of eyelid (C49.0)*

✓6th **C44.10 Unspecified malignant neoplasm of skin of eyelid, including canthus**

C44.101 Unspecified malignant neoplasm of skin of unspecified eyelid, including canthus

C44.102 Unspecified malignant neoplasm of skin of right eyelid, including canthus

C44.109 Unspecified malignant neoplasm of skin of left eyelid, including canthus

✓6th **C44.11 Basal cell carcinoma of skin of eyelid, including canthus**

C44.111 Basal cell carcinoma of skin of unspecified eyelid, including canthus

C44.112 Basal cell carcinoma of skin of right eyelid, including canthus

C44.119 Basal cell carcinoma of skin of left eyelid, including canthus

✓6th **C44.12 Squamous cell carcinoma of skin of eyelid, including canthus**

C44.121 Squamous cell carcinoma of skin of unspecified eyelid, including canthus

C44.122 Squamous cell carcinoma of skin of right eyelid, including canthus

C44.129 Squamous cell carcinoma of skin of left eyelid, including canthus

✓6th **C44.19 Other specified malignant neoplasm of skin of eyelid, including canthus**

C44.191 Other specified malignant neoplasm of skin of unspecified eyelid, including canthus

C44.192 Other specified malignant neoplasm of skin of right eyelid, including canthus

C44.199 Other specified malignant neoplasm of skin of left eyelid, including canthus

✓5th **C44.2 Other and unspecified malignant neoplasm of skin of ear and external auricular canal**

EXCLUDES 1 *connective tissue of ear (C49.0)*

✓6th **C44.20 Unspecified malignant neoplasm of skin of ear and external auricular canal**

C44.201 Unspecified malignant neoplasm of skin of unspecified ear and external auricular canal

C44.202 Unspecified malignant neoplasm of skin of right ear and external auricular canal

C44.209 Unspecified malignant neoplasm of skin of left ear and external auricular canal

✓6th **C44.21 Basal cell carcinoma of skin of ear and external auricular canal**

C44.211 Basal cell carcinoma of skin of unspecified ear and external auricular canal

C44.212 Basal cell carcinoma of skin of right ear and external auricular canal

C44.219 Basal cell carcinoma of skin of left ear and external auricular canal

✓6th **C44.22 Squamous cell carcinoma of skin of ear and external auricular canal**

C44.221 Squamous cell carcinoma of skin of unspecified ear and external auricular canal

C44.222 Squamous cell carcinoma of skin of right ear and external auricular canal

C44.229 Squamous cell carcinoma of skin of left ear and external auricular canal

✓6th C44.29 Other specified malignant neoplasm of skin of ear and external auricular canal

C44.291 Other specified malignant neoplasm of skin of unspecified ear and external auricular canal

C44.292 Other specified malignant neoplasm of skin of right ear and external auricular canal

C44.299 Other specified malignant neoplasm of skin of left ear and external auricular canal

✓5th C44.3 Other and unspecified malignant neoplasm of skin of other and unspecified parts of face

✓6th C44.30 Unspecified malignant neoplasm of skin of other and unspecified parts of face

C44.300 Unspecified malignant neoplasm of skin of unspecified part of face

C44.301 Unspecified malignant neoplasm of skin of nose

C44.309 Unspecified malignant neoplasm of skin of other parts of face

✓6th C44.31 Basal cell carcinoma of skin of other and unspecified parts of face

C44.310 Basal cell carcinoma of skin of unspecified parts of face

C44.311 Basal cell carcinoma of skin of nose

C44.319 Basal cell carcinoma of skin of other parts of face

✓6th C44.32 Squamous cell carcinoma of skin of other and unspecified parts of face

C44.320 Squamous cell carcinoma of skin of unspecified parts of face

C44.321 Squamous cell carcinoma of skin of nose

C44.329 Squamous cell carcinoma of skin of other parts of face

✓6th C44.39 Other specified malignant neoplasm of skin of other and unspecified parts of face

C44.390 Other specified malignant neoplasm of skin of unspecified parts of face

C44.391 Other specified malignant neoplasm of skin of nose

C44.399 Other specified malignant neoplasm of skin of other parts of face

✓5th C44.4 Other and unspecified malignant neoplasm of skin of scalp and neck

C44.40 Unspecified malignant neoplasm of skin of scalp and neck

C44.41 Basal cell carcinoma of skin of scalp and neck

C44.42 Squamous cell carcinoma of skin of scalp and neck

C44.49 Other specified malignant neoplasm of skin of scalp and neck

✓5th C44.5 Other and unspecified malignant neoplasm of skin of trunk

EXCLUDES 1 *anus NOS (C21.0)*
scrotum (C63.2)

✓6th C44.50 Unspecified malignant neoplasm of skin of trunk

C44.500 Unspecified malignant neoplasm of anal skin
Unspecified malignant neoplasm of anal margin
Unspecified malignant neoplasm of perianal skin

C44.501 Unspecified malignant neoplasm of skin of breast

C44.509 Unspecified malignant neoplasm of skin of other part of trunk

✓6th C44.51 Basal cell carcinoma of skin of trunk

C44.510 Basal cell carcinoma of anal skin
Basal cell carcinoma of anal margin
Basal cell carcinoma of perianal skin

C44.511 Basal cell carcinoma of skin of breast

C44.519 Basal cell carcinoma of skin of other part of trunk

✓6th C44.52 Squamous cell carcinoma of skin of trunk

C44.520 Squamous cell carcinoma of anal skin
Squamous cell carcinoma of anal margin
Squamous cell carcinoma of perianal skin

C44.521 Squamous cell carcinoma of skin of breast

C44.529 Squamous cell carcinoma of skin of other part of trunk

✓6th C44.59 Other specified malignant neoplasm of skin of trunk

C44.590 Other specified malignant neoplasm of anal skin
Other specified malignant neoplasm of anal margin
Other specified malignant neoplasm of perianal skin

C44.591 Other specified malignant neoplasm of skin of breast

C44.599 Other specified malignant neoplasm of skin of other part of trunk

✓5th C44.6 Other and unspecified malignant neoplasm of skin of upper limb, including shoulder

✓6th C44.60 Unspecified malignant neoplasm of skin of upper limb, including shoulder

C44.601 Unspecified malignant neoplasm of skin of unspecified upper limb, including shoulder

C44.602 Unspecified malignant neoplasm of skin of right upper limb, including shoulder

C44.609 Unspecified malignant neoplasm of skin of left upper limb, including shoulder

✓6th C44.61 Basal cell carcinoma of skin of upper limb, including shoulder

C44.611 Basal cell carcinoma of skin of unspecified upper limb, including shoulder

C44.612 Basal cell carcinoma of skin of right upper limb, including shoulder

C44.619 Basal cell carcinoma of skin of left upper limb, including shoulder

✓6th C44.62 Squamous cell carcinoma of skin of upper limb, including shoulder

C44.621 Squamous cell carcinoma of skin of unspecified upper limb, including shoulder

C44.622 Squamous cell carcinoma of skin of right upper limb, including shoulder

C44.629 Squamous cell carcinoma of skin of left upper limb, including shoulder

✓6th C44.69 Other specified malignant neoplasm of skin of upper limb, including shoulder

C44.691 Other specified malignant neoplasm of skin of unspecified upper limb, including shoulder

C44.692 Other specified malignant neoplasm of skin of right upper limb, including shoulder

C44.699 Other specified malignant neoplasm of skin of left upper limb, including shoulder

✓5th C44.7 Other and unspecified malignant neoplasm of skin of lower limb, including hip

✓6th C44.70 Unspecified malignant neoplasm of skin of lower limb, including hip

C44.701 Unspecified malignant neoplasm of skin of unspecified lower limb, including hip

C44.702 Unspecified malignant neoplasm of skin of right lower limb, including hip

C44.709 Unspecified malignant neoplasm of skin of left lower limb, including hip

✓6th C44.71 Basal cell carcinoma of skin of lower limb, including hip

C44.711 Basal cell carcinoma of skin of unspecified lower limb, including hip

C44.712 Basal cell carcinoma of skin of right lower limb, including hip

C44.719 Basal cell carcinoma of skin of left lower limb, including hip

✓6th C44.72 Squamous cell carcinoma of skin of lower limb, including hip

C44.721 Squamous cell carcinoma of skin of unspecified lower limb, including hip

C44.722 Squamous cell carcinoma of skin of right lower limb, including hip

C44.729 Squamous cell carcinoma of skin of left lower limb, including hip

✓6th **C44.79 Other specified malignant neoplasm of skin of lower limb, including hip**
- **C44.791 Other specified malignant neoplasm of skin of unspecified lower limb, including hip**
- **C44.792 Other specified malignant neoplasm of skin of right lower limb, including hip**
- **C44.799 Other specified malignant neoplasm of skin of left lower limb, including hip**

✓5th **C44.8 Other and unspecified malignant neoplasm of overlapping sites of skin**
- **C44.80 Unspecified malignant neoplasm of overlapping sites of skin**
- **C44.81 Basal cell carcinoma of overlapping sites of skin**
- **C44.82 Squamous cell carcinoma of overlapping sites of skin**
- **C44.89 Other specified malignant neoplasm of overlapping sites of skin**

✓5th **C44.9 Other and unspecified malignant neoplasm of skin, unspecified**
- **C44.90 Unspecified malignant neoplasm of skin, unspecified**
  Malignant neoplasm of unspecified site of skin
- **C44.91 Basal cell carcinoma of skin, unspecified**
- **C44.92 Squamous cell carcinoma of skin, unspecified**
- **C44.99 Other specified malignant neoplasm of skin, unspecified**

Malignant neoplasms of mesothelial and soft tissue (C45-C49)

✓4th **C45 Mesothelioma**

C45.0 Mesothelioma of pleura CC
EXCLUDES 1 *other malignant neoplasm of pleura (C38.4)*
CC Excl: C38.4, C39.9, C45.0, C45.7-C45.9, C76.8, C7A.00, C7A.098-C7B.00, C7B.1, C80.0-C80.2, D49.1, D49.81-D49.9

C45.1 Mesothelioma of peritoneum CC
Mesothelioma of cul-de-sac
Mesothelioma of mesentery
Mesothelioma of mesocolon
Mesothelioma of omentum
Mesothelioma of peritoneum (parietal) (pelvic)
EXCLUDES 1 *other malignant neoplasm of soft tissue of peritoneum (C48.-)*
CC Excl: C45.1, C48.0-C48.8, Z51.0

C45.2 Mesothelioma of pericardium CC
EXCLUDES 1 *other malignant neoplasm of pericardium (C38.0)*
CC Excl: C38.0, C45.2

C45.7 Mesothelioma of other sites

C45.9 Mesothelioma, unspecified

✓4th **C46 Kaposi's sarcoma**
Code first any human immunodeficiency virus [HIV] disease (B20)

C46.0 Kaposi's sarcoma of skin HIV CC
CC Excl: C46.0, C46.7-C46.9, Z51.0

C46.1 Kaposi's sarcoma of soft tissue HIV CC
Kaposi's sarcoma of blood vessel
Kaposi's sarcoma of connective tissue
Kaposi's sarcoma of fascia
Kaposi's sarcoma of ligament
Kaposi's sarcoma of lymphatic(s) NEC
Kaposi's sarcoma of muscle
EXCLUDES 2 *Kaposi's sarcoma of lymph glands and nodes (C46.3)*
CC Excl: C46.1, C46.7-C46.9, Z51.0

C46.2 Kaposi's sarcoma of palate HIV CC
CC Excl: C46.2, C46.7-C46.9, Z51.0

C46.3 Kaposi's sarcoma of lymph nodes HIV CC
CC Excl: C45.7-C45.9, C46.3, C76.8-C77.9, C7A.00, C7A.098-C7B.01, C7B.1, C80.0-C80.2, D49.81-D49.9

C46.4 Kaposi's sarcoma of gastrointestinal sites HIV CC
CC Excl: C46.4, C46.7-C46.9, Z51.0

✓5th **C46.5 Kaposi's sarcoma of lung**

CC Excl: For CC codes in subcategory C46.5, unless otherwise noted: C34.80-C34.92, C39.9, C45.7-C45.9, C46.50-C46.52, C76.8, C7A.00, C7A.090, C7A.098-C7B.00, C7B.1, C80.0-C80.2, D49.1, D49.81-D49.9

- **C46.50 Kaposi's sarcoma of unspecified lung** HIV CC
- **C46.51 Kaposi's sarcoma of right lung** HIV CC
- **C46.52 Kaposi's sarcoma of left lung** HIV CC

C46.7 Kaposi's sarcoma of other sites HIV CC
CC Excl: See code: C46.0

C46.9 Kaposi's sarcoma, unspecified HIV CC
Kaposi's sarcoma of unspecified site
CC Excl: C45.7-C46.9, C51.0-C55, C56.1-C63.9, C64.1-C64.9, C65.1-C65.9, C66.1-C72.9, C76.0-C76.52, C76.8-C7A.00, C7A.093, C7A.098-C80.2, D00.00-D02.4, D04.0-D05.02, D05.10-D05.12, D05.80-D05.92, D06.0-D09.3, D09.8-D09.9, D37.01-D37.6, D37.8-D39.2, D39.8-D39.9, D40.0-D40.12, D40.8-D41.4, D41.8-D43.4, D43.8-D44.7, D44.9, D48.0-D48.62, D48.7-D49.9, Z51.0

✓4th **C47 Malignant neoplasm of peripheral nerves and autonomic nervous system**
INCLUDES malignant neoplasm of sympathetic and parasympathetic nerves and ganglia
EXCLUDES 1 *Kaposi's sarcoma of soft tissue (C46.1)*

CC Excl: For CC codes in category C47, unless otherwise noted: Z51.0

C47.0 Malignant neoplasm of peripheral nerves of head, face and neck CC
EXCLUDES 1 *malignant neoplasm of peripheral nerves of orbit (C69.6-)*

✓5th **C47.1 Malignant neoplasm of peripheral nerves of upper limb, including shoulder**
- **C47.10 Malignant neoplasm of peripheral nerves of unspecified upper limb, including shoulder** CC
- **C47.11 Malignant neoplasm of peripheral nerves of right upper limb, including shoulder** CC
- **C47.12 Malignant neoplasm of peripheral nerves of left upper limb, including shoulder** CC

✓5th **C47.2 Malignant neoplasm of peripheral nerves of lower limb, including hip**
- **C47.20 Malignant neoplasm of peripheral nerves of unspecified lower limb, including hip** CC
- **C47.21 Malignant neoplasm of peripheral nerves of right lower limb, including hip** CC
- **C47.22 Malignant neoplasm of peripheral nerves of left lower limb, including hip** CC

C47.3 Malignant neoplasm of peripheral nerves of thorax CC

C47.4 Malignant neoplasm of peripheral nerves of abdomen CC

C47.5 Malignant neoplasm of peripheral nerves of pelvis CC

C47.6 Malignant neoplasm of peripheral nerves of trunk, unspecified CC
Malignant neoplasm of peripheral nerves of unspecified part of trunk

C47.8 Malignant neoplasm of overlapping sites of peripheral nerves and autonomic nervous system CC

C47.9 Malignant neoplasm of peripheral nerves and autonomic nervous system, unspecified CC
Malignant neoplasm of unspecified site of peripheral nerves and autonomic nervous system

✓4th **C48 Malignant neoplasm of retroperitoneum and peritoneum**
EXCLUDES 1 *Kaposi's sarcoma of connective tissue (C46.1)*
mesothelioma (C45.-)

C48.0 Malignant neoplasm of retroperitoneum CC
CC Excl: C48.0-Z51.0

C48.1 Malignant neoplasm of specified parts of peritoneum CC
Malignant neoplasm of cul-de-sac
Malignant neoplasm of mesentery
Malignant neoplasm of mesocolon
Malignant neoplasm of omentum
Malignant neoplasm of parietal peritoneum
Malignant neoplasm of pelvic peritoneum
CC Excl: C45.1, C48.0-C48.8, Z51.0

C48.2 Malignant neoplasm of peritoneum, unspecified CC
CC Excl: See code: C48.1

C48.8 Malignant neoplasm of overlapping sites of retroperitoneum and peritoneum CC
CC Excl: See code: C48.1

C49 Malignant neoplasm of other connective and soft tissue

INCLUDES malignant neoplasm of blood vessel
malignant neoplasm of bursa
malignant neoplasm of cartilage
malignant neoplasm of fascia
malignant neoplasm of fat
malignant neoplasm of ligament, except uterine
malignant neoplasm of lymphatic vessel
malignant neoplasm of muscle
malignant neoplasm of synovia
malignant neoplasm of tendon (sheath)

EXCLUDES 1 *malignant neoplasm of cartilage (of):*
articular (C40-C41)
larynx (C32.3)
nose (C30.0)
malignant neoplasm of connective tissue of breast (C50.-)

EXCLUDES 2 *Kaposi's sarcoma of soft tissue (C46.1)*
malignant neoplasm of heart (C38.0)
malignant neoplasm of peripheral nerves and autonomic nervous system (C47.-)
malignant neoplasm of peritoneum (C48.2)
malignant neoplasm of retroperitoneum (C48.0)
malignant neoplasm of uterine ligament (C57.3)
mesothelioma (C45.-)

CC Excl: For CC codes in category C49, unless otherwise noted:
Z51.0

C49.0 Malignant neoplasm of connective and soft tissue of head, face and neck CC
Malignant neoplasm of connective tissue of ear
Malignant neoplasm of connective tissue of eyelid
EXCLUDES 1 *connective tissue of orbit (C69.6-)*

C49.1 Malignant neoplasm of connective and soft tissue of upper limb, including shoulder

C49.10 Malignant neoplasm of connective and soft tissue of unspecified upper limb, including shoulder CC

C49.11 Malignant neoplasm of connective and soft tissue of right upper limb, including shoulder CC

C49.12 Malignant neoplasm of connective and soft tissue of left upper limb, including shoulder CC

C49.2 Malignant neoplasm of connective and soft tissue of lower limb, including hip

C49.20 Malignant neoplasm of connective and soft tissue of unspecified lower limb, including hip CC

C49.21 Malignant neoplasm of connective and soft tissue of right lower limb, including hip CC

C49.22 Malignant neoplasm of connective and soft tissue of left lower limb, including hip CC

C49.3 Malignant neoplasm of connective and soft tissue of thorax CC
Malignant neoplasm of axilla
Malignant neoplasm of diaphragm
Malignant neoplasm of great vessels
EXCLUDES 1 *malignant neoplasm of breast (C50.-)*
malignant neoplasm of heart (C38.0)
malignant neoplasm of mediastinum (C38.1-C38.3)
malignant neoplasm of thymus (C37)

C49.4 Malignant neoplasm of connective and soft tissue of abdomen CC
Malignant neoplasm of abdominal wall
Malignant neoplasm of hypochondrium

C49.5 Malignant neoplasm of connective and soft tissue of pelvis CC
Malignant neoplasm of buttock
Malignant neoplasm of groin
Malignant neoplasm of perineum

C49.6 Malignant neoplasm of connective and soft tissue of trunk, unspecified CC
Malignant neoplasm of back NOS

C49.8 Malignant neoplasm of overlapping sites of connective and soft tissue CC
Primary malignant neoplasm of two or more contiguous sites of connective and soft tissue

C49.9 Malignant neoplasm of connective and soft tissue, unspecified CC

Malignant neoplasms of breast (C50)

C50 Malignant neoplasm of breast

INCLUDES connective tissue of breast
Paget's disease of breast
Paget's disease of nipple

Use additional code to identify estrogen receptor status (Z17.0, Z17.1)

EXCLUDES 1 *skin of breast (C44.501, C44.511, C44.521, C44.591)*

C50.0 Malignant neoplasm of nipple and areola

C50.01 Malignant neoplasm of nipple and areola, female

C50.011 Malignant neoplasm of nipple and areola, right female breast ♀

C50.012 Malignant neoplasm of nipple and areola, left female breast ♀

C50.019 Malignant neoplasm of nipple and areola, unspecified female breast ♀

C50.02 Malignant neoplasm of nipple and areola, male

C50.021 Malignant neoplasm of nipple and areola, right male breast ♂

C50.022 Malignant neoplasm of nipple and areola, left male breast ♂

C50.029 Malignant neoplasm of nipple and areola, unspecified male breast ♂

C50.1 Malignant neoplasm of central portion of breast

C50.11 Malignant neoplasm of central portion of breast, female

C50.111 Malignant neoplasm of central portion of right female breast ♀

C50.112 Malignant neoplasm of central portion of left female breast ♀

C50.119 Malignant neoplasm of central portion of unspecified female breast ♀

C50.12 Malignant neoplasm of central portion of breast, male

C50.121 Malignant neoplasm of central portion of right male breast ♂

C50.122 Malignant neoplasm of central portion of left male breast ♂

C50.129 Malignant neoplasm of central portion of unspecified male breast ♂

C50.2 Malignant neoplasm of upper-inner quadrant of breast

C50.21 Malignant neoplasm of upper-inner quadrant of breast, female

C50.211 Malignant neoplasm of upper-inner quadrant of right female breast ♀

C50.212 Malignant neoplasm of upper-inner quadrant of left female breast ♀

C50.219 Malignant neoplasm of upper-inner quadrant of unspecified female breast ♀

C50.22 Malignant neoplasm of upper-inner quadrant of breast, male

C50.221 Malignant neoplasm of upper-inner quadrant of right male breast ♂

C50.222 Malignant neoplasm of upper-inner quadrant of left male breast ♂

C50.229 Malignant neoplasm of upper-inner quadrant of unspecified male breast ♂

C50.3 Malignant neoplasm of lower-inner quadrant of breast

C50.31 Malignant neoplasm of lower-inner quadrant of breast, female

C50.311 Malignant neoplasm of lower-inner quadrant of right female breast ♀

C50.312 Malignant neoplasm of lower-inner quadrant of left female breast ♀

C50.319 Malignant neoplasm of lower-inner quadrant of unspecified female breast ♀

C50.32 Malignant neoplasm of lower-inner quadrant of breast, male

C50.321 Malignant neoplasm of lower-inner quadrant of right male breast ♂

C50.322 Malignant neoplasm of lower-inner quadrant of left male breast ♂

C50.329 Malignant neoplasm of lower-inner quadrant of unspecified male breast ♂

√5th **C50.4 Malignant neoplasm of upper-outer quadrant of breast**

√6th **C50.41 Malignant neoplasm of upper-outer quadrant of breast, female**

C50.411 Malignant neoplasm of upper-outer quadrant of right female breast ♀

C50.412 Malignant neoplasm of upper-outer quadrant of left female breast ♀

C50.419 Malignant neoplasm of upper-outer quadrant of unspecified female breast ♀

√6th **C50.42 Malignant neoplasm of upper-outer quadrant of breast, male**

C50.421 Malignant neoplasm of upper-outer quadrant of right male breast ♂

C50.422 Malignant neoplasm of upper-outer quadrant of left male breast ♂

C50.429 Malignant neoplasm of upper-outer quadrant of unspecified male breast ♂

√5th **C50.5 Malignant neoplasm of lower-outer quadrant of breast**

√6th **C50.51 Malignant neoplasm of lower-outer quadrant of breast, female**

C50.511 Malignant neoplasm of lower-outer quadrant of right female breast ♀

C50.512 Malignant neoplasm of lower-outer quadrant of left female breast ♀

C50.519 Malignant neoplasm of lower-outer quadrant of unspecified female breast ♀

√6th **C50.52 Malignant neoplasm of lower-outer quadrant of breast, male**

C50.521 Malignant neoplasm of lower-outer quadrant of right male breast ♂

C50.522 Malignant neoplasm of lower-outer quadrant of left male breast ♂

C50.529 Malignant neoplasm of lower-outer quadrant of unspecified male breast ♂

√5th **C50.6 Malignant neoplasm of axillary tail of breast**

√6th **C50.61 Malignant neoplasm of axillary tail of breast, female**

C50.611 Malignant neoplasm of axillary tail of right female breast ♀

C50.612 Malignant neoplasm of axillary tail of left female breast ♀

C50.619 Malignant neoplasm of axillary tail of unspecified female breast ♀

√6th **C50.62 Malignant neoplasm of axillary tail of breast, male**

C50.621 Malignant neoplasm of axillary tail of right male breast ♂

C50.622 Malignant neoplasm of axillary tail of left male breast ♂

C50.629 Malignant neoplasm of axillary tail of unspecified male breast ♂

√5th **C50.8 Malignant neoplasm of overlapping sites of breast**

√6th **C50.81 Malignant neoplasm of overlapping sites of breast, female**

C50.811 Malignant neoplasm of overlapping sites of right female breast ♀

C50.812 Malignant neoplasm of overlapping sites of left female breast ♀

C50.819 Malignant neoplasm of overlapping sites of unspecified female breast ♀

√6th **C50.82 Malignant neoplasm of overlapping sites of breast, male**

C50.821 Malignant neoplasm of overlapping sites of right male breast ♂

C50.822 Malignant neoplasm of overlapping sites of left male breast ♂

C50.829 Malignant neoplasm of overlapping sites of unspecified male breast ♂

√5th **C50.9 Malignant neoplasm of breast of unspecified site**

√6th **C50.91 Malignant neoplasm of breast of unspecified site, female**

C50.911 Malignant neoplasm of unspecified site of right female breast ♀

C50.912 Malignant neoplasm of unspecified site of left female breast ♀

C50.919 Malignant neoplasm of unspecified site of unspecified female breast ♀

√6th **C50.92 Malignant neoplasm of breast of unspecified site, male**

C50.921 Malignant neoplasm of unspecified site of right male breast ♂

C50.922 Malignant neoplasm of unspecified site of left male breast ♂

C50.929 Malignant neoplasm of unspecified site of unspecified male breast ♂

Malignant neoplasms of female genital organs (C51-C58)

INCLUDES malignant neoplasm of skin of female genital organs

√4th **C51 Malignant neoplasm of vulva**

EXCLUDES 1 *carcinoma in situ of vulva (D07.1)*

C51.0 Malignant neoplasm of labium majus ♀
Malignant neoplasm of Bartholin's [greater vestibular] gland

C51.1 Malignant neoplasm of labium minus ♀

C51.2 Malignant neoplasm of clitoris ♀

C51.8 Malignant neoplasm of overlapping sites of vulva ♀

C51.9 Malignant neoplasm of vulva, unspecified ♀
Malignant neoplasm of external female genitalia NOS
Malignant neoplasm of pudendum

C52 Malignant neoplasm of vagina ♀

EXCLUDES 1 *carcinoma in situ of vagina (D07.2)*

√4th **C53 Malignant neoplasm of cervix uteri**

EXCLUDES 1 *carcinoma in situ of cervix uteri (D06.-)*

C53.0 Malignant neoplasm of endocervix ♀

C53.1 Malignant neoplasm of exocervix ♀

C53.8 Malignant neoplasm of overlapping sites of cervix uteri ♀

C53.9 Malignant neoplasm of cervix uteri, unspecified ♀

√4th **C54 Malignant neoplasm of corpus uteri**

C54.0 Malignant neoplasm of isthmus uteri ♀
Malignant neoplasm of lower uterine segment

C54.1 Malignant neoplasm of endometrium ♀

C54.2 Malignant neoplasm of myometrium ♀

C54.3 Malignant neoplasm of fundus uteri ♀

C54.8 Malignant neoplasm of overlapping sites of corpus uteri ♀

C54.9 Malignant neoplasm of corpus uteri, unspecified ♀

C55 Malignant neoplasm of uterus, part unspecified ♀

√4th **C56 Malignant neoplasm of ovary**

Use additional code to identify any functional activity

CC Excl: For CC codes in category C56, unless otherwise noted: C45.9, C56.1-C57.4, C7A.00, C7A.098-C7B.00, C7B.1, C76.3, C79.60-C79.62, C80.0-C80.2

C56.1 Malignant neoplasm of right ovary CC ♀

C56.2 Malignant neoplasm of left ovary CC ♀

C56.9 Malignant neoplasm of unspecified ovary CC ♀

√4th **C57 Malignant neoplasm of other and unspecified female genital organs**

√5th **C57.0 Malignant neoplasm of fallopian tube**
Malignant neoplasm of oviduct
Malignant neoplasm of uterine tube

C57.00 Malignant neoplasm of unspecified fallopian tube ♀

C57.01 Malignant neoplasm of right fallopian tube ♀

C57.02 Malignant neoplasm of left fallopian tube ♀

√5th **C57.1 Malignant neoplasm of broad ligament**

C57.10 Malignant neoplasm of unspecified broad ligament ♀

C57.11 Malignant neoplasm of right broad ligament ♀

C57.12 Malignant neoplasm of left broad ligament ♀

√5th **C57.2 Malignant neoplasm of round ligament**

C57.20 Malignant neoplasm of unspecified round ligament ♀

C57.21 Malignant neoplasm of right round ligament ♀

C57.22 Malignant neoplasm of left round ligament ♀

C57.3 Malignant neoplasm of parametrium ♀
Malignant neoplasm of uterine ligament NOS

C57.4 Malignant neoplasm of uterine adnexa, unspecified ♀

C57.7 Malignant neoplasm of other specified female genital organs ♀
Malignant neoplasm of wolffian body or duct

C57.8 Malignant neoplasm of overlapping sites of female genital organs ♀
Primary malignant neoplasm of two or more contiguous sites of the female genital organs whose point of origin cannot be determined
Primary tubo-ovarian malignant neoplasm whose point of origin cannot be determined
Primary utero-ovarian malignant neoplasm whose point of origin cannot be determined

C57.9 Malignant neoplasm of female genital organ, unspecified ♀
Malignant neoplasm of female genitourinary tract NOS

C58 Malignant neoplasm of placenta ♀
INCLUDES choriocarcinoma NOS
chorionepithelioma NOS
EXCLUDES 1 *chorioadenoma (destruens) (D39.2)*
hydatidiform mole NOS (O01.9)
invasive hydatidiform mole (D39.2)
male choriocarcinoma NOS (C62.9-)
malignant hydatidiform mole (D39.2)

Malignant neoplasms of male genital organs (C60-C63)

INCLUDES malignant neoplasm of skin of male genital organs

✓4th **C60 Malignant neoplasm of penis**

C60.0 Malignant neoplasm of prepuce ♂
Malignant neoplasm of foreskin

C60.1 Malignant neoplasm of glans penis ♂

C60.2 Malignant neoplasm of body of penis ♂
Malignant neoplasm of corpus cavernosum

C60.8 Malignant neoplasm of overlapping sites of penis ♂

C60.9 Malignant neoplasm of penis, unspecified ♂
Malignant neoplasm of skin of penis NOS

C61 Malignant neoplasm of prostate ♂
EXCLUDES 1 *malignant neoplasm of seminal vesicle (C63.7)*

✓4th **C62 Malignant neoplasm of testis**
Use additional code to identify any functional activity

✓5th **C62.0 Malignant neoplasm of undescended testis**
Malignant neoplasm of ectopic testis
Malignant neoplasm of retained testis

C62.00 Malignant neoplasm of unspecified undescended testis ♂

C62.01 Malignant neoplasm of undescended right testis ♂

C62.02 Malignant neoplasm of undescended left testis ♂

✓5th **C62.1 Malignant neoplasm of descended testis**
Malignant neoplasm of scrotal testis

C62.10 Malignant neoplasm of unspecified descended testis ♂

C62.11 Malignant neoplasm of descended right testis ♂

C62.12 Malignant neoplasm of descended left testis ♂

✓5th **C62.9 Malignant neoplasm of testis, unspecified whether descended or undescended**

C62.90 Malignant neoplasm of unspecified testis, unspecified whether descended or undescended ♂
Malignant neoplasm of testis NOS

C62.91 Malignant neoplasm of right testis, unspecified whether descended or undescended ♂

C62.92 Malignant neoplasm of left testis, unspecified whether descended or undescended ♂

✓4th **C63 Malignant neoplasm of other and unspecified male genital organs**

✓5th **C63.0 Malignant neoplasm of epididymis**

C63.00 Malignant neoplasm of unspecified epididymis ♂

C63.01 Malignant neoplasm of right epididymis ♂

C63.02 Malignant neoplasm of left epididymis ♂

✓5th **C63.1 Malignant neoplasm of spermatic cord**

C63.10 Malignant neoplasm of unspecified spermatic cord ♂

C63.11 Malignant neoplasm of right spermatic cord ♂

C63.12 Malignant neoplasm of left spermatic cord ♂

C63.2 Malignant neoplasm of scrotum ♂
Malignant neoplasm of skin of scrotum

C63.7 Malignant neoplasm of other specified male genital organs ♂
Malignant neoplasm of seminal vesicle
Malignant neoplasm of tunica vaginalis

C63.8 Malignant neoplasm of overlapping sites of male genital organs ♂
Primary malignant neoplasm of two or more contiguous sites of male genital organs whose point of origin cannot be determined

C63.9 Malignant neoplasm of male genital organ, unspecified ♂
Malignant neoplasm of male genitourinary tract NOS

Malignant neoplasms of urinary tract (C64-C68)

✓4th **C64 Malignant neoplasm of kidney, except renal pelvis**
EXCLUDES 1 *malignant carcinoid tumor of the kidney (C7A.093)*
malignant neoplasm of renal calyces (C65.-)
malignant neoplasm of renal pelvis (C65.-)

CC Excl: For CC codes in category C64, unless otherwise noted: C45.7-C45.9, C64.1-C64.9, C65.1-C65.9, C68.8-C68.9, C76.8, C7A.00, C7A.093, C7A.098-C7B.00, C7B.1, C80.0-C80.2, D49.5, D49.81-D49.9

C64.1 Malignant neoplasm of right kidney, except renal pelvis CC

C64.2 Malignant neoplasm of left kidney, except renal pelvis CC

C64.9 Malignant neoplasm of unspecified kidney, except renal pelvis CC

✓4th **C65 Malignant neoplasm of renal pelvis**
INCLUDES malignant neoplasm of pelviureteric junction
malignant neoplasm of renal calyces

CC Excl: For CC codes in category C65, unless otherwise noted: C45.7-C45.9, C64.1-C64.9, C65.1-C65.9, C68.8-C68.9, C76.8, C7A.00, C7A.093, C7A.098-C7B.00, C7B.1, C80.0-C80.2, D49.5, D49.81-D49.9

C65.1 Malignant neoplasm of right renal pelvis CC

C65.2 Malignant neoplasm of left renal pelvis CC

C65.9 Malignant neoplasm of unspecified renal pelvis CC

✓4th **C66 Malignant neoplasm of ureter**
EXCLUDES 1 *malignant neoplasm of ureteric orifice of bladder (C67.6)*

CC Excl: For CC codes in category C66, unless otherwise noted: C45.7-C45.9, C66.1-C66.9, C68.8-C68.9, C76.8, C7A.00, C7A.098-C7B.00, C7B.1, C80.0-C80.2, D49.5, D49.81-D49.9

C66.1 Malignant neoplasm of right ureter CC

C66.2 Malignant neoplasm of left ureter CC

C66.9 Malignant neoplasm of unspecified ureter CC

✓4th **C67 Malignant neoplasm of bladder**

C67.0 Malignant neoplasm of trigone of bladder

C67.1 Malignant neoplasm of dome of bladder

C67.2 Malignant neoplasm of lateral wall of bladder

C67.3 Malignant neoplasm of anterior wall of bladder

C67.4 Malignant neoplasm of posterior wall of bladder

C67.5 Malignant neoplasm of bladder neck
Malignant neoplasm of internal urethral orifice

C67.6 Malignant neoplasm of ureteric orifice

C67.7 Malignant neoplasm of urachus

C67.8 Malignant neoplasm of overlapping sites of bladder

C67.9 Malignant neoplasm of bladder, unspecified

✓4th **C68 Malignant neoplasm of other and unspecified urinary organs**
EXCLUDES 1 *malignant neoplasm of female genitourinary tract NOS (C57.9)*
malignant neoplasm of male genitourinary tract NOS (C63.9)

C68.0 Malignant neoplasm of urethra CC
EXCLUDES 1 *malignant neoplasm of urethral orifice of bladder (C67.5)*
CC Excl: C68.0-C68.9, C79.82

C68.1 Malignant neoplasm of paraurethral glands CC
CC Excl: See code: C68.0

C68.8 Malignant neoplasm of overlapping sites of urinary organs CC
Primary malignant neoplasm of two or more contiguous sites of urinary organs whose point of origin cannot be determined
CC Excl: C64.1-C64.9, C65.1-C65.9, C66.1-C66.9, C68.0-C68.9, C76.3, C79.00-C79.19, C7A.093

C68.9 Malignant neoplasm of urinary organ, unspecified CC
Malignant neoplasm of urinary system NOS
CC Excl: See code: C68.8

Neoplasms

Malignant neoplasms of eye, brain and other parts of central nervous system (C69-C72)

C69 Malignant neoplasm of eye and adnexa
EXCLUDES 1 *malignant neoplasm of connective tissue of eyelid (C49.Ø)*
malignant neoplasm of eyelid (skin) (C43.1-, C44.1-)
malignant neoplasm of optic nerve (C72.3-)

C69.Ø Malignant neoplasm of conjunctiva
C69.ØØ Malignant neoplasm of unspecified conjunctiva
C69.Ø1 Malignant neoplasm of right conjunctiva
C69.Ø2 Malignant neoplasm of left conjunctiva

C69.1 Malignant neoplasm of cornea
C69.1Ø Malignant neoplasm of unspecified cornea
C69.11 Malignant neoplasm of right cornea
C69.12 Malignant neoplasm of left cornea

C69.2 Malignant neoplasm of retina
EXCLUDES 1 *dark area on retina (D49.81)*
neoplasm of unspecified behavior of retina and choroid (D49.81)
retinal freckle (D49.81)
C69.2Ø Malignant neoplasm of unspecified retina
C69.21 Malignant neoplasm of right retina
C69.22 Malignant neoplasm of left retina

C69.3 Malignant neoplasm of choroid
C69.3Ø Malignant neoplasm of unspecified choroid
C69.31 Malignant neoplasm of right choroid
C69.32 Malignant neoplasm of left choroid

C69.4 Malignant neoplasm of ciliary body
C69.4Ø Malignant neoplasm of unspecified ciliary body
C69.41 Malignant neoplasm of right ciliary body
C69.42 Malignant neoplasm of left ciliary body

C69.5 Malignant neoplasm of lacrimal gland and duct
Malignant neoplasm of lacrimal sac
Malignant neoplasm of nasolacrimal duct
C69.5Ø Malignant neoplasm of unspecified lacrimal gland and duct
C69.51 Malignant neoplasm of right lacrimal gland and duct
C69.52 Malignant neoplasm of left lacrimal gland and duct

C69.6 Malignant neoplasm of orbit
Malignant neoplasm of connective tissue of orbit
Malignant neoplasm of extraocular muscle
Malignant neoplasm of peripheral nerves of orbit
Malignant neoplasm of retrobulbar tissue
Malignant neoplasm of retro-ocular tissue
EXCLUDES 1 *malignant neoplasm of orbital bone (C41.Ø)*
C69.6Ø Malignant neoplasm of unspecified orbit
C69.61 Malignant neoplasm of right orbit
C69.62 Malignant neoplasm of left orbit

C69.8 Malignant neoplasm of overlapping sites of eye and adnexa
C69.8Ø Malignant neoplasm of overlapping sites of unspecified eye and adnexa
C69.81 Malignant neoplasm of overlapping sites of right eye and adnexa
C69.82 Malignant neoplasm of overlapping sites of left eye and adnexa

C69.9 Malignant neoplasm of unspecified site of eye
Malignant neoplasm of eyeball
C69.9Ø Malignant neoplasm of unspecified site of unspecified eye
C69.91 Malignant neoplasm of unspecified site of right eye
C69.92 Malignant neoplasm of unspecified site of left eye

C7Ø Malignant neoplasm of meninges
C7Ø.Ø Malignant neoplasm of cerebral meninges CC
CC Excl: C45.7-C45.9, C7Ø.Ø, C7Ø.9, C72.9, C76.8, C7A.ØØ, C7A.Ø98-C7B.ØØ, C7B.1, C8Ø.Ø-C8Ø.2, D49.6-D49.9
C7Ø.1 Malignant neoplasm of spinal meninges CC
CC Excl: C45.7-C45.9, C7Ø.1, C72.9, C76.8, C7A.ØØ, C7A.Ø98-C7B.ØØ, C7B.1, C8Ø.Ø-C8Ø.2, D49.6-D49.9
C7Ø.9 Malignant neoplasm of meninges, unspecified CC
CC Excl: See code: C7Ø.Ø

C71 Malignant neoplasm of brain
EXCLUDES 1 *malignant neoplasm of cranial nerves (C72.2-C72.5)*
retrobulbar malignant neoplasm (C69.6-)

CC Excl: For CC codes in category C71, unless otherwise noted: C45.7-C45.9, C7Ø.Ø, C7Ø.9-C71.9, C72.2Ø-C72.9, C76.8, C7A.ØØ, C7A.Ø98-C7B.ØØ, C7B.1, C8Ø.Ø-C8Ø.2, D49.6-D49.9

C71.Ø Malignant neoplasm of cerebrum, except lobes and ventricles CC
Malignant neoplasm of supratentorial NOS
C71.1 Malignant neoplasm of frontal lobe CC
C71.2 Malignant neoplasm of temporal lobe CC
C71.3 Malignant neoplasm of parietal lobe CC
C71.4 Malignant neoplasm of occipital lobe CC
C71.5 Malignant neoplasm of cerebral ventricle CC
EXCLUDES 1 *malignant neoplasm of fourth cerebral ventricle (C71.7)*
C71.6 Malignant neoplasm of cerebellum CC
C71.7 Malignant neoplasm of brain stem CC
Malignant neoplasm of fourth cerebral ventricle
Infratentorial malignant neoplasm NOS
C71.8 Malignant neoplasm of overlapping sites of brain CC
C71.9 Malignant neoplasm of brain, unspecified CC

C72 Malignant neoplasm of spinal cord, cranial nerves and other parts of central nervous system
EXCLUDES 1 *malignant neoplasm of meninges (C7Ø.-)*
malignant neoplasm of peripheral nerves and autonomic nervous system (C47.-)

C72.Ø Malignant neoplasm of spinal cord CC
CC Excl: C45.7-C45.9, C72.Ø-C72.1, C72.9, C76.8, C7A.ØØ, C7A.Ø98-C7B.ØØ, C7B.1, C8Ø.Ø-C8Ø.2, D49.6-D49.9
C72.1 Malignant neoplasm of cauda equina CC
CC Excl: See code: C72.Ø

C72.2 Malignant neoplasm of olfactory nerve
Malignant neoplasm of olfactory bulb

CC Excl: For CC codes in subcategory C72.2, unless otherwise noted: C45.7-C45.9, C72.2Ø-C72.9, C76.8, C7A.ØØ, C7A.Ø98-C7B.ØØ, C7B.1, C8Ø.Ø-C8Ø.2, D49.6-D49.9

C72.2Ø Malignant neoplasm of unspecified olfactory nerve CC
C72.21 Malignant neoplasm of right olfactory nerve CC
C72.22 Malignant neoplasm of left olfactory nerve CC

C72.3 Malignant neoplasm of optic nerve

CC Excl: For CC codes in subcategory C72.3, unless otherwise noted: C45.7-C45.9, C72.2Ø-C72.9, C76.8, C7A.ØØ, C7A.Ø98-C7B.ØØ, C7B.1, C8Ø.Ø-C8Ø.2, D49.6-D49.9

C72.3Ø Malignant neoplasm of unspecified optic nerve CC
C72.31 Malignant neoplasm of right optic nerve CC
C72.32 Malignant neoplasm of left optic nerve CC

C72.4 Malignant neoplasm of acoustic nerve

CC Excl: For CC codes in subcategory C72.4, unless otherwise noted: C45.7-C45.9, C72.2Ø-C72.9, C76.8, C7A.ØØ, C7A.Ø98-C7B.ØØ, C7B.1, C8Ø.Ø-C8Ø.2, D49.6-D49.9

C72.4Ø Malignant neoplasm of unspecified acoustic nerve CC
C72.41 Malignant neoplasm of right acoustic nerve CC
C72.42 Malignant neoplasm of left acoustic nerve CC

C72.5 Malignant neoplasm of other and unspecified cranial nerves

CC Excl: For CC codes in subcategory C72.5, unless otherwise noted: C45.7-C45.9, C72.2Ø-C72.9, C76.8, C7A.ØØ, C7A.Ø98-C7B.ØØ, C7B.1, C8Ø.Ø-C8Ø.2, D49.6-D49.9

C72.5Ø Malignant neoplasm of unspecified cranial nerve CC
Malignant neoplasm of cranial nerve NOS
C72.59 Malignant neoplasm of other cranial nerves CC
C72.9 Malignant neoplasm of central nervous system, unspecified CC
Malignant neoplasm of unspecified site of central nervous system
Malignant neoplasm of nervous system NOS
CC Excl: C45.7-C45.9, C7Ø.Ø-C72.9, C7A.ØØ, C7A.Ø98-C7B.ØØ, C7B.1, C76.8, C79.31-C79.49, C8Ø.Ø-C8Ø.2, D49.6-D49.9

Malignant neoplasms of thyroid and other endocrine glands (C73-C75)

C73 Malignant neoplasm of thyroid gland
Use additional code to identify any functional activity

✓4th **C74 Malignant neoplasm of adrenal gland**

CC Excl: For CC codes in category C74, unless otherwise noted: C45.7-C45.9, C74.00-C74.92, C75.9-C7A.00, C7A.098-C7B.00, C7B.1, C76.2, C76.8, C79.70-C79.72, C80.0-C80.2

✓5th **C74.0 Malignant neoplasm of cortex of adrenal gland**
- **C74.00 Malignant neoplasm of cortex of unspecified adrenal gland** CC
- **C74.01 Malignant neoplasm of cortex of right adrenal gland** CC
- **C74.02 Malignant neoplasm of cortex of left adrenal gland** CC

✓5th **C74.1 Malignant neoplasm of medulla of adrenal gland**
- **C74.10 Malignant neoplasm of medulla of unspecified adrenal gland** CC
- **C74.11 Malignant neoplasm of medulla of right adrenal gland** CC
- **C74.12 Malignant neoplasm of medulla of left adrenal gland** CC

✓5th **C74.9 Malignant neoplasm of unspecified part of adrenal gland**
- **C74.90 Malignant neoplasm of unspecified part of unspecified adrenal gland** CC
- **C74.91 Malignant neoplasm of unspecified part of right adrenal gland** CC
- **C74.92 Malignant neoplasm of unspecified part of left adrenal gland** CC

✓4th **C75 Malignant neoplasm of other endocrine glands and related structures**

EXCLUDES 1 *malignant carcinoid tumors (C7A.0-)*
malignant neoplasm of adrenal gland (C74.-)
malignant neoplasm of endocrine pancreas (C25.4)
malignant neoplasm of islets of Langerhans (C25.4)
malignant neoplasm of ovary (C56.-)
malignant neoplasm of testis (C62.-)
malignant neoplasm of thymus (C37)
malignant neoplasm of thyroid gland (C73)
malignant neuroendocrine tumors (C7A.-)

C75.0 Malignant neoplasm of parathyroid gland CC
CC Excl: C75.0-C75.9

C75.1 Malignant neoplasm of pituitary gland CC
CC Excl: C75.1-C75.2, Z51.0

C75.2 Malignant neoplasm of craniopharyngeal duct CC
CC Excl: See code: C75.1

C75.3 Malignant neoplasm of pineal gland CC
CC Excl: C75.3-Z51.0

C75.4 Malignant neoplasm of carotid body CC
CC Excl: C75.4-C75.9

C75.5 Malignant neoplasm of aortic body and other paraganglia CC
CC Excl: See code: C75.4

C75.8 Malignant neoplasm with pluriglandular involvement, unspecified CC
CC Excl: C74.00-C75.9

C75.9 Malignant neoplasm of endocrine gland, unspecified CC
CC Excl: See code: C75.8

Malignant neuroendocrine tumors (C7A)

✓4th **C7A Malignant neuroendocrine tumors**
Code also any associated multiple endocrine neoplasia [MEN] syndromes (E31.2-)
Use additional code to identify any associated endocrine syndrome, such as:
carcinoid syndrome (E34.0)

EXCLUDES 2 *malignant pancreatic islet cell tumors (C25.4)*
Merkel cell carcinoma (C4A.-)

✓5th **C7A.0 Malignant carcinoid tumors**

C7A.00 Malignant carcinoid tumor of unspecified site CC
CC Excl: C45.7-C45.9, C76.8, C79.89-C7B.00, C7B.09-C80.2, D49.81-D49.9

✓6th **C7A.01 Malignant carcinoid tumors of the small intestine**

C7A.010 Malignant carcinoid tumor of the duodenum CC
CC Excl: C17.0-C17.9, C26.0, C26.9, C45.7-C45.9, C46.4, C76.8, C7A.00-C7B.00, C7B.1, C80.0-C80.2, D49.0, D49.81-D49.9

C7A.011 Malignant carcinoid tumor of the jejunum CC
CC Excl: C17.1-C17.9, C26.0, C26.9, C45.7-C45.9, C46.4, C76.8, C7A.00-C7B.00, C7B.1, C80.0-C80.2, D49.0, D49.81-D49.9

C7A.012 Malignant carcinoid tumor of the ileum CC
CC Excl: C17.2-C17.9, C26.0, C26.9, C45.7-C45.9, C46.4, C76.8, C7A.00-C7B.00, C7B.1, C80.0-C80.2, D49.0, D49.81-D49.9

C7A.019 Malignant carcinoid tumor of the small intestine, unspecified portion CC
CC Excl: C17.8-C17.9, C26.0, C26.9, C45.7-C45.9, C46.4, C76.8, C7A.00-C7B.00, C7B.1, C80.0-C80.2, D49.0, D49.81-D49.9

✓6th **C7A.02 Malignant carcinoid tumors of the appendix, large intestine, and rectum**

C7A.020 Malignant carcinoid tumor of the appendix CC
CC Excl: C18.1-C18.9, C26.0, C26.9, C45.7-C45.9, C46.4, C76.8, C7A.00-C7B.00, C7B.1, C80.0-C80.2, D49.0, D49.81-D49.9

C7A.021 Malignant carcinoid tumor of the cecum CC
CC Excl: C18.0-C18.9, C26.0, C26.9, C45.7-C45.9, C46.4, C76.8, C7A.00-C7B.00, C7B.1, C80.0-C80.2, D49.0, D49.81-D49.9

C7A.022 Malignant carcinoid tumor of the ascending colon CC
CC Excl: C18.2-C18.9, C26.0, C26.9, C45.7-C45.9, C46.4, C76.8, C7A.00-C7B.00, C7B.1, C80.0-C80.2, D49.0, D49.81-D49.9

C7A.023 Malignant carcinoid tumor of the transverse colon CC
CC Excl: C18.4-C18.9, C26.0, C26.9, C45.7-C45.9, C46.4, C76.8, C7A.00-C7B.00, C7B.1, C80.0-C80.2, D49.0, D49.81-D49.9

C7A.024 Malignant carcinoid tumor of the descending colon CC
CC Excl: C18.6-C18.9, C26.0, C26.9, C45.7-C45.9, C46.4, C76.8, C7A.00-C7B.00, C7B.1, C80.0-C80.2, D49.0, D49.81-D49.9

C7A.025 Malignant carcinoid tumor of the sigmoid colon CC
CC Excl: C18.7-C18.9, C26.0, C26.9, C45.7-C45.9, C46.4, C76.8, C7A.00-C7B.00, C7B.1, C80.0-C80.2, D49.0, D49.81-D49.9

C7A.026 Malignant carcinoid tumor of the rectum CC
CC Excl: C20-C21.8, C26.0, C26.9, C45.7-C45.9, C46.4, C76.8, C7A.00-C7B.00, C7B.1, C80.0-C80.2, D49.0, D49.81-D49.9

C7A.029 Malignant carcinoid tumor of the large intestine, unspecified portion CC
Malignant carcinoid tumor of the colon NOS
CC Excl: C18.8-C18.9, C26.0, C26.9, C45.7-C45.9, C46.4, C76.8, C7A.00-C7B.00, C7B.1, C80.0-C80.2, D49.0, D49.81-D49.9

✓6th **C7A.09 Malignant carcinoid tumors of other sites**

C7A.090 Malignant carcinoid tumor of the bronchus and lung CC
CC Excl: C34.80-C34.92, C39.9, C45.7-C45.9, C46.50-C46.52, C76.8, C7A.00-C7B.00, C7B.1, C80.0-C80.2, D49.1, D49.81-D49.9

C7A.091 Malignant carcinoid tumor of the thymus CC
CC Excl: C37-C7A.8

C7A.092 Malignant carcinoid tumor of the stomach CC
CC Excl: C16.0-C16.9, C26.0, C26.9, C45.7-C45.9, C46.4, C76.8, C7A.00-C7B.00, C7B.1, C80.0-C80.2, D49.0, D49.81-D49.9

C7A.093 Malignant carcinoid tumor of the kidney CC
CC Excl: C45.7-C45.9, C64.1-C64.9, C65.1-C65.9, C68.8-C68.9, C76.8, C7A.00-C7B.00, C7B.1, C80.0-C80.2, D49.5, D49.81-D49.9

C7A.094 **Malignant carcinoid tumor of the foregut NOS** CC
CC Excl: See code: C7A.092

C7A.095 **Malignant carcinoid tumor of the midgut NOS** CC
CC Excl: See code: C7A.092

C7A.096 **Malignant carcinoid tumor of the hindgut NOS** CC
CC Excl: See code: C7A.092

C7A.098 **Malignant carcinoid tumors of other sites** CC
CC Excl: See code: C7A.00

C7A.1 **Malignant poorly differentiated neuroendocrine tumors** CC
High grade neuroendocrine carcinoma, any site
Malignant poorly differentiated neuroendocrine tumor NOS
Malignant poorly differentiated neuroendocrine carcinoma, any site
CC Excl: See code: C7A.00

C7A.8 **Other malignant neuroendocrine tumors** CC
CC Excl: See code: C7A.00

Secondary neuroendocrine tumors (C7B)

4th C7B **Secondary neuroendocrine tumors**
Use additional code to identify any functional activity

5th C7B.0 **Secondary carcinoid tumors**

C7B.00 **Secondary carcinoid tumors, unspecified site**

C7B.01 **Secondary carcinoid tumors of distant lymph nodes** CC
CC Excl: C45.7-C45.9, C46.3, C76.8-C77.9, C7A.00, C7A.098-C80.2, D49.81-D49.9

C7B.02 **Secondary carcinoid tumors of liver** CC
CC Excl: C45.7-C45.9, C76.8, C78.7-C78.89, C79.89-C7A.00, C7A.098-C80.2, D49.81-D49.9

C7B.03 **Secondary carcinoid tumors of bone** CC
CC Excl: C45.7-C45.9, C76.8, C79.51-C79.52, C79.89-C7A.00, C7A.098-C80.2, D49.81-D49.9

C7B.04 **Secondary carcinoid tumors of peritoneum** CC
Mesentery metastasis of carcinoid tumor
CC Excl: C45.7-C45.9, C76.8, C78.6, C78.80-C78.89, C79.89-C7A.00, C7A.098-C80.2, D49.81-D49.9

C7B.09 **Secondary carcinoid tumors of other sites** CC
CC Excl: C45.7-C45.9, C76.8, C79.89-C7A.00, C7A.098-C80.2, D49.81-D49.9

C7B.1 **Secondary Merkel cell carcinoma**
Merkel cell carcinoma nodal presentation
Merkel cell carcinoma visceral metastatic presentation

C7B.8 **Other secondary neuroendocrine tumors** CC
CC Excl: See code: C7B.09

Malignant neoplasms of ill-defined, other secondary and unspecified sites (C76-C80)

4th C76 **Malignant neoplasm of other and ill-defined sites**
EXCLUDES 1 *malignant neoplasm of female genitourinary tract NOS (C57.9)*
malignant neoplasm of male genitourinary tract NOS (C63.9)
malignant neoplasm of lymphoid, hematopoietic and related tissue (C81-C96)
malignant neoplasm of skin (C44.-)
malignant neoplasm of unspecified site NOS (C80.1)

C76.0 **Malignant neoplasm of head, face and neck**
Malignant neoplasm of cheek NOS
Malignant neoplasm of nose NOS

C76.1 **Malignant neoplasm of thorax**
Intrathoracic malignant neoplasm NOS
Malignant neoplasm of axilla NOS
Thoracic malignant neoplasm NOS

C76.2 **Malignant neoplasm of abdomen**

C76.3 **Malignant neoplasm of pelvis**
Malignant neoplasm of groin NOS
Malignant neoplasm of sites overlapping systems within the pelvis
Rectovaginal (septum) malignant neoplasm
Rectovesical (septum) malignant neoplasm

5th C76.4 **Malignant neoplasm of upper limb**

C76.40 **Malignant neoplasm of unspecified upper limb**

C76.41 **Malignant neoplasm of right upper limb**

C76.42 **Malignant neoplasm of left upper limb**

5th C76.5 **Malignant neoplasm of lower limb**

C76.50 **Malignant neoplasm of unspecified lower limb**

C76.51 **Malignant neoplasm of right lower limb**

C76.52 **Malignant neoplasm of left lower limb**

C76.8 **Malignant neoplasm of other specified ill-defined sites**
Malignant neoplasm of overlapping ill-defined sites

4th C77 **Secondary and unspecified malignant neoplasm of lymph nodes**
EXCLUDES 1 *malignant neoplasm of lymph nodes, specified as primary (C81-C86, C88, C96.-)*
mesentery metastasis of carcinoid tumor (C7B.04)
secondary carcinoid tumors of distant lymph nodes (C7B.01)

CC Excl: For CC codes in category C77, unless otherwise noted: C45.7-C45.9, C46.3, C76.8-C77.9, C7A.00, C7A.098-C7B.01, C7B.1, C80.0-C80.2, D49.81-D49.9

C77.0 **Secondary and unspecified malignant neoplasm of lymph nodes of head, face and neck** CC
Secondary and unspecified malignant neoplasm of supraclavicular lymph nodes

C77.1 **Secondary and unspecified malignant neoplasm of intrathoracic lymph nodes** CC

C77.2 **Secondary and unspecified malignant neoplasm of intra-abdominal lymph nodes** CC

C77.3 **Secondary and unspecified malignant neoplasm of axilla and upper limb lymph nodes** CC
Secondary and unspecified malignant neoplasm of pectoral lymph nodes

C77.4 **Secondary and unspecified malignant neoplasm of inguinal and lower limb lymph nodes** CC

C77.5 **Secondary and unspecified malignant neoplasm of intrapelvic lymph nodes** CC

C77.8 **Secondary and unspecified malignant neoplasm of lymph nodes of multiple regions** CC

C77.9 **Secondary and unspecified malignant neoplasm of lymph node, unspecified** CC

4th C78 **Secondary malignant neoplasm of respiratory and digestive organs**
EXCLUDES 1 *lymph node metastases (C77.0)*
secondary carcinoid tumors of liver (C7B.02)
secondary carcinoid tumors of peritoneum (C7B.04)

5th C78.0 **Secondary malignant neoplasm of lung**

C78.00 **Secondary malignant neoplasm of unspecified lung** CC
CC Excl: C45.7-C45.9, C76.8, C78.00-C78.02, C78.30-C78.39, C79.89-C7A.00, C7A.098-C7B.00, C7B.09-C80.2, D49.81-D49.9

C78.01 **Secondary malignant neoplasm of right lung** CC
CC Excl: See code: C78.00

C78.02 **Secondary malignant neoplasm of left lung** CC
CC Excl: See code: C78.00

C78.1 **Secondary malignant neoplasm of mediastinum** CC
CC Excl: C45.7-C45.9, C76.8, C78.1, C78.30-C78.39, C79.89-C7A.00, C7A.098-C7B.00, C7B.09-C80.2, D49.81-D49.9

C78.2 **Secondary malignant neoplasm of pleura** CC
CC Excl: C45.7-C45.9, C76.8, C78.2-C78.39, C79.89-C7A.00, C7A.098-C7B.00, C7B.09-C80.2, D49.81-D49.9, J91.0

5th C78.3 **Secondary malignant neoplasm of other and unspecified respiratory organs**

C78.30 **Secondary malignant neoplasm of unspecified respiratory organ** CC
CC Excl: C45.7-C45.9, C76.8, C78.00-C78.39, C79.89-C7A.00, C7A.098-C7B.00, C7B.09-C80.2, D49.81-D49.9

C78.39 **Secondary malignant neoplasm of other respiratory organs** CC
CC Excl: See code: C78.30

C78.4 **Secondary malignant neoplasm of small intestine** CC
CC Excl: C45.7-C45.9, C76.8, C78.4, C78.80-C78.89, C79.89-C7A.00, C7A.098-C7B.00, C7B.09-C80.2, D49.81-D49.9

C78.5 **Secondary malignant neoplasm of large intestine and rectum** CC
CC Excl: C45.7-C45.9, C76.8, C78.5, C78.80-C78.89, C79.89-C7A.00, C7A.098-C7B.00, C7B.09-C80.2, D49.81-D49.9

C78.6 **Secondary malignant neoplasm of retroperitoneum and peritoneum** CC
CC Excl: C45.7-C45.9, C76.8, C78.6, C78.80-C78.89, C79.89-C7A.00, C7A.098-C7B.00, C7B.04-C80.2, D49.81-D49.9

C78.7 **Secondary malignant neoplasm of liver and intrahepatic bile duct** CC
CC Excl: C45.7-C45.9, C76.8, C78.7-C78.89, C79.89-C7A.00, C7A.098-C7B.00, C7B.02, C7B.09-C80.2, D49.81-D49.9

C78.8 Secondary malignant neoplasm of other and unspecified digestive organs

C78.80 Secondary malignant neoplasm of unspecified digestive organ CC
CC Excl: C45.7-C45.9, C76.8, C78.4-C78.89, C79.89-C7A.00, C7A.098-C7B.00, C7B.02, C7B.04-C80.2, D49.81-D49.9

C78.89 Secondary malignant neoplasm of other digestive organs CC
CC Excl: See code: C78.80

C79 Secondary malignant neoplasm of other and unspecified sites
EXCLUDES 1 *lymph node metastases (C77.0)*
secondary carcinoid tumors (C7B.-)
secondary neuroendocrine tumors (C7B.-)

C79.0 Secondary malignant neoplasm of kidney and renal pelvis

CC Excl: For CC codes in subcategory C79.0, unless otherwise noted: C45.7-C45.9, C76.8, C79.00-C79.19, C79.89-C7A.00, C7A.098-C7B.00, C7B.09-C80.2, D49.81-D49.9

C79.00 Secondary malignant neoplasm of unspecified kidney and renal pelvis CC

C79.01 Secondary malignant neoplasm of right kidney and renal pelvis CC

C79.02 Secondary malignant neoplasm of left kidney and renal pelvis CC

C79.1 Secondary malignant neoplasm of bladder and other and unspecified urinary organs

CC Excl: For CC codes in subcategory C79.1, unless otherwise noted: C45.7-C45.9, C76.8, C79.00-C79.19, C79.89-C7A.00, C7A.098-C7B.00, C7B.09-C80.2, D49.81-D49.9

C79.10 Secondary malignant neoplasm of unspecified urinary organs CC

C79.11 Secondary malignant neoplasm of bladder CC

C79.19 Secondary malignant neoplasm of other urinary organs CC

C79.2 Secondary malignant neoplasm of skin CC
EXCLUDES 1 *secondary Merkel cell carcinoma (C7B.1)*
CC Excl: C45.7-C45.9, C76.8, C79.2, C79.89-C7A.00, C7A.098-C7B.00, C7B.09-C80.2, D49.81-D49.9

C79.3 Secondary malignant neoplasm of brain and cerebral meninges

C79.31 Secondary malignant neoplasm of brain CC
CC Excl: C45.7-C45.9, C76.8, C79.31, C79.89-C7A.00, C7A.098-C7B.00, C7B.09-C80.2, D49.81-D49.9

C79.32 Secondary malignant neoplasm of cerebral meninges CC
CC Excl: C45.7-C45.9, C76.8, C79.32-C79.49, C79.89-C7A.00, C7A.098-C7B.00, C7B.09-C80.2, D49.81-D49.9

C79.4 Secondary malignant neoplasm of other and unspecified parts of nervous system

C79.40 Secondary malignant neoplasm of unspecified part of nervous system CC
CC Excl: See code: C79.32

C79.49 Secondary malignant neoplasm of other parts of nervous system CC
CC Excl: See code: C79.32

C79.5 Secondary malignant neoplasm of bone and bone marrow
EXCLUDES 1 *secondary carcinoid tumors of bone (C7B.03)*

C79.51 Secondary malignant neoplasm of bone CC
CC Excl: C45.7-C45.9, C76.8, C79.51-C79.52, C79.89-C7A.00, C7A.098-C7B.00, C7B.03, C7B.09-C80.2, D49.81-D49.9

C79.52 Secondary malignant neoplasm of bone marrow CC
CC Excl: See code: C79.51

C79.6 Secondary malignant neoplasm of ovary

CC Excl: For CC codes in subcategory C79.6, unless otherwise noted: C45.7-C45.9, C76.8, C79.60-C79.62, C79.89-C7A.00, C7A.098-C7B.00, C7B.09-C80.2, D49.81-D49.9

C79.60 Secondary malignant neoplasm of unspecified ovary CC ♀

C79.61 Secondary malignant neoplasm of right ovary CC ♀

C79.62 Secondary malignant neoplasm of left ovary CC ♀

C79.7 Secondary malignant neoplasm of adrenal gland

CC Excl: For CC codes in subcategory C79.7, unless otherwise noted: C45.7-C45.9, C76.8, C79.70-C79.72, C79.89-C7A.00, C7A.098-C7B.00, C7B.09-C80.2, D49.81-D49.9

C79.70 Secondary malignant neoplasm of unspecified adrenal gland CC

C79.71 Secondary malignant neoplasm of right adrenal gland CC

C79.72 Secondary malignant neoplasm of left adrenal gland CC

C79.8 Secondary malignant neoplasm of other specified sites

C79.81 Secondary malignant neoplasm of breast CC
CC Excl: C45.7-C45.9, C76.8, C79.81, C79.89-C7A.00, C7A.098-C7B.00, C7B.09-C80.2, D49.81-D49.9

C79.82 Secondary malignant neoplasm of genital organs CC
CC Excl: C45.7-C45.9, C76.8, C79.82-C7A.00, C7A.098-C7B.00, C7B.09-C80.2, D49.81-D49.9

C79.89 Secondary malignant neoplasm of other specified sites CC
CC Excl: C45.7-C45.9, C76.8, C79.89-C7A.00, C7A.098-C7B.00, C7B.09-C80.2, D49.81-D49.9

C79.9 Secondary malignant neoplasm of unspecified site CC
Metastatic cancer NOS
Metastatic disease NOS
EXCLUDES 1 *carcinomatosis NOS (C80.0)*
generalized cancer NOS (C80.0)
malignant (primary) neoplasm of unspecified site (C80.1)
CC Excl: See code: C79.89

C80 Malignant neoplasm without specification of site
EXCLUDES 1 *malignant carcinoid tumor of unspecified site (C7A.00)*
malignant neoplasm of specified multiple sites—code to each site

C80.0 Disseminated malignant neoplasm, unspecified CC
Carcinomatosis NOS
Generalized cancer, unspecified site (primary) (secondary)
Generalized malignancy, unspecified site (primary) (secondary)
CC Excl: See code: C79.89

C80.1 Malignant (primary) neoplasm, unspecified
Cancer NOS
Cancer unspecified site (primary)
Carcinoma unspecified site (primary)
Malignancy unspecified site (primary)
EXCLUDES 1 *secondary malignant neoplasm of unspecified site (C79.9)*

C80.2 Malignant neoplasm associated with transplanted organ CC
Code first complication of transplanted organ (T86.-)
Use additional code to identify the specific malignancy
CC Excl: See code: C79.89

Malignant neoplasms of lymphoid, hematopoietic and related tissue (C81-C96)

EXCLUDES 2 *Kaposi's sarcoma of lymph nodes (C46.3)*
secondary and unspecified neoplasm of lymph nodes (C77.-)
secondary neoplasm of bone marrow (C79.52)
secondary neoplasm of spleen (C78.89)

C81 Hodgkin lymphoma
EXCLUDES 1 *personal history of Hodgkin lymphoma (Z85.71)*

C81.0 Nodular lymphocyte predominant Hodgkin lymphoma

C81.00 Nodular lymphocyte predominant Hodgkin lymphoma, unspecified site CC
CC Excl: C81.00-C81.09, C81.40-C81.49, C81.90, C81.98, D49.81-D49.9

C81.01 Nodular lymphocyte predominant Hodgkin lymphoma, lymph nodes of head, face, and neck CC
CC Excl: C81.00-C81.01, C81.08-C81.09, C81.40-C81.41, C81.48-C81.49, C81.90-C81.91, C81.98, D49.81-D49.9

C81.02 Nodular lymphocyte predominant Hodgkin lymphoma, intrathoracic lymph nodes CC
CC Excl: C81.00-C81.02, C81.08-C81.09, C81.40, C81.42, C81.48-C81.49, C81.90, C81.92, C81.98, D49.81-D49.9

C81.03 Nodular lymphocyte predominant Hodgkin lymphoma, intra-abdominal lymph nodes CC
CC Excl: C81.00, C81.03, C81.08-C81.09, C81.40, C81.43, C81.48-C81.49, C81.90, C81.93, C81.98, D49.81-D49.9

C81.04 Nodular lymphocyte predominant Hodgkin lymphoma, lymph nodes of axilla and upper limb CC
CC Excl: C81.00, C81.04, C81.08-C81.09, C81.40, C81.44, C81.48-C81.49, C81.90, C81.94, C81.98, D49.81-D49.9

C81.05 **Nodular lymphocyte predominant Hodgkin lymphoma, lymph nodes of inguinal region and lower limb** CC
CC Excl: C81.00, C81.05, C81.08-C81.09, C81.40, C81.45, C81.48-C81.49, C81.90, C81.95, C81.98, D49.81-D49.9

C81.06 **Nodular lymphocyte predominant Hodgkin lymphoma, intrapelvic lymph nodes** CC
CC Excl: C81.00, C81.06, C81.08-C81.09, C81.40, C81.46, C81.48-C81.49, C81.90, C81.96, C81.98, D49.81-D49.9

C81.07 **Nodular lymphocyte predominant Hodgkin lymphoma, spleen** CC
CC Excl: C81.00, C81.07-C81.09, C81.40, C81.47-C81.49, C81.90, C81.97-C81.98, D49.81-D49.99

C81.08 **Nodular lymphocyte predominant Hodgkin lymphoma, lymph nodes of multiple sites** CC
CC Excl: C81.00-C81.09, C81.40-C81.49, C81.90, C81.98, D49.81-D49.9

C81.09 **Nodular lymphocyte predominant Hodgkin lymphoma, extranodal and solid organ sites** CC
CC Excl: See code: C81.08

✓5th **C81.1** **Nodular sclerosis classical Hodgkin lymphoma**

C81.10 **Nodular sclerosis classical Hodgkin lymphoma, unspecified site** CC
CC Excl: C81.10-C81.19, C81.90, C81.98, D49.81-D49.9

C81.11 **Nodular sclerosis classical Hodgkin lymphoma, lymph nodes of head, face, and neck** CC
CC Excl: C81.10-C81.11, C81.18-C81.19, C81.90-C81.91, C81.98, D49.81-D49.9

C81.12 **Nodular sclerosis classical Hodgkin lymphoma, intrathoracic lymph nodes** CC
CC Excl: C81.10, C81.12, C81.18-C81.19, C81.90, C81.92, C81.98, D49.81-D49.9

C81.13 **Nodular sclerosis classical Hodgkin lymphoma, intra-abdominal lymph nodes** CC
CC Excl: C81.10, C81.13, C81.18-C81.19, C81.90, C81.93, C81.98, D49.81-D49.9

C81.14 **Nodular sclerosis classical Hodgkin lymphoma, lymph nodes of axilla and upper limb** CC
CC Excl: C81.10, C81.14, C81.18-C81.19, C81.90, C81.94, C81.98, D49.81-D49.9

C81.15 **Nodular sclerosis classical Hodgkin lymphoma, lymph nodes of inguinal region and lower limb** CC
CC Excl: C81.10, C81.15, C81.18-C81.19, C81.90, C81.95, C81.98, D49.81-D49.9

C81.16 **Nodular sclerosis classical Hodgkin lymphoma, intrapelvic lymph nodes** CC
CC Excl: C81.10, C81.16, C81.18-C81.19, C81.90, C81.96, C81.98, D49.81-D49.9

C81.17 **Nodular sclerosis classical Hodgkin lymphoma, spleen** CC
CC Excl: C81.10, C81.17-C81.19, C81.90, C81.97-C81.98, D49.81-D49.9

C81.18 **Nodular sclerosis classical Hodgkin lymphoma, lymph nodes of multiple sites** CC
CC Excl: C81.10-C81.19, C81.90, C81.98, D49.81-D49.9

C81.19 **Nodular sclerosis classical Hodgkin lymphoma, extranodal and solid organ sites** CC
CC Excl: See code: C81.18

✓5th **C81.2** **Mixed cellularity classical Hodgkin lymphoma**

C81.20 **Mixed cellularity classical Hodgkin lymphoma, unspecified site** CC
CC Excl: C81.20-C81.29, C81.90, C81.98, D49.81-D49.9

C81.21 **Mixed cellularity classical Hodgkin lymphoma, lymph nodes of head, face, and neck** CC
CC Excl: C81.20-C81.21, C81.28-C81.29, C81.90-C81.91, C81.98, D49.81-D49.9

C81.22 **Mixed cellularity classical Hodgkin lymphoma, intrathoracic lymph nodes** CC
CC Excl: C81.20, C81.22, C81.28-C81.29, C81.90, C81.92, C81.98, D49.81-D49.9

C81.23 **Mixed cellularity classical Hodgkin lymphoma, intra-abdominal lymph nodes** CC
CC Excl: C81.20, C81.23, C81.28-C81.29, C81.90, C81.93, C81.98, D49.81-D49.9

C81.24 **Mixed cellularity classical Hodgkin lymphoma, lymph nodes of axilla and upper limb** CC
CC Excl: C81.20, C81.24, C81.28-C81.29, C81.90, C81.94, C81.98, D49.81-D49.9

C81.25 **Mixed cellularity classical Hodgkin lymphoma, lymph nodes of inguinal region and lower limb** CC
CC Excl: C81.20, C81.25, C81.28-C81.29, C81.90, C81.95, C81.98, D49.81-D49.9

C81.26 **Mixed cellularity classical Hodgkin lymphoma, intrapelvic lymph nodes** CC
CC Excl: C81.20, C81.26, C81.28-C81.29, C81.90, C81.96, C81.98, D49.81-D49.9

C81.27 **Mixed cellularity classical Hodgkin lymphoma, spleen** CC
CC Excl: C81.20, C81.27-C81.29, C81.90, C81.97-C81.98, D49.81-D49.9

C81.28 **Mixed cellularity classical Hodgkin lymphoma, lymph nodes of multiple sites** CC
CC Excl: See code: C81.20

C81.29 **Mixed cellularity classical Hodgkin lymphoma, extranodal and solid organ sites** CC
CC Excl: See code: C81.20

✓5th **C81.3** **Lymphocyte-depleted classical Hodgkin lymphoma**

C81.30 **Lymphocyte-depleted classical Hodgkin lymphoma, unspecified site** CC
CC Excl: C81.30-C81.39, C81.90, C81.98, D49.81-D49.9

C81.31 **Lymphocyte-depleted classical Hodgkin lymphoma, lymph nodes of head, face, and neck** CC
CC Excl: C81.30-C81.31, C81.38-C81.39, C81.91, C81.98, D49.81-D49.9

C81.32 **Lymphocyte-depleted classical Hodgkin lymphoma, intrathoracic lymph nodes** CC
CC Excl: C81.30, C81.32, C81.38-C81.39, C81.92, C81.98, D49.81-D49.9

C81.33 **Lymphocyte-depleted classical Hodgkin lymphoma, intra-abdominal lymph nodes** CC
CC Excl: C81.30, C81.33, C81.38-C81.39, C81.93, C81.98, D49.81-D49.9

C81.34 **Lymphocyte-depleted classical Hodgkin lymphoma, lymph nodes of axilla and upper limb** CC
CC Excl: C81.30, C81.34, C81.38-C81.39, C81.94, C81.98, D49.81-D49.9

C81.35 **Lymphocyte-depleted classical Hodgkin lymphoma, lymph nodes of inguinal region and lower limb** CC
CC Excl: C81.30, C81.35, C81.38-C81.39, C81.95, C81.98, D49.81-D49.9

C81.36 **Lymphocyte-depleted classical Hodgkin lymphoma, intrapelvic lymph nodes** CC
CC Excl: C81.30, C81.36, C81.38-C81.39, C81.96, C81.98, D49.81-D49.9

C81.37 **Lymphocyte-depleted classical Hodgkin lymphoma, spleen** CC
CC Excl: C81.30, C81.37-C81.39, C81.97-C81.98, D49.81-D49.9

C81.38 **Lymphocyte-depleted classical Hodgkin lymphoma, lymph nodes of multiple sites** CC
CC Excl: C81.30-C81.39, C81.98, D49.81-D49.9

C81.39 **Lymphocyte-depleted classical Hodgkin lymphoma, extranodal and solid organ sites** CC
CC Excl: See code: C81.38

✓5th **C81.4** **Lymphocyte-rich classical Hodgkin lymphoma**
EXCLUDES 1 *nodular lymphocyte predominant Hodgkin lymphoma (C81.0-)*

C81.40 **Lymphocyte-rich classical Hodgkin lymphoma, unspecified site** CC
CC Excl: C81.00-C81.09, C81.40-C81.49, C81.90, C81.98, D49.81-D49.9

C81.41 **Lymphocyte-rich classical Hodgkin lymphoma, lymph nodes of head, face, and neck** CC
CC Excl: C81.00-C81.01, C81.08-C81.09, C81.40-C81.41, C81.48-C81.49, C81.90-C81.91, C81.98, D49.81-D49.9

C81.42 **Lymphocyte-rich classical Hodgkin lymphoma, intrathoracic lymph nodes** CC
CC Excl: C81.00, C81.02, C81.08-C81.09, C81.40, C81.42, C81.48-C81.49, C81.90, C81.92, C81.98, D49.81-D49.9

C81.43 **Lymphocyte-rich classical Hodgkin lymphoma, intra-abdominal lymph nodes** CC
CC Excl: C81.00, C81.03, C81.08-C81.09, C81.40, C81.43, C81.48-C81.49, C81.90, C81.93, C81.98, D49.81-D49.9

C81.44 **Lymphocyte-rich classical Hodgkin lymphoma, lymph nodes of axilla and upper limb** CC
CC Excl: C81.00, C81.04, C81.08-C81.09, C81.40, C81.44, C81.48-C81.49, C81.90, C81.94, C81.98, D49.81-D49.9

C81.45 **Lymphocyte-rich classical Hodgkin lymphoma, lymph nodes of inguinal region and lower limb** CC
CC Excl: C81.00, C81.05, C81.08-C81.09, C81.40, C81.45, C81.48-C81.49, C81.90, C81.95, C81.98, D49.81-D49.9

C81.46 Lymphocyte-rich classical Hodgkin lymphoma, intrapelvic lymph nodes CC
CC Excl: C81.00, C81.06, C81.08-C81.09, C81.40, C81.46, C81.48-C81.49, C81.90, C81.96, C81.98, D49.81-D49.9

C81.47 Lymphocyte-rich classical Hodgkin lymphoma, spleen CC
CC Excl: C81.00, C81.07-C81.09, C81.40, C81.47-C81.49, C81.90, C81.97-C81.98, D49.81-D49.9

C81.48 Lymphocyte-rich classical Hodgkin lymphoma, lymph nodes of multiple sites CC
CC Excl: See code: C81.40

C81.49 Lymphocyte-rich classical Hodgkin lymphoma, extranodal and solid organ sites CC
CC Excl: See code: C81.40

✓5th **C81.7 Other classical Hodgkin lymphoma**
Classical Hodgkin lymphoma NOS

C81.70 Other classical Hodgkin lymphoma, unspecified site CC
CC Excl: C81.70-C81.90, C81.98, D49.81-D49.9

C81.71 Other classical Hodgkin lymphoma, lymph nodes of head, face, and neck CC
CC Excl: C81.70-C81.71, C81.78-C81.91, C81.98, D49.81-D49.9

C81.72 Other classical Hodgkin lymphoma, intrathoracic lymph nodes CC
CC Excl: C81.70, C81.72, C81.78-C81.90, C81.92, C81.98, D49.81-D49.9

C81.73 Other classical Hodgkin lymphoma, intra-abdominal lymph nodes CC
CC Excl: C81.70, C81.73, C81.78-C81.90, C81.93, C81.98, D49.81-D49.9

C81.74 Other classical Hodgkin lymphoma, lymph nodes of axilla and upper limb CC
CC Excl: C81.70, C81.74, C81.78-C81.90, C81.94, C81.98, D49.81-D49.9

C81.75 Other classical Hodgkin lymphoma, lymph nodes of inguinal region and lower limb CC
CC Excl: C81.70, C81.75, C81.78-C81.90, C81.95, C81.98, D49.81-D49.9

C81.76 Other classical Hodgkin lymphoma, intrapelvic lymph nodes CC
CC Excl: C81.70, C81.76, C81.78-C81.90, C81.96, C81.98, D49.81-D49.9

C81.77 Other classical Hodgkin lymphoma, spleen CC
CC Excl: C81.70, C81.77-C81.90, C81.97-C81.98, D49.81-D49.

C81.78 Other classical Hodgkin lymphoma, lymph nodes of multiple sites CC
CC Excl: See code: C81.70

C81.79 Other classical Hodgkin lymphoma, extranodal and solid organ sites CC
CC Excl: See code: C81.70

✓5th **C81.9 Hodgkin lymphoma, unspecified**

C81.90 Hodgkin lymphoma, unspecified, unspecified site CC
CC Excl: C81.90-C81.98, D49.81-D49.9

C81.91 Hodgkin lymphoma, unspecified, lymph nodes of head, face, and neck CC
CC Excl: C81.90-C81.91, C81.98, D49.81-D49.9

C81.92 Hodgkin lymphoma, unspecified, intrathoracic lymph nodes CC
CC Excl: C81.9, C81.92, C81.98, D49.81-D49.9

C81.93 Hodgkin lymphoma, unspecified, intra-abdominal lymph nodes CC
CC Excl: C81.90, C81.93, C81.98, D49.81-D49.9

C81.94 Hodgkin lymphoma, unspecified, lymph nodes of axilla and upper limb CC
CC Excl: C81.90, C81.94, C81.98, D49.81-D49.9

C81.95 Hodgkin lymphoma, unspecified, lymph nodes of inguinal region and lower limb CC
CC Excl: C81.90, C81.95, C81.98, D49.81-D49.9

C81.96 Hodgkin lymphoma, unspecified, intrapelvic lymph nodes CC
CC Excl: C81.90, C81.96, C81.98, D49.81-D49.9

C81.97 Hodgkin lymphoma, unspecified, spleen CC
CC Excl: C81.90, C81.97-C81.98, D49.81-D49.9

C81.98 Hodgkin lymphoma, unspecified, lymph nodes of multiple sites CC
CC Excl: See code: C81.90

C81.99 Hodgkin lymphoma, unspecified, extranodal and solid organ sites CC
CC Excl: No Excl

✓4th **C82 Follicular lymphoma**
INCLUDES follicular lymphoma with or without diffuse areas
EXCLUDES 1 *mature T/NK-cell lymphomas (C84.-)*
personal history of non-Hodgkin lymphoma (Z85.72)

✓5th **C82.0 Follicular lymphoma grade I**

C82.00 Follicular lymphoma grade I, unspecified site CC
CC Excl: C82.00-C82.50, C82.59-C82.69, C82.80-C82.99, C83.10, C83.19, C84.40, C84.49, C84.60, C84.69-C84.70, C84.79-C84.90, C84.99-C84.A0, C84.A9-C84.Z0, C84.Z9, C85.10, C85.19-C85.20, C85.29, C85.80, C85.89-C85.90, C85.99, C86.4, C88.4, C96.4, C96.9, C96.Z, D49.81-D49.9

C82.01 Follicular lymphoma grade I, lymph nodes of head, face, and neck CC
CC Excl: C82.00-C82.01, C82.08-C82.11, C82.18-C82.21, C82.28-C82.31, C82.38-C82.41, C82.48-C82.49, C82.51, C82.60-C82.61, C82.68-C82.69, C82.80-C82.81, C82.88-C82.91, C82.98-C82.99, C83.11, C84.41, C84.61, C84.71, C84.91, C84.A1, C84.Z1, C85.11, C85.21, C85.81, C85.91, C86.0, D49.81-D49.9

C82.02 Follicular lymphoma grade I, intrathoracic lymph nodes CC
CC Excl: C82.00, C82.02, C82.08-C82.10, C82.12, C82.18-C82.20, C82.22, C82.28-C82.30, C82.32, C82.38-C82.40, C82.42 C82.48-C82.49, C82.52, C82.60, C82.62, C82.68-C82.69, C82.80, C82.82, C82.88-C82.90, C82.92, C82.98-C82.99, C83.12, C84.42, C84.62, C84.72 C84.92, C84.A2, C84.Z2, C85.12, C85.22, C85.82, C85.92, D49.81-D49.9

C82.03 Follicular lymphoma grade I, intra-abdominal lymph nodes CC
CC Excl: C82.00, C82.03, C82.08-C82.10, C82.13, C82.18-C82.20, C82.23, C82.28-C82.30, C82.33, C82.38-C82.40, C82.43 C82.48-C82.49, C82.53, C82.60, C82.63, C82.68-C82.69, C82.80, C82.83, C82.88-C82.90, C82.93, C82.98-C82.99, C83.13, C84.43, C84.63, C84.73 C84.93, C84.A3, C84.Z3, C85.13, C85.23, C85.83, C85.93, C86.2-C86.3, D49.81-D49.9

C82.04 Follicular lymphoma grade I, lymph nodes of axilla and upper limb CC
CC Excl: C82.00, C82.04, C82.08-C82.10, C82.14, C82.18-C82.20, C82.24, C82.28-C82.30, C82.34, C82.38-C82.40, C82.44 C82.48-C82.49, C82.54, C82.60, C82.64, C82.68-C82.69, C82.80, C82.84, C82.88-C82.90, C82.94, C82.98-C82.99, C83.14, C84.44, C84.64, C84.74 C84.94, C84.A4, C84.Z4, C85.14, C85.24, C85.84, C85.94, D49.81-D49.9

C82.05 Follicular lymphoma grade I, lymph nodes of inguinal region and lower limb CC
CC Excl: C82.00, C82.05, C82.08-C82.10, C82.15, C82.18-C82.20, C82.25, C82.28-C82.30, C82.35, C82.38-C82.40, C82.45 C82.48-C82.49, C82.55, C82.60, C82.65, C82.68-C82.69, C82.80, C82.85, C82.88-C82.90, C82.95, C82.98-C82.99, C83.15, C84.45, C84.65, C84.75 C84.95, C84.A5, C84.Z5, C85.15, C85.25, C85.85, C85.95, D49.81-D49.9

C82.06 Follicular lymphoma grade I, intrapelvic lymph nodes CC
CC Excl: C82.00, C82.06, C82.08-C82.10, C82.16, C82.18-C82.20, C82.26, C82.28-C82.30, C82.36, C82.38-C82.40, C82.46 C82.48-C82.49, C82.56, C82.60, C82.66, C82.68-C82.69, C82.80, C82.86, C82.88-C82.90, C82.96, C82.98-C82.99, C83.16, C84.46, C84.66, C84.76 C84.96, C84.A6, C84.Z6, C85.16, C85.26, C85.86, C85.96, D49.81-D49.9

C82.07 Follicular lymphoma grade I, spleen CC
CC Excl: C82.00, C82.07-C82.10, C82.17-C82.20, C82.27-C82.30, C82.37-C82.40, C82.47-C82.49, C82.57, C82.60, C82.67-C82.80, C82.87-C82.90, C82.97-C82.99, C83.17, C84.47, C84.67, C84.77, C84.A7, C84.Z7, C84.97, C85.17, C85.27, C85.87, C85.97, C86.1, D49.81-D49.9

C82.08 Follicular lymphoma grade I, lymph nodes of multiple sites CC
CC Excl: C82.00-C82.49, C82.58, C82.60-C82.69, C82.80-C82.99, C83.18, C84.48, C84.68, C84.78, C84.98, C84.A8, C84.Z8, C85.18 C85.28, C85.88, C85.98, D49.81-D49.9

C82.09 Follicular lymphoma grade I, extranodal and solid organ sites CC
CC Excl: C82.00-C82.50, C82.59-C82.99, C83.10, C83.19, C84.40, C84.49-C84.60, C84.69-C84.70, C84.79-C84.A0, C84.A9-C84.Z0, C84.Z9-C84.90, C84.99-C85.10, C85.19-C85.20, C85.29-C85.80, C85.89-C85.90, C85.99, C86.4, C88.4, C96.4, C96.Z-C96.9, D49.81-D49.9

✓5th **C82.1 Follicular lymphoma grade II**

C82.10 Follicular lymphoma grade II, unspecified site CC
CC Excl: See code: C82.00

C82.11 Follicular lymphoma grade II, lymph nodes of head, face, and neck CC
CC Excl: See code: C82.01

Neoplasms C81.46–C82.11

C82.12 **Follicular lymphoma grade II, intrathoracic lymph nodes** CC
CC Excl: See code: C82.02

C82.13 **Follicular lymphoma grade II, intra-abdominal lymph nodes** CC
CC Excl: See code: C82.03

C82.14 **Follicular lymphoma grade II, lymph nodes of axilla and upper limb** CC
CC Excl: See code: C82.04

C82.15 **Follicular lymphoma grade II, lymph nodes of inguinal region and lower limb** CC
CC Excl: See code: C82.05

C82.16 **Follicular lymphoma grade II, intrapelvic lymph nodes** CC
CC Excl: See code: C82.06

C82.17 **Follicular lymphoma grade II, spleen** CC
CC Excl: See code: C82.07

C82.18 **Follicular lymphoma grade II, lymph nodes of multiple sites** CC
CC Excl: See code: C82.08

C82.19 **Follicular lymphoma grade II, extranodal and solid organ sites** CC
CC Excl: See code: C82.00

✓5th **C82.2** **Follicular lymphoma grade III, unspecified**

C82.20 **Follicular lymphoma grade III, unspecified, unspecified site** CC
CC Excl: See code: C82.00

C82.21 **Follicular lymphoma grade III, unspecified, lymph nodes of head, face, and neck** CC
CC Excl: See code: C82.01

C82.22 **Follicular lymphoma grade III, unspecified, intrathoracic lymph nodes** CC
CC Excl: See code: C82.02

C82.23 **Follicular lymphoma grade III, unspecified, intra-abdominal lymph nodes** CC
CC Excl: See code: C82.03

C82.24 **Follicular lymphoma grade III, unspecified, lymph nodes of axilla and upper limb** CC
CC Excl: See code: C82.04

C82.25 **Follicular lymphoma grade III, unspecified, lymph nodes of inguinal region and lower limb** CC
CC Excl: See code: C82.05

C82.26 **Follicular lymphoma grade III, unspecified, intrapelvic lymph nodes** CC
CC Excl: See code: C82.06

C82.27 **Follicular lymphoma grade III, unspecified, spleen** CC
CC Excl: See code: C82.07

C82.28 **Follicular lymphoma grade III, unspecified, lymph nodes of multiple sites** CC
CC Excl: See code: C82.08

C82.29 **Follicular lymphoma grade III, unspecified, extranodal and solid organ sites** CC
CC Excl: See code: C82.00

✓5th **C82.3** **Follicular lymphoma grade IIIa**

C82.30 **Follicular lymphoma grade IIIa, unspecified sitespleen** CC
CC Excl: See code: C82.00

C82.31 **Follicular lymphoma grade IIIa, lymph nodes of head, face, and neck** CC
CC Excl: See code: C82.01

C82.32 **Follicular lymphoma grade IIIa, intrathoracic lymph nodes** CC
CC Excl: See code: C82.02

C82.33 **Follicular lymphoma grade IIIa, intra-abdominal lymph nodes** CC
CC Excl: See code: C82.03

C82.34 **Follicular lymphoma grade IIIa, lymph nodes of axilla and upper limb** CC
CC Excl: See code: C82.04

C82.35 **Follicular lymphoma grade IIIa, lymph nodes of inguinal region and lower limb** CC
CC Excl: See code: C82.05

C82.36 **Follicular lymphoma grade IIIa, intrapelvic lymph nodes** CC
CC Excl: See code: C82.06

C82.37 **Follicular lymphoma grade IIIa, spleen** CC
CC Excl: See code: C82.07

C82.38 **Follicular lymphoma grade IIIa, lymph nodes of multiple sites** CC
CC Excl: See code: C82.08

C82.39 **Follicular lymphoma grade IIIa, extranodal and solid organ sites** CC
CC Excl: See code: C82.00

✓5th **C82.4** **Follicular lymphoma grade IIIb**

C82.40 **Follicular lymphoma grade IIIb, unspecified site** CC
CC Excl: See code: C82.00

C82.41 **Follicular lymphoma grade IIIb, lymph nodes of head, face, and neck** CC
CC Excl: See code: C82.01

C82.42 **Follicular lymphoma grade IIIb, intrathoracic lymph nodes** CC
CC Excl: See code: C82.02

C82.43 **Follicular lymphoma grade IIIb, intra-abdominal lymph nodes** CC
CC Excl: See code: C82.03

C82.44 **Follicular lymphoma grade IIIb, lymph nodes of axilla and upper limb** CC
CC Excl: See code: C82.04

C82.45 **Follicular lymphoma grade IIIb, lymph nodes of inguinal region and lower limb** CC
CC Excl: See code: C82.05

C82.46 **Follicular lymphoma grade IIIb, intrapelvic lymph nodes** CC
CC Excl: See code: C82.06

C82.47 **Follicular lymphoma grade IIIb, spleen** CC
CC Excl: See code: C82.07

C82.48 **Follicular lymphoma grade IIIb, lymph nodes of multiple sites** CC
CC Excl: See code: C82.08

C82.49 **Follicular lymphoma grade IIIb, extranodal and solid organ sites** CC
CC Excl: See code: C82.00

✓5th **C82.5** **Diffuse follicle center lymphoma**

C82.50 **Diffuse follicle center lymphoma, unspecified site** HIV CC
CC Excl: C82.50-C82.59, C83.10-C83.19, C84.40-C84.49, C84.60-C84.Z9, C85.10-C85.29, C85.80-C86.4, C88.4, C96.4, C96.9, C96.Z, D49.81-D49.9

C82.51 **Diffuse follicle center lymphoma, lymph nodes of head, face, and neck** HIV CC
CC Excl: C82.50-C82.51, C82.58-C82.59, C83.10-C83.11, C83.18-C83.19, C84.40-C84.41, C84.48-C84.49, C84.60-C84.61, C84.68-C84.71, C84.78-C84.91, C84.98-C84.A1, C84.A8-C84.Z1, C84.Z8-C84.Z9, C85.10-C85.11, C85.18-C85.21, C85.28-C85.29, C85.80-C85.81 C85.88-C85.91, C85.98-C86.0, C86.4, C88.4, D49.81-D49.9

C82.52 **Diffuse follicle center lymphoma, intrathoracic lymph nodes** HIV CC
CC Excl: C82.50-C82.52, C82.58-C82.59, C83.10, C83.12, C83.18-C83.19, C84.40, C84.42, C84.48-C84.49, C84.60, C84.62, C84.68-C84.70, C84.72, C84.78-C84.90, C84.92, C84.98-C84.A0, C84.A2, C84.A8-C84.Z0, C84.Z2, C84.Z8-C84.Z9, C85.10, C85.12, C85.18-C85.20, C85.22 C85.28-C85.29, C85.80, C85.82, C85.88-C85.90, C85.92, C85.98-C85.99, C86.4, C88.4, D49.81-D49.9

C82.53 **Diffuse follicle center lymphoma, intra-abdominal lymph nodes** HIV CC
CC Excl: C82.50-C82.53, C82.58-C82.59, C83.10, C83.13, C83.18-C83.19, C84.40, C84.43, C84.48-C84.49, C84.60, C84.63, C84.68-C84.70, C84.73, C84.78-C84.90, C84.93, C84.98-C84.A0, C84.A3, C84.A8-C84.Z0, C84.Z3, C84.Z8-C84.Z9, C85.10, C85.13, C85.18-C85.20, C85.23 C85.28-C85.29, C85.80, C85.83, C85.88-C85.90, C85.93, C85.98-C85.99, C86.2-C86.4, C88.4, D49.81-D49.9

C82.54 **Diffuse follicle center lymphoma, lymph nodes of axilla and upper limb** HIV CC
CC Excl: C82.50-C82.54, C82.58-C82.59, C83.10, C83.14, C83.18-C83.19, C84.40, C84.44, C84.48-C84.49, C84.60, C84.64, C84.68-C84.70, C84.74, C84.78-C84.90, C84.94, C84.98-C84.A0, C84.A4, C84.A8-C84.Z0, C84.Z4, C84.Z8-C84.Z9, C85.10, C85.14, C85.18-C85.20, C85.24 C85.28-C85.29, C85.80, C85.84, C85.88-C85.90, C85.94, C85.98-C85.99, C86.4, C88.4, D49.81-D49.9

C82.55 **Diffuse follicle center lymphoma, lymph nodes of inguinal region and lower limb** HIV CC
CC Excl: C82.50-C82.55, C82.58-C82.59, C83.10, C83.15, C83.18-C83.19, C84.40, C84.45, C84.48-C84.49, C84.60, C84.65, C84.68-C84.70, C84.75, C84.78-C84.90, C84.95, C84.98-C84.A0, C84.A5, C84.A8-C84.Z0, C84.Z5, C84.Z8-C84.Z9, C85.10, C85.15, C85.18-C85.20, C85.25 C85.28-C85.29, C85.80, C85.85, C85.88-C85.90, C85.95, C85.98-C85.99, C86.4, C88.4, D49.81-D49.9

C82.56 Diffuse follicle center lymphoma, intrapelvic lymph nodes HIV CC
CC Excl: C82.50-C82.56, C82.58-C82.59, C83.10, C83.16, C83.18-C83.19, C84.40, C84.46, C84.48-C84.49, C84.60, C84.66, C84.68-C84.70, C84.76, C84.78-C84.90, C84.96, C84.98-C84.A0, C84.A6, C84.A8-C84.Z0, C84.Z6, C84.Z8-C84.Z9, C85.10, C85.16, C85.18-C85.20, C85.26 C85.28-C85.29, C85.80, C85.86, C85.88-C85.90, C85.96, C85.98-C85.99, C86.4, C88.4, D49.81-D49.9

C82.57 Diffuse follicle center lymphoma, spleen HIV CC
CC Excl: C82.50, C82.57-C82.59, C83.10, C83.17-C83.19, C84.40, C84.47-C84.60, C84.67-C84.70, C84.77-C84.A0, C84.A7-C84.Z0, C84.Z7-C84.90, C84.97-C85.10, C85.17-C85.20, C85.27-C85.80, C85.87-C85.90, C85.97-C85.99, C86.1, C86.4, C88.4, D49.81-D49.9

C82.58 Diffuse follicle center lymphoma, lymph nodes of multiple sites HIV CC
CC Excl: C82.50-C82.59, C83.10-C83.19, C84.40-C84.49, C84.60-C84.Z9, C85.10-C85.29, C85.80-C86.4, C88.4, D49.81-D49.9

C82.59 Diffuse follicle center lymphoma, extranodal and solid organ sites HIV CC
CC Excl: See code: C82.50

✓5th **C82.6 Cutaneous follicle center lymphoma**

C82.60 Cutaneous follicle center lymphoma, unspecified site CC
CC Excl: See code: C82.00

C82.61 Cutaneous follicle center lymphoma, lymph nodes of head, face, and neck CC
CC Excl: See code: C82.01

C82.62 Cutaneous follicle center lymphoma, intrathoracic lymph nodes CC
CC Excl: See code: C82.02

C82.63 Cutaneous follicle center lymphoma, intra-abdominal lymph nodes CC
CC Excl: See code: C82.03

C82.64 Cutaneous follicle center lymphoma, lymph nodes of axilla and upper limb CC
CC Excl: See code: C82.04

C82.65 Cutaneous follicle center lymphoma, lymph nodes of inguinal region and lower limb CC
CC Excl: See code: C82.05

C82.66 Cutaneous follicle center lymphoma, intrapelvic lymph nodes CC
CC Excl: See code: C82.06

C82.67 Cutaneous follicle center lymphoma, spleen CC
CC Excl: See code: C82.07

C82.68 Cutaneous follicle center lymphoma, lymph nodes of multiple sites CC
CC Excl: See code: C82.08

C82.69 Cutaneous follicle center lymphoma, extranodal and solid organ sites CC
CC Excl: See code: C82.00

✓5th **C82.8 Other types of follicular lymphoma**

C82.80 Other types of follicular lymphoma, unspecified site CC
CC Excl: See code: C82.00

C82.81 Other types of follicular lymphoma, lymph nodes of head, face, and neck CC
CC Excl: See code: C82.01

C82.82 Other types of follicular lymphoma, intrathoracic lymph nodes CC
CC Excl: See code: C82.02

C82.83 Other types of follicular lymphoma, intra-abdominal lymph nodes CC
CC Excl: See code: C82.03

C82.84 Other types of follicular lymphoma, lymph nodes of axilla and upper limb CC
CC Excl: See code: C82.04

C82.85 Other types of follicular lymphoma, lymph nodes of inguinal region and lower limb CC
CC Excl: See code: C82.05

C82.86 Other types of follicular lymphoma, intrapelvic lymph nodes CC
CC Excl: See code: C82.06

C82.87 Other types of follicular lymphoma, spleen CC
CC Excl: See code: C82.07

C82.88 Other types of follicular lymphoma, lymph nodes of multiple sites CC
CC Excl: See code: C82.08

C82.89 Other types of follicular lymphoma, extranodal and solid organ sites CC
CC Excl: See code: C82.00

✓5th **C82.9 Follicular lymphoma, unspecified**

C82.90 Follicular lymphoma, unspecified, unspecified site CC
CC Excl: See code: C82.00

C82.91 Follicular lymphoma, unspecified, lymph nodes of head, face, and neck CC
CC Excl: See code: C82.01

C82.92 Follicular lymphoma, unspecified, intrathoracic lymph nodes CC
CC Excl: See code: C82.02

C82.93 Follicular lymphoma, unspecified, intra-abdominal lymph nodes CC
CC Excl: See code: C82.03

C82.94 Follicular lymphoma, unspecified, lymph nodes of axilla and upper limb CC
CC Excl: See code: C82.04

C82.95 Follicular lymphoma, unspecified, lymph nodes of inguinal region and lower limb CC
CC Excl: See code: C82.05

C82.96 Follicular lymphoma, unspecified, intrapelvic lymph nodes CC
CC Excl: See code: C82.06

C82.97 Follicular lymphoma, unspecified, spleen CC
CC Excl: See code: C82.07

C82.98 Follicular lymphoma, unspecified, lymph nodes of multiple sites CC
CC Excl: See code: C82.08

C82.99 Follicular lymphoma, unspecified, extranodal and solid organ sites CC
CC Excl: See code: C82.00

✓4th **C83 Non-follicular lymphoma**

EXCLUDES 1 *personal history of non-Hodgkin lymphoma (Z85.72)*

✓5th **C83.0 Small cell B-cell lymphoma**

Lymphoplasmacytic lymphoma
Nodal marginal zone lymphoma
Non-leukemic variant of B-CLL
Splenic marginal zone lymphoma

EXCLUDES 1 *chronic lymphocytic leukemia (C91.1)*
mature T/NK-cell lymphomas (C84.-)
Waldenström macroglobulinemia (C88.0)

C83.00 Small cell B-cell lymphoma, unspecified site HIV CC
CC Excl: C83.00-C83.09, C83.80-C83.99, C86.5-C86.6, D49.81-D49.9

C83.01 Small cell B-cell lymphoma, lymph nodes of head, face, and neck HIV CC
CC Excl: C83.00-C83.01, C83.08-C83.09, C83.80-C83.81, C83.88-C83.91, C83.98-C83.99, C86.5-C86.6, D49.81-D49.9

C83.02 Small cell B-cell lymphoma, intrathoracic lymph nodes HIV CC
CC Excl: C83.00-C83.02, C83.08-C83.09, C83.80, C83.82, C83.88-C83.90, C83.92, C83.98-C83.99, C86.5-C86.6, D49.81-D49.9

C83.03 Small cell B-cell lymphoma, intra-abdominal lymph nodes HIV CC
CC Excl: C83.00-C83.03, C83.08-C83.09, C83.80, C83.83, C83.88-C83.90, C83.93, C83.98-C83.99, C86.5-C86.6, D49.81-D49.9

C83.04 Small cell B-cell lymphoma, lymph nodes of axilla and upper limb HIV CC
CC Excl: C83.00-C83.04, C83.08-C83.09, C83.80, C83.84, C83.88-C83.90, C83.94, C83.98-C83.99, C86.5-C86.6, D49.81-D49.9

C83.05 Small cell B-cell lymphoma, lymph nodes of inguinal region and lower limb HIV CC
CC Excl: C83.00-C83.05, C83.08-C83.09, C83.80, C83.85, C83.88-C83.90, C83.95, C83.98-C83.99, C86.5-C86.6, D49.81-D49.9

C83.06 Small cell B-cell lymphoma, intrapelvic lymph nodes HIV CC
CC Excl: C83.00-C83.06, C83.08-C83.09, C83.80, C83.86, C83.88-C83.90, C83.96, C83.98-C83.99, C86.5-C86.6, D49.81-D49.9

C83.07 Small cell B-cell lymphoma, spleen HIV CC
CC Excl: C83.00, C83.07-C83.09, C83.80, C83.87-C83.90, C83.97-C83.99, C86.5-C86.6, D49.81-D49.9

C83.08 Small cell B-cell lymphoma, lymph nodes of multiple sites HIV CC
CC Excl: C83.00-C83.09, C83.80-C83.99, C86.5-C86.6, D49.81-D49.9

C83.09 Small cell B-cell lymphoma, extranodal and solid organ sites HIV CC
CC Excl: See code: C83.00

C83.1 Mantle cell lymphoma
Centrocytic lymphoma
Malignant lymphomatous polyposis

C83.10 Mantle cell lymphoma, unspecified site HIV CC
CC Excl: See code: C82.50

C83.11 Mantle cell lymphoma, lymph nodes of head, face, and neck HIV CC
CC Excl: See code: C82.51

C83.12 Mantle cell lymphoma, intrathoracic lymph nodes HIV CC
CC Excl: See code: C82.52

C83.13 Mantle cell lymphoma, intra-abdominal lymph nodes HIV CC
CC Excl: See code: C82.53

C83.14 Mantle cell lymphoma, lymph nodes of axilla and upper limb HIV CC
CC Excl: See code: C82.54

C83.15 Mantle cell lymphoma, lymph nodes of inguinal region and lower limb HIV CC
CC Excl: See code: C82.55

C83.16 Mantle cell lymphoma, intrapelvic lymph nodes HIV CC
CC Excl: See code: C82.56

C83.17 Mantle cell lymphoma, spleen HIV CC
CC Excl: See code: C82.57

C83.18 Mantle cell lymphoma, lymph nodes of multiple sites HIV CC
CC Excl: See code: C82.58

C83.19 Mantle cell lymphoma, extranodal and solid organ sites HIV CC
CC Excl: See code: C82.50

C83.3 Diffuse large B-cell lymphoma
Anaplastic diffuse large B-cell lymphoma
CD30-positive diffuse large B-cell lymphoma
Centroblastic diffuse large B-cell lymphoma
Diffuse large B-cell lymphoma, subtype not specified
Immunoblastic diffuse large B-cell lymphoma
Plasmablastic diffuse large B-cell lymphoma
T-cell rich diffuse large B-cell lymphoma

EXCLUDES 1 *mature T/NK-cell lymphomas (C84.-)*
mediastinal (thymic) large B-cell lymphoma (C85.2-)

C83.30 Diffuse large B-cell lymphoma, unspecified site HIV CC
CC Excl: C83.30-C83.39, D49.81-D49.9

C83.31 Diffuse large B-cell lymphoma, lymph nodes of head, face, and neck HIV CC
CC Excl: C83.30-C83.31, C83.38-C83.39, D49.81-D49.9

C83.32 Diffuse large B-cell lymphoma, intrathoracic lymph nodes HIV CC
CC Excl: C83.30-C83.32, C83.38-C83.39, D49.81-D49.9

C83.33 Diffuse large B-cell lymphoma, intra-abdominal lymph nodes HIV CC
CC Excl: C83.30-C83.33, C83.38-C83.39, D49.81-D49.9

C83.34 Diffuse large B-cell lymphoma, lymph nodes of axilla and upper limb HIV CC
CC Excl: C83.30-C83.34, C83.38-C83.39, D49.81-D49.9

C83.35 Diffuse large B-cell lymphoma, lymph nodes of inguinal region and lower limb HIV CC
CC Excl: C83.30-C83.35, C83.38-C83.39, D49.81-D49.9

C83.36 Diffuse large B-cell lymphoma, intrapelvic lymph nodes HIV CC
CC Excl: C83.30-C83.36, C83.38-C83.39, D49.81-D49.9

C83.37 Diffuse large B-cell lymphoma, spleen HIV CC
CC Excl: C83.30, C83.37-C83.39, D49.81-D49.9

C83.38 Diffuse large B-cell lymphoma, lymph nodes of multiple sites HIV CC
CC Excl: C83.30-C83.39, D49.81-D49.9

C83.39 Diffuse large B-cell lymphoma, extranodal and solid organ sites HIV CC
CC Excl: See code: C83.38

C83.5 Lymphoblastic (diffuse) lymphoma
B-precursor lymphoma
Lymphoblastic B-cell lymphoma
Lymphoblastic lymphoma NOS
Lymphoblastic T-cell lymphoma
T-precursor lymphoma

C83.50 Lymphoblastic (diffuse) lymphoma, unspecified site CC
CC Excl: C83.50-C83.59, D49.81-D49.9

C83.51 Lymphoblastic (diffuse) lymphoma, lymph nodes of head, face, and neck CC
CC Excl: C83.50-C83.51, C83.58-C83.59, D49.81-D49.9

C83.52 Lymphoblastic (diffuse) lymphoma, intrathoracic lymph nodes CC
CC Excl: C83.50, C83.52, C83.58-C83.59, D49.81-D49.9

C83.53 Lymphoblastic (diffuse) lymphoma, intra-abdominal lymph nodes CC
CC Excl: C83.50, C83.53, C83.58-C83.59, D49.81-D49.9

C83.54 Lymphoblastic (diffuse) lymphoma, lymph nodes of axilla and upper limb CC
CC Excl: C83.50, C83.54, C83.58-C83.59, D49.81-D49.9

C83.55 Lymphoblastic (diffuse) lymphoma, lymph nodes of inguinal region and lower limb CC
CC Excl: C83.50, C83.55, C83.58-C83.59, D49.81-D49.9

C83.56 Lymphoblastic (diffuse) lymphoma, intrapelvic lymph nodes CC
CC Excl: C83.50, C83.56, C83.58-C83.59, D49.81-D49.9

C83.57 Lymphoblastic (diffuse) lymphoma, spleen CC
CC Excl: C83.50, C83.57-C83.59, D49.81-D49.9

C83.58 Lymphoblastic (diffuse) lymphoma, lymph nodes of multiple sites CC
CC Excl: See code: C83.50

C83.59 Lymphoblastic (diffuse) lymphoma, extranodal and solid organ sites CC
CC Excl: See code: C83.50

C83.7 Burkitt lymphoma
Atypical Burkitt lymphoma
Burkitt-like lymphoma

EXCLUDES 1 *mature B-cell leukemia Burkitt type (C91.A-)*

C83.70 Burkitt lymphoma, unspecified site HIV CC
CC Excl: C83.70-C83.79, D49.81-D49.9

C83.71 Burkitt lymphoma, lymph nodes of head, face, and neck HIV CC
CC Excl: C83.70-C83.71, C83.78-C83.79, D49.81-D49.9

C83.72 Burkitt lymphoma, intrathoracic lymph nodes HIV CC
CC Excl: C83.70, C83.72, C83.78-C83.79, D49.81-D49.9

C83.73 Burkitt lymphoma, intra-abdominal lymph nodes HIV CC
CC Excl: C83.70, C83.73, C83.78-C83.79, D49.81-D49.9

C83.74 Burkitt lymphoma, lymph nodes of axilla and upper limb HIV CC
CC Excl: C83.70, C83.74, C83.78-C83.79, D49.81-D49.9

C83.75 Burkitt lymphoma, lymph nodes of inguinal region and lower limb HIV CC
CC Excl: C83.70, C83.75, C83.78-C83.79, D49.81-D49.9

C83.76 Burkitt lymphoma, intrapelvic lymph nodes HIV CC
CC Excl: C83.70, C83.76, C83.78-C83.79, D49.81-D49.9

C83.77 Burkitt lymphoma, spleen HIV CC
CC Excl: C83.70, C83.77-C83.79, D49.81-D49.9

C83.78 Burkitt lymphoma, lymph nodes of multiple sites HIV CC
CC Excl: See code: C83.70

C83.79 Burkitt lymphoma, extranodal and solid organ sites HIV CC
CC Excl: See code: C83.70

C83.8 Other non-follicular lymphoma
Intravascular large B-cell lymphoma
Lymphoid granulomatosis
Primary effusion B-cell lymphoma

EXCLUDES 1 *mediastinal (thymic) large B-cell lymphoma (C85.2-)*
T-cell rich B-cell lymphoma (C83.3-)

C83.80 Other non-follicular lymphoma, unspecified site HIV CC
CC Excl: See code: C83.00

C83.81 Other non-follicular lymphoma, lymph nodes of head, face, and neck HIV CC
CC Excl: See code: C83.01

C83.82 Other non-follicular lymphoma, intrathoracic lymph nodes HIV CC
CC Excl: See code: C83.02

C83.83 Other non-follicular lymphoma, intra-abdominal lymph nodes HIV CC
CC Excl: See code: C83.03

C83.84 Other non-follicular lymphoma, lymph nodes of axilla and upper limb HIV CC
CC Excl: See code: C83.04

C83.85 Other non-follicular lymphoma, lymph nodes of inguinal region and lower limb HIV CC
CC Excl: See code: C83.05

C83.86 Other non-follicular lymphoma, intrapelvic lymph nodes HIV CC
CC Excl: See code: C83.Ø6

C83.87 Other non-follicular lymphoma, spleen HIV CC
CC Excl: See code: C83.Ø7

C83.88 Other non-follicular lymphoma, lymph nodes of multiple sites HIV CC
CC Excl: See code: C83.ØØ

C83.89 Other non-follicular lymphoma, extranodal and solid organ sites HIV CC
CC Excl: See code: C83.ØØ

✓5th **C83.9 Non-follicular (diffuse) lymphoma, unspecified**

C83.9Ø Non-follicular (diffuse) lymphoma, unspecified, unspecified site HIV CC
CC Excl: See code: C83.ØØ

C83.91 Non-follicular (diffuse) lymphoma, unspecified, lymph nodes of head, face, and neck HIV CC
CC Excl: See code: C83.Ø1

C83.92 Non-follicular (diffuse) lymphoma, unspecified, intrathoracic lymph nodes HIV CC
CC Excl: See code: C83.Ø2

C83.93 Non-follicular (diffuse) lymphoma, unspecified, intra-abdominal lymph nodes HIV CC
CC Excl: See code: C83.Ø3

C83.94 Non-follicular (diffuse) lymphoma, unspecified, lymph nodes of axilla and upper limb HIV CC
CC Excl: See code: C83.Ø4

C83.95 Non-follicular (diffuse) lymphoma, unspecified, lymph nodes of inguinal region and lower limb HIV CC
CC Excl: See code: C83.Ø5

C83.96 Non-follicular (diffuse) lymphoma, unspecified, intrapelvic lymph nodes HIV CC
CC Excl: See code: C83.Ø6

C83.97 Non-follicular (diffuse) lymphoma, unspecified, spleen HIV CC
CC Excl: See code: C83.Ø7

C83.98 Non-follicular (diffuse) lymphoma, unspecified, lymph nodes of multiple sites HIV CC
CC Excl: See code: C83.ØØ

C83.99 Non-follicular (diffuse) lymphoma, unspecified, extranodal and solid organ sites HIV CC
CC Excl: See code: C83.ØØ

✓4th **C84 Mature T/NK-cell lymphomas**
EXCLUDES 1 *personal history of non-Hodgkin lymphoma (Z85.72)*

✓5th **C84.Ø Mycosis fungoides**
EXCLUDES 1 *peripheral T-cell lymphoma, not classified (C84.4-)*

C84.ØØ Mycosis fungoides, unspecified site CC
CC Excl: C82.5Ø, C82.59, C83.1Ø, C83.19, C84.ØØ-C84.Ø9, C84.4Ø, C84.49, C84.6Ø, C84.69-C84.7Ø, C84.79-C84.9Ø, C84.99-C84.AØ, C84.A9-C84.ZØ, C84.Z9, C85.1Ø, C85.19-C85.2Ø, C85.29, C85.8Ø, C85.89-C85.9Ø, C85.99, C86.4, C88.4, C96.4, C96.9, C96.Z, D49.81-D49.9

C84.Ø1 Mycosis fungoides, lymph nodes of head, face, and neck CC
CC Excl: C82.51, C83.11, C84.ØØ-C84.Ø1, C84.Ø8-C84.Ø9, C84.41, C84.61, C84.71, C84.91, C84.A1, C84.Z1, C85.11, C85.21, C85.81, C85.91, C86.Ø, D49.81-D49.9

C84.Ø2 Mycosis fungoides, intrathoracic lymph nodes CC
CC Excl: C82.52, C83.12, C84.ØØ, C84.Ø2, C84.Ø8-C84.Ø9, C84.42, C84.62, C84.72, C84.92, C84.A2, C84.Z2, C85.12, C85.22, C85.82, C85.92, D49.81-D49.9

C84.Ø3 Mycosis fungoides, intra-abdominal lymph nodes CC
CC Excl: C82.53, C83.13, C84.ØØ, C84.Ø3, C84.Ø8-C84.Ø9, C84.43, C84.63, C84.73, C84.93, C84.A3, C84.Z3, C85.13, C85.23, C85.83, C85.93, C86.2-C86.3, D49.81-D49.9

C84.Ø4 Mycosis fungoides, lymph nodes of axilla and upper limb CC
CC Excl: C82.54, C83.14, C84.ØØ, C84.Ø4, C84.Ø8-C84.Ø9, C84.44, C84.64, C84.74, C84.94, C84.A4, C84.Z4, C85.14, C85.24, C85.84, C85.94, D49.81-D49.9

C84.Ø5 Mycosis fungoides, lymph nodes of inguinal region and lower limb CC
CC Excl: C82.55, C83.15, C84.ØØ, C84.Ø5, C84.Ø8-C84.Ø9, C84.45, C84.65, C84.75, C84.95, C84.A5, C84.Z5, C85.15, C85.25, C85.85, C85.95, D49.81-D49.9

C84.Ø6 Mycosis fungoides, intrapelvic lymph nodes CC
CC Excl: C82.56, C83.16, C84.ØØ, C84.Ø6, C84.Ø8-C84.Ø9, C84.46, C84.66, C84.76, C84.96, C84.A6, C84.Z6, C85.16, C85.26, C85.86, C85.96, D49.81-D49.9

C84.Ø7 Mycosis fungoides, spleen CC
CC Excl: C82.57, C83.17, C84.ØØ, C84.Ø7-C84.Ø9, C84.47, C84.67, C84.77, C84.97, C84.A7, C84.Z7, C85.17, C85.27, C85.87, C85.97, C86.1, D49.81-D49.9

C84.Ø8 Mycosis fungoides, lymph nodes of multiple sites CC
CC Excl: C82.58, C83.18, C84.ØØ-C84.Ø9, C84.48, C84.68, C84.78, C84.98, C84.A8, C84.Z8, C85.18, C85.28, C85.88, C85.98, D49.81-D49.9

C84.Ø9 Mycosis fungoides, extranodal and solid organ sites CC
CC Excl: See code: C84.ØØ

✓5th **C84.1 Sézary disease**

C84.1Ø Sézary disease, unspecified site CC
CC Excl: C82.5Ø, C82.59, C83.1Ø, C83.19, C84.1Ø-C84.19, C84.4Ø, C84.49, C84.6Ø, C84.69-C84.7Ø, C84.79-C84.9Ø, C84.99-C84.AØ, C84.A9-C84.ZØ, C84.Z9, C85.1Ø, C85.19-C85.2Ø, C85.29, C85.8Ø, C85.89-C85.9Ø, C85.99, C86.4, C88.4, C96.4, C96.9, C96.Z, D49.81-D49.9

C84.11 Sézary disease, lymph nodes of head, face, and neck CC
CC Excl: C82.51, C83.11, C84.1Ø-C84.11, C84.18-C84.19, C84.41, C84.61, C84.71, C84.91, C84.A1, C84.Z1, C85.11, C85.21, C85.81, C85.91, C86.Ø, D49.81-D49.9

C84.12 Sézary disease, intrathoracic lymph nodes CC
CC Excl: C82.52, C83.12, C84.1Ø, C84.12, C84.18-C84.19, C84.42, C84.62, C84.72, C84.92, C84.A2, C84.Z2, C85.12, C85.22, C85.82, C85.92, D49.81-D49.9

C84.13 Sézary disease, intra-abdominal lymph nodes CC
CC Excl: C82.53, C83.13, C84.1Ø, C84.13, C84.18-C84.19, C84.43, C84.63, C84.73, C84.93, C84.A3, C84.Z3, C85.13, C85.23, C85.83, C85.93, C86.2-C86.3, D49.81-D49.9

C84.14 Sézary disease, lymph nodes of axilla and upper limb CC
CC Excl: C82.54, C83.14, C84.1Ø, C84.14, C84.18-C84.19, C84.44, C84.64, C84.74, C84.94, C84.A4, C84.Z4, C85.14, C85.24, C85.84, C85.94, D49.81-D49.9

C84.15 Sézary disease, lymph nodes of inguinal region and lower limb CC
CC Excl: C82.55, C83.15, C84.1Ø, C84.15, C84.18-C84.19, C84.45, C84.65, C84.75, C84.95, C84.A5, C84.Z5, C85.15, C85.25, C85.85, C85.95, D49.81-D49.9

C84.16 Sézary disease, intrapelvic lymph nodes CC
CC Excl: C82.56, C83.16, C84.1Ø, C84.16, C84.18-C84.19, C84.46, C84.66, C84.76, C84.96, C84.A6, C84.Z6, C85.16, C85.26, C85.86, C85.96, D49.81-D49.9

C84.17 Sézary disease, spleen CC
CC Excl: C82.57, C83.17, C84.1Ø, C84.17-C84.19, C84.47, C84.67, C84.77, C84.97, C84.A7, C84.Z7, C85.17, C85.27, C85.87, C85.97, C86.1, D49.81-D49.9

C84.18 Sézary disease, lymph nodes of multiple sites CC
CC Excl: C82.58, C83.18, C84.1Ø-C84.19, C84.48, C84.68, C84.78, C84.98, C84.A8, C84.Z8, C85.18, C85.28, C85.88, C85.98, D49.81-D49.9

C84.19 Sézary disease, extranodal and solid organ sites CC
CC Excl: See code: C84.1Ø

✓5th **C84.4 Peripheral T-cell lymphoma, not classified**
Lennert's lymphoma
Lymphoepithelioid lymphoma
Mature T-cell lymphoma, not elsewhere classified

C84.4Ø Peripheral T-cell lymphoma, not classified, unspecified site HIV CC
CC Excl: See code: C82.5Ø

C84.41 Peripheral T-cell lymphoma, not classified, lymph nodes of head, face, and neck HIV CC
CC Excl: See code: C82.51

C84.42 Peripheral T-cell lymphoma, not classified, intrathoracic lymph nodes HIV CC
CC Excl: See code: C82.52

C84.43 Peripheral T-cell lymphoma, not classified, intra-abdominal lymph nodes HIV CC
CC Excl: See code: C82.53

C84.44 Peripheral T-cell lymphoma, not classified, lymph nodes of axilla and upper limb HIV CC
CC Excl: See code: C82.54

C84.45 Peripheral T-cell lymphoma, not classified, lymph nodes of inguinal region and lower limb HIV CC
CC Excl: See code: C82.55

C84.46 Peripheral T-cell lymphoma, not classified, intrapelvic lymph nodes HIV CC
CC Excl: See code: C82.56

C84.47 Peripheral T-cell lymphoma, not classified, spleen HIV CC
CC Excl: See code: C82.57

C84.48 **Peripheral T-cell lymphoma, not classified, lymph nodes of multiple sites** HIV CC
CC Excl: See code: C82.58

C84.49 **Peripheral T-cell lymphoma, not classified, extranodal and solid organ sites** HIV CC
CC Excl: See code: C82.50

✓5th **C84.6** **Anaplastic large cell lymphoma, ALK-positive**
Anaplastic large cell lymphoma, CD30-positive

C84.60 **Anaplastic large cell lymphoma, ALK-positive, unspecified site** HIV CC
CC Excl: See code: C82.50

C84.61 **Anaplastic large cell lymphoma, ALK-positive, lymph nodes of head, face, and neck** HIV CC
CC Excl: See code: C82.51

C84.62 **Anaplastic large cell lymphoma, ALK-positive, intrathoracic lymph nodes** HIV CC
CC Excl: See code: C82.52

C84.63 **Anaplastic large cell lymphoma, ALK-positive, intra-abdominal lymph nodes** HIV CC
CC Excl: See code: C82.53

C84.64 **Anaplastic large cell lymphoma, ALK-positive, lymph nodes of axilla and upper limb** HIV CC
CC Excl: See code: C82.54

C84.65 **Anaplastic large cell lymphoma, ALK-positive, lymph nodes of inguinal region and lower limb** HIV CC
CC Excl: See code: C82.55

C84.66 **Anaplastic large cell lymphoma, ALK-positive, intrapelvic lymph nodes** HIV CC
CC Excl: See code: C82.56

C84.67 **Anaplastic large cell lymphoma, ALK-positive, spleen** HIV CC
CC Excl: See code: C82.57

C84.68 **Anaplastic large cell lymphoma, ALK-positive, lymph nodes of multiple sites** HIV CC
CC Excl: See code: C82.58

C84.69 **Anaplastic large cell lymphoma, ALK-positive, extranodal and solid organ sites** HIV CC
CC Excl: See code: C82.50

✓5th **C84.7** **Anaplastic large cell lymphoma, ALK-negative**
EXCLUDES 1 *primary cutaneous CD30-positive T-cell proliferations (C86.6-)*

C84.70 **Anaplastic large cell lymphoma, ALK-negative, unspecified site** HIV CC
CC Excl: See code: C82.50

C84.71 **Anaplastic large cell lymphoma, ALK-negative, lymph nodes of head, face, and neck** HIV CC
CC Excl: See code: C82.51

C84.72 **Anaplastic large cell lymphoma, ALK-negative, intrathoracic lymph nodes** HIV CC
CC Excl: See code: C82.52

C84.73 **Anaplastic large cell lymphoma, ALK-negative, intra-abdominal lymph nodes** HIV CC
CC Excl: See code: C82.53

C84.74 **Anaplastic large cell lymphoma, ALK-negative, lymph nodes of axilla and upper limb** HIV CC
CC Excl: See code: C82.54

C84.75 **Anaplastic large cell lymphoma, ALK-negative, lymph nodes of inguinal region and lower limb** HIV CC
CC Excl: See code: C82.55

C84.76 **Anaplastic large cell lymphoma, ALK-negative, intrapelvic lymph nodes** HIV CC
CC Excl: See code: C82.56

C84.77 **Anaplastic large cell lymphoma, ALK-negative, spleen** HIV CC
CC Excl: See code: C82.57

C84.78 **Anaplastic large cell lymphoma, ALK-negative, lymph nodes of multiple sites** HIV CC
CC Excl: See code: C82.58

C84.79 **Anaplastic large cell lymphoma, ALK-negative, extranodal and solid organ sites** HIV CC
CC Excl: See code: C82.50

✓5th **C84.A** **Cutaneous T-cell lymphoma, unspecified**

C84.A0 **Cutaneous T-cell lymphoma, unspecified, unspecified site** HIV CC
CC Excl: See code: C82.50

C84.A1 **Cutaneous T-cell lymphoma, unspecified lymph nodes of head, face, and neck** HIV CC
CC Excl: See code: C82.51

C84.A2 **Cutaneous T-cell lymphoma, unspecified, intrathoracic lymph nodes** HIV CC
CC Excl: See code: C82.52

C84.A3 **Cutaneous T-cell lymphoma, unspecified, intra-abdominal lymph nodes** HIV CC
CC Excl: See code: C82.53

C84.A4 **Cutaneous T-cell lymphoma, unspecified, lymph nodes of axilla and upper limb** HIV CC
CC Excl: See code: C82.54

C84.A5 **Cutaneous T-cell lymphoma, unspecified, lymph nodes of inguinal region and lower limb** HIV CC
CC Excl: See code: C82.55

C84.A6 **Cutaneous T-cell lymphoma, unspecified, intrapelvic lymph nodes** HIV CC
CC Excl: See code: C82.56

C84.A7 **Cutaneous T-cell lymphoma, unspecified, spleen** HIV CC
CC Excl: See code: C82.57

C84.A8 **Cutaneous T-cell lymphoma, unspecified, lymph nodes of multiple sites** HIV CC
CC Excl: See code: C82.58

C84.A9 **Cutaneous T-cell lymphoma, unspecified, extranodal and solid organ sites** HIV CC
CC Excl: See code: C82.50

✓5th **C84.Z** **Other mature T/NK-cell lymphomas**
NOTE If T-cell lineage or involvement is mentioned in conjunction with a specific lymphoma, code to the more specific description.
EXCLUDES 1 *angioimmunoblastic T-cell lymphoma (C86.5)*
blastic NK-cell lymphoma (C86.4)
enteropathy-type T-cell lymphoma (C86.2)
extranodal NK-cell lymphoma, nasal type (C86.0)
hepatosplenic T-cell lymphoma (C86.1)
primary cutaneous CD30-positive T-cell proliferations (C86.6)
subcutaneous panniculitis-like T-cell lymphoma (C86.3)
T-cell leukemia (C91.1-)

C84.Z0 **Other mature T/NK-cell lymphomas, unspecified site** HIV CC
CC Excl: See code: C82.50

C84.Z1 **Other mature T/NK-cell lymphomas, lymph nodes of head, face, and neck** HIV CC
CC Excl: See code: C82.51

C84.Z2 **Other mature T/NK-cell lymphomas, intrathoracic lymph nodes** HIV CC
CC Excl: See code: C82.52

C84.Z3 **Other mature T/NK-cell lymphomas, intra-abdominal lymph nodes** HIV CC
CC Excl: See code: C82.53

C84.Z4 **Other mature T/NK-cell lymphomas, lymph nodes of axilla and upper limb** HIV CC
CC Excl: See code: C82.54

C84.Z5 **Other mature T/NK-cell lymphomas, lymph nodes of inguinal region and lower limb** HIV CC
CC Excl: See code: C82.55

C84.Z6 **Other mature T/NK-cell lymphomas, intrapelvic lymph nodes** HIV CC
CC Excl: See code: C82.56

C84.Z7 **Other mature T/NK-cell lymphomas, spleen** HIV CC
CC Excl: See code: C82.57

C84.Z8 **Other mature T/NK-cell lymphomas, lymph ndoes of multiple sites** HIV CC
CC Excl: See code: C82.58

C84.Z9 **Other mature T/NK-cell lymphomas, extranodal and solid organ sites** HIV CC
CC Excl: See code: C82.50

✓5th **C84.9** **Mature T/NK-cell lymphomas, unspecified**
NK/T cell lymphoma NOS
EXCLUDES 1 *mature T-cell lymphoma, not elsewhere classified (C84.4-)*

C84.90 **Mature T/NK-cell lymphomas, unspecified, unspecified site** HIV CC
CC Excl: See code: C82.50

C84.91 **Mature T/NK-cell lymphomas, unspecified, lymph nodes of head, face, and neck** HIV CC
CC Excl: See code: C82.51

C84.92 **Mature T/NK-cell lymphomas, unspecified, intrathoracic lymph nodes** HIV CC
CC Excl: See code: C82.52

C84.93 **Mature T/NK-cell lymphomas, unspecified, intra-abdominal lymph nodes** HIV CC
CC Excl: See code: C82.53

C84.94 Mature T/NK-cell lymphomas, unspecified, lymph nodes of axilla and upper limb HIV CC
CC Excl: See code: C82.54

C84.95 Mature T/NK-cell lymphomas, unspecified, lymph nodes of inguinal region and lower limb HIV CC
CC Excl: See code: C82.55

C84.96 Mature T/NK-cell lymphomas, unspecified, intrapelvic lymph nodes HIV CC
CC Excl: See code: C82.56

C84.97 Mature T/NK-cell lymphomas, unspecified, spleen HIV CC
CC Excl: See code: C82.57

C84.98 Mature T/NK-cell lymphomas, unspecified, lymph nodes of multiple sites HIV CC
CC Excl: See code: C82.58

C84.99 Mature T/NK-cell lymphomas, unspecified, extranodal and solid organ sites HIV CC
CC Excl: See code: C82.50

✓4th C85 Other specified and unspecified types of non-Hodgkin lymphoma

EXCLUDES 1 *other specified types of T/NK-cell lymphoma (C86.-)*
personal history of non-Hodgkin lymphoma (Z85.72)

✓5th C85.1 Unspecified B-cell lymphoma

NOTE If B-cell lineage or involvement is mentioned in conjunction with a specific lymphoma, code to the more specific description.

C85.10 Unspecified B-cell lymphoma, unspecified site HIV CC
CC Excl: See code: C82.50

C85.11 Unspecified B-cell lymphoma, lymph nodes of head, face, and neck HIV CC
CC Excl: See code: C82.51

C85.12 Unspecified B-cell lymphoma, intrathoracic lymph nodes HIV CC
CC Excl: See code: C82.52

C85.13 Unspecified B-cell lymphoma, intra-abdominal lymph nodes HIV CC
CC Excl: See code: C82.53

C85.14 Unspecified B-cell lymphoma, lymph nodes of axilla and upper limb HIV CC
CC Excl: See code: C82.54

C85.15 Unspecified B-cell lymphoma, lymph nodes of inguinal region and lower limb HIV CC
CC Excl: See code: C82.55

C85.16 Unspecified B-cell lymphoma, intrapelvic lymph nodes HIV CC
CC Excl: See code: C82.56

C85.17 Unspecified B-cell lymphoma, spleen HIV CC
CC Excl: See code: C82.57

C85.18 Unspecified B-cell lymphoma, lymph nodes of multiple sites HIV CC
CC Excl: See code: C82.58

C85.19 Unspecified B-cell lymphoma, extranodal and solid organ sites HIV CC
CC Excl: See code: C82.50

✓5th C85.2 Mediastinal (thymic) large B-cell lymphoma

C85.20 Mediastinal (thymic) large B-cell lymphoma, unspecified site HIV CC
CC Excl: See code: C82.50

C85.21 Mediastinal (thymic) large B-cell lymphoma, lymph nodes of head, face, and neck HIV CC
CC Excl: See code: C82.51

C85.22 Mediastinal (thymic) large B-cell lymphoma, intrathoracic lymph nodes HIV CC
CC Excl: See code: C82.52

C85.23 Mediastinal (thymic) large B-cell lymphoma, intra-abdominal lymph nodes HIV CC
CC Excl: See code: C82.53

C85.24 Mediastinal (thymic) large B-cell lymphoma, lymph nodes of axilla and upper limb HIV CC
CC Excl: See code: C82.54

C85.25 Mediastinal (thymic) large B-cell lymphoma, lymph nodes of inguinal region and lower limb HIV CC
CC Excl: See code: C82.55

C85.26 Mediastinal (thymic) large B-cell lymphoma, intrapelvic lymph nodes HIV CC
CC Excl: See code: C82.56

C85.27 Mediastinal (thymic) large B-cell lymphoma, spleen HIV CC
CC Excl: See code: C82.57

C85.28 Mediastinal (thymic) large B-cell lymphoma, lymph nodes of multiple sites HIV CC
CC Excl: See code: C82.58

C85.29 Mediastinal (thymic) large B-cell lymphoma, extranodal and solid organ sites HIV CC
CC Excl: See code: C82.50

✓5th C85.8 Other specified types of non-Hodgkin lymphoma

C85.80 Other specified types of non-Hodgkin lymphoma, unspecified site HIV CC
CC Excl: See code: C82.50

C85.81 Other specified types of non-Hodgkin lymphoma, lymph nodes of head, face, and neck HIV CC
CC Excl: See code: C82.51

C85.82 Other specified types of non-Hodgkin lymphoma, intrathoracic lymph nodes HIV CC
CC Excl: See code: C82.52

C85.83 Other specified types of non-Hodgkin lymphoma, intra-abdominal lymph nodes HIV CC
CC Excl: See code: C82.53

C85.84 Other specified types of non-Hodgkin lymphoma, lymph nodes of axilla and upper limb HIV CC
CC Excl: See code: C82.54

C85.85 Other specified types of non-Hodgkin lymphoma, lymph nodes of inguinal region and lower limb HIV CC
CC Excl: See code: C82.55

C85.86 Other specified types of non-Hodgkin lymphoma, intrapelvic lymph nodes HIV CC
CC Excl: See code: C82.56

C85.87 Other specified types of non-Hodgkin lymphoma, spleen HIV CC
CC Excl: See code: C82.57

C85.88 Other specified types of non-Hodgkin lymphoma, lymph nodes of multiple sites HIV CC
CC Excl: See code: C82.58

C85.89 Other specified types of non-Hodgkin lymphoma, extranodal and solid organ sites HIV CC
CC Excl: See code: C82.50

✓5th C85.9 Non-Hodgkin lymphoma, unspecified

Lymphoma NOS
Malignant lymphoma NOS
Non-Hodgkin lymphoma NOS

C85.90 Non-Hodgkin lymphoma, unspecified, unspecified site HIV CC
CC Excl: See code: C82.50

C85.91 Non-Hodgkin lymphoma, unspecified, lymph nodes of head, face, and neck HIV CC
CC Excl: See code: C82.51

C85.92 Non-Hodgkin lymphoma, unspecified, intrathoracic lymph nodes HIV CC
CC Excl: See code: C82.52

C85.93 Non-Hodgkin lymphoma, unspecified, intra-abdominal lymph nodes HIV CC
CC Excl: See code: C82.53

C85.94 Non-Hodgkin lymphoma, unspecified, lymph nodes of axilla and upper limb HIV CC
CC Excl: See code: C82.54

C85.95 Non-Hodgkin lymphoma, unspecified, lymph nodes of inguinal region and lower limb HIV CC
CC Excl: See code: C82.55

C85.96 Non-Hodgkin lymphoma, unspecified, intrapelvic lymph nodes HIV CC
CC Excl: See code: C82.56

C85.97 Non-Hodgkin lymphoma, unspecified, spleen HIV CC
CC Excl: See code: C82.57

C85.98 Non-Hodgkin lymphoma, unspecified, lymph nodes of multiple sites HIV CC
CC Excl: See code: C82.58

C85.99 Non-Hodgkin lymphoma, unspecified, extranodal and solid organ sites HIV CC
CC Excl: See code: C82.50

✓4th C86 Other specified types of T/NK-cell lymphoma

EXCLUDES 1 *anaplastic large cell lymphoma, ALK negative (C84.7-)*
anaplastic large cell lymphoma, ALK positive (C84.6-)
mature T/NK-cell lymphomas (C84.-)
other specified types of non-Hodgkin lymphoma (C85.8-)

C86.0 Extranodal NK/T-cell lymphoma, nasal type HIV CC
CC Excl: See code: C82.51

C86.1 Hepatosplenic T-cell lymphoma HIV CC
Alpha-beta and gamma delta types
CC Excl: See code: C82.57

C86.2 Enteropathy-type (intestinal) T-cell lymphoma HIV CC
Enteropathy associated T-cell lymphoma
CC Excl: See code: C82.53

C86.3 Subcutaneous panniculitis-like T-cell lymphoma HIV CC
CC Excl: See code: C82.53

C86.4 Blastic NK-cell lymphoma HIV CC
CC Excl: See code: C82.50

C86.5 Angioimmunoblastic T-cell lymphoma HIV CC
Angioimmunoblastic lymphadenopathy with dysproteinemia [AILD]
CC Excl: See code: C83.00

C86.6 Primary cutaneous CD30-positive T-cell proliferations HIV CC
Lymphomatoid papulosis
Primary cutaneous anaplastic large cell lymphoma
Primary cutaneous CD30-positive large T-cell lymphoma
CC Excl: See code: C83.00

✓4th C88 Malignant immunoproliferative diseases and certain other B-cell lymphomas

EXCLUDES 1 *B-cell lymphoma, unspecified (C85.1-)*
personal history of other malignant neoplasms of lymphoid, hematopoietic and related tissues (Z85.79)

C88.0 Waldenström macroglobulinemia
Lymphoplasmacytic lymphoma with IgM-production
Macroglobulinemia (idiopathic) (primary)
EXCLUDES 1 *small cell B-cell lymphoma (C83.0)*

C88.2 Heavy chain disease CC
Franklin disease
Gamma heavy chain disease
Mu heavy chain disease
CC Excl: C88.2-C88.3, C88.8-C91.32, C91.50-C94.32, C94.80-C95.92, D49.81-D49.9

C88.3 Immunoproliferative small intestinal disease CC
Alpha heavy chain disease
Mediterranean lymphoma
CC Excl: See code: C88.2

C88.4 Extranodal marginal zone B-cell lymphoma of mucosa-associated lymphoid tissue [MALT-lymphoma] HIV CC
Lymphoma of skin-associated lymphoid tissue [SALT-lymphoma]
Lymphoma of bronchial-associated lymphoid tissue [BALT-lymphoma]
EXCLUDES 1 *high malignant (diffuse large B-cell) lymphoma (C83.3-)*
CC Excl: C82.50-C82.59, C83.10-C83.19, C84.40-C86.4, C88.4, C96.4, C96.Z-C96.9, D49.81-D49.9

C88.8 Other malignant immunoproliferative diseases CC
CC Excl: C88.2-C88.3, C88.8-C95.92, D45-D47.1, D47.3, D47.Z9-D47.9, D48.7-D48.9, D49.81-D49.9

C88.9 Malignant immunoproliferative disease, unspecified CC
Immunoproliferative disease NOS
CC Excl: See code: C88.2

✓4th C90 Multiple myeloma and malignant plasma cell neoplasms

EXCLUDES 1 *personal history of other malignant neoplasms of lymphoid, hematopoietic and related tissues (Z85.79)*

CC Excl: For CC codes in category C90, unless otherwise noted: C88.2-C88.3, C88.8-C95.92, D45-D47.1, D47.3, D47.Z9-D47.9, D48.7-D48.9, D49.81-D49.9

✓5th **C90.0 Multiple myeloma**
Kahler's disease
Medullary plasmacytoma
Myelomatosis
Plasma cell myeloma
EXCLUDES 1 *solitary myeloma (C90.3-)*
solitary plasmactyoma (C90.3-)

C90.00 Multiple myeloma not having achieved remission CC
Multiple myeloma with failed remission
Multiple myeloma NOS

C90.01 Multiple myeloma in remission CC

C90.02 Multiple myeloma in relapse CC

✓5th **C90.1 Plasma cell leukemia**
Plasmacytic leukemia

C90.10 Plasma cell leukemia not having achieved remission CC
Plasma cell leukemia with failed remission
Plasma cell leukemia NOS

C90.11 Plasma cell leukemia in remission CC

C90.12 Plasma cell leukemia in relapse CC

✓5th **C90.2 Extramedullary plasmacytoma**

C90.20 Extramedullary plasmacytoma not having achieved remission CC
Extramedullary plasmacytoma with failed remission
Extramedullary plasmacytoma NOS

C90.21 Extramedullary plasmacytoma in remission CC

C90.22 Extramedullary plasmacytoma in relapse CC

✓5th **C90.3 Solitary plasmacytoma**
Localized malignant plasma cell tumor NOS
Plasmacytoma NOS
Solitary myeloma

C90.30 Solitary plasmacytoma not having achieved remission CC
Solitary plasmacytoma with failed remission
Solitary plasmacytoma NOS

C90.31 Solitary plasmacytoma in remission CC

C90.32 Solitary plasmacytoma in relapse CC

✓4th C91 Lymphoid leukemia

EXCLUDES 1 *personal history of leukemia (Z85.6)*

CC Excl: For CC codes in category C91, unless otherwise noted: C88.2-C88.3, C88.8-C95.92, D45-D47.1, D47.3, D47.Z9-D47.9, D48.7-D48.9, D49.81-D49.9

✓5th **C91.0 Acute lymphoblastic leukemia [ALL]**
NOTE Code C91.0 should only be used for T-cell and B-cell precursor leukemia

C91.00 Acute lymphoblastic leukemia not having achieved remission CC
Acute lymphoblastic leukemia with failed remission
Acute lymphoblastic leukemia NOS

C91.01 Acute lymphoblastic leukemia, in remission CC

C91.02 Acute lymphoblastic leukemia, in relapse CC

✓5th **C91.1 Chronic lymphocytic leukemia of B-cell type**
Lymphoplasmacytic leukemia
Richter syndrome
EXCLUDES 1 *lymphoplasmacytic lymphoma (C83.0-)*

C91.10 Chronic lymphocytic leukemia of B-cell type not having achieved remission CC
Chronic lymphocytic leukemia of B-cell type with failed remission
Chronic lymphocytic leukemia of B-cell type NOS

C91.11 Chronic lymphocytic leukemia of B-cell type in remission CC

C91.12 Chronic lymphocytic leukemia of B-cell type in relapse CC

✓5th **C91.3 Prolymphocytic leukemia of B-cell type**

C91.30 Prolymphocytic leukemia of B-cell type not having achieved remission CC
Prolymphocytic leukemia of B-cell type with failed remission
Prolymphocytic leukemia of B-cell type NOS

C91.31 Prolymphocytic leukemia of B-cell type, in remission CC

C91.32 Prolymphocytic leukemia of B-cell type, in relapse CC

✓5th **C91.4 Hairy cell leukemia**
Leukemic reticuloendotheliosis

C91.40 Hairy cell leukemia not having achieved remission CC
Hairy cell leukemia with failed remission
Hairy cell leukemia NOS
CC Excl: C82.50, C82.59, C83.10, C83.19, C84.40, C84.49, C84.60, C84.69-C84.70, C84.79-C84.90, C84.99-C84.A0, C84.A9-C84.Z0, C84.Z9, C85.10, C85.19-C85.20, C85.29, C85.80, C85.89-C85.90, C85.99, C86.4, C88.4, C91.40-C91.42, C96.4, C96.9, C96.Z, D49.81-D49.9

C91.41 Hairy cell leukemia, in remission CC
CC Excl: See code: C91.40

C91.42 Hairy cell leukemia, in relapse CC
CC Excl: See code: C91.40

C91.5 Adult T-cell lymphoma/leukemia (HTLV-1-associated)
Acute variant of adult T-cell lymphoma/leukemia (HTLV-1-associated)
Chronic variant of adult T-cell lymphoma/leukemia (HTLV-1-associated)
Lymphomatoid variant of adult T-cell lymphoma/leukemia (HTLV-1-associated)
Smouldering variant of adult T-cell lymphoma/leukemia (HTLV-1-associated)

C91.50 Adult T-cell lymphoma/leukemia (HTLV-1-associated) not having achieved remission CC A
Adult T-cell lymphoma/leukemia (HTLV-1-associated) with failed remission
Adult T-cell lymphoma/leukemia (HTLV-1-associated) NOS
CC Excl: C88.2-C88.3, C88.8-C91.32, C91.50-C94.32, C94.80-C95.92, D49.81-D49.9

C91.51 Adult T-cell lymphoma/leukemia (HTLV-1-associated), in remission CC A
CC Excl: See code: C91.50

C91.52 Adult T-cell lymphoma/leukemia (HTLV-1-associated), in relapse CC A
CC Excl: See code: C91.50

C91.6 Prolymphocytic leukemia of T-cell type

C91.60 Prolymphocytic leukemia of T-cell type not having achieved remission CC
Prolymphocytic leukemia of T-cell type with failed remission
Prolymphocytic leukemia of T-cell type NOS
CC Excl: See code: C91.50

C91.61 Prolymphocytic leukemia of T-cell type, in remission CC
CC Excl: See code: C91.50

C91.62 Prolymphocytic leukemia of T-cell type, in relapse CC
CC Excl: See code: C91.50

C91.A Mature B-cell leukemia Burkitt-type
EXCLUDES 1 *Burkitt lymphoma (C83.7-)*

C91.A0 Mature B-cell leukemia Burkitt-type not having achieved remission CC
Mature B-cell leukemia Burkitt-type with failed remission
Mature B-cell leukemia Burkitt-type NOS
CC Excl: See code: C91.50

C91.A1 Mature B-cell leukemia Burkitt-type, in remission CC
CC Excl: See code: C91.50

C91.A2 Mature B-cell leukemia Burkitt-type, in relapse CC
CC Excl: See code: C91.50

C91.Z Other lymphoid leukemia
T-cell large granular lymphocytic leukemia (associated with rheumatoid arthritis)

C91.Z0 Other lymphoid leukemia not having achieved remission CC
Other lymphoid leukemia with failed remission
Other lymphoid leukemia NOS
CC Excl: See code: C91.50

C91.Z1 Other lymphoid leukemia, in remission CC
CC Excl: See code: C91.50

C91.Z2 Other lymphoid leukemia, in relapse CC
CC Excl: See code: C91.50

C91.9 Lymphoid leukemia, unspecified

C91.90 Lymphoid leukemia, unspecified not having achieved remission CC
Lymphoid leukemia with failed remission
Lymphoid leukemia NOS
CC Excl: See code: C91.50

C91.91 Lymphoid leukemia, unspecified, in remission CC
CC Excl: See code: C91.50

C91.92 Lymphoid leukemia, unspecified, in relapse CC
CC Excl: See code: C91.50

C92 Myeloid leukemia
INCLUDES granulocytic leukemia
myelogenous leukemia
EXCLUDES 1 *personal history of leukemia (Z85.6)*

CC Excl: For CC codes in category C92, unless otherwise noted: C88.2-C88.3, C88.8-C91.32, C91.50-C94.32, C94.80-C95.92, D49.81-D49.9

C92.0 Acute myeloblastic leukemia
Acute myeloblastic leukemia, minimal differentiation
Acute myeloblastic leukemia (with maturation)
Acute myeloblastic leukemia 1/ETO
Acute myeloblastic leukemia M0
Acute myeloblastic leukemia M1
Acute myeloblastic leukemia M2
Acute myeloblastic leukemia with t(8;21)
Acute myeloblastic leukemia (without a FAB classification) NOS
Refractory anemia with excess blasts in transformation [RAEB T]
EXCLUDES 1 *acute exacerbation of chronic myeloid leukemia (C92.10)*
refractory anemia with excess of blasts not in transformation (D46.2-)

C92.00 Acute myeloblastic leukemia, not having achieved remission CC
Acute myeloblastic leukemia with failed remission
Acute myeloblastic leukemia NOS

C92.01 Acute myeloblastic leukemia, in remission CC

C92.02 Acute myeloblastic leukemia, in relapse CC

C92.1 Chronic myeloid leukemia, BCR/ABL-positive
Chronic myelogenous leukemia, Philadelphia chromosome (Ph1) positive
Chronic myelogenous leukemia, t(9;22) (q34;q11)
Chronic myelogenous leukemia with crisis of blast cells
EXCLUDES 1 *atypical chronic myeloid leukemia BCR/ABL-negative (C92.2-)*
chronic myelomonocytic leukemia (C93.1-)
chronic myeloproliferative disease (D47.1)

C92.10 Chronic myeloid leukemia, BCR/ABL-positive, not having achieved remission CC
Chronic myeloid leukemia, BCR/ABL-positive with failed remission
Chronic myeloid leukemia, BCR/ABL-positive NOS

C92.11 Chronic myeloid leukemia, BCR/ABL-positive, in remission CC

C92.12 Chronic myeloid leukemia, BCR/ABL-positive, in relapse CC

C92.2 Atypical chronic myeloid leukemia, BCR/ABL-negative

C92.20 Atypical chronic myeloid leukemia, BCR/ABL-negative, not having achieved remission CC
Atypical chronic myeloid leukemia, BCR/ABL-negative with failed remission
Atypical chronic myeloid leukemia, BCR/ABL-negative NOS

C92.21 Atypical chronic myeloid leukemia, BCR/ABL-negative, in remission CC

C92.22 Atypical chronic myeloid leukemia, BCR/ABL-negative, in relapse CC

C92.3 Myeloid sarcoma
A malignant tumor of immature myeloid cells
Chloroma
Granulocytic sarcoma

C92.30 Myeloid sarcoma, not having achieved remission CC
Myeloid sarcoma with failed remission
Myeloid sarcoma NOS

C92.31 Myeloid sarcoma, in remission CC

C92.32 Myeloid sarcoma, in relapse CC

C92.4 Acute promyelocytic leukemia
AML M3
AML Me with t(15;17) and variants

C92.40 Acute promyelocytic leukemia, not having achieved remission CC
Acute promyelocytic leukemia with failed remission
Acute promyelocytic leukemia NOS

C92.41 Acute promyelocytic leukemia, in remission CC

C92.42 Acute promyelocytic leukemia, in relapse CC

✓5th **C92.5 Acute myelomonocytic leukemia**
AML M4
AML M4 Eo with inv(16) or t(16;16)
C92.50 Acute myelomonocytic leukemia, not having achieved remission CC
Acute myelomonocytic leukemia with failed remission
Acute myelomonocytic leukemia NOS
C92.51 Acute myelomonocytic leukemia, in remission CC
C92.52 Acute myelomonocytic leukemia, in relapse CC

✓5th **C92.6 Acute myeloid leukemia with 11q23-abnormality**
Acute myeloid leukemia with variation of MLL-gene
C92.60 Acute myeloid leukemia with 11q23-abnormality not having achieved remission CC
Acute myeloid leukemia with 11q23-abnormality with failed remission
Acute myeloid leukemia with 11q23-abnormality NOS
C92.61 Acute myeloid leukemia with 11q23-abnormality in remission CC
C92.62 Acute myeloid leukemia with 11q23-abnormality in relapse CC

✓5th **C92.A Acute myeloid leukemia with multilineage dysplasia**
Acute myeloid leukemia with dysplasia of remaining hematopoesis and/or myelodysplastic disease in its history
C92.A0 Acute myeloid leukemia with multilineage dysplasia, not having achieved remission CC
Acute myeloid leukemia with multilineage dysplasia with failed remission
Acute myeloid leukemia with multilineage dysplasia NOS
C92.A1 Acute myeloid leukemia with multilineage dysplasia, in remission CC
C92.A2 Acute myeloid leukemia with multilineage dysplasia, in relapse CC

✓5th **C92.Z Other myeloid leukemia**
C92.Z0 Other myeloid leukemia not having achieved remission CC
Myeloid leukemia NEC with failed remission
Myeloid leukemia NEC
C92.Z1 Other myeloid leukemia, in remission CC
C92.Z2 Other myeloid leukemia, in relapse CC

✓5th **C92.9 Myeloid leukemia, unspecified**
C92.90 Myeloid leukemia, unspecified, not having achieved remission CC
Myeloid leukemia, unspecified with failed remission
Myeloid leukemia, unspecified NOS
C92.91 Myeloid leukemia, unspecified in remission CC
C92.92 Myeloid leukemia, unspecified in relapse CC

✓4th **C93 Monocytic leukemia**
INCLUDES monocytoid leukemia
EXCLUDES 1 *personal history of leukemia (Z85.6))*

CC Excl: For CC codes in category C93, unless otherwise noted: C88.2-C88.3, C88.8-C91.32, C91.50-C94.32, C94.80-C95.92, D49.81-D49.9

✓5th **C93.0 Acute monoblastic/monocytic leukemia**
AML M5 AML M5b
AML M5a
C93.00 Acute monoblastic/monocytic leukemia, not having achieved remission CC
Acute monoblastic/monocytic leukemia with failed remission
Acute monoblastic/monocytic leukemia NOS
C93.01 Acute monoblastic/monocytic leukemia, in remission CC
C93.02 Acute monoblastic/monocytic leukemia, in relapse CC

✓5th **C93.1 Chronic myelomonocytic leukemia**
Chronic monocytic leukemia
CMML-1
CMML-2
CMML with eosinophilia
C93.10 Chronic myelomonocytic leukemia not having achieved remission CC
Chronic myelomonocytic leukemia with failed remission
Chronic myelomonocytic leukemia NOS
C93.11 Chronic myelomonocytic leukemia, in remission CC
C93.12 Chronic myelomonocytic leukemia, in relapse CC

✓5th **C93.3 Juvenile myelomonocytic leukemia**
C93.30 Juvenile myelomonocytic leukemia, not having achieved remission CC P
Juvenile myelomonocytic leukemia with failed remission
Juvenile myelomonocytic leukemia NOS
C93.31 Juvenile myelomonocytic leukemia, in remission CC P
C93.32 Juvenile myelomonocytic leukemia, in relapse CC P

✓5th **C93.Z Other monocytic leukemia**
C93.Z0 Other monocytic leukemia, not having achieved remission CC
Other monocytic leukemia NOS
C93.Z1 Other monocytic leukemia, in remission CC
C93.Z2 Other monocytic leukemia, in relapse CC

✓5th **C93.9 Monocytic leukemia, unspecified**
C93.90 Monocytic leukemia, unspecified, not having achieved remission CC
Monocytic leukemia, unspecified with failed remission
Monocytic leukemia, unspecified NOS
C93.91 Monocytic leukemia, unspecified in remission CC
C93.92 Monocytic leukemia, unspecified in relapse CC

✓4th **C94 Other leukemias of specified cell type**
EXCLUDES 1 *leukemic reticuloendotheliosis (C91.4-)*
myelodysplastic syndromes (D46.-)
personal history of leukemia (Z85.6)
plasma cell leukemia (C90.1-)

CC Excl: For CC codes in category C94, unless otherwise noted: C88.2-C88.3, C88.8-C91.32, C91.50-C94.32, C94.80-C95.92, D49.81-D49.9

✓5th **C94.0 Acute erythroid leukemia**
Acute myeloid leukemia M6(a)(b)
Erythroleukemia
C94.00 Acute erythroid leukemia, not having achieved remission CC
Acute erythroid leukemia with failed remission
Acute erythroid leukemia NOS
C94.01 Acute erythroid leukemia, in remission CC
C94.02 Acute erythroid leukemia, in relapse CC

✓5th **C94.2 Acute megakaryoblastic leukemia**
Acute myeloid leukemia M7
Acute megakaryocytic leukemia
C94.20 Acute megakaryoblastic leukemia not having achieved remission CC
Acute megakaryoblastic leukemia with failied remission
Acute megakaryoblastic leukemia NOS
C94.21 Acute megakaryoblastic leukemia, in remission CC
C94.22 Acute megakaryoblastic leukemia, in relapse CC

✓5th **C94.3 Mast cell leukemia**
C94.30 Mast cell leukemia not having achieved remission CC
Mast cell leukemia with failed remission
Mast cell leukemia NOS
C94.31 Mast cell leukemia, in remission CC
C94.32 Mast cell leukemia, in relapse CC

✓5th **C94.4 Acute panmyelosis with myelofibrosis**
Acute myelofibrosis
EXCLUDES 1 *myelofibrosis NOS (D75.81)*
secondary myelofibrosis NOS (D75.81)
C94.40 Acute panmyelosis with myelofibrosis not having achieved remission CC
Acute myelofibrosis NOS
Acute panmyelosis with myelofibrosis with failed remission
Acute panmyelosis NOS
CC Excl: C88.2-C88.3, C88.8-C88.9, C90.10-C90.11, C90.20-C90.21, C90.30-C90.31, C91.00-C95.92, D45-D47.1, D47.3, D47.Z9-D47.9, D48.7-D48.9
C94.41 Acute panmyelosis with myelofibrosis, in remission CC
CC Excl: See code: C94.40
C94.42 Acute panmyelosis with myelofibrosis, in relapse CC
CC Excl: See code: C94.40

C94.6 Myelodysplastic disease, not classified CC
Myeloproliferative disease, not classified
CC Excl: See code: C94.40

C94.8 Other specified leukemias
Aggressive NK-cell leukemia
Acute basophilic leukemia

C94.80 Other specified leukemias not having achieved remission CC
Other specified leukemia with failed remission
Other specified leukemias NOS

C94.81 Other specified leukemias, in remission CC

C94.82 Other specified leukemias, in relapse CC

C95 Leukemia of unspecified cell type
EXCLUDES 1 *personal history of leukemia (Z85.6)*

CC Excl: For CC codes in category C95, unless otherwise noted: C88.2-C88.3, C88.8-C91.32, C91.50-C94.32, C94.80-C95.92, D49.81-D49.9

C95.0 Acute leukemia of unspecified cell type
Acute bilineal leukemia
Acute mixed lineage leukemia
Biphenotypic acute leukemia
Stem cell leukemia of unclear lineage
EXCLUDES 1 *acute exacerbation of unspecified chronic leukemia (C95.10)*

C95.00 Acute leukemia of unspecified cell type not having achieved remission CC
Acute leukemia of unspecified cell type with failed remission
Acute leukemia NOS

C95.01 Acute leukemia of unspecified cell type, in remission CC

C95.02 Acute leukemia of unspecified cell type, in relapse CC

C95.1 Chronic leukemia of unspecified cell type

C95.10 Chronic leukemia of unspecified cell type not having achieved remission CC
Chronic leukemia of unspecified cell type with failed remission
Chronic leukemia NOS

C95.11 Chronic leukemia of unspecified cell type, in remission CC

C95.12 Chronic leukemia of unspecified cell type, in relapse CC

C95.9 Leukemia, unspecified

C95.90 Leukemia, unspecified not having achieved remission CC
Leukemia, unspecified with failed remission
Leukemia NOS

C95.91 Leukemia, unspecified, in remission CC

C95.92 Leukemia, unspecified, in relapse CC

C96 Other and unspecified malignant neoplasms of lymphoid, hematopoietic and related tissue
EXCLUDES 1 *personal history of other malignant neoplasms of lymphoid, hematopoietic and related tissues (Z85.79)*

C96.0 Multifocal and multisystemic (disseminated) Langerhans-cell histiocytosis CC
Histiocytosis X, multisystemic
Letterer-Siwe disease
EXCLUDES 1 *adult pulmonary Langerhans cell histiocytosis (J84.82)*
multifocal and unisystemic Langerhans-cell histiocytosis (C96.5)
unifocal Langerhans-cell histiocytosis (C96.6)
CC Excl: C82.50, C82.59, C83.10, C83.19, C84.40, C84.49, C84.60, C84.69-C84.70, C84.79-C84.90, C84.99-C84.A0, C84.A9-C84.Z0, C84.Z9, C85.10, C85.19-C85.20, C85.29, C85.80, C85.89-C85.90, C85.99, C86.4, C88.4, C96.0, C96.4, C96.9, C96.Z, D49.81-D49.9

C96.2 Malignant mast cell tumor CC
Aggressive systemic mastocytosis
Mast cell sarcoma
EXCLUDES 1 *indolent mastocytosis (D47.0)*
mast cell leukemia (C94.30)
mastocytosis (congenital) (cutaneous) (Q82.2)
CC Excl: C82.50, C82.59, C83.10, C83.19, C84.40, C84.49, C84.60, C84.69-C84.70, C84.79-C84.90, C84.99-C84.A0, C84.A9-C84.Z0, C84.Z9, C85.10, C85.19-C85.20, C85.29, C85.80, C85.89-C85.90, C85.99, C86.4, C88.4, C96.2, C96.4, C96.9, C96.Z, D49.81-D49.9

C96.4 Sarcoma of dendritic cells (accessory cells) CC
Follicular dendritic cell sarcoma
Interdigitating dendritic cell sarcoma
Langerhans cell sarcoma
CC Excl: C96.4, C96.9, C96.Z, D49.81-D49.9

C96.5 Multifocal and unisystemic Langerhans-cell histiocytosis CC
Hand-Schüller-Christian disease
Histiocytosis X, multifocal
EXCLUDES 1 *multifocal and multisystemic (disseminated) Langerhans-cell histiocytosis (C96.0)*
unifocal Langerhans-cell histiocytosis (C96.6)
CC Excl: E71.310-E71.32, E71.40-E71.548, E80.4-E80.7, E88.40-E88.49, H49.811-H49.819

C96.6 Unifocal Langerhans-cell histiocytosis CC
Eosinophilic granuloma CC
Histiocytosis X, unifocal
Histiocytosis X NOS
Langerhans-cell histiocytosis NOS
EXCLUDES 1 *multifocal and multisysemic (disseminated) Langerhans-cell histiocytosis (C96.0)*
multifocal and unisystemic Langerhans-cell histiocytosis (C96.5)
CC Excl: See code: C96.5

C96.A Histiocytic sarcoma CC
Malignant histiocytosis
CC Excl: C82.50, C82.59, C83.10, C83.19, C84.40, C84.49, C84.60, C84.69-C84.70, C84.79-C84.90, C84.99-C84.A0, C84.A9-C84.Z0, C84.Z9, C85.10, C85.19-C85.20, C85.29, C85.80, C85.89-C85.90, C85.99, C86.4, C88.4, C96.4, C96.9-C96.Z, D49.81-D49.9

C96.Z Other specified malignant neoplasms of lymphoid, hematopoietic and related tissue CC
CC Excl: See code: C96.4

C96.9 Malignant neoplasm of lymphoid, hematopoietic and related tissue, unspecified CC
CC Excl: See code: C96.4

In situ neoplasms (D00-D09)

INCLUDES Bowen's disease
erythroplasia
grade III intraepithelial neoplasia
Queyrat's erythroplasia

D00 Carcinoma in situ of oral cavity, esophagus and stomach
EXCLUDES 1 *melanoma in situ (D03.-)*

D00.0 Carcinoma in situ of lip, oral cavity and pharynx
Use additional code to identify:
exposure to environmental tobacco smoke (Z77.22)
exposure to tobacco smoke in the perinatal period (P96.81)
history of tobacco use (Z87.891)
occupational exposure to environmental tobacco smoke (Z57.31)
tobacco dependence (F17.-)
tobacco use (Z72.0)
EXCLUDES 1 *carcinoma in situ of aryepiglottic fold or interarytenoid fold, laryngeal aspect (D02.0)*
carcinoma in situ of epiglottis NOS (D02.0)
carcinoma in situ of epiglottis suprahyoid portion (D02.0)
carcinoma in situ of skin of lip (D03.0, D04.0)

D00.00 Carcinoma in situ of oral cavity, unspecified site

D00.01 Carcinoma in situ of labial mucosa and vermilion border

D00.02 Carcinoma in situ of buccal mucosa

D00.03 Carcinoma in situ of gingiva and edentulous alveolar ridge

D00.04 Carcinoma in situ of soft palate

D00.05 Carcinoma in situ of hard palate

D00.06 Carcinoma in situ of floor of mouth

D00.07 Carcinoma in situ of tongue

D00.08 Carcinoma in situ of pharynx
Carcinoma in situ of aryepiglottic fold NOS
Carcinoma in situ of hypopharyngeal aspect of aryepiglottic fold
Carcinoma in situ of marginal zone of aryepiglottic fold

D00.1 Carcinoma in situ of esophagus

D00.2 Carcinoma in situ of stomach

D01 Carcinoma in situ of other and unspecified digestive organs
EXCLUDES 1 *melanoma in situ (D03.-)*

D01.0 Carcinoma in situ of colon
EXCLUDES 1 *carcinoma in situ of rectosigmoid junction (D01.1)*

D01.1 Carcinoma in situ of rectosigmoid junction

D01.2 Carcinoma in situ of rectum

D01.3 Carcinoma in situ of anus and anal canal
EXCLUDES 1 *carcinoma in situ of anal margin (D04.5)*
carcinoma in situ of anal skin (D04.5)
carcinoma in situ of perianal skin (D04.5)

✓5th **D01.4 Carcinoma in situ of other and unspecified parts of intestine**
EXCLUDES 1 *carcinoma in situ of ampulla of Vater (D01.5)*

D01.40 Carcinoma in situ of unspecified part of intestine

D01.49 Carcinoma in situ of other parts of intestine

D01.5 Carcinoma in situ of liver, gallbladder and bile ducts
Carcinoma in situ of ampulla of Vater

D01.7 Carcinoma in situ of other specified digestive organs
Carcinoma in situ of pancreas

D01.9 Carcinoma in situ of digestive organ, unspecified

✓4th **D02 Carcinoma in situ of middle ear and respiratory system**
Use additional code to identify:
exposure to environmental tobacco smoke (Z77.22)
exposure to tobacco smoke in the perinatal period (P96.81)
history of tobacco use (Z87.891)
occupational exposure to environmental tobacco smoke (Z57.31)
tobacco dependence (F17.-)
tobacco use (Z72.0)
EXCLUDES 1 *melanoma in situ (D03.-)*

D02.0 Carcinoma in situ of larynx
Carcinoma in situ of aryepiglottic fold or interarytenoid fold, laryngeal aspect
Carcinoma in situ of epiglottis (suprahyoid portion)
EXCLUDES 1 *carcinoma in situ of aryepiglottic fold or interarytenoid fold NOS (D00.08)*
carcinoma in situ of hypopharyngeal aspect (D00.08)
carcinoma in situ of marginal zone (D00.08)

D02.1 Carcinoma in situ of trachea

✓5th **D02.2 Carcinoma in situ of bronchus and lung**

D02.20 Carcinoma in situ of unspecified bronchus and lung

D02.21 Carcinoma in situ of right bronchus and lung

D02.22 Carcinoma in situ of left bronchus and lung

D02.3 Carcinoma in situ of other parts of respiratory system
Carcinoma in situ of accessory sinuses
Carcinoma in situ of middle ear
Carcinoma in situ of nasal cavities
EXCLUDES 1 *carcinoma in situ of ear (external) (skin) (D04.2-)*
carcinoma in situ of nose NOS (D09.8)
carcinoma in situ of skin of nose (D04.3)

D02.4 Carcinoma in situ of respiratory system, unspecified

✓4th **D03 Melanoma in situ**

D03.0 Melanoma in situ of lip

✓5th **D03.1 Melanoma in situ of eyelid, including canthus**

D03.10 Melanoma in situ of unspecified eyelid, including canthus

D03.11 Melanoma in situ of right eyelid, including canthus

D03.12 Melanoma in situ of left eyelid, including canthus

✓5th **D03.2 Melanoma in situ of ear and external auricular canal**

D03.20 Melanoma in situ of unspecified ear and external auricular canal

D03.21 Melanoma in situ of right ear and external auricular canal

D03.22 Melanoma in situ of left ear and external auricular canal

✓5th **D03.3 Melanoma in situ of other and unspecified parts of face**

D03.30 Melanoma in situ of unspecified part of face

D03.39 Melanoma in situ of other parts of face

D03.4 Melanoma in situ of scalp and neck

✓5th **D03.5 Melanoma in situ of trunk**

D03.51 Melanoma in situ of anal skin
Melanoma in situ of anal margin
Melanoma in situ of perianal skin

D03.52 Melanoma in situ of breast (skin) (soft tissue)

D03.59 Melanoma in situ of other part of trunk

✓5th **D03.6 Melanoma in situ of upper limb, including shoulder**

D03.60 Melanoma in situ of unspecified upper limb, including shoulder

D03.61 Melanoma in situ of right upper limb, including shoulder

D03.62 Melanoma in situ of left upper limb, including shoulder

✓5th **D03.7 Melanoma in situ of lower limb, including hip**

D03.70 Melanoma in situ of unspecified lower limb, including hip

D03.71 Melanoma in situ of right lower limb, including hip

D03.72 Melanoma in situ of left lower limb, including hip

D03.8 Melanoma in situ of other sites
Melanoma in situ of scrotum
EXCLUDES 1 *carcinoma in situ of scrotum (D07.61)*

D03.9 Melanoma in situ, unspecified

✓4th **D04 Carcinoma in situ of skin**
EXCLUDES 1 *erythroplasia of Queyrat (penis) NOS (D07.4)*
melanoma in situ (D03.-)

D04.0 Carcinoma in situ of skin of lip
EXCLUDES 1 *carcinoma in situ of vermilion border of lip (D00.01)*

✓5th **D04.1 Carcinoma in situ of skin of eyelid, including canthus**

D04.10 Carcinoma in situ of skin of unspecified eyelid, including canthus

D04.11 Carcinoma in situ of skin of right eyelid, including canthus

D04.12 Carcinoma in situ of skin of left eyelid, including canthus

✓5th **D04.2 Carcinoma in situ of skin of ear and external auricular canal**

D04.20 Carcinoma in situ of skin of unspecified ear and external auricular canal

D04.21 Carcinoma in situ of skin of right ear and external auricular canal

D04.22 Carcinoma in situ of skin of left ear and external auricular canal

✓5th **D04.3 Carcinoma in situ of skin of other and unspecified parts of face**

D04.30 Carcinoma in situ of skin of unspecified part of face

D04.39 Carcinoma in situ of skin of other parts of face

D04.4 Carcinoma in situ of skin of scalp and neck

D04.5 Carcinoma in situ of skin of trunk
Carcinoma in situ of anal margin
Carcinoma in situ of anal skin
Carcinoma in situ of perianal skin
Carcinoma in situ of skin of breast
EXCLUDES 1 *carcinoma in situ of anus NOS (D01.3)*
carcinoma in situ of scrotum (D07.61)
carcinoma in situ of skin of genital organs (D07.-)

✓5th **D04.6 Carcinoma in situ of skin of upper limb, including shoulder**

D04.60 Carcinoma in situ of skin of unspecified upper limb, including shoulder

D04.61 Carcinoma in situ of skin of right upper limb, including shoulder

D04.62 Carcinoma in situ of skin of left upper limb, including shoulder

✓5th **D04.7 Carcinoma in situ of skin of lower limb, including hip**

D04.70 Carcinoma in situ of skin of unspecified lower limb, including hip

D04.71 Carcinoma in situ of skin of right lower limb, including hip

D04.72 Carcinoma in situ of skin of left lower limb, including hip

D04.8 Carcinoma in situ of skin of other sites

D04.9 Carcinoma in situ of skin, unspecified

✓4th **D05 Carcinoma in situ of breast**
EXCLUDES 1 *carcinoma in situ of skin of breast (D04.5)*
melanoma in situ of breast (skin) (D03.5)
Paget's disease of breast or nipple (C50.-)

✓5th **D05.0 Lobular carcinoma in situ of breast**

D05.00 Lobular carcinoma in situ of unspecified breast

D05.01 Lobular carcinoma in situ of right breast

D05.02 Lobular carcinoma in situ of left breast

✓5th **D05.1 Intraductal carcinoma in situ of breast**

D05.10 Intraductal carcinoma in situ of unspecified breast

D05.11 Intraductal carcinoma in situ of right breast

D05.12 Intraductal carcinoma in situ of left breast

✓5th **D05.8 Other specified type of carcinoma in situ of breast**

D05.80 Other specified type of carcinoma in situ of unspecified breast

D05.81 Other specified type of carcinoma in situ of right breast

D05.82 **Other specified type of carcinoma in situ of left breast**

✓5th D05.9 **Unspecified type of carcinoma in situ of breast**

D05.90 **Unspecified type of carcinoma in situ of unspecified breast**

D05.91 **Unspecified type of carcinoma in situ of right breast**

D05.92 **Unspecified type of carcinoma in situ of left breast**

✓4th **D06 Carcinoma in situ of cervix uteri**

INCLUDES cervical adenocarcinoma in situ
cervical intraepithelial glandular neoplasia
cervical intraepithelial neoplasia III [CIN III]
severe dysplasia of cervix uteri

EXCLUDES 1 *cervical intraepithelial neoplasia II [CIN II] (N87.1)*
cytologic evidence of malignancy of cervix without histologic confirmation (R87.614)
high grade squamous intraepithelial lesion (HGSIL) of cervix (R87.613)
melanoma in situ of cervix (D03.5)
moderate cervical dysplasia (N87.1)

D06.0 **Carcinoma in situ of endocervix** ♀

D06.1 **Carcinoma in situ of exocervix** ♀

D06.7 **Carcinoma in situ of other parts of cervix** ♀

D06.9 **Carcinoma in situ of cervix, unspecified** ♀

✓4th **D07 Carcinoma in situ of other and unspecified genital organs**

EXCLUDES 1 *melanoma in situ of trunk (D03.5)*

D07.0 **Carcinoma in situ of endometrium** ♀

D07.1 **Carcinoma in situ of vulva** ♀
Severe dysplasia of vulva
Vulvar intraepithelial neoplasia III [VIN III]
EXCLUDES 1 *moderate dysplasia of vulva (N90.1)*
vulvar intraepithelial neoplasia II [VIN II] (N90.1)

D07.2 **Carcinoma in situ of vagina** ♀
Severe dysplasia of vagina
Vaginal intraepithelial neoplasia III [VAIN III]
EXCLUDES 1 *moderate dysplasia of vagina (N89.1)*
vaginal intraepithelial neoplasia II [VIN II] (N89.1)

✓5th D07.3 **Carcinoma in situ of other and unspecified female genital organs**

D07.30 **Carcinoma in situ of unspecified female genital organs** ♀

D07.39 **Carcinoma in situ of other female genital organs** ♀

D07.4 **Carcinoma in situ of penis** ♂
Erythroplasia of Queyrat NOS

D07.5 **Carcinoma in situ of prostate** ♂
Prostatic intraepithelial neoplasia III (PIN III)
Severe dysplasia of prostate
EXCLUDES 1 *dysplasia (mild) (moderate) of prostate (N42.3)*

✓5th D07.6 **Carcinoma in situ of other and unspecified male genital organs**

D07.60 **Carcinoma in situ of unspecified male genital organs** ♂

D07.61 **Carcinoma in situ of scrotum** ♂

D07.69 **Carcinoma in situ of other male genital organs** ♂

✓4th **D09 Carcinoma in situ of other and unspecified sites**

EXCLUDES 1 *melanoma in situ (D03.-)*

D09.0 **Carcinoma in situ of bladder**

✓5th D09.1 **Carcinoma in situ of other and unspecified urinary organs**

D09.10 **Carcinoma in situ of unspecified urinary organ**

D09.19 **Carcinoma in situ of other urinary organs**

✓5th D09.2 **Carcinoma in situ of eye**
EXCLUDES 1 *carcinoma in situ of skin of eyelid (D04.1-)*

D09.20 **Carcinoma in situ of unspecified eye**

D09.21 **Carcinoma in situ of right eye**

D09.22 **Carcinoma in situ of left eye**

D09.3 **Carcinoma in situ of thyroid and other endocrine glands**
EXCLUDES 1 *carcinoma in situ of endocrine pancreas (D01.7)*
carcinoma in situ of ovary (D07.39)
carcinoma in situ of testis (D07.69)

D09.8 **Carcinoma in situ of other specified sites**

D09.9 **Carcinoma in situ, unspecified**

Benign neoplasms, except benign neuroendocrine tumors (D10-D36)

✓4th **D10 Benign neoplasm of mouth and pharynx**

D10.0 **Benign neoplasm of lip**
Benign neoplasm of lip (frenulum) (inner aspect) (mucosa) (vermilion border)
EXCLUDES 1 *benign neoplasm of skin of lip (D22.0, D23.0)*

D10.1 **Benign neoplasm of tongue**
Benign neoplasm of lingual tonsil

D10.2 **Benign neoplasm of floor of mouth**

✓5th D10.3 **Other and unspecified parts of mouth**

D10.30 **Benign neoplasm of unspecified part of mouth**

D10.39 **Benign neoplasm of other parts of mouth**
Benign neoplasm of minor salivary gland NOS
EXCLUDES 1 *benign odontogenic neoplasms (D16.4-D16.5)*
benign neoplasm of mucosa of lip (D10.0)
benign neoplasm of nasopharyngeal surface of soft palate (D10.6)

D10.4 **Benign neoplasm of tonsil**
Benign neoplasm of tonsil (faucial) (palatine)
EXCLUDES 1 *benign neoplasm of lingual tonsil (D10.1)*
benign neoplasm of pharyngeal tonsil (D10.6)
benign neoplasm of tonsillar fossa (D10.5)
benign neoplasm of tonsillar pillars (D10.5)

D10.5 **Benign neoplasm of other parts of oropharynx**
Benign neoplasm of epiglottis, anterior aspect
Benign neoplasm of tonsillar fossa
Benign neoplasm of tonsillar pillars
Benign neoplasm of vallecula
EXCLUDES 1 *benign neoplasm of epiglottis NOS (D14.1)*
benign neoplasm of epiglottis, suprahyoid portion (D14.1)

D10.6 **Benign neoplasm of nasopharynx**
Benign neoplasm of pharyngeal tonsil
Benign neoplasm of posterior margin of septum and choanae

D10.7 **Benign neoplasm of hypopharynx**

D10.9 **Benign neoplasm of pharynx, unspecified**

✓4th **D11 Benign neoplasm of major salivary glands**

EXCLUDES 1 *benign neoplasms of specified minor salivary glands which are classified according to their anatomical location*
benign neoplasms of minor salivary glands NOS (D10.39)

D11.0 **Benign neoplasm of parotid gland**

D11.7 **Benign neoplasm of other major salivary glands**
Benign neoplasm of sublingual salivary gland
Benign neoplasm of submandibular salivary gland

D11.9 **Benign neoplasm of major salivary gland, unspecified**

✓4th **D12 Benign neoplasm of colon, rectum, anus and anal canal**

EXCLUDES 1 *benign carcinoid tumors of the large intestine, and rectum (D3A.02-)*

D12.0 **Benign neoplasm of cecum**
Benign neoplasm of ileocecal valve

D12.1 **Benign neoplasm of appendix**
EXCLUDES 1 *benign carcinoid tumor of the appendix (D3A.020)*

D12.2 **Benign neoplasm of ascending colon**

D12.3 **Benign neoplasm of transverse colon**
Benign neoplasm of hepatic flexure
Benign neoplasm of splenic flexure

D12.4 **Benign neoplasm of descending colon**

D12.5 **Benign neoplasm of sigmoid colon**

D12.6 **Benign neoplasm of colon, unspecified**
Adenomatosis of colon
Benign neoplasm of large intestine NOS
Polyposis (hereditary) of colon
EXCLUDES 1 *inflammatory polyp of colon (K51.4-)*
polyp of colon NOS (K63.5)

D12.7 **Benign neoplasm of rectosigmoid junction**

D12.8 **Benign neoplasm of rectum**
EXCLUDES 1 *benign carcinoid tumor of the rectum (D3A.026)*

D12.9 **Benign neoplasm of anus and anal canal**
Benign neoplasm of anus NOS
EXCLUDES 1 *benign neoplasm of anal margin (D22.5, D23.5)*
benign neoplasm of anal skin (D22.5, D23.5)
benign neoplasm of perianal skin (D22.5, D23.5)

✓4th **D13 Benign neoplasm of other and ill-defined parts of digestive system**
EXCLUDES 1 *benign stromal tumors of digestive system (D21.4)*

D13.Ø Benign neoplasm of esophagus

D13.1 Benign neoplasm of stomach
EXCLUDES 1 *benign carcinoid tumor of the stomach (D3A.Ø92)*

D13.2 Benign neoplasm of duodenum
EXCLUDES 1 *benign carcinoid tumor of the duodenum (D3A.Ø1Ø)*

✓5th **D13.3 Benign neoplasm of other and unspecified parts of small intestine**
EXCLUDES 1 *benign carcinoid tumors of the small intestine (D3A.Ø1)*
benign neoplasm of ileocecal valve (D12.Ø)

D13.3Ø Benign neoplasm of unspecified part of small intestine

D13.39 Benign neoplasm of other parts of small intestine

D13.4 Benign neoplasm of liver
Benign neoplasm of intrahepatic bile ducts

D13.5 Benign neoplasm of extrahepatic bile ducts

D13.6 Benign neoplasm of pancreas
EXCLUDES 1 *benign neoplasm of endocrine pancreas (D13.7)*

D13.7 Benign neoplasm of endocrine pancreas
Islet cell tumor
Benign neoplasm of islets of Langerhans
Use additional code to identify any functional activity

D13.9 Benign neoplasm of ill-defined sites within the digestive system
Benign neoplasm of digestive system NOS
Benign neoplasm of intestine NOS
Benign neoplasm of spleen

✓4th **D14 Benign neoplasm of middle ear and respiratory system**

D14.Ø Benign neoplasm of middle ear, nasal cavity and accessory sinuses
Benign neoplasm of cartilage of nose
EXCLUDES 1 *benign neoplasm of auricular canal (external) (D22.2-, D23.2-)*
benign neoplasm of bone of ear (D16.4)
benign neoplasm of bone of nose (D16.4)
benign neoplasm of cartilage of ear (D21.Ø)
benign neoplasm of ear (external)(skin) (D22.2-, D23.2-)
benign neoplasm of nose NOS (D36.7)
benign neoplasm of skin of nose (D22.39, D23.39)
benign neoplasm of olfactory bulb (D33.3)
benign neoplasm of posterior margin of septum and choanae (D1Ø.6)
polyp of accessory sinus (J33.8)
polyp of ear (middle) (H74.4)
polyp of nasal (cavity) (J33.-)

D14.1 Benign neoplasm of larynx
Adenomatous polyp of larynx
Benign neoplasm of epiglottis (suprahyoid portion)
EXCLUDES 1 *benign neoplasm of epiglottis, anterior aspect (D1Ø.5)*
polyp (nonadenomatous) of vocal cord or larynx (J38.1)

D14.2 Benign neoplasm of trachea

✓5th **D14.3 Benign neoplasm of bronchus and lung**
EXCLUDES 1 *benign carcinoid tumor of the bronchus and lung (D3A.Ø9Ø)*

D14.3Ø Benign neoplasm of unspecified bronchus and lung

D14.31 Benign neoplasm of right bronchus and lung

D14.32 Benign neoplasm of left bronchus and lung

D14.4 Benign neoplasm of respiratory system, unspecified

✓4th **D15 Benign neoplasm of other and unspecified intrathoracic organs**
EXCLUDES 1 *benign neoplasm of mesothelial tissue (D19.-)*

D15.Ø Benign neoplasm of thymus
EXCLUDES 1 *benign carcinoid tumor of the thymus (D3A.Ø91)*

D15.1 Benign neoplasm of heart
EXCLUDES 1 *benign neoplasm of great vessels (D21.3)*

D15.2 Benign neoplasm of mediastinum

D15.7 Benign neoplasm of other specified intrathoracic organs

D15.9 Benign neoplasm of intrathoracic organ, unspecified

✓4th **D16 Benign neoplasm of bone and articular cartilage**
EXCLUDES 1 *benign neoplasm of connective tissue of ear (D21.Ø)*
benign neoplasm of connective tissue of eyelid (D21.Ø)
benign neoplasm of connective tissue of larynx (D14.1)
benign neoplasm of connective tissue of nose (D14.Ø)
benign neoplasm of synovia (D21.-)

✓5th **D16.Ø Benign neoplasm of scapula and long bones of upper limb**

D16.ØØ Benign neoplasm of scapula and long bones of unspecified upper limb

D16.Ø1 Benign neoplasm of scapula and long bones of right upper limb

D16.Ø2 Benign neoplasm of scapula and long bones of left upper limb

✓5th **D16.1 Benign neoplasm of short bones of upper limb**

D16.1Ø Benign neoplasm of short bones of unspecified upper limb

D16.11 Benign neoplasm of short bones of right upper limb

D16.12 Benign neoplasm of short bones of left upper limb

✓5th **D16.2 Benign neoplasm of long bones of lower limb**

D16.2Ø Benign neoplasm of long bones of unspecified lower limb

D16.21 Benign neoplasm of long bones of right lower limb

D16.22 Benign neoplasm of long bones of left lower limb

✓5th **D16.3 Benign neoplasm of short bones of lower limb**

D16.3Ø Benign neoplasm of short bones of unspecified lower limb

D16.31 Benign neoplasm of short bones of right lower limb

D16.32 Benign neoplasm of short bones of left lower limb

D16.4 Benign neoplasm of bones of skull and face
Benign neoplasm of maxilla (superior)
Benign neoplasm of orbital bone
Keratocyst of maxilla
Keratocystic odontogenic tumor of maxilla
EXCLUDES 1 *benign neoplasm of lower jaw bone (D16.5)*

D16.5 Benign neoplasm of lower jaw bone
Keratocyst of mandible
Keratocystic odontogenic tumor of mandible

D16.6 Benign neoplasm of vertebral column
EXCLUDES 1 *benign neoplasm of sacrum and coccyx (D16.8)*

D16.7 Benign neoplasm of ribs, sternum and clavicle

D16.8 Benign neoplasm of pelvic bones, sacrum and coccyx

D16.9 Benign neoplasm of bone and articular cartilage, unspecified

✓4th **D17 Benign lipomatous neoplasm**

D17.Ø Benign lipomatous neoplasm of skin and subcutaneous tissue of head, face and neck

D17.1 Benign lipomatous neoplasm of skin and subcutaneous tissue of trunk

✓5th **D17.2 Benign lipomatous neoplasm of skin and subcutaneous tissue of limb**

D17.2Ø Benign lipomatous neoplasm of skin and subcutaneous tissue of unspecified limb

D17.21 Benign lipomatous neoplasm of skin and subcutaneous tissue of right arm

D17.22 Benign lipomatous neoplasm of skin and subcutaneous tissue of left arm

D17.23 Benign lipomatous neoplasm of skin and subcutaneous tissue of right leg

D17.24 Benign lipomatous neoplasm of skin and subcutaneous tissue of left leg

✓5th **D17.3 Benign lipomatous neoplasm of skin and subcutaneous tissue of other and unspecified sites**

D17.3Ø Benign lipomatous neoplasm of skin and subcutaneous tissue of unspecified sites

D17.39 Benign lipomatous neoplasm of skin and subcutaneous tissue of other sites

D17.4 Benign lipomatous neoplasm of intrathoracic organs

D17.5 Benign lipomatous neoplasm of intra-abdominal organs
EXCLUDES 1 *benign lipomatous neoplasm of peritoneum and retroperitoneum (D17.79)*

D17.6 Benign lipomatous neoplasm of spermatic cord ♂

✓5th **D17.7 Benign lipomatous neoplasm of other sites**

D17.71 Benign lipomatous neoplasm of kidney

D17.72 Benign lipomatous neoplasm of other genitourinary organ

D17.79 Benign lipomatous neoplasm of other sites
Benign lipomatous neoplasm of peritoneum
Benign lipomatous neoplasm of retroperitoneum

D17.9 Benign lipomatous neoplasm, unspecified
Lipoma NOS

D18 Hemangioma and lymphangioma, any site
EXCLUDES 1 *benign neoplasm of glomus jugulare (D35.6)*
blue or pigmented nevus (D22.-)
nevus NOS (D22.-)
vascular nevus (Q82.5)

D18.0 Hemangioma
Angioma NOS
Cavernous nevus

D18.00 Hemangioma unspecified site
D18.01 Hemangioma of skin and subcutaneous tissue
D18.02 Hemangioma of intracranial structures
D18.03 Hemangioma of intra-abdominal structures
D18.09 Hemangioma of other sites
D18.1 Lymphangioma, any site

D19 Benign neoplasm of mesothelial tissue
D19.0 Benign neoplasm of mesothelial tissue of pleura
D19.1 Benign neoplasm of mesothelial tissue of peritoneum
D19.7 Benign neoplasm of mesothelial tissue of other sites
D19.9 Benign neoplasm of mesothelial tissue, unspecified
Benign mesothelioma NOS

D20 Benign neoplasm of soft tissue of retroperitoneum and peritoneum
EXCLUDES 1 *benign lipomatous neoplasm of peritoneum and retroperitoneum (D17.79)*
benign neoplasm of mesothelial tissue (D19.-)

D20.0 Benign neoplasm of soft tissue of retroperitoneum
D20.1 Benign neoplasm of soft tissue of peritoneum

D21 Other benign neoplasms of connective and other soft tissue
INCLUDES benign neoplasm of blood vessel
benign neoplasm of bursa
benign neoplasm of cartilage
benign neoplasm of fascia
benign neoplasm of fat
benign neoplasm of ligament, except uterine
benign neoplasm of lymphatic channel
benign neoplasm of muscle
benign neoplasm of synovia
benign neoplasm of tendon (sheath)
benign stromal tumors
EXCLUDES 1 *benign neoplasm of articular cartilage (D16.-)*
benign neoplasm of cartilage of larynx (D14.1)
benign neoplasm of cartilage of nose (D14.0)
benign neoplasm of connective tissue of breast (D24.-)
benign neoplasm of peripheral nerves and autonomic nervous system (D36.1-)
benign neoplasm of peritoneum (D20.1)
benign neoplasm of retroperitoneum (D20.0)
benign neoplasm of uterine ligament, any (D28.2)
benign neoplasm of vascular tissue (D18.-)
hemangioma (D18.0-)
lipomatous neoplasm (D17.-)
lymphangioma (D18.1)
uterine leiomyoma (D25.-)

D21.0 Benign neoplasm of connective and other soft tissue of head, face and neck
Benign neoplasm of connective tissue of ear
Benign neoplasm of connective tissue of eyelid
EXCLUDES 1 *benign neoplasm of connective tissue of orbit (D31.6-)*

D21.1 Benign neoplasm of connective and other soft tissue of upper limb, including shoulder
D21.10 Benign neoplasm of connective and other soft tissue of unspecified upper limb, including shoulder
D21.11 Benign neoplasm of connective and other soft tissue of right upper limb, including shoulder
D21.12 Benign neoplasm of connective and other soft tissue of left upper limb, including shoulder

D21.2 Benign neoplasm of connective and other soft tissue of lower limb, including hip
D21.20 Benign neoplasm of connective and other soft tissue of unspecified lower limb, including hip
D21.21 Benign neoplasm of connective and other soft tissue of right lower limb, including hip
D21.22 Benign neoplasm of connective and other soft tissue of left lower limb, including hip

D21.3 Benign neoplasm of connective and other soft tissue of thorax
Benign neoplasm of axilla
Benign neoplasm of diaphragm
Benign neoplasm of great vessels
EXCLUDES 1 *benign neoplasm of heart (D15.1)*
benign neoplasm of mediastinum (D15.2)
benign neoplasm of thymus (D15.0)

D21.4 Benign neoplasm of connective and other soft tissue of abdomen
Benign stromal tumors of abdomen

D21.5 Benign neoplasm of connective and other soft tissue of pelvis
EXCLUDES 1 *benign neoplasm of any uterine ligament (D28.2)*
uterine leiomyoma (D25.-)

D21.6 Benign neoplasm of connective and other soft tissue of trunk, unspecified
Benign neoplasm of back NOS

D21.9 Benign neoplasm of connective and other soft tissue, unspecified

D22 Melanocytic nevi
INCLUDES atypical nevus
blue hairy pigmented nevus
nevus NOS

D22.0 Melanocytic nevi of lip

D22.1 Melanocytic nevi of eyelid, including canthus
D22.10 Melanocytic nevi of unspecified eyelid, including canthus
D22.11 Melanocytic nevi of right eyelid, including canthus
D22.12 Melanocytic nevi of left eyelid, including canthus

D22.2 Melanocytic nevi of ear and external auricular canal
D22.20 Melanocytic nevi of unspecified ear and external auricular canal
D22.21 Melanocytic nevi of right ear and external auricular canal
D22.22 Melanocytic nevi of left ear and external auricular canal

D22.3 Melanocytic nevi of other and unspecified parts of face
D22.30 Melanocytic nevi of unspecified part of face
D22.39 Melanocytic nevi of other parts of face
D22.4 Melanocytic nevi of scalp and neck
D22.5 Melanocytic nevi of trunk
Melanocytic nevi of anal margin
Melanocytic nevi of anal skin
Melanocytic nevi of perianal skin
Melanocytic nevi of skin of breast

D22.6 Melanocytic nevi of upper limb, including shoulder
D22.60 Melanocytic nevi of unspecified upper limb, including shoulder
D22.61 Melanocytic nevi of right upper limb, including shoulder
D22.62 Melanocytic nevi of left upper limb, including shoulder

D22.7 Melanocytic nevi of lower limb, including hip
D22.70 Melanocytic nevi of unspecified lower limb, including hip
D22.71 Melanocytic nevi of right lower limb, including hip
D22.72 Melanocytic nevi of left lower limb, including hip
D22.9 Melanocytic nevi, unspecified

D23 Other benign neoplasms of skin
INCLUDES benign neoplasm of hair follicles
benign neoplasm of sebaceous glands
benign neoplasm of sweat glands
EXCLUDES 1 *benign lipomatous neoplasms of skin (D17.0-D17.3)*
melanocytic nevi (D22.-)

D23.0 Other benign neoplasm of skin of lip
EXCLUDES 1 *benign neoplasm of vermilion border of lip (D10.0)*

D23.1 Other benign neoplasm of skin of eyelid, including canthus
D23.10 Other benign neoplasm of skin of unspecified eyelid, including canthus
D23.11 Other benign neoplasm of skin of right eyelid, including canthus
D23.12 Other benign neoplasm of skin of left eyelid, including canthus

✓5th **D23.2 Other benign neoplasm of skin of ear and external auricular canal**
- **D23.20 Other benign neoplasm of skin of unspecified ear and external auricular canal**
- **D23.21 Other benign neoplasm of skin of right ear and external auricular canal**
- **D23.22 Other benign neoplasm of skin of left ear and external auricular canal**

✓5th **D23.3 Other benign neoplasm of skin of other and unspecified parts of face**
- **D23.30 Other benign neoplasm of skin of unspecified part of face**
- **D23.39 Other benign neoplasm of skin of other parts of face**

D23.4 Other benign neoplasm of skin of scalp and neck

D23.5 Other benign neoplasm of skin of trunk
Other benign neoplasm of anal margin
Other benign neoplasm of anal skin
Other benign neoplasm of perianal skin
Other benign neoplasm of skin of breast
EXCLUDES 1 *benign neoplasm of anus NOS (D12.9)*

✓5th **D23.6 Other benign neoplasm of skin of upper limb, including shoulder**
- **D23.60 Other benign neoplasm of skin of unspecified upper limb, including shoulder**
- **D23.61 Other benign neoplasm of skin of right upper limb, including shoulder**
- **D23.62 Other benign neoplasm of skin of left upper limb, including shoulder**

✓5th **D23.7 Other benign neoplasm of skin of lower limb, including hip**
- **D23.70 Other benign neoplasm of skin of unspecified lower limb, including hip**
- **D23.71 Other benign neoplasm of skin of right lower limb, including hip**
- **D23.72 Other benign neoplasm of skin of left lower limb, including hip**

D23.9 Other benign neoplasm of skin, unspecified

✓4th D24 Benign neoplasm of breast
INCLUDES benign neoplasm of connective tissue of breast
benign neoplasm of soft parts of breast
fibroadenoma of breast
EXCLUDES 2 *adenofibrosis of breast (N60.2)*
benign cyst of breast (N60.-)
benign mammary dysplasia (N60.-)
benign neoplasm of skin of breast (D22.5, D23.5)
fibrocystic disease of breast (N60.-)

- **D24.1 Benign neoplasm of right breast**
- **D24.2 Benign neoplasm of left breast**
- **D24.9 Benign neoplasm of unspecified breast**

✓4th D25 Leiomyoma of uterus
INCLUDES uterine fibroid
uterine fibromyoma
uterine myoma

- **D25.0 Submucous leiomyoma of uterus** ♀
- **D25.1 Intramural leiomyoma of uterus** ♀
  Interstitial leiomyoma of uterus
- **D25.2 Subserosal leiomyoma of uterus** ♀
  Subperitoneal leiomyoma of uterus
- **D25.9 Leiomyoma of uterus, unspecified** ♀

✓4th D26 Other benign neoplasms of uterus
- **D26.0 Other benign neoplasm of cervix uteri** ♀
- **D26.1 Other benign neoplasm of corpus uteri** ♀
- **D26.7 Other benign neoplasm of other parts of uterus** ♀
- **D26.9 Other benign neoplasm of uterus, unspecified** ♀

✓4th D27 Benign neoplasm of ovary
Use additional code to identify any functional activity
EXCLUDES 2 *corpus albicans cyst (N83.2)*
corpus luteum cyst (N83.1)
endometrial cyst (N80.1)
follicular (atretic) cyst (N83.0)
graafian follicle cyst (N83.0)
ovarian cyst NEC (N83.2)
ovarian retention cyst (N83.2)

- **D27.0 Benign neoplasm of right ovary** ♀
- **D27.1 Benign neoplasm of left ovary** ♀
- **D27.9 Benign neoplasm of unspecified ovary** ♀

✓4th D28 Benign neoplasm of other and unspecified female genital organs
INCLUDES adenomatous polyp
benign neoplasm of skin of female genital organs
benign teratoma
EXCLUDES 1 *epoophoron cyst (Q50.5)*
fimbrial cyst (Q50.4)
Gartner's duct cyst (Q52.4)
parovarian cyst (Q50.5)

- **D28.0 Benign neoplasm of vulva** ♀
- **D28.1 Benign neoplasm of vagina** ♀
- **D28.2 Benign neoplasm of uterine tubes and ligaments** ♀
  Benign neoplasm of fallopian tube
  Benign neoplasm of uterine ligament (broad) (round)
- **D28.7 Benign neoplasm of other specified female genital organs** ♀
- **D28.9 Benign neoplasm of female genital organ, unspecified** ♀

✓4th D29 Benign neoplasm of male genital organs
INCLUDES benign neoplasm of skin of male genital organs

- **D29.0 Benign neoplasm of penis** ♂
- **D29.1 Benign neoplasm of prostate** ♂
  EXCLUDES 1 *enlarged prostate (N40.-)*

✓5th **D29.2 Benign neoplasm of testis**
Use additional code to identify any functional activity
- **D29.20 Benign neoplasm of unspecified testis** ♂
- **D29.21 Benign neoplasm of right testis** ♂
- **D29.22 Benign neoplasm of left testis** ♂

✓5th **D29.3 Benign neoplasm of epididymis**
- **D29.30 Benign neoplasm of unspecified epididymis** ♂
- **D29.31 Benign neoplasm of right epididymis** ♂
- **D29.32 Benign neoplasm of left epididymis** ♂

D29.4 Benign neoplasm of scrotum ♂
Benign neoplasm of skin of scrotum

D29.8 Benign neoplasm of other specified male genital organs ♂
Benign neoplasm of seminal vesicle
Benign neoplasm of spermatic cord
Benign neoplasm of tunica vaginalis

D29.9 Benign neoplasm of male genital organ, unspecified ♂

✓4th D30 Benign neoplasm of urinary organs

✓5th **D30.0 Benign neoplasm of kidney**
EXCLUDES 1 *benign carcinoid tumor of the kidney (D3A.093)*
benign neoplasm of renal calyces (D30.1-)
benign neoplasm of renal pelvis (D30.1-)
- **D30.00 Benign neoplasm of unspecified kidney**
- **D30.01 Benign neoplasm of right kidney**
- **D30.02 Benign neoplasm of left kidney**

✓5th **D30.1 Benign neoplasm of renal pelvis**
- **D30.10 Benign neoplasm of unspecified renal pelvis**
- **D30.11 Benign neoplasm of right renal pelvis**
- **D30.12 Benign neoplasm of left renal pelvis**

✓5th **D30.2 Benign neoplasm of ureter**
EXCLUDES 1 *benign neoplasm of ureteric orifice of bladder (D30.3)*
- **D30.20 Benign neoplasm of unspecified ureter**
- **D30.21 Benign neoplasm of right ureter**
- **D30.22 Benign neoplasm of left ureter**

D30.3 Benign neoplasm of bladder
Benign neoplasm of ureteric orifice of bladder
Benign neoplasm of urethral orifice of bladder

D30.4 Benign neoplasm of urethra
EXCLUDES 1 *benign neoplasm of urethral orifice of bladder (D30.3)*

D30.8 Benign neoplasm of other specified urinary organs
Benign neoplasm of paraurethral glands

D30.9 Benign neoplasm of urinary organ, unspecified
Benign neoplasm of urinary system NOS

✓4th D31 Benign neoplasm of eye and adnexa
EXCLUDES 1 *benign neoplasm of connective tissue of eyelid (D21.0)*
benign neoplasm of optic nerve (D33.3)
benign neoplasm of skin of eyelid (D22.1-, D23.1-)

✓5th **D31.0 Benign neoplasm of conjunctiva**
- **D31.00 Benign neoplasm of unspecified conjunctiva**
- **D31.01 Benign neoplasm of right conjunctiva**
- **D31.02 Benign neoplasm of left conjunctiva**

✓5th **D31.1 Benign neoplasm of cornea**
- **D31.10 Benign neoplasm of unspecified cornea**

D31.11 Benign neoplasm of right cornea

D31.12 Benign neoplasm of left cornea

✓5th **D31.2 Benign neoplasm of retina**

EXCLUDES 1 *dark area on retina (D49.81)*
hemangioma of retina (D49.81)
neoplasm of unspecified behavior of retina and choroid (D49.81)
retinal freckle (D49.81)

D31.2Ø Benign neoplasm of unspecified retina

D31.21 Benign neoplasm of right retina

D31.22 Benign neoplasm of left retina

✓5th **D31.3 Benign neoplasm of choroid**

D31.3Ø Benign neoplasm of unspecified choroid

D31.31 Benign neoplasm of right choroid

D31.32 Benign neoplasm of left choroid

✓5th **D31.4 Benign neoplasm of ciliary body**

D31.4Ø Benign neoplasm of unspecified ciliary body

D31.41 Benign neoplasm of right ciliary body

D31.42 Benign neoplasm of left ciliary body

✓5th **D31.5 Benign neoplasm of lacrimal gland and duct**

Benign neoplasm of lacrimal sac
Benign neoplasm of nasolacrimal duct

D31.5Ø Benign neoplasm of unspecified lacrimal gland and duct

D31.51 Benign neoplasm of right lacrimal gland and duct

D31.52 Benign neoplasm of left lacrimal gland and duct

✓5th **D31.6 Benign neoplasm of unspecified site of orbit**

Benign neoplasm of connective tissue of orbit
Benign neoplasm of extraocular muscle
Benign neoplasm of peripheral nerves of orbit
Benign neoplasm of retrobulbar tissue
Benign neoplasm of retro-ocular tissue

EXCLUDES 1 *benign neoplasm of orbital bone (D16.4)*

D31.6Ø Benign neoplasm of unspecified site of unspecified orbit

D31.61 Benign neoplasm of unspecified site of right orbit

D31.62 Benign neoplasm of unspecified site of left orbit

✓5th **D31.9 Benign neoplasm of unspecified part of eye**

Benign neoplasm of eyeball

D31.9Ø Benign neoplasm of unspecified part of unspecified eye

D31.91 Benign neoplasm of unspecified part of right eye

D31.92 Benign neoplasm of unspecified part of left eye

✓4th **D32 Benign neoplasm of meninges**

D32.Ø Benign neoplasm of cerebral meninges

D32.1 Benign neoplasm of spinal meninges

D32.9 Benign neoplasm of meninges, unspecified

Meningioma NOS

✓4th **D33 Benign neoplasm of brain and other parts of central nervous system**

EXCLUDES 1 *angioma (D18.Ø-)*
benign neoplasm of meninges (D32.-)
benign neoplasm of peripheral nerves and autonomic nervous system (D36.1-)
hemangioma (D18.Ø-)
neurofibromatosis (Q85.Ø-)
retro-ocular benign neoplasm (D31.6-)

D33.Ø Benign neoplasm of brain, supratentorial

Benign neoplasm of cerebral ventricle
Benign neoplasm of cerebrum
Benign neoplasm of frontal lobe
Benign neoplasm of occipital lobe
Benign neoplasm of parietal lobe
Benign neoplasm of temporal lobe

EXCLUDES 1 *benign neoplasm of fourth ventricle (D33.1)*

D33.1 Benign neoplasm of brain, infratentorial

Benign neoplasm of brain stem
Benign neoplasm of cerebellum
Benign neoplasm of fourth ventricle

D33.2 Benign neoplasm of brain, unspecified

D33.3 Benign neoplasm of cranial nerves

Benign neoplasm of olfactory bulb

D33.4 Benign neoplasm of spinal cord

D33.7 Benign neoplasm of other specified parts of central nervous system

D33.9 Benign neoplasm of central nervous system, unspecified

Benign neoplasm of nervous system (central) NOS

D34 Benign neoplasm of thyroid gland

Use additional code to identify any functional activity

✓4th **D35 Benign neoplasm of other and unspecified endocrine glands**

Use additional code to identify any functional activity

EXCLUDES 1 *benign neoplasm of endocrine pancreas (D13.7)*
benign neoplasm of ovary (D27.-)
benign neoplasm of testis (D29.2-)
benign neoplasm of thymus (D15.Ø)

✓5th **D35.Ø Benign neoplasm of adrenal gland**

D35.ØØ Benign neoplasm of unspecified adrenal gland

D35.Ø1 Benign neoplasm of right adrenal gland

D35.Ø2 Benign neoplasm of left adrenal gland

D35.1 Benign neoplasm of parathyroid gland

D35.2 Benign neoplasm of pituitary gland

D35.3 Benign neoplasm of craniopharyngeal duct

D35.4 Benign neoplasm of pineal gland

D35.5 Benign neoplasm of carotid body

D35.6 Benign neoplasm of aortic body and other paraganglia

Benign tumor of glomus jugulare

D35.7 Benign neoplasm of other specified endocrine glands

D35.9 Benign neoplasm of endocrine gland, unspecified

Benign neoplasm of unspecified endocrine gland

✓4th **D36 Benign neoplasm of other and unspecified sites**

D36.Ø Benign neoplasm of lymph nodes

EXCLUDES 1 *lymphangioma (D18.1)*

✓5th **D36.1 Benign neoplasm of peripheral nerves and autonomic nervous system**

EXCLUDES 1 *benign neoplasm of peripheral nerves of orbit (D31.6-)*
neurofibromatosis (Q85.Ø-)

D36.1Ø Benign neoplasm of peripheral nerves and autonomic nervous system, unspecified

D36.11 Benign neoplasm of peripheral nerves and autonomic nervous system of face, head, and neck

D36.12 Benign neoplasm of peripheral nerves and autonomic nervous system, upper limb, including shoulder

D36.13 Benign neoplasm of peripheral nerves and autonomic nervous system of lower limb, including hip

D36.14 Benign neoplasm of peripheral nerves and autonomic nervous system of thorax

D36.15 Benign neoplasm of peripheral nerves and autonomic nervous system of abdomen

D36.16 Benign neoplasm of peripheral nerves and autonomic nervous system of pelvis

D36.17 Benign neoplasm of peripheral nerves and autonomic nervous system of trunk, unspecified

D36.7 Benign neoplasm of other specified sites

Benign neoplasm of nose NOS

D36.9 Benign neoplasm, unspecified site

Benign neuroendocrine tumors (D3A)

✓4th **D3A Benign neuroendocrine tumors**

Code also any associated multiple endocrine neoplasia [MEN] syndromes (E31.2-)
Use additional code to identify any associated endocrine syndrome, such as:
carcinoid syndrome (E34.Ø)

EXCLUDES 2 *benign pancreatic islet cell tumors (D13.7)*

✓5th **D3A.Ø Benign carcinoid tumors**

D3A.ØØ Benign carcinoid tumor of unspecified site

Carcinoid tumor NOS

✓6th **D3A.Ø1 Benign carcinoid tumors of the small intestine**

D3A.Ø1Ø Benign carcinoid tumor of the duodenum

D3A.Ø11 Benign carcinoid tumor of the jejunum

D3A.Ø12 Benign carcinoid tumor of the ileum

D3A.Ø19 Benign carcinoid tumor of the small intestine, unspecified portion

✓6th **D3A.Ø2 Benign carcinoid tumors of the appendix, large intestine, and rectum**

D3A.Ø2Ø Benign carcinoid tumor of the appendix

D3A.Ø21 Benign carcinoid tumor of the cecum

D3A.022 **Benign carcinoid tumor of the ascending colon**

D3A.023 **Benign carcinoid tumor of the transverse colon**

D3A.024 **Benign carcinoid tumor of the descending colon**

D3A.025 **Benign carcinoid tumor of the sigmoid colon**

D3A.026 **Benign carcinoid tumor of the rectum**

D3A.029 **Benign carcinoid tumor of the large intestine, unspecified portion**
Benign carcinoid tumor of the colon NOS

✓6th D3A.09 **Benign carcinoid tumors of other sites**

D3A.090 **Benign carcinoid tumor of the bronchus and lung**

D3A.091 **Benign carcinoid tumor of the thymus**

D3A.092 **Benign carcinoid tumor of the stomach**

D3A.093 **Benign carcinoid tumor of the kidney**

D3A.094 **Benign carcinoid tumor of the foregut NOS**

D3A.095 **Benign carcinoid tumor of the midgut NOS**

D3A.096 **Benign carcinoid tumor of the hindgut NOS**

D3A.098 **Benign carcinoid tumors of other sites**

D3A.8 **Other benign neuroendocrine tumors**
Neuroendocrine tumor NOS

Neoplasms of uncertain behavior, polycythemia vera and myelodysplastic syndromes (D37-D48)

NOTE Categories D37-D44, and D48 classify by site neoplasms of uncertain behavior, i.e., histologic confirmation whether the neoplasm is malignant or benign cannot be made.

EXCLUDES 1 *neoplasms of unspecified behavior (D49.-)*

✓4th **D37 Neoplasm of uncertain behavior of oral cavity and digestive organs**

EXCLUDES 1 *stromal tumors of uncertain behavior of digestive system (D48.1)*

✓5th D37.0 **Neoplasm of uncertain behavior of lip, oral cavity and pharynx**

EXCLUDES 1 *neoplasm of uncertain behavior of aryepiglottic fold or interarytenoid fold, laryngeal aspect (D38.0)*
neoplasm of uncertain behavior of epiglottis NOS (D38.0)
neoplasm of uncertain behavior of skin of lip (D48.5)
neoplasm of uncertain behavior of suprahyoid portion of epiglottis (D38.0)

D37.01 **Neoplasm of uncertain behavior of lip**
Neoplasm of uncertain behavior of vermilion border of lip

D37.02 **Neoplasm of uncertain behavior of tongue**

✓6th D37.03 **Neoplasm of uncertain behavior of the major salivary glands**

D37.030 **Neoplasm of uncertain behavior of the parotid salivary glands**

D37.031 **Neoplasm of uncertain behavior of the sublingual salivary glands**

D37.032 **Neoplasm of uncertain behavior of the submandibular salivary glands**

D37.039 **Neoplasm of uncertain behavior of the major salivary glands, unspecified**

D37.04 **Neoplasm of uncertain behavior of the minor salivary glands**
Neoplasm of uncertain behavior of submucosal salivary glands of lip
Neoplasm of uncertain behavior of submucosal salivary glands of cheek
Neoplasm of uncertain behavior of submucosal salivary glands of hard palate
Neoplasm of uncertain behavior of submucosal salivary glands of soft palate

D37.05 **Neoplasm of uncertain behavior of pharynx**
Neoplasm of uncertain behavior of aryepiglottic fold of pharynx NOS
Neoplasm of uncertain behavior of hypopharyngeal aspect of aryepiglottic fold of pharynx
Neoplasm of uncertain behavior of marginal zone of aryepiglottic fold of pharynx

D37.09 **Neoplasm of uncertain behavior of other specified sites of the oral cavity**

D37.1 **Neoplasm of uncertain behavior of stomach**

D37.2 **Neoplasm of uncertain behavior of small intestine**

D37.3 **Neoplasm of uncertain behavior of appendix**

D37.4 **Neoplasm of uncertain behavior of colon**

D37.5 **Neoplasm of uncertain behavior of rectum**
Neoplasm of uncertain behavior of rectosigmoid junction

D37.6 **Neoplasm of uncertain behavior of liver, gallbladder and bile ducts**
Neoplasm of uncertain behavior of ampulla of Vater

D37.8 **Neoplasm of uncertain behavior of other specified digestive organs**
Neoplasm of uncertain behavior of anal canal
Neoplasm of uncertain behavior of anal sphincter
Neoplasm of uncertain behavior of anus NOS
Neoplasm of uncertain behavior of esophagus
Neoplasm of uncertain behavior of intestine NOS
Neoplasm of uncertain behavior of pancreas

EXCLUDES 1 *neoplasm of uncertain behavior of anal margin (D48.5)*
neoplasm of uncertain behavior of anal skin (D48.5)
neoplasm of uncertain behavior of perianal skin (D48.5)

D37.9 **Neoplasm of uncertain behavior of digestive organ, unspecified**

✓4th **D38 Neoplasm of uncertain behavior of middle ear and respiratory and intrathoracic organs**

EXCLUDES 1 *neoplasm of uncertain behavior of heart (D48.7)*

D38.0 **Neoplasm of uncertain behavior of larynx**
Neoplasm of uncertain behavior of aryepiglottic fold or interarytenoid fold, laryngeal aspect
Neoplasm of uncertain behavior of epiglottis (suprahyoid portion)

EXCLUDES 1 *neoplasm of uncertain behavior of aryepiglottic fold or interarytenoid fold NOS (D37.05)*
neoplasm of uncertain behavior of hypopharyngeal aspect of aryepiglottic fold (D37.05)
neoplasm of uncertain behavior of marginal zone of aryepiglottic fold (D37.05)

D38.1 **Neoplasm of uncertain behavior of trachea, bronchus and lung**

D38.2 **Neoplasm of uncertain behavior of pleura**

D38.3 **Neoplasm of uncertain behavior of mediastinum**

D38.4 **Neoplasm of uncertain behavior of thymus**

D38.5 **Neoplasm of uncertain behavior of other respiratory organs**
Neoplasm of uncertain behavior of accessory sinuses
Neoplasm of uncertain behavior of cartilage of nose
Neoplasm of uncertain behavior of middle ear
Neoplasm of uncertain behavior of nasal cavities

EXCLUDES 1 *neoplasm of uncertain behavior of ear (external) (skin) (D48.5)*
neoplasm of uncertain behavior of nose NOS (D48.7)
neoplasm of uncertain behavior of skin of nose (D48.5)

D38.6 **Neoplasm of uncertain behavior of respiratory organ, unspecified**

✓4th **D39 Neoplasm of uncertain behavior of female genital organs**

D39.0 **Neoplasm of uncertain behavior of uterus** ♀

✓5th D39.1 **Neoplasm of uncertain behavior of ovary**
Use additional code to identify any functional activity

D39.10 **Neoplasm of uncertain behavior of unspecified ovary** ♀

D39.11 **Neoplasm of uncertain behavior of right ovary** ♀

D39.12 **Neoplasm of uncertain behavior of left ovary** ♀

D39.2 **Neoplasm of uncertain behavior of placenta** ♀
Chorioadenoma destruens
Invasive hydatidiform mole
Malignant hydatidiform mole

EXCLUDES 1 *hydatidiform mole NOS (O01.9)*

D39.8 **Neoplasm of uncertain behavior of other specified female genital organs** ♀
Neoplasm of uncertain behavior of skin of female genital organs

D39.9 **Neoplasm of uncertain behavior of female genital organ, unspecified** ♀

✓4th **D40 Neoplasm of uncertain behavior of male genital organs**

D40.0 **Neoplasm of uncertain behavior of prostate** ♂

✓5th D40.1 **Neoplasm of uncertain behavior of testis**

D40.10 **Neoplasm of uncertain behavior of unspecified testis** ♂

D40.11 **Neoplasm of uncertain behavior of right testis** ♂

D40.12 **Neoplasm of uncertain behavior of left testis** ♂

D40.8 Neoplasm of uncertain behavior of other specified male genital organs ♂
Neoplasm of uncertain behavior of skin of male genital organs

D40.9 Neoplasm of uncertain behavior of male genital organ, unspecified ♂

✓4th **D41 Neoplasm of uncertain behavior of urinary organs**

✓5th **D41.0 Neoplasm of uncertain behavior of kidney**
EXCLUDES 1 *neoplasm of uncertain behavior of renal pelvis (D41.1-)*

D41.00 Neoplasm of uncertain behavior of unspecified kidney

D41.01 Neoplasm of uncertain behavior of right kidney

D41.02 Neoplasm of uncertain behavior of left kidney

✓5th **D41.1 Neoplasm of uncertain behavior of renal pelvis**

D41.10 Neoplasm of uncertain behavior of unspecified renal pelvis

D41.11 Neoplasm of uncertain behavior of right renal pelvis

D41.12 Neoplasm of uncertain behavior of left renal pelvis

✓5th **D41.2 Neoplasm of uncertain behavior of ureter**

D41.20 Neoplasm of uncertain behavior of unspecified ureter

D41.21 Neoplasm of uncertain behavior of right ureter

D41.22 Neoplasm of uncertain behavior of left ureter

D41.3 Neoplasm of uncertain behavior of urethra

D41.4 Neoplasm of uncertain behavior of bladder

D41.8 Neoplasm of uncertain behavior of other specified urinary organs

D41.9 Neoplasm of uncertain behavior of unspecified urinary organ

✓4th **D42 Neoplasm of uncertain behavior of meninges**

D42.0 Neoplasm of uncertain behavior of cerebral meninges

D42.1 Neoplasm of uncertain behavior of spinal meninges

D42.9 Neoplasm of uncertain behavior of meninges, unspecified

✓4th **D43 Neoplasm of uncertain behavior of brain and central nervous system**
EXCLUDES 1 *neoplasm of uncertain behavior of peripheral nerves and autonomic nervous system (D48.2)*

D43.0 Neoplasm of uncertain behavior of brain, supratentorial
Neoplasm of uncertain behavior of cerebral ventricle
Neoplasm of uncertain behavior of cerebrum
Neoplasm of uncertain behavior of frontal lobe
Neoplasm of uncertain behavior of occipital lobe
Neoplasm of uncertain behavior of parietal lobe
Neoplasm of uncertain behavior of temporal lobe
EXCLUDES 1 *neoplasm of uncertain behavior of fourth ventricle (D43.1)*

D43.1 Neoplasm of uncertain behavior of brain, infratentorial
Neoplasm of uncertain behavior of brain stem
Neoplasm of uncertain behavior of cerebellum
Neoplasm of uncertain behavior of fourth ventricle

D43.2 Neoplasm of uncertain behavior of brain, unspecified

D43.3 Neoplasm of uncertain behavior of cranial nerves

D43.4 Neoplasm of uncertain behavior of spinal cord

D43.8 Neoplasm of uncertain behavior of other specified parts of central nervous system

D43.9 Neoplasm of uncertain behavior of central nervous system, unspecified
Neoplasm of uncertain behavior of nervous system (central) NOS

✓4th **D44 Neoplasm of uncertain behavior of endocrine glands**
EXCLUDES 1 *multiple endocrine adenomatosis (E31.2-)*
multiple endocrine neoplasia (E31.2-)
neoplasm of uncertain behavior of endocrine pancreas (D37.8)
neoplasm of uncertain behavior of ovary (D39.1-)
neoplasm of uncertain behavior of testis (D40.1-)
neoplasm of uncertain behavior of thymus (D38.4)

D44.0 Neoplasm of uncertain behavior of thyroid gland

✓5th **D44.1 Neoplasm of uncertain behavior of adrenal gland**
Use additional code to identify any functional activity

D44.10 Neoplasm of uncertain behavior of unspecified adrenal gland

D44.11 Neoplasm of uncertain behavior of right adrenal gland

D44.12 Neoplasm of uncertain behavior of left adrenal gland

D44.2 Neoplasm of uncertain behavior of parathyroid gland

D44.3 Neoplasm of uncertain behavior of pituitary gland
Use additional code to identify any functional activity

D44.4 Neoplasm of uncertain behavior of craniopharyngeal duct

D44.5 Neoplasm of uncertain behavior of pineal gland

D44.6 Neoplasm of uncertain behavior of carotid body

D44.7 Neoplasm of uncertain behavior of aortic body and other paraganglia

D44.9 Neoplasm of uncertain behavior of unspecified endocrine gland

D45 Polycythemia vera
EXCLUDES 1 *familial polycythemia (D75.0)*
secondary polycythemia (D75.1)

✓4th **D46 Myelodysplastic syndromes**
Use additional code for adverse effect, if applicable, to identify drug (T36-T50 with fifth or sixth character 5)
EXCLUDES 2 *drug-induced aplastic anemia (D61.1)*

D46.0 Refractory anemia without ring sideroblasts, so stated
Refractory anemia without sideroblasts, without excess of blasts

D46.1 Refractory anemia with ring sideroblasts
RARS

✓5th **D46.2 Refractory anemia with excess of blasts**

D46.20 Refractory anemia with excess of blasts, unspecified
RAEB NOS

D46.21 Refractory anemia with excess of blasts 1
RAEB 1

D46.22 Refractory anemia with excess of blasts 2 CC
RAEB 2
CC Excl: C88.2-C88.3, C88.8-C88.9, C90.10-C90.11, C90.20-C90.21, C90.30-C90.31, C91.00-C95.92, D45-D47.1, D47.3, D47.Z9-D47.9, D48.7-D48.9

D46.A Refractory cytopenia with multilineage dysplasia

D46.B Refractory cytopenia with multilineage dysplasia and ring sideroblasts
RCMD RS

D46.C Myelodysplastic syndrome with isolated del(5q) chromosomal abnormality CC
Myelodysplastic syndrome with 5q deletion
5q minus syndrome NOS
CC Excl: See code: D46.22

D46.4 Refractory anemia, unspecified

D46.Z Other myelodysplastic syndromes
EXCLUDES 1 *chronic myelomonocytic leukemia (C93.1-)*

D46.9 Myelodysplastic syndrome, unspecified
Myelodysplasia NOS

✓4th **D47 Other neoplasms of uncertain behavior of lymphoid, hematopoietic and related tissue**

D47.0 Histiocytic and mast cell tumors of uncertain behavior CC
Indolent systemic mastocytosis
Mast cell tumor NOS
Mastocytoma NOS
EXCLUDES 1 *malignant mast cell tumor (C96.2)*
mastocytosis (congenital) (cutaneous) (Q82.2)
CC Excl: C88.8, C94.40-C94.6, D45-D47.1, D47.3, D47.Z9-D47.9, D75.81, Z51.0

D47.1 Chronic myeloproliferative disease CC
Chronic neutrophilic leukemia
Myeloproliferative disease, unspecified
EXCLUDES 1 *atypical chronic myeloid leukemia BCR/ABL-negative (C92.2-)*
chronic myeloid leukemia BCR/ABL-positive (C92.1-)
myelofibrosis NOS (D75.81)
myelophthisic anemia (D61.82)
myelophthisis (D61.82)
secondary myelofibrosis NOS (D75.81)
CC Excl: See code: D46.22

D47.2 Monoclonal gammopathy
Monoclonal gammopathy of undetermined significance [MGUS]

D47.3 Essential (hemorrhagic) thrombocythemia
Essential thrombocytosis
Idiopathic hemorrhagic thrombocythemia

D47.4 Osteomyelofibrosis
Chronic idiopathic myelofibrosis
Myelofibrosis (idiopathic) (with myeloid metaplasia)
Myelosclerosis (megakaryocytic) with myeloid metaplasia
Secondary myelofibrosis in myeloproliferative disease
EXCLUDES 1 *acute myelofibrosis (C94.4-)*

✓5th **D47.Z Other specified neoplasms of uncertain behavior of lymphoid, hematopoietic and related tissue**

D47.Z1 Post-transplant lymphoproliferative disorder (PTLD) CC

Code first complications of transplanted organs and tissue (T86.-)

CC Excl: D47.Z1, D78.81-D78.89, E89.810-E89.89, H59.011-H59.019, H59.031-H59.099, H59.811-H59.89, H95.811-H95.89, I97.3, M96.89, N98.1-N98.9, T86.850-T86.859, T86.90-T86.99

D47.Z9 Other specified neoplasms of uncertain behavior of lymphoid, hematopoietic and related tissue CC

Histiocytic tumors of uncertain behavior

CC Excl: C88.2-C88.3, C88.8-C88.9, C90.10-C90.11, C90.20-C90.21, C90.30-C90.31, C91.00-C95.92, D45-D47.1, D47.3, D47.Z9-D47.9, D48.7-D48.9

D47.9 Neoplasm of uncertain behavior of lymphoid, hematopoietic and related tissue, unspecified CC

Lymphoproliferative disease NOS

CC Excl: See code: D47.Z9

✓4th **D48 Neoplasm of uncertain behavior of other and unspecified sites**

EXCLUDES 1 *neurofibromatosis (nonmalignant) (Q85.0-)*

D48.0 Neoplasm of uncertain behavior of bone and articular cartilage

EXCLUDES 1 *neoplasm of uncertain behavior of cartilage of ear (D48.1)*
neoplasm of uncertain behavior of cartilage of larynx (D38.0)
neoplasm of uncertain behavior of cartilage of nose (D38.5)
neoplasm of uncertain behavior of connective tissue of eyelid (D48.1)
neoplasm of uncertain behavior of synovia (D48.1)

D48.1 Neoplasm of uncertain behavior of connective and other soft tissue

Neoplasm of uncertain behavior of connective tissue of ear
Neoplasm of uncertain behavior of connective tissue of eyelid
Stromal tumors of uncertain behavior of digestive system

EXCLUDES 1 *neoplasm of uncertain behavior of articular cartilage (D48.0)*
neoplasm of uncertain behavior of cartilage of larynx (D38.0)
neoplasm of uncertain behavior of cartilage of nose (D38.5)
neoplasm of uncertain behavior of connective tissue of breast (D48.6-)

D48.2 Neoplasm of uncertain behavior of peripheral nerves and autonomic nervous system

EXCLUDES 1 *neoplasm of uncertain behavior of peripheral nerves of orbit (D48.7)*

D48.3 Neoplasm of uncertain behavior of retroperitoneum

D48.4 Neoplasm of uncertain behavior of peritoneum

D48.5 Neoplasm of uncertain behavior of skin

Neoplasm of uncertain behavior of anal margin
Neoplasm of uncertain behavior of anal skin
Neoplasm of uncertain behavior of perianal skin
Neoplasm of uncertain behavior of skin of breast

EXCLUDES 1 *neoplasm of uncertain behavior of anus NOS (D37.8)*
neoplasm of uncertain behavior of skin of genital organs (D39.8, D40.8)
neoplasm of uncertain behavior of vermilion border of lip (D37.0)

✓5th **D48.6 Neoplasm of uncertain behavior of breast**

Neoplasm of uncertain behavior of connective tissue of breast
Cystosarcoma phyllodes

EXCLUDES 1 *neoplasm of uncertain behavior of skin of breast (D48.5)*

D48.60 Neoplasm of uncertain behavior of unspecified breast

D48.61 Neoplasm of uncertain behavior of right breast

D48.62 Neoplasm of uncertain behavior of left breast

D48.7 Neoplasm of uncertain behavior of other specified sites

Neoplasm of uncertain behavior of eye
Neoplasm of uncertain behavior of heart
Neoplasm of uncertain behavior of peripheral nerves of orbit

EXCLUDES 1 *neoplasm of uncertain behavior of connective tissue (D48.1)*
neoplasm of uncertain behavior of skin of eyelid (D48.5)

D48.9 Neoplasm of uncertain behavior, unspecified

Neoplasms of unspecified behavior (D49)

✓4th **D49 Neoplasms of unspecified behavior**

NOTE Category D49 classifies by site neoplasms of unspecified morphology and behavior. The term "mass", unless otherwise stated, is not to be regarded as a neoplastic growth.

INCLUDES "growth" NOS
neoplasm NOS
new growth NOS
tumor NOS

EXCLUDES 1 *neoplasms of uncertain behavior (D37-D44, D48)*

D49.0 Neoplasm of unspecified behavior of digestive system

EXCLUDES 1 *neoplasm of unspecified behavior of margin of anus (D49.2)*
neoplasm of unspecified behavior of perianal skin (D49.2)
neoplasm of unspecified behavior of skin of anus (D49.2)

D49.1 Neoplasm of unspecified behavior of respiratory system

D49.2 Neoplasm of unspecified behavior of bone, soft tissue, and skin

EXCLUDES 1 *neoplasm of unspecified behavior of anal canal (D49.0)*
neoplasm of unspecified behavior of anus NOS (D49.0)
neoplasm of unspecified behavior of bone marrow (D49.89)
neoplasm of unspecified behavior of cartilage of larynx (D49.1)
neoplasm of unspecified behavior of cartilage of nose (D49.1)
neoplasm of unspecified behavior of connective tissue of breast (D49.3)
neoplasm of unspecified behavior of skin of genital organs (D49.5)
neoplasm of unspecified behavior of vermilion border of lip (D49.0)

D49.3 Neoplasm of unspecified behavior of breast

EXCLUDES 1 *neoplasm of unspecified behavior of skin of breast (D49.2)*

D49.4 Neoplasm of unspecified behavior of bladder

D49.5 Neoplasm of unspecified behavior of other genitourinary organs

D49.6 Neoplasm of unspecified behavior of brain

EXCLUDES 1 *neoplasm of unspecified behavior of cerebral meninges (D49.7)*
neoplasm of unspecified behavior of cranial nerves (D49.7)

D49.7 Neoplasm of unspecified behavior of endocrine glands and other parts of nervous system

EXCLUDES 1 *neoplasm of unspecified behavior of peripheral, sympathetic, and parasympathetic nerves and ganglia (D49.2)*

✓5th **D49.8 Neoplasm of unspecified behavior of other specified sites**

EXCLUDES 1 *neoplasm of unspecified behavior of eyelid (skin) (D49.2)*
neoplasm of unspecified behavior of eyelid cartilage (D49.2)
neoplasm of unspecified behavior of great vessels (D49.2)
neoplasm of unspecified behavior of optic nerve (D49.7)

D49.81 Neoplasm of unspecified behavior of retina and choroid

Dark area on retina
Retinal freckle

D49.89 Neoplasm of unspecified behavior of other specified sites

D49.9 Neoplasm of unspecified behavior of unspecified site

Chapter 3. Diseases of the Blood and Blood-forming Organs and Certain Disorders Involving the Immune Mechanism (D50-D89)

EXCLUDES 2 *autoimmune disease (systemic) NOS (M35.9)*
certain conditions originating in the perinatal period (P00-P96)
complications of pregnancy, childbirth and the puerperium (O00-O9A)
congenital malformations, deformations and chromosomal abnormalities (Q00-Q99)
endocrine, nutritional and metabolic diseases (E00-E88)
human immunodeficiency virus [HIV] disease (B20)
injury, poisoning and certain other consequences of external causes (S00-T88)
neoplasms (C00-D49)
symptoms, signs and abnormal clinical and laboratory findings, not elsewhere classified (R00-R94)

This chapter contains the following blocks:

D50-D53	Nutritional anemias
D55-D59	Hemolytic anemias
D60-D64	Aplastic and other anemias and other bone marrow failure syndromes
D65-D69	Coagulation defects, purpura and other hemorrhagic conditions
D70-D77	Other disorders of blood and blood-forming organs
D78	Intraoperative and postprocedural complications of the spleen
D80-D89	Certain disorders involving the immune mechanism

Nutritional anemias (D50-D53)

✓4th **D50 Iron deficiency anemia**
INCLUDES asiderotic anemia
hypochromic anemia

D50.0 Iron deficiency anemia secondary to blood loss (chronic)
Posthemorrhagic anemia (chronic)
EXCLUDES 1 *acute posthemorrhagic anemia (D62)*
congenital anemia from fetal blood loss (P61.3)

D50.1 Sideropenic dysphagia
Kelly-Paterson syndrome
Plummer-Vinson syndrome

D50.8 Other iron deficiency anemias
Iron deficiency anemia due to inadequate dietary iron intake

D50.9 Iron deficiency anemia, unspecified

✓4th **D51 Vitamin B12 deficiency anemia**
EXCLUDES 1 *vitamin B12 deficiency (E53.8)*

D51.0 Vitamin B12 deficiency anemia due to intrinsic factor deficiency
Addison anemia
Biermer anemia
Pernicious (congenital) anemia
Congenital intrinsic factor deficiency

D51.1 Vitamin B12 deficiency anemia due to selective vitamin B12 malabsorption with proteinuria
Imerslund (Gräsbeck) syndrome
Megaloblastic hereditary anemia

D51.2 Transcobalamin II deficiency

D51.3 Other dietary vitamin B12 deficiency anemia
Vegan anemia

D51.8 Other vitamin B12 deficiency anemias

D51.9 Vitamin B12 deficiency anemia, unspecified

✓4th **D52 Folate deficiency anemia**
EXCLUDES 1 *folate deficiency without anemia (E53.8)*

D52.0 Dietary folate deficiency anemia
Nutritional megaloblastic anemia

D52.1 Drug-induced folate deficiency anemia
Use additional code for adverse effect, if applicable, to identify drug (T36-T50 with fifth or sixth character 5)

D52.8 Other folate deficiency anemias

D52.9 Folate deficiency anemia, unspecified
Folic acid deficiency anemia NOS

✓4th **D53 Other nutritional anemias**
INCLUDES megaloblastic anemia unresponsive to vitamin B12 or folate therapy

D53.0 Protein deficiency anemia
Amino-acid deficiency anemia
Orotaciduric anemia
EXCLUDES 1 *Lesch-Nyhan syndrome (E79.1)*

D53.1 Other megaloblastic anemias, not elsewhere classified
Megaloblastic anemia NOS
EXCLUDES 1 *Di Guglielmo's disease (C94.0)*

D53.2 Scorbutic anemia
EXCLUDES 1 *scurvy (E54)*

D53.8 Other specified nutritional anemias
Anemia associated with deficiency of copper
Anemia associated with deficiency of molybdenum
Anemia associated with deficiency of zinc
EXCLUDES 1 *nutritional deficiencies without anemia, such as:*
copper deficiency NOS (E61.0)
molybdenum deficiency NOS (E61.5)
zinc deficiency NOS (E60)

D53.9 Nutritional anemia, unspecified
Simple chronic anemia
EXCLUDES 1 *anemia NOS (D64.9)*

Hemolytic anemias (D55-D59)

✓4th **D55 Anemia due to enzyme disorders**
EXCLUDES 1 *drug-induced enzyme deficiency anemia (D59.2)*

D55.0 Anemia due to glucose-6-phosphate dehydrogenase [G6PD] deficiency
Favism
G6PD deficiency anemia

D55.1 Anemia due to other disorders of glutathione metabolism
Anemia (due to) enzyme deficiencies, except G6PD, related to the hexose monophosphate [HMP] shunt pathway
Anemia (due to) hemolytic nonspherocytic (hereditary), type I

D55.2 Anemia due to disorders of glycolytic enzymes
Hemolytic nonspherocytic (hereditary) anemia, type II
Hexokinase deficiency anemia
Pyruvate kinase [PK] deficiency anemia
Triose-phosphate isomerase deficiency anemia
EXCLUDES 1 *disorders of glycolysis not associated with anemia (E74.8)*

D55.3 Anemia due to disorders of nucleotide metabolism

D55.8 Other anemias due to enzyme disorders

D55.9 Anemia due to enzyme disorder, unspecified

✓4th **D56 Thalassemia**
EXCLUDES 1 *sickle-cell thalassemia (D57.4-)*

D56.0 Alpha thalassemia
Alpha thalassemia major
Hemoglobin H Constant Spring
Hemoglobin H disease
Hydrops fetalis due to alpha thalassemia
Severe alpha thalassemia
Triple gene defect alpha thalassemia
Use additional code, if applicable, for hydrops fetalis due to alpha thalassemia (P56.99)
EXCLUDES 1 *alpha thalassemia trait or minor (D56.3)*
asymptomatic alpha thalassemia (D56.3)
hydrops fetalis due to isoimmunization (P56.0)
hydrops fetalis not due to immune hemolysis (P83.2)

D56.1 Beta thalassemia
Beta thalassemia major
Cooley's anemia
Homozygous beta thalassemia
Severe beta thalassemia
Thalassemia intermedia
Thalassemia major
EXCLUDES 1 *beta thalassemia minor (D56.3)*
beta thalassemia trait (D56.3)
delta-beta thalassemia (D56.2)
hemoglobin E-beta thalassemia (D56.5)
sickle-cell beta thalassemia (D57.4-)

D56.2 Delta-beta thalassemia
Homozygous delta-beta thalassemia
EXCLUDES 1 *delta-beta thalassemia minor (D56.3)*
delta-beta thalassemia trait (D56.3)

D56.3 Thalassemia minor
- Alpha thalassemia minor
- Alpha thalassemia silent carrier
- Alpha thalassemia trait
- Beta thalassemia minor
- Beta thalassemia trait
- Delta-beta thalassemia minor
- Delta-beta thalassemia trait
- Thalassemia trait NOS

EXCLUDES 1 *alpha thalassemia (D56.Ø)*
beta thalassemia (D56.1)
delta-beta thalassemia (D56.2)
hemoglobin E-beta thalassemia (D56.5)
sickle-cell trait (D57.3)

D56.4 Hereditary persistence of fetal hemoglobin [HPFH]

D56.5 Hemoglobin E-beta thalassemia

EXCLUDES 1 *beta thalassemia (D56.1)*
beta thalassemia minor (D56.3)
beta thalassemia trait (D56.3)
delta-beta thalassemia (D56.2)
delta-beta thalassemia trait (D56.3)
hemoglobin E disease (D58.2)
other hemoglobinopathies (D58.2)
sickle-cell beta thalassemia (D57.4-)

D56.8 Other thalassemias
- Dominant thalassemia
- Hemoglobin C thalassemia
- Mixed thalassemia
- Thalassemia with other hemoglobinopathy

EXCLUDES 1 *hemoglobin C disease (D58.2)*
hemoglobin E disease (D58.2)
other hemoglobinopathies (D58.2)
sickle-cell anemia (D57.-)
sickle-cell thalassemia (D57.4)

D56.9 Thalassemia, unspecified
- Mediterranean anemia (with other hemoglobinopathy)

✓4th **D57 Sickle-cell disorders**

Use additional code for any associated fever (R5Ø.81)

EXCLUDES 1 *other hemoglobinopathies (D58.-)*

CC Excl: For MCC codes in category D57, unless otherwise noted: D47.4, D5Ø.Ø-D64.9, D68.312, D68.51-D68.69, D75.81, D75.89-D75.9, D77, D89.2

✓5th **D57.Ø Hb-SS disease with crisis**
- Sickle-cell disease NOS with crisis
- Hb-SS disease with vasoocclusive pain

D57.ØØ Hb-SS disease with crisis, unspecified MCC

D57.Ø1 Hb-SS disease with acute chest syndrome MCC

D57.Ø2 Hb-SS disease with splenic sequestration MCC

D57.1 Sickle-cell disease without crisis
- Hb-SS disease without crisis
- Sickle-cell anemia NOS
- Sickle-cell disease NOS
- Sickle-cell disorder NOS

✓5th **D57.2 Sickle-cell/Hb-C disease**
- Hb-SC disease
- Hb-S/Hb-C disease

D57.2Ø Sickle-cell/Hb-C disease without crisis

✓6th **D57.21 Sickle-cell/Hb-C disease with crisis**

D57.211 Sickle-cell/Hb-C disease with acute chest syndrome PDx CC MCC

D57.212 Sickle-cell/Hb-C disease with splenic sequestration MCC

D57.219 Sickle-cell/Hb-C disease with crisis, unspecified MCC
- Sickle-cell/Hb-C disease with crisis NOS

D57.3 Sickle-cell trait
- Hb-S trait
- Heterozygous hemoglobin S

✓5th **D57.4 Sickle-cell thalassemia**
- Sickle-cell beta thalassemia
- Thalassemia Hb-S disease

D57.4Ø Sickle-cell thalassemia without crisis
- Microdrepanocytosis
- Sickle-cell thalassemia NOS

✓6th **D57.41 Sickle-cell thalassemia with crisis**
- Sickle-cell thalassemia with vasoocclusive pain

D57.411 Sickle-cell thalassemia with acute chest syndrome PDx CC MCC

D57.412 Sickle-cell thalassemia with splenic sequestration MCC

D57.419 Sickle-cell thalassemia with crisis, unspecified MCC
- Sickle-cell thalassemia with crisis NOS

✓5th **D57.8 Other sickle-cell disorders**
- Hb-SD disease
- Hb-SE disease

D57.8Ø Other sickle-cell disorders without crisis

✓6th **D57.81 Other sickle-cell disorders with crisis**

D57.811 Other sickle-cell disorders with acute chest syndrome MCC

D57.812 Other sickle-cell disorders with splenic sequestration MCC

D57.819 Other sickle-cell disorders with crisis, unspecified MCC
- Other sickle-cell disorders with crisis NOS

✓4th **D58 Other hereditary hemolytic anemias**

EXCLUDES 1 *hemolytic anemia of the newborn (P55.-)*

D58.Ø Hereditary spherocytosis
- Acholuric (familial) jaundice
- Congenital (spherocytic) hemolytic icterus
- Minkowski-Chauffard syndrome

D58.1 Hereditary elliptocytosis
- Elliptocytosis (congenital)
- Ovalocytosis (congenital) (hereditary)

D58.2 Other hemoglobinopathies
- Abnormal hemoglobin NOS
- Congenital Heinz body anemia
- Hb-C disease
- Hb-D disease
- Hb-E disease
- Hemoglobinopathy NOS
- Unstable hemoglobin hemolytic disease

EXCLUDES 1 *familial polycythemia (D75.Ø)*
Hb-M disease (D74.Ø)
hemoglobin E-beta thalassemia (D56.5)
hereditary persistence of fetal hemoglobin [HPFH] (D56.4)
high-altitude polycythemia (D75.1)
methemoglobinemia (D74.-)
other hemoglobinopathies with thalassemia (D56.8)

D58.8 Other specified hereditary hemolytic anemias CC
- Stomatocytosis

CC Excl: D5Ø.Ø-D64.9, D75.9, P61.2-P61.4

D58.9 Hereditary hemolytic anemia, unspecified CC

CC Excl: See code: D58.8

✓4th **D59 Acquired hemolytic anemia**

CC Excl: For CC/MCC codes in category D59, unless otherwise noted: D47.4, D5Ø.Ø-D64.9, D68.312, D68.51-D68.69, D75.81, D75.89-D75.9, D77, D89.2

D59.Ø Drug-induced autoimmune hemolytic anemia CC

Use additional code for adverse effect, if applicable, to identify drug (T36-T5Ø with fifth or sixth character 5)

D59.1 Other autoimmune hemolytic anemias CC
- Autoimmune hemolytic disease (cold type) (warm type)
- Chronic cold hemagglutinin disease
- Cold agglutinin disease
- Cold agglutinin hemoglobinuria
- Cold type (secondary) (symptomatic) hemolytic anemia
- Warm type (secondary) (symptomatic) hemolytic anemia

EXCLUDES 1 *Evans syndrome (D69.41)*
hemolytic disease of newborn (P55.-)
paroxysmal cold hemoglobinuria (D59.6)

D59.2 Drug-induced nonautoimmune hemolytic anemia CC
- Drug-induced enzyme deficiency anemia

Use additional code for adverse effect, if applicable, to identify drug (T36-T5Ø with fifth or sixth character 5)

D59.3 Hemolytic-uremic syndrome MCC

Use additional code to identify associated:
- E. coli infection (B96.2-)
- Pneumococcal pneumonia (J13)
- Shigella dysenteriae (AØ3.9)

D59.4 Other nonautoimmune hemolytic anemias CC
- Mechanical hemolytic anemia
- Microangiopathic hemolytic anemia
- Toxic hemolytic anemia

D59.5 Paroxysmal nocturnal hemoglobinuria [Marchiafava-Micheli]

EXCLUDES 1 *hemoglobinuria NOS (R82.3)*

D59.6 Hemoglobinuria due to hemolysis from other external causes
Hemoglobinuria from exertion
March hemoglobinuria
Paroxysmal cold hemoglobinuria
Use additional code (Chapter 20) to identify external cause
EXCLUDES 1 *hemoglobinuria NOS (R82.3)*

D59.8 Other acquired hemolytic anemias

D59.9 Acquired hemolytic anemia, unspecified CC
Idiopathic hemolytic anemia, chronic

Aplastic and other anemias and other bone marrow failure syndromes (D60-D64)

D60 Acquired pure red cell aplasia [erythroblastopenia]
INCLUDES red cell aplasia (acquired) (adult) (with thymoma)
EXCLUDES 1 *congenital red cell aplasia (D61.01)*

CC Excl: For CC/MCC codes in category D60, unless otherwise noted: D47.4, D50.0-D64.9, D68.312, D68.51-D68.69, D75.81, D75.89-D75.9, D77, D89.2

D60.0 Chronic acquired pure red cell aplasia MCC

D60.1 Transient acquired pure red cell aplasia MCC

D60.8 Other acquired pure red cell aplasias MCC

D60.9 Acquired pure red cell aplasia, unspecified MCC

D61 Other aplastic anemias and other bone marrow failure syndromes
EXCLUDES 1 *neutropenia (D70.-)*

D61.0 Constitutional aplastic anemia

D61.01 Constitutional (pure) red blood cell aplasia CC
Blackfan-Diamond syndrome
Congenital (pure) red cell aplasia
Familial hypoplastic anemia
Primary (pure) red cell aplasia
Red cell (pure) aplasia of infants
EXCLUDES 1 *acquired red cell aplasia (D60.9)*
CC Excl: D50.0-D61.3, D61.89-D64.9, D75.9, P61.2-P61.4

D61.09 Other constitutional aplastic anemia CC
Fanconi's anemia
Pancytopenia with malformations
CC Excl: D50.0-D61.3, D61.89-D64.9, D69.3-D69.49, D75.9, P61.2-P61.4

D61.1 Drug-induced aplastic anemia MCC
Use additional code for adverse effect, if applicable, to identify drug (T36-T50 with fifth or sixth character 5)
CC Excl: D47.4, D50.0-D64.9, D68.312, D68.51-D68.69, D75.81, D75.89-D75.9, D77, D89.2

D61.2 Aplastic anemia due to other external agents MCC
Code first, if applicable, toxic effects of substances chiefly nonmedicinal as to source (T51-T65)
CC Excl: See code: D61.1

D61.3 Idiopathic aplastic anemia MCC
CC Excl: See code: D61.1

D61.8 Other specified aplastic anemias and other bone marrow failure syndromes

CC Excl: For CC/MCC codes in subcategory D61.8, unless otherwise noted: D60.0-D60.9, D61.1-D64.9, D70.0-D70.9, D72.810-D72.820, D72.823, D72.825-D72.829, D75.9, D76.1-D76.3, P61.2

D61.81 Pancytopenia
EXCLUDES 1 *pancytopenia (due to) (with) aplastic anemia (D61.9)*
pancytopenia (due to) (with) bone marrow infiltration (D61.82)
pancytopenia (due to) (with) congenital (pure) red cell aplasia (D61.01)
pancytopenia (due to) (with) hairy cell leukemia (C91.4-)
pancytopenia (due to) (with) human immunodeficiency virus disease (B20)
pancytopenia (due to) (with) leukoerythroblastic anemia (D61.82)
pancytopenia (due to) (with) myelodysplastic syndromes (D46.-)
pancytopenia (due to) (with) myeloproliferative disease (D47.1)

D61.810 Antineoplastic chemotherapy induced pancytopenia MCC
EXCLUDES 2 *aplastic anemia due to antineoplastic chemotherapy (D61.1)*

D61.811 Other drug-induced pancytopenia MCC
EXCLUDES 2 *aplastic anemia due to drugs (D61.1)*

D61.818 Other pancytopenia CC

D61.82 Myelophthisis CC
Leukoerythroblastic anemia
Myelophthisic anemia
Panmyelophthisis
Code also the underlying disorder, such as:
malignant neoplasm of breast (C50.-)
tuberculosis (A15.-)
EXCLUDES 1 *idiopathic myelofibrosis (D47.1)*
myelofibrosis NOS (D75.81)
myelofibrosis with myeloid metaplasia (D47.4)
primary myelofibrosis (D47.1)
secondary myelofibrosis (D75.81)

D61.89 Other specified aplastic anemias and other bone marrow failure syndromes MCC
CC Excl: See code: D61.1

D61.9 Aplastic anemia, unspecified CC
Hypoplastic anemia NOS
Medullary hypoplasia
CC Excl: See code: D61.1

D62 Acute posthemorrhagic anemia CC
EXCLUDES 1 *anemia due to chronic blood loss (D50.0)*
blood loss anemia NOS (D50.0)
congenital anemia from fetal blood loss (P61.3)
CC Excl: D47.4, D50.0-D64.9, D68.312, D68.51-D68.69, D75.81, D75.89-D75.9, D77, D89.2, T79.2XXA

D63 Anemia in chronic diseases classified elsewhere

D63.0 Anemia in neoplastic disease
Code first neoplasm (C00-D49)
EXCLUDES 1 *anemia due to antineoplastic chemotherapy (D64.81)*
aplastic anemia due to antineoplastic chemotherapy (D61.1)

D63.1 Anemia in chronic kidney disease
Erythropoietin resistant anemia (EPO resistant anemia)
Code first underlying chronic kidney disease (CKD) (N18.-)

D63.8 Anemia in other chronic diseases classified elsewhere
Code first underlying disease, such as:
diphyllobothriasis (B70.0)
hookworm disease (B76.0-B76.9)
hypothyroidism (E00.0-E03.9)
malaria (B50.0-B54)
symptomatic late syphilis (A52.79)
tuberculosis (A18.89)

D64 Other anemias
EXCLUDES 1 *refractory anemia (D46.-)*
refractory anemia with excess blasts in transformation [RAEB T] (C92.0-)

D64.0 Hereditary sideroblastic anemia
Sex-linked hypochromic sideroblastic anemia

D64.1 Secondary sideroblastic anemia due to disease
Code first underlying disease

D64.2 Secondary sideroblastic anemia due to drugs and toxins
Code first poisoning due to drug or toxin, if applicable (T36-T65 with fifth or sixth character 1-4 or 6)
Use additional code for adverse effect, if applicable, to identify drug (T36-T50 with fifth or sixth character 5)

D64.3 Other sideroblastic anemias
Sideroblastic anemia NOS
Pyridoxine-responsive sideroblastic anemia NEC

D64.4 Congenital dyserythropoietic anemia
Dyshematopoietic anemia (congenital)
EXCLUDES 1 *Blackfan-Diamond syndrome (D61.01)*
Di Guglielmo's disease (C94.0)

D64.8 Other specified anemias

D64.81 Anemia due to antineoplastic chemotherapy
Antineoplastic chemotherapy induced anemia
EXCLUDES 1 *anemia in neoplastic disease (D63.0)*
aplastic anemia due to antineoplastic chemotherapy (D61.1)

D64.89 Other specified anemias
Infantile pseudoleukemia

D64.9 Anemia, unspecified

Coagulation defects, purpura and other hemorrhagic conditions (D65-D69)

D65 Disseminated intravascular coagulation [defibrination syndrome] MCC
Afibrinogenemia, acquired
Consumption coagulopathy
Diffuse or disseminated intravascular coagulation [DIC]
Fibrinolytic hemorrhage, acquired
Fibrinolytic purpura
Purpura fulminans
EXCLUDES 1 *disseminated intravascular coagulation (complicating):*
abortion or ectopic or molar pregnancy (O00-O07, O08.1)
in newborn (P60)
pregnancy, childbirth and the puerperium (O45.0, O46.0, O67.0, O72.3)
CC Excl: D47.4, D65-D69.9, D75.81-D75.9, D77, D89.2

D66 Hereditary factor VIII deficiency MCC
Classical hemophilia
Deficiency factor VIII (with functional defect)
Hemophilia A
Hemophilia NOS
EXCLUDES 1 *factor VIII deficiency with vascular defect (D68.0)*
CC Excl: See code: D65

D67 Hereditary factor IX deficiency MCC
Christmas disease
Factor IX deficiency (with functional defect)
Hemophilia B
Plasma thromboplastin component [PTC] deficiency
CC Excl: See code: D65

4th **D68 Other coagulation defects**
EXCLUDES 1 *abnormal coagulation profile (R79.1)*
coagulation defects complicating abortion or ectopic or molar pregnancy (O00-O07, O08.1)
coagulation defects complicating pregnancy, childbirth and the puerperium (O45.0, O46.0, O67.0, O72.3)

D68.0 Von Willebrand's disease CC
Angiohemophilia
Factor VIII deficiency with vascular defect
Vascular hemophilia
EXCLUDES 1 *capillary fragility (hereditary) (D69.8)*
factor VIII deficiency NOS (D66)
factor VIII deficiency with functional defect (D66)
CC Excl: See code: D65

D68.1 Hereditary factor XI deficiency CC
Hemophilia C
Plasma thromboplastin antecedent [PTA] deficiency
Rosenthal's disease
CC Excl: See code: D65

D68.2 Hereditary deficiency of other clotting factors CC
AC globulin deficiency
Congenital afibrinogenemia
Deficiency of factor I [fibrinogen]
Deficiency of factor II [prothrombin]
Deficiency of factor V [labile]
Deficiency of factor VII [stable]
Deficiency of factor X [Stuart-Prower]
Deficiency of factor XII [Hageman]
Deficiency of factor XIII [fibrin stabilizing]
Dysfibrinogenemia (congenital)
Hypoproconvertinemia
Owren's disease
Proaccelerin deficiency
CC Excl: See code: D65

5th **D68.3 Hemorrhagic disorder due to circulating anticoagulants**

6th **D68.31 Hemorrhagic disorder due to intrinsic circulating anticoagulants, antibodies, or inhibitors**

D68.311 Acquired hemophilia CC
Autoimmune hemophilia
Autoimmune inhibitors to clotting factors
Secondary hemophilia
CC Excl: D47.4, D65-D69.9, D75.82-D75.9, D77, D89.2

D68.312 Antiphospholipid antibody with hemorrhagic disorder CC
Lupus anticoagulant (LAC) with hemorrhagic disorder
Systemic lupus erythematosus [SLE] inhibitor with hemorrhagic disorder
EXCLUDES 1 *antiphospholipid antibody, finding without diagnosis (R76.0)*
antiphospholipid antibody syndrome (D68.61)
antiphospholipid antibody with hypercoagulable state (D68.61)
lupus anticoagulant (LAC) finding without diagnosis (R76.0)
lupus anticoagulant (LAC) with hypercoagulable state (D68.62)
systemic lupus erythematosus [SLE] inhibitor finding without diagnosis (R76.0)
systemic lupus erythematosus [SLE] inhibitor with hypercoagulable state (D68.62)
CC Excl: D47.4, D68.311-D68.318, D68.51-D68.69, D70.0-D72.9, D73.81, D75.81, D75.89-D77, D89.2

D68.318 Other hemorrhagic disorder due to intrinsic circulating anticoagulants, antibodies, or inhibitors CC
Antithromboplastinemia
Antithromboplastinogenemia
Hemorrhagic disorder due to intrinsic increase in antithrombin
Hemorrhagic disorder due to intrinsic increase in anti-VIIIa
Hemorrhagic disorder due to intrinsic increase in anti-IXa
Hemorrhagic disorder due to intrinsic increase in anti-XIa
CC Excl: See code: D68.311

D68.32 Hemorrhagic disorder due to extrinsic circulating anticoagulants CC
Drug-induced hemorrhagic disorder
Hemorrhagic disorder due to increase in anti-IIa
Hemorrhagic disorder due to increase in anti-Xa
Hyperheparinemia
Use additional code for adverse effect, if applicable, to identify drug (T45.515, T45.525)
CC Excl: D47.4, D65-D69.9, D75.81-D75.9, D77, D89.2

D68.4 Acquired coagulation factor deficiency CC
Deficiency of coagulation factor due to liver disease
Deficiency of coagulation factor due to vitamin K deficiency
EXCLUDES 1 *vitamin K deficiency of newborn (P53)*
CC Excl: See code: D68.32

5th **D68.5 Primary thrombophilia**
Primary hypercoagulable states
EXCLUDES 1 *antiphospholipid syndrome (D68.61)*
lupus anticoagulant (D68.62)
secondary activated protein C resistance (D68.69)
secondary antiphospholipid antibody syndrome (D68.69)
secondary lupus anticoagulant with hypercoagulable state (D68.69)
secondary systemic lupus erythematosus [SLE] inhibitor with hypercoagulable state (D68.69)
systemic lupus erythematosus [SLE] inhibitor finding without diagnosis (R76.0)
systemic lupus erythematosus [SLE] inhibitor with hemorrhagic disorder (D68.312)
thrombotic thrombocytopenic purpura (M31.1)

CC Excl: For CC codes in subcategory D68.5, unless otherwise noted: D47.4, D68.312, D68.51-D68.69, D70.0-D72.9, D73.81, D75.81, D75.89-D75.9, D76.1-D77, D89.2

D68.51 Activated protein C resistance CC
Factor V Leiden mutation

D68.52 Prothrombin gene mutation CC

DRAFT

D68.59 Other primary thrombophilia CC
Antithrombin III deficiency
Hypercoagulable state NOS
Primary hypercoagulable state NEC
Primary thrombophilia NEC
Protein C deficiency
Protein S deficiency
Thrombophilia NOS

✓5th **D68.6 Other thrombophilia**
Other hypercoagulable states
EXCLUDES 1 *diffuse or disseminated intravascular coagulation [DIC] (D65)*
heparin induced thrombocytopenia (HIT) (D75.82)
hyperhomocysteinemia (E72.11)

CC Excl: For CC codes in subcategory D68.6, unless otherwise noted: D47.4, D68.312, D68.51-D68.69, D70.0-D72.9, D73.81, D75.81, D75.89-D75.9, D76.1-D77, D89.2

D68.61 Antiphospholipid syndrome CC
Anticardiolipin syndrome
Antiphospholipid antibody syndrome
EXCLUDES 1 *antiphospholipid antibody, finding without diagnosis (R76.0)*
antiphospholipid antibody with hemorrhagic disorder (D68.312)
lupus anticoagulant syndrome (D68.62)

D68.62 Lupus anticoagulant syndrome CC
Lupus anticoagulant
Presence of systemic lupus erythematosus [SLE] inhibitor
EXCLUDES 1 *anticardiolipin syndrome (D68.61)*
antiphospholipid syndrome (D68.61)
lupus anticoagulant (LAC) finding without diagnosis (R79.0)
lupus anticoagulant (LAC) with hemorrhagic disorder (D68.312)

D68.69 Other thrombophilia CC
Hypercoagulable states NEC
Secondary hypercoagulable state NOS

D68.8 Other specified coagulation defects CC
EXCLUDES 1 *hemorrhagic disease of newborn (P53)*
CC Excl: See code: D68.32

D68.9 Coagulation defect, unspecified CC
CC Excl: See code: D68.32

✓4th **D69 Purpura and other hemorrhagic conditions**
EXCLUDES 1 *benign hypergammaglobulinemic purpura (D89.0)*
cryoglobulinemic purpura (D89.1)
essential (hemorrhagic) thrombocythemia (D47.3)
hemorrhagic thrombocythemia (D47.3)
purpura fulminans (D65)
thrombotic thrombocytopenic purpura (M31.1)
Waldenström hypergammaglobulinemic purpura (D89.0)

CC Excl: For CC codes in category D69, unless otherwise noted: D47.4, D65-D69.9, D75.81-D75.9, D77, D89.2

D69.0 Allergic purpura CC
Allergic vasculitis
Nonthrombocytopenic hemorrhagic purpura
Nonthrombocytopenic idiopathic purpura
Purpura anaphylactoid
Purpura Henoch(-Schönlein)
Purpura rheumatica
Vascular purpura
EXCLUDES 1 *thrombocytopenic hemorrhagic purpura (D69.3)*

D69.1 Qualitative platelet defects
Bernard-Soulier [giant platelet] syndrome
Glanzmann's disease
Grey platelet syndrome
Thromboasthenia (hemorrhagic) (hereditary)
Thrombocytopathy
EXCLUDES 1 *von Willebrand's disease (D68.0)*

D69.2 Other nonthrombocytopenic purpura
Purpura NOS
Purpura simplex
Senile purpura

D69.3 Immune thrombocytopenic purpura CC
Hemorrhagic (thrombocytopenic) purpura
Idiopathic thrombocytopenic purpura
Tidal platelet dysgenesis

✓5th **D69.4 Other primary thrombocytopenia**
EXCLUDES 1 *transient neonatal thrombocytopenia (P61.0)*
Wiskott-Aldrich syndrome (D82.0)

D69.41 Evans syndrome CC

D69.42 Congenital and hereditary thrombocytopenia purpura CC
Congenital thrombocytopenia
Hereditary thrombocytopenia
Code first congenital or hereditary disorder, such as: thrombocytopenia with absent radius (TAR syndrome) (Q87.2)

D69.49 Other primary thrombocytopenia
Megakaryocytic hypoplasia
Primary thrombocytopenia NOS

✓5th **D69.5 Secondary thrombocytopenia**
EXCLUDES 1 *heparin induced thrombocytopenia (HIT) (D75.82)*
transient thrombocytopenia of newborn (P61.0)

D69.51 Posttransfusion purpura
Posttransfusion purpura from whole blood (fresh) or blood products
PTP

D69.59 Other secondary thrombocytopenia

D69.6 Thrombocytopenia, unspecified

D69.8 Other specified hemorrhagic conditions
Capillary fragility (hereditary)
Vascular pseudohemophilia

D69.9 Hemorrhagic condition, unspecified

Other disorders of blood and blood-forming organs (D70-D77)

✓4th **D70 Neutropenia**
INCLUDES agranulocytosis
decreased absolute neurophile count (ANC)
Use additional code for any associated:
fever (R50.81)
mucositis (J34.81, K12.3-, K92.81, N76.81)
EXCLUDES 1 *neutropenic splenomegaly (D73.81)*
transient neonatal neutropenia (P61.5)

D70.0 Congenital agranulocytosis
Congenital neutropenia
Infantile genetic agranulocytosis
Kostmann's disease

D70.1 Agranulocytosis secondary to cancer chemotherapy
Code also underlying neoplasm
Use additional code for adverse effect, if applicable, to identify drug (T45.1X5)

D70.2 Other drug-induced agranulocytosis
Use additional code for adverse effect, if applicable, to identify drug (T36-T50 with fifth or sixth character 5)

D70.3 Neutropenia due to infection

D70.4 Cyclic neutropenia
Cyclic hematopoiesis
Periodic neutropenia

D70.8 Other neutropenia

D70.9 Neutropenia, unspecified

D71 Functional disorders of polymorphonuclear neutrophils
Cell membrane receptor complex [CR3] defect
Chronic (childhood) granulomatous disease
Congenital dysphagocytosis
Progressive septic granulomatosis

✓4th **D72 Other disorders of white blood cells**
EXCLUDES 1 *basophilia (D72.824)*
immunity disorders (D80-D89)
neutropenia (D70)
preleukemia (syndrome) (D46.9)

D72.0 Genetic anomalies of leukocytes
Alder (granulation) (granulocyte) anomaly
Alder syndrome
Hereditary leukocytic hypersegmentation
Hereditary leukocytic hyposegmentation
Hereditary leukomelanopathy
May-Hegglin (granulation) (granulocyte) anomaly
May-Hegglin syndrome
Pelger-Huët (granulation) (granulocyte) anomaly
Pelger-Huët syndrome
EXCLUDES 1 *Chédiak (-Steinbrinck)-Higashi syndrome (E70.330)*

D72.1 Eosinophilia
Allergic eosinophilia
Hereditary eosinophilia
EXCLUDES 1 *Löffler's syndrome (J82)*
pulmonary eosinophilia (J82)

✓5th **D72.8 Other specified disorders of white blood cells**
EXCLUDES 1 *leukemia (C91-C95)*

✓6th **D72.81 Decreased white blood cell count**
EXCLUDES 1 *neutropenia (D70.-)*

D72.810 Lymphocytopenia
Decreased lymphocytes

D72.818 Other decreased white blood cell count
Basophilic leukopenia
Eosinophilic leukopenia
Monocytopenia
Other decreased leukocytes
Plasmacytopenia

D72.819 Decreased white blood cell count, unspecified
Decreased leukocytes, unspecified
Leukocytopenia, unspecified
Leukopenia
EXCLUDES 1 *malignant leukopenia (D70.9)*

✓6th **D72.82 Elevated white blood cell count**
EXCLUDES 1 *eosinophilia (D72.1)*

D72.820 Lymphocytosis (symptomatic)
Elevated lymphocytes

D72.821 Monocytosis (symptomatic)
EXCLUDES 1 *infectious mononucleosis (B27.-)*

D72.822 Plasmacytosis

D72.823 Leukemoid reaction
Basophilic leukemoid reaction
Leukemoid reaction NOS
Lymphocytic leukemoid reaction
Monocytic leukemoid reaction
Myelocytic leukemoid reaction
Neutrophilic leukemoid reaction

D72.824 Basophilia

D72.825 Bandemia
Bandemia without diagnosis of specific infection
EXCLUDES 1 *confirmed infection—code to infection*
leukemia (C91.-, C92.-, C93.-, C94.-, C95.-)

D72.828 Other elevated white blood cell count

D72.829 Elevated white blood cell count, unspecified
Elevated leukocytes, unspecified
Leukocytosis, unspecified

D72.89 Other specified disorders of white blood cells
Abnormality of white blood cells NEC

D72.9 Disorder of white blood cells, unspecified
Abnormal leukocyte differential NOS

✓4th **D73 Diseases of spleen**

D73.0 Hyposplenism
Atrophy of spleen
EXCLUDES 1 *asplenia (congenital) (Q89.01)*
postsurgical absence of spleen (Z90.81)

D73.1 Hypersplenism
EXCLUDES 1 *neutropenic splenomegaly (D73.81)*
primary splenic neutropenia (D73.81)
splenitis, splenomegaly in late syphilis (A52.79)
splenitis, splenomegaly in tuberculosis (A18.85)
splenomegaly NOS (R16.1)
splenomegaly congenital (Q89.0)

D73.2 Chronic congestive splenomegaly

D73.3 Abscess of spleen

D73.4 Cyst of spleen

D73.5 Infarction of spleen
Splenic rupture, nontraumatic
Torsion of spleen
EXCLUDES 1 *rupture of spleen due to Plasmodium vivax malaria (B51.0)*
traumatic rupture of spleen (S36.03-)

✓5th **D73.8 Other diseases of spleen**

D73.81 Neutropenic splenomegaly
Werner-Schultz disease

D73.89 Other diseases of spleen
Fibrosis of spleen NOS
Perisplenitis
Splenitis NOS

D73.9 Disease of spleen, unspecified

✓4th **D74 Methemoglobinemia**

CC Excl: For CC codes in category D74, unless otherwise noted: D56.4, D58.2-D59.2, D59.4-D59.9, D64.4-D64.9, D74.0-D74.9, D75.9

D74.0 Congenital methemoglobinemia CC
Congenital NADH-methemoglobin reductase deficiency
Hemoglobin-M [Hb-M] disease
Methemoglobinemia, hereditary

D74.8 Other methemoglobinemias CC
Acquired methemoglobinemia (with sulfhemoglobinemia)
Toxic methemoglobinemia

D74.9 Methemoglobinemia, unspecified CC

✓4th **D75 Other and unspecified diseases of blood and blood-forming organs**
EXCLUDES 2 *acute lymphadenitis (L04.-)*
chronic lymphadenitis (I88.1)
enlarged lymph nodes (R59.-)
hypergammaglobulinemia NOS (D89.2)
lymphadenitis NOS (I88.9)
mesenteric lymphadenitis (acute) (chronic) (I88.0)

D75.0 Familial erythrocytosis
Benign polycythemia
Familial polycythemia
EXCLUDES 1 *hereditary ovalocytosis (D58.1)*

D75.1 Secondary polycythemia
Acquired polycythemia
Emotional polycythemia
Erythrocytosis NOS
Hypoxemic polycythemia
Nephrogenous polycythemia
Polycythemia due to erythropoietin
Polycythemia due to fall in plasma volume
Polycythemia due to high altitude
Polycythemia due to stress
Polycythemia NOS
Relative polycythemia
EXCLUDES 1 *polycythemia neonatorum (P61.1)*
polycythemia vera (D45)

✓5th **D75.8 Other specified diseases of blood and blood-forming organs**

D75.81 Myelofibrosis CC
Myelofibrosis NOS
Secondary myelofibrosis NOS
Code first the underlying disorder, such as:
malignant neoplasm of breast (C50.-)
Use additional code, if applicable, for associated therapy-related myelodysplastic syndrome (D46.-)
Use additional code for adverse effect, if applicable, to identify drug (T45.1X5)
EXCLUDES 1 *acute myelofibrosis (C94.4-)*
idiopathic myelofibrosis (D47.1)
leukoerythroblastic anemia (D61.82)
myelofibrosis with myeloid metaplasia (D47.4)
myelophthisic anemia (D61.82)
myelophthisis (D61.82)
primary myelofibrosis (D47.1)
CC Excl: C88.2-C88.3, C88.8-C88.9, C90.10-C90.11, C90.20-C90.21, C90.30-C90.31, C91.00-C95.92, D45-D47.1, D47.3, D47.Z9-D47.9, D48.7-D48.9

D75.82 Heparin induced thrombocytopenia (HIT)

D75.89 Other specified diseases of blood and blood-forming organs

D75.9 Disease of blood and blood-forming organs, unspecified

D76 Other specified diseases with participation of lymphoreticular and reticulohistiocytic tissue

EXCLUDES 1 *(Abt-) Letterer-Siwe disease (C96.0)*
eosinophilic granuloma (C96.6)
Hand-Schüller-Christian disease (C96.5)
histiocytic sarcoma (C96.A)
histiocytosis X, multifocal (C96.5)
histiocytosis X, unifocal (C96.6)
Langerhans-cell histiocytosis, multifocal (C96.5)
Langerhans-cell histiocytosis NOS (C96.6)
Langerhans-cell histiocytosis, unifocal (C96.6)
leukemic reticuloendotheliosis or reticulosis (C91.4-)
lipomelanotic reticuloendotheliosis or reticulosis (I89.8)
malignant histiocytosis (C96.A)

D76.1 Hemophagocytic lymphohistiocytosis CC
Familial hemophagocytic reticulosis
Histiocytoses of mononuclear phagocytes
CC Excl: D60.0-D60.9, D61.1-D61.9, D65, D69.3-D70.9, D72.818-D72.819, D75.82, D75.9

D76.2 Hemophagocytic syndrome, infection-associated CC
Use additional code to identify infectious agent or disease
CC Excl: See code: D76.1

D76.3 Other histiocytosis syndromes CC
Reticulohistiocytoma (giant-cell)
Sinus histiocytosis with massive lymphadenopathy
Xanthogranuloma
CC Excl: See code: D76.1

D77 Other disorders of blood and blood-forming organs in diseases classified elsewhere

Code first underlying disease, such as:
amyloidosis (E85.-)
congenital early syphilis (A50.0)
echinococcosis (B67.0-B67.9)
malaria (B50.0-B54)
schistosomiasis [bilharziasis] (B65.0-B65.9)
vitamin C deficiency (E54)

EXCLUDES 1 *rupture of spleen due to Plasmodium vivax malaria (B51.0)*
splenitis, splenomegaly in late syphilis (A52.79)
splenitis, splenomegaly in tuberculosis (A18.85)

Intraoperative and postprocedural complications of the spleen (D78)

D78 Intraoperative and postprocedural complications of the spleen

D78.0 Intraoperative hemorrhage and hematoma of the spleen complicating a procedure

EXCLUDES 1 *intraoperative hemorrhage and hematoma of the spleen due to accidental puncture or laceration during a procedure (D78.1-)*

D78.01 Intraoperative hemorrhage and hematoma of the spleen complicating a procedure on the spleen CC
CC Excl: D78.01-D78.02, D78.21-D78.89, H95.811-H95.89, I85.01, I85.11, I97.3, K21.9, K22.8, K23-K25.0, K25.2, K25.4, K25.6, K26.0, K26.2, K26.4, K26.6, K27.0, K27.2, K27.4, K27.6, K28.0, K28.2, K28.4, K28.6, K29.01, K29.21, K29.31, K29.41, K29.51, K29.61, K29.71, K29.81, K29.91, K31.811, K55.21, K57.01, K57.11, K57.13, K57.21, K57.31, K57.33, K57.41, K57.51, K57.53, K57.81, K57.91, K57.93, K62.5, K92.0-K92.2, M96.89, N98.1-N98.9, P54.1-P54.3, T81.10XA, T81.11XA, T81.12XA, T81.19XA, T81.82XA, T81.89XA, T81.9XXA

D78.02 Intraoperative hemorrhage and hematoma of the spleen complicating other procedure CC
CC Excl: See code: D78.01

D78.1 Accidental puncture and laceration of the spleen during a procedure

D78.11 Accidental puncture and laceration of the spleen during a procedure on the spleen CC
CC Excl: D78.11-D78.12, D78.81-D78.89, E36.11-E36.8, E89.810-E89.89, G96.11, G97.41-G97.49, H59.011-H59.019, H59.031-H59.099, H59.211-H59.229, H59.811-H59.89, H95.31-H95.32, H95.811-H95.89, I97.3, I97.51-I97.52, J95.71-J95.72, K91.71-K91.72, L76.11-L76.12, L76.81-L76.82, M96.820-M96.821, M96.89, N98.1-N98.9, N99.71-N99.72, T81.82XXA, T81.89XX1, T81.9XXA

D78.12 Accidental puncture and laceration of the spleen during other procedure CC
CC Excl: See code: D78.11

D78.2 Postprocedural hemorrhage and hematoma of the spleen following a procedure

D78.21 Postprocedural hemorrhage and hematoma of the spleen following a procedure on the spleen CC
CC Excl: See code: D78.01

D78.22 Postprocedural hemorrhage and hematoma of the spleen following other procedure CC
CC Excl: See code: D78.01

D78.8 Other intraoperative and postprocedural complications of the spleen
Use additional code, if applicable, to further specify disorder

D78.81 Other intraoperative complications of the spleen CC
CC Excl: D78.81-D78.89, H95.811-H95.89, I97.3, M96.89, N98.1-N98.9, T81.82XA, T81.89XA, T81.9XXA

D78.89 Other postprocedural complications of the spleen CC
CC Excl: See code: D78.81

Certain disorders involving the immune mechanism (D80-D89)

INCLUDES defects in the complement system
immunodeficiency disorders, except human immunodeficiency virus [HIV] disease
sarcoidosis

EXCLUDES 1 *autoimmune disease (systemic) NOS (M35.9)*
functional disorders of polymorphonuclear neutrophils (D71)
human immunodeficiency virus [HIV] disease (B20)

D80 Immunodeficiency with predominantly antibody defects

CC Excl: For CC codes in category D80, unless otherwise noted: D80.0, D80.3-D81.2, D81.4, D81.6-D81.7, D81.89-D84.0, D84.8-D84.9, D89.3, D89.82-D89.9

D80.0 Hereditary hypogammaglobulinemia CC
Autosomal recessive agammaglobulinemia (Swiss type)
X-linked agammaglobulinemia [Bruton] (with growth hormone deficiency)

D80.1 Nonfamilial hypogammaglobulinemia CC
Agammaglobulinemia with immunoglobulin-bearing B-lymphocytes
Common variable agammaglobulinemia [CVAgamma]
Hypogammaglobulinemia NOS
CC Excl: D80.0-D81.2, D81.4, D81.6-D81.7, D81.89-D84.0, D84.8-D84.9, D89.3, D89.82-D89.9

D80.2 Selective deficiency of immunoglobulin A [IgA] CC
D80.3 Selective deficiency of immunoglobulin G [IgG] subclasses CC
D80.4 Selective deficiency of immunoglobulin M [IgM] CC
D80.5 Immunodeficiency with increased immunoglobulin M [IgM] CC
D80.6 Antibody deficiency with near-normal immunoglobulins or with hyperimmunoglobulinemia CC
D80.7 Transient hypogammaglobulinemia of infancy CC N
D80.8 Other immunodeficiencies with predominantly antibody defects CC
Kappa light chain deficiency
D80.9 Immunodeficiency with predominantly antibody defects, unspecified CC

D81 Combined immunodeficiencies

EXCLUDES 1 *autosomal recessive agammaglobulinemia (Swiss type) (D80.0)*

CC Excl: For CC codes in category D81, unless otherwise noted: D80.0, D80.3-D81.2, D81.4, D81.6-D81.7, D81.89-D84.0, D84.8-D84.9, D89.3, D89.82-D89.9

D81.0 Severe combined immunodeficiency [SCID] with reticular dysgenesis CC
D81.1 Severe combined immunodeficiency [SCID] with low T- and B-cell numbers CC
D81.2 Severe combined immunodeficiency [SCID] with low or normal B-cell numbers CC
D81.3 Adenosine deaminase [ADA] deficiency CC
CC Excl: D81.3, D81.5, D81.810, D84.1, E76.01-E76.9, E79.1-E80.29, E80.4-E80.7, E88.81
D81.4 Nezelof's syndrome CC
D81.5 Purine nucleoside phosphorylase [PNP] deficiency CC
CC Excl: See code: D81.3
D81.6 Major histocompatibility complex class I deficiency CC
Bare lymphocyte syndrome
D81.7 Major histocompatibility complex class II deficiency CC

D81.8 Other combined immunodeficiencies

D81.81 Biotin-dependent carboxylase deficiency
Multiple carboxylase deficiency
EXCLUDES 1 *biotin-dependent carboxylase deficiency due to dietary deficiency of biotin (E53.8)*

D81.810 Biotinidase deficiency

D81.818 Other biotin-dependent carboxylase deficiency
Holocarboxylase synthetase deficiency
Other multiple carboxylase deficiency

D81.819 Biotin-dependent carboxylase deficiency, unspecified
Multiple carboxylase deficiency, unspecified

D81.89 Other combined immunodeficiencies CC

D81.9 Combined immunodeficiency, unspecified CC
Severe combined immunodeficiency disorder [SCID] NOS

D82 Immunodeficiency associated with other major defects
EXCLUDES 1 *ataxia telangiectasia [Louis-Bar] (G11.3)*

D82.0 Wiskott-Aldrich syndrome CC
Immunodeficiency with thrombocytopenia and eczema
CC Excl: See code: D80

D82.1 Di George's syndrome CC
Pharyngeal pouch syndrome
Thymic alymphoplasia
Thymic aplasia or hypoplasia with immunodeficiency
CC Excl: See code: D80

D82.2 Immunodeficiency with short-limbed stature

D82.3 Immunodeficiency following hereditary defective response to Epstein-Barr virus
X-linked lymphoproliferative disease

D82.4 Hyperimmunoglobulin E [IgE] syndrome

D82.8 Immunodeficiency associated with other specified major defects

D82.9 Immunodeficiency associated with major defect, unspecified

D83 Common variable immunodeficiency

CC Excl: For CC codes in category D83, unless otherwise noted: D80.0, D80.3-D81.2, D81.4, D81.6-D81.7, D81.89-D84.0, D84.8-D84.9, D89.3, D89.82-D89.9

D83.0 Common variable immunodeficiency with predominant abnormalities of B-cell numbers and function CC

D83.1 Common variable immunodeficiency with predominant immunoregulatory T-cell disorders CC

D83.2 Common variable immunodeficiency with autoantibodies to B- or T-cells CC

D83.8 Other common variable immunodeficiencies CC

D83.9 Common variable immunodeficiency, unspecified CC

D84 Other immunodeficiencies

D84.0 Lymphocyte function antigen-1 [LFA-1] defect

D84.1 Defects in the complement system
C1 esterase inhibitor [C1-INH] deficiency

D84.8 Other specified immunodeficiencies CC
CC Excl: See code: D83

D84.9 Immunodeficiency, unspecified CC
CC Excl: See code: D83

D86 Sarcoidosis

D86.0 Sarcoidosis of lung

D86.1 Sarcoidosis of lymph nodes

D86.2 Sarcoidosis of lung with sarcoidosis of lymph nodes

D86.3 Sarcoidosis of skin

D86.8 Sarcoidosis of other sites

D86.81 Sarcoid meningitis

D86.82 Multiple cranial nerve palsies in sarcoidosis

D86.83 Sarcoid iridocyclitis

D86.84 Sarcoid pyelonephritis
Tubulo-interstitial nephropathy in sarcoidosis

D86.85 Sarcoid myocarditis

D86.86 Sarcoid arthropathy
Polyarthritis in sarcoidosis

D86.87 Sarcoid myositis

D86.89 Sarcoidosis of other sites
Hepatic granuloma
Uveoparotid fever [Heerfordt]

D86.9 Sarcoidosis, unspecified

D89 Other disorders involving the immune mechanism, not elsewhere classified
EXCLUDES 1 *hyperglobulinemia NOS (R77.1)*
monoclonal gammopathy (of undetermined significance) (D47.2)
EXCLUDES 2 *transplant failure and rejection (T86.-)*

D89.0 Polyclonal hypergammaglobulinemia
Benign hypergammaglobulinemic purpura
Polyclonal gammopathy NOS

D89.1 Cryoglobulinemia
Cryoglobulinemic purpura
Cryoglobulinemic vasculitis
Essential cryoglobulinemia
Idiopathic cryoglobulinemia
Mixed cryoglobulinemia
Primary cryoglobulinemia
Secondary cryoglobulinemia

D89.2 Hypergammaglobulinemia, unspecified

D89.3 Immune reconstitution syndrome
Immune reconstitution inflammatory syndrome [IRIS]
Use additional code for adverse effect, if applicable, to identify drug (T36-T50 with fifth or sixth character 5)

D89.8 Other specified disorders involving the immune mechanism, not elsewhere classified

D89.81 Graft-versus-host disease
Code first underlying cause, such as:
complications of transplanted organs and tissue (T86.-)
complications of blood transfusion (T80.89)
Use additional code to identify associated manifestations, such as:
desquamative dermatitis (L30.8)
diarrhea (R19.7)
elevated bilirubin (R17)
hair loss (L65.9)

CC Excl: For CC codes in subcategory D89.81, unless otherwise noted: D78.81-D78.89, D89.810-D89.813, E89.810-E89.89, H59.011-H59.019, H59.031-H59.099, H59.811-H59.89, H95.811-H95.89, I97.3, M96.89, N98.1-N98.9, T86.00-T86.09

D89.810 Acute graft-versus-host disease CC

D89.811 Chronic graft-versus-host disease CC

D89.812 Acute on chronic graft-versus-host disease CC

D89.813 Graft-versus-host disease, unspecified CC

D89.82 Autoimmune lymphoproliferative syndrome [ALPS]

D89.89 Other specified disorders involving the immune mechanism, not elsewhere classified
EXCLUDES 1 *human immunodeficiency virus disease (B20)*

D89.9 Disorder involving the immune mechanism, unspecified
Immune disease NOS

Chapter 4. Endocrine, Nutritional and Metabolic Diseases (E00-E89)

NOTE All neoplasms, whether functionally active or not, are classified in Chapter 2. Appropriate codes in this chapter (i.e. E05.8, E07.0, E16-E31, E34-) may be used as additional codes to indicate either functional activity by neoplasms and ectopic endocrine tissue or hyperfunction and hypofunction of endocrine glands associated with neoplasms and other conditions classified elsewhere.

EXCLUDES 1 *transitory endocrine and metabolic disorders specific to newborn (P70-P74)*

This chapter contains the following blocks:

- E00-E07 Disorders of thyroid gland
- E08-E13 Diabetes mellitus
- E15-E16 Other disorders of glucose regulation and pancreatic internal secretion
- E20-E35 Disorders of other endocrine glands
- E36 Intraoperative complications of endocrine system
- E40-E46 Malnutrition
- E50-E64 Other nutritional deficiencies
- E65-E68 Overweight, obesity and other hyperalimentation
- E70-E88 Metabolic disorders
- E89 Postprocedural endocrine and metabolic complications and disorders, not elsewhere classified

Disorders of thyroid gland (E00-E07)

✓4th E00 Congenital iodine-deficiency syndrome
Use additional code (F70-F79) to identify associated intellectual disabilities
EXCLUDES 1 *subclinical iodine-deficiency hypothyroidism (E02)*

E00.0 Congenital iodine-deficiency syndrome, neurological type
Endemic cretinism, neurological type

E00.1 Congenital iodine-deficiency syndrome, myxedematous type
Endemic hypothyroid cretinism
Endemic cretinism, myxedematous type

E00.2 Congenital iodine-deficiency syndrome, mixed type
Endemic cretinism, mixed type

E00.9 Congenital iodine-deficiency syndrome, unspecified
Congenital iodine-deficiency hypothyroidism NOS
Endemic cretinism NOS

✓4th E01 Iodine-deficiency related thyroid disorders and allied conditions
EXCLUDES 1 *congenital iodine-deficiency syndrome (E00.-)*
subclinical iodine-deficiency hypothyroidism (E02)

E01.0 Iodine-deficiency related diffuse (endemic) goiter

E01.1 Iodine-deficiency related multinodular (endemic) goiter
Iodine-deficiency related nodular goiter

E01.2 Iodine-deficiency related (endemic) goiter, unspecified
Endemic goiter NOS

E01.8 Other iodine-deficiency related thyroid disorders and allied conditions
Acquired iodine-deficiency hypothyroidism NOS

E02 Subclinical iodine-deficiency hypothyroidism

✓4th E03 Other hypothyroidism
EXCLUDES 1 *iodine-deficiency related hypothyroidism (E00-E02)*
postprocedural hypothyroidism (E89.0)

E03.0 Congenital hypothyroidism with diffuse goiter
Congenital parenchymatous goiter (nontoxic)
Congenital goiter (nontoxic) NOS
EXCLUDES 1 *transitory congenital goiter with normal function (P72.0)*

E03.1 Congenital hypothyroidism without goiter
Aplasia of thyroid (with myxedema)
Congenital atrophy of thyroid
Congenital hypothyroidism NOS

E03.2 Hypothyroidism due to medicaments and other exogenous substances
Code first poisoning due to drug or toxin, if applicable (T36-T65 with fifth or sixth character 1-4 or 6)
Use additional code for adverse effect, if applicable, to identify drug (T36-T50 with fifth or sixth character 5)

E03.3 Postinfectious hypothyroidism

E03.4 Atrophy of thyroid (acquired)
EXCLUDES 1 *congenital atrophy of thyroid (E03.1)*

E03.5 Myxedema coma MCC
CC Excl: B15.0-B19.9, E03.5, E08.00-E08.59, E08.618-E08.638, E08.641-E09.59, E09.618-E09.638, E09.641-E10.59, E10.618-E10.638, E10.641-E10.649, E10.69-E11.59, E11.618-E11.638, E11.641-E11.649, E11.69-E13.59, E13.618-E13.638, E13.641-E16.2, E89.1, G32.89, G89.0-G89.4, G93.81-G93.9, G96.8-G96.9, G98.0-G98.8, G99.8, I60.00- I62.9, K72.91, R40.0-R40.2124, R40.2210-R40.2224, R40.2310- R40.2324, R40.2340-R40.2344, R40.3-R41.3, R41.82, R41.9-R42, R44.8-R44.9, R45.83-R45.84, R46.0-R46.89, R52, R55, R68.0-R68.19, R68.81-R68.83, R68.89-R69; S02.0XX-S06.9X9 with 7th character A

E03.8 Other specified hypothyroidism

E03.9 Hypothyroidism, unspecified
Myxedema NOS

✓4th E04 Other nontoxic goiter
EXCLUDES 1 *congenital goiter (NOS) (diffuse) (parenchymatous) (E03.0)*
iodine-deficiency related goiter (E00-E02)

E04.0 Nontoxic diffuse goiter
Diffuse (colloid) nontoxic goiter
Simple nontoxic goiter

E04.1 Nontoxic single thyroid nodule
Colloid nodule (cystic) (thyroid)
Nontoxic uninodular goiter
Thyroid (cystic) nodule NOS

E04.2 Non toxic multinodular goiter
Cystic goiter NOS
Multinodular (cystic) goiter NOS

E04.8 Other specified nontoxic goiter

E04.9 Nontoxic goiter, unspecified
Goiter NOS
Nodular goiter (nontoxic) NOS

✓4th E05 Thyrotoxicosis [hyperthyroidism]
EXCLUDES 1 *chronic thyroiditis with transient thyrotoxicosis (E06.2)*
neonatal thyrotoxicosis (P72.1)

CC Excl: For MCC codes in category E05, unless otherwise noted: A17.9-A18.82, A18.84, A18.89, E00.0-E03.4, E03.8-E07.1, E07.89-E07.9, E30.9, E34.1, E34.50-E35, E89.0

✓5th E05.0 Thyrotoxicosis with diffuse goiter
Exophthalmic or toxic goiter NOS
Graves' disease
Toxic diffuse goiter

E05.00 Thyrotoxicosis with diffuse goiter without thyrotoxic crisis or storm

E05.01 Thyrotoxicosis with diffuse goiter with thyrotoxic crisis or storm MCC

✓5th E05.1 Thyrotoxicosis with toxic single thyroid nodule
Thyrotoxicosis with toxic uninodular goiter

E05.10 Thyrotoxicosis with toxic single thyroid nodule without thyrotoxic crisis or storm

E05.11 Thyrotoxicosis with toxic single thyroid nodule with thyrotoxic crisis or storm MCC

✓5th E05.2 Thyrotoxicosis with toxic multinodular goiter
Toxic nodular goiter NOS

E05.20 Thyrotoxicosis with toxic multinodular goiter without thyrotoxic crisis or storm

E05.21 Thyrotoxicosis with toxic multinodular goiter with thyrotoxic crisis or storm MCC

✓5th E05.3 Thyrotoxicosis from ectopic thyroid tissue

E05.30 Thyrotoxicosis from ectopic thyroid tissue without thyrotoxic crisis or storm

E05.31 Thyrotoxicosis from ectopic thyroid tissue with thyrotoxic crisis or storm MCC

✓5th E05.4 Thyrotoxicosis factitia

E05.40 Thyrotoxicosis factitia without thyrotoxic crisis or storm

E05.41 Thyrotoxicosis factitia with thyrotoxic crisis or storm MCC

✓5th E05.8 Other thyrotoxicosis
Overproduction of thyroid-stimulating hormone

E05.80 Other thyrotoxicosis without thyrotoxic crisis or storm

E05.81 Other thyrotoxicosis with thyrotoxic crisis or storm MCC

✓5th E05.9 Thyrotoxicosis, unspecified
Hyperthyroidism NOS

E05.90 Thyrotoxicosis, unspecified without thyrotoxic crisis or storm

E05.91 Thyrotoxicosis, unspecified with thyrotoxic crisis or storm MCC

✓4th **E06 Thyroiditis**

EXCLUDES 1 *postpartum thyroiditis (O90.5)*

E06.0 Acute thyroiditis CC
- Abscess of thyroid
- Pyogenic thyroiditis
- Suppurative thyroiditis

Use additional code (B95-B97) to identify infectious agent

CC Excl: E06.0-E06.9

E06.1 Subacute thyroiditis
- de Quervain thyroiditis
- Giant-cell thyroiditis
- Granulomatous thyroiditis
- Nonsuppurative thyroiditis
- Viral thyroiditis

EXCLUDES 1 *autoimmune thyroiditis (E06.3)*

E06.2 Chronic thyroiditis with transient thyrotoxicosis

EXCLUDES 1 *autoimmune thyroiditis (E06.3)*

E06.3 Autoimmune thyroiditis
- Hashimoto's thyroiditis
- Hashitoxicosis (transient)
- Lymphadenoid goiter
- Lymphocytic thyroiditis
- Struma lymphomatosa

E06.4 Drug-induced thyroiditis

Use additional code for adverse effect, if applicable, to identify drug (T36-T50 with fifth or sixth character 5)

E06.5 Other chronic thyroiditis
- Chronic fibrous thyroiditis
- Chronic thyroiditis NOS
- Ligneous thyroiditis
- Riedel thyroiditis

E06.9 Thyroiditis, unspecified

✓4th **E07 Other disorders of thyroid**

E07.0 Hypersecretion of calcitonin
- C-cell hyperplasia of thyroid
- Hypersecretion of thyrocalcitonin

E07.1 Dyshormogenetic goiter
- Familial dyshormogenetic goiter
- Pendred's syndrome

EXCLUDES 1 *transitory congenital goiter with normal function (P72.0)*

✓5th **E07.8 Other specified disorders of thyroid**

E07.81 Sick-euthyroid syndrome
- Euthyroid sick-syndrome

E07.89 Other specified disorders of thyroid
- Abnormality of thyroid-binding globulin
- Hemorrhage of thyroid
- Infarction of thyroid

E07.9 Disorder of thyroid, unspecified

Diabetes mellitus (E08-E13)

✓4th **E08 Diabetes mellitus due to underlying condition**

Code first the underlying condition, such as:
- congenital rubella (P35.0)
- cushing's syndrome (E24.-)
- cystic fibrosis (E84.-)
- malignant neoplasm (C00-C96)
- malnutrition (E40-E46)
- pancreatitis and other diseases of the pancreas (K85.-, K86.-)

Use additional code to identify any insulin use (Z79.4)

EXCLUDES 1
- *drug or chemical induced diabetes mellitus (E09.-)*
- *gestational diabetes (O24.4-)*
- *neonatal diabetes mellitus (P70.2)*
- *postpancreatectomy diabetes mellitus (E13.-)*
- *postprocedural diabetes mellitus (E13.-)*
- *secondary diabetes mellitus NEC (E13.-)*
- *type 1 diabetes mellitus (E10.-)*
- *type 2 diabetes mellitus (E11.-)*

AHA: 2013, 4Q, 114; 2013, 3Q, 20

CC Excl: For MCC codes in category E08, unless otherwise noted: E08.00-E08.59, E08.618-E08.638, E08.641-E09.59, E09.618-E09.638, E09.641-E10.59, E10.618-E10.638, E10.641-E10.649, E10.69-E11.59, E11.618-E11.638, E11.641-E11.649, E11.69-E13.59, E13.618-E13.638, E13.641-E16.2, E30.9, E34.1, E34.8-E35, E89.1

✓5th **E08.0 Diabetes mellitus due to underlying condition with hyperosmolarity**

E08.00 Diabetes mellitus due to underlying condition with hyperosmolarity without nonketotic hyperglycemic-hyperosmolar coma (NKHHC) MCC

E08.01 Diabetes mellitus due to underlying condition with hyperosmolarity with coma MCC

✓5th **E08.1 Diabetes mellitus due to underlying condition with ketoacidosis**

E08.10 Diabetes mellitus due to underlying condition with ketoacidosis without coma MCC

E08.11 Diabetes mellitus due to underlying condition with ketoacidosis with coma MCC

✓5th **E08.2 Diabetes mellitus due to underlying condition with kidney complications**

E08.21 Diabetes mellitus due to underlying condition with diabetic nephropathy
- Diabetes mellitus due to underlying condition with intercapillary glomerulosclerosis
- Diabetes mellitus due to underlying condition with intracapillary glomerulonephrosis
- Diabetes mellitus due to underlying condition with Kimmelstiel-Wilson disease

E08.22 Diabetes mellitus due to underlying condition with diabetic chronic kidney disease

Use additional code to identify stage of chronic kidney disease (N18.1-N18.6)

E08.29 Diabetes mellitus due to underlying condition with other diabetic kidney complication
- Renal tubular degeneration in diabetes mellitus due to underlying condition

✓5th **E08.3 Diabetes mellitus due to underlying condition with ophthalmic complications**

✓6th **E08.31 Diabetes mellitus due to underlying condition with unspecified diabetic retinopathy**

E08.311 Diabetes mellitus due to underlying condition with unspecified diabetic retinopathy with macular edema

E08.319 Diabetes mellitus due to underlying condition with unspecified diabetic retinopathy without macular edema

✓6th **E08.32 Diabetes mellitus due to underlying condition with mild nonproliferative diabetic retinopathy**
- Diabetes mellitus due to underlying condition with nonproliferative diabetic retinopathy NOS

E08.321 Diabetes mellitus due to underlying condition with mild nonproliferative diabetic retinopathy with macular edema

E08.329 Diabetes mellitus due to underlying condition with mild nonproliferative diabetic retinopathy without macular edema

✓6th **E08.33 Diabetes mellitus due to underlying condition with moderate nonproliferative diabetic retinopathy**

E08.331 Diabetes mellitus due to underlying condition with moderate nonproliferative diabetic retinopathy with macular edema

E08.339 Diabetes mellitus due to underlying condition with moderate nonproliferative diabetic retinopathy without macular edema

✓6th **E08.34 Diabetes mellitus due to underlying condition with severe nonproliferative diabetic retinopathy**

E08.341 Diabetes mellitus due to underlying condition with severe nonproliferative diabetic retinopathy with macular edema

E08.349 Diabetes mellitus due to underlying condition with severe nonproliferative diabetic retinopathy without macular edema

✓6th **E08.35 Diabetes mellitus due to underlying condition with proliferative diabetic retinopathy**

E08.351 Diabetes mellitus due to underlying condition with proliferative diabetic retinopathy with macular edema

E08.359 Diabetes mellitus due to underlying condition with proliferative diabetic retinopathy without macular edema

E08.36 Diabetes mellitus due to underlying condition with diabetic cataract

E08.39 Diabetes mellitus due to underlying condition with other diabetic ophthalmic complication
Use additional code to identify manifestation, such as: diabetic glaucoma (H40-H42)

✓5th **E08.4 Diabetes mellitus due to underlying condition with neurological complications**

E08.40 Diabetes mellitus due to underlying condition with diabetic neuropathy, unspecified

E08.41 Diabetes mellitus due to underlying condition with diabetic mononeuropathy

E08.42 Diabetes mellitus due to underlying condition with diabetic polyneuropathy
Diabetes mellitus due to underlying condition with diabetic neuralgia

E08.43 Diabetes mellitus due to underlying condition with diabetic autonomic (poly)neuropathy
Diabetes mellitus due to underlying condition with diabetic gastroparesis
AHA: 2013, 4Q, 114

E08.44 Diabetes mellitus due to underlying condition with diabetic amyotrophy

E08.49 Diabetes mellitus due to underlying condition with other diabetic neurological complication

✓5th **E08.5 Diabetes mellitus due to underlying condition with circulatory complications**

E08.51 Diabetes mellitus due to underlying condition with diabetic peripheral angiopathy without gangrene

E08.52 Diabetes mellitus due to underlying condition with diabetic peripheral angiopathy with gangrene PDx CC CC
Diabetes mellitus due to underlying condition with diabetic gangrene
CC Excl: G89.0-G89.4, I70.261-I70.269, I96, R41.0-R41.3, R41.82, R41.9, R44.8-R44.9, R45.83-R45.84, R46.0-R46.89, R52, R68.0-R68.19, R68.81-R68.83, R68.89-R69

E08.59 Diabetes mellitus due to underlying condition with other circulatory complications

✓5th **E08.6 Diabetes mellitus due to underlying condition with other specified complications**

✓6th **E08.61 Diabetes mellitus due to underlying condition with diabetic arthropathy**

E08.610 Diabetes mellitus due to underlying condition with diabetic neuropathic arthropathy
Diabetes mellitus due to underlying condition with Charcôt's joints

E08.618 Diabetes mellitus due to underlying condition with other diabetic arthropathy

✓6th **E08.62 Diabetes mellitus due to underlying condition with skin complications**

E08.620 Diabetes mellitus due to underlying condition with diabetic dermatitis
Diabetes mellitus due to underlying condition with diabetic necrobiosis lipoidica

E08.621 Diabetes mellitus due to underlying condition with foot ulcer
Use additional code to identify site of ulcer (L97.4-, L97.5-)

E08.622 Diabetes mellitus due to underlying condition with other skin ulcer
Use additional code to identify site of ulcer (L97.1-L97.9, L98.41-L98.49)

E08.628 Diabetes mellitus due to underlying condition with other skin complications

✓6th **E08.63 Diabetes mellitus due to underlying condition with oral complications**

E08.630 Diabetes mellitus due to underlying condition with periodontal disease

E08.638 Diabetes mellitus due to underlying condition with other oral complications

✓6th **E08.64 Diabetes mellitus due to underlying condition with hypoglycemia**

E08.641 Diabetes mellitus due to underlying condition with hypoglycemia with coma MCC

E08.649 Diabetes mellitus due to underlying condition with hypoglycemia without coma

E08.65 Diabetes mellitus due to underlying condition with hyperglycemia

E08.69 Diabetes mellitus due to underlying condition with other specified complication
Use additional code to identify complication

E08.8 Diabetes mellitus due to underlying condition with unspecified complications

E08.9 Diabetes mellitus due to underlying condition without complications

✓4th **E09 Drug or chemical induced diabetes mellitus**
Code first poisoning due to drug or toxin, if applicable (T36-T65 with fifth or sixth character 1-4 or 6)
Use additional code for adverse effect, if applicable, to identify drug (T36-T50 with fifth or sixth character 5)
Use additional code to identify any insulin use (Z79.4)
EXCLUDES 1 *diabetes mellitus due to underlying condition (E08.-)*
gestational diabetes (O24.4-)
neonatal diabetes mellitus (P70.2)
postpancreatectomy diabetes mellitus (E13.-)
postprocedural diabetes mellitus (E13.-)
secondary diabetes mellitus NEC (E13.-)
type 1 diabetes mellitus (E10.-)
type 2 diabetes mellitus (E11.-)
AHA: 2013, 4Q, 114; 2013, 3Q, 20

CC Excl: For MCC codes in category E09, unless otherwise noted: E08.00-E08.59, E08.618-E08.638, E08.641-E09.59, E09.618-E09.638, E09.641-E10.59, E10.618-E10.638, E10.641-E10.649, E10.69-E11.59, E11.618-E11.638, E11.641-E11.649, E11.69-E13.59, E13.618-E13.638, E13.641-E16.2, E30.9, E34.1, E34.8-E35, E89.1

✓5th **E09.0 Drug or chemical induced diabetes mellitus with hyperosmolarity**

E09.00 Drug or chemical induced diabetes mellitus with hyperosmolarity without nonketotic hyperglycemic-hyperosmolar coma (NKHHC) MCC

E09.01 Drug or chemical induced diabetes mellitus with hyperosmolarity with coma MCC

✓5th **E09.1 Drug or chemical induced diabetes mellitus with ketoacidosis**

E09.10 Drug or chemical induced diabetes mellitus with ketoacidosis without coma MCC

E09.11 Drug or chemical induced diabetes mellitus with ketoacidosis with coma MCC

✓5th **E09.2 Drug or chemical induced diabetes mellitus with kidney complications**

E09.21 Drug or chemical induced diabetes mellitus with diabetic nephropathy
Drug or chemical induced diabetes mellitus with intercapillary glomerulosclerosis
Drug or chemical induced diabetes mellitus with intracapillary glomerulonephrosis
Drug or chemical induced diabetes mellitus with Kimmelstiel-Wilson disease

E09.22 Drug or chemical induced diabetes mellitus with diabetic chronic kidney disease
Use additional code to identify stage of chronic kidney disease (N18.1-N18.6)

E09.29 Drug or chemical induced diabetes mellitus with other diabetic kidney complication
Drug or chemical induced diabetes mellitus with renal tubular degeneration

✓5th **E09.3 Drug or chemical induced diabetes mellitus with ophthalmic complications**

✓6th **E09.31 Drug or chemical induced diabetes mellitus with unspecified diabetic retinopathy**

E09.311 Drug or chemical induced diabetes mellitus with unspecified diabetic retinopathy with macular edema

E09.319 Drug or chemical induced diabetes mellitus with unspecified diabetic retinopathy without macular edema

✓6th **E09.32 Drug or chemical induced diabetes mellitus with mild nonproliferative diabetic retinopathy**
Drug or chemical induced diabetes mellitus with nonproliferative diabetic retinopathy NOS

E09.321 Drug or chemical induced diabetes mellitus with mild nonproliferative diabetic retinopathy with macular edema

E09.329 Drug or chemical induced diabetes mellitus with mild nonproliferative diabetic retinopathy without macular edema

✓6th **E09.33 Drug or chemical induced diabetes mellitus with moderate nonproliferative diabetic retinopathy**

EØ9.331 Drug or chemical induced diabetes mellitus with moderate nonproliferative diabetic retinopathy with macular edema

EØ9.339 Drug or chemical induced diabetes mellitus with moderate nonproliferative diabetic retinopathy without macular edema

✓6th **EØ9.34 Drug or chemical induced diabetes mellitus with severe nonproliferative diabetic retinopathy**

EØ9.341 Drug or chemical induced diabetes mellitus with severe nonproliferative diabetic retinopathy with macular edema

EØ9.349 Drug or chemical induced diabetes mellitus with severe nonproliferative diabetic retinopathy without macular edema

✓6th **EØ9.35 Drug or chemical induced diabetes mellitus with proliferative diabetic retinopathy**

EØ9.351 Drug or chemical induced diabetes mellitus with proliferative diabetic retinopathy with macular edema

EØ9.359 Drug or chemical induced diabetes mellitus with proliferative diabetic retinopathy without macular edema

EØ9.36 Drug or chemical induced diabetes mellitus with diabetic cataract

EØ9.39 Drug or chemical induced diabetes mellitus with other diabetic ophthalmic complication

Use additional code to identify manifestation, such as: diabetic glaucoma (H4Ø-H42)

✓5th **EØ9.4 Drug or chemical induced diabetes mellitus with neurological complications**

EØ9.4Ø Drug or chemical induced diabetes mellitus with neurological complications with diabetic neuropathy, unspecified

EØ9.41 Drug or chemical induced diabetes mellitus with neurological complications with diabetic mononeuropathy

EØ9.42 Drug or chemical induced diabetes mellitus with neurological complications with diabetic polyneuropathy

Drug or chemical induced diabetes mellitus with diabetic neuralgia

EØ9.43 Drug or chemical induced diabetes mellitus with neurological complications with diabetic autonomic (poly)neuropathy

Drug or chemical induced diabetes mellitus with diabetic gastroparesis

AHA: 2Ø13, 4Q, 114

EØ9.44 Drug or chemical induced diabetes mellitus with neurological complications with diabetic amyotrophy

EØ9.49 Drug or chemical induced diabetes mellitus with neurological complications with other diabetic neurological complication

✓5th **EØ9.5 Drug or chemical induced diabetes mellitus with circulatory complications**

EØ9.51 Drug or chemical induced diabetes mellitus with diabetic peripheral angiopathy without gangrene

EØ9.52 Drug or chemical induced diabetes mellitus with diabetic peripheral angiopathy with gangrene PDx CC CC

Drug or chemical induced diabetes mellitus with diabetic gangrene

CC Excl: G89.Ø-G89.4, I7Ø.261-I7Ø.269, I96, R41.Ø-R41.3, R41.82, R41.9, R44.8-R44.9, R45.83-R45.84, R46.Ø-R46.89, R52, R68.Ø-R68.19, R68.81-R68.83, R68.89-R69

EØ9.59 Drug or chemical induced diabetes mellitus with other circulatory complications

✓5th **EØ9.6 Drug or chemical induced diabetes mellitus with other specified complications**

✓6th **EØ9.61 Drug or chemical induced diabetes mellitus with diabetic arthropathy**

EØ9.61Ø Drug or chemical induced diabetes mellitus with diabetic neuropathic arthropathy

Drug or chemical induced diabetes mellitus with Charcôt's joints

EØ9.618 Drug or chemical induced diabetes mellitus with other diabetic arthropathy

✓6th **EØ9.62 Drug or chemical induced diabetes mellitus with skin complications**

EØ9.62Ø Drug or chemical induced diabetes mellitus with diabetic dermatitis

Drug or chemical induced diabetes mellitus with diabetic necrobiosis lipoidica

EØ9.621 Drug or chemical induced diabetes mellitus with foot ulcer

Use additional code to identify site of ulcer (L97.4-, L97.5-)

EØ9.622 Drug or chemical induced diabetes mellitus with other skin ulcer

Use additional code to identify site of ulcer (L97.1-L97.9, L98.41-L98.49)

EØ9.628 Drug or chemical induced diabetes mellitus with other skin complications

✓6th **EØ9.63 Drug or chemical induced diabetes mellitus with oral complications**

EØ9.63Ø Drug or chemical induced diabetes mellitus with periodontal disease

EØ9.638 Drug or chemical induced diabetes mellitus with other oral complications

✓6th **EØ9.64 Drug or chemical induced diabetes mellitus with hypoglycemia**

EØ9.641 Drug or chemical induced diabetes mellitus with hypoglycemia with coma MCC

EØ9.649 Drug or chemical induced diabetes mellitus with hypoglycemia without coma

EØ9.65 Drug or chemical induced diabetes mellitus with hyperglycemia

EØ9.69 Drug or chemical induced diabetes mellitus with other specified complication

Use additional code to identify complication

EØ9.8 Drug or chemical induced diabetes mellitus with unspecified complications

EØ9.9 Drug or chemical induced diabetes mellitus without complications

✓4th **E1Ø Type 1 diabetes mellitus**

INCLUDES brittle diabetes (mellitus)
diabetes (mellitus) due to autoimmune process
diabetes (mellitus) due to immune mediated pancreatic islet beta-cell destruction
idiopathic diabetes (mellitus)
juvenile onset diabetes (mellitus)
ketosis-prone diabetes (mellitus)

EXCLUDES 1 *diabetes mellitus due to underlying condition (EØ8.-)*
drug or chemical induced diabetes mellitus (EØ9.-)
gestational diabetes (O24.4-)
hyperglycemia NOS (R73.9)
neonatal diabetes mellitus (P7Ø.2)
postpancreatectomy diabetes mellitus (E13.-)
postprocedural diabetes mellitus (E13.-)
secondary diabetes mellitus NEC (E13.-)
type 2 diabetes mellitus (E11.-)

AHA: 2Ø13, 4Q, 114; 2Ø13, 3Q, 2Ø

CC Excl: For MCC codes in category E1Ø, unless otherwise noted: EØ8.ØØ-EØ8.59, EØ8.618-EØ8.638, EØ8.641-EØ9.59, EØ9.618-EØ9.638, EØ9.641-E1Ø.59, E1Ø.618-E1Ø.638, E1Ø.641-E1Ø.649, E1Ø.69-E11.59, E11.618-E11.638, E11.641-E11.649, E11.69-E13.59, E13.618-E13.638, E13.641-E16.2, E3Ø.9, E34.1, E34.5Ø-E35, E89.1

✓5th **E1Ø.1 Type 1 diabetes mellitus with ketoacidosis**

AHA: 2Ø13, 3Q, 2Ø

E1Ø.1Ø Type 1 diabetes mellitus with ketoacidosis without coma MCC

E1Ø.11 Type 1 diabetes mellitus with ketoacidosis with coma MCC

✓5th **E1Ø.2 Type 1 diabetes mellitus with kidney complications**

E1Ø.21 Type 1 diabetes mellitus with diabetic nephropathy

Type 1 diabetes mellitus with intercapillary glomerulosclerosis
Type 1 diabetes mellitus with intracapillary glomerulonephrosis
Type 1 diabetes mellitus with Kimmelstiel-Wilson disease

E1Ø.22 Type 1 diabetes mellitus with diabetic chronic kidney disease

Use additional code to identify stage of chronic kidney disease (N18.1-N18.6)

E10.29 Type 1 diabetes mellitus with other diabetic kidney complication
Type 1 diabetes mellitus with renal tubular degeneration

E10.3 Type 1 diabetes mellitus with ophthalmic complications

E10.31 Type 1 diabetes mellitus with unspecified diabetic retinopathy

E10.311 Type 1 diabetes mellitus with unspecified diabetic retinopathy with macular edema

E10.319 Type 1 diabetes mellitus with unspecified diabetic retinopathy without macular edema

E10.32 Type 1 diabetes mellitus with mild nonproliferative diabetic retinopathy
Type 1 diabetes mellitus with nonproliferative diabetic retinopathy NOS

E10.321 Type 1 diabetes mellitus with mild nonproliferative diabetic retinopathy with macular edema

E10.329 Type 1 diabetes mellitus with mild nonproliferative diabetic retinopathy without macular edema

E10.33 Type 1 diabetes mellitus with moderate nonproliferative diabetic retinopathy

E10.331 Type 1 diabetes mellitus with moderate nonproliferative diabetic retinopathy with macular edema

E10.339 Type 1 diabetes mellitus with moderate nonproliferative diabetic retinopathy without macular edema

E10.34 Type 1 diabetes mellitus with severe nonproliferative diabetic retinopathy

E10.341 Type 1 diabetes mellitus with severe nonproliferative diabetic retinopathy with macular edema

E10.349 Type 1 diabetes mellitus with severe nonproliferative diabetic retinopathy without macular edema

E10.35 Type 1 diabetes mellitus with proliferative diabetic retinopathy

E10.351 Type 1 diabetes mellitus with proliferative diabetic retinopathy with macular edema

E10.359 Type 1 diabetes mellitus with proliferative diabetic retinopathy without macular edema

E10.36 Type 1 diabetes mellitus with diabetic cataract

E10.39 Type 1 diabetes mellitus with other diabetic ophthalmic complication
Use additional code to identify manifestation, such as: diabetic glaucoma (H40-H42)

E10.4 Type 1 diabetes mellitus with neurological complications

E10.40 Type 1 diabetes mellitus with diabetic neuropathy, unspecified

E10.41 Type 1 diabetes mellitus with diabetic mononeuropathy

E10.42 Type 1 diabetes mellitus with diabetic polyneuropathy
Type 1 diabetes mellitus with diabetic neuralgia

E10.43 Type 1 diabetes mellitus with diabetic autonomic (poly)neuropathy
Type 1 diabetes mellitus with diabetic gastroparesis
AHA: 2013, 4Q, 114

E10.44 Type 1 diabetes mellitus with diabetic amyotrophy

E10.49 Type 1 diabetes mellitus with other diabetic neurological complication

E10.5 Type 1 diabetes mellitus with circulatory complications

E10.51 Type 1 diabetes mellitus with diabetic peripheral angiopathy without gangrene

E10.52 Type 1 diabetes mellitus with diabetic peripheral angiopathy with gangrene PDx CC CC
Type 1 diabetes mellitus with diabetic gangrene
CC Excl: G89.0-G89.4, I70.261-I70.269, I96, R41.0-R41.3, R41.82, R41.9, R44.8-R44.9, R45.83-R45.84, R46.0-R46.89, R52, R68.0-R68.19, R68.81-R68.83, R68.89-R69

E10.59 Type 1 diabetes mellitus with other circulatory complications

E10.6 Type 1 diabetes mellitus with other specified complications

E10.61 Type 1 diabetes mellitus with diabetic arthropathy

E10.610 Type 1 diabetes mellitus with diabetic neuropathic arthropathy
Type 1 diabetes mellitus with Charcôt's joints

E10.618 Type 1 diabetes mellitus with other diabetic arthropathy

E10.62 Type 1 diabetes mellitus with skin complications

E10.620 Type 1 diabetes mellitus with diabetic dermatitis
Type 1 diabetes mellitus with diabetic necrobiosis lipoidica

E10.621 Type 1 diabetes mellitus with foot ulcer
Use additional code to identify site of ulcer (L97.4-, L97.5-)

E10.622 Type 1 diabetes mellitus with other skin ulcer
Use additional code to identify site of ulcer (L97.1-L97.9, L98.41-L98.49)

E10.628 Type 1 diabetes mellitus with other skin complications

E10.63 Type 1 diabetes mellitus with oral complications

E10.630 Type 1 diabetes mellitus with periodontal disease

E10.638 Type 1 diabetes mellitus with other oral complications

E10.64 Type 1 diabetes mellitus with hypoglycemia

E10.641 Type 1 diabetes mellitus with hypoglycemia with coma MCC

E10.649 Type 1 diabetes mellitus with hypoglycemia without coma

E10.65 Type 1 diabetes mellitus with hyperglycemia
AHA: 2013, 3Q, 20

E10.69 Type 1 diabetes mellitus with other specified complication
Use additional code to identify complication

E10.8 Type 1 diabetes mellitus with unspecified complications

E10.9 Type 1 diabetes mellitus without complications

E11 Type 2 diabetes mellitus
INCLUDES diabetes (mellitus) due to insulin secretory defect
diabetes NOS
insulin resistant diabetes (mellitus)
Use additional code to identify any insulin use (Z79.4)
EXCLUDES 1 *diabetes mellitus due to underlying condition (E08.-)*
drug or chemical induced diabetes mellitus (E09.-)
gestational diabetes (O24.4-)
neonatal diabetes mellitus (P70.2)
postpancreatectomy diabetes mellitus (E13.-)
postprocedural diabetes mellitus (E13.-)
secondary diabetes mellitus NEC (E13.-)
type 1 diabetes mellitus (E10.-)
AHA: 2013, 4Q, 114; 2013, 3Q, 20; 2013, 1Q, 26

CC Excl: For MCC codes in category E11, unless otherwise noted: E08.00-E08.59, E08.618-E08.638, E08.641-E09.59, E09.618-E09.638, E09.641-E10.59, E10.618-E10.638, E10.641-E10.649, E10.69-E11.59, E11.618-E11.638, E11.641-E11.649, E11.69-E13.59, E13.618-E13.638, E13.641-E16.2, E30.9, E34.1, E34.8-E35, E89.1

E11.0 Type 2 diabetes mellitus with hyperosmolarity

E11.00 Type 2 diabetes mellitus with hyperosmolarity without nonketotic hyperglycemic-hyperosmolar coma (NKHHC) MCC

E11.01 Type 2 diabetes mellitus with hyperosmolarity with coma MCC

E11.2 Type 2 diabetes mellitus with kidney complications

E11.21 Type 2 diabetes mellitus with diabetic nephropathy
Type 2 diabetes mellitus with intercapillary glomerulosclerosis
Type 2 diabetes mellitus with intracapillary glomerulonephrosis
Type 2 diabetes mellitus with Kimmelstiel-Wilson disease

E11.22 Type 2 diabetes mellitus with diabetic chronic kidney disease
Use additional code to identify stage of chronic kidney disease (N18.1-N18.6)

E11.29 Type 2 diabetes mellitus with other diabetic kidney complication
Type 2 diabetes mellitus with renal tubular degeneration

✓5th **E11.3 Type 2 diabetes mellitus with ophthalmic complications**

✓6th **E11.31 Type 2 diabetes mellitus with unspecified diabetic retinopathy**
- **E11.311 Type 2 diabetes mellitus with unspecified diabetic retinopathy with macular edema**
- **E11.319 Type 2 diabetes mellitus with unspecified diabetic retinopathy without macular edema**

✓6th **E11.32 Type 2 diabetes mellitus with mild nonproliferative diabetic retinopathy**
Type 2 diabetes mellitus with nonproliferative diabetic retinopathy NOS
- **E11.321 Type 2 diabetes mellitus with mild nonproliferative diabetic retinopathy with macular edema**
- **E11.329 Type 2 diabetes mellitus with mild nonproliferative diabetic retinopathy without macular edema**

✓6th **E11.33 Type 2 diabetes mellitus with moderate nonproliferative diabetic retinopathy**
- **E11.331 Type 2 diabetes mellitus with moderate nonproliferative diabetic retinopathy with macular edema**
- **E11.339 Type 2 diabetes mellitus with moderate nonproliferative diabetic retinopathy without macular edema**

✓6th **E11.34 Type 2 diabetes mellitus with severe nonproliferative diabetic retinopathy**
- **E11.341 Type 2 diabetes mellitus with severe nonproliferative diabetic retinopathy with macular edema**
- **E11.349 Type 2 diabetes mellitus with severe nonproliferative diabetic retinopathy without macular edema**

✓6th **E11.35 Type 2 diabetes mellitus with proliferative diabetic retinopathy**
- **E11.351 Type 2 diabetes mellitus with proliferative diabetic retinopathy with macular edema**
- **E11.359 Type 2 diabetes mellitus with proliferative diabetic retinopathy without macular edema**

E11.36 Type 2 diabetes mellitus with diabetic cataract

E11.39 Type 2 diabetes mellitus with other diabetic ophthalmic complication
Use additional code to identify manifestation, such as: diabetic glaucoma (H40-H42)

✓5th **E11.4 Type 2 diabetes mellitus with neurological complications**

E11.40 Type 2 diabetes mellitus with diabetic neuropathy, unspecified
AHA: 2013, 4Q, 129

E11.41 Type 2 diabetes mellitus with diabetic mononeuropathy

E11.42 Type 2 diabetes mellitus with diabetic polyneuropathy
Type 2 diabetes mellitus with diabetic neuralgia

E11.43 Type 2 diabetes mellitus with diabetic autonomic (poly)neuropathy
Type 2 diabetes mellitus with diabetic gastroparesis
AHA: 2013, 4Q, 114

E11.44 Type 2 diabetes mellitus with diabetic amyotrophy

E11.49 Type 2 diabetes mellitus with other diabetic neurological complication

✓5th **E11.5 Type 2 diabetes mellitus with circulatory complications**

E11.51 Type 2 diabetes mellitus with diabetic peripheral angiopathy without gangrene

E11.52 Type 2 diabetes mellitus with diabetic peripheral angiopathy with gangrene PDx CC CC
Type 2 diabetes mellitus with diabetic gangrene
CC Excl: G89.0-G89.4, I70.261-I70.269, I96, R41.0-R41.3, R41.82, R41.9, R44.8-R44.9, R45.83-R45.84, R46.0-R46.89, R52, R68.0-R68.19, R68.81-R68.83, R68.89-R69

E11.59 Type 2 diabetes mellitus with other circulatory complications

✓5th **E11.6 Type 2 diabetes mellitus with other specified complications**

✓6th **E11.61 Type 2 diabetes mellitus with diabetic arthropathy**
- **E11.610 Type 2 diabetes mellitus with diabetic neuropathic arthropathy**
  Type 2 diabetes mellitus with Charcôt's joints
- **E11.618 Type 2 diabetes mellitus with other diabetic arthropathy**

✓6th **E11.62 Type 2 diabetes mellitus with skin complications**
- **E11.620 Type 2 diabetes mellitus with diabetic dermatitis**
  Type 2 diabetes mellitus with diabetic necrobiosis lipoidica
- **E11.621 Type 2 diabetes mellitus with foot ulcer**
  Use additional code to identify site of ulcer (L97.4-, L97.5-)
- **E11.622 Type 2 diabetes mellitus with other skin ulcer**
  Use additional code to identify site of ulcer (L97.1-L97.9, L98.41-L98.49)
- **E11.628 Type 2 diabetes mellitus with other skin complications**

✓6th **E11.63 Type 2 diabetes mellitus with oral complications**
- **E11.630 Type 2 diabetes mellitus with periodontal disease**
- **E11.638 Type 2 diabetes mellitus with other oral complications**

✓6th **E11.64 Type 2 diabetes mellitus with hypoglycemia**
- **E11.641 Type 2 diabetes mellitus with hypoglycemia with coma** MCC
- **E11.649 Type 2 diabetes mellitus with hypoglycemia without coma**

E11.65 Type 2 diabetes mellitus with hyperglycemia
AHA: 2013, 3Q, 20

E11.69 Type 2 diabetes mellitus with other specified complication
Use additional code to identify complication

E11.8 Type 2 diabetes mellitus with unspecified complications

13 **E11.9 Type 2 diabetes mellitus without complications**

✓4th **E13 Other specified diabetes mellitus**
Diabetes mellitus due to genetic defects of beta-cell function
Diabetes mellitus due to genetic defects in insulin action
Postpancreatectomy diabetes mellitus
Postprocedural diabetes mellitus
Secondary diabetes mellitus NEC
Use additional code to identify any insulin use (Z79.4)

EXCLUDES 1 *diabetes (mellitus) due to autoimmune process (E10.-)*
diabetes (mellitus) due to immune mediated pancreatic islet beta-cell destruction (E10.-)
diabetes mellitus due to underlying condition (E08.-)
drug or chemical induced diabetes mellitus (E09.-)
gestational diabetes (O24.4-)
neonatal diabetes mellitus (P70.2)
type 2 diabetes mellitus (E11.-)

AHA: 2013, 4Q, 114; 2013, 3Q, 20

CC Excl: For MCC codes in category E13, unless otherwise noted: E08.00-E08.59, E08.618-E08.638, E08.641-E09.59, E09.618-E09.638, E09.641-E10.59, E10.618-E10.638, E10.641-E10.649, E10.69-E11.59, E11.618-E11.638, E11.641-E11.649, E11.69-E13.59, E13.618-E13.638, E13.641-E16.2, E30.9, E34.1, E34.8-E35, E89.1

✓5th **E13.0 Other specified diabetes mellitus with hyperosmolarity**
- **E13.00 Other specified diabetes mellitus with hyperosmolarity without nonketotic hyperglycemic-hyperosmolar coma (NKHHC)** MCC
- **E13.01 Other specified diabetes mellitus with hyperosmolarity with coma** MCC

✓5th **E13.1 Other specified diabetes mellitus with ketoacidosis**
AHA: 2013, 1Q, 26
- **E13.10 Other specified diabetes mellitus with ketoacidosis without coma** MCC
- **E13.11 Other specified diabetes mellitus with ketoacidosis with coma** MCC

13 Questionable admission when used as PDx.

✓5th **E13.2 Other specified diabetes mellitus with kidney complications**

E13.21 Other specified diabetes mellitus with diabetic nephropathy
Other specified diabetes mellitus with intercapillary glomerulosclerosis
Other specified diabetes mellitus with intracapillary glomerulonephrosis
Other specified diabetes mellitus with Kimmelstiel-Wilson disease

E13.22 Other specified diabetes mellitus with diabetic chronic kidney disease
Use additional code to identify stage of chronic kidney disease (N18.1-N18.6)

E13.29 Other specified diabetes mellitus with other diabetic kidney complication
Other specified diabetes mellitus with renal tubular degeneration

✓5th **E13.3 Other specified diabetes mellitus with ophthalmic complications**

✓6th **E13.31 Other specified diabetes mellitus with unspecified diabetic retinopathy**

E13.311 Other specified diabetes mellitus with unspecified diabetic retinopathy with macular edema

E13.319 Other specified diabetes mellitus with unspecified diabetic retinopathy without macular edema

✓6th **E13.32 Other specified diabetes mellitus with mild nonproliferative diabetic retinopathy**
Other specified diabetes mellitus with nonproliferative diabetic retinopathy NOS

E13.321 Other specified diabetes mellitus with mild nonproliferative diabetic retinopathy with macular edema

E13.329 Other specified diabetes mellitus with mild nonproliferative diabetic retinopathy without macular edema

✓6th **E13.33 Other specified diabetes mellitus with moderate nonproliferative diabetic retinopathy**

E13.331 Other specified diabetes mellitus with moderate nonproliferative diabetic retinopathy with macular edema

E13.339 Other specified diabetes mellitus with moderate nonproliferative diabetic retinopathy without macular edema

✓6th **E13.34 Other specified diabetes mellitus with severe nonproliferative diabetic retinopathy**

E13.341 Other specified diabetes mellitus with severe nonproliferative diabetic retinopathy with macular edema

E13.349 Other specified diabetes mellitus with severe nonproliferative diabetic retinopathy without macular edema

✓6th **E13.35 Other specified diabetes mellitus with proliferative diabetic retinopathy**

E13.351 Other specified diabetes mellitus with proliferative diabetic retinopathy with macular edema

E13.359 Other specified diabetes mellitus with proliferative diabetic retinopathy without macular edema

E13.36 Other specified diabetes mellitus with diabetic cataract

E13.39 Other specified diabetes mellitus with other diabetic ophthalmic complication
Use additional code to identify manifestation, such as: diabetic glaucoma (H4Ø-H42)

✓5th **E13.4 Other specified diabetes mellitus with neurological complications**

E13.4Ø Other specified diabetes mellitus with diabetic neuropathy, unspecified

E13.41 Other specified diabetes mellitus with diabetic mononeuropathy

E13.42 Other specified diabetes mellitus with diabetic polyneuropathy
Other specified diabetes mellitus with diabetic neuralgia

E13.43 Other specified diabetes mellitus with diabetic autonomic (poly)neuropathy
Other specified diabetes mellitus with diabetic gastroparesis
AHA: 2Ø13, 4Q, 114

E13.44 Other specified diabetes mellitus with diabetic amyotrophy

E13.49 Other specified diabetes mellitus with other diabetic neurological complication

✓5th **E13.5 Other specified diabetes mellitus with circulatory complications**

E13.51 Other specified diabetes mellitus with diabetic peripheral angiopathy without gangrene

E13.52 Other specified diabetes mellitus with diabetic peripheral angiopathy with gangrene PDx CC CC
Other specified diabetes mellitus with diabetic gangrene
CC Excl: G89.Ø-G89.4, I7Ø.261-I7Ø.269, I96, R41.Ø-R41.3, R41.82, R41.9, R44.8-R44.9, R45.83-R45.84, R46.Ø-R46.89, R52, R68.Ø-R68.19, R68.81-R68.83, R68.89-R69

E13.59 Other specified diabetes mellitus with other circulatory complications

✓5th **E13.6 Other specified diabetes mellitus with other specified complications**

✓6th **E13.61 Other specified diabetes mellitus with diabetic arthropathy**

E13.61Ø Other specified diabetes mellitus with diabetic neuropathic arthropathy
Other specified diabetes mellitus with Charcôt's joints

E13.618 Other specified diabetes mellitus with other diabetic arthropathy

✓6th **E13.62 Other specified diabetes mellitus with skin complications**

E13.62Ø Other specified diabetes mellitus with diabetic dermatitis
Other specified diabetes mellitus with diabetic necrobiosis lipoidica

E13.621 Other specified diabetes mellitus with foot ulcer
Use additional code to identify site of ulcer (L97.4-, L97.5-)

E13.622 Other specified diabetes mellitus with other skin ulcer
Use additional code to identify site of ulcer (L97.1-L97.9, L98.41-L98.49)

E13.628 Other specified diabetes mellitus with other skin complications

✓6th **E13.63 Other specified diabetes mellitus with oral complications**

E13.63Ø Other specified diabetes mellitus with periodontal disease

E13.638 Other specified diabetes mellitus with other oral complications

✓6th **E13.64 Other specified diabetes mellitus with hypoglycemia**

E13.641 Other specified diabetes mellitus with hypoglycemia with coma MCC

E13.649 Other specified diabetes mellitus with hypoglycemia without coma

E13.65 Other specified diabetes mellitus with hyperglycemia

E13.69 Other specified diabetes mellitus with other specified complication
Use additional code to identify complication

E13.8 Other specified diabetes mellitus with unspecified complications

13 **E13.9 Other specified diabetes mellitus without complications**

13 Questionable admission when used as PDx.

Other disorders of glucose regulation and pancreatic internal secretion (E15-E16)

E15 Nondiabetic hypoglycemic coma CC
INCLUDES drug-induced insulin coma in nondiabetic
hyperinsulinism with hypoglycemic coma
hypoglycemic coma NOS
CC Excl: E08.00-E08.59, E08.618-E08.638, E08.641-E09.59, E09.618-E09.638, E09.641-E10.59, E10.618-E10.638, E10.641-E10.649, E10.69-E11.59, E11.618-E11.638, E11.641-E11.649, E11.69-E13.59, E13.618-E13.638, E13.641-E16.2, E30.9, E34.1, E34.50-E35, E89.1

✓4th **E16 Other disorders of pancreatic internal secretion**

E16.0 Drug-induced hypoglycemia without coma
Use additional code for adverse effect, if applicable, to identify drug (T36-T50 with fifth or sixth character 5)

E16.1 Other hypoglycemia
Functional hyperinsulinism
Functional nonhyperinsulinemic hypoglycemia
Hyperinsulinism NOS
Hyperplasia of pancreatic islet beta cells NOS
EXCLUDES 1 *hypoglycemia in infant of diabetic mother (P70.1)*
neonatal hypoglycemia (P70.4)

E16.2 Hypoglycemia, unspecified

E16.3 Increased secretion of glucagon
Hyperplasia of pancreatic endocrine cells with glucagon excess

E16.4 Increased secretion of gastrin
Hypergastrinemia
Hyperplasia of pancreatic endocrine cells with gastrin excess
Zollinger-Ellison syndrome

E16.8 Other specified disorders of pancreatic internal secretion
Increased secretion from endocrine pancreas of growth hormone-releasing hormone
Increased secretion from endocrine pancreas of pancreatic polypeptide
Increased secretion from endocrine pancreas of somatostatin
Increased secretion from endocrine pancreas of vasoactive-intestinal polypeptide

E16.9 Disorder of pancreatic internal secretion, unspecified
Islet-cell hyperplasia NOS
Pancreatic endocrine cell hyperplasia NOS

Disorders of other endocrine glands (E20-E35)

EXCLUDES 1 *galactorrhea (N64.3)*
gynecomastia (N62)

✓4th **E20 Hypoparathyroidism**
EXCLUDES 1 *Di George's syndrome (D82.1)*
postprocedural hypoparathyroidism (E89.2)
tetany NOS (R29.0)
transitory neonatal hypoparathyroidism (P71.4)

E20.0 Idiopathic hypoparathyroidism

E20.1 Pseudohypoparathyroidism

E20.8 Other hypoparathyroidism

E20.9 Hypoparathyroidism, unspecified
Parathyroid tetany

✓4th **E21 Hyperparathyroidism and other disorders of parathyroid gland**
EXCLUDES 1 *adult osteomalacia (M83.-)*
ectopic hyperparathyroidism (E34.2)
familial hypocalciuric hypercalcemia (E83.52)
hungry bone syndrome (E83.81)
infantile and juvenile osteomalacia (E55.0)

E21.0 Primary hyperparathyroidism
Hyperplasia of parathyroid
Osteitis fibrosa cystica generalisata [von Recklinghausen's disease of bone]

E21.1 Secondary hyperparathyroidism, not elsewhere classified
EXCLUDES 1 *secondary hyperparathyroidism of renal origin (N25.81)*

E21.2 Other hyperparathyroidism
Tertiary hyperparathyroidism
EXCLUDES 1 *familial hypocalciuric hypercalcemia (E83.52)*

E21.3 Hyperparathyroidism, unspecified

E21.4 Other specified disorders of parathyroid gland

E21.5 Disorder of parathyroid gland, unspecified

✓4th **E22 Hyperfunction of pituitary gland**
EXCLUDES 1 *Cushing's syndrome (E24.-)*
Nelson's syndrome (E24.1)
overproduction of ACTH not associated with Cushing's disease (E27.0)
overproduction of pituitary ACTH (E24.0)
overproduction of thyroid-stimulating hormone (E05.8-)

E22.0 Acromegaly and pituitary gigantism
Overproduction of growth hormone
EXCLUDES 1 *constitutional gigantism (E34.4)*
constitutional tall stature (E34.4)
increased secretion from endocrine pancreas of growth hormone-releasing hormone (E16.8)

E22.1 Hyperprolactinemia CC
Use additional code for adverse effect, if applicable, to identify drug (T36-T50 with fifth or sixth character 5)
CC Excl: E22.1-E22.9

E22.2 Syndrome of inappropriate secretion of antidiuretic hormone CC
CC Excl: E22.0-E23.7, E24.1, E30.9, E34.1, E34.4, E34.8-E35, E89.3

E22.8 Other hyperfunction of pituitary gland CC
Central precocious puberty
CC Excl: See code: E22.1

E22.9 Hyperfunction of pituitary gland, unspecified CC
CC Excl: See code: E22.1

✓4th **E23 Hypofunction and other disorders of the pituitary gland**
INCLUDES the listed conditions whether the disorder is in the pituitary or the hypothalamus
EXCLUDES 1 *postprocedural hypopituitarism (E89.3)*

E23.0 Hypopituitarism CC
Fertile eunuch syndrome
Hypogonadotropic hypogonadism
Idiopathic growth hormone deficiency
Isolated deficiency of gonadotropin
Isolated deficiency of growth hormone
Isolated deficiency of pituitary hormone
Kallmann's syndrome
Lorain-Levi short stature
Necrosis of pituitary gland (postpartum)
Panhypopituitarism
Pituitary cachexia
Pituitary insufficiency NOS
Pituitary short stature
Sheehan's syndrome
Simmonds' disease
CC Excl: E22.0-E23.7, E24.1, E30.9, E34.1, E34.4-E35, E89.3

E23.1 Drug-induced hypopituitarism
Use additional code for adverse effect, if applicable, to identify drug (T36-T50 with fifth or sixth character 5)

E23.2 Diabetes insipidus CC
EXCLUDES 1 *nephrogenic diabetes insipidus (N25.1)*
CC Excl: E22.1-E23.7, E24.1, E30.9, E34.1, E34.50-E35, E89.3

E23.3 Hypothalamic dysfunction, not elsewhere classified
EXCLUDES 1 *Prader-Willi syndrome (Q87.1)*
Russell-Silver syndrome (Q87.1)

E23.6 Other disorders of pituitary gland
Abscess of pituitary
Adiposogenital dystrophy

E23.7 Disorder of pituitary gland, unspecified

✓4th **E24 Cushing's syndrome**
EXCLUDES 1 *congenital adrenal hyperplasia (E25.0)*

CC Excl: For CC codes in category E24, unless otherwise noted: E24.0, E24.2-E26.9, E30.9, E34.1, E34.50-E35

E24.0 Pituitary-dependent Cushing's disease CC
Overproduction of pituitary ACTH
Pituitary-dependent hypercorticalism

E24.1 Nelson's syndrome

E24.2 Drug-induced Cushing's syndrome CC
Use additional code for adverse effect, if applicable, to identify drug (T36-T50 with fifth or sixth character 5)

E24.3 Ectopic ACTH syndrome CC

E24.4 Alcohol-induced pseudo-Cushing's syndrome CC

E24.8 Other Cushing's syndrome CC

E24.9 Cushing's syndrome, unspecified CC

E25 Adrenogenital disorders

INCLUDES adrenogenital syndromes, virilizing or feminizing, whether acquired or due to adrenal hyperplasia consequent on inborn enzyme defects in hormone synthesis
female adrenal pseudohermaphroditism
female heterosexual precocious pseudopuberty
male isosexual precocious pseudopuberty
male macrogenitosomia praecox
male sexual precocity with adrenal hyperplasia
male virilization (female)

EXCLUDES 1 *indeterminate sex and pseudohermaphroditism (Q56)*
chromosomal abnormalities (Q90-Q99)

E25.0 Congenital adrenogenital disorders associated with enzyme deficiency
Congenital adrenal hyperplasia
21-Hydroxylase deficiency
Salt-losing congenital adrenal hyperplasia

E25.8 Other adrenogenital disorders
Idiopathic adrenogenital disorder
Use additional code for adverse effect, if applicable, to identify drug (T36-T50 with fifth or sixth character 5)

E25.9 Adrenogenital disorder, unspecified
Adrenogenital syndrome NOS

E26 Hyperaldosteronism

E26.0 Primary hyperaldosteronism

E26.01 Conn's syndrome
Code also adrenal adenoma (D35.0-)

E26.02 Glucocorticoid-remediable aldosteronism
Familial aldosteronism type I

E26.09 Other primary hyperaldosteronism
Primary aldosteronism due to adrenal hyperplasia (bilateral)

E26.1 Secondary hyperaldosteronism

E26.8 Other hyperaldosteronism

E26.81 Bartter's syndrome

E26.89 Other hyperaldosteronism

E26.9 Hyperaldosteronism, unspecified
Aldosteronism NOS
Hyperaldosteronism NOS

E27 Other disorders of adrenal gland

CC Excl: For CC codes in category E27, unless otherwise noted: A17.9, A18.7, A18.82, A18.84, A18.89, E27.0-E27.9, E30.9, E34.1, E34.50-E35, E89.6

E27.0 Other adrenocortical overactivity CC
Overproduction of ACTH, not associated with Cushing's disease
Premature adrenarche
EXCLUDES 1 *Cushing's syndrome (E24.-)*

E27.1 Primary adrenocortical insufficiency CC
Addison's disease
Autoimmune adrenalitis
EXCLUDES 1 *Addison only phenotype adrenoleukodystrophy (E71.528)*
amyloidosis (E85.-)
tuberculous Addison's disease (A18.7)
Waterhouse-Friderichsen syndrome (A39.1)

E27.2 Addisonian crisis CC
Adrenal crisis
Adrenocortical crisis

E27.3 Drug-induced adrenocortical insufficiency CC
Use additional code for adverse effect, if applicable, to identify drug (T36-T50 with fifth or sixth character 5)

E27.4 Other and unspecified adrenocortical insufficiency
EXCLUDES 1 *adrenoleukodystrophy [Addison-Schilder] (E71.528)*
Waterhouse-Friderichsen syndrome (A39.1)

E27.40 Unspecified adrenocortical insufficiency CC
Adrenocortical insufficiency NOS
Hypoaldosteronism

E27.49 Other adrenocortical insufficiency CC
Adrenal hemorrhage
Adrenal infarction

E27.5 Adrenomedullary hyperfunction CC
Adrenomedullary hyperplasia
Catecholamine hypersecretion

E27.8 Other specified disorders of adrenal gland
Abnormality of cortisol-binding globulin

E27.9 Disorder of adrenal gland, unspecified

E28 Ovarian dysfunction
EXCLUDES 1 *isolated gonadotropin deficiency (E23.0)*
postprocedural ovarian failure (E89.4-)

E28.0 Estrogen excess ♀
Use additional code for adverse effect, if applicable, to identify drug (T36-T50 with fifth or sixth character 5)

E28.1 Androgen excess ♀
Hypersecretion of ovarian androgens
Use additional code for adverse effect, if applicable, to identify drug (T36-T50 with fifth or sixth character 5)

E28.2 Polycystic ovarian syndrome ♀
Sclerocystic ovary syndrome
Stein-Leventhal syndrome

E28.3 Primary ovarian failure
EXCLUDES 1 *pure gonadal dysgenesis (Q99.1)*
Turner's syndrome (Q96.-)

E28.31 Premature menopause

E28.310 Symptomatic premature menopause A ♀
Symptoms such as flushing, sleeplessness, headache, lack of concentration, associated with premature menopause

E28.319 Asymptomatic premature menopause A ♀
Premature menopause NOS

E28.39 Other primary ovarian failure ♀
Decreased estrogen
Resistant ovary syndrome

E28.8 Other ovarian dysfunction ♀
Ovarian hyperfunction NOS
EXCLUDES 1 *postprocedural ovarian failure (E89.4-)*

E28.9 Ovarian dysfunction, unspecified ♀

E29 Testicular dysfunction
EXCLUDES 1 *androgen insensitivity syndrome (E34.5-)*
azoospermia or oligospermia NOS (N46.0-N46.1)
isolated gonadotropin deficiency (E23.0)
Klinefelter's syndrome (Q98.0-Q98.2, Q98.4)

E29.0 Testicular hyperfunction ♂
Hypersecretion of testicular hormones

E29.1 Testicular hypofunction ♂
Defective biosynthesis of testicular androgen NOS
5-delta-Reductase deficiency (with male pseudohermaphroditism)
Testicular hypogonadism NOS
Use additional code for adverse effect, if applicable, to identify drug (T36-T50 with fifth or sixth character 5)
EXCLUDES 1 *postprocedural testicular hypofunction (E89.5)*

E29.8 Other testicular dysfunction ♂

E29.9 Testicular dysfunction, unspecified ♂

E30 Disorders of puberty, not elsewhere classified

E30.0 Delayed puberty
Constitutional delay of puberty
Delayed sexual development

E30.1 Precocious puberty P
Precocious menstruation
EXCLUDES 1 *Albright (-McCune) (-Sternberg) syndrome (Q78.1)*
central precocious puberty (E22.8)
congenital adrenal hyperplasia (E25.0)
female heterosexual precocious pseudopuberty (E25.-)
male isosexual precocious pseudopuberty (E25.-)

E30.8 Other disorders of puberty P
Premature thelarche

E30.9 Disorder of puberty, unspecified

E31 Polyglandular dysfunction
EXCLUDES 1 *ataxia telangiectasia [Louis-Bar] (G11.3)*
dystrophia myotonica [Steinert] (G71.11)
pseudohypoparathyroidism (E20.1)

E31.0 Autoimmune polyglandular failure
Schmidt's syndrome

E31.1 Polyglandular hyperfunction
EXCLUDES 1 *multiple endocrine adenomatosis (E31.2-)*
multiple endocrine neoplasia (E31.2-)

✓5th **E31.2 Multiple endocrine neoplasia [MEN] syndromes**
Multiple endocrine adenomatosis
Code also any associated malignancies and other conditions associated with the syndromes

E31.20 Multiple endocrine neoplasia [MEN] syndrome, unspecified
Multiple endocrine adenomatosis NOS
Multiple endocrine neoplasia [MEN] syndrome NOS

E31.21 Multiple endocrine neoplasia [MEN] type I
Wermer's syndrome

E31.22 Multiple endocrine neoplasia [MEN] type IIA
Sipple's syndrome

E31.23 Multiple endocrine neoplasia [MEN] type IIB

E31.8 Other polyglandular dysfunction

E31.9 Polyglandular dysfunction, unspecified

✓4th **E32 Diseases of thymus**
EXCLUDES 1 *aplasia or hypoplasia of thymus with immunodeficiency (D82.1)*
myasthenia gravis (G70.0)

E32.0 Persistent hyperplasia of thymus
Hypertrophy of thymus

E32.1 Abscess of thymus CC
CC Excl: E30.9, E32.0-E32.9, E34.1, E34.50-E35

E32.8 Other diseases of thymus
EXCLUDES 1 *aplasia or hypoplasia with immunodeficiency (D82.1)*
thymoma (D15.0)

E32.9 Disease of thymus, unspecified

✓4th **E34 Other endocrine disorders**
EXCLUDES 1 *pseudohypoparathyroidism (E20.1)*

E34.0 Carcinoid syndrome CC
NOTE May be used as an additional code to identify functional activity associated with a carcinoid tumor.
CC Excl: E30.9, E34.0-E34.2, E34.50-E35

E34.1 Other hypersecretion of intestinal hormones

E34.2 Ectopic hormone secretion, not elsewhere classified
EXCLUDES 1 *ectopic ACTH syndrome (E24.3)*

E34.3 Short stature due to endocrine disorder
Constitutional short stature
Laron-type short stature
EXCLUDES 1 *achondroplastic short stature (Q77.4)*
hypochondroplastic short stature (Q77.4)
nutritional short stature (E45)
pituitary short stature (E23.0)
progeria (E34.8)
renal short stature (N25.0)
Russell-Silver syndrome (Q87.1)
short-limbed stature with immunodeficiency (D82.2)
short stature in specific dysmorphic syndromes— code to syndrome—see Alphabetical Index
short stature NOS (R62.52)

E34.4 Constitutional tall stature
Constitutional gigantism

✓5th **E34.5 Androgen insensitivity syndrome**

E34.50 Androgen insensitivity syndrome, unspecified
Androgen insensitivity NOS

E34.51 Complete androgen insensitivity syndrome
Complete androgen insensitivity
de Quervain syndrome
Goldberg-Maxwell syndrome

E34.52 Partial androgen insensitivity syndrome
Partial androgen insensitivity
Reifenstein syndrome

E34.8 Other specified endocrine disorders
Pineal gland dysfunction
Progeria
EXCLUDES 2 *pseudohypoparathyroidism (E20.1)*

E34.9 Endocrine disorder, unspecified
Endocrine disturbance NOS
Hormone disturbance NOS

E35 Disorders of endocrine glands in diseases classified elsewhere
Code first underlying disease, such as:
late congenital syphilis of thymus gland [Dubois disease] (A50.5)
Use additional code, if applicable, to identify:
sequelae of tuberculosis of other organs (B90.8)
EXCLUDES 1 *Echinococcus granulosus infection of thyroid gland (B67.3)*
meningococcal hemorrhagic adrenalitis (A39.1)
syphilis of endocrine gland (A52.79)
tuberculosis of adrenal gland, except calcification (A18.7)
tuberculosis of endocrine gland NEC (A18.82)
tuberculosis of thyroid gland (A18.81)
Waterhouse-Friderichsen syndrome (A39.1)

✓4th **E36 Intraoperative complications of endocrine system**
EXCLUDES 2 *postprocedural endocrine and metabolic complications and disorders, not elsewhere classified (E89.-)*

✓5th **E36.0 Intraoperative hemorrhage and hematoma of an endocrine system organ or structure complicating a procedure**
EXCLUDES 1 *intraoperative hemorrhage and hematoma of an endocrine system organ or structure due to accidental puncture or laceration during a procedure (E36.1-)*

E36.01 Intraoperative hemorrhage and hematoma of an endocrine system organ or structure complicating an endocrine system procedure CC
CC Excl: E36.01-E36.02, E36.8, E89.810-E89.89, H95.811-H95.89, I85.01, I85.11, I97.3, K21.9, K22.8, K23-K25.0, K25.2, K25.4, K25.6, K26.0, K26.2, K26.4, K26.6, K27.0, K27.2, K27.4, K27.6, K28.0, K28.2, K28.4, K28.6, K29.01, K29.21, K29.31, K29.41, K29.51, K29.61, K29.71, K29.81, K29.91, K31.811, K55.21, K57.01, K57.11, K57.13, K57.21, K57.31, K57.33, K57.41, K57.51, K57.53, K57.81, K57.91, K57.93, K62.5, K92.0-K92.2, M96.89, N98.1-N98.9, P54.1-P54.3, T81.10XA, T81.11XA, T81.12XA, T81.19XA, T81.82XA, T81.89XA, T81.9XXA

E36.02 Intraoperative hemorrhage and hematoma of an endocrine system organ or structure complicating other procedure CC
CC Excl: See code: E36.01

✓5th **E36.1 Accidental puncture and laceration of an endocrine system organ or structure during a procedure**

E36.11 Accidental puncture and laceration of an endocrine system organ or structure during an endocrine system procedure CC
CC Excl: D78.11-D78.12, D78.81-D78.89, E36.11-E36.8, E89.810-E89.89, G96.11, G97.41, G97.48-G97.49, H59.011-H59.019, H59.031-H59.099, H59.211-H59.229, H59.811-H59.89, H95.31-H95.32, H95.811-H95.89, I97.3, I97.51-I97.52, J95.71-J95.72, K91.71-K91.72, L76.11-L76.12, L76.81-L76.82, M96.820-M96.821, M96.89, N98.1-N98.9, N99.71-N99.72, T81.82XA, T81.89XA, T81.9XXA

E36.12 Accidental puncture and laceration of an endocrine system organ or structure during other procedure CC
CC Excl: See code: E36.11

E36.8 Other intraoperative complications of endocrine system
Use additional code, if applicable, to further specify disorder

Malnutrition (E40-E46)

EXCLUDES 1 *intestinal malabsorption (K90.-)*
sequelae of protein-calorie malnutrition (E64.0)
EXCLUDES 2 *nutritional anemias (D50-D53)*
starvation (T73.0)

E40 Kwashiorkor MCC
Severe malnutrition with nutritional edema with dyspigmentation of skin and hair
EXCLUDES 1 *marasmic kwashiorkor (E42)*
CC Excl: E40-E46, E64.0

E41 Nutritional marasmus MCC
Severe malnutrition with marasmus
EXCLUDES 1 *marasmic kwashiorkor (E42)*
CC Excl: See code: E40

E42 Marasmic kwashiorkor MCC
Intermediate form severe protein-calorie malnutrition
Severe protein-calorie malnutrition with signs of both kwashiorkor and marasmus
CC Excl: See code: E40

E43 Unspecified severe protein-calorie malnutrition MCC
Starvation edema
CC Excl: See code: E40

✓4th **E44 Protein-calorie malnutrition of moderate and mild degree**
E44.0 Moderate protein-calorie malnutrition CC
E44.1 Mild protein-calorie malnutrition CC

E45 Retarded development following protein-calorie malnutrition CC
Nutritional short stature
Nutritional stunting
Physical retardation due to malnutrition
CC Excl: See code: E40

E46 Unspecified protein-calorie malnutrition CC
Malnutrition NOS
Protein-calorie imbalance NOS
EXCLUDES 1 *nutritional deficiency NOS (E63.9)*
CC Excl: See code: E40

Other nutritional deficiencies (E50-E64)

EXCLUDES 2 *nutritional anemias (D50-D53)*

✓4th **E50 Vitamin A deficiency**
EXCLUDES 1 *sequelae of vitamin A deficiency (E64.1)*
E50.0 Vitamin A deficiency with conjunctival xerosis
E50.1 Vitamin A deficiency with Bitot's spot and conjunctival xerosis
Bitot's spot in the young child
E50.2 Vitamin A deficiency with corneal xerosis
E50.3 Vitamin A deficiency with corneal ulceration and xerosis
E50.4 Vitamin A deficiency with keratomalacia
E50.5 Vitamin A deficiency with night blindness
E50.6 Vitamin A deficiency with xerophthalmic scars of cornea
E50.7 Other ocular manifestations of vitamin A deficiency
Xerophthalmia NOS
E50.8 Other manifestations of vitamin A deficiency
Follicular keratosis
Xeroderma
E50.9 Vitamin A deficiency, unspecified
Hypovitaminosis A NOS

✓4th **E51 Thiamine deficiency**
EXCLUDES 1 *sequelae of thiamine deficiency (E64.8)*

CC Excl: For CC codes in category E51, unless otherwise noted:
D81.818-D81.819, E51.11-E53.9, E56.0, E56.8-E63.9, E64.8-E64.9

✓5th **E51.1 Beriberi**
E51.11 Dry beriberi CC
Beriberi NOS
Beriberi with polyneuropathy
E51.12 Wet beriberi CC
Beriberi with cardiovascular manifestations
Cardiovascular beriberi
Shoshin disease
E51.2 Wernicke's encephalopathy CC
E51.8 Other manifestations of thiamine deficiency CC
E51.9 Thiamine deficiency, unspecified CC

E52 Niacin deficiency [pellagra]
Niacin (-tryptophan) deficiency
Nicotinamide deficiency
Pellagra (alcoholic)
EXCLUDES 1 *sequelae of niacin deficiency (E64.8)*

✓4th **E53 Deficiency of other B group vitamins**
EXCLUDES 1 *sequelae of vitamin B deficiency (E64.8)*
E53.0 Riboflavin deficiency CC
Ariboflavinosis
Vitamin B2 deficiency
CC Excl: See code: E51
E53.1 Pyridoxine deficiency
Vitamin B6 deficiency
EXCLUDES 1 *pyridoxine-responsive sideroblastic anemia (D64.3)*
E53.8 Deficiency of other specified B group vitamins
Biotin deficiency
Cyanocobalamin deficiency
Folate deficiency
Folic acid deficiency
Pantothenic acid deficiency
Vitamin B12 deficiency
EXCLUDES 1 *folate deficiency anemia (D52.-)*
vitamin B12 deficiency anemia (D51.-)
E53.9 Vitamin B deficiency, unspecified

E54 Ascorbic acid deficiency
Deficiency of vitamin C
Scurvy
EXCLUDES 1 *scorbutic anemia (D53.2)*
sequelae of vitamin C deficiency (E64.2)

✓4th **E55 Vitamin D deficiency**
EXCLUDES 1 *adult osteomalacia (M83.-)*
osteoporosis (M80.-)
sequelae of rickets (E64.3)
E55.0 Rickets, active CC
Infantile osteomalacia
Juvenile osteomalacia
EXCLUDES 1 *celiac rickets (K90.0)*
Crohn's rickets (K50.-)
hereditary vitamin D-dependent rickets (E83.32)
inactive rickets (E64.3)
renal rickets (N25.0)
sequelae of rickets (E64.3)
vitamin D-resistant rickets (E83.31)
CC Excl: E55.0-E63.9, E64.3-E64.9, M83.0-M83.9
E55.9 Vitamin D deficiency, unspecified
Avitaminosis D

✓4th **E56 Other vitamin deficiencies**
EXCLUDES 1 *sequelae of other vitamin deficiencies (E64.8)*
E56.0 Deficiency of vitamin E
E56.1 Deficiency of vitamin K
EXCLUDES 1 *deficiency of coagulation factor due to vitamin K deficiency (D68.4)*
vitamin K deficiency of newborn (P53)
E56.8 Deficiency of other vitamins
E56.9 Vitamin deficiency, unspecified

E58 Dietary calcium deficiency
EXCLUDES 1 *disorders of calcium metabolism (E83.5-)*
sequelae of calcium deficiency (E64.8)

E59 Dietary selenium deficiency
Keshan disease
EXCLUDES 1 *sequelae of selenium deficiency (E64.8)*

E60 Dietary zinc deficiency

✓4th **E61 Deficiency of other nutrient elements**
Use additional code for adverse effect, if applicable, to identify drug (T36-T50 with fifth or sixth character 5)
EXCLUDES 1 *disorders of mineral metabolism (E83.-)*
iodine deficiency related thyroid disorders (E00-E02)
sequelae of malnutrition and other nutritional deficiencies (E64.-)
E61.0 Copper deficiency
E61.1 Iron deficiency
EXCLUDES 1 *iron deficiency anemia (D50.-)*
E61.2 Magnesium deficiency
E61.3 Manganese deficiency
E61.4 Chromium deficiency
E61.5 Molybdenum deficiency
E61.6 Vanadium deficiency
E61.7 Deficiency of multiple nutrient elements
E61.8 Deficiency of other specified nutrient elements
E61.9 Deficiency of nutrient element, unspecified

✓4th **E63 Other nutritional deficiencies**
EXCLUDES 1 *dehydration (E86.0)*
failure to thrive, adult (R62.7)
failure to thrive, child (R62.51)
feeding problems in newborn (P92.-)
sequelae of malnutrition and other nutritional deficiencies (E64.-)
E63.0 Essential fatty acid [EFA] deficiency
E63.1 Imbalance of constituents of food intake
E63.8 Other specified nutritional deficiencies
E63.9 Nutritional deficiency, unspecified

E64 Sequelae of malnutrition and other nutritional deficiencies ✓4th

NOTE This category is to be used to indicate conditions in categories E43, E44, E46, E50-E63 as the cause of sequelae, which are themselves classified elsewhere. The 'sequelae' include conditions specified as such; they also include the late effects of diseases classifiable to the above categories if the disease itself is no longer present

Code first condition resulting from (sequela) of malnutrition and other nutritional deficiencies

E64.0 Sequelae of protein-calorie malnutrition CC

EXCLUDES 2 *retarded development following protein-calorie malnutrition (E45)*

CC Excl: E40-E46, E64.0

E64.1 Sequelae of vitamin A deficiency

E64.2 Sequelae of vitamin C deficiency

E64.3 Sequelae of rickets

E64.8 Sequelae of other nutritional deficiencies

E64.9 Sequelae of unspecified nutritional deficiency

Overweight, obesity and other hyperalimentation (E65-E68)

E65 Localized adiposity

Fat pad

E66 Overweight and obesity ✓4th

Code first obesity complicating pregnancy, childbirth and the puerperium, if applicable (O99.21-)

Use additional code to identify body mass index (BMI), if known (Z68.-)

EXCLUDES 1 *adiposogenital dystrophy (E23.6)*
lipomatosis NOS (E88.2)
lipomatosis dolorosa [Dercum] (E88.2)
Prader-Willi syndrome (Q87.1)

E66.0 Obesity due to excess calories ✓5th

2 **E66.01 Morbid (severe) obesity due to excess calories**

EXCLUDES 1 *morbid (severe) obesity with alveolar hypoventilation (E66.2)*

13 **E66.09 Other obesity due to excess calories**

13 **E66.1 Drug-induced obesity**

Use additional code for adverse effect, if applicable, to identify drug (T36-T50 with fifth or sixth character 5)

E66.2 Morbid (severe) obesity with alveolar hypoventilation CC

Pickwickian syndrome

CC Excl: E66.2-I27.81, I27.89-I27.9

E66.3 Overweight

13 **E66.8 Other obesity**

13 **E66.9 Obesity, unspecified**

Obesity NOS

E67 Other hyperalimentation ✓4th

EXCLUDES 1 *hyperalimentation NOS (R63.2)*
sequelae of hyperalimentation (E68)

E67.0 Hypervitaminosis A

E67.1 Hypercarotinemia

E67.2 Megavitamin-B6 syndrome

E67.3 Hypervitaminosis D

E67.8 Other specified hyperalimentation

E68 Sequelae of hyperalimentation

Code first condition resulting from (sequela) of hyperalimentation

Metabolic disorders (E70-E88)

EXCLUDES 1 *androgen insensitivity syndrome (E34.5-)*
congenital adrenal hyperplasia (E25.0)
Ehlers-Danlos syndrome (Q79.6)
hemolytic anemias attributable to enzyme disorders (D55.-)
Marfan's syndrome (Q87.4)
5-alpha-reductase deficiency (E29.1)

E70 Disorders of aromatic amino-acid metabolism ✓4th

CC Excl: For CC codes in category E70, unless otherwise noted: C88.0, D47.2, D89.0-D89.1, E70.0-E71.30, E72.00-E72.02, E72.04-E74.9, E75.21-E75.22, E75.240-E75.249, E75.3, E75.5-E75.6, E77.0-E78.70, E78.79-E78.9, E88.09-E88.2, E88.89

E70.0 Classical phenylketonuria CC

E70.1 Other hyperphenylalaninemias CC

E70.2 Disorders of tyrosine metabolism ✓5th

EXCLUDES 1 *transitory tyrosinemia of newborn (P74.5)*

E70.20 Disorder of tyrosine metabolism, unspecified CC

E70.21 Tyrosinemia CC

Hypertyrosinemia

E70.29 Other disorders of tyrosine metabolism CC

Alkaptonuria
Ochronosis

E70.3 Albinism ✓5th

E70.30 Albinism, unspecified CC

E70.31 Ocular albinism ✓6th

E70.310 X-linked ocular albinism CC

E70.311 Autosomal recessive ocular albinism CC

E70.318 Other ocular albinism CC

E70.319 Ocular albinism, unspecified CC

E70.32 Oculocutaneous albinism ✓6th

EXCLUDES 1 *Chediak-Higashi syndrome (E70.330)*
Hermansky-Pudlak syndrome (E70.331)

E70.320 Tyrosinase negative oculocutaneous albinism CC

Albinism I
Oculocutaneous albinism ty-neg

E70.321 Tyrosinase positive oculocutaneous albinism CC

Albinism II
Oculocutaneous albinism ty-pos

E70.328 Other oculocutaneous albinism CC

Cross syndrome

E70.329 Oculocutaneous albinism, unspecified CC

E70.33 Albinism with hematologic abnormality ✓6th

E70.330 Chediak-Higashi syndrome CC

E70.331 Hermansky-Pudlak syndrome CC

E70.338 Other albinism with hematologic abnormality CC

E70.339 Albinism with hematologic abnormality, unspecified CC

E70.39 Other specified albinism CC

Piebaldism

E70.4 Disorders of histidine metabolism ✓5th

E70.40 Disorders of histidine metabolism, unspecified CC

E70.41 Histidinemia CC

E70.49 Other disorders of histidine metabolism CC

E70.5 Disorders of tryptophan metabolism CC

E70.8 Other disorders of aromatic amino-acid metabolism CC

E70.9 Disorder of aromatic amino-acid metabolism, unspecified CC

E71 Disorders of branched-chain amino-acid metabolism and fatty-acid metabolism ✓4th

E71.0 Maple-syrup-urine disease CC

CC Excl: See code: E70

E71.1 Other disorders of branched-chain amino-acid metabolism ✓5th

CC Excl: For CC codes in subcategory E71.1, unless otherwise noted: C88.0, D47.2, D89.0-D89.1, E70.0-E71.30, E72.00-E72.02, E72.04-E74.9, E75.21-E75.22, E75.240-E75.249, E75.3, E75.5-E75.6, E77.0-E78.70, E78.79-E78.9, E88.09-E88.2, E88.89

E71.11 Branched-chain organic acidurias ✓6th

E71.110 Isovaleric acidemia CC

E71.111 3-methylglutaconic aciduria CC

E71.118 Other branched-chain organic acidurias CC

E71.12 Disorders of propionate metabolism ✓6th

E71.120 Methylmalonic acidemia CC

E71.121 Propionic acidemia CC

E71.128 Other disorders of propionate metabolism CC

E71.19 Other disorders of branched-chain amino-acid metabolism CC

Hyperleucine-isoleucinemia
Hypervalinemia

E71.2 Disorder of branched-chain amino-acid metabolism, unspecified CC

CC Excl: See code: E70

2 HAC = as PDx in combination with one of the following procedure codes: 0D16[0,4,8][7,J,K,Z][9,A,B,L] or 0DV64CZ **AND** in combination with SDx, not POA, of K68.11, K95.01, K95.81 or T81.4XXA.

13 Questionable admission when used as PDx.

E71.3 Disorders of fatty-acid metabolism
EXCLUDES 1 *peroxisomal disorders (E71.5)*
Refsum's disease (G60.1)
Schilder's disease (G37.0)
EXCLUDES 2 *carnitine deficiency due to inborn error of metabolism (E71.42)*

CC Excl: For CC codes in subcategory E71.3, unless otherwise noted: C96.5-C96.6, E71.39-E71.548, E80.3, E88.40-E88.49, E88.89, H49.811-H49.819

E71.30 Disorder of fatty-acid metabolism, unspecified
E71.31 Disorders of fatty-acid oxidation
E71.310 Long chain/very long chain acyl CoA dehydrogenase deficiency CC
LCAD
VLCAD
E71.311 Medium chain acyl CoA dehydrogenase deficiency CC
MCAD
E71.312 Short chain acyl CoA dehydrogenase deficiency CC
SCAD
E71.313 Glutaric aciduria type II CC
Glutaric aciduria type II A
Glutaric aciduria type II B
Glutaric aciduria type II C
EXCLUDES 1 *glutaric aciduria (type 1) NOS (E72.3)*
E71.314 Muscle carnitine palmitoyltransferase deficiency CC
E71.318 Other disorders of fatty-acid oxidation CC
E71.32 Disorders of ketone metabolism CC
E71.39 Other disorders of fatty-acid metabolism CC
CC Excl: E71.310-E71.32, E71.40-E71.548, E80.4-E80.7, E88.40-E88.49, H49.811-H49.819

E71.4 Disorders of carnitine metabolism
EXCLUDES 1 *muscle carnitine palmitoyltransferase deficiency (E71.314)*
E71.40 Disorder of carnitine metabolism, unspecified
E71.41 Primary carnitine deficiency
E71.42 Carnitine deficiency due to inborn errors of metabolism
Code also associated inborn error or metabolism
E71.43 Iatrogenic carnitine deficiency
Carnitine deficiency due to hemodialysis
Carnitine deficiency due to Valproic acid therapy
E71.44 Other secondary carnitine deficiency
E71.440 Ruvalcaba-Myhre-Smith syndrome
E71.448 Other secondary carnitine deficiency

E71.5 Peroxisomal disorders
EXCLUDES 1 *Schilder's disease (G37.0)*

CC Excl: For CC codes in subcategory E71.5, unless otherwise noted: C96.5-C96.6, E71.310-E71.448, E80.3-E80.7, E88.40-E88.49, E88.89, H49.811-H49.819

E71.50 Peroxisomal disorder, unspecified CC
E71.51 Disorders of peroxisome biogenesis
Group 1 peroxisomal disorders
EXCLUDES 1 *Refsum's disease (G60.1)*
E71.510 Zellweger syndrome CC
E71.511 Neonatal adrenoleukodystrophy CC N
EXCLUDES 1 *X-linked adrenoleukodystrophy (E71.52-)*
E71.518 Other disorders of peroxisome biogenesis CC
E71.52 X-linked adrenoleukodystrophy
E71.520 Childhood cerebral X-linked adrenoleukodystrophy CC
E71.521 Adolescent X-linked adrenoleukodystrophy CC
E71.522 Adrenomyeloneuropathy CC
E71.528 Other X-linked adrenoleukodystrophy CC
Addison only phenotype adrenoleukodystrophy
Addison-Schilder adrenoleukodystrophy
E71.529 X-linked adrenoleukodystrophy, unspecified type CC
E71.53 Other group 2 peroxisomal disorders CC
E71.54 Other peroxisomal disorders
E71.540 Rhizomelic chondrodysplasia punctata CC
EXCLUDES 1 *chondrodysplasia punctata NOS (Q77.3)*
E71.541 Zellweger-like syndrome CC
E71.542 Other group 3 peroxisomal disorders CC
E71.548 Other peroxisomal disorders CC

E72 Other disorders of amino-acid metabolism
EXCLUDES 1 *disorders of:*
aromatic amino-acid metabolism (E70.-)
branched-chain amino-acid metabolism (E71.0-E71.2)
fatty-acid metabolism (E71.3)
purine and pyrimidine metabolism (E79.-)
gout (M1A.-, M10.-)

CC Excl: For CC codes in category E72, unless otherwise noted: C88.0, D47.2, D89.0-D89.1, E70.0-E71.30, E72.00-E72.02, E72.04-E74.9, E75.21-E75.22, E75.240-E75.249, E75.3, E75.5-E75.6, E77.0-E78.70, E78.79-E78.9, E88.09-E88.2, E88.89

E72.0 Disorders of amino-acid transport
EXCLUDES 1 *disorders of tryptophan metabolism (E70.5)*
E72.00 Disorders of amino-acid transport, unspecified CC
E72.01 Cystinuria CC
E72.02 Hartnup's disease CC
E72.03 Lowe's syndrome CC
Use additional code for associated glaucoma (H42)
CC Excl: No Excl
E72.04 Cystinosis CC
Fanconi (-de Toni) (-Debré) syndrome with cystinosis
EXCLUDES 1 *Fanconi (-de Toni) (-Debré) syndrome without cystinosis (E72.09)*
E72.09 Other disorders of amino-acid transport CC
Fanconi (-de Toni) (-Debré) syndrome, unspecified

E72.1 Disorders of sulfur-bearing amino-acid metabolism
EXCLUDES 1 *cystinosis (E72.04)*
cystinuria (E72.01)
transcobalamin II deficiency (D51.2)
E72.10 Disorders of sulfur-bearing amino-acid metabolism, unspecified CC
E72.11 Homocystinuria CC
Cystathionine synthase deficiency
E72.12 Methylenetetrahydrofolate reductase deficiency CC
E72.19 Other disorders of sulfur-bearing amino-acid metabolism CC
Cystathioninuria
Methioninemia
Sulfite oxidase deficiency

E72.2 Disorders of urea cycle metabolism
EXCLUDES 1 *disorders of ornithine metabolism (E72.4)*
E72.20 Disorder of urea cycle metabolism, unspecified CC
Hyperammonemia
EXCLUDES 1 *hyperammonemia- hyperornithinemia-homocitrullinemia syndrome (E72.4)*
transient hyperammonemia of newborn (P74.6)
E72.21 Argininemia CC
E72.22 Arginosuccinic aciduria CC
E72.23 Citrullinemia CC
E72.29 Other disorders of urea cycle metabolism CC

E72.3 Disorders of lysine and hydroxylysine metabolism CC
Glutaric aciduria NOS
Glutaric aciduria (type I)
Hydroxylysinemia
Hyperlysinemia
EXCLUDES 1 *glutaric aciduria type II (E71.313)*
Refsum's disease (G60.1)
Zellweger syndrome (E71.510)

E72.4 Disorders of ornithine metabolism CC
Hyperammonemia-hyperornithinemia-homocitrullinemia syndrome
Ornithinemia (types I, II)
Ornithine transcarbamylase deficiency
EXCLUDES 1 *hereditary choroidal dystrophy (H31.2-)*

E72.5 Disorders of glycine metabolism
E72.50 Disorder of glycine metabolism, unspecified CC
E72.51 Non-ketotic hyperglycinemia CC
E72.52 Trimethylaminuria CC

E72.53 **Hyperoxaluria** CC
Oxalosis
Oxaluria

E72.59 **Other disorders of glycine metabolism** CC
D-glycericacidemia
Hyperhydroxyprolinemia
Hyperprolinemia (types I, II)
Sarcosinemia

E72.8 **Other specified disorders of amino-acid metabolism** CC
Disorders of beta-amino-acid metabolism
Disorders of gamma-glutamyl cycle

E72.9 **Disorder of amino-acid metabolism, unspecified** CC

✓4th **E73 Lactose intolerance**

E73.0 **Congenital lactase deficiency**

E73.1 **Secondary lactase deficiency**

E73.8 **Other lactose intolerance**

E73.9 **Lactose intolerance, unspecified**

✓4th **E74 Other disorders of carbohydrate metabolism**

EXCLUDES 1 *diabetes mellitus (E08-E13)*
hypoglycemia NOS (E16.2)
increased secretion of glucagon (E16.3)
mucopolysaccharidosis (E76.0-E76.3)

CC Excl: For CC codes in category E74, unless otherwise noted: C88.0, D47.2, D89.0-D89.1, E70.0-E71.30, E72.00-E72.02, E72.04-E74.9, E75.21-E75.22, E75.240-E75.249, E75.3, E75.5-E75.6, E77.0-E78.70, E78.79-E78.9, E88.09-E88.2, E88.89

✓5th E74.0 **Glycogen storage disease**

E74.00 **Glycogen storage disease, unspecified** CC

E74.01 **von Gierke disease** CC
Type I glycogen storage disease

E74.02 **Pompe disease** CC
Cardiac glycogenosis
Type II glycogen storage disease

E74.03 **Cori disease** CC
Forbes disease
Type III glycogen storage disease

E74.04 **McArdle disease** CC
Type V glycogen storage disease

E74.09 **Other glycogen storage disease** CC
Andersen disease
Hers disease
Tauri disease
Glycogen storage disease, types 0, IV, VI-XI
Liver phosphorylase deficiency
Muscle phosphofructokinase deficiency

✓5th E74.1 **Disorders of fructose metabolism**

EXCLUDES 1 *muscle phosphofructokinase deficiency (E74.09)*

E74.10 **Disorder of fructose metabolism, unspecified**

E74.11 **Essential fructosuria**
Fructokinase deficiency

E74.12 **Hereditary fructose intolerance**
Fructosemia

E74.19 **Other disorders of fructose metabolism**
Fructose-1, 6-diphosphatase deficiency

✓5th E74.2 **Disorders of galactose metabolism**

E74.20 **Disorders of galactose metabolism, unspecified** CC

E74.21 **Galactosemia** CC

E74.29 **Other disorders of galactose metabolism** CC
Galactokinase deficiency

✓5th E74.3 **Other disorders of intestinal carbohydrate absorption**

EXCLUDES 2 *lactose intolerance (E73.-)*

E74.31 **Sucrase-isomaltase deficiency**

E74.39 **Other disorders of intestinal carbohydrate absorption**
Disorder of intestinal carbohydrate absorption NOS
Glucose-galactose malabsorption
Sucrase deficiency

E74.4 **Disorders of pyruvate metabolism and gluconeogenesis** CC
Deficiency of phosphoenolpyruvate carboxykinase
Deficiency of pyruvate carboxylase
Deficiency of pyruvate dehydrogenase

EXCLUDES 1 *disorders of pyruvate metabolism and gluconeogenesis with anemia (D55.-)*
Leigh's syndrome (G31.82)

E74.8 **Other specified disorders of carbohydrate metabolism** CC
Essential pentosuria
Renal glycosuria

E74.9 **Disorder of carbohydrate metabolism, unspecified**

✓4th **E75 Disorders of sphingolipid metabolism and other lipid storage disorders**

EXCLUDES 1 *mucolipidosis, types I-III (E77.0-E77.1)*
Refsum's disease (G60.1)

✓5th E75.0 **GM2 gangliosidosis**

CC Excl: For CC codes in subcategory E75.0, unless otherwise noted: E75.00-E75.19, E75.4, F84.2, G13.2-G13.8, G30.0-G31.82, G31.84-G31.9, G91.4, G94

E75.00 **GM2 gangliosidosis, unspecified** CC

E75.01 **Sandhoff disease** CC

E75.02 **Tay-Sachs disease** CC

E75.09 **Other GM2 gangliosidosis** CC
Adult GM2 gangliosidosis
Juvenile GM2 gangliosidosis

✓5th E75.1 **Other and unspecified gangliosidosis**

CC Excl: For CC codes in subcategory E75.1, unless otherwise noted: E75.00-E75.19, E75.4, F84.2, G13.2-G13.8, G30.0-G31.82, G31.84-G31.9, G91.4, G94

E75.10 **Unspecified gangliosidosis** CC
Gangliosidosis NOS

E75.11 **Mucolipidosis IV** CC

E75.19 **Other gangliosidosis** CC
GM1 gangliosidosis
GM3 gangliosidosis

✓5th E75.2 **Other sphingolipidosis**

EXCLUDES 1 *adrenoleukodystrophy [Addison-Schilder] (E71.528)*

CC Excl: For CC codes in subcategory E75.2, unless otherwise noted: E75.00-E75.19, E75.23, E75.25-E75.29, E75.4, F84.2, G13.2-G13.8, G31.2-G31.82, G32.89, G91.4, G93.81, G93.89-G94, G96.8-G96.9, G98.0-G98.8, G99.8

E75.21 **Fabry (-Anderson) disease**

E75.22 **Gaucher disease**

E75.23 **Krabbe disease** CC

✓6th E75.24 **Niemann-Pick disease**

E75.240 **Niemann-Pick disease type A**

E75.241 **Niemann-Pick disease type B**

E75.242 **Niemann-Pick disease type C**

E75.243 **Niemann-Pick disease type D**

E75.248 **Other Niemann-Pick disease**

E75.249 **Niemann-Pick disease, unspecified**

E75.25 **Metachromatic leukodystrophy** CC

E75.29 **Other sphingolipidosis** CC
Farber's syndrome
Sulfatase deficiency
Sulfatide lipidosis

E75.3 **Sphingolipidosis, unspecified**

E75.4 **Neuronal ceroid lipofuscinosis** CC
Batten disease
Bielschowsky-Jansky disease
Kufs disease
Spielmeyer-Vogt disease
CC Excl: See code: E75.0

E75.5 **Other lipid storage disorders**
Cerebrotendinous cholesterosis [van Bogaert-Scherer-Epstein]
Wolman's disease

E75.6 **Lipid storage disorder, unspecified**

✓4th **E76 Disorders of glycosaminoglycan metabolism**

CC Excl: For CC codes in category E76, unless otherwise noted: D81.3, D81.5, D81.810, D84.1, E76.01-E76.9, E79.1-E80.29, E80.4-E80.7, E85.0, E85.9, E88.81

✓5th E76.0 **Mucopolysaccharidosis, type I**

E76.01 **Hurler's syndrome** CC

E76.02 **Hurler-Scheie syndrome** CC

E76.03 **Scheie's syndrome** CC

E76.1 **Mucopolysaccharidosis, type II** CC
Hunter's syndrome

✓5th E76.2 **Other mucopolysaccharidoses**

✓6th E76.21 **Morquio mucopolysaccharidoses**

E76.210 **Morquio A mucopolysaccharidoses** CC
Classic Morquio syndrome
Morquio syndrome A
Mucopolysaccharidosis, type IVA

E76.211 **Morquio B mucopolysaccharidoses** CC
Morquio-like mucopolysaccharidoses
Morquio-like syndrome
Morquio syndrome B
Mucopolysaccharidosis, type IVB

E76.219 **Morquio mucopolysaccharidoses, unspecified** CC
Morquio syndrome
Mucopolysaccharidosis, type IV

E76.22 **Sanfilippo mucopolysaccharidoses** CC
Mucopolysaccharidosis, type III (A) (B) (C) (D)
Sanfilippo A syndrome
Sanfilippo B syndrome
Sanfilippo C syndrome
Sanfilippo D syndrome

E76.29 **Other mucopolysaccharidoses** CC
beta-Glucuronidase deficiency
Maroteaux-Lamy (mild) (severe) syndrome
Mucopolysaccharidosis, types VI, VII

E76.3 **Mucopolysaccharidosis, unspecified** CC

E76.8 **Other disorders of glucosaminoglycan metabolism** CC

E76.9 **Glucosaminoglycan metabolism disorder, unspecified** CC

E77 Disorders of glycoprotein metabolism

E77.0 **Defects in post-translational modification of lysosomal enzymes**
Mucolipidosis II [I-cell disease]
Mucolipidosis III [pseudo-Hurler polydystrophy]

E77.1 **Defects in glycoprotein degradation**
Aspartylglucosaminuria
Fucosidosis
Mannosidosis
Sialidosis [mucolipidosis I]
CC Excl: See code: E76

E77.8 **Other disorders of glycoprotein metabolism**

E77.9 **Disorder of glycoprotein metabolism, unspecified**

E78 Disorders of lipoprotein metabolism and other lipidemias
EXCLUDES 1 *sphingolipidosis (E75.0-E75.3)*

E78.0 **Pure hypercholesterolemia**
Familial hypercholesterolemia
Fredrickson's hyperlipoproteinemia, type IIa
Hyperbetalipoproteinemia
Hyperlipidemia, Group A
Low-density-lipoprotein-type [LDL] hyperlipoproteinemia

E78.1 **Pure hyperglyceridemia**
Elevated fasting triglycerides
Endogenous hyperglyceridemia
Fredrickson's hyperlipoproteinemia, type IV
Hyperlipidemia, group B
Hyperprebetalipoproteinemia
Very-low-density-lipoprotein-type [VLDL] hyperlipoproteinemia

E78.2 **Mixed hyperlipidemia**
Broad- or floating-betalipoproteinemia
Combined hyperlipidemia NOS
Elevated cholesterol with elevated triglycerides NEC
Fredrickson's hyperlipoproteinemia, type IIb or III
Hyperbetalipoproteinemia with prebetalipoproteinemia
Hypercholesteremia with endogenous hyperglyceridemia
Hyperlipidemia, group C
Tubo-eruptive xanthoma
Xanthoma tuberosum
EXCLUDES 1 *cerebrotendinous cholesterosis [van Bogaert-Scherer-Epstein] (E75.5)*
familial combined hyperlipidemia (E78.4)

E78.3 **Hyperchylomicronemia**
Chylomicron retention disease
Fredrickson's hyperlipoproteinemia, type I or V
Hyperlipidemia, group D
Mixed hyperglyceridemia

E78.4 **Other hyperlipidemia**
Familial combined hyperlipidemia

E78.5 **Hyperlipidemia, unspecified**

E78.6 **Lipoprotein deficiency**
Abetalipoproteinemia
Depressed HDL cholesterol
High-density lipoprotein deficiency
Hypoalphalipoproteinemia
Hypobetalipoproteinemia (familial)
Lecithin cholesterol acyltransferase deficiency
Tangier disease

E78.7 **Disorders of bile acid and cholesterol metabolism**
EXCLUDES 1 *Niemann-Pick disease type C (E75.242)*

E78.70 **Disorder of bile acid and cholesterol metabolism, unspecified**

E78.71 **Barth syndrome** CC
CC Excl: E78.71-E78.72, Q87.1-Q87.89, Q89.8, Q99.2

E78.72 **Smith-Lemli-Opitz syndrome** CC
CC Excl: See code: E78.71

E78.79 **Other disorders of bile acid and cholesterol metabolism**

E78.8 **Other disorders of lipoprotein metabolism**

E78.81 **Lipoid dermatoarthritis**

E78.89 **Other lipoprotein metabolism disorders**

E78.9 **Disorder of lipoprotein metabolism, unspecified**

E79 Disorders of purine and pyrimidine metabolism
EXCLUDES 1 *Ataxia-telangiectasia (Q87.1)*
Bloom's syndrome (Q82.8)
Cockayne's syndrome (Q87.1)
calculus of kidney (N20.0)
combined immunodeficiency disorders (D81.-)
Fanconi's anemia (D61.09)
gout (M1A.-, M10.-)
orotaciduric anemia (D53.0)
progeria (E34.8)
Werner's syndrome (E34.8)
xeroderma pigmentosum (Q82.1)

CC Excl: For CC codes in category E79, unless otherwise noted: D81.3, D81.5, D81.810, D84.1, E76.01-E76.9, E79.1-E80.29, E80.4-E80.7, E88.81

E79.0 **Hyperuricemia without signs of inflammatory arthritis and tophaceous disease**
Asymptomatic hyperuricemia

E79.1 **Lesch-Nyhan syndrome** CC
HGPRT deficiency

E79.2 **Myoadenylate deaminase deficiency** CC

E79.8 **Other disorders of purine and pyrimidine metabolism** CC
Hereditary xanthinuria

E79.9 **Disorder of purine and pyrimidine metabolism, unspecified** CC

E80 Disorders of porphyrin and bilirubin metabolism
INCLUDES defects of catalase and peroxidase

CC Excl: For CC codes in category E80, unless otherwise noted: D81.3, D81.5, D81.810, D84.1, E76.01-E76.9, E79.1-E80.29, E80.4-E80.7, E88.81

E80.0 **Hereditary erythropoietic porphyria** CC
Congenital erythropoietic porphyria
Erythropoietic protoporphyria

E80.1 **Porphyria cutanea tarda** CC

E80.2 **Other and unspecified porphyria**

E80.20 **Unspecified porphyria** CC
Porphyria NOS

E80.21 **Acute intermittent (hepatic) porphyria** CC

E80.29 **Other porphyria** CC
Hereditary coproporphyria

E80.3 **Defects of catalase and peroxidase** CC
Acatalasia [Takahara]
CC Excl: E71.310-E71.32, E71.40-E71.548, E80.4-E80.7, E88.40-E88.49, H49.811-H49.819

E80.4 **Gilbert syndrome**

E80.5 **Crigler-Najjar syndrome**

E80.6 **Other disorders of bilirubin metabolism**
Dubin-Johnson syndrome
Rotor's syndrome

E80.7 **Disorder of bilirubin metabolism, unspecified**

E83 Disorders of mineral metabolism
EXCLUDES 1 *dietary mineral deficiency (E58-E61)*
parathyroid disorders (E20-E21)
vitamin D deficiency (E55.-)

E83.0 **Disorders of copper metabolism**

E83.00 **Disorder of copper metabolism, unspecified**

E83.01 **Wilson's disease**
Code also associated Kayser Fleischer ring (H18.04-)

E83.09 **Other disorders of copper metabolism**
Menkes' (kinky hair) (steely hair) disease

5th **E83.1 Disorders of iron metabolism**
EXCLUDES 1 *iron deficiency anemia (D50.-)*
sideroblastic anemia (D64.0-D64.3)
E83.10 Disorder of iron metabolism, unspecified
6th **E83.11 Hemochromatosis**
E83.110 Hereditary hemochromatosis
Bronzed diabetes
Pigmentary cirrhosis (of liver)
Primary (hereditary) hemochromatosis
E83.111 Hemochromatosis due to repeated red blood cell transfusions
Iron overload due to repeated red blood cell transfusions
Transfusion (red blood cell) associated hemochromatosis
E83.118 Other hemochromatosis
E83.119 Hemochromatosis, unspecified
E83.19 Other disorders of iron metabolism
Use additional code, if applicable, for idiopathic pulmonary hemosiderosis (J84.03)
E83.2 Disorders of zinc metabolism
Acrodermatitis enteropathica
5th **E83.3 Disorders of phosphorus metabolism and phosphatases**
EXCLUDES 1 *adult osteomalacia (M83.-)*
osteoporosis (M80.-)
E83.30 Disorder of phosphorus metabolism, unspecified
E83.31 Familial hypophosphatemia
Vitamin D-resistant osteomalacia
Vitamin D-resistant rickets
EXCLUDES 1 *vitamin D-deficiency rickets (E55.0)*
E83.32 Hereditary vitamin D-dependent rickets (type 1) (type 2)
25-hydroxyvitamin D 1-alpha-hydroxylase deficiency
Pseudovitamin D deficiency
Vitamin D receptor defect
E83.39 Other disorders of phosphorus metabolism
Acid phosphatase deficiency
Hypophosphatasia
5th **E83.4 Disorders of magnesium metabolism**
E83.40 Disorders of magnesium metabolism, unspecified
E83.41 Hypermagnesemia
E83.42 Hypomagnesemia
E83.49 Other disorders of magnesium metabolism
5th **E83.5 Disorders of calcium metabolism**
EXCLUDES 1 *chondrocalcinosis (M11.1-M11.2)*
hungry bone syndrome (E83.81)
hyperparathyroidism (E21.0-E21.3)
E83.50 Unspecified disorder of calcium metabolism
E83.51 Hypocalcemia
E83.52 Hypercalcemia
Familial hypocalciuric hypercalcemia
E83.59 Other disorders of calcium metabolism
Idiopathic hypercalciuria
5th **E83.8 Other disorders of mineral metabolism**
E83.81 Hungry bone syndrome
E83.89 Other disorders of mineral metabolism
E83.9 Disorder of mineral metabolism, unspecified

4th **E84 Cystic fibrosis**
INCLUDES mucoviscidosis

CC Excl: For CC/MCC codes in category E84, unless otherwise noted: E84.0-E84.9

E84.0 Cystic fibrosis with pulmonary manifestations MCC
Use additional code to identify any infectious organism present, such as:
Pseudomonas (B96.5)
5th **E84.1 Cystic fibrosis with intestinal manifestations**
E84.11 Meconium ileus in cystic fibrosis MCC N
EXCLUDES 1 *meconium ileus not due to cystic fibrosis (P76.0)*
E84.19 Cystic fibrosis with other intestinal manifestations CC
Distal intestinal obstruction syndrome
E84.8 Cystic fibrosis with other manifestations CC
E84.9 Cystic fibrosis, unspecified CC

4th **E85 Amyloidosis**
EXCLUDES 1 *Alzheimer's disease (G30.0-)*

CC Excl: For CC codes in category E85, unless otherwise noted: E85.0-E85.9, E88.81

E85.0 Non-neuropathic heredofamilial amyloidosis CC
Familial Mediterranean fever
Hereditary amyloid nephropathy
AHA: 2012, 4Q, 99
E85.1 Neuropathic heredofamilial amyloidosis CC
Amyloid polyneuropathy (Portuguese)
E85.2 Heredofamilial amyloidosis, unspecified CC
E85.3 Secondary systemic amyloidosis CC
Hemodialysis-associated amyloidosis
E85.4 Organ-limited amyloidosis CC
Localized amyloidosis
E85.8 Other amyloidosis CC
E85.9 Amyloidosis, unspecified CC

4th **E86 Volume depletion**
EXCLUDES 1 *dehydration of newborn (P74.1)*
hypovolemic shock NOS (R57.1)
postprocedural hypovolemic shock (T81.19)
traumatic hypovolemic shock (T79.4)
E86.0 Dehydration
AHA: 2014, 1Q, 7
E86.1 Hypovolemia
Depletion of volume of plasma
E86.9 Volume depletion, unspecified

4th **E87 Other disorders of fluid, electrolyte and acid-base balance**
EXCLUDES 1 *diabetes insipidus (E23.2)*
electrolyte imbalance associated with hyperemesis gravidarum (O21.1)
electrolyte imbalance following ectopic or molar pregnancy (O08.5)
familial periodic paralysis (G72.3)

CC Excl: For CC codes in category E87, unless otherwise noted: E86.0-E87.8

E87.0 Hyperosmolality and hypernatremia CC
Sodium [Na] excess
Sodium [Na] overload
AHA: 2014, 1Q, 7
E87.1 Hypo-osmolality and hyponatremia CC
Sodium [Na] deficiency
EXCLUDES 1 *syndrome of inappropriate secretion of antidiuretic hormone (E22.2)*
AHA: 2014, 1Q, 7
E87.2 Acidosis CC
Acidosis NOS
Lactic acidosis
Metabolic acidosis
Respiratory acidosis
EXCLUDES 1 *diabetic acidosis—see categories E08-E10, E13 with ketoacidosis*
E87.3 Alkalosis CC
Alkalosis NOS
Metabolic alkalosis
Respiratory alkalosis
E87.4 Mixed disorder of acid-base balance CC
E87.5 Hyperkalemia
Potassium [K] excess
Potassium [K] overload
E87.6 Hypokalemia
Potassium [K] deficiency
5th **E87.7 Fluid overload**
EXCLUDES 1 *edema NOS (R60.9)*
fluid retention (R60.9)
E87.70 Fluid overload, unspecified
E87.71 Transfusion associated circulatory overload
Fluid overload due to transfusion (blood) (blood components)
TACO
E87.79 Other fluid overload
E87.8 Other disorders of electrolyte and fluid balance, not elsewhere classified
Electrolyte imbalance NOS
Hyperchloremia
Hypochloremia

E88 Other and unspecified metabolic disorders
Use additional codes for associated conditions
EXCLUDES 1 *histiocytosis X (chronic) (C96.6)*

E88.0 Disorders of plasma-protein metabolism, not elsewhere classified
EXCLUDES 1 *disorder of lipoprotein metabolism (E78.-)*
monoclonal gammopathy (of undetermined significance) (D47.2)
polyclonal hypergammaglobulinemia (D89.0)
Waldenström's macroglobulinemia (C88.0)

E88.01 Alpha-1-antitrypsin deficiency
AAT deficiency

E88.09 Other disorders of plasma-protein metabolism, not elsewhere classified
Bisalbuminemia

E88.1 Lipodystrophy, not elsewhere classified
Lipodystrophy NOS
EXCLUDES 1 *Whipple's disease (K90.81)*

E88.2 Lipomatosis, not elsewhere classified
Lipomatosis NOS
Lipomatosis (Check) dolorosa [Dercum]

E88.3 Tumor lysis syndrome MCC
Tumor lysis syndrome (spontaneous)
Tumor lysis syndrome following antineoplastic drug chemotherapy
Use additional code for adverse effect, if applicable, to identify drug (T45.1X5)
CC Excl: E08.21-E08.29, E09.21-E09.29, E88.3, N00.0-N01.9, N02.8-N02.9, N04.7-N05.1, N05.6-N06.1, N06.6-N07.1, N07.6-N08, N14.0-N15.0, N15.8-N17.9

E88.4 Mitochondrial metabolism disorders
EXCLUDES 1 *disorders of pyruvate metabolism (E74.4)*
Kearns-Sayre syndrome (H49.81)
Leber's disease (H47.22)
Leigh's encephalopathy (G31.82)
Mitochondrial myopathy, NEC (G71.3)
Reye's syndrome (G93.7)

CC Excl: For CC codes in subcategory E88.4, unless otherwise noted: C96.5-C96.6, E71.310-E71.548, E80.3-E80.7, E88.89

E88.40 Mitochondrial metabolism disorder, unspecified CC

E88.41 MELAS syndrome CC
Mitochondrial myopathy, encephalopathy, lactic acidosis and stroke-like episodes

E88.42 MERRF syndrome CC
Myoclonic epilepsy associated with ragged-red fibers
Code also myoclonic epilepsy (G40.3-)

E88.49 Other mitochondrial metabolism disorders CC

E88.8 Other specified metabolic disorders

E88.81 Metabolic syndrome
Dysmetabolic syndrome X
Use additional codes for associated manifestations, such as:
obesity (E66.-)

E88.89 Other specified metabolic disorders CC
Launois-Bensaude adenolipomatosis
EXCLUDES 1 *adult pulmonary Langerhans cell histiocytosis (J84.82)*
CC Excl: E71.310-E71.32, E71.40-E71.548, E80.4-E80.7, E88.40-E88.49, H49.811-H49.819

E88.9 Metabolic disorder, unspecified

E89 Postprocedural endocrine and metabolic complications and disorders, not elsewhere classified
EXCLUDES 2 *intraoperative complications of endocrine system organ or structure (E36.0-, E36.1-, E36.8)*

E89.0 Postprocedural hypothyroidism
Postirradiation hypothyroidism
Postsurgical hypothyroidism

E89.1 Postprocedural hypoinsulinemia CC
Postpancreatectomy hyperglycemia
Postsurgical hypoinsulinemia
Use additional code, if applicable, to identify:
acquired absence of pancreas (Z90.41-)
diabetes mellitus (postpancreatectomy) (postprocedural) (E13.-)
insulin use (Z79.4)
EXCLUDES 1 *transient postprocedural hyperglycemia (R73.9)*
transient postprocedural hypoglycemia (E16.2)
CC Excl: E08.00-E08.59, E08.618-E08.638, E08.641-E09.59, E09.618-E09.638, E09.641-E10.59, E10.618-E10.638, E10.641-E10.649, E10.69-E11.59, E11.618-E11.638, E11.641-E11.649, E11.69-E13.59, E13.618-E13.638, E13.641-E16.2, E30.9, E34.1, E34.50-E35, E89.1

E89.2 Postprocedural hypoparathyroidism
Parathyroprival tetany

E89.3 Postprocedural hypopituitarism
Postirradiation hypopituitarism

E89.4 Postprocedural ovarian failure

E89.40 Asymptomatic postprocedural ovarian failure ♀
Postprocedural ovarian failure NOS

E89.41 Symptomatic postprocedural ovarian failure ♀
Symptoms such as flushing, sleeplessness, headache, lack of concentration, associated with postprocedural menopause

E89.5 Postprocedural testicular hypofunction ♂

E89.6 Postprocedural adrenocortical (-medullary) hypofunction CC
CC Excl: A17.9, A18.7, A18.82, A18.84, A18.89, E27.0-E27.9, E30.9, E34.1, E34.50-E35, E89.6

E89.8 Other postprocedural endocrine and metabolic complications and disordersd

E89.81 Postprocedural hemorrhage and hematoma of an endocrine system organ or structure following a procedure

E89.810 Postprocedural hemorrhage and hematoma of an endocrine system organ or structure following an endocrine system procedure CC
CC Excl: E36.8, E89.810-E89.89, H95.811-H95.89, I97.3, M96.89, N98.1-N98.9, T81.82 with 7th character A, T81.89X-T81.9XX with 7th A

E89.811 Postprocedural hemorrhage and hematoma of an endocrine system organ or structure following other procedure CC
CC Excl: See code E89.810

E89.89 Other postprocedural endocrine and metabolic complications and disorders CC
Use additional code, if applicable, to further specify disorder
CC Excl: See code E89.810

Chapter 5. Mental, Behavioral, and Neurodevelopmental Disorders (F01-F99)

INCLUDES disorders of psychological development
EXCLUDES 2 *symptoms, signs and abnormal clinical laboratory findings, not elsewhere classified (R00-R99)*

This chapter contains the following blocks:

F01-F09 Mental disorders due to known physiological conditions
F10-F19 Mental and behavioral disorders due to psychoactive substance use
F20-F29 Schizophrenia, schizotypal, delusional, and other non-mood psychotic disorders
F30-F39 Mood [affective] disorders
F40-F48 Anxiety, dissociative, stress-related, somatoform and other nonpsychotic mental disorders
F50-F59 Behavioral syndromes associated with physiological disturbances and physical factors
F60-F69 Disorders of adult personality and behavior
F70-F79 Intellectual disabilities
F80-F89 Pervasive and specific developmental disorders
F90-F98 Behavioral and emotional disorders with onset usually occurring in childhood and adolescence
F99 Unspecified mental disorder

Mental disorders due to known physiological conditions (F01-F09)

NOTE This block comprises a range of mental disorders grouped together on the basis of their having in common a demonstrable etiology in cerebral disease, brain injury, or other insult leading to cerebral dysfunction. The dysfunction may be primary, as in diseases, injuries, and insults that affect the brain directly and selectively; or secondary, as in systemic diseases and disorders that attack the brain only as one of the multiple organs or systems of the body that are involved.

√4th **F01 Vascular dementia**
Vascular demdentia as a result of infarction of the brain due to vascular disease, including hypertensive cerebrovascular disease.
INCLUDES arteriosclerotic dementia
Code first the underlying physiological condition or sequelae of cerebrovascular disease.

√5th **F01.5 Vascular dementia**

F01.50 Vascular dementia without behavioral disturbance A

F01.51 Vascular dementia with behavioral disturbance CC A
Vascular dementia with aggressive behavior
Vascular dementia with combative behavior
Vascular dementia with violent behavior
Use additional code, if applicable, to identify wandering in vascular dementia (Z91.83)
CC Excl: F01.51

√4th **F02 Dementia in other diseases classified elsewhere**
Code first the underlying physiological condition, such as:
Alzheimer's (G30.-)
cerebral lipidosis (E75.4)
Creutzfeldt-Jakob disease (A81.0-)
dementia with Lewy bodies (G31.83)
epilepsy and recurrent seizures (G40.-)
frontotemporal dementia (G31.09)
hepatolenticular degeneration (E83.0)
human immunodeficiency virus [HIV] disease (B20)
hypercalcemia (E83.52)
hypothyroidism, acquired (E00-E03.-)
intoxications (T36-T65)
Jakob-Creutzfeldt disease (A81.0-)
multiple sclerosis (G35)
neurosyphilis (A52.17)
niacin deficiency [pellagra] (E52)
Parkinson's disease (G20)
Pick's disease (G31.01)
polyarteritis nodosa (M30.0)
systemic lupus erythematosus (M32.-)
trypanosomiasis (B56.-, B57.-)
vitamin B deficiency (E53.8)
EXCLUDES 1 *dementia with Parkinsonism (G31.83)*
EXCLUDES 2 *dementia in alcohol and psychoactive substance disorders (F10-F19, with .17, .27, .97)*
vascular dementia (F01.5-)

√5th **F02.8 Dementia in other diseases classified elsewhere**

F02.80 Dementia in other diseases classified elsewhere without behavioral disturbance
Dementia in other diseases classified elsewhere NOS

***F02.81 Dementia in other diseases classified elsewhere** with behavioral disturbance* CC
Dementia in other diseases classified elsewhere with aggressive behavior
Dementia in other diseases classified elsewhere with combative behavior
Dementia in other diseases classified elsewhere with violent behavior
Use additional code, if applicable, to identify wandering in dementia in conditions classified elsewhere (Z91.83)
CC Excl: F02.81, F03.91

√4th **F03 Unspecified dementia**
Presenile dementia NOS
Presenile psychosis NOS
Primary degenerative dementia NOS
Senile dementia NOS
Senile dementia NOS
Senile dementia depressed or paranoid type
Senile psychosis NOS
EXCLUDES 1 *senility NOS (R41.81)*
EXCLUDES 2 *mild memory disturbance due to known physiological condition (F06.8)*
senile dementia with delirium or acute confusional state (F05)

√5th **F03.9 Unspecified dementia**

F03.90 Unspecified dementia without behavioral disturbance HIV A
Dementia NOS
AHA: 2012, 4Q, 92

F03.91 Unspecified dementia with behavioral disturbance CC A
Unspecified dementia with aggressive behavior
Unspecified dementia with combative behavior
Unspecified dementia with violent behavior
Use additional code, if applicable, to identify wandering in unspecified dementia (Z91.83)
CC Excl: See code: F02.81

F04 Amnestic disorder due to known physiological condition
Korsakov's psychosis or syndrome, nonalcoholic
Code first the underlying physiological condition
EXCLUDES 1 *amnesia NOS (R41.3)*
anterograde amnesia (R41.1)
dissociative amnesia (F44.0)
retrograde amnesia (R41.2)
EXCLUDES 2 *alcohol-induced or unspecified Korsakov's syndrome (F10.26, F10.96)*
Korsakov's syndrome induced by other psychoactive substances (F13.26, F13.96, F19.16, F19.26, F19.96)

F05 Delirium due to known physiological condition CC
Acute or subacute brain syndrome
Acute or subacute confusional state (nonalcoholic)
Acute or subacute infective psychosis
Acute or subacute organic reaction
Acute or subacute psycho-organic syndrome
Delirium of mixed etiology
Delirium superimposed on dementia
Sundowning
Code first the underlying physiological condition
EXCLUDES 1 *delirium NOS (R41.0)*
EXCLUDES 2 *delirium tremens alcohol-induced or unspecified (F10.231, F10.921)*
CC Excl: F05, R45.851

√4th **F06 Other mental disorders due to known physiological condition**
INCLUDES mental disorders due to endocrine disorder
mental disorders due to exogenous hormone
mental disorders due to exogenous toxic substance
mental disorders due to primary cerebral disease
mental disorders due to somatic illness
mental disorders due to systemic disease affecting the brain
Code first the underlying physiological condition
EXCLUDES 1 *unspecified dementia (F03)*
EXCLUDES 2 *delirium due to known physiological condition (F05)*
dementia as classified in F01-F02
other mental disorders associated with alcohol and other psychoactive substances (F10-F19)

F06.0 Psychotic disorder with hallucinations **due to known physiological condition** CC
Organic hallucinatory state (nonalcoholic)
EXCLUDES 2 *hallucinations and perceptual disturbance induced by alcohol and other psychoactive substances (F10-F19 with .151, .251, .951)*
schizophrenia (F20.-)
CC Excl: F02.80-F02.81, F04-F06.8, F10.10-F11.19, F11.21-F13.19, F13.21-F14.19, F14.21-F15.19, F15.21-F16.19, F16.21-F16.99, F17.203-F17.209, F17.213-F17.219, F17.223-F17.229, F17.293-F18.19, F18.21-F19.19, F19.21-F19.99, F53, F55.0-F55.8, R78.0

FØ6.1 Catatonic disorder due to known physiological condition
EXCLUDES 1 *catatonic stupor (R4Ø.1)*
stupor NOS (R4Ø.1)
EXCLUDES 2 *catatonic schizophrenia (F2Ø.2)*
dissociative stupor (F44.2)

FØ6.2 Psychotic disorder with delusions due to known physiological condition CC
Paranoid and paranoid-hallucinatory organic states
Schizophrenia-like psychosis in epilepsy
EXCLUDES 2 *alcohol and drug-induced psychotic disorder (F1Ø-F19 with .15Ø, .25Ø, .95Ø)*
brief psychotic disorder (F23)
delusional disorder (F22)
schizophrenia (F2Ø.-)
CC Excl: See code: FØ6.Ø

✓5th **FØ6.3 Mood disorder due to known physiological condition**
EXCLUDES 2 *mood disorders due to alcohol and other psychoactive substances (F1Ø-F19 with .14, .24, .94)*
mood disorders, not due to known physiological condition or unspecified (F3Ø-F39)

FØ6.3Ø Mood disorder due to known physiological condition, unspecified

FØ6.31 Mood disorder due to known physiological condition with depressive features

FØ6.32 Mood disorder due to known physiological condition with major depressive-like episode

FØ6.33 Mood disorder due to known physiological condition with manic features

FØ6.34 Mood disorder due to known physiological condition with mixed features

FØ6.4 Anxiety disorder due to known physiological condition
EXCLUDES 2 *anxiety disorders due to alcohol and other psychoactive substances (F1Ø-F19 with .18Ø, .28Ø, .98Ø)*
anxiety disorders, not due to known physiological condition or unspecified (F4Ø.-, F41.-)

FØ6.8 Other specified mental disorders due to known physiological condition HIV
Epileptic psychosis NOS
Organic dissociative disorder
Organic emotionally labile [asthenic] disorder

✓4th **FØ7 Personality and behavioral disorders due to known physiological condition**
Code first the underlying physiological condition

FØ7.Ø Personality change due to known physiological condition
Frontal lobe syndrome
Limbic epilepsy personality syndrome
Lobotomy syndrome
Organic personality disorder
Organic pseudopsychopathic personality
Organic pseudoretarded personality
Postleucotomy syndrome
Code first underlying physiological condition
EXCLUDES 1 *mild cognitive impairment (G31.84)*
postconcussional syndrome (FØ7.81)
postencephalitic syndrome (FØ7.89)
signs and symptoms involving emotional state (R45.-)
EXCLUDES 2 *specific personality disorder (F6Ø.-)*

✓5th **FØ7.8 Other personality and behavioral disorders due to known physiological condition**

FØ7.81 Postconcussional syndrome
Postcontusional syndrome (encephalopathy)
Post-traumatic brain syndrome, nonpsychotic
Use additional code to identify associated post-traumatic headache, if applicable (G44.3-)
EXCLUDES 1 *current concussion (brain) (SØ6.Ø-)*
postencephalitic syndrome (FØ7.89)

FØ7.89 Other personality and behavioral disorders due to known physiological condition
Postencephalitic syndrome
Right hemispheric organic affective disorder

FØ7.9 Unspecified personality and behavioral disorder due to known physiological condition HIV
Organic psychosyndrome

FØ9 Unspecified mental disorder due to known physiological condition HIV
Mental disorder NOS due to known physiological condition
Organic brain syndrome NOS
Organic mental disorder NOS
Organic psychosis NOS
Symptomatic psychosis NOS
Code first the underlying physiological condition
EXCLUDES 1 *psychosis NOS (F29)*

Mental and behavioral disorders due to psychoactive substance use (F1Ø-F19)

✓4th **F1Ø Alcohol related disorders**
Use additional code for blood alcohol level, if applicable (Y9Ø.-)

CC Excl: For CC codes in category F1Ø, unless otherwise noted: FØ2.8Ø-FØ2.81, FØ4-FØ6.8, F1Ø.1Ø-F11.19, F11.21-F13.19, F13.21-F14.19, F14.21-F15.19, F15.21-F16.19, F16.21-F16.99, F17.2Ø3-F17.2Ø9, F17.213-F17.219, F17.223-F17.229, F17.293-F18.19, F18.21-F19.19, F19.21-F19.99, F53, F55.Ø-F55.8, R78.Ø

✓5th **F1Ø.1 Alcohol abuse**
EXCLUDES 1 *alcohol dependence (F1Ø.2-)*
alcohol use, unspecified (F1Ø.9-)

F1Ø.1Ø Alcohol abuse, uncomplicated

✓6th **F1Ø.12 Alcohol abuse with intoxication**

F1Ø.12Ø Alcohol abuse with intoxication, uncomplicated

F1Ø.121 Alcohol abuse with intoxication delirium CC

F1Ø.129 Alcohol abuse with intoxication, unspecified

F1Ø.14 Alcohol abuse with alcohol-induced mood disorder CC

✓6th **F1Ø.15 Alcohol abuse with alcohol-induced psychotic disorder**

F1Ø.15Ø Alcohol abuse with alcohol-induced psychotic disorder with delusions

F1Ø.151 Alcohol abuse with alcohol-induced psychotic disorder with hallucinations CC

F1Ø.159 Alcohol abuse with alcohol-induced psychotic disorder, unspecified CC

✓6th **F1Ø.18 Alcohol abuse with other alcohol-induced disorders**

F1Ø.18Ø Alcohol abuse with alcohol-induced anxiety disorder CC

F1Ø.181 Alcohol abuse with alcohol-induced sexual dysfunction CC

F1Ø.182 Alcohol abuse with alcohol-induced sleep disorder

F1Ø.188 Alcohol abuse with other alcohol-induced disorder CC

F1Ø.19 Alcohol abuse with unspecified alcohol-induced disorder CC

✓5th **F1Ø.2 Alcohol dependence**
EXCLUDES 1 *alcohol abuse (F1Ø.1-)*
alcohol use, unspecified (F1Ø.9-)
EXCLUDES 2 *toxic effect of alcohol (T51.Ø-)*

F1Ø.2Ø Alcohol dependence, uncomplicated

F1Ø.21 Alcohol dependence, in remission

✓6th **F1Ø.22 Alcohol dependence with intoxication**
Acute drunkenness (in alcoholism)
EXCLUDES 1 *alcohol dependence with withdrawal (F1Ø.23-)*

F1Ø.22Ø Alcohol dependence with intoxication, uncomplicated

F1Ø.221 Alcohol dependence with intoxication delirium CC

F1Ø.229 Alcohol dependence with intoxication, unspecified

✓6th **F1Ø.23 Alcohol dependence with withdrawal**
EXCLUDES 1 *Alcohol dependence with intoxication (F1Ø.22-)*

F1Ø.23Ø Alcohol dependence with withdrawal, uncomplicated CC

F1Ø.231 Alcohol dependence with withdrawal delirium CC

F1Ø.232 Alcohol dependence with withdrawal with perceptual disturbance CC

Mental, Behavioral, and Neurodevelopmental Disorders
FØ6.1–F1Ø.232

F10.239 Alcohol dependence with withdrawal, unspecified CC

F10.24 Alcohol dependence with alcohol-induced mood disorder CC

✓6th F10.25 Alcohol dependence with alcohol-induced psychotic disorder

F10.250 Alcohol dependence with alcohol-induced psychotic disorder with delusions

F10.251 Alcohol dependence with alcohol-induced psychotic disorder with hallucinations CC

F10.259 Alcohol dependence with alcohol-induced psychotic disorder, unspecified CC

F10.26 Alcohol dependence with alcohol-induced persisting amnestic disorder

F10.27 Alcohol dependence with alcohol-induced persisting dementia CC

✓6th F10.28 Alcohol dependence with other alcohol-induced disorders

F10.280 Alcohol dependence with alcohol-induced anxiety disorder CC

F10.281 Alcohol dependence with alcohol-induced sexual dysfunction CC

F10.282 Alcohol dependence with alcohol-induced sleep disorder

F10.288 Alcohol dependence with other alcohol-induced disorder CC

F10.29 Alcohol dependence with unspecified alcohol-induced disorder CC

✓5th F10.9 Alcohol use, unspecified

EXCLUDES 1 *alcohol abuse (F10.1-)*
alcohol dependence (F10.2-)

✓6th F10.92 Alcohol use, unspecified with intoxication

F10.920 Alcohol use, unspecified with intoxication, uncomplicated

F10.921 Alcohol use, unspecified with intoxication delirium CC

F10.929 Alcohol use, unspecified with intoxication, unspecified

F10.94 Alcohol use, unspecified with alcohol-induced mood disorder CC

✓6th F10.95 Alcohol use, unspecified with alcohol-induced psychotic disorder

F10.950 Alcohol use, unspecified with alcohol-induced psychotic disorder with delusions

F10.951 Alcohol use, unspecified with alcohol-induced psychotic disorder with hallucinations CC

F10.959 Alcohol use, unspecified with alcohol-induced psychotic disorder, unspecified CC

F10.96 Alcohol use, unspecified with alcohol-induced persisting amnestic disorder

F10.97 Alcohol use, unspecified with alcohol-induced persisting dementia

✓6th F10.98 Alcohol use, unspecified with other alcohol-induced disorders

F10.980 Alcohol use, unspecified with alcohol-induced anxiety disorder CC

F10.981 Alcohol use, unspecified with alcohol-induced sexual dysfunction CC

F10.982 Alcohol use, unspecified with alcohol-induced sleep disorder

F10.988 Alcohol use, unspecified with other alcohol-induced disorder CC

F10.99 Alcohol use, unspecified with unspecified alcohol-induced disorder CC

✓4th F11 Opioid related disorders

CC Excl: For CC codes in category F11, unless otherwise noted: F02.80-F02.81, F04-F06.8, F10.10-F11.19, F11.21-F13.19, F13.21-F14.19, F14.21-F15.19, F15.21-F16.19, F16.21-F16.99, F17.203-F17.209, F17.213-F17.219, F17.223-F17.229, F17.293-F18.19, F18.21-F19.19, F19.21-F19.99, F53, F55.0-F55.8, R78.0

✓5th F11.1 Opioid abuse

EXCLUDES 1 *opioid dependence (F11.2-)*
opioid use, unspecified (F11.9-)

F11.10 Opioid abuse, uncomplicated

✓6th F11.12 Opioid abuse with intoxication

F11.120 Opioid abuse with intoxication, uncomplicated

F11.121 Opioid abuse with intoxication delirium CC

F11.122 Opioid abuse with intoxication with perceptual disturbance

F11.129 Opioid abuse with intoxication, unspecified

F11.14 Opioid abuse with opioid-induced mood disorder

✓6th F11.15 Opioid abuse with opioid-induced psychotic disorder

F11.150 Opioid abuse with opioid-induced psychotic disorder with delusions CC

F11.151 Opioid abuse with opioid-induced psychotic disorder with hallucinations CC

F11.159 Opioid abuse with opioid-induced psychotic disorder, unspecified

✓6th F11.18 Opioid abuse with other opioid-induced disorder

F11.181 Opioid abuse with opioid-induced sexual dysfunction

F11.182 Opioid abuse with opioid-induced sleep disorder

F11.188 Opioid abuse with other opioid-induced disorder

F11.19 Opioid abuse with unspecified opioid-induced disorder

✓5th F11.2 Opioid dependence

EXCLUDES 1 *opioid abuse (F11.1-)*
opioid use, unspecified (F11.9-)

EXCLUDES 2 *opioid poisoning (T40.0-T40.2-)*

F11.20 Opioid dependence, uncomplicated CC
CC Excl: No excl

F11.21 Opioid dependence, in remission

✓6th F11.22 Opioid dependence with intoxication

EXCLUDES 1 *opioid dependence with withdrawal (F11.23)*

F11.220 Opioid dependence with intoxication, uncomplicated
CC Excl: No excl

F11.221 Opioid dependence with intoxication delirium CC
CC Excl: F02.80-F02.81, F04- F06.8, F10.10-F11.19, F11.21-F13.19, F13.21- F14.19, F14.21-F15.19, F15.21-F16.19, F16.21-F16.99, F17.203-F17.209, F17.213- F17.219, F17.223-F17.229, F17.293-F18.19, F18.21-F19.19, F19.21-F19.99, F53, F55.0-F55.8, R78.0

F11.222 Opioid dependence with intoxication with perceptual disturbance CC
CC Excl: No excl

F11.229 Opioid dependence with intoxication, unspecified
CC Excl: No excl

F11.23 Opioid dependence with withdrawal CC

EXCLUDES 1 *opioid dependence with intoxication (F11.22-)*

CC Excl: See code: F11.221

F11.24 Opioid dependence with opioid-induced mood disorder

✓6th F11.25 Opioid dependence with opioid-induced psychotic disorder

F11.250 Opioid dependence with opioid-induced psychotic disorder with delusions CC
CC Excl: See code: F11.221

F11.251 Opioid dependence with opioid-induced psychotic disorder with hallucinations CC
CC Excl: See code: F11.221

F11.259 Opioid dependence with opioid-induced psychotic disorder, unspecified CC
CC Excl: No excl

✓6th F11.28 Opioid dependence with other opioid-induced disorder

F11.281 Opioid dependence with opioid-induced sexual dysfunction CC
CC Excl: No excl

F11.282 Opioid dependence with opioid-induced sleep disorder CC
CC Excl: No excl

F11.288 Opioid dependence with other opioid-induced disorder CC
CC Excl: No excl

F11.29 Opioid dependence with unspecified opioid-induced disorder
CC Excl: No excl

✓5th F11.9 Opioid use, unspecified
EXCLUDES 1 *opioid abuse (F11.1-)*
opioid dependence (F11.2-)

F11.90 Opioid use, unspecified, uncomplicated

✓6th F11.92 Opioid use, unspecified with intoxication
EXCLUDES 1 *opioid use, unspecified with withdrawal (F11.93)*

F11.920 Opioid use, unspecified with intoxication, uncomplicated

F11.921 Opioid use, unspecified with intoxication delirium CC
CC Excl: See code: F11.221

F11.922 Opioid use, unspecified with intoxication with perceptual disturbance

F11.929 Opioid use, unspecified with intoxication, unspecified

F11.93 Opioid use, unspecified with withdrawal CC
EXCLUDES 1 *opioid use, unspecified with intoxication (F11.92-)*
CC Excl: See code: F11.221

F11.94 Opioid use, unspecified with opioid-induced mood disorder

✓6th F11.95 Opioid use, unspecified with opioid-induced psychotic disorder

F11.950 Opioid use, unspecified with opioid-induced psychotic disorder with delusions CC
CC Excl: See code: F11.221

F11.951 Opioid use, unspecified with opioid-induced psychotic disorder with hallucinations CC
CC Excl: See code: F11.221

F11.959 Opioid use, unspecified with opioid-induced psychotic disorder, unspecified

✓6th F11.98 Opioid use, unspecified with other specified opioid-induced disorder

F11.981 Opioid use, unspecified with opioid-induced sexual dysfunction

F11.982 Opioid use, unspecified with opioid-induced sleep disorder

F11.988 Opioid use, unspecified with other opioid-induced disorder

F11.99 Opioid use, unspecified with unspecified opioid-induced disorder

✓4th F12 Cannabis related disorders
INCLUDES marijuana

CC Excl: For CC codes in category F12, unless otherwise noted:
F02.80-F02.81, F04-F06.8, F10.10-F11.19, F11.21-F13.19, F13.21-F14.19, F14.21-F15.19, F15.21-F16.19, F16.21-F16.99, F17.203-F17.209, F17.213-F17.219, F17.223-F17.229, F17.293-F18.19, F18.21-F19.19, F19.21-F19.99, F53, F55.0-F55.8, R78.0

✓5th F12.1 Cannabis abuse
EXCLUDES 1 *cannabis dependence (F12.2-)*
cannabis use, unspecified (F12.9-)

F12.10 Cannabis abuse, uncomplicated

✓6th F12.12 Cannabis abuse with intoxication

F12.120 Cannabis abuse with intoxication, uncomplicated

F12.121 Cannabis abuse with intoxication delirium CC

F12.122 Cannabis abuse with intoxication with perceptual disturbance

F12.129 Cannabis abuse with intoxication, unspecified

✓6th F12.15 Cannabis abuse with psychotic disorder

F12.150 Cannabis abuse with psychotic disorder with delusions CC

F12.151 Cannabis abuse with psychotic disorder with hallucinations CC

F12.159 Cannabis abuse with psychotic disorder, unspecified

✓6th F12.18 Cannabis abuse with other cannabis-induced disorder

F12.180 Cannabis abuse with cannabis-induced anxiety disorder

F12.188 Cannabis abuse with other cannabis-induced disorder

F12.19 Cannabis abuse with unspecified cannabis-induced disorder

✓5th F12.2 Cannabis dependence
EXCLUDES 1 *cannabis abuse (F12.1-)*
cannabis use, unspecified (F12.9-)
EXCLUDES 2 *cannabis poisoning (T40.7-)*

F12.20 Cannabis dependence, uncomplicated

F12.21 Cannabis dependence, in remission

✓6th F12.22 Cannabis dependence with intoxication

F12.220 Cannabis dependence with intoxication, uncomplicated

F12.221 Cannabis dependence with intoxication delirium CC

F12.222 Cannabis dependence with intoxication with perceptual disturbance

F12.229 Cannabis dependence with intoxication, unspecified

✓6th F12.25 Cannabis dependence with psychotic disorder

F12.250 Cannabis dependence with psychotic disorder with delusions CC

F12.251 Cannabis dependence with psychotic disorder with hallucinations CC

F12.259 Cannabis dependence with psychotic disorder, unspecified

✓6th F12.28 Cannabis dependence with other cannabis-induced disorder

F12.280 Cannabis dependence with cannabis-induced anxiety disorder

F12.288 Cannabis dependence with other cannabis-induced disorder

F12.29 Cannabis dependence with unspecified cannabis-induced disorder

✓5th F12.9 Cannabis use, unspecified
EXCLUDES 1 *cannabis abuse (F12.1-)*
cannabis dependence (F12.2-)

F12.90 Cannabis use, unspecified, uncomplicated

✓6th F12.92 Cannabis use, unspecified with intoxication

F12.920 Cannabis use, unspecified with intoxication, uncomplicated

F12.921 Cannabis use, unspecified with intoxication delirium CC

F12.922 Cannabis use, unspecified with intoxication with perceptual disturbance

F12.929 Cannabis use, unspecified with intoxication, unspecified

✓6th F12.95 Cannabis use, unspecified with psychotic disorder

F12.950 Cannabis use, unspecified with psychotic disorder with delusions CC

F12.951 Cannabis use, unspecified with psychotic disorder with hallucinations CC

F12.959 Cannabis use, unspecified with psychotic disorder, unspecified

✓6th F12.98 Cannabis use, unspecified with other cannabis-induced disorder

F12.980 Cannabis use, unspecified with anxiety disorder

F12.988 Cannabis use, unspecified with other cannabis-induced disorder

F12.99 **Cannabis use, unspecified with unspecified cannabis-induced disorder**

✓4th **F13 Sedative, hypnotic, or anxiolytic related disorders**

CC Excl: For CC codes in category F13, unless otherwise noted: FØ2.8Ø-FØ2.81, FØ4-FØ6.8, F1Ø.1Ø-F11.19, F11.21-F13.19, F13.21-F14.19, F14.21-F15.19, F15.21-F16.19, F16.21-F16.99, F17.2Ø3-F17.2Ø9, F17.213-F17.219, F17.223-F17.229, F17.293- F18.19, F18.21-F19.19, F19.21-F19.99, F53, F55.Ø-F55.8, R78.Ø

✓5th **F13.1 Sedative, hypnotic or anxiolytic-related abuse**

EXCLUDES 1 *sedative, hypnotic or anxiolytic-related dependence (F13.2-)*
sedative, hypnotic, or anxiolytic use, unspecified (F13.9-)

F13.1Ø **Sedative, hypnotic or anxiolytic abuse, uncomplicated**

✓6th F13.12 **Sedative, hypnotic or anxiolytic abuse with intoxication**

F13.12Ø **Sedative, hypnotic or anxiolytic abuse with intoxication, uncomplicated**

F13.121 **Sedative, hypnotic or anxiolytic abuse with intoxication delirium** CC

F13.129 **Sedative, hypnotic or anxiolytic abuse with intoxication, unspecified**

F13.14 **Sedative, hypnotic or anxiolytic abuse with sedative, hypnotic or anxiolytic-induced mood disorder**

✓6th F13.15 **Sedative, hypnotic or anxiolytic abuse with sedative, hypnotic or anxiolytic-induced psychotic disorder**

F13.15Ø **Sedative, hypnotic or anxiolytic abuse with sedative, hypnotic or anxiolytic-induced psychotic disorder with delusions** CC

F13.151 **Sedative, hypnotic or anxiolytic abuse with sedative, hypnotic or anxiolytic-induced psychotic disorder with hallucinations** CC

F13.159 **Sedative, hypnotic or anxiolytic abuse with sedative, hypnotic or anxiolytic-induced psychotic disorder, unspecified**

✓6th F13.18 **Sedative, hypnotic or anxiolytic abuse with other sedative, hypnotic or anxiolytic-induced disorders**

F13.18Ø **Sedative, hypnotic or anxiolytic abuse with sedative, hypnotic or anxiolytic-induced anxiety disorder**

F13.181 **Sedative, hypnotic or anxiolytic abuse with sedative, hypnotic or anxiolytic-induced sexual dysfunction**

F13.182 **Sedative, hypnotic or anxiolytic abuse with sedative, hypnotic or anxiolytic-induced sleep disorder**

F13.188 **Sedative, hypnotic or anxiolytic abuse with other sedative, hypnotic or anxiolytic-induced disorder**

F13.19 **Sedative, hypnotic or anxiolytic abuse with unspecified sedative, hypnotic or anxiolytic-induced disorder**

✓5th **F13.2 Sedative, hypnotic or anxiolytic-related dependence**

EXCLUDES 1 *sedative, hypnotic or anxiolytic-related abuse (F13.1-)*
sedative, hypnotic, or anxiolytic use, unspecified (F13.9-)

EXCLUDES 2 *sedative, hypnotic, or anxiolytic poisoning (T42.-)*

F13.2Ø **Sedative, hypnotic or anxiolytic dependence, uncomplicated** CC
CC Excl: No excl

F13.21 **Sedative, hypnotic or anxiolytic dependence, in remission**

✓6th F13.22 **Sedative, hypnotic or anxiolytic dependence with intoxication**

EXCLUDES 1 *sedative, hypnotic or anxiolytic dependence with withdrawal (F13.23-)*

F13.22Ø **Sedative, hypnotic or anxiolytic dependence with intoxication, uncomplicated**

F13.221 **Sedative, hypnotic or anxiolytic dependence with intoxication delirium** CC
CC Excl: See code: F13

F13.229 **Sedative, hypnotic or anxiolytic dependence with intoxication, unspecified**
CC Excl: No Excl

✓6th F13.23 **Sedative, hypnotic or anxiolytic dependence with withdrawal**

EXCLUDES 1 *sedative, hypnotic or anxiolytic dependence with intoxication (F13.22-)*

F13.23Ø **Sedative, hypnotic or anxiolytic dependence with withdrawal, uncomplicated** CC
CC Excl: See code: F13

F13.231 **Sedative, hypnotic or anxiolytic dependence with withdrawal delirium** CC
CC Excl: See code: F13

F13.232 **Sedative, hypnotic or anxiolytic dependence with withdrawal with perceptual disturbance** CC
CC Excl: See code: F13

F13.239 **Sedative, hypnotic or anxiolytic dependence with withdrawal, unspecified** CC
CC Excl: See code: F13

F13.24 **Sedative, hypnotic or anxiolytic dependence with sedative, hypnotic or anxiolytic-induced mood disorder**

✓6th F13.25 **Sedative, hypnotic or anxiolytic dependence with sedative, hypnotic or anxiolytic-induced psychotic disorder**

F13.25Ø **Sedative, hypnotic or anxiolytic dependence with sedative, hypnotic or anxiolytic-induced psychotic disorder with delusions** CC
CC Excl: See code: F13

F13.251 **Sedative, hypnotic or anxiolytic dependence with sedative, hypnotic or anxiolytic-induced psychotic disorder with hallucinations** CC
CC Excl: See code: F13

F13.259 **Sedative, hypnotic or anxiolytic dependence with sedative, hypnotic or anxiolytic-induced psychotic disorder, unspecified** CC
CC Excl: No Excl

F13.26 **Sedative, hypnotic or anxiolytic dependence with sedative, hypnotic or anxiolytic-induced persisting amnestic disorder** CC
CC Excl: No Excl

F13.27 **Sedative, hypnotic or anxiolytic dependence with sedative, hypnotic or anxiolytic-induced persisting dementia** CC
CC Excl: See code: F13

✓6th F13.28 **Sedative, hypnotic or anxiolytic dependence with other sedative, hypnotic or anxiolytic-induced disorders**

F13.28Ø **Sedative, hypnotic or anxiolytic dependence with sedative, hypnotic or anxiolytic-induced anxiety disorder** CC
CC Excl: No Excl

F13.281 **Sedative, hypnotic or anxiolytic dependence with sedative, hypnotic or anxiolytic-induced sexual dysfunction** CC
CC Excl: No Excl

F13.282 **Sedative, hypnotic or anxiolytic dependence with sedative, hypnotic or anxiolytic-induced sleep disorder** CC
CC Excl: No Excl

F13.288 **Sedative, hypnotic or anxiolytic dependence with other sedative, hypnotic or anxiolytic-induced disorder** CC
CC Excl: No Excl

F13.29 **Sedative, hypnotic or anxiolytic dependence with unspecified sedative, hypnotic or anxiolytic-induced disorder**
CC Excl: No Excl

✓5th **F13.9 Sedative, hypnotic or anxiolytic-related use, unspecified**

EXCLUDES 1 *sedative, hypnotic or anxiolytic-related abuse (F13.1-)*
sedative, hypnotic or anxiolytic-related dependence (F13.2-)

F13.9Ø **Sedative, hypnotic, or anxiolytic use, unspecified, uncomplicated**

√6th **F13.92 Sedative, hypnotic or anxiolytic use, unspecified with intoxication**
EXCLUDES 1 *sedative, hypnotic or anxiolytic use, unspecified with withdrawal (F13.93-)*
F13.920 Sedative, hypnotic or anxiolytic use, unspecified with intoxication, uncomplicated
F13.921 Sedative, hypnotic or anxiolytic use, unspecified with intoxication delirium CC
F13.929 Sedative, hypnotic or anxiolytic use, unspecified with intoxication, unspecified

√6th **F13.93 Sedative, hypnotic or anxiolytic use, unspecified with withdrawal**
EXCLUDES 1 *sedative, hypnotic or anxiolytic use, unspecified with intoxication (F13.92-)*
F13.930 Sedative, hypnotic or anxiolytic use, unspecified with withdrawal, uncomplicated CC
F13.931 Sedative, hypnotic or anxiolytic use, unspecified with withdrawal delirium CC
F13.932 Sedative, hypnotic or anxiolytic use, unspecified with withdrawal with perceptual disturbances CC
F13.939 Sedative, hypnotic or anxiolytic use, unspecified with withdrawal, unspecified CC

F13.94 Sedative, hypnotic or anxiolytic use, unspecified with sedative, hypnotic or anxiolytic-induced mood disorder

√6th **F13.95 Sedative, hypnotic or anxiolytic use, unspecified with sedative, hypnotic or anxiolytic-induced psychotic disorder**
F13.950 Sedative, hypnotic or anxiolytic use, unspecified with sedative, hypnotic or anxiolytic-induced psychotic disorder with delusions CC
F13.951 Sedative, hypnotic or anxiolytic use, unspecified with sedative, hypnotic or anxiolytic-induced psychotic disorder with hallucinations CC
F13.959 Sedative, hypnotic or anxiolytic use, unspecified with sedative, hypnotic or anxiolytic-induced psychotic disorder, unspecified

F13.96 Sedative, hypnotic or anxiolytic use, unspecified with sedative, hypnotic or anxiolytic-induced persisting amnestic disorder

F13.97 Sedative, hypnotic or anxiolytic use, unspecified with sedative, hypnotic or anxiolytic-induced persisting dementia CC

√6th **F13.98 Sedative, hypnotic or anxiolytic use, unspecified with other sedative, hypnotic or anxiolytic-induced disorders**
F13.980 Sedative, hypnotic or anxiolytic use, unspecified with sedative, hypnotic or anxiolytic-induced anxiety disorder
F13.981 Sedative, hypnotic or anxiolytic use, unspecified with sedative, hypnotic or anxiolytic-induced sexual dysfunction
F13.982 Sedative, hypnotic or anxiolytic use, unspecified with sedative, hypnotic or anxiolytic-induced sleep disorder
F13.988 Sedative, hypnotic or anxiolytic use, unspecified with other sedative, hypnotic or anxiolytic-induced disorder

F13.99 Sedative, hypnotic or anxiolytic use, unspecified with unspecified sedative, hypnotic or anxiolytic-induced disorder

√4th **F14 Cocaine related disorders**
EXCLUDES 2 *other stimulant-related disorders (F15.-)*

CC Excl: For CC codes in category F14, unless otherwise noted: F02.80-F02.81, F04-F06.8, F10.10-F11.19, F11.21-F13.19, F13.21-F14.19, F14.21-F15.19, F15.21-F16.19, F16.21-F16.99, F17.203-F17.209, F17.213-F17.219, F17.223-F17.229, F17.293-F18.19, F18.21-F19.19, F19.21-F19.99, F53, F55.0-F55.8, R78.0

√5th **F14.1 Cocaine abuse**
EXCLUDES 1 *cocaine dependence (F14.2-)*
cocaine use, unspecified (F14.9-)
F14.10 Cocaine abuse, uncomplicated

√6th **F14.12 Cocaine abuse with intoxication**
F14.120 Cocaine abuse with intoxication, uncomplicated
F14.121 Cocaine abuse with intoxication with delirium CC
F14.122 Cocaine abuse with intoxication with perceptual disturbance
F14.129 Cocaine abuse with intoxication, unspecified

F14.14 Cocaine abuse with cocaine-induced mood disorder

√6th **F14.15 Cocaine abuse with cocaine-induced psychotic disorder**
F14.150 Cocaine abuse with cocaine-induced psychotic disorder with delusions CC
F14.151 Cocaine abuse with cocaine-induced psychotic disorder with hallucinations CC
F14.159 Cocaine abuse with cocaine-induced psychotic disorder, unspecified

√6th **F14.18 Cocaine abuse with other cocaine-induced disorder**
F14.180 Cocaine abuse with cocaine-induced anxiety disorder
F14.181 Cocaine abuse with cocaine-induced sexual dysfunction
F14.182 Cocaine abuse with cocaine-induced sleep disorder
F14.188 Cocaine abuse with other cocaine-induced disorder

F14.19 Cocaine abuse with unspecified cocaine-induced disorder

√5th **F14.2 Cocaine dependence**
EXCLUDES 1 *cocaine abuse (F14.1-)*
cocaine use, unspecified (F14.9-)
EXCLUDES 2 *cocaine poisoning (T40.5-)*

F14.20 Cocaine dependence, uncomplicated CC
CC Excl: No Excl

F14.21 Cocaine dependence, in remission

√6th **F14.22 Cocaine dependence with intoxication**
EXCLUDES 1 *cocaine dependence with withdrawal (F14.23)*
F14.220 Cocaine dependence with intoxication, uncomplicated
F14.221 Cocaine dependence with intoxication delirium CC
F14.222 Cocaine dependence with intoxication with perceptual disturbance CC
CC Excl: No Excl
F14.229 Cocaine dependence with intoxication, unspecified CC
CC Excl: No Excl

F14.23 Cocaine dependence with withdrawal CC
EXCLUDES 1 *cocaine dependence with intoxication (F14.22-)*

F14.24 Cocaine dependence with cocaine-induced mood disorder

√6th **F14.25 Cocaine dependence with cocaine-induced psychotic disorder**
F14.250 Cocaine dependence with cocaine-induced psychotic disorder with delusions CC
F14.251 Cocaine dependence with cocaine-induced psychotic disorder with hallucinations CC
F14.259 Cocaine dependence with cocaine-induced psychotic disorder, unspecified CC
CC Excl: No Excl

√6th **F14.28 Cocaine dependence with other cocaine-induced disorder**
F14.280 Cocaine dependence with cocaine-induced anxiety disorder CC
CC Excl: No Excl
F14.281 Cocaine dependence with cocaine-induced sexual dysfunction CC
CC Excl: No Excl
F14.282 Cocaine dependence with cocaine-induced sleep disorder CC
CC Excl: No Excl

F14.288 Cocaine dependence with other cocaine-induced disorder CC
CC Excl: No Excl

F14.29 Cocaine dependence with unspecified cocaine-induced disorder

✓5th F14.9 Cocaine use, unspecified
EXCLUDES 1 *cocaine abuse (F14.1-)*
cocaine dependence (F14.2-)

F14.90 Cocaine use, unspecified, uncomplicated

✓6th F14.92 Cocaine use, unspecified with intoxication

F14.920 Cocaine use, unspecified with intoxication, uncomplicated

F14.921 Cocaine use, unspecified with intoxication delirium CC

F14.922 Cocaine use, unspecified with intoxication with perceptual disturbance

F14.929 Cocaine use, unspecified with intoxication, unspecified

F14.94 Cocaine use, unspecified with cocaine-induced mood disorder

✓6th F14.95 Cocaine use, unspecified with cocaine-induced psychotic disorder

F14.950 Cocaine use, unspecified with cocaine-induced psychotic disorder with delusions CC

F14.951 Cocaine use, unspecified with cocaine-induced psychotic disorder with hallucinations CC

F14.959 Cocaine use, unspecified with cocaine-induced psychotic disorder, unspecified

✓6th F14.98 Cocaine use, unspecified with other specified cocaine-induced disorder

F14.980 Cocaine use, unspecified with cocaine-induced anxiety disorder

F14.981 Cocaine use, unspecified with cocaine-induced sexual dysfunction

F14.982 Cocaine use, unspecified with cocaine-induced sleep disorder

F14.988 Cocaine use, unspecified with other cocaine-induced disorder

F14.99 Cocaine use, unspecified with unspecified cocaine-induced disorder

✓4th **F15 Other stimulant related disorders**
INCLUDES amphetamine-related disorders
caffeine
EXCLUDES 2 *cocaine-related disorders (F14.-)*

CC Excl: For CC codes in category F15, unless otherwise noted: F02.80-F02.81, F04-F06.8, F10.10-F11.19, F11.21-F13.19, F13.21-F14.19, F14.21-F15.19, F15.21-F16.19, F16.21-F16.99, F17.203-F17.209, F17.213-F17.219, F17.223-F17.229, F17.293-F18.19, F18.21-F19.19, F19.21-F19.99, F53, F55.0-F55.8, R78.0

✓5th F15.1 Other stimulant abuse
EXCLUDES 1 *other stimulant dependence (F15.2-)*
other stimulant use, unspecified (F15.9-)

F15.10 Other stimulant abuse, uncomplicated

✓6th F15.12 Other stimulant abuse with intoxication

F15.120 Other stimulant abuse with intoxication, uncomplicated

F15.121 Other stimulant abuse with intoxication delirium CC

F15.122 Other stimulant abuse with intoxication with perceptual disturbance

F15.129 Other stimulant abuse with intoxication, unspecified

F15.14 Other stimulant abuse with stimulant-induced mood disorder

✓6th F15.15 Other stimulant abuse with stimulant-induced psychotic disorder

F15.150 Other stimulant abuse with stimulant-induced psychotic disorder with delusions CC

F15.151 Other stimulant abuse with stimulant-induced psychotic disorder with hallucinations CC

F15.159 Other stimulant abuse with stimulant-induced psychotic disorder, unspecified

✓6th F15.18 Other stimulant abuse with other stimulant-induced disorder

F15.180 Other stimulant abuse with stimulant-induced anxiety disorder

F15.181 Other stimulant abuse with stimulant-induced sexual dysfunction

F15.182 Other stimulant abuse with stimulant-induced sleep disorder

F15.188 Other stimulant abuse with other stimulant-induced disorder

F15.19 Other stimulant abuse with unspecified stimulant-induced disorder

✓5th F15.2 Other stimulant dependence
EXCLUDES 1 *other stimulant abuse (F15.1-)*
other stimulant use, unspecified (F15.9-)

F15.20 Other stimulant dependence, uncomplicated CC
CC Excl: No Excl

F15.21 Other stimulant dependence, in remission

✓6th F15.22 Other stimulant dependence with intoxication
EXCLUDES 1 *other stimulant dependence with withdrawal (F15.23)*

F15.220 Other stimulant dependence with intoxication, uncomplicated

F15.221 Other stimulant dependence with intoxication delirium CC

F15.222 Other stimulant dependence with intoxication with perceptual disturbance CC
CC Excl: No Excl

F15.229 Other stimulant dependence with intoxication, unspecified

F15.23 Other stimulant dependence with withdrawal CC
EXCLUDES 1 *other stimulant dependence with intoxication (F15.22-)*

F15.24 Other stimulant dependence with stimulant-induced mood disorder

✓6th F15.25 Other stimulant dependence with stimulant-induced psychotic disorder

F15.250 Other stimulant dependence with stimulant-induced psychotic disorder with delusions CC

F15.251 Other stimulant dependence with stimulant-induced psychotic disorder with hallucinations CC

F15.259 Other stimulant dependence with stimulant-induced psychotic disorder, unspecified CC
CC Excl: No Excl

✓6th F15.28 Other stimulant dependence with other stimulant-induced disorder

F15.280 Other stimulant dependence with stimulant-induced anxiety disorder CC
CC Excl: No Excl

F15.281 Other stimulant dependence with stimulant-induced sexual dysfunction CC
CC Excl: No Excl

F15.282 Other stimulant dependence with stimulant-induced sleep disorder CC
CC Excl: No Excl

F15.288 Other stimulant dependence with other stimulant-induced disorder CC
CC Excl: No Excl

F15.29 Other stimulant dependence with unspecified stimulant-induced disorder

✓5th F15.9 Other stimulant use, unspecified
EXCLUDES 1 *other stimulant abuse (F15.1-)*
other stimulant dependence (F15.2-)

F15.90 Other stimulant use, unspecified, uncomplicated

✓6th F15.92 Other stimulant use, unspecified with intoxication
EXCLUDES 1 *other stimulant use, unspecified with withdrawal (F15.93)*

F15.920 Other stimulant use, unspecified with intoxication, uncomplicated

F15.921 Other stimulant use, unspecified with intoxication delirium CC

F15.922 Other stimulant use, unspecified with intoxication with perceptual disturbance

F15.929 Other stimulant use, unspecified with intoxication, unspecified

F15.93 **Other stimulant use, unspecified with withdrawal** CC
EXCLUDES 1 *other stimulant use, unspecified with intoxication (F15.92-)*

F15.94 **Other stimulant use, unspecified with stimulant-induced mood disorder**

✓6th F15.95 **Other stimulant use, unspecified with stimulant-induced psychotic disorder**

F15.950 **Other stimulant use, unspecified with stimulant-induced psychotic disorder with delusions** CC

F15.951 **Other stimulant use, unspecified with stimulant-induced psychotic disorder with hallucinations** CC

F15.959 **Other stimulant use, unspecified with stimulant-induced psychotic disorder, unspecified**

✓6th F15.98 **Other stimulant use, unspecified with other stimulant-induced disorder**

F15.980 **Other stimulant use, unspecified with stimulant-induced anxiety disorder**

F15.981 **Other stimulant use, unspecified with stimulant-induced sexual dysfunction**

F15.982 **Other stimulant use, unspecified with stimulant-induced sleep disorder**

F15.988 **Other stimulant use, unspecified with other stimulant-induced disorder**

F15.99 **Other stimulant use, unspecified with unspecified stimulant-induced disorder**

✓4th F16 Hallucinogen related disorders

INCLUDES ecstasy
PCP
phencyclidine

CC Excl: For CC codes in category F16, unless otherwise noted: F02.80-F02.81, F04-F06.8, F10.10-F11.19, F11.21-F13.19, F13.21-F14.19, F14.21-F15.19, F15.21-F16.19, F16.21-F16.99, F17.203-F17.209, F17.213-F17.219, F17.223-F17.229, F17.293-F18.19, F18.21-F19.19, F19.21-F19.99, F53, F55.0-F55.8, R78.0

✓5th F16.1 **Hallucinogen abuse**
EXCLUDES 1 *hallucinogen dependence (F16.2-)*
hallucinogen use, unspecified (F16.9-)

F16.10 **Hallucinogen abuse, uncomplicated**

✓6th F16.12 **Hallucinogen abuse with intoxication**

F16.120 **Hallucinogen abuse with intoxication, uncomplicated**

F16.121 **Hallucinogen abuse with intoxication with delirium** CC

F16.122 **Hallucinogen abuse with intoxication with perceptual disturbance**

F16.129 **Hallucinogen abuse with intoxication, unspecified**

F16.14 **Hallucinogen abuse with hallucinogen-induced mood disorder**

✓6th F16.15 **Hallucinogen abuse with hallucinogen-induced psychotic disorder**

F16.150 **Hallucinogen abuse with hallucinogen-induced psychotic disorder with delusions** CC

F16.151 **Hallucinogen abuse with hallucinogen-induced psychotic disorder with hallucinations** CC

F16.159 **Hallucinogen abuse with hallucinogen-induced psychotic disorder, unspecified**

✓6th F16.18 **Hallucinogen abuse with other hallucinogen-induced disorder**

F16.180 **Hallucinogen abuse with hallucinogen-induced anxiety disorder**

F16.183 **Hallucinogen abuse with hallucinogen-induced persisting perception disorder (flashbacks)**

F16.188 **Hallucinogen abuse with other hallucinogen-induced disorder**

F16.19 **Hallucinogen abuse with unspecified hallucinogen-induced disorder**

✓5th F16.2 **Hallucinogen dependence**
EXCLUDES 1 *hallucinogen abuse (F16.1-)*
hallucinogen use, unspecified (F16.9-)

F16.20 **Hallucinogen dependence, uncomplicated** CC
CC Excl: No Excl

F16.21 **Hallucinogen dependence, in remission**

✓6th F16.22 **Hallucinogen dependence with intoxication**

F16.220 **Hallucinogen dependence with intoxication, uncomplicated**

F16.221 **Hallucinogen dependence with intoxication with delirium** CC

F16.229 **Hallucinogen dependence with intoxication, unspecified**

F16.24 **Hallucinogen dependence with hallucinogen-induced mood disorder**

✓6th F16.25 **Hallucinogen dependence with hallucinogen-induced psychotic disorder**

F16.250 **Hallucinogen dependence with hallucinogen-induced psychotic disorder with delusions** CC

F16.251 **Hallucinogen dependence with hallucinogen-induced psychotic disorder with hallucinations** CC

F16.259 **Hallucinogen dependence with hallucinogen-induced psychotic disorder, unspecified** CC
CC Excl: No Excl

✓6th F16.28 **Hallucinogen dependence with other hallucinogen-induced disorder**

F16.280 **Hallucinogen dependence with hallucinogen-induced anxiety disorder** CC
CC Excl: No Excl

F16.283 **Hallucinogen dependence with hallucinogen persisting perception disorder (flashbacks)** CC
CC Excl: No Excl

F16.288 **Hallucinogen dependence with other hallucinogen-induced disorder** CC
CC Excl: No Excl

F16.29 **Hallucinogen dependence with unspecified hallucinogen-induced disorder**

✓5th F16.9 **Hallucinogen use, unspecified**
EXCLUDES 1 *hallucinogen abuse (F16.1-)*
hallucinogen dependence (F16.2-)

F16.90 **Hallucinogen use, unspecified, uncomplicated**

✓6th F16.92 **Hallucinogen use, unspecified with intoxication**

F16.920 **Hallucinogen use, unspecified with intoxication, uncomplicated**

F16.921 **Hallucinogen use, unspecified with intoxication with delirium** CC

F16.929 **Hallucinogen use, unspecified with intoxication, unspecified**

F16.94 **Hallucinogen use, unspecified with hallucinogen-induced mood disorder**

✓6th F16.95 **Hallucinogen use, unspecified with hallucinogen-induced psychotic disorder**

F16.950 **Hallucinogen use, unspecified with hallucinogen-induced psychotic disorder with delusions** CC

F16.951 **Hallucinogen use, unspecified with hallucinogen-induced psychotic disorder with hallucinations** CC

F16.959 **Hallucinogen use, unspecified with hallucinogen-induced psychotic disorder, unspecified**

✓6th F16.98 **Hallucinogen use, unspecified with other specified hallucinogen-induced disorder**

F16.980 **Hallucinogen use, unspecified with hallucinogen-induced anxiety disorder**

F16.983 **Hallucinogen use, unspecified with hallucinogen persisting perception disorder (flashbacks)**

F16.988 **Hallucinogen use, unspecified with other hallucinogen-induced disorder**

F16.99 **Hallucinogen use, unspecified with unspecified hallucinogen-induced disorder**

F17 Nicotine dependence

EXCLUDES 1 *history of tobacco dependence (Z87.891)*
tobacco use NOS (Z72.0)

EXCLUDES 2 *tobacco use (smoking) during pregnancy, childbirth and the puerperium (O99.33-)*
toxic effect of nicotine (T65.2-)

AHA: 2013, 4Q, 108-109

CC Excl: For CC codes in category F17, unless otherwise noted: F02.80-F02.81, F04-F06.8, F10.10-F11.19, F11.21-F13.19, F13.21-F14.19, F14.21-F15.19, F15.21-F16.19, F16.21-F16.99, F17.203-F17.209, F17.213-F17.219, F17.223-F17.229, F17.293-F18.19, F18.21-F19.19, F19.21-F19.99, F53, F55.0-F55.8, R78.0

F17.2 Nicotine dependence

F17.20 Nicotine dependence, unspecified
- **F17.200** Nicotine dependence, unspecified, uncomplicated
- **F17.201** Nicotine dependence, unspecified, in remission
- **F17.203** Nicotine dependence unspecified, withdrawal CC
- **F17.208** Nicotine dependence, unspecified, with other nicotine-induced disorders
- **F17.209** Nicotine dependence, unspecified, with unspecified nicotine-induced disorders

F17.21 Nicotine dependence, cigarettes
- **F17.210** Nicotine dependence, cigarettes, uncomplicated
- **F17.211** Nicotine dependence, cigarettes, in remission
- **F17.213** Nicotine dependence, cigarettes, with withdrawal CC
- **F17.218** Nicotine dependence, cigarettes, with other nicotine-induced disorders
- **F17.219** Nicotine dependence, cigarettes, with unspecified nicotine-induced disorders

F17.22 Nicotine dependence, chewing tobacco
- **F17.220** Nicotine dependence, chewing tobacco, uncomplicated
- **F17.221** Nicotine dependence, chewing tobacco, in remission
- **F17.223** Nicotine dependence, chewing tobacco, with withdrawal CC
- **F17.228** Nicotine dependence, chewing tobacco, with other nicotine-induced disorders
- **F17.229** Nicotine dependence, chewing tobacco, with unspecified nicotine-induced disorders

F17.29 Nicotine dependence, other tobacco product
- **F17.290** Nicotine dependence, other tobacco product, uncomplicated
- **F17.291** Nicotine dependence, other tobacco product, in remission
- **F17.293** Nicotine dependence, other tobacco product, with withdrawal CC
- **F17.298** Nicotine dependence, other tobacco product, with other nicotine-induced disorders
- **F17.299** Nicotine dependence, other tobacco product, with unspecified nicotine-induced disorders

F18 Inhalant related disorders

INCLUDES volatile solvents

CC Excl: For CC codes in category F18, unless otherwise noted: F02.80-F02.81, F04-F06.8, F10.10-F11.19, F11.21-F13.19, F13.21-F14.19, F14.21-F15.19, F15.21-F16.19, F16.21-F16.99, F17.203-F17.209, F17.213-F17.219, F17.223-F17.229, F17.293-F18.19, F18.21-F19.19, F19.21-F19.99, F53, F55.0-F55.8, R78.0

F18.1 Inhalant abuse

EXCLUDES 1 *inhalant dependence (F18.2-)*
inhalant use, unspecified (F18.9-)

F18.10 Inhalant abuse, uncomplicated

F18.12 Inhalant abuse with intoxication
- **F18.120** Inhalant abuse with intoxication, uncomplicated
- **F18.121** Inhalant abuse with intoxication delirium CC
- **F18.129** Inhalant abuse with intoxication, unspecified

F18.14 Inhalant abuse with inhalant-induced mood disorder

F18.15 Inhalant abuse with inhalant-induced psychotic disorder
- **F18.150** Inhalant abuse with inhalant-induced psychotic disorder with delusions CC
- **F18.151** Inhalant abuse with inhalant-induced psychotic disorder with hallucinations CC
- **F18.159** Inhalant abuse with inhalant-induced psychotic disorder, unspecified

F18.17 Inhalant abuse with inhalant-induced dementia CC

F18.18 Inhalant abuse with other inhalant-induced disorders
- **F18.180** Inhalant abuse with inhalant-induced anxiety disorder
- **F18.188** Inhalant abuse with other inhalant-induced disorder

F18.19 Inhalant abuse with unspecified inhalant-induced disorder

F18.2 Inhalant dependence

EXCLUDES 1 *inhalant abuse (F18.1-)*
inhalant use, unspecified (F18.9-)

F18.20 Inhalant dependence, uncomplicated CC
CC Excl: No Excl

F18.21 Inhalant dependence, in remission

F18.22 Inhalant dependence with intoxication
- **F18.220** Inhalant dependence with intoxication, uncomplicated
- **F18.221** Inhalant dependence with intoxication delirium CC
- **F18.229** Inhalant dependence with intoxication, unspecified

F18.24 Inhalant dependence with inhalant-induced mood disorder

F18.25 Inhalant dependence with inhalant-induced psychotic disorder
- **F18.250** Inhalant dependence with inhalant-induced psychotic disorder with delusions CC
- **F18.251** Inhalant dependence with inhalant-induced psychotic disorder with hallucinations CC
- **F18.259** Inhalant dependence with inhalant-induced psychotic disorder, unspecified CC
  CC Excl: No Excl

F18.27 Inhalant dependence with inhalant-induced dementia CC

F18.28 Inhalant dependence with other inhalant-induced disorders
- **F18.280** Inhalant dependence with inhalant-induced anxiety disorder CC
  CC Excl: No Excl
- **F18.288** Inhalant dependence with other inhalant-induced disorder CC
  CC Excl: No Excl

F18.29 Inhalant dependence with unspecified inhalant-induced disorder
CC Excl: No Excl

F18.9 Inhalant use, unspecified

EXCLUDES 1 *inhalant abuse (F18.1-)*
inhalant dependence (F18.2-)

F18.90 Inhalant use, unspecified, uncomplicated

F18.92 Inhalant use, unspecified with intoxication
- **F18.920** Inhalant use, unspecified with intoxication, uncomplicated
- **F18.921** Inhalant use, unspecified with intoxication with delirium CC
- **F18.929** Inhalant use, unspecified with intoxication, unspecified

F18.94 Inhalant use, unspecified with inhalant-induced mood disorder

F18.95 Inhalant use, unspecified with inhalant-induced psychotic disorder
- **F18.950** Inhalant use, unspecified with inhalant-induced psychotic disorder with delusions CC

F18.951 Inhalant use, unspecified with inhalant-induced psychotic disorder with hallucinations CC

F18.959 Inhalant use, unspecified with inhalant-induced psychotic disorder, unspecified

F18.97 Inhalant use, unspecified with inhalant-induced persisting dementia CC

✓6th F18.98 Inhalant use, unspecified with other inhalant-induced disorders

F18.980 Inhalant use, unspecified with inhalant-induced anxiety disorder

F18.988 Inhalant use, unspecified with other inhalant-induced disorder

F18.99 Inhalant use, unspecified with unspecified inhalant-induced disorder

✓4th **F19 Other psychoactive substance related disorders**

INCLUDES polysubstance drug use (indiscriminate drug use)

CC Excl: For CC codes in category F19, unless otherwise noted: F02.80-F02.81, F04-F06.8, F10.10-F11.19, F11.21-F13.19, F13.21-F14.19, F14.21-F15.19, F15.21-F16.19, F16.21-F16.99, F17.203-F17.209, F17.213-F17.219, F17.223-F17.229, F17.293-F18.19, F18.21-F19.19, F19.21-F19.99, F53, F55.0-F55.8, R78.0

✓5th F19.1 Other psychoactive substance abuse

EXCLUDES 1 *other psychoactive substance dependence (F19.2-)*
other psychoactive substance use, unspecified (F19.9-)

F19.10 Other psychoactive substance abuse, uncomplicated

✓6th F19.12 Other psychoactive substance abuse with intoxication

F19.120 Other psychoactive substance abuse with intoxication, uncomplicated

F19.121 Other psychoactive substance abuse with intoxication delirium CC

F19.122 Other psychoactive substance abuse with intoxication with perceptual disturbances

F19.129 Other psychoactive substance abuse with intoxication, unspecified

F19.14 Other psychoactive substance abuse with psychoactive substance-induced mood disorder

✓6th F19.15 Other psychoactive substance abuse with psychoactive substance-induced psychotic disorder

F19.150 Other psychoactive substance abuse with psychoactive substance-induced psychotic disorder with delusions CC

F19.151 Other psychoactive substance abuse with psychoactive substance-induced psychotic disorder with hallucinations CC

F19.159 Other psychoactive substance abuse with psychoactive substance-induced psychotic disorder, unspecified

F19.16 Other psychoactive substance abuse with psychoactive substance-induced persisting amnestic disorder

F19.17 Other psychoactive substance abuse with psychoactive substance-induced persisting dementia CC

✓6th F19.18 Other psychoactive substance abuse with other psychoactive substance-induced disorders

F19.180 Other psychoactive substance abuse with psychoactive substance-induced anxiety disorder

F19.181 Other psychoactive substance abuse with psychoactive substance-induced sexual dysfunction

F19.182 Other psychoactive substance abuse with psychoactive substance-induced sleep disorder

F19.188 Other psychoactive substance abuse with other psychoactive substance-induced disorder

F19.19 Other psychoactive substance abuse with unspecified psychoactive substance-induced disorder

✓5th F19.2 Other psychoactive substance dependence

EXCLUDES 1 *other psychoactive substance abuse (F19.1-)*
other psychoactive substance use, unspecified (F19.9-)

F19.20 Other psychoactive substance dependence, uncomplicated CC
CC Excl: No Excl

F19.21 Other psychoactive substance dependence, in remission

✓6th F19.22 Other psychoactive substance dependence with intoxication

EXCLUDES 1 *other psychoactive substance dependence with withdrawal (F19.23-)*

F19.220 Other psychoactive substance dependence with intoxication, uncomplicated

F19.221 Other psychoactive substance dependence with intoxication delirium CC

F19.222 Other psychoactive substance dependence with intoxication with perceptual disturbance CC
CC Excl: No Excl

F19.229 Other psychoactive substance dependence with intoxication, unspecified

✓6th F19.23 Other psychoactive substance dependence with withdrawal

EXCLUDES 1 *other psychoactive substance dependence with intoxication (F19.22-)*

F19.230 Other psychoactive substance dependence with withdrawal, uncomplicated CC

F19.231 Other psychoactive substance dependence with withdrawal delirium CC

F19.232 Other psychoactive substance dependence with withdrawal with perceptual disturbance CC

F19.239 Other psychoactive substance dependence with withdrawal, unspecified CC

F19.24 Other psychoactive substance dependence with psychoactive substance-induced mood disorder

✓6th F19.25 Other psychoactive substance dependence with psychoactive substance-induced psychotic disorder

F19.250 Other psychoactive substance dependence with psychoactive substance-induced psychotic disorder with delusions CC

F19.251 Other psychoactive substance dependence with psychoactive substance-induced psychotic disorder with hallucinations CC

F19.259 Other psychoactive substance dependence with psychoactive substance-induced psychotic disorder, unspecified CC
CC Excl: No Excl

F19.26 Other psychoactive substance dependence with psychoactive substance-induced persisting amnestic disorder CC
CC Excl: No Excl

F19.27 Other psychoactive substance dependence with psychoactive substance-induced persisting dementia CC

✓6th F19.28 Other psychoactive substance dependence with other psychoactive substance-induced disorders

F19.280 Other psychoactive substance dependence with psychoactive substance-induced anxiety disorder CC
CC Excl: No Excl

F19.281 Other psychoactive substance dependence with psychoactive substance-induced sexual dysfunction CC
CC Excl: No Excl

F19.282 Other psychoactive substance dependence with psychoactive substance-induced sleep disorder CC
CC Excl: No Excl

F19.288 Other psychoactive substance dependence with other psychoactive substance-induced disorder CC
CC Excl: No Excl

F19.29 Other psychoactive substance dependence with unspecified psychoactive substance-induced disorder

✓5th **F19.9 Other psychoactive substance use, unspecified**
EXCLUDES 1 *other psychoactive substance abuse (F19.1-)*
other psychoactive substance dependence (F19.2-)

F19.90 Other psychoactive substance use, unspecified, uncomplicated

✓6th **F19.92 Other psychoactive substance use, unspecified with intoxication**
EXCLUDES 1 *other psychoactive substance use, unspecified with withdrawal (F19.93)*

F19.920 Other psychoactive substance use, unspecified with intoxication, uncomplicated

F19.921 Other psychoactive substance use, unspecified with intoxication with delirium CC

F19.922 Other psychoactive substance use, unspecified with intoxication with perceptual disturbance

F19.929 Other psychoactive substance use, unspecified with intoxication, unspecified

✓6th **F19.93 Other psychoactive substance use, unspecified with withdrawal**
EXCLUDES 1 *other psychoactive substance use, unspecified with intoxication (F19.92-)*

F19.930 Other psychoactive substance use, unspecified with withdrawal, uncomplicated CC

F19.931 Other psychoactive substance use, unspecified with withdrawal delirium CC

F19.932 Other psychoactive substance use, unspecified with withdrawal with perceptual disturbance CC

F19.939 Other psychoactive substance use, unspecified with withdrawal, unspecified CC

F19.94 Other psychoactive substance use, unspecified with psychoactive substance-induced mood disorder

✓6th **F19.95 Other psychoactive substance use, unspecified with psychoactive substance-induced psychotic disorder**

F19.950 Other psychoactive substance use, unspecified with psychoactive substance-induced psychotic disorder with delusions CC

F19.951 Other psychoactive substance use, unspecified with psychoactive substance-induced psychotic disorder with hallucinations CC

F19.959 Other psychoactive substance use, unspecified with psychoactive substance-induced psychotic disorder, unspecified

F19.96 Other psychoactive substance use, unspecified with psychoactive substance-induced persisting amnestic disorder

F19.97 Other psychoactive substance use, unspecified with psychoactive substance-induced persisting dementia CC

✓6th **F19.98 Other psychoactive substance use, unspecified with other psychoactive substance-induced disorders**

F19.980 Other psychoactive substance use, unspecified with psychoactive substance-induced anxiety disorder

F19.981 Other psychoactive substance use, unspecified with psychoactive substance-induced sexual dysfunction

F19.982 Other psychoactive substance use, unspecified with psychoactive substance-induced sleep disorder

F19.988 Other psychoactive substance use, unspecified with other psychoactive substance-induced disorder

F19.99 Other psychoactive substance use, unspecified with unspecified psychoactive substance-induced disorder

Schizophrenia, schizotypal, delusional, and other non-mood psychotic disorders (F20-F29)

✓4th **F20 Schizophrenia**
EXCLUDES 1 *brief psychotic disorder (F23)*
cyclic schizophrenia (F25.0)
mood [affective] disorders with psychotic symptoms (F30.2, F31.2, F31.5, F31.64, F32.3, F33.3)
schizoaffective disorder (F25.-)
schizophrenic reaction NOS (F23)
EXCLUDES 2 *schizophrenic reaction in:*
alcoholism (F10.15-, F10.25-, F10.95-)
brain disease (F06.2)
epilepsy (F06.2)
psychoactive drug use (F11-F19 with .15..25, .95)
schizotypal disorder (F21)

CC Excl: For CC codes in category F20, unless otherwise noted: F07.0-F07.81, F07.9-F09, F20.0-F48.1, F48.8-F51.03, F51.12, F51.19, F51.3-F51.9, F52.5, F54, F59-F63.2, F63.81-F63.9, F68.10-F80.2, F80.4, F80.89-F84.0, F84.3-F99, G44.201-G44.229, H93.25, R45.1-R45.2, R45.5-R45.82, R45.86-R45.87

F20.0 Paranoid schizophrenia CC
Paraphrenic schizophrenia
EXCLUDES 1 *involutional paranoid state (F22)*
paranoia (F22)

F20.1 Disorganized schizophrenia CC
Hebephrenic schizophrenia
Hebephrenia

F20.2 Catatonic schizophrenia CC
Schizophrenic catalepsy
Schizophrenic catatonia
Schizophrenic flexibilitas cerea
EXCLUDES 1 *catatonic stupor (R40.1)*

F20.3 Undifferentiated schizophrenia
Atypical schizophrenia
EXCLUDES 1 *acute schizophrenia-like psychotic disorder (F23)*
EXCLUDES 2 *post-schizophrenic depression (F32.8)*

F20.5 Residual schizophrenia CC
Restzustand (schizophrenic)
Schizophrenic residual state

✓5th **F20.8 Other schizophrenia**

F20.81 Schizophreniform disorder CC
Schizophreniform psychosis NOS

F20.89 Other schizophrenia CC
Cenesthopathic schizophrenia
Simple schizophrenia

F20.9 Schizophrenia, unspecified

F21 Schizotypal disorder
Borderline schizophrenia
Latent schizophrenia
Latent schizophrenic reaction
Prepsychotic schizophrenia
Prodromal schizophrenia
Pseudoneurotic schizophrenia
Pseudopsychopathic schizophrenia
Schizotypal personality disorder
EXCLUDES 2 *Asperger's syndrome (F84.5)*
schizoid personality disorder (F60.1)

F22 Delusional disorders
Delusional dysmorphophobia
Involutional paranoid state
Paranoia
Paranoia querulans
Paranoid psychosis
Paranoid state
Paraphrenia (late)
Sensitiver Beziehungswahn
EXCLUDES 1 *mood [affective] disorders with psychotic symptoms (F30.2, F31.2, F31.5, F31.64, F32.3, F33.3)*
paranoid schizophrenia (F20.0)
EXCLUDES 2 *paranoid personality disorder (F60.0)*
paranoid psychosis, psychogenic (F23)
paranoid reaction (F23)

F23 Brief psychotic disorder CC
Paranoid reaction
Psychogenic paranoid psychosis
EXCLUDES 2 *mood [affective] disorders with psychotic symptoms (F30.2, F31.2, F31.5, F31.64, F32.3, F33.3)*

CC Excl: No Excl

F24 Shared psychotic disorder
Folie à deux
Induced paranoid disorder
Induced psychotic disorder

✓4th **F25 Schizoaffective disorders**
EXCLUDES 1 *mood [affective] disorders with psychotic symptoms (F3Ø.2, F31.2, F31.5, F31.64, F32.3, F33.3)*
schizophrenia (F2Ø.-)

F25.Ø Schizoaffective disorder, bipolar type
Cyclic schizophrenia
Schizoaffective disorder, manic type
Schizoaffective disorder, mixed type
Schizoaffective psychosis, bipolar type
Schizophreniform psychosis, manic type

F25.1 Schizoaffective disorder, depressive type
Schizoaffective psychosis, depressive type
Schizophreniform psychosis, depressive type

F25.8 Other schizoaffective disorders

F25.9 Schizoaffective disorder, unspecified
Schizoaffective psychosis NOS

F28 Other psychotic disorder not due to a substance or known physiological condition HIV
Chronic hallucinatory psychosis

F29 Unspecified psychosis not due to a substance or known physiological condition HIV
Psychosis NOS
EXCLUDES 1 *mental disorder NOS (F99)*
unspecified mental disorder due to known physiological condition (FØ9)

Mood [affective] disorders (F3Ø-F39)

✓4th **F3Ø Manic episode**
INCLUDES bipolar disorder, single manic episode
mixed affective episode
EXCLUDES 1 *bipolar disorder (F31.-)*
major depressive disorder, recurrent (F33.-)
major depressive disorder, single episode (F32.-)

CC Excl: For CC codes in category F3Ø, unless otherwise noted: FØ7.Ø-FØ7.81, FØ7.9-FØ9, F2Ø.Ø-F48.1, F48.8-F51.Ø3, F51.12, F51.19, F51.3-F51.9, F52.5, F54, F59-F63.2, F63.81-F63.9, F68.1Ø-F8Ø.2, F8Ø.4, F8Ø.89-F84.Ø, F84.3-F99, G44.2Ø1-G44.229, H93.25, R45.1-R45.2, R45.5-R45.82, R45.86-R45.87

✓5th **F3Ø.1 Manic episode without psychotic symptoms**

F3Ø.1Ø Manic episode without psychotic symptoms, unspecified CC

F3Ø.11 Manic episode without psychotic symptoms, mild CC

F3Ø.12 Manic episode without psychotic symptoms, moderate CC

F3Ø.13 Manic episode, severe, without psychotic symptoms CC
CC Excl: F3Ø.13-F3Ø.2, F31.13-F31.2, F31.4-F31.5, F31.63-F31.64

F3Ø.2 Manic episode, severe with psychotic symptoms CC
Manic stupor
Mania with mood-congruent psychotic symptoms
Mania with mood-incongruent psychotic symptoms

F3Ø.3 Manic episode in partial remission

F3Ø.4 Manic episode in full remission

F3Ø.8 Other manic episodes
Hypomania

F3Ø.9 Manic episode, unspecified CC
Mania NOS

✓4th **F31 Bipolar disorder**
INCLUDES manic-depressive illness
manic-depressive psychosis
manic-depressive reaction
EXCLUDES 1 *bipolar disorder, single manic episode (F3Ø.-)*
major depressive disorder, single episode (F32.-)
major depressive disorder, recurrent (F33.-)
EXCLUDES 2 *cyclothymia (F34.Ø)*

CC Excl: For CC codes in category F31, unless otherwise noted: FØ7.Ø-FØ7.81, FØ7.9-FØ9, F2Ø.Ø-F48.1, F48.8-F51.Ø3, F51.12, F51.19, F51.3-F51.9, F52.5, F54, F59-F63.2, F63.81-F63.9, F68.1Ø-F8Ø.2, F8Ø.4, F8Ø.89-F84.Ø, F84.3-F99, G44.2Ø1-G44.229, H93.25, R45.1-R45.2, R45.5-R45.82, R45.86-R45.87

F31.Ø Bipolar disorder, current episode hypomanic CC

✓5th **F31.1 Bipolar disorder, current episode manic without psychotic features**

F31.1Ø Bipolar disorder, current episode manic without psychotic features, unspecified CC

F31.11 Bipolar disorder, current episode manic without psychotic features, mild CC

F31.12 Bipolar disorder, current episode manic without psychotic features, moderate CC

F31.13 Bipolar disorder, current episode manic without psychotic features, severe CC
CC Excl: F31.13-F31.2, F31.63-F31.64

F31.2 Bipolar disorder, current episode manic severe with psychotic features CC
Bipolar disorder, current episode manic with mood-congruent psychotic symptoms
Bipolar disorder, current episode manic with mood-incongruent psychotic symptoms

✓5th **F31.3 Bipolar disorder, current episode depressed, mild or moderate severity**

F31.3Ø Bipolar disorder, current episode depressed, mild or moderate severity, unspecified CC

F31.31 Bipolar disorder, current episode depressed, mild CC

F31.32 Bipolar disorder, current episode depressed, moderate CC

F31.4 Bipolar disorder, current episode depressed, severe, without psychotic features CC
CC Excl: F31.13-F31.2, F31.4-F31.5, F31.63-F31.64

F31.5 Bipolar disorder, current episode depressed, severe, with psychotic features CC
Bipolar disorder, current episode depressed with mood-incongruent psychotic symptoms
Bipolar disorder, current episode depressed with mood-congruent psychotic symptoms

✓5th **F31.6 Bipolar disorder, current episode mixed**

F31.6Ø Bipolar disorder, current episode mixed, unspecified CC

F31.61 Bipolar disorder, current episode mixed, mild CC

F31.62 Bipolar disorder, current episode mixed, moderate CC

F31.63 Bipolar disorder, current episode mixed, severe, without psychotic features CC
CC Excl: See code: F31.4

F31.64 Bipolar disorder, current episode mixed, severe, with psychotic features CC
Bipolar disorder, current episode mixed with mood-congruent psychotic symptoms
Bipolar disorder, current episode mixed with mood-incongruent psychotic symptoms

✓5th **F31.7 Bipolar disorder, currently in remission**

F31.7Ø Bipolar disorder, currently in remission, most recent episode unspecified

F31.71 Bipolar disorder, in partial remission, most recent episode hypomanic

F31.72 Bipolar disorder, in full remission, most recent episode hypomanic

F31.73 Bipolar disorder, in partial remission, most recent episode manic

F31.74 Bipolar disorder, in full remission, most recent episode manic

F31.75 Bipolar disorder, in partial remission, most recent episode depressed

F31.76 Bipolar disorder, in full remission, most recent episode depressed

F31.77 Bipolar disorder, in partial remission, most recent episode mixed

F31.78 Bipolar disorder, in full remission, most recent episode mixed

✓5th **F31.8 Other bipolar disorders**

F31.81 Bipolar II disorder CC

F31.89 Other bipolar disorder CC
Recurrent manic episodes NOS

F31.9 Bipolar disorder, unspecified

F32 Major depressive disorder, single episode
INCLUDES single episode of agitated depression
single episode of depressive reaction
single episode of major depression
single episode of psychogenic depression
single episode of reactive depression
single episode of vital depression
EXCLUDES 1 *bipolar disorder (F31.-)*
manic episode (F30.-)
recurrent depressive disorder (F33.-)
EXCLUDES 2 *adjustment disorder (F43.2)*

CC Excl: For CC codes in category F32, unless otherwise noted: F32.0-F32.3, F33.0-F33.40, F33.9

F32.0 Major depressive disorder, single episode, mild CC
F32.1 Major depressive disorder, single episode, moderate CC
F32.2 Major depressive disorder, single episode, severe without psychotic features CC
F32.3 Major depressive disorder, single episode, severe with psychotic features CC
Single episode of major depression with mood-congruent psychotic symptoms
Single episode of major depression with mood-incongruent psychotic symptoms
Single episode of major depression with psychotic symptoms
Single episode of psychogenic depressive psychosis
Single episode of psychotic depression
Single episode of reactive depressive psychosis
F32.4 Major depressive disorder, single episode, in partial remission
F32.5 Major depressive disorder, single episode, in full remission
F32.8 Other depressive episodes
Atypical depression
Post-schizophrenic depression
Single episode of 'masked' depression NOS
F32.9 Major depressive disorder, single episode, unspecified
Depression NOS
Depressive disorder NOS
Major depression NOS
AHA: 2013, 4Q, 107

F33 Major depressive disorder, recurrent
Recurrent episodes of depressive reaction
Recurrent episodes of endogenous depression
Recurrent episodes of major depression
Recurrent episodes of psychogenic depression
Recurrent episodes of reactive depression
Recurrent episodes of seasonal depressive disorder
Recurrent episodes of vital depression
EXCLUDES 1 *bipolar disorder (F31.-)*
manic episode (F30.-)

F33.0 Major depressive disorder, recurrent, mild CC
CC Excl: See code: F32
F33.1 Major depressive disorder, recurrent, moderate CC
CC Excl: See code: F32
F33.2 Major depressive disorder, recurrent, severe without psychotic features CC
CC Excl: See code: F32
F33.3 Major depressive disorder, recurrent, severe with psychotic symptoms CC
Endogenous depression with psychotic symptoms
Recurrent severe episodes of major depression with mood-congruent psychotic symptoms
Recurrent severe episodes of major depression with mood-incongruent psychotic symptoms
Recurrent severe episodes of major depression with psychotic symptoms
Recurrent severe episodes of psychogenic depressive psychosis
Recurrent severe episodes of psychotic depression
Recurrent severe episodes of reactive depressive psychosis
CC Excl: F07.0-F07.81, F07.9-F09, F20.0-F48.1, F48.8-F51.03, F51.12, F51.19, F51.3-F51.9, F52.5, F54, F59-F63.2, F63.81-F63.9, F68.10-F80.4, F80.89-F84.0, F84.3-F99, G44.201-G44.229, H93.25, R45.1-R45.2, R45.5-R45.82, R45.86-R45.87
F33.4 Major depressive disorder, recurrent, in remission
F33.40 Major depressive disorder, recurrent, in remission, unspecified CC
CC Excl: See code: F32
F33.41 Major depressive disorder, recurrent, in partial remission
F33.42 Major depressive disorder, recurrent, in full remission
F33.8 Other recurrent depressive disorders CC
Recurrent brief depressive episodes
CC Excl: See code: F33.3
F33.9 Major depressive disorder, recurrent, unspecified CC
Monopolar depression NOS
CC Excl: See code: F32

F34 Persistent mood [affective] disorders
F34.0 Cyclothymic disorder
Affective personality disorder
Cycloid personality
Cyclothymia
Cyclothymic personality
F34.1 Dysthymic disorder
Depressive neurosis
Depressive personality disorder
Dysthymia
Neurotic depression
Persistent anxiety depression
EXCLUDES 2 *anxiety depression (mild or not persistent) (F41.8)*
F34.8 Other persistent mood [affective] disorders CC
CC Excl: See code: F33.3
F34.9 Persistent mood [affective] disorder, unspecified CC
CC Excl: See code: F33.3

F39 Unspecified mood [affective] disorder
Affective psychosis NOS

Anxiety, dissociative, stress-related, somatoform and other nonpsychotic mental disorders (F40-F48)

F40 Phobic anxiety disorders
F40.0 Agoraphobia
F40.00 Agoraphobia, unspecified
F40.01 Agoraphobia with panic disorder
Panic disorder with agoraphobia
EXCLUDES 1 *panic disorder without agoraphobia (F41.0)*
F40.02 Agoraphobia without panic disorder
F40.1 Social phobias
Anthropophobia
Social anxiety disorder of childhood
Social neurosis
F40.10 Social phobia, unspecified
F40.11 Social phobia, generalized
F40.2 Specific (isolated) phobias
EXCLUDES 2 *dysmorphophobia (nondelusional) (F45.22)*
nosophobia (F45.22)
F40.21 Animal type phobia
F40.210 Arachnophobia
Fear of spiders
F40.218 Other animal type phobia
F40.22 Natural environment type phobia
F40.220 Fear of thunderstorms
F40.228 Other natural environment type phobia
F40.23 Blood, injection, injury type phobia
F40.230 Fear of blood
F40.231 Fear of injections and transfusions
F40.232 Fear of other medical care
F40.233 Fear of injury
F40.24 Situational type phobia
F40.240 Claustrophobia
F40.241 Acrophobia
F40.242 Fear of bridges
F40.243 Fear of flying
F40.248 Other situational type phobia
F40.29 Other specified phobia
F40.290 Androphobia
Fear of men
F40.291 Gynephobia
Fear of women
F40.298 Other specified phobia
F40.8 Other phobic anxiety disorders
Phobic anxiety disorder of childhood
F40.9 Phobic anxiety disorder, unspecified
Phobia NOS
Phobic state NOS

F41 Other anxiety disorders

EXCLUDES 2 *anxiety in:*
acute stress reaction (F43.0)
transient adjustment reaction (F43.2)
neurasthenia (F48.8)
psychophysiologic disorders (F45.-)
separation anxiety (F93.0)

F41.0 Panic disorder [episodic paroxysmal anxiety] without agoraphobia
Panic attack
Panic state
EXCLUDES 1 *panic disorder with agoraphobia (F40.01)*

F41.1 Generalized anxiety disorder
Anxiety neurosis
Anxiety reaction
Anxiety state
Overanxious disorder
EXCLUDES 2 *neurasthenia (F48.8)*

F41.3 Other mixed anxiety disorders

F41.8 Other specified anxiety disorders
Anxiety depression (mild or not persistent)
Anxiety hysteria
Mixed anxiety and depressive disorder

F41.9 Anxiety disorder, unspecified
Anxiety NOS

F42 Obsessive-compulsive disorder
Anancastic neurosis
Obsessive-compulsive neurosis
EXCLUDES 2 *obsessive-compulsive personality (disorder) (F60.5)*
obsessive-compulsive symptoms occurring in depression (F32-F33)
obsessive-compulsive symptoms occurring in schizophrenia (F20.-)

F43 Reaction to severe stress, and adjustment disorders

F43.0 Acute stress reaction
Acute crisis reaction
Acute reaction to stress
Combat and operational stress reaction
Combat fatigue
Crisis state
Psychic shock

F43.1 Post-traumatic stress disorder (PTSD)
Traumatic neurosis

F43.10 Post-traumatic stress disorder, unspecified
F43.11 Post-traumatic stress disorder, acute
F43.12 Post-traumatic stress disorder, chronic

F43.2 Adjustment disorders
Culture shock
Grief reaction
Hospitalism in children
EXCLUDES 2 *separation anxiety disorder of childhood (F93.0)*

F43.20 Adjustment disorder, unspecified
F43.21 Adjustment disorder with depressed mood
AHA: 2014, 1Q, 25
F43.22 Adjustment disorder with anxiety
F43.23 Adjustment disorder with mixed anxiety and depressed mood
F43.24 Adjustment disorder with disturbance of conduct
F43.25 Adjustment disorder with mixed disturbance of emotions and conduct
F43.29 Adjustment disorder with other symptoms

F43.8 Other reactions to severe stress
F43.9 Reaction to severe stress, unspecified

F44 Dissociative and conversion disorders

INCLUDES conversion hysteria
conversion reaction
hysteria
hysterical psychosis
EXCLUDES 2 *malingering [conscious simulation] (Z76.5)*

F44.0 Dissociative amnesia
EXCLUDES 1 *amnesia NOS (R41.3)*
anterograde amnesia (R41.1)
retrograde amnesia (R41.2)
EXCLUDES 2 *alcohol-or other psychoactive substance-induced amnestic disorder (F10, F13, F19 with .26, .96)*
amnestic disorder due to known physiological condition (F04)
postictal amnesia in epilepsy (G40.-)

F44.1 Dissociative fugue
EXCLUDES 2 *postictal fugue in epilepsy (G40.-)*

F44.2 Dissociative stupor
EXCLUDES 1 *catatonic stupor (R40.1)*
stupor NOS (R40.1)
EXCLUDES 2 *catatonic disorder due to known physiological condition (F06.1)*
depressive stupor (F32, F33)
manic stupor (F30, F31)

F44.4 Conversion disorder with motor symptom or deficit
Dissociative motor disorders
Psychogenic aphonia
Psychogenic dysphonia

F44.5 Conversion disorder with seizures or convulsions
Dissociative convulsions

F44.6 Conversion disorder with sensory symptom or deficit
Dissociative anesthesia and sensory loss
Psychogenic deafness

F44.7 Conversion disorder with mixed symptom presentation

F44.8 Other dissociative and conversion disorders

F44.81 Dissociative identity disorder
Multiple personality disorder

F44.89 Other dissociative and conversion disorders
Ganser's syndrome
Psychogenic confusion
Psychogenic twilight state
Trance and possession disorders

F44.9 Dissociative and conversion disorder, unspecified
Dissociative disorder NOS

F45 Somatoform disorders

EXCLUDES 2 *dissociative and conversion disorders (F44.-)*
factitious disorders (F68.1-)
hair-plucking (F63.3)
lalling (F80.0)
lisping (F80.0)
malingering [conscious simulation] (Z76.5)
nail-biting (F98.8)
psychological or behavioral factors associated with disorders or diseases classified elsewhere (F54)
sexual dysfunction, not due to a substance or known physiological condition (F52.-)
thumb-sucking (F98.8)
tic disorders (in childhood and adolescence) (F95.-)
Tourette's syndrome (F95.2)
trichotillomania (F63.3)

F45.0 Somatization disorder
Briquet's disorder
Multiple psychosomatic disorder

F45.1 Undifferentiated somatoform disorder
Undifferentiated psychosomatic disorder

F45.2 Hypochondriacal disorders
EXCLUDES 2 *delusional dysmorphophobia (F22)*
fixed delusions about bodily functions or shape (F22)

F45.20 Hypochondriacal disorder, unspecified
F45.21 Hypochondriasis
Hypochondriacal neurosis
F45.22 Body dysmorphic disorder
Dysmorphophobia (nondelusional)
Nosophobia
F45.29 Other hypochondriacal disorders

F45.4 Pain disorders related to psychological factors
EXCLUDES 1 *pain NOS (R52)*

F45.41 Pain disorder exclusively related to psychological factors
Somatoform pain disorder (persistent)
F45.42 Pain disorder with related psychological factors
Code also associated acute or chronic pain (G89.-)

F45.8 Other somatoform disorders
Psychogenic dysmenorrhea
Psychogenic dysphagia, including "globus hystericus"
Psychogenic pruritus
Psychogenic torticollis
Somatoform autonomic dysfunction
Teeth grinding
EXCLUDES 1 *sleep related teeth grinding (G47.63)*

F45.9 Somatoform disorder, unspecified
Psychosomatic disorder NOS

√4th F48 Other nonpsychotic mental disorders

F48.1 Depersonalization-derealization syndrome

F48.2 Pseudobulbar affect
Involuntary emotional expression disorder
Code first underlying cause, if known, such as:
amyotrophic lateral sclerosis (G12.21)
multiple sclerosis (G35)
sequelae of cerebrovascular disease (I69.-)
sequelae of traumatic intracranial injury (S06.-)

F48.8 Other specified nonpsychotic mental disorders
Dhat syndrome
Neurasthenia
Occupational neurosis, including writer's cramp
Psychasthenia
Psychasthenic neurosis
Psychogenic syncope

F48.9 Nonpsychotic mental disorder, unspecified
Neurosis NOS

Behavioral syndromes associated with physiological disturbances and physical factors (F50-F59)

√4th F50 Eating disorders
EXCLUDES 1 *anorexia NOS (R63.0)*
feeding difficulties (R63.3)
polyphagia (R63.2)
EXCLUDES 2 *feeding disorder in infancy or childhood (F98.2-)*

CC Excl: For CC codes in category F50, unless otherwise noted:
F45.9, F50.00-F50.9, F59, F98.21-F98.3

√5th F50.0 Anorexia nervosa
EXCLUDES 1 *loss of appetite (R63.0)*
psychogenic loss of appetite (F50.8)

F50.00 Anorexia nervosa, unspecified CC

F50.01 Anorexia nervosa, restricting type CC

F50.02 Anorexia nervosa, binge eating/purging type CC
EXCLUDES 1 *bulimia nervosa (F50.2)*

F50.2 Bulimia nervosa CC
Bulimia NOS
Hyperorexia nervosa
EXCLUDES 1 *anorexia nervosa, binge eating/purging type (F50.02)*
CC Excl: F50.00-F50.9, F98.21-F98.29

F50.8 Other eating disorders
Pica in adults
Psychogenic loss of appetite
EXCLUDES 2 *pica of infancy and childhood (F98.3)*

F50.9 Eating disorder, unspecified
Atypical anorexia nervosa
Atypical bulimia nervosa

√4th F51 Sleep disorders not due to a substance or known physiological condition
EXCLUDES 2 *organic sleep disorders (G47.-)*

√5th F51.0 Insomnia not due to a substance or known physiological condition
EXCLUDES 2 *alcohol related insomnia (F10.182, F10.282, F10.982)*
drug-related insomnia (F11.182, F11.282, F11.982, F13.182, F13.282, F13.982, F14.182, F14.282, F14.982, F15.182, F15.282, F15.982, F19.182, F19.282, F19.982)
insomnia NOS (G47.0-)
insomnia due to known physiological condition (G47.0-)
organic insomnia (G47.0-)
sleep deprivation (Z72.820)

F51.01 Primary insomnia
Idiopathic insomnia

F51.02 Adjustment insomnia

F51.03 Paradoxical insomnia

F51.04 Psychophysiologic insomnia

F51.05 Insomnia due to other mental disorder
Code also associated mental disorder

F51.09 Other insomnia not due to a substance or known physiological condition

√5th F51.1 Hypersomnia not due to a substance or known physiological condition
EXCLUDES 2 *alcohol related hypersomnia (F10.182, F10.282, F10.982)*
drug-related hypersomnia (F11.182, F11.282, F11.982, F13.182, F13.282, F13.982, F14.182, F14.282, F14.982, F15.182, F15.282, F15.982, F19.182, F19.282, F19.982)
hypersomnia NOS (G47.10)
hypersomnia due to known physiological condition (G47.10)
idiopathic hypersomnia (G47.11, G47.12)
narcolepsy (G47.4-)

F51.11 Primary hypersomnia

F51.12 Insufficient sleep syndrome
EXCLUDES 1 *sleep deprivation (Z72.820)*

F51.13 Hypersomnia due to other mental disorder
Code also associated mental disorder

F51.19 Other hypersomnia not due to a substance or known physiological condition

F51.3 Sleepwalking [somnambulism]

F51.4 Sleep terrors [night terrors]

F51.5 Nightmare disorder
Dream anxiety disorder

F51.8 Other sleep disorders not due to a substance or known physiological condition

F51.9 Sleep disorder not due to a substance or known physiological condition, unspecified
Emotional sleep disorder NOS

√4th F52 Sexual dysfunction not due to a substance or known physiological condition
EXCLUDES 2 *Dhat syndrome (F48.8)*

F52.0 Hypoactive sexual desire disorder
Anhedonia (sexual)
Lack or loss of sexual desire
EXCLUDES 1 *decreased libido (R68.82)*

F52.1 Sexual aversion disorder
Sexual aversion and lack of sexual enjoyment

√5th F52.2 Sexual arousal disorders
Failure of genital response

F52.21 Male erectile disorder ♂
Psychogenic impotence
EXCLUDES 1 *impotence of organic origin (N52.-)*
impotence NOS (N52.-)

F52.22 Female sexual arousal disorder ♀
Frigidity

√5th F52.3 Orgasmic disorder
Inhibited orgasm
Psychogenic anorgasmy

F52.31 Female orgasmic disorder ♀

F52.32 Male orgasmic disorder ♂

F52.4 Premature ejaculation ♂

F52.5 Vaginismus not due to a substance or known physiological condition ♀
Psychogenic vaginismus
EXCLUDES 2 *vaginismus (due to a known physiological condition) (N94.2)*

F52.6 Dyspareunia not due to a substance or known physiological condition ♀
Psychogenic dyspareunia
EXCLUDES 2 *dyspareunia (due to a known physiological condition) (N94.1)*

F52.8 Other sexual dysfunction not due to a substance or known physiological condition
Excessive sexual drive
Nymphomania
Satyriasis

F52.9 Unspecified sexual dysfunction not due to a substance or known physiological condition
Sexual dysfunction NOS

F53 Puerperal psychosis ♀
Postpartum depression
EXCLUDES 1 *mood disorders with psychotic features (F30.2, F31.2, F31.5, F31.64, F32.3, F33.3)*
postpartum dysphoria (O90.6)
psychosis in schizophrenia, schizotypal, delusional, and other psychotic disorders (F20-F29)

F54 Psychological and behavioral factors associated with disorders or diseases classified elsewhere
Psychological factors affecting physical conditions
Code first the associated physical disorder, such as:
asthma (J45.-)
dermatitis (L23-L25)
gastric ulcer (K25.-)
mucous colitis (K58.-)
ulcerative colitis (K51.-)
urticaria (L50.-)
EXCLUDES 2 *tension-type headache (G44.2)*

✓4th **F55 Abuse of non-psychoactive substances**
EXCLUDES 2 *abuse of psychoactive substances (F10-F19)*
F55.0 Abuse of antacids
F55.1 Abuse of herbal or folk remedies
F55.2 Abuse of laxatives
F55.3 Abuse of steroids or hormones
F55.4 Abuse of vitamins
F55.8 Abuse of other non-psychoactive substances

F59 Unspecified behavioral syndromes associated with physiological disturbances and physical factors
Psychogenic physiological dysfunction NOS

Disorders of adult personality and behavior (F60-F69)

✓4th **F60 Specific personality disorders**
F60.0 Paranoid personality disorder
Expansive paranoid personality (disorder)
Fanatic personality (disorder)
Paranoid personality (disorder)
Querulant personality (disorder)
Sensitive paranoid personality (disorder)
EXCLUDES 2 *paranoia (F22)*
paranoia querulans (F22)
paranoid psychosis (F22)
paranoid schizophrenia (F20.0)
paranoid state (F22)
F60.1 Schizoid personality disorder
EXCLUDES 2 *Asperger's syndrome (F84.5)*
delusional disorder (F22)
schizoid disorder of childhood (F84.5)
schizophrenia (F20.-)
schizotypal disorder (F21)
F60.2 Antisocial personality disorder
Amoral personality (disorder)
Asocial personality (disorder)
Dissocial personality disorder
Psychopathic personality (disorder)
Sociopathic personality (disorder)
EXCLUDES 1 *conduct disorders (F91.-)*
EXCLUDES 2 *borderline personality disorder (F60.3)*
F60.3 Borderline personality disorder
Aggressive personality (disorder)
Emotionally unstable personality disorder
Explosive personality (disorder)
EXCLUDES 2 *antisocial personality disorder (F60.2)*
F60.4 Histrionic personality disorder
Hysterical personality (disorder)
Psychoinfantile personality (disorder)
F60.5 Obsessive-compulsive personality disorder
Anankastic personality (disorder)
Compulsive personality (disorder)
Obsessional personality (disorder)
EXCLUDES 2 *obsessive-compulsive disorder (F42)*
F60.6 Avoidant personality disorder
Anxious personality disorder
F60.7 Dependent personality disorder
Asthenic personality (disorder)
Inadequate personality (disorder)
Passive personality (disorder)
✓5th **F60.8 Other specific personality disorders**
F60.81 Narcissistic personality disorder
F60.89 Other specific personality disorders
Eccentric personality disorder
"Haltlose" type personality disorder
Immature personality disorder
Passive-aggressive personality disorder
Psychoneurotic personality disorder
Self-defeating personality disorder
F60.9 Personality disorder, unspecified
Character disorder NOS
Character neurosis NOS
Pathological personality NOS

✓4th **F63 Impulse disorders**
EXCLUDES 2 *habitual excessive use of alcohol or psychoactive substances (F10-F19)*
impulse disorders involving sexual behavior (F65.-)
F63.0 Pathological gambling
Compulsive gambling
EXCLUDES 1 *gambling and betting NOS (Z72.6)*
EXCLUDES 2 *excessive gambling by manic patients (F30, F31)*
gambling in antisocial personality disorder (F60.2)
F63.1 Pyromania
Pathological fire-setting
EXCLUDES 2 *fire-setting (by) (in):*
adult with antisocial personality disorder (F60.2)
alcohol or psychoactive substance intoxication (F10-F19)
conduct disorders (F91.-)
mental disorders due to known physiological condition (F01-F09)
schizophrenia (F20.-)
F63.2 Kleptomania
Pathological stealing
EXCLUDES 1 *shoplifting as the reason for observation for suspected mental disorder (Z03.8)*
EXCLUDES 2 *depressive disorder with stealing (F31-F33)*
stealing due to underlying mental condition—code to mental condition
stealing in mental disorders due to known physiological condition (F01-F09)
F63.3 Trichotillomania
Hair plucking
EXCLUDES 2 *other stereotyped movement disorder (F98.4)*
✓5th **F63.8 Other impulse disorders**
F63.81 Intermittent explosive disorder
F63.89 Other impulse disorders
F63.9 Impulse disorder, unspecified
Impulse control disorder NOS

✓4th **F64 Gender identity disorders**
F64.1 Gender identity disorder in adolescence and adulthood
Dual role transvestism
Transsexualism
Use additional code to identify sex reassignment status (Z87.890)
EXCLUDES 1 *gender identity disorder in childhood (F64.2)*
EXCLUDES 2 *fetishistic transvestism (F65.1)*
F64.2 Gender identity disorder of childhood P
EXCLUDES 1 *gender identity disorder in adolescence and adulthood (F64.1)*
EXCLUDES 2 *sexual maturation disorder (F66)*
F64.8 Other gender identity disorders
F64.9 Gender identity disorder, unspecified
Gender-role disorder NOS

✓4th **F65 Paraphilias**
F65.0 Fetishism
F65.1 Transvestic fetishism
Fetishistic transvestism
F65.2 Exhibitionism
F65.3 Voyeurism
F65.4 Pedophilia
✓5th **F65.5 Sadomasochism**
F65.50 Sadomasochism, unspecified
F65.51 Sexual masochism
F65.52 Sexual sadism
✓5th **F65.8 Other paraphilias**
F65.81 Frotteurism
F65.89 Other paraphilias
Necrophilia
F65.9 Paraphilia, unspecified
Sexual deviation NOS

F66 Other sexual disorders
Sexual maturation disorder
Sexual relationship disorder

✓4th F68 Other disorders of adult personality and behavior

✓5th F68.1 Factitious disorder

Compensation neurosis
Elaboration of physical symptoms for psychological reasons
Hospital hopper syndrome
Münchhausen's syndrome
Peregrinating patient

EXCLUDES 2 *factitial dermatitis (L98.1)*
person feigning illness (with obvious motivation) (Z76.5)

F68.1Ø Factitious disorder, unspecified CC

CC Excl: FØ7.Ø-FØ7.81, FØ7.9-FØ9, F2Ø.Ø-F48.1, F48.8-F51.Ø3, F51.12, F51.19, F51.3-F51.9, F52.5, F54, F59-F63.2, F63.81-F63.9, F68.1Ø-F8Ø.2, F8Ø.4, F8Ø.89-F84.Ø, F84.3-F99, G44.2Ø1-G44.229, H93.25, R45.1-R45.2, R45.5-R45.82, R45.86-R45.87

F68.11 Factitious disorder with predominantly psychological signs and symptoms

F68.12 Factitious disorder with predominantly physical signs and symptoms CC

CC Excl: See code: F68.1Ø

F68.13 Factitious disorder with combined psychological and physical signs and symptoms

F68.8 Other specified disorders of adult personality and behavior

F69 Unspecified disorder of adult personality and behavior A

Intellectual Disabilities (F7Ø-F79)

Code first any associated physical or developmental disorders

EXCLUDES 1 *borderline intellectual functioning, IQ above 7Ø to 84 (R41.83)*

F7Ø Mild intellectual disabilities

IQ level 5Ø-55 to approximately 7Ø
Mild mental subnormality

F71 Moderate intellectual disabilities

IQ level 35-4Ø to 5Ø-55
Moderate mental subnormality

F72 Severe intellectual disabilities CC

IQ 2Ø-25 to 35-4Ø
Severe mental subnormality
CC Excl: F72-F73

F73 Profound intellectual disabilities CC

IQ level below 2Ø-25
Profound mental subnormality
CC Excl: See code: F72

F78 Other intellectual disabilities

F79 Unspecified intellectual disabilities

Mental deficiency NOS
Mental subnormality NOS

Pervasive and specific developmental disorders (F8Ø-F89)

✓4th F8Ø Specific developmental disorders of speech and language

F8Ø.Ø Phonological disorder

Dyslalia
Functional speech articulation disorder
Lalling
Lisping
Phonological developmental disorder
Speech articulation developmental disorder

EXCLUDES 1 *speech articulation impairment due to aphasia NOS (R47.Ø1)*
speech articulation impairment due to apraxia (R48.2)

EXCLUDES 2 *speech articulation impairment due to hearing loss (F8Ø.4)*
speech articulation impairment due to intellectual disabilities (F7Ø-F79)
speech articulation impairment with expressive language developmental disorder (F8Ø.1)
speech articulation impairment with mixed receptive expressive language developmental disorder (F8Ø.2)

F8Ø.1 Expressive language disorder

Developmental dysphasia or aphasia, expressive type

EXCLUDES 1 *dysphasia and aphasia NOS (R47.-)*
mixed receptive-expressive language disorder (F8Ø.2)

EXCLUDES 2 *acquired aphasia with epilepsy [Landau-Kleffner] (G4Ø.8Ø-)*
intellectual disabilities (F7Ø-F79)
pervasive developmental disorders (F84.-)
selective mutism (F94.Ø)

F8Ø.2 Mixed receptive-expressive language disorder

Developmental dysphasia or aphasia, receptive type
Developmental Wernicke's aphasia

EXCLUDES 1 *central auditory processing disorder (H93.25)*
dysphasia or aphasia NOS (R47.-)
expressive language disorder (F8Ø.1)
expressive type dysphasia or aphasia (F8Ø.1)
word deafness (H93.25)

EXCLUDES 2 *acquired aphasia with epilepsy [Landau-Kleffner] (G4Ø.8Ø-)*
intellectual disabilities (F7Ø-F79)
pervasive developmental disorders (F84.-)
selective mutism (F94.Ø)

F8Ø.4 Speech and language development delay due to hearing loss

Code also type of hearing loss (H9Ø.-, H91.-)

✓5th F8Ø.8 Other developmental disorders of speech and language

F8Ø.81 Childhood onset fluency disorder

Cluttering NOS
Stuttering NOS

EXCLUDES 1 *adult onset fluency disorder (F98.5)*
fluency disorder in conditions classified elsewhere (R47.82)
fluency disorder (stuttering) following cerebrovascular disease (I69. with final characters-23)

F8Ø.89 Other developmental disorders of speech and language

F8Ø.9 Developmental disorder of speech and language, unspecified

Communication disorder NOS
Language disorder NOS

✓4th F81 Specific developmental disorders of scholastic skills

F81.Ø Specific reading disorder

"Backward reading"
Developmental dyslexia
Specific reading retardation

EXCLUDES 1 *alexia NOS (R48.Ø)*
dyslexia NOS (R48.Ø)

F81.2 Mathematics disorder

Developmental acalculia
Developmental arithmetical disorder
Developmental Gerstmann's syndrome

EXCLUDES 1 *acalculia NOS (R48.8)*

EXCLUDES 2 *arithmetical difficulties associated with a reading disorder (F81.Ø)*
arithmetical difficulties associated with a spelling disorder (F81.81)
arithmetical difficulties due to inadequate teaching (Z55.8)

✓5th F81.8 Other developmental disorders of scholastic skills

F81.81 Disorder of written expression

Specific spelling disorder

F81.89 Other developmental disorders of scholastic skills

F81.9 Developmental disorder of scholastic skills, unspecified

Knowledge acquisition disability NOS
Learning disability NOS
Learning disorder NOS

F82 Specific developmental disorder of motor function

Clumsy child syndrome
Developmental coordination disorder
Developmental dyspraxia

EXCLUDES 1 *abnormalities of gait and mobility (R26.-)*
lack of coordination (R27.-)

EXCLUDES 2 *lack of coordination secondary to intellectual disabilities (F7Ø-F79)*

✓4th F84 Pervasive developmental disorders

Use additional code to identify any associated medical condition and intellectual disabilities

CC Excl: For CC codes in category F84, unless otherwise noted: FØ7.Ø-FØ7.81, FØ7.9-FØ9, F2Ø.Ø-F48.1, F48.8-F51.Ø3, F51.12, F51.19, F51.3-F51.9, F52.5, F54, F59-F63.2, F63.81-F63.9, F68.1Ø-F8Ø.2, F8Ø.4, F8Ø.89-F84.Ø, F84.3-F99, G44.2Ø1-G44.229, H93.25, R45.1-R45.2, R45.5-R45.82, R45.86-R45.87

F84.Ø Autistic disorder CC

Infantile autism
Infantile psychosis
Kanner's syndrome

EXCLUDES 1 *Asperger's syndrome (F84.5)*

F84.2 Rett's syndrome CC
EXCLUDES 1 *Asperger's syndrome (F84.5)*
Autistic disorder (F84.0)
Other childhood disintegrative disorder (F84.3)
CC Excl: E75.00-E75.19, E75.4, F84.2, G13.2-G13.8, G30.0-G31.82, G31.84-G31.9, G91.4, G94

F84.3 Other childhood disintegrative disorder CC P
Dementia infantilis
Disintegrative psychosis
Heller's syndrome
Symbiotic psychosis
Use additional code to identify any associated neurological condition
EXCLUDES 1 *Asperger's syndrome (F84.5)*
Autistic disorder (F84.0)
Rett's syndrome (F84.2)

F84.5 Asperger's syndrome CC
Asperger's disorder
Autistic psychopathy
Schizoid disorder of childhood

F84.8 Other pervasive developmental disorders CC
Overactive disorder associated with intellectual disabilities and stereotyped movements

F84.9 Pervasive developmental disorder, unspecified CC
Atypical autism

F88 Other disorders of psychological development
Developmental agnosia

F89 Unspecified disorder of psychological development
Developmental disorder NOS

Behavioral and emotional disorders with onset usually occurring in childhood and adolescence (F90-F98)

NOTE Codes within categories F90-F98 may be used regardless of the age of a patient. These disorders generally have onset within the childhood or adolescent years, but may continue throughout life or not be diagnosed until adulthood

✓4th **F90 Attention-deficit hyperactivity disorders**
INCLUDES attention deficit disorder with hyperactivity
attention deficit syndrome with hyperactivity
EXCLUDES 2 *anxiety disorders (F40.-, F41.-)*
mood [affective] disorders (F30-F39)
pervasive developmental disorders (F84.-)
schizophrenia (F20.-)

F90.0 Attention-deficit hyperactivity disorder, predominantly inattentive type

F90.1 Attention-deficit hyperactivity disorder, predominantly hyperactive type

F90.2 Attention-deficit hyperactivity disorder, combined type

F90.8 Attention-deficit hyperactivity disorder, other type

F90.9 Attention-deficit hyperactivity disorder, unspecified type
Attention-deficit hyperactivity disorder of childhood or adolescence NOS
Attention-deficit hyperactivity disorder NOS

✓4th **F91 Conduct disorders**
EXCLUDES 1 *antisocial behavior (Z72.81-)*
antisocial personality disorder (F60.2)
EXCLUDES 2 *conduct problems associated with attention-deficit hyperactivity disorder (F90.-)*
mood [affective] disorders (F30-F39)
pervasive developmental disorders (F84.-)
schizophrenia (F20.-)

F91.0 Conduct disorder confined to family context

F91.1 Conduct disorder, childhood-onset type
Unsocialized conduct disorder
Conduct disorder, solitary aggressive type
Unsocialized aggressive disorder

F91.2 Conduct disorder, adolescent-onset type
Socialized conduct disorder
Conduct disorder, group type

F91.3 Oppositional defiant disorder

F91.8 Other conduct disorders

F91.9 Conduct disorder, unspecified
Behavioral disorder NOS
Conduct disorder NOS
Disruptive behavior disorder NOS

✓4th **F93 Emotional disorders with onset specific to childhood**

F93.0 Separation anxiety disorder of childhood P
EXCLUDES 2 *mood [affective] disorders (F30-F39)*
nonpsychotic mental disorders (F40-F48)
phobic anxiety disorder of childhood (F40.8)
social phobia (F40.1)

F93.8 Other childhood emotional disorders P
Identity disorder
EXCLUDES 2 *gender identity disorder of childhood (F64.2)*

F93.9 Childhood emotional disorder, unspecified P

✓4th **F94 Disorders of social functioning with onset specific to childhood and adolescence**

F94.0 Selective mutism
Elective mutism
EXCLUDES 2 *pervasive developmental disorders (F84.-)*
schizophrenia (F20.-)
specific developmental disorders of speech and language (F80.-)
transient mutism as part of separation anxiety in young children (F93.0)

F94.1 Reactive attachment disorder of childhood P
Use additional code to identify any associated failure to thrive or growth retardation
EXCLUDES 1 *disinhibited attachment disorder of childhood (F94.1)*
normal variation in pattern of selective attachment
EXCLUDES 2 *Asperger's syndrome (F84.5)*
maltreatment syndromes (T74.-)
sexual or physical abuse in childhood, resulting in psychosocial problems (Z62.81-)

F94.2 Disinhibited attachment disorder of childhood P
Affectionless psychopathy
Institutional syndrome
EXCLUDES 1 *reactive attachment disorder of childhood (F94.1)*
EXCLUDES 2 *Asperger's syndrome (F84.5)*
attention-deficit hyperactivity disorders (F90.-)
hospitalism in children (F43.2-)

F94.8 Other childhood disorders of social functioning P

F94.9 Childhood disorder of social functioning, unspecified P

✓4th **F95 Tic disorder**

F95.0 Transient tic disorder

F95.1 Chronic motor or vocal tic disorder

F95.2 Tourette's disorder
Combined vocal and multiple motor tic disorder [de la Tourette]
Tourette's syndrome

F95.8 Other tic disorders

F95.9 Tic disorder, unspecified
Tic NOS

✓4th **F98 Other behavioral and emotional disorders with onset usually occurring in childhood and adolescence**
EXCLUDES 2 *breath-holding spells (R06.89)*
gender identity disorder of childhood (F64.2)
Kleine-Levin syndrome (G47.13)
obsessive-compulsive disorder (F42)
sleep disorders not due to a substance or known physiological condition (F51.-)

F98.0 Enuresis not due to a substance or known physiological condition
Enuresis (primary) (secondary) of nonorganic origin
Functional enuresis
Psychogenic enuresis
Urinary incontinence of nonorganic origin
EXCLUDES 1 *enuresis NOS (R32)*

F98.1 Encopresis not due to a substance or known physiological condition
Functional encopresis
Incontinence of feces of nonorganic origin
Psychogenic encopresis
Use additional code to identify the cause of any coexisting constipation
EXCLUDES 1 *encopresis NOS (R15.-)*

✓5th **F98.2 Other feeding disorders of infancy and childhood**
EXCLUDES 1 *feeding difficulties (R63.3)*
EXCLUDES 2 *anorexia nervosa and other eating disorders (F50.-)*
feeding problems of newborn (P92.-)
pica of infancy or childhood (F98.3)

F98.21 Rumination disorder of infancy P

F98.29 Other feeding disorders of infancy and early childhood P

F98.3 Pica of infancy and childhood P

F98.4 Stereotyped movement disorders

Stereotype/habit disorder

EXCLUDES 1 *abnormal involuntary movements (R25.-)*

EXCLUDES 2 *compulsions in obsessive-compulsive disorder (F42)*
hair plucking (F63.3)
movement disorders of organic origin (G20-G25)
nail-biting (F98.8)
nose-picking (F98.8)
stereotypies that are part of a broader psychiatric condition (F01-F95)
thumb-sucking (F98.8)
tic disorders (F95.-)
trichotillomania (F63.3)

F98.5 Adult onset fluency disorder

EXCLUDES 1 *childhood onset fluency disorder (F80.81)*
dysphasia (R47.02)
fluency disorder in conditions classified elsewhere (R47.82)
fluency disorder (stuttering) following cerebrovascular disease (I69. with final characters -23)
tic disorders (F95.-)

F98.8 Other specified behavioral and emotional disorders with onset usually occurring in childhood and adolescence P

Excessive masturbation
Nail-biting
Nose-picking
Thumb-sucking

F98.9 Unspecified behavioral and emotional disorders with onset usually occurring in childhood and adolescence P

Unspecified mental disorder (F99)

F99 Mental disorder, not otherwise specified

Mental illness NOS

EXCLUDES 1 *unspecified mental disorder due to known physiological condition (F09)*

Chapter 6. Diseases of the Nervous System (GØØ-G99)

EXCLUDES 2 *certain conditions originating in the perinatal period (PØ4-P96)*
certain infectious and parasitic diseases (AØØ-B99)
complications of pregnancy, childbirth and the puerperium (OØØ-O9A)
congenital malformations, deformations, and chromosomal abnormalities (QØØ-Q99)
endocrine, nutritional and metabolic diseases (EØØ-E88)
injury, poisoning and certain other consequences of external causes (SØØ-T88)
neoplasms (CØØ-D49)
symptoms, signs and abnormal clinical and laboratory findings, not elsewhere classified (RØØ-R94)

This chapter contains the following blocks:

GØØ-GØ9 Inflammatory diseases of the central nervous system
G1Ø-G14 Systemic atrophies primarily affecting the central nervous system
G2Ø-G26 Extrapyramidal and movement disorders
G3Ø-G32 Other degenerative diseases of the nervous system
G35-G37 Demyelinating diseases of the central nervous system
G4Ø-G47 Episodic and paroxysmal disorders
G5Ø-G59 Nerve, nerve root and plexus disorders
G6Ø-G65 Polyneuropathies and other disorders of the peripheral nervous system
G7Ø-G73 Diseases of myoneural junction and muscle
G8Ø-G83 Cerebral palsy and other paralytic syndromes
G89-G99 Other disorders of the nervous system

Inflammatory diseases of the central nervous system (GØØ-GØ9)

✓4th **GØØ Bacterial meningitis, not elsewhere classified**
INCLUDES bacterial arachnoiditis
bacterial leptomeningitis
bacterial meningitis
bacterial pachymeningitis
EXCLUDES 1 *bacterial:*
meningoencephalitis (GØ4.2)
meningomyelitis (GØ4.2)

CC Excl: For MCC codes in category GØØ, unless otherwise noted: AØ2.21, A17.Ø-A17.1, A27.81, A39.Ø, A5Ø.41, A51.41, A52.13, A54.82, A54.84, A54.89-A54.9, A87.Ø-A87.9, BØØ.3, BØ2.1, B26.1, B37.5, B38.4, B45.1, B58.2, EØ8.4Ø-EØ8.49, EØ8.618-EØ8.638, EØ8.649-EØ8.8, EØ9.4Ø-EØ9.49, EØ9.618-EØ9.638, EØ9.649-EØ9.8, E1Ø.4Ø-E1Ø.49, E1Ø.618-E1Ø.638, E1Ø.649, E1Ø.69-E1Ø.8, E11.4Ø-E11.49, E11.618-E11.638, E11.649, E11.69-E11.8, E13.4Ø-E13.49, E13.618-E13.638, E13.649-E13.8, GØØ.Ø-GØ3.9, GØ4.2, G32.89, G61.Ø, G96.8-G96.9, G98.Ø-G98.8, G99.8

GØØ.Ø Hemophilus meningitis MCC
Meningitis due to Hemophilus influenzae

GØØ.1 Pneumococcal meningitis MCC

GØØ.2 Streptococcal meningitis MCC
Use additional code to further identify organism (B95.Ø-B95.5)

GØØ.3 Staphylococcal meningitis MCC
Use additional code to further identify organism (B95.61-B95.8)

GØØ.8 Other bacterial meningitis MCC
Meningitis due to Escherichia coli
Meningitis due to Friedländer's bacillus
Meningitis due to Klebsiella
Use additional code to further identify organism (B96.-)

GØØ.9 Bacterial meningitis, unspecified MCC
Meningitis due to gram-negative bacteria, unspecified
Purulent meningitis NOS
Pyogenic meningitis NOS
Suppurative meningitis NOS

GØ1 Meningitis in bacterial diseases classified elsewhere MCC
Code first underlying disease
EXCLUDES 1 *meningitis (in):*
gonococcal (A54.81)
leptospirosis (A27.81)
listeriosis (A32.11)
Lyme disease (A69.21)
meningococcal (A39.Ø)
neurosyphilis (A52.13)
tuberculosis (A17.Ø)
meningoencephalitis and meningomyelitis in bacterial diseases classified elsewhere (GØ5)
CC Excl: See code: GØØ

GØ2 Meningitis in other infectious and parasitic diseases classified elsewhere MCC
Code first underlying disease, such as:
African trypanosomiasis (B56.-)
poliovirus infection (A8Ø.-)
EXCLUDES 1 *candidal meningitis (B37.5)*
coccidioidomycosis meningitis (B38.4)
cryptococcal meningitis (B45.1)
herpesviral [herpes simplex] meningitis (BØØ.3)
infectious mononucleosis complicated by meningitis (B27.- with fourth character 2)
measles complicated by meningitis (BØ5.1)
meningoencephalitis and meningomyelitis in other infectious and parasitic diseases classified elsewhere (GØ5)
mumps meningitis (B26.1)
rubella meningitis (BØ6.Ø2)
varicella [chickenpox] meningitis (BØ1.Ø)
zoster meningitis (BØ2.1)
CC Excl: AØ2.21, A17.Ø-A17.1, A27.81, A39.Ø, A5Ø.41, A51.41, A52.13, A54.82, A54.84, A54.89-A54.9, A87.Ø-A87.9, BØØ.3, BØ2.1, B26.1, B37.5, B38.4, B45.1, B58.2, GØØ.Ø-GØ3.9, GØ4.2, G32.89, G61.Ø, G96.8-G96.9, G98.Ø-G98.8, G99.8

✓4th **GØ3 Meningitis due to other and unspecified causes**
INCLUDES arachnoiditis NOS
leptomeningitis NOS
meningitis NOS
pachymeningitis NOS
EXCLUDES 1 *meningoencephalitis (GØ4.-)*
meningomyelitis (GØ4.-)

GØ3.Ø Nonpyogenic meningitis MCC
Aseptic meningitis
Nonbacterial meningitis
CC Excl: See code: GØØ

GØ3.1 Chronic meningitis CC
CC Excl: See code: GØØ

GØ3.2 Benign recurrent meningitis [Mollaret] CC
CC Excl: AØ2.21, A17.Ø-A17.1, A27.81, A39.Ø, A5Ø.41, A51.41, A52.13, A54.82, A54.84, A54.89-A54.9, A74.81-A74.9, A87.Ø-A87.9, A96.2, A98.3-A98.4, B26.1, B33.24, B33.4-B33.8, B34.1-B34.2, B34.4-B34.8, B37.5, B38.4, B45.1, B58.2, B92, B94.2-B94.9, B97.1Ø, B97.19, B97.29, B97.5-B97.6, B97.81-B97.89, GØØ.Ø-GØ3.9, GØ4.2, G32.89, G61.Ø, G96.8-G96.9, G98.Ø-G98.8, G99.8

GØ3.8 Meningitis due to other specified causes MCC
CC Excl: See code: GØØ

GØ3.9 Meningitis, unspecified MCC
Arachnoiditis (spinal) NOS
CC Excl: See code: GØØ

✓4th **GØ4 Encephalitis, myelitis and encephalomyelitis**
INCLUDES acute ascending myelitis
meningoencephalitis
meningomyelitis
EXCLUDES 1 *encephalopathy NOS (G93.4Ø)*
EXCLUDES 2 *acute transverse myelitis (G37.3-)*
alcoholic encephalopathy (G31.2)
benign myalgic encephalomyelitis (G93.3)
multiple sclerosis (G35)
subacute necrotizing myelitis (G37.4)
toxic encephalitis (G92)
toxic encephalopathy (G92)

✓5th **GØ4.Ø Acute disseminated encephalitis and encephalomyelitis (ADEM)**
EXCLUDES 1 *acute necrotizing hemorrhagic encephalopathy (GØ4.3-)*
other noninfectious acute disseminated encephalomyelitis (noninfectious ADEM) (GØ4.81)

GØ4.ØØ Acute disseminated encephalitis and encephalomyelitis, unspecified MCC
CC Excl: AØ2.21, A17.Ø-A17.1, A17.82, A27.81, A39.Ø, A5Ø.41-A5Ø.42, A51.41, A52.13-A52.14, A54.82, A54.84, A54.89-A54.9, A81.1, A81.82-A81.89, A83.Ø-A85.8, A87.Ø-A88.Ø, A88.8, A92.1-A92.8, A93.Ø, A96.2, A98.3-A98.4, BØØ.3-BØØ.4, BØØ.89-BØ1.11, BØ1.81-BØ2.23, BØ2.29, BØ2.7-BØ2.9, BØ4, BØ6.Ø1, BØ8.Ø4-BØ8.Ø9, BØ8.2Ø-BØ8.22, BØ8.6Ø-BØ8.79, BØ9-B1Ø.89, B26.1-B26.2, B27.ØØ-B27.99, B33.1, B33.24, B33.4-B33.8, B34.1-B34.2, B34.4-B34.8, B37.5, B38.4, B45.1, B58.2, B92, B94.2-B94.9, B97.1Ø, B97.19-B97.29, B97.5-B97.6, B97.81-B97.89, GØØ.Ø-GØ4.Ø1, GØ4.2, GØ4.31, GØ4.81-GØ5.4, G32.89, G37.Ø, G37.4-G37.5, G61.Ø, G96.8-G96.9, G98.Ø-G98.8, G99.8, JØ9.X3-JØ9.X9, J1Ø.2-J1Ø.89, J11.2-J11.89, L44.4, P35.2-P35.9, P37.Ø-P37.4, P37.8-P37.9

GØ4.Ø1 Postinfectious acute disseminated encephalitis and encephalomyelitis (postinfectious ADEM) MCC
EXCLUDES 1 *post chickenpox encephalitis (BØ1.1)*
post measles encephalitis (BØ5.Ø)
post measles myelitis (BØ5.1)
CC Excl: See code: GØ4.ØØ

GØ4.Ø2 Postimmunization acute disseminated encephalitis, myelitis and encephalomyelitis MCC
Encephalitis, postimmunization
Encephalomyelitis, postimmunization
Use additional code to identify the vaccine (T5Ø.A-, T5Ø.B-, T5ØZ-)
CC Excl: No Excl

GØ4.1 Tropical spastic paraplegia CC
CC Excl: GØ4.1, G11.Ø-G12.9, G32.Ø-G37.3, G37.5-G37.9, G8Ø.Ø-G8Ø.2, G8Ø.4-G83.9, G9Ø.Ø1-G9Ø.Ø9, G9Ø.2, G9Ø.4-G9Ø.9, G92, G93.4Ø-G93.49, G93.81, G93.89-G93.9, G95.Ø-G95.9, G96.8-G96.9, G98.Ø-G99.8, I67.83, R53.2

GØ4.2 Bacterial meningoencephalitis and meningomyelitis, not elsewhere classified MCC
CC Excl: See code: GØØ

✓5th **GØ4.3 Acute necrotizing hemorrhagic encephalopathy**
EXCLUDES 1 *acute disseminated encephalitis and encephalomyelitis (GØ4.Ø-)*

GØ4.3Ø Acute necrotizing hemorrhagic encephalopathy, unspecified MCC
CC Excl: No Excl

GØ4.31 Postinfectious acute necrotizing hemorrhagic encephalopathy MCC
CC Excl: See code: GØ4.ØØ

GØ4.32 Postimmunization acute necrotizing hemorrhagic encephalopathy MCC
Use additional code to identify the vaccine (T5Ø.A-, T5Ø.B-, T5ØZ-)
CC Excl: No Excl

GØ4.39 Other acute necrotizing hemorrhagic encephalopathy MCC
Code also underlying etiology, if applicable
CC Excl: No Excl

✓5th **GØ4.8 Other encephalitis, myelitis and encephalomyelitis**
Code also any associated seizure (G4Ø.-, R56.9)

GØ4.81 Other encephalitis and encephalomyelitis HIV MCC
Noninfectious acute disseminated encephalomyelitis (noninfectious ADEM)
CC Excl: See code: GØ4.ØØ

GØ4.89 Other myelitis HIV MCC
CC Excl: See code: GØ4.ØØ

✓5th **GØ4.9 Encephalitis, myelitis and encephalomyelitis, unspecified**

GØ4.9Ø Encephalitis and encephalomyelitis, unspecified HIV MCC
Ventriculitis (cerebral) NOS
CC Excl: A17.82, A28.1, A5Ø.42, A52.14, A75.9, A79.9, A81.1, A81.82-A81.89, A83.Ø-A85.8, A87.2, A88.Ø, A88.8, A92.1-A92.8, A93.Ø, BØØ.4, BØØ.82, BØ1.11-BØ1.12, BØ4, BØ6.Ø1, BØ8.Ø9, BØ8.2Ø-BØ8.22, BØ8.6Ø-BØ8.79, BØ9-B1Ø.Ø9, B26.2, B27.ØØ-B27.99, B33.1, B45.Ø, B45.2-B45.9, B54, B58.2, B75, B97.1Ø, B97.21, GØ4.ØØ-GØ4.Ø1, GØ4.31, GØ4.81-GØ5.4, G37.Ø, G37.4-G37.5, H66.4Ø-H66.43, JØ9.X3-JØ9.X9, J1Ø.2-J1Ø.89, J11.2-J11.89, L44.4, M1A.1ØXØ-M1A.19X1, M32.Ø-M32.9, P35.2-P35.9, P37.Ø-P37.4, P37.8-P37.9, T56.ØX1A, T56.ØX2A, T56.ØX3A, T56.ØX4A

GØ4.91 Myelitis, unspecified HIV MCC
CC Excl: See code: GØ4.9Ø

✓4th **GØ5 Encephalitis, myelitis and encephalomyelitis in diseases classified elsewhere**
Code first underlying disease, such as:
human immunodeficiency virus [HIV] disease (B2Ø)
poliovirus (A8Ø.-)
suppurative otitis media (H66.Ø1-H66.4)
trichinellosis (B75)
EXCLUDES 1 *adenoviral encephalitis, myelitis and encephalomyelitis (A85.1)*
congenital toxoplasmosis encephalitis, myelitis and encephalomyelitis (P37.1)
cytomegaloviral encephalitis, myelitis and encephalomyelitis (B25.8)
encephalitis, myelitis and encephalomyelitis (in) measles (BØ5.Ø)
encephalitis, myelitis and encephalomyelitis (in) systemic lupus erythematosus (M32.19)
enteroviral encephalitis, myelitis and encephalomyelitis (A85.Ø)
eosinophilic meningoencephalitis (B83.2)
herpesviral [herpes simplex] encephalitis, myelitis and encephalomyelitis (BØØ.4)
listerial encephalitis, myelitis and encephalomyelitis (A32.12)
meningococcal encephalitis, myelitis and encephalomyelitis (A39.81)
mumps encephalitis, myelitis and encephalomyelitis (B26.2)
postchickenpox encephalitis, myelitis and encephalomyelitis (BØ1.1-)
rubella encephalitis, myelitis and encephalomyelitis (BØ6.Ø1)
toxoplasmosis encephalitis, myelitis and encephalomyelitis (B58.2)
zoster encephalitis, myelitis and encephalomyelitis (BØ2.Ø)

GØ5.3 Encephalitis and encephalomyelitis in diseases classified elsewhere MCC
Meningoencephalitis in diseases classified elsewhere
CC Excl: See code: GØ4.ØØ

GØ5.4 Myelitis in diseases classified elsewhere MCC
Meningomyelitis in diseases classified elsewhere
CC Excl: See code: GØ4.ØØ

✓4th **GØ6 Intracranial and intraspinal abscess and granuloma**
Use additional code (B95-B97) to identify infectious agent

GØ6.Ø Intracranial abscess and granuloma MCC
Brain [any part] abscess (embolic)
Cerebellar abscess (embolic)
Cerebral abscess (embolic)
Intracranial epidural abscess or granuloma
Intracranial extradural abscess or granuloma
Intracranial subdural abscess or granuloma
Otogenic abscess (embolic)
EXCLUDES 1 *tuberculous intracranial abscess and granuloma (A17.81)*
CC Excl: AØ6.6, A17.81, EØ8.4Ø-EØ8.49, EØ8.618-EØ8.638, EØ8.649-EØ8.8, EØ9.4Ø-EØ9.49, EØ9.618-EØ9.638, EØ9.649-EØ9.8, E1Ø.4Ø-E1Ø.49, E1Ø.618-E1Ø.638, E1Ø.649, E1Ø.69-E1Ø.8, E11.4Ø-E11.49, E11.618-E11.638, E11.649, E11.69-E11.8, E13.4Ø-E13.49, E13.618-E13.638, E13.649-E13.8, GØ6.Ø-GØ8, G93.81, G93.89-G93.9

GØ6.1 Intraspinal abscess and granulom MCC
Abscess (embolic) of spinal cord [any part]
Intraspinal epidural abscess or granuloma
Intraspinal extradural abscess or granuloma
Intraspinal subdural abscess or granuloma
EXCLUDES 1 *tuberculous intraspinal abscess and granuloma (A17.81)*
CC Excl: AØ6.6, A17.81, EØ8.4Ø-EØ8.49, EØ8.618-EØ8.638, EØ8.649-EØ8.8, EØ9.4Ø-EØ9.49, EØ9.618-EØ9.638, EØ9.649-EØ9.8, E1Ø.4Ø-E1Ø.49, E1Ø.618-E1Ø.638, E1Ø.649, E1Ø.69-E1Ø.8, E11.4Ø-E11.49, E11.618-E11.638, E11.649, E11.69-E11.8, E13.4Ø-E13.49, E13.618-E13.638, E13.649-E13.8, GØ6.1

GØ6.2 Extradural and subdural abscess, unspecified MCC
CC Excl: AØ6.6, A17.81, EØ8.4Ø-EØ8.49, EØ8.618-EØ8.638, EØ8.649-EØ8.8, EØ9.4Ø-EØ9.49, EØ9.618-EØ9.638, EØ9.649-EØ9.8, E1Ø.4Ø-E1Ø.49, E1Ø.618-E1Ø.638, E1Ø.649, E1Ø.69-E1Ø.8, E11.4Ø-E11.49, E11.618-E11.638, E11.649, E11.69-E11.8, E13.4Ø-E13.49, E13.618-E13.638, E13.649-E13.8, GØ6.Ø-GØ8

GØ7 Intracranial and intraspinal abscess and granuloma in diseases classified elsewhere MCC
Code first underlying disease, such as:
schistosomiasis granuloma of brain (B65.-)
EXCLUDES 1 *abscess of brain:*
amebic (AØ6.6)
chromomycotic (B43.1)
gonococcal (A54.82)
tuberculous (A17.81)
tuberculoma of meninges (A17.1)
CC Excl: See code: GØ6.2

GØ8 Intracranial and intraspinal phlebitis and thrombophlebitis MCC
Septic embolism of intracranial or intraspinal venous sinuses and veins
Septic endophlebitis of intracranial or intraspinal venous sinuses and veins
Septic phlebitis of intracranial or intraspinal venous sinuses and veins
Septic thrombophlebitis of intracranial or intraspinal venous sinuses and veins
Septic thrombosis of intracranial or intraspinal venous sinuses and veins
EXCLUDES 1 *intracranial phlebitis and thrombophlebitis complicating:*
abortion, ectopic or molar pregnancy (OØØ-OØ7, OØ8.7)
pregnancy, childbirth and the puerperium (O22.5, O87.3)
nonpyogenic intracranial phlebitis and thrombophlebitis (I67.6)
EXCLUDES 2 *intracranial phlebitis and thrombophlebitis complicating nonpyogenic intraspinal phlebitis and thrombophlebitis (G95.1)*
CC Excl: See code: GØ6.2

GØ9 Sequelae of inflammatory diseases of central nervous system
NOTE Category GØ9 is to be used to indicate conditions whose primary classification is to GØØ-GØ8 as the cause of sequelae, themselves classifiable elsewhere. The "sequelae" include conditions specified as residuals.
Code first condition resulting from (sequela) of inflammatory diseases of central nervous system

Systemic atrophies primarily affecting the central nervous system (G1Ø-G14)

G1Ø Huntington's disease CC
Huntington's chorea
Huntington's dementia
CC Excl: GØ4.1, G2Ø, G21.11-G21.9, G32.89-G37.2, G37.5-G37.9, G8Ø.Ø-G8Ø.2, G8Ø.4-G8Ø.9, G82.2Ø-G83.Ø, G92, G93.1, G93.4Ø-G93.6, G93.81, G93.89-G93.9, G96.8-G96.9, G98.Ø-G98.8, G99.8, I67.83, R53.2

✓4th **G11 Hereditary ataxia**
EXCLUDES 2 *cerebral palsy (G8Ø.-)*
hereditary and idiopathic neuropathy (G6Ø.-)
metabolic disorders (E7Ø-E88)

CC Excl: For CC codes in category G11, unless otherwise noted: GØ4.1, G1Ø-G12.9, G21.Ø, G23.Ø-G25.79, G25.82-G26, G32.Ø-G37.3, G37.5-G37.9, G8Ø.Ø-G83.9, G9Ø.Ø1-G9Ø.Ø9, G9Ø.2-G9Ø.9, G92-G93.1, G93.4Ø-G93.49, G93.81, G93.89-G93.9, G95.Ø-G95.9, G96.8-G96.9, G98.Ø-G99.8, I67.83, R53.2

G11.Ø Congenital nonprogressive ataxia CC
G11.1 Early-onset cerebellar ataxia CC
Early-onset cerebellar ataxia with essential tremor
Early-onset cerebellar ataxia with myoclonus [Hunt's ataxia]
Early-onset cerebellar ataxia with retained tendon reflexes
Friedreich's ataxia (autosomal recessive)
X-linked recessive spinocerebellar ataxia
G11.2 Late-onset cerebellar ataxia CC A
G11.3 Cerebellar ataxia with defective DNA repair CC
Ataxia telangiectasia [Louis-Bar]
EXCLUDES 2 *Cockayne's syndrome (Q87.1)*
other disorders of purine and pyrimidine metabolism (E79.-)
xeroderma pigmentosum (Q82.1)
G11.4 Hereditary spastic paraplegia CC
CC Excl: GØ4.1, G1Ø-G12.9, G21.Ø, G23.Ø-G25.79, G25.82-G26, G32.Ø-G37.3, G37.5-G37.9, G8Ø.Ø-G83.9, G9Ø.Ø1-G9Ø.Ø9, G9Ø.2-G9Ø.9, G92, G93.1, G93.4Ø-G93.49, G93.81, G93.89-G93.9, G95.Ø-G95.9, G96.12-G96.9, G97.1, G98.Ø-G99.8, I67.83, R53.2
G11.8 Other hereditary ataxias CC
G11.9 Hereditary ataxia, unspecified CC
Hereditary cerebellar ataxia NOS
Hereditary cerebellar degeneration
Hereditary cerebellar disease
Hereditary cerebellar syndrome
CC Excl: G11.Ø-G11.9, G32.81

✓4th **G12 Spinal muscular atrophy and related syndromes**

CC Excl: For CC codes in category G12, unless otherwise noted: EØ8.4Ø-EØ8.49, EØ8.618-EØ8.638, EØ8.649-EØ8.8, EØ9.4Ø-EØ9.49, EØ9.618-EØ9.638, EØ9.649-EØ9.8, E1Ø.4Ø-E1Ø.49, E1Ø.618-E1Ø.638, E1Ø.649, E1Ø.69-E1Ø.8, E11.4Ø-E11.49, E11.618-E11.638, E11.649, E11.69-E11.8, E13.4Ø-E13.49, E13.618-E13.638, E13.649-E13.8, G11.3, G11.8-G12.9, G32.Ø, G32.89, G9Ø.Ø1-G9Ø.Ø9, G9Ø.2, G9Ø.4-G9Ø.9, G95.Ø-G95.9, G96.8-G96.9, G98.Ø-G99.8

G12.Ø Infantile spinal muscular atrophy, type I [Werdnig-Hoffman] CC
G12.1 Other inherited spinal muscular atrophy CC
Adult form spinal muscular atrophy
Childhood form, type II spinal muscular atrophy
Distal spinal muscular atrophy
Juvenile form, type III spinal muscular atrophy [Kugelberg-Welander]
Progressive bulbar palsy of childhood [Fazio-Londe]
Scapuloperoneal form spinal muscular atrophy
✓5th **G12.2 Motor neuron disease**
G12.2Ø Motor neuron disease, unspecified CC
G12.21 Amyotrophic lateral sclerosis CC A
Progressive spinal muscle atrophy
G12.22 Progressive bulbar palsy CC
G12.29 Other motor neuron disease CC
Familial motor neuron disease
Primary lateral sclerosis
G12.8 Other spinal muscular atrophies and related syndromes CC
G12.9 Spinal muscular atrophy, unspecified CC

✓4th **G13 Systemic atrophies primarily affecting central nervous system in diseases classified elsewhere**
G13.Ø Paraneoplastic neuromyopathy and neuropathy
Carcinomatous neuromyopathy
Sensorial paraneoplastic neuropathy [Denny Brown]
Code first underlying neoplasm (CØØ-D49)
G13.1 Other systemic atrophy primarily affecting central nervous system in neoplastic disease
Paraneoplastic limbic encephalopathy
Code first underlying neoplasm (CØØ-D49)
G13.2 *Systemic atrophy primarily affecting the central nervous system in myxedema*
Code first underlying disease, such as:
hypothyroidism (EØ3.-)
myxedematous congenital iodine deficiency (EØØ.1)
G13.8 Systemic atrophy primarily affecting central nervous system in other diseases classified elsewhere
Code first underlying disease

G14 Postpolio syndrome
Postpolio myelitic syndrome
EXCLUDES 1 *sequelae of poliomyelitis (B91)*

Extrapyramidal and movement disorders (G2Ø-G26)

G2Ø Parkinson's disease
Hemiparkinsonism
Idiopathic Parkinsonism or Parkinson's disease
Paralysis agitans
Parkinsonism or Parkinson's disease NOS
Primary Parkinsonism or Parkinson's disease
EXCLUDES 1 *dementia with Parkinsonism (G31.83)*

✓4th **G21 Secondary parkinsonism**
EXCLUDES 1 *dementia with Parkinsonism (G31.83)*
Huntington's disease (G1Ø)
Shy-Drager syndrome (G9Ø.3)
syphilitic Parkinsonism (A52.19)
G21.Ø Malignant neuroleptic syndrome MCC
Use additional code for adverse effect, if applicable, to identify drug (T43.3X5, T43.4X5, T43.5Ø5, T43.595)
EXCLUDES 1 *neuroleptic induced parkinsonism (G21.11)*
CC Excl: G1Ø, G21.Ø, G23.Ø-G25.79, G25.82-G26, G8Ø.3, G81.ØØ-G81.94, G9Ø.3, G93.2, G93.4Ø-G93.49, I67.83
✓5th **G21.1 Other drug-induced secondary parkinsonism**
G21.11 Neuroleptic induced parkinsonism CC
Use additional code for adverse effect, if applicable, to identify drug (T43.3X5, T43.4X5, T43.5Ø5, T43.595)
EXCLUDES 1 *malignant neuroleptic syndrome (G21.Ø)*
CC Excl: G2Ø-G21.9
G21.19 Other drug induced secondary parkinsonism CC
Use additional code for adverse effect, if applicable, to identify drug (T36-T5Ø with fifth or sixth character 5)
CC Excl: See code: G21.11
G21.2 Secondary parkinsonism due to other external agents CC
Code first (T51-T65) to identify external agent
CC Excl: See code: G21.11
G21.3 Postencephalitic parkinsonism CC
CC Excl: See code: G21.11
G21.4 Vascular parkinsonism

G21.8 Other secondary parkinsonism CC
CC Excl: See code: G21.11

G21.9 Secondary parkinsonism, unspecified CC
CC Excl: See code: G21.11

4th G23 Other degenerative diseases of basal ganglia
EXCLUDES 2 *multi-system degeneration of the autonomic nervous system (G90.3)*

CC Excl: For CC codes in category G23, unless otherwise noted:
G20, G21.11-G21.9, G90.01-G90.09, G93.40-G93.49, I67.83

G23.0 Hallervorden-Spatz disease CC
Pigmentary pallidal degeneration

G23.1 Progressive supranuclear ophthalmoplegia [Steele-Richardson-Olszewski] CC
Progressive supranuclear palsy

G23.2 Striatonigral degeneration CC

G23.8 Other specified degenerative diseases of basal ganglia CC
Calcification of basal ganglia

G23.9 Degenerative disease of basal ganglia, unspecified CC

4th G24 Dystonia
INCLUDES dyskinesia
EXCLUDES 2 *athetoid cerebral palsy (G80.3)*

CC Excl: For CC codes in category G24, unless otherwise noted:
G20, G21.11-G21.9, G25.70-G25.79, G25.89-G26, G80.3, G93.40-G93.49, I67.8

5th G24.0 Drug induced dystonia
Use additional code code for adverse effect, if applicable, to identify drug (T36-T50 with fifth or sixth character5)

G24.01 Drug induced subacute dyskinesia
Drug induced blepharospasm
Drug induced orofacial dyskinesia
Neuroleptic induced tardive dyskinesia
Tardive dyskinesia

G24.02 Drug induced acute dystonia CC
Acute dystonic reaction to drugs
Neuroleptic induced acute dystonia

G24.09 Other drug induced dystonia CC

G24.1 Genetic torsion dystonia
Dystonia deformans progressiva
Dystonia musculorum deformans
Familial torsion dystonia
Idiopathic familial dystonia
Idiopathic (torsion) dystonia NOS
(Schwalbe-) Ziehen-Oppenheim disease

G24.2 Idiopathic nonfamilial dystonia CC

G24.3 Spasmodic torticollis
EXCLUDES 1 *congenital torticollis (Q68.0)*
hysterical torticollis (F44.4)
ocular torticollis (R29.891)
psychogenic torticollis (F45.8)
torticollis NOS (M43.6)
traumatic recurrent torticollis (S13.4)

G24.4 Idiopathic orofacial dystonia
Orofacial dyskinesia
EXCLUDES 1 *drug induced orofacial dyskinesia (G24.01)*

G24.5 Blepharospasm
EXCLUDES 1 *drug induced blepharospasm (G24.01)*

G24.8 Other dystonia CC
Acquired torsion dystonia NOS

G24.9 Dystonia, unspecified
Dyskinesia NOS

4th G25 Other extrapyramidal and movement disorders
EXCLUDES 2 *sleep related movement disorders (G47.6-)*

G25.0 Essential tremor
Familial tremor
EXCLUDES 1 *tremor NOS (R25.1)*

G25.1 Drug-induced tremor
Use additional code for adverse effect, if applicable, to identify drug (T36-T50 with fifth or sixth character 5)

G25.2 Other specified forms of tremor
Intention tremor

G25.3 Myoclonus
Drug-induced myoclonus
Palatal myoclonus
Use additional code for adverse effect, if applicable, to identify drug (T36-T50 with fifth or sixth character 5)
EXCLUDES 1 *facial myokymia (G51.4)*
myoclonic epilepsy (G40.-)

G25.4 Drug-induced chorea
Use additional code for adverse effect, if applicable, to identify drug (T36-T50 with fifth or sixth character 5)

G25.5 Other chorea
Chorea NOS
EXCLUDES 1 *chorea NOS with heart involvement (I02.0)*
Huntington's chorea (G10)
rheumatic chorea (I02.-)
Sydenham's chorea (I02.-)

5th G25.6 Drug induced tics and other tics of organic origin

G25.61 Drug induced tics
Use additional code for adverse effect, if applicable, to identify drug (T36-T50 with fifth or sixth character 5)

G25.69 Other tics of organic origin
EXCLUDES 1 *habit spasm (F95.9)*
tic NOS (F95.9)
Tourette's syndrome (F95.2)

5th G25.7 Other and unspecified drug induced movement disorders
Use additional code for adverse effect, if applicable, to identify drug (T36-T50 with fifth or sixth character 5)

G25.70 Drug induced movement disorder, unspecified

G25.71 Drug induced akathisia
Drug induced acathisia
Neuroleptic induced acute akathisia

G25.79 Other drug induced movement disorders

5th G25.8 Other specified extrapyramidal and movement disorders

G25.81 Restless legs syndrome

G25.82 Stiff-man syndrome CC
CC Excl: G04.1, G10, G12.22, G20-G21.9, G24.01-G25.79, G25.82-G26, G32.89-G37.2, G37.5-G37.9, G80.0-G80.9, G82.20-G83.0, G92, G93.1, G93.40-G93.6, G93.81, G93.89-G93.9, G96.8-G96.9

G25.83 Benign shuddering attacks

G25.89 Other specified extrapyramidal and movement disorders

G25.9 Extrapyramidal and movement disorder, unspecified CC
CC Excl: See code: G25.82

G26 Extrapyramidal and movement disorders in diseases classified elsewhere
Code first underlying disease

Other degenerative diseases of the nervous system (G30-G32)

4th G30 Alzheimer's disease
INCLUDES Alzheimer's dementia senile and presenile forms
Use additional code to identify:
delirium, if applicable (F05)
dementia with behavioral disturbance (F02.81)
dementia without behavioral disturbance (F02.80)
EXCLUDES 1 *senile degeneration of brain NEC (G31.1)*
senile dementia NOS (F03)
senility NOS (R41.81)

G30.0 Alzheimer's disease with early onset

G30.1 Alzheimer's disease with late onset A

G30.8 Other Alzheimer's disease

G30.9 Alzheimer's disease, unspecified
AHA: 2012, 4Q, 95

4th G31 Other degenerative diseases of nervous system, not elsewhere classified
Use additional code to identify:
dementia with behavioral disturbance (F02.81)
dementia without behavioral disturbance (F02.80)
EXCLUDES 2 *Reye's syndrome (G93.7)*

5th G31.0 Frontotemporal dementia

G31.01 Pick's disease
Primary progressive aphasia
Progressive isolated aphasia

G31.09 Other frontotemporal dementia
Frontal dementia

G31.1 Senile degeneration of brain, not elsewhere classified
EXCLUDES 1 *Alzheimer's disease (G30.-)*
senility NOS (R41.81)

G31.2 Degeneration of nervous system due to alcohol
Alcoholic cerebellar ataxia
Alcoholic cerebellar degeneration
Alcoholic cerebral degeneration
Alcoholic encephalopathy
Dysfunction of the autonomic nervous system due to alcohol
Code also associated alcoholism (F10.-)

✓5th **G31.8 Other specified degenerative diseases of nervous system**

CC Excl: For CC codes in subcategory G31.8, unless otherwise noted: E75.00-E75.19, E75.4, F84.2, G13.2-G13.8, G30.0-G31.82, G31.84-G31.9, G91.4, G94

G31.81 Alpers disease CC
Grey-matter degeneration

G31.82 Leigh's disease CC
Subacute necrotizing encephalopathy

G31.83 Dementia with Lewy bodies
Dementia with Parkinsonism
Lewy body disease
Lewy body dementia

G31.84 Mild cognitive impairment, so stated
EXCLUDES 1 *age related cognitive decline (R41.81)*
altered mental status (R41.82)
cerebral degeneration (G31.9)
change in mental status (R41.82)
cognitive deficits following (sequelae of) cerebral hemorrhage or infarction (I69.01, I69.11, I69.21, I69.31, I69.81, I69.91)
cognitive impairment due to intracranial or head injury (S06.-)
dementia (F01.-, F02.-, F03)
mild memory disturbance (F06.8)
neurologic neglect syndrome (R41.4)
personality change, nonpsychotic (F68.8)

G31.85 Corticobasal degeneration

G31.89 Other specified degenerative diseases of nervous system

G31.9 Degenerative disease of nervous system, unspecified

✓4th **G32 Other degenerative disorders of nervous system in diseases classified elsewhere**

G32.0 Subacute combined degeneration of spinal cord in diseases elsewhere CC
Dana-Putnam syndrome
Sclerosis of spinal cord (combined) (dorsolateral) (posterolateral)
Code first underlying disease, such as:
vitamin B12 deficiency (E53.8)
vitamin B12 deficiency:
anemia (D51.9)
dietary (D51.3)
pernicious (D51.0)
EXCLUDES 1 *syphilitic combined degeneration of spinal cord (A52.11)*
CC Excl: G04.1, G11.3, G11.8-G12.9, G32.0, G32.89-G37.3, G37.5-G37.9, G80.0-G80.2, G80.4-G83.9, G90.01-G90.09, G90.2, G90.4-G90.9, G93.1, G93.40-G93.49, G95.0-G95.9, G96.12-G96.9, G97.1, G98.0-G99.8, I67.83, R53.2

✓5th **G32.8 Other specified degenerative disorders of nervous system in diseases classified elsewhere**
Code first underlying disease, such as:
amyloidosis cerebral degeneration (E85.-)
cerebral degeneration (due to) hypothyroidism (E00.0-E03.9)
cerebral degeneration (due to) neoplasm (C00-D49)
cerebral degeneration (due to) vitamin B deficiency, except thiamine (E52-E53.-)
EXCLUDES 1 *superior hemorrhagic polioencephalitis [Wernicke's encephalopathy] (E51.2)*

G32.81 Cerebellar ataxia in diseases classified elsewhere CC
Code first underlying disease, such as:
celiac disease (with gluten ataxia) (K90.0)
cerebellar ataxia (in) neoplastic disease (paraneoplastic cerebellar degeneration) (C00-D49)
non-celiac gluten ataxia (M35.9)
EXCLUDES 1 *systemic atrophy primarily affecting the central nervous system in alcoholic cerebellar ataxia (G31.2)*
systemic atrophy primarily affecting the central nervous system in myxedema (G13.2)
CC Excl: G04.1, G10-G12.9, G21.0, G23.0-G25.79, G25.82-G26, G32.0-G37.3, G37.5-G37.9, G80.0-G83.9, G90.01-G90.09, G90.2-G90.9, G92-G93.1, G93.40-G93.49, G93.81, G93.89-G93.9, G95.0-G95.9, G96.8-G96.9, G98.0-G99.8, I67.83, R53.2

G32.89 Other specified degenerative disorders of nervous system in diseases classified elsewhere
Degenerative encephalopathy in diseases classified elsewhere

Demyelinating diseases of the central nervous system (G35-G37)

G35 Multiple sclerosis
Disseminated multiple sclerosis
Generalized multiple sclerosis
Multiple sclerosis NOS
Multiple sclerosis of brain stem
Multiple sclerosis of cord

✓4th **G36 Other acute disseminated demyelination**
EXCLUDES 1 *postinfectious encephalitis and encephalomyelitis NOS (G04.01)*

G36.0 Neuromyelitis optica [Devic] CC
Demyelination in optic neuritis
EXCLUDES 1 *optic neuritis NOS (H46)*
CC Excl: G36.0, G93.40-G93.49, I67.83

G36.1 Acute and subacute hemorrhagic leuko encephalitis [Hurst] CC
CC Excl: G04.1, G10-G12.9, G21.0, G24.01-G25.79, G25.82-G26, G32.0-G37.3, G37.5-G37.9, G80.0-G83.9, G90.01-G90.09, G90.2, G90.4-G90.9, G92, G93.40-G93.49, G93.81, G93.89-G93.9, G95.0-G95.9, G96.8-G96.9, G98.0-G99.8, I67.83, R53.2

G36.8 Other specified acute disseminated demyelination CC
CC Excl: See code: G36.1

G36.9 Acute disseminated demyelination, unspecified HIV CC
CC Excl: See code: G36.1

✓4th **G37 Other demyelinating diseases of central nervous system**

G37.0 Diffuse sclerosis of central nervous system CC
Periaxial encephalitis
Schilder's disease
EXCLUDES 1 *X linked adrenoleukodystrophy (E71.52-)*
CC Excl: A92.30-A92.39, B97.21, G93.40-G93.49, I67.83

G37.1 Central demyelination of corpus callosum CC
CC Excl: See code: G36.1

G37.2 Central pontine myelinolysis CC
CC Excl: See code: G36.1

G37.3 Acute transverse myelitis in demyelinating disease of central nervous system CC
Acute transverse myelitis NOS
Acute transverse myelopathy
EXCLUDES 1 *multiple sclerosis (G35)*
neuromyelitis optica [Devic] (G36.0)
CC Excl: A02.21, A17.0-A17.1, A27.81, A39.0, A50.41, A51.41, A52.13, A54.82, A54.84, A54.89-A54.9, A87.0-A87.9, A96.2, A98.3-A98.4, B00.3, B00.89-B00.9, B02.0-B02.23, B02.29, B02.7-B02.9, B10.81-B10.89, B26.1, B33.24, B33.4-B33.8, B34.1-B34.2, B34.4-B34.8, B37.5, B38.4, B45.1, B58.2, B92, B94.2-B94.9, B97.10, B97.19, B97.29, B97.5-B97.6, B97.81-B97.89, E08.40-E08.49, E09.40-E09.49, E10.40-E10.49, E11.40-E11.49, E13.40-E13.49, G00.0-G03.9, G04.1-G04.2, G11.3, G11.8-G12.9, G32.0, G32.89-G37.2, G37.5-G37.9, G61.0, G80.0-G80.2, G80.4-G83.9, G90.01-G90.09, G90.2, G90.4-G90.9, G93.1, G93.40-G93.49, G95.0-G95.9, G96.12-G96.9, G97.1, G98.0-G99.8, I67.83, R53.2

G37.4 Subacute necrotizing myelitis of central nervous system HIV MCC
CC Excl: A17.82, A28.1, A50.42, A52.14, A75.9, A79.9, A81.1, A81.82-A81.89, A83.0-A85.8, A87.2, A88.0, A88.8, A92.1-A92.8, A93.0, B00.4, B00.82, B01.11-B01.12, B04, B06.01, B08.09, B08.20-B08.22, B08.60-B08.79, B09-B10.09, B26.2, B27.00-B27.99, B33.1, B45.0, B45.2-B45.9, B54, B58.2, B75, B97.10, B97.21, G04.00-G04.01, G04.31, G04.81-G05.4, G37.0, G37.4-G37.5, H66.40-H66.43, J09.X3-J09.X9, J10.2-J10.89, J11.2-J11.89, L44.4, M1A.10X0-M1A.19X1, M32.0-M32.9, P35.2-P35.9, P37.0-P37.4, P37.8-P37.9, T56.0X1A, T56.0X2A, T56.0X3A, T56.0X4A

G37.5 Concentric sclerosis [Balo] of central nervous system CC
CC Excl: See code: G37.0

G37.8 Other specified demyelinating diseases of central nervous system CC
CC Excl: See code: G36.1

G37.9 Demyelinating disease of central nervous system, unspecified HIV CC
CC Excl: See code: G36.1

Episodic and paroxysmal disorders (G40-G47)

✓4th **G40 Epilepsy and recurrent seizures**

NOTE The following terms are to be considered equivalent to intractable: pharmacoresistant (pharmacologically resistant), treatment resistant, refractory (medically) and poorly controlled

EXCLUDES 1 *conversion disorder with seizures (F44.5)*
convulsions NOS (R56.9)
hippocampal sclerosis (G93.81)
mesial temporal sclerosis (G93.81)
post traumatic seizures (R56.1)
seizure (convulsive) NOS (R56.9)
seizure of newborn (P90)
temporal sclerosis (G93.81)
Todd's paralysis (G83.8)

✓5th **G40.0 Localization-related (focal) (partial) idiopathic epilepsy and epileptic syndromes with seizures of localized onset**
Benign childhood epilepsy with centrotemporal EEG spikes
Childhood epilepsy with occipital EEG paroxysms
EXCLUDES 1 *adult onset localization-related epilepsy (G40.1-, G40.2-)*

✓6th **G40.00 Localization-related (focal) (partial) idiopathic epilepsy and epileptic syndromes with seizures of localized onset, not intractable**
Localization-related (focal) (partial) idiopathic epilepsy and epileptic syndromes with seizures of localized onset without intractability

G40.001 Localization-related (focal) (partial) idiopathic epilepsy and epileptic syndromes with seizures of localized onset, not intractable, with status epilepticus CC
CC Excl: G32.89, G40.001-G40.919, G93.40-G93.49, G93.9, G96.8-G96.9, G98.0-G98.8, G99.8, I67.83, R56.1

G40.009 Localization-related (focal) (partial) idiopathic epilepsy and epileptic syndromes with seizures of localized onset, not intractable, without status epilepticus CC
Localization-related (focal) (partial) idiopathic epilepsy and epileptic syndromes with seizures of localized onset NOS
CC Excl: See code: G40.001

✓6th **G40.01 Localization-related (focal) (partial) idiopathic epilepsy and epileptic syndromes with seizures of localized onset, intractable**

CC Excl: For CC codes in subcategory G40.01, unless otherwise noted: E08.40-E08.49, E09.40-E09.49, E10.40-E10.49, E11.40-E11.49, E13.40-E13.49, G32.89, G40.001-G40.919, G93.81, G93.89-G93.9, G96.8-G96.9, G98.0-G98.8, G99.8, R56.1

G40.011 Localization-related (focal) (partial) idiopathic epilepsy and epileptic syndromes with seizures of localized onset, intractable, with status epilepticus CC

G40.019 Localization-related (focal) (partial) idiopathic epilepsy and epileptic syndromes with seizures of localized onset, intractable, without status epilepticus CC

✓5th **G40.1 Localization-related (focal) (partial) symptomatic epilepsy and epileptic syndromes with simple partial seizures**
Attacks without alteration of consciousness
Epilepsia partialis continua [Kozhevnikof]
Simple partial seizures developing into secondarily generalized seizures

✓6th **G40.10 Localization-related (focal) (partial) symptomatic epilepsy and epileptic syndromes with simple partial seizures, not intractable**
Localization-related (focal) (partial) symptomatic epilepsy and epileptic syndromes with simple partial seizures without intractability

CC Excl: For CC codes in subcategory G40.10, unless otherwise noted: G32.89, G40.001-G40.919, G93.40-G93.49, G93.9, G96.8-G96.9, G98.0-G98.8, G99.8, I67.83, R56.1

G40.101 Localization-related (focal) (partial) symptomatic epilepsy and epileptic syndromes with simple partial seizures, not intractable, with status epilepticus CC

G40.109 Localization-related (focal) (partial) symptomatic epilepsy and epileptic syndromes with simple partial seizures, not intractable, without status epilepticus CC
Localization-related (focal) (partial) symptomatic epilepsy and epileptic syndromes with simple partial seizures NOS

✓6th **G40.11 Localization-related (focal) (partial) symptomatic epilepsy and epileptic syndromes with simple partial seizures, intractable**

CC Excl: For CC codes in subcategory G40.11, unless otherwise noted: E08.40-E08.49, E09.40-E09.49, E10.40-E10.49, E11.40-E11.49, E13.40-E13.49, G32.89, G40.001-G40.919, G93.81, G93.89-G93.9, G96.8-G96.9, G98.0-G98.8, G99.8, R56.1

G40.111 Localization-related (focal) (partial) symptomatic epilepsy and epileptic syndromes with simple partial seizures, intractable, with status epilepticus CC

G40.119 Localization-related (focal) (partial) symptomatic epilepsy and epileptic syndromes with simple partial seizures, intractable, without status epilepticus CC

✓5th **G40.2 Localization-related (focal) (partial) symptomatic epilepsy and epileptic syndromes with complex partial seizures**
Attacks with alteration of consciousness, often with automatisms
Complex partial seizures developing into secondarily generalized seizures

✓6th **G40.20 Localization-related (focal) (partial) symptomatic epilepsy and epileptic syndromes with complex partial seizures, not intractable**
Localization-related (focal) (partial) symptomatic epilepsy and epileptic syndromes with complex partial seizures without intractability

CC Excl: For CC codes in subcategory G40.20, unless otherwise noted: G32.89, G40.001-G40.919, G93.40-G93.49, G93.9, G96.8-G96.9, G98.0-G98.8, G99.8, I67.83, R56.1

G40.201 Localization-related (focal) (partial) symptomatic epilepsy and epileptic syndromes with complex partial seizures, not intractable, with status epilepticus CC

G40.209 Localization-related (focal) (partial) symptomatic epilepsy and epileptic syndromes with complex partial seizures, not intractable, without status epilepticus CC
Localization-related (focal) (partial) symptomatic epilepsy and epileptic syndromes with complex partial seizures NOS

✓6th **G40.21 Localization-related (focal) (partial) symptomatic epilepsy and epileptic syndromes with complex partial seizures, intractable**

CC Excl: For CC codes in subcategory G40.21, unless otherwise noted: E08.40-E08.49, E09.40-E09.49, E10.40-E10.49, E11.40-E11.49, E13.40-E13.49, G32.89, G40.001-G40.919, G93.81, G93.89-G93.9, G96.8-G96.9, G98.0-G98.8, G99.8, R56.1

G40.211 Localization-related (focal) (partial) symptomatic epilepsy and epileptic syndromes with complex partial seizures, intractable, with status epilepticus CC

G40.219 Localization-related (focal) (partial) symptomatic epilepsy and epileptic syndromes with complex partial seizures, intractable, without status epilepticus CC

✓5th **G40.3 Generalized idiopathic epilepsy and epileptic syndromes**
Code also MERRF syndrome, if applicable (E88.42)

CC Excl: For MCC codes in subcategory G40.3, unless otherwise noted: E08.40-E08.49, E08.618-E08.638, E08.649-E08.8, E09.40-E09.49, E09.618-E09.638, E09.649-E09.8, E10.40-E10.49, E10.618-E10.638, E10.649, E10.69-E10.8, E11.40-E11.49, E11.618-E11.638, E11.649, E11.69-E11.8, E13.40-E13.49, E13.618-E13.638, E13.649-E13.8, G32.89, G40.001-G40.919, G93.81, G93.89-G93.9, G96.8-G96.9, G98.0-G98.8, G99.8, R56.1

✓6th **G40.30 Generalized idiopathic epilepsy and epileptic syndromes, not intractable**
Generalized idiopathic epilepsy and epileptic syndromes without intractability

G40.301 Generalized idiopathic epilepsy and epileptic syndromes, not intractable, with status epilepticus MCC

G40.309 Generalized idiopathic epilepsy and epileptic syndromes, not intractable, without status epilepticus
Generalized idiopathic epilepsy and epileptic syndromes NOS

✓6th **G40.31 Generalized idiopathic epilepsy and epileptic syndromes, intractable**

G40.311 Generalized idiopathic epilepsy and epileptic syndromes, intractable, with status epilepticus MCC

G40.319 Generalized idiopathic epilepsy and epileptic syndromes, intractable, without status epilepticus MCC

✓5th **G40.A Absence epileptic syndrome**
Childhood absence epilepsy [pyknolepsy]
Juvenile absence epilepsy
Absence epileptic syndrome, NOS

CC Excl: For CC codes in subcategory G40.A, unless otherwise noted: E08.40-E08.49, E09.40-E09.49, E10.40-E10.49, E11.40-E11.49, E13.40-E13.49, G32.89, G40.001-G40.919, G93.81, G93.89-G93.9, G96.8-G96.9, G98.0-G98.8, G99.8, R56.1

✓6th **G40.A0 Absence epileptic syndrome, not intractable**

G40.A01 Absence epileptic syndrome, not intractable, with status epilepticus

G40.A09 Absence epileptic syndrome, not intractable, without status epilepticus

✓6th **G40.A1 Absence epileptic syndrome, intractable**

G40.A11 Absence epileptic syndrome, intractable, with status epilepticus CC

G40.A19 Absence epileptic syndrome, intractable, without status epilepticus CC

✓5th **G40.B Juvenile myoclonic epilepsy [impulsive petit mal]**

CC Excl: For CC codes in subcategory G40.B, unless otherwise noted: E08.40-E08.49, E09.40-E09.49, E10.40-E10.49, E11.40-E11.49, E13.40-E13.49, G32.89, G40.001-G40.919, G93.81, G93.89-G93.9, G96.8-G96.9, G98.0-G98.8, G99.8, R56.1

✓6th **G40.B0 Juvenile myoclonic epilepsy, not intractable**

G40.B01 Juvenile myoclonic epilepsy, not intractable, with status epilepticus CC

G40.B09 Juvenile myoclonic epilepsy, not intractable, without status epilepticus CC

✓6th **G40.B1 Juvenile myoclonic epilepsy, intractable**

G40.B11 Juvenile myoclonic epilepsy, intractable, with status epilepticus CC

G40.B19 Juvenile myoclonic epilepsy, intractable, without status epilepticus CC

✓5th **G40.4 Other generalized epilepsy and epileptic syndromes**
Epilepsy with grand mal seizures on awakening
Epilepsy with myoclonic absences
Epilepsy with myoclonic-astatic seizures
Grand mal seizure NOS
Nonspecific atonic epileptic seizures
Nonspecific clonic epileptic seizures
Nonspecific myoclonic epileptic seizures
Nonspecific tonic epileptic seizures
Nonspecific tonic-clonic epileptic seizures
Symptomatic early myoclonic encephalopathy

✓6th **G40.40 Other generalized epilepsy and epileptic syndromes, not intractable**
Other generalized epilepsy and epileptic syndromes without intractability
Other generalized epilepsy and epileptic syndromes NOS

G40.401 Other generalized epilepsy and epileptic syndromes, not intractable, with status epilepticus
CC Excl: See code: G40.001

G40.409 Other generalized epilepsy and epileptic syndromes, not intractable, without status epilepticus
CC Excl: See code: G40.001

✓6th **G40.41 Other generalized epilepsy and epileptic syndromes, intractable**

CC Excl: For CC codes in subcategory G40.41, unless otherwise noted: E08.40-E08.49, E09.40-E09.49, E10.40-E10.49, E11.40-E11.49, E13.40-E13.49, G32.89, G40.001-G40.919, G93.81, G93.89-G93.9, G96.8-G96.9, G98.0-G98.8, G99.8, R56.1

G40.411 Other generalized epilepsy and epileptic syndromes, intractable, with status epilepticus CC

G40.419 Other generalized epilepsy and epileptic syndromes, intractable, without status epilepticus CC

✓5th **G40.5 Epileptic seizures related to external causes**
Epileptic seizures related to alcohol
Epileptic seizures related to drugs
Epileptic seizures related to hormonal changes
Epileptic seizures related to sleep deprivation
Epileptic seizures related to stress
Use additional code for adverse effect, if applicable, to identify drug (T36-T50 with fifth or sixth character 5)
Code also, if applicable, associated epilepsy and recurrent seizures (G40.-)

CC Excl: For CC codes in subcategory G40.5, unless otherwise noted: E08.40-E08.49, E09.40-E09.49, E10.40-E10.49, E11.40-E11.49, E13.40-E13.49, G32.89, G40.001-G40.919, G93.81, G93.89-G93.9, G96.8-G96.9, G98.0-G98.8, G99.8, R56.1

✓6th **G40.50 Epileptic seizures related to external causes, not intractable**

G40.501 Epileptic seizures related to external causes, not intractable, with status epilepticus CC

G40.509 Epileptic seizures related to external causes, not intractable, without status epilepticus CC
Epileptic seizures related to external causes, NOS

✓5th **G40.8 Other epilepsy and recurrent seizures**
Epilepsies and epileptic syndromes undetermined as to whether they are focal or generalized
Landau-Kleffner syndrome

CC Excl: For CC codes in subcategory G40.8, unless otherwise noted: E08.40-E08.49, E09.40-E09.49, E10.40-E10.49, E11.40-E11.49, E13.40-E13.49, G32.89, G40.001-G40.919, G93.81, G93.89-G93.9, G96.8-G96.9, G98.0-G98.8, G99.8, R56.1

✓6th **G40.80 Other epilepsy**

G40.801 Other epilepsy, not intractable, with status epilepticus CC
Other epilepsy without intractability with status epilepticus

G40.802 Other epilepsy, not intractable, without status epilepticus CC
Other epilepsy without intractability without status epilepticus

G40.803 Other epilepsy, intractable, with status epilepticus CC

G40.804 Other epilepsy, intractable, without status epilepticus CC

✓6th **G40.81 Lennox-Gastaut syndrome**

G40.811 Lennox-Gastaut syndrome, not intractable, with status epilepticus CC

G40.812 Lennox-Gastaut syndrome, not intractable, without status epilepticus CC

G40.813 Lennox-Gastaut syndrome, intractable, with status epilepticus CC

G40.814 Lennox-Gastaut syndrome, intractable, without status epilepticus CC

✓6th **G40.82 Epileptic spasms**
Infantile spasms
Salaam attacks
West's syndrome

G40.821 Epileptic spasms, not intractable, with status epilepticus CC

G40.822 Epileptic spasms, not intractable, without status epilepticus CC

G40.823 Epileptic spasms, intractable, with status epilepticus CC

G40.824 Epileptic spasms, intractable, without status epilepticus CC

G40.89 Other seizures CC
EXCLUDES 1 *post traumatic seizures (R56.1)*
recurrent seizures NOS (G40.909)
seizure NOS (R56.9)

✓5th **G40.9 Epilepsy, unspecified**

CC Excl: For CC codes in subcategory G40.9, unless otherwise noted: E08.40-E08.49, E09.40-E09.49, E10.40-E10.49, E11.40-E11.49, E13.40-E13.49, G32.89, G40.001-G40.919, G93.81, G93.89-G93.9, G96.8-G96.9, G98.0-G98.8, G99.8, R56.1

✓6th **G40.90 Epilepsy, unspecified, not intractable**
Epilepsy, unspecified, without intractability

G40.901 Epilepsy, unspecified, not intractable, with status epilepticus

G40.909 Epilepsy, unspecified, not intractable, without status epilepticus
Epilepsy NOS
Epileptic convulsions NOS
Epileptic fits NOS
Epileptic seizures NOS
Recurrent seizures NOS
Seizure disorder NOS

✓6th **G40.91 Epilepsy, unspecified, intractable**
Intractable seizure disorder NOS

G40.911 Epilepsy, unspecified, intractable, with status epilepticus CC

G40.919 Epilepsy, unspecified, intractable, without status epilepticus CC

✓4th **G43 Migraine**
NOTE The following terms are to be considered equivalent to intractable: pharmacoresistant (pharmacologically resistant), treatment resistant, refractory (medically) and poorly controlled
Use additional code for adverse effect, if applicable, to identify drug (T36-T50 with fifth or sixth character 5)
EXCLUDES 1 *headache NOS (R51)*
lower half migraine (G44.00)
EXCLUDES 2 *headache syndromes (G44.-)*

✓5th **G43.0 Migraine without aura**
Common migraine
EXCLUDES 1 *chronic migraine without aura (G43.7-)*

✓6th **G43.00 Migraine without aura, not intractable**
Migraine without aura without mention of refractory migraine

G43.001 Migraine without aura, not intractable, with status migrainosus

G43.009 Migraine without aura, not intractable, without status migrainosus
Migraine without aura NOS

✓6th **G43.01 Migraine without aura, intractable**
Migraine without aura with refractory migraine

G43.011 Migraine without aura, intractable, with status migrainosus

G43.019 Migraine without aura, intractable, without status migrainosus

✓5th **G43.1 Migraine with aura**
Basilar migraine
Classical migraine
Migraine equivalents
Migraine preceded or accompanied by transient focal neurological phenomena
Migraine triggered seizures
Migraine with acute-onset aura
Migraine with aura without headache (migraine equivalents)
Migraine with prolonged aura
Migraine with typical aura
Retinal migraine
Code also any associated seizure (G40.-, R56.9)
EXCLUDES 1 *persistent migraine aura (G43.5-, G43.6-)*

✓6th **G43.10 Migraine with aura, not intractable**
Migraine with aura without mention of refractory migraine

G43.101 Migraine with aura, not intractable, with status migrainosus

G43.109 Migraine with aura, not intractable, without status migrainosus
Migraine with aura NOS

✓6th **G43.11 Migraine with aura, intractable**
Migraine with aura with refractory migraine

G43.111 Migraine with aura, intractable, with status migrainosus

G43.119 Migraine with aura, intractable, without status migrainosus

✓5th **G43.4 Hemiplegic migraine**
Familial migraine
Sporadic migraine

✓6th **G43.40 Hemiplegic migraine, not intractable**
Hemiplegic migraine without refractory migraine

G43.401 Hemiplegic migraine, not intractable, with status migrainosus

G43.409 Hemiplegic migraine, not intractable, without status migrainosus
Hemiplegic migraine NOS

✓6th **G43.41 Hemiplegic migraine, intractable**
Hemiplegic migraine with refractory migraine

G43.411 Hemiplegic migraine, intractable, with status migrainosus

G43.419 Hemiplegic migraine, intractable, without status migrainosus

✓5th **G43.5 Persistent migraine aura without cerebral infarction**

✓6th **G43.50 Persistent migraine aura without cerebral infarction, not intractable**
Persistent migraine aura without cerebral infarction, without refractory migraine

G43.501 Persistent migraine aura without cerebral infarction, not intractable, with status migrainosus

G43.509 Persistent migraine aura without cerebral infarction, not intractable, without status migrainosus
Persistent migraine aura NOS

✓6th **G43.51 Persistent migraine aura without cerebral infarction, intractable**
Persistent migraine aura without cerebral infarction, with refractory migraine

G43.511 Persistent migraine aura without cerebral infarction, intractable, with status migrainosus

G43.519 Persistent migraine aura without cerebral infarction, intractable, without status migrainosus

G43.6 Persistent migraine aura with cerebral infarction (5th)
Code also the type of cerebral infarction (I63.-)

CC Excl: For CC codes in subcategory G43.6, unless otherwise noted: G43.601-G43.619, I63.00-I66.9

G43.60 Persistent migraine aura with cerebral infarction, not intractable (6th)
Persistent migraine aura with cerebral infarction, without refractory migraine

G43.601 Persistent migraine aura with cerebral infarction, not intractable, with status migrainosus CC

G43.609 Persistent migraine aura with cerebral infarction, not intractable, without status migrainosus CC

G43.61 Persistent migraine aura with cerebral infarction, intractable (6th)
Persistent migraine aura with cerebral infarction, with refractory migraine

G43.611 Persistent migraine aura with cerebral infarction, intractable, with status migrainosus CC

G43.619 Persistent migraine aura with cerebral infarction, intractable, without status migrainosus CC

G43.7 Chronic migraine without aura (5th)
Transformed migraine
EXCLUDES 1 *migraine without aura (G43.0-)*

G43.70 Chronic migraine without aura, not intractable (6th)
Chronic migraine without aura, without refractory migraine

G43.701 Chronic migraine without aura, not intractable, with status migrainosus

G43.709 Chronic migraine without aura, not intractable, without status migrainosus
Chronic migraine without aura NOS

G43.71 Chronic migraine without aura, intractable (6th)
Chronic migraine without aura, with refractory migraine

G43.711 Chronic migraine without aura, intractable, with status migrainosus

G43.719 Chronic migraine without aura, intractable, without status migrainosus

G43.A Cyclical vomiting (5th)

G43.A0 Cyclical vomiting, not intractable
Cyclical vomiting, without refractory migraine

G43.A1 Cyclical vomiting, intractable
Cyclical vomiting, with refractory migraine

G43.B Ophthalmoplegic migraine (5th)

G43.B0 Ophthalmoplegic migraine, not intractable
Ophthalmoplegic migraine, without refractory migraine

G43.B1 Ophthalmoplegic migraine, intractable
Ophthalmoplegic migraine, with refractory migraine

G43.C Periodic headache syndromes in child or adult (5th)

G43.C0 Periodic headache syndromes in child or adult, not intractable
Periodic headache syndromes in child or adult, without refractory migraine

G43.C1 Periodic headache syndromes in child or adult, intractable
Periodic headache syndromes in child or adult, with refractory migraine

G43.D Abdominal migraine (5th)

G43.D0 Abdominal migraine, not intractable
Abdominal migraine, without refractory migraine

G43.D1 Abdominal migraine, intractable
Abdominal migraine, with refractory migraine

G43.8 Other migraine (5th)

G43.80 Other migraine, not intractable (6th)
Other migraine, without refractory migraine

G43.801 Other migraine, not intractable, with status migrainosus

G43.809 Other migraine, not intractable, without status migrainosus

G43.81 Other migraine, intractable (6th)
Other migraine, with refractory migraine

G43.811 Other migraine, intractable, with status migrainosus

G43.819 Other migraine, intractable, without status migrainosus

G43.82 Menstrual migraine, not intractable (6th)
Menstrual headache, not intractable
Menstrual migraine, without refractory migraine
Menstrually related migraine, not intractable
Pre-menstrual headache, not intractable
Pre-menstrual migraine, not intractable
Pure menstrual migraine, not intractable
Code also associated premenstrual tension syndrome (N94.3)

G43.821 Menstrual migraine, not intractable, with status migrainosus ♀

G43.829 Menstrual migraine, not intractable, without status migrainosus ♀
Menstrual migraine NOS

G43.83 Menstrual migraine, intractable (6th)
Menstrual headache, intractable
Menstrual migraine, with refractory migraine
Menstrually related migraine, intractable
Pre-menstrual headache, intractable
Pre-menstrual migraine, intractable
Pure menstrual migraine, intractable
Code also associated premenstrual tension syndrome (N94.3)

G43.831 Menstrual migraine, intractable, with status migrainosus ♀

G43.839 Menstrual migraine, intractable, without status migrainosus ♀

G43.9 Migraine, unspecified (5th)

G43.90 Migraine, unspecified, not intractable (6th)
Migraine, unspecified, without refractory migraine

G43.901 Migraine, unspecified, not intractable, with status migrainosus
Status migrainosus NOS

G43.909 Migraine, unspecified, not intractable, without status migrainosus
Migraine NOS

G43.91 Migraine, unspecified, intractable (6th)
Migraine, unspecified, with refractory migraine

G43.911 Migraine, unspecified, intractable, with status migrainosus

G43.919 Migraine, unspecified, intractable, without status migrainosus

G44 Other headache syndromes (4th)
EXCLUDES 1 *headache NOS (R51)*
EXCLUDES 2 *atypical facial pain (G50.1)*
headache due to lumbar puncture (G97.1)
migraines (G43.-)
trigeminal neuralgia (G50.0)

G44.0 Cluster headaches and other trigeminal autonomic cephalgias (TAC) (5th)

G44.00 Cluster headache syndrome, unspecified (6th)
Ciliary neuralgia
Cluster headache NOS
Histamine cephalgia
Lower half migraine
Migrainous neuralgia

G44.001 Cluster headache syndrome, unspecified, intractable

G44.009 Cluster headache syndrome, unspecified, not intractable
Cluster headache syndrome NOS

G44.01 Episodic cluster headache (6th)

G44.011 Episodic cluster headache, intractable

G44.019 Episodic cluster headache, not intractable
Episodic cluster headache NOS

G44.02 Chronic cluster headache (6th)

G44.021 Chronic cluster headache, intractable

G44.029 Chronic cluster headache, not intractable
Chronic cluster headache NOS

G44.03 Episodic paroxysmal hemicrania (6th)
Paroxysmal hemicrania NOS

G44.031 Episodic paroxysmal hemicrania, intractable

G44.039 Episodic paroxysmal hemicrania, not intractable
Episodic paroxysmal hemicrania NOS

✓6th **G44.04 Chronic paroxysmal hemicrania**

G44.041 Chronic paroxysmal hemicrania, intractable

G44.049 Chronic paroxysmal hemicrania, not intractable
Chronic paroxysmal hemicrania NOS

✓6th **G44.05 Short lasting unilateral neuralgiform headache with conjunctival injection and tearing (SUNCT)**

G44.051 Short lasting unilateral neuralgiform headache with conjunctival injection and tearing (SUNCT), intractable

G44.059 Short lasting unilateral neuralgiform headache with conjunctival injection and tearing (SUNCT), not intractable
Short lasting unilateral neuralgiform headache with conjunctival injection and tearing (SUNCT) NOS

✓6th **G44.09 Other trigeminal autonomic cephalgias (TAC)**

G44.091 Other trigeminal autonomic cephalgias (TAC), intractable

G44.099 Other trigeminal autonomic cephalgias (TAC), not intractable

G44.1 Vascular headache, not elsewhere classified
EXCLUDES 2 *cluster headache (G44.Ø)*
complicated headache syndromes (G44.5-)
drug-induced headache (G44.4-)
migraine (G43.-)
other specified headache syndromes (G44.8-)
post-traumatic headache (G44.3-)
tension-type headache (G44.2-)

✓5th **G44.2 Tension-type headache**

✓6th **G44.2Ø Tension-type headache, unspecified**

G44.2Ø1 Tension-type headache, unspecified, intractable

G44.2Ø9 Tension-type headache, unspecified, not intractable
Tension headache NOS

✓6th **G44.21 Episodic tension-type headache**

G44.211 Episodic tension-type headache, intractable

G44.219 Episodic tension-type headache, not intractable
Episodic tension-type headache NOS

✓6th **G44.22 Chronic tension-type headache**

G44.221 Chronic tension-type headache, intractable

G44.229 Chronic tension-type headache, not intractable
Chronic tension-type headache NOS

✓5th **G44.3 Post-traumatic headache**

✓6th **G44.3Ø Post-traumatic headache, unspecified**

G44.3Ø1 Post-traumatic headache, unspecified, intractable

G44.3Ø9 Post-traumatic headache, unspecified, not intractable
Post-traumatic headache NOS

✓6th **G44.31 Acute post-traumatic headache**

G44.311 Acute post-traumatic headache, intractable

G44.319 Acute post-traumatic headache, not intractable
Acute post-traumatic headache NOS

✓6th **G44.32 Chronic post-traumatic headache**

G44.321 Chronic post-traumatic headache, intractable

G44.329 Chronic post-traumatic headache, not intractable
Chronic post-traumatic headache NOS

✓5th **G44.4 Drug-induced headache, not elsewhere classified**
Medication overuse headache
Use additional code for adverse effect, if applicable, to identify drug (T36-T5Ø with fifth or sixth character 5)

G44.4Ø Drug-induced headache, not elsewhere classified, not intractable

G44.41 Drug-induced headache, not elsewhere classified, intractable

✓5th **G44.5 Complicated headache syndromes**

G44.51 Hemicrania continua

G44.52 New daily persistent headache (NDPH)

G44.53 Primary thunderclap headache

G44.59 Other complicated headache syndrome

✓5th **G44.8 Other specified headache syndromes**

G44.81 Hypnic headache

G44.82 Headache associated with sexual activity
Orgasmic headache
Preorgasmic headache

G44.83 Primary cough headache

G44.84 Primary exertional headache

G44.85 Primary stabbing headache

G44.89 Other headache syndrome

✓4th **G45 Transient cerebral ischemic attacks and related syndromes**
EXCLUDES 1 *neonatal cerebral ischemia (P91.Ø)*
transient retinal artery occlusion (H34.Ø-)

CC Excl: For CC codes in category G45, unless otherwise noted:
EØ8.51-EØ8.59, EØ8.618-EØ8.638, EØ8.649-EØ8.8, EØ9.51-EØ9.59, EØ9.618-EØ9.638, EØ9.649-EØ9.8, E1Ø.51-E1Ø.59, E1Ø.618-E1Ø.638, E1Ø.649, E1Ø.69-E1Ø.8, E11.51-E11.59, E11.618-E11.638, E11.649, E11.69-E11.8, E13.51-E13.59, E13.618-E13.638, E13.649-E13.8, G45.Ø-G45.2, G45.8-G46.2, I63.ØØ-I63.29, I65.Ø1-I65.9, I67.841-I67.848, I87.8, I99.8-I99.9

G45.Ø Vertebro-basilar artery syndrome CC

G45.1 Carotid artery syndrome (hemispheric) CC

G45.2 Multiple and bilateral precerebral artery syndromes CC

G45.3 Amaurosis fugax CC
CC Excl: G45.3-H34.9

G45.4 Transient global amnesia
EXCLUDES 1 *amnesia NOS (R41.3)*

G45.8 Other transient cerebral ischemic attacks and related syndromes CC

G45.9 Transient cerebral ischemic attack, unspecified CC
Spasm of cerebral artery
TIA
Transient cerebral ischemia NOS

✓4th **G46 Vascular syndromes of brain in cerebrovascular diseases**
Code first underlying cerebrovascular disease (I6Ø-I69)

CC Excl: For CC codes in category G46, unless otherwise noted:
EØ8.51-EØ8.59, EØ8.618-EØ8.638, EØ8.649-EØ8.8, EØ9.51-EØ9.59, EØ9.618-EØ9.638, EØ9.649-EØ9.8, E1Ø.51-E1Ø.59, E1Ø.618-E1Ø.638, E1Ø.649, E1Ø.69-E1Ø.8, E11.51-E11.59, E11.618-E11.638, E11.649, E11.69-E11.8, E13.51-E13.59, E13.618-E13.638, E13.649-E13.8, G45.Ø-G45.2, G45.8-G46.2, I63.ØØ-I63.29, I65.Ø1-I65.9, I67.841-I67.848, I87.8, I99.8-I99.9

G46.Ø Middle cerebral artery syndrome CC

G46.1 Anterior cerebral artery syndrome CC

G46.2 Posterior cerebral artery syndrome CC

G46.3 Brain stem stroke syndrome
Benedikt syndrome
Claude syndrome
Foville syndrome
Millard-Gubler syndrome
Wallenberg syndrome
Weber syndrome

G46.4 Cerebellar stroke syndrome

G46.5 Pure motor lacunar syndrome

G46.6 Pure sensory lacunar syndrome

G46.7 Other lacunar syndromes

G46.8 Other vascular syndromes of brain in cerebrovascular diseases

✓4th **G47 Sleep disorders**
EXCLUDES 2 *nightmares (F51.5)*
nonorganic sleep disorders (F51.-)
sleep terrors (F51.4)
sleepwalking (F51.3)

G47.0 Insomnia
EXCLUDES 2 *alcohol related insomnia (F10.182, F10.282, F10.982)*
drug-related insomnia (F11.182, F11.282, F11.982, F13.182, F13.282, F13.982, F14.182, F14.282,F14.982, F15.182, F15.282, F15.982, F19.182, F19.282, F19.982)
idiopathic insomnia (F51.01)
insomnia due to a mental disorder (F51.05)
insomnia not due to a substance or known physiological condition (F51.0-)
nonorganic insomnia (F51.0-)
primary insomnia (F51.01)
sleep apnea (G47.3-)

G47.00 Insomnia, unspecified
Insomnia NOS

G47.01 Insomnia due to medical condition
Code also associated medical condition

G47.09 Other insomnia

G47.1 Hypersomnia
EXCLUDES 2 *alcohol-related hypersomnia (F10.182, F10.282, F10.982)*
drug-related hypersomnia (F11.182, F11.282, F11.982, F13.182, F13.282, F13.982, F14.182,F14.282, F14.982, F15.182, F15.282, F15.982, F19.182, F19.282, F19.982)
hypersomnia due to a mental disorder (F51.13)
hypersomnia not due to a substance or known physiological condition (F51.1-)
primary hypersomnia (F51.11)
sleep apnea (G47.3-)

G47.10 Hypersomnia, unspecified
Hypersomnia NOS

G47.11 Idiopathic hypersomnia with long sleep time
Idiopathic hypersomnia NOS

G47.12 Idiopathic hypersomnia without long sleep time

G47.13 Recurrent hypersomnia
Kleine-Levin syndrome
Menstrual related hypersomnia

G47.14 Hypersomnia due to medical condition
Code also associated medical condition

G47.19 Other hypersomnia

G47.2 Circadian rhythm sleep disorders
Disorders of the sleep wake schedule
Inversion of nyctohemeral rhythm
Inversion of sleep rhythm

G47.20 Circadian rhythm sleep disorder, unspecified type
Sleep wake schedule disorder NOS

G47.21 Circadian rhythm sleep disorder, delayed sleep phase type
Delayed sleep phase syndrome

G47.22 Circadian rhythm sleep disorder, advanced sleep phase type

G47.23 Circadian rhythm sleep disorder, irregular sleep wake type
Irregular sleep-wake pattern

G47.24 Circadian rhythm sleep disorder, free running type

G47.25 Circadian rhythm sleep disorder, jet lag type

G47.26 Circadian rhythm sleep disorder, shift work type

G47.27 Circadian rhythm sleep disorder in conditions classified elsewhere
Code first underlying condition

G47.29 Other circadian rhythm sleep disorder

G47.3 Sleep apnea
Code also any associated underlying condition
EXCLUDES 1 *apnea NOS (R06.81)*
Cheyne-Stokes breathing (R06.3)
pickwickian syndrome (E66.2)
sleep apnea of newborn (P28.3)

G47.30 Sleep apnea, unspecified
Sleep apnea NOS

G47.31 Primary central sleep apnea

G47.32 High altitude periodic breathing

G47.33 Obstructive sleep apnea (adult) (pediatric)
EXCLUDES 1 *obstructive sleep apnea of newborn (P28.3)*

G47.34 Idiopathic sleep related nonobstructive alveolar hypoventilation
Sleep related hypoxia

G47.35 Congenital central alveolar hypoventilation syndrome

G47.36 Sleep related hypoventilation in conditions classified elsewhere
Sleep related hypoxemia in conditions classified elsewhere
Code first underlying condition

G47.37 Central sleep apnea in conditions classified elsewhere
Code first underlying condition

G47.39 Other sleep apnea

G47.4 Narcolepsy and cataplexy

G47.41 Narcolepsy

G47.411 Narcolepsy with cataplexy

G47.419 Narcolepsy without cataplexy
Narcolepsy NOS

G47.42 Narcolepsy in conditions classified elsewhere
Code first underlying condition

G47.421 Narcolepsy in conditions classified elsewhere with cataplexy

G47.429 Narcolepsy in conditions classified elsewhere without cataplexy

G47.5 Parasomnia
EXCLUDES 1 *alcohol induced parasomnia (F10.182, F10.282, F10.982)*
drug induced parasomnia (F11.182, F11.282, F11.982, F13.182, F13.282, F13.982, F14.182, F14.282, F14.982, F15.182, F15.282, F15.982, F19.182, F19.282, F19.982)
parasomnia not due to a substance or known physiological condition (F51.8)

G47.50 Parasomnia, unspecified
Parasomnia NOS

G47.51 Confusional arousals

G47.52 REM sleep behavior disorder

G47.53 Recurrent isolated sleep paralysis

G47.54 Parasomnia in conditions classified elsewhere
Code first underlying condition

G47.59 Other parasomnia

G47.6 Sleep related movement disorders
EXCLUDES 2 *restless legs syndrome (G25.81)*

G47.61 Periodic limb movement disorder

G47.62 Sleep related leg cramps

G47.63 Sleep related bruxism
EXCLUDES 1 *psychogenic bruxism (F45.8)*

G47.69 Other sleep related movement disorders

G47.8 Other sleep disorders

G47.9 Sleep disorder, unspecified
Sleep disorder NOS

Nerve, nerve root and plexus disorders (G50-G59)

EXCLUDES 1 *current traumatic nerve, nerve root and plexus disorders—see Injury, nerve by body region*
neuralgia NOS (M79.2)
neuritis NOS (M79.2)
peripheral neuritis in pregnancy (O26.82-)
radiculitis NOS (M54.1-)

G50 Disorders of trigeminal nerve
INCLUDES disorders of 5th cranial nerve

G50.0 Trigeminal neuralgia
Syndrome of paroxysmal facial pain
Tic douloureux

G50.1 Atypical facial pain

G50.8 Other disorders of trigeminal nerve

G50.9 Disorder of trigeminal nerve, unspecified

G51 Facial nerve disorders
INCLUDES disorders of 7th cranial nerve

G51.0 Bell's palsy
Facial palsy

G51.1 Geniculate ganglionitis
EXCLUDES 1 *postherpetic geniculate ganglionitis (B02.21)*

G51.2 Melkersson's syndrome
Melkersson-Rosenthal syndrome

G51.3 Clonic hemifacial spasm

G51.4 Facial myokymia

G51.8 Other disorders of facial nerve

G51.9 Disorder of facial nerve, unspecified

✓4th G52 Disorders of other cranial nerves

EXCLUDES 2 *disorders of acoustic [8th] nerve (H93.3)*
disorders of optic [2nd] nerve (H46, H47.0)
paralytic strabismus due to nerve palsy (H49.0-H49.2)

G52.0 Disorders of olfactory nerve
Disorders of 1st cranial nerve

G52.1 Disorders of glossopharyngeal nerve
Disorder of 9th cranial nerve
Glossopharyngeal neuralgia

G52.2 Disorders of vagus nerve
Disorders of pneumogastric [10th] nerve

G52.3 Disorders of hypoglossal nerve
Disorders of 12th cranial nerve

G52.7 Disorders of multiple cranial nerves
Polyneuritis cranialis

G52.8 Disorders of other specified cranial nerves

G52.9 Cranial nerve disorder, unspecified

G53 Cranial nerve disorders in diseases classified elsewhere

Code first underlying disease, such as:
neoplasm (C00-D49)

EXCLUDES 1 *multiple cranial nerve palsy in sarcoidosis (D86.82)*
multiple cranial nerve palsy in syphilis (A52.15)
postherpetic geniculate ganglionitis (B02.21)
postherpetic trigeminal neuralgia (B02.22)

✓4th G54 Nerve root and plexus disorders

EXCLUDES 1 *current traumatic nerve root and plexus disorders—see nerve injury by body region*
intervertebral disc disorders (M50-M51)
neuritis or radiculitis brachial NOS (M54.13)
neuritis or radiculitis lumbar NOS (M54.16)
neuritis or radiculitis lumbosacral NOS (M54.17)
neuritis or radiculitis thoracic NOS (M54.14)
radiculitis NOS (M54.10)
radiculopathy NOS (M54.10)
spondylosis (M47.-)

G54.0 Brachial plexus disorders
Thoracic outlet syndrome

G54.1 Lumbosacral plexus disorders

G54.2 Cervical root disorders, not elsewhere classified

G54.3 Thoracic root disorders, not elsewhere classified

G54.4 Lumbosacral root disorders, not elsewhere classified

G54.5 Neuralgic amyotrophy
Parsonage-Aldren-Turner syndrome
Shoulder-girdle neuritis

EXCLUDES 1 *neuralgic amyotrophy in diabetes mellitus (E08-E13 with .44)*

G54.6 Phantom limb syndrome with pain

G54.7 Phantom limb syndrome without pain
Phantom limb syndrome NOS

G54.8 Other nerve root and plexus disorders

G54.9 Nerve root and plexus disorder, unspecified

G55 Nerve root and plexus compressions in diseases classified elsewhere

Code first underlying disease, such as:
neoplasm (C00-D49)

EXCLUDES 1 *nerve root compression (due to) (in) ankylosing spondylitis (M45.-)*
nerve root compression (due to) (in) dorsopathies (M53.-, M54.-)
nerve root compression (due to) (in) intervertebral disc disorders (M50.1-, M51.1-)
nerve root compression (due to) (in) spondylopathies (M46.-, M48.-)

✓4th G56 Mononeuropathies of upper limb

EXCLUDES 1 *current traumatic nerve disorder—see nerve injury by body region*

✓5th G56.0 Carpal tunnel syndrome

G56.00 Carpal tunnel syndrome, unspecified upper limb
G56.01 Carpal tunnel syndrome, right upper limb
G56.02 Carpal tunnel syndrome, left upper limb

✓5th G56.1 Other lesions of median nerve

G56.10 Other lesions of median nerve, unspecified upper limb
G56.11 Other lesions of median nerve, right upper limb
G56.12 Other lesions of median nerve, left upper limb

✓5th G56.2 Lesion of ulnar nerve
Tardy ulnar nerve palsy

G56.20 Lesion of ulnar nerve, unspecified upper limb
G56.21 Lesion of ulnar nerve, right upper limb
G56.22 Lesion of ulnar nerve, left upper limb

✓5th G56.3 Lesion of radial nerve

G56.30 Lesion of radial nerve, unspecified upper limb
G56.31 Lesion of radial nerve, right upper limb
G56.32 Lesion of radial nerve, left upper limb

✓5th G56.4 Causalgia of upper limb
Complex regional pain syndrome II of upper limb

EXCLUDES 1 *complex regional pain syndrome I of lower limb (G90.52-)*
complex regional pain syndrome I of upper limb (G90.51-)
complex regional pain syndrome II of lower limb (G57.7-)
reflex sympathetic dystrophy of lower limb (G90.52-)
reflex sympathetic dystrophy of upper limb (G90.51-)

G56.40 Causalgia of unspecified upper limb
G56.41 Causalgia of right upper limb
G56.42 Causalgia of left upper limb

✓5th G56.8 Other specified mononeuropathies of upper limb
Interdigital neuroma of upper limb

G56.80 Other specified mononeuropathies of unspecified upper limb
G56.81 Other specified mononeuropathies of right upper limb
G56.82 Other specified mononeuropathies of left upper limb

✓5th G56.9 Unspecified mononeuropathy of upper limb

G56.90 Unspecified mononeuropathy of unspecified upper limb
G56.91 Unspecified mononeuropathy of right upper limb
G56.92 Unspecified mononeuropathy of left upper limb

✓4th G57 Mononeuropathies of lower limb

EXCLUDES 1 *current traumatic nerve disorder—see nerve injury by body region*

✓5th G57.0 Lesion of sciatic nerve

EXCLUDES 1 *sciatica NOS (M54.3-)*

EXCLUDES 2 *sciatica attributed to intervertebral disc disorder (M51.1-)*

G57.00 Lesion of sciatic nerve, unspecified lower limb
G57.01 Lesion of sciatic nerve, right lower limb
G57.02 Lesion of sciatic nerve, left lower limb

✓5th G57.1 Meralgia paresthetica
Lateral cutaneous nerve of thigh syndrome

G57.10 Meralgia paresthetica, unspecified lower limb
G57.11 Meralgia paresthetica, right lower limb
G57.12 Meralgia paresthetica, left lower limb

✓5th G57.2 Lesion of femoral nerve

G57.20 Lesion of femoral nerve, unspecified lower limb
G57.21 Lesion of femoral nerve, right lower limb
G57.22 Lesion of femoral nerve, left lower limb

✓5th G57.3 Lesion of lateral popliteal nerve
Peroneal nerve palsy

G57.30 Lesion of lateral popliteal nerve, unspecified lower limb
G57.31 Lesion of lateral popliteal nerve, right lower limb
G57.32 Lesion of lateral popliteal nerve, left lower limb

✓5th G57.4 Lesion of medial popliteal nerve

G57.40 Lesion of medial popliteal nerve, unspecified lower limb
G57.41 Lesion of medial popliteal nerve, right lower limb
G57.42 Lesion of medial popliteal nerve, left lower limb

✓5th G57.5 Tarsal tunnel syndrome

G57.50 Tarsal tunnel syndrome, unspecified lower limb
G57.51 Tarsal tunnel syndrome, right lower limb
G57.52 Tarsal tunnel syndrome, left lower limb

✓5th G57.6 Lesion of plantar nerve
Morton's metatarsalgia

G57.60 Lesion of plantar nerve, unspecified lower limb
G57.61 Lesion of plantar nerve, right lower limb

G57.62 **Lesion of plantar nerve, left lower limb**

✓5th G57.7 **Causalgia of lower limb**
Complex regional pain syndrome II of lower limb
EXCLUDES 1 *complex regional pain syndrome I of lower limb (G90.52-)*
complex regional pain syndrome I of upper limb (G90.51-)
complex regional pain syndrome II of upper limb (G56.4-)
reflex sympathetic dystrophy of lower limb (G90.52-)
reflex sympathetic dystrophy of upper limb (G90.51-)

G57.70 **Causalgia of unspecified lower limb**
G57.71 **Causalgia of right lower limb**
G57.72 **Causalgia of left lower limb**

✓5th G57.8 **Other specified mononeuropathies of lower limb**
Interdigital neuroma of lower limb
G57.80 **Other specified mononeuropathies of unspecified lower limb**
G57.81 **Other specified mononeuropathies of right lower limb**
G57.82 **Other specified mononeuropathies of left lower limb**

✓5th G57.9 **Unspecified mononeuropathy of lower limb**
G57.90 **Unspecified mononeuropathy of unspecified lower limb**
G57.91 **Unspecified mononeuropathy of right lower limb**
G57.92 **Unspecified mononeuropathy of left lower limb**

✓4th **G58 Other mononeuropathies**
G58.0 **Intercostal neuropathy**
G58.7 **Mononeuritis multiplex**
G58.8 **Other specified mononeuropathies**
G58.9 **Mononeuropathy, unspecified**

G59 Mononeuropathy in diseases classified elsewhere
Code first underlying disease
EXCLUDES 1 *diabetic mononeuropathy (E08-E13 with .41)*
syphilitic nerve paralysis (A52.19)
syphilitic neuritis (A52.15)
tuberculous mononeuropathy (A17.83)

Polyneuropathies and other disorders of the peripheral nervous system (G60-G65)

EXCLUDES 1 *neuralgia NOS (M79.2)*
neuritis NOS (M79.2)
peripheral neuritis in pregnancy (O26.82-)
radiculitis NOS (M54.10)

✓4th **G60 Hereditary and idiopathic neuropathy**
G60.0 **Hereditary motor and sensory neuropathy**
Charcôt-Marie-Tooth disease
Déjérine-Sottas disease
Hereditary motor and sensory neuropathy, types I-IV
Hypertrophic neuropathy of infancy
Peroneal muscular atrophy (axonal type) (hypertrophic type)
Roussy-Levy syndrome
G60.1 **Refsum's disease** CC
Infantile Refsum disease
AHA: 2014, 2Q, 4
CC Excl: E11.42, G13.0-G13.1, G50.0-G65.2, M34.83
G60.2 **Neuropathy in association with hereditary ataxia**
G60.3 **Idiopathic progressive neuropathy**
G60.8 **Other hereditary and idiopathic neuropathies**
Dominantly inherited sensory neuropathy
Morvan's disease
Nelaton's syndrome
Recessively inherited sensory neuropathy
G60.9 **Hereditary and idiopathic neuropathy, unspecified**

✓4th **G61 Inflammatory polyneuropathy**
G61.0 **Guillain-Barre syndrome** CC
Acute (post-)infective polyneuritis
Miller Fisher syndrome
AHA: 2014, 2Q, 4
CC Excl: A02.21, A17.0-A17.1, A27.81, A39.0, A39.89-A39.9, A49.3-A49.9, A50.41, A51.41, A52.13, A54.82, A54.84, A54.89-A54.9, A87.0-A87.9, B00.3, B02.1, B26.1, B37.5, B38.4, B45.1, B58.2, B92, B94.2-B94.9, B96.0, B96.6-B96.89, G00.0-G03.9, G04.2, G32.89, G61.0, G96.8-G96.9, G98.0-G98.8, G99.8
G61.1 **Serum neuropathy**
Use additional code for adverse effect, if applicable, to identify serum (T50.-)

✓5th G61.8 **Other inflammatory polyneuropathies**
G61.81 **Chronic inflammatory demyelinating polyneuritis** CC
CC Excl: G51.0-G54.5, G54.8-G60.9, G61.81-G61.89, G62.81, G62.89, G64
G61.89 **Other inflammatory polyneuropathies**
G61.9 **Inflammatory polyneuropathy, unspecified**

✓4th **G62 Other and unspecified polyneuropathies**
G62.0 **Drug-induced polyneuropathy**
Use additional code for adverse effect, if applicable, to identify drug (T36-T50 with fifth or sixth character 5)
G62.1 **Alcoholic polyneuropathy**
G62.2 **Polyneuropathy due to other toxic agents**
Code first (T51-T65) to identify toxic agent
✓5th G62.8 **Other specified polyneuropathies**
G62.81 **Critical illness polyneuropathy** CC
Acute motor neuropathy
CC Excl: G51.0-G54.5, G54.8-G60.9, G61.81-G61.9, G62.81, G62.89-G62.9, G64
G62.82 **Radiation-induced polyneuropathy**
Use additional external cause code (W88-W90, X39.0-) to identify cause
G62.89 **Other specified polyneuropathies**
G62.9 **Polyneuropathy, unspecified**
Neuropathy NOS

G63 Polyneuropathy in diseases classified elsewhere
Code first underlying disease, such as:
amyloidosis (E85.-)
endocrine disease, except diabetes (E00-E07, E15-E16, E20-E34)
metabolic diseases (E70-E88)
neoplasm (C00-D49)
nutritional deficiency (E40-E64)
EXCLUDES 1 *polyneuropathy (in):*
diabetes mellitus (E08-E13 with .42)
diphtheria (A36.83)
infectious mononucleosis (B27.0-B27.9 with 1)
Lyme disease (A69.22)
mumps (B26.84)
postherpetic (B02.23)
rheumatoid arthritis (M05.33)
scleroderma (M34.83)
systemic lupus erythematosus (M32.19)
AHA: 2012, 4Q, 99

G64 Other disorders of peripheral nervous system
Disorder of peripheral nervous system NOS

✓4th **G65 Sequelae of inflammatory and toxic polyneuropathies**
Code first condition resulting from (sequela) of inflammatory and toxic polyneuropathies
G65.0 **Sequelae of Guillain-Barré syndrome**
G65.1 **Sequelae of other inflammatory polyneuropathy**
G65.2 **Sequelae of toxic polyneuropathy**

Diseases of myoneural junction and muscle (G70-G73)

✓4th **G70 Myasthenia gravis and other myoneural disorders**
EXCLUDES 1 *botulism (A05.1, A48.51-A48.52)*
transient neonatal myasthenia gravis (P94.0)

CC Excl: For CC/MCC codes in category G70, unless otherwise noted: E08.40-E08.49, E08.618-E08.638, E08.649-E08.8, E09.40-E09.49, E09.618-E09.638, E09.649-E09.8, E10.40-E10.49, E10.618-E10.638, E10.649, E10.69-E10.8, E11.40-E11.49, E11.618-E11.638, E11.649, E11.69-E11.8, E13.40-E13.49, E13.618-E13.638, E13.649-E13.8, G32.89, G70.00-G70.01, G70.80-G70.81, G73.1-G73.3, G96.8-G96.9, G98.0-G98.8, G99.8

✓5th G70.0 **Myasthenia gravis**
G70.00 **Myasthenia gravis without (acute) exacerbation**
Myasthenia gravis NOS
G70.01 **Myasthenia gravis with (acute) exacerbation** MCC
Myasthenia gravis in crisis
G70.1 **Toxic myoneural disorders**
Code first (T51-T65) to identify toxic agent
G70.2 **Congenital and developmental myasthenia**
✓5th G70.8 **Other specified myoneural disorders**
G70.80 **Lambert-Eaton syndrome, unspecified** CC
Lambert-Eaton syndrome NOS

G70.81 ***Lambert-Eaton syndrome in disease classified elsewhere*** CC
Code first underlying disease
EXCLUDES 1 *Lambert-Eaton syndrome in neoplastic disease (G73.1)*

G70.89 Other specified myoneural disorders

G70.9 Myoneural disorder, unspecified

4th **G71 Primary disorders of muscles**

EXCLUDES 2 *arthrogryposis multiplex congenita (Q74.3)*
metabolic disorders (E70-E88)
myositis (M60.-)

G71.0 Muscular dystrophy CC
Autosomal recessive, childhood type, muscular dystrophy resembling Duchenne or Becker muscular dystrophy
Benign [Becker] muscular dystrophy
Benign scapuloperoneal muscular dystrophy with early contractures [Emery-Dreifuss]
Congenital muscular dystrophy NOS
Congenital muscular dystrophy with specific morphological abnormalities of the muscle fiber
Distal muscular dystrophy
Facioscapulohumeral muscular dystrophy
Limb-girdle muscular dystrophy
Ocular muscular dystrophy
Oculopharyngeal muscular dystrophy
Scapuloperoneal muscular dystrophy
Severe [Duchenne] muscular dystrophy
CC Excl: E08.40-E08.49, E08.618-E08.638, E08.649-E08.8, E09.40-E09.49, E09.618-E09.638, E09.649-E09.8, E10.40-E10.49, E10.618-E10.638, E10.649, E10.69-E10.8, E11.40-E11.49, E11.618-E11.638, E11.649, E11.69-E11.8, E13.40-E13.49, E13.618-E13.638, E13.649-E13.8, G32.89, G71.0, G71.2, G96.8-G96.9, G98.0-G98.8, G99.8

5th **G71.1 Myotonic disorders**

G71.11 Myotonic muscular dystrophy
Dystrophia myotonica [Steinert]
Myotonia atrophica
Myotonic dystrophy
Proximal myotonic myopathy (PROMM)
Steinert disease

G71.12 Myotonia congenita
Acetazolamide responsive myotonia congenita
Dominant myotonia congenita [Thomsen disease]
Myotonia levior
Recessive myotonia congenita [Becker disease]

G71.13 Myotonic chondrodystrophy
Chondrodystrophic myotonia
Congenital myotonic chondrodystrophy
Schwartz-Jampel disease

G71.14 Drug induced myotonia
Use additional code for adverse effect, if applicable, to identify drug (T36-T50 with fifth or sixth character 5)

G71.19 Other specified myotonic disorders
Myotonia fluctuans
Myotonia permanens
Neuromyotonia [Isaacs]
Paramyotonia congenita (of von Eulenburg)
Pseudomyotonia
Symptomatic myotonia

G71.2 Congenital myopathies CC
Central core disease
Fiber-type disproportion
Minicore disease
Multicore disease
Myotubular (centronuclear) myopathy
Nemaline myopathy
EXCLUDES 1 *arthrogryposis multiplex congenita (Q74.3)*
CC Excl: See code: G71.0

G71.3 Mitochondrial myopathy, not elsewhere classified
EXCLUDES 1 *Kearns-Sayre syndrome (H49.81)*
Leber's disease (H47.21)
Leigh's encephalopathy (G31.82)
mitochondrial metabolism disorders (E88.4-)
Reye's syndrome (G93.7)

G71.8 Other primary disorders of muscles

G71.9 Primary disorder of muscle, unspecified
Hereditary myopathy NOS

4th **G72 Other and unspecified myopathies**

EXCLUDES 1 *arthrogryposis multiplex congenita (Q74.3)*
dermatopolymyositis (M33.-)
ischemic infarction of muscle (M62.2-)
myositis (M60.-)
polymyositis (M33.2-)

G72.0 Drug-induced myopathy CC
Use additional code for adverse effect, if applicable, to identify drug (T36-T50 with fifth or sixth character 5)
CC Excl: G32.89, G70.00-G72.3, G72.81-G73.7, G96.8-G96.9, G98.0-G98.8, G99.8

G72.1 Alcoholic myopathy CC
Use additional code to identify alcoholism (F10.-)
CC Excl: See code: G72.0

G72.2 Myopathy due to other toxic agents CC
Code first (T51-T65) to identify toxic agent
CC Excl: See code: G72.0

G72.3 Periodic paralysis
Familial periodic paralysis
Hyperkalemic periodic paralysis (familial)
Hypokalemic periodic paralysis (familial)
Myotonic periodic paralysis (familial)
Normokalemic paralysis (familial)
Potassium sensitive periodic paralysis
EXCLUDES 1 *paramyotonia congenita (of von Eulenburg) (G71.19)*

5th **G72.4 Inflammatory and immune myopathies, not elsewhere classified**

G72.41 Inclusion body myositis [IBM]

G72.49 Other inflammatory and immune myopathies, not elsewhere classified
Inflammatory myopathy NOS

5th **G72.8 Other specified myopathies**

G72.81 Critical illness myopathy CC
Acute necrotizing myopathy
Acute quadriplegic myopathy
Intensive care (ICU) myopathy
Myopathy of critical illness
CC Excl: G70.1-G72.3, G72.81-G73.7

G72.89 Other specified myopathies

G72.9 Myopathy, unspecified

4th **G73 Disorders of myoneural junction and muscle in diseases classified elsewhere**

G73.1 ***Lambert-Eaton syndrome in neoplastic disease*** CC
Code first underlying neoplasm (C00-D49)
EXCLUDES 1 *Lambert-Eaton syndrome not associated with neoplasm (G70.80-G70.81)*
CC Excl: E08.40-E08.49, E08.618-E08.638, E08.649-E08.8, E09.40-E09.49, E09.618-E09.638, E09.649-E09.8, E10.40-E10.49, E10.618-E10.638, E10.649, E10.69-E10.8, E11.40-E11.49, E11.618-E11.638, E11.649, E11.69-E11.8, E13.40-E13.49, E13.618-E13.638, E13.649-E13.8, G32.89, G70.00-G70.01, G70.80-G70.81, G73.1-G73.3, G96.8-G96.9, G98.0-G98.8, G99.8

G73.3 ***Myasthenic syndromes in other diseases classified elsewhere*** CC
Code first underlying disease, such as:
neoplasm (C00-D49)
thyrotoxicosis (E05.-)
CC Excl: See code: G73.1

G73.7 ***Myopathy in diseases classified elsewhere***
Code first underlying disease, such as:
hyperparathyroidism (E21.0, E21.3)
hypoparathyroidism (E20.-)
glycogen storage disease (E74.0)
lipid storage disorders (E75.-)
EXCLUDES 1 *myopathy in:*
rheumatoid arthritis (M05.4-)
sarcoidosis (D86.87)
scleroderma (M34.82)
sicca syndrome [Sjögren] (M35.03)
systemic lupus erythematosus (M32.19)

Cerebral palsy and other paralytic syndromes (G80-G83)

4th **G80 Cerebral palsy**

EXCLUDES 1 *hereditary spastic paraplegia (G11.4)*

G80.0 Spastic quadriplegic cerebral palsy MCC
Congenital spastic paralysis (cerebral)
CC Excl: E08.40-E08.49, E08.618-E08.638, E08.649-E08.8, E09.40-E09.49, E09.618-E09.638, E09.649-E09.8, E10.40-E10.49, E10.618-E10.638, E10.649, E10.69-E10.8, E11.40-E11.49, E11.618-E11.638, E11.649, E11.69-E11.8, E13.40-E13.49, E13.618-E13.638, E13.649-E13.8, G04.1, G32.89, G80.0-G80.2, G80.4-G83.9, G90.1, G93.81, G93.89-G93.9, G96.8-G96.9, G98.0-G98.8, G99.8, Q06.0-Q06.1, Q06.3, Q06.8-Q06.9, Q07.8-Q07.9, R53.2

G80.1 Spastic diplegic cerebral palsy CC
Spastic cerebral palsy NOS
CC Excl: G80.1, G93.40-G93.49, I67.83

G80.2 Spastic hemiplegic **cerebral palsy** CC
CC Excl: G80.2, G93.40-G93.49, I67.83

G80.3 Athetoid **cerebral palsy** CC
Double athetosis (syndrome)
Dyskinetic cerebral palsy
Dystonic cerebral palsy
Vogt disease
CC Excl: G20, G21.11-G21.9, G25.70-G25.79, G25.89-G26, G80.0-G80.9, G93.40-G93.49, I67.83

G80.4 Ataxic **cerebral palsy**

G80.8 Other **cerebral palsy**
Mixed cerebral palsy syndromes

G80.9 **Cerebral palsy,** unspecified
Cerebral palsy NOS

✓4th G81 Hemiplegia and hemiparesis

NOTE This category is to be used only when hemiplegia (complete)(incomplete) is reported without further specification, or is stated to be old or longstanding but of unspecified cause. The category is also for use in multiple coding to identify these types of hemiplegia resulting from any cause.

EXCLUDES 1 *congenital cerebral palsy (G80.-)*
hemiplegia and hemiparesis due to sequela of cerebrovascular disease (I69.05-, I69.15-, I69.25-, I69.35-, I69.85-, I69.95-)

CC Excl: For CC codes in category G81, unless otherwise noted: G04.1, G11.0-G12.9, G32.0-G37.3, G37.5-G37.9, G80.0-G80.2, G80.4-G83.9, G90.01-G90.09, G90.2, G90.4-G90.9, G92, G93.40-G93.49, G93.81, G93.89-G93.9, G95.0-G95.9, G96.8-G96.9, G98.0-G99.8, I67.83, R53.2

✓5th **G81.0** Flaccid **hemiplegia**
- **G81.00** **Flaccid hemiplegia affecting** unspecified **side** CC
- **G81.01** **Flaccid hemiplegia affecting** right dominant **side** CC
- **G81.02** **Flaccid hemiplegia affecting** left dominant **side** CC
- **G81.03** **Flaccid hemiplegia affecting** right nondominant **side** CC
- **G81.04** **Flaccid hemiplegia affecting** left nondominant **side** CC

✓5th **G81.1** Spastic **hemiplegia**
- **G81.10** **Spastic hemiplegia affecting** unspecified **side** CC
- **G81.11** **Spastic hemiplegia affecting** right dominant **side** CC
- **G81.12** **Spastic hemiplegia affecting** left dominant **side** CC
- **G81.13** **Spastic hemiplegia affecting** right nondominant **side** CC
- **G81.14** **Spastic hemiplegia affecting** left nondominant **side** CC

✓5th **G81.9** Hemiplegia**, unspecified**
AHA: 2014, 1Q, 23
- **G81.90** **Hemiplegia, unspecified affecting** unspecified **side** CC
- **G81.91** **Hemiplegia, unspecified affecting** right dominant **side** CC
- **G81.92** **Hemiplegia, unspecified affecting** left dominant **side** CC
- **G81.93** **Hemiplegia, unspecified affecting** right nondominant **side** CC
- **G81.94** **Hemiplegia, unspecified affecting** left nondominant **side** CC

✓4th G82 Paraplegia (paraparesis) and quadriplegia (quadriparesis)

NOTE This category is to be used only when the listed conditions are reported without further specification, or are stated to be old or longstanding but of unspecified cause. The category is also for use in multiple coding to identify these conditions resulting from any cause

EXCLUDES 1 *congenital cerebral palsy (G80.-)*
functional quadriplegia (R53.2)
hysterical paralysis (F44.4)

✓5th **G82.2** Paraplegia
Paralysis of both lower limbs NOS
Paraparesis (lower) NOS
Paraplegia (lower) NOS

CC Excl: For CC codes in subcategory G82.2, unless otherwise noted: See code: G81

- **G82.20** **Paraplegia,** unspecified CC
- **G82.21** **Paraplegia,** complete CC
- **G82.22** **Paraplegia,** incomplete CC

✓5th **G82.5** Quadriplegia

CC Excl: For MCC codes in subcategory G82.5, unless otherwise noted: See code: G80.0

- **G82.50** **Quadriplegia,** unspecified MCC
- **G82.51** **Quadriplegia,** C1-C4 complete MCC
- **G82.52** **Quadriplegia,** C1-C4 incomplete MCC
- **G82.53** **Quadriplegia,** C5-C7 complete MCC
- **G82.54** **Quadriplegia,** C5-C7 incomplete MCC

✓4th G83 Other paralytic syndromes

NOTE This category is to be used only when the listed conditions are reported without further specification, or are stated to be old or longstanding but of unspecified cause. The category is also for use in multiple coding to identify these conditions resulting from any cause.

INCLUDES paralysis (complete) (incomplete), except as in G80-G82

G83.0 Diplegia **of upper limbs** CC
Diplegia (upper) Paralysis of both upper limbs
CC Excl: G32.89, G82.50-G83.0, G83.5-G83.9, G96.8-G96.9, G98.0-G98.8, G99.8, R53.2

✓5th **G83.1** Monoplegia of lower limb
Paralysis of lower limb
EXCLUDES 1 *monoplegia of lower limbs due to sequela of cerebrovascular disease (I69.04-, I69.14-, I69.24-, I69.34-, I69.84-, I69.94-)*
- **G83.10** **Monoplegia of lower limb affecting** unspecified **side**
- **G83.11** **Monoplegia of lower limb affecting** right dominant **side**
- **G83.12** **Monoplegia of lower limb affecting** left dominant **side**
- **G83.13** **Monoplegia of lower limb affecting** right nondominant **side**
- **G83.14** **Monoplegia of lower limb affecting** left nondominant **side**

✓5th **G83.2** Monoplegia **of** upper limb
Paralysis of upper limb
EXCLUDES 1 *monoplegia of upper limbs due to sequela of cerebrovascular disease (I69.03-, I69.13-, I69.23-, I69.33-, I69.83-, I69.93-)*
- **G83.20** **Monoplegia of upper limb affecting** unspecified **side**
- **G83.21** **Monoplegia of upper limb affecting** right dominant **side**
- **G83.22** **Monoplegia of upper limb affecting** left dominant **side**
- **G83.23** **Monoplegia of upper limb affecting** right nondominant **side**
- **G83.24** **Monoplegia of upper limb affecting** left nondominant **side**

✓5th **G83.3** **Monoplegia,** unspecified
- **G83.30** **Monoplegia, unspecified affecting** unspecified **side**
- **G83.31** **Monoplegia, unspecified affecting** right dominant **side**
- **G83.32** **Monoplegia, unspecified affecting** left | dominant **side**
- **G83.33** **Monoplegia, unspecified affecting** right nondominant **side**
- **G83.34** **Monoplegia, unspecified affecting** left nondominant **side**

G83.4 **Cauda equina syndrome** CC
Neurogenic bladder due to cauda equina syndrome
EXCLUDES 1 *cord bladder NOS (G95.89)*
neurogenic bladder NOS (N31.9)
CC Excl: G04.1, G32.89, G82.20-G82.54, G83.10-G83.14, G83.4-G83.9, G96.8-G96.9, G98.0-G98.8, G99.8, R53.2

G83.5 **Locked-in state** MCC
CC Excl: G04.1, G32.89, G80.0-G80.2, G80.4-G83.9, G92, G93.40-G93.49, G93.81, G93.89-G93.9, G96.8-G96.9, G98.0-G98.8, G99.8, I67.83, R53.2

✓5th **G83.8** **Other specified paralytic syndromes**
EXCLUDES 1 *paralytic syndromes due to current spinal cord injury—code to spinal cord injury (S14, S24, S34)*
- **G83.81** **Brown-Séquard syndrome**
- **G83.82** **Anterior cord syndrome**
- **G83.83** **Posterior cord syndrome**
- **G83.84** **Todd's paralysis (postepileptic)**
- **G83.89** **Other specified paralytic syndromes**

G83.9 **Paralytic syndrome, unspecified**

Other disorders of the nervous system (G89-G99)

✓4th G89 Pain, not elsewhere classified

Code also related psychological factors associated with pain (F45.42)

EXCLUDES 1 *generalized pain NOS (R52)*
pain disorders exclusively related to psychological factors (F45.41)
pain NOS (R52)

EXCLUDES 2 *atypical face pain (G5Ø.1)*
headache syndromes (G44.-)
localized pain, unspecified type—code to pain by site, such as:
- *abdomen pain (R1Ø.-)*
- *back pain (M54.9)*
- *breast pain (N64.4)*
- *chest pain (RØ7.1-RØ7.9)*
- *ear pain (H92.Ø-)*
- *eye pain (H57.1)*
- *headache (R51)*
- *joint pain (M25.5-)*
- *limb pain (M79.6-)*
- *lumbar region pain (M54.5)*
- *painful urination (R3Ø.9)*
- *pelvic and perineal pain (R1Ø.2)*
- *renal colic (N23)*
- *shoulder pain (M25.51-)*
- *spine pain (M54.-)*
- *throat pain (RØ7.Ø)*
- *tongue pain (K14.6)*
- *tooth pain (KØ8.8)*

migraines (G43.-)
myalgia (M79.1)
pain from prosthetic devices, implants, and grafts (T82.84, T83.84, T84.84, T85.84)
phantom limb syndrome with pain (G54.6)
vulvar vestibulitis (N94.81Ø)
vulvodynia (N94.81-)

G89.Ø Central pain syndrome
Déjérine-Roussy syndrome
Myelopathic pain syndrome
Thalamic pain syndrome (hyperesthetic)

✓5th G89.1 Acute pain, not elsewhere classified

G89.11 Acute pain due to trauma

G89.12 Acute post-thoracotomy pain
Post-thoracotomy pain NOS

G89.18 Other acute postprocedural pain
Postoperative pain NOS
Postprocedural pain NOS

✓5th G89.2 Chronic pain, not elsewhere classified

EXCLUDES 1 *causalgia, lower limb (G57.7-)*
causalgia, upper limb (G56.4-)
central pain syndrome (G89.Ø)
chronic pain syndrome (G89.4)
complex regional pain syndrome II, lower limb (G57.7-)
complex regional pain syndrome II, upper limb (G56.4-)
neoplasm related chronic pain (G89.3)
reflex sympathetic dystrophy (G9Ø.5-)

G89.21 Chronic pain due to trauma

G89.22 Chronic post-thoracotomy pain

G89.28 Other chronic postprocedural pain
Other chronic postoperative pain

G89.29 Other chronic pain

G89.3 Neoplasm related pain (acute) (chronic)
Cancer associated pain
Pain due to malignancy (primary) (secondary)
Tumor associated pain

G89.4 Chronic pain syndrome
Chronic pain associated with significant psychosocial dysfunction

✓4th G9Ø Disorders of autonomic nervous system

EXCLUDES 1 *dysfunction of the autonomic nervous system due to alcohol (G31.2)*

✓5th G9Ø.Ø Idiopathic peripheral autonomic neuropathy

G9Ø.Ø1 Carotid sinus syncope
Carotid sinus syndrome

G9Ø.Ø9 Other idiopathic peripheral autonomic neuropathy
Idiopathic peripheral autonomic neuropathy NOS

G9Ø.1 Familial dysautonomia [Riley-Day]

G9Ø.2 Horner's syndrome
Bernard(-Horner) syndrome
Cervical sympathetic dystrophy or paralysis

G9Ø.3 Multi-system degeneration of the autonomic nervous system CC
Neurogenic orthostatic hypotension [Shy-Drager]
EXCLUDES 1 *orthostatic hypotension NOS (I95.1)*
CC Excl: G2Ø-G21.9, G9Ø.Ø1-G9Ø.Ø9, G93.4Ø-G93.49, I67.83

G9Ø.4 Autonomic dysreflexia
Use additional code to identify the cause, such as:
- fecal impaction (K56.41)
- pressure ulcer (pressure area) (L89.-)
- urinary tract infection (N39.Ø)

✓5th G9Ø.5 Complex regional pain syndrome I (CRPS I)
Reflex sympathetic dystrophy

EXCLUDES 1 *causalgia of lower limb (G57.7-)*
causalgia of upper limb (G56.4-)
complex regional pain syndrome II of lower limb (G57.7-)
complex regional pain syndrome II of upper limb (G56.4-)

G9Ø.5Ø Complex regional pain syndrome I, unspecified CC
CC Excl: G9Ø.5Ø-G9Ø.59

✓6th G9Ø.51 Complex regional pain syndrome I of upper limb

CC Excl: For CC codes in subcategory G9Ø.51, unless otherwise noted: EØ8.4Ø-EØ8.49, EØ9.4Ø-EØ9.49, E1Ø.4Ø-E1Ø.49, E11.4Ø-E11.49, E13.4Ø-E13.49, GØ4.1, G11.3, G11.8-G12.9, G32.Ø, G32.89-G37.3, G37.5-G37.9, G8Ø.Ø-G8Ø.2, G8Ø.4-G83.9, G9Ø.Ø1-G9Ø.Ø9, G9Ø.2, G9Ø.4-G9Ø.9, G93.1, G93.4Ø-G93.49, G95.Ø-G95.9, G96.12-G96.9, G97.1, G98.Ø-G99.8, I67.83, R53.2

G9Ø.511 Complex regional pain syndrome I of right upper limb CC

G9Ø.512 Complex regional pain syndrome I of left upper limb CC

G9Ø.513 Complex regional pain syndrome I of upper limb, bilateral CC

G9Ø.519 Complex regional pain syndrome I of unspecified upper limb CC

✓6th G9Ø.52 Complex regional pain syndrome I of lower limb

CC Excl: For CC codes in subcategory G9Ø.52, unless otherwise noted: EØ8.4Ø-EØ8.49, EØ9.4Ø-EØ9.49, E1Ø.4Ø-E1Ø.49, E11.4Ø-E11.49, E13.4Ø-E13.49, GØ4.1, G11.3, G11.8-G12.9, G32.Ø, G32.89-G37.3, G37.5-G37.9, G8Ø.Ø-G8Ø.2, G8Ø.4-G83.9, G9Ø.Ø1-G9Ø.Ø9, G9Ø.2, G9Ø.4-G9Ø.9, G93.1, G93.4Ø-G93.49, G95.Ø-G95.9, G96.12-G96.9, G97.1, G98.Ø-G99.8, I67.83, R53.2

G9Ø.521 Complex regional pain syndrome I of right lower limb CC

G9Ø.522 Complex regional pain syndrome I of left lower limb CC

G9Ø.523 Complex regional pain syndrome I of lower limb, bilateral CC

G9Ø.529 Complex regional pain syndrome I of unspecified lower limb CC

G9Ø.59 Complex regional pain syndrome I of other specified site CC
CC Excl: See code: G9Ø.52

G9Ø.8 Other disorders of autonomic nervous system

G9Ø.9 Disorder of the autonomic nervous system, unspecified

✓4th G91 Hydrocephalus

INCLUDES acquired hydrocephalus

EXCLUDES 1 *Arnold-Chiari syndrome with hydrocephalus (QØ7.-)*
congenital hydrocephalus (QØ3.-)
spina bifida with hydrocephalus (QØ5.-)

CC Excl: For CC codes in subcategories G91.Ø & G91.2, unless otherwise noted: G91.Ø-G91.3, G91.8-G91.9
For CC codes in subcategories G91.1, G91.3-G91.9, unless otherwise noted: EØ8.4Ø-EØ8.49, EØ8.618-EØ8.638, EØ8.649-EØ8.8, EØ9.4Ø-EØ9.49, EØ9.618-EØ9.638, EØ9.649-EØ9.8, E1Ø.4Ø-E1Ø.49, E1Ø.618-E1Ø.638, E1Ø.649, E1Ø.69-E1Ø.8, E11.4Ø-E11.49, E11.618-E11.638, E11.649, E11.69-E11.8, E13.4Ø-E13.49, E13.618-E13.638, E13.649-E13.8, G13.2-G13.8, G31.2, G31.83-G31.9, G9Ø.1, G91.Ø-G91.9, G93.81, G93.89-G94, QØ3.Ø-QØ3.9, QØ4.4-QØ4.8, QØ5.Ø-QØ5.4, QØ5.9-QØ6.1, QØ6.3, QØ6.8-QØ6.9, QØ7.Ø2-QØ7.9

G91.Ø Communicating hydrocephalus CC
Secondary normal pressure hydrocephalus

G91.1 Obstructive hydrocephalus CC

G91.2 (Idiopathic) normal pressure hydrocephalus CC
Normal pressure hydrocephalus NOS

G91.3 Post-traumatic hydrocephalus, unspecified CC

G91.4 Hydrocephalus in diseases classified elsewhere
Code first underlying condition, such as:
congenital syphilis (A50.4-)
neoplasm (C00-D49)
EXCLUDES 1 *hydrocephalus due to congenital toxoplasmosis (P37.1)*

G91.8 Other hydrocephalus CC

G91.9 Hydrocephalus, unspecified CC

G92 Toxic encephalopathy MCC
Toxic encephalitis
Toxic metabolic encephalopathy
Code first (T51-T65) to identify toxic agent
CC Excl: A17.82, A17.9, A18.82, A18.84, A18.89, A39.81, A50.42, A52.14, A83.0-A85.1, A85.8-A86, A88.8-A89, B00.4, B01.11, B10.01-B10.09, B26.2, B58.2, E08.40-E08.49, E08.618-E08.638, E08.649-E08.8, E09.40-E09.49, E09.618-E09.638, E09.649-E09.8, E10.40-E10.49, E10.618-E10.638, E10.649, E10.69-E10.8, E11.40-E11.49, E11.618-E11.638, E11.649, E11.69- E11.8, E13.40-E13.49, E13.618-E13.638, E13.649-E13.8, G04.00-G04.01, G04.31, G04.81-G05.4, G32.89, G37.3-G37.4, G92, G93.40-G93.49, G93.81, G93.89-G93.9, G96.8-G96.9, G98.0-G98.8, G99.8, I67.83

✓4th **G93 Other disorders of brain**

G93.0 Cerebral cysts
Arachnoid cyst
Porencephalic cyst, acquired
EXCLUDES 1 *acquired periventricular cysts of newborn (P91.1)*
congenital cerebral cysts (Q04.6)

G93.1 Anoxic brain damage, not elsewhere classified CC
EXCLUDES 1 *cerebral anoxia due to anesthesia during labor and delivery (O74.3)*
cerebral anoxia due to anesthesia during the puerperium (O89.2)
neonatal anoxia (P84)
CC Excl: E08.40-E08.49, E08.618-E08.638, E08.649-E08.8, E09.40-E09.49, E09.618-E09.638, E09.649-E09.8, E10.40-E10.49, E10.618-E10.638, E10.649, E10.69-E10.8, E11.40-E11.49, E11.618-E11.638, E11.649, E11.69-E11.8, E13.40-E13.49, E13.618-E13.638, E13.649-E13.8, G32.89, G93.1-G93.2, G96.8-G96.9, G98.0-G98.8, G99.8

G93.2 Benign intracranial hypertension
EXCLUDES 1 *hypertensive encephalopathy (I67.4)*

G93.3 Postviral fatigue syndrome
Benign myalgic encephalomyelitis
EXCLUDES 1 *chronic fatigue syndrome NOS (R53.82)*

✓5th **G93.4 Other and unspecified encephalopathy**
EXCLUDES 1 *alcoholic encephalopathy (G31.2)*
encephalopathy in diseases classified elsewhere (G94)
hypertensive encephalopathy (I67.4)
toxic (metabolic) encephalopathy (G92)

G93.40 Encephalopathy, unspecified HIV MCC
CC Excl: G21.0, G83.5, G93.41-G93.49, I67.83

G93.41 Metabolic encephalopathy HIV MCC
Septic encephalopathy
CC Excl: G21.0, G83.5, G93.40, G93.49, I67.83

G93.49 Other encephalopathy HIV MCC
Encephalopathy NEC
CC Excl: G21.0, G83.5, G93.40-G93.41

G93.5 Compression of brain MCC
Arnold-Chiari type 1 compression of brain
Compression of brain (stem)
Herniation of brain (stem)
EXCLUDES 1 *diffuse traumatic compression of brain (S06.2-)*
focal traumatic compression of brain (S06.3-)
CC Excl: G81.90, G93.82

G93.6 Cerebral edema MCC
EXCLUDES 1 *cerebral edema due to birth injury (P11.0)*
traumatic cerebral edema (S06.1-)
CC Excl: G93.6, G93.82

G93.7 Reye's syndrome MCC P
Code first (T39.0-), if salicylates-induced
CC Excl: G93.7

✓5th **G93.8 Other specified disorders of brain**

G93.81 Temporal sclerosis
Hippocampal sclerosis
Mesial temporal sclerosis

G93.82 Brain death MCC
CC Excl: B15.0-B19.9, E03.5, E08.00-E08.59, E08.618-E09.59, E09.618-E10.59, E10.618-E10.649, E10.69-E11.59, E11.618-E11.649, E11.69-E13.59, E13.618-E16.2, E89.1, G32.89, G89.0-G89.4, G93.81-G93.9, G96.8-G96.9, G98.0-G98.8, G99.8, I60.00-I62.9, K72.91, R40.0-R40.2124, R40.2210-R40.2224, R40.2310-R40.2324, R40.2340-R40.2344, R40.3-R41.3, R41.82, R41.9-R42, R44.8-R44.9, R45.83-R45.84, R46.0-R46.89, R52, R55, R68.0-R68.19, R68.81-R68.83, R68.89-R69, S02.0XX-S02.19X with 7th [A, B], S02.91X with 7th [A, B], S06.0X0-S06.9X9 with 7th A

G93.89 Other specified disorders of brain
Postradiation encephalopathy

G93.9 Disorder of brain, unspecified HIV

G94 Other disorders of brain in diseases classified elsewhere
Code first underlying disease
EXCLUDES 1 *encephalopathy in congenital syphilis (A50.49)*
encephalopathy in influenza (J09.X9, J10.81, J11.81)
encephalopathy in syphilis (A52.19)
hydrocephalus in diseases classified elsewhere (G91.4)

✓4th **G95 Other and unspecified diseases of spinal cord**
EXCLUDES 2 *myelitis (G04.-)*

G95.0 Syringomyelia and syringobulbia CC
CC Excl: G04.1, G11.3, G11.8-G12.9, G32.0, G32.89-G37.3, G37.5-G37.9, G80.0-G80.2, G80.4-G83.9, G90.01-G90.09, G90.2, G90.4-G90.9, G93.40-G93.49, G93.81, G93.89-G93.9, G95.0-G95.9, G96.12-G96.9, G97.1, G98.0-G99.8, I67.83, R53.2

✓5th **G95.1 Vascular myelopathies**
EXCLUDES 2 *intraspinal phlebitis and thrombophlebitis, except non-pyogenic (G08)*

G95.11 Acute infarction of spinal cord (embolic) (nonembolic) MCC
Anoxia of spinal cord
Arterial thrombosis of spinal cord
CC Excl: E08.40-E08.49, E09.40-E09.49, E10.40-E10.49, E11.40-E11.49, E13.40-E13.49, G04.1, G11.3, G11.8-G12.9, G32.0, G32.89-G37.3, G37.5-G37.9, G80.0-G80.2, G80.4-G83.9, G90.01-G90.09, G90.2, G90.4-G90.9, G93.1, G93.40-G93.49, G95.0-G95.9, G96.12-G96.9, G97.1, G98.0-G99.8, I67.83, R53.2

G95.19 Other vascular myelopathies MCC
Edema of spinal cord
Hematomyelia
Nonpyogenic intraspinal phlebitis and thrombophlebitis
Subacute necrotic myelopathy
CC Excl: See code: G95.11

✓5th **G95.2 Other and unspecified cord compression**

G95.20 Unspecified cord compression HIV CC
CC Excl: E08.40-E08.49, E09.40-E09.49, E10.40-E10.49, E11.40-E11.49, E13.40-E13.49, G04.1, G11.3-G12.9, G32.0, G32.89-G37.3, G37.5-G37.9, G80.0-G80.2, G80.4-G83.9, G90.01-G90.09, G90.2, G90.4-G90.9, G93.1, G93.40-G93.49, G95.0-G95.9, G96.12-G96.9, G97.1, G98.0-G99.8, I67.83, R53.2

G95.29 Other cord compression HIV CC
CC Excl: See code: G95.20

✓5th **G95.8 Other specified diseases of spinal cord**
EXCLUDES 1 *neurogenic bladder NOS (N31.9)*
neurogenic bladder due to cauda equina syndrome (G83.4)
neuromuscular dysfunction of bladder without spinal cord lesion (N31.-)

G95.81 Conus medullaris syndrome CC
CC Excl: See code: G90.51

G95.89 Other specified diseases of spinal cord CC
Cord bladder NOS
Drug-induced myelopathy
Radiation-induced myelopathy
EXCLUDES 1 *myelopathy NOS (G95.9)*
CC Excl: See code: G90.51

G95.9 Disease of spinal cord, unspecified HIV CC
Myelopathy NOS
CC Excl: See code: G95.20

DRAFT

4th G96 Other disorders of central nervous system

G96.0 Cerebrospinal fluid leak CC

EXCLUDES 1 *cerebrospinal fluid leak from spinal puncture (G97.0)*

CC Excl: E08.40-E08.49, E08.618-E08.638, E08.649-E08.8, E09.40-E09.49, E09.618-E09.638, E09.649-E09.8, E10.40-E10.49, E10.618-E10.638, E10.649, E10.69-E10.8, E11.40-E11.49, E11.618-E11.638, E11.649, E11.69-E11.8, E13.40-E13.49, E13.618-E13.638, E13.649-E13.8, G32.89, G96.0, G96.8-G96.9, G98.0-G98.8, G99.8

5th G96.1 Disorders of meninges, not elsewhere classified

G96.11 Dural tear CC

EXCLUDES 1 *accidental puncture or laceration of dura during a procedure (G97.41)*

CC Excl: D78.11-D78.12, D78.81-D78.89, E36.11-E36.8, E89.810-E89.89, G96.11, G97.41, G97.48-G97.49, H59.011-H59.019, H59.031-H59.099, H59.211-H59.229, H59.811-H59.89, H95.31-H95.32, H95.811-H95.89, I97.3, I97.51-I97.52, J95.71-J95.72, K91.71-K91.72, L76.11-L76.12, L76.81-L76.82, M96.820-M96.821, M96.89, N98.1-N98.9, N99.71-N99.72, T81.82XA, T81.89XA, T81.9XXA

G96.12 Meningeal adhesions (cerebral) (spinal)

G96.19 Other disorders of meninges, not elsewhere classified

G96.8 Other specified disorders of central nervous system

G96.9 Disorder of central nervous system, unspecified HIV

4th G97 Intraoperative and postprocedural complications and disorders of nervous system, not elsewhere classified

EXCLUDES 2 *intraoperative and postprocedural cerebrovascular infarction (I97.81-, I97.82-)*

G97.0 Cerebrospinal fluid leak from spinal puncture CC

CC Excl: D78.81-D78.89, E36.8, E89.810-E89.89, G97.0, G97.2-G97.32, G97.81-G97.82, H59.011-H59.019, H59.031-H59.099, H59.811-H59.89, H95.811-H95.89, I97.3, I97.810-I97.821, L76.81-L76.82, M96.89, N98.1-N98.9, T81.82XA, T81.89XA, T81.9XXA

G97.1 Other reaction to spinal and lumbar puncture

Headache due to lumbar puncture

G97.2 Intracranial hypotension following ventricular shunting CC

CC Excl: See code: G97.0

5th G97.3 Intraoperative hemorrhage and hematoma of a nervous system organ or structure complicating a procedure

EXCLUDES 1 *intraoperative hemorrhage and hematoma of a nervous system organ or structure due to accidental puncture and laceration during a procedure (G97.4-)*

G97.31 Intraoperative hemorrhage and hematoma of a nervous system organ or structure complicating a nervous system procedure CC

CC Excl: G97.4, G97.2-G97.32, G97.81-G97.82, H95.811-H95.89, I97.3, I97.810-I97.821, M96.89, N98.1-N98.9, T81.82XA, T81.89XA, T81.9XXA

G97.32 Intraoperative hemorrhage and hematoma of a nervous system organ or structure complicating other procedure CC

CC Excl: See code: G97.31

5th G97.4 Accidental puncture and laceration of a nervous system organ or structure during a procedure

CC Excl: For CC codes in subcategory G97.4, unless otherwise noted: D78.11-D78.12, D78.81-D78.89, E36.11-E36.8, E89.810-E89.89, G96.11, G97.41, G97.48-G97.49, H59.011-H59.019, H59.031-H59.099, H59.211-H59.229, H59.811-H59.89, H95.31-H95.32, H95.811-H95.89, I97.3, I97.51-I97.52, J95.71-J95.72, K91.71-K91.72, L76.11-L76.12, L76.81-L76.82, M96.820-M96.821, M96.89, N98.1-N98.9, N99.71-N99.72, T81.82XA, T81.89XA, T81.9XXA

G97.41 Accidental puncture or laceration of dura during a procedure CC

Incidental (inadvertent) durotomy

G97.48 Accidental puncture and laceration of other nervous system organ or structure during a nervous system procedure CC

G97.49 Accidental puncture and laceration of other nervous system organ or structure during other procedure CC

5th G97.5 Postprocedural hemorrhage and hematoma of a nervous system organ or structure following a procedure

G97.51 Postprocedural hemorrhage and hematoma of a nervous system organ or structure following a nervous system procedure CC

CC Excl: G97.51-G97.52, H95.811-H95.89, I85.01, I85.11, I97.3, K21.9, K22.8, K23-K25.0, K25.2, K25.4, K25.6, K26.0, K26.2, K26.4, K26.6, K27.0, K27.2, K27.4, K27.6, K28.0, K28.2, K28.4, K28.6, K29.01, K29.21, K29.31, K29.41, K29.51, K29.61, K29.71, K29.81, K29.91, K31.811, K55.21, K57.01, K57.11, K57.13, K57.21, K57.31, K57.33, K57.41, K57.51, K57.53, K57.81, K57.91, K57.93, K62.5, K92.0-K92.2, M96.89, N98.1-N98.9, P54.1-P54.3, T81.10XA, T81.11XA, T81.12XA, T81.19XA, T81.82XA, T81.89XA, T81.9XXA

G97.52 Postprocedural hemorrhage and hematoma of a nervous system organ or structure following other procedure CC

CC Excl: See code: G97.51

5th G97.8 Other intraoperative and postprocedural complications and disorders of nervous system

Use additional code to further specify disorder

G97.81 Other intraoperative complications of nervous system CC

CC Excl: See code: G97.0

G97.82 Other postprocedural complications and disorders of nervous system CC

CC Excl: See code: G97.0

4th G98 Other disorders of nervous system not elsewhere classified

INCLUDES nervous system disorder NOS

G98.0 Neurogenic arthritis, not elsewhere classified

Nonsyphilitic neurogenic arthropathy NEC
Nonsyphilitic neurogenic spondylopathy NEC

EXCLUDES 1 *spondylopathy (in):*
syringomyelia and syringobulbia (G95.0)
tabes dorsalis (A52.11)

G98.8 Other disorders of nervous system HIV

Nervous system disorder NOS

4th G99 Other disorders of nervous system in diseases classified elsewhere

G99.0 Autonomic neuropathy in diseases classified elsewhere CC

Code first underlying disease, such as:
amyloidosis (E85.-)
gout (M1A.-, M10.-)
hyperthyroidism (E05.-)

EXCLUDES 1 *diabetic autonomic neuropathy (E08-E13 with .43)*

CC Excl: G90.01-G90.09, G90.2, G90.50-G90.9, G93.40-G93.49, G99.0, I67.83

G99.2 Myelopathy in diseases classified elsewhere CC

Code first underlying disease, such as:
neoplasm (C00-D49)

EXCLUDES 1 *myelopathy in:*
intervertebral disease (M50.0-, M51.0-)
spondylosis (M47.0-, M47.1-)

CC Excl: E08.40-E08.49, E09.40-E09.49, E10.40-E10.49, E11.40-E11.49, E13.40-E13.49, G04.1, G11.3, G11.8-G12.9, G32.0, G32.89-G37.3, G37.5-G37.9, G80.0-G80.2, G80.4-G83.9, G90.01-G90.09, G90.2, G90.4-G90.9, G93.1, G93.40-G93.49, G95.0-G95.9, G96.12-G96.9, G97.1, G98.0-G99.8, I67.83, R53.2

G99.8 Other specified disorders of nervous system in diseases classified elsewhere

Code first underlying disorder, such as:
amyloidosis (E85.-)
avitaminosis (E56.9)

EXCLUDES 1 *nervous system involvement in:*
cysticercosis (B69.0)
rubella (B06.0-)
syphilis (A52.1-)

Chapter 7. Diseases of the Eye and Adnexa (H00-H59)

NOTE Use an external cause code following the code for the eye condition, if applicable, to identify the cause of the eye condition.

EXCLUDES 2 *certain conditions originating in the perinatal period (P04-P96)*
certain infectious and parasitic diseases (A00-B99)
complications of pregnancy, childbirth and the puerperium (O00-O9A)
congenital malformations, deformations, and chromosomal abnormalities (Q00-Q99)
diabetes mellitus related eye conditions (E09.3-, E10.3-, E11.3-, E13.3-)
endocrine, nutritional and metabolic diseases (E00-E88)
injury (trauma) of eye and orbit (S05.-)
injury, poisoning and certain other consequences of external causes (S00-T88)
neoplasms (C00-D49)
symptoms, signs and abnormal clinical and laboratory findings, not elsewhere classified (R00-R94)
syphilis related eye disorders (A50.01, A50.3-, A51.43, A52.71)

This chapter contains the following blocks:

H00-H05	Disorders of eyelid, lacrimal system and orbit
H10-H11	Disorders of conjunctiva
H15-H22	Disorders of sclera, cornea, iris and ciliary body
H25-H28	Disorders of lens
H30-H36	Disorders of choroid and retina
H40-H42	Glaucoma
H43-H44	Disorders of vitreous body and globe
H46-H47	Disorders of optic nerve and visual pathways
H49-H52	Disorders of ocular muscles, binocular movement, accommodation and refraction
H53-H54	Visual disturbances and blindness
H55-H57	Other disorders of eye and adnexa
H59	Intraoperative and postprocedural complications and disorders of eye and adnexa, not elsewhere classified

Disorders of eyelid, lacrimal system and orbit (H00-H05)

EXCLUDES 2 *open wound of eyelid (S01.1-)*
superficial injury of eyelid (S00.1-, S00.2-)

✓4th **H00 Hordeolum and chalazion**

✓5th **H00.0 Hordeolum (externum) (internum) of eyelid**

✓6th **H00.01 Hordeolum externum**
Hordeolum NOS
Stye

- **H00.011 Hordeolum externum right upper eyelid**
- **H00.012 Hordeolum externum right lower eyelid**
- **H00.013 Hordeolum externum right eye, unspecified eyelid**
- **H00.014 Hordeolum externum left upper eyelid**
- **H00.015 Hordeolum externum left lower eyelid**
- **H00.016 Hordeolum externum left eye, unspecified eyelid**
- **H00.019 Hordeolum externum unspecified eye, unspecified eyelid**

✓6th **H00.02 Hordeolum internum**
Infection of meibomian gland

- **H00.021 Hordeolum internum right upper eyelid**
- **H00.022 Hordeolum internum right lower eyelid**
- **H00.023 Hordeolum internum right eye, unspecified eyelid**
- **H00.024 Hordeolum internum left upper eyelid**
- **H00.025 Hordeolum internum left lower eyelid**
- **H00.026 Hordeolum internum left eye, unspecified eyelid**
- **H00.029 Hordeolum internum unspecified eye, unspecified eyelid**

✓6th **H00.03 Abscess of eyelid**
Furuncle of eyelid

- **H00.031 Abscess of right upper eyelid**
- **H00.032 Abscess of right lower eyelid**
- **H00.033 Abscess of eyelid right eye, unspecified eyelid**
- **H00.034 Abscess of left upper eyelid**
- **H00.035 Abscess of left lower eyelid**
- **H00.036 Abscess of eyelid left eye, unspecified eyelid**
- **H00.039 Abscess of eyelid unspecified eye, unspecified eyelid**

✓5th **H00.1 Chalazion**
Meibomian (gland) cyst
EXCLUDES 2 *infected meibomian gland (H00.02-)*

- **H00.11 Chalazion right upper eyelid**
- **H00.12 Chalazion right lower eyelid**
- **H00.13 Chalazion right eye, unspecified eyelid**
- **H00.14 Chalazion left upper eyelid**
- **H00.15 Chalazion left lower eyelid**
- **H00.16 Chalazion left eye, unspecified eyelid**
- **H00.19 Chalazion unspecified eye, unspecified eyelid**

✓4th **H01 Other inflammation of eyelid**

✓5th **H01.0 Blepharitis**
EXCLUDES 1 *blepharoconjunctivitis (H10.5-)*

✓6th **H01.00 Unspecified blepharitis**

- **H01.001 Unspecified blepharitis right upper eyelid**
- **H01.002 Unspecified blepharitis right lower eyelid**
- **H01.003 Unspecified blepharitis right eye, unspecified eyelid**
- **H01.004 Unspecified blepharitis left upper eyelid**
- **H01.005 Unspecified blepharitis left lower eyelid**
- **H01.006 Unspecified blepharitis left eye, unspecified eyelid**
- **H01.009 Unspecified blepharitis unspecified eye, unspecified eyelid**

✓6th **H01.01 Ulcerative blepharitis**

- **H01.011 Ulcerative blepharitis right upper eyelid**
- **H01.012 Ulcerative blepharitis right lower eyelid**
- **H01.013 Ulcerative blepharitis right eye, unspecified eyelid**
- **H01.014 Ulcerative blepharitis left upper eyelid**
- **H01.015 Ulcerative blepharitis left lower eyelid**
- **H01.016 Ulcerative blepharitis left eye, unspecified eyelid**
- **H01.019 Ulcerative blepharitis unspecified eye, unspecified eyelid**

✓6th **H01.02 Squamous blepharitis**

- **H01.021 Squamous blepharitis right upper eyelid**
- **H01.022 Squamous blepharitis right lower eyelid**
- **H01.023 Squamous blepharitis right eye, unspecified eyelid**
- **H01.024 Squamous blepharitis left upper eyelid**
- **H01.025 Squamous blepharitis left lower eyelid**
- **H01.026 Squamous blepharitis left eye, unspecified eyelid**
- **H01.029 Squamous blepharitis unspecified eye, unspecified eyelid**

✓5th **H01.1 Noninfectious dermatoses of eyelid**

✓6th **H01.11 Allergic dermatitis of eyelid**
Contact dermatitis of eyelid

- **H01.111 Allergic dermatitis of right upper eyelid**
- **H01.112 Allergic dermatitis of right lower eyelid**
- **H01.113 Allergic dermatitis of right eye, unspecified eyelid**
- **H01.114 Allergic dermatitis of left upper eyelid**
- **H01.115 Allergic dermatitis of left lower eyelid**
- **H01.116 Allergic dermatitis of left eye, unspecified eyelid**
- **H01.119 Allergic dermatitis of unspecified eye, unspecified eyelid**

✓6th **H01.12 Discoid lupus erythematosus of eyelid**

- **H01.121 Discoid lupus erythematosus of right upper eyelid**
- **H01.122 Discoid lupus erythematosus of right lower eyelid**
- **H01.123 Discoid lupus erythematosus of right eye, unspecified eyelid**
- **H01.124 Discoid lupus erythematosus of left upper eyelid**
- **H01.125 Discoid lupus erythematosus of left lower eyelid**
- **H01.126 Discoid lupus erythematosus of left eye, unspecified eyelid**
- **H01.129 Discoid lupus erythematosus of unspecified eye, unspecified eyelid**

✓6th **H01.13 Eczematous dermatitis of eyelid**
- **H01.131 Eczematous dermatitis of right upper eyelid**
- **H01.132 Eczematous dermatitis of right lower eyelid**
- **H01.133 Eczematous dermatitis of right eye, unspecified eyelid**
- **H01.134 Eczematous dermatitis of left upper eyelid**
- **H01.135 Eczematous dermatitis of left lower eyelid**
- **H01.136 Eczematous dermatitis of left eye, unspecified eyelid**
- **H01.139 Eczematous dermatitis of unspecified eye, unspecified eyelid**

✓6th **H01.14 Xeroderma of eyelid**
- **H01.141 Xeroderma of right upper eyelid**
- **H01.142 Xeroderma of right lower eyelid**
- **H01.143 Xeroderma of right eye, unspecified eyelid**
- **H01.144 Xeroderma of left upper eyelid**
- **H01.145 Xeroderma of left lower eyelid**
- **H01.146 Xeroderma of left eye, unspecified eyelid**
- **H01.149 Xeroderma of unspecified eye, unspecified eyelid**

H01.8 Other specified inflammations of eyelid

H01.9 Unspecified inflammation of eyelid
Inflammation of eyelid NOS

✓4th **H02 Other disorders of eyelid**
EXCLUDES1 *congenital malformations of eyelid (Q10.0-Q10.3)*

✓5th **H02.0 Entropion and trichiasis of eyelid**

✓6th **H02.00 Unspecified entropion of eyelid**
- **H02.001 Unspecified entropion of right upper eyelid**
- **H02.002 Unspecified entropion of right lower eyelid**
- **H02.003 Unspecified entropion of right eye, unspecified eyelid**
- **H02.004 Unspecified entropion of left upper eyelid**
- **H02.005 Unspecified entropion of left lower eyelid**
- **H02.006 Unspecified entropion of left eye, unspecified eyelid**
- **H02.009 Unspecified entropion of unspecified eye, unspecified eyelid**

✓6th **H02.01 Cicatricial entropion of eyelid**
- **H02.011 Cicatricial entropion of right upper eyelid**
- **H02.012 Cicatricial entropion of right lower eyelid**
- **H02.013 Cicatricial entropion of right eye, unspecified eyelid**
- **H02.014 Cicatricial entropion of left upper eyelid**
- **H02.015 Cicatricial entropion of left lower eyelid**
- **H02.016 Cicatricial entropion of left eye, unspecified eyelid**
- **H02.019 Cicatricial entropion of unspecified eye, unspecified eyelid**

✓6th **H02.02 Mechanical entropion of eyelid**
- **H02.021 Mechanical entropion of right upper eyelid**
- **H02.022 Mechanical entropion of right lower eyelid**
- **H02.023 Mechanical entropion of right eye, unspecified eyelid**
- **H02.024 Mechanical entropion of left upper eyelid**
- **H02.025 Mechanical entropion of left lower eyelid**
- **H02.026 Mechanical entropion of left eye, unspecified eyelid**
- **H02.029 Mechanical entropion of unspecified eye, unspecified eyelid**

✓6th **H02.03 Senile entropion of eyelid**
- **H02.031 Senile entropion of right upper eyelid** A
- **H02.032 Senile entropion of right lower eyelid** A
- **H02.033 Senile entropion of right eye, unspecified eyelid** A
- **H02.034 Senile entropion of left upper eyelid** A
- **H02.035 Senile entropion of left lower eyelid** A
- **H02.036 Senile entropion of left eye, unspecified eyelid** A
- **H02.039 Senile entropion of unspecified eye, unspecified eyelid** A

✓6th **H02.04 Spastic entropion of eyelid**
- **H02.041 Spastic entropion of right upper eyelid**
- **H02.042 Spastic entropion of right lower eyelid**
- **H02.043 Spastic entropion of right eye, unspecified eyelid**
- **H02.044 Spastic entropion of left upper eyelid**
- **H02.045 Spastic entropion of left lower eyelid**
- **H02.046 Spastic entropion of left eye, unspecified eyelid**
- **H02.049 Spastic entropion of unspecified eye, unspecified eyelid**

✓6th **H02.05 Trichiasis without entropian**
- **H02.051 Trichiasis without entropian right upper eyelid**
- **H02.052 Trichiasis without entropian right lower eyelid**
- **H02.053 Trichiasis without entropian right eye, unspecified eyelid**
- **H02.054 Trichiasis without entropian left upper eyelid**
- **H02.055 Trichiasis without entropian left lower eyelid**
- **H02.056 Trichiasis without entropian left eye, unspecified eyelid**
- **H02.059 Trichiasis without entropian unspecified eye, unspecified eyelid**

✓5th **H02.1 Ectropion of eyelid**

✓6th **H02.10 Unspecified ectropion of eyelid**
- **H02.101 Unspecified ectropion of right upper eyelid**
- **H02.102 Unspecified ectropion of right lower eyelid**
- **H02.103 Unspecified ectropion of right eye, unspecified eyelid**
- **H02.104 Unspecified ectropion of left upper eyelid**
- **H02.105 Unspecified ectropion of left lower eyelid**
- **H02.106 Unspecified ectropion of left eye, unspecified eyelid**
- **H02.109 Unspecified ectropion of unspecified eye, unspecified eyelid**

✓6th **H02.11 Cicatricial ectropion of eyelid**
- **H02.111 Cicatricial ectropion of right upper eyelid**
- **H02.112 Cicatricial ectropion of right lower eyelid**
- **H02.113 Cicatricial ectropion of right eye, unspecified eyelid**
- **H02.114 Cicatricial ectropion of left upper eyelid**
- **H02.115 Cicatricial ectropion of left lower eyelid**
- **H02.116 Cicatricial ectropion of left eye, unspecified eyelid**
- **H02.119 Cicatricial ectropion of unspecified eye, unspecified eyelid**

✓6th **H02.12 Mechanical ectropion of eyelid**
- **H02.121 Mechanical ectropion of right upper eyelid**
- **H02.122 Mechanical ectropion of right lower eyelid**
- **H02.123 Mechanical ectropion of right eye, unspecified eyelid**
- **H02.124 Mechanical ectropion of left upper eyelid**
- **H02.125 Mechanical ectropion of left lower eyelid**
- **H02.126 Mechanical ectropion of left eye, unspecified eyelid**
- **H02.129 Mechanical ectropion of unspecified eye, unspecified eyelid**

✓6th **H02.13 Senile ectropion of eyelid**
- **H02.131 Senile ectropion of right upper eyelid** A
- **H02.132 Senile ectropion of right lower eyelid** A
- **H02.133 Senile ectropion of right eye, unspecified eyelid** A
- **H02.134 Senile ectropion of left upper eyelid** A
- **H02.135 Senile ectropion of left lower eyelid** A
- **H02.136 Senile ectropion of left eye, unspecified eyelid** A
- **H02.139 Senile ectropion of unspecified eye, unspecified eyelid** A

✓6th **H02.14 Spastic ectropion of eyelid**
- **H02.141 Spastic ectropion of right upper eyelid**
- **H02.142 Spastic ectropion of right lower eyelid**

H02.143 Spastic ectropion of right eye, unspecified eyelid
H02.144 Spastic ectropion of left upper eyelid
H02.145 Spastic ectropion of left lower eyelid
H02.146 Spastic ectropion of left eye, unspecified eyelid
H02.149 Spastic ectropion of unspecified eye, unspecified eyelid

✓5th H02.2 Lagophthalmos

✓6th H02.20 Unspecified lagophthalmos
H02.201 Unspecified lagophthalmos right upper eyelid
H02.202 Unspecified lagophthalmos right lower eyelid
H02.203 Unspecified lagophthalmos right eye, unspecified eyelid
H02.204 Unspecified lagophthalmos left upper eyelid
H02.205 Unspecified lagophthalmos left lower eyelid
H02.206 Unspecified lagophthalmos left eye, unspecified eyelid
H02.209 Unspecified lagophthalmos unspecified eye, unspecified eyelid

✓6th H02.21 Cicatricial lagophthalmos
H02.211 Cicatricial lagophthalmos right upper eyelid
H02.212 Cicatricial lagophthalmos right lower eyelid
H02.213 Cicatricial lagophthalmos right eye, unspecified eyelid
H02.214 Cicatricial lagophthalmos left upper eyelid
H02.215 Cicatricial lagophthalmos left lower eyelid
H02.216 Cicatricial lagophthalmos left eye, unspecified eyelid
H02.219 Cicatricial lagophthalmos unspecified eye, unspecified eyelid

✓6th H02.22 Mechanical lagophthalmos
H02.221 Mechanical lagophthalmos right upper eyelid
H02.222 Mechanical lagophthalmos right lower eyelid
H02.223 Mechanical lagophthalmos right eye, unspecified eyelid
H02.224 Mechanical lagophthalmos left upper eyelid
H02.225 Mechanical lagophthalmos left lower eyelid
H02.226 Mechanical lagophthalmos left eye, unspecified eyelid
H02.229 Mechanical lagophthalmos unspecified eye, unspecified eyelid

✓6th H02.23 Paralytic lagophthalmos
H02.231 Paralytic lagophthalmos right upper eyelid
H02.232 Paralytic lagophthalmos right lower eyelid
H02.233 Paralytic lagophthalmos right eye, unspecified eyelid
H02.234 Paralytic lagophthalmos left upper eyelid
H02.235 Paralytic lagophthalmos left lower eyelid
H02.236 Paralytic lagophthalmos left eye, unspecified eyelid
H02.239 Paralytic lagophthalmos unspecified eye, unspecified eyelid

✓5th H02.3 Blepharochalasis
Pseudoptosis
H02.30 Blepharochalasis unspecified eye, unspecified eyelid
H02.31 Blepharochalasis right upper eyelid
H02.32 Blepharochalasis right lower eyelid
H02.33 Blepharochalasis right eye, unspecified eyelid
H02.34 Blepharochalasis left upper eyelid
H02.35 Blepharochalasis left lower eyelid
H02.36 Blepharochalasis left eye, unspecified eyelid

✓5th H02.4 Ptosis of eyelid

✓6th H02.40 Unspecified ptosis of eyelid
H02.401 Unspecified ptosis of right eyelid
H02.402 Unspecified ptosis of left eyelid
H02.403 Unspecified ptosis of bilateral eyelids
H02.409 Unspecified ptosis of unspecified eyelid

✓6th H02.41 Mechanical ptosis of eyelid
H02.411 Mechanical ptosis of right eyelid
H02.412 Mechanical ptosis of left eyelid
H02.413 Mechanical ptosis of bilateral eyelids
H02.419 Mechanical ptosis of unspecified eyelid

✓6th H02.42 Myogenic ptosis of eyelid
H02.421 Myogenic ptosis of right eyelid
H02.422 Myogenic ptosis of left eyelid
H02.423 Myogenic ptosis of bilateral eyelids
H02.429 Myogenic ptosis of unspecified eyelid

✓6th H02.43 Paralytic ptosis of eyelid
Neurogenic ptosis of eyelid
H02.431 Paralytic ptosis of right eyelid
H02.432 Paralytic ptosis of left eyelid
H02.433 Paralytic ptosis of bilateral eyelids
H02.439 Paralytic ptosis unspecified eyelid

✓5th H02.5 Other disorders affecting eyelid function
EXCLUDES 2 *blepharospasm (G24.5)*
organic tic (G25.69)
psychogenic tic (F95.-)

✓6th H02.51 Abnormal innervation syndrome
H02.511 Abnormal innervation syndrome right upper eyelid
H02.512 Abnormal innervation syndrome right lower eyelid
H02.513 Abnormal innervation syndrome right eye, unspecified eyelid
H02.514 Abnormal innervation syndrome left upper eyelid
H02.515 Abnormal innervation syndrome left lower eyelid
H02.516 Abnormal innervation syndrome left eye, unspecified eyelid
H02.519 Abnormal innervation syndrome unspecified eye, unspecified eyelid

✓6th H02.52 Blepharophimosis
Ankyloblepharon
H02.521 Blepharophimosis right upper eyelid
H02.522 Blepharophimosis right lower eyelid
H02.523 Blepharophimosis right eye, unspecified eyelid
H02.524 Blepharophimosis left upper eyelid
H02.525 Blepharophimosis left lower eyelid
H02.526 Blepharophimosis left eye, unspecified eyelid
H02.529 Blepharophimosis unspecified eye, unspecified lid

✓6th H02.53 Eyelid retraction
Eyelid lag
H02.531 Eyelid retraction right upper eyelid
H02.532 Eyelid retraction right lower eyelid
H02.533 Eyelid retraction right eye, unspecified eyelid
H02.534 Eyelid retraction left upper eyelid
H02.535 Eyelid retraction left lower eyelid
H02.536 Eyelid retraction left eye, unspecified eyelid
H02.539 Eyelid retraction unspecified eye, unspecified lid

H02.59 Other disorders affecting eyelid function
Deficient blink reflex
Sensory disorders

✓5th H02.6 Xanthelasma of eyelid
H02.60 Xanthelasma of unspecified eye, unspecified eyelid
H02.61 Xanthelasma of right upper eyelid
H02.62 Xanthelasma of right lower eyelid
H02.63 Xanthelasma of right eye, unspecified eyelid
H02.64 Xanthelasma of left upper eyelid

H02.65 **Xanthelasma of left lower eyelid**

H02.66 **Xanthelasma of left eye, unspecified eyelid**

✓5th **H02.7 Other and unspecified degenerative disorders of eyelid and periocular area**

H02.70 **Unspecified degenerative disorders of eyelid and periocular area**

✓6th **H02.71 Chloasma of eyelid and periocular area**

Dyspigmentation of eyelid
Hyperpigmentation of eyelid

H02.711 **Chloasma of right upper eyelid and periocular area**

H02.712 **Chloasma of right lower eyelid and periocular area**

H02.713 **Chloasma of right eye, unspecified eyelid and periocular area**

H02.714 **Chloasma of left upper eyelid and periocular area**

H02.715 **Chloasma of left lower eyelid and periocular area**

H02.716 **Chloasma of left eye, unspecified eyelid and periocular area**

H02.719 **Chloasma of unspecified eye, unspecified eyelid and periocular area**

✓6th **H02.72 Madarosis of eyelid and periocular area**

Hypotrichosis of eyelid

H02.721 **Madarosis of right upper eyelid and periocular area**

H02.722 **Madarosis of right lower eyelid and periocular area**

H02.723 **Madarosis of right eye, unspecified eyelid and periocular area**

H02.724 **Madarosis of left upper eyelid and periocular area**

H02.725 **Madarosis of left lower eyelid and periocular area**

H02.726 **Madarosis of left eye, unspecified eyelid and periocular area**

H02.729 **Madarosis of unspecified eye, unspecified eyelid and periocular area**

✓6th **H02.73 Vitiligo of eyelid and periocular area**

Hypopigmentation of eyelid

H02.731 **Vitiligo of right upper eyelid and periocular area**

H02.732 **Vitiligo of right lower eyelid and periocular area**

H02.733 **Vitiligo of right eye, unspecified eyelid and periocular area**

H02.734 **Vitiligo of left upper eyelid and periocular area**

H02.735 **Vitiligo of left lower eyelid and periocular area**

H02.736 **Vitiligo of left eye, unspecified eyelid and periocular area**

H02.739 **Vitiligo of unspecified eye, unspecified eyelid and periocular area**

H02.79 **Other degenerative disorders of eyelid and periocular area**

✓5th **H02.8 Other specified disorders of eyelid**

✓6th **H02.81 Retained foreign body in eyelid**

Use additional code to identify the type of retained foreign body (Z18.-)

EXCLUDES 1 *laceration of eyelid with foreign body (S01.12-)*
retained intraocular foreign body (H44.6-, H44.7-)
superficial foreign body of eyelid and periocular area (S00.25-)

H02.811 **Retained foreign body in right upper eyelid**

H02.812 **Retained foreign body in right lower eyelid**

H02.813 **Retained foreign body in right eye, unspecified eyelid**

H02.814 **Retained foreign body in left upper eyelid**

H02.815 **Retained foreign body in left lower eyelid**

H02.816 **Retained foreign body in left eye, unspecified eyelid**

H02.819 **Retained foreign body in unspecified eye, unspecified eyelid**

✓6th **H02.82 Cysts of eyelid**

Sebaceous cyst of eyelid

H02.821 **Cysts of right upper eyelid**

H02.822 **Cysts of right lower eyelid**

H02.823 **Cysts of right eye, unspecified eyelid**

H02.824 **Cysts of left upper eyelid**

H02.825 **Cysts of left lower eyelid**

H02.826 **Cysts of left eye, unspecified eyelid**

H02.829 **Cysts of unspecified eye, unspecified eyelid**

✓6th **H02.83 Dermatochalasis of eyelid**

H02.831 **Dermatochalasis of right upper eyelid**

H02.832 **Dermatochalasis of right lower eyelid**

H02.833 **Dermatochalasis of right eye, unspecified eyelid**

H02.834 **Dermatochalasis of left upper eyelid**

H02.835 **Dermatochalasis of left lower eyelid**

H02.836 **Dermatochalasis of left eye, unspecified eyelid**

H02.839 **Dermatochalasis of unspecified eye, unspecified eyelid**

✓6th **H02.84 Edema of eyelid**

Hyperemia of eyelid

H02.841 **Edema of right upper eyelid**

H02.842 **Edema of right lower eyelid**

H02.843 **Edema of right eye, unspecified eyelid**

H02.844 **Edema of left upper eyelid**

H02.845 **Edema of left lower eyelid**

H02.846 **Edema of left eye, unspecified eyelid**

H02.849 **Edema of unspecified eye, unspecified eyelid**

✓6th **H02.85 Elephantiasis of eyelid**

H02.851 **Elephantiasis of right upper eyelid**

H02.852 **Elephantiasis of right lower eyelid**

H02.853 **Elephantiasis of right eye, unspecified eyelid**

H02.854 **Elephantiasis of left upper eyelid**

H02.855 **Elephantiasis of left lower eyelid**

H02.856 **Elephantiasis of left eye, unspecified eyelid**

H02.859 **Elephantiasis of unspecified eye, unspecified eyelid**

✓6th **H02.86 Hypertrichosis of eyelid**

H02.861 **Hypertrichosis of right upper eyelid**

H02.862 **Hypertrichosis of right lower eyelid**

H02.863 **Hypertrichosis of right eye, unspecified eyelid**

H02.864 **Hypertrichosis of left upper eyelid**

H02.865 **Hypertrichosis of left lower eyelid**

H02.866 **Hypertrichosis of left eye, unspecified eyelid**

H02.869 **Hypertrichosis of unspecified eye, unspecified eyelid**

✓6th **H02.87 Vascular anomalies of eyelid**

H02.871 **Vascular anomalies of right upper eyelid**

H02.872 **Vascular anomalies of right lower eyelid**

H02.873 **Vascular anomalies of right eye, unspecified eyelid**

H02.874 **Vascular anomalies of left upper eyelid**

H02.875 **Vascular anomalies of left lower eyelid**

H02.876 **Vascular anomalies of left eye, unspecified eyelid**

H02.879 **Vascular anomalies of unspecified eye, unspecified eyelid**

H02.89 **Other specified disorders of eyelid**

Hemorrhage of eyelid

H02.9 Unspecified disorder of eyelid

Disorder of eyelid NOS

✓4th **H04 Disorders of lacrimal system**

EXCLUDES 1 *congenital malformations of lacrimal system (Q10.4-Q10.6)*

✓5th **H04.0 Dacryoadenitis**

✓6th **H04.00 Unspecified dacryoadenitis**

H04.001 **Unspecified dacryoadenitis, right lacrimal gland**

H04.002 Unspecified dacryoadenitis, left lacrimal gland
H04.003 Unspecified dacryoadenitis, bilateral lacrimal glands
H04.009 Unspecified dacryoadenitis, unspecified lacrimal gland

✓6th H04.01 Acute dacryoadenitis
H04.011 Acute dacryoadenitis, right lacrimal gland
H04.012 Acute dacryoadenitis, left lacrimal gland
H04.013 Acute dacryoadenitis, bilateral lacrimal glands
H04.019 Acute dacryoadenitis, unspecified lacrimal gland

✓6th H04.02 Chronic dacryoadenitis
H04.021 Chronic dacryoadenitis, right lacrimal gland
H04.022 Chronic dacryoadenitis, left lacrimal gland
H04.023 Chronic dacryoadenitis, bilateral lacrimal glands
H04.029 Chronic dacryoadenitis, unspecified lacrimal gland

✓6th H04.03 Chronic enlargement of lacrimal gland
H04.031 Chronic enlargement of right lacrimal gland
H04.032 Chronic enlargement of left lacrimal gland
H04.033 Chronic enlargement of bilateral lacrimal glands
H04.039 Chronic enlargement of unspecified lacrimal gland

✓5th H04.1 Other disorders of lacrimal gland

✓6th H04.11 Dacryops
H04.111 Dacryops of right lacrimal gland
H04.112 Dacryops of left lacrimal gland
H04.113 Dacryops of bilateral lacrimal glands
H04.119 Dacryops of unspecified lacrimal gland

✓6th H04.12 Dry eye syndrome
Tear film insufficiency, NOS
H04.121 Dry eye syndrome of right lacrimal gland
H04.122 Dry eye syndrome of left lacrimal gland
H04.123 Dry eye syndrome of bilateral lacrimal glands
H04.129 Dry eye syndrome of unspecified lacrimal gland

✓6th H04.13 Lacrimal cyst
Lacrimal cystic degeneration
H04.131 Lacrimal cyst, right lacrimal gland
H04.132 Lacrimal cyst, left lacrimal gland
H04.133 Lacrimal cyst, bilateral lacrimal glands
H04.139 Lacrimal cyst, unspecified lacrimal gland

✓6th H04.14 Primary lacrimal gland atrophy
H04.141 Primary lacrimal gland atrophy, right lacrimal gland
H04.142 Primary lacrimal gland atrophy, left lacrimal gland
H04.143 Primary lacrimal gland atrophy, bilateral lacrimal glands
H04.149 Primary lacrimal gland atrophy, unspecified lacrimal gland

✓6th H04.15 Secondary lacrimal gland atrophy
H04.151 Secondary lacrimal gland atrophy, right lacrimal gland
H04.152 Secondary lacrimal gland atrophy, left lacrimal gland
H04.153 Secondary lacrimal gland atrophy, bilateral lacrimal glands
H04.159 Secondary lacrimal gland atrophy, unspecified lacrimal gland

✓6th H04.16 Lacrimal gland dislocation
H04.161 Lacrimal gland dislocation, right lacrimal gland
H04.162 Lacrimal gland dislocation, left lacrimal gland
H04.163 Lacrimal gland dislocation, bilateral lacrimal glands
H04.169 Lacrimal gland dislocation, unspecified lacrimal gland

H04.19 Other specified disorders of lacrimal gland

✓5th H04.2 Epiphora

✓6th H04.20 Unspecified epiphora
H04.201 Unspecified epiphora, right lacrimal gland
H04.202 Unspecified epiphora, left lacrimal gland
H04.203 Unspecified epiphora, bilateral lacrimal glands
H04.209 Unspecified epiphora, unspecified lacrimal gland

✓6th H04.21 Epiphora due to excess lacrimation
H04.211 Epiphora due to excess lacrimation, right lacrimal gland
H04.212 Epiphora due to excess lacrimation, left lacrimal gland
H04.213 Epiphora due to excess lacrimation, bilateral lacrimal glands
H04.219 Epiphora due to excess lacrimation, unspecified lacrimal gland

✓6th H04.22 Epiphora due to insufficient drainage
H04.221 Epiphora due to insufficient drainage, right lacrimal gland
H04.222 Epiphora due to insufficient drainage, left lacrimal gland
H04.223 Epiphora due to insufficient drainage, bilateral lacrimal glands
H04.229 Epiphora due to insufficient drainage, unspecified lacrimal gland

✓5th H04.3 Acute and unspecified inflammation of lacrimal passages
EXCLUDES 1 *neonatal dacryocystitis (P39.1)*

✓6th H04.30 Unspecified dacryocystitis
H04.301 Unspecified dacryocystitis of right lacrimal passage
H04.302 Unspecified dacryocystitis of left lacrimal passage
H04.303 Unspecified dacryocystitis of bilateral lacrimal passages
H04.309 Unspecified dacryocystitis of unspecified lacrimal passage

✓6th H04.31 Phlegmonous dacryocystitis
H04.311 Phlegmonous dacryocystitis of right lacrimal passage
H04.312 Phlegmonous dacryocystitis of left lacrimal passage
H04.313 Phlegmonous dacryocystitis of bilateral lacrimal passages
H04.319 Phlegmonous dacryocystitis of unspecified lacrimal passage

✓6th H04.32 Acute dacryocystitis
Acute dacryopericystitis
H04.321 Acute dacryocystitis of right lacrimal passage
H04.322 Acute dacryocystitis of left lacrimal passage
H04.323 Acute dacryocystitis of bilateral lacrimal passages
H04.329 Acute dacryocystitis of unspecified lacrimal passage

✓6th H04.33 Acute lacrimal canaliculitis
H04.331 Acute lacrimal canaliculitis of right lacrimal passage
H04.332 Acute lacrimal canaliculitis of left lacrimal passage
H04.333 Acute lacrimal canaliculitis of bilateral lacrimal passages
H04.339 Acute lacrimal canaliculitis of unspecified lacrimal passage

✓5th H04.4 Chronic inflammation of lacrimal passages

✓6th H04.41 Chronic dacryocystitis
H04.411 Chronic dacryocystitis of right lacrimal passage
H04.412 Chronic dacryocystitis of left lacrimal passage

H04.413 Chronic dacryocystitis of bilateral lacrimal passages
H04.419 Chronic dacryocystitis of unspecified lacrimal passage

✓6th H04.42 Chronic lacrimal canaliculitis
H04.421 Chronic lacrimal canaliculitis of right lacrimal passage
H04.422 Chronic lacrimal canaliculitis of left lacrimal passage
H04.423 Chronic lacrimal canaliculitis of bilateral lacrimal passages
H04.429 Chronic lacrimal canaliculitis of unspecified lacrimal passage

✓6th H04.43 Chronic lacrimal mucocele
H04.431 Chronic lacrimal mucocele of right lacrimal passage
H04.432 Chronic lacrimal mucocele of left lacrimal passage
H04.433 Chronic lacrimal mucocele of bilateral lacrimal passages
H04.439 Chronic lacrimal mucocele of unspecified lacrimal passage

✓5th H04.5 Stenosis and insufficiency of lacrimal passages

✓6th H04.51 Dacryolith
H04.511 Dacryolith of right lacrimal passage
H04.512 Dacryolith of left lacrimal passage
H04.513 Dacryolith of bilateral lacrimal passages
H04.519 Dacryolith of unspecified lacrimal passage

✓6th H04.52 Eversion of lacrimal punctum
H04.521 Eversion of right lacrimal punctum
H04.522 Eversion of left lacrimal punctum
H04.523 Eversion of bilateral lacrimal punctum
H04.529 Eversion of unspecified lacrimal punctum

✓6th H04.53 Neonatal obstruction of nasolacrimal duct
EXCLUDES 1 *congenital stenosis and stricture of lacrimal duct (Q10.5)*
H04.531 Neonatal obstruction of right nasolacrimal duct N
H04.532 Neonatal obstruction of left nasolacrimal duct N
H04.533 Neonatal obstruction of bilateral nasolacrimal duct N
H04.539 Neonatal obstruction of unspecified nasolacrimal duct N

✓6th H04.54 Stenosis of lacrimal canaliculi
H04.541 Stenosis of right lacrimal canaliculi
H04.542 Stenosis of left lacrimal canaliculi
H04.543 Stenosis of bilateral lacrimal canaliculi
H04.549 Stenosis of unspecified lacrimal canaliculi

✓6th H04.55 Acquired stenosis of nasolacrimal duct
H04.551 Acquired stenosis of right nasolacrimal duct
H04.552 Acquired stenosis of left nasolacrimal duct
H04.553 Acquired stenosis of bilateral nasolacrimal duct
H04.559 Acquired stenosis of unspecified nasolacrimal duct

✓6th H04.56 Stenosis of lacrimal punctum
H04.561 Stenosis of right lacrimal punctum
H04.562 Stenosis of left lacrimal punctum
H04.563 Stenosis of bilateral lacrimal punctum
H04.569 Stenosis of unspecified lacrimal punctum

✓6th H04.57 Stenosis of lacrimal sac
H04.571 Stenosis of right lacrimal sac
H04.572 Stenosis of left lacrimal sac
H04.573 Stenosis of bilateral lacrimal sac
H04.579 Stenosis of unspecified lacrimal sac

✓5th H04.6 Other changes of lacrimal passages

✓6th H04.61 Lacrimal fistula
H04.611 Lacrimal fistula right lacrimal passage
H04.612 Lacrimal fistula left lacrimal passage
H04.613 Lacrimal fistula bilateral lacrimal passages
H04.619 Lacrimal fistula unspecified lacrimal passage

H04.69 Other changes of lacrimal passages

✓5th H04.8 Other disorders of lacrimal system

✓6th H04.81 Granuloma of lacrimal passages
H04.811 Granuloma of right lacrimal passage
H04.812 Granuloma of left lacrimal passage
H04.813 Granuloma of bilateral lacrimal passages
H04.819 Granuloma of unspecified lacrimal passage

H04.89 Other disorders of lacrimal system

H04.9 Disorder of lacrimal system, unspecified

✓4th H05 Disorders of orbit
EXCLUDES 1 *congenital malformation of orbit (Q10.7)*

✓5th H05.0 Acute inflammation of orbit

H05.00 Unspecified acute inflammation of orbit

✓6th H05.01 Cellulitis of orbit
Abscess of orbit

CC Excl: For CC codes in subcategory H05.01, unless otherwise noted: H05.00-H05.049

H05.011 Cellulitis of right orbit CC
H05.012 Cellulitis of left orbit CC
H05.013 Cellulitis of bilateral orbits CC
H05.019 Cellulitis of unspecified orbit CC

✓6th H05.02 Osteomyelitis of orbit

CC Excl: For CC codes in subcategory H05.02, unless otherwise noted: A02.24, A17.9, A18.03-A18.09, A18.82, A18.84, A18.89, H05.021-H05.029, M46.20-M46.39, M86.00-M86.9

H05.021 Osteomyelitis of right orbit CC
H05.022 Osteomyelitis of left orbit CC
H05.023 Osteomyelitis of bilateral orbits CC
H05.029 Osteomyelitis of unspecified orbit CC

✓6th H05.03 Periostitis of orbit

CC Excl: For CC codes in subcategory H05.03, unless otherwise noted: A02.24, A17.9, A18.03-A18.09, A18.82, A18.84, A18.89, H05.031-H05.039, M46.20-M46.39, M86.00-M86.9

H05.031 Periostitis of right orbit CC
H05.032 Periostitis of left orbit CC
H05.033 Periostitis of bilateral orbits CC
H05.039 Periostitis of unspecified orbit CC

✓6th H05.04 Tenonitis of orbit
H05.041 Tenonitis of right orbit
H05.042 Tenonitis of left orbit
H05.043 Tenonitis of bilateral orbits
H05.049 Tenonitis of unspecified orbit

✓5th H05.1 Chronic inflammatory disorders of orbit

H05.10 Unspecified chronic inflammatory disorders of orbit

✓6th H05.11 Granuloma of orbit
Pseudotumor (inflammatory) of orbit
H05.111 Granuloma of right orbit
H05.112 Granuloma of left orbit
H05.113 Granuloma of bilateral orbits
H05.119 Granuloma of unspecified orbit

✓6th H05.12 Orbital myositis
H05.121 Orbital myositis, right orbit
H05.122 Orbital myositis, left orbit
H05.123 Orbital myositis, bilateral
H05.129 Orbital myositis, unspecified orbit

✓5th H05.2 Exophthalmic conditions

H05.20 Unspecified exophthalmos

✓6th H05.21 Displacement (lateral) of globe
H05.211 Displacement (lateral) of globe, right eye
H05.212 Displacement (lateral) of globe, left eye
H05.213 Displacement (lateral) of globe, bilateral
H05.219 Displacement (lateral) of globe, unspecified eye

✓6th H05.22 Edema of orbit
Orbital congestion
H05.221 Edema of right orbit
H05.222 Edema of left orbit
H05.223 Edema of bilateral orbit
H05.229 Edema of unspecified orbit

✓6th **HØ5.23 Hemorrhage of orbit**
- **HØ5.231 Hemorrhage of right orbit**
- **HØ5.232 Hemorrhage of left orbit**
- **HØ5.233 Hemorrhage of bilateral orbit**
- **HØ5.239 Hemorrhage of unspecified orbit**

✓6th **HØ5.24 Constant exophthalmos**
- **HØ5.241 Constant exophthalmos, right eye**
- **HØ5.242 Constant exophthalmos, left eye**
- **HØ5.243 Constant exophthalmos, bilateral**
- **HØ5.249 Constant exophthalmos, unspecified eye**

✓6th **HØ5.25 Intermittent exophthalmos**
- **HØ5.251 Intermittent exophthalmos, right eye**
- **HØ5.252 Intermittent exophthalmos, left eye**
- **HØ5.253 Intermittent exophthalmos, bilateral**
- **HØ5.259 Intermittent exophthalmos, unspecified eye**

✓6th **HØ5.26 Pulsating exophthalmos**
- **HØ5.261 Pulsating exophthalmos, right eye**
- **HØ5.262 Pulsating exophthalmos, left eye**
- **HØ5.263 Pulsating exophthalmos, bilateral**
- **HØ5.269 Pulsating exophthalmos, unspecified eye**

✓5th **HØ5.3 Deformity of orbit**

EXCLUDES 1 *congenital deformity of orbit (Q1Ø.7)*
hypertelorism (Q75.2)

HØ5.3Ø Unspecified deformity of orbit

✓6th **HØ5.31 Atrophy of orbit**
- **HØ5.311 Atrophy of right orbit**
- **HØ5.312 Atrophy of left orbit**
- **HØ5.313 Atrophy of bilateral orbit**
- **HØ5.319 Atrophy of unspecified orbit**

✓6th **HØ5.32 Deformity of orbit due to bone disease**

Code also associated bone disease
- **HØ5.321 Deformity of right orbit due to bone disease**
- **HØ5.322 Deformity of left orbit due to bone disease**
- **HØ5.323 Deformity of bilateral orbits due to bone disease**
- **HØ5.329 Deformity of unspecified orbit due to bone disease**

✓6th **HØ5.33 Deformity of orbit due to trauma or surgery**
- **HØ5.331 Deformity of right orbit due to trauma or surgery**
- **HØ5.332 Deformity of left orbit due to trauma or surgery**
- **HØ5.333 Deformity of bilateral orbits due to trauma or surgery**
- **HØ5.339 Deformity of unspecified orbit due to trauma or surgery**

✓6th **HØ5.34 Enlargement of orbit**
- **HØ5.341 Enlargement of right orbit**
- **HØ5.342 Enlargement of left orbit**
- **HØ5.343 Enlargement of bilateral orbits**
- **HØ5.349 Enlargement of unspecified orbit**

✓6th **HØ5.35 Exostosis of orbit**
- **HØ5.351 Exostosis of right orbit**
- **HØ5.352 Exostosis of left orbit**
- **HØ5.353 Exostosis of bilateral orbits**
- **HØ5.359 Exostosis of unspecified orbit**

✓5th **HØ5.4 Enophthalmos**

✓6th **HØ5.4Ø Unspecified enophthalmos**
- **HØ5.4Ø1 Unspecified enophthalmos, right eye**
- **HØ5.4Ø2 Unspecified enophthalmos, left eye**
- **HØ5.4Ø3 Unspecified enophthalmos, bilateral**
- **HØ5.4Ø9 Unspecified enophthalmos, unspecified eye**

✓6th **HØ5.41 Enophthalmos due to atrophy of orbital tissue**
- **HØ5.411 Enophthalmos due to atrophy of orbital tissue, right eye**
- **HØ5.412 Enophthalmos due to atrophy of orbital tissue, left eye**
- **HØ5.413 Enophthalmos due to atrophy of orbital tissue, bilateral**
- **HØ5.419 Enophthalmos due to atrophy of orbital tissue, unspecified eye**

✓6th **HØ5.42 Enophthalmos due to trauma or surgery**
- **HØ5.421 Enophthalmos due to trauma or surgery, right eye**
- **HØ5.422 Enophthalmos due to trauma or surgery, left eye**
- **HØ5.423 Enophthalmos due to trauma or surgery, bilateral**
- **HØ5.429 Enophthalmos due to trauma or surgery, unspecified eye**

✓5th **HØ5.5 Retained (old) foreign body following penetrating wound of orbit**

Retrobulbar foreign body

Use additional code to identify the type of retained foreign body (Z18.-)

EXCLUDES 1 *current penetrating wound of orbit (SØ5.4-)*

EXCLUDES 2 *retained foreign body of eyelid (HØ2.81-)*
retained intraocular foreign body (H44.6-, H44.7-)

- **HØ5.5Ø Retained (old) foreign body following penetrating wound of unspecified orbit**
- **HØ5.51 Retained (old) foreign body following penetrating wound of right orbit**
- **HØ5.52 Retained (old) foreign body following penetrating wound of left orbit**
- **HØ5.53 Retained (old) foreign body following penetrating wound of bilateral orbits**

✓5th **HØ5.8 Other disorders of orbit**

✓6th **HØ5.81 Cyst of orbit**

Encephalocele of orbit
- **HØ5.811 Cyst of right orbit**
- **HØ5.812 Cyst of left orbit**
- **HØ5.813 Cyst of bilateral orbits**
- **HØ5.819 Cyst of unspecified orbit**

✓6th **HØ5.82 Myopathy of extraocular muscles**
- **HØ5.821 Myopathy of extraocular muscles, right orbit**
- **HØ5.822 Myopathy of extraocular muscles, left orbit**
- **HØ5.823 Myopathy of extraocular muscles, bilateral**
- **HØ5.829 Myopathy of extraocular muscles, unspecified orbit**

HØ5.89 Other disorders of orbit

HØ5.9 Unspecified disorder of orbit

Disorders of conjunctiva (H1Ø-H11)

✓4th **H1Ø Conjunctivitis**

EXCLUDES 1 *keratoconjunctivitis (H16.2-)*

✓5th **H1Ø.Ø Mucopurulent conjunctivitis**

✓6th **H1Ø.Ø1 Acute follicular conjunctivitis**
- **H1Ø.Ø11 Acute follicular conjunctivitis, right eye**
- **H1Ø.Ø12 Acute follicular conjunctivitis, left eye**
- **H1Ø.Ø13 Acute follicular conjunctivitis, bilateral**
- **H1Ø.Ø19 Acute follicular conjunctivitis, unspecified eye**

✓6th **H1Ø.Ø2 Other mucopurulent conjunctivitis**
- **H1Ø.Ø21 Other mucopurulent conjunctivitis, right eye**
- **H1Ø.Ø22 Other mucopurulent conjunctivitis, left eye**
- **H1Ø.Ø23 Other mucopurulent conjunctivitis, bilateral**
- **H1Ø.Ø29 Other mucopurulent conjunctivitis, unspecified eye**

✓5th **H1Ø.1 Acute atopic conjunctivitis**

Acute papillary conjunctivitis
- **H1Ø.1Ø Acute atopic conjunctivitis, unspecified eye**
- **H1Ø.11 Acute atopic conjunctivitis, right eye**
- **H1Ø.12 Acute atopic conjunctivitis, left eye**
- **H1Ø.13 Acute atopic conjunctivitis, bilateral**

H10.2 Other acute conjunctivitis

H10.21 Acute toxic conjunctivitis
Acute chemical conjunctivitis
Code first (T51-T65) to identify chemical and intent
EXCLUDES 1 *burn and corrosion of eye and adnexa (T26.-)*
- **H10.211 Acute toxic conjunctivitis, right eye**
- **H10.212 Acute toxic conjunctivitis, left eye**
- **H10.213 Acute toxic conjunctivitis, bilateral**
- **H10.219 Acute toxic conjunctivitis, unspecified eye**

H10.22 Pseudomembranous conjunctivitis
- **H10.221 Pseudomembranous conjunctivitis, right eye**
- **H10.222 Pseudomembranous conjunctivitis, left eye**
- **H10.223 Pseudomembranous conjunctivitis, bilateral**
- **H10.229 Pseudomembranous conjunctivitis, unspecified eye**

H10.23 Serous conjunctivitis, except viral
EXCLUDES 1 *viral conjunctivitis (B30.-)*
- **H10.231 Serous conjunctivitis, except viral, right eye**
- **H10.232 Serous conjunctivitis, except viral, left eye**
- **H10.233 Serous conjunctivitis, except viral, bilateral**
- **H10.239 Serous conjunctivitis, except viral, unspecified eye**

H10.3 Unspecified acute conjunctivitis
EXCLUDES 1 *ophthalmia neonatorum NOS (P39.1)*
- **H10.30 Unspecified acute conjunctivitis, unspecified eye**
- **H10.31 Unspecified acute conjunctivitis, right eye**
- **H10.32 Unspecified acute conjunctivitis, left eye**
- **H10.33 Unspecified acute conjunctivitis, bilateral**

H10.4 Chronic conjunctivitis

H10.40 Unspecified chronic conjunctivitis
- **H10.401 Unspecified chronic conjunctivitis, right eye**
- **H10.402 Unspecified chronic conjunctivitis, left eye**
- **H10.403 Unspecified chronic conjunctivitis, bilateral**
- **H10.409 Unspecified chronic conjunctivitis, unspecified eye**

H10.41 Chronic giant papillary conjunctivitis
- **H10.411 Chronic giant papillary conjunctivitis, right eye**
- **H10.412 Chronic giant papillary conjunctivitis, left eye**
- **H10.413 Chronic giant papillary conjunctivitis, bilateral**
- **H10.419 Chronic giant papillary conjunctivitis, unspecified eye**

H10.42 Simple chronic conjunctivitis
- **H10.421 Simple chronic conjunctivitis, right eye**
- **H10.422 Simple chronic conjunctivitis, left eye**
- **H10.423 Simple chronic conjunctivitis, bilateral**
- **H10.429 Simple chronic conjunctivitis, unspecified eye**

H10.43 Chronic follicular conjunctivitis
- **H10.431 Chronic follicular conjunctivitis, right eye**
- **H10.432 Chronic follicular conjunctivitis, left eye**
- **H10.433 Chronic follicular conjunctivitis, bilateral**
- **H10.439 Chronic follicular conjunctivitis, unspecified eye**

H10.44 Vernal conjunctivitis
EXCLUDES 1 *vernal keratoconjunctivitis with limbar and corneal involvement (H16.26-)*

H10.45 Other chronic allergic conjunctivitis

H10.5 Blepharoconjunctivitis

H10.50 Unspecified blepharoconjunctivitis
- **H10.501 Unspecified blepharoconjunctivitis, right eye**
- **H10.502 Unspecified blepharoconjunctivitis, left eye**
- **H10.503 Unspecified blepharoconjunctivitis, bilateral**
- **H10.509 Unspecified blepharoconjunctivitis, unspecified eye**

H10.51 Ligneous conjunctivitis
- **H10.511 Ligneous conjunctivitis, right eye**
- **H10.512 Ligneous conjunctivitis, left eye**
- **H10.513 Ligneous conjunctivitis, bilateral**
- **H10.519 Ligneous conjunctivitis, unspecified eye**

H10.52 Angular blepharoconjunctivitis
- **H10.521 Angular blepharoconjunctivitis, right eye**
- **H10.522 Angular blepharoconjunctivitis, left eye**
- **H10.523 Angular blepharoconjunctivitis, bilateral**
- **H10.529 Angular blepharoconjunctivitis, unspecified eye**

H10.53 Contact blepharoconjunctivitis
- **H10.531 Contact blepharoconjunctivitis, right eye**
- **H10.532 Contact blepharoconjunctivitis, left eye**
- **H10.533 Contact blepharoconjunctivitis, bilateral**
- **H10.539 Contact blepharoconjunctivitis, unspecified eye**

H10.8 Other conjunctivitis

H10.81 Pingueculitis
EXCLUDES 1 *pinguecula (H11.15-)*
- **H10.811 Pingueculitis, right eye**
- **H10.812 Pingueculitis, left eye**
- **H10.813 Pingueculitis, bilateral**
- **H10.819 Pingueculitis, unspecified eye**

H10.89 Other conjunctivitis

H10.9 Unspecified conjunctivitis

H11 Other disorders of conjunctiva
EXCLUDES 1 *keratoconjunctivitis (H16.2-)*

H11.0 Pterygium of eye
EXCLUDES 1 *pseudopterygium (H11.81-)*

H11.00 Unspecified pterygium of eye
- **H11.001 Unspecified pterygium of right eye**
- **H11.002 Unspecified pterygium of left eye**
- **H11.003 Unspecified pterygium of eye, bilateral**
- **H11.009 Unspecified pterygium of unspecified eye**

H11.01 Amyloid pterygium
- **H11.011 Amyloid pterygium of right eye**
- **H11.012 Amyloid pterygium of left eye**
- **H11.013 Amyloid pterygium of eye, bilateral**
- **H11.019 Amyloid pterygium of unspecified eye**

H11.02 Central pterygium of eye
- **H11.021 Central pterygium of right eye**
- **H11.022 Central pterygium of left eye**
- **H11.023 Central pterygium of eye, bilateral**
- **H11.029 Central pterygium of unspecified eye**

H11.03 Double pterygium of eye
- **H11.031 Double pterygium of right eye**
- **H11.032 Double pterygium of left eye**
- **H11.033 Double pterygium of eye, bilateral**
- **H11.039 Double pterygium of unspecified eye**

H11.04 Peripheral pterygium of eye, stationary
- **H11.041 Peripheral pterygium, stationary, right eye**
- **H11.042 Peripheral pterygium, stationary, left eye**
- **H11.043 Peripheral pterygium, stationary, bilateral**
- **H11.049 Peripheral pterygium, stationary, unspecified eye**

H11.05 Peripheral pterygium of eye, progressive
- **H11.051 Peripheral pterygium, progressive, right eye**
- **H11.052 Peripheral pterygium, progressive, left eye**
- **H11.053 Peripheral pterygium, progressive, bilateral**
- **H11.059 Peripheral pterygium, progressive, unspecified eye**

✓6th H11.06 Recurrent pterygium of eye
H11.061 Recurrent pterygium of right eye
H11.062 Recurrent pterygium of left eye
H11.063 Recurrent pterygium of eye, bilateral
H11.069 Recurrent pterygium of unspecified eye

✓5th H11.1 Conjunctival degenerations and deposits
EXCLUDES 2 *pseudopterygium (H11.81)*
H11.10 Unspecified conjunctival degenerations
✓6th H11.11 Conjunctival deposits
H11.111 Conjunctival deposits, right eye
H11.112 Conjunctival deposits, left eye
H11.113 Conjunctival deposits, bilateral
H11.119 Conjunctival deposits, unspecified eye
✓6th H11.12 Conjunctival concretions
H11.121 Conjunctival concretions, right eye
H11.122 Conjunctival concretions, left eye
H11.123 Conjunctival concretions, bilateral
H11.129 Conjunctival concretions, unspecified eye
✓6th H11.13 Conjunctival pigmentations
Conjunctival argyrosis [argyria]
H11.131 Conjunctival pigmentations, right eye
H11.132 Conjunctival pigmentations, left eye
H11.133 Conjunctival pigmentations, bilateral
H11.139 Conjunctival pigmentations, unspecified eye
✓6th H11.14 Conjunctival xerosis, unspecified
EXCLUDES 1 *xerosis of conjunctiva due to vitamin A deficiency (E50.0, E50.1)*
H11.141 Conjunctival xerosis, unspecified, right eye
H11.142 Conjunctival xerosis , unspecified, left eye
H11.143 Conjunctival xerosis, unspecified, bilateral
H11.149 Conjunctival xerosis, unspecified, unspecified eye
✓6th H11.15 Pinguecula
EXCLUDES 1 *pingueculitis (H10.81-)*
H11.151 Pinguecula, right eye
H11.152 Pinguecula, left eye
H11.153 Pinguecula, bilateral
H11.159 Pinguecula, unspecified eye

✓5th H11.2 Conjunctival scars
✓6th H11.21 Conjunctival adhesions and strands (localized)
H11.211 Conjunctival adhesions and strands (localized), right eye
H11.212 Conjunctival adhesions and strands (localized), left eye
H11.213 Conjunctival adhesions and strands (localized), bilateral
H11.219 Conjunctival adhesions and strands (localized), unspecified eye
✓6th H11.22 Conjunctival granuloma
H11.221 Conjunctival granuloma, right eye
H11.222 Conjunctival granuloma, left eye
H11.223 Conjunctival granuloma, bilateral
H11.229 Conjunctival granuloma, unspecified
✓6th H11.23 Symblepharon
H11.231 Symblepharon, right eye
H11.232 Symblepharon, left eye
H11.233 Symblepharon, bilateral
H11.239 Symblepharon, unspecified eye
✓6th H11.24 Scarring of conjunctiva
H11.241 Scarring of conjunctiva, right eye
H11.242 Scarring of conjunctiva, left eye
H11.243 Scarring of conjunctiva, bilateral
H11.249 Scarring of conjunctiva, unspecified eye

✓5th H11.3 Conjunctival hemorrhage
Subconjunctival hemorrhage
H11.30 Conjunctival hemorrhage, unspecified eye
H11.31 Conjunctival hemorrhage, right eye
H11.32 Conjunctival hemorrhage, left eye
H11.33 Conjunctival hemorrhage, bilateral

✓5th H11.4 Other conjunctival vascular disorders and cysts
✓6th H11.41 Vascular abnormalities of conjunctiva
Conjunctival aneurysm
H11.411 Vascular abnormalities of conjunctiva, right eye
H11.412 Vascular abnormalities of conjunctiva, left eye
H11.413 Vascular abnormalities of conjunctiva, bilateral
H11.419 Vascular abnormalities of conjunctiva, unspecified eye
✓6th H11.42 Conjunctival edema
H11.421 Conjunctival edema, right eye
H11.422 Conjunctival edema, left eye
H11.423 Conjunctival edema, bilateral
H11.429 Conjunctival edema, unspecified eye
✓6th H11.43 Conjunctival hyperemia
H11.431 Conjunctival hyperemia, right eye
H11.432 Conjunctival hyperemia, left eye
H11.433 Conjunctival hyperemia, bilateral
H11.439 Conjunctival hyperemia, unspecified eye
✓6th H11.44 Conjunctival cysts
H11.441 Conjunctival cysts, right eye
H11.442 Conjunctival cysts, left eye
H11.443 Conjunctival cysts, bilateral
H11.449 Conjunctival cysts, unspecified eye

✓5th H11.8 Other specified disorders of conjunctiva
✓6th H11.81 Pseudopterygium of conjunctiva
H11.811 Pseudopterygium of conjunctiva, right eye
H11.812 Pseudopterygium of conjunctiva, left eye
H11.813 Pseudopterygium of conjunctiva, bilateral
H11.819 Pseudopterygium of conjunctiva, unspecified eye
✓6th H11.82 Conjunctivochalasis
H11.821 Conjunctivochalasis, right eye
H11.822 Conjunctivochalasis, left eye
H11.823 Conjunctivochalasis, bilateral
H11.829 Conjunctivochalasis, unspecified eye
H11.89 Other specified disorders of conjunctiva
H11.9 Unspecified disorder of conjunctiva

Disorders of sclera, cornea, iris and ciliary body (H15-H22)

✓4th H15 Disorders of sclera
✓5th H15.0 Scleritis
✓6th H15.00 Unspecified scleritis
H15.001 Unspecified scleritis, right eye
H15.002 Unspecified scleritis, left eye
H15.003 Unspecified scleritis, bilateral
H15.009 Unspecified scleritis, unspecified eye
✓6th H15.01 Anterior scleritis
H15.011 Anterior scleritis, right eye
H15.012 Anterior scleritis, left eye
H15.013 Anterior scleritis, bilateral
H15.019 Anterior scleritis, unspecified eye
✓6th H15.02 Brawny scleritis
H15.021 Brawny scleritis, right eye
H15.022 Brawny scleritis, left eye
H15.023 Brawny scleritis, bilateral
H15.029 Brawny scleritis, unspecified eye
✓6th H15.03 Posterior scleritis
Sclerotenonitis
H15.031 Posterior scleritis, right eye
H15.032 Posterior scleritis, left eye
H15.033 Posterior scleritis, bilateral
H15.039 Posterior scleritis, unspecified eye
✓6th H15.04 Scleritis with corneal involvement
H15.041 Scleritis with corneal involvement, right eye
H15.042 Scleritis with corneal involvement, left eye
H15.043 Scleritis with corneal involvement, bilateral

H15.049 Scleritis with corneal involvement, unspecified eye
✓6th H15.05 Scleromalacia perforans
H15.051 Scleromalacia perforans, right eye
H15.052 Scleromalacia perforans, left eye
H15.053 Scleromalacia perforans, bilateral
H15.059 Scleromalacia perforans, unspecified eye
✓6th H15.09 Other scleritis
Scleral abscess
H15.091 Other scleritis, right eye
H15.092 Other scleritis, left eye
H15.093 Other scleritis, bilateral
H15.099 Other scleritis, unspecified eye
✓5th H15.1 Episcleritis
✓6th H15.10 Unspecified episcleritis
H15.101 Unspecified episcleritis, right eye
H15.102 Unspecified episcleritis, left eye
H15.103 Unspecified episcleritis, bilateral
H15.109 Unspecified episcleritis, unspecified eye
✓6th H15.11 Episcleritis periodica fugax
H15.111 Episcleritis periodica fugax, right eye
H15.112 Episcleritis periodica fugax, left eye
H15.113 Episcleritis periodica fugax, bilateral
H15.119 Episcleritis periodica fugax, unspecified eye
✓6th H15.12 Nodular episcleritis
H15.121 Nodular episcleritis, right eye
H15.122 Nodular episcleritis, left eye
H15.123 Nodular episcleritis, bilateral
H15.129 Nodular episcleritis, unspecified eye
✓5th H15.8 Other disorders of sclera
EXCLUDES 2 *blue sclera (Q13.5)*
degenerative myopia (H44.2-)
✓6th H15.81 Equatorial staphyloma
H15.811 Equatorial staphyloma, right eye
H15.812 Equatorial staphyloma, left eye
H15.813 Equatorial staphyloma, bilateral
H15.819 Equatorial staphyloma, unspecified eye
✓6th H15.82 Localized anterior staphyloma
H15.821 Localized anterior staphyloma, right eye
H15.822 Localized anterior staphyloma, left eye
H15.823 Localized anterior staphyloma, bilateral
H15.829 Localized anterior staphyloma, unspecified eye
✓6th H15.83 Staphyloma posticum
H15.831 Staphyloma posticum, right eye
H15.832 Staphyloma posticum, left eye
H15.833 Staphyloma posticum, bilateral
H15.839 Staphyloma posticum, unspecified eye
✓6th H15.84 Scleral ectasia
H15.841 Scleral ectasia, right eye
H15.842 Scleral ectasia, left eye
H15.843 Scleral ectasia, bilateral
H15.849 Scleral ectasia, unspecified eye
✓6th H15.85 Ring staphyloma
H15.851 Ring staphyloma, right eye
H15.852 Ring staphyloma, left eye
H15.853 Ring staphyloma, bilateral
H15.859 Ring staphyloma, unspecified eye
H15.89 Other disorders of sclera
H15.9 Unspecified disorder of sclera
✓4th H16 Keratitis
✓5th H16.0 Corneal ulcer
✓6th H16.00 Unspecified corneal ulcer
H16.001 Unspecified corneal ulcer, right eye
H16.002 Unspecified corneal ulcer, left eye
H16.003 Unspecified corneal ulcer, bilateral
H16.009 Unspecified corneal ulcer, unspecified eye
✓6th H16.01 Central corneal ulcer
H16.011 Central corneal ulcer, right eye
H16.012 Central corneal ulcer, left eye
H16.013 Central corneal ulcer, bilateral
H16.019 Central corneal ulcer, unspecified eye
✓6th H16.02 Ring corneal ulcer
H16.021 Ring corneal ulcer, right eye
H16.022 Ring corneal ulcer, left eye
H16.023 Ring corneal ulcer, bilateral
H16.029 Ring corneal ulcer, unspecified eye
✓6th H16.03 Corneal ulcer with hypopyon
H16.031 Corneal ulcer with hypopyon, right eye
H16.032 Corneal ulcer with hypopyon, left eye
H16.033 Corneal ulcer with hypopyon, bilateral
H16.039 Corneal ulcer with hypopyon, unspecified eye
✓6th H16.04 Marginal corneal ulcer
H16.041 Marginal corneal ulcer, right eye
H16.042 Marginal corneal ulcer, left eye
H16.043 Marginal corneal ulcer, bilateral
H16.049 Marginal corneal ulcer, unspecified eye
✓6th H16.05 Mooren's corneal ulcer
H16.051 Mooren's corneal ulcer, right eye
H16.052 Mooren's corneal ulcer, left eye
H16.053 Mooren's corneal ulcer, bilateral
H16.059 Mooren's corneal ulcer, unspecified eye
✓6th H16.06 Mycotic corneal ulcer
H16.061 Mycotic corneal ulcer, right eye
H16.062 Mycotic corneal ulcer, left eye
H16.063 Mycotic corneal ulcer, bilateral
H16.069 Mycotic corneal ulcer, unspecified eye
✓6th H16.07 Perforated corneal ulcer
H16.071 Perforated corneal ulcer, right eye
H16.072 Perforated corneal ulcer, left eye
H16.073 Perforated corneal ulcer, bilateral
H16.079 Perforated corneal ulcer, unspecified eye
✓5th H16.1 Other and unspecified superficial keratitis without conjunctivitis
✓6th H16.10 Unspecified superficial keratitis
H16.101 Unspecified superficial keratitis, right eye
H16.102 Unspecified superficial keratitis, left eye
H16.103 Unspecified superficial keratitis, bilateral
H16.109 Unspecified superficial keratitis, unspecified eye
✓6th H16.11 Macular keratitis
Areolar keratitis
Nummular keratitis
Stellate keratitis
Striate keratitis
H16.111 Macular keratitis, right eye
H16.112 Macular keratitis, left eye
H16.113 Macular keratitis, bilateral
H16.119 Macular keratitis, unspecified eye
✓6th H16.12 Filamentary keratitis
H16.121 Filamentary keratitis, right eye
H16.122 Filamentary keratitis, left eye
H16.123 Filamentary keratitis, bilateral
H16.129 Filamentary keratitis, unspecified eye
✓6th H16.13 Photokeratitis
Snow blindness
Welders keratitis
H16.131 Photokeratitis, right eye
H16.132 Photokeratitis, left eye
H16.133 Photokeratitis, bilateral
H16.139 Photokeratitis, unspecified eye
✓6th H16.14 Punctate keratitis
H16.141 Punctate keratitis, right eye
H16.142 Punctate keratitis, left eye
H16.143 Punctate keratitis, bilateral
H16.149 Punctate keratitis, unspecified eye
✓5th H16.2 Keratoconjunctivitis
✓6th H16.20 Unspecified keratoconjunctivitis
Superficial keratitis with conjunctivitis NOS
H16.201 Unspecified keratoconjunctivitis, right eye
H16.202 Unspecified keratoconjunctivitis, left eye

H16.203 Unspecified keratoconjunctivitis, bilateral
H16.209 Unspecified keratoconjunctivitis, unspecified eye

✓6th H16.21 Exposure keratoconjunctivitis
H16.211 Exposure keratoconjunctivitis, right eye
H16.212 Exposure keratoconjunctivitis, left eye
H16.213 Exposure keratoconjunctivitis, bilateral
H16.219 Exposure keratoconjunctivitis, unspecified eye

✓6th H16.22 Keratoconjunctivitis sicca, not specified as Sjögren's
EXCLUDES 1 *Sjögren's syndrome (M35.01)*
H16.221 Keratoconjunctivitis sicca, not specified as Sjögren's, right eye
H16.222 Keratoconjunctivitis sicca, not specified as Sjögren's, left eye
H16.223 Keratoconjunctivitis sicca, not specified as Sjögren's, bilateral
H16.229 Keratoconjunctivitis sicca, not specified as Sjögren's, unspecified eye

✓6th H16.23 Neurotrophic keratoconjunctivitis
H16.231 Neurotrophic keratoconjunctivitis, right eye
H16.232 Neurotrophic keratoconjunctivitis, left eye
H16.233 Neurotrophic keratoconjunctivitis, bilateral
H16.239 Neurotrophic keratoconjunctivitis, unspecified eye

✓6th H16.24 Ophthalmia nodosa
H16.241 Ophthalmia nodosa, right eye
H16.242 Ophthalmia nodosa, left eye
H16.243 Ophthalmia nodosa, bilateral
H16.249 Ophthalmia nodosa, unspecified eye

✓6th H16.25 Phlyctenular keratoconjunctivitis
H16.251 Phlyctenular keratoconjunctivitis, right eye
H16.252 Phlyctenular keratoconjunctivitis, left eye
H16.253 Phlyctenular keratoconjunctivitis, bilateral
H16.259 Phlyctenular keratoconjunctivitis, unspecified eye

✓6th H16.26 Vernal keratoconjunctivitis, with limbar and corneal involvement
EXCLUDES 1 *vernal conjunctivitis without limbar and corneal involvement (H10.44)*
H16.261 Vernal keratoconjunctivitis, with limbar and corneal involvement, right eye
H16.262 Vernal keratoconjunctivitis, with limbar and corneal involvement, left eye
H16.263 Vernal keratoconjunctivitis, with limbar and corneal involvement, bilateral
H16.269 Vernal keratoconjunctivitis, with limbar and corneal involvement, unspecified eye

✓6th H16.29 Other keratoconjunctivitis
H16.291 Other keratoconjunctivitis, right eye
H16.292 Other keratoconjunctivitis, left eye
H16.293 Other keratoconjunctivitis, bilateral
H16.299 Other keratoconjunctivitis, unspecified eye

✓5th H16.3 Interstitial and deep keratitis

✓6th H16.30 Unspecified interstitial keratitis
H16.301 Unspecified interstitial keratitis, right eye
H16.302 Unspecified interstitial keratitis, left eye
H16.303 Unspecified interstitial keratitis, bilateral
H16.309 Unspecified interstitial keratitis, unspecified eye

✓6th H16.31 Corneal abscess
H16.311 Corneal abscess, right eye
H16.312 Corneal abscess, left eye
H16.313 Corneal abscess, bilateral
H16.319 Corneal abscess, unspecified eye

✓6th H16.32 Diffuse interstitial keratitis
Cogan's syndrome
H16.321 Diffuse interstitial keratitis, right eye
H16.322 Diffuse interstitial keratitis, left eye
H16.323 Diffuse interstitial keratitis, bilateral
H16.329 Diffuse interstitial keratitis, unspecified eye

✓6th H16.33 Sclerosing keratitis
H16.331 Sclerosing keratitis, right eye
H16.332 Sclerosing keratitis, left eye
H16.333 Sclerosing keratitis, bilateral
H16.339 Sclerosing keratitis, unspecified eye

✓6th H16.39 Other interstitial and deep keratitis
H16.391 Other interstitial and deep keratitis, right eye
H16.392 Other interstitial and deep keratitis, left eye
H16.393 Other interstitial and deep keratitis, bilateral
H16.399 Other interstitial and deep keratitis, unspecified eye

✓5th H16.4 Corneal neovascularization

✓6th H16.40 Unspecified corneal neovascularization
H16.401 Unspecified corneal neovascularization, right eye
H16.402 Unspecified corneal neovascularization, left eye
H16.403 Unspecified corneal neovascularization, bilateral
H16.409 Unspecified corneal neovascularization, unspecified eye

✓6th H16.41 Ghost vessels (corneal)
H16.411 Ghost vessels (corneal), right eye
H16.412 Ghost vessels (corneal), left eye
H16.413 Ghost vessels (corneal), bilateral
H16.419 Ghost vessels (corneal), unspecified eye

✓6th H16.42 Pannus (corneal)
H16.421 Pannus (corneal), right eye
H16.422 Pannus (corneal), left eye
H16.423 Pannus (corneal), bilateral
H16.429 Pannus (corneal), unspecified eye

✓6th H16.43 Localized vascularization of cornea
H16.431 Localized vascularization of cornea, right eye
H16.432 Localized vascularization of cornea, left eye
H16.433 Localized vascularization of cornea, bilateral
H16.439 Localized vascularization of cornea, unspecified eye

✓6th H16.44 Deep vascularization of cornea
H16.441 Deep vascularization of cornea, right eye
H16.442 Deep vascularization of cornea, left eye
H16.443 Deep vascularization of cornea, bilateral
H16.449 Deep vascularization of cornea, unspecified eye

H16.8 Other keratitis
H16.9 Unspecified keratitis

✓4th H17 Corneal scars and opacities

✓5th H17.0 Adherent leukoma
H17.00 Adherent leukoma, unspecified eye
H17.01 Adherent leukoma, right eye
H17.02 Adherent leukoma, left eye
H17.03 Adherent leukoma, bilateral

✓5th H17.1 Central corneal opacity
H17.10 Central corneal opacity, unspecified eye
H17.11 Central corneal opacity, right eye
H17.12 Central corneal opacity, left eye
H17.13 Central corneal opacity, bilateral

✓5th H17.8 Other corneal scars and opacities

✓6th H17.81 Minor opacity of cornea
Corneal nebula
H17.811 Minor opacity of cornea, right eye
H17.812 Minor opacity of cornea, left eye
H17.813 Minor opacity of cornea, bilateral
H17.819 Minor opacity of cornea, unspecified eye

✓6th **H17.82 Peripheral opacity of cornea**
- **H17.821 Peripheral opacity of cornea, right eye**
- **H17.822 Peripheral opacity of cornea, left eye**
- **H17.823 Peripheral opacity of cornea, bilateral**
- **H17.829 Peripheral opacity of cornea, unspecified eye**

H17.89 Other corneal scars and opacities

H17.9 Unspecified corneal scar and opacity

✓4th **H18 Other disorders of cornea**

✓5th **H18.0 Corneal pigmentations and deposits**

✓6th **H18.00 Unspecified corneal deposit**
- **H18.001 Unspecified corneal deposit, right eye**
- **H18.002 Unspecified corneal deposit, left eye**
- **H18.003 Unspecified corneal deposit, bilateral**
- **H18.009 Unspecified corneal deposit, unspecified eye**

✓6th **H18.01 Anterior corneal pigmentations**
Staehli's line
- **H18.011 Anterior corneal pigmentations, right eye**
- **H18.012 Anterior corneal pigmentations, left eye**
- **H18.013 Anterior corneal pigmentations, bilateral**
- **H18.019 Anterior corneal pigmentations, unspecified eye**

✓6th **H18.02 Argentous corneal deposits**
- **H18.021 Argentous corneal deposits, right eye**
- **H18.022 Argentous corneal deposits, left eye**
- **H18.023 Argentous corneal deposits, bilateral**
- **H18.029 Argentous corneal deposits, unspecified eye**

✓6th **H18.03 Corneal deposits in metabolic disorders**
Code also associated metabolic disorder
- **H18.031 Corneal deposits in metabolic disorders, right eye**
- **H18.032 Corneal deposits in metabolic disorders, left eye**
- **H18.033 Corneal deposits in metabolic disorders, bilateral**
- **H18.039 Corneal deposits in metabolic disorders, unspecified eye**

✓6th **H18.04 Kayser-Fleischer ring**
Code also associated Wilson's disease (E83.01)
- **H18.041 Kayser-Fleischer ring, right eye**
- **H18.042 Kayser-Fleischer ring, left eye**
- **H18.043 Kayser-Fleischer ring, bilateral**
- **H18.049 Kayser-Fleischer ring, unspecified eye**

✓6th **H18.05 Posterior corneal pigmentations**
Krukenberg's spindle
- **H18.051 Posterior corneal pigmentations, right eye**
- **H18.052 Posterior corneal pigmentations, left eye**
- **H18.053 Posterior corneal pigmentations, bilateral**
- **H18.059 Posterior corneal pigmentations, unspecified eye**

✓6th **H18.06 Stromal corneal pigmentations**
Hematocornea
- **H18.061 Stromal corneal pigmentations, right eye**
- **H18.062 Stromal corneal pigmentations, left eye**
- **H18.063 Stromal corneal pigmentations, bilateral**
- **H18.069 Stromal corneal pigmentations, unspecified eye**

✓5th **H18.1 Bullous keratopathy**
- **H18.10 Bullous keratopathy, unspecified eye**
- **H18.11 Bullous keratopathy, right eye**
- **H18.12 Bullous keratopathy, left eye**
- **H18.13 Bullous keratopathy, bilateral**

✓5th **H18.2 Other and unspecified corneal edema**

H18.20 Unspecified corneal edema

✓6th **H18.21 Corneal edema secondary to contact lens**
EXCLUDES 2 *other corneal disorders due to contact lens (H18.82-)*
- **H18.211 Corneal edema secondary to contact lens, right eye**
- **H18.212 Corneal edema secondary to contact lens, left eye**
- **H18.213 Corneal edema secondary to contact lens, bilateral**
- **H18.219 Corneal edema secondary to contact lens, unspecified eye**

✓6th **H18.22 Idiopathic corneal edema**
- **H18.221 Idiopathic corneal edema, right eye**
- **H18.222 Idiopathic corneal edema, left eye**
- **H18.223 Idiopathic corneal edema, bilateral**
- **H18.229 Idiopathic corneal edema, unspecified eye**

✓6th **H18.23 Secondary corneal edema**
- **H18.231 Secondary corneal edema, right eye**
- **H18.232 Secondary corneal edema, left eye**
- **H18.233 Secondary corneal edema, bilateral**
- **H18.239 Secondary corneal edema, unspecified eye**

✓5th **H18.3 Changes of corneal membranes**

H18.30 Unspecified corneal membrane change

✓6th **H18.31 Folds and rupture in Bowman's membrane**
- **H18.311 Folds and rupture in Bowman's membrane, right eye**
- **H18.312 Folds and rupture in Bowman's membrane, left eye**
- **H18.313 Folds and rupture in Bowman's membrane, bilateral**
- **H18.319 Folds and rupture in Bowman's membrane, unspecified eye**

✓6th **H18.32 Folds in Descemet's membrane**
- **H18.321 Folds in Descemet's membrane, right eye**
- **H18.322 Folds in Descemet's membrane, left eye**
- **H18.323 Folds in Descemet's membrane, bilateral**
- **H18.329 Folds in Descemet's membrane, unspecified eye**

✓6th **H18.33 Rupture in Descemet's membrane**
- **H18.331 Rupture in Descemet's membrane, right eye**
- **H18.332 Rupture in Descemet's membrane, left eye**
- **H18.333 Rupture in Descemet's membrane, bilateral**
- **H18.339 Rupture in Descemet's membrane, unspecified eye**

✓5th **H18.4 Corneal degeneration**
EXCLUDES 1 *Mooren's ulcer (H16.0-)*
recurrent erosion of cornea (H18.83-)

H18.40 Unspecified corneal degeneration

✓6th **H18.41 Arcus senilis**
Senile corneal changes
- **H18.411 Arcus senilis, right eye**
- **H18.412 Arcus senilis, left eye**
- **H18.413 Arcus senilis, bilateral**
- **H18.419 Arcus senilis, unspecified eye**

✓6th **H18.42 Band keratopathy**
- **H18.421 Band keratopathy, right eye**
- **H18.422 Band keratopathy, left eye**
- **H18.423 Band keratopathy, bilateral**
- **H18.429 Band keratopathy, unspecified eye**

H18.43 Other calcerous corneal degeneration

✓6th **H18.44 Keratomalacia**
EXCLUDES 1 *keratomalacia due to vitamin A deficiency (E50.4)*
- **H18.441 Keratomalacia, right eye**
- **H18.442 Keratomalacia, left eye**
- **H18.443 Keratomalacia, bilateral**
- **H18.449 Keratomalacia, unspecified eye**

✓6th **H18.45 Nodular corneal degeneration**
- **H18.451 Nodular corneal degeneration, right eye**
- **H18.452 Nodular corneal degeneration, left eye**
- **H18.453 Nodular corneal degeneration, bilateral**
- **H18.459 Nodular corneal degeneration, unspecified eye**

✓6th **H18.46 Peripheral corneal degeneration**
- **H18.461 Peripheral corneal degeneration, right eye**
- **H18.462 Peripheral corneal degeneration, left eye**
- **H18.463 Peripheral corneal degeneration, bilateral**

H18.469 Peripheral corneal degeneration, unspecified eye
H18.49 Other corneal degeneration
✓5th H18.5 Hereditary corneal dystrophies
H18.50 Unspecified hereditary corneal dystrophies
H18.51 Endothelial corneal dystrophy
Fuchs' dystrophy
H18.52 Epithelial (juvenile) corneal dystrophy
H18.53 Granular corneal dystrophy
H18.54 Lattice corneal dystrophy
H18.55 Macular corneal dystrophy
H18.59 Other hereditary corneal dystrophies
✓5th H18.6 Keratoconus
✓6th H18.60 Keratoconus, unspecified
H18.601 Keratoconus, unspecified, right eye
H18.602 Keratoconus, unspecified, left eye
H18.603 Keratoconus, unspecified, bilateral
H18.609 Keratoconus, unspecified, unspecified eye
✓6th H18.61 Keratoconus, stable
H18.611 Keratoconus, stable, right eye
H18.612 Keratoconus, stable, left eye
H18.613 Keratoconus, stable, bilateral
H18.619 Keratoconus, stable, unspecified eye
✓6th H18.62 Keratoconus, unstable
Acute hydrops
H18.621 Keratoconus, unstable, right eye
H18.622 Keratoconus, unstable, left eye
H18.623 Keratoconus, unstable, bilateral
H18.629 Keratoconus, unstable, unspecified eye
✓5th H18.7 Other and unspecified corneal deformities
EXCLUDES 1 *congenital malformations of cornea (Q13.3-Q13.4)*
H18.70 Unspecified corneal deformity
✓6th H18.71 Corneal ectasia
H18.711 Corneal ectasia, right eye
H18.712 Corneal ectasia, left eye
H18.713 Corneal ectasia, bilateral
H18.719 Corneal ectasia, unspecified eye
✓6th H18.72 Corneal staphyloma
H18.721 Corneal staphyloma, right eye
H18.722 Corneal staphyloma, left eye
H18.723 Corneal staphyloma, bilateral
H18.729 Corneal staphyloma, unspecified eye
✓6th H18.73 Descemetocele
H18.731 Descemetocele, right eye
H18.732 Descemetocele, left eye
H18.733 Descemetocele, bilateral
H18.739 Descemetocele, unspecified eye
✓6th H18.79 Other corneal deformities
H18.791 Other corneal deformities, right eye
H18.792 Other corneal deformities, left eye
H18.793 Other corneal deformities, bilateral
H18.799 Other corneal deformities, unspecified eye
✓5th H18.8 Other specified disorders of cornea
✓6th H18.81 Anesthesia and hypoesthesia of cornea
H18.811 Anesthesia and hypoesthesia of cornea, right eye
H18.812 Anesthesia and hypoesthesia of cornea, left eye
H18.813 Anesthesia and hypoesthesia of cornea, bilateral
H18.819 Anesthesia and hypoesthesia of cornea, unspecified eye
✓6th H18.82 Corneal disorder due to contact lens
EXCLUDES 2 *corneal edema due to contact lens (H18.21-)*
H18.821 Corneal disorder due to contact lens, right eye
H18.822 Corneal disorder due to contact lens, left eye
H18.823 Corneal disorder due to contact lens, bilateral
H18.829 Corneal disorder due to contact lens, unspecified eye
✓6th H18.83 Recurrent erosion of cornea
H18.831 Recurrent erosion of cornea, right eye
H18.832 Recurrent erosion of cornea, left eye
H18.833 Recurrent erosion of cornea, bilateral
H18.839 Recurrent erosion of cornea, unspecified eye
✓6th H18.89 Other specified disorders of cornea
H18.891 Other specified disorders of cornea, right eye
H18.892 Other specified disorders of cornea, left eye
H18.893 Other specified disorders of cornea, bilateral
H18.899 Other specified disorders of cornea, unspecified eye
H18.9 Unspecified disorder of cornea

✓4th **H20 Iridocyclitis**

CC Excl: For CC codes in category H20, unless otherwise noted: A18.54, H20.00-H20.9

✓5th H20.0 Acute and subacute iridocyclitis
Acute anterior uveitis
Acute cyclitis
Acute iritis
Subacute anterior uveitis
Subacute cyclitis
Subacute iritis
EXCLUDES 1 *iridocyclitis, iritis, uveitis (due to) (in) diabetes mellitus (E08-E13 with .39)*
iridocyclitis, iritis, uveitis (due to) (in) diphtheria (A36.89)
iridocyclitis, iritis, uveitis (due to) (in) gonococcal (A54.32)
iridocyclitis, iritis, uveitis (due to) (in) herpes (simplex) (B00.51)
iridocyclitis, iritis, uveitis (due to) (in) herpes zoster (B02.32)
iridocyclitis, iritis, uveitis (due to) (in) late congenital syphilis (A50.39)
iridocyclitis, iritis, uveitis (due to) (in) late syphilis (A52.71)
iridocyclitis, iritis, uveitis (due to) (in) sarcoidosis (D86.83)
iridocyclitis, iritis, uveitis (due to) (in) syphilis (A51.43)
iridocyclitis, iritis, uveitis (due to) (in) toxoplasmosis (B58.09)
iridocyclitis, iritis, uveitis (due to) (in) tuberculosis (A18.54)
H20.00 Unspecified acute and subacute iridocyclitis CC
✓6th H20.01 Primary iridocyclitis
H20.011 Primary iridocyclitis, right eye CC
H20.012 Primary iridocyclitis, left eye CC
H20.013 Primary iridocyclitis, bilateral CC
H20.019 Primary iridocyclitis, unspecified eye CC
✓6th H20.02 Recurrent acute iridocyclitis
H20.021 Recurrent acute iridocyclitis, right eye CC
H20.022 Recurrent acute iridocyclitis, left eye CC
H20.023 Recurrent acute iridocyclitis, bilateral CC
H20.029 Recurrent acute iridocyclitis, unspecified eye CC
✓6th H20.03 Secondary infectious iridocyclitis
H20.031 Secondary infectious iridocyclitis, right eye CC
H20.032 Secondary infectious iridocyclitis, left eye CC
H20.033 Secondary infectious iridocyclitis, bilateral CC
H20.039 Secondary infectious iridocyclitis, unspecified eye CC
✓6th H20.04 Secondary noninfectious iridocyclitis
H20.041 Secondary noninfectious iridocyclitis, right eye
H20.042 Secondary noninfectious iridocyclitis, left eye
H20.043 Secondary noninfectious iridocyclitis, bilateral
H20.049 Secondary noninfectious iridocyclitis, unspecified eye

✓6th **H20.05 Hypopyon**
- **H20.051 Hypopyon, right eye**
- **H20.052 Hypopyon, left eye**
- **H20.053 Hypopyon, bilateral**
- **H20.059 Hypopyon, unspecified eye**

✓5th **H20.1 Chronic iridocyclitis**

Use additional code for any associated cataract (H26.21-)

EXCLUDES 2 *posterior cyclitis (H30.2-)*
- **H20.10 Chronic iridocyclitis, unspecified eye**
- **H20.11 Chronic iridocyclitis, right eye**
- **H20.12 Chronic iridocyclitis, left eye**
- **H20.13 Chronic iridocyclitis, bilateral**

✓5th **H20.2 Lens-induced iridocyclitis**
- **H20.20 Lens-induced iridocyclitis, unspecified eye**
- **H20.21 Lens-induced iridocyclitis, right eye**
- **H20.22 Lens-induced iridocyclitis, left eye**
- **H20.23 Lens-induced iridocyclitis, bilateral**

✓5th **H20.8 Other iridocyclitis**

EXCLUDES 2 *glaucomatocyclitis crises (H40.4-)*
posterior cyclitis (H30.2-)
sympathetic uveitis (H44.13-)

✓6th **H20.81 Fuchs' heterochromic cyclitis**
- **H20.811 Fuchs' heterochromic cyclitis, right eye**
- **H20.812 Fuchs' heterochromic cyclitis, left eye**
- **H20.813 Fuchs' heterochromic cyclitis, bilateral**
- **H20.819 Fuchs' heterochromic cyclitis, unspecified eye**

✓6th **H20.82 Vogt-Koyanagi syndrome**
- **H20.821 Vogt-Koyanagi syndrome, right eye**
- **H20.822 Vogt-Koyanagi syndrome, left eye**
- **H20.823 Vogt-Koyanagi syndrome, bilateral**
- **H20.829 Vogt-Koyanagi syndrome, unspecified eye** CC

H20.9 Unspecified iridocyclitis

Uveitis NOS

✓4th **H21 Other disorders of iris and ciliary body**

EXCLUDES 2 *sympathetic uveitis (H44.1-)*

✓5th **H21.0 Hyphema**

EXCLUDES 1 *traumatic hyphema (S05.1-)*
- **H21.00 Hyphema, unspecified eye**
- **H21.01 Hyphema, right eye**
- **H21.02 Hyphema, left eye**
- **H21.03 Hyphema, bilateral**

✓5th **H21.1 Other vascular disorders of iris and ciliary body**

Neovascularization of iris or ciliary body
Rubeosis iridis
Rubeosis of iris

✓6th **H21.1X Other vascular disorders of iris and ciliary body**
- **H21.1X1 Other vascular disorders of iris and ciliary body, right eye**
- **H21.1X2 Other vascular disorders of iris and ciliary body, left eye**
- **H21.1X3 Other vascular disorders of iris and ciliary body, bilateral**
- **H21.1X9 Other vascular disorders of iris and ciliary body, unspecified eye**

✓5th **H21.2 Degeneration of iris and ciliary body**

✓6th **H21.21 Degeneration of chamber angle**
- **H21.211 Degeneration of chamber angle, right eye**
- **H21.212 Degeneration of chamber angle, left eye**
- **H21.213 Degeneration of chamber angle, bilateral**
- **H21.219 Degeneration of chamber angle, unspecified eye**

✓6th **H21.22 Degeneration of ciliary body**
- **H21.221 Degeneration of ciliary body, right eye**
- **H21.222 Degeneration of ciliary body, left eye**
- **H21.223 Degeneration of ciliary body, bilateral**
- **H21.229 Degeneration of ciliary body, unspecified eye**

✓6th **H21.23 Degeneration of iris (pigmentary)**

Translucency of iris
- **H21.231 Degeneration of iris (pigmentary), right eye**
- **H21.232 Degeneration of iris (pigmentary), left eye**
- **H21.233 Degeneration of iris (pigmentary), bilateral**
- **H21.239 Degeneration of iris (pigmentary), unspecified eye**

✓6th **H21.24 Degeneration of pupillary margin**
- **H21.241 Degeneration of pupillary margin, right eye**
- **H21.242 Degeneration of pupillary margin, left eye**
- **H21.243 Degeneration of pupillary margin, bilateral**
- **H21.249 Degeneration of pupillary margin, unspecified eye**

✓6th **H21.25 Iridoschisis**
- **H21.251 Iridoschisis, right eye**
- **H21.252 Iridoschisis, left eye**
- **H21.253 Iridoschisis, bilateral**
- **H21.259 Iridoschisis, unspecified eye**

✓6th **H21.26 Iris atrophy (essential) (progressive)**
- **H21.261 Iris atrophy (essential) (progressive), right eye**
- **H21.262 Iris atrophy (essential) (progressive), left eye**
- **H21.263 Iris atrophy (essential) (progressive), bilateral**
- **H21.269 Iris atrophy (essential) (progressive), unspecified eye**

✓6th **H21.27 Miotic pupillary cyst**
- **H21.271 Miotic pupillary cyst, right eye**
- **H21.272 Miotic pupillary cyst, left eye**
- **H21.273 Miotic pupillary cyst, bilateral**
- **H21.279 Miotic pupillary cyst, unspecified eye**

H21.29 Other iris atrophy

✓5th **H21.3 Cyst of iris, ciliary body and anterior chamber**

EXCLUDES 2 *miotic pupillary cyst (H21.27-)*

✓6th **H21.30 Idiopathic cysts of iris, ciliary body or anterior chamber**

Cyst of iris, ciliary body or anterior chamber NOS
- **H21.301 Idiopathic cysts of iris, ciliary body or anterior chamber, right eye**
- **H21.302 Idiopathic cysts of iris, ciliary body or anterior chamber, left eye**
- **H21.303 Idiopathic cysts of iris, ciliary body or anterior chamber, bilateral**
- **H21.309 Idiopathic cysts of iris, ciliary body or anterior chamber, unspecified eye**

✓6th **H21.31 Exudative cysts of iris or anterior chamber**
- **H21.311 Exudative cysts of iris or anterior chamber, right eye**
- **H21.312 Exudative cysts of iris or anterior chamber, left eye**
- **H21.313 Exudative cysts of iris or anterior chamber, bilateral**
- **H21.319 Exudative cysts of iris or anterior chamber, unspecified eye**

✓6th **H21.32 Implantation cysts of iris, ciliary body or anterior chamber**
- **H21.321 Implantation cysts of iris, ciliary body or anterior chamber, right eye**
- **H21.322 Implantation cysts of iris, ciliary body or anterior chamber, left eye**
- **H21.323 Implantation cysts of iris, ciliary body or anterior chamber, bilateral**
- **H21.329 Implantation cysts of iris, ciliary body or anterior chamber, unspecified eye**

✓6th **H21.33 Parasitic cyst of iris, ciliary body or anterior chamber**

CC Excl: For CC codes in subcategory H21.33, unless otherwise noted: H20.051-H20.059, H21.331-H21.339, H33.121-H33.129, H44.001-H44.029, H44.121-H44.129, H44.19

- **H21.331 Parasitic cyst of iris, ciliary body or anterior chamber, right eye** CC
- **H21.332 Parasitic cyst of iris, ciliary body or anterior chamber, left eye** CC

H21.333 Parasitic cyst of iris, ciliary body or anterior chamber, bilateral CC

H21.339 Parasitic cyst of iris, ciliary body or anterior chamber, unspecified eye CC

✓6th H21.34 Primary cyst of pars plana

H21.341 Primary cyst of pars plana, right eye

H21.342 Primary cyst of pars plana, left eye

H21.343 Primary cyst of pars plana, bilateral

H21.349 Primary cyst of pars plana, unspecified eye

✓6th H21.35 Exudative cyst of pars plana

H21.351 Exudative cyst of pars plana, right eye

H21.352 Exudative cyst of pars plana, left eye

H21.353 Exudative cyst of pars plana, bilateral

H21.359 Exudative cyst of pars plana, unspecified eye

✓5th H21.4 Pupillary membranes

Iris bombé

Pupillary occlusion

Pupillary seclusion

EXCLUDES 1 *congenital pupillary membranes (Q13.8)*

H21.40 Pupillary membranes, unspecified eye

H21.41 Pupillary membranes, right eye

H21.42 Pupillary membranes, left eye

H21.43 Pupillary membranes, bilateral

✓5th H21.5 Other and unspecified adhesions and disruptions of iris and ciliary body

EXCLUDES 1 *corectopia (Q13.2)*

✓6th H21.50 Unspecified adhesions of iris

Synechia (iris) NOS

H21.501 Unspecified adhesions of iris, right eye

H21.502 Unspecified adhesions of iris, left eye

H21.503 Unspecified adhesions of iris, bilateral

H21.509 Unspecified adhesions of iris and ciliary body, unspecified eye

✓6th H21.51 Anterior synechiae (iris)

H21.511 Anterior synechiae (iris), right eye

H21.512 Anterior synechiae (iris), left eye

H21.513 Anterior synechiae (iris), bilateral

H21.519 Anterior synechiae (iris), unspecified eye

✓6th H21.52 Goniosynechiae

H21.521 Goniosynechiae, right eye

H21.522 Goniosynechiae, left eye

H21.523 Goniosynechiae, bilateral

H21.529 Goniosynechiae, unspecified eye

✓6th H21.53 Iridodialysis

H21.531 Iridodialysis, right eye

H21.532 Iridodialysis, left eye

H21.533 Iridodialysis, bilateral

H21.539 Iridodialysis, unspecified eye

✓6th H21.54 Posterior synechiae (iris)

H21.541 Posterior synechiae (iris), right eye

H21.542 Posterior synechiae (iris), left eye

H21.543 Posterior synechiae (iris), bilateral

H21.549 Posterior synechiae (iris), unspecified eye

✓6th H21.55 Recession of chamber angle

H21.551 Recession of chamber angle, right eye

H21.552 Recession of chamber angle, left eye

H21.553 Recession of chamber angle, bilateral

H21.559 Recession of chamber angle, unspecified eye

✓6th H21.56 Pupillary abnormalities

Deformed pupil

Ectopic pupil

Rupture of sphincter, pupil

EXCLUDES 1 *congenital deformity of pupil (Q13.2-)*

H21.561 Pupillary abnormality, right eye

H21.562 Pupillary abnormality, left eye

H21.563 Pupillary abnormality, bilateral

H21.569 Pupillary abnormality, unspecified eye

✓5th H21.8 Other specified disorders of iris and ciliary body

H21.81 Floppy iris syndrome

Intraoperative floppy iris syndrome (IFIS)

Use additional code for adverse effect, if applicable, to identify drug (T36-T50 with fifth or sixth character 5)

H21.82 Plateau iris syndrome (post-iridectomy) (postprocedural)

H21.89 Other specified disorders of iris and ciliary body

H21.9 Unspecified disorder of iris and ciliary body

H22 ***Disorders of iris and ciliary body in diseases classified elsewhere***

Code first underlying disease, such as:

gout (M1A.-, M10.-)

leprosy (A30.-)

parasitic disease (B89)

Disorders of lens (H25-H28)

✓4th **H25 Age-related cataract**

Senile cataract

EXCLUDES 2 *capsular glaucoma with pseudoexfoliation of lens (H40.1-)*

✓5th H25.0 Age-related incipient cataract

✓6th H25.01 Cortical age-related cataract

H25.011 Cortical age-related cataract, right eye A

H25.012 Cortical age-related cataract, left eye A

H25.013 Cortical age-related cataract, bilateral A

H25.019 Cortical age-related cataract, unspecified eye A

✓6th H25.03 Anterior subcapsular polar age-related cataract

H25.031 Anterior subcapsular polar age-related cataract, right eye A

H25.032 Anterior subcapsular polar age-related cataract, left eye A

H25.033 Anterior subcapsular polar age-related cataract, bilateral A

H25.039 Anterior subcapsular polar age-related cataract, unspecified eye A

✓6th H25.04 Posterior subcapsular polar age-related cataract

H25.041 Posterior subcapsular polar age-related cataract, right eye A

H25.042 Posterior subcapsular polar age-related cataract, left eye A

H25.043 Posterior subcapsular polar age-related cataract, bilateral A

H25.049 Posterior subcapsular polar age-related cataract, unspecified eye A

✓6th H25.09 Other age-related incipient cataract

Coronary age-related cataract

Punctate age-related cataract

Water clefts

H25.091 Other age-related incipient cataract, right eye A

H25.092 Other age-related incipient cataract, left eye A

H25.093 Other age-related incipient cataract, bilateral A

H25.099 Other age-related incipient cataract, unspecified eye A

✓5th H25.1 Age-related nuclear cataract

Cataracta brunescens

Nuclear sclerosis cataract

H25.10 Age-related nuclear cataract, unspecified eye A

H25.11 Age-related nuclear cataract, right eye A

H25.12 Age-related nuclear cataract, left eye A

H25.13 Age-related nuclear cataract, bilateral A

✓5th H25.2 Age-related cataract, morgagnian type

Age-related hypermature cataract

H25.20 Age-related cataract, morgagnian type, unspecified eye A

H25.21 Age-related cataract, morgagnian type, right eye A

H25.22 Age-related cataract, morgagnian type, left eye A

H25.23 Age-related cataract, morgagnian type, bilateral A

✓5th **H25.8 Other age-related cataract**

✓6th **H25.81 Combined forms of age-related cataract**

- **H25.811 Combined forms of age-related cataract, right eye** A
- **H25.812 Combined forms of age-related cataract, left eye** A
- **H25.813 Combined forms of age-related cataract, bilateral** A
- **H25.819 Combined forms of age-related cataract, unspecified eye** A

H25.89 Other age-related cataract A

H25.9 Unspecified age-related cataract A

✓4th **H26 Other cataract**

EXCLUDES 1 *congenital cataract (Q12.0)*

✓5th **H26.0 Infantile and juvenile cataract**

✓6th **H26.00 Unspecified infantile and juvenile cataract**

- **H26.001 Unspecified infantile and juvenile cataract, right eye** P
- **H26.002 Unspecified infantile and juvenile cataract, left eye** P
- **H26.003 Unspecified infantile and juvenile cataract, bilateral** P
- **H26.009 Unspecified infantile and juvenile cataract, unspecified eye** P

✓6th **H26.01 Infantile and juvenile cortical, lamellar, or zonular cataract**

- **H26.011 Infantile and juvenile cortical, lamellar, or zonular cataract, right eye** P
- **H26.012 Infantile and juvenile cortical, lamellar, or zonular cataract, left eye** P
- **H26.013 Infantile and juvenile cortical, lamellar, or zonular cataract, bilateral** P
- **H26.019 Infantile and juvenile cortical, lamellar, or zonular cataract, unspecified eye** P

✓6th **H26.03 Infantile and juvenile nuclear cataract**

- **H26.031 Infantile and juvenile nuclear cataract, right eye** P
- **H26.032 Infantile and juvenile nuclear cataract, left eye** P
- **H26.033 Infantile and juvenile nuclear cataract, bilateral** P
- **H26.039 Infantile and juvenile nuclear cataract, unspecified eye** P

✓6th **H26.04 Anterior subcapsular polar infantile and juvenile cataract**

- **H26.041 Anterior subcapsular polar infantile and juvenile cataract, right eye** P
- **H26.042 Anterior subcapsular polar infantile and juvenile cataract, left eye** P
- **H26.043 Anterior subcapsular polar infantile and juvenile cataract, bilateral** P
- **H26.049 Anterior subcapsular polar infantile and juvenile cataract, unspecified eye** P

✓6th **H26.05 Posterior subcapsular polar infantile and juvenile cataract**

- **H26.051 Posterior subcapsular polar infantile and juvenile cataract, right eye** P
- **H26.052 Posterior subcapsular polar infantile and juvenile cataract, left eye** P
- **H26.053 Posterior subcapsular polar infantile and juvenile cataract, bilateral** P
- **H26.059 Posterior subcapsular polar infantile and juvenile cataract, unspecified eye** P

✓6th **H26.06 Combined forms of infantile and juvenile cataract**

- **H26.061 Combined forms of infantile and juvenile cataract, right eye** P
- **H26.062 Combined forms of infantile and juvenile cataract, left eye** P
- **H26.063 Combined forms of infantile and juvenile cataract, bilateral** P
- **H26.069 Combined forms of infantile and juvenile cataract, unspecified eye** P

H26.09 Other infantile and juvenile cataract P

✓5th **H26.1 Traumatic cataract**

Use additional code (Chapter 20) to identify external cause

✓6th **H26.10 Unspecified traumatic cataract**

- **H26.101 Unspecified traumatic cataract, right eye**
- **H26.102 Unspecified traumatic cataract, left eye**
- **H26.103 Unspecified traumatic cataract, bilateral**
- **H26.109 Unspecified traumatic cataract, unspecified eye**

✓6th **H26.11 Localized traumatic opacities**

- **H26.111 Localized traumatic opacities, right eye**
- **H26.112 Localized traumatic opacities, left eye**
- **H26.113 Localized traumatic opacities, bilateral**
- **H26.119 Localized traumatic opacities, unspecified eye**

✓6th **H26.12 Partially resolved traumatic cataract**

- **H26.121 Partially resolved traumatic cataract, right eye**
- **H26.122 Partially resolved traumatic cataract, left eye**
- **H26.123 Partially resolved traumatic cataract, bilateral**
- **H26.129 Partially resolved traumatic cataract, unspecified eye**

✓6th **H26.13 Total traumatic cataract**

- **H26.131 Total traumatic cataract, right eye**
- **H26.132 Total traumatic cataract, left eye**
- **H26.133 Total traumatic cataract, bilateral**
- **H26.139 Total traumatic cataract, unspecified eye**

✓5th **H26.2 Complicated cataract**

H26.20 Unspecified complicated cataract

Cataracta complicata NOS

✓6th **H26.21 Cataract with neovascularization**

Code also associated condition, such as:
chronic iridocyclitis (H20.1-)

- **H26.211 Cataract with neovascularization, right eye**
- **H26.212 Cataract with neovascularization, left eye**
- **H26.213 Cataract with neovascularization, bilateral**
- **H26.219 Cataract with neovascularization, unspecified eye**

✓6th **H26.22 Cataract secondary to ocular disorders (degenerative) (inflammatory)**

Code also associated ocular disorder

- **H26.221 Cataract secondary to ocular disorders (degenerative) (inflammatory), right eye**
- **H26.222 Cataract secondary to ocular disorders (degenerative) (inflammatory), left eye**
- **H26.223 Cataract secondary to ocular disorders (degenerative) (inflammatory), bilateral**
- **H26.229 Cataract secondary to ocular disorders (degenerative) (inflammatory), unspecified eye**

✓6th **H26.23 Glaucomatous flecks (subcapsular)**

Code first underlying glaucoma (H40-H42)

- **H26.231 Glaucomatous flecks (subcapsular), right eye**
- **H26.232 Glaucomatous flecks (subcapsular), left eye**
- **H26.233 Glaucomatous flecks (subcapsular), bilateral**
- **H26.239 Glaucomatous flecks (subcapsular), unspecified eye**

✓5th **H26.3 Drug-induced cataract**

Toxic cataract

Use additional code for adverse effect, if applicable, to identify drug (T36-T50 with fifth or sixth character 5)

- **H26.30 Drug-induced cataract, unspecified eye**
- **H26.31 Drug-induced cataract, right eye**
- **H26.32 Drug-induced cataract, left eye**
- **H26.33 Drug-induced cataract, bilateral**

✓5th **H26.4 Secondary cataract**

H26.40 Unspecified secondary cataract

✓6th **H26.41 Soemmering's ring**

- **H26.411 Soemmering's ring, right eye**
- **H26.412 Soemmering's ring, left eye**

H26.413 Soemmering's ring, bilateral
H26.419 Soemmering's ring, unspecified eye

H26.49 Other secondary cataract
H26.491 Other secondary cataract, right eye
H26.492 Other secondary cataract, left eye
H26.493 Other secondary cataract, bilateral
H26.499 Other secondary cataract, unspecified eye

H26.8 Other specified cataract
H26.9 Unspecified cataract

H27 Other disorders of lens
EXCLUDES 1 *congenital lens malformations (Q12.-)*
mechanical complications of intraocular lens implant (T85.2)
pseudophakia (Z96.1)

H27.0 Aphakia
Acquired absence of lens
Acquired aphakia
Aphakia due to trauma
EXCLUDES 1 *cataract extraction status (Z98.4-)*
congenital absence of lens (Q12.3)
congenital aphakia (Q12.3)

H27.00 Aphakia, unspecified eye
H27.01 Aphakia, right eye
H27.02 Aphakia, left eye
H27.03 Aphakia, bilateral

H27.1 Dislocation of lens
H27.10 Unspecified dislocation of lens
H27.11 Subluxation of lens
H27.111 Subluxation of lens, right eye
H27.112 Subluxation of lens, left eye
H27.113 Subluxation of lens, bilateral
H27.119 Subluxation of lens, unspecified eye
H27.12 Anterior dislocation of lens
H27.121 Anterior dislocation of lens, right eye
H27.122 Anterior dislocation of lens, left eye
H27.123 Anterior dislocation of lens, bilateral
H27.129 Anterior dislocation of lens, unspecified eye
H27.13 Posterior dislocation of lens
H27.131 Posterior dislocation of lens, right eye
H27.132 Posterior dislocation of lens, left eye
H27.133 Posterior dislocation of lens, bilateral
H27.139 Posterior dislocation of lens, unspecified eye

H27.8 Other specified disorders of lens
H27.9 Unspecified disorder of lens

H28 Cataract in diseases classified elsewhere
Code first underlying disease, such as:
hypoparathyroidism (E20.-)
myotonia (G71.1-)
myxedema (E03.-)
protein-calorie malnutrition (E40-E46)
EXCLUDES 1 *cataract in diabetes mellitus (E08.36, E09.36, E10.36, E11.36, E13.36)*

Disorders of choroid and retina (H30-H36)

H30 Chorioretinal inflammation

CC Excl: For CC codes in category H30, unless otherwise noted: H30.001-H30.93

H30.0 Focal chorioretinal inflammation
Focal chorioretinitis
Focal choroiditis
Focal retinitis
Focal retinochoroiditis

H30.00 Unspecified focal chorioretinal inflammation
Focal chorioretinitis NOS
Focal choroiditis NOS
Focal retinitis NOS
Focal retinochoroiditis NOS
H30.001 Unspecified focal chorioretinal inflammation, right eye
H30.002 Unspecified focal chorioretinal inflammation, left eye
H30.003 Unspecified focal chorioretinal inflammation, bilateral
H30.009 Unspecified focal chorioretinal inflammation, unspecified eye

H30.01 Focal chorioretinal inflammation, juxtapapillary
H30.011 Focal chorioretinal inflammation, juxtapapillary, right eye
H30.012 Focal chorioretinal inflammation, juxtapapillary, left eye
H30.013 Focal chorioretinal inflammation, juxtapapillary, bilateral
H30.019 Focal chorioretinal inflammation, juxtapapillary, unspecified eye

H30.02 Focal chorioretinal inflammation of posterior pole
H30.021 Focal chorioretinal inflammation of posterior pole, right eye
H30.022 Focal chorioretinal inflammation of posterior pole, left eye
H30.023 Focal chorioretinal inflammation of posterior pole, bilateral
H30.029 Focal chorioretinal inflammation of posterior pole, unspecified eye

H30.03 Focal chorioretinal inflammation, peripheral
H30.031 Focal chorioretinal inflammation, peripheral, right eye
H30.032 Focal chorioretinal inflammation, peripheral, left eye
H30.033 Focal chorioretinal inflammation, peripheral, bilateral
H30.039 Focal chorioretinal inflammation, peripheral, unspecified eye

H30.04 Focal chorioretinal inflammation, macular or paramacular
H30.041 Focal chorioretinal inflammation, macular or paramacular, right eye
H30.042 Focal chorioretinal inflammation, macular or paramacular, left eye
H30.043 Focal chorioretinal inflammation, macular or paramacular, bilateral
H30.049 Focal chorioretinal inflammation, macular or paramacular, unspecified eye

H30.1 Disseminated chorioretinal inflammation
Disseminated chorioretinitis
Disseminated choroiditis
Disseminated retinitis
Disseminated retinochoroiditis
EXCLUDES 2 *exudative retinopathy (H35.02-)*

H30.10 Unspecified disseminated chorioretinal inflammation
Disseminated chorioretinitis NOS
Disseminated choroiditis NOS
Disseminated retinitis NOS
Disseminated retinochoroiditis NOS
H30.101 Unspecified disseminated chorioretinal inflammation, right eye CC
H30.102 Unspecified disseminated chorioretinal inflammation, left eye CC
H30.103 Unspecified disseminated chorioretinal inflammation, bilateral CC
H30.109 Unspecified disseminated chorioretinal inflammation, unspecified eye CC

H30.11 Disseminated chorioretinal inflammation of posterior pole
H30.111 Disseminated chorioretinal inflammation of posterior pole, right eye CC
H30.112 Disseminated chorioretinal inflammation of posterior pole, left eye CC
H30.113 Disseminated chorioretinal inflammation of posterior pole, bilateral CC
H30.119 Disseminated chorioretinal inflammation of posterior pole, unspecified eye CC

H30.12 Disseminated chorioretinal inflammation, peripheral
H30.121 Disseminated chorioretinal inflammation, peripheral right eye CC

H30.122 Disseminated chorioretinal inflammation, peripheral, left eye CC
H30.123 Disseminated chorioretinal inflammation, peripheral, bilateral CC
H30.129 Disseminated chorioretinal inflammation, peripheral, unspecified eye CC

✓6th H30.13 Disseminated chorioretinal inflammation, generalized
H30.131 Disseminated chorioretinal inflammation, generalized, right eye CC
H30.132 Disseminated chorioretinal inflammation, generalized, left eye CC
H30.133 Disseminated chorioretinal inflammation, generalized, bilateral CC
H30.139 Disseminated chorioretinal inflammation, generalized, unspecified eye CC

✓6th H30.14 Acute posterior multifocal placoid pigment epitheliopathy
H30.141 Acute posterior multifocal placoid pigment epitheliopathy, right eye CC
H30.142 Acute posterior multifocal placoid pigment epitheliopathy, left eye CC
H30.143 Acute posterior multifocal placoid pigment epitheliopathy, bilateral CC
H30.149 Acute posterior multifocal placoid pigment epitheliopathy, unspecified eye CC

✓5th H30.2 Posterior cyclitis
Pars planitis
H30.20 Posterior cyclitis, unspecified eye
H30.21 Posterior cyclitis, right eye
H30.22 Posterior cyclitis, left eye
H30.23 Posterior cyclitis, bilateral

✓5th H30.8 Other chorioretinal inflammations

✓6th H30.81 Harada's disease
H30.811 Harada's disease, right eye
H30.812 Harada's disease, left eye
H30.813 Harada's disease, bilateral
H30.819 Harada's disease, unspecified eye

✓6th H30.89 Other chorioretinal inflammations
H30.891 Other chorioretinal inflammations, right eye CC
H30.892 Other chorioretinal inflammations, left eye CC
H30.893 Other chorioretinal inflammations, bilateral CC
H30.899 Other chorioretinal inflammations, unspecified eye CC

✓5th H30.9 Unspecified chorioretinal inflammation
Chorioretinitis NOS
Choroiditis NOS
Neuroretinitis NOS
Retinitis NOS
Retinochoroiditis NOS
H30.90 Unspecified chorioretinal inflammation, unspecified eye CC
H30.91 Unspecified chorioretinal inflammation, right eye CC
H30.92 Unspecified chorioretinal inflammation, left eye CC
H30.93 Unspecified chorioretinal inflammation, bilateral CC

✓4th H31 Other disorders of choroid

CC Excl: For CC codes in category H31, unless otherwise noted: H31.301-H32

✓5th H31.0 Chorioretinal scars
EXCLUDES 2 *postsurgical chorioretinal scars (H59.81-)*

✓6th H31.00 Unspecified chorioretinal scars
H31.001 Unspecified chorioretinal scars, right eye
H31.002 Unspecified chorioretinal scars, left eye
H31.003 Unspecified chorioretinal scars, bilateral
H31.009 Unspecified chorioretinal scars, unspecified eye

✓6th H31.01 Macula scars of posterior pole (postinflammatory) (post-traumatic)
EXCLUDES 1 *postprocedural choriorentinal scar (H59.81-)*
H31.011 Macula scars of posterior pole (postinflammatory) (post-traumatic), right eye
H31.012 Macula scars of posterior pole (postinflammatory) (post-traumatic), left eye
H31.013 Macula scars of posterior pole (postinflammatory) (post-traumatic), bilateral
H31.019 Macula scars of posterior pole (postinflammatory) (post-traumatic), unspecified eye

✓6th H31.02 Solar retinopathy
H31.021 Solar retinopathy, right eye
H31.022 Solar retinopathy, left eye
H31.023 Solar retinopathy, bilateral
H31.029 Solar retinopathy, unspecified eye

✓6th H31.09 Other chorioretinal scars
H31.091 Other chorioretinal scars, right eye
H31.092 Other chorioretinal scars, left eye
H31.093 Other chorioretinal scars, bilateral
H31.099 Other chorioretinal scars, unspecified eye

✓5th H31.1 Choroidal degeneration
EXCLUDES 2 *angioid streaks of macula (H35.33)*

✓6th H31.10 Unspecified choroidal degeneration
Choroidal sclerosis NOS
H31.101 Choroidal degeneration, unspecified, right eye
H31.102 Choroidal degeneration, unspecified, left eye
H31.103 Choroidal degeneration, unspecified, bilateral
H31.109 Choroidal degeneration, unspecified, unspecified eye

✓6th H31.11 Age-related choroidal atrophy
H31.111 Age-related choroidal atrophy, right eye A
H31.112 Age-related choroidal atrophy, left eye A
H31.113 Age-related choroidal atrophy, bilateral A
H31.119 Age-related choroidal atrophy, unspecified eye A

✓6th H31.12 Diffuse secondary atrophy of choroid
H31.121 Diffuse secondary atrophy of choroid, right eye
H31.122 Diffuse secondary atrophy of choroid, left eye
H31.123 Diffuse secondary atrophy of choroid, bilateral
H31.129 Diffuse secondary atrophy of choroid, unspecified eye

✓5th H31.2 Hereditary choroidal dystrophy
EXCLUDES 2 *hyperornithinemia (E72.4)*
ornithinemia (E72.4)
H31.20 Hereditary choroidal dystrophy, unspecified
H31.21 Choroideremia
H31.22 Choroidal dystrophy (central areolar) (generalized) (peripapillary)
H31.23 Gyrate atrophy, choroid
H31.29 Other hereditary choroidal dystrophy

✓5th H31.3 Choroidal hemorrhage and rupture

✓6th H31.30 Unspecified choroidal hemorrhage
H31.301 Unspecified choroidal hemorrhage, right eye
H31.302 Unspecified choroidal hemorrhage, left eye
H31.303 Unspecified choroidal hemorrhage, bilateral
H31.309 Unspecified choroidal hemorrhage, unspecified eye

✓6th H31.31 Expulsive choroidal hemorrhage
H31.311 Expulsive choroidal hemorrhage, right eye
H31.312 Expulsive choroidal hemorrhage, left eye

DRAFT

H31.313 **Expulsive choroidal hemorrhage, bilateral**
H31.319 **Expulsive choroidal hemorrhage, unspecified eye**

✓6th **H31.32** **Choroidal rupture**
H31.321 **Choroidal rupture, right eye** CC
H31.322 **Choroidal rupture, left eye** CC
H31.323 **Choroidal rupture, bilateral** CC
H31.329 **Choroidal rupture, unspecified eye** CC

✓5th **H31.4** **Choroidal detachment**

✓6th **H31.40** **Unspecified choroidal detachment**
H31.401 **Unspecified choroidal detachment, right eye** CC
H31.402 **Unspecified choroidal detachment, left eye** CC
H31.403 **Unspecified choroidal detachment, bilateral** CC
H31.409 **Unspecified choroidal detachment, unspecified eye** CC

✓6th **H31.41** **Hemorrhagic choroidal detachment**
H31.411 **Hemorrhagic choroidal detachment, right eye** CC
H31.412 **Hemorrhagic choroidal detachment, left eye** CC
H31.413 **Hemorrhagic choroidal detachment, bilateral** CC
H31.419 **Hemorrhagic choroidal detachment, unspecified eye** CC

✓6th **H31.42** **Serous choroidal detachment**
H31.421 **Serous choroidal detachment, right eye** CC
H31.422 **Serous choroidal detachment, left eye** CC
H31.423 **Serous choroidal detachment, bilateral** CC
H31.429 **Serous choroidal detachment, unspecified eye** CC

H31.8 **Other specified disorders of choroid**
H31.9 **Unspecified disorder of choroid**

H32 ***Chorioretinal disorders in diseases classified elsewhere***

Code first underlying disease, such as:
congenital toxoplasmosis (P37.1)
histoplasmosis (B39.-)
leprosy (A30.-)

EXCLUDES 1 *chorioretinitis (in):*
toxoplasmosis (acquired) (B58.01)
tuberculosis (A18.53)

✓4th **H33** **Retinal detachments and breaks**

CC Excl: For CC codes in category H33, unless otherwise noted: H33.001-H33.119, H33.191-H33.8, H35.70-H35.739

EXCLUDES 1 *detachment of retinal pigment epithelium (H35.72-, H35.73-)*

✓5th **H33.0** **Retinal detachment with retinal break**
Rhegmatogenous retinal detachment
EXCLUDES 1 *serous retinal detachment (without retinal break) (H33.2-)*

✓6th **H33.00** **Unspecified retinal detachment with retinal break**
H33.001 **Unspecified retinal detachment with retinal break, right eye**
H33.002 **Unspecified retinal detachment with retinal break, left eye**
H33.003 **Unspecified retinal detachment with retinal break, bilateral**
H33.009 **Unspecified retinal detachment with retinal break, unspecified eye**

✓6th **H33.01** **Retinal detachment with single break**
H33.011 **Retinal detachment with single break, right eye**
H33.012 **Retinal detachment with single break, left eye**
H33.013 **Retinal detachment with single break, bilateral**
H33.019 **Retinal detachment with single break, unspecified eye**

✓6th **H33.02** **Retinal detachment with multiple breaks**
H33.021 **Retinal detachment with multiple breaks, right eye**
H33.022 **Retinal detachment with multiple breaks, left eye**
H33.023 **Retinal detachment with multiple breaks, bilateral**
H33.029 **Retinal detachment with multiple breaks, unspecified eye**

✓6th **H33.03** **Retinal detachment with giant retinal tear**
H33.031 **Retinal detachment with giant retinal tear, right eye**
H33.032 **Retinal detachment with giant retinal tear, left eye**
H33.033 **Retinal detachment with giant retinal tear, bilateral**
H33.039 **Retinal detachment with giant retinal tear, unspecified eye**

✓6th **H33.04** **Retinal detachment with retinal dialysis**
H33.041 **Retinal detachment with retinal dialysis, right eye**
H33.042 **Retinal detachment with retinal dialysis, left eye**
H33.043 **Retinal detachment with retinal dialysis, bilateral**
H33.049 **Retinal detachment with retinal dialysis, unspecified eye**

✓6th **H33.05** **Total retinal detachment**
H33.051 **Total retinal detachment, right eye**
H33.052 **Total retinal detachment, left eye**
H33.053 **Total retinal detachment, bilateral**
H33.059 **Total retinal detachment, unspecified eye**

✓5th **H33.1** **Retinoschisis and retinal cysts**
EXCLUDES 1 *congenital retinoschisis (Q14.1)*
microcystoid degeneration of retina (H35.42-)

✓6th **H33.10** **Unspecified retinoschisis**
H33.101 **Unspecified retinoschisis, right eye**
H33.102 **Unspecified retinoschisis, left eye**
H33.103 **Unspecified retinoschisis, bilateral**
H33.109 **Unspecified retinoschisis, unspecified eye**

✓6th **H33.11** **Cyst of ora serrata**
H33.111 **Cyst of ora serrata, right eye**
H33.112 **Cyst of ora serrata, left eye**
H33.113 **Cyst of ora serrata, bilateral**
H33.119 **Cyst of ora serrata, unspecified eye**

✓6th **H33.12** **Parasitic cyst of retina**

CC Excl: For CC codes in subcategory H33.12, unless otherwise noted: H20.051-H20.059, H21.331-H21.339, H33.121-H33.129, H44.001-H44.029, H44.121-H44.129, H44.19

H33.121 **Parasitic cyst of retina, right eye** CC
H33.122 **Parasitic cyst of retina, left eye** CC
H33.123 **Parasitic cyst of retina, bilateral** CC
H33.129 **Parasitic cyst of retina, unspecified eye** CC

✓6th **H33.19** **Other retinoschisis and retinal cysts**
Pseudocyst of retina
H33.191 **Other retinoschisis and retinal cysts, right eye**
H33.192 **Other retinoschisis and retinal cysts, left eye**
H33.193 **Other retinoschisis and retinal cysts, bilateral**
H33.199 **Other retinoschisis and retinal cysts, unspecified eye**

✓5th **H33.2** **Serous retinal detachment**
Retinal detachment NOS
Retinal detachment without retinal break
EXCLUDES 1 *central serous chorioretinopathy (H35.71-)*

H33.20 **Serous retinal detachment, unspecified eye** CC
H33.21 **Serous retinal detachment, right eye** CC
H33.22 **Serous retinal detachment, left eye** CC
H33.23 **Serous retinal detachment, bilateral** CC

✓5th **H33.3 Retinal breaks without detachment**

EXCLUDES 1 *chorioretinal scars after surgery for detachment (H59.81-)*
peripheral retinal degeneration without break (H35.4-)

✓6th **H33.3Ø Unspecified retinal break**

H33.3Ø1 Unspecified retinal break, right eye
H33.3Ø2 Unspecified retinal break, left eye
H33.3Ø3 Unspecified retinal break, bilateral
H33.3Ø9 Unspecified retinal break, unspecified eye

✓6th **H33.31 Horseshoe tear of retina without detachment**

Operculum of retina without detachment

H33.311 Horseshoe tear of retina without detachment, right eye
H33.312 Horseshoe tear of retina without detachment, left eye
H33.313 Horseshoe tear of retina without detachment, bilateral
H33.319 Horseshoe tear of retina without detachment, unspecified eye

✓6th **H33.32 Round hole of retina without detachment**

H33.321 Round hole, right eye
H33.322 Round hole, left eye
H33.323 Round hole, bilateral
H33.329 Round hole, unspecified eye

✓6th **H33.33 Multiple defects of retina without detachment**

H33.331 Multiple defects of retina without detachment, right eye
H33.332 Multiple defects of retina without detachment, left eye
H33.333 Multiple defects of retina without detachment, bilateral
H33.339 Multiple defects of retina without detachment, unspecified eye

✓5th **H33.4 Traction detachment of retina**

Proliferative vitreo-retinopathy with retinal detachment

H33.4Ø Traction detachment of retina, unspecified eye CC
H33.41 Traction detachment of retina, right eye CC
H33.42 Traction detachment of retina, left eye CC
H33.43 Traction detachment of retina, bilateral CC

H33.8 Other retinal detachments CC

✓4th **H34 Retinal vascular occlusions**

CC Excl: For CC codes in category H34, unless otherwise noted:
G45.3, H34.ØØ-H34.9

EXCLUDES 1 *amaurosis fugax (G45.3)*

✓5th **H34.Ø Transient retinal artery occlusion**

H34.ØØ Transient retinal artery occlusion, unspecified eye CC
H34.Ø1 Transient retinal artery occlusion, right eye CC
H34.Ø2 Transient retinal artery occlusion, left eye CC
H34.Ø3 Transient retinal artery occlusion, bilateral CC

✓5th **H34.1 Central retinal artery occlusion**

H34.1Ø Central retinal artery occlusion, unspecified eye CC
H34.11 Central retinal artery occlusion, right eye CC
H34.12 Central retinal artery occlusion, left eye CC
H34.13 Central retinal artery occlusion, bilateral CC

✓5th **H34.2 Other retinal artery occlusions**

✓6th **H34.21 Partial retinal artery occlusion**

Hollenhorst's plaque
Retinal microembolism

H34.211 Partial retinal artery occlusion, right eye CC
H34.212 Partial retinal artery occlusion, left eye CC
H34.213 Partial retinal artery occlusion, bilateral CC
H34.219 Partial retinal artery occlusion, unspecified eye CC

✓6th **H34.23 Retinal artery branch occlusion**

H34.231 Retinal artery branch occlusion, right eye CC
H34.232 Retinal artery branch occlusion, left eye CC
H34.233 Retinal artery branch occlusion, bilateral CC
H34.239 Retinal artery branch occlusion, unspecified eye CC

✓5th **H34.8 Other retinal vascular occlusions**

✓6th **H34.81 Central retinal vein occlusion**

H34.811 Central retinal vein occlusion, right eye CC
H34.812 Central retinal vein occlusion, left eye CC
H34.813 Central retinal vein occlusion, bilateral CC
H34.819 Central retinal vein occlusion, unspecified eye CC

✓6th **H34.82 Venous engorgement**

Incipient retinal vein occlusion
Partial retinal vein occlusion

H34.821 Venous engorgement, right eye
H34.822 Venous engorgement, left eye
H34.823 Venous engorgement, bilateral
H34.829 Venous engorgement, unspecified eye

✓6th **H34.83 Tributary (branch) retinal vein occlusion**

H34.831 Tributary (branch) retinal vein occlusion, right eye
H34.832 Tributary (branch) retinal vein occlusion, left eye
H34.833 Tributary (branch) retinal vein occlusion, bilateral
H34.839 Tributary (branch) retinal vein occlusion, unspecified eye

H34.9 Unspecified retinal vascular occlusion CC

✓4th **H35 Other retinal disorders**

EXCLUDES 2 *diabetic retinal disorders (EØ8.311- EØ8.359, EØ9.311- EØ9.359, E1Ø.311- E1Ø.359, E11.311- E11.359, E13.311- E13.359)*

✓5th **H35.Ø Background retinopathy and retinal vascular changes**

Code also any associated hypertension (I1Ø.-)

H35.ØØ Unspecified background retinopathy

✓6th **H35.Ø1 Changes in retinal vascular appearance**

Retinal vascular sheathing

H35.Ø11 Changes in retinal vascular appearance, right eye
H35.Ø12 Changes in retinal vascular appearance, left eye
H35.Ø13 Changes in retinal vascular appearance, bilateral
H35.Ø19 Changes in retinal vascular appearance, unspecified eye

✓6th **H35.Ø2 Exudative retinopathy**

Coats retinopathy

H35.Ø21 Exudative retinopathy, right eye
H35.Ø22 Exudative retinopathy, left eye
H35.Ø23 Exudative retinopathy, bilateral
H35.Ø29 Exudative retinopathy, unspecified eye

✓6th **H35.Ø3 Hypertensive retinopathy**

H35.Ø31 Hypertensive retinopathy, right eye
H35.Ø32 Hypertensive retinopathy, left eye
H35.Ø33 Hypertensive retinopathy, bilateral
H35.Ø39 Hypertensive retinopathy, unspecified eye

✓6th **H35.Ø4 Retinal micro-aneurysms, unspecified**

H35.Ø41 Retinal micro-aneurysms, unspecified, right eye
H35.Ø42 Retinal micro-aneurysms, unspecified, left eye
H35.Ø43 Retinal micro-aneurysms, unspecified, bilateral
H35.Ø49 Retinal micro-aneurysms, unspecified, unspecified eye

✓6th **H35.Ø5 Retinal neovascularization, unspecified**

H35.Ø51 Retinal neovascularization, unspecified, right eye
H35.Ø52 Retinal neovascularization, unspecified, left eye
H35.Ø53 Retinal neovascularization, unspecified, bilateral
H35.Ø59 Retinal neovascularization, unspecified, unspecified eye

√6th H35.06 Retinal vasculitis
Eales disease
Retinal perivasculitis
H35.061 Retinal vasculitis, right eye
H35.062 Retinal vasculitis, left eye
H35.063 Retinal vasculitis, bilateral
H35.069 Retinal vasculitis, unspecified eye
√6th H35.07 Retinal telangiectasis
H35.071 Retinal telangiectasis, right eye
H35.072 Retinal telangiectasis, left eye
H35.073 Retinal telangiectasis, bilateral
H35.079 Retinal telangiectasis, unspecified eye
H35.09 Other intraretinal microvascular abnormalities
Retinal varices
√5th H35.1 Retinopathy of prematurity
√6th H35.10 Retinopathy of prematurity, unspecified
Retinopathy of prematurity NOS
H35.101 Retinopathy of prematurity, unspecified, right eye
H35.102 Retinopathy of prematurity, unspecified, left eye
H35.103 Retinopathy of prematurity, unspecified, bilateral
H35.109 Retinopathy of prematurity, unspecified, unspecified eye
√6th H35.11 Retinopathy of prematurity, stage 0
H35.111 Retinopathy of prematurity, stage 0, right eye
H35.112 Retinopathy of prematurity, stage 0, left eye
H35.113 Retinopathy of prematurity, stage 0, bilateral
H35.119 Retinopathy of prematurity, stage 0, unspecified eye
√6th H35.12 Retinopathy of prematurity, stage 1
H35.121 Retinopathy of prematurity, stage 1, right eye
H35.122 Retinopathy of prematurity, stage 1, left eye
H35.123 Retinopathy of prematurity, stage 1, bilateral
H35.129 Retinopathy of prematurity, stage 1, unspecified eye
√6th H35.13 Retinopathy of prematurity, stage 2
H35.131 Retinopathy of prematurity, stage 2, right eye
H35.132 Retinopathy of prematurity, stage 2, left eye
H35.133 Retinopathy of prematurity, stage 2, bilateral
H35.139 Retinopathy of prematurity, stage 2, unspecified eye
√6th H35.14 Retinopathy of prematurity, stage 3
H35.141 Retinopathy of prematurity, stage 3, right eye
H35.142 Retinopathy of prematurity, stage 3, left eye
H35.143 Retinopathy of prematurity, stage 3, bilateral
H35.149 Retinopathy of prematurity, stage 3, unspecified eye
√6th H35.15 Retinopathy of prematurity, stage 4
H35.151 Retinopathy of prematurity, stage 4, right eye
H35.152 Retinopathy of prematurity, stage 4, left eye
H35.153 Retinopathy of prematurity, stage 4, bilateral
H35.159 Retinopathy of prematurity, stage 4, unspecified eye
√6th H35.16 Retinopathy of prematurity, stage 5
H35.161 Retinopathy of prematurity, stage 5, right eye
H35.162 Retinopathy of prematurity, stage 5, left eye
H35.163 Retinopathy of prematurity, stage 5, bilateral
H35.169 Retinopathy of prematurity, stage 5, unspecified eye
√6th H35.17 Retrolental fibroplasia
H35.171 Retrolental fibroplasia, right eye
H35.172 Retrolental fibroplasia, left eye
H35.173 Retrolental fibroplasia, bilateral
H35.179 Retrolental fibroplasia, unspecified eye
√5th H35.2 Other non-diabetic proliferative retinopathy
Proliferative vitreo-retinopathy
EXCLUDES 1 *proliferative vitreo-retinopathy with retinal detachment (H33.4-)*
H35.20 Other non-diabetic proliferative retinopathy, unspecified eye
H35.21 Other non-diabetic proliferative retinopathy, right eye
H35.22 Other non-diabetic proliferative retinopathy, left eye
H35.23 Other non-diabetic proliferative retinopathy, bilateral
√5th H35.3 Degeneration of macula and posterior pole
H35.30 Unspecified macular degeneration A
Age-related macular degeneration
H35.31 Nonexudative age-related macular degeneration A
Atrophic age-related macular degeneration
H35.32 Exudative age-related macular degeneration A
H35.33 Angioid streaks of macula
√6th H35.34 Macular cyst, hole, or pseudohole
H35.341 Macular cyst, hole, or pseudohole, right eye
H35.342 Macular cyst, hole, or pseudohole, left eye
H35.343 Macular cyst, hole, or pseudohole, bilateral
H35.349 Macular cyst, hole, or pseudohole, unspecified eye
√6th H35.35 Cystoid macular degeneration
EXCLUDES 1 *cystoid macular edema following cataract surgery (H59.03-)*
H35.351 Cystoid macular degeneration, right eye
H35.352 Cystoid macular degeneration, left eye
H35.353 Cystoid macular degeneration, bilateral
H35.359 Cystoid macular degeneration, unspecified eye
√6th H35.36 Drusen (degenerative) of macula
H35.361 Drusen (degenerative) of macula, right eye
H35.362 Drusen (degenerative) of macula, left eye
H35.363 Drusen (degenerative) of macula, bilateral
H35.369 Drusen (degenerative) of macula, unspecified eye
√6th H35.37 Puckering of macula
H35.371 Puckering of macula, right eye
H35.372 Puckering of macula, left eye
H35.373 Puckering of macula, bilateral
H35.379 Puckering of macula, unspecified eye
√6th H35.38 Toxic maculopathy
Code first poisoning due to drug or toxin, if applicable (T36-T65 with fifth or sixth character 1-4 or 6)
Use additional code for adverse effect, if applicable, to identify drug (T36-T50 with fifth or sixth character 5)
H35.381 Toxic maculopathy, right eye
H35.382 Toxic maculopathy, left eye
H35.383 Toxic maculopathy, bilateral
H35.389 Toxic maculopathy, unspecified eye
√5th H35.4 Peripheral retinal degeneration
EXCLUDES 1 *hereditary retinal degeneration (dystrophy) (H35.5-)*
peripheral retinal degeneration with retinal break (H33.3-)
H35.40 Unspecified peripheral retinal degeneration
√6th H35.41 Lattice degeneration of retina
Palisade degeneration of retina
H35.411 Lattice degeneration of retina, right eye
H35.412 Lattice degeneration of retina, left eye
H35.413 Lattice degeneration of retina, bilateral

H35.419 **Lattice degeneration of retina, unspecified eye**

✓6th H35.42 **Microcystoid degeneration of retina**

H35.421 **Microcystoid degeneration of retina, right eye**

H35.422 **Microcystoid degeneration of retina, left eye**

H35.423 **Microcystoid degeneration of retina, bilateral**

H35.429 **Microcystoid degeneration of retina, unspecified eye**

✓6th H35.43 **Paving stone degeneration of retina**

H35.431 **Paving stone degeneration of retina, right eye**

H35.432 **Paving stone degeneration of retina, left eye**

H35.433 **Paving stone degeneration of retina, bilateral**

H35.439 **Paving stone degeneration of retina, unspecified eye**

✓6th H35.44 **Age-related reticular degeneration of retina**

H35.441 **Age-related reticular degeneration of retina, right eye** A

H35.442 **Age-related reticular degeneration of retina, left eye** A

H35.443 **Age-related reticular degeneration of retina, bilateral** A

H35.449 **Age-related reticular degeneration of retina, unspecified eye** A

✓6th H35.45 **Secondary pigmentary degeneration**

H35.451 **Secondary pigmentary degeneration, right eye**

H35.452 **Secondary pigmentary degeneration, left eye**

H35.453 **Secondary pigmentary degeneration, bilateral**

H35.459 **Secondary pigmentary degeneration, unspecified eye**

✓6th H35.46 **Secondary vitreoretinal degeneration**

H35.461 **Secondary vitreoretinal degeneration, right eye**

H35.462 **Secondary vitreoretinal degeneration, left eye**

H35.463 **Secondary vitreoretinal degeneration, bilateral**

H35.469 **Secondary vitreoretinal degeneration, unspecified eye**

✓5th H35.5 **Hereditary retinal dystrophy**

EXCLUDES 1 *dystrophies primarily involving Bruch's membrane (H31.1-)*

H35.5Ø **Unspecified hereditary retinal dystrophy**

H35.51 **Vitreoretinal dystrophy**

H35.52 **Pigmentary retinal dystrophy**

Albipunctate retinal dystrophy
Retinitis pigmentosa
Tapetoretinal dystrophy

H35.53 **Other dystrophies primarily involving the sensory retina**

Stargardt's disease

H35.54 **Dystrophies primarily involving the retinal pigment epithelium**

Vitelliform retinal dystrophy

✓5th H35.6 **Retinal hemorrhage**

H35.6Ø **Retinal hemorrhage, unspecified eye**

H35.61 **Retinal hemorrhage, right eye**

H35.62 **Retinal hemorrhage, left eye**

H35.63 **Retinal hemorrhage, bilateral**

✓5th H35.7 **Separation of retinal layers**

EXCLUDES 1 *retinal detachment (serous) (H33.2-)*
rhegmatogenous retinal detachment (H33.Ø-)

CC Excl: For CC codes in subcategory H35.7, unless otherwise noted: H33.ØØ1-H33.119, H33.191-H33.8, H35.7Ø-H35.739

H35.7Ø **Unspecified separation of retinal layers** CC

✓6th H35.71 **Central serous chorioretinopathy**

H35.711 **Central serous chorioretinopathy, right eye**

H35.712 **Central serous chorioretinopathy, left eye**

H35.713 **Central serous chorioretinopathy, bilateral**

H35.719 **Central serous chorioretinopathy, unspecified eye**

✓6th H35.72 **Serous detachment of retinal pigment epithelium**

H35.721 **Serous detachment of retinal pigment epithelium, right eye** CC

H35.722 **Serous detachment of retinal pigment epithelium, left eye** CC

H35.723 **Serous detachment of retinal pigment epithelium, bilateral** CC

H35.729 **Serous detachment of retinal pigment epithelium, unspecified eye** CC

✓6th H35.73 **Hemorrhagic detachment of retinal pigment epithelium**

H35.731 **Hemorrhagic detachment of retinal pigment epithelium, right eye** CC

H35.732 **Hemorrhagic detachment of retinal pigment epithelium, left eye** CC

H35.733 **Hemorrhagic detachment of retinal pigment epithelium, bilateral** CC

H35.739 **Hemorrhagic detachment of retinal pigment epithelium, unspecified eye** CC

✓5th H35.8 **Other specified retinal disorders**

EXCLUDES 2 *retinal hemorrhage (H35.6-)*

H35.81 **Retinal edema**

Retinal cotton wool spots

H35.82 **Retinal ischemia** CC

CC Excl: H35.6Ø-H35.63, H35.81-H35.89

H35.89 **Other specified retinal disorders**

H35.9 **Unspecified retinal disorder**

H36 Retinal disorders in diseases classified elsewhere

Code first underlying disease, such as:
lipid storage disorders (E75.-)
sickle-cell disorders (D57.-)

EXCLUDES 1 *arteriosclerotic retinopathy (H35.Ø-)*
diabetic retinopathy (EØ8.3-, EØ9.3-, E1Ø.3-, E11.3-, E13.3-)

Glaucoma (H4Ø-H42)

✓4th **H4Ø Glaucoma**

EXCLUDES 1 *absolute glaucoma (H44.51-)*
congenital glaucoma (Q15.Ø)
traumatic glaucoma due to birth injury (P15.3)

✓5th H4Ø.Ø **Glaucoma suspect**

✓6th H4Ø.ØØ **Preglaucoma, unspecified**

H4Ø.ØØ1 **Preglaucoma, unspecified, right eye**

H4Ø.ØØ2 **Preglaucoma, unspecified, left eye**

H4Ø.ØØ3 **Preglaucoma, unspecified, bilateral**

H4Ø.ØØ9 **Preglaucoma, unspecified, unspecified eye**

✓6th H4Ø.Ø1 **Open angle with borderline findings, low risk**

Open angle, low risk

H4Ø.Ø11 **Open angle with borderline findings, low risk, right eye**

H4Ø.Ø12 **Open angle with borderline findings, low risk, left eye**

H4Ø.Ø13 **Open angle with borderline findings, low risk, bilateral**

H4Ø.Ø19 **Open angle with borderline findings, low risk, unspecified eye**

✓6th H4Ø.Ø2 **Open angle with borderline findings, high risk**

Open angle, high risk

H4Ø.Ø21 **Open angle with borderline findings, high risk, right eye**

H4Ø.Ø22 **Open angle with borderline findings, high risk, left eye**

H4Ø.Ø23 **Open angle with borderline findings, high risk, bilateral**

H4Ø.Ø29 **Open angle with borderline findings, high risk, unspecified eye**

√6th **H40.03 Anatomical narrow angle**
Primary angle closure suspect
- **H40.031 Anatomical narrow angle, right eye**
- **H40.032 Anatomical narrow angle, left eye**
- **H40.033 Anatomical narrow angle, bilateral**
- **H40.039 Anatomical narrow angle, unspecified eye**

√6th **H40.04 Steroid responder**
- **H40.041 Steroid responder, right eye**
- **H40.042 Steroid responder, left eye**
- **H40.043 Steroid responder, bilateral**
- **H40.049 Steroid responder, unspecified eye**

√6th **H40.05 Ocular hypertension**
- **H40.051 Ocular hypertension, right eye**
- **H40.052 Ocular hypertension, left eye**
- **H40.053 Ocular hypertension, bilateral**
- **H40.059 Ocular hypertension, unspecified eye**

√6th **H40.06 Primary angle closure without glaucoma damage**
- **H40.061 Primary angle closure without glaucoma damage, right eye**
- **H40.062 Primary angle closure without glaucoma damage, left eye**
- **H40.063 Primary angle closure without glaucoma damage, bilateral**
- **H40.069 Primary angle closure without glaucoma damage, unspecified eye**

√5th **H40.1 Open-angle glaucoma**

One of the following 7th characters is to be assigned to each code in subcategories H40.10, H40.11, H40.12-, H40.13-, and H40.14- to designate the stage of glaucoma.
0 stage unspecified
1 mild stage
2 moderate stage
3 severe stage
4 indeterminate stage

√x7th **H40.10 Unspecified open-angle glaucoma**

√x7th **H40.11 Primary open-angle glaucoma**
Chronic simple glaucoma

√6th **H40.12 Low-tension glaucoma**
- √7th **H40.121 Low-tension glaucoma, right eye**
- √7th **H40.122 Low-tension glaucoma, left eye**
- √7th **H40.123 Low-tension glaucoma, bilateral**
- √7th **H40.129 Low-tension glaucoma, unspecified eye**

√6th **H40.13 Pigmentary glaucoma**
- √7th **H40.131 Pigmentary glaucoma, right eye**
- √7th **H40.132 Pigmentary glaucoma, left eye**
- √7th **H40.133 Pigmentary glaucoma, bilateral**
- √7th **H40.139 Pigmentary glaucoma, unspecified eye**

√6th **H40.14 Capsular glaucoma with pseudoexfoliation of lens**
- √7th **H40.141 Capsular glaucoma with pseudoexfoliation of lens, right eye**
- √7th **H40.142 Capsular glaucoma with pseudoexfoliation of lens, left eye**
- √7th **H40.143 Capsular glaucoma with pseudoexfoliation of lens, bilateral**
- √7th **H40.149 Capsular glaucoma with pseudoexfoliation of lens, unspecified eye**

√6th **H40.15 Residual stage of open-angle glaucoma**
- **H40.151 Residual stage of open-angle glaucoma, right eye**
- **H40.152 Residual stage of open-angle glaucoma, left eye**
- **H40.153 Residual stage of open-angle glaucoma, bilateral**
- **H40.159 Residual stage of open-angle glaucoma, unspecified eye**

√5th **H40.2 Primary angle-closure glaucoma**
EXCLUDES1 *aqueous misdirection (H40.83-)*
malignant glaucoma (H40.83-)

One of the following 7th characters is to be assigned to each code in subcategories H40.20 and H40.22- to designate the stage of glaucoma.
0 stage unspecified
1 mild stage
2 moderate stage
3 severe stage
4 indeterminate stage

CC Excl: For CC codes in subcategory H40.2, unless otherwise noted: H40.211-H40.219

√x7th **H40.20 Unspecified primary angle-closure glaucoma**

√6th **H40.21 Acute angle-closure glaucoma**
Acute angle-closure glaucoma attack
Acute angle-closure glaucoma crisis
- **H40.211 Acute angle-closure glaucoma, right eye** CC
- **H40.212 Acute angle-closure glaucoma, left eye** CC
- **H40.213 Acute angle-closure glaucoma, bilateral** CC
- **H40.219 Acute angle-closure glaucoma, unspecified eye** CC

√6th **H40.22 Chronic angle-closure glaucoma**
Chronic primary angle-closure glaucoma
- √7th **H40.221 Chronic angle-closure glaucoma, right eye**
- √7th **H40.222 Chronic angle-closure glaucoma, left eye**
- √7th **H40.223 Chronic angle-closure glaucoma, bilateral**
- √7th **H40.229 Chronic angle-closure glaucoma, unspecified eye**

√6th **H40.23 Intermittent angle-closure glaucoma**
- **H40.231 Intermittent angle-closure glaucoma, right eye**
- **H40.232 Intermittent angle-closure glaucoma, left eye**
- **H40.233 Intermittent angle-closure glaucoma, bilateral**
- **H40.239 Intermittent angle-closure glaucoma, unspecified eye**

√6th **H40.24 Residual stage of angle-closure glaucoma**
- **H40.241 Residual stage of angle-closure glaucoma, right eye**
- **H40.242 Residual stage of angle-closure glaucoma, left eye**
- **H40.243 Residual stage of angle-closure glaucoma, bilateral**
- **H40.249 Residual stage of angle-closure glaucoma, unspecified eye**

√5th **H40.3 Glaucoma secondary to eye trauma**
Code also underlying condition

One of the following 7th characters is to be assigned to each code in subcategory H40.3- to designate the stage of glaucoma.
0 stage unspecified
1 mild stage
2 moderate stage
3 severe stage
4 indeterminate stage

- √x7th **H40.30 Glaucoma secondary to eye trauma, unspecified eye**
- √x7th **H40.31 Glaucoma secondary to eye trauma, right eye**
- √x7th **H40.32 Glaucoma secondary to eye trauma, left eye**
- √x7th **H40.33 Glaucoma secondary to eye trauma, bilateral**

√5th **H40.4 Glaucoma secondary to eye inflammation**
Code also underlying condition

One of the following 7th characters is to be assigned to each code in subcategory H40.4- to designate the stage of glaucoma.
0 stage unspecified
1 mild stage
2 moderate stage
3 severe stage
4 indeterminate stage

√x7th **H40.40 Glaucoma secondary to eye inflammation, unspecified eye**

√x7th **H40.41 Glaucoma secondary to eye inflammation, right eye**

√x7th **H40.42 Glaucoma secondary to eye inflammation, left eye**

√x7th **H40.43 Glaucoma secondary to eye inflammation, bilateral**

√5th **H40.5 Glaucoma secondary to other eye disorders**

Code also underlying eye disorder

One of the following 7th characters is to be assigned to each code in subcategory H40.5- to designate the stage of glaucoma.
- 0 stage unspecified
- 1 mild stage
- 2 moderate stage
- 3 severe stage
- 4 indeterminate stage

√x7th **H40.50 Glaucoma secondary to other eye disorders, unspecified eye**

√x7th **H40.51 Glaucoma secondary to other eye disorders, right eye**

√x7th **H40.52 Glaucoma secondary to other eye disorders, left eye**

√x7th **H40.53 Glaucoma secondary to other eye disorders, bilateral**

√5th **H40.6 Glaucoma secondary to drugs**

Use additional code for adverse effect, if applicable, to identify drug (T36-T50 with fifth or sixth character 5)

One of the following 7th characters is to be assigned to each code in subcategory H40.6- to designate the stage of glaucoma.
- 0 stage unspecified
- 1 mild stage
- 2 moderate stage
- 3 severe stage
- 4 indeterminate stage

√x7th **H40.60 Glaucoma secondary to drugs, unspecified eye**

√x7th **H40.61 Glaucoma secondary to drugs, right eye**

√x7th **H40.62 Glaucoma secondary to drugs, left eye**

√x7th **H40.63 Glaucoma secondary to drugs, bilateral**

√5th **H40.8 Other glaucoma**

√6th **H40.81 Glaucoma with increased episcleral venous pressure**

H40.811 Glaucoma with increased episcleral venous pressure, right eye

H40.812 Glaucoma with increased episcleral venous pressure, left eye

H40.813 Glaucoma with increased episcleral venous pressure, bilateral

H40.819 Glaucoma with increased episcleral venous pressure, unspecified eye

√6th **H40.82 Hypersecretion glaucoma**

H40.821 Hypersecretion glaucoma, right eye

H40.822 Hypersecretion glaucoma, left eye

H40.823 Hypersecretion glaucoma, bilateral

H40.829 Hypersecretion glaucoma, unspecified eye

√6th **H40.83 Aqueous misdirection**

Malignant glaucoma

H40.831 Aqueous misdirection, right eye

H40.832 Aqueous misdirection, left eye

H40.833 Aqueous misdirection, bilateral

H40.839 Aqueous misdirection, unspecified eye

H40.89 Other specified glaucoma

H40.9 Unspecified glaucoma

H42 Glaucoma in diseases classified elsewhere

Code first underlying condition, such as:
- *amyloidosis (E85.-)*
- *aniridia (Q13.1)*
- *Lowe's syndrome (E72.03)*
- *Reiger's anomaly (Q13.81)*
- *specified metabolic disorder (E70-E88)*

EXCLUDES 1 *glaucoma (in):*
- *diabetes mellitus (E08.39, E09.39, E10.39, E11.39, E13.39)*
- *onchocerciasis (B73.02)*
- *syphilis (A52.71)*
- *tuberculous (A18.59)*

Disorders of vitreous body and globe (H43-H44)

√4th **H43 Disorders of vitreous body**

√5th **H43.0 Vitreous prolapse**

EXCLUDES 1 *traumatic vitreous prolapse (S05.2-)*
vitreous syndrome following cataract surgery (H59.0-)

H43.00 Vitreous prolapse, unspecified eye

H43.01 Vitreous prolapse, right eye

H43.02 Vitreous prolapse, left eye

H43.03 Vitreous prolapse, bilateral

√5th **H43.1 Vitreous hemorrhage**

H43.10 Vitreous hemorrhage, unspecified eye

H43.11 Vitreous hemorrhage, right eye

H43.12 Vitreous hemorrhage, left eye

H43.13 Vitreous hemorrhage, bilateral

√5th **H43.2 Crystalline deposits in vitreous body**

H43.20 Crystalline deposits in vitreous body, unspecified eye

H43.21 Crystalline deposits in vitreous body, right eye

H43.22 Crystalline deposits in vitreous body, left eye

H43.23 Crystalline deposits in vitreous body, bilateral

√5th **H43.3 Other vitreous opacities**

√6th **H43.31 Vitreous membranes and strands**

H43.311 Vitreous membranes and strands, right eye

H43.312 Vitreous membranes and strands, left eye

H43.313 Vitreous membranes and strands, bilateral

H43.319 Vitreous membranes and strands, unspecified eye

√6th **H43.39 Other vitreous opacities**

Vitreous floaters

H43.391 Other vitreous opacities, right eye

H43.392 Other vitreous opacities, left eye

H43.393 Other vitreous opacities, bilateral

H43.399 Other vitreous opacities, unspecified eye

√5th **H43.8 Other disorders of vitreous body**

EXCLUDES 1 *proliferative vitreo-retinopathy with retinal detachment (H33.4-)*

EXCLUDES 2 *vitreous abscess (H44.02-)*

√6th **H43.81 Vitreous degeneration**

Vitreous detachment

H43.811 Vitreous degeneration, right eye

H43.812 Vitreous degeneration, left eye

H43.813 Vitreous degeneration, bilateral

H43.819 Vitreous degeneration, unspecified eye

√6th **H43.82 Vitreomacular adhesion**

Vitreomacular traction

H43.821 Vitreomacular adhesion, right eye A

H43.822 Vitreomacular adhesion, left eye A

H43.823 Vitreomacular adhesion, bilateral A

H43.829 Vitreomacular adhesion, unspecified eye A

H43.89 Other disorders of vitreous body

H43.9 Unspecified disorder of vitreous body

√4th **H44 Disorders of globe**

INCLUDES disorders affecting multiple structures of eye

√5th **H44.0 Purulent endophthalmitis**

Use additional code to identify organism

EXCLUDES 1 *bleb associated endophthalmitis (H59.4-)*

√6th **H44.00 Unspecified purulent endophthalmitis**

CC Excl: For CC codes in subcategory H44.00, unless otherwise noted: H20.051-H20.059, H21.331-H21.339, H33.121-H33.129, H44.001-H44.029, H44.121-H44.129, H44.19

H44.001 Unspecified purulent endophthalmitis, right eye CC

H44.002 Unspecified purulent endophthalmitis, left eye CC

H44.003 Unspecified purulent endophthalmitis, bilateral CC

H44.009 Unspecified purulent endophthalmitis, unspecified eye CC

DRAFT

H44.01 Panophthalmitis (acute)

CC Excl: For CC codes in subcategory H44.01, unless otherwise noted: H20.051-H20.059, H21.331-H21.339, H33.121-H33.129, H44.001-H44.029, H44.121-H44.129, H44.19

H44.011 Panophthalmitis (acute), right eye CC
H44.012 Panophthalmitis (acute), left eye CC
H44.013 Panophthalmitis (acute), bilateral CC
H44.019 Panophthalmitis (acute), unspecified eye CC

H44.02 Vitreous abscess (chronic)

CC Excl: For CC codes in subcategory H44.02, unless otherwise noted: H16.241-H16.249, H21.331-H21.339, H33.121-H33.129, H44.001-H44.19

H44.021 Vitreous abscess (chronic), right eye CC
H44.022 Vitreous abscess (chronic), left eye CC
H44.023 Vitreous abscess (chronic), bilateral CC
H44.029 Vitreous abscess (chronic), unspecified eye CC

H44.1 Other endophthalmitis
EXCLUDES 1 *bleb associated endophthalmitis (H59.4-)*
EXCLUDES 2 *ophthalmia nodosa (H16.2-)*

H44.11 Panuveitis

CC Excl: For CC codes in subcategory H44.11, unless otherwise noted: H44.111-H44.119, H44.131-H44.139

H44.111 Panuveitis, right eye CC
H44.112 Panuveitis, left eye CC
H44.113 Panuveitis, bilateral CC
H44.119 Panuveitis, unspecified eye CC

H44.12 Parasitic endophthalmitis, unspecified

CC Excl: For CC codes in subcategory H44.12, unless otherwise noted: H20.051-H20.059, H21.331-H21.339, H33.121-H33.129, H44.001-H44.029, H44.121-H44.129, H44.19

H44.121 Parasitic endophthalmitis, unspecified, right eye CC
H44.122 Parasitic endophthalmitis, unspecified, left eye CC
H44.123 Parasitic endophthalmitis, unspecified, bilateral CC
H44.129 Parasitic endophthalmitis, unspecified, unspecified eye CC

H44.13 Sympathetic uveitis

CC Excl: For CC codes in subcategory H44.13 unless otherwise noted: H44.111-H44.119, H44.131-H44.139

H44.131 Sympathetic uveitis, right eye CC
H44.132 Sympathetic uveitis, left eye CC
H44.133 Sympathetic uveitis, bilateral CC
H44.139 Sympathetic uveitis, unspecified eye CC

H44.19 Other endophthalmitis CC
CC Excl: H20.051-H20.059, H21.331-H21.339, H33.121-H33.129, H44.001-H44.029, H44.121-H44.129, H44.19

H44.2 Degenerative myopia
Malignant myopia
H44.20 Degenerative myopia, unspecified eye
H44.21 Degenerative myopia, right eye
H44.22 Degenerative myopia, left eye
H44.23 Degenerative myopia, bilateral

H44.3 Other and unspecified degenerative disorders of globe
H44.30 Unspecified degenerative disorder of globe

H44.31 Chalcosis
H44.311 Chalcosis, right eye
H44.312 Chalcosis, left eye
H44.313 Chalcosis, bilateral
H44.319 Chalcosis, unspecified eye

H44.32 Siderosis of eye
H44.321 Siderosis of eye, right eye
H44.322 Siderosis of eye, left eye
H44.323 Siderosis of eye, bilateral
H44.329 Siderosis of eye, unspecified eye

H44.39 Other degenerative disorders of globe
H44.391 Other degenerative disorders of globe, right eye
H44.392 Other degenerative disorders of globe, left eye
H44.393 Other degenerative disorders of globe, bilateral
H44.399 Other degenerative disorders of globe, unspecified eye

H44.4 Hypotony of eye
H44.40 Unspecified hypotony of eye

H44.41 Flat anterior chamber hypotony of eye
H44.411 Flat anterior chamber hypotony of right eye
H44.412 Flat anterior chamber hypotony of left eye
H44.413 Flat anterior chamber hypotony of eye, bilateral
H44.419 Flat anterior chamber hypotony of unspecified eye

H44.42 Hypotony of eye due to ocular fistula
H44.421 Hypotony of right eye due to ocular fistula
H44.422 Hypotony of left eye due to ocular fistula
H44.423 Hypotony of eye due to ocular fistula, bilateral
H44.429 Hypotony of unspecified eye due to ocular fistula

H44.43 Hypotony of eye due to other ocular disorders
H44.431 Hypotony of eye due to other ocular disorders, right eye
H44.432 Hypotony of eye due to other ocular disorders, left eye
H44.433 Hypotony of eye due to other ocular disorders, bilateral
H44.439 Hypotony of eye due to other ocular disorders, unspecified eye

H44.44 Primary hypotony of eye
H44.441 Primary hypotony of right eye
H44.442 Primary hypotony of left eye
H44.443 Primary hypotony of eye, bilateral
H44.449 Primary hypotony of unspecified eye

H44.5 Degenerated conditions of globe
H44.50 Unspecified degenerated conditions of globe

H44.51 Absolute glaucoma
H44.511 Absolute glaucoma, right eye
H44.512 Absolute glaucoma, left eye
H44.513 Absolute glaucoma, bilateral
H44.519 Absolute glaucoma, unspecified eye

H44.52 Atrophy of globe
Phthisis bulbi
H44.521 Atrophy of globe, right eye
H44.522 Atrophy of globe, left eye
H44.523 Atrophy of globe, bilateral
H44.529 Atrophy of globe, unspecified eye

H44.53 Leucocoria
H44.531 Leucocoria, right eye
H44.532 Leucocoria, left eye
H44.533 Leucocoria, bilateral
H44.539 Leucocoria, unspecified eye

H44.6 Retained (old) intraocular foreign body, magnetic
Use additional code to identify magnetic foreign body (Z18.11)
EXCLUDES 1 *current intraocular foreign body (S05.-)*
EXCLUDES 2 *retained foreign body in eyelid (H02.81-)*
retained (old) foreign body following penetrating wound of orbit (H05.5-)
retained (old) intraocular foreign body, nonmagnetic (H44.7-)

H44.60 Unspecified retained (old) intraocular foreign body, magnetic
H44.601 Unspecified retained (old) intraocular foreign body, magnetic, right eye

H44.602 Unspecified retained (old) intraocular foreign body, magnetic, left eye

H44.603 Unspecified retained (old) intraocular foreign body, magnetic, bilateral

H44.609 Unspecified retained (old) intraocular foreign body, magnetic, unspecified eye

✓6th H44.61 Retained (old) magnetic foreign body in anterior chamber

H44.611 Retained (old) magnetic foreign body in anterior chamber, right eye

H44.612 Retained (old) magnetic foreign body in anterior chamber, left eye

H44.613 Retained (old) magnetic foreign body in anterior chamber, bilateral

H44.619 Retained (old) magnetic foreign body in anterior chamber, unspecified eye

✓6th H44.62 Retained (old) magnetic foreign body in iris or ciliary body

H44.621 Retained (old) magnetic foreign body in iris or ciliary body, right eye

H44.622 Retained (old) magnetic foreign body in iris or ciliary body, left eye

H44.623 Retained (old) magnetic foreign body in iris or ciliary body, bilateral

H44.629 Retained (old) magnetic foreign body in iris or ciliary body, unspecified eye

✓6th H44.63 Retained (old) magnetic foreign body in lens

H44.631 Retained (old) magnetic foreign body in lens, right eye

H44.632 Retained (old) magnetic foreign body in lens, left eye

H44.633 Retained (old) magnetic foreign body in lens, bilateral

H44.639 Retained (old) magnetic foreign body in lens, unspecified eye

✓6th H44.64 Retained (old) magnetic foreign body in posterior wall of globe

H44.641 Retained (old) magnetic foreign body in posterior wall of globe, right eye

H44.642 Retained (old) magnetic foreign body in posterior wall of globe, left eye

H44.643 Retained (old) magnetic foreign body in posterior wall of globe, bilateral

H44.649 Retained (old) magnetic foreign body in posterior wall of globe, unspecified eye

✓6th H44.65 Retained (old) magnetic foreign body in vitreous body

H44.651 Retained (old) magnetic foreign body in vitreous body, right eye

H44.652 Retained (old) magnetic foreign body in vitreous body, left eye

H44.653 Retained (old) magnetic foreign body in vitreous body, bilateral

H44.659 Retained (old) magnetic foreign body in vitreous body, unspecified eye

✓6th H44.69 Retained (old) intraocular foreign body, magnetic, in other or multiple sites

H44.691 Retained (old) intraocular foreign body, magnetic, in other or multiple sites, right eye

H44.692 Retained (old) intraocular foreign body, magnetic, in other or multiple sites, left eye

H44.693 Retained (old) intraocular foreign body, magnetic, in other or multiple sites, bilateral

H44.699 Retained (old) intraocular foreign body, magnetic, in other or multiple sites, unspecified eye

✓5th H44.7 Retained (old) intraocular foreign body, nonmagnetic

Use additional code to identify nonmagnetic foreign body (Z18.01-Z18.10, Z18.12, Z18.2-Z18.9)

EXCLUDES 1 *current intraocular foreign body (S05.-)*

EXCLUDES 2 *retained foreign body in eyelid (H02.81-)*
retained (old) foreign body following penetrating wound of orbit (H05.5-)
retained (old) intraocular foreign body, magnetic (H44.6-)

✓6th H44.70 Unspecified retained (old) intraocular foreign body, nonmagnetic

H44.701 Unspecified retained (old) intraocular foreign body, nonmagnetic, right eye

H44.702 Unspecified retained (old) intraocular foreign body, nonmagnetic, left eye

H44.703 Unspecified retained (old) intraocular foreign body, nonmagnetic, bilateral

H44.709 Unspecified retained (old) intraocular foreign body, nonmagnetic, unspecified eye

Retained (old) intraocular foreign body NOS

✓6th H44.71 Retained (nonmagnetic) (old) foreign body in anterior chamber

H44.711 Retained (nonmagnetic) (old) foreign body in anterior chamber, right eye

H44.712 Retained (nonmagnetic) (old) foreign body in anterior chamber, left eye

H44.713 Retained (nonmagnetic) (old) foreign body in anterior chamber, bilateral

H44.719 Retained (nonmagnetic) (old) foreign body in anterior chamber, unspecified eye

✓6th H44.72 Retained (nonmagnetic) (old) foreign body in iris or ciliary body

H44.721 Retained (nonmagnetic) (old) foreign body in iris or ciliary body, right eye

H44.722 Retained (nonmagnetic) (old) foreign body in iris or ciliary body, left eye

H44.723 Retained (nonmagnetic) (old) foreign body in iris or ciliary body, bilateral

H44.729 Retained (nonmagnetic) (old) foreign body in iris or ciliary body, unspecified eye

✓6th H44.73 Retained (nonmagnetic) (old) foreign body in lens

H44.731 Retained (nonmagnetic) (old) foreign body in lens, right eye

H44.732 Retained (nonmagnetic) (old) foreign body in lens, left eye

H44.733 Retained (nonmagnetic) (old) foreign body in lens, bilateral

H44.739 Retained (nonmagnetic) (old) foreign body in lens, unspecified eye

✓6th H44.74 Retained (nonmagnetic) (old) foreign body in posterior wall of globe

H44.741 Retained (nonmagnetic) (old) foreign body in posterior wall of globe, right eye

H44.742 Retained (nonmagnetic) (old) foreign body in posterior wall of globe, left eye

H44.743 Retained (nonmagnetic) (old) foreign body in posterior wall of globe, bilateral

H44.749 Retained (nonmagnetic) (old) foreign body in posterior wall of globe, unspecified eye

✓6th H44.75 Retained (nonmagnetic) (old) foreign body in vitreous body

H44.751 Retained (nonmagnetic) (old) foreign body in vitreous body, right eye

H44.752 Retained (nonmagnetic) (old) foreign body in vitreous body, left eye

H44.753 Retained (nonmagnetic) (old) foreign body in vitreous body, bilateral

H44.759 Retained (nonmagnetic) (old) foreign body in vitreous body, unspecified eye

✓6th H44.79 Retained (old) intraocular foreign body, nonmagnetic, in other or multiple sites

H44.791 Retained (old) intraocular foreign body, nonmagnetic, in other or multiple sites, right eye

H44.792 Retained (old) intraocular foreign body, nonmagnetic, in other or multiple sites, left eye
H44.793 Retained (old) intraocular foreign body, nonmagnetic, in other or multiple sites, bilateral
H44.799 Retained (old) intraocular foreign body, nonmagnetic, in other or multiple sites, unspecified eye

✓5th H44.8 Other disorders of globe
✓6th H44.81 Hemophthalmos
H44.811 Hemophthalmos, right eye
H44.812 Hemophthalmos, left eye
H44.813 Hemophthalmos, bilateral
H44.819 Hemophthalmos, unspecified eye
✓6th H44.82 Luxation of globe
H44.821 Luxation of globe, right eye
H44.822 Luxation of globe, left eye
H44.823 Luxation of globe, bilateral
H44.829 Luxation of globe, unspecified eye
H44.89 Other disorders of globe
H44.9 Unspecified disorder of globe

Disorders of optic nerve and visual pathways (H46-H47)

✓4th **H46 Optic neuritis**
EXCLUDES 2 *ischemic optic neuropathy (H47.01-)*
neuromyelitis optica [Devic] (G36.0)

CC Excl: For CC codes in category H46, unless otherwise noted: H46.00-H46.9

✓5th H46.0 Optic papillitis
H46.00 Optic papillitis, unspecified eye CC
H46.01 Optic papillitis, right eye CC
H46.02 Optic papillitis, left eye CC
H46.03 Optic papillitis, bilateral CC
✓5th H46.1 Retrobulbar neuritis
Retrobulbar neuritis NOS
EXCLUDES 1 *syphilitic retrobulbar neuritis (A52.15)*
H46.10 Retrobulbar neuritis, unspecified eye CC
H46.11 Retrobulbar neuritis, right eye CC
H46.12 Retrobulbar neuritis, left eye CC
H46.13 Retrobulbar neuritis, bilateral CC
H46.2 Nutritional optic neuropathy
H46.3 Toxic optic neuropathy
Code first (T51-T65) to identify cause
H46.8 Other optic neuritis CC
H46.9 Unspecified optic neuritis CC

✓4th **H47 Other disorders of optic [2nd] nerve and visual pathways**
✓5th H47.0 Disorders of optic nerve, not elsewhere classified
✓6th H47.01 Ischemic optic neuropathy
H47.011 Ischemic optic neuropathy, right eye
H47.012 Ischemic optic neuropathy, left eye
H47.013 Ischemic optic neuropathy, bilateral
H47.019 Ischemic optic neuropathy, unspecified eye
✓6th H47.02 Hemorrhage in optic nerve sheath
H47.021 Hemorrhage in optic nerve sheath, right eye
H47.022 Hemorrhage in optic nerve sheath, left eye
H47.023 Hemorrhage in optic nerve sheath, bilateral
H47.029 Hemorrhage in optic nerve sheath, unspecified eye
✓6th H47.03 Optic nerve hypoplasia
H47.031 Optic nerve hypoplasia, right eye
H47.032 Optic nerve hypoplasia, left eye
H47.033 Optic nerve hypoplasia, bilateral
H47.039 Optic nerve hypoplasia, unspecified eye
✓6th H47.09 Other disorders of optic nerve, not elsewhere classified
Compression of optic nerve
H47.091 Other disorders of optic nerve, not elsewhere classified, right eye
H47.092 Other disorders of optic nerve, not elsewhere classified, left eye
H47.093 Other disorders of optic nerve, not elsewhere classified, bilateral
H47.099 Other disorders of optic nerve, not elsewhere classified, unspecified eye
✓5th H47.1 Papilledema
H47.10 Unspecified papilledema CC
CC Excl: A17.9, A18.50-A18.59, A18.82, A18.84, A18.89, A39.82, E08.311-E08.39, E08.618-E08.638, E08.649-E08.8, E09.311-E09.39, E09.618-E09.638, E09.649-E09.8, E10.311-E10.39, E10.618-E10.638, E10.649, E10.69-E10.8, E11.311-E11.39, E11.618-E11.638, E11.649, E11.69-E11.8, E13.311-E13.39, E13.618-E13.638, E13.649-E13.8, H47.10-H47.13, H47.231-H47.239, H47.331-H47.339, H57.8-H57.9, H59.40-H59.43, Q11.3, Q15.8-Q15.9
H47.11 Papilledema associated with increased intracranial pressure CC
CC Excl: See code: H47.10
H47.12 Papilledema associated with decreased ocular pressure
H47.13 Papilledema associated with retinal disorder
✓6th H47.14 Foster-Kennedy syndrome
H47.141 Foster-Kennedy syndrome, right eye
H47.142 Foster-Kennedy syndrome, left eye
H47.143 Foster-Kennedy syndrome, bilateral
H47.149 Foster-Kennedy syndrome, unspecified eye
✓5th H47.2 Optic atrophy
H47.20 Unspecified optic atrophy
✓6th H47.21 Primary optic atrophy
H47.211 Primary optic atrophy, right eye
H47.212 Primary optic atrophy, left eye
H47.213 Primary optic atrophy, bilateral
H47.219 Primary optic atrophy, unspecified eye
H47.22 Hereditary optic atrophy
Leber's optic atrophy
✓6th H47.23 Glaucomatous optic atrophy
H47.231 Glaucomatous optic atrophy, right eye
H47.232 Glaucomatous optic atrophy, left eye
H47.233 Glaucomatous optic atrophy, bilateral
H47.239 Glaucomatous optic atrophy, unspecified eye
✓6th H47.29 Other optic atrophy
Temporal pallor of optic disc
H47.291 Other optic atrophy, right eye
H47.292 Other optic atrophy, left eye
H47.293 Other optic atrophy, bilateral
H47.299 Other optic atrophy, unspecified eye
✓5th H47.3 Other disorders of optic disc
✓6th H47.31 Coloboma of optic disc
H47.311 Coloboma of optic disc, right eye
H47.312 Coloboma of optic disc, left eye
H47.313 Coloboma of optic disc, bilateral
H47.319 Coloboma of optic disc, unspecified eye
✓6th H47.32 Drusen of optic disc
H47.321 Drusen of optic disc, right eye
H47.322 Drusen of optic disc, left eye
H47.323 Drusen of optic disc, bilateral
H47.329 Drusen of optic disc, unspecified eye
✓6th H47.33 Pseudopapilledema of optic disc
H47.331 Pseudopapilledema of optic disc, right eye
H47.332 Pseudopapilledema of optic disc, left eye
H47.333 Pseudopapilledema of optic disc, bilateral
H47.339 Pseudopapilledema of optic disc, unspecified eye
✓6th H47.39 Other disorders of optic disc
H47.391 Other disorders of optic disc, right eye
H47.392 Other disorders of optic disc, left eye
H47.393 Other disorders of optic disc, bilateral
H47.399 Other disorders of optic disc, unspecified eye

✓5th H47.4 Disorders of optic chiasm
Code also underlying condition

CC Excl: For CC codes in subcategory H47.4, unless otherwise noted: H47.41-H47.539

H47.41 Disorders of optic chiasm in (due to) inflammatory disorders CC
H47.42 Disorders of optic chiasm in (due to) neoplasm CC
H47.43 Disorders of optic chiasm in (due to) vascular disorders CC
H47.49 Disorders of optic chiasm in (due to) other disorders CC

✓5th H47.5 Disorders of other visual pathways
Disorders of optic tracts, geniculate nuclei and optic radiations
Code also underlying condition

CC Excl: For CC codes in subcategory H47.5, unless otherwise noted: H47.41-H47.539

✓6th H47.51 Disorders of visual pathways in (due to) inflammatory disorders
H47.511 Disorders of visual pathways in (due to) inflammatory disorders, right side CC
H47.512 Disorders of visual pathways in (due to) inflammatory disorders, left side CC
H47.519 Disorders of visual pathways in (due to) inflammatory disorders, unspecified side CC

✓6th H47.52 Disorders of visual pathways in (due to) neoplasm
H47.521 Disorders of visual pathways in (due to) neoplasm, right side CC
H47.522 Disorders of visual pathways in (due to) neoplasm, left side CC
H47.529 Disorders of visual pathways in (due to) neoplasm, unspecified side CC

✓6th H47.53 Disorders of visual pathways in (due to) vascular disorders
H47.531 Disorders of visual pathways in (due to) vascular disorders, right side CC
H47.532 Disorders of visual pathways in (due to) vascular disorders, left side CC
H47.539 Disorders of visual pathways in (due to) vascular disorders, unspecified side CC

✓5th H47.6 Disorders of visual cortex
Code also underlying condition
EXCLUDES 1 *injury to visual cortex S04.04*

CC Excl: For CC codes in subcategory H47.6, unless otherwise noted: H47.611-H47.9

✓6th H47.61 Cortical blindness
H47.611 Cortical blindness, right side of brain
H47.612 Cortical blindness, left side of brain
H47.619 Cortical blindness, unspecified side of brain

✓6th H47.62 Disorders of visual cortex in (due to) inflammatory disorders
H47.621 Disorders of visual cortex in (due to) inflammatory disorders, right side of brain CC
H47.622 Disorders of visual cortex in (due to) inflammatory disorders, left side of brain CC
H47.629 Disorders of visual cortex in (due to) inflammatory disorders, unspecified side of brain CC

✓6th H47.63 Disorders of visual cortex in (due to) neoplasm
H47.631 Disorders of visual cortex in (due to) neoplasm, right side of brain CC
H47.632 Disorders of visual cortex in (due to) neoplasm, left side of brain CC
H47.639 Disorders of visual cortex in (due to) neoplasm, unspecified side of brain CC

✓6th H47.64 Disorders of visual cortex in (due to) vascular disorders
H47.641 Disorders of visual cortex in (due to) vascular disorders, right side of brain CC
H47.642 Disorders of visual cortex in (due to) vascular disorders, left side of brain CC
H47.649 Disorders of visual cortex in (due to) vascular disorders, unspecified side of brain CC

H47.9 Unspecified disorder of visual pathways

Disorders of ocular muscles, binocular movement, accommodation and refraction (H49-H52)

EXCLUDES 2 *nystagmus and other irregular eye movements (H55)*

✓4th H49 Paralytic strabismus
EXCLUDES 2 *internal ophthalmoplegia (H52.51-)*
internuclear ophthalmoplegia (H51.2-)
progressive supranuclear ophthalmoplegia (G23.1)

✓5th H49.0 Third [oculomotor] nerve palsy
H49.00 Third [oculomotor] nerve palsy, unspecified eye
H49.01 Third [oculomotor] nerve palsy, right eye
H49.02 Third [oculomotor] nerve palsy, left eye
H49.03 Third [oculomotor] nerve palsy, bilateral

✓5th H49.1 Fourth [trochlear] nerve palsy
H49.10 Fourth [trochlear] nerve palsy, unspecified eye
H49.11 Fourth [trochlear] nerve palsy, right eye
H49.12 Fourth [trochlear] nerve palsy, left eye
H49.13 Fourth [trochlear] nerve palsy, bilateral

✓5th H49.2 Sixth [abducent] nerve palsy
H49.20 Sixth [abducent] nerve palsy, unspecified eye
H49.21 Sixth [abducent] nerve palsy, right eye
H49.22 Sixth [abducent] nerve palsy, left eye
H49.23 Sixth [abducent] nerve palsy, bilateral

✓5th H49.3 Total (external) ophthalmoplegia
H49.30 Total (external) ophthalmoplegia, unspecified eye
H49.31 Total (external) ophthalmoplegia, right eye
H49.32 Total (external) ophthalmoplegia, left eye
H49.33 Total (external) ophthalmoplegia, bilateral

✓5th H49.4 Progressive external ophthalmoplegia
EXCLUDES 1 *Kearns-Sayre syndrome (H49.81-)*
H49.40 Progressive external ophthalmoplegia, unspecified eye
H49.41 Progressive external ophthalmoplegia, right eye
H49.42 Progressive external ophthalmoplegia, left eye
H49.43 Progressive external ophthalmoplegia, bilateral

✓5th H49.8 Other paralytic strabismus

CC Excl: For CC codes in subcategory H49.8, unless otherwise noted: C96.5-C96.6, E71.310-E71.548, E80.3-E80.7, E88.89

✓6th H49.81 Kearns-Sayre syndrome
Progressive external ophthalmoplegia with pigmentary retinopathy
Use additional code for other manifestation, such as: heart block (I45.9)
H49.811 Kearns-Sayre syndrome, right eye CC
H49.812 Kearns-Sayre syndrome, left eye CC
H49.813 Kearns-Sayre syndrome, bilateral CC
H49.819 Kearns-Sayre syndrome, unspecified eye CC

✓6th H49.88 Other paralytic strabismus
External ophthalmoplegia NOS
H49.881 Other paralytic strabismus, right eye
H49.882 Other paralytic strabismus, left eye
H49.883 Other paralytic strabismus, bilateral
H49.889 Other paralytic strabismus, unspecified eye

H49.9 Unspecified paralytic strabismus

✓4th H50 Other strabismus

✓5th H50.0 Esotropia
Convergent concomitant strabismus
EXCLUDES 1 *intermittent esotropia (H50.31-, H50.32)*
H50.00 Unspecified esotropia
✓6th H50.01 Monocular esotropia
H50.011 Monocular esotropia, right eye
H50.012 Monocular esotropia, left eye

✓6th H50.02 Monocular esotropia with A pattern
H50.021 Monocular esotropia with A pattern, right eye
H50.022 Monocular esotropia with A pattern, left eye
✓6th H50.03 Monocular esotropia with V pattern
H50.031 Monocular esotropia with V pattern, right eye
H50.032 Monocular esotropia with V pattern, left eye
✓6th H50.04 Monocular esotropia with other noncomitancies
H50.041 Monocular esotropia with other noncomitancies, right eye
H50.042 Monocular esotropia with other noncomitancies, left eye
H50.05 Alternating esotropia
H50.06 Alternating esotropia with A pattern
H50.07 Alternating esotropia with V pattern
H50.08 Alternating esotropia with other noncomitancies
✓5th H50.1 Exotropia
Divergent concomitant strabismus
EXCLUDES 1 *intermittent exotropia (H50.33-, H50.34)*
H50.10 Unspecified exotropia
✓6th H50.11 Monocular exotropia
H50.111 Monocular exotropia, right eye
H50.112 Monocular exotropia, left eye
✓6th H50.12 Monocular exotropia with A pattern
H50.121 Monocular exotropia with A pattern, right eye
H50.122 Monocular exotropia with A pattern, left eye
✓6th H50.13 Monocular exotropia with V pattern
H50.131 Monocular exotropia with V pattern, right eye
H50.132 Monocular exotropia with V pattern, left eye
✓6th H50.14 Monocular exotropia with other noncomitancies
H50.141 Monocular exotropia with other noncomitancies, right eye
H50.142 Monocular exotropia with other noncomitancies, left eye
H50.15 Alternating exotropia
H50.16 Alternating exotropia with A pattern
H50.17 Alternating exotropia with V pattern
H50.18 Alternating exotropia with other noncomitancies
✓5th H50.2 Vertical strabismus
Hypertropia
H50.21 Vertical strabismus, right eye
H50.22 Vertical strabismus, left eye
✓5th H50.3 Intermittent heterotropia
H50.30 Unspecified intermittent heterotropia
✓6th H50.31 Intermittent monocular esotropia
H50.311 Intermittent monocular esotropia, right eye
H50.312 Intermittent monocular esotropia, left eye
H50.32 Intermittent alternating esotropia
✓6th H50.33 Intermittent monocular exotropia
H50.331 Intermittent monocular exotropia, right eye
H50.332 Intermittent monocular exotropia, left eye
H50.34 Intermittent alternating exotropia
✓5th H50.4 Other and unspecified heterotropia
H50.40 Unspecified heterotropia
✓6th H50.41 Cyclotropia
H50.411 Cyclotropia, right eye
H50.412 Cyclotropia, left eye
H50.42 Monofixation syndrome
H50.43 Accommodative component in esotropia
✓5th H50.5 Heterophoria
H50.50 Unspecified heterophoria
H50.51 Esophoria
H50.52 Exophoria
H50.53 Vertical heterophoria
H50.54 Cyclophoria
H50.55 Alternating heterophoria
✓5th H50.6 Mechanical strabismus
H50.60 Mechanical strabismus, unspecified
✓6th H50.61 Brown's sheath syndrome
H50.611 Brown's sheath syndrome, right eye
H50.612 Brown's sheath syndrome, left eye
H50.69 Other mechanical strabismus
Strabismus due to adhesions
Traumatic limitation of duction of eye muscle
✓5th H50.8 Other specified strabismus
✓6th H50.81 Duane's syndrome
H50.811 Duane's syndrome, right eye
H50.812 Duane's syndrome, left eye
H50.89 Other specified strabismus
H50.9 Unspecified strabismus

✓4th **H51 Other disorders of binocular movement**
H51.0 Palsy (spasm) of conjugate gaze
✓5th H51.1 Convergence insufficiency and excess
H51.11 Convergence insufficiency
H51.12 Convergence excess
✓5th H51.2 Internuclear ophthalmoplegia
H51.20 Internuclear ophthalmoplegia, unspecified eye
H51.21 Internuclear ophthalmoplegia, right eye
H51.22 Internuclear ophthalmoplegia, left eye
H51.23 Internuclear ophthalmoplegia, bilateral
H51.8 Other specified disorders of binocular movement
H51.9 Unspecified disorder of binocular movement

✓4th **H52 Disorders of refraction and accommodation**
✓5th H52.0 Hypermetropia
H52.00 Hypermetropia, unspecified eye
H52.01 Hypermetropia, right eye
H52.02 Hypermetropia, left eye
H52.03 Hypermetropia, bilateral
✓5th H52.1 Myopia
EXCLUDES 1 *degenerative myopia (H44.2-)*
H52.10 Myopia, unspecified eye
H52.11 Myopia, right eye
H52.12 Myopia, left eye
H52.13 Myopia, bilateral
✓5th H52.2 Astigmatism
✓6th H52.20 Unspecified astigmatism
H52.201 Unspecified astigmatism, right eye
H52.202 Unspecified astigmatism, left eye
H52.203 Unspecified astigmatism, bilateral
H52.209 Unspecified astigmatism, unspecified eye
✓6th H52.21 Irregular astigmatism
H52.211 Irregular astigmatism, right eye
H52.212 Irregular astigmatism, left eye
H52.213 Irregular astigmatism, bilateral
H52.219 Irregular astigmatism, unspecified eye
✓6th H52.22 Regular astigmatism
H52.221 Regular astigmatism, right eye
H52.222 Regular astigmatism, left eye
H52.223 Regular astigmatism, bilateral
H52.229 Regular astigmatism, unspecified eye
✓5th H52.3 Anisometropia and aniseikonia
H52.31 Anisometropia
H52.32 Aniseikonia
H52.4 Presbyopia
✓5th H52.5 Disorders of accommodation
✓6th H52.51 Internal ophthalmoplegia (complete) (total)
H52.511 Internal ophthalmoplegia (complete) (total), right eye
H52.512 Internal ophthalmoplegia (complete) (total), left eye
H52.513 Internal ophthalmoplegia (complete) (total), bilateral
H52.519 Internal ophthalmoplegia (complete) (total), unspecified eye

√6th H52.52 Paresis of accommodation
H52.521 Paresis of accommodation, right eye
H52.522 Paresis of accommodation, left eye
H52.523 Paresis of accommodation, bilateral
H52.529 Paresis of accommodation, unspecified eye

√6th H52.53 Spasm of accommodation
H52.531 Spasm of accommodation, right eye
H52.532 Spasm of accommodation, left eye
H52.533 Spasm of accommodation, bilateral
H52.539 Spasm of accommodation, unspecified eye

H52.6 Other disorders of refraction
H52.7 Unspecified disorder of refraction

Visual disturbances and blindness (H53-H54)

√4th **H53 Visual disturbances**

√5th H53.0 Amblyopia ex anopsia
EXCLUDES 1 *amblyopia due to vitamin A deficiency (E50.5)*

√6th H53.00 Unspecified amblyopia
H53.001 Unspecified amblyopia, right eye
H53.002 Unspecified amblyopia, left eye
H53.003 Unspecified amblyopia, bilateral
H53.009 Unspecified amblyopia, unspecified eye

√6th H53.01 Deprivation amblyopia
H53.011 Deprivation amblyopia, right eye
H53.012 Deprivation amblyopia, left eye
H53.013 Deprivation amblyopia, bilateral
H53.019 Deprivation amblyopia, unspecified eye

√6th H53.02 Refractive amblyopia
H53.021 Refractive amblyopia, right eye
H53.022 Refractive amblyopia, left eye
H53.023 Refractive amblyopia, bilateral
H53.029 Refractive amblyopia, unspecified eye

√6th H53.03 Strabismic amblyopia
EXCLUDES 1 *strabismus (H50.-)*
H53.031 Strabismic amblyopia, right eye
H53.032 Strabismic amblyopia, left eye
H53.033 Strabismic amblyopia, bilateral
H53.039 Strabismic amblyopia, unspecified eye

√5th H53.1 Subjective visual disturbances
CC Excl: For CC codes in subcategory H53.1, unless otherwise noted: H53.10-H53.139, H53.16, R44.1, R48.3
EXCLUDES 1 *subjective visual disturbances due to vitamin A deficiency (E50.5)*
visual hallucinations (R44.1)

H53.10 Unspecified subjective visual disturbances
H53.11 Day blindness
Hemeralopia

√6th H53.12 Transient visual loss
Scintillating scotoma
EXCLUDES 1 *amaurosis fugax (G45.3-)*
transient retinal artery occlusion (H34.0-)
H53.121 Transient visual loss, right eye CC
H53.122 Transient visual loss, left eye CC
H53.123 Transient visual loss, bilateral CC
H53.129 Transient visual loss, unspecified eye CC

√6th H53.13 Sudden visual loss
H53.131 Sudden visual loss, right eye CC
H53.132 Sudden visual loss, left eye CC
H53.133 Sudden visual loss, bilateral CC
H53.139 Sudden visual loss, unspecified eye CC

√6th H53.14 Visual discomfort
Asthenopia
Photophobia
H53.141 Visual discomfort, right eye
H53.142 Visual discomfort, left eye
H53.143 Visual discomfort, bilateral
H53.149 Visual discomfort, unspecified

H53.15 Visual distortions of shape and size
Metamorphopsia
H53.16 Psychophysical visual disturbances

H53.19 Other subjective visual disturbances
Visual halos

H53.2 Diplopia
Double vision

√5th H53.3 Other and unspecified disorders of binocular vision
H53.30 Unspecified disorder of binocular vision
H53.31 Abnormal retinal correspondence
H53.32 Fusion with defective stereopsis
H53.33 Simultaneous visual perception without fusion
H53.34 Suppression of binocular vision

√5th H53.4 Visual field defects
H53.40 Unspecified visual field defects

√6th H53.41 Scotoma involving central area
Central scotoma
H53.411 Scotoma involving central area, right eye
H53.412 Scotoma involving central area, left eye
H53.413 Scotoma involving central area, bilateral
H53.419 Scotoma involving central area, unspecified eye

√6th H53.42 Scotoma of blind spot area
Enlarged blind spot
H53.421 Scotoma of blind spot area, right eye
H53.422 Scotoma of blind spot area, left eye
H53.423 Scotoma of blind spot area, bilateral
H53.429 Scotoma of blind spot area, unspecified eye

√6th H53.43 Sector or arcuate defects
Arcuate scotoma
Bjerrum scotoma
H53.431 Sector or arcuate defects, right eye
H53.432 Sector or arcuate defects, left eye
H53.433 Sector or arcuate defects, bilateral
H53.439 Sector or arcuate defects, unspecified eye

√6th H53.45 Other localized visual field defect
Peripheral visual field defect
Ring scotoma NOS
Scotoma NOS
H53.451 Other localized visual field defect, right eye
H53.452 Other localized visual field defect, left eye
H53.453 Other localized visual field defect, bilateral
H53.459 Other localized visual field defect, unspecified eye

√6th H53.46 Homonymous bilateral field defects
Homonymous hemianopia
Homonymous hemianopsia
Quadrant anopia
Quadrant anopsia
H53.461 Homonymous bilateral field defects, right side
H53.462 Homonymous bilateral field defects, left side
H53.469 Homonymous bilateral field defects, unspecified side
Homonymous bilateral field defects NOS

H53.47 Heteronymous bilateral field defects
Heteronymous hemianop(s)ia

√6th H53.48 Generalized contraction of visual field
H53.481 Generalized contraction of visual field, right eye
H53.482 Generalized contraction of visual field, left eye
H53.483 Generalized contraction of visual field, bilateral
H53.489 Generalized contraction of visual field, unspecified eye

√5th H53.5 Color vision deficiencies
Color blindness
EXCLUDES 2 *day blindness (H53.11)*
H53.50 Unspecified color vision deficiencies
Color blindness NOS
H53.51 Achromatopsia
H53.52 Acquired color vision deficiency
H53.53 Deuteranomaly
Deuteranopia

H53.54 **Protanomaly**
Protanopia
H53.55 **Tritanomaly**
Tritanopia
H53.59 **Other color vision deficiencies**

✓5th **H53.6 Night blindness**
EXCLUDES 1 *night blindness due to vitamin A deficiency (E50.5)*
H53.60 **Unspecified night blindness**
H53.61 **Abnormal dark adaptation curve**
H53.62 **Acquired night blindness**
H53.63 **Congenital night blindness**
H53.69 **Other night blindness**

✓5th **H53.7 Vision sensitivity deficiencies**
H53.71 **Glare sensitivity**
H53.72 **Impaired contrast sensitivity**

H53.8 Other visual disturbances
H53.9 Unspecified visual disturbance

✓4th **H54 Blindness and low vision**
NOTE For definition of visual impairment categories see table below
Code first any associated underlying cause of the blindness
EXCLUDES 1 *amaurosis fugax (G45.3)*

H54.0 Blindness, both eyes
Visual impairment categories 3, 4, 5 in both eyes.

✓5th **H54.1 Blindness, one eye, low vision other eye**
Visual impairment categories 3, 4, 5 in one eye, with categories 1 or 2 in the other eye.
H54.10 **Blindness, one eye, low vision other eye, unspecified eyes**
H54.11 **Blindness, right eye, low vision left eye**
H54.12 **Blindness, left eye, low vision right eye**

H54.2 Low vision, both eyes
Visual impairment categories 1 or 2 in both eyes.

H54.3 Unqualified visual loss, both eyes
Visual impairment category 9 in both eyes.

✓5th **H54.4 Blindness, one eye**
Visual impairment categories 3, 4, 5 in one eye [normal vision in other eye]
H54.40 **Blindness, one eye, unspecified eye**
H54.41 **Blindness, right eye, normal vision left eye**
H54.42 **Blindness, left eye, normal vision right eye**

✓5th **H54.5 Low vision, one eye**
Visual impairment categories 1 or 2 in one eye [normal vision in other eye].
H54.50 **Low vision, one eye, unspecified eye**
H54.51 **Low vision, right eye, normal vision left eye**
H54.52 **Low vision, left eye, normal vision right eye**

✓5th **H54.6 Unqualified visual loss, one eye**
Visual impairment category 9 in one eye [normal vision in other eye].
H54.60 **Unqualified visual loss, one eye, unspecified**
H54.61 **Unqualified visual loss, right eye, normal vision left eye**
H54.62 **Unqualified visual loss, left eye, normal vision right eye**

H54.7 Unspecified visual loss
Visual impairment category 9 NOS

H54.8 Legal blindness, as defined in USA
Blindness NOS according to USA definition
EXCLUDES 1 *legal blindness with specification of impairment level (H54.0-H54.7)*

NOTE The following table gives a classification of severity of visual impairment recommended by a WHO Study Group on the Prevention of Blindness, Geneva, 6-10 November 1972.

The term "low vision" in category H54 comprises categories 1 and 2 of the table, the term "blindness" categories 3, 4 and 5, and the term "unqualified visual loss" category 9.

If the extent of the visual field is taken into account, patients with a field no greater than 10 but greater than 5 around central fixation should be placed in category 3 and patients with a field nocategory greater than 5 around central fixation should be placed in 4, even if the central acuity is not impaired.

Category of visual impairment	Visual acuity with best possible correction	
	Maximum less than:	Minimum equal to or better than:
1	6/18 3/10 (0.3) 20/70	6/60 1/10 (0.1) 20/200
2	6/60 1/10 (0.1) 20/200	3/60 1/20 (0.5) 20/400
3	3/60 1/20 (0.05) 20/400	1/60 (finger counting at one meter) 1/50 (0.02) 5/300 (20/1200)
4	1/60 (finger counting at one meter) 1/50 (0.02) 5/300	Light perception
5	No light perception	
9	Undetermined or unspecified	

Other disorders of eye and adnexa (H55-H59)

✓4th **H55 Nystagmus and other irregular eye movements**

✓5th **H55.0 Nystagmus**
H55.00 **Unspecified nystagmus**
H55.01 **Congenital nystagmus**
H55.02 **Latent nystagmus**
H55.03 **Visual deprivation nystagmus**
H55.04 **Dissociated nystagmus**
H55.09 **Other forms of nystagmus**

✓5th **H55.8 Other irregular eye movements**
H55.81 **Saccadic eye movements**
H55.89 **Other irregular eye movements**

✓4th **H57 Other disorders of eye and adnexa**

✓5th **H57.0 Anomalies of pupillary function**
H57.00 **Unspecified anomaly of pupillary function**
H57.01 **Argyll Robertson pupil, atypical**
EXCLUDES 1 *syphilitic Argyll Robertson pupil (A52.19)*
H57.02 **Anisocoria**
H57.03 **Miosis**
H57.04 **Mydriasis**
✓6th H57.05 **Tonic pupil**
H57.051 **Tonic pupil, right eye**
H57.052 **Tonic pupil, left eye**
H57.053 **Tonic pupil, bilateral**
H57.059 **Tonic pupil, unspecified eye**
H57.09 **Other anomalies of pupillary function**

✓5th **H57.1 Ocular pain**
H57.10 **Ocular pain, unspecified eye**
H57.11 **Ocular pain, right eye**
H57.12 **Ocular pain, left eye**
H57.13 **Ocular pain, bilateral**

H57.8 Other specified disorders of eye and adnexa
H57.9 Unspecified disorder of eye and adnexa

✓4th H59 Intraoperative and postprocedural complications and disorders of eye and adnexa, not elsewhere classified

EXCLUDES 1 *mechanical complication of intraocular lens (T85.2)*
mechanical complication of other ocular prosthetic devices, implants and grafts (T85.3)
pseudophakia (Z96.1)
secondary cataracts (H26.4-)

✓5th H59.0 Disorders of the eye following cataract surgery

CC Excl: For CC codes in subcategory H59.0, unless otherwise noted: H59.011-H59.019, H59.031-H59.099, H59.811-H59.89, H95.811-H95.89, I97.3, M96.89, N98.1-N98.9, T81.82XA, T81.89XA, T81.9XXA

✓6th H59.01 Keratopathy (bullous aphakic) following cataract surgery
Vitreal corneal syndrome
Vitreous (touch) syndrome

- **H59.011 Keratopathy (bullous aphakic) following cataract surgery, right eye** CC
- **H59.012 Keratopathy (bullous aphakic) following cataract surgery, left eye** CC
- **H59.013 Keratopathy (bullous aphakic) following cataract surgery, bilateral** CC
- **H59.019 Keratopathy (bullous aphakic) following cataract surgery, unspecified eye** CC

✓6th H59.02 Cataract (lens) fragments in eye following cataract surgery

- **H59.021 Cataract (lens) fragments in eye following cataract surgery, right eye**
- **H59.022 Cataract (lens) fragments in eye following cataract surgery, left eye**
- **H59.023 Cataract (lens) fragments in eye following cataract surgery, bilateral**
- **H59.029 Cataract (lens) fragments in eye following cataract surgery, unspecified eye**

✓6th H59.03 Cystoid macular edema following cataract surgery

- **H59.031 Cystoid macular edema following cataract surgery, right eye** CC
- **H59.032 Cystoid macular edema following cataract surgery, left eye** CC
- **H59.033 Cystoid macular edema following cataract surgery, bilateral** CC
- **H59.039 Cystoid macular edema following cataract surgery, unspecified eye** CC

✓6th H59.09 Other disorders of the eye following cataract surgery

- **H59.091 Other disorders of the right eye following cataract surgery** CC
- **H59.092 Other disorders of the left eye following cataract surgery** CC
- **H59.093 Other disorders of the eye following cataract surgery, bilateral** CC
- **H59.099 Other disorders of unspecified eye following cataract surgery** CC

✓5th H59.1 Intraoperative hemorrhage and hematoma of eye and adnexa complicating a procedure

EXCLUDES 1 *intraoperative hemorrhage and hematoma of eye and adnexa due to accidental puncture or laceration during a procedure (H59.2-)*

CC Excl: For CC codes in subcategory H59.1, unless otherwise noted: H59.011-H59.019, H59.031-H59.129, H59.311-H59.329, H59.811-H59.89, H95.811-H95.89, I85.01, I85.11, I97.3, K21.9, K22.8, K23-K25.0, K25.2, K25.4, K25.6, K26.0, K26.2, K26.4, K26.6, K27.0, K27.2, K27.4, K27.6, K28.0, K28.2, K28.4, K28.6, K29.01, K29.21, K29.31, K29.41, K29.51, K29.61, K29.71, K29.81, K29.91, K31.811, K55.21, K57.01, K57.11, K57.13, K57.21, K57.31, K57.33, K57.41, K57.51, K57.53, K57.81, K57.91, K57.93, K62.5, K92.0-K92.2, M96.89, N98.1-N98.9, P54.1-P54.3, T81.10XA, T81.11XA, T81.12XA, T81.19XA, T81.82XA, T81.89XA, T81.9XXA

✓6th H59.11 Intraoperative hemorrhage and hematoma of eye and adnexa complicating an ophthalmic procedure

- **H59.111 Intraoperative hemorrhage and hematoma of right eye and adnexa complicating an ophthalmic procedure** CC
- **H59.112 Intraoperative hemorrhage and hematoma of left eye and adnexa complicating an ophthalmic procedure** CC
- **H59.113 Intraoperative hemorrhage and hematoma of eye and adnexa complicating an ophthalmic procedure, bilateral** CC
- **H59.119 Intraoperative hemorrhage and hematoma of unspecified eye and adnexa complicating an ophthalmic procedure** CC

✓6th H59.12 Intraoperative hemorrhage and hematoma of eye and adnexa complicating other procedure

- **H59.121 Intraoperative hemorrhage and hematoma of right eye and adnexa complicating other procedure** CC
- **H59.122 Intraoperative hemorrhage and hematoma of left eye and adnexa complicating other procedure** CC
- **H59.123 Intraoperative hemorrhage and hematoma of eye and adnexa complicating other procedure, bilateral** CC
- **H59.129 Intraoperative hemorrhage and hematoma of unspecified eye and adnexa complicating other procedure** CC

✓5th H59.2 Accidental puncture and laceration of eye and adnexa during a procedure

CC Excl: For CC codes in subcategory H59.2, unless otherwise noted: D78.11-D78.12, D78.81-D78.89, E36.11-E36.8, E89.810-E89.89, G96.11, G97.41, G97.48-G97.49, H59.011-H59.019, H59.031-H59.099, H59.211-H59.229, H59.811-H59.89, H95.31-H95.32, H95.811-H95.89, I97.3, I97.51-I97.52, J95.71-J95.72, K91.71-K91.72, L76.11-L76.12, L76.81-L76.82, M96.820-M96.821, M96.89, N98.1-N98.9, N99.71-N99.72, T81.82XA, T81.89XA, T81.9XXA

✓6th H59.21 Accidental puncture and laceration of eye and adnexa during an ophthalmic procedure

- **H59.211 Accidental puncture and laceration of right eye and adnexa during an ophthalmic procedure** CC
- **H59.212 Accidental puncture and laceration of left eye and adnexa during an ophthalmic procedure** CC
- **H59.213 Accidental puncture and laceration of eye and adnexa during an ophthalmic procedure, bilateral** CC
- **H59.219 Accidental puncture and laceration of unspecified eye and adnexa during an ophthalmic procedure** CC

✓6th H59.22 Accidental puncture and laceration of eye and adnexa during other procedure

- **H59.221 Accidental puncture and laceration of right eye and adnexa during other procedure** CC
- **H59.222 Accidental puncture and laceration of left eye and adnexa during other procedure** CC
- **H59.223 Accidental puncture and laceration of eye and adnexa during other procedure, bilateral** CC
- **H59.229 Accidental puncture and laceration of unspecified eye and adnexa during other procedure** CC

✓5th H59.3 Postprocedural hemorrhage and hematoma of eye and adnexa following a procedure

CC Excl: For CC codes in subcategory H59.3, unless otherwise noted: See code: H59.1

✓6th H59.31 Postprocedural hemorrhage and hematoma of eye and adnexa following an ophthalmic procedure

- **H59.311 Postprocedural hemorrhage and hematoma of right eye and adnexa following an ophthalmic procedure** CC
- **H59.312 Postprocedural hemorrhage and hematoma of left eye and adnexa following an ophthalmic procedure** CC
- **H59.313 Postprocedural hemorrhage and hematoma of eye and adnexa following an ophthalmic procedure, bilateral** CC
- **H59.319 Postprocedural hemorrhage and hematoma of unspecified eye and adnexa following an ophthalmic procedure** CC

✓6th **H59.32 Postprocedural hemorrhage and hematoma of eye and adnexa following other procedure**

H59.321 Postprocedural hemorrhage and hematoma of right eye and adnexa following other procedure CC

H59.322 Postprocedural hemorrhage and hematoma of left eye and adnexa following other procedure CC

H59.323 Postprocedural hemorrhage and hematoma of eye and adnexa following other procedure, bilateral CC

H59.329 Postprocedural hemorrhage and hematoma of unspecified eye and adnexa following other procedure CC

✓5th **H59.4 Inflammation (infection) of postprocedural bleb**

Postprocedural blebitis

EXCLUDES 1 *filtering (vitreous) bleb after glaucoma surgery status (Z98.83)*

H59.40 Inflammation (infection) of postprocedural bleb, unspecified

H59.41 Inflammation (infection) of postprocedural bleb, stage 1

H59.42 Inflammation (infection) of postprocedural bleb, stage 2

H59.43 Inflammation (infection) of postprocedural bleb, stage 3

Bleb endophthalmitis

✓5th **H59.8 Other intraoperative and postprocedural complications and disorders of eye and adnexa, not elsewhere classified**

CC Excl: For CC codes in subcategory H59.8, unless otherwise noted: H59.011-H59.019, H59.031-H59.099, H59.811-H59.89, H95.811-H95.89, I97.3, M96.89, N98.1-N98.9, T81.82XA, T81.89XA, T81.9XXA

✓6th **H59.81 Chorioretinal scars after surgery for detachment**

H59.811 Chorioretinal scars after surgery for detachment, right eye CC

H59.812 Chorioretinal scars after surgery for detachment, left eye CC

H59.813 Chorioretinal scars after surgery for detachment, bilateral CC

H59.819 Chorioretinal scars after surgery for detachment, unspecified eye CC

H59.88 Other intraoperative complications of eye and adnexa, not elsewhere classified CC

H59.89 Other postprocedural complications and disorders of eye and adnexa, not elsewhere classified CC

Chapter 8. Diseases of the Ear and Mastoid Process (H60-H95)

NOTE Use an external cause code following the code for the ear condition, if applicable, to identify the cause of the ear condition.

EXCLUDES 2 *certain conditions originating in the perinatal period (P04-P96)*
certain infectious and parasitic diseases (A00-B99)
complications of pregnancy, childbirth and the puerperium (O00-O9A)
congenital malformations, deformations and chromosomal abnormalities (Q00-Q99)
endocrine, nutritional and metabolic diseases (E00-E88)
injury, poisoning and certain other consequences of external causes (S00-T88)
neoplasms (C00-D49)
symptoms, signs and abnormal clinical and laboratory findings, not elsewhere classified (R00-R94)

This chapter contains the following blocks:

H60-H62	Diseases of external ear
H65-H75	Diseases of middle ear and mastoid
H80-H83	Diseases of inner ear
H90-H94	Other disorders of ear
H95	Intraoperative and postprocedural complications and disorders of ear and mastoid process, not elsewhere classified

Diseases of external ear (H60-H62)

√4th **H60 Otitis externa**

√5th **H60.0 Abscess of external ear**
Boil of external ear
Carbuncle of auricle or external auditory canal
Furuncle of external ear
H60.00 Abscess of external ear, unspecified ear
H60.01 Abscess of right external ear
H60.02 Abscess of left external ear
H60.03 Abscess of external ear, bilateral

√5th **H60.1 Cellulitis of external ear**
Cellulitis of auricle
Cellulitis of external auditory canal
H60.10 Cellulitis of external ear, unspecified ear
H60.11 Cellulitis of right external ear
H60.12 Cellulitis of left external ear
H60.13 Cellulitis of external ear, bilateral

√5th **H60.2 Malignant otitis externa**

CC Excl: For CC codes in subcategory H60.2, unless otherwise noted: H60.20-H60.23, H70.001-H70.13

H60.20 Malignant otitis externa, unspecified ear CC
H60.21 Malignant otitis externa, right ear CC
H60.22 Malignant otitis externa, left ear CC
H60.23 Malignant otitis externa, bilateral CC

√5th **H60.3 Other infective otitis externa**

√6th **H60.31 Diffuse otitis externa**
H60.311 Diffuse otitis externa, right ear
H60.312 Diffuse otitis externa, left ear
H60.313 Diffuse otitis externa, bilateral
H60.319 Diffuse otitis externa, unspecified ear

√6th **H60.32 Hemorrhagic otitis externa**
H60.321 Hemorrhagic otitis externa, right ear
H60.322 Hemorrhagic otitis externa, left ear
H60.323 Hemorrhagic otitis externa, bilateral
H60.329 Hemorrhagic otitis externa, unspecified ear

√6th **H60.33 Swimmer's ear**
H60.331 Swimmer's ear, right ear
H60.332 Swimmer's ear, left ear
H60.333 Swimmer's ear, bilateral
H60.339 Swimmer's ear, unspecified ear

√6th **H60.39 Other infective otitis externa**
H60.391 Other infective otitis externa, right ear
H60.392 Other infective otitis externa, left ear
H60.393 Other infective otitis externa, bilateral
H60.399 Other infective otitis externa, unspecified ear

√5th **H60.4 Cholesteatoma of external ear**
Keratosis obturans of external ear (canal)
EXCLUDES 2 *cholesteatoma of middle ear (H71.-)*
recurrent cholesteatoma of postmastoidectomy cavity (H95.0-)
H60.40 Cholesteatoma of external ear, unspecified ear
H60.41 Cholesteatoma of right external ear
H60.42 Cholesteatoma of left external ear
H60.43 Cholesteatoma of external ear, bilateral

√5th **H60.5 Acute noninfective otitis externa**

√6th **H60.50 Unspecified acute noninfective otitis externa**
Acute otitis externa NOS
H60.501 Unspecified acute noninfective otitis externa, right ear
H60.502 Unspecified acute noninfective otitis externa, left ear
H60.503 Unspecified acute noninfective otitis externa, bilateral
H60.509 Unspecified acute noninfective otitis externa, unspecified ear

√6th **H60.51 Acute actinic otitis externa**
H60.511 Acute actinic otitis externa, right ear
H60.512 Acute actinic otitis externa, left ear
H60.513 Acute actinic otitis externa, bilateral
H60.519 Acute actinic otitis externa, unspecified ear

√6th **H60.52 Acute chemical otitis externa**
H60.521 Acute chemical otitis externa, right ear
H60.522 Acute chemical otitis externa, left ear
H60.523 Acute chemical otitis externa, bilateral
H60.529 Acute chemical otitis externa, unspecified ear

√6th **H60.53 Acute contact otitis externa**
H60.531 Acute contact otitis externa, right ear
H60.532 Acute contact otitis externa, left ear
H60.533 Acute contact otitis externa, bilateral
H60.539 Acute contact otitis externa, unspecified ear

√6th **H60.54 Acute eczematoid otitis externa**
H60.541 Acute eczematoid otitis externa, right ear
H60.542 Acute eczematoid otitis externa, left ear
H60.543 Acute eczematoid otitis externa, bilateral
H60.549 Acute eczematoid otitis externa, unspecified ear

√6th **H60.55 Acute reactive otitis externa**
H60.551 Acute reactive otitis externa, right ear
H60.552 Acute reactive otitis externa, left ear
H60.553 Acute reactive otitis externa, bilateral
H60.559 Acute reactive otitis externa, unspecified ear

√6th **H60.59 Other noninfective acute otitis externa**
H60.591 Other noninfective acute otitis externa, right ear
H60.592 Other noninfective acute otitis externa, left ear
H60.593 Other noninfective acute otitis externa, bilateral
H60.599 Other noninfective acute otitis externa, unspecified ear

√5th **H60.6 Unspecified chronic otitis externa**
H60.60 Unspecified chronic otitis externa, unspecified ear
H60.61 Unspecified chronic otitis externa, right ear
H60.62 Unspecified chronic otitis externa, left ear
H60.63 Unspecified chronic otitis externa, bilateral

√5th **H60.8 Other otitis externa**

√6th **H60.8X Other otitis externa**
H60.8X1 Other otitis externa, right ear
H60.8X2 Other otitis externa, left ear
H60.8X3 Other otitis externa, bilateral
H60.8X9 Other otitis externa, unspecified ear

√5th **H60.9 Unspecified otitis externa**
H60.90 Unspecified otitis externa, unspecified ear
H60.91 Unspecified otitis externa, right ear

H60.92 Unspecified otitis externa, left ear
H60.93 Unspecified otitis externa, bilateral

H61 Other disorders of external ear

H61.0 Chondritis and perichondritis of external ear
Chondrodermatitis nodularis chronica helicis
Perichondritis of auricle
Perichondritis of pinna

H61.00 Unspecified perichondritis of external ear
- H61.001 Unspecified perichondritis of right external ear
- H61.002 Unspecified perichondritis of left external ear
- H61.003 Unspecified perichondritis of external ear, bilateral
- H61.009 Unspecified perichondritis of external ear, unspecified ear

H61.01 Acute perichondritis of external ear
- H61.011 Acute perichondritis of right external ear
- H61.012 Acute perichondritis of left external ear
- H61.013 Acute perichondritis of external ear, bilateral
- H61.019 Acute perichondritis of external ear, unspecified ear

H61.02 Chronic perichondritis of external ear
- H61.021 Chronic perichondritis of right external ear
- H61.022 Chronic perichondritis of left external ear
- H61.023 Chronic perichondritis of external ear, bilateral
- H61.029 Chronic perichondritis of external ear, unspecified ear

H61.03 Chondritis of external ear
Chondritis of auricle Chondritis of pinna
- H61.031 Chondritis of right external ear
- H61.032 Chondritis of left external ear
- H61.033 Chondritis of external ear, bilateral
- H61.039 Chondritis of external ear, unspecified ear

H61.1 Noninfective disorders of pinna
EXCLUDES 2 *cauliflower ear (M95.1-)*
gouty tophi of ear (M1A.-)

H61.10 Unspecified noninfective disorders of pinna
Disorder of pinna NOS
- H61.101 Unspecified noninfective disorders of pinna, right ear
- H61.102 Unspecified noninfective disorders of pinna, left ear
- H61.103 Unspecified noninfective disorders of pinna, bilateral
- H61.109 Unspecified noninfective disorders of pinna, unspecified ear

H61.11 Acquired deformity of pinna
Acquired deformity of auricle
EXCLUDES 2 *cauliflower ear (M95.1-)*
- H61.111 Acquired deformity of pinna, right ear
- H61.112 Acquired deformity of pinna, left ear
- H61.113 Acquired deformity of pinna, bilateral
- H61.119 Acquired deformity of pinna, unspecified ear

H61.12 Hematoma of pinna
Hematoma of auricle
- H61.121 Hematoma of pinna, right ear
- H61.122 Hematoma of pinna, left ear
- H61.123 Hematoma of pinna, bilateral
- H61.129 Hematoma of pinna, unspecified ear

H61.19 Other noninfective disorders of pinna
- H61.191 Noninfective disorders of pinna, right ear
- H61.192 Noninfective disorders of pinna, left ear
- H61.193 Noninfective disorders of pinna, bilateral
- H61.199 Noninfective disorders of pinna, unspecified ear

H61.2 Impacted cerumen
Wax in ear
- [13] H61.20 Impacted cerumen, unspecified ear
- [13] H61.21 Impacted cerumen, right ear
- [13] H61.22 Impacted cerumen, left ear
- [13] H61.23 Impacted cerumen, bilateral

H61.3 Acquired stenosis of external ear canal
Collapse of external ear canal
EXCLUDES 1 *postprocedural stenosis of external ear canal (H95.81-)*

H61.30 Acquired stenosis of external ear canal, unspecified
- H61.301 Acquired stenosis of right external ear canal, unspecified
- H61.302 Acquired stenosis of left external ear canal, unspecified
- H61.303 Acquired stenosis of external ear canal, unspecified, bilateral
- H61.309 Acquired stenosis of external ear canal, unspecified, unspecified ear

H61.31 Acquired stenosis of external ear canal secondary to trauma
- H61.311 Acquired stenosis of right external ear canal secondary to trauma
- H61.312 Acquired stenosis of left external ear canal secondary to trauma
- H61.313 Acquired stenosis of external ear canal secondary to trauma, bilateral
- H61.319 Acquired stenosis of external ear canal secondary to trauma, unspecified ear

H61.32 Acquired stenosis of external ear canal secondary to inflammation and infection
- H61.321 Acquired stenosis of right external ear canal secondary to inflammation and infection
- H61.322 Acquired stenosis of left external ear canal secondary to inflammation and infection
- H61.323 Acquired stenosis of external ear canal secondary to inflammation and infection, bilateral
- H61.329 Acquired stenosis of external ear canal secondary to inflammation and infection, unspecified ear

H61.39 Other acquired stenosis of external ear canal
- H61.391 Other acquired stenosis of right external ear canal
- H61.392 Other acquired stenosis of left external ear canal
- H61.393 Other acquired stenosis of external ear canal, bilateral
- H61.399 Other acquired stenosis of external ear canal, unspecified ear

H61.8 Other specified disorders of external ear

H61.81 Exostosis of external canal
- H61.811 Exostosis of right external canal
- H61.812 Exostosis of left external canal
- H61.813 Exostosis of external canal, bilateral
- H61.819 Exostosis of external canal, unspecified ear

H61.89 Other specified disorders of external ear
- H61.891 Other specified disorders of right external ear
- H61.892 Other specified disorders of left external ear
- H61.893 Other specified disorders of external ear, bilateral
- H61.899 Other specified disorders of external ear, unspecified ear

H61.9 Disorder of external ear, unspecified
- H61.90 Disorder of external ear, unspecified, unspecified ear
- H61.91 Disorder of right external ear, unspecified
- H61.92 Disorder of left external ear, unspecified
- H61.93 Disorder of external ear, unspecified, bilateral

13 Questionable admission when used as PDx.

4th H62 Disorders of external ear in diseases classified elsewhere

5th H62.4 Otitis externa in other diseases classified elsewhere

Code first underlying disease, such as:
erysipelas (A46)
impetigo (LØ1.Ø)

EXCLUDES 1 *otitis externa (in):*
candidiasis (B37.84)
herpes viral [herpes simplex] (BØØ.1)
herpes zoster (BØ2.8)

H62.4Ø Otitis externa in other diseases classified elsewhere, unspecified ear
H62.41 Otitis externa in other diseases classified elsewhere, right ear
H62.42 Otitis externa in other diseases classified elsewhere, left ear
H62.43 Otitis externa in other diseases classified elsewhere, bilateral

5th H62.8 Other disorders of external ear in diseases classified elsewhere

Code first underlying disease, such as:
gout (M1A.-, M1Ø.-)

6th H62.8X Other disorders of external ear in diseases classified elsewhere

H62.8X1 Other disorders of right external ear in diseases classified elsewhere
H62.8X2 Other disorders of left external ear in diseases classified elsewhere
H62.8X3 Other disorders of external ear in diseases classified elsewhere, bilateral
H62.8X9 Other disorders of external ear in diseases classified elsewhere, unspecified ear

Diseases of middle ear and mastoid (H65-H75)

4th H65 Nonsuppurative otitis media

INCLUDES nonsuppurative otitis media with myringitis

Use additional code for any associated perforated tympanic membrane (H72.-)

Use additional code to identify:
exposure to environmental tobacco smoke (Z77.22)
exposure to tobacco smoke in the perinatal period (P96.81)
history of tobacco use (Z87.891)
occupational exposure to environmental tobacco smoke (Z57.31)
tobacco dependence (F17.-)
tobacco use (Z72.Ø)

5th H65.Ø Acute serous otitis media

Acute and subacute secretory otitis

H65.ØØ Acute serous otitis media, unspecified ear
H65.Ø1 Acute serous otitis media, right ear
H65.Ø2 Acute serous otitis media, left ear
H65.Ø3 Acute serous otitis media, bilateral
H65.Ø4 Acute serous otitis media, recurrent, right ear
H65.Ø5 Acute serous otitis media, recurrent, left ear
H65.Ø6 Acute serous otitis media, recurrent, bilateral
H65.Ø7 Acute serous otitis media, recurrent, unspecified ear

5th H65.1 Other acute nonsuppurative otitis media

EXCLUDES 1 *otitic barotrauma (T7Ø.Ø)*
otitis media (acute) NOS (H66.9)

6th H65.11 Acute and subacute allergic otitis media (mucoid) (sanguinous) (serous)

H65.111 Acute and subacute allergic otitis media (mucoid) (sanguinous) (serous), right ear
H65.112 Acute and subacute allergic otitis media (mucoid) (sanguinous) (serous), left ear
H65.113 Acute and subacute allergic otitis media (mucoid) (sanguinous) (serous), bilateral
H65.114 Acute and subacute allergic otitis media (mucoid) (sanguinous) (serous), recurrent, right ear
H65.115 Acute and subacute allergic otitis media (mucoid) (sanguinous) (serous), recurrent, left ear
H65.116 Acute and subacute allergic otitis media (mucoid) (sanguinous) (serous), recurrent, bilateral
H65.117 Acute and subacute allergic otitis media (mucoid) (sanguinous) (serous), recurrent, unspecified ear
H65.119 Acute and subacute allergic otitis media (mucoid) (sanguinous) (serous), unspecified ear

6th H65.19 Other acute nonsuppurative otitis media

Acute and subacute mucoid otitis media
Acute and subacute nonsuppurative otitis media NOS
Acute and subacute sanguinous otitis media
Acute and subacute seromucinous otitis media

H65.191 Other acute nonsuppurative otitis media, right ear
H65.192 Other acute nonsuppurative otitis media, left ear
H65.193 Other acute nonsuppurative otitis media, bilateral
H65.194 Other acute nonsuppurative otitis media, recurrent, right ear
H65.195 Other acute nonsuppurative otitis media, recurrent, left ear
H65.196 Other acute nonsuppurative otitis media, recurrent, bilateral
H65.197 Other acute nonsuppurative otitis media recurrent, unspecified ear
H65.199 Other acute nonsuppurative otitis media, unspecified ear

5th H65.2 Chronic serous otitis media

Chronic tubotympanal catarrh

H65.2Ø Chronic serous otitis media, unspecified ear
H65.21 Chronic serous otitis media, right ear
H65.22 Chronic serous otitis media, left ear
H65.23 Chronic serous otitis media, bilateral

5th H65.3 Chronic mucoid otitis media

Chronic mucinous otitis media
Chronic secretory otitis media
Chronic transudative otitis media
Glue ear

EXCLUDES 1 *adhesive middle ear disease (H74.1)*

H65.3Ø Chronic mucoid otitis media, unspecified ear
H65.31 Chronic mucoid otitis media, right ear
H65.32 Chronic mucoid otitis media, left ear
H65.33 Chronic mucoid otitis media, bilateral

5th H65.4 Other chronic nonsuppurative otitis media

6th H65.41 Chronic allergic otitis media

H65.411 Chronic allergic otitis media, right ear
H65.412 Chronic allergic otitis media, left ear
H65.413 Chronic allergic otitis media, bilateral
H65.419 Chronic allergic otitis media, unspecified ear

6th H65.49 Other chronic nonsuppurative otitis media

Chronic exudative otitis media
Chronic nonsuppurative otitis media NOS
Chronic otitis media with effusion (nonpurulent)
Chronic seromucinous otitis media

H65.491 Other chronic nonsuppurative otitis media, right ear
H65.492 Other chronic nonsuppurative otitis media, left ear
H65.493 Other chronic nonsuppurative otitis media, bilateral
H65.499 Other chronic nonsuppurative otitis media, unspecified ear

5th H65.9 Unspecified nonsuppurative otitis media

Allergic otitis media NOS
Catarrhal otitis media NOS
Exudative otitis media NOS
Mucoid otitis media NOS
Otitis media with effusion (nonpurulent) NOS
Secretory otitis media NOS
Seromucinous otitis media NOS
Serous otitis media NOS
Transudative otitis media NOS

H65.9Ø Unspecified nonsuppurative otitis media, unspecified ear
H65.91 Unspecified nonsuppurative otitis media, right ear
H65.92 Unspecified nonsuppurative otitis media, left ear
H65.93 Unspecified nonsuppurative otitis media, bilateral

H66 Suppurative and unspecified otitis media
INCLUDES suppurative and unspecified otitis media with myringitis
Use additional code to identify:
exposure to environmental tobacco smoke (Z77.22)
exposure to tobacco smoke in the perinatal period (P96.81)
history of tobacco use (Z87.891)
occupational exposure to environmental tobacco smoke (Z57.31)
tobacco dependence (F17.-)
tobacco use (Z72.0)

H66.0 Acute suppurative otitis media

H66.00 Acute suppurative otitis media without spontaneous rupture of ear drum
H66.001 Acute suppurative otitis media without spontaneous rupture of ear drum, right ear
H66.002 Acute suppurative otitis media without spontaneous rupture of ear drum, left ear
H66.003 Acute suppurative otitis media without spontaneous rupture of ear drum, bilateral
H66.004 Acute suppurative otitis media without spontaneous rupture of ear drum, recurrent, right ear
H66.005 Acute suppurative otitis media without spontaneous rupture of ear drum, recurrent, left ear
H66.006 Acute suppurative otitis media without spontaneous rupture of ear drum, recurrent, bilateral
H66.007 Acute suppurative otitis media without spontaneous rupture of ear drum, recurrent, unspecified ear
H66.009 Acute suppurative otitis media without spontaneous rupture of ear drum, unspecified ear

H66.01 Acute suppurative otitis media with spontaneous rupture of ear drum
H66.011 Acute suppurative otitis media with spontaneous rupture of ear drum, right ear
H66.012 Acute suppurative otitis media with spontaneous rupture of ear drum, left ear
H66.013 Acute suppurative otitis media with spontaneous rupture of ear drum, bilateral
H66.014 Acute suppurative otitis media with spontaneous rupture of ear drum, recurrent, right ear
H66.015 Acute suppurative otitis media with spontaneous rupture of ear drum, recurrent, left ear
H66.016 Acute suppurative otitis media with spontaneous rupture of ear drum, recurrent, bilateral
H66.017 Acute suppurative otitis media with spontaneous rupture of ear drum, recurrent, unspecified ear
H66.019 Acute suppurative otitis media with spontaneous rupture of ear drum, unspecified ear

H66.1 Chronic tubotympanic suppurative otitis media
Benign chronic suppurative otitis media
Chronic tubotympanic disease
Use additional code for any associated perforated tympanic membrane (H72.-)
H66.10 Chronic tubotympanic suppurative otitis media, unspecified
H66.11 Chronic tubotympanic suppurative otitis media, right ear
H66.12 Chronic tubotympanic suppurative otitis media, left ear
H66.13 Chronic tubotympanic suppurative otitis media, bilateral

H66.2 Chronic atticoantral suppurative otitis media
Chronic atticoantral disease
Use additional code for any associated perforated tympanic membrane (H72.-)
H66.20 Chronic atticoantral suppurative otitis media, unspecified ear
H66.21 Chronic atticoantral suppurative otitis media, right ear
H66.22 Chronic atticoantral suppurative otitis media, left ear
H66.23 Chronic atticoantral suppurative otitis media, bilateral

H66.3 Other chronic suppurative otitis media
Chronic suppurative otitis media NOS
Use additional code for any associated perforated tympanic membrane (H72.-)
EXCLUDES 1 *tuberculous otitis media (A18.6)*

H66.3X Other chronic suppurative otitis media
H66.3X1 Other chronic suppurative otitis media, right ear
H66.3X2 Other chronic suppurative otitis media, left ear
H66.3X3 Other chronic suppurative otitis media, bilateral
H66.3X9 Other chronic suppurative otitis media, unspecified ear

H66.4 Suppurative otitis media, unspecified
Purulent otitis media NOS
Use additional code for any associated perforated tympanic membrane (H72.-)
H66.40 Suppurative otitis media, unspecified, unspecified ear
H66.41 Suppurative otitis media, unspecified, right ear
H66.42 Suppurative otitis media, unspecified, left ear
H66.43 Suppurative otitis media, unspecified, bilateral

H66.9 Otitis media, unspecified
Otitis media NOS
Acute otitis media NOS
Chronic otitis media NOS
Use additional code for any associated perforated tympanic membrane (H72.-)
H66.90 Otitis media, unspecified, unspecified ear
H66.91 Otitis media, unspecified, right ear
H66.92 Otitis media, unspecified, left ear
H66.93 Otitis media, unspecified, bilateral

H67 Otitis media in diseases classified elsewhere
Code first underlying disease, such as:
viral disease NEC (B00-B34)
Use additional code for any associated perforated tympanic membrane (H72.-)
EXCLUDES 1 *otitis media in:*
influenza (J09.X9, J10.83, J11.83)
measles (B05.3)
scarlet fever (A38.0)
tuberculosis (A18.6)
H67.1 ***Otitis media in diseases classified elsewhere, right ear***
H67.2 ***Otitis media in diseases classified elsewhere, left ear***
H67.3 ***Otitis media in diseases classified elsewhere, bilateral***
H67.9 ***Otitis media in diseases classified elsewhere, unspecified ear***

H68 Eustachian salpingitis and obstruction

H68.0 Eustachian salpingitis

H68.00 Unspecified Eustachian salpingitis
H68.001 Unspecified Eustachian salpingitis, right ear
H68.002 Unspecified Eustachian salpingitis, left ear
H68.003 Unspecified Eustachian salpingitis, bilateral
H68.009 Unspecified Eustachian salpingitis, unspecified ear

H68.01 Acute Eustachian salpingitis
H68.011 Acute Eustachian salpingitis, right ear
H68.012 Acute Eustachian salpingitis, left ear
H68.013 Acute Eustachian salpingitis, bilateral
H68.019 Acute Eustachian salpingitis, unspecified ear

H68.02 Chronic Eustachian salpingitis
H68.021 Chronic Eustachian salpingitis, right ear
H68.022 Chronic Eustachian salpingitis, left ear
H68.023 Chronic Eustachian salpingitis, bilateral
H68.029 Chronic Eustachian salpingitis, unspecified ear

5th **H68.1 Obstruction of Eustachian tube**
Stenosis of Eustachian tube
Stricture of Eustachian tube

6th **H68.10 Unspecified obstruction of Eustachian tube**
H68.101 Unspecified obstruction of Eustachian tube, right ear
H68.102 Unspecified obstruction of Eustachian tube, left ear
H68.103 Unspecified obstruction of Eustachian tube, bilateral
H68.109 Unspecified obstruction of Eustachian tube, unspecified ear

6th **H68.11 Osseous obstruction of Eustachian tube**
H68.111 Osseous obstruction of Eustachian tube, right ear
H68.112 Osseous obstruction of Eustachian tube, left ear
H68.113 Osseous obstruction of Eustachian tube, bilateral
H68.119 Osseous obstruction of Eustachian tube, unspecified ear

6th **H68.12 Intrinsic cartilagenous obstruction of Eustachian tube**
H68.121 Intrinsic cartilagenous obstruction of Eustachian tube, right ear
H68.122 Intrinsic cartilagenous obstruction of Eustachian tube, left ear
H68.123 Intrinsic cartilagenous obstruction of Eustachian tube, bilateral
H68.129 Intrinsic cartilagenous obstruction of Eustachian tube, unspecified ear

6th **H68.13 Extrinsic cartilagenous obstruction of Eustachian tube**
Compression of Eustachian tube
H68.131 Extrinsic cartilagenous obstruction of Eustachian tube, right ear
H68.132 Extrinsic cartilagenous obstruction of Eustachian tube, left ear
H68.133 Extrinsic cartilagenous obstruction of Eustachian tube, bilateral
H68.139 Extrinsic cartilagenous obstruction of Eustachian tube, unspecified ear

4th **H69 Other and unspecified disorders of Eustachian tube**

5th **H69.0 Patulous Eustachian tube**
H69.00 Patulous Eustachian tube, unspecified ear
H69.01 Patulous Eustachian tube, right ear
H69.02 Patulous Eustachian tube, left ear
H69.03 Patulous Eustachian tube, bilateral

5th **H69.8 Other specified disorders of Eustachian tube**
H69.80 Other specified disorders of Eustachian tube, unspecified ear
H69.81 Other specified disorders of Eustachian tube, right ear
H69.82 Other specified disorders of Eustachian tube, left ear
H69.83 Other specified disorders of Eustachian tube, bilateral

5th **H69.9 Unspecified Eustachian tube disorder**
H69.90 Unspecified Eustachian tube disorder, unspecified ear
H69.91 Unspecified Eustachian tube disorder, right ear
H69.92 Unspecified Eustachian tube disorder, left ear
H69.93 Unspecified Eustachian tube disorder, bilateral

4th **H70 Mastoiditis and related conditions**

5th **H70.0 Acute mastoiditis**
Abscess of mastoid
Empyema of mastoid

CC Excl: For CC codes in subcategory H70.0, unless otherwise noted: A17.9, A18.6, A18.82, A18.84, A18.89, H70.001-H70.93, H75.00-H75.83, H93.8X1-H93.93, H94.80-H95.199, Q16.1, Q16.9, Q17.3-Q17.9

6th **H70.00 Acute mastoiditis without complications**
H70.001 Acute mastoiditis without complications, right ear CC
H70.002 Acute mastoiditis without complications, left ear CC
H70.003 Acute mastoiditis without complications, bilateral CC
H70.009 Acute mastoiditis without complications, unspecified eard CC

6th **H70.01 Subperiosteal abscess of mastoid**
H70.011 Subperiosteal abscess of mastoid, right ear CC
H70.012 Subperiosteal abscess of mastoid, left ear CC
H70.013 Subperiosteal abscess of mastoid, bilateral CC
H70.019 Subperiosteal abscess of mastoid, unspecified ear CC

6th **H70.09 Acute mastoiditis with other complications**
H70.091 Acute mastoiditis with other complications, right ear CC
H70.092 Acute mastoiditis with other complications, left ear CC
H70.093 Acute mastoiditis with other complications, bilateral CC
H70.099 Acute mastoiditis with other complications, unspecified ear CC

5th **H70.1 Chronic mastoiditis**
Caries of mastoid
Fistula of mastoid
EXCLUDES 1 *tuberculous mastoiditis (A18.03)*
H70.10 Chronic mastoiditis, unspecified ear
H70.11 Chronic mastoiditis, right ear
H70.12 Chronic mastoiditis, left ear
H70.13 Chronic mastoiditis, bilateral

5th **H70.2 Petrositis**
Inflammation of petrous bone

6th **H70.20 Unspecified petrositis**
H70.201 Unspecified petrositis, right ear
H70.202 Unspecified petrositis, left ear
H70.203 Unspecified petrositis, bilateral
H70.209 Unspecified petrositis, unspecified ear

6th **H70.21 Acute petrositis**
H70.211 Acute petrositis, right ear
H70.212 Acute petrositis, left ear
H70.213 Acute petrositis, bilateral
H70.219 Acute petrositis, unspecified ear

6th **H70.22 Chronic petrositis**
H70.221 Chronic petrositis, right ear
H70.222 Chronic petrositis, left ear
H70.223 Chronic petrositis, bilateral
H70.229 Chronic petrositis, unspecified ear

5th **H70.8 Other mastoiditis and related conditions**
EXCLUDES 1 *preauricular sinus and cyst (Q18.1)*
sinus, fistula, and cyst of branchial cleft (Q18.0)

6th **H70.81 Postauricular fistula**
H70.811 Postauricular fistula, right ear
H70.812 Postauricular fistula, left ear
H70.813 Postauricular fistula, bilateral
H70.819 Postauricular fistula, unspecified ear

6th **H70.89 Other mastoiditis and related conditions**
H70.891 Other mastoiditis and related conditions, right ear
H70.892 Other mastoiditis and related conditions, left ear
H70.893 Other mastoiditis and related conditions, bilateral
H70.899 Other mastoiditis and related conditions, unspecified ear

5th **H70.9 Unspecified mastoiditis**
H70.90 Unspecified mastoiditis, unspecified ear
H70.91 Unspecified mastoiditis, right ear
H70.92 Unspecified mastoiditis, left ear
H70.93 Unspecified mastoiditis, bilateral

H71 Cholesteatoma of middle ear
EXCLUDES 2 *cholesteatoma of external ear (H60.4-)*
recurrent cholesteatoma of postmastoidectomy cavity (H95.0-)

H71.0 Cholesteatoma of attic
- **H71.00 Cholesteatoma of attic, unspecified ear**
- **H71.01 Cholesteatoma of attic, right ear**
- **H71.02 Cholesteatoma of attic, left ear**
- **H71.03 Cholesteatoma of attic, bilateral**

H71.1 Cholesteatoma of tympanum
- **H71.10 Cholesteatoma of tympanum, unspecified ear**
- **H71.11 Cholesteatoma of tympanum, right ear**
- **H71.12 Cholesteatoma of tympanum, left ear**
- **H71.13 Cholesteatoma of tympanum, bilateral**

H71.2 Cholesteatoma of mastoid
- **H71.20 Cholesteatoma of mastoid, unspecified ear**
- **H71.21 Cholesteatoma of mastoid, right ear**
- **H71.22 Cholesteatoma of mastoid, left ear**
- **H71.23 Cholesteatoma of mastoid, bilateral**

H71.3 Diffuse cholesteatosis
- **H71.30 Diffuse cholesteatosis, unspecified ear**
- **H71.31 Diffuse cholesteatosis, right ear**
- **H71.32 Diffuse cholesteatosis, left ear**
- **H71.33 Diffuse cholesteatosis, bilateral**

H71.9 Unspecified cholesteatoma
- **H71.90 Unspecified cholesteatoma, unspecified ear**
- **H71.91 Unspecified cholesteatoma, right ear**
- **H71.92 Unspecified cholesteatoma, left ear**
- **H71.93 Unspecified cholesteatoma, bilateral**

H72 Perforation of tympanic membrane
INCLUDES persistent post-traumatic perforation of ear drum
postinflammatory perforation of ear drum
Code first any associated otitis media (H65.-, H66.1-, H66.2-, H66.3-, H66.4-, H66.9-, H67.-)
EXCLUDES 1 *acute suppurative otitis media with rupture of the tympanic membrane (H66.01-)*
traumatic rupture of ear drum (S09.2-)

H72.0 Central perforation of tympanic membrane
- **H72.00 Central perforation of tympanic membrane, unspecified ear**
- **H72.01 Central perforation of tympanic membrane, right ear**
- **H72.02 Central perforation of tympanic membrane, left ear**
- **H72.03 Central perforation of tympanic membrane, bilateral**

H72.1 Attic perforation of tympanic membrane
Perforation of pars flaccida
- **H72.10 Attic perforation of tympanic membrane, unspecified ear**
- **H72.11 Attic perforation of tympanic membrane, right ear**
- **H72.12 Attic perforation of tympanic membrane, left ear**
- **H72.13 Attic perforation of tympanic membrane, bilateral**

H72.2 Other marginal perforations of tympanic membrane

H72.2X Other marginal perforations of tympanic membrane
- **H72.2X1 Other marginal perforations of tympanic membrane, right ear**
- **H72.2X2 Other marginal perforations of tympanic membrane, left ear**
- **H72.2X3 Other marginal perforations of tympanic membrane, bilateral**
- **H72.2X9 Other marginal perforations of tympanic membrane, unspecified ear**

H72.8 Other perforations of tympanic membrane

H72.81 Multiple perforations of tympanic membrane
- **H72.811 Multiple perforations of tympanic membrane, right ear**
- **H72.812 Multiple perforations of tympanic membrane, left ear**
- **H72.813 Multiple perforations of tympanic membrane, bilateral**
- **H72.819 Multiple perforations of tympanic membrane, unspecified ear**

H72.82 Total perforations of tympanic membrane
- **H72.821 Total perforations of tympanic membrane, right ear**
- **H72.822 Total perforations of tympanic membrane, left ear**
- **H72.823 Total perforations of tympanic membrane, bilateral**
- **H72.829 Total perforations of tympanic membrane, unspecified ear**

H72.9 Unspecified perforation of tympanic membrane
- **H72.90 Unspecified perforation of tympanic membrane, unspecified ear**
- **H72.91 Unspecified perforation of tympanic membrane, right ear**
- **H72.92 Unspecified perforation of tympanic membrane, left ear**
- **H72.93 Unspecified perforation of tympanic membrane, bilateral**

H73 Other disorders of tympanic membrane

H73.0 Acute myringitis
EXCLUDES 1 *acute myringitis with otitis media (H65, H66)*

H73.00 Unspecified acute myringitis
Acute tympanitis NOS
- **H73.001 Acute myringitis, right ear**
- **H73.002 Acute myringitis, left ear**
- **H73.003 Acute myringitis, bilateral**
- **H73.009 Acute myringitis, unspecified ear**

H73.01 Bullous myringitis
- **H73.011 Bullous myringitis, right ear**
- **H73.012 Bullous myringitis, left ear**
- **H73.013 Bullous myringitis, bilateral**
- **H73.019 Bullous myringitis, unspecified ear**

H73.09 Other acute myringitis
- **H73.091 Other acute myringitis, right ear**
- **H73.092 Other acute myringitis, left ear**
- **H73.093 Other acute myringitis, bilateral**
- **H73.099 Other acute myringitis, unspecified ear**

H73.1 Chronic myringitis
Chronic tympanitis
EXCLUDES 1 *chronic myringitis with otitis media (H65, H66)*
- **H73.10 Chronic myringitis, unspecified ear**
- **H73.11 Chronic myringitis, right ear**
- **H73.12 Chronic myringitis, left ear**
- **H73.13 Chronic myringitis, bilateral**

H73.2 Unspecified myringitis
- **H73.20 Unspecified myringitis, unspecified ear**
- **H73.21 Unspecified myringitis, right ear**
- **H73.22 Unspecified myringitis, left ear**
- **H73.23 Unspecified myringitis, bilateral**

H73.8 Other specified disorders of tympanic membrane

H73.81 Atrophic flaccid tympanic membrane
- **H73.811 Atrophic flaccid tympanic membrane, right ear**
- **H73.812 Atrophic flaccid tympanic membrane, left ear**
- **H73.813 Atrophic flaccid tympanic membrane, bilateral**
- **H73.819 Atrophic flaccid tympanic membrane, unspecified ear**

H73.82 Atrophic nonflaccid tympanic membrane
- **H73.821 Atrophic nonflaccid tympanic membrane, right ear**
- **H73.822 Atrophic nonflaccid tympanic membrane, left ear**
- **H73.823 Atrophic nonflaccid tympanic membrane, bilateral**
- **H73.829 Atrophic nonflaccid tympanic membrane, unspecified ear**

H73.89 Other specified disorders of tympanic membrane
- **H73.891 Other specified disorders of tympanic membrane, right ear**
- **H73.892 Other specified disorders of tympanic membrane, left ear**

H73.893 Other specified disorders of tympanic membrane, bilateral
H73.899 Other specified disorders of tympanic membrane, unspecified ear

5th H73.9 Unspecified disorder of tympanic membrane
H73.90 Unspecified disorder of tympanic membrane, unspecified ear
H73.91 Unspecified disorder of tympanic membrane, right ear
H73.92 Unspecified disorder of tympanic membrane, left ear
H73.93 Unspecified disorder of tympanic membrane, bilateral

4th **H74 Other disorders of middle ear mastoid**
EXCLUDES 2 *mastoiditis (H70.-)*

5th H74.0 Tympanosclerosis
H74.01 Tympanosclerosis, right ear
H74.02 Tympanosclerosis, left ear
H74.03 Tympanosclerosis, bilateral
H74.09 Tympanosclerosis, unspecified ear

5th H74.1 Adhesive middle ear disease
Adhesive otitis
EXCLUDES 1 *glue ear (H65.3-)*
H74.11 Adhesive right middle ear disease
H74.12 Adhesive left middle ear disease
H74.13 Adhesive middle ear disease, bilateral
H74.19 Adhesive middle ear disease, unspecified ear

5th H74.2 Discontinuity and dislocation of ear ossicles
H74.20 Discontinuity and dislocation of ear ossicles, unspecified ear
H74.21 Discontinuity and dislocation of right ear ossicles
H74.22 Discontinuity and dislocation of left ear ossicles
H74.23 Discontinuity and dislocation of ear ossicles, bilateral

5th H74.3 Other acquired abnormalities of ear ossicles
6th H74.31 Ankylosis of ear ossicles
H74.311 Ankylosis of ear ossicles, right ear
H74.312 Ankylosis of ear ossicles, left ear
H74.313 Ankylosis of ear ossicles, bilateral
H74.319 Ankylosis of ear ossicles, unspecified ear
6th H74.32 Partial loss of ear ossicles
H74.321 Partial loss of ear ossicles, right ear
H74.322 Partial loss of ear ossicles, left ear
H74.323 Partial loss of ear ossicles, bilateral
H74.329 Partial loss of ear ossicles, unspecified ear
6th H74.39 Other acquired abnormalities of ear ossicles
H74.391 Other acquired abnormalities of right ear ossicles
H74.392 Other acquired abnormalities of left ear ossicles
H74.393 Other acquired abnormalities of ear ossicles, bilateral
H74.399 Other acquired abnormalities of ear ossicles, unspecified ear

5th H74.4 Polyp of middle ear
H74.40 Polyp of middle ear, unspecified ear
H74.41 Polyp of right middle ear
H74.42 Polyp of left middle ear
H74.43 Polyp of middle ear, bilateral

5th H74.8 Other specified disorders of middle ear and mastoid
6th H74.8X Other specified disorders of middle ear and mastoid
H74.8X1 Other specified disorders of right middle ear and mastoid
H74.8X2 Other specified disorders of left middle ear and mastoid
H74.8X3 Other specified disorders of middle ear and mastoid, bilateral
H74.8X9 Other specified disorders of middle ear and mastoid, unspecified ear

5th H74.9 Unspecified disorder of middle ear and mastoid
H74.90 Unspecified disorder of middle ear and mastoid, unspecified ear
H74.91 Unspecified disorder of right middle ear and mastoid
H74.92 Unspecified disorder of left middle ear and mastoid
H74.93 Unspecified disorder of middle ear and mastoid, bilateral

4th **H75 Other disorders of middle ear and mastoid in diseases classified elsewhere**
Code first underlying disease

5th H75.0 Mastoiditis in infectious and parasitic diseases classified elsewhere
EXCLUDES 1 *mastoiditis (in):*
syphilis (A52.77)
tuberculosis (A18.03)
H75.00 *Mastoiditis in infectious and parasitic diseases classified elsewhere, unspecified ear*
H75.01 *Mastoiditis in infectious and parasitic diseases classified elsewhere, right ear*
H75.02 *Mastoiditis in infectious and parasitic diseases classified elsewhere, left ear*
H75.03 *Mastoiditis in infectious and parasitic diseases classified elsewhere, bilateral*

5th H75.8 Other specified disorders of middle ear and mastoid in diseases classified elsewhere
H75.80 *Other specified disorders of middle ear and mastoid in diseases classified elsewhere, unspecified ear*
H75.81 *Other specified disorders of right middle ear and mastoid in diseases classified elsewhere*
H75.82 *Other specified disorders of left middle ear and mastoid in diseases classified elsewhere*
H75.83 *Other specified disorders of middle ear and mastoid in diseases classified elsewhere, bilateral*

Diseases of inner ear (H80-H83)

4th **H80 Otosclerosis**
INCLUDES Otospongiosis

5th H80.0 Otosclerosis involving oval window, nonobliterative
H80.00 Otosclerosis involving oval window, nonobliterative, unspecified ear
H80.01 Otosclerosis involving oval window, nonobliterative, right ear
H80.02 Otosclerosis involving oval window, nonobliterative, left ear
H80.03 Otosclerosis involving oval window, nonobliterative, bilateral

5th H80.1 Otosclerosis involving oval window, obliterative
H80.10 Otosclerosis involving oval window, obliterative, unspecified ear
H80.11 Otosclerosis involving oval window, obliterative, right ear
H80.12 Otosclerosis involving oval window, obliterative, left ear
H80.13 Otosclerosis involving oval window, obliterative, bilateral

5th H80.2 Cochlear otosclerosis
Otosclerosis involving otic capsule
Otosclerosis involving round window
H80.20 Cochlear otosclerosis, unspecified ear
H80.21 Cochlear otosclerosis, right ear
H80.22 Cochlear otosclerosis, left ear
H80.23 Cochlear otosclerosis, bilateral

5th H80.8 Other otosclerosis
H80.80 Other otosclerosis, unspecified ear
H80.81 Other otosclerosis, right ear
H80.82 Other otosclerosis, left ear
H80.83 Other otosclerosis, bilateral

5th H80.9 Unspecified otosclerosis
H80.90 Unspecified otosclerosis, unspecified ear
H80.91 Unspecified otosclerosis, right ear
H80.92 Unspecified otosclerosis, left ear
H80.93 Unspecified otosclerosis, bilateral

H81 Disorders of vestibular function
EXCLUDES 1 *epidemic vertigo (A88.1)*
vertigo NOS (R42)

H81.0 Ménière's disease
Labyrinthine hydrops
Ménière's syndrome or vertigo
H81.01 Ménière's disease, right ear
H81.02 Ménière's disease, left ear
H81.03 Ménière's disease, bilateral
H81.09 Ménière's disease, unspecified ear

H81.1 Benign paroxysmal vertigo
H81.10 Benign paroxysmal vertigo, unspecified ear
H81.11 Benign paroxysmal vertigo, right ear
H81.12 Benign paroxysmal vertigo, left ear
H81.13 Benign paroxysmal vertigo, bilateral

H81.2 Vestibular neuronitis
H81.20 Vestibular neuronitis, unspecified ear
H81.21 Vestibular neuronitis, right ear
H81.22 Vestibular neuronitis, left ear
H81.23 Vestibular neuronitis, bilateral

H81.3 Other peripheral vertigo
H81.31 Aural vertigo
H81.311 Aural vertigo, right ear
H81.312 Aural vertigo, left ear
H81.313 Aural vertigo, bilateral
H81.319 Aural vertigo, unspecified ear
H81.39 Other peripheral vertigo
Lermoyez' syndrome
Otogenic vertigo
Peripheral vertigo NOS
H81.391 Other peripheral vertigo, right ear
H81.392 Other peripheral vertigo, left ear
H81.393 Other peripheral vertigo, bilateral
H81.399 Other peripheral vertigo, unspecified ear

H81.4 Vertigo of central origin
Central positional nystagmus
H81.41 Vertigo of central origin, right ear
H81.42 Vertigo of central origin, left ear
H81.43 Vertigo of central origin, bilateral
H81.49 Vertigo of central origin, unspecified ear

H81.8 Other disorders of vestibular function
H81.8X Other disorders of vestibular function
H81.8X1 Other disorders of vestibular function, right ear
H81.8X2 Other disorders of vestibular function, left ear
H81.8X3 Other disorders of vestibular function, bilateral
H81.8X9 Other disorders of vestibular function, unspecified ear

H81.9 Unspecified disorder of vestibular function
Vertiginous syndrome NOS
H81.90 Unspecified disorder of vestibular function, unspecified ear
H81.91 Unspecified disorder of vestibular function, right ear
H81.92 Unspecified disorder of vestibular function, left ear
H81.93 Unspecified disorder of vestibular function, bilateral

H82 Vertiginous syndromes in diseases classified elsewhere
Code first underlying disease
EXCLUDES 1 *epidemic vertigo (A88.1)*
H82.1 *Vertiginous syndromes in diseases classified elsewhere, right ear*
H82.2 *Vertiginous syndromes in diseases classified elsewhere, left ear*
H82.3 *Vertiginous syndromes in diseases classified elsewhere, bilateral*
H82.9 *Vertiginous syndromes in diseases classified elsewhere, unspecified ear*

H83 Other diseases of inner ear
H83.0 Labyrinthitis
H83.01 Labyrinthitis, right ear
H83.02 Labyrinthitis, left ear
H83.03 Labyrinthitis, bilateral
H83.09 Labyrinthitis, unspecified ear

H83.1 Labyrinthine fistula
H83.11 Labyrinthine fistula, right ear
H83.12 Labyrinthine fistula, left ear
H83.13 Labyrinthine fistula, bilateral
H83.19 Labyrinthine fistula, unspecified ear

H83.2 Labyrinthine dysfunction
Labyrinthine hypersensitivity
Labyrinthine hypofunction
Labyrinthine loss of function
H83.2X Labyrinthine dysfunction
H83.2X1 Labyrinthine dysfunction, right ear
H83.2X2 Labyrinthine dysfunction, left ear
H83.2X3 Labyrinthine dysfunction, bilateral
H83.2X9 Labyrinthine dysfunction, unspecified ear

H83.3 Noise effects on inner ear
Acoustic trauma of inner ear
Noise-induced hearing loss of inner ear
H83.3X Noise effects on inner ear
H83.3X1 Noise effects on right inner ear
H83.3X2 Noise effects on left inner ear
H83.3X3 Noise effects on inner ear, bilateral
H83.3X9 Noise effects on inner ear, unspecified ear

H83.8 Other specified diseases of inner ear
H83.8X Other specified diseases of inner ear
H83.8X1 Other specified diseases of right inner ear
H83.8X2 Other specified diseases of left inner ear
H83.8X3 Other specified diseases of inner ear, bilateral
H83.8X9 Other specified diseases of inner ear, unspecified ear

H83.9 Unspecified disease of inner ear
H83.90 Unspecified disease of inner ear, unspecified ear
H83.91 Unspecified disease of right inner ear
H83.92 Unspecified disease of left inner ear
H83.93 Unspecified disease of inner ear, bilateral

Other disorders of ear (H90-H94)

H90 Conductive and sensorineural hearing loss
EXCLUDES 1 *deaf nonspeaking NEC (H91.3)*
deafness NOS (H91.9-)
hearing loss NOS (H91.9-)
noise-induced hearing loss (H83.3-)
ototoxic hearing loss (H91.0-)
sudden (idiopathic) hearing loss (H91.2-)
H90.0 Conductive hearing loss, bilateral
H90.1 Conductive hearing loss, unilateral with unrestricted hearing on the contralateral side
H90.11 Conductive hearing loss, unilateral, right ear, with unrestricted hearing on the contralateral side
H90.12 Conductive hearing loss, unilateral, left ear, with unrestricted hearing on the contralateral side
H90.2 Conductive hearing loss, unspecified
Conductive deafness NOS
H90.3 Sensorineural hearing loss, bilateral
H90.4 Sensorineural hearing loss, unilateral with unrestricted hearing on the contralateral side
H90.41 Sensorineural hearing loss, unilateral, right ear, with unrestricted hearing on the contralateral side
H90.42 Sensorineural hearing loss, unilateral, left ear, with unrestricted hearing on the contralateral side
H90.5 Unspecified sensorineural hearing loss
Central hearing loss NOS
Congenital deafness NOS
Neural hearing loss NOS
Perceptive hearing loss NOS
Sensorineural deafness NOS
Sensory hearing loss NOS
EXCLUDES 1 *abnormal auditory perception (H93.2-)*
psychogenic deafness (F44.6)
H90.6 Mixed conductive and sensorineural hearing loss, bilateral
H90.7 Mixed conductive and sensorineural hearing loss, unilateral with unrestricted hearing on the contralateral side
H90.71 Mixed conductive and sensorineural hearing loss, unilateral, right ear, with unrestricted hearing on the contralateral side

H90.72 **Mixed conductive and sensorineural hearing loss, unilateral, left ear, with unrestricted hearing on the contralateral side**

H90.8 **Mixed conductive and sensorineural hearing loss, unspecified**

√4th **H91 Other and unspecified hearing loss**

EXCLUDES 1 *abnormal auditory perception (H93.2-)*
hearing loss as classified in H90-
impacted cerumen (H61.2-)
noise-induced hearing loss (H83.3-)
psychogenic deafness (F44.6)
transient ischemic deafness (H93.01-)

√5th **H91.0 Ototoxic hearing loss**

Code first poisoning due to drug or toxin, if applicable (T36-T65 with fifth or sixth character 1-4 or 6)

Use additional code for adverse effect, if applicable, to identify drug (T36-T50 with fifth or sixth character 5)

H91.01 **Ototoxic hearing loss, right ear**
H91.02 **Ototoxic hearing loss, left ear**
H91.03 **Ototoxic hearing loss, bilateral**
H91.09 **Ototoxic hearing loss, unspecified ear**

√5th **H91.1 Presbycusis**

Presbyacusia

H91.10 **Presbycusis, unspecified ear**
H91.11 **Presbycusis, right ear**
H91.12 **Presbycusis, left ear**
H91.13 **Presbycusis, bilateral**

√5th **H91.2 Sudden idiopathic hearing loss**

Sudden hearing loss NOS

H91.20 **Sudden idiopathic hearing loss, unspecified ear**
H91.21 **Sudden idiopathic hearing loss, right ear**
H91.22 **Sudden idiopathic hearing loss, left ear**
H91.23 **Sudden idiopathic hearing loss, bilateral**

H91.3 **Deaf nonspeaking, not elsewhere classified**

√5th **H91.8 Other specified hearing loss**

√6th **H91.8X Other specified hearing loss**

H91.8X1 **Other specified hearing loss, right ear**
H91.8X2 **Other specified hearing loss, left ear**
H91.8X3 **Other specified hearing loss, bilateral**
H91.8X9 **Other specified hearing loss, unspecified ear**

√5th **H91.9 Unspecified hearing loss**

Deafness NOS
High frequency deafness
Low frequency deafness

H91.90 **Unspecified hearing loss, unspecified ear**
H91.91 **Unspecified hearing loss, right ear**
H91.92 **Unspecified hearing loss, left ear**
H91.93 **Unspecified hearing loss, bilateral**

√4th **H92 Otalgia and effusion of ear**

√5th **H92.0 Otalgia**

H92.01 **Otalgia, right ear**
H92.02 **Otalgia, left ear**
H92.03 **Otalgia, bilateral**
H92.09 **Otalgia, unspecified ear**

√5th **H92.1 Otorrhea**

EXCLUDES 1 *leakage of cerebrospinal fluid through ear (G96.0)*

H92.10 **Otorrhea, unspecified ear**
H92.11 **Otorrhea, right ear**
H92.12 **Otorrhea, left ear**
H92.13 **Otorrhea, bilateral**

√5th **H92.2 Otorrhagia**

EXCLUDES 1 *traumatic otorrhagia—code to injury*

H92.20 **Otorrhagia, unspecified ear**
H92.21 **Otorrhagia, right ear**
H92.22 **Otorrhagia, left ear**
H92.23 **Otorrhagia, bilateral**

√4th **H93 Other disorders of ear, not elsewhere classified**

√5th **H93.0 Degenerative and vascular disorders of ear**

EXCLUDES 1 *presbycusis (H91.1)*

√6th **H93.01 Transient ischemic deafness**

H93.011 **Transient ischemic deafness, right ear**
H93.012 **Transient ischemic deafness, left ear**
H93.013 **Transient ischemic deafness, bilateral**
H93.019 **Transient ischemic deafness, unspecified ear**

√6th **H93.09 Unspecified degenerative and vascular disorders of ear**

H93.091 **Unspecified degenerative and vascular disorders of right ear**
H93.092 **Unspecified degenerative and vascular disorders of left ear**
H93.093 **Unspecified degenerative and vascular disorders of ear, bilateral**
H93.099 **Unspecified degenerative and vascular disorders of unspecified ear**

√5th **H93.1 Tinnitus**

H93.11 **Tinnitus, right ear**
H93.12 **Tinnitus, left ear**
H93.13 **Tinnitus, bilateral**
H93.19 **Tinnitus, unspecified ear**

√5th **H93.2 Other abnormal auditory perceptions**

EXCLUDES 2 *auditory hallucinations (R44.0)*

√6th **H93.21 Auditory recruitment**

H93.211 **Auditory recruitment, right ear**
H93.212 **Auditory recruitment, left ear**
H93.213 **Auditory recruitment, bilateral**
H93.219 **Auditory recruitment, unspecified ear**

√6th **H93.22 Diplacusis**

H93.221 **Diplacusis, right ear**
H93.222 **Diplacusis, left ear**
H93.223 **Diplacusis, bilateral**
H93.229 **Diplacusis, unspecified ear**

√6th **H93.23 Hyperacusis**

H93.231 **Hyperacusis, right ear**
H93.232 **Hyperacusis, left ear**
H93.233 **Hyperacusis, bilateral**
H93.239 **Hyperacusis, unspecified ear**

√6th **H93.24 Temporary auditory threshold shift**

H93.241 **Temporary auditory threshold shift, right ear**
H93.242 **Temporary auditory threshold shift, left ear**
H93.243 **Temporary auditory threshold shift, bilateral**
H93.249 **Temporary auditory threshold shift, unspecified ear**

H93.25 **Central auditory processing disorder**

Congenital auditory imperception
Word deafness

EXCLUDES 1 *mixed receptive-expressive language disorder (F80.2)*

√6th **H93.29 Other abnormal auditory perceptions**

H93.291 **Other abnormal auditory perceptions, right ear**
H93.292 **Other abnormal auditory perceptions, left ear**
H93.293 **Other abnormal auditory perceptions, bilateral**
H93.299 **Other abnormal auditory perceptions, unspecified ear**

√5th **H93.3 Disorders of acoustic nerve**

Disorder of 8th cranial nerve

EXCLUDES 1 *acoustic neuroma (D33.3)*
syphilitic acoustic neuritis (A52.15)

√6th **H93.3X Disorders of acoustic nerve**

H93.3X1 **Disorders of right acoustic nerve**
H93.3X2 **Disorders of left acoustic nerve**
H93.3X3 **Disorders of bilateral acoustic nerves**
H93.3X9 **Disorders of unspecified acoustic nerve**

√5th **H93.8 Other specified disorders of ear**

√6th **H93.8X Other specified disorders of ear**

H93.8X1 **Other specified disorders of right ear**
H93.8X2 **Other specified disorders of left ear**
H93.8X3 **Other specified disorders of ear, bilateral**
H93.8X9 **Other specified disorders of ear, unspecified ear**

✓5th **H93.9 Unspecified disorder of ear**

H93.90 Unspecified disorder of ear, unspecified ear

H93.91 Unspecified disorder of right ear

H93.92 Unspecified disorder of left ear

H93.93 Unspecified disorder of ear, bilateral

✓4th **H94 Other disorders of ear in diseases classified elsewhere**

✓5th **H94.0 Acoustic neuritis in infectious and parasitic diseases classified elsewhere**

Code first underlying disease, such as:
parasitic disease (B65-B89)

EXCLUDES 1 *acoustic neuritis (in):*
herpes zoster (B02.29)
syphilis (A52.15)

H94.00 Acoustic neuritis in infectious and parasitic diseases classified elsewhere, unspecified ear

H94.01 Acoustic neuritis in infectious and parasitic diseases classified elsewhere, right ear

H94.02 Acoustic neuritis in infectious and parasitic diseases classified elsewhere, left ear

H94.03 Acoustic neuritis in infectious and parasitic diseases classified elsewhere, bilateral

✓5th **H94.8 Other specified disorders of ear in diseases classified elsewhere**

Code first underlying disease, such as:
congenital syphilis (A50.0)

EXCLUDES 1 *aural myiasis (B87.4)*
syphilitic labyrinthitis (A52.79)

H94.80 Other specified disorders of ear in diseases classified elsewhere, unspecified ear

H94.81 Other specified disorders of right ear in diseases classified elsewhere

H94.82 Other specified disorders of left ear in diseases classified elsewhere

H94.83 Other specified disorders of ear in diseases classified elsewhere, bilateral

Intraoperative and postprocedural complications and disorders of ear and mastoid process, not elsewhere classified (H95)

✓4th **H95 Intraoperative and postprocedural complications and disorders of ear and mastoid process, not elsewhere classified**

✓5th **H95.0 Recurrent cholesteatoma of postmastoidectomy cavity**

H95.00 Recurrent cholesteatoma of postmastoidectomy cavity, unspecified ear

H95.01 Recurrent cholesteatoma of postmastoidectomy cavity, right ear

H95.02 Recurrent cholesteatoma of postmastoidectomy cavity, left ear

H95.03 Recurrent cholesteatoma of postmastoidectomy cavity, bilateral ears

✓5th **H95.1 Other disorders of ear and mastoid process following mastoidectomy**

✓6th **H95.11 Chronic inflammation of postmastoidectomy cavity**

H95.111 Chronic inflammation of postmastoidectomy cavity, right ear

H95.112 Chronic inflammation of postmastoidectomy cavity, left ear

H95.113 Chronic inflammation of postmastoidectomy cavity, bilateral ears

H95.119 Chronic inflammation of postmastoidectomy cavity, unspecified ear

✓6th **H95.12 Granulation of postmastoidectomy cavity**

H95.121 Granulation of postmastoidectomy cavity, right ear

H95.122 Granulation of postmastoidectomy cavity, left ear

H95.123 Granulation of postmastoidectomy cavity, bilateral ears

H95.129 Granulation of postmastoidectomy cavity, unspecified ear

✓6th **H95.13 Mucosal cyst of postmastoidectomy cavity**

H95.131 Mucosal cyst of postmastoidectomy cavity, right ear

H95.132 Mucosal cyst of postmastoidectomy cavity, left ear

H95.133 Mucosal cyst of postmastoidectomy cavity, bilateral ears

H95.139 Mucosal cyst of postmastoidectomy cavity, unspecified ear

✓6th **H95.19 Other disorders following mastoidectomy**

H95.191 Other disorders following mastoidectomy, right ear

H95.192 Other disorders following mastoidectomy, left ear

H95.193 Other disorders following mastoidectomy, bilateral ears

H95.199 Other disorders following mastoidectomy, unspecified ear

✓5th **H95.2 Intraoperative hemorrhage and hematoma of ear and mastoid process complicating a procedure**

EXCLUDES 1 *intraoperative hemorrhage and hematoma of ear and mastoid process due to accidental puncture or laceration during a procedure (H95.3-)*

H95.21 Intraoperative hemorrhage and hematoma of ear and mastoid process complicating a procedure on the ear and mastoid process CC

CC Excl: H95.21-H95.22, H95.41-H95.89, I85.01, I85.11, I97.3, K21.9, K22.8, K23-K25.0, K25.2, K25.4, K25.6, K26.0, K26.2, K26.4, K26.6, K27.0, K27.2, K27.4, K27.6, K28.0, K28.2, K28.4, K28.6, K29.01, K29.21, K29.31, K29.41, K29.51, K29.61, K29.71, K29.81, K29.91, K31.811, K55.21, K57.01, K57.11, K57.13, K57.21, K57.31, K57.33, K57.41, K57.51, K57.53, K57.81, K57.91, K57.93, K62.5, K92.0-K92.2, M96.89, N98.1-N98.9, P54.1-P54.3, T81.10XA, T81.11XA, T81.12XA, T81.19XA, T81.82XA, T81.89XA, T81.9XXA

H95.22 Intraoperative hemorrhage and hematoma of ear and mastoid process complicating other procedure CC

CC Excl: See code: H95.21

✓5th **H95.3 Accidental puncture and laceration of ear and mastoid process during a procedure**

CC Excl: For CC codes in subcategory H95.3, unless otherwise noted: D78.11-D78.12, D78.81-D78.89, E36.11-E36.8, E89.810-E89.89, G96.11, G97.41, G97.48-G97.49, H59.011-H59.019, H59.031-H59.099, H59.211-H59.229, H59.811-H59.89, H95.31-H95.32, H95.811-H95.89, I97.3, I97.51-I97.52, J95.71-J95.72, K91.71-K91.72, L76.11-L76.12, L76.81-L76.82, M96.820-M96.821, M96.89, N98.1-N98.9, N99.71-N99.72, T81.82XA, T81.89XA, T81.9XXA

H95.31 Accidental puncture and laceration of the ear and mastoid process during a procedure on the ear and mastoid process CC

H95.32 Accidental puncture and laceration of the ear and mastoid process during other procedure CC

✓5th **H95.4 Postprocedural hemorrhage and hematoma of ear and mastoid process following a procedure**

H95.41 Postprocedural hemorrhage and hematoma of ear and mastoid process following a procedure on the ear and mastoid process CC

CC Excl: See code: H95.21

H95.42 Postprocedural hemorrhage and hematoma of ear and mastoid process following other procedure CC

CC Excl: See code: H95.21

✓5th **H95.8 Other intraoperative and postprocedural complications and disorders of the ear and mastoid process, not elsewhere classified**

EXCLUDES 2 *postprocedural complications and disorders following mastoidectomy (H95.0-, H95.1-)*

CC Excl: For CC codes in subcategory H95.8, unless otherwise noted: D78.81-D78.89, E36.8, E89.810-E89.89, H59.011-H59.019, H59.031-H59.099, H59.811-H59.89, H95.811-H95.89, I97.3, L76.81-L76.82, M96.89, N98.1-N98.9, T81.82XA, T81.89XA, T81.9XXA

✓6th **H95.81 Postprocedural stenosis of external ear canal**

H95.811 Postprocedural stenosis of right external ear canal CC

H95.812 Postprocedural stenosis of left external ear canal CC

H95.813 Postprocedural stenosis of external ear canal, bilateral CC

H95.819 Postprocedural stenosis of unspecified external ear canal CC

H95.88 Other intraoperative complications and disorders of the ear and mastoid process, not elsewhere classified CC

Use additional code, if applicable, to further specify disorder

H95.89 Other postprocedural complications and disorders of the ear and mastoid process, not elsewhere classified CC

Use additional code, if applicable, to further specify disorder

Chapter 9. Diseases of the Circulatory System (I00-I99)

EXCLUDES 2 *certain conditions originating in the perinatal period (P04-P96)*
certain infectious and parasitic diseases (A00-B99)
complications of pregnancy, childbirth and the puerperium (O00-O9A)
congenital malformations, deformations, and chromosomal abnormalities (Q00-Q99)
endocrine, nutritional and metabolic diseases (E00-E88)
injury, poisoning and certain other consequences of external causes (S00-T88)
neoplasms (C00-D49)
symptoms, signs and abnormal clinical and laboratory findings, not elsewhere classified (R00-R94)
systemic connective tissue disorders (M30-M36)
transient cerebral ischemic attacks and related syndromes (G45.-)

This chapter contains the following blocks:

I00-I02	Acute rheumatic fever
I05-I09	Chronic rheumatic heart diseases
I10-I15	Hypertensive diseases
I20-I25	Ischemic heart diseases
I26-I28	Pulmonary heart disease and diseases of pulmonary circulation
I30-I52	Other forms of heart disease
I60-I69	Cerebrovascular diseases
I70-I79	Diseases of arteries, arterioles and capillaries
I80-I89	Diseases of veins, lymphatic vessels and lymph nodes, not elsewhere classified
I95-I99	Other and unspecified disorders of the circulatory system

Acute rheumatic fever (I00-I02)

I00 Rheumatic fever without heart involvement
INCLUDES arthritis, rheumatic, acute or subacute
EXCLUDES 1 *rheumatic fever with heart involvement (I01.0-I01.9)*

✓4th **I01 Rheumatic fever with heart involvement**
EXCLUDES 1 *chronic diseases of rheumatic origin (I05-I09) unless rheumatic fever is also present or there is evidence of reactivation or activity of the rheumatic process.*

I01.0 Acute rheumatic pericarditis CC
Any condition in I00 with pericarditis
Rheumatic pericarditis (acute)
EXCLUDES 1 *acute pericarditis not specified as rheumatic (I30.-)*
CC Excl: B33.23, I01.0, I09.2, I30.0-I30.9, I31.3-I32, I87.8, I99.8-I99.9

I01.1 Acute rheumatic endocarditis CC
Any condition in I00 with endocarditis or valvulitis
Acute rheumatic valvulitis
CC Excl: A01.00-A01.09, A39.51, A52.03, A78, B33.21, B37.6, I00, I01.1, I01.8-I02.0, I05.0-I07.9, I08.1-I08.3, I08.9, I09.1, I09.89-I09.9, I33.0-I39, I42.4, I87.8, I99.8-I99.9, Q22.2, Q23.8-Q23.9, Q24.8, T82.6XXA

I01.2 Acute rheumatic myocarditis CC
Any condition in I00 with myocarditis
CC Excl: A52.06, B33.22, I00, I01.2-I01.9, I09.0, I09.9, I23.0-I23.3, I23.6-I23.8, I40.0-I41, I51.0, I51.4, I87.8, I99.8-I99.9

I01.8 Other acute rheumatic heart disease CC
Any condition in I00 with other or multiple types of heart involvement
Acute rheumatic pancarditis
CC Excl: I01.0-I09.9, I50.20-I50.43

I01.9 Acute rheumatic heart disease, unspecified CC
Any condition in I00 with unspecified type of heart involvement
Rheumatic carditis, acute
Rheumatic heart disease, active or acute
CC Excl: I01.0-I09.9

✓4th **I02 Rheumatic chorea**
INCLUDES Sydenham's chorea
EXCLUDES 1 *chorea NOS (G25.5)*
Huntington's chorea (G10)

I02.0 Rheumatic chorea with heart involvement CC
Chorea NOS with heart involvement
Rheumatic chorea with heart involvement of any type classifiable under I01-
CC Excl: See code: I01.8

I02.9 Rheumatic chorea without heart involvement CC
Rheumatic chorea NOS
CC Excl: See code: I01.9

Chronic rheumatic heart diseases (I05-I09)

✓4th **I05 Rheumatic mitral valve diseases**
INCLUDES conditions classifiable to both I05.0 and I05.2-I05.9, whether specified as rheumatic or not
EXCLUDES 1 *mitral valve disease specified as nonrheumatic (I34.-)*
mitral valve disease with aortic and/or tricuspid valve involvement (I08.-)

I05.0 Rheumatic mitral stenosis
Mitral (valve) obstruction (rheumatic)

I05.1 Rheumatic mitral insufficiency
Rheumatic mitral incompetence
Rheumatic mitral regurgitation
EXCLUDES 1 *mitral insufficiency not specified as rheumatic (I34.0)*

I05.2 Rheumatic mitral stenosis with insufficiency
Rheumatic mitral stenosis with incompetence or regurgitation

I05.8 Other rheumatic mitral valve diseases
Rheumatic mitral (valve) failure

I05.9 Rheumatic mitral valve disease, unspecified
Rheumatic mitral (valve) disorder (chronic) NOS

✓4th **I06 Rheumatic aortic valve diseases**
EXCLUDES 1 *aortic valve disease not specified as rheumatic (I35.-)*
aortic valve disease with mitral and/or tricuspid valve involvement (I08.-)

I06.0 Rheumatic aortic stenosis
Rheumatic aortic (valve) obstruction

I06.1 Rheumatic aortic insufficiency
Rheumatic aortic incompetence
Rheumatic aortic regurgitation

I06.2 Rheumatic aortic stenosis with insufficiency
Rheumatic aortic stenosis with incompetence or regurgitation

I06.8 Other rheumatic aortic valve diseases

I06.9 Rheumatic aortic valve disease, unspecified
Rheumatic aortic (valve) disease NOS

✓4th **I07 Rheumatic tricuspid valve diseases**
INCLUDES rheumatic tricuspid valve diseases specified as rheumatic or unspecified
EXCLUDES 1 *tricuspid valve disease specified as nonrheumatic (I36.-)*
tricuspid valve disease with aortic and/or mitral valve involvement (I08.-)

I07.0 Rheumatic tricuspid stenosis
Tricuspid (valve) stenosis (rheumatic)

I07.1 Rheumatic tricuspid insufficiency
Tricuspid (valve) insufficiency (rheumatic)

I07.2 Rheumatic tricuspid stenosis and insufficiency

I07.8 Other rheumatic tricuspid valve diseases

I07.9 Rheumatic tricuspid valve disease, unspecified
Rheumatic tricuspid valve disorder NOS

✓4th **I08 Multiple valve diseases**
INCLUDES multiple valve diseases specified as rheumatic or unspecified
EXCLUDES 1 *endocarditis, valve unspecified (I38)*
multiple valve disease specified a nonrheumatic (I34.-, I35.-, I36.-, I37.-, I38.-, Q22.-, Q23.-, Q24.8-)
rheumatic valve disease NOS (I09.1)

I08.0 Rheumatic disorders of both mitral and aortic valves
Involvement of both mitral and aortic valves specified as rheumatic or unspecified

I08.1 Rheumatic disorders of both mitral and tricuspid valves

I08.2 Rheumatic disorders of both aortic and tricuspid valves

I08.3 Combined rheumatic disorders of mitral, aortic and tricuspid valves

I08.8 Other rheumatic multiple valve diseases

I08.9 Rheumatic multiple valve disease, unspecified

✓4th **I09 Other rheumatic heart diseases**

I09.0 Rheumatic myocarditis CC
EXCLUDES 1 *myocarditis not specified as rheumatic (I51.4)*
CC Excl: I00, I01.2-I01.9, I09.0, I09.9, I23.0-I23.3, I23.6-I23.8, I40.0-I41, I51.0, I51.4, I87.8, I99.8-I99.9

I09.1 Rheumatic diseases of endocardium, valve unspecified
Rheumatic endocarditis (chronic)
Rheumatic valvulitis (chronic)
EXCLUDES 1 *endocarditis, valve unspecified (I38)*

I09.2 Chronic rheumatic pericarditis CC
Adherent pericardium, rheumatic
Chronic rheumatic mediastinopericarditis
Chronic rheumatic myopericarditis
EXCLUDES 1 *chronic pericarditis not specified as rheumatic (I31.-)*
CC Excl: B33.23, I01.0, I09.2, I30.0-I30.9, I31.3-I32, I87.8, I99.8-I99.9

✓5th **I09.8 Other specified rheumatic heart diseases**

I09.81 Rheumatic heart failure CC
Use additional code to identify type of heart failure (I50.-)
CC Excl: I09.81, I09.9, I11.0, I50.1-I50.9, I87.8, I99.8-I99.9

I09.89 Other specified rheumatic heart diseases
Rheumatic disease of pulmonary valve

I09.9 Rheumatic heart disease, unspecified
Rheumatic carditis
EXCLUDES 1 *rheumatoid carditis (M05.31)*

Hypertensive diseases (I10-I15)

Use additional code to identify:
exposure to environmental tobacco smoke (Z77.22)
history of tobacco use (Z87.891)
occupational exposure to environmental tobacco smoke (Z57.31)
tobacco dependence (F17.-)
tobacco use (Z72.0)

EXCLUDES 1 *hypertensive disease complicating pregnancy, childbirth and the puerperium (O10-O11, O13-O16)*
neonatal hypertension (P29.2)
primary pulmonary hypertension (I27.0)

13 **I10 Essential (primary) hypertension**
INCLUDES high blood pressure
hypertension (arterial) (benign) (essential) (malignant) (primary) (systemic)
EXCLUDES 1 *hypertensive disease complicating pregnancy, childbirth and the puerperium (O10-O11, O13-O16)*
EXCLUDES 2 *essential (primary) hypertension involving vessels of brain (I60-I69)*
essential (primary) hypertension involving vessels of eye (H35.0-)

✓4th **I11 Hypertensive heart disease**
INCLUDES any condition in I51.4-I51.9 due to hypertension

I11.0 Hypertensive heart disease with heart failure
Hypertensive heart failure
Use additional code to identify type of heart failure (I50.-)

I11.9 Hypertensive heart disease without heart failure
Hypertensive heart disease NOS

✓4th **I12 Hypertensive chronic kidney disease**
INCLUDES any condition in N18- and N26- due to hypertension
arteriosclerosis of kidney
arteriosclerotic nephritis (chronic) (interstitial)
hypertensive nephropathy
nephrosclerosis
EXCLUDES 1 *hypertension due to kidney disease (I15.0, I15.1)*
renovascular hypertension (I15.0)
secondary hypertension (I15.-)
EXCLUDES 2 *acute kidney failure (N17.-)*

I12.0 Hypertensive chronic kidney disease with stage 5 chronic kidney disease or end stage renal disease CC
Use additional code to identify the stage of chronic kidney disease (N18.5, N18.6)
CC Excl: I10-I15.9, I87.8, I99.8-I99.9, N18.6, N26.2

I12.9 Hypertensive chronic kidney disease with stage 1 through stage 4 chronic kidney disease, or unspecified chronic kidney disease
Hypertensive chronic kidney disease NOS
Hypertensive renal disease NOS
Use additional code to identify the stage of chronic kidney disease (N18.1-N18.4, N18.9)

✓4th **I13 Hypertensive heart and chronic kidney disease**
INCLUDES any condition in I11- with any condition in I12-
cardiorenal disease
cardiovascular renal disease

CC Excl: For CC codes in category I13, unless otherwise noted:
I10-I15.9, I87.8, I99.8-I99.9, N26.2

I13.0 Hypertensive heart and chronic kidney disease with heart failure and stage 1 through stage 4 chronic kidney disease, or unspecified chronic kidney disease CC
Use additional code to identify type of heart failure (I50.-)
Use additional code to identify stage of chronic kidney disease (N18.1-N18.4, N18.9)

✓5th **I13.1 Hypertensive heart and chronic kidney disease without heart failure**

I13.10 Hypertensive heart and chronic kidney disease without heart failure, with stage 1 through stage 4 chronic kidney disease, or unspecified chronic kidney disease
Hypertensive heart disease and hypertensive chronic kidney disease NOS
Use additional code to identify the stage of chronic kidney disease (N18.1-N18.4, N18.9)

I13.11 Hypertensive heart and chronic kidney disease without heart failure, with stage 5 chronic kidney disease, or end stage renal disease CC
Use additional code to identify the stage of chronic kidney disease (N18.5, N18.6)

I13.2 Hypertensive heart and chronic kidney disease with heart failure and with stage 5 chronic kidney disease, or end stage renal disease CC
Use additional code to identify type of heart failure (I50.-)
Use additional code to identify the stage of chronic kidney disease (N18.5, N18.6)

✓4th **I15 Secondary hypertension**
Code also underlying condition
EXCLUDES 1 *postprocedural hypertension (I97.3)*
EXCLUDES 2 *secondary hypertension involving vessels of brain (I60-I69)*
secondary hypertension involving vessels of eye (H35.0-)

I15.0 Renovascular hypertension
I15.1 Hypertension secondary to other renal disorders
I15.2 Hypertension secondary to endocrine disorders
I15.8 Other secondary hypertension
I15.9 Secondary hypertension, unspecified

Ischemic heart diseases (I20-I25)

Use additional code to identify presence of hypertension (I10-I15)

✓4th **I20 Angina pectoris**
Use additional code to identify:
exposure to environmental tobacco smoke (Z77.22)
history of tobacco use (Z87.891)
occupational exposure to environmental tobacco smoke (Z57.31)
tobacco dependence (F17.-)
tobacco use (Z72.0)
EXCLUDES 1 *angina pectoris with atherosclerotic heart disease of native coronary arteries (I25.1-)*
atherosclerosis of coronary artery bypass graft(s) and coronary artery of transplanted heart with angina pectoris (I25.7-)
postinfarction angina (I23.7)

I20.0 Unstable angina CC
Accelerated angina
Crescendo angina
De novo effort angina
Intermediate coronary syndrome
Preinfarction syndrome
Worsening effort angina
CC Excl: I09.81, I11.0, I13.0, I13.2, I20.0-I22.9, I24.0, I24.8-I24.9, I25.5-I25.6, I25.82-I25.83, I25.89-I25.9, I50.1, I50.9, I87.8, I99.8-I99.9, R57.0, R57.9

I20.1 Angina pectoris with documented spasm CC
Angiospastic angina
Prinzmetal angina
Spasm-induced angina
Variant angina
CC Excl: I20.0-I22.9, I24.0, I24.8-I24.9, I25.5-I25.6, I25.89-I25.9, I87.8, I99.8-I99.9

I20.8 Other forms of angina pectoris
Angina equivalent
Angina of effort
Coronary slow flow syndrome
Stenocardia
Use additional code(s) for symptoms associated with angina equivalent

I20.9 Angina pectoris, unspecified
Angina NOS
Anginal syndrome
Cardiac angina
Ischemic chest pain

13 Questionable admission when used as PDx.

✓4th I21 ST elevation (STEMI) and non-ST elevation (NSTEMI) myocardial infarction

INCLUDES cardiac infarction
coronary (artery) embolism
coronary (artery) occlusion
coronary (artery) rupture
coronary (artery) thrombosis
infarction of heart, myocardium, or ventricle
myocardial infarction specified as acute or with a stated duration of 4 weeks (28 days) or less from onset

Use additional code, if applicable, to identify:
exposure to environmental tobacco smoke (Z77.22)
history of tobacco use (Z87.891)
occupational exposure to environmental tobacco smoke (Z57.31)
status post administration of tPA (rtPA) in a different facility within the last 24 hours prior to admission to current facility (Z92.82)
tobacco dependence (F17.-)
tobacco use (Z72.0)

EXCLUDES 2 *old myocardial infarction (I25.2)*
postmyocardial infarction syndrome (I24.1)
subsequent myocardial infarction (I22.-)

AHA: 2013, 1Q, 25; 2012, 4Q, 96, 102-103

CC Excl: For MCC codes in category I21, unless otherwise noted:
I21.01-I22.9, I87.8, I99.8-I99.9

✓5th I21.0 ST elevation (STEMI) myocardial infarction of anterior wall

I21.01 ST elevation (STEMI) myocardial infarction involving left main coronary artery MCC

I21.02 ST elevation (STEMI) myocardial infarction involving left anterior descending coronary artery MCC
ST elevation (STEMI) myocardial infarction involving diagonal coronary artery
AHA: 2013, 1Q, 25

I21.09 ST elevation (STEMI) myocardial infarction involving other coronary artery of anterior wall MCC
Acute transmural myocardial infarction of anterior wall
Anteroapical transmural (Q wave) infarction (acute)
Anterolateral transmural (Q wave) infarction (acute)
Anteroseptal transmural (Q wave) infarction (acute)
Transmural (Q wave) infarction (acute) (of) anterior (wall) NOS
AHA: 2012, 4Q, 102-103

✓5th I21.1 ST elevation (STEMI) myocardial infarction of inferior wall

I21.11 ST elevation (STEMI) myocardial infarction involving right coronary artery MCC
Inferoposterior transmural (Q wave) infarction (acute)

I21.19 ST elevation (STEMI) myocardial infarction involving other coronary artery of inferior wall MCC
Acute transmural myocardial infarction of inferior wall
Inferolateral transmural (Q wave) infarction (acute)
Transmural (Q wave) infarction (acute) (of) diaphragmatic wall
Transmural (Q wave) infarction (acute) (of) inferior (wall) NOS
EXCLUDES 2 *ST elevation (STEMI) myocardial infarction involving left circumflex coronary artery (I21.21)*
AHA: 2012, 4Q, 96

✓5th I21.2 ST elevation (STEMI) myocardial infarction of other sites

I21.21 ST elevation (STEMI) myocardial infarction involving left circumflex coronary artery MCC
ST elevation (STEMI) myocardial infarction involving oblique marginal coronary artery

I21.29 ST elevation (STEMI) myocardial infarction involving other sites MCC
Acute transmural myocardial infarction of other sites
Apical-lateral transmural (Q wave) infarction (acute)
Basal-lateral transmural (Q wave) infarction (acute)
High lateral transmural (Q wave) infarction (acute)
Lateral (wall) NOS transmural (Q wave) infarction (acute)
Posterior (true) transmural (Q wave) infarction (acute)
Posterobasal transmural (Q wave) infarction (acute)
Posterolateral transmural (Q wave) infarction (acute)
Posteroseptal transmural (Q wave) infarction (acute)
Septal transmural (Q wave) infarction (acute) NOS

I21.3 ST elevation (STEMI) myocardial infarction of unspecified site MCC
Acute transmural myocardial infarction of unspecified site
Myocardial infarction (acute) NOS
Transmural (Q wave) myocardial infarction NOS

I21.4 Non-ST elevation (NSTEMI) myocardial infarction MCC
Acute subendocardial myocardial infarction
Non-Q wave myocardial infarction NOS
Nontransmural myocardial infarction NOS

✓4th I22 Subsequent ST elevation (STEMI) and non-ST elevation (NSTEMI) myocardial infarction

INCLUDES acute myocardial infarction occurring within four weeks (28 days) of a previous acute myocardial infarction, regardless of site
cardiac infarction
coronary (artery) embolism
coronary (artery) occlusion
coronary (artery) rupture
coronary (artery) thrombosis
infarction of heart, myocardium, or ventricle
recurrent myocardial infarction
reinfarction of myocardium
rupture of heart, myocardium, or ventricle

Use additional code, if applicable, to identify:
exposure to environmental tobacco smoke (Z77.22)
history of tobacco use (Z87.891)
occupational exposure to environmental tobacco smoke (Z57.31)
status post administration of tPA (rtPA) in a different facility within the last 24 hours prior to admission to current facility (Z92.82)
tobacco dependence (F17.-)
tobacco use (Z72.0))

AHA: 2013, 1Q, 25; 2012, 4Q, 97, 102-103

CC Excl: For MCC codes in category I22, unless otherwise noted:
See code: I21

I22.0 Subsequent ST elevation (STEMI) myocardial infarction of anterior wall MCC
Subsequent acute transmural myocardial infarction of anterior wall
Subsequent transmural (Q wave) infarction (acute)(of) anterior (wall) NOS
Subsequent anteroapical transmural (Q wave) infarction (acute)
Subsequent anterolateral transmural (Q wave) infarction (acute)
Subsequent anteroseptal transmural (Q wave) infarction (acute)

I22.1 Subsequent ST elevation (STEMI) myocardial infarction of inferior wall MCC
Subsequent acute transmural myocardial infarction of inferior wall
Subsequent transmural (Q wave) infarction (acute)(of) diaphragmatic wall
Subsequent transmural (Q wave) infarction (acute)(of) inferior (wall) NOS
Subsequent inferolateral transmural (Q wave) infarction (acute)
Subsequent inferoposterior transmural (Q wave) infarction (acute)
AHA: 2012, 4Q, 102

I22.2 Subsequent non-ST elevation (NSTEMI) myocardial infarction MCC
Subsequent acute subendocardial myocardial infarction
Subsequent non-Q wave myocardial infarction NOS
Subsequent nontransmural myocardial infarction NOS

I22.8 Subsequent ST elevation (STEMI) myocardial infarction of other sites MCC
Subsequent acute transmural myocardial infarction of other sites
Subsequent apical-lateral transmural (Q wave) myocardial infarction (acute)
Subsequent basal-lateral transmural (Q wave) myocardial infarction (acute)
Subsequent high lateral transmural (Q wave) myocardial infarction (acute)
Subsequent transmural (Q wave) myocardial infarction (acute)(of) lateral (wall) NOS
Subsequent posterior (true)transmural (Q wave) myocardial infarction (acute)
Subsequent posterobasal transmural (Q wave) myocardial infarction (acute)
Subsequent posterolateral transmural (Q wave) myocardial infarction (acute)
Subsequent posteroseptal transmural (Q wave) myocardial infarction (acute)
Subsequent septal NOS transmural (Q wave) myocardial infarction (acute)

I22.9 Subsequent ST elevation (STEMI) myocardial infarction of unspecified site MCC
Subsequent acute myocardial infarction of unspecified site
Subsequent myocardial infarction (acute) NOS

✓4th I23 Certain current complications following ST elevation (STEMI) and non-ST elevation (NSTEMI) myocardial infarction (within the 28 day period)

CC Excl: For CC/MCC codes in category I23, unless otherwise noted: E78.71-E78.72, I23.0-I23.8, I40.0-I41, I51.0-I51.2, I51.4, I87.8, I97.0-I97.191, I99.8-I99.9, P29.3, Q20.0-Q21.9, Q23.8-Q23.9, Q24.8-Q24.9, Q27.30, Q27.4, Q28.0-Q28.1, Q28.8-Q28.9, Q87.1-Q87.89, Q89.7-Q89.8, Q99.2

I23.0 Hemopericardium as current complication following acute myocardial infarction CC A
EXCLUDES 1 *hemopericardium not specified as current complication following acute myocardial infarction (I31.2)*

I23.1 Atrial septal defect as current complication following acute myocardial infarction CC A
EXCLUDES 1 *acquired atrial septal defect not specified as current complication following acute myocardial infarction (I51.0)*

I23.2 Ventricular septal defect as current complication following acutemyocardial infarction CC A
EXCLUDES 1 *acquired ventricular septal defect not specified as current complication following acute myocardial infarction (I51.0)*

I23.3 Rupture of cardiac wall without hemopericardium as current complication following acute myocardial infarction CC A

I23.4 Rupture of chordae tendineae as current complication following acute myocardial infarction MCC
EXCLUDES 1 *rupture of chordae tendineae not specified as current complication following acute myocardial infarction (I51.1)*
CC Excl: I23.0-I23.4, I23.6-I23.8, I51.0-I51.1, I87.8, I99.8-I99.9

I23.5 Rupture of papillary muscle as current complication following acute myocardial infarction MCC
EXCLUDES 1 *rupture of papillary muscle not specified as current complication following acute myocardial infarction (I51.2)*
CC Excl: I23.0-I23.3, I23.5-I23.8, I51.0, I51.2, I87.8, I99.8-I99.9

I23.6 Thrombosis of atrium, auricular appendage, and ventricle as current complications following acute myocardial infarction CC A
EXCLUDES 1 *thrombosis of atrium, auricular appendage, and ventricle not specified as current complication following acute myocardial infarction (I51.3)*

I23.7 Postinfarction angina CC A

I23.8 Other current complications following acute myocardial infarction CC A

✓4th I24 Other acute ischemic heart diseases
EXCLUDES 1 *angina pectoris (I20.-)*
transient myocardial ischemia in newborn (P29.4)

CC Excl: For CC codes in category I24, unless otherwise noted: I20.0-I22.9, I24.0-I24.9, I25.5-I25.6, I25.89-I25.9, I87.8, I99.8-I99.9

I24.0 Acute coronary thrombosis not resulting in myocardial infarction CC
Acute coronary (artery) (vein) embolism not resulting in myocardial infarction
Acute coronary (artery) (vein) occlusion not resulting in myocardial infarction
Acute coronary (artery) (vein) thromboembolism not resulting in myocardial infarction
EXCLUDES 1 *atherosclerotic heart disease (I25.1-)*
AHA: 2013, 1Q, 24

I24.1 Dressler's syndrome CC
Postmyocardial infarction syndrome
EXCLUDES 1 *postinfarction angina (I23.7)*
CC Excl: I24.0-I24.9, I87.8, I99.8-I99.9

I24.8 Other forms of acute ischemic heart disease CC

I24.9 Acute ischemic heart disease, unspecified CC
EXCLUDES 1 *ischemic heart disease (chronic) NOS (I25.9)*

✓4th I25 Chronic ischemic heart disease
Use additional code to identify:
- chronic total occlusion of coronary artery (I25.82)
- exposure to environmental tobacco smoke (Z77.22)
- history of tobacco use (Z87.891)
- occupational exposure to environmental tobacco smoke (Z57.31)
- tobacco dependence (F17.-)
- tobacco use (Z72.0)

I25.1 Atherosclerotic heart disease of native coronary artery
Atherosclerotic cardiovascular disease
Coronary (artery) atheroma
Coronary (artery) atherosclerosis
Coronary (artery) disease
Coronary (artery) sclerosis
Use additional code, if applicable, to identify:
- coronary atherosclerosis due to calcified coronary lesion (I25.84)
- coronary atherosclerosis due to lipid rich plaque (I25.83)

EXCLUDES 2 *atheroembolism (I75.-)*
atherosclerosis of coronary artery bypass graft(s) and transplanted heart (I25.7-)

I25.10 Atherosclerotic heart disease of native coronary artery without angina pectoris A
Atherosclerotic heart disease NOS
AHA: 2012, 4Q, 92

✓6th I25.11 Atherosclerotic heart disease of native coronary artery with angina pectoris

I25.110 Atherosclerotic heart disease of native coronary artery with unstable angina pectoris PDx CC CC A
EXCLUDES 1 *unstable angina without atherosclerotic heart disease (I20.0)*
CC Excl: I09.81, I11.0, I13.0, I13.2, I20.0-I22.9, I24.0, I24.8-I24.9, I25.5-I25.6, I25.82-I25.83, I25.89-I25.9, I50.1, I50.9, I87.8, I99.8-I99.9, R57.0, R57.9

I25.111 Atherosclerotic heart disease of native coronary artery with angina pectoris with documented spasm A
EXCLUDES 1 *angina pectoris with documented spasm without atherosclerotic heart disease (I20.1)*

I25.118 Atherosclerotic heart disease of native coronary artery with other forms of angina pectoris A
EXCLUDES 1 *other forms of angina pectoris without atherosclerotic heart disease (I20.8)*

I25.119 Atherosclerotic heart disease of native coronary artery with unspecified angina pectoris A
Atherosclerotic heart disease with angina NOS
Atherosclerotic heart disease with ischemic chest pain
EXCLUDES 1 *unspecified angina pectoris without atherosclerotic heart disease (I20.9)*

I25.2 Old myocardial infarction
Healed myocardial infarction
Past myocardial infarction diagnosed by ECG or other investigation, but currently presenting no symptoms

I25.3 Aneurysm of heart CC
Mural aneurysm
Ventricular aneurysm
CC Excl: I25.3-I25.41

✓5th I25.4 Coronary artery aneurysm and dissection

I25.41 Coronary artery aneurysm
Coronary arteriovenous fistula, acquired
EXCLUDES 1 *congenital coronary (artery) aneurysm (Q24.5)*

I25.42 Coronary artery dissection MCC
CC Excl: I25.42, I67.0, I77.2-I77.3, I77.5-I77.6, I77.79, I77.89-I77.9, M31.8-M31.9

I25.5 Ischemic cardiomyopathy
EXCLUDES 2 *coronary atherosclerosis (I25.1-, I25.7-)*

I25.6 Silent myocardial ischemia

I25.7 Atherosclerosis of coronary artery bypass graft(s) and coronary artery of transplanted heart with angina pectoris

Use additional code, if applicable, to identify:
coronary atherosclerosis due to calcified coronary lesion (I25.84)
coronary atherosclerosis due to lipid rich plaque (I25.83)

EXCLUDES 1 *atherosclerosis of bypass graft(s) of transplanted heart without angina pectoris (I25.812)*
atherosclerosis of coronary artery bypass graft(s) without angina pectoris (I25.810)
atherosclerosis of native coronary artery of transplanted heart without angina pectoris (I25.811)
embolism or thrombus of coronary artery bypass graft(s) (T82.8-)

I25.70 Atherosclerosis of coronary artery bypass graft(s), unspecified, with angina pectoris

I25.700 Atherosclerosis of coronary artery bypass graft(s), unspecified, with unstable angina pectoris PDx CC CC A

EXCLUDES 1 *unstable angina pectoris without atherosclerosis of coronary artery bypass graft (I20.0)*

CC Excl: I09.81, I11.0, I13.0, I13.2, I20.0-I22.9, I24.0, I24.8-I24.9, I25.5-I25.6, I25.82-I25.83, I25.89-I25.9, I50.1, I50.9, I87.8, I99.8-I99.9, R57.0, R57.9

I25.701 Atherosclerosis of coronary artery bypass graft(s), unspecified, with angina pectoris with documented spasm A

EXCLUDES 1 *angina pectoris with documented spasm without atherosclerosis of coronary artery bypass graft (I20.1)*

I25.708 Atherosclerosis of coronary artery bypass graft(s), unspecified, with other forms of angina pectoris A

EXCLUDES 1 *other forms of angina pectoris without atherosclerosis of coronary artery bypass graft (I20.8)*

I25.709 Atherosclerosis of coronary artery bypass graft(s), unspecified, with unspecified angina pectoris A

EXCLUDES 1 *unspecified angina pectoris without atherosclerosis of coronary artery bypass graft (I20.9)*

I25.71 Atherosclerosis of autologous vein coronary artery bypass graft(s) with angina pectoris

CC Excl: For CC codes in subcategory I25.71, unless otherwise noted: I25.10-I25.119, I25.700-I25.799, I25.811-I25.84

I25.710 Atherosclerosis of autologous vein coronary artery bypass graft(s) with unstable angina pectoris PDx CC CC A

EXCLUDES 1 *unstable angina without atherosclerosis of autologous vein coronary artery bypass graft(s) (I20.0)*

CC Excl: I09.81-I11.0, I13.0, I13.2, I20.0-I22.9, I24.0, I24.8-I25.119, I25.5-I25.739, I25.760-I25.799, I25.812-I25.9, I50.1, I50.9, I87.8, I99.8-I99.9, R57.0, R57.9

I25.711 Atherosclerosis of autologous vein coronary artery bypass graft(s) with angina pectoris with documented spasm CC A

EXCLUDES 1 *angina pectoris with documented spasm without atherosclerosis of autologous vein coronary artery bypass graft(s) (I20.1)*

I25.718 Atherosclerosis of autologous vein coronary artery bypass graft(s) with other forms of angina pectoris CC A

EXCLUDES 1 *other forms of angina pectoris without atherosclerosis of autologous vein coronary artery bypass graft(s) (I20.8)*

I25.719 Atherosclerosis of autologous vein coronary artery bypass graft(s) with unspecified angina pectoris CC A

EXCLUDES 1 *unspecified angina pectoris without atherosclerosis of autologous vein coronary artery bypass graft(s) (I20.9)*

I25.72 Atherosclerosis of autologous artery coronary artery bypass graft(s) with angina pectoris

Atherosclerosis of internal mammary artery graft with angina pectoris

CC Excl: For CC codes in subcategories I25.72, unless otherwise noted: I25.10-I25.119, I25.700-I25.738

I25.720 Atherosclerosis of autologous artery coronary artery bypass graft(s) with unstable angina pectoris PDx CC CC A

EXCLUDES 1 *unstable angina without atherosclerosis of autologous artery coronary artery bypass graft(s) (I20.0)*

CC Excl: See code: I25.710

I25.721 Atherosclerosis of autologous artery coronary artery bypass graft(s) with angina pectoris with documented spasm CC A

EXCLUDES 1 *angina pectoris with documented spasm without atherosclerosis of autologous artery coronary artery bypass graft(s) (I20.1)*

I25.728 Atherosclerosis of autologous artery coronary artery bypass graft(s) with other forms of angina pectoris CC A

EXCLUDES 1 *other forms of angina pectoris without atherosclerosis of autologous artery coronary artery bypass graft(s) (I20.8)*

I25.729 Atherosclerosis of autologous artery coronary artery bypass graft(s) with unspecified angina pectoris CC A

EXCLUDES 1 *unspecified angina pectoris without atherosclerosis of autologous artery coronary artery bypass graft(s) (I20.9)*

I25.73 Atherosclerosis of nonautologous biological coronary artery bypass graft(s) with angina pectoris

CC Excl: For CC codes in subcategories I25.73, unless otherwise noted: I25.10-I25.119, I25.700-I25.738

I25.730 Atherosclerosis of nonautologous biological coronary artery bypass graft(s) with unstable angina pectoris PDx CC CC A

EXCLUDES 1 *unstable angina without atherosclerosis of nonautologous biological coronary artery bypass graft(s) (I20.0)*

CC Excl: See code: I25.710

I25.731 Atherosclerosis of nonautologous biological coronary artery bypass graft(s) with angina pectoris with documented spasm CC A

EXCLUDES 1 *angina pectoris with documented spasm without atherosclerosis of nonautologous biological coronary artery bypass graft(s) (I20.1)*

I25.738 Atherosclerosis of nonautologous biological coronary artery bypass graft(s) with other forms of angina pectoris CC A

EXCLUDES 1 *other forms of angina pectoris without atherosclerosis of nonautologous biological coronary artery bypass graft(s) (I20.8)*

I25.739 Atherosclerosis of nonautologous biological coronary artery bypass graft(s) with unspecified angina pectoris CC A

EXCLUDES 1 *unspecified angina pectoris without atherosclerosis of nonautologous biological coronary artery bypass graft(s) (I20.9)*

✓6th **I25.75 Atherosclerosis of native coronary artery of transplanted heart with angina pectoris**

EXCLUDES 1 *atherosclerosis of native coronary artery of transplanted heart without angina pectoris (I25.811)*

CC Excl: For CC codes in subcategory I25.75, unless otherwise noted: I25.10-I25.119, I25.700-I25.799, I25.811-I25.84

I25.750 Atherosclerosis of native coronary artery of transplanted heart with unstable angina PDx CC CC

CC Excl: I09.81, I11.0, I13.0, I13.2, I20.0-I22.9, I24.8-I25.119, I25.5-I25.799, I25.811-I25.9, I50.1, I50.9, I87.8, I99.8-I99.9, R57.0, R57.9

I25.751 Atherosclerosis of native coronary artery of transplanted heart with angina pectoris with documented spasm CC

I25.758 Atherosclerosis of native coronary artery of transplanted heart with other forms of angina pectoris CC

I25.759 Atherosclerosis of native coronary artery of transplanted heart with unspecified angina pectoris CC

✓6th **I25.76 Atherosclerosis of bypass graft of coronary artery of transplanted heart with angina pectoris**

EXCLUDES 1 *atherosclerosis of bypass graft of coronary artery of transplanted heart without angina pectoris (I25.812)*

CC Excl: For CC codes in subcategory I25.76, unless otherwise noted: I25.10-I25.119, I25.700-I25.759, I25.790-I25.799, I25.811, I25.82-I25.84

I25.760 Atherosclerosis of bypass graft of coronary artery of transplanted heart with unstable angina PDx CC CC A

CC Excl: I09.81-I11.0, I13.0, I13.2, I20.0-I22.9, I24.0, I24.8-I25.119, I25.5-I25.759, I25.790-I25.799, I25.811, I25.82-I25.9, I50.1, I50.9, I87.8, I99.8-I99.9, R57.0, R57.9

I25.761 Atherosclerosis of bypass graft of coronary artery of transplanted heart with angina pectoris with documented spasm CC A

I25.768 Atherosclerosis of bypass graft of coronary artery of transplanted heart with other forms of angina pectoris CC A

I25.769 Atherosclerosis of bypass graft of coronary artery of transplanted heart with unspecified angina pectoris CC A

✓6th **I25.79 Atherosclerosis of other coronary artery bypass graft(s) with angina pectoris**

CC Excl: For CC codes in subcategory I25.79, unless otherwise noted: No exclusion

I25.790 Atherosclerosis of other coronary artery bypass graft(s) with unstable angina pectoris PDx CC CC A

EXCLUDES 1 *unstable angina without atherosclerosis of other coronary artery bypass graft(s) (I20.0)*

CC Excl: I09.81, I11.0, I13.0, I13.2, I20.0-I22.9, I24.0, I24.8-I24.9, I25.5-I25.6, I25.82-I25.83, I25.89-I25.9, I50.1, I50.9, I87.8, I99.8-I99.9, R57.0, R57.9

I25.791 Atherosclerosis of other coronary artery bypass graft(s) with angina pectoris with documented spasm CC A

EXCLUDES 1 *angina pectoris with documented spasm without atherosclerosis of other coronary artery bypass graft(s) (I20.1)*

I25.798 Atherosclerosis of other coronary artery bypass graft(s) with other forms of angina pectoris CC A

EXCLUDES 1 *other forms of angina pectoris without atherosclerosis of other coronary artery bypass graft(s) (I20.8)*

I25.799 Atherosclerosis of other coronary artery bypass graft(s) with unspecified angina pectoris CC A

EXCLUDES 1 *unspecified angina pectoris without atherosclerosis of other coronary artery bypass graft(s) (I20.9)*

✓5th **I25.8 Other forms of chronic ischemic heart disease**

✓6th **I25.81 Atherosclerosis of other coronary vessels without angina pectoris**

Use additional code, if applicable, to identify:
- coronary atherosclerosis due to calcified coronary lesion (I25.84)
- coronary atherosclerosis due to lipid rich plaque (I25.83)

EXCLUDES 1 *atherosclerotic heart disease of native coronary artery without angina pectoris (I25.10)*

I25.810 Atherosclerosis of coronary artery bypass graft(s) without angina pectoris CC A

Atherosclerosis of coronary artery bypass graft NOS

EXCLUDES 1 *atherosclerosis of coronary bypass graft(s) with angina pectoris (I25.70--I25.73-, I25.79-)*

CC Excl: No excl

I25.811 Atherosclerosis of native coronary artery of transplanted heart without angina pectoris CC

Atherosclerosis of native coronary artery of transplanted heart NOS

EXCLUDES 1 *atherosclerosis of native coronary artery of transplanted heart with angina pectoris (I25.75-)*

CC Excl: See code: I25.75

I25.812 Atherosclerosis of bypass graft of coronary artery of transplanted heart without angina pectoris CC A

Atherosclerosis of bypass graft of transplanted heart NOS

EXCLUDES 1 *atherosclerosis of bypass graft of transplanted heart with angina pectoris (I25.76)*

CC Excl: See code: I25.76

I25.82 Chronic total occlusion of coronary artery

Complete occlusion of coronary artery
Total occlusion of coronary artery
Code first coronary atherosclerosis (I25.1-, I25.7-, I25.81-)

EXCLUDES 1 *acute coronary occulsion with myocardial infarction (I21.-, I22.-)*
acute coronary occulsion without myocardial infarction (I24.0)

I25.83 Coronary atherosclerosis due to lipid rich plaque A

Code first coronary atherosclerosis (I25.1-, I25.7-, I25.81-)

I25.84 Coronary atherosclerosis due to calcified coronary lesion

Coronary atherosclerosis due to severely calcified coronary lesion
Code first coronary atherosclerosis (I25.1-, I25.7-, I25.81-)

I25.89 Other forms of chronic ischemic heart disease

I25.9 Chronic ischemic heart disease, unspecified

Ischemic heart disease (chronic) NOS

Pulmonary heart disease and diseases of pulmonary circulation (I26-I28)

I26 Pulmonary embolism
Pulmonary (acute) (artery)(vein) infarction
Pulmonary (acute) (artery)(vein) thromboembolism
Pulmonary (acute) (artery)(vein) thrombosis
EXCLUDES 2 *chronic pulmonary embolism (I27.82)*
personal history of pulmonary embolism (Z86.711)
pulmonary embolism due to trauma (T79.0, T79.1)
pulmonary embolism due to complications of surgical and medical care (T80.0, T81.7-, T82.8-)
pulmonary embolism complicating abortion, ectopic or molar pregnancy (O00-O07, O08.2)
pulmonary embolism complicating pregnancy, childbirth and the puerperium (O88.-)
septic (non-pulmonary) arterial embolism (I76)

I26.0 Pulmonary embolism with acute cor pulmonale

I26.01 Septic pulmonary embolism with acute cor pulmonale PDx MCC MCC
Code first underlying infection
CC Excl: I26.01-I26.99, I27.2-I27.9, I74.01-I74.10, I74.19, I87.8, I99.8-I99.9

3 **I26.02 Saddle embolus of pulmonary artery with acute cor pulmonale** PDx MCC MCC
CC Excl: See code: I26.01

3 **I26.09 Other pulmonary embolism with acute cor pulmonale** PDx MCC MCC
Acute cor pulmonale NOS
CC Excl: See code: I26.01

I26.9 Pulmonary embolism without acute cor pulmonale

I26.90 Septic pulmonary embolism without acute cor pulmonale MCC
Code first underlying infection
CC Excl: I26.01-I26.99, I27.82, I74.01-I74.10, I74.19, I87.8, I99.8-I99.9, T80.0XXA, T81.718A, T81.72XA, T82.817A, T82.818A

3 **I26.92 Saddle embolus of pulmonary artery without acute cor pulmonale** MCC
CC Excl: I26.01-I26.99, I27.82, I74.01-I74.10, I74.19, I87.8, I99.8-I99.9

3 **I26.99 Other pulmonary embolism without acute cor pulmonale** MCC
Acute pulmonary embolism NOS
Pulmonary embolism NOS
CC Excl: See code: I26.90

I27 Other pulmonary heart diseases

I27.0 Primary pulmonary hypertension CC
EXCLUDES 1 *pulmonary hypertension NOS (I27.2)*
secondary pulmonary hypertension (I27.2)
CC Excl: E66.2, I27.0, I27.2-I27.81, I27.89-I27.9, I28.8-I28.9, I87.8, I99.8-I99.9

I27.1 Kyphoscoliotic heart disease CC
CC Excl: E66.2, I27.0-I27.81, I27.89-I27.9

I27.2 Other secondary pulmonary hypertension
Pulmonary hypertension NOS
Code also associated underlying condition

I27.8 Other specified pulmonary heart diseases

I27.81 Cor pulmonale (chronic)
Cor pulmonale NOS
EXCLUDES 1 *acute cor pulmonale (I26.0-)*

I27.82 Chronic pulmonary embolism CC
Use additional code, if applicable, for associated long-term (current) use of anticoagulants (Z79.01)
EXCLUDES 1 *personal history of pulmonary embolism (Z86.711)*
CC Excl: I26.01-I26.99, I27.82, I74.01-I74.10, I74.19, I87.8, I99.8-I99.9

I27.89 Other specified pulmonary heart diseases
Eisenmenger's complex
Eisenmenger's syndrome
EXCLUDES 1 *Eisenmenger's defect (Q21.8)*

I27.9 Pulmonary heart disease, unspecified
Chronic cardiopulmonary disease

I28 Other diseases of pulmonary vessels

I28.0 Arteriovenous fistula of pulmonary vessels CC
EXCLUDES 1 *congenital arteriovenous fistula (Q25.72)*
CC Excl: I28.0-I28.9

I28.1 Aneurysm of pulmonary artery CC
EXCLUDES 1 *congenital aneurysm (Q25.79)*
congenital arteriovenous aneurysm (Q25.72)
CC Excl: See code: I28.0

I28.8 Other diseases of pulmonary vessels
Pulmonary arteritis
Pulmonary endarteritis
Rupture of pulmonary vessels
Stenosis of pulmonary vessels
Stricture of pulmonary vessels

I28.9 Disease of pulmonary vessels, unspecified

Other forms of heart disease (I30-I52)

I30 Acute pericarditis
INCLUDES acute mediastinopericarditis
acute myopericarditis
acute pericardial effusion
acute pleuropericarditis
acute pneumopericarditis
EXCLUDES 1 *Dressler's syndrome (I24.1)*
rheumatic pericarditis (acute) (I01.0)

CC Excl: For CC codes in category I30, unless otherwise noted: I01.0, I09.2, I30.0-I30.9, I31.3-I32, I87.8, I99.8-I99.9

I30.0 Acute nonspecific idiopathic pericarditis CC

I30.1 Infective pericarditis CC
Pneumococcal pericarditis
Pneumopyopericardium
Purulent pericarditis
Pyopericarditis
Pyopericardium
Pyopneumopericardium
Staphylococcal pericarditis
Streptococcal pericarditis
Suppurative pericarditis
Viral pericarditis
Use additional code (B95-B97) to identify infectious agent

I30.8 Other forms of acute pericarditis CC

I30.9 Acute pericarditis, unspecified CC

I31 Other diseases of pericardium
EXCLUDES 1 *diseases of pericardium specified as rheumatic (I09.2)*
postcardiotomy syndrome (I97.0)
traumatic injury to pericardium (S26.-)

I31.0 Chronic adhesive pericarditis CC
Accretio cordis
Adherent pericardium
Adhesive mediastinopericarditis
CC Excl: I31.0-I31.9, I87.8, I99.8-I99.9

I31.1 Chronic constrictive pericarditis CC
Concretio cordis
Pericardial calcification
CC Excl: See code: I31.0

I31.2 Hemopericardium, not elsewhere classified CC
EXCLUDES 1 *hemopericardium as current complication following acute myocardial infarction (I23.0)*
CC Excl: See code: I31.0

I31.3 Pericardial effusion (noninflammatory) CC
Chylopericardium
EXCLUDES 1 *acute pericardial effusion (I30.9)*
CC Excl: B33.23, I01.0, I09.2, I30.0-I30.9, I31.3-I32, I87.8, I99.8-I99.9

I31.4 Cardiac tamponade CC
Code first underlying cause
CC Excl: See code: I31.3

I31.8 Other specified diseases of pericardium CC
Epicardial plaques
Focal pericardial adhesions
CC Excl: See code: I31.3

I31.9 Disease of pericardium, unspecified CC
Pericarditis (chronic) NOS
CC Excl: See code: I31.3

I32 Pericarditis in diseases classified elsewhere CC
Code first underlying disease
EXCLUDES 1 *pericarditis (in):*
coxsackie (virus) (B33.23)
gonococcal (A54.83)
meningococcal (A39.53)
rheumatoid (arthritis) (M05.31)
syphilitic (A52.06)
systemic lupus erythematosus (M32.12)
tuberculosis (A18.84)
CC Excl: I01.0, I09.2, I30.0-I30.9, I31.3-I32, I87.8, I99.8-I99.9

3 These codes, although not unacceptable as PDx, would be considered questionable as a PDx for acute care hospital admissions.

I33 Acute and subacute endocarditis

EXCLUDES 1 *acute rheumatic endocarditis (I01.1)*
endocarditis NOS (I38)

I33.0 Acute and subacute infective endocarditis HIV MCC
Bacterial endocarditis (acute) (subacute)
Infective endocarditis (acute) (subacute) NOS
Endocarditis lenta (acute) (subacute)
Malignant endocarditis (acute) (subacute)
Purulent endocarditis (acute) (subacute)
Septic endocarditis (acute) (subacute)
Ulcerative endocarditis (acute) (subacute)
Vegetative endocarditis (acute) (subacute)
Use additional code (B95-B97) to identify infectious agent
CC Excl: I01.1-I08.3, I09.1, I33.0-I33.9, I38-I39, I87.8, I99.8-I99.9

I33.9 Acute and subacute endocarditis, unspecified HIV MCC
Acute endocarditis NOS
Acute myoendocarditis NOS
Acute periendocarditis NOS
Subacute endocarditis NOS
Subacute myoendocarditis NOS
Subacute periendocarditis NOS
CC Excl: See code: I33.0

I34 Nonrheumatic mitral valve disorders

EXCLUDES 1 *mitral valve disease (I05.9)*
mitral valve failure (I05.8)
mitral valve stenosis (I05.0)
mitral valve disorder of unspecified cause with diseases of aortic and/or tricuspid valve(s) (I08.-)
mitral valve disorder of unspecified cause with mitral stenosis or obstruction (I05.0)
mitral valve disorder specified as congenital (Q23.2, Q23.3)
mitral valve disorder specified as rheumatic (I05.-)

I34.0 Nonrheumatic mitral (valve) insufficiency
Nonrheumatic mitral (valve) incompetence NOS
Nonrheumatic mitral (valve) regurgitation NOS

I34.1 Nonrheumatic mitral (valve) prolapse
Floppy nonrheumatic mitral valve syndrome
EXCLUDES 1 *Marfan's syndrome (Q87.4-)*

I34.2 Nonrheumatic mitral (valve) stenosis

I34.8 Other nonrheumatic mitral valve disorders

I34.9 Nonrheumatic mitral valve disorder, unspecified

I35 Nonrheumatic aortic valve disorders

EXCLUDES 1 *aortic valve disorder of unspecified cause but with diseases of mitral and/or tricuspid valve(s) (I08.-)*
aortic valve disorder specified as congenital (Q23.0, Q23.1)
aortic valve disorder specified as rheumatic (I06.-)
hypertrophic subaortic stenosis (I42.1)

I35.0 Nonrheumatic aortic (valve) stenosis

I35.1 Nonrheumatic aortic (valve) insufficiency
Nonrheumatic aortic (valve) incompetence NOS
Nonrheumatic aortic (valve) regurgitation NOS

I35.2 Nonrheumatic aortic (valve) stenosis with insufficiency

I35.8 Other nonrheumatic aortic valve disorders

I35.9 Nonrheumatic aortic valve disorder, unspecified

I36 Nonrheumatic tricuspid valve disorders

EXCLUDES 1 *tricuspid valve disorders of unspecified cause (I07.-)*
tricuspid valve disorders specified as congenital (Q22.4, Q22.8, Q22.9)
tricuspid valve disorders specified as rheumatic (I07.-)
tricuspid valve disorders with aortic and/or mitral valve involvement (I08.-)

I36.0 Nonrheumatic tricuspid (valve) stenosis

I36.1 Nonrheumatic tricuspid (valve) insufficiency
Nonrheumatic tricuspid (valve) incompetence
Nonrheumatic tricuspid (valve) regurgitation

I36.2 Nonrheumatic tricuspid (valve) stenosis with insufficiency

I36.8 Other nonrheumatic tricuspid valve disorders

I36.9 Nonrheumatic tricuspid valve disorder, unspecified

I37 Nonrheumatic pulmonary valve disorders

EXCLUDES 1 *pulmonary valve disorder specified as congenital (Q22.1, Q22.2, Q22.3)*
pulmonary valve disorder specified as rheumatic (I09.89)

I37.0 Nonrheumatic pulmonary valve stenosis

I37.1 Nonrheumatic pulmonary valve insufficiency
Nonrheumatic pulmonary valve incompetence
Nonrheumatic pulmonary valve regurgitation

I37.2 Nonrheumatic pulmonary valve stenosis with insufficiency

I37.8 Other nonrheumatic pulmonary valve disorders

I37.9 Nonrheumatic pulmonary valve disorder, unspecified

I38 Endocarditis, valve unspecified CC

INCLUDES endocarditis (chronic) NOS
valvular incompetence NOS
valvular insufficiency NOS
valvular regurgitation NOS
valvular stenosis NOS
valvulitis (chronic) NOS

EXCLUDES 1 *congenital insufficiency of cardiac valve NOS (Q24.8)*
congenital stenosis of cardiac valve NOS (Q24.8)
endocardial fibroelastosis (I42.4)
endocarditis specified as rheumatic (I09.1)

CC Excl: I38-I39, I87.8, I99.8-I99.9

I39 Endocarditis and heart valve disorders in diseases classified elsewhere CC

Code first underlying disease, such as:
Q fever (A78)

EXCLUDES 1 *endocardial involvement in:*
candidiasis (B37.6)
gonococcal infection (A54.83)
Libman-Sacks disease (M32.11)
listerosis (A32.82)
meningococcal infection (A39.51)
rheumatoid arthritis (M05.31)
syphilis (A52.03)
tuberculosis (A18.84)
typhoid fever (A01.02)

CC Excl: See code: I38

I40 Acute myocarditis

INCLUDES subacute myocarditis

EXCLUDES 1 *acute rheumatic myocarditis (I01.2)*

CC Excl: For MCC codes in category I40, unless otherwise noted: I01.2, I09.0, I23.0-I23.3, I23.6-I23.8, I40.0-I41, I51.0, I51.4, I87.8, I99.8-I99.9

I40.0 Infective myocarditis HIV MCC
Septic myocarditis
Use additional code (B95-B97) to identify infectious agent

I40.1 Isolated myocarditis HIV MCC
Fiedler's myocarditis
Giant cell myocarditis
Idiopathic myocarditis

I40.8 Other acute myocarditis HIV MCC

I40.9 Acute myocarditis, unspecified HIV MCC

I41 Myocarditis in diseases classified elsewhere MCC

Code first underlying disease, such as:
typhus (A75.0-A75.9)

EXCLUDES 1 *myocarditis (in):*
Chagas' disease (chronic) (B57.2)
acute (B57.0)
coxsackie (virus) infection (B33.22)
diphtheritic (A36.81)
gonococcal (A54.83)
influenzal (J09.X9, J10.82, J11.82)
meningococcal (A39.52)
mumps (B26.82)
rheumatoid arthritis (M05.31)
sarcoid (D86.85)
syphilis (A52.06)
toxoplasmosis (B58.81)
tuberculous (A18.84)

CC Excl: See code: I40

I42 Cardiomyopathy

INCLUDES myocardiopathy

Code first pre-existing cardiomyopathy complicating pregnancy and puerperium (O99.4)

EXCLUDES 1 *ischemic cardiomyopathy (I25.5)*
peripartum cardiomyopathy (O90.3)

EXCLUDES 2 *ventricular hypertrophy (I51.7)*

CC Excl: For CC codes in category I42, unless otherwise noted: I09.81, I11.0, I13.0, I13.2, I25.10-I25.119, I25.5-I25.799, I25.811-I25.9, I42.0-I44.1, I44.30-I44.39, I45.2-I45.4, I45.81-I45.89, I48.0-I49.1, I49.3-I49.8, I50.1, I50.9, I87.8, I99.8-I99.9, Q24.6, R00.0-R00.2, R57.0, R57.9

I42.0 Dilated cardiomyopathy CC
Congestive cardiomyopathy

I42.1 Obstructive hypertrophic cardiomyopathy CC
Hypertrophic subaortic stenosis (idiopathic)

I42.2 Other hypertrophic cardiomyopathy CC
Nonobstructive hypertrophic cardiomyopathy

I42.3 Endomyocardial (eosinophilic) disease CC
Endomyocardial (tropical) fibrosis
Löffler's endocarditis

I42.4 Endocardial fibroelastosis CC
Congenital cardiomyopathy
Elastomyofibrosis

I42.5 Other restrictive cardiomyopathy CC
Constrictive cardiomyopathy NOS

I42.6 Alcoholic cardiomyopathy CC
Code also presence of alcoholism (F1Ø.-)

I42.7 Cardiomyopathy due to drug and external agent CC
Code first poisoning due to drug or toxin, if applicable (T36-T65 with fifth or sixth character 1-4 or 6)
Use additional code for adverse effect, if applicable, to identify drug (T36-T5Ø with fifth or sixth character 5)

I42.8 Other cardiomyopathies CC

I42.9 Cardiomyopathy, unspecified CC
Cardiomyopathy (primary) (secondary) NOS

I43 Cardiomyopathy in diseases classified elsewhere CC
Code first underlying disease, such as:
amyloidosis (E85.-)
glycogen storage disease (E74.Ø)
gout (M1Ø.Ø-)
thyrotoxicosis (EØ5.Ø-EØ5.9-)
EXCLUDES 1 *cardiomyopathy (in):*
coxsackie (virus) (B33.24)
diphtheria (A36.81)
sarcoidosis (D86.85)
tuberculosis (A18.84)
CC Excl: See code: I42

✓4th **I44 Atrioventricular and left bundle-branch block**

I44.Ø Atrioventricular block, first degree

I44.1 Atrioventricular block, second degree
Atrioventricular block, type I and II
Möbitz block, type I and II
Second degree block, type I and II
Wenckebach's block

I44.2 Atrioventricular block, complete CC
Complete heart block NOS
Third degree block
CC Excl: I44.Ø-I49.Ø2, I49.2, I49.8, I87.8, I99.8-I99.9, RØØ.1

✓5th **I44.3 Other and unspecified atrioventricular block**
Atrioventricular block NOS

I44.3Ø Unspecified atrioventricular block

I44.39 Other atrioventricular block

13 **I44.4 Left anterior fascicular block**

13 **I44.5 Left posterior fascicular block**

✓5th **I44.6 Other and unspecified fascicular block**

13 **I44.6Ø Unspecified fascicular block**
Left bundle-branch hemiblock NOS

13 **I44.69 Other fascicular block**

13 **I44.7 Left bundle-branch block, unspecified**

✓4th **I45 Other conduction disorders**

CC Excl: For CC codes in category I45, unless otherwise noted: I44.Ø-I49.Ø2, I49.2, I49.8, I87.8, I99.8-I99.9, RØØ.1

13 **I45.Ø Right fascicular block**

✓5th **I45.1 Other and unspecified right bundle-branch block**

13 **I45.1Ø Unspecified right bundle-branch block**
Right bundle-branch block NOS

13 **I45.19 Other right bundle-branch block**

I45.2 Bifascicular block CC

I45.3 Trifascicular block CC

I45.4 Nonspecific intraventricular block
Bundle-branch block NOS

I45.5 Other specified heart block
Sinoatrial block Sinoauricular block
EXCLUDES 1 *heart block NOS (I45.9)*

I45.6 Pre-excitation syndrome
Accelerated atrioventricular conduction
Accessory atrioventricular conduction
Anomalous atrioventricular excitation
Lown-Ganong-Levine syndrome
Pre-excitation atrioventricular conduction
Wolff-Parkinson-White syndrome

✓5th **I45.8 Other specified conduction disorders**

I45.81 Long QT syndrome

I45.89 Other specified conduction disorders CC
Atrioventricular [AV] dissociation
Interference dissociation
Isorhythmic dissociation
Nonparoxysmal AV nodal tachycardia
AHA: 2Ø13, 2Q, 31

I45.9 Conduction disorder, unspecified
Heart block NOS
Stokes-Adams syndrome

✓4th **I46 Cardiac arrest**
EXCLUDES 1 *cardiogenic shock (R57.Ø)*

CC Excl: For MCC codes in category I46, unless otherwise noted: I46.2-I49.Ø2, I49.2, I87.8, I99.8-I99.9

10 **I46.2 Cardiac arrest due to underlying cardiac condition** MCC
Code first underlying cardiac condition

10 **I46.8 Cardiac arrest due to other underlying condition** MCC
Code first underlying condition

10 **I46.9 Cardiac arrest, cause unspecified** MCC

✓4th **I47 Paroxysmal tachycardia**
Code first tachycardia complicating:
abortion or ectopic or molar pregnancy (OØØ-OØ7, OØ8.8)
obstetric surgery and procedures (O75.4)
EXCLUDES 1 *tachycardia NOS (RØØ.Ø)*
sinoauricular tachycardia NOS (RØØ.Ø)
sinus [sinusal] tachycardia NOS (RØØ.Ø)

CC Excl: For CC codes in category I47, unless otherwise noted: See code: I45

I47.Ø Re-entry ventricular arrhythmia CC

I47.1 Supraventricular tachycardia CC
Atrial (paroxysmal) tachycardia
Atrioventricular [AV] (paroxysmal) tachycardia
Atrioventricular re-entrant (nodal) tachycardia [AVNRT] [AVRT]
Junctional (paroxysmal) tachycardia
Nodal (paroxysmal) tachycardia

I47.2 Ventricular tachycardia CC
AHA: 2Ø13, 3Q, 23

I47.9 Paroxysmal tachycardia, unspecified
Bouveret (-Hoffman) syndrome

✓4th **I48 Atrial fibrillation and flutter**

CC Excl: For CC codes in category I48, unless otherwise noted: See code: I45

I48.Ø Paroxysmal atrial fibrillation

I48.1 Persistent atrial fibrillation CC

I48.2 Chronic atrial fibrillation
Permanent atrial fibrillation

I48.3 Typical atrial flutter CC
Type I atrial flutter

I48.4 Atypical atrial flutter CC
Type II atrial flutter

✓5th **I48.9 Unspecified atrial fibrillation and atrial flutter**

I48.91 Unspecified atrial fibrillation

I48.92 Unspecified atrial flutter CC

✓4th **I49 Other cardiac arrhythmias**

CC Excl: For MCC codes in category I49, unless otherwise noted: See code: I45

Code first cardiac arrhythmia complicating:
abortion or ectopic or molar pregnancy (OØØ-OØ7, OØ8.8)
obstetric surgery and procedures (O75.4)
EXCLUDES 1 *bradycardia NOS (RØØ.1)*
neonatal dysrhythmia (P29.1-)
sinoatrial bradycardia (RØØ.1)
sinus bradycardia (RØØ.1)
vagal bradycardia (RØØ.1)

✓5th **I49.Ø Ventricular fibrillation and flutter**

10 **I49.Ø1 Ventricular fibrillation** MCC

I49.Ø2 Ventricular flutter MCC

I49.1 Atrial premature depolarization
Atrial premature beats

I49.2 Junctional premature depolarization CC

10 MCC only if patient is discharged alive.
13 Questionable admission when used as PDx.

I49.3 **Ventricular premature depolarization**

5th **I49.4 Other and unspecified premature depolarization**

I49.40 Unspecified premature depolarization
Premature beats NOS

I49.49 Other premature depolarization
Ectopic beats
Extrasystoles
Extrasystolic arrhythmias
Premature contractions

I49.5 Sick sinus syndrome
Tachycardia-bradycardia syndrome

I49.8 Other specified cardiac arrhythmias
Coronary sinus rhythm disorder
Ectopic rhythm disorder
Nodal rhythm disorder

I49.9 Cardiac arrhythmia, unspecified
Arrhythmia (cardiac) NOS

4th **I5Ø Heart failure**
Code first:
heart failure complicating abortion or ectopic or molar pregnancy (OØØ-OØ7, OØ8.8)
heart failure following surgery (I97.13-)
heart failure due to hypertension (I11.Ø)
heart failure due to hypertension with chronic kidney disease (I13.-)
obstetric surgery and procedures (O75.4)
rheumatic heart failure (IØ9.81)

EXCLUDES 1 *cardiac arrest (I46.-)*
neonatal cardiac failure (P29.Ø)

AHA: 2Ø14, 1Q, 25; 2Ø13, 2Q, 33

CC Excl: For CC/MCC codes in category I5Ø, unless otherwise noted: IØ9.81, I11.Ø, I5Ø.1-I5Ø.9, I87.8, I99.8-I99.9, J81.Ø

I5Ø.1 Left ventricular failure CC
Cardiac asthma
Edema of lung with heart disease NOS
Edema of lung with heart failure
Left heart failure
Pulmonary edema with heart disease NOS
Pulmonary edema with heart failure

EXCLUDES 1 *edema of lung without heart disease or heart failure (J81.-)*
pulmonary edema without heart disease or failure (J81.-)

CC Excl: IØ9.81, I11.Ø, I5Ø.1-I5Ø.9, I87.8, I99.8-I99.9

5th **I5Ø.2 Systolic (congestive) heart failure**
EXCLUDES 1 *combined systolic (congestive) and diastolic (congestive) heart failure (I5Ø.4-)*

I5Ø.2Ø Unspecified systolic (congestive) heart failure CC
I5Ø.21 Acute systolic (congestive) heart failure MCC
I5Ø.22 Chronic systolic (congestive) heart failure CC
I5Ø.23 Acute on chronic systolic (congestive) heart failure MCC

5th **I5Ø.3 Diastolic (congestive) heart failure**
EXCLUDES 1 *combined systolic (congestive) and diastolic (congestive) heart failure (I5Ø.4-)*

I5Ø.3Ø Unspecified diastolic (congestive) heart failure CC
I5Ø.31 Acute diastolic (congestive) heart failure MCC
I5Ø.32 Chronic diastolic (congestive) heart failure CC
I5Ø.33 Acute on chronic diastolic (congestive) heart failure MCC

5th **I5Ø.4 Combined systolic (congestive) and diastolic (congestive) heart failure**

I5Ø.4Ø Unspecified combined systolic (congestive) and diastolic (congestive) heart failure CC
I5Ø.41 Acute combined systolic (congestive) and diastolic (congestive) heart failure MCC
I5Ø.42 Chronic combined systolic (congestive) and diastolic (congestive) heart failure CC
I5Ø.43 Acute on chronic combined systolic (congestive) and diastolic (congestive) heart failure MCC

I5Ø.9 Heart failure, unspecified
Biventricular (heart) failure NOS
Cardiac, heart or myocardial failure NOS
Congestive heart disease
Congestive heart failure NOS
Right ventricular failure (secondary to left heart failure)

EXCLUDES 1 *fluid overload (E87.7Ø)*

AHA: 2Ø12, 4Q, 92

4th **I51 Complications and ill-defined descriptions of heart disease**
EXCLUDES 1 *any condition in I51.4-I51.9 due to hypertension (I11.-)*
any condition in I51.4-I51.9 due to hypertension and chronic kidney disease (I13.-)
heart disease specified as rheumatic (IØØ-IØ9)

I51.Ø Cardiac septal defect, acquired CC A
Acquired septal atrial defect (old)
Acquired septal auricular defect (old)
Acquired septal ventricular defect (old)

EXCLUDES 1 *cardiac septal defect as current complication following acute myocardial infarction (I23.1, I23.2)*

CC Excl: E78.71-E78.72, I23.Ø-I23.8, I4Ø.Ø-I41, I51.Ø-I51.2, I51.4, I87.8, I97.Ø-I97.191, I99.8-I99.9, P29.3, Q2Ø.Ø-Q21.9, Q23.8-Q23.9, Q24.8-Q24.9, Q27.3Ø, Q27.4, Q28.Ø-Q28.1, Q28.8-Q28.9, Q87.1-Q87.89, Q89.7-Q89.8, Q99.2

I51.1 Rupture of chordae tendineae, not elsewhere classified MCC
EXCLUDES 1 *rupture of chordae tendineae as current complication following acute myocardial infarction (I23.4)*

CC Excl: I23.Ø-I23.4, I23.6-I23.8, I51.Ø-I51.1, I87.8, I99.8-I99.9

I51.2 Rupture of papillary muscle, not elsewhere classified MCC
EXCLUDES 1 *rupture of papillary muscle as current complication following acute myocardial infarction (I23.5)*

CC Excl: I23.Ø-I23.3, I23.5-I23.8, I51.Ø, I51.2, I87.8, I99.8-I99.9

I51.3 Intracardiac thrombosis, not elsewhere classified A
Apical thrombosis (old)
Atrial thrombosis (old)
Auricular thrombosis (old)
Mural thrombosis (old)
Ventricular thrombosis (old)

EXCLUDES 1 *intracardiac thrombosis as current complication following acute myocardial infarction (I23.6)*

AHA: 2Ø13, 1Q, 24

I51.4 Myocarditis, unspecified
Chronic (interstitial) myocarditis
Myocardial fibrosis
Myocarditis NOS

EXCLUDES 1 *acute or subacute myocarditis (I4Ø.-)*

I51.5 Myocardial degeneration
Fatty degeneration of heart or myocardium
Myocardial disease
Senile degeneration of heart or myocardium

I51.7 Cardiomegaly
Cardiac dilatation
Cardiac hypertrophy
Ventricular dilatation

5th **I51.8 Other ill-defined heart diseases**

I51.81 Takotsubo syndrome CC
Reversible left ventricular dysfunction following sudden emotional stress
Stress induced cardiomyopathy
Takotsubo cardiomyopathy
Transient left ventricular apical ballooning syndrome
CC Excl: IØ9.81, I11.Ø, I5Ø.1-I5Ø.9, I51.81, I51.9-I52, I87.8, I99.8-I99.9

I51.89 Other ill-defined heart diseases
Carditis (acute)(chronic)
Pancarditis (acute)(chronic)

I51.9 Heart disease, unspecified

I52 Other heart disorders in diseases classified elsewhere
Code first underlying disease, such as:
congenital syphilis (A5Ø.5)
mucopolysaccharidosis (E76.3)
schistosomiasis (B65.Ø-B65.9)

EXCLUDES 1 *heart disease (in):*
gonococcal infection (A54.83)
meningococcal infection (A39.5Ø)
rheumatoid arthritis (MØ5.31)
syphilis (A52.Ø6)

Cerebrovascular diseases (I6Ø-I69)

Use additional code to identify presence of:
alcohol abuse and dependence (F1Ø.-)
exposure to environmental tobacco smoke (Z77.22)
history of tobacco use (Z87.891)
hypertension (I1Ø-I15)
occupational exposure to environmental tobacco smoke (Z57.31)
tobacco dependence (F17.-)
tobacco use (Z72.Ø)

EXCLUDES 1 *transient cerebral ischemic attacks and related syndromes (G45.-)*
traumatic intracranial hemorrhage (SØ6.-)

AHA: 2Ø12, 4Q, 91-92

✓4th I6Ø Nontraumatic subarachnoid hemorrhage

INCLUDES ruptured cerebral aneurysm

EXCLUDES 1 *sequelae of subarachnoid hemorrhage (I69.Ø-)*
syphilitic ruptured cerebral aneurysm (A52.Ø5)

CC Excl: For MCC codes in category I6Ø, unless otherwise noted: EØ3.5, G93.82, I6Ø.ØØ-I62.9, I87.8, I99.8-I99.9, R4Ø.Ø-R4Ø.2124, R4Ø.221Ø-R4Ø.2224, R4Ø.231Ø-R4Ø.2324, R4Ø.234Ø-R4Ø.2344, R4Ø.3-R4Ø.4, SØ2.ØXX-SØ2.19X with 7th [A, B], SØ2.91X with 7th [A, B], SØ6.ØXØ-SØ6.9X9 with 7th A

✓5th I6Ø.Ø Nontraumatic subarachnoid hemorrhage from carotid siphon and bifurcation

- **I6Ø.ØØ Nontraumatic subarachnoid hemorrhage from unspecified carotid siphon and bifurcation** MCC
- **I6Ø.Ø1 Nontraumatic subarachnoid hemorrhage from right carotid siphon and bifurcation** MCC
- **I6Ø.Ø2 Nontraumatic subarachnoid hemorrhage from left carotid siphon and bifurcation** MCC

✓5th I6Ø.1 Nontraumatic subarachnoid hemorrhage from middle cerebral artery

- **I6Ø.1Ø Nontraumatic subarachnoid hemorrhage from unspecified middle cerebral artery** MCC
- **I6Ø.11 Nontraumatic subarachnoid hemorrhage from right middle cerebral artery** MCC
- **I6Ø.12 Nontraumatic subarachnoid hemorrhage from left middle cerebral artery** MCC

✓5th I6Ø.2 Nontraumatic subarachnoid hemorrhage from anterior communicating artery

- **I6Ø.2Ø Nontraumatic subarachnoid hemorrhage from unspecified anterior communicating artery** MCC
- **I6Ø.21 Nontraumatic subarachnoid hemorrhage from right anterior communicating artery** MCC
- **I6Ø.22 Nontraumatic subarachnoid hemorrhage from left anterior communicating artery** MCC

✓5th I6Ø.3 Nontraumatic subarachnoid hemorrhage from posterior communicating artery

- **I6Ø.3Ø Nontraumatic subarachnoid hemorrhage from unspecified posterior communicating artery** MCC
- **I6Ø.31 Nontraumatic subarachnoid hemorrhage from right posterior communicating artery** MCC
- **I6Ø.32 Nontraumatic subarachnoid hemorrhage from left posterior communicating artery** MCC

I6Ø.4 Nontraumatic subarachnoid hemorrhage from basilar artery MCC

✓5th I6Ø.5 Nontraumatic subarachnoid hemorrhage from vertebral artery

- **I6Ø.5Ø Nontraumatic subarachnoid hemorrhage from unspecified vertebral artery** MCC
- **I6Ø.51 Nontraumatic subarachnoid hemorrhage from right vertebral artery** MCC
- **I6Ø.52 Nontraumatic subarachnoid hemorrhage from left vertebral artery** MCC

I6Ø.6 Nontraumatic subarachnoid hemorrhage from other intracranial arteries MCC

I6Ø.7 Nontraumatic subarachnoid hemorrhage from unspecified intracranial artery MCC

Ruptured (congenital) berry aneurysm
Ruptured (congenital) cerebral aneurysm
Subarachnoid hemorrhage (nontraumatic) from cerebral artery NOS
Subarachnoid hemorrhage (nontraumatic) from communicating artery NOS

EXCLUDES 1 *berry aneurysm, nonruptured (I67.1)*

I6Ø.8 Other nontraumatic subarachnoid hemorrhage MCC

Meningeal hemorrhage
Rupture of cerebral arteriovenous malformation

I6Ø.9 Nontraumatic subarachnoid hemorrhage, unspecified MCC

✓4th I61 Nontraumatic intracerebral hemorrhage

EXCLUDES 1 *sequelae of intracerebral hemorrhage (I69.1-)*

CC Excl: For MCC codes in category I61, unless otherwise noted: See code: I6Ø

I61.Ø Nontraumatic intracerebral hemorrhage in hemisphere, subcortical MCC

Deep intracerebral hemorrhage (nontraumatic)

I61.1 Nontraumatic intracerebral hemorrhage in hemisphere, cortical MCC

Cerebral lobe hemorrhage (nontraumatic)
Superficial intracerebral hemorrhage (nontraumatic)

I61.2 Nontraumatic intracerebral hemorrhage in hemisphere, unspecified MCC

I61.3 Nontraumatic intracerebral hemorrhage in brain stem MCC

I61.4 Nontraumatic intracerebral hemorrhage in cerebellum MCC

I61.5 Nontraumatic intracerebral hemorrhage, intraventricular MCC

I61.6 Nontraumatic intracerebral hemorrhage, multiple localized MCC

I61.8 Other nontraumatic intracerebral hemorrhage MCC

I61.9 Nontraumatic intracerebral hemorrhage, unspecified MCC

✓4th I62 Other and unspecified nontraumatic intracranial hemorrhage

EXCLUDES 1 *sequelae of intracranial hemorrhage (I69.2)*

CC Excl: For CC/MCC codes in category I62, unless otherwise noted: See code: I6Ø

✓5th I62.Ø Nontraumatic subdural hemorrhage

- **I62.ØØ Nontraumatic subdural hemorrhage, unspecified** MCC
- **I62.Ø1 Nontraumatic acute subdural hemorrhage** MCC
- **I62.Ø2 Nontraumatic subacute subdural hemorrhage** MCC
- **I62.Ø3 Nontraumatic chronic subdural hemorrhage** MCC

I62.1 Nontraumatic extradural hemorrhage MCC

Nontraumatic epidural hemorrhage

I62.9 Nontraumatic intracranial hemorrhage, unspecified CC

✓4th I63 Cerebral infarction

INCLUDES occlusion and stenosis of cerebral and precerebral arteries, resulting in cerebral infarction

Use additional code, if applicable, to identify status post administration of tPA (rtPA) in a different facility within the last 24 hours prior to admission to current facility (Z92.82)

EXCLUDES 1 *sequelae of cerebral infarction (I69.3-)*

AHA: 2Ø14, 1Q, 23

✓5th I63.Ø Cerebral infarction due to thrombosis of precerebral arteries

CC Excl: For MCC codes in subcategory I63.Ø, unless otherwise noted: EØ8.51-EØ8.59, EØ8.618-EØ8.638, EØ8.649-EØ8.8, EØ9.51-EØ9.59, EØ9.618-EØ9.638, EØ9.649-EØ9.8, E1Ø.51-E1Ø.59, E1Ø.618-E1Ø.638, E1Ø.649, E1Ø.69-E1Ø.8, E11.51-E11.59, E11.618-E11.638, E11.649, E11.69-E11.8, E13.51-E13.59, E13.618-E13.638, E13.649-E13.8, G43.6Ø1-G43.619, I63.ØØ-I63.29, I65.Ø1-I65.9, I87.8, I99.8-I99.9

I63.ØØ Cerebral infarction due to thrombosis of unspecified precerebral artery MCC

✓6th I63.Ø1 Cerebral infarction due to thrombosis of vertebral artery

- **I63.Ø11 Cerebral infarction due to thrombosis of right vertebral artery** MCC
- **I63.Ø12 Cerebral infarction due to thrombosis of left vertebral artery** MCC
- **I63.Ø19 Cerebral infarction due to thrombosis of unspecified vertebral artery** MCC

I63.Ø2 Cerebral infarction due to thrombosis of basilar artery MCC

✓6th I63.Ø3 Cerebral infarction due to thrombosis of carotid artery

- **I63.Ø31 Cerebral infarction due to thrombosis of right carotid artery** MCC
- **I63.Ø32 Cerebral infarction due to thrombosis of left carotid artery** MCC
- **I63.Ø39 Cerebral infarction due to thrombosis of unspecified carotid artery** MCC

I63.Ø9 Cerebral infarction due to thrombosis of other precerebral artery MCC

✓5th I63.1 Cerebral infarction due to embolism of precerebral arteries

CC Excl: For MCC codes in subcategory I63.1, unless otherwise noted: EØ8.51-EØ8.59, EØ8.618-EØ8.638, EØ8.649-EØ8.8, EØ9.51-EØ9.59, EØ9.618-EØ9.638, EØ9.649-EØ9.8, E1Ø.51-E1Ø.59, E1Ø.618-E1Ø.638, E1Ø.649, E1Ø.69-E1Ø.8, E11.51-E11.59, E11.618-E11.638, E11.649, E11.69-E11.8, E13.51-E13.59, E13.618-E13.638, E13.649-E13.8, G43.6Ø1-G43.619, I63.ØØ-I63.29, I65.Ø1-I65.9, I87.8, I99.8-I99.9

I63.1Ø Cerebral infarction due to embolism of unspecified precerebral artery MCC

✓6th I63.11 Cerebral infarction due to embolism of vertebral artery

- **I63.111 Cerebral infarction due to embolism of right vertebral artery** MCC

I63.112 Cerebral infarction due to embolism of left vertebral artery MCC

I63.119 Cerebral infarction due to embolism of unspecified vertebral artery MCC

I63.12 Cerebral infarction due to embolism of basilar artery MCC

✓6th **I63.13** Cerebral infarction due to embolism of carotid artery

I63.131 Cerebral infarction due to embolism of right carotid artery MCC

I63.132 Cerebral infarction due to embolism of left carotid artery MCC

I63.139 Cerebral infarction due to embolism of unspecified carotid artery MCC

I63.19 Cerebral infarction due to embolism of other precerebral artery MCC

✓5th **I63.2** Cerebral infarction due to unspecified occlusion or stenosis of precerebral arteries

CC Excl: For MCC codes in subcategory I63.2, unless otherwise noted: EØ8.51-EØ8.59, EØ8.618-EØ8.638, EØ8.649-EØ8.8, EØ9.51-EØ9.59, EØ9.618-EØ9.638, EØ9.649-EØ9.8, E1Ø.51-E1Ø.59, E1Ø.618-E1Ø.638, E1Ø.649, E1Ø.69-E1Ø.8, E11.51-E11.59, E11.618-E11.638, E11.649, E11.69-E11.8, E13.51-E13.59, E13.618-E13.638, E13.649-E13.8, G43.6Ø1-G43.619, I63.ØØ-I63.29, I65.Ø1-I65.9, I87.8, I99.8-I99.9

I63.2Ø Cerebral infarction due to unspecified occlusion or stenosis of unspecified precerebral arteries MCC

✓6th **I63.21** Cerebral infarction due to unspecified occlusion or stenosis of vertebral arteries

I63.211 Cerebral infarction due to unspecified occlusion or stenosis of right vertebral arteries MCC

I63.212 Cerebral infarction due to unspecified occlusion or stenosis of left vertebral arteries MCC

I63.219 Cerebral infarction due to unspecified occlusion or stenosis of unspecified vertebral arteries MCC

I63.22 Cerebral infarction due to unspecified occlusion or stenosis of basilar arteries MCC

✓6th **I63.23** Cerebral infarction due to unspecified occlusion or stenosis of carotid arteries

I63.231 Cerebral infarction due to unspecified occlusion or stenosis of right carotid arteries MCC

I63.232 Cerebral infarction due to unspecified occlusion or stenosis of left carotid arteries MCC

I63.239 Cerebral infarction due to unspecified occlusion or stenosis of unspecified carotid arteries MCC

I63.29 Cerebral infarction due to unspecified occlusion or stenosis of other precerebral arteries MCC

✓5th **I63.3** Cerebral infarction due to thrombosis of cerebral arteries

CC Excl: For MCC codes in subcategory I63.3, unless otherwise noted: EØ8.51-EØ8.59, EØ8.618-EØ8.638, EØ8.649-EØ8.8, EØ9.51-EØ9.59, EØ9.618-EØ9.638, EØ9.649-EØ9.8, E1Ø.51-E1Ø.59, E1Ø.618-E1Ø.638, E1Ø.649, E1Ø.69-E1Ø.8, E11.51-E11.59, E11.618-E11.638, E11.649, E11.69-E11.8, E13.51-E13.59, E13.618-E13.638, E13.649-E13.8, G43.6Ø1-G43.619, I63.3Ø-I63.9, I66.Ø1-I66.9, I87.8, I99.8-I99.9

I63.3Ø Cerebral infarction due to thrombosis of unspecified cerebral artery MCC

✓6th **I63.31** Cerebral infarction due to thrombosis of middle cerebral artery

I63.311 Cerebral infarction due to thrombosis of right middle cerebral artery MCC

I63.312 Cerebral infarction due to thrombosis of left middle cerebral artery MCC

I63.319 Cerebral infarction due to thrombosis of unspecified middle cerebral artery MCC

✓6th **I63.32** Cerebral infarction due to thrombosis of anterior cerebral artery

I63.321 Cerebral infarction due to thrombosis of right anterior cerebral artery MCC

I63.322 Cerebral infarction due to thrombosis of left anterior cerebral artery MCC

I63.329 Cerebral infarction due to thrombosis of unspecified anterior cerebral artery MCC

✓6th **I63.33** Cerebral infarction due to thrombosis of posterior cerebral artery

I63.331 Cerebral infarction due to thrombosis of right posterior cerebral artery MCC

I63.332 Cerebral infarction due to thrombosis of left posterior cerebral artery MCC

I63.339 Cerebral infarction due to thrombosis of unspecified posterior cerebral artery MCC

✓6th **I63.34** Cerebral infarction due to thrombosis of cerebellar artery

I63.341 Cerebral infarction due to thrombosis of right cerebellar artery MCC

I63.342 Cerebral infarction due to thrombosis of left cerebellar artery MCC

I63.349 Cerebral infarction due to thrombosis of unspecified cerebellar artery MCC

I63.39 Cerebral infarction due to thrombosis of other cerebral artery MCC

✓5th **I63.4** Cerebral infarction due to embolism of cerebral arteries

CC Excl: For MCC codes in subcategory I63.4, unless otherwise noted: EØ8.51-EØ8.59, EØ8.618-EØ8.638, EØ8.649-EØ8.8, EØ9.51-EØ9.59, EØ9.618-EØ9.638, EØ9.649-EØ9.8, E1Ø.51-E1Ø.59, E1Ø.618-E1Ø.638, E1Ø.649, E1Ø.69-E1Ø.8, E11.51-E11.59, E11.618-E11.638, E11.649, E11.69-E11.8, E13.51-E13.59, E13.618-E13.638, E13.649-E13.8, G43.6Ø1-G43.619, I63.3Ø-I63.9, I66.Ø1-I66.9, I87.8, I99.8-I99.9

I63.4Ø Cerebral infarction due to embolism of unspecified cerebral artery MCC

✓6th **I63.41** Cerebral infarction due to embolism of middle cerebral artery

I63.411 Cerebral infarction due to embolism of right middle cerebral artery MCC

I63.412 Cerebral infarction due to embolism of left middle cerebral artery MCC

I63.419 Cerebral infarction due to embolism of unspecified middle cerebral artery MCC

✓6th **I63.42** Cerebral infarction due to embolism of anterior cerebral artery

I63.421 Cerebral infarction due to embolism of right anterior cerebral artery MCC

I63.422 Cerebral infarction due to embolism of left anterior cerebral artery MCC

I63.429 Cerebral infarction due to embolism of unspecified anterior cerebral artery MCC

✓6th **I63.43** Cerebral infarction due to embolism of posterior cerebral artery

I63.431 Cerebral infarction due to embolism of right posterior cerebral artery MCC

I63.432 Cerebral infarction due to embolism of left posterior cerebral artery MCC

I63.439 Cerebral infarction due to embolism of unspecified posterior cerebral artery MCC

✓6th **I63.44** Cerebral infarction due to embolism of cerebellar artery

I63.441 Cerebral infarction due to embolism of right cerebellar artery MCC

I63.442 Cerebral infarction due to embolism of left cerebellar artery MCC

I63.449 Cerebral infarction due to embolism of unspecified cerebellar artery MCC

I63.49 Cerebral infarction due to embolism of other cerebral artery MCC

✓5th **I63.5** Cerebral infarction due to unspecified occlusion or stenosis of cerebral arteries

CC Excl: For MCC codes in subcategory I63.5, unless otherwise noted: EØ8.51-EØ8.59, EØ8.618-EØ8.638, EØ8.649-EØ8.8, EØ9.51-EØ9.59, EØ9.618-EØ9.638, EØ9.649-EØ9.8, E1Ø.51-E1Ø.59, E1Ø.618-E1Ø.638, E1Ø.649, E1Ø.69-E1Ø.8, E11.51-E11.59, E11.618-E11.638, E11.649, E11.69-E11.8, E13.51-E13.59, E13.618-E13.638, E13.649-E13.8, G43.6Ø1-G43.619, I63.3Ø-I63.9, I66.Ø1-I66.9, I87.8, I99.8-I99.9

I63.5Ø Cerebral infarction due to unspecified occlusion or stenosis of unspecified cerebral artery MCC

✓6th **I63.51 Cerebral infarction due to unspecified occlusion or stenosis of middle cerebral artery**

I63.511 Cerebral infarction due to unspecified occlusion or stenosis of right middle cerebral artery MCC

I63.512 Cerebral infarction due to unspecified occlusion or stenosis of left middle cerebral artery MCC

I63.519 Cerebral infarction due to unspecified occlusion or stenosis of unspecified middle cerebral artery MCC

✓6th **I63.52 Cerebral infarction due to unspecified occlusion or stenosis of anterior cerebral artery**

I63.521 Cerebral infarction due to unspecified occlusion or stenosis of right anterior cerebral artery MCC

I63.522 Cerebral infarction due to unspecified occlusion or stenosis of left anterior cerebral artery MCC

I63.529 Cerebral infarction due to unspecified occlusion or stenosis of unspecified anterior cerebral artery MCC

✓6th **I63.53 Cerebral infarction due to unspecified occlusion or stenosis of posterior cerebral artery**

I63.531 Cerebral infarction due to unspecified occlusion or stenosis of right posterior cerebral artery MCC

I63.532 Cerebral infarction due to unspecified occlusion or stenosis of left posterior cerebral artery MCC

I63.539 Cerebral infarction due to unspecified occlusion or stenosis of unspecified posterior cerebral artery MCC

✓6th **I63.54 Cerebral infarction due to unspecified occlusion or stenosis of cerebellar artery**

I63.541 Cerebral infarction due to unspecified occlusion or stenosis of right cerebellar artery MCC

I63.542 Cerebral infarction due to unspecified occlusion or stenosis of left cerebellar artery MCC

I63.549 Cerebral infarction due to unspecified occlusion or stenosis of unspecified cerebellar artery MCC

I63.59 Cerebral infarction due to unspecified occlusion or stenosis of other cerebral artery MCC

I63.6 Cerebral infarction due to cerebral venous thrombosis, nonpyogenic MCC
CC Excl: See code: I63.5

I63.8 Other cerebral infarction MCC
CC Excl: See code: I63.5

I63.9 Cerebral infarction, unspecified MCC
Stroke NOS
CC Excl: See code: I63.5

✓4th **I65 Occlusion and stenosis of precerebral arteries, not resulting in cerebral infarction**

INCLUDES embolism of precerebral artery
narrowing of precerebral artery
obstruction (complete) (partial) of precerebral artery
thrombosis of precerebral artery

EXCLUDES 1 *insufficiency, NOS, of precerebral artery (G45.-)*
insufficiency of precerebral arteries causing cerebral infarction (I63.Ø-I63.2)

✓5th **I65.Ø Occlusion and stenosis of vertebral artery**

I65.Ø1 Occlusion and stenosis of right vertebral artery

I65.Ø2 Occlusion and stenosis of left vertebral artery

I65.Ø3 Occlusion and stenosis of bilateral vertebral arteries

I65.Ø9 Occlusion and stenosis of unspecified vertebral artery

I65.1 Occlusion and stenosis of basilar artery

✓5th **I65.2 Occlusion and stenosis of carotid artery**

I65.21 Occlusion and stenosis of right carotid artery

I65.22 Occlusion and stenosis of left carotid artery

I65.23 Occlusion and stenosis of bilateral carotid arteries

I65.29 Occlusion and stenosis of unspecified carotid artery

I65.8 Occlusion and stenosis of other precerebral arteries

I65.9 Occlusion and stenosis of unspecified precerebral artery
Occlusion and stenosis of precerebral artery NOS

✓4th **I66 Occlusion and stenosis of cerebral arteries, not resulting in cerebral infarction**

INCLUDES embolism of cerebral artery
narrowing of cerebral artery
obstruction (complete) (partial) of cerebral artery
thrombosis of cerebral artery

EXCLUDES 1 *occlusion and stenosis of cerebral artery causing cerebral infarction (I63.3-I63.5)*

✓5th **I66.Ø Occlusion and stenosis of middle cerebral artery**

I66.Ø1 Occlusion and stenosis of right middle cerebral artery

I66.Ø2 Occlusion and stenosis of left middle cerebral artery

I66.Ø3 Occlusion and stenosis of bilateral middle cerebral arteries

I66.Ø9 Occlusion and stenosis of unspecified middle cerebral artery

✓5th **I66.1 Occlusion and stenosis of anterior cerebral artery**

I66.11 Occlusion and stenosis of right anterior cerebral artery

I66.12 Occlusion and stenosis of left anterior cerebral artery

I66.13 Occlusion and stenosis of bilateral anterior cerebral arteries

I66.19 Occlusion and stenosis of unspecified anterior cerebral artery

✓5th **I66.2 Occlusion and stenosis of posterior cerebral artery**

I66.21 Occlusion and stenosis of right posterior cerebral artery

I66.22 Occlusion and stenosis of left posterior cerebral artery

I66.23 Occlusion and stenosis of bilateral posterior cerebral arteries

I66.29 Occlusion and stenosis of unspecified posterior cerebral artery

I66.3 Occlusion and stenosis of cerebellar arteries

I66.8 Occlusion and stenosis of other cerebral arteries
Occlusion and stenosis of perforating arteries

I66.9 Occlusion and stenosis of unspecified cerebral artery

✓4th **I67 Other cerebrovascular diseases**

EXCLUDES 1 *sequelae of the listed conditions (I69.8)*

I67.Ø Dissection of cerebral arteries, nonruptured MCC
EXCLUDES 1 *ruptured cerebral arteries (I6Ø.7)*
CC Excl: I77.2-I77.3, I77.5-I77.6, I77.89-I77.9, M31.8-M31.9

I67.1 Cerebral aneurysm, nonruptured
Cerebral aneurysm NOS
Cerebral arteriovenous fistula, acquired
Internal carotid artery aneurysm, intracranial portion
Internal carotid artery aneurysm, NOS
EXCLUDES 1 *congenital cerebral aneurysm, nonruptured (Q28.-)*
ruptured cerebral aneurysm (I6Ø.7)

I67.2 Cerebral atherosclerosis A
Atheroma of cerebral and precerebral arteries

I67.3 Progressive vascular leukoencephalopathy HIV CC
Binswanger's disease
CC Excl: A17.82, A5Ø.42, A52.14, A75.9, A79.9, A81.ØØ-A81.9, A83.Ø-A85.8, A87.2, A88.Ø, A88.8, A92.1-A92.2, A92.4-A92.8, A93.Ø, BØØ.4, BØØ.82, BØ1.11-BØ1.12, BØ4, BØ6.Ø1, BØ8.Ø9, BØ8.2Ø-BØ8.22, BØ8.6Ø-BØ8.79, BØ9-B1Ø.Ø9, B26.2, B27.ØØ-B27.99, B33.1, B45.Ø, B45.2-B45.9, B58.2, B75, GØ4.ØØ-GØ4.Ø1, GØ4.31, GØ4.81-GØ5.4, G37.Ø, G37.4-G37.5, I67.3, JØ9.X3-JØ9.X9, J1Ø.2-J1Ø.89, J11.2-J11.89, L44.4, M1A.1ØXØ-M1A.19X1, P35.2-P35.9, P37.Ø-P37.4, P37.8-P37.9, T56.ØX1A, T56.ØX2A, T56.ØX3A, T56.ØX4A

I67.4 Hypertensive encephalopathy CC
CC Excl: EØ8.51-EØ8.59, EØ8.618-EØ8.638, EØ8.649-EØ8.8, EØ9.51-EØ9.59, EØ9.618-EØ9.638, EØ9.649-EØ9.8, E1Ø.51-E1Ø.59, E1Ø.618-E1Ø.638, E1Ø.649, E1Ø.69-E1Ø.8, E11.51-E11.59, E11.618-E11.638, E11.649, E11.69-E11.8, E13.51-E13.59, E13.618-E13.638, E13.649-E13.8, I67.4, I87.8, I99.8-I99.9

I67.5 Moyamoya disease CC
CC Excl: EØ8.51-EØ8.59, EØ8.618-EØ8.638, EØ8.649-EØ8.8, EØ9.51-EØ9.59, EØ9.618-EØ9.638, EØ9.649-EØ9.8, E1Ø.51-E1Ø.59, E1Ø.618-E1Ø.638, E1Ø.649, E1Ø.69-E1Ø.8, E11.51-E11.59, E11.618-E11.638, E11.649, E11.69-E11.8, E13.51-E13.59, E13.618-E13.638, E13.649-E13.8, I67.5, I87.8, I99.8-I99.9

I67.6 Nonpyogenic thrombosis of intracranial venous system CC
Nonpyogenic thrombosis of cerebral vein
Nonpyogenic thrombosis of intracranial venous sinus
EXCLUDES 1 *nonpyogenic thrombosis of intracranial venous system causing infarction (I63.6)*
CC Excl: EØ8.51-EØ8.59, EØ8.618-EØ8.638, EØ8.649-EØ8.8, EØ9.51-EØ9.59, EØ9.618-EØ9.638, EØ9.649-EØ9.8, E1Ø.51-E1Ø.59, E1Ø.618-E1Ø.638, E1Ø.649, E1Ø.69-E1Ø.8, E11.51-E11.59, E11.618-E11.638, E11.649, E11.69-E11.8, E13.51-E13.59, E13.618-E13.638, E13.649-E13.8, I67.6, I87.8, I99.8-I99.9

I67.7 Cerebral arteritis, not elsewhere classified CC
Granulomatous angiitis of the nervous system
EXCLUDES 1 *allergic granulomatous angiitis (M3Ø.1)*
CC Excl: EØ8.51-EØ8.59, EØ8.618-EØ8.638, EØ8.649-EØ8.8, EØ9.51-EØ9.59, EØ9.618-EØ9.638, EØ9.649-EØ9.8, E1Ø.51-E1Ø.59, E1Ø.618-E1Ø.638, E1Ø.649, E1Ø.69-E1Ø.8, E11.51-E11.59, E11.618-E11.638, E11.649, E11.69-E11.8, E13.51-E13.59, E13.618-E13.638, E13.649-E13.8, I67.7, I68.2, I87.8, I99.8-I99.9

✓5th **I67.8 Other specified cerebrovascular diseases**

I67.81 Acute cerebrovascular insufficiency CC
Acute cerebrovascular insufficiency unspecified as to location or reversibility
CC Excl: EØ8.51-EØ8.59, EØ8.618-EØ8.638, EØ8.649-EØ8.8, EØ9.51-EØ9.59, EØ9.618-EØ9.638, EØ9.649-EØ9.8, E1Ø.51-E1Ø.59, E1Ø.618-E1Ø.638, E1Ø.649, E1Ø.69-E1Ø.8, E11.51-E11.59, E11.618-E11.638, E11.649, E11.69-E11.8, E13.51-E13.59, E13.618-E13.638, E13.649-E13.8, G45.Ø-G45.2, G45.8-G46.2, I6Ø.ØØ-I62.9, I63.3Ø-I63.9, I66.Ø1-I66.9, I67.81-I67.82, I67.841-I67.89, I87.8, I99.8-I99.9

I67.82 Cerebral ischemia CC
Chronic cerebral ischemia
CC Excl: See code: I67.81

I67.83 Posterior reversible encephalopathy syndrome HIV MCC
PRES
CC Excl: G21.Ø, G83.5, G93.4Ø-G93.41

✓6th **I67.84 Cerebral vasospasm and vasoconstriction**

I67.841 Reversible cerebrovascular vasoconstriction syndrome CC
Call-Fleming syndrome
Code first underlying condition, if applicable, such as eclampsia (O15.ØØ-O15.9)
CC Excl: EØ8.51-EØ8.59, EØ8.618-EØ8.638, EØ8.649-EØ8.8, EØ9.51-EØ9.59, EØ9.618-EØ9.638, EØ9.649-EØ9.8, E1Ø.51-E1Ø.59, E1Ø.618-E1Ø.638, E1Ø.649, E1Ø.69-E1Ø.8, E11.51-E11.59, E11.618-E11.638, E11.649, E11.69-E11.8, E13.51-E13.59, E13.618-E13.638, E13.649-E13.8, G45.Ø-G45.2, G45.8-G46.2, I63.ØØ-I63.29, I65.Ø1-I65.9, I67.841-I67.848, I87.8, I99.8-I99.9

I67.848 Other cerebrovascular vasospasm and vasoconstriction CC
CC Excl: See code: I67.841

I67.89 Other cerebrovascular disease CC
CC Excl: See code: I67.81

I67.9 Cerebrovascular disease, unspecified

✓4th **I68 Cerebrovascular disorders in diseases classified elsewhere**

I68.Ø Cerebral amyloid angiopathy
Code first underlying amyloidosis (E85.-)

I68.2 Cerebral arteritis in other diseases classified elsewhere CC
Code first underlying disease
EXCLUDES 1 *cerebral arteritis (in):*
listerosis (A32.89)
systemic lupus erythematosus (M32.19)
syphilis (A52.Ø4)
tuberculosis (A18.89)
CC Excl: See code: I67.7

I68.8 Other cerebrovascular disorders in diseases classified elsewhere
Code first underlying disease
EXCLUDES 1 *syphilitic cerebral aneurysm (A52.Ø5)*

✓4th **I69 Sequelae of cerebrovascular disease**
NOTE Category I69 is to be used to indicate conditions in I6Ø-I67 as the cause of sequelae. The "sequelae" include conditions specified as such or as residuals which may occur at any time after the onset of the causal condition
EXCLUDES 1 *personal history of cerebral infarction without residual deficit (Z86.73)*
personal history of prolonged reversible ischemic neurologic deficit (PRIND) (Z86.73)
personal history of reversible ischemic neurologcial deficit (RIND) (Z86.73)
sequelae of traumatic intracranial injury (SØ6.-)
transient ischemic attack (TIA) (G45.9)
AHA: 2Ø12, 4Q, 1Ø6

✓5th **I69.Ø Sequelae of nontraumatic subarachnoid hemorrhage**

I69.ØØ Unspecified sequelae of nontraumatic subarachnoid hemorrhage

I69.Ø1 Cognitive deficits following nontraumatic subarachnoid hemorrhage

✓6th **I69.Ø2 Speech and language deficits following nontraumatic subarachnoid hemorrhage**

I69.Ø2Ø Aphasia following nontraumatic subarachnoid hemorrhage

I69.Ø21 Dysphasia following nontraumatic subarachnoid hemorrhage

I69.Ø22 Dysarthria following nontraumatic subarachnoid hemorrhage

I69.Ø23 Fluency disorder following nontraumatic subarachnoid hemorrhage
Stuttering following nontraumatic subarachnoid hemorrhage

I69.Ø28 Other speech and language deficits following nontraumatic subarachnoid hemorrhage

✓6th **I69.Ø3 Monoplegia of upper limb following nontraumatic subarachnoid hemorrhage**

I69.Ø31 Monoplegia of upper limb following nontraumatic subarachnoid hemorrhage affecting right dominant side

I69.Ø32 Monoplegia of upper limb following nontraumatic subarachnoid hemorrhage affecting left dominant side

I69.Ø33 Monoplegia of upper limb following nontraumatic subarachnoid hemorrhage affecting right non-dominant side

I69.Ø34 Monoplegia of upper limb following nontraumatic subarachnoid hemorrhage affecting left non-dominant side

I69.Ø39 Monoplegia of upper limb following nontraumatic subarachnoid hemorrhage affecting unspecified side

✓6th **I69.Ø4 Monoplegia of lower limb following nontraumatic subarachnoid hemorrhage**

I69.Ø41 Monoplegia of lower limb following nontraumatic subarachnoid hemorrhage affecting right dominant side

I69.Ø42 Monoplegia of lower limb following nontraumatic subarachnoid hemorrhage affecting left dominant side

I69.Ø43 Monoplegia of lower limb following nontraumatic subarachnoid hemorrhage affecting right non-dominant side

I69.Ø44 Monoplegia of lower limb following nontraumatic subarachnoid hemorrhage affecting left non-dominant side

I69.Ø49 Monoplegia of lower limb following nontraumatic subarachnoid hemorrhage affecting unspecified side

✓6th **I69.Ø5 Hemiplegia and hemiparesis following nontraumatic subarachnoid hemorrhage**

I69.Ø51 Hemiplegia and hemiparesis following nontraumatic subarachnoid hemorrhage affecting right dominant side CC
CC Excl: I69.Ø51-I69.Ø52, I69.151-I69.152, I69.251-I69.252, I69.351-I69.352, I69.851-I69.852, I69.951-I69.952

I69.Ø52 Hemiplegia and hemiparesis following nontraumatic subarachnoid hemorrhage affecting left dominant side CC
CC Excl: See code: I69.Ø51

I69.053 Hemiplegia and hemiparesis following nontraumatic subarachnoid hemorrhage affecting right non-dominant side CC
CC Excl: I69.053-I69.054, I69.153-I69.154, I69.253-I69.254, I69.353-I69.354, I69.853-I69.854, I69.953-I69.954

I69.054 Hemiplegia and hemiparesis following nontraumatic subarachnoid hemorrhage affecting left non-dominant side CC
CC Excl: See code: I69.053

I69.059 Hemiplegia and hemiparesis following nontraumatic subarachnoid hemorrhage affecting unspecified side CC
CC Excl: I69.059-I69.159, I69.259, I69.359, I69.859, I69.959

✓6th **I69.06 Other paralytic syndrome following nontraumatic subarachnoid hemorrhage**
Use additional code to identify type of paralytic syndrome, such as:
locked-in state (G83.5)
quadriplegia (G82.5-)
EXCLUDES 1 *hemiplegia/hemiparesis following nontraumatic subarachnoid hemorrhage (I69.05-)*
monoplegia of lower limb following nontraumatic subarachnoid hemorrhage (I69.04-)
monoplegia of upper limb following nontraumatic subarachnoid hemorrhage (I69.03-)

I69.061 Other paralytic syndrome following nontraumatic subarachnoid hemorrhage affecting right dominant side

I69.062 Other paralytic syndrome following nontraumatic subarachnoid hemorrhage affecting left dominant side

I69.063 Other paralytic syndrome following nontraumatic subarachnoid hemorrhage affecting right non-dominant side

I69.064 Other paralytic syndrome following nontraumatic subarachnoid hemorrhage affecting left non-dominant side

I69.065 Other paralytic syndrome following nontraumatic subarachnoid hemorrhage, bilateral

I69.069 Other paralytic syndrome following nontraumatic subarachnoid hemorrhage affecting unspecified side

✓6th **I69.09 Other sequelae of nontraumatic subarachnoid hemorrhage**

I69.090 Apraxia following nontraumatic subarachnoid hemorrhage

I69.091 Dysphagia following nontraumatic subarachnoid hemorrhage
Use additional code to identify the type of dysphagia, if known (R13.1-)

I69.092 Facial weakness following nontraumatic subarachnoid hemorrhage
Facial droop following nontraumatic subarachnoid hemorrhage

I69.093 Ataxia following nontraumatic subarachnoid hemorrhage

I69.098 Other sequelae following nontraumatic subarachnoid hemorrhage
Alterations of sensation following nontraumatic subarachnoid hemorrhage
Disturbance of vision following nontraumatic subarachnoid hemorrhage
Use additional code to identify the sequelae

✓5th **I69.1 Sequelae of nontraumatic intracerebral hemorrhage**

I69.10 Unspecified sequelae of nontraumatic intracerebral hemorrhage

I69.11 Cognitive deficits following nontraumatic intracerebral hemorrhage

✓6th **I69.12 Speech and language deficits following nontraumatic intracerebral hemorrhage**

I69.120 Aphasia following nontraumatic intracerebral hemorrhage

I69.121 Dysphasia following nontraumatic intracerebral hemorrhage

I69.122 Dysarthria following nontraumatic intracerebral hemorrhage

I69.123 Fluency disorder following nontraumatic intracerebral hemorrhage
Stuttering following nontraumatic subarachnoid hemorrhage

I69.128 Other speech and language deficits following nontraumatic intracerebral hemorrhage

✓6th **I69.13 Monoplegia of upper limb following nontraumatic intracerebral hemorrhage**

I69.131 Monoplegia of upper limb following nontraumatic intracerebral hemorrhage affecting right dominant side

I69.132 Monoplegia of upper limb following nontraumatic intracerebral hemorrhage affecting left dominant side

I69.133 Monoplegia of upper limb following nontraumatic intracerebral hemorrhage affecting right non-dominant side

I69.134 Monoplegia of upper limb following nontraumatic intracerebral hemorrhage affecting left non-dominant side

I69.139 Monoplegia of upper limb following nontraumatic intracerebral hemorrhage affecting unspecified side

✓6th **I69.14 Monoplegia of lower limb following nontraumatic intracerebral hemorrhage**

I69.141 Monoplegia of lower limb following nontraumatic intracerebral hemorrhage affecting right dominant side

I69.142 Monoplegia of lower limb following nontraumatic intracerebral hemorrhage affecting left dominant side

I69.143 Monoplegia of lower limb following nontraumatic intracerebral hemorrhage affecting right non-dominant side

I69.144 Monoplegia of lower limb following nontraumatic intracerebral hemorrhage affecting left non-dominant side

I69.149 Monoplegia of lower limb following nontraumatic intracerebral hemorrhage affecting unspecified side

✓6th **I69.15 Hemiplegia and hemiparesis following nontraumatic intracerebral hemorrhage**

I69.151 Hemiplegia and hemiparesis following nontraumatic intracerebral hemorrhage affecting right dominant side CC
CC Excl: I69.051-I69.052, I69.151-I69.152, I69.251-I69.252, I69.351-I69.352, I69.851-I69.852, I69.951-I69.952

I69.152 Hemiplegia and hemiparesis following nontraumatic intracerebral hemorrhage affecting left dominant side CC
CC Excl: See code: I69.151

I69.153 Hemiplegia and hemiparesis following nontraumatic intracerebral hemorrhage affecting right non-dominant side CC
CC Excl: I69.053-I69.054, I69.153-I69.154, I69.253-I69.254, I69.353-I69.354, I69.853-I69.854, I69.953-I69.954

I69.154 Hemiplegia and hemiparesis following nontraumatic intracerebral hemorrhage affecting left non-dominant side CC
CC Excl: See code: I69.153

I69.159 Hemiplegia and hemiparesis following nontraumatic intracerebral hemorrhage affecting unspecified side CC
CC Excl: I69.059, I69.159, I69.259, I69.359, I69.859, I69.959

✓6th **I69.16 Other paralytic syndrome following nontraumatic intracerebral hemorrhage**
Use additional code to identify type of paralytic syndrome, such as:
locked-in state (G83.5)
quadriplegia (G82.5-)
EXCLUDES 1 *hemiplegia/hemiparesis following nontraumatic intracerebral hemorrhage (I69.15-)*
monoplegia of lower limb following nontraumatic intracerebral hemorrhage (I69.14-)
monoplegia of upper limb following nontraumatic intracerebral hemorrhage (I69.13-)

I69.161 Other paralytic syndrome following nontraumatic intracerebral hemorrhage affecting right dominant side

I69.162 Other paralytic syndrome following nontraumatic intracerebral hemorrhage affecting left dominant side

I69.163 Other paralytic syndrome following nontraumatic intracerebral hemorrhage affecting right non-dominant side

I69.164 Other paralytic syndrome following nontraumatic intracerebral hemorrhage affecting left non-dominant side

I69.165 Other paralytic syndrome following nontraumatic intracerebral hemorrhage, bilateral

I69.169 Other paralytic syndrome following nontraumatic intracerebral hemorrhage affecting unspecified side

✓6th **I69.19 Other sequelae of nontraumatic intracerebral hemorrhage**

I69.190 Apraxia following nontraumatic intracerebral hemorrhage

I69.191 Dysphagia following nontraumatic intracerebral hemorrhage
Use additional code to identify the type of dysphagia, if known (R13.1-)

I69.192 Facial weakness following nontraumatic intracerebral hemorrhage
Facial droop following nontraumatic intracerebral hemorrhage

I69.193 Ataxia following nontraumatic intracerebral hemorrhage

I69.198 Other sequelae of nontraumatic intracerebral hemorrhage
Alteration of sensations following nontraumatic intracerebral hemorrhage
Disturbance of vision following nontraumatic intracerebral hemorrhage
Use additional code to identify the sequelae

✓5th **I69.2 Sequelae of other nontraumatic intracranial hemorrhage**

I69.20 Unspecified sequelae of other nontraumatic intracranial hemorrhage

I69.21 Cognitive deficits following other nontraumatic intracranial hemorrhage

✓6th **I69.22 Speech and language deficits following other nontraumatic intracranial hemorrhage**

I69.220 Aphasia following other nontraumatic intracranial hemorrhage

I69.221 Dysphasia following other nontraumatic intracranial hemorrhage

I69.222 Dysarthria following other nontraumatic intracranial hemorrhage

I69.223 Fluency disorder following other nontraumatic intracranial hemorrhage
Stuttering following nontraumatic subarachnoid hemorrhage

I69.228 Other speech and language deficits following other nontraumatic intracranial hemorrhage

✓6th **I69.23 Monoplegia of upper limb following other nontraumatic intracranial hemorrhage**

I69.231 Monoplegia of upper limb following other nontraumatic intracranial hemorrhage affecting right dominant side

I69.232 Monoplegia of upper limb following other nontraumatic intracranial hemorrhage affecting left dominant side

I69.233 Monoplegia of upper limb following other nontraumatic intracranial hemorrhage affecting right non-dominant side

I69.234 Monoplegia of upper limb following other nontraumatic intracranial hemorrhage affecting left non-dominant side

I69.239 Monoplegia of upper limb following other nontraumatic intracranial hemorrhage affecting unspecified side

✓6th **I69.24 Monoplegia of lower limb following other nontraumatic intracranial hemorrhage**

I69.241 Monoplegia of lower limb following other nontraumatic intracranial hemorrhage affecting right dominant side

I69.242 Monoplegia of lower limb following other nontraumatic intracranial hemorrhage affecting left dominant side

I69.243 Monoplegia of lower limb following other nontraumatic intracranial hemorrhage affecting right non-dominant side

I69.244 Monoplegia of lower limb following other nontraumatic intracranial hemorrhage affecting left non-dominant side

I69.249 Monoplegia of lower limb following other nontraumatic intracranial hemorrhage affecting unspecified side

✓6th **I69.25 Hemiplegia and hemiparesis following other nontraumatic intracranial hemorrhage**

I69.251 Hemiplegia and hemiparesis following other nontraumatic intracranial hemorrhage affecting right dominant side CC
CC Excl: See code: I69.151

I69.252 Hemiplegia and hemiparesis following other nontraumatic intracranial hemorrhage affecting left dominant side CC
CC Excl: See code: I69.151

I69.253 Hemiplegia and hemiparesis following other nontraumatic intracranial hemorrhage affecting right non-dominant side CC
CC Excl: See code: I69.153

I69.254 Hemiplegia and hemiparesis following other nontraumatic intracranial hemorrhage affecting left non-dominant side CC
CC Excl: See code: I69.153

I69.259 Hemiplegia and hemiparesis following other nontraumatic intracranial hemorrhage affecting unspecified side CC
CC Excl: See code: I69.159

✓6th **I69.26 Other paralytic syndrome following other nontraumatic intracranial hemorrhage**
Use additional code to identify type of paralytic syndrome, such as:
locked-in state (G83.5)
quadriplegia (G82.5-)
EXCLUDES 1 *hemiplegia/hemiparesis following other nontraumatic intracranial hemorrhage (I69.25-)*
monoplegia of lower limb following other nontraumatic intracranial hemorrhage (I69.24-)
monoplegia of upper limb following other nontraumatic intracranial hemorrhage (I69.23-)

I69.261 Other paralytic syndrome following other nontraumatic intracranial hemorrhage affecting right dominant side

I69.262 Other paralytic syndrome following other nontraumatic intracranial hemorrhage affecting left dominant side

I69.263 **Other paralytic syndrome following other nontraumatic intracranial hemorrhage affecting right non-dominant side**

I69.264 **Other paralytic syndrome following other nontraumatic intracranial hemorrhage affecting left non-dominant side**

I69.265 **Other paralytic syndrome following other nontraumatic intracranial hemorrhage, bilateral**

I69.269 **Other paralytic syndrome following other nontraumatic intracranial hemorrhage affecting unspecified side**

✓6th I69.29 **Other sequelae of other nontraumatic intracranial hemorrhage**

I69.290 **Apraxia following other nontraumatic intracranial hemorrhage**

I69.291 **Dysphagia following other nontraumatic intracranial hemorrhage**
Use additional code to identify the type of dysphagia, if known (R13.1-)

I69.292 **Facial weakness following other nontraumatic intracranial hemorrhage**
Facial droop following other nontraumatic intracranial hemorrhage

I69.293 **Ataxia following other nontraumatic intracranial hemorrhage**

I69.298 **Other sequelae of other nontraumatic intracranial hemorrhage**
Alteration of sensation following other nontraumatic intracranial hemorrhage
Disturbance of vision following other nontraumatic intracranial hemorrhage
Use additional code to identify the sequelae

✓5th I69.3 **Sequelae of cerebral infarction**
Sequelae of stroke NOS
AHA: 2013, 4Q, 127-128; 2012, 4Q, 92, 94

I69.30 **Unspecified sequelae of cerebral infarction**

I69.31 **Cognitive deficits following cerebral infarction**

✓6th I69.32 **Speech and language deficits following cerebral infarction**

I69.320 **Aphasia following cerebral infarction**

I69.321 **Dysphasia following cerebral infarction**
AHA: 2012, 4Q, 91

I69.322 **Dysarthria following cerebral infarction**

I69.323 **Fluency disorder following cerebral infarction**
Stuttering following nontraumatic subarachnoid hemorrhage

I69.328 **Other speech and language deficits following cerebral infarction**

✓6th I69.33 **Monoplegia of upper limb following cerebral infarction**

I69.331 **Monoplegia of upper limb following cerebral infarction affecting right dominant side**

I69.332 **Monoplegia of upper limb following cerebral infarction affecting left dominant side**

I69.333 **Monoplegia of upper limb following cerebral infarction affecting right non-dominant side**

I69.334 **Monoplegia of upper limb following cerebral infarction affecting left non-dominant side**

I69.339 **Monoplegia of upper limb following cerebral infarction affecting unspecified side**

✓6th I69.34 **Monoplegia of lower limb following cerebral infarction**

I69.341 **Monoplegia of lower limb following cerebral infarction affecting right dominant side**

I69.342 **Monoplegia of lower limb following cerebral infarction affecting left dominant side**

I69.343 **Monoplegia of lower limb following cerebral infarction affecting right non-dominant side**

I69.344 **Monoplegia of lower limb following cerebral infarction affecting left non-dominant side**

I69.349 **Monoplegia of lower limb following cerebral infarction affecting unspecified side**

✓6th I69.35 **Hemiplegia and hemiparesis following cerebral infarction**

I69.351 **Hemiplegia and hemiparesis following cerebral infarction affecting right dominant side** CC
CC Excl: I69.051-I69.052, I69.151-I69.152, I69.251-I69.252, I69.351-I69.352, I69.851-I69.852, I69.951-I69.952

I69.352 **Hemiplegia and hemiparesis following cerebral infarction affecting left dominant side** CC
CC Excl: See code: I69.351

I69.353 **Hemiplegia and hemiparesis following cerebral infarction affecting right non-dominant side** CC
CC Excl: I69.053-I69.054, I69.153-I69.154, I69.253-I69.254, I69.353-I69.354, I69.853-I69.854, I69.953-I69.954

I69.354 **Hemiplegia and hemiparesis following cerebral infarction affecting left non-dominant side** CC
CC Excl: See code: I69.353
AHA: 2012, 4Q, 91

I69.359 **Hemiplegia and hemiparesis following cerebral infarction affecting unspecified side** CC
CC Excl: I69.059, I69.159, I69.259, I69.359, I69.859, I69.959

✓6th I69.36 **Other paralytic syndrome following cerebral infarction**
Use additional code to identify type of paralytic syndrome, such as:
locked-in state (G83.5)
quadriplegia (G82.5-)

EXCLUDES 1 *hemiplegia/hemiparesis following cerebral infarction (I69.35-)*
monoplegia of lower limb following cerebral infarction (I69.34-)
monoplegia of upper limb following cerebral infarction (I69.33-)

I69.361 **Other paralytic syndrome following cerebral infarction affecting right dominant side**

I69.362 **Other paralytic syndrome following cerebral infarction affecting left dominant side**

I69.363 **Other paralytic syndrome following cerebral infarction affecting right non-dominant side**

I69.364 **Other paralytic syndrome following cerebral infarction affecting left non-dominant side**

I69.365 **Other paralytic syndrome following cerebral infarction, bilateral**

I69.369 **Other paralytic syndrome following cerebral infarction affecting unspecified side**

✓6th I69.39 **Other sequelae of cerebral infarction**

I69.390 **Apraxia following cerebral infarction**

I69.391 **Dysphagia following cerebral infarction**
Use additional code to identify the type of dysphagia, if known (R13.1-)

I69.392 **Facial weakness following cerebral infarction**
Facial droop following cerebral infarction

I69.393 **Ataxia following cerebral infarction**

I69.398 **Other sequelae of cerebral infarction**
Alteration of sensation following cerebral infarction
Disturbance of vision following cerebral infarction
Use additional code to identify the sequelae

✓5th **I69.8 Sequelae of other cerebrovascular diseases**
EXCLUDES 1 *sequelae of traumatic intracranial injury (SØ6.-)*

I69.8Ø Unspecified sequelae of other cerebrovascular disease

I69.81 Cognitive deficits following other cerebrovascular disease

✓6th **I69.82 Speech and language deficits following other cerebrovascular disease**

I69.82Ø Aphasia following other cerebrovascular disease

I69.821 Dysphasia following other cerebrovascular disease

I69.822 Dysarthria following other cerebrovascular disease

I69.823 Fluency disorder following other cerebrovascular disease
Stuttering following nontraumatic subarachnoid hemorrhage

I69.828 Other speech and language deficits following other cerebrovascular disease

✓6th **I69.83 Monoplegia of upper limb following other cerebrovascular disease**

I69.831 Monoplegia of upper limb following other cerebrovascular disease affecting right dominant side

I69.832 Monoplegia of upper limb following other cerebrovascular disease affecting left dominant side

I69.833 Monoplegia of upper limb following other cerebrovascular disease affecting right non-dominant side

I69.834 Monoplegia of upper limb following other cerebrovascular disease affecting left non-dominant side

I69.839 Monoplegia of upper limb following other cerebrovascular disease affecting unspecified side

✓6th **I69.84 Monoplegia of lower limb following other cerebrovascular disease**

I69.841 Monoplegia of lower limb following other cerebrovascular disease affecting right dominant side

I69.842 Monoplegia of lower limb following other cerebrovascular disease affecting left dominant side

I69.843 Monoplegia of lower limb following other cerebrovascular disease affecting right non-dominant side

I69.844 Monoplegia of lower limb following other cerebrovascular disease affecting left non-dominant side

I69.849 Monoplegia of lower limb following other cerebrovascular disease affecting unspecified side

✓6th **I69.85 Hemiplegia and hemiparesis following other cerebrovascular disease**

I69.851 Hemiplegia and hemiparesis following other cerebrovascular disease affecting right dominant side CC
CC Excl: See code: I69.Ø51

I69.852 Hemiplegia and hemiparesis following other cerebrovascular disease affecting left dominant side CC
CC Excl: See code: I69.Ø51

I69.853 Hemiplegia and hemiparesis following other cerebrovascular disease affecting right non-dominant side CC
CC Excl: See code: I69.Ø53

I69.854 Hemiplegia and hemiparesis following other cerebrovascular disease affecting left non-dominant side CC
CC Excl: See code: I69.Ø53

I69.859 Hemiplegia and hemiparesis following other cerebrovascular disease affecting unspecified side CC
CC Excl: See code: I69.Ø59

✓6th **I69.86 Other paralytic syndrome following other cerebrovascular disease**
Use additional code to identify type of paralytic syndrome, such as:
locked-in state (G83.5)
quadriplegia (G82.5-)
EXCLUDES 1 *hemiplegia/hemiparesis following other cerebrovascular disease (I69.85-)*
monoplegia of lower limb following other cerebrovascular disease (I69.84-)
monoplegia of upper limb following other cerebrovascular disease (I69.83-)

I69.861 Other paralytic syndrome following other cerebrovascular disease affecting right dominant side

I69.862 Other paralytic syndrome following other cerebrovascular disease affecting left dominant side

I69.863 Other paralytic syndrome following other cerebrovascular disease affecting right non-dominant side

I69.864 Other paralytic syndrome following other cerebrovascular disease affecting left non-dominant side

I69.865 Other paralytic syndrome following other cerebrovascular disease, bilateral

I69.869 Other paralytic syndrome following other cerebrovascular disease affecting unspecified side

✓6th **I69.89 Other sequelae of other cerebrovascular disease**

I69.89Ø Apraxia following other cerebrovascular disease

I69.891 Dysphagia following other cerebrovascular disease
Use additional code to identify the type of dysphagia, if known (R13.1-)

I69.892 Facial weakness following other cerebrovascular disease
Facial droop following other cerebrovascular disease

I69.893 Ataxia following other cerebrovascular disease

I69.898 Other sequelae of other cerebrovascular disease
Alteration of sensation following other cerebrovascular disease
Disturbance of vision following other cerebrovascular disease
Use additional code to identify the sequelae

✓5th **I69.9 Sequelae of unspecified cerebrovascular diseases**
EXCLUDES 1 *sequelae of stroke (I69.3)*
sequelae of traumatic intracranial injury (SØ6.-)

I69.9Ø Unspecified sequelae of unspecified cerebrovascular disease

I69.91 Cognitive deficits following unspecified cerebrovascular disease

✓6th **I69.92 Speech and language deficits following unspecified cerebrovascular disease**

I69.92Ø Aphasia following unspecified cerebrovascular disease

I69.921 Dysphasia following unspecified cerebrovascular disease

I69.922 Dysarthria following unspecified cerebrovascular disease

I69.923 Fluency disorder following unspecified cerebrovascular disease
Stuttering following nontraumatic subarachnoid hemorrhage

I69.928 Other speech and language deficits following unspecified cerebrovascular disease

✓6th **I69.93 Monoplegia of upper limb following unspecified cerebrovascular disease**

I69.931 Monoplegia of upper limb following unspecified cerebrovascular disease affecting right dominant side

I69.932 Monoplegia of upper limb following unspecified cerebrovascular disease affecting left dominant side

I69.933 **Monoplegia of upper limb following unspecified cerebrovascular disease affecting right non-dominant side**

I69.934 **Monoplegia of upper limb following unspecified cerebrovascular disease affecting left non-dominant side**

I69.939 **Monoplegia of upper limb following unspecified cerebrovascular disease affecting unspecified side**

✓6th **I69.94** **Monoplegia of lower limb following unspecified cerebrovascular disease**

I69.941 **Monoplegia of lower limb following unspecified cerebrovascular disease affecting right dominant side**

I69.942 **Monoplegia of lower limb following unspecified cerebrovascular disease affecting left dominant side**

I69.943 **Monoplegia of lower limb following unspecified cerebrovascular disease affecting right non-dominant side**

I69.944 **Monoplegia of lower limb following unspecified cerebrovascular disease affecting left non-dominant side**

I69.949 **Monoplegia of lower limb following unspecified cerebrovascular disease affecting unspecified side**

✓6th **I69.95** **Hemiplegia and hemiparesis following unspecified cerebrovascular disease**

I69.951 **Hemiplegia and hemiparesis following unspecified cerebrovascular disease affecting right dominant side** CC
CC Excl: I69.051-I69.052, I69.151-I69.152, I69.251-I69.252, I69.351-I69.352, I69.851-I69.852, I69.951-I69.952

I69.952 **Hemiplegia and hemiparesis following unspecified cerebrovascular disease affecting left dominant side** CC
CC Excl: See code: I69.951

I69.953 **Hemiplegia and hemiparesis following unspecified cerebrovascular disease affecting right non-dominant side** CC
CC Excl: I69.053-I69.054, I69.153-I69.154, I69.253-I69.254, I69.353-I69.354, I69.853-I69.854, I69.953-I69.954

I69.954 **Hemiplegia and hemiparesis following unspecified cerebrovascular disease affecting left non-dominant side** CC
CC Excl: See code: I69.953

I69.959 **Hemiplegia and hemiparesis following unspecified cerebrovascular disease affecting unspecified side** CC
CC Excl: I69.059, I69.159, I69.259, I69.359, I69.859, I69.959

✓6th **I69.96** **Other paralytic syndrome following unspecified cerebrovascular disease**
Use additional code to identify type of paralytic syndrome, such as:
locked-in state (G83.5)
quadriplegia (G82.5-)
EXCLUDES 1 *hemiplegia/hemiparesis following unspecified cerebrovascular disease (I69.95-)*
monoplegia of lower limb following unspecified cerebrovascular disease (I69.94-)
monoplegia of upper limb following unspecified cerebrovascular disease (I69.93-)

I69.961 **Other paralytic syndrome following unspecified cerebrovascular disease affecting right dominant side**

I69.962 **Other paralytic syndrome following unspecified cerebrovascular disease affecting left dominant side**

I69.963 **Other paralytic syndrome following unspecified cerebrovascular disease affecting right non-dominant side**

I69.964 **Other paralytic syndrome following unspecified cerebrovascular disease affecting left non-dominant side**

I69.965 **Other paralytic syndrome following unspecified cerebrovascular disease, bilateral**

I69.969 **Other paralytic syndrome following unspecified cerebrovascular disease affecting unspecified side**

✓6th **I69.99** **Other sequelae of unspecified cerebrovascular disease**

I69.990 **Apraxia following unspecified cerebrovascular disease**

I69.991 **Dysphagia following unspecified cerebrovascular disease**
Use additional code to identify the type of dysphagia, if known (R13.1-)

I69.992 **Facial weakness following unspecified cerebrovascular disease**
Facial droop following unspecified cerebrovascular disease

I69.993 **Ataxia following unspecified cerebrovascular disease**

I69.998 **Other sequelae following unspecified cerebrovascular disease**
Alteration in sensation following unspecified cerebrovascular disease
Disturbance of vision following unspecified cerebrovascular disease
Use additional code to identify the sequelae

Diseases of arteries, arterioles and capillaries (I70-I79)

✓4th **I70** **Atherosclerosis**
INCLUDES arteriolosclerosis
arterial degeneration
arteriosclerosis
arteriosclerotic vascular disease
arteriovascular degeneration
atheroma
endarteritis deformans or obliterans
senile arteritis
senile endarteritis
vascular degeneration
Use additional code to identify:
exposure to environmental tobacco smoke (Z77.22)
history of tobacco use (Z87.891)
occupational exposure to environmental tobacco smoke (Z57.31)
tobacco dependence (F17.-)
tobacco use (Z72.0)
EXCLUDES 2 *arteriosclerotic cardiovascular disease (I25.1-)*
arteriosclerotic heart disease (I25.1-)
atheroembolism (I75.-)
cerebral atherosclerosis (I67.2)
coronary atherosclerosis (I25.1-)
mesenteric atherosclerosis (K55.1)
precerebral atherosclerosis (I67.2)
primary pulmonary atherosclerosis (I27.0)

I70.0 **Atherosclerosis of aorta** A

I70.1 **Atherosclerosis of renal artery** A
Goldblatt's kidney
EXCLUDES 2 *atherosclerosis of renal arterioles (I12.-)*

✓5th **I70.2** **Atherosclerosis of native arteries of the extremities**
Mönckeberg's (medial) sclerosis
Use additional code, if applicable, to identify chronic total occlusion of artery of extremity (I70.92)
EXCLUDES 2 *atherosclerosis of bypass graft of extremities (I70.30-I70.79)*

✓6th **I70.20** **Unspecified atherosclerosis of native arteries of extremities**

I70.201 **Unspecified atherosclerosis of native arteries of extremities, right leg** A

I70.202 **Unspecified atherosclerosis of native arteries of extremities, left leg** A

I70.203 **Unspecified atherosclerosis of native arteries of extremities, bilateral legs** A

I70.208 **Unspecified atherosclerosis of native arteries of extremities, other extremity** A

I70.209 **Unspecified atherosclerosis of native arteries of extremities, unspecified extremity** A

✓6th **I70.21** **Atherosclerosis of native arteries of extremities with intermittent claudication**

I70.211 **Atherosclerosis of native arteries of extremities with intermittent claudication, right leg** A

Diseases of the Circulatory System I69.933–I70.211

I70.212 **Atherosclerosis of native arteries of extremities with intermittent claudication, left leg** A

I70.213 **Atherosclerosis of native arteries of extremities with intermittent claudication, bilateral legs** A

I70.218 **Atherosclerosis of native arteries of extremities with intermittent claudication, other extremity** A

I70.219 **Atherosclerosis of native arteries of extremities with intermittent claudication, unspecified extremity** A

✓6th **I70.22** **Atherosclerosis of native arteries of extremities with rest pain**

INCLUDES any condition classifiable to I70.21-

I70.221 **Atherosclerosis of native arteries of extremities with rest pain, right leg** A

I70.222 **Atherosclerosis of native arteries of extremities with rest pain, left leg** A

I70.223 **Atherosclerosis of native arteries of extremities with rest pain, bilateral legs** A

I70.228 **Atherosclerosis of native arteries of extremities with rest pain, other extremity** A

I70.229 **Atherosclerosis of native arteries of extremities with rest pain, unspecified extremity** A

✓6th **I70.23** **Atherosclerosis of native arteries of right leg with ulceration**

INCLUDES any condition classifiable to I70.211 and I70.221

Use additional code to identify severity of ulcer (L97.-)

I70.231 **Atherosclerosis of native arteries of right leg with ulceration of thigh** A

I70.232 **Atherosclerosis of native arteries of right leg with ulceration of calf** A

I70.233 **Atherosclerosis of native arteries of right leg with ulceration of ankle** A

I70.234 **Atherosclerosis of native arteries of right leg with ulceration of heel and midfoot** A

Atherosclerosis of native arteries of right leg with ulceration of plantar surface of midfoot

I70.235 **Atherosclerosis of native arteries of right leg with ulceration of other part of foot** A

Atherosclerosis of native arteries of right leg extremities with ulceration of toe

I70.238 **Atherosclerosis of native arteries of right leg with ulceration of other part of lower right leg** A

I70.239 **Atherosclerosis of native arteries of right leg with ulceration of unspecified site** A

✓6th **I70.24** **Atherosclerosis of native arteries of left leg with ulceration**

INCLUDES any condition classifiable to I70.212 and I70.222

Use additional code to identify severity of ulcer (L97.-)

I70.241 **Atherosclerosis of native arteries of left leg with ulceration of thigh** A

I70.242 **Atherosclerosis of native arteries of left leg with ulceration of calf** A

I70.243 **Atherosclerosis of native arteries of left leg with ulceration of ankle** A

I70.244 **Atherosclerosis of native arteries of left leg with ulceration of heel and midfoot** A

Atherosclerosis of native arteries of left leg with ulceration of plantar surface of midfoot

I70.245 **Atherosclerosis of native arteries of left leg with ulceration of other part of foot** A

Atherosclerosis of native arteries of left leg extremities with ulceration of toe

I70.248 **Atherosclerosis of native arteries of left leg with ulceration of other part of lower left leg** A

I70.249 **Atherosclerosis of native arteries of left leg with ulceration of unspecified site** A

I70.25 **Atherosclerosis of native arteries of other extremities with ulceration** A

INCLUDES any condition classifiable to I70.218 and I70.228

Use additional code to identify the severity of the ulcer (L98.49-)

✓6th **I70.26** **Atherosclerosis of native arteries of extremities with gangrene**

INCLUDES any condition classifiable to I70.21-, I70.22-, I70.23-, I70.24-, and I70.25-

Use additional code to identify the severity of any ulcer (L97.-, L98.49-), if applicable

CC Excl: For CC codes in subcategory I70.26, unless otherwise noted: G89.0-G89.4, I70.261-I70.269, I96, R41.0-R41.3, R41.82, R41.9, R44.8-R44.9, R45.83-R45.84, R46.0-R46.89, R52, R68.0-R68.19, R68.81-R68.83, R68.89-R69

I70.261 **Atherosclerosis of native arteries of extremities with gangrene, right leg** CC A

I70.262 **Atherosclerosis of native arteries of extremities with gangrene, left leg** CC A

I70.263 **Atherosclerosis of native arteries of extremities with gangrene, bilateral legs** CC A

I70.268 **Atherosclerosis of native arteries of extremities with gangrene, other extremity** CC A

I70.269 **Atherosclerosis of native arteries of extremities with gangrene, unspecified extremity** CC A

✓6th **I70.29** **Other atherosclerosis of native arteries of extremities**

I70.291 **Other atherosclerosis of native arteries of extremities, right leg** A

I70.292 **Other atherosclerosis of native arteries of extremities, left leg** A

I70.293 **Other atherosclerosis of native arteries of extremities, bilateral legs** A

I70.298 **Other atherosclerosis of native arteries of extremities, other extremity** A

I70.299 **Other atherosclerosis of native arteries of extremities, unspecified extremity** A

✓5th **I70.3** **Atherosclerosis of unspecified type of bypass graft(s) of the extremities**

Use additional code, if applicable, to identify chronic total occlusion of artery of extremity (I70.92)

EXCLUDES 1 *embolism or thrombus of bypass graft(s) of extremities (T82.8-)*

✓6th **I70.30** **Unspecified atherosclerosis of unspecified type of bypass graft(s) of the extremities**

I70.301 **Unspecified atherosclerosis of unspecified type of bypass graft(s) of the extremities, right leg** A

I70.302 **Unspecified atherosclerosis of unspecified type of bypass graft(s) of the extremities, left leg** A

I70.303 **Unspecified atherosclerosis of unspecified type of bypass graft(s) of the extremities, bilateral legs** A

I70.308 **Unspecified atherosclerosis of unspecified type of bypass graft(s) of the extremities, other extremity** A

I70.309 **Unspecified atherosclerosis of unspecified type of bypass graft(s) of the extremities, unspecified extremity** A

✓6th **I70.31** **Atherosclerosis of unspecified type of bypass graft(s) of the extremities with intermittent claudication**

I70.311 **Atherosclerosis of unspecified type of bypass graft(s) of the extremities with intermittent claudication, right leg** A

I70.312 **Atherosclerosis of unspecified type of bypass graft(s) of the extremities with intermittent claudication, left leg** A

I70.313 Atherosclerosis of unspecified type of bypass graft(s) of the extremities with intermittent claudication, bilateral legs A

I70.318 Atherosclerosis of unspecified type of bypass graft(s) of the extremities with intermittent claudication, other extremity A

I70.319 Atherosclerosis of unspecified type of bypass graft(s) of the extremities with intermittent claudication, unspecified extremity A

✓6th I70.32 Atherosclerosis of unspecified type of bypass graft(s) of the extremities with rest pain

INCLUDES any condition classifiable to I70.31-

I70.321 Atherosclerosis of unspecified type of bypass graft(s) of the extremities with rest pain, right leg A

I70.322 Atherosclerosis of unspecified type of bypass graft(s) of the extremities with rest pain, left leg A

I70.323 Atherosclerosis of unspecified type of bypass graft(s) of the extremities with rest pain, bilateral legs A

I70.328 Atherosclerosis of unspecified type of bypass graft(s) of the extremities with rest pain, other extremity A

I70.329 Atherosclerosis of unspecified type of bypass graft(s) of the extremities with rest pain, unspecified extremity A

✓6th I70.33 Atherosclerosis of unspecified type of bypass graft(s) of the right leg with ulceration

INCLUDES any condition classifiable to I70.311 and I70.321

Use additional code to identify severity of ulcer (L97.-)

CC Excl: For CC codes in subcategory I70.33, unless otherwise noted: I70.231-I70.25, L44.8-L45, L94.2, L94.4, L97.101-L97.929, L98.411-L98.499, L98.8, L99

I70.331 Atherosclerosis of unspecified type of bypass graft(s) of the right leg with ulceration of thigh PDx CC CC A

I70.332 Atherosclerosis of unspecified type of bypass graft(s) of the right leg with ulceration of calf PDx CC CC A

I70.333 Atherosclerosis of unspecified type of bypass graft(s) of the right leg with ulceration of ankle PDx CC CC A

I70.334 Atherosclerosis of unspecified type of bypass graft(s) of the right leg with ulceration of heel and midfoot PDx CC CC A

Atherosclerosis of unspecified type of bypass graft(s) of right leg with ulceration of plantar surface of midfoot

I70.335 Atherosclerosis of unspecified type of bypass graft(s) of the right leg with ulceration of other part of foot A

Atherosclerosis of unspecified type of bypass graft(s) of the right leg with ulceration of toe

I70.338 Atherosclerosis of unspecified type of bypass graft(s) of the right leg with ulceration of other part of lower leg PDx CC CC A

I70.339 Atherosclerosis of unspecified type of bypass graft(s) of the right leg with ulceration of unspecified site PDx CC CC A

✓6th I70.34 Atherosclerosis of unspecified type of bypass graft(s) of the left leg with ulceration

INCLUDES any condition classifiable to I70.312 and I70.322

Use additional code to identify severity of ulcer (L97.-)

I70.341 Atherosclerosis of unspecified type of bypass graft(s) of the left leg with ulceration of thigh PDx CC CC A

I70.342 Atherosclerosis of unspecified type of bypass graft(s) of the left leg with ulceration of calf PDx CC CC A

I70.343 Atherosclerosis of unspecified type of bypass graft(s) of the left leg with ulceration of ankle PDx CC CC A

I70.344 Atherosclerosis of unspecified type of bypass graft(s) of the left leg with ulceration of heel and midfoot PDx CC CC A

Atherosclerosis of unspecified type of bypass graft(s) of left leg with ulceration of plantar surface of midfoot

I70.345 Atherosclerosis of unspecified type of bypass graft(s) of the left leg with ulceration of other part of foot A

Atherosclerosis of unspecified type of bypass graft(s) of the left leg with ulceration of toe

I70.348 Atherosclerosis of unspecified type of bypass graft(s) of the left leg with ulceration of other part of lower leg PDx CC CC A

I70.349 Atherosclerosis of unspecified type of bypass graft(s) of the left leg with ulceration of unspecified site PDx CC CC A

I70.35 Atherosclerosis of unspecified type of bypass graft(s) of other extremity with ulceration A

INCLUDES any condition classifiable to I70.318 and I70.328

Use additional code to identify severity of ulcer (L98.49-)

✓6th I70.36 Atherosclerosis of unspecified type of bypass graft(s) of the extremities with gangrene

INCLUDES any condition classifiable to I70.31-, I70.32-, I70.33-, I70.34-, I70.35

Use additional code to identify the severity of any ulcer (L97.-, L98.49-), if applicable

I70.361 Atherosclerosis of unspecified type of bypass graft(s) of the extremities with gangrene, right leg PDx CC CC A

CC Excl: G89.0-G89.4, I70.261-I70.269, I96, R41.0-R41.3, R41.82, R41.9, R44.8-R44.9, R45.83-R45.84, R46.0-R46.89, R52, R68.0-R68.19, R68.81-R68.83, R68.89-R69

I70.362 Atherosclerosis of unspecified type of bypass graft(s) of the extremities with gangrene, left leg PDx CC CC A

CC Excl: See code: I70.361

I70.363 Atherosclerosis of unspecified type of bypass graft(s) of the extremities with gangrene, bilateral legs PDx CC CC A

CC Excl: See code: I70.361

I70.368 Atherosclerosis of unspecified type of bypass graft(s) of the extremities with gangrene, other extremity PDx CC CC A

CC Excl: See code: I70.361

I70.369 Atherosclerosis of unspecified type of bypass graft(s) of the extremities with gangrene, unspecified extremity PDx CC CC A

CC Excl: See code: I70.361

✓6th I70.39 Other atherosclerosis of unspecified type of bypass graft(s) of the extremities

I70.391 Other atherosclerosis of unspecified type of bypass graft(s) of the extremities, right leg A

I70.392 Other atherosclerosis of unspecified type of bypass graft(s) of the extremities, left leg A

I70.393 Other atherosclerosis of unspecified type of bypass graft(s) of the extremities, bilateral legs A

I70.398 Other atherosclerosis of unspecified type of bypass graft(s) of the extremities, other extremity A

I70.399 Other atherosclerosis of unspecified type of bypass graft(s) of the extremities, unspecified extremity A

I70.4 Atherosclerosis of autologous vein bypass graft(s) of the extremities
Use additional code, if applicable, to identify chronic total occlusion of artery of extremity (I70.92)

I70.40 Unspecified atherosclerosis of autologous vein bypass graft(s) of the extremities

I70.401 Unspecified atherosclerosis of autologous vein bypass graft(s) of the extremities, right leg A

I70.402 Unspecified atherosclerosis of autologous vein bypass graft(s) of the extremities, left leg A

I70.403 Unspecified atherosclerosis of autologous vein bypass graft(s) of the extremities, bilateral legs A

I70.408 Unspecified atherosclerosis of autologous vein bypass graft(s) of the extremities, other extremity A

I70.409 Unspecified atherosclerosis of autologous vein bypass graft(s) of the extremities, unspecified extremity A

I70.41 Atherosclerosis of autologous vein bypass graft(s) of the extremities with intermittent claudication

I70.411 Atherosclerosis of autologous vein bypass graft(s) of the extremities with intermittent claudication, right leg A

I70.412 Atherosclerosis of autologous vein bypass graft(s) of the extremities with intermittent claudication, left leg A

I70.413 Atherosclerosis of autologous vein bypass graft(s) of the extremities with intermittent claudication, bilateral legs A

I70.418 Atherosclerosis of autologous vein bypass graft(s) of the extremities with intermittent claudication, other extremity A

I70.419 Atherosclerosis of autologous vein bypass graft(s) of the extremities with intermittent claudication, unspecified extremity A

I70.42 Atherosclerosis of autologous vein bypass graft(s) of the extremities with rest pain
INCLUDES any condition classifiable to I70.41-

I70.421 Atherosclerosis of autologous vein bypass graft(s) of the extremities with rest pain, right leg A

I70.422 Atherosclerosis of autologous vein bypass graft(s) of the extremities with rest pain, left leg A

I70.423 Atherosclerosis of autologous vein bypass graft(s) of the extremities with rest pain, bilateral legs A

I70.428 Atherosclerosis of autologous vein bypass graft(s) of the extremities with rest pain, other extremity A

I70.429 Atherosclerosis of autologous vein bypass graft(s) of the extremities with rest pain, unspecified extremity A

I70.43 Atherosclerosis of autologous vein bypass graft(s) of the right leg with ulceration
INCLUDES any condition classifiable to I70.411 and I70.421
Use additional code to identify severity of ulcer (L97.-)

CC Excl: For CC codes in subcategory I70.43, unless otherwise noted: I70.231-I70.25, L44.8-L45, L94.2, L94.4, L97.101-L97.929, L98.411-L98.499, L98.8, L99

I70.431 Atherosclerosis of autologous vein bypass graft(s) of the right leg with ulceration of thigh PDx CC CC A

I70.432 Atherosclerosis of autologous vein bypass graft(s) of the right leg with ulceration of calf PDx CC CC A

I70.433 Atherosclerosis of autologous vein bypass graft(s) of the right leg with ulceration of ankle PDx CC CC A

I70.434 Atherosclerosis of autologous vein bypass graft(s) of the right leg with ulceration of heel and midfoot PDx CC CC A
Atherosclerosis of autologous vein bypass graft(s) of right leg with ulceration of plantar surface of midfoot

I70.435 Atherosclerosis of autologous vein bypass graft(s) of the right leg with ulceration of other part of foot A
Atherosclerosis of autologous vein bypass graft(s) of right leg with ulceration of toe

I70.438 Atherosclerosis of autologous vein bypass graft(s) of the right leg with ulceration of other part of lower leg PDx CC CC A

I70.439 Atherosclerosis of autologous vein bypass graft(s) of the right leg with ulceration of unspecified site PDx CC CC A

I70.44 Atherosclerosis of autologous vein bypass graft(s) of the left leg with ulceration
INCLUDES any condition classifiable to I70.412 and I70.422
Use additional code to identify severity of ulcer (L97.-)

I70.441 Atherosclerosis of autologous vein bypass graft(s) of the left leg with ulceration of thigh PDx CC CC A

I70.442 Atherosclerosis of autologous vein bypass graft(s) of the left leg with ulceration of calf PDx CC CC A

I70.443 Atherosclerosis of autologous vein bypass graft(s) of the left leg with ulceration of ankle PDx CC CC A

I70.444 Atherosclerosis of autologous vein bypass graft(s) of the left leg with ulceration of heel and midfoot PDx CC CC A
Atherosclerosis of autologous vein bypass graft(s) of left leg with ulceration of plantar surface of midfoot

I70.445 Atherosclerosis of autologous vein bypass graft(s) of the left leg with ulceration of other part of foot A
Atherosclerosis of autologous vein bypass graft(s) of left leg with ulceration of toe

I70.448 Atherosclerosis of autologous vein bypass graft(s) of the left leg with ulceration of other part of lower leg PDx CC CC A

I70.449 Atherosclerosis of autologous vein bypass graft(s) of the left leg with ulceration of unspecified site PDx CC CC A

I70.45 Atherosclerosis of autologous vein bypass graft(s) of other extremity with ulceration A
INCLUDES any condition classifiable to I70.418, I70.428, and I70.438
Use additional code to identify severity of ulcer (L98.49)

I70.46 Atherosclerosis of autologous vein bypass graft(s) of the extremities with gangrene
INCLUDES any condition classifiable to I70.41-, I70.42-, and I70.43-, I70.44-, I70.45
Use additional code to identify the severity of any ulcer (L97.-, L98.49-), if applicable

I70.461 Atherosclerosis of autologous vein bypass graft(s) of the extremities with gangrene, right leg PDx CC CC A
CC Excl: G89.0-G89.4, I70.261-I70.269, I96, R41.0-R41.3, R41.82, R41.9, R44.8-R44.9, R45.83-R45.84, R46.0-R46.89, R52, R68.0-R68.19, R68.81-R68.83, R68.89-R69

I70.462 Atherosclerosis of autologous vein bypass graft(s) of the extremities with gangrene, left leg PDx CC CC A
CC Excl: See code: I70.461

I70.463 Atherosclerosis of autologous vein bypass graft(s) of the extremities with gangrene, bilateral legs PDx CC CC A
CC Excl: See code: I70.461

I70.468 Atherosclerosis of autologous vein bypass graft(s) of the extremities with gangrene, other extremity PDx CC CC A
CC Excl: See code: I70.461

I70.469 Atherosclerosis of autologous vein bypass graft(s) of the extremities with gangrene, unspecified extremity PDx CC CC A
CC Excl: See code: I70.461

✓6th **I70.49 Other atherosclerosis of autologous vein bypass graft(s) of the extremities**

I70.491 Other atherosclerosis of autologous vein bypass graft(s) of the extremities, right leg A

I70.492 Other atherosclerosis of autologous vein bypass graft(s) of the extremities, left leg A

I70.493 Other atherosclerosis of autologous vein bypass graft(s) of the extremities, bilateral legs A

I70.498 Other atherosclerosis of autologous vein bypass graft(s) of the extremities, other extremity A

I70.499 Other atherosclerosis of autologous vein bypass graft(s) of the extremities, unspecified extremity A

✓5th **I70.5 Atherosclerosis of nonautologous biological bypass graft(s) of the extremities**
Use additional code, if applicable, to identify chronic total occlusion of artery of extremity (I70.92)

✓6th **I70.50 Unspecified atherosclerosis of nonautologous biological bypass graft(s) of the extremities**

I70.501 Unspecified atherosclerosis of nonautologous biological bypass graft(s) of the extremities, right leg A

I70.502 Unspecified atherosclerosis of nonautologous biological bypass graft(s) of the extremities, left leg A

I70.503 Unspecified atherosclerosis of nonautologous biological bypass graft(s) of the extremities, bilateral legs A

I70.508 Unspecified atherosclerosis of nonautologous biological bypass graft(s) of the extremities, other extremity A

I70.509 Unspecified atherosclerosis of nonautologous biological bypass graft(s) of the extremities, unspecified extremity A

✓6th **I70.51 Atherosclerosis of nonautologous biological bypass graft(s) of the extremities with intermittent claudication**

I70.511 Atherosclerosis of nonautologous biological bypass graft(s) of the extremities with intermittent claudication, right leg A

I70.512 Atherosclerosis of nonautologous biological bypass graft(s) of the extremities with intermittent claudication, left leg A

I70.513 Atherosclerosis of nonautologous biological bypass graft(s) of the extremities with intermittent claudication, bilateral legs A

I70.518 Atherosclerosis of nonautologous biological bypass graft(s) of the extremities with intermittent claudication, other extremity A

I70.519 Atherosclerosis of nonautologous biological bypass graft(s) of the extremities with intermittent claudication, unspecified extremity A

✓6th **I70.52 Atherosclerosis of nonautologous biological bypass graft(s) of the extremities with rest pain**
INCLUDES any condition classifiable to I70.51-

I70.521 Atherosclerosis of nonautologous biological bypass graft(s) of the extremities with rest pain, right leg A

I70.522 Atherosclerosis of nonautologous biological bypass graft(s) of the extremities with rest pain, left leg A

I70.523 Atherosclerosis of nonautologous biological bypass graft(s) of the extremities with rest pain, bilateral legs A

I70.528 Atherosclerosis of nonautologous biological bypass graft(s) of the extremities with rest pain, other extremity A

I70.529 Atherosclerosis of nonautologous biological bypass graft(s) of the extremities with rest pain, unspecified extremity A

✓6th **I70.53 Atherosclerosis of nonautologous biological bypass graft(s) of the right leg with ulceration**
INCLUDES any condition classifiable to I70.511 and I70.521
Use additional code to identify severity of ulcer (L97.-)

CC Excl: For CC codes in subcategory I70.53, unless otherwise noted: I70.231-I70.25, L44.8-L45, L94.2, L94.4, L97.101-L97.929, L98.411-L98.499, L98.8, L99

I70.531 Atherosclerosis of biological nonautologous bypass graft(s) of the right leg with ulceration of thigh PDx CC CC A

I70.532 Atherosclerosis of biological nonautologous bypass graft(s) of the right leg with ulceration of calf PDx CC CC A

I70.533 Atherosclerosis of nonautologous biological bypass graft(s) of the right leg with ulceration of ankle PDx CC CC A

I70.534 Atherosclerosis of nonautologous biological bypass graft(s) of the right leg with ulceration of heel and midfoot PDx CC CC A
Atherosclerosis of nonautologous biological bypass graft(s) of right leg with ulceration of plantar surface of midfoot

I70.535 Atherosclerosis of nonautologous biological bypass graft(s) of the right leg with ulceration of other part of foot A
Atherosclerosis of nonautologous biological bypass graft(s) of the right leg with ulceration of toe

I70.538 Atherosclerosis of nonautologous biological bypass graft(s) of the right leg with ulceration of other part of lower leg PDx CC CC A

I70.539 Atherosclerosis of nonautologous biological bypass graft(s) of the right leg with ulceration of unspecified site PDx CC CC A

✓6th **I70.54 Atherosclerosis of nonautologous biological bypass graft(s) of the left leg with ulceration**
INCLUDES any condition classifiable to I70.512 and I70.522
Use additional code to identify severity of ulcer (L97.-)

I70.541 Atherosclerosis of nonautologous biological bypass graft(s) of the left leg with ulceration of thigh PDx CC CC A

I70.542 Atherosclerosis of nonautologous biological bypass graft(s) of the left leg with ulceration of calf PDx CC CC A

I70.543 Atherosclerosis of nonautologous biological bypass graft(s) of the left leg with ulceration of ankle PDx CC CC A

I70.544 Atherosclerosis of nonautologous biological bypass graft(s) of the left leg with ulceration of heel and midfoot PDx CC CC A
Atherosclerosis of nonautologous biological bypass graft(s) of left leg with ulceration of plantar surface of midfoot

I70.545 Atherosclerosis of nonautologous biological bypass graft(s) of the left leg with ulceration of other part of foot A
Atherosclerosis of nonautologous biological bypass graft(s) of the left leg with ulceration of toe

I70.548 Atherosclerosis of nonautologous biological bypass graft(s) of the left leg with ulceration of other part of lower leg PDx CC CC A

I70.549 Atherosclerosis of nonautologous biological bypass graft(s) of the left leg with ulceration of unspecified site PDx CC CC A

I7Ø.55 Atherosclerosis of nonautologous biological bypass graft(s) of other extremity with ulceration A
INCLUDES any condition classifiable to I7Ø.518, I7Ø.528, and I7Ø.538
Use additional code to identify severity of ulcer (L98.49)

√6th **I7Ø.56 Atherosclerosis of nonautologous biological bypass graft(s) of the extremities with gangrene**
INCLUDES any condition classifiable to I7Ø.51-, I7Ø.52-, and I7Ø.53-, I7Ø.54-, I7Ø.55
Use additional code to identify the severity of any ulcer (L97.-, L98.49-), if applicable

I7Ø.561 Atherosclerosis of nonautologous biological bypass graft(s) of the extremities with gangrene, right leg PDx CC CC A
CC Excl: G89.Ø-G89.4, I7Ø.261-I7Ø.269, I96, R41.Ø-R41.3, R41.82, R41.9, R44.8-R44.9, R45.83-R45.84, R46.Ø-R46.89, R52, R68.Ø-R68.19, R68.81-R68.83, R68.89-R69

I7Ø.562 Atherosclerosis of nonautologous biological bypass graft(s) of the extremities with gangrene, left leg PDx CC CC A
CC Excl: See code: I7Ø.561

I7Ø.563 Atherosclerosis of nonautologous biological bypass graft(s) of the extremities with gangrene, bilateral legs PDx CC CC A
CC Excl: See code: I7Ø.561

I7Ø.568 Atherosclerosis of nonautologous biological bypass graft(s) of the extremities with gangrene, other extremity PDx CC CC A
CC Excl: See code: I7Ø.561

I7Ø.569 Atherosclerosis of nonautologous biological bypass graft(s) of the extremities with gangrene, unspecified extremity PDx CC CC A
CC Excl: See code: I7Ø.561

√6th **I7Ø.59 Other atherosclerosis of nonautologous biological bypass graft(s) of the extremities**

I7Ø.591 Other atherosclerosis of biological nonautologous bypass graft(s) of the extremities, right leg A

I7Ø.592 Other atherosclerosis of nonautologous biological bypass graft(s) of the extremities, left leg A

I7Ø.593 Other atherosclerosis of nonautologous biological bypass graft(s) of the extremities, bilateral legs A

I7Ø.598 Other atherosclerosis of nonautologous biological bypass graft(s) of the extremities, other extremity A

I7Ø.599 Other atherosclerosis of nonautologous biological bypass graft(s) of the extremities, unspecified extremity A

√5th **I7Ø.6 Atherosclerosis of nonbiological bypass graft(s) of the extremities**
Use additional code, if applicable, to identify chronic total occlusion of artery of extremity (I7Ø.92)

√6th **I7Ø.6Ø Unspecified atherosclerosis of nonbiological bypass graft(s) of the extremities**

I7Ø.6Ø1 Unspecified atherosclerosis of nonbiological bypass graft(s) of the extremities, right leg A

I7Ø.6Ø2 Unspecified atherosclerosis of nonbiological bypass graft(s) of the extremities, left leg A

I7Ø.6Ø3 Unspecified atherosclerosis of nonbiological bypass graft(s) of the extremities, bilateral legs A

I7Ø.6Ø8 Unspecified atherosclerosis of nonbiological bypass graft(s) of the extremities, other extremity A

I7Ø.6Ø9 Unspecified atherosclerosis of nonbiological bypass graft(s) of the extremities, unspecified extremity A

√6th **I7Ø.61 Atherosclerosis of nonbiological bypass graft(s) of the extremities with intermittent claudication**

I7Ø.611 Atherosclerosis of nonbiological bypass graft(s) of the extremities with intermittent claudication, right leg A

I7Ø.612 Atherosclerosis of nonbiological bypass graft(s) of the extremities with intermittent claudication, left leg A

I7Ø.613 Atherosclerosis of nonbiological bypass graft(s) of the extremities with intermittent claudication, bilateral legs A

I7Ø.618 Atherosclerosis of nonbiological bypass graft(s) of the extremities with intermittent claudication, other extremity A

I7Ø.619 Atherosclerosis of nonbiological bypass graft(s) of the extremities with intermittent claudication, unspecified extremity A

√6th **I7Ø.62 Atherosclerosis of nonbiological bypass graft(s) of the extremities with rest pain**
INCLUDES any condition classifiable to I7Ø.61-

I7Ø.621 Atherosclerosis of nonbiological bypass graft(s) of the extremities with rest pain, right leg A

I7Ø.622 Atherosclerosis of nonbiological bypass graft(s) of the extremities with rest pain, left leg A

I7Ø.623 Atherosclerosis of nonbiological bypass graft(s) of the extremities with rest pain, bilateral legs A

I7Ø.628 Atherosclerosis of nonbiological bypass graft(s) of the extremities with rest pain, other extremity A

I7Ø.629 Atherosclerosis of nonbiological bypass graft(s) of the extremities with rest pain, unspecified extremity A

√6th **I7Ø.63 Atherosclerosis of nonbiological bypass graft(s) of the right leg with ulceration**
INCLUDES any condition classifiable to I7Ø.611 and I7Ø.621
Use additional code to identify severity of ulcer (L97.-)

CC Excl: For CC codes in subcategory I7Ø.63, unless otherwise noted: I7Ø.231-I7Ø.25, L44.8-L45, L94.2, L94.4, L97.1Ø1-L97.929, L98.411-L98.499, L98.8, L99

I7Ø.631 Atherosclerosis of nonbiological bypass graft(s) of the right leg with ulceration of thigh PDx CC CC A

I7Ø.632 Atherosclerosis of nonbiological bypass graft(s) of the right leg with ulceration of calf PDx CC CC A

I7Ø.633 Atherosclerosis of nonbiological bypass graft(s) of the right leg with ulceration of ankle PDx CC CC A

I7Ø.634 Atherosclerosis of nonbiological bypass graft(s) of the right leg with ulceration of heel and midfoot PDx CC CC A
Atherosclerosis of nonbiological bypass graft(s) of right leg with ulceration of plantar surface of midfoot

I7Ø.635 Atherosclerosis of nonbiological bypass graft(s) of the right leg with ulceration of other part of foot A
Atherosclerosis of nonbiological bypass graft(s) of the right leg with ulceration of toe

I7Ø.638 Atherosclerosis of nonbiological bypass graft(s) of the right leg with ulceration of other part of lower leg PDx CC CC A

I7Ø.639 Atherosclerosis of nonbiological bypass graft(s) of the right leg with ulceration of unspecified site PDx CC CC A

✓6th **I70.64 Atherosclerosis of nonbiological bypass graft(s) of the left leg with ulceration**
INCLUDES any condition classifiable to I70.612 and I70.622
Use additional code to identify severity of ulcer (L97.-)

I70.641 Atherosclerosis of nonbiological bypass graft(s) of the left leg with ulceration of thigh PDx CC CC A

I70.642 Atherosclerosis of nonbiological bypass graft(s) of the left leg with ulceration of calf PDx CC CC A

I70.643 Atherosclerosis of nonbiological bypass graft(s) of the left leg with ulceration of ankle PDx CC CC A

I70.644 Atherosclerosis of nonbiological bypass graft(s) of the left leg with ulceration of heel and midfoot PDx CC CC A
Atherosclerosis of nonbiological bypass graft(s) of left leg with ulceration of plantar surface of midfoot

I70.645 Atherosclerosis of nonbiological bypass graft(s) of the left leg with ulceration of other part of foot A
Atherosclerosis of nonbiological bypass graft(s) of the left leg with ulceration of toe

I70.648 Atherosclerosis of nonbiological bypass graft(s) of the left leg with ulceration of other part of lower leg PDx CC CC A

I70.649 Atherosclerosis of nonbiological bypass graft(s) of the left leg with ulceration of unspecified site PDx CC CC A

I70.65 Atherosclerosis of nonbiological bypass graft(s) of other extremity with ulceration A
INCLUDES any condition classifiable to I70.618 and I70.628
Use additional code to identify severity of ulcer (L98.49)

✓6th **I70.66 Atherosclerosis of nonbiological bypass graft(s) of the extremities with gangrene**
INCLUDES any condition classifiable to I70.61-, I70.62-, I70.63-, I70.64-, I70.65
Use additional code to identify the severity of any ulcer (L97.-, L98.49-), if applicable

I70.661 Atherosclerosis of nonbiological bypass graft(s) of the extremities with gangrene, right leg PDx CC CC A
CC Excl: G89.0-G89.4, I70.261-I70.269, I96, R41.0-R41.3, R41.82, R41.9, R44.8-R44.9, R45.83-R45.84, R46.0-R46.89, R52, R68.0-R68.19, R68.81-R68.83, R68.89-R69

I70.662 Atherosclerosis of nonbiological bypass graft(s) of the extremities with gangrene, left leg PDx CC CC A
CC Excl: See code: I70.661

I70.663 Atherosclerosis of nonbiological bypass graft(s) of the extremities with gangrene, bilateral legs PDx CC CC A
CC Excl: See code: I70.661

I70.668 Atherosclerosis of nonbiological bypass graft(s) of the extremities with gangrene, other extremity PDx CC CC A
CC Excl: See code: I70.661

I70.669 Atherosclerosis of nonbiological bypass graft(s) of the extremities with gangrene, unspecified extremity PDx CC CC A
CC Excl: See code: I70.661

✓6th **I70.69 Other atherosclerosis of nonbiological bypass graft(s) of the extremities**

I70.691 Other atherosclerosis of nonbiological bypass graft(s) of the extremities, right leg A

I70.692 Other atherosclerosis of nonbiological bypass graft(s) of the extremities, left leg A

I70.693 Other atherosclerosis of nonbiological bypass graft(s) of the extremities, bilateral legs A

I70.698 Other atherosclerosis of nonbiological bypass graft(s) of the extremities, other extremity A

I70.699 Other atherosclerosis of nonbiological bypass graft(s) of the extremities, unspecified extremity A

✓5th **I70.7 Atherosclerosis of other type of bypass graft(s) of the extremities**
Use additional code, if applicable, to identify chronic total occlusion of artery of extremity (I70.92)

✓6th **I70.70 Unspecified atherosclerosis of other type of bypass graft(s) of the extremities**

I70.701 Unspecified atherosclerosis of other type of bypass graft(s) of the extremities, right leg A

I70.702 Unspecified atherosclerosis of other type of bypass graft(s) of the extremities, left leg A

I70.703 Unspecified atherosclerosis of other type of bypass graft(s) of the extremities, bilateral legs A

I70.708 Unspecified atherosclerosis of other type of bypass graft(s) of the extremities, other extremity A

I70.709 Unspecified atherosclerosis of other type of bypass graft(s) of the extremities, unspecified extremity A

✓6th **I70.71 Atherosclerosis of other type of bypass graft(s) of the extremities with intermittent claudication**

I70.711 Atherosclerosis of other type of bypass graft(s) of the extremities with intermittent claudication, right leg A

I70.712 Atherosclerosis of other type of bypass graft(s) of the extremities with intermittent claudication, left leg A

I70.713 Atherosclerosis of other type of bypass graft(s) of the extremities with intermittent claudication, bilateral legs A

I70.718 Atherosclerosis of other type of bypass graft(s) of the extremities with intermittent claudication, other extremity A

I70.719 Atherosclerosis of other type of bypass graft(s) of the extremities with intermittent claudication, unspecified extremity A

✓6th **I70.72 Atherosclerosis of other type of bypass graft(s) of the extremities with rest pain**
INCLUDES any condition classifiable to I70.71-

I70.721 Atherosclerosis of other type of bypass graft(s) of the extremities with rest pain, right leg A

I70.722 Atherosclerosis of other type of bypass graft(s) of the extremities with rest pain, left leg A

I70.723 Atherosclerosis of other type of bypass graft(s) of the extremities with rest pain, bilateral legs A

I70.728 Atherosclerosis of other type of bypass graft(s) of the extremities with rest pain, other extremity A

I70.729 Atherosclerosis of other type of bypass graft(s) of the extremities with rest pain, unspecified extremity A

✓6th **I70.73 Atherosclerosis of other type of bypass graft(s) of the right leg with ulceration**
INCLUDES any condition classifiable to I70.711 and I70.721
Use additional code to identify severity of ulcer (L97.-)

CC Excl: For CC codes in subcategory I70.73, unless otherwise noted: I70.231-I70.25, L44.8-L45, L94.2, L94.4, L97.101-L97.929, L98.411-L98.499, L98.8, L99

I70.731 Atherosclerosis of other type of bypass graft(s) of the right leg with ulceration of thigh PDx CC CC A

I70.732 Atherosclerosis of other type of bypass graft(s) of the right leg with ulceration of calf PDx CC CC A

I70.733 Atherosclerosis of other type of bypass graft(s) of the right leg with ulceration of ankle PDx CC CC A

I70.734 Atherosclerosis of other type of bypass graft(s) of the right leg with ulceration of heel and midfoot PDx CC CC A
Atherosclerosis of other type of bypass graft(s) of right leg with ulceration of plantar surface of midfoot

I70.735 Atherosclerosis of other type of bypass graft(s) of the right leg with ulceration of other part of foot A
Atherosclerosis of other type of bypass graft(s) of right leg with ulceration of toe

I70.738 Atherosclerosis of other type of bypass graft(s) of the right leg with ulceration of other part of lower leg PDx CC CC A

I70.739 Atherosclerosis of other type of bypass graft(s) of the right leg with ulceration of unspecified site PDx CC CC A

✓6th **I70.74 Atherosclerosis of other type of bypass graft(s) of the left leg with ulceration**
INCLUDES any condition classifiable to I70.712 and I70.722
Use additional code to identify severity of ulcer (L97.-)

I70.741 Atherosclerosis of other type of bypass graft(s) of the left leg with ulceration of thigh PDx CC CC A

I70.742 Atherosclerosis of other type of bypass graft(s) of the left leg with ulceration of calf PDx CC CC A

I70.743 Atherosclerosis of other type of bypass graft(s) of the left leg with ulceration of ankle PDx CC CC A

I70.744 Atherosclerosis of other type of bypass raft(s) of the left leg with ulceration of heel and midfoot PDx CC CC A
Atherosclerosis of other type of bypass graft(s) of left leg with ulceration of plantar surface of midfoot

I70.745 Atherosclerosis of other type of bypass graft(s) of the left leg with ulceration of other part of foot A
Atherosclerosis of other type of bypass graft(s) of left leg with ulceration of toe

I70.748 Atherosclerosis of other type of bypass graft(s) of the left leg with ulceration of other part of lower leg PDx CC CC A

I70.749 Atherosclerosis of other type of bypass graft(s) of the left leg with ulceration of unspecified site PDx CC CC A

I70.75 Atherosclerosis of other type of bypass graft(s) of other extremity with ulceration A
INCLUDES any condition classifiable to I70.718 and I70.728
Use additional code to identify severity of ulcer (L98.49)

✓6th **I70.76 Atherosclerosis of other type of bypass graft(s) of the extremities with gangrene**
INCLUDES any condition classifiable to I70.71-, I70.72-, I70.73-, I70.74-, I70.75
Use additional code to identify the severity of any ulcer (L97.-, L98.49-), if applicable

I70.761 Atherosclerosis of other type of bypass graft(s) of the extremities with gangrene, right leg PDx CC CC A
CC Excl: G89.0-G89.4, I70.261-I70.269, I96, R41.0-R41.3, R41.82, R41.9, R44.8-R44.9, R45.83-R45.84, R46.0-R46.89, R52, R68.0-R68.19, R68.81-R68.83, R68.89-R69

I70.762 Atherosclerosis of other type of bypass graft(s) of the extremities with gangrene, left leg PDx CC CC A
CC Excl: See code: I70.761

I70.763 Atherosclerosis of other type of bypass graft(s) of the extremities with gangrene, bilateral legs PDx CC CC A
CC Excl: See code: I70.761

I70.768 Atherosclerosis of other type of bypass graft(s) of the extremities with gangrene, other extremity PDx CC CC A
CC Excl: See code: I70.761

I70.769 Atherosclerosis of other type of bypass graft(s) of the extremities with gangrene, unspecified extremity PDx CC CC A
CC Excl: See code: I70.761

✓6th **I70.79 Other atherosclerosis of other type of bypass graft(s) of the extremities**

I70.791 Other atherosclerosis of other type of bypass graft(s) of the extremities, right leg A

I70.792 Other atherosclerosis of other type of bypass graft(s) of the extremities, left leg A

I70.793 Other atherosclerosis of other type of bypass graft(s) of the extremities, bilateral legs A

I70.798 Other atherosclerosis of other type of bypass graft(s) of the extremities, other extremity A

I70.799 Other atherosclerosis of other type of bypass graft(s) of the extremities, unspecified extremity A

I70.8 Atherosclerosis of other arteries A

✓5th **I70.9 Other and unspecified atherosclerosis**

I70.90 Unspecified atherosclerosis A

I70.91 Generalized atherosclerosis A

I70.92 Chronic total occlusion of artery of the extremities CC A
Complete occlusion of artery of the extremities
Total occlusion of artery of the extremities
Code first atherosclerosis of arteries of the extremities (I70.2-, I70.3-, I70.4-, I70.5-, I70.6-, I70.7-)
CC Excl: I67.0, I70.201-I70.799, I70.92-I71.9, I72.1, I72.3-I72.4, I72.9, I73.81-I77.2, I77.5-I77.6, I77.72, I77.79-I77.819, I79.0-I79.8, M31.8-M31.9

✓4th **I71 Aortic aneurysm and dissection**
EXCLUDES 1 *aortic ectasia (I77.81-)*
syphilitic aortic aneurysm (A52.01)
traumatic aortic aneurysm (S25.09, S35.09)

CC Excl: For MCC codes in category I71, unless otherwise noted: E08.51-E08.59, E08.618-E08.638, E08.649-E08.8, E09.51-E09.59, E09.618-E09.638, E09.649-E09.8, E10.51-E10.59, E10.618-E10.638, E10.649, E10.69-E10.8, E11.51-E11.59, E11.618-E11.638, E11.649, E11.69-E11.8, E13.51-E13.59, E13.618-E13.638, E13.649-E13.8, I71.00-I71.9, I77.810-I77.819, I79.0, I87.8, I99.8-I99.9

✓5th **I71.0 Dissection of aorta**

I71.00 Dissection of unspecified site of aorta MCC

I71.01 Dissection of thoracic aorta MCC

I71.02 Dissection of abdominal aorta MCC

I71.03 Dissection of thoracoabdominal aorta MCC

I71.1 Thoracic aortic aneurysm, ruptured MCC

I71.2 Thoracic aortic aneurysm, without rupture

I71.3 Abdominal aortic aneurysm, ruptured MCC

I71.4 Abdominal aortic aneurysm, without rupture

I71.5 Thoracoabdominal aortic aneurysm, ruptured MCC

I71.6 Thoracoabdominal aortic aneurysm, without rupture

I71.8 Aortic aneurysm of unspecified site, ruptured MCC
Rupture of aorta NOS

I71.9 Aortic aneurysm of unspecified site, without rupture
Aneurysm of aorta
Dilatation of aorta
Hyaline necrosis of aorta

I72 Other aneurysm

INCLUDES aneurysm (cirsoid) (false) (ruptured)

EXCLUDES 2 *acquired aneurysm (I77.0)*
aneurysm (of) aorta (I71.-)
aneurysm (of) arteriovenous NOS (Q27.3-)
carotid artery dissection (I77.71)
cerebral (nonruptured) aneurysm (I67.1)
coronary aneurysm (I25.4)
coronary artery dissection (I25.42)
dissection of artery NEC (I77.79)
heart aneurysm (I25.3)
iliac artery dissection (I77.72)
pulmonary artery aneurysm (I28.1)
renal artery dissection (I77.73)
retinal aneurysm (H35.0)
ruptured cerebral aneurysm (I60.7)
varicose aneurysm (I77.0)
vertebral artery dissection (I77.74)

I72.0 Aneurysm of carotid artery
Aneurysm of common carotid artery
Aneurysm of external carotid artery
Aneurysm of internal carotid artery, extracranial portion
EXCLUDES 1 *aneurysm of internal carotid artery, intracranial portion (I67.1)*
aneurysm of internal carotid artery NOS (I67.1)

I72.1 Aneurysm of artery of upper extremity

I72.2 Aneurysm of renal artery

I72.3 Aneurysm of iliac artery

I72.4 Aneurysm of artery of lower extremity

I72.8 Aneurysm of other specified arteries

I72.9 Aneurysm of unspecified site

I73 Other peripheral vascular diseases

EXCLUDES 2 *chilblains (T69.1)*
frostbite (T33-T34)
immersion hand or foot (T69.0-)
spasm of cerebral artery (G45.9)

I73.0 Raynaud's syndrome
Raynaud's disease
Raynaud's phenomenon (secondary)

I73.00 Raynaud's syndrome without gangrene

I73.01 Raynaud's syndrome with gangrene PDx CC CC
CC Excl: G89.0-G89.4, I70.261-I70.269, I96, R41.0-R41.3, R41.82, R41.9, R44.8-R44.9, R45.83-R45.84, R46.0-R46.89, R52, R68.0-R68.19, R68.81-R68.83, R68.89-R69

I73.1 Thromboangiitis obliterans [Buerger's disease]

I73.8 Other specified peripheral vascular diseases
EXCLUDES 1 *diabetic (peripheral) angiopathy (E08-E13 with .51-.52)*

I73.81 Erythromelalgia

I73.89 Other specified peripheral vascular diseases
Acrocyanosis
Erythrocyanosis
Simple acroparesthesia [Schultze's type]
Vasomotor acroparesthesia [Nothnagel's type]

I73.9 Peripheral vascular disease, unspecified
Intermittent claudication
Peripheral angiopathy NOS
Spasm of artery
EXCLUDES 1 *atherosclerosis of the extremities (I70.2--I70.7-)*

I74 Arterial embolism and thrombosis
Embolic infarction
Embolic occlusion
Thrombotic infarction
Thrombotic occlusion

Code first:
embolism and thrombosis complicating abortion or ectopic or molar pregnancy (O00-O07, O08.2)
embolism and thrombosis complicating pregnancy, childbirth and the puerperium (O88.-)

EXCLUDES 2 *atheroembolism (I75.-)*
basilar embolism and thrombosis (I63.0-I63.2, I65.1)
carotid embolism and thrombosis (I63.0-I63.2, I65.2)
cerebral embolism and thrombosis (I63.3-I63.5, I66-)
coronary embolism and thrombosis (I21-I25)
mesenteric embolism and thrombosis (K55.0)
ophthalmic embolism and thrombosis (H34.-)
precerebral embolism and thrombosis NOS (I63.0-I63.2, I65.9)
pulmonary embolism and thrombosis (I26.-)
renal embolism and thrombosis (N28.0)
retinal embolism and thrombosis (H34.-)
septic embolism and thrombosis (I76)
vertebral embolism and thrombosis (I63.0-I63.2, I65.0)

I74.0 Embolism and thrombosis of abdominal aorta

I74.01 Saddle embolus of abdominal aorta MCC
CC Excl: I26.01-I26.99, I27.82, I74.01-I74.10, I74.19, I87.8, I99.8-I99.9

I74.09 Other arterial embolism and thrombosis of abdominal aorta CC
Aortic bifurcation syndrome
Leriche's syndrome
Aortoiliac obstruction
CC Excl: See code: I74.01

I74.1 Embolism and thrombosis of other and unspecified parts of aorta

I74.10 Embolism and thrombosis of unspecified parts of aorta CC
CC Excl: See code: I74.01

I74.11 Embolism and thrombosis of thoracic aorta CC
CC Excl: E08.51-E08.59, E08.618-E08.638, E08.649-E08.8, E09.51-E09.59, E09.618-E09.638, E09.649-E09.8, E10.51-E10.59, E10.618-E10.638, E10.649, E10.69-E10.8, E11.51-E11.59, E11.618-E11.638, E11.649, E11.69-E11.8, E13.51-E13.59, E13.618-E13.638, E13.649-E13.8, I74.11, I74.8-I74.9, I76, I87.8, I99.8-I99.9

I74.19 Embolism and thrombosis of other parts of aorta CC
CC Excl: I26.01-I26.99, I27.82, I74.01-I74.10, I74.19, I87.8, I99.8-I99.9

I74.2 Embolism and thrombosis of arteries of the upper extremities CC
CC Excl: E08.51-E08.59, E08.618-E08.638, E08.649-E08.8, E09.51-E09.59, E09.618-E09.638, E09.649-E09.8, E10.51-E10.59, E10.618-E10.638, E10.649, E10.69-E10.8, E11.51-E11.59, E11.618-E11.638, E11.649, E11.69-E11.8, E13.51-E13.59, E13.618-E13.638, E13.649-E13.8, I74.2, I74.8-I74.9, I76, I87.8, I99.8-I99.9

I74.3 Embolism and thrombosis of arteries of the lower extremities CC
CC Excl: E08.51-E08.59, E08.618-E08.638, E08.649-E08.8, E09.51-E09.59, E09.618-E09.638, E09.649-E09.8, E10.51-E10.59, E10.618-E10.638, E10.649, E10.69-E10.8, E11.51-E11.59, E11.618-E11.638, E11.649, E11.69-E11.8, E13.51-E13.59, E13.618-E13.638, E13.649-E13.8, I74.3-I74.4, I74.8-I74.9, I76, I87.8, I99.8-I99.9

I74.4 Embolism and thrombosis of arteries of extremities, unspecified CC
Peripheral arterial embolism NOS
CC Excl: See code: I74.3

I74.5 Embolism and thrombosis of iliac artery CC
CC Excl: E08.51-E08.59, E08.618-E08.638, E08.649-E08.8, E09.51-E09.59, E09.618-E09.638, E09.649-E09.8, E10.51-E10.59, E10.618-E10.638, E10.649, E10.69-E10.8, E11.51-E11.59, E11.618-E11.638, E11.649, E11.69-E11.8, E13.51-E13.59, E13.618-E13.638, E13.649-E13.8, I74.5-I74.9, I76, I87.8, I99.8-I99.9

I74.8 Embolism and thrombosis of other arteries CC
CC Excl: E08.51-E08.59, E08.618-E08.638, E08.649-E08.8, E09.51-E09.59, E09.618-E09.638, E09.649-E09.8, E10.51-E10.59, E10.618-E10.638, E10.649, E10.69-E10.8, E11.51-E11.59, E11.618-E11.638, E11.649, E11.69-E11.8, E13.51-E13.59, E13.618-E13.638, E13.649-E13.8, I74.8-I74.9, I76, I87.8, I99.8-I99.9

I74.9 Embolism and thrombosis of unspecified artery CC
CC Excl: See code: I74.8

I75 Atheroembolism
Atherothrombotic microembolism
Cholesterol embolism

I75.0 Atheroembolism of extremities

I75.01 Atheroembolism of upper extremity

CC Excl: For CC codes in subcategory I75.01, unless otherwise noted: E08.51-E08.59, E08.618-E08.638, E08.649-E08.8, E09.51-E09.59, E09.618-E09.638, E09.649-E09.8, E10.51-E10.59, E10.618-E10.638, E10.649, E10.69-E10.8, E11.51-E11.59, E11.618-E11.638, E11.649, E11.69-E11.8, E13.51-E13.59, E13.618-E13.638, E13.649-E13.8, I74.8-I75.019, I76, I87.8, I99.8-I99.9

I75.011 Atheroembolism of right upper extremity CC

I75.012 Atheroembolism of left upper extremity CC

I75.013 Atheroembolism of bilateral upper extremities CC

I75.019 Atheroembolism of unspecified upper extremity CC

✓6th **I75.Ø2 Atheroembolism of lower extremity**

CC Excl: For CC codes in subcategory I75.Ø2, unless otherwise noted: EØ8.51-EØ8.59, EØ8.618-EØ8.638, EØ8.649-EØ8.8, EØ9.51-EØ9.59, EØ9.618-EØ9.638, EØ9.649-EØ9.8, E1Ø.51-E1Ø.59, E1Ø.618-E1Ø.638, E1Ø.649, E1Ø.69-E1Ø.8, E11.51-E11.59, E11.618-E11.638, E11.649, E11.69-E11.8, E13.51-E13.59, E13.618-E13.638, E13.649-E13.8, I74.8-I74.9, I75.Ø21-I75.Ø29, I76, I87.8, I99.8-I99.9

I75.Ø21 Atheroembolism of right lower extremity CC

I75.Ø22 Atheroembolism of left lower extremity CC

I75.Ø23 Atheroembolism of bilateral lower extremities CC

I75.Ø29 Atheroembolism of unspecified lower extremity CC

✓5th **I75.8 Atheroembolism of other sites**

I75.81 Atheroembolism of kidney CC

Use additional code for any associated acute kidney failure and chronic kidney disease (N17.-, N18.-)

CC Excl: EØ8.51-EØ8.59, EØ8.618-EØ8.638, EØ8.649-EØ8.8, EØ9.51-EØ9.59, EØ9.618-EØ9.638, EØ9.649-EØ9.8, E1Ø.51-E1Ø.59, E1Ø.618-E1Ø.638, E1Ø.649, E1Ø.69-E1Ø.8, E11.51-E11.59, E11.618-E11.638, E11.649, E11.69-E11.8, E13.51-E13.59, E13.618-E13.638, E13.649-E13.8, I74.8-I74.9, I75.81, I76, I87.8, I99.8-I99.9

I75.89 Atheroembolism of other site CC

CC Excl: EØ8.51-EØ8.59, EØ8.618-EØ8.638, EØ8.649-EØ8.8, EØ9.51-EØ9.59, EØ9.618-EØ9.638, EØ9.649-EØ9.8, E1Ø.51-E1Ø.59, E1Ø.618-E1Ø.638, E1Ø.649, E1Ø.69-E1Ø.8, E11.51-E11.59, E11.618-E11.638, E11.649, E11.69-E11.8, E13.51-E13.59, E13.618-E13.638, E13.649-E13.8, I74.8-I74.9, I75.89-I76, I87.8, I99.8-I99.9

I76 Septic arterial embolism CC

Code first underlying infection, such as:
infective endocarditis (I33.Ø)
lung abscess (J85.-)

Use additional code to identify the site of the embolism (I74.-)

EXCLUDES 2 *septic pulmonary embolism (I26.Ø1, I26.9Ø)*

CC Excl: See code: I74.8

✓4th **I77 Other disorders of arteries and arterioles**

EXCLUDES 2 *collagen (vascular) diseases (M3Ø-M36)*
hypersensitivity angiitis (M31.Ø)
pulmonary artery (I28.-)

I77.Ø Arteriovenous fistula, acquired

Aneurysmal varix
Arteriovenous aneurysm, acquired

EXCLUDES 1 *arteriovenous aneurysm NOS (Q27.3-)*
presence of arteriovenous shunt (fistula) for dialysis (Z99.2)
traumatic—see injury of blood vessel by body region

EXCLUDES 2 *cerebral (I67.1)*
coronary (I25.4)

I77.1 Stricture of artery

Narrowing of artery

I77.2 Rupture of artery CC

Erosion of artery
Fistula of artery
Ulcer of artery

EXCLUDES 1 *traumatic rupture of artery—see injury of blood vessel by body region*

CC Excl: I25.42, I67.Ø, I77.2, I77.72-I77.79

I77.3 Arterial fibromuscular dysplasia

Fibromuscular hyperplasia (of) carotid artery
Fibromuscular hyperplasia (of) renal artery

I77.4 Celiac artery compression syndrome CC

CC Excl: I77.4

I77.5 Necrosis of artery CC

CC Excl: I77.5, M31.8-M31.9

I77.6 Arteritis, unspecified

Aortitis NOS
Endarteritis NOS

EXCLUDES 1 *arteritis or endarteritis:*
aortic arch (M31.4)
cerebral NEC (I67.7)
coronary (I25.89)
deformans (I7Ø.-)
giant cell (M31.5., M31.6)
obliterans (I7Ø.-)
senile (I7Ø.-)

✓5th **I77.7 Other arterial dissection**

EXCLUDES 2 *dissection of aorta (I71.Ø-)*
dissection of coronary artery (I25.42)

CC Excl: For MCC codes in subcategory I77.7, unless otherwise noted: I77.2-I77.3, I77.5-I77.6, I77.89-I77.9, M31.8-M31.9

I77.71 Dissection of carotid artery MCC

I77.72 Dissection of iliac artery MCC

I77.73 Dissection of renal artery MCC

I77.74 Dissection of vertebral artery MCC

I77.79 Dissection of other artery MCC

✓5th **I77.8 Other specified disorders of arteries and arterioles**

✓6th **I77.81 Aortic ectasia**

Ectasis aorta

EXCLUDES 1 *aortic aneurysm and dissection (I71.Ø-)*

I77.81Ø Thoracic aortic ectasia

I77.811 Abdominal aortic ectasia

I77.812 Thoracoabdominal aortic ectasia

I77.819 Aortic ectasia, unspecified site

I77.89 Other specified disorders of arteries and arterioles

I77.9 Disorder of arteries and arterioles, unspecified

✓4th **I78 Diseases of capillaries**

I78.Ø Hereditary hemorrhagic telangiectasia

Rendu-Osler-Weber disease

I78.1 Nevus, non-neoplastic

Araneus nevus
Senile nevus
Spider nevus
Stellar nevus

EXCLUDES 1 *nevus NOS (D22.-)*
vascular NOS (Q82.5)

EXCLUDES 2 *blue nevus (D22.-)*
flammeus nevus (Q82.5)
hairy nevus (D22.-)
melanocytic nevus (D22.-)
pigmented nevus (D22.-)
portwine nevus (Q82.5)
sanguineous nevus (Q82.5)
strawberry nevus (Q82.5)
verrucous nevus (Q82.5)

I78.8 Other diseases of capillaries

I78.9 Disease of capillaries, unspecified

✓4th **I79 Disorders of arteries, arterioles and capillaries in diseases classified elsewhere**

I79.Ø Aneurysm of aorta in diseases classified elsewhere

Code first underlying disease

EXCLUDES 1 *syphilitic aneurysm (A52.Ø1)*

I79.1 Aortitis in diseases classified elsewhere

Code first underlying disease

EXCLUDES 1 *syphilitic aortitis (A52.Ø2)*

I79.8 Other disorders of arteries, arterioles and capillaries in diseases classified elsewhere

Code first underlying disease, such as:
amyloidosis (E85.-)

EXCLUDES 1 *diabetic (peripheral) angiopathy (EØ8-E13 with .51-.52)*
syphilitic endarteritis (A52.Ø9)
tuberculous endarteritis (A18.89)

Diseases of veins, lymphatic vessels and lymph nodes, not elsewhere classified. (I80-I89)

I80 Phlebitis and thrombophlebitis (4th)
INCLUDES endophlebitis
inflammation, vein
periphlebitis
suppurative phlebitis
Code first:
phlebitis and thrombophlebitis complicating abortion, ectopic or molar pregnancy (O00-O07, O08.7)
phlebitis and thrombophlebitis complicating pregnancy, childbirth and the puerperium (O22.-, O87.-)
EXCLUDES 1 *venous embolism and thrombosis of lower extremities ((I82.4-, I82.5-, I82.81-)*

CC Excl: For CC codes in category I80, unless otherwise noted: E08.51-E08.59, E08.618-E08.638, E08.649-E08.8, E09.51-E09.59, E09.618-E09.638, E09.649-E09.8, E10.51-E10.59, E10.618-E10.638, E10.649, E10.69-E10.8, E11.51-E11.59, E11.618-E11.638, E11.649, E11.69-E11.8, E13.51-E13.59, E13.618-E13.638, E13.649-E13.8, I80.00-I80.9, I87.8, I99.8-I99.9

I80.0 Phlebitis and thrombophlebitis of superficial vessels of lower extremities (5th)
Phlebitis and thrombophlebitis of femoropopliteal vein
I80.00 Phlebitis and thrombophlebitis of superficial vessels of unspecified lower extremity
I80.01 Phlebitis and thrombophlebitis of superficial vessels of right lower extremity
I80.02 Phlebitis and thrombophlebitis of superficial vessels of left lower extremity
I80.03 Phlebitis and thrombophlebitis of superficial vessels of lower extremities, bilateral

I80.1 Phlebitis and thrombophlebitis of femoral vein (5th)
I80.10 Phlebitis and thrombophlebitis of unspecified femoral vein CC
I80.11 Phlebitis and thrombophlebitis of right femoral vein CC
I80.12 Phlebitis and thrombophlebitis of left femoral vein CC
I80.13 Phlebitis and thrombophlebitis of femoral vein, bilateral CC

I80.2 Phlebitis and thrombophlebitis of other and unspecified deep vessels of lower extremities (5th)
I80.20 Phlebitis and thrombophlebitis of unspecified deep vessels of lower extremities (6th)
I80.201 Phlebitis and thrombophlebitis of unspecified deep vessels of right lower extremity CC
I80.202 Phlebitis and thrombophlebitis of unspecified deep vessels of left lower extremity CC
I80.203 Phlebitis and thrombophlebitis of unspecified deep vessels of lower extremities, bilateral CC
I80.209 Phlebitis and thrombophlebitis of unspecified deep vessels of unspecified lower extremity CC
I80.21 Phlebitis and thrombophlebitis of iliac vein (6th)
I80.211 Phlebitis and thrombophlebitis of right iliac vein CC
I80.212 Phlebitis and thrombophlebitis of left iliac vein CC
I80.213 Phlebitis and thrombophlebitis of iliac vein, bilateral CC
I80.219 Phlebitis and thrombophlebitis of unspecified iliac vein CC
I80.22 Phlebitis and thrombophlebitis of popliteal vein (6th)
I80.221 Phlebitis and thrombophlebitis of right popliteal vein CC
I80.222 Phlebitis and thrombophlebitis of left popliteal vein CC
I80.223 Phlebitis and thrombophlebitis of popliteal vein, bilateral CC
I80.229 Phlebitis and thrombophlebitis of unspecified popliteal vein CC
I80.23 Phlebitis and thrombophlebitis of tibial vein (6th)
I80.231 Phlebitis and thrombophlebitis of right tibial vein CC
I80.232 Phlebitis and thrombophlebitis of left tibial vein CC
I80.233 Phlebitis and thrombophlebitis of tibial vein, bilateral CC
I80.239 Phlebitis and thrombophlebitis of unspecified tibial vein CC
I80.29 Phlebitis and thrombophlebitis of other deep vessels of lower extremities (6th)
I80.291 Phlebitis and thrombophlebitis of other deep vessels of right lower extremity CC
I80.292 Phlebitis and thrombophlebitis of other deep vessels of left lower extremity CC
I80.293 Phlebitis and thrombophlebitis of other deep vessels of lower extremity, bilateral CC
I80.299 Phlebitis and thrombophlebitis of other deep vessels of unspecified lower extremity CC
I80.3 Phlebitis and thrombophlebitis of lower extremities, unspecified
I80.8 Phlebitis and thrombophlebitis of other sites
I80.9 Phlebitis and thrombophlebitis of unspecified site

I81 Portal vein thrombosis MCC
Portal (vein) obstruction
EXCLUDES 2 *hepatic vein thrombosis (I82.0)*
phlebitis of portal vein (K75.1)
CC Excl: E08.51-E08.59, E08.618-E08.638, E08.649-E08.8, E09.51-E09.59, E09.618-E09.638, E09.649-E09.8, E10.51-E10.59, E10.618-E10.638, E10.649, E10.69-E10.8, E11.51-E11.59, E11.618-E11.638, E11.649, E11.69-E11.8, E13.51-E13.59, E13.618-E13.638, E13.649-E13.8, I81, I82.210-I82.211, I82.290-I82.291, I82.401-I82.91, I87.8, I99.8-I99.9

I82 Other venous embolism and thrombosis (4th)
Code first venous embolism and thrombosis complicating:
abortion, ectopic or molar pregnancy (O00-O07, O08.7)
pregnancy, childbirth and the puerperium (O22.-, O87.-)
EXCLUDES 2 *venous embolism and thrombosis (of):*
cerebral (I63.6, I67.6)
coronary (I21-I25)
intracranial and intraspinal, septic or NOS (G08)
intracranial, nonpyogenic (I67.6)
intraspinal, nonpyogenic (G95.1)
mesenteric (K55.0)
portal (I81)
pulmonary (I26.-)

I82.0 Budd-Chiari syndrome MCC
Hepatic vein thrombosis
CC Excl: E08.51-E08.59, E08.618-E08.638, E08.649-E08.8, E09.51-E09.59, E09.618-E09.638, E09.649-E09.8, E10.51-E10.59, E10.618-E10.638, E10.649, E10.69-E10.8, E11.51-E11.59, E11.618-E11.638, E11.649, E11.69-E11.8, E13.51-E13.59, E13.618-E13.638, E13.649-E13.8, I82.0, I82.210-I82.211, I82.290-I82.291, I82.401-I82.91, I87.8, I99.8-I99.9

I82.1 Thrombophlebitis migrans CC
CC Excl: E08.51-E08.59, E08.618-E08.638, E08.649-E08.8, E09.51-E09.59, E09.618-E09.638, E09.649-E09.8, E10.51-E10.59, E10.618-E10.638, E10.649, E10.69-E10.8, E11.51-E11.59, E11.618-E11.638, E11.649, E11.69-E11.8, E13.51-E13.59, E13.618-E13.638, E13.649-E13.8, I82.1-I82.211, I82.290-I82.291, I82.401-I82.91, I87.8, I99.8-I99.9

I82.2 Embolism and thrombosis of vena cava and other thoracic veins (5th)
I82.21 Embolism and thrombosis of superior vena cava (6th)
I82.210 Acute embolism and thrombosis of superior vena cava CC
Embolism and thrombosis of superior vena cava NOS
CC Excl: E08.51-E08.59, E08.618-E08.638, E08.649-E08.8, E09.51-E09.59, E09.618-E09.638, E09.649-E09.8, E10.51-E10.59, E10.618-E10.638, E10.649, E10.69-E10.8, E11.51-E11.59, E11.618-E11.638, E11.649, E11.69-E11.8, E13.51-E13.59, E13.618-E13.638, E13.649-E13.8, I82.210-I82.211, I82.290-I82.291, I82.401-I82.91, I87.8, I99.8-I99.9
I82.211 Chronic embolism and thrombosis of superior vena cava CC
CC Excl: See code: I82.210

✓6th I82.22 Embolism and thrombosis of inferior vena cava

I82.220 Acute embolism and thrombosis of inferior vena cava MCC

Embolism and thrombosis of inferior vena cava NOS

CC Excl: E08.51-E08.59, E08.618-E08.638, E08.649-E08.8, E09.51-E09.59, E09.618-E09.638, E09.649-E09.8, E10.51-E10.59, E10.618-E10.638, E10.649, E10.69-E10.8, E11.51-E11.59, E11.618-E11.638, E11.649, E11.69-E11.8, E13.51-E13.59, E13.618-E13.638, E13.649-E13.8, I82.210-I82.291, I82.401-I82.91, I87.8, I99.8-I99.9

I82.221 Chronic embolism and thrombosis of inferior vena cava MCC

CC Excl: See code: I82.220

✓6th I82.29 Embolism and thrombosis of other thoracic veins

Embolism and thrombosis of brachiocephalic (innominate) vein

I82.290 Acute embolism and thrombosis of other thoracic veins CC

CC Excl: See code: I82.210

I82.291 Chronic embolism and thrombosis of other thoracic veins CC

CC Excl: See code: I82.210

I82.3 Embolism and thrombosis of renal vein CC

CC Excl: E08.51-E08.59, E08.618-E08.638, E08.649-E08.8, E09.51-E09.59, E09.618-E09.638, E09.649-E09.8, E10.51-E10.59, E10.618-E10.638, E10.649, E10.69-E10.8, E11.51-E11.59, E11.618-E11.638, E11.649, E11.69-E11.8, E13.51-E13.59, E13.618-E13.638, E13.649-E13.8, I82.210-I82.211, I82.290-I82.91, I87.8, I99.8-I99.9

✓5th I82.4 Acute embolism and thrombosis of deep veins of lower extremity

CC Excl: For CC codes in subcategory I82.4, unless otherwise noted: E08.51-E08.59, E08.618-E08.638, E08.649-E08.8, E09.51-E09.59, E09.618-E09.638, E09.649-E09.8, E10.51-E10.59, E10.618-E10.638, E10.649, E10.69-E10.8, E11.51-E11.59, E11.618-E11.638, E11.649, E11.69-E11.8, E13.51-E13.59, E13.618-E13.638, E13.649-E13.8, I82.210-I82.211, I82.290-I82.291, I82.401-I82.91, I87.8, I99.8-I99.9

✓6th I82.40 Acute embolism and thrombosis of unspecified deep veins of lower extremity

Deep vein thrombosis NOS

DVT NOS

EXCLUDES 1 *acute embolism and thrombosis of unspecified deep veins of distal lower extremity (I82.4Z-)*

acute embolism and thrombosis of unspecified deep veins of proximal lower extremity (I82.4Y-)

3 **I82.401 Acute embolism and thrombosis of unspecified deep veins of right lower extremity** CC

3 **I82.402 Acute embolism and thrombosis of unspecified deep veins of left lower extremity** CC

3 **I82.403 Acute embolism and thrombosis of unspecified deep veins of lower extremity, bilateral** CC

3 **I82.409 Acute embolism and thrombosis of unspecified deep veins of unspecified lower extremity** CC

✓6th I82.41 Acute embolism and thrombosis of femoral vein

3 **I82.411 Acute embolism and thrombosis of right femoral vein** CC

3 **I82.412 Acute embolism and thrombosis of left femoral vein** CC

3 **I82.413 Acute embolism and thrombosis of femoral vein, bilateral** CC

3 **I82.419 Acute embolism and thrombosis of unspecified femoral vein** CC

✓6th I82.42 Acute embolism and thrombosis of iliac vein

3 **I82.421 Acute embolism and thrombosis of right iliac vein** CC

3 **I82.422 Acute embolism and thrombosis of left iliac vein** CC

3 **I82.423 Acute embolism and thrombosis of iliac vein, bilateral** CC

3 **I82.429 Acute embolism and thrombosis of unspecified iliac vein** CC

✓6th I82.43 Acute embolism and thrombosis of popliteal vein

3 **I82.431 Acute embolism and thrombosis of right popliteal vein** CC

3 **I82.432 Acute embolism and thrombosis of left popliteal vein** CC

3 **I82.433 Acute embolism and thrombosis of popliteal vein, bilateral** CC

3 **I82.439 Acute embolism and thrombosis of unspecified popliteal vein** CC

✓6th I82.44 Acute embolism and thrombosis of tibial vein

3 **I82.441 Acute embolism and thrombosis of right tibial vein** CC

3 **I82.442 Acute embolism and thrombosis of left tibial vein** CC

3 **I82.443 Acute embolism and thrombosis of tibial vein, bilateral** CC

3 **I82.449 Acute embolism and thrombosis of unspecified tibial vein** CC

✓6th I82.49 Acute embolism and thrombosis of other specified deep vein of lower extremity

3 **I82.491 Acute embolism and thrombosis of other specified deep vein of right lower extremity** CC

3 **I82.492 Acute embolism and thrombosis of other specified deep vein of left lower extremity** CC

3 **I82.493 Acute embolism and thrombosis of other specified deep vein of lower extremity, bilateral** CC

3 **I82.499 Acute embolism and thrombosis of other specified deep vein of unspecified lower extremity** CC

✓6th I82.4Y Acute embolism and thrombosis of unspecified deep veins of proximal lower extremity

Acute embolism and thrombosis of deep vein of thigh NOS

Acute embolism and thrombosis of deep vein of upper leg NOS

3 **I82.4Y1 Acute embolism and thrombosis of unspecified deep veins of right proximal lower extremity** CC

3 **I82.4Y2 Acute embolism and thrombosis of unspecified deep veins of left proximal lower extremity** CC

3 **I82.4Y3 Acute embolism and thrombosis of unspecified deep veins of proximal lower extremity, bilateral** CC

3 **I82.4Y9 Acute embolism and thrombosis of unspecified deep veins of unspecified proximal lower extremity** CC

✓6th I82.4Z Acute embolism and thrombosis of unspecified deep veins of distal lower extremity

Acute embolism and thrombosis of deep vein of calf NOS

Acute embolism and thrombosis of deep vein of lower leg NOS

3 **I82.4Z1 Acute embolism and thrombosis of unspecified deep veins of right distal lower extremity** CC

3 **I82.4Z2 Acute embolism and thrombosis of unspecified deep veins of left distal lower extremity** CC

3 **I82.4Z3 Acute embolism and thrombosis of unspecified deep veins of distal lower extremity, bilateral** CC

3 **I82.4Z9 Acute embolism and thrombosis of unspecified deep veins of unspecified distal lower extremity** CC

3 HAC = as SDx not POA, in combination with one of the following procedure codes: 0SR[9,B]0[1,2,3,4,J][9,A,Z]; 0SR[9,B]0[7,K]Z; 0SR[A,E]0[0,1,3,J][9,A,Z]; 0SR[A,E]0[7,K]Z; 0SR[C,D,T,U,V,W]0[7,K]Z; 0SR[C,D,T,U,V,W]0J[9,A,Z]; 0SR[R,S]0[1,3,J][9,A,Z]; 0SR[R,S]0[7,K]Z; 0SU[9,B]0BZ; 0SU[A,E,R,S]0BZ.

5th I82.5 Chronic embolism and thrombosis of deep veins of lower extremity
Use additional code, if applicable, for associated long-term (current) use of anticoagulants (Z79.01)
EXCLUDES 1 *personal history of venous embolism and thrombosis (Z86.718)*

CC Excl: For CC codes in subcategory I82.5, unless otherwise noted: See code: I82.4

6th I82.50 Chronic embolism and thrombosis of unspecified deep veins of lower extremity
EXCLUDES 1 *chronic embolism and thrombosis of unspecified deep veins of distal lower extremity (I82.5Z-)*
chronic embolism and thrombosis of unspecified deep veins of proximal lower extremity (I82.5Y-)

I82.501 Chronic embolism and thrombosis of unspecified deep veins of right lower extremity CC
I82.502 Chronic embolism and thrombosis of unspecified deep veins of left lower extremity CC
I82.503 Chronic embolism and thrombosis of unspecified deep veins of lower extremity, bilateral CC
I82.509 Chronic embolism and thrombosis of unspecified deep veins of unspecified lower extremity CC

6th I82.51 Chronic embolism and thrombosis of femoral vein
I82.511 Chronic embolism and thrombosis of right femoral vein CC
I82.512 Chronic embolism and thrombosis of left femoral vein CC
I82.513 Chronic embolism and thrombosis of femoral vein, bilateral CC
I82.519 Chronic embolism and thrombosis of unspecified femoral vein CC

6th I82.52 Chronic embolism and thrombosis of iliac vein
I82.521 Chronic embolism and thrombosis of right iliac vein CC
I82.522 Chronic embolism and thrombosis of left iliac vein CC
I82.523 Chronic embolism and thrombosis of iliac vein, bilateral CC
I82.529 Chronic embolism and thrombosis of unspecified iliac vein CC

6th I82.53 Chronic embolism and thrombosis of popliteal vein
I82.531 Chronic embolism and thrombosis of right popliteal vein CC
I82.532 Chronic embolism and thrombosis of left popliteal vein CC
I82.533 Chronic embolism and thrombosis of popliteal vein, bilateral CC
I82.539 Chronic embolism and thrombosis of unspecified popliteal vein CC

6th I82.54 Chronic embolism and thrombosis of tibial vein
I82.541 Chronic embolism and thrombosis of right tibial vein CC
I82.542 Chronic embolism and thrombosis of left tibial vein CC
I82.543 Chronic embolism and thrombosis of tibial vein, bilateral CC
I82.549 Chronic embolism and thrombosis of unspecified tibial vein CC

6th I82.59 Chronic embolism and thrombosis of other specified deep vein of lower extremity
I82.591 Chronic embolism and thrombosis of other specified deep vein of right lower extremity CC
I82.592 Chronic embolism and thrombosis of other specified deep vein of left lower extremity CC
I82.593 Chronic embolism and thrombosis of other specified deep vein of lower extremity, bilateral CC
I82.599 Chronic embolism and thrombosis of other specified deep vein of unspecified lower extremity CC

6th I82.5Y Chronic embolism and thrombosis of unspecified deep veins of proximal lower extremity
Chronic embolism and thrombosis of deep veins of thigh NOS
Chronic embolism and thrombosis of deep veins of upper leg NOS
I82.5Y1 Chronic embolism and thrombosis of unspecified deep veins of right proximal lower extremity CC
I82.5Y2 Chronic embolism and thrombosis of unspecified deep veins of left proximal lower extremity CC
I82.5Y3 Chronic embolism and thrombosis of unspecified deep veins of proximal lower extremity, bilateral CC
I82.5Y9 Chronic embolism and thrombosis of unspecified deep veins of unspecified proximal lower extremity CC

6th I82.5Z Chronic embolism and thrombosis of unspecified deep veins of distal lower extremity
Chronic embolism and thrombosis of deep veins of calf NOS
Chronic embolism and thrombosis of deep veins of lower leg NOS
I82.5Z1 Chronic embolism and thrombosis of unspecified deep veins of right distal lower extremity CC
I82.5Z2 Chronic embolism and thrombosis of unspecified deep veins of left distal lower extremity CC
I82.5Z3 Chronic embolism and thrombosis of unspecified deep veins of distal lower extremity, bilateral CC
I82.5Z9 Chronic embolism and thrombosis of unspecified deep veins of unspecified distal lower extremity CC

5th I82.6 Acute embolism and thrombosis of veins of upper extremity

CC Excl: For CC codes in subcategory I82.6, unless otherwise noted: See code: I82.4

6th I82.60 Acute embolism and thrombosis of unspecified veins of upper extremity
I82.601 Acute embolism and thrombosis of unspecified veins of right upper extremity CC
I82.602 Acute embolism and thrombosis of unspecified veins of left upper extremity CC
I82.603 Acute embolism and thrombosis of unspecified veins of upper extremity, bilateral CC
I82.609 Acute embolism and thrombosis of unspecified veins of unspecified upper extremity CC

6th I82.61 Acute embolism and thrombosis of superficial veins of upper extremity
Acute embolism and thrombosis of antecubital vein
Acute embolism and thrombosis of basilic vein
Acute embolism and thrombosis of cephalic vein
I82.611 Acute embolism and thrombosis of superficial veins of right upper extremity CC
I82.612 Acute embolism and thrombosis of superficial veins of left upper extremity CC
I82.613 Acute embolism and thrombosis of superficial veins of upper extremity, bilateral CC
I82.619 Acute embolism and thrombosis of superficial veins of unspecified upper extremity CC

6th I82.62 Acute embolism and thrombosis of deep veins of upper extremity
Acute embolism and thrombosis of brachial vein
Acute embolism and thrombosis of radial vein
Acute embolism and thrombosis of ulnar vein
I82.621 Acute embolism and thrombosis of deep veins of right upper extremity CC
I82.622 Acute embolism and thrombosis of deep veins of left upper extremity CC

I82.623 **Acute embolism and thrombosis of deep veins of upper extremity, bilateral** CC

I82.629 **Acute embolism and thrombosis of deep veins of unspecified upper extremity** CC

✓5th **I82.7** **Chronic embolism and thrombosis of veins of upper extremity**

Use additional code, if applicable, for associated long-term (current) use of anticoagulants (Z79.01)

EXCLUDES 1 *personal history of venous embolism and thrombosis (Z86.718)*

CC Excl: For CC codes in subcategory I82.7, unless otherwise noted: See code: I82.4

✓6th **I82.70** **Chronic embolism and thrombosis of unspecified veins of upper extremity**

I82.701 **Chronic embolism and thrombosis of unspecified veins of right upper extremity** CC

I82.702 **Chronic embolism and thrombosis of unspecified veins of left upper extremity** CC

I82.703 **Chronic embolism and thrombosis of unspecified veins of upper extremity, bilateral** CC

I82.709 **Chronic embolism and thrombosis of unspecified veins of unspecified upper extremity** CC

✓6th **I82.71** **Chronic embolism and thrombosis of superficial veins of upper extremity**

Chronic embolism and thrombosis of antecubital vein
Chronic embolism and thrombosis of basilic vein
Chronic embolism and thrombosis of cephalic vein

I82.711 **Chronic embolism and thrombosis of superficial veins of right upper extremity** CC

I82.712 **Chronic embolism and thrombosis of superficial veins of left upper extremity** CC

I82.713 **Chronic embolism and thrombosis of superficial veins of upper extremity, bilateral** CC

I82.719 **Chronic embolism and thrombosis of superficial veins of unspecified upper extremity** CC

✓6th **I82.72** **Chronic embolism and thrombosis of deep veins of upper extremity**

Chronic embolism and thrombosis of brachial vein
Chronic embolism and thrombosis of radial vein
Chronic embolism and thrombosis of ulnar vein

I82.721 **Chronic embolism and thrombosis of deep veins of right upper extremity** CC

I82.722 **Chronic embolism and thrombosis of deep veins of left upper extremity** CC

I82.723 **Chronic embolism and thrombosis of deep veins of upper extremity, bilateral** CC

I82.729 **Chronic embolism and thrombosis of deep veins of unspecified upper extremity** CC

✓5th **I82.A** **Embolism and thrombosis of axillary vein**

CC Excl: For CC codes in subcategory I82.A, unless otherwise noted: See code: I82.4

✓6th **I82.A1** **Acute embolism and thrombosis of axillary vein**

I82.A11 **Acute embolism and thrombosis of right axillary vein** CC

I82.A12 **Acute embolism and thrombosis of left axillary vein** CC

I82.A13 **Acute embolism and thrombosis of axillary vein, bilateral** CC

I82.A19 **Acute embolism and thrombosis of unspecified axillary vein** CC

✓6th **I82.A2** **Chronic embolism and thrombosis of axillary vein**

I82.A21 **Chronic embolism and thrombosis of right axillary vein** CC

I82.A22 **Chronic embolism and thrombosis of left axillary vein** CC

I82.A23 **Chronic embolism and thrombosis of axillary vein, bilateral** CC

I82.A29 **Chronic embolism and thrombosis of unspecified axillary vein** CC

✓5th **I82.B** **Embolism and thrombosis of subclavian vein**

CC Excl: For CC codes in subcategory I82.B, unless otherwise noted: E08.51-E08.59, E08.618-E08.638, E08.649-E08.8, E09.51-E09.59, E09.618-E09.638, E09.649-E09.8, E10.51-E10.59, E10.618-E10.638, E10.649, E10.69-E10.8, E11.51-E11.59, E11.618-E11.638, E11.649, E11.69-E11.8, E13.51-E13.59, E13.618-E13.638, E13.649-E13.8, I82.210-I82.211, I82.290-I82.291, I82.401-I82.91, I87.8, I99.8-I99.9

✓6th **I82.B1** **Acute embolism and thrombosis of subclavian vein**

I82.B11 **Acute embolism and thrombosis of right subclavian vein** CC

I82.B12 **Acute embolism and thrombosis of left subclavian vein** CC

I82.B13 **Acute embolism and thrombosis of subclavian vein, bilateral** CC

I82.B19 **Acute embolism and thrombosis of unspecified subclavian vein** CC

✓6th **I82.B2** **Chronic embolism and thrombosis of subclavian vein**

I82.B21 **Chronic embolism and thrombosis of right subclavian vein** CC

I82.B22 **Chronic embolism and thrombosis of left subclavian vein** CC

I82.B23 **Chronic embolism and thrombosis of subclavian vein, bilateral** CC

I82.B29 **Chronic embolism and thrombosis of unspecified subclavian vein** CC

✓5th **I82.C** **Embolism and thrombosis of internal jugular vein**

CC Excl: For CC codes in subcategory I82.C, unless otherwise noted: See code: I82.B

✓6th **I82.C1** **Acute embolism and thrombosis of internal jugular vein**

I82.C11 **Acute embolism and thrombosis of right internal jugular vein** CC

I82.C12 **Acute embolism and thrombosis of left internal jugular vein** CC

I82.C13 **Acute embolism and thrombosis of internal jugular vein, bilateral** CC

I82.C19 **Acute embolism and thrombosis of unspecified internal jugular vein** CC

✓6th **I82.C2** **Chronic embolism and thrombosis of internal jugular vein**

I82.C21 **Chronic embolism and thrombosis of right internal jugular vein** CC

I82.C22 **Chronic embolism and thrombosis of left internal jugular vein** CC

I82.C23 **Chronic embolism and thrombosis of internal jugular vein, bilateral** CC

I82.C29 **Chronic embolism and thrombosis of unspecified internal jugular vein** CC

✓5th **I82.8** **Embolism and thrombosis of other specified veins**

Use additional code, if applicable, for associated long-term (current) use of anticoagulants (Z79.01)

CC Excl: For CC codes in subcategory I82.8, unless otherwise noted: See code: I82.B

✓6th **I82.81** **Embolism and thrombosis of superficial veins of lower extremities**

Embolism and thrombosis of saphenous vein (greater) (lesser)

I82.811 **Embolism and thrombosis of superficial veins of right lower extremities** CC

I82.812 **Embolism and thrombosis of superficial veins of left lower extremities** CC

I82.813 **Embolism and thrombosis of superficial veins of lower extremities, bilateral** CC

I82.819 **Embolism and thrombosis of superficial veins of unspecified lower extremities** CC

✓6th **I82.89** **Embolism and thrombosis of other specified veins**

I82.890 **Acute embolism and thrombosis of other specified veins** CC

I82.891 Chronic embolism and thrombosis of other specified veins CC

✓5th I82.9 Embolism and thrombosis of unspecified vein

CC Excl: For CC codes in subcategory I82.9, unless otherwise noted: See code: I82B

I82.90 Acute embolism and thrombosis of unspecified vein CC
Embolism of vein NOS
Thrombosis (vein) NOS

I82.91 Chronic embolism and thrombosis of unspecified vein CC

✓4th **I83 Varicose veins of lower extremities**

EXCLUDES 1 *varicose veins complicating pregnancy (O22.0-)*
varicose veins complicating the puerperium (O87.4)

✓5th I83.0 Varicose veins of lower extremities with ulcer
Use additional code to identify severity of ulcer (L97.-)

✓6th I83.00 Varicose veins of unspecified lower extremity with ulcer

I83.001 Varicose veins of unspecified lower extremity with ulcer of thigh A

I83.002 Varicose veins of unspecified lower extremity with ulcer of calf A

I83.003 Varicose veins of unspecified lower extremity with ulcer of ankle A

I83.004 Varicose veins of unspecified lower extremity with ulcer of heel and midfoot A
Varicose veins of unspecified lower extremity with ulcer of plantar surface of midfoot

I83.005 Varicose veins of unspecified lower extremity with ulcer other part of foot A
Varicose veins of unspecified lower extremity with ulcer of toe

I83.008 Varicose veins of unspecified lower extremity with ulcer other part of lower leg A

I83.009 Varicose veins of unspecified lower extremity with ulcer of unspecified site A

✓6th I83.01 Varicose veins of right lower extremity with ulcer

I83.011 Varicose veins of right lower extremity with ulcer of thigh A

I83.012 Varicose veins of right lower extremity with ulcer of calf A

I83.013 Varicose veins of right lower extremity with ulcer of ankle A

I83.014 Varicose veins of right lower extremity with ulcer of heel and midfoot A
Varicose veins of right lower extremity with ulcer of plantar surface of midfoot

I83.015 Varicose veins of right lower extremity with ulcer other part of foot A
Varicose veins of right lower extremity with ulcer of toe

I83.018 Varicose veins of right lower extremity with ulcer other part of lower leg A

I83.019 Varicose veins of right lower extremity with ulcer of unspecified site A

✓6th I83.02 Varicose veins of left lower extremity with ulcer

I83.021 Varicose veins of left lower extremity with ulcer of thigh A

I83.022 Varicose veins of left lower extremity with ulcer of calf A

I83.023 Varicose veins of left lower extremity with ulcer of ankle A

I83.024 Varicose veins of left lower extremity with ulcer of heel and midfoot A
Varicose veins of left lower extremity with ulcer of plantar surface of midfoot

I83.025 Varicose veins of left lower extremity with ulcer other part of foot A
Varicose veins of left lower extremity with ulcer of toe

I83.028 Varicose veins of left lower extremity with ulcer other part of lower leg A

I83.029 Varicose veins of left lower extremity with ulcer of unspecified site A

✓5th I83.1 Varicose veins of lower extremities with inflammation
Stasis dermatitis

I83.10 Varicose veins of unspecified lower extremity with inflammation A

I83.11 Varicose veins of right lower extremity with inflammation A

I83.12 Varicose veins of left lower extremity with inflammation A

✓5th I83.2 Varicose veins of lower extremities with both ulcer and inflammation

CC Excl: For CC codes in subcategory I83.2, unless otherwise noted: I83.001-I83.229, I83.90-I83.93

Use additional code to identify severity of ulcer (L97.-)

✓6th I83.20 Varicose veins of unspecified lower extremity with both ulcer and inflammation

I83.201 Varicose veins of unspecified lower extremity with both ulcer of thigh and inflammation CC A

I83.202 Varicose veins of unspecified lower extremity with both ulcer of calf and inflammation CC A

I83.203 Varicose veins of unspecified lower extremity with both ulcer of ankle and inflammation CC A

I83.204 Varicose veins of unspecified lower extremity with both ulcer of heel and midfoot and inflammation CC A
Varicose veins of unspecified lower extremity with both ulcer of plantar surface of midfoot and inflammation

I83.205 Varicose veins of unspecified lower extremity with both ulcer of other part of foot and inflammation CC A
Varicose veins of unspecified lower extremity with both ulcer of toe and inflammation

I83.208 Varicose veins of unspecified lower extremity with both ulcer of other part of lower extremity and inflammation CC A

I83.209 Varicose veins of unspecified lower extremity with both ulcer of unspecified site and inflammation CC A

✓6th I83.21 Varicose veins of right lower extremity with both ulcer and inflammation

I83.211 Varicose veins of right lower extremity with both ulcer of thigh and inflammation CC A

I83.212 Varicose veins of right lower extremity with both ulcer of calf and inflammation CC A

I83.213 Varicose veins of right lower extremity with both ulcer of ankle and inflammation CC A

I83.214 Varicose veins of right lower extremity with both ulcer of heel and midfoot and inflammation CC A
Varicose veins of right lower extremity with both ulcer of plantar surface of midfoot and inflammation

I83.215 Varicose veins of right lower extremity with both ulcer other part of foot and inflammation CC A
Varicose veins of right lower extremity with both ulcer of toe and inflammation

I83.218 Varicose veins of right lower extremity with both ulcer of other part of lower extremity and inflammation CC A

I83.219 Varicose veins of right lower extremity with both ulcer of unspecified site and inflammation CC A

✓6th I83.22 Varicose veins of left lower extremity with both ulcer and inflammation

I83.221 Varicose veins of left lower extremity with both ulcer of thigh and inflammation CC A

I83.222 Varicose veins of left lower extremity with both ulcer of calf and inflammation CC A

I83.223 Varicose veins of left lower extremity with both ulcer of ankle and inflammation CC A

I83.224 Varicose veins of left lower extremity with both ulcer of heel and midfoot and inflammation CC A
Varicose veins of left lower extremity with both ulcer of plantar surface of midfoot and inflammation

I83.225 Varicose veins of left lower extremity with both ulcer other part of foot and inflammation CC A
Varicose veins of left lower extremity with both ulcer of toe and inflammation

I83.228 Varicose veins of left lower extremity with both ulcer of other part of lower extremity and inflammation CC A

I83.229 Varicose veins of left lower extremity with both ulcer of unspecified site and inflammation CC A

✓5th **I83.8 Varicose veins of lower extremities with other complications**

✓6th **I83.81 Varicose veins of lower extremities with pain**

I83.811 Varicose veins of right lower extremities with pain A

I83.812 Varicose veins of left lower extremities with pain A

I83.813 Varicose veins of bilateral lower extremities with pain A

I83.819 Varicose veins of unspecified lower extremities with pain A

✓6th **I83.89 Varicose veins of lower extremities with other complications**
Varicose veins of lower extremities with edema
Varicose veins of lower extremities with swelling

I83.891 Varicose veins of right lower extremities with other complications A

I83.892 Varicose veins of left lower extremities with other complications A

I83.893 Varicose veins of bilateral lower extremities with other complications A

I83.899 Varicose veins of unspecified lower extremities with other complications A

✓5th **I83.9 Asymptomatic varicose veins of lower extremities**
Phlebectasia of lower extremities
Varicose veins of lower extremities
Varix of lower extremities

I83.90 Asymptomatic varicose veins of unspecified lower extremity A
Varicose veins NOS

I83.91 Asymptomatic varicose veins of right lower extremity A

I83.92 Asymptomatic varicose veins of left lower extremity A

I83.93 Asymptomatic varicose veins of bilateral lower extremities A

✓4th **I85 Esophageal varices**
Use additional code to identify:
alcohol abuse and dependence (F10.-)

✓5th **I85.0 Esophageal varices**
Idiopathic esophageal varices
Primary esophageal varices

I85.00 Esophageal varices without bleeding CC
Esophageal varices NOS
CC Excl: E16.4, I85.00-I85.01, I85.11, I87.8, I99.8-I99.9, K22.6, K25.0-K28.9, K29.01, K29.21, K29.31, K29.41, K29.51, K29.61, K29.71, K29.81, K29.91, K31.811, K92.0-K92.2

I85.01 Esophageal varices with bleeding MCC
CC Excl: E16.4, I85.01, I85.11, I87.8, I99.8-I99.9, K22.10-K22.11, K22.6-K22.719, K25.0-K28.9, K29.01, K29.21, K29.31, K29.41, K29.51, K29.61, K29.71, K29.81, K29.91, K31.811, K55.21, K57.01, K57.11, K57.13, K57.21, K57.31, K57.33, K57.41, K57.51, K57.53, K57.81, K57.91, K57.93, K62.5, K92.0-K92.2

✓5th **I85.1 Secondary esophageal varices**
Esophageal varices secondary to alcoholic liver disease
Esophageal varices secondary to cirrhosis of liver
Esophageal varices secondary to schistosomiasis
Esophageal varices secondary to toxic liver disease
Code first underlying disease

I85.10 Secondary esophageal varices without bleeding CC
CC Excl: E16.4, I85.01-I85.11, I87.8, I99.8-I99.9, K22.6, K25.0-K28.9, K29.01, K29.21, K29.31, K29.41, K29.51, K29.61, K29.71, K29.81, K29.91, K31.811, K92.0-K92.2

I85.11 Secondary esophageal varices with bleeding MCC
CC Excl: I85.01, I85.11, I87.8, I99.8-I99.9

✓4th **I86 Varicose veins of other sites**
EXCLUDES 1 *varicose veins of unspecified site (I83.9-)*
EXCLUDES 2 *retinal varices (H35.0-)*

I86.0 Sublingual varices

I86.1 Scrotal varices ♂
Varicocele

I86.2 Pelvic varices

I86.3 Vulval varices ♀
EXCLUDES 1 *vulval varices complicating childbirth and the puerperium (O87.8)*
vulval varices complicating pregnancy (O22.1-)

I86.4 Gastric varices

I86.8 Varicose veins of other specified sites A
Varicose ulcer of nasal septum

✓4th **I87 Other disorders of veins**

✓5th **I87.0 Postthrombotic syndrome**
Chronic venous hypertension due to deep vein thrombosis
Postphlebitic syndrome
EXCLUDES 1 *chronic venous hypertension without deep vein thrombosis (I87.3-)*

CC Excl: For CC codes in subcategory I87.0, unless otherwise noted: I80.00-I80.9

✓6th **I87.00 Postthrombotic syndrome without complications**
Asymptomatic postthrombotic syndrome

I87.001 Postthrombotic syndrome without complications of right lower extremity

I87.002 Postthrombotic syndrome without complications of left lower extremity

I87.003 Postthrombotic syndrome without complications of bilateral lower extremity

I87.009 Postthrombotic syndrome without complications of unspecified extremity
Postthrombotic syndrome NOS

✓6th **I87.01 Postthrombotic syndrome with ulcer**
Use additional code to specify site and severity of ulcer (L97.-)

I87.011 Postthrombotic syndrome with ulcer of right lower extremity CC

I87.012 Postthrombotic syndrome with ulcer of left lower extremity CC

I87.013 Postthrombotic syndrome with ulcer of bilateral lower extremity CC

I87.019 Postthrombotic syndrome with ulcer of unspecified lower extremity CC

✓6th **I87.02 Postthrombotic syndrome with inflammation**

I87.021 Postthrombotic syndrome with inflammation of right lower extremity

I87.022 Postthrombotic syndrome with inflammation of left lower extremity

I87.023 Postthrombotic syndrome with inflammation of bilateral lower extremity

I87.029 Postthrombotic syndrome with inflammation of unspecified lower extremity

✓6th **I87.03 Postthrombotic syndrome with ulcer and inflammation**
Use additional code to specify site and severity of ulcer (L97.-)

I87.031 Postthrombotic syndrome with ulcer and inflammation of right lower extremity CC

I87.032 Postthrombotic syndrome with ulcer and inflammation of left lower extremity CC

I87.033 Postthrombotic syndrome with ulcer and inflammation of bilateral lower extremity CC

I87.039 Postthrombotic syndrome with ulcer and inflammation of unspecified lower extremity CC

✓6th **I87.09 Postthrombotic syndrome with other complications**

I87.091 Postthrombotic syndrome with other complications of right lower extremity

I87.092 **Postthrombotic syndrome with other complications of left lower extremity**

I87.093 **Postthrombotic syndrome with other complications of bilateral lower extremity**

I87.099 **Postthrombotic syndrome with other complications of unspecified lower extremity**

I87.1 **Compression of vein** CC
Stricture of vein
Vena cava syndrome (inferior) (superior)
EXCLUDES 2 *compression of pulmonary vein (I28.8)*
CC Excl: I87.1

I87.2 **Venous insufficiency (chronic) (peripheral)**

✓5th I87.3 **Chronic venous hypertension (idiopathic)**
Stasis edema
EXCLUDES 1 *chronic venous hypertension due to deep vein thrombosis (I87.0-)*
varicose veins of lower extremities (I83.-)

CC Excl: For CC codes in subcategory I87.3, unless otherwise noted: I83.001-I83.229, I83.90-I83.93, I87.2, I87.8-I87.9, I99.8-I99.9

✓6th I87.30 **Chronic venous hypertension (idiopathic) without complications**
Asymptomatic chronic venous hypertension (idiopathic)

I87.301 **Chronic venous hypertension (idiopathic) without complications of right lower extremity**

I87.302 **Chronic venous hypertension (idiopathic) without complications of left lower extremity**

I87.303 **Chronic venous hypertension (idiopathic) without complications of bilateral lower extremity**

I87.309 **Chronic venous hypertension (idiopathic) without complications of unspecified lower extremity**
Chronic venous hypertension NOS

✓6th I87.31 **Chronic venous hypertension (idiopathic) with ulcer**
Use additional code to specify site and severity of ulcer (L97.-)

I87.311 **Chronic venous hypertension (idiopathic) with ulcer of right lower extremity** CC

I87.312 **Chronic venous hypertension (idiopathic) with ulcer of left lower extremity** CC

I87.313 **Chronic venous hypertension (idiopathic) with ulcer of bilateral lower extremity** CC

I87.319 **Chronic venous hypertension (idiopathic) with ulcer of unspecified lower extremity** CC

✓6th I87.32 **Chronic venous hypertension (idiopathic) with inflammation**

I87.321 **Chronic venous hypertension (idiopathic) with inflammation of right lower extremity**

I87.322 **Chronic venous hypertension (idiopathic) with inflammation of left lower extremity**

I87.323 **Chronic venous hypertension (idiopathic) with inflammation of bilateral lower extremity**

I87.329 **Chronic venous hypertension (idiopathic) with inflammation of unspecified lower extremity**

✓6th I87.33 **Chronic venous hypertension (idiopathic) with ulcer and inflammation**
Use additional code to specify site and severity of ulcer (L97.-)

I87.331 **Chronic venous hypertension (idiopathic) with ulcer and inflammation of right lower extremity** CC

I87.332 **Chronic venous hypertension (idiopathic) with ulcer and inflammation of left lower extremity** CC

I87.333 **Chronic venous hypertension (idiopathic) with ulcer and inflammation of bilateral lower extremity** CC

I87.339 **Chronic venous hypertension (idiopathic) with ulcer and inflammation of unspecified lower extremity** CC

✓6th I87.39 **Chronic venous hypertension (idiopathic) with other complications**

I87.391 **Chronic venous hypertension (idiopathic) with other complications of right lower extremity**

I87.392 **Chronic venous hypertension (idiopathic) with other complications of left lower extremity**

I87.393 **Chronic venous hypertension (idiopathic) with other complications of bilateral lower extremity**

I87.399 **Chronic venous hypertension (idiopathic) with other complications of unspecified lower extremity**

I87.8 **Other specified disorders of veins**
Phlebosclerosis
Venofibrosis

I87.9 **Disorder of vein, unspecified**

✓4th I88 **Nonspecific lymphadenitis**
EXCLUDES 1 *acute lymphadenitis, except mesenteric (L04.-)*
enlarged lymph nodes NOS (R59.-)
human immunodeficiency virus [HIV] disease resulting in generalized lymphadenopathy (B20)

I88.0 **Nonspecific mesenteric lymphadenitis**
Mesenteric lymphadenitis (acute)(chronic)

I88.1 **Chronic lymphadenitis, except mesenteric**
Adenitis
Lymphadenitis

I88.8 **Other nonspecific lymphadenitis**

I88.9 **Nonspecific lymphadenitis, unspecified**
Lymphadenitis NOS

✓4th I89 **Other noninfective disorders of lymphatic vessels and lymph nodes**
EXCLUDES 1 *chylocele, tunica vaginalis (nonfilarial) NOS (N50.8)*
enlarged lymph nodes NOS (R59.-)
filarial chylocele (B74.-)
hereditary lymphedema (Q82.0)

I89.0 **Lymphedema, not elsewhere classified**
Elephantiasis (nonfilarial) NOS
Lymphangiectasis
Obliteration, lymphatic vessel
Praecox lymphedema
Secondary lymphedema
EXCLUDES 1 *postmastectomy lymphedema (I97.2)*

I89.1 **Lymphangitis**
Chronic lymphangitis
Lymphangitis NOS
Subacute lymphangitis
EXCLUDES 1 *acute lymphangitis (L03.-)*

I89.8 **Other specified noninfective disorders of lymphatic vessels and lymph nodes**
Chylocele (nonfilarial)
Chylous ascites
Chylous cyst
Lipomelanotic reticulosis
Lymph node or vessel fistula
Lymph node or vessel infarction
Lymph node or vessel rupture

I89.9 **Noninfective disorder of lymphatic vessels and lymph nodes, unspecified**
Disease of lymphatic vessels NOS

Other and unspecified disorders of the circulatory system (I95-I99)

✓4th I95 **Hypotension**
EXCLUDES 1 *cardiovascular collapse (R57.9)*
maternal hypotension syndrome (O26.5-)
nonspecific low blood pressure reading NOS (R03.1)

I95.0 **Idiopathic hypotension**

I95.1 **Orthostatic hypotension**
Hypotension, postural
EXCLUDES 1 *neurogenic orthostatic hypotension [Shy-Drager] (G90.3)*
orthostatic hypotension due to drugs (I95.2)

I95.2 Hypotension due to drugs
Orthostatic hypotension due to drugs
Use additional code for adverse effect, if applicable, to identify drug (T36-T50 with fifth or sixth character 5)

I95.3 Hypotension of hemodialysis
Intra-dialytic hypotension

✓5th **I95.8 Other hypotension**

I95.81 Postprocedural hypotension

I95.89 Other hypotension
Chronic hypotension

I95.9 Hypotension, unspecified

I96 Gangrene, not elsewhere classified CC
Gangrenous cellulitis
EXCLUDES 1 *gangrene in atherosclerosis of native arteries of the extremities (I70.26)*
gangrene in diabetes mellitus (E08-E13)
gangrene in hernia (K40.1, K40.4, K41.1, K41.4, K42.1, K43.1-, K44.1, K45.1, K46.1)
gangrene in other peripheral vascular diseases (I73.-)
gangrene of certain specified sites—see Alphabetical Index
gas gangrene (A48.0)
pyoderma gangrenosum (L88)
AHA: 2013, 2Q, 34
CC Excl: G89.0-G89.4, I70.261-I70.269, I96, R41.0-R41.3, R41.82, R41.9, R44.8-R44.9, R45.83-R45.84, R46.0-R46.89, R52, R68.0-R68.19, R68.81-R68.83, R68.89-R69

✓4th **I97 Intraoperative and postprocedural complications and disorders of circulatory system, not elsewhere classified**
EXCLUDES 2 *postprocedural shock (T81.1-)*

I97.0 Postcardiotomy syndrome

✓5th **I97.1 Other postprocedural cardiac functional disturbances**
EXCLUDES 2 *acute pulmonary insufficiency following thoracic surgery (J95.1)*
intraoperative cardiac functional disturbances (I97.7-)

CC Excl: For CC codes in subcategory I97.1, unless otherwise noted: D78.81-D78.89, E36.8, E89.810-E89.89, H59.011-H59.019, H59.031-H59.099, H59.811-H59.89, H95.811-H95.89, I97.110-I97.191, I97.3, I97.710-I97.791, I97.88-I97.89, L76.81-L76.82, M96.89, N98.1-N98.9, T81.82XA, T81.89XA, T81.9XXA

✓6th **I97.11 Postprocedural cardiac insufficiency**

I97.110 Postprocedural cardiac insufficiency following cardiac surgery CC

I97.111 Postprocedural cardiac insufficiency following other surgery CC

✓6th **I97.12 Postprocedural cardiac arrest**

I97.120 Postprocedural cardiac arrest following cardiac surgery CC

I97.121 Postprocedural cardiac arrest following other surgery CC

✓6th **I97.13 Postprocedural heart failure**
Use additional code to identify the heart failure (I50.-)

I97.130 Postprocedural heart failure following cardiac surgery CC

I97.131 Postprocedural heart failure following other surgery CC

✓6th **I97.19 Other postprocedural cardiac functional disturbances**
Use additional code, if applicable, to further specify disorder

I97.190 Other postprocedural cardiac functional disturbances following cardiac surgery CC

I97.191 Other postprocedural cardiac functional disturbances following other surgery CC

I97.2 Postmastectomy lymphedema syndrome A
Elephantiasis due to mastectomy
Obliteration of lymphatic vessels

I97.3 Postprocedural hypertension

✓5th **I97.4 Intraoperative hemorrhage and hematoma of a circulatory system organ or structure complicating a procedure**
EXCLUDES 1 *intraoperative hemorrhage and hematoma of a circulatory system organ or structure due to accidental puncture and laceration during a procedure (I97.5-)*
EXCLUDES 2 *intraoperative cerebrovascular hemorrhage complicating a procedure (G97.3-)*

CC Excl: For CC codes in subcategory I97.4, unless otherwise noted: H95.811-H95.89, I85.01, I85.11, I97.3-I97.42, I97.610-I97.62, K21.9, K22.8, K23-K25.0, K25.2, K25.4, K25.6, K26.0, K26.2, K26.4, K26.6, K27.0, K27.2, K27.4, K27.6, K28.0, K28.2, K28.4, K28.6, K29.01, K29.21, K29.31, K29.41, K29.51, K29.61, K29.71, K29.81, K29.91, K31.811, K55.21, K57.01, K57.11, K57.13, K57.21, K57.31, K57.33, K57.41, K57.51, K57.53, K57.81, K57.91, K57.93, K62.5, K92.0-K92.2, M96.89, N98.1-N98.9, P54.1-P54.3, T81.10XA, T81.11XA,T81.12XA, T81.19XA,T81.82XA, T81.89XA, T81.9XXA

✓6th **I97.41 Intraoperative hemorrhage and hematoma of a circulatory system organ or structure complicating a circulatory system procedure**

I97.410 Intraoperative hemorrhage and hematoma of a circulatory system organ or structure complicating a cardiac catheterization CC

I97.411 Intraoperative hemorrhage and hematoma of a circulatory system organ or structure complicating a cardiac bypass CC

I97.418 Intraoperative hemorrhage and hematoma of a circulatory system organ or structure complicating other circulatory system procedure CC

I97.42 Intraoperative hemorrhage and hematoma of a circulatory system organ or structure complicating other procedure CC

✓5th **I97.5 Accidental puncture and laceration of a circulatory system organ or structure during a procedure**
EXCLUDES 2 *accidental puncture and laceration of brain during a procedure (G97.4-)*

I97.51 Accidental puncture and laceration of a circulatory system organ or structure during a circulatory system procedure CC
CC Excl: D78.11-D78.12, D78.81-D78.89, E36.11-E36.8, E89.810-E89.89, G96.11, G97.41-G97.49, H59.011-H59.019, H59.031-H59.099, H59.211-H59.229, H59.811-H59.89, H95.31-H95.32, H95.811-H95.89, I97.3, I97.51-I97.52, J95.71-J95.72, K91.71-K91.72, L76.11-L76.12, L76.81-L76.82, M96.820-M96.821, M96.89, N98.1-N98.9, N99.71-N99.72, T81.10XA, T81.11XA,T81.12XA, T81.19XA,T81.82XA, T81.89XA, T81.9XXA

I97.52 Accidental puncture and laceration of a circulatory system organ or structure during other procedure CC
CC Excl: See code: I97.51

✓5th **I97.6 Postprocedural hemorrhage and hematoma of a circulatory system organ or structure following a procedure**
EXCLUDES 2 *postprocedural cerebrovascular hemorrhage complicating a procedure (G97.5-)*

CC Excl: For CC codes in subcategory I97.6, unless otherwise noted: See code: I97.4

✓6th **I97.61 Postprocedural hemorrhage and hematoma of a circulatory system organ or structure following a circulatory system procedure**

I97.610 Postprocedural hemorrhage and hematoma of a circulatory system organ or structure following a cardiac catheterization CC

I97.611 Postprocedural hemorrhage and hematoma of a circulatory system organ or structure following cardiac bypass CC

I97.618 Postprocedural hemorrhage and hematoma of a circulatory system organ or structure following other circulatory system procedure CC

I97.62 Postprocedural hemorrhage and hematoma of a circulatory system organ or structure following other procedure CC

✓5th **I97.7 Intraoperative cardiac functional disturbances**

EXCLUDES 2 *acute pulmonary insufficiency following thoracic surgery (J95.1)*
postprocedural cardiac functional disturbances (I97.1-)

CC Excl: For CC codes in subcategory I97.7, unless otherwise noted: D78.81-D78.89, E36.8, E89.810-E89.89, H59.011-H59.019, H59.031-H59.099, H59.811-H59.89, H95.811-H95.89, I97.110-I97.191, I97.3, I97.710-I97.791, I97.88-I97.89, L76.81-L76.82, M96.89, N98.1-N98.9, T81.82XA,T81.89XA,T81.9XXA

✓6th **I97.71 Intraoperative cardiac arrest**

I97.710 Intraoperative cardiac arrest during cardiac surgery CC

I97.711 Intraoperative cardiac arrest during other surgery CC

✓6th **I97.79 Other intraoperative cardiac functional disturbances**

Use additional code, if applicable, to further specify disorder

I97.790 Other intraoperative cardiac functional disturbances during cardiac surgery CC

I97.791 Other intraoperative cardiac functional disturbances during other surgery CC

✓5th **I97.8 Other intraoperative and postprocedural complications and disorders of the circulatory system, not elsewhere classified**

Use additional code, if applicable, to further specify disorder

✓6th **I97.81 Intraoperative cerebrovascular infarction**

I97.810 Intraoperative cerebrovascular infarction during cardiac surgery CC

CC Excl: D78.81-D78.89, E36.8, E89.810-E89.89, G97.0, G97.2-G97.32, G97.81-G97.82, H59.011-H59.019, H59.031-H59.099, H59.811-H59.89, H95.811-H95.89, I97.3, I97.810-I97.821, L76.81-L76.82, M96.89, N98.1-N98.9, T81.10XA, T81.11XA,T81.12XA, T81.19XA,T81.82XA, T81.89XA, T81.9XXA

I97.811 Intraoperative cerebrovascular infarction during other surgery CC

CC Excl: See code: I97.810

✓6th **I97.82 Postprocedural cerebrovascular infarction**

I97.820 Postprocedural cerebrovascular infarction during cardiac surgery CC

CC Excl: See code: I97.810

I97.821 Postprocedural cerebrovascular infarction during other surgery CC

CC Excl: See code: I97.810

I97.88 Other intraoperative complications of the circulatory system, not elsewhere classified CC

CC Excl: See code: I97.1

I97.89 Other postprocedural complications and disorders of the circulatory system, not elsewhere classified CC

CC Excl: See code: I97.1

✓4th **I99 Other and unspecified disorders of circulatory system**

I99.8 Other disorder of circulatory system

I99.9 Unspecified disorder of circulatory system

Chapter 10. Diseases of the Respiratory System (J00-J99)

NOTE When a respiratory condition is described as occurring in more than one site and is not specifically indexed, it should be classified to the lower anatomic site (e.g. tracheobronchitis to bronchitis in J40).

Use additional code, where applicable, to identify:
exposure to environmental tobacco smoke (Z77.22)
exposure to tobacco smoke in the perinatal period (P96.81)
history of tobacco use (Z87.891)
occupational exposure to environmental tobacco smoke (Z57.31)
tobacco dependence (F17.-)
tobacco use (Z72.0)

EXCLUDES 2 *certain conditions originating in the perinatal period (P04-P96)*
certain infectious and parasitic diseases (A00-B99)
complications of pregnancy, childbirth and the puerperium (O00-O9A)
congenital malformations, deformations and chromosomal abnormalities (Q00-Q99)
endocrine, nutritional and metabolic diseases (E00-E88)
injury, poisoning and certain other consequences of external causes (S00-T88)
neoplasms (C00-D49)
smoke inhalation (T59.81-)
symptoms, signs and abnormal clinical and laboratory findings, not elsewhere classified (R00-R94)

This chapter contains the following blocks:

J00-J06	Acute upper respiratory infections
J09-J18	Influenza and pneumonia
J20-J22	Other acute lower respiratory infections
J30-J39	Other diseases of upper respiratory tract
J40-J47	Chronic lower respiratory diseases
J60-J70	Lung diseases due to external agents
J80-J84	Other respiratory diseases principally affecting the interstitium
J85-J86	Suppurative and necrotic conditions of the lower respiratory tract
J90-J94	Other diseases of the pleura
J95	Intraoperative and postprocedural complications and disorders of respiratory system, not elsewhere classified
J96-J99	Other diseases of the respiratory system

Acute upper respiratory infections (J00-J06)

EXCLUDES 1 *chronic obstructive pulmonary disease with acute lower respiratory infection (J44.0)*
influenza virus with other respiratory manifestations (J09.X2, J10.1, J11.1)

J00 Acute nasopharyngitis (common cold)
Acute rhinitis
Coryza (acute)
Infective nasopharyngitis NOS
Infective rhinitis
Nasal catarrh, acute
Nasopharyngitis NOS

EXCLUDES 1 *acute pharyngitis (J02.-)*
acute sore throat NOS (J02.9)
pharyngitis NOS (J02.9)
rhinitis NOS (J31.0)
sore throat NOS (J02.9)

EXCLUDES 2 *allergic rhinitis (J30.1-J30.9)*
chronic pharyngitis (J31.2)
chronic rhinitis (J31.0)
chronic sore throat (J31.2)
nasopharyngitis, chronic (J31.1)
vasomotor rhinitis (J30.0)

✓4th **J01 Acute sinusitis**
INCLUDES acute abscess of sinus
acute empyema of sinus
acute infection of sinus
acute inflammation of sinus
acute suppuration of sinus

Use additional code (B95-B97) to identify infectious agent

EXCLUDES 1 *sinusitis NOS (J32.9)*

EXCLUDES 2 *chronic sinusitis (J32.0-J32.8)*

✓5th **J01.0 Acute maxillary sinusitis**
Acute antritis
J01.00 Acute maxillary sinusitis, unspecified
J01.01 Acute recurrent maxillary sinusitis

✓5th **J01.1 Acute frontal sinusitis**
J01.10 Acute frontal sinusitis, unspecified
J01.11 Acute recurrent frontal sinusitis

✓5th **J01.2 Acute ethmoidal sinusitis**
J01.20 Acute ethmoidal sinusitis, unspecified
J01.21 Acute recurrent ethmoidal sinusitis

✓5th **J01.3 Acute sphenoidal sinusitis**
J01.30 Acute sphenoidal sinusitis, unspecified
J01.31 Acute recurrent sphenoidal sinusitis

✓5th **J01.4 Acute pansinusitis**
J01.40 Acute pansinusitis, unspecified
J01.41 Acute recurrent pansinusitis

✓5th **J01.8 Other acute sinusitis**
J01.80 Other acute sinusitis
Acute sinusitis involving more than one sinus but not pansinusitis
J01.81 Other acute recurrent sinusitis
Acute recurrent sinusitis involving more than one sinus but not pansinusitis

✓5th **J01.9 Acute sinusitis, unspecified**
J01.90 Acute sinusitis, unspecified
J01.91 Acute recurrent sinusitis, unspecified

✓4th **J02 Acute pharyngitis**
INCLUDES acute sore throat

EXCLUDES 1 *acute laryngopharyngitis (J06.0)*
peritonsillar abscess (J36)
pharyngeal abscess (J39.1)
retropharyngeal abscess (J39.0)

EXCLUDES 2 *chronic pharyngitis (J31.2)*

J02.0 Streptococcal pharyngitis
Septic pharyngitis
Streptococcal sore throat
EXCLUDES 2 *scarlet fever (A38.-)*

J02.8 Acute pharyngitis due to other specified organisms
Use additional code (B95-B97) to identify infectious agent
EXCLUDES 1 *acute pharyngitis due to coxsackie virus (B08.5)*
acute pharyngitis due to gonococcus (A54.5)
acute pharyngitis due to herpes [simplex] virus (B00.2)
acute pharyngitis due to infectious mononucleosis (B27.-)
enteroviral vesicular pharyngitis (B08.5)

J02.9 Acute pharyngitis, unspecified
Gangrenous pharyngitis (acute)
Infective pharyngitis (acute) NOS
Pharyngitis (acute) NOS
Sore throat (acute) NOS
Suppurative pharyngitis (acute)
Ulcerative pharyngitis (acute)

✓4th **J03 Acute tonsillitis**
EXCLUDES 1 *acute sore throat (J02.-)*
hypertrophy of tonsils (J35.1)
peritonsillar abscess (J36)
sore throat NOS (J02.9)
streptococcal sore throat (J02.0)

EXCLUDES 2 *chronic tonsillitis (J35.0)*

✓5th **J03.0 Streptococcal tonsillitis**
J03.00 Acute streptococcal tonsillitis, unspecified
J03.01 Acute recurrent streptococcal tonsillitis

✓5th **J03.8 Acute tonsillitis due to other specified organisms**
Use additional code (B95-B97) to identify infectious agent
EXCLUDES 1 *diphtheritic tonsillitis (A36.0)*
herpesviral pharyngotonsillitis (B00.2)
streptococcal tonsillitis (J03.0)
tuberculous tonsillitis (A15.8)
Vincent's tonsillitis (A69.1)
J03.80 Acute tonsillitis due to other specified organisms
J03.81 Acute recurrent tonsillitis due to other specified organisms

✓5th **J03.9 Acute tonsillitis, unspecified**
Follicular tonsillitis (acute)
Gangrenous tonsillitis (acute)
Infective tonsillitis (acute)
Tonsillitis (acute) NOS
Ulcerative tonsillitis (acute)
J03.90 Acute tonsillitis, unspecified
J03.91 Acute recurrent tonsillitis, unspecified

✓4th **J04 Acute laryngitis and tracheitis**
Use additional code (B95-B97) to identify infectious agent
EXCLUDES 1 *acute obstructive laryngitis [croup] and epiglottitis (J05.-)*
EXCLUDES 2 *laryngismus (stridulus) (J38.5)*

J04.Ø Acute laryngitis
Edematous laryngitis (acute)
Laryngitis (acute) NOS
Subglottic laryngitis (acute)
Suppurative laryngitis (acute)
Ulcerative laryngitis (acute)
EXCLUDES 1 *acute obstructive laryngitis (J05.Ø)*
EXCLUDES 2 *chronic laryngitis (J37.Ø)*

✓5th **J04.1 Acute tracheitis**
Acute viral tracheitis
Catarrhal tracheitis (acute)
Tracheitis (acute) NOS
EXCLUDES 2 *chronic tracheitis (J42)*

J04.1Ø Acute tracheitis without obstruction

J04.11 Acute tracheitis with obstruction MCC
CC Excl: A15.8-A15.9, A17.9, A18.82, A18.84, A18.89, J04.1Ø-J04.2, J05.1Ø-J05.11, J22, J98.8-J98.9

J04.2 Acute laryngotracheitis
Laryngotracheitis NOS
Tracheitis (acute) with laryngitis (acute)
EXCLUDES 1 *acute obstructive laryngotracheitis (J05.Ø)*
EXCLUDES 2 *chronic laryngotracheitis (J37.1)*

✓5th **J04.3 Supraglottitis, unspecified**

J04.3Ø Supraglottitis, unspecified, without obstruction

J04.31 Supraglottitis, unspecified, with obstruction MCC
CC Excl: A15.8-A15.9, A17.9, A18.82, A18.84, A18.89, J04.Ø-J04.2, J05.1Ø-J05.11, J22, J98.8-J98.9

✓4th **J05 Acute obstructive laryngitis [croup] and epiglottitis**
Use additional code (B95-B97) to identify infectious agent

J05.Ø Acute obstructive laryngitis [croup]
Obstructive laryngitis (acute) NOS
Obstructive laryngotracheitis NOS

✓5th **J05.1 Acute epiglottitis**
EXCLUDES 2 *epiglottitis, chronic (J37.Ø)*

J05.1Ø Acute epiglottitis without obstruction CC
Epiglottitis NOS
CC Excl: J04.31, J05.1Ø-J05.11

J05.11 Acute epiglottitis with obstruction MCC
CC Excl: See code: J04.31

✓4th **J06 Acute upper respiratory infections of multiple and unspecified sites**
EXCLUDES 1 *acute respiratory infection NOS (J22)*
streptococcal pharyngitis (J02.Ø)3

J06.Ø Acute laryngopharyngitis

J06.9 Acute upper respiratory infection, unspecified
Upper respiratory disease, acute
Upper respiratory infection NOS

Influenza and pneumonia (J09-J18)

EXCLUDES 2 *allergic or eosinophilic pneumonia (J82)*
aspiration pneumonia NOS (J69.Ø)
congenital pneumonia (P23.9)
lipid pneumonia (J69.1)
meconium pneumonia (P24.Ø1)
neonatal aspiration pneumonia (P24.-)
pneumonia due to solids and liquids (J69.-)
rheumatic pneumonia (IØØ)
ventilator associated pneumonia (J95.851)

✓4th **J09 Influenza due to certain identified influenza viruses**
EXCLUDES 1 *seasonal influenza due to other identified influenza virus (J1Ø.-)*
seasonal influenza due to unidentified influenza virus (J11.-)

✓5th **J09.X Influenza due to identified novel influenza A virus**
Avian influenza
Bird influenza
Influenza A/H5N1
Influenza of other animal origin, not bird or swine
Swine influenza virus (viruses that normally cause infections in pigs)

J09.X1 Influenza due to identified novel influenza A virus with pneumonia HIV MCC
Code also, if applicable, associated:
lung abscess (J85.1)
other specified type of pneumonia
CC Excl: A15.Ø-A15.6, A15.8-A15.9, A17.9, A18.82, A18.84, A18.89, A21.2, A22.1, A31.Ø, A37.Ø1, A37.11, A37.81, A37.91, A42.Ø, A43.Ø, A48.1, B25.Ø, B39.Ø-B39.2, B44.Ø, B58.3, B59, B67.1, J09.X1-J09.X2, J1Ø.ØØ-J1Ø.1, J11.ØØ-J11.1, J12.Ø-J12.3, J12.89-J18.1, J18.8-J18.9, J22, J44.9, J47.Ø-J7Ø.4, J7Ø.8-J7Ø.9, J98.4, J98.8-J99, Q33.4, R91.1

J09.X2 Influenza due to identified novel influenza A virus with other respiratory manifestations
Influenza due to identified novel influenza A virus NOS
Influenza due to identified novel influenza A virus with laryngitis
Influenza due to identified novel influenza A virus with pharyngitis
Influenza due to identified novel influenza A virus with upper respiratory symptoms
Use additional code, if applicable, for associated:
pleural effusion (J91.8)
sinusitis (JØ1.-)

J09.X3 Influenza due to identified novel influenza A virus with gastrointestinal manifestations
Influenza due to identified novel influenza A virus gastroenteritis
EXCLUDES 1 *'intestinal flu' [viral gastroenteritis] (AØ8.-)*

J09.X9 Influenza due to identified novel influenza A virus with other manifestations
Influenza due to identified novel influenza A virus with encephalopathy
Influenza due to identified novel influenza A virus with myocarditis
Influenza due to identified novel influenza A virus with otitis media
Use additional code to identify manifestation

✓4th **J1Ø Influenza due to other identified influenza virus**
EXCLUDES 1 *influenza due to avian influenza virus (J09.X-)*
influenza due to swine flu (J09.X-)
influenza due to unidentifed influenza virus (J11.-)

✓5th **J1Ø.Ø Influenza due to other identified influenza virus with pneumonia**
Code also associated lung abscess, if applicable (J85.1)

J1Ø.ØØ Influenza due to other identified influenza virus with unspecified type of pneumonia MCC
CC Excl: See code: J09.X1

J1Ø.Ø1 Influenza due to other identified influenza virus with the same other identified influenza virus pneumonia MCC
CC Excl: See code: J09.X1

J1Ø.Ø8 Influenza due to other identified influenza virus with other specified pneumonia HIV MCC
Code also other specified type of pneumonia
CC Excl: See code: J09.X1

J1Ø.1 Influenza due to other identified influenza virus with other respiratory manifestations
Influenza due to other identified influenza virus NOS
Influenza due to other identified influenza virus with laryngitis
Influenza due to other identified influenza virus with pharyngitis
Influenza due to other identified influenza virus with upper respiratory symptoms
Use additional code for associated pleural effusion, if applicable (J91.8)
Use additional code for associated sinusitis, if applicable (JØ1.-)

J1Ø.2 Influenza due to other identified influenza virus with gastrointestinal manifestations
Influenza due to other identified influenza virus gastroenteritis
EXCLUDES 1 *'intestinal flu' [viral gastroenteritis] (AØ8.-)*

✓5th **J1Ø.8 Influenza due to other identified influenza virus with other manifestations**

J1Ø.81 Influenza due to other identified influenza virus with encephalopathy

J1Ø.82 Influenza due to other identified influenza virus with myocarditis

J1Ø.83 Influenza due to other identified influenza virus with otitis media
Use additional code for any associated perforated tympanic membrane (H72.-)

J1Ø.89 Influenza due to other identified influenza virus with other manifestations
Use additional codes to identify the manifestations

✓4th **J11 Influenza due to unidentified influenza virus**

✓5th **J11.Ø Influenza due to unidentified influenza virus with pneumonia**
Code also associated lung abscess, if applicable (J85.1)

J11.ØØ Influenza due to unidentified influenza virus with unspecified type of pneumonia MCC
Influenza with pneumonia NOS
CC Excl: See code: J09.X1

J11.08 Influenza due to unidentified influenza virus with specified pneumonia MCC
Code also other specified type of pneumonia
CC Excl: See code: J09.X1

J11.1 Influenza due to unidentified influenza virus with other respiratory manifestations
Influenza NOS
Influenzal laryngitis NOS
Influenzal pharyngitis NOS
Influenza with upper respiratory symptoms NOS
Use additional code for associated pleural effusion, if applicable (J91.8)
Use additional code for associated sinusitis, if applicable (J01.-)

J11.2 Influenza due to unidentified influenza virus with gastrointestinal manifestations
Influenza gastroenteritis NOS
EXCLUDES 1 *'intestinal flu' [viral gastroenteritis] (A08.-)*

✓5th **J11.8 Influenza due to unidentified influenza virus with other manifestations**

J11.81 Influenza due to unidentified influenza virus with encephalopathy
Influenzal encephalopathy NOS

J11.82 Influenza due to unidentified influenza virus with myocarditis
Influenzal myocarditis NOS

J11.83 Influenza due to unidentified influenza virus with otitis media
Influenzal otitis media NOS
Use additional code for any associated perforated tympanic membrane (H72.-)

J11.89 Influenza due to unidentified influenza virus with other manifestations
Use additional codes to identify the manifestations

✓4th **J12 Viral pneumonia, not elsewhere classified**
INCLUDES bronchopneumonia due to viruses other than influenza viruses
Code first associated influenza, if applicable (J09.X1, J10.0-, J11.0-)
Code also associated abscess, if applicable (J85.1)
EXCLUDES 1 *aspiration pneumonia due to anesthesia during labor and delivery (O74.0)*
aspiration pneumonia due to anesthesia during pregnancy (O29)
aspiration pneumonia due to anesthesia during puerperium (O89.0)
aspiration pneumonia due to solids and liquids (J69.-)
aspiration pneumonia NOS (J69.0)
congenital pneumonia (P23.0)
congenital rubella pneumonitis (P35.0)
interstitial pneumonia NOS (J84.9)
lipid pneumonia (J69.1)
neonatal aspiration pneumonia (P24.-)
AHA: 2013, 4Q, 118

CC Excl: For MCC codes in category J12, unless otherwise noted: A15.0-A15.6, A15.8-A15.9, A17.9, A18.82, A18.84, A18.89, A20.2, A21.1, A22.1, A31.0, A37.01, A37.11, A37.81, A37.91, A42.0, A43.0, A48.1, B25.0, B39.0-B39.2, B44.0, B58.3, B59, B67.1, J09.X1-J09.X2, J10.00-J10.1, J11.00-J11.1, J12.0-J18.1, J18.8-J18.9, J22, J60-J70.4, J70.8-J70.9, J98.4, J98.8-J99, R91.1

J12.0 Adenoviral pneumonia MCC
J12.1 Respiratory syncytial virus pneumonia MCC
J12.2 Parainfluenza virus pneumonia MCC
J12.3 Human metapneumovirus pneumonia HIV MCC

✓5th **J12.8 Other viral pneumonia**

J12.81 Pneumonia due to SARS-associated coronavirus HIV MCC
Severe acute respiratory syndrome NOS
CC Excl: A15.0-A15.6, A15.8-A15.9, A17.9, A18.82, A18.84, A18.89, A21.2, A22.1, A31.0, A37.01, A37.11, A37.81, A37.91, A42.0, A43.0, A48.1, B25.0, B39.0-B39.2, B44.0, B58.3, B59, B67.1, J09.X1-J09.X2, J10.00-J10.1, J11.00-J11.1, J12.0-J18.1, J18.8-J18.9, J22, J44.9, J47.0-J70.4, J70.8-J70.9, J98.4, J98.8-J99, Q33.4, R91.1

J12.89 Other viral pneumonia HIV MCC

J12.9 Viral pneumonia, unspecified HIV MCC

J13 Pneumonia due to Streptococcus pneumoniae HIV MCC
Bronchopneumonia due to S. pneumoniae
Code first associated influenza, if applicable (J09.X1, J10.0-, J11.0-)
Code also associated lung abscess, if applicable (J85.1)
EXCLUDES 1 *congenital pneumonia due to S. pneumoniae (P23.6)*
lobar pneumonia, unspecified organism (J18.1)
pneumonia due to other streptococci (J15.3-J15.4)
AHA: 2013, 4Q, 118
CC Excl: See code: J09.X1

J14 Pneumonia due to Hemophilus influenzae HIV MCC
Bronchopneumonia due to H. influenzae
Code first associated influenza, if applicable (J09.X1, J10.0-, J11.0-)
Code also associated lung abscess, if applicable (J85.1)
EXCLUDES 1 *congenital pneumonia due to H. influenzae (P23.6)*
AHA: 2013, 4Q, 118
CC Excl: See code: J09.X1

✓4th **J15 Bacterial pneumonia, not elsewhere classified**
Bronchopneumonia due to bacteria other than S. pneumoniae and H. influenzae
Code first associated influenza, if applicable (J09.X1, J10.0-, J11.0-)
Code also associated lung abscess, if applicable (J85.1)
EXCLUDES 1 *chlamydial pneumonia (J16.0)*
congenital pneumonia (P23.-)
Legionnaires' disease (A48.1)
spirochetal pneumonia (A69.8)
AHA: 2013, 4Q, 118

CC Excl: For MCC codes in category J15, unless otherwise noted: See code: J09.X1

J15.0 Pneumonia due to Klebsiella pneumoniae HIV MCC
J15.1 Pneumonia due to Pseudomonas HIV MCC

✓5th **J15.2 Pneumonia due to staphylococcus**

J15.20 Pneumonia due to staphylococcus, unspecified HIV MCC

✓6th **J15.21 Pneumonia due to Staphylococcus aureus**

J15.211 Pneumonia due to methicillin susceptible Staphylococcus aureus HIV MCC
MSSA pneumonia
Pneumonia due to Staphylococcus aureus NOS

J15.212 Pneumonia due to methicillin resistant Staphylococcus aureus HIV MCC

J15.29 Pneumonia due to other staphylococcus HIV MCC

J15.3 Pneumonia due to streptococcus, group B HIV MCC
J15.4 Pneumonia due to other streptococci HIV MCC
EXCLUDES 1 *pneumonia due to streptococcus, group B (J15.3)*
pneumonia due to Streptococcus pneumoniae (J13)
J15.5 Pneumonia due to Escherichia coli HIV MCC
J15.6 Pneumonia due to other aerobic Gram-negative bacteria HIV MCC
Pneumonia due to Serratia marcescens
J15.7 Pneumonia due to Mycoplasma pneumoniae MCC
J15.8 Pneumonia due to other specified bacteria HIV MCC
J15.9 Unspecified bacterial pneumonia HIV MCC
Pneumonia due to gram-positive bacteria

✓4th **J16 Pneumonia due to other infectious organisms, not elsewhere classified**
Code first associated influenza, if applicable (J09.X1, J10.0-, J11.0-)
Code also associated lung abscess, if applicable (J85.1)
EXCLUDES 1 *congenital pneumonia (P23.-)*
ornithosis (A70)
pneumocystosis (B59)
pneumonia NOS (J18.9)
AHA: 2013, 4Q, 118

J16.0 Chlamydial pneumonia MCC
CC Excl: See code: J09.X1

J16.8 Pneumonia due to other specified infectious organisms MCC
CC Excl: See code: J09.X1

J17 Pneumonia in diseases classified elsewhere MCC

Code first underlying disease, such as:
Q fever (A78)
rheumatic fever (I00)
schistosomiasis (B65.0-B65.9)

EXCLUDES 1 candidial pneumonia (B37.1)
chlamydial pneumonia (J16.0)
gonorrheal pneumonia (A54.84)
histoplasmosis pneumonia (B39.0-B39.2)
measles pneumonia (B05.2)
nocardiosis pneumonia (A43.0)
pneumocystosis (B59)
pneumonia due to Pneumocystis carinii (B59)
pneumonia due to Pneumocystis jiroveci (B59)
pneumonia in actinomycosis (A42.0)
pneumonia in anthrax (A22.1)
pneumonia in ascariasis (B77.81)
pneumonia in aspergillosis (B44.0-B44.1)
pneumonia in coccidioidomycosis (B38.0-B38.2)
pneumonia in cytomegalovirus disease (B25.0)
pneumonia in toxoplasmosis (B58.3)
rubella pneumonia (B06.81)
salmonella pneumonia (A02.22)
spirochetal infection NEC with pneumonia (A69.8)
tularemia pneumonia (A21.2)
typhoid fever with pneumonia (A01.03)
varicella pneumonia (B01.2)
whooping cough with pneumonia (A37 with fifth-character 1)

AHA: 2013, 4Q, 118

CC Excl: A15.0-A15.6, A15.8-A15.9, A17.9, A18.82, A18.84, A18.89, A21.2, A22.1, A31.0, A37.01, A37.11, A37.81, A37.91, A42.0, A43.0, A48.1, B25.0, B39.0-B39.2, B44.0, B58.3, B59, B67.1, J09.X1-J09.X2, J10.00-J10.1, J11.00-J11.1, J12.0-J12.3, J12.89-J18.1, J18.8-J18.9, J22, J44.9, J47.0-J70.4, J70.8-J70.9, J98.4, J98.8-J99, Q33.4, R91.1

✓4th **J18 Pneumonia, unspecified organism**

Code first associated influenza, if applicable (J09.X1, J10.0-, J11.0-)

EXCLUDES 1 abscess of lung with pneumonia (J85.1)
aspiration pneumonia due to anesthesia during labor and delivery (O74.0)
aspiration pneumonia due to anesthesia during pregnancy (O29)
aspiration pneumonia due to anesthesia during puerperium (O89.0)
aspiration pneumonia due to solids and liquids (J69.-)
aspiration pneumonia NOS (J69.0)
congenital pneumonia (P23.0)
drug-induced interstitial lung disorder (J70.2-J70.4)
interstitial pneumonia NOS (J84.9)
lipid pneumonia (J69.1)
neonatal aspiration pneumonia (P24.-)
pneumonitis due to external agents (J67-J70)
pneumonitis due to fumes and vapors (J68.0)
usual interstitial pneumonia (J84.17)

AHA: 2013, 4Q, 118

CC Excl: For CC/MCC codes in category J18, unless otherwise noted: See code: J17

J18.0 Bronchopneumonia, unspecified organism MCC

EXCLUDES 1 hypostatic bronchopneumonia (J18.2)
lipid pneumonia (J69.1)

EXCLUDES 2 acute bronchiolitis (J21.-)
chronic bronchiolitis (J44.9)

J18.1 Lobar pneumonia, unspecified organism HIV MCC

J18.2 Hypostatic pneumonia, unspecified organism CC

Hypostatic bronchopneumonia
Passive pneumonia

CC Excl: J18.2, J22, J81.1, J98.4, J98.8-J99, R91.1

J18.8 Other pneumonia, unspecified organism HIV MCC

J18.9 Pneumonia, unspecified organism HIV MCC

AHA: 2013, 4Q, 119; 2012, 4Q, 94

Other acute lower respiratory infections (J20-J22)

EXCLUDES 2 chronic obstructive pulmonary disease with acute lower respiratory infection (J44.0)

✓4th **J20 Acute bronchitis**

INCLUDES acute and subacute bronchitis (with) bronchospasm
acute and subacute bronchitis (with) tracheitis
acute and subacute bronchitis (with) tracheobronchitis, acute
acute and subacute fibrinous bronchitis
acute and subacute membranous bronchitis
acute and subacute purulent bronchitis
acute and subacute septic bronchitis

EXCLUDES 1 bronchitis NOS (J40)
tracheobronchitis NOS (J40)

EXCLUDES 2 acute bronchitis with bronchiectasis (J47.0)
acute bronchitis with chronic obstructive asthma (J44.0)
acute bronchitis with chronic obstructive pulmonary disease (J44.0)
allergic bronchitis NOS (J45.909)
bronchitis due to chemicals, fumes and vapors (J68.0)
chronic bronchitis NOS (J42)
chronic mucopurulent bronchitis (J41.1)
chronic obstructive bronchitis (J44.-)
chronic obstructive tracheobronchitis (J44.-)
chronic simple bronchitis (J41.0)
chronic tracheobronchitis (J42)

J20.0 Acute bronchitis due to Mycoplasma pneumoniae
J20.1 Acute bronchitis due to Hemophilus influenzae
J20.2 Acute bronchitis due to streptococcus
J20.3 Acute bronchitis due to coxsackievirus
J20.4 Acute bronchitis due to parainfluenza virus
J20.5 Acute bronchitis due to respiratory syncytial virus
J20.6 Acute bronchitis due to rhinovirus
J20.7 Acute bronchitis due to echovirus
J20.8 Acute bronchitis due to other specified organisms
J20.9 Acute bronchitis, unspecified

✓4th **J21 Acute bronchiolitis**

Acute bronchiolitis with bronchospasm

EXCLUDES 2 respiratory bronchiolitis interstitial lung disease (J84.115)

CC Excl: For CC codes in category J21, unless otherwise noted: J20.0-J21.9

J21.0 Acute bronchiolitis due to respiratory syncytial virus CC

CC Excl: J21.0

J21.1 Acute bronchiolitis due to human metapneumovirus CC
J21.8 Acute bronchiolitis due to other specified organisms CC
J21.9 Acute bronchiolitis, unspecified CC

Bronchiolitis (acute)

EXCLUDES 1 chronic bronchiolitis (J44.-)

J22 Unspecified acute lower respiratory infection

Acute (lower) respiratory (tract) infection NOS

EXCLUDES 1 upper respiratory infection (acute) (J06.9)

Other diseases of upper respiratory tract (J30-J39)

✓4th **J30 Vasomotor and allergic rhinitis**

INCLUDES spasmodic rhinorrhea

EXCLUDES 1 allergic rhinitis with asthma (bronchial) (J45.909)
rhinitis NOS (J31.0)

J30.0 Vasomotor rhinitis

J30.1 Allergic rhinitis due to pollen

Allergy NOS due to pollen
Hay fever
Pollinosis

J30.2 Other seasonal allergic rhinitis

J30.5 Allergic rhinitis due to food

✓5th **J30.8 Other allergic rhinitis**

J30.81 Allergic rhinitis due to animal (cat) (dog) hair and dander

J30.89 Other allergic rhinitis

Perennial allergic rhinitis

J30.9 Allergic rhinitis, unspecified

✓4th J31 Chronic rhinitis, nasopharyngitis and pharyngitis
Use additional code to identify:
exposure to environmental tobacco smoke (Z77.22)
exposure to tobacco smoke in the perinatal period (P96.81)
history of tobacco use (Z87.891)
occupational exposure to environmental tobacco smoke (Z57.31)
tobacco dependence (F17.-)
tobacco use (Z72.Ø)

J31.Ø Chronic rhinitis
Atrophic rhinitis (chronic)
Granulomatous rhinitis (chronic)
Hypertrophic rhinitis (chronic)
Obstructive rhinitis (chronic)
Ozena
Purulent rhinitis (chronic)
Rhinitis (chronic) NOS
Ulcerative rhinitis (chronic)
EXCLUDES 1 *allergic rhinitis (J3Ø.1-J3Ø.9)*
vasomotor rhinitis (J3Ø.Ø)

J31.1 Chronic nasopharyngitis
EXCLUDES 2 *acute nasopharyngitis (JØØ)*

J31.2 Chronic pharyngitis
Atrophic pharyngitis (chronic)
Chronic sore throat
Granular pharyngitis (chronic)
Hypertrophic pharyngitis (chronic)
EXCLUDES 2 *acute pharyngitis (JØ2.9)*

✓4th J32 Chronic sinusitis
INCLUDES sinus abscess
sinus empyema
sinus infection
sinus suppuration
Use additional code to identify:
exposure to environmental tobacco smoke (Z77.22)
exposure to tobacco smoke in the perinatal period (P96.81)
history of tobacco use (Z87.891)
infectious agent (B95-B97)
occupational exposure to environmental tobacco smoke (Z57.31)
tobacco dependence (F17.-)
tobacco use (Z72.Ø)
EXCLUDES 2 *acute sinusitis (JØ1.-)*

J32.Ø Chronic maxillary sinusitis
Antritis (chronic)
Maxillary sinusitis NOS

J32.1 Chronic frontal sinusitis
Frontal sinusitis NOS

J32.2 Chronic ethmoidal sinusitis
Ethmoidal sinusitis NOS
EXCLUDES 1 *Woakes' ethmoiditis (J33.1)*

J32.3 Chronic sphenoidal sinusitis
Sphenoidal sinusitis NOS

J32.4 Chronic pansinusitis
Pansinusitis NOS

J32.8 Other chronic sinusitis
Sinusitis (chronic) involving more than one sinus but not pansinusitis

J32.9 Chronic sinusitis, unspecified
Sinusitis (chronic) NOS

✓4th J33 Nasal polyp
Use additional code to identify:
exposure to environmental tobacco smoke (Z77.22)
exposure to tobacco smoke in the perinatal period (P96.81)
history of tobacco use (Z87.891)
occupational exposure to environmental tobacco smoke (Z57.31)
tobacco dependence (F17.-)
tobacco use (Z72.Ø)
EXCLUDES 1 *adenomatous polyps (D14.Ø)*

J33.Ø Polyp of nasal cavity
Choanal polyp
Nasopharyngeal polyp

J33.1 Polypoid sinus degeneration
Woakes' syndrome or ethmoiditis

J33.8 Other polyp of sinus
Accessory polyp of sinus
Ethmoidal polyp of sinus
Maxillary polyp of sinus
Sphenoidal polyp of sinus

J33.9 Nasal polyp, unspecified

✓4th J34 Other and unspecified disorders of nose and nasal sinuses
EXCLUDES 2 *varicose ulcer of nasal septum (I86.8)*

J34.Ø Abscess, furuncle and carbuncle of nose
Cellulitis of nose
Ulceration of nose
Necrosis of nose

J34.1 Cyst and mucocele of nose and nasal sinus

J34.2 Deviated nasal septum
Deflection or deviation of septum (nasal) (acquired)
EXCLUDES 1 *congenital deviated nasal septum (Q67.4)*

J34.3 Hypertrophy of nasal turbinates

✓5th J34.8 Other specified disorders of nose and nasal sinuses

J34.81 Nasal mucositis (ulcerative)
Code also type of associated therapy, such as:
antineoplastic and immunosuppressive drugs (T45.1X-)
radiological procedure and radiotherapy (Y84.2)
EXCLUDES 2 *gastrointestinal mucositis (ulcerative) (K92.81)*
mucositis (ulcerative) of vagina and vulva (N76.81)
oral mucositis (ulcerative) (K12.3-)

J34.89 Other specified disorders of nose and nasal sinuses
Perforation of nasal septum NOS
Rhinolith

J34.9 Unspecified disorder of nose and nasal sinuses

✓4th J35 Chronic diseases of tonsils and adenoids
Use additional code to identify:
exposure to environmental tobacco smoke (Z77.22)
exposure to tobacco smoke in the perinatal period (P96.81)
history of tobacco use (Z87.891)
occupational exposure to environmental tobacco smoke (Z57.31)
tobacco dependence (F17.-)
tobacco use (Z72.Ø)

✓5th J35.Ø Chronic tonsillitis and adenoiditis
EXCLUDES 2 *acute tonsillitis (JØ3.-)*

J35.Ø1 Chronic tonsillitis

J35.Ø2 Chronic adenoiditis

J35.Ø3 Chronic tonsillitis and adenoiditis

J35.1 Hypertrophy of tonsils
Enlargement of tonsils
EXCLUDES 1 *hypertrophy of tonsils with tonsillitis (J35.Ø-)*

J35.2 Hypertrophy of adenoids
Enlargement of adenoids
EXCLUDES 1 *hypertrophy of adenoids with adenoiditis (J35.Ø-)*

J35.3 Hypertrophy of tonsils with hypertrophy of adenoids
EXCLUDES 1 *hypertrophy of tonsils and adenoids with tonsillitis and adenoiditis (J35.Ø3)*

J35.8 Other chronic diseases of tonsils and adenoids
Adenoid vegetations
Tonsillar tag
Amygdalolith
Ulcer of tonsil
Calculus, tonsil
Cicatrix of tonsil (and adenoid)

J35.9 Chronic disease of tonsils and adenoids, unspecified
Disease (chronic) of tonsils and adenoids NOS

J36 Peritonsillar abscess CC
INCLUDES abscess of tonsil
peritonsillar cellulitis
quinsy
Use additional code (B95-B97) to identify infectious agent
EXCLUDES 1 *acute tonsillitis (JØ3.-)*
chronic tonsillitis (J35.Ø)
retropharyngeal abscess (J39.Ø)
tonsillitis NOS (JØ3.9-)
CC Excl: J22, J36, J98.8-J98.9

✓4th J37 Chronic laryngitis and laryngotracheitis
Use additional code to identify:
exposure to environmental tobacco smoke (Z77.22)
exposure to tobacco smoke in the perinatal period (P96.81)
history of tobacco use (Z87.891)
infectious agent (B95-B97)
occupational exposure to environmental tobacco smoke (Z57.31)
tobacco dependence (F17.-)
tobacco use (Z72.Ø)

J37.Ø Chronic laryngitis
Catarrhal laryngitis
Hypertrophic laryngitis
Sicca laryngitis
EXCLUDES 2 *acute laryngitis (JØ4.Ø)*
obstructive (acute) laryngitis (JØ5.Ø)

J37.1 Chronic laryngotracheitis
Laryngitis, chronic, with tracheitis (chronic)
Tracheitis, chronic, with laryngitis
EXCLUDES 1 *chronic tracheitis (J42)*
EXCLUDES 2 *acute laryngotracheitis (J04.2)*
acute tracheitis (J04.1)

✓4th **J38 Diseases of vocal cords and larynx, not elsewhere classified**
Use additional code to identify:
exposure to environmental tobacco smoke (Z77.22)
exposure to tobacco smoke in the perinatal period (P96.81)
history of tobacco use (Z87.891)
occupational exposure to environmental tobacco smoke (Z57.31)
tobacco dependence (F17.-)
tobacco use (Z72.0)
EXCLUDES 1 *congenital laryngeal stridor (P28.89)*
obstructive laryngitis (acute) (J05.0)
postprocedural subglottic stenosis (J95.5)
stridor (R06.1)
ulcerative laryngitis (J04.0)

✓5th **J38.0 Paralysis of vocal cords and larynx**
Laryngoplegia
Paralysis of glottis

J38.00 Paralysis of vocal cords and larynx, unspecified
J38.01 Paralysis of vocal cords and larynx, unilateral
J38.02 Paralysis of vocal cords and larynx, bilateral

J38.1 Polyp of vocal cord and larynx
EXCLUDES 1 *adenomatous polyps (D14.1)*

J38.2 Nodules of vocal cords
Chorditis (fibrinous)(nodosa)(tuberosa)
Singer's nodes
Teacher's nodes

J38.3 Other diseases of vocal cords
Abscess of vocal cords
Cellulitis of vocal cords
Granuloma of vocal cords
Leukokeratosis of vocal cords
Leukoplakia of vocal cords

J38.4 Edema of larynx
Edema (of) glottis
Subglottic edema
Supraglottic edema
EXCLUDES 1 *acute obstructive laryngitis [croup] (J05.0)*
edematous laryngitis (J04.0)

J38.5 Laryngeal spasm
Laryngismus (stridulus)

J38.6 Stenosis of larynx

J38.7 Other diseases of larynx
Abscess of larynx
Cellulitis of larynx
Disease of larynx NOS
Necrosis of larynx
Pachyderma of larynx
Perichondritis of larynx
Ulcer of larynx

✓4th **J39 Other diseases of upper respiratory tract**
EXCLUDES 1 *acute respiratory infection NOS (J22)*
acute upper respiratory infection (J06.9)
upper respiratory inflammation due to chemicals, gases, fumes or vapors (J68.2)

J39.0 Retropharyngeal and parapharyngeal abscess CC
Peripharyngeal abscess
EXCLUDES 1 *peritonsillar abscess (J36)*
CC Excl: J22, J39.0-J39.1, J98.8-J98.9

J39.1 Other abscess of pharynx CC
Cellulitis of pharynx
Nasopharyngeal abscess
CC Excl: See code: J39.0

J39.2 Other diseases of pharynx
Cyst of pharynx
Edema of pharynx
EXCLUDES 2 *chronic pharyngitis (J31.2)*
ulcerative pharyngitis (J02.9)

J39.3 Upper respiratory tract hypersensitivity reaction, site unspecified
EXCLUDES 1 *hypersensitivity reaction of upper respiratory tract, such as:*
extrinsic allergic alveolitis (J67.9)
pneumoconiosis (J60-J67.9)

J39.8 Other specified diseases of upper respiratory tract
J39.9 Disease of upper respiratory tract, unspecified

Chronic lower respiratory diseases (J40-J47)

EXCLUDES 1 *bronchitis due to chemicals, gases, fumes and vapors (J68.0)*
EXCLUDES 2 *cystic fibrosis (E84.-)*

J40 Bronchitis, not specified as acute or chronic
Bronchitis NOS
Bronchitis with tracheitis NOS
Catarrhal bronchitis
Tracheobronchitis NOS
Use additional code to identify:
exposure to environmental tobacco smoke (Z77.22)
exposure to tobacco smoke in the perinatal period (P96.81)
history of tobacco use (Z87.891)
occupational exposure to environmental tobacco smoke (Z57.31)
tobacco dependence (F17.-)
tobacco use (Z72.0)
EXCLUDES 1 *acute bronchitis (J20.-)*
allergic bronchitis NOS (J45.909)
asthmatic bronchitis NOS (J45.9-)
bronchitis due to chemicals, gases, fumes and vapors (J68.0)

✓4th **J41 Simple and mucopurulent chronic bronchitis**
Use additional code to identify:
exposure to environmental tobacco smoke (Z77.22)
exposure to tobacco smoke in the perinatal period (P96.81)
history of tobacco use (Z87.891)
occupational exposure to environmental tobacco smoke (Z57.31)
tobacco dependence (F17.-)
tobacco use (Z72.0)
EXCLUDES 1 *chronic bronchitis NOS (J42)*
chronic obstructive bronchitis (J44.-)

J41.0 Simple chronic bronchitis
J41.1 Mucopurulent chronic bronchitis
J41.8 Mixed simple and mucopurulent chronic bronchitis

J42 Unspecified chronic bronchitis
Chronic bronchitis NOS
Chronic tracheitis
Chronic tracheobronchitis
Use additional code to identify:
exposure to environmental tobacco smoke (Z77.22)
exposure to tobacco smoke in the perinatal period (P96.81)
history of tobacco use (Z87.891)
occupational exposure to environmental tobacco smoke (Z57.31)
tobacco dependence (F17.-)
tobacco use (Z72.0)
EXCLUDES 1 *chronic asthmatic bronchitis (J44.-)*
chronic bronchitis with airways obstruction (J44.-)
chronic emphysematous bronchitis (J44.-)
chronic obstructive pulmonary disease NOS (J44.9)
simple and mucopurulent chronic bronchitis (J41.-)

✓4th **J43 Emphysema**
Use additional code to identify:
exposure to environmental tobacco smoke (Z77.22)
history of tobacco use (Z87.891)
occupational exposure to environmental tobacco smoke (Z57.31)
tobacco dependence (F17.-)
tobacco use (Z72.0)
EXCLUDES 1 *compensatory emphysema (J98.3)*
emphysema due to inhalation of chemicals, gases, fumes or vapors (J68.4)
emphysema with chronic (obstructive) bronchitis (J44.-)
emphysematous (obstructive) bronchitis (J44.-)
interstitial emphysema (J98.2)
mediastinal emphysema (J98.2)
neonatal interstitial emphysema (P25.0)
surgical (subcutaneous) emphysema (T81.82)
traumatic subcutaneous emphysema (T79.7)

J43.0 Unilateral pulmonary emphysema [MacLeod's syndrome]
Swyer-James syndrome
Unilateral emphysema
Unilateral hyperlucent lung
Unilateral pulmonary artery functional hypoplasia
Unilateral transparency of lung

J43.1 Panlobular emphysema
Panacinar emphysema

J43.2 Centrilobular emphysema
J43.8 Other emphysema
J43.9 Emphysema, unspecified
Bullous emphysema (lung)(pulmonary)
Emphysema (lung)(pulmonary) NOS
Emphysematous bleb
Vesicular emphysema (lung)(pulmonary)

✓4th **J44 Other chronic obstructive pulmonary disease**
INCLUDES asthma with chronic obstructive pulmonary disease
chronic asthmatic (obstructive) bronchitis
chronic bronchitis with airways obstruction
chronic bronchitis with emphysema
chronic emphysematous bronchitis
chronic obstructive asthma
chronic obstructive bronchitis
chronic obstructive tracheobronchitis
Code also type of asthma, if applicable (J45.-)
Use additional code to identify:
exposure to environmental tobacco smoke (Z77.22)
history of tobacco use (Z87.891)
occupational exposure to environmental tobacco smoke (Z57.31)
tobacco dependence (F17.-)
tobacco use (Z72.Ø)
EXCLUDES 1 *bronchiectasis (J47.-)*
chronic bronchitis NOS (J42)
chronic simple and mucopurulent bronchitis (J41.-)
chronic tracheitis (J42)
chronic tracheobronchitis (J42)
emphysema without chronic bronchitis (J43.-)
lung diseases due to external agents (J6Ø-J7Ø)
AHA: 2Ø13, 4Q, 1Ø9

J44.Ø Chronic obstructive pulmonary disease with acute lower respiratory infection CC
Use additional code to identify the infection
CC Excl: J1Ø.Ø8, J41.1-J42, J44.Ø-J44.1

J44.1 Chronic obstructive pulmonary disease with (acute) exacerbation CC
Decompensated COPD
Decompensated COPD with (acute) exacerbation
EXCLUDES 2 *chronic obstructive pulmonary disease [COPD] with acute bronchitis (J44.Ø)*
CC Excl: See code: J44.Ø

J44.9 Chronic obstructive pulmonary disease, unspecified
Chronic obstructive airway disease NOS
Chronic obstructive lung disease NOS
AHA: 2Ø13, 4Q, 129

✓4th **J45 Asthma**
INCLUDES allergic (predominantly) asthma
allergic bronchitis NOS
allergic rhinitis with asthma
atopic asthma
extrinsic allergic asthma
hay fever with asthma
idiosyncratic asthma
intrinsic nonallergic asthma
nonallergic asthma
Use additional code to identify:
exposure to environmental tobacco smoke (Z77.22)
exposure to tobacco smoke in the perinatal period (P96.81)
history of tobacco use (Z87.891)
occupational exposure to environmental tobacco smoke (Z57.31)
tobacco dependence (F17.-)
tobacco use (Z72.Ø)
EXCLUDES 1 *detergent asthma (J69.8)*
eosinophilic asthma (J82)
lung diseases due to external agents (J6Ø-J7Ø)
miner's asthma (J6Ø)
wheezing NOS (RØ6.2)
wood asthma (J67.8)
EXCLUDES 2 *asthma with chronic obstructive pulmonary disease (J44.9)*
chronic asthmatic (obstructive) bronchitis (J44.9)
chronic obstructive asthma (J44.9)

CC Excl: For CC codes in category J45, unless otherwise noted:
J1Ø.Ø8, J22, J45.998, J98.4, J98.8-J99, R91.1

✓5th **J45.2 Mild intermittent asthma**
J45.2Ø Mild intermittent asthma, uncomplicated
Mild intermittent asthma NOS
J45.21 Mild intermittent asthma with (acute) exacerbation CC
J45.22 Mild intermittent asthma with status asthmaticus CC

✓5th **J45.3 Mild persistent asthma**
J45.3Ø Mild persistent asthma, uncomplicated
Mild persistent asthma NOS
J45.31 Mild persistent asthma with (acute) exacerbation CC
J45.32 Mild persistent asthma with status asthmaticus CC

✓5th **J45.4 Moderate persistent asthma**
J45.4Ø Moderate persistent asthma, uncomplicated
Moderate persistent asthma NOS
J45.41 Moderate persistent asthma with (acute) exacerbation CC
J45.42 Moderate persistent asthma with status asthmaticus CC

✓5th **J45.5 Severe persistent asthma**
J45.5Ø Severe persistent asthma, uncomplicated
Severe persistent asthma NOS
J45.51 Severe persistent asthma with (acute) exacerbation CC
J45.52 Severe persistent asthma with status asthmaticus CC

✓5th **J45.9 Other and unspecified asthma**
✓6th **J45.9Ø Unspecified asthma**
Asthmatic bronchitis NOS
Childhood asthma NOS
Late onset asthma
J45.9Ø1 Unspecified asthma with (acute) exacerbation CC
J45.9Ø2 Unspecified asthma with status asthmaticus CC
J45.9Ø9 Unspecified asthma, uncomplicated
Asthma NOS

✓6th **J45.99 Other asthma**
J45.99Ø Exercise induced bronchospasm
J45.991 Cough variant asthma
J45.998 Other asthma

✓4th **J47 Bronchiectasis**
INCLUDES bronchiolectasis
Use additional code to identify:
exposure to environmental tobacco smoke (Z77.22)
exposure to tobacco smoke in the perinatal period (P96.81)
history of tobacco use (Z87.891)
occupational exposure to environmental tobacco smoke (Z57.31)
tobacco dependence (F17.-)
tobacco use (Z72.Ø)
EXCLUDES 1 *congenital bronchiectasis (Q33.4)*
tuberculous bronchiectasis (current disease) (A15.Ø)

J47.Ø Bronchiectasis with acute lower respiratory infection CC
Bronchiectasis with acute bronchitis
CC Excl: A17.9, A18.82, A18.84, A18.89, JØ9.X2, J1Ø.1, J11.1, J44.9, J47.Ø-J47.1, J68.1, J68.4-J68.9, Q33.4

J47.1 Bronchiectasis with (acute) exacerbation CC
CC Excl: See code: J47.Ø

J47.9 Bronchiectasis, uncomplicated
Bronchiectasis NOS

Lung diseases due to external agents (J6Ø-J7Ø)

EXCLUDES 2 *asthma (J45.-)*
malignant neoplasm of bronchus and lung (C34.-)

J6Ø Coalworker's pneumoconiosis A
Anthracosilicosis
Anthracosis
Black lung disease
Coalworker's lung
EXCLUDES 1 *coalworker pneumoconiosis with tuberculosis, any type in A15 (J65)*

J61 Pneumoconiosis due to asbestos and other mineral fibers A
Asbestosis
EXCLUDES 1 *pleural plaque with asbestosis (J92.Ø)*
pneumoconiosis with tuberculosis, any type in A15 (J65)

✓4th **J62 Pneumoconiosis due to dust containing silica**
INCLUDES silicotic fibrosis (massive) of lung
EXCLUDES 1 *pneumoconiosis with tuberculosis, any type in A15 (J65)*
J62.Ø Pneumoconiosis due to talc dust
J62.8 Pneumoconiosis due to other dust containing silica
Silicosis NOS

✓4th **J63 Pneumoconiosis due to other inorganic dusts**
EXCLUDES 1 *pneumoconiosis with tuberculosis, any type in A15 (J65)*
J63.Ø Aluminosis (of lung)
J63.1 Bauxite fibrosis (of lung)
J63.2 Berylliosis
J63.3 Graphite fibrosis (of lung)
J63.4 Siderosis

J63.5 Stannosis

J63.6 Pneumoconiosis due to other specified inorganic dusts

J64 Unspecified pneumoconiosis

EXCLUDES 1 *pneumonoconiosis with tuberculosis, any type in A15 (J65)*

J65 Pneumoconiosis associated with tuberculosis

Any condition in J60-J64 with tuberculosis, any type in A15

Silicotuberculosis

✓4th **J66 Airway disease due to specific organic dust**

EXCLUDES 2 *allergic alveolitis (J67.-)*
asbestosis (J61)
bagassosis (J67.1)
farmer's lung (J67.0)
hypersensitivity pneumonitis due to organic dust (J67.-)
reactive airways dysfunction syndrome (J68.3)

J66.0 Byssinosis

Airway disease due to cotton dust

J66.1 Flax-dressers' disease

J66.2 Cannabinosis

J66.8 Airway disease due to other specific organic dusts

✓4th **J67 Hypersensitivity pneumonitis due to organic dust**

INCLUDES allergic alveolitis and pneumonitis due to inhaled organic dust and particles of fungal, actinomycetic or other origin

EXCLUDES 1 *pneumonitis due to inhalation of chemicals, gases, fumes or vapors (J68.0)*

CC Excl: For CC codes in category J67, unless otherwise noted: A15.0-A15.6, A15.8-A15.9, A17.9, A18.82, A18.84, A18.89, A21.2, A22.1, A31.0, A37.01, A37.11, A37.81, A37.91, A42.0, A43.0, A48.1, B25.0, B39.0-B39.2, B44.0, B58.3, B59, B67.1, J09.X1-J09.X2, J10.00-J10.1, J11.00-J11.1, J12.0-J12.3, J12.89-J18.1, J18.8-J18.9, J22, J44.9, J47.0-J70.4, J70.8-J70.9, J98.4, J98.8-J99, Q33.4, R91.1

J67.0 Farmer's lung

Harvester's lung
Haymaker's lung
Moldy hay disease

J67.1 Bagassosis

Bagasse disease
Bagasse pneumonitis

J67.2 Bird fancier's lung

Budgerigar fancier's disease or lung
Pigeon fancier's disease or lung

J67.3 Suberosis

Corkhandler's disease or lung
Corkworker's disease or lung

J67.4 Maltworker's lung

Alveolitis due to Aspergillus clavatus

J67.5 Mushroom-worker's lung

J67.6 Maple-bark-stripper's lung

Alveolitis due to Cryptostroma corticale
Cryptostromosis

J67.7 Air conditioner and humidifier lung CC

Allergic alveolitis due to fungal, thermophilic actinomycetes and other organisms growing in ventilation [air conditioning] systems

J67.8 Hypersensitivity pneumonitis due to other organic dusts CC

Cheese-washer's lung
Coffee-worker's lung
Fish-meal worker's lung
Furrier's lung
Sequoiosis

J67.9 Hypersensitivity pneumonitis due to unspecified organic dust CC

Allergic alveolitis (extrinsic) NOS
Hypersensitivity pneumonitis NOS

✓4th **J68 Respiratory conditions due to inhalation of chemicals, gases, fumes and vapors**

Code first (T51-T65) to identify cause

Use additional code to identify associated respiratory conditions, such as:
acute respiratory failure (J96.0-)

CC Excl: For CC/MCC codes in category J68, unless otherwise noted: See code: J67

J68.0 Bronchitis and pneumonitis due to chemicals, gases, fumes and vapors CC

Chemical bronchitis (acute)

J68.1 Pulmonary edema due to chemicals, gases, fumes and vapors MCC

Chemical pulmonary edema (acute) (chronic)

EXCLUDES 1 *pulmonary edema (acute) (chronic) NOS (J81.-)*

J68.2 Upper respiratory inflammation due to chemicals, gases, fumes and vapors, not elsewhere classified

J68.3 Other acute and subacute respiratory conditions due to chemicals, gases, fumes and vapors

Reactive airways dysfunction syndrome

J68.4 Chronic respiratory conditions due to chemicals, gases, fumes and vapors

Emphysema (diffuse) (chronic) due to inhalation of chemicals, gases, fumes and vapors
Obliterative bronchiolitis (chronic) (subacute) due to inhalation of chemicals, gases, fumes and vapors
Pulmonary fibrosis (chronic) due to inhalation of chemicals, gases, fumes and vapors

EXCLUDES 1 *chronic pulmonary edema due to chemicals, gases, fumes and vapors (J68.1)*

J68.8 Other respiratory conditions due to chemicals, gases, fumes and vapors

J68.9 Unspecified respiratory condition due to chemicals, gases, fumes and vapors

✓4th **J69 Pneumonitis due to solids and liquids**

EXCLUDES 1 *neonatal aspiration syndromes (P24.-)*
postprocedural pneumonitis (J95.4)

CC Excl: For MCC codes in category J69, unless otherwise noted: See code: J67

J69.0 Pneumonitis due to inhalation of food and vomit MCC

Aspiration pneumonia NOS
Aspiration pneumonia (due to) food (regurgitated)
Aspiration pneumonia (due to) gastric secretions
Aspiration pneumonia (due to) milk
Aspiration pneumonia (due to) vomit

Code also any associated foreign body in respiratory tract (T17.-)

EXCLUDES 1 *chemical pneumonitis due to anesthesia (J95.4)*
obstetric aspiration pneumonitis (O74.0)

J69.1 Pneumonitis due to inhalation of oils and essences MCC

Exogenous lipoid pneumonia
Lipid pneumonia NOS

Code first (T51-T65) to identify substance

EXCLUDES 1 *endogenous lipoid pneumonia (J84.89)*

J69.8 Pneumonitis due to inhalation of other solids and liquids MCC

Pneumonitis due to aspiration of blood
Pneumonitis due to aspiration of detergent

Code first (T51-T65) to identify substance

✓4th **J70 Respiratory conditions due to other external agents**

CC Excl: For CC codes in category J70, unless otherwise noted: See code: J67

J70.0 Acute pulmonary manifestations due to radiation CC

Radiation pneumonitis

Use additional code (W88-W90, X39.0-) to identify the external cause

J70.1 Chronic and other pulmonary manifestations due to radiation CC

Fibrosis of lung following radiation

Use additional code (W88-W90, X39.0-) to identify the external cause

J70.2 Acute drug-induced interstitial lung disorders

Use additional code for adverse effect, if applicable, to identify drug (T36-T50 with fifth or sixth character 5)

EXCLUDES 1 *interstitial pneumonia NOS (J84.9)*
lymphoid interstitial pneumonia (J84.2)

J70.3 Chronic drug-induced interstitial lung disorders

Use additional code for adverse effect, if applicable, to identify drug (T36-T50 with fifth or sixth character 5)

EXCLUDES 1 *interstitial pneumonia NOS (J84.9)*
lymphoid interstitial pneumonia (J84.2)

J70.4 Drug-induced interstitial lung disorders, unspecified

Use additional code for adverse effect, if applicable, to identify drug (T36-T50 with fifth or sixth character 5)

EXCLUDES 1 *interstitial pneumonia NOS (J84.9)*
lymphoid interstitial pneumonia (J84.2)

J70.5 Respiratory conditions due to smoke inhalation

Smoke inhalation NOS

EXCLUDES 1 *smoke inhalation due to chemicals, gases, fumes and vapors (J68.9)*

AHA: 2013, 4Q, 121

J70.8 Respiratory conditions due to other specified external agents
Code first (T51-T65) to identify the external agent

J70.9 Respiratory conditions due to unspecified external agent
Code first (T51-T65) to identify the external agent

Other respiratory diseases principally affecting the interstitium (J80-J84)

J80 Acute respiratory distress syndrome CC
Acute respiratory distress syndrome in adult or child
Adult hyaline membrane disease
EXCLUDES 1 *respiratory distress syndrome in newborn (perinatal) (P22.0)*
CC Excl: J22, J80, J96.00-J96.92, J98.8-J98.9, R09.2

✓4th **J81 Pulmonary edema**
Use additional code to identify:
exposure to environmental tobacco smoke (Z77.22)
history of tobacco use (Z87.891)
occupational exposure to environmental tobacco smoke (Z57.31)
tobacco dependence (F17.-)
tobacco use (Z72.0)
EXCLUDES 1 *chemical (acute) pulmonary edema (J68.1)*
hypostatic pneumonia (J18.2)
passive pneumonia (J18.2)
pulmonary edema due to external agents (J60-J70)
pulmonary edema with heart disease NOS (I50.1)
pulmonary edema with heart failure (I50.1)

J81.0 Acute pulmonary edema MCC
Acute edema of lung
CC Excl: I09.81, I50.9, J22, J81.0, J98.8-J98.9

J81.1 Chronic pulmonary edema CC
Pulmonary congestion (chronic) (passive)
Pulmonary edema NOS
CC Excl: J18.2, J22, J81.1, J98.4, J98.8-J99, R91.1

J82 Pulmonary eosinophilia, not elsewhere classified CC
Allergic pneumonia
Eosinophilic asthma
Eosinophilic pneumonia
Löffler's pneumonia
Tropical (pulmonary) eosinophilia NOS
EXCLUDES 1 *pulmonary eosinophilia due to aspergillosis (B44.-)*
pulmonary eosinophilia due to drugs (J70.2-J70.4)
pulmonary eosinophilia due to specified parasitic infection (B50-B83)
pulmonary eosinophilia due to systemic connective tissue disorders (M30-M36)
pulmonary infiltrate NOS (R91.8)
CC Excl: A15.0-A15.6, A15.8-A15.9, A17.9, A18.82, A18.84, A18.89, A20.2, A21.1, A22.1, A31.0, A37.01, A37.11, A37.81, A37.91, A42.0, A43.0, A48.1, B25.0, B39.0-B39.2, B44.0, B58.3, B59, B67.1, J09.X1-J09.X2, J10.00-J10.1, J11.00-J11.1, J12.0-J12.3, J12.89-J18.1, J18.8-J18.9, J22, J47.0-J70.4, J70.8-J70.9, J82, J98.4, J98.8-J99, Q33.4, R91.1

✓4th **J84 Other interstitial pulmonary diseases**
EXCLUDES 1 *drug-induced interstitial lung disorders (J70.2-J70.4)*
interstitial emphysema (J98.2)
lung diseases due to external agents (J60-J70)

✓5th **J84.0 Alveolar and parieto-alveolar conditions**
CC Excl: For CC codes in subcategory J84.0, unless otherwise noted: A15.0-A15.6, A15.8-A15.9, A17.9, A18.82, A18.84, A18.89, J22, J44.9, J47.0-J70.4, J70.8-J70.9, J84.01-J84.82, J84.89-J84.9, J98.4, J98.8-J99, Q33.4, R91.1

J84.01 Alveolar proteinosis CC
J84.02 Pulmonary alveolar microlithiasis CC
J84.03 Idiopathic pulmonary hemosiderosis CC
Essential brown induration of lung
Code first underlying disease, such as:
disorders of iron metabolism (E83.1-)
EXCLUDES 1 *acute idiopathic pulmonary hemorrhage in infants [AIPHI] (R04.81)*

J84.09 Other alveolar and parieto-alveolar conditions CC

✓5th **J84.1 Other interstitial pulmonary diseases with fibrosis**
EXCLUDES 1 *pulmonary fibrosis (chronic) due to inhalation of chemicals, gases, fumes or vapors (J68.4)*
pulmonary fibrosis (chronic) following radiation (J70.1)
CC Excl: For CC codes in subcategory J84.1, unless otherwise noted: See code: J84.0

J84.10 Pulmonary fibrosis, unspecified
Capillary fibrosis of lung
Cirrhosis of lung (chronic) NOS
Fibrosis of lung (atrophic) (chronic) (confluent) (massive) (perialveolar) (peribronchial) NOS
Induration of lung (chronic) NOS
Postinflammatory pulmonary fibrosis

✓6th **J84.11 Idiopathic interstitial pneumonia**
EXCLUDES 1 *lymphoid interstitial pneumonia (J84.2)*
pneumocystis pneumonia (B59)

J84.111 Idiopathic interstitial pneumonia, not otherwise specified

J84.112 Idiopathic pulmonary fibrosis
Cryptogenic fibrosing alveolitis
Idiopathic fibrosing alveolitis

J84.113 Idiopathic non-specific interstitial pneumonitis
EXCLUDES 1 *non-specific interstitial pneumonia NOS, or due to known underlying cause (J84.89)*

J84.114 Acute interstitial pneumonitis CC
Hamman-Rich syndrome
EXCLUDES 1 *pneumocystis pneumonia (B59)*

J84.115 Respiratory bronchiolitis interstitial lung disease

J84.116 Cryptogenic organizing pneumonia CC
EXCLUDES 1 *organizing pneumonia NOS, or due to known underlying cause (J84.89)*

J84.117 Desquamative interstitial pneumonia CC

J84.17 Other interstitial pulmonary diseases with fibrosis in diseases classified elsewhere
Interstitial pneumonia (nonspecific) (usual) due to collagen vascular disease
Interstitial pneumonia (nonspecific) (usual) in diseases classified elsewhere
Organizing pneumonia due to collagen vascular disease
Organizing pneumonia in diseases classified elsewhere
Code first underlying disease, such as:
progressive systemic sclerosis (M34.0)
rheumatoid arthritis (M05.00-M06.9)
systemic lupus erythematosis (M32.0-M32.9)

J84.2 Lymphoid interstitial pneumonia CC
Lymphoid interstitial pneumonitis
CC Excl: See code: J84.0

✓5th **J84.8 Other specified interstitial pulmonary diseases**
EXCLUDES 1 *exogenous lipoid pneumonia (J69.1)*
unspecified lipoid pneumonia (J69.1)

J84.81 Lymphangioleiomyomatosis MCC ♀
Lymphangiomyomatosis
CC Excl: See code: J84.0

J84.82 Adult pulmonary Langerhans cell histiocytosis CC A
Adult PLCH
CC Excl: See code: J84.0

J84.83 Surfactant mutations of the lung MCC
CC Excl: J84.83-J84.848, P22.0-P28.5, P28.89-P29.2, P29.4, P29.89-P29.9, P84, P94.1-P94.9, P96.0, P96.3-P96.5, P96.82-P96.89

✓6th **J84.84 Other interstitial lung diseases of childhood**
CC Excl: For MCC codes in subcategory J84.84, unless otherwise noted: See code: J84.83

J84.841 Neuroendocrine cell hyperplasia of infancy MCC
J84.842 Pulmonary interstitial glycogenosis MCC
J84.843 Alveolar capillary dysplasia with vein misalignment MCC
J84.848 Other interstitial lung diseases of childhood MCC

J84.89 **Other specified interstitial pulmonary diseases**
Endogenous lipoid pneumonia
Interstitial pneumonitis
Non-specific interstitial pneumonitis NOS
Organizing pneumonia due to known underlying cause
Organizing pneumonia NOS
Code first, if applicable:
poisoning due to drug or toxin (T51-T65 with fifth or sixth character to indicate intent), for toxic pneumonopathy
underlying cause of pneumonopathy, if known
Use additional code, for adverse effect, to identify drug (T36-T5Ø with fifth or sixth character 5), if drug-induced
EXCLUDES 1 *cryptogenic organizing pneumonia (J84.116)*
idiopathic non-specific interstitial pneumonitis (J84.113)
lipoid pneumonia, exogenous or unspecified (J69.1)
lymphoid interstitial pneumonia (J84.2)

J84.9 **Interstitial pulmonary disease, unspecified** CC
Interstitial pneumonia NOS
CC Excl: See code: J84.Ø

Suppurative and necrotic conditions of the lower respiratory tract (J85-J86)

4th **J85 Abscess of lung and mediastinum**
Use additional code (B95-B97) to identify infectious agent.

J85.Ø **Gangrene and necrosis of lung** MCC
CC Excl: AØ6.5, A15.6, A15.8-A15.9, A17.9, A18.82, A18.84, A18.89, J22, J85.Ø-J85.2, J98.8-J98.9

J85.1 **Abscess of lung with pneumonia** MCC
Code also the type of pneumonia
CC Excl: See code: J85.Ø

J85.2 **Abscess of lung without pneumonia** MCC
Abscess of lung NOS
CC Excl: See code: J85.Ø

J85.3 **Abscess of mediastinum** MCC
CC Excl: J22, J85.3, J98.8-J98.9

4th **J86 Pyothorax**
Use additional code (B95-B97) to identify infectious agent
EXCLUDES 1 *abscess of lung (J85.-)*
pyothorax due to tuberculosis (A15.6)

J86.Ø **Pyothorax with fistula** MCC
Bronchocutaneous fistula
Bronchopleural fistula
Hepatopleural fistula
Mediastinal fistula
Pleural fistula
Thoracic fistula
Any condition classifiable to J86.9 with fistula
CC Excl: J22-J86.9, J98.4, J98.8-J99, R91.1

J86.9 **Pyothorax without fistula** MCC
Abscess of pleura
Abscess of thorax
Empyema (chest) (lung) (pleura)
Fibrinopurulent pleurisy
Purulent pleurisy
Pyopneumothorax
Septic pleurisy
Seropurulent pleurisy
Suppurative pleurisy
CC Excl: See code: J86.Ø

Other diseases of the pleura (J9Ø-J94)

J9Ø Pleural effusion, not elsewhere classified CC
Encysted pleurisy
Pleural effusion NOS
Pleurisy with effusion (exudative) (serous)
EXCLUDES 1 *chylous (pleural) effusion (J94.Ø)*
malignant pleural effusion (J91.Ø))
pleurisy NOS (RØ9.1)
tuberculous pleural effusion (A15.6)
CC Excl: A15.Ø-A15.6, A15.8-A15.9, A17.9, A18.82, A18.84, A18.89, J22, J9Ø-J92.9, J94.Ø-J94.9, J98.4, J98.8-J99, RØ9.1, R91.1

4th **J91 Pleural effusion in conditions classified elsewhere**
EXCLUDES 2 *pleural effusion in heart failure (I5Ø.-)*
pleural effusion in systemic lupus erythematosus (M32.13)

J91.Ø ***Malignant pleural effusion*** CC
Code first underlying neoplasm
CC Excl: C45.7-C45.9, C76.8, C78.2-C78.39, C79.89-C7A.ØØ, C7A.Ø98-C7B.ØØ, C7B.Ø9-C8Ø.2, D49.81-D49.9, J9Ø-J91.Ø, J94.Ø, J94.2

J91.8 ***Pleural effusion in other conditions classified elsewhere*** CC
Code first underlying disease, such as:
filariasis (B74.Ø-B74.9)
influenza (JØ9.X2, J1Ø.1, J11.1)
CC Excl: See code: J9Ø

4th **J92 Pleural plaque**
INCLUDES pleural thickening

J92.Ø **Pleural plaque with presence of asbestos**

J92.9 **Pleural plaque without asbestos**
Pleural plaque NOS

4th **J93 Pneumothorax and air leak**
EXCLUDES 1 *congenital or perinatal pneumothorax (P25.1)*
postprocedural air leak (J95.812)
postprocedural pneumothorax (J95.811)
traumatic pneumothorax (S27.Ø)
tuberculous (current disease) pneumothorax (A15.-)
pyopneumothorax (J86.-)

CC Excl: For CC/MCC codes in category J93, unless otherwise noted: J22, J93.9, J95.811-J95.812, J98.4, J98.8-J99, R91.1

J93.Ø **Spontaneous tension pneumothorax** MCC

5th J93.1 **Other spontaneous pneumothorax**

J93.11 **Primary spontaneous pneumothorax** CC

J93.12 **Secondary spontaneous pneumothorax** CC
Code first underlying condition, such as:
catamenial pneumothorax due to endometriosis (N8Ø.8)
cystic fibrosis (E84.-)
eosinophilic pneumonia (J82)
lymphangioleiomyomatosis (J84.81)
malignant neoplasm of bronchus and lung (C34.-)
Marfan's syndrome (Q87.4)
pneumonia due to Pneumocystis carinii (B59)
secondary malignant neoplasm of lung (C78.Ø-)
spontaneous rupture of the esophagus (K22.3)

5th J93.8 **Other pneumothorax and air leak**

J93.81 **Chronic pneumothorax** CC

J93.82 **Other air leak** CC
Persistent air leak

J93.83 **Other pneumothorax** CC
Acute pneumothorax
Spontaneous pneumothorax NOS

J93.9 **Pneumothorax, unspecified** CC
Pneumothorax NOS

4th **J94 Other pleural conditions**
EXCLUDES 1 *pleurisy NOS (RØ9.1)*
traumatic hemopneumothorax (S27.2)
traumatic hemothorax (S27.1)
tuberculous pleural conditions (current disease) (A15.-)

J94.Ø **Chylous effusion** CC
Chyliform effusion
CC Excl: See code: J9Ø

J94.1 **Fibrothorax**

J94.2 **Hemothorax** CC
Hemopneumothorax
CC Excl: See code: J9Ø

J94.8 **Other specified pleural conditions** CC
Hydropneumothorax
Hydrothorax
CC Excl: No excl

J94.9 **Pleural condition, unspecified**

Intraoperative and postprocedural complications and disorders of respiratory system, not elsewhere classified (J95)

✓4th J95 Intraoperative and postprocedural complications and disorders of respiratory system, not elsewhere classified

EXCLUDES 2 *aspiration pneumonia (J69.-)*
emphysema (subcutaneous) resulting from a procedure (T81.82)
hypostatic pneumonia (J18.2)
pulmonary manifestations due to radiation (J7Ø.Ø- J7Ø.1)

✓5th J95.Ø Tracheostomy complications

CC Excl: For CC codes in subcategory J95.Ø, unless otherwise noted: J22, J39.8, J95.ØØ-J95.Ø9, J98.Ø1-J98.Ø9, J98.8-J98.9

J95.ØØ Unspecified tracheostomy complication CC

J95.Ø1 Hemorrhage from tracheostomy stoma CC

J95.Ø2 Infection of tracheostomy stoma CC
Use additional code to identify type of infection, such as:
cellulitis of neck (LØ3.8)
sepsis (A4Ø, A41-)

J95.Ø3 Malfunction of tracheostomy stoma CC
Mechanical complication of tracheostomy stoma
Obstruction of tracheostomy airway
Tracheal stenosis due to tracheostomy

J95.Ø4 Tracheo-esophageal fistula following tracheostomy CC

J95.Ø9 Other tracheostomy complication CC

J95.1 Acute pulmonary insufficiency following thoracic surgery MCC
EXCLUDES 2 *functional disturbances following cardiac surgery (I97.Ø, I97.1-)*
CC Excl: J22, J95.3, J95.821-J95.822, J98.8-J98.9

J95.2 Acute pulmonary insufficiency following nonthoracic surgery MCC
EXCLUDES 2 *functional disturbances following cardiac surgery (I97.Ø, I97.1-)*
CC Excl: See code: J95.1

J95.3 Chronic pulmonary insufficiency following surgery MCC
EXCLUDES 2 *functional disturbances following cardiac surgery (I97.Ø, I97.1-)*
CC Excl: See code: J95.1

J95.4 Chemical pneumonitis due to anesthesia CC
Mendelson's syndrome
Postprocedural aspiration pneumonia
Use additional code for adverse effect, if applicable, to identify drug (T41.- with fifth or sixth character 5)
EXCLUDES 1 *aspiration pneumonitis due to anesthesia complicating labor and delivery (O74.Ø)*
aspiration pneumonitis due to anesthesia complicating pregnancy (O29)
aspiration pneumonitis due to anesthesia complicating the puerperium (O89.Ø1)
CC Excl: D78.81-D78.89, E36.8, E89.81Ø-E89.89, H59.Ø11-H59.Ø19, H59.Ø31-H59.Ø99, H59.811-H59.89, H95.811-H95.89, I97.3, J95.4-J95.5, J95.84, J95.851-J95.89, L76.81-L76.82, M96.89, N98.1-N98.9, T81.82XA, T81.89XA, T81.9XXA

J95.5 Postprocedural subglottic stenosis CC
CC Excl: See code: J95.4

✓5th J95.6 Intraoperative hemorrhage and hematoma of a respiratory system organ or structure complicating a procedure
EXCLUDES 1 *intraoperative hemorrhage and hematoma of a respiratory system organ or structure due to accidental puncture and laceration during procedure (J95.7-)*

J95.61 Intraoperative hemorrhage and hematoma of a respiratory system organ or structure complicating a respiratory system procedure CC
CC Excl: H95.811-H95.89, I85.Ø1, I85.11, I97.3, J95.61-J95.62, J95.83Ø-J95.831, K21.9, K22.8, K23-K25.Ø, K25.2, K25.4, K25.6, K26.Ø, K26.2, K26.4, K26.6, K27.Ø, K27.2, K27.4, K27.6, K28.Ø, K28.2, K28.4, K28.6, K29.Ø1, K29.21, K29.31, K29.41, K29.51, K29.61, K29.71, K29.81, K29.91, K31.811, K55.21, K57.Ø1, K57.11, K57.13, K57.21, K57.31, K57.33, K57.41, K57.51, K57.53, K57.81, K57.91, K57.93, K62.5, K92.Ø-K92.2, M96.89, N98.1-N98.9, P54.1-P54.3, T81.1ØXA, T81.11XA, T81.12XA, T81.19XA, T81.82XA, T81.89XA, T81.9XXA

J95.62 Intraoperative hemorrhage and hematoma of a respiratory system organ or structure complicating other procedure CC
CC Excl: See code: J95.61

✓5th J95.7 Accidental puncture and laceration of a respiratory system organ or structure during a procedure
EXCLUDES 2 *postprocedural pneumothorax (J95.811)*

J95.71 Accidental puncture and laceration of a respiratory system organ or structure during a respiratory system procedure CC
CC Excl: D78.11-D78.12, D78.81-D78.89, E36.11-E36.8, E89.81Ø-E89.89, G96.11, G97.41-G97.49, H59.Ø11-H59.Ø19, H59.Ø31-H59.Ø99, H59.211-H59.229, H59.811-H59.89, H95.31-H95.32, H95.811-H95.89, I97.3, I97.51-I97.52, J95.71-J95.72, K91.71-K91.72, L76.11-L76.12, L76.81-L76.82, M96.82Ø-M96.821, M96.89, N98.1-N98.9, N99.71-N99.72, T81.1ØXA, T81.11XA, T81.12XA, T81.19XA, T81.82XA, T81.89XA, T81.9XXA

J95.72 Accidental puncture and laceration of a respiratory system organ or structure during other procedure CC
CC Excl: See code: J95.71

✓5th J95.8 Other intraoperative and postprocedural complications and disorders of respiratory system, not elsewhere classified

✓6th J95.81 Postprocedural pneumothorax and air leak

9 **J95.811 Postprocedural pneumothorax** CC
CC Excl: J22, J93.9, J95.811-J95.812, J98.4, J98.8-J99, R91.1

J95.812 Postprocedural air leak CC
CC Excl: See code: J95.811

✓6th J95.82 Postprocedural respiratory failure
EXCLUDES 1 *respiratory failure in other conditions (J96.-)*

J95.821 Acute postprocedural respiratory failure MCC
Postprocedural respiratory failure NOS
CC Excl: See code: J95.1

J95.822 Acute and chronic postprocedural respiratory failure MCC
CC Excl: See code: J95.1

✓6th J95.83 Postprocedural hemorrhage and hematoma of a respiratory system organ or structure following a procedure

J95.83Ø Postprocedural hemorrhage and hematoma of a respiratory system organ or structure following a respiratory system procedure CC
CC Excl: See code: J95.61

J95.831 Postprocedural hemorrhage and hematoma of a respiratory system organ or structure following other procedure CC
CC Excl: See code: J95.61

J95.84 Transfusion-related acute lung injury (TRALI) CC
CC Excl: See code: J95.4

✓6th J95.85 Complication of respirator [ventilator]

CC Excl: For CC codes in subcategory J95.Ø, unless otherwise noted: See code: J95.4

J95.85Ø Mechanical complication of respirator CC
EXCLUDES 1 *encounter for respirator [ventilator] dependence during power failure (Z99.12)*
CC Excl: J95.85Ø, Z99.12, Z99.81-Z99.89

J95.851 Ventilator associated pneumonia CC
Ventilator associated pneumonitis
Use additional code to identify the organism, if known (B95.-, B96.-, B97.-)
EXCLUDES 1 *ventilator lung in newborn (P27.8)*

J95.859 Other complication of respirator [ventilator] CC

J95.88 Other intraoperative complications of respiratory system, not elsewhere classified CC
CC Excl: See code: J95.4

9 HAC = as SDx not POA, in combination with one of the following procedure codes: Ø5H[M,N,P,Q]33Z or ØJH63XZ.

J95.89 Other postprocedural complications and disorders of respiratory system, not elsewhere classified CC

Use additional code to identify disorder, such as:
- aspiration pneumonia (J69.-)
- bacterial or viral pneumonia (J12-J18)

EXCLUDES 2 *acute pulmonary insufficiency following thoracic surgery (J95.1)*
postprocedural subglottic stenosis (J95.5)

CC Excl: See code: J95.4

Other diseases of the respiratory system (J96-J99)

✓4th **J96 Respiratory failure, not elsewhere classified**

EXCLUDES 1 *acute respiratory distress syndrome (J8Ø)*
cardiorespiratory failure (RØ9.2)
newborn respiratory distress syndrome (P22.Ø)
postprocedural respiratory failure (J95.82-)
respiratory arrest (RØ9.2)
respiratory arrest of newborn (P28.81)
respiratory failure of newborn (P28.5)

CC Excl: For CC/MCC codes in category J96, unless otherwise noted: J22, J8Ø, J96.ØØ-J96.92, J98.8-J98.9, RØ9.2

✓5th **J96.Ø Acute respiratory failure**

J96.ØØ Acute respiratory failure, unspecified whether with hypoxia or hypercapnia MCC
AHA: 2Ø13, 4Q, 121

J96.Ø1 Acute respiratory failure with hypoxia MCC

J96.Ø2 Acute respiratory failure with hypercapnia MCC

✓5th **J96.1 Chronic respiratory failure**

J96.1Ø Chronic respiratory failure, unspecified whether with hypoxia or hypercapnia CC

J96.11 Chronic respiratory failure with hypoxia CC
AHA: 2Ø13, 4Q, 129

J96.12 Chronic respiratory failure with hypercapnia CC

✓5th **J96.2 Acute and chronic respiratory failure**
Acute on chronic respiratory failure

J96.2Ø Acute and chronic respiratory failure, unspecified whether with hypoxia or hypercapnia MCC

J96.21 Acute and chronic respiratory failure with hypoxia MCC

J96.22 Acute and chronic respiratory failure with hypercapnia MCC

✓5th **J96.9 Respiratory failure, unspecified**

J96.9Ø Respiratory failure, unspecified, unspecified whether with hypoxia or hypercapnia MCC

J96.91 Respiratory failure, unspecified with hypoxia MCC

J96.92 Respiratory failure, unspecified with hypercapnia MCC

✓4th **J98 Other respiratory disorders**

Use additional code to identify:
- exposure to environmental tobacco smoke (Z77.22)
- exposure to tobacco smoke in the perinatal period (P96.81)
- history of tobacco use (Z87.891)
- occupational exposure to environmental tobacco smoke (Z57.31)
- tobacco dependence (F17.-)
- tobacco use (Z72.Ø)

EXCLUDES 1 *newborn apnea (P28.4)*
newborn sleep apnea (P28.3)

EXCLUDES 2 *apnea NOS (RØ6.81)*
sleep apnea (G47.3-)

✓5th **J98.Ø Diseases of bronchus, not elsewhere classified**

J98.Ø1 Acute bronchospasm

EXCLUDES 1 *acute bronchiolitis with bronchospasm (J21.-)*
acute bronchitis with bronchospasm (J2Ø.-)
asthma (J45.-)
exercise induced bronchospasm (J45.99Ø)

J98.Ø9 Other diseases of bronchus, not elsewhere classified
Broncholithiasis
Calcification of bronchus
Stenosis of bronchus
Tracheobronchial collapse
Tracheobronchial dyskinesia
Ulcer of bronchus

✓5th **J98.1 Pulmonary collapse**

EXCLUDES 1 *therapeutic collapse of lung status (Z98.3)*

J98.11 Atelectasis CC

EXCLUDES 1 *newborn atelectasis*
tuberculous atelectasis (current disease) (A15)

CC Excl: J22, J98.19, J98.8-J98.9

J98.19 Other pulmonary collapse CC
CC Excl: See code: J98.11

J98.2 Interstitial emphysema
Mediastinal emphysema

EXCLUDES 1 *emphysema NOS (J43.9)*
emphysema in newborn (P25.Ø)
surgical emphysema (subcutaneous) (T81.82)
traumatic subcutaneous emphysema (T79.7)

J98.3 Compensatory emphysema

J98.4 Other disorders of lung
Calcification of lung
Cystic lung disease (acquired)
Lung disease NOS
Pulmolithiasis

EXCLUDES 1 *acute interstitial pneumonitis (J84.114)*
pulmonary insufficiency following surgery (J95.1-J95.2)

5 **J98.5 Diseases of mediastinum, not elsewhere classified** MCC
Fibrosis of mediastinum
Hernia of mediastinum
Retraction of mediastinum
Mediastinitis

EXCLUDES 2 *abscess of mediastinum (J85.3)*

CC Excl: No excl

J98.6 Disorders of diaphragm
Diaphragmatitis
Paralysis of diaphragm
Relaxation of diaphragm

EXCLUDES 1 *congenital malformation of diaphragm NEC (Q79.1)*
congenital diaphragmatic hernia (Q79.Ø)

EXCLUDES 2 *diaphragmatic hernia (K44.-)*

J98.8 Other specified respiratory disorders

J98.9 Respiratory disorder, unspecified
Respiratory disease (chronic) NOS

J99 Respiratory disorders in diseases classified elsewhere

Code first underlying disease, such as:
- *amyloidosis (E85.-)*
- *ankylosing spondylitis (M45)*
- *congenital syphilis (A5Ø.5)*
- *cryoglobulinemia (D89.1)*
- *early congenital syphilis (A5Ø.Ø)*
- *schistosomiasis (B65.Ø-B65.9)*

EXCLUDES 1 *respiratory disorders in:*
amebiasis (AØ6.5)
blastomycosis (B4Ø.Ø-B4Ø.2)
candidiasis (B37.1)
coccidioidomycosis (B38.Ø-B38.2)
cystic fibrosis with pulmonary manifestations (E84.Ø)
dermatomyositis (M33.Ø1, M33.11)
histoplasmosis (B39.Ø-B39.2)
late syphilis (A52.72, A52.73)
polymyositis (M33.21)
sicca syndrome (M35.Ø2)
systemic lupus erythematosus (M32.13)
systemic sclerosis (M34.81)
Wegener's granulomatosis (M31.3Ø-M31.31)

5 HAC = as SDx not POA, in combination with one of the following procedure codes: Ø21[Ø,1,2,3][Ø,4][9,A,J,K][3,8,9,C,F,W]; Ø21[Ø,1,2,3][Ø,4]Z[3,8,9,C,F].

Chapter 11. Diseases of the Digestive System (K00-K95)

EXCLUDES 2 *certain conditions originating in the perinatal period (P04-P96)*
certain infectious and parasitic diseases (A00-B99)
complications of pregnancy, childbirth and the puerperium (O00-O9A)
congenital malformations, deformations and chromosomal abnormalities (Q00-Q99)
endocrine, nutritional and metabolic diseases (E00-E88)
injury, poisoning and certain other consequences of external causes (S00-T88)
neoplasms (C00-D49)
symptoms, signs and abnormal clinical and laboratory findings, not elsewhere classified (R00-R94)

This chapter contains the following blocks:

K00-K14	Diseases of oral cavity and salivary glands
K20-K31	Diseases of esophagus, stomach and duodenum
K35-K38	Diseases of appendix
K40-K46	Hernia
K50-K52	Noninfective enteritis and colitis
K55-K64	Other diseases of intestines
K65-K68	Diseases of peritoneum and retroperitoneum
K70-K77	Diseases of liver
K80-K87	Disorders of gallbladder, biliary tract and pancreas
K90-K95	Other diseases of the digestive system

Diseases of oral cavity and salivary glands (K00-K14)

✓4th K00 Disorders of tooth development and eruption
EXCLUDES 2 *embedded and impacted teeth (K01.-)*

K00.0 Anodontia
Hypodontia
Oligodontia
EXCLUDES 1 *acquired absence of teeth (K08.1-)*

K00.1 Supernumerary teeth
Distomolar
Fourth molar
Mesiodens
Paramolar
Supplementary teeth
EXCLUDES 2 *supernumerary roots (K00.2)*

K00.2 Abnormalities of size and form of teeth
Concrescence of teeth
Dens evaginatus
Dens in dente
Dens invaginatus
Enamel pearls
Fusion of teeth
Gemination of teeth
Macrodontia
Microdontia
Peg-shaped [conical] teeth
Supernumerary roots
Taurodontism
Tuberculum paramolare
EXCLUDES 1 *abnormalities of teeth due to congenital syphilis (A50.5)*
tuberculum Carabelli, which is regarded as a normal variation and should not be coded

K00.3 Mottled teeth
Dental fluorosis
Mottling of enamel
Nonfluoride enamel opacities
EXCLUDES 2 *deposits [accretions] on teeth (K03.6)*

K00.4 Disturbances in tooth formation
Aplasia and hypoplasia of cementum
Dilaceration of tooth
Enamel hypoplasia (neonatal) (postnatal) (prenatal)
Regional odontodysplasia
Turner's tooth
EXCLUDES 1 *Hutchinson's teeth and mulberry molars in congenital syphilis (A50.5)*
EXCLUDES 2 *mottled teeth (K00.3)*

K00.5 Hereditary disturbances in tooth structure, not elsewhere classified
Amelogenesis imperfecta
Dentinogenesis imperfecta
Odontogenesis imperfecta
Dentinal dysplasia
Shell teeth

K00.6 Disturbances in tooth eruption
Dentia praecox
Natal tooth
Neonatal tooth
Premature eruption of tooth
Premature shedding of primary [deciduous] tooth
Prenatal teeth
Retained [persistent] primary tooth
EXCLUDES 2 *embedded and impacted teeth (K01.-)*

K00.7 Teething syndrome

K00.8 Other disorders of tooth development
Color changes during tooth formation
Intrinsic staining of teeth NOS
EXCLUDES 2 *posteruptive color changes (K03.7)*

K00.9 Disorder of tooth development, unspecified
Disorder of odontogenesis NOS

✓4th K01 Embedded and impacted teeth
EXCLUDES 1 *abnormal position of fully erupted teeth (M26.3-)*

K01.0 Embedded teeth

K01.1 Impacted teeth

✓4th K02 Dental caries
Dental cavities
Tooth decay

K02.3 Arrested dental caries
Arrested coronal and root caries

✓5th K02.5 Dental caries on pit and fissure surface
Dental caries on chewing surface of tooth

K02.51 Dental caries on pit and fissure surface limited to enamel
White spot lesions [initial caries] on pit and fissure surface of tooth

K02.52 Dental caries on pit and fissure surface penetrating into dentin

K02.53 Dental caries on pit and fissure surface penetrating into pulp

✓5th K02.6 Dental caries on smooth surface

K02.61 Dental caries on smooth surface limited to enamel
White spot lesions [initial caries] on smooth surface of tooth

K02.62 Dental caries on smooth surface penetrating into dentin

K02.63 Dental caries on smooth surface penetrating into pulp

K02.7 Dental root caries

K02.9 Dental caries, unspecified

✓4th K03 Other diseases of hard tissues of teeth
EXCLUDES 2 *bruxism (F45.8)*
dental caries (K02.-)
teeth-grinding NOS (F45.8)

K03.0 Excessive attrition of teeth
Approximal wear of teeth
Occlusal wear of teeth

K03.1 Abrasion of teeth
Dentifrice abrasion of teeth
Habitual abrasion of teeth
Occupational abrasion of teeth
Ritual abrasion of teeth
Traditional abrasion of teeth
Wedge defect NOS

K03.2 Erosion of teeth
Erosion of teeth due to diet
Erosion of teeth due to drugs and medicaments
Erosion of teeth due to persistent vomiting
Erosion of teeth NOS
Idiopathic erosion of teeth
Occupational erosion of teeth

K03.3 Pathological resorption of teeth
Internal granuloma of pulp
Resorption of teeth (external)

K03.4 Hypercementosis
Cementation hyperplasia

K03.5 Ankylosis of teeth

K03.6 Deposits [accretions] on teeth
Betel deposits [accretions] on teeth
Black deposits [accretions] on teeth
Extrinsic staining of teeth NOS
Green deposits [accretions] on teeth
Materia alba deposits [accretions] on teeth
Orange deposits [accretions] on teeth
Staining of teeth NOS
Subgingival dental calculus
Supragingival dental calculus
Tobacco deposits [accretions] on teeth

K03.7 Posteruptive color changes of dental hard tissues
EXCLUDES 2 *deposits [accretions] on teeth (K03.6)*

✓5th **K03.8 Other specified diseases of hard tissues of teeth**

K03.81 Cracked tooth
EXCLUDES 1 *asymptomatic craze lines in enamel—omit code*
broken or fractured tooth due to trauma (S02.5)

K03.89 Other specified diseases of hard tissues of teeth

K03.9 Disease of hard tissues of teeth, unspecified

✓4th **K04 Diseases of pulp and periapical tissues**

K04.0 Pulpitis CC
Acute pulpitis
Chronic (hyperplastic) (ulcerative) pulpitis
Irreversible pulpitis
Reversible pulpitis
CC Excl: K00.0-K08.9, M26.00-M26.9, M27.61-M27.69

K04.1 Necrosis of pulp
Pulpal gangrene

K04.2 Pulp degeneration
Denticles
Pulpal calcifications
Pulpal stones

K04.3 Abnormal hard tissue formation in pulp
Secondary or irregular dentine

K04.4 Acute apical periodontitis of pulpal origin CC
Acute apical periodontitis NOS
EXCLUDES 1 *acute periodontitis (K05.2-)*
CC Excl: See code: K04.0

K04.5 Chronic apical periodontitis
Apical or periapical granuloma
Apical periodontitis NOS
EXCLUDES 1 *chronic periodontitis (K05.3-)*

K04.6 Periapical abscess with sinus
Dental abscess with sinus
Dentoalveolar abscess with sinus

K04.7 Periapical abscess without sinus
Dental abscess without sinus
Dentoalveolar abscess without sinus
Periapical abscess without sinus

K04.8 Radicular cyst
Apical (periodontal) cyst
Periapical cyst
Residual radicular cyst
EXCLUDES 2 *lateral periodontal cyst (K09.0)*

✓5th **K04.9 Other and unspecified diseases of pulp and periapical tissues**

K04.90 Unspecified diseases of pulp and periapical tissues

K04.99 Other diseases of pulp and periapical tissues

✓4th **K05 Gingivitis and periodontal diseases**
Use additional code to identify:
alcohol abuse and dependence (F10.-)
exposure to environmental tobacco smoke (Z77.22)
exposure to tobacco smoke in the perinatal period (P96.81)
history of tobacco use (Z87.891)
occupational exposure to environmental tobacco smoke (Z57.31)
tobacco dependence (F17.-)
tobacco use (Z72.0)

✓5th **K05.0 Acute gingivitis**
EXCLUDES 1 *acute necrotizing ulcerative gingivitis (A69.1)*
herpesviral [herpes simplex] gingivostomatitis (B00.2)

K05.00 Acute gingivitis, plaque induced
Acute gingivitis NOS

K05.01 Acute gingivitis, non-plaque induced

✓5th **K05.1 Chronic gingivitis**
Desquamative gingivitis (chronic)
Gingivitis (chronic) NOS
Hyperplastic gingivitis (chronic)
Simple marginal gingivitis (chronic)
Ulcerative gingivitis (chronic)

K05.10 Chronic gingivitis, plaque induced
Chronic gingivitis NOS
Gingivitis NOS

K05.11 Chronic gingivitis, non-plaque induced

✓5th **K05.2 Aggressive periodontitis**
Acute pericoronitis
EXCLUDES 1 *acute apical periodontitis (K04.4)*
periapical abscess (K04.7)
periapical abscess with sinus (K04.6)

K05.20 Aggressive periodontitis, unspecified

K05.21 Aggressive periodontitis, localized
Periodontal abscess

K05.22 Aggressive periodontitis, generalized

✓5th **K05.3 Chronic periodontitis**
Chronic pericoronitis
Complex periodontitis
Periodontitis NOS
Simplex periodontitis
EXCLUDES 1 *chronic apical periodontitis (K04.5)*

K05.30 Chronic periodontitis, unspecified

K05.31 Chronic periodontitis, localized

K05.32 Chronic periodontitis, generalized

K05.4 Periodontosis
Juvenile periodontosis

K05.5 Other periodontal diseases
EXCLUDES 2 *leukoplakia of gingiva (K13.21)*

K05.6 Periodontal disease, unspecified

✓4th **K06 Other disorders of gingiva and edentulous alveolar ridge**
EXCLUDES 2 *acute gingivitis (K05.0)*
atrophy of edentulous alveolar ridge (K08.2)
chronic gingivitis (K05.1)
gingivitis NOS (K05.1)

K06.0 Gingival recession
Gingival recession (generalized) (localized) (postinfective) (postprocedural)

K06.1 Gingival enlargement
Gingival fibromatosis

K06.2 Gingival and edentulous alveolar ridge lesions associated with trauma
Irritative hyperplasia of edentulous ridge [denture hyperplasia]
Use additional code (Chapter 20) to identify external cause or denture status (Z97.2)

K06.8 Other specified disorders of gingiva and edentulous alveolar ridge
Fibrous epulis
Flabby alveolar ridge
Giant cell epulis
Peripheral giant cell granuloma of gingiva
Pyogenic granuloma of gingiva
EXCLUDES 2 *gingival cyst (K09.0)*

K06.9 Disorder of gingiva and edentulous alveolar ridge, unspecified

✓4th **K08 Other disorders of teeth and supporting structures**
EXCLUDES 2 *dentofacial anomalies [including malocclusion] (M26.-)*
disorders of jaw (M27.-)

K08.0 Exfoliation of teeth due to systemic causes
Code also underlying systemic condition

✓5th **K08.1 Complete loss of teeth**
Acquired loss of teeth, complete
EXCLUDES 1 *congenital absence of teeth (K00.0)*
exfoliation of teeth due to systemic causes (K08.0)
partial loss of teeth (K08.4-)

✓6th **K08.10 Complete loss of teeth, unspecified cause**

K08.101 Complete loss of teeth, unspecified cause, class I

K08.102 Complete loss of teeth, unspecified cause, class II

K08.103 Complete loss of teeth, unspecified cause, class III

K08.104 Complete loss of teeth, unspecified cause, class IV

KØ8.1Ø9 Complete loss of teeth, unspecified cause, unspecified class
Edentulism NOS

✓6th **KØ8.11 Complete loss of teeth due to trauma**
KØ8.111 Complete loss of teeth due to trauma, class I
KØ8.112 Complete loss of teeth due to trauma, class II
KØ8.113 Complete loss of teeth due to trauma, class III
KØ8.114 Complete loss of teeth due to trauma, class IV
KØ8.119 Complete loss of teeth due to trauma, unspecified class

✓6th **KØ8.12 Complete loss of teeth due to periodontal diseases**
KØ8.121 Complete loss of teeth due to periodontal diseases, class I
KØ8.122 Complete loss of teeth due to periodontal diseases, class II
KØ8.123 Complete loss of teeth due to periodontal diseases, class III
KØ8.124 Complete loss of teeth due to periodontal diseases, class IV
KØ8.129 Complete loss of teeth due to periodontal diseases, unspecified class

✓6th **KØ8.13 Complete loss of teeth due to caries**
KØ8.131 Complete loss of teeth due to caries, class I
KØ8.132 Complete loss of teeth due to caries, class II
KØ8.133 Complete loss of teeth due to caries, class III
KØ8.134 Complete loss of teeth due to caries, class IV
KØ8.139 Complete loss of teeth due to caries, unspecified class

✓6th **KØ8.19 Complete loss of teeth due to other specified cause**
KØ8.191 Complete loss of teeth due to other specified cause, class I
KØ8.192 Complete loss of teeth due to other specified cause, class II
KØ8.193 Complete loss of teeth due to other specified cause, class III
KØ8.194 Complete loss of teeth due to other specified cause, class IV
KØ8.199 Complete loss of teeth due to other specified cause, unspecified class

✓5th **KØ8.2 Atrophy of edentulous alveolar ridge**
KØ8.2Ø Unspecified atrophy of edentulous alveolar ridge
Atrophy of the mandible NOS
Atrophy of the maxilla NOS
KØ8.21 Minimal atrophy of the mandible
Minimal atrophy of the edentulous mandible
KØ8.22 Moderate atrophy of the mandible
Moderate atrophy of the edentulous mandible
KØ8.23 Severe atrophy of the mandible
Severe atrophy of the edentulous mandible
KØ8.24 Minimal atrophy of maxilla
Minimal atrophy of the edentulous maxilla
KØ8.25 Moderate atrophy of the maxilla
Moderate atrophy of the edentulous maxilla
KØ8.26 Severe atrophy of the maxilla
Severe atrophy of the edentulous maxilla

KØ8.3 Retained dental root

✓5th **KØ8.4 Partial loss of teeth**
Acquired loss of teeth, partial
EXCLUDES 1 *complete loss of teeth (KØ8.1-)*
congenital absence of teeth (KØØ.Ø)
EXCLUDES 2 *exfoliation of teeth due to systemic causes (KØ8.Ø)*

✓6th **KØ8.4Ø Partial loss of teeth, unspecified cause**
KØ8.4Ø1 Partial loss of teeth, unspecified cause, class I
KØ8.4Ø2 Partial loss of teeth, unspecified cause, class II
KØ8.4Ø3 Partial loss of teeth, unspecified cause, class III
KØ8.4Ø4 Partial loss of teeth, unspecified cause, class IV
KØ8.4Ø9 Partial loss of teeth, unspecified cause, unspecified class
Tooth extraction status NOS

✓6th **KØ8.41 Partial loss of teeth due to trauma**
KØ8.411 Partial loss of teeth due to trauma, class I
KØ8.412 Partial loss of teeth due to trauma, class II
KØ8.413 Partial loss of teeth due to trauma, class III
KØ8.414 Partial loss of teeth due to trauma, class IV
KØ8.419 Partial loss of teeth due to trauma, unspecified class

✓6th **KØ8.42 Partial loss of teeth due to periodontal diseases**
KØ8.421 Partial loss of teeth due to periodontal diseases, class I
KØ8.422 Partial loss of teeth due to periodontal diseases, class II
KØ8.423 Partial loss of teeth due to periodontal diseases, class III
KØ8.424 Partial loss of teeth due to periodontal diseases, class IV
KØ8.429 Partial loss of teeth due to periodontal diseases, unspecified class

✓6th **KØ8.43 Partial loss of teeth due to caries**
KØ8.431 Partial loss of teeth due to caries, class I
KØ8.432 Partial loss of teeth due to caries, class II
KØ8.433 Partial loss of teeth due to caries, class III
KØ8.434 Partial loss of teeth due to caries, class IV
KØ8.439 Partial loss of teeth due to caries, unspecified class

✓6th **KØ8.49 Partial loss of teeth due to other specified cause**
KØ8.491 Partial loss of teeth due to other specified cause, class I
KØ8.492 Partial loss of teeth due to other specified cause, class II
KØ8.493 Partial loss of teeth due to other specified cause, class III
KØ8.494 Partial loss of teeth due to other specified cause, class IV
KØ8.499 Partial loss of teeth due to other specified cause, unspecified class

✓5th **KØ8.5 Unsatisfactory restoration of tooth**
Defective bridge, crown, filling
Defective dental restoration
EXCLUDES 1 *dental restoration status (Z98.811)*
EXCLUDES 2 *endosseous dental implant failure (M27.6-)*
unsatisfactory endodontic treatment (M27.5-)

KØ8.5Ø Unsatisfactory restoration of tooth, unspecified
Defective dental restoration NOS
KØ8.51 Open restoration margins of tooth
Dental restoration failure of marginal integrity
Open margin on tooth restoration
Poor gingival margin to tooth restoration
KØ8.52 Unrepairable overhanging of dental restorative materials
Overhanging of tooth restoration

✓6th **KØ8.53 Fractured dental restorative material**
EXCLUDES 1 *cracked tooth (KØ3.81)*
traumatic fracture of tooth (SØ2.5)
KØ8.53Ø Fractured dental restorative material without loss of material
KØ8.531 Fractured dental restorative material with loss of material
KØ8.539 Fractured dental restorative material, unspecified

KØ8.54 Contour of existing restoration of tooth biologically incompatible with oral health
Dental restoration failure of periodontal anatomical integrity
Unacceptable contours of existing restoration of tooth
Unacceptable morphology of existing restoration of tooth
KØ8.55 Allergy to existing dental restorative material
Use additional code to identify the specific type of allergy

K08.56 Poor aesthetic of existing restoration of tooth
Dental restoration aesthetically inadequate or displeasing

K08.59 Other unsatisfactory restoration of tooth
Other defective dental restoration

K08.8 Other specified disorders of teeth and supporting structures
Enlargement of alveolar ridge NOS
Irregular alveolar process
Toothache NOS

K08.9 Disorder of teeth and supporting structures, unspecified

✓4th **K09 Cysts of oral region, not elsewhere classified**
INCLUDES lesions showing histological features both of aneurysmal cyst and of another fibro-osseous lesion
EXCLUDES 2 *cysts of jaw (M27.0-, M27.4-)*
radicular cyst (K04.8)

K09.0 Developmental odontogenic cysts
Dentigerous cyst
Eruption cyst
Follicular cyst
Gingival cyst
Lateral periodontal cyst
Primordial cyst
EXCLUDES 2 *keratocysts (D16.4, D16.5)*
odontogenic keratocystic tumors (D16.4, D16.5)

K09.1 Developmental (nonodontogenic) cysts of oral region
Cyst (of) incisive canal
Cyst (of) palatine of papilla
Globulomaxillary cyst
Median palatal cyst
Nasoalveolar cyst
Nasolabial cyst
Nasopalatine duct cyst

K09.8 Other cysts of oral region, not elsewhere classified
Dermoid cyst
Epidermoid cyst
Lymphoepithelial cyst
Epstein's pearl

K09.9 Cyst of oral region, unspecified

✓4th **K11 Diseases of salivary glands**
Use additional code to identify:
alcohol abuse and dependence (F10.-)
exposure to environmental tobacco smoke (Z77.22)
exposure to tobacco smoke in the perinatal period (P96.81)
history of tobacco use (Z87.891)
occupational exposure to environmental tobacco smoke (Z57.31)
tobacco dependence (F17.-)
tobacco use (Z72.0)

K11.0 Atrophy of salivary gland

K11.1 Hypertrophy of salivary gland

✓5th **K11.2 Sialoadenitis**
Parotitis
EXCLUDES 1 *epidemic parotitis (B26.-)*
mumps (B26.-)
uveoparotid fever [Heerfordt] (D86.89)

K11.20 Sialoadenitis, unspecified

K11.21 Acute sialoadenitis
EXCLUDES 1 *acute recurrent sialoadenitis (K11.22)*

K11.22 Acute recurrent sialoadenitis

K11.23 Chronic sialoadenitis

K11.3 Abscess of salivary gland CC
CC Excl: K11.0-K11.9, K31.89-K31.9, K92.81, R68.2

K11.4 Fistula of salivary gland CC
EXCLUDES 1 *congenital fistula of salivary gland (Q38.4)*
CC Excl: See code: K11.3

K11.5 Sialolithiasis
Calculus of salivary gland or duct
Stone of salivary gland or duct

K11.6 Mucocele of salivary gland
Mucous extravasation cyst of salivary gland
Mucous retention cyst of salivary gland
Ranula

K11.7 Disturbances of salivary secretion
Hypoptyalism
Ptyalism
Xerostomia
EXCLUDES 2 *dry mouth NOS (R68.2)*

K11.8 Other diseases of salivary glands
Benign lymphoepithelial lesion of salivary gland
Mikulicz' disease
Necrotizing sialometaplasia
Sialectasia
Stenosis of salivary duct
Stricture of salivary duct
EXCLUDES 1 *sicca syndrome [Sjögren] (M35.0-)*

K11.9 Disease of salivary gland, unspecified
Sialoadenopathy NOS

✓4th **K12 Stomatitis and related lesions**
Use additional code to identify:
alcohol abuse and dependence (F10.-)
exposure to environmental tobacco smoke (Z77.22)
exposure to tobacco smoke in the perinatal period (P96.81)
history of tobacco use (Z87.891)
occupational exposure to environmental tobacco smoke (Z57.31)
tobacco dependence (F17.-)
tobacco use (Z72.0)
EXCLUDES 1 *cancrum oris (A69.0)*
cheilitis (K13.0)
gangrenous stomatitis (A69.0)
herpesviral [herpes simplex] gingivostomatitis (B00.2)
noma (A69.0)

K12.0 Recurrent oral aphthae
Aphthous stomatitis (major) (minor)
Bednar's aphthae
Periadenitis mucosa necrotica recurrens
Recurrent aphthous ulcer
Stomatitis herpetiformis

K12.1 Other forms of stomatitis
Stomatitis NOS
Denture stomatitis
Ulcerative stomatitis
Vesicular stomatitis
EXCLUDES 1 *acute necrotizing ulcerative stomatitis (A69.1)*
Vincent's stomatitis (A69.1)

K12.2 Cellulitis and abscess of mouth CC
Cellulitis of mouth (floor)
Submandibular abscess
EXCLUDES 2 *abscess of salivary gland (K11.3)*
abscess of tongue (K14.0)
periapical abscess (K04.6-K04.7)
periodontal abscess (K05.21)
peritonsillar abscess (J36)
CC Excl: K12.1-K12.39, K14.0, K14.2

✓5th **K12.3 Oral mucositis (ulcerative)**
Mucositis (oral) (oropharyneal)
EXCLUDES 2 *gastrointestinal mucositis (ulcerative) (K92.81)*
mucositis (ulcerative) of vagina and vulva (N76.81)
nasal mucositis (ulcerative) (J34.81)

K12.30 Oral mucositis (ulcerative), unspecified

K12.31 Oral mucositis (ulcerative) due to antineoplastic therapy
Use additional code for adverse effect, if applicable, to identify antineoplastic and immunosuppressive drugs (T45.1X5)
Use additional code for other antineoplastic therapy, such as:
radiological procedure and radiotherapy (Y84.2)

K12.32 Oral mucositis (ulcerative) due to other drugs
Use additional code for adverse effect, if applicable, to identify drug (T36-T50 with fifth or sixth character 5)

K12.33 Oral mucositis (ulcerative) due to radiation
Use additional external cause code (W88-W90, X39.0-) to identify cause

K12.39 Other oral mucositis (ulcerative)
Viral oral mucositis (ulcerative)

K13 Other diseases of lip and oral mucosa

INCLUDES epithelial disturbances of tongue

Use additional code to identify:
alcohol abuse and dependence (F1Ø.-)
exposure to environmental tobacco smoke (Z77.22)
exposure to tobacco smoke in the perinatal period (P96.81)
history of tobacco use (Z87.891)
occupational exposure to environmental tobacco smoke (Z57.31)
tobacco dependence (F17.-)
tobacco use (Z72.Ø)

EXCLUDES 2 *certain disorders of gingiva and edentulous alveolar ridge (KØ5-KØ6)*
cysts of oral region (KØ9.-)
diseases of tongue (K14.-)
stomatitis and related lesions (K12.-)

K13.Ø Diseases of lips
Abscess of lips
Angular cheilitis
Cellulitis of lips
Cheilitis NOS
Cheilodynia
Cheilosis
Exfoliative cheilitis
Fistula of lips
Glandular cheilitis
Hypertrophy of lips
Perlèche NEC

EXCLUDES 1 *ariboflavinosis (E53.Ø)*
cheilitis due to radiation-related disorders (L55-L59)
congenital fistula of lips (Q38.Ø)
congenital hypertrophy of lips (Q18.6)
Perlèche due to candidiasis (B37.83)
Perlèche due to riboflavin deficiency (E53.Ø)

K13.1 Cheek and lip biting

K13.2 Leukoplakia and other disturbances of oral epithelium, including tongue

EXCLUDES 1 *carcinoma in situ of oral epithelium (DØØ.Ø-)*
hairy leukoplakia (K13.3)

K13.21 Leukoplakia of oral mucosa, including tongue
Leukokeratosis of oral mucosa
Leukoplakia of gingiva, lips, tongue

EXCLUDES 1 *hairy leukoplakia (K13.3)*
leukokeratosis nicotina palati (K13.24)

K13.22 Minimal keratinized residual ridge mucosa
Minimal keratinization of alveolar ridge mucosa

K13.23 Excessive keratinized residual ridge mucosa
Excessive keratinization of alveolar ridge mucosa

K13.24 Leukokeratosis nicotina palati
Smoker's palate

K13.29 Other disturbances of oral epithelium, including tongue
Erythroplakia of mouth or tongue
Focal epithelial hyperplasia of mouth or tongue
Leukoedema of mouth or tongue
Other oral epithelium disturbances

K13.3 Hairy leukoplakia

K13.4 Granuloma and granuloma-like lesions of oral mucosa
Eosinophilic granuloma
Granuloma pyogenicum
Verrucous xanthoma

K13.5 Oral submucous fibrosis
Submucous fibrosis of tongue

K13.6 Irritative hyperplasia of oral mucosa

EXCLUDES 2 *irritative hyperplasia of edentulous ridge [denture hyperplasia] (KØ6.2)*

K13.7 Other and unspecified lesions of oral mucosa

K13.7Ø Unspecified lesions of oral mucosa

K13.79 Other lesions of oral mucosa
Focal oral mucinosis

K14 Diseases of tongue

Use additional code to identify:
alcohol abuse and dependence (F1Ø.-)
exposure to environmental tobacco smoke (Z77.22)
history of tobacco use (Z87.891)
occupational exposure to environmental tobacco smoke (Z57.31)
tobacco dependence (F17.-)
tobacco use (Z72.Ø)

EXCLUDES 2 *erythroplakia (K13.29)*
focal epithelial hyperplasia (K13.29)
leukedema of tongue (K13.29)
leukoplakia of tongue (K13.21)
hairy leukoplakia (K13.3)
macroglossia (congenital) (Q38.2)
submucous fibrosis of tongue (K13.5)

K14.Ø Glossitis
Abscess of tongue
Ulceration (traumatic) of tongue

EXCLUDES 1 *atrophic glossitis (K14.4)*

K14.1 Geographic tongue
Benign migratory glossitis
Glossitis areata exfoliativa

K14.2 Median rhomboid glossitis

K14.3 Hypertrophy of tongue papillae
Black hairy tongue
Coated tongue
Hypertrophy of foliate papillae
Lingua villosa nigra

K14.4 Atrophy of tongue papillae
Atrophic glossitis

K14.5 Plicated tongue
Fissured tongue
Furrowed tongue
Scrotal tongue

EXCLUDES 1 *fissured tongue, congenital (Q38.3)*

K14.6 Glossodynia
Glossopyrosis
Painful tongue

K14.8 Other diseases of tongue
Atrophy of tongue
Crenated tongue
Enlargement of tongue
Glossocele
Glossoptosis
Hypertrophy of tongue

K14.9 Disease of tongue, unspecified
Glossopathy NOS

Diseases of esophagus, stomach and duodenum (K2Ø-K31)

EXCLUDES 2 *hiatus hernia (K44.-)*

K2Ø Esophagitis

Use additional code to identify:
alcohol abuse and dependence (F1Ø.-)

EXCLUDES 1 *erosion of esophagus (K22.1-)*
esophagitis with gastro-esophageal reflux disease (K21.Ø)
reflux esophagitis (K21.Ø)
ulcerative esophagitis (K22.1-)

EXCLUDES 2 *eosinophilic gastritis or gastroenteritis (K52.81)*

K2Ø.Ø Eosinophilic esophagitis

K2Ø.8 Other esophagitis
Abscess of esophagus

K2Ø.9 Esophagitis, unspecified
Esophagitis NOS

K21 Gastro-esophageal reflux disease

EXCLUDES 1 *newborn esophageal reflux (P78.83)*

K21.Ø Gastro-esophageal reflux disease with esophagitis
Reflux esophagitis

K21.9 Gastro-esophageal reflux disease without esophagitis
Esophageal reflux NOS

K22 Other diseases of esophagus

EXCLUDES 2 *esophageal varices (I85.-)*

K22.Ø Achalasia of cardia
Achalasia NOS
Cardiospasm

EXCLUDES 1 *congenital cardiospasm (Q39.5)*

✓5th K22.1 Ulcer of esophagus
- Barrett's ulcer
- Erosion of esophagus
- Fungal ulcer of esophagus
- Peptic ulcer of esophagus
- Ulcer of esophagus due to ingestion of chemicals
- Ulcer of esophagus due to ingestion of drugs and medicaments
- Ulcerative esophagitis

Code first poisoning due to drug or toxin, if applicable (T36-T65 with fifth or sixth character 1-4 or 6)

Use additional code for adverse effect, if applicable, to identify drug (T36-T50 with fifth or sixth character 5)

EXCLUDES 1 *Barrett's esophagus (K22.7-)*

K22.10 Ulcer of esophagus without bleeding CC
- Ulcer of esophagus NOS
- **CC Excl:** K22.11, K22.8-K23, K31.82

K22.11 Ulcer of esophagus with bleeding MCC
- EXCLUDES 2 *bleeding esophageal varices (I85.01, I85.11)*
- **CC Excl:** E16.4, I85.01, K22.10-K22.11, K22.6-K22.719, K25.0-K28.9, K29.01, K29.21, K29.31, K29.41, K29.51, K29.61, K29.71, K29.81, K29.91, K31.811, K31.89-K31.9, K55.21, K57.01, K57.11, K57.13, K57.21, K57.31, K57.33, K57.41, K57.51, K57.53, K57.81, K57.91, K57.93, K62.5, K92.0-K92.81

K22.2 Esophageal obstruction
- Compression of esophagus
- Constriction of esophagus
- Stenosis of esophagus
- Stricture of esophagus
- EXCLUDES 1 *congenital stenosis or stricture of esophagus (Q39.3)*

K22.3 Perforation of esophagus MCC
- Rupture of esophagus
- EXCLUDES 1 *traumatic perforation of (thoracic) esophagus (S27.8-)*
- **CC Excl:** K21.9, K22.3, K22.6, K22.8-K23

K22.4 Dyskinesia of esophagus
- Corkscrew esophagus
- Diffuse esophageal spasm
- Spasm of esophagus
- EXCLUDES 1 *cardiospasm (K22.0)*

K22.5 Diverticulum of esophagus, acquired
- Esophageal pouch, acquired
- EXCLUDES 1 *diverticulum of esophagus (congenital) (Q39.6)*

K22.6 Gastro-esophageal laceration-hemorrhage syndrome MCC
- Mallory-Weiss syndrome
- **CC Excl:** E16.4, I85.01, K21.9, K22.10-K22.11, K22.3, K22.6-K28.9, K29.01, K29.21, K29.31, K29.41, K29.51, K29.61, K29.71, K29.81, K29.91, K31.811, K55.21, K57.01, K57.11, K57.13, K57.21, K57.31, K57.33, K57.41, K57.51, K57.53, K57.81, K57.91, K57.93, K62.5, K92.0-K92.2

✓5th K22.7 Barrett's esophagus
- Barrett's disease
- Barrett's syndrome
- EXCLUDES 1 *Barrett's ulcer (K22.1)*
  malignant neoplasm of esophagus (C15.-)

K22.70 Barrett's esophagus without dysplasia
- Barrett's esophagus NOS

✓6th K22.71 Barrett's esophagus with dysplasia
- **K22.710 Barrett's esophagus with low grade dysplasia**
- **K22.711 Barrett's esophagus with high grade dysplasia**
- **K22.719 Barrett's esophagus with dysplasia, unspecified**

K22.8 Other specified diseases of esophagus
- Hemorrhage of esophagus NOS
- EXCLUDES 2 *esophageal varices (I85.-)*
  Paterson-Kelly syndrome (D50.1)

K22.9 Disease of esophagus, unspecified

K23 Disorders of esophagus in diseases classified elsewhere

Code first underlying disease, such as:
congenital syphilis (A50.5)

EXCLUDES 1 *late syphilis (A52.79)*
megaesophagus due to Chagas' disease (B57.31)
tuberculosis (A18.83)

✓4th K25 Gastric ulcer

INCLUDES erosion (acute) of stomach
pylorus ulcer (peptic)
stomach ulcer (peptic)

Use additional code to identify:
alcohol abuse and dependence (F10.-)

EXCLUDES 1 *acute gastritis (K29.0-)*
peptic ulcer NOS (K27.-)

CC Excl: For CC/MCC codes in category K25, unless otherwise noted: See code: K22.11

- **K25.0 Acute gastric ulcer with hemorrhage** MCC
- **K25.1 Acute gastric ulcer with perforation** MCC
- **K25.2 Acute gastric ulcer with both hemorrhage and perforation** MCC
- **K25.3 Acute gastric ulcer without hemorrhage or perforation** CC
- **K25.4 Chronic or unspecified gastric ulcer with hemorrhage** MCC
- **K25.5 Chronic or unspecified gastric ulcer with perforation** MCC
- **K25.6 Chronic or unspecified gastric ulcer with both hemorrhage and perforation** MCC
- **K25.7 Chronic gastric ulcer without hemorrhage or perforation**
- **K25.9 Gastric ulcer, unspecified as acute or chronic, without hemorrhage or perforation**

✓4th K26 Duodenal ulcer

INCLUDES erosion (acute) of duodenum
duodenum ulcer (peptic)
postpyloric ulcer (peptic)

Use additional code to identify:
alcohol abuse and dependence (F10.-)

EXCLUDES 1 *peptic ulcer NOS (K27.-)*

CC Excl: For CC/MCC codes in category K26, unless otherwise noted: E16.4, I85.01, K22.10-K22.11, K22.6-K22.719, K25.0-K28.9, K29.01, K29.21, K29.31, K29.41, K29.51, K29.61, K29.71, K29.81, K29.91, K31.5, K31.811, K31.89-K31.9, K55.21, K57.01, K57.11, K57.13, K57.21, K57.31, K57.33, K57.41, K57.51, K57.53, K57.81, K57.91, K57.93, K62.5, K92.0-K92.81

- **K26.0 Acute duodenal ulcer with hemorrhage** MCC
- **K26.1 Acute duodenal ulcer with perforation** MCC
- **K26.2 Acute duodenal ulcer with both hemorrhage and perforation** MCC
- **K26.3 Acute duodenal ulcer without hemorrhage or perforation** CC
  - **CC Excl:** E16.4, I85.01, K22.6, K25.0-K28.9, K29.01, K29.21, K29.31, K29.41, K29.51, K29.61, K29.71, K29.81, K29.91, K31.5, K31.811, K31.82, K31.89-K31.9, K55.21, K57.01, K57.11, K57.13, K57.21, K57.31, K57.33, K57.41, K57.51, K57.53, K57.81, K57.91, K57.93, K62.5, K92.0-K92.81
- **K26.4 Chronic or unspecified duodenal ulcer with hemorrhage** MCC
- **K26.5 Chronic or unspecified duodenal ulcer with perforation** MCC
- **K26.6 Chronic or unspecified duodenal ulcer with both hemorrhage and perforation** MCC
- **K26.7 Chronic duodenal ulcer without hemorrhage or perforation**
- **K26.9 Duodenal ulcer, unspecified as acute or chronic, without hemorrhage or perforation**

✓4th K27 Peptic ulcer, site unspecified

INCLUDES gastroduodenal ulcer NOS
peptic ulcer NOS

Use additional code to identify:
alcohol abuse and dependence (F10.-)

EXCLUDES 1 *peptic ulcer of newborn (P78.82)*

CC Excl: For CC/MCC codes in category K27, unless otherwise noted: See code: K26

- **K27.0 Acute peptic ulcer, site unspecified, with hemorrhage** MCC
- **K27.1 Acute peptic ulcer, site unspecified, with perforation** MCC
- **K27.2 Acute peptic ulcer, site unspecified, with both hemorrhage and perforation** MCC
- **K27.3 Acute peptic ulcer, site unspecified, without hemorrhage or perforation** CC
- **K27.4 Chronic or unspecified peptic ulcer, site unspecified, with hemorrhage** MCC
- **K27.5 Chronic or unspecified peptic ulcer, site unspecified, with perforation** MCC
- **K27.6 Chronic or unspecified peptic ulcer, site unspecified, with both hemorrhage and perforation** MCC
- **K27.7 Chronic peptic ulcer, site unspecified, without hemorrhage or perforation**
- **K27.9 Peptic ulcer, site unspecified, unspecified as acute or chronic, without hemorrhage or perforation**

4th K28 Gastrojejunal ulcer

INCLUDES anastomotic ulcer (peptic) or erosion
gastrocolic ulcer (peptic) or erosion
gastrointestinal ulcer (peptic) or erosion
gastrojejunal ulcer (peptic) or erosion
jejunal ulcer (peptic) or erosion
marginal ulcer (peptic) or erosion
stomal ulcer (peptic) or erosion

Use additional code to identify:
alcohol abuse and dependence (F1Ø.-)

EXCLUDES 1 *primary ulcer of small intestine (K63.3)*

CC Excl: For CC/MCC codes in category K28, unless otherwise noted: See code: K22.11

K28.Ø Acute gastrojejunal ulcer with hemorrhage MCC

K28.1 Acute gastrojejunal ulcer with perforation MCC

K28.2 Acute gastrojejunal ulcer with both hemorrhage and perforation MCC

K28.3 Acute gastrojejunal ulcer without hemorrhage or perforation CC

K28.4 Chronic or unspecified gastrojejunal ulcer with hemorrhage MCC

K28.5 Chronic or unspecified gastrojejunal ulcer with perforation MCC

K28.6 Chronic or unspecified gastrojejunal ulcer with both hemorrhage and perforation MCC

K28.7 Chronic gastrojejunal ulcer without hemorrhage or perforation

K28.9 Gastrojejunal ulcer, unspecified as acute or chronic, without hemorrhage or perforation

4th K29 Gastritis and duodenitis

EXCLUDES 1 *eosinophilic gastritis or gastroenteritis (K52.81)*
Zollinger-Ellison syndrome (E16.4)

CC Excl: For MCC codes in category K29, unless otherwise noted: E16.4, I85.Ø1, K22.1Ø-K22.11, K22.6-K22.719, K25.Ø-K28.9, K29.Ø1, K29.21, K29.31, K29.41, K29.51, K29.61, K29.71, K29.81, K29.91, K31.811, K55.21, K57.Ø1, K57.11, K57.13, K57.21, K57.31, K57.33, K57.41, K57.51, K57.53, K57.81, K57.91, K57.93, K62.5, K92.Ø-K92.2

5th K29.Ø Acute gastritis

Use additional code to identify:
alcohol abuse and dependence (F1Ø.-)

EXCLUDES 1 *erosion (acute) of stomach (K25.-)*

K29.ØØ Acute gastritis without bleeding

K29.Ø1 Acute gastritis with bleeding MCC

5th K29.2 Alcoholic gastritis

Use additional code to identify:
alcohol abuse and dependence (F1Ø.-)

K29.2Ø Alcoholic gastritis without bleeding

K29.21 Alcoholic gastritis with bleeding MCC

5th K29.3 Chronic superficial gastritis

K29.3Ø Chronic superficial gastritis without bleeding

K29.31 Chronic superficial gastritis with bleeding MCC

5th K29.4 Chronic atrophic gastritis

Gastric atrophy

K29.4Ø Chronic atrophic gastritis without bleeding

K29.41 Chronic atrophic gastritis with bleeding MCC

5th K29.5 Unspecified chronic gastritis

Chronic antral gastritis
Chronic fundal gastritis

K29.5Ø Unspecified chronic gastritis without bleeding

K29.51 Unspecified chronic gastritis with bleeding MCC

5th K29.6 Other gastritis

Giant hypertrophic gastritis
Granulomatous gastritis
Ménétrier's disease

K29.6Ø Other gastritis without bleeding

K29.61 Other gastritis with bleeding MCC

5th K29.7 Gastritis, unspecified

K29.7Ø Gastritis, unspecified, without bleeding

K29.71 Gastritis, unspecified, with bleeding MCC

5th K29.8 Duodenitis

K29.8Ø Duodenitis without bleeding

K29.81 Duodenitis with bleeding MCC

5th K29.9 Gastroduodenitis, unspecified

K29.9Ø Gastroduodenitis, unspecified, without bleeding

K29.91 Gastroduodenitis, unspecified, with bleeding MCC

K3Ø Functional dyspepsia

Indigestion

EXCLUDES 1 *dyspepsia NOS (R1Ø.13)*
heartburn (R12)
nervous dyspepsia (F45.8)
neurotic dyspepsia (F45.8)
psychogenic dyspepsia (F45.8)

4th K31 Other diseases of stomach and duodenum

INCLUDES functional disorders of stomach

EXCLUDES 2 *diabetic gastroparesis (EØ8.43, EØ9.43, E1Ø.43, E11.43, E13.43)*
diverticulum of duodenum (K57.ØØ-K57.13)

K31.Ø Acute dilatation of stomach CC

Acute distention of stomach
CC Excl: K31.Ø

K31.1 Adult hypertrophic pyloric stenosis CC A

Pyloric stenosis NOS

EXCLUDES 1 *congenital or infantile pyloric stenosis (Q4Ø.Ø)*

CC Excl: K3Ø, K31.1, K31.5, K31.84, Q38.5, Q4Ø.Ø, Q4Ø.8-Q41.9, Q43.4-Q43.9

K31.2 Hourglass stricture and stenosis of stomach

EXCLUDES 1 *congenital hourglass stomach (Q4Ø.2)*
hourglass contraction of stomach (K31.89)

K31.3 Pylorospasm, not elsewhere classified

EXCLUDES 1 *congenital or infantile pylorospasm (Q4Ø.Ø)*
neurotic pylorospasm (F45.8)
psychogenic pylorospasm (F45.8)

K31.4 Gastric diverticulum

EXCLUDES 1 *congenital diverticulum of stomach (Q4Ø.2)*

K31.5 Obstruction of duodenum CC

Constriction of duodenum
Duodenal ileus (chronic)
Stenosis of duodenum
Stricture of duodenum
Volvulus of duodenum

EXCLUDES 1 *congenital stenosis of duodenum (Q41.Ø)*

CC Excl: K31.5, Q38.5, Q4Ø.8-Q41.9, Q43.4-Q43.9

K31.6 Fistula of stomach and duodenum CC

Gastrocolic fistula
Gastrojejunocolic fistula
CC Excl: K31.6, Q38.5, Q4Ø.8-Q4Ø.9, Q43.4-Q43.9

K31.7 Polyp of stomach and duodenum

EXCLUDES 1 *adenomatous polyp of stomach (D13.1)*

5th K31.8 Other specified diseases of stomach and duodenum

6th K31.81 Angiodysplasia of stomach and duodenum

K31.811 Angiodysplasia of stomach and duodenum with bleeding MCC

CC Excl: See code: K29

K31.819 Angiodysplasia of stomach and duodenum without bleeding

Angiodysplasia of stomach and duodenum NOS

K31.82 Dieulafoy lesion (hemorrhagic) of stomach and duodenum MCC

EXCLUDES 2 *Dieulafoy lesion of intestine (K63.81)*

CC Excl: E16.4, I85.Ø1, K22.1Ø-K22.11, K22.6-K22.719, K25.Ø-K28.9, K29.Ø1, K29.21, K29.31, K29.41, K29.51, K29.61, K29.71, K29.81, K29.91, K31.811, K31.82, K55.21, K57.Ø1, K57.11, K57.13, K57.21, K57.31, K57.33, K57.41, K57.51, K57.53, K57.81, K57.91, K57.93, K62.5, K92.Ø-K92.2

K31.83 Achlorhydria

K31.84 Gastroparesis

Gastroparalysis

Code first underlying disease, if known, such as:
anorexia nervosa (F5Ø.Ø-)
diabetes mellitus (EØ8.43, EØ9.43, E1Ø.43, E11.43, E13.43)
scleroderma (M34.-)

AHA: 2Ø13, 4Q, 114

K31.89 Other diseases of stomach and duodenum

K31.9 Disease of stomach and duodenum, unspecified

Diseases of appendix (K35-K38)

✓4th **K35 Acute appendicitis**

CC Excl: For CC/MCC codes in category K35, unless otherwise noted: K31.89-K38.9, K92.81

K35.2 Acute appendicitis with generalized peritonitis MCC
Appendicitis (acute) with generalized (diffuse) peritonitis following rupture or perforation of appendix
Perforated appendix NOS
Ruptured appendix NOS

K35.3 Acute appendicitis with localized peritonitis MCC
Acute appendicitis with or without perforation or rupture NOS
Acute appendicitis with or without perforation or rupture with localized peritonitis
Acute appendicitis with peritoneal abscess

✓5th **K35.8 Other and unspecified acute appendicitis**

K35.80 Unspecified acute appendicitis CC
Acute appendicitis NOS
Acute appendicitis without (localized) (generalized) peritonitis

K35.89 Other acute appendicitis CC

K36 Other appendicitis
Chronic appendicitis
Recurrent appendicitis

K37 Unspecified appendicitis
EXCLUDES1 *unspecified appendicitis with peritonitis (K35.2-K35.3)*

✓4th **K38 Other diseases of appendix**

K38.0 Hyperplasia of appendix

K38.1 Appendicular concretions
Fecalith of appendix
Stercolith of appendix

K38.2 Diverticulum of appendix

K38.3 Fistula of appendix

K38.8 Other specified diseases of appendix
Intussusception of appendix

K38.9 Disease of appendix, unspecified

Hernia (K40-K46)

NOTE Hernia with both gangrene and obstruction is classified to hernia with gangrene.

INCLUDES acquired hernia
congenital [except diaphragmatic or hiatus] hernia
recurrent hernia

✓4th **K40 Inguinal hernia**
INCLUDES bubonocele
direct inguinal hernia
double inguinal hernia
indirect inguinal hernia
inguinal hernia NOS
oblique inguinal hernia
scrotal hernia

CC Excl: For CC/MCC codes in category K40, unless otherwise noted: K31.89-K31.9, K40.00-K40.91, K45.0, K45.8-K46.0, K92.81

✓5th **K40.0 Bilateral inguinal hernia, with obstruction, without gangrene**
Inguinal hernia (bilateral) causing obstruction without gangrene
Incarcerated inguinal hernia (bilateral) without gangrene
Irreducible inguinal hernia (bilateral) without gangrene
Strangulated inguinal hernia (bilateral) without gangrene

K40.00 Bilateral inguinal hernia, with obstruction, without gangrene, not specified as recurrent CC
Bilateral inguinal hernia, with obstruction, without gangrene NOS

K40.01 Bilateral inguinal hernia, with obstruction, without gangrene, recurrent CC

✓5th **K40.1 Bilateral inguinal hernia, with gangrene**

K40.10 Bilateral inguinal hernia, with gangrene, not specified as recurrent MCC
Bilateral inguinal hernia, with gangrene NOS

K40.11 Bilateral inguinal hernia, with gangrene, recurrent MCC

✓5th **K40.2 Bilateral inguinal hernia, without obstruction or gangrene**

K40.20 Bilateral inguinal hernia, without obstruction or gangrene, not specified as recurrent
Bilateral inguinal hernia NOS

K40.21 Bilateral inguinal hernia, without obstruction or gangrene, recurrent

✓5th **K40.3 Unilateral inguinal hernia, with obstruction, without gangrene**
Inguinal hernia (unilateral) causing obstruction without gangrene
Incarcerated inguinal hernia (unilateral) without gangrene
Irreducible inguinal hernia (unilateral) without gangrene
Strangulated inguinal hernia (unilateral) without gangrene

K40.30 Unilateral inguinal hernia, with obstruction, without gangrene, not specified as recurrent CC
Inguinal hernia, with obstruction NOS
Unilateral inguinal hernia, with obstruction, without gangrene NOS

K40.31 Unilateral inguinal hernia, with obstruction, without gangrene, recurrent CC

✓5th **K40.4 Unilateral inguinal hernia, with gangrene**

K40.40 Unilateral inguinal hernia, with gangrene, not specified as recurrent MCC
Inguinal hernia with gangrene NOS
Unilateral inguinal hernia with gangrene NOS

K40.41 Unilateral inguinal hernia, with gangrene, recurrent MCC

✓5th **K40.9 Unilateral inguinal hernia, without obstruction or gangrene**

K40.90 Unilateral inguinal hernia, without obstruction or gangrene, not specified as recurrent
Inguinal hernia NOS
Unilateral inguinal hernia NOS

K40.91 Unilateral inguinal hernia, without obstruction or gangrene, recurrent

✓4th **K41 Femoral hernia**

CC Excl: For CC/MCC codes in category K41, unless otherwise noted: K31.89-K31.9, K41.00-K41.91, K45.0, K45.8-K46.0, K92.81

✓5th **K41.0 Bilateral femoral hernia, with obstruction, without gangrene**
Femoral hernia (bilateral) causing obstruction, without gangrene
Incarcerated femoral hernia (bilateral), without gangrene
Irreducible femoral hernia (bilateral), without gangrene
Strangulated femoral hernia (bilateral), without gangrene

K41.00 Bilateral femoral hernia, with obstruction, without gangrene, not specified as recurrent CC
Bilateral femoral hernia, with obstruction, without gangrene NOS

K41.01 Bilateral femoral hernia, with obstruction, without gangrene, recurrent CC

✓5th **K41.1 Bilateral femoral hernia, with gangrene**

K41.10 Bilateral femoral hernia, with gangrene, not specified as recurrent MCC
Bilateral femoral hernia, with gangrene NOS
CC Excl: K31.89-K31.9, K41.10-K41.21, K41.40-K41.91, K45.0, K45.8-K46.0, K92.81

K41.11 Bilateral femoral hernia, with gangrene, recurrent MCC
CC Excl: See code: K41.10

✓5th **K41.2 Bilateral femoral hernia, without obstruction or gangrene**

K41.20 Bilateral femoral hernia, without obstruction or gangrene, not specified as recurrent
Bilateral femoral hernia NOS

K41.21 Bilateral femoral hernia, without obstruction or gangrene, recurrent

✓5th **K41.3 Unilateral femoral hernia, with obstruction, without gangrene**
Femoral hernia (unilateral) causing obstruction, without gangrene
Incarcerated femoral hernia (unilateral), without gangrene
Irreducible femoral hernia (unilateral), without gangrene
Strangulated femoral hernia (unilateral), without gangrene

K41.30 Unilateral femoral hernia, with obstruction, without gangrene, not specified as recurrent CC
Femoral hernia, with obstruction NOS
Unilateral femoral hernia, with obstruction NOS

K41.31 Unilateral femoral hernia, with obstruction, without gangrene, recurrent CC

✓5th **K41.4 Unilateral femoral hernia, with gangrene**

K41.40 Unilateral femoral hernia, with gangrene, not specified as recurrent MCC
Femoral hernia, with gangrene NOS
Unilateral femoral hernia, with gangrene NOS
CC Excl: See code: K41.10

K41.41 **Unilateral femoral hernia, with gangrene, recurrent** MCC
CC Excl: See code: K41.10

✓5th **K41.9 Unilateral femoral hernia, without obstruction or gangrene**

K41.90 **Unilateral femoral hernia, without obstruction or gangrene, not specified as recurrent**
Femoral hernia NOS
Unilateral femoral hernia NOS

K41.91 **Unilateral femoral hernia, without obstruction or gangrene, recurrent**

✓4th **K42 Umbilical hernia**
INCLUDES paraumbilical hernia
EXCLUDES 1 *omphalocele (Q79.2)*

K42.0 **Umbilical hernia with obstruction, without gangrene** CC
Umbilical hernia causing obstruction, without gangrene
Incarcerated umbilical hernia, without gangrene
Irreducible umbilical hernia, without gangrene
Strangulated umbilical hernia, without gangrene
CC Excl: K42.0-K42.1, K43.0, K43.1, K43.3-K43.4, K43.6-K43.7, K45.0, K45.8-K46.0

K42.1 **Umbilical hernia with gangrene** MCC
Gangrenous umbilical hernia
CC Excl: K31.89-K31.9, K42.0-K43.0, K43.1, K43.2-K43.9, K45.0, K45.8-K46.0, K46.9, K92.81

K42.9 **Umbilical hernia without obstruction or gangrene**
Umbilical hernia NOS

✓4th **K43 Ventral hernia**

K43.0 **Incisional hernia with obstruction, without gangrene** CC
Incisional hernia causing obstruction, without gangrene
Incarcerated incisional hernia, without gangrene
Irreducible incisional hernia, without gangrene
Strangulated incisional hernia, without gangrene
CC Excl: See code: K42.0

K43.1 **Incisional hernia with gangrene** MCC
Gangrenous incisional hernia
CC Excl: See code: K42.1

K43.2 **Incisional hernia without obstruction or gangrene**
Incisional hernia NOS

K43.3 **Parastomal hernia with obstruction, without gangrene** CC
Incarcerated parastomal hernia, without gangrene
Irreducible parastomal hernia, without gangrene
Parastomal hernia causing obstruction, without gangrene
Strangulated parastomal hernia, without gangrene
CC Excl: See code: K42.0

K43.4 **Parastomal hernia with gangrene** MCC
Gangrenous parastomal hernia
CC Excl: See code: K42.1

K43.5 **Parastomal hernia without obstruction or gangrene**
Parastomal hernia NOS

K43.6 **Other and unspecified ventral hernia with obstruction, without gangrene** CC
Epigastric hernia causing obstruction, without gangrene
Hypogastric hernia causing obstruction, without gangrene
Incarcerated epigastric hernia without gangrene
Incarcerated hypogastric hernia without gangrene
Incarcerated midline hernia without gangrene
Incarcerated spigelian hernia without gangrene
Incarcerated subxiphoid hernia without gangrene
Irreducible epigastric hernia without gangrene
Irreducible hypogastric hernia without gangrene
Irreducible midline hernia without gangrene
Irreducible spigelian hernia without gangrene
Irreducible subxiphoid hernia without gangrene
Midline hernia causing obstruction, without gangrene
Spigelian hernia causing obstruction, without gangrene
Strangulated epigastric hernia without gangrene
Strangulated hypogastric hernia without gangrene
Strangulated midline hernia without gangrene
Strangulated spigelian hernia without gangrene
Strangulated subxiphoid hernia without gangrene
Subxiphoid hernia causing obstruction, without gangrene
CC Excl: See code: K42.0

K43.7 **Other and unspecified ventral hernia with gangrene** MCC
Any condition listed under K43.6 specified as gangrenous
CC Excl: See code: K42.1

K43.9 **Ventral hernia without obstruction or gangrene**
Epigastric hernia
Ventral hernia NOS

✓4th **K44 Diaphragmatic hernia**
INCLUDES hiatus hernia (esophageal) (sliding)
paraesophageal hernia
EXCLUDES 1 *congenital diaphragmatic hernia (Q79.0)*
congenital hiatus hernia (Q40.1)

K44.0 **Diaphragmatic hernia with obstruction, without gangrene** CC
Diaphragmatic hernia causing obstruction
Incarcerated diaphragmatic hernia
Irreducible diaphragmatic hernia
Strangulated diaphragmatic hernia
CC Excl: K44.0-K45.0, K45.8-K46.0

K44.1 **Diaphragmatic hernia with gangrene** MCC
Gangrenous diaphragmatic hernia
CC Excl: See code: K44.0

K44.9 **Diaphragmatic hernia without obstruction or gangrene**
Diaphragmatic hernia NOS

✓4th **K45 Other abdominal hernia**
INCLUDES abdominal hernia, specified site NEC
lumbar hernia
obturator hernia
pudendal hernia
retroperitoneal hernia
sciatic hernia

K45.0 **Other specified abdominal hernia with obstruction, without gangrene** CC
Other specified abdominal hernia causing obstruction
Other specified incarcerated abdominal hernia
Other specified irreducible abdominal hernia
Other specified strangulated abdominal hernia
CC Excl: K40.00-K43.0, K43.1, K43.2-K43.9, K44.0-K46.9

K45.1 **Other specified abdominal hernia with gangrene** MCC
Any condition listed under K45 specified as gangrenous
CC Excl: K31.89-K31.9, K40.00-K43.0, K43.1, K43.2-K43.9, K44.0-K46.9, K92.81

K45.8 **Other specified abdominal hernia without obstruction or gangrene**

✓4th **K46 Unspecified abdominal hernia**
INCLUDES enterocele
epiplocele
hernia NOS
interstitial hernia
intestinal hernia
intra-abdominal hernia
EXCLUDES 1 *vaginal enterocele (N81.5)*

K46.0 **Unspecified abdominal hernia with obstruction, without gangrene** CC
Unspecified abdominal hernia causing obstruction
Unspecified incarcerated abdominal hernia
Unspecified irreducible abdominal hernia
Unspecified strangulated abdominal hernia
CC Excl: See code: K45.0

K46.1 **Unspecified abdominal hernia with gangrene** MCC
Any condition listed under K46 specified as gangrenous
CC Excl: See code: K45.1

K46.9 **Unspecified abdominal hernia without obstruction or gangrene**
Abdominal hernia NOS

Noninfective enteritis and colitis (K50-K52)

INCLUDES noninfective inflammatory bowel disease
EXCLUDES 1 *irritable bowel syndrome (K58.-)*
megacolon (K59.3)

✓4th **K50 Crohn's disease [regional enteritis]**
INCLUDES granulomatous enteritis
Use additional code to identify manifestations, such as:
pyoderma gangrenosum (L88)
EXCLUDES 1 *ulcerative colitis (K51.-)*
AHA: 2012, 4Q, 104

CC Excl: For CC codes in category K50, unless otherwise noted: K50.00-K51.919

✓5th **K50.0 Crohn's disease of small intestine**
Crohn's disease [regional enteritis] of duodenum
Crohn's disease [regional enteritis] of ileum
Crohn's disease [regional enteritis] of jejunum
Regional ileitis
Terminal ileitis
EXCLUDES 1 *Crohn's disease of both small and large intestine (K50.8-)*

K50.00 Crohn's disease of small intestine without complications CC

K50.01 Crohn's disease of small intestine with complications
- K50.011 Crohn's disease of small intestine with rectal bleeding CC
- K50.012 Crohn's disease of small intestine with intestinal obstruction PDx CC CC
- K50.013 Crohn's disease of small intestine with fistula PDx CC CC
- K50.014 Crohn's disease of small intestine with abscess PDx CC CC
  AHA: 2012, 4Q, 104
- K50.018 Crohn's disease of small intestine with other complication CC
- K50.019 Crohn's disease of small intestine with unspecified complications CC

K50.1 Crohn's disease of large intestine
Crohn's disease [regional enteritis] of colon
Crohn's disease [regional enteritis] of large bowel
Crohn's disease [regional enteritis] of rectum
Granulomatous colitis
Regional colitis
EXCLUDES 1 *Crohn's disease of both small and large intestine (K50.8)*

K50.10 Crohn's disease of large intestine without complications CC

K50.11 Crohn's disease of large intestine with complications
- K50.111 Crohn's disease of large intestine with rectal bleeding CC
- K50.112 Crohn's disease of large intestine with intestinal obstruction PDx CC CC
- K50.113 Crohn's disease of large intestine with fistula PDx CC CC
- K50.114 Crohn's disease of large intestine with abscess PDx CC CC
- K50.118 Crohn's disease of large intestine with other complication CC
- K50.119 Crohn's disease of large intestine with unspecified complications CC

K50.8 Crohn's disease of both small and large intestine

K50.80 Crohn's disease of both small and large intestine without complications CC

K50.81 Crohn's disease of both small and large intestine with complications
- K50.811 Crohn's disease of both small and large intestine with rectal bleeding CC
- K50.812 Crohn's disease of both small and large intestine with intestinal obstruction PDx CC CC
- K50.813 Crohn's disease of both small and large intestine with fistula PDx CC CC
- K50.814 Crohn's disease of both small and large intestine with abscess PDx CC CC
- K50.818 Crohn's disease of both small and large intestine with other complication CC
- K50.819 Crohn's disease of both small and large intestine with unspecified complications CC

K50.9 Crohn's disease, unspecified

CC Excl: For CC codes in subcategory K50.9, unless otherwise noted: K50.00-K50.919

K50.90 Crohn's disease, unspecified, without complications CC
Crohn's disease NOS
Regional enteritis NOS

K50.91 Crohn's disease, unspecified, with complications
- K50.911 Crohn's disease, unspecified, with rectal bleeding CC
- K50.912 Crohn's disease, unspecified, with intestinal obstruction PDx CC CC
- K50.913 Crohn's disease, unspecified, with fistula PDx CC CC
- K50.914 Crohn's disease, unspecified, with abscess PDx CC CC
- K50.918 Crohn's disease, unspecified, with other complication CC
- K50.919 Crohn's disease, unspecified, with unspecified complications CC

K51 Ulcerative colitis
Use additional code to identify manifestations, such as:
pyoderma gangrenosum (L88)
EXCLUDES 1 *Crohn's disease [regional enteritis] (K50.-)*

CC Excl: For CC codes in category K51, unless otherwise noted: See code: K50.9

K51.0 Ulcerative (chronic) pancolitis
Backwash ileitis

K51.00 Ulcerative (chronic) pancolitis without complications CC
Ulcerative (chronic) pancolitis NOS

K51.01 Ulcerative (chronic) pancolitis with complications
- K51.011 Ulcerative (chronic) pancolitis with rectal bleeding CC
- K51.012 Ulcerative (chronic) pancolitis with intestinal obstruction PDx CC CC
- K51.013 Ulcerative (chronic) pancolitis with fistula PDx CC CC
- K51.014 Ulcerative (chronic) pancolitis with abscess PDx CC CC
- K51.018 Ulcerative (chronic) pancolitis with other complication CC
- K51.019 Ulcerative (chronic) pancolitis with unspecified complications CC

K51.2 Ulcerative (chronic) proctitis

K51.20 Ulcerative (chronic) proctitis without complications CC
Ulcerative (chronic) proctitis NOS

K51.21 Ulcerative (chronic) proctitis with complications
- K51.211 Ulcerative (chronic) proctitis with rectal bleeding CC
- K51.212 Ulcerative (chronic) proctitis with intestinal obstruction PDx CC CC
- K51.213 Ulcerative (chronic) proctitis with fistula PDx CC CC
- K51.214 Ulcerative (chronic) proctitis with abscess PDx CC CC
- K51.218 Ulcerative (chronic) proctitis with other complication CC
- K51.219 Ulcerative (chronic) proctitis with unspecified complications CC

K51.3 Ulcerative (chronic) rectosigmoiditis

K51.30 Ulcerative (chronic) rectosigmoiditis without complications CC
Ulcerative (chronic) rectosigmoiditis NOS

K51.31 Ulcerative (chronic) rectosigmoiditis with complications
- K51.311 Ulcerative (chronic) rectosigmoiditis with rectal bleeding CC
- K51.312 Ulcerative (chronic) rectosigmoiditis with intestinal obstruction PDx CC CC
- K51.313 Ulcerative (chronic) rectosigmoiditis with fistula PDx CC CC
- K51.314 Ulcerative (chronic) rectosigmoiditis with abscess PDx CC CC
- K51.318 Ulcerative (chronic) rectosigmoiditis with other complication CC
- K51.319 Ulcerative (chronic) rectosigmoiditis with unspecified complications CC

K51.4 Inflammatory polyps of colon
EXCLUDES 1 *adenomatous polyp of colon (D12.6)*
polyposis of colon (D12.6)
polyps of colon NOS (K63.5)

K51.40 Inflammatory polyps of colon without complications CC
Inflammatory polyps of colon NOS

K51.41 Inflammatory polyps of colon with complications
- K51.411 Inflammatory polyps of colon with rectal bleeding CC
- K51.412 Inflammatory polyps of colon with intestinal obstruction PDx CC CC
- K51.413 Inflammatory polyps of colon with fistula PDx CC CC
- K51.414 Inflammatory polyps of colon with abscess PDx CC CC

K51.418 Inflammatory polyps of colon with other complication CC

K51.419 Inflammatory polyps of colon with unspecified complications CC

✓5th **K51.5 Left sided colitis**
Left hemicolitis

K51.50 Left sided colitis without complications CC
Left sided colitis NOS

✓6th **K51.51 Left sided colitis with complications**

K51.511 Left sided colitis with rectal bleeding CC

K51.512 Left sided colitis with intestinal obstruction PDx CC CC

K51.513 Left sided colitis with fistula PDx CC CC

K51.514 Left sided colitis with abscess PDx CC CC

K51.518 Left sided colitis with other complication CC

K51.519 Left sided colitis with unspecified complications CC

✓5th **K51.8 Other ulcerative colitis**

K51.80 Other ulcerative colitis without complications CC

✓6th **K51.81 Other ulcerative colitis with complications**

K51.811 Other ulcerative colitis with rectal bleeding CC

K51.812 Other ulcerative colitis with intestinal obstruction PDx CC CC

K51.813 Other ulcerative colitis with fistula PDx CC CC

K51.814 Other ulcerative colitis with abscess PDx CC CC

K51.818 Other ulcerative colitis with other complication CC

K51.819 Other ulcerative colitis with unspecified complications CC

✓5th **K51.9 Ulcerative colitis, unspecified**

CC Excl: For CC codes in subcategory K51.9, unless otherwise noted: K51.00-K51.919

K51.90 Ulcerative colitis, unspecified, without complications CC

✓6th **K51.91 Ulcerative colitis, unspecified, with complications**

K51.911 Ulcerative colitis, unspecified with rectal bleeding CC

K51.912 Ulcerative colitis, unspecified with intestinal obstruction PDx CC CC

K51.913 Ulcerative colitis, unspecified with fistula PDx CC CC

K51.914 Ulcerative colitis, unspecified with abscess PDx CC CC

K51.918 Ulcerative colitis, unspecified with other complication CC

K51.919 Ulcerative colitis, unspecified with unspecified complications CC

✓4th **K52 Other and unspecified noninfective gastroenteritis and colitis**

K52.0 Gastroenteritis and colitis due to radiation CC
CC Excl: K52.0

K52.1 Toxic gastroenteritis and colitis CC
Drug-induced gastroenteritis and colitis
Code first (T51-T65) to identify toxic agent
Use additional code for adverse effect, if applicable, to identify drug (T36-T50 with fifth or sixth character 5)
CC Excl: K52.1

K52.2 Allergic and dietetic gastroenteritis and colitis
Food hypersensitivity gastroenteritis or colitis
Use additional code to identify type of food allergy (Z91.01-, Z91.02-)

✓5th **K52.8 Other specified noninfective gastroenteritis and colitis**

K52.81 Eosinophilic gastritis or gastroenteritis
Eosinophilic enteritis
EXCLUDES 1 *eosinophilic esophagitis (K20.0)*

K52.82 Eosinophilic colitis

K52.89 Other specified noninfective gastroenteritis and colitis
Collagenous colitis
Lymphocytic colitis
Microscopic colitis (collagenous or lymphocytic)

K52.9 Noninfective gastroenteritis and colitis, unspecified
Colitis NOS
Enteritis NOS
Gastroenteritis NOS
Ileitis NOS
Jejunitis NOS
Sigmoiditis NOS
EXCLUDES 1 *diarrhea NOS (R19.7)*
functional diarrhea (K59.1)
infectious gastroenteritis and colitis NOS (A09)
neonatal diarrhea (noninfective) (P78.3)
psychogenic diarrhea (F45.8)

Other diseases of intestines (K55-K64)

✓4th **K55 Vascular disorders of intestine**
EXCLUDES 1 *necrotizing enterocolitis of newborn (P77.-)*

K55.0 Acute vascular disorders of intestine MCC
Acute fulminant ischemic colitis
Acute intestinal infarction
Acute small intestine ischemia
Infarction of appendices epiploicae
Mesenteric (artery) (vein) embolism
Mesenteric (artery) (vein) infarction
Mesenteric (artery) (vein) thrombosis
Necrosis of intestine
Subacute ischemic colitis
CC Excl: K55.0-K55.1

K55.1 Chronic vascular disorders of intestine CC
Chronic ischemic colitis
Chronic ischemic enteritis
Chronic ischemic enterocolitis
Ischemic stricture of intestine
Mesenteric atherosclerosis
Mesenteric vascular insufficiency
CC Excl: K55.0-K55.1, K55.8-K55.9

✓5th **K55.2 Angiodysplasia of colon**

K55.20 Angiodysplasia of colon without hemorrhage

K55.21 Angiodysplasia of colon with hemorrhage MCC
CC Excl: E16.4, I85.01, K22.10-K22.11, K22.6-K22.719, K25.0-K28.9, K29.01, K29.21, K29.31, K29.41, K29.51, K29.61, K29.71, K29.81, K29.91, K31.811, K55.21, K57.01, K57.11, K57.13, K57.21, K57.31, K57.33, K57.41, K57.51, K57.53, K57.81, K57.91, K57.93, K62.5, K92.0-K92.2

K55.8 Other vascular disorders of intestine CC
CC Excl: See code: K55.1

K55.9 Vascular disorder of intestine, unspecified CC
Ischemic colitis
Ischemic enteritis
Ischemic enterocolitis
CC Excl: See code: K55.1

✓4th **K56 Paralytic ileus and intestinal obstruction without hernia**
EXCLUDES 1 *congenital stricture or stenosis of intestine (Q41-Q42)*
cystic fibrosis with meconium ileus (E84.11)
intestinal obstruction with hernia (K40-K46)
ischemic stricture of intestine (K55.1)
meconium ileus NOS (P76.0)
neonatal intestinal obstructions classifiable to P76-
obstruction of duodenum (K31.5)
postprocedural intestinal obstruction (K91.3)
stenosis of anus or rectum (K62.4)

CC Excl: For CC/MCC codes in category K56, unless otherwise noted: K56.0-K56.3, K56.49-K56.7, K63.4, K63.89-K63.9, K92.89-K92.9, R11.13

K56.0 Paralytic ileus CC
Paralysis of bowel
Paralysis of colon
Paralysis of intestine
EXCLUDES 1 *gallstone ileus (K56.3)*
ileus NOS (K56.7)
obstructive ileus NOS (K56.69)

K56.1 Intussusception CC
Intussusception or invagination of bowel
Intussusception or invagination of colon
Intussusception or invagination of intestine
Intussusception or invagination of rectum
EXCLUDES 2 *intussusception of appendix (K38.8)*

K56.2 Volvulus MCC
Strangulation of colon or intestine
Torsion of colon or intestine
Twist of colon or intestine
EXCLUDES 2 *volvulus of duodenum (K31.5)*

K56.3 Gallstone ileus CC
Obstruction of intestine by gallstone

✓5th **K56.4 Other impaction of intestine**

K56.41 Fecal impaction

EXCLUDES 1 *constipation (K59.0-)*
incomplete defecation (R15.0)

K56.49 Other impaction of intestine CC

K56.5 Intestinal adhesions [bands] with obstruction (postprocedural) (postinfection) CC

Abdominal hernia due to adhesions with obstruction
Peritoneal adhesions [bands] with intestinal obstruction (postprocedural) (postinfection)

✓5th **K56.6 Other and unspecified intestinal obstruction**

K56.60 Unspecified intestinal obstruction CC

Intestinal obstruction NOS

EXCLUDES 1 *intestinal obstruction due to specified condition—code to condition*

K56.69 Other intestinal obstruction CC

Enterostenosis NOS
Obstructive ileus NOS
Occlusion of colon or intestine NOS
Stenosis of colon or intestine NOS
Stricture of colon or intestine NOS

EXCLUDES 1 *intestinal obstruction due to specified condition—code to condition*

K56.7 Ileus, unspecified CC

EXCLUDES 1 *obstructive ileus (K56.69)*

✓4th **K57 Diverticular disease of intestine**

EXCLUDES 1 *congenital diverticulum of intestine (Q43.8)*
Meckel's diverticulum (Q43.0)

EXCLUDES 2 *diverticulum of appendix (K38.2)*

CC Excl: For CC/MCC codes in category K57, unless otherwise noted: E16.4, I85.01, K22.10-K22.11, K22.6-K22.719, K25.0-K28.9, K29.01, K29.21, K29.31, K29.41, K29.51, K29.61, K29.71, K29.81, K29.91, K31.811, K55.21, K57.01, K57.11, K57.13, K57.21, K57.31, K57.33, K57.41, K57.51, K57.53, K57.81, K57.91, K57.93, K62.5, K92.0-K92.2

✓5th **K57.0 Diverticulitis of small intestine with perforation and abscess**

Diverticulitis of small intestine with peritonitis

EXCLUDES 1 *diverticulitis of both small and large intestine with perforation and abscess (K57.4-)*

K57.00 Diverticulitis of small intestine with perforation and abscess without bleeding PDx CC CC

CC Excl: K57.00-K57.13

K57.01 Diverticulitis of small intestine with perforation and abscess with bleeding PDx CC MCC

✓5th **K57.1 Diverticular disease of small intestine without perforation or abscess**

EXCLUDES 1 *diverticular disease of both small and large intestine without perforation or abscess (K57.5-)*

K57.10 Diverticulosis of small intestine without perforation or abscess without bleeding

Diverticular disease of small intestine NOS

K57.11 Diverticulosis of small intestine without perforation or abscess with bleeding MCC

K57.12 Diverticulitis of small intestine without perforation or abscess without bleeding CC

CC Excl: See code: K57.00

K57.13 Diverticulitis of small intestine without perforation or abscess with bleeding MCC

✓5th **K57.2 Diverticulitis of large intestine with perforation and abscess**

Diverticulitis of colon with peritonitis

EXCLUDES 1 *diverticulitis of both small and large intestine with perforation and abscess (K57.4-)*

K57.20 Diverticulitis of large intestine with perforation and abscess without bleeding PDx CC CC

CC Excl: K57.20-K57.93

K57.21 Diverticulitis of large intestine with perforation and abscess with bleeding PDx CC MCC

✓5th **K57.3 Diverticular disease of large intestine without perforation or abscess**

EXCLUDES 1 *diverticular disease of both small and large intestine without perforation or abscess (K57.5-)*

K57.30 Diverticulosis of large intestine without perforation or abscess without bleeding

Diverticular disease of colon NOS

K57.31 Diverticulosis of large intestine without perforation or abscess with bleeding MCC

K57.32 Diverticulitis of large intestine without perforation or abscess without bleeding CC

CC Excl: See code: K57.20

K57.33 Diverticulitis of large intestine without perforation or abscess with bleeding MCC

✓5th **K57.4 Diverticulitis of both small and large intestine with perforation and abscess**

Diverticulitis of both small and large intestine with peritonitis

K57.40 Diverticulitis of both small and large intestine with perforation and abscess without bleeding PDx CC CC

CC Excl: See code: K57.20

K57.41 Diverticulitis of both small and large intestine with perforation and abscess with bleeding PDx CC MCC

✓5th **K57.5 Diverticular disease of both small and large intestine without perforation or abscess**

K57.50 Diverticulosis of both small and large intestine without perforation or abscess without bleeding

Diverticular disease of both small and large intestine NOS

K57.51 Diverticulosis of both small and large intestine without perforation or abscess with bleeding MCC

K57.52 Diverticulitis of both small and large intestine without perforation or abscess without bleeding PDx CC CC

CC Excl: See code: K57.20

K57.53 Diverticulitis of both small and large intestine without perforation or abscess with bleeding MCC

✓5th **K57.8 Diverticulitis of intestine, part unspecified, with perforation and abscess**

Diverticulitis of intestine NOS with peritonitis

K57.80 Diverticulitis of intestine, part unspecified, with perforation and abscess without bleeding PDx CC CC

CC Excl: See code: K57.20

K57.81 Diverticulitis of intestine, part unspecified, with perforation and abscess with bleeding PDx CC MCC

✓5th **K57.9 Diverticular disease of intestine, part unspecified, without perforation or abscess**

K57.90 Diverticulosis of intestine, part unspecified, without perforation or abscess without bleeding

Diverticular disease of intestine NOS

K57.91 Diverticulosis of intestine, part unspecified, without perforation or abscess with bleeding MCC

K57.92 Diverticulitis of intestine, part unspecified, without perforation or abscess without bleeding CC

CC Excl: See code: K57.20

K57.93 Diverticulitis of intestine, part unspecified, without perforation or abscess with bleeding MCC

✓4th **K58 Irritable bowel syndrome**

INCLUDES irritable colon
spastic colon

K58.0 Irritable bowel syndrome with diarrhea

K58.9 Irritable bowel syndrome without diarrhea

Irritable bowel syndrome NOS

✓4th **K59 Other functional intestinal disorders**

EXCLUDES 1 *change in bowel habit NOS (R19.4)*
intestinal malabsorption (K90.-)
psychogenic intestinal disorders (F45.8)

EXCLUDES 2 *functional disorders of stomach (K31.-)*

✓5th **K59.0 Constipation**

EXCLUDES 1 *fecal impaction (K56.41)*
incomplete defecation (R15.0)

K59.00 Constipation, unspecified

K59.01 Slow transit constipation

K59.02 Outlet dysfunction constipation

K59.09 Other constipation

K59.1 Functional diarrhea

EXCLUDES 1 *diarrhea NOS (R19.7)*
irritable bowel syndrome with diarrhea (K58.0)

K59.2 Neurogenic bowel, not elsewhere classified CC

CC Excl: K58.0-K58.9, K59.1-K59.9, K91.0-K91.1

K59.3 Megacolon, not elsewhere classified CC
Dilatation of colon
Toxic megacolon
Code first (T51-T65) to identify toxic agent
EXCLUDES 1 *congenital megacolon (aganglionic) (Q43.1)*
megacolon (due to) (in) Chagas' disease (B57.32)
megacolon (due to) (in) Clostridium difficile (A04.7)
megacolon (due to) (in) Hirschsprung's disease (Q43.1)
CC Excl: See code: K59.2

K59.4 Anal spasm
Proctalgia fugax

K59.8 Other specified functional intestinal disorders
Atony of colon
Pseudo-obstruction (acute) (chronic) of intestine

K59.9 Functional intestinal disorder, unspecified

✓4th K60 Fissure and fistula of anal and rectal regions
EXCLUDES 1 *fissure and fistula of anal and rectal regions with abscess or cellulitis (K61.-)*
EXCLUDES 2 *anal sphincter tear (healed) (nontraumatic) (old) (K62.81)*

K60.0 Acute anal fissure
K60.1 Chronic anal fissure
K60.2 Anal fissure, unspecified
K60.3 Anal fistula
K60.4 Rectal fistula
Fistula of rectum to skin
EXCLUDES 1 *rectovaginal fistula (N82.3)*
vesicorectal fistual (N32.1)
K60.5 Anorectal fistula

✓4th K61 Abscess of anal and rectal regions
INCLUDES abscess of anal and rectal regions
cellulitis of anal and rectal regions

CC Excl: For CC codes in category K61, unless otherwise noted: K61.0-K61.4

K61.0 Anal abscess CC
Perianal abscess
EXCLUDES 1 *intrasphincteric abscess (K61.4)*

K61.1 Rectal abscess CC
Perirectal abscess
EXCLUDES 1 *ischiorectal abscess (K61.3)*
AHA: 2012, 4Q, 104

K61.2 Anorectal abscess CC
K61.3 Ischiorectal abscess CC
Abscess of ischiorectal fossa
K61.4 Intrasphincteric abscess CC

✓4th K62 Other diseases of anus and rectum
INCLUDES anal canal
EXCLUDES 2 *colostomy and enterostomy malfunction (K94.0-, K94.1-)*
fecal incontinence (R15.-)
hemorrhoids (K64.-)

K62.0 Anal polyp
K62.1 Rectal polyp
EXCLUDES 1 *adenomatous polyp (D12.8)*
K62.2 Anal prolapse
Prolapse of anal canal
K62.3 Rectal prolapse
Prolapse of rectal mucosa
K62.4 Stenosis of anus and rectum
Stricture of anus (sphincter)
K62.5 Hemorrhage of anus and rectum CC
EXCLUDES 1 *gastrointestinal bleeding NOS (K92.2)*
melena (K92.1)
neonatal rectal hemorrhage (P54.2)
CC Excl: E16.4, I85.01, K22.10-K22.11, K22.6-K22.719, K25.0-K28.9, K29.01, K29.21, K29.31, K29.41, K29.51, K29.61, K29.71, K29.81, K29.91, K31.811, K55.21, K57.01, K57.11, K57.13, K57.21, K57.31, K57.33, K57.41, K57.51, K57.53, K57.81, K57.91, K57.93, K62.5, K92.0-K92.2
K62.6 Ulcer of anus and rectum CC
Solitary ulcer of anus and rectum
Stercoral ulcer of anus and rectum
EXCLUDES 1 *fissure and fistula of anus and rectum (K60.-)*
ulcerative colitis (K51.-)
CC Excl: K62.6
K62.7 Radiation proctitis
Use additional code to identify the type of radiation (W90.-)

✓5th K62.8 Other specified diseases of anus and rectum
EXCLUDES 2 *ulcerative proctitis (K51.2)*

K62.81 Anal sphincter tear (healed) (nontraumatic) (old)
Tear of anus, nontraumatic
Use additional code for any associated fecal incontinence (R15.-)
EXCLUDES 2 *anal fissure (K60.-)*
anal sphincter tear (healed) (old) complicating delivery (O34.7-)
traumatic tear of anal sphincter (S31.831)

K62.82 Dysplasia of anus
Anal intraepithelial neoplasia I and II (AIN I and II) (histologically confirmed)
Dysplasia of anus NOS
Mild and moderate dysplasia of anus (histologically confirmed)
EXCLUDES 1 *abnormal results from anal cytologic examination without histologic confirmation (R85.61-)*
anal intraepithelial neoplasia III (D01.3)
carcinoma in situ of anus (D01.3)
HGSIL of anus (R85.613)
severe dysplasia of anus (D01.3)

K62.89 Other specified diseases of anus and rectum
Proctitis NOS
Use additional code for any associated fecal incontinence (R15.-)

K62.9 Disease of anus and rectum, unspecified

✓4th K63 Other diseases of intestine

K63.0 Abscess of intestine CC
EXCLUDES 1 *abscess of intestine with Crohn's disease (K50.014, K50.114, K50.814, K50.914)*
abscess of intestine with diverticular disease (K57.0, K57.2, K57.4, K57.8)
abscess of intestine with ulcerative colitis (K51.014, K51.214, K51.314, K51.414, K51.514, K51.814, K51.914)
EXCLUDES 2 *abscess of anal and rectal regions (K61.-)*
abscess of appendix (K35.3)
CC Excl: K63.0

K63.1 Perforation of intestine (nontraumatic) MCC
Perforation (nontraumatic) of rectum
EXCLUDES 1 *perforation (nontraumatic) of duodenum (K26.-)*
perforation (nontraumatic) of intestine with diverticular disease (K57.0, K57.2, K57.4, K57.8)
EXCLUDES 2 *perforation (nontraumatic) of appendix (K35.2, K35.3)*
CC Excl: K63.1

K63.2 Fistula of intestine CC
EXCLUDES 1 *fistula of duodenum (K31.6)*
fistula of intestine with Crohn's disease (K50.013, K50.113, K50.813, K50.913)
fistula of intestine with ulcerative colitis (K51.013, K51.213, K51.313, K51.413, K51.513, K51.813, K51.913)
EXCLUDES 2 *fistula of anal and rectal regions (K60.-)*
fistula of appendix (K38.3)
intestinal-genital fistula, female (N82.2-N82.4)
vesicointestinal fistula (N32.1)
CC Excl: K63.2

K63.3 Ulcer of intestine CC
Primary ulcer of small intestine
EXCLUDES 1 *duodenal ulcer (K26.-)*
gastrointestinal ulcer (K28.-)
gastrojejunal ulcer (K28.-)
jejunal ulcer (K28.-)
peptic ulcer, site unspecified (K27.-)
ulcer of intestine with perforation (K63.1)
ulcer of anus or rectum (K62.6)
ulcerative colitis (K51.-)
CC Excl: K63.3

K63.4 Enteroptosis

K63.5 Polyp of colon
EXCLUDES 1 *adenomatous polyp of colon (D12.6)*
inflammatory polyp of colon (K51.4-)
polyposis of colon (D12.6)

✓5th **K63.8 Other specified diseases of intestine**

K63.81 Dieulafoy lesion of intestine MCC
EXCLUDES 2 *Dieulafoy lesion of stomach and duodenum (K31.82)*
CC Excl: E16.4, I85.01, K22.10-K22.11, K22.6-K22.719, K25.0-K28.9, K29.01, K29.21, K29.31, K29.41, K29.51, K29.61, K29.71, K29.81, K29.91, K31.811, K55.21, K57.01, K57.11, K57.13, K57.21, K57.31, K57.33, K57.41, K57.51, K57.53, K57.81, K57.91, K57.93, K62.5, K63.81, K92.0-K92.2

K63.89 Other specified diseases of intestine
AHA: 2013, 2Q, 31

K63.9 Disease of intestine, unspecified

✓4th **K64 Hemorrhoids and perianal venous thrombosis**
INCLUDES piles
EXCLUDES 1 *hemorrhoids complicating childbirth and the puerperium (O87.2)*
hemorrhoids complicating pregnancy (O22.4)

K64.0 First degree hemorrhoids
Grade/stage I hemorrhoids
Hemorrhoids (bleeding) without prolapse outside of anal canal

K64.1 Second degree hemorrhoids
Grade/stage II hemorrhoids
Hemorrhoids (bleeding) that prolapse with straining, but retract spontaneously

K64.2 Third degree hemorrhoids
Grade/stage III hemorrhoids
Hemorrhoids (bleeding) that prolapse with straining and require manual replacement back inside anal canal

K64.3 Fourth degree hemorrhoids
Grade/stage IV hemorrhoids
Hemorrhoids (bleeding) with prolapsed tissue that cannot be manually replaced

K64.4 Residual hemorrhoidal skin tags
External hemorrhoids, NOS
Skin tags of anus

K64.5 Perianal venous thrombosis
External hemorrhoids with thrombosis
Perianal hematoma
Thrombosed hemorrhoids NOS

K64.8 Other hemorrhoids
Internal hemorrhoids, without mention of degree
Prolapsed hemorrhoids, degree not specified

K64.9 Unspecified hemorrhoids
Hemorrhoids (bleeding) NOS
Hemorrhoids (bleeding) without mention of degree

Diseases of peritoneum and retroperitoneum (K65-K68)

✓4th **K65 Peritonitis**
Use additional code (B95-B97), to identify infectious agent
EXCLUDES 1 *acute appendicitis with generalized peritonitis (K35.2)*
aseptic peritonitis (T81.6)
benign paroxysmal peritonitis (E85.0)
chemical peritonitis (T81.6)
diverticulitis of both small and large intestine with peritonitis (K57.4-)
diverticulitis of colon with peritonitis (K57.2-)
diverticulitis of intestine, NOS, with peritonitis (K57.8-)
diverticulitis of small intestine with peritonitis (K57.0-)
gonococcal peritonitis (A54.85)
neonatal peritonitis (P78.0-P78.1)
pelvic peritonitis, female (N73.3-N73.5)
periodic familial peritonitis (E85.0)
peritonitis due to talc or other foreign substance (T81.6)
peritonitis in chlamydia (A74.81)
peritonitis in diphtheria (A36.89)
peritonitis in syphilis (late) (A52.74)
peritonitis in tuberculosis (A18.31)
peritonitis with or following abortion or ectopic or molar pregnancy (O00-O07, O08.0)
peritonitis with or following appendicitis (K35.-)
peritonitis with or following diverticular disease of intestine (K57.-)
puerperal peritonitis (O85)
retroperitoneal infections (K68.-)

CC Excl: For MCC codes in category K65, unless otherwise noted:
K63.4, K63.89-K63.9, K65.0-K65.9, K67, K68.19-K68.9, K92.89-K92.9, R11.13

K65.0 Generalized (acute) peritonitis MCC
Pelvic peritonitis (acute), male
Subphrenic peritonitis (acute)
Suppurative peritonitis (acute)

K65.1 Peritoneal abscess MCC
Abdominopelvic abscess
Abscess (of) omentum
Abscess (of) peritoneum
Mesenteric abscess
Retrocecal abscess
Subdiaphragmatic abscess
Subhepatic abscess
Subphrenic abscess

K65.2 Spontaneous bacterial peritonitis MCC
EXCLUDES 1 *bacterial peritonitis NOS (K65.9)*

K65.3 Choleperitonitis MCC
Peritonitis due to bile

K65.4 Sclerosing mesenteritis CC
Fat necrosis of peritoneum
(Idiopathic) sclerosing mesenteric fibrosis
Mesenteric lipodystrophy
Mesenteric panniculitis
Retractile mesenteritis

K65.8 Other peritonitis MCC
Chronic proliferative peritonitis
Peritonitis due to urine

K65.9 Peritonitis, unspecified MCC
Bacterial peritonitis NOS
AHA: 2013, 2Q, 31

✓4th **K66 Other disorders of peritoneum**
EXCLUDES 2 *ascites (R18.-)*
peritoneal effusion (chronic) (R18.8)

K66.0 Peritoneal adhesions (postprocedural) (postinfection)
Adhesions (of) abdominal (wall)
Adhesions (of) diaphragm
Adhesions (of) intestine
Adhesions (of) male pelvis
Adhesions (of) omentum
Adhesions (of) stomach
Adhesive bands
Mesenteric adhesions
EXCLUDES 1 *female pelvic adhesions [bands] (N73.6)*
peritoneal adhesions with intestinal obstruction (K56.5)

K66.1 Hemoperitoneum MCC
EXCLUDES 1 *traumatic hemoperitoneum (S36.8-)*
CC Excl: K66.1

K66.8 Other specified disorders of peritoneum

K66.9 Disorder of peritoneum, unspecified

K67 Disorders of peritoneum in infectious diseases classified elsewhere MCC
Code first underlying disease, such as:
congenital syphilis (A50.0)
helminthiasis (B65.0-B83.9)
EXCLUDES 1 *peritonitis in chlamydia (A74.81)*
peritonitis in diphtheria (A36.89)
peritonitis in gonococcal (A54.85)
peritonitis in syphilis (late) (A52.74)
peritonitis in tuberculosis (A18.31)
CC Excl: See code: K65

✓4th **K68 Disorders of retroperitoneum**

✓5th **K68.1 Retroperitoneal abscess**

4, 6, 8 **K68.11 Postprocedural retroperitoneal abscess** CC
CC Excl: D78.81-D78.89, E36.8, E89.810-E89.89, H59.011-H59.019, H59.031-H59.099, H59.811-H59.89, H95.811-H95.89, I97.3, K68.11, L76.81-L76.82, M96.89, N98.1-N98.9, T81.4XXA, T81.82XA, T81.89XA, T81.9XXA

K68.12 Psoas muscle abscess MCC
CC Excl: K68.12, M60.000-M60.19, M61.00-M61.19, M61.30-M61.59, M62.3, M62.50-M62.59, M62.89, M72.6

K68.19 Other retroperitoneal abscess MCC
CC Excl: See code: K65

K68.9 Other disorders of retroperitoneum MCC
CC Excl: See code: K65

4 HAC = as SDx not POA, in combination with PDx E66.01 **AND** one of the following procedure codes: 0D16[0,4,8][7,J,K,Z][9,A,B,L] or 0DV64CZ.
6 HAC = as SDx not POA, in combination with one of the following procedure codes: 0RG[0,1,2,4,6,7,8,A][0,3,4][7,A,J,K,Z][0,1,J]; 0RG[E,F,G,H,J,K][0,3,4][4,7,J,K,Z]Z; 0RG[L,M][0,3,4][4,5,7,J,K,Z]Z; 0RQ[E,F,G,H,J,K,L,M][0,3,4,X]ZZ; 0RU[E,F,G,H,J,K,L,M][0,3,4][7,J,K]Z; 0SG[0,1,3][0,3,4][7,A,J,K,Z][0,1,J]; 0SG[7,8][0,3,4[4,7,J,K,Z]Z.
8 HAC = as SDx not POA, in combination with one of the following procedure codes: 02H43[J,K,M]Z; 02H[6,7]3[J,M]Z; 02H[K,L]3JZ; 02HN[0,3,4][J,M]Z; 02PA[0,3,4]MZ; 02PAXMZ; 02WA[0,3,4]MZ; 0JH[6,8][0,3][4,5,6,7,8,9,P]Z; 0J[P,W]T[0,3]PZ.

Diseases of liver (K70-K77)

EXCLUDES 1 *jaundice NOS (R17)*
EXCLUDES 2 *hemochromatosis (E83.11-)*
Reye's syndrome (G93.7)
viral hepatitis (B15-B19)
Wilson's disease (E83.0)

✓4th **K70 Alcoholic liver disease**
Use additional code to identify:
alcohol abuse and dependence (F10.-)

K70.0 Alcoholic fatty liver A
✓5th **K70.1 Alcoholic hepatitis**
K70.10 Alcoholic hepatitis without ascites A
K70.11 Alcoholic hepatitis with ascites A
K70.2 Alcoholic fibrosis and sclerosis of liver A
✓5th **K70.3 Alcoholic cirrhosis of liver**
Alcoholic cirrhosis NOS
K70.30 Alcoholic cirrhosis of liver without ascites A
K70.31 Alcoholic cirrhosis of liver with ascites A
✓5th **K70.4 Alcoholic hepatic failure**
Acute alcoholic hepatic failure
Alcoholic hepatic failure NOS
Chronic alcoholic hepatic failure
Subacute alcoholic hepatic failure
K70.40 Alcoholic hepatic failure without coma A
K70.41 Alcoholic hepatic failure with coma PDx MCC MCC A
CC Excl: K72.91, K76.5, K76.89-K76.9
K70.9 Alcoholic liver disease, unspecified A

✓4th **K71 Toxic liver disease**
INCLUDES drug-induced idiosyncratic (unpredictable) liver disease
drug-induced toxic (predictable) liver disease
Code first poisoning due to drug or toxin, if applicable (T36-T65 with fifth or sixth character 1-4 or 6)
Use additional code for adverse effect, if applicable, to identify drug (T36-T50 with fifth or sixth character 5)
EXCLUDES 2 *alcoholic liver disease (K70.-)*
Budd-Chiari syndrome (I82.0)

K71.0 Toxic liver disease with cholestasis
Cholestasis with hepatocyte injury
"Pure" cholestasis
✓5th **K71.1 Toxic liver disease with hepatic necrosis**
Hepatic failure (acute) (chronic) due to drugs
K71.10 Toxic liver disease with hepatic necrosis, without coma
K71.11 Toxic liver disease with hepatic necrosis, with coma PDx MCC MCC
CC Excl: See code: K70.41
K71.2 Toxic liver disease with acute hepatitis
K71.3 Toxic liver disease with chronic persistent hepatitis
K71.4 Toxic liver disease with chronic lobular hepatitis
✓5th **K71.5 Toxic liver disease with chronic active hepatitis**
Toxic liver disease with lupoid hepatitis
K71.50 Toxic liver disease with chronic active hepatitis without ascites
K71.51 Toxic liver disease with chronic active hepatitis with ascites
K71.6 Toxic liver disease with hepatitis, not elsewhere classified
K71.7 Toxic liver disease with fibrosis and cirrhosis of liver
K71.8 Toxic liver disease with other disorders of liver
Toxic liver disease with focal nodular hyperplasia
Toxic liver disease with hepatic granulomas
Toxic liver disease with peliosis hepatis
Toxic liver disease with veno-occlusive disease of liver
K71.9 Toxic liver disease, unspecified

✓4th **K72 Hepatic failure, not elsewhere classified**
INCLUDES acute hepatitis NEC, with hepatic failure
fulminant hepatitis NEC, with hepatic failure
hepatic encephalopathy NOS
liver (cell) necrosis with hepatic failure
malignant hepatitis NEC, with hepatic failure
yellow liver atrophy or dystrophy
EXCLUDES 1 *alcoholic hepatic failure (K70.4)*
hepatic failure with toxic liver disease (K71.1-)
icterus of newborn (P55-P59)
postprocedural hepatic failure (K91.82)
viral hepatitis with hepatic coma (B15-B19)
EXCLUDES 2 *hepatic failure complicating abortion or ectopic or molar pregnancy (O00-O07, O08.8)*
hepatic failure complicating pregnancy, childbirth and the puerperium (O26.6-)

✓5th **K72.0 Acute and subacute hepatic failure**
AHA: 2014, 2Q, 13
K72.00 Acute and subacute hepatic failure without coma MCC
CC Excl: K72.00-K72.01, K76.2-K76.3, K76.5, K76.89-K76.9
K72.01 Acute and subacute hepatic failure with coma PDx MCC MCC
CC Excl: See code: K72.00
✓5th **K72.1 Chronic hepatic failure**
K72.10 Chronic hepatic failure without coma
K72.11 Chronic hepatic failure with coma PDx MCC MCC
CC Excl: K72.91, K76.5, K76.89-K76.9
✓5th **K72.9 Hepatic failure, unspecified**
K72.90 Hepatic failure, unspecified without coma
CC Excl: No Excl
K72.91 Hepatic failure, unspecified with coma MCC
Hepatic coma NOS
CC Excl: K72.91-K76.5, K76.89-K76.9

✓4th **K73 Chronic hepatitis, not elsewhere classified**
EXCLUDES 1 *alcoholic hepatitis (chronic) (K70.1-)*
drug-induced hepatitis (chronic) (K71.-)
granulomatous hepatitis (chronic) NEC (K75.3)
reactive, nonspecific hepatitis (chronic) (K75.2)
viral hepatitis (chronic) (B15-B19)

K73.0 Chronic persistent hepatitis, not elsewhere classified
K73.1 Chronic lobular hepatitis, not elsewhere classified
K73.2 Chronic active hepatitis, not elsewhere classified
K73.8 Other chronic hepatitis, not elsewhere classified
K73.9 Chronic hepatitis, unspecified

✓4th **K74 Fibrosis and cirrhosis of liver**
Code also, if applicable, viral hepatitis (acute) (chronic) (B15-B19)
EXCLUDES 1 *alcoholic cirrhosis (of liver) (K70.3)*
alcoholic fibrosis of liver (K70.2)
cardiac sclerosis of liver (K76.1)
cirrhosis (of liver) with toxic liver disease (K71.7)
congenital cirrhosis (of liver) (P78.81)
pigmentary cirrhosis (of liver) (E83.110)

K74.0 Hepatic fibrosis
K74.1 Hepatic sclerosis
K74.2 Hepatic fibrosis with hepatic sclerosis
K74.3 Primary biliary cirrhosis
Chronic nonsuppurative destructive cholangitis
K74.4 Secondary biliary cirrhosis
K74.5 Biliary cirrhosis, unspecified
✓5th **K74.6 Other and unspecified cirrhosis of liver**
K74.60 Unspecified cirrhosis of liver
Cirrhosis (of liver) NOS
K74.69 Other cirrhosis of liver
Cryptogenic cirrhosis (of liver)
Macronodular cirrhosis (of liver)
Micronodular cirrhosis (of liver)
Mixed type cirrhosis (of liver)
Portal cirrhosis (of liver)
Postnecrotic cirrhosis (of liver)

✓4th K75 Other inflammatory liver diseases
EXCLUDES 2 *toxic liver disease (K71.-)*

K75.Ø Abscess of liver MCC
Cholangitic hepatic abscess
Hematogenic hepatic abscess
Hepatic abscess NOS
Lymphogenic hepatic abscess
Pylephlebitic hepatic abscess
EXCLUDES 1 *amebic liver abscess (AØ6.4)*
cholangitis without liver abscess (K83.Ø)
pylephlebitis without liver abscess (K75.1)
CC Excl: AØ6.4, K75.1, K76.5, K76.89-K76.9

K75.1 Phlebitis of portal vein MCC
Pylephlebitis
EXCLUDES 1 *pylephlebitic liver abscess (K75.Ø)*
CC Excl: See code: K75.Ø

K75.2 Nonspecific reactive hepatitis
EXCLUDES 1 *acute or subacute hepatitis (K72.Ø-)*
chronic hepatitis NEC (K73.-)
viral hepatitis (B15-B19)

K75.3 Granulomatous hepatitis, not elsewhere classified
EXCLUDES 1 *acute or subacute hepatitis (K72.Ø-)*
chronic hepatitis NEC (K73.-)
viral hepatitis (B15-B19)

K75.4 Autoimmune hepatitis
Lupoid hepatitis NEC

✓5th K75.8 Other specified inflammatory liver diseases
K75.81 Nonalcoholic steatohepatitis (NASH)
K75.89 Other specified inflammatory liver diseases

K75.9 Inflammatory liver disease, unspecified
Hepatitis NOS
EXCLUDES 1 *acute or subacute hepatitis (K72.Ø-)*
chronic hepatitis NEC (K73.-)
viral hepatitis (B15-B19)

✓4th K76 Other diseases of liver
EXCLUDES 2 *alcoholic liver disease (K7Ø.-)*
amyloid degeneration of liver (E85.-)
cystic disease of liver (congenital) (Q44.6)
hepatic vein thrombosis (I82.Ø)
hepatomegaly NOS (R16.Ø)
pigmentary cirrhosis (of liver) (E83.11Ø)
portal vein thrombosis (I81)
toxic liver disease (K71.-)

K76.Ø Fatty (change of) liver, not elsewhere classified
Nonalcoholic fatty liver disease (NAFLD)
EXCLUDES 1 *nonalcoholic steatohepatitis (NASH) (K75.81)*

K76.1 Chronic passive congestion of liver
Cardiac cirrhosis
Cardiac sclerosis

K76.2 Central hemorrhagic necrosis of liver MCC
EXCLUDES 1 *liver necrosis with hepatic failure (K72.-)*
CC Excl: K72.ØØ-K72.Ø1, K76.2-K76.3, K76.5, K76.89-K76.9

K76.3 Infarction of liver MCC
CC Excl: See code: K76.2

K76.4 Peliosis hepatis
Hepatic angiomatosis

K76.5 Hepatic veno-occlusive disease
EXCLUDES 1 *Budd-Chiari syndrome (I82.Ø)*

K76.6 Portal hypertension CC
Use additional code for any associated complications, such as:
portal hypertensive gastropathy (K31.89)
CC Excl: K72.91-K76.6, K76.89-K76.9

K76.7 Hepatorenal syndrome MCC
EXCLUDES 1 *hepatorenal syndrome following labor and delivery (O9Ø.4)*
postprocedural hepatorenal syndrome (K91.82)
CC Excl: K76.5-K76.7, K76.89-K76.9

✓5th K76.8 Other specified diseases of liver
K76.81 Hepatopulmonary syndrome
Code first underlying liver disease, such as:
alcoholic cirrhosis of liver (K7Ø.3-)
cirrhosis of liver without mention of alcohol (K74.6-)
K76.89 Other specified diseases of liver
Cyst (simple) of liver
Focal nodular hyperplasia of liver
Hepatoptosis

K76.9 Liver disease, unspecified

K77 Liver disorders in diseases classified elsewhere CC
Code first underlying disease, such as:
amyloidosis (E85.-)
congenital syphilis (A5Ø.Ø, A5Ø.5)
congenital toxoplasmosis (P37.1)
schistosomiasis (B65.Ø-B65.9)
EXCLUDES 1 *alcoholic hepatitis (K7Ø.1-)*
alcoholic liver disease (K7Ø-.)
cytomegaloviral hepatitis (B25.1)
herpesviral [herpes simplex] hepatitis (BØØ.81)
infectious mononucleosis with liver disease (B27.Ø-B27.9 with .9)
mumps hepatitis (B26.81)
sarcoidosis with liver disease (D86.89)
secondary syphilis with liver disease (A51.45)
syphilis (late) with liver disease (A52.74)
toxoplasmosis (acquired) hepatitis (B58.1)
tuberculosis with liver disease (A18.83)
CC Excl: No Excl

Disorders of gallbladder, biliary tract and pancreas (K8Ø-K87)

✓4th K8Ø Cholelithiasis
EXCLUDES 1 *retained cholelithiasis following cholecystectomy (K91.86)*

✓5th K8Ø.Ø Calculus of gallbladder with acute cholecystitis
Any condition listed in K8Ø.2 with acute cholecystitis
K8Ø.ØØ Calculus of gallbladder with acute cholecystitis without obstruction CC
CC Excl: K8Ø.ØØ-K8Ø.21, K8Ø.4Ø, K8Ø.44, K8Ø.62-K8Ø.63, K8Ø.66-K8Ø.67, K8Ø.8Ø, K81.Ø-K81.9, K82.9, K83.5-K83.9, K87
K8Ø.Ø1 Calculus of gallbladder with acute cholecystitis with obstruction CC
CC Excl: K8Ø.ØØ-K8Ø.21, K8Ø.62-K8Ø.63, K8Ø.66-K8Ø.67, K8Ø.8Ø, K81.Ø-K81.9, K82.9, K83.5-K83.9, K87

✓5th K8Ø.1 Calculus of gallbladder with other cholecystitis
CC Excl: For CC codes in subcategory K8Ø.1, unless otherwise noted: See code: K8Ø.Ø1
K8Ø.1Ø Calculus of gallbladder with chronic cholecystitis without obstruction CC
Cholelithiasis with cholecystitis NOS
K8Ø.11 Calculus of gallbladder with chronic cholecystitis with obstruction CC
K8Ø.12 Calculus of gallbladder with acute and chronic cholecystitis without obstruction CC
CC Excl: See code: K8Ø.ØØ
K8Ø.13 Calculus of gallbladder with acute and chronic cholecystitis with obstruction CC
K8Ø.18 Calculus of gallbladder with other cholecystitis without obstruction CC
K8Ø.19 Calculus of gallbladder with other cholecystitis with obstruction CC

✓5th K8Ø.2 Calculus of gallbladder without cholecystitis
Cholecystolithiasis without cholecystitis
Cholelithiasis (without cholecystitis)
Colic (recurrent) of gallbladder (without cholecystitis)
Gallstone (impacted) of cystic duct (without cholecystitis)
Gallstone (impacted) of gallbladder (without cholecystitis)
K8Ø.2Ø Calculus of gallbladder without cholecystitis without obstruction
K8Ø.21 Calculus of gallbladder without cholecystitis with obstruction CC
CC Excl: See code: K8Ø.Ø1

✓5th K8Ø.3 Calculus of bile duct with cholangitis
Any condition listed in K8Ø.5 with cholangitis
CC Excl: For CC codes in subcategory K8Ø.3, unless otherwise noted: K83.Ø, K83.5-K83.9, K87
K8Ø.3Ø Calculus of bile duct with cholangitis, unspecified, without obstruction PDx CC
K8Ø.31 Calculus of bile duct with cholangitis, unspecified, with obstruction PDx CC CC
CC Excl: K8Ø.3Ø-K8Ø.71, K8Ø.81-K81.9, K83.5-K83.9, K87
K8Ø.32 Calculus of bile duct with acute cholangitis without obstruction PDx CC
K8Ø.33 Calculus of bile duct with acute cholangitis with obstruction PDx CC CC
CC Excl: See code: K8Ø.31
K8Ø.34 Calculus of bile duct with chronic cholangitis without obstruction PDx CC

K8Ø.35 Calculus of bile duct with chronic cholangitis with obstruction PDx CC CC
CC Excl: See code: K8Ø.31

K8Ø.36 Calculus of bile duct with acute and chronic cholangitis without obstruction PDx CC

K8Ø.37 Calculus of bile duct with acute and chronic cholangitis with obstruction PDx CC CC
CC Excl: See code: K8Ø.31

5th **K8Ø.4 Calculus of bile duct with cholecystitis**
Any condition listed in K8Ø.5 with cholecystitis (with cholangitis)

CC Excl: For CC codes in subcategory K8Ø.4, unless otherwise noted: K8Ø.3Ø-K8Ø.71, K8Ø.81-K81.9, K83.5-K83.9, K87

K8Ø.4Ø Calculus of bile duct with cholecystitis, unspecified, without obstruction CC

K8Ø.41 Calculus of bile duct with cholecystitis, unspecified, with obstruction CC

K8Ø.42 Calculus of bile duct with acute cholecystitis without obstruction CC

K8Ø.43 Calculus of bile duct with acute cholecystitis with obstruction CC

K8Ø.44 Calculus of bile duct with chronic cholecystitis without obstruction CC

K8Ø.45 Calculus of bile duct with chronic cholecystitis with obstruction CC

K8Ø.46 Calculus of bile duct with acute and chronic cholecystitis without obstruction CC

K8Ø.47 Calculus of bile duct with acute and chronic cholecystitis with obstruction CC

5th **K8Ø.5 Calculus of bile duct without cholangitis or cholecystitis**
Choledocholithiasis (without cholangitis or cholecystitis)
Gallstone (impacted) of bile duct NOS (without cholangitis or cholecystitis)
Gallstone (impacted) of common duct (without cholangitis or cholecystitis)
Gallstone (impacted) of hepatic duct (without cholangitis or cholecystitis)
Hepatic cholelithiasis (without cholangitis or cholecystitis)
Hepatic colic (recurrent) (without cholangitis or cholecystitis)

K8Ø.5Ø Calculus of bile duct without cholangitis or cholecystitis without obstruction

K8Ø.51 Calculus of bile duct without cholangitis or cholecystitis with obstruction CC
CC Excl: K8Ø.3Ø-K8Ø.71, K8Ø.81-K81.9, K83.5-K83.9, K87

5th **K8Ø.6 Calculus of gallbladder and bile duct with cholecystitis**

CC Excl: For CC codes in subcategory K8Ø.6, unless otherwise noted: See code: K8Ø.51

K8Ø.6Ø Calculus of gallbladder and bile duct with cholecystitis, unspecified, without obstruction CC

K8Ø.61 Calculus of gallbladder and bile duct with cholecystitis, unspecified, with obstruction CC

K8Ø.62 Calculus of gallbladder and bile duct with acute cholecystitis without obstruction CC
CC Excl: K8Ø.62-K8Ø.63, K81.Ø-K81.9, K82.9, K83.5-K83.9, K87

K8Ø.63 Calculus of gallbladder and bile duct with acute cholecystitis with obstruction CC
CC Excl: See code: K8Ø.62

K8Ø.64 Calculus of gallbladder and bile duct with chronic cholecystitis without obstruction CC

K8Ø.65 Calculus of gallbladder and bile duct with chronic cholecystitis with obstruction CC

K8Ø.66 Calculus of gallbladder and bile duct with acute and chronic cholecystitis without obstruction CC
CC Excl: K8Ø.66-K8Ø.67, K81.Ø-K81.9, K82.9, K83.5-K83.9, K87

K8Ø.67 Calculus of gallbladder and bile duct with acute and chronic cholecystitis with obstruction MCC
CC Excl: See code: K8Ø.66

5th **K8Ø.7 Calculus of gallbladder and bile duct without cholecystitis**

K8Ø.7Ø Calculus of gallbladder and bile duct without cholecystitis without obstruction

K8Ø.71 Calculus of gallbladder and bile duct without cholecystitis with obstruction CC
CC Excl: See code: K8Ø.51

5th **K8Ø.8 Other cholelithiasis**

K8Ø.8Ø Other cholelithiasis without obstruction

K8Ø.81 Other cholelithiasis with obstruction CC
CC Excl: See code: K8Ø.51

4th **K81 Cholecystitis**
EXCLUDES 1 *cholecystitis with cholelithiasis (K8Ø.-)*

K81.Ø Acute cholecystitis CC
Abscess of gallbladder
Angiocholecystitis
Emphysematous (acute) cholecystitis
Empyema of gallbladder
Gangrene of gallbladder
Gangrenous cholecystitis
Suppurative cholecystitis
CC Excl: K8Ø.62-K8Ø.63, K8Ø.66-K8Ø.67, K81.Ø-K81.9, K82.9, K83.5-K83.9, K87

K81.1 Chronic cholecystitis

K81.2 Acute cholecystitis with chronic cholecystitis CC
CC Excl: K81.Ø-K81.9, K82.9, K83.5-K83.9, K87

K81.9 Cholecystitis, unspecified

4th **K82 Other diseases of gallbladder**
EXCLUDES 1 *nonvisualization of gallbladder (R93.2)*
postcholecystectomy syndrome (K91.5)

CC Excl: For CC/MCC codes in category K82, unless otherwise noted: K82.Ø-K82.9, K83.5-K83.9, K87

K82.Ø Obstruction of gallbladder CC
Occlusion of cystic duct or gallbladder without cholelithiasis
Stenosis of cystic duct or gallbladder without cholelithiasis
Stricture of cystic duct or gallbladder without cholelithiasis
EXCLUDES 1 *obstruction of gallbladder with cholelithiasis (K8Ø.-)*

K82.1 Hydrops of gallbladder CC
Mucocele of gallbladder

K82.2 Perforation of gallbladder MCC
Rupture of cystic duct or gallbladder

K82.3 Fistula of gallbladder CC
Cholecystocolic fistula
Cholecystoduodenal fistula

K82.4 Cholesterolosis of gallbladder
Strawberry gallbladder
EXCLUDES 1 *cholesterolosis of gallbladder with cholecystitis (K81.-)*
cholesterolosis of gallbladder with cholelithiasis (K8Ø.-)

K82.8 Other specified diseases of gallbladder
Adhesions of cystic duct or gallbladder
Atrophy of cystic duct or gallbladder
Cyst of cystic duct or gallbladder
Dyskinesia of cystic duct or gallbladder
Hypertrophy of cystic duct or gallbladder
Nonfunctioning of cystic duct or gallbladder
Ulcer of cystic duct or gallbladder

K82.9 Disease of gallbladder, unspecified

4th **K83 Other diseases of biliary tract**
EXCLUDES 1 *postcholecystectomy syndrome (K91.5)*
EXCLUDES 2 *conditions involving the gallbladder (K81-K82)*
conditions involving the cystic duct (K81-K82)

K83.Ø Cholangitis CC
Ascending cholangitis
Cholangitis NOS
Primary cholangitis
Recurrent cholangitis
Sclerosing cholangitis
Secondary cholangitis
Stenosing cholangitis
Suppurative cholangitis
EXCLUDES 1 *cholangitic liver abscess (K75.Ø)*
cholangitis with choledocholithiasis (K8Ø.3-, K8Ø.4-)
chronic nonsuppurative destructive cholangitis (K74.3)
CC Excl: K83.Ø, K83.5-K83.9, K87

K83.1 Obstruction of bile duct MCC
Occlusion of bile duct without cholelithiasis
Stenosis of bile duct without cholelithiasis
Stricture of bile duct without cholelithiasis
EXCLUDES 1 *congenital obstruction of bile duct (Q44.3)*
obstruction of bile duct with cholelithiasis (K8Ø.-)
CC Excl: K8Ø.31, K8Ø.33, K8Ø.35, K8Ø.37, K8Ø.41, K8Ø.43, K8Ø.45, K8Ø.47, K8Ø.51, K8Ø.81, K83.1, K83.5-K83.9, K87, Q44.2-Q44.3

K83.2 Perforation of bile duct MCC
Rupture of bile duct
CC Excl: K83.2-K83.3, K83.5-K83.9, K87

K83.3 Fistula of bile duct CC
Choledochoduodenal fistula
CC Excl: See code: K83.2

K83.4 Spasm of sphincter of Oddi

K83.5 Biliary cyst

K83.8 Other specified diseases of biliary tract
Adhesions of biliary tract
Atrophy of biliary tract
Hypertrophy of biliary tract
Ulcer of biliary tract

K83.9 Disease of biliary tract, unspecified

K85 Acute pancreatitis
Abscess of pancreas
Acute necrosis of pancreas
Acute (recurrent) pancreatitis
Gangrene of (gangrenous) pancreas
Hemorrhagic pancreatitis
Infective necrosis of pancreas
Subacute pancreatitis
Suppurative pancreatitis

CC Excl: For MCC codes in category K85, unless otherwise noted: B25.2, K86.1, K86.8-K86.9

K85.0 Idiopathic acute pancreatitis MCC

K85.1 Biliary acute pancreatitis MCC
Gallstone pancreatitis

K85.2 Alcohol induced acute pancreatitis MCC
EXCLUDES 2 *alcohol induced chronic pancreatitis (K86.0)*

K85.3 Drug induced acute pancreatitis MCC
Use additional code for adverse effect, if applicable, to identify drug (T36-T50 with fifth or sixth character 5)
Use additional code to identify drug abuse and dependence (F11.– F17.-)

K85.8 Other acute pancreatitis MCC

K85.9 Acute pancreatitis, unspecified MCC
Pancreatitis NOS

K86 Other diseases of pancreas
EXCLUDES 2 *fibrocystic disease of pancreas (E84.-)*
islet cell tumor (of pancreas) (D13.7)
pancreatic steatorrhea (K90.3)

K86.0 Alcohol-induced chronic pancreatitis CC
Use additional code to identify:
alcohol abuse and dependence (F10.-)
EXCLUDES 2 *alcohol induced acute pancreatitis (K85.2)*
CC Excl: B25.2, E16.8, K85.0-K86.9

K86.1 Other chronic pancreatitis CC
Chronic pancreatitis NOS
Infectious chronic pancreatitis
Recurrent chronic pancreatitis
Relapsing chronic pancreatitis
CC Excl: See code: K86.0

K86.2 Cyst of pancreas CC
CC Excl: K86.2-K86.9

K86.3 Pseudocyst of pancreas CC
CC Excl: See code: K86.2

K86.8 Other specified diseases of pancreas
Aseptic pancreatic necrosis
Atrophy of pancreas
Calculus of pancreas
Cirrhosis of pancreas
Fibrosis of pancreas
Pancreatic fat necrosis
Pancreatic infantilism
Pancreatic necrosis NOS

K86.9 Disease of pancreas, unspecified

K87 Disorders of gallbladder, biliary tract and pancreas in diseases classified elsewhere
Code first underlying disease
EXCLUDES 1 *cytomegaloviral pancreatitis (B25.2)*
mumps pancreatitis (B26.3)
syphilitic gallbladder (A52.74)
syphilitic pancreas (A52.74)
tuberculosis of gallbladder (A18.83)
tuberculosis of pancreas (A18.83)

Other diseases of the digestive system (K90-K95)

K90 Intestinal malabsorption
EXCLUDES 1 *intestinal malabsorption following gastrointestinal surgery (K91.2)*

CC Excl: For CC codes in category K90, unless otherwise noted: E84.19, K90.0-K90.4, K90.89-K90.9, K91.2

K90.0 Celiac disease
Gluten-sensitive enteropathy
Idiopathic steatorrhea
Nontropical sprue
Use additional code for associated disorders including:
dermatitis herpetiformis (L13.0)
gluten ataxia (G32.81)

K90.1 Tropical sprue CC
Sprue NOS
Tropical steatorrhea

K90.2 Blind loop syndrome, not elsewhere classified CC
Blind loop syndrome NOS
EXCLUDES 1 *congenital blind loop syndrome (Q43.8)*
postsurgical blind loop syndrome (K91.2)

K90.3 Pancreatic steatorrhea CC

K90.4 Malabsorption due to intolerance, not elsewhere classified CC
Malabsorption due to intolerance to carbohydrate
Malabsorption due to intolerance to fat
Malabsorption due to intolerance to protein
Malabsorption due to intolerance to starch
EXCLUDES 2 *gluten-sensitive enteropathy (K90.0)*
lactose intolerance (E73.-)

K90.8 Other intestinal malabsorption

K90.81 Whipple's disease CC
CC Excl: K90.81

K90.89 Other intestinal malabsorption CC

K90.9 Intestinal malabsorption, unspecified CC

K91 Intraoperative and postprocedural complications and disorders of digestive system, not elsewhere classified
EXCLUDES 2 *complications of artificial opening of digestive system (K94.-)*
complications of bariatric procedures (K95.-)
gastrojejunal ulcer (K28.-)
postprocedural (radiation) retroperitoneal abscess (K68.11)
radiation colitis (K52.0)
radiation gastroenteritis (K52.0)
radiation proctitis (K62.7)

K91.0 Vomiting following gastrointestinal surgery

K91.1 Postgastric surgery syndromes
Dumping syndrome
Postgastrectomy syndrome
Postvagotomy syndrome

K91.2 Postsurgical malabsorption, not elsewhere classified CC
Postsurgical blind loop syndrome
EXCLUDES 1 *malabsorption osteomalacia in adults (M83.2)*
malabsorption osteoporosis, postsurgical (M80.8-, M81.8)
CC Excl: K90.3-K90.4, K90.89-K90.9, K91.2

K91.3 Postprocedural intestinal obstruction CC
CC Excl: D78.81-D78.89, E36.8, E89.810-E89.89, H59.011-H59.019, H59.031-H59.099, H59.811-H59.89, H95.811-H95.89, I97.3, K91.3, K91.81-K91.83, K91.850-K91.89, K94.20-K95.89, L76.81-L76.82, M96.89, N98.1-N98.9, T81.710A, T81.82XA, T81.89XA, T81.9XXA

K91.5 Postcholecystectomy syndrome

K91.6 Intraoperative hemorrhage and hematoma of a digestive system organ or structure complicating a procedure
EXCLUDES 1 *intraoperative hemorrhage and hematoma of a digestive system organ or structure due to accidental puncture and laceration during a procedure (K91.7-)*

K91.61 Intraoperative hemorrhage and hematoma of a digestive system organ or structure complicating a digestive sytem procedure CC
CC Excl: H95.811-H95.89, I85.01, I85.11, I97.3, K21.9, K22.8, K23-K25.0, K25.2, K25.4, K25.6, K26.0, K26.2, K26.4, K26.6, K27.0, K27.2, K27.4, K27.6, K28.0, K28.2, K28.4, K28.6, K29.01, K29.21, K29.31, K29.41, K29.51, K29.61, K29.71, K29.81, K29.91, K31.811, K55.21, K57.01, K57.11, K57.13, K57.21, K57.31, K57.33, K57.41, K57.51, K57.53, K57.81, K57.91, K57.93, K62.5, K91.61-K91.62, K91.840-K91.841, K92.0-K92.2, M96.89, N98.1-N98.9, P54.1-P54.3, T81.10XA, T81.11XA, T81.12XA, T81.19XA, T81.82XA, T81.89XA, T81.9XXA

K91.62 Intraoperative hemorrhage and hematoma of a digestive system organ or structure complicating other procedure CC
CC Excl: See code: K91.61

✓5th **K91.7 Accidental puncture and laceration of a digestive system organ or structure during a procedure**

K91.71 Accidental puncture and laceration of a digestive system organ or structure during a digestive system procedure CC
CC Excl: D78.11-D78.12, D78.81-D78.89, E36.11-E36.8, E89.810-E89.89, G96.11, G97.41-G97.49, H59.011-H59.019, H59.031-H59.099, H59.211-H59.229, H59.811-H59.89, H95.31-H95.32, H95.811-H95.89, I97.3, I97.51-I97.52, J95.71-J95.72, K91.71-K91.72, L76.11-L76.12, L76.81-L76.82, M96.820-M96.821, M96.89, N98.1-N98.9, N99.71-N99.72, T81.82XA, T81.89XA, T81.9XXA

K91.72 Accidental puncture and laceration of a digestive system organ or structure during other procedure CC
CC Excl: See code: K91.71

✓5th **K91.8 Other intraoperative and postprocedural complications and disorders of digestive system**

CC Excl: For CC codes in subcategory K91.8, unless otherwise noted: See code: K91.3

K91.81 Other intraoperative complications of digestive system CC

K91.82 Postprocedural hepatic failure CC

K91.83 Postprocedural hepatorenal syndrome CC

✓6th **K91.84 Postprocedural hemorrhage and hematoma of a digestive system organ or structure following a procedure**

K91.840 Postprocedural hemorrhage and hematoma of a digestive system organ or structure following a digestive system procedure CC
CC Excl: See code: K91.61

K91.841 Postprocedural hemorrhage and hematoma of a digestive system organ or structure following other procedure CC
CC Excl: See code: K91.61

✓6th **K91.85 Complications of intestinal pouch**

K91.850 Pouchitis CC
Inflammation of internal ileoanal pouch

K91.858 Other complications of intestinal pouch CC

K91.86 Retained cholelithiasis following cholecystectomy CC

K91.89 Other postprocedural complications and disorders of digestive system CC
Use additional code, if applicable, to further specify disorder
EXCLUDES 2 *postprocedural retroperitoneal abscess (K68.11)*

✓4th **K92 Other diseases of digestive system**
EXCLUDES 1 *neonatal gastrointestinal hemorrhage (P54.0-P54.3)*

K92.0 Hematemesis CC
CC Excl: E16.4, I85.01, K22.10-K22.11, K22.6-K22.719, K25.0-K28.9, K29.01, K29.21, K29.31, K29.41, K29.51, K29.61, K29.71, K29.81, K29.91, K31.811, K55.21, K57.01, K57.11, K57.13, K57.21, K57.31, K57.33, K57.41, K57.51, K57.53, K57.81, K57.91, K57.93, K62.5, K92.0-K92.2

K92.1 Melena CC
EXCLUDES 1 *occult blood in feces (R19.5)*
CC Excl: See code: K92.0

K92.2 Gastrointestinal hemorrhage, unspecified CC
Gastric hemorrhage NOS
Intestinal hemorrhage NOS
EXCLUDES 1 *acute hemorrhagic gastritis (K29.01)*
hemorrhage of anus and rectum (K62.5)
angiodysplasia of stomach with hemorrhage (K31.811)
diverticular disease with hemorrhage (K57.-)
gastritis and duodenitis with hemorrhage (K29.-)
peptic ulcer with hemorrhage (K25-K28)
CC Excl: See code: K92.0

✓5th **K92.8 Other specified diseases of the digestive system**

K92.81 Gastrointestinal mucositis (ulcerative) CC
Code also type of associated therapy, such as:
antineoplastic and immunosuppressive drugs (T45.1X-)
radiological procedure and radiotherapy (Y84.2)
EXCLUDES 2 *mucositis (ulcerative) of vagina and vulva (N76.81)*
nasal mucositis (ulcerative) (J34.81)
oral mucositis (ulcerative) (K12.3-)
CC Excl: E16.4, I85.01, K22.10-K22.11, K22.6-K22.719, K25.0-K28.9, K29.01, K29.21, K29.31, K29.41, K29.51, K29.61, K29.71, K29.81, K29.91, K31.811, K31.89-K31.9, K55.21, K57.01, K57.11, K57.13, K57.21, K57.31, K57.33, K57.41, K57.51, K57.53, K57.81, K57.91, K57.93, K62.5, K92.0-K92.81

K92.89 Other specified diseases of the digestive system

K92.9 Disease of digestive system, unspecified

✓4th **K94 Complications of artificial openings of the digestive system**

✓5th **K94.0 Colostomy complications**

K94.00 Colostomy complication, unspecified

K94.01 Colostomy hemorrhage CC
CC Excl: K94.00-K94.19

K94.02 Colostomy infection CC
Use additional code to specify type of infection, such as:
cellulitis of abdominal wall (L03.311)
sepsis (A40-, A41-)
CC Excl: See code: K94.01

K94.03 Colostomy malfunction CC
Mechanical complication of colostomy
CC Excl: D78.81-D78.89, E36.8, E89.810-E89.89, H59.011-H59.019, H59.031-H59.099, H59.811-H59.89, H95.811-H95.89, I97.3, K91.3, K91.81-K91.83, K91.850-K91.89, K94.00-K95.89, L76.81-L76.82, M96.89, N98.1-N98.9, T81.710A, T81.82XA, T81.89XA, T81.9XXA

K94.09 Other complications of colostomy CC
CC Excl: See code: K94.01

✓5th **K94.1 Enterostomy complications**

K94.10 Enterostomy complication, unspecified

K94.11 Enterostomy hemorrhage CC
CC Excl: See code: K94.01

K94.12 Enterostomy infection CC
Use additional code to specify type of infection, such as:
cellulitis of abdominal wall (L03.311)
sepsis (A40-, A41-)
CC Excl: See code: K94.01

K94.13 Enterostomy malfunction CC
Mechanical complication of enterostomy
CC Excl: See code: K94.03

K94.19 Other complications of enterostomy CC
CC Excl: See code: K94.01

✓5th **K94.2 Gastrostomy complications**

K94.20 Gastrostomy complication, unspecified

K94.21 Gastrostomy hemorrhage

K94.22 Gastrostomy infection CC
Use additional code to specify type of infection, such as:
cellulitis of abdominal wall (L03.311)
sepsis (A40-, A41-)
CC Excl: See code: K91.3

K94.23 Gastrostomy malfunction CC
Mechanical complication of gastrostomy
CC Excl: See code: K91.3

K94.29 Other complications of gastrostomy

✓5th **K94.3 Esophagostomy complications**

CC Excl: For CC codes in subcategory K94.3, unless otherwise noted:D78.81-D78.89, E36.8, E89.810-E89.89, H59.011-H59.019, H59.031-H59.099, H59.811-H59.89, H95.811-H95.89, I97.3, K91.3, K91.81-K91.83, K91.850-K91.89, K94.20-K95.89, L76.81-L76.82, M96.89, N98.1-N98.9, T81.710A, T81.82XA, T81.89XA,T81.9XXA

K94.30 Esophagostomy complications, unspecified CC

K94.31 Esophagostomy hemorrhage CC

K94.32 Esophagostomy infection CC
Use additional code to identify the infection

K94.33 Esophagostomy malfunction CC
Mechanical complication of esophagostomy

K94.39 Other complications of esophagostom CC

✓4th K95 Complications of bariatric procedures

CC Excl: For CC codes in category K95, unless otherwise noted:
See code: K94.3

✓5th K95.0 Complications of gastric band procedure

4 **K95.01 Infection due to gastric band procedure** CC
Use additional code to specify type of infection or organism, such as:
bacterial and viral infectious agents (B95.-, B96.-)
cellulitis of abdominal wall (L03.311)
sepsis (A40.-, A41.-)

K95.09 Other complications of gastric band procedure CC
Use additional code, if applicable, to further specify complication

✓5th K95.8 Complications of other bariatric procedure

EXCLUDES 1 *complications of gastric band surgery (K95.0-)*

4 **K95.81 Infection due to other bariatric procedure** CC
Use additional code to specify type of infection or organism, such as:
bacterial and viral infectious agents (B95.-, B96.-)
cellulitis of abdominal wall (L03.311)
sepsis (A40.-, A41.-)

K95.89 Other complications of other bariatric procedure CC
Use additional code, if applicable, to further specify complication

4 HAC = as SDx not POA, in combination with PDx E66.01 **AND** one of the following procedure codes: 0D16[0,4,8][7,J,K,Z][9,A,B,L] or 0DV64CZ.

Chapter 12. Diseases of the Skin and Subcutaneous Tissue (LØØ-L99)

EXCLUDES 2 *certain conditions originating in the perinatal period (PØ4-P96)*
certain infectious and parasitic diseases (AØØ-B99)
complications of pregnancy, childbirth and the puerperium (OØØ-O9A)
congenital malformations, deformations, and chromosomal abnormalities (QØØ-Q99)
endocrine, nutritional and metabolic diseases (EØØ-E88)
lipomelanotic reticulosis (I89.8)
neoplasms (CØØ-D49)
symptoms, signs and abnormal clinical and laboratory findings, not elsewhere classified (RØØ-R94)
systemic connective tissue disorders (M3Ø-M36)
viral warts (BØ7.-)

This chapter contains the following blocks:

LØØ-LØ8	Infections of the skin and subcutaneous tissue
L1Ø-L14	Bullous disorders
L2Ø-L3Ø	Dermatitis and eczema
L4Ø-L45	Papulosquamous disorders
L49-L54	Urticaria and erythema
L55-L59	Radiation-related disorders of the skin and subcutaneous tissue
L6Ø-L75	Disorders of skin appendages
L76	Intraoperative and postprocedural complications of skin and subcutaneous tissue
L8Ø-L99	Other disorders of the skin and subcutaneous tissue

Infections of the skin and subcutaneous tissue (LØØ-LØ8)

Use additional code (B95-B97) to identify infectious agent

EXCLUDES 2 *hordeolum (HØØ.Ø)*
infective dermatitis (L3Ø.3)
local infections of skin classified in Chapter 1
lupus panniculitis (L93.2)
panniculitis NOS (M79.3)
panniculitis of neck and back (M54.Ø-)
Perlèche NOS (K13.Ø)
Perlèche due to candidiasis (B37.Ø)
Perlèche due to riboflavin deficiency (E53.Ø)
pyogenic granuloma (L98.Ø)
relapsing panniculitis [Weber-Christian] (M35.6)
viral warts (BØ7.-)
zoster (BØ2.-)

LØØ Staphylococcal scalded skin syndrome
Ritter's disease
Use additional code to identify percentage of skin exfoliation (L49.-)
EXCLUDES 1 *bullous impetigo (LØ1.Ø3)*
pemphigus neonatorum (LØ1.Ø3)
toxic epidermal necrolysis [Lyell] (L51.2)

✓4th **LØ1 Impetigo**
EXCLUDES 1 *impetigo herpetiformis (L4Ø.1)*

✓5th **LØ1.Ø Impetigo**
Impetigo contagiosa — Impetigo vulgaris

LØ1.ØØ Impetigo, unspecified
Impetigo NOS

LØ1.Ø1 Non-bullous impetigo

LØ1.Ø2 Bockhart's impetigo
Impetigo follicularis
Perifolliculitis NOS
Superficial pustular perifolliculitis

LØ1.Ø3 Bullous impetigo
Impetigo neonatorum — Pemphigus neonatorum

LØ1.Ø9 Other impetigo
Ulcerative impetigo

LØ1.1 Impetiginization of other dermatoses

✓4th **LØ2 Cutaneous abscess, furuncle and carbuncle**
Use additional code to identify organism (B95-B96)
EXCLUDES 2 *abscess of anus and rectal regions (K61.-)*
abscess of female genital organs (external) (N76.4)
abscess of male genital organs (external) (N48.2, N49-)

✓5th **LØ2.Ø Cutaneous abscess, furuncle and carbuncle of face**
EXCLUDES 2 *abscess of ear, external (H6Ø.Ø)*
abscess of eyelid (HØØ.Ø)
abscess of head [any part, except face] (LØ2.8)
abscess of lacrimal gland (HØ4.Ø)
abscess of lacrimal passages (HØ4.3)
abscess of mouth (K12.2)
abscess of nose (J34.Ø)
abscess of orbit (HØ5.Ø)
submandibular abscess (K12.2)

LØ2.Ø1 Cutaneous abscess of face CC

LØ2.Ø2 Furuncle of face
Boil of faceFolliculitis of face

LØ2.Ø3 Carbuncle of face

✓5th **LØ2.1 Cutaneous abscess, furuncle and carbuncle of neck**
CC Excl: No Excl

LØ2.11 Cutaneous abscess of neck CC
CC Excl: A17.9, A18.4, A18.82, A18.84, A18.89, A48.2-A48.4, A48.8-A49.9, B78.1, B95.Ø-B96.89, E83.2, LØ2.11, LØ2.811-LØ2.818, LØ2.91, LØ3.221-LØ3.222, LØ3.811-LØ3.91, LØ8.Ø, LØ8.81-LØ8.9, L44.8-L45, L73.2, L88, L92.8, L94.2, L94.4, L98.Ø, L98.3, L98.8, L99, MØØ.Ø11-MØØ.Ø12, MØØ.Ø21-MØØ.Ø22,MØØ.Ø31-MØØ.Ø32, MØØ.Ø41-MØØ.Ø42, MØØ.Ø51-MØØ.Ø52, MØØ.Ø61-MØØ.Ø62, MØØ.Ø71-MØØ.Ø72, Z16.1Ø-Z16.39

LØ2.12 Furuncle of neck
Boil of neck
Folliculitis of neck

LØ2.13 Carbuncle of neck

✓5th **LØ2.2 Cutaneous abscess, furuncle and carbuncle of trunk**
EXCLUDES 1 *non-newborn omphalitis (LØ8.82)*
omphalitis of newborn (P38.-)
EXCLUDES 2 *abscess of breast (N61)*
abscess of buttocks (LØ2.3)
abscess of female external genital organs (N76.4)
abscess of hip (LØ2.4)
abscess of male external genital organs (N48.2, N49-)

CC Excl: For CC codes in subcategory LØ2.2, unless otherwise noted: A17.9, A18.4, A18.82, A18.84, A18.89, A48.2-A48.4, A48.8-A49.9, B78.1, B95.Ø-B96.89, E83.2, LØ2.211-LØ2.219, LØ2.811-LØ2.818, LØ2.91, LØ3.311-LØ3.316, LØ3.319-LØ3.326, LØ3.329-LØ3.91, LØ8.Ø, LØ8.81-LØ8.9, L44.8-L45, L73.2, L88, L92.8, L94.2, L94.4, L98.Ø, L98.3, L98.8, L99, MØØ.Ø11-MØØ.Ø12, MØØ.Ø21-MØØ.Ø22,MØØ.Ø31-MØØ.Ø32, MØØ.Ø41-MØØ.Ø42, MØØ.Ø51-MØØ.Ø52, MØØ.Ø61-MØØ.Ø62, MØØ.Ø71-MØØ.Ø72, Z16.1Ø-Z16.39

✓6th **LØ2.21 Cutaneous abscess of trunk**
LØ2.211 Cutaneous abscess of abdominal wall CC
LØ2.212 Cutaneous abscess of back [any part, except buttock] CC
LØ2.213 Cutaneous abscess of chest wall CC
LØ2.214 Cutaneous abscess of groin CC
LØ2.215 Cutaneous abscess of perineum CC
LØ2.216 Cutaneous abscess of umbilicus CC
LØ2.219 Cutaneous abscess of trunk, unspecified CC

✓6th **LØ2.22 Furuncle of trunk**
Boil of trunkFolliculitis of trunk
LØ2.221 Furuncle of abdominal wall
LØ2.222 Furuncle of back [any part, except buttock]
LØ2.223 Furuncle of chest wall
LØ2.224 Furuncle of groin
LØ2.225 Furuncle of perineum
LØ2.226 Furuncle of umbilicus
LØ2.229 Furuncle of trunk, unspecified

✓6th **LØ2.23 Carbuncle of trunk**
LØ2.231 Carbuncle of abdominal wall
LØ2.232 Carbuncle of back [any part, except buttock]
LØ2.233 Carbuncle of chest wall
LØ2.234 Carbuncle of groin
LØ2.235 Carbuncle of perineum
LØ2.236 Carbuncle of umbilicus
LØ2.239 Carbuncle of trunk, unspecified

✓5th **LØ2.3 Cutaneous abscess, furuncle and carbuncle of buttock**
EXCLUDES 1 *pilonidal cyst with abscess (LØ5.Ø1)*

LØ2.31 Cutaneous abscess of buttock CC
Cutaneous abscess of gluteal region
CC Excl: A17.9, A18.4, A18.82, A18.84, A18.89, A48.2-A48.4, A48.8-A49.9, B78.1, B95.Ø-B96.89, E83.2, LØ2.31, LØ2.811-LØ2.818, LØ2.91, LØ3.317, LØ3.327, LØ3.811-LØ3.91, LØ8.Ø, LØ8.81-LØ8.9, L44.8-L45, L73.2, L88, L92.8, L94.2, L94.4, L98.Ø, L98.3, L98.8, L99, MØØ.Ø11-MØØ.Ø12, MØØ.Ø21-MØØ.Ø22,MØØ.Ø31-MØØ.Ø32, MØØ.Ø41-MØØ.Ø42, MØØ.Ø51-MØØ.Ø52, MØØ.Ø61-MØØ.Ø62, MØØ.Ø71-MØØ.Ø72, Z16.1Ø-Z16.39

L02.32 Furuncle of buttock
Boil of buttock
Furuncle of gluteal region
Folliculitis of buttock

L02.33 Carbuncle of buttock
Carbuncle of gluteal region

L02.4 Cutaneous abscess, furuncle and carbuncle of limb
EXCLUDES 2 *cutaneous abscess, furuncle and carbuncle of groin (L02.214, L02.224, L02.234)*
cutaneous abscess, furuncle and carbuncle of hand (L02.5-)
cutaneous abscess, furuncle and carbuncle of foot (L02.6-)

CC Excl: For CC codes in subcategory L02.4, unless otherwise noted: A17.9, A18.4, A18.82, A18.84, A18.89, A48.2-A48.4, A48.8-A49.9, B78.1, B95.0-B96.89, E83.2, L02.411-L02.414, L02.811-L02.818, L02.91, L03.111-L03.114, L03.121-L03.124, L03.811-L03.91, L08.0, L08.81-L08.9, L44.8-L45, L73.2, L88, L92.8, L94.2, L94.4, L98.0, L98.3, L98.8, L99, M00.011-M00.012, M00.021-M00.022,M00.031-M00.032, M00.041-M00.042, M00.051-M00.052, M00.061-M00.062, M00.071-M00.072, Z16.10-Z16.39

L02.41 Cutaneous abscess of limb
L02.411 Cutaneous abscess of right axilla CC
L02.412 Cutaneous abscess of left axilla CC
L02.413 Cutaneous abscess of right upper limb CC
L02.414 Cutaneous abscess of left upper limb CC
L02.415 Cutaneous abscess of right lower limb CC
CC Excl: A17.9-A18.4, A18.82, A18.84, A18.89, A48.2-A48.4, A48.8-A49.9, B78.1, B95.0-B96.89, E83.2, L02.415-L02.419, L02.811-L02.818, L02.91, L03.115-L03.119, L03.125-L03.129, L03.811-L03.91, L08.0, L08.81-L08.9, L44.8-L45, L73.2, L88, L92.8, L94.2, L94.4, L98.0, L98.3, L98.8, L99, M00.011-M00.012, M00.021-M00.022, M00.031-M00.032, M00.041-M00.042, M00.051-M00.052, M00.061-M00.062, M00.071-M00.072, Z16.10-Z16.39
L02.416 Cutaneous abscess of left lower limb CC
CC Excl: See code: L02.415
L02.419 Cutaneous abscess of limb, unspecified CC
CC Excl: See code: L02.415

L02.42 Furuncle of limb
Boil of limbFolliculitis of limb
L02.421 Furuncle of right axilla
L02.422 Furuncle of left axilla
L02.423 Furuncle of right upper limb
L02.424 Furuncle of left upper limb
L02.425 Furuncle of right lower limb
L02.426 Furuncle of left lower limb
L02.429 Furuncle of limb, unspecified

L02.43 Carbuncle of limb
L02.431 Carbuncle of right axilla
L02.432 Carbuncle of left axilla
L02.433 Carbuncle of right upper limb
L02.434 Carbuncle of left upper limb
L02.435 Carbuncle of right lower limb
L02.436 Carbuncle of left lower limb
L02.439 Carbuncle of limb, unspecified

L02.5 Cutaneous abscess, furuncle and carbuncle of hand

CC Excl: For CC codes in subcategory L02.5, unless otherwise noted: A17.9, A18.4, A18.82, A18.84, A18.89, A48.2-A48.4, A48.8-A49.9, B78.1, B95.0-B96.89, E83.2, L02.511-L02.519, L02.811-L02.818, L02.91, L03.811-L03.91, L08.0, L08.81-L08.9, L44.8-L45, L73.2, L88, L92.8, L94.2, L94.4, L98.0, L98.3, L98.8, L99, M00.011-M00.012, M00.021-M00.022, M00.031-M00.032, M00.041-M00.042, M00.051-M00.052, M00.061-M00.062, M00.071-M00.072, Z16.10-Z16.39

L02.51 Cutaneous abscess of hand
L02.511 Cutaneous abscess of right hand CC
L02.512 Cutaneous abscess of left hand CC
L02.519 Cutaneous abscess of unspecified hand CC

L02.52 Furuncle hand
Boil of handFolliculitis of hand
L02.521 Furuncle right hand
L02.522 Furuncle left hand
L02.529 Furuncle unspecified hand

L02.53 Carbuncle of hand
L02.531 Carbuncle of right hand
L02.532 Carbuncle of left hand
L02.539 Carbuncle of unspecified hand

L02.6 Cutaneous abscess, furuncle and carbuncle of foot

CC Excl: For CC codes in subcategory L02.6, unless otherwise noted: A17.9, A18.4, A18.82, A18.84, A18.89, A48.2-A48.4, A48.8-A49.9, B78.1, B95.0-B96.89, E83.2, L02.611-L02.619, L02.811-L02.818, L02.91, L03.811-L03.91, L08.0, L08.81-L08.9, L44.8-L45, L73.2, L88, L92.8, L94.2, L98.0, L98.3, L98.8, L99, M00.011-M00.012, M00.021-M00.022, M00.031-M00.032, M00.041-M00.042, M00.051-M00.052, M00.061-M00.062, M00.071-M00.072, Z16.10-Z16.39

L02.61 Cutaneous abscess of foot
L02.611 Cutaneous abscess of right foot CC
L02.612 Cutaneous abscess of left foot CC
L02.619 Cutaneous abscess of unspecified foot CC

L02.62 Furuncle of foot
Boil of footFolliculitis of foot
L02.621 Furuncle of right foot
L02.622 Furuncle of left foot
L02.629 Furuncle of unspecified foot

L02.63 Carbuncle of foot
L02.631 Carbuncle of right foot
L02.632 Carbuncle of left foot
L02.639 Carbuncle of unspecified foot

L02.8 Cutaneous abscess, furuncle and carbuncle of other sites

L02.81 Cutaneous abscess of other sites
L02.811 Cutaneous abscess of head [any part, except face] CC
CC Excl: A17.9, A18.4, A18.82, A18.84, A18.89, A48.2-A48.4, A48.8-A49.9, B78.1, B95.0-B96.89, E83.2, L02.811-L02.818, L02.91, L03.811-L03.91, L08.0, L08.81-L08.9, L44.8-L45, L73.2, L88, L92.8, L94.2, L94.4, L98.0, L98.3, L98.8, L99, M00.011-M00.012, M00.021-M00.022,M00.031-M00.032, M00.041-M00.042, M00.051-M00.052, M00.061-M00.062, M00.071-M00.07, Z16.10-Z16.39
L02.818 Cutaneous abscess of other sites CC
CC Excl: See code: L02.811

L02.82 Furuncle of other sites
Boil of other sites Folliculitis of other sites
L02.821 Furuncle of head [any part, except face]
L02.828 Furuncle of other sites

L02.83 Carbuncle of other sites
L02.831 Carbuncle of head [any part, except face]
L02.838 Carbuncle of other sites

L02.9 Cutaneous abscess, furuncle and carbuncle, unspecified
L02.91 Cutaneous abscess, unspecified CC
CC Excl: See code: L02.811
L02.92 Furuncle, unspecified
Boil NOS
Furunculosis NOS
L02.93 Carbuncle, unspecified

L03 Cellulitis and acute lymphangitis
EXCLUDES 2 *cellulitis of anal and rectal region (K61.-)*
cellulitis of external auditory canal (H60.1)
cellulitis of eyelid (H00.03-)
cellulitis of female external genital organs (N76.4)
cellulitis of lacrimal apparatus (H04.3)
cellulitis of male external genital organs (N48.2, N49-)
cellulitis of mouth (K12.2)
cellulitis of nose (J34.0)
eosinophilic cellulitis [Wells] (L98.3)
febrile neutrophilic dermatosis [Sweet] (L98.2)
lymphangitis (chronic) (subacute) (I89.1)

L03.0 Cellulitis and acute lymphangitis of finger and toe
Infection of nail
Onychia
Paronychia
Perionychia

L03.01 Cellulitis of finger
Felon
Whitlow
EXCLUDES 1 *herpetic whitlow (B00.89)*
L03.011 Cellulitis of right finger
L03.012 Cellulitis of left finger
L03.019 Cellulitis of unspecified finger

✓6th **LØ3.Ø2 Acute lymphangitis of finger**
Hangnail with lymphangitis of finger
LØ3.Ø21 Acute lymphangitis of right finger
LØ3.Ø22 Acute lymphangitis of left finger
LØ3.Ø29 Acute lymphangitis of unspecified finger

✓6th **LØ3.Ø3 Cellulitis of toe**
LØ3.Ø31 Cellulitis of right toe
LØ3.Ø32 Cellulitis of left toe
LØ3.Ø39 Cellulitis of unspecified toe

✓6th **LØ3.Ø4 Acute lymphangitis of toe**
Hangnail with lymphangitis of toe
LØ3.Ø41 Acute lymphangitis of right toe
LØ3.Ø42 Acute lymphangitis of left toe
LØ3.Ø49 Acute lymphangitis of unspecified toe

✓5th **LØ3.1 Cellulitis and acute lymphangitis of other parts of limb**

CC Excl: For CC codes in subcategory LØ3.1, unless otherwise noted: A17.9, A18.4, A18.82, A18.84, A18.89, A48.2-A48.4, A48.8-A49.9, B78.1, B95.Ø-B96.89, E83.2, LØ2.411-LØ2.414, LØ2.811-LØ2.818, LØ2.91, LØ3.111-LØ3.114, LØ3.121-LØ3.124, LØ3.811-LØ3.91, LØ8.Ø, LØ8.81-LØ8.9, L44.8-L45, L73.2, L88, L92.8, L94.2, L94.4, L98.Ø, L98.3, L98.8, L99, MØØ.Ø11-MØØ.Ø12, MØØ.Ø21-MØØ.Ø22, MØØ.Ø31-MØØ.Ø32, MØØ.Ø41-MØØ.Ø42, MØØ.Ø51-MØØ.Ø52, MØØ.Ø61-MØØ.Ø62, MØØ.Ø71-MØØ.Ø72, Z16.1Ø-Z16.39

✓6th **LØ3.11 Cellulitis of other parts of limb**
EXCLUDES 2 *cellulitis of fingers (LØ3.Ø1-)*
cellulitis of toes (LØ3.Ø3-)
groin (LØ3.314)
LØ3.111 Cellulitis of right axilla CC
LØ3.112 Cellulitis of left axilla CC
LØ3.113 Cellulitis of right upper limb CC
LØ3.114 Cellulitis of left upper limb CC
LØ3.115 Cellulitis of right lower limb CC
CC Excl: See code: LØ2.415
LØ3.116 Cellulitis of left lower limb CC
CC Excl: See code: LØ2.415
LØ3.119 Cellulitis of unspecified part of limb CC
CC Excl: See code: LØ2.415

✓6th **LØ3.12 Acute lymphangitis of other parts of limb**
EXCLUDES 2 *acute lymphangitis of fingers (LØ3.Ø2-)*
acute lymphangitis of groin (LØ3.324)
acute lymphangitis of toes (LØ3.Ø4-)
LØ3.121 Acute lymphangitis of right axilla CC
LØ3.122 Acute lymphangitis of left axilla CC
LØ3.123 Acute lymphangitis of right upper limb CC
LØ3.124 Acute lymphangitis of left upper limb CC
LØ3.125 Acute lymphangitis of right lower limb CC
CC Excl: See code: LØ2.415
LØ3.126 Acute lymphangitis of left lower limb CC
CC Excl: See code: LØ2.415
LØ3.129 Acute lymphangitis of unspecified part of limb CC
CC Excl: See code: LØ2.415

✓5th **LØ3.2 Cellulitis and acute lymphangitis of face and neck**

✓6th **LØ3.21 Cellulitis and acute lymphangitis of face**
LØ3.211 Cellulitis of face CC
EXCLUDES 2 *cellulitis of ear (H6Ø.1-)*
cellulitis of eyelid (HØØ.Ø3-)
cellulitis of head (LØ3.811)
cellulitis of lacrimal apparatus (HØ4.3)
cellulitis of lip (K13.Ø)
cellulitis of mouth (K12.2)
cellulitis of nose (internal) (J34.Ø)
cellulitis of orbit (HØ5.Ø)
cellulitis of scalp (LØ3.811)
AHA: 2013, 4Q, 123
CC Excl: A17.9, A18.4, A18.82, A18.84, A18.89, A48.2-A48.4, A48.8-A49.9, B78.1, B95.Ø-B96.89, E83.2, LØ2.811-LØ2.818, LØ2.91, LØ3.211, LØ3.811-LØ3.91, LØ8.Ø, LØ8.81-LØ8.9, L44.8-L45, L73.2, L88, L92.8, L94.2, L94.4, L98.Ø, L98.3, L98.8, L99, MØØ.Ø11-MØØ.Ø12, MØØ.Ø21-MØØ.Ø22, MØØ.Ø31-MØØ.Ø32, MØØ.Ø41-MØØ.Ø42, MØØ.Ø51-MØØ.Ø52, MØØ.Ø61-MØØ.Ø62, MØØ.Ø71-MØØ.Ø72, Z16.1Ø-Z16.39
LØ3.212 Acute lymphangitis of face CC
CC Excl: No Excl

✓6th **LØ3.22 Cellulitis and acute lymphangitis of neck**
LØ3.221 Cellulitis of neck CC
CC Excl: A17.9, A18.4, A18.82, A18.84, A18.89, A48.2-A48.4, A48.8-A49.9, B78.1, B95.Ø-B96.89, E83.2, LØ2.11, LØ2.811-LØ2.818, LØ2.91, LØ3.221-LØ3.222, LØ3.811-LØ3.91, LØ8.Ø, LØ8.81-LØ8.9, L44.8-L45, L73.2, L88, L92.8, L94.2, L94.4, L98.Ø, L98.3, L98.8, L99, MØØ.Ø11-MØØ.Ø12, MØØ.Ø21-MØØ.Ø22, MØØ.Ø31-MØØ.Ø32, MØØ.Ø41-MØØ.Ø42, MØØ.Ø51-MØØ.Ø52, MØØ.Ø61-MØØ.Ø62, MØØ.Ø71-MØØ.Ø72, Z16.1Ø-Z16.39
LØ3.222 Acute lymphangitis of neck CC
CC Excl: See code: LØ3.221

✓5th **LØ3.3 Cellulitis and acute lymphangitis of trunk**

CC Excl: For CC codes in subcategory LØ3.3, unless otherwise noted: A17.9, A18.4, A18.82, A18.84, A18.89, A48.2-A48.4, A48.8-A49.9, B78.1, B95.Ø-B96.89, E83.2, LØ2.211-LØ2.219, LØ2.811-LØ2.818, LØ2.91, LØ3.311-LØ3.316, LØ3.319-LØ3.326, LØ3.329-LØ3.91, LØ8.Ø, LØ8.81-LØ8.9, L44.8-L45, L73.2, L88, L92.8, L94.2, L94.4, L98.Ø, L98.3, L98.8, L99, MØØ.Ø11-MØØ.Ø12, MØØ.Ø21-MØØ.Ø22, MØØ.Ø31-MØØ.Ø32, MØØ.Ø41-MØØ.Ø42, MØØ.Ø51-MØØ.Ø52, MØØ.Ø61-MØØ.Ø62, MØØ.Ø71-MØØ.Ø72, Z16.1Ø-Z16.39

✓6th **LØ3.31 Cellulitis of trunk**
EXCLUDES 2 *cellulitis of anal and rectal regions (K61.-)*
cellulitis of breast NOS (N61)
cellulitis of female external genital organs (N76.4)
cellulitis of male external genital organs (N48.2, N49.-)
omphalitis of newborn (P38.-)
puerperal cellulitis of breast (O91.2)
LØ3.311 Cellulitis of abdominal wall CC
EXCLUDES 2 *cellulitis of umbilicus (LØ3.316)*
cellulitis of groin (LØ3.314)
LØ3.312 Cellulitis of back [any part except buttock] CC
LØ3.313 Cellulitis of chest wall CC
LØ3.314 Cellulitis of groin CC
LØ3.315 Cellulitis of perineum CC
LØ3.316 Cellulitis of umbilicus CC
LØ3.317 Cellulitis of buttock CC
CC Excl: A17.9, A18.4, A18.82, A18.84, A18.89, A48.2-A48.4, A48.8-A49.9, B78.1, B95.Ø-B96.89, E83.2, LØ2.31, LØ2.811-LØ2.818, LØ2.91, LØ3.317, LØ3.327, LØ3.811-LØ3.91, LØ8.Ø, LØ8.81-LØ8.9, L44.8-L45, L73.2, L88, L92.8, L94.2, L94.4, L98.Ø, L98.3, L98.8, L99, MØØ.Ø11-MØØ.Ø12, MØØ.Ø21-MØØ.Ø22, MØØ.Ø31-MØØ.Ø32, MØØ.Ø41-MØØ.Ø42, MØØ.Ø51-MØØ.Ø52, MØØ.Ø61-MØØ.Ø62, MØØ.Ø71-MØØ.Ø72, Z16.1Ø-Z16.39
LØ3.319 Cellulitis of trunk, unspecified CC

✓6th **LØ3.32 Acute lymphangitis of trunk**
LØ3.321 Acute lymphangitis of abdominal wall CC
LØ3.322 Acute lymphangitis of back [any part except buttock] CC
LØ3.323 Acute lymphangitis of chest wall CC
LØ3.324 Acute lymphangitis of groin CC
LØ3.325 Acute lymphangitis of perineum CC
LØ3.326 Acute lymphangitis of umbilicus CC
LØ3.327 Acute lymphangitis of buttock CC
CC Excl: See code: LØ3.317
LØ3.329 Acute lymphangitis of trunk, unspecified CC

✓5th **LØ3.8 Cellulitis and acute lymphangitis of other sites**

CC Excl: For CC codes in subcategory LØ3.8, unless otherwise noted: A17.9, A18.4, A18.82, A18.84, A18.89, A48.2-A48.4, A48.8-A49.9, B78.1, B95.Ø-B96.89, E83.2, LØ2.811-LØ2.818, LØ2.91, LØ3.811-LØ3.91, LØ8.Ø, LØ8.81-LØ8.9, L44.8-L45, L73.2, L88, L92.8, L94.2, L94.4, L98.Ø, L98.3, L98.8, L99, MØØ.Ø11-MØØ.Ø12, MØØ.Ø21-MØØ.Ø22, MØØ.Ø31-MØØ.Ø32, MØØ.Ø41-MØØ.Ø42, MØØ.Ø51-MØØ.Ø52, MØØ.Ø61-MØØ.Ø62, MØØ.Ø71-MØØ.Ø72, Z16.1Ø-Z16.39

✓6th **LØ3.81 Cellulitis of other sites**
LØ3.811 Cellulitis of head [any part, except face] CC
Cellulitis of scalp
EXCLUDES 2 *cellulitis of face (LØ3.211)*
LØ3.818 Cellulitis of other sites CC

✓6th **L03.89 Acute lymphangitis of other sites**

L03.891 Acute lymphangitis of head [any part, except face] CC

L03.898 Acute lymphangitis of other sites CC

✓5th **L03.9 Cellulitis and acute lymphangitis, unspecified**

CC Excl: For CC codes in subcategory L03.9, unless otherwise noted: See code: L03.8

L03.90 Cellulitis, unspecified CC

L03.91 Acute lymphangitis, unspecified CC

EXCLUDES 1 *lymphangitis NOS (I89.1)*

✓4th **L04 Acute lymphadenitis**

INCLUDES abscess (acute) of lymph nodes, except mesenteric
acute lymphadenitis, except mesenteric

EXCLUDES 1 *chronic or subacute lymphadenitis, except mesenteric (I88.1)*
enlarged lymph nodes (R59.-)
human immunodeficiency virus [HIV] disease resulting in generalized lymphadenopathy (B20)
lymphadenitis NOS (I88.9)
nonspecific mesenteric lymphadenitis (I88.0)

L04.0 Acute lymphadenitis of face, head and neck

L04.1 Acute lymphadenitis of trunk

L04.2 Acute lymphadenitis of upper limb
Acute lymphadenitis of axilla Acute lymphadenitis of shoulder

L04.3 Acute lymphadenitis of lower limb
Acute lymphadenitis of hip
EXCLUDES 2 *acute lymphadenitis of groin (L04.1)*

L04.8 Acute lymphadenitis of other sites

L04.9 Acute lymphadenitis, unspecified

✓4th **L05 Pilonidal cyst and sinus**

✓5th **L05.0 Pilonidal cyst and sinus with abscess**

L05.01 Pilonidal cyst with abscess CC
Parasacral dimple with abscess
Pilonidal abscess
Pilonidal dimple with abscess
Postanal dimple with abscess
CC Excl: L05.01-L05.92, L44.8-L45, L94.2, L94.4, L98.8, L99

L05.02 Pilonidal sinus with abscess CC
Coccygeal fistula with abscess
Coccygeal sinus with abscess
Pilonidal fistula with abscess
CC Excl: See code: L05.01

✓5th **L05.9 Pilonidal cyst and sinus without abscess**

L05.91 Pilonidal cyst without abscess
Parasacral dimplePostanal dimple
Pilonidal dimple Pilonidal cyst NOS

L05.92 Pilonidal sinus without abscess
Coccygeal fistula
Coccygeal sinus without abscess
Pilonidal fistula

✓4th **L08 Other local infections of skin and subcutaneous tissue**

L08.0 Pyoderma
Dermatitis gangrenosa Septic dermatitis
Purulent dermatitis Suppurative dermatitis
EXCLUDES 1 *pyoderma gangrenosum (L88)*
pyoderma vegetans (L08.81)

L08.1 Erythrasma HIV CC
CC Excl: A42.81-A42.9, A43.1-A43.9, B47.1, L08.1

✓5th **L08.8 Other specified local infections of the skin and subcutaneous tissue**

L08.81 Pyoderma vegetans
EXCLUDES 1 *pyoderma gangrenosum (L88)*
pyoderma NOS (L08.0)

L08.82 Omphalitis not of newborn
EXCLUDES 1 *omphalitis of newborn (P38.-)*

L08.89 Other specified local infections of the skin and subcutaneous tissue

L08.9 Local infection of the skin and subcutaneous tissue, unspecified

Bullous disorders (L10-L14)

EXCLUDES 1 *benign familial pemphigus [Hailey-Hailey] (Q82.8)*
staphylococcal scalded skin syndrome (L00)
toxic epidermal necrolysis [Lyell] (L51.2)

✓4th **L10 Pemphigus**

EXCLUDES 1 *pemphigus neonatorum (L01.03)*

CC Excl: For CC codes in category L10, unless otherwise noted: L10.0-L10.9, L12.0-L12.1, L12.8-L12.9, L13.8-L14, L44.8-L45, L94.2, L94.4, L98.8, L99

L10.0 Pemphigus vulgaris CC

L10.1 Pemphigus vegetans CC

L10.2 Pemphigus foliaceous CC

L10.3 Brazilian pemphigus [fogo selvagem] CC

L10.4 Pemphigus erythematosus CC
Senear-Usher syndrome

L10.5 Drug-induced pemphigus CC
Use additional code for adverse effect, if applicable, to identify drug (T36-T50 with fifth or sixth character 5)

✓5th **L10.8 Other pemphigus**

L10.81 Paraneoplastic pemphigus CC

L10.89 Other pemphigus CC

L10.9 Pemphigus, unspecified CC

✓4th **L11 Other acantholytic disorders**

L11.0 Acquired keratosis follicularis
EXCLUDES 1 *keratosis follicularis (congenital) [Darier-White] (Q82.8)*

L11.1 Transient acantholytic dermatosis [Grover]

L11.8 Other specified acantholytic disorders

L11.9 Acantholytic disorder, unspecified

✓4th **L12 Pemphigoid**

EXCLUDES 1 *herpes gestationis (O26.4-)*
impetigo herpetiformis (L40.1)

CC Excl: For CC codes in category L12, unless otherwise noted: See code: L10

L12.0 Bullous pemphigoid CC

L12.1 Cicatricial pemphigoid CC
Benign mucous membrane pemphigoid

L12.2 Chronic bullous disease of childhood P
Juvenile dermatitis herpetiformis

✓5th **L12.3 Acquired epidermolysis bullosa**
EXCLUDES 1 *epidermolysis bullosa (congenital) (Q81.-)*

L12.30 Acquired epidermolysis bullosa, unspecified CC
CC Excl: L00, L12.30-L12.35, L26, L30.4, L44.8-L45, L51.0-L54, L71.0-L71.9, L92.0, L93.0-L93.2, L94.2, L94.4, L95.1, L98.2, L98.8, L99

L12.31 Epidermolysis bullosa due to drug CC
Use additional code for adverse effect, if applicable, to identify drug (T36-T50 with fifth or sixth character 5)
CC Excl: See code: L12.30

L12.35 Other acquired epidermolysis bullosa CC
CC Excl: See code: L12.30

L12.8 Other pemphigoid CC

L12.9 Pemphigoid, unspecified CC

✓4th **L13 Other bullous disorders**

L13.0 Dermatitis herpetiformis
Duhring's disease
Hydroa herpetiformis
EXCLUDES 1 *juvenile dermatitis herpetiformis (L12.2)*
senile dermatitis herpetiformis (L12.0)

L13.1 Subcorneal pustular dermatitis
Sneddon-Wilkinson disease

L13.8 Other specified bullous disorders

L13.9 Bullous disorder, unspecified

L14 Bullous disorders in diseases classified elsewhere
Code first underlying disease

Dermatitis and eczema (L20-L30)

NOTE In this block the terms dermatitis and eczema are used synonymously and interchangeably.

EXCLUDES 2 *chronic (childhood) granulomatous disease (D71)*
dermatitis gangrenosa (L08.0)
dermatitis herpetiformis (L13.0)
dry skin dermatitis (L85.3)
factitial dermatitis (L98.1)
perioral dermatitis (L71.0)
radiation-related disorders of the skin and subcutaneous tissue (L55-L59)
stasis dermatitis (I83.1-I83.2)

✓4th **L20 Atopic dermatitis**
L20.0 Besnier's prurigo
✓5th **L20.8 Other atopic dermatitis**
EXCLUDES 2 *circumscribed neurodermatitis (L28.0)*
L20.81 Atopic neurodermatitis
Diffuse neurodermatitis
L20.82 Flexural eczema
L20.83 Infantile (acute) (chronic) eczema P
L20.84 Intrinsic (allergic) eczema
L20.89 Other atopic dermatitis
L20.9 Atopic dermatitis, unspecified

✓4th **L21 Seborrheic dermatitis**
EXCLUDES 2 *infective dermatitis (L30.3)*
seborrheic keratosis (L82.-)
L21.0 Seborrhea capitis P
Cradle cap
L21.1 Seborrheic infantile dermatitis P
L21.8 Other seborrheic dermatitis
L21.9 Seborrheic dermatitis, unspecified
Seborrhea NOS

L22 Diaper dermatitis
Diaper erythema
Diaper rash
Psoriasiform diaper rash

✓4th **L23 Allergic contact dermatitis**
EXCLUDES 1 *allergy NOS (T78.40)*
contact dermatitis NOS (L25.9)
dermatitis NOS (L30.9)
EXCLUDES 2 *dermatitis due to substances taken internally (L27.-)*
dermatitis of eyelid (H01.1-)
diaper dermatitis (L22)
eczema of external ear (H60.5-)
irritant contact dermatitis (L24.-)
perioral dermatitis (L71.0)
radiation-related disorders of the skin and subcutaneous tissue (L55-L59)
L23.0 Allergic contact dermatitis due to metals
Allergic contact dermatitis due to chromium
Allergic contact dermatitis due to nickel
L23.1 Allergic contact dermatitis due to adhesives
L23.2 Allergic contact dermatitis due to cosmetics
L23.3 Allergic contact dermatitis due to drugs in contact with skin
Use additional code for adverse effect, if applicable, to identify drug (T36-T50 with fifth or sixth character 5)
EXCLUDES 2 *dermatitis due to ingested drugs and medicaments (L27.0-L27.1)*
L23.4 Allergic contact dermatitis due to dyes
L23.5 Allergic contact dermatitis due to other chemical products
Allergic contact dermatitis due to cement
Allergic contact dermatitis due to insecticide
Allergic contact dermatitis due to plastic
Allergic contact dermatitis due to rubber
L23.6 Allergic contact dermatitis due to food in contact with the skin
EXCLUDES 2 *dermatitis due to ingested food (L27.2)*
L23.7 Allergic contact dermatitis due to plants, except food
EXCLUDES 2 *allergy NOS due to pollen (J30.1)*
✓5th **L23.8 Allergic contact dermatitis due to other agents**
L23.81 Allergic contact dermatitis due to animal (cat) (dog) dander
Allergic contact dermatitis due to animal (cat) (dog) hair
L23.89 Allergic contact dermatitis due to other agents
L23.9 Allergic contact dermatitis, unspecified cause
Allergic contact eczema NOS

✓4th **L24 Irritant contact dermatitis**
EXCLUDES 1 *allergy NOS (T78.40)*
contact dermatitis NOS (L25.9)
dermatitis NOS (L30.9)
EXCLUDES 2 *allergic contact dermatitis (L23.-)*
dermatitis due to substances taken internally (L27.-)
dermatitis of eyelid (H01.1-)
diaper dermatitis (L22)
eczema of external ear (H60.5-)
perioral dermatitis (L71.0)
radiation-related disorders of the skin and subcutaneous tissue (L55-L59)
L24.0 Irritant contact dermatitis due to detergents
L24.1 Irritant contact dermatitis due to oils and greases
L24.2 Irritant contact dermatitis due to solvents
Irritant contact dermatitis due to chlorocompound
Irritant contact dermatitis due to cyclohexane
Irritant contact dermatitis due to ester
Irritant contact dermatitis due to glycol
Irritant contact dermatitis due to hydrocarbon
Irritant contact dermatitis due to ketone
L24.3 Irritant contact dermatitis due to cosmetics
L24.4 Irritant contact dermatitis due to drugs in contact with skin
Use additional code for adverse effect, if applicable, to identify drug (T36-T50 with fifth or sixth character 5)
L24.5 Irritant contact dermatitis due to other chemical products
Irritant contact dermatitis due to cement
Irritant contact dermatitis due to insecticide
Irritant contact dermatitis due to plastic
Irritant contact dermatitis due to rubber
L24.6 Irritant contact dermatitis due to food in contact with skin
EXCLUDES 2 *dermatitis due to ingested food (L27.2)*
L24.7 Irritant contact dermatitis due to plants, except food
EXCLUDES 2 *allergy NOS to pollen (J30.1)*
✓5th **L24.8 Irritant contact dermatitis due to other agents**
L24.81 Irritant contact dermatitis due to metals
Irritant contact dermatitis due to chromium
Irritant contact dermatitis due to nickel
L24.89 Irritant contact dermatitis due to other agents
Irritant contact dermatitis due to dyes
L24.9 Irritant contact dermatitis, unspecified cause
Irritant contact eczema NOS

✓4th **L25 Unspecified contact dermatitis**
EXCLUDES 1 *allergic contact dermatitis (L23.-)*
allergy NOS (T78.40)
dermatitis NOS (L30.9)
irritant contact dermatitis (L24.-)
EXCLUDES 2 *dermatitis due to ingested substances (L27.-)*
dermatitis of eyelid (H01.1-)
eczema of external ear (H60.5-)
perioral dermatitis (L71.0)
radiation-related disorders of the skin and subcutaneous tissue (L55-L59)
L25.0 Unspecified contact dermatitis due to cosmetics
L25.1 Unspecified contact dermatitis due to drugs in contact with skin
Use additional code for adverse effect, if applicable, to identify drug (T36-T50 with fifth or sixth character 5)
EXCLUDES 2 *dermatitis due to ingested drugs and medicaments (L27.0-L27.1)*
L25.2 Unspecified contact dermatitis due to dyes
L25.3 Unspecified contact dermatitis due to other chemical products
Unspecified contact dermatitis due to cement
Unspecified contact dermatitis due to insecticide
L25.4 Unspecified contact dermatitis due to food in contact with skin
EXCLUDES 2 *dermatitis due to ingested food (L27.2)*
L25.5 Unspecified contact dermatitis due to plants, except food
EXCLUDES 1 *nettle rash (L50.9)*
EXCLUDES 2 *allergy NOS due to pollen (J30.1)*
L25.8 Unspecified contact dermatitis due to other agents
L25.9 Unspecified contact dermatitis, unspecified cause
Contact dermatitis (occupational) NOS
Contact eczema (occupational) NOS

L26 Exfoliative dermatitis
Hebra's pityriasis
EXCLUDES 1 *Ritter's disease (L00)*

L27 Dermatitis due to substances taken internally
EXCLUDES 1 *allergy NOS (T78.40)*
EXCLUDES 2 *adverse food reaction, except dermatitis (T78.0-T78.1)*
contact dermatitis (L23-L25)
drug photoallergic response (L56.1)
drug phototoxic response (L56.0)
urticaria (L50.-)

L27.0 Generalized skin eruption due to drugs and medicaments taken internally
Use additional code for adverse effect, if applicable, to identify drug (T36-T50 with fifth or sixth character 5)

L27.1 Localized skin eruption due to drugs and medicaments taken internally
Use additional code for adverse effect, if applicable, to identify drug (T36-T50 with fifth or sixth character 5)

L27.2 Dermatitis due to ingested food
EXCLUDES 2 *dermatitis due to food in contact with skin (L23.6, L24.6, L25.4)*

L27.8 Dermatitis due to other substances taken internally
L27.9 Dermatitis due to unspecified substance taken internally

L28 Lichen simplex chronicus and prurigo
L28.0 Lichen simplex chronicus
Circumscribed neurodermatitis
Lichen NOS
L28.1 Prurigo nodularis
L28.2 Other prurigo
Prurigo NOS
Prurigo Hebra
Prurigo mitis
Urticaria papulosa

L29 Pruritus
EXCLUDES 1 *neurotic excoriation (L98.1)*
psychogenic pruritus (F45.8)
L29.0 Pruritus ani
L29.1 Pruritus scroti ♂
L29.2 Pruritus vulvae ♀
L29.3 Anogenital pruritus, unspecified
L29.8 Other pruritus
L29.9 Pruritus, unspecified
Itch NOS

L30 Other and unspecified dermatitis
EXCLUDES 2 *contact dermatitis (L23-L25)*
dry skin dermatitis (L85.3)
small plaque parapsoriasis (L41.3)
stasis dermatitis (I83.1-.2)
L30.0 Nummular dermatitis
L30.1 Dyshidrosis [pompholyx]
L30.2 Cutaneous autosensitization
Candidid [levurid]
Dermatophytid
Eczematid
L30.3 Infective dermatitis
Infectious eczematoid dermatitis
L30.4 Erythema intertrigo
L30.5 Pityriasis alba
L30.8 Other specified dermatitis
L30.9 Dermatitis, unspecified
Eczema NOS

Papulosquamous disorders (L40-L45)

L40 Psoriasis
L40.0 Psoriasis vulgaris
Nummular psoriasis
Plaque psoriasis
L40.1 Generalized pustular psoriasis
Impetigo herpetiformis
Von Zumbusch's disease
L40.2 Acrodermatitis continua
L40.3 Pustulosis palmaris et plantaris
L40.4 Guttate psoriasis
L40.5 Arthropathic psoriasis
L40.50 Arthropathic psoriasis, unspecified
L40.51 Distal interphalangeal psoriatic arthropathy
L40.52 Psoriatic arthritis mutilans
L40.53 Psoriatic spondylitis
L40.54 Psoriatic juvenile arthropathy
L40.59 Other psoriatic arthropathy
L40.8 Other psoriasis
Flexural psoriasis
L40.9 Psoriasis, unspecified

L41 Parapsoriasis
EXCLUDES 1 *poikiloderma vasculare atrophicans (L94.5)*
L41.0 Pityriasis lichenoides et varioliformis acuta
Mucha-Habermann disease
L41.1 Pityriasis lichenoides chronica
L41.3 Small plaque parapsoriasis
L41.4 Large plaque parapsoriasis
L41.5 Retiform parapsoriasis
L41.8 Other parapsoriasis
L41.9 Parapsoriasis, unspecified

L42 Pityriasis rosea

L43 Lichen planus
EXCLUDES 1 *lichen planopilaris (L66.1)*
L43.0 Hypertrophic lichen planus
L43.1 Bullous lichen planus
L43.2 Lichenoid drug reaction
Use additional code for adverse effect, if applicable, to identify drug (T36-T50 with fifth or sixth character 5)
L43.3 Subacute (active) lichen planus
Lichen planus tropicus
L43.8 Other lichen planus
L43.9 Lichen planus, unspecified

L44 Other papulosquamous disorders
L44.0 Pityriasis rubra pilaris
L44.1 Lichen nitidus
L44.3 Lichen ruber moniliformis
L44.4 Infantile papular acrodermatitis [Gianotti-Crosti] P
L44.8 Other specified papulosquamous disorders
L44.9 Papulosquamous disorder, unspecified

L45 Papulosquamous disorders in diseases classified elsewhere
Code first underlying disease

Urticaria and erythema (L49-L54)

EXCLUDES 1 *Lyme disease (A69.2-)*
rosacea (L71.-)

L49 Exfoliation due to erythematous conditions according to extent of body surface involved
Code first erythematous condition causing exfoliation, such as:
Ritter's disease (L00)
(Staphylococcal) scalded skin syndrom (L00)
Stevens-Johnson syndrome (L51.1)
Stevens-Johnson syndrome-toxic epidermal necrolysis overlap syndrome (L51.3)
toxic epidermal necrolysis (L51.2)
L49.0 Exfoliation due to erythematous condition involving less than 10 percent of body surface
Exfoliation due to erythematous condition NOS
L49.1 Exfoliation due to erythematous condition involving 10-19 percent of body surface
L49.2 Exfoliation due to erythematous condition involving 20-29 percent of body surface
L49.3 Exfoliation due to erythematous condition involving 30-39 percent of body surface CC
CC Excl: L49.3
L49.4 Exfoliation due to erythematous condition involving 40-49 percent of body surface CC
CC Excl: L49.4
L49.5 Exfoliation due to erythematous condition involving 50-59 percent of body surface CC
CC Excl: L49.5
L49.6 Exfoliation due to erythematous condition involving 60-69 percent of body surface CC
CC Excl: L49.6
L49.7 Exfoliation due to erythematous condition involving 70-79 percent of body surface CC
CC Excl: L49.7
L49.8 Exfoliation due to erythematous condition involving 80-89 percent of body surface CC
CC Excl: L49.8
L49.9 Exfoliation due to erythematous condition involving 90 or more percent of body surface CC
CC Excl: L49.9

✓4th L5Ø Urticaria

EXCLUDES 1 *allergic contact dermatitis (L23.-)*
angioneurotic edema (T78.3)
giant urticaria (T78.3)
hereditary angio-edema (D84.1)
Quincke's edema (T78.3)
serum urticaria (T8Ø.6-)
solar urticaria (L56.3)
urticaria neonatorum (P83.8)
urticaria papulosa (L28.2)
urticaria pigmentosa (Q82.2)

L5Ø.Ø Allergic urticaria
L5Ø.1 Idiopathic urticaria
L5Ø.2 Urticaria due to cold and heat
L5Ø.3 Dermatographic urticaria
L5Ø.4 Vibratory urticaria
L5Ø.5 Cholinergic urticaria
L5Ø.6 Contact urticaria
L5Ø.8 Other urticaria
Chronic urticaria
Recurrent periodic urticaria
L5Ø.9 Urticaria, unspecified

✓4th L51 Erythema multiforme

Use additional code for adverse effect, if applicable, to identify drug (T36-T5Ø with fifth or sixth character 5)
Use additional code to identify associated manifestations, such as:
arthropathy associated with dermatological disorders (M14.8-)
conjunctival edema (H11.42)
conjunctivitis (H1Ø.22-)
corneal scars and opacities (H17.-)
corneal ulcer (H16.Ø-)
edema of eyelid (HØ2.84)
inflammation of eyelid (HØ1.8)
keratoconjunctivitis sicca (H16.22-)
mechanical lagophthalmos (HØ2.22-)
stomatitis (K12.-)
symblepharon (H11.23-)
Use additional code to identify percentage of skin exfoliation (L49.-)

EXCLUDES 1 *staphylococcal scalded skin syndrome (LØØ)*
Ritter's disease (LØØ)

L51.Ø Nonbullous erythema multiforme CC
L51.1 Stevens-Johnson syndrome
CC Excl: LØØ, L12.3Ø-L12.35, L26, L3Ø.4, L44.8-L45, L51.Ø-L54, L71.Ø-L71.9, L92.Ø, L93.Ø-L93.2, L94.2, L94.4, L95.1, L98.2, L98.8, L99
L51.2 Toxic epidermal necrolysis [Lyell] CC
CC Excl: See code: L51.1
L51.3 Stevens-Johnson syndrome-toxic epidermal necrolysis overlap syndrome CC
SJS-TEN overlap syndrome
CC Excl: See code: L51.1
L51.8 Other erythema multiforme
L51.9 Erythema multiforme, unspecified
Erythema iris
Erythema multiforme major NOS
Erythema multiforme minor NOS
Herpes iris

L52 Erythema nodosum

EXCLUDES 1 *tuberculous erythema nodosum (A18.4)*

✓4th L53 Other erythematous conditions

EXCLUDES 1 *erythema ab igne (L59.Ø)*
erythema due to external agents in contact with skin (L23-L25)
erythema intertrigo (L3Ø.4)

CC Excl: For CC codes in category L53, unless otherwise noted: L12.3Ø-L12.35, L44.8-L45, L51.Ø-L53.3, L71.Ø-L71.9, L93.Ø-L93.2, L94.2, L94.4, L98.8, L99

L53.Ø Toxic erythema CC
Code first poisoning due to drug or toxin, if applicable (T36-T65 with fifth or sixth character 1-4 or 6)
Use additional code for adverse effect, if applicable, to identify drug (T36-T5Ø with fifth or sixth character 5)
EXCLUDES 1 *neonatal erythema toxicum (P83.1)*
L53.1 Erythema annulare centrifugum CC
L53.2 Erythema marginatum CC
L53.3 Other chronic figurate erythema CC
L53.8 Other specified erythematous conditions
L53.9 Erythematous condition, unspecified
Erythema NOS
Erythroderma NOS

L54 Erythema in diseases classified elsewhere

Code first underlying disease

Radiation-related disorders of the skin and subcutaneous tissue (L55-L59)

✓4th L55 Sunburn

L55.Ø Sunburn of first degree
L55.1 Sunburn of second degree
L55.2 Sunburn of third degree
L55.9 Sunburn, unspecified

✓4th L56 Other acute skin changes due to ultraviolet radiation

Use additional code to identify the source of the ultraviolet radiation (W89, X32)

L56.Ø Drug phototoxic response
Use additional code for adverse effect, if applicable, to identify drug (T36-T5Ø with fifth or sixth character 5)
L56.1 Drug photoallergic response
Use additional code for adverse effect, if applicable, to identify drug (T36-T5Ø with fifth or sixth character 5)
L56.2 Photocontact dermatitis [berloque dermatitis]
L56.3 Solar urticaria
L56.4 Polymorphous light eruption
L56.5 Disseminated superficial actinic porokeratosis (DSAP)
L56.8 Other specified acute skin changes due to ultraviolet radiation
L56.9 Acute skin change due to ultraviolet radiation, unspecified

✓4th L57 Skin changes due to chronic exposure to nonionizing radiation

Use additional code to identify the source of the ultraviolet radiation (W89, X32)

L57.Ø Actinic keratosis
Keratosis NOS
Senile keratosis
Solar keratosis
L57.1 Actinic reticuloid
L57.2 Cutis rhomboidalis nuchae
L57.3 Poikiloderma of Civatte
L57.4 Cutis laxa senilis
Elastosis senilis
L57.5 Actinic granuloma
L57.8 Other skin changes due to chronic exposure to nonionizing radiation
Farmer's skin
Sailor's skin
Solar dermatitis
L57.9 Skin changes due to chronic exposure to nonionizing radiation, unspecified

✓4th L58 Radiodermatitis

Use additional code to identify the source of the radiation (W88, W9Ø)

L58.Ø Acute radiodermatitis
L58.1 Chronic radiodermatitis
L58.9 Radiodermatitis, unspecified

✓4th L59 Other disorders of skin and subcutaneous tissue related to radiation

L59.Ø Erythema ab igne [dermatitis ab igne]
L59.8 Other specified disorders of the skin and subcutaneous tissue related to radiation
L59.9 Disorder of the skin and subcutaneous tissue related to radiation, unspecified

Disorders of skin appendages (L6Ø-L75)

EXCLUDES 1 *congenital malformations of integument (Q84.-)*

✓4th L6Ø Nail disorders

EXCLUDES 2 *clubbing of nails (R68.3)*
onychia and paronychia (LØ3.Ø-)

L6Ø.Ø Ingrowing nail
L6Ø.1 Onycholysis
L6Ø.2 Onychogryphosis
L6Ø.3 Nail dystrophy
L6Ø.4 Beau's lines
L6Ø.5 Yellow nail syndrome
L6Ø.8 Other nail disorders
L6Ø.9 Nail disorder, unspecified

L62 Nail disorders in diseases classified elsewhere

Code first underlying disease, such as:
pachydermoperiostosis (M89.4-)

✓4th L63 Alopecia areata
- **L63.0 Alopecia (capitis) totalis**
- **L63.1 Alopecia universalis**
- **L63.2 Ophiasis**
- **L63.8 Other alopecia areata**
- **L63.9 Alopecia areata, unspecified**

✓4th L64 Androgenic alopecia

INCLUDES male-pattern baldness
- **L64.0 Drug-induced androgenic alopecia**
  Use additional code for adverse effect, if applicable, to identify drug (T36-T50 with fifth or sixth character 5)
- **L64.8 Other androgenic alopecia**
- **L64.9 Androgenic alopecia, unspecified**

✓4th L65 Other nonscarring hair loss

Use additional code for adverse effect, if applicable, to identify drug (T36-T50 with fifth or sixth character 5)

EXCLUDES 1 *trichotillomania (F63.3)*
- **L65.0 Telogen effluvium**
- **L65.1 Anagen effluvium**
- **L65.2 Alopecia mucinosa**
- **L65.8 Other specified nonscarring hair loss**
- **L65.9 Nonscarring hair loss, unspecified**
  Alopecia NOS

✓4th L66 Cicatricial alopecia [scarring hair loss]
- **L66.0 Pseudopelade**
- **L66.1 Lichen planopilaris**
  Follicular lichen planus
- **L66.2 Folliculitis decalvans**
- **L66.3 Perifolliculitis capitis abscedens**
- **L66.4 Folliculitis ulerythematosa reticulata**
- **L66.8 Other cicatricial alopecia**
- **L66.9 Cicatricial alopecia, unspecified**

✓4th L67 Hair color and hair shaft abnormalities

EXCLUDES 1 *monilethrix (Q84.1)*
pili annulati (Q84.1)
telogen effluvium (L65.0)
- **L67.0 Trichorrhexis nodosa**
- **L67.1 Variations in hair color**
  Canities
  Greyness, hair (premature)
  Heterochromia of hair
  Poliosis circumscripta, acquired
  Poliosis NOS
- **L67.8 Other hair color and hair shaft abnormalities**
  Fragilitas crinium
- **L67.9 Hair color and hair shaft abnormality, unspecified**

✓4th L68 Hypertrichosis

INCLUDES excess hair

EXCLUDES 1 *congenital hypertrichosis (Q84.2)*
persistent lanugo (Q84.2)
- **L68.0 Hirsutism**
- **L68.1 Acquired hypertrichosis lanuginosa**
- **L68.2 Localized hypertrichosis**
- **L68.3 Polytrichia**
- **L68.8 Other hypertrichosis**
- **L68.9 Hypertrichosis, unspecified**

✓4th L70 Acne

EXCLUDES 2 *acne keloid (L73.0)*
- **L70.0 Acne vulgaris**
- **L70.1 Acne conglobata**
- **L70.2 Acne varioliformis**
  Acne necrotica miliaris
- **L70.3 Acne tropica**
- **L70.4 Infantile acne** P
- **L70.5 Acné excoriée des jeunes filles**
  Picker's acne
- **L70.8 Other acne**
- **L70.9 Acne, unspecified**

✓4th L71 Rosacea

Use additional code for adverse effect, if applicable, to identify drug (T36-T50 with fifth or sixth character 5)
- **L71.0 Perioral dermatitis**
- **L71.1 Rhinophyma**
- **L71.8 Other rosacea**
- **L71.9 Rosacea, unspecified**

✓4th L72 Follicular cysts of skin and subcutaneous tissue
- **L72.0 Epidermal cyst**
- **✓5th L72.1 Pilar and trichodermal cyst**
  - **L72.11 Pilar cyst**
  - **L72.12 Trichodermal cyst**
    Trichilemmal (proliferating) cyst
- **L72.2 Steatocystoma multiplex**
- **L72.3 Sebaceous cyst**
  EXCLUDES 2 *pilar cyst (L72.11)*
  trichilemmal (proliferating) cyst (L72.12)
- **L72.8 Other follicular cysts of the skin and subcutaneous tissue**
- **L72.9 Follicular cyst of the skin and subcutaneous tissue, unspecified**

✓4th L73 Other follicular disorders
- **L73.0 Acne keloid**
- **L73.1 Pseudofolliculitis barbae**
- **L73.2 Hidradenitis suppurativa**
- **L73.8 Other specified follicular disorders**
  Sycosis barbae
- **L73.9 Follicular disorder, unspecified**

✓4th L74 Eccrine sweat disorders

EXCLUDES 2 *generalized hyperhidrosis (R61)*
- **L74.0 Miliaria rubra**
- **L74.1 Miliaria crystallina**
- **L74.2 Miliaria profunda**
  Miliaria tropicalis
- **L74.3 Miliaria, unspecified**
- **L74.4 Anhidrosis**
  Hypohidrosis
- **✓5th L74.5 Focal hyperhidrosis**
  - **✓6th L74.51 Primary focal hyperhidrosis**
    - **L74.510 Primary focal hyperhidrosis, axilla**
    - **L74.511 Primary focal hyperhidrosis, face**
    - **L74.512 Primary focal hyperhidrosis, palms**
    - **L74.513 Primary focal hyperhidrosis, soles**
    - **L74.519 Primary focal hyperhidrosis, unspecified**
  - **L74.52 Secondary focal hyperhidrosis**
    Frey's syndrome
- **L74.8 Other eccrine sweat disorders**
- **L74.9 Eccrine sweat disorder, unspecified**
  Sweat gland disorder NOS

✓4th L75 Apocrine sweat disorders

EXCLUDES 1 *dyshidrosis (L30.1)*
hidradenitis suppurativa (L73.2)
- **L75.0 Bromhidrosis**
- **L75.1 Chromhidrosis**
- **L75.2 Apocrine miliaria**
  Fox-Fordyce disease
- **L75.8 Other apocrine sweat disorders**
- **L75.9 Apocrine sweat disorder, unspecified**

Intraoperative and postprocedural complications of skin and subcutaneous tissue (L76)

✓4th L76 Intraoperative and postprocedural complications of skin and subcutaneous tissue

CC Excl: For CC codes in category L76, unless otherwise noted:
H95.811-H95.89, I85.01, I85.11, I97.3, K21.9, K22.8, K23-K25.0, K25.2, K25.4, K25.6, K26.0, K26.2, K26.4, K26.6, K27.0, K27.2, K27.4, K27.6, K28.0, K28.2, K28.4, K28.6, K29.01, K29.21, K29.31, K29.41, K29.51, K29.61, K29.71, K29.81, K29.91, K31.811, K55.21, K57.01, K57.11, K57.13, K57.21, K57.31, K57.33, K57.41, K57.51, K57.53, K57.81, K57.91, K57.93, K62.5, K92.0-K92.2, L76.01-L76.02, L76.21-L76.82, M96.89, N98.1-N98.9, P54.1-P54.3, T81.10XA, T81.11XA, T81.12XA, T81.19XA, T81.82XA, T81.89XA, T81.9XXA

√5th **L76.Ø Intraoperative hemorrhage and hematoma of skin and subcutaneous tissue complicating a procedure**
EXCLUDES 1 *intraoperative hemorrhage and hematoma of skin and subcutaneous tissue due to accidental puncture and laceration during a procedure (L76.1-)*

L76.Ø1 Intraoperative hemorrhage and hematoma of skin and subcutaneous tissue complicating a dermatologic procedure CC

L76.Ø2 Intraoperative hemorrhage and hematoma of skin and subcutaneous tissue complicating other procedure CC

√5th **L76.1 Accidental puncture and laceration of skin and subcutaneous tissue during a procedure**

L76.11 Accidental puncture and laceration of skin and subcutaneous tissue during a dermatologic procedure CC
CC Excl: D78.11-D78.12, D78.81-D78.89, E36.11-E36.8, E89.81Ø-E89.89, G96.11, G97.41, G97.48-G97.49, H59.Ø11-H59.Ø19, H59.Ø31-H59.Ø99, H59.211-H59.229, H59.811-H59.89, H95.31-H95.32, H95.811-H95.89, I97.3, I97.51-I97.52, J95.71-J95.72, K91.71-K91.72, L76.11-L76.12, L76.81-L76.82, M96.82Ø-M96.821, M96.89, N98.1-N98.9, N99.71-N99.72, T81.82XA, T81.89XA, T81.9XXA

L76.12 Accidental puncture and laceration of skin and subcutaneous tissue during other procedure CC
CC Excl: See code: D76.11

√5th **L76.2 Postprocedural hemorrhage and hematoma of skin and subcutaneous tissue following a procedure**

L76.21 Postprocedural hemorrhage and hematoma of skin and subcutaneous tissue following a dermatologic procedure CC

L76.22 Postprocedural hemorrhage and hematoma of skin and subcutaneous tissue following other procedure CC

√5th **L76.8 Other intraoperative and postprocedural complications of skin and subcutaneous tissue**
Use additional code, if applicable, to further specify disorder

L76.81 Other intraoperative complications of skin and subcutaneous tissue

L76.82 Other postprocedural complications of skin and subcutaneous tissue

Other disorders of the skin and subcutaneous tissue (L8Ø-L99)

L8Ø Vitiligo
EXCLUDES 2 *vitiligo of eyelids (HØ2.73-)*
vitiligo of vulva (N9Ø.89)

√4th **L81 Other disorders of pigmentation**
EXCLUDES 1 *birthmark NOS (Q82.5)*
Peutz-Jeghers syndrome (Q85.8)
EXCLUDES 2 *nevus—see Alphabetical Index*

L81.Ø Postinflammatory hyperpigmentation

L81.1 Chloasma

L81.2 Freckles

L81.3 Café au lait spots

L81.4 Other melanin hyperpigmentation
Lentigo

L81.5 Leukoderma, not elsewhere classified

L81.6 Other disorders of diminished melanin formation

L81.7 Pigmented purpuric dermatosis
Angioma serpiginosum

L81.8 Other specified disorders of pigmentation
Iron pigmentation
Tattoo pigmentation

L81.9 Disorder of pigmentation, unspecified

√4th **L82 Seborrheic keratosis**
INCLUDES dermatosis papulosa nigra
Leser-Trélat disease
EXCLUDES 2 *seborrheic dermatitis (L21.-)*

L82.Ø Inflamed seborrheic keratosis

L82.1 Other seborrheic keratosis
Seborrheic keratosis NOS

L83 Acanthosis nigricans
Confluent and reticulated papillomatosis

L84 Corns and callosities
Callus
Clavus

√4th **L85 Other epidermal thickening**
EXCLUDES 2 *hypertrophic disorders of the skin (L91.-)*

L85.Ø Acquired ichthyosis
EXCLUDES 1 *congenital ichthyosis (Q8Ø.-)*

L85.1 Acquired keratosis [keratoderma] palmaris et plantaris
EXCLUDES 1 *inherited keratosis palmaris et plantaris (Q82.8)*

L85.2 Keratosis punctata (palmaris et plantaris)

L85.3 Xerosis cutis
Dry skin dermatitis

L85.8 Other specified epidermal thickening
Cutaneous horn

L85.9 Epidermal thickening, unspecified

L86 Keratoderma in diseases classified elsewhere
Code first underlying disease, such as:
Reiter's disease (MØ2.3-)
EXCLUDES 1 *gonococcal keratoderma (A54.89)*
gonococcal keratosis (A54.89)
keratoderma due to vitamin A deficiency (E5Ø.8)
keratosis due to vitamin A deficiency (E5Ø.8)
xeroderma due to vitamin A deficiency (E5Ø.8)

√4th **L87 Transepidermal elimination disorders**
EXCLUDES 1 *granuloma annulare (perforating) (L92.Ø)*

L87.Ø Keratosis follicularis et parafollicularis in cutem penetrans
Hyperkeratosis follicularis penetrans
Kyrle disease

L87.1 Reactive perforating collagenosis

L87.2 Elastosis perforans serpiginosa

L87.8 Other transepidermal elimination disorders

L87.9 Transepidermal elimination disorder, unspecified

L88 Pyoderma gangrenosum CC
Phagedenic pyoderma
EXCLUDES 1 *dermatitis gangrenosa (LØ8.Ø)*
CC Excl: LØ8.Ø, LØ8.81, L88

√4th **L89 Pressure ulcer**
Bed sore
Decubitus ulcer
Plaster ulcer
Pressure area
Pressure sore
Code first any associated gangrene (I96)
EXCLUDES 2 *decubitus (trophic) ulcer of cervix (uteri) (N86)*
diabetic ulcers (EØ8.621, EØ8.622, EØ9.621, EØ9.622, E1Ø.621, E1Ø.622, E11.621, E11.622, E13.621, E13.622)
non-pressure chronic ulcer of skin (L97.-)
skin infections (LØØ-LØ8)
varicose ulcer (I83.Ø, I83.2)

CC Excl: For MCC codes in category L89, unless otherwise noted:
L89.ØØØ-L89.95, L97.1Ø1-L97.929, L98.411-L98.499

√5th **L89.Ø Pressure ulcer of elbow**

√6th **L89.ØØ Pressure ulcer of unspecified elbow**

L89.ØØØ Pressure ulcer of unspecified elbow, unstageable

L89.ØØ1 Pressure ulcer of unspecified elbow, stage 1
Healing pressure ulcer of unspecified elbow, stage 1
Pressure pre-ulcer skin changes limited to persistent focal edema, unspecified elbow

L89.ØØ2 Pressure ulcer of unspecified elbow, stage 2
Healing pressure ulcer of unspecified elbow, stage 2
Pressure ulcer with abrasion, blister, partial thickness skin loss involving epidermis and/or dermis, unspecified elbow

L89.ØØ3 Pressure ulcer of unspecified elbow, stage 3 PDx MCC MCC
Healing pressure ulcer of unspecified elbow, stage 3
Pressure ulcer with full thickness skin loss involving damage or necrosis of subcutaneous tissue, unspecified elbow

L89.004 Pressure ulcer of unspecified elbow, stage 4 PDx MCC MCC
Healing pressure ulcer of unspecified elbow, stage 4
Pressure ulcer with necrosis of soft tissues through to underlying muscle, tendon, or bone, unspecified elbow

L89.009 Pressure ulcer of unspecified elbow, unspecified stage
Healing pressure ulcer of elbow NOS
Healing pressure ulcer of unspecified elbow, unspecified stage

✓6th **L89.01 Pressure ulcer of right elbow**

L89.010 Pressure ulcer of right elbow, unstageable

L89.011 Pressure ulcer of right elbow, stage 1
Healing pressure ulcer of right elbow, stage 1
Pressure pre-ulcer skin changes limited to persistent focal edema, right elbow

L89.012 Pressure ulcer of right elbow, stage 2
Healing pressure ulcer of right elbow, stage 2
Pressure ulcer with abrasion, blister, partial thickness skin loss involving epidermis and/or dermis, right elbow

L89.013 Pressure ulcer of right elbow, stage 3 PDx MCC MCC
Healing pressure ulcer of right elbow, stage 3
Pressure ulcer with full thickness skin loss involving damage or necrosis of subcutaneous tissue, right elbow

L89.014 Pressure ulcer of right elbow, stage 4 PDx MCC MCC
Healing pressure ulcer of right elbow, stage 4
Pressure ulcer with necrosis of soft tissues through to underlying muscle, tendon, or bone, right elbow

L89.019 Pressure ulcer of right elbow, unspecified stage
Healing pressure right of elbow NOS
Healing pressure ulcer of unspecified elbow, unspecified stage

✓6th **L89.02 Pressure ulcer of left elbow**

L89.020 Pressure ulcer of left elbow, unstageable

L89.021 Pressure ulcer of left elbow, stage 1
Healing pressure ulcer of left elbow, stage 1
Pressure pre-ulcer skin changes limited to persistent focal edema, left elbow

L89.022 Pressure ulcer of left elbow, stage 2
Healing pressure ulcer of left elbow, stage 2
Pressure ulcer with abrasion, blister, partial thickness skin loss involving epidermis and/or dermis, left elbow

L89.023 Pressure ulcer of left elbow, stage 3 PDx MCC MCC
Healing pressure ulcer of left elbow, stage 3
Pressure ulcer with full thickness skin loss involving damage or necrosis of subcutaneous tissue, left elbow

L89.024 Pressure ulcer of left elbow, stage 4 PDx MCC MCC
Healing pressure ulcer of left elbow, stage 4
Pressure ulcer with necrosis of soft tissues through to underlying muscle, tendon, or bone, left elbow

L89.029 Pressure ulcer of left elbow, unspecified stage
Healing pressure ulcer of left of elbow NOS
Healing pressure ulcer of unspecified elbow, unspecified stage

✓5th **L89.1 Pressure ulcer of back**

✓6th **L89.10 Pressure ulcer of unspecified part of back**

L89.100 Pressure ulcer of unspecified part of back, unstageable

L89.101 Pressure ulcer of unspecified part of back, stage 1
Healing pressure ulcer of unspecified part of back, stage 1
Pressure pre-ulcer skin changes limited to persistent focal edema, unspecified part of back

L89.102 Pressure ulcer of unspecified part of back, stage 2
Healing pressure ulcer of unspecified part of back, stage 2
Pressure ulcer with abrasion, blister, partial thickness skin loss involving epidermis and/or dermis, unspecified part of back

L89.103 Pressure ulcer of unspecified part of back, stage 3 PDx MCC MCC
Healing pressure ulcer of unspecified part of back, stage 3
Pressure ulcer with full thickness skin loss involving damage or necrosis of subcutaneous tissue, unspecified part of back

L89.104 Pressure ulcer of unspecified part of back, stage 4 PDx MCC MCC
Healing pressure ulcer of unspecified part of back, stage 4
Pressure ulcer with necrosis of soft tissues through to underlying muscle, tendon, or bone, unspecified part of back

L89.109 Pressure ulcer of unspecified part of back, unspecified stage
Healing pressure ulcer of unspecified part of back NOS
Healing pressure ulcer of unspecified part of back, unspecified stage

✓6th **L89.11 Pressure ulcer of right upper back**
Pressure ulcer of right shoulder blade

L89.110 Pressure ulcer of right upper back, unstageable

L89.111 Pressure ulcer of right upper back, stage 1
Healing pressure ulcer of right upper back, stage 1
Pressure pre-ulcer skin changes limited to persistent focal edema, right upper back

L89.112 Pressure ulcer of right upper back, stage 2
Healing pressure ulcer of right upper back, stage 2
Pressure ulcer with abrasion, blister, partial thickness skin loss involving epidermis and/or dermis, right upper back

L89.113 Pressure ulcer of right upper back, stage 3 PDx MCC MCC
Healing pressure ulcer of right upper back, stage 3
Pressure ulcer with full thickness skin loss involving damage or necrosis of subcutaneous tissue, right upper back

L89.114 Pressure ulcer of right upper back, stage 4 PDx MCC MCC
Healing pressure ulcer of right upper back, stage 4
Pressure ulcer with necrosis of soft tissues through to underlying muscle, tendon, or bone, right upper back

L89.119 Pressure ulcer of right upper back, unspecified stage
Healing pressure ulcer of right upper back NOS
Healing pressure ulcer of right upper back, unspecified stage

✓6th **L89.12 Pressure ulcer of left upper back**
Pressure ulcer of left shoulder blade

L89.120 Pressure ulcer of left upper back, unstageable

L89.121 Pressure ulcer of left upper back, stage 1
Healing pressure ulcer of left upper back, stage 1
Pressure pre-ulcer skin changes limited to persistent focal edema, left upper back

L89.122 Pressure ulcer of left upper back, stage 2
Healing pressure ulcer of left upper back, stage 2
Pressure ulcer with abrasion, blister, partial thickness skin loss involving epidermis and/or dermis, left upper back

L89.123 **Pressure ulcer of left upper back, stage 3** PDx MCC MCC
Healing pressure ulcer of left upper back, stage 3
Pressure ulcer with full thickness skin loss involving damage or necrosis of subcutaneous tissue, left upper back

L89.124 **Pressure ulcer of left upper back, stage 4** PDx MCC MCC
Healing pressure ulcer of left upper back, stage 4
Pressure ulcer with necrosis of soft tissues through to underlying muscle, tendon, or bone, left upper back

L89.129 **Pressure ulcer of left upper back, unspecified stage**
Healing pressure ulcer of left upper back NOS
Healing pressure ulcer of left upper back, unspecified stage

✓6th L89.13 **Pressure ulcer of right lower back**

L89.13Ø **Pressure ulcer of right lower back, unstageable**

L89.131 **Pressure ulcer of right lower back, stage 1**
Healing pressure ulcer of right lower back, stage 1
Pressure pre-ulcer skin changes limited to persistent focal edema, right lower back

L89.132 **Pressure ulcer of right lower back, stage 2**
Healing pressure ulcer of right lower back, stage 2
Pressure ulcer with abrasion, blister, partial thickness skin loss involving epidermis and/or dermis, right lower back

L89.133 **Pressure ulcer of right lower back, stage 3** PDx MCC MCC
Healing pressure ulcer of right lower back, stage 3
Pressure ulcer with full thickness skin loss involving damage or necrosis of subcutaneous tissue, right lower back

L89.134 **Pressure ulcer of right lower back, stage 4** PDx MCC MCC
Healing pressure ulcer of right lower back, stage 4
Pressure ulcer with necrosis of soft tissues through to underlying muscle, tendon, or bone, right lower back

L89.139 **Pressure ulcer of right lower back, unspecified stage**
Healing pressure ulcer of right lower back NOS
Healing pressure ulcer of right lower back, unspecified stage

✓6th L89.14 **Pressure ulcer of left lower back**

L89.14Ø **Pressure ulcer of left lower back, unstageable**

L89.141 **Pressure ulcer of left lower back, stage 1**
Healing pressure ulcer of left lower back, stage 1
Pressure pre-ulcer skin changes limited to persistent focal edema, left lower back

L89.142 **Pressure ulcer of left lower back, stage 2**
Healing pressure ulcer of left lower back, stage 2
Pressure ulcer with abrasion, blister, partial thickness skin loss involving epidermis and/or dermis, left lower back

L89.143 **Pressure ulcer of left lower back, stage 3** PDx MCC MCC
Healing pressure ulcer of left lower back, stage 3
Pressure ulcer with full thickness skin loss involving damage or necrosis of subcutaneous tissue, left lower back

L89.144 **Pressure ulcer of left lower back, stage 4** PDx MCC MCC
Healing pressure ulcer of left lower back, stage 4
Pressure ulcer with necrosis of soft tissues through to underlying muscle, tendon, or bone, left lower back

L89.149 **Pressure ulcer of left lower back, unspecified stage**
Healing pressure ulcer of left lower back NOS
Healing pressure ulcer of left lower back, unspecified stage

✓6th L89.15 **Pressure ulcer of sacral region**
Pressure ulcer of coccyx
Pressure ulcer of tailbone

L89.15Ø **Pressure ulcer of sacral region, unstageable**

L89.151 **Pressure ulcer of sacral region, stage 1**
Healing pressure ulcer of sacral region, stage 1
Pressure pre-ulcer skin changes limited to persistent focal edema, sacral region

L89.152 **Pressure ulcer of sacral region, stage 2**
Healing pressure ulcer of sacral region, stage 2
Pressure ulcer with abrasion, blister, partial thickness skin loss involving epidermis and/or dermis, sacral region

L89.153 **Pressure ulcer of sacral region, stage 3** PDx MCC MCC
Healing pressure ulcer of sacral region, stage 3
Pressure ulcer with full thickness skin loss involving damage or necrosis of subcutaneous tissue, sacral region

L89.154 **Pressure ulcer of sacral region, stage 4** PDx MCC MCC
Healing pressure ulcer of sacral region, stage 4
Pressure ulcer with necrosis of soft tissues through to underlying muscle, tendon, or bone, sacral region

L89.159 **Pressure ulcer of sacral region, unspecified stage**
Healing pressure ulcer of sacral region NOS
Healing pressure ulcer of sacral region, unspecified stage

✓5th L89.2 **Pressure ulcer of hip**

✓6th L89.20 **Pressure ulcer of unspecified hip**

L89.2ØØ **Pressure ulcer of unspecified hip, unstageable**

L89.2Ø1 **Pressure ulcer of unspecified hip, stage 1**
Healing pressure ulcer of unspecified hip back, stage 1
Pressure pre-ulcer skin changes limited to persistent focal edema, unspecified hip

L89.2Ø2 **Pressure ulcer of unspecified hip, stage 2**
Healing pressure ulcer of unspecified hip, stage 2
Pressure ulcer with abrasion, blister, partial thickness skin loss involving epidermis and/or dermis, unspecified hip

L89.2Ø3 **Pressure ulcer of unspecified hip, stage 3** PDx MCC MCC
Healing pressure ulcer of unspecified hip, stage 3
Pressure ulcer with full thickness skin loss involving damage or necrosis of subcutaneous tissue, unspecified hip

L89.2Ø4 **Pressure ulcer of unspecified hip, stage 4** PDx MCC MCC
Healing pressure ulcer of unspecified hip, stage 4
Pressure ulcer with necrosis of soft tissues through to underlying muscle, tendon, or bone, unspecified hip

L89.2Ø9 **Pressure ulcer of unspecified hip, unspecified stage**
Healing pressure ulcer of unspecified hip NOS
Healing pressure ulcer of unspecified hip, unspecified stage

✓6th L89.21 **Pressure ulcer of right hip**

L89.21Ø **Pressure ulcer of right hip, unstageable**

L89.211 Pressure ulcer of right hip, stage 1
Healing pressure ulcer of right hip back, stage 1
Pressure pre-ulcer skin changes limited to persistent focal edema, right hip

L89.212 Pressure ulcer of right hip, stage 2
Healing pressure ulcer of right hip, stage 2
Pressure ulcer with abrasion, blister, partial thickness skin loss involving epidermis and/or dermis, right hip

L89.213 Pressure ulcer of right hip, stage 3 PDx MCC MCC
Healing pressure ulcer of right hip, stage 3
Pressure ulcer with full thickness skin loss involving damage or necrosis of subcutaneous tissue, right hip

L89.214 Pressure ulcer of right hip, stage 4 PDx MCC MCC
Healing pressure ulcer of right hip, stage 4
Pressure ulcer with necrosis of soft tissues through to underlying muscle, tendon, or bone, right hip

L89.219 Pressure ulcer of right hip, unspecified stage
Healing pressure ulcer of right hip NOS
Healing pressure ulcer of right hip, unspecified stage

✓6th **L89.22 Pressure ulcer of left hip**

L89.220 Pressure ulcer of left hip, unstageable

L89.221 Pressure ulcer of left hip, stage 1
Healing pressure ulcer of left hip back, stage 1
Pressure pre-ulcer skin changes limited to persistent focal edema, left hip

L89.222 Pressure ulcer of left hip, stage 2
Healing pressure ulcer of left hip, stage 2
Pressure ulcer with abrasion, blister, partial thickness skin loss involving epidermis and/or dermis, left hip

L89.223 Pressure ulcer of left hip, stage 3 PDx MCC MCC
Healing pressure ulcer of left hip, stage 3
Pressure ulcer with full thickness skin loss involving damage or necrosis of subcutaneous tissue, left hip

L89.224 Pressure ulcer of left hip, stage 4 PDx MCC MCC
Healing pressure ulcer of left hip, stage 4
Pressure ulcer with necrosis of soft tissues through to underlying muscle, tendon, or bone, left hip

L89.229 Pressure ulcer of left hip, unspecified stage
Healing pressure ulcer of left hip NOS
Healing pressure ulcer of left hip, unspecified stage

✓5th **L89.3 Pressure ulcer of buttock**

✓6th **L89.30 Pressure ulcer of unspecified buttock**

L89.300 Pressure ulcer of unspecified buttock, unstageable

L89.301 Pressure ulcer of unspecified buttock, stage 1
Healing pressure ulcer of unspecified buttock, stage 1
Pressure pre-ulcer skin changes limited to persistent focal edema, unspecified buttock

L89.302 Pressure ulcer of unspecified buttock, stage 2
Healing pressure ulcer of unspecified buttock, stage 2
Pressure ulcer with abrasion, blister, partial thickness skin loss involving epidermis and/or dermis, unspecified buttock

L89.303 Pressure ulcer of unspecified buttock, stage 3 PDx MCC MCC
Healing pressure ulcer of unspecified buttock, stage 3
Pressure ulcer with full thickness skin loss involving damage or necrosis of subcutaneous tissue, unspecified buttock

L89.304 Pressure ulcer of unspecified buttock, stage 4 PDx MCC MCC
Healing pressure ulcer of unspecified buttock, stage 4
Pressure ulcer with necrosis of soft tissues through to underlying muscle, tendon, or bone, unspecified buttock

L89.309 Pressure ulcer of unspecified buttock, unspecified stage
Healing pressure ulcer of unspecified buttock NOS
Healing pressure ulcer of unspecified buttock, unspecified stage

✓6th **L89.31 Pressure ulcer of right buttock**

L89.310 Pressure ulcer of right buttock, unstageable

L89.311 Pressure ulcer of right buttock, stage 1
Healing pressure ulcer of right buttock, stage 1
Pressure pre-ulcer skin changes limited to persistent focal edema, right buttock

L89.312 Pressure ulcer of right buttock, stage 2
Healing pressure ulcer of right buttock, stage 2
Pressure ulcer with abrasion, blister, partial thickness skin loss involving epidermis and/or dermis, right buttock

L89.313 Pressure ulcer of right buttock, stage 3 PDx MCC MCC
Healing pressure ulcer of right buttock, stage 3
Pressure ulcer with full thickness skin loss involving damage or necrosis of subcutaneous tissue, right buttock

L89.314 Pressure ulcer of right buttock, stage 4 PDx MCC MCC
Healing pressure ulcer of right buttock, stage 4
Pressure ulcer with necrosis of soft tissues through to underlying muscle, tendon, or bone, right buttock

L89.319 Pressure ulcer of right buttock, unspecified stage
Healing pressure ulcer of right buttock NOS
Healing pressure ulcer of right buttock, unspecified stage

✓6th **L89.32 Pressure ulcer of left buttock**

L89.320 Pressure ulcer of left buttock, unstageable

L89.321 Pressure ulcer of left buttock, stage 1
Healing pressure ulcer of left buttock, stage 1
Pressure pre-ulcer skin changes limited to persistent focal edema, left buttock

L89.322 Pressure ulcer of left buttock, stage 2
Healing pressure ulcer of left buttock, stage 2
Pressure ulcer with abrasion, blister, partial thickness skin loss involving epidermis and/or dermis, left buttock

L89.323 Pressure ulcer of left buttock, stage 3 PDx MCC MCC
Healing pressure ulcer of left buttock, stage 3
Pressure ulcer with full thickness skin loss involving damage or necrosis of subcutaneous tissue, left buttock

L89.324 Pressure ulcer of left buttock, stage 4 PDx MCC MCC
Healing pressure ulcer of left buttock, stage 4
Pressure ulcer with necrosis of soft tissues through to underlying muscle, tendon, or bone, left buttock

L89.329 Pressure ulcer of left buttock, unspecified stage
Healing pressure ulcer of left buttock NOS
Healing pressure ulcer of left buttock, unspecified stage

✓5th L89.4 Pressure ulcer of contiguous site of back, buttock and hip

L89.4Ø Pressure ulcer of contiguous site of back, buttock and hip, unspecified stage
Healing pressure ulcer of contiguous site of back, buttock and hip NOS
Healing pressure ulcer of contiguous site of back, buttock and hip, unspecified stage

L89.41 Pressure ulcer of contiguous site of back, buttock and hip, stage 1
Healing pressure ulcer of contiguous site of back, buttock and hip, stage 1
Pressure pre-ulcer skin changes limited to persistent focal edema, contiguous site of back, buttock and hip

L89.42 Pressure ulcer of contiguous site of back, buttock and hip, stage 2
Healing pressure ulcer of contiguous site of back, buttock and hip, stage 2
Pressure ulcer with abrasion, blister, partial thickness skin loss involving epidermis and/or dermis, contiguous site of back, buttock and hip

L89.43 Pressure ulcer of contiguous site of back, buttock and hip, stage 3 PDx MCC MCC
Healing pressure ulcer of contiguous site of back, buttock and hip, stage 3
Pressure ulcer with full thickness skin loss involving damage or necrosis of subcutaneous tissue, contiguous site of back, buttock and hip

L89.44 Pressure ulcer of contiguous site of back, buttock and hip, stage 4 PDx MCC MCC
Healing pressure ulcer of contiguous site of back, buttock and hip, stage 4
Pressure ulcer with necrosis of soft tissues through to underlying muscle, tendon, or bone, contiguous site of back, buttock and hip

L89.45 Pressure ulcer of contiguous site of back, buttock and hip, unstageable

✓5th L89.5 Pressure ulcer of ankle

✓6th L89.5Ø Pressure ulcer of unspecified ankle

L89.5ØØ Pressure ulcer of unspecified ankle, unstageable

L89.5Ø1 Pressure ulcer of unspecified ankle, stage 1
Healing pressure ulcer of unspecified ankle, stage 1
Pressure pre-ulcer skin changes limited to persistent focal edema, unspecified ankle

L89.5Ø2 Pressure ulcer of unspecified ankle, stage 2
Healing pressure ulcer of unspecified ankle, stage 2
Pressure ulcer with abrasion, blister, partial thickness skin loss involving epidermis and/or dermis, unspecified ankle

L89.5Ø3 Pressure ulcer of unspecified ankle, stage 3 PDx MCC MCC
Healing pressure ulcer of unspecified ankle, stage 3
Pressure ulcer with full thickness skin loss involving damage or necrosis of subcutaneous tissue, unspecified ankle

L89.5Ø4 Pressure ulcer of unspecified ankle, stage 4 PDx MCC MCC
Healing pressure ulcer of unspecified ankle, stage 4
Pressure ulcer with necrosis of soft tissues through to underlying muscle, tendon, or bone, unspecified ankle

L89.5Ø9 Pressure ulcer of unspecified ankle, unspecified stage
Healing pressure ulcer of unspecified ankle NOS
Healing pressure ulcer of unspecified ankle, unspecified stage

✓6th L89.51 Pressure ulcer of right ankle

L89.51Ø Pressure ulcer of right ankle, unstageable

L89.511 Pressure ulcer of right ankle, stage 1
Healing pressure ulcer of right ankle, stage 1
Pressure pre-ulcer skin changes limited to persistent focal edema, right ankle

L89.512 Pressure ulcer of right ankle, stage 2
Healing pressure ulcer of right ankle, stage 2
Pressure ulcer with abrasion, blister, partial thickness skin loss involving epidermis and/or dermis, right ankle

L89.513 Pressure ulcer of right ankle, stage 3 PDx MCC MCC
Healing pressure ulcer of right ankle, stage 3
Pressure ulcer with full thickness skin loss involving damage or necrosis of subcutaneous tissue, right ankle

L89.514 Pressure ulcer of right ankle, stage 4 PDx MCC MCC
Healing pressure ulcer of right ankle, stage 4
Pressure ulcer with necrosis of soft tissues through to underlying muscle, tendon, or bone, right ankle

L89.519 Pressure ulcer of right ankle, unspecified stage
Healing pressure ulcer of right ankle NOS
Healing pressure ulcer of right ankle, unspecified stage

✓6th L89.52 Pressure ulcer of left ankle

L89.52Ø Pressure ulcer of left ankle, unstageable

L89.521 Pressure ulcer of left ankle, stage 1
Healing pressure ulcer of left ankle, stage 1
Pressure pre-ulcer skin changes limited to persistnt focal edema, left ankle

L89.522 Pressure ulcer of left ankle, stage 2
Healing pressure ulcer of left ankle, stage 2
Pressure ulcer with abrasion, blister, partial thickness skin loss involving epidermis and/or dermis, left ankle

L89.523 Pressure ulcer of left ankle, stage 3 PDx MCC MCC
Healing pressure ulcer of left ankle, stage 3
Pressure ulcer with full thickness skin loss involving damage or necrosis of subcutaneous tissue, left ankle

L89.524 Pressure ulcer of left ankle, stage 4 PDx MCC MCC
Healing pressure ulcer of left ankle, stage 4
Pressure ulcer with necrosis of soft tissues through to underlying muscle, tendon, or bone, left ankle

L89.529 Pressure ulcer of left ankle, unspecified stage
Healing pressure ulcer of left ankle NOS
Healing pressure ulcer of left ankle, unspecified stage

✓5th L89.6 Pressure ulcer of heel

✓6th L89.6Ø Pressure ulcer of unspecified heel

L89.6ØØ Pressure ulcer of unspecified heel, unstageable

L89.6Ø1 Pressure ulcer of unspecified heel, stage 1
Healing pressure ulcer of unspecified heel, stage 1
Pressure pre-ulcer skin changes limited to persistent focal edema, unspecified heel

L89.6Ø2 Pressure ulcer of unspecified heel, stage 2
Healing pressure ulcer of unspecified heel, stage 2
Pressure ulcer with abrasion, blister, partial thickness skin loss involving epidermis and/or dermis, unspecified heel

L89.6Ø3 Pressure ulcer of unspecified heel, stage 3 PDx MCC MCC
Healing pressure ulcer of unspecified heel, stage 3
Pressure ulcer with full thickness skin loss involving damage or necrosis of subcutaneous tissue, unspecified heel

L89.6Ø4 Pressure ulcer of unspecified heel, stage 4 PDx MCC MCC
Healing pressure ulcer of unspecified heel, stage 4
Pressure ulcer with necrosis of soft tissues through to underlying muscle, tendon, or bone, unspecified heel

L89.609 Pressure ulcer of unspecified heel, unspecified stage
Healing pressure ulcer of unspecified heel NOS
Healing pressure ulcer of unspecified heel, unspecified stage

✓6th **L89.61 Pressure ulcer of right heel**

L89.610 Pressure ulcer of right heel, unstageable

L89.611 Pressure ulcer of right heel, stage 1
Healing pressure ulcer of right heel, stage 1
Pressure pre-ulcer skin changes limited to persistent focal edema, right heel

L89.612 Pressure ulcer of right heel, stage 2
Healing pressure ulcer of right heel, stage 2
Pressure ulcer with abrasion, blister, partial thickness skin loss involving epidermis and/or dermis, right heel

L89.613 Pressure ulcer of right heel, stage 3 PDx MCC MCC
Healing pressure ulcer of right heel, stage 3
Pressure ulcer with full thickness skin loss involving damage or necrosis of subcutaneous tissue, right heel

L89.614 Pressure ulcer of right heel, stage 4 PDx MCC MCC
Healing pressure ulcer of right heel, stage 4
Pressure ulcer with necrosis of soft tissues through to underlying muscle, tendon, or bone, right heel

L89.619 Pressure ulcer of right heel, unspecified stage
Healing pressure ulcer of right heel NOS
Healing pressure ulcer of unspecified heel, right stage

✓6th **L89.62 Pressure ulcer of left heel**

L89.620 Pressure ulcer of left heel, unstageable

L89.621 Pressure ulcer of left heel, stage 1
Healing pressure ulcer of left heel, stage 1
Pressure pre-ulcer skin changes limited to persistent focal edema, left heel

L89.622 Pressure ulcer of left heel, stage 2
Healing pressure ulcer of left heel, stage 2
Pressure ulcer with abrasion, blister, partial thickness skin loss involving epidermis and/or dermis, left heel

L89.623 Pressure ulcer of left heel, stage 3 PDx MCC MCC
Healing pressure ulcer of left heel, stage 3
Pressure ulcer with full thickness skin loss involving damage or necrosis of subcutaneous tissue, left heel

L89.624 Pressure ulcer of left heel, stage 4 PDx MCC MCC
Healing pressure ulcer of left heel, stage 4
Pressure ulcer with necrosis of soft tissues through to underlying muscle, tendon, or bone, left heel

L89.629 Pressure ulcer of left heel, unspecified stage
Healing pressure ulcer of left heel NOS
Healing pressure ulcer of left heel, unspecified stage

✓5th **L89.8 Pressure ulcer of other site**

✓6th **L89.81 Pressure ulcer of head**
Pressure ulcer of face

L89.810 Pressure ulcer of head, unstageable

L89.811 Pressure ulcer of head, stage 1
Healing pressure ulcer of head, stage 1
Pressure pre-ulcer skin changes limited to persistent focal edema, head

L89.812 Pressure ulcer of head, stage 2
Healing pressure ulcer of head, stage 2
Pressure ulcer with abrasion, blister, partial thickness skin loss involving epidermis and/or dermis, head

L89.813 Pressure ulcer of head, stage 3 PDx MCC MCC
Healing pressure ulcer of head, stage 3
Pressure ulcer with full thickness skin loss involving damage or necrosis of subcutaneous tissue, head

L89.814 Pressure ulcer of head, stage 4 PDx MCC MCC
Healing pressure ulcer of head, stage 4
Pressure ulcer with necrosis of soft tissues through to underlying muscle, tendon, or bone, head

L89.819 Pressure ulcer of head, unspecified stage
Healing pressure ulcer of head NOS
Healing pressure ulcer of head, unspecified stage

✓6th **L89.89 Pressure ulcer of other site**

L89.890 Pressure ulcer of other site, unstageable

L89.891 Pressure ulcer of other site, stage 1
Healing pressure ulcer of other site, stage 1
Pressure pre-ulcer skin changes limited to persistent focal edema, other site

L89.892 Pressure ulcer of other site, stage 2
Healing pressure ulcer of other site, stage 2
Pressure ulcer with abrasion, blister, partial thickness skin loss involving epidermis and/or dermis, other site

L89.893 Pressure ulcer of other site, stage 3 PDx MCC MCC
Healing pressure ulcer of other site, stage 3
Pressure ulcer with full thickness skin loss involving damage or necrosis of subcutaneous tissue, other site

L89.894 Pressure ulcer of other site, stage 4 PDx MCC MCC
Healing pressure ulcer of other site, stage 4
Pressure ulcer with necrosis of soft tissues through to underlying muscle, tendon, or bone, other site

L89.899 Pressure ulcer of other site, unspecified stage
Healing pressure ulcer of other site NOS
Healing pressure ulcer of other site, unspecified stage

✓5th **L89.9 Pressure ulcer of unspecified site**

L89.90 Pressure ulcer of unspecified site, unspecified stage
Healing pressure ulcer of unspecified site NOS
Healing pressure ulcer of unspecified site, unspecified stage

L89.91 Pressure ulcer of unspecified site, stage 1
Healing pressure ulcer of unspecified site, stage 1
Pressure pre-ulcer skin changes limited to persistent focal edema, unspecified site

L89.92 Pressure ulcer of unspecified site, stage 2
Healing pressure ulcer of unspecified site, stage 2
Pressure ulcer with abrasion, blister, partial thickness skin loss involving epidermis and/or dermis, unspecified site

L89.93 Pressure ulcer of unspecified site, stage 3 PDx MCC MCC
Healing pressure ulcer of unspecified site, stage 3
Pressure ulcer with full thickness skin loss involving damage or necrosis of subcutaneous tissue, unspecified site

L89.94 Pressure ulcer of unspecified site, stage 4 PDx MCC MCC
Healing pressure ulcer of unspecified site, stage 4
Pressure ulcer with necrosis of soft tissues through to underlying muscle, tendon, or bone, unspecified site

L89.95 Pressure ulcer of unspecified site, unstageable

✓4th **L90 Atrophic disorders of skin**

L90.0 Lichen sclerosus et atrophicus
EXCLUDES 2 *lichen sclerosus of external female genital organs (N90.4)*
lichen sclerosus of external male genital organs (N48.0)

L90.1 Anetoderma of Schweninger-Buzzi

L90.2 Anetoderma of Jadassohn-Pellizzari

L90.3 Atrophoderma of Pasini and Pierini

L90.4 Acrodermatitis chronica atrophicans

L90.5 Scar conditions and fibrosis of skin
Adherent scar (skin)
Cicatrix
Disfigurement of skin due to scar
Fibrosis of skin NOS
Scar NOS
EXCLUDES 2 *hypertrophic scar (L91.0)*
keloid scar (L91.0)

L90.6 Striae atrophicae

L90.8 Other atrophic disorders of skin

L90.9 Atrophic disorder of skin, unspecified

4th L91 Hypertrophic disorders of skin

L91.0 Hypertrophic scar
Keloid Keloid scar
EXCLUDES 2 *acne keloid (L73.0)*
scar NOS (L90.5)

L91.8 Other hypertrophic disorders of the skin

L91.9 Hypertrophic disorder of the skin, unspecified

4th L92 Granulomatous disorders of skin and subcutaneous tissue
EXCLUDES 2 *actinic granuloma (L57.5)*

L92.0 Granuloma annulare
Perforating granuloma annulare

L92.1 Necrobiosis lipoidica, not elsewhere classified
EXCLUDES 1 *necrobiosis lipoidica associated with diabetes mellitus (E08-E13 with .620)*

L92.2 Granuloma faciale [eosinophilic granuloma of skin]

L92.3 Foreign body granuloma of the skin and subcutaneous tissue
Use additional code to identify the type of retained foreign body (Z18.-)

L92.8 Other granulomatous disorders of the skin and subcutaneous tissue

L92.9 Granulomatous disorder of the skin and subcutaneous tissue, unspecified

4th L93 Lupus erythematosus
Use additional code for adverse effect, if applicable, to identify drug (T36-T50 with fifth or sixth character 5)
EXCLUDES 1 *lupus exedens (A18.4)*
lupus vulgaris (A18.4)
scleroderma (M34.-)
systemic lupus erythematosus (M32.-)

L93.0 Discoid lupus erythematosus
Lupus erythematosus NOS

L93.1 Subacute cutaneous lupus erythematosus

L93.2 Other local lupus erythematosus
Lupus erythematosus profundus
Lupus panniculitis

4th L94 Other localized connective tissue disorders
EXCLUDES 1 *systemic connective tissue disorders (M30-M36)*

L94.0 Localized scleroderma [morphea]
Circumscribed scleroderma

L94.1 Linear scleroderma
En coup de sabre lesion

L94.2 Calcinosis cutis

L94.3 Sclerodactyly

L94.4 Gottron's papules

L94.5 Poikiloderma vasculare atrophicans

L94.6 Ainhum

L94.8 Other specified localized connective tissue disorders

L94.9 Localized connective tissue disorder, unspecified

4th L95 Vasculitis limited to skin, not elsewhere classified
EXCLUDES 1 *angioma serpiginosum (L81.7)*
Henoch(-Schönlein) purpura (D69.0)
hypersensitivity angiitis (M31.0)
lupus panniculitis (L93.2)
panniculitis NOS (M79.3)
panniculitis of neck and back (M54.0-)
polyarteritis nodosa (M30.0)
relapsing panniculitis (M35.6)
rheumatoid vasculitis (M05.2)
serum sickness (T80.6-)
urticaria (L50.-)
Wegener's granulomatosis (M31.3-)

L95.0 Livedoid vasculitis
Atrophie blanche (en plaque)

L95.1 Erythema elevatum diutinum

L95.8 Other vasculitis limited to the skin

L95.9 Vasculitis limited to the skin, unspecified

4th L97 Non-pressure chronic ulcer of lower limb, not elsewhere classified
INCLUDES chronic ulcer of skin of lower limb NOS
non-healing ulcer of skin
non-infected sinus of skin
trophic ulcer NOS
tropical ulcer NOS
ulcer of skin of lower limb NOS

Code first any associated underlying condition, such as:
atherosclerosis of the lower extremities (I70.23-, I70.24-, I70.33-, I70.34-, I70.43-, I70.44-, I70.53-, I70.54-, I70.63-, I70.64-, I70.73-, I70.74-)
chronic venous hypertension (I87.31-, I87.33-)
diabetic ulcers (E08.621, E08.622, E09.621, E09.622, E10.621, E10.622, E11.621, E11.622, E13.621, E13.622)
postphlebitic syndrome (I87.01-, I87.03-)
postthrombotic syndrome (I87.01-, I87.03-)
varicose ulcer (I83.0-, I83.2-)
Code first any associated gangrene (I96)
EXCLUDES 2 *pressure ulcer (pressure area) (L89.-)*
skin infections (L00-L08)
specific infections classified to A00-B99

CC Excl: For CC codes in category L97, unless otherwise noted: I70.231-I70.25, L44.8-L45, L94.2, L94.4, L97.101-L97.929, L98.411-L98.499, L98.8, L99

5th L97.1 Non-pressure chronic ulcer of thigh

6th L97.10 Non-pressure chronic ulcer of unspecified thigh

L97.101 Non-pressure chronic ulcer of unspecified thigh limited to breakdown of skin CC

L97.102 Non-pressure chronic ulcer of unspecified thigh with fat layer exposed CC

L97.103 Non-pressure chronic ulcer of unspecified thigh with necrosis of muscle CC

L97.104 Non-pressure chronic ulcer of unspecified thigh with necrosis of bone CC

L97.109 Non-pressure chronic ulcer of unspecified thigh with unspecified severity CC

6th L97.11 Non-pressure chronic ulcer of right thigh

L97.111 Non-pressure chronic ulcer of right thigh limited to breakdown of skin CC

L97.112 Non-pressure chronic ulcer of right thigh with fat layer exposed CC

L97.113 Non-pressure chronic ulcer of right thigh with necrosis of muscle CC

L97.114 Non-pressure chronic ulcer of right thigh with necrosis of bone CC

L97.119 Non-pressure chronic ulcer of right thigh with unspecified severity CC

6th L97.12 Non-pressure chronic ulcer of left thigh

L97.121 Non-pressure chronic ulcer of left thigh limited to breakdown of skin CC

L97.122 Non-pressure chronic ulcer of left thigh with fat layer exposed CC

L97.123 Non-pressure chronic ulcer of left thigh with necrosis of muscle CC

L97.124 Non-pressure chronic ulcer of left thigh with necrosis of bone CC

L97.129 Non-pressure chronic ulcer of left thigh with unspecified severity CC

5th L97.2 Non-pressure chronic ulcer of calf

6th L97.20 Non-pressure chronic ulcer of unspecified calf

L97.201 Non-pressure chronic ulcer of unspecified calf limited to breakdown of skin CC

L97.202 Non-pressure chronic ulcer of unspecified calf with fat layer exposed CC

L97.203 Non-pressure chronic ulcer of unspecified calf with necrosis of muscle CC

L97.204 Non-pressure chronic ulcer of unspecified calf with necrosis of bone CC

L97.209 Non-pressure chronic ulcer of unspecified calf with unspecified severity CC

6th L97.21 Non-pressure chronic ulcer of right calf

L97.211 Non-pressure chronic ulcer of right calf limited to breakdown of skin CC

L97.212 Non-pressure chronic ulcer of right calf with fat layer exposed CC

L97.213 Non-pressure chronic ulcer of right calf with necrosis of muscle CC
L97.214 Non-pressure chronic ulcer of right calf with necrosis of bone CC
L97.219 Non-pressure chronic ulcer of right calf with unspecified severity CC

✓6th L97.22 Non-pressure chronic ulcer of left calf
L97.221 Non-pressure chronic ulcer of left calf limited to breakdown of skin CC
L97.222 Non-pressure chronic ulcer of left calf with fat layer exposed CC
L97.223 Non-pressure chronic ulcer of left calf with necrosis of muscle CC
L97.224 Non-pressure chronic ulcer of left calf with necrosis of bone CC
L97.229 Non-pressure chronic ulcer of left calf with unspecified severity CC

✓5th L97.3 Non-pressure chronic ulcer of ankle

✓6th L97.30 Non-pressure chronic ulcer of unspecified ankle
L97.301 Non-pressure chronic ulcer of unspecified ankle limited to breakdown of skin CC
L97.302 Non-pressure chronic ulcer of unspecified ankle with fat layer exposed CC
L97.303 Non-pressure chronic ulcer of unspecified ankle with necrosis of muscle CC
L97.304 Non-pressure chronic ulcer of unspecified ankle with necrosis of bone CC
L97.309 Non-pressure chronic ulcer of unspecified ankle with unspecified severity CC

✓6th L97.31 Non-pressure chronic ulcer of right ankle
L97.311 Non-pressure chronic ulcer of right ankle limited to breakdown of skin CC
L97.312 Non-pressure chronic ulcer of right ankle with fat layer exposed CC
L97.313 Non-pressure chronic ulcer of right ankle with necrosis of muscle CC
L97.314 Non-pressure chronic ulcer of right ankle with necrosis of bone CC
L97.319 Non-pressure chronic ulcer of right ankle with unspecified severity CC

✓6th L97.32 Non-pressure chronic ulcer of left ankle
L97.321 Non-pressure chronic ulcer of left ankle limited to breakdown of skin CC
L97.322 Non-pressure chronic ulcer of left ankle with fat layer exposed CC
L97.323 Non-pressure chronic ulcer of left ankle with necrosis of muscle CC
L97.324 Non-pressure chronic ulcer of left ankle with necrosis of bone CC
L97.329 Non-pressure chronic ulcer of left ankle with unspecified severity CC

✓5th L97.4 Non-pressure chronic ulcer of heel and midfoot
Non-pressure chronic ulcer of plantar surface of midfoot

✓6th L97.40 Non-pressure chronic ulcer of unspecified heel and midfoot
L97.401 Non-pressure chronic ulcer of unspecified heel and midfoot limited to breakdown of skin CC
L97.402 Non-pressure chronic ulcer of unspecified heel and midfoot with fat layer exposed CC
L97.403 Non-pressure chronic ulcer of unspecified heel and midfoot with necrosis of muscle CC
L97.404 Non-pressure chronic ulcer of unspecified heel and midfoot with necrosis of bone CC
L97.409 Non-pressure chronic ulcer of unspecified heel and midfoot with unspecified severity CC

✓6th L97.41 Non-pressure chronic ulcer of right heel and midfoot
L97.411 Non-pressure chronic ulcer of right heel and midfoot limited to breakdown of skin CC
L97.412 Non-pressure chronic ulcer of right heel and midfoot with fat layer exposed CC
L97.413 Non-pressure chronic ulcer of right heel and midfoot with necrosis of muscle CC
L97.414 Non-pressure chronic ulcer of right heel and midfoot with necrosis of bone CC
L97.419 Non-pressure chronic ulcer of right heel and midfoot with unspecified severity CC

✓6th L97.42 Non-pressure chronic ulcer of left heel and midfoot
L97.421 Non-pressure chronic ulcer of left heel and midfoot limited to breakdown of skin CC
L97.422 Non-pressure chronic ulcer of left heel and midfoot with fat layer exposed CC
L97.423 Non-pressure chronic ulcer of left heel and midfoot with necrosis of muscle CC
L97.424 Non-pressure chronic ulcer of left heel and midfoot with necrosis of bone CC
L97.429 Non-pressure chronic ulcer of left heel and midfoot with unspecified severity CC

✓5th L97.5 Non-pressure chronic ulcer of other part of foot
Non-pressure chronic ulcer of toe

✓6th L97.50 Non-pressure chronic ulcer of other part of unspecified foot
L97.501 Non-pressure chronic ulcer of other part of unspecified foot limited to breakdown of skin
L97.502 Non-pressure chronic ulcer of other part of unspecified foot with fat layer exposed
L97.503 Non-pressure chronic ulcer of other part of unspecified foot with necrosis of muscle
L97.504 Non-pressure chronic ulcer of other part of unspecified foot with necrosis of bone
L97.509 Non-pressure chronic ulcer of other part of unspecified foot with unspecified severity

✓6th L97.51 Non-pressure chronic ulcer of other part of right foot
L97.511 Non-pressure chronic ulcer of other part of right foot limited to breakdown of skin
L97.512 Non-pressure chronic ulcer of other part of right foot with fat layer exposed
L97.513 Non-pressure chronic ulcer of other part of right foot with necrosis of muscle
L97.514 Non-pressure chronic ulcer of other part of right foot with necrosis of bone
L97.519 Non-pressure chronic ulcer of other part of right foot with unspecified severity

✓6th L97.52 Non-pressure chronic ulcer of other part of left foot
L97.521 Non-pressure chronic ulcer of other part of left foot limited to breakdown of skin
L97.522 Non-pressure chronic ulcer of other part of left foot with fat layer exposed
L97.523 Non-pressure chronic ulcer of other part of left foot with necrosis of muscle
L97.524 Non-pressure chronic ulcer of other part of left foot with necrosis of bone
L97.529 Non-pressure chronic ulcer of other part of left foot with unspecified severity

✓5th L97.8 Non-pressure chronic ulcer of other part of lower leg

✓6th L97.80 Non-pressure chronic ulcer of other part of unspecified lower leg
L97.801 Non-pressure chronic ulcer of other part of unspecified lower leg limited to breakdown of skin CC
L97.802 Non-pressure chronic ulcer of other part of unspecified lower leg with fat layer exposed CC
L97.803 Non-pressure chronic ulcer of other part of unspecified lower leg with necrosis of muscle CC
L97.804 Non-pressure chronic ulcer of other part of unspecified lower leg with necrosis of bone CC
L97.809 Non-pressure chronic ulcer of other part of unspecified lower leg with unspecified severity CC

✓6th L97.81 Non-pressure chronic ulcer of other part of right lower leg
L97.811 Non-pressure chronic ulcer of other part of right lower leg limited to breakdown of skin CC

L97.812 Non-pressure chronic ulcer of other part of right lower leg with fat layer exposed CC

L97.813 Non-pressure chronic ulcer of other part of right lower leg with necrosis of muscle CC

L97.814 Non-pressure chronic ulcer of other part of right lower leg with necrosis of bone CC

L97.819 Non-pressure chronic ulcer of other part of right lower leg with unspecified severity CC

6th **L97.82 Non-pressure chronic ulcer of other part of left lower leg**

L97.821 Non-pressure chronic ulcer of other part of left lower leg limited to breakdown of skin CC

L97.822 Non-pressure chronic ulcer of other part of left lower leg with fat layer exposed CC

L97.823 Non-pressure chronic ulcer of other part of left lower leg with necrosis of muscle CC

L97.824 Non-pressure chronic ulcer of other part of left lower leg with necrosis of bone CC

L97.829 Non-pressure chronic ulcer of other part of left lower leg with unspecified severity CC

5th **L97.9 Non-pressure chronic ulcer of unspecified part of lower leg**

6th **L97.90 Non-pressure chronic ulcer of unspecified part of unspecified lower leg**

L97.901 Non-pressure chronic ulcer of unspecified part of unspecified lower leg limited to breakdown of skin CC

L97.902 Non-pressure chronic ulcer of unspecified part of unspecified lower leg with fat layer exposed CC

L97.903 Non-pressure chronic ulcer of unspecified part of unspecified lower leg with necrosis of muscle CC

L97.904 Non-pressure chronic ulcer of unspecified part of unspecified lower leg with necrosis of bone CC

L97.909 Non-pressure chronic ulcer of unspecified part of unspecified lower leg with unspecified severity CC

6th **L97.91 Non-pressure chronic ulcer of unspecified part of right lower leg**

L97.911 Non-pressure chronic ulcer of unspecified part of right lower leg limited to breakdown of skin CC

L97.912 Non-pressure chronic ulcer of unspecified part of right lower leg with fat layer exposed CC

L97.913 Non-pressure chronic ulcer of unspecified part of right lower leg with necrosis of muscle CC

L97.914 Non-pressure chronic ulcer of unspecified part of right lower leg with necrosis of bone CC

L97.919 Non-pressure chronic ulcer of unspecified part of right lower leg with unspecified severity CC

6th **L97.92 Non-pressure chronic ulcer of unspecified part of left lower leg**

L97.921 Non-pressure chronic ulcer of unspecified part of left lower leg limited to breakdown of skin CC

L97.922 Non-pressure chronic ulcer of unspecified part of left lower leg with fat layer exposed CC

L97.923 Non-pressure chronic ulcer of unspecified part of left lower leg with necrosis of muscle CC

L97.924 Non-pressure chronic ulcer of unspecified part of left lower leg with necrosis of bone CC

L97.929 Non-pressure chronic ulcer of unspecified part of left lower leg with unspecified severity CC

4th **L98 Other disorders of skin and subcutaneous tissue, not elsewhere classified**

L98.0 Pyogenic granuloma

EXCLUDES 2 *pyogenic granuloma of gingiva (K06.8)*
pyogenic granuloma of maxillary alveolar ridge (K04.5)
pyogenic granuloma of oral mucosa (K13.4)

L98.1 Factitial dermatitis

Neurotic excoriation

L98.2 Febrile neutrophilic dermatosis [Sweet]

L98.3 Eosinophilic cellulitis [Wells] CC

CC Excl: A17.9, A18.4, A18.82, A18.84, A18.89, A48.2-A48.4, A48.8-A49.9, B78.1, B95.0-B96.89, E83.2, L02.811-L02.818, L02.91, L03.811-L03.91, L08.0, L08.81-L08.9, L44.8-L45, L73.2, L88, L92.8, L94.2, L94.4, L98.0, L98.3, L98.8, L99, M00.011-M00.012, M00.021-M00.022, M00.031-M00.032, M00.041-M00.042, M00.051-M00.052, M00.061-M00.062, M00.071-M00.072, Z16.10-Z16.39

5th **L98.4 Non-pressure chronic ulcer of skin, not elsewhere classified**

Chronic ulcer of skin NOS
Ulcer of skin NOS
Tropical ulcer NOS

EXCLUDES 2 *pressure ulcer (pressure area) (L89.-)*
gangrene (I96)
skin infections (L00-L08)
specific infections classified to A00-B99
ulcer of lower limb NEC (L97.-)
varicose ulcer (I83.0-I82.2)

6th **L98.41 Non-pressure chronic ulcer of buttock**

L98.411 Non-pressure chronic ulcer of buttock limited to breakdown of skin

L98.412 Non-pressure chronic ulcer of buttock with fat layer exposed

L98.413 Non-pressure chronic ulcer of buttock with necrosis of muscle

L98.414 Non-pressure chronic ulcer of buttock with necrosis of bone

L98.419 Non-pressure chronic ulcer of buttock with unspecified severity

6th **L98.42 Non-pressure chronic ulcer of back**

L98.421 Non-pressure chronic ulcer of back limited to breakdown of skin

L98.422 Non-pressure chronic ulcer of back with fat layer exposed

L98.423 Non-pressure chronic ulcer of back with necrosis of muscle

L98.424 Non-pressure chronic ulcer of back with necrosis of bone

L98.429 Non-pressure chronic ulcer of back with unspecified severity

6th **L98.49 Non-pressure chronic ulcer of skin of other sites**

Non-pressure chronic ulcer of skin NOS

L98.491 Non-pressure chronic ulcer of skin of other sites limited to breakdown of skin

L98.492 Non-pressure chronic ulcer of skin of other sites with fat layer exposed

L98.493 Non-pressure chronic ulcer of skin of other sites with necrosis of muscle

L98.494 Non-pressure chronic ulcer of skin of other sites with necrosis of bone

L98.499 Non-pressure chronic ulcer of skin of other sites with unspecified severity

L98.5 Mucinosis of the skin

Focal mucinosis
Reticular erythematous mucinosis
Lichen myxedematosus

EXCLUDES 1 *focal oral mucinosis (K13.79)*
myxedema (E03.9)

L98.6 Other infiltrative disorders of the skin and subcutaneous tissue

EXCLUDES 1 *hyalinosis cutis et mucosae (E78.89)*

L98.8 Other specified disorders of the skin and subcutaneous tissue

AHA: 2013, 2Q, 32

L98.9 Disorder of the skin and subcutaneous tissue, unspecified

L99 Other disorders of skin and subcutaneous tissue in diseases classified elsewhere

Code first underlying disease, such as:
amyloidosis (E85.-)

EXCLUDES 1 *skin disorders in diabetes (E08-E13 with .62)*
skin disorders in gonorrhea (A54.89)
skin disorders in syphilis (A51.31, A52.79)

DRAFT

Chapter 13. Diseases of the Musculoskeletal System and Connective Tissue (MØØ-M99)

NOTE Use an external cause code following the code for the musculoskeletal condition, if applicable, to identify the cause of the musculoskeletal condition.

EXCLUDES 2 *arthropathic psoriasis (L4Ø.5-)*
certain conditions originating in the perinatal period (PØ4-P96)
certain infectious and parasitic diseases (AØØ-B99)
compartment syndrome (traumatic) (T79.A-)
complications of pregnancy, childbirth and the puerperium (OØØ-O9A)
congenital malformations, deformations, and chromosomal abnormalities (QØØ-Q99)
endocrine, nutritional and metabolic diseases (EØØ-E88)
injury, poisoning and certain other consequences of external causes (SØØ-T88)
neoplasms (CØØ-D49)
symptoms, signs and abnormal clinical and laboratory findings, not elsewhere classified (RØØ-R94)

This chapter contains the following blocks:

MØØ-MØ2	Infectious arthropathies
MØ5-M14	Inflammatory polyarthropathies
M15-M19	Osteoarthritis
M2Ø-M25	Other joint disorders
M26-M27	Dentofacial anomalies [including malocclusion] and other disorders of jaw
M3Ø-M36	Systemic connective tissue disorders
M4Ø-M43	Deforming dorsopathies
M45-M49	Spondylopathies
M5Ø-M54	Other dorsopathies
M6Ø-M63	Disorders of muscles
M65-M67	Disorders of synovium and tendon
M7Ø-M79	Other soft tissue disorders
M8Ø-M85	Disorders of bone density and structure
M86-M9Ø	Other osteopathies
M91-M94	Chondropathies
M95	Other disorders of the musculoskeletal system and connective tissue
M96	Intraoperative and postprocedural complications and disorders of musculoskeletal system, not elsewhere classified
M99	Biomechanical lesions, not elsewhere classified

ARTHROPATHIES (MØØ-M25)

INCLUDES disorders affecting predominantly peripheral (limb) joints

Infectious arthropathies (MØØ-MØ2)

NOTE This block comprises arthropathies due to microbiological agents. Distinction is made between the following types of etiological relationship:

a) direct infection of joint, where organisms invade synovial tissue and microbial antigen is present in the joint;

b) indirect infection, which may be of two types: a reactive arthropathy, where microbial infection of the body is established but neither organisms nor antigens can be identified in the joint, and a postinfective arthropathy, where microbial antigen is present but recovery of an organism is inconstant and evidence of local multiplication is lacking.

✓4th **MØØ Pyogenic arthritis**

✓5th **MØØ.Ø Staphylococcal arthritis and polyarthritis**

Use additional code (B95.61-B95.8) to identify bacterial agent

EXCLUDES 2 *infection and inflammatory reaction due to internal joint prosthesis (T84.5-)*

MØØ.ØØ Staphylococcal arthritis, unspecified joint CC

CC Excl: A17.9, A18.Ø2, A18.Ø9, A18.82, A18.84, A18.89, A39.83-A39.84, A54.4Ø, A54.42-A54.43, A54.82, A54.84, A54.89-A54.9, BØ6.82, MØØ.ØØ, MØØ.Ø19, MØØ.Ø29, MØØ.Ø39, MØØ.Ø49, MØØ.Ø59, MØØ.Ø69, MØØ.Ø79, MØØ.Ø8-MØ2.3Ø, MØ2.319, MØ2.329, MØ2.339, MØ2.349, MØ2.359, MØ2.369, MØ2.379-MØ2.9, MØ5.4Ø-MØ5.59, MØ5.7Ø-MØ6.Ø9, MØ6.2Ø-MØ6.39, MØ6.8Ø-MØ7.69, M11.ØØ-M11.9, M12.1Ø-M15.Ø, M15.3-M15.9, M16.2-M16.9, M17.2-M17.9, M18.2-M18.9, M19.111-M19.93, M24.1Ø-M24.176, M25.ØØ, M25.Ø8-M25.18, M25.4Ø-M25.676, M25.8Ø-M25.9, M35.2, M36.1-M36.4, R26.2, R29.4

✓6th **MØØ.Ø1 Staphylococcal arthritis, shoulder**

MØØ.Ø11 Staphylococcal arthritis, right shoulder

MØØ.Ø12 Staphylococcal arthritis, left shoulder

MØØ.Ø19 Staphylococcal arthritis, unspecified shoulder CC

CC Excl: A17.9, A18.Ø2, A18.Ø9, A18.82, A18.84, A18.89, A39.83-A39.84, A54.4Ø, A54.42-A54.43, A54.82, A54.84, A54.89-A54.9, BØ6.82, MØØ.ØØ, MØØ.Ø19, MØØ.Ø8-MØØ.119, MØØ.18-MØØ.219, MØØ.28-MØØ.819, MØØ.88-MØ1.X19, MØ1.X8-MØ2.119, MØ2.18-MØ2.3Ø, MØ2.319, MØ2.38-MØ2.819, MØ2.88-MØ2.9, MØ5.4Ø-MØ5.59, MØ5.7Ø-MØ6.Ø9, MØ6.2Ø-MØ6.39, MØ6.8Ø-MØ7.619, MØ7.68-MØ7.69, M11.ØØ-M11.Ø19, M11.Ø8-M11.119, M11.18-M11.219, M11.28-M11.819, M11.88-M11.9, M12.1Ø-M12.119, M12.18-M12.219, M12.28-M12.319, M12.38-M12.419, M12.48-M12.519, M12.58-M12.819, M12.88-M13.119, M13.8Ø-M13.819, M13.88-M15.Ø, M15.3-M15.9, M19.Ø11-M19.Ø19, M19.111-M19.119, M19.211-M19.219, M19.9Ø-M19.93, M24.1Ø-M24.119, M25.ØØ-M25.Ø19, M25.Ø8-M25.119, M25.18, M25.4Ø-M25.419, M25.48-M25.519, M25.6Ø-M25.619, M25.8Ø-M25.819, M25.9, M35.2, M36.1-M36.4, R26.2

✓6th **MØØ.Ø2 Staphylococcal arthritis, elbow**

MØØ.Ø21 Staphylococcal arthritis, right elbow

MØØ.Ø22 Staphylococcal arthritis, left elbow

MØØ.Ø29 Staphylococcal arthritis, unspecified elbow CC

CC Excl: A17.9, A18.Ø2, A18.Ø9, A18.82, A18.84, A18.89, A39.83-A39.84, A54.4Ø, A54.42-A54.43, A54.82, A54.84, A54.89-A54.9, BØ6.82, MØØ.ØØ, MØØ.Ø29, MØØ.Ø8-MØØ.1Ø, MØØ.121-MØØ.129, MØØ.18-MØØ.2Ø, MØØ.221-MØØ.229, MØØ.28-MØØ.8Ø, MØØ.821-MØØ.829, MØØ.88-MØ1.XØ, MØ1.X21-MØ1.X29, MØ1.X8, MØ1.X9, MØ2.ØØ-MØ2.1, MØ2.121-MØ2.129, MØ2.18-MØ2.3Ø, MØ2.329, MØ2.38-MØ2.8Ø, MØ2.821-MØ2.829, MØ2.88-MØ2.9, MØ5.4Ø-MØ5.59, MØ5.7Ø-MØ6.Ø9, MØ6.2Ø-MØ6.39, MØ6.8Ø-MØ7.6Ø, MØ7.621-MØ7.629, MØ7.68-MØ7.69, M11.ØØ, M11.Ø21-M11.Ø29, M11.Ø8-M11.1Ø, M11.121-M11.129, M11.18-M11.2Ø, M11.221-M11.229, M11.28-M11.8Ø, M11.821-M11.829, M11.88-M11.9, M12.1Ø, M12.121-M12.129, M12.18-M12.2Ø, M12.221-M12.229, M12.28-M12.3Ø, M12.321-M12.329, M12.38-M12.4Ø, M12.421-M12.429, M12.48-M12.5Ø, M12.521-M12.529, M12.58-M12.8Ø, M12.821-M12.829, M12.88-M13.1Ø, M13.121-M13.129, M13.8Ø, M13.821-M13.829, M13.88-M15.Ø, M15.3-M15.9, M19.Ø21-M19.Ø29, M19.121-M19.129, M19.221-M19.229, M19.9Ø-M19.93, M24.1Ø, M24.121-M24.129, M25.ØØ, M25.Ø21-M25.Ø29, M25.Ø8-M25.1Ø, M25.121-M25.129, M25.18, M25.4Ø, M25.421-M25.429, M25.48-M25.5Ø, M25.521-M25.529, M25.6Ø, M25.621-M25.629, M25.8Ø, M25.821-M25.829, M25.9, M35.2, M36.1-M36.4, R26.2

✓6th **MØØ.Ø3 Staphylococcal arthritis, wrist**
Staphylococcal arthritis of carpal bones

MØØ.Ø31 Staphylococcal arthritis, right wrist

MØØ.Ø32 Staphylococcal arthritis, left wrist

MØØ.Ø39 Staphylococcal arthritis, unspecified wrist CC

CC Excl: A17.9, A18.Ø2, A18.Ø9, A18.82, A18.84, A18.89, A39.83-A39.84, A54.4Ø, A54.42-A54.43, A54.82, A54.84, A54.89-A54.9, BØ6.82, MØØ.ØØ, MØØ.Ø39, MØØ.Ø8-MØØ.1Ø, MØØ.131-MØØ.139, MØØ.18-MØØ.2Ø, MØØ.231-MØØ.239, MØØ.28-MØØ.8Ø, MØØ.831-MØØ.839, MØØ.88-MØ1.XØ, MØ1.X31-MØ1.X39, MØ1.X8-MØ2.1Ø, MØ2.131-MØ2.139, MØ2.18-MØ2.3Ø, MØ2.339, MØ2.38-MØ2.8Ø, MØ2.831-MØ2.839, MØ2.88-MØ2.9, MØ5.4Ø-MØ5.59, MØ5.7Ø-MØ6.Ø9, MØ6.2Ø-MØ6.39, MØ6.8Ø-MØ7.6Ø, MØ7.631-MØ7.639, MØ7.68-MØ7.69, M11.ØØ, M11.Ø31-M11.Ø39, M11.Ø8-M11.1Ø, M11.131-M11.139, M11.18-M11.2Ø, M11.231-M11.239, M11.28-M11.8Ø, M11.831-M11.839, M11.88-M11.9, M12.1Ø, M12.131-M12.139, M12.18-M12.2Ø, M12.231-M12.239, M12.28-M12.3Ø, M12.331-M12.339, M12.38-M12.4Ø, M12.431-M12.439, M12.48-M12.5Ø, M12.531-M12.539, M12.58-M12.8Ø, M12.831-M12.839, M12.88-M13.1Ø, M13.131-M13.139, M13.8Ø, M13.831-M13.839, M13.88-M15.Ø, M15.3-M15.9, M19.Ø31-M19.Ø39, M19.131-M19.139, M19.231-M19.239, M19.9Ø-M19.93, M24.1Ø, M24.131-M24.139, M25.ØØ, M25.Ø31-M25.Ø39, M25.Ø8-M25.1Ø, M25.131-M25.139, M25.18, M25.4Ø, M25.431-M25.439, M25.48-M25.5Ø, M25.531-M25.539, M25.6Ø, M25.631-M25.639, M25.8Ø, M25.831-M25.839, M25.9, M35.2, M36.1-M36.4, R26.2

✓6th **MØØ.Ø4 Staphylococcal arthritis, hand**
Staphylococcal arthritis of metacarpus and phalanges

MØØ.Ø41 Staphylococcal arthritis, right hand

MØØ.Ø42 Staphylococcal arthritis, left hand

MØØ.Ø49 Staphylococcal arthritis, unspecified hand CC

CC Excl: A17.9, A18.Ø2, A18.Ø9, A18.82, A18.84, A18.89, A39.83-A39.84, A54.4Ø, A54.42-A54.43, A54.82, A54.84, A54.89-A54.9, BØ6.82, MØØ.ØØ, MØØ.Ø49, MØØ.Ø8-MØØ.1Ø, MØØ.141-MØØ.149, MØØ.18-MØØ.2Ø, MØØ.241-MØØ.249, MØØ.28-MØØ.8Ø, MØØ.841-MØØ.849, MØØ.88-MØ1.XØ, MØ1.X41-MØ1.X49, MØ1.X8-MØ2.1Ø, MØ2.141-MØ2.149, MØ2.18-MØ2.3Ø, MØ2.349, MØ2.38-MØ2.8Ø, MØ2.841-MØ2.849, MØ2.88-MØ2.9, MØ5.4Ø-MØ5.59, MØ5.7Ø-MØ6.Ø9, MØ6.2Ø-MØ6.39, MØ6.8Ø-MØ7.6Ø, MØ7.641-MØ7.649, MØ7.68-MØ7.69, M11.ØØ, M11.Ø41-M11.Ø49, M11.Ø8-M11.1Ø, M11.141-M11.149, M11.18-M11.2Ø, M11.241-M11.249, M11.28-M11.8Ø, M11.841-M11.849, M11.88-M11.9, M12.1Ø, M12.141-M12.149, M12.18-M12.2Ø, M12.241-M12.249, M12.28-M12.3Ø, M12.341-M12.349, M12.38-M12.4Ø, M12.441-M12.449, M12.48-M12.5Ø, M12.541-M12.549, M12.58-M12.8Ø, M12.841-M12.849, M12.88-M13.1Ø, M13.141-M13.149, M13.8Ø, M13.841-M13.849, M13.88-M15.9, M18.Ø-M18.9, M19.Ø41-M19.Ø49, M19.141-M19.149, M19.241-M19.249, M19.9Ø-M19.93, M24.1Ø, M24.141-M24.149, M25.ØØ, M25.Ø41-M25.Ø49, M25.Ø8-M25.1Ø, M25.141-M25.149, M25.18, M25.4Ø, M25.441-M25.449, M25.48-M25.5Ø, M25.6Ø, M25.641-M25.649, M25.8Ø, M25.841-M25.849, M25.9, M35.2, M36.1-M36.4, R26.2

✓6th **MØØ.Ø5 Staphylococcal arthritis, hip**

MØØ.Ø51 Staphylococcal arthritis, right hip

MØØ.Ø52 Staphylococcal arthritis, left hip

MØØ.Ø59 Staphylococcal arthritis, unspecified hip CC

CC Excl: A17.9, A18.Ø2, A18.Ø9, A18.82, A18.84, A18.89, A39.83-A39.84, A54.4Ø, A54.42-A54.43, A54.82, A54.84, A54.89-A54.9, BØ6.82, MØØ.ØØ, MØØ.Ø59, MØØ.Ø8-MØØ.1Ø, MØØ.151-MØØ.159, MØØ.18-MØØ.2Ø, MØØ.251-MØØ.259, MØØ.28-MØØ.8Ø, MØØ.851-MØØ.859, MØØ.88-MØ1.XØ, MØ1.X51-MØ1.X59, MØ1.X8-MØ2.1Ø, MØ2.151-MØ2.159, MØ2.18-MØ2.3Ø, MØ2.359, MØ2.38-MØ2.8Ø, MØ2.851-MØ2.859, MØ2.88-MØ2.9, MØ5.4Ø-MØ5.59, MØ5.7Ø-MØ6.Ø9, MØ6.2Ø-MØ6.39, MØ6.8Ø-MØ7.6Ø, MØ7.651-MØ7.659, MØ7.68-MØ7.69, M11.ØØ, M11.Ø51-M11.Ø59, M11.Ø8-M11.1Ø, M11.151-M11.159, M11.18-M11.2Ø, M11.251-M11.259, M11.28-M11.8Ø, M11.851-M11.859, M11.88-M11.9, M12.1Ø, M12.151-M12.159, M12.18-M12.2Ø, M12.251-M12.259, M12.28-M12.3Ø, M12.351-M12.359, M12.38-M12.4Ø, M12.451-M12.459, M12.48-M12.5Ø, M12.551-M12.559, M12.58-M12.8Ø, M12.851-M12.859, M12.88-M13.1Ø, M13.151-M13.159, M13.8Ø, M13.851-M13.859, M13.88-M15.Ø, M15.3-M16.9, M19.9Ø-M19.93, M24.1Ø, M24.151-M24.159, M25.ØØ, M25.Ø51-M25.Ø59, M25.Ø8-M25.1Ø, M25.151-M25.159, M25.18, M25.4Ø, M25.451-M25.459, M25.48-M25.5Ø, M25.551-M25.559, M25.6Ø, M25.651-M25.659, M25.8Ø, M25.851-M25.859, M25.9, M35.2, M36.1-M36.4, R26.2, R29.4

✓6th **MØØ.Ø6 Staphylococcal arthritis, knee**

MØØ.Ø61 Staphylococcal arthritis, right knee

MØØ.Ø62 Staphylococcal arthritis, left knee

MØØ.Ø69 Staphylococcal arthritis, unspecified knee CC

CC Excl: A17.9, A18.Ø2, A18.Ø9, A18.82, A18.84, A18.89, A39.83-A39.84, A54.4Ø, A54.42-A54.43, A54.82, A54.84, A54.89-A54.9, BØ6.82, MØØ.ØØ, MØØ.Ø69, MØØ.Ø8-MØØ.1Ø, MØØ.161-MØØ.169, MØØ.18-MØØ.2Ø, MØØ.261-MØØ.269, MØØ.28-MØØ.8Ø, MØØ.861-MØØ.869, MØØ.88-MØ1.XØ, MØ1.X61-MØ1.X69, MØ1.X8-MØ2.1Ø, MØ2.161-MØ2.169, MØ2.18-MØ2.3Ø, MØ2.369, MØ2.38-MØ2.8Ø, MØ2.861-MØ2.869, MØ2.88-MØ2.9, MØ5.4Ø-MØ5.59, MØ5.7Ø-MØ6.Ø9, MØ6.2Ø-MØ6.39, MØ6.8Ø-MØ7.6Ø, MØ7.661-MØ7.669, MØ7.68-MØ7.69, M11.ØØ, M11.Ø61-M11.Ø69, M11.Ø8-M11.1Ø, M11.161-M11.169, M11.18-M11.2Ø, M11.261-M11.269, M11.28-M11.8Ø, M11.861-M11.869, M11.88-M11.9, M12.1Ø, M12.161-M12.169, M12.18-M12.2Ø, M12.261-M12.269, M12.28-M12.3Ø, M12.361-M12.369, M12.38-M12.4Ø, M12.461-M12.469, M12.48-M12.5Ø, M12.561-M12.569, M12.58-M12.8Ø, M12.861-M12.869, M12.88-M13.1Ø, M13.161-M13.169, M13.8Ø, M13.861-M13.869, M13.88-M15.Ø, M15.3-M15.9, M17.Ø-M17.9, M19.9Ø-M19.93, M24.1Ø, M25.ØØ, M25.Ø61-M25.Ø69, M25.Ø8-M25.1Ø, M25.161-M25.169, M25.18, M25.4Ø, M25.461-M25.469, M25.48-M25.5Ø, M25.561-M25.569, M25.6Ø, M25.661-M25.669, M25.8Ø, M25.861-M25.869, M25.9, M35.2, M36.1-M36.4, R26.2

M00.07 Staphylococcal arthritis, ankle and foot
Staphylococcal arthritis, tarsus, metatarsus and phalanges

M00.071 Staphylococcal arthritis, right ankle and foot

M00.072 Staphylococcal arthritis, left ankle and foot

M00.079 Staphylococcal arthritis, unspecified ankle and foot CC
CC Excl: A17.9, A18.02, A18.09, A18.82, A18.84, A18.89, A39.83-A39.84, A54.40, A54.42-A54.43, A54.82, A54.84, A54.89-A54.9, B06.82, M00.00, M00.10, M00.171-M00.20, M00.271-M00.80, M00.871-M01.X0, M01.X71-M02.10, M02.171-M02.30, M02.379-M02.80, M02.871-M02.9, M05.40-M05.59, M05.70-M06.09, M06.20-M06.39, M06.80-M07.60, M07.671-M07.69, M11.00, M11.071-M11.10, M11.171-M11.20, M11.271-M11.80, M11.871-M11.9, M12.10, M12.171-M12.20, M12.271-M12.30, M12.371-M12.40, M12.471-M12.50, M12.571-M12.80, M12.871-M13.10, M13.171-M13.80, M13.871-M15.0, M15.3-M15.9, M19.071-M19.079, M19.171-M19.179, M19.271-M19.93, M24.10, M24.171-M24.176, M25.00, M25.071-M25.10, M25.171-M25.18, M25.40, M25.471-M25.50, M25.571-M25.60, M25.671-M25.676, M25.80, M25.871-M25.9, M35.2, M36.1-M36.4, R26.2

M00.08 Staphylococcal arthritis, vertebrae CC
CC Excl: A17.9, A18.02, A18.09, A18.82, A18.84, A18.89, A39.83-A39.84, A54.40, A54.42-A54.43, A54.82, A54.84, A54.89-A54.9, B06.82, M00.00, M00.019, M00.029, M00.039, M00.049, M00.059, M00.069, M00.079, M00.08-M02.30, M02.319, M02.329, M02.339, M02.349, M02.359, M02.369, M02.379-M02.9, M05.40-M05.59, M05.70-M06.09, M06.20-M06.39, M06.80-M07.69, M11.00-M11.9, M12.10-M15.0, M15.3-M15.9, M16.2-M16.9, M17.2-M17.9, M18.2-M18.9, M19.111-M19.93, M24.10-M24.176, M25.00, M25.08-M25.18, M25.40-M25.676, M25.80-M25.9, M35.2, M36.1-M36.4, R26.2, R29.4

M00.09 Staphylococcal polyarthritis CC
CC Excl: See code: M00.08

M00.1 Pneumococcal arthritis and polyarthritis

M00.10 Pneumococcal arthritis, unspecified joint CC
CC Excl: See code: M00.08

M00.11 Pneumococcal arthritis, shoulder

M00.111 Pneumococcal arthritis, right shoulder CC
CC Excl: A17.9, A18.02, A18.09, A18.82, A18.84, A18.89, A39.83-A39.84, A54.40, A54.42-A54.43, A54.82, A54.84, A54.89-A54.9, B06.82, M00.00, M00.019, M00.08-M00.119, M00.18-M00.219, M00.28-M00.819, M00.88-M01.X19, M01.X8-M02.119, M02.18-M02.211

M00.112 Pneumococcal arthritis, left shoulder CC
CC Excl: See code: M00.111

M00.119 Pneumococcal arthritis, unspecified shoulder CC
CC Excl: See code: M00.111

M00.12 Pneumococcal arthritis, elbow

M00.121 Pneumococcal arthritis, right elbow CC
CC Excl: A17.9, A18.02, A18.09, A18.82, A18.84, A18.89, A39.83-A39.84, A54.40, A54.42-A54.43, A54.82, A54.84, A54.89-A54.9, B06.82, M00.00, M00.029, M00.08-M00.10, M00.121-M00.129, M00.18-M00.20, M00.221-M00.229, M00.28-M00.80, M00.821-M00.829, M00.88-M01.X0, M01.X21-M01.X29, M01.X8-M02.10, M02.121-M02.129, M02.18-M02.30, M02.329, M02.38-M02.80, M02.821-M02.829, M02.88-M02.9, M05.40-M05.59, M05.70-M06.09, M06.20-M06.39, M06.80-M07.60, M07.621-M07.629, M07.68-M07.69, M11.00, M11.021-M11.029, M11.08-M11.10, M11.121-M11.129, M11.18-M11.20, M11.221-M11.229, M11.28-M11.80, M11.821-M11.829, M11.88-M11.9, M12.10, M12.121-M12.129, M12.18-M12.20, M12.221-M12.229, M12.28-M12.30, M12.321-M12.329, M12.38-M12.40, M12.421-M12.429, M12.48-M12.50, M12.521-M12.529, M12.58-M12.80, M12.821-M12.829, M12.88-M13.10, M13.121-M13.129, M13.80, M13.821-M13.829, M13.88-M15.0, M15.3-M15.9, M19.021-M19.029, M19.121-M19.129, M19.221-M19.229, M19.90-M19.93, M24.10, M24.121-M24.129, M25.00, M25.021-M25.029, M25.08-M25.10, M25.121-M25.129, M25.18, M25.40, M25.421-M25.429, M25.48-M25.50, M25.521-M25.529, M25.60, M25.621-M25.629, M25.80, M25.821-M25.829, M25.9, M35.2, M36.1-M36.4, R26.2

M00.122 Pneumococcal arthritis, left elbow CC
CC Excl: See code: M00.121

M00.129 Pneumococcal arthritis, unspecified elbow CC
CC Excl: See code: M00.121

M00.13 Pneumococcal arthritis, wrist
Pneumococcal arthritis of carpal bones

M00.131 Pneumococcal arthritis, right wrist CC
CC Excl: A17.9, A18.02, A18.09, A18.82, A18.84, A18.89, A39.83-A39.84, A54.40, A54.42-A54.43, A54.82, A54.84, A54.89-A54.9, B06.82, M00.00, M00.039, M00.08-M00.10, M00.131-M00.139, M00.18-M00.20, M00.231-M00.239, M00.28-M00.80, M00.831-M00.839, M00.88-M01.X0, M01.X31-M01.X39, M01.X8-M02.10, M02.131-M02.139, M02.18-M02.30, M02.339, M02.38-M02.80, M02.831-M02.839, M02.88-M02.9, M05.40-M05.59, M05.70-M06.09, M06.20-M06.39, M06.80-M07.60, M07.631-M07.639, M07.68-M07.69, M11.00, M11.031-M11.039, M11.08-M11.10, M11.131-M11.139, M11.18-M11.20, M11.231-M11.239, M11.28-M11.80, M11.831-M11.839, M11.88-M11.9, M12.10, M12.131-M12.139, M12.18-M12.20, M12.231-M12.239, M12.28-M12.30, M12.331-M12.339, M12.38-M12.40, M12.431-M12.439, M12.48-M12.50, M12.531-M12.539, M12.58-M12.80, M12.831-M12.839, M12.88-M13.10, M13.131-M13.139, M13.80, M13.831-M13.839, M13.88-M15.0, M15.3-M15.9, M19.031-M19.039, M19.131-M19.139, M19.231-M19.239, M19.90-M19.93, M24.10, M24.131-M24.139, M25.00, M25.031-M25.039, M25.08-M25.10, M25.131-M25.139, M25.18, M25.40, M25.431-M25.439, M25.48-M25.50, M25.531-M25.539, M25.60, M25.631-M25.639, M25.80, M25.831-M25.839, M25.9, M35.2, M36.1-M36.4, R26.2

M00.132 Pneumococcal arthritis, left wrist CC
CC Excl: See code: M00.131

M00.139 Pneumococcal arthritis, unspecified wrist CC
CC Excl: See code: M00.131

✓6th **MØØ.14 Pneumococcal arthritis, hand**
Pneumococcal arthritis of metacarpus and phalanges

MØØ.141 Pneumococcal arthritis, right hand CC
CC Excl: A17.9, A18.Ø2, A18.Ø9, A18.82, A18.84, A18.89, A39.83-A39.84, A54.4Ø, A54.42-A54.43, A54.82, A54.84, A54.89-A54.9, BØ6.82, MØØ.ØØ, MØØ.Ø49, MØØ.Ø8-MØØ.1Ø, MØØ.141-MØØ.149, MØØ.18-MØØ.2Ø, MØØ.241-MØØ.249, MØØ.28-MØØ.8Ø, MØØ.841-MØØ.849, MØØ.88-MØ1.XØ, MØ1.X41-MØ1.X49, MØ1.X8-MØ2.1Ø, MØ2.141-MØ2.149, MØ2.18-MØ2.3Ø, MØ2.349, MØ2.38-MØ2.8Ø, MØ2.841-MØ2.849, MØ2.88-MØ2.9, MØ5.4Ø-MØ5.59, MØ5.7Ø-MØ6.Ø9, MØ6.2Ø-MØ6.39, MØ6.8Ø-MØ7.6Ø, MØ7.641-MØ7.649, MØ7.68-MØ7.69, M11.ØØ, M11.Ø41-M11.Ø49, M11.Ø8-M11.1Ø, M11.141-M11.149, M11.18-M11.2Ø, M11.241-M11.249, M11.28-M11.8Ø, M11.841-M11.849, M11.88-M11.9, M12.1Ø, M12.141-M12.149, M12.18-M12.2Ø, M12.241-M12.249, M12.28-M12.3Ø, M12.341-M12.349, M12.38-M12.4Ø, M12.441-M12.449, M12.48-M12.5Ø, M12.541-M12.549, M12.58-M12.8Ø, M12.841-M12.849, M12.88-M13.1Ø, M13.141-M13.149, M13.8Ø, M13.841-M13.849, M13.88-M15.9, M18.Ø-M18.9, M19.Ø41-M19.Ø49, M19.141-M19.149, M19.241-M19.249, M19.9Ø-M19.93, M24.1Ø, M24.141-M24.149, M25.ØØ, M25.Ø41-M25.Ø49, M25.Ø8-M25.1Ø, M25.141-M25.149, M25.18, M25.4Ø, M25.441-M25.449, M25.48-M25.5Ø, M25.6Ø, M25.641-M25.649, M25.8Ø, M25.841-M25.849, M25.9, M35.2, M36.1-M36.4, R26.2

MØØ.142 Pneumococcal arthritis, left hand CC
CC Excl: See code: MØØ.141

MØØ.149 Pneumococcal arthritis, unspecified hand CC
CC Excl: See code: MØØ.141

✓6th **MØØ.15 Pneumococcal arthritis, hip**

MØØ.151 Pneumococcal arthritis, right hip CC
CC Excl: A17.9, A18.Ø2, A18.Ø9, A18.82, A18.84, A18.89, A39.83-A39.84, A54.4Ø, A54.42-A54.43, A54.82, A54.84, A54.89-A54.9, BØ6.82, MØØ.ØØ, MØØ.Ø59, MØØ.Ø8-MØØ.1Ø, MØØ.151-MØØ.159, MØØ.18-MØØ.2Ø, MØØ.251-MØØ.259, MØØ.28-MØØ.8Ø, MØØ.851-MØØ.859, MØØ.88-MØ1.XØ, MØ1.X51-MØ1.X59, MØ1.X8-MØ2.1Ø, MØ2.151-MØ2.159, MØ2.18-MØ2.3Ø, MØ2.359, MØ2.38-MØ2.8Ø, MØ2.851-MØ2.859, MØ2.88-MØ2.9, MØ5.4Ø-MØ5.59, MØ5.7Ø-MØ6.Ø9, MØ6.2Ø-MØ6.39, MØ6.8Ø-MØ7.6Ø, MØ7.651-MØ7.659, MØ7.68-MØ7.69, M11.ØØ, M11.Ø51-M11.Ø59, M11.Ø8-M11.1Ø, M11.151-M11.159, M11.18-M11.2Ø, M11.251-M11.259, M11.28-M11.8Ø, M11.851-M11.859, M11.88-M11.9, M12.1Ø, M12.151-M12.159, M12.18-M12.2Ø, M12.251-M12.259, M12.28-M12.3Ø, M12.351-M12.359, M12.38-M12.4Ø, M12.451-M12.459, M12.48-M12.5Ø, M12.551-M12.559, M12.58-M12.8Ø, M12.851-M12.859, M12.88-M13.1Ø, M13.151-M13.159, M13.8Ø, M13.851-M13.859, M13.88-M15.Ø, M15.3-M16.9, M19.9Ø-M19.93, M24.1Ø, M24.151-M24.159, M25.ØØ, M25.Ø51-M25.Ø59, M25.Ø8-M25.1Ø, M25.151-M25.159, M25.18, M25.4Ø, M25.451-M25.459, M25.48-M25.5Ø, M25.551-M25.559, M25.6Ø, M25.651-M25.659, M25.8Ø, M25.851-M25.859, M25.9, M35.2, M36.1-M36.4, R26.2, R29.4

MØØ.152 Pneumococcal arthritis, left hip CC
CC Excl: See code: MØØ.151

MØØ.159 Pneumococcal arthritis, unspecified hip CC
CC Excl: See code: MØØ.151

✓6th **MØØ.16 Pneumococcal arthritis, knee**

MØØ.161 Pneumococcal arthritis, right knee CC
CC Excl: A17.9, A18.Ø2, A18.Ø9, A18.82, A18.84, A18.89, A39.83-A39.84, A54.4Ø, A54.42-A54.43, A54.82, A54.84, A54.89-A54.9, BØ6.82, MØØ.ØØ, MØØ.Ø69, MØØ.Ø8-MØØ.1Ø, MØØ.161-MØØ.169, MØØ.18-MØØ.2Ø, MØØ.261-MØØ.269, MØØ.28-MØØ.8Ø, MØØ.861-MØØ.869, MØØ.88-MØ1.XØ, MØ1.X61-MØ1.X69, MØ1.X8-MØ2.1Ø, MØ2.161-MØ2.169, MØ2.18-MØ2.3Ø, MØ2.369, MØ2.38-MØ2.8Ø, MØ2.861-MØ2.869, MØ2.88-MØ2.9, MØ5.4Ø-MØ5.59, MØ5.7Ø-MØ6.Ø9, MØ6.2Ø-MØ6.39, MØ6.8Ø-MØ7.6Ø, MØ7.661-MØ7.669, MØ7.68-MØ7.69, M11.ØØ, M11.Ø61-M11.Ø69, M11.Ø8-M11.1Ø, M11.161-M11.169, M11.18-M11.2Ø, M11.261-M11.269, M11.28-M11.8Ø, M11.861-M11.869, M11.88-M11.9, M12.1Ø, M12.161-M12.169, M12.18-M12.2Ø, M12.261-M12.269, M12.28-M12.3Ø, M12.361-M12.369, M12.38-M12.4Ø, M12.461-M12.469, M12.48-M12.5Ø, M12.561-M12.569, M12.58-M12.8Ø, M12.861-M12.869, M12.88-M13.1Ø, M13.161-M13.169, M13.8Ø, M13.861-M13.869, M13.88-M15.Ø, M15.3 -M15.9, M17.Ø-M17.9, M19.9Ø-M19.93, M24.1Ø, M25.ØØ, M25.Ø61-M25.Ø69, M25.Ø8-M25.1Ø, M25.161-M25.169, M25.18, M25.4Ø, M25.461-M25.469, M25.48-M25.5Ø, M25.561-M25.569, M25.6Ø, M25.661-M25.669, M25.8Ø, M25.861-M25.869, M25.9, M35.2, M36.1-M36.4, R26.2

MØØ.162 Pneumococcal arthritis, left knee CC
CC Excl: See code: MØØ.161

MØØ.169 Pneumococcal arthritis, unspecified knee CC
CC Excl: See code: MØØ.161

✓6th **MØØ.17 Pneumococcal arthritis, ankle and foot**
Pneumococcal arthritis, tarsus, metatarsus and phalanges

MØØ.171 Pneumococcal arthritis, right ankle and foot CC
CC Excl: A17.9, A18.Ø2, A18.Ø9, A18.82, A18.84, A18.89, A39.83-A39.84, A54.4Ø, A54.42-A54.43, A54.82, A54.84, A54.89-A54.9, BØ6.82, MØØ.ØØ, MØØ.Ø79-MØØ.2Ø, MØØ.271-MØØ.8Ø, MØØ.871-MØ1.XØ, MØ1.X71-MØ2.1Ø, MØ2.171-MØ2.3Ø, MØ2.379-MØ2.8Ø, MØ2.871-MØ2.9, MØ5.4Ø-MØ5.59, MØ5.7Ø-MØ6.Ø9, MØ6.2Ø-MØ6.39, MØ6.8Ø-MØ7.6Ø, MØ7.671-MØ7.69, M11.ØØ, M11.Ø71-M11.1Ø, M11.171-M11.2Ø, M11.271-M11.8Ø, M11.871-M11.9, M12.1Ø, M12.171-M12.2Ø, M12.271-M12.3Ø, M12.371-M12.4Ø, M12.471-M12.5Ø, M12.571-M12.8Ø, M12.871-M13.1Ø, M13.171-M13.8Ø, M13.871-M15.Ø, M15.3-M15.9, M19.Ø71-M19.Ø79, M19.171-M19.179, M19.271-M19.93, M24.1Ø, M24.171-M24.176, M25.ØØ, M25.Ø71-M25.1Ø, M25.171-M25.18, M25.4Ø, M25.471-M25.5Ø, M25.571-M25.6Ø, M25.671-M25.676, M25.8Ø, M25.871-M25.9, M35.2, M36.1-M36.4, R26.2

MØØ.172 Pneumococcal arthritis, left ankle and foot CC
CC Excl: See code: MØØ.171

MØØ.179 Pneumococcal arthritis, unspecified ankle and foot CC
CC Excl: See code: MØØ.171

MØØ.18 Pneumococcal arthritis, vertebrae CC
CC Excl: A17.9, A18.Ø2, A18.Ø9, A18.82, A18.84, A18.89, A39.83-A39.84, A54.4Ø, A54.42-A54.43, A54.82, A54.84, A54.89-A54.9, BØ6.82, MØØ.ØØ, MØØ.Ø19, MØØ.Ø29, MØØ.Ø39, MØØ.Ø49, MØØ.Ø59, MØØ.Ø69, MØØ.Ø79, MØØ.Ø8-MØ2.3Ø, MØ2.319, MØ2.329, MØ2.339, MØ2.349, MØ2.359, MØ2.369, MØ2.379-MØ2.9, MØ5.4Ø-MØ5.59, MØ5.7Ø-MØ6.Ø9, MØ6.2Ø-MØ6.39, MØ6.8Ø-MØ7.69, M11.ØØ-M11.9, M12.1Ø-M15.Ø, M15.3-M15.9, M16.2-M16.9, M17.2-M17.9, M18.2-M18.9, M19.111-M19.93, M24.1Ø-M24.176, M25.ØØ, M25.Ø8-M25.18, M25.4Ø-M25.676, M25.8Ø-M25.9, M35.2, M36.1-M36.4, R26.2, R29.4

MØØ.19 Pneumococcal polyarthritis CC
CC Excl: See code: MØØ.18

✓5th **MØØ.2 Other streptococcal arthritis and polyarthritis**
Use additional code (B95.Ø-B95.2, B95.4-B95.5) to identify bacterial agent

MØØ.2Ø Other streptococcal arthritis, unspecified joint CC
CC Excl: See code: MØØ.18

✓6th **MØØ.21 Other streptococcal arthritis, shoulder**

MØØ.211 Other streptococcal arthritis, right shoulder CC

CC Excl: A17.9, A18.Ø2, A18.Ø9, A18.82, A18.84, A18.89, A39.83-A39.84, A54.4Ø, A54.42-A54.43, A54.82, A54.84, A54.89-A54.9, BØ6.82, MØØ.ØØ, MØØ.Ø19, MØØ.Ø8-MØØ.119, MØØ.18-MØØ.219, MØØ.28-MØØ.819, MØØ.88-MØ1.X19, MØ1.X8-MØ2.119, MØ2.18-MØ2.211

MØØ.212 Other streptococcal arthritis, left shoulder CC

CC Excl: See code: MØØ.211

MØØ.219 Other streptococcal arthritis, unspecified shoulder CC

CC Excl: See code: MØØ.211

✓6th **MØØ.22 Other streptococcal arthritis, elbow**

MØØ.221 Other streptococcal arthritis, right elbow CC

CC Excl: A17.9, A18.Ø2, A18.Ø9, A18.82, A18.84, A18.89, A39.83-A39.84, A54.4Ø, A54.42-A54.43, A54.82, A54.84, A54.89-A54.9, BØ6.82, MØØ.ØØ, MØØ.Ø29, MØØ.Ø8-MØØ.1Ø, MØØ.121-MØØ.129, MØØ.18-MØØ.2Ø, MØØ.221-MØØ.229, MØØ.28-MØØ.8Ø, MØØ.821-MØØ.829, MØØ.88-MØ1.XØ, MØ1.X21-MØ1.X29, MØ1.X8-MØ2.1Ø, MØ2.121-MØ2.129, MØ2.18-MØ2.3Ø, MØ2.329, MØ2.38-MØ2.8Ø, MØ2.821-MØ2.829, MØ2.88-MØ2.9, MØ5.4Ø-MØ5.59, MØ5.7Ø-MØ6.Ø9, MØ6.2Ø-MØ6.39, MØ6.8Ø-MØ7.6Ø, MØ7.621-MØ7.629, MØ7.68-MØ7.69, M11.ØØ, M11.Ø21-M11.Ø29, M11.Ø8-M11.1Ø, M11.121-M11.129, M11.18-M11.2Ø, M11.221-M11.229, M11.28-M11.8Ø, M11.821-M11.829, M11.88-M11.9, M12.1Ø, M12.121-M12.129, M12.18-M12.2Ø, M12.221-M12.229, M12.28-M12.3Ø, M12.321-M12.329, M12.38-M12.4Ø, M12.421-M12.429, M12.48-M12.5Ø, M12.521-M12.529, M12.58-M12.8Ø, M12.821-M12.829, M12.88-M13.1Ø, M13.121-M13.129, M13.8Ø, M13.821-M13.829, M13.88-M15.Ø, M15.3-M15.9, M19.Ø21-M19.Ø29, M19.121-M19.129, M19.221-M19.229, M19.9Ø-M19.93, M24.1Ø, M24.121-M24.129, M25.ØØ, M25.Ø21-M25.Ø29, M25.Ø8-M25.1Ø, M25.121-M25.129, M25.18, M25.4Ø, M25.421-M25.429, M25.48-M25.5Ø, M25.521-M25.529, M25.6Ø, M25.621-M25.629, M25.8Ø, M25.821-M25.829, M25.9, M35.2, M36.1-M36.4, R26.2

MØØ.222 Other streptococcal arthritis, left elbow CC

CC Excl: See code: MØØ.221

MØØ.229 Other streptococcal arthritis, unspecified elbow CC

CC Excl: See code: MØØ.221

✓6th **MØØ.23 Other streptococcal arthritis, wrist**

Other streptococcal arthritis of carpal bones

MØØ.231 Other streptococcal arthritis, right wrist CC

CC Excl: A17.9, A18.Ø2, A18.Ø9, A18.82, A18.84, A18.89, A39.83-A39.84, A54.4Ø, A54.42-A54.43, A54.82, A54.84, A54.89-A54.9, BØ6.82, MØØ.ØØ, MØØ.Ø39, MØØ.Ø8-MØØ.1Ø, MØØ.131-MØØ.139, MØØ.18-MØØ.2Ø, MØØ.231-MØØ.239, MØØ.28-MØØ.8Ø, MØØ.831-MØØ.839, MØØ.88-MØ1.XØ, MØ1.X31-MØ1.X39, MØ1.X8-MØ2.1Ø, MØ2.131-MØ2.139, MØ2.18-MØ2.3Ø, MØ2.339, MØ2.38-MØ2.8Ø, MØ2.831-MØ2.839, MØ2.88-MØ2.9, MØ5.4Ø-MØ5.59, MØ5.7Ø-MØ6.Ø9, MØ6.2Ø-MØ6.39, MØ6.8Ø-MØ7.6Ø, MØ7.631-MØ7.639, MØ7.68-MØ7.69, M11.ØØ, M11.Ø31-M11.Ø39, M11.Ø8-M11.1Ø, M11.131-M11.139, M11.18-M11.2Ø, M11.231-M11.239, M11.28-M11.8Ø, M11.831-M11.839, M11.88-M11.9, M12.1Ø, M12.131-M12.139, M12.18-M12.2Ø, M12.231-M12.239, M12.28-M12.3Ø, M12.331-M12.339, M12.38-M12.4Ø, M12.431-M12.439, M12.48-M12.5Ø, M12.531-M12.539, M12.58-M12.8Ø, M12.831-M12.839, M12.88-M13.1Ø, M13.131-M13.139, M13.8Ø, M13.831-M13.839, M13.88-M15.Ø, M15.3-M15.9, M19.Ø31-M19.Ø39, M19.131-M19.139, M19.231-M19.239, M19.9Ø-M19.93, M24.1Ø, M24.131-M24.139, M25.ØØ, M25.Ø31-M25.Ø39, M25.Ø8-M25.1Ø, M25.131-M25.139, M25.18, M25.4Ø, M25.431-M25.439, M25.48-M25.5Ø, M25.531-M25.539, M25.6Ø, M25.631-M25.639, M25.8Ø, M25.831-M25.839, M25.9, M35.2, M36.1-M36.4, R26.2

MØØ.232 Other streptococcal arthritis, left wrist CC

CC Excl: See code: MØØ.231

MØØ.239 Other streptococcal arthritis, unspecified wrist CC

CC Excl: See code: MØØ.231

✓6th **MØØ.24 Other streptococcal arthritis, hand**

Other streptococcal arthritis metacarpus and phalanges

MØØ.241 Other streptococcal arthritis, right hand CC

CC Excl: A17.9, A18.Ø2, A18.Ø9, A18.82, A18.84, A18.89, A39.83-A39.84, A54.4Ø, A54.42-A54.43, A54.82, A54.84, A54.89-A54.9, BØ6.82, MØØ.ØØ, MØØ.Ø49, MØØ.Ø8-MØØ.1Ø, MØØ.141-MØØ.149, MØØ.18-MØØ.2Ø, MØØ.241-MØØ.249, MØØ.28-MØØ.8Ø, MØØ.841-MØØ.849, MØØ.88-MØ1.XØ, MØ1.X41-MØ1.X49, MØ1.X8-MØ2.1Ø, MØ2.141-MØ2.149, MØ2.18-MØ2.3Ø, MØ2.349, MØ2.38-MØ2.8Ø, MØ2.841-MØ2.849, MØ2.88-MØ2.9, MØ5.4Ø-MØ5.59, MØ5.7Ø-MØ6.Ø9, MØ6.2Ø-MØ6.39, MØ6.8Ø-MØ7.6Ø, MØ7.641-MØ7.649, MØ7.68-MØ7.69, M11.ØØ, M11.Ø41-M11.Ø49, M11.Ø8-M11.1Ø, M11.141-M11.149, M11.18-M11.2Ø, M11.241-M11.249, M11.28-M11.8Ø, M11.841-M11.849, M11.88-M11.9, M12.1Ø, M12.141-M12.149, M12.18-M12.2Ø, M12.241-M12.249, M12.28-M12.3Ø, M12.341-M12.349, M12.38-M12.4Ø, M12.441-M12.449, M12.48-M12.5Ø, M12.541-M12.549, M12.58-M12.8Ø, M12.841-M12.849, M12.88-M13.1Ø, M13.141-M13.149, M13.8Ø, M13.841-M13.849, M13.88-M15.9, M18.Ø-M18.9, M19.Ø41-M19.Ø49, M19.141-M19.149, M19.241-M19.249, M19.9Ø-M19.93, M24.1Ø, M24.141-M24.149, M25.ØØ, M25.Ø41-M25.Ø49, M25.Ø8-M25.1Ø, M25.141-M25.149, M25.18, M25.4Ø, M25.441-M25.449, M25.48-M25.5Ø, M25.6Ø, M25.641-M25.649, M25.8Ø, M25.841-M25.849, M25.9, M35.2, M36.1-M36.4, R26.2

MØØ.242 Other streptococcal arthritis, left hand CC

CC Excl: See code: MØØ.241

MØØ.249 Other streptococcal arthritis, unspecified hand CC

CC Excl: See code: MØØ.241

✓6th **MØØ.25 Other streptococcal arthritis, hip**

MØØ.251 Other streptococcal arthritis, right hip CC

CC Excl: A17.9, A18.Ø2, A18.Ø9, A18.82, A18.84, A18.89, A39.83-A39.84, A54.4Ø, A54.42-A54.43, A54.82, A54.84, A54.89-A54.9, BØ6.82, MØØ.ØØ, MØØ.Ø59, MØØ.Ø8-MØØ.1Ø, MØØ.151-MØØ.159, MØØ.18-MØØ.2Ø, MØØ.251-MØØ.259, MØØ.28-MØØ.8Ø, MØØ.851-MØØ.859, MØØ.88-MØ1.XØ, MØ1.X51-MØ1.X59, MØ1.X8-MØ2.1Ø, MØ2.151-MØ2.159, MØ2.18-MØ2.3Ø, MØ2.359, MØ2.38-MØ2.8Ø, MØ2.851-MØ2.859, MØ2.88-MØ2.9, MØ5.4Ø-MØ5.59, MØ5.7Ø-MØ6.Ø9, MØ6.2Ø-MØ6.39, MØ6.8Ø-MØ7.6Ø, MØ7.651-MØ7.659, MØ7.68-MØ7.69, M11.ØØ, M11.Ø51-M11.Ø59, M11.Ø8-M11.1Ø, M11.151-M11.159, M11.18-M11.2Ø, M11.251-M11.259, M11.28-M11.8Ø, M11.851-M11.859, M11.88-M11.9, M12.1Ø, M12.151-M12.159, M12.18-M12.2Ø, M12.251-M12.259, M12.28-M12.3Ø, M12.351-M12.359, M12.38-M12.4Ø, M12.451-M12.459, M12.48-M12.5Ø, M12.551-M12.559, M12.58-M12.8Ø, M12.851-M12.859, M12.88-M13.1Ø, M13.151-M13.159, M13.8Ø, M13.851-M13.859, M13.88-M15.Ø, M15.3-M16.9, M19.9Ø-M19.93, M24.1Ø, M24.151-M24.159, M25.ØØ, M25.Ø51-M25.Ø59, M25.Ø8-M25.1Ø, M25.151-M25.159, M25.18, M25.4Ø, M25.451-M25.459, M25.48-M25.5Ø, M25.551-M25.559, M25.6Ø, M25.651-M25.659, M25.8Ø, M25.851-M25.859, M25.9, M35.2, M36.1-M36.4, R26.2, R29.4

MØØ.252 Other streptococcal arthritis, left hip CC

CC Excl: See code: MØØ.251

MØØ.259 Other streptococcal arthritis, unspecified hip CC

CC Excl: See code: MØØ.251

✓6th **MØØ.26 Other streptococcal arthritis, knee**

MØØ.261 Other streptococcal arthritis, right knee CC

CC Excl: A17.9, A18.Ø2, A18.Ø9, A18.82, A18.84, A18.89, A39.83-A39.84, A54.4Ø, A54.42-A54.43, A54.82, A54.84, A54.89-A54.9, BØ6.82, MØØ.ØØ, MØØ.Ø69, MØØ.Ø8-MØØ.1Ø, MØØ.161-MØØ.169, MØØ.18-MØØ.2Ø, MØØ.261-MØØ.269, MØØ.28-MØØ.8Ø, MØØ.861-MØØ.869, MØØ.88-MØ1.XØ, MØ1.X61-MØ1.X69, MØ1.X8-MØ2.1Ø, MØ2.161-MØ2.169, MØ2.18-MØ2.3Ø, MØ2.369, MØ2.38-MØ2.8Ø, MØ2.861-MØ2.869, MØ2.88-MØ2.9, MØ5.4Ø-MØ5.59, MØ5.7Ø-MØ6.Ø9, MØ6.2Ø-MØ6.39, MØ6.8Ø-MØ7.6Ø, MØ7.661-MØ7.669, MØ7.68-MØ7.69, M11.ØØ, M11.Ø61-M11.Ø69, M11.Ø8-M11.1Ø, M11.161-M11.169, M11.18-M11.2Ø, M11.261-M11.269, M11.28-M11.8Ø, M11.861-M11.869, M11.88-M11.9, M12.1Ø, M12.161-M12.169, M12.18-M12.2Ø, M12.261-M12.269, M12.28-M12.3Ø, M12.361-M12.369, M12.38-M12.4Ø, M12.461-M12.469, M12.48-M12.5Ø, M12.561-M12.569, M12.58-M12.8Ø, M12.861-M12.869, M12.88-M13.1Ø, M13.161-M13.169, M13.8Ø, M13.861-M13.869, M13.88-M15.Ø, M15.3-M15.9, M17.Ø-M17.9, M19.9Ø-M19.93, M24.1Ø, M25.ØØ, M25.Ø61-M25.Ø69, M25.Ø8-M25.1Ø, M25.161-M25.169, M25.18, M25.4Ø, M25.461-M25.469, M25.48-M25.5Ø, M25.561-M25.569, M25.6Ø, M25.661-M25.669, M25.8Ø, M25.861-M25.869, M25.9, M35.2, M36.1-M36.4, R26.2

MØØ.262 Other streptococcal arthritis, left knee CC

CC Excl: See code: MØØ.261

MØØ.269 Other streptococcal arthritis, unspecified knee CC

CC Excl: See code: MØØ.261

✓6th **MØØ.27 Other streptococcal arthritis, ankle and foot**

Other streptococcal arthritis, tarsus, metatarsus and phalanges

MØØ.271 Other streptococcal arthritis, right ankle and foot CC

CC Excl: A17.9, A18.Ø2, A18.Ø9, A18.82, A18.84, A18.89, A39.83-A39.84, A54.4Ø, A54.42-A54.43, A54.82, A54.84, A54.89-A54.9, BØ6.82, MØØ.ØØ, MØØ.Ø79–MØØ.1Ø, MØØ.171-MØØ.2Ø, MØØ.271-MØØ.8Ø, MØØ.871-MØ1.XØ, MØ1.X71-MØ2.1Ø, MØ2.171-MØ2.3Ø, MØ2.379-MØ2.8Ø, MØ2.871-MØ2.9, MØ5.4Ø-MØ5.59, MØ5.7Ø-MØ6.Ø9, MØ6.2Ø-MØ6.39, MØ6.8Ø-MØ7.6Ø, MØ7.671-MØ7.69, M11.ØØ, M11.Ø71-M11.1Ø, M11.171-M11.2Ø, M11.271-M11.8Ø, M11.871-M11.9, M12.1Ø, M12.171-M12.2Ø, M12.271-M12.3Ø, M12.371-M12.4Ø, M12.471-M12.5Ø, M12.571-M12.8Ø, M12.871-M13.1Ø, M13.171-M13.8Ø, M13.871-M15.Ø, M15.3-M15.9, M19.Ø71-M19.Ø79, M19.171-M19.179, M19.271-M19.93, M24.1Ø, M24.171-M24.176, M25.ØØ, M25.Ø71-M25.1Ø, M25.171-M25.18, M25.4Ø, M25.471-M25.5Ø, M25.571-M25.6Ø, M25.671-M25.676, M25.8Ø, M25.871-M25.9, M35.2, M36.1-M36.4, R26.2

MØØ.272 Other streptococcal arthritis, left ankle and foot CC

CC Excl: See code: MØØ.271

MØØ.279 Other streptococcal arthritis, unspecified ankle and foot CC

CC Excl: See code: MØØ.271

MØØ.28 Other streptococcal arthritis, vertebrae CC

CC Excl: A17.9, A18.Ø2, A18.Ø9, A18.82, A18.84, A18.89, A39.83-A39.84, A54.4Ø, A54.42-A54.43, A54.82, A54.84, A54.89-A54.9, BØ6.82, MØØ.ØØ, MØØ.Ø19, MØØ.Ø29, MØØ.Ø39, MØØ.Ø49, MØØ.Ø59, MØØ.Ø69, MØØ.Ø79, MØØ.Ø8-MØ2.3Ø, MØ2.319, MØ2.329, MØ2.339, MØ2.349, MØ2.359, MØ2.369, MØ2.379-MØ2.9, MØ5.4Ø-MØ5.59, MØ5.7Ø-MØ6.Ø9, MØ6.2Ø-MØ6.39, MØ6.8Ø-MØ7.69, M11.ØØ-M11.9, M12.1Ø-M15.Ø, M15.3-M15.9, M16.2-M16.9, M17.2-M17.9, M18.2-M18.9, M19.111-M19.93, M24.1Ø-M24.176, M25.ØØ, M25.Ø8-M25.18, M25.4Ø-M25.676, M25.8Ø-M25.9, M35.2, M36.1-M36.4, R26.2, R29.4

MØØ.29 Other streptococcal polyarthritis CC

CC Excl: See code: MØØ.28

✓5th **MØØ.8 Arthritis and polyarthritis due to other bacteria**

Use additional code (B96) to identify bacteria

MØØ.8Ø Arthritis due to other bacteria, unspecified joint CC

CC Excl: See code: MØØ.28

✓6th **MØØ.81 Arthritis due to other bacteria, shoulder**

MØØ.811 Arthritis due to other bacteria, right shoulder CC

CC Excl: A17.9, A18.Ø2, A18.Ø9, A18.82, A18.84, A18.89, A39.83-A39.84, A54.4Ø, A54.42-A54.43, A54.82, A54.84, A54.89-A54.9, BØ6.82, MØØ.ØØ, MØØ.Ø19, MØØ.Ø8-MØØ.119, MØØ.18-MØØ.219, MØØ.28-MØØ.819, MØØ.88-MØ1.X19, MØ1.X8-MØ2.119, MØ2.18-MØ2.211

MØØ.812 Arthritis due to other bacteria, left shoulder CC

CC Excl: See code: MØØ.811

MØØ.819 Arthritis due to other bacteria, unspecified shoulder CC

CC Excl: See code: MØØ.811

✓6th **MØØ.82 Arthritis due to other bacteria, elbow**

MØØ.821 Arthritis due to other bacteria, right elbow CC

CC Excl: A17.9, A18.Ø2, A18.Ø9, A18.82, A18.84, A18.89, A39.83-A39.84, A54.4Ø, A54.42-A54.43, A54.82, A54.84, A54.89-A54.9, BØ6.82, MØØ.ØØ, MØØ.Ø29, MØØ.Ø8-MØØ.1Ø, MØØ.121-MØØ.129, MØØ.18-MØØ.2Ø, MØØ.221-MØØ.229, MØØ.28-MØØ.8Ø, MØØ.821-MØØ.829, MØØ.88-MØ1.XØ, MØ1.X21-MØ1.X29, MØ1.X8-MØ2.1Ø, MØ2.121-MØ2.129, MØ2.18-MØ2.3Ø, MØ2.329, MØ2.38-MØ2.8Ø, MØ2.821-MØ2.829, MØ2.88-MØ2.9, MØ5.4Ø-MØ5.59, MØ5.7Ø-MØ6.Ø9, MØ6.2Ø-MØ6.39, MØ6.8Ø-MØ7.6Ø, MØ7.621-MØ7.629, MØ7.68-MØ7.69, M11.ØØ, M11.Ø21-M11.Ø29, M11.Ø8-M11.1Ø, M11.121-M11.129, M11.18-M11.2Ø, M11.221-M11.229, M11.28-M11.8Ø, M11.821-M11.829, M11.88-M11.9, M12.1Ø, M12.121-M12.129, M12.18-M12.2Ø, M12.221-M12.229, M12.28-M12.3Ø, M12.321-M12.329, M12.38-M12.4Ø, M12.421-M12.429, M12.48-M12.5Ø, M12.521-M12.529, M12.58-M12.8Ø, M12.821-M12.829, M12.88-M13.1Ø, M13.121-M13.129, M13.8Ø, M13.821-M13.829, M13.88-M15.Ø, M15.3-M15.9, M19.Ø21-M19.Ø29, M19.121-M19.129, M19.221-M19.229, M19.9Ø-M19.93, M24.1Ø, M24.121-M24.129, M25.ØØ, M25.Ø21-M25.Ø29, M25.Ø8-M25.1Ø, M25.121-M25.129, M25.18, M25.4Ø, M25.421-M25.429, M25.48-M25.5Ø, M25.521-M25.529, M25.6Ø, M25.621-M25.629, M25.8Ø, M25.821-M25.829, M25.9, M35.2, M36.1-M36.4, R26.2

MØØ.822 Arthritis due to other bacteria, left elbow CC

CC Excl: See code: MØØ.821

MØØ.829 Arthritis due to other bacteria, unspecified elbow CC

CC Excl: See code: MØØ.821

✓6th **MØØ.83 Arthritis due to other bacteria, wrist**

Arthritis due to other bacteria, carpal bones

MØØ.831 Arthritis due to other bacteria, right wrist CC

CC Excl: A17.9, A18.Ø2, A18.Ø9, A18.82, A18.84, A18.89, A39.83-A39.84, A54.4Ø, A54.42-A54.43, A54.82, A54.84, A54.89-A54.9, BØ6.82, MØØ.ØØ, MØØ.Ø39, MØØ.Ø8-MØØ.1Ø, MØØ.131-MØØ.139, MØØ.18-MØØ.2Ø, MØØ.231-MØØ.239, MØØ.28-MØØ.8Ø, MØØ.831-MØØ.839, MØØ.88-MØ1.XØ, MØ1.X31-MØ1.X39, MØ1.X8-MØ2.1Ø, MØ2.131-MØ2.139, MØ2.18-MØ2.3Ø, MØ2.339, MØ2.38-MØ2.8Ø, MØ2.831-MØ2.839, MØ2.88-MØ2.9, MØ5.4Ø-MØ5.59, MØ5.7Ø-MØ6.Ø9, MØ6.2Ø-MØ6.39, MØ6.8Ø-MØ7.6Ø, MØ7.631-MØ7.639, MØ7.68-MØ7.69, M11.ØØ, M11.Ø31-M11.Ø39, M11.Ø8-M11.1Ø, M11.131-M11.139, M11.18-M11.2Ø, M11.231-M11.239, M11.28-M11.8Ø, M11.831-M11.839, M11.88-M11.9, M12.1Ø, M12.131-M12.139, M12.18-M12.2Ø, M12.231-M12.239, M12.28-M12.3Ø, M12.331-M12.339, M12.38-M12.4Ø, M12.431-M12.439, M12.48-M12.5Ø, M12.531-M12.539, M12.58-M12.8Ø, M12.831-M12.839, M12.88-M13.1Ø, M13.131-M13.139, M13.8Ø, M13.831-M13.839, M13.88-M15.Ø, M15.3-M15.9, M19.Ø31-M19.Ø39, M19.131-M19.139, M19.231-M19.239, M19.9Ø-M19.93, M24.1Ø, M24.131-M24.139, M25.ØØ, M25.Ø31-M25.Ø39, M25.Ø8-M25.1Ø, M25.131-M25.139, M25.18, M25.4Ø, M25.431-M25.439, M25.48-M25.5Ø, M25.531-M25.539, M25.6Ø, M25.631-M25.639, M25.8Ø, M25.831-M25.839, M25.9, M35.2, M36.1-M36.4, R26.2

MØØ.832 Arthritis due to other bacteria, left wrist CC
CC Excl: See code: MØØ.831

MØØ.839 Arthritis due to other bacteria, unspecified wrist CC
CC Excl: See code: MØØ.831

✓6th **MØØ.84 Arthritis due to other bacteria, hand**
Arthritis due to other bacteria, metacarpus and phalanges

MØØ.841 Arthritis due to other bacteria, right hand CC
CC Excl: A17.9, A18.Ø2, A18.Ø9, A18.82, A18.84, A18.89, A39.83-A39.84, A54.4Ø, A54.42-A54.43, A54.82, A54.84, A54.89-A54.9, BØ6.82, MØØ.ØØ, MØØ.Ø49, MØØ.Ø8-MØØ.1Ø, MØØ.141-MØØ.149, MØØ.18-MØØ.2Ø, MØØ.241-MØØ.249, MØØ.28-MØØ.8Ø, MØØ.841-MØØ.849, MØØ.88-MØ1.XØ, MØ1.X41-MØ1.X49, MØ1.X8-MØ2.1Ø, MØ2.141-MØ2.149, MØ2.18-MØ2.3Ø, MØ2.349, MØ2.38-MØ2.8Ø, MØ2.841-MØ2.849, MØ2.88-MØ2.9, MØ5.4Ø-MØ5.59, MØ5.7Ø-MØ6.Ø9, MØ6.2Ø-MØ6.39, MØ6.8Ø-MØ7.6Ø, MØ7.641-MØ7.649, MØ7.68-MØ7.69, M11.ØØ, M11.Ø41-M11.Ø49, M11.Ø8-M11.1Ø, M11.141-M11.149, M11.18-M11.2Ø, M11.241-M11.249, M11.28-M11.8Ø, M11.841-M11.849, M11.88-M11.9, M12.1Ø, M12.141-M12.149, M12.18-M12.2Ø, M12.241-M12.249, M12.28-M12.3Ø, M12.341-M12.349, M12.38-M12.4Ø, M12.441-M12.449, M12.48-M12.5Ø, M12.541-M12.549, M12.58-M12.8Ø, M12.841-M12.849, M12.88-M13.1Ø, M13.141-M13.149, M13.8Ø, M13.841-M13.849, M13.88-M15.9, M18.Ø-M18.9, M19.Ø41-M19.Ø49, M19.141-M19.149, M19.241-M19.249, M19.9Ø-M19.93, M24.1Ø, M24.141-M24.149, M25.ØØ, M25.Ø41-M25.Ø49, M25.Ø8-M25.1Ø, M25.141-M25.149, M25.18, M25.4Ø, M25.441-M25.449, M25.48-M25.5Ø, M25.6Ø, M25.641-M25.649, M25.8Ø, M25.841-M25.849, M25.9, M35.2, M36.1-M36.4, R26.2

MØØ.842 Arthritis due to other bacteria, left hand CC
CC Excl: See code: MØØ.841

MØØ.849 Arthritis due to other bacteria, unspecified hand CC
CC Excl: See code: MØØ.841

✓6th **MØØ.85 Arthritis due to other bacteria, hip**

MØØ.851 Arthritis due to other bacteria, right hip CC
CC Excl: A17.9, A18.Ø2, A18.Ø9, A18.82, A18.84, A18.89, A39.83-A39.84, A54.4Ø, A54.42-A54.43, A54.82, A54.84, A54.89-A54.9, BØ6.82, MØØ.ØØ, MØØ.Ø59, MØØ.Ø8-MØØ.1Ø, MØØ.151-MØØ.159, MØØ.18-MØØ.2Ø, MØØ.251-MØØ.259, MØØ.28-MØØ.8Ø, MØØ.851-MØØ.859, MØØ.88-MØ1.XØ, MØ1.X51-MØ1.X59, MØ1.X8-MØ2.1Ø, MØ2.151-MØ2.159, MØ2.18-MØ2.3Ø, MØ2.359, MØ2.38-MØ2.8Ø, MØ2.851-MØ2.859, MØ2.88-MØ2.9, MØ5.4Ø-MØ5.59, MØ5.7Ø-MØ6.Ø9, MØ6.2Ø-MØ6.39, MØ6.8Ø-MØ7.6Ø, MØ7.651-MØ7.659, MØ7.68-MØ7.69, M11.ØØ, M11.Ø51-M11.Ø59, M11.Ø8-M11.1Ø, M11.151-M11.159, M11.18-M11.2Ø, M11.251-M11.259, M11.28-M11.8Ø, M11.851-M11.859, M11.88-M11.9, M12.1Ø, M12.151-M12.159, M12.18-M12.2Ø, M12.251-M12.259, M12.28-M12.3Ø, M12.351-M12.359, M12.38-M12.4Ø, M12.451-M12.459, M12.48-M12.5Ø, M12.551-M12.559, M12.58-M12.8Ø, M12.851-M12.859, M12.88-M13.1Ø, M13.151-M13.159, M13.8Ø, M13.851-M13.859, M13.88-M15.Ø, M15.3-M16.9, M19.9Ø-M19.93, M24.1Ø, M24.151-M24.159, M25.ØØ, M25.Ø51-M25.Ø59, M25.Ø8-M25.1Ø, M25.151-M25.159, M25.18, M25.4Ø, M25.451-M25.459, M25.48-M25.5Ø, M25.551-M25.559, M25.6Ø, M25.651-M25.659, M25.8Ø, M25.851-M25.859, M25.9, M35.2, M36.1-M36.4, R26.2, R29.4

MØØ.852 Arthritis due to other bacteria, left hip CC
CC Excl: See code: MØØ.851

MØØ.859 Arthritis due to other bacteria, unspecified hip CC
CC Excl: See code: MØØ.851

✓6th **MØØ.86 Arthritis due to other bacteria, knee**

MØØ.861 Arthritis due to other bacteria, right knee CC
CC Excl: A17.9, A18.Ø2, A18.Ø9, A18.82, A18.84, A18.89, A39.83-A39.84, A54.4Ø, A54.42-A54.43, A54.82, A54.84, A54.89-A54.9, BØ6.82, MØØ.ØØ, MØØ.Ø69, MØØ.Ø8-MØØ.1Ø, MØØ.161-MØØ.169, MØØ.18-MØØ.2Ø, MØØ.261-MØØ.269, MØØ.28-MØØ.8Ø, MØØ.861-MØØ.869, MØØ.88-MØ1.XØ, MØ1.X61-MØ1.X69, MØ1.X8-MØ2.1Ø, MØ2.161-MØ2.169, MØ2.18-MØ2.3Ø, MØ2.369, MØ2.38-MØ2.8Ø, MØ2.861-MØ2.869, MØ2.88-MØ2.9, MØ5.4Ø-MØ5.59, MØ5.7Ø-MØ6.Ø9, MØ6.2Ø-MØ6.39, MØ6.8Ø-MØ7.6Ø, MØ7.661-MØ7.669, MØ7.68-MØ7.69, M11.ØØ, M11.Ø61-M11.Ø69, M11.Ø8-M11.1Ø, M11.161-M11.169, M11.18-M11.2Ø, M11.261-M11.269, M11.28-M11.8Ø, M11.861-M11.869, M11.88-M11.9, M12.1Ø, M12.161-M12.169, M12.18-M12.2Ø, M12.261-M12.269, M12.28-M12.3Ø, M12.361-M12.369, M12.38-M12.4Ø, M12.461-M12.469, M12.48-M12.5Ø, M12.561-M12.569, M12.58-M12.8Ø, M12.861-M12.869, M12.88-M13.1Ø, M13.161-M13.169, M13.8Ø, M13.861-M13.869, M13.88-M15.Ø, M15.3-M15.9, M17.Ø-M17.9, M19.9Ø-M19.93, M24.1Ø, M25.ØØ, M25.Ø61-M25.Ø69, M25.Ø8-M25.1Ø, M25.161-M25.169, M25.18, M25.4Ø, M25.461-M25.469, M25.48-M25.5Ø, M25.561-M25.569, M25.6Ø, M25.661-M25.669, M25.8Ø, M25.861-M25.869, M25.9, M35.2, M36.1-M36.4, R26.2

MØØ.862 Arthritis due to other bacteria, left knee CC
CC Excl: See code: MØØ.861

MØØ.869 Arthritis due to other bacteria, unspecified knee CC
CC Excl: See code: MØØ.861

✓6th **MØØ.87 Arthritis due to other bacteria, ankle and foot**
Arthritis due to other bacteria, tarsus, metatarsus, and phalanges

MØØ.871 Arthritis due to other bacteria, right ankle and foot CC
CC Excl: A17.9, A18.Ø2, A18.Ø9, A18.82, A18.84, A18.89, A39.83-A39.84, A54.4Ø, A54.42-A54.43, A54.82, A54.84, A54.89-A54.9, BØ6.82, MØØ.ØØ, MØØ.Ø71-MØØ.1Ø, MØØ.171-MØØ.2Ø, MØØ.271-MØØ.8Ø, MØØ.871-MØ1.XØ, MØ1.X71-MØ2.1Ø, MØ2.171-MØ2.3Ø, MØ2.379-MØ2.8Ø, MØ2.871-MØ2.9, MØ5.4Ø-MØ5.59, MØ5.7Ø-MØ6.Ø9, MØ6.2Ø-MØ6.39, MØ6.8Ø-MØ7.6Ø, MØ7.671-MØ7.69, M11.ØØ, M11.Ø71-M11.1Ø, M11.171-M11.2Ø, M11.271-M11.8Ø, M11.871-M11.9, M12.1Ø, M12.171-M12.2Ø, M12.271-M12.3Ø, M12.371-M12.4Ø, M12.471-M12.5Ø, M12.571-M12.8Ø, M12.871-M13.1Ø, M13.171-M13.8Ø, M13.871-M15.Ø, M15.3-M15.9, M19.Ø71-M19.Ø79, M19.171-M19.179, M19.271-M19.93, M24.1Ø, M24.171-M24.176, M25.ØØ, M25.Ø71-M25.1Ø, M25.171-M25.18, M25.4Ø, M25.471-M25.5Ø, M25.571-M25.6Ø, M25.671-M25.676, M25.8Ø, M25.871-M25.9, M35.2, M36.1-M36.4, R26.2

MØØ.872 Arthritis due to other bacteria, left ankle and foot CC
CC Excl: See code: MØØ.871

MØØ.879 Arthritis due to other bacteria, unspecified ankle and foot CC
CC Excl: See code: MØØ.871

MØØ.88 Arthritis due to other bacteria, vertebrae CC
CC Excl: A17.9, A18.Ø2, A18.Ø9, A18.82, A18.84, A18.89, A39.83-A39.84, A54.4Ø, A54.42-A54.43, A54.82, A54.84, A54.89-A54.9, BØ6.82, MØØ.ØØ, MØØ.Ø19, MØØ.Ø29, MØØ.Ø39, MØØ.Ø49, MØØ.Ø59, MØØ.Ø69, MØØ.Ø79, MØØ.Ø8-MØ2.3Ø, MØ2.319, MØ2.329, MØ2.339, MØ2.349, MØ2.359, MØ2.369, MØ2.379-MØ2.9, MØ5.4Ø-MØ5.59, MØ5.7Ø-MØ6.Ø9, MØ6.2Ø-MØ6.39, MØ6.8Ø-MØ7.69, M11.ØØ-M11.9, M12.1Ø-M15.Ø, M15.3-M15.9, M16.2-M16.9, M17.2-M17.9, M18.2-M18.9, M19.111-M19.93, M24.1Ø-M24.176, M25.ØØ, M25.Ø8-M25.18, M25.4Ø-M25.676, M25.8Ø-M25.9, M35.2, M36.1-M36.4, R26.2, R29.4

MØØ.89 Polyarthritis due to other bacteria CC
CC Excl: See code: MØØ.88

MØØ.9 Pyogenic arthritis, unspecified CC
Infective arthritis NOS
CC Excl:See code: MØØ.88

MØ1 Direct infections of joint in infectious and parasitic diseases classified elsewhere

Code first underlying disease, such as:
leprosy [Hansen's disease] (A3Ø.-)
mycoses (B35-B49)
O'nyong-nyong fever (A92.1)
paratyphoid fever (AØ1.1-AØ1.4)

EXCLUDES 1 *arthropathy in Lyme disease (A69.23)*
gonococcal arthritis (A54.42)
meningococcal arthritis (A39.83)
mumps arthritis (B26.85)
postinfective arthropathy (MØ2.-)
postmeningococcal arthritis (A39.84)
reactive arthritis (MØ2.3)
rubella arthritis (BØ6.82)
sarcoidosis arthritis (D86.86)
typhoid fever arthritis (AØ1.Ø4)
tuberculosis arthritis (A18.Ø1-A18.Ø2)

MØ1.X Direct infection of joint in infectious and parasitic diseases classified elsewhere

MØ1.XØ Direct infection of unspecified joint in infectious and parasitic diseases classified elsewhere CC
CC Excl: AØ2.23, A17.9, A18.Ø2, A18.Ø9, A18.82, A18.84, A18.89, A39.83-A39.84, A54.4Ø, A54.42-A54.43, A54.82, A54.84, A54.89-A54.9, BØ6.82, MØØ.ØØ, MØØ.Ø19, MØØ.Ø29, MØØ.Ø39, MØØ.Ø49, MØØ.Ø59, MØØ.Ø69, MØØ.Ø79, MØØ.Ø8-MØ2.3Ø, MØ2.319, MØ2.329, MØ2.339, MØ2.349, MØ2.359, MØ2.369, MØ2.379-MØ2.9, MØ5.4Ø-MØ5.59, MØ5.7Ø-MØ6.Ø9, MØ6.2Ø-MØ6.39, MØ6.8Ø-MØ7.69, M11.ØØ-M11.9, M12.1Ø-M15.Ø, M15.3-M15.9, M16.2-M16.9, M17.2-M17.9, M18.2-M18.9, M19.111-M19.93, M24.1Ø-M24.176, M25.ØØ, M25.Ø8-M25.18, M25.4Ø-M25.676, M25.8Ø-M25.9, M35.2, M36.1-M36.4, R29.4

MØ1.X1 Direct infection of shoulder joint in infectious and parasitic diseases classified elsewhere

MØ1.X11 Direct infection of right shoulder in infectious and parasitic diseases classified elsewhere CC
CC Excl: AØ2.23, A17.9, A18.Ø2, A18.Ø9, A18.82, A18.84, A18.89, A39.83-A39.84, A54.4Ø, A54.42-A54.43, A54.82, A54.84, A54.89-A54.9, BØ6.82, MØØ.ØØ, MØØ.Ø19, MØØ.Ø29, MØØ.Ø39, MØØ.Ø49, MØØ.Ø59, MØØ.Ø69, MØØ.Ø79, MØØ.Ø8-MØ2.3Ø, MØ2.319, MØ2.329, MØ2.339, MØ2.349, MØ2.359, MØ2.369, MØ2.379-MØ2.9, MØ5.4Ø-MØ5.59, MØ5.7Ø-MØ6.Ø9, MØ6.2Ø-MØ6.39, MØ6.8Ø-MØ7.69, M11.ØØ-M11.9, M12.1Ø-M12.419

MØ1.X12 Direct infection of left shoulder in infectious and parasitic diseases classified elsewhere CC
CC Excl: See code: MØ1.X11

MØ1.X19 Direct infection of unspecified shoulder in infectious and parasitic diseases classified elsewhere CC
CC Excl: See code: MØ1.X11

MØ1.X2 Direct infection of elbow in infectious and parasitic diseases classified elsewhere

MØ1.X21 Direct infection of right elbow in infectious and parasitic diseases classified elsewhere CC
CC Excl: See code: MØ1.XØ

MØ1.X22 Direct infection of left elbow in infectious and parasitic diseases classified elsewhere CC
CC Excl: See code: MØ1.XØ

MØ1.X29 Direct infection of unspecified elbow in infectious and parasitic diseases classified elsewhere CC
CC Excl: See code: MØ1.XØ

MØ1.X3 Direct infection of wrist in infectious and parasitic diseases classified elsewhere
Direct infection of carpal bones in infectious and parasitic diseases classified elsewhere

MØ1.X31 Direct infection of right wrist in infectious and parasitic diseases classified elsewhere CC
CC Excl: See code: MØ1.XØ

MØ1.X32 Direct infection of left wrist in infectious and parasitic diseases classified elsewhere CC
CC Excl: See code: MØ1.XØ

MØ1.X39 Direct infection of unspecified wrist in infectious and parasitic diseases classified elsewhere CC
CC Excl: See code: MØ1.XØ

MØ1.X4 Direct infection of hand in infectious and parasitic diseases classified elsewhere
Direct infection of metacarpus and phalanges in infectious and parasitic diseases classified elsewhere

MØ1.X41 Direct infection of right hand in infectious and parasitic diseases classified elsewhere CC
CC Excl: See code: MØ1.XØ

MØ1.X42 Direct infection of left hand in infectious and parasitic diseases classified elsewhere CC
CC Excl: See code: MØ1.XØ

MØ1.X49 Direct infection of unspecified hand in infectious and parasitic diseases classified elsewhere CC
CC Excl: See code: MØ1.XØ

MØ1.X5 Direct infection of hip in infectious and parasitic diseases classified elsewhere

MØ1.X51 Direct infection of right hip in infectious and parasitic diseases classified elsewhere CC
CC Excl: See code: MØ1.XØ

MØ1.X52 Direct infection of left hip in infectious and parasitic diseases classified elsewhere CC
CC Excl: See code: MØ1.XØ

MØ1.X59 Direct infection of unspecified hip in infectious and parasitic diseases classified elsewhere CC
CC Excl: See code: MØ1.XØ

MØ1.X6 Direct infection of knee in infectious and parasitic diseases classified elsewhere

MØ1.X61 Direct infection of right knee in infectious and parasitic diseases classified elsewhere CC
CC Excl: See code: MØ1.XØ

MØ1.X62 Direct infection of left knee in infectious and parasitic diseases classified elsewhere CC
CC Excl: See code: MØ1.XØ

MØ1.X69 Direct infection of unspecified knee in infectious and parasitic diseases classified elsewhere CC
CC Excl: See code: MØ1.XØ

MØ1.X7 Direct infection of ankle and foot in infectious and parasitic diseases classified elsewhere
Direct infection of tarsus, metatarsus and phalanges in infectious and parasitic diseases classified elsewhere

MØ1.X71 Direct infection of right ankle and foot in infectious and parasitic diseases classified elsewhere CC
CC Excl: See code: MØ1.XØ

MØ1.X72 Direct infection of left ankle and foot in infectious and parasitic diseases classified elsewhere CC
CC Excl: See code: MØ1.XØ

MØ1.X79 Direct infection of unspecified ankle and foot in infectious and parasitic diseases classified elsewhere CC
CC Excl: See code: MØ1.XØ

MØ1.X8 Direct infection of vertebrae in infectious and parasitic diseases classified elsewhere CC
CC Excl: See code: MØ1.XØ

MØ1.X9 Direct infection of multiple joints in infectious and parasitic diseases classified elsewhere CC
CC Excl: See code: MØ1.XØ

M02 Postinfective and reactive arthropathies

Code first underlying disease, such as:
congenital syphilis [Clutton's joints] (A50.5)
enteritis due to Yersinia enterocolitica (A04.6)
infective endocarditis (I33.0)
viral hepatitis (B15-B19)

EXCLUDES 1 *Behçet's disease (M35.2)*
direct infections of joint in infectious and parasitic diseases classified elsewhere (M01.-)
mumps arthritis (B26.85)
postmeningococcal arthritis (A39.84)
rheumatic fever (I00)
rubella arthritis (B06.82)
syphilis arthritis (late) (A52.77)
tabetic arthropathy [Charcôt's] (A52.16)

M02.0 Arthropathy following intestinal bypass
M02.00 Arthropathy following intestinal bypass, unspecified site
M02.01 Arthropathy following intestinal bypass, shoulder
M02.011 Arthropathy following intestinal bypass, right shoulder
M02.012 Arthropathy following intestinal bypass, left shoulder
M02.019 Arthropathy following intestinal bypass, unspecified shoulder
M02.02 Arthropathy following intestinal bypass, elbow
M02.021 Arthropathy following intestinal bypass, right elbow
M02.022 Arthropathy following intestinal bypass, left elbow
M02.029 Arthropathy following intestinal bypass, unspecified elbow
M02.03 Arthropathy following intestinal bypass, wrist
Arthropathy following intestinal bypass, carpal bones
M02.031 Arthropathy following intestinal bypass, right wrist
M02.032 Arthropathy following intestinal bypass, left wrist
M02.039 Arthropathy following intestinal bypass, unspecified wrist
M02.04 Arthropathy following intestinal bypass, hand
Arthropathy following intestinal bypass, metacarpals and phalanges
M02.041 Arthropathy following intestinal bypass, right hand
M02.042 Arthropathy following intestinal bypass, left hand
M02.049 Arthropathy following intestinal bypass, unspecified hand
M02.05 Arthropathy following intestinal bypass, hip
M02.051 Arthropathy following intestinal bypass, right hip
M02.052 Arthropathy following intestinal bypass, left hip
M02.059 Arthropathy following intestinal bypass, unspecified hip
M02.06 Arthropathy following intestinal bypass, knee
M02.061 Arthropathy following intestinal bypass, right knee
M02.062 Arthropathy following intestinal bypass, left knee
M02.069 Arthropathy following intestinal bypass, unspecified knee
M02.07 Arthropathy following intestinal bypass, ankle and foot
Arthropathy following intestinal bypass, tarsus, metatarsus and phalanges
M02.071 Arthropathy following intestinal bypass, right ankle and foot
M02.072 Arthropathy following intestinal bypass, left ankle and foot
M02.079 Arthropathy following intestinal bypass, unspecified ankle and foot
M02.08 Arthropathy following intestinal bypass, vertebrae
M02.09 Arthropathy following intestinal bypass, multiple sites

M02.1 Postdysenteric arthropathy
M02.10 Postdysenteric arthropathy, unspecified site CC
CC Excl: A02.23, A17.9, A18.02, A18.09, A18.82, A18.84, A18.89, A39.83-A39.84, A54.40, A54.42-A54.43, A54.82, A54.84, A54.89-A54.9, B06.82, M00.00, M00.019, M00.029, M00.039, M00.049, M00.059, M00.069, M00.079, M00.08-M02.30, M02.319, M02.329, M02.339, M02.349, M02.359, M02.369, M02.379-M02.9, M05.40-M05.59, M05.70-M06.09, M06.20-M06.39, M06.80-M07.69, M11.00-M11.9, M12.10-M15.0, M15.3-M15.9, M16.2-M16.9, M17.2-M17.9, M18.2-M18.9, M19.111-M19.93, M24.10-M24.176, M25.00, M25.08-M25.18, M25.40-M25.676, M25.80-M25.9, M35.2, M36.1-M36.4, R29.4
M02.11 Postdysenteric arthropathy, shoulder
M02.111 Postdysenteric arthropathy, right shoulder CC
CC Excl: See code: M02.10
M02.112 Postdysenteric arthropathy, left shoulder CC
CC Excl: See code: M02.10
M02.119 Postdysenteric arthropathy, unspecified shoulder CC
CC Excl: See code: M02.10
M02.12 Postdysenteric arthropathy, elbow
M02.121 Postdysenteric arthropathy, right elbow CC
CC Excl: See code: M02.10
M02.122 Postdysenteric arthropathy, left elbow CC
CC Excl: See code: M02.10
M02.129 Postdysenteric arthropathy, unspecified elbow CC
CC Excl: See code: M02.10
M02.13 Postdysenteric arthropathy, wrist
Postdysenteric arthropathy, carpal bones
M02.131 Postdysenteric arthropathy, right wrist CC
CC Excl: See code: M02.10
M02.132 Postdysenteric arthropathy, left wrist CC
CC Excl: See code: M02.10
M02.139 Postdysenteric arthropathy, unspecified wrist CC
CC Excl: See code: M02.10
M02.14 Postdysenteric arthropathy, hand
Postdysenteric arthropathy, metacarpus and phalanges
M02.141 Postdysenteric arthropathy, right hand CC
CC Excl: See code: M02.10
M02.142 Postdysenteric arthropathy, left hand CC
CC Excl: See code: M02.10
M02.149 Postdysenteric arthropathy, unspecified hand CC
CC Excl: See code: M02.10
M02.15 Postdysenteric arthropathy, hip
M02.151 Postdysenteric arthropathy, right hip CC
CC Excl: See code: M02.10
M02.152 Postdysenteric arthropathy, left hip CC
CC Excl: See code: M02.10
M02.159 Postdysenteric arthropathy, unspecified hip CC
CC Excl: See code: M02.10
M02.16 Postdysenteric arthropathy, knee
M02.161 Postdysenteric arthropathy, right knee CC
CC Excl: A02.23, A17.9, A18.02, A18.09, A18.82, A18.84, A18.89, A39.83-A39.84, A54.40, A54.42-A54.43, A54.82, A54.84, A54.89-A54.9, B06.82, M00.00, M00.019, M00.029, M00.039, M00.049, M00.059, M00.069, M00.079, M00.08-M02.30, M02.319, M02.329, M02.339, M02.349, M02.359, M02.369, M02.379-M02.9, M05.40-M05.59, M05.70-M06.09, M06.20-M06.39, M06.80-M07.69, M11.00-M11.9, M12.10-M12.179, M12.19-M15.0, M15.3-M15.9, M16.2-M16.9, M17.2-M17.9, M18.2-M18.9, M19.111-M19.93, M24.10-M24.176, M25.00, M25.08-M25.18, M25.40-M25.676, M25.80-M25.9, M35.2, M36.1-M36.4, R29.4
M02.162 Postdysenteric arthropathy, left knee CC
CC Excl: See code: M02.161
M02.169 Postdysenteric arthropathy, unspecified knee CC
CC Excl: See code: M02.161

✓6th **MØ2.17 Postdysenteric arthropathy, ankle and foot**
Postdysenteric arthropathy, tarsus, metatarsus and phalanges

MØ2.171 Postdysenteric arthropathy, right ankle and foot CC
CC Excl: See code: MØ2.1Ø

MØ2.172 Postdysenteric arthropathy, left ankle and foot CC
CC Excl: See code: MØ2.1Ø

MØ2.179 Postdysenteric arthropathy, unspecified ankle and foot CC
CC Excl: See code: MØ2.1Ø

MØ2.18 Postdysenteric arthropathy, vertebrae CC
CC Excl: See code: MØ2.1Ø

MØ2.19 Postdysenteric arthropathy, multiple sites CC
CC Excl: See code: MØ2.1Ø

✓5th **MØ2.2 Postimmunization arthropathy**

MØ2.2Ø Postimmunization arthropathy, unspecified site

✓6th **MØ2.21 Postimmunization arthropathy, shoulder**

MØ2.211 Postimmunization arthropathy, right shoulder

MØ2.212 Postimmunization arthropathy, left shoulder

MØ2.219 Postimmunization arthropathy, unspecified shoulder

✓6th **MØ2.22 Postimmunization arthropathy, elbow**

MØ2.221 Postimmunization arthropathy, right elbow

MØ2.222 Postimmunization arthropathy, left elbow

MØ2.229 Postimmunization arthropathy, unspecified elbow

✓6th **MØ2.23 Postimmunization arthropathy, wrist**
Postimmunization arthropathy, carpal bones

MØ2.231 Postimmunization arthropathy, right wrist

MØ2.232 Postimmunization arthropathy, left wrist

MØ2.239 Postimmunization arthropathy, unspecified wrist

✓6th **MØ2.24 Postimmunization arthropathy, hand**
Postimmunization arthropathy, metacarpus and phalanges

MØ2.241 Postimmunization arthropathy, right hand

MØ2.242 Postimmunization arthropathy, left hand

MØ2.249 Postimmunization arthropathy, unspecified hand

✓6th **MØ2.25 Postimmunization arthropathy, hip**

MØ2.251 Postimmunization arthropathy, right hip

MØ2.252 Postimmunization arthropathy, left hip

MØ2.259 Postimmunization arthropathy, unspecified hip

✓6th **MØ2.26 Postimmunization arthropathy, knee**

MØ2.261 Postimmunization arthropathy, right knee

MØ2.262 Postimmunization arthropathy, left knee

MØ2.269 Postimmunization arthropathy, unspecified knee

✓6th **MØ2.27 Postimmunization arthropathy, ankle and foot**
Postimmunization arthropathy, tarsus, metatarsus and phalanges

MØ2.271 Postimmunization arthropathy, right ankle and foot

MØ2.272 Postimmunization arthropathy, left ankle and foot

MØ2.279 Postimmunization arthropathy, unspecified ankle and foot

MØ2.28 Postimmunization arthropathy, vertebrae

MØ2.29 Postimmunization arthropathy, multiple sites

✓5th **MØ2.3 Reiter's disease**
Reactive arthritis

MØ2.3Ø Reiter's disease, unspecified site PDx CC CC
CC Excl: AØ2.23, A17.9, A18.Ø2, A18.Ø9, A18.82, A18.84, A18.89, A39.83-A39.84, A54.4Ø, A54.42-A54.43, A54.82, A54.84, A54.89-A54.9, BØ6.82, MØØ.ØØ, MØØ.Ø19, MØØ.Ø29, MØØ.Ø39, MØØ.Ø49, MØØ.Ø59, MØØ.Ø69, MØØ.Ø79, MØØ.Ø8-MØ2.3Ø, MØ2.319, MØ2.329, MØ2.339, MØ2.349, MØ2.359, MØ2.369, MØ2.379-MØ2.9, MØ5.4Ø-MØ5.59, MØ5.7Ø-MØ6.Ø9, MØ6.2Ø-MØ6.39, MØ6.8Ø-MØ7.69, M11.ØØ-M11.9, M12.1Ø-M15.Ø, M15.3-M15.9, M16.2-M16.9, M17.2-M17.9, M18.2-M18.9, M19.111-M19.93, M24.1Ø-M24.176, M25.ØØ, M25.Ø8-M25.18, M25.4Ø-M25.676, M25.8Ø-M25.9, M35.2, M36.1-M36.4, R29.4

✓6th **MØ2.31 Reiter's disease, shoulder**

MØ2.311 Reiter's disease, right shoulder PDx CC CC
CC Excl: See code: MØ2.3Ø

MØ2.312 Reiter's disease, left shoulder PDx CC CC
CC Excl: See code: MØ2.3Ø

MØ2.319 Reiter's disease, unspecified shoulder PDx CC CC
CC Excl: See code: MØ2.3Ø

✓6th **MØ2.32 Reiter's disease, elbow**

MØ2.321 Reiter's disease, right elbow PDx CC CC
CC Excl: See code: MØ2.3Ø

MØ2.322 Reiter's disease, left elbow PDx CC CC
CC Excl: See code: MØ2.3Ø

MØ2.329 Reiter's disease, unspecified elbow PDx CC CC
CC Excl: See code: MØ2.3Ø

✓6th **MØ2.33 Reiter's disease, wrist**
Reiter's disease, carpal bones

MØ2.331 Reiter's disease, right wrist PDx CC CC
CC Excl: See code: MØ2.3Ø

MØ2.332 Reiter's disease, left wrist PDx CC CC
CC Excl: See code: MØ2.3Ø

MØ2.339 Reiter's disease, unspecified wrist PDx CC CC
CC Excl: See code: MØ2.3Ø

✓6th **MØ2.34 Reiter's disease, hand**
Reiter's disease, metacarpus and phalanges

MØ2.341 Reiter's disease, right hand PDx CC CC
CC Excl: See code: MØ2.3Ø

MØ2.342 Reiter's disease, left hand PDx CC CC
CC Excl: See code: MØ2.3Ø

MØ2.349 Reiter's disease, unspecified hand PDx CC CC
CC Excl: See code: MØ2.3Ø

✓6th **MØ2.35 Reiter's disease, hip**

MØ2.351 Reiter's disease, right hip PDx CC CC
CC Excl: See code: MØ2.3Ø

MØ2.352 Reiter's disease, left hip PDx CC CC
CC Excl: See code: MØ2.3Ø

MØ2.359 Reiter's disease, unspecified hip PDx CC CC
CC Excl: See code: MØ2.3Ø

✓6th **MØ2.36 Reiter's disease, knee**

MØ2.361 Reiter's disease, right knee PDx CC CC
CC Excl: See code: MØ2.3Ø

MØ2.362 Reiter's disease, left knee PDx CC CC
CC Excl: See code: MØ2.3Ø

MØ2.369 Reiter's disease, unspecified knee PDx CC CC
CC Excl: See code: MØ2.3Ø

✓6th **MØ2.37 Reiter's disease, ankle and foot**
Reiter's disease, tarsus, metatarsus and phalanges

MØ2.371 Reiter's disease, right ankle and foot PDx CC CC
CC Excl: See code: MØ2.3Ø

MØ2.372 Reiter's disease, left ankle and foot PDx CC CC
CC Excl: See code: MØ2.3Ø

MØ2.379 Reiter's disease, unspecified ankle and foot PDx CC CC
CC Excl: See code: MØ2.3Ø

MØ2.38 Reiter's disease, vertebrae PDx CC CC
CC Excl: See code: MØ2.3Ø

MØ2.39 Reiter's disease, multiple sites PDx CC CC
CC Excl: See code: MØ2.3Ø

✓5th **M02.8 Other reactive arthropathies**

M02.80 Other reactive arthropathies, unspecified site CC
CC Excl: See code: M02.30

✓6th **M02.81 Other reactive arthropathies, shoulder**

M02.811 Other reactive arthropathies, right shoulder CC
CC Excl: A02.23, A17.9, A18.02, A18.09, A18.82, A18.84, A18.89, A39.83-A39.84, A54.40, A54.42-A54.43, A54.82, A54.84, A54.89-A54.9, B06.82, M00.00, M00.019, M00.029, M00.039, M00.049, M00.059, M00.069, M00.079, M00.08-M02.30, M02.319, M02.329, M02.339, M02.349, M02.359, M02.369, M02.379-M02.9, M05.40-M05.59, M05.70-M06.09, M06.20-M06.39, M06.80-M07.69, M11.00-M11.9, M12.10-M12.419

M02.812 Other reactive arthropathies, left shoulder CC
CC Excl: See code: M02.811

M02.819 Other reactive arthropathies, unspecified shoulder CC
CC Excl: See code: M02.811

✓6th **M02.82 Other reactive arthropathies, elbow**

M02.821 Other reactive arthropathies, right elbow CC
CC Excl: A02.23, A17.9, A18.02, A18.09, A18.82, A18.84, A18.89, A39.83-A39.84, A54.40, A54.42-A54.43, A54.82, A54.84, A54.89-A54.9, B06.82, M00.00, M00.019, M00.029, M00.039, M00.049, M00.059, M00.069, M00.079, M00.08-M02.30, M02.319, M02.329, M02.339, M02.349, M02.359, M02.369, M02.379-M02.9, M05.40-M05.59, M05.70-M06.09, M06.20-M06.39, M06.80-M07.69, M11.00-M11.9, M12.10-M15.0, M15.3-M15.9, M16.2-M16.9, M17.2-M17.9, M18.2-M18.9, M19.111-M19.93, M24.10-M24.176, M25.00, M25.08-M25.18, M25.40-M25.676, M25.80-M25.9, M35.2, M36.1-M36.4, R29.4

M02.822 Other reactive arthropathies, left elbow CC
CC Excl: See code: M02.821

M02.829 Other reactive arthropathies, unspecified elbow CC
CC Excl: See code: M02.821

✓6th **M02.83 Other reactive arthropathies, wrist**
Other reactive arthropathies, carpal bones

M02.831 Other reactive arthropathies, right wrist CC
CC Excl: See code: M02.821

M02.832 Other reactive arthropathies, left wrist CC
CC Excl: See code: M02.821

M02.839 Other reactive arthropathies, unspecified wrist CC
CC Excl: See code: M02.821

✓6th **M02.84 Other reactive arthropathies, hand**
Other reactive arthropathies, metacarpus and phalanges

M02.841 Other reactive arthropathies, right hand CC
CC Excl: See code: M02.821

M02.842 Other reactive arthropathies, left hand CC
CC Excl: See code: M02.821

M02.849 Other reactive arthropathies, unspecified hand CC
CC Excl: See code: M02.821

✓6th **M02.85 Other reactive arthropathies, hip**

M02.851 Other reactive arthropathies, right hip CC
CC Excl: See code: M02.821

M02.852 Other reactive arthropathies, left hip CC
CC Excl: See code: M02.821

M02.859 Other reactive arthropathies, unspecified hip CC
CC Excl: See code: M02.821

✓6th **M02.86 Other reactive arthropathies, knee**

M02.861 Other reactive arthropathies, right knee CC
CC Excl: See code: M02.821

M02.862 Other reactive arthropathies, left knee CC
CC Excl: See code: M02.821

M02.869 Other reactive arthropathies, unspecified knee CC
CC Excl: See code: M02.821

✓6th **M02.87 Other reactive arthropathies, ankle and foot**
Other reactive arthropathies, tarsus, metatarsus and phalanges

M02.871 Other reactive arthropathies, right ankle and foot CC
CC Excl: See code: M02.821

M02.872 Other reactive arthropathies, left ankle and foot CC
CC Excl: See code: M02.821

M02.879 Other reactive arthropathies, unspecified ankle and foot CC
CC Excl: See code: M02.821

M02.88 Other reactive arthropathies, vertebrae CC
CC Excl: See code: M02.821

M02.89 Other reactive arthropathies, multiple sites CC
CC Excl: See code: M02.821

M02.9 Reactive arthropathy, unspecified

Inflammatory polyarthropathies (M05-M14)

✓4th **M05 Rheumatoid arthritis with rheumatoid factor**
EXCLUDES 1 *rheumatic fever (I00)*
juvenile rheumatoid arthritis (M08.-)
rheumatoid arthritis of spine (M45.-)

✓5th **M05.0 Felty's syndrome**
Rheumatoid arthritis with splenoadenomegaly and leukopenia

M05.00 Felty's syndrome, unspecified site

✓6th **M05.01 Felty's syndrome, shoulder**

M05.011 Felty's syndrome, right shoulder
M05.012 Felty's syndrome, left shoulder
M05.019 Felty's syndrome, unspecified shoulder

✓6th **M05.02 Felty's syndrome, elbow**

M05.021 Felty's syndrome, right elbow
M05.022 Felty's syndrome, left elbow
M05.029 Felty's syndrome, unspecified elbow

✓6th **M05.03 Felty's syndrome, wrist**
Felty's syndrome, carpal bones

M05.031 Felty's syndrome, right wrist
M05.032 Felty's syndrome, left wrist
M05.039 Felty's syndrome, unspecified wrist

✓6th **M05.04 Felty's syndrome, hand**
Felty's syndrome, metacarpus and phalanges

M05.041 Felty's syndrome, right hand
M05.042 Felty's syndrome, left hand
M05.049 Felty's syndrome, unspecified hand

✓6th **M05.05 Felty's syndrome, hip**

M05.051 Felty's syndrome, right hip
M05.052 Felty's syndrome, left hip
M05.059 Felty's syndrome, unspecified hip

✓6th **M05.06 Felty's syndrome, knee**

M05.061 Felty's syndrome, right knee
M05.062 Felty's syndrome, left knee
M05.069 Felty's syndrome, unspecified knee

✓6th **M05.07 Felty's syndrome, ankle and foot**
Felty's syndrome, tarsus, metatarsus and phalanges

M05.071 Felty's syndrome, right ankle and foot
M05.072 Felty's syndrome, left ankle and foot
M05.079 Felty's syndrome, unspecified ankle and foot

M05.09 Felty's syndrome, multiple sites

✓5th **M05.1 Rheumatoid lung disease with rheumatoid arthritis**

M05.10 Rheumatoid lung disease with rheumatoid arthritis of unspecified site

✓6th **M05.11 Rheumatoid lung disease with rheumatoid arthritis of shoulder**

M05.111 Rheumatoid lung disease with rheumatoid arthritis of right shoulder
M05.112 Rheumatoid lung disease with rheumatoid arthritis of left shoulder

M05.119 Rheumatoid lung disease with rheumatoid arthritis of unspecified shoulder

✓6th M05.12 Rheumatoid lung disease with rheumatoid arthritis of elbow
- M05.121 Rheumatoid lung disease with rheumatoid arthritis of right elbow
- M05.122 Rheumatoid lung disease with rheumatoid arthritis of left elbow
- M05.129 Rheumatoid lung disease with rheumatoid arthritis of unspecified elbow

✓6th M05.13 Rheumatoid lung disease with rheumatoid arthritis of wrist
Rheumatoid lung disease with rheumatoid arthritis, carpal bones
- M05.131 Rheumatoid lung disease with rheumatoid arthritis of right wrist
- M05.132 Rheumatoid lung disease with rheumatoid arthritis of left wrist
- M05.139 Rheumatoid lung disease with rheumatoid arthritis of unspecified wrist

✓6th M05.14 Rheumatoid lung disease with rheumatoid arthritis of hand
Rheumatoid lung disease with rheumatoid arthritis, metacarpus and phalanges
- M05.141 Rheumatoid lung disease with rheumatoid arthritis of right hand
- M05.142 Rheumatoid lung disease with rheumatoid arthritis of left hand
- M05.149 Rheumatoid lung disease with rheumatoid arthritis of unspecified hand

✓6th M05.15 Rheumatoid lung disease with rheumatoid arthritis of hip
- M05.151 Rheumatoid lung disease with rheumatoid arthritis of right hip
- M05.152 Rheumatoid lung disease with rheumatoid arthritis of left hip
- M05.159 Rheumatoid lung disease with rheumatoid arthritis of unspecified hip

✓6th M05.16 Rheumatoid lung disease with rheumatoid arthritis of knee
- M05.161 Rheumatoid lung disease with rheumatoid arthritis of right knee
- M05.162 Rheumatoid lung disease with rheumatoid arthritis of left knee
- M05.169 Rheumatoid lung disease with rheumatoid arthritis of unspecified knee

✓6th M05.17 Rheumatoid lung disease with rheumatoid arthritis of ankle and foot
Rheumatoid lung disease with rheumatoid arthritis, tarsus, metatarsus and phalanges
- M05.171 Rheumatoid lung disease with rheumatoid arthritis of right ankle and foot
- M05.172 Rheumatoid lung disease with rheumatoid arthritis of left ankle and foot
- M05.179 Rheumatoid lung disease with rheumatoid arthritis of unspecified ankle and foot

M05.19 Rheumatoid lung disease with rheumatoid arthritis of multiple sites

✓5th M05.2 Rheumatoid vasculitis with rheumatoid arthritis

M05.20 Rheumatoid vasculitis with rheumatoid arthritis of unspecified site

✓6th M05.21 Rheumatoid vasculitis with rheumatoid arthritis of shoulder
- M05.211 Rheumatoid vasculitis with rheumatoid arthritis of right shoulder
- M05.212 Rheumatoid vasculitis with rheumatoid arthritis of left shoulder
- M05.219 Rheumatoid vasculitis with rheumatoid arthritis of unspecified shoulder

✓6th M05.22 Rheumatoid vasculitis with rheumatoid arthritis of elbow
- M05.221 Rheumatoid vasculitis with rheumatoid arthritis of right elbow
- M05.222 Rheumatoid vasculitis with rheumatoid arthritis of left elbow
- M05.229 Rheumatoid vasculitis with rheumatoid arthritis of unspecified elbow

✓6th M05.23 Rheumatoid vasculitis with rheumatoid arthritis of wrist
Rheumatoid vasculitis with rheumatoid arthritis, carpal bones
- M05.231 Rheumatoid vasculitis with rheumatoid arthritis of right wrist
- M05.232 Rheumatoid vasculitis with rheumatoid arthritis of left wrist
- M05.239 Rheumatoid vasculitis with rheumatoid arthritis of unspecified wrist

✓6th M05.24 Rheumatoid vasculitis with rheumatoid arthritis of hand
Rheumatoid vasculitis with rheumatoid arthritis, metacarpus and phalanges
- M05.241 Rheumatoid vasculitis with rheumatoid arthritis of right hand
- M05.242 Rheumatoid vasculitis with rheumatoid arthritis of left hand
- M05.249 Rheumatoid vasculitis with rheumatoid arthritis of unspecified hand

✓6th M05.25 Rheumatoid vasculitis with rheumatoid arthritis of hip
- M05.251 Rheumatoid vasculitis with rheumatoid arthritis of right hip
- M05.252 Rheumatoid vasculitis with rheumatoid arthritis of left hip
- M05.259 Rheumatoid vasculitis with rheumatoid arthritis of unspecified hip

✓6th M05.26 Rheumatoid vasculitis with rheumatoid arthritis of knee
- M05.261 Rheumatoid vasculitis with rheumatoid arthritis of right knee
- M05.262 Rheumatoid vasculitis with rheumatoid arthritis of left knee
- M05.269 Rheumatoid vasculitis with rheumatoid arthritis of unspecified knee

✓6th M05.27 Rheumatoid vasculitis with rheumatoid arthritis of ankle and foot
Rheumatoid vasculitis with rheumatoid arthritis, tarsus, metatarsus and phalanges
- M05.271 Rheumatoid vasculitis with rheumatoid arthritis of right ankle and foot
- M05.272 Rheumatoid vasculitis with rheumatoid arthritis of left ankle and foot
- M05.279 Rheumatoid vasculitis with rheumatoid arthritis of unspecified ankle and foot

M05.29 Rheumatoid vasculitis with rheumatoid arthritis of multiple sites

✓5th M05.3 Rheumatoid heart disease with rheumatoid arthritis
Rheumatoid carditis
Rheumatoid endocarditis
Rheumatoid myocarditis
Rheumatoid pericarditis

M05.30 Rheumatoid heart disease with rheumatoid arthritis of unspecified site

✓6th M05.31 Rheumatoid heart disease with rheumatoid arthritis of shoulder
- M05.311 Rheumatoid heart disease with rheumatoid arthritis of right shoulder
- M05.312 Rheumatoid heart disease with rheumatoid arthritis of left shoulder
- M05.319 Rheumatoid heart disease with rheumatoid arthritis of unspecified shoulder

✓6th M05.32 Rheumatoid heart disease with rheumatoid arthritis of elbow
- M05.321 Rheumatoid heart disease with rheumatoid arthritis of right elbow
- M05.322 Rheumatoid heart disease with rheumatoid arthritis of left elbow
- M05.329 Rheumatoid heart disease with rheumatoid arthritis of unspecified elbow

✓6th M05.33 Rheumatoid heart disease with rheumatoid arthritis of wrist
Rheumatoid heart disease with rheumatoid arthritis, carpal bones
- M05.331 Rheumatoid heart disease with rheumatoid arthritis of right wrist

M05.332 **Rheumatoid heart disease with rheumatoid arthritis of left wrist**

M05.339 **Rheumatoid heart disease with rheumatoid arthritis of unspecified wrist**

✓6th **M05.34 Rheumatoid heart disease with rheumatoid arthritis of hand**

Rheumatoid heart disease with rheumatoid arthritis, metacarpus and phalanges

M05.341 **Rheumatoid heart disease with rheumatoid arthritis of right hand**

M05.342 **Rheumatoid heart disease with rheumatoid arthritis of left hand**

M05.349 **Rheumatoid heart disease with rheumatoid arthritis of unspecified hand**

✓6th **M05.35 Rheumatoid heart disease with rheumatoid arthritis of hip**

M05.351 **Rheumatoid heart disease with rheumatoid arthritis of right hip**

M05.352 **Rheumatoid heart disease with rheumatoid arthritis of left hip**

M05.359 **Rheumatoid heart disease with rheumatoid arthritis of unspecified hip**

✓6th **M05.36 Rheumatoid heart disease with rheumatoid arthritis of knee**

M05.361 **Rheumatoid heart disease with rheumatoid arthritis of right knee**

M05.362 **Rheumatoid heart disease with rheumatoid arthritis of left knee**

M05.369 **Rheumatoid heart disease with rheumatoid arthritis of unspecified knee**

✓6th **M05.37 Rheumatoid heart disease with rheumatoid arthritis of ankle and foot**

Rheumatoid heart disease with rheumatoid arthritis, tarsus, metatarsus and phalanges

M05.371 **Rheumatoid heart disease with rheumatoid arthritis of right ankle and foot**

M05.372 **Rheumatoid heart disease with rheumatoid arthritis of left ankle and foot**

M05.379 **Rheumatoid heart disease with rheumatoid arthritis of unspecified ankle and foot**

M05.39 **Rheumatoid heart disease with rheumatoid arthritis of multiple sites**

✓5th **M05.4 Rheumatoid myopathy with rheumatoid arthritis**

CC Excl: For all CC codes in subcategory M05.4, unless otherwise noted: E08.40-E08.49, E08.618-E08.638, E08.649-E08.8, E09.40-E09.49, E09.618-E09.638, E09.649-E09.8, E10.40-E10.49, E10.618-E10.638, E10.649, E10.69-E10.8, E11.40-E11.49, E11.618-E11.638, E11.649, E11.69-E11.8, E13.40-E13.49, E13.618-E13.638, E13.649-E13.8, G32.89, G70.00-G72.3, G72.81-G73.7, G96.8-G96.9, G98.0-G98.8, G99.8

M05.40 **Rheumatoid myopathy with rheumatoid arthritis of unspecified site** PDx CC CC

✓6th **M05.41 Rheumatoid myopathy with rheumatoid arthritis of shoulder**

M05.411 **Rheumatoid myopathy with rheumatoid arthritis of right shoulder** PDx CC CC

M05.412 **Rheumatoid myopathy with rheumatoid arthritis of left shoulder** PDx CC CC

M05.419 **Rheumatoid myopathy with rheumatoid arthritis of unspecified shoulder** PDx CC CC

✓6th **M05.42 Rheumatoid myopathy with rheumatoid arthritis of elbow**

M05.421 **Rheumatoid myopathy with rheumatoid arthritis of right elbow** PDx CC CC

M05.422 **Rheumatoid myopathy with rheumatoid arthritis of left elbow** PDx CC CC

M05.429 **Rheumatoid myopathy with rheumatoid arthritis of unspecified elbow** PDx CC CC

✓6th **M05.43 Rheumatoid myopathy with rheumatoid arthritis of wrist**

Rheumatoid myopathy with rheumatoid arthritis, carpal bones

M05.431 **Rheumatoid myopathy with rheumatoid arthritis of right wrist** PDx CC CC

M05.432 **Rheumatoid myopathy with rheumatoid arthritis of left wrist** PDx CC CC

M05.439 **Rheumatoid myopathy with rheumatoid arthritis of unspecified wrist** PDx CC CC

✓6th **M05.44 Rheumatoid myopathy with rheumatoid arthritis of hand**

Rheumatoid myopathy with rheumatoid arthritis, metacarpus and phalanges

M05.441 **Rheumatoid myopathy with rheumatoid arthritis of right hand** PDx CC CC

M05.442 **Rheumatoid myopathy with rheumatoid arthritis of left hand** PDx CC CC

M05.449 **Rheumatoid myopathy with rheumatoid arthritis of unspecified hand** PDx CC CC

✓6th **M05.45 Rheumatoid myopathy with rheumatoid arthritis of hip**

M05.451 **Rheumatoid myopathy with rheumatoid arthritis of right hip** PDx CC CC

M05.452 **Rheumatoid myopathy with rheumatoid arthritis of left hip** PDx CC CC

M05.459 **Rheumatoid myopathy with rheumatoid arthritis of unspecified hip** PDx CC CC

✓6th **M05.46 Rheumatoid myopathy with rheumatoid arthritis of knee**

M05.461 **Rheumatoid myopathy with rheumatoid arthritis of right knee** PDx CC CC

M05.462 **Rheumatoid myopathy with rheumatoid arthritis of left knee** PDx CC CC

M05.469 **Rheumatoid myopathy with rheumatoid arthritis of unspecified knee** PDx CC CC

✓6th **M05.47 Rheumatoid myopathy with rheumatoid arthritis of ankle and foot**

Rheumatoid myopathy with rheumatoid arthritis, tarsus, metatarsus and phalanges

M05.471 **Rheumatoid myopathy with rheumatoid arthritis of right ankle and foot** PDx CC CC

M05.472 **Rheumatoid myopathy with rheumatoid arthritis of left ankle and foot** PDx CC CC

M05.479 **Rheumatoid myopathy with rheumatoid arthritis of unspecified ankle and foot** PDx CC CC

M05.49 **Rheumatoid myopathy with rheumatoid arthritis of multiple sites** PDx CC CC

✓5th **M05.5 Rheumatoid polyneuropathy with rheumatoid arthritis**

M05.50 **Rheumatoid polyneuropathy with rheumatoid arthritis of unspecified site**

✓6th **M05.51 Rheumatoid polyneuropathy with rheumatoid arthritis of shoulder**

M05.511 **Rheumatoid polyneuropathy with rheumatoid arthritis of right shoulder**

M05.512 **Rheumatoid polyneuropathy with rheumatoid arthritis of left shoulder**

M05.519 **Rheumatoid polyneuropathy with rheumatoid arthritis of unspecified shoulder**

✓6th **M05.52 Rheumatoid polyneuropathy with rheumatoid arthritis of elbow**

M05.521 **Rheumatoid polyneuropathy with rheumatoid arthritis of right elbow**

M05.522 **Rheumatoid polyneuropathy with rheumatoid arthritis of left elbow**

M05.529 **Rheumatoid polyneuropathy with rheumatoid arthritis of unspecified elbow**

✓6th **M05.53 Rheumatoid polyneuropathy with rheumatoid arthritis of wrist**

Rheumatoid polyneuropathy with rheumatoid arthritis, carpal bones

M05.531 **Rheumatoid polyneuropathy with rheumatoid arthritis of right wrist**

M05.532 **Rheumatoid polyneuropathy with rheumatoid arthritis of left wrist**

M05.539 **Rheumatoid polyneuropathy with rheumatoid arthritis of unspecified wrist**

√6th **MØ5.54 Rheumatoid polyneuropathy with rheumatoid arthritis of hand**
Rheumatoid polyneuropathy with rheumatoid arthritis, metacarpus and phalanges
MØ5.541 Rheumatoid polyneuropathy with rheumatoid arthritis of right hand
MØ5.542 Rheumatoid polyneuropathy with rheumatoid arthritis of left hand
MØ5.549 Rheumatoid polyneuropathy with rheumatoid arthritis of unspecified hand

√6th **MØ5.55 Rheumatoid polyneuropathy with rheumatoid arthritis of hip**
MØ5.551 Rheumatoid polyneuropathy with rheumatoid arthritis of right hip
MØ5.552 Rheumatoid polyneuropathy with rheumatoid arthritis of left hip
MØ5.559 Rheumatoid polyneuropathy with rheumatoid arthritis of unspecified hip

√6th **MØ5.56 Rheumatoid polyneuropathy with rheumatoid arthritis of knee**
MØ5.561 Rheumatoid polyneuropathy with rheumatoid arthritis of right knee
MØ5.562 Rheumatoid polyneuropathy with rheumatoid arthritis of left knee
MØ5.569 Rheumatoid polyneuropathy with rheumatoid arthritis of unspecified knee

√6th **MØ5.57 Rheumatoid polyneuropathy with rheumatoid arthritis of ankle and foot**
Rheumatoid polyneuropathy with rheumatoid arthritis, tarsus, metatarsus and phalanges
MØ5.571 Rheumatoid polyneuropathy with rheumatoid arthritis of right ankle and foot
MØ5.572 Rheumatoid polyneuropathy with rheumatoid arthritis of left ankle and foot
MØ5.579 Rheumatoid polyneuropathy with rheumatoid arthritis of unspecified ankle and foot

MØ5.59 Rheumatoid polyneuropathy with rheumatoid arthritis of multiple sites

√5th **MØ5.6 Rheumatoid arthritis with involvement of other organs and systems**
MØ5.6Ø Rheumatoid arthritis of unspecified site with involvement of other organs and systems

√6th **MØ5.61 Rheumatoid arthritis of shoulder with involvement of other organs and systems**
MØ5.611 Rheumatoid arthritis of right shoulder with involvement of other organs and systems
MØ5.612 Rheumatoid arthritis of left shoulder with involvement of other organs and systems
MØ5.619 Rheumatoid arthritis of unspecified shoulder with involvement of other organs and systems

√6th **MØ5.62 Rheumatoid arthritis of elbow with involvement of other organs and systems**
MØ5.621 Rheumatoid arthritis of right elbow with involvement of other organs and systems
MØ5.622 Rheumatoid arthritis of left elbow with involvement of other organs and systems
MØ5.629 Rheumatoid arthritis of unspecified elbow with involvement of other organs and systems

√6th **MØ5.63 Rheumatoid arthritis of wrist with involvement of other organs and systems**
Rheumatoid arthritis of carpal bones with involvement of other organs and systems
MØ5.631 Rheumatoid arthritis of right wrist with involvement of other organs and systems
MØ5.632 Rheumatoid arthritis of left wrist with involvement of other organs and systems
MØ5.639 Rheumatoid arthritis of unspecified wrist with involvement of other organs and systems

√6th **MØ5.64 Rheumatoid arthritis of hand with involvement of other organs and systems**
Rheumatoid arthritis of metacarpus and phalanges with involvement of other organs and systems
MØ5.641 Rheumatoid arthritis of right hand with involvement of other organs and systems
MØ5.642 Rheumatoid arthritis of left hand with involvement of other organs and systems
MØ5.649 Rheumatoid arthritis of unspecified hand with involvement of other organs and systems

√6th **MØ5.65 Rheumatoid arthritis of hip with involvement of other organs and systems**
MØ5.651 Rheumatoid arthritis of right hip with involvement of other organs and systems
MØ5.652 Rheumatoid arthritis of left hip with involvement of other organs and systems
MØ5.659 Rheumatoid arthritis of unspecified hip with involvement of other organs and systems

√6th **MØ5.66 Rheumatoid arthritis of knee with involvement of other organs and systems**
MØ5.661 Rheumatoid arthritis of right knee with involvement of other organs and systems
MØ5.662 Rheumatoid arthritis of left knee with involvement of other organs and systems
MØ5.669 Rheumatoid arthritis of unspecified knee with involvement of other organs and systems

√6th **MØ5.67 Rheumatoid arthritis of ankle and foot with involvement of other organs and systems**
Rheumatoid arthritis of tarsus, metatarsus and phalanges with involvement of other organs and systems
MØ5.671 Rheumatoid arthritis of right ankle and foot with involvement of other organs and systems
MØ5.672 Rheumatoid arthritis of left ankle and foot with involvement of other organs and systems
MØ5.679 Rheumatoid arthritis of unspecified ankle and foot with involvement of other organs and systems

MØ5.69 Rheumatoid arthritis of multiple sites with involvement of other organs and systems

√5th **MØ5.7 Rheumatoid arthritis with rheumatoid factor without organ or systems involvement**
MØ5.7Ø Rheumatoid arthritis with rheumatoid factor of unspecified site without organ or systems involvement

√6th **MØ5.71 Rheumatoid arthritis with rheumatoid factor of shoulder without organ or systems involvement**
MØ5.711 Rheumatoid arthritis with rheumatoid factor of right shoulder without organ or systems involvement
MØ5.712 Rheumatoid arthritis with rheumatoid factor of left shoulder without organ or systems involvement
MØ5.719 Rheumatoid arthritis with rheumatoid factor of unspecified shoulder without organ or systems involvement

√6th **MØ5.72 Rheumatoid arthritis with rheumatoid factor of elbow without organ or systems involvement**
MØ5.721 Rheumatoid arthritis with rheumatoid factor of right elbow without organ or systems involvement
MØ5.722 Rheumatoid arthritis with rheumatoid factor of left elbow without organ or systems involvement
MØ5.729 Rheumatoid arthritis with rheumatoid factor of unspecified elbow without organ or systems involvement

√6th **MØ5.73 Rheumatoid arthritis with rheumatoid factor of wrist without organ or systems involvement**
MØ5.731 Rheumatoid arthritis with rheumatoid factor of right wrist without organ or systems involvement
MØ5.732 Rheumatoid arthritis with rheumatoid factor of left wrist without organ or systems involvement

M05.739 Rheumatoid arthritis with rheumatoid factor of unspecified wrist without organ or systems involvement

✓6th M05.74 Rheumatoid arthritis with rheumatoid factor of hand without organ or systems involvement
M05.741 Rheumatoid arthritis with rheumatoid factor of right hand without organ or systems involvement
M05.742 Rheumatoid arthritis with rheumatoid factor of left hand without organ or systems involvement
M05.749 Rheumatoid arthritis with rheumatoid factor of unspecified hand without organ or systems involvement

✓6th M05.75 Rheumatoid arthritis with rheumatoid factor of hip without organ or systems involvement
M05.751 Rheumatoid arthritis with rheumatoid factor of right hip without organ or systems involvement
M05.752 Rheumatoid arthritis with rheumatoid factor of left hip without organ or systems involvement
M05.759 Rheumatoid arthritis with rheumatoid factor of unspecified hip without organ or systems involvement

✓6th M05.76 Rheumatoid arthritis with rheumatoid factor of knee without organ or systems involvement
M05.761 Rheumatoid arthritis with rheumatoid factor of right knee without organ or systems involvement
M05.762 Rheumatoid arthritis with rheumatoid factor of left knee without organ or systems involvement
M05.769 Rheumatoid arthritis with rheumatoid factor of unspecified knee without organ or systems involvement

✓6th M05.77 Rheumatoid arthritis with rheumatoid factor of ankle and foot without organ or systems involvement
M05.771 Rheumatoid arthritis with rheumatoid factor of right ankle and foot without organ or systems involvement
M05.772 Rheumatoid arthritis with rheumatoid factor of left ankle and foot without organ or systems involvement
M05.779 Rheumatoid arthritis with rheumatoid factor of unspecified ankle and foot without organ or systems involvement

M05.79 Rheumatoid arthritis with rheumatoid factor of multiple sites without organ or systems involvement

✓5th M05.8 Other rheumatoid arthritis with rheumatoid factor
M05.80 Other rheumatoid arthritis with rheumatoid factor of unspecified site

✓6th M05.81 Other rheumatoid arthritis with rheumatoid factor of shoulder
M05.811 Other rheumatoid arthritis with rheumatoid factor of right shoulder
M05.812 Other rheumatoid arthritis with rheumatoid factor of left shoulder
M05.819 Other rheumatoid arthritis with rheumatoid factor of unspecified shoulder

✓6th M05.82 Other rheumatoid arthritis with rheumatoid factor of elbow
M05.821 Other rheumatoid arthritis with rheumatoid factor of right elbow
M05.822 Other rheumatoid arthritis with rheumatoid factor of left elbow
M05.829 Other rheumatoid arthritis with rheumatoid factor of unspecified elbow

✓6th M05.83 Other rheumatoid arthritis with rheumatoid factor of wrist
M05.831 Other rheumatoid arthritis with rheumatoid factor of right wrist
M05.832 Other rheumatoid arthritis with rheumatoid factor of left wrist
M05.839 Other rheumatoid arthritis with rheumatoid factor of unspecified wrist

✓6th M05.84 Other rheumatoid arthritis with rheumatoid factor of hand
M05.841 Other rheumatoid arthritis with rheumatoid factor of right hand
M05.842 Other rheumatoid arthritis with rheumatoid factor of left hand
M05.849 Other rheumatoid arthritis with rheumatoid factor of unspecified hand

✓6th M05.85 Other rheumatoid arthritis with rheumatoid factor of hip
M05.851 Other rheumatoid arthritis with rheumatoid factor of right hip
M05.852 Other rheumatoid arthritis with rheumatoid factor of left hip
M05.859 Other rheumatoid arthritis with rheumatoid factor of unspecified hip

✓6th M05.86 Other rheumatoid arthritis with rheumatoid factor of knee
M05.861 Other rheumatoid arthritis with rheumatoid factor of right knee
M05.862 Other rheumatoid arthritis with rheumatoid factor of left knee
M05.869 Other rheumatoid arthritis with rheumatoid factor of unspecified knee

✓6th M05.87 Other rheumatoid arthritis with rheumatoid factor of ankle and foot
M05.871 Other rheumatoid arthritis with rheumatoid factor of right ankle and foot
M05.872 Other rheumatoid arthritis with rheumatoid factor of left ankle and foot
M05.879 Other rheumatoid arthritis with rheumatoid factor of unspecified ankle and foot

M05.89 Other rheumatoid arthritis with rheumatoid factor of multiple sites

M05.9 Rheumatoid arthritis with rheumatoid factor, unspecified

✓4th **M06 Other rheumatoid arthritis**

✓5th M06.0 Rheumatoid arthritis without rheumatoid factor
M06.00 Rheumatoid arthritis without rheumatoid factor, unspecified site

✓6th M06.01 Rheumatoid arthritis without rheumatoid factor, shoulder
M06.011 Rheumatoid arthritis without rheumatoid factor, right shoulder
M06.012 Rheumatoid arthritis without rheumatoid factor, left shoulder
M06.019 Rheumatoid arthritis without rheumatoid factor, unspecified shoulder

✓6th M06.02 Rheumatoid arthritis without rheumatoid factor, elbow
M06.021 Rheumatoid arthritis without rheumatoid factor, right elbow
M06.022 Rheumatoid arthritis without rheumatoid factor, left elbow
M06.029 Rheumatoid arthritis without rheumatoid factor, unspecified elbow

✓6th M06.03 Rheumatoid arthritis without rheumatoid factor, wrist
M06.031 Rheumatoid arthritis without rheumatoid factor, right wrist
M06.032 Rheumatoid arthritis without rheumatoid factor, left wrist
M06.039 Rheumatoid arthritis without rheumatoid factor, unspecified wrist

✓6th M06.04 Rheumatoid arthritis without rheumatoid factor, hand
M06.041 Rheumatoid arthritis without rheumatoid factor, right hand
M06.042 Rheumatoid arthritis without rheumatoid factor, left hand
M06.049 Rheumatoid arthritis without rheumatoid factor, unspecified hand

✓6th M06.05 Rheumatoid arthritis without rheumatoid factor, hip
M06.051 Rheumatoid arthritis without rheumatoid factor, right hip
M06.052 Rheumatoid arthritis without rheumatoid factor, left hip

MØ6.Ø59 Rheumatoid arthritis without rheumatoid factor, unspecified hip

✓6th **MØ6.Ø6** Rheumatoid arthritis without rheumatoid factor, knee

MØ6.Ø61 Rheumatoid arthritis without rheumatoid factor, right knee

MØ6.Ø62 Rheumatoid arthritis without rheumatoid factor, left knee

MØ6.Ø69 Rheumatoid arthritis without rheumatoid factor, unspecified knee

✓6th **MØ6.Ø7** Rheumatoid arthritis without rheumatoid factor, ankle and foot

MØ6.Ø71 Rheumatoid arthritis without rheumatoid factor, right ankle and foot

MØ6.Ø72 Rheumatoid arthritis without rheumatoid factor, left ankle and foot

MØ6.Ø79 Rheumatoid arthritis without rheumatoid factor, unspecified ankle and foot

MØ6.Ø8 Rheumatoid arthritis without rheumatoid factor, vertebrae

MØ6.Ø9 Rheumatoid arthritis without rheumatoid factor, multiple sites

MØ6.1 Adult-onset Still's disease A

EXCLUDES 1 *Still's disease NOS (MØ8.2-)*

✓5th **MØ6.2** Rheumatoid bursitis

MØ6.2Ø Rheumatoid bursitis, unspecified site

✓6th **MØ6.21** Rheumatoid bursitis, shoulder

MØ6.211 Rheumatoid bursitis, right shoulder

MØ6.212 Rheumatoid bursitis, left shoulder

MØ6.219 Rheumatoid bursitis, unspecified shoulder

✓6th **MØ6.22** Rheumatoid bursitis, elbow

MØ6.221 Rheumatoid bursitis, right elbow

MØ6.222 Rheumatoid bursitis, left elbow

MØ6.229 Rheumatoid bursitis, unspecified elbow

✓6th **MØ6.23** Rheumatoid bursitis, wrist

MØ6.231 Rheumatoid bursitis, right wrist

MØ6.232 Rheumatoid bursitis, left wrist

MØ6.239 Rheumatoid bursitis, unspecified wrist

✓6th **MØ6.24** Rheumatoid bursitis, hand

MØ6.241 Rheumatoid bursitis, right hand

MØ6.242 Rheumatoid bursitis, left hand

MØ6.249 Rheumatoid bursitis, unspecified hand

✓6th **MØ6.25** Rheumatoid bursitis, hip

MØ6.251 Rheumatoid bursitis, right hip

MØ6.252 Rheumatoid bursitis, left hip

MØ6.259 Rheumatoid bursitis, unspecified hip

✓6th **MØ6.26** Rheumatoid bursitis, knee

MØ6.261 Rheumatoid bursitis, right knee

MØ6.262 Rheumatoid bursitis, left knee

MØ6.269 Rheumatoid bursitis, unspecified knee

✓6th **MØ6.27** Rheumatoid bursitis, ankle and foot

MØ6.271 Rheumatoid bursitis, right ankle and foot

MØ6.272 Rheumatoid bursitis, left ankle and foot

MØ6.279 Rheumatoid bursitis, unspecified ankle and foot

MØ6.28 Rheumatoid bursitis, vertebrae

MØ6.29 Rheumatoid bursitis, multiple sites

✓5th **MØ6.3** Rheumatoid nodule

MØ6.3Ø Rheumatoid nodule, unspecified site

✓6th **MØ6.31** Rheumatoid nodule, shoulder

MØ6.311 Rheumatoid nodule, right shoulder

MØ6.312 Rheumatoid nodule, left shoulder

MØ6.319 Rheumatoid nodule, unspecified shoulder

✓6th **MØ6.32** Rheumatoid nodule, elbow

MØ6.321 Rheumatoid nodule, right elbow

MØ6.322 Rheumatoid nodule, left elbow

MØ6.329 Rheumatoid nodule, unspecified elbow

✓6th **MØ6.33** Rheumatoid nodule, wrist

MØ6.331 Rheumatoid nodule, right wrist

MØ6.332 Rheumatoid nodule, left wrist

MØ6.339 Rheumatoid nodule, unspecified wrist

✓6th **MØ6.34** Rheumatoid nodule, hand

MØ6.341 Rheumatoid nodule, right hand

MØ6.342 Rheumatoid nodule, left hand

MØ6.349 Rheumatoid nodule, unspecified hand

✓6th **MØ6.35** Rheumatoid nodule, hip

MØ6.351 Rheumatoid nodule, right hip

MØ6.352 Rheumatoid nodule, left hip

MØ6.359 Rheumatoid nodule, unspecified hip

✓6th **MØ6.36** Rheumatoid nodule, knee

MØ6.361 Rheumatoid nodule, right knee

MØ6.362 Rheumatoid nodule, left knee

MØ6.369 Rheumatoid nodule, unspecified knee

✓6th **MØ6.37** Rheumatoid nodule, ankle and foot

MØ6.371 Rheumatoid nodule, right ankle and foot

MØ6.372 Rheumatoid nodule, left ankle and foot

MØ6.379 Rheumatoid nodule, unspecified ankle and foot

MØ6.38 Rheumatoid nodule, vertebrae

MØ6.39 Rheumatoid nodule, multiple sites

MØ6.4 Inflammatory polyarthropathy

EXCLUDES 1 *polyarthritis NOS (M13.Ø)*

✓5th **MØ6.8** Other specified rheumatoid arthritis

MØ6.8Ø Other specified rheumatoid arthritis, unspecified site

✓6th **MØ6.81** Other specified rheumatoid arthritis, shoulder

MØ6.811 Other specified rheumatoid arthritis, right shoulder

MØ6.812 Other specified rheumatoid arthritis, left shoulder

MØ6.819 Other specified rheumatoid arthritis, unspecified shoulder

✓6th **MØ6.82** Other specified rheumatoid arthritis, elbow

MØ6.821 Other specified rheumatoid arthritis, right elbow

MØ6.822 Other specified rheumatoid arthritis, left elbow

MØ6.829 Other specified rheumatoid arthritis, unspecified elbow

✓6th **MØ6.83** Other specified rheumatoid arthritis, wrist

MØ6.831 Other specified rheumatoid arthritis, right wrist

MØ6.832 Other specified rheumatoid arthritis, left wrist

MØ6.839 Other specified rheumatoid arthritis, unspecified wrist

✓6th **MØ6.84** Other specified rheumatoid arthritis, hand

MØ6.841 Other specified rheumatoid arthritis, right hand

MØ6.842 Other specified rheumatoid arthritis, left hand

MØ6.849 Other specified rheumatoid arthritis, unspecified hand

✓6th **MØ6.85** Other specified rheumatoid arthritis, hip

MØ6.851 Other specified rheumatoid arthritis, right hip

MØ6.852 Other specified rheumatoid arthritis, left hip

MØ6.859 Other specified rheumatoid arthritis, unspecified hip

✓6th **MØ6.86** Other specified rheumatoid arthritis, knee

MØ6.861 Other specified rheumatoid arthritis, right knee

MØ6.862 Other specified rheumatoid arthritis, left knee

MØ6.869 Other specified rheumatoid arthritis, unspecified knee

✓6th **MØ6.87** Other specified rheumatoid arthritis, ankle and foot

MØ6.871 Other specified rheumatoid arthritis, right ankle and foot

MØ6.872 Other specified rheumatoid arthritis, left ankle and foot

MØ6.879 Other specified rheumatoid arthritis, unspecified ankle and foot

MØ6.88 Other specified rheumatoid arthritis, vertebrae

MØ6.89 Other specified rheumatoid arthritis, multiple sites

MØ6.9 Rheumatoid arthritis, unspecified

M07 Enteropathic arthropathies
Code also associated enteropathy, such as:
regional enteritis [Crohn's disease] (K50.-)
ulcerative colitis (K51.-)
EXCLUDES 1 *psoriatic arthropathies (L40.5-)*

M07.6 Enteropathic arthropathies
M07.60 Enteropathic arthropathies, unspecified site
M07.61 Enteropathic arthropathies, shoulder
M07.611 Enteropathic arthropathies, right shoulder
M07.612 Enteropathic arthropathies, left shoulder
M07.619 Enteropathic arthropathies, unspecified shoulder
M07.62 Enteropathic arthropathies, elbow
M07.621 Enteropathic arthropathies, right elbow
M07.622 Enteropathic arthropathies, left elbow
M07.629 Enteropathic arthropathies, unspecified elbow
M07.63 Enteropathic arthropathies, wrist
M07.631 Enteropathic arthropathies, right wrist
M07.632 Enteropathic arthropathies, left wrist
M07.639 Enteropathic arthropathies, unspecified wrist
M07.64 Enteropathic arthropathies, hand
M07.641 Enteropathic arthropathies, right hand
M07.642 Enteropathic arthropathies, left hand
M07.649 Enteropathic arthropathies, unspecified hand
M07.65 Enteropathic arthropathies, hip
M07.651 Enteropathic arthropathies, right hip
M07.652 Enteropathic arthropathies, left hip
M07.659 Enteropathic arthropathies, unspecified hip
M07.66 Enteropathic arthropathies, knee
M07.661 Enteropathic arthropathies, right knee
M07.662 Enteropathic arthropathies, left knee
M07.669 Enteropathic arthropathies, unspecified knee
M07.67 Enteropathic arthropathies, ankle and foot
M07.671 Enteropathic arthropathies, right ankle and foot
M07.672 Enteropathic arthropathies, left ankle and foot
M07.679 Enteropathic arthropathies, unspecified ankle and foot
M07.68 Enteropathic arthropathies, vertebrae
M07.69 Enteropathic arthropathies, multiple sites

M08 Juvenile arthritis
Code also any associated underlying condition, such as:
regional enteritis [Crohn's disease] (K50.-)
ulcerative colitis (K51.-)
EXCLUDES 1 *arthropathy in Whipple's disease (M14.8)*
Felty's syndrome (M05.0)
juvenile dermatomyositis (M33.0-)
psoriatic juvenile arthropathy (L40.54)

M08.0 Unspecified juvenile rheumatoid arthritis
Juvenile rheumatoid arthritis with or without rheumatoid factor
M08.00 Unspecified juvenile rheumatoid arthritis of unspecified site
M08.01 Unspecified juvenile rheumatoid arthritis, shoulder
M08.011 Unspecified juvenile rheumatoid arthritis, right shoulder
M08.012 Unspecified juvenile rheumatoid arthritis, left shoulder
M08.019 Unspecified juvenile rheumatoid arthritis, unspecified shoulder
M08.02 Unspecified juvenile rheumatoid arthritis of elbow
M08.021 Unspecified juvenile rheumatoid arthritis, right elbow
M08.022 Unspecified juvenile rheumatoid arthritis, left elbow
M08.029 Unspecified juvenile rheumatoid arthritis, unspecified elbow
M08.03 Unspecified juvenile rheumatoid arthritis, wrist
M08.031 Unspecified juvenile rheumatoid arthritis, right wrist
M08.032 Unspecified juvenile rheumatoid arthritis, left wrist
M08.039 Unspecified juvenile rheumatoid arthritis, unspecified wrist
M08.04 Unspecified juvenile rheumatoid arthritis, hand
M08.041 Unspecified juvenile rheumatoid arthritis, right hand
M08.042 Unspecified juvenile rheumatoid arthritis, left hand
M08.049 Unspecified juvenile rheumatoid arthritis, unspecified hand
M08.05 Unspecified juvenile rheumatoid arthritis, hip
M08.051 Unspecified juvenile rheumatoid arthritis, right hip
M08.052 Unspecified juvenile rheumatoid arthritis, left hip
M08.059 Unspecified juvenile rheumatoid arthritis, unspecified hip
M08.06 Unspecified juvenile rheumatoid arthritis, knee
M08.061 Unspecified juvenile rheumatoid arthritis, right knee
M08.062 Unspecified juvenile rheumatoid arthritis, left knee
M08.069 Unspecified juvenile rheumatoid arthritis, unspecified knee
M08.07 Unspecified juvenile rheumatoid arthritis, ankle and foot
M08.071 Unspecified juvenile rheumatoid arthritis, right ankle and foot
M08.072 Unspecified juvenile rheumatoid arthritis, left ankle and foot
M08.079 Unspecified juvenile rheumatoid arthritis, unspecified ankle and foot
M08.08 Unspecified juvenile rheumatoid arthritis, vertebrae
M08.09 Unspecified juvenile rheumatoid arthritis, multiple sites

M08.1 Juvenile ankylosing spondylitis
EXCLUDES 1 *ankylosing spondylitis in adults (M45.0-)*

M08.2 Juvenile rheumatoid arthritis with systemic onset
Still's disease NOS
EXCLUDES 1 *adult-onset Still's disease (M06.1-)*
M08.20 Juvenile rheumatoid arthritis with systemic onset, unspecified site
M08.21 Juvenile rheumatoid arthritis with systemic onset, shoulder
M08.211 Juvenile rheumatoid arthritis with systemic onset, right shoulder
M08.212 Juvenile rheumatoid arthritis with systemic onset, left shoulder
M08.219 Juvenile rheumatoid arthritis with systemic onset, unspecified shoulder
M08.22 Juvenile rheumatoid arthritis with systemic onset, elbow
M08.221 Juvenile rheumatoid arthritis with systemic onset, right elbow
M08.222 Juvenile rheumatoid arthritis with systemic onset, left elbow
M08.229 Juvenile rheumatoid arthritis with systemic onset, unspecified elbow
M08.23 Juvenile rheumatoid arthritis with systemic onset, wrist
M08.231 Juvenile rheumatoid arthritis with systemic onset, right wrist
M08.232 Juvenile rheumatoid arthritis with systemic onset, left wrist
M08.239 Juvenile rheumatoid arthritis with systemic onset, unspecified wrist
M08.24 Juvenile rheumatoid arthritis with systemic onset, hand
M08.241 Juvenile rheumatoid arthritis with systemic onset, right hand
M08.242 Juvenile rheumatoid arthritis with systemic onset, left hand

MØ8.249 Juvenile rheumatoid arthritis with systemic onset, unspecified hand

✓6th MØ8.25 Juvenile rheumatoid arthritis with systemic onset, hip

MØ8.251 Juvenile rheumatoid arthritis with systemic onset, right hip

MØ8.252 Juvenile rheumatoid arthritis with systemic onset, left hip

MØ8.259 Juvenile rheumatoid arthritis with systemic onset, unspecified hip

✓6th MØ8.26 Juvenile rheumatoid arthritis with systemic onset, knee

MØ8.261 Juvenile rheumatoid arthritis with systemic onset, right knee

MØ8.262 Juvenile rheumatoid arthritis with systemic onset, left knee

MØ8.269 Juvenile rheumatoid arthritis with systemic onset, unspecified knee

✓6th MØ8.27 Juvenile rheumatoid arthritis with systemic onset, ankle and foot

MØ8.271 Juvenile rheumatoid arthritis with systemic onset, right ankle and foot

MØ8.272 Juvenile rheumatoid arthritis with systemic onset, left ankle and foot

MØ8.279 Juvenile rheumatoid arthritis with systemic onset, unspecified ankle and foot

MØ8.28 Juvenile rheumatoid arthritis with systemic onset, vertebrae

MØ8.29 Juvenile rheumatoid arthritis with systemic onset, multiple sites

MØ8.3 Juvenile rheumatoid polyarthritis (seronegative)

✓5th MØ8.4 Pauciarticular juvenile rheumatoid arthritis

MØ8.40 Pauciarticular juvenile rheumatoid arthritis, unspecified site

✓6th MØ8.41 Pauciarticular juvenile rheumatoid arthritis, shoulder

MØ8.411 Pauciarticular juvenile rheumatoid arthritis, right shoulder

MØ8.412 Pauciarticular juvenile rheumatoid arthritis, left shoulder

MØ8.419 Pauciarticular juvenile rheumatoid arthritis, unspecified shoulder

✓6th MØ8.42 Pauciarticular juvenile rheumatoid arthritis, elbow

MØ8.421 Pauciarticular juvenile rheumatoid arthritis, right elbow

MØ8.422 Pauciarticular juvenile rheumatoid arthritis, left elbow

MØ8.429 Pauciarticular juvenile rheumatoid arthritis, unspecified elbow

✓6th MØ8.43 Pauciarticular juvenile rheumatoid arthritis, wrist

MØ8.431 Pauciarticular juvenile rheumatoid arthritis, right wrist

MØ8.432 Pauciarticular juvenile rheumatoid arthritis, left wrist

MØ8.439 Pauciarticular juvenile rheumatoid arthritis, unspecified wrist

✓6th MØ8.44 Pauciarticular juvenile rheumatoid arthritis, hand

MØ8.441 Pauciarticular juvenile rheumatoid arthritis, right hand

MØ8.442 Pauciarticular juvenile rheumatoid arthritis, left hand

MØ8.449 Pauciarticular juvenile rheumatoid arthritis, unspecified hand

✓6th MØ8.45 Pauciarticular juvenile rheumatoid arthritis, hip

MØ8.451 Pauciarticular juvenile rheumatoid arthritis, right hip

MØ8.452 Pauciarticular juvenile rheumatoid arthritis, left hip

MØ8.459 Pauciarticular juvenile rheumatoid arthritis, unspecified hip

✓6th MØ8.46 Pauciarticular juvenile rheumatoid arthritis, knee

MØ8.461 Pauciarticular juvenile rheumatoid arthritis, right knee

MØ8.462 Pauciarticular juvenile rheumatoid arthritis, left knee

MØ8.469 Pauciarticular juvenile rheumatoid arthritis, unspecified knee

✓6th MØ8.47 Pauciarticular juvenile rheumatoid arthritis, ankle and foot

MØ8.471 Pauciarticular juvenile rheumatoid arthritis, right ankle and foot

MØ8.472 Pauciarticular juvenile rheumatoid arthritis, left ankle and foot

MØ8.479 Pauciarticular juvenile rheumatoid arthritis, unspecified ankle and foot

MØ8.48 Pauciarticular juvenile rheumatoid arthritis, vertebrae

✓5th MØ8.8 Other juvenile arthritis

MØ8.80 Other juvenile arthritis, unspecified site

✓6th MØ8.81 Other juvenile arthritis, shoulder

MØ8.811 Other juvenile arthritis, right shoulder

MØ8.812 Other juvenile arthritis, left shoulder

MØ8.819 Other juvenile arthritis, unspecified shoulder

✓6th MØ8.82 Other juvenile arthritis, elbow

MØ8.821 Other juvenile arthritis, right elbow

MØ8.822 Other juvenile arthritis, left elbow

MØ8.829 Other juvenile arthritis, unspecified elbow

✓6th MØ8.83 Other juvenile arthritis, wrist

MØ8.831 Other juvenile arthritis, right wrist

MØ8.832 Other juvenile arthritis, left wrist

MØ8.839 Other juvenile arthritis, unspecified wrist

✓6th MØ8.84 Other juvenile arthritis, hand

MØ8.841 Other juvenile arthritis, right hand

MØ8.842 Other juvenile arthritis, left hand

MØ8.849 Other juvenile arthritis, unspecified hand

✓6th MØ8.85 Other juvenile arthritis, hip

MØ8.851 Other juvenile arthritis, right hip

MØ8.852 Other juvenile arthritis, left hip

MØ8.859 Other juvenile arthritis, unspecified hip

✓6th MØ8.86 Other juvenile arthritis, knee

MØ8.861 Other juvenile arthritis, right knee

MØ8.862 Other juvenile arthritis, left knee

MØ8.869 Other juvenile arthritis, unspecified knee

✓6th MØ8.87 Other juvenile arthritis, ankle and foot

MØ8.871 Other juvenile arthritis, right ankle and foot

MØ8.872 Other juvenile arthritis, left ankle and foot

MØ8.879 Other juvenile arthritis, unspecified ankle and foot

MØ8.88 Other juvenile arthritis, other specified site

Other juvenile arthritis, vertebrae

MØ8.89 Other juvenile arthritis, multiple sites

✓5th MØ8.9 Juvenile arthritis, unspecified

EXCLUDES 1 *juvenile rheumatoid arthritis, unspecified (MØ8.Ø-)*

MØ8.90 Juvenile arthritis, unspecified, unspecified site

✓6th MØ8.91 Juvenile arthritis, unspecified, shoulder

MØ8.911 Juvenile arthritis, unspecified, right shoulder

MØ8.912 Juvenile arthritis, unspecified, left shoulder

MØ8.919 Juvenile arthritis, unspecified, unspecified shoulder

✓6th MØ8.92 Juvenile arthritis, unspecified, elbow

MØ8.921 Juvenile arthritis, unspecified, right elbow

MØ8.922 Juvenile arthritis, unspecified, left elbow

MØ8.929 Juvenile arthritis, unspecified, unspecified elbow

✓6th MØ8.93 Juvenile arthritis, unspecified, wrist

MØ8.931 Juvenile arthritis, unspecified, right wrist

MØ8.932 Juvenile arthritis, unspecified, left wrist

MØ8.939 Juvenile arthritis, unspecified, unspecified wrist

✓6th MØ8.94 Juvenile arthritis, unspecified, hand

MØ8.941 Juvenile arthritis, unspecified, right hand

MØ8.942 Juvenile arthritis, unspecified, left hand

MØ8.949 Juvenile arthritis, unspecified, unspecified hand

✓6th MØ8.95 Juvenile arthritis, unspecified, hip

MØ8.951 Juvenile arthritis, unspecified, right hip

M08.952 Juvenile arthritis, unspecified, left hip
M08.959 Juvenile arthritis, unspecified, unspecified hip
✓6th M08.96 Juvenile arthritis, unspecified, knee
M08.961 Juvenile arthritis, unspecified, right knee
M08.962 Juvenile arthritis, unspecified, left knee
M08.969 Juvenile arthritis, unspecified, unspecified knee
✓6th M08.97 Juvenile arthritis, unspecified, ankle and foot
M08.971 Juvenile arthritis, unspecified, right ankle and foot
M08.972 Juvenile arthritis, unspecified, left ankle and foot
M08.979 Juvenile arthritis, unspecified, unspecified ankle and foot
M08.98 Juvenile arthritis, unspecified, vertebrae
M08.99 Juvenile arthritis, unspecified, multiple sites

✓4th **M1A Chronic gout**

Use additional code to identify:
autonomic neuropathy in diseases classified elsewhere (G99.0)
calculus of urinary tract in diseases classified elsewhere (N22)
cardiomyopathy in diseases classified elsewhere (I43)
disorders of external ear in diseases classified elsewhere (H61.1-, H62.8-)
disorders of iris and ciliary body in diseases classified elsewhere (H22)
glomerular disorders in diseases classified elsewhere (N08)

EXCLUDES 1 *acute gout (M10.-)*
gout NOS (M10.-)

The appropriate 7th character is to be added to each code from category M1A.
0 without tophus (tophi)
1 with tophus (tophi)

✓5th M1A.0 Idiopathic chronic gout
Chronic gouty bursitis
Primary chronic gout
✓x7th M1A.00 Idiopathic chronic gout, unspecified site
✓6th M1A.01 Idiopathic chronic gout, shoulder
✓7th M1A.011 Idiopathic chronic gout, right shoulder
✓7th M1A.012 Idiopathic chronic gout, left shoulder
✓7th M1A.019 Idiopathic chronic gout, unspecified shoulder
✓6th M1A.02 Idiopathic chronic gout, elbow
✓7th M1A.021 Idiopathic chronic gout, right elbow
✓7th M1A.022 Idiopathic chronic gout, left elbow
✓7th M1A.029 Idiopathic chronic gout, unspecified elbow
✓6th M1A.03 Idiopathic chronic gout, wrist
✓7th M1A.031 Idiopathic chronic gout, right wrist
✓7th M1A.032 Idiopathic chronic gout, left wrist
✓7th M1A.039 Idiopathic chronic gout, unspecified wrist
✓6th M1A.04 Idiopathic chronic gout, hand
✓7th M1A.041 Idiopathic chronic gout, right hand
✓7th M1A.042 Idiopathic chronic gout, left hand
✓7th M1A.049 Idiopathic chronic gout, unspecified hand
✓6th M1A.05 Idiopathic chronic gout, hip
✓7th M1A.051 Idiopathic chronic gout, right hip
✓7th M1A.052 Idiopathic chronic gout, left hip
✓7th M1A.059 Idiopathic chronic gout, unspecified hip
✓6th M1A.06 Idiopathic chronic gout, knee
✓7th M1A.061 Idiopathic chronic gout, right knee
✓7th M1A.062 Idiopathic chronic gout, left knee
✓7th M1A.069 Idiopathic chronic gout, unspecified knee
✓6th M1A.07 Idiopathic chronic gout, ankle and foot
✓7th M1A.071 Idiopathic chronic gout, right ankle and foot
✓7th M1A.072 Idiopathic chronic gout, left ankle and foot
✓7th M1A.079 Idiopathic chronic gout, unspecified ankle and foot
✓x7th M1A.08 Idiopathic chronic gout, vertebrae
✓x7th M1A.09 Idiopathic chronic gout, multiple sites

✓5th M1A.1 Lead-induced chronic gout
Code first toxic effects of lead and its compounds (T56.0-)
✓x7th M1A.10 Lead-induced chronic gout, unspecified site
✓6th M1A.11 Lead-induced chronic gout, shoulder
✓7th M1A.111 Lead-induced chronic gout, right shoulder
✓7th M1A.112 Lead-induced chronic gout, left shoulder
✓7th M1A.119 Lead-induced chronic gout, unspecified shoulder
✓6th M1A.12 Lead-induced chronic gout, elbow
✓7th M1A.121 Lead-induced chronic gout, right elbow
✓7th M1A.122 Lead-induced chronic gout, left elbow
✓7th M1A.129 Lead-induced chronic gout, unspecified elbow
✓6th M1A.13 Lead-induced chronic gout, wrist
✓7th M1A.131 Lead-induced chronic gout, right wrist
✓7th M1A.132 Lead-induced chronic gout, left wrist
✓7th M1A.139 Lead-induced chronic gout, unspecified wrist
✓6th M1A.14 Lead-induced chronic gout, hand
✓7th M1A.141 Lead-induced chronic gout, right hand
✓7th M1A.142 Lead-induced chronic gout, left hand
✓7th M1A.149 Lead-induced chronic gout, unspecified hand
✓6th M1A.15 Lead-induced chronic gout, hip
✓7th M1A.151 Lead-induced chronic gout, right hip
✓7th M1A.152 Lead-induced chronic gout, left hip
✓7th M1A.159 Lead-induced chronic gout, unspecified hip
✓6th M1A.16 Lead-induced chronic gout, knee
✓7th M1A.161 Lead-induced chronic gout, right knee
✓7th M1A.162 Lead-induced chronic gout, left knee
✓7th M1A.169 Lead-induced chronic gout, unspecified knee
✓6th M1A.17 Lead-induced chronic gout, ankle and foot
✓7th M1A.171 Lead-induced chronic gout, right ankle and foot
✓7th M1A.172 Lead-induced chronic gout, left ankle and foot
✓7th M1A.179 Lead-induced chronic gout, unspecified ankle and foot
✓x7th M1A.18 Lead-induced chronic gout, vertebrae
✓x7th M1A.19 Lead-induced chronic gout, multiple sites

✓5th M1A.2 Drug-induced chronic gout
Use additional code for adverse effect, if applicable, to identify drug (T36-T50 with fifth or sixth character 5)
✓x7th M1A.20 Drug-induced chronic gout, unspecified site
✓6th M1A.21 Drug-induced chronic gout, shoulder
✓7th M1A.211 Drug-induced chronic gout, right shoulder
✓7th M1A.212 Drug-induced chronic gout, left shoulder
✓7th M1A.219 Drug-induced chronic gout, unspecified shoulder
✓6th M1A.22 Drug-induced chronic gout, elbow
✓7th M1A.221 Drug-induced chronic gout, right elbow
✓7th M1A.222 Drug-induced chronic gout, left elbow
✓7th M1A.229 Drug-induced chronic gout, unspecified elbow
✓6th M1A.23 Drug-induced chronic gout, wrist
✓7th M1A.231 Drug-induced chronic gout, right wrist
✓7th M1A.232 Drug-induced chronic gout, left wrist
✓7th M1A.239 Drug-induced chronic gout, unspecified wrist
✓6th M1A.24 Drug-induced chronic gout, hand
✓7th M1A.241 Drug-induced chronic gout, right hand
✓7th M1A.242 Drug-induced chronic gout, left hand
✓7th M1A.249 Drug-induced chronic gout, unspecified hand
✓6th M1A.25 Drug-induced chronic gout, hip
✓7th M1A.251 Drug-induced chronic gout, right hip
✓7th M1A.252 Drug-induced chronic gout, left hip

✓7th **M1A.259 Drug-induced chronic gout, unspecified hip**

✓6th **M1A.26 Drug-induced chronic gout, knee**

✓7th **M1A.261 Drug-induced chronic gout, right knee**

✓7th **M1A.262 Drug-induced chronic gout, left knee**

✓7th **M1A.269 Drug-induced chronic gout, unspecified knee**

✓6th **M1A.27 Drug-induced chronic gout, ankle and foot**

✓7th **M1A.271 Drug-induced chronic gout, right ankle and foot**

✓7th **M1A.272 Drug-induced chronic gout, left ankle and foot**

✓7th **M1A.279 Drug-induced chronic gout, unspecified ankle and foot**

✓x7th **M1A.28 Drug-induced chronic gout, vertebrae**

✓x7th **M1A.29 Drug-induced chronic gout, multiple sites**

✓5th **M1A.3 Chronic gout due to renal impairment**

Code first associated renal disease

✓x7th **M1A.30 Chronic gout due to renal impairment, unspecified site**

✓6th **M1A.31 Chronic gout due to renal impairment, shoulder**

✓7th **M1A.311 Chronic gout due to renal impairment, right shoulder**

✓7th **M1A.312 Chronic gout due to renal impairment, left shoulder**

✓7th **M1A.319 Chronic gout due to renal impairment, unspecified shoulder**

✓6th **M1A.32 Chronic gout due to renal impairment, elbow**

✓7th **M1A.321 Chronic gout due to renal impairment, right elbow**

✓7th **M1A.322 Chronic gout due to renal impairment, left elbow**

✓7th **M1A.329 Chronic gout due to renal impairment, unspecified elbow**

✓6th **M1A.33 Chronic gout due to renal impairment, wrist**

✓7th **M1A.331 Chronic gout due to renal impairment, right wrist**

✓7th **M1A.332 Chronic gout due to renal impairment, left wrist**

✓7th **M1A.339 Chronic gout due to renal impairment, unspecified wrist**

✓6th **M1A.34 Chronic gout due to renal impairment, hand**

✓7th **M1A.341 Chronic gout due to renal impairment, right hand**

✓7th **M1A.342 Chronic gout due to renal impairment, left hand**

✓7th **M1A.349 Chronic gout due to renal impairment, unspecified hand**

✓6th **M1A.35 Chronic gout due to renal impairment, hip**

✓7th **M1A.351 Chronic gout due to renal impairment, right hip**

✓7th **M1A.352 Chronic gout due to renal impairment, left hip**

✓7th **M1A.359 Chronic gout due to renal impairment, unspecified hip**

✓6th **M1A.36 Chronic gout due to renal impairment, knee**

✓7th **M1A.361 Chronic gout due to renal impairment, right knee**

✓7th **M1A.362 Chronic gout due to renal impairment, left knee**

✓7th **M1A.369 Chronic gout due to renal impairment, unspecified knee**

✓6th **M1A.37 Chronic gout due to renal impairment, ankle and foot**

✓7th **M1A.371 Chronic gout due to renal impairment, right ankle and foot**

✓7th **M1A.372 Chronic gout due to renal impairment, left ankle and foot**

✓7th **M1A.379 Chronic gout due to renal impairment, unspecified ankle and foot**

✓x7th **M1A.38 Chronic gout due to renal impairment, vertebrae**

✓x7th **M1A.39 Chronic gout due to renal impairment, multiple sites**

✓5th **M1A.4 Other secondary chronic gout**

Code first associated condition

✓x7th **M1A.40 Other secondary chronic gout, unspecified site**

✓6th **M1A.41 Other secondary chronic gout, shoulder**

✓7th **M1A.411 Other secondary chronic gout, right shoulder**

✓7th **M1A.412 Other secondary chronic gout, left shoulder**

✓7th **M1A.419 Other secondary chronic gout, unspecified shoulder**

✓6th **M1A.42 Other secondary chronic gout, elbow**

✓7th **M1A.421 Other secondary chronic gout, right elbow**

✓7th **M1A.422 Other secondary chronic gout, left elbow**

✓7th **M1A.429 Other secondary chronic gout, unspecified elbow**

✓6th **M1A.43 Other secondary chronic gout, wrist**

✓7th **M1A.431 Other secondary chronic gout, right wrist**

✓7th **M1A.432 Other secondary chronic gout, left wrist**

✓7th **M1A.439 Other secondary chronic gout, unspecified wrist**

✓6th **M1A.44 Other secondary chronic gout, hand**

✓7th **M1A.441 Other secondary chronic gout, right hand**

✓7th **M1A.442 Other secondary chronic gout, left hand**

✓7th **M1A.449 Other secondary chronic gout, unspecified hand**

✓6th **M1A.45 Other secondary chronic gout, hip**

✓7th **M1A.451 Other secondary chronic gout, right hip**

✓7th **M1A.452 Other secondary chronic gout, left hip**

✓7th **M1A.459 Other secondary chronic gout, unspecified hip**

✓6th **M1A.46 Other secondary chronic gout, knee**

✓7th **M1A.461 Other secondary chronic gout, right knee**

✓7th **M1A.462 Other secondary chronic gout, left knee**

✓7th **M1A.469 Other secondary chronic gout, unspecified knee**

✓6th **M1A.47 Other secondary chronic gout, ankle and foot**

✓7th **M1A.471 Other secondary chronic gout, right ankle and foot**

✓7th **M1A.472 Other secondary chronic gout, left ankle and foot**

✓7th **M1A.479 Other secondary chronic gout, unspecified ankle and foot**

✓x7th **M1A.48 Other secondary chronic gout, vertebrae**

✓x7th **M1A.49 Other secondary chronic gout, multiple sites**

✓x7th **M1A.9 Chronic gout, unspecified**

✓4th **M10 Gout**

Acute gout
Gout attack
Gout flare
Gout NOS
Podagra

Use additional code to identify:
- autonomic neuropathy in diseases classified elsewhere (G99.0)
- calculus of urinary tract in diseases classified elsewhere (N22)
- cardiomyopathy in diseases classified elsewhere (I43)
- disorders of external ear in diseases classified elsewhere (H61.1-, H62.8-)
- disorders of iris and ciliary body in diseases classified elsewhere (H22)
- glomerular disorders in diseases classified elsewhere (N08)

EXCLUDES 1 *chronic gout (M1A.-)*

✓5th **M10.0 Idiopathic gout**

Gouty bursitis
Primary gout

M10.00 Idiopathic gout, unspecified site

✓6th **M10.01 Idiopathic gout, shoulder**

M10.011 Idiopathic gout, right shoulder

M10.012 Idiopathic gout, left shoulder

M10.019 Idiopathic gout, unspecified shoulder

✓6th **M10.02 Idiopathic gout, elbow**

M10.021 Idiopathic gout, right elbow

M10.022 Idiopathic gout, left elbow

M10.029 Idiopathic gout, unspecified elbow

✓6th **M10.03 Idiopathic gout, wrist**

M10.031 Idiopathic gout, right wrist

M10.032 Idiopathic gout, left wrist

M10.039 Idiopathic gout, unspecified wrist
√6th M10.04 Idiopathic gout, hand
M10.041 Idiopathic gout, right hand
M10.042 Idiopathic gout, left hand
M10.049 Idiopathic gout, unspecified hand
√6th M10.05 Idiopathic gout, hip
M10.051 Idiopathic gout, right hip
M10.052 Idiopathic gout, left hip
M10.059 Idiopathic gout, unspecified hip
√6th M10.06 Idiopathic gout, knee
M10.061 Idiopathic gout, right knee
M10.062 Idiopathic gout, left knee
M10.069 Idiopathic gout, unspecified knee
√6th M10.07 Idiopathic gout, ankle and foot
M10.071 Idiopathic gout, right ankle and foot
M10.072 Idiopathic gout, left ankle and foot
M10.079 Idiopathic gout, unspecified ankle and foot
M10.08 Idiopathic gout, vertebrae
M10.09 Idiopathic gout, multiple sites
√5th M10.1 Lead-induced gout
Code first toxic effects of lead and its compounds (T56.0-)
M10.10 Lead-induced gout, unspecified site
√6th M10.11 Lead-induced gout, shoulder
M10.111 Lead-induced gout, right shoulder
M10.112 Lead-induced gout, left shoulder
M10.119 Lead-induced gout, unspecified shoulder
√6th M10.12 Lead-induced gout, elbow
M10.121 Lead-induced gout, right elbow
M10.122 Lead-induced gout, left elbow
M10.129 Lead-induced gout, unspecified elbow
√6th M10.13 Lead-induced gout, wrist
M10.131 Lead-induced gout, right wrist
M10.132 Lead-induced gout, left wrist
M10.139 Lead-induced gout, unspecified wrist
√6th M10.14 Lead-induced gout, hand
M10.141 Lead-induced gout, right hand
M10.142 Lead-induced gout, left hand
M10.149 Lead-induced gout, unspecified hand
√6th M10.15 Lead-induced gout, hip
M10.151 Lead-induced gout, right hip
M10.152 Lead-induced gout, left hip
M10.159 Lead-induced gout, unspecified hip
√6th M10.16 Lead-induced gout, knee
M10.161 Lead-induced gout, right knee
M10.162 Lead-induced gout, left knee
M10.169 Lead-induced gout, unspecified knee
√6th M10.17 Lead-induced gout, ankle and foot
M10.171 Lead-induced gout, right ankle and foot
M10.172 Lead-induced gout, left ankle and foot
M10.179 Lead-induced gout, unspecified ankle and foot
M10.18 Lead-induced gout, vertebrae
M10.19 Lead-induced gout, multiple sites
√5th M10.2 Drug-induced gout
Use additional code for adverse effect, if applicable, to identify drug (T36-T50 with fifth or sixth character 5)
M10.20 Drug-induced gout, unspecified site
√6th M10.21 Drug-induced gout, shoulder
M10.211 Drug-induced gout, right shoulder
M10.212 Drug-induced gout, left shoulder
M10.219 Drug-induced gout, unspecified shoulder
√6th M10.22 Drug-induced gout, elbow
M10.221 Drug-induced gout, right elbow
M10.222 Drug-induced gout, left elbow
M10.229 Drug-induced gout, unspecified elbow
√6th M10.23 Drug-induced gout, wrist
M10.231 Drug-induced gout, right wrist
M10.232 Drug-induced gout, left wrist
M10.239 Drug-induced gout, unspecified wrist
√6th M10.24 Drug-induced gout, hand
M10.241 Drug-induced gout, right hand
M10.242 Drug-induced gout, left hand
M10.249 Drug-induced gout, unspecified hand
√6th M10.25 Drug-induced gout, hip
M10.251 Drug-induced gout, right hip
M10.252 Drug-induced gout, left hip
M10.259 Drug-induced gout, unspecified hip
√6th M10.26 Drug-induced gout, knee
M10.261 Drug-induced gout, right knee
M10.262 Drug-induced gout, left knee
M10.269 Drug-induced gout, unspecified knee
√6th M10.27 Drug-induced gout, ankle and foot
M10.271 Drug-induced gout, right ankle and foot
M10.272 Drug-induced gout, left ankle and foot
M10.279 Drug-induced gout, unspecified ankle and foot
M10.28 Drug-induced gout, vertebrae
M10.29 Drug-induced gout, multiple sites
√5th M10.3 Gout due to renal impairment
Code first associated renal disease
M10.30 Gout due to renal impairment, unspecified site
√6th M10.31 Gout due to renal impairment, shoulder
M10.311 Gout due to renal impairment, right shoulder
M10.312 Gout due to renal impairment, left shoulder
M10.319 Gout due to renal impairment, unspecified shoulder
√6th M10.32 Gout due to renal impairment, elbow
M10.321 Gout due to renal impairment, right elbow
M10.322 Gout due to renal impairment, left elbow
M10.329 Gout due to renal impairment, unspecified elbow
√6th M10.33 Gout due to renal impairment, wrist
M10.331 Gout due to renal impairment, right wrist
M10.332 Gout due to renal impairment, left wrist
M10.339 Gout due to renal impairment, unspecified wrist
√6th M10.34 Gout due to renal impairment, hand
M10.341 Gout due to renal impairment, right hand
M10.342 Gout due to renal impairment, left hand
M10.349 Gout due to renal impairment, unspecified hand
√6th M10.35 Gout due to renal impairment, hip
M10.351 Gout due to renal impairment, right hip
M10.352 Gout due to renal impairment, left hip
M10.359 Gout due to renal impairment, unspecified hip
√6th M10.36 Gout due to renal impairment, knee
M10.361 Gout due to renal impairment, right knee
M10.362 Gout due to renal impairment, left knee
M10.369 Gout due to renal impairment, unspecified knee
√6th M10.37 Gout due to renal impairment, ankle and foot
M10.371 Gout due to renal impairment, right ankle and foot
M10.372 Gout due to renal impairment, left ankle and foot
M10.379 Gout due to renal impairment, unspecified ankle and foot
M10.38 Gout due to renal impairment, vertebrae
M10.39 Gout due to renal impairment, multiple sites
√5th M10.4 Other secondary gout
Code first associated condition
M10.40 Other secondary gout, unspecified site
√6th M10.41 Other secondary gout, shoulder
M10.411 Other secondary gout, right shoulder
M10.412 Other secondary gout, left shoulder
M10.419 Other secondary gout, unspecified shoulder
√6th M10.42 Other secondary gout, elbow
M10.421 Other secondary gout, right elbow

M10.422 Other secondary gout, left elbow
M10.429 Other secondary gout, unspecified elbow
√6th M10.43 Other secondary gout, wrist
M10.431 Other secondary gout, right wrist
M10.432 Other secondary gout, left wrist
M10.439 Other secondary gout, unspecified wrist
√6th M10.44 Other secondary gout, hand
M10.441 Other secondary gout, right hand
M10.442 Other secondary gout, left hand
M10.449 Other secondary gout, unspecified hand
√6th M10.45 Other secondary gout, hip
M10.451 Other secondary gout, right hip
M10.452 Other secondary gout, left hip
M10.459 Other secondary gout, unspecified hip
√6th M10.46 Other secondary gout, knee
M10.461 Other secondary gout, right knee
M10.462 Other secondary gout, left knee
M10.469 Other secondary gout, unspecified knee
√6th M10.47 Other secondary gout, ankle and foot
M10.471 Other secondary gout, right ankle and foot
M10.472 Other secondary gout, left ankle and foot
M10.479 Other secondary gout, unspecified ankle and foot
M10.48 Other secondary gout, vertebrae
M10.49 Other secondary gout, multiple sites
M10.9 Gout, unspecified
Gout NOS

√4th **M11 Other crystal arthropathies**

√5th M11.0 Hydroxyapatite deposition disease
M11.00 Hydroxyapatite deposition disease, unspecified site
√6th M11.01 Hydroxyapatite deposition disease, shoulder
M11.011 Hydroxyapatite deposition disease, right shoulder
M11.012 Hydroxyapatite deposition disease, left shoulder
M11.019 Hydroxyapatite deposition disease, unspecified shoulder
√6th M11.02 Hydroxyapatite deposition disease, elbow
M11.021 Hydroxyapatite deposition disease, right elbow
M11.022 Hydroxyapatite deposition disease, left elbow
M11.029 Hydroxyapatite deposition disease, unspecified elbow
√6th M11.03 Hydroxyapatite deposition disease, wrist
M11.031 Hydroxyapatite deposition disease, right wrist
M11.032 Hydroxyapatite deposition disease, left wrist
M11.039 Hydroxyapatite deposition disease, unspecified wrist
√6th M11.04 Hydroxyapatite deposition disease, hand
M11.041 Hydroxyapatite deposition disease, right hand
M11.042 Hydroxyapatite deposition disease, left hand
M11.049 Hydroxyapatite deposition disease, unspecified hand
√6th M11.05 Hydroxyapatite deposition disease, hip
M11.051 Hydroxyapatite deposition disease, right hip
M11.052 Hydroxyapatite deposition disease, left hip
M11.059 Hydroxyapatite deposition disease, unspecified hip
√6th M11.06 Hydroxyapatite deposition disease, knee
M11.061 Hydroxyapatite deposition disease, right knee
M11.062 Hydroxyapatite deposition disease, left knee
M11.069 Hydroxyapatite deposition disease, unspecified knee
√6th M11.07 Hydroxyapatite deposition disease, ankle and foot
M11.071 Hydroxyapatite deposition disease, right ankle and foot
M11.072 Hydroxyapatite deposition disease, left ankle and foot
M11.079 Hydroxyapatite deposition disease, unspecified ankle and foot
M11.08 Hydroxyapatite deposition disease, vertebrae
M11.09 Hydroxyapatite deposition disease, multiple sites
√5th M11.1 Familial chondrocalcinosis
M11.10 Familial chondrocalcinosis, unspecified site
√6th M11.11 Familial chondrocalcinosis, shoulder
M11.111 Familial chondrocalcinosis, right shoulder
M11.112 Familial chondrocalcinosis, left shoulder
M11.119 Familial chondrocalcinosis, unspecified shoulder
√6th M11.12 Familial chondrocalcinosis, elbow
M11.121 Familial chondrocalcinosis, right elbow
M11.122 Familial chondrocalcinosis, left elbow
M11.129 Familial chondrocalcinosis, unspecified elbow
√6th M11.13 Familial chondrocalcinosis, wrist
M11.131 Familial chondrocalcinosis, right wrist
M11.132 Familial chondrocalcinosis, left wrist
M11.139 Familial chondrocalcinosis, unspecified wrist
√6th M11.14 Familial chondrocalcinosis, hand
M11.141 Familial chondrocalcinosis, right hand
M11.142 Familial chondrocalcinosis, left hand
M11.149 Familial chondrocalcinosis, unspecified hand
√6th M11.15 Familial chondrocalcinosis, hip
M11.151 Familial chondrocalcinosis, right hip
M11.152 Familial chondrocalcinosis, left hip
M11.159 Familial chondrocalcinosis, unspecified hip
√6th M11.16 Familial chondrocalcinosis, knee
M11.161 Familial chondrocalcinosis, right knee
M11.162 Familial chondrocalcinosis, left knee
M11.169 Familial chondrocalcinosis, unspecified knee
√6th M11.17 Familial chondrocalcinosis, ankle and foot
M11.171 Familial chondrocalcinosis, right ankle and foot
M11.172 Familial chondrocalcinosis, left ankle and foot
M11.179 Familial chondrocalcinosis, unspecified ankle and foot
M11.18 Familial chondrocalcinosis, vertebrae
M11.19 Familial chondrocalcinosis, multiple sites
√5th M11.2 Other chondrocalcinosis
Chondrocalcinosis NOS
M11.20 Other chondrocalcinosis, unspecified site
√6th M11.21 Other chondrocalcinosis, shoulder
M11.211 Other chondrocalcinosis, right shoulder
M11.212 Other chondrocalcinosis, left shoulder
M11.219 Other chondrocalcinosis, unspecified shoulder
√6th M11.22 Other chondrocalcinosis, elbow
M11.221 Other chondrocalcinosis, right elbow
M11.222 Other chondrocalcinosis, left elbow
M11.229 Other chondrocalcinosis, unspecified elbow
√6th M11.23 Other chondrocalcinosis, wrist
M11.231 Other chondrocalcinosis, right wrist
M11.232 Other chondrocalcinosis, left wrist
M11.239 Other chondrocalcinosis, unspecified wrist
√6th M11.24 Other chondrocalcinosis, hand
M11.241 Other chondrocalcinosis, right hand
M11.242 Other chondrocalcinosis, left hand
M11.249 Other chondrocalcinosis, unspecified hand

✓6th **M11.25 Other chondrocalcinosis, hip**
- **M11.251 Other chondrocalcinosis, right hip**
- **M11.252 Other chondrocalcinosis, left hip**
- **M11.259 Other chondrocalcinosis, unspecified hip**

✓6th **M11.26 Other chondrocalcinosis, knee**
- **M11.261 Other chondrocalcinosis, right knee**
- **M11.262 Other chondrocalcinosis, left knee**
- **M11.269 Other chondrocalcinosis, unspecified knee**

✓6th **M11.27 Other chondrocalcinosis, ankle and foot**
- **M11.271 Other chondrocalcinosis, right ankle and foot**
- **M11.272 Other chondrocalcinosis, left ankle and foot**
- **M11.279 Other chondrocalcinosis, unspecified ankle and foot**

M11.28 Other chondrocalcinosis, vertebrae

M11.29 Other chondrocalcinosis, multiple sites

✓5th **M11.8 Other specified crystal arthropathies**

M11.80 Other specified crystal arthropathies, unspecified site

✓6th **M11.81 Other specified crystal arthropathies, shoulder**
- **M11.811 Other specified crystal arthropathies, right shoulder**
- **M11.812 Other specified crystal arthropathies, left shoulder**
- **M11.819 Other specified crystal arthropathies, unspecified shoulder**

✓6th **M11.82 Other specified crystal arthropathies, elbow**
- **M11.821 Other specified crystal arthropathies, right elbow**
- **M11.822 Other specified crystal arthropathies, left elbow**
- **M11.829 Other specified crystal arthropathies, unspecified elbow**

✓6th **M11.83 Other specified crystal arthropathies, wrist**
- **M11.831 Other specified crystal arthropathies, right wrist**
- **M11.832 Other specified crystal arthropathies, left wrist**
- **M11.839 Other specified crystal arthropathies, unspecified wrist**

✓6th **M11.84 Other specified crystal arthropathies, hand**
- **M11.841 Other specified crystal arthropathies, right hand**
- **M11.842 Other specified crystal arthropathies, left hand**
- **M11.849 Other specified crystal arthropathies, unspecified hand**

✓6th **M11.85 Other specified crystal arthropathies, hip**
- **M11.851 Other specified crystal arthropathies, right hip**
- **M11.852 Other specified crystal arthropathies, left hip**
- **M11.859 Other specified crystal arthropathies, unspecified hip**

✓6th **M11.86 Other specified crystal arthropathies, knee**
- **M11.861 Other specified crystal arthropathies, right knee**
- **M11.862 Other specified crystal arthropathies, left knee**
- **M11.869 Other specified crystal arthropathies, unspecified knee**

✓6th **M11.87 Other specified crystal arthropathies, ankle and foot**
- **M11.871 Other specified crystal arthropathies, right ankle and foot**
- **M11.872 Other specified crystal arthropathies, left ankle and foot**
- **M11.879 Other specified crystal arthropathies, unspecified ankle and foot**

M11.88 Other specified crystal arthropathies, vertebrae

M11.89 Other specified crystal arthropathies, multiple sites

M11.9 Crystal arthropathy, unspecified

✓4th **M12 Other and unspecified arthropathy**

EXCLUDES 1 *arthrosis (M15-M19)*
cricoarytenoid arthropathy (J38.7)

✓5th **M12.0 Chronic postrheumatic arthropathy [Jaccoud]**

M12.00 Chronic postrheumatic arthropathy [Jaccoud], unspecified site

✓6th **M12.01 Chronic postrheumatic arthropathy [Jaccoud], shoulder**
- **M12.011 Chronic postrheumatic arthropathy [Jaccoud], right shoulder**
- **M12.012 Chronic postrheumatic arthropathy [Jaccoud], left shoulder**
- **M12.019 Chronic postrheumatic arthropathy [Jaccoud], unspecified shoulder**

✓6th **M12.02 Chronic postrheumatic arthropathy [Jaccoud], elbow**
- **M12.021 Chronic postrheumatic arthropathy [Jaccoud], right elbow**
- **M12.022 Chronic postrheumatic arthropathy [Jaccoud], left elbow**
- **M12.029 Chronic postrheumatic arthropathy [Jaccoud], unspecified elbow**

✓6th **M12.03 Chronic postrheumatic arthropathy [Jaccoud], wrist**
- **M12.031 Chronic postrheumatic arthropathy [Jaccoud], right wrist**
- **M12.032 Chronic postrheumatic arthropathy [Jaccoud], left wrist**
- **M12.039 Chronic postrheumatic arthropathy [Jaccoud], unspecified wrist**

✓6th **M12.04 Chronic postrheumatic arthropathy [Jaccoud], hand**
- **M12.041 Chronic postrheumatic arthropathy [Jaccoud], right hand**
- **M12.042 Chronic postrheumatic arthropathy [Jaccoud], left hand**
- **M12.049 Chronic postrheumatic arthropathy [Jaccoud], unspecified hand**

✓6th **M12.05 Chronic postrheumatic arthropathy [Jaccoud], hip**
- **M12.051 Chronic postrheumatic arthropathy [Jaccoud], right hip**
- **M12.052 Chronic postrheumatic arthropathy [Jaccoud], left hip**
- **M12.059 Chronic postrheumatic arthropathy [Jaccoud], unspecified hip**

✓6th **M12.06 Chronic postrheumatic arthropathy [Jaccoud], knee**
- **M12.061 Chronic postrheumatic arthropathy [Jaccoud], right knee**
- **M12.062 Chronic postrheumatic arthropathy [Jaccoud], left knee**
- **M12.069 Chronic postrheumatic arthropathy [Jaccoud], unspecified knee**

✓6th **M12.07 Chronic postrheumatic arthropathy [Jaccoud], ankle and foot**
- **M12.071 Chronic postrheumatic arthropathy [Jaccoud], right ankle and foot**
- **M12.072 Chronic postrheumatic arthropathy [Jaccoud], left ankle and foot**
- **M12.079 Chronic postrheumatic arthropathy [Jaccoud], unspecified ankle and foot**

M12.08 Chronic postrheumatic arthropathy [Jaccoud], other specified site

Chronic postrheumatic arthropathy [Jaccoud], vertebrae

M12.09 Chronic postrheumatic arthropathy [Jaccoud], multiple sites

✓5th **M12.1 Kaschin-Beck disease**

Osteochondroarthrosis deformans endemica

M12.10 Kaschin-Beck disease, unspecified site

✓6th **M12.11 Kaschin-Beck disease, shoulder**
- **M12.111 Kaschin-Beck disease, right shoulder**
- **M12.112 Kaschin-Beck disease, left shoulder**
- **M12.119 Kaschin-Beck disease, unspecified shoulder**

✓6th **M12.12 Kaschin-Beck disease, elbow**
- **M12.121 Kaschin-Beck disease, right elbow**
- **M12.122 Kaschin-Beck disease, left elbow**
- **M12.129 Kaschin-Beck disease, unspecified elbow**

✓6th **M12.13 Kaschin-Beck disease, wrist**
M12.131 Kaschin-Beck disease, right wrist
M12.132 Kaschin-Beck disease, left wrist
M12.139 Kaschin-Beck disease, unspecified wrist

✓6th **M12.14 Kaschin-Beck disease, hand**
M12.141 Kaschin-Beck disease, right hand
M12.142 Kaschin-Beck disease, left hand
M12.149 Kaschin-Beck disease, unspecified hand

✓6th **M12.15 Kaschin-Beck disease, hip**
M12.151 Kaschin-Beck disease, right hip
M12.152 Kaschin-Beck disease, left hip
M12.159 Kaschin-Beck disease, unspecified hip

✓6th **M12.16 Kaschin-Beck disease, knee**
M12.161 Kaschin-Beck disease, right knee
M12.162 Kaschin-Beck disease, left knee
M12.169 Kaschin-Beck disease, unspecified knee

✓6th **M12.17 Kaschin-Beck disease, ankle and foot**
M12.171 Kaschin-Beck disease, right ankle and foot
M12.172 Kaschin-Beck disease, left ankle and foot
M12.179 Kaschin-Beck disease, unspecified ankle and foot

M12.18 Kaschin-Beck disease, vertebrae
M12.19 Kaschin-Beck disease, multiple sites

✓5th **M12.2 Villonodular synovitis (pigmented)**
M12.20 Villonodular synovitis (pigmented), unspecified site

✓6th **M12.21 Villonodular synovitis (pigmented), shoulder**
M12.211 Villonodular synovitis (pigmented), right shoulder
M12.212 Villonodular synovitis (pigmented), left shoulder
M12.219 Villonodular synovitis (pigmented), unspecified shoulder

✓6th **M12.22 Villonodular synovitis (pigmented), elbow**
M12.221 Villonodular synovitis (pigmented), right elbow
M12.222 Villonodular synovitis (pigmented), left elbow
M12.229 Villonodular synovitis (pigmented), unspecified elbow

✓6th **M12.23 Villonodular synovitis (pigmented), wrist**
M12.231 Villonodular synovitis (pigmented), right wrist
M12.232 Villonodular synovitis (pigmented), left wrist
M12.239 Villonodular synovitis (pigmented), unspecified wrist

✓6th **M12.24 Villonodular synovitis (pigmented), hand**
M12.241 Villonodular synovitis (pigmented), right hand
M12.242 Villonodular synovitis (pigmented), left hand
M12.249 Villonodular synovitis (pigmented), unspecified hand

✓6th **M12.25 Villonodular synovitis (pigmented), hip**
M12.251 Villonodular synovitis (pigmented), right hip
M12.252 Villonodular synovitis (pigmented), left hip
M12.259 Villonodular synovitis (pigmented), unspecified hip

✓6th **M12.26 Villonodular synovitis (pigmented), knee**
M12.261 Villonodular synovitis (pigmented), right knee
M12.262 Villonodular synovitis (pigmented), left knee
M12.269 Villonodular synovitis (pigmented), unspecified knee

✓6th **M12.27 Villonodular synovitis (pigmented), ankle and foot**
M12.271 Villonodular synovitis (pigmented), right ankle and foot
M12.272 Villonodular synovitis (pigmented), left ankle and foot
M12.279 Villonodular synovitis (pigmented), unspecified ankle and foot

M12.28 Villonodular synovitis (pigmented), other specified site
Villonodular synovitis (pigmented), vertebrae
M12.29 Villonodular synovitis (pigmented), multiple sites

✓5th **M12.3 Palindromic rheumatism**
M12.30 Palindromic rheumatism, unspecified site

✓6th **M12.31 Palindromic rheumatism, shoulder**
M12.311 Palindromic rheumatism, right shoulder
M12.312 Palindromic rheumatism, left shoulder
M12.319 Palindromic rheumatism, unspecified shoulder

✓6th **M12.32 Palindromic rheumatism, elbow**
M12.321 Palindromic rheumatism, right elbow
M12.322 Palindromic rheumatism, left elbow
M12.329 Palindromic rheumatism, unspecified elbow

✓6th **M12.33 Palindromic rheumatism, wrist**
M12.331 Palindromic rheumatism, right wrist
M12.332 Palindromic rheumatism, left wrist
M12.339 Palindromic rheumatism, unspecified wrist

✓6th **M12.34 Palindromic rheumatism, hand**
M12.341 Palindromic rheumatism, right hand
M12.342 Palindromic rheumatism, left hand
M12.349 Palindromic rheumatism, unspecified hand

✓6th **M12.35 Palindromic rheumatism, hip**
M12.351 Palindromic rheumatism, right hip
M12.352 Palindromic rheumatism, left hip
M12.359 Palindromic rheumatism, unspecified hip

✓6th **M12.36 Palindromic rheumatism, knee**
M12.361 Palindromic rheumatism, right knee
M12.362 Palindromic rheumatism, left knee
M12.369 Palindromic rheumatism, unspecified knee

✓6th **M12.37 Palindromic rheumatism, ankle and foot**
M12.371 Palindromic rheumatism, right ankle and foot
M12.372 Palindromic rheumatism, left ankle and foot
M12.379 Palindromic rheumatism, unspecified ankle and foot

M12.38 Palindromic rheumatism, other specified site
Palindromic rheumatism, vertebrae
M12.39 Palindromic rheumatism, multiple sites

✓5th **M12.4 Intermittent hydrarthrosis**
M12.40 Intermittent hydrarthrosis, unspecified site

✓6th **M12.41 Intermittent hydrarthrosis, shoulder**
M12.411 Intermittent hydrarthrosis, right shoulder
M12.412 Intermittent hydrarthrosis, left shoulder
M12.419 Intermittent hydrarthrosis, unspecified shoulder

✓6th **M12.42 Intermittent hydrarthrosis, elbow**
M12.421 Intermittent hydrarthrosis, right elbow
M12.422 Intermittent hydrarthrosis, left elbow
M12.429 Intermittent hydrarthrosis, unspecified elbow

✓6th **M12.43 Intermittent hydrarthrosis, wrist**
M12.431 Intermittent hydrarthrosis, right wrist
M12.432 Intermittent hydrarthrosis, left wrist
M12.439 Intermittent hydrarthrosis, unspecified wrist

✓6th **M12.44 Intermittent hydrarthrosis, hand**
M12.441 Intermittent hydrarthrosis, right hand
M12.442 Intermittent hydrarthrosis, left hand
M12.449 Intermittent hydrarthrosis, unspecified hand

✓6th **M12.45 Intermittent hydrarthrosis, hip**
M12.451 Intermittent hydrarthrosis, right hip
M12.452 Intermittent hydrarthrosis, left hip
M12.459 Intermittent hydrarthrosis, unspecified hip

M12.46 Intermittent hydrarthrosis, knee
M12.461 Intermittent hydrarthrosis, right knee
M12.462 Intermittent hydrarthrosis, left knee
M12.469 Intermittent hydrarthrosis, unspecified knee
M12.47 Intermittent hydrarthrosis, ankle and foot
M12.471 Intermittent hydrarthrosis, right ankle and foot
M12.472 Intermittent hydrarthrosis, left ankle and foot
M12.479 Intermittent hydrarthrosis, unspecified ankle and foot
M12.48 Intermittent hydrarthrosis, other site
M12.49 Intermittent hydrarthrosis, multiple sites

M12.5 Traumatic arthropathy

EXCLUDES 1 *current injury-see Alphabetic Index*
post-traumatic osteoarthritis NOS (M19.1-)
post-traumatic osteoarthritis of first carpometacarpal joint (M18.2-M18.3)
post-traumatic osteoarthritis of hip (M16.4-M16.5)
post-traumatic osteoarthritis of knee (M17.2-M17.3)
post-traumatic osteoarthritis of other single joints (M19.1-)

M12.50 Traumatic arthropathy, unspecified site
M12.51 Traumatic arthropathy, shoulder
M12.511 Traumatic arthropathy, right shoulder
M12.512 Traumatic arthropathy, left shoulder
M12.519 Traumatic arthropathy, unspecified shoulder
M12.52 Traumatic arthropathy, elbow
M12.521 Traumatic arthropathy, right elbow
M12.522 Traumatic arthropathy, left elbow
M12.529 Traumatic arthropathy, unspecified elbow
M12.53 Traumatic arthropathy, wrist
M12.531 Traumatic arthropathy, right wrist
M12.532 Traumatic arthropathy, left wrist
M12.539 Traumatic arthropathy, unspecified wrist
M12.54 Traumatic arthropathy, hand
M12.541 Traumatic arthropathy, right hand
M12.542 Traumatic arthropathy, left hand
M12.549 Traumatic arthropathy, unspecified hand
M12.55 Traumatic arthropathy, hip
M12.551 Traumatic arthropathy, right hip
M12.552 Traumatic arthropathy, left hip
M12.559 Traumatic arthropathy, unspecified hip
M12.56 Traumatic arthropathy, knee
M12.561 Traumatic arthropathy, right knee
M12.562 Traumatic arthropathy, left knee
M12.569 Traumatic arthropathy, unspecified knee
M12.57 Traumatic arthropathy, ankle and foot
M12.571 Traumatic arthropathy, right ankle and foot
M12.572 Traumatic arthropathy, left ankle and foot
M12.579 Traumatic arthropathy, unspecified ankle and foot
M12.58 Traumatic arthropathy, other specified site
Traumatic arthropathy, vertebrae
M12.59 Traumatic arthropathy, multiple sites

M12.8 Other specific arthropathies, not elsewhere classified

Transient arthropathy

M12.80 Other specific arthropathies, not elsewhere classified, unspecified site
M12.81 Other specific arthropathies, not elsewhere classified, shoulder
M12.811 Other specific arthropathies, not elsewhere classified, right shoulder
M12.812 Other specific arthropathies, not elsewhere classified, left shoulder
M12.819 Other specific arthropathies, not elsewhere classified, unspecified shoulder
M12.82 Other specific arthropathies, not elsewhere classified, elbow
M12.821 Other specific arthropathies, not elsewhere classified, right elbow
M12.822 Other specific arthropathies, not elsewhere classified, left elbow
M12.829 Other specific arthropathies, not elsewhere classified, unspecified elbow
M12.83 Other specific arthropathies, not elsewhere classified, wrist
M12.831 Other specific arthropathies, not elsewhere classified, right wrist
M12.832 Other specific arthropathies, not elsewhere classified, left wrist
M12.839 Other specific arthropathies, not elsewhere classified, unspecified wrist
M12.84 Other specific arthropathies, not elsewhere classified, hand
M12.841 Other specific arthropathies, not elsewhere classified, right hand
M12.842 Other specific arthropathies, not elsewhere classified, left hand
M12.849 Other specific arthropathies, not elsewhere classified, unspecified hand
M12.85 Other specific arthropathies, not elsewhere classified, hip
M12.851 Other specific arthropathies, not elsewhere classified, right hip
M12.852 Other specific arthropathies, not elsewhere classified, left hip
M12.859 Other specific arthropathies, not elsewhere classified, unspecified hip
M12.86 Other specific arthropathies, not elsewhere classified, knee
M12.861 Other specific arthropathies, not elsewhere classified, right knee
M12.862 Other specific arthropathies, not elsewhere classified, left knee
M12.869 Other specific arthropathies, not elsewhere classified, unspecified knee
M12.87 Other specific arthropathies, not elsewhere classified, ankle and foot
M12.871 Other specific arthropathies, not elsewhere classified, right ankle and foot
M12.872 Other specific arthropathies, not elsewhere classified, left ankle and foot
M12.879 Other specific arthropathies, not elsewhere classified, unspecified ankle and foot
M12.88 Other specific arthropathies, not elsewhere classified, other specified site
Other specific arthropathies, not elsewhere classified, vertebrae
M12.89 Other specific arthropathies, not elsewhere classified, multiple sites

M12.9 Arthropathy, unspecified

M13 Other arthritis

EXCLUDES 1 *arthrosis (M15-M19)*
osteoarthritis (M15-M19)

M13.0 Polyarthritis, unspecified

M13.1 Monoarthritis, not elsewhere classified

M13.10 Monoarthritis, not elsewhere classified, unspecified site
M13.11 Monoarthritis, not elsewhere classified, shoulder
M13.111 Monoarthritis, not elsewhere classified, right shoulder
M13.112 Monoarthritis, not elsewhere classified, left shoulder
M13.119 Monoarthritis, not elsewhere classified, unspecified shoulder
M13.12 Monoarthritis, not elsewhere classified, elbow
M13.121 Monoarthritis, not elsewhere classified, right elbow
M13.122 Monoarthritis, not elsewhere classified, left elbow
M13.129 Monoarthritis, not elsewhere classified, unspecified elbow
M13.13 Monoarthritis, not elsewhere classified, wrist
M13.131 Monoarthritis, not elsewhere classified, right wrist

M13.132 Monoarthritis, not elsewhere classified, left wrist
M13.139 Monoarthritis, not elsewhere classified, unspecified wrist

√6th M13.14 Monoarthritis, not elsewhere classified, hand
M13.141 Monoarthritis, not elsewhere classified, right hand
M13.142 Monoarthritis, not elsewhere classified, left hand
M13.149 Monoarthritis, not elsewhere classified, unspecified hand

√6th M13.15 Monoarthritis, not elsewhere classified, hip
M13.151 Monoarthritis, not elsewhere classified, right hip
M13.152 Monoarthritis, not elsewhere classified, left hip
M13.159 Monoarthritis, not elsewhere classified, unspecified hip

√6th M13.16 Monoarthritis, not elsewhere classified, knee
M13.161 Monoarthritis, not elsewhere classified, right knee
M13.162 Monoarthritis, not elsewhere classified, left knee
M13.169 Monoarthritis, not elsewhere classified, unspecified knee

√6th M13.17 Monoarthritis, not elsewhere classified, ankle and foot
M13.171 Monoarthritis, not elsewhere classified, right ankle and foot
M13.172 Monoarthritis, not elsewhere classified, left ankle and foot
M13.179 Monoarthritis, not elsewhere classified, unspecified ankle and foot

√5th M13.8 Other specified arthritis
Allergic arthritis
EXCLUDES 1 *osteoarthritis (M15-M19)*
M13.80 Other specified arthritis, unspecified site

√6th M13.81 Other specified arthritis, shoulder
M13.811 Other specified arthritis, right shoulder
M13.812 Other specified arthritis, left shoulder
M13.819 Other specified arthritis, unspecified shoulder

√6th M13.82 Other specified arthritis, elbow
M13.821 Other specified arthritis, right elbow
M13.822 Other specified arthritis, left elbow
M13.829 Other specified arthritis, unspecified elbow

√6th M13.83 Other specified arthritis, wrist
M13.831 Other specified arthritis, right wrist
M13.832 Other specified arthritis, left wrist
M13.839 Other specified arthritis, unspecified wrist

√6th M13.84 Other specified arthritis, hand
M13.841 Other specified arthritis, right hand
M13.842 Other specified arthritis, left hand
M13.849 Other specified arthritis, unspecified hand

√6th M13.85 Other specified arthritis, hip
M13.851 Other specified arthritis, right hip
M13.852 Other specified arthritis, left hip
M13.859 Other specified arthritis, unspecified hip

√6th M13.86 Other specified arthritis, knee
M13.861 Other specified arthritis, right knee
M13.862 Other specified arthritis, left knee
M13.869 Other specified arthritis, unspecified knee

√6th M13.87 Other specified arthritis, ankle and foot
M13.871 Other specified arthritis, right ankle and foot
M13.872 Other specified arthritis, left ankle and foot
M13.879 Other specified arthritis, unspecified ankle and foot
M13.88 Other specified arthritis, other site
M13.89 Other specified arthritis, multiple sites

√4th **M14 Arthropathies in other diseases classified elsewhere**
EXCLUDES 1 *arthropathy in:*
diabetes mellitus (E08-E13 with .61-)
hematological disorders (M36.2-M36.3)
hypersensitivity reactions (M36.4)
neoplastic disease (M36.1)
neurosyphillis (A52.16)
sarcoidosis (D86.86)
enteropathic arthropathies (M07.-)
juvenile psoriatic arthropathy (L40.54)
lipoid dermatoarthritis (E78.81)

√5th M14.6 Charcôt's joint
Neuropathic arthropathy
EXCLUDES 1 *Charcôt's joint in diabetes mellitus (E08-E13 with .610-)*
Charcôt's joint in tabes dorsalis (A52.16)
M14.60 Charcôt's joint, unspecified site

√6th M14.61 Charcôt's joint, shoulder
M14.611 Charcôt's joint, right shoulder
M14.612 Charcôt's joint, left shoulder
M14.619 Charcôt's joint, unspecified shoulder

√6th M14.62 Charcôt's joint, elbow
M14.621 Charcôt's joint, right elbow
M14.622 Charcôt's joint, left elbow
M14.629 Charcôt's joint, unspecified elbow

√6th M14.63 Charcôt's joint, wrist
M14.631 Charcôt's joint, right wrist
M14.632 Charcôt's joint, left wrist
M14.639 Charcôt's joint, unspecified wrist

√6th M14.64 Charcôt's joint, hand
M14.641 Charcôt's joint, right hand
M14.642 Charcôt's joint, left hand
M14.649 Charcôt's joint, unspecified hand

√6th M14.65 Charcôt's joint, hip
M14.651 Charcôt's joint, right hip
M14.652 Charcôt's joint, left hip
M14.659 Charcôt's joint, unspecified hip

√6th M14.66 Charcôt's joint, knee
M14.661 Charcôt's joint, right knee
M14.662 Charcôt's joint, left knee
M14.669 Charcôt's joint, unspecified knee

√6th M14.67 Charcôt's joint, ankle and foot
M14.671 Charcôt's joint, right ankle and foot
M14.672 Charcôt's joint, left ankle and foot
M14.679 Charcôt's joint, unspecified ankle and foot
M14.68 Charcôt's joint, vertebrae
M14.69 Charcôt's joint, multiple sites

√5th M14.8 Arthropathies in other specified diseases classified elsewhere
Code first underlying disease, such as:
amyloidosis (E85.-)
erythema multiforme (L51.-)
erythema nodosum (L52)
hemochromatosis (E83.11-)
hyperparathyroidism (E21.-)
hypothyroidism (E00-E03)
sickle-cell disorders (D57.-)
thyrotoxicosis [hyperthyroidism] (E05.-)
Whipple's disease (K90.81)
M14.80 *Arthropathies in other specified diseases classified elsewhere, unspecified site*

√6th M14.81 Arthropathies in other specified diseases classified elsewhere, shoulder
M14.811 *Arthropathies in other specified diseases classified elsewhere, right shoulder*
M14.812 *Arthropathies in other specified diseases classified elsewhere, left shoulder*
M14.819 *Arthropathies in other specified diseases classified elsewhere, unspecified shoulder*

√6th M14.82 Arthropathies in other specified diseases classified elsewhere, elbow
M14.821 *Arthropathies in other specified diseases classified elsewhere, right elbow*
M14.822 *Arthropathies in other specified diseases classified elsewhere, left elbow*
M14.829 *Arthropathies in other specified diseases classified elsewhere, unspecified elbow*

M14.83 Arthropathies in other specified diseases classified elsewhere, wrist
- *M14.831 Arthropathies in other specified diseases classified elsewhere, right wrist*
- *M14.832 Arthropathies in other specified diseases classified elsewhere, left wrist*
- *M14.839 Arthropathies in other specified diseases classified elsewhere, unspecified wrist*

M14.84 Arthropathies in other specified diseases classified elsewhere, hand
- *M14.841 Arthropathies in other specified diseases classified elsewhere, right hand*
- *M14.842 Arthropathies in other specified diseases classified elsewhere, left hand*
- *M14.849 Arthropathies in other specified diseases classified elsewhere, unspecified hand*

M14.85 Arthropathies in other specified diseases classified elsewhere, hip
- *M14.851 Arthropathies in other specified diseases classified elsewhere, right hip*
- *M14.852 Arthropathies in other specified diseases classified elsewhere, left hip*
- *M14.859 Arthropathies in other specified diseases classified elsewhere, unspecified hip*

M14.86 Arthropathies in other specified diseases classified elsewhere, knee
- *M14.861 Arthropathies in other specified diseases classified elsewhere, right knee*
- *M14.862 Arthropathies in other specified diseases classified elsewhere, left knee*
- *M14.869 Arthropathies in other specified diseases classified elsewhere, unspecified knee*

M14.87 Arthropathies in other specified diseases classified elsewhere, ankle and foot
- *M14.871 Arthropathies in other specified diseases classified elsewhere, right ankle and foot*
- *M14.872 Arthropathies in other specified diseases classified elsewhere, left ankle and foot*
- *M14.879 Arthropathies in other specified diseases classified elsewhere, unspecified ankle and foot*

M14.88 Arthropathies in other specified diseases classified elsewhere, vertebrae

M14.89 Arthropathies in other specified diseases classified elsewhere, multiple sites

Osteoarthritis (M15-M19)

EXCLUDES 2 *osteoarthritis of spine (M47.-)*

M15 Polyosteoarthritis
INCLUDES arthritis of multiple sites

EXCLUDES 1 *bilateral involvement of single joint (M16-M19)*

- **M15.0 Primary generalized (osteo)arthritis**
- **M15.1 Heberden's nodes (with arthropathy)**
  Interphalangeal distal osteoarthritis
- **M15.2 Bouchard's nodes (with arthropathy)**
  Juxtaphalangeal distal osteoarthritis
- **M15.3 Secondary multiple arthritis**
  Post-traumatic polyosteoarthritis
- **M15.4 Erosive (osteo)arthritis**
- **M15.8 Other polyosteoarthritis**
- **M15.9 Polyosteoarthritis, unspecified**
  Generalized osteoarthritis NOS

M16 Osteoarthritis of hip
- **M16.0 Bilateral primary osteoarthritis of hip**
- **M16.1 Unilateral primary osteoarthritis of hip**
  Primary osteoarthritis of hip NOS
  - **M16.10 Unilateral primary osteoarthritis, unspecified hip**
  - **M16.11 Unilateral primary osteoarthritis, right hip**
  - **M16.12 Unilateral primary osteoarthritis, left hip**
- **M16.2 Bilateral osteoarthritis resulting from hip dysplasia**
- **M16.3 Unilateral osteoarthritis resulting from hip dysplasia**
  Dysplastic osteoarthritis of hip NOS
  - **M16.30 Unilateral osteoarthritis resulting from hip dysplasia, unspecified hip**
  - **M16.31 Unilateral osteoarthritis resulting from hip dysplasia, right hip**
  - **M16.32 Unilateral osteoarthritis resulting from hip dysplasia, left hip**
- **M16.4 Bilateral post-traumatic osteoarthritis of hip**
- **M16.5 Unilateral post-traumatic osteoarthritis of hip**
  Post-traumatic osteoarthritis of hip NOS
  - **M16.50 Unilateral post-traumatic osteoarthritis, unspecified hip**
  - **M16.51 Unilateral post-traumatic osteoarthritis, right hip**
  - **M16.52 Unilateral post-traumatic osteoarthritis, left hip**
- **M16.6 Other bilateral secondary osteoarthritis of hip**
- **M16.7 Other unilateral secondary osteoarthritis of hip**
  Secondary osteoarthritis of hip NOS
- **M16.9 Osteoarthritis of hip, unspecified**

M17 Osteoarthritis of knee
- **M17.0 Bilateral primary osteoarthritis of knee**
- **M17.1 Unilateral primary osteoarthritis of knee**
  Primary osteoarthritis of knee NOS
  - **M17.10 Unilateral primary osteoarthritis, unspecified knee**
  - **M17.11 Unilateral primary osteoarthritis, right knee**
  - **M17.12 Unilateral primary osteoarthritis, left knee**
- **M17.2 Bilateral post-traumatic osteoarthritis of knee**
- **M17.3 Unilateral post-traumatic osteoarthritis of knee**
  Post-traumatic osteoarthritis of knee NOS
  - **M17.30 Unilateral post-traumatic osteoarthritis, unspecified knee**
  - **M17.31 Unilateral post-traumatic osteoarthritis, right knee**
  - **M17.32 Unilateral post-traumatic osteoarthritis, left knee**
- **M17.4 Other bilateral secondary osteoarthritis of knee**
- **M17.5 Other unilateral secondary osteoarthritis of knee**
  Secondary osteoarthritis of knee NOS
- **M17.9 Osteoarthritis of knee, unspecified**

M18 Osteoarthritis of first carpometacarpal joint
- **M18.0 Bilateral primary osteoarthritis of first carpometacarpal joints**
- **M18.1 Unilateral primary osteoarthritis of first carpometacarpal joint**
  Primary osteoarthritis of first carpometacarpal joint NOS
  - **M18.10 Unilateral primary osteoarthritis of first carpometacarpal joint, unspecified hand**
  - **M18.11 Unilateral primary osteoarthritis of first carpometacarpal joint, right hand**
  - **M18.12 Unilateral primary osteoarthritis of first carpometacarpal joint, left hand**
- **M18.2 Bilateral post-traumatic osteoarthritis of first carpometacarpal joints**
- **M18.3 Unilateral post-traumatic osteoarthritis of first carpometacarpal joint**
  Post-traumatic osteoarthritis of first carpometacarpal joint NOS
  - **M18.30 Unilateral post-traumatic osteoarthritis of first carpometacarpal joint, unspecified hand**
  - **M18.31 Unilateral post-traumatic osteoarthritis of first carpometacarpal joint, right hand**
  - **M18.32 Unilateral post-traumatic osteoarthritis of first carpometacarpal joint, left hand**
- **M18.4 Other bilateral secondary osteoarthritis of first carpometacarpal joints**
- **M18.5 Other unilateral secondary osteoarthritis of first carpometacarpal joint**
  Secondary osteoarthritis of first carpometacarpal joint NOS
  - **M18.50 Other unilateral secondary osteoarthritis of first carpometacarpal joint, unspecified hand**
  - **M18.51 Other unilateral secondary osteoarthritis of first carpometacarpal joint, right hand**
  - **M18.52 Other unilateral secondary osteoarthritis of first carpometacarpal joint, left hand**
- **M18.9 Osteoarthritis of first carpometacarpal joint, unspecified**

M19 Other and unspecified osteoarthritis
EXCLUDES 1 *polyarthritis (M15.-)*

EXCLUDES 2 *arthrosis of spine (M47.-)*
hallux rigidus (M20.2)
osteoarthritis of spine (M47.-)

- **M19.0 Primary osteoarthritis of other joints**
  - **M19.01 Primary osteoarthritis, shoulder**
    - **M19.011 Primary osteoarthritis, right shoulder**

M19.012 Primary osteoarthritis, left shoulder
M19.019 Primary osteoarthritis, unspecified shoulder

✓6th M19.02 Primary osteoarthritis, elbow
M19.021 Primary osteoarthritis, right elbow
M19.022 Primary osteoarthritis, left elbow
M19.029 Primary osteoarthritis, unspecified elbow

✓6th M19.03 Primary osteoarthritis, wrist
M19.031 Primary osteoarthritis, right wrist
M19.032 Primary osteoarthritis, left wrist
M19.039 Primary osteoarthritis, unspecified wrist

✓6th M19.04 Primary osteoarthritis, hand
EXCLUDES 2 *primary osteoarthritis of first carpometacarpal joint (M18.0-, M18.1-)*
M19.041 Primary osteoarthritis, right hand
M19.042 Primary osteoarthritis, left hand
M19.049 Primary osteoarthritis, unspecified hand

✓6th M19.07 Primary osteoarthritis ankle and foot
M19.071 Primary osteoarthritis, right ankle and foot
M19.072 Primary osteoarthritis, left ankle and foot
M19.079 Primary osteoarthritis, unspecified ankle and foot

✓5th M19.1 Post-traumatic osteoarthritis of other joints

✓6th M19.11 Post-traumatic osteoarthritis, shoulder
M19.111 Post-traumatic osteoarthritis, right shoulder
M19.112 Post-traumatic osteoarthritis, left shoulder
M19.119 Post-traumatic osteoarthritis, unspecified shoulder

✓6th M19.12 Post-traumatic osteoarthritis, elbow
M19.121 Post-traumatic osteoarthritis, right elbow
M19.122 Post-traumatic osteoarthritis, left elbow
M19.129 Post-traumatic osteoarthritis, unspecified elbow

✓6th M19.13 Post-traumatic osteoarthritis, wrist
M19.131 Post-traumatic osteoarthritis, right wrist
M19.132 Post-traumatic osteoarthritis, left wrist
M19.139 Post-traumatic osteoarthritis, unspecified wrist

✓6th M19.14 Post-traumatic osteoarthritis, hand
EXCLUDES 2 *post-traumatic osteoarthritis of first carpometacarpal joint (M18.2-, M18.3-)*
M19.141 Post-traumatic osteoarthritis, right hand
M19.142 Post-traumatic osteoarthritis, left hand
M19.149 Post-traumatic osteoarthritis, unspecified hand

✓6th M19.17 Post-traumatic osteoarthritis, ankle and foot
M19.171 Post-traumatic osteoarthritis, right ankle and foot
M19.172 Post-traumatic osteoarthritis, left ankle and foot
M19.179 Post-traumatic osteoarthritis, unspecified ankle and foot

✓5th M19.2 Secondary osteoarthritis of other joints

✓6th M19.21 Secondary osteoarthritis, shoulder
M19.211 Secondary osteoarthritis, right shoulder
M19.212 Secondary osteoarthritis, left shoulder
M19.219 Secondary osteoarthritis, unspecified shoulder

✓6th M19.22 Secondary osteoarthritis, elbow
M19.221 Secondary osteoarthritis, right elbow
M19.222 Secondary osteoarthritis, left elbow
M19.229 Secondary osteoarthritis, unspecified elbow

✓6th M19.23 Secondary osteoarthritis, wrist
M19.231 Secondary osteoarthritis, right wrist
M19.232 Secondary osteoarthritis, left wrist
M19.239 Secondary osteoarthritis, unspecified wrist

✓6th M19.24 Secondary osteoarthritis, hand
M19.241 Secondary osteoarthritis, right hand
M19.242 Secondary osteoarthritis, left hand
M19.249 Secondary osteoarthritis, unspecified hand

✓6th M19.27 Secondary osteoarthritis, ankle and foot
M19.271 Secondary osteoarthritis, right ankle and foot
M19.272 Secondary osteoarthritis, left ankle and foot
M19.279 Secondary osteoarthritis, unspecified ankle and foot

✓5th M19.9 Osteoarthritis, unspecified site
M19.90 Unspecified osteoarthritis, unspecified site
Arthrosis NOS
Arthritis NOS
Osteoarthritis NOS
M19.91 Primary osteoarthritis, unspecified site
Primary osteoarthritis NOS
M19.92 Post-traumatic osteoarthritis, unspecified site
Post-traumatic osteoarthritis NOS
M19.93 Secondary osteoarthritis, unspecified site
Secondary osteoarthritis NOS

Other joint disorders (M20-M25)

EXCLUDES 2 *joints of the spine (M40-M54)*

✓4th **M20 Acquired deformities of fingers and toes**
EXCLUDES 1 *acquired absence of fingers and toes (Z89.-)*
congenital absence of fingers and toes (Q71.3-, Q72.3-)
congenital deformities and malformations of fingers and toes (Q66-, Q68-Q70, Q74-)

✓5th M20.0 Deformity of finger(s)
EXCLUDES 1 *clubbing of fingers (R68.3)*
palmar fascial fibromatosis [Dupuytren] (M72.0)
trigger finger (M65.3)

✓6th M20.00 Unspecified deformity of finger(s)
M20.001 Unspecified deformity of right finger(s)
M20.002 Unspecified deformity of left finger(s)
M20.009 Unspecified deformity of unspecified finger(s)

✓6th M20.01 Mallet finger
M20.011 Mallet finger of right finger(s)
M20.012 Mallet finger of left finger(s)
M20.019 Mallet finger of unspecified finger(s)

✓6th M20.02 Boutonnière deformity
M20.021 Boutonnière deformity of right finger(s)
M20.022 Boutonnière deformity of left finger(s)
M20.029 Boutonnière deformity of unspecified finger(s)

✓6th M20.03 Swan-neck deformity
M20.031 Swan-neck deformity of right finger(s)
M20.032 Swan-neck deformity of left finger(s)
M20.039 Swan-neck deformity of unspecified finger(s)

✓6th M20.09 Other deformity of finger(s)
M20.091 Other deformity of right finger(s)
M20.092 Other deformity of left finger(s)
M20.099 Other deformity of finger(s), unspecified finger(s)

✓5th M20.1 Hallux valgus (acquired)
Bunion
M20.10 Hallux valgus (acquired), unspecified foot
M20.11 Hallux valgus (acquired), right foot
M20.12 Hallux valgus (acquired), left foot

✓5th M20.2 Hallux rigidus
M20.20 Hallux rigidus, unspecified foot
M20.21 Hallux rigidus, right foot
M20.22 Hallux rigidus, left foot

✓5th M20.3 Hallux varus (acquired)
M20.30 Hallux varus (acquired), unspecified foot
M20.31 Hallux varus (acquired), right foot
M20.32 Hallux varus (acquired), left foot

✓5th M20.4 Other hammer toe(s) (acquired)
M20.40 Other hammer toe(s) (acquired), unspecified foot
M20.41 Other hammer toe(s) (acquired), right foot
M20.42 Other hammer toe(s) (acquired), left foot

✓5th **M20.5 Other deformities of toe(s) (acquired)**
✓6th **M20.5X Other deformities of toe(s) (acquired)**
M20.5X1 Other deformities of toe(s) (acquired), right foot
M20.5X2 Other deformities of toe(s) (acquired), left foot
M20.5X9 Other deformities of toe(s) (acquired), unspecified foot
✓5th **M20.6 Acquired deformities of toe(s), unspecified**
M20.60 Acquired deformities of toe(s), unspecified, unspecified foot
M20.61 Acquired deformities of toe(s), unspecified, right foot
M20.62 Acquired deformities of toe(s), unspecified, left foot

✓4th **M21 Other acquired deformities of limbs**
EXCLUDES 1 *acquired absence of limb (Z89.-)*
congenital absence of limbs (Q71-Q73)
congenital deformities and malformations of limbs (Q65-Q66, Q68-Q74)
EXCLUDES 2 *acquired deformities of fingers or toes (M20.-)*
coxa plana (M91.2)
✓5th **M21.0 Valgus deformity, not elsewhere classified**
EXCLUDES 1 *metatarsus valgus (Q66.6)*
talipes calcaneovalgus (Q66.4)
M21.00 Valgus deformity, not elsewhere classified, unspecified site
✓6th **M21.02 Valgus deformity, not elsewhere classified, elbow**
Cubitus valgus
M21.021 Valgus deformity, not elsewhere classified, right elbow
M21.022 Valgus deformity, not elsewhere classified, left elbow
M21.029 Valgus deformity, not elsewhere classified, unspecified elbow
✓6th **M21.05 Valgus deformity, not elsewhere classified, hip**
M21.051 Valgus deformity, not elsewhere classified, right hip
M21.052 Valgus deformity, not elsewhere classified, left hip
M21.059 Valgus deformity, not elsewhere classified, unspecified hip
✓6th **M21.06 Valgus deformity, not elsewhere classified, knee**
Genu valgum
Knock knee
M21.061 Valgus deformity, not elsewhere classified, right knee
M21.062 Valgus deformity, not elsewhere classified, left knee
M21.069 Valgus deformity, not elsewhere classified, unspecified knee
✓6th **M21.07 Valgus deformity, not elsewhere classified, ankle**
M21.071 Valgus deformity, not elsewhere classified, right ankle
M21.072 Valgus deformity, not elsewhere classified, left ankle
M21.079 Valgus deformity, not elsewhere classified, unspecified ankle
✓5th **M21.1 Varus deformity, not elsewhere classified**
EXCLUDES 1 *metatarsus varus (Q66.2)*
tibia vara (M92.5)
M21.10 Varus deformity, not elsewhere classified, unspecified site
✓6th **M21.12 Varus deformity, not elsewhere classified, elbow**
Cubitus varus, elbow
M21.121 Varus deformity, not elsewhere classified, right elbow
M21.122 Varus deformity, not elsewhere classified, left elbow
M21.129 Varus deformity, not elsewhere classified, unspecified elbow
✓6th **M21.15 Varus deformity, not elsewhere classified, hip**
M21.151 Varus deformity, not elsewhere classified, right hip
M21.152 Varus deformity, not elsewhere classified, left hip
M21.159 Varus deformity, not elsewhere classified, unspecified
✓6th **M21.16 Varus deformity, not elsewhere classified, knee**
Bow leg
Genu varum
M21.161 Varus deformity, not elsewhere classified, right knee
M21.162 Varus deformity, not elsewhere classified, left knee
M21.169 Varus deformity, not elsewhere classified, unspecified knee
✓6th **M21.17 Varus deformity, not elsewhere classified, ankle**
M21.171 Varus deformity, not elsewhere classified, right ankle
M21.172 Varus deformity, not elsewhere classified, left ankle
M21.179 Varus deformity, not elsewhere classified, unspecified ankle
✓5th **M21.2 Flexion deformity**
M21.20 Flexion deformity, unspecified site
✓6th **M21.21 Flexion deformity, shoulder**
M21.211 Flexion deformity, right shoulder
M21.212 Flexion deformity, left shoulder
M21.219 Flexion deformity, unspecified shoulder
✓6th **M21.22 Flexion deformity, elbow**
M21.221 Flexion deformity, right elbow
M21.222 Flexion deformity, left elbow
M21.229 Flexion deformity, unspecified elbow
✓6th **M21.23 Flexion deformity, wrist**
M21.231 Flexion deformity, right wrist
M21.232 Flexion deformity, left wrist
M21.239 Flexion deformity, unspecified wrist
✓6th **M21.24 Flexion deformity, finger joints**
M21.241 Flexion deformity, right finger joints
M21.242 Flexion deformity, left finger joints
M21.249 Flexion deformity, unspecified finger joints
✓6th **M21.25 Flexion deformity, hip**
M21.251 Flexion deformity, right hip
M21.252 Flexion deformity, left hip
M21.259 Flexion deformity, unspecified hip
✓6th **M21.26 Flexion deformity, knee**
M21.261 Flexion deformity, right knee
M21.262 Flexion deformity, left knee
M21.269 Flexion deformity, unspecified knee
✓6th **M21.27 Flexion deformity, ankle and toes**
M21.271 Flexion deformity, right ankle and toes
M21.272 Flexion deformity, left ankle and toes
M21.279 Flexion deformity, unspecified ankle and toes
✓5th **M21.3 Wrist or foot drop (acquired)**
✓6th **M21.33 Wrist drop (acquired)**
M21.331 Wrist drop, right wrist
M21.332 Wrist drop, left wrist
M21.339 Wrist drop, unspecified wrist
✓6th **M21.37 Foot drop (acquired)**
M21.371 Foot drop, right foot
M21.372 Foot drop, left foot
M21.379 Foot drop, unspecified foot
✓5th **M21.4 Flat foot [pes planus] (acquired)**
EXCLUDES 1 *congenital pes planus (Q66.5-)*
M21.40 Flat foot [pes planus] (acquired), unspecified foot
M21.41 Flat foot [pes planus] (acquired), right foot
M21.42 Flat foot [pes planus] (acquired), left foot
✓5th **M21.5 Acquired clawhand, clubhand, clawfoot and clubfoot**
EXCLUDES 1 *clubfoot, not specified as acquired (Q66.89)*
✓6th **M21.51 Acquired clawhand**
M21.511 Acquired clawhand, right hand
M21.512 Acquired clawhand, left hand
M21.519 Acquired clawhand, unspecified hand
✓6th **M21.52 Acquired clubhand**
M21.521 Acquired clubhand, right hand
M21.522 Acquired clubhand, left hand
M21.529 Acquired clubhand, unspecified hand

✓6th **M21.53 Acquired clawfoot**
M21.531 Acquired clawfoot, right foot
M21.532 Acquired clawfoot, left foot
M21.539 Acquired clawfoot, unspecified foot

✓6th **M21.54 Acquired clubfoot**
M21.541 Acquired clubfoot, right foot
M21.542 Acquired clubfoot, left foot
M21.549 Acquired clubfoot, unspecified foot

✓5th **M21.6 Other acquired deformities of foot**
EXCLUDES 2 *deformities of toe (acquired) (M20.1-M20.6)*

✓6th **M21.6X Other acquired deformities of foot**
M21.6X1 Other acquired deformities of right foot
M21.6X2 Other acquired deformities of left foot
M21.6X9 Other acquired deformities of unspecified foot

✓5th **M21.7 Unequal limb length (acquired)**
NOTE The site used should correspond to the shorter limb.
M21.70 Unequal limb length (acquired), unspecified site

✓6th **M21.72 Unequal limb length (acquired), humerus**
M21.721 Unequal limb length (acquired), right humerus
M21.722 Unequal limb length (acquired), left humerus
M21.729 Unequal limb length (acquired), unspecified humerus

✓6th **M21.73 Unequal limb length (acquired), ulna and radius**
M21.731 Unequal limb length (acquired), right ulna
M21.732 Unequal limb length (acquired), left ulna
M21.733 Unequal limb length (acquired), right radius
M21.734 Unequal limb length (acquired), left radius
M21.739 Unequal limb length (acquired), unspecified ulna and radius

✓6th **M21.75 Unequal limb length (acquired), femur**
M21.751 Unequal limb length (acquired), right femur
M21.752 Unequal limb length (acquired), left femur
M21.759 Unequal limb length (acquired), unspecified femur

✓6th **M21.76 Unequal limb length (acquired), tibia and fibula**
M21.761 Unequal limb length (acquired), right tibia
M21.762 Unequal limb length (acquired), left tibia
M21.763 Unequal limb length (acquired), right fibula
M21.764 Unequal limb length (acquired), left fibula
M21.769 Unequal limb length (acquired), unspecified tibia and fibula

✓5th **M21.8 Other specified acquired deformities of limbs**
EXCLUDES 2 *coxa plana (M91.2)*
M21.80 Other specified acquired deformities of unspecified limb

✓6th **M21.82 Other specified acquired deformities of upper arm**
M21.821 Other specified acquired deformities of right upper arm
M21.822 Other specified acquired deformities of left upper arm
M21.829 Other specified acquired deformities of unspecified upper arm

✓6th **M21.83 Other specified acquired deformities of forearm**
M21.831 Other specified acquired deformities of right forearm
M21.832 Other specified acquired deformities of left forearm
M21.839 Other specified acquired deformities of unspecified forearm

✓6th **M21.85 Other specified acquired deformities of thigh**
M21.851 Other specified acquired deformities of right thigh
M21.852 Other specified acquired deformities of left thigh
M21.859 Other specified acquired deformities of unspecified thigh

✓6th **M21.86 Other specified acquired deformities of lower leg**
M21.861 Other specified acquired deformities of right lower leg
M21.862 Other specified acquired deformities of left lower leg
M21.869 Other specified acquired deformities of unspecified lower leg

✓5th **M21.9 Unspecified acquired deformity of limb and hand**
M21.90 Unspecified acquired deformity of unspecified limb

✓6th **M21.92 Unspecified acquired deformity of upper arm**
M21.921 Unspecified acquired deformity of right upper arm
M21.922 Unspecified acquired deformity of left upper arm
M21.929 Unspecified acquired deformity of unspecified upper arm

✓6th **M21.93 Unspecified acquired deformity of forearm**
M21.931 Unspecified acquired deformity of right forearm
M21.932 Unspecified acquired deformity of left forearm
M21.939 Unspecified acquired deformity of unspecified forearm

✓6th **M21.94 Unspecified acquired deformity of hand**
M21.941 Unspecified acquired deformity of hand, right hand
M21.942 Unspecified acquired deformity of hand, left hand
M21.949 Unspecified acquired deformity of hand, unspecified hand

✓6th **M21.95 Unspecified acquired deformity of thigh**
M21.951 Unspecified acquired deformity of right thigh
M21.952 Unspecified acquired deformity of left thigh
M21.959 Unspecified acquired deformity of unspecified thigh

✓6th **M21.96 Unspecified acquired deformity of lower leg**
M21.961 Unspecified acquired deformity of right lower leg
M21.962 Unspecified acquired deformity of left lower leg
M21.969 Unspecified acquired deformity of unspecified lower leg

✓4th **M22 Disorder of patella**
EXCLUDES 1 *traumatic dislocation of patella (S83.0-)*

✓5th **M22.0 Recurrent dislocation of patella**
M22.00 Recurrent dislocation of patella, unspecified knee
M22.01 Recurrent dislocation of patella, right knee
M22.02 Recurrent dislocation of patella, left knee

✓5th **M22.1 Recurrent subluxation of patella**
Incomplete dislocation of patella
M22.10 Recurrent subluxation of patella, unspecified knee
M22.11 Recurrent subluxation of patella, right knee
M22.12 Recurrent subluxation of patella, left knee

✓5th **M22.2 Patellofemoral disorders**

✓6th **M22.2X Patellofemoral disorders**
M22.2X1 Patellofemoral disorders, right knee
M22.2X2 Patellofemoral disorders, left knee
M22.2X9 Patellofemoral disorders, unspecified knee

✓5th **M22.3 Other derangements of patella**

✓6th **M22.3X Other derangements of patella**
M22.3X1 Other derangements of patella, right knee
M22.3X2 Other derangements of patella, left knee
M22.3X9 Other derangements of patella, unspecified knee

✓5th **M22.4 Chondromalacia patellae**
M22.40 Chondromalacia patellae, unspecified knee
M22.41 Chondromalacia patellae, right knee
M22.42 Chondromalacia patellae, left knee

✓5th **M22.8 Other disorders of patella**

✓6th **M22.8X Other disorders of patella**
M22.8X1 Other disorders of patella, right knee
M22.8X2 Other disorders of patella, left knee
M22.8X9 Other disorders of patella, unspecified knee

5th **M22.9 Unspecified disorder of patella**
- **M22.90 Unspecified disorder of patella, unspecified knee**
- **M22.91 Unspecified disorder of patella, right knee**
- **M22.92 Unspecified disorder of patella, left knee**

4th **M23 Internal derangement of knee**

EXCLUDES 1 *ankylosis (M24.66)*
current injury—see injury of knee and lower leg (S80-S89)
deformity of knee (M21.-)
osteochondritis dissecans (M93.2)
recurrent dislocation or subluxation of joints (M24.4)
recurrent dislocation or subluxation of patella (M22.0-M22.1)

5th **M23.0 Cystic meniscus**

6th **M23.00 Cystic meniscus, unspecified meniscus**
Cystic meniscus, unspecified lateral meniscus
Cystic meniscus, unspecified medial meniscus
- **M23.000 Cystic meniscus, unspecified lateral meniscus, right knee**
- **M23.001 Cystic meniscus, unspecified lateral meniscus, left knee**
- **M23.002 Cystic meniscus, unspecified lateral meniscus, unspecified knee**
- **M23.003 Cystic meniscus, unspecified medial meniscus, right knee**
- **M23.004 Cystic meniscus, unspecified medial meniscus, left knee**
- **M23.005 Cystic meniscus, unspecified medial meniscus, unspecified knee**
- **M23.006 Cystic meniscus, unspecified meniscus, right knee**
- **M23.007 Cystic meniscus, unspecified meniscus, left knee**
- **M23.009 Cystic meniscus, unspecified meniscus, unspecified knee**

6th **M23.01 Cystic meniscus, anterior horn of medial meniscus**
- **M23.011 Cystic meniscus, anterior horn of medial meniscus, right knee**
- **M23.012 Cystic meniscus, anterior horn of medial meniscus, left knee**
- **M23.019 Cystic meniscus, anterior horn of medial meniscus, unspecified knee**

6th **M23.02 Cystic meniscus, posterior horn of medial meniscus**
- **M23.021 Cystic meniscus, posterior horn of medial meniscus, right knee**
- **M23.022 Cystic meniscus, posterior horn of medial meniscus, left knee**
- **M23.029 Cystic meniscus, posterior horn of medial meniscus, unspecified knee**

6th **M23.03 Cystic meniscus, other medial meniscus**
- **M23.031 Cystic meniscus, other medial meniscus, right knee**
- **M23.032 Cystic meniscus, other medial meniscus, left knee**
- **M23.039 Cystic meniscus, other medial meniscus, unspecified knee**

6th **M23.04 Cystic meniscus, anterior horn of lateral meniscus**
- **M23.041 Cystic meniscus, anterior horn of lateral meniscus, right knee**
- **M23.042 Cystic meniscus, anterior horn of lateral meniscus, left knee**
- **M23.049 Cystic meniscus, anterior horn of lateral meniscus, unspecified knee**

6th **M23.05 Cystic meniscus, posterior horn of lateral meniscus**
- **M23.051 Cystic meniscus, posterior horn of lateral meniscus, right knee**
- **M23.052 Cystic meniscus, posterior horn of lateral meniscus, left knee**
- **M23.059 Cystic meniscus, posterior horn of lateral meniscus, unspecified knee**

6th **M23.06 Cystic meniscus, other lateral meniscus**
- **M23.061 Cystic meniscus, other lateral meniscus, right knee**
- **M23.062 Cystic meniscus, other lateral meniscus, left knee**
- **M23.069 Cystic meniscus, other lateral meniscus, unspecified knee**

5th **M23.2 Derangement of meniscus due to old tear or injury**
Old bucket-handle tear

6th **M23.20 Derangement of unspecified meniscus due to old tear or injury**
Derangement of unspecified lateral meniscus due to old tear or injury
Derangement of unspecified medial meniscus due to old tear or injury
- **M23.200 Derangement of unspecified lateral meniscus due to old tear or injury, right knee**
- **M23.201 Derangement of unspecified lateral meniscus due to old tear or injury, left knee**
- **M23.202 Derangement of unspecified lateral meniscus due to old tear or injury, unspecified knee**
- **M23.203 Derangement of unspecified medial meniscus due to old tear or injury, right knee**
- **M23.204 Derangement of unspecified medial meniscus due to old tear or injury, left knee**
- **M23.205 Derangement of unspecified medial meniscus due to old tear or injury, unspecified knee**
- **M23.206 Derangement of unspecified meniscus due to old tear or injury, right knee**
- **M23.207 Derangement of unspecified meniscus due to old tear or injury, left knee**
- **M23.209 Derangement of unspecified meniscus due to old tear or injury, unspecified knee**

6th **M23.21 Derangement of anterior horn of medial meniscus due to old tear or injury**
- **M23.211 Derangement of anterior horn of medial meniscus due to old tear or injury, right knee**
- **M23.212 Derangement of anterior horn of medial meniscus due to old tear or injury, left knee**
- **M23.219 Derangement of anterior horn of medial meniscus due to old tear or injury, unspecified knee**

6th **M23.22 Derangement of posterior horn of medial meniscus due to old tear or injury**
- **M23.221 Derangement of posterior horn of medial meniscus due to old tear or injury, right knee**
- **M23.222 Derangement of posterior horn of medial meniscus due to old tear or injury, left knee**
- **M23.229 Derangement of posterior horn of medial meniscus due to old tear or injury, unspecified knee**

6th **M23.23 Derangement of other medial meniscus due to old tear or injury**
- **M23.231 Derangement of other medial meniscus due to old tear or injury, right knee**
- **M23.232 Derangement of other medial meniscus due to old tear or injury, left knee**
- **M23.239 Derangement of other medial meniscus due to old tear or injury, unspecified knee**

6th **M23.24 Derangement of anterior horn of lateral meniscus due to old tear or injury**
- **M23.241 Derangement of anterior horn of lateral meniscus due to old tear or injury, right knee**
- **M23.242 Derangement of anterior horn of lateral meniscus due to old tear or injury, left knee**
- **M23.249 Derangement of anterior horn of lateral meniscus due to old tear or injury, unspecified knee**

6th **M23.25 Derangement of posterior horn of lateral meniscus due to old tear or injury**
- **M23.251 Derangement of posterior horn of lateral meniscus due to old tear or injury, right knee**

M23.252 Derangement of posterior horn of lateral meniscus due to old tear or injury, left knee

M23.259 Derangement of posterior horn of lateral meniscus due to old tear or injury, unspecified knee

✓6th **M23.26 Derangement of other lateral meniscus due to old tear or injury**

M23.261 Derangement of other lateral meniscus due to old tear or injury, right knee

M23.262 Derangement of other lateral meniscus due to old tear or injury, left knee

M23.269 Derangement of other lateral meniscus due to old tear or injury, unspecified knee

✓5th **M23.3 Other meniscus derangements**

Degenerate meniscus
Detached meniscus
Retained meniscus

✓6th **M23.30 Other meniscus derangements, unspecified meniscus**

Other meniscus derangements, unspecified lateral meniscus
Other meniscus derangements, unspecified medial meniscus

M23.300 Other meniscus derangements, unspecified lateral meniscus, right knee

M23.301 Other meniscus derangements, unspecified lateral meniscus, left knee

M23.302 Other meniscus derangements, unspecified lateral meniscus, unspecified knee

M23.303 Other meniscus derangements, unspecified medial meniscus, right knee

M23.304 Other meniscus derangements, unspecified medial meniscus, left knee

M23.305 Other meniscus derangements, unspecified medial meniscus, unspecified knee

M23.306 Other meniscus derangements, unspecified meniscus, right knee

M23.307 Other meniscus derangements, unspecified meniscus, left knee

M23.309 Other meniscus derangements, unspecified meniscus, unspecified knee

✓6th **M23.31 Other meniscus derangements, anterior horn of medial meniscus**

M23.311 Other meniscus derangements, anterior horn of medial meniscus, right knee

M23.312 Other meniscus derangements, anterior horn of medial meniscus, left knee

M23.319 Other meniscus derangements, anterior horn of medial meniscus, unspecified knee

✓6th **M23.32 Other meniscus derangements, posterior horn of medial meniscus**

M23.321 Other meniscus derangements, posterior horn of medial meniscus, right knee

M23.322 Other meniscus derangements, posterior horn of medial meniscus, left knee

M23.329 Other meniscus derangements, posterior horn of medial meniscus, unspecified knee

✓6th **M23.33 Other meniscus derangements, other medial meniscus**

M23.331 Other meniscus derangements, other medial meniscus, right knee

M23.332 Other meniscus derangements, other medial meniscus, left knee

M23.339 Other meniscus derangements, other medial meniscus, unspecified knee

✓6th **M23.34 Other meniscus derangements, anterior horn of lateral meniscus**

M23.341 Other meniscus derangements, anterior horn of lateral meniscus, right knee

M23.342 Other meniscus derangements, anterior horn of lateral meniscus, left knee

M23.349 Other meniscus derangements, anterior horn of lateral meniscus, unspecified knee

✓6th **M23.35 Other meniscus derangements, posterior horn of lateral meniscus**

M23.351 Other meniscus derangements, posterior horn of lateral meniscus, right knee

M23.352 Other meniscus derangements, posterior horn of lateral meniscus, left knee

M23.359 Other meniscus derangements, posterior horn of lateral meniscus, unspecified knee

✓6th **M23.36 Other meniscus derangements, other lateral meniscus**

M23.361 Other meniscus derangements, other lateral meniscus, right knee

M23.362 Other meniscus derangements, other lateral meniscus, left knee

M23.369 Other meniscus derangements, other lateral meniscus, unspecified knee

✓5th **M23.4 Loose body in knee**

M23.40 Loose body in knee, unspecified knee

M23.41 Loose body in knee, right knee

M23.42 Loose body in knee, left knee

✓5th **M23.5 Chronic instability of knee**

M23.50 Chronic instability of knee, unspecified knee

M23.51 Chronic instability of knee, right knee

M23.52 Chronic instability of knee, left knee

✓5th **M23.6 Other spontaneous disruption of ligament(s) of knee**

✓6th **M23.60 Other spontaneous disruption of unspecified ligament of knee**

M23.601 Other spontaneous disruption of unspecified ligament of right knee

M23.602 Other spontaneous disruption of unspecified ligament of left knee

M23.609 Other spontaneous disruption of unspecified ligament of unspecified knee

✓6th **M23.61 Other spontaneous disruption of anterior cruciate ligament of knee**

M23.611 Other spontaneous disruption of anterior cruciate ligament of right knee

M23.612 Other spontaneous disruption of anterior cruciate ligament of left knee

M23.619 Other spontaneous disruption of anterior cruciate ligament of unspecified knee

✓6th **M23.62 Other spontaneous disruption of posterior cruciate ligament of knee**

M23.621 Other spontaneous disruption of posterior cruciate ligament of right knee

M23.622 Other spontaneous disruption of posterior cruciate ligament of left knee

M23.629 Other spontaneous disruption of posterior cruciate ligament of unspecified knee

✓6th **M23.63 Other spontaneous disruption of medial collateral ligament of knee**

M23.631 Other spontaneous disruption of medial collateral ligament of right knee

M23.632 Other spontaneous disruption of medial collateral ligament of left knee

M23.639 Other spontaneous disruption of medial collateral ligament of unspecified knee

✓6th **M23.64 Other spontaneous disruption of lateral collateral ligament of knee**

M23.641 Other spontaneous disruption of lateral collateral ligament of right knee

M23.642 Other spontaneous disruption of lateral collateral ligament of left knee

M23.649 Other spontaneous disruption of lateral collateral ligament of unspecified knee

✓6th **M23.67 Other spontaneous disruption of capsular ligament of knee**

M23.671 Other spontaneous disruption of capsular ligament of right knee

M23.672 Other spontaneous disruption of capsular ligament of left knee

M23.679 Other spontaneous disruption of capsular ligament of unspecified knee

M23.8 Other internal derangements of knee
Laxity of ligament of knee
Snapping knee

M23.8X Other internal derangements of knee
- **M23.8X1** Other internal derangements of right knee
- **M23.8X2** Other internal derangements of left knee
- **M23.8X9** Other internal derangements of unspecified knee

M23.9 Unspecified internal derangement of knee
- **M23.90** Unspecified internal derangement of unspecified knee
- **M23.91** Unspecified internal derangement of right knee
- **M23.92** Unspecified internal derangement of left knee

M24 Other specific joint derangements

EXCLUDES 1 *current injury—see injury of joint by body region*
EXCLUDES 2 *ganglion (M67.4)*
snapping knee (M23.8-)
temporomandibular joint disorders (M26.6-)

M24.0 Loose body in joint
EXCLUDES 2 *loose body in knee (M23.4)*
- **M24.00** Loose body in unspecified joint

M24.01 Loose body in shoulder
- **M24.011** Loose body in right shoulder
- **M24.012** Loose body in left shoulder
- **M24.019** Loose body in unspecified shoulder

M24.02 Loose body in elbow
- **M24.021** Loose body in right elbow
- **M24.022** Loose body in left elbow
- **M24.029** Loose body in unspecified elbow

M24.03 Loose body in wrist
- **M24.031** Loose body in right wrist
- **M24.032** Loose body in left wrist
- **M24.039** Loose body in unspecified wrist

M24.04 Loose body in finger joints
- **M24.041** Loose body in right finger joint(s)
- **M24.042** Loose body in left finger joint(s)
- **M24.049** Loose body in unspecified finger joint(s)

M24.05 Loose body in hip
- **M24.051** Loose body in right hip
- **M24.052** Loose body in left hip
- **M24.059** Loose body in unspecified hip

M24.07 Loose body in ankle and toe joints
- **M24.071** Loose body in right ankle
- **M24.072** Loose body in left ankle
- **M24.073** Loose body in unspecified ankle
- **M24.074** Loose body in right toe joint(s)
- **M24.075** Loose body in left toe joint(s)
- **M24.076** Loose body in unspecified toe joints

M24.08 Loose body, other site

M24.1 Other articular cartilage disorders
EXCLUDES 2 *chondrocalcinosis (M11.1, M11.2-)*
internal derangement of knee (M23.-)
metastatic calcification (E83.5)
ochronosis (E70.2)
- **M24.10** Other articular cartilage disorders, unspecified site

M24.11 Other articular cartilage disorders, shoulder
- **M24.111** Other articular cartilage disorders, right shoulder
- **M24.112** Other articular cartilage disorders, left shoulder
- **M24.119** Other articular cartilage disorders, unspecified shoulder

M24.12 Other articular cartilage disorders, elbow
- **M24.121** Other articular cartilage disorders, right elbow
- **M24.122** Other articular cartilage disorders, left elbow
- **M24.129** Other articular cartilage disorders, unspecified elbow

M24.13 Other articular cartilage disorders, wrist
- **M24.131** Other articular cartilage disorders, right wrist
- **M24.132** Other articular cartilage disorders, left wrist
- **M24.139** Other articular cartilage disorders, unspecified wrist

M24.14 Other articular cartilage disorders, hand
- **M24.141** Other articular cartilage disorders, right hand
- **M24.142** Other articular cartilage disorders, left hand
- **M24.149** Other articular cartilage disorders, unspecified hand

M24.15 Other articular cartilage disorders, hip
- **M24.151** Other articular cartilage disorders, right hip
- **M24.152** Other articular cartilage disorders, left hip
- **M24.159** Other articular cartilage disorders, unspecified hip

M24.17 Other articular cartilage disorders, ankle and foot
- **M24.171** Other articular cartilage disorders, right ankle
- **M24.172** Other articular cartilage disorders, left ankle
- **M24.173** Other articular cartilage disorders, unspecified ankle
- **M24.174** Other articular cartilage disorders, right foot
- **M24.175** Other articular cartilage disorders, left foot
- **M24.176** Other articular cartilage disorders, unspecified foot

M24.2 Disorder of ligament
Instability secondary to old ligament injury
Ligamentous laxity NOS
EXCLUDES 1 *familial ligamentous laxity (M35.7)*
EXCLUDES 2 *internal derangement of knee (M23.5-M23.89)*
- **M24.20** Disorder of ligament, unspecified site

M24.21 Disorder of ligament, shoulder
- **M24.211** Disorder of ligament, right shoulder
- **M24.212** Disorder of ligament, left shoulder
- **M24.219** Disorder of ligament, unspecified shoulder

M24.22 Disorder of ligament, elbow
- **M24.221** Disorder of ligament, right elbow
- **M24.222** Disorder of ligament, left elbow
- **M24.229** Disorder of ligament, unspecified elbow

M24.23 Disorder of ligament, wrist
- **M24.231** Disorder of ligament, right wrist
- **M24.232** Disorder of ligament, left wrist
- **M24.239** Disorder of ligament, unspecified wrist

M24.24 Disorder of ligament, hand
- **M24.241** Disorder of ligament, right hand
- **M24.242** Disorder of ligament, left hand
- **M24.249** Disorder of ligament, unspecified hand

M24.25 Disorder of ligament, hip
- **M24.251** Disorder of ligament, right hip
- **M24.252** Disorder of ligament, left hip
- **M24.259** Disorder of ligament, unspecified hip

M24.27 Disorder of ligament, ankle and foot
- **M24.271** Disorder of ligament, right ankle
- **M24.272** Disorder of ligament, left ankle
- **M24.273** Disorder of ligament, unspecified ankle
- **M24.274** Disorder of ligament, right foot
- **M24.275** Disorder of ligament, left foot
- **M24.276** Disorder of ligament, unspecified foot

M24.28 Disorder of ligament, vertebrae

M24.3 Pathological dislocation of joint, not elsewhere classified
EXCLUDES 1 *congenital dislocation or displacement of joint—see congenital malformations and deformations of the musculoskeletal system (Q65-Q79)*
current injury—see injury of joints and ligaments by body region
recurrent dislocation of joint (M24.4-)
- **M24.30** Pathological dislocation of unspecified joint, not elsewhere classified

✓6th **M24.31 Pathological dislocation of shoulder, not elsewhere classified**
- **M24.311 Pathological dislocation of right shoulder, not elsewhere classified**
- **M24.312 Pathological dislocation of left shoulder, not elsewhere classified**
- **M24.319 Pathological dislocation of unspecified shoulder, not elsewhere classified**

✓6th **M24.32 Pathological dislocation of elbow, not elsewhere classified**
- **M24.321 Pathological dislocation of right elbow, not elsewhere classified**
- **M24.322 Pathological dislocation of left elbow, not elsewhere classified**
- **M24.329 Pathological dislocation of unspecified elbow, not elsewhere classified**

✓6th **M24.33 Pathological dislocation of wrist, not elsewhere classified**
- **M24.331 Pathological dislocation of right wrist, not elsewhere classified**
- **M24.332 Pathological dislocation of left wrist, not elsewhere classified**
- **M24.339 Pathological dislocation of unspecified wrist, not elsewhere classified**

✓6th **M24.34 Pathological dislocation of hand, not elsewhere classified**
- **M24.341 Pathological dislocation of right hand, not elsewhere classified**
- **M24.342 Pathological dislocation of left hand, not elsewhere classified**
- **M24.349 Pathological dislocation of unspecified hand, not elsewhere classified**

✓6th **M24.35 Pathological dislocation of hip, not elsewhere classified**
- **M24.351 Pathological dislocation of right hip, not elsewhere classified**
- **M24.352 Pathological dislocation of left hip, not elsewhere classified**
- **M24.359 Pathological dislocation of unspecified hip, not elsewhere classified**

✓6th **M24.36 Pathological dislocation of knee, not elsewhere classified**
- **M24.361 Pathological dislocation of right knee, not elsewhere classified**
- **M24.362 Pathological dislocation of left knee, not elsewhere classified**
- **M24.369 Pathological dislocation of unspecified knee, not elsewhere classified**

✓6th **M24.37 Pathological dislocation of ankle and foot, not elsewhere classified**
- **M24.371 Pathological dislocation of right ankle, not elsewhere classified**
- **M24.372 Pathological dislocation of left ankle, not elsewhere classified**
- **M24.373 Pathological dislocation of unspecified ankle, not elsewhere classified**
- **M24.374 Pathological dislocation of right foot, not elsewhere classified**
- **M24.375 Pathological dislocation of left foot, not elsewhere classified**
- **M24.376 Pathological dislocation of unspecified foot, not elsewhere classified**

✓5th **M24.4 Recurrent dislocation of joint**

Recurrent subluxation of joint

EXCLUDES 2 *recurrent dislocation of patella (M22.Ø-M22.1)*
recurrent vertebral dislocation (M43.3-, M43.4, M43.5-)

M24.4Ø Recurrent dislocation, unspecified joint

✓6th **M24.41 Recurrent dislocation, shoulder**
- **M24.411 Recurrent dislocation, right shoulder**
- **M24.412 Recurrent dislocation, left shoulder**
- **M24.419 Recurrent dislocation, unspecified shoulder**

✓6th **M24.42 Recurrent dislocation, elbow**
- **M24.421 Recurrent dislocation, right elbow**
- **M24.422 Recurrent dislocation, left elbow**
- **M24.429 Recurrent dislocation, unspecified elbow**

✓6th **M24.43 Recurrent dislocation, wrist**
- **M24.431 Recurrent dislocation, right wrist**
- **M24.432 Recurrent dislocation, left wrist**
- **M24.439 Recurrent dislocation, unspecified wrist**

✓6th **M24.44 Recurrent dislocation, hand and finger(s)**
- **M24.441 Recurrent dislocation, right hand**
- **M24.442 Recurrent dislocation, left hand**
- **M24.443 Recurrent dislocation, unspecified hand**
- **M24.444 Recurrent dislocation, right finger**
- **M24.445 Recurrent dislocation, left finger**
- **M24.446 Recurrent dislocation, unspecified finger**

✓6th **M24.45 Recurrent dislocation, hip**
- **M24.451 Recurrent dislocation, right hip**
- **M24.452 Recurrent dislocation, left hip**
- **M24.459 Recurrent dislocation, unspecified hip**

✓6th **M24.46 Recurrent dislocation, knee**
- **M24.461 Recurrent dislocation, right knee**
- **M24.462 Recurrent dislocation, left knee**
- **M24.469 Recurrent dislocation, unspecified knee**

✓6th **M24.47 Recurrent dislocation, ankle, foot and toes**
- **M24.471 Recurrent dislocation, right ankle**
- **M24.472 Recurrent dislocation, left ankle**
- **M24.473 Recurrent dislocation, unspecified ankle**
- **M24.474 Recurrent dislocation, right foot**
- **M24.475 Recurrent dislocation, left foot**
- **M24.476 Recurrent dislocation, unspecified foot**
- **M24.477 Recurrent dislocation, right toe(s)**
- **M24.478 Recurrent dislocation, left toe(s)**
- **M24.479 Recurrent dislocation, unspecified toe(s)**

✓5th **M24.5 Contracture of joint**

EXCLUDES 1 *contracture of muscle without contracture of joint (M62.4-)*
contracture of tendon (sheath) without contracture of joint (M62.4-)
Dupuytren's contracture (M72.Ø)

EXCLUDES 2 *acquired deformities of limbs (M2Ø-M21)*

M24.5Ø Contracture, unspecified joint

✓6th **M24.51 Contracture, shoulder**
- **M24.511 Contracture, right shoulder**
- **M24.512 Contracture, left shoulder**
- **M24.519 Contracture, unspecified shoulder**

✓6th **M24.52 Contracture, elbow**
- **M24.521 Contracture, right elbow**
- **M24.522 Contracture, left elbow**
- **M24.529 Contracture, unspecified elbow**

✓6th **M24.53 Contracture, wrist**
- **M24.531 Contracture, right wrist**
- **M24.532 Contracture, left wrist**
- **M24.539 Contracture, unspecified wrist**

✓6th **M24.54 Contracture, hand**
- **M24.541 Contracture, right hand**
- **M24.542 Contracture, left hand**
- **M24.549 Contracture, unspecified hand**

✓6th **M24.55 Contracture, hip**
- **M24.551 Contracture, right hip**
- **M24.552 Contracture, left hip**
- **M24.559 Contracture, unspecified hip**

✓6th **M24.56 Contracture, knee**
- **M24.561 Contracture, right knee**
- **M24.562 Contracture, left knee**
- **M24.569 Contracture, unspecified knee**

✓6th **M24.57 Contracture, ankle and foot**
- **M24.571 Contracture, right ankle**
- **M24.572 Contracture, left ankle**
- **M24.573 Contracture, unspecified ankle**
- **M24.574 Contracture, right foot**
- **M24.575 Contracture, left foot**
- **M24.576 Contracture, unspecified foot**

✓5th **M24.6 Ankylosis of joint**

EXCLUDES 1 *stiffness of joint without ankylosis (M25.6-)*

EXCLUDES 2 *spine (M43.2-)*

M24.6Ø Ankylosis, unspecified joint

M24.61 Ankylosis, shoulder
- M24.611 Ankylosis, right shoulder
- M24.612 Ankylosis, left shoulder
- M24.619 Ankylosis, unspecified shoulder

M24.62 Ankylosis, elbow
- M24.621 Ankylosis, right elbow
- M24.622 Ankylosis, left elbow
- M24.629 Ankylosis, unspecified elbow

M24.63 Ankylosis, wrist
- M24.631 Ankylosis, right wrist
- M24.632 Ankylosis, left wrist
- M24.639 Ankylosis, unspecified wrist

M24.64 Ankylosis, hand
- M24.641 Ankylosis, right hand
- M24.642 Ankylosis, left hand
- M24.649 Ankylosis, unspecified hand

M24.65 Ankylosis, hip
- M24.651 Ankylosis, right hip
- M24.652 Ankylosis, left hip
- M24.659 Ankylosis, unspecified hip

M24.66 Ankylosis, knee
- M24.661 Ankylosis, right knee
- M24.662 Ankylosis, left knee
- M24.669 Ankylosis, unspecified knee

M24.67 Ankylosis, ankle and foot
- M24.671 Ankylosis, right ankle
- M24.672 Ankylosis, left ankle
- M24.673 Ankylosis, unspecified ankle
- M24.674 Ankylosis, right foot
- M24.675 Ankylosis, left foot
- M24.676 Ankylosis, unspecified foot

M24.7 Protrusio acetabuli

M24.8 Other specific joint derangements, not elsewhere classified
EXCLUDES 2 *iliotibial band syndrome (M76.3)*

M24.80 Other specific joint derangements of unspecified joint, not elsewhere classified

M24.81 Other specific joint derangements of shoulder, not elsewhere classified
- M24.811 Other specific joint derangements of right shoulder, not elsewhere classified
- M24.812 Other specific joint derangements of left shoulder, not elsewhere classified
- M24.819 Other specific joint derangements of unspecified shoulder, not elsewhere classified

M24.82 Other specific joint derangements of elbow, not elsewhere classified
- M24.821 Other specific joint derangements of right elbow, not elsewhere classified
- M24.822 Other specific joint derangements of left elbow, not elsewhere classified
- M24.829 Other specific joint derangements of unspecified elbow, not elsewhere classified

M24.83 Other specific joint derangements of wrist, not elsewhere classified
- M24.831 Other specific joint derangements of right wrist, not elsewhere classified
- M24.832 Other specific joint derangements of left wrist, not elsewhere classified
- M24.839 Other specific joint derangements of unspecified wrist, not elsewhere classified

M24.84 Other specific joint derangements of hand, not elsewhere classified
- M24.841 Other specific joint derangements of right hand, not elsewhere classified
- M24.842 Other specific joint derangements of left hand, not elsewhere classified
- M24.849 Other specific joint derangements of unspecified hand, not elsewhere classified

M24.85 Other specific joint derangements of hip, not elsewhere classified
Irritable hip
- M24.851 Other specific joint derangements of right hip, not elsewhere classified
- M24.852 Other specific joint derangements of left hip, not elsewhere classified
- M24.859 Other specific joint derangements of unspecified hip, not elsewhere classified

M24.87 Other specific joint derangements of ankle and foot, not elsewhere classified
- M24.871 Other specific joint derangements of right ankle, not elsewhere classified
- M24.872 Other specific joint derangements of left ankle, not elsewhere classified
- M24.873 Other specific joint derangements of unspecified ankle, not elsewhere classified
- M24.874 Other specific joint derangements of right foot, not elsewhere classified
- M24.875 Other specific joint derangements left foot, not elsewhere classified
- M24.876 Other specific joint derangements of unspecified foot, not elsewhere classified

M24.9 Joint derangement, unspecified

M25 Other joint disorder, not elsewhere classified

EXCLUDES 2
- *abnormality of gait and mobility (R26.-)*
- *acquired deformities of limb (M20-M21)*
- *calcification of bursa (M71.4-)*
- *calcification of shoulder (joint) (M75.3)*
- *calcification of tendon (M65.2-)*
- *difficulty in walking (R26.2)*
- *temporomandibular joint disorder (M26.6-)*

M25.0 Hemarthrosis

EXCLUDES 1
- *current injury—see injury of joint by body region*
- *hemophilic arthropathy (M36.2)*

M25.00 Hemarthrosis, unspecified joint CC
CC Excl: M25.00-M25.08, T79.A11A, T79.A12A, T79.A19A, T79.A21A, T79.A22A, T79.A29A

M25.01 Hemarthrosis, shoulder
- M25.011 Hemarthrosis, right shoulder CC
  CC Excl: M25.00-M25.039, M25.08, T79.A11A, T79.A12A, T79.A19A
- M25.012 Hemarthrosis, left shoulder CC
  CC Excl: See code: M25.011
- M25.019 Hemarthrosis, unspecified shoulder CC
  CC Excl: See code: M25.011

M25.02 Hemarthrosis, elbow
- M25.021 Hemarthrosis, right elbow CC
  CC Excl: M25.00-M25.029, M25.08, T79.A11A, T79.A12A, T79.A19A
- M25.022 Hemarthrosis, left elbow CC
  CC Excl: See code: M25.022
- M25.029 Hemarthrosis, unspecified elbow CC
  CC Excl: See code: M25.022

M25.03 Hemarthrosis, wrist
- M25.031 Hemarthrosis, right wrist CC
  CC Excl: M25.00, M25.021-M25.049, M25.08, T79.A11-T79.A19 with 7th character A
- M25.032 Hemarthrosis, left wrist CC
  CC Excl: See code: M25.031
- M25.039 Hemarthrosis, unspecified wrist CC
  CC Excl: See code: M25.031

M25.04 Hemarthrosis, hand
- M25.041 Hemarthrosis, right hand CC
  CC Excl: M25.00, M25.031-M25.049, M25.08, T79.A11-T79.A19 with 7th character A
- M25.042 Hemarthrosis, left hand CC
  CC Excl: See code: M25.041
- M25.049 Hemarthrosis, unspecified hand CC
  CC Excl: See code: M25.041

M25.05 Hemarthrosis, hip
- M25.051 Hemarthrosis, right hip CC
  CC Excl: M25.00-M25.08, T79.A11A, T79.A12A, T79.A19A, T79.A21A, T79.A22A, T79.A29A
- M25.052 Hemarthrosis, left hip CC
  CC Excl: See code: M25.051
- M25.059 Hemarthrosis, unspecified hip CC
  CC Excl: See code: M25.051

M25.06 Hemarthrosis, knee
- M25.061 Hemarthrosis, right knee CC
  CC Excl: M25.00, M25.061-M25.08, T79.A21-T79.A29 with 7th character A

M25.Ø62 Hemarthrosis, left knee CC
CC Excl: See code: M25.Ø61

M25.Ø69 Hemarthrosis, unspecified knee CC
CC Excl: See code: M25.Ø61

✓6th **M25.Ø7 Hemarthrosis, ankle and foot**

M25.Ø71 Hemarthrosis, right ankle CC
CC Excl: See code: M25.Ø61

M25.Ø72 Hemarthrosis, left ankle CC
CC Excl: See code: M25.Ø61

M25.Ø73 Hemarthrosis, unspecified ankle CC
CC Excl: See code: M25.Ø61

M25.Ø74 Hemarthrosis, right foot CC
CC Excl: See code: M25.Ø61

M25.Ø75 Hemarthrosis, left foot CC
CC Excl: See code: M25.Ø61

M25.Ø76 Hemarthrosis, unspecified foot CC
CC Excl: See code: M25.Ø61

M25.Ø8 Hemarthrosis, other specified site
Hemarthrosis, vertebrae
CC Excl: M25.ØØ-M25.Ø8, T79.A11A, T79.A12A, T79.A19A, T79.A21A, T79.A22A, T79.A29A

✓5th **M25.1 Fistula of joint**

M25.1Ø Fistula, unspecified joint

✓6th **M25.11 Fistula, shoulder**

M25.111 Fistula, right shoulder
M25.112 Fistula, left shoulder
M25.119 Fistula, unspecified shoulder

✓6th **M25.12 Fistula, elbow**

M25.121 Fistula, right elbow
M25.122 Fistula, left elbow
M25.129 Fistula, unspecified elbow

✓6th **M25.13 Fistula, wrist**

M25.131 Fistula, right wrist
M25.132 Fistula, left wrist
M25.139 Fistula, unspecified wrist

✓6th **M25.14 Fistula, hand**

M25.141 Fistula, right hand
M25.142 Fistula, left hand
M25.149 Fistula, unspecified hand

✓6th **M25.15 Fistula, hip**

M25.151 Fistula, right hip
M25.152 Fistula, left hip
M25.159 Fistula, unspecified hip

✓6th **M25.16 Fistula, knee**

M25.161 Fistula, right knee
M25.162 Fistula, left knee
M25.169 Fistula, unspecified knee

✓6th **M25.17 Fistula, ankle and foot**

M25.171 Fistula, right ankle
M25.172 Fistula, left ankle
M25.173 Fistula, unspecified ankle
M25.174 Fistula, right foot
M25.175 Fistula, left foot
M25.176 Fistula, unspecified foot

M25.18 Fistula, other specified site
Fistula, vertebrae

✓5th **M25.2 Flail joint**

M25.2Ø Flail joint, unspecified joint

✓6th **M25.21 Flail joint, shoulder**

M25.211 Flail joint, right shoulder
M25.212 Flail joint, left shoulder
M25.219 Flail joint, unspecified shoulder

✓6th **M25.22 Flail joint, elbow**

M25.221 Flail joint, right elbow
M25.222 Flail joint, left elbow
M25.229 Flail joint, unspecified elbow

✓6th **M25.23 Flail joint, wrist**

M25.231 Flail joint, right wrist
M25.232 Flail joint, left wrist
M25.239 Flail joint, unspecified wrist

✓6th **M25.24 Flail joint, hand**

M25.241 Flail joint, right hand
M25.242 Flail joint, left hand
M25.249 Flail joint, unspecified hand

✓6th **M25.25 Flail joint, hip**

M25.251 Flail joint, right hip
M25.252 Flail joint, left hip
M25.259 Flail joint, unspecified hip

✓6th **M25.26 Flail joint, knee**

M25.261 Flail joint, right knee
M25.262 Flail joint, left knee
M25.269 Flail joint, unspecified knee

✓6th **M25.27 Flail joint, ankle and foot**

M25.271 Flail joint, right ankle and foot
M25.272 Flail joint, left ankle and foot
M25.279 Flail joint, unspecified ankle and foot

M25.28 Flail joint, other site

✓5th **M25.3 Other instability of joint**

EXCLUDES 1 *instability of joint secondary to old ligament injury (M24.2-)*
instability of joint secondary to removal of joint prosthesis (M96.8-)

EXCLUDES 2 *spinal instabilities (M53.2-)*

M25.3Ø Other instability, unspecified joint

✓6th **M25.31 Other instability, shoulder**

M25.311 Other instability, right shoulder
M25.312 Other instability, left shoulder
M25.319 Other instability, unspecified shoulder

✓6th **M25.32 Other instability, elbow**

M25.321 Other instability, right elbow
M25.322 Other instability, left elbow
M25.329 Other instability, unspecified elbow

✓6th **M25.33 Other instability, wrist**

M25.331 Other instability, right wrist
M25.332 Other instability, left wrist
M25.339 Other instability, unspecified wrist

✓6th **M25.34 Other instability, hand**

M25.341 Other instability, right hand
M25.342 Other instability, left hand
M25.349 Other instability, unspecified hand

✓6th **M25.35 Other instability, hip**

M25.351 Other instability, right hip
M25.352 Other instability, left hip
M25.359 Other instability, unspecified hip

✓6th **M25.36 Other instability, knee**

M25.361 Other instability, right knee
M25.362 Other instability, left knee
M25.369 Other instability, unspecified knee

✓6th **M25.37 Other instability, ankle and foot**

M25.371 Other instability, right ankle
M25.372 Other instability, left ankle
M25.373 Other instability, unspecified ankle
M25.374 Other instability, right foot
M25.375 Other instability, left foot
M25.376 Other instability, unspecified foot

✓5th **M25.4 Effusion of joint**

EXCLUDES 1 *hydrarthrosis in yaws (A66.6)*
intermittent hydrarthrosis (M12.4-)
other infective (teno)synovitis (M65.1-)

M25.4Ø Effusion, unspecified joint

✓6th **M25.41 Effusion, shoulder**

M25.411 Effusion, right shoulder
M25.412 Effusion, left shoulder
M25.419 Effusion, unspecified shoulder

✓6th **M25.42 Effusion, elbow**

M25.421 Effusion, right elbow
M25.422 Effusion, left elbow
M25.429 Effusion, unspecified elbow

✓6th **M25.43 Effusion, wrist**

M25.431 Effusion, right wrist
M25.432 Effusion, left wrist
M25.439 Effusion, unspecified wrist

✓6th **M25.44 Effusion, hand**

M25.441 Effusion, right hand
M25.442 Effusion, left hand

M25.449 Effusion, unspecified hand
✓6th M25.45 Effusion, hip
M25.451 Effusion, right hip
M25.452 Effusion, left hip
M25.459 Effusion, unspecified hip
✓6th M25.46 Effusion, knee
M25.461 Effusion, right knee
M25.462 Effusion, left knee
M25.469 Effusion, unspecified knee
✓6th M25.47 Effusion, ankle and foot
M25.471 Effusion, right ankle
M25.472 Effusion, left ankle
M25.473 Effusion, unspecified ankle
M25.474 Effusion, right foot
M25.475 Effusion, left foot
M25.476 Effusion, unspecified foot
M25.48 Effusion, other site
✓5th M25.5 Pain in joint
EXCLUDES 2 *pain in hand (M79.64-)*
pain in fingers (M79.64-)
pain in foot (M79.67-)
pain in limb (M79.6-)
pain in toes (M79.67-)
M25.50 Pain in unspecified joint
✓6th M25.51 Pain in shoulder
M25.511 Pain in right shoulder
M25.512 Pain in left shoulder
M25.519 Pain in unspecified shoulder
✓6th M25.52 Pain in elbow
M25.521 Pain in right elbow
M25.522 Pain in left elbow
M25.529 Pain in unspecified elbow
✓6th M25.53 Pain in wrist
M25.531 Pain in right wrist
M25.532 Pain in left wrist
M25.539 Pain in unspecified wrist
✓6th M25.55 Pain in hip
M25.551 Pain in right hip
M25.552 Pain in left hip
M25.559 Pain in unspecified hip
✓6th M25.56 Pain in knee
M25.561 Pain in right knee
M25.562 Pain in left knee
M25.569 Pain in unspecified knee
✓6th M25.57 Pain in ankle and joints of foot
M25.571 Pain in right ankle and joints of right foot
M25.572 Pain in left ankle and joints of left foot
M25.579 Pain in unspecified ankle and joints of unspecified foot
✓5th M25.6 Stiffness of joint, not elsewhere classified
EXCLUDES 1 *ankylosis of joint (M24.6-)*
contracture of joint (M24.5-)
M25.60 Stiffness of unspecified joint, not elsewhere classified
✓6th M25.61 Stiffness of shoulder, not elsewhere classified
M25.611 Stiffness of right shoulder, not elsewhere classified
M25.612 Stiffness of left shoulder, not elsewhere classified
M25.619 Stiffness of unspecified shoulder, not elsewhere classified
✓6th M25.62 Stiffness of elbow, not elsewhere classified
M25.621 Stiffness of right elbow, not elsewhere classified
M25.622 Stiffness of left elbow, not elsewhere classified
M25.629 Stiffness of unspecified elbow, not elsewhere classified
✓6th M25.63 Stiffness of wrist, not elsewhere classified
M25.631 Stiffness of right wrist, not elsewhere classified
M25.632 Stiffness of left wrist, not elsewhere classified
M25.639 Stiffness of unspecified wrist, not elsewhere classified
✓6th M25.64 Stiffness of hand, not elsewhere classified
M25.641 Stiffness of right hand, not elsewhere classified
M25.642 Stiffness of left hand, not elsewhere classified
M25.649 Stiffness of unspecified hand, not elsewhere classified
✓6th M25.65 Stiffness of hip, not elsewhere classified
M25.651 Stiffness of right hip, not elsewhere classified
M25.652 Stiffness of left hip, not elsewhere classified
M25.659 Stiffness of unspecified hip, not elsewhere classified
✓6th M25.66 Stiffness of knee, not elsewhere classified
M25.661 Stiffness of right knee, not elsewhere classified
M25.662 Stiffness of left knee, not elsewhere classified
M25.669 Stiffness of unspecified knee, not elsewhere classified
✓6th M25.67 Stiffness of ankle and foot, not elsewhere classified
M25.671 Stiffness of right ankle, not elsewhere classified
M25.672 Stiffness of left ankle, not elsewhere classified
M25.673 Stiffness of unspecified ankle, not elsewhere classified
M25.674 Stiffness of right foot, not elsewhere classified
M25.675 Stiffness of left foot, not elsewhere classified
M25.676 Stiffness of unspecified foot, not elsewhere classified
✓5th M25.7 Osteophyte
M25.70 Osteophyte, unspecified joint
✓6th M25.71 Osteophyte, shoulder
M25.711 Osteophyte, right shoulder
M25.712 Osteophyte, left shoulder
M25.719 Osteophyte, unspecified shoulder
✓6th M25.72 Osteophyte, elbow
M25.721 Osteophyte, right elbow
M25.722 Osteophyte, left elbow
M25.729 Osteophyte, unspecified elbow
✓6th M25.73 Osteophyte, wrist
M25.731 Osteophyte, right wrist
M25.732 Osteophyte, left wrist
M25.739 Osteophyte, unspecified wrist
✓6th M25.74 Osteophyte, hand
M25.741 Osteophyte, right hand
M25.742 Osteophyte, left hand
M25.749 Osteophyte, unspecified hand
✓6th M25.75 Osteophyte, hip
M25.751 Osteophyte, right hip
M25.752 Osteophyte, left hip
M25.759 Osteophyte, unspecified hip
✓6th M25.76 Osteophyte, knee
M25.761 Osteophyte, right knee
M25.762 Osteophyte, left knee
M25.769 Osteophyte, unspecified knee
✓6th M25.77 Osteophyte, ankle and foot
M25.771 Osteophyte, right ankle
M25.772 Osteophyte, left ankle
M25.773 Osteophyte, unspecified ankle
M25.774 Osteophyte, right foot
M25.775 Osteophyte, left foot
M25.776 Osteophyte, unspecified foot
M25.78 Osteophyte, vertebrae
✓5th M25.8 Other specified joint disorders
M25.80 Other specified joint disorders, unspecified joint

✓6th M25.81 Other specified joint disorders, shoulder
M25.811 Other specified joint disorders, right shoulder
M25.812 Other specified joint disorders, left shoulder
M25.819 Other specified joint disorders, unspecified shoulder

✓6th M25.82 Other specified joint disorders, elbow
M25.821 Other specified joint disorders, right elbow
M25.822 Other specified joint disorders, left elbow
M25.829 Other specified joint disorders, unspecified elbow

✓6th M25.83 Other specified joint disorders, wrist
M25.831 Other specified joint disorders, right wrist
M25.832 Other specified joint disorders, left wrist
M25.839 Other specified joint disorders, unspecified wrist

✓6th M25.84 Other specified joint disorders, hand
M25.841 Other specified joint disorders, right hand
M25.842 Other specified joint disorders, left hand
M25.849 Other specified joint disorders, unspecified hand

✓6th M25.85 Other specified joint disorders, hip
M25.851 Other specified joint disorders, right hip
M25.852 Other specified joint disorders, left hip
M25.859 Other specified joint disorders, unspecified hip

✓6th M25.86 Other specified joint disorders, knee
M25.861 Other specified joint disorders, right knee
M25.862 Other specified joint disorders, left knee
M25.869 Other specified joint disorders, unspecified knee

✓6th M25.87 Other specified joint disorders, ankle and foot
M25.871 Other specified joint disorders, right ankle and foot
M25.872 Other specified joint disorders, left ankle and foot
M25.879 Other specified joint disorders, unspecified ankle and foot

M25.9 Joint disorder, unspecified

Dentofacial anomalies [including malocclusion] and other disorders of jaw (M26-M27)

EXCLUDES 1 *hemifacial atrophy or hypertrophy (Q67.4)*
unilateral condylar hyperplasia or hypoplasia (M27.8)

✓4th **M26 Dentofacial anomalies [including malocclusion]**

✓5th M26.0 Major anomalies of jaw size
EXCLUDES 1 *acromegaly (E22.0)*
Robin's syndrome (Q87.0)
M26.00 Unspecified anomaly of jaw size
M26.01 Maxillary hyperplasia
M26.02 Maxillary hypoplasia
M26.03 Mandibular hyperplasia
M26.04 Mandibular hypoplasia
M26.05 Macrogenia
M26.06 Microgenia
M26.07 Excessive tuberosity of jaw
Entire maxillary tuberosity
M26.09 Other specified anomalies of jaw size

✓5th M26.1 Anomalies of jaw-cranial base relationship
M26.10 Unspecified anomaly of jaw-cranial base relationship
M26.11 Maxillary asymmetry
M26.12 Other jaw asymmetry
M26.19 Other specified anomalies of jaw-cranial base relationship

✓5th M26.2 Anomalies of dental arch relationship
M26.20 Unspecified anomaly of dental arch relationship
✓6th M26.21 Malocclusion, Angle's class
M26.211 Malocclusion, Angle's class I
Neutro-occlusion
M26.212 Malocclusion, Angle's class II
Disto-occlusion Division I
Disto-occlusion Division II
M26.213 Malocclusion, Angle's class III
Mesio-occlusion
M26.219 Malocclusion, Angle's class, unspecified
✓6th M26.22 Open occlusal relationship
M26.220 Open anterior occlusal relationship
Anterior openbite
M26.221 Open posterior occlusal relationship
Posterior openbite
M26.23 Excessive horizontal overlap
Excessive horizontal overjet
M26.24 Reverse articulation
Crossbite (anterior) (posterior)
M26.25 Anomalies of interarch distance
M26.29 Other anomalies of dental arch relationship
Midline deviation of dental arch
Overbite (excessive) deep
Overbite (excessive) horizontal
Overbite (excessive) vertical
Posterior lingual occlusion of mandibular teeth

✓5th M26.3 Anomalies of tooth position of fully erupted tooth or teeth
EXCLUDES 2 *embedded and impacted teeth (K01.-)*
M26.30 Unspecified anomaly of tooth position of fully erupted tooth or teeth
Abnormal spacing of fully erupted tooth or teeth NOS
Displacement of fully erupted tooth or teeth NOS
Transposition of fully erupted tooth or teeth NOS
M26.31 Crowding of fully erupted teeth
M26.32 Excessive spacing of fully erupted teeth
Diastema of fully erupted tooth or teeth NOS
M26.33 Horizontal displacement of fully erupted tooth or teeth
Tipped tooth or teeth
Tipping of fully erupted tooth
M26.34 Vertical displacement of fully erupted tooth or teeth
Extruded tooth
Infraeruption of tooth or teeth
Supraeruption of tooth or teeth
M26.35 Rotation of fully erupted tooth or teeth
M26.36 Insufficient interocclusal distance of fully erupted teeth (ridge)
Lack of adequate intermaxillary vertical dimension of fully erupted teeth
M26.37 Excessive interocclusal distance of fully erupted teeth
Excessive intermaxillary vertical dimension of fully erupted teeth
Loss of occlusal vertical dimension of fully erupted teeth
M26.39 Other anomalies of tooth position of fully erupted tooth or teeth

M26.4 Malocclusion, unspecified

✓5th M26.5 Dentofacial functional abnormalities
EXCLUDES 1 *bruxism (F45.8)*
teeth-grinding NOS (F45.8)
M26.50 Dentofacial functional abnormalities, unspecified
M26.51 Abnormal jaw closure
M26.52 Limited mandibular range of motion
M26.53 Deviation in opening and closing of the mandible
M26.54 Insufficient anterior guidance
Insufficient anterior occlusal guidance
M26.55 Centric occlusion maximum intercuspation discrepancy
EXCLUDES 1 *centric occlusion NOS (M26.59)*
M26.56 Non-working side interference
Balancing side interference
M26.57 Lack of posterior occlusal support
M26.59 Other dentofacial functional abnormalities
Centric occlusion (of teeth) NOS
Malocclusion due to abnormal swallowing
Malocclusion due to mouth breathing
Malocclusion due to tongue, lip or finger habits

✓5th M26.6 Temporomandibular joint disorders
EXCLUDES 2 *current temporomandibular joint dislocation (S03.0)*
current temporomandibular joint sprain (S03.4)
M26.60 Temporomandibular joint disorder, unspecified

M26.61 Adhesions and ankylosis of temporomandibular joint

M26.62 Arthralgia of temporomandibular joint

M26.63 Articular disc disorder of temporomandibular joint

M26.69 Other specified disorders of temporomandibular joint

✓5th **M26.7 Dental alveolar anomalies**

M26.70 Unspecified alveolar anomaly

M26.71 Alveolar maxillary hyperplasia

M26.72 Alveolar mandibular hyperplasia

M26.73 Alveolar maxillary hypoplasia

M26.74 Alveolar mandibular hypoplasia

M26.79 Other specified alveolar anomalies

✓5th **M26.8 Other dentofacial anomalies**

M26.81 Anterior soft tissue impingement
Anterior soft tissue impingement on teeth

M26.82 Posterior soft tissue impingement
Posterior soft tissue impingement on teeth

M26.89 Other dentofacial anomalies

M26.9 Dentofacial anomaly, unspecified

✓4th **M27 Other diseases of jaws**

M27.0 Developmental disorders of jaws
Latent bone cyst of jaw
Stafne's cyst
Torus mandibularis
Torus palatinus

M27.1 Giant cell granuloma, central
Giant cell granuloma NOS
EXCLUDES 1 *peripheral giant cell granuloma (K06.8)*

M27.2 Inflammatory conditions of jaws
Osteitis of jaw(s)
Osteomyelitis (neonatal) jaw(s)
Osteoradionecrosis jaw(s)
Periostitis jaw(s)
Sequestrum of jaw bone
Use additional code (W88-W90, X39.0) to identify radiation, if radiation-induced
EXCLUDES 2 *osteonecrosis of jaw due to drug (M87.180)*

M27.3 Alveolitis of jaws
Alveolar osteitis
Dry socket

✓5th **M27.4 Other and unspecified cysts of jaw**
EXCLUDES 1 *cysts of oral region (K09.-)*
latent bone cyst of jaw (M27.0)
Stafne's cyst (M27.0)

M27.40 Unspecified cyst of jaw
Cyst of jaw NOS

M27.49 Other cysts of jaw
Aneurysmal cyst of jaw
Hemorrhagic cyst of jaw
Traumatic cyst of jaw

✓5th **M27.5 Periradicular pathology associated with previous endodontic treatment**

M27.51 Perforation of root canal space due to endodontic treatment

M27.52 Endodontic overfill

M27.53 Endodontic underfill

M27.59 Other periradicular pathology associated with previous endodontic treatment

✓5th **M27.6 Endosseous dental implant failure**

M27.61 Osseointegration failure of dental implant
Hemorrhagic complications of dental implant placement
Iatrogenic osseointegration failure of dental implant
Osseointegration failure of dental implant due to complications of systemic disease
Osseointegration failure of dental implant due to poor bone quality
Pre-integration failure of dental implant NOS
Pre-osseointegration failure of dental implant

M27.62 Post-osseointegration biological failure of dental implant
Failure of dental implant due to lack of attached gingiva
Failure of dental implant due to occlusal trauma (caused by poor prosthetic design)
Failure of dental implant due to parafunctional habits
Failure of dental implant due to periodontal infection (peri-implantitis)
Failure of dental implant due to poor oral hygiene
Iatrogenic post-osseointegration failure of dental implant
Post-osseointegration failure of dental implant due to complications of systemic disease

M27.63 Post-osseointegration mechanical failure of dental implant
Failure of dental prosthesis causing loss of dental implant
Fracture of dental implant
EXCLUDES 2 *cracked tooth (K03.81)*
fractured dental restorative material with loss of material (K08.531)
fractured dental restorative material without loss of material (K08.530)
fractured tooth (S02.5)

M27.69 Other endosseous dental implant failure
Dental implant failure NOS

M27.8 Other specified diseases of jaws
Cherubism
Exostosis
Fibrous dysplasia
Unilateral condylar hyperplasia
Unilateral condylar hypoplasia
EXCLUDES 1 *jaw pain (R68.84)*

M27.9 Disease of jaws, unspecified

Systemic connective tissue disorders (M30-M36)

INCLUDES autoimmune disease NOS
collagen (vascular) disease NOS
systemic autoimmune disease
systemic collagen (vascular) disease

EXCLUDES 1 *autoimmune disease, single organ or single cell-type—code to relevant condition category*

✓4th **M30 Polyarteritis nodosa and related conditions**
EXCLUDES 1 *microscopic polyarteritis (M31.7)*

M30.0 Polyarteritis nodosa CC
CC Excl: E08.51-E08.59, E08.618-E08.638, E08.649-E08.8, E09.51-E09.59, E09.618-E09.638, E09.649-E09.8, E10.51-E10.59, E10.618-E10.638, E10.649, E10.69-E10.8, E11.51-E11.59, E11.618-E11.638, E11.649, E11.69-E11.8, E13.51-E13.59, E13.618-E13.638, E13.649-E13.8, I87.8, I99.8-I99.9, M30.0-M31.7

M30.1 Polyarteritis with lung involvement [Churg-Strauss] CC
Allergic granulomatous angiitis
CC Excl: See code: M30.0

M30.2 Juvenile polyarteritis CC
CC Excl: See code: M30.0

M30.3 Mucocutaneous lymph node syndrome [Kawasaki] CC
CC Excl: I87.8, I99.8-I99.9, M30.0-M31.1, M31.30-M31.7

M30.8 Other conditions related to polyarteritis nodosa CC
Polyangiitis overlap syndrome
CC Excl: See code: M30.0

✓4th **M31 Other necrotizing vasculopathies**

M31.0 Hypersensitivity angiitis CC
Goodpasture's syndrome
CC Excl: See code: M30.0

M31.1 Thrombotic microangiopathy MCC
Thrombotic thrombocytopenic purpura
CC Excl: See code: M30.0

M31.2 Lethal midline granuloma CC
CC Excl: See code: M30.0

✓5th **M31.3 Wegener's granulomatosis**
Necrotizing respiratory granulomatosis

M31.30 Wegener's granulomatosis without renal involvement CC
Wegener's granulomatosis NOS
CC Excl: See code: M30.0

M31.31 Wegener's granulomatosis with renal involvement CC
CC Excl: See code: M30.0

M31.4 Aortic arch syndrome [Takayasu] CC
CC Excl: See code: M30.0

M31.5 Giant cell arteritis with polymyalgia rheumatica

M31.6 Other giant cell arteritis

M31.7 Microscopic polyangiitis CC
Microscopic polyarteritis
EXCLUDES 1 *polyarteritis nodosa (M30.0)*
CC Excl: See code: M30.0

M31.8 Other specified necrotizing vasculopathies CC
Hypocomplementemic vasculitis
Septic vasculitis
CC Excl: I77.5, M31.8-M31.9

M31.9 Necrotizing vasculopathy, unspecified CC
CC Excl: See code: M31.8

M32 Systemic lupus erythematosus (SLE)
EXCLUDES 1 *lupus erythematosus (discoid) (NOS) (L93.0)*

M32.0 Drug-induced systemic lupus erythematosus
Use additional code for adverse effect, if applicable, to identify drug (T36-T50 with fifth or sixth character 5)

M32.1 Systemic lupus erythematosus with organ or system involvement

M32.10 Systemic lupus erythematosus, organ or system involvement unspecified

M32.11 Endocarditis in systemic lupus erythematosus PDx CC CC
Libman-Sacks disease
CC Excl: I38-I39, I87.8, I99.8-I99.9

M32.12 Pericarditis in systemic lupus erythematosus PDx CC CC
Lupus pericarditis
CC Excl: I01.0, I09.2, I30.0-I30.9, I31.3-I32, I87.8, I99.8-I99.9

M32.13 Lung involvement in systemic lupus erythematosus
Pleural effusion due to systemic lupus erythematosus

M32.14 Glomerular disease in systemic lupus erythematosus
Lupus renal disease NOS
AHA: 2013, 4Q, 125

M32.15 Tubulo-interstitial nephropathy in systemic lupus erythematosus

M32.19 Other organ or system involvement in systemic lupus erythematosus

M32.8 Other forms of systemic lupus erythematosus

M32.9 Systemic lupus erythematosus, unspecified
SLE NOS
Systemic lupus erythematosus NOS
Systemic lupus erythematosus without organ involvement

M33 Dermatopolymyositis

M33.0 Juvenile dermatopolymyositis

M33.00 Juvenile dermatopolymyositis, organ involvement unspecified CC
CC Excl: M33.00-M33.19, M33.90-M33.99, M36.0

M33.01 Juvenile dermatopolymyositis with respiratory involvement CC
CC Excl: See code: M33.00

M33.02 Juvenile dermatopolymyositis with myopathy PDx CC CC
CC Excl: E08.40-E08.49, E08.618-E08.638, E08.649-E08.8, E09.40-E09.49, E09.618-E09.638, E09.649-E09.8, E10.40-E10.49, E10.618-E10.638, E10.649, E10.69-E10.8, E11.40-E11.49, E11.618-E11.638, E11.649, E11.69-E11.8, E13.40-E13.49, E13.618-E13.638, E13.649-E13.8, G32.89, G70.00-G72.3, G72.81-G73.7, G96.8-G96.9, G98.0-G98.8, G99.8, M33.00-M33.19, M33.90-M33.99, M36.0

M33.09 Juvenile dermatopolymyositis with other organ involvement CC
CC Excl: See code: M33.00

M33.1 Other dermatopolymyositis

M33.10 Other dermatopolymyositis, organ involvement unspecified CC
CC Excl: See code: M33.00

M33.11 Other dermatopolymyositis with respiratory involvement CC
CC Excl: See code: M33.00

M33.12 Other dermatopolymyositis with myopathy PDx CC CC
CC Excl: See code: M33.02

M33.19 Other dermatopolymyositis with other organ involvement CC
CC Excl: See code: M33.00

M33.2 Polymyositis

M33.20 Polymyositis, organ involvement unspecified CC
CC Excl: M33.20-M33.29

M33.21 Polymyositis with respiratory involvement CC
CC Excl: See code: M33.20

M33.22 Polymyositis with myopathy PDx CC CC
CC Excl: E08.40-E08.49, E08.618-E08.638, E08.649-E08.8, E09.40-E09.49, E09.618-E09.638, E09.649-E09.8, E10.40-E10.49, E10.618-E10.638, E10.649, E10.69-E10.8, E11.40-E11.49, E11.618-E11.638, E11.649, E11.69-E11.8, E13.40-E13.49, E13.618-E13.638, E13.649-E13.8, G32.89, G70.00-G72.3, G72.81-G73.7, G96.8-G96.9, G98.0-G98.8, G99.8, M33.20-M33.29

M33.29 Polymyositis with other organ involvement CC
CC Excl: See code: M33.20

M33.9 Dermatopolymyositis, unspecified

M33.90 Dermatopolymyositis, unspecified, organ involvement unspecified CC
CC Excl: See code: M33.19

M33.91 Dermatopolymyositis, unspecified with respiratory involvement CC
CC Excl: See code: M33.19

M33.92 Dermatopolymyositis, unspecified with myopathy PDx CC CC
CC Excl: See code: M33.12

M33.99 Dermatopolymyositis, unspecified with other organ involvement CC
CC Excl: See code: M33.19

M34 Systemic sclerosis [scleroderma]
EXCLUDES 1 *circumscribed scleroderma (L94.0)*
neonatal scleroderma (P83.8)

M34.0 Progressive systemic sclerosis

M34.1 CR(E)ST syndrome
Combination of calcinosis, Raynaud's phenomenon, esophageal dysfunction, sclerodactyly, telangiectasia

M34.2 Systemic sclerosis induced by drug and chemical
Code first poisoning due to drug or toxin, if applicable (T36-T65 with fifth or sixth character 1-4 or 6)
Use additional code for adverse effect, if applicable, to identify drug (T36-T50 with fifth or sixth character 5)

M34.8 Other forms of systemic sclerosis

M34.81 Systemic sclerosis with lung involvement PDx CC CC
CC Excl: No excl

M34.82 Systemic sclerosis with myopathy PDx CC CC
CC Excl: E08.40-E08.49, E08.618-E08.638, E08.649-E08.8, E09.40-E09.49, E09.618-E09.638, E09.649-E09.8, E10.40-E10.49, E10.618-E10.638, E10.649, E10.69-E10.8, E11.40-E11.49, E11.618-E11.638, E11.649, E11.69-E11.8, E13.40-E13.49, E13.618-E13.638, E13.649-E13.8, G32.89, G70.00-G72.3, G72.81-G73.7, G96.8-G96.9, G98.0-G98.8, G99.8

M34.83 Systemic sclerosis with polyneuropathy

M34.89 Other systemic sclerosis

M34.9 Systemic sclerosis, unspecified

M35 Other systemic involvement of connective tissue
EXCLUDES 1 *reactive perforating collagenosis (L87.1)*

M35.0 Sicca syndrome [Sjögren]

M35.00 Sicca syndrome, unspecified

M35.01 Sicca syndrome with keratoconjunctivitis

M35.02 Sicca syndrome with lung involvement

M35.03 Sicca syndrome with myopathy PDx CC CC
CC Excl: See code M34.82

M35.04 Sicca syndrome with tubulo-interstitial nephropathy
Renal tubular acidosis in sicca syndrome

M35.09 Sicca syndrome with other organ involvement

M35.1 Other overlap syndromes CC
Mixed connective tissue disease
EXCLUDES 1 *polyangiitis overlap syndrome (M30.8)*
CC Excl: G72.41-G72.49, M35.1, M35.5, M35.8

M35.2 Behçet's disease CC
CC Excl: A02.23, A17.9, A18.02, A18.09, A18.82, A18.84, A18.89, A39.83-A39.84, A54.40, A54.42-A54.43, A54.82, A54.84, A54.89-A54.9, B06.82, M00.00, M00.019, M00.029, M00.039, M00.049, M00.059, M00.069, M00.079, M00.08-M02.30, M02.319, M02.329, M02.339, M02.349, M02.359, M02.369, M02.379-M02.9, M05.40-M05.59, M05.70-M06.09, M06.20-M06.39, M06.80-M07.69, M11.00-M11.9, M12.10-M15.0, M15.3-M15.9, M16.2-M16.9, M17.2-M17.9, M18.2-M18.9, M19.111-M19.93, M24.10-M24.176, M25.00, M25.08-M25.18, M25.40-M25.676, M25.80-M25.9, M35.2, M36.1-M36.4, R29.4

M35.3 Polymyalgia rheumatica
EXCLUDES 1 *polymyalgia rheumatica with giant cell arteritis (M31.5)*

M35.4 Diffuse (eosinophilic) fasciitis

M35.5 Multifocal fibrosclerosis CC
CC Excl: G72.41-G72.49, M35.1, M35.5, M35.8

M35.6 Relapsing panniculitis [Weber-Christian]
EXCLUDES 1 *lupus panniculitis (L93.2)*
panniculitis NOS (M79.3-)

M35.7 Hypermobility syndrome
Familial ligamentous laxity
EXCLUDES 1 *Ehlers-Danlos syndrome (Q79.6)*
ligamentous laxity, NOS (M24.2-)

M35.8 Other specified systemic involvement of connective tissue CC
CC Excl: G72.41-G72.49, M35.1, M35.5, M35.8

M35.9 Systemic involvement of connective tissue, unspecified
Autoimmune disease (systemic) NOS
Collagen (vascular) disease NOS

✓4th **M36 Systemic disorders of connective tissue in diseases classified elsewhere**
EXCLUDES 2 *arthropathies in diseases classified elsewhere (M14.-)*

M36.Ø Dermato(poly)myositis in neoplastic disease CC
Code first underlying neoplasm (CØØ-D49)
CC Excl: M33.ØØ-M33.19, M33.9Ø-M33.99, M36.Ø

M36.1 Arthropathy in neoplastic disease
Code first underlying neoplasm, such as:
leukemia (C91-C95)
malignant histiocytosis (C96.A)
multiple myeloma (C9Ø.Ø)

M36.2 Hemophilic arthropathy
Hemarthrosis in hemophilic arthropathy
Code first underlying disease, such as:
factor VIII deficiency (D66)
with vascular defect (D68.Ø)
factor IX deficiency (D67)
hemophilia (classical) (D66)
hemophilia B (D67)
hemophilia C (D68.1)

M36.3 Arthropathy in other blood disorders

M36.4 Arthropathy in hypersensitivity reactions classified elsewhere
Code first underlying disease, such as:
Henoch (-Schönlein) purpura (D69.Ø)
serum sickness (T8Ø.6-)

M36.8 Systemic disorders of connective tissue in other diseases classified elsewhere
Code first underlying disease, such as:
alkaptonuria (E7Ø.2)
hypogammaglobulinemia (D8Ø.-)
ochronosis (E7Ø.2)

DORSOPATHIES (M4Ø-M54)

Deforming dorsopathies (M4Ø-M43)

✓4th **M4Ø Kyphosis and lordosis**
EXCLUDES 1 *congenital kyphosis and lordosis (Q76.4)*
kyphoscoliosis (M41.-)
postprocedural kyphosis and lordosis (M96.-)

✓5th **M4Ø.Ø Postural kyphosis**
EXCLUDES 1 *osteochondrosis of spine (M42.-)*
M4Ø.ØØ Postural kyphosis, site unspecified
M4Ø.Ø3 Postural kyphosis, cervicothoracic region
M4Ø.Ø4 Postural kyphosis, thoracic region
M4Ø.Ø5 Postural kyphosis, thoracolumbar region

✓5th **M4Ø.1 Other secondary kyphosis**
M4Ø.1Ø Other secondary kyphosis, site unspecified
M4Ø.12 Other secondary kyphosis, cervical region
M4Ø.13 Other secondary kyphosis, cervicothoracic region
M4Ø.14 Other secondary kyphosis, thoracic region
M4Ø.15 Other secondary kyphosis, thoracolumbar region

✓5th **M4Ø.2 Other and unspecified kyphosis**
✓6th **M4Ø.2Ø Unspecified kyphosis**
M4Ø.2Ø2 Unspecified kyphosis, cervical region
M4Ø.2Ø3 Unspecified kyphosis, cervicothoracic region
M4Ø.2Ø4 Unspecified kyphosis, thoracic region
M4Ø.2Ø5 Unspecified kyphosis, thoracolumbar region
M4Ø.2Ø9 Unspecified kyphosis, site unspecified

✓6th **M4Ø.29 Other kyphosis**
M4Ø.292 Other kyphosis, cervical region
M4Ø.293 Other kyphosis, cervicothoracic region
M4Ø.294 Other kyphosis, thoracic region
M4Ø.295 Other kyphosis, thoracolumbar region
M4Ø.299 Other kyphosis, site unspecified

✓5th **M4Ø.3 Flatback syndrome**
M4Ø.3Ø Flatback syndrome, site unspecified
M4Ø.35 Flatback syndrome, thoracolumbar region
M4Ø.36 Flatback syndrome, lumbar region
M4Ø.37 Flatback syndrome, lumbosacral region

✓5th **M4Ø.4 Postural lordosis**
Acquired lordosis
M4Ø.4Ø Postural lordosis, site unspecified
M4Ø.45 Postural lordosis, thoracolumbar region
M4Ø.46 Postural lordosis, lumbar region
M4Ø.47 Postural lordosis, lumbosacral region

✓5th **M4Ø.5 Lordosis, unspecified**
M4Ø.5Ø Lordosis, unspecified, site unspecified
M4Ø.55 Lordosis, unspecified, thoracolumbar region
M4Ø.56 Lordosis, unspecified, lumbar region
M4Ø.57 Lordosis, unspecified, lumbosacral region

✓4th **M41 Scoliosis**
INCLUDES kyphoscoliosis
EXCLUDES 1 *congenital scoliosis due to bony malformation (Q76.3)*
congenital scoliosis NOS (Q67.5)
kyphoscoliotic heart disease (I27.1)
postprocedural scoliosis (M96.-)
postural congenital scoliosis (Q67.5)

✓5th **M41.Ø Infantile idiopathic scoliosis**
M41.ØØ Infantile idiopathic scoliosis, site unspecified
M41.Ø2 Infantile idiopathic scoliosis, cervical region
M41.Ø3 Infantile idiopathic scoliosis, cervicothoracic region
M41.Ø4 Infantile idiopathic scoliosis, thoracic region
M41.Ø5 Infantile idiopathic scoliosis, thoracolumbar region
M41.Ø6 Infantile idiopathic scoliosis, lumbar region
M41.Ø7 Infantile idiopathic scoliosis, lumbosacral region
M41.Ø8 Infantile idiopathic scoliosis, sacral and sacrococcygeal region

✓5th **M41.1 Juvenile and adolescent idiopathic scoliosis**
✓6th **M41.11 Juvenile idiopathic scoliosis**
M41.112 Juvenile idiopathic scoliosis, cervical region
M41.113 Juvenile idiopathic scoliosis, cervicothoracic region
M41.114 Juvenile idiopathic scoliosis, thoracic region
M41.115 Juvenile idiopathic scoliosis, thoracolumbar region
M41.116 Juvenile idiopathic scoliosis, lumbar region
M41.117 Juvenile idiopathic scoliosis, lumbosacral region
M41.119 Juvenile idiopathic scoliosis, site unspecified

✓6th **M41.12 Adolescent scoliosis**
M41.122 Adolescent idiopathic scoliosis, cervical region
M41.123 Adolescent idiopathic scoliosis, cervicothoracic region
M41.124 Adolescent idiopathic scoliosis, thoracic region
M41.125 Adolescent idiopathic scoliosis, thoracolumbar region
M41.126 Adolescent idiopathic scoliosis, lumbar region
M41.127 Adolescent idiopathic scoliosis, lumbosacral region
M41.129 Adolescent idiopathic scoliosis, site unspecified

✓5th **M41.2 Other idiopathic scoliosis**
M41.2Ø Other idiopathic scoliosis, site unspecified
M41.22 Other idiopathic scoliosis, cervical region
M41.23 Other idiopathic scoliosis, cervicothoracic region

M41.24 Other idiopathic scoliosis, thoracic region
M41.25 Other idiopathic scoliosis, thoracolumbar region
M41.26 Other idiopathic scoliosis, lumbar region
M41.27 Other idiopathic scoliosis, lumbosacral region

✓5th **M41.3 Thoracogenic scoliosis**
M41.30 Thoracogenic scoliosis, site unspecified
M41.34 Thoracogenic scoliosis, thoracic region
M41.35 Thoracogenic scoliosis, thoracolumbar region

✓5th **M41.4 Neuromuscular scoliosis**
Scoliosis secondary to cerebral palsy, Friedreich's ataxia, poliomyelitis and other neuromuscular disorders
Code also underlying condition
M41.40 Neuromuscular scoliosis, site unspecified
M41.41 Neuromuscular scoliosis, occipito-atlanto-axial region
M41.42 Neuromuscular scoliosis, cervical region
M41.43 Neuromuscular scoliosis, cervicothoracic region
M41.44 Neuromuscular scoliosis, thoracic region
M41.45 Neuromuscular scoliosis, thoracolumbar region
M41.46 Neuromuscular scoliosis, lumbar region
M41.47 Neuromuscular scoliosis, lumbosacral region

✓5th **M41.5 Other secondary scoliosis**
M41.50 Other secondary scoliosis, site unspecified
M41.52 Other secondary scoliosis, cervical region
M41.53 Other secondary scoliosis, cervicothoracic region
M41.54 Other secondary scoliosis, thoracic region
M41.55 Other secondary scoliosis, thoracolumbar region
M41.56 Other secondary scoliosis, lumbar region
M41.57 Other secondary scoliosis, lumbosacral region

✓5th **M41.8 Other forms of scoliosis**
M41.80 Other forms of scoliosis, site unspecified
M41.82 Other forms of scoliosis, cervical region
M41.83 Other forms of scoliosis, cervicothoracic region
M41.84 Other forms of scoliosis, thoracic region
M41.85 Other forms of scoliosis, thoracolumbar region
M41.86 Other forms of scoliosis, lumbar region
M41.87 Other forms of scoliosis, lumbosacral region

M41.9 Scoliosis, unspecified

✓4th **M42 Spinal osteochondrosis**

✓5th **M42.Ø Juvenile osteochondrosis of spine**
Calvé's disease
Scheuermann's disease
EXCLUDES 1 *postural kyphosis (M40.Ø)*
M42.ØØ Juvenile osteochondrosis of spine, site unspecified
M42.Ø1 Juvenile osteochondrosis of spine, occipito-atlanto-axial region
M42.Ø2 Juvenile osteochondrosis of spine, cervical region
M42.Ø3 Juvenile osteochondrosis of spine, cervicothoracic region
M42.Ø4 Juvenile osteochondrosis of spine, thoracic region
M42.Ø5 Juvenile osteochondrosis of spine, thoracolumbar region
M42.Ø6 Juvenile osteochondrosis of spine, lumbar region
M42.Ø7 Juvenile osteochondrosis of spine, lumbosacral region
M42.Ø8 Juvenile osteochondrosis of spine, sacral and sacrococcygeal region
M42.Ø9 Juvenile osteochondrosis of spine, multiple sites in spine

✓5th **M42.1 Adult osteochondrosis of spine**
M42.1Ø Adult osteochondrosis of spine, site unspecified A
M42.11 Adult osteochondrosis of spine, occipito-atlanto-axial region A
M42.12 Adult osteochondrosis of spine, cervical region A
M42.13 Adult osteochondrosis of spine, cervicothoracic region A
M42.14 Adult osteochondrosis of spine, thoracic region A
M42.15 Adult osteochondrosis of spine, thoracolumbar region A
M42.16 Adult osteochondrosis of spine, lumbar region A
M42.17 Adult osteochondrosis of spine, lumbosacral region A
M42.18 Adult osteochondrosis of spine, sacral and sacrococcygeal region A
M42.19 Adult osteochondrosis of spine, multiple sites in spine A

M42.9 Spinal osteochondrosis, unspecified

✓4th **M43 Other deforming dorsopathies**
EXCLUDES 1 *congenital spondylolysis and spondylolisthesis (Q76.2)*
hemivertebra (Q76.3-Q76.4)
Klippel-Feil syndrome (Q76.1)
lumbarization and sacralization (Q76.4)
platyspondylisis (Q76.4)
spina bifida occulta (Q76.Ø)
spinal curvature in osteoporosis (M8Ø.-)
spinal curvature in Paget's disease of bone [osteitis deformans] (M88.-)

✓5th **M43.Ø Spondylolysis**
EXCLUDES 1 *congenital spondylolysis (Q76.2)*
spondylolisthesis (M43.1)
M43.ØØ Spondylolysis, site unspecified
M43.Ø1 Spondylolysis, occipito-atlanto-axial region
M43.Ø2 Spondylolysis, cervical region
M43.Ø3 Spondylolysis, cervicothoracic region
M43.Ø4 Spondylolysis, thoracic region
M43.Ø5 Spondylolysis, thoracolumbar region
M43.Ø6 Spondylolysis, lumbar region
M43.Ø7 Spondylolysis, lumbosacral region
M43.Ø8 Spondylolysis, sacral and sacrococcygeal region
M43.Ø9 Spondylolysis, multiple sites in spine

✓5th **M43.1 Spondylolisthesis**
EXCLUDES 1 *acute traumatic of lumbosacral region (S33.1)*
acute traumatic of sites other than lumbosacral— code to Fracture, vertebra, by region
congenital spondylolisthesis (Q76.2)
M43.1Ø Spondylolisthesis, site unspecified
M43.11 Spondylolisthesis, occipito-atlanto-axial region
M43.12 Spondylolisthesis, cervical region
M43.13 Spondylolisthesis, cervicothoracic region
M43.14 Spondylolisthesis, thoracic region
M43.15 Spondylolisthesis, thoracolumbar region
M43.16 Spondylolisthesis, lumbar region
M43.17 Spondylolisthesis, lumbosacral region
M43.18 Spondylolisthesis, sacral and sacrococcygeal region
M43.19 Spondylolisthesis, multiple sites in spine

✓5th **M43.2 Fusion of spine**
Ankylosis of spinal joint
EXCLUDES 1 *ankylosing spondylitis (M45.Ø-)*
congenital fusion of spine (Q76.4)
EXCLUDES 2 *arthrodesis status (Z98.1)*
pseudoarthrosis after fusion or arthrodesis (M96.Ø)
M43.2Ø Fusion of spine, site unspecified
M43.21 Fusion of spine, occipito-atlanto-axial region
M43.22 Fusion of spine, cervical region
M43.23 Fusion of spine, cervicothoracic region
M43.24 Fusion of spine, thoracic region
M43.25 Fusion of spine, thoracolumbar region
M43.26 Fusion of spine, lumbar region
M43.27 Fusion of spine, lumbosacral region
M43.28 Fusion of spine, sacral and sacrococcygeal region

M43.3 Recurrent atlantoaxial dislocation with myelopathy
M43.4 Other recurrent atlantoaxial dislocation

✓5th **M43.5 Other recurrent vertebral dislocation**
EXCLUDES 1 *biomechanical lesions NEC (M99.-)*

✓6th **M43.5X Other recurrent vertebral dislocation**
M43.5X2 Other recurrent vertebral dislocation, cervical region
M43.5X3 Other recurrent vertebral dislocation, cervicothoracic region
M43.5X4 Other recurrent vertebral dislocation, thoracic region
M43.5X5 Other recurrent vertebral dislocation, thoracolumbar region
M43.5X6 Other recurrent vertebral dislocation, lumbar region

M43.5X7 Other recurrent vertebral dislocation, lumbosacral region
M43.5X8 Other recurrent vertebral dislocation, sacral and sacrococcygeal region
M43.5X9 Other recurrent vertebral dislocation, site unspecified

M43.6 Torticollis
EXCLUDES 1 *congenital (sternomastoid) torticollis (Q68.0)*
current injury—see Injury, of spine, by body region
ocular torticollis (R29.891)
psychogenic torticollis (F45.8)
spasmodic torticollis (G24.3)
torticollis due to birth injury (P15.2)

✓5th M43.8 Other specified deforming dorsopathies
EXCLUDES 2 *kyphosis and lordosis (M40.-)*
scoliosis (M41.-)

✓6th M43.8X Other specified deforming dorsopathies
M43.8X1 Other specified deforming dorsopathies, occipito-atlanto-axial region
M43.8X2 Other specified deforming dorsopathies, cervical region
M43.8X3 Other specified deforming dorsopathies, cervicothoracic region
M43.8X4 Other specified deforming dorsopathies, thoracic region
M43.8X5 Other specified deforming dorsopathies, thoracolumbar region
M43.8X6 Other specified deforming dorsopathies, lumbar region
M43.8X7 Other specified deforming dorsopathies, lumbosacral region
M43.8X8 Other specified deforming dorsopathies, sacral and sacrococcygeal region
M43.8X9 Other specified deforming dorsopathies, site unspecified

M43.9 Deforming dorsopathy, unspecified
Curvature of spine NOS

Spondylopathies (M45-M49)

✓4th M45 Ankylosing spondylitis
Rheumatoid arthritis of spine
EXCLUDES 1 *arthropathy in Reiter's disease (M02.3-)*
juvenile (ankylosing) spondylitis (M08.1)
EXCLUDES 2 *Behçet's disease (M35.2)*

M45.0 Ankylosing spondylitis of multiple sites in spine
M45.1 Ankylosing spondylitis of occipito-atlanto-axial region
M45.2 Ankylosing spondylitis of cervical region
M45.3 Ankylosing spondylitis of cervicothoracic region
M45.4 Ankylosing spondylitis of thoracic region
M45.5 Ankylosing spondylitis of thoracolumbar region
M45.6 Ankylosing spondylitis lumbar region
M45.7 Ankylosing spondylitis of lumbosacral region
M45.8 Ankylosing spondylitis sacral and sacrococcygeal region
M45.9 Ankylosing spondylitis of unspecified sites in spine

✓4th M46 Other inflammatory spondylopathies

✓5th M46.0 Spinal enthesopathy
Disorder of ligamentous or muscular attachments of spine
M46.00 Spinal enthesopathy, site unspecified
M46.01 Spinal enthesopathy, occipito-atlanto-axial region
M46.02 Spinal enthesopathy, cervical region
M46.03 Spinal enthesopathy, cervicothoracic region
M46.04 Spinal enthesopathy, thoracic region
M46.05 Spinal enthesopathy, thoracolumbar region
M46.06 Spinal enthesopathy, lumbar region
M46.07 Spinal enthesopathy, lumbosacral region
M46.08 Spinal enthesopathy, sacral and sacrococcygeal region
M46.09 Spinal enthesopathy, multiple sites in spine

M46.1 Sacroiliitis, not elsewhere classified

✓5th M46.2 Osteomyelitis of vertebra
CC Excl: For CC codes in subcategory M46.20, unless otherwise noted: A02.24, A17.9, A18.03-A18.09, A18.82, A18.84, A18.89, M46.20-M46.39, M86.00-M86.9
M46.20 Osteomyelitis of vertebra, site unspecified CC
M46.21 Osteomyelitis of vertebra, occipito-atlanto-axial region CC
M46.22 Osteomyelitis of vertebra, cervical region CC
M46.23 Osteomyelitis of vertebra, cervicothoracic region CC
M46.24 Osteomyelitis of vertebra, thoracic region CC
M46.25 Osteomyelitis of vertebra, thoracolumbar region CC
M46.26 Osteomyelitis of vertebra, lumbar region CC
M46.27 Osteomyelitis of vertebra, lumbosacral region CC
M46.28 Osteomyelitis of vertebra, sacral and sacrococcygeal region CC

✓5th M46.3 Infection of intervertebral disc (pyogenic)
Use additional code (B95-B97) to identify infectious agent
M46.30 Infection of intervertebral disc (pyogenic), site unspecified CC
CC Excl: A17.9-A18.01, A18.03-A18.09, A18.82, A18.84, A18.89, M46.20-M46.39, M86.00-M86.9
M46.31 Infection of intervertebral disc (pyogenic), occipito-atlanto-axial region CC
CC Excl: See code: M46.30
M46.32 Infection of intervertebral disc (pyogenic), cervical region CC
CC Excl: See code: M46.30
M46.33 Infection of intervertebral disc (pyogenic), cervicothoracic region CC
CC Excl: See code: M46.30
M46.34 Infection of intervertebral disc (pyogenic), thoracic region CC
CC Excl: See code: M46.30
M46.35 Infection of intervertebral disc (pyogenic), thoracolumbar region CC
CC Excl: See code: M46.30
M46.36 Infection of intervertebral disc (pyogenic), lumbar region CC
CC Excl: See code: M46.30
M46.37 Infection of intervertebral disc (pyogenic), lumbosacral region CC
CC Excl: See code: M46.30
M46.38 Infection of intervertebral disc (pyogenic), sacral and sacrococcygeal region CC
CC Excl: See code: M46.30
M46.39 Infection of intervertebral disc (pyogenic), multiple sites in spine CC
CC Excl: See code: M46.30

✓5th M46.4 Discitis, unspecified
M46.40 Discitis, unspecified, site unspecified
M46.41 Discitis, unspecified, occipito-atlanto-axial region
M46.42 Discitis, unspecified, cervical region
M46.43 Discitis, unspecified, cervicothoracic region
M46.44 Discitis, unspecified, thoracic region
M46.45 Discitis, unspecified, thoracolumbar region
M46.46 Discitis, unspecified, lumbar region
M46.47 Discitis, unspecified, lumbosacral region
M46.48 Discitis, unspecified, sacral and sacrococcygeal region
M46.49 Discitis, unspecified, multiple sites in spine

✓5th M46.5 Other infective spondylopathies
M46.50 Other infective spondylopathies, site unspecified
M46.51 Other infective spondylopathies, occipito-atlanto-axial region
M46.52 Other infective spondylopathies, cervical region
M46.53 Other infective spondylopathies, cervicothoracic region
M46.54 Other infective spondylopathies, thoracic region
M46.55 Other infective spondylopathies, thoracolumbar region
M46.56 Other infective spondylopathies, lumbar region
M46.57 Other infective spondylopathies, lumbosacral region
M46.58 Other infective spondylopathies, sacral and sacrococcygeal region
M46.59 Other infective spondylopathies, multiple sites in spine

✓5th M46.8 Other specified inflammatory spondylopathies
M46.80 Other specified inflammatory spondylopathies, site unspecified

M46.81 Other specified inflammatory spondylopathies, occipito-atlanto-axial region

M46.82 Other specified inflammatory spondylopathies, cervical region

M46.83 Other specified inflammatory spondylopathies, cervicothoracic region

M46.84 Other specified inflammatory spondylopathies, thoracic region

M46.85 Other specified inflammatory spondylopathies, thoracolumbar region

M46.86 Other specified inflammatory spondylopathies, lumbar region

M46.87 Other specified inflammatory spondylopathies, lumbosacral region

M46.88 Other specified inflammatory spondylopathies, sacral and sacrococcygeal region

M46.89 Other specified inflammatory spondylopathies, multiple sites in spine

✓5th **M46.9 Unspecified inflammatory spondylopathy**

M46.90 Unspecified inflammatory spondylopathy, site unspecified

M46.91 Unspecified inflammatory spondylopathy, occipito-atlanto-axial region

M46.92 Unspecified inflammatory spondylopathy, cervical region

M46.93 Unspecified inflammatory spondylopathy, cervicothoracic region

M46.94 Unspecified inflammatory spondylopathy, thoracic region

M46.95 Unspecified inflammatory spondylopathy, thoracolumbar region

M46.96 Unspecified inflammatory spondylopathy, lumbar region

M46.97 Unspecified inflammatory spondylopathy, lumbosacral region

M46.98 Unspecified inflammatory spondylopathy, sacral and sacrococcygeal region

M46.99 Unspecified inflammatory spondylopathy, multiple sites in spine

✓4th **M47 Spondylosis**

INCLUDES arthrosis or osteoarthritis of spine
degeneration of facet joints

✓5th **M47.0 Anterior spinal and vertebral artery compression syndromes**

✓6th **M47.01 Anterior spinal artery compression syndromes**

CC Excl: For CC codes in subcategory M47.01, unless otherwise noted: M47.011-M47.029, M47.11-M47.13, M47.21-M47.23, M47.811-M47.813, M47.891-M47.893

M47.011 Anterior spinal artery compression syndromes, occipito-atlanto-axial region CC

M47.012 Anterior spinal artery compression syndromes, cervical region CC

M47.013 Anterior spinal artery compression syndromes, cervicothoracic region CC

M47.014 Anterior spinal artery compression syndromes, thoracic region CC

M47.015 Anterior spinal artery compression syndromes, thoracolumbar region CC

M47.016 Anterior spinal artery compression syndromes, lumbar region CC

M47.019 Anterior spinal artery compression syndromes, site unspecified CC

✓6th **M47.02 Vertebral artery compression syndromes**

M47.021 Vertebral artery compression syndromes, occipito-atlanto-axial region CC

M47.022 Vertebral artery compression syndromes, cervical region CC

M47.029 Vertebral artery compression syndromes, site unspecified CC

✓5th **M47.1 Other spondylosis with myelopathy**

Spondylogenic compression of spinal cord

EXCLUDES 1 *vertebral subluxation (M43.3-M43.5X9)*

M47.10 Other spondylosis with myelopathy, site unspecified CC

CC Excl: M25.78, M47.011-M47.9, M48.10-M48.38, M48.9

M47.11 Other spondylosis with myelopathy, occipito-atlanto-axial region CC

CC Excl: M47.011-M47.029, M47.11-M47.13, M47.21-M47.23, M47.811-M47.813, M47.891-M47.893

M47.12 Other spondylosis with myelopathy, cervical region CC

CC Excl: See code: M47.11

M47.13 Other spondylosis with myelopathy, cervicothoracic region CC

CC Excl: See code: M47.11

M47.14 Other spondylosis with myelopathy, thoracic region CC

CC Excl: M47.14-M47.15

M47.15 Other spondylosis with myelopathy, thoracolumbar region CC

CC Excl: See code: M47.14

M47.16 Other spondylosis with myelopathy, lumbar region CC

CC Excl: M46.40, M46.46-M46.49, M47.16-M47.18, M47.26-M47.28, M47.816-M47.818, M47.896-M47.898, M51.06-M51.07, M51.26-M51.27, M51.36-M51.37, M51.46-M51.47, M51.86-M51.9

✓5th **M47.2 Other spondylosis with radiculopathy**

M47.20 Other spondylosis with radiculopathy, site unspecified

M47.21 Other spondylosis with radiculopathy, occipito-atlanto-axial region

M47.22 Other spondylosis with radiculopathy, cervical region

M47.23 Other spondylosis with radiculopathy, cervicothoracic region

M47.24 Other spondylosis with radiculopathy, thoracic region

M47.25 Other spondylosis with radiculopathy, thoracolumbar region

M47.26 Other spondylosis with radiculopathy, lumbar region

M47.27 Other spondylosis with radiculopathy, lumbosacral region

M47.28 Other spondylosis with radiculopathy, sacral and sacrococcygeal region

✓5th **M47.8 Other spondylosis**

✓6th **M47.81 Spondylosis without myelopathy or radiculopathy**

M47.811 Spondylosis without myelopathy or radiculopathy, occipito-atlanto-axial region

M47.812 Spondylosis without myelopathy or radiculopathy, cervical region

M47.813 Spondylosis without myelopathy or radiculopathy, cervicothoracic region

M47.814 Spondylosis without myelopathy or radiculopathy, thoracic region

M47.815 Spondylosis without myelopathy or radiculopathy, thoracolumbar region

M47.816 Spondylosis without myelopathy or radiculopathy, lumbar region

M47.817 Spondylosis without myelopathy or radiculopathy, lumbosacral region

M47.818 Spondylosis without myelopathy or radiculopathy, sacral and sacrococcygeal region

M47.819 Spondylosis without myelopathy or radiculopathy, site unspecified

✓6th **M47.89 Other spondylosis**

M47.891 Other spondylosis, occipito-atlanto-axial region

M47.892 Other spondylosis, cervical region

M47.893 Other spondylosis, cervicothoracic region

M47.894 Other spondylosis, thoracic region

M47.895 Other spondylosis, thoracolumbar region

M47.896 Other spondylosis, lumbar region

M47.897 Other spondylosis, lumbosacral region

M47.898 **Other spondylosis, sacral and sacrococcygeal region**

M47.899 **Other spondylosis, site unspecified**

M47.9 **Spondylosis, unspecified**

M48 Other spondylopathies

M48.0 Spinal stenosis
Caudal stenosis

M48.00 **Spinal stenosis, site unspecified**
M48.01 **Spinal stenosis, occipito-atlanto-axial region**
M48.02 **Spinal stenosis, cervical region**
M48.03 **Spinal stenosis, cervicothoracic region**
M48.04 **Spinal stenosis, thoracic region**
M48.05 **Spinal stenosis, thoracolumbar region**
M48.06 **Spinal stenosis, lumbar region**
M48.07 **Spinal stenosis, lumbosacral region**
M48.08 **Spinal stenosis, sacral and sacrococcygeal region**

M48.1 Ankylosing hyperostosis [Forestier]
Diffuse idiopathic skeletal hyperostosis [DISH]

M48.10 **Ankylosing hyperostosis [Forestier], site unspecified**
M48.11 **Ankylosing hyperostosis [Forestier], occipito-atlanto-axial region**
M48.12 **Ankylosing hyperostosis [Forestier], cervical region**
M48.13 **Ankylosing hyperostosis [Forestier], cervicothoracic region**
M48.14 **Ankylosing hyperostosis [Forestier], thoracic region**
M48.15 **Ankylosing hyperostosis [Forestier], thoracolumbar region**
M48.16 **Ankylosing hyperostosis [Forestier], lumbar region**
M48.17 **Ankylosing hyperostosis [Forestier], lumbosacral region**
M48.18 **Ankylosing hyperostosis [Forestier], sacral and sacrococcygeal region**
M48.19 **Ankylosing hyperostosis [Forestier], multiple sites in spine**

M48.2 Kissing spine

M48.20 **Kissing spine, site unspecified**
M48.21 **Kissing spine, occipito-atlanto-axial region**
M48.22 **Kissing spine, cervical region**
M48.23 **Kissing spine, cervicothoracic region**
M48.24 **Kissing spine, thoracic region**
M48.25 **Kissing spine, thoracolumbar region**
M48.26 **Kissing spine, lumbar region**
M48.27 **Kissing spine, lumbosacral region**

M48.3 Traumatic spondylopathy

CC Excl: For CC codes in subcategory M48.3, unless otherwise noted: M48.30-M48.38

M48.30 **Traumatic spondylopathy, site unspecified** CC
M48.31 **Traumatic spondylopathy, occipito-atlanto-axial region** CC
M48.32 **Traumatic spondylopathy, cervical region** CC
M48.33 **Traumatic spondylopathy, cervicothoracic region** CC
M48.34 **Traumatic spondylopathy, thoracic region** CC
M48.35 **Traumatic spondylopathy, thoracolumbar region** CC
M48.36 **Traumatic spondylopathy, lumbar region** CC
M48.37 **Traumatic spondylopathy, lumbosacral region** CC
M48.38 **Traumatic spondylopathy, sacral and sacrococcygeal region** CC

M48.4 Fatigue fracture of vertebra
Stress fracture of vertebra

EXCLUDES 1
pathological fracture NOS (M84.4-)
pathological fracture of vertebra due to neoplasm (M84.58)
pathological fracture of vertebra due to other diagnosis (M84.68)
pathological fracture of vertebra due to osteoporosis (M80.-)
traumatic fracture of vertebrae (S12.0-S12.3-, S22.0-, S32.0-)

The appropriate 7th character is to be added to each code from subcategory M48.4.
A initial encounter for fracture
D subsequent encounter for fracture with routine healing
G subsequent encounter for fracture with delayed healing
S sequela of fracture

M48.40 **Fatigue fracture of vertebra, site unspecified**
M48.41 **Fatigue fracture of vertebra, occipito-atlanto-axial region**
M48.42 **Fatigue fracture of vertebra, cervical region**
M48.43 **Fatigue fracture of vertebra, cervicothoracic region**
M48.44 **Fatigue fracture of vertebra, thoracic region**
M48.45 **Fatigue fracture of vertebra, thoracolumbar region**
M48.46 **Fatigue fracture of vertebra, lumbar region**
M48.47 **Fatigue fracture of vertebra, lumbosacral region**
M48.48 **Fatigue fracture of vertebra, sacral and sacrococcygeal region**

M48.5 Collapsed vertebra, not elsewhere classified
Collapsed vertebra NOS
Wedging of vertebra NOS

EXCLUDES 1
current injury—see Injury of spine, by body region
fatigue fracture of vertebra (M48.4)
pathological fracture of vertebra due to neoplasm (M84.58)
pathological fracture of vertebra due to other diagnosis (M84.68)
pathological fracture of vertebra due to osteoporosis (M80.-)
pathological fracture NOS (M84.4-)
stress fracture of vertebra (M48.4-)
traumatic fracture of vertebra (S12-, S22-, S32-)

The appropriate 7th character is to be added to each code from subcategory M48.5.
A initial encounter for fracture
D subsequent encounter for fracture with routine healing
G subsequent encounter for fracture with delayed healing
S sequela of fracture

CC Excl: For CC codes in subcategory M48.5 with 7th character A, unless otherwise noted: M48.40X-M48.58X with 7th A, M80.00X-M84.68X with 7th A

M48.50 **Collapsed vertebra, not elsewhere classified, site unspecified** CC
M48.51 **Collapsed vertebra, not elsewhere classified, occipito-atlanto-axial region** CC
M48.52 **Collapsed vertebra, not elsewhere classified, cervical region** CC
M48.53 **Collapsed vertebra, not elsewhere classified, cervicothoracic region** CC
M48.54 **Collapsed vertebra, not elsewhere classified, thoracic region** CC
M48.55 **Collapsed vertebra, not elsewhere classified, thoracolumbar region** CC
M48.56 **Collapsed vertebra, not elsewhere classified, lumbar region** CC
M48.57 **Collapsed vertebra, not elsewhere classified, lumbosacral region** CC
M48.58 **Collapsed vertebra, not elsewhere classified, sacral and sacrococcygeal region** CC

M48.8 Other specified spondylopathies
Ossification of posterior longitudinal ligament

M48.8X Other specified spondylopathies

M48.8X1 Other specified spondylopathies, occipito-atlanto-axial region

M48.8X2 Other specified spondylopathies, cervical region

M48.8X3 Other specified spondylopathies, cervicothoracic region

M48.8X4 Other specified spondylopathies, thoracic region

M48.8X5 Other specified spondylopathies, thoracolumbar region

M48.8X6 Other specified spondylopathies, lumbar region

M48.8X7 Other specified spondylopathies, lumbosacral region

M48.8X8 Other specified spondylopathies, sacral and sacrococcygeal region

M48.8X9 Other specified spondylopathies, site unspecified

M48.9 Spondylopathy, unspecified

M49 Spondylopathies in diseases classified elsewhere

INCLUDES curvature of spine in diseases classified elsewhere
deformity of spine in diseases classified elsewhere
kyphosis in diseases classified elsewhere
scoliosis in diseases classified elsewhere
spondylopathy in diseases classified elsewhere

Code first underlying disease, such as:
brucellosis (A23.-)
Charcôt-Marie-Tooth disease (G60.0)
enterobacterial infections (A01-A04)
osteitis fibrosa cystica (E21.0)

EXCLUDES 1 *curvature of spine in tuberculosis [Pott's] (A18.01)*
enteropathic arthropathies (M07.-)
gonococcal spondylitis (A54.41)
neuropathic [tabes dorsalis] spondylitis (A52.11)
neuropathic spondylopathy in syringomyelia (G95.0)
neuropathic spondylopathy in tabes dorsalis (A52.11)
nonsyphilitic neuropathic spondylopathy NEC (G98.0)
spondylitis in syphilis (acquired) (A52.77)
tuberculous spondylitis (A18.01)
typhoid fever spondylitis (A01.05)

M49.8 Spondylopathy in diseases classified elsewhere

M49.80 Spondylopathy in diseases classified elsewhere, site unspecified

M49.81 Spondylopathy in diseases classified elsewhere, occipito-atlanto-axial region

M49.82 Spondylopathy in diseases classified elsewhere, cervical region

M49.83 Spondylopathy in diseases classified elsewhere, cervicothoracic region

M49.84 Spondylopathy in diseases classified elsewhere, thoracic region

M49.85 Spondylopathy in diseases classified elsewhere, thoracolumbar region

M49.86 Spondylopathy in diseases classified elsewhere, lumbar region

M49.87 Spondylopathy in diseases classified elsewhere, lumbosacral region

M49.88 Spondylopathy in diseases classified elsewhere, sacral and sacrococcygeal region

M49.89 Spondylopathy in diseases classified elsewhere, multiple sites in spine

Other dorsopathies (M50-M54)

EXCLUDES 1 *current injury—see injury of spine by body region*
discitis NOS (M46.4-)

M50 Cervical disc disorders

NOTE Code to the most superior level of disorder.

INCLUDES cervicothoracic disc disorders with cervicalgia
cervicothoracic disc disorders

M50.0 Cervical disc disorder with myelopathy

M50.00 Cervical disc disorder with myelopathy, unspecified cervical region CC
CC Excl: M50.00-M50.03, M50.20-M50.23

M50.01 Cervical disc disorder with myelopathy, high cervical region CC
C2-C3 disc disorder with myelopathy
C3-C4 disc disorder with myelopathy
CC Excl: See code: M50.00

M50.02 Cervical disc disorder with myelopathy, mid-cervical region CC
C4-C5 disc disorder with myelopathy
C5-C6 disc disorder with myelopathy
C6-C7 disc disorder with myelopathy
CC Excl: See code: M50.00

M50.03 Cervical disc disorder with myelopathy, cervicothoracic region CC
C7-T1 disc disorder with myelopathy
CC Excl: See code: M50.00

M50.1 Cervical disc disorder with radiculopathy

EXCLUDES 2 *brachial radiculitis NOS (M54.13)*

M50.10 Cervical disc disorder with radiculopathy, unspecified cervical region

M50.11 Cervical disc disorder with radiculopathy, high cervical region
C2-C3 disc disorder with radiculopathy
C3 radiculopathy due to disc disorder
C3-C4 disc disorder with radiculopathy
C4 radiculopathy due to disc disorder

M50.12 Cervical disc disorder with radiculopathy, mid-cervical region
C4-C5 disc disorder with radiculopathy
C5 radiculopathy due to disc disorder
C5-C6 disc disorder with radiculopathy
C6 radiculopathy due to disc disorder
C6-C7 disc disorder with radiculopathy
C7 radiculopathy due to disc disorder

M50.13 Cervical disc disorder with radiculopathy, cervicothoracic region
C7-T1 disc disorder with radiculopathy
C8 radiculopathy due to disc disorder

M50.2 Other cervical disc displacement

M50.20 Other cervical disc displacement, unspecified cervical region

M50.21 Other cervical disc displacement, high cervical region
Other C2-C3 cervical disc displacement
Other C3-C4 cervical disc displacement

M50.22 Other cervical disc displacement, mid-cervical region
Other C4-C5 cervical disc displacement
Other C5-C6 cervical disc displacement
Other C6-C7 cervical disc displacement

M50.23 Other cervical disc displacement, cervicothoracic region
Other C7-T1 cervical disc displacement

M50.3 Other cervical disc degeneration

M50.30 Other cervical disc degeneration, unspecified cervical region

M50.31 Other cervical disc degeneration, high cervical region
Other C2-C3 cervical disc degeneration
Other C3-C4 cervical disc degeneration

M50.32 Other cervical disc degeneration, mid-cervical region
Other C4-C5 cervical disc degeneration
Other C5-C6 cervical disc degeneration
Other C6-C7 cervical disc degeneration

M50.33 Other cervical disc degeneration, cervicothoracic region
Other C7-T1 cervical disc degeneration

M50.8 Other cervical disc disorders

M50.80 Other cervical disc disorders, unspecified cervical region

M50.81 Other cervical disc disorders, high cervical region
Other C2-C3 cervical disc disorders
Other C3-C4 cervical disc disorders

M50.82 Other cervical disc disorders, mid-cervical region
Other C4-C5 cervical disc disorders
Other C5-C6 cervical disc disorders
Other C6-C7 cervical disc disorders

M50.83 Other cervical disc disorders, cervicothoracic region
Other C7-T1 cervical disc disorders

√5th **M50.9 Cervical disc disorder, unspecified**

M50.90 Cervical disc disorder, unspecified, unspecified cervical region

M50.91 Cervical disc disorder, unspecified, high cervical region
C2-C3 cervical disc disorder, unspecified
C3-C4 cervical disc disorder, unspecified

M50.92 Cervical disc disorder, unspecified, mid-cervical region
C4-C5 cervical disc disorder, unspecified
C5-C6 cervical disc disorder, unspecified
C6-C7 cervical disc disorder, unspecified

M50.93 Cervical disc disorder, unspecified, cervicothoracic region
C7-T1 cervical disc disorder, unspecified

√4th **M51 Thoracic, thoracolumbar, and lumbosacral intervertebral disc disorders**
EXCLUDES 2 *cervical and cervicothoracic disc disorders (M50.-)*
sacral and sacrococcygeal disorders (M53.3)

√5th **M51.0 Thoracic, thoracolumbar and lumbosacral intervertebral disc disorders with myelopathy**

M51.04 Intervertebral disc disorders with myelopathy, thoracic region CC
CC Excl: M51.04-M51.05, M51.24-M51.25

M51.05 Intervertebral disc disorders with myelopathy, thoracolumbar region CC
CC Excl: See code: M51.04

M51.06 Intervertebral disc disorders with myelopathy, lumbar region CC
CC Excl: M51.06-M51.07, M51.24-M51.25

√5th **M51.1 Thoracic, thoracolumbar and lumbosacral intervertebral disc disorders with radiculopathy**
Sciatica due to intervertebral disc disorder
EXCLUDES 1 *lumbar radiculitis NOS (M54.16)*
sciatica NOS (M54.3)

M51.14 Intervertebral disc disorders with radiculopathy, thoracic region

M51.15 Intervertebral disc disorders with radiculopathy, thoracolumbar region

M51.16 Intervertebral disc disorders with radiculopathy, lumbar region

M51.17 Intervertebral disc disorders with radiculopathy, lumbosacral region

√5th **M51.2 Other thoracic, thoracolumbar and lumbosacral intervertebral disc displacement**
Lumbago due to displacement of intervertebral disc

M51.24 Other intervertebral disc displacement, thoracic region

M51.25 Other intervertebral disc displacement, thoracolumbar region

M51.26 Other intervertebral disc displacement, lumbar region

M51.27 Other intervertebral disc displacement, lumbosacral region

√5th **M51.3 Other thoracic, thoracolumbar and lumbosacral intervertebral disc degeneration**
AHA: 2013, 3Q, 22

M51.34 Other intervertebral disc degeneration, thoracic region

M51.35 Other intervertebral disc degeneration, thoracolumbar region

M51.36 Other intervertebral disc degeneration, lumbar region

M51.37 Other intervertebral disc degeneration, lumbosacral region

√5th **M51.4 Schmorl's nodes**

M51.44 Schmorl's nodes, thoracic region

M51.45 Schmorl's nodes, thoracolumbar region

M51.46 Schmorl's nodes, lumbar region

M51.47 Schmorl's nodes, lumbosacral region

√5th **M51.8 Other thoracic, thoracolumbar and lumbosacral intervertebral disc disorders**

M51.84 Other intervertebral disc disorders, thoracic region

M51.85 Other intervertebral disc disorders, thoracolumbar region

M51.86 Other intervertebral disc disorders, lumbar region

M51.87 Other intervertebral disc disorders, lumbosacral region

M51.9 Unspecified thoracic, thoracolumbar and lumbosacral intervertebral disc disorder

√4th **M53 Other and unspecified dorsopathies, not elsewhere classified**

M53.0 Cervicocranial syndrome
Posterior cervical sympathetic syndrome

M53.1 Cervicobrachial syndrome
EXCLUDES 2 *cervical disc disorder (M50.-)*
thoracic outlet syndrome (G54.0)

√5th **M53.2 Spinal instabilities**

√6th **M53.2X Spinal instabilities**

M53.2X1 Spinal instabilities, occipito-atlanto-axial region

M53.2X2 Spinal instabilities, cervical region

M53.2X3 Spinal instabilities, cervicothoracic region

M53.2X4 Spinal instabilities, thoracic region

M53.2X5 Spinal instabilities, thoracolumbar region

M53.2X6 Spinal instabilities, lumbar region

M53.2X7 Spinal instabilities, lumbosacral region

M53.2X8 Spinal instabilities, sacral and sacrococcygeal region

M53.2X9 Spinal instabilities, site unspecified

M53.3 Sacrococcygeal disorders, not elsewhere classified
Coccygodynia

√5th **M53.8 Other specified dorsopathies**

M53.80 Other specified dorsopathies, site unspecified

M53.81 Other specified dorsopathies, occipito-atlanto-axial region

M53.82 Other specified dorsopathies, cervical region

M53.83 Other specified dorsopathies, cervicothoracic region

M53.84 Other specified dorsopathies, thoracic region

M53.85 Other specified dorsopathies, thoracolumbar region

M53.86 Other specified dorsopathies, lumbar region

M53.87 Other specified dorsopathies, lumbosacral region

M53.88 Other specified dorsopathies, sacral and sacrococcygeal region

M53.9 Dorsopathy, unspecified

√4th **M54 Dorsalgia**
EXCLUDES 1 *psychogenic dorsalgia (F45.41)*

√5th **M54.0 Panniculitis affecting regions of neck and back**
EXCLUDES 1 *lupus panniculitis (L93.2)*
panniculitis NOS (M79.3)
relapsing [Weber-Christian] panniculitis (M35.6)

M54.00 Panniculitis affecting regions of neck and back, site unspecified

M54.01 Panniculitis affecting regions of neck and back, occipito-atlanto-axial region

M54.02 Panniculitis affecting regions of neck and back, cervical region

M54.03 Panniculitis affecting regions of neck and back, cervicothoracic region

M54.04 Panniculitis affecting regions of neck and back, thoracic region

M54.05 Panniculitis affecting regions of neck and back, thoracolumbar region

M54.06 Panniculitis affecting regions of neck and back, lumbar region

M54.07 Panniculitis affecting regions of neck and back, lumbosacral region

M54.08 Panniculitis affecting regions of neck and back, sacral and sacrococcygeal region

M54.09 Panniculitis affecting regions, neck and back, multiple sites in spine

M54.1 Radiculopathy
Brachial neuritis or radiculitis NOS
Lumbar neuritis or radiculitis NOS
Lumbosacral neuritis or radiculitis NOS
Thoracic neuritis or radiculitis NOS
Radiculitis NOS
EXCLUDES 1 *neuralgia and neuritis NOS (M79.2)*
radiculopathy with cervical disc disorder (M5Ø.1)
radiculopathy with lumbar and other intervertebral disc disorder (M51.1-)
radiculopathy with spondylosis (M47.2-)

M54.1Ø Radiculopathy, site unspecified
M54.11 Radiculopathy, occipito-atlanto-axial region
M54.12 Radiculopathy, cervical region
M54.13 Radiculopathy, cervicothoracic region
M54.14 Radiculopathy, thoracic region
M54.15 Radiculopathy, thoracolumbar region
M54.16 Radiculopathy, lumbar region
M54.17 Radiculopathy, lumbosacral region
M54.18 Radiculopathy, sacral and sacrococcygeal region

M54.2 Cervicalgia
EXCLUDES 1 *cervicalgia due to intervertebral cervical disc disorder (M5Ø.-)*

M54.3 Sciatica
EXCLUDES 1 *lesion of sciatic nerve (G57.Ø)*
sciatica due to intervertebral disc disorder (M51.1-)
sciatica with lumbago (M54.4-)

M54.3Ø Sciatica, unspecified side
M54.31 Sciatica, right side
M54.32 Sciatica, left side

M54.4 Lumbago with sciatica
EXCLUDES 1 *lumbago with sciatica due to intervertebral disc disorder (M51.1-)*

M54.4Ø Lumbago with sciatica, unspecified side
M54.41 Lumbago with sciatica, right side
M54.42 Lumbago with sciatica, left side

M54.5 Low back pain
Loin pain
Lumbago NOS
EXCLUDES 1 *low back strain (S39.Ø12)*
lumbago due to intervertebral disc displacement (M51.2-)
lumbago with sciatica (M54.4-)

M54.6 Pain in thoracic spine
EXCLUDES 1 *pain in thoracic spine due to intervertebral disc disorder (M51.-)*

M54.8 Other dorsalgia
EXCLUDES 1 *dorsalgia in thoracic region (M54.6)*
low back pain (M54.5)

M54.81 Occipital neuralgia
M54.89 Other dorsalgia

M54.9 Dorsalgia, unspecified
Backache NOS
Back pain NOS

SOFT TISSUE DISORDERS (M6Ø-M79)

Disorders of muscles (M6Ø-M63)

EXCLUDES 1 *dermatopolymyositis (M33.-)*
muscular dystrophies and myopathies (G71-G72)
myopathy in amyloidosis (E85.-)
myopathy in polyarteritis nodosa (M3Ø.Ø)
myopathy in rheumatoid arthritis (MØ5.32)
myopathy in scleroderma (M34.-)
myopathy in Sjögren's syndrome (M35.Ø3)
myopathy in systemic lupus erythematosus (M32.-)

M6Ø Myositis
EXCLUDES 2 *inclusion body myositis [IBM] (G72.41)*

M6Ø.Ø Infective myositis
Tropical pyomyositis
Use additional code (B95-B97) to identify infectious agent

CC Excl: For CC codes in subcategory M6Ø.Ø, unless otherwise noted: K68.12, M6Ø.ØØØ-M6Ø.19, M61.ØØ-M61.19, M61.3Ø-M61.59, M62.3, M62.5Ø-M62.59, M62.89, M72.6

M6Ø.ØØ Infective myositis, unspecified site
M6Ø.ØØØ Infective myositis, unspecified right arm CC
Infective myositis, right upper limb NOS
M6Ø.ØØ1 Infective myositis, unspecified left arm CC
Infective myositis, left upper limb NOS
M6Ø.ØØ2 Infective myositis, unspecified arm CC
Infective myositis, upper limb NOS
M6Ø.ØØ3 Infective myositis, unspecified right leg CC
Infective myositis, right lower limb NOS
M6Ø.ØØ4 Infective myositis, unspecified left leg CC
Infective myositis, left lower limb NOS
M6Ø.ØØ5 Infective myositis, unspecified leg CC
Infective myositis, lower limb NOS
M6Ø.ØØ9 Infective myositis, unspecified site CC

M6Ø.Ø1 Infective myositis, shoulder
M6Ø.Ø11 Infective myositis, right shoulder CC
M6Ø.Ø12 Infective myositis, left shoulder CC
M6Ø.Ø19 Infective myositis, unspecified shoulder CC

M6Ø.Ø2 Infective myositis, upper arm
M6Ø.Ø21 Infective myositis, right upper arm CC
M6Ø.Ø22 Infective myositis, left upper arm CC
M6Ø.Ø29 Infective myositis, unspecified upper arm CC

M6Ø.Ø3 Infective myositis, forearm
M6Ø.Ø31 Infective myositis, right forearm CC
M6Ø.Ø32 Infective myositis, left forearm CC
M6Ø.Ø39 Infective myositis, unspecified forearm CC

M6Ø.Ø4 Infective myositis, hand and fingers
M6Ø.Ø41 Infective myositis, right hand CC
M6Ø.Ø42 Infective myositis, left hand CC
M6Ø.Ø43 Infective myositis, unspecified hand CC
M6Ø.Ø44 Infective myositis, right finger(s) CC
M6Ø.Ø45 Infective myositis, left finger(s) CC
M6Ø.Ø46 Infective myositis, unspecified finger(s) CC

M6Ø.Ø5 Infective myositis, thigh
M6Ø.Ø51 Infective myositis, right thigh CC
M6Ø.Ø52 Infective myositis, left thigh CC
M6Ø.Ø59 Infective myositis, unspecified thigh CC

M6Ø.Ø6 Infective myositis, lower leg
M6Ø.Ø61 Infective myositis, right lower leg CC
M6Ø.Ø62 Infective myositis, left lower leg CC
M6Ø.Ø69 Infective myositis, unspecified lower leg CC

M6Ø.Ø7 Infective myositis, ankle, foot and toes
M6Ø.Ø7Ø Infective myositis, right ankle CC
M6Ø.Ø71 Infective myositis, left ankle CC
M6Ø.Ø72 Infective myositis, unspecified ankle CC
M6Ø.Ø73 Infective myositis, right foot CC
M6Ø.Ø74 Infective myositis, left foot CC
M6Ø.Ø75 Infective myositis, unspecified foot CC
M6Ø.Ø76 Infective myositis, right toe(s) CC
M6Ø.Ø77 Infective myositis, left toe(s) CC
M6Ø.Ø78 Infective myositis, unspecified toe(s) CC

M6Ø.Ø8 Infective myositis, other site CC
M6Ø.Ø9 Infective myositis, multiple sites CC

M6Ø.1 Interstitial myositis
M6Ø.1Ø Interstitial myositis of unspecified site

M6Ø.11 Interstitial myositis, shoulder
M6Ø.111 Interstitial myositis, right shoulder
M6Ø.112 Interstitial myositis, left shoulder
M6Ø.119 Interstitial myositis, unspecified shoulder

M6Ø.12 Interstitial myositis, upper arm
M6Ø.121 Interstitial myositis, right upper arm
M6Ø.122 Interstitial myositis, left upper arm
M6Ø.129 Interstitial myositis, unspecified upper arm

M6Ø.13 Interstitial myositis, forearm
M6Ø.131 Interstitial myositis, right forearm

M60.132 Interstitial myositis, left forearm
M60.139 Interstitial myositis, unspecified forearm
✓6th M60.14 Interstitial myositis, hand
M60.141 Interstitial myositis, right hand
M60.142 Interstitial myositis, left hand
M60.149 Interstitial myositis, unspecified hand
✓6th M60.15 Interstitial myositis, thigh
M60.151 Interstitial myositis, right thigh
M60.152 Interstitial myositis, left thigh
M60.159 Interstitial myositis, unspecified thigh
✓6th M60.16 Interstitial myositis, lower leg
M60.161 Interstitial myositis, right lower leg
M60.162 Interstitial myositis, left lower leg
M60.169 Interstitial myositis, unspecified lower leg
✓6th M60.17 Interstitial myositis, ankle and foot
M60.171 Interstitial myositis, right ankle and foot
M60.172 Interstitial myositis, left ankle and foot
M60.179 Interstitial myositis, unspecified ankle and foot
M60.18 Interstitial myositis, other site
M60.19 Interstitial myositis, multiple sites
✓5th M60.2 Foreign body granuloma of soft tissue, not elsewhere classified
Use additional code to identify the type of retained foreign body (Z18.-)
EXCLUDES 1 *foreign body granuloma of skin and subcutaneous tissue (L92.3)*
M60.20 Foreign body granuloma of soft tissue, not elsewhere classified, unspecified site
✓6th M60.21 Foreign body granuloma of soft tissue, not elsewhere classified, shoulder
M60.211 Foreign body granuloma of soft tissue, not elsewhere classified, right shoulder
M60.212 Foreign body granuloma of soft tissue, not elsewhere classified, left shoulder
M60.219 Foreign body granuloma of soft tissue, not elsewhere classified, unspecified shoulder
✓6th M60.22 Foreign body granuloma of soft tissue, not elsewhere classified, upper arm
M60.221 Foreign body granuloma of soft tissue, not elsewhere classified, right upper arm
M60.222 Foreign body granuloma of soft tissue, not elsewhere classified, left upper arm
M60.229 Foreign body granuloma of soft tissue, not elsewhere classified, unspecified upper arm
✓6th M60.23 Foreign body granuloma of soft tissue, not elsewhere classified, forearm
M60.231 Foreign body granuloma of soft tissue, not elsewhere classified, right forearm
M60.232 Foreign body granuloma of soft tissue, not elsewhere classified, left forearm
M60.239 Foreign body granuloma of soft tissue, not elsewhere classified, unspecified forearm
✓6th M60.24 Foreign body granuloma of soft tissue, not elsewhere classified, hand
M60.241 Foreign body granuloma of soft tissue, not elsewhere classified, right hand
M60.242 Foreign body granuloma of soft tissue, not elsewhere classified, left hand
M60.249 Foreign body granuloma of soft tissue, not elsewhere classified, unspecified hand
✓6th M60.25 Foreign body granuloma of soft tissue, not elsewhere classified, thigh
M60.251 Foreign body granuloma of soft tissue, not elsewhere classified, right thigh
M60.252 Foreign body granuloma of soft tissue, not elsewhere classified, left thigh
M60.259 Foreign body granuloma of soft tissue, not elsewhere classified, unspecified thigh
✓6th M60.26 Foreign body granuloma of soft tissue, not elsewhere classified, lower leg
M60.261 Foreign body granuloma of soft tissue, not elsewhere classified, right lower leg
M60.262 Foreign body granuloma of soft tissue, not elsewhere classified, left lower leg
M60.269 Foreign body granuloma of soft tissue, not elsewhere classified, unspecified lower leg
✓6th M60.27 Foreign body granuloma of soft tissue, not elsewhere classified, ankle and foot
M60.271 Foreign body granuloma of soft tissue, not elsewhere classified, right ankle and foot
M60.272 Foreign body granuloma of soft tissue, not elsewhere classified, left ankle and foot
M60.279 Foreign body granuloma of soft tissue, not elsewhere classified, unspecified ankle and foot
M60.28 Foreign body granuloma of soft tissue, not elsewhere classified, other site
✓5th M60.8 Other myositis
M60.80 Other myositis, unspecified site
✓6th M60.81 Other myositis shoulder
M60.811 Other myositis, right shoulder
M60.812 Other myositis, left shoulder
M60.819 Other myositis, unspecified shoulder
✓6th M60.82 Other myositis, upper arm
M60.821 Other myositis, right upper arm
M60.822 Other myositis, left upper arm
M60.829 Other myositis, unspecified upper arm
✓6th M60.83 Other myositis, forearm
M60.831 Other myositis, right forearm
M60.832 Other myositis, left forearm
M60.839 Other myositis, unspecified forearm
✓6th M60.84 Other myositis, hand
M60.841 Other myositis, right hand
M60.842 Other myositis, left hand
M60.849 Other myositis, unspecified hand
✓6th M60.85 Other myositis, thigh
M60.851 Other myositis, right thigh
M60.852 Other myositis, left thigh
M60.859 Other myositis, unspecified thigh
✓6th M60.86 Other myositis, lower leg
M60.861 Other myositis, right lower leg
M60.862 Other myositis, left lower leg
M60.869 Other myositis, unspecified lower leg
✓6th M60.87 Other myositis, ankle and foot
M60.871 Other myositis, right ankle and foot
M60.872 Other myositis, left ankle and foot
M60.879 Other myositis, unspecified ankle and foot
M60.88 Other myositis, other site
M60.89 Other myositis, multiple sites
M60.9 Myositis, unspecified

✓4th M61 Calcification and ossification of muscle

✓5th M61.0 Myositis ossificans traumatica
M61.00 Myositis ossificans traumatica, unspecified site
✓6th M61.01 Myositis ossificans traumatica, shoulder
M61.011 Myositis ossificans traumatica, right shoulder
M61.012 Myositis ossificans traumatica, left shoulder
M61.019 Myositis ossificans traumatica, unspecified shoulder
✓6th M61.02 Myositis ossificans traumatica, upper arm
M61.021 Myositis ossificans traumatica, right upper arm
M61.022 Myositis ossificans traumatica, left upper arm
M61.029 Myositis ossificans traumatica, unspecified upper arm
✓6th M61.03 Myositis ossificans traumatica, forearm
M61.031 Myositis ossificans traumatica, right forearm
M61.032 Myositis ossificans traumatica, left forearm
M61.039 Myositis ossificans traumatica, unspecified forearm
✓6th M61.04 Myositis ossificans traumatica, hand
M61.041 Myositis ossificans traumatica, right hand
M61.042 Myositis ossificans traumatica, left hand

M61.049 Myositis ossificans traumatica, unspecified hand

✓6th M61.05 Myositis ossificans traumatica, thigh
M61.051 Myositis ossificans traumatica, right thigh
M61.052 Myositis ossificans traumatica, left thigh
M61.059 Myositis ossificans traumatica, unspecified thigh

✓6th M61.06 Myositis ossificans traumatica, lower leg
M61.061 Myositis ossificans traumatica, right lower leg
M61.062 Myositis ossificans traumatica, left lower leg
M61.069 Myositis ossificans traumatica, unspecified lower leg

✓6th M61.07 Myositis ossificans traumatica, ankle and foot
M61.071 Myositis ossificans traumatica, right ankle and foot
M61.072 Myositis ossificans traumatica, left ankle and foot
M61.079 Myositis ossificans traumatica, unspecified ankle and foot

M61.08 Myositis ossificans traumatica, other site
M61.09 Myositis ossificans traumatica, multiple sites

✓5th M61.1 Myositis ossificans progressiva
Fibrodysplasia ossificans progressiva
M61.10 Myositis ossificans progressiva, unspecified site

✓6th M61.11 Myositis ossificans progressiva, shoulder
M61.111 Myositis ossificans progressiva, right shoulder
M61.112 Myositis ossificans progressiva, left shoulder
M61.119 Myositis ossificans progressiva, unspecified shoulder

✓6th M61.12 Myositis ossificans progressiva, upper arm
M61.121 Myositis ossificans progressiva, right upper arm
M61.122 Myositis ossificans progressiva, left upper arm
M61.129 Myositis ossificans progressiva, unspecified arm

✓6th M61.13 Myositis ossificans progressiva, forearm
M61.131 Myositis ossificans progressiva, right forearm
M61.132 Myositis ossificans progressiva, left forearm
M61.139 Myositis ossificans progressiva, unspecified forearm

✓6th M61.14 Myositis ossificans progressiva, hand and finger(s)
M61.141 Myositis ossificans progressiva, right hand
M61.142 Myositis ossificans progressiva, left hand
M61.143 Myositis ossificans progressiva, unspecified hand
M61.144 Myositis ossificans progressiva, right finger(s)
M61.145 Myositis ossificans progressiva, left finger(s)
M61.146 Myositis ossificans progressiva, unspecified finger(s)

✓6th M61.15 Myositis ossificans progressiva, thigh
M61.151 Myositis ossificans progressiva, right thigh
M61.152 Myositis ossificans progressiva, left thigh
M61.159 Myositis ossificans progressiva, unspecified thigh

✓6th M61.16 Myositis ossificans progressiva, lower leg
M61.161 Myositis ossificans progressiva, right lower leg
M61.162 Myositis ossificans progressiva, left lower leg
M61.169 Myositis ossificans progressiva, unspecified lower leg

✓6th M61.17 Myositis ossificans progressiva, ankle, foot and toe(s)
M61.171 Myositis ossificans progressiva, right ankle
M61.172 Myositis ossificans progressiva, left ankle
M61.173 Myositis ossificans progressiva, unspecified ankle
M61.174 Myositis ossificans progressiva, right foot
M61.175 Myositis ossificans progressiva, left foot
M61.176 Myositis ossificans progressiva, unspecified foot
M61.177 Myositis ossificans progressiva, right toe(s)
M61.178 Myositis ossificans progressiva, left toe(s)
M61.179 Myositis ossificans progressiva, unspecified toe(s)

M61.18 Myositis ossificans progressiva, other site
M61.19 Myositis ossificans progressiva, multiple sites

✓5th M61.2 Paralytic calcification and ossification of muscle
Myositis ossificans associated with quadriplegia or paraplegia
M61.20 Paralytic calcification and ossification of muscle, unspecified site

✓6th M61.21 Paralytic calcification and ossification of muscle, shoulder
M61.211 Paralytic calcification and ossification of muscle, right shoulder
M61.212 Paralytic calcification and ossification of muscle, left shoulder
M61.219 Paralytic calcification and ossification of muscle, unspecified shoulder

✓6th M61.22 Paralytic calcification and ossification of muscle, upper arm
M61.221 Paralytic calcification and ossification of muscle, right upper arm
M61.222 Paralytic calcification and ossification of muscle, left upper arm
M61.229 Paralytic calcification and ossification of muscle, unspecified upper arm

✓6th M61.23 Paralytic calcification and ossification of muscle, forearm
M61.231 Paralytic calcification and ossification of muscle, right forearm
M61.232 Paralytic calcification and ossification of muscle, left forearm
M61.239 Paralytic calcification and ossification of muscle, unspecified forearm

✓6th M61.24 Paralytic calcification and ossification of muscle, hand
M61.241 Paralytic calcification and ossification of muscle, right hand
M61.242 Paralytic calcification and ossification of muscle, left hand
M61.249 Paralytic calcification and ossification of muscle, unspecified hand

✓6th M61.25 Paralytic calcification and ossification of muscle, thigh
M61.251 Paralytic calcification and ossification of muscle, right thigh
M61.252 Paralytic calcification and ossification of muscle, left thigh
M61.259 Paralytic calcification and ossification of muscle, unspecified thigh

✓6th M61.26 Paralytic calcification and ossification of muscle, lower leg
M61.261 Paralytic calcification and ossification of muscle, right lower leg
M61.262 Paralytic calcification and ossification of muscle, left lower leg
M61.269 Paralytic calcification and ossification of muscle, unspecified lower leg

✓6th M61.27 Paralytic calcification and ossification of muscle, ankle and foot
M61.271 Paralytic calcification and ossification of muscle, right ankle and foot
M61.272 Paralytic calcification and ossification of muscle, left ankle and foot
M61.279 Paralytic calcification and ossification of muscle, unspecified ankle and foot

M61.28 Paralytic calcification and ossification of muscle, other site
M61.29 Paralytic calcification and ossification of muscle, multiple sites

✓5th **M61.3 Calcification and ossification of muscles associated with burns**
Myositis ossificans associated with burns
M61.30 Calcification and ossification of muscles associated with burns, unspecified site
✓6th **M61.31 Calcification and ossification of muscles associated with burns, shoulder**
M61.311 Calcification and ossification of muscles associated with burns, right shoulder
M61.312 Calcification and ossification of muscles associated with burns, left shoulder
M61.319 Calcification and ossification of muscles associated with burns, unspecified shoulder
✓6th **M61.32 Calcification and ossification of muscles associated with burns, upper arm**
M61.321 Calcification and ossification of muscles associated with burns, right upper arm
M61.322 Calcification and ossification of muscles associated with burns, left upper arm
M61.329 Calcification and ossification of muscles associated with burns, unspecified upper arm
✓6th **M61.33 Calcification and ossification of muscles associated with burns, forearm**
M61.331 Calcification and ossification of muscles associated with burns, right forearm
M61.332 Calcification and ossification of muscles associated with burns, left forearm
M61.339 Calcification and ossification of muscles associated with burns, unspecified forearm
✓6th **M61.34 Calcification and ossification of muscles associated with burns, hand**
M61.341 Calcification and ossification of muscles associated with burns, right hand
M61.342 Calcification and ossification of muscles associated with burns, left hand
M61.349 Calcification and ossification of muscles associated with burns, unspecified hand
✓6th **M61.35 Calcification and ossification of muscles associated with burns, thigh**
M61.351 Calcification and ossification of muscles associated with burns, right thigh
M61.352 Calcification and ossification of muscles associated with burns, left thigh
M61.359 Calcification and ossification of muscles associated with burns, unspecified thigh
✓6th **M61.36 Calcification and ossification of muscles associated with burns, lower leg**
M61.361 Calcification and ossification of muscles associated with burns, right lower leg
M61.362 Calcification and ossification of muscles associated with burns, left lower leg
M61.369 Calcification and ossification of muscles associated with burns, unspecified lower leg
✓6th **M61.37 Calcification and ossification of muscles associated with burns, ankle and foot**
M61.371 Calcification and ossification of muscles associated with burns, right ankle and foot
M61.372 Calcification and ossification of muscles associated with burns, left ankle and foot
M61.379 Calcification and ossification of muscles associated with burns, unspecified ankle and foot
M61.38 Calcification and ossification of muscles associated with burns, other site
M61.39 Calcification and ossification of muscles associated with burns, multiple sites
✓5th **M61.4 Other calcification of muscle**
EXCLUDES 1 *calcific tendinitis NOS (M65.2-)*
calcific tendinitis of shoulder (M75.3)
M61.40 Other calcification of muscle, unspecified site
✓6th **M61.41 Other calcification of muscle, shoulder**
M61.411 Other calcification of muscle, right shoulder
M61.412 Other calcification of muscle, left shoulder
M61.419 Other calcification of muscle, unspecified shoulder
✓6th **M61.42 Other calcification of muscle, upper arm**
M61.421 Other calcification of muscle, right upper arm
M61.422 Other calcification of muscle, left upper arm
M61.429 Other calcification of muscle, unspecified upper arm
✓6th **M61.43 Other calcification of muscle, forearm**
M61.431 Other calcification of muscle, right forearm
M61.432 Other calcification of muscle, left forearm
M61.439 Other calcification of muscle, unspecified forearm
✓6th **M61.44 Other calcification of muscle, hand**
M61.441 Other calcification of muscle, right hand
M61.442 Other calcification of muscle, left hand
M61.449 Other calcification of muscle, unspecified hand
✓6th **M61.45 Other calcification of muscle, thigh**
M61.451 Other calcification of muscle, right thigh
M61.452 Other calcification of muscle, left thigh
M61.459 Other calcification of muscle, unspecified thigh
✓6th **M61.46 Other calcification of muscle, lower leg**
M61.461 Other calcification of muscle, right lower leg
M61.462 Other calcification of muscle, left lower leg
M61.469 Other calcification of muscle, unspecified lower leg
✓6th **M61.47 Other calcification of muscle, ankle and foot**
M61.471 Other calcification of muscle, right ankle and foot
M61.472 Other calcification of muscle, left ankle and foot
M61.479 Other calcification of muscle, unspecified ankle and foot
M61.48 Other calcification of muscle, other site
M61.49 Other calcification of muscle, multiple sites
✓5th **M61.5 Other ossification of muscle**
M61.50 Other ossification of muscle, unspecified site
✓6th **M61.51 Other ossification of muscle, shoulder**
M61.511 Other ossification of muscle, right shoulder
M61.512 Other ossification of muscle, left shoulder
M61.519 Other ossification of muscle, unspecified shoulder
✓6th **M61.52 Other ossification of muscle, upper arm**
M61.521 Other ossification of muscle, right upper arm
M61.522 Other ossification of muscle, left upper arm
M61.529 Other ossification of muscle, unspecified upper arm
✓6th **M61.53 Other ossification of muscle, forearm**
M61.531 Other ossification of muscle, right forearm
M61.532 Other ossification of muscle, left forearm
M61.539 Other ossification of muscle, unspecified forearm
✓6th **M61.54 Other ossification of muscle, hand**
M61.541 Other ossification of muscle, right hand
M61.542 Other ossification of muscle, left hand
M61.549 Other ossification of muscle, unspecified hand
✓6th **M61.55 Other ossification of muscle, thigh**
M61.551 Other ossification of muscle, right thigh
M61.552 Other ossification of muscle, left thigh
M61.559 Other ossification of muscle, unspecified thigh
✓6th **M61.56 Other ossification of muscle, lower leg**
M61.561 Other ossification of muscle, right lower leg
M61.562 Other ossification of muscle, left lower leg

M61.569 Other ossification of muscle, unspecified lower leg

✓6th **M61.57 Other ossification of muscle, ankle and foot**

M61.571 Other ossification of muscle, right ankle and foot

M61.572 Other ossification of muscle, left ankle and foot

M61.579 Other ossification of muscle, unspecified ankle and foot

M61.58 Other ossification of muscle, other site

M61.59 Other ossification of muscle, multiple sites

M61.9 Calcification and ossification of muscle, unspecified

✓4th **M62 Other disorders of muscle**

EXCLUDES 1 *alcoholic myopathy (G72.1)*
cramp and spasm (R25.2)
drug-induced myopathy (G72.0)
myalgia (M79.1)
stiff-man syndrome (G25.82)

EXCLUDES 2 *nontraumatic hematoma of muscle (M79.81)*

✓5th **M62.0 Separation of muscle (nontraumatic)**

Diastasis of muscle

EXCLUDES 1 *diastasis recti complicating pregnancy, labor and delivery (O71.8)*
traumatic separation of muscle—see strain of muscle by body region

M62.00 Separation of muscle (nontraumatic), unspecified site

✓6th **M62.01 Separation of muscle (nontraumatic), shoulder**

M62.011 Separation of muscle (nontraumatic), right shoulder

M62.012 Separation of muscle (nontraumatic), left shoulder

M62.019 Separation of muscle (nontraumatic), unspecified shoulder

✓6th **M62.02 Separation of muscle (nontraumatic), upper arm**

M62.021 Separation of muscle (nontraumatic), right upper arm

M62.022 Separation of muscle (nontraumatic), left upper arm

M62.029 Separation of muscle (nontraumatic), unspecified upper arm

✓6th **M62.03 Separation of muscle (nontraumatic), forearm**

M62.031 Separation of muscle (nontraumatic), right forearm

M62.032 Separation of muscle (nontraumatic), left forearm

M62.039 Separation of muscle (nontraumatic), unspecified forearm

✓6th **M62.04 Separation of muscle (nontraumatic), hand**

M62.041 Separation of muscle (nontraumatic), right hand

M62.042 Separation of muscle (nontraumatic), left hand

M62.049 Separation of muscle (nontraumatic), unspecified hand

✓6th **M62.05 Separation of muscle (nontraumatic), thigh**

M62.051 Separation of muscle (nontraumatic), right thigh

M62.052 Separation of muscle (nontraumatic), left thigh

M62.059 Separation of muscle (nontraumatic), unspecified thigh

✓6th **M62.06 Separation of muscle (nontraumatic), lower leg**

M62.061 Separation of muscle (nontraumatic), right lower leg

M62.062 Separation of muscle (nontraumatic), left lower leg

M62.069 Separation of muscle (nontraumatic), unspecified lower leg

✓6th **M62.07 Separation of muscle (nontraumatic), ankle and foot**

M62.071 Separation of muscle (nontraumatic), right ankle and foot

M62.072 Separation of muscle (nontraumatic), left ankle and foot

M62.079 Separation of muscle (nontraumatic), unspecified ankle and foot

M62.08 Separation of muscle (nontraumatic), other site

✓5th **M62.1 Other rupture of muscle (nontraumatic)**

EXCLUDES 1 *traumatic rupture of muscle—see strain of muscle by body region*

EXCLUDES 2 *rupture of tendon (M66.-)*

M62.10 Other rupture of muscle (nontraumatic), unspecified site

✓6th **M62.11 Other rupture of muscle (nontraumatic), shoulder**

M62.111 Other rupture of muscle (nontraumatic), right shoulder

M62.112 Other rupture of muscle (nontraumatic), left shoulder

M62.119 Other rupture of muscle (nontraumatic), unspecified shoulder

✓6th **M62.12 Other rupture of muscle (nontraumatic), upper arm**

M62.121 Other rupture of muscle (nontraumatic), right upper arm

M62.122 Other rupture of muscle (nontraumatic), left upper arm

M62.129 Other rupture of muscle (nontraumatic), unspecified upper arm

✓6th **M62.13 Other rupture of muscle (nontraumatic), forearm**

M62.131 Other rupture of muscle (nontraumatic), right forearm

M62.132 Other rupture of muscle (nontraumatic), left forearm

M62.139 Other rupture of muscle (nontraumatic), unspecified forearm

✓6th **M62.14 Other rupture of muscle (nontraumatic), hand**

M62.141 Other rupture of muscle (nontraumatic), right hand

M62.142 Other rupture of muscle (nontraumatic), left hand

M62.149 Other rupture of muscle (nontraumatic), unspecified hand

✓6th **M62.15 Other rupture of muscle (nontraumatic), thigh**

M62.151 Other rupture of muscle (nontraumatic), right thigh

M62.152 Other rupture of muscle (nontraumatic), left thigh

M62.159 Other rupture of muscle (nontraumatic), unspecified thigh

✓6th **M62.16 Other rupture of muscle (nontraumatic), lower leg**

M62.161 Other rupture of muscle (nontraumatic), right lower leg

M62.162 Other rupture of muscle (nontraumatic), left lower leg

M62.169 Other rupture of muscle (nontraumatic), unspecified lower leg

✓6th **M62.17 Other rupture of muscle (nontraumatic), ankle and foot**

M62.171 Other rupture of muscle (nontraumatic), right ankle and foot

M62.172 Other rupture of muscle (nontraumatic), left ankle and foot

M62.179 Other rupture of muscle (nontraumatic), unspecified ankle and foot

M62.18 Other rupture of muscle (nontraumatic), other site

✓5th **M62.2 Nontraumatic ischemic infarction of muscle**

EXCLUDES 1 *compartment syndrome (traumatic) (T79.A-)*
nontraumatic compartment syndrome (M79.A-)
rhabdomyolysis (M62.82)
traumatic ischemia of muscle (T79.6)
Volkmann's ischemic contracture (T79.6)

M62.20 Nontraumatic ischemic infarction of muscle, unspecified site

✓6th **M62.21 Nontraumatic ischemic infarction of muscle, shoulder**

M62.211 Nontraumatic ischemic infarction of muscle, right shoulder

M62.212 Nontraumatic ischemic infarction of muscle, left shoulder

M62.219 Nontraumatic ischemic infarction of muscle, unspecified shoulder

✓6th **M62.22 Nontraumatic ischemic infarction of muscle, upper arm**

M62.221 Nontraumatic ischemic infarction of muscle, right upper arm

M62.222 Nontraumatic ischemic infarction of muscle, left upper arm
M62.229 Nontraumatic ischemic infarction of muscle, unspecified upper arm

✓6th M62.23 Nontraumatic ischemic infarction of muscle, forearm
M62.231 Nontraumatic ischemic infarction of muscle, right forearm
M62.232 Nontraumatic ischemic infarction of muscle, left forearm
M62.239 Nontraumatic ischemic infarction of muscle, unspecified forearm

✓6th M62.24 Nontraumatic ischemic infarction of muscle, hand
M62.241 Nontraumatic ischemic infarction of muscle, right hand
M62.242 Nontraumatic ischemic infarction of muscle, left hand
M62.249 Nontraumatic ischemic infarction of muscle, unspecified hand

✓6th M62.25 Nontraumatic ischemic infarction of muscle, thigh
M62.251 Nontraumatic ischemic infarction of muscle, right thigh
M62.252 Nontraumatic ischemic infarction of muscle, left thigh
M62.259 Nontraumatic ischemic infarction of muscle, unspecified thigh

✓6th M62.26 Nontraumatic ischemic infarction of muscle, lower leg
M62.261 Nontraumatic ischemic infarction of muscle, right lower leg
M62.262 Nontraumatic ischemic infarction of muscle, left lower leg
M62.269 Nontraumatic ischemic infarction of muscle, unspecified lower leg

✓6th M62.27 Nontraumatic ischemic infarction of muscle, ankle and foot
M62.271 Nontraumatic ischemic infarction of muscle, right ankle and foot
M62.272 Nontraumatic ischemic infarction of muscle, left ankle and foot
M62.279 Nontraumatic ischemic infarction of muscle, unspecified ankle and foot

M62.28 Nontraumatic ischemic infarction of muscle, other site

M62.3 Immobility syndrome (paraplegic)

✓5th M62.4 Contracture of muscle
Contracture of tendon (sheath)
EXCLUDES 1 *contracture of joint (M24.5-)*

M62.40 Contracture of muscle, unspecified site

✓6th M62.41 Contracture of muscle, shoulder
M62.411 Contracture of muscle, right shoulder
M62.412 Contracture of muscle, left shoulder
M62.419 Contracture of muscle, unspecified shoulder

✓6th M62.42 Contracture of muscle, upper arm
M62.421 Contracture of muscle, right upper arm
M62.422 Contracture of muscle, left upper arm
M62.429 Contracture of muscle, unspecified upper arm

✓6th M62.43 Contracture of muscle, forearm
M62.431 Contracture of muscle, right forearm
M62.432 Contracture of muscle, left forearm
M62.439 Contracture of muscle, unspecified forearm

✓6th M62.44 Contracture of muscle, hand
M62.441 Contracture of muscle, right hand
M62.442 Contracture of muscle, left hand
M62.449 Contracture of muscle, unspecified hand

✓6th M62.45 Contracture of muscle, thigh
M62.451 Contracture of muscle, right thigh
M62.452 Contracture of muscle, left thigh
M62.459 Contracture of muscle, unspecified thigh

✓6th M62.46 Contracture of muscle, lower leg
M62.461 Contracture of muscle, right lower leg
M62.462 Contracture of muscle, left lower leg
M62.469 Contracture of muscle, unspecified lower leg

✓6th M62.47 Contracture of muscle, ankle and foot
M62.471 Contracture of muscle, right ankle and foot
M62.472 Contracture of muscle, left ankle and foot
M62.479 Contracture of muscle, unspecified ankle and foot

M62.48 Contracture of muscle, other site
M62.49 Contracture of muscle, multiple sites

✓5th M62.5 Muscle wasting and atrophy, not elsewhere classified
Disuse atrophy NEC
EXCLUDES 1 *neuralgic amyotrophy (G54.5)*
progressive muscular atrophy (G12.29)
EXCLUDES 2 *pelvic muscle wasting (N81.84)*

M62.50 Muscle wasting and atrophy, not elsewhere classified, unspecified site

✓6th M62.51 Muscle wasting and atrophy, not elsewhere classified, shoulder
M62.511 Muscle wasting and atrophy, not elsewhere classified, right shoulder
M62.512 Muscle wasting and atrophy, not elsewhere classified, left shoulder
M62.519 Muscle wasting and atrophy, not elsewhere classified, unspecified shoulder

✓6th M62.52 Muscle wasting and atrophy, not elsewhere classified, upper arm
M62.521 Muscle wasting and atrophy, not elsewhere classified, right upper arm
M62.522 Muscle wasting and atrophy, not elsewhere classified, left upper arm
M62.529 Muscle wasting and atrophy, not elsewhere classified, unspecified upper arm

✓6th M62.53 Muscle wasting and atrophy, not elsewhere classified, forearm
M62.531 Muscle wasting and atrophy, not elsewhere classified, right forearm
M62.532 Muscle wasting and atrophy, not elsewhere classified, left forearm
M62.539 Muscle wasting and atrophy, not elsewhere classified, unspecified forearm

✓6th M62.54 Muscle wasting and atrophy, not elsewhere classified, hand
M62.541 Muscle wasting and atrophy, not elsewhere classified, right hand
M62.542 Muscle wasting and atrophy, not elsewhere classified, left hand
M62.549 Muscle wasting and atrophy, not elsewhere classified, unspecified hand

✓6th M62.55 Muscle wasting and atrophy, not elsewhere classified, thigh
M62.551 Muscle wasting and atrophy, not elsewhere classified, right thigh
M62.552 Muscle wasting and atrophy, not elsewhere classified, left thigh
M62.559 Muscle wasting and atrophy, not elsewhere classified, unspecified thigh

✓6th M62.56 Muscle wasting and atrophy, not elsewhere classified, lower leg
M62.561 Muscle wasting and atrophy, not elsewhere classified, right lower leg
M62.562 Muscle wasting and atrophy, not elsewhere classified, left lower leg
M62.569 Muscle wasting and atrophy, not elsewhere classified, unspecified lower leg

✓6th M62.57 Muscle wasting and atrophy, not elsewhere classified, ankle and foot
M62.571 Muscle wasting and atrophy, not elsewhere classified, right ankle and foot
M62.572 Muscle wasting and atrophy, not elsewhere classified, left ankle and foot
M62.579 Muscle wasting and atrophy, not elsewhere classified, unspecified ankle and foot

M62.58 Muscle wasting and atrophy, not elsewhere classified, other site

M62.59 Muscle wasting and atrophy, not elsewhere classified, multiple sites

5th M62.8 Other specified disorders of muscle
EXCLUDES 2 *nontraumatic hematoma of muscle (M79.81)*

M62.81 Muscle weakness (generalized)

M62.82 Rhabdomyolysis CC
EXCLUDES 1 *traumatic rhabdomyolysis (T79.6)*
CC Excl: K68.12, M60.000-M60.19, M61.00-M61.19, M61.30-M61.59, M62.3, M62.50-M62.59, M62.82, M62.89, M72.6

6th M62.83 Muscle spasm
M62.830 Muscle spasm of back
M62.831 Muscle spasm of calf
Charley-horse
M62.838 Other muscle spasm

M62.89 Other specified disorders of muscle
Muscle (sheath) hernia

M62.9 Disorder of muscle, unspecified

4th M63 Disorders of muscle in diseases classified elsewhere
Code first underlying disease, such as:
leprosy (A30.-)
neoplasm (C49-, C79.89, D21-, D48.1)
schistosomiasis (B65.-)
trichinellosis (B75)
EXCLUDES 1 *myopathy in cysticercosis (B69.81)*
myopathy in endocrine diseases (G73.7)
myopathy in metabolic diseases (G73.7)
myopathy in sarcoidosis (D86.87)
myopathy in secondary syphilis (A51.49)
myopathy in syphilis (late) (A52.78)
myopathy in toxoplasmosis (B58.82)
myopathy in tuberculosis (A18.09)

5th M63.8 Disorders of muscle in diseases classified elsewhere
M63.80 Disorders of muscle in diseases classified elsewhere, unspecified site

6th M63.81 Disorders of muscle in diseases classified elsewhere, shoulder
M63.811 Disorders of muscle in diseases classified elsewhere, right shoulder
M63.812 Disorders of muscle in diseases classified elsewhere, left shoulder
M63.819 Disorders of muscle in diseases classified elsewhere, unspecified shoulder

6th M63.82 Disorders of muscle in diseases classified elsewhere, upper arm
M63.821 Disorders of muscle in diseases classified elsewhere, right upper arm
M63.822 Disorders of muscle in diseases classified elsewhere, left upper arm
M63.829 Disorders of muscle in diseases classified elsewhere, unspecified upper arm

6th M63.83 Disorders of muscle in diseases classified elsewhere, forearm
M63.831 Disorders of muscle in diseases classified elsewhere, right forearm
M63.832 Disorders of muscle in diseases classified elsewhere, left forearm
M63.839 Disorders of muscle in diseases classified elsewhere, unspecified forearm

6th M63.84 Disorders of muscle in diseases classified elsewhere, hand
M63.841 Disorders of muscle in diseases classified elsewhere, right hand
M63.842 Disorders of muscle in diseases classified elsewhere, left hand
M63.849 Disorders of muscle in diseases classified elsewhere, unspecified hand

6th M63.85 Disorders of muscle in diseases classified elsewhere, thigh
M63.851 Disorders of muscle in diseases classified elsewhere, right thigh
M63.852 Disorders of muscle in diseases classified elsewhere, left thigh
M63.859 Disorders of muscle in diseases classified elsewhere, unspecified thigh

6th M63.86 Disorders of muscle in diseases classified elsewhere, lower leg
M63.861 Disorders of muscle in diseases classified elsewhere, right lower leg
M63.862 Disorders of muscle in diseases classified elsewhere, left lower leg
M63.869 Disorders of muscle in diseases classified elsewhere, unspecified lower leg

6th M63.87 Disorders of muscle in diseases classified elsewhere, ankle and foot
M63.871 Disorders of muscle in diseases classified elsewhere, right ankle and foot
M63.872 Disorders of muscle in diseases classified elsewhere, left ankle and foot
M63.879 Disorders of muscle in diseases classified elsewhere, unspecified ankle and foot

M63.88 Disorders of muscle in diseases classified elsewhere, other site

M63.89 Disorders of muscle in diseases classified elsewhere, multiple sites

Disorders of synovium and tendon (M65-M67)

4th M65 Synovitis and tenosynovitis
EXCLUDES 1 *chronic crepitant synovitis of hand and wrist (M70.0-)*
current injury—see injury of ligament or tendon by body region
soft tissue disorders related to use, overuse and pressure (M70.-)

5th M65.0 Abscess of tendon sheath
Use additional code (B95-B96) to identify bacterial agent.

M65.00 Abscess of tendon sheath, unspecified site

6th M65.01 Abscess of tendon sheath, shoulder
M65.011 Abscess of tendon sheath, right shoulder
M65.012 Abscess of tendon sheath, left shoulder
M65.019 Abscess of tendon sheath, unspecified shoulder

6th M65.02 Abscess of tendon sheath, upper arm
M65.021 Abscess of tendon sheath, right upper arm
M65.022 Abscess of tendon sheath, left upper arm
M65.029 Abscess of tendon sheath, unspecified upper arm

6th M65.03 Abscess of tendon sheath, forearm
M65.031 Abscess of tendon sheath, right forearm
M65.032 Abscess of tendon sheath, left forearm
M65.039 Abscess of tendon sheath, unspecified forearm

6th M65.04 Abscess of tendon sheath, hand
M65.041 Abscess of tendon sheath, right hand
M65.042 Abscess of tendon sheath, left hand
M65.049 Abscess of tendon sheath, unspecified hand

6th M65.05 Abscess of tendon sheath, thigh
M65.051 Abscess of tendon sheath, right thigh
M65.052 Abscess of tendon sheath, left thigh
M65.059 Abscess of tendon sheath, unspecified thigh

6th M65.06 Abscess of tendon sheath, lower leg
M65.061 Abscess of tendon sheath, right lower leg
M65.062 Abscess of tendon sheath, left lower leg
M65.069 Abscess of tendon sheath, unspecified lower leg

6th M65.07 Abscess of tendon sheath, ankle and foot
M65.071 Abscess of tendon sheath, right ankle and foot
M65.072 Abscess of tendon sheath, left ankle and foot
M65.079 Abscess of tendon sheath, unspecified ankle and foot

M65.08 Abscess of tendon sheath, other site

5th M65.1 Other infective (teno)synovitis
M65.10 Other infective (teno)synovitis, unspecified site

6th M65.11 Other infective (teno)synovitis, shoulder
M65.111 Other infective (teno)synovitis, right shoulder
M65.112 Other infective (teno)synovitis, left shoulder

M65.119 Other infective (teno)synovitis, unspecified shoulder
✓6th M65.12 Other infective (teno)synovitis, elbow
M65.121 Other infective (teno)synovitis, right elbow
M65.122 Other infective (teno)synovitis, left elbow
M65.129 Other infective (teno)synovitis, unspecified elbow
✓6th M65.13 Other infective (teno)synovitis, wrist
M65.131 Other infective (teno)synovitis, right wrist
M65.132 Other infective (teno)synovitis, left wrist
M65.139 Other infective (teno)synovitis, unspecified wrist
✓6th M65.14 Other infective (teno)synovitis, hand
M65.141 Other infective (teno)synovitis, right hand
M65.142 Other infective (teno)synovitis, left hand
M65.149 Other infective (teno)synovitis, unspecified hand
✓6th M65.15 Other infective (teno)synovitis, hip
M65.151 Other infective (teno)synovitis, right hip
M65.152 Other infective (teno)synovitis, left hip
M65.159 Other infective (teno)synovitis, unspecified hip
✓6th M65.16 Other infective (teno)synovitis, knee
M65.161 Other infective (teno)synovitis, right knee
M65.162 Other infective (teno)synovitis, left knee
M65.169 Other infective (teno)synovitis, unspecified knee
✓6th M65.17 Other infective (teno)synovitis, ankle and foot
M65.171 Other infective (teno)synovitis, right ankle and foot
M65.172 Other infective (teno)synovitis, left ankle and foot
M65.179 Other infective (teno)synovitis, unspecified ankle and foot
M65.18 Other infective (teno)synovitis, other site
M65.19 Other infective (teno)synovitis, multiple sites
✓5th M65.2 Calcific tendinitis
EXCLUDES1 *tendinitis as classified in M75-M77*
calcified tendinitis of shoulder (M75.3)
M65.20 Calcific tendinitis, unspecified site
✓6th M65.22 Calcific tendinitis, upper arm
M65.221 Calcific tendinitis, right upper arm
M65.222 Calcific tendinitis, left upper arm
M65.229 Calcific tendinitis, unspecified upper arm
✓6th M65.23 Calcific tendinitis, forearm
M65.231 Calcific tendinitis, right forearm
M65.232 Calcific tendinitis, left forearm
M65.239 Calcific tendinitis, unspecified forearm
✓6th M65.24 Calcific tendinitis, hand
M65.241 Calcific tendinitis, right hand
M65.242 Calcific tendinitis, left hand
M65.249 Calcific tendinitis, unspecified hand
✓6th M65.25 Calcific tendinitis, thigh
M65.251 Calcific tendinitis, right thigh
M65.252 Calcific tendinitis, left thigh
M65.259 Calcific tendinitis, unspecified thigh
✓6th M65.26 Calcific tendinitis, lower leg
M65.261 Calcific tendinitis, right lower leg
M65.262 Calcific tendinitis, left lower leg
M65.269 Calcific tendinitis, unspecified lower leg
✓6th M65.27 Calcific tendinitis, ankle and foot
M65.271 Calcific tendinitis, right ankle and foot
M65.272 Calcific tendinitis, left ankle and foot
M65.279 Calcific tendinitis, unspecified ankle and foot
M65.28 Calcific tendinitis, other site
M65.29 Calcific tendinitis, multiple sites
M65.3 Trigger finger
Nodular tendinous disease
M65.30 Trigger finger, unspecified finger
✓6th M65.31 Trigger thumb
M65.311 Trigger thumb, right thumb
M65.312 Trigger thumb, left thumb
M65.319 Trigger thumb, unspecified thumb
✓6th M65.32 Trigger finger, index finger
M65.321 Trigger finger, right index finger
M65.322 Trigger finger, left index finger
M65.329 Trigger finger, unspecified index finger
✓6th M65.33 Trigger finger, middle finger
M65.331 Trigger finger, right middle finger
M65.332 Trigger finger, left middle finger
M65.339 Trigger finger, unspecified middle finger
✓6th M65.34 Trigger finger, ring finger
M65.341 Trigger finger, right ring finger
M65.342 Trigger finger, left ring finger
M65.349 Trigger finger, unspecified ring finger
✓6th M65.35 Trigger finger, little finger
M65.351 Trigger finger, right little finger
M65.352 Trigger finger, left little finger
M65.359 Trigger finger, unspecified little finger
M65.4 Radial styloid tenosynovitis [de Quervain]
✓5th M65.8 Other synovitis and tenosynovitis
M65.80 Other synovitis and tenosynovitis, unspecified site
✓6th M65.81 Other synovitis and tenosynovitis, shoulder
M65.811 Other synovitis and tenosynovitis, right shoulder
M65.812 Other synovitis and tenosynovitis, left shoulder
M65.819 Other synovitis and tenosynovitis, unspecified shoulder
✓6th M65.82 Other synovitis and tenosynovitis, upper arm
M65.821 Other synovitis and tenosynovitis, right upper arm
M65.822 Other synovitis and tenosynovitis, left upper arm
M65.829 Other synovitis and tenosynovitis, unspecified upper arm
✓6th M65.83 Other synovitis and tenosynovitis, forearm
M65.831 Other synovitis and tenosynovitis, right forearm
M65.832 Other synovitis and tenosynovitis, left forearm
M65.839 Other synovitis and tenosynovitis, unspecified forearm
✓6th M65.84 Other synovitis and tenosynovitis, hand
M65.841 Other synovitis and tenosynovitis, right hand
M65.842 Other synovitis and tenosynovitis, left hand
M65.849 Other synovitis and tenosynovitis, unspecified hand
✓6th M65.85 Other synovitis and tenosynovitis, thigh
M65.851 Other synovitis and tenosynovitis, right thigh
M65.852 Other synovitis and tenosynovitis, left thigh
M65.859 Other synovitis and tenosynovitis, unspecified thigh
✓6th M65.86 Other synovitis and tenosynovitis, lower leg
M65.861 Other synovitis and tenosynovitis, right lower leg
M65.862 Other synovitis and tenosynovitis, left lower leg
M65.869 Other synovitis and tenosynovitis, unspecified lower leg
✓6th M65.87 Other synovitis and tenosynovitis, ankle and foot
M65.871 Other synovitis and tenosynovitis, right ankle and foot
M65.872 Other synovitis and tenosynovitis, left ankle and foot
M65.879 Other synovitis and tenosynovitis, unspecified ankle and foot
M65.88 Other synovitis and tenosynovitis, other site
M65.89 Other synovitis and tenosynovitis, multiple sites
M65.9 Synovitis and tenosynovitis, unspecified

✓4th M66 Spontaneous rupture of synovium and tendon

INCLUDES rupture that occurs when a normal force is applied to tissues that are inferred to have less than normal strength

EXCLUDES 2 *rotator cuff syndrome (M75.1-)*
rupture where an abnormal force is applied to normal tissue—see injury of tendon by body region

M66.0 Rupture of popliteal cyst

✓5th M66.1 Rupture of synovium
Rupture of synovial cyst
EXCLUDES 2 *rupture of popliteal cyst (M66.0)*

M66.10 Rupture of synovium, unspecified joint

✓6th M66.11 Rupture of synovium, shoulder
- **M66.111 Rupture of synovium, right shoulder**
- **M66.112 Rupture of synovium, left shoulder**
- **M66.119 Rupture of synovium, unspecified shoulder**

✓6th M66.12 Rupture of synovium, elbow
- **M66.121 Rupture of synovium, right elbow**
- **M66.122 Rupture of synovium, left elbow**
- **M66.129 Rupture of synovium, unspecified elbow**

✓6th M66.13 Rupture of synovium, wrist
- **M66.131 Rupture of synovium, right wrist**
- **M66.132 Rupture of synovium, left wrist**
- **M66.139 Rupture of synovium, unspecified wrist**

✓6th M66.14 Rupture of synovium, hand and fingers
- **M66.141 Rupture of synovium, right hand**
- **M66.142 Rupture of synovium, left hand**
- **M66.143 Rupture of synovium, unspecified hand**
- **M66.144 Rupture of synovium, right finger(s)**
- **M66.145 Rupture of synovium, left finger(s)**
- **M66.146 Rupture of synovium, unspecified finger(s)**

✓6th M66.15 Rupture of synovium, hip
- **M66.151 Rupture of synovium, right hip**
- **M66.152 Rupture of synovium, left hip**
- **M66.159 Rupture of synovium, unspecified hip**

✓6th M66.17 Rupture of synovium, ankle, foot and toes
- **M66.171 Rupture of synovium, right ankle**
- **M66.172 Rupture of synovium, left ankle**
- **M66.173 Rupture of synovium, unspecified ankle**
- **M66.174 Rupture of synovium, right foot**
- **M66.175 Rupture of synovium, left foot**
- **M66.176 Rupture of synovium, unspecified foot**
- **M66.177 Rupture of synovium, right toe(s)**
- **M66.178 Rupture of synovium, left toe(s)**
- **M66.179 Rupture of synovium, unspecified toe(s)**

M66.18 Rupture of synovium, other site

✓5th M66.2 Spontaneous rupture of extensor tendons

M66.20 Spontaneous rupture of extensor tendons, unspecified site

✓6th M66.21 Spontaneous rupture of extensor tendons, shoulder
- **M66.211 Spontaneous rupture of extensor tendons, right shoulder**
- **M66.212 Spontaneous rupture of extensor tendons, left shoulder**
- **M66.219 Spontaneous rupture of extensor tendons, unspecified shoulder**

✓6th M66.22 Spontaneous rupture of extensor tendons, upper arm
- **M66.221 Spontaneous rupture of extensor tendons, right upper arm**
- **M66.222 Spontaneous rupture of extensor tendons, left upper arm**
- **M66.229 Spontaneous rupture of extensor tendons, unspecified upper arm**

✓6th M66.23 Spontaneous rupture of extensor tendons, forearm
- **M66.231 Spontaneous rupture of extensor tendons, right forearm**
- **M66.232 Spontaneous rupture of extensor tendons, left forearm**
- **M66.239 Spontaneous rupture of extensor tendons, unspecified forearm**

✓6th M66.24 Spontaneous rupture of extensor tendons, hand
- **M66.241 Spontaneous rupture of extensor tendons, right hand**
- **M66.242 Spontaneous rupture of extensor tendons, left hand**
- **M66.249 Spontaneous rupture of extensor tendons, unspecified hand**

✓6th M66.25 Spontaneous rupture of extensor tendons, thigh
- **M66.251 Spontaneous rupture of extensor tendons, right thigh**
- **M66.252 Spontaneous rupture of extensor tendons, left thigh**
- **M66.259 Spontaneous rupture of extensor tendons, unspecified thigh**

✓6th M66.26 Spontaneous rupture of extensor tendons, lower leg
- **M66.261 Spontaneous rupture of extensor tendons, right lower leg**
- **M66.262 Spontaneous rupture of extensor tendons, left lower leg**
- **M66.269 Spontaneous rupture of extensor tendons, unspecified lower leg**

✓6th M66.27 Spontaneous rupture of extensor tendons, ankle and foot
- **M66.271 Spontaneous rupture of extensor tendons, right ankle and foot**
- **M66.272 Spontaneous rupture of extensor tendons, left ankle and foot**
- **M66.279 Spontaneous rupture of extensor tendons, unspecified ankle and foot**

M66.28 Spontaneous rupture of extensor tendons, other site

M66.29 Spontaneous rupture of extensor tendons, multiple sites

✓5th M66.3 Spontaneous rupture of flexor tendons

M66.30 Spontaneous rupture of flexor tendons, unspecified site

✓6th M66.31 Spontaneous rupture of flexor tendons, shoulder
- **M66.311 Spontaneous rupture of flexor tendons, right shoulder**
- **M66.312 Spontaneous rupture of flexor tendons, left shoulder**
- **M66.319 Spontaneous rupture of flexor tendons, unspecified shoulder**

✓6th M66.32 Spontaneous rupture of flexor tendons, upper arm
- **M66.321 Spontaneous rupture of flexor tendons, right upper arm**
- **M66.322 Spontaneous rupture of flexor tendons, left upper arm**
- **M66.329 Spontaneous rupture of flexor tendons, unspecified upper arm**

✓6th M66.33 Spontaneous rupture of flexor tendons, forearm
- **M66.331 Spontaneous rupture of flexor tendons, right forearm**
- **M66.332 Spontaneous rupture of flexor tendons, left forearm**
- **M66.339 Spontaneous rupture of flexor tendons, unspecified forearm**

✓6th M66.34 Spontaneous rupture of flexor tendons, hand
- **M66.341 Spontaneous rupture of flexor tendons, right hand**
- **M66.342 Spontaneous rupture of flexor tendons, left hand**
- **M66.349 Spontaneous rupture of flexor tendons, unspecified hand**

✓6th M66.35 Spontaneous rupture of flexor tendons, thigh
- **M66.351 Spontaneous rupture of flexor tendons, right thigh**
- **M66.352 Spontaneous rupture of flexor tendons, left thigh**
- **M66.359 Spontaneous rupture of flexor tendons, unspecified thigh**

✓6th M66.36 Spontaneous rupture of flexor tendons, lower leg
- **M66.361 Spontaneous rupture of flexor tendons, right lower leg**
- **M66.362 Spontaneous rupture of flexor tendons, left lower leg**
- **M66.369 Spontaneous rupture of flexor tendons, unspecified lower leg**

6th **M66.37 Spontaneous rupture of flexor tendons, ankle and foot**
M66.371 Spontaneous rupture of flexor tendons, right ankle and foot
M66.372 Spontaneous rupture of flexor tendons, left ankle and foot
M66.379 Spontaneous rupture of flexor tendons, unspecified ankle and foot
M66.38 Spontaneous rupture of flexor tendons, other site
M66.39 Spontaneous rupture of flexor tendons, multiple sites

5th **M66.8 Spontaneous rupture of other tendons**
M66.80 Spontaneous rupture of other tendons, unspecified site
6th **M66.81 Spontaneous rupture of other tendons, shoulder**
M66.811 Spontaneous rupture of other tendons, right shoulder
M66.812 Spontaneous rupture of other tendons, left shoulder
M66.819 Spontaneous rupture of other tendons, unspecified shoulder
6th **M66.82 Spontaneous rupture of other tendons, upper arm**
M66.821 Spontaneous rupture of other tendons, right upper arm
M66.822 Spontaneous rupture of other tendons, left upper arm
M66.829 Spontaneous rupture of other tendons, unspecified upper arm
6th **M66.83 Spontaneous rupture of other tendons, forearm**
M66.831 Spontaneous rupture of other tendons, right forearm
M66.832 Spontaneous rupture of other tendons, left forearm
M66.839 Spontaneous rupture of other tendons, unspecified forearm
6th **M66.84 Spontaneous rupture of other tendons, hand**
M66.841 Spontaneous rupture of other tendons, right hand
M66.842 Spontaneous rupture of other tendons, left hand
M66.849 Spontaneous rupture of other tendons, unspecified hand
6th **M66.85 Spontaneous rupture of other tendons, thigh**
M66.851 Spontaneous rupture of other tendons, right thigh
M66.852 Spontaneous rupture of other tendons, left thigh
M66.859 Spontaneous rupture of other tendons, unspecified thigh
6th **M66.86 Spontaneous rupture of other tendons, lower leg**
M66.861 Spontaneous rupture of other tendons, right lower leg
M66.862 Spontaneous rupture of other tendons, left lower leg
M66.869 Spontaneous rupture of other tendons, unspecified lower leg
6th **M66.87 Spontaneous rupture of other tendons, ankle and foot**
M66.871 Spontaneous rupture of other tendons, right ankle and foot
M66.872 Spontaneous rupture of other tendons, left ankle and foot
M66.879 Spontaneous rupture of other tendons, unspecified ankle and foot
M66.88 Spontaneous rupture of other tendons, other
M66.89 Spontaneous rupture of other tendons, multiple sites

M66.9 Spontaneous rupture of unspecified tendon
Rupture at musculotendinous junction, nontraumatic

4th **M67 Other disorders of synovium and tendon**
EXCLUDES 1 *palmar fascial fibromatosis [Dupuytren] (M72.0)*
tendinitis NOS (M77.9-)
xanthomatosis localized to tendons (E78.2)

5th **M67.0 Short Achilles tendon (acquired)**
M67.00 Short Achilles tendon (acquired), unspecified ankle
M67.01 Short Achilles tendon (acquired), right ankle
M67.02 Short Achilles tendon (acquired), left ankle

5th **M67.2 Synovial hypertrophy, not elsewhere classified**
EXCLUDES 1 *villonodular synovitis (pigmented) (M12.2-)*
M67.20 Synovial hypertrophy, not elsewhere classified, unspecified site
6th **M67.21 Synovial hypertrophy, not elsewhere classified, shoulder**
M67.211 Synovial hypertrophy, not elsewhere classified, right shoulder
M67.212 Synovial hypertrophy, not elsewhere classified, left shoulder
M67.219 Synovial hypertrophy, not elsewhere classified, unspecified shoulder
6th **M67.22 Synovial hypertrophy, not elsewhere classified, upper arm**
M67.221 Synovial hypertrophy, not elsewhere classified, right upper arm
M67.222 Synovial hypertrophy, not elsewhere classified, left upper arm
M67.229 Synovial hypertrophy, not elsewhere classified, unspecified upper arm
6th **M67.23 Synovial hypertrophy, not elsewhere classified, forearm**
M67.231 Synovial hypertrophy, not elsewhere classified, right forearm
M67.232 Synovial hypertrophy, not elsewhere classified, left forearm
M67.239 Synovial hypertrophy, not elsewhere classified, unspecified forearm
6th **M67.24 Synovial hypertrophy, not elsewhere classified, hand**
M67.241 Synovial hypertrophy, not elsewhere classified, right hand
M67.242 Synovial hypertrophy, not elsewhere classified, left hand
M67.249 Synovial hypertrophy, not elsewhere classified, unspecified hand
6th **M67.25 Synovial hypertrophy, not elsewhere classified, thigh**
M67.251 Synovial hypertrophy, not elsewhere classified, right thigh
M67.252 Synovial hypertrophy, not elsewhere classified, left thigh
M67.259 Synovial hypertrophy, not elsewhere classified, unspecified thigh
6th **M67.26 Synovial hypertrophy, not elsewhere classified, lower leg**
M67.261 Synovial hypertrophy, not elsewhere classified, right lower leg
M67.262 Synovial hypertrophy, not elsewhere classified, left lower leg
M67.269 Synovial hypertrophy, not elsewhere classified, unspecified lower leg
6th **M67.27 Synovial hypertrophy, not elsewhere classified, ankle and foot**
M67.271 Synovial hypertrophy, not elsewhere classified, right ankle and foot
M67.272 Synovial hypertrophy, not elsewhere classified, left ankle and foot
M67.279 Synovial hypertrophy, not elsewhere classified, unspecified ankle and foot
M67.28 Synovial hypertrophy, not elsewhere classified, other site
M67.29 Synovial hypertrophy, not elsewhere classified, multiple sites

5th **M67.3 Transient synovitis**
Toxic synovitis
EXCLUDES 1 *palindromic rheumatism (M12.3-)*
M67.30 Transient synovitis, unspecified site
6th **M67.31 Transient synovitis, shoulder**
M67.311 Transient synovitis, right shoulder
M67.312 Transient synovitis, left shoulder
M67.319 Transient synovitis, unspecified shoulder
6th **M67.32 Transient synovitis, elbow**
M67.321 Transient synovitis, right elbow
M67.322 Transient synovitis, left elbow
M67.329 Transient synovitis, unspecified elbow

✓6th **M67.33 Transient synovitis, wrist**
- **M67.331 Transient synovitis, right wrist**
- **M67.332 Transient synovitis, left wrist**
- **M67.339 Transient synovitis, unspecified wrist**

✓6th **M67.34 Transient synovitis, hand**
- **M67.341 Transient synovitis, right hand**
- **M67.342 Transient synovitis, left hand**
- **M67.349 Transient synovitis, unspecified hand**

✓6th **M67.35 Transient synovitis, hip**
- **M67.351 Transient synovitis, right hip**
- **M67.352 Transient synovitis, left hip**
- **M67.359 Transient synovitis, unspecified hip**

✓6th **M67.36 Transient synovitis, knee**
- **M67.361 Transient synovitis, right knee**
- **M67.362 Transient synovitis, left knee**
- **M67.369 Transient synovitis, unspecified knee**

✓6th **M67.37 Transient synovitis, ankle and foot**
- **M67.371 Transient synovitis, right ankle and foot**
- **M67.372 Transient synovitis, left ankle and foot**
- **M67.379 Transient synovitis, unspecified ankle and foot**

M67.38 Transient synovitis, other site

M67.39 Transient synovitis, multiple sites

✓5th **M67.4 Ganglion**

Ganglion of joint or tendon (sheath)

EXCLUDES 1 *ganglion in yaws (A66.6)*

EXCLUDES 2 *cyst of bursa (M71.2-M71.3)*
cyst of synovium (M71.2-M71.3)

M67.40 Ganglion, unspecified site

✓6th **M67.41 Ganglion, shoulder**
- **M67.411 Ganglion, right shoulder**
- **M67.412 Ganglion, left shoulder**
- **M67.419 Ganglion, unspecified shoulder**

✓6th **M67.42 Ganglion, elbow**
- **M67.421 Ganglion, right elbow**
- **M67.422 Ganglion, left elbow**
- **M67.429 Ganglion, unspecified elbow**

✓6th **M67.43 Ganglion, wrist**
- **M67.431 Ganglion, right wrist**
- **M67.432 Ganglion, left wrist**
- **M67.439 Ganglion, unspecified wrist**

✓6th **M67.44 Ganglion, hand**
- **M67.441 Ganglion, right hand**
- **M67.442 Ganglion, left hand**
- **M67.449 Ganglion, unspecified hand**

✓6th **M67.45 Ganglion, hip**
- **M67.451 Ganglion, right hip**
- **M67.452 Ganglion, left hip**
- **M67.459 Ganglion, unspecified hip**

✓6th **M67.46 Ganglion, knee**
- **M67.461 Ganglion, right knee**
- **M67.462 Ganglion, left knee**
- **M67.469 Ganglion, unspecified knee**

✓6th **M67.47 Ganglion, ankle and foot**
- **M67.471 Ganglion, right ankle and foot**
- **M67.472 Ganglion, left ankle and foot**
- **M67.479 Ganglion, unspecified ankle and foot**

M67.48 Ganglion, other site

M67.49 Ganglion, multiple sites

✓5th **M67.5 Plica syndrome**

Plica knee

M67.50 Plica syndrome, unspecified knee

M67.51 Plica syndrome, right knee

M67.52 Plica syndrome, left knee

✓5th **M67.8 Other specified disorders of synovium and tendon**

M67.80 Other specified disorders of synovium and tendon, unspecified site

✓6th **M67.81 Other specified disorders of synovium and tendon, shoulder**
- **M67.811 Other specified disorders of synovium, right shoulder**
- **M67.812 Other specified disorders of synovium, left shoulder**
- **M67.813 Other specified disorders of tendon, right shoulder**
- **M67.814 Other specified disorders of tendon, left shoulder**
- **M67.819 Other specified disorders of synovium and tendon, unspecified shoulder**

✓6th **M67.82 Other specified disorders of synovium and tendon, elbow**
- **M67.821 Other specified disorders of synovium, right elbow**
- **M67.822 Other specified disorders of synovium, left elbow**
- **M67.823 Other specified disorders of tendon, right elbow**
- **M67.824 Other specified disorders of tendon, left elbow**
- **M67.829 Other specified disorders of synovium and tendon, unspecified elbow**

✓6th **M67.83 Other specified disorders of synovium and tendon, wrist**
- **M67.831 Other specified disorders of synovium, right wrist**
- **M67.832 Other specified disorders of synovium, left wrist**
- **M67.833 Other specified disorders of tendon, right wrist**
- **M67.834 Other specified disorders of tendon, left wrist**
- **M67.839 Other specified disorders of synovium and tendon, unspecified forearm**

✓6th **M67.84 Other specified disorders of synovium and tendon, hand**
- **M67.841 Other specified disorders of synovium, right hand**
- **M67.842 Other specified disorders of synovium, left hand**
- **M67.843 Other specified disorders of tendon, right hand**
- **M67.844 Other specified disorders of tendon, left hand**
- **M67.849 Other specified disorders of synovium and tendon, unspecified hand**

✓6th **M67.85 Other specified disorders of synovium and tendon, hip**
- **M67.851 Other specified disorders of synovium, right hip**
- **M67.852 Other specified disorders of synovium, left hip**
- **M67.853 Other specified disorders of tendon, right hip**
- **M67.854 Other specified disorders of tendon, left hip**
- **M67.859 Other specified disorders of synovium and tendon, unspecified hip**

✓6th **M67.86 Other specified disorders of synovium and tendon, knee**
- **M67.861 Other specified disorders of synovium, right knee**
- **M67.862 Other specified disorders of synovium, left knee**
- **M67.863 Other specified disorders of tendon, right knee**
- **M67.864 Other specified disorders of tendon, left knee**
- **M67.869 Other specified disorders of synovium and tendon, unspecified knee**

✓6th **M67.87 Other specified disorders of synovium and tendon, ankle and foot**
- **M67.871 Other specified disorders of synovium, right ankle and foot**
- **M67.872 Other specified disorders of synovium, left ankle and foot**
- **M67.873 Other specified disorders of tendon, right ankle and foot**
- **M67.874 Other specified disorders of tendon, left ankle and foot**

M67.879 Other specified disorders of synovium and tendon, unspecified ankle and foot
M67.88 Other specified disorders of synovium and tendon, other site
M67.89 Other specified disorders of synovium and tendon, multiple sites
✓5th M67.9 Unspecified disorder of synovium and tendon
M67.90 Unspecified disorder of synovium and tendon, unspecified site
✓6th M67.91 Unspecified disorder of synovium and tendon, shoulder
M67.911 Unspecified disorder of synovium and tendon, right shoulder
M67.912 Unspecified disorder of synovium and tendon, left shoulder
M67.919 Unspecified disorder of synovium and tendon, unspecified shoulder
✓6th M67.92 Unspecified disorder of synovium and tendon, upper arm
M67.921 Unspecified disorder of synovium and tendon, right upper arm
M67.922 Unspecified disorder of synovium and tendon, left upper arm
M67.929 Unspecified disorder of synovium and tendon, unspecified upper arm
✓6th M67.93 Unspecified disorder of synovium and tendon, forearm
M67.931 Unspecified disorder of synovium and tendon, right forearm
M67.932 Unspecified disorder of synovium and tendon, left forearm
M67.939 Unspecified disorder of synovium and tendon, unspecified forearm
✓6th M67.94 Unspecified disorder of synovium and tendon, hand
M67.941 Unspecified disorder of synovium and tendon, right hand
M67.942 Unspecified disorder of synovium and tendon, left hand
M67.949 Unspecified disorder of synovium and tendon, unspecified hand
✓6th M67.95 Unspecified disorder of synovium and tendon, thigh
M67.951 Unspecified disorder of synovium and tendon, right thigh
M67.952 Unspecified disorder of synovium and tendon, left thigh
M67.959 Unspecified disorder of synovium and tendon, unspecified thigh
✓6th M67.96 Unspecified disorder of synovium and tendon, lower leg
M67.961 Unspecified disorder of synovium and tendon, right lower leg
M67.962 Unspecified disorder of synovium and tendon, left lower leg
M67.969 Unspecified disorder of synovium and tendon, unspecified lower leg
✓6th M67.97 Unspecified disorder of synovium and tendon, ankle and foot
M67.971 Unspecified disorder of synovium and tendon, right ankle and foot
M67.972 Unspecified disorder of synovium and tendon, left ankle and foot
M67.979 Unspecified disorder of synovium and tendon, unspecified ankle and foot
M67.98 Unspecified disorder of synovium and tendon, other site
M67.99 Unspecified disorder of synovium and tendon, multiple sites

Other soft tissue disorders (M70-M79)

✓4th **M70 Soft tissue disorders related to use, overuse and pressure**
INCLUDES soft tissue disorders of occupational origin
Use additional external cause code to identify activity causing disorder (Y93.-)
EXCLUDES 1 *bursitis NOS (M71.9-)*
EXCLUDES 2 *bursitis of shoulder (M75.5)*
enthesopathies (M76-M77)
pressure ulcer (pressure area) (L89.-)

✓5th M70.0 Crepitant synovitis (acute) (chronic) of hand and wrist
✓6th M70.03 Crepitant synovitis (acute) (chronic), wrist
M70.031 Crepitant synovitis (acute) (chronic), right wrist
M70.032 Crepitant synovitis (acute) (chronic), left wrist
M70.039 Crepitant synovitis (acute) (chronic), unspecified wrist
✓6th M70.04 Crepitant synovitis (acute) (chronic), hand
M70.041 Crepitant synovitis (acute) (chronic), right hand
M70.042 Crepitant synovitis (acute) (chronic), left hand
M70.049 Crepitant synovitis (acute) (chronic), unspecified hand
✓5th M70.1 Bursitis of hand
M70.10 Bursitis, unspecified hand
M70.11 Bursitis, right hand
M70.12 Bursitis, left hand
✓5th M70.2 Olecranon bursitis
M70.20 Olecranon bursitis, unspecified elbow
M70.21 Olecranon bursitis, right elbow
M70.22 Olecranon bursitis, left elbow
✓5th M70.3 Other bursitis of elbow
M70.30 Other bursitis of elbow, unspecified elbow
M70.31 Other bursitis of elbow, right elbow
M70.32 Other bursitis of elbow, left elbow
✓5th M70.4 Prepatellar bursitis
M70.40 Prepatellar bursitis, unspecified knee
M70.41 Prepatellar bursitis, right knee
M70.42 Prepatellar bursitis, left knee
✓5th M70.5 Other bursitis of knee
M70.50 Other bursitis of knee, unspecified knee
M70.51 Other bursitis of knee, right knee
M70.52 Other bursitis of knee, left knee
✓5th M70.6 Trochanteric bursitis
Trochanteric tendinitis
M70.60 Trochanteric bursitis, unspecified hip
M70.61 Trochanteric bursitis, right hip
M70.62 Trochanteric bursitis, left hip
✓5th M70.7 Other bursitis of hip
Ischial bursitis
M70.70 Other bursitis of hip, unspecified hip
M70.71 Other bursitis of hip, right hip
M70.72 Other bursitis of hip, left hip
✓5th M70.8 Other soft tissue disorders related to use, overuse and pressure
M70.80 Other soft tissue disorders related to use, overuse and pressure of unspecified site
✓6th M70.81 Other soft tissue disorders related to use, overuse and pressure of shoulder
M70.811 Other soft tissue disorders related to use, overuse and pressure, right shoulder
M70.812 Other soft tissue disorders related to use, overuse and pressure, left shoulder
M70.819 Other soft tissue disorders related to use, overuse and pressure, unspecified shoulder
✓6th M70.82 Other soft tissue disorders related to use, overuse and pressure of upper arm
M70.821 Other soft tissue disorders related to use, overuse and pressure, right upper arm
M70.822 Other soft tissue disorders related to use, overuse and pressure, left upper arm
M70.829 Other soft tissue disorders related to use, overuse and pressure, unspecified upper arms
✓6th M70.83 Other soft tissue disorders related to use, overuse and pressure of forearm
M70.831 Other soft tissue disorders related to use, overuse and pressure, right forearm
M70.832 Other soft tissue disorders related to use, overuse and pressure, left forearm

M7Ø.839 Other soft tissue disorders related to use, overuse and pressure, unspecified forearm

✓6th **M7Ø.84** Other soft tissue disorders related to use, overuse and pressure of hand

M7Ø.841 Other soft tissue disorders related to use, overuse and pressure, right hand

M7Ø.842 Other soft tissue disorders related to use, overuse and pressure, left hand

M7Ø.849 Other soft tissue disorders related to use, overuse and pressure, unspecified hand

✓6th **M7Ø.85** Other soft tissue disorders related to use, overuse and pressure of thigh

M7Ø.851 Other soft tissue disorders related to use, overuse and pressure, right thigh

M7Ø.852 Other soft tissue disorders related to use, overuse and pressure, left thigh

M7Ø.859 Other soft tissue disorders related to use, overuse and pressure, unspecified thigh

✓6th **M7Ø.86** Other soft tissue disorders related to use, overuse and pressure lower leg

M7Ø.861 Other soft tissue disorders related to use, overuse and pressure, right lower leg

M7Ø.862 Other soft tissue disorders related to use, overuse and pressure, left lower leg

M7Ø.869 Other soft tissue disorders related to use, overuse and pressure, unspecified leg

✓6th **M7Ø.87** Other soft tissue disorders related to use, overuse and pressure of ankle and foot

M7Ø.871 Other soft tissue disorders related to use, overuse and pressure, right ankle and foot

M7Ø.872 Other soft tissue disorders related to use, overuse and pressure, left ankle and foot

M7Ø.879 Other soft tissue disorders related to use, overuse and pressure, unspecified ankle and foot

M7Ø.88 Other soft tissue disorders related to use, overuse and pressure other site

M7Ø.89 Other soft tissue disorders related to use, overuse and pressure multiple sites

✓5th **M7Ø.9** Unspecified soft tissue disorder related to use, overuse and pressure

M7Ø.9Ø Unspecified soft tissue disorder related to use, overuse and pressure of unspecified site

✓6th **M7Ø.91** Unspecified soft tissue disorder related to use, overuse and pressure of shoulder

M7Ø.911 Unspecified soft tissue disorder related to use, overuse and pressure, right shoulder

M7Ø.912 Unspecified soft tissue disorder related to use, overuse and pressure, left shoulder

M7Ø.919 Unspecified soft tissue disorder related to use, overuse and pressure, unspecified shoulder

✓6th **M7Ø.92** Unspecified soft tissue disorder related to use, overuse and pressure of upper arm

M7Ø.921 Unspecified soft tissue disorder related to use, overuse and pressure, right upper arm

M7Ø.922 Unspecified soft tissue disorder related to use, overuse and pressure, left upper arm

M7Ø.929 Unspecified soft tissue disorder related to use, overuse and pressure, unspecified upper arm

✓6th **M7Ø.93** Unspecified soft tissue disorder related to use, overuse and pressure of forearm

M7Ø.931 Unspecified soft tissue disorder related to use, overuse and pressure, right forearm

M7Ø.932 Unspecified soft tissue disorder related to use, overuse and pressure, left forearm

M7Ø.939 Unspecified soft tissue disorder related to use, overuse and pressure, unspecified forearm

✓6th **M7Ø.94** Unspecified soft tissue disorder related to use, overuse and pressure of hand

M7Ø.941 Unspecified soft tissue disorder related to use, overuse and pressure, right hand

M7Ø.942 Unspecified soft tissue disorder related to use, overuse and pressure, left hand

M7Ø.949 Unspecified soft tissue disorder related to use, overuse and pressure, unspecified hand

✓6th **M7Ø.95** Unspecified soft tissue disorder related to use, overuse and pressure of thigh

M7Ø.951 Unspecified soft tissue disorder related to use, overuse and pressure, right thigh

M7Ø.952 Unspecified soft tissue disorder related to use, overuse and pressure, left thigh

M7Ø.959 Unspecified soft tissue disorder related to use, overuse and pressure, unspecified thigh

✓6th **M7Ø.96** Unspecified soft tissue disorder related to use, overuse and pressure lower leg

M7Ø.961 Unspecified soft tissue disorder related to use, overuse and pressure, right lower leg

M7Ø.962 Unspecified soft tissue disorder related to use, overuse and pressure, left lower leg

M7Ø.969 Unspecified soft tissue disorder related to use, overuse and pressure, unspecified lower leg

✓6th **M7Ø.97** Unspecified soft tissue disorder related to use, overuse and pressure of ankle and foot

M7Ø.971 Unspecified soft tissue disorder related to use, overuse and pressure, right ankle and foot

M7Ø.972 Unspecified soft tissue disorder related to use, overuse and pressure, left ankle and foot

M7Ø.979 Unspecified soft tissue disorder related to use, overuse and pressure, unspecified ankle and foot

M7Ø.98 Unspecified soft tissue disorder related to use, overuse and pressure other

M7Ø.99 Unspecified soft tissue disorder related to use, overuse and pressure multiple sites

✓4th **M71 Other bursopathies**

EXCLUDES 1 *bunion (M2Ø.1)*
bursitis related to use, overuse or pressure (M7Ø.-)
enthesopathies (M76-M77)

✓5th **M71.Ø** Abscess of bursa

Use additional code (B95.-, B96.-) to identify causative organism

M71.ØØ Abscess of bursa, unspecified site

✓6th **M71.Ø1** Abscess of bursa, shoulder

M71.Ø11 Abscess of bursa, right shoulder

M71.Ø12 Abscess of bursa, left shoulder

M71.Ø19 Abscess of bursa, unspecified shoulder

✓6th **M71.Ø2** Abscess of bursa, elbow

M71.Ø21 Abscess of bursa, right elbow

M71.Ø22 Abscess of bursa, left elbow

M71.Ø29 Abscess of bursa, unspecified elbow

✓6th **M71.Ø3** Abscess of bursa, wrist

M71.Ø31 Abscess of bursa, right wrist

M71.Ø32 Abscess of bursa, left wrist

M71.Ø39 Abscess of bursa, unspecified wrist

✓6th **M71.Ø4** Abscess of bursa, hand

M71.Ø41 Abscess of bursa, right hand

M71.Ø42 Abscess of bursa, left hand

M71.Ø49 Abscess of bursa, unspecified hand

✓6th **M71.Ø5** Abscess of bursa, hip

M71.Ø51 Abscess of bursa, right hip

M71.Ø52 Abscess of bursa, left hip

M71.Ø59 Abscess of bursa, unspecified hip

✓6th **M71.Ø6** Abscess of bursa, knee

M71.Ø61 Abscess of bursa, right knee

M71.Ø62 Abscess of bursa, left knee

M71.Ø69 Abscess of bursa, unspecified knee

✓6th **M71.Ø7** Abscess of bursa, ankle and foot

M71.Ø71 Abscess of bursa, right ankle and foot

M71.Ø72 Abscess of bursa, left ankle and foot

M71.Ø79 Abscess of bursa, unspecified ankle and foot

M71.Ø8 Abscess of bursa, other site

M71.Ø9 Abscess of bursa, multiple sites

✓5th **M71.1 Other infective bursitis**
Use additional code (B95.-, B96.-) to identify causative organism
M71.10 Other infective bursitis, unspecified site
✓6th **M71.11 Other infective bursitis,** shoulder
M71.111 Other infective bursitis, right **shoulder**
M71.112 Other infective bursitis, left **shoulder**
M71.119 Other infective bursitis, unspecified **shoulder**
✓6th **M71.12 Other infective bursitis,** elbow
M71.121 Other infective bursitis, right **elbow**
M71.122 Other infective bursitis, left **elbow**
M71.129 Other infective bursitis, unspecified **elbow**
✓6th **M71.13 Other infective bursitis,** wrist
M71.131 Other infective bursitis, right **wrist**
M71.132 Other infective bursitis, left **wrist**
M71.139 Other infective bursitis, unspecified **wrist**
✓6th **M71.14 Other infective bursitis,** hand
M71.141 Other infective bursitis, right **hand**
M71.142 Other infective bursitis, left **hand**
M71.149 Other infective bursitis, unspecified **hand**
✓6th **M71.15 Other infective bursitis,** hip
M71.151 Other infective bursitis, right **hip**
M71.152 Other infective bursitis, left **hip**
M71.159 Other infective bursitis, unspecified **hip**
✓6th **M71.16 Other infective bursitis,** knee
M71.161 Other infective bursitis, right **knee**
M71.162 Other infective bursitis, left **knee**
M71.169 Other infective bursitis, unspecified **knee**
✓6th **M71.17 Other infective bursitis,** ankle and foot
M71.171 Other infective bursitis, right **ankle and foot**
M71.172 Other infective bursitis, left **ankle and foot**
M71.179 Other infective bursitis, unspecified **ankle and foot**
M71.18 Other infective bursitis, other site
M71.19 Other infective bursitis, multiple sites

✓5th **M71.2 Synovial cyst of popliteal space [Baker]**
EXCLUDES 1 *synovial cyst of popliteal space with rupture (M66.0)*
M71.20 Synovial cyst of popliteal space [Baker], unspecified **knee**
M71.21 Synovial cyst of popliteal space [Baker], right **knee**
M71.22 Synovial cyst of popliteal space [Baker], left **knee**

✓5th **M71.3 Other bursal cyst**
Synovial cyst NOS
EXCLUDES 1 *synovial cyst with rupture (M66.1-)*
M71.30 Other bursal cyst, unspecified **site**
✓6th **M71.31 Other bursal cyst,** shoulder
M71.311 Other bursal cyst, right **shoulder**
M71.312 Other bursal cyst, left **shoulder**
M71.319 Other bursal cyst, unspecified **shoulder**
✓6th **M71.32 Other bursal cyst,** elbow
M71.321 Other bursal cyst, right **elbow**
M71.322 Other bursal cyst, left **elbow**
M71.329 Other bursal cyst, unspecified **elbow**
✓6th **M71.33 Other bursal cyst,** wrist
M71.331 Other bursal cyst, right **wrist**
M71.332 Other bursal cyst, left **wrist**
M71.339 Other bursal cyst, unspecified **wrist**
✓6th **M71.34 Other bursal cyst,** hand
M71.341 Other bursal cyst, right **hand**
M71.342 Other bursal cyst, left **hand**
M71.349 Other bursal cyst, unspecified **hand**
✓6th **M71.35 Other bursal cyst,** hip
M71.351 Other bursal cyst, right **hip**
M71.352 Other bursal cyst, left **hip**
M71.359 Other bursal cyst, unspecified **hip**
✓6th **M71.37 Other bursal cyst,** ankle and foot
M71.371 Other bursal cyst, right **ankle and foot**
M71.372 Other bursal cyst, left **ankle and foot**
M71.379 Other bursal cyst, unspecified **ankle and foot**
M71.38 Other bursal cyst, other site
M71.39 Other bursal cyst, multiple sites

✓5th **M71.4 Calcium deposit in bursa**
EXCLUDES 2 *calcium deposit in bursa of shoulder (M75.3)*
M71.40 Calcium deposit in bursa, unspecified **site**
✓6th **M71.42 Calcium deposit in bursa,** elbow
M71.421 Calcium deposit in bursa, right **elbow**
M71.422 Calcium deposit in bursa, left **elbow**
M71.429 Calcium deposit in bursa, unspecified **elbow**
✓6th **M71.43 Calcium deposit in bursa,** wrist
M71.431 Calcium deposit in bursa, right **wrist**
M71.432 Calcium deposit in bursa, left **wrist**
M71.439 Calcium deposit in bursa, unspecified **wrist**
✓6th **M71.44 Calcium deposit in bursa,** hand
M71.441 Calcium deposit in bursa, right **hand**
M71.442 Calcium deposit in bursa, left **hand**
M71.449 Calcium deposit in bursa, unspecified **hand**
✓6th **M71.45 Calcium deposit in bursa,** hip
M71.451 Calcium deposit in bursa, right **hip**
M71.452 Calcium deposit in bursa, left **hip**
M71.459 Calcium deposit in bursa, unspecified **hip**
✓6th **M71.46 Calcium deposit in bursa,** knee
M71.461 Calcium deposit in bursa, right **knee**
M71.462 Calcium deposit in bursa, left **knee**
M71.469 Calcium deposit in bursa, unspecified **knee**
✓6th **M71.47 Calcium deposit in bursa,** ankle and foot
M71.471 Calcium deposit in bursa, right **ankle and foot**
M71.472 Calcium deposit in bursa, left **ankle and foot**
M71.479 Calcium deposit in bursa, unspecified **ankle and foot**
M71.48 Calcium deposit in bursa, other site
M71.49 Calcium deposit in bursa, multiple sites

✓5th **M71.5 Other bursitis, not elsewhere classified**
EXCLUDES 1 *bursitis NOS (M71.9-)*
EXCLUDES 2 *bursitis of shoulder (M75.5)*
bursitis of tibial collateral [Pellegrini-Stieda] (M76.4)
M71.50 Other bursitis, not elsewhere classified, unspecified site
✓6th **M71.52 Other bursitis, not elsewhere classified,** elbow
M71.521 Other bursitis, not elsewhere classified, right **elbow**
M71.522 Other bursitis, not elsewhere classified, left **elbow**
M71.529 Other bursitis, not elsewhere classified, unspecified **elbow**
✓6th **M71.53 Other bursitis, not elsewhere classified,** wrist
M71.531 Other bursitis, not elsewhere classified, right **wrist**
M71.532 Other bursitis, not elsewhere classified, left **wrist**
M71.539 Other bursitis, not elsewhere classified, unspecified **wrist**
✓6th **M71.54 Other bursitis, not elsewhere classified,** hand
M71.541 Other bursitis, not elsewhere classified, right **hand**
M71.542 Other bursitis, not elsewhere classified, left **hand**
M71.549 Other bursitis, not elsewhere classified, unspecified **hand**
✓6th **M71.55 Other bursitis, not elsewhere classified,** hip
M71.551 Other bursitis, not elsewhere classified, right **hip**
M71.552 Other bursitis, not elsewhere classified, left **hip**
M71.559 Other bursitis, not elsewhere classified, unspecified **hip**
✓6th **M71.56 Other bursitis, not elsewhere classified,** knee
M71.561 Other bursitis, not elsewhere classified, right **knee**

M71.562 Other bursitis, not elsewhere classified, left knee

M71.569 Other bursitis, not elsewhere classified, unspecified knee

√6th **M71.57 Other bursitis, not elsewhere classified, ankle and foot**

M71.571 Other bursitis, not elsewhere classified, right ankle and foot

M71.572 Other bursitis, not elsewhere classified, left ankle and foot

M71.579 Other bursitis, not elsewhere classified, unspecified ankle and foot

M71.58 Other bursitis, not elsewhere classified, other site

√5th **M71.8 Other specified bursopathies**

M71.80 Other specified bursopathies, unspecified site

√6th **M71.81 Other specified bursopathies, shoulder**

M71.811 Other specified bursopathies, right shoulder

M71.812 Other specified bursopathies, left shoulder

M71.819 Other specified bursopathies, unspecified shoulder

√6th **M71.82 Other specified bursopathies, elbow**

M71.821 Other specified bursopathies, right elbow

M71.822 Other specified bursopathies, left elbow

M71.829 Other specified bursopathies, unspecified elbow

√6th **M71.83 Other specified bursopathies, wrist**

M71.831 Other specified bursopathies, right wrist

M71.832 Other specified bursopathies, left wrist

M71.839 Other specified bursopathies, unspecified wrist

√6th **M71.84 Other specified bursopathies, hand**

M71.841 Other specified bursopathies, right hand

M71.842 Other specified bursopathies, left hand

M71.849 Other specified bursopathies, unspecified hand

√6th **M71.85 Other specified bursopathies, hip**

M71.851 Other specified bursopathies, right hip

M71.852 Other specified bursopathies, left hip

M71.859 Other specified bursopathies, unspecified hip

√6th **M71.86 Other specified bursopathies, knee**

M71.861 Other specified bursopathies, right knee

M71.862 Other specified bursopathies, left knee

M71.869 Other specified bursopathies, unspecified knee

√6th **M71.87 Other specified bursopathies, ankle and foot**

M71.871 Other specified bursopathies, right ankle and foot

M71.872 Other specified bursopathies, left ankle and foot

M71.879 Other specified bursopathies, unspecified ankle and foot

M71.88 Other specified bursopathies, other site

M71.89 Other specified bursopathies, multiple sites

M71.9 Bursopathy, unspecified
Bursitis NOS

√4th **M72 Fibroblastic disorders**

EXCLUDES 2 *retroperitoneal fibromatosis (D48.3)*

M72.0 Palmar fascial fibromatosis [Dupuytren] A

M72.1 Knuckle pads

M72.2 Plantar fascial fibromatosis
Plantar fasciitis

M72.4 Pseudosarcomatous fibromatosis
Nodular fasciitis

M72.6 Necrotizing fasciitis MCC
Use additional code (B95.-, B96.-) to identify causative organism
CC Excl: K68.12, M60.000-M60.19, M61.00-M61.19, M61.30-M61.59, M62.3, M62.50-M62.59, M62.89, M72.6

M72.8 Other fibroblastic disorders
Abscess of fascia
Fasciitis NEC
Other infective fasciitis
Use additional code to (B95.-, B96.-) identify causative organism

EXCLUDES 1 *diffuse (eosinophilic) fasciitis (M35.4)*
necrotizing fasciitis (M72.6)
nodular fasciitis (M72.4)
perirenal fasciitis NOS (N13.5)
perirenal fasciitis with infection (N13.6)
plantar fasciitis (M72.2)

M72.9 Fibroblastic disorder, unspecified
Fasciitis NOS
Fibromatosis NOS

√4th **M75 Shoulder lesions**

EXCLUDES 2 *shoulder-hand syndrome (M89.0-)*

√5th **M75.0 Adhesive capsulitis of shoulder**
Frozen shoulder
Periarthritis of shoulder

M75.00 Adhesive capsulitis of unspecified shoulder

M75.01 Adhesive capsulitis of right shoulder

M75.02 Adhesive capsulitis of left shoulder

√5th **M75.1 Rotator cuff tear or rupture, not specified as traumatic**
Rotator cuff syndrome
Supraspinatus syndrome
Supraspinatus tear or rupture, not specified as traumatic

EXCLUDES 1 *tear of rotator cuff, traumatic (S46.01-)*

√6th **M75.10 Unspecified rotator cuff tear or rupture, not specified as traumatic**

M75.100 Unspecified rotator cuff tear or rupture of unspecified shoulder, not specified as traumatic

M75.101 Unspecified rotator cuff tear or rupture of right shoulder, not specified as traumatic

M75.102 Unspecified rotator cuff tear or rupture of left shoulder, not specified as traumatic

√6th **M75.11 Incomplete rotator cuff tear or rupture not specified as traumatic**

M75.110 Incomplete rotator cuff tear or rupture of unspecified shoulder, not specified as traumatic

M75.111 Incomplete rotator cuff tear or rupture of right shoulder, not specified as traumatic

M75.112 Incomplete rotator cuff tear or rupture of left shoulder, not specified as traumatic

√6th **M75.12 Complete rotator cuff tear or rupture not specified as traumatic**

M75.120 Complete rotator cuff tear or rupture of unspecified shoulder, not specified as traumatic

M75.121 Complete rotator cuff tear or rupture of right shoulder, not specified as traumatic

M75.122 Complete rotator cuff tear or rupture of left shoulder, not specified as traumatic

√5th **M75.2 Bicipital tendinitis**

M75.20 Bicipital tendinitis, unspecified shoulder

M75.21 Bicipital tendinitis, right shoulder

M75.22 Bicipital tendinitis, left shoulder

√5th **M75.3 Calcific tendinitis of shoulder**
Calcified bursa of shoulder

M75.30 Calcific tendinitis of unspecified shoulder

M75.31 Calcific tendinitis of right shoulder

M75.32 Calcific tendinitis of left shoulder

√5th **M75.4 Impingement syndrome of shoulder**

M75.40 Impingement syndrome of unspecified shoulder

M75.41 Impingement syndrome of right shoulder

M75.42 Impingement syndrome of left shoulder

√5th **M75.5 Bursitis of shoulder**

M75.50 Bursitis of unspecified shoulder

M75.51 Bursitis of right shoulder

M75.52 Bursitis of left shoulder

√5th **M75.8 Other shoulder lesions**

M75.80 Other shoulder lesions, unspecified shoulder

M75.81 Other shoulder lesions, right shoulder

M75.82 Other shoulder lesions, left shoulder

√5th **M75.9 Shoulder lesion, unspecified**
- **M75.90 Shoulder lesion, unspecified, unspecified shoulder**
- **M75.91 Shoulder lesion, unspecified, right shoulder**
- **M75.92 Shoulder lesion, unspecified, left shoulder**

√4th **M76 Enthesopathies, lower limb, excluding foot**

EXCLUDES 2 *bursitis due to use, overuse and pressure (M70.-)*
enthesopathies of ankle and foot (M77.5-)

√5th **M76.0 Gluteal tendinitis**
- **M76.00 Gluteal tendinitis, unspecified hip**
- **M76.01 Gluteal tendinitis, right hip**
- **M76.02 Gluteal tendinitis, left hip**

√5th **M76.1 Psoas tendinitis**
- **M76.10 Psoas tendinitis, unspecified hip**
- **M76.11 Psoas tendinitis, right hip**
- **M76.12 Psoas tendinitis, left hip**

√5th **M76.2 Iliac crest spur**
- **M76.20 Iliac crest spur, unspecified hip**
- **M76.21 Iliac crest spur, right hip**
- **M76.22 Iliac crest spur, left hip**

√5th **M76.3 Iliotibial band syndrome**
- **M76.30 Iliotibial band syndrome, unspecified leg**
- **M76.31 Iliotibial band syndrome, right leg**
- **M76.32 Iliotibial band syndrome, left leg**

√5th **M76.4 Tibial collateral bursitis [Pellegrini-Stieda]**
- **M76.40 Tibial collateral bursitis [Pellegrini-Stieda], unspecified leg**
- **M76.41 Tibial collateral bursitis [Pellegrini-Stieda], right leg**
- **M76.42 Tibial collateral bursitis [Pellegrini-Stieda], left leg**

√5th **M76.5 Patellar tendinitis**
- **M76.50 Patellar tendinitis, unspecified knee**
- **M76.51 Patellar tendinitis, right knee**
- **M76.52 Patellar tendinitis, left knee**

√5th **M76.6 Achilles tendinitis**

Achilles bursitis
- **M76.60 Achilles tendinitis, unspecified leg**
- **M76.61 Achilles tendinitis, right leg**
- **M76.62 Achilles tendinitis, left leg**

√5th **M76.7 Peroneal tendinitis**
- **M76.70 Peroneal tendinitis, unspecified leg**
- **M76.71 Peroneal tendinitis, right leg**
- **M76.72 Peroneal tendinitis, left leg**

√5th **M76.8 Other specified enthesopathies of lower limb, excluding foot**

√6th **M76.81 Anterior tibial syndrome**
- **M76.811 Anterior tibial syndrome, right leg**
- **M76.812 Anterior tibial syndrome, left leg**
- **M76.819 Anterior tibial syndrome, unspecified leg**

√6th **M76.82 Posterior tibial tendinitis**
- **M76.821 Posterior tibial tendinitis, right leg**
- **M76.822 Posterior tibial tendinitis, left leg**
- **M76.829 Posterior tibial tendinitis, unspecified leg**

√6th **M76.89 Other specified enthesopathies of lower limb, excluding foot**
- **M76.891 Other specified enthesopathies of right lower limb, excluding foot**
- **M76.892 Other specified enthesopathies of left lower limb, excluding foot**
- **M76.899 Other specified enthesopathies of unspecified lower limb, excluding foot**

M76.9 Unspecified enthesopathy, lower limb, excluding foot

√4th **M77 Other enthesopathies**

EXCLUDES 1 *bursitis NOS (M71.9-)*

EXCLUDES 2 *bursitis due to use, overuse and pressure (M70.-)*
osteophyte (M25.7)
spinal enthesopathy (M46.0-)

√5th **M77.0 Medial epicondylitis**
- **M77.00 Medial epicondylitis, unspecified elbow**
- **M77.01 Medial epicondylitis, right elbow**
- **M77.02 Medial epicondylitis, left elbow**

√5th **M77.1 Lateral epicondylitis**

Tennis elbow
- **M77.10 Lateral epicondylitis, unspecified elbow**
- **M77.11 Lateral epicondylitis, right elbow**
- **M77.12 Lateral epicondylitis, left elbow**

√5th **M77.2 Periarthritis of wrist**
- **M77.20 Periarthritis, unspecified wrist**
- **M77.21 Periarthritis, right wrist**
- **M77.22 Periarthritis, left wrist**

√5th **M77.3 Calcaneal spur**
- **M77.30 Calcaneal spur, unspecified foot**
- **M77.31 Calcaneal spur, right foot**
- **M77.32 Calcaneal spur, left foot**

√5th **M77.4 Metatarsalgia**

EXCLUDES 1 *Morton's metatarsalgia (G57.6)*
- **M77.40 Metatarsalgia, unspecified foot**
- **M77.41 Metatarsalgia, right foot**
- **M77.42 Metatarsalgia, left foot**

√5th **M77.5 Other enthesopathy of foot**
- **M77.50 Other enthesopathy of unspecified foot**
- **M77.51 Other enthesopathy of right foot**
- **M77.52 Other enthesopathy of left foot**

M77.8 Other enthesopathies, not elsewhere classified

M77.9 Enthesopathy, unspecified

Bone spur NOS
Capsulitis NOS
Periarthritis NOS
Tendinitis NOS

√4th **M79 Other and unspecified soft tissue disorders, not elsewhere classified**

EXCLUDES 1 *psychogenic rheumatism (F45.8)*
soft tissue pain, psychogenic (F45.41)

M79.0 Rheumatism, unspecified

EXCLUDES 1 *fibromyalgia (M79.7)*
palindromic rheumatism (M12.3-)

M79.1 Myalgia

Myofascial pain syndrome

EXCLUDES 1 *fibromyalgia (M79.7)*
myositis (M60.-)

M79.2 Neuralgia and neuritis, unspecified

EXCLUDES 1 *brachial radiculitis NOS (M54.1)*
lumbosacral radiculitis NOS (M54.1)
mononeuropathies (G56-G58)
radiculitis NOS (M54.1)
sciatica (M54.3-M54.4)

M79.3 Panniculitis, unspecified

EXCLUDES 1 *lupus panniculitis (L93.2)*
neck and back panniculitis (M54.0-)
relapsing [Weber-Christian] panniculitis (M35.6)

M79.4 Hypertrophy of (infrapatellar) fat pad

M79.5 Residual foreign body in soft tissue

EXCLUDES 1 *foreign body granuloma of skin and subcutaneous tissue (L92.3)*
foreign body granuloma of soft tissue (M60.2-)

√5th **M79.6 Pain in limb, hand, foot, fingers and toes**

EXCLUDES 2 *pain in joint (M25.5-)*

√6th **M79.60 Pain in limb, unspecified**
- **M79.601 Pain in right arm**
  Pain in right upper limb NOS
- **M79.602 Pain in left arm**
  Pain in left upper limb NOS
- **M79.603 Pain in arm, unspecified**
  Pain in upper limb NOS
- **M79.604 Pain in right leg**
  Pain in right lower limb NOS
- **M79.605 Pain in left leg**
  Pain in left lower limb NOS
- **M79.606 Pain in leg, unspecified**
  Pain in lower limb NOS
- **M79.609 Pain in unspecified limb**
  Pain in limb NOS

√6th **M79.62 Pain in upper arm**

Pain in axillary region
- **M79.621 Pain in right upper arm**
- **M79.622 Pain in left upper arm**
- **M79.629 Pain in unspecified upper arm**

✓6th **M79.63 Pain in forearm**
- **M79.631 Pain in right forearm**
- **M79.632 Pain in left forearm**
- **M79.639 Pain in unspecified forearm**

✓6th **M79.64 Pain in hand and fingers**
- **M79.641 Pain in right hand**
- **M79.642 Pain in left hand**
- **M79.643 Pain in unspecified hand**
- **M79.644 Pain in right finger(s)**
- **M79.645 Pain in left finger(s)**
- **M79.646 Pain in unspecified finger(s)**

✓6th **M79.65 Pain in thigh**
- **M79.651 Pain in right thigh**
- **M79.652 Pain in left thigh**
- **M79.659 Pain in unspecified thigh**

✓6th **M79.66 Pain in lower leg**
- **M79.661 Pain in right lower leg**
- **M79.662 Pain in left lower leg**
- **M79.669 Pain in unspecified lower leg**

✓6th **M79.67 Pain in foot and toes**
- **M79.671 Pain in right foot**
- **M79.672 Pain in left foot**
- **M79.673 Pain in unspecified foot**
- **M79.674 Pain in right toe(s)**
- **M79.675 Pain in left toe(s)**
- **M79.676 Pain in unspecified toe(s)**

M79.7 Fibromyalgia
Fibromyositis
Fibrositis
Myofibrositis

✓5th **M79.A Nontraumatic compartment syndrome**
Code first, if applicable, associated postprocedural complication
EXCLUDES 1 *compartment syndrome NOS (T79.A-)*
fibromyalgia (M79.7)
nontraumatic ischemic infarction of muscle (M62.2-)
traumatic compartment syndrome (T79.A-)

✓6th **M79.A1 Nontraumatic compartment syndrome of upper extremity**
Nontraumatic compartment syndrome of shoulder, arm, forearm, wrist, hand, and fingers

CC Excl: M70.80-M70.99, M79.81-M79.9, R29.898, S45.301-S45.899 with 7th A, S55.201-S55.899 with 7th A, S65.801-S65.899 with 7th A

- **M79.A11 Nontraumatic compartment syndrome of right upper extremity** CC
- **M79.A12 Nontraumatic compartment syndrome of left upper extremity** CC
- **M79.A19 Nontraumatic compartment syndrome of unspecified upper extremity** CC

✓6th **M79.A2 Nontraumatic compartment syndrome of lower extremity**
Nontraumatic compartment syndrome of hip, buttock, thigh, leg, foot, and toes

CC Excl: M70.80-M70.99, M79.81-M79.9, R29.898, S75.801-S75.899 with 7th A, S85.201-S85.299 with 7th A, S85.801-S85.899 with 7th A, S95.001-S95.099 with 7th A, S95.201-S95.899 with 7th A

- **M79.A21 Nontraumatic compartment syndrome of right lower extremity** CC
- **M79.A22 Nontraumatic compartment syndrome of left lower extremity** CC
- **M79.A29 Nontraumatic compartment syndrome of unspecified lower extremity** CC

M79.A3 Nontraumatic compartment syndrome of abdomen CC
CC Excl: S31.001 with 7th A, S31.011 with 7th A, S31.021 with 7th A, S31.031 with 7th A, S31.041 with 7th A, S31.051-S31.159 with 7th A, S31.600-S31.659 with 7th A, S31.831-S31.839 with 7th A, S36.00-S37.99 with 7th A, S38.3XX-S39.023 with 7th A, T14.8-T14.91, T79.8XX-T79.9XX with 7th A

M79.A9 Nontraumatic compartment syndrome of other sites CC
CC Excl: S31.001 with 7th A, S31.011 with 7th A, S31.021 with 7th A, S31.031 with 7th A, S31.041 with 7th A, S31.051 with 7th A, S31.600-S31.659 with 7th A, S36.81X-S36.899 with 7th A

✓5th **M79.8 Other specified soft tissue disorders**
- **M79.81 Nontraumatic hematoma of soft tissue**
  Nontraumatic hematoma of muscle
  Nontraumatic seroma of muscle and soft tissue
- **M79.89 Other specified soft tissue disorders**
  Polyalgia

M79.9 Soft tissue disorder, unspecified

OSTEOPATHIES AND CHONDROPATHIES (M80-M94)

Disorders of bone density and structure (M80-M85)

✓4th **M80 Osteoporosis with current pathological fracture**
INCLUDES osteoporosis with current fragility fracture
Use additional code to identify major osseous defect, if applicable (M89.7-)
EXCLUDES 1 *collapsed vertebra NOS (M48.5)*
pathological fracture NOS (M84.4)
wedging of vertebra NOS (M48.5)
EXCLUDES 2 *personal history of (healed) osteoporosis fracture (Z87.310)*

The appropriate 7th character is to be added to each code from category M80.
- A initial encounter for fracture
- D subsequent encounter for fracture with routine healing
- G subsequent encounter for fracture with delayed healing
- K subsequent encounter for fracture with nonunion
- P subsequent encounter for fracture with malunion
- S sequela

CC Excl: For codes M80, CC with 7th character A, unless otherwise noted: M48.40X-M48.58X with 7th A, M80.00X-M84.68X with 7th A
CC codes with 7th character K or P: M80.00X-M84.68X with 7th [K, P], S02.0XX-S02.92X with 7th K, S12.000-S12.691 with 7th K, S22.000-S22.9XX with 7th K, S32.000-S32.9XX with 7th K, S42.001-S42.92 with 7th [K, P], S49.001-S49.199 with 7th [K, P], S52.001-S52.92X with 7th [K, M, N, P, Q, R], S59.001-S59.299 with 7th [K, P], S62.001-S62.92X with 7th [K, P], S72.001-S72.92X with 7th [K, M, N, P, Q, R], S79.001-S79.199 with 7th [K, P], S82.001-S82.92X with 7th [K, M, N, P, Q, R], S89.001-S89.399 with 7th [K, P], S92.001-S92.919 with 7th [K, P]

✓5th **M80.0 Age-related osteoporosis with current pathological fracture**
Involutional osteoporosis with current pathological fracture
Osteoporosis NOS with current pathological fracture
Postmenopausal osteoporosis with current pathological fracture
Senile osteoporosis with current pathological fracture

✓x7th **M80.00 Age-related osteoporosis with current pathological fracture, unspecified site** CC A

✓6th **M80.01 Age-related osteoporosis with current pathological fracture, shoulder**
- ✓7th **M80.011 Age-related osteoporosis with current pathological fracture, right shoulder** CC A
- ✓7th **M80.012 Age-related osteoporosis with current pathological fracture, left shoulder** CC A
- ✓7th **M80.019 Age-related osteoporosis with current pathological fracture, unspecified shoulder** CC A

✓6th **M80.02 Age-related osteoporosis with current pathological fracture, humerus**
- ✓7th **M80.021 Age-related osteoporosis with current pathological fracture, right humerus** CC A
- ✓7th **M80.022 Age-related osteoporosis with current pathological fracture, left humerus** CC A
- ✓7th **M80.029 Age-related osteoporosis with current pathological fracture, unspecified humerus** CC A

✓6th **M80.03 Age-related osteoporosis with current pathological fracture, forearm**
Age-related osteoporosis with current pathological fracture of wrist
- ✓7th **M80.031 Age-related osteoporosis with current pathological fracture, right forearm** CC A
- ✓7th **M80.032 Age-related osteoporosis with current pathological fracture, left forearm** CC A

M80.039 Age-related osteoporosis with current pathological fracture, unspecified forearm CC A

M80.04 Age-related osteoporosis with current pathological fracture, hand

M80.041 Age-related osteoporosis with current pathological fracture, right hand CC A

M80.042 Age-related osteoporosis with current pathological fracture, left hand CC A

M80.049 Age-related osteoporosis with current pathological fracture, unspecified hand CC A

M80.05 Age-related osteoporosis with current pathological fracture, femur

Age-related osteoporosis with current pathological fracture of hip

M80.051 Age-related osteoporosis with current pathological fracture, right femur CC A

M80.052 Age-related osteoporosis with current pathological fracture, left femur CC A

M80.059 Age-related osteoporosis with current pathological fracture, unspecified femur CC A

M80.06 Age-related osteoporosis with current pathological fracture, lower leg

M80.061 Age-related osteoporosis with current pathological fracture, right lower leg CC A

M80.062 Age-related osteoporosis with current pathological fracture, left lower leg CC A

M80.069 Age-related osteoporosis with current pathological fracture, unspecified lower leg CC A

M80.07 Age-related osteoporosis with current pathological fracture, ankle and foot

M80.071 Age-related osteoporosis with current pathological fracture, right ankle and foot CC A

M80.072 Age-related osteoporosis with current pathological fracture, left ankle and foot CC A

M80.079 Age-related osteoporosis with current pathological fracture, unspecified ankle and foot CC A

M80.08 Age-related osteoporosis with current pathological fracture, vertebra(e) CC A

M80.8 Other osteoporosis with current pathological fracture

Drug-induced osteoporosis with current pathological fracture
Idiopathic osteoporosis with current pathological fracture
Osteoporosis of disuse with current pathological fracture
Postoophorectomy osteoporosis with current pathological fracture
Postsurgical malabsorption osteoporosis with current pathological fracture
Post-traumatic osteoporosis with current pathological fracture

Use additional code for adverse effect, if applicable, to identify drug (T36-T50 with fifth or sixth character 5)

M80.80 Other osteoporosis with current pathological fracture, unspecified site CC

M80.81 Other osteoporosis with pathological fracture, shoulder

M80.811 Other osteoporosis with current pathological fracture, right shoulder CC

M80.812 Other osteoporosis with current pathological fracture, left shoulder CC

M80.819 Other osteoporosis with current pathological fracture, unspecified shoulder CC

M80.82 Other osteoporosis with current pathological fracture, humerus

M80.821 Other osteoporosis with current pathological fracture, right humerus CC

M80.822 Other osteoporosis with current pathological fracture, left humerus CC

M80.829 Other osteoporosis with current pathological fracture, unspecified humerus CC

M80.83 Other osteoporosis with current pathological fracture, forearm

Other osteoporosis with current pathological fracture of wrist

M80.831 Other osteoporosis with current pathological fracture, right forearm CC

M80.832 Other osteoporosis with current pathological fracture, left forearm CC

M80.839 Other osteoporosis with current pathological fracture, unspecified forearm CC

M80.84 Other osteoporosis with current pathological fracture, hand

M80.841 Other osteoporosis with current pathological fracture, right hand CC

M80.842 Other osteoporosis with current pathological fracture, left hand CC

M80.849 Other osteoporosis with current pathological fracture, unspecified hand CC

M80.85 Other osteoporosis with current pathological fracture, femur

Other osteoporosis with current pathological fracture of hip

M80.851 Other osteoporosis with current pathological fracture, right femur CC

M80.852 Other osteoporosis with current pathological fracture, left femur CC

M80.859 Other osteoporosis with current pathological fracture, unspecified femur CC

M80.86 Other osteoporosis with current pathological fracture, lower leg

M80.861 Other osteoporosis with current pathological fracture, right lower leg CC

M80.862 Other osteoporosis with current pathological fracture, left lower leg CC

M80.869 Other osteoporosis with current pathological fracture, unspecified lower leg CC

M80.87 Other osteoporosis with current pathological fracture, ankle and foot

M80.871 Other osteoporosis with current pathological fracture, right ankle and foot CC

M80.872 Other osteoporosis with current pathological fracture, left ankle and foot CC

M80.879 Other osteoporosis with current pathological fracture, unspecified ankle and foot CC

M80.88 Other osteoporosis with current pathological fracture, vertebra(e) CC

M81 Osteoporosis without current pathological fracture

Use additional code to identify:
major osseous defect, if applicable (M89.7-)
personal history of (healed) osteoporosis fracture, if applicable (Z87.310)

EXCLUDES1 *osteoporosis with current pathological fracture (M80.-)*
Sudeck's atrophy (M89.0)

M81.0 Age-related osteoporosis without current pathological fracture A

Involutional osteoporosis without current pathological fracture
Osteoporosis NOS
Postmenopausal osteoporosis without current pathological fracture
Senile osteoporosis without current pathological fracture

M81.6 Localized osteoporosis [Lequesne]

EXCLUDES1 *Sudeck's atrophy (M89.0)*

Additional Character Required | Xtension Alert | Unacceptable PDx | Manifestation | Hospital Acquired Condition | EXCLUDES1 Not Coded Here | EXCLUDES2 Not Included Here

M81.8 Other osteoporosis without current pathological fracture
Drug-induced osteoporosis without current pathological fracture
Idiopathic osteoporosis without current pathological fracture
Osteoporosis of disuse without current pathological fracture
Postoophorectomy osteoporosis without current pathological fracture
Postsurgical malabsorption osteoporosis without current pathological fracture
Post-traumatic osteoporosis without current pathological fracture
Use additional code for adverse effect, if applicable, to identify drug (T36-T50 with fifth or sixth character 5)

✓4th M83 Adult osteomalacia
EXCLUDES 1 *infantile and juvenile osteomalacia (E55.Ø)*
renal osteodystrophy (N25.Ø)
rickets (active) (E55.Ø)
rickets (active) sequelae (E64.3)
vitamin D-resistant osteomalacia (E83.3)
vitamin D-resistant rickets (active) (E83.3)

M83.Ø Puerperal osteomalacia M♀
M83.1 Senile osteomalacia A
M83.2 Adult osteomalacia due to malabsorption A
Postsurgical malabsorption osteomalacia in adults
M83.3 Adult osteomalacia due to malnutrition A
M83.4 Aluminum bone disease
M83.5 Other drug-induced osteomalacia in adults A
Use additional code for adverse effect, if applicable, to identify drug (T36-T50 with fifth or sixth character 5)
M83.8 Other adult osteomalacia A
M83.9 Adult osteomalacia, unspecified A

✓4th M84 Disorder of continuity of bone
EXCLUDES 2 *traumatic fracture of bone-see fracture, by site*

✓5th M84.3 Stress fracture
Fatigue fracture
March fracture
Stress fracture NOS
Stress reaction
Use additional external cause code(s) to identify the cause of the stress fracture
EXCLUDES 1 *pathological fracture NOS (M84.4-)*
pathological fracture due to osteoporosis (M8Ø.-)
traumatic fracture (S12-, S22-, S32-, S42-, S52-, S62-, S72-, S82-, S92-)
EXCLUDES 2 *personal history of (healed) stress (fatigue) fracture (Z87.312)*
stress fracture of vertebra (M48.4-)

The appropriate 7th character is to be added to each code from subcategory M84.3.
A initial encounter for fracture
D subsequent encounter for fracture with routine healing
G subsequent encounter for fracture with delayed healing
K subsequent encounter for fracture with nonunion
P subsequent encounter for fracture with malunion
S sequela

CC Excl: For CC codes in subcatagory M84.3, unless otherwise noted: For CC codes with 7th character K or P: M8Ø.ØØX-M84.68X with 7th [K, P], SØ2.ØXX-SØ2.92X with 7th K, S12.ØØØ-S12.691 with 7th K, S22.ØØØ-S22.9XX with 7th K, S32ØØØ-S32.9XX with 7th K, S42.ØØ1-S42.92X with 7th [K, P], S49.ØØ1-S49.199 with 7th [K, P], S52.ØØ1-S52.92X with 7th [K, M, N, P, Q, R], S59.ØØ1-S59.299 with 7th [K, P], S62.ØØ1-S62.92X with 7th [K, P], S72.ØØ1-S72.92X with 7th [K, M, N, P, Q, R], S79.ØØ1-S79.199 with 7th [K, P], S82.ØØ1-S82.92X with 7th [K, M, N, P, Q, R], S89.ØØ1-S89.399 with 7th [K, P], S92.ØØ1-S92.919 with 7th [K, P]

✓x7th **M84.3Ø Stress fracture, unspecified site** CC
✓6th **M84.31 Stress fracture, shoulder**
✓7th **M84.311 Stress fracture, right shoulder** CC
✓7th **M84.312 Stress fracture, left shoulder** CC
✓7th **M84.319 Stress fracture, unspecified shoulder** CC
✓6th **M84.32 Stress fracture, humerus**
✓7th **M84.321 Stress fracture, right humerus** CC
✓7th **M84.322 Stress fracture, left humerus** CC
✓7th **M84.329 Stress fracture, unspecified humerus** CC
✓6th **M84.33 Stress fracture, ulna and radius**
✓7th **M84.331 Stress fracture, right ulna** CC
✓7th **M84.332 Stress fracture, left ulna** CC
✓7th **M84.333 Stress fracture, right radius** CC
✓7th **M84.334 Stress fracture, left radius** CC
✓7th **M84.339 Stress fracture, unspecified ulna and radius** CC
✓6th **M84.34 Stress fracture, hand and fingers**
✓7th **M84.341 Stress fracture, right hand** CC
✓7th **M84.342 Stress fracture, left hand** CC
✓7th **M84.343 Stress fracture, unspecified hand** CC
✓7th **M84.344 Stress fracture, right finger(s)** CC
✓7th **M84.345 Stress fracture, left finger(s)** CC
✓7th **M84.346 Stress fracture, unspecified finger(s)** CC
✓6th **M84.35 Stress fracture, pelvis and femur**
Stress fracture, hip
✓7th **M84.35Ø Stress fracture, pelvis** CC
✓7th **M84.351 Stress fracture, right femur** CC
✓7th **M84.352 Stress fracture, left femur** CC
✓7th **M84.353 Stress fracture, unspecified femur** CC
✓7th **M84.359 Stress fracture, hip, unspecified** CC
✓6th **M84.36 Stress fracture, tibia and fibula**
✓7th **M84.361 Stress fracture, right tibia** CC
✓7th **M84.362 Stress fracture, left tibia** CC
✓7th **M84.363 Stress fracture, right fibula** CC
✓7th **M84.364 Stress fracture, left fibula** CC
✓7th **M84.369 Stress fracture, unspecified tibia and fibula** CC
✓6th **M84.37 Stress fracture, ankle, foot and toes**
✓7th **M84.371 Stress fracture, right ankle** CC
✓7th **M84.372 Stress fracture, left ankle** CC
✓7th **M84.373 Stress fracture, unspecified ankle** CC
✓7th **M84.374 Stress fracture, right foot** CC
✓7th **M84.375 Stress fracture, left foot** CC
✓7th **M84.376 Stress fracture, unspecified foot** CC
✓7th **M84.377 Stress fracture, right toe(s)** CC
✓7th **M84.378 Stress fracture, left toe(s)** CC
✓7th **M84.379 Stress fracture, unspecified toe(s)** CC
✓x7th **M84.38 Stress fracture, other site** CC
EXCLUDES 2 *stress fracture of vertebra (M48.4-)*

✓5th M84.4 Pathological fracture, not elsewhere classified
Chronic fracture
Pathological fracture NOS
EXCLUDES 1 *collapsed vertebra NEC (M48.5)*
pathological fracture in neoplastic disease (M84.5-)
pathological fracture in osteoporosis (M8Ø.-)
pathological fracture in other disease (M84.6-)
stress fracture (M84.3-)
traumatic fracture (S12.-, S22.-, S32.-, S42.-, S52.-, S62.-, S72.-, S82.-, S92.-)
EXCLUDES 2 *personal history of (healed) pathological fracture (Z87.311)*

The appropriate 7th character is to be added to each code from subcategory M84.4.
A initial encounter for fracture
D subsequent encounter for fracture with routine healing
G subsequent encounter for fracture with delayed healing
K subsequent encounter for fracture with nonunion
P subsequent encounter for fracture with malunion
S sequela

CC Excl: For codes M84.4, CC with 7th character A, unless otherwise noted: M48.4ØX-M48.58X with 7th A, M8Ø.ØØX-M84.68X with 7th A
CC with 7th character K or P: M8Ø.ØØX-M84.68X with 7th [K, P], SØ2.ØXX-SØ2.92Xwith 7th K, S12.ØØØ-S12.691 with 7th K, S22.ØØØ-S22.9XX with 7th K, S32.ØØØ-S32.9XX with 7th K, S42.ØØ1-S42.92X with 7th [K, P], S49.ØØ1-S49.199 with 7th [K, P], S52.ØØ1-S52.92X with 7th [K, M, N, P, Q, R], S59.ØØ1-S59.299 with 7th [K, P], S62.ØØ1-S62.92X with 7th [K, P], S72.ØØ1-S72.92X with 7th [K, M, N, P, Q, R], S79.ØØ1-S79.199 with 7th [K, P], S82.ØØ1-S82.92X with 7th [K, M, N, P, Q, R], S89.ØØ1-S89.399 with 7th [K, P], S92.ØØ1-S92.919 with 7th [K, P]

✓x7th **M84.4Ø Pathological fracture, unspecified site** CC
✓6th **M84.41 Pathological fracture, shoulder**
✓7th **M84.411 Pathological fracture, right shoulder** CC
✓7th **M84.412 Pathological fracture, left shoulder** CC

✓7th **M84.419 Pathological fracture, unspecified shoulder** CC

✓6th **M84.42 Pathological fracture, humerus**

✓7th **M84.421 Pathological fracture, right humerus** CC

✓7th **M84.422 Pathological fracture, left humerus** CC

✓7th **M84.429 Pathological fracture, unspecified humerus** CC

✓6th **M84.43 Pathological fracture, ulna and radius**

✓7th **M84.431 Pathological fracture, right ulna** CC

✓7th **M84.432 Pathological fracture, left ulna** CC

✓7th **M84.433 Pathological fracture, right radius** CC

✓7th **M84.434 Pathological fracture, left radius** CC

✓7th **M84.439 Pathological fracture, unspecified ulna and radius** CC

✓6th **M84.44 Pathological fracture, hand and fingers**

✓7th **M84.441 Pathological fracture, right hand** CC

✓7th **M84.442 Pathological fracture, left hand** CC

✓7th **M84.443 Pathological fracture, unspecified hand** CC

✓7th **M84.444 Pathological fracture, right finger(s)** CC

✓7th **M84.445 Pathological fracture, left finger(s)** CC

✓7th **M84.446 Pathological fracture, unspecified finger(s)** CC

✓6th **M84.45 Pathological fracture, femur and pelvis**

✓7th **M84.451 Pathological fracture, right femur** CC

✓7th **M84.452 Pathological fracture, left femur** CC

✓7th **M84.453 Pathological fracture, unspecified femur** CC

✓7th **M84.454 Pathological fracture, pelvis** CC

✓7th **M84.459 Pathological fracture, hip, unspecified** CC

✓6th **M84.46 Pathological fracture, tibia and fibula**

✓7th **M84.461 Pathological fracture, right tibia** CC

✓7th **M84.462 Pathological fracture, left tibia** CC

✓7th **M84.463 Pathological fracture, right fibula** CC

✓7th **M84.464 Pathological fracture, left fibula** CC

✓7th **M84.469 Pathological fracture, unspecified tibia and fibula** CC

✓6th **M84.47 Pathological fracture, ankle, foot and toes**

✓7th **M84.471 Pathological fracture, right ankle** CC

✓7th **M84.472 Pathological fracture, left ankle** CC

✓7th **M84.473 Pathological fracture, unspecified ankle** CC

✓7th **M84.474 Pathological fracture, right foot** CC

✓7th **M84.475 Pathological fracture, left foot** CC

✓7th **M84.476 Pathological fracture, unspecified foot** CC

✓7th **M84.477 Pathological fracture, right toe(s)** CC

✓7th **M84.478 Pathological fracture, left toe(s)** CC

✓7th **M84.479 Pathological fracture, unspecified toe(s)** CC

✓x7th **M84.48 Pathological fracture, other site** CC

✓5th **M84.5 Pathological fracture in neoplastic disease**

Code also underlying neoplasm

The appropriate 7th character is to be added to each code from subcategory M84.5.

- A initial encounter for fracture
- D subsequent encounter for fracture with routine healing
- G subsequent encounter for fracture with delayed healing
- K subsequent encounter for fracture with nonunion
- P subsequent encounter for fracture with malunion
- S sequela

CC Excl: For codes M84.5, CC with 7th character A, unless otherwise noted: M48.40X-M48.58X with 7th A, M80.00X-M84.68X with 7th A

CC with 7th character K or P: M80.00X-M84.68X with 7th [K, P], S02.0XX-S02.92X with 7th K, S12.000-S12.691 with 7th K, S22.000-S22.9XX with 7th K, S32.000-S32.9XX with 7th K, S42.001-S42.92X with 7th [K, P], S49.001-S49.199 with 7th [K, P], S52.001-S52.92X with 7th [K, M, N, P, Q, R], S59.001-S59.299 with 7th [K, P], S62.001-S62.92X with 7th [K, P], S72.001-S72.92X with 7th [K, M, N, P, Q, R], S79.001-S79.199 with 7th [K, P], S82.001-S82.92X with 7th [K, M, N, P, Q, R], S89.001-S89.399 with 7th [K, P], S92.001-S92.919 with 7th [K, P]

✓x7th **M84.50 Pathological fracture in neoplastic disease, unspecified site** CC

✓6th **M84.51 Pathological fracture in neoplastic disease, shoulder**

✓7th **M84.511 Pathological fracture in neoplastic disease, right shoulder** CC

✓7th **M84.512 Pathological fracture in neoplastic disease, left shoulder** CC

✓7th **M84.519 Pathological fracture in neoplastic disease, unspecified shoulder** CC

✓6th **M84.52 Pathological fracture in neoplastic disease, humerus**

✓7th **M84.521 Pathological fracture in neoplastic disease, right humerus** CC

✓7th **M84.522 Pathological fracture in neoplastic disease, left humerus** CC

✓7th **M84.529 Pathological fracture in neoplastic disease, unspecified humerus** CC

✓6th **M84.53 Pathological fracture in neoplastic disease, ulna and radius**

✓7th **M84.531 Pathological fracture in neoplastic disease, right ulna** CC

✓7th **M84.532 Pathological fracture in neoplastic disease, left ulna** CC

✓7th **M84.533 Pathological fracture in neoplastic disease, right radius** CC

✓7th **M84.534 Pathological fracture in neoplastic disease, left radius** CC

✓7th **M84.539 Pathunspecifiedological fracture in neoplastic disease, ulna and radius** CC

✓6th **M84.54 Pathological fracture in neoplastic disease, hand**

✓7th **M84.541 Pathological fracture in neoplastic disease, right hand** CC

✓7th **M84.542 Pathological fracture in neoplastic disease, left hand** CC

✓7th **M84.549 Pathological fracture in neoplastic disease, unspecified hand** CC

✓6th **M84.55 Pathological fracture in neoplastic disease, pelvis and femur**

✓7th **M84.550 Pathological fracture in neoplastic disease, pelvis** CC

✓7th **M84.551 Pathological fracture in neoplastic disease, right femur** CC

✓7th **M84.552 Pathological fracture in neoplastic disease, left femur** CC

✓7th **M84.553 Pathological fracture in neoplastic disease, unspecified femur** CC

✓7th **M84.559 Pathological fracture in neoplastic disease, hip, unspecified** CC

✓6th **M84.56 Pathological fracture in neoplastic disease, tibia and fibula**

✓7th **M84.561 Pathological fracture in neoplastic disease, right tibia** CC

✓7th **M84.562 Pathological fracture in neoplastic disease, left tibia** CC

√7th **M84.563 Pathological fracture in neoplastic disease, right fibula** CC

√7th **M84.564 Pathological fracture in neoplastic disease, left fibula** CC

√7th **M84.569 Pathological fracture in neoplastic disease, unspecified tibia and fibula** CC

√6th **M84.57 Pathological fracture in neoplastic disease, ankle and foot**

√7th **M84.571 Pathological fracture in neoplastic disease, right ankle** CC

√7th **M84.572 Pathological fracture in neoplastic disease, left ankle** CC

√7th **M84.573 Pathological fracture in neoplastic disease, unspecified ankle** CC

√7th **M84.574 Pathological fracture in neoplastic disease, right foot** CC

√7th **M84.575 Pathological fracture in neoplastic disease, left foot** CC

√7th **M84.576 Pathological fracture in neoplastic disease, unspecified foot** CC

√x7th **M84.58 Pathological fracture in neoplastic disease, other specified site** CC
Pathological fracture in neoplastic disease, vertebrae

√5th **M84.6 Pathological fracture in other disease**
Code also underlying condition
EXCLUDES 1 *pathological fracture in osteoporosis (M8Ø.-)*

The appropriate 7th character is to be added to each code from subcategory M84.6.
A initial encounter for fracture
D subsequent encounter for fracture with routine healing
G subsequent encounter for fracture with delayed healing
K subsequent encounter for fracture with nonunion
P subsequent encounter for fracture with malunion
S sequela

CC Excl: For codes M84.6, CC with 7th character A, unless otherwise noted: M48.40X-M48.58X with 7th A, M8Ø.ØØX-M84.68X with 7th A.
CC with 7th character K or P: M8Ø.ØØX-M84.68X with 7th [K, P], SØ2.ØXX-SØ2.92X with 7th K, S12.ØØØ-S12.691 with 7th K, S22.ØØØ-S22.9XX with 7th K, S32.ØØØ-S32.9XX with 7th K, S42.ØØ1-S42.92X with 7th [K, P], S49.ØØ1-S49.199 with 7th [K, P], S52.ØØ1-S52.92X with 7th [K, M, N, P, Q, R], S59.ØØ1-S59.299 with 7th [K, P], S62.ØØ1-S62.92X with 7th [K, P], S72.ØØ1-S72.92X with 7th [K, M, N, P, Q, R], S79.ØØ1-S79.199 with 7th [K, P], S82.ØØ1-S82.92X with 7th [K, M, N, P, Q, R], S89.ØØ1-S89.399 with 7th [K, P], S92.ØØ1-S92.919 with 7th [K, P]

√x7th **M84.6Ø Pathological fracture in other disease, unspecified site** CC

√6th **M84.61 Pathological fracture in other disease, shoulder**

√7th **M84.611 Pathological fracture in other disease, right shoulder** CC

√7th **M84.612 Pathological fracture in other disease, left shoulder** CC

√7th **M84.619 Pathological fracture in other disease, unspecified shoulder** CC

√6th **M84.62 Pathological fracture in other disease, humerus**

√7th **M84.621 Pathological fracture in other disease, right humerus** CC

√7th **M84.622 Pathological fracture in other disease, left humerus** CC

√7th **M84.629 Pathological fracture in other disease, unspecified humerus** CC

√6th **M84.63 Pathological fracture in other disease, ulna and radius**

√7th **M84.631 Pathological fracture in other disease, right ulna** CC

√7th **M84.632 Pathological fracture in other disease, left ulna** CC

√7th **M84.633 Pathological fracture in other disease, right radius** CC

√7th **M84.634 Pathological fracture in other disease, left radius** CC

√7th **M84.639 Pathological fracture in other disease, unspecified ulna and radius** CC

√6th **M84.64 Pathological fracture in other disease, hand**

√7th **M84.641 Pathological fracture in other disease, right hand** CC

√7th **M84.642 Pathological fracture in other disease, left hand** CC

√7th **M84.649 Pathological fracture in other disease, unspecified hand** CC

√6th **M84.65 Pathological fracture in other disease, pelvis and femur**

√7th **M84.65Ø Pathological fracture in other disease, pelvis** CC

√7th **M84.651 Pathological fracture in other disease, right femur** CC

√7th **M84.652 Pathological fracture in other disease, left femur** CC

√7th **M84.653 Pathological fracture in other disease, unspecified femur** CC

√7th **M84.659 Pathological fracture in other disease, hip, unspecified** CC

√6th **M84.66 Pathological fracture in other disease, tibia and fibula**

√7th **M84.661 Pathological fracture in other disease, right tibia** CC

√7th **M84.662 Pathological fracture in other disease, left tibia** CC

√7th **M84.663 Pathological fracture in other disease, right fibula** CC

√7th **M84.664 Pathological fracture in other disease, left fibula** CC

√7th **M84.669 Pathological fracture in other disease, unspecified tibia and fibula** CC

√6th **M84.67 Pathological fracture in other disease, ankle and foot**

√7th **M84.671 Pathological fracture in other disease, right ankle** CC

√7th **M84.672 Pathological fracture in other disease, left ankle** CC

√7th **M84.673 Pathological fracture in other disease, unspecified ankle** CC

√7th **M84.674 Pathological fracture in other disease, right foot** CC

√7th **M84.675 Pathological fracture in other disease, left foot** CC

√7th **M84.676 Pathological fracture in other disease, unspecified foot** CC

√x7th **M84.68 Pathological fracture in other disease, other site** CC

√5th **M84.8 Other disorders of continuity of bone**

M84.8Ø Other disorders of continuity of bone, unspecified site

√6th **M84.81 Other disorders of continuity of bone, shoulder**

M84.811 Other disorders of continuity of bone, right shoulder

M84.812 Other disorders of continuity of bone, left shoulder

M84.819 Other disorders of continuity of bone, unspecified shoulder

√6th **M84.82 Other disorders of continuity of bone, humerus**

M84.821 Other disorders of continuity of bone, right humerus

M84.822 Other disorders of continuity of bone, left humerus

M84.829 Other disorders of continuity of bone, unspecified humerus

√6th **M84.83 Other disorders of continuity of bone, ulna and radius**

M84.831 Other disorders of continuity of bone, right ulna

M84.832 Other disorders of continuity of bone, left ulna

M84.833 Other disorders of continuity of bone, right radius

M84.834 Other disorders of continuity of bone, left radius

M84.839 Other disorders of continuity of bone, unspecified ulna and radius

✓6th M84.84 Other disorders of continuity of bone, hand
M84.841 Other disorders of continuity of bone, right hand
M84.842 Other disorders of continuity of bone, left hand
M84.849 Other disorders of continuity of bone, unspecified hand
✓6th M84.85 Other disorders of continuity of bone, pelvic region and thigh
M84.851 Other disorders of continuity of bone, right pelvic region and thigh
M84.852 Other disorders of continuity of bone, left pelvic region and thigh
M84.859 Other disorders of continuity of bone, unspecified pelvic region and thigh
✓6th M84.86 Other disorders of continuity of bone, tibia and fibula
M84.861 Other disorders of continuity of bone, right tibia
M84.862 Other disorders of continuity of bone, left tibia
M84.863 Other disorders of continuity of bone, right fibula
M84.864 Other disorders of continuity of bone, left fibula
M84.869 Other disorders of continuity of bone, unspecified tibia and fibula
✓6th M84.87 Other disorders of continuity of bone, ankle and foot
M84.871 Other disorders of continuity of bone, right ankle and foot
M84.872 Other disorders of continuity of bone, left ankle and foot
M84.879 Other disorders of continuity of bone, unspecified ankle and foot
M84.88 Other disorders of continuity of bone, other site
M84.9 Disorder of continuity of bone, unspecified

✓4th **M85 Other disorders of bone density and structure**
EXCLUDES 1 *osteogenesis imperfecta (Q78.0)*
osteopetrosis (Q78.2)
osteopoikilosis (Q78.8)
polyostotic fibrous dysplasia (Q78.1)
✓5th M85.0 Fibrous dysplasia (monostotic)
EXCLUDES 2 *fibrous dysplasia of jaw (M27.8)*
M85.00 Fibrous dysplasia (monostotic), unspecified site
✓6th M85.01 Fibrous dysplasia (monostotic), shoulder
M85.011 Fibrous dysplasia (monostotic), right shoulder
M85.012 Fibrous dysplasia (monostotic), left shoulder
M85.019 Fibrous dysplasia (monostotic), unspecified shoulder
✓6th M85.02 Fibrous dysplasia (monostotic), upper arm
M85.021 Fibrous dysplasia (monostotic), right upper arm
M85.022 Fibrous dysplasia (monostotic), left upper arm
M85.029 Fibrous dysplasia (monostotic), unspecified upper arm
✓6th M85.03 Fibrous dysplasia (monostotic), forearm
M85.031 Fibrous dysplasia (monostotic), right forearm
M85.032 Fibrous dysplasia (monostotic), left forearm
M85.039 Fibrous dysplasia (monostotic), unspecified forearm
✓6th M85.04 Fibrous dysplasia (monostotic), hand
M85.041 Fibrous dysplasia (monostotic), right hand
M85.042 Fibrous dysplasia (monostotic), left hand
M85.049 Fibrous dysplasia (monostotic), unspecified hand
✓6th M85.05 Fibrous dysplasia (monostotic), thigh
M85.051 Fibrous dysplasia (monostotic), right thigh
M85.052 Fibrous dysplasia (monostotic), left thigh
M85.059 Fibrous dysplasia (monostotic), unspecified thigh
✓6th M85.06 Fibrous dysplasia (monostotic), lower leg
M85.061 Fibrous dysplasia (monostotic), right lower leg
M85.062 Fibrous dysplasia (monostotic), left lower leg
M85.069 Fibrous dysplasia (monostotic), unspecified lower leg
✓6th M85.07 Fibrous dysplasia (monostotic), ankle and foot
M85.071 Fibrous dysplasia (monostotic), right ankle and foot
M85.072 Fibrous dysplasia (monostotic), left ankle and foot
M85.079 Fibrous dysplasia (monostotic), unspecified ankle and foot
M85.08 Fibrous dysplasia (monostotic), other site
M85.09 Fibrous dysplasia (monostotic), multiple sites
✓5th M85.1 Skeletal fluorosis
M85.10 Skeletal fluorosis, unspecified site
✓6th M85.11 Skeletal fluorosis, shoulder
M85.111 Skeletal fluorosis, right shoulder
M85.112 Skeletal fluorosis, left shoulder
M85.119 Skeletal fluorosis, unspecified shoulder
✓6th M85.12 Skeletal fluorosis, upper arm
M85.121 Skeletal fluorosis, right upper arm
M85.122 Skeletal fluorosis, left upper arm
M85.129 Skeletal fluorosis, unspecified upper arm
✓6th M85.13 Skeletal fluorosis, forearm
M85.131 Skeletal fluorosis, right forearm
M85.132 Skeletal fluorosis, left forearm
M85.139 Skeletal fluorosis, unspecified forearm
✓6th M85.14 Skeletal fluorosis, hand
M85.141 Skeletal fluorosis, right hand
M85.142 Skeletal fluorosis, left hand
M85.149 Skeletal fluorosis, unspecified hand
✓6th M85.15 Skeletal fluorosis, thigh
M85.151 Skeletal fluorosis, right thigh
M85.152 Skeletal fluorosis, left thigh
M85.159 Skeletal fluorosis, unspecified thigh
✓6th M85.16 Skeletal fluorosis, lower leg
M85.161 Skeletal fluorosis, right lower leg
M85.162 Skeletal fluorosis, left lower leg
M85.169 Skeletal fluorosis, unspecified lower leg
✓6th M85.17 Skeletal fluorosis, ankle and foot
M85.171 Skeletal fluorosis, right ankle and foot
M85.172 Skeletal fluorosis, left ankle and foot
M85.179 Skeletal fluorosis, unspecified ankle and foot
M85.18 Skeletal fluorosis, other site
M85.19 Skeletal fluorosis, multiple sites
M85.2 Hyperostosis of skull
✓5th M85.3 Osteitis condensans
M85.30 Osteitis condensans, unspecified site
✓6th M85.31 Osteitis condensans, shoulder
M85.311 Osteitis condensans, right shoulder
M85.312 Osteitis condensans, left shoulder
M85.319 Osteitis condensans, unspecified shoulder
✓6th M85.32 Osteitis condensans, upper arm
M85.321 Osteitis condensans, right upper arm
M85.322 Osteitis condensans, left upper arm
M85.329 Osteitis condensans, unspecified upper arm
✓6th M85.33 Osteitis condensans, forearm
M85.331 Osteitis condensans, right forearm
M85.332 Osteitis condensans, left forearm
M85.339 Osteitis condensans, unspecified forearm
✓6th M85.34 Osteitis condensans, hand
M85.341 Osteitis condensans, right hand
M85.342 Osteitis condensans, left hand
M85.349 Osteitis condensans, unspecified hand
✓6th M85.35 Osteitis condensans, thigh
M85.351 Osteitis condensans, right thigh
M85.352 Osteitis condensans, left thigh

M85.359 Osteitis condensans, unspecified thigh

✓6th **M85.36** Osteitis condensans, lower leg
- **M85.361** Osteitis condensans, right lower leg
- **M85.362** Osteitis condensans, left lower leg
- **M85.369** Osteitis condensans, unspecified lower leg

✓6th **M85.37** Osteitis condensans, ankle and foot
- **M85.371** Osteitis condensans, right ankle and foot
- **M85.372** Osteitis condensans, left ankle and foot
- **M85.379** Osteitis condensans, unspecified ankle and foot

M85.38 Osteitis condensans, other site

M85.39 Osteitis condensans, multiple sites

✓5th **M85.4 Solitary bone cyst**

EXCLUDES 2 *solitary cyst of jaw (M27.4)*

M85.40 Solitary bone cyst, unspecified site

✓6th **M85.41** Solitary bone cyst, shoulder
- **M85.411** Solitary bone cyst, right shoulder
- **M85.412** Solitary bone cyst, left shoulder
- **M85.419** Solitary bone cyst, unspecified shoulder

✓6th **M85.42** Solitary bone cyst, humerus
- **M85.421** Solitary bone cyst, right humerus
- **M85.422** Solitary bone cyst, left humerus
- **M85.429** Solitary bone cyst, unspecified humerus

✓6th **M85.43** Solitary bone cyst, ulna and radius
- **M85.431** Solitary bone cyst, right ulna and radius
- **M85.432** Solitary bone cyst, left ulna and radius
- **M85.439** Solitary bone cyst, unspecified ulna and radius

✓6th **M85.44** Solitary bone cyst, hand
- **M85.441** Solitary bone cyst, right hand
- **M85.442** Solitary bone cyst, left hand
- **M85.449** Solitary bone cyst, unspecified hand

✓6th **M85.45** Solitary bone cyst, pelvis
- **M85.451** Solitary bone cyst, right pelvis
- **M85.452** Solitary bone cyst, left pelvis
- **M85.459** Solitary bone cyst, unspecified pelvis

✓6th **M85.46** Solitary bone cyst, tibia and fibula
- **M85.461** Solitary bone cyst, right tibia and fibula
- **M85.462** Solitary bone cyst, left tibia and fibula
- **M85.469** Solitary bone cyst, unspecified tibia and fibula

✓6th **M85.47** Solitary bone cyst, ankle and foot
- **M85.471** Solitary bone cyst, right ankle and foot
- **M85.472** Solitary bone cyst, left ankle and foot
- **M85.479** Solitary bone cyst, unspecified ankle and foot

M85.48 Solitary bone cyst, other site

✓5th **M85.5 Aneurysmal bone cyst**

EXCLUDES 2 *aneurysmal cyst of jaw (M27.4)*

M85.50 Aneurysmal bone cyst, unspecified site

✓6th **M85.51** Aneurysmal bone cyst, shoulder
- **M85.511** Aneurysmal bone cyst, right shoulder
- **M85.512** Aneurysmal bone cyst, left shoulder
- **M85.519** Aneurysmal bone cyst, unspecified shoulder

✓6th **M85.52** Aneurysmal bone cyst, upper arm
- **M85.521** Aneurysmal bone cyst, right upper arm
- **M85.522** Aneurysmal bone cyst, left upper arm
- **M85.529** Aneurysmal bone cyst, unspecified upper arm

✓6th **M85.53** Aneurysmal bone cyst, forearm
- **M85.531** Aneurysmal bone cyst, right forearm
- **M85.532** Aneurysmal bone cyst, left forearm
- **M85.539** Aneurysmal bone cyst, unspecified forearm

✓6th **M85.54** Aneurysmal bone cyst, hand
- **M85.541** Aneurysmal bone cyst, right hand
- **M85.542** Aneurysmal bone cyst, left hand
- **M85.549** Aneurysmal bone cyst, unspecified hand

✓6th **M85.55** Aneurysmal bone cyst, thigh
- **M85.551** Aneurysmal bone cyst, right thigh
- **M85.552** Aneurysmal bone cyst, left thigh
- **M85.559** Aneurysmal bone cyst, unspecified thigh

✓6th **M85.56** Aneurysmal bone cyst, lower leg
- **M85.561** Aneurysmal bone cyst, right lower leg
- **M85.562** Aneurysmal bone cyst, left lower leg
- **M85.569** Aneurysmal bone cyst, unspecified lower leg

✓6th **M85.57** Aneurysmal bone cyst, ankle and foot
- **M85.571** Aneurysmal bone cyst, right ankle and foot
- **M85.572** Aneurysmal bone cyst, left ankle and foot
- **M85.579** Aneurysmal bone cyst, unspecified ankle and foot

M85.58 Aneurysmal bone cyst, other site

M85.59 Aneurysmal bone cyst, multiple sites

✓5th **M85.6 Other cyst of bone**

EXCLUDES 1 *cyst of jaw NEC (M27.4)*
osteitis fibrosa cystica generalisata [von Recklinghausen's disease of bone] (E21.0)

M85.60 Other cyst of bone, unspecified site

✓6th **M85.61** Other cyst of bone, shoulder
- **M85.611** Other cyst of bone, right shoulder
- **M85.612** Other cyst of bone, left shoulder
- **M85.619** Other cyst of bone, unspecified shoulder

✓6th **M85.62** Other cyst of bone, upper arm
- **M85.621** Other cyst of bone, right upper arm
- **M85.622** Other cyst of bone, left upper arm
- **M85.629** Other cyst of bone, unspecified upper arm

✓6th **M85.63** Other cyst of bone, forearm
- **M85.631** Other cyst of bone, right forearm
- **M85.632** Other cyst of bone, left forearm
- **M85.639** Other cyst of bone, unspecified forearm

✓6th **M85.64** Other cyst of bone, hand
- **M85.641** Other cyst of bone, right hand
- **M85.642** Other cyst of bone, left hand
- **M85.649** Other cyst of bone, unspecified hand

✓6th **M85.65** Other cyst of bone, thigh
- **M85.651** Other cyst of bone, right thigh
- **M85.652** Other cyst of bone, left thigh
- **M85.659** Other cyst of bone, unspecified thigh

✓6th **M85.66** Other cyst of bone, lower leg
- **M85.661** Other cyst of bone, right lower leg
- **M85.662** Other cyst of bone, left lower leg
- **M85.669** Other cyst of bone, unspecified lower leg

✓6th **M85.67** Other cyst of bone, ankle and foot
- **M85.671** Other cyst of bone, right ankle and foot
- **M85.672** Other cyst of bone, left ankle and foot
- **M85.679** Other cyst of bone, unspecified ankle and foot

M85.68 Other cyst of bone, other site

M85.69 Other cyst of bone, multiple sites

✓5th **M85.8 Other specified disorders of bone density and structure**

Hyperostosis of bones, except skull
Osteosclerosis, acquired

EXCLUDES 1 *diffuse idiopathic skeletal hyperostosis [DISH] (M48.1)*
osteosclerosis congenita (Q77.4)
osteosclerosis fragilitas (generalista) (Q78.2)
osteosclerosis myelofibrosis (D75.81)

M85.80 Other specified disorders of bone density and structure, unspecified site

✓6th **M85.81** Other specified disorders of bone density and structure, shoulder
- **M85.811** Other specified disorders of bone density and structure, right shoulder
- **M85.812** Other specified disorders of bone density and structure, left shoulder
- **M85.819** Other specified disorders of bone density and structure, unspecified shoulder

✓6th **M85.82** Other specified disorders of bone density and structure, upper arm
- **M85.821** Other specified disorders of bone density and structure, right upper arm
- **M85.822** Other specified disorders of bone density and structure, left upper arm

M85.829 Other specified disorders of bone density and structure, unspecified upper arm

✓6th M85.83 Other specified disorders of bone density and structure, forearm

M85.831 Other specified disorders of bone density and structure, right forearm

M85.832 Other specified disorders of bone density and structure, left forearm

M85.839 Other specified disorders of bone density and structure, unspecified forearm

✓6th M85.84 Other specified disorders of bone density and structure, hand

M85.841 Other specified disorders of bone density and structure, right hand

M85.842 Other specified disorders of bone density and structure, left hand

M85.849 Other specified disorders of bone density and structure, unspecified hand

✓6th M85.85 Other specified disorders of bone density and structure, thigh

M85.851 Other specified disorders of bone density and structure, right thigh

M85.852 Other specified disorders of bone density and structure, left thigh

M85.859 Other specified disorders of bone density and structure, unspecified thigh

✓6th M85.86 Other specified disorders of bone density and structure, lower leg

M85.861 Other specified disorders of bone density and structure, right lower leg

M85.862 Other specified disorders of bone density and structure, left lower leg

M85.869 Other specified disorders of bone density and structure, unspecified lower leg

✓6th M85.87 Other specified disorders of bone density and structure, ankle and foot

M85.871 Other specified disorders of bone density and structure, right ankle and foot

M85.872 Other specified disorders of bone density and structure, left ankle and foot

M85.879 Other specified disorders of bone density and structure, unspecified ankle and foot

M85.88 Other specified disorders of bone density and structure, other site

M85.89 Other specified disorders of bone density and structure, multiple sites

M85.9 Disorder of bone density and structure, unspecified

Other osteopathies (M86-M9Ø)

EXCLUDES1 *postprocedural osteopathies (M96.-)*

✓4th **M86 Osteomyelitis**

Use additional code (B95-B97) to identify infectious agent

Use additional code to identify major osseous defect, if applicable (M89.7-)

EXCLUDES1 *osteomyelitis due to:*
echinococcus (B67.2)
gonococcus (A54.43)
salmonella (AØ2.24)

EXCLUDES2 *ostemyelitis of:*
orbit (HØ5.Ø-)
petrous bone (H7Ø.2-)
vertebra (M46.2-)

✓5th M86.Ø Acute hematogenous osteomyelitis

M86.ØØ Acute hematogenous osteomyelitis, unspecified site CC
CC Excl: A17.9, A18.Ø3-A18.Ø9, A18.82, A18.84, A18.89, M46.2Ø-M46.39, M86.ØØ-M86.9

✓6th M86.Ø1 Acute hematogenous osteomyelitis, shoulder

M86.Ø11 Acute hematogenous osteomyelitis, right shoulder CC
CC Excl: A17.9, A18.Ø3-A18.Ø9, A18.82, A18.84, A18.89, M46.2Ø-M46.39, M86.ØØ, M86.Ø8-M86.1Ø, M86.18-M86.2Ø, M86.28-M86.319, M86.38-M86.419, M86.48-M86.519, M86.58-M86.619, M86.68-M86.8X1, M86.8X8-M86.9

M86.Ø12 Acute hematogenous osteomyelitis, left shoulder CC
CC Excl: See code: M86.Ø11

M86.Ø19 Acute hematogenous osteomyelitis, unspecified shoulder CC
CC Excl: See code: M86.Ø11

✓6th M86.Ø2 Acute hematogenous osteomyelitis, humerus

M86.Ø21 Acute hematogenous osteomyelitis, right humerus CC
CC Excl: A17.9, A18.Ø3-A18.Ø9, A18.82, A18.84, A18.89, M46.2Ø-M46.39, M86.ØØ, M86.Ø8-M86.1Ø, M86.18-M86.2Ø, M86.28-M86.3Ø, M86.321-M86.329, M86.38-M86.4Ø, M86.421-M86.429, M86.48-M86.5Ø, M86.521-M86.529, M86.58-M86.6Ø, M86.621-M86.629, M86.68-M86.8XØ, M86.8X2, M86.8X8-M86.9

M86.Ø22 Acute hematogenous osteomyelitis, left humerus CC
CC Excl: See code: M86.Ø21

M86.Ø29 Acute hematogenous osteomyelitis, unspecified humerus CC
CC Excl: See code: M86.Ø21

✓6th M86.Ø3 Acute hematogenous osteomyelitis, radius and ulna

M86.Ø31 Acute hematogenous osteomyelitis, right radius and ulna CC
CC Excl: A17.9, A18.Ø3-A18.Ø9, A18.82, A18.84, A18.89, M46.2Ø-M46.39, M86.ØØ, M86.Ø8-M86.1Ø, M86.18-M86.2Ø, M86.28-M86.3Ø, M86.331-M86.339, M86.38-M86.4Ø, M86.431-M86.439, M86.48-M86.5Ø, M86.531-M86.539, M86.58-M86.6Ø, M86.631-M86.639, M86.68-M86.8XØ, M86.8X3, M86.8X8-M86.9

M86.Ø32 Acute hematogenous osteomyelitis, left radius and ulna CC
CC Excl: See code: M86.Ø31

M86.Ø39 Acute hematogenous osteomyelitis, unspecified radius and ulna CC
CC Excl: See code: M86.Ø31

✓6th M86.Ø4 Acute hematogenous osteomyelitis, hand

M86.Ø41 Acute hematogenous osteomyelitis, right hand CC
CC Excl: A17.9, A18.Ø3-A18.Ø9, A18.82, A18.84, A18.89, M46.2Ø-M46.39, M86.ØØ, M86.Ø8-M86.1Ø, M86.18-M86.2Ø, M86.28-M86.3Ø, M86.341-M86.349, M86.38-M86.4Ø, M86.441-M86.449, M86.48-M86.5Ø, M86.541-M86.549, M86.58-M86.6Ø, M86.641-M86.649, M86.68-M86.8XØ, M86.8X4, M86.8X8-M86.9

M86.Ø42 Acute hematogenous osteomyelitis, left hand CC
CC Excl: See code: M86.Ø41

M86.Ø49 Acute hematogenous osteomyelitis, unspecified hand CC
CC Excl: See code: M86.Ø41

✓6th M86.Ø5 Acute hematogenous osteomyelitis, femur

M86.Ø51 Acute hematogenous osteomyelitis, right femur CC
CC Excl: A17.9, A18.Ø3-A18.Ø9, A18.82, A18.84, A18.89, M46.2Ø-M46.39, M86.ØØ, M86.Ø8-M86.1Ø, M86.18-M86.2Ø, M86.28-M86.3Ø, M86.351-M86.359, M86.38-M86.4Ø, M86.451-M86.459, M86.48-M86.5Ø, M86.551-M86.559, M86.58-M86.6Ø, M86.651-M86.659, M86.68-M86.8XØ, M86.8X5, M86.8X8-M86.9

M86.Ø52 Acute hematogenous osteomyelitis, left femur CC
CC Excl: See code: M86.Ø51

M86.Ø59 Acute hematogenous osteomyelitis, unspecified femur CC
CC Excl: See code: M86.Ø51

✓6th M86.Ø6 Acute hematogenous osteomyelitis, tibia and fibula

M86.Ø61 Acute hematogenous osteomyelitis, right tibia and fibula CC
CC Excl: A17.9, A18.Ø3-A18.Ø9, A18.82, A18.84, A18.89, M46.2Ø-M46.39, M86.ØØ, M86.Ø8-M86.1Ø, M86.18-M86.2Ø, M86.28-M86.3Ø, M86.361-M86.369, M86.38-M86.4Ø, M86.461-M86.469, M86.48-M86.5Ø, M86.561-M86.569, M86.58-M86.6Ø, M86.661-M86.669, M86.68-M86.8XØ, M86.8X6, M86.8X8-M86.9

M86.Ø62 Acute hematogenous osteomyelitis, left tibia and fibula CC
CC Excl: See code: M86.Ø61

M86.Ø69 Acute hematogenous osteomyelitis, unspecified tibia and fibula CC
CC Excl: See code: M86.Ø61

✓6th **M86.Ø7 Acute hematogenous osteomyelitis, ankle and foot**

M86.Ø71 Acute hematogenous osteomyelitis, right ankle and foot CC
CC Excl: A17.9, A18.Ø3-A18.Ø9, A18.82, A18.84, A18.89, M46.2Ø-M46.39, M86.ØØ, M86.Ø8-M86.1Ø, M86.18-M86.2Ø, M86.28-M86.3Ø, M86.371-M86.4Ø, M86.471-M86.5Ø, M86.571-M86.6Ø, M86.671-M86.8XØ, M86.8X7-M86.9

M86.Ø72 Acute hematogenous osteomyelitis, left ankle and foot CC
CC Excl: See code: M86.Ø71

M86.Ø79 Acute hematogenous osteomyelitis, unspecified ankle and foot CC
CC Excl: See code: M86.Ø71

M86.Ø8 Acute hematogenous osteomyelitis, other sites CC
CC Excl: A17.9-A18.Ø1, A18.Ø3-A18.Ø9, A18.82, A18.84, A18.89, M46.2Ø-M46.39, M86.ØØ-M86.9

M86.Ø9 Acute hematogenous osteomyelitis, multiple sites CC
CC Excl: A17.9, A18.Ø3-A18.Ø9, A18.82, A18.84, A18.89, M46.2Ø-M46.39, M86.ØØ-M86.9

✓5th **M86.1 Other acute osteomyelitis**

M86.1Ø Other acute osteomyelitis, unspecified site CC
CC Excl: See code: 86.Ø9

✓6th **M86.11 Other acute osteomyelitis, shoulder**

M86.111 Other acute osteomyelitis, right shoulder CC
CC Excl: See code: M86.Ø71

M86.112 Other acute osteomyelitis, left shoulder CC
CC Excl: See code: M86.Ø71

M86.119 Other acute osteomyelitis, unspecified shoulder CC
CC Excl: See code: M86.Ø71

✓6th **M86.12 Other acute osteomyelitis, humerus**

M86.121 Other acute osteomyelitis, right humerus CC
CC Excl: See code: M86.Ø21

M86.122 Other acute osteomyelitis, left humerus CC
CC Excl: See code: M86.Ø21

M86.129 Other acute osteomyelitis, unspecified humerus CC
CC Excl: See code: M86.Ø21

✓6th **M86.13 Other acute osteomyelitis, radius and ulna**

M86.131 Other acute osteomyelitis, right radius and ulna CC
CC Excl: See code: M86.Ø31

M86.132 Other acute osteomyelitis, left radius and ulna CC
CC Excl: See code: M86.Ø31

M86.139 Other acute osteomyelitis, unspecified radius and ulna CC
CC Excl: See code: M86.Ø31

✓6th **M86.14 Other acute osteomyelitis, hand**

M86.141 Other acute osteomyelitis, right hand CC
CC Excl: See code: M86.Ø41

M86.142 Other acute osteomyelitis, left hand CC
CC Excl: See code: M86.Ø41

M86.149 Other acute osteomyelitis, unspecified hand CC
CC Excl: See code: M86.Ø41

✓6th **M86.15 Other acute osteomyelitis, femur**

M86.151 Other acute osteomyelitis, right femur CC
CC Excl: See code: M86.Ø51

M86.152 Other acute osteomyelitis, left femur CC
CC Excl: See code: M86.Ø51

M86.159 Other acute osteomyelitis, unspecified femur CC
CC Excl: See code: M86.Ø51

✓6th **M86.16 Other acute osteomyelitis, tibia and fibula**

M86.161 Other acute osteomyelitis, right tibia and fibula CC
CC Excl: See code: M86.Ø61

M86.162 Other acute osteomyelitis, left tibia and fibula CC
CC Excl: See code: M86.Ø61

M86.169 Other acute osteomyelitis, unspecified tibia and fibula CC
CC Excl: See code: M86.Ø61

✓6th **M86.17 Other acute osteomyelitis, ankle and foot**

M86.171 Other acute osteomyelitis, right ankle and foot CC
CC Excl: See code: M86.Ø71

M86.172 Other acute osteomyelitis, left ankle and foot CC
CC Excl: See code: M86.Ø71

M86.179 Other acute osteomyelitis, unspecified ankle and foot CC
CC Excl: See code: M86.Ø71

M86.18 Other acute osteomyelitis, other site CC
CC Excl: A17.9-A18.Ø1, A18.Ø3-A18.Ø9, A18.82, A18.84, A18.89, M46.2Ø-M46.39, M86.ØØ-M86.9

M86.19 Other acute osteomyelitis, multiple sites CC
CC Excl: A17.9, A18.Ø3-A18.Ø9, A18.82, A18.84, A18.89, M46.2Ø-M46.39, M86.ØØ-M86.9

✓5th **M86.2 Subacute osteomyelitis**

M86.2Ø Subacute osteomyelitis, unspecified site CC
CC Excl: See code: M86.19

✓6th **M86.21 Subacute osteomyelitis, shoulder**

M86.211 Subacute osteomyelitis, right shoulder CC
CC Excl: A17.9, A18.Ø3-A18.Ø9, A18.82, A18.84, A18.89, M46.2Ø-M46.39, M86.ØØ, M86.Ø8-M86.1Ø, M86.18-M86.2Ø, M86.28-M86.319, M86.38-M86.419, M86.48-M86.519, M86.58-M86.619, M86.68-M86.8X1, M86.8X8-M86.9

M86.212 Subacute osteomyelitis, left shoulder CC
CC Excl: See code: M86.211

M86.219 Subacute osteomyelitis, unspecified shoulder CC
CC Excl: See code: M86.211

✓6th **M86.22 Subacute osteomyelitis, humerus**

M86.221 Subacute osteomyelitis, right humerus CC
CC Excl: A17.9, A18.Ø3-A18.Ø9, A18.82, A18.84, A18.89, M46.2Ø-M46.39, M86.ØØ, M86.Ø8-M86.1Ø, M86.18-M86.2Ø, M86.28-M86.3Ø, M86.321-M86.329, M86.38-M86.4Ø, M86.421-M86.429, M86.48-M86.5Ø, M86.521-M86.529, M86.58-M86.6Ø, M86.621-M86.629, M86.68-M86.8XØ, M86.8X2, M86.8X8-M86.9

M86.222 Subacute osteomyelitis, left humerus CC
CC Excl: See code: M86.221

M86.229 Subacute osteomyelitis, unspecified humerus CC
CC Excl: See code: M86.221

✓6th **M86.23 Subacute osteomyelitis, radius and ulna**

M86.231 Subacute osteomyelitis, right radius and ulna CC
CC Excl: A17.9, A18.Ø3-A18.Ø9, A18.82, A18.84, A18.89, M46.2Ø-M46.39, M86.ØØ, M86.Ø8-M86.1Ø, M86.18-M86.2Ø, M86.28-M86.3Ø, M86.331-M86.339, M86.38-M86.4Ø, M86.431-M86.439, M86.48-M86.5Ø, M86.531-M86.539, M86.58-M86.6Ø, M86.631-M86.639, M86.68-M86.8XØ, M86.8X3, M86.8X8-M86.9

M86.232 Subacute osteomyelitis, left radius and ulna CC
CC Excl: See code: M86.231

M86.239 Subacute osteomyelitis, unspecified radius and ulna CC
CC Excl: See code: M86.231

✓6th **M86.24 Subacute osteomyelitis, hand**

M86.241 Subacute osteomyelitis, right hand CC
CC Excl: A17.9, A18.Ø3-A18.Ø9, A18.82, A18.84, A18.89, M46.2Ø-M46.39, M86.ØØ, M86.Ø8-M86.1Ø, M86.18-M86.2Ø, M86.28-M86.3Ø, M86.341-M86.349, M86.38-M86.4Ø, M86.441-M86.449, M86.48-M86.5Ø, M86.541-M86.549, M86.58-M86.6Ø, M86.641-M86.649, M86.68-M86.8XØ, M86.8X4, M86.8X8-M86.9

M86.242 Subacute osteomyelitis, left hand CC
CC Excl: See code: M86.241

M86.249 Subacute osteomyelitis, unspecified hand CC
CC Excl: See code: M86.241

✓6th **M86.25 Subacute osteomyelitis, femur**

M86.251 Subacute osteomyelitis, right femur CC
CC Excl: A17.9, A18.03-A18.09, A18.82, A18.84, A18.89, M46.20-M46.39, M86.00, M86.08-M86.10, M86.18-M86.20, M86.28-M86.30, M86.351-M86.359, M86.38-M86.40, M86.451-M86.459, M86.48-M86.50, M86.551-M86.559, M86.58-M86.60, M86.651-M86.659, M86.68-M86.8X0, M86.8X5, M86.8X8-M86.9

M86.252 Subacute osteomyelitis, left femur CC
CC Excl: See code: M86.251

M86.259 Subacute osteomyelitis, unspecified femur CC
CC Excl: See code: M86.251

✓6th **M86.26 Subacute osteomyelitis, tibia and fibula**

M86.261 Subacute osteomyelitis, right tibia and fibula CC
CC Excl: A17.9, A18.03-A18.09, A18.82, A18.84, A18.89, M46.20-M46.39, M86.00, M86.08-M86.10, M86.18-M86.20, M86.28-M86.30, M86.361-M86.369, M86.38-M86.40, M86.461-M86.469, M86.48-M86.50, M86.561-M86.569, M86.58-M86.60, M86.661-M86.669, M86.68-M86.8X0, M86.8X6, M86.8X8-M86.9

M86.262 Subacute osteomyelitis, left tibia and fibula CC
CC Excl: See code: M86.261

M86.269 Subacute osteomyelitis, unspecified tibia and fibula CC
CC Excl: See code: M86.261

✓6th **M86.27 Subacute osteomyelitis, ankle and foot**

M86.271 Subacute osteomyelitis, right ankle and foot CC
CC Excl: A17.9, A18.03-A18.09, A18.82, A18.84, A18.89, M46.20-M46.39, M86.00, M86.08-M86.10, M86.18-M86.20, M86.28-M86.30, M86.371-M86.40, M86.471-M86.50, M86.571-M86.60, M86.671-M86.8X0, M86.8X7-M86.9

M86.272 Subacute osteomyelitis, left ankle and foot CC
CC Excl: See code: M86.271

M86.279 Subacute osteomyelitis, unspecified ankle and foot CC
CC Excl: See code: M86.271

M86.28 Subacute osteomyelitis, other site CC
CC Excl: A17.9-A18.01, A18.03-A18.09, A18.82, A18.84, A18.89, M46.20-M46.39, M86.00-M86.9

M86.29 Subacute osteomyelitis, multiple sites CC
CC Excl: A17.9, A18.03-A18.09, A18.82, A18.84, A18.89, M46.20-M46.39, M86.00-M86.9

✓5th **M86.3 Chronic multifocal osteomyelitis**

M86.30 Chronic multifocal osteomyelitis, unspecified site CC
CC Excl: M46.20-M46.39, M86.30-M86.9, M88.0-M88.9, M90.60-M90.69

✓6th **M86.31 Chronic multifocal osteomyelitis, shoulder**

M86.311 Chronic multifocal osteomyelitis, right shoulder CC
CC Excl: A02.24, A17.9, A18.03-A18.09, A18.82, A18.84, A18.89, M46.20-M46.39, M86.00-M86.9

M86.312 Chronic multifocal osteomyelitis, left shoulder CC
CC Excl: See code: M86.311

M86.319 Chronic multifocal osteomyelitis, unspecified shoulder CC
CC Excl: See code: M86.311

✓6th **M86.32 Chronic multifocal osteomyelitis, humerus**

M86.321 Chronic multifocal osteomyelitis, right humerus CC
CC Excl: See code: M86.311

M86.322 Chronic multifocal osteomyelitis, left humerus CC
CC Excl: See code: M86.311

M86.329 Chronic multifocal osteomyelitis, unspecified humerus CC
CC Excl: See code: M86.311

✓6th **M86.33 Chronic multifocal osteomyelitis, radius and ulna**

M86.331 Chronic multifocal osteomyelitis, right radius and ulna CC
CC Excl: See code: M86.311

M86.332 Chronic multifocal osteomyelitis, left radius and ulna CC
CC Excl: See code: M86.311

M86.339 Chronic multifocal osteomyelitis, unspecified radius and ulna CC
CC Excl: See code: M86.311

✓6th **M86.34 Chronic multifocal osteomyelitis, hand**

M86.341 Chronic multifocal osteomyelitis, right hand CC
CC Excl: See code: M86.311

M86.342 Chronic multifocal osteomyelitis, left hand CC
CC Excl: See code: M86.311

M86.349 Chronic multifocal osteomyelitis, unspecified hand CC
CC Excl: See code: M86.311

✓6th **M86.35 Chronic multifocal osteomyelitis, femur**

M86.351 Chronic multifocal osteomyelitis, right femur CC
CC Excl: See code: M86.311

M86.352 Chronic multifocal osteomyelitis, left femur CC
CC Excl: See code: M86.311

M86.359 Chronic multifocal osteomyelitis, unspecified femur CC
CC Excl: See code: M86.311

✓6th **M86.36 Chronic multifocal osteomyelitis, tibia and fibula**

M86.361 Chronic multifocal osteomyelitis, right tibia and fibula CC
CC Excl: See code: M86.311

M86.362 Chronic multifocal osteomyelitis, left tibia and fibula CC
CC Excl: See code: M86.311

M86.369 Chronic multifocal osteomyelitis, unspecified tibia and fibula CC
CC Excl: See code: M86.311

✓6th **M86.37 Chronic multifocal osteomyelitis, ankle and foot**

M86.371 Chronic multifocal osteomyelitis, right ankle and foot CC
CC Excl: See code: M86.311

M86.372 Chronic multifocal osteomyelitis, left ankle and foot CC
CC Excl: See code: M86.311

M86.379 Chronic multifocal osteomyelitis, unspecified ankle and foot CC
CC Excl: See code: M86.311

M86.38 Chronic multifocal osteomyelitis, other site CC
CC Excl: See code: 86.311

M86.39 Chronic multifocal osteomyelitis, multiple sites CC
CC Excl: See code: 86.311

✓5th **M86.4 Chronic osteomyelitis with draining sinus**

CC Excl: For CC codes in subcategory M86.4, M86.5, M86.6, M86.8, M86.9, unless otherwise noted: A02.24, A17.9, A18.03-A18.09, A18.82, A18.84, A18.89, M46.20-M46.39, M86.00-M86.9

M86.40 Chronic osteomyelitis with draining sinus, unspecified site CC
CC Excl: M46.20-M46.39, M86.30-M86.9, M88.0-M88.9, M90.60-M90.69

✓6th **M86.41 Chronic osteomyelitis with draining sinus, shoulder**

M86.411 Chronic osteomyelitis with draining sinus, right shoulder CC

M86.412 Chronic osteomyelitis with draining sinus, left shoulder CC

M86.419 Chronic osteomyelitis with draining sinus, unspecified shoulder CC

✓6th **M86.42 Chronic osteomyelitis with draining sinus, humerus**

M86.421 Chronic osteomyelitis with draining sinus, right humerus CC

M86.422 Chronic osteomyelitis with draining sinus, left humerus CC

M86.429 Chronic osteomyelitis with draining sinus, unspecified humerus CC

✓6th **M86.43 Chronic osteomyelitis with draining sinus, radius and ulna**

M86.431 Chronic osteomyelitis with draining sinus, right radius and ulna CC

M86.432 Chronic osteomyelitis with draining sinus, left radius and ulna CC

M86.439 Chronic osteomyelitis with draining sinus, unspecified radius and ulna CC

✓6th M86.44 Chronic osteomyelitis with draining sinus, hand

M86.441 Chronic osteomyelitis with draining sinus, right hand CC

M86.442 Chronic osteomyelitis with draining sinus, left hand CC

M86.449 Chronic osteomyelitis with draining sinus, unspecified hand CC

✓6th M86.45 Chronic osteomyelitis with draining sinus, femur

M86.451 Chronic osteomyelitis with draining sinus, right femur CC

M86.452 Chronic osteomyelitis with draining sinus, left femur CC

M86.459 Chronic osteomyelitis with draining sinus, unspecified femur CC

✓6th M86.46 Chronic osteomyelitis with draining sinus, tibia and fibula

M86.461 Chronic osteomyelitis with draining sinus, right tibia and fibula CC

M86.462 Chronic osteomyelitis with draining sinus, left tibia and fibula CC

M86.469 Chronic osteomyelitis with draining sinus, unspecified tibia and fibula CC

✓6th M86.47 Chronic osteomyelitis with draining sinus, ankle and foot

M86.471 Chronic osteomyelitis with draining sinus, right ankle and foot CC

M86.472 Chronic osteomyelitis with draining sinus, left ankle and foot CC

M86.479 Chronic osteomyelitis with draining sinus, unspecified ankle and foot CC

M86.48 Chronic osteomyelitis with draining sinus, other site CC

M86.49 Chronic osteomyelitis with draining sinus, multiple sites CC

✓5th M86.5 Other chronic hematogenous osteomyelitis

M86.50 Other chronic hematogenous osteomyelitis, unspecified site CC

CC Excl: M46.20-M46.39, M86.30-M86.9, M88.0-M88.9, M90.60-M90.69

✓6th M86.51 Other chronic hematogenous osteomyelitis, shoulder

M86.511 Other chronic hematogenous osteomyelitis, right shoulder CC

M86.512 Other chronic hematogenous osteomyelitis, left shoulder CC

M86.519 Other chronic hematogenous osteomyelitis, unspecified shoulder CC

✓6th M86.52 Other chronic hematogenous osteomyelitis, humerus

M86.521 Other chronic hematogenous osteomyelitis, right humerus CC

M86.522 Other chronic hematogenous osteomyelitis, left humerus CC

M86.529 Other chronic hematogenous osteomyelitis, unspecified humerus CC

✓6th M86.53 Other chronic hematogenous osteomyelitis, radius and ulna

M86.531 Other chronic hematogenous osteomyelitis, right radius and ulna CC

M86.532 Other chronic hematogenous osteomyelitis, left radius and ulna CC

M86.539 Other chronic hematogenous osteomyelitis, unspecified radius and ulna CC

✓6th M86.54 Other chronic hematogenous osteomyelitis, hand

M86.541 Other chronic hematogenous osteomyelitis, right hand CC

M86.542 Other chronic hematogenous osteomyelitis, left hand CC

M86.549 Other chronic hematogenous osteomyelitis, unspecified hand CC

✓6th M86.55 Other chronic hematogenous osteomyelitis, femur

M86.551 Other chronic hematogenous osteomyelitis, right femur CC

M86.552 Other chronic hematogenous osteomyelitis, left femur CC

M86.559 Other chronic hematogenous osteomyelitis, unspecified femur CC

✓6th M86.56 Other chronic hematogenous osteomyelitis, tibia and fibula

M86.561 Other chronic hematogenous osteomyelitis, right tibia and fibula CC

M86.562 Other chronic hematogenous osteomyelitis, left tibia and fibula CC

M86.569 Other chronic hematogenous osteomyelitis, unspecified tibia and fibula CC

✓6th M86.57 Other chronic hematogenous osteomyelitis, ankle and foot

M86.571 Other chronic hematogenous osteomyelitis, right ankle and foot CC

M86.572 Other chronic hematogenous osteomyelitis, left ankle and foot CC

M86.579 Other chronic hematogenous osteomyelitis, unspecified ankle and foot CC

M86.58 Other chronic hematogenous osteomyelitis, other site CC

M86.59 Other chronic hematogenous osteomyelitis, multiple sites CC

✓5th M86.6 Other chronic osteomyelitis

M86.60 Other chronic osteomyelitis, unspecified site CC

CC Excl: M46.20-M46.39, M86.30-M86.9, M88.0-M88.9, M90.60-M90.69

✓6th M86.61 Other chronic osteomyelitis, shoulder

M86.611 Other chronic osteomyelitis, right shoulder CC

M86.612 Other chronic osteomyelitis, left shoulder CC

M86.619 Other chronic osteomyelitis, unspecified shoulder CC

✓6th M86.62 Other chronic osteomyelitis, humerus

M86.621 Other chronic osteomyelitis, right humerus CC

M86.622 Other chronic osteomyelitis, left humerus CC

M86.629 Other chronic osteomyelitis, unspecified humerus CC

✓6th M86.63 Other chronic osteomyelitis, radius and ulna

M86.631 Other chronic osteomyelitis, right radius and ulna CC

M86.632 Other chronic osteomyelitis, left radius and ulna CC

M86.639 Other chronic osteomyelitis, unspecified radius and ulna CC

✓6th M86.64 Other chronic osteomyelitis, hand

M86.641 Other chronic osteomyelitis, right hand CC

M86.642 Other chronic osteomyelitis, left hand CC

M86.649 Other chronic osteomyelitis, unspecified hand CC

✓6th M86.65 Other chronic osteomyelitis, thigh

M86.651 Other chronic osteomyelitis, right thigh CC

M86.652 Other chronic osteomyelitis, left thigh CC

M86.659 Other chronic osteomyelitis, unspecified thigh CC

✓6th M86.66 Other chronic osteomyelitis, tibia and fibula

M86.661 Other chronic osteomyelitis, right tibia and fibula CC

M86.662 Other chronic osteomyelitis, left tibia and fibula CC

M86.669 Other chronic osteomyelitis, unspecified tibia and fibula CC

✓6th M86.67 Other chronic osteomyelitis, ankle and foot

M86.671 Other chronic osteomyelitis, right ankle and foot CC

M86.672 Other chronic osteomyelitis, left ankle and foot CC

M86.679 Other chronic osteomyelitis, unspecified ankle and foot CC

M86.68 Other chronic osteomyelitis, other site CC

M86.69 Other chronic osteomyelitis, multiple sites CC

✓5th **M86.8 Other osteomyelitis**
Brodie's abscess

✓6th **M86.8X Other osteomyelitis**

M86.8XØ Other osteomyelitis, multiple sites CC
M86.8X1 Other osteomyelitis, shoulder CC
M86.8X2 Other osteomyelitis, upper arm CC
M86.8X3 Other osteomyelitis, forearm CC
M86.8X4 Other osteomyelitis, hand CC
M86.8X5 Other osteomyelitis, thigh CC
M86.8X6 Other osteomyelitis, lower leg CC
M86.8X7 Other osteomyelitis, ankle and foot CC
M86.8X8 Other osteomyelitis, other site CC
M86.8X9 Other osteomyelitis, unspecified sites CC
CC Excl: M46.2Ø-M46.39, M86.3Ø-M86.9, M88.Ø-M88.9, M9Ø.6Ø-M9Ø.69

M86.9 Osteomyelitis, unspecified CC
Infection of bone NOS
Periostitis without osteomyelitis
CC Excl: See code: M86.8X9

✓4th **M87 Osteonecrosis**

INCLUDES avascular necrosis of bone

Use additional code to identify major osseous defect, if applicable (M89.7-)

EXCLUDES 1 *juvenile osteonecrosis (M91-M92)*
osteochondropathies (M9Ø-M93)

✓5th **M87.Ø Idiopathic aseptic necrosis of bone**

M87.ØØ Idiopathic aseptic necrosis of unspecified bone CC
CC Excl: M87.ØØ-M87.9, M9Ø.5Ø-M9Ø.59

✓6th **M87.Ø1 Idiopathic aseptic necrosis of shoulder**
Idiopathic aseptic necrosis of clavicle and scapula

M87.Ø11 Idiopathic aseptic necrosis of right shoulder CC
CC Excl: M87.ØØ-M87.Ø5Ø, M87.Ø61-M87.Ø73, M87.Ø77-M87.146, M87.161-M87.173, M87.177-M87.25Ø, M87.261-M87.273, M87.277-M87.346, M87.361-M87.373, M87.377-M87.849, M87.861-M87.873, M87.877-M87.9, M9Ø.5Ø-M9Ø.549, M9Ø.561-M9Ø.59

M87.Ø12 Idiopathic aseptic necrosis of left shoulder CC
CC Excl: See code: M87.Ø11

M87.Ø19 Idiopathic aseptic necrosis of unspecified shoulder CC
CC Excl: See code: M87.Ø11

✓6th **M87.Ø2 Idiopathic aseptic necrosis of humerus**

M87.Ø21 Idiopathic aseptic necrosis of right humerus CC
CC Excl: See code: M87.Ø11

M87.Ø22 Idiopathic aseptic necrosis of left humerus CC
CC Excl: See code: M87.Ø11

M87.Ø29 Idiopathic aseptic necrosis of unspecified humerus CC
CC Excl: See code: M87.Ø11

✓6th **M87.Ø3 Idiopathic aseptic necrosis of radius, ulna and carpus**

M87.Ø31 Idiopathic aseptic necrosis of right radius CC
CC Excl: M87.ØØ-M87.9, M9Ø.5Ø-M9Ø.59

M87.Ø32 Idiopathic aseptic necrosis of left radius CC
CC Excl: See code: M87.31

M87.Ø33 Idiopathic aseptic necrosis of unspecified radius CC
CC Excl: See code: M87.31

M87.Ø34 Idiopathic aseptic necrosis of right ulna CC
CC Excl: See code: M87.31

M87.Ø35 Idiopathic aseptic necrosis of left ulna CC
CC Excl: See code: M87.31

M87.Ø36 Idiopathic aseptic necrosis of unspecified ulna CC
CC Excl: See code: M87.31

M87.Ø37 Idiopathic aseptic necrosis of right carpus CC
CC Excl: See code: M87.31

M87.Ø38 Idiopathic aseptic necrosis of left carpus CC
CC Excl: See code: M87.31

M87.Ø39 Idiopathic aseptic necrosis of unspecified carpus CC
CC Excl: See code: M87.31

✓6th **M87.Ø4 Idiopathic aseptic necrosis of hand and fingers**
Idiopathic aseptic necrosis of metacarpals and phalanges of hands

M87.Ø41 Idiopathic aseptic necrosis of right hand CC
CC Excl: See code: M87.31

M87.Ø42 Idiopathic aseptic necrosis of left hand CC
CC Excl: See code: M87.31

M87.Ø43 Idiopathic aseptic necrosis of unspecified hand CC
CC Excl: See code: M87.31

M87.Ø44 Idiopathic aseptic necrosis of right finger(s) CC
CC Excl: See code: M87.31

M87.Ø45 Idiopathic aseptic necrosis of left finger(s) CC
CC Excl: See code: M87.31

M87.Ø46 Idiopathic aseptic necrosis of unspecified finger(s) CC
CC Excl: See code: M87.31

✓6th **M87.Ø5 Idiopathic aseptic necrosis of pelvis and femur**

M87.Ø5Ø Idiopathic aseptic necrosis of pelvis CC
CC Excl: See code: M87.31

M87.Ø51 Idiopathic aseptic necrosis of right femur CC
CC Excl: M87.ØØ, M87.Ø31-M87.Ø73, M87.Ø77-M87.119, M87.131-M87.173, M87.177-M87.219, M87.231-M87.273, M87.277-M87.319, M87.331-M87.373, M87.377-M87.819, M87.831-M87.873, M87.877-M87.9, M9Ø.5Ø, M9Ø.521-M9Ø.59

M87.Ø52 Idiopathic aseptic necrosis of left femur CC
CC Excl: See code: M87.Ø51

M87.Ø59 Idiopathic aseptic necrosis of unspecified femur CC
Idiopathic aseptic necrosis of hip NOS
CC Excl: See code: M87.Ø51

✓6th **M87.Ø6 Idiopathic aseptic necrosis of tibia and fibula**

M87.Ø61 Idiopathic aseptic necrosis of right tibia CC
CC Excl: M87.ØØ-M87.9, M9Ø.5Ø-M9Ø.59

M87.Ø62 Idiopathic aseptic necrosis of left tibia CC
CC Excl: See code: M87.61

M87.Ø63 Idiopathic aseptic necrosis of unspecified tibia CC
CC Excl: See code: M87.61

M87.Ø64 Idiopathic aseptic necrosis of right fibula CC
CC Excl: See code: M87.61

M87.Ø65 Idiopathic aseptic necrosis of left fibula CC
CC Excl: See code: M87.61

M87.Ø66 Idiopathic aseptic necrosis of unspecified fibula CC
CC Excl: See code: M87.61

✓6th **M87.Ø7 Idiopathic aseptic necrosis of ankle, foot and toes**
Idiopathic aseptic necrosis of metatarsus, tarsus, and phalanges of toes

M87.Ø71 Idiopathic aseptic necrosis of right ankle CC
CC Excl: See code: M87.61

M87.Ø72 Idiopathic aseptic necrosis of left ankle CC
CC Excl: See code: M87.61

M87.Ø73 Idiopathic aseptic necrosis of unspecified ankle CC
CC Excl: See code: M87.61

M87.Ø74 Idiopathic aseptic necrosis of right foot CC
CC Excl: M87.ØØ, M87.Ø31-M87.Ø5Ø, M87.Ø61-M87.119, M87.131-M87.146, M87.161-M87.219, M87.231-M87.25Ø, M87.261-M87.319, M87.331-M87.346, M87.361-M87.819, M87.831-M87.849, M87.861-M87.9, M9Ø.5Ø, M9Ø.521-M9Ø.549, M9Ø.561-M9Ø.59

M87.Ø75 Idiopathic aseptic necrosis of left foot CC
CC Excl: See code: M87.Ø74

M87.Ø76 Idiopathic aseptic necrosis of unspecified foot CC
CC Excl: See code: M87.Ø74

M87.Ø77 Idiopathic aseptic necrosis of right toe(s) CC
CC Excl: M87.ØØ-M87.9, M9Ø.5Ø-M9Ø.59

M87.Ø78 Idiopathic aseptic necrosis of left toe(s) CC
CC Excl: See code: M87.Ø77

M87.Ø79 Idiopathic aseptic necrosis of unspecified toe(s) CC
CC Excl: See code: M87.Ø77

M87.Ø8 Idiopathic aseptic necrosis of bone, other site CC
CC Excl: See code: M87.Ø77

M87.Ø9 Idiopathic aseptic necrosis of bone, multiple sites CC
CC Excl: See code: M87.Ø77

5th **M87.1 Osteonecrosis due to drugs**
Use additional code for adverse effect, if applicable, to identify drug (T36-T5Ø with fifth or sixth character 5)

M87.1Ø Osteonecrosis due to drugs, unspecified bone CC
CC Excl: See code: M87.ØØ

6th **M87.11 Osteonecrosis due to drugs, shoulder**

M87.111 Osteonecrosis due to drugs, right shoulder CC
CC Excl: See code: M87.77

M87.112 Osteonecrosis due to drugs, left shoulder CC
CC Excl: See code: M87.77

M87.119 Osteonecrosis due to drugs, unspecified shoulder CC
CC Excl: See code: M87.77

6th **M87.12 Osteonecrosis due to drugs, humerus**

M87.121 Osteonecrosis due to drugs, right humerus CC
CC Excl: M87.ØØ-M87.Ø5Ø, M87.Ø61-M87.Ø73, M87.Ø77-M87.146, M87.161-M87.173, M87.177-M87.25Ø, M87.261-M87.273, M87.277-M87.346, M87.361-M87.373, M87.377-M87.849, M87.861-M87.873, M87.877-M87.9, M9Ø.5Ø-M9Ø.549, M9Ø.561-M9Ø.59

M87.122 Osteonecrosis due to drugs, left humerus CC
CC Excl: See code: M87.121

M87.129 Osteonecrosis due to drugs, unspecified humerus CC
CC Excl: See code: M87.121

6th **M87.13 Osteonecrosis due to drugs of radius, ulna and carpus**

M87.131 Osteonecrosis due to drugs of right radius CC
CC Excl: See code: M87.Ø77

M87.132 Osteonecrosis due to drugs of left radius CC
CC Excl: See code: M87.Ø77

M87.133 Osteonecrosis due to drugs of unspecified radius CC
CC Excl: See code: M87.Ø77

M87.134 Osteonecrosis due to drugs of right ulna CC
CC Excl: See code: M87.Ø77

M87.135 Osteonecrosis due to drugs of left ulna CC
CC Excl: See code: M87.Ø77

M87.136 Osteonecrosis due to drugs of unspecified ulna CC
CC Excl: See code: M87.Ø77

M87.137 Osteonecrosis due to drugs of right carpus CC
CC Excl: See code: M87.Ø77

M87.138 Osteonecrosis due to drugs of left carpus CC
CC Excl: See code: M87.Ø77

M87.139 Osteonecrosis due to drugs of unspecified carpus CC
CC Excl: See code: M87.Ø77

6th **M87.14 Osteonecrosis due to drugs, hand and fingers**

M87.141 Osteonecrosis due to drugs, right hand CC
CC Excl: See code: M87.Ø77

M87.142 Osteonecrosis due to drugs, left hand CC
CC Excl: See code: M87.Ø77

M87.143 Osteonecrosis due to drugs, unspecified hand CC
CC Excl: See code: M87.Ø77

M87.144 Osteonecrosis due to drugs, right finger(s) CC
CC Excl: See code: M87.Ø77

M87.145 Osteonecrosis due to drugs, left finger(s) CC
CC Excl: See code: M87.Ø77

M87.146 Osteonecrosis due to drugs, unspecified finger(s) CC
CC Excl: See code: M87.Ø77

6th **M87.15 Osteonecrosis due to drugs, pelvis and femur**

M87.15Ø Osteonecrosis due to drugs, pelvis CC
CC Excl: M87.ØØ, M87.Ø31-M87.Ø73, M87.Ø77-M87.119, M87.131-M87.173, M87.177-M87.219, M87.231-M87.273, M87.277-M87.319, M87.331-M87.373, M87.377-M87.819, M87.831-M87.873, M87.877-M87.9, M9Ø.5Ø, M9Ø.521-M9Ø.59

M87.151 Osteonecrosis due to drugs, right femur CC
CC Excl: See code: M87.15Ø

M87.152 Osteonecrosis due to drugs, left femur CC
CC Excl: See code: M87.15Ø

M87.159 Osteonecrosis due to drugs, unspecified femur CC
CC Excl: See code: M87.15Ø

6th **M87.16 Osteonecrosis due to drugs, tibia and fibula**

M87.161 Osteonecrosis due to drugs, right tibia CC
CC Excl: M87.ØØ-M87.9, M9Ø.5Ø-M9Ø.59

M87.162 Osteonecrosis due to drugs, left tibia CC
CC Excl: See code: M87.161

M87.163 Osteonecrosis due to drugs, unspecified tibia CC
CC Excl: See code: M87.161

M87.164 Osteonecrosis due to drugs, right fibula CC
CC Excl: See code: M87.161

M87.165 Osteonecrosis due to drugs, left fibula CC
CC Excl: See code: M87.161

M87.166 Osteonecrosis due to drugs, unspecified fibula CC
CC Excl: See code: M87.161

6th **M87.17 Osteonecrosis due to drugs, ankle, foot and toes**

M87.171 Osteonecrosis due to drugs, right ankle CC
CC Excl: See code: M87.161

M87.172 Osteonecrosis due to drugs, left ankle CC
CC Excl: See code: M87.161

M87.173 Osteonecrosis due to drugs, unspecified ankle CC
CC Excl: See code: M87.161

M87.174 Osteonecrosis due to drugs, right foot CC
CC Excl: M87.ØØ, M87.Ø31-M87.Ø5Ø, M87.Ø61-M87.119, M87.131-M87.146, M87.161-M87.219, M87.231-M87.25Ø, M87.261-M87.319, M87.331-M87.346, M87.361-M87.819, M87.831-M87.849, M87.861-M87.9, M9Ø.5Ø, M9Ø.521-M9Ø.549, M9Ø.561-M9Ø.59

M87.175 Osteonecrosis due to drugs, left foot CC
CC Excl: See code: M87.174

M87.176 Osteonecrosis due to drugs, unspecified foot CC
CC Excl: See code: M87.174

M87.177 Osteonecrosis due to drugs, right toe(s) CC
CC Excl: See code: M87.161

M87.178 Osteonecrosis due to drugs, left toe(s) CC
CC Excl: See code: M87.161

M87.179 Osteonecrosis due to drugs, unspecified toe(s) CC
CC Excl: See code: M87.161

6th **M87.18 Osteonecrosis due to drugs, other site**

M87.18Ø Osteonecrosis due to drugs, jaw CC
CC Excl: See code: M87.161

M87.188 Osteonecrosis due to drugs, other site CC
CC Excl: See code: M87.161

M87.19 Osteonecrosis due to drugs, multiple sites CC
CC Excl: See code: M87.161

✓5th **M87.2 Osteonecrosis due to previous trauma**

M87.20 Osteonecrosis due to previous trauma, unspecified bone CC
CC Excl: See code: M87.161

✓6th **M87.21 Osteonecrosis due to previous trauma, shoulder**

M87.211 Osteonecrosis due to previous trauma, right shoulder CC
CC Excl: See code: M87.161

M87.212 Osteonecrosis due to previous trauma, left shoulder CC
CC Excl: See code: M87.161

M87.219 Osteonecrosis due to previous trauma, unspecified shoulder CC
CC Excl: See code: M87.161

✓6th **M87.22 Osteonecrosis due to previous trauma, humerus**

M87.221 Osteonecrosis due to previous trauma, right humerus CC
CC Excl: M87.00-M87.050, M87.061-M87.073, M87.077-M87.146, M87.161-M87.173, M87.177-M87.250, M87.261-M87.273, M87.277-M87.346, M87.361-M87.373, M87.377-M87.849, M87.861-M87.873, M87.877-M87.9, M90.50-M90.549, M90.561-M90.59

M87.222 Osteonecrosis due to previous trauma, left humerus CC
CC Excl: See code: M87.221

M87.229 Osteonecrosis due to previous trauma, unspecified humerus CC
CC Excl: See code: M87.221

✓6th **M87.23 Osteonecrosis due to previous trauma of radius, ulna and carpus**

M87.231 Osteonecrosis due to previous trauma of right radius CC
CC Excl: See code: M87.161

M87.232 Osteonecrosis due to previous trauma of left radius CC
CC Excl: See code: M87.161

M87.233 Osteonecrosis due to previous trauma of unspecified radius CC
CC Excl: See code: M87.161

M87.234 Osteonecrosis due to previous trauma of right ulna CC
CC Excl: See code: M87.161

M87.235 Osteonecrosis due to previous trauma of left ulna CC
CC Excl: See code: M87.161

M87.236 Osteonecrosis due to previous trauma of unspecified ulna CC
CC Excl: See code: M87.161

M87.237 Osteonecrosis due to previous trauma of right carpus CC
CC Excl: See code: M87.161

M87.238 Osteonecrosis due to previous trauma of left carpus CC
CC Excl: See code: M87.161

M87.239 Osteonecrosis due to previous trauma of unspecified carpus CC
CC Excl: See code: M87.161

✓6th **M87.24 Osteonecrosis due to previous trauma, hand and fingers**

M87.241 Osteonecrosis due to previous trauma, right hand CC
CC Excl: See code: M87.161

M87.242 Osteonecrosis due to previous trauma, left hand CC
CC Excl: See code: M87.161

M87.243 Osteonecrosis due to previous trauma, unspecified hand CC
CC Excl: See code: M87.161

M87.244 Osteonecrosis due to previous trauma, right finger(s) CC
CC Excl: See code: M87.161

M87.245 Osteonecrosis due to previous trauma, left finger(s) CC
CC Excl: See code: M87.161

M87.246 Osteonecrosis due to previous trauma, unspecified finger(s) CC
CC Excl: See code: M87.161

✓6th **M87.25 Osteonecrosis due to previous trauma, pelvis and femur**

M87.250 Osteonecrosis due to previous trauma, pelvis CC
CC Excl: M87.00-M87.9, M90.50-M90.59

M87.251 Osteonecrosis due to previous trauma, right femur CC
CC Excl: M87.00, M87.031-M87.073, M87.077-M87.119, M87.131-M87.173, M87.177-M87.219, M87.231-M87.273, M87.277-M87.319, M87.331-M87.373, M87.377-M87.819, M87.831-M87.873, M87.877-M87.9, M90.50, M90.521-M90.59

M87.252 Osteonecrosis due to previous trauma, left femur CC
CC Excl: See code: M87.251

M87.256 Osteonecrosis due to previous trauma, unspecified femur CC
CC Excl: See code: M87.251

✓6th **M87.26 Osteonecrosis due to previous trauma, tibia and fibula**

M87.261 Osteonecrosis due to previous trauma, right tibia CC
CC Excl: See code: M87.250

M87.262 Osteonecrosis due to previous trauma, left tibia CC
CC Excl: See code: M87.250

M87.263 Osteonecrosis due to previous trauma, unspecified tibia CC
CC Excl: See code: M87.250

M87.264 Osteonecrosis due to previous trauma, right fibula CC
CC Excl: See code: M87.250

M87.265 Osteonecrosis due to previous trauma, left fibula CC
CC Excl: See code: M87.250

M87.266 Osteonecrosis due to previous trauma, unspecified fibula CC
CC Excl: See code: M87.250

✓6th **M87.27 Osteonecrosis due to previous trauma, ankle, foot and toes**

M87.271 Osteonecrosis due to previous trauma, right ankle CC
CC Excl: See code: M87.250

M87.272 Osteonecrosis due to previous trauma, left ankle CC
CC Excl: See code: M87.250

M87.273 Osteonecrosis due to previous trauma, unspecified ankle CC
CC Excl: See code: M87.250

M87.274 Osteonecrosis due to previous trauma, right foot CC
CC Excl: M87.00, M87.031-M87.050, M87.061-M87.119, M87.131-M87.146, M87.161-M87.219, M87.231-M87.250, M87.261-M87.319, M87.331-M87.346, M87.361-M87.819, M87.831-M87.849, M87.861-M87.9, M90.50, M90.521-M90.549, M90.561-M90.59

M87.275 Osteonecrosis due to previous trauma, left foot CC
CC Excl: See code: M87.274

M87.276 Osteonecrosis due to previous trauma, unspecified foot CC
CC Excl: See code: M87.274

M87.277 Osteonecrosis due to previous trauma, right toe(s) CC
CC Excl: See code: M87.250

M87.278 Osteonecrosis due to previous trauma, left toe(s) CC
CC Excl: See code: M87.250

M87.279 Osteonecrosis due to previous trauma, unspecified toe(s) CC
CC Excl: See code: M87.250

M87.28 Osteonecrosis due to previous trauma, other site CC
CC Excl: See code: M87.250

M87.29 Osteonecrosis due to previous trauma, multiple sites CC
CC Excl: See code: M87.250

✓5th **M87.3 Other secondary osteonecrosis**

M87.3Ø Other secondary osteonecrosis, unspecified bone CC
CC Excl: M87.ØØ-M87.9, M9Ø.5Ø-M9Ø.59

✓6th **M87.31 Other secondary osteonecrosis, shoulder**

M87.311 Other secondary osteonecrosis, right shoulder CC
CC Excl: See code: M87.3Ø

M87.312 Other secondary osteonecrosis, left shoulder CC
CC Excl: See code: M87.3Ø

M87.319 Other secondary osteonecrosis, unspecified shoulder CC
CC Excl: See code: M87.3Ø

✓6th **M87.32 Other secondary osteonecrosis, humerus**

M87.321 Other secondary osteonecrosis, right humerus CC
CC Excl: M87.ØØ-M87.Ø5Ø, M87.Ø61-M87.Ø73, M87.Ø77-M87.146, M87.161-M87.173, M87.177-M87.25Ø, M87.261-M87.273, M87.277-M87.346, M87.361-M87.373, M87.377-M87.849, M87.861-M87.873, M87.877-M87.9, M9Ø.5Ø-M9Ø.549, M9Ø.561-M9Ø.59

M87.322 Other secondary osteonecrosis, left humerus CC
CC Excl: See code: M87.321

M87.329 Other secondary osteonecrosis, unspecified humerus CC
CC Excl: See code: M87.321

✓6th **M87.33 Other secondary osteonecrosis of radius, ulna and carpus**

M87.331 Other secondary osteonecrosis of right radius CC
CC Excl: See code: M87.3Ø

M87.332 Other secondary osteonecrosis of left radius CC
CC Excl: See code: M87.3Ø

M87.333 Other secondary osteonecrosis of unspecified radius CC
CC Excl: See code: M87.3Ø

M87.334 Other secondary osteonecrosis of right ulna CC
CC Excl: See code: M87.3Ø

M87.335 Other secondary osteonecrosis of left ulna CC
CC Excl: See code: M87.3Ø

M87.336 Other secondary osteonecrosis of unspecified ulna CC
CC Excl: See code: M87.3Ø

M87.337 Other secondary osteonecrosis of right carpus CC
CC Excl: See code: M87.3Ø

M87.338 Other secondary osteonecrosis of left carpus CC
CC Excl: See code: M87.3Ø

M87.339 Other secondary osteonecrosis of unspecified carpus CC
CC Excl: See code: M87.3Ø

✓6th **M87.34 Other secondary osteonecrosis, hand and fingers**

M87.341 Other secondary osteonecrosis, right hand CC
CC Excl: See code: M87.3Ø

M87.342 Other secondary osteonecrosis, left hand CC
CC Excl: See code: M87.3Ø

M87.343 Other secondary osteonecrosis, unspecified hand CC
CC Excl: See code: M87.3Ø

M87.344 Other secondary osteonecrosis, right finger(s) CC
CC Excl: See code: M87.3Ø

M87.345 Other secondary osteonecrosis, left finger(s) CC
CC Excl: See code: M87.3Ø

M87.346 Other secondary osteonecrosis, unspecified finger(s) CC
CC Excl: See code: M87.3Ø

✓6th **M87.35 Other secondary osteonecrosis, pelvis and femur**

M87.35Ø Other secondary osteonecrosis, pelvis CC
CC Excl: M87.ØØ, M87.Ø31-M87.Ø73, M87.Ø77-M87.119, M87.131-M87.173, M87.177-M87.219, M87.231-M87.273, M87.277-M87.319, M87.331-M87.373, M87.377-M87.819, M87.831-M87.873, M87.877-M87.9, M9Ø.5Ø, M9Ø.521-M9Ø.59

M87.351 Other secondary osteonecrosis, right femur CC
CC Excl: See code: M87.35Ø

M87.352 Other secondary osteonecrosis, left femur CC
CC Excl: See code: M87.35Ø

M87.353 Other secondary osteonecrosis, unspecified femur CC
CC Excl: See code: M87.35Ø

✓6th **M87.36 Other secondary osteonecrosis, tibia and fibula**

M87.361 Other secondary osteonecrosis, right tibia CC
CC Excl: M87.ØØ-M87.9, M9Ø.5Ø-M9Ø.59

M87.362 Other secondary osteonecrosis, left tibia CC
CC Excl: See code: M87.361

M87.363 Other secondary osteonecrosis, unspecified tibia CC
CC Excl: See code: M87.361

M87.364 Other secondary osteonecrosis, right fibula CC
CC Excl: See code: M87.361

M87.365 Other secondary osteonecrosis, left fibula CC
CC Excl: See code: M87.361

M87.366 Other secondary osteonecrosis, unspecified fibula CC
CC Excl: See code: M87.361

✓6th **M87.37 Other secondary osteonecrosis, ankle and foot**

M87.371 Other secondary osteonecrosis, right ankle CC
CC Excl: See code: M87.361

M87.372 Other secondary osteonecrosis, left ankle CC
CC Excl: See code: M87.361

M87.373 Other secondary osteonecrosis, unspecified ankle CC
CC Excl: See code: M87.361

M87.374 Other secondary osteonecrosis, right foot CC
CC Excl: M87.ØØ, M87.Ø31-M87.Ø5Ø, M87.Ø61-M87.119, M87.131-M87.146, M87.161-M87.219, M87.231-M87.25Ø, M87.261-M87.319, M87.331-M87.346, M87.361-M87.819, M87.831-M87.849, M87.861-M87.9, M9Ø.5Ø, M9Ø.521-M9Ø.549, M9Ø.561-M9Ø.59

M87.375 Other secondary osteonecrosis, left foot CC
CC Excl: See code: M87.374

M87.376 Other secondary osteonecrosis, unspecified foot CC
CC Excl: See code: M87.374

M87.377 Other secondary osteonecrosis, right toe(s) CC
CC Excl: See code: M87.361

M87.378 Other secondary osteonecrosis, left toe(s) CC
CC Excl: See code: M87.361

M87.379 Other secondary osteonecrosis, unspecified toe(s) CC
CC Excl: See code: M87.361

M87.38 Other secondary osteonecrosis, other site CC
CC Excl: See code: M87.361

M87.39 Other secondary osteonecrosis, multiple sites CC
CC Excl: See code: M87.361

✓5th **M87.8 Other osteonecrosis**

M87.8Ø Other osteonecrosis, unspecified bone CC
CC Excl: See code: M87.361

✓6th **M87.81 Other osteonecrosis, shoulder**

M87.811 Other osteonecrosis, right shoulder CC
CC Excl: See code: M87.361

M87.812 Other osteonecrosis, left shoulder CC
CC Excl: See code: M87.361

M87.819 Other osteonecrosis, unspecified shoulder CC
CC Excl: See code: M87.361

M87.82 Other osteonecrosis, humerus

M87.821 Other osteonecrosis, right humerus CC
CC Excl: M87.00-M87.050, M87.061-M87.073, M87.077-M87.146, M87.161-M87.173, M87.177-M87.250, M87.261-M87.273, M87.277-M87.346, M87.361-M87.373, M87.377-M87.849, M87.861-M87.873, M87.877-M87.9, M90.50-M90.549, M90.561-M90.59

M87.822 Other osteonecrosis, left humerus CC
CC Excl: See code: M87.821

M87.829 Other osteonecrosis, unspecified humerus CC
CC Excl: See code: M87.821

M87.83 Other osteonecrosis of radius, ulna and carpus

M87.831 Other osteonecrosis of right radius CC
CC Excl: See code: M87.361

M87.832 Other osteonecrosis of left radius CC
CC Excl: See code: M87.361

M87.833 Other osteonecrosis of unspecified radius CC
CC Excl: See code: M87.361

M87.834 Other osteonecrosis of right ulna CC
CC Excl: See code: M87.361

M87.835 Other osteonecrosis of left ulna CC
CC Excl: See code: M87.361

M87.836 Other osteonecrosis of unspecified ulna CC
CC Excl: See code: M87.361

M87.837 Other osteonecrosis of right carpus CC
CC Excl: See code: M87.361

M87.838 Other osteonecrosis of left carpus CC
CC Excl: See code: M87.361

M87.839 Other osteonecrosis of unspecified carpus CC
CC Excl: See code: M87.361

M87.84 Other osteonecrosis, hand and fingers

M87.841 Other osteonecrosis, right hand CC
CC Excl: See code: M87.361

M87.842 Other osteonecrosis, left hand CC
CC Excl: See code: M87.361

M87.843 Other osteonecrosis, unspecified hand CC
CC Excl: See code: M87.361

M87.844 Other osteonecrosis, right finger(s) CC
CC Excl: See code: M87.361

M87.845 Other osteonecrosis, left finger(s) CC
CC Excl: See code: M87.361

M87.849 Other osteonecrosis, unspecified finger(s) CC
CC Excl: See code: M87.361

M87.85 Other osteonecrosis, pelvis and femur

M87.850 Other osteonecrosis, pelvis CC
CC Excl: M87.00, M87.031-M87.073, M87.077-M87.119, M87.131-M87.173, M87.177-M87.219, M87.231-M87.273, M87.277-M87.319, M87.331-M87.373, M87.377-M87.819, M87.831-M87.873, M87.877-M87.9, M90.50, M90.521-M90.59

M87.851 Other osteonecrosis, right femur CC
CC Excl: See code: M87.850

M87.852 Other osteonecrosis, left femur CC
CC Excl: See code: M87.850

M87.859 Other osteonecrosis, unspecified femur CC
CC Excl: See code: M87.850

M87.86 Other osteonecrosis, tibia and fibula

M87.861 Other osteonecrosis, right tibia CC
CC Excl: See code: M87.361

M87.862 Other osteonecrosis, left tibia CC
CC Excl: See code: M87.361

M87.863 Other osteonecrosis, unspecified tibia CC
CC Excl: See code: M87.361

M87.864 Other osteonecrosis, right fibula CC
CC Excl: See code: M87.361

M87.865 Other osteonecrosis, left fibula CC
CC Excl: See code: M87.361

M87.869 Other osteonecrosis, unspecified fibula CC
CC Excl: See code: M87.361

M87.87 Other osteonecrosis, ankle, foot and toes

M87.871 Other osteonecrosis, right ankle CC
CC Excl: See code: M87.361

M87.872 Other osteonecrosis, left ankle CC
CC Excl: See code: M87.361

M87.873 Other osteonecrosis, unspecified ankle CC
CC Excl: See code: M87.361

M87.874 Other osteonecrosis, right foot CC
CC Excl: M87.00, M87.031-M87.050, M87.061-M87.119, M87.131-M87.146, M87.161-M87.219, M87.231-M87.250, M87.261-M87.319, M87.331-M87.346, M87.361-M87.819, M87.831-M87.849, M87.861-M87.9, M90.50, M90.521-M90.549, M90.561-M90.59

M87.875 Other osteonecrosis, left foot CC
CC Excl: See code: M87.874

M87.876 Other osteonecrosis, unspecified foot CC
CC Excl: See code: M87.874

M87.877 Other osteonecrosis, right toe(s) CC
CC Excl: See code: M87.361

M87.878 Other osteonecrosis, left toe(s) CC
CC Excl: See code: M87.361

M87.879 Other osteonecrosis, unspecified toe(s) CC
CC Excl: See code: M87.361

M87.88 Other osteonecrosis, other site CC
CC Excl: See code: M87.361

M87.89 Other osteonecrosis, multiple sites CC
CC Excl: See code: M87.361

M87.9 Osteonecrosis, unspecified CC
Necrosis of bone NOS
CC Excl: See code: M87.361

M88 Osteitis deformans [Paget's disease of bone]
EXCLUDES 1 *osteitis deformans in neoplastic disease (M90.6)*

M88.0 Osteitis deformans of skull

M88.1 Osteitis deformans of vertebrae

M88.8 Osteitis deformans of other bones

M88.81 Osteitis deformans of shoulder
M88.811 Osteitis deformans of right shoulder
M88.812 Osteitis deformans of left shoulder
M88.819 Osteitis deformans of unspecified shoulder

M88.82 Osteitis deformans of upper arm
M88.821 Osteitis deformans of right upper arm
M88.822 Osteitis deformans of left upper arm
M88.829 Osteitis deformans of unspecified upper arm

M88.83 Osteitis deformans of forearm
M88.831 Osteitis deformans of right forearm
M88.832 Osteitis deformans of left forearm
M88.839 Osteitis deformans of unspecified forearm

M88.84 Osteitis deformans of hand
M88.841 Osteitis deformans of right hand
M88.842 Osteitis deformans of left hand
M88.849 Osteitis deformans of unspecified hand

M88.85 Osteitis deformans of thigh
M88.851 Osteitis deformans of right thigh
M88.852 Osteitis deformans of left thigh
M88.859 Osteitis deformans of unspecified thigh

M88.86 Osteitis deformans of lower leg
M88.861 Osteitis deformans of right lower leg
M88.862 Osteitis deformans of left lower leg
M88.869 Osteitis deformans of unspecified lower leg

M88.87 Osteitis deformans of ankle and foot
M88.871 Osteitis deformans of right ankle and foot
M88.872 Osteitis deformans of left ankle and foot
M88.879 Osteitis deformans of unspecified ankle and foot

M88.88 Osteitis deformans of other bones
EXCLUDES 2 *osteitis deformans of skull (M88.0)*
osteitis deformans of vertebrae (M88.1)

M88.89 Osteitis deformans of multiple sites

M88.9 Osteitis deformans of unspecified bone

✓4th **M89 Other disorders of bone**

✓5th **M89.0 Algoneurodystrophy**
Shoulder-hand syndrome
Sudeck's atrophy

EXCLUDES 1 *causalgia, lower limb (G57.7-)*
causalgia, upper limb (G56.4-)
complex regional pain syndrome II, lower limb (G57.7-)
complex regional pain syndrome II, upper limb (G56.4-)
reflex sympathetic dystrophy (G90.5-)

M89.00 Algoneurodystrophy, unspecified site

✓6th **M89.01 Algoneurodystrophy, shoulder**
- **M89.011 Algoneurodystrophy, right shoulder**
- **M89.012 Algoneurodystrophy, left shoulder**
- **M89.019 Algoneurodystrophy, unspecified shoulder**

✓6th **M89.02 Algoneurodystrophy, upper arm**
- **M89.021 Algoneurodystrophy, right upper arm**
- **M89.022 Algoneurodystrophy, left upper arm**
- **M89.029 Algoneurodystrophy, unspecified upper arm**

✓6th **M89.03 Algoneurodystrophy, forearm**
- **M89.031 Algoneurodystrophy, right forearm**
- **M89.032 Algoneurodystrophy, left forearm**
- **M89.039 Algoneurodystrophy, unspecified forearm**

✓6th **M89.04 Algoneurodystrophy, hand**
- **M89.041 Algoneurodystrophy, right hand**
- **M89.042 Algoneurodystrophy, left hand**
- **M89.049 Algoneurodystrophy, unspecified hand**

✓6th **M89.05 Algoneurodystrophy, thigh**
- **M89.051 Algoneurodystrophy, right thigh**
- **M89.052 Algoneurodystrophy, left thigh**
- **M89.059 Algoneurodystrophy, unspecified thigh**

✓6th **M89.06 Algoneurodystrophy, lower leg**
- **M89.061 Algoneurodystrophy, right lower leg**
- **M89.062 Algoneurodystrophy, left lower leg**
- **M89.069 Algoneurodystrophy, unspecified lower leg**

✓6th **M89.07 Algoneurodystrophy, ankle and foot**
- **M89.071 Algoneurodystrophy, right ankle and foot**
- **M89.072 Algoneurodystrophy, left ankle and foot**
- **M89.079 Algoneurodystrophy, unspecified ankle and foot**

M89.08 Algoneurodystrophy, other site

M89.09 Algoneurodystrophy, multiple sites

✓5th **M89.1 Physeal arrest**
Arrest of growth plate
Epiphyseal arrest
Growth plate arrest

✓6th **M89.12 Physeal arrest, humerus**
- **M89.121 Complete physeal arrest, right proximal humerus**
- **M89.122 Complete physeal arrest, left proximal humerus**
- **M89.123 Partial physeal arrest, right proximal humerus**
- **M89.124 Partial physeal arrest, left proximal humerus**
- **M89.125 Complete physeal arrest, right distal humerus**
- **M89.126 Complete physeal arrest, left distal humerus**
- **M89.127 Partial physeal arrest, right distal humerus**
- **M89.128 Partial physeal arrest, left distal humerus**
- **M89.129 Physeal arrest, humerus, unspecified**

✓6th **M89.13 Physeal arrest, forearm**
- **M89.131 Complete physeal arrest, right distal radius**
- **M89.132 Complete physeal arrest, left distal radius**
- **M89.133 Partial physeal arrest, right distal radius**
- **M89.134 Partial physeal arrest, left distal radius**
- **M89.138 Other physeal arrest of forearm**
- **M89.139 Physeal arrest, forearm, unspecified**

✓6th **M89.15 Physeal arrest, femur**
- **M89.151 Complete physeal arrest, right proximal femur**
- **M89.152 Complete physeal arrest, left proximal femur**
- **M89.153 Partial physeal arrest, right proximal femur**
- **M89.154 Partial physeal arrest, left proximal femur**
- **M89.155 Complete physeal arrest, right distal femur**
- **M89.156 Complete physeal arrest, left distal femur**
- **M89.157 Partial physeal arrest, right distal femur**
- **M89.158 Partial physeal arrest, left distal femur**
- **M89.159 Physeal arrest, femur, unspecified**

✓6th **M89.16 Physeal arrest, lower leg**
- **M89.160 Complete physeal arrest, right proximal tibia**
- **M89.161 Complete physeal arrest, left proximal tibia**
- **M89.162 Partial physeal arrest, right proximal tibia**
- **M89.163 Partial physeal arrest, left proximal tibia**
- **M89.164 Complete physeal arrest, right distal tibia**
- **M89.165 Complete physeal arrest, left distal tibia**
- **M89.166 Partial physeal arrest, right distal tibia**
- **M89.167 Partial physeal arrest, left distal tibia**
- **M89.168 Other physeal arrest of lower leg**
- **M89.169 Physeal arrest, lower leg, unspecified**

M89.18 Physeal arrest, other site

✓5th **M89.2 Other disorders of bone development and growth**

M89.20 Other disorders of bone development and growth, unspecified site

✓6th **M89.21 Other disorders of bone development and growth, shoulder**
- **M89.211 Other disorders of bone development and growth, right shoulder**
- **M89.212 Other disorders of bone development and growth, left shoulder**
- **M89.219 Other disorders of bone development and growth, unspecified shoulder**

✓6th **M89.22 Other disorders of bone development and growth, humerus**
- **M89.221 Other disorders of bone development and growth, right humerus**
- **M89.222 Other disorders of bone development and growth, left humerus**
- **M89.229 Other disorders of bone development and growth, unspecified humerus**

✓6th **M89.23 Other disorders of bone development and growth, ulna and radius**
- **M89.231 Other disorders of bone development and growth, right ulna**
- **M89.232 Other disorders of bone development and growth, left ulna**
- **M89.233 Other disorders of bone development and growth, right radius**
- **M89.234 Other disorders of bone development and growth, left radius**
- **M89.239 Other disorders of bone development and growth, unspecified ulna and radius**

✓6th **M89.24 Other disorders of bone development and growth, hand**
- **M89.241 Other disorders of bone development and growth, right hand**
- **M89.242 Other disorders of bone development and growth, left hand**
- **M89.249 Other disorders of bone development and growth, unspecified hand**

✓6th **M89.25 Other disorders of bone development and growth, femur**
- **M89.251 Other disorders of bone development and growth, right femur**
- **M89.252 Other disorders of bone development and growth, left femur**
- **M89.259 Other disorders of bone development and growth, unspecified femur**

✓6th M89.26 Other disorders of bone development and growth, tibia and fibula
M89.261 Other disorders of bone development and growth, right tibia
M89.262 Other disorders of bone development and growth, left tibia
M89.263 Other disorders of bone development and growth, right fibula
M89.264 Other disorders of bone development and growth, left fibula
M89.269 Other disorders of bone development and growth, unspecified lower leg
✓6th M89.27 Other disorders of bone development and growth, ankle and foot
M89.271 Other disorders of bone development and growth, right ankle and foot
M89.272 Other disorders of bone development and growth, left ankle and foot
M89.279 Other disorders of bone development and growth, unspecified ankle and foot
M89.28 Other disorders of bone development and growth, other site
M89.29 Other disorders of bone development and growth, multiple sites
✓5th M89.3 Hypertrophy of bone
M89.30 Hypertrophy of bone, unspecified site
✓6th M89.31 Hypertrophy of bone, shoulder
M89.311 Hypertrophy of bone, right shoulder
M89.312 Hypertrophy of bone, left shoulder
M89.319 Hypertrophy of bone, unspecified shoulder
✓6th M89.32 Hypertrophy of bone, humerus
M89.321 Hypertrophy of bone, right humerus
M89.322 Hypertrophy of bone, left humerus
M89.329 Hypertrophy of bone, unspecified humerus
✓6th M89.33 Hypertrophy of bone, ulna and radius
M89.331 Hypertrophy of bone, right ulna
M89.332 Hypertrophy of bone, left ulna
M89.333 Hypertrophy of bone, right radius
M89.334 Hypertrophy of bone, left radius
M89.339 Hypertrophy of bone, unspecified ulna and radius
✓6th M89.34 Hypertrophy of bone, hand
M89.341 Hypertrophy of bone, right hand
M89.342 Hypertrophy of bone, left hand
M89.349 Hypertrophy of bone, unspecified hand
✓6th M89.35 Hypertrophy of bone, femur
M89.351 Hypertrophy of bone, right femur
M89.352 Hypertrophy of bone, left femur
M89.359 Hypertrophy of bone, unspecified femur
✓6th M89.36 Hypertrophy of bone, tibia and fibula
M89.361 Hypertrophy of bone, right tibia
M89.362 Hypertrophy of bone, left tibia
M89.363 Hypertrophy of bone, right fibula
M89.364 Hypertrophy of bone, left fibula
M89.369 Hypertrophy of bone, unspecified tibia and fibula
✓6th M89.37 Hypertrophy of bone, ankle and foot
M89.371 Hypertrophy of bone, right ankle and foot
M89.372 Hypertrophy of bone, left ankle and foot
M89.379 Hypertrophy of bone, unspecified ankle and foot
M89.38 Hypertrophy of bone, other site
M89.39 Hypertrophy of bone, multiple sites
✓5th M89.4 Other hypertrophic osteoarthropathy
Marie-Bamberger disease
Pachydermoperiostosis
M89.40 Other hypertrophic osteoarthropathy, unspecified site
✓6th M89.41 Other hypertrophic osteoarthropathy, shoulder
M89.411 Other hypertrophic osteoarthropathy, right shoulder
M89.412 Other hypertrophic osteoarthropathy, left shoulder
M89.419 Other hypertrophic osteoarthropathy, unspecified shoulder
✓6th M89.42 Other hypertrophic osteoarthropathy, upper arm
M89.421 Other hypertrophic osteoarthropathy, right upper arm
M89.422 Other hypertrophic osteoarthropathy, left upper arm
M89.429 Other hypertrophic osteoarthropathy, unspecified upper arm
✓6th M89.43 Other hypertrophic osteoarthropathy, forearm
M89.431 Other hypertrophic osteoarthropathy, right forearm
M89.432 Other hypertrophic osteoarthropathy, left forearm
M89.439 Other hypertrophic osteoarthropathy, unspecified forearm
✓6th M89.44 Other hypertrophic osteoarthropathy, hand
M89.441 Other hypertrophic osteoarthropathy, right hand
M89.442 Other hypertrophic osteoarthropathy, left hand
M89.449 Other hypertrophic osteoarthropathy, unspecified hand
✓6th M89.45 Other hypertrophic osteoarthropathy, thigh
M89.451 Other hypertrophic osteoarthropathy, right thigh
M89.452 Other hypertrophic osteoarthropathy, left thigh
M89.459 Other hypertrophic osteoarthropathy, unspecified thigh
✓6th M89.46 Other hypertrophic osteoarthropathy, lower leg
M89.461 Other hypertrophic osteoarthropathy, right lower leg
M89.462 Other hypertrophic osteoarthropathy, left lower leg
M89.469 Other hypertrophic osteoarthropathy, unspecified lower leg
✓6th M89.47 Other hypertrophic osteoarthropathy, ankle and foot
M89.471 Other hypertrophic osteoarthropathy, right ankle and foot
M89.472 Other hypertrophic osteoarthropathy, left ankle and foot
M89.479 Other hypertrophic osteoarthropathy, unspecified ankle and foot
M89.48 Other hypertrophic osteoarthropathy, other site
M89.49 Other hypertrophic osteoarthropathy, multiple sites
✓5th M89.5 Osteolysis
Use additional code to identify major osseous defect, if applicable (M89.7-)
EXCLUDES 2 *periprosthetic osteolysis of internal prosthetic joint (T84.05-)*
M89.50 Osteolysis, unspecified site
✓6th M89.51 Osteolysis, shoulder
M89.511 Osteolysis, right shoulder
M89.512 Osteolysis, left shoulder
M89.519 Osteolysis, unspecified shoulder
✓6th M89.52 Osteolysis, upper arm
M89.521 Osteolysis, right upper arm
M89.522 Osteolysis, left upper arm
M89.529 Osteolysis, unspecified upper arm
✓6th M89.53 Osteolysis, forearm
M89.531 Osteolysis, right forearm
M89.532 Osteolysis, left forearm
M89.539 Osteolysis, unspecified forearm
✓6th M89.54 Osteolysis, hand
M89.541 Osteolysis, right hand
M89.542 Osteolysis, left hand
M89.549 Osteolysis, unspecified hand
✓6th M89.55 Osteolysis, thigh
M89.551 Osteolysis, right thigh
M89.552 Osteolysis, left thigh
M89.559 Osteolysis, unspecified thigh

√6th **M89.56 Osteolysis, lower leg**
- **M89.561 Osteolysis, right lower leg**
- **M89.562 Osteolysis, left lower leg**
- **M89.569 Osteolysis, unspecified lower leg**

√6th **M89.57 Osteolysis, ankle and foot**
- **M89.571 Osteolysis, right ankle and foot**
- **M89.572 Osteolysis, left ankle and foot**
- **M89.579 Osteolysis, unspecified ankle and foot**

M89.58 Osteolysis, other site

M89.59 Osteolysis, multiple sites

√5th **M89.6 Osteopathy after poliomyelitis**

Use additional code (B91) to identify previous poliomyelitis

EXCLUDES1 *postpolio syndrome (G14)*

M89.60 Osteopathy after poliomyelitis, unspecified site

√6th **M89.61 Osteopathy after poliomyelitis, shoulder**
- **M89.611 Osteopathy after poliomyelitis, right shoulder**
- **M89.612 Osteopathy after poliomyelitis, left shoulder**
- **M89.619 Osteopathy after poliomyelitis, unspecified shoulder**

√6th **M89.62 Osteopathy after poliomyelitis, upper arm**
- **M89.621 Osteopathy after poliomyelitis, right upper arm**
- **M89.622 Osteopathy after poliomyelitis, left upper arm**
- **M89.629 Osteopathy after poliomyelitis, unspecified upper arm**

√6th **M89.63 Osteopathy after poliomyelitis, forearm**
- **M89.631 Osteopathy after poliomyelitis, right forearm**
- **M89.632 Osteopathy after poliomyelitis, left forearm**
- **M89.639 Osteopathy after poliomyelitis, unspecified forearm**

√6th **M89.64 Osteopathy after poliomyelitis, hand**
- **M89.641 Osteopathy after poliomyelitis, right hand**
- **M89.642 Osteopathy after poliomyelitis, left hand**
- **M89.649 Osteopathy after poliomyelitis, unspecified hand**

√6th **M89.65 Osteopathy after poliomyelitis, thigh**
- **M89.651 Osteopathy after poliomyelitis, right thigh**
- **M89.652 Osteopathy after poliomyelitis, left thigh**
- **M89.659 Osteopathy after poliomyelitis, unspecified thigh**

√6th **M89.66 Osteopathy after poliomyelitis, lower leg**
- **M89.661 Osteopathy after poliomyelitis, right lower leg**
- **M89.662 Osteopathy after poliomyelitis, left lower leg**
- **M89.669 Osteopathy after poliomyelitis, unspecified lower leg**

√6th **M89.67 Osteopathy after poliomyelitis, ankle and foot**
- **M89.671 Osteopathy after poliomyelitis, right ankle and foot**
- **M89.672 Osteopathy after poliomyelitis, left ankle and foot**
- **M89.679 Osteopathy after poliomyelitis, unspecified ankle and foot**

M89.68 Osteopathy after poliomyelitis, other site

M89.69 Osteopathy after poliomyelitis, multiple sites

√5th **M89.7 Major osseous defect**

Code first underlying disease, if known, such as:
- aseptic necrosis of bone (M87.-)
- malignant neoplasm of bone (C4Ø.-)
- osteolysis (M89.5)
- osteomyelitis (M86.-)
- osteonecrosis (M87.-)
- osteoporosis (M8Ø.-, M81.-)
- periprosthetic osteolysis (T84.Ø5-)

M89.7Ø Major osseous defect, unspecified site

√6th **M89.71 Major osseous defect, shoulder region**

Major osseous defect clavicle or scapula
- **M89.711 Major osseous defect, right shoulder region**
- **M89.712 Major osseous defect, left shoulder region**
- **M89.719 Major osseous defect, unspecified shoulder region**

√6th **M89.72 Major osseous defect, humerus**
- **M89.721 Major osseous defect, right humerus**
- **M89.722 Major osseous defect, left humerus**
- **M89.729 Major osseous defect, unspecified humerus**

√6th **M89.73 Major osseous defect, forearm**

Major osseous defect of radius and ulna
- **M89.731 Major osseous defect, right forearm**
- **M89.732 Major osseous defect, left forearm**
- **M89.739 Major osseous defect, unspecified forearm**

√6th **M89.74 Major osseous defect, hand**

Major osseous defect of carpus, fingers, metacarpus
- **M89.741 Major osseous defect, right hand**
- **M89.742 Major osseous defect, left hand**
- **M89.749 Major osseous defect, unspecified hand**

√6th **M89.75 Major osseous defect, pelvic region and thigh**

Major osseous defect of femur and pelvis
- **M89.751 Major osseous defect, right pelvic region and thigh**
- **M89.752 Major osseous defect, left pelvic region and thigh**
- **M89.759 Major osseous defect, unspecified pelvic region and thigh**

√6th **M89.76 Major osseous defect, lower leg**

Major osseous defect of fibula and tibia
- **M89.761 Major osseous defect, right lower leg**
- **M89.762 Major osseous defect, left lower leg**
- **M89.769 Major osseous defect, unspecified lower leg**

√6th **M89.77 Major osseous defect, ankle and foot**

Major osseous defect of metatarsus, tarsus, toes
- **M89.771 Major osseous defect, right ankle and foot**
- **M89.772 Major osseous defect, left ankle and foot**
- **M89.779 Major osseous defect, unspecified ankle and foot**

M89.78 Major osseous defect, other site

M89.79 Major osseous defect, multiple sites

√5th **M89.8 Other specified disorders of bone**

Infantile cortical hyperostoses

Post-traumatic subperiosteal ossification

√6th **M89.8X Other specified disorders of bone**
- **M89.8XØ Other specified disorders of bone, multiple sites**
- **M89.8X1 Other specified disorders of bone, shoulder**
- **M89.8X2 Other specified disorders of bone, upper arm**
- **M89.8X3 Other specified disorders of bone, forearm**
- **M89.8X4 Other specified disorders of bone, hand**
- **M89.8X5 Other specified disorders of bone, thigh**
- **M89.8X6 Other specified disorders of bone, lower leg**
- **M89.8X7 Other specified disorders of bone, ankle and foot**
- **M89.8X8 Other specified disorders of bone, other site**
- **M89.8X9 Other specified disorders of bone, unspecified site**

M89.9 Disorder of bone, unspecified

M90 Osteopathies in diseases classified elsewhere

EXCLUDES 1 *osteochondritis, osteomyelitis, and osteopathy (in):*
cryptococcosis (B45.3)
diabetes mellitus (E08-E13 with .61-)
gonococcal (A54.43)
neurogenic syphilis (A52.11)
renal osteodystrophy (N25.0)
salmonellosis (A02.24)
secondary syphilis (A51.46)
syphilis (late) (A52.77)

M90.5 Osteonecrosis in diseases classified elsewhere

Code first underlying disease, such as:
caisson disease (T70.3)
hemoglobinopathy (D50-D64)

CC Excl: For CC codes in subcategory M90.5, unless otherwise noted: M87.00-M87.9, M90.50-M90.59

M90.50 ***Osteonecrosis in diseases classified elsewhere, unspecified site*** PDx CC CC

M90.51 Osteonecrosis in diseases classified elsewhere, shoulder

M90.511 ***Osteonecrosis in diseases classified elsewhere, right shoulder*** PDx CC CC
CC Excl: M87.00-M87.050, M87.061-M87.073, M87.077-M87.146, M87.161-M87.173, M87.177-M87.250, M87.261-M87.273, M87.277-M87.346, M87.361-M87.373, M87.377-M87.849, M87.861-M87.873, M87.877-M87.9, M90.50-M90.549, M90.561-M90.59

M90.512 ***Osteonecrosis in diseases classified elsewhere, left shoulder*** PDx CC CC
CC Excl: See code: M90.511

M90.519 ***Osteonecrosis in diseases classified elsewhere, unspecified shoulder*** PDx CC CC
CC Excl: See code: M90.511

M90.52 Osteonecrosis in diseases classified elsewhere, upper arm

M90.521 ***Osteonecrosis in diseases classified elsewhere, right upper arm*** PDx CC CC

M90.522 ***Osteonecrosis in diseases classified elsewhere, left upper arm*** PDx CC CC

M90.529 ***Osteonecrosis in diseases classified elsewhere, unspecified upper arm*** PDx CC CC

M90.53 Osteonecrosis in diseases classified elsewhere, forearm

M90.531 ***Osteonecrosis in diseases classified elsewhere, right forearm*** PDx CC CC

M90.532 ***Osteonecrosis in diseases classified elsewhere, left forearm*** PDx CC CC

M90.539 ***Osteonecrosis in diseases classified elsewhere, unspecified forearm*** PDx CC CC

M90.54 Osteonecrosis in diseases classified elsewhere, hand

M90.541 ***Osteonecrosis in diseases classified elsewhere, right hand*** PDx CC CC

M90.542 ***Osteonecrosis in diseases classified elsewhere, left hand*** PDx CC CC

M90.549 ***Osteonecrosis in diseases classified elsewhere, unspecified hand*** PDx CC CC

M90.55 Osteonecrosis in diseases classified elsewhere, thigh

M90.551 ***Osteonecrosis in diseases classified elsewhere, right thigh*** PDx CC CC
CC Excl: M87.00, M87.031-M87.073, M87.077-M87.119, M87.131-M87.173, M87.177-M87.219, M87.231-M87.273, M87.277-M87.319, M87.331-M87.373, M87.377-M87.819, M87.831-M87.873, M87.877-M87.9, M90.50, M90.521-M90.59

M90.552 ***Osteonecrosis in diseases classified elsewhere, left thigh*** PDx CC CC
CC Excl: See code: M90.551

M90.559 ***Osteonecrosis in diseases classified elsewhere, unspecified thigh*** PDx CC CC
CC Excl: See code: M90.551

M90.56 Osteonecrosis in diseases classified elsewhere, lower leg

M90.561 ***Osteonecrosis in diseases classified elsewhere, right lower leg*** PDx CC CC

M90.562 ***Osteonecrosis in diseases classified elsewhere, left lower leg*** PDx CC CC

M90.569 ***Osteonecrosis in diseases classified elsewhere, unspecified lower leg*** PDx CC CC

M90.57 Osteonecrosis in diseases classified elsewhere, ankle and foot

M90.571 ***Osteonecrosis in diseases classified elsewhere, right ankle and foot*** PDx CC CC

M90.572 ***Osteonecrosis in diseases classified elsewhere, left ankle and foot*** PDx CC CC

M90.579 ***Osteonecrosis in diseases classified elsewhere, unspecified ankle and foot*** PDx CC CC

M90.58 ***Osteonecrosis in diseases classified elsewhere, other site*** PDx CC CC

M90.59 ***Osteonecrosis in diseases classified elsewhere, multiple sites*** PDx CC CC

M90.6 Osteitis deformans in neoplastic diseases

Osteitis deformans in malignant neoplasm of bone
Code first the neoplasm (C40-, C41-)
EXCLUDES 1 *osteitis deformans [Paget's disease of bone] (M88.-)*

M90.60 ***Osteitis deformans in neoplastic diseases, unspecified site***

M90.61 Osteitis deformans in neoplastic diseases, shoulder

M90.611 ***Osteitis deformans in neoplastic diseases, right shoulder***

M90.612 ***Osteitis deformans in neoplastic diseases, left shoulder***

M90.619 ***Osteitis deformans in neoplastic diseases, unspecified shoulder***

M90.62 Osteitis deformans in neoplastic diseases, upper arm

M90.621 ***Osteitis deformans in neoplastic diseases, right upper arm***

M90.622 ***Osteitis deformans in neoplastic diseases, left upper arm***

M90.629 ***Osteitis deformans in neoplastic diseases, unspecified upper arm***

M90.63 Osteitis deformans in neoplastic diseases, forearm

M90.631 ***Osteitis deformans in neoplastic diseases, right forearm***

M90.632 ***Osteitis deformans in neoplastic diseases, left forearm***

M90.639 ***Osteitis deformans in neoplastic diseases, unspecified forearm***

M90.64 Osteitis deformans in neoplastic diseases, hand

M90.641 ***Osteitis deformans in neoplastic diseases, right hand***

M90.642 ***Osteitis deformans in neoplastic diseases, left hand***

M90.649 ***Osteitis deformans in neoplastic diseases, unspecified hand***

M90.65 Osteitis deformans in neoplastic diseases, thigh

M90.651 ***Osteitis deformans in neoplastic diseases, right thigh***

M90.652 ***Osteitis deformans in neoplastic diseases, left thigh***

M90.659 ***Osteitis deformans in neoplastic diseases, unspecified thigh***

M90.66 Osteitis deformans in neoplastic diseases, lower leg

M90.661 ***Osteitis deformans in neoplastic diseases, right lower leg***

M90.662 ***Osteitis deformans in neoplastic diseases, left lower leg***

M90.669 ***Osteitis deformans in neoplastic diseases, unspecified lower leg***

M90.67 Osteitis deformans in neoplastic diseases, ankle and foot

M90.671 ***Osteitis deformans in neoplastic diseases, right ankle and foot***

M90.672 ***Osteitis deformans in neoplastic diseases, left ankle and foot***

M90.679 ***Osteitis deformans in neoplastic diseases, unspecified ankle and foot***

M90.68 *Osteitis deformans in neoplastic diseases, other site*

M90.69 *Osteitis deformans in neoplastic diseases, multiple sites*

✓5th **M90.8 Osteopathy in diseases classified elsewhere**

Code first underlying disease, such as:
rickets (E55.0)
vitamin-D-resistant rickets (E83.3)

M90.80 *Osteopathy in diseases classified elsewhere, unspecified site*

✓6th **M90.81 Osteopathy in diseases classified elsewhere, shoulder**

M90.811 *Osteopathy in diseases classified elsewhere, right shoulder*

M90.812 *Osteopathy in diseases classified elsewhere, left shoulder*

M90.819 *Osteopathy in diseases classified elsewhere, unspecified shoulder*

✓6th **M90.82 Osteopathy in diseases classified elsewhere, upper arm**

M90.821 *Osteopathy in diseases classified elsewhere, right upper arm*

M90.822 *Osteopathy in diseases classified elsewhere, left upper arm*

M90.829 *Osteopathy in diseases classified elsewhere, unspecified upper arm*

✓6th **M90.83 Osteopathy in diseases classified elsewhere, forearm**

M90.831 *Osteopathy in diseases classified elsewhere, right forearm*

M90.832 *Osteopathy in diseases classified elsewhere, left forearm*

M90.839 *Osteopathy in diseases classified elsewhere, unspecified forearm*

✓6th **M90.84 Osteopathy in diseases classified elsewhere, hand**

M90.841 *Osteopathy in diseases classified elsewhere, right hand*

M90.842 *Osteopathy in diseases classified elsewhere, left hand*

M90.849 *Osteopathy in diseases classified elsewhere, unspecified hand*

✓6th **M90.85 Osteopathy in diseases classified elsewhere, thigh**

M90.851 *Osteopathy in diseases classified elsewhere, right thigh*

M90.852 *Osteopathy in diseases classified elsewhere, left thigh*

M90.859 *Osteopathy in diseases classified elsewhere, unspecified thigh*

✓6th **M90.86 Osteopathy in diseases classified elsewhere, lower leg**

M90.861 *Osteopathy in diseases classified elsewhere, right lower leg*

M90.862 *Osteopathy in diseases classified elsewhere, left lower leg*

M90.869 *Osteopathy in diseases classified elsewhere, unspecified lower leg*

✓6th **M90.87 Osteopathy in diseases classified elsewhere, ankle and foot**

M90.871 *Osteopathy in diseases classified elsewhere, right ankle and foot*

M90.872 *Osteopathy in diseases classified elsewhere, left ankle and foot*

M90.879 *Osteopathy in diseases classified elsewhere, unspecified ankle and foot*

M90.88 *Osteopathy in diseases classified elsewhere, other site*

M90.89 *Osteopathy in diseases classified elsewhere, multiple sites*

Chondropathies (M91-M94)

EXCLUDES 1 *postprocedural chondropathies (M96.-)*

✓4th **M91 Juvenile osteochondrosis of hip and pelvis**

EXCLUDES 1 *slipped upper femoral epiphysis (nontraumatic) (M93.0)*

M91.0 Juvenile osteochondrosis of pelvis

Osteochondrosis (juvenile) of acetabulum
Osteochondrosis (juvenile) of iliac crest [Buchanan]
Osteochondrosis (juvenile) of ischiopubic synchondrosis [van Neck]
Osteochondrosis (juvenile) of symphysis pubis [Pierson]

✓5th **M91.1 Juvenile osteochondrosis of head of femur [Legg-Calvé-Perthes]**

M91.10 Juvenile osteochondrosis of head of femur [Legg-Calvé-Perthes], unspecified leg

M91.11 Juvenile osteochondrosis of head of femur [Legg-Calvé-Perthes], right leg

M91.12 Juvenile osteochondrosis of head of femur [Legg-Calvé-Perthes], left leg

✓5th **M91.2 Coxa plana**

Hip deformity due to previous juvenile osteochondrosis

M91.20 Coxa plana, unspecified hip

M91.21 Coxa plana, right hip

M91.22 Coxa plana, left hip

✓5th **M91.3 Pseudocoxalgia**

M91.30 Pseudocoxalgia, unspecified hip

M91.31 Pseudocoxalgia, right hip

M91.32 Pseudocoxalgia, left hip

✓5th **M91.4 Coxa magna**

M91.40 Coxa magna, unspecified hip

M91.41 Coxa magna, right hip

M91.42 Coxa magna, left hip

✓5th **M91.8 Other juvenile osteochondrosis of hip and pelvis**

Juvenile osteochondrosis after reduction of congenital dislocation of hip

M91.80 Other juvenile osteochondrosis of hip and pelvis, unspecified leg

M91.81 Other juvenile osteochondrosis of hip and pelvis, right leg

M91.82 Other juvenile osteochondrosis of hip and pelvis, left leg

✓5th **M91.9 Juvenile osteochondrosis of hip and pelvis, unspecified**

M91.90 Juvenile osteochondrosis of hip and pelvis, unspecified, unspecified leg

M91.91 Juvenile osteochondrosis of hip and pelvis, unspecified, right leg

M91.92 Juvenile osteochondrosis of hip and pelvis, unspecified, left leg

✓4th **M92 Other juvenile osteochondrosis**

✓5th **M92.0 Juvenile osteochondrosis of humerus**

Osteochondrosis (juvenile) of capitulum of humerus [Panner]
Osteochondrosis (juvenile) of head of humerus [Haas]

M92.00 Juvenile osteochondrosis of humerus, unspecified arm

M92.01 Juvenile osteochondrosis of humerus, right arm

M92.02 Juvenile osteochondrosis of humerus, left arm

✓5th **M92.1 Juvenile osteochondrosis of radius and ulna**

Osteochondrosis (juvenile) of lower ulna [Burns]
Osteochondrosis (juvenile) of radial head [Brailsford]

M92.10 Juvenile osteochondrosis of radius and ulna, unspecified arm

M92.11 Juvenile osteochondrosis of radius and ulna, right arm

M92.12 Juvenile osteochondrosis of radius and ulna, left arm

✓5th **M92.2 Juvenile osteochondrosis, hand**

✓6th **M92.20 Unspecified juvenile osteochondrosis, hand**

M92.201 Unspecified juvenile osteochondrosis, right hand

M92.202 Unspecified juvenile osteochondrosis, left hand

M92.209 Unspecified juvenile osteochondrosis, unspecified hand

✓6th M92.21 Osteochondrosis (juvenile) of carpal lunate [Kienböck]
- M92.211 Osteochondrosis (juvenile) of carpal lunate [Kienböck], right hand
- M92.212 Osteochondrosis (juvenile) of carpal lunate [Kienböck], left hand
- M92.219 Osteochondrosis (juvenile) of carpal lunate [Kienböck], unspecified hand

✓6th M92.22 Osteochondrosis (juvenile) of metacarpal heads [Mauclaire]
- M92.221 Osteochondrosis (juvenile) of metacarpal heads [Mauclaire], right hand
- M92.222 Osteochondrosis (juvenile) of metacarpal heads [Mauclaire], left hand
- M92.229 Osteochondrosis (juvenile) of metacarpal heads [Mauclaire], unspecified hand

✓6th M92.29 Other juvenile osteochondrosis, hand
- M92.291 Other juvenile osteochondrosis, right hand
- M92.292 Other juvenile osteochondrosis, left hand
- M92.299 Other juvenile osteochondrosis, unspecified hand

✓5th M92.3 Other juvenile osteochondrosis, upper limb
- M92.30 Other juvenile osteochondrosis, unspecified upper limb
- M92.31 Other juvenile osteochondrosis, right upper limb
- M92.32 Other juvenile osteochondrosis, left upper limb

✓5th M92.4 Juvenile osteochondrosis of patella

Osteochondrosis (juvenile) of primary patellar center [Köhler]
Osteochondrosis (juvenile) of secondary patellar centre [Sinding Larsen]

- M92.40 Juvenile osteochondrosis of patella, unspecified knee
- M92.41 Juvenile osteochondrosis of patella, right knee
- M92.42 Juvenile osteochondrosis of patella, left knee

✓5th M92.5 Juvenile osteochondrosis of tibia and fibula

Osteochondrosis (juvenile) of proximal tibia [Blount]
Osteochondrosis (juvenile) of tibial tubercle [Osgood-Schlatter]
Tibia vara

- M92.50 Juvenile osteochondrosis of tibia and fibula, unspecified leg
- M92.51 Juvenile osteochondrosis of tibia and fibula, right leg
- M92.52 Juvenile osteochondrosis of tibia and fibula, left leg

✓5th M92.6 Juvenile osteochondrosis of tarsus

Osteochondrosis (juvenile) of calcaneum [Sever]
Osteochondrosis (juvenile) of os tibiale externum [Haglund]
Osteochondrosis (juvenile) of talus [Diaz]
Osteochondrosis (juvenile) of tarsal navicular [Köhler]

- M92.60 Juvenile osteochondrosis of tarsus, unspecified ankle
- M92.61 Juvenile osteochondrosis of tarsus, right ankle
- M92.62 Juvenile osteochondrosis of tarsus, left ankle

✓5th M92.7 Juvenile osteochondrosis of metatarsus

Osteochondrosis (juvenile) of fifth metatarsus [Iselin]
Osteochondrosis (juvenile) of second metatarsus [Freiberg]

- M92.70 Juvenile osteochondrosis of metatarsus, unspecified foot
- M92.71 Juvenile osteochondrosis of metatarsus, right foot
- M92.72 Juvenile osteochondrosis of metatarsus, left foot

M92.8 Other specified juvenile osteochondrosis

Calcaneal apophysitis

M92.9 Juvenile osteochondrosis, unspecified

Juvenile apophysitis NOS
Juvenile epiphysitis NOS
Juvenile osteochondritis NOS
Juvenile osteochondrosis NOS

✓4th M93 Other osteochondropathies

EXCLUDES 2 *osteochondrosis of spine (M42.-)*

✓5th M93.0 Slipped upper femoral epiphysis (nontraumatic)

Use additional code for associated chondrolysis (M94.3)

✓6th M93.00 Unspecified slipped upper femoral epiphysis (nontraumatic)
- M93.001 Unspecified slipped upper femoral epiphysis (nontraumatic), right hip
- M93.002 Unspecified slipped upper femoral epiphysis (nontraumatic), left hip
- M93.003 Unspecified slipped upper femoral epiphysis (nontraumatic), unspecified hip

✓6th M93.01 Acute slipped upper femoral epiphysis (nontraumatic)
- M93.011 Acute slipped upper femoral epiphysis (nontraumatic), right hip
- M93.012 Acute slipped upper femoral epiphysis (nontraumatic), left hip
- M93.013 Acute slipped upper femoral epiphysis (nontraumatic), unspecified hip

✓6th M93.02 Chronic slipped upper femoral epiphysis (nontraumatic)
- M93.021 Chronic slipped upper femoral epiphysis (nontraumatic), right hip
- M93.022 Chronic slipped upper femoral epiphysis (nontraumatic), left hip
- M93.023 Chronic slipped upper femoral epiphysis (nontraumatic), unspecified hip

✓6th M93.03 Acute on chronic slipped upper femoral epiphysis (nontraumatic)
- M93.031 Acute on chronic slipped upper femoral epiphysis (nontraumatic), right hip
- M93.032 Acute on chronic slipped upper femoral epiphysis (nontraumatic), left hip
- M93.033 Acute on chronic slipped upper femoral epiphysis (nontraumatic), unspecified hip

M93.1 Kienböck's disease of adults A

Adult osteochondrosis of carpal lunates

✓5th M93.2 Osteochondritis dissecans
- M93.20 Osteochondritis dissecans of unspecified site

✓6th M93.21 Osteochondritis dissecans of shoulder
- M93.211 Osteochondritis dissecans, right shoulder
- M93.212 Osteochondritis dissecans, left shoulder
- M93.219 Osteochondritis dissecans, unspecified shoulder

✓6th M93.22 Osteochondritis dissecans of elbow
- M93.221 Osteochondritis dissecans, right elbow
- M93.222 Osteochondritis dissecans, left elbow
- M93.229 Osteochondritis dissecans, unspecified elbow

✓6th M93.23 Osteochondritis dissecans of wrist
- M93.231 Osteochondritis dissecans, right wrist
- M93.232 Osteochondritis dissecans, left wrist
- M93.239 Osteochondritis dissecans, unspecified wrist

✓6th M93.24 Osteochondritis dissecans of joints of hand
- M93.241 Osteochondritis dissecans, joints of right hand
- M93.242 Osteochondritis dissecans, joints of left hand
- M93.249 Osteochondritis dissecans, joints of unspecified hand

✓6th M93.25 Osteochondritis dissecans of hip
- M93.251 Osteochondritis dissecans, right hip
- M93.252 Osteochondritis dissecans, left hip
- M93.259 Osteochondritis dissecans, unspecified hip

✓6th M93.26 Osteochondritis dissecans knee
- M93.261 Osteochondritis dissecans, right knee
- M93.262 Osteochondritis dissecans, left knee
- M93.269 Osteochondritis dissecans, unspecified knee

✓6th M93.27 Osteochondritis dissecans of ankle and joints of foot
- M93.271 Osteochondritis dissecans, right ankle and joints of right foot
- M93.272 Osteochondritis dissecans, left ankle and joints of left foot
- M93.279 Osteochondritis dissecans, unspecified ankle and joints of foot

- M93.28 Osteochondritis dissecans other site
- M93.29 Osteochondritis dissecans multiple sites

✓5th M93.8 Other specified osteochondropathies
- M93.80 Other specified osteochondropathies of unspecified site

✓6th **M93.81 Other specified osteochondropathies of shoulder**
- **M93.811 Other specified osteochondropathies, right shoulder**
- **M93.812 Other specified osteochondropathies, left shoulder**
- **M93.819 Other specified osteochondropathies, unspecified shoulder**

✓6th **M93.82 Other specified osteochondropathies of upper arm**
- **M93.821 Other specified osteochondropathies, right upper arm**
- **M93.822 Other specified osteochondropathies, left upper arm**
- **M93.829 Other specified osteochondropathies, unspecified upper arm**

✓6th **M93.83 Other specified osteochondropathies of forearm**
- **M93.831 Other specified osteochondropathies, right forearm**
- **M93.832 Other specified osteochondropathies, left forearm**
- **M93.839 Other specified osteochondropathies, unspecified forearm**

✓6th **M93.84 Other specified osteochondropathies of hand**
- **M93.841 Other specified osteochondropathies, right hand**
- **M93.842 Other specified osteochondropathies, left hand**
- **M93.849 Other specified osteochondropathies, unspecified hand**

✓6th **M93.85 Other specified osteochondropathies of thigh**
- **M93.851 Other specified osteochondropathies, right thigh**
- **M93.852 Other specified osteochondropathies, left thigh**
- **M93.859 Other specified osteochondropathies, unspecified thigh**

✓6th **M93.86 Other specified osteochondropathies lower leg**
- **M93.861 Other specified osteochondropathies, right lower leg**
- **M93.862 Other specified osteochondropathies, left lower leg**
- **M93.869 Other specified osteochondropathies, unspecified lower leg**

✓6th **M93.87 Other specified osteochondropathies of ankle and foot**
- **M93.871 Other specified osteochondropathies, right ankle and foot**
- **M93.872 Other specified osteochondropathies, left ankle and foot**
- **M93.879 Other specified osteochondropathies, unspecified ankle and foot**

M93.88 Other specified osteochondropathies other site

M93.89 Other specified osteochondropathies multiple sites

✓5th **M93.9 Osteochondropathy, unspecified**

Apophysitis NOS
Epiphysitis NOS
Osteochondritis NOS
Osteochondrosis NOS

M93.9Ø Osteochondropathy, unspecified of unspecified site

✓6th **M93.91 Osteochondropathy, unspecified of shoulder**
- **M93.911 Osteochondropathy, unspecified, right shoulder**
- **M93.912 Osteochondropathy, unspecified, left shoulder**
- **M93.919 Osteochondropathy, unspecified, unspecified shoulder**

✓6th **M93.92 Osteochondropathy, unspecified of upper arm**
- **M93.921 Osteochondropathy, unspecified, right upper arm**
- **M93.922 Osteochondropathy, unspecified, left upper arm**
- **M93.929 Osteochondropathy, unspecified, unspecified upper arm**

✓6th **M93.93 Osteochondropathy, unspecified of forearm**
- **M93.931 Osteochondropathy, unspecified, right forearm**
- **M93.932 Osteochondropathy, unspecified, left forearm**
- **M93.939 Osteochondropathy, unspecified, unspecified forearm**

✓6th **M93.94 Osteochondropathy, unspecified of hand**
- **M93.941 Osteochondropathy, unspecified, right hand**
- **M93.942 Osteochondropathy, unspecified, left hand**
- **M93.949 Osteochondropathy, unspecified, unspecified hand**

✓6th **M93.95 Osteochondropathy, unspecified of thigh**
- **M93.951 Osteochondropathy, unspecified, right thigh**
- **M93.952 Osteochondropathy, unspecified, left thigh**
- **M93.959 Osteochondropathy, unspecified, unspecified thigh**

✓6th **M93.96 Osteochondropathy, unspecified lower leg**
- **M93.961 Osteochondropathy, unspecified, right lower leg**
- **M93.962 Osteochondropathy, unspecified, left lower leg**
- **M93.969 Osteochondropathy, unspecified, unspecified lower leg**

✓6th **M93.97 Osteochondropathy, unspecified of ankle and foot**
- **M93.971 Osteochondropathy, unspecified, right ankle and foot**
- **M93.972 Osteochondropathy, unspecified, left ankle and foot**
- **M93.979 Osteochondropathy, unspecified, unspecified ankle and foot**

M93.98 Osteochondropathy, unspecified other site

M93.99 Osteochondropathy, unspecified multiple sites

✓4th M94 Other disorders of cartilage

M94.Ø Chondrocostal junction syndrome [Tietze]

Costochondritis

M94.1 Relapsing polychondritis

✓5th **M94.2 Chondromalacia**

EXCLUDES 1 *chondromalacia patellae (M22.4)*

M94.2Ø Chondromalacia, unspecified site

✓6th **M94.21 Chondromalacia, shoulder**
- **M94.211 Chondromalacia, right shoulder**
- **M94.212 Chondromalacia, left shoulder**
- **M94.219 Chondromalacia, unspecified shoulder**

✓6th **M94.22 Chondromalacia, elbow**
- **M94.221 Chondromalacia, right elbow**
- **M94.222 Chondromalacia, left elbow**
- **M94.229 Chondromalacia, unspecified elbow**

✓6th **M94.23 Chondromalacia, wrist**
- **M94.231 Chondromalacia, right wrist**
- **M94.232 Chondromalacia, left wrist**
- **M94.239 Chondromalacia, unspecified wrist**

✓6th **M94.24 Chondromalacia, joints of hand**
- **M94.241 Chondromalacia, joints of right hand**
- **M94.242 Chondromalacia, joints of left hand**
- **M94.249 Chondromalacia, joints of unspecified hand**

✓6th **M94.25 Chondromalacia, hip**
- **M94.251 Chondromalacia, right hip**
- **M94.252 Chondromalacia, left hip**
- **M94.259 Chondromalacia, unspecified hip**

✓6th **M94.26 Chondromalacia, knee**
- **M94.261 Chondromalacia, right knee**
- **M94.262 Chondromalacia, left knee**
- **M94.269 Chondromalacia, unspecified knee**

✓6th **M94.27 Chondromalacia, ankle and joints of foot**
- **M94.271 Chondromalacia, right ankle and joints of right foot**
- **M94.272 Chondromalacia, left ankle and joints of left foot**
- **M94.279 Chondromalacia, unspecified ankle and joints of foot**

M94.28 Chondromalacia, other site

M94.29 Chondromalacia, multiple sites

M94.3 Chondrolysis
Code first any associated slipped upper femoral epiphysis (nontraumatic) (M93.0-)

M94.35 Chondrolysis, hip

M94.351 Chondrolysis, right hip

M94.352 Chondrolysis, left hip

M94.359 Chondrolysis, unspecified hip

M94.8 Other specified disorders of cartilage

M94.8X Other specified disorders of cartilage

M94.8X0 Other specified disorders of cartilage, multiple sites

M94.8X1 Other specified disorders of cartilage, shoulder

M94.8X2 Other specified disorders of cartilage, upper arm

M94.8X3 Other specified disorders of cartilage, forearm

M94.8X4 Other specified disorders of cartilage, hand

M94.8X5 Other specified disorders of cartilage, thigh

M94.8X6 Other specified disorders of cartilage, lower leg

M94.8X7 Other specified disorders of cartilage, ankle and foot

M94.8X8 Other specified disorders of cartilage, other site

M94.8X9 Other specified disorders of cartilage, unspecified sites

M94.9 Disorder of cartilage, unspecified

Other disorders of the musculoskeletal system and connective tissue (M95)

M95 Other acquired deformities of musculoskeletal system and connective tissue
EXCLUDES 2 *acquired absence of limbs and organs (Z89-Z90)*
acquired deformities of limbs (M20-M21)
congenital malformations and deformations of the musculoskeletal system (Q65-Q79)
deforming dorsopathies (M40-M43)
dentofacial anomalies [including malocclusion] (M26.-)
postprocedural musculoskeletal disorders (M96.-)

M95.0 Acquired deformity of nose
EXCLUDES 2 *deviated nasal septum (J34.2)*

M95.1 Cauliflower ear
EXCLUDES 2 *other acquired deformities of ear (H61.1)*

M95.10 Cauliflower ear, unspecified ear

M95.11 Cauliflower ear, right ear

M95.12 Cauliflower ear, left ear

M95.2 Other acquired deformity of head

M95.3 Acquired deformity of neck

M95.4 Acquired deformity of chest and rib

M95.5 Acquired deformity of pelvis
EXCLUDES 1 *maternal care for known or suspected disproportion (O33.-)*

M95.8 Other specified acquired deformities of musculoskeletal system

M95.9 Acquired deformity of musculoskeletal system, unspecified

Intraoperative and postprocedural complications and disorders of musculoskeletal system, not elsewhere classified (M96)

M96 Intraoperative and postprocedural complications and disorders of musculoskeletal system, not elsewhere classified
EXCLUDES 2 *arthropathy following intestinal bypass (M02.0-)*
complications of internal orthopedic prosthetic devices, implants and grafts (T84.-)
disorders associated with osteoporosis (M80)
presence of functional implants and other devices (Z96-Z97)

M96.0 Pseudarthrosis after fusion or arthrodesis CC

M96.1 Postlaminectomy syndrome, not elsewhere classified

M96.2 Postradiation kyphosis

M96.3 Postlaminectomy kyphosis

M96.4 Postsurgical lordosis

M96.5 Postradiation scoliosis

M96.6 Fracture of bone following insertion of orthopedic implant, joint prosthesis, or bone plate
Intraoperative fracture of bone during insertion of orthopedic implant, joint prosthesis, or bone plate
EXCLUDES 2 *complication of internal orthopedic devices, implants or grafts (T84.-)*

M96.62 Fracture of humerus following insertion of orthopedic implant, joint prosthesis, or bone plate

M96.621 Fracture of humerus following insertion of orthopedic implant, joint prosthesis, or bone plate, right arm CC
CC Excl: D78.81-D78.89, E36.8, E89.810-E89.89, H59.011-H59.019, H59.031-H59.099, H59.811-H59.89, H95.811-H95.89, I97.3, L76.81-L76.82, M96.621-M96.69, M96.89, N98.1-N98.9, T84.010-T84.9XX with 7th A; T81.82XA, T81.89XA, T81.9XXA, T84.9

M96.622 Fracture of humerus following insertion of orthopedic implant, joint prosthesis, or bone plate, left arm CC
CC Excl: See code: M96.621

M96.629 Fracture of humerus following insertion of orthopedic implant, joint prosthesis, or bone plate, unspecified arm CC
CC Excl: See code: M96.621

M96.63 Fracture of radius or ulna following insertion of orthopedic implant, joint prosthesis, or bone plate

M96.631 Fracture of radius or ulna following insertion of orthopedic implant, joint prosthesis, or bone plate, right arm CC
CC Excl: See code: M96.621

M96.632 Fracture of radius or ulna following insertion of orthopedic implant, joint prosthesis, or bone plate, left arm CC
CC Excl: See code: M96.621

M96.639 Fracture of radius or ulna following insertion of orthopedic implant, joint prosthesis, or bone plate, unspecified arm CC
CC Excl: See code: M96.621

M96.65 Fracture of pelvis following insertion of orthopedic implant, joint prosthesis, or bone plate CC
CC Excl: See code: M96.621

M96.66 Fracture of femur following insertion of orthopedic implant, joint prosthesis, or bone plate

M96.661 Fracture of femur following insertion of orthopedic implant, joint prosthesis, or bone plate, right leg CC
CC Excl: See code: M96.621

M96.662 Fracture of femur following insertion of orthopedic implant, joint prosthesis, or bone plate, left leg CC
CC Excl: See code: M96.621

M96.669 Fracture of femur following insertion of orthopedic implant, joint prosthesis, or bone plate, unspecified leg CC
CC Excl: See code: M96.621

M96.67 Fracture of tibia or fibula following insertion of orthopedic implant, joint prosthesis, or bone plate

M96.671 Fracture of tibia or fibula following insertion of orthopedic implant, joint prosthesis, or bone plate, right leg CC
CC Excl: See code: M96.621

M96.672 Fracture of tibia or fibula following insertion of orthopedic implant, joint prosthesis, or bone plate, left leg CC
CC Excl: See code: M96.621

M96.679 Fracture of tibia or fibula following insertion of orthopedic implant, joint prosthesis, or bone plate, unspecified leg CC
CC Excl: See code: M96.621

M96.69 Fracture of other bone following insertion of orthopedic implant, joint prosthesis, or bone plate CC
CC Excl: See code: M96.621

M96.8 Other intraoperative and postprocedural complications and disorders of musculoskeletal system, not elsewhere classified

M96.81 Intraoperative hemorrhage and hematoma of a musculoskeletal structure complicating a procedure

EXCLUDES 1 *intraoperative hemorrhage and hematoma of a musculoskeletal structure due to accidental puncture and laceration during a procedure (M96.82-)*

M96.810 Intraoperative hemorrhage and hematoma of a musculoskeletal structure complicating a musculoskeletal system procedure CC

CC Excl: H95.811-H95.89, I85.01, I85.11, I97.3, K21.9, K22.8, K23-K25.0, K25.2, K25.4, K25.6, K26.0, K26.2, K26.4, K26.6, K27.0, K27.2, K27.4, K27.6, K28.0, K28.2, K28.4, K28.6, K29.01, K29.21, K29.31, K29.41, K29.51, K29.61, K29.71, K29.81, K29.91, K31.811, K55.21, K57.01, K57.11, K57.13, K57.21, K57.31, K57.33, K57.41, K57.51, K57.53, K57.81, K57.91, K57.93, K62.5, K92.0-K92.2, M96.810-M96.811, M96.830-M96.89, N98.1-N98.9, P54.1-P54.3, T81.10XA, T81.11XA, T81.12XA, T81.19XA, T81.82XA, T81.89XA, T81.9XXA

M96.811 Intraoperative hemorrhage and hematoma of a musculoskeletal structure complicating other procedure CC

CC Excl: See code: M96.810

M96.82 Accidental puncture and laceration of a musculoskeletal structure during a procedure

M96.820 Accidental puncture and laceration of a musculoskeletal structure during a musculoskeletal system procedure CC

CC Excl: D78.11-D78.12, D78.81-D78.89, E36.11-E36.8, E89.810-E89.89, G96.11, G97.41-G97.49, H59.011-H59.019, H59.031-H59.099, H59.211-H59.229, H59.811-H59.89, H95.31-H95.32, H95.811-H95.89, I97.3, I97.51-I97.52, J95.71-J95.72, K91.71-K91.72, L76.11-L76.12, L76.81-L76.82, M96.820-M96.821, M96.89, N98.1-N98.9, N99.71-N99.72, T81.82XA, T81.89XA, T81.9XXA

M96.821 Accidental puncture and laceration of a musculoskeletal structure during other procedure CC

CC Excl: See code: M96.820

M96.83 Postprocedural hemorrhage and hematoma of a musculoskeletal structure following a procedure

M96.830 Postprocedural hemorrhage and hematoma of a musculoskeletal structure following a musculoskeletal system procedure CC

CC Excl: See code: M96.810

M96.831 Postprocedural hemorrhage and hematoma of a musculoskeletal structure following other procedure CC

CC Excl: See code: M96.810

M96.89 Other intraoperative and postprocedural complications and disorders of the musculoskeletal system CC

Instability of joint secondary to removal of joint prosthesis

Use additional code, if applicable, to further specify disorder

CC Excl: D78.81-D78.89, E36.8, E89.810-E89.89, H59.011-H59.019, H59.031-H59.099, H59.811-H59.89, H95.811-H95.89, I97.3, L76.81-L76.82, M96.89, N98.1-N98.9, T81.82XA, T81.89XA, T81.9XXA

Biomechanical lesions, not elsewhere classified (M99)

M99 Biomechanical lesions, not elsewhere classified

NOTE This category should not be used if the condition can be classified elsewhere.

M99.0 Segmental and somatic dysfunction

M99.00 Segmental and somatic dysfunction of head region

M99.01 Segmental and somatic dysfunction of cervical region

M99.02 Segmental and somatic dysfunction of thoracic region

M99.03 Segmental and somatic dysfunction of lumbar region

M99.04 Segmental and somatic dysfunction of sacral region

M99.05 Segmental and somatic dysfunction of pelvic region

M99.06 Segmental and somatic dysfunction of lower extremity

M99.07 Segmental and somatic dysfunction of upper extremity

M99.08 Segmental and somatic dysfunction of rib cage

M99.09 Segmental and somatic dysfunction of abdomen and other regions

M99.1 Subluxation complex (vertebral)

CC Excl: For CC codes in subcategory M99.1, unless otherwise noted: M99.10-M99.11, S03.8XX-S03.9XX with 7th A, S12.000-S12.691 with 7th [A, B], S12.9XX-S13.4XX with 7th A, S13.8XXA, S14.0XX-S14.108 with 7th A, S14.111-S14.118 with 7th A, S14.121-S14.128 with 7th A, S14.131-S14.138 with 7th A, S14.141-S14.148 with 7th A, S14.151-S14.158 with 7th A, S16.1XX A, S29.011-S29.019 with 7th A, S38.3XX-S39.013 with 7th A, T14.8-T14.91, T79.A0X-T79.9XX with 7th A

M99.10 Subluxation complex (vertebral) of head region CC

M99.11 Subluxation complex (vertebral) of cervical region CC

M99.12 Subluxation complex (vertebral) of thoracic region

M99.13 Subluxation complex (vertebral) of lumbar region

M99.14 Subluxation complex (vertebral) of sacral region

M99.15 Subluxation complex (vertebral) of pelvic region

M99.16 Subluxation complex (vertebral) of lower extremity

M99.17 Subluxation complex (vertebral) of upper extremity

M99.18 Subluxation complex (vertebral) of rib cage CC

CC Excl: M99.18, S43.201-S43.226 with 7th character A

M99.19 Subluxation complex (vertebral) of abdomen and other regions

M99.2 Subluxation stenosis of neural canal

M99.20 Subluxation stenosis of neural canal of head region

M99.21 Subluxation stenosis of neural canal of cervical region

M99.22 Subluxation stenosis of neural canal of thoracic region

M99.23 Subluxation stenosis of neural canal of lumbar region

M99.24 Subluxation stenosis of neural canal of sacral region

M99.25 Subluxation stenosis of neural canal of pelvic region

M99.26 Subluxation stenosis of neural canal of lower extremity

M99.27 Subluxation stenosis of neural canal of upper extremity

M99.28 Subluxation stenosis of neural canal of rib cage

M99.29 Subluxation stenosis of neural canal of abdomen and other regions

M99.3 Osseous stenosis of neural canal

M99.30 Osseous stenosis of neural canal of head region

M99.31 Osseous stenosis of neural canal of cervical region

M99.32 Osseous stenosis of neural canal of thoracic region

M99.33 Osseous stenosis of neural canal of lumbar region

M99.34 Osseous stenosis of neural canal of sacral region

M99.35 Osseous stenosis of neural canal of pelvic region

M99.36 Osseous stenosis of neural canal of lower extremity

M99.37 Osseous stenosis of neural canal of upper extremity

M99.38 Osseous stenosis of neural canal of rib cage

M99.39 Osseous stenosis of neural canal of abdomen and other regions

M99.4 Connective tissue stenosis of neural canal

M99.40 Connective tissue stenosis of neural canal of head region

M99.41 Connective tissue stenosis of neural canal of cervical region

M99.42 Connective tissue stenosis of neural canal of thoracic region

M99.43 Connective tissue stenosis of neural canal of lumbar region

M99.44 Connective tissue stenosis of neural canal of sacral region

M99.45 Connective tissue stenosis of neural canal of pelvic region

M99.46 Connective tissue stenosis of neural canal of lower extremity

M99.47 Connective tissue stenosis of neural canal of upper extremity

M99.48 Connective tissue stenosis of neural canal of rib cage

M99.49 Connective tissue stenosis of neural canal of abdomen and other regions

√5th M99.5 Intervertebral disc stenosis of neural canal

M99.50 Intervertebral disc stenosis of neural canal of head region

M99.51 Intervertebral disc stenosis of neural canal of cervical region

M99.52 Intervertebral disc stenosis of neural canal of thoracic region

M99.53 Intervertebral disc stenosis of neural canal of lumbar region

M99.54 Intervertebral disc stenosis of neural canal of sacral region

M99.55 Intervertebral disc stenosis of neural canal of pelvic region

M99.56 Intervertebral disc stenosis of neural canal of lower extremity

M99.57 Intervertebral disc stenosis of neural canal of upper extremity

M99.58 Intervertebral disc stenosis of neural canal of rib cage

M99.59 Intervertebral disc stenosis of neural canal of abdomen and other regions

√5th M99.6 Osseous and subluxation stenosis of intervertebral foramina

M99.60 Osseous and subluxation stenosis of intervertebral foramina of head region

M99.61 Osseous and subluxation stenosis of intervertebral foramina of cervical region

M99.62 Osseous and subluxation stenosis of intervertebral foramina of thoracic region

M99.63 Osseous and subluxation stenosis of intervertebral foramina of lumbar region

M99.64 Osseous and subluxation stenosis of intervertebral foramina of sacral region

M99.65 Osseous and subluxation stenosis of intervertebral foramina of pelvic region

M99.66 Osseous and subluxation stenosis of intervertebral foramina of lower extremity

M99.67 Osseous and subluxation stenosis of intervertebral foramina of upper extremity

M99.68 Osseous and subluxation stenosis of intervertebral foramina of rib cage

M99.69 Osseous and subluxation stenosis of intervertebral foramina of abdomen and other regions

√5th M99.7 Connective tissue and disc stenosis of intervertebral foramina

M99.70 Connective tissue and disc stenosis of intervertebral foramina of head region

M99.71 Connective tissue and disc stenosis of intervertebral foramina of cervical region

M99.72 Connective tissue and disc stenosis of intervertebral foramina of thoracic region

M99.73 Connective tissue and disc stenosis of intervertebral foramina of lumbar region

M99.74 Connective tissue and disc stenosis of intervertebral foramina of sacral region

M99.75 Connective tissue and disc stenosis of intervertebral foramina of pelvic region

M99.76 Connective tissue and disc stenosis of intervertebral foramina of lower extremity

M99.77 Connective tissue and disc stenosis of intervertebral foramina of upper extremity

M99.78 Connective tissue and disc stenosis of intervertebral foramina of rib cage

M99.79 Connective tissue and disc stenosis of intervertebral foramina of abdomen and other regions

√5th M99.8 Other biomechanical lesions

M99.80 Other biomechanical lesions of head region

M99.81 Other biomechanical lesions of cervical region

M99.82 Other biomechanical lesions of thoracic region

M99.83 Other biomechanical lesions of lumbar region

M99.84 Other biomechanical lesions of sacral region

M99.85 Other biomechanical lesions of pelvic region

M99.86 Other biomechanical lesions of lower extremity

M99.87 Other biomechanical lesions of upper extremity

M99.88 Other biomechanical lesions of rib cage

M99.89 Other biomechanical lesions of abdomen and other regions

M99.9 Biomechanical lesion, unspecified

Chapter 14. Diseases of the Genitourinary System (NØØ-N99)

EXCLUDES 2 *certain conditions originating in the perinatal period (PØ4-P96)*
certain infectious and parasitic diseases (AØØ-B99)
complications of pregnancy, childbirth and the puerperium (OØØ-O9A)
congenital malformations, deformations and chromosomal abnormalities (QØØ-Q99)
endocrine, nutritional and metabolic diseases (EØØ-E88)
injury, poisoning and certain other consequences of external causes (SØØ-T88)
neoplasms (CØØ-D49)
symptoms, signs and abnormal clinical and laboratory findings, not elsewhere classified (RØØ-R94)

This chapter contains the following blocks:

NØØ-NØ8	Glomerular diseases
N1Ø-N16	Renal tubulo-interstitial diseases
N17-N19	Acute kidney failure and chronic kidney disease
N2Ø-N23	Urolithiasis
N25-N29	Other disorders of kidney and ureter
N3Ø-N39	Other diseases of the urinary system
N4Ø-N53	Diseases of male genital organs
N6Ø-N65	Disorders of breast
N7Ø-N77	Inflammatory diseases of female pelvic organs
N8Ø-N98	Noninflammatory disorders of female genital tract
N99	Intraoperative and postprocedural complications and disorders of genitourinary system, not elsewhere classified

Glomerular diseases (NØØ-NØ8)

Code also any associated kidney failure (N17-N19).

EXCLUDES 1 *hypertensive chronic kidney disease (I12.-)*

✓4th NØØ Acute nephritic syndrome

INCLUDES acute glomerular disease
acute glomerulonephritis
acute nephritis

EXCLUDES 1 *acute tubulo-interstitial nephritis (N1Ø)*
nephritic syndrome NOS (NØ5.-)

CC Excl: For MCC codes in category NØØ, unless otherwise noted: A17.9, A18.1Ø-A18.11, A18.13, A18.82, A18.84, A18.89, A54.21, A54.29, A54.82, A54.84, A54.89-A54.9, A59.ØØ, A59.8-A59.9, B37.41-B37.49, EØ8.21-EØ8.29, EØ8.618-EØ8.638, EØ8.649-EØ8.8, EØ9.21-EØ9.29, EØ9.618-EØ9.638, EØ9.649-EØ9.8, E1Ø.21-E1Ø.29, E1Ø.618-E1Ø.638, E1Ø.649, E1Ø.69-E1Ø.8, E11.21-E11.29, E11.618-E11.638, E11.649, E11.69-E11.8, E13.21-E13.29, E13.618-E13.638, E13.649-E13.8, E88.3, M1Ø.3Ø-M1Ø.39, NØØ.Ø-N11.Ø, N11.8-N13.39, N13.6, N14.Ø-N19, N25.Ø-N26.1, N26.9-N27.9, N28.1-N29, N36.41-N36.43, N36.8-N36.9, N39.8-N39.9, R31.Ø-R31.9

NØØ.Ø Acute nephritic syndrome with minor glomerular abnormality MCC
Acute nephritic syndrome with minimal change lesion

NØØ.1 Acute nephritic syndrome with focal and segmental glomerular lesions MCC
Acute nephritic syndrome with focal and segmental hyalinosis
Acute nephritic syndrome with focal and segmental sclerosis
Acute nephritic syndrome with focal glomerulonephritis

NØØ.2 Acute nephritic syndrome with diffuse membranous glomerulonephritis MCC

NØØ.3 Acute nephritic syndrome with diffuse mesangial proliferative glomerulonephritis MCC

NØØ.4 Acute nephritic syndrome with diffuse endocapillary proliferative glomerulonephritis MCC

NØØ.5 Acute nephritic syndrome with diffuse mesangiocapillary glomerulonephritis MCC
Acute nephritic syndrome with membranoproliferative glomerulonephritis, types 1 and 3, or NOS

NØØ.6 Acute nephritic syndrome with dense deposit disease MCC
Acute nephritic syndrome with membranoproliferative glomerulonephritis, type 2

NØØ.7 Acute nephritic syndrome with diffuse crescentic glomerulonephritis MCC
Acute nephritic syndrome with extracapillary glomerulonephritis

NØØ.8 Acute nephritic syndrome with other morphologic changes MCC
Acute nephritic syndrome with proliferative glomerulonephritis NOS
CC Excl: A17.9, A18.1Ø-A18.11, A18.13, A18.82, A18.84, A18.89, A54.21, A54.29, A54.82, A54.84, A54.89-A54.9, A59.ØØ, A59.8-A59.9, B37.41-B37.49, EØ8.21-EØ8.29, EØ9.21-EØ9.29, E88.3, M1Ø.3Ø-M1Ø.39, NØØ.Ø-N11.Ø, N11.8-N13.39, N13.6, N14.Ø-N19, N25.Ø-N26.1, N26.9-N27.9, N28.1-N29, N36.41-N36.43, N36.8-N36.9, N39.8-N39.9, R31.Ø-R31.9

NØØ.9 Acute nephritic syndrome with unspecified morphologic changes MCC

✓4th NØ1 Rapidly progressive nephritic syndrome

INCLUDES rapidly progressive glomerular disease
rapidly progressive glomerulonephritis
rapidly progressive nephritis

EXCLUDES 1 *nephritic syndrome NOS (NØ5.-)*

CC Excl: For MCC codes in category NØ1, unless otherwise noted: See code: NØØ

NØ1.Ø Rapidly progressive nephritic syndrome with minor glomerular abnormality MCC
Rapidly progressive nephritic syndrome with minimal change lesion

NØ1.1 Rapidly progressive nephritic syndrome with focal and segmental glomerular lesions MCC
Rapidly progressive nephritic syndrome with focal and segmental hyalinosis
Rapidly progressive nephritic syndrome with focal and segmental sclerosis
Rapidly progressive nephritic syndrome with focal glomerulonephritis

NØ1.2 Rapidly progressive nephritic syndrome with diffuse membranous glomerulonephritis MCC

NØ1.3 Rapidly progressive nephritic syndrome with diffuse mesangial proliferative glomerulonephritis MCC

NØ1.4 Rapidly progressive nephritic syndrome with diffuse endocapillary proliferative glomerulonephritis MCC

NØ1.5 Rapidly progressive nephritic syndrome with diffuse mesangiocapillary glomerulonephritis MCC
Rapidly progressive nephritic syndrome with membranoproliferative glomerulonephritis, types 1 and 3, or NOS

NØ1.6 Rapidly progressive nephritic syndrome with dense deposit disease MCC
Rapidly progressive nephritic syndrome with membranoproliferative glomerulonephritis, type 2

NØ1.7 Rapidly progressive nephritic syndrome with diffuse crescentic glomerulonephritis MCC
Rapidly progressive nephritic syndrome with extracapillary glomerulonephritis

NØ1.8 Rapidly progressive nephritic syndrome with other morphologic changes MCC
Rapidly progressive nephritic syndrome with proliferative glomerulonephritis NOS

NØ1.9 Rapidly progressive nephritic syndrome with unspecified morphologic changes MCC

✓4th NØ2 Recurrent and persistent hematuria

EXCLUDES 1 *acute cystitis with hematuria (N3Ø.Ø1)*
hematuria NOS (R31.9)
hematuria not associated with specified morphologic lesions (R31.-)

CC Excl: For CC codes in category NØ2, unless otherwise noted: See code: NØØ

NØ2.Ø Recurrent and persistent hematuria with minor glomerular abnormality CC
Recurrent and persistent hematuria with minimal change lesion

NØ2.1 Recurrent and persistent hematuria with focal and segmental glomerular lesions CC
Recurrent and persistent hematuria with focal and segmental hyalinosis
Recurrent and persistent hematuria with focal and segmental sclerosis
Recurrent and persistent hematuria with focal glomerulonephritis

NØ2.2 Recurrent and persistent hematuria with diffuse membranous glomerulonephritis CC

NØ2.3 Recurrent and persistent hematuria with diffuse mesangial proliferative glomerulonephritis CC

NØ2.4 Recurrent and persistent hematuria with diffuse endocapillary proliferative glomerulonephritis CC

NØ2.5 Recurrent and persistent hematuria with diffuse mesangiocapillary glomerulonephritis CC
Recurrent and persistent hematuria with membranoproliferative glomerulonephritis, types 1 and 3, or NOS

N02.6 Recurrent and persistent hematuria with dense deposit disease CC
Recurrent and persistent hematuria with membranoproliferative glomerulonephritis, type 2

N02.7 Recurrent and persistent hematuria with diffuse crescentic glomerulonephritis CC
Recurrent and persistent hematuria with extracapillary glomerulonephritis

N02.8 Recurrent and persistent hematuria with other morphologic changes CC
Recurrent and persistent hematuria with proliferative glomerulonephritis NOS
CC Excl: A17.9, A18.10-A18.11, A18.13, A18.82, A18.84, A18.89, A54.21, A54.29, A54.82, A54.84, A54.89-A54.9, A59.00, A59.8-A59.9, B37.41-B37.49, E08.21-E08.29, E08.618-E08.638, E08.649-E08.8, E09.21-E09.29, E09.618-E09.638, E09.649-E09.8, E10.21-E10.29, E10.618-E10.638, E10.649, E10.69-E10.8, E11.21-E11.29, E11.618-E11.638, E11.649, E11.69-E11.8, E13.21-E13.29, E13.618-E13.638, E13.649-E13.8, E88.3, M10.30-M10.39, N00.0-N11.0, N11.8-N13.39, N13.6, N14.0-N19, N25.0-N26.1, N26.9-N27.9, N28.1-N29, N36.41-N36.43, N36.8-N36.9, N39.8-N39.9, R31.0-R31.9

N02.9 Recurrent and persistent hematuria with unspecified morphologic changes CC

✓4th N03 Chronic nephritic syndrome

INCLUDES chronic glomerular disease
chronic glomerulonephritis
chronic nephritis

EXCLUDES 1 *chronic tubulo-interstitial nephritis (N11.-)*
diffuse sclerosing glomerulonephritis (N05.8-)
nephritic syndrome NOS (N05.-)

CC Excl: For CC codes in catagory N03, unless otherwise noted: A17.9, A18.10-A18.11, A18.13, A18.82, A18.84, A18.89, A54.21, A54.29, A54.82, A54.84, A54.89-A54.9, A59.00, A59.8-A59.9, A98.5, B37.41-B37.49, E08.21-E08.29, E08.618-E08.638, E08.649-E08.8, E09.21-E09.29, E09.618-E09.638, E09.649-E09.8, E10.21-E10.29, E10.618-E10.638, E10.649, E10.69-E10.8, E11.21-E11.29, E11.618-E11.638, E11.649, E11.69-E11.8, E13.21-E13.29, E13.618-E13.638, E13.649-E13.8, M10.30-M10.39, N00.0-N11.0, N11.8-N13.39, N13.6, N14.0-N17.9, N19, N25.0-N26.1, N26.9-N27.9, N28.1-N29, N36.41-N36.43, N36.8-N36.9, N39.8-N39.9, R31.0-R31.9

N03.0 Chronic nephritic syndrome with minor glomerular abnormality CC
Chronic nephritic syndrome with minimal change lesion

N03.1 Chronic nephritic syndrome with focal and segmental glomerular lesions CC
Chronic nephritic syndrome with focal and segmental hyalinosis
Chronic nephritic syndrome with focal and segmental sclerosis
Chronic nephritic syndrome with focal glomerulonephritis

N03.2 Chronic nephritic syndrome with diffuse membranous glomerulonephritis CC

N03.3 Chronic nephritic syndrome with diffuse mesangial proliferative glomerulonephritis CC

N03.4 Chronic nephritic syndrome with diffuse endocapillary proliferative glomerulonephritis CC

N03.5 Chronic nephritic syndrome with diffuse mesangiocapillary glomerulonephritis CC
Chronic nephritic syndrome with membranoproliferative glomerulonephritis, types 1 and 3, or NOS

N03.6 Chronic nephritic syndrome with dense deposit disease CC
Chronic nephritic syndrome with membranoproliferative glomerulonephritis, type 2

N03.7 Chronic nephritic syndrome with diffuse crescentic glomerulonephritis CC
Chronic nephritic syndrome with extracapillary glomerulonephritis

N03.8 Chronic nephritic syndrome with other morphologic changes CC
Chronic nephritic syndrome with proliferative glomerulonephritis NOS

N03.9 Chronic nephritic syndrome with unspecified morphologic changes CC

✓4th N04 Nephrotic syndrome

INCLUDES congenital nephrotic syndrome
lipoid nephrosis

CC Excl: For CC codes in category N04, unless otherwise noted: A17.9, A18.10-A18.11, A18.13, A18.82, A18.84, A18.89, A54.21, A54.29, A54.82, A54.84, A54.89-A54.9, A59.00, A59.8-A59.9, B37.41-B37.49, E08.21-E08.29, E08.618-E08.638, E08.649-E08.8, E09.21-E09.29, E09.618-E09.638, E09.649-E09.8, E10.21-E10.29, E10.618-E10.638, E10.649, E10.69-E10.8, E11.21-E11.29, E11.618-E11.638, E11.649, E11.69-E11.8, E13.21-E13.29, E13.618-E13.638, E13.649-E13.8, M10.30-M10.39, N00.0-N11.0, N11.8-N13.39, N13.6, N14.0-N19, N25.0-N26.1, N26.9-N27.9, N28.1-N29, N36.41-N36.43, N36.8-N36.9, N39.8-N39.9, R31.0-R31.9

N04.0 Nephrotic syndrome with minor glomerular abnormality CC
Nephrotic syndrome with minimal change lesion

N04.1 Nephrotic syndrome with focal and segmental glomerular lesions CC
Nephrotic syndrome with focal and segmental hyalinosis
Nephrotic syndrome with focal and segmental sclerosis
Nephrotic syndrome with focal glomerulonephritis

N04.2 Nephrotic syndrome with diffuse membranous glomerulonephritis CC

N04.3 Nephrotic syndrome with diffuse mesangial proliferative glomerulonephritis CC

N04.4 Nephrotic syndrome with diffuse endocapillary proliferative glomerulonephritis CC

N04.5 Nephrotic syndrome with diffuse mesangiocapillary glomerulonephritis CC
Nephrotic syndrome with membranoproliferative glomerulonephritis, types 1 and 3, or NOS

N04.6 Nephrotic syndrome with dense deposit disease CC
Nephrotic syndrome with membranoproliferative glomerulonephritis, type 2

N04.7 Nephrotic syndrome with diffuse crescentic glomerulonephritis CC
Nephrotic syndrome with extracapillary glomerulonephritis
CC Excl: A17.9, A18.10-A18.11, A18.13, A18.82, A18.84, A18.89, A54.21, A54.29, A54.82, A54.84, A54.89-A54.9, A59.00, A59.8-A59.9, B37.41-B37.49, E08.21-E08.29, E08.618-E08.638, E08.649-E08.8, E09.21-E09.29, E09.618-E09.638, E09.649-E09.8, E10.21-E10.29, E10.618-E10.638, E10.649, E10.69-E10.8, E11.21-E11.29, E11.618-E11.638, E11.649, E11.69-E11.8, E13.21-E13.29, E13.618-E13.638, E13.649-E13.8, E88.3, M10.30-M10.39, N00.0-N11.0, N11.8-N13.39, N13.6, N14.0-N19, N25.0-N26.1, N26.9-N27.9, N28.1-N29, N36.41-N36.43, N36.8-N36.9, N39.8-N39.9, R31.0-R31.9

N04.8 Nephrotic syndrome with other morphologic changes CC
Nephrotic syndrome with proliferative glomerulonephritis NOS
CC Excl: See code: N04.7

N04.9 Nephrotic syndrome with unspecified morphologic changes CC
CC Excl: See code: N04.7

✓4th N05 Unspecified nephritic syndrome

INCLUDES glomerular disease NOS
glomerulonephritis NOS
nephritis NOS
nephropathy NOS and renal disease NOS with morphological lesion specified in .0-.8

EXCLUDES 1 *nephropathy NOS with no stated morphological lesion (N28.9)*
renal disease NOS with no stated morphological lesion (N28.9)
tubulo-interstitial nephritis NOS (N12)

CC Excl: For CC codes in category N05, unless otherwise noted: A17.9, A18.10-A18.11, A18.13, A18.82, A18.84, A18.89, A54.21, A54.29, A54.82, A54.84, A54.89-A54.9, A59.00, A59.8-A59.9, A98.5, B37.41-B37.49, E08.21-E08.29, E08.618-E08.638, E08.649-E08.8, E09.21-E09.29, E09.618-E09.638, E09.649-E09.8, E10.21-E10.29, E10.618-E10.638, E10.649, E10.69-E10.8, E11.21-E11.29, E11.618-E11.638, E11.649, E11.69-E11.8, E13.21-E13.29, E13.618-E13.638, E13.649-E13.8, M10.30-M10.39, N00.0-N11.0, N11.8-N13.39, N13.6, N14.0-N17.9, N19, N25.0-N26.1, N26.9-N27.9, N28.1-N29, N36.41-N36.43, N36.8-N36.9, N39.8-N39.9, R31.0-R31.9

N05.0 Unspecified nephritic syndrome with minor glomerular abnormality
Unspecified nephritic syndrome with minimal change lesion

N05.1 Unspecified nephritic syndrome with focal and segmental glomerular lesions
Unspecified nephritic syndrome with focal and segmental hyalinosis
Unspecified nephritic syndrome with focal and segmental sclerosis
Unspecified nephritic syndrome with focal glomerulonephritis

N05.2 Unspecified nephritic syndrome with diffuse membranous glomerulonephritis CC

NØ5.3 Unspecified nephritic syndrome with diffuse mesangial proliferative glomerulonephritis CC

NØ5.4 Unspecified nephritic syndrome with diffuse endocapillary proliferative glomerulonephritis CC

NØ5.5 Unspecified nephritic syndrome with diffuse mesangiocapillary glomerulonephritis CC
Unspecified nephritic syndrome with membranoproliferative glomerulonephritis, types 1 and 3, or NOS

NØ5.6 Unspecified nephritic syndrome with dense deposit disease
Unspecified nephritic syndrome with membranoproliferative glomerulonephritis, type 2

NØ5.7 Unspecified nephritic syndrome with diffuse crescentic glomerulonephritis
Unspecified nephritic syndrome with extracapillary glomerulonephritis

NØ5.8 Unspecified nephritic syndrome with other morphologic changes
Unspecified nephritic syndrome with proliferative glomerulonephritis NOS

NØ5.9 Unspecified nephritic syndrome with unspecified morphologic changes

✓4th NØ6 Isolated proteinuria with specified morphological lesion

EXCLUDES 1 *proteinuria not associated with specific morphologic lesions (R8Ø.Ø)*

CC Excl: For CC codes in category NØ6, unless otherwise noted:
See code: NØ3

NØ6.Ø Isolated proteinuria with minor glomerular abnormality
Isolated proteinuria with minimal change lesion

NØ6.1 Isolated proteinuria with focal and segmental glomerular lesions
Isolated proteinuria with focal and segmental hyalinosis
Isolated proteinuria with focal and segmental sclerosis
Isolated proteinuria with focal glomerulonephritis

NØ6.2 Isolated proteinuria with diffuse membranous glomerulonephritis CC

NØ6.3 Isolated proteinuria with diffuse mesangial proliferative glomerulonephritis CC

NØ6.4 Isolated proteinuria with diffuse endocapillary proliferative glomerulonephritis CC

NØ6.5 Isolated proteinuria with diffuse mesangiocapillary glomerulonephritis CC
Isolated proteinuria with membranoproliferative glomerulonephritis, types 1 and 3, or NOS

NØ6.6 Isolated proteinuria with dense deposit disease
Isolated proteinuria with membranoproliferative glomerulonephritis, type 2

NØ6.7 Isolated proteinuria with diffuse crescentic glomerulonephritis
Isolated proteinuria with extracapillary glomerulonephritis

NØ6.8 Isolated proteinuria with other morphologic lesion
Isolated proteinuria with proliferative glomerulonephritis NOS

NØ6.9 Isolated proteinuria with unspecified morphologic lesion

✓4th NØ7 Hereditary nephropathy, not elsewhere classified

EXCLUDES 2 *Alport's syndrome (Q87.81-)*
hereditary amyloid nephropathy (E85.-)
nail patella syndrome (Q87.2)
non-neuropathic heredofamilial amyloidosis (E85.-)

CC Excl: For CC codes in category NØ7, unless otherwise noted:
A17.9, A18.1Ø-A18.11, A18.13, A18.82, A18.84, A18.89, A54.21, A54.29, A54.82, A54.84, A54.89-A54.9, A59.ØØ, A59.8-A59.9, A98.5, B37.41-B37.49, EØ8.21-EØ8.29, EØ8.618-EØ8.638, EØ8.649-EØ8.8, EØ9.21-EØ9.29, EØ9.618-EØ9.638, EØ9.649-EØ9.8, E1Ø.21-E1Ø.29, E1Ø.618-E1Ø.638, E1Ø.649, E1Ø.69-E1Ø.8, E11.21-E11.29, E11.618-E11.638, E11.649, E11.69-E11.8, E13.21-E13.29, E13.618-E13.638, E13.649-E13.8, M1Ø.3Ø-M1Ø.39, NØØ.Ø-N11.Ø, N11.8-N13.39, N13.6, N14.Ø-N17.9, N19, N25.Ø-N26.1, N26.9-N27.9, N28.1-N29, N36.41-N36.43, N36.8-N36.9, N39.8-N39.9, R31.Ø-R31.9

NØ7.Ø Hereditary nephropathy, not elsewhere classified with minor glomerular abnormality
Hereditary nephropathy, not elsewhere classified with minimal change lesion

NØ7.1 Hereditary nephropathy, not elsewhere classified with focal and segmental glomerular lesions
Hereditary nephropathy, not elsewhere classified with focal and segmental hyalinosis
Hereditary nephropathy, not elsewhere classified with focal and segmental sclerosis
Hereditary nephropathy, not elsewhere classified with focal glomerulonephritis

NØ7.2 Hereditary nephropathy, not elsewhere classified with diffuse membranous glomerulonephritis CC

NØ7.3 Hereditary nephropathy, not elsewhere classified with diffuse mesangial proliferative glomerulonephritis CC

NØ7.4 Hereditary nephropathy, not elsewhere classified with diffuse endocapillary proliferative glomerulonephritis CC

NØ7.5 Hereditary nephropathy, not elsewhere classified with diffuse mesangiocapillary glomerulonephritis CC
Hereditary nephropathy, not elsewhere classified with membranoproliferative glomerulonephritis, types 1 and 3, or NOS

NØ7.6 Hereditary nephropathy, not elsewhere classified with dense deposit disease
Hereditary nephropathy, not elsewhere classified with membranoproliferative glomerulonephritis, type 2

NØ7.7 Hereditary nephropathy, not elsewhere classified with diffuse crescentic glomerulonephritis
Hereditary nephropathy, not elsewhere classified with extracapillary glomerulonephritis

NØ7.8 Hereditary nephropathy, not elsewhere classified with other morphologic lesions
Hereditary nephropathy, not elsewhere classified with proliferative glomerulonephritis NOS

NØ7.9 Hereditary nephropathy, not elsewhere classified with unspecified morphologic lesions

NØ8 Glomerular disorders in diseases classified elsewhere

Glomerulonephritis
Nephritis
Nephropathy

Code first underlying disease, such as:
amyloidosis (E85.-)
congenital syphilis (A5Ø.5)
cryoglobulinemia (D89.1)
disseminated intravascular coagulation (D65)
gout (M1A.-, M1Ø.-)
microscopic polyangiitis (M31.7)
multiple myeloma (C9Ø.Ø-)
sepsis (A4Ø.Ø-A41.9)
sickle-cell disease (D57.Ø-D57.8)

EXCLUDES 1 *glomerulonephritis, nephritis and nephropathy (in):*
antiglomerular basement membrane disease (M31.Ø)
diabetes (EØ8-E13 with .21)
gonococcal (A54.21)
Goodpasture's syndrome (M31.Ø)
hemolytic-uremic syndrome (D59.3)
lupus (M32.14)
mumps (B26.83)
syphilis (A52.75)
systemic lupus erythematosus (M32.14)
Wegener's granulomatosis (M31.31)
pyelonephritis in diseases classified elsewhere (N16)
renal tubulo-interstitial disorders classified elsewhere (N16)

Renal tubulo-interstitial diseases (N1Ø-N16)

INCLUDES pyelonephritis

EXCLUDES 1 *pyeloureteritis cystica (N28.85)*

1 **N1Ø Acute tubulo-interstitial nephritis** CC

Acute infectious interstitial nephritis
Acute pyelitis
Acute pyelonephritis
Hemoglobin nephrosis
Myoglobin nephrosis

Use additional code (B95-B97), to identify infectious agent

CC Excl: A17.9, A18.1Ø-A18.11, A18.13, A18.82, A18.84, A18.89, A54.21, A54.29, A54.82, A54.84, A54.89-A54.9, A59.ØØ, A59.8-A59.9, B37.41-B37.49, EØ8.21-EØ8.29, EØ8.618-EØ8.638, EØ8.649-EØ8.8, EØ9.21-EØ9.29, EØ9.618-EØ9.638, EØ9.649-EØ9.8, E1Ø.21-E1Ø.29, E1Ø.618-E1Ø.638, E1Ø.649, E1Ø.69-E1Ø.8, E11.21-E11.29, E11.618-E11.638, E11.649, E11.69-E11.8, E13.21-E13.29, E13.618-E13.638, E13.649-E13.8, M1Ø.3Ø-M1Ø.39, NØØ.Ø-N11.Ø, N11.8-N13.39, N13.6, N14.Ø-N19, N25.Ø-N26.1, N26.9-N27.9, N28.1-N29, N36.41-N36.43, N36.8-N36.9, N39.Ø, N39.8-N39.9, R31.Ø-R31.9

1 HAC = as SDx not POA, in combination with SDx code T83.51XA also not POA.

N11 Chronic tubulo-interstitial nephritis (4th)
INCLUDES chronic infectious interstitial nephritis
chronic pyelitis
chronic pyelonephritis
Use additional code (B95-B97), to identify infectious agent

N11.Ø Nonobstructive reflux-associated chronic pyelonephritis
Pyelonephritis (chronic) associated with (vesicoureteral) reflux
EXCLUDES 1 *vesicoureteral reflux NOS (N13.7Ø)*

N11.1 Chronic obstructive pyelonephritis PDx CC CC
Pyelonephritis (chronic) associated with anomaly of pelviureteric junction
Pyelonephritis (chronic) associated with anomaly of pyeloureteric junction
Pyelonephritis (chronic) associated with crossing of vessel
Pyelonephritis (chronic) associated with kinking of ureter
Pyelonephritis (chronic) associated with obstruction of ureter
Pyelonephritis (chronic) associated with stricture of pelviureteric junction
Pyelonephritis (chronic) associated with stricture of ureter
EXCLUDES 1 *calculous pyelonephritis (N2Ø.9)*
obstructive uropathy (N13.-)
CC Excl: N11.1, N13.4-N13.5, N13.8-N13.9, N28.82, N28.89-N3Ø.91, N32.89-N33, N36.41-N36.43, N36.8-N36.9, N39.Ø, N39.8-N39.9, Q62.4-Q62.8, Q64.1Ø-Q64.19, Q64.8-Q64.9, R31.Ø-R31.9, Z9Ø.6

N11.8 Other chronic tubulo-interstitial nephritis CC
Nonobstructive chronic pyelonephritis NOS
CC Excl: A17.9, A18.1Ø-A18.11, A18.13, A18.82, A18.84, A18.89, A54.21, A54.29, A54.82, A54.84, A54.89-A54.9, A59.ØØ, A59.8-A59.9, A98.5, B37.41-B37.49, EØ8.21-EØ8.29, EØ8.618-EØ8.638, EØ8.649-EØ8.8, EØ9.21-EØ9.29, EØ9.618-EØ9.638, EØ9.649-EØ9.8, E1Ø.21-E1Ø.29, E1Ø.618-E1Ø.638, E1Ø.649, E1Ø.69-E1Ø.8, E11.21-E11.29, E11.618-E11.638, E11.649, E11.69-E11.8, E13.21-E13.29, E13.618-E13.638, E13.649-E13.8, M1Ø.3Ø-M1Ø.39, NØØ.Ø-N11.Ø, N11.8-N13.39, N13.6, N14.Ø-N17.9, N19, N25.Ø-N26.1, N26.9-N27.9, N28.1-N29, N36.41-N36.43, N36.8-N36.9, N39.8-N39.9, O23.Ø1-O23.Ø3, O23.11-O23.13, O23.21-O23.23, O23.31-O23.33, O23.41-O23.513, O23.521-O23.523, O23.591-O23.593, O23.91-O23.93, O86.11, O86.13-O86.29, R31.Ø-R31.9

1 **N11.9 Chronic tubulo-interstitial nephritis, unspecified** CC
Chronic interstitial nephritis NOS
Chronic pyelitis NOS
Chronic pyelonephritis NOS
CC Excl: A17.9, A18.1Ø-A18.11, A18.13, A18.82, A18.84, A18.89, A54.21, A54.29, A54.82, A54.84, A54.89-A54.9, A59.ØØ, A59.8-A59.9, B37.41-B37.49, EØ8.21-EØ8.29, EØ9.21-EØ9.29, M1Ø.3Ø-M1Ø.39, NØØ.Ø-N11.Ø, N11.8-N13.39, N13.6, N14.Ø-N19, N25.Ø-N26.1, N26.9-N27.9, N28.1-N29, N36.41-N36.43, N36.8-N36.9, N39.Ø, N39.8-N39.9, R31.Ø-R31.9

1 **N12 Tubulo-interstitial nephritis, not specified as acute or chronic** CC
Interstitial nephritis NOS
Pyelitis NOS
Pyelonephritis NOS
EXCLUDES 1 *calculous pyelonephritis (N2Ø.9)*
CC Excl: See code: N11.9

N13 Obstructive and reflux uropathy (4th)
EXCLUDES 2 *calculus of kidney and ureter without hydronephrosis (N2Ø.-)*
congenital obstructive defects of renal pelvis and ureter (Q62.Ø-Q62.3)
hydronephrosis with ureteropelvic junction obstruction (Q62.1)
obstructive pyelonephritis (N11.1)

CC Excl: For CC codes in category N13, unless otherwise noted:
See code: N11.9

N13.1 Hydronephrosis with ureteral stricture, not elsewhere classified CC
EXCLUDES 1 *hydronephrosis with ureteral stricture with infection (N13.6)*

N13.2 Hydronephrosis with renal and ureteral calculous obstruction CC
EXCLUDES 1 *hydronephrosis with renal and ureteral calculous obstruction with infection (N13.6)*

N13.3 Other and unspecified hydronephrosis (5th)
EXCLUDES 1 *hydronephrosis with infection (N13.6)*

N13.3Ø Unspecified hydronephrosis CC

N13.39 Other hydronephrosis CC

N13.4 Hydroureter CC
EXCLUDES 1 *congenital hydroureter (Q62.3-)*
hydroureter with infection (N13.6)
vesicoureteral-reflux with hydroureter (N13.73-)
CC Excl: N11.1, N13.4-N13.5, N13.8-N13.9, N28.82, N28.89-N3Ø.91, N32.89-N33, N36.41-N36.43, N36.8-N36.9, N39.Ø, N39.8-N39.9, Q62.4-Q62.8, Q64.1Ø-Q64.19, Q64.8-Q64.9, R31.Ø-R31.9

N13.5 Crossing vessel and stricture of ureter without hydronephrosis
Kinking and stricture of ureter without hydronephrosis
EXCLUDES 1 *crossing vessel and stricture of ureter without hydronephrosis with infection (N13.6)*

1 **N13.6 Pyonephrosis** CC
Conditions in N13.1-N13.5 with infection
Obstructive uropathy with infection
Use additional code (B95-B97), to identify infectious agent

N13.7 Vesicoureteral-reflux (5th)
EXCLUDES 1 *reflux-associated pyelonephritis (N11.Ø)*

N13.7Ø Vesicoureteral-reflux, unspecified
Vesicoureteral-reflux NOS

N13.71 Vesicoureteral-reflux without reflux nephropathy

N13.72 Vesicoureteral-reflux with reflux nephropathy without hydroureter (6th)

N13.721 Vesicoureteral-reflux with reflux nephropathy without hydroureter, unilateral

N13.722 Vesicoureteral-reflux with reflux nephropathy without hydroureter, bilateral

N13.729 Vesicoureteral-reflux with reflux nephropathy without hydroureter, unspecified

N13.73 Vesicoureteral-reflux with reflux nephropathy with hydroureter (6th)

N13.731 Vesicoureteral-reflux with reflux nephropathy with hydroureter, unilateral

N13.732 Vesicoureteral-reflux with reflux nephropathy with hydroureter, bilateral

N13.739 Vesicoureteral-reflux with reflux nephropathy with hydroureter, unspecified

N13.8 Other obstructive and reflux uropathy CC
Urinary tract obstruction due to specified cause
Code first, if applicable, any causal condition, such as: enlarged prostate (N4Ø.1)
CC Excl: See code: N11.1

N13.9 Obstructive and reflux uropathy, unspecified
Urinary tract obstruction NOS

N14 Drug- and heavy-metal-induced tubulo-interstitial and tubular conditions (4th)
Code first poisoning due to drug or toxin, if applicable (T36-T65 with fifth or sixth character 1-4 or 6)
Use additional code for adverse effect, if applicable, to identify drug (T36-T5Ø with fifth or sixth character 5)

N14.Ø Analgesic nephropathy

N14.1 Nephropathy induced by other drugs, medicaments and biological substances

N14.2 Nephropathy induced by unspecified drug, medicament or biological substance

N14.3 Nephropathy induced by heavy metals

N14.4 Toxic nephropathy, not elsewhere classified

N15 Other renal tubulo-interstitial diseases (4th)

N15.Ø Balkan nephropathy
Balkan endemic nephropathy

1 **N15.1 Renal and perinephric abscess** MCC
CC Excl: A17.9, A18.1Ø-A18.11, A18.13, A18.82, A18.84, A18.89, A54.21, A54.29, A54.82, A54.84, A54.89-A54.9, A59.ØØ, A59.8-A59.9, B37.41-B37.49, EØ8.21-EØ8.29, EØ8.618-EØ8.638, EØ8.649-EØ8.8, EØ9.21-EØ9.29, EØ9.618-EØ9.638, EØ9.649-EØ9.8, E1Ø.21-E1Ø.29, E1Ø.618-E1Ø.638, E1Ø.649, E1Ø.69-E1Ø.8, E11.21-E11.29, E11.618-E11.638, E11.649, E11.69-E11.8, E13.21-E13.29, E13.618-E13.638, E13.649-E13.8, M1Ø.3Ø-M1Ø.39, NØØ.Ø-N11.Ø, N11.8-N13.39, N13.6, N14.Ø-N19, N25.Ø-N26.1, N26.9-N27.9, N28.1-N29, N36.41-N36.43, N36.8-N36.9, N39.Ø, N39.8-N39.9, R31.Ø-R31.9

N15.8 Other specified renal tubulo-interstitial diseases

N15.9 Renal tubulo-interstitial disease, unspecified
Infection of kidney NOS
EXCLUDES 1 *urinary tract infection NOS (N39.Ø)*

1 HAC = as SDx not POA, in combination with SDx code T83.51XA also not POA.

N16 *Renal tubulo-interstitial disorders in diseases classified elsewhere*
Pyelonephritis
Tubulo-interstitial nephritis
Code first underlying disease, such as:
brucellosis (A23.0-A23.9)
cryoglobulinemia (D89.1)
glycogen storage disease (E74.0)
leukemia (C91-C95)
lymphoma (C81.0-C85.9, C96.0-C96.9)
multiple myeloma (C90.0-)
sepsis (A40.0-A41.9)
Wilson's disease (E83.0)
EXCLUDES 1 *diphtheritic pyelonephritis and tubulo-interstitial nephritis (A36.84)*
pyelonephritis and tubulo-interstitial nephritis in candidiasis (B37.49)
pyelonephritis and tubulo-interstitial nephritis in cystinosis (E72.04)
pyelonephritis and tubulo-interstitial nephritis in salmonella infection (A02.25)
pyelonephritis and tubulo-interstitial nephritis in sarcoidosis (D86.84)
pyelonephritis and tubulo-interstitial nephritis in sicca syndrome [Sjogren's] (M35.04)
pyelonephritis and tubulo-interstitial nephritis in systemic lupus erythematosus (M32.15)
pyelonephritis and tubulo-interstitial nephritis in toxoplasmosis (B58.83)
renal tubular degeneration in diabetes (E08-E13 with .29)
syphilitic pyelonephritis and tubulo-interstitial nephritis (A52.75)

Acute kidney failure and chronic kidney disease (N17-N19)

EXCLUDES 2 *congenital renal failure (P96.0)*
drug- and heavy-metal-induced tubulo-interstitial and tubular conditions (N14.-)
extrarenal uremia (R39.2)
hemolytic-uremic syndrome (D59.3)
hepatorenal syndrome (K76.7)
postpartum hepatorenal syndrome (O90.4)
posttraumatic renal failure (T79.5)
prerenal uremia (R39.2)
renal failure complicating abortion or ectopic or molar pregnancy (O00-O07, O08.4)
renal failure following labor and delivery (O90.4)
renal failure postprocedural (N99.0)

✓4th **N17 Acute kidney failure**
Code also associated underlying condition
EXCLUDES 1 *posttraumatic renal failure (T79.5)*
AHA: 2013, 4Q, 124

CC Excl: For CC/MCC codes in category N17, unless otherwise noted: E08.21-E08.29, E08.618-E08.638, E08.649-E08.8, E09.21-E09.29, E09.618-E09.638, E09.649-E09.8, E10.21-E10.29, E10.618-E10.638, E10.649, E10.69-E10.8, E11.21-E11.29, E11.618-E11.638, E11.649, E11.69-E11.8, E13.21-E13.29, E13.618-E13.638, E13.649-E13.8, E88.3, M10.30-M10.39, N00.0-N11.0, N11.8-N13.39, N13.6, N14.0-N19, N25.0-N26.1, N26.9-N27.9, N28.1-N29, N36.41-N36.43, N36.8-N36.9, N39.8-N39.9, Q60.0-Q62.39, Q63.0-Q63.9, Q64.8-Q64.9, R31.0-R31.9

N17.0 Acute kidney failure with tubular necrosis MCC
Acute tubular necrosis
Renal tubular necrosis
Tubular necrosis NOS

N17.1 Acute kidney failure with acute cortical necrosis MCC
Acute cortical necrosis
Cortical necrosis NOS
Renal cortical necrosis

N17.2 Acute kidney failure with medullary necrosis MCC
Medullary [papillary] necrosis NOS
Acute medullary [papillary] necrosis
Renal medullary [papillary] necrosis

N17.8 Other acute kidney failure CC
CC Excl: E08.21-E08.29, E08.618-E08.638, E08.649-E08.8, E09.21-E09.29, E09.618-E09.638, E09.649-E09.8, E10.21-E10.29, E10.618-E10.638, E10.649, E10.69-E10.8, E11.21-E11.29, E11.618-E11.638, E11.649, E11.69-E11.8, E13.21-E13.29, E13.618-E13.638, E13.649-E13.8, E88.3, M10.30-M10.39, N00.0-N11.0, N11.8-N13.39, N13.6, N14.0-N19, N25.0-N26.1, N26.9-N27.9, N28.1-N29, N36.41-N36.43, N36.8-N36.9, N39.8-N39.9, R31.0-R31.9

N17.9 Acute kidney failure, unspecified CC
Acute kidney injury (nontraumatic)
EXCLUDES 2 *traumatic kidney injury (S37.0-)*

✓4th **N18 Chronic kidney disease (CKD)**
Code first any associated:
diabetic chronic kidney disease (E08.22, E09.22, E10.22, E11.22, E13.22)
hypertensive chronic kidney disease (I12-, I13-)
Use additional code to identify kidney transplant status, if applicable, (Z94.0)
AHA: 2013, 1Q, 24

N18.1 Chronic kidney disease, stage 1

N18.2 Chronic kidney disease, stage 2 (mild)

N18.3 Chronic kidney disease, stage 3 (moderate)

N18.4 Chronic kidney disease, stage 4 (severe) CC
CC Excl: E08.21-E08.29, E08.618-E08.638, E08.649-E08.8, E09.21-E09.29, E09.618-E09.638, E09.649-E09.8, E10.21-E10.29, E10.618-E10.638, E10.649, E10.69-E10.8, E11.21-E11.29, E11.618-E11.638, E11.649, E11.69-E11.8, E13.21-E13.29, E13.618-E13.638, E13.649-E13.8, M10.30-M10.39, N00.0-N11.0, N11.8-N13.39, N13.6, N14.0-N19, N25.0-N26.1, N26.9-N27.9, N28.1-N29, N36.41-N36.43, N36.8-N36.9, N39.8-N39.9, Q60.0-Q62.39, Q63.0-Q63.9, Q64.8-Q64.9, R31.0-R31.9

N18.5 Chronic kidney disease, stage 5 CC
EXCLUDES 1 *chronic kidney disease, stage 5 requiring chronic dialysis (N18.6)*
CC Excl: See code: N18.4

N18.6 End stage renal disease MCC
Chronic kidney disease requiring chronic dialysis
Use additional code to identify dialysis status (Z99.2)
AHA: 2013, 4Q, 124-125
CC Excl: E08.21-E08.29, E08.618-E08.638, E08.649-E08.8, E09.21-E09.29, E09.618-E09.638, E09.649-E09.8, E10.21-E10.29, E10.618-E10.638, E10.649, E10.69-E10.8, E11.21-E11.29, E11.618-E11.638, E11.649, E11.69-E11.8, E13.21-E13.29, E13.618-E13.638, E13.649-E13.8, I12.9, M10.30-M10.39, N00.0-N11.0, N11.8-N13.39, N13.6, N14.0-N19, N25.0-N26.1, N26.9-N27.9, N28.1-N29, N36.41-N36.43, N36.8-N36.9, N39.8-N39.9, Q60.0-Q62.39, Q63.0-Q63.9, Q64.8-Q64.9, R31.0-R31.9

N18.9 Chronic kidney disease, unspecified
Chronic renal disease
Chronic renal failure NOS
Chronic renal insufficiency
Chronic uremia

N19 Unspecified kidney failure
Uremia NOS
EXCLUDES 1 *acute kidney failure (N17.-)*
chronic kidney disease (N18.-)
chronic uremia (N18.9)
extrarenal uremia (R39.2)
prerenal uremia (R39.2)
renal insufficiency (acute) (N28.9)
uremia of newborn (P96.0)

Urolithiasis (N20-N23)

✓4th **N20 Calculus of kidney and ureter**
Calculous pyelonephritis
EXCLUDES 1 *nephrocalcinosis (E83.5)*
that with hydronephrosis (N13.2)

N20.0 Calculus of kidney
Nephrolithiasis NOS
Renal calculus
Renal stone
Staghorn calculus
Stone in kidney

N20.1 Calculus of ureter CC
Ureteric stone
CC Excl: N11.1, N13.4-N13.5, N13.8-N13.9, N20.0-N22, N28.82, N28.89-N29, N36.41-N36.43, N36.8-N36.9, N39.8-N39.9, R31.0-R31.9

N20.2 Calculus of kidney with calculus of ureter CC

N20.9 Urinary calculus, unspecified

✓4th **N21 Calculus of lower urinary tract**
Calculus of lower urinary tract with cystitis and urethritis

N21.0 Calculus in bladder
Calculus in diverticulum of bladder
Urinary bladder stone
EXCLUDES 2 *staghorn calculus (N20.0)*

N21.1 Calculus in urethra
EXCLUDES 2 *calculus of prostate (N42.0)*

N21.8 Other lower urinary tract calculus

N21.9 Calculus of lower urinary tract, unspecified
EXCLUDES 1 *calculus of urinary tract NOS (N20.9)*

N22 *Calculus of urinary tract in diseases classified elsewhere*
Code first underlying disease, such as:
gout (M1A.-, M10.-)
schistosomiasis (B65.0-B65.9)

N23 Unspecified renal colic

Other disorders of kidney and ureter (N25-N29)

EXCLUDES 2 *disorders of kidney and ureter with urolithiasis (N20-N23)*

N25 Disorders resulting from impaired renal tubular function

EXCLUDES 1 *metabolic disorders classifiable to E70-E88*

N25.0 Renal osteodystrophy

Azotemic osteodystrophy
Phosphate-losing tubular disorders
Renal rickets
Renal short stature

N25.1 Nephrogenic diabetes insipidus CC

EXCLUDES 1 *diabetes insipidus NOS (E23.2)*

CC Excl: A17.9, A18.10-A18.11, A18.13, A18.82, A18.84, A18.89, A54.21, A54.29, A54.82, A54.84, A54.89-A54.9, A59.00, A59.8-A59.9, A98.5, B37.41-B37.49, E08.21-E08.29, E08.618-E08.638, E08.649-E08.8, E09.21-E09.29, E09.618-E09.638, E09.649-E09.8, E10.21-E10.29, E10.618-E10.638, E10.649, E10.69-E10.8, E11.21-E11.29, E11.618-E11.638, E11.649, E11.69-E11.8, E13.21-E13.29, E13.618-E13.638, E13.649-E13.8, M10.30-M10.39, N00.0-N11.0, N11.8-N13.39, N13.6, N14.0-N17.9, N18.3-N18.6, N19, N25.0-N26.1, N26.9-N27.9, N28.1-N29, N36.41-N36.43, N36.8-N36.9, N39.8-N39.9, R31.0-R31.9

N25.8 Other disorders resulting from impaired renal tubular function

N25.81 Secondary hyperparathyroidism of renal origin CC

EXCLUDES 1 *secondary hyperparathyroidism, non-renal (E21.1)*

CC Excl: A17.9, A18.10-A18.11, A18.13, A18.82, A18.84, A18.89, A54.21, A54.29, A54.82, A54.84, A54.89-A54.9, A59.00, A59.8-A59.9, A98.5, B37.41-B37.49, E08.21-E08.29, E08.618-E08.638, E08.649-E08.8, E09.21-E09.29, E09.618-E09.638, E09.649-E09.8, E10.21-E10.29, E10.618-E10.638, E10.649, E10.69-E10.8, E11.21-E11.29, E11.618-E11.638, E11.649, E11.69-E11.8, E13.21-E13.29, E13.618-E13.638, E13.649-E13.8, M10.30-M10.39, N00.0-N11.0, N11.8-N13.39, N13.6, N14.0-N17.9, N19, N25.0-N25.1, N25.89-N26.1, N26.9-N27.9, N28.1-N29, N36.41-N36.43, N36.8-N36.9, N39.8-N39.9, R31.0-R31.9

N25.89 Other disorders resulting from impaired renal tubular function

Hypokalemic nephropathy
Lightwood-Albright syndrome
Renal tubular acidosis NOS

N25.9 Disorder resulting from impaired renal tubular function, unspecified

N26 Unspecified contracted kidney

EXCLUDES 1 *contracted kidney due to hypertension (I12.-)*
diffuse sclerosing glomerulonephritis (N05.8-)
hypertensive nephrosclerosis (arteriolar) (arteriosclerotic) (I12.-)
small kidney of unknown cause (N27.-)

N26.1 Atrophy of kidney (terminal)

N26.2 Page kidney

N26.9 Renal sclerosis, unspecified

N27 Small kidney of unknown cause

INCLUDES oligonephronia

N27.0 Small kidney, unilateral

N27.1 Small kidney, bilateral

N27.9 Small kidney, unspecified

N28 Other disorders of kidney and ureter, not elsewhere classified

N28.0 Ischemia and infarction of kidney CC

Renal artery embolism
Renal artery obstruction
Renal artery occlusion
Renal artery thrombosis
Renal infarct

EXCLUDES 1 *atherosclerosis of renal artery (extrarenal part) (I70.1)*
congenital stenosis of renal artery (Q27.1)
Goldblatt's kidney (I70.1)

CC Excl: N13.70-N13.739, N28.0, N28.9-N29

N28.1 Cyst of kidney, acquired

Cyst (multiple)(solitary) of kidney, acquired

EXCLUDES 1 *cystic kidney disease (congenital) (Q61.-)*

N28.8 Other specified disorders of kidney and ureter

EXCLUDES 1 *hydroureter (N13.4)*
ureteric stricture with hydronephrosis (N13.1)
ureteric stricture without hydronephrosis (N13.5)

CC Excl: For CC codes in subcategory N28.8, unless otherwise noted: A17.9, A18.10-A18.11, A18.13, A18.82, A18.84, A18.89, A54.21, A54.29, A54.82, A54.84, A54.89-A54.9, A59.00, A59.8-A59.9, B37.41-B37.49, E08.21-E08.29, E09.21-E09.29, M10.30-M10.39, N00.0-N11.0, N11.8-N13.39, N13.6, N14.0-N19, N25.0-N26.1, N26.9-N27.9, N28.1-N29, N36.41-N36.43, N36.8-N36.9, N39.0, N39.8-N39.9, R31.0-R31.9

N28.81 Hypertrophy of kidney

N28.82 Megaloureter

N28.83 Nephroptosis

1 **N28.84 Pyelitis cystica** CC

1 **N28.85 Pyeloureteritis cystica** CC

1 **N28.86 Ureteritis cystica** CC

N28.89 Other specified disorders of kidney and ureter

N28.9 Disorder of kidney and ureter, unspecified

Nephropathy NOS
Renal disease (acute) NOS
Renal insufficiency (acute)

EXCLUDES 1 *chronic renal insufficiency (N18.9)*
unspecified nephritic syndrome (N05.-)

N29 Other disorders of kidney and ureter in diseases classified elsewhere

Code first underlying disease, such as:
amyloidosis (E85.-)
nephrocalcinosis (E83.5)
schistosomiasis (B65.0-B65.9)

EXCLUDES 1 *disorders of kidney and ureter in:*
cystinosis (E72.0)
gonorrhea (A54.21)
syphilis (A52.75)
tuberculosis (A18.11)

Other diseases of the urinary system (N30-N39)

EXCLUDES 1 *urinary infection (complicating):*
abortion or ectopic or molar pregnancy (O00-O07, O08.8)
pregnancy, childbirth and the puerperium (O23-, O75.3, O86.2-)

N30 Cystitis

Use additional code to identify infectious agent (B95-B97)

EXCLUDES 1 *prostatocystitis (N41.3)*

CC Excl: For CC codes in category N30, unless otherwise noted: A17.9, A18.10, A18.12-A18.13, A18.82, A18.84, A18.89, A54.00-A54.02, A54.09-A54.1, A54.82, A54.84, A54.89-A54.9, A59.00, A59.8-A59.9, B37.41-B37.49, N11.1, N13.4-N13.5, N13.8-N13.9, N28.82, N28.89-N30.91, N32.89-N33, N36.41-N36.43, N36.8-N36.9, N39.0, N39.8-N39.9, R31.0-R31.9

N30.0 Acute cystitis

EXCLUDES 1 *irradiation cystitis (N30.4-)*
trigonitis (N30.3-)

1 **N30.00 Acute cystitis without hematuria** CC

1 **N30.01 Acute cystitis with hematuria** CC

N30.1 Interstitial cystitis (chronic)

N30.10 Interstitial cystitis (chronic) without hematuria

N30.11 Interstitial cystitis (chronic) with hematuria

N30.2 Other chronic cystitis

N30.20 Other chronic cystitis without hematuria

N30.21 Other chronic cystitis with hematuria

N30.3 Trigonitis

Urethrotrigonitis

N30.30 Trigonitis without hematuria

N30.31 Trigonitis with hematuria

N30.4 Irradiation cystitis

N30.40 Irradiation cystitis without hematuria CC

N30.41 Irradiation cystitis with hematuria CC

N30.8 Other cystitis

Abscess of bladder

N30.80 Other cystitis without hematuria

N30.81 Other cystitis with hematuria

N30.9 Cystitis, unspecified

N30.90 Cystitis, unspecified without hematuria

1 HAC = as SDx not POA, in combination with SDx code T83.51XA also not POA.

N3Ø.91 Cystitis, unspecified with hematuria

✓4th **N31 Neuromuscular dysfunction of bladder, not elsewhere classified**
Use additional code to identify any associated urinary incontinence (N39.3-N39.4-)
EXCLUDES 1 *cord bladder NOS (G95.89)*
neurogenic bladder due to cauda equina syndrome (G83.4)
neuromuscular dysfunction due to spinal cord lesion (G95.89)

N31.Ø Uninhibited neuropathic bladder, not elsewhere classified

N31.1 Reflex neuropathic bladder, not elsewhere classified

N31.2 Flaccid neuropathic bladder, not elsewhere classified
Atonic (motor) (sensory) neuropathic bladder
Autonomous neuropathic bladder
Nonreflex neuropathic bladder

N31.8 Other neuromuscular dysfunction of bladder

N31.9 Neuromuscular dysfunction of bladder, unspecified
Neurogenic bladder dysfunction NOS

✓4th **N32 Other disorders of bladder**
EXCLUDES 2 *calculus of bladder (N21.Ø)*
cystocele (N81.1-)
hernia or prolapse of bladder, female (N81.1-)

N32.Ø Bladder-neck obstruction
Bladder-neck stenosis (acquired)
EXCLUDES 1 *congenital bladder-neck obstruction (Q64.3-)*

N32.1 Vesicointestinal fistula CC
Vesicorectal fistula
CC Excl: A54.ØØ, A54.Ø2, A54.Ø9-A54.1, A54.82, A54.84, A54.89-A54.9, N32.1-N32.2, N32.89-N33, N36.41-N36.43, N36.8-N36.9, N39.8-N39.9, R3Ø.Ø, R3Ø.9-R31.9

N32.2 Vesical fistula, not elsewhere classified CC
EXCLUDES 1 *fistula between bladder and female genital tract (N82.Ø-N82.1)*
CC Excl: See code: N32.1

N32.3 Diverticulum of bladder
EXCLUDES 1 *congenital diverticulum of bladder (Q64.6)*
diverticulitis of bladder (N3Ø.8-)

✓5th **N32.8 Other specified disorders of bladder**

N32.81 Overactive bladder
Detrusor muscle hyperactivity
EXCLUDES 1 *frequent urination due to specified bladder condition—code to condition*

N32.89 Other specified disorders of bladder
Bladder hemorrhage
Bladder hypertrophy
Calcified bladder
Contracted bladder

N32.9 Bladder disorder, unspecified

N33 Bladder disorders in diseases classified elsewhere
Code first underlying disease, such as:
schistosomiasis (B65.Ø-B65.9)
EXCLUDES 1 *bladder disorder in syphilis (A52.76)*
bladder disorder in tuberculosis (A18.12)
candidal cystitis (B37.41)
chlamydial cystitis (A56.Ø1)
cystitis in gonorrhea (A54.Ø1)
cystitis in neurogenic bladder (N31.-)
diphtheritic cystitis (A36.85)
neurogenic bladder (N31.-)
syphilitic cystitis (A52.76)
trichomonal cystitis (A59.Ø3)

✓4th **N34 Urethritis and urethral syndrome**
Use additional code (B95-B97), to identify infectious agent
EXCLUDES 2 *Reiter's disease (MØ2.3-)*
urethritis in diseases with a predominantly sexual mode of transmission (A5Ø-A64)
urethrotrigonitis (N3Ø.3-)

1 **N34.Ø Urethral abscess** CC
Abscess (of) Cowper's gland
Abscess (of) Littrés gland
Abscess (of) urethral (gland)
Periurethral abscess
EXCLUDES 1 *urethral caruncle (N36.2)*
CC Excl: A54.ØØ, A54.Ø2, A54.Ø9-A54.1, A54.82, A54.84, A54.89-A54.9, A59.ØØ, A59.Ø3, A59.8-A59.9, B37.41-B37.49, N13.9, N34.Ø-N34.3, N35.111-N35.9, N36.41-N36.43, N36.8-N39.Ø, N39.8-N39.9, N44.1-N44.8, N47.6, N48.1-N48.9, N49.1-N49.9, N5Ø.3-N5Ø.8, N51, N53.11-N53.9, Q54.Ø-Q55.21, Q55.23-Q55.9, Q64.Ø, Q64.2-Q64.9, R3Ø.Ø, R3Ø.9-R31.9

N34.1 Nonspecific urethritis
Nongonococcal urethritis
Nonvenereal urethritis

N34.2 Other urethritis
Meatitis, urethral
Postmenopausal urethritis
Ulcer of urethra (meatus)
Urethritis NOS

N34.3 Urethral syndrome, unspecified

✓4th **N35 Urethral stricture**
EXCLUDES 1 *congenital urethral stricture (Q64.3-)*
postprocedural urethral stricture (N99.1-)

✓5th **N35.Ø Post-traumatic urethral stricture**
Urethral stricture due to injury
EXCLUDES 1 *postprocedural urethral stricture (N99.1-)*

✓6th **N35.Ø1 Post-traumatic urethral stricture, male**

N35.Ø1Ø Post-traumatic urethral stricture, male, meatal ♂

N35.Ø11 Post-traumatic bulbous urethral stricture

N35.Ø12 Post-traumatic membranous urethral stricture

N35.Ø13 Post-traumatic anterior urethral stricture

N35.Ø14 Post-traumatic urethral stricture, male, unspecified ♂

✓6th **N35.Ø2 Post-traumatic urethral stricture, female**

N35.Ø21 Urethral stricture due to childbirth ♀

N35.Ø28 Other post-traumatic urethral stricture, female ♀

✓5th **N35.1 Postinfective urethral stricture, not elsewhere classified**
EXCLUDES 1 *urethral stricture associated with schistosomiasis (B65-, N29)*
gonococcal urethral stricture (A54.Ø1)
syphilitic urethral stricture (A52.76)

✓6th **N35.11 Postinfective urethral stricture, not elsewhere classified, male**

N35.111 Postinfective urethral stricture, not elsewhere classified, male, meatal ♂

N35.112 Postinfective bulbous urethral stricture, not elsewhere classified

N35.113 Postinfective membranous urethral stricture, not elsewhere classified

N35.114 Postinfective anterior urethral stricture, not elsewhere classified

N35.119 Postinfective urethral stricture, not elsewhere classified, male, unspecified ♂

N35.12 Postinfective urethral stricture, not elsewhere classified, female ♀

N35.8 Other urethral stricture
EXCLUDES 1 *postprocedural urethral stricture (N99.1-)*

N35.9 Urethral stricture, unspecified

✓4th **N36 Other disorders of urethra**

N36.Ø Urethral fistula CC
Urethroperineal fistula
Urethrorectal fistula
Urinary fistula NOS
EXCLUDES 1 *urethroscrotal fistula (N5Ø.8)*
urethrovaginal fistula (N82.1)
urethrovesicovaginal fistula (N82.1)
CC Excl: N13.9, N34.Ø, N34.2-N36.43, N36.5-N37, N39.8-N39.9, N44.1-N44.8, N47.6, N48.1-N48.9, N49.1-N49.9, N5Ø.3-N5Ø.8, N51, N53.11-N53.9, N99.11Ø-N99.12, Q54.Ø-Q55.21, Q55.23-Q55.9, Q64.Ø, Q64.8-Q64.9, R3Ø.Ø, R3Ø.9-R31.9

N36.1 Urethral diverticulum

N36.2 Urethral caruncle

✓5th **N36.4 Urethral functional and muscular disorders**
Use additional code to identify associated urinary stress incontinence (N39.3)

N36.41 Hypermobility of urethra

N36.42 Intrinsic sphincter deficiency (ISD)

N36.43 Combined hypermobility of urethra and intrinsic sphincter deficiency

N36.44 Muscular disorders of urethra
Bladder sphincter dyssynergy

N36.5 Urethral false passage

N36.8 Other specified disorders of urethra

N36.9 Urethral disorder, unspecified

1 HAC = as SDx not POA, in combination with SDx code T83.51XA also not POA.

N37 Urethral disorders in diseases classified elsewhere
Code first underlying disease
EXCLUDES 1 *urethritis (in):*
candidal infection (B37.41)
chlamydial (A56.01)
gonorrhea (A54.01)
syphilis (A52.76)
trichomonal infection (A59.03)
tuberculosis (A18.13)

✓4th **N39 Other disorders of urinary system**
EXCLUDES 2 *hematuria NOS (R31.-)*
recurrent or persistent hematuria (N02.-)
recurrent or persistent hematuria with specified morphological lesion (N02.-)
proteinuria NOS (R80.-)

1 **N39.0 Urinary tract infection, site not specified** CC
Use additional code (B95-B97), to identify infectious agent
EXCLUDES 1 *candidiasis of urinary tract (B37.4-)*
neonatal urinary tract infection (P39.3)
urinary tract infection of specified site, such as:
cystitis (N30.-)
urethritis (N34.-)
AHA: 2012, 4Q, 94
CC Excl: A54.82, A54.84, A54.89-A54.9, A59.00, A59.8-A59.9, B37.41-B37.49, N10, N11.9-N13.39, N13.6, N13.9, N15.1, N28.82, N28.84-N30.91, N34.1, N36.41-N36.43, N36.8-N36.9, N39.0, N39.8-N39.9, N99.511, R30.0, R30.9-R31.9, T83.51XA

N39.3 Stress incontinence (female) (male)
Code also any associated overactive bladder (N32.81)
EXCLUDES 1 *mixed incontinence (N39.46)*

✓5th **N39.4 Other specified urinary incontinence**
Code also any associated overactive bladder (N32.81)
EXCLUDES 1 *enuresis NOS (R32)*
functional urinary incontinence (R39.81)
urinary incontinence associated with cognitive impairment (R39.81)
urinary incontinence NOS (R32)
urinary incontinence of nonorganic origin (F98.0)

N39.41 Urge incontinence
EXCLUDES 1 *mixed incontinence (N39.46)*
N39.42 Incontinence without sensory awareness
N39.43 Post-void dribbling
N39.44 Nocturnal enuresis
N39.45 Continuous leakage
N39.46 Mixed incontinence
Urge and stress incontinence

✓6th **N39.49 Other specified urinary incontinence**
N39.490 Overflow incontinence
N39.498 Other specified urinary incontinence
Reflex incontinence
Total incontinence

N39.8 Other specified disorders of urinary system
N39.9 Disorder of urinary system, unspecified

Diseases of male genital organs (N40-N53)

✓4th **N40 Enlarged prostate**
Adenofibromatous hypertrophy of prostate
Benign hypertrophy of the prostate
Benign prostatic hyperplasia
Benign prostatic hypertrophy
BPH
Nodular prostate
Polyp of prostate
EXCLUDES 1 *benign neoplasms of prostate (adenoma, benign) (fibroadenoma) (fibroma) (myoma) (D29.1)*
EXCLUDES 2 *malignant neoplasm of prostate (C61)*

N40.0 Enlarged prostate without lower urinary tract symptoms A♂
Enlarged prostate NOS
Enlarged prostate without LUTS

N40.1 Enlarged prostate with lower urinary tract symptoms A♂
Enlarged prostate with LUTS
Use additional code for associated symptoms, when specified:
incomplete bladder emptying (R39.14)
nocturia (R35.1)
straining on urination (R39.16)
urinary frequency (R35.0)
urinary hesitancy (R39.11)
urinary incontinence (N39.4-)
urinary obstruction (N13.8)
urinary retention (R33.8)
urinary urgency (R39.15)
weak urinary stream (R39.12)

1 HAC = as SDx not POA, in combination with SDx code T83.51XA also not POA.

N40.2 Nodular prostate without lower urinary tract symptoms A♂
Nodular prostate without LUTS

N40.3 Nodular prostate with lower urinary tract symptoms A♂
Use additional code for associated symptoms, when specified:
incomplete bladder emptying (R39.14)
nocturia (R35.1)
straining on urination (R39.16)
urinary frequency (R35.0)
urinary hesitancy (R39.11)
urinary incontinence (N39.4-)
urinary obstruction (N13.8)
urinary retention (R33.8)
urinary urgency (R39.15)
weak urinary stream (R39.12)

✓4th **N41 Inflammatory diseases of prostate**
Use additional code (B95-B97), to identify infectious agent

N41.0 Acute prostatitis CC A♂
CC Excl: A18.14, A54.22, A54.82, A54.84, A54.89-A54.9, A59.00, A59.02, A59.8-A59.9, B37.41-B37.49, N40.0-N41.0, N41.1, N41.2-N42.9
N41.1 Chronic prostatitis A♂
N41.2 Abscess of prostate CC A♂
CC Excl: See code: N41.0
N41.3 Prostatocystitis A♂
N41.4 Granulomatous prostatitis A♂
N41.8 Other inflammatory diseases of prostate A♂
N41.9 Inflammatory disease of prostate, unspecified A♂
Prostatitis NOS

✓4th **N42 Other and unspecified disorders of prostate**
N42.0 Calculus of prostate A♂
Prostatic stone
N42.1 Congestion and hemorrhage of prostate A♂
EXCLUDES 1 *enlarged prostate (N40.-)*
hematuria (R31.-)
hyperplasia of prostate (N40.-)
inflammatory diseases of prostate (N41.-)
N42.3 Dysplasia of prostate ♂
Prostatic intraepithelial neoplasia I (PIN I)
Prostatic intraepithelial neoplasia II (PIN II)
EXCLUDES 1 *prostatic intraepithelial neoplasia III (PIN III) (D07.5)*

✓5th **N42.8 Other specified disorders of prostate**
N42.81 Prostatodynia syndrome A♂
Painful prostate syndrome
N42.82 Prostatosis syndrome A♂
N42.83 Cyst of prostate A♂
N42.89 Other specified disorders of prostate A♂
N42.9 Disorder of prostate, unspecified A♂

✓4th **N43 Hydrocele and spermatocele**
INCLUDES hydrocele of spermatic cord, testis or tunica vaginalis
EXCLUDES 1 *congenital hydrocele (P83.5)*
N43.0 Encysted hydrocele ♂
N43.1 Infected hydrocele CC ♂
Use additional code (B95-B97), to identify infectious agent
CC Excl: A59.00, A59.8-A59.9, B37.41-B37.49, N43.0-N43.3
N43.2 Other hydrocele ♂
N43.3 Hydrocele, unspecified ♂

✓5th **N43.4 Spermatocele of epididymis**
Spermatic cyst
N43.40 Spermatocele of epididymis, unspecified ♂
N43.41 Spermatocele of epididymis, single ♂
N43.42 Spermatocele of epididymis, multiple ♂

✓4th **N44 Noninflammatory disorders of testis**
CC Excl: For CC codes in category N44, unless otherwise noted: N44.00-N44.04

✓5th **N44.0 Torsion of testis**
N44.00 Torsion of testis, unspecified CC ♂
N44.01 Extravaginal torsion of spermatic cord CC ♂
N44.02 Intravaginal torsion of spermatic cord CC ♂
Torsion of spermatic cord NOS
N44.03 Torsion of appendix testis CC ♂
N44.04 Torsion of appendix epididymis CC ♂
N44.1 Cyst of tunica albuginea testis ♂
N44.2 Benign cyst of testis ♂

N44.8 Other noninflammatory disorders of the testis ♂

✓4th **N45 Orchitis and epididymitis**
Use additional code (B95-B97), to identify infectious agent
- **N45.1 Epididymitis** ♂
- **N45.2 Orchitis** ♂
- **N45.3 Epididymo-orchitis** ♂
- **N45.4 Abscess of epididymis or testis** CC ♂
  CC Excl: A54.23, A54.82, A54.84, A54.89-A54.9, A59.ØØ, A59.8-A59.9, B26.Ø, B37.41-B37.49, N45.1-N45.4

✓4th **N46 Male infertility**
EXCLUDES 1 *vasectomy status (Z98.52)*

✓5th **N46.Ø Azoospermia**
Absolute male infertility
Male infertility due to germinal (cell) aplasia
Male infertility due to spermatogenic arrest (complete)
- **N46.Ø1 Organic azoospermia** A ♂
  Azoospermia NOS
- ✓6th **N46.Ø2 Azoospermia due to extratesticular causes**
  Code also associated cause
  - **N46.Ø21 Azoospermia due to drug therapy** A ♂
  - **N46.Ø22 Azoospermia due to infection** A ♂
  - **N46.Ø23 Azoospermia due to obstruction of efferent ducts** A ♂
  - **N46.Ø24 Azoospermia due to radiation** A ♂
  - **N46.Ø25 Azoospermia due to systemic disease** A ♂
  - **N46.Ø29 Azoospermia due to other extratesticular causes** A ♂

✓5th **N46.1 Oligospermia**
Male infertility due to germinal cell desquamation
Male infertility due to hypospermatogenesis
Male infertility due to incomplete spermatogenic arrest
- **N46.11 Organic oligospermia** A ♂
  Oligospermia NOS
- ✓6th **N46.12 Oligospermia due to extratesticular causes**
  Code also associated cause
  - **N46.121 Oligospermia due to drug therapy** A ♂
  - **N46.122 Oligospermia due to infection** A ♂
  - **N46.123 Oligospermia due to obstruction of efferent ducts** A ♂
  - **N46.124 Oligospermia due to radiation** A ♂
  - **N46.125 Oligospermia due to systemic disease** A ♂
  - **N46.129 Oligospermia due to other extratesticular causes** A ♂

N46.8 Other male infertility A ♂
N46.9 Male infertility, unspecified A ♂

✓4th **N47 Disorders of prepuce**
- **N47.Ø Adherent prepuce, newborn** N ♂
- **N47.1 Phimosis** ♂
- **N47.2 Paraphimosis** ♂
- **N47.3 Deficient foreskin** ♂
- **N47.4 Benign cyst of prepuce** ♂
- **N47.5 Adhesions of prepuce and glans penis** ♂
- **N47.6 Balanoposthitis** ♂
  Use additional code (B95-B97), to identify infectious agent
  EXCLUDES 1 *balanitis (N48.1)*
- **N47.7 Other inflammatory diseases of prepuce** ♂
  Use additional code (B95-B97), to identify infectious agent
- **N47.8 Other disorders of prepuce** ♂

✓4th **N48 Other disorders of penis**
- **N48.Ø Leukoplakia of penis** ♂
  Balanitis xerotica obliterans
  Kraurosis of penis
  Lichen sclerosus of external male genital organs
  EXCLUDES 1 *carcinoma in situ of penis (DØ7.4)*
- **N48.1 Balanitis** ♂
  Use additional code (B95-B97), to identify infectious agent
  EXCLUDES 1 *amebic balanitis (AØ6.8)*
  balanitis xerotica obliterans (N48.Ø)
  candidal balanitis (B37.42)
  gonococcal balanitis (A54.23)
  herpesviral [herpes simplex] balanitis (A6Ø.Ø1)

✓5th **N48.2 Other inflammatory disorders of penis**
Use additional code (B95-B97), to identify infectious agent
EXCLUDES 1 *balanitis (N48.1)*
balanitis xerotica obliterans (N48.Ø)
balanoposthitis (N47.6)
- **N48.21 Abscess of corpus cavernosum and penis** ♂
- **N48.22 Cellulitis of corpus cavernosum and penis** ♂
- **N48.29 Other inflammatory disorders of penis** ♂

✓5th **N48.3 Priapism**
Painful erection
Code first underlying cause
CC Excl: For CC codes in subcategory N48.3, unless otherwise noted: N47.6, N48.Ø-N48.9, N52.Ø1-N52.9
- **N48.3Ø Priapism, unspecified** CC ♂
- **N48.31 Priapism due to trauma** CC ♂
- *N48.32* ***Priapism due to disease classified elsewhere*** CC ♂
- **N48.33 Priapism, drug-induced** CC ♂
- **N48.39 Other priapism** CC ♂

N48.5 Ulcer of penis ♂
N48.6 Induration penis plastica ♂
Peyronie's disease
Plastic induration of penis

✓5th **N48.8 Other specified disorders of penis**
- **N48.81 Thrombosis of superficial vein of penis** ♂
- **N48.82 Acquired torsion of penis** ♂
  Acquired torsion of penis NOS
  EXCLUDES 1 *congenital torsion of penis (Q55.63)*
- **N48.83 Acquired buried penis** ♂
  EXCLUDES 1 *congenital hidden penis (Q55.64)*
- **N48.89 Other specified disorders of penis** ♂

N48.9 Disorder of penis, unspecified ♂

✓4th **N49 Inflammatory disorders of male genital organs, not elsewhere classified**
Use additional code (B95-B97), to identify infectious agent
EXCLUDES 1 *inflammation of penis (N48.1, N48.2-)*
orchitis and epididymitis (N45.-)
- **N49.Ø Inflammatory disorders of seminal vesicle** ♂
  Vesiculitis NOS
- **N49.1 Inflammatory disorders of spermatic cord, tunica vaginalis and vas deferens** ♂
  Vasitis
- **N49.2 Inflammatory disorders of scrotum** ♂
- **N49.3 Fournier gangrene** ♂
- **N49.8 Inflammatory disorders of other specified male genital organs** ♂
  Inflammation of multiple sites in male genital organs
- **N49.9 Inflammatory disorder of unspecified male genital organ** ♂
  Abscess of unspecified male genital organ
  Boil of unspecified male genital organ
  Carbuncle of unspecified male genital organ
  Cellulitis of unspecified male genital organ

✓4th **N5Ø Other and unspecified disorders of male genital organs**
EXCLUDES 2 *torsion of testis (N44.Ø-)*
- **N5Ø.Ø Atrophy of testis** ♂
- **N5Ø.1 Vascular disorders of male genital organs** ♂
  Hematocele, NOS, of male genital organs
  Hemorrhage of male genital organs
  Thrombosis of male genital organs
- **N5Ø.3 Cyst of epididymis** ♂
- **N5Ø.8 Other specified disorders of male genital organs** ♂
  Atrophy of scrotum, seminal vesicle, spermatic cord, tunica vaginalis and vas deferens
  Chylocele, tunica vaginalis (nonfilarial) NOS
  Edema of scrotum, seminal vesicle, spermatic cord, testis, tunica vaginalis and vas deferens
  Hypertrophy of scrotum, seminal vesicle, spermatic cord, testis, tunica vaginalis and vas deferens
  Stricture of spermatic cord, tunica vaginalis, and vas deferens
  Ulcer of scrotum, seminal vesicle, spermatic cord, testis, tunica vaginalis and vas deferens
  Urethroscrotal fistula
- **N5Ø.9 Disorder of male genital organs, unspecified** ♂

N51 Disorders of male genital organs in diseases classified elsewhere ♂

Code first underlying disease, such as:
filariasis (B74.0-B74.9)

EXCLUDES 1 *amebic balanitis (A06.8)*
candidal balanitis (B37.42)
gonococcal balanitis (A54.23)
gonococcal prostatitis (A54.22)
herpesviral [herpes simplex] balanitis (A60.01)
trichomonal prostatitis (A59.02)
tuberculous prostatitis (A18.14)

N52 Male erectile dysfunction

EXCLUDES 1 *psychogenic impotence (F52.21)*

N52.0 Vasculogenic erectile dysfunction
- **N52.01 Erectile dysfunction due to arterial insufficiency** A ♂
- **N52.02 Corporo-venous occlusive erectile dysfunction** A ♂
- **N52.03 Combined arterial insufficiency and corporo-venous occlusive erectile dysfunction** A ♂

N52.1 Erectile dysfunction due to diseases classified elsewhere A ♂

Code first underlying disease

N52.2 Drug-induced erectile dysfunction A ♂

N52.3 Post-surgical erectile dysfunction
- **N52.31 Erectile dysfunction following radical prostatectomy** A ♂
- **N52.32 Erectile dysfunction following radical cystectomy** A ♂
- **N52.33 Erectile dysfunction following urethral surgery** A ♂
- **N52.34 Erectile dysfunction following simple prostatectomy** A ♂
- **N52.39 Other post-surgical erectile dysfunction** A ♂

N52.8 Other male erectile dysfunction A ♂

N52.9 Male erectile dysfunction, unspecified A ♂

Impotence NOS

N53 Other male sexual dysfunction

EXCLUDES 1 *psychogenic sexual dysfunction (F52.-)*

N53.1 Ejaculatory dysfunction

EXCLUDES 1 *premature ejaculation (F52.4)*

- **N53.11 Retarded ejaculation** ♂
- **N53.12 Painful ejaculation** ♂
- **N53.13 Anejaculatory orgasm** ♂
- **N53.14 Retrograde ejaculation** ♂
- **N53.19 Other ejaculatory dysfunction** ♂
  Ejaculatory dysfunction NOS

N53.8 Other male sexual dysfunction ♂

N53.9 Unspecified male sexual dysfunction ♂

Disorders of breast (N60-N65)

EXCLUDES 1 *disorders of breast associated with childbirth (O91-O92)*

N60 Benign mammary dysplasia

INCLUDES fibrocystic mastopathy

N60.0 Solitary cyst of breast

Cyst of breast

- **N60.01 Solitary cyst of right breast**
- **N60.02 Solitary cyst of left breast**
- **N60.09 Solitary cyst of unspecified breast**

N60.1 Diffuse cystic mastopathy

Cystic breast
Fibrocystic disease of breast

EXCLUDES 1 *diffuse cystic mastopathy with epithelial proliferation (N60.3-)*

- **N60.11 Diffuse cystic mastopathy of right breast** A
- **N60.12 Diffuse cystic mastopathy of left breast** A
- **N60.19 Diffuse cystic mastopathy of unspecified breast** A

N60.2 Fibroadenosis of breast

Adenofibrosis of breast

EXCLUDES 2 *fibroadenoma of breast (D24.-)*

- **N60.21 Fibroadenosis of right breast**
- **N60.22 Fibroadenosis of left breast**
- **N60.29 Fibroadenosis of unspecified breast**

N60.3 Fibrosclerosis of breast

Cystic mastopathy with epithelial proliferation

- **N60.31 Fibrosclerosis of right breast**
- **N60.32 Fibrosclerosis of left breast**
- **N60.39 Fibrosclerosis of unspecified breast**

N60.4 Mammary duct ectasia
- **N60.41 Mammary duct ectasia of right breast**
- **N60.42 Mammary duct ectasia of left breast**
- **N60.49 Mammary duct ectasia of unspecified breast**

N60.8 Other benign mammary dysplasias
- **N60.81 Other benign mammary dysplasias of right breast**
- **N60.82 Other benign mammary dysplasias of left breast**
- **N60.89 Other benign mammary dysplasias of unspecified breast**

N60.9 Unspecified benign mammary dysplasia
- **N60.91 Unspecified benign mammary dysplasia of right breast**
- **N60.92 Unspecified benign mammary dysplasia of left breast**
- **N60.99 Unspecified benign mammary dysplasia of unspecified breast**

N61 Inflammatory disorders of breast

Abscess (acute) (chronic) (nonpuerperal) of areola
Abscess (acute) (chronic) (nonpuerperal) of breast
Carbuncle of breast
Infective mastitis (acute) (subacute) (nonpuerperal)
Mastitis (acute) (subacute) (nonpuerperal) NOS

EXCLUDES 1 *inflammatory carcinoma of breast (C50.9)*
inflammatory disorder of breast associated with childbirth (O91.-)
neonatal infective mastitis (P39.0)
thrombophlebitis of breast [Mondor's disease] (I80.8)

N62 Hypertrophy of breast

Gynecomastia
Hypertrophy of breast NOS
Massive pubertal hypertrophy of breast

EXCLUDES 1 *breast engorgement of newborn (P83.4)*
disproportion of reconstructed breast (N65.1)

N63 Unspecified lump in breast

Nodule(s) NOS in breast

N64 Other disorders of breast

EXCLUDES 2 *mechanical complication of breast prosthesis and implant (T85.4-)*

N64.0 Fissure and fistula of nipple

N64.1 Fat necrosis of breast

Fat necrosis (segmental) of breast
Code first breast necrosis due to breast graft (T85.89)

N64.2 Atrophy of breast

N64.3 Galactorrhea not associated with childbirth

N64.4 Mastodynia

N64.5 Other signs and symptoms in breast

EXCLUDES 2 *abnormal findings on diagnostic imaging of breast (R92.-)*

- **N64.51 Induration of breast**
- **N64.52 Nipple discharge**
  EXCLUDES 1 *abnormal findings in nipple discharge (R89.-)*
- **N64.53 Retraction of nipple**
- **N64.59 Other signs and symptoms in breast**

N64.8 Other specified disorders of breast
- **N64.81 Ptosis of breast** A
  EXCLUDES 1 *ptosis of native breast in relation to reconstructed breast (N65.1)*
- **N64.82 Hypoplasia of breast** A
  Micromastia
  EXCLUDES 1 *congenital absence of breast (Q83.0)*
  hypoplasia of native breast in relation to reconstructed breast (N65.1)
- **N64.89 Other specified disorders of breast**
  Galactocele
  Subinvolution of breast (postlactational)

N64.9 Disorder of breast, unspecified

N65 Deformity and disproportion of reconstructed breast

N65.0 Deformity of reconstructed breast A

Contour irregularity in reconstructed breast
Excess tissue in reconstructed breast
Misshapen reconstructed breast

N65.1 Disproportion of reconstructed breast A
Breast asymmetry between native breast and reconstructed breast
Disproportion between native breast and reconstructed breast

Inflammatory diseases of female pelvic organs (N7Ø-N77)

EXCLUDES 1 *inflammatory diseases of female pelvic organs complicating:*
abortion or ectopic or molar pregnancy (OØØ-OØ7, OØ8.Ø)
pregnancy, childbirth and the puerperium (O23-, O75.3, O85, O86-)

4th **N7Ø Salpingitis and oophoritis**
INCLUDES abscess (of) fallopian tube
abscess (of) ovary
pyosalpinx
salpingo-oophoritis
tubo-ovarian abscess
tubo-ovarian inflammatory disease
Use additional code (B95-B97), to identify infectious agent
EXCLUDES 1 *gonococcal infection (A54.24)*
tuberculous infection (A18.17)

CC Excl: For CC codes in subcategory N7Ø.Ø, unless otherwise noted: A17.9, A18.1Ø, A18.16-A18.18, A18.82, A18.84, A18.89, A54.Ø3, A54.24, A54.82, A54.84, A54.89-A54.9, A59.ØØ, A59.8-A59.9, B37.41-B37.49, N7Ø.Ø1-N71.9, N73.Ø-N74, N75.9, N76.5, N76.81-N76.89, N9Ø.81Ø-N9Ø.818, N94.818-N94.9, N96, Q55.Ø-Q55.21, Q55.23-Q55.4, Q55.7-Q55.9

5th **N7Ø.Ø Acute salpingitis and oophoritis**
N7Ø.Ø1 Acute salpingitis CC ♀
N7Ø.Ø2 Acute oophoritis CC ♀
N7Ø.Ø3 Acute salpingitis and oophoritis CC ♀

5th **N7Ø.1 Chronic salpingitis and oophoritis**
Hydrosalpinx
N7Ø.11 Chronic salpingitis ♀
N7Ø.12 Chronic oophoritis ♀
N7Ø.13 Chronic salpingitis and oophoritis ♀

5th **N7Ø.9 Salpingitis and oophoritis, unspecified**
N7Ø.91 Salpingitis, unspecified ♀
N7Ø.92 Oophoritis, unspecified ♀
N7Ø.93 Salpingitis and oophoritis, unspecified ♀

4th **N71 Inflammatory disease of uterus, except cervix**
Endo (myo) metritis
Metritis
Myometritis
Pyometra
Uterine abscess
Use additional code (B95-B97), to identify infectious agent
EXCLUDES 1 *hyperplastic endometritis (N85.Ø-)*
infection of uterus following delivery (O85, O86.-)

N71.Ø Acute inflammatory disease of uterus CC ♀
CC Excl: A17.9, A18.1Ø, A18.16-A18.18, A18.82, A18.84, A18.89, A54.Ø3, A54.24, A54.82, A54.84, A54.89-A54.9, A59.ØØ, A59.8-A59.9, B37.41-B37.49, N7Ø.Ø1-N74, N75.9, N76.5, N76.81-N76.89, N85.8-N85.9, N9Ø.81Ø-N9Ø.818, N94.818-N94.9, N96, Q55.Ø-Q55.21, Q55.23-Q55.4, Q55.7-Q55.9

N71.1 Chronic inflammatory disease of uterus ♀
N71.9 Inflammatory disease of uterus, unspecified ♀

N72 Inflammatory disease of cervix uteri ♀
Cervicitis (with or without erosion or ectropion)
Endocervicitis (with or without erosion or ectropion)
Exocervicitis (with or without erosion or ectropion)
Use additional code (B95-B97), to identify infectious agent
EXCLUDES 1 *erosion and ectropion of cervix without cervicitis (N86)*

4th **N73 Other female pelvic inflammatory diseases**
Use additional code (B95-B97), to identify infectious agent

CC Excl: For CC/MCC codes in category N73, unless otherwise noted: A17.9, A18.1Ø, A18.16-A18.18, A18.82, A18.84, A18.89, A54.Ø3, A54.24, A54.82, A54.84, A54.89-A54.9, A59.ØØ, A59.8-A59.9, B37.41-B37.49, N7Ø.Ø1-N71.9, N73.Ø-N74, N75.9, N76.5, N76.81-N76.89, N9Ø.81Ø-N9Ø.818, N94.818-N94.9, N96, Q55.Ø-Q55.21, Q55.23-Q55.4, Q55.7-Q55.9

N73.Ø Acute parametritis and pelvic cellulitis CC ♀
Abscess of broad ligament
Abscess of parametrium
Pelvic cellulitis, female

N73.1 Chronic parametritis and pelvic cellulitis ♀
Any condition in N73.Ø specified as chronic
EXCLUDES 1 *tuberculous parametritis and pelvic cellultis (A18.17)*

N73.2 Unspecified parametritis and pelvic cellulitis ♀
Any condition in N73.Ø unspecified whether acute or chronic

N73.3 Female acute pelvic peritonitis MCC ♀

N73.4 Female chronic pelvic peritonitis CC ♀
EXCLUDES 1 *tuberculous pelvic (female) peritonitis (A18.17)*

N73.5 Female pelvic peritonitis, unspecified ♀

N73.6 Female pelvic peritoneal adhesions (postinfective) ♀
EXCLUDES 2 *postprocedural pelvic peritoneal adhesions (N99.4)*
AHA: 2Ø14, 1Q, 6

N73.8 Other specified female pelvic inflammatory diseases ♀

N73.9 Female pelvic inflammatory disease, unspecified ♀
Female pelvic infection or inflammation NOS

N74 Female pelvic inflammatory disorders in diseases classified elsewhere ♀
Code first underlying disease
EXCLUDES 1 *chlamydial cervicitis (A56.Ø2)*
chlamydial pelvic inflammatory disease (A56.11)
gonococcal cervicitis (A54.Ø3)
gonococcal pelvic inflammatory disease (A54.24)
herpesviral [herpes simplex] cervicitis (A6Ø.Ø3)
herpesviral [herpes simplex] pelvic inflammatory disease (A6Ø.Ø9)
syphilitic cervicitis (A52.76)
syphilitic pelvic inflammatory disease (A52.76)
trichomonal cervicitis (A59.Ø9)
tuberculous cervicitis (A18.16)
tuberculous pelvic inflammatory disease (A18.17)

4th **N75 Diseases of Bartholin's gland**

N75.Ø Cyst of Bartholin's gland ♀

N75.1 Abscess of Bartholin's gland CC ♀
CC Excl: A17.9, A18.1Ø, A18.16-A18.18, A18.82, A18.84, A18.89, A59.ØØ-A59.Ø1, A59.8-A59.9, B37.3-B37.49, N75.Ø-N77.1, N84.3, N9Ø.3, N9Ø.6-N9Ø.9, N94.81Ø-N94.9, N96, Q55.Ø-Q55.21, Q55.23-Q55.4, Q55.7-Q55.9

N75.8 Other diseases of Bartholin's gland ♀
Bartholinitis

N75.9 Disease of Bartholin's gland, unspecified ♀

4th **N76 Other inflammation of vagina and vulva**
Use additional code (B95-B97), to identify infectious agent
EXCLUDES 2 *senile (atrophic) vaginitis (N95.2)*
vulvar vestibulitis (N94.81Ø)

N76.Ø Acute vaginitis ♀
Acute vulvovaginitis
Vaginitis NOS
Vulvovaginitis NOS

N76.1 Subacute and chronic vaginitis ♀
Chronic vulvovaginitis
Subacute vulvovaginitis

N76.2 Acute vulvitis ♀
Vulvitis NOS

N76.3 Subacute and chronic vulvitis ♀

N76.4 Abscess of vulva CC ♀
Furuncle of vulva
CC Excl: See code: N75.1

N76.5 Ulceration of vagina ♀

N76.6 Ulceration of vulva ♀

5th **N76.8 Other specified inflammation of vagina and vulva**

N76.81 Mucositis (ulcerative) of vagina and vulva CC ♀
Code also type of associated therapy, such as:
antineoplastic and immunosuppressive drugs (T45.1X-)
radiological procedure and radiotherapy (Y84.2)
EXCLUDES 2 *gastrointestinal mucositis (ulcerative) (K92.81)*
nasal mucositis (ulcerative) (J34.81)
oral mucositis (ulcerative) (K12.3-)
CC Excl: N72, N75.9, N76.5, N76.81-N76.89

N76.89 Other specified inflammation of vagina and vulva ♀

4th **N77 Vulvovaginal ulceration and inflammation in diseases classified elsewhere**

N77.Ø Ulceration of vulva in diseases classified elsewhere ♀
Code first underlying disease, such as:
Behçet's disease (M35.2)
EXCLUDES 1 *ulceration of vulva in gonococcal infection (A54.Ø2)*
ulceration of vulva in herpesviral [herpes simplex] infection (A6Ø.Ø4)
ulceration of vulva in syphilis (A51.Ø)
ulceration of vulva in tuberculosis (A18.18)

N77.1 Vaginitis, vulvitis and vulvovaginitis in diseases classified elsewhere ♀
Code first underlying disease, such as:
pinworm (B80)
EXCLUDES 1 candidal vulvovaginitis (B37.3)
chlamydial vulvovaginitis (A56.02)
gonococcal vulvovaginitis (A54.02)
herpesviral [herpes simplex] vulvovaginitis (A60.04)
trichomonal vulvovaginitis (A59.01)
tuberculous vulvovaginitis (A18.18)
vulvovaginitis in early syphilis (A51.0)
vulvovaginitis in late syphilis (A52.76)

Noninflammatory disorders of female genital tract (N80-N98)

N80 Endometriosis
- **N80.0 Endometriosis of uterus** ♀
  Adenomyosis
  EXCLUDES 1 stromal endometriosis (D39.0)
- **N80.1 Endometriosis of ovary** ♀
- **N80.2 Endometriosis of fallopian tube** ♀
- **N80.3 Endometriosis of pelvic peritoneum** ♀
- **N80.4 Endometriosis of rectovaginal septum and vagina** ♀
- **N80.5 Endometriosis of intestine** ♀
- **N80.6 Endometriosis in cutaneous scar** ♀
- **N80.8 Other endometriosis** ♀
- **N80.9 Endometriosis, unspecified** ♀

N81 Female genital prolapse
EXCLUDES 1 genital prolapse complicating pregnancy, labor or delivery (O34.5-)
prolapse and hernia of ovary and fallopian tube (N83.4)
prolapse of vaginal vault after hysterectomy (N99.3)
- **N81.0 Urethrocele** ♀
  EXCLUDES 1 urethrocele with cystocele (N81.1-)
  urethrocele with prolapse of uterus (N81.2-N81.4)
- **N81.1 Cystocele**
  Cystocele with urethrocele
  Cystourethrocele
  EXCLUDES 1 cystocele with prolapse of uterus (N81.2-N81.4)
  - **N81.10 Cystocele, unspecified** ♀
    Prolapse of (anterior) vaginal wall NOS
  - **N81.11 Cystocele, midline** ♀
  - **N81.12 Cystocele, lateral** ♀
    Paravaginal cystocele
- **N81.2 Incomplete uterovaginal prolapse** ♀
  First degree uterine prolapse
  Prolapse of cervix NOS
  Second degree uterine prolapse
  EXCLUDES 1 cervical stump prolaspe (N81.85)
- **N81.3 Complete uterovaginal prolapse** ♀
  Procidentia (uteri) NOS
  Third degree uterine prolapse
- **N81.4 Uterovaginal prolapse, unspecified** ♀
  Prolapse of uterus NOS
- **N81.5 Vaginal enterocele** ♀
  EXCLUDES 1 enterocele with prolapse of uterus (N81.2-N81.4)
- **N81.6 Rectocele** ♀
  Prolapse of posterior vaginal wall
  Use additional code for any associated fecal incontinence, if applicable (R15.-)
  EXCLUDES 2 perineocele (N81.81)
  rectal prolapse (K62.3)
  rectocele with prolapse of uterus (N81.2-N81.4)
- **N81.8 Other female genital prolapse**
  - **N81.81 Perineocele** ♀
  - **N81.82 Incompetence or weakening of pubocervical tissue** ♀
  - **N81.83 Incompetence or weakening of rectovaginal tissue** ♀
  - **N81.84 Pelvic muscle wasting** ♀
    Disuse atrophy of pelvic muscles and anal sphincter
  - **N81.85 Cervical stump prolapse** ♀
  - **N81.89 Other female genital prolapse** ♀
    Deficient perineum
    Old laceration of muscles of pelvic floor
- **N81.9 Female genital prolapse, unspecified** ♀

N82 Fistulae involving female genital tract
EXCLUDES 1 vesicointestinal fistulae (N32.1)

CC Excl: For CC codes in category N82, unless otherwise noted: N82.0-N82.9

- **N82.0 Vesicovaginal fistula** CC ♀
- **N82.1 Other female urinary-genital tract fistulae** CC ♀
  Cervicovesical fistula
  Ureterovaginal fistula
  Urethrovaginal fistula
  Uteroureteric fistula
  Uterovesical fistula
- **N82.2 Fistula of vagina to small intestine** CC ♀
- **N82.3 Fistula of vagina to large intestine** CC ♀
  Rectovaginal fistula
- **N82.4 Other female intestinal-genital tract fistulae** CC ♀
  Intestinouterine fistula
- **N82.5 Female genital tract-skin fistulae** CC ♀
  Uterus to abdominal wall fistula
  Vaginoperineal fistula
- **N82.8 Other female genital tract fistulae** CC ♀
- **N82.9 Female genital tract fistula, unspecified** CC ♀

N83 Noninflammatory disorders of ovary, fallopian tube and broad ligament
EXCLUDES 2 hydrosalpinx (N70.1-)
- **N83.0 Follicular cyst of ovary** ♀
  Cyst of graafian follicle
  Hemorrhagic follicular cyst (of ovary)
- **N83.1 Corpus luteum cyst** ♀
  Hemorrhagic corpus luteum cyst
- **N83.2 Other and unspecified ovarian cysts**
  EXCLUDES 1 developmental ovarian cyst (Q50.1)
  neoplastic ovarian cyst (D27.-)
  polycystic ovarian syndrome (E28.2)
  Stein-Leventhal syndrome (E28.2)
  - **N83.20 Unspecified ovarian cysts** ♀
  - **N83.29 Other ovarian cysts** ♀
    Retention cyst of ovary
    Simple cyst of ovary
- **N83.3 Acquired atrophy of ovary and fallopian tube**
  - **N83.31 Acquired atrophy of ovary** ♀
  - **N83.32 Acquired atrophy of fallopian tube** ♀
  - **N83.33 Acquired atrophy of ovary and fallopian tube** ♀
- **N83.4 Prolapse and hernia of ovary and fallopian tube** ♀
- **N83.5 Torsion of ovary, ovarian pedicle and fallopian tube**
  Torsion of accessory tube

  CC Excl: For CC codes in subcategory N83.5, unless otherwise noted: N83.0-N83.9, N99.83

  - **N83.51 Torsion of ovary and ovarian pedicle** CC ♀
  - **N83.52 Torsion of fallopian tube** CC ♀
    Torsion of hydatid of Morgagni
  - **N83.53 Torsion of ovary, ovarian pedicle and fallopian tube** CC ♀
- **N83.6 Hematosalpinx** ♀
  EXCLUDES 1 hematosalpinx (with) (in):
  hematocolpos (N89.7)
  hematometra (N85.7)
  tubal pregnancy (O00.1)
- **N83.7 Hematoma of broad ligament** ♀
- **N83.8 Other noninflammatory disorders of ovary, fallopian tube and broad ligament** ♀
  Broad ligament laceration syndrome [Allen-Masters]
- **N83.9 Noninflammatory disorder of ovary, fallopian tube and broad ligament, unspecified** ♀

N84 Polyp of female genital tract
EXCLUDES 1 adenomatous polyp (D28.-)
placental polyp (O90.89)
- **N84.0 Polyp of corpus uteri** ♀
  Polyp of endometrium
  Polyp of uterus NOS
  EXCLUDES 1 polypoid endometrial hyperplasia (N85.0-)
- **N84.1 Polyp of cervix uteri** ♀
  Mucous polyp of cervix
- **N84.2 Polyp of vagina** ♀
- **N84.3 Polyp of vulva** ♀
  Polyp of labia
- **N84.8 Polyp of other parts of female genital tract** ♀
- **N84.9 Polyp of female genital tract, unspecified** ♀

✓4th N85 Other noninflammatory disorders of uterus, except cervix
EXCLUDES 1 *endometriosis (N80.-)*
inflammatory diseases of uterus (N71.-)
noninflammatory disorders of cervix, except malposition (N86-N88)
polyp of corpus uteri (N84.0)
uterine prolapse (N81.-)

✓5th N85.0 Endometrial hyperplasia

N85.00 Endometrial hyperplasia, unspecified ♀
Hyperplasia (adenomatous) (cystic) (glandular) of endometrium
Hyperplastic endometritis

N85.01 Benign endometrial hyperplasia ♀
Endometrial hyperplasia (complex) (simple) without atypia

N85.02 Endometrial intraepithelial neoplasia [EIN] ♀
Endometrial hyperplasia with atypia
EXCLUDES 1 *malignant neoplasm of endometrium (with endometrial intraepithelial neoplasia [EIN]) (C54.1)*

N85.2 Hypertrophy of uterus ♀
Bulky or enlarged uterus
EXCLUDES 1 *puerperal hypertrophy of uterus (O90.89)*

N85.3 Subinvolution of uterus ♀
EXCLUDES 1 *puerperal subinvolution of uterus (O90.89)*

N85.4 Malposition of uterus ♀
Anteversion of uterus
Retroflexion of uterus
Retroversion of uterus
EXCLUDES 1 *malposition of uterus complicating pregnancy, labor or delivery (O34.5-, O65.5)*

N85.5 Inversion of uterus ♀
EXCLUDES 1 *current obstetric trauma (O71.2)*
postpartum inversion of uterus (O71.2)

N85.6 Intrauterine synechiae ♀

N85.7 Hematometra ♀
Hematosalpinx with hematometra
EXCLUDES 1 *hematometra with hematocolpos (N89.7)*

N85.8 Other specified noninflammatory disorders of uterus ♀
Atrophy of uterus, acquired
Fibrosis of uterus NOS

N85.9 Noninflammatory disorder of uterus, unspecified ♀
Disorder of uterus NOS

N86 Erosion and ectropion of cervix uteri ♀
Decubitus (trophic) ulcer of cervix
Eversion of cervix
EXCLUDES 1 *erosion and ectropion of cervix with cervicitis (N72)*

✓4th N87 Dysplasia of cervix uteri
EXCLUDES 1 *abnormal results from cervical cytologic examination without histologic confirmation (R87.61-)*
carcinoma in situ of cervix uteri (D06.-)
cervical intraepithelial neoplasia III [CIN III] (D06.-)
HGSIL of cervix (R87.613)
severe dysplasia of cervix uteri (D06.-)

N87.0 Mild cervical dysplasia ♀
Cervical intraepithelial neoplasia I [CIN I]

N87.1 Moderate cervical dysplasia ♀
Cervical intraepithelial neoplasia II [CIN II]

N87.9 Dysplasia of cervix uteri, unspecified ♀
Anaplasia of cervix
Cervical atypism
Cervical dysplasia NOS

✓4th N88 Other noninflammatory disorders of cervix uteri
EXCLUDES 2 *inflammatory disease of cervix (N72)*
polyp of cervix (N84.1)

N88.0 Leukoplakia of cervix uteri ♀

N88.1 Old laceration of cervix uteri ♀
Adhesions of cervix
EXCLUDES 1 *current obstetric trauma (O71.3)*

N88.2 Stricture and stenosis of cervix uteri ♀
EXCLUDES 1 *stricture and stenosis of cervix uteri complicating labor (O65.5)*

N88.3 Incompetence of cervix uteri ♀
Investigation and management of (suspected) cervical incompetence in a nonpregnant woman
EXCLUDES 1 *cervical incompetence complicating pregnancy (O34.3-)*

N88.4 Hypertrophic elongation of cervix uteri ♀

N88.8 Other specified noninflammatory disorders of cervix uteri ♀
EXCLUDES 1 *current obstetric trauma (O71.3)*

N88.9 Noninflammatory disorder of cervix uteri, unspecified ♀

✓4th N89 Other noninflammatory disorders of vagina
EXCLUDES 1 *abnormal results from vaginal cytologic examination without histologic confirmation (R87.62-)*
carcinoma in situ of vagina (D07.2)
HGSIL of vagina (R87.623)
inflammation of vagina (N76.-)
senile (atrophic) vaginitis (N95.2)
severe dysplasia of vagina (D07.2)
trichomonal leukorrhea (A59.00)
vaginal intraepithelial neoplasia [VAIN], grade III (D07.2)

N89.0 Mild vaginal dysplasia ♀
Vaginal intraepithelial neoplasia [VAIN], grade I

N89.1 Moderate vaginal dysplasia ♀
Vaginal intraepithelial neoplasia [VAIN], grade II

N89.3 Dysplasia of vagina, unspecified ♀

N89.4 Leukoplakia of vagina ♀

N89.5 Stricture and atresia of vagina ♀
Vaginal adhesions
Vaginal stenosis
EXCLUDES 1 *congenital atresia or stricture (Q52.4)*
postprocedural adhesions of vagina (N99.2)

N89.6 Tight hymenal ring ♀
Rigid hymen
Tight introitus
EXCLUDES 1 *imperforate hymen (Q52.3)*

N89.7 Hematocolpos ♀
Hematocolpos with hematometra or hematosalpinx

N89.8 Other specified noninflammatory disorders of vagina ♀
Leukorrhea NOS
Old vaginal laceration
Pessary ulcer of vagina
EXCLUDES 1 *current obstetric trauma (O70-, O71.4, O71.7-O71.8)*
old laceration involving muscles of pelvic floor (N81.8)

N89.9 Noninflammatory disorder of vagina, unspecified ♀

✓4th N90 Other noninflammatory disorders of vulva and perineum
EXCLUDES 1 *anogenital (venereal) warts (A63.0)*
carcinoma in situ of vulva (D07.1)
condyloma acuminatum (A63.0)
current obstetric trauma (O70-, O71.7-O71.8)
inflammation of vulva (N76.-)
severe dysplasia of vulva (D07.1)
vulvar intraepithelial neoplasm III [VIN III] (D07.1)

N90.0 Mild vulvar dysplasia ♀
Vulvar intraepithelial neoplasia [VIN], grade I

N90.1 Moderate vulvar dysplasia ♀
Vulvar intraepithelial neoplasia [VIN], grade II

N90.3 Dysplasia of vulva, unspecified ♀

N90.4 Leukoplakia of vulva ♀
Dystrophy of vulva
Kraurosis of vulva
Lichen sclerosus of external female genital organs

N90.5 Atrophy of vulva ♀
Stenosis of vulva

N90.6 Hypertrophy of vulva ♀
Hypertrophy of labia

N90.7 Vulvar cyst ♀

✓5th N90.8 Other specified noninflammatory disorders of vulva and perineum

✓6th N90.81 Female genital mutilation status
Female genital cutting status

N90.810 Female genital mutilation status, unspecified ♀
Female genital cutting status, unspecified
Female genital mutilation status NOS

N90.811 Female genital mutilation Type I status ♀
Clitorectomy status
Female genital cutting Type I status

N90.812 Female genital mutilation Type II status ♀
Clitorectomy with excision of labia minora status
Female genital cutting Type II status

N90.813 Female genital mutilation Type III status ♀
Female genital cutting Type III status
Infibulation status

N90.818 Other female genital mutilation status ♀
Female genital cutting Type IV status
Female genital mutilation Type IV status
Other female genital cutting status

N90.89 **Other specified noninflammatory disorders of vulva and perineum** ♀
Adhesions of vulva
Hypertrophy of clitoris

N90.9 **Noninflammatory disorder of vulva and perineum, unspecified** ♀

✓4th **N91 Absent, scanty and rare menstruation**
EXCLUDES 1 *ovarian dysfunction (E28.-)*

N91.0 **Primary amenorrhea** ♀
N91.1 **Secondary amenorrhea** ♀
N91.2 **Amenorrhea, unspecified** ♀
N91.3 **Primary oligomenorrhea** ♀
N91.4 **Secondary oligomenorrhea** ♀
N91.5 **Oligomenorrhea, unspecified** ♀
Hypomenorrhea NOS

✓4th **N92 Excessive, frequent and irregular menstruation**
EXCLUDES 1 *postmenopausal bleeding (N95.0)*
precocious puberty (menstruation) (E30.1)

N92.0 **Excessive and frequent menstruation with regular cycle** ♀
Heavy periods NOS
Menorrhagia NOS
Polymenorrhea

N92.1 **Excessive and frequent menstruation with irregular cycle** ♀
Irregular intermenstrual bleeding
Irregular, shortened intervals between menstrual bleeding
Menometrorrhagia
Metrorrhagia

N92.2 **Excessive menstruation at puberty** P ♀
Excessive bleeding associated with onset of menstrual periods
Pubertal menorrhagia
Puberty bleeding

N92.3 **Ovulation bleeding** ♀
Regular intermenstrual bleeding

N92.4 **Excessive bleeding in the premenopausal period** ♀
Climacteric menorrhagia or metrorrhagia
Menopausal menorrhagia or metrorrhagia
Preclimacteric menorrhagia or metrorrhagia
Premenopausal menorrhagia or metrorrhagia

N92.5 **Other specified irregular menstruation** ♀

N92.6 **Irregular menstruation, unspecified** ♀
Irregular bleeding NOS
Irregular periods NOS
EXCLUDES 1 *irregular menstruation with:*
lengthened intervals or scanty bleeding (N91.3-N91.5)
shortened intervals or excessive bleeding (N92.1)

✓4th **N93 Other abnormal uterine and vaginal bleeding**
EXCLUDES 1 *neonatal vaginal hemorrhage (P54.6)*
precocious puberty (menstruation) (E30.1)
pseudomenses (P54.6)

N93.0 **Postcoital and contact bleeding** ♀
N93.8 **Other specified abnormal uterine and vaginal bleeding** ♀
Dysfunctional or functional uterine or vaginal bleeding NOS
N93.9 **Abnormal uterine and vaginal bleeding, unspecified** ♀

✓4th **N94 Pain and other conditions associated with female genital organs and menstrual cycle**

N94.0 **Mittelschmerz** ♀
N94.1 **Dyspareunia** ♀
EXCLUDES 1 *psychogenic dyspareunia (F52.6)*
N94.2 **Vaginismus** ♀
EXCLUDES 1 *psychogenic vaginismus (F52.5)*
N94.3 **Premenstrual tension syndrome** ♀
Premenstrual dysphoric disorder
Code also associated menstrual migraine (G43.82-, G43.83-)
N94.4 **Primary dysmenorrhea** ♀
N94.5 **Secondary dysmenorrhea** ♀
N94.6 **Dysmenorrhea, unspecified** ♀
EXCLUDES 1 *psychogenic dysmenorrhea (F45.8)*

✓5th N94.8 **Other specified conditions associated with female genital organs and menstrual cycle**

✓6th N94.81 **Vulvodynia**
N94.810 **Vulvar vestibulitis** ♀
N94.818 **Other vulvodynia** ♀
N94.819 **Vulvodynia, unspecified** ♀
Vulvodynia NOS

N94.89 **Other specified conditions associated with female genital organs and menstrual cycle** ♀

N94.9 **Unspecified condition associated with female genital organs and menstrual cycle** ♀

✓4th **N95 Menopausal and other perimenopausal disorders**
Menopausal and other perimenopausal disorders due to naturally occurring (age-related) menopause and perimenopause
EXCLUDES 1 *excessive bleeding in the premenopausal period (N92.4)*
menopausal and perimenopausal disorders due to artificial or premature menopause (E89.4-, E28.31-)
premature menopause (E28.31-)
EXCLUDES 2 *postmenopausal osteoporosis (M81.0-)*
postmenopausal osteoporosis with current pathological fracture (M80.0-)
postmenopausal urethritis (N34.2)

N95.0 **Postmenopausal bleeding** ♀
N95.1 **Menopausal and female climacteric states** ♀
Symptoms such as flushing, sleeplessness, headache, lack of concentration, associated with natural (age-related) menopause
Use additional code for associated symptoms
EXCLUDES 1 *asymptomatic menopausal state (Z78.0)*
symptoms associated with artificial menopause (E89.41)
symptoms associated with premature menopause (E28.310)
N95.2 **Postmenopausal atrophic vaginitis** ♀
Senile (atrophic) vaginitis
N95.8 **Other specified menopausal and perimenopausal disorders** ♀
N95.9 **Unspecified menopausal and perimenopausal disorder** ♀

N96 Recurrent pregnancy loss ♀
Investigation or care in a nonpregnant woman with history of recurrent pregnancy loss
EXCLUDES 1 *recurrent pregnancy loss with current pregnancy (O26.2-)*

✓4th **N97 Female infertility**
INCLUDES inability to achieve a pregnancy
sterility, female NOS
EXCLUDES 1 *female infertility associated with:*
hypopituitarism (E23.0)
Stein-Leventhal syndrome (E28.2)
EXCLUDES 2 *incompetence of cervix uteri (N88.3)*

N97.0 **Female infertility associated with anovulation** ♀
N97.1 **Female infertility of tubal origin** ♀
Female infertility associated with congenital anomaly of tube
Female infertility due to tubal block
Female infertility due to tubal occlusion
Female infertility due to tubal stenosis
N97.2 **Female infertility of uterine origin** ♀
Female infertility associated with congenital anomaly of uterus
Female infertility due to nonimplantation of ovum
N97.8 **Female infertility of other origin** ♀
N97.9 **Female infertility, unspecified** ♀

✓4th **N98 Complications associated with artificial fertilization**

N98.0 **Infection associated with artificial insemination** CC ♀
CC Excl: N98.0, T80.211A, T80.212A, T80.218A, T80.219A, T80.22XA, T80.29XA, T82.7XXA, T88.0XXA
N98.1 **Hyperstimulation of ovaries** CC ♀
Hyperstimulation of ovaries NOS
Hyperstimulation of ovaries associated with induced ovulation
CC Excl: D78.81-D78.89, E36.8, E89.810-E89.89, H59.011-H59.019, H59.031-H59.099, H59.811-H59.89, H95.811-H95.89, I97.3, L76.81-L76.82, M96.89, N98.1-N98.9, T81.8[2,9]XA, T81.9XXA
N98.2 **Complications of attempted introduction of fertilized ovum following in vitro fertilization** CC ♀
CC Excl: See code: N98.1
N98.3 **Complications of attempted introduction of embryo in embryo transfer** CC ♀
CC Excl: See code: N98.1
N98.8 **Other complications associated with artificial fertilization** CC ♀
CC Excl: See code: N98.1
N98.9 **Complication associated with artificial fertilization, unspecified** CC ♀
CC Excl: See code: N98.1

Intraoperative and postprocedural complications and disorders of genitourinary system, not elsewhere classified (N99)

√4th **N99 Intraoperative and postprocedural complications and disorders of genitourinary system, not elsewhere classified**

EXCLUDES 2 *irradiation cystitis (N3Ø.4-)*
postoophorectomy osteoporosis with current pathological fracture (M8Ø.8-)
postoophorectomy osteoporosis without current pathological fracture (M81.8)

N99.Ø Postprocedural (acute) (chronic) kidney failure
Use additional code for type of kidney disease

√5th **N99.1 Postprocedural urethral stricture**
Postcatheterization urethral stricture

√6th **N99.11 Postprocedural urethral stricture, male**

N99.11Ø Postprocedural urethral stricture, male, meatal ♂

N99.111 Postprocedural bulbous urethral stricture

N99.112 Postprocedural membranous urethral stricture

N99.113 Postprocedural anterior urethral stricture

N99.114 Postprocedural urethral stricture, male, unspecified ♂

N99.12 Postprocedural urethral stricture, female ♀

N99.2 Postprocedural adhesions of vagina ♀

N99.3 Prolapse of vaginal vault after hysterectomy ♀

N99.4 Postprocedural pelvic peritoneal adhesions

EXCLUDES 2 *pelvic peritoneal adhesions NOS (N73.6)*
postinfective pelvic peritoneal adhesions (N73.6)

√5th **N99.5 Complications of stoma of urinary tract**

EXCLUDES 2 *mechanical complication of urinary (indwelling) catheter (T83.Ø-)*

√6th **N99.51 Complication of cystostomy**

N99.51Ø Cystostomy hemorrhage CC
CC Excl: D78.81-D78.89, E36.8, E89.81Ø-E89.89, H59.Ø11-H59.Ø19, H59.Ø31-H59.Ø99, H59.811-H59.89, H95.811-H95.89, I97.3, L76.81-L76.82, M96.89, N32.89, N33, N98.1-N98.9, N99.51Ø-N99.518, T81.82A, T81.89X-T81.9XX with 7th A, T83.Ø1ØA, T83.Ø2ØA, T83.Ø3ØA, T83.Ø9ØA, T83.11Ø-T83.29X with 7th A, T83.41Ø-T83.718 with 7th A, T83.728-T83.9XX with 7th A, T85.31Ø-T85.311 with 7th A, T85.32Ø-T85.321 with 7th A, T85.39Ø-T85.391 with 7th A, T85.51Ø-T85.9XX with 7th A, T86.82Ø-T86.829, T86.842-T86.849

N99.511 Cystostomy infection CC
CC Excl: D78.81-D78.89, E36.8, E89.81Ø-E89.89, H59.Ø11-H59.Ø19, H59.Ø31-H59.Ø99, H59.811-H59.89, H95.811-H95.89, I97.3, L76.81-L76.82, M96.89, N32.89, N33, N39.Ø, N98.1-N98.9, N99.51Ø-N99.518, T81.82A, T81.89X-T81.9XX with 7th A, T83.Ø1ØA, T83.Ø2ØA, T83.Ø3ØA, T83.Ø9ØA, T83.11Ø-T83.29X with 7th A, T83.41Ø-T83.718 with 7th A, T83.728-T83.9XX with 7th A, T85.31Ø-T85.311 with 7th A, T85.32Ø-T85.321 with 7th A, T85.39Ø-T85.391 with 7th A, T85.51Ø-T85.612 with 7th A, T85.614-T85.622 with 7th A, T85.624-T85.692 with 7th A, T85.694-T85.9XX with 7th A, T86.842-T86.849

N99.512 Cystostomy malfunction CC
CC Excl: D78.81-D78.89, E36.8, E89.81Ø-E89.89, H59.Ø11-H59.Ø19, H59.Ø31-H59.Ø99, H59.811-H59.89, H95.811-H95.89, I97.3, L76.81-L76.82, M96.89, N32.89, N33, N98.1-N98.9, N99.51Ø-N99.518, T81.82XA, T81.89XA, T81.9XXA, T83.Ø1ØA, T83.Ø2ØA, T83.Ø3ØA, T83.Ø9ØA, T83.11ØA, T83.111A, T83.112A, T83.118A, T83.12ØA, T83.121A, T83.122A, T83.128A, T83.19ØA, T83.191A, T83.192A, T83.198A, T83.21XA, T83.22XA, T83.23XA, T83.29XA, T83.41ØA, T83.418A, T83.42ØA, T83.428A, T83.49ØA, T83.498A, T83.51XA, T83.59XA, T83.6XXA, T83.718A, T83.728A, T83.81XA, T83.82XA, T83.83XA, T83.84XA, T83.85XA, T83.86XA, T83.89XA, T83.9XXA

N99.518 Other cystostomy complication CC
CC Excl: See code: N99.51Ø

√6th **N99.52 Complication of other external stoma of urinary tract**

N99.52Ø Hemorrhage of other external stoma of urinary tract

N99.521 Infection of other external stoma of urinary tract

N99.522 Malfunction of other external stoma of urinary tract

N99.528 Other complication of other external stoma of urinary tract

√6th **N99.53 Complication of other stoma of urinary tract**

N99.53Ø Hemorrhage of other stoma of urinary tract

N99.531 Infection of other stoma of urinary tract

N99.532 Malfunction of other stoma of urinary tract

N99.538 Other complication of other stoma of urinary tract

√5th **N99.6 Intraoperative hemorrhage and hematoma of a genitourinary system organ or structure complicating a procedure**

EXCLUDES 1 *intraoperative hemorrhage and hematoma of a genitourinary system organ or structure due to accidental puncture or laceration during a procedure (N99.7-)*

N99.61 Intraoperative hemorrhage and hematoma of a genitourinary system organ or structure complicating a genitourinary system procedure CC
CC Excl: H95.811-H95.89, I85.Ø1, I85.11, I97.3, K21.9, K22.8, K23-K25.Ø, K25.2, K25.4, K25.6, K26.Ø, K26.2, K26.4, K26.6, K27.Ø, K27.2, K27.4, K27.6, K28.Ø, K28.2, K28.4, K28.6, K29.Ø1, K29.21, K29.31, K29.41, K29.51, K29.61, K29.71, K29.81, K29.91, K31.811, K55.21, K57.Ø1, K57.11, K57.13, K57.21, K57.31, K57.33, K57.41, K57.51, K57.53, K57.81, K57.91, K57.93, K62.5, K92.Ø-K92.2, M96.89, N98.1-N98.9, N99.61-N99.62, N99.82Ø-N99.821, P54.1-P54.3, T81.1ØXA, T81.11XA, T81.12XA, T81.19XA, T81.82XA, T81.89XA, T81.9XXA

N99.62 Intraoperative hemorrhage and hematoma of a genitourinary system organ or structure complicating other procedure CC
CC Excl: See code: N99.61

√5th **N99.7 Accidental puncture and laceration of a genitourinary system organ or structure during a procedure**

N99.71 Accidental puncture and laceration of a genitourinary system organ or structure during a genitourinary system procedure CC
CC Excl: D78.11-D78.12, D78.81-D78.89, E36.11-E36.8, E89.81Ø-E89.89, G96.11, G97.41, G97.48-G97.49, H59.Ø11-H59.Ø19, H59.Ø31-H59.Ø99, H59.211-H59.229, H59.811-H59.89, H95.31-H95.32, H95.811-H95.89, I97.3, I97.51-I97.52, J95.71-J95.72, K91.71-K91.72, L76.11-L76.12, L76.81-L76.82, M96.82Ø-M96.821, M96.89, N98.1-N98.9, N99.71-N99.72, T81.8[2,9]XA, T81.9XXA

N99.72 Accidental puncture and laceration of a genitourinary system organ or structure during other procedure CC
CC Excl: See code: N99.71

√5th **N99.8 Other intraoperative and postprocedural complications and disorders of genitourinary system**

N99.81 Other intraoperative complications of genitourinary system

√6th **N99.82 Postprocedural hemorrhage and hematoma of a genitourinary system organ or structure following a procedure**

N99.82Ø Postprocedural hemorrhage and hematoma of a genitourinary system organ or structure following a genitourinary system procedure CC
CC Excl: See code: N99.61

N99.821 Postprocedural hemorrhage and hematoma of a genitourinary system organ or structure following other procedure CC
CC Excl: See code: N99.61

N99.83 Residual ovary syndrome ♀

N99.89 Other postprocedural complications and disorders of genitourinary system

Chapter 15. Pregnancy, Childbirth and the Puerperium (OØØ-O9A)

NOTE CODES FROM THIS CHAPTER ARE FOR USE ONLY ON MATERNAL RECORDS, NEVER ON NEWBORN RECORDS.

Codes from this chapter are for use for conditions related to or aggravated by the pregnancy, childbirth, or by the puerperium (maternal causes or obstetric causes).

NOTE Trimesters are counted from the first day of the last menstrual period. They are defined as follows:

1st trimester- less than 14 weeks Ø days
2nd trimester- 14 weeks Ø days to less than 28 weeks Ø days
3rd trimester- 28 weeks Ø days until delivery

Use additional code from category Z3A, Weeks of gestation, to identify the specific week of the pregnancy

EXCLUDES 1 *supervision of normal pregnancy (Z34.-)*
EXCLUDES 2 *mental and behavioral disorders associated with the puerperium (F53)*
dobstetrical tetanus (A34)
postpartum necrosis of pituitary gland (E23.Ø)
puerperal osteomalacia (M83.Ø)

This chapter contains the following blocks:

OØØ-OØ8	Pregnancy with abortive outcome
OØ9	Supervision of high risk pregnancy
O1Ø-O16	Edema, proteinuria and hypertensive disorders in pregnancy, childbirth and the puerperium
O2Ø-O29	Other maternal disorders predominantly related to pregnancy
O3Ø-O48	Maternal care related to the fetus and amniotic cavity and possible delivery problems
O6Ø-O77	Complications of labor and delivery
O8Ø, O82	Encounter for delivery
O85-O92	Complications predominantly related to the puerperium
O94-O9A	Other obstetric conditions, not elsewhere classified

Pregnancy with abortive outcome (OØØ-OØ8)

EXCLUDES 1 *continuing pregnancy in multiple gestation after abortion of one fetus or more (O31.1-, O31.3-)*

✓4th OØØ Ectopic pregnancy

INCLUDES ruptured ectopic pregnancy

Use additional code from category OØ8 to identify any associated complication

CC Excl: For CC codes in category OØØ, unless otherwise noted: OØØ.Ø-OØØ.9

OØØ.Ø Abdominal pregnancy CC M ♀
EXCLUDES 1 *maternal care for viable fetus in abdominal pregnancy (O36.7-)*

OØØ.1 Tubal pregnancy CC M ♀
Fallopian pregnancy
Rupture of (fallopian) tube due to pregnancy
Tubal abortion

OØØ.2 Ovarian pregnancy CC M ♀

OØØ.8 Other ectopic pregnancy CC M ♀
Cervical pregnancy
Cornual pregnancy
Intraligamentous pregnancy
Mural pregnancy

OØØ.9 Ectopic pregnancy, unspecified CC M ♀

✓4th OØ1 Hydatidiform mole

Use additional code from category OØ8 to identify any associated complication

EXCLUDES 1 *chorioadenoma (destruens) (D39.2)*
malignant hydatidiform mole (D39.2)

OØ1.Ø Classical hydatidiform mole M ♀
Complete hydatidiform mole

OØ1.1 Incomplete and partial hydatidiform mole M ♀

OØ1.9 Hydatidiform mole, unspecified M ♀
Trophoblastic disease NOS
Vesicular mole NOS

✓4th OØ2 Other abnormal products of conception

Use additional code from category OØ8 to identify any associated complication

EXCLUDES 1 *papyraceous fetus (O31.Ø-)*

OØ2.Ø Blighted ovum and nonhydatidiform mole M ♀
Carneous mole
Fleshy mole
Intrauterine mole NOS
Molar pregnancy NEC
Pathological ovum

OØ2.1 Missed abortion M ♀
Early fetal death, before completion of 2Ø weeks of gestation, with retention of dead fetus
EXCLUDES 1 *failed induced abortion (OØ7.-)*
fetal death (intrauterine) (late) (O36.4)
missed abortion with blighted ovum (OØ2.Ø)
missed abortion with hydatidiform mole (OØ1.-)
missed abortion with nonhydatidiform (OØ2.Ø)
missed abortion with other abnormal products of conception (OØ2.8-)
missed delivery (O36.4)
stillbirth (P95)

✓5th **OØ2.8 Other specified abnormal products of conception**
EXCLUDES 1 *abnormal products of conception with blighted ovum (OØ2.Ø)*
abnormal products of conception with hydatidiform mole (OØ1.-)
abnormal products of conception with nonhydatidiform mole (OØ2.Ø)

OØ2.81 Inappropriate change in quantitative human chorionic gonadotropin (hCG) in early pregnancy M ♀
Biochemical pregnancy
Chemical pregnancy
Inappropriate level of quantitative human chorionic gonadotropin (hCG) for gestational age in early pregnancy

OØ2.89 Other abnormal products of conception M ♀

OØ2.9 Abnormal product of conception, unspecified M ♀

✓4th OØ3 Spontaneous abortion

NOTE Incomplete abortion includes retained products of conception following spontaneous abortion.

INCLUDES miscarriage

CC Excl: For CC/MCC codes in category OØ3, unless otherwise noted: OØ3.Ø-OØ7.4, O2Ø.Ø-O2Ø.9, O25.1Ø-O25.3, O26.1Ø-O26.13, O26.3Ø-O26.43, O26.63-O26.819, O26.841-O26.86, O26.891-O26.93, O29.Ø11-O29.93, O35.7XXØ-O35.7XX9, O44.ØØ-O44.13, O45.8X1-O45.93, O75.4, O75.81, O75.89-O75.9, O8Ø, O9Ø.89, O99.111-O99.285, O99.33Ø-O99.335, O99.35Ø-O99.355, O99.511-O99.73, O99.82Ø-O99.825, O99.84Ø-O9A.53, Z33.2

OØ3.Ø Genital tract and pelvic infection following incomplete spontaneous abortion CC M ♀
Endometritis following incomplete spontaneous abortion
Oophoritis following incomplete spontaneous abortion
Parametritis following incomplete spontaneous abortion
Pelvic peritonitis following incomplete spontaneous abortion
Salpingitis following incomplete spontaneous abortion
Salpingo-oophoritis following incomplete spontaneous abortion
EXCLUDES 1 *sepsis following incomplete spontaneous abortion (OØ3.37)*
urinary tract infection following incomplete spontaneous abortion (OØ3.38)

OØ3.1 Delayed or excessive hemorrhage following incomplete spontaneous abortion M ♀
Afibrinogenemia following incomplete spontaneous abortion
Defibrination syndrome following incomplete spontaneous abortion
Hemolysis following incomplete spontaneous abortion
Intravascular coagulation following incomplete spontaneous abortion

OØ3.2 Embolism following incomplete spontaneous abortion MCC M ♀
Air embolism following incomplete spontaneous abortion
Amniotic fluid embolism following incomplete spontaneous abortion
Blood-clot embolism following incomplete spontaneous abortion
Embolism NOS following incomplete spontaneous abortion
Fat embolism following incomplete spontaneous abortion
Pulmonary embolism following incomplete spontaneous abortion
Pyemic embolism following incomplete spontaneous abortion
Septic or septicopyemic embolism following incomplete spontaneous abortion
Soap embolism following incomplete spontaneous abortion

✓5th **OØ3.3 Other and unspecified complications following incomplete spontaneous abortion**

OØ3.3Ø Unspecified complication following incomplete spontaneous abortion CC M ♀

O03.31 Shock following incomplete spontaneous abortion MCC M ♀
Circulatory collapse following incomplete spontaneous abortion
Shock (postprocedural) following incomplete spontaneous abortion
EXCLUDES 1 *shock due to infection following incomplete spontaneous abortion (O03.37)*

O03.32 Renal failure following incomplete spontaneous abortion MCC M ♀
Kidney failure (acute) following incomplete spontaneous abortion
Oliguria following incomplete spontaneous abortion
Renal shutdown following incomplete spontaneous abortion
Renal tubular necrosis following incomplete spontaneous abortion
Uremia following incomplete spontaneous abortion

O03.33 Metabolic disorder following incomplete spontaneous abortion CC M ♀

O03.34 Damage to pelvic organs following incompletespontaneous abortion CC M ♀
Laceration, perforation, tear or chemical damage of bladder following incomplete spontaneous abortion
Laceration, perforation, tear or chemical damage of bowel following incomplete spontaneous abortion
Laceration, perforation, tear or chemical damage of broad ligament following incomplete spontaneous abortion
Laceration, perforation, tear or chemical damage of cervix following incomplete spontaneous abortion
Laceration, perforation, tear or chemical damage of periurethral tissue following incomplete spontaneous abortion
Laceration, perforation, tear or chemical damage of uterus following incomplete spontaneous abortion
Laceration, perforation, tear or chemical damage of vagina following incomplete spontaneous abortion

O03.35 Other venous complications following incomplete spontaneous abortion CC M ♀

O03.36 Cardiac arrest following incomplete spontaneous abortion CC M ♀

O03.37 Sepsis following incomplete spontaneous abortion CC M ♀
Use additional code to identify infectious agent (B95-B97)
Use additional code to identify severe sepsis, if applicable (R65.2-)
EXCLUDES 1 *septic or septicopyemic embolism following incomplete spontaneous abortion (O03.2)*

O03.38 Urinary tract infection following incomplete spontaneous abortion CC M ♀
Cystitis following incomplete spontaneous abortion

O03.39 Incomplete spontaneous abortion with other complications CC M ♀

O03.4 Incomplete spontaneous abortion without complication M ♀

O03.5 Genital tract and pelvic infection following complete or unspecified spontaneous abortion CC M ♀
Endometritis following complete or unspecified spontaneous abortion
Oophoritis following complete or unspecified spontaneous abortion
Parametritis following complete or unspecified spontaneous abortion
Pelvic peritonitis following complete or unspecified spontaneous abortion
Salpingitis following complete or unspecified spontaneous abortion
Salpingo-oophoritis following complete or unspecified spontaneous abortion
EXCLUDES 1 *sepsis following complete or unspecified spontaneous abortion (O03.87)*
urinary tract infection following complete or unspecified spontaneous abortion (O03.88)

O03.6 Delayed or excessive hemorrhage following complete or unspecified spontaneous abortion M ♀
Afibrinogenemia following complete or unspecified spontaneous abortion
Defibrination syndrome following complete or unspecified spontaneous abortion
Hemolysis following complete or unspecified spontaneous abortion
Intravascular coagulation following complete or unspecified spontaneous abortion

O03.7 Embolism following complete or unspecified spontaneous abortion CC M ♀
Air embolism following complete or unspecified spontaneous abortion
Amniotic fluid embolism following complete or unspecified spontaneous abortion
Blood-clot embolism following complete or unspecified spontaneous abortion
Embolism NOS following complete or unspecified spontaneous abortion
Fat embolism following complete or unspecified spontaneous abortion
Pulmonary embolism following complete or unspecified spontaneous abortion
Pyemic embolism following complete or unspecified spontaneous abortion
Septic or septicopyemic embolism following complete or unspecified spontaneous abortion
Soap embolism following complete or unspecified spontaneous abortion

✓5th **O03.8 Other and unspecified complications following complete or unspecified spontaneous abortion**

O03.80 Unspecified complication following complete or unspecified spontaneous abortion CC M ♀

O03.81 Shock following complete or unspecified spontaneous abortion MCC M ♀
Circulatory collapse following complete or unspecified spontaneous abortion
Shock (postprocedural) following complete or unspecified spontaneous abortion
EXCLUDES 1 *shock due to infection following complete or unspecified spontaneous abortion (O03.87)*

O03.82 Renal failure following complete or unspecified spontaneous abortion MCC M ♀
Kidney failure (acute) following complete or unspecified spontaneous abortion
Oliguria following complete or unspecified spontaneous abortion
Renal shutdown following complete or unspecified spontaneous abortion
Renal tubular necrosis following complete or unspecified spontaneous abortion
Uremia following complete or unspecified spontaneous abortion

O03.83 Metabolic disorder following complete or unspecified spontaneous abortion CC M ♀

O03.84 Damage to pelvic organs following complete or unspecified spontaneous abortion CC M ♀
Laceration, perforation, tear or chemical damage of bladder following complete or unspecified spontaneous abortion
Laceration, perforation, tear or chemical damage of bowel following complete or unspecified spontaneous abortion
Laceration, perforation, tear or chemical damage of broad ligament following complete or unspecified spontaneous abortion
Laceration, perforation, tear or chemical damage of cervix following complete or unspecified spontaneous abortion
Laceration, perforation, tear or chemical damage of periurethral tissue following complete or unspecified spontaneous abortion
Laceration, perforation, tear or chemical damage of uterus following complete or unspecified spontaneous abortion
Laceration, perforation, tear or chemical damage of vagina following complete or unspecified spontaneous abortion

O03.85 Other venous complications following complete or unspecified spontaneous abortion CC M ♀

O03.86 Cardiac arrest following complete or unspecified spontaneous abortion CC M ♀

O03.87 Sepsis following complete or unspecified spontaneous abortion CC M ♀
Use additional code to identify infectious agent (B95-B97)
Use additional code to identify severe sepsis, if applicable (R65.2-)
EXCLUDES 1 *septic or septicopyemic embolism following complete or unspecified spontaneous abortion (O03.7)*

O03.88 Urinary tract infection following complete or unspecified spontaneous abortion CC M ♀
Cystitis following complete or unspecified spontaneous abortion

O03.89 Complete or unspecified spontaneous abortion with other complications CC M ♀

O03.9 Complete or unspecified spontaneous abortion without complication M ♀
Miscarriage NOS
Spontaneous abortion NOS

✓4th O04 Complications following (induced) termination of pregnancy
INCLUDES complications following (induced) termination of pregnancy
EXCLUDES 1 *encounter for elective termination of pregnancy, uncomplicated (Z33.2)*
failed attempted termination of pregnancy (O07.-)

CC Excl: For CC/MCC codes in category O04, unless otherwise noted: See code: O03

O04.5 Genital tract and pelvic infection following (induced) termination of pregnancy CC M ♀
Endometritis following (induced) termination of pregnancy
Oophoritis following (induced) termination of pregnancy
Parametritis following (induced) termination of pregnancy
Pelvic peritonitis following (induced) termination of pregnancy
Salpingitis following (induced) termination of pregnancy
Salpingo-oophoritis following (induced) termination of pregnancy
EXCLUDES 1 *sepsis following (induced) termination of pregnancy (O04.87)*
urinary tract infection following (induced) termination of pregnancy (O04.88)

O04.6 Delayed or excessive hemorrhage following (induced) termination of pregnancy M ♀
Afibrinogenemia following (induced) termination of pregnancy
Defibrination syndrome following (induced) termination of pregnancy
Hemolysis following (induced) termination of pregnancy
Intravascular coagulation following (induced) termination of pregnancy

O04.7 Embolism following (induced) termination of pregnancy MCC M ♀
Air embolism following (induced) termination of pregnancy
Amniotic fluid embolism following (induced) termination of pregnancy
Blood-clot embolism following (induced) termination of pregnancy
Embolism NOS following (induced) termination of pregnancy
Fat embolism following (induced) termination of pregnancy
Pulmonary embolism following (induced) termination of pregnancy
Pyemic embolism following (induced) termination of pregnancy
Septic or septicopyemic embolism following (induced) termination of pregnancy
Soap embolism following (induced) termination of pregnancy

✓5th O04.8 (Induced) termination of pregnancy with other and unspecified complications

O04.80 (Induced) termination of pregnancy with unspecified complications CC M ♀

O04.81 Shock following (induced) termination of pregnancy MCC M ♀
Circulatory collapse following (induced) termination of pregnancy
Shock (postprocedural) following (induced) termination of pregnancy
EXCLUDES 1 *shock due to infection following (induced) termination of pregnancy (O04.87)*

O04.82 Renal failure following (induced) termination of pregnancy MCC M ♀
Kidney failure (acute) following (induced) termination of pregnancy
Oliguria following (induced) termination of pregnancy
Renal shutdown following (induced) termination of pregnancy
Renal tubular necrosis following (induced) termination of pregnancy
Uremia following (induced) termination of pregnancy

O04.83 Metabolic disorder following (induced) termination of pregnancy CC M ♀

O04.84 Damage to pelvic organs following (induced) termination of pregnancy CC M ♀
Laceration, perforation, tear or chemical damage of bladder following (induced) termination of pregnancy
Laceration, perforation, tear or chemical damage of bowel following (induced) termination of pregnancy
Laceration, perforation, tear or chemical damage of broad ligament following (induced) termination of pregnancy
Laceration, perforation, tear or chemical damage of cervix following (induced) termination of pregnancy
Laceration, perforation, tear or chemical damage of periurethral tissue following (induced) termination of pregnancy
Laceration, perforation, tear or chemical damage of uterus following (induced) termination of pregnancy
Laceration, perforation, tear or chemical damage of vagina following (induced) termination of pregnancy

O04.85 Other venous complications following (induced) termination of pregnancy CC M ♀

O04.86 Cardiac arrest following (induced) termination of pregnancy CC M ♀

O04.87 Sepsis following (induced) termination of pregnancy CC M ♀
Use additional code to identify infectious agent (B95-B97)
Use additional code to identify severe sepsis, if applicable (R65.2-)
EXCLUDES 1 *septic or septicopyemic embolism following (induced) termination of pregnancy (O04.7)*
CC Excl: O03.0-O07.4, O20.0-O20.9, O25.10-O25.3, O26.10-O26.13, O26.30-O26.43, O26.63-O26.819, O26.841-O26.86, O26.891-O26.93, O29.011-O29.93, O35.7X-O35.7X, O44.00-O44.13, O45.8X1-O45.93, O75.4, O75.81, O75.89-O75.9, O80, O90.89, O99.111-O99.285, O99.330-O99.335, O99.350-O99.355, O99.511-O99.73, O99.820-O99.825, O99.840-O9A.53, Z33.2

O04.88 Urinary tract infection following (induced) termination of pregnancy CC M ♀
Cystitis following (induced) termination of pregnancy
CC Excl: O03.0-O07.4, O20.0-O20.9, O25.10-O25.3, O26.10-O26.13, O26.30-O26.43, O26.63-O26.819, O26.841-O26.86, O26.891-O26.93, O29.011-O29.93, O35.7X-O35.7X, O44.00-O44.13, O45.8X1-O45.93, O75.4, O75.81, O75.89-O75.9, O80, O90.89, O99.111-O99.285, O99.330-O99.335, O99.350-O99.355, O99.511-O99.73, O99.820-O99.825, O99.840-O9A.53, Z33.2

O04.89 (Induced) termination of pregnancy with other complications CC M ♀
CC Excl: See code O04.88

O07 Failed attempted termination of pregnancy (4th)

INCLUDES failure of attempted induction of termination of pregnancy
incomplete elective abortion

EXCLUDES 1 *incomplete spontaneous abortion (O03.0-)*

O07.0 Genital tract and pelvic infection following failed attempted termination of pregnancy CC M ♀

Endometritis following failed attempted termination of pregnancy
Oophoritis following failed attempted termination of pregnancy
Parametritis following failed attempted termination of pregnancy
Pelvic peritonitis following failed attempted termination of pregnancy
Salpingitis following failed attempted termination of pregnancy
Salpingo-oophoritis following failed attempted termination of pregnancy

EXCLUDES 1 *sepsis following failed attempted termination of pregnancy (O07.37)*
urinary tract infection following failed attempted termination of pregnancy (O07.38)

CC Excl: O03.0-O04.89, O07.1, O07.30, O07.35-O07.36, O07.38-O07.4, O20.0-O20.9, O25.10-O25.3, O26.10-O26.13, O26.30-O26.43, O26.63-O26.819, O26.841-O26.86, O26.891-O26.93, O29.011-O29.93, O35.7XX0-O35.7XX9, O44.00-O44.13, O45.8X1-O45.93, O75.4, O75.81, O75.89-O75.9, O80, O90.89, O99.111-O99.285, O99.330-O99.335, O99.350-O99.355, O99.511-O99.73, O99.820-O99.825, O99.840-O9A.53, Z33.2

O07.1 Delayed or excessive hemorrhage following failed attempted termination of pregnancy CC M ♀

Afibrinogenemia following failed attempted termination of pregnancy
Defibrination syndrome following failed attempted termination of pregnancy
Hemolysis following failed attempted termination of pregnancy
Intravascular coagulation following failed attempted termination of pregnancy

CC Excl: O03.0-O04.89, O07.1, O07.30, O07.35-O07.36, O07.38-O07.4, O20.0-O20.9, O25.10-O25.3, O26.10-O26.13, O26.30-O26.43, O26.63-O26.819, O26.841-O26.86, O26.891-O26.93, O29.011-O29.93, O35.7XX0-O35.7XX9, O44.00-O44.13, O45.8X1-O45.93, O75.4, O75.81, O75.89-O75.9, O80, O90.89, O99.111-O99.285, O99.330-O99.335, O99.350-O99.355, O99.511-O99.73, O99.820-O99.825, O99.840-O9A.53, Z33.2

O07.2 Embolism following failed attempted termination of pregnancy MCC M ♀

Air embolism following failed attempted termination of pregnancy
Amniotic fluid embolism following failed attempted termination of pregnancy
Blood-clot embolism following failed attempted termination of pregnancy
Embolism NOS following failed attempted termination of pregnancy
Fat embolism following failed attempted termination of pregnancy
Pulmonary embolism following failed attempted termination of pregnancy
Pyemic embolism following failed attempted termination of pregnancy
Septic or septicopyemic embolism following failed attempted termination of pregnancy
Soap embolism following failed attempted termination of pregnancy

CC Excl: O03.0-O04.89, O07.2-O07.30, O07.35-O07.36, O07.38-O07.4, O20.0-O20.9, O25.10-O25.3, O26.10-O26.13, O26.30-O26.43, O26.63-O26.819, O26.841-O26.86, O26.891-O26.93, O29.011-O29.93, O35.7XX0-O35.7XX9, O44.00-O44.13, O45.8X1-O45.93, O75.4, O75.81, O75.89-O75.9, O80, O90.89, O99.111-O99.285, O99.330-O99.335, O99.350-O99.355, O99.511-O99.73, O99.820-O99.825, O99.840-O9A.53, Z33.2

O07.3 Failed attempted termination of pregnancy with other and unspecified complications (5th)

O07.30 Failed attempted termination of pregnancy with unspecified complications CC M ♀

CC Excl: O03.0-O07.4, O20.0-O20.9, O25.10-O25.3, O26.10-O26.13, O26.30-O26.43, O26.63-O26.819, O26.841-O26.86, O26.891-O26.93, O29.011-O29.93, O35.7X-O35.7X, O44.00-O44.13, O45.8X1-O45.93, O75.4, O75.81, O75.89-O75.9, O80, O90.89, O99.111-O99.285, O99.330-O99.335, O99.350-O99.355, O99.511-O99.73, O99.820-O99.825, O99.840-O9A.53, Z33.2

O07.31 Shock following failed attempted termination of pregnancy MCC M ♀

Circulatory collapse following failed attempted termination of pregnancy
Shock (postprocedural) following failed attempted termination of pregnancy

EXCLUDES 1 *shock due to infection following failed attempted termination of pregnancy (O07.37)*

CC Excl: O03.0-O04.89, O07.30-O07.31, O07.33, O07.35-O07.36, O07.38-O07.4, O20.0-O20.9, O25.10-O25.3, O26.10-O26.13, O26.30-O26.43, O26.63-O26.819, O26.841-O26.86, O26.891-O26.93, O29.011-O29.93, O35.7XX0-O35.7XX9, O44.00-O44.13, O45.8X1-O45.93, O75.4, O75.81, O75.89-O75.9, O80, O90.89, O99.111-O99.285, O99.330-O99.335, O99.350-O99.355, O99.511-O99.73, O99.820-O99.825, O99.840-O9A.53, Z33.2

O07.32 Renal failure following failed attempted termination of pregnancy MCC M ♀

Kidney failure (acute) following failed attempted termination of pregnancy
Oliguria following failed attempted termination of pregnancy
Renal shutdown following failed attempted termination of pregnancy
Renal tubular necrosis following failed attempted termination of pregnancy
Uremia following failed attempted termination of pregnancy

CC Excl: O03.0-O04.89, O07.30, O07.32, O07.35-O07.36, O07.38-O07.4, O20.0-O20.9, O25.10-O25.3, O26.10-O26.13, O26.30-O26.43, O26.63-O26.819, O26.841-O26.86, O26.891-O26.93, O29.011-O29.93, O35.7XX0-O35.7XX9, O44.00-O44.13, O45.8X1-O45.93, O75.4, O75.81, O75.89-O75.9, O80, O90.89, O99.111-O99.285, O99.330-O99.335, O99.350-O99.355, O99.511-O99.73, O99.820-O99.825, O99.840-O9A.53, Z33.2

O07.33 Metabolic disorder following failed attempted termination of pregnancy CC M ♀

CC Excl: See code: O07.30

O07.34 Damage to pelvic organs following failed attempted termination of pregnancy CC M ♀

Laceration, perforation, tear or chemical damage of bladder following failed attempted termination of pregnancy
Laceration, perforation, tear or chemical damage of bowel following failed attempted termination of pregnancy
Laceration, perforation, tear or chemical damage of broad ligament following failed attempted termination of pregnancy
Laceration, perforation, tear or chemical damage of cervix following failed attempted termination of pregnancy
Laceration, perforation, tear or chemical damage of periurethral tissue following failed attempted termination of pregnancy
Laceration, perforation, tear or chemical damage of uterus following failed attempted termination of pregnancy
Laceration, perforation, tear or chemical damage of vagina following failed attempted termination of pregnancy

CC Excl: O03.0-O04.89, O07.30, O07.34-O07.36, O07.38-O07.4, O20.0-O20.9, O25.10-O25.3, O26.10-O26.13, O26.30-O26.43, O26.63-O26.819, O26.841-O26.86, O26.891-O26.93, O29.011-O29.93, O35.7XX0-O35.7XX9, O44.00-O44.13, O45.8X1-O45.93, O75.4, O75.81, O75.89-O75.9, O80, O90.89, O99.111-O99.285, O99.330-O99.335, O99.350-O99.355, O99.511-O99.73, O99.820-O99.825, O99.840-O9A.53, Z33.2

O07.35 Other venous complications following failed attempted termination of pregnancy CC M ♀

CC Excl: See code: O07.30

O07.36 Cardiac arrest following failed attempted termination of pregnancy CC M ♀

CC Excl: See code: O07.30

O07.37 Sepsis following failed attempted termination of pregnancy CC M ♀
Use additional code to identify infectious agent (B95-B97)
Use additional code to identify severe sepsis, if applicable (R65.2-)
EXCLUDES 1 *septic or septicopyemic embolism following failed attempted termination of pregnancy (O07.2)*
CC Excl: O03.0-O07.0, O07.30, O07.35-O07.4, O20.0-O20.9, O25.10-O25.3, O26.10-O26.13, O26.30-O26.43, O26.63-O26.819, O26.841-O26.86, O26.891-O26.93, O29.011-O29.93, O35.7X-O35.7X, O44.00-O44.13, O45.8X1-O45.93, O75.4, O75.81, O75.89-O75.9, O80, O90.89, O99.111-O99.285, O99.330-O99.335, O99.350-O99.355, O99.511-O99.73, O99.820-O99.825, O99.840-O9A.53, Z33.2

O07.38 Urinary tract infection following failed attempted termination of pregnancy CC M ♀
Cystitis following failed attempted termination of pregnancy
CC Excl: See code: O07.30

O07.39 Failed attempted termination of pregnancy with other complications CC M ♀
CC Excl: See code: O07.30

O07.4 Failed attempted termination of pregnancy without complication M ♀

4th O08 Complications following ectopic and molar pregnancy
This category is for use with categories O00-O02 to identify any associated complications

CC Excl: For CC/MCC codes in category O08, unless otherwise noted: O08.2-O08.81, O08.83-O08.9, O20.0-O20.9, O25.10-O25.3, O26.10-O26.13, O26.30-O26.43, O26.63-O26.819, O26.841-O26.86, O26.891-O26.93, O29.011-O29.93, O35.7XX0-O35.7XX9, O44.00-O44.13, O45.8X1-O45.93, O75.4, O75.81, O75.89-O75.9, O80, O90.89, O99.111-O99.285, O99.330-O99.335, O99.350-O99.355, O99.511-O99.73, O99.820-O99.825, O99.840-O9A.53

O08.0 Genital tract and pelvic infection following ectopic and molar pregnancy CC M ♀
Endometritis following ectopic and molar pregnancy
Oophoritis following ectopic and molar pregnancy
Parametritis following ectopic and molar pregnancy
Pelvic peritonitis following ectopic and molar pregnancy
Salpingitis following ectopic and molar pregnancy
Salpingo-oophoritis following ectopic and molar pregnancy
EXCLUDES 1 *sepsis following ectopic and molar pregnancy (O08.82)*
urinary tract infection (O08.83)
CC Excl: A34, O08.0, O08.2-O08.9, O20.0-O20.9, O25.10-O25.3, O26.10-O26.13, O26.30-O26.43, O26.63-O26.819, O26.841-O26.86, O26.891-O26.93, O29.011-O29.93, O35.7XX0-O35.7XX9, O44.00-O44.13, O45.8X1-O45.93, O75.4, O75.81, O75.89-O75.9, O80, O90.89, O99.111-O99.285, O99.330-O99.335, O99.350-O99.355, O99.511-O99.73, O99.820-O99.825, O99.840-O9A.53

O08.1 Delayed or excessive hemorrhage following ectopic and molar pregnancy CC M ♀
Afibrinogenemia following ectopic and molar pregnancy
Defibrination syndrome following ectopic and molar pregnancy
Hemolysis following ectopic and molar pregnancy
Intravascular coagulation following ectopic and molar pregnancy
EXCLUDES 1 *delayed or excessive hemorrhage due to incomplete abortion (O03.1)*
CC Excl: O08.1-O08.81, O08.83-O08.9, O20.0-O20.9, O25.10-O25.3, O26.10-O26.13, O26.30-O26.43, O26.63-O26.819, O26.841-O26.86, O26.891-O26.93, O29.011-O29.93, O35.7XX0-O35.7XX9, O44.00-O44.13, O45.8X1-O45.93, O75.4, O75.81, O75.89-O75.9, O80, O90.89, O99.111-O99.285, O99.330-O99.335, O99.350-O99.355, O99.511-O99.73, O99.820-O99.825, O99.840-O9A.53

O08.2 Embolism following ectopic and molar pregnancy MCC M ♀
Air embolism following ectopic and molar pregnancy
Amniotic fluid embolism following ectopic and molar pregnancy
Blood-clot embolism following ectopic and molar pregnancy
Embolism NOS following ectopic and molar pregnancy
Fat embolism following ectopic and molar pregnancy
Pulmonary embolism following ectopic and molar pregnancy
Pyemic embolism following ectopic and molar pregnancy
Septic or septicopyemic embolism following ectopic and molar pregnancy
Soap embolism following ectopic and molar pregnancy

O08.3 Shock following ectopic and molar pregnancy MCC M ♀
Circulatory collapse following ectopic and molar pregnancy
Shock (postprocedural) following ectopic and molar pregnancy
EXCLUDES 1 *shock due to infection following ectopic and molar pregnancy (O08.82)*

O08.4 Renal failure following ectopic and molar pregnancy MCC M ♀
Kidney failure (acute) following ectopic and molar pregnancy
Oliguria following ectopic and molar pregnancy
Renal shutdown following ectopic and molar pregnancy
Renal tubular necrosis following ectopic and molar pregnancy
Uremia following ectopic and molar pregnancy

O08.5 Metabolic disorders following an ectopic and molar pregnancy CC M ♀

O08.6 Damage to pelvic organs and tissues following an ectopic and molar pregnancy CC M ♀
Laceration, perforation, tear or chemical damage of bladder following an ectopic and molar pregnancy
Laceration, perforation, tear or chemical damage of bowel following an ectopic and molar pregnancy
Laceration, perforation, tear or chemical damage of broad ligament following an ectopic and molar pregnancy
Laceration, perforation, tear or chemical damage of cervix following an ectopic and molar pregnancy
Laceration, perforation, tear or chemical damage of periurethral tissue following an ectopic and molar pregnancy
Laceration, perforation, tear or chemical damage of uterus following an ectopic and molar pregnancy
Laceration, perforation, tear or chemical damage of vagina following an ectopic and molar pregnancy

O08.7 Other venous complications following an ectopic and molar pregnancy CC M ♀

5th O08.8 Other complications following an ectopic and molar pregnancy

O08.81 Cardiac arrest following an ectopic and molar pregnancy CC M ♀

O08.82 Sepsis following ectopic and molar pregnancy CC M ♀
Use additional code to identify infectious agent (B95-B97)
Use additional code to identify severe sepsis, if applicable (R65.2-)
EXCLUDES 1 *septic or septicopyemic embolism following ectopic and molar pregnancy (O08.2)*
CC Excl: See code: O08.0

O08.83 Urinary tract infection following an ectopic and molar pregnancy CC M ♀
Cystitis following an ectopic and molar pregnancy
CC Excl: O08.2-O08.81, O08.83-O08.9, O20.0-O20.9, O25.10-O25.3, O26.10-O26.13, O26.30-O26.43, O26.63-O26.819, O26.841-O26.86, O26.891-O26.93, O29.011-O29.93, O35.7XX0-O35.7XX9, O44.00-O44.13, O45.8X1-O45.93, O75.4, O75.81, O75.89-O75.9, O80, O90.89, O99.111-O99.285, O99.330-O99.335, O99.350-O99.355, O99.511-O99.73, O99.820-O99.825, O99.840-O9A.53

O08.89 Other complications following an ectopic and molar pregnancy CC M ♀
CC Excl: See code: O08.83

O08.9 Unspecified complication following an ectopic and molar pregnancy CC M ♀
CC Excl: See code: O08.83

Supervision of high risk pregnancy (O09)

4th O09 Supervision of high risk pregnancy

5th O09.0 Supervision of pregnancy with history of infertility

O09.00 Supervision of pregnancy with history of infertility, unspecified trimester M ♀

O09.01 Supervision of pregnancy with history of infertility, first trimester M ♀

O09.02 Supervision of pregnancy with history of infertility, second trimester M ♀

O09.03 Supervision of pregnancy with history of infertility, third trimester M ♀

5th O09.1 Supervision of pregnancy with history of ectopic or molar pregnancy

O09.10 Supervision of pregnancy with history of ectopic or molar pregnancy, unspecified trimester M ♀

O09.11 Supervision of pregnancy with history of ectopic or molar pregnancy, first trimester M ♀

O09.12 Supervision of pregnancy with history of ectopic or molar pregnancy, second trimester M ♀

O09.13 Supervision of pregnancy with history of ectopic or molar pregnancy, third trimester M ♀

O09.2 Supervision of pregnancy with other poor reproductive or obstetric history (5th)

EXCLUDES 2 *pregnancy care for patient with history of recurrent pregnancy loss (O26.2-)*

O09.21 Supervision of pregnancy with history of pre-term labor (6th)

- **O09.211 Supervision of pregnancy with history of pre-term labor, first trimester** M♀
- **O09.212 Supervision of pregnancy with history of pre-term labor, second trimester** M♀
- **O09.213 Supervision of pregnancy with history of pre-term labor, third trimester** M♀
- **O09.219 Supervision of pregnancy with history of pre-term labor, unspecified trimester** M♀

O09.29 Supervision of pregnancy with other poor reproductive or obstetric history (6th)

Supervision of pregnancy with history of neonatal death

Supervision of pregnancy with history of stillbirth

- **O09.291 Supervision of pregnancy with other poor reproductive or obstetric history, first trimester** M♀
- **O09.292 Supervision of pregnancy with other poor reproductive or obstetric history, second trimester** M♀
- **O09.293 Supervision of pregnancy with other poor reproductive or obstetric history, third trimester** M♀
- **O09.299 Supervision of pregnancy with other poor reproductive or obstetric history, unspecified trimester** M♀

O09.3 Supervision of pregnancy with insufficient antenatal care (5th)

Supervision of concealed pregnancy

Supervision of hidden pregnancy

- **O09.30 Supervision of pregnancy with insufficient antenatal care, unspecified trimester** M♀
- **O09.31 Supervision of pregnancy with insufficient antenatal care, first trimester** M♀
- **O09.32 Supervision of pregnancy with insufficient antenatal care, second trimester** M♀
- **O09.33 Supervision of pregnancy with insufficient antenatal care, third trimester** M♀

O09.4 Supervision of pregnancy with grand multiparity (5th)

- **O09.40 Supervision of pregnancy with grand multiparity, unspecified trimester** M♀
- **O09.41 Supervision of pregnancy with grand multiparity, first trimester** M♀
- **O09.42 Supervision of pregnancy with grand multiparity, second trimester** M♀
- **O09.43 Supervision of pregnancy with grand multiparity, third trimester** M♀

O09.5 Supervision of elderly primigravida and multigravida (5th)

Pregnancy for a female 35 years and older at expected date of delivery

O09.51 Supervision of elderly primigravida (6th)

- **O09.511 Supervision of elderly primigravida, first trimester** M♀
- **O09.512 Supervision of elderly primigravida, second trimester** M♀
- **O09.513 Supervision of elderly primigravida, third trimester** M♀
- **O09.519 Supervision of elderly primigravida, unspecified trimester** M♀

O09.52 Supervision of elderly multigravida (6th)

- **O09.521 Supervision of elderly multigravida, first trimester** M♀
- **O09.522 Supervision of elderly multigravida, second trimester** M♀
- **O09.523 Supervision of elderly multigravida, third trimester** M♀
- **O09.529 Supervision of elderly multigravida, unspecified trimester** M♀

O09.6 Supervision of young primigravida and multigravida (5th)

Supervision of pregnancy for a female less than 16 years old at expected date of delivery

O09.61 Supervision of young primigravida (6th)

- **O09.611 Supervision of young primigravida, first trimester** M♀
- **O09.612 Supervision of young primigravida, second trimester** M♀
- **O09.613 Supervision of young primigravida, third trimester** M♀
- **O09.619 Supervision of young primigravida, unspecified trimester** M♀

O09.62 Supervision of young multigravida (6th)

- **O09.621 Supervision of young multigravida, first trimester** M♀
- **O09.622 Supervision of young multigravida, second trimester** M♀
- **O09.623 Supervision of young multigravida, third trimester** M♀
- **O09.629 Supervision of young multigravida, unspecified trimester** M♀

O09.7 Supervision of high risk pregnancy due to social problems (5th)

- **O09.70 Supervision of high risk pregnancy due to social problems, unspecified trimester** M♀
- **O09.71 Supervision of high risk pregnancy due to social problems, first trimester** M♀
- **O09.72 Supervision of high risk pregnancy due to social problems, second trimester** M♀
- **O09.73 Supervision of high risk pregnancy due to social problems, third trimester** M♀

O09.8 Supervision of other high risk pregnancies (5th)

O09.81 Supervision of pregnancy resulting from assisted reproductive technology (6th)

Supervision of pregnancy resulting from in-vitro fertilization

- **O09.811 Supervision of pregnancy resulting from assisted reproductive technology, first trimester** M♀
- **O09.812 Supervision of pregnancy resulting from assisted reproductive technology, second trimester** M♀
- **O09.813 Supervision of pregnancy resulting from assisted reproductive technology, third trimester** M♀
- **O09.819 Supervision of pregnancy resulting from assisted reproductive technology, unspecified trimester** M♀

O09.82 Supervision of pregnancy with history of in utero procedure during previous pregnancy (6th)

- **O09.821 Supervision of pregnancy with history of in utero procedure during previous pregnancy, first trimester** M♀
- **O09.822 Supervision of pregnancy with history of in utero procedure during previous pregnancy, second trimester** M♀
- **O09.823 Supervision of pregnancy with history of in utero procedure during previous pregnancy, third trimester** M♀
- **O09.829 Supervision of pregnancy with history of in utero procedure during previous pregnancy, unspecified trimester** M♀

EXCLUDES 1 *supervision of pregnancy affected by in utero procedure during current pregnancy (O35.7)*

O09.89 Supervision of other high risk pregnancies (6th)

- **O09.891 Supervision of other high risk pregnancies, first trimester** M♀
- **O09.892 Supervision of other high risk pregnancies, second trimester** M♀
- **O09.893 Supervision of other high risk pregnancies, third trimester** M♀
- **O09.899 Supervision of other high risk pregnancies, unspecified trimester** M♀

O09.9 Supervision of high risk pregnancy, unspecified (5th)

- **O09.90 Supervision of high risk pregnancy, unspecified, unspecified trimester** M♀
- **O09.91 Supervision of high risk pregnancy, unspecified, first trimester** M♀
- **O09.92 Supervision of high risk pregnancy, unspecified, second trimester** M♀
- **O09.93 Supervision of high risk pregnancy, unspecified, third trimester** M♀

Edema, proteinuria and hypertensive disorders in pregnancy, childbirth and the puerperium (O10-O16)

✓4th **O10 Pre-existing hypertension complicating pregnancy, childbirth and the puerperium**
Pre-existing hypertension with pre-existing proteinuria complicating pregnancy, childbirth and the puerperium
EXCLUDES 2 *pre-existing hypertension with superimposed pre-eclampsia complicating pregnancy, childbirth and the puerperium (O11.-)*

CC Excl: For CC/MCC codes in category O10, unless otherwise noted: O10.011-O12.03, O12.20-O16.9, O25.10-O26.13, O26.30-O26.43, O26.63-O26.819, O26.841-O26.86, O26.891-O26.93, O29.011-O29.93, O35.7XX0-O35.7XX9, O75.4, O75.81, O75.89-O75.9, O80, O90.89, O99.111-O99.285, O99.330-O99.335, O99.350-O99.355, O99.511-O99.73, O99.820-O99.825, O99.840-O9A.53

✓5th **O10.0 Pre-existing essential hypertension complicating pregnancy, childbirth and the puerperium**
Any condition in I10 specified as a reason for obstetric care during pregnancy, childbirth or the puerperium

✓6th **O10.01 Pre-existing essential hypertension complicating pregnancy**
O10.011 Pre-existing essential hypertension complicating pregnancy, first trimester CC M ♀
O10.012 Pre-existing essential hypertension complicating pregnancy, second trimester CC M ♀
O10.013 Pre-existing essential hypertension complicating pregnancy, third trimester CC M ♀
O10.019 Pre-existing essential hypertension complicating pregnancy, unspecified trimester M ♀
O10.02 Pre-existing essential hypertension complicating childbirth CC M ♀
O10.03 Pre-existing essential hypertension complicating the puerperium M ♀

✓5th **O10.1 Pre-existing hypertensive heart disease complicating pregnancy, childbirth and the puerperium**
Any condition in I11 specified as a reason for obstetric care during pregnancy, childbirth or the puerperium
Use additional code from I11 to identify the type of hypertensive heart disease

✓6th **O10.11 Pre-existing hypertensive heart disease complicating pregnancy**
O10.111 Pre-existing hypertensive heart disease complicating pregnancy, first trimester M ♀
O10.112 Pre-existing hypertensive heart disease complicating pregnancy, second trimester M ♀
O10.113 Pre-existing hypertensive heart disease complicating pregnancy, third trimester M ♀
O10.119 Pre-existing hypertensive heart disease complicating pregnancy, unspecified trimester M ♀
O10.12 Pre-existing hypertensive heart disease complicating childbirth M ♀
O10.13 Pre-existing hypertensive heart disease complicating the puerperium M ♀

✓5th **O10.2 Pre-existing hypertensive chronic kidney disease complicating pregnancy, childbirth and the puerperium**
Any condition in I12 specified as a reason for obstetric care during pregnancy, childbirth or the puerperium
Use additional code from I12 to identify the type of hypertensive chronic kidney disease

✓6th **O10.21 Pre-existing hypertensive chronic kidney disease complicating pregnancy**
O10.211 Pre-existing hypertensive chronic kidney disease complicating pregnancy, first trimester M ♀
O10.212 Pre-existing hypertensive chronic kidney disease complicating pregnancy, second trimester M ♀
O10.213 Pre-existing hypertensive chronic kidney disease complicating pregnancy, third trimester M ♀
O10.219 Pre-existing hypertensive chronic kidney disease complicating pregnancy, unspecified trimester M ♀
O10.22 Pre-existing hypertensive chronic kidney disease complicating childbirth M ♀
O10.23 Pre-existing hypertensive chronic kidney disease complicating the puerperium M ♀

✓5th **O10.3 Pre-existing hypertensive heart and chronic kidney disease complicating pregnancy, childbirth and the puerperium**
Any condition in I13 specified as a reason for obstetric care during pregnancy, childbirth or the puerperium
Use additional code from I13 to identify the type of hypertensive heart and chronic kidney disease

✓6th **O10.31 Pre-existing hypertensive heart and chronic kidney disease complicating pregnancy**
O10.311 Pre-existing hypertensive heart and chronic kidney disease complicating pregnancy, first trimester M ♀
O10.312 Pre-existing hypertensive heart and chronic kidney disease complicating pregnancy, second trimester M ♀
O10.313 Pre-existing hypertensive heart and chronic kidney disease complicating pregnancy, third trimester M ♀
O10.319 Pre-existing hypertensive heart and chronic kidney disease complicating pregnancy, unspecified trimester M ♀
O10.32 Pre-existing hypertensive heart and chronic kidney disease complicating childbirth M ♀
O10.33 Pre-existing hypertensive heart and chronic kidney disease complicating the puerperium M ♀

✓5th **O10.4 Pre-existing secondary hypertension complicating pregnancy, childbirth and the puerperium**
Any condition in I15 specified as a reason for obstetric care during pregnancy, childbirth or the puerperium
Use additional code from I15 to identify the type of secondary hypertension

✓6th **O10.41 Pre-existing secondary hypertension complicating pregnancy**
O10.411 Pre-existing secondary hypertension complicating pregnancy, first trimester CC M ♀
O10.412 Pre-existing secondary hypertension complicating pregnancy, second trimester CC M ♀
O10.413 Pre-existing secondary hypertension complicating pregnancy, third trimester CC M ♀
O10.419 Pre-existing secondary hypertension complicating pregnancy, unspecified trimester M ♀
O10.42 Pre-existing secondary hypertension complicating childbirth MCC M ♀
O10.43 Pre-existing secondary hypertension complicating the puerperium CC M ♀

✓5th **O10.9 Unspecified pre-existing hypertension complicating pregnancy, childbirth and the puerperium**

✓6th **O10.91 Unspecified pre-existing hypertension complicating pregnancy**
O10.911 Unspecified pre-existing hypertension complicating pregnancy, first trimester CC M ♀
O10.912 Unspecified pre-existing hypertension complicating pregnancy, second trimester CC M ♀
O10.913 Unspecified pre-existing hypertension complicating pregnancy, third trimester CC M ♀
O10.919 Unspecified pre-existing hypertension complicating pregnancy, unspecified trimester M ♀
O10.92 Unspecified pre-existing hypertension complicating childbirth CC M ♀
O10.93 Unspecified pre-existing hypertension complicating the puerperium M ♀

4th **O11 Pre-existing hypertension with pre-eclampsia**
Conditions in O1Ø complicated by pre-eclampsia
Pre-eclampsia superimposed pre-existing hypertension
Use additional code from O1Ø to identify the type of hypertension

CC Excl: For MCC codes in category O11, unless otherwise noted:
See code: O1Ø

O11.1 Pre-existing hypertension with pre-eclampsia, first trimester MCC M ♀
O11.2 Pre-existing hypertension with pre-eclampsia, second trimester MCC M ♀
O11.3 Pre-existing hypertension with pre-eclampsia, third trimester MCC M ♀
O11.9 Pre-existing hypertension with pre-eclampsia, unspecified trimester M ♀

4th **O12 Gestational [pregnancy-induced] edema and proteinuria without hypertension**

CC Excl: For CC codes in category O12, unless otherwise noted:
O12.11-O12.13, O12.21-O12.23, O26.831-O26.833, O9Ø.89

5th **O12.Ø Gestational edema**
O12.ØØ Gestational edema, unspecified trimester M ♀
O12.Ø1 Gestational edema, first trimester M ♀
O12.Ø2 Gestational edema, second trimester M ♀
O12.Ø3 Gestational edema, third trimester M ♀

5th **O12.1 Gestational proteinuria**
O12.1Ø Gestational proteinuria, unspecified trimester M ♀
O12.11 Gestational proteinuria, first trimester CC M ♀
O12.12 Gestational proteinuria, second trimester CC M ♀
O12.13 Gestational proteinuria, third trimester CC M ♀

5th **O12.2 Gestational edema with proteinuria**
O12.2Ø Gestational edema with proteinuria, unspecified trimester M ♀
O12.21 Gestational edema with proteinuria, first trimester PDx CC CC M ♀
O12.22 Gestational edema with proteinuria, second trimester PDx CC CC M ♀
O12.23 Gestational edema with proteinuria, third trimester PDx CC CC M ♀

4th **O13 Gestational [pregnancy-induced] hypertension without significant proteinuria**
INCLUDES gestational hypertension NOS

CC Excl: For CC codes in category O13, unless otherwise noted:
See code: O1Ø

O13.1 Gestational [pregnancy-induced] hypertension without significant proteinuria, first trimester M ♀
O13.2 Gestational [pregnancy-induced] hypertension without significant proteinuria, second trimester M ♀
O13.3 Gestational [pregnancy-induced] hypertension without significant proteinuria, third trimester M ♀
O13.9 Gestational [pregnancy-induced] hypertension without significant proteinuria, unspecified trimester M ♀

4th **O14 Pre-eclampsia**
EXCLUDES 1 *pre-existing hypertension with pre-eclampsia (O11)*

CC Excl: For CC codes in category O14, unless otherwise noted:
See code: O1Ø

5th **O14.Ø Mild to moderate pre-eclampsia**
O14.ØØ Mild to moderate pre-eclampsia, unspecified trimester M ♀
O14.Ø2 Mild to moderate pre-eclampsia, second trimester CC M ♀
O14.Ø3 Mild to moderate pre-eclampsia, third trimester CC M ♀

5th **O14.1 Severe pre-eclampsia**
EXCLUDES 1 *HELLP syndrome (O14.2-)*
O14.1Ø Severe pre-eclampsia, unspecified trimester M ♀
O14.12 Severe pre-eclampsia, second trimester MCC M ♀
O14.13 Severe pre-eclampsia, third trimester MCC M ♀

5th **O14.2 HELLP syndrome**
Severe pre-eclampsia with hemolysis, elevated liver enzymes and low platelet count (HELLP)
O14.2Ø HELLP syndrome (HELLP), unspecified trimester M ♀
O14.22 HELLP syndrome (HELLP), second trimester MCC M ♀
O14.23 HELLP syndrome (HELLP), third trimester MCC M ♀

5th **O14.9 Unspecified pre-eclampsia**
O14.9Ø Unspecified pre-eclampsia, unspecified trimester M ♀
O14.92 Unspecified pre-eclampsia, second trimester CC M ♀
O14.93 Unspecified pre-eclampsia, third trimester CC M ♀

4th **O15 Eclampsia**
INCLUDES convulsions following conditions in O1Ø-O14 and O16

CC Excl: For MCC codes in category O15, unless otherwise noted:
See code: O1Ø

5th **O15.Ø Eclampsia in pregnancy**
O15.ØØ Eclampsia in pregnancy, unspecified trimester M ♀
O15.Ø2 Eclampsia in pregnancy, second trimester MCC M ♀
O15.Ø3 Eclampsia in pregnancy, third trimester MCC M ♀
O15.1 Eclampsia in labor MCC M ♀
O15.2 Eclampsia in the puerperium MCC M ♀
O15.9 Eclampsia, unspecified as to time period M ♀
Eclampsia NOS

4th **O16 Unspecified maternal hypertension**

CC Excl: For CC codes in category O16, unless otherwise noted:
See code: O1Ø

O16.1 Unspecified maternal hypertension, first trimester CC M ♀
O16.2 Unspecified maternal hypertension, second trimester CC M ♀
O16.3 Unspecified maternal hypertension, third trimester CC M ♀
O16.9 Unspecified maternal hypertension, unspecified trimester M ♀

Other maternal disorders predominantly related to pregnancy (O2Ø-O29)

EXCLUDES 2 *maternal care related to the fetus and amniotic cavity and possible delivery problems (O3Ø-O48)*
maternal diseases classifiable elsewhere but complicating pregnancy, labor and delivery, and the puerperium (O98-O99)

4th **O2Ø Hemorrhage in early pregnancy**
Hemorrhage before completion of 2Ø weeks gestation
EXCLUDES 1 *pregnancy with abortive outcome (OØØ-OØ8)*

O2Ø.Ø Threatened abortion CC M ♀
Hemorrhage specified as due to threatened abortion
CC Excl: O2Ø.Ø-O2Ø.9, O25.1Ø-O25.3, O26.1Ø-O26.13, O26.3Ø-O26.43, O26.63-O26.819, O26.841-O26.86, O26.891-O26.93, O29.Ø11-O29.93, O35.7XXØ-O35.7XX9, O44.ØØ-O44.13, O75.4, O75.81, O75.89-O75.9, O8Ø, O9Ø.89, O99.111-O99.285, O99.33Ø-O99.335, O99.35Ø-O99.355, O99.511-O99.73, O99.82Ø-O99.825, O99.84Ø-O9A.53
O2Ø.8 Other hemorrhage in early pregnancy M ♀
O2Ø.9 Hemorrhage in early pregnancy, unspecified CC M ♀
CC Excl: See code: O2Ø.Ø

4th **O21 Excessive vomiting in pregnancy**

O21.Ø Mild hyperemesis gravidarum M ♀
Hyperemesis gravidarum, mild or unspecified, starting before the end of the 2Øth week of gestation

O21.1 Hyperemesis gravidarum with metabolic disturbance M ♀
Hyperemesis gravidarum, starting before the end of the 2Øth week of gestation, with metabolic disturbance such as carbohydrate depletion
Hyperemesis gravidarum, starting before the end of the 2Øth week of gestation, with metabolic disturbance such as dehydration
Hyperemesis gravidarum, starting before the end of the 2Øth week of gestation, with metabolic disturbance such as electrolyte imbalance

O21.2 Late vomiting of pregnancy M ♀
Excessive vomiting starting after 2Ø completed weeks of gestation

O21.8 Other vomiting complicating pregnancy M ♀
Vomiting due to diseases classified elsewhere, complicating pregnancy
Use additional code to identify cause

O21.9 Vomiting of pregnancy, unspecified M ♀

O22 Venous complications and hemorrhoids in pregnancy

EXCLUDES 1 *venous complications of:*
abortion NOS (O03.9)
ectopic or molar pregnancy (O08.7)
failed attempted abortion (O07.35)
induced abortion (O04.85)
spontaneous abortion (O03.89)

EXCLUDES 2 *obstetric pulmonary embolism (O88.-)*
venous complications and hemorrhoids of childbirth and the puerperium (O87.-)

CC Excl: For CC/MCC codes in category O22, unless otherwise noted: O22.20-O22.93, O25.10-O25.3, O26.10-O26.13, O26.30-O26.43, O26.63-O26.819, O26.841-O26.86, O26.891-O26.93, O29.011-O29.93, O35.7XX0-O35.7XX9, O75.4, O75.81, O75.89-O75.9, O80, O87.0-O87.3, O87.8-O87.9, O90.89, O99.111-O99.285, O99.330-O99.335, O99.350-O99.355, O99.511-O99.73, O99.820-O99.825, O99.840-O9A.53

O22.0 Varicose veins of lower extremity in pregnancy
Varicose veins NOS in pregnancy

- **O22.00 Varicose veins of lower extremity in pregnancy, unspecified trimester** M♀
- **O22.01 Varicose veins of lower extremity in pregnancy, first trimester** M♀
- **O22.02 Varicose veins of lower extremity in pregnancy, second trimester** M♀
- **O22.03 Varicose veins of lower extremity in pregnancy, third trimester** M♀

O22.1 Genital varices in pregnancy
Perineal varices in pregnancy
Vaginal varices in pregnancy
Vulval varices in pregnancy

- **O22.10 Genital varices in pregnancy, unspecified trimester** M♀
- **O22.11 Genital varices in pregnancy, first trimester** M♀
- **O22.12 Genital varices in pregnancy, second trimester** M♀
- **O22.13 Genital varices in pregnancy, third trimester** M♀

O22.2 Superficial thrombophlebitis in pregnancy
Phlebitis in pregnancy NOS
Thrombophlebitis of legs in pregnancy
Thrombosis in pregnancy NOS
Use additional code to identify the superficial thrombophlebitis (I80.0-)

- **O22.20 Superficial thrombophlebitis in pregnancy, unspecified trimester** CC M♀
- **O22.21 Superficial thrombophlebitis in pregnancy, first trimester** CC M♀
- **O22.22 Superficial thrombophlebitis in pregnancy, second trimester** CC M♀
- **O22.23 Superficial thrombophlebitis in pregnancy, third trimester** CC M♀

O22.3 Deep phlebothrombosis in pregnancy
Deep vein thrombosis, antepartum
Use additional code to identify the deep vein thrombosis (I82.4-, I82.5-, I82.62-, I82.72-)
Use additional code, if applicable, for associated long-term (current) use of anticoagulants (Z79.01)

- **O22.30 Deep phlebothrombosis in pregnancy, unspecified trimester** CC M♀
- **O22.31 Deep phlebothrombosis in pregnancy, first trimester** MCC M♀
- **O22.32 Deep phlebothrombosis in pregnancy, second trimester** MCC M♀
- **O22.33 Deep phlebothrombosis in pregnancy, third trimester** MCC M♀

O22.4 Hemorrhoids in pregnancy

- **O22.40 Hemorrhoids in pregnancy, unspecified trimester** CC M♀
- **O22.41 Hemorrhoids in pregnancy, first trimester** CC M♀
- **O22.42 Hemorrhoids in pregnancy, second trimester** CC M♀
- **O22.43 Hemorrhoids in pregnancy, third trimester** CC M♀

O22.5 Cerebral venous thrombosis in pregnancy
Cerebrovenous sinus thrombosis in pregnancy

- **O22.50 Cerebral venous thrombosis in pregnancy, unspecified trimester** CC M♀
- **O22.51 Cerebral venous thrombosis in pregnancy, first trimester** CC M♀
- **O22.52 Cerebral venous thrombosis in pregnancy, second trimester** CC M♀
- **O22.53 Cerebral venous thrombosis in pregnancy, third trimester** CC M♀

O22.8 Other venous complications in pregnancy

O22.8X Other venous complications in pregnancy

- **O22.8X1 Other venous complications in pregnancy, first trimester** CC M♀
- **O22.8X2 Other venous complications in pregnancy, second trimester** CC M♀
- **O22.8X3 Other venous complications in pregnancy, third trimester** CC M♀
- **O22.8X9 Other venous complications in pregnancy, unspecified trimester** CC M♀

O22.9 Venous complication in pregnancy, unspecified
Gestational phlebitis NOS
Gestational phlebopathy NOS
Gestational thrombosis NOS

- **O22.90 Venous complication in pregnancy, unspecified, unspecified trimester** CC M♀
- **O22.91 Venous complication in pregnancy, unspecified, first trimester** M♀
- **O22.92 Venous complication in pregnancy, unspecified, second trimester** M♀
- **O22.93 Venous complication in pregnancy, unspecified, third trimester** M♀

O23 Infections of genitourinary tract in pregnancy
Use additional code to identify organism (B95.-, B96.-)

EXCLUDES 2 *gonococcal infections complicating pregnancy, childbirth and the puerperium (O98.2)*
infections with a predominantly sexual mode of transmission NOS complicating pregnancy, childbirth and the puerperium (O98.3)
syphilis complicating pregnancy, childbirth and the puerperium (O98.1)
tuberculosis of genitourinary system complicating pregnancy, childbirth and the puerperium (O98.0)
venereal disease NOS complicating pregnancy, childbirth and the puerperium (O98.3)

CC Excl: For CC codes in category O23, unless otherwise noted: O23.00-O23.93, O25.10-O25.3, O26.10-O26.13, O26.30-O26.43, O26.63-O26.819, O26.841-O26.86, O26.891-O26.93, O29.011-O29.93, O35.7XX0-O35.7XX9, O75.4, O75.81, O75.89-O75.9, O80, O86.11, O86.13-O86.29, O90.89, O99.111-O99.285, O99.330-O99.335, O99.350-O99.355, O99.511-O99.73, O99.820-O99.825, O99.840-O9A.53

O23.0 Infections of kidney in pregnancy
Pyelonephritis in pregnancy

- **O23.00 Infections of kidney in pregnancy, unspecified trimester** M♀
- **O23.01 Infections of kidney in pregnancy, first trimester** CC M♀
- **O23.02 Infections of kidney in pregnancy, second trimester** CC M♀
- **O23.03 Infections of kidney in pregnancy, third trimester** CC M♀

O23.1 Infections of bladder in pregnancy

- **O23.10 Infections of bladder in pregnancy, unspecified trimester** M♀
- **O23.11 Infections of bladder in pregnancy, first trimester** CC M♀
- **O23.12 Infections of bladder in pregnancy, second trimester** CC M♀
- **O23.13 Infections of bladder in pregnancy, third trimester** CC M♀

O23.2 Infections of urethra in pregnancy

- **O23.20 Infections of urethra in pregnancy, unspecified trimester** M♀
- **O23.21 Infections of urethra in pregnancy, first trimester** CC M♀
- **O23.22 Infections of urethra in pregnancy, second trimester** CC M♀
- **O23.23 Infections of urethra in pregnancy, third trimester** CC M♀

O23.3 Infections of other parts of urinary tract in pregnancy

- **O23.30 Infections of other parts of urinary tract in pregnancy, unspecified trimester** M♀
- **O23.31 Infections of other parts of urinary tract in pregnancy, first trimester** CC M♀

O23.32 Infections of other parts of urinary tract in pregnancy, second trimester CC M ♀

O23.33 Infections of other parts of urinary tract in pregnancy, third trimester CC M ♀

✓5th **O23.4 Unspecified infection of urinary tract in pregnancy**

O23.40 Unspecified infection of urinary tract in pregnancy, unspecified trimester M ♀

O23.41 Unspecified infection of urinary tract in pregnancy, first trimester CC M ♀

O23.42 Unspecified infection of urinary tract in pregnancy, second trimester CC M ♀

O23.43 Unspecified infection of urinary tract in pregnancy, third trimester CC M ♀

✓5th **O23.5 Infections of the genital tract in pregnancy**

✓6th **O23.51 Infection of cervix in pregnancy**

O23.511 Infections of cervix in pregnancy, first trimester CC M ♀

O23.512 Infections of cervix in pregnancy, second trimester CC M ♀

O23.513 Infections of cervix in pregnancy, third trimester CC M ♀

O23.519 Infections of cervix in pregnancy, unspecified trimester M ♀

✓6th **O23.52 Salpingo-oophoritis in pregnancy**

Oophoritis in pregnancy
Salpingitis in pregnancy

O23.521 Salpingo-oophoritis in pregnancy, first trimester CC M ♀

O23.522 Salpingo-oophoritis in pregnancy, second trimester CC M ♀

O23.523 Salpingo-oophoritis in pregnancy, third trimester CC M ♀

O23.529 Salpingo-oophoritis in pregnancy, unspecified trimester M ♀

✓6th **O23.59 Infection of other part of genital tract in pregnancy**

O23.591 Infection of other part of genital tract in pregnancy, first trimester CC M ♀

O23.592 Infection of other part of genital tract in pregnancy, second trimester CC M ♀

O23.593 Infection of other part of genital tract in pregnancy, third trimester CC M ♀

O23.599 Infection of other part of genital tract in pregnancy, unspecified trimester M ♀

✓5th **O23.9 Unspecified genitourinary tract infection in pregnancy**

Genitourinary tract infection in pregnancy NOS

O23.90 Unspecified genitourinary tract infection in pregnancy, unspecified trimester M ♀

O23.91 Unspecified genitourinary tract infection in pregnancy, first trimester CC M ♀

O23.92 Unspecified genitourinary tract infection in pregnancy, second trimester CC M ♀

O23.93 Unspecified genitourinary tract infection in pregnancy, third trimester CC M ♀

✓4th **O24 Diabetes mellitus in pregnancy, childbirth, and the puerperium**

CC Excl: For CC/MCC codes in category O24, unless otherwise noted: O24.011-O24.33, O24.811-O25.3, O26.10-O26.13, O26.30-O26.43, O26.63-O26.819, O26.841-O26.86, O26.891-O26.93, O29.011-O29.93, O35.7XX0-O35.7XX9, O75.4, O75.81, O75.89-O75.9, O80, O90.89, O99.111-O99.285, O99.330-O99.335, O99.350-O99.355, O99.511-O99.73, O99.820-O99.825, O99.840-O9A.53

✓5th **O24.0 Pre-existing diabetes mellitus, type 1, in pregnancy, childbirth and the puerperium**

Juvenile onset diabetes mellitus, in pregnancy, childbirth and the puerperium
Ketosis-prone diabetes mellitus in pregnancy, childbirth and the puerperium

Use additional code from category E10 to further identify any manifestations

✓6th **O24.01 Pre-existing diabetes mellitus, type 1, in pregnancy**

O24.011 Pre-existing diabetes mellitus, type 1, in pregnancy, first trimester CC M ♀

O24.012 Pre-existing diabetes mellitus, type 1, in pregnancy, second trimester CC M ♀

O24.013 Pre-existing diabetes mellitus, type 1, in pregnancy, third trimester CC M ♀

O24.019 Pre-existing diabetes mellitus, type 1, in pregnancy, unspecified trimester CC M ♀

O24.02 Pre-existing diabetes mellitus, type 1, in childbirth MCC M ♀

O24.03 Pre-existing diabetes mellitus, type 1, in the puerperium CC M ♀

✓5th **O24.1 Pre-existing diabetes mellitus, type 2, in pregnancy, childbirth and the puerperium**

Insulin-resistant diabetes mellitus in pregnancy, childbirth and the puerperium

Use additional code (for):
from category E11 to further identify any manifestations
long-term (current) use of insulin (Z79.4)

✓6th **O24.11 Pre-existing diabetes mellitus, type 2, in pregnancy**

O24.111 Pre-existing diabetes mellitus, type 2, in pregnancy, first trimester CC M ♀

O24.112 Pre-existing diabetes mellitus, type 2, in pregnancy, second trimester CC M ♀

O24.113 Pre-existing diabetes mellitus, type 2, in pregnancy, third trimester CC M ♀

O24.119 Pre-existing diabetes mellitus, type 2, in pregnancy, unspecified trimester CC M ♀

O24.12 Pre-existing diabetes mellitus, type 2, in childbirth MCC M ♀

O24.13 Pre-existing diabetes mellitus, type 2, in the puerperium CC M ♀

✓5th **O24.3 Unspecified pre-existing diabetes mellitus in pregnancy, childbirth and the puerperium**

Use additional code (for):
from category E11 to further identify any manifestation
long-term (current) use of insulin (Z79.4)

✓6th **O24.31 Unspecified pre-existing diabetes mellitus in pregnancy**

O24.311 Unspecified pre-existing diabetes mellitus in pregnancy, first trimester CC M ♀

O24.312 Unspecified pre-existing diabetes mellitus in pregnancy, second trimester CC M ♀

O24.313 Unspecified pre-existing diabetes mellitus in pregnancy, third trimester CC M ♀

O24.319 Unspecified pre-existing diabetes mellitus in pregnancy, unspecified trimester CC M ♀

O24.32 Unspecified pre-existing diabetes mellitus in childbirth MCC M ♀

O24.33 Unspecified pre-existing diabetes mellitus in the puerperium CC M ♀

✓5th **O24.4 Gestational diabetes mellitus**

Diabetes mellitus arising in pregnancy
Gestational diabetes mellitus NOS

✓6th **O24.41 Gestational diabetes mellitus in pregnancy**

O24.410 Gestational diabetes mellitus in pregnancy, diet controlled M ♀

O24.414 Gestational diabetes mellitus in pregnancy, insulin controlled M ♀

O24.419 Gestational diabetes mellitus in pregnancy, unspecified control M ♀

✓6th **O24.42 Gestational diabetes mellitus in childbirth**

O24.420 Gestational diabetes mellitus in childbirth, diet controlled M ♀

O24.424 Gestational diabetes mellitus in childbirth, insulin controlled M ♀

O24.429 Gestational diabetes mellitus in childbirth, unspecified control M ♀

✓6th **O24.43 Gestational diabetes mellitus in the puerperium**

O24.430 Gestational diabetes mellitus in the puerperium, diet controlled M ♀

O24.434 Gestational diabetes mellitus in the puerperium, insulin controlled M ♀

O24.439 Gestational diabetes mellitus in the puerperium, unspecified control M ♀

✓5th **O24.8 Other pre-existing diabetes mellitus in pregnancy, childbirth, and the puerperium**

Use additional code (for):
from categories E08, E09 and E13 to further identify any manifestation
long-term (current) use of insulin (Z79.4)

✓6th **O24.81 Other pre-existing diabetes mellitus in pregnancy**
- **O24.811 Other pre-existing diabetes mellitus in pregnancy, first trimester** CC M ♀
- **O24.812 Other pre-existing diabetes mellitus in pregnancy, second trimester** CC M ♀
- **O24.813 Other pre-existing diabetes mellitus in pregnancy, third trimester** CC M ♀
- **O24.819 Other pre-existing diabetes mellitus in pregnancy, unspecified trimester** CC M ♀

O24.82 Other pre-existing diabetes mellitus in childbirth MCC M ♀

O24.83 Other pre-existing diabetes mellitus in the puerperium CC M ♀

✓5th **O24.9 Unspecified diabetes mellitus in pregnancy, childbirth and the puerperium**

Use additional code for long-term (current) use of insulin (Z79.4)

✓6th **O24.91 Unspecified diabetes mellitus in pregnancy**
- **O24.911 Unspecified diabetes mellitus in pregnancy, first trimester** CC M ♀
- **O24.912 Unspecified diabetes mellitus in pregnancy, second trimester** CC M ♀
- **O24.913 Unspecified diabetes mellitus in pregnancy, third trimester** CC M ♀
- **O24.919 Unspecified diabetes mellitus in pregnancy, unspecified trimester** CC M ♀

O24.92 Unspecified diabetes mellitus in childbirth M ♀

O24.93 Unspecified diabetes mellitus in the puerperium CC M ♀

✓4th O25 Malnutrition in pregnancy, childbirth and the puerperium

✓5th **O25.1 Malnutrition in pregnancy**
- **O25.10 Malnutrition in pregnancy, unspecified trimester** M ♀
- **O25.11 Malnutrition in pregnancy, first trimester** M ♀
- **O25.12 Malnutrition in pregnancy, second trimester** M ♀
- **O25.13 Malnutrition in pregnancy, third trimester** M ♀

O25.2 Malnutrition in childbirth M ♀

O25.3 Malnutrition in the puerperium M ♀

✓4th O26 Maternal care for other conditions predominantly related to pregnancy

✓5th **O26.0 Excessive weight gain in pregnancy**

EXCLUDES 2 *gestational edema (O12.0, O12.2)*

- **O26.00 Excessive weight gain in pregnancy, unspecified trimester** M ♀
- **O26.01 Excessive weight gain in pregnancy, first trimester** M ♀
- **O26.02 Excessive weight gain in pregnancy, second trimester** M ♀
- **O26.03 Excessive weight gain in pregnancy, third trimester** M ♀

✓5th **O26.1 Low weight gain in pregnancy**
- **O26.10 Low weight gain in pregnancy, unspecified trimester** M ♀
- **O26.11 Low weight gain in pregnancy, first trimester** M ♀
- **O26.12 Low weight gain in pregnancy, second trimester** M ♀
- **O26.13 Low weight gain in pregnancy, third trimester** M ♀

✓5th **O26.2 Pregnancy care for patient with recurrent pregnancy loss**

CC Excl: For CC codes in subcategory O26.2, unless otherwise noted: O26.21-O26.23

- **O26.20 Pregnancy care for patient with recurrent pregnancy loss, unspecified trimester** M ♀
- **O26.21 Pregnancy care for patient with recurrent pregnancy loss, first trimester** M ♀
- **O26.22 Pregnancy care for patient with recurrent pregnancy loss, second trimester** M ♀
- **O26.23 Pregnancy care for patient with recurrent pregnancy loss, third trimester** M ♀

✓5th **O26.3 Retained intrauterine contraceptive device in pregnancy**
- **O26.30 Retained intrauterine contraceptive device in pregnancy, unspecified trimester** M ♀
- **O26.31 Retained intrauterine contraceptive device in pregnancy, first trimester** M ♀
- **O26.32 Retained intrauterine contraceptive device in pregnancy, second trimester** M ♀
- **O26.33 Retained intrauterine contraceptive device in pregnancy, third trimester** M ♀

✓5th **O26.4 Herpes gestationis**
- **O26.40 Herpes gestationis, unspecified trimester** M ♀
- **O26.41 Herpes gestationis, first trimester** M ♀
- **O26.42 Herpes gestationis, second trimester** M ♀
- **O26.43 Herpes gestationis, third trimester** M ♀

✓5th **O26.5 Maternal hypotension syndrome**

Supine hypotensive syndrome

CC Excl: For MCC codes in subcategory O26.5, unless otherwise noted: O25.10-O25.3, O26.10-O26.13, O26.30-O26.43, O26.51-O26.53, O26.63-O26.819, O26.841-O26.86, O26.891-O26.93, O29.011-O29.93, O35.7XX0-O35.7XX9, O75.1, O75.4, O75.81, O75.89-O75.9, O80, O90.89, O99.111-O99.285, O99.330-O99.335, O99.350-O99.355, O99.511-O99.73, O99.820-O99.825, O99.840-O9A.53

- **O26.50 Maternal hypotension syndrome, unspecified trimester** M ♀
- **O26.51 Maternal hypotension syndrome, first trimester** M ♀
- **O26.52 Maternal hypotension syndrome, second trimester** M ♀
- **O26.53 Maternal hypotension syndrome, third trimester** M ♀

✓5th **O26.6 Liver and biliary tract disorders in pregnancy, childbirth and the puerperium**

Use additional code to identify the specific disorder

EXCLUDES 2 *hepatorenal syndrome following labor and delivery (O90.4)*

CC Excl: For CC codes in subcategory O26.6, unless otherwise noted: O25.10-O25.3, O26.10-O26.13, O26.30-O26.43, O26.611-O26.819, O26.841-O26.86, O26.891-O26.93, O29.011-O29.93, O35.7XX0-O35.7XX9, O75.4, O75.81, O75.89-O75.9, O80, O90.89, O99.111-O99.285, O99.330-O99.335, O99.350-O99.355, O99.511-O99.73, O99.820-O99.825, O99.840-O9A.53

✓6th **O26.61 Liver and biliary tract disorders in pregnancy**
- **O26.611 Liver and biliary tract disorders in pregnancy, first trimester** CC M ♀
- **O26.612 Liver and biliary tract disorders in pregnancy, second trimester** CC M ♀
- **O26.613 Liver and biliary tract disorders in pregnancy, third trimester** CC M ♀
- **O26.619 Liver and biliary tract disorders in pregnancy, unspecified trimester** M ♀

O26.62 Liver and biliary tract disorders in childbirth CC M ♀

O26.63 Liver and biliary tract disorders in the puerperium M ♀

✓5th **O26.7 Subluxation of symphysis (pubis) in pregnancy, childbirth and the puerperium**

EXCLUDES 1 *traumatic separation of symphysis (pubis) during childbirth (O71.6)*

✓6th **O26.71 Subluxation of symphysis (pubis) in pregnancy**
- **O26.711 Subluxation of symphysis (pubis) in pregnancy, first trimester** M ♀
- **O26.712 Subluxation of symphysis (pubis) in pregnancy, second trimester** M ♀
- **O26.713 Subluxation of symphysis (pubis) in pregnancy, third trimester** M ♀
- **O26.719 Subluxation of symphysis (pubis) in pregnancy, unspecified trimester** M ♀

O26.72 Subluxation of symphysis (pubis) in childbirth M ♀

O26.73 Subluxation of symphysis (pubis) in the puerperium M ♀

✓5th **O26.8 Other specified pregnancy related conditions**

✓6th **O26.81 Pregnancy related exhaustion and fatigue**
- **O26.811 Pregnancy related exhaustion and fatigue, first trimester** M ♀
- **O26.812 Pregnancy related exhaustion and fatigue, second trimester** M ♀
- **O26.813 Pregnancy related exhaustion and fatigue, third trimester** M ♀
- **O26.819 Pregnancy related exhaustion and fatigue, unspecified trimester** M ♀

✓6th **O26.82 Pregnancy related peripheral neuritis**
- **O26.821 Pregnancy related peripheral neuritis, first trimester** M ♀

O26.822 Pregnancy related peripheral neuritis, second trimester M♀

O26.823 Pregnancy related peripheral neuritis, third trimester M♀

O26.829 Pregnancy related peripheral neuritis, unspecified trimester M♀

✓6th O26.83 Pregnancy related renal disease

Use additional code to identify the specific disorder

CC Excl: For CC codes in subcategory O26.83, unless otherwise noted: O12.11-O12.13, O12.21-O12.23, O26.831-O26.833, O90.89

O26.831 Pregnancy related renal disease, first trimester CC M♀

O26.832 Pregnancy related renal disease, second trimester CC M♀

O26.833 Pregnancy related renal disease, third trimester CC M♀

O26.839 Pregnancy related renal disease, unspecified trimester M♀

✓6th O26.84 Uterine size-date discrepancy complicating pregnancy

EXCLUDES 1 *encounter for suspected problem with fetal growth ruled out (Z03.74)*

O26.841 Uterine size-date discrepancy, first trimester M♀

O26.842 Uterine size-date discrepancy, second trimester M♀

O26.843 Uterine size-date discrepancy, third trimester M♀

O26.849 Uterine size-date discrepancy, unspecified trimester M♀

✓6th O26.85 Spotting complicating pregnancy

O26.851 Spotting complicating pregnancy, first trimester M♀

O26.852 Spotting complicating pregnancy, second trimester M♀

O26.853 Spotting complicating pregnancy, third trimester M♀

O26.859 Spotting complicating pregnancy, unspecified trimester M♀

O26.86 Pruritic urticarial papules and plaques of pregnancy (PUPPP) M♀

Polymorphic eruption of pregnancy

✓6th O26.87 Cervical shortening

EXCLUDES 1 *encounter for suspected cervical shortening ruled out (Z03.75)*

CC Excl: For CC codes in subcategory O26.87, unless otherwise noted: O26.872-O26.879, O34.31-O34.33

O26.872 Cervical shortening, second trimester CC M♀

O26.873 Cervical shortening, third trimester CC M♀

O26.879 Cervical shortening, unspecified trimester CC M♀

✓6th O26.89 Other specified pregnancy related conditions

O26.891 Other specified pregnancy related conditions, first trimester M♀

O26.892 Other specified pregnancy related conditions, second trimester M♀

O26.893 Other specified pregnancy related conditions, third trimester M♀

O26.899 Other specified pregnancy related conditions, unspecified trimester M♀

✓5th O26.9 Pregnancy related conditions, unspecified

O26.90 Pregnancy related conditions, unspecified, unspecified trimester M♀

O26.91 Pregnancy related conditions, unspecified, first trimester M♀

O26.92 Pregnancy related conditions, unspecified, second trimester M♀

O26.93 Pregnancy related conditions, unspecified, third trimester M♀

✓4th **O28 Abnormal findings on antenatal screening of mother**

EXCLUDES 1 *diagnostic findings classified elsewhere—see Alphabetical Index*

O28.0 Abnormal hematological finding on antenatal screening of mother M♀

O28.1 Abnormal biochemical finding on antenatal screening of mother M♀

O28.2 Abnormal cytological finding on antenatal screening of mother M♀

O28.3 Abnormal ultrasonic finding on antenatal screening of mother M♀

O28.4 Abnormal radiological finding on antenatal screening of mother M♀

O28.5 Abnormal chromosomal and genetic finding on antenatal screening of mother M♀

O28.8 Other abnormal findings on antenatal screening of mother M♀

O28.9 Unspecified abnormal findings on antenatal screening of mother M♀

✓4th **O29 Complications of anesthesia during pregnancy**

INCLUDES maternal complications arising from the administration of a general, regional or local anesthetic, analgesic or other sedation during pregnancy

Use additional code, if necessary, to identify the complication

EXCLUDES 2 *complications of anesthesia during labor and delivery (O74.-)*
complications of anesthesia during the puerperium (O89.-)

✓5th O29.0 Pulmonary complications of anesthesia during pregnancy

✓6th O29.01 Aspiration pneumonitis due to anesthesia during pregnancy

Inhalation of stomach contents or secretions NOS due to anesthesia during pregnancy

Mendelson's syndrome due to anesthesia during pregnancy

O29.011 Aspiration pneumonitis due to anesthesia during pregnancy, first trimester M♀

O29.012 Aspiration pneumonitis due to anesthesia during pregnancy, second trimester M♀

O29.013 Aspiration pneumonitis due to anesthesia during pregnancy, third trimester M♀

O29.019 Aspiration pneumonitis due to anesthesia during pregnancy, unspecified trimester M♀

✓6th O29.02 Pressure collapse of lung due to anesthesia during pregnancy

O29.021 Pressure collapse of lung due to anesthesia during pregnancy, first trimester M♀

O29.022 Pressure collapse of lung due to anesthesia during pregnancy, second trimester M♀

O29.023 Pressure collapse of lung due to anesthesia during pregnancy, third trimester M♀

O29.029 Pressure collapse of lung due to anesthesia during pregnancy, unspecified trimester M♀

✓6th O29.09 Other pulmonary complications of anesthesia during pregnancy

O29.091 Other pulmonary complications of anesthesia during pregnancy, first trimester M♀

O29.092 Other pulmonary complications of anesthesia during pregnancy, second trimester M♀

O29.093 Other pulmonary complications of anesthesia during pregnancy, third trimester M♀

O29.099 Other pulmonary complications of anesthesia during pregnancy, unspecified trimester M♀

✓5th O29.1 Cardiac complications of anesthesia during pregnancy

✓6th O29.11 Cardiac arrest due to anesthesia during pregnancy

O29.111 Cardiac arrest due to anesthesia during pregnancy, first trimester M♀

O29.112 Cardiac arrest due to anesthesia during pregnancy, second trimester M♀

O29.113 Cardiac arrest due to anesthesia during pregnancy, third trimester M♀

O29.119 Cardiac arrest due to anesthesia during pregnancy, unspecified trimester M♀

✓6th O29.12 Cardiac failure due to anesthesia during pregnancy

O29.121 Cardiac failure due to anesthesia during pregnancy, first trimester M♀

O29.122 Cardiac failure due to anesthesia during pregnancy, second trimester M♀

O29.123 Cardiac failure due to anesthesia during pregnancy, third trimester M♀

O29.129 Cardiac failure due to anesthesia during pregnancy, unspecified trimester M♀

✓6th O29.19 Other cardiac complications of anesthesia during pregnancy

O29.191 Other cardiac complications of anesthesia during pregnancy, first trimester M♀

O29.192 Other cardiac complications of anesthesia during pregnancy, second trimester M♀

O29.193 Other cardiac complications of anesthesia during pregnancy, third trimester M♀

O29.199 Other cardiac complications of anesthesia during pregnancy, unspecified trimester M♀

✓5th O29.2 Central nervous system complications of anesthesia during pregnancy

✓6th O29.21 Cerebral anoxia due to anesthesia during pregnancy

O29.211 Cerebral anoxia due to anesthesia during pregnancy, first trimester M♀

O29.212 Cerebral anoxia due to anesthesia during pregnancy, second trimester M♀

O29.213 Cerebral anoxia due to anesthesia during pregnancy, third trimester M♀

O29.219 Cerebral anoxia due to anesthesia during pregnancy, unspecified trimester M♀

✓6th O29.29 Other central nervous system complications of anesthesia during pregnancy

O29.291 Other central nervous system complications of anesthesia during pregnancy, first trimester M♀

O29.292 Other central nervous system complications of anesthesia during pregnancy, second trimester M♀

O29.293 Other central nervous system complications of anesthesia during pregnancy, third trimester M♀

O29.299 Other central nervous system complications of anesthesia during pregnancy, unspecified trimester M♀

✓5th O29.3 Toxic reaction to local anesthesia during pregnancy

✓6th O29.3X Toxic reaction to local anesthesia during pregnancy

O29.3X1 Toxic reaction to local anesthesia during pregnancy, first trimester M♀

O29.3X2 Toxic reaction to local anesthesia during pregnancy, second trimester M♀

O29.3X3 Toxic reaction to local anesthesia during pregnancy, third trimester M♀

O29.3X9 Toxic reaction to local anesthesia during pregnancy, unspecified trimester M♀

✓5th O29.4 Spinal and epidural anesthesia induced headache during pregnancy

O29.40 Spinal and epidural anesthesia induced headache during pregnancy, unspecified trimester M♀

O29.41 Spinal and epidural anesthesia induced headache during pregnancy, first trimester M♀

O29.42 Spinal and epidural anesthesia induced headache during pregnancy, second trimester M♀

O29.43 Spinal and epidural anesthesia induced headache during pregnancy, third trimester M♀

✓5th O29.5 Other complications of spinal and epidural anesthesia during pregnancy

✓6th O29.5X Other complications of spinal and epidural anesthesia during pregnancy

O29.5X1 Other complications of spinal and epidural anesthesia during pregnancy, first trimester M♀

O29.5X2 Other complications of spinal and epidural anesthesia during pregnancy, second trimester M♀

O29.5X3 Other complications of spinal and epidural anesthesia during pregnancy, third trimester M♀

O29.5X9 Other complications of spinal and epidural anesthesia during pregnancy, unspecified trimester M♀

✓5th O29.6 Failed or difficult intubation for anesthesia during pregnancy

O29.60 Failed or difficult intubation for anesthesia during pregnancy, unspecified trimester M♀

O29.61 Failed or difficult intubation for anesthesia during pregnancy, first trimester M♀

O29.62 Failed or difficult intubation for anesthesia during pregnancy, second trimester M♀

O29.63 Failed or difficult intubation for anesthesia during pregnancy, third trimester M♀

✓5th O29.8 Other complications of anesthesia during pregnancy

✓6th O29.8X Other complications of anesthesia during pregnancy

O29.8X1 Other complications of anesthesia during pregnancy, first trimester M♀

O29.8X2 Other complications of anesthesia during pregnancy, second trimester M♀

O29.8X3 Other complications of anesthesia during pregnancy, third trimester M♀

O29.8X9 Other complications of anesthesia during pregnancy, unspecified trimester M♀

✓5th O29.9 Unspecified complication of anesthesia during pregnancy

O29.90 Unspecified complication of anesthesia during pregnancy, unspecified trimester M♀

O29.91 Unspecified complication of anesthesia during pregnancy, first trimester M♀

O29.92 Unspecified complication of anesthesia during pregnancy, second trimester M♀

O29.93 Unspecified complication of anesthesia during pregnancy, third trimester M♀

Maternal care related to the fetus and amniotic cavity and possible delivery problems (O30-O48)

✓4th **O30 Multiple gestation**

Code also any complications specific to multiple gestation

CC Excl: For CC codes in category O30, unless otherwise noted: O30.001-O30.019, O30.031-O30.93, O31.10X0-O31.23X9, O31.31X0-O32.9XX9, O80

✓5th O30.0 Twin pregnancy

✓6th O30.00 Twin pregnancy, unspecified number of placenta and unspecified number of amniotic sacs

O30.001 Twin pregnancy, unspecified number of placenta and unspecified number of amniotic sacs, first trimester M♀

O30.002 Twin pregnancy, unspecified number of placenta and unspecified number of amniotic sacs, second trimester M♀

O30.003 Twin pregnancy, unspecified number of placenta and unspecified number of amniotic sacs, third trimester M♀

O30.009 Twin pregnancy, unspecified number of placenta and unspecified number of amniotic sacs, unspecified trimester M♀

✓6th O30.01 Twin pregnancy, monochorionic/monoamniotic

Twin pregnancy, one placenta, one amniotic sac

EXCLUDES 1 *conjoined twins (O30.02-)*

O30.011 Twin pregnancy, monochorionic/monoamniotic, first trimester M♀

O30.012 Twin pregnancy, monochorionic/monoamniotic, second trimester M♀

O30.013 Twin pregnancy, monochorionic/monoamniotic, third trimester M♀

O30.019 Twin pregnancy, monochorionic/monoamniotic, unspecified trimester M♀

✓6th O30.02 Conjoined twin pregnancy

O30.021 Conjoined twin pregnancy, first trimester M♀

O30.022 Conjoined twin pregnancy, second trimester M♀

O30.023 **Conjoined twin pregnancy, third trimester** M♀

O30.029 **Conjoined twin pregnancy, unspecified trimester** M♀

✓6th O30.03 **Twin pregnancy, monochorionic/diamniotic**
Twin pregnancy, one placenta, two amniotic sacs

O30.031 **Twin pregnancy, monochorionic/diamniotic, first trimester** M♀

O30.032 **Twin pregnancy, monochorionic/diamniotic, second trimester** M♀

O30.033 **Twin pregnancy, monochorionic/diamniotic, third trimester** M♀

O30.039 **Twin pregnancy, monochorionic/diamniotic, unspecified trimester** M♀

✓6th O30.04 **Twin pregnancy, dichorionic/diamniotic**
Twin pregnancy, two placentae, two amniotic sacs

O30.041 **Twin pregnancy, dichorionic/diamniotic, first trimester** M♀

O30.042 **Twin pregnancy, dichorionic/diamniotic, second trimester** M♀

O30.043 **Twin pregnancy, dichorionic/diamniotic, third trimester** M♀

O30.049 **Twin pregnancy, dichorionic/diamniotic, unspecified trimester** M♀

✓6th O30.09 **Twin pregnancy, unable to determine number of placenta and number of amniotic sacs**

O30.091 **Twin pregnancy, unable to determine number of placenta and number of amniotic sacs, first trimester** M♀

O30.092 **Twin pregnancy, unable to determine number of placenta and number of amniotic sacs, second trimester** M♀

O30.093 **Twin pregnancy, unable to determine number of placenta and number of amniotic sacs, third trimester** M♀

O30.099 **Twin pregnancy, unable to determine number of placenta and number of amniotic sacs, unspecified trimester** M♀

✓5th O30.1 **Triplet pregnancy**

✓6th O30.10 **Triplet pregnancy, unspecified number of placenta and unspecified number of amniotic sacs**

O30.101 **Triplet pregnancy, unspecified number of placenta and unspecified number of amniotic sacs, first trimester** CC M♀

O30.102 **Triplet pregnancy, unspecified number of placenta and unspecified number of amniotic sacs, second trimester** CC M♀

O30.103 **Triplet pregnancy, unspecified number of placenta and unspecified number of amniotic sacs, third trimester** CC M♀

O30.109 **Triplet pregnancy, unspecified number of placenta and unspecified number of amniotic sacs, unspecified trimester** M♀

✓6th O30.11 **Triplet pregnancy with two or more monochorionic fetuses**

O30.111 **Triplet pregnancy with two or more monochorionic fetuses, first trimester** CC M♀

O30.112 **Triplet pregnancy with two or more monochorionic fetuses, second trimester** CC M♀

O30.113 **Triplet pregnancy with two or more monochorionic fetuses, third trimester** CC M♀

O30.119 **Triplet pregnancy with two or more monochorionic fetuses, unspecified trimester** M♀

✓6th O30.12 **Triplet pregnancy with two or more monoamniotic fetuses**

O30.121 **Triplet pregnancy with two or more monoamniotic fetuses, first trimester** CC M♀

O30.122 **Triplet pregnancy with two or more monoamniotic fetuses, second trimester** CC M♀

O30.123 **Triplet pregnancy with two or more monoamniotic fetuses, third trimester** CC M♀

O30.129 **Triplet pregnancy with two or more monoamniotic fetuses, unspecified trimester** M♀

✓6th O30.19 **Triplet pregnancy, unable to determine number of placenta and number of amniotic sacs**

O30.191 **Triplet pregnancy, unable to determine number of placenta and number of amniotic sacs, first trimester** CC M♀

O30.192 **Triplet pregnancy, unable to determine number of placenta and number of amniotic sacs, second trimester** CC M♀

O30.193 **Triplet pregnancy, unable to determine number of placenta and number of amniotic sacs, third trimester** CC M♀

O30.199 **Triplet pregnancy, unable to determine number of placenta and number of amniotic sacs, unspecified trimester** M♀

✓6th O30.2 **Quadruplet pregnancy**

✓6th O30.20 **Quadruplet pregnancy, unspecified number of placenta and unspecified number of amniotic sacs**

O30.201 **Quadruplet pregnancy, unspecified number of placenta and unspecified number of amniotic sacs, first trimester** CC M♀

O30.202 **Quadruplet pregnancy, unspecified number of placenta and unspecified number of amniotic sacs, second trimester** CC M♀

O30.203 **Quadruplet pregnancy, unspecified number of placenta and unspecified number of amniotic sacs, third trimester** CC M♀

O30.209 **Quadruplet pregnancy, unspecified number of placenta and unspecified number of amniotic sacs, unspecified trimester** M♀

✓6th O30.21 **Quadruplet pregnancy with two or more monochorionic fetuses**

O30.211 **Quadruplet pregnancy with two or more monochorionic fetuses, first trimester** CC M♀

O30.212 **Quadruplet pregnancy with two or more monochorionic fetuses, second trimester** CC M♀

O30.213 **Quadruplet pregnancy with two or more monochorionic fetuses, third trimester** CC M♀

O30.219 **Quadruplet pregnancy with two or more monochorionic fetuses, unspecified trimester** M♀

✓6th O30.22 **Quadruplet pregnancy with two or more monoamniotic fetuses**

O30.221 **Quadruplet pregnancy with two or more monoamniotic fetuses, first trimester** CC M♀

O30.222 **Quadruplet pregnancy with two or more monoamniotic fetuses, second trimester** CC M♀

O30.223 **Quadruplet pregnancy with two or more monoamniotic fetuses, third trimester** CC M♀

O30.229 **Quadruplet pregnancy with two or more monoamniotic fetuses, unspecified trimester** M♀

✓6th O30.29 **Quadruplet pregnancy, unable to determine number of placenta and number of amniotic sacs**

O30.291 **Quadruplet pregnancy, unable to determine number of placenta and number of amniotic sacs, first trimester** CC M♀

O30.292 Quadruplet pregnancy, unable to determine number of placenta and number of amniotic sacs, second trimester CC M ♀

O30.293 Quadruplet pregnancy, unable to determine number of placenta and number of amniotic sacs, third trimester CC M ♀

O30.299 Quadruplet pregnancy, unable to determine number of placenta and number of amniotic sacs, unspecified trimester M ♀

✓5th **O30.8 Other specified multiple gestation**
Multiple gestation pregnancy greater than quadruplets

✓6th **O30.80 Other specified multiple gestation, unspecified number of placenta and unspecified number of amniotic sacs**

O30.801 Other specified multiple gestation, unspecified number of placenta and unspecified number of amniotic sacs, first trimester CC M ♀

O30.802 Other specified multiple gestation, unspecified number of placenta and unspecified number of amniotic sacs, second trimester CC M ♀

O30.803 Other specified multiple gestation, unspecified number of placenta and unspecified number of amniotic sacs, third trimester CC M ♀

O30.809 Other specified multiple gestation, unspecified number of placenta and unspecified number of amniotic sacs, unspecified trimester M ♀

✓6th **O30.81 Other specified multiple gestation with two or more monochorionic fetuses**

O30.811 Other specified multiple gestation with two or more monochorionic fetuses, first trimester CC M ♀

O30.812 Other specified multiple gestation with two or more monochorionic fetuses, second trimester CC M ♀

O30.813 Other specified multiple gestation with two or more monochorionic fetuses, third trimester CC M ♀

O30.819 Other specified multiple gestation with two or more monochorionic fetuses, unspecified trimester M ♀

✓6th **O30.82 Other specified multiple gestation with two or more monoamniotic fetuses**

O30.821 Other specified multiple gestation with two or more monoamniotic fetuses, first trimester CC M ♀

O30.822 Other specified multiple gestation with two or more monoamniotic fetuses, second trimester CC M ♀

O30.823 Other specified multiple gestation with two or more monoamniotic fetuses, third trimester CC M ♀

O30.829 Other specified multiple gestation with two or more monoamniotic fetuses, unspecified trimester M ♀

✓6th **O30.89 Other specified multiple gestation, unable to determine number of placenta and number of amniotic sacs**

O30.891 Other specified multiple gestation, unable to determine number of placenta and number of amniotic sacs, first trimester CC M ♀

O30.892 Other specified multiple gestation, unable to determine number of placenta and number of amniotic sacs, second trimester CC M ♀

O30.893 Other specified multiple gestation, unable to determine number of placenta and number of amniotic sacs, third trimester CC M ♀

O30.899 Other specified multiple gestation, unable to determine number of placenta and number of amniotic sacs, unspecified trimester M ♀

✓5th **O30.9 Multiple gestation, unspecified**
Multiple pregnancy NOS

O30.90 Multiple gestation, unspecified, unspecified trimester M ♀

O30.91 Multiple gestation, unspecified, first trimester M ♀

O30.92 Multiple gestation, unspecified, second trimester M ♀

O30.93 Multiple gestation, unspecified, third trimester M ♀

✓4th **O31 Complications specific to multiple gestation**

EXCLUDES 2 *delayed delivery of second twin, triplet, etc. (O63.2)*
malpresentation of one fetus or more (O32.9)
placental transfusion syndromes (O43.0-)

AHA: 2012, 4Q, 107

One of the following 7th characters is to be assigned to each code under category O31. 7th character 0 is for single gestations and multiple gestations where the fetus is unspecified. 7th characters 1 through 9 are for cases of multiple gestations to identify the fetus for which the code applies. The appropriate code from category O30, Multiple gestation, must also be assigned when assigning a code from category O31 that has a 7th character of 1 through 9.

0	not applicable or unspecified	3	fetus 3
1	fetus 1	4	fetus 4
2	fetus 2	5	fetus 5
		9	other fetus

✓5th **O31.0 Papyraceous fetus**
Fetus compressus

✓x7th O31.00 Papyraceous fetus, unspecified trimester M ♀

✓x7th O31.01 Papyraceous fetus, first trimester M ♀

✓x7th O31.02 Papyraceous fetus, second trimester M ♀

✓x7th O31.03 Papyraceous fetus, third trimester M ♀

✓5th **O31.1 Continuing pregnancy after spontaneous abortion of one fetus or more**

✓x7th O31.10 Continuing pregnancy after spontaneous abortion of one fetus or more, unspecified trimester M ♀

✓x7th O31.11 Continuing pregnancy after spontaneous abortion of one fetus or more, first trimester M ♀

✓x7th O31.12 Continuing pregnancy after spontaneous abortion of one fetus or more, second trimester M ♀

✓x7th O31.13 Continuing pregnancy after spontaneous abortion of one fetus or more, third trimester M ♀

✓5th **O31.2 Continuing pregnancy after intrauterine death of one fetus or more**

✓x7th O31.20 Continuing pregnancy after intrauterine death of one fetus or more, unspecified trimester M ♀

✓x7th O31.21 Continuing pregnancy after intrauterine death of one fetus or more, first trimester M ♀

✓x7th O31.22 Continuing pregnancy after intrauterine death of one fetus or more, second trimester M ♀

✓x7th O31.23 Continuing pregnancy after intrauterine death of one fetus or more, third trimester M ♀

✓5th **O31.3 Continuing pregnancy after elective fetal reduction of one fetus or more**
Continuing pregnancy after selective termination of one fetus or more

✓x7th O31.30 Continuing pregnancy after elective fetal reduction of one fetus or more, unspecified trimester M ♀

✓x7th O31.31 Continuing pregnancy after elective fetal reduction of one fetus or more, first trimester M ♀

✓x7th O31.32 Continuing pregnancy after elective fetal reduction of one fetus or more, second trimester M ♀

✓x7th O31.33 Continuing pregnancy after elective fetal reduction of one fetus or more, third trimester M ♀

✓5th **O31.8 Other complications specific to multiple gestation**

✓6th **O31.8X Other complications specific to multiple gestation**

CC Excl: For CC codes in subcategory O31.8X, unless otherwise noted: See code: O30

✓7th O31.8X1 Other complications specific to multiple gestation, first trimester CC M ♀

✓7th O31.8X2 Other complications specific to multiple gestation, second trimester CC M ♀

DRAFT

√7th **O31.8X3 Other complications specific to multiple gestation, third trimester** CC M♀

√7th **O31.8X9 Other complications specific to multiple gestation, unspecified trimester** M♀

√4th **O32 Maternal care for malpresentation of fetus**

INCLUDES the listed conditions as a reason for observation, hospitalization or other obstetric care of the mother, or for cesarean delivery before onset of labor

EXCLUDES 1 *malpresentation of fetus with obstructed labor (O64.-)*

AHA: 2Ø12, 4Q, 1Ø7

One of the following 7th characters is to be assigned to each code under category O32. 7th character Ø is for single gestations and multiple gestations where the fetus is unspecified. 7th characters 1 through 9 are for cases of multiple gestations to identify the fetus for which the code applies. The appropriate code from category O3Ø, Multiple gestation, must also be assigned when assigning a code from category O32 that has a 7th character of 1 through 9.

Ø	not applicable or unspecified	3	fetus 3
		4	fetus 4
1	fetus 1	5	fetus 5
2	fetus 2	9	other fetus

√x7th **O32.Ø Maternal care for unstable lie** M♀

√x7th **O32.1 Maternal care for breech presentation** M♀

Maternal care for buttocks presentation
Maternal care for complete breech
Maternal care for frank breech

EXCLUDES 1 *footling presentation (O32.8)*
incomplete breech (O32.8)

√x7th **O32.2 Maternal care for transverse and oblique lie** M♀

Maternal care for oblique presentation
Maternal care for transverse presentation

√x7th **O32.3 Maternal care for face, brow and chin presentation** M♀

√x7th **O32.4 Maternal care for high head at term** M♀

Maternal care for failure of head to enter pelvic brim

√x7th **O32.6 Maternal care for compound presentation** M♀

√x7th **O32.8 Maternal care for other malpresentation of fetus** M♀

Maternal care for footling presentation
Maternal care for incomplete breech

√x7th **O32.9 Maternal care for malpresentation of fetus, unspecified** M♀

√4th **O33 Maternal care for disproportion**

INCLUDES the listed conditions as a reason for observation, hospitalization or other obstetric care of the mother, or for cesarean delivery before onset of labor

EXCLUDES 1 *disproportion with obstructed labor (O65-O66)*

O33.Ø Maternal care for disproportion due to deformity of maternal pelvic bones CC M♀

Maternal care for disproportion due to pelvic deformity causing disproportion NOS

CC Excl: O33.Ø

O33.1 Maternal care for disproportion due to generally contracted pelvis M♀

Maternal care for disproportion due to contracted pelvis NOS causing disproportion

O33.2 Maternal care for disproportion due to inlet contraction of pelvis M♀

Maternal care for disproportion due to inlet contraction (pelvis) causing disproportion

√x7th **O33.3 Maternal care for disproportion due to outlet contraction of pelvis** M♀

Maternal care for disproportion due to mid-cavity contraction (pelvis)

Maternal care for disproportion due to outlet contraction (pelvis)

One of the following 7th characters is to be assigned to code O33.3. 7th character Ø is for single gestations and multiple gestations where the fetus is unspecified. 7th characters 1 through 9 are for cases of multiple gestations to identify the fetus for which the code applies. The appropriate code from category O3Ø, Multiple gestation, must also be assigned when assigning code O33.3 with a 7th character of 1 through 9.

Ø	not applicable or unspecified	3	fetus 3
		4	fetus 4
1	fetus 1	5	fetus 5
2	fetus 2	9	other fetus

√x7th **O33.4 Maternal care for disproportion of mixed maternal and fetal origin** M♀

One of the following 7th characters is to be assigned to code O33.4. 7th character Ø is for single gestations and multiple gestations where the fetus is unspecified. 7th characters 1 through 9 are for cases of multiple gestations to identify the fetus for which the code applies. The appropriate code from category O3Ø, Multiple gestation, must also be assigned when assigning code O33.4 with a 7th character of 1 through 9.

Ø	not applicable or unspecified	3	fetus 3
		4	fetus 4
1	fetus 1	5	fetus 5
2	fetus 2	9	other fetus

√x7th **O33.5 Maternal care for disproportion due to unusually large fetus** M♀

Maternal care for disproportion due to disproportion of fetal origin with normally formed fetus
Maternal care for disproportion due to fetal disproportion NOS

One of the following 7th characters is to be assigned to code O33.5. 7th character Ø is for single gestations and multiple gestations where the fetus is unspecified. 7th characters 1 through 9 are for cases of multiple gestations to identify the fetus for which the code applies. The appropriate code from category O3Ø, Multiple gestation, must also be assigned when assigning code O33.5 with a 7th character of 1 through 9.

Ø	not applicable or unspecified	3	fetus 3
		4	fetus 4
1	fetus 1	5	fetus 5
2	fetus 2	9	other fetus

√x7th **O33.6 Maternal care for disproportion due to hydrocephalic fetus** M♀

One of the following 7th characters is to be assigned to code O33.6. 7th character Ø is for single gestations and multiple gestations where the fetus is unspecified. 7th characters 1 through 9 are for cases of multiple gestations to identify the fetus for which the code applies. The appropriate code from category O3Ø, Multiple gestation, must also be assigned when assigning code O33.6 with a 7th character of 1 through 9.

Ø	not applicable or unspecified	3	fetus 3
		4	fetus 4
1	fetus 1	5	fetus 5
2	fetus 2	9	other fetus

O33.7 Maternal care for disproportion due to other fetal deformities M♀

Maternal care for disproportion due to fetal ascites
Maternal care for disproportion due to fetal hydrops
Maternal care for disproportion due to fetal meningomyelocele
Maternal care for disproportion due to fetal sacral teratoma
Maternal care for disproportion due to fetal tumor

EXCLUDES 1 *obstructed labor due to other fetal deformities (O66.3)*

O33.8 Maternal care for disproportion of other origin M♀

O33.9 Maternal care for disproportion, unspecified M♀

Maternal care for disproportion due to cephalopelvic disproportion NOS
Maternal care for disproportion due to fetopelvic disproportion NOS

√4th **O34 Maternal care for abnormality of pelvic organs**

INCLUDES the listed conditions as a reason for hospitalization or other obstetric care of the mother, or for cesarean delivery before onset of labor

Code first any associated obstructed labor (O65.5)
Use additional code for specific condition

√5th **O34.Ø Maternal care for congenital malformation of uterus**

O34.ØØ Maternal care for unspecified congenital malformation of uterus, unspecified trimester M♀

O34.Ø1 Maternal care for unspecified congenital malformation of uterus, first trimester M♀

O34.02 Maternal care for unspecified congenital malformation of uterus, second trimester M♀

O34.03 Maternal care for unspecified congenital malformation of uterus, third trimester M♀

✓5th **O34.1 Maternal care for benign tumor of corpus uteri**

EXCLUDES 2 *maternal care for benign tumor of cervix (O34.4-)*
maternal care for malignant neoplasm of uterus (O9A.1-)

O34.10 Maternal care for benign tumor of corpus uteri, unspecified trimester M♀

O34.11 Maternal care for benign tumor of corpus uteri, first trimester M♀

O34.12 Maternal care for benign tumor of corpus uteri, second trimester M♀

O34.13 Maternal care for benign tumor of corpus uteri, third trimester M♀

✓5th **O34.2 Maternal care due to uterine scar from previous surgery**

O34.21 Maternal care for scar from previous cesarean delivery M♀

O34.29 Maternal care due to uterine scar from other previous surgery M♀

✓5th **O34.3 Maternal care for cervical incompetence**

Maternal care for cerclage with or without cervical incompetence
Maternal care for Shirodkar suture with or without cervical incompetence

CC Excl: For MCC codes in subcategory O34.3, unless otherwise noted: O26.872-O26.879, O34.31-O34.33

O34.30 Maternal care for cervical incompetence, unspecified trimester M♀

O34.31 Maternal care for cervical incompetence, first trimester MCC M♀

O34.32 Maternal care for cervical incompetence, second trimester MCC M♀

O34.33 Maternal care for cervical incompetence, third trimester MCC M♀

✓5th **O34.4 Maternal care for other abnormalities of cervix**

O34.40 Maternal care for other abnormalities of cervix, unspecified trimester M♀

O34.41 Maternal care for other abnormalities of cervix, first trimester M♀

O34.42 Maternal care for other abnormalities of cervix, second trimester M♀

O34.43 Maternal care for other abnormalities of cervix, third trimester M♀

✓5th **O34.5 Maternal care for other abnormalities of gravid uterus**

✓6th **O34.51 Maternal care for incarceration of gravid uterus**

O34.511 Maternal care for incarceration of gravid uterus, first trimester M♀

O34.512 Maternal care for incarceration of gravid uterus, second trimester M♀

O34.513 Maternal care for incarceration of gravid uterus, third trimester M♀

O34.519 Maternal care for incarceration of gravid uterus, unspecified trimester M♀

✓6th **O34.52 Maternal care for prolapse of gravid uterus**

O34.521 Maternal care for prolapse of gravid uterus, first trimester M♀

O34.522 Maternal care for prolapse of gravid uterus, second trimester M♀

O34.523 Maternal care for prolapse of gravid uterus, third trimester M♀

O34.529 Maternal care for prolapse of gravid uterus, unspecified trimester M♀

✓6th **O34.53 Maternal care for retroversion of gravid uterus**

O34.531 Maternal care for retroversion of gravid uterus, first trimester M♀

O34.532 Maternal care for retroversion of gravid uterus, second trimester M♀

O34.533 Maternal care for retroversion of gravid uterus, third trimester M♀

O34.539 Maternal care for retroversion of gravid uterus, unspecified trimester M♀

✓6th **O34.59 Maternal care for other abnormalities of gravid uterus**

O34.591 Maternal care for other abnormalities of gravid uterus, first trimester M♀

O34.592 Maternal care for other abnormalities of gravid uterus, second trimester M♀

O34.593 Maternal care for other abnormalities of gravid uterus, third trimester M♀

O34.599 Maternal care for other abnormalities of gravid uterus, unspecified trimester M♀

✓5th **O34.6 Maternal care for abnormality of vagina**

EXCLUDES 2 *maternal care for vaginal varices in pregnancy (O22.1-)*

O34.60 Maternal care for abnormality of vagina, unspecified trimester M♀

O34.61 Maternal care for abnormality of vagina, first trimester M♀

O34.62 Maternal care for abnormality of vagina, second trimester M♀

O34.63 Maternal care for abnormality of vagina, third trimester M♀

✓5th **O34.7 Maternal care for abnormality of vulva and perineum**

EXCLUDES 2 *maternal care for perineal and vulval varices in pregnancy (O22.1-)*

O34.70 Maternal care for abnormality of vulva and perineum, unspecified trimester M♀

O34.71 Maternal care for abnormality of vulva and perineum, first trimester M♀

O34.72 Maternal care for abnormality of vulva and perineum, second trimester M♀

O34.73 Maternal care for abnormality of vulva and perineum, third trimester M♀

✓5th **O34.8 Maternal care for other abnormalities of pelvic organs**

O34.80 Maternal care for other abnormalities of pelvic organs, unspecified trimester M♀

O34.81 Maternal care for other abnormalities of pelvic organs, first trimester M♀

O34.82 Maternal care for other abnormalities of pelvic organs, second trimester M♀

O34.83 Maternal care for other abnormalities of pelvic organs, third trimester M♀

✓5th **O34.9 Maternal care for abnormality of pelvic organ, unspecified**

O34.90 Maternal care for abnormality of pelvic organ, unspecified, unspecified trimester M♀

O34.91 Maternal care for abnormality of pelvic organ, unspecified, first trimester M♀

O34.92 Maternal care for abnormality of pelvic organ, unspecified, second trimester M♀

O34.93 Maternal care for abnormality of pelvic organ, unspecified, third trimester M♀

✓4th **O35 Maternal care for known or suspected fetal abnormality and damage**

INCLUDES the listed conditions in the fetus as a reason for hospitalization or other obstetric care to the mother, or for termination of pregnancy

Code also any associated maternal condition

EXCLUDES 1 *encounter for suspected maternal and fetal conditions ruled out (Z03.7-)*

One of the following 7th characters is to be assigned to each code under category O35. 7th character 0 is for single gestations and multiple gestations where the fetus is unspecified. 7th characters 1 through 9 are for cases of multiple gestations to identify the fetus for which the code applies. The appropriate code from category O30, Multiple gestation, must also be assigned when assigning a code from category O35 that has a 7th character of 1 through 9.

0	not applicable or unspecified	3	fetus 3
		4	fetus 4
1	fetus 1	5	fetus 5
2	fetus 2	9	other fetus

✓x7th **O35.0 Maternal care for (suspected) central nervous system malformation in fetus** M♀

Maternal care for fetal anencephaly
Maternal care for fetal hydrocephalus
Maternal care for fetal spina bifida

EXCLUDES 2 *chromosomal abnormality in fetus (O35.1)*

✓x7th **O35.1 Maternal care for (suspected) chromosomal abnormality in fetus** M♀

√x7th **O35.2 Maternal care for (suspected) hereditary disease in fetus** M♀
EXCLUDES 2 *chromosomal abnormality in fetus (O35.1)*

√x7th **O35.3 Maternal care for (suspected) damage to fetus from viral disease in mother** M♀
Maternal care for damage to fetus from maternal cytomegalovirus infection
Maternal care for damage to fetus from maternal rubella

√x7th **O35.4 Maternal care for (suspected) damage to fetus from alcohol** M♀

√x7th **O35.5 Maternal care for (suspected) damage to fetus by drugs** M♀
Maternal care for damage to fetus from drug addiction

√x7th **O35.6 Maternal care for (suspected) damage to fetus by radiation** M♀

√x7th **O35.7 Maternal care for (suspected) damage to fetus by other medical procedures** M♀
Maternal care for damage to fetus by amniocentesis
Maternal care for damage to fetus by biopsy procedures
Maternal care for damage to fetus by hematological investigation
Maternal care for damage to fetus by intrauterine contraceptive device
Maternal care for damage to fetus by intrauterine surgery

√x7th **O35.8 Maternal care for other (suspected) fetal abnormality and damage** M♀
Maternal care for damage to fetus from maternal listeriosis
Maternal care for damage to fetus from maternal toxoplasmosis

√x7th **O35.9 Maternal care for (suspected) fetal abnormality and damage, unspecified** M♀

√4th **O36 Maternal care for other fetal problems**
INCLUDES the listed conditions in the fetus as a reason for hospitalization or other obstetric care of the mother, or for termination of pregnancy
EXCLUDES 1 *encounter for suspected maternal and fetal conditions ruled out (ZØ3.7-)*
placental transfusion syndromes (O43.Ø-)
EXCLUDES 2 *labor and delivery complicated by fetal stress (O77.-)*

One of the following 7th characters is to be assigned to each code under category O36. 7th character Ø is for single gestations and multiple gestations where the fetus is unspecified. 7th characters 1 through 9 are for cases of multiple gestations to identify the fetus for which the code applies. The appropriate code from category O3Ø, Multiple gestation, must also be assigned when assigning a code from category O36 that has a 7th character of 1 through 9.

Ø	not applicable or unspecified	3	fetus 3
		4	fetus 4
1	fetus 1	5	fetus 5
2	fetus 2	9	other fetus

√5th **O36.Ø Maternal care for rhesus isoimmunization**
Maternal care for Rh incompatibility (with hydrops fetalis)

CC Excl: For CC codes in subcategory O36.Ø, unless otherwise noted: O36.Ø11Ø-O36.Ø139, O36.Ø91Ø-O36.Ø939

√6th **O36.Ø1 Maternal care for anti-D [Rh] antibodies**

√7th **O36.Ø11 Maternal care for anti-D [Rh] antibodies, first trimester** CC M♀

√7th **O36.Ø12 Maternal care for anti-D [Rh] antibodies, second trimester** CC M♀

√7th **O36.Ø13 Maternal care for anti-D [Rh] antibodies, third trimester** CC M♀

√7th **O36.Ø19 Maternal care for anti-D [Rh] antibodies, unspecified trimester** M♀

√6th **O36.Ø9 Maternal care for other rhesus isoimmunization**

√7th **O36.Ø91 Maternal care for other rhesus isoimmunization, first trimester** CC M♀

√7th **O36.Ø92 Maternal care for other rhesus isoimmunization, second trimester** CC M♀

√7th **O36.Ø93 Maternal care for other rhesus isoimmunization, third trimester** CC M♀

√7th **O36.Ø99 Maternal care for other rhesus isoimmunization, unspecified trimester** M♀

√5th **O36.1 Maternal care for other isoimmunization**
Maternal care for ABO isoimmunization

√6th **O36.11 Maternal care for Anti-A sensitization**
Maternal care for isoimmunization NOS (with hydrops fetalis)

√7th **O36.111 Maternal care for Anti-A sensitization, first trimester** M♀

√7th **O36.112 Maternal care for Anti-A sensitization, second trimester** M♀

√7th **O36.113 Maternal care for Anti-A sensitization, third trimester** M♀

√7th **O36.119 Maternal care for Anti-A sensitization, unspecified trimester** M♀

√6th **O36.19 Maternal care for other isoimmunization**
Maternal care for Anti-B sensitization

√7th **O36.191 Maternal care for other isoimmunization, first trimester** M♀

√7th **O36.192 Maternal care for other isoimmunization, second trimester** M♀

√7th **O36.193 Maternal care for other isoimmunization, third trimester** M♀

√7th **O36.199 Maternal care for other isoimmunization, unspecified trimester** M♀

√5th **O36.2 Maternal care for hydrops fetalis**
Maternal care for hydrops fetalis NOS
Maternal care for hydrops fetalis not associated with isoimmunization
EXCLUDES 1 *hydrops fetalis associated with ABO isoimmunization (O36.1-)*
hydrops fetalis associated with rhesus isoimmunization (O36.Ø-)

√x7th **O36.2Ø Maternal care for hydrops fetalis, unspecified trimester** M♀

√x7th **O36.21 Maternal care for hydrops fetalis, first trimester** M♀

√x7th **O36.22 Maternal care for hydrops fetalis, second trimester** M♀

√x7th **O36.23 Maternal care for hydrops fetalis, third trimester** M♀

√x7th **O36.4 Maternal care for intrauterine death** CC M♀
Maternal care for intrauterine fetal death NOS
Maternal care for intrauterine fetal death after completion of 2Ø weeks of gestation
Maternal care for late fetal death
Maternal care for missed delivery
EXCLUDES 1 *missed abortion (OØ2.1)*
stillbirth (P95)
CC Excl: O36.4XXØ-O36.4XX9

√5th **O36.5 Maternal care for known or suspected poor fetal growth**

CC Excl: For CC codes in subcategory O36.5, unless otherwise noted: O36.511Ø-O36.5139, O36.591Ø-O36.5939

√6th **O36.51 Maternal care for known or suspected placental insufficiency**

√7th **O36.511 Maternal care for known or suspected placental insufficiency, first trimester** M♀

√7th **O36.512 Maternal care for known or suspected placental insufficiency, second trimester** M♀

√7th **O36.513 Maternal care for known or suspected placental insufficiency, third trimester** M♀

√7th **O36.519 Maternal care for known or suspected placental insufficiency, unspecified trimester** M♀

√6th **O36.59 Maternal care for other known or suspected poor fetal growth**
Maternal care for known or suspected light-for-dates NOS
Maternal care for known or suspected small-for-dates NOS

√7th **O36.591 Maternal care for other known or suspected poor fetal growth, first trimester** M♀

√7th **O36.592 Maternal care for other known or suspected poor fetal growth, second trimester** M♀

√7th **O36.593 Maternal care for other known or suspected poor fetal growth, third trimester** M♀

√7th **O36.599 Maternal care for other known or suspected poor fetal growth, unspecified trimester** M♀

√5th **O36.6 Maternal care for excessive fetal growth**
Maternal care for known or suspected large-for-dates

√x7th **O36.60 Maternal care for excessive fetal growth,** unspecified trimester M♀

√x7th **O36.61 Maternal care for excessive fetal growth,** first trimester M♀

√x7th **O36.62 Maternal care for excessive fetal growth,** second trimester M♀

√x7th **O36.63 Maternal care for excessive fetal growth,** third trimester M♀

√5th **O36.7 Maternal care for viable fetus in abdominal pregnancy**

√x7th **O36.70 Maternal care for viable fetus in abdominal pregnancy,** unspecified trimester M♀

√x7th **O36.71 Maternal care for viable fetus in abdominal pregnancy,** first trimester M♀

√x7th **O36.72 Maternal care for viable fetus in abdominal pregnancy,** second trimester M♀

√x7th **O36.73 Maternal care for viable fetus in abdominal pregnancy,** third trimester M♀

√5th **O36.8 Maternal care for other specified fetal problems**

√x7th **O36.80 Pregnancy with inconclusive fetal viability** M♀
Encounter to determine fetal viability of pregnancy

√6th **O36.81 Decreased fetal movements**

√7th **O36.812 Decreased fetal movements,** second trimester M♀

√7th **O36.813 Decreased fetal movements,** third trimester M♀

√7th **O36.819 Decreased fetal movements,** unspecified trimester M♀

√6th **O36.82 Fetal anemia and thrombocytopenia**

√7th **O36.821 Fetal anemia and thrombocytopenia,** first trimester M♀

√7th **O36.822 Fetal anemia and thrombocytopenia,** second trimester M♀

√7th **O36.823 Fetal anemia and thrombocytopenia,** third trimester M♀

√7th **O36.829 Fetal anemia and thrombocytopenia,** unspecified trimester M♀

√6th **O36.89 Maternal care for other specified fetal problems**

√7th **O36.891 Maternal care for other specified fetal problems,** first trimester M♀

√7th **O36.892 Maternal care for other specified fetal problems,** second trimester M♀

√7th **O36.893 Maternal care for other specified fetal problems,** third trimester M♀

√7th **O36.899 Maternal care for other specified fetal problems,** unspecified trimester M♀

√5th **O36.9 Maternal care for fetal problem, unspecified**

√x7th **O36.90 Maternal care for fetal problem, unspecified,** unspecified trimester M♀

√x7th **O36.91 Maternal care for fetal problem, unspecified,** first trimester M♀

√x7th **O36.92 Maternal care for fetal problem, unspecified,** second trimester M♀

√x7th **O36.93 Maternal care for fetal problem, unspecified,** third trimester M♀

√4th **O40 Polyhydramnios**
Hydramnios
EXCLUDES 1 *encounter for suspected maternal and fetal conditions ruled out (Z03.7-)*

One of the following 7th characters is to be assigned to each code under category O40. 7th character 0 is for single gestations and multiple gestations where the fetus is unspecified. 7th characters 1 through 9 are for cases of multiple gestations to identify the fetus for which the code applies. The appropriate code from category O30, Multiple gestation, must also be assigned when assigning a code from category O40 that has a 7th character of 1 through 9.

0	not applicable or unspecified	3	fetus 3
		4	fetus 4
1	fetus 1	5	fetus 5
2	fetus 2	9	other fetus

√x7th **O40.1 Polyhydramnios,** first trimester M♀

√x7th **O40.2 Polyhydramnios,** second trimester M♀

√x7th **O40.3 Polyhydramnios,** third trimester M♀

√x7th **O40.9 Polyhydramnios,** unspecified trimester M♀

√4th **O41 Other disorders of amniotic fluid and membranes**
EXCLUDES 1 *encounter for suspected maternal and fetal conditions ruled out (Z03.7-)*

One of the following 7th characters is to be assigned to each code under category O41. 7th character 0 is for single gestations and multiple gestations where the fetus is unspecified. 7th characters 1 through 9 are for cases of multiple gestations to identify the fetus for which the code applies. The appropriate code from category O30, Multiple gestation, must also be assigned when assigning a code from category O41 that has a 7th character of 1 through 9.

0	not applicable or unspecified	3	fetus 3
		4	fetus 4
1	fetus 1	5	fetus 5
2	fetus 2	9	other fetus

√5th **O41.0 Oligohydramnios**
Oligohydramnios without rupture of membranes

CC Excl: For CC codes in subcategory O41.0, unless otherwise noted: O41.01X0-O41.03X9

√x7th **O41.00 Oligohydramnios,** unspecified trimester M♀

√x7th **O41.01 Oligohydramnios,** first trimester CC M♀

√x7th **O41.02 Oligohydramnios,** second trimester CC M♀

√x7th **O41.03 Oligohydramnios,** third trimester CC M♀

√5th **O41.1 Infection of amniotic sac and membranes**

CC Excl: For MCC codes in subcategory O41.1, unless otherwise noted: O41.1010-O41.1039, O41.1210-O41.1239, O41.1410-O41.1439

√6th **O41.10 Infection of amniotic sac and membranes, unspecified**

√7th **O41.101 Infection of amniotic sac and membranes, unspecified,** first trimester MCC M♀

√7th **O41.102 Infection of amniotic sac and membranes, unspecified,** second trimester MCC M♀

√7th **O41.103 Infection of amniotic sac and membranes, unspecified,** third trimester MCC M♀

√7th **O41.109 Infection of amniotic sac and membranes, unspecified,** unspecified trimester M♀

√6th **O41.12 Chorioamnionitis**

√7th **O41.121 Chorioamnionitis,** first trimester MCC M♀

√7th **O41.122 Chorioamnionitis,** second trimester MCC M♀

√7th **O41.123 Chorioamnionitis,** third trimester MCC M♀

√7th **O41.129 Chorioamnionitis,** unspecified trimester M♀

√6th **O41.14 Placentitis**

√7th **O41.141 Placentitis,** first trimester MCC M♀

√7th **O41.142 Placentitis,** second trimester MCC M♀

√7th **O41.143 Placentitis,** third trimester MCC M♀

√7th **O41.149 Placentitis,** unspecified trimester M♀

√5th **O41.8 Other specified disorders of amniotic fluid and membranes**

CC Excl: For CC codes in subcategory O41.8, unless otherwise noted: O41.8X10-O41.8X39

√6th **O41.8X Other specified disorders of amniotic fluid and membranes**

√7th **O41.8X1 Other specified disorders of amniotic fluid and membranes,** first trimester M♀

√7th **O41.8X2 Other specified disorders of amniotic fluid and membranes,** second trimester M♀

√7th **O41.8X3 Other specified disorders of amniotic fluid and membranes,** third trimester M♀

√7th **O41.8X9 Other specified disorders of amniotic fluid and membranes,** unspecified trimester M♀

√5th **O41.9 Disorder of amniotic fluid and membranes, unspecified**

√x7th **O41.90 Disorder of amniotic fluid and membranes, unspecified,** unspecified trimester M♀

✓x7th **O41.91 Disorder of amniotic fluid and membranes, unspecified, first trimester** M♀

✓x7th **O41.92 Disorder of amniotic fluid and membranes, unspecified, second trimester** M♀

✓x7th **O41.93 Disorder of amniotic fluid and membranes, unspecified, third trimester** M♀

✓4th **O42 Premature rupture of membranes**

✓5th **O42.0 Premature rupture of membranes, onset of labor within 24 hours of rupture**

O42.00 Premature rupture of membranes, onset of labor within 24 hours of rupture, unspecified weeks of gestation M♀

✓6th **O42.01 Preterm premature rupture of membranes, onset of labor within 24 hours of rupture**
Premature rupture of membranes before 37 completed weeks of gestation

O42.011 Preterm premature rupture of membranes, onset of labor within 24 hours of rupture, first trimester M♀

O42.012 Preterm premature rupture of membranes, onset of labor within 24 hours of rupture, second trimester M♀

O42.013 Preterm premature rupture of membranes, onset of labor within 24 hours of rupture, third trimester M♀

O42.019 Preterm premature rupture of membranes, onset of labor within 24 hours of rupture, unspecified trimester M♀

O42.02 Full-term premature rupture of membranes, onset of labor within 24 hours of rupture M♀
Premature rupture of membranes after 37 completed weeks of gestation

✓5th **O42.1 Premature rupture of membranes, onset of labor more than 24 hours following rupture**

O42.10 Premature rupture of membranes, onset of labor more than 24 hours following rupture, unspecified weeks of gestation M♀

✓6th **O42.11 Preterm premature rupture of membranes, onset of labor more than 24 hours following rupture**
Premature rupture of membranes before 37 completed weeks of gestation

O42.111 Preterm premature rupture of membranes, onset of labor more than 24 hours following rupture, first trimester M♀

O42.112 Preterm premature rupture of membranes, onset of labor more than 24 hours following rupture, second trimester M♀

O42.113 Preterm premature rupture of membranes, onset of labor more than 24 hours following rupture, third trimester M♀

O42.119 Preterm premature rupture of membranes, onset of labor more than 24 hours following rupture, unspecified trimester M♀

O42.12 Full-term premature rupture of membranes, onset of labor more than 24 hours following rupture M♀
Premature rupture of membranes after 37 completed weeks of gestation

✓5th **O42.9 Premature rupture of membranes, unspecified as to length of time between rupture and onset of labor**

O42.90 Premature rupture of membranes, unspecified as to length of time between rupture and onset of labor, unspecified weeks of gestation M♀

✓6th **O42.91 Preterm premature rupture of membranes, unspecified as to length of time between rupture and onset of labor**
Premature rupture of membranes before 37 completed weeks of gestation

O42.911 Preterm premature rupture of membranes, unspecified as to length of time between rupture and onset of labor, first trimester M♀

O42.912 Preterm premature rupture of membranes, unspecified as to length of time between rupture and onset of abor, second trimester M♀

O42.913 Preterm premature rupture of membranes, unspecified as to length of time between rupture and onset of labor, third trimester M♀

O42.919 Preterm premature rupture of membranes, unspecified as to length of time between rupture and onset of labor, unspecified trimester M♀

O42.92 Full-term premature rupture of membranes, unspecified as to length of time between rupture and onset of labor M♀
Premature rupture of membranes after 37 completed weeks of gestation

✓4th **O43 Placental disorders**

EXCLUDES 2 *maternal care for poor fetal growth due to placental insufficiency (O36.5-)*
placenta previa (O44.-)
placental polyp (O90.89)
placentitis (O41.14-)
premature separation of placenta [abruptio placentae] (O45.-)

✓5th **O43.0 Placental transfusion syndromes**

✓6th **O43.01 Fetomaternal placental transfusion syndrome**
Maternofetal placental transfusion syndrome

O43.011 Fetomaternal placental transfusion syndrome, first trimester M♀

O43.012 Fetomaternal placental transfusion syndrome, second trimester M♀

O43.013 Fetomaternal placental transfusion syndrome, third trimester M♀

O43.019 Fetomaternal placental transfusion syndrome, unspecified trimester M♀

✓6th **O43.02 Fetus-to-fetus placental transfusion syndrome**

O43.021 Fetus-to-fetus placental transfusion syndrome, first trimester M♀

O43.022 Fetus-to-fetus placental transfusion syndrome, second trimester M♀

O43.023 Fetus-to-fetus placental transfusion syndrome, third trimester M♀

O43.029 Fetus-to-fetus placental transfusion syndrome, unspecified trimester M♀

✓5th **O43.1 Malformation of placenta**

✓6th **O43.10 Malformation of placenta, unspecified**
Abnormal placenta NOS

O43.101 Malformation of placenta, unspecified, first trimester M♀

O43.102 Malformation of placenta, unspecified, second trimester M♀

O43.103 Malformation of placenta, unspecified, third trimester M♀

O43.109 Malformation of placenta, unspecified, unspecified trimester M♀

✓6th **O43.11 Circumvallate placenta**

O43.111 Circumvallate placenta, first trimester M♀

O43.112 Circumvallate placenta, second trimester M♀

O43.113 Circumvallate placenta, third trimester M♀

O43.119 Circumvallate placenta, unspecified trimester M♀

✓6th **O43.12 Velamentous insertion of umbilical cord**

O43.121 Velamentous insertion of umbilical cord, first trimester M♀

O43.122 Velamentous insertion of umbilical cord, second trimester M♀

O43.123 Velamentous insertion of umbilical cord, third trimester M♀

O43.129 Velamentous insertion of umbilical cord, unspecified trimester M♀

✓6th **O43.19 Other malformation of placenta**

O43.191 Other malformation of placenta, first trimester M♀

O43.192 Other malformation of placenta, second trimester M♀

O43.193 Other malformation of placenta, third trimester M♀

O43.199 Other malformation of placenta, unspecified trimester M♀

✓5th **O43.2 Morbidly adherent placenta**
Code also associated third stage postpartum hemorrhage, if applicable (O72.0)
EXCLUDES 1 *retained placenta (O73.-)*

✓6th **O43.21 Placenta accreta**
O43.211 Placenta accreta, first trimester M♀
O43.212 Placenta accreta, second trimester M♀
O43.213 Placenta accreta, third trimester M♀
O43.219 Placenta accreta, unspecified trimester M♀

✓6th **O43.22 Placenta increta**
O43.221 Placenta increta, first trimester M♀
O43.222 Placenta increta, second trimester M♀
O43.223 Placenta increta, third trimester M♀
O43.229 Placenta increta, unspecified trimester M♀

✓6th **O43.23 Placenta percreta**
O43.231 Placenta percreta, first trimester M♀
O43.232 Placenta percreta, second trimester M♀
O43.233 Placenta percreta, third trimester M♀
O43.239 Placenta percreta, unspecified trimester M♀

✓5th **O43.8 Other placental disorders**

✓6th **O43.81 Placental infarction**
O43.811 Placental infarction, first trimester M♀
O43.812 Placental infarction, second trimester M♀
O43.813 Placental infarction, third trimester M♀
O43.819 Placental infarction, unspecified trimester M♀

✓6th **O43.89 Other placental disorders**
Placental dysfunction
O43.891 Other placental disorders, first trimester M♀
O43.892 Other placental disorders, second trimester M♀
O43.893 Other placental disorders, third trimester M♀
O43.899 Other placental disorders, unspecified trimester M♀

✓5th **O43.9 Unspecified placental disorder**
O43.90 Unspecified placental disorder, unspecified trimester M♀
O43.91 Unspecified placental disorder, first trimester M♀
O43.92 Unspecified placental disorder, second trimester M♀
O43.93 Unspecified placental disorder, third trimester M♀

✓4th **O44 Placenta previa**

CC Excl: For CC/MCC codes in category O44, unless otherwise noted: O20.0-O20.9, O25.10-O25.3, O26.10-O26.13, O26.30-O26.43, O26.63-O26.819, O26.841-O26.86, O26.891-O26.93, O29.011-O29.93, O35.7XX0-O35.7XX9, O44.00-O44.13, O75.4, O75.81, O75.89-O75.9, O80, O90.89, O99.111-O99.285, O99.330-O99.335, O99.350-O99.355, O99.511-O99.73, O99.820-O99.825, O99.840-O9A.53

✓5th **O44.0 Placenta previa specified as without hemorrhage**
Low implantation of placenta specified as without hemorrhage
O44.00 Placenta previa specified as without hemorrhage, unspecified trimester M♀
O44.01 Placenta previa specified as without hemorrhage, first trimester CC M♀
O44.02 Placenta previa specified as without hemorrhage, second trimester CC M♀
O44.03 Placenta previa specified as without hemorrhage, third trimester CC M♀

✓5th **O44.1 Placenta previa with hemorrhage**
Low implantation of placenta, NOS or with hemorrhage
Marginal placenta previa, NOS or with hemorrhage
Partial placenta previa, NOS or with hemorrhage
Total placenta previa, NOS or with hemorrhage
EXCLUDES 1 *labor and delivery complicated by hemorrhage from vasa previa (O69.4)*
O44.10 Placenta previa with hemorrhage, unspecified trimester M♀
O44.11 Placenta previa with hemorrhage, first trimester MCC M♀
O44.12 Placenta previa with hemorrhage, second trimester MCC M♀
O44.13 Placenta previa with hemorrhage, third trimester MCC M♀

✓4th **O45 Premature separation of placenta [abruptio placentae]**

✓5th **O45.0 Premature separation of placenta with coagulation defect**

CC Excl: For MCC codes in subcategory O45.0, unless otherwise noted: O25.10-O25.3, O26.10-O26.13, O26.30-O26.43, O26.63-O26.819, O26.841-O26.86, O26.891-O26.93, O29.011-O29.93, O35.7XX0-O35.7XX9, O45.001-O45.099, O46.001-O46.93, O67.0-O67.9, O75.4, O75.81, O75.89-O75.9, O80, O90.89, O99.111-O99.285, O99.330-O99.335, O99.350-O99.355, O99.511-O99.73, O99.820-O99.825, O99.840-O9A.53

✓6th **O45.00 Premature separation of placenta with coagulation defect, unspecified**
O45.001 Premature separation of placenta with coagulation defect, unspecified, first trimester MCC M♀
O45.002 Premature separation of placenta with coagulation defect, unspecified, second trimester MCC M♀
O45.003 Premature separation of placenta with coagulation defect, unspecified, third trimester MCC M♀
O45.009 Premature separation of placenta with coagulation defect, unspecified, unspecified trimester M♀

✓6th **O45.01 Premature separation of placenta with afibrinogenemia**
Premature separation of placenta with hypofibrinogenemia
O45.011 Premature separation of placenta with afibrinogenemia, first trimester MCC M♀
O45.012 Premature separation of placenta with afibrinogenemia, second trimester MCC M♀
O45.013 Premature separation of placenta with afibrinogenemia, third trimester MCC M♀
O45.019 Premature separation of placenta with afibrinogenemia, unspecified trimester M♀

✓6th **O45.02 Premature separation of placenta with disseminated intravascular coagulation**
O45.021 Premature separation of placenta with disseminated intravascular coagulation, first trimester MCC M♀
O45.022 Premature separation of placenta with disseminated intravascular coagulation, second trimester MCC M♀
O45.023 Premature separation of placenta with disseminated intravascular coagulation, third trimester MCC M♀
O45.029 Premature separation of placenta with disseminated intravascular coagulation, unspecified trimester M♀

✓6th **O45.09 Premature separation of placenta with other coagulation defect**
O45.091 Premature separation of placenta with other coagulation defect, first trimester MCC M♀
O45.092 Premature separation of placenta with other coagulation defect, second trimester MCC M♀
O45.093 Premature separation of placenta with other coagulation defect, third trimester MCC M♀
O45.099 Premature separation of placenta with other coagulation defect, unspecified trimester M♀

O45.8 Other premature separation of placenta

> **CC Excl: For MCC codes in subcategory O45.8, unless otherwise noted:** O20.0-O20.9, O25.10-O25.3, O26.10-O26.13, O26.30-O26.43, O26.63-O26.819, O26.841-O26.86, O26.891-O26.93, O29.011-O29.93, O35.7XX0-O35.7XX9, O44.00-O44.13, O45.8X1-O45.8X3, O45.91-O45.93, O75.4, O75.81, O75.89-O75.9, O80, O90.89, O99.111-O99.285, O99.330-O99.335, O99.350-O99.355, O99.511-O99.73, O99.820-O99.825, O99.840-O9A.53

O45.8X Other premature separation of placenta

- **O45.8X1 Other premature separation of placenta, first trimester** MCC M ♀
- **O45.8X2 Other premature separation of placenta, second trimester** MCC M ♀
- **O45.8X3 Other premature separation of placenta, third trimester** MCC M ♀
- **O45.8X9 Other premature separation of placenta, unspecified trimester** M ♀

O45.9 Premature separation of placenta, unspecified
Abruptio placentae NOS

> **CC Excl: For MCC codes in subcategory O45.9, unless otherwise noted:** See code: O45.8

- **O45.90 Premature separation of placenta, unspecified, unspecified trimester** M ♀
- **O45.91 Premature separation of placenta, unspecified, first trimester** MCC M ♀
- **O45.92 Premature separation of placenta, unspecified, second trimester** MCC M ♀
- **O45.93 Premature separation of placenta, unspecified, third trimester** MCC M ♀

O46 Antepartum hemorrhage, not elsewhere classified

EXCLUDES 1 *hemorrhage in early pregnancy (O20.-)*
intrapartum hemorrhage NEC (O67.-)
placenta previa (O44.-)
premature separation of placenta [abruptio placentae] (O45.-)

O46.0 Antepartum hemorrhage with coagulation defect

> **CC Excl: For MCC codes in subcategory O46.0, unless otherwise noted:** See code: O45.0

O46.00 Antepartum hemorrhage with coagulation defect, unspecified

- **O46.001 Antepartum hemorrhage with coagulation defect, unspecified, first trimester** MCC M ♀
- **O46.002 Antepartum hemorrhage with coagulation defect, unspecified, second trimester** MCC M ♀
- **O46.003 Antepartum hemorrhage with coagulation defect, unspecified, third trimester** MCC M ♀
- **O46.009 Antepartum hemorrhage with coagulation defect, unspecified, unspecified trimester** M ♀

O46.01 Antepartum hemorrhage with afibrinogenemia
Antepartum hemorrhage with hypofibrinogenemia

- **O46.011 Antepartum hemorrhage with afibrinogenemia, first trimester** MCC M ♀
- **O46.012 Antepartum hemorrhage with afibrinogenemia, second trimester** MCC M ♀
- **O46.013 Antepartum hemorrhage with afibrinogenemia, third trimester** MCC M ♀
- **O46.019 Antepartum hemorrhage with afibrinogenemia, unspecified trimester** M ♀

O46.02 Antepartum hemorrhage with disseminated intravascular coagulation

- **O46.021 Antepartum hemorrhage with disseminated intravascular coagulation, first trimester** MCC M ♀
- **O46.022 Antepartum hemorrhage with disseminated intravascular coagulation, second trimester** MCC M ♀
- **O46.023 Antepartum hemorrhage with disseminated intravascular coagulation, third trimester** MCC M ♀
- **O46.029 Antepartum hemorrhage with disseminated intravascular coagulation, unspecified trimester** M ♀

O46.09 Antepartum hemorrhage with other coagulation defect

- **O46.091 Antepartum hemorrhage with other coagulation defect, first trimester** MCC M ♀
- **O46.092 Antepartum hemorrhage with other coagulation defect, second trimester** MCC M ♀
- **O46.093 Antepartum hemorrhage with other coagulation defect, third trimester** MCC M ♀
- **O46.099 Antepartum hemorrhage with other coagulation defect, unspecified trimester** M ♀

O46.8 Other antepartum hemorrhage

O46.8X Other antepartum hemorrhage

- **O46.8X1 Other antepartum hemorrhage, first trimester** M ♀
- **O46.8X2 Other antepartum hemorrhage, second trimester** M ♀
- **O46.8X3 Other antepartum hemorrhage, third trimester** M ♀
- **O46.8X9 Other antepartum hemorrhage, unspecified trimester** M ♀

O46.9 Antepartum hemorrhage, unspecified

- **O46.90 Antepartum hemorrhage, unspecified, unspecified trimester** M ♀
- **O46.91 Antepartum hemorrhage, unspecified, first trimester** M ♀
- **O46.92 Antepartum hemorrhage, unspecified, second trimester** M ♀
- **O46.93 Antepartum hemorrhage, unspecified, third trimester** M ♀

O47 False labor
Braxton Hicks contractions
Threatened labor

EXCLUDES 1 *preterm labor (O60.-)*

> **CC Excl: For CC codes in catagory O47, unless otherwise noted:** O25.10-O25.3, O26.10-O26.13, O26.30-O26.43, O26.63-O26.819, O26.841-O26.86, O26.891-O26.93, O29.011-O29.93, O35.7XX0-O35.7XX9, O47.00-O47.9, O60.00-O60.23, O75.4, O75.81, O75.89-O75.9, O80, O90.89, O99.111-O99.285, O99.330-O99.335, O99.350-O99.355, O99.511-O99.73, O99.820-O99.825, O99.840-O9A.53

O47.0 False labor before 37 completed weeks of gestation

- **O47.00 False labor before 37 completed weeks of gestation, unspecified trimester** M ♀
- **O47.02 False labor before 37 completed weeks of gestation, second trimester** CC M ♀
- **O47.03 False labor before 37 completed weeks of gestation, third trimester** CC M ♀

O47.1 False labor at or after 37 completed weeks of gestation CC M ♀

O47.9 False labor, unspecified M ♀

O48 Late pregnancy

O48.0 Post-term pregnancy M ♀
Pregnancy over 40 completed weeks to 42 completed weeks gestation

O48.1 Prolonged pregnancy M ♀
Pregnancy which has advanced beyond 42 completed weeks gestation

Complications of labor and delivery (O60-O77)

O60 Preterm labor

INCLUDES onset (spontaneous) of labor before 37 completed weeks of gestation

EXCLUDES 1 *false labor (O47.0-)*
threatened labor NOS (O47.0-)

> **CC Excl: For CC/MCC codes in category O60, unless otherwise noted:** See code: O47

O60.0 Preterm labor without delivery

- **O60.00 Preterm labor without delivery, unspecified trimester** M ♀
- **O60.02 Preterm labor without delivery, second trimester** MCC M ♀
- **O60.03 Preterm labor without delivery, third trimester** MCC M ♀

√5th **O60.1 Preterm labor with preterm delivery**

One of the following 7th characters is to be assigned to each code under subcategory O60.1. 7th character 0 is for single gestations and multiple gestations where the fetus is unspecified. 7th characters 1 through 9 are for cases of multiple gestations to identify the fetus for which the code applies. The appropriate code from category O30, Multiple gestation, must also be assigned when assigning a code from subcategory O60.1 that has a 7th character of 1 through 9.

0	not applicable or unspecified	3	fetus 3
		4	fetus 4
1	fetus 1	5	fetus 5
2	fetus 2	9	other fetus

√x7th **O60.10 Preterm labor with preterm delivery, unspecified trimester** CC M ♀
Preterm labor with delivery NOS

√x7th **O60.12 Preterm labor second trimester with preterm delivery second trimester** MCC M ♀

√x7th **O60.13 Preterm labor second trimester with preterm delivery third trimester** MCC M ♀

√x7th **O60.14 Preterm labor third trimester with preterm delivery third trimester** MCC M ♀

√5th **O60.2 Term delivery with preterm labor**

One of the following 7th characters is to be assigned to each code under subcategory O60.2. 7th character 0 is for single gestations and multiple gestations where the fetus is unspecified. 7th characters 1 through 9 are for cases of multiple gestations to identify the fetus for which the code applies. The appropriate code from category O30, Multiple gestation, must also be assigned when assigning a code from subcategory O60.2 that has a 7th character of 1 through 9.

0	not applicable or unspecified	3	fetus 3
		4	fetus 4
1	fetus 1	5	fetus 5
2	fetus 2	9	other fetus

√x7th **O60.20 Term delivery with preterm labor, unspecified trimester** CC M ♀

√x7th **O60.22 Term delivery with preterm labor, second trimester** MCC M ♀

√x7th **O60.23 Term delivery with preterm labor, third trimester** MCC M ♀

√4th **O61 Failed induction of labor**

O61.0 Failed medical induction of labor M ♀
Failed induction (of labor) by oxytocin
Failed induction (of labor) by prostaglandins

O61.1 Failed instrumental induction of labor M ♀
Failed mechanical induction (of labor)
Failed surgical induction (of labor)

O61.8 Other failed induction of labor M ♀

O61.9 Failed induction of labor, unspecified M ♀

√4th **O62 Abnormalities of forces of labor**

O62.0 Primary inadequate contractions M ♀
Failure of cervical dilatation
Primary hypotonic uterine dysfunction
Uterine inertia during latent phase of labor

O62.1 Secondary uterine inertia M ♀
Arrested active phase of labor
Secondary hypotonic uterine dysfunction

O62.2 Other uterine inertia M ♀
Atony of uterus without hemorrhage
Atony of uterus NOS
Desultory labor
Hypotonic uterine dysfunction NOS
Irregular labor
Poor contractions
Slow slope active phase of labor
Uterine inertia NOS
EXCLUDES 1 *atony of uterus with hemorrhage (postpartum) (O72.1)*
postpartum atony of uterus without hemorrhage (O75.89)

O62.3 Precipitate labor M ♀

O62.4 Hypertonic, incoordinate, and prolonged uterine contractions M ♀
Cervical spasm
Contraction ring dystocia
Dyscoordinate labor
Hour-glass contraction of uterus
Hypertonic uterine dysfunction
Incoordinate uterine action
Tetanic contractions
Uterine dystocia NOS
Uterine spasm
EXCLUDES 1 *dystocia (fetal) (maternal) NOS (O66.9)*

O62.8 Other abnormalities of forces of labor M ♀

O62.9 Abnormality of forces of labor, unspecified M ♀

√4th **O63 Long labor**

O63.0 Prolonged first stage (of labor) M ♀

O63.1 Prolonged second stage (of labor) M ♀

O63.2 Delayed delivery of second twin, triplet, etc. M ♀

O63.9 Long labor, unspecified CC M ♀
Prolonged labor NOS
CC Excl: O25.10-O25.3, O26.10-O26.13, O26.30-O26.43, O26.63-O26.819, O26.841-O26.86, O26.891-O26.93, O29.011-O29.93, O35.7XX0-O35.7XX9, O36.8120-O36.8199, O63.9, O71.00-O71.1, O71.5, O71.81, O71.89-O71.9, O75.4, O75.81, O75.89-O75.9, O80, O90.89, O99.111-O99.285, O99.330-O99.335, O99.350-O99.355, O99.511-O99.73, O99.820-O99.825, O99.840-O9A.53

√4th **O64 Obstructed labor due to malposition and malpresentation of fetus**

One of the following 7th characters is to be assigned to each code under category O64. 7th character 0 is for single gestations and multiple gestations where the fetus is unspecified. 7th characters 1 through 9 are for cases of multiple gestations to identify the fetus for which the code applies. The appropriate code from category O30, Multiple gestation, must also be assigned when assigning a code from category O64 that has a 7th character of 1 through 9.

0	not applicable or unspecified	3	fetus 3
		4	fetus 4
1	fetus 1	5	fetus 5
2	fetus 2	9	other fetus

√x7th **O64.0 Obstructed labor due to incomplete rotation of fetal head** M ♀
Deep transverse arrest
Obstructed labor due to persistent occipitoiliac (position)
Obstructed labor due to persistent occipitoposterior (position)
Obstructed labor due to persistent occipitosacral (position)
Obstructed labor due to persistent occipitotransverse (position)

√x7th **O64.1 Obstructed labor due to breech presentation** M ♀
Obstructed labor due to buttocks presentation
Obstructed labor due to complete breech presentation
Obstructed labor due to frank breech presentation

√x7th **O64.2 Obstructed labor due to face presentation** M ♀
Obstructed labor due to chin presentation

√x7th **O64.3 Obstructed labor due to brow presentation** M ♀

√x7th **O64.4 Obstructed labor due to shoulder presentation** M ♀
Prolapsed arm
EXCLUDES 1 *impacted shoulders (O66.0)*
shoulder dystocia (O66.0)

√x7th **O64.5 Obstructed labor due to compound presentation** M ♀

√x7th **O64.8 Obstructed labor due to other malposition and malpresentation** M ♀
Obstructed labor due to footling presentation
Obstructed labor due to incomplete breech presentation

√x7th **O64.9 Obstructed labor due to malposition and malpresentation, unspecified** M ♀

√4th **O65 Obstructed labor due to maternal pelvic abnormality**

O65.0 Obstructed labor due to deformed pelvis M ♀

O65.1 Obstructed labor due to generally contracted pelvis M ♀

O65.2 Obstructed labor due to pelvic inlet contraction M ♀

O65.3 Obstructed labor due to pelvic outlet and mid-cavity contraction M ♀

O65.4 Obstructed labor due to fetopelvic disproportion, unspecified M ♀
EXCLUDES 1 *dystocia due to abnormality of fetus (O66.2-O66.3)*

O65.5 Obstructed labor due to abnormality of maternal pelvic organs M ♀
Obstructed labor due to conditions listed in O34-
Use additional code to identify abnormality of pelvic organs (O34.-)

O65.8 Obstructed labor due to other maternal pelvic abnormalities M ♀

O65.9 Obstructed labor due to maternal pelvic abnormality, unspecified M ♀

√4th **O66 Other obstructed labor**

O66.0 Obstructed labor due to shoulder dystocia M ♀
Impacted shoulders

O66.1 Obstructed labor due to locked twins M ♀

O66.2 Obstructed labor due to unusually large fetus M ♀

O66.3 Obstructed labor due to other abnormalities of fetus M♀
Dystocia due to fetal ascites
Dystocia due to fetal hydrops
Dystocia due to fetal meningomyelocele
Dystocia due to fetal sacral teratoma
Dystocia due to fetal tumor
Dystocia due to hydrocephalic fetus
Use additional code to identify cause of obstruction

√5th **O66.4 Failed trial of labor**

O66.4Ø Failed trial of labor, unspecified M♀

O66.41 Failed attempted vaginal birth after previous cesarean delivery M♀
Code first rupture of uterus, if applicable (O71.Ø-, O71.1)

O66.5 Attempted application of vacuum extractor and forceps M♀
Attempted application of vacuum or forceps, with subsequent delivery by forceps or cesarean delivery

O66.6 Obstructed labor due to other multiple fetuses M♀

O66.8 Other specified obstructed labor M♀
Use additional code to identify cause of obstruction

O66.9 Obstructed labor, unspecified M♀
Dystocia NOS
Maternal dystocia NOS
Fetal dystocia NOS

√4th **O67 Labor and delivery complicated by intrapartum hemorrhage, not elsewhere classified**

EXCLUDES 1 *antepartum hemorrhage NEC (O46.-)*
placenta previa (O44.-)
premature separation of placenta [abruptio placentae] (O45.-)

EXCLUDES 2 *postpartum hemorrhage (O72.-)*

O67.Ø Intrapartum hemorrhage with coagulation defect MCC M♀
Intrapartum hemorrhage (excessive) associated with afibrinogenemia
Intrapartum hemorrhage (excessive) associated with disseminated intravascular coagulation
Intrapartum hemorrhage (excessive) associated with hyperfibrinolysis
Intrapartum hemorrhage (excessive) associated with hypofibrinogenemia
CC Excl: O25.1Ø-O25.3, O26.1Ø-O26.13, O26.3Ø-O26.43, O26.63-O26.819, O26.841-O26.86, O26.891-O26.93, O29.Ø11-O29.93, O35.7X-O35.7X, O45.ØØ1-O45.Ø99, O46.ØØ1-O46.93, O67.Ø-O67.9, O75.4, O75.81, O75.89-O75.9, O8Ø, O9Ø.89, O99.111-O99.285, O99.33Ø-O99.335, O99.35Ø-O99.355, O99.511-O99.73, O99.82Ø-O99.825, O99.84Ø-O9A.53

O67.8 Other intrapartum hemorrhage M♀
Excessive intrapartum hemorrhage

O67.9 Intrapartum hemorrhage, unspecified M♀

O68 Labor and delivery complicated by abnormality of fetal acid-base balance CC M♀
Fetal acidemia complicating labor and delivery
Fetal acidosis complicating labor and delivery
Fetal alkalosis complicating labor and delivery
Fetal metabolic acidemia complicating labor and delivery

EXCLUDES 1 *fetal stress NOS (O77.9)*
labor and delivery complicated by electrocardiographic evidence of fetal stress (O77.8)
labor and delivery complicated by ultrasonic evidence of fetal stress (O77.8)

EXCLUDES 2 *abnormality in fetal heart rate or rhythm (O76)*
labor and delivery complicated by meconium in amniotic fluid (O77.Ø)

CC Excl: O68-O76, PØ3.811

√4th **O69 Labor and delivery complicated by umbilical cord complications**

One of the following 7th characters is to be assigned to each code under category O69. 7th character Ø is for single gestations and multiple gestations where the fetus is unspecified. 7th characters 1 through 9 are for cases of multiple gestations to identify the fetus for which the code applies. The appropriate code from category O3Ø, Multiple gestation, must also be assigned when assigning a code from category O69 that has a 7th character of 1 through 9.

Ø	not applicable or unspecified	3	fetus 3
		4	fetus 4
1	fetus 1	5	fetus 5
2	fetus 2	9	other fetus

√x7th **O69.Ø Labor and delivery complicated by prolapse of cord** M♀

√x7th **O69.1 Labor and delivery complicated by cord around neck, with compression** M♀

EXCLUDES 1 *labor and delivery complicated by cord around neck, without compression (O69.81)*

√x7th **O69.2 Labor and delivery complicated by other cord entanglement, with compression** M♀
Labor and delivery complicated by compression of cord NOS
Labor and delivery complicated by entanglement of cords of twins in monoamniotic sac
Labor and delivery complicated by knot in cord

EXCLUDES 1 *labor and delivery complicated by other cord entanglement, without compression (O69.82)*

√x7th **O69.3 Labor and delivery complicated by short cord** M♀

√x7th **O69.4 Labor and delivery complicated by vasa previa** M♀
Labor and delivery complicated by hemorrhage from vasa previa

√x7th **O69.5 Labor and delivery complicated by vascular lesion of cord** M♀
Labor and delivery complicated by cord bruising
Labor and delivery complicated by cord hematoma
Labor and delivery complicated by thrombosis of umbilical vessels

√5th **O69.8 Labor and delivery complicated by other cord complications**

√x7th **O69.81 Labor and delivery complicated by cord around neck, without compression** M♀

√x7th **O69.82 Labor and delivery complicated by other cord entanglement, without compression** M♀

√x7th **O69.89 Labor and delivery complicated by other cord complications** M♀

√x7th **O69.9 Labor and delivery complicated by cord complication, unspecified** M♀

√4th **O7Ø Perineal laceration during delivery**
Episiotomy extended by laceration

EXCLUDES 1 *obstetric high vaginal laceration alone (O71.4)*

O7Ø.Ø First degree perineal laceration during delivery M♀
Perineal laceration, rupture or tear involving fourchette during delivery
Perineal laceration, rupture or tear involving labia during delivery
Perineal laceration, rupture or tear involving skin during delivery
Perineal laceration, rupture or tear involving vagina during delivery
Perineal laceration, rupture or tear involving vulva during delivery
Slight perineal laceration, rupture or tear during delivery

O7Ø.1 Second degree perineal laceration during delivery M♀
Perineal laceration, rupture or tear during delivery as in O7Ø.Ø, also involving pelvic floor
Perineal laceration, rupture or tear during delivery as in O7Ø.Ø, also involving perineal muscles
Perineal laceration, rupture or tear during delivery as in O7Ø.Ø, also involving vaginal muscles

EXCLUDES 1 *perineal laceration involving anal sphincter (O7Ø.2)*

O7Ø.2 Third degree perineal laceration during delivery CC M♀
Perineal laceration, rupture or tear during delivery as in O7Ø.1, also involving anal sphincter
Perineal laceration, rupture or tear during delivery as in O7Ø.1, also involving rectovaginal septum
Perineal laceration, rupture or tear during delivery as in O7Ø.1, also involving sphincter NOS

EXCLUDES 1 *anal sphincter tear during delivery without third degree perineal laceration (O7Ø.4)*
perineal laceration involving anal or rectal mucosa (O7Ø.3)

CC Excl: O25.1Ø-O25.3, O26.1Ø-O26.13, O26.3Ø-O26.43, O26.63-O26.819, O26.841-O26.86, O26.891-O26.93, O29.Ø11-O29.93, O35.7XXØ-O35.7XX9, O36.812Ø-O36.8199, O7Ø.2, O7Ø.4, O71.ØØ-O71.1, O71.5, O71.81, O71.89-O71.9, O75.4, O75.81, O75.89-O75.9, O8Ø, O9Ø.89, O99.111-O99.285, O99.33Ø-O99.335, O99.35Ø-O99.355, O99.511-O99.73, O99.82Ø-O99.825, O99.84Ø-O9A.53

O7Ø.3 Fourth degree perineal laceration during delivery CC M♀
Perineal laceration, rupture or tear during delivery as in O7Ø.2, also involving anal mucosa
Perineal laceration, rupture or tear during delivery as in O7Ø.2, also involving rectal mucosa
CC Excl: O25.1Ø-O25.3, O26.1Ø-O26.13, O26.3Ø-O26.43, O26.63-O26.819, O26.841-O26.86, O26.891-O26.93, O29.Ø11-O29.93, O35.7XXØ-O35.7XX9, O36.812Ø-O36.8199, O7Ø.3, O71.ØØ-O71.1, O71.5, O71.81, O71.89-O71.9, O75.4, O75.81, O75.89-O75.9, O8Ø, O9Ø.89, O99.111-O99.285, O99.33Ø-O99.335, O99.35Ø-O99.355, O99.511-O99.73, O99.82Ø-O99.825, O99.84Ø-O9A.53

O7Ø.4 Anal sphincter tear complicating delivery, not associated with third degree laceration CC M♀

EXCLUDES 1 *anal sphincter tear with third degree perineal laceration (O7Ø.2)*

CC Excl: See code: O7Ø.2

O7Ø.9 Perineal laceration during delivery, unspecified M♀

N Newborn: Ø P Pediatric: Ø-17 M Maternity: 12-55 A Adult: 15-124 MCC Major CC Condition PDx MCC PDx acts as own MCC CC CC Condition PDx CC PDx acts as own CC

O71 Other obstetric trauma
Obstetric damage from instruments

O71.0 Rupture of uterus (spontaneous) before onset of labor
EXCLUDES 1 *disruption of (current) cesarean delivery wound (O90.0)*
laceration of uterus, NEC (O71.81)

O71.00 Rupture of uterus before onset of labor, unspecified trimester M♀

O71.02 Rupture of uterus before onset of labor, second trimester MCC M♀
CC Excl: O25.10-O25.3, O26.10-O26.13, O26.30-O26.43, O26.63-O26.819, O26.841-O26.86, O26.891-O26.93, O29.011-O29.93, O35.7XX0-O35.7XX9, O36.8120-O36.8199, O71.00-O71.1, O71.5, O71.81, O71.89-O71.9, O75.4, O75.81, O75.89-O75.9, O80, O90.89, O99.111-O99.285, O99.330-O99.335, O99.350-O99.355, O99.511-O99.73, O99.820-O99.825, O99.840-O9A.53

O71.03 Rupture of uterus before onset of labor, third trimester MCC M♀
CC Excl: See code: O71.02

O71.1 Rupture of uterus during labor MCC M♀
Rupture of uterus not stated as occurring before onset of labor
EXCLUDES 1 *disruption of cesarean delivery wound (O90.0)*
laceration of uterus, NEC (O71.81)
CC Excl: See code: O71.02

O71.2 Postpartum inversion of uterus CC M♀
CC Excl: O25.10-O25.3, O26.10-O26.13, O26.30-O26.43, O26.63-O26.819, O26.841-O26.86, O26.891-O26.93, O29.011-O29.93, O35.7XX0-O35.7XX9, O36.8120-O36.8199, O71.00-O71.2, O71.5, O71.81, O71.89-O71.9, O75.4, O75.81, O75.89-O75.9, O80, O90.89, O99.111-O99.285, O99.330-O99.335, O99.350-O99.355, O99.511-O99.73, O99.820-O99.825, O99.840-O9A.53

O71.3 Obstetric laceration of cervix CC M♀
Annular detachment of cervix
CC Excl: O25.10-O25.3, O26.10-O26.13, O26.30-O26.43, O26.63-O26.819, O26.841-O26.86, O26.891-O26.93, O29.011-O29.93, O35.7XX0-O35.7XX9, O36.8120-O36.8199, O71.00-O71.1, O71.3, O71.5, O71.81, O71.89-O71.9, O75.4, O75.81, O75.89-O75.9, O80, O90.89, O99.111-O99.285, O99.330-O99.335, O99.350-O99.355, O99.511-O99.73, O99.820-O99.825, O99.840-O9A.53

O71.4 Obstetric high vaginal laceration alone CC M♀
Laceration of vaginal wall without perineal laceration
EXCLUDES 1 *obstetric high vaginal laceration with perineal laceration (O70.-)*
CC Excl: O25.10-O25.3, O26.10-O26.13, O26.30-O26.43, O26.63-O26.819, O26.841-O26.86, O26.891-O26.93, O29.011-O29.93, O35.7XX0-O35.7XX9, O36.8120-O36.8199, O71.00-O71.1, O71.4-O71.5, O71.81, O71.89-O71.9, O75.4, O75.81, O75.89-O75.9, O80, O90.89, O99.111-O99.285, O99.330-O99.335, O99.350-O99.355, O99.511-O99.73, O99.820-O99.825, O99.840-O9A.53

O71.5 Other obstetric injury to pelvic organs CC M♀
Obstetric injury to bladder
Obstetric injury to urethra
EXCLUDES 2 *obstetric periurethral trauma (O71.82)*
CC Excl: O25.10-O25.3, O26.10-O26.13, O26.30-O26.43, O26.63-O26.819, O26.841-O26.86, O26.891-O26.93, O29.011-O29.93, O35.7XX0-O35.7XX9, O36.8120-O36.8199, O71.00-O71.1, O71.5, O71.81, O71.89-O71.9, O75.4, O75.81, O75.89-O75.9, O80, O90.89, O99.111-O99.285, O99.330-O99.335, O99.350-O99.355, O99.511-O99.73, O99.820-O99.825, O99.840-O9A.53

O71.6 Obstetric damage to pelvic joints and ligaments CC M♀
Obstetric avulsion of inner symphyseal cartilage
Obstetric damage to coccyx
Obstetric traumatic separation of symphysis (pubis)
CC Excl: O25.10-O25.3, O26.10-O26.13, O26.30-O26.43, O26.63-O26.819, O26.841-O26.86, O26.891-O26.93, O29.011-O29.93, O35.7XX0-O35.7XX9, O36.8120-O36.8199, O71.00-O71.1, O71.5-O71.6, O71.81, O71.89-O71.9, O75.4, O75.81, O75.89-O75.9, O80, O90.89, O99.111-O99.285, O99.330-O99.335, O99.350-O99.355, O99.511-O99.73, O99.820-O99.825, O99.840-O9A.53

O71.7 Obstetric hematoma of pelvis CC M♀
Obstetric hematoma of perineum
Obstetric hematoma of vagina
Obstetric hematoma of vulva
CC Excl: O25.10-O25.3, O26.10-O26.13, O26.30-O26.43, O26.63-O26.819, O26.841-O26.86, O26.891-O26.93, O29.011-O29.93, O35.7XX0-O35.7XX9, O36.8120-O36.8199, O71.00-O71.1, O71.5, O71.7-O71.81, O71.89-O71.9, O75.4, O75.81, O75.89-O75.9, O80, O90.89, O99.111-O99.285, O99.330-O99.335, O99.350-O99.355, O99.511-O99.73, O99.820-O99.825, O99.840-O9A.53

O71.8 Other specified obstetric trauma

O71.81 Laceration of uterus, not elsewhere classified M♀

O71.82 Other specified trauma to perineum and vulva M♀
Obstetric periurethral trauma

O71.89 Other specified obstetric trauma M♀

O71.9 Obstetric trauma, unspecified M♀

O72 Postpartum hemorrhage
INCLUDES hemorrhage after delivery of fetus or infant

O72.0 Third-stage hemorrhage CC M♀
Hemorrhage associated with retained, trapped or adherent placenta
Retained placenta NOS
Code also type of adherent placenta (O43.2-)
CC Excl: O25.10-O25.3, O26.10-O26.13, O26.30-O26.43, O26.63-O26.819, O26.841-O26.86, O26.891-O26.93, O29.011-O29.93, O35.7XX0-O35.7XX9, O36.8120-O36.8199, O71.00-O71.1, O71.5, O71.81, O71.89-O72.0, O75.4, O75.81, O75.89-O75.9, O80, O90.89, O99.111-O99.285, O99.330-O99.335, O99.350-O99.355, O99.511-O99.73, O99.820-O99.825, O99.840-O9A.12

O72.1 Other immediate postpartum hemorrhage CC M♀
Hemorrhage following delivery of placenta
Postpartum hemorrhage (atonic) NOS
Uterine atony with hemorrhage
EXCLUDES 1 *uterine atony NOS (O62.2)*
uterine atony without hemorrhage (O62.2)
postpartum atony of uterus without hemorrhage (O75.89)
CC Excl: O25.10-O25.3, O26.10-O26.13, O26.30-O26.43, O26.63-O26.819, O26.841-O26.86, O26.891-O26.93, O29.011-O29.93, O35.7XX0-O35.7XX9, O36.8120-O36.8199, O71.00-O71.1, O71.5, O71.81, O71.89-O71.9, O72.1, O75.4, O75.81, O75.89-O75.9, O80, O90.89, O99.111-O99.285, O99.330-O99.335, O99.350-O99.355, O99.511-O99.73, O99.820-O99.825, O99.840-O9A.53

O72.2 Delayed and secondary postpartum hemorrhage CC M♀
Hemorrhage associated with retained portions of placenta or membranes after the first 24 hours following delivery of placenta
Retained products of conception NOS, following delivery
CC Excl: O25.10-O25.3, O26.10-O26.13, O26.30-O26.43, O26.63-O26.819, O26.841-O26.86, O26.891-O26.93, O29.011-O29.93, O35.7XX0-O35.7XX9, O36.8120-O36.8199, O71.00-O71.1, O71.5, O71.81, O71.89-O71.9, O72.2, O75.4, O75.81, O75.89-O75.9, O80, O90.89, O99.111-O99.285, O99.330-O99.335, O99.350-O99.355, O99.511-O99.73, O99.820-O99.825, O99.840-O9A.53

O72.3 Postpartum coagulation defects M♀
Postpartum afibrinogenemia
Postpartum fibrinolysis

O73 Retained placenta and membranes, without hemorrhage
EXCLUDES 1 *placenta accreta (O43.21-)*
placenta increta (O43.22-)
placenta percreta (O43.23-)

O73.0 Retained placenta without hemorrhage M♀
Adherent placenta, without hemorrhage
Trapped placenta without hemorrhage

O73.1 Retained portions of placenta and membranes, without hemorrhage M♀
Retained products of conception following delivery, without hemorrhage

O74 Complications of anesthesia during labor and delivery
INCLUDES maternal complications arising from the administration of a general, regional or local anesthetic, analgesic or other sedation during labor and delivery
Use additional code, if applicable, to identify specific complication

O74.0 Aspiration pneumonitis due to anesthesia during labor and delivery M♀
Inhalation of stomach contents or secretions NOS due to anesthesia during labor and delivery
Mendelson's syndrome due to anesthesia during labor and delivery

O74.1 Other pulmonary complications of anesthesia during labor and delivery M♀

O74.2 Cardiac complications of anesthesia during labor and delivery M♀

O74.3 Central nervous system complications of anesthesia during labor and delivery M♀

O74.4 Toxic reaction to local anesthesia during labor and delivery M♀

O74.5 Spinal and epidural anesthesia-induced headache during labor and delivery M♀

O74.6 Other complications of spinal and epidural anesthesia during labor and delivery M♀

O74.7 Failed or difficult intubation for anesthesia during labor and delivery M♀

O74.8 Other complications of anesthesia during labor and delivery M♀

O74.9 Complication of anesthesia during labor and delivery, unspecified M♀

O75 Other complications of labor and delivery, not elsewhere classified

EXCLUDES 2 *puerperal (postpartum) infection (O86.-)*
puerperal (postpartum) sepsis (O85)

O75.Ø Maternal distress during labor and delivery M ♀

O75.1 Shock during or following labor and delivery MCC M ♀
Obstetric shock following labor and delivery
CC Excl: O25.1Ø-O25.3, O26.1Ø-O26.13, O26.3Ø-O26.43, O26.63-O26.819, O26.841-O26.86, O26.891-O26.93, O29.Ø11-O29.93, O35.7XXØ-O35.7XX9, O75.1, O75.4, O75.81, O75.89-O75.9, O8Ø, O9Ø.89, O99.111-O99.285, O99.33Ø-O99.335, O99.35Ø-O99.355, O99.511-O99.73, O99.82Ø-O99.825, O99.84Ø-O9A.53

O75.2 Pyrexia during labor, not elsewhere classified CC M ♀
CC Excl: O75.2

O75.3 Other infection during labor MCC M ♀
Sepsis during labor
Use additional code (B95-B97), to identify infectious agent
CC Excl: O25.1Ø-O25.3, O26.1Ø-O26.13, O26.3Ø-O26.43, O26.63-O26.819, O26.841-O26.86, O26.891-O26.93, O29.Ø11-O29.93, O35.7XXØ-O35.7XX9, O75.3-O75.4, O75.81, O75.89-O75.9, O8Ø, O9Ø.89, O99.111-O99.285, O99.33Ø-O99.335, O99.35Ø-O99.355, O99.511-O99.73, O99.82Ø-O99.825, O99.84Ø-O9A.53

O75.4 Other complications of obstetric surgery and procedures M ♀
Cardiac arrest following obstetric surgery or procedures
Cardiac failure following obstetric surgery or procedures
Cerebral anoxia following obstetric surgery or procedures
Pulmonary edema following obstetric surgery or procedures
Use additional code to identify specific complication
EXCLUDES 2 *complications of anesthesia during labor and delivery (O74.-)*
disruption of obstetrical (surgical) wound (O9Ø.Ø-O9Ø.1)
hematoma of obstetrical (surgical) wound (O9Ø.2)
infection of obstetrical (surgical) wound (O86.Ø)

O75.5 Delayed delivery after artificial rupture of membranes M ♀

O75.8 Other specified complications of labor and delivery

O75.81 Maternal exhaustion complicating labor and delivery M ♀

O75.82 Onset (spontaneous) of labor after 37 completed weeks of gestation but before 39 completed weeks gestation, with delivery by (planned) cesarean section M ♀
Delivery by (planned) cesarean section occurring after 37 completed weeks of gestation but before 39 completed weeks gestation due to (spontaneous) onset of labor
Code first to specify reason for planned cesarean section such as:
cephalopelvic disproportion (normally formed fetus) (O33.9)
previous cesarean delivery (O34.21)

O75.89 Other specified complications of labor and delivery M ♀

O75.9 Complication of labor and delivery, unspecified M ♀

O76 Abnormality in fetal heart rate and rhythm complicating labor and delivery M ♀
Depressed fetal heart rate tones complicating labor and delivery
Fetal bradycardia complicating labor and delivery
Fetal heart rate abnormal variability complicating labor and delivery
Fetal heart rate decelerations complicating labor and delivery
Fetal heart rate irregularity complicating labor and delivery
Fetal tachycardia complicating labor and delivery
Non-reassuring fetal heart rate or rhythm complicating labor and delivery
EXCLUDES 1 *fetal stress NOS (O77.9)*
labor and delivery complicated by electrocardiographic evidence of fetal stress (O77.8)
labor and delivery complicated by ultrasonic evidence of fetal stress (O77.8)
EXCLUDES 2 *fetal metabolic acidemia (O68)*
other fetal stress (O77.Ø-O77.1)
AHA: 2Ø13, 4Q, 118

O77 Other fetal stress complicating labor and delivery

O77.Ø Labor and delivery complicated by meconium in amniotic fluid M ♀
AHA: 2Ø13, 4Q, 117-118

O77.1 Fetal stress in labor or delivery due to drug administration M ♀

O77.8 Labor and delivery complicated by other evidence of fetal stress M ♀
Labor and delivery complicated by electrocardiographic evidence of fetal stress
Labor and delivery complicated by ultrasonic evidence of fetal stress
EXCLUDES 1 *abnormality in fetal heart rate or rhythm (O76)*
abnormality of fetal acid-base balance (O68)
fetal metabolic acidemia (O68)

O77.9 Labor and delivery complicated by fetal stress, unspecified M ♀
EXCLUDES 1 *abnormality in fetal heart rate or rhythm (O76)*
abnormality of fetal acid-base balance (O68)
fetal metabolic acidemia (O68)

Encounter for delivery (O8Ø, O82)

O8Ø Encounter for full-term uncomplicated delivery M ♀
NOTE Delivery requiring minimal or no assistance, with or without episiotomy, without fetal manipulation [e.g., rotation version] or instrumentation [forceps] of a spontaneous, cephalic, vaginal, full-term, single, live-born infant. This code is for use as a single diagnosis code and is not to be used with any other code from chapter 15.
Use additional code to indicate outcome of delivery (Z37.Ø)
AHA: 2Ø14, 2Q, 9

O82 Encounter for cesarean delivery without indication M ♀
Use additional code to indicate outcome of delivery (Z37.Ø)

Complications predominantly related to the puerperium (O85-O92)

EXCLUDES 2 *mental and behavioral disorders associated with the puerperium (F53)*
obstetrical tetanus (A34)
puerperal osteomalacia (M83.Ø)

O85 Puerperal sepsis MCC M ♀
Postpartum sepsis
Puerperal peritonitis
Puerperal pyemia
Use additional code (B95-B97), to identify infectious agent
Use additional code (R65.2-) to identify severe sepsis, if applicable
EXCLUDES 1 *fever of unknown origin following delivery (O86.4)*
genital tract infection following delivery (O86.1-)
obstetric pyemic and septic embolism (O88.3-)
puerperal septic thrombophlebitis (O86.81)
urinary tract infection following delivery (O86.2-)
EXCLUDES 2 *sepsis during labor (O75.3)*
CC Excl: O25.1Ø-O25.3, O26.1Ø-O26.13, O26.3Ø-O26.43, O26.63-O26.819, O26.841-O26.86, O26.891-O26.93, O29.Ø11-O29.93, O35.7XXØ-O35.7XX9, O75.4, O75.81, O75.89-O75.9, O8Ø, O85, O86.12, O86.81-O86.89, O9Ø.89, O99.111-O99.285, O99.33Ø-O99.335, O99.35Ø-O99.355, O99.511-O99.73, O99.82Ø-O99.825, O99.84Ø-O9A.53

O86 Other puerperal infections
Use additional code (B95-B97), to identify infectious agent
EXCLUDES 2 *infection during labor (O75.3)*
obstetrical tetanus (A34)

CC Excl: For CC/MCC codes in category O86, unless otherwise noted: O23.ØØ-O23.93, O25.1Ø-O25.3, O26.1Ø-O26.13, O26.3Ø-O26.43, O26.63-O26.819, O26.841-O26.86, O26.891-O26.93, O29.Ø11-O29.93, O35.7XXØ-O35.7XX9, O75.4, O75.81, O75.89-O75.9, O8Ø, O86.11, O86.13-O86.29, O9Ø.89, O99.111-O99.285, O99.33Ø-O99.335, O99.35Ø-O99.355, O99.511-O99.73, O99.82Ø-O99.825, O99.84Ø-O9A.53

O86.Ø Infection of obstetric surgical wound M ♀
Infected cesarean delivery wound following delivery
Infected perineal repair following delivery

O86.1 Other infection of genital tract following delivery

O86.11 Cervicitis following delivery CC M ♀

O86.12 Endometritis following delivery CC M ♀
CC Excl: O25.1Ø-O25.3, O26.1Ø-O26.13, O26.3Ø-O26.43, O26.63-O26.819, O26.841-O26.86, O26.891-O26.93, O29.Ø11-O29.93, O35.7XXØ-O35.7XX9, O75.4, O75.81, O75.89-O75.9, O8Ø, O85, O86.12, O86.81-O86.89, O9Ø.89, O99.111-O99.285, O99.33Ø-O99.335, O99.35Ø-O99.355, O99.511-O99.73, O99.82Ø-O99.825, O99.84Ø-O9A.53

O86.13 Vaginitis following delivery CC M ♀

O86.19 Other infection of genital tract following delivery CC M ♀

✓5th **O86.2 Urinary tract infection following delivery**

- **O86.20 Urinary tract infection following delivery, unspecified** CC M ♀
  Puerperal urinary tract infection NOS
- **O86.21 Infection of kidney following delivery** CC M ♀
- **O86.22 Infection of bladder following delivery** CC M ♀
  Infection of urethra following delivery
- **O86.29 Other urinary tract infection following delivery** CC M ♀

O86.4 Pyrexia of unknown origin following delivery CC M ♀
Puerperal infection NOS following delivery
Puerperal pyrexia NOS following delivery
EXCLUDES 2 *pyrexia during labor (O75.2)*
CC Excl: O22.20-O22.93, O25.10-O25.3, O26.10-O26.13, O26.30-O26.43, O26.63-O26.819, O26.841-O26.86, O26.891-O26.93, O29.011-O29.93, O35.7XX0-O35.7XX9, O75.4, O75.81, O75.89-O75.9, O80, O86.4, O87.0-O87.3, O87.8-O87.9, O90.89, O99.111-O99.285, O99.330-O99.335, O99.350-O99.355, O99.511-O99.73, O99.820-O99.825, O99.840-O9A.53

✓5th **O86.8 Other specified puerperal infections**

- **O86.81 Puerperal septic thrombophlebitis** MCC M ♀
  CC Excl: See code: O85
- **O86.89 Other specified puerperal infections** MCC M ♀
  CC Excl: See code: O85

✓4th O87 Venous complications and hemorrhoids in the puerperium

Venous complications in labor, delivery and the puerperium
EXCLUDES 2 *obstetric embolism (O88.-)*
puerperal septic thrombophlebitis (O86.81)
venous complications in pregnancy (O22.-)

CC Excl: For CC/MCC codes in category O87, unless otherwise noted: O22.20-O22.93, O25.10-O25.3, O26.10-O26.13, O26.30-O26.43, O26.63-O26.819, O26.841-O26.86, O26.891-O26.93, O29.011-O29.93, O35.7XX0-O35.7XX9, O75.4, O75.81, O75.89-O75.9, O80, O87.0-O87.3, O87.8-O87.9, O90.89, O99.111-O99.285, O99.330-O99.335, O99.350-O99.355, O99.511-O99.73, O99.820-O99.825, O99.840-O9A.53

O87.0 Superficial thrombophlebitis in the puerperium CC M ♀
Puerperal phlebitis NOS
Puerperal thrombosis NOS

O87.1 Deep phlebothrombosis in the puerperium MCC M ♀
Deep vein thrombosis, postpartum
Pelvic thrombophlebitis, postpartum
Use additional code to identify the deep vein thrombosis (I82.4-, I82.5-, I82.62-, I82.72-)
Use additional code, if applicable, for associated long-term (current) use of anticoagulants (Z79.01)

O87.2 Hemorrhoids in the puerperium CC M ♀

O87.3 Cerebral venous thrombosis in the puerperium CC M ♀
Cerebrovenous sinus thrombosis in the puerperium

O87.4 Varicose veins of lower extremity in the puerperium M ♀

O87.8 Other venous complications in the puerperium CC M ♀
Genital varices in the puerperium

O87.9 Venous complication in the puerperium, unspecified M ♀
Puerperal phlebopathy NOS

✓4th O88 Obstetric embolism

EXCLUDES 1 *embolism complicating abortion NOS (O03.2)*
embolism complicating ectopic or molar pregnancy (O08.2)
embolism complicating failed attempted abortion (O07.2)
embolism complicating induced abortion (O04.7)
embolism complicating spontaneous abortion (O03.2, O03.7)

CC Excl: For CC/MCC codes in category O88, unless otherwise noted: O25.10-O25.3, O26.10-O26.13, O26.30-O26.43, O26.63-O26.819, O26.841-O26.86, O26.891-O26.93, O29.011-O29.93, O35.7XX0-O35.7XX9, O75.4, O75.81, O75.89-O75.9, O80, O88.011-O88.83, O90.89, O99.111-O99.285, O99.330-O99.335, O99.350-O99.355, O99.511-O99.73, O99.820-O99.825, O99.840-O9A.53

✓5th **O88.0 Obstetric air embolism**

✓6th **O88.01 Obstetric air embolism in pregnancy**

- **O88.011 Air embolism in pregnancy, first trimester** MCC M ♀
- **O88.012 Air embolism in pregnancy, second trimester** MCC M ♀
- **O88.013 Air embolism in pregnancy, third trimester** MCC M ♀
- **O88.019 Air embolism in pregnancy, unspecified trimester** M ♀

O88.02 Air embolism in childbirth MCC M ♀
O88.03 Air embolism in the puerperium MCC M ♀

✓5th **O88.1 Amniotic fluid embolism**
Anaphylactoid syndrome in pregnancy

✓6th **O88.11 Amniotic fluid embolism in pregnancy**

- **O88.111 Amniotic fluid embolism in pregnancy, first trimester** MCC M ♀
- **O88.112 Amniotic fluid embolism in pregnancy, second trimester** MCC M ♀
- **O88.113 Amniotic fluid embolism in pregnancy, third trimester** MCC M ♀
- **O88.119 Amniotic fluid embolism in pregnancy, unspecified trimester** M ♀

O88.12 Amniotic fluid embolism in childbirth MCC M ♀
O88.13 Amniotic fluid embolism in the puerperium MCC M ♀

✓5th **O88.2 Obstetric thromboembolism**

✓6th **O88.21 Thromboembolism in pregnancy**
Obstetric (pulmonary) embolism NOS

- **O88.211 Thromboembolism in pregnancy, first trimester** MCC M ♀
- **O88.212 Thromboembolism in pregnancy, second trimester** MCC M ♀
- **O88.213 Thromboembolism in pregnancy, third trimester** MCC M ♀
- **O88.219 Thromboembolism in pregnancy, unspecified trimester** M ♀

O88.22 Thromboembolism in childbirth MCC M ♀
O88.23 Thromboembolism in the puerperium MCC M ♀
Puerperal (pulmonary) embolism NOS

✓5th **O88.3 Obstetric pyemic and septic embolism**

✓6th **O88.31 Pyemic and septic embolism in pregnancy**

- **O88.311 Pyemic and septic embolism in pregnancy, first trimester** MCC M ♀
- **O88.312 Pyemic and septic embolism in pregnancy, second trimester** MCC M ♀
- **O88.313 Pyemic and septic embolism in pregnancy, third trimester** MCC M ♀
- **O88.319 Pyemic and septic embolism in pregnancy, unspecified trimester** CC M ♀

O88.32 Pyemic and septic embolism in childbirth MCC M ♀
O88.33 Pyemic and septic embolism in the puerperium MCC M ♀

✓5th **O88.8 Other obstetric embolism**
Obstetric fat embolism

✓6th **O88.81 Other embolism in pregnancy**

- **O88.811 Other embolism in pregnancy, first trimester** MCC M ♀
- **O88.812 Other embolism in pregnancy, second trimester** MCC M ♀
- **O88.813 Other embolism in pregnancy, third trimester** MCC M ♀
- **O88.819 Other embolism in pregnancy, unspecified trimester** M ♀

O88.82 Other embolism in childbirth MCC M ♀
O88.83 Other embolism in the puerperium MCC M ♀

✓4th O89 Complications of anesthesia during the puerperium

INCLUDES maternal complications arising from the administration of a general, regional or local anesthetic, analgesic or other sedation during the puerperium
Use additional code, if applicable, to identify specific complication

✓5th **O89.0 Pulmonary complications of anesthesia during the puerperium**

- **O89.01 Aspiration pneumonitis due to anesthesia during the puerperium** M ♀
  Inhalation of stomach contents or secretions NOS due to anesthesia during the puerperium
  Mendelson's syndrome due to anesthesia during the puerperium
- **O89.09 Other pulmonary complications of anesthesia during the puerperium** M ♀

O89.1 Cardiac complications of anesthesia during the puerperium M ♀
O89.2 Central nervous system complications of anesthesia during the puerperium M ♀
O89.3 Toxic reaction to local anesthesia during the puerperium M ♀
O89.4 Spinal and epidural anesthesia-induced headache during the puerperium M ♀

O89.5 **Other complications of spinal and epidural anesthesia during the puerperium** M♀

O89.6 **Failed or difficult intubation for anesthesia during the puerperium** M♀

O89.8 **Other complications of anesthesia during the puerperium** M♀

O89.9 **Complication of anesthesia during the puerperium, unspecified** M♀

✓4th O9Ø Complications of the puerperium, not elsewhere classified

O9Ø.Ø **Disruption of cesarean delivery wound** M♀
Dehiscence of cesarean delivery wound
EXCLUDES 1 *rupture of uterus (spontaneous) before onset of labor (O71.Ø-)*
rupture of uterus during labor (O71.1)

O9Ø.1 **Disruption of perineal obstetric wound** M♀
Disruption of wound of episiotomy
Disruption of wound of perineal laceration
Secondary perineal tear

O9Ø.2 **Hematoma of obstetric wound** M♀

O9Ø.3 **Peripartum cardiomyopathy** MCC M♀
Conditions in I42- arising during pregnancy and the puerperium
EXCLUDES 1 *pre-existing heart disease complicating pregnancy and the puerperium (O99.4-)*
CC Excl: O25.1Ø-O25.3, O26.1Ø-O26.13, O26.3Ø-O26.43, O26.63-O26.819, O26.841-O26.86, O26.891-O26.93, O29.Ø11-O29.93, O35.7XXØ-O35.7XX9, O75.4, O75.81, O75.89-O75.9, O8Ø, O9Ø.3, O9Ø.89, O99.111-O99.285, O99.33Ø-O99.335, O99.35Ø-O99.73, O99.82Ø-O99.825, O99.84Ø-O9A.53

O9Ø.4 **Postpartum acute kidney failure** MCC M♀
Hepatorenal syndrome following labor and delivery
CC Excl: O25.1Ø-O25.3, O26.1Ø-O26.13, O26.3Ø-O26.43, O26.63-O26.819, O26.841-O26.86, O26.891-O26.93, O29.Ø11-O29.93, O35.7XXØ-O35.7XX9, O75.4, O75.81, O75.89-O75.9, O8Ø, O9Ø.4, O9Ø.89, O99.111-O99.285, O99.33Ø-O99.335, O99.35Ø-O99.355, O99.511-O99.73, O99.82Ø-O99.825, O99.84Ø-O9A.53

O9Ø.5 **Postpartum thyroiditis** M♀

O9Ø.6 **Postpartum mood disturbance** M♀
Postpartum blues
Postpartum dysphoria
Postpartum sadness
EXCLUDES 1 *postpartum depression (F53)*
puerperal psychosis (F53)

✓5th O9Ø.8 **Other complications of the puerperium, not elsewhere classified**

O9Ø.81 **Anemia of the puerperium** M♀
Postpartum anemia NOS
EXCLUDES 1 *pre-existing anemia complicating the puerperium (O99.Ø3)*

O9Ø.89 **Other complications of the puerperium, not elsewhere classified** M♀
Placental polyp

O9Ø.9 **Complication of the puerperium, unspecified** M♀

✓4th O91 Infections of breast associated with pregnancy, the puerperium and lactation
Use additional code to identify infection

✓5th O91.Ø **Infection of nipple associated with pregnancy, the puerperium and lactation**

✓6th O91.Ø1 **Infection of nipple associated with pregnancy**
Gestational abscess of nipple

O91.Ø11 **Infection of nipple associated with pregnancy, first trimester** M♀

O91.Ø12 **Infection of nipple associated with pregnancy, second trimester** M♀

O91.Ø13 **Infection of nipple associated with pregnancy, third trimester** M♀

O91.Ø19 **Infection of nipple associated with pregnancy, unspecified trimester** M♀

O91.Ø2 **Infection of nipple associated with the puerperium** M♀
Puerperal abscess of nipple

O91.Ø3 **Infection of nipple associated with lactation** M♀
Abscess of nipple associated with lactation

✓5th O91.1 **Abscess of breast associated with pregnancy, the puerperium and lactation**

✓6th O91.11 **Abscess of breast associated with pregnancy**
Gestational mammary abscess
Gestational purulent mastitis
Gestational subareolar abscess

O91.111 **Abscess of breast associated with pregnancy, first trimester** M♀

O91.112 **Abscess of breast associated with pregnancy, second trimester** M♀

O91.113 **Abscess of breast associated with pregnancy, third trimester** M♀

O91.119 **Abscess of breast associated with pregnancy, unspecified trimester** M♀

O91.12 **Abscess of breast associated with the puerperium** M♀
Puerperal mammary abscess
Puerperal purulent mastitis
Puerperal subareolar abscess

O91.13 **Abscess of breast associated with lactation** M♀
Mammary abscess associated with lactation
Purulent mastitis associated with lactation
Subareolar abscess associated with lactation

✓5th O91.2 **Nonpurulent mastitis associated with pregnancy, the puerperium and lactation**

✓6th O91.21 **Nonpurulent mastitis associated with pregnancy**
Gestational interstitial mastitis
Gestational lymphangitis of breast
Gestational mastitis NOS
Gestational parenchymatous mastitis

O91.211 **Nonpurulent mastitis associated with pregnancy, first trimester** M♀

O91.212 **Nonpurulent mastitis associated with pregnancy, second trimester** M♀

O91.213 **Nonpurulent mastitis associated with pregnancy, third trimester** M♀

O91.219 **Nonpurulent mastitis associated with pregnancy, unspecified trimester** M♀

O91.22 **Nonpurulent mastitis associated with the puerperium** M♀
Puerperal interstitial mastitis
Puerperal lymphangitis of breast
Puerperal mastitis NOS
Puerperal parenchymatous mastitis

O91.23 **Nonpurulent mastitis associated with lactation** M♀
Interstitial mastitis associated with lactation
Lymphangitis of breast associated with lactation
Mastitis NOS associated with lactation
Parenchymatous mastitis associated with lactation

✓4th O92 Other disorders of breast and disorders of lactation associated with pregnancy and the puerperium

✓5th O92.Ø **Retracted nipple associated with pregnancy, the puerperium, and lactation**

✓6th O92.Ø1 **Retracted nipple associated with pregnancy**

O92.Ø11 **Retracted nipple associated with pregnancy, first trimester** M♀

O92.Ø12 **Retracted nipple associated with pregnancy, second trimester** M♀

O92.Ø13 **Retracted nipple associated with pregnancy, third trimester** M♀

O92.Ø19 **Retracted nipple associated with pregnancy, unspecified trimester** M♀

O92.Ø2 **Retracted nipple associated with the puerperium** M♀

O92.Ø3 **Retracted nipple associated with lactation** M♀

✓5th O92.1 **Cracked nipple associated with pregnancy, the puerperium, and lactation**
Fissure of nipple, gestational or puerperal

✓6th O92.11 **Cracked nipple associated with pregnancy**

O92.111 **Cracked nipple associated with pregnancy, first trimester** M♀

O92.112 **Cracked nipple associated with pregnancy, second trimester** M♀

O92.113 **Cracked nipple associated with pregnancy, third trimester** M♀

O92.119 **Cracked nipple associated with pregnancy, unspecified trimester** M♀

O92.12 **Cracked nipple associated with the puerperium** M♀

O92.13 **Cracked nipple associated with lactation** M♀

✓5th O92.2 **Other and unspecified disorders of breast associated with pregnancy and the puerperium**

O92.2Ø **Unspecified disorder of breast associated with pregnancy and the puerperium** M♀

O92.29 **Other disorders of breast associated with pregnancy and the puerperium** M♀

O92.3 Agalactia M♀
Primary agalactia
EXCLUDES 1 *elective agalactia (O92.5)*
secondary agalactia (O92.5)
therapeutic agalactia (O92.5)

O92.4 Hypogalactia M♀

O92.5 Suppressed lactation M♀
Elective agalactia
Secondary agalactia
Therapeutic agalactia
EXCLUDES 1 *primary agalactia (O92.3)*

O92.6 Galactorrhea M♀

✓5th **O92.7 Other and unspecified disorders of lactation**
O92.70 Unspecified disorders of lactation M♀
O92.79 Other disorders of lactation M♀
Puerperal galactocele

Other obstetric conditions, not elsewhere classified (O94-O9A)

O94 Sequelae of complication of pregnancy, childbirth, and the puerperium M♀
NOTE This category is to be used to indicate conditions in O00-O77.-, O85-O94 and O98-O9A.- as the cause of late effects. The sequelae include conditions specified as such, or as late effects, which may occur at any time after the puerperium.
Code first condition resulting from (sequela) of complication of pregnancy, childbirth, and the puerperium

✓4th **O98 Maternal infectious and parasitic diseases classifiable elsewhere but complicating pregnancy, childbirth and the puerperium**
INCLUDES the listed conditions when complicating the pregnant state, when aggravated by the pregnancy, or as a reason for obstetric care
Use additional code (Chapter 1), to identify specific infectious or parasitic disease
EXCLUDES 2 *herpes gestationis (O26.4-)*
infectious carrier state (O99.82-, O99.83-)
obstetrical tetanus (A34)
puerperal infection (O86.-)
puerperal sepsis (O85)
when the reason for maternal care is that the disease is known or suspected to have affected the fetus (O35-O36)

✓5th **O98.0 Tuberculosis complicating pregnancy, childbirth and the puerperium**
Conditions in A15-A19

CC Excl: For CC codes in subcategory O98.0, unless otherwise noted: O25.10-O25.3, O26.10-O26.13, O26.30-O26.43, O26.63-O26.819, O26.841-O26.86, O26.891-O26.93, O29.011-O29.93, O35.7XX0-O35.7XX9, O75.4, O75.81, O75.89-O75.9, O80, O90.89, O98.011-O98.03, O99.111-O99.285, O99.330-O99.335, O99.350-O99.355, O99.511-O99.73, O99.820-O99.825, O99.840-O9A.53

✓6th **O98.01 Tuberculosis complicating pregnancy**
O98.011 Tuberculosis complicating pregnancy, first trimester CC M♀
O98.012 Tuberculosis complicating pregnancy, second trimester CC M♀
O98.013 Tuberculosis complicating pregnancy, third trimester CC M♀
O98.019 Tuberculosis complicating pregnancy, unspecified trimester M♀

O98.02 Tuberculosis complicating childbirth CC M♀
O98.03 Tuberculosis complicating the puerperium CC M♀

✓5th **O98.1 Syphilis complicating pregnancy, childbirth and the puerperium**
Conditions in A50-A53

CC Excl: For CC codes in subcategory O98.1, unless otherwise noted: O26.11-O26.13, O26.31-O26.33, O26.41-O26.43, O26.63-O26.713, O26.72-O26.813, O26.86, O26.891-O26.893, O26.90-O26.93, O29.011-O29.013, O29.021-O29.023, O29.091-O29.093, O29.111-O29.113, O29.121-O29.123, O29.191-O29.193, O29.211-O29.213, O29.291-O29.293, O29.3X1-O29.3X3, O29.41-O29.5X3, O29.61-O29.8X3, O29.91-O29.93, O35.7XX0-O35.7XX9, O98.111-O98.33, O99.351-O99.353, O99.355, O99.89

✓6th **O98.11 Syphilis complicating pregnancy**
O98.111 Syphilis complicating pregnancy, first trimester CC M♀
O98.112 Syphilis complicating pregnancy, second trimester CC M♀
O98.113 Syphilis complicating pregnancy, third trimester CC M♀
O98.119 Syphilis complicating pregnancy, unspecified trimester M♀

O98.12 Syphilis complicating childbirth CC M♀
O98.13 Syphilis complicating the puerperium CC M♀

✓5th **O98.2 Gonorrhea complicating pregnancy, childbirth and the puerperium**
Conditions in A54-

CC Excl: For CC codes in subcategory O98.2, unless otherwise noted: See code: O98.1

✓6th **O98.21 Gonorrhea complicating pregnancy**
O98.211 Gonorrhea complicating pregnancy, first trimester CC M♀
O98.212 Gonorrhea complicating pregnancy, second trimester CC M♀
O98.213 Gonorrhea complicating pregnancy, third trimester CC M♀
O98.219 Gonorrhea complicating pregnancy, unspecified trimester M♀

O98.22 Gonorrhea complicating childbirth CC M♀
O98.23 Gonorrhea complicating the puerperium CC M♀

✓5th **O98.3 Other infections with a predominantly sexual mode of transmission complicating pregnancy, childbirth and the puerperium**
Conditions in A55-A64

CC Excl: For CC codes in subcategory O98.3, unless otherwise noted: See code: O98.1

✓6th **O98.31 Other infections with a predominantly sexual mode of transmission complicating pregnancy**
O98.311 Other infections with a predominantly sexual mode of transmission complicating pregnancy, first trimester CC M♀
O98.312 Other infections with a predominantly sexual mode of transmission complicating pregnancy, second trimester CC M♀
O98.313 Other infections with a predominantly sexual mode of transmission complicating pregnancy, third trimester CC M♀
O98.319 Other infections with a predominantly sexual mode of transmission complicating pregnancy, unspecified trimester M♀

O98.32 Other infections with a predominantly sexual mode of transmission complicating childbirth CC M♀
O98.33 Other infections with a predominantly sexual mode of transmission complicating the puerperium CC M♀

✓5th **O98.4 Viral hepatitis complicating pregnancy, childbirth and the puerperium**
Conditions in B15-B19

CC Excl: For CC codes in subcategory O98.4, unless otherwise noted: O98.411-O98.613, O98.711-O98.93, O99.830-O99.835

✓6th **O98.41 Viral hepatitis complicating pregnancy**
O98.411 Viral hepatitis complicating pregnancy, first trimester CC M♀
O98.412 Viral hepatitis complicating pregnancy, second trimester CC M♀
O98.413 Viral hepatitis complicating pregnancy, third trimester CC M♀
O98.419 Viral hepatitis complicating pregnancy, unspecified trimester M♀

O98.42 Viral hepatitis complicating childbirth CC M♀
O98.43 Viral hepatitis complicating the puerperium CC M♀

✓5th **O98.5 Other viral diseases complicating pregnancy, childbirth and the puerperium**
Conditions in A80-B09, B25-B34, R87.81-, R87.82-
EXCLUDES 1 *human immunodeficiency virus [HIV] disease complicating pregnancy, childbirth and the puerperium (O98.7-)*

CC Excl: For CC codes in subcategory O98.5, unless otherwise noted: See code: O98.4

✓6th **O98.51 Other viral diseases complicating pregnancy**
O98.511 Other viral diseases complicating pregnancy, first trimester CC M♀

O98.512 Other viral diseases complicating pregnancy, second trimester CC M ♀

O98.513 Other viral diseases complicating pregnancy, third trimester CC M ♀

O98.519 Other viral diseases complicating pregnancy, unspecified trimester M ♀

O98.52 Other viral diseases complicating childbirth CC M ♀

O98.53 Other viral diseases complicating the puerperium CC M ♀

✓5th **O98.6 Protozoal diseases complicating pregnancy, childbirth and the puerperium**

Conditions in B5Ø-B64

CC Excl: For CC codes in subcategory O98.6, unless otherwise noted: O25.1Ø-O25.3, O26.1Ø-O26.13, O26.3Ø-O26.43, O26.63-O26.819, O26.841-O26.86, O26.891-O26.93, O29.Ø11-O29.93, O35.7XXØ-O35.7XX9, O75.4, O75.81, O75.89-O75.9, O8Ø, O9Ø.89, O98.411-O98.93, O99.111-O99.285, O99.33Ø-O99.335, O99.35Ø-O99.355, O99.511-O99.73, O99.82Ø-O9A.53

✓6th **O98.61 Protozoal diseases complicating pregnancy**

O98.611 Protozoal diseases complicating pregnancy, first trimester CC M ♀

O98.612 Protozoal diseases complicating pregnancy, second trimester CC M ♀

O98.613 Protozoal diseases complicating pregnancy, third trimester CC M ♀

O98.619 Protozoal diseases complicating pregnancy, unspecified trimester M ♀

O98.62 Protozoal diseases complicating childbirth CC M ♀

CC Excl: O25.1Ø-O25.3, O26.1Ø-O26.13, O26.3Ø-O26.43, O26.63-O26.819, O26.841-O26.86, O26.891-O26.93, O29.Ø11-O29.93, O35.7XXØ-O35.7XX9, O75.4, O75.81, O75.89-O75.9, O8Ø, O9Ø.89, O98.611-O98.63, O99.111-O99.285, O99.33Ø-O99.335, O99.35Ø-O99.355, O99.511-O99.73, O99.82Ø-O99.825, O99.84Ø-O9A.53

O98.63 Protozoal diseases complicating the puerperium CC M ♀

CC Excl: See code: O98.62

✓5th **O98.7 Human immunodeficiency virus [HIV] disease complicating pregnancy, childbirth and the puerperium**

Use additional code to identify the type of HIV disease:
- acquired immune deficiency syndrome (AIDS) (B2Ø)
- asymptomatic HIV status (Z21)
- HIV positive NOS (Z21)
- symptomatic HIV disease (B2Ø)

CC Excl: For CC codes in subcategory O98.7, unless otherwise noted: O98.411-O98.613, O98.711-O98.93, O99.83Ø-O99.835

✓6th **O98.71 Human immunodeficiency virus [HIV] disease complicating pregnancy**

O98.711 Human immunodeficiency virus [HIV] disease complicating pregnancy, first trimester CC M ♀

O98.712 Human immunodeficiency virus [HIV] disease complicating pregnancy, second trimester CC M ♀

O98.713 Human immunodeficiency virus [HIV] disease complicating pregnancy, third trimester CC M ♀

O98.719 Human immunodeficiency virus [HIV] disease complicating pregnancy, unspecified trimester M ♀

O98.72 Human immunodeficiency virus [HIV] disease complicating childbirth CC M ♀

O98.73 Human immunodeficiency virus [HIV] disease complicating the puerperium CC M ♀

✓5th **O98.8 Other maternal infectious and parasitic diseases complicating pregnancy, childbirth and the puerperium**

CC Excl: For CC codes in subcategory O98.8, unless otherwise noted: See code: O98.7

✓6th **O98.81 Other maternal infectious and parasitic diseases complicating pregnancy**

O98.811 Other maternal infectious and parasitic diseases complicating pregnancy, first trimester CC M ♀

O98.812 Other maternal infectious and parasitic diseases complicating pregnancy, second trimester CC M ♀

O98.813 Other maternal infectious and parasitic diseases complicating pregnancy, third trimester CC M ♀

O98.819 Other maternal infectious and parasitic diseases complicating pregnancy, unspecified trimester M ♀

O98.82 Other maternal infectious and parasitic diseases complicating childbirth CC M ♀

O98.83 Other maternal infectious and parasitic diseases complicating the puerperium CC M ♀

✓5th **O98.9 Unspecified maternal infectious and parasitic disease complicating pregnancy, childbirth and the puerperium**

CC Excl: For CC codes in subcategory O98.9, unless otherwise noted: See code: O98.7

✓6th **O98.91 Unspecified maternal infectious and parasitic disease complicating pregnancy**

O98.911 Unspecified maternal infectious and parasitic disease complicating pregnancy, first trimester CC M ♀

O98.912 Unspecified maternal infectious and parasitic disease complicating pregnancy, second trimester CC M ♀

O98.913 Unspecified maternal infectious and parasitic disease complicating pregnancy, third trimester CC M ♀

O98.919 Unspecified maternal infectious and parasitic disease complicating pregnancy, unspecified trimester M ♀

O98.92 Unspecified maternal infectious and parasitic disease complicating childbirth CC M ♀

O98.93 Unspecified maternal infectious and parasitic disease complicating the puerperium CC M ♀

✓4th **O99 Other maternal diseases classifiable elsewhere but complicating pregnancy, childbirth and the puerperium**

INCLUDES conditions which complicate the pregnant state, are aggravated by the pregnancy or are a main reason for obstetric care

Use additional code to identify specific condition

EXCLUDES 2 *when the reason for maternal care is that the condition is known or suspected to have affected the fetus (O35-O36)*

✓5th **O99.Ø Anemia complicating pregnancy, childbirth and the puerperium**

Conditions in D5Ø-D64

EXCLUDES 1 *anemia arising in the puerperium (O9Ø.81)*
postpartum anemia NOS (O9Ø.81)

✓6th **O99.Ø1 Anemia complicating pregnancy**

O99.Ø11 Anemia complicating pregnancy, first trimester M ♀

O99.Ø12 Anemia complicating pregnancy, second trimester M ♀

O99.Ø13 Anemia complicating pregnancy, third trimester M ♀

O99.Ø19 Anemia complicating pregnancy, unspecified trimester M ♀

O99.Ø2 Anemia complicating childbirth M ♀

O99.Ø3 Anemia complicating the puerperium M ♀

EXCLUDES 1 *postpartum anemia not pre-existing prior to delivery (O9Ø.81)*

✓5th **O99.1 Other diseases of the blood and blood-forming organs and certain disorders involving the immune mechanism complicating pregnancy, childbirth and the puerperium**

Conditions in D65-D89

EXCLUDES 2 *hemorrhage with coagulation defects (O45.-, O46.Ø-, O67.Ø, O72.3)*

CC Excl: For CC codes in subcategory O99.1, unless otherwise noted: O25.11-O25.3, O99.281-O99.285, O99.511-O99.513, O99.52-O99.613, O99.62-O99.713, O99.72-O99.73, O99.82Ø-O99.825, O9A.111-O9A.113, O9A.12-O9A.213, O9A.22-O9A.313, O9A.32-O9A.413, O9A.42-O9A.513, O9A.52-O9A.53

✓6th **O99.11 Other diseases of the blood and blood-forming organs and certain disorders involving the immune mechanism complicating pregnancy**

O99.111 Other diseases of the blood and blood-forming organs and certain disorders involving the immune mechanism complicating pregnancy, first trimester CC M ♀

O99.112 **Other diseases of the blood and blood-forming organs and certain disorders involving the immune mechanism complicating pregnancy, second trimester** CC M ♀

O99.113 **Other diseases of the blood and blood-forming organs and certain disorders involving the immune mechanism complicating pregnancy, third trimester** CC M ♀

O99.119 **Other diseases of the blood and blood-forming organs and certain disorders involving the immune mechanism complicating pregnancy, unspecified trimester** CC M ♀
CC Excl: O25.10-O99.280, O99.519, O99.619, O99.719, O9A.119, O9A.219, O9A.319, O9A.419, O9A.519

O99.12 **Other diseases of the blood and blood-forming organs and certain disorders involving the immune mechanism complicating childbirth** CC M ♀

O99.13 **Other diseases of the blood and blood-forming organs and certain disorders involving the immune mechanism complicating the puerperium** CC M ♀

✓5th **O99.2 Endocrine, nutritional and metabolic diseases complicating pregnancy, childbirth and the puerperium**
Conditions in E00-E88
EXCLUDES 2 *diabetes mellitus (O24.-)*
malnutrition (O25.-)
postpartum thyroiditis (O90.5)

✓6th **O99.21 Obesity complicating pregnancy, childbirth, and the puerperium**
Use additional code to identify the type of obesity (E66.-)

O99.210 **Obesity complicating pregnancy, unspecified trimester** M ♀

O99.211 **Obesity complicating pregnancy, first trimester** M ♀

O99.212 **Obesity complicating pregnancy, second trimester** M ♀

O99.213 **Obesity complicating pregnancy, third trimester** M ♀

O99.214 **Obesity complicating childbirth** M ♀

O99.215 **Obesity complicating the puerperium** M ♀

✓6th **O99.28 Other endocrine, nutritional and metabolic diseases complicating pregnancy, childbirth and the puerperium**

O99.280 **Endocrine, nutritional and metabolic diseases complicating pregnancy, unspecified trimester** M ♀

O99.281 **Endocrine, nutritional and metabolic diseases complicating pregnancy, first trimester** M ♀

O99.282 **Endocrine, nutritional and metabolic diseases complicating pregnancy, second trimester** M ♀

O99.283 **Endocrine, nutritional and metabolic diseases complicating pregnancy, third trimester** M ♀

O99.284 **Endocrine, nutritional and metabolic diseases complicating childbirth** M ♀

O99.285 **Endocrine, nutritional and metabolic diseases complicating the puerperium** M ♀

✓5th **O99.3 Mental disorders and diseases of the nervous system complicating pregnancy, childbirth and the puerperium**

CC Excl: For CC codes in subcategory O99.3, unless otherwise noted: O25.10-O25.3, O26.10-O26.13, O26.30-O26.43, O26.63-O26.819, O26.841-O26.86, O26.891-O26.93, O29.011-O29.93, O35.7XX0-O35.7XX9, O75.4, O75.81, O75.89-O75.9, O80, O90.89, O99.111-O99.285, O99.320-O99.335, O99.350-O99.355, O99.511-O99.73, O99.820-O99.825, O99.840-O9A.53

✓6th **O99.31 Alcohol use complicating pregnancy, childbirth, and the puerperium**
Use additional code(s) from F10 to identify manifestations of the alcohol use

O99.310 **Alcohol use complicating pregnancy, unspecified trimester** M ♀

O99.311 **Alcohol use complicating pregnancy, first trimester** M ♀

O99.312 **Alcohol use complicating pregnancy, second trimester** M ♀

O99.313 **Alcohol use complicating pregnancy, third trimester** M ♀

O99.314 **Alcohol use complicating childbirth** M ♀

O99.315 **Alcohol use complicating the puerperium** M ♀

✓6th **O99.32 Drug use complicating pregnancy, childbirth, and the puerperium**
Use additional code(s) from F11-F16 and F18-F19 to identify manifestations of the drug use

O99.320 **Drug use complicating pregnancy, unspecified trimester** M ♀

O99.321 **Drug use complicating pregnancy, first trimester** CC M ♀

O99.322 **Drug use complicating pregnancy, second trimester** CC M ♀

O99.323 **Drug use complicating pregnancy, third trimester** CC M ♀

O99.324 **Drug use complicating childbirth** CC M ♀

O99.325 **Drug use complicating the puerperium** CC M ♀

✓6th **O99.33 Smoking (tobacco) complicating pregnancy, childbirth, and the puerperium**
Use additional code from F17 to identify type of tobacco

O99.330 **Smoking (tobacco) complicating pregnancy, unspecified trimester** M ♀

O99.331 **Smoking (tobacco) complicating pregnancy, first trimester** M ♀

O99.332 **Smoking (tobacco) complicating pregnancy, second trimester** M ♀

O99.333 **Smoking (tobacco) complicating pregnancy, third trimester** M ♀

O99.334 **Smoking (tobacco) complicating childbirth** M ♀

O99.335 **Smoking (tobacco) complicating the puerperium** M ♀

✓6th **O99.34 Other mental disorders complicating pregnancy, childbirth, and the puerperium**
Conditions in F01-F09 and F20-F99
EXCLUDES 2 *postpartum mood disturbance (O90.6)*
postnatal psychosis (F53)
puerperal psychosis (F53)

O99.340 **Other mental disorders complicating pregnancy, unspecified trimester** M ♀

O99.341 **Other mental disorders complicating pregnancy, first trimester** M ♀

O99.342 **Other mental disorders complicating pregnancy, second trimester** M ♀

O99.343 **Other mental disorders complicating pregnancy, third trimester** M ♀

O99.344 **Other mental disorders complicating childbirth** M ♀

O99.345 **Other mental disorders complicating the puerperium** M ♀

✓6th **O99.35 Diseases of the nervous system complicating pregnancy, childbirth, and the puerperium**
Conditions in G00-G99
EXCLUDES 2 *pregnancy related peripheral neuritis (O26.8-)*

O99.350 **Diseases of the nervous system complicating pregnancy, unspecified trimester** M ♀

O99.351 **Diseases of the nervous system complicating pregnancy, first trimester** M ♀

O99.352 **Diseases of the nervous system complicating pregnancy, second trimester** M ♀

O99.353 **Diseases of the nervous system complicating pregnancy, third trimester** M ♀

O99.354 **Diseases of the nervous system complicating childbirth** CC M ♀
CC Excl: See code: O99.1

O99.355 **Diseases of the nervous system complicating the puerperium** CC M ♀
CC Excl: See code: O99.1

✓5th **O99.4 Diseases of the circulatory system complicating pregnancy, childbirth and the puerperium**
Conditions in IØØ-I99
EXCLUDES 1 *peripartum cardiomyopathy (O9Ø.3)*
EXCLUDES 2 *hypertensive disorders (O1Ø-O16)*
obstetric embolism (O88.-)
venous complications and cerebrovenous sinus thrombosis in labor, childbirth and the puerperium (O87.-)
venous complications and cerebrovenous sinus thrombosis in pregnancy (O22.-)

CC Excl: For CC codes in subcategory O99.4, unless otherwise noted: O25.1Ø-O25.3, O26.1Ø-O26.13, O26.3Ø-O26.43, O26.63-O26.819, O26.841-O26.86, O26.891-O26.93, O29.Ø11-O29.93, O35.7XXØ-O35.7XX9, O75.4, O75.81, O75.89-O75.9, O8Ø, O9Ø.3, O9Ø.89, O99.111-O99.285, O99.33Ø-O99.335, O99.35Ø-O99.73, O99.82Ø-O99.825, O99.84Ø-O9A.53

✓6th **O99.41 Diseases of the circulatory system complicating pregnancy**
O99.411 **Diseases of the circulatory system complicating pregnancy, first trimester** CC M ♀
O99.412 **Diseases of the circulatory system complicating pregnancy, second trimester** CC M ♀
O99.413 **Diseases of the circulatory system complicating pregnancy, third trimester** CC M ♀
O99.419 **Diseases of the circulatory system complicating pregnancy, unspecified trimester** M ♀

O99.42 **Diseases of the circulatory system complicating childbirth** MCC M ♀
CC Excl: See code: O9Ø.3

O99.43 **Diseases of the circulatory system complicating the puerperium** CC M ♀

✓5th **O99.5 Diseases of the respiratory system complicating pregnancy, childbirth and the puerperium**
Conditions in JØØ-J99

✓6th **O99.51 Diseases of the respiratory system complicating pregnancy**
O99.511 **Diseases of the respiratory system complicating pregnancy, first trimester** M ♀
O99.512 **Diseases of the respiratory system complicating pregnancy, second trimester** M ♀
O99.513 **Diseases of the respiratory system complicating pregnancy, third trimester** M ♀
O99.519 **Diseases of the respiratory system complicating pregnancy, unspecified trimester** M ♀

O99.52 **Diseases of the respiratory system complicating childbirth** M ♀
O99.53 **Diseases of the respiratory system complicating the puerperium** M ♀

✓5th **O99.6 Diseases of the digestive system complicating pregnancy, childbirth and the puerperium**
Conditions in KØØ-K93
EXCLUDES 2 *liver and biliary tract disorders in pregnancy, childbirth and the puerperium (O26.6-)*

✓6th **O99.61 Diseases of the digestive system complicating pregnancy**
O99.611 **Diseases of the digestive system complicating pregnancy, first trimester** M ♀
O99.612 **Diseases of the digestive system complicating pregnancy, second trimester** M ♀
O99.613 **Diseases of the digestive system complicating pregnancy, third trimester** M ♀
O99.619 **Diseases of the digestive system complicating pregnancy, unspecified trimester** M ♀

O99.62 **Diseases of the digestive system complicating childbirth** M ♀
O99.63 **Diseases of the digestive system complicating the puerperium** M ♀

✓5th **O99.7 Diseases of the skin and subcutaneous tissue complicating pregnancy, childbirth and the puerperium**
Conditions in LØØ-L99
EXCLUDES 2 *herpes gestationis (O26.4)*
pruritic urticarial papules and plaques of pregnancy (PUPPP) (O26.86)

✓6th **O99.71 Diseases of the skin and subcutaneous tissue complicating pregnancy**
O99.711 **Diseases of the skin and subcutaneous tissue complicating pregnancy, first trimester** M ♀
O99.712 **Diseases of the skin and subcutaneous tissue complicating pregnancy, second trimester** M ♀
O99.713 **Diseases of the skin and subcutaneous tissue complicating pregnancy, third trimester** M ♀
O99.719 **Diseases of the skin and subcutaneous tissue complicating pregnancy, unspecified trimester** M ♀

O99.72 **Diseases of the skin and subcutaneous tissue complicating childbirth** M ♀
O99.73 **Diseases of the skin and subcutaneous tissue complicating the puerperium** M ♀

✓5th **O99.8 Other specified diseases and conditions complicating pregnancy, childbirth and the puerperium**
Conditions in DØØ-D48, HØØ-H95, MØØ-N99, and QØØ-Q99
Use additional code to identify condition
EXCLUDES 2 *genitourinary infections in pregnancy (O23.-)*
infection of genitourinary tract following delivery (O86.1-O86.3)
malignant neoplasm complicating pregnancy, childbirth and the puerperium (O9A.1-)
maternal care for known or suspected abnormality of maternal pelvic organs (O34.-)
postpartum acute kidney failure (O9Ø.4)
traumatic injuries in pregnancy (O9A.2)

CC Excl: For CC codes in subcategory O99.8, unless otherwise noted: O98.411-O98.613, O98.711-O98.93, O99.83Ø-O99.835

✓6th **O99.81 Abnormal glucose complicating pregnancy, childbirth and the puerperium**
EXCLUDES 1 *gestational diabetes (O24.4-)*
O99.81Ø **Abnormal glucose complicating pregnancy** M ♀
O99.814 **Abnormal glucose complicating childbirth** M ♀
O99.815 **Abnormal glucose complicating the puerperium** M ♀

✓6th **O99.82 Streptococcus B carrier state complicating pregnancy, childbirth and the puerperium**
O99.82Ø **Streptococcus B carrier state complicating pregnancy** M ♀
O99.824 **Streptococcus B carrier state complicating childbirth** M ♀
O99.825 **Streptococcus B carrier state complicating the puerperium** M ♀

✓6th **O99.83 Other infection carrier state complicating pregnancy, childbirth and the puerperium**
Use additional code to identify the carrier state (Z22.-)
O99.83Ø **Other infection carrier state complicating pregnancy** CC M ♀
O99.834 **Other infection carrier state complicating childbirth** CC M ♀
O99.835 **Other infection carrier state complicating the puerperium** CC M ♀

✓6th **O99.84 Bariatric surgery status complicating pregnancy, childbirth and the puerperium**
Gastric banding status complicating pregnancy, childbirth and the puerperium
Gastric bypass status for obesity complicating pregnancy, childbirth and the puerperium
Obesity surgery status complicating pregnancy, childbirth and the puerperium
O99.84Ø **Bariatric surgery status complicating pregnancy, unspecified trimester** M ♀

O99.841 Bariatric surgery status complicating pregnancy, first trimester M♀

O99.842 Bariatric surgery status complicating pregnancy, second trimester M♀

O99.843 Bariatric surgery status complicating pregnancy, third trimester M♀

O99.844 Bariatric surgery status complicating childbirth M♀

O99.845 Bariatric surgery status complicating the puerperium M♀

O99.89 Other specified diseases and conditions complicating pregnancy, childbirth and the puerperium M♀

✓4th O9A Maternal malignant neoplasms, traumatic injuries and abuse classifiable elsewhere but complicating pregnancy, childbirth and the puerperium

✓5th O9A.1 Malignant neoplasm complicating pregnancy, childbirth and the puerperium

Conditions in C00-C96

Use additional code to identify neoplasm

EXCLUDES 2 *maternal care for benign tumor of corpus uteri (O34.1-)*
maternal care for benign tumor of cervix (O34.4-)

✓6th O9A.11 Malignant neoplasm complicating pregnancy

O9A.111 Malignant neoplasm complicating pregnancy, first trimester M♀

O9A.112 Malignant neoplasm complicating pregnancy, second trimester M♀

O9A.113 Malignant neoplasm complicating pregnancy, third trimester M♀

O9A.119 Malignant neoplasm complicating pregnancy, unspecified trimester M♀

O9A.12 Malignant neoplasm complicating childbirth M♀

O9A.13 Malignant neoplasm complicating the puerperium M♀

✓5th O9A.2 Injury, poisoning and certain other consequences of external causes complicating pregnancy, childbirth and the puerperium

Conditions in S00-T88, except T74 and T76

Use additional code(s) to identify the injury or poisoning

EXCLUDES 2 *physical, sexual and psychological abuse complicating pregnancy, childbirth and the puerperium (O9A.3-, O9A.4-, O9A.5-)*

✓6th O9A.21 Injury, poisoning and certain other consequences of external causes complicating pregnancy

O9A.211 Injury, poisoning and certain other consequences of external causes complicating pregnancy, first trimester M♀

O9A.212 Injury, poisoning and certain other consequences of external causes complicating pregnancy, second trimester M♀

O9A.213 Injury, poisoning and certain other consequences of external causes complicating pregnancy, third trimester M♀

O9A.219 Injury, poisoning and certain other consequences of external causes complicating pregnancy, unspecified trimester M♀

O9A.22 Injury, poisoning and certain other consequences of external causes complicating childbirth M♀

O9A.23 Injury, poisoning and certain other consequences of external causes complicating the puerperium M♀

✓5th O9A.3 Physical abuse complicating pregnancy, childbirth and the puerperium

Conditions in T74.11 or T76.11

Use additional code (if applicable):
to identify any associated current injury due to physical abuse
to identify the perpetrator of abuse (Y07.-)

EXCLUDES 2 *sexual abuse complicating pregnancy, childbirth and the puerperium (O9A.4)*

✓6th O9A.31 Physical abuse complicating pregnancy

O9A.311 Physical abuse complicating pregnancy, first trimester M♀

O9A.312 Physical abuse complicating pregnancy, second trimester M♀

O9A.313 Physical abuse complicating pregnancy, third trimester M♀

O9A.319 Physical abuse complicating pregnancy, unspecified trimester M♀

O9A.32 Physical abuse complicating childbirth M♀

O9A.33 Physical abuse complicating the puerperium M♀

✓5th O9A.4 Sexual abuse complicating pregnancy, childbirth and the puerperium

Conditions in T74.21 or T76.21

Use additional code (if applicable):
to identify any associated current injury due to sexual abuse
to identify the perpetrator of abuse (Y07.-)

✓6th O9A.41 Sexual abuse complicating pregnancy

O9A.411 Sexual abuse complicating pregnancy, first trimester M♀

O9A.412 Sexual abuse complicating pregnancy, second trimester M♀

O9A.413 Sexual abuse complicating pregnancy, third trimester M♀

O9A.419 Sexual abuse complicating pregnancy, unspecified trimester M♀

O9A.42 Sexual abuse complicating childbirth M♀

O9A.43 Sexual abuse complicating the puerperium M♀

✓5th O9A.5 Psychological abuse complicating pregnancy, childbirth and the puerperium

Conditions in T74.31 or T76.31

Use additional code to identify the perpetrator of abuse (Y07.-)

✓6th O9A.51 Psychological abuse complicating pregnancy

O9A.511 Psychological abuse complicating pregnancy, first trimester M♀

O9A.512 Psychological abuse complicating pregnancy, second trimester M♀

O9A.513 Psychological abuse complicating pregnancy, third trimester M♀

O9A.519 Psychological abuse complicating pregnancy, unspecified trimester M♀

O9A.52 Psychological abuse complicating childbirth M♀

O9A.53 Psychological abuse complicating the puerperium M♀

Chapter 16. Certain Conditions Originating in the Perinatal Period (P00-P96)

NOTE Codes from this chapter are for use on newborn records only, never on maternal records.

INCLUDES conditions that have their origin in the fetal or perinatal period (before birth through the first 28 days after birth) even if morbidity occurs later

EXCLUDES 2 *congenital malformations, deformations and chromosomal abnormalities (Q00-Q99)*
endocrine, nutritional and metabolic diseases (E00-E88)
injury, poisoning and certain other consequences of external causes (S00-T88)
neoplasms (C00-D49)
tetanus neonatorum (A33)

This chapter contains the following blocks:

- P00-P04 Newborn affected by maternal factors and by complications of pregnancy, labor, and delivery
- P05-P08 Disorders of newborn related to length of gestation and fetal growth
- P09 Abnormal findings on neonatal screening
- P10-P15 Birth trauma
- P19-P29 Respiratory and cardiovascular disorders specific to the perinatal period
- P35-P39 Infections specific to the perinatal period
- P50-P61 Hemorrhagic and hematological disorders of newborn
- P70-P74 Transitory endocrine and metabolic disorders specific to newborn
- P76-P78 Digestive system disorders of newborn
- P80-P83 Conditions involving the integument and temperature regulation of newborn
- P84 Other problems with newborn
- P90-P96 Other disorders originating in the perinatal period

Newborn affected by maternal factors and by complications of pregnancy, labor, and delivery (P00-P04)

NOTE These codes are for use when the listed maternal conditions are specified as the cause of confirmed morbidity or potential morbidity which have their origin in the perinatal period (before birth through the first 28 days after birth). Codes from these categories are also for use for newborns who are suspected of having an abnormal condition resulting from exposure from the mother or the birth process, but without signs or symptoms, and, which after examination and observation, is found not to exist. These codes may be used even if treatment is begun for a suspected condition that is ruled out.

✓4th **P00 Newborn (suspected to be) affected by maternal conditions that may be unrelated to present pregnancy**
Code first any current condition in newborn
EXCLUDES 2 *newborn (suspected to be) affected by maternal complications of pregnancy (P01.-)*
newborn affected by maternal endocrine and metabolic disorders (P70-P74)
newborn affected by noxious substances transmitted via placenta or breast milk (P04.-)

P00.0 Newborn (suspected to be) affected by maternal hypertensive disorders N
Newborn (suspected to be) affected by maternal conditions classifiable to O10-O11, O13-O16

P00.1 Newborn (suspected to be) affected by maternal renal and urinary tract diseases N
Newborn (suspected to be) affected by maternal conditions classifiable to N00-N39

P00.2 Newborn (suspected to be) affected by maternal infectious and parasitic diseases N
Newborn (suspected to be) affected by maternal infectious disease classifiable to A00-B99, J09 and J10
EXCLUDES 1 *infections specific to the perinatal period (P35-P39)*
maternal genital tract or other localized infections (P00.8)

P00.3 Newborn (suspected to be) affected by other maternal circulatory and respiratory diseases N
Newborn (suspected to be) affected by maternal conditions classifiable to I00-I99, J00-J99, Q20-Q34 and not included in P00.0, P00.2

P00.4 Newborn (suspected to be) affected by maternal nutritional disorders N
Newborn (suspected to be) affected by maternal disorders classifiable to E40-E64
Maternal malnutrition NOS

P00.5 Newborn (suspected to be) affected by maternal injury N
Newborn (suspected to be) affected by maternal conditions classifiable to O9A.2-

P00.6 Newborn (suspected to be) affected by surgical procedure on mother N
Newborn (suspected to be) affected by amniocentesis
EXCLUDES 1 *Cesarean delivery for present delivery (P03.4)*
damage to placenta from amniocentesis, Cesarean delivery or surgical induction (P02.1)
previous surgery to uterus or pelvic organs (P03.89)
EXCLUDES 2 *newborn affected by complication of (fetal) intrauterine procedure (P96.5)*

P00.7 Newborn (suspected to be) affected by other medical procedures on mother, not elsewhere classified N
Newborn (suspected to be) affected by radiation to mother
EXCLUDES 1 *damage to placenta from amniocentesis, cesarean delivery or surgical induction (P02.1)*
newborn affected by other complications of labor and delivery (P03.-)

✓5th **P00.8 Newborn (suspected to be) affected by other maternal conditions**

P00.81 Newborn (suspected to be) affected by periodontal disease in mother N

P00.89 Newborn (suspected to be) affected by other maternal conditions N
Newborn (suspected to be) affected by conditions classifiable to T80-T88
Newborn (suspected to be) affected by maternal genital tract or other localized infections
Newborn (suspected to be) affected by maternal systemic lupus erythematosus

P00.9 Newborn (suspected to be) affected by unspecified maternal condition N

✓4th **P01 Newborn (suspected to be) affected by maternal complications of pregnancy**
Code first any current condition in newborn

P01.0 Newborn (suspected to be) affected by incompetent cervix N

P01.1 Newborn (suspected to be) affected by premature rupture of membranes N

P01.2 Newborn (suspected to be) affected by oligohydramnios N
EXCLUDES 1 *oligohydramnios due to premature rupture of membranes (P01.1)*

P01.3 Newborn (suspected to be) affected by polyhydramnios N
Newborn (suspected to be) affected by hydramnios

P01.4 Newborn (suspected to be) affected by ectopic pregnancy N
Newborn (suspected to be) affected by abdominal pregnancy

P01.5 Newborn (suspected to be) affected by multiple pregnancy N
Newborn (suspected to be) affected by triplet (pregnancy)
Newborn (suspected to be) affected by twin (pregnancy)

P01.6 Newborn (suspected to be) affected by maternal death N

P01.7 Newborn (suspected to be) affected by malpresentation before labor N
Newborn (suspected to be) affected by breech presentation before labor
Newborn (suspected to be) affected by external version before labor
Newborn (suspected to be) affected by face presentation before labor
Newborn (suspected to be) affected by transverse lie before labor
Newborn (suspected to be) affected by unstable lie before labor

P01.8 Newborn (suspected to be) affected by other maternal complications of pregnancy N

P01.9 Newborn (suspected to be) affected by maternal complication of pregnancy, unspecified N

✓4th **P02 Newborn (suspected to be) affected by complications of placenta, cord and membranes**
Code first any current condition in newborn

P02.0 Newborn (suspected to be) affected by placenta previa N

P02.1 Newborn (suspected to be) affected by other forms of placental separation and hemorrhage N
Newborn (suspected to be) affected by abruptio placenta
Newborn (suspected to be) affected by accidental hemorrhage
Newborn (suspected to be) affected by antepartum hemorrhage
Newborn (suspected to be) affected by damage to placenta from amniocentesis, cesarean delivery or surgical induction
Newborn (suspected to be) affected by maternal blood loss
Newborn (suspected to be) affected by premature separation of placenta

P02.2 Newborn (suspected to be) affected by other and unspecified morphological and functional abnormalities of placenta

P02.20 Newborn (suspected to be) affected by unspecified morphological and functional abnormalities of placenta N

P02.29 Newborn (suspected to be) affected by other morphological and functional abnormalities of placenta N

Newborn (suspected to be) affected by placental dysfunction

Newborn (suspected to be) affected by placental infarction

Newborn (suspected to be) affected by placental insufficiency

P02.3 Newborn (suspected to be) affected by placental transfusion syndromes N

Newborn (suspected to be) affected by placental and cord abnormalities resulting in twin-to-twin or other transplacental transfusion

P02.4 Newborn (suspected to be) affected by prolapsed cord N

P02.5 Newborn (suspected to be) affected by other compression of umbilical cord N

Newborn (suspected to be) affected by umbilical cord (tightly) around neck

Newborn (suspected to be) affected by entanglement of umbilical cord

Newborn (suspected to be) affected by knot in umbilical cord

P02.6 Newborn (suspected to be) affected by other and unspecified conditions of umbilical cord

P02.60 Newborn (suspected to be) affected by unspecified conditions of umbilical cord N

P02.69 Newborn (suspected to be) affected by other conditions of umbilical cord N

Newborn (suspected to be) affected by short umbilical cord

Newborn (suspected to be) affected by vasa previa

EXCLUDES 1 *newborn affected by single umbilical artery (Q27.0)*

P02.7 Newborn (suspected to be) affected by chorioamnionitis N

Newborn (suspected to be) affected by amnionitis

Newborn (suspected to be) affected by membranitis

Newborn (suspected to be) affected by placentitis

P02.8 Newborn (suspected to be) affected by other abnormalities of membranes N

P02.9 Newborn (suspected to be) affected by abnormality of membranes, unspecified N

P03 Newborn (suspected to be) affected by other complications of labor and delivery

Code first any current condition in newborn

P03.0 Newborn (suspected to be) affected by breech delivery and extraction N

P03.1 Newborn (suspected to be) affected by other malpresentation, malposition and disproportion during labor and delivery N

Newborn (suspected to be) affected by contracted pelvis

Newborn (suspected to be) affected by conditions classifiable to O64-O66

Newborn (suspected to be) affected by persistent occipitoposterior

Newborn (suspected to be) affected by transverse lie

P03.2 Newborn (suspected to be) affected by forceps delivery N

P03.3 Newborn (suspected to be) affected by delivery by vacuum extractor [ventouse] N

P03.4 Newborn (suspected to be) affected by Cesarean delivery N

P03.5 Newborn (suspected to be) affected by precipitate delivery N

Newborn (suspected to be) affected by rapid second stage

P03.6 Newborn (suspected to be) affected by abnormal uterine contractions N

Newborn (suspected to be) affected by conditions classifiable to O62-, except O62.3

Newborn (suspected to be) affected by hypertonic labor

Newborn (suspected to be) affected by uterine inertia

P03.8 Newborn (suspected to be) affected by other specified complications of labor and delivery

P03.81 Newborn (suspected to be) affected by abnormality in fetal (intrauterine) heart rate or rhythm

EXCLUDES 1 *neonatal cardiac dysrhythmia (P29.1-)*

P03.810 Newborn (suspected to be) affected by abnormality in fetal (intrauterine) heart rate or rhythm before the onset of labor N

P03.811 Newborn (suspected to be) affected by abnormality in fetal (intrauterine) heart rate or rhythm during labor N

P03.819 Newborn (suspected to be) affected by abnormality in fetal (intrauterine) heart rate or rhythm, unspecified as to time of onset N

P03.82 Meconium passage during delivery N

EXCLUDES 1 *meconium aspiration (P24.00, P24.01)*
meconium staining (P96.83)

P03.89 Newborn (suspected to be) affected by other specified complications of labor and delivery N

Newborn (suspected to be) affected by abnormality of maternal soft tissues

Newborn (suspected to be) affected by conditions classifiable to O60-O75 and by procedures used in labor and delivery not included in P02- and P03.0-P03.6

Newborn (suspected to be) affected by induction of labor

P03.9 Newborn (suspected to be) affected by complication of labor and delivery, unspecified N

P04 Newborn (suspected to be) affected by noxious substances transmitted via placenta or breast milk

INCLUDES nonteratogenic effects of substances transmitted via placenta

EXCLUDES 2 *congenital malformations (Q00-Q99)*
neonatal jaundice from excessive hemolysis due to drugs or toxins transmitted from mother (P58.4)
newborn in contact with and (suspected) exposures hazardous to health not transmitted via placenta or breast milk (Z77.-)

P04.0 Newborn (suspected to be) affected by maternal anesthesia and analgesia in pregnancy, labor and delivery N

Newborn (suspected to be) affected by reactions and intoxications from maternal opiates and tranquilizers administered during labor and delivery

P04.1 Newborn (suspected to be) affected by other maternal medication N

Newborn (suspected to be) affected by cancer chemotherapy

Newborn (suspected to be) affected by cytotoxic drugs

EXCLUDES 1 *dysmorphism due to warfarin (Q86.2)*
fetal hydantoin syndrome (Q86.1)
maternal use of drugs of addiction (P04.4-)

P04.2 Newborn (suspected to be) affected by maternal use of tobacco N

Newborn (suspected to be) affected by exposure in utero to tobacco smoke

EXCLUDES 2 *newborn exposure to environmental tobacco smoke (P96.81)*

P04.3 Newborn (suspected to be) affected by maternal use of alcohol N

EXCLUDES 1 *fetal alcohol syndrome (Q86.0)*

P04.4 Newborn (suspected to be) affected by maternal use of drugs of addiction

P04.41 Newborn (suspected to be) affected by maternal use of cocaine N

"Crack baby"

P04.49 Newborn (suspected to be) affected by maternal use of other drugs of addiction N

EXCLUDES 2 *newborn (suspected to be) affected by maternal anesthesia and analgesia (P04.0)*
withdrawal symptoms from maternal use of drugs of addiction (P96.1)

P04.5 Newborn (suspected to be) affected by maternal use of nutritional chemical substances N

P04.6 Newborn (suspected to be) affected by maternal exposure to environmental chemical substances N

P04.8 Newborn (suspected to be) affected by other maternal noxious substances N

P04.9 Newborn (suspected to be) affected by maternal noxious substance, unspecified N

Disorders of newborn related to length of gestation and fetal growth (P05-P08)

P05 Disorders of newborn related to slow fetal growth and fetal malnutrition

P05.0 Newborn light for gestational age
Newborn light-for-dates

P05.00 Newborn light for gestational age, unspecified weight N
P05.01 Newborn light for gestational age, less than 500 grams N
P05.02 Newborn light for gestational age, 500-749 grams N
P05.03 Newborn light for gestational age, 750-999 grams N
P05.04 Newborn light for gestational age, 1000-1249 grams N
P05.05 Newborn light for gestational age, 1250-1499 grams N
P05.06 Newborn light for gestational age, 1500-1749 grams N
P05.07 Newborn light for gestational age, 1750-1999 grams N
P05.08 Newborn light for gestational age, 2000-2499 grams N

P05.1 Newborn small for gestational age
Newborn small-and-light-for-dates
Newborn small-for-dates

P05.10 Newborn small for gestational age, unspecified weight N
P05.11 Newborn small for gestational age, less than 500 grams N
P05.12 Newborn small for gestational age, 500-749 grams N
P05.13 Newborn small for gestational age, 750-999 grams N
P05.14 Newborn small for gestational age, 1000-1249 grams N
P05.15 Newborn small for gestational age, 1250-1499 grams N
P05.16 Newborn small for gestational age, 1500-1749 grams N
P05.17 Newborn small for gestational age, 1750-1999 grams N
P05.18 Newborn small for gestational age, 2000-2499 grams N

P05.2 Newborn affected by fetal (intrauterine) malnutrition not light or small for gestational age N
Infant, not light or small for gestational age, showing signs of fetal malnutrition, such as dry, peeling skin and loss of subcutaneous tissue
EXCLUDES 1 *newborn affected by fetal malnutrition with light for gestational age (P05.0-)*
newborn affected by fetal malnutrition with small for gestational age (P05.1-)

P05.9 Newborn affected by slow intrauterine growth, unspecified N
Newborn affected by fetal growth retardation NOS

P07 Disorders of newborn related to short gestation and low birth weight, not elsewhere classified
NOTE When both birth weight and gestational age of the newborn are available, both should be coded with birth weight sequenced before gestational age
INCLUDES the listed conditions, without further specification, as the cause of morbidity or additional care, in newborn
EXCLUDES 1 *low birth weight due to slow fetal growth and fetal malnutrition (P05.-)*

P07.0 Extremely low birth weight newborn
Newborn birth weight 999 g. or less

P07.00 Extremely low birth weight newborn, unspecified weight N
P07.01 Extremely low birth weight newborn, less than 500 grams N
P07.02 Extremely low birth weight newborn, 500-749 grams N
P07.03 Extremely low birth weight newborn, 750-999 grams N

P07.1 Other low birth weight newborn
Newborn birth weight 1000-2499 g.

P07.10 Other low birth weight newborn, unspecified weight N
P07.14 Other low birth weight newborn, 1000-1249 grams N
P07.15 Other low birth weight newborn, 1250-1499 grams N
P07.16 Other low birth weight newborn, 1500-1749 grams N
P07.17 Other low birth weight newborn, 1750-1999 grams N
P07.18 Other low birth weight newborn, 2000-2499 grams N

P07.2 Extreme immaturity of newborn
Less than 28 completed weeks (less than 196 completed days) of gestation.

P07.20 Extreme immaturity of newborn, unspecified weeks of gestation N
Gestational age less than 28 completed weeks NOS
P07.21 Extreme immaturity of newborn, gestational age less than 23 completed weeks N
Extreme immaturity of newborn, gestational age less than 23 weeks, 0 days
P07.22 Extreme immaturity of newborn, gestational age 23 completed weeks N
Extreme immaturity of newborn, gestational age 23 weeks, 0 days through 23 weeks, 6 days
P07.23 Extreme immaturity of newborn, gestational age 24 completed weeks N
Extreme immaturity of newborn, gestational age 24 weeks, 0 days through 24 weeks, 6 days
P07.24 Extreme immaturity of newborn, gestational age 25 completed weeks N
Extreme immaturity of newborn, gestational age 25 weeks, 0 days through 25 weeks, 6 days
P07.25 Extreme immaturity of newborn, gestational age 26 completed weeks N
Extreme immaturity of newborn, gestational age 26 weeks, 0 days through 26 weeks, 6 days
P07.26 Extreme immaturity of newborn, gestational age 27 completed weeks N
Extreme immaturity of newborn, gestational age 27 weeks, 0 days through 27 weeks, 6 days

P07.3 Preterm [premature] newborn [other]
28 completed weeks or more but less than 37 completed weeks (196 completed days but less than 259 completed days) of gestation
Prematurity NOS

P07.30 Preterm newborn, unspecified weeks of gestation N
P07.31 Preterm newborn, gestational age 28 completed weeks N
Preterm newborn, gestational age 28 weeks, 0 days through 28 weeks, 6 days
P07.32 Preterm newborn, gestational age 29 completed weeks N
Preterm newborn, gestational age 29 weeks, 0 days through 29 weeks, 6 days
P07.33 Preterm newborn, gestational age 30 completed weeks N
Preterm newborn, gestational age 30 weeks, 0 days through 30 weeks, 6 days
P07.34 Preterm newborn, gestational age 31 completed weeks N
Preterm newborn, gestational age 31 weeks, 0 days through 31 weeks, 6 days
P07.35 Preterm newborn, gestational age 32 completed weeks N
Preterm newborn, gestational age 32 weeks, 0 days through 32 weeks, 6 days
P07.36 Preterm newborn, gestational age 33 completed weeks N
Preterm newborn, gestational age 33 weeks, 0 days through 33 weeks, 6 days
P07.37 Preterm newborn, gestational age 34 completed weeks N
Preterm newborn, gestational age 34 weeks, 0 days through 34 weeks, 6 days

P07.38 Preterm newborn, gestational age 35 completed weeks N
Preterm newborn, gestational age 35 weeks, 0 days through 35 weeks, 6 days

P07.39 Preterm newborn, gestational age 36 completed weeks N
Preterm newborn, gestational age 36 weeks, 0 days through 36 weeks, 6 days

✓4th P08 Disorders of newborn related to long gestation and high birth weight
NOTE When both birth weight and gestational age of the newborn are available, priority of assignment should be given to birth weight
INCLUDES the listed conditions, without further specification, as causes of morbidity or additional care, in newborn

P08.0 Exceptionally large newborn baby N
Usually implies a birth weight of 4500 g. or more
EXCLUDES 1 *syndrome of infant of diabetic mother (P70.1)*
syndrome of infant of mother with gestational diabetes (P70.0)

P08.1 Other heavy for gestational age newborn N
Other newborn heavy- or large-for-dates regardless of period of gestation
Usually implies a birth weight of 4000 g. to 4499 g.
EXCLUDES 1 *newborn with a birth weight of 4500 or more (P08.0)*
syndrome of infant of diabetic mother (P70.1)
syndrome of infant of mother with gestational diabetes (P70.0).

✓5th P08.2 Late newborn, not heavy for gestational age
AHA: 2014, 1Q, 14

P08.21 Post-term newborn N
Newborn with gestation period over 40 completed weeks to 42 completed weeks

P08.22 Prolonged gestation of newborn N
Newborn with gestation period over 42 completed weeks (294 days or more), not heavy- or large-for-dates.
Postmaturity NOS

Abnormal findings on neonatal screening (P09)

P09 Abnormal findings on neonatal screening N
Use additional code to identify signs, symptoms and conditions associated with the screening
EXCLUDES 2 *nonspecific serologic evidence of human immunodeficiency virus [HIV] (R75)*

Birth trauma (P10-P15)

✓4th P10 Intracranial laceration and hemorrhage due to birth injury
EXCLUDES 1 *intracranial hemorrhage of newborn NOS (P52.9)*
intracranial hemorrhage of newborn due to anoxia or hypoxia (P52.-)
nontraumatic intracranial hemorrhage of newborn (P52.-)

P10.0 Subdural hemorrhage due to birth injury MCC N
Subdural hematoma (localized) due to birth injury
EXCLUDES 1 *subdural hemorrhage accompanying tentorial tear (P10.4)*
CC Excl: P10.0-P10.1, P10.4-P11.2, P11.9, P15.0-P15.9, P29.0-P29.2, P29.4, P29.89-P29.9, P52.4, P52.6-P52.9, P94.1-P94.9, P96.0, P96.3-P96.5, P96.82-P96.89

P10.1 Cerebral hemorrhage due to birth injury MCC N
CC Excl: See code P10.0

P10.2 Intraventricular hemorrhage due to birth injury CC N
CC Excl: P10.2-P10.3, P29.0-P29.2, P29.4, P29.89-P29.9, P50.0-P50.9, P52.0-P52.3, P52.5, P53-P54.0, P54.6-P54.9, P60-P61.9, P94.1-P94.9, P96.0, P96.3-P96.5, P96.82-P96.89

P10.3 Subarachnoid hemorrhage due to birth injury MCC N
CC Excl: P10.2-P10.3, P29.0-P29.2, P29.4, P29.89-P29.9, P50.0-P50.9, P52.0-P52.3, P52.5, P53-P54.0, P54.6-P54.9, P60-P61.9, P91.2, P94.1-P94.9, P96.0, P96.3-P96.5, P96.82-P96.89

P10.4 Tentorial tear due to birth injury MCC N
CC Excl: See code P10.0

P10.8 Other intracranial lacerations and hemorrhages due to birth injury MCC N
CC Excl: See code P10.0

P10.9 Unspecified intracranial laceration and hemorrhage due to birth injury MCC N
CC Excl: See code P10.0

✓4th P11 Other birth injuries to central nervous system

P11.0 Cerebral edema due to birth injury MCC N
CC Excl: See code P10.0

P11.1 Other specified brain damage due to birth injury N

P11.2 Unspecified brain damage due to birth injury MCC N
CC Excl: See code P10.0

P11.3 Birth injury to facial nerve N
Facial palsy due to birth injury

P11.4 Birth injury to other cranial nerves N

P11.5 Birth injury to spine and spinal cord N
Fracture of spine due to birth injury

P11.9 Birth injury to central nervous system, unspecified MCC N
CC Excl: See code P10.0

✓4th P12 Birth injury to scalp

P12.0 Cephalhematoma due to birth injury N

P12.1 Chignon (from vacuum extraction) due to birth injury N

P12.2 Epicranial subaponeurotic hemorrhage due to birth injury CC N
Subgaleal hemorrhage
CC Excl: P10.0-P10.1, P10.4-P11.2, P11.9, P12.2, P15.0-P15.9, P29.0-P29.2, P29.4, P29.89-P29.9, P52.4, P52.6-P52.9, P94.1-P94.9, P96.0, P96.3-P96.5, P96.82-P96.89

P12.3 Bruising of scalp due to birth injury N

P12.4 Injury of scalp of newborn due to monitoring equipment N
Sampling incision of scalp of newborn
Scalp clip (electrode) injury of newborn

✓5th P12.8 Other birth injuries to scalp

P12.81 Caput succedaneum N

P12.89 Other birth injuries to scalp N

P12.9 Birth injury to scalp, unspecified N

✓4th P13 Birth injury to skeleton
EXCLUDES 2 *birth injury to spine (P11.5)*

P13.0 Fracture of skull due to birth injury N

P13.1 Other birth injuries to skull N
EXCLUDES 1 *cephalhematoma (P12.0)*

P13.2 Birth injury to femur N

P13.3 Birth injury to other long bones N

P13.4 Fracture of clavicle due to birth injury N

P13.8 Birth injuries to other parts of skeleton N

P13.9 Birth injury to skeleton, unspecified N

✓4th P14 Birth injury to peripheral nervous system

P14.0 Erb's paralysis due to birth injury N

P14.1 Klumpke's paralysis due to birth injury N

P14.2 Phrenic nerve paralysis due to birth injury N

P14.3 Other brachial plexus birth injuries N

P14.8 Birth injuries to other parts of peripheral nervous system N

P14.9 Birth injury to peripheral nervous system, unspecified N

✓4th P15 Other birth injuries

P15.0 Birth injury to liver N
Rupture of liver due to birth injury

P15.1 Birth injury to spleen N
Rupture of spleen due to birth injury

P15.2 Sternomastoid injury due to birth injury N

P15.3 Birth injury to eye N
Subconjunctival hemorrhage due to birth injury
Traumatic glaucoma due to birth injury

P15.4 Birth injury to face N
Facial congestion due to birth injury

P15.5 Birth injury to external genitalia N

P15.6 Subcutaneous fat necrosis due to birth injury N

P15.8 Other specified birth injuries N

P15.9 Birth injury, unspecified N

Respiratory and cardiovascular disorders specific to the perinatal period (P19-P29)

✓4th P19 Metabolic acidemia in newborn
Metabolic acidemia in newborn

P19.0 Metabolic acidemia in newborn first noted before onset of labor N

P19.1 Metabolic acidemia in newborn first noted during labor N

P19.2 Metabolic acidemia noted at birth N

P19.9 Metabolic acidemia, unspecified N

✓4th P22 Respiratory distress of newborn
EXCLUDES 1 *respiratory arrest of newborn (P28.81)*
respiratory failure of newborn NOS (P28.5)

P22.0 Respiratory distress syndrome of newborn MCC N
Cardiorespiratory distress syndrome of newborn
Hyaline membrane disease
Idiopathic respiratory distress syndrome [IRDS or RDS] of newborn
Pulmonary hypoperfusion syndrome
Respiratory distress syndrome, type I
CC Excl: J84.83-J84.848, P22.0-P28.5, P28.89-P29.2, P29.4, P29.89-P29.9, P84, P94.1-P94.9, P96.0, P96.3-P96.5, P96.82-P96.89

P22.1 Transient tachypnea of newborn N
Idiopathic tachypnea of newborn
Respiratory distress syndrome, type II
Wet lung syndrome

P22.8 Other respiratory distress of newborn N

P22.9 Respiratory distress of newborn, unspecified N

✓4th P23 Congenital pneumonia
INCLUDES infective pneumonia acquired in utero or during birth
EXCLUDES 1 *neonatal pneumonia resulting from aspiration (P24.-)*

CC Excl: For MCC codes in subcategory P23, unless otherwise noted: J84.83-J84.848, P22.0-P28.5, P28.89-P29.2, P29.4, P29.89-P29.9, P84, P94.1-P94.9, P96.0, P96.3-P96.5, P96.82-P96.89

P23.0 Congenital pneumonia due to viral agent MCC N
Use additional code (B97) to identify organism
EXCLUDES 1 *congenital rubella pneumonitis (P35.0)*

P23.1 Congenital pneumonia due to Chlamydia MCC N

P23.2 Congenital pneumonia due to staphylococcus MCC N

P23.3 Congenital pneumonia due to streptococcus, group B MCC N

P23.4 Congenital pneumonia due to Escherichia coli MCC N

P23.5 Congenital pneumonia due to Pseudomonas MCC N

P23.6 Congenital pneumonia due to other bacterial agents MCC N
Congenital pneumonia due to Hemophilus influenzae
Congenital pneumonia due to Klebsiella pneumoniae
Congenital pneumonia due to Mycoplasma
Congenital pneumonia due to Streptococcus, except group B
Use additional code (B95-B96) to identify organism

P23.8 Congenital pneumonia due to other organisms MCC N

P23.9 Congenital pneumonia, unspecified MCC N

✓4th P24 Neonatal aspiration
INCLUDES aspiration in utero and during delivery

✓5th P24.0 Meconium aspiration
EXCLUDES 1 *meconium passage (without aspiration) during delivery (P03.82)*
meconium staining (P96.83)

P24.00 Meconium aspiration without respiratory symptoms N
Meconium aspiration NOS

P24.01 Meconium aspiration with respiratory symptoms MCC N
Meconium aspiration pneumonia
Meconium aspiration pneumonitis
Meconium aspiration syndrome NOS
Use additional code to identify any secondary pulmonary hypertension, if applicable (I27.2)
CC Excl: See code P23

✓5th P24.1 Neonatal aspiration of (clear) amniotic fluid and mucus
Neonatal aspiration of liquor (amnii)

P24.10 Neonatal aspiration of (clear) amniotic fluid and mucus without respiratory symptoms N
Neonatal aspiration of amniotic fluid and mucus NOS

P24.11 Neonatal aspiration of (clear) amniotic fluid and mucus with respiratory symptoms MCC N
Neonatal aspiration of amniotic fluid and mucus with pneumonia
Neonatal aspiration of amniotic fluid and mucus with pneumonitis
Use additional code to identify any secondary pulmonary hypertension, if applicable (I27.2)
CC Excl: See code P23

✓5th P24.2 Neonatal aspiration of blood

P24.20 Neonatal aspiration of blood without respiratory symptoms N
Neonatal aspiration of blood NOS

P24.21 Neonatal aspiration of blood with respiratory symptoms MCC N
Neonatal aspiration of blood with pneumonia
Neonatal aspiration of blood with pneumonitis
Use additional code to identify any secondary pulmonary hypertension, if applicable (I27.2)
CC Excl: See code P23

✓5th P24.3 Neonatal aspiration of milk and regurgitated food
Neonatal aspiration of stomach contents

P24.30 Neonatal aspiration of milk and regurgitated food without respiratory symptoms N
Neonatal aspiration of milk and regurgitated food NOS

P24.31 Neonatal aspiration of milk and regurgitated food with respiratory symptoms MCC N
Neonatal aspiration of milk and regurgitated food with pneumonia
Neonatal aspiration of milk and regurgitated food with pneumonitis
Use additional code to identify any secondary pulmonary hypertension, if applicable (I27.2)
CC Excl: See code P23

✓5th P24.8 Other neonatal aspiration

P24.80 Other neonatal aspiration without respiratory symptoms N
Neonatal aspiration NEC

P24.81 Other neonatal aspiration with respiratory symptoms MCC N
Neonatal aspiration pneumonia NEC
Neonatal aspiration with pneumonitis NEC
Neonatal aspiration with pneumonia NOS
Neonatal aspiration with pneumonitis NOS
Use additional code to identify any secondary pulmonary hypertension, if applicable (I27.2)
CC Excl: See code P23

P24.9 Neonatal aspiration, unspecified N

✓4th P25 Interstitial emphysema and related conditions originating in the perinatal period

CC Excl: For MCC codes in subcategory P25, unless otherwise noted: J84.83-J84.848, P22.0-P28.5, P28.89-P29.2, P29.4, P29.89-P29.9, P84, P94.1-P94.9, P96.0, P96.3-P96.5, P96.82-P96.89

P25.0 Interstitial emphysema originating in the perinatal period MCC N

P25.1 Pneumothorax originating in the perinatal period MCC N

P25.2 Pneumomediastinum originating in the perinatal period MCC N

P25.3 Pneumopericardium originating in the perinatal period MCC N

P25.8 Other conditions related to interstitial emphysema originating in the perinatal period MCC N

✓4th P26 Pulmonary hemorrhage originating in the perinatal period
EXCLUDES 1 *acute idiopathic hemorrhage in infants over 28 days old (R04.81)*

CC Excl: For MCC codes in subcategory P26, unless otherwise noted: J84.83-J84.848, P22.0-P28.5, P28.89-P29.2, P29.4, P29.89-P29.9, P84, P94.1-P94.9, P96.0, P96.3-P96.5, P96.82-P96.89

P26.0 Tracheobronchial hemorrhage originating in the perinatal period MCC N

P26.1 Massive pulmonary hemorrhage originating in the perinatal period MCC N

P26.8 Other pulmonary hemorrhages originating in the perinatal period MCC N

P26.9 Unspecified pulmonary hemorrhage originating in the perinatal period MCC N

✓4th P27 Chronic respiratory disease originating in the perinatal period
EXCLUDES 1 *respiratory distress of newborn (P22.0-P22.9)*

CC Excl: For MCC codes in subcategory P27, unless otherwise noted: J84.83-J84.848, P22.0-P28.5, P28.89-P29.2, P29.4, P29.89-P29.9, P84, P94.1-P94.9, P96.0, P96.3-P96.5, P96.82-P96.89

P27.0 Wilson-Mikity syndrome MCC
Pulmonary dysmaturity

P27.1 Bronchopulmonary dysplasia originating in the perinatal period MCC

P27.8 Other chronic respiratory diseases originating in the perinatal period MCC
Congenital pulmonary fibrosis
Ventilator lung in newborn

P27.9 Unspecified chronic respiratory disease originating in the perinatal period MCC

✓4th **P28 Other respiratory conditions originating in the perinatal period**
EXCLUDES 1 *congenital malformations of the respiratory system (Q30-Q34)*

P28.0 Primary atelectasis of newborn CC N
Primary failure to expand terminal respiratory units
Pulmonary hypoplasia associated with short gestation
Pulmonary immaturity NOS
CC Excl: See code P27

✓5th **P28.1 Other and unspecified atelectasis of newborn**

P28.10 Unspecified atelectasis of newborn CC N
Atelectasis of newborn NOS
CC Excl: See code P27

P28.11 Resorption atelectasis without respiratory distress syndrome CC N
EXCLUDES 1 *resorption atelectasis with respiratory distress syndrome (P22.0)*
CC Excl: See code P27

P28.19 Other atelectasis of newborn CC N
Partial atelectasis of newborn
Secondary atelectasis of newborn
CC Excl: See code P27

P28.2 Cyanotic attacks of newborn CC N
EXCLUDES 1 *apnea of newborn (P28.3-P28.4)*
CC Excl: P22.8-P22.9, P28.2-P28.4, P28.81-P28.9, R06.81, R23.0

P28.3 Primary sleep apnea of newborn CC N
Central sleep apnea of newborn
Obstructive sleep apnea of newborn
Sleep apnea of newborn NOS
CC Excl: P22.8-P22.9, P28.2, P28.4, P28.81-P28.9, R06.81

P28.4 Other apnea of newborn CC N
Apnea of prematurity
Obstructive apnea of newborn
EXCLUDES 1 *obstructive sleep apnea of newborn (P28.3)*
CC Excl: P22.8-P22.9, P28.2-P28.4, P28.81-P28.9, R06.81

P28.5 Respiratory failure of newborn MCC N
EXCLUDES 1 *respiratory arrest of newborn (P28.81)*
respiratory distress of newborn (P22.0-)
CC Excl: See code P27

✓5th **P28.8 Other specified respiratory conditions of newborn**

P28.81 Respiratory arrest of newborn MCC N
CC Excl: P22.1-P22.9, P24.00, P24.10, P24.20, P24.30, P24.80, Code P28.2-P28.5, P28.89-P28.9, P29.81, R06.81, R09.2

P28.89 Other specified respiratory conditions of newborn N
Congenital laryngeal stridor
Sniffles in newborn
Snuffles in newborn
EXCLUDES 1 *early congenital syphilitic rhinitis (A50.05)*

P28.9 Respiratory condition of newborn, unspecified N
Respiratory depression in newborn

✓4th **P29 Cardiovascular disorders originating in the perinatal period**
EXCLUDES 1 *congenital malformations of the circulatory system (Q20-Q28)*

P29.0 Neonatal cardiac failure N

✓5th **P29.1 Neonatal cardiac dysrhythmia**

P29.11 Neonatal tachycardia N

P29.12 Neonatal bradycardia N

P29.2 Neonatal hypertension N

P29.3 Persistent fetal circulation MCC N
Delayed closure of ductus arteriosus
(Persistent) pulmonary hypertension of newborn
CC Excl: I27.0, I27.2-I27.81, I27.89-I27.9

P29.4 Transient myocardial ischemia in newborn N

✓5th **P29.8 Other cardiovascular disorders originating in the perinatal period**

P29.81 Cardiac arrest of newborn MCC N
CC Excl: P29.81

P29.89 Other cardiovascular disorders originating in the perinatal period N

P29.9 Cardiovascular disorder originating in the perinatal period, unspecified N

Infections specific to the perinatal period (P35-P39)

Infections acquired in utero, during birth via the umbilicus, or during the first 28 days after birth

EXCLUDES 2 *asymptomatic human immunodeficiency virus [HIV] infection status (Z21)*
congenital gonococcal infection (A54.-)
congenital pneumonia (P23.-)
congenital syphilis (A50.-)
human immunodeficiency virus [HIV] disease (B20)
infant botulism (A48.51)
infectious diseases not specific to the perinatal period (A00-B99, J09, J10-)
intestinal infectious disease (A00-A09)
laboratory evidence of human immunodeficiency virus [HIV] (R75)
tetanus neonatorum (A33)

✓4th **P35 Congenital viral diseases**
INCLUDES infections acquired in utero or during birth

P35.0 Congenital rubella syndrome CC N
Congenital rubella pneumonitis
CC Excl: P29.0-P29.2, P29.4, P29.89-P35.9, P37.0-P37.4, P37.8-P37.9, P94.1-P94.9, P96.0, P96.3-P96.5, P96.82-P96.89

P35.1 Congenital cytomegalovirus infection MCC N
CC Excl: See code P35.0

P35.2 Congenital herpesviral [herpes simplex] infection MCC N
CC Excl: A17.82, A28.1, A50.42, A52.14, A75.9, A79.9, A81.1, A81.82-A81.89, A83.0-A85.8, A87.2, A88.0, A88.8, A92.1-A92.8, A93.0, B00.4, B00.82, B01.11-B01.12, B04, B06.01, B08.09, B08.20-B08.22, B08.60-B08.79, B09-B10.09, B26.2, B27.00-B27.99, B33.1, B45.0, B45.2-B45.9, B54, B58.2, B75, B97.10, B97.21, G04.00-G04.01, G04.31, G04.81-G05.4, G37.0, G37.4-G37.5, H66.40-H66.43, J09.X3-J09.X9, J10.2-J10.89, J11.2-J11.89, L44.4, M1A.10X0-M1A.19X1, M32.0-M32.9, P35.2-P35.9, P37.0-P37.4, P37.8-P37.9, T56.0X1A, T56.0X2A, T56.0X3A, T56.0X4A

P35.3 Congenital viral hepatitis MCC N
CC Excl: See code P35.2

P35.8 Other congenital viral diseases MCC N
Congenital varicella [chickenpox]
CC Excl: See code P35.2

P35.9 Congenital viral disease, unspecified MCC N
CC Excl: See code P35.2

✓4th **P36 Bacterial sepsis of newborn**
INCLUDES congenital sepsis
Use additional code(s), if applicable, to identify severe sepsis (R65.2-) and associated acute organ dysfunction(s)

CC Excl: For MCC codes in subcategory P36, unless otherwise noted: P29.0-P29.2, P29.4, P29.89-P29.9, P36.0-P36.9, P37.5, P38.1-P39.9, P53, P60-P61.9, P94.1-P94.9, P96.0, P96.3-P96.5, P96.82-P96.89

P36.0 Sepsis of newborn due to streptococcus, group B MCC N

✓5th **P36.1 Sepsis of newborn due to other and unspecified streptococci**

P36.10 Sepsis of newborn due to unspecified streptococci MCC N

P36.19 Sepsis of newborn due to other streptococci MCC N

P36.2 Sepsis of newborn due to Staphylococcus aureus MCC N

✓5th **P36.3 Sepsis of newborn due to other and unspecified staphylococci**

P36.30 Sepsis of newborn due to unspecified staphylococci MCC N

P36.39 Sepsis of newborn due to other staphylococci MCC N

P36.4 Sepsis of newborn due to Escherichia coli MCC N

P36.5 Sepsis of newborn due to anaerobes MCC N

P36.8 Other bacterial sepsis of newborn MCC N
Use additional code from category B96 to identify organism

P36.9 Bacterial sepsis of newborn, unspecified MCC N

✓4th P37 Other congenital infectious and parasitic diseases

EXCLUDES 2 *congenital syphilis (A5Ø.-)*
infectious neonatal diarrhea (AØØ-AØ9)
necrotizing enterocolitis in newborn (P77.-)
noninfectious neonatal diarrhea (P78.3)
ophthalmia neonatorum due to gonococcus (A54.31)
tetanus neonatorum (A33)

CC Excl: For MCC codes in subcategory P37, unless otherwise noted: A17.82, A28.1, A5Ø.42, A52.14, A75.9, A79.9, A81.1, A81.82-A81.89, A83.Ø-A85.8, A87.2, A88.Ø, A88.8, A92.1-A92.8, A93.Ø, BØØ.4, BØØ.82, BØ1.11-BØ1.12, BØ4, BØ6.Ø1, BØ8.Ø9, BØ8.2Ø-BØ8.22, BØ8.6Ø-BØ8.79, BØ9-B1Ø.Ø9, B26.2, B27.ØØ-B27.99, B33.1, B45.Ø, B45.2-B45.9, B54, B58.2, B75, B97.1Ø, B97.21, GØ4.ØØ-GØ4.Ø1, GØ4.31, GØ4.81-GØ5.4, G37.Ø, G37.4-G37.5, H66.4Ø-H66.43, JØ9.X3-JØ9.X9, J1Ø.2-J1Ø.89, J11.2-J11.89, L44.4, M1A.1ØXØ-M1A.19X1, M32.Ø-M32.9, P35.2-P35.9, P37.Ø-P37.4, P37.8-P37.9, T56.ØX1A, T56.ØX2A, T56.ØX3A, T56.ØX4A

P37.Ø Congenital tuberculosis MCC N

P37.1 Congenital toxoplasmosis MCC N
Hydrocephalus due to congenital toxoplasmosis

P37.2 Neonatal (disseminated) listeriosis MCC N

P37.3 Congenital falciparum malaria MCC N

P37.4 Other congenital malaria MCC N

P37.5 Neonatal candidiasis N

P37.8 Other specified congenital infectious and parasitic diseases MCC N

P37.9 Congenital infectious or parasitic disease, unspecified MCC N

✓4th P38 Omphalitis of newborn

EXCLUDES 1 *omphalitis not of newborn (LØ8.82)*
tetanus omphalitis (A33)
umbilical hemorrhage of newborn (P51.-)

P38.1 Omphalitis with mild hemorrhage CC N
CC Excl: P39.2-P39.9

P38.9 Omphalitis without hemorrhage CC N
Omphalitis of newborn NOS
CC Excl: See code P38.1

✓4th P39 Other infections specific to the perinatal period

Use additional code to identify organism or specific infection

P39.Ø Neonatal infective mastitis CC N
EXCLUDES 1 *breast engorgement of newborn (P83.4)*
noninfective mastitis of newborn (P83.4)
CC Excl: See code P38.1

P39.1 Neonatal conjunctivitis and dacryocystitis N
Neonatal chlamydial conjunctivitis
Ophthalmia neonatorum NOS
EXCLUDES 1 *gonococcal conjunctivitis (A54.31)*

P39.2 Intra-amniotic infection affecting newborn, not elsewhere classified CC N
CC Excl: AØ2.1, A2Ø.7, A22.7, A39.2-A39.4, A4Ø.9-A41.9, A42.7, A48.2, A48.4, A48.8-A49.9, BØØ.7, B92, B94.2-B96.89, MØØ.Ø11-MØØ.Ø12, MØØ.Ø21-MØØ.Ø22, MØØ.Ø31- MØØ.Ø32, MØØ.Ø41-MØØ.Ø42, MØØ.Ø51- MØØ.Ø52, MØØ.Ø61-MØØ.Ø62, MØØ.Ø71-MØØ.Ø72, P39.2-P39.9, P95, P96.9, R78.81

P39.3 Neonatal urinary tract infection CC N
CC Excl: A49.9, N1Ø-N11.Ø, N11.8-N12, N13.6, N15.1, N28.82, N28.84-N3Ø.31, N3Ø.8Ø-N3Ø.91, N36.9, N39.Ø, N39.9, N99.511, P39.2, P39.4-P39.9, R3Ø.Ø, R3Ø.9, T83.51XA

P39.4 Neonatal skin infection CC N
Neonatal pyoderma
EXCLUDES 1 *pemphigus neonatorum (LØØ)*
staphylococcal scalded skin syndrome (LØØ)
CC Excl: See code P39.2

P39.8 Other specified infections specific to the perinatal period CC N
CC Excl: See code P39.2

P39.9 Infection specific to the perinatal period, unspecified CC N
CC Excl: See code P39.2

Hemorrhagic and hematological disorders of newborn (P5Ø-P61)

EXCLUDES 1 *congenital stenosis and stricture of bile ducts (Q44.3)*
Crigler-Najjar syndrome (E8Ø.5)
Dubin-Johnson syndrome (E8Ø.6)
Gilbert syndrome (E8Ø.4)
hereditary hemolytic anemias (D55-D58)

✓4th P5Ø Newborn affected by intrauterine (fetal) blood loss

EXCLUDES 1 *congenital anemia from intrauterine (fetal) blood loss (P61.3)*

P5Ø.Ø Newborn affected by intrauterine (fetal) blood loss from vasa previa N

P5Ø.1 Newborn affected by intrauterine (fetal) blood loss from ruptured cord N

P5Ø.2 Newborn affected by intrauterine (fetal) blood loss from placenta N

P5Ø.3 Newborn affected by hemorrhage into co-twin N

P5Ø.4 Newborn affected by hemorrhage into maternal circulation N

P5Ø.5 Newborn affected by intrauterine (fetal) blood loss from cut end of co-twin's cord N

P5Ø.8 Newborn affected by other intrauterine (fetal) blood loss N

P5Ø.9 Newborn affected by intrauterine (fetal) blood loss, unspecified N
Newborn affected by fetal hemorrhage NOS

✓4th P51 Umbilical hemorrhage of newborn

EXCLUDES 1 *omphalitis with mild hemorrhage (P38.1)*
umbilical hemorrhage from cut end of co-twins cord (P5Ø.5)

P51.Ø Massive umbilical hemorrhage of newborn N

P51.8 Other umbilical hemorrhages of newborn N
Slipped umbilical ligature NOS

P51.9 Umbilical hemorrhage of newborn, unspecified N

✓4th P52 Intracranial nontraumatic hemorrhage of newborn

Intracranial hemorrhage due to anoxia or hypoxia

EXCLUDES 1 *intracranial hemorrhage due to birth injury (P1Ø.-)*
intracranial hemorrhage due to other injury (SØ6.-)

P52.Ø Intraventricular (nontraumatic) hemorrhage, grade 1, of newborn CC N
Subependymal hemorrhage (without intraventricular extension)
Bleeding into germinal matrix
CC Excl: P1Ø.2-P1Ø.3, P29.Ø-P29.2, P29.4, P29.89-P29.9, P5Ø.Ø-P5Ø.9, P52.Ø-P52.3, P52.5, P53-P54.Ø, P54.6-P54.9, P6Ø-P61.9, P94.1-P94.9, P96.Ø, P96.3-P96.5, P96.82-P96.89

P52.1 Intraventricular (nontraumatic) hemorrhage, grade 2, of newborn CC N
Subependymal hemorrhage with intraventricular extension
Bleeding into ventricle
CC Excl: See code P52.Ø

✓5th P52.2 Intraventricular (nontraumatic) hemorrhage, grade 3 and grade 4, of newborn

P52.21 Intraventricular (nontraumatic) hemorrhage, grade 3, of newborn MCC N
Subependymal hemorrhage with intraventricular extension with enlargement of ventricle
CC Excl: See code P52.Ø

P52.22 Intraventricular (nontraumatic) hemorrhage, grade 4, of newborn MCC N
Bleeding into cerebral cortex
Subependymal hemorrhage with intracerebral extension
CC Excl: See code P52.Ø

P52.3 Unspecified intraventricular (nontraumatic) hemorrhage of newborn CC N
CC Excl: See code P52.Ø

P52.4 Intracerebral (nontraumatic) hemorrhage of newborn MCC N
CC Excl: P1Ø.Ø-P1Ø.1, P1Ø.4-P11.2, P11.9, P15.Ø-P15.9, P29.Ø-P29.2, P29.4, P29.89-P29.9, P52.4, P52.6-P52.9, P94.1-P94.9, P96.Ø, P96.3-P96.5, P96.82-P96.89

P52.5 Subarachnoid (nontraumatic) hemorrhage of newborn MCC N
CC Excl: P1Ø.2-P1Ø.3, P29.Ø-P29.2, P29.4, P29.89-P29.9, P5Ø.Ø-P5Ø.9, P52.Ø-P52.3, P52.5, P53-P54.Ø, P54.6-P54.9, P6Ø-P61.9, P91.2, P94.1-P94.9, P96.Ø, P96.3-P96.5, P96.82-P96.89

P52.6 Cerebellar (nontraumatic) and posterior fossa hemorrhage of newborn MCC N
CC Excl: See code P52.4

P52.8 Other intracranial (nontraumatic) hemorrhages of newborn MCC N
CC Excl: See code P52.4

P52.9 Intracranial (nontraumatic) hemorrhage of newborn, unspecified MCC N
CC Excl: See code P52.4

P53 Hemorrhagic disease of newborn CC N
Vitamin K deficiency of newborn
CC Excl: P29.Ø-P29.2, P29.4, P29.89-P29.9, P53, P6Ø-P61.9, P94.1-P94.9, P96.Ø, P96.3-P96.5, P96.82-P96.89

✓4th P54 Other neonatal hemorrhages

EXCLUDES 1 *newborn affected by (intrauterine) blood loss (P5Ø.-)*
pulmonary hemorrhage originating in the perinatal period (P26.-)

P54.Ø Neonatal hematemesis N
EXCLUDES 1 *neonatal hematemesis due to swallowed maternal blood (P78.2)*

P54.1 Neonatal melena MCC N
EXCLUDES 1 *neonatal melena due to swallowed maternal blood (P78.2)*
CC Excl: P29.0-P29.2, P29.4, P29.89-P29.9, P50.0-P50.9, P53-P54.4, P54.6-P54.9, P60-P61.9, P94.1-P94.9, P96.0, P96.3-P96.5, P96.82-P96.89

P54.2 Neonatal rectal hemorrhage MCC N
CC Excl: See code P54.1

P54.3 Other neonatal gastrointestinal hemorrhage MCC N
CC Excl: See code P54.1

P54.4 Neonatal adrenal hemorrhage CC N
CC Excl: See code P54.1

P54.5 Neonatal cutaneous hemorrhage N
Neonatal bruising
Neonatal ecchymoses
Neonatal petechiae
Neonatal superficial hematomata
EXCLUDES 2 *bruising of scalp due to birth injury (P12.3)*
cephalhematoma due to birth injury (P12.0)

P54.6 Neonatal vaginal hemorrhage N ♀
Neonatal pseudomenses

P54.8 Other specified neonatal hemorrhages N

P54.9 Neonatal hemorrhage, unspecified N

✓4th P55 Hemolytic disease of newborn

P55.0 Rh isoimmunization of newborn N

P55.1 ABO isoimmunization of newborn N

P55.8 Other hemolytic diseases of newborn N

P55.9 Hemolytic disease of newborn, unspecified N

✓4th P56 Hydrops fetalis due to hemolytic disease
EXCLUDES 1 *hydrops fetalis NOS (P83.2)*

P56.0 Hydrops fetalis due to isoimmunization MCC N
CC Excl: P29.0-P29.2, P29.4, P29.89-P29.9, P55.0-P57.0, P94.1-P94.9, P96.0, P96.3-P96.5, P96.82-P96.89

✓5th P56.9 Hydrops fetalis due to other and unspecified hemolytic disease

P56.90 Hydrops fetalis due to unspecified hemolytic disease MCC N
CC Excl: See code P56.0

P56.99 Hydrops fetalis due to other hemolytic disease MCC N
CC Excl: See code P56.0

✓4th P57 Kernicterus

P57.0 Kernicterus due to isoimmunization MCC N
CC Excl: See code P56.0

P57.8 Other specified kernicterus MCC N
EXCLUDES 1 *Crigler-Najjar syndrome (E80.5)*
CC Excl: P29.0-P29.2, P29.4, P29.89-P29.9, P57.8-P59.9, P94.1-P94.9, P96.0, P96.3-P96.5, P96.82-P96.89

P57.9 Kernicterus, unspecified MCC N
CC Excl: See code P57.8

✓4th P58 Neonatal jaundice due to other excessive hemolysis
EXCLUDES 1 *jaundice due to isoimmunization (P55-P57)*

P58.0 Neonatal jaundice due to bruising N

P58.1 Neonatal jaundice due to bleeding N

P58.2 Neonatal jaundice due to infection N

P58.3 Neonatal jaundice due to polycythemia N

✓5th P58.4 Neonatal jaundice due to drugs or toxins transmitted from mother or given to newborn
Code first poisoning due to drug or toxin, if applicable (T36-T65 with fifth or sixth character 1-4 or 6)
Use additional code for adverse effect, if applicable, to identify drug (T36-T50 with fifth or sixth character 5)

P58.41 Neonatal jaundice due to drugs or toxins transmitted from mother N

P58.42 Neonatal jaundice due to drugs or toxins given to newborn N

P58.5 Neonatal jaundice due to swallowed maternal blood N

P58.8 Neonatal jaundice due to other specified excessive hemolysis N

P58.9 Neonatal jaundice due to excessive hemolysis, unspecified N

✓4th P59 Neonatal jaundice from other and unspecified causes
EXCLUDES 1 *jaundice due to inborn errors of metabolism (E70-E88)*
kernicterus (P57.-)

P59.0 Neonatal jaundice associated with preterm delivery N
Hyperbilirubinemia of prematurity
Jaundice due to delayed conjugation associated with preterm delivery

P59.1 Inspissated bile syndrome MCC N
CC Excl: See code P57.8

✓5th P59.2 Neonatal jaundice from other and unspecified hepatocellular damage
EXCLUDES 1 *congenital viral hepatitis (P35.3)*

P59.20 Neonatal jaundice from unspecified hepatocellular damage MCC N
CC Excl: See code P57.8

P59.29 Neonatal jaundice from other hepatocellular damage MCC N
Neonatal giant cell hepatitis
Neonatal (idiopathic) hepatitis
CC Excl: See code P57.8

P59.3 Neonatal jaundice from breast milk inhibitor N

P59.8 Neonatal jaundice from other specified causes N

P59.9 Neonatal jaundice, unspecified N
Neonatal physiological jaundice (intense)(prolonged) NOS

P60 Disseminated intravascular coagulation of newborn MCC N
Defibrination syndrome of newborn
CC Excl: P29.0-P29.2, P29.4, P29.89-P29.9, P53, P60-P61.9, P94.1-P94.9, P96.0, P96.3-P96.5, P96.82-P96.89

✓4th P61 Other perinatal hematological disorders
EXCLUDES 1 *transient hypogammaglobulinemia of infancy (D80.7)*

P61.0 Transient neonatal thrombocytopenia MCC N
Neonatal thrombocytopenia due to exchange transfusion
Neonatal thrombocytopenia due to idiopathic maternal thrombocytopenia
Neonatal thrombocytopenia due to isoimmunization
CC Excl: See code P60

P61.1 Polycythemia neonatorum N

P61.2 Anemia of prematurity CC N
CC Excl: D50.0-D55.9, D56.4, D57.00-D57.3, D57.80-D64.9, D75.9, P61.2-P61.4

P61.3 Congenital anemia from fetal blood loss CC N
CC Excl: See code P61.2

P61.4 Other congenital anemias, not elsewhere classified CC N
Congenital anemia NOS
CC Excl: See code P61.2

P61.5 Transient neonatal neutropenia MCC N
EXCLUDES 1 *congenital neutropenia (nontransient) (D70.0)*
CC Excl: D50.1-D53.9, D56.4, D57.00-D57.20, D57.3, D57.811-D57.819, D58.2, D59.0-D59.1, D59.3, D60.0-D61.9, D63.0-D64.9, D75.9, P61.5, P61.8-P61.9

P61.6 Other transient neonatal disorders of coagulation CC N
CC Excl: P29.0-P29.2, P29.4, P29.89-P29.9, P53, P60-P61.9, P94.1-P94.9, P96.0, P96.3-P96.5, P96.82-P96.89

P61.8 Other specified perinatal hematological disorders N

P61.9 Perinatal hematological disorder, unspecified N

Transitory endocrine and metabolic disorders specific to newborn (P70-P74)

INCLUDES transitory endocrine and metabolic disturbances caused by the infant's response to maternal endocrine and metabolic factors, or its adjustment to extrauterine environment

✓4th P70 Transitory disorders of carbohydrate metabolism specific to newborn

P70.0 Syndrome of infant of mother with gestational diabetes N
Newborn (with hypoglycemia) affected by maternal gestational diabetes
EXCLUDES 1 *newborn (with hypoglycemia) affected by maternal (pre-existing) diabetes mellitus (P70.1)*
syndrome of infant of a diabetic mother (P70.1)

P70.1 Syndrome of infant of a diabetic mother N
Newborn (with hypoglycemia) affected by maternal (pre-existing) diabetes mellitus
EXCLUDES 1 *newborn (with hypoglycemia) affected by maternal gestational diabetes (P70.0)*
syndrome of infant of mother with gestational diabetes (P70.0)

P70.2 Neonatal diabetes mellitus CC N
CC Excl: P29.0-P29.2, P29.4, P29.89-P29.9, P70.0-P70.4, P70.9-P71.9, P72.1, P72.9-P74.4, P74.9, P94.0-P94.9, P96.0, P96.3-P96.5, P96.82-P96.89

P70.3 Iatrogenic neonatal hypoglycemia N

P70.4 Other neonatal hypoglycemia N
Transitory neonatal hypoglycemia

P70.8 Other transitory disorders of carbohydrate metabolism of newborn CC N
CC Excl: P70.0-P70.4, P70.9-P71.9, P72.1, P72.9-P74.4, P74.9, P94.0

P70.9 Transitory disorder of carbohydrate metabolism of newborn, unspecified N

✓4th P71 Transitory neonatal disorders of calcium and magnesium metabolism

CC Excl: For CC codes in subcategory P71, unless otherwise noted: P29.0-P29.2, P29.4, P29.89-P29.9, P70.0-P70.4, P70.9-P71.9, P72.1, P72.9-P74.4, P74.9, P94.0-P94.9, P96.0, P96.3-P96.5, P96.82-P96.89

P71.0 Cow's milk hypocalcemia in newborn CC N

P71.1 Other neonatal hypocalcemia CC N
EXCLUDES 1 *neonatal hypoparathyroidism (P71.4)*

P71.2 Neonatal hypomagnesemia CC N

P71.3 Neonatal tetany without calcium or magnesium deficiency CC N
Neonatal tetany NOS

P71.4 Transitory neonatal hypoparathyroidism CC N

P71.8 Other transitory neonatal disorders of calcium and magnesium metabolism CC N

P71.9 Transitory neonatal disorder of calcium and magnesium metabolism, unspecified CC N

✓4th P72 Other transitory neonatal endocrine disorders
EXCLUDES 1 *congenital hypothyroidism with or without goiter (E03.0-E03.1)*
dyshormogenetic goiter (E07.1)
Pendred's syndrome (E07.1)

CC Excl: For CC codes in subcategory P72, unless otherwise noted: P70.0-P70.4, P70.9-P71.9, P72.1, P72.9-P74.4, P74.9, P94.0

P72.0 Neonatal goiter, not elsewhere classified CC N
Transitory congenital goiter with normal functioning

P72.1 Transitory neonatal hyperthyroidism CC N
Neonatal thyrotoxicosis
CC Excl: P29.0-P29.2, P29.4, P29.89-P29.9, P70.0-P70.4, P70.9-P71.9, P72.1, P72.9-P74.4, P74.9, P94.0-P94.9, P96.0, P96.3-P96.5, P96.82-P96.89

P72.2 Other transitory neonatal disorders of thyroid function, not elsewhere classified CC N
Transitory neonatal hypothyroidism

P72.8 Other specified transitory neonatal endocrine disorders CC N

P72.9 Transitory neonatal endocrine disorder, unspecified N

✓4th P74 Other transitory neonatal electrolyte and metabolic disturbances

P74.0 Late metabolic acidosis of newborn MCC N
EXCLUDES 1 *(fetal) metabolic acidosis of newborn (P19)*
CC Excl: P29.0-P29.2, P29.4, P29.89-P29.9, P70.0-P70.4, P70.9-P71.9, P72.1, P72.9-P74.4, P74.9, P94.0-P94.9, P96.0, P96.3-P96.5, P96.82-P96.89

P74.1 Dehydration of newborn N

P74.2 Disturbances of sodium balance of newborn N

P74.3 Disturbances of potassium balance of newborn N

P74.4 Other transitory electrolyte disturbances of newborn N

P74.5 Transitory tyrosinemia of newborn CC N
CC Excl: P70.0-P70.4, P70.9-P71.9, P72.1, P72.9-P74.4, P74.9, P94.0

P74.6 Transitory hyperammonemia of newborn CC N
CC Excl: See code: P70.8

P74.8 Other transitory metabolic disturbances of newborn CC N
Amino-acid metabolic disorders described as transitory
CC Excl: See code: P70.8

P74.9 Transitory metabolic disturbance of newborn, unspecified N

Digestive system disorders of newborn (P76-P78)

✓4th P76 Other intestinal obstruction of newborn

P76.0 Meconium plug syndrome N
Meconium ileus NOS
EXCLUDES 1 *meconium ileus in cystic fibrosis (E84.11)*

P76.1 Transitory ileus of newborn CC N
EXCLUDES 1 *Hirschsprung's disease (Q43.1)*
CC Excl: P76.0-P78.9

P76.2 Intestinal obstruction due to inspissated milk N

P76.8 Other specified intestinal obstruction of newborn N
EXCLUDES 1 *intestinal obstruction classifiable to K56-*

P76.9 Intestinal obstruction of newborn, unspecified N

✓4th P77 Necrotizing enterocolitis of newborn

P77.1 Stage 1 necrotizing enterocolitis in newborn MCC N
Necrotizing enterocolitis without pneumatosis, without perforation
CC Excl: P29.0-P29.2, P29.4, P29.89-P29.9, P76.0-P78.9, P94.1-P94.9, P96.0, P96.3-P96.5, P96.82-P96.89

P77.2 Stage 2 necrotizing enterocolitis in newborn MCC N
Necrotizing enterocolitis with pneumatosis, without perforation
CC Excl: See code P77.1

P77.3 Stage 3 necrotizing enterocolitis in newborn MCC N
Necrotizing enterocolitis with perforation
Necrotizing enterocolitis with pneumatosis and perforation
CC Excl: See code P77.1

P77.9 Necrotizing enterocolitis in newborn, unspecified MCC N
Necrotizing enterocolitis in newborn, NOS
CC Excl: See code P77.1

✓4th P78 Other perinatal digestive system disorders
EXCLUDES 1 *cystic fibrosis (E84.0-E84.9)*
neonatal gastrointestinal hemorrhages (P54.0-P54.3)

P78.0 Perinatal intestinal perforation MCC N
Meconium peritonitis
CC Excl: See code P77.1

P78.1 Other neonatal peritonitis N
Neonatal peritonitis NOS

P78.2 Neonatal hematemesis and melena due to swallowed maternal blood N

P78.3 Noninfective neonatal diarrhea N
Neonatal diarrhea NOS

✓5th P78.8 Other specified perinatal digestive system disorders

P78.81 Congenital cirrhosis (of liver) N

P78.82 Peptic ulcer of newborn N

P78.83 Newborn esophageal reflux N
Neonatal esophageal reflux

P78.89 Other specified perinatal digestive system disorders N

P78.9 Perinatal digestive system disorder, unspecified N

Conditions involving the integument and temperature regulation of newborn (P80-P83)

✓4th P80 Hypothermia of newborn

P80.0 Cold injury syndrome N
Severe and usually chronic hypothermia associated with a pink flushed appearance, edema and neurological and biochemical abnormalities.
EXCLUDES 1 *mild hypothermia of newborn (P80.8)*

P80.8 Other hypothermia of newborn N
Mild hypothermia of newborn

P80.9 Hypothermia of newborn, unspecified N

✓4th P81 Other disturbances of temperature regulation of newborn

P81.0 Environmental hyperthermia of newborn N

P81.8 Other specified disturbances of temperature regulation of newborn N

P81.9 Disturbance of temperature regulation of newborn, unspecified N
Fever of newborn NOS

P83 Other conditions of integument specific to newborn
EXCLUDES 1 *congenital malformations of skin and integument (Q80-Q84)*
hydrops fetalis due to hemolytic disease (P56.-)
neonatal skin infection (P39.4)
staphylococcal scalded skin syndrome (L00)
EXCLUDES 2 *cradle cap (L21.0)*
diaper [napkin] dermatitis (L22)

P83.0 Sclerema neonatorum CC N
CC Excl: P83.0, P83.30-P83.39

P83.1 Neonatal erythema toxicum N

P83.2 Hydrops fetalis not due to hemolytic disease MCC N
Hydrops fetalis NOS
CC Excl: P29.0-P29.2, P29.4, P29.89-P29.9, P83.2, P94.1-P94.9, P96.0, P96.3-P96.5, P96.82-P96.89

P83.3 Other and unspecified edema specific to newborn

P83.30 Unspecified edema specific to newborn CC N
CC Excl: P80.0-P83.0, P83.30-P83.39

P83.39 Other edema specific to newborn CC N
CC Excl: See code P83.30

P83.4 Breast engorgement of newborn N
Noninfective mastitis of newborn

P83.5 Congenital hydrocele ♂

P83.6 Umbilical polyp of newborn N

P83.8 Other specified conditions of integument specific to newborn N
Bronze baby syndrome
Neonatal scleroderma
Urticaria neonatorum

P83.9 Condition of the integument specific to newborn, unspecified N

Other problems with newborn (P84)

P84 Other problems with newborn N
Acidemia of newborn
Acidosis of newborn
Anoxia of newborn NOS
Asphyxia of newborn NOS
Hypercapnia of newborn
Hypoxemia of newborn
Hypoxia of newborn NOS
Mixed metabolic and respiratory acidosis of newborn
EXCLUDES 1 *intracranial hemorrhage due to anoxia or hypoxia (P52.-)*
hypoxic ischemic encephalopathy [HIE] (P91.6-)
late metabolic acidosis of newborn (P74.0)
CC Excl: No Excl

Other disorders originating in the perinatal period (P90-P96)

P90 Convulsions of newborn MCC N
EXCLUDES 1 *benign myoclonic epilepsy in infancy (G40.3-)*
benign neonatal convulsions (familial) (G40.3-)
CC Excl: P29.0-P29.2, P29.4, P29.89-P29.9, P90, P91.8-P91.9, P94.1-P94.9, P96.0, P96.3-P96.5, P96.82-P96.89

P91 Other disturbances of cerebral status of newborn

P91.0 Neonatal cerebral ischemia MCC N
CC Excl: P90-P91.1, P91.3-P91.5, P91.8-P91.9

P91.1 Acquired periventricular cysts of newborn MCC N
CC Excl: See code P91.0

P91.2 Neonatal cerebral leukomalacia MCC N
Periventricular leukomalacia
CC Excl: P10.2-P10.3, P29.0-P29.2, P29.4, P29.89-P29.9, P50.0-P50.9, P52.0-P52.3, P52.5, P53-P54.0, P54.6-P54.9, P60-P61.9, P91.2, P94.1-P94.9, P96.0, P96.3-P96.5, P96.82-P96.89

P91.3 Neonatal cerebral irritability MCC N
CC Excl: See code P91.0

P91.4 Neonatal cerebral depression MCC N
CC Excl: See code P91.0

P91.5 Neonatal coma MCC N
CC Excl: See code P91.0

P91.6 Hypoxic ischemic encephalopathy [HIE]

P91.60 Hypoxic ischemic encephalopathy [HIE], unspecified CC N
CC Excl: P84, P91.60-P91.63

P91.61 Mild hypoxic ischemic encephalopathy [HIE] CC N
CC Excl: See code P91.60

P91.62 Moderate hypoxic ischemic encephalopathy [HIE] CC N
CC Excl: See code P91.60

P91.63 Severe hypoxic ischemic encephalopathy [HIE] MCC N
CC Excl: See code P91.60

P91.8 Other specified disturbances of cerebral status of newborn N

P91.9 Disturbance of cerebral status of newborn, unspecified N

P92 Feeding problems of newborn
EXCLUDES 1 *feeding problems in child over 28 days old (R63.3)*

P92.0 Vomiting of newborn
EXCLUDES 1 *vomiting of child over 28 days old (R11.-)*

P92.01 Bilious vomiting of newborn MCC N
EXCLUDES 1 *bilious vomiting in child over 28 days old (R11.14)*
CC Excl: P92.01-P92.09

P92.09 Other vomiting of newborn N
EXCLUDES 1 *regurgitation of food in newborn (P92.1)*

P92.1 Regurgitation and rumination of newborn N

P92.2 Slow feeding of newborn N

P92.3 Underfeeding of newborn N

P92.4 Overfeeding of newborn N

P92.5 Neonatal difficulty in feeding at breast N

P92.6 Failure to thrive in newborn N
EXCLUDES 1 *failure to thrive in child over 28 days old (R62.51)*

P92.8 Other feeding problems of newborn N

P92.9 Feeding problem of newborn, unspecified N

P93 Reactions and intoxications due to drugs administered to newborn
INCLUDES reactions and intoxications due to drugs administered to fetus affecting newborn
EXCLUDES 1 *jaundice due to drugs or toxins transmitted from mother or given to newborn (P58.4-)*
reactions and intoxications from maternal opiates, tranquilizers and other medication (P04.0-P04.1, P04.4)
withdrawal symptoms from maternal use of drugs of addiction (P96.1)
withdrawal symptoms from therapeutic use of drugs in newborn (P96.2)

P93.0 Grey baby syndrome CC N
Grey syndrome from chloramphenicol administration in newborn
CC Excl: P93.0-P93.8, P96.1-P96.2

P93.8 Other reactions and intoxications due to drugs administered to newborn CC N
Use additional code for adverse effect, if applicable, to identify drug (T36-T50 with fifth or sixth character 5)
CC Excl: See code P93.0

P94 Disorders of muscle tone of newborn

P94.0 Transient neonatal myasthenia gravis CC N
EXCLUDES 1 *myasthenia gravis (G70.0)*
CC Excl: P29.0-P29.2, P29.4, P29.89-P29.9, P70.0-P70.4, P70.9-P71.9, P72.1, P72.9-P74.4, P74.9, P94.0-P94.9, P96.0, P96.3-P96.5, P96.82-P96.89

P94.1 Congenital hypertonia N

P94.2 Congenital hypotonia N
Floppy baby syndrome, unspecified

P94.8 Other disorders of muscle tone of newborn N

P94.9 Disorder of muscle tone of newborn, unspecified N

P95 Stillbirth N
Deadborn fetus NOS
Fetal death of unspecified cause
Stillbirth NOS
EXCLUDES 1 *maternal care for intrauterine death (O36.4)*
missed abortion (O02.1)
outcome of delivery, stillbirth (Z37.1, Z37.3, Z37.4, Z37.7)

P96 Other conditions originating in the perinatal period

P96.0 Congenital renal failure N
Uremia of newborn

P96.1 Neonatal withdrawal symptoms from maternal use of drugs of addiction CC N
Drug withdrawal syndrome in infant of dependent mother
Neonatal abstinence syndrome
EXCLUDES 1 *reactions and intoxications from maternal opiates and tranquilizers administered during labor and delivery (P04.0)*
CC Excl: P93.0-P93.8, P96.1-P96.2

P96.2 Withdrawal symptoms from therapeutic use of drugs in newborn CC N
CC Excl: See code P96.1

P96.3 Wide cranial sutures of newborn N
Neonatal craniotabes

P96.5 Complication to newborn due to (fetal) intrauterine procedure N
EXCLUDES 2 *newborn (suspected to be) affected by amniocentesis (P00.6)*

✓5th **P96.8 Other specified conditions originating in the perinatal period**

P96.81 Exposure to (parental) (environmental) tobacco smoke in the perinatal period
EXCLUDES 2 *newborn affected by in utero exposure to tobacco (P04.2)*
exposure to environmental tobacco smoke after the perinatal period (Z77.22)

P96.82 Delayed separation of umbilical cord N

P96.83 Meconium staining N
EXCLUDES 1 *meconium aspiration (P24.00, P24.01)*
meconium passage during delivery (P03.82)

P96.89 Other specified conditions originating in the perinatal period N
Use additional code to specify condition

P96.9 Condition originating in the perinatal period, unspecified N
Congenital debility NOS

Chapter 17. Congenital Malformations, Deformations and Chromosomal Abnormalities(Q00-Q99)

NOTE Codes from this chapter are not for use on maternal or fetal records.

EXCLUDES 2 *inborn errors of metabolism (E70-E88)*

This chapter contains the following blocks:

- Q00-Q07 Congenital malformations of the nervous system
- Q10-Q18 Congenital malformations of eye, ear, face and neck
- Q20-Q28 Congenital malformations of the circulatory system
- Q30-Q34 Congenital malformations of the respiratory system
- Q35-Q37 Cleft lip and cleft palate
- Q38-Q45 Other congenital malformations of the digestive system
- Q50-Q56 Congenital malformations of genital organs
- Q60-Q64 Congenital malformations of the urinary system
- Q65-Q79 Congenital malformations and deformations of the musculoskeletal system
- Q80-Q89 Other congenital malformations
- Q90-Q99 Chromosomal abnormalities, not elsewhere classified

Congenital malformations of the nervous system (Q00-Q07)

✓4th **Q00 Anencephaly and similar malformations**

CC Excl: For MCC codes in category Q00, unless otherwise noted: Q00.0-Q00.2

Q00.0 Anencephaly MCC
- Acephaly
- Acrania
- Amyelencephaly
- Hemianencephaly
- Hemicephaly

Q00.1 Craniorachischisis MCC

Q00.2 Iniencephaly MCC

✓4th **Q01 Encephalocele**

INCLUDES Arnold-Chiari syndrome, type III
- encephalocystocele
- encephalomyelocele
- hydroencephalocele
- hydromeningocele, cranial
- meningocele, cerebral
- meningoencephalocele

EXCLUDES 1 *Meckel-Gruber syndrome (Q61.9)*

CC Excl: For CC codes in category Q01, unless otherwise noted: Q01.0-Q02, Q04.0-Q04.8

Q01.0 Frontal encephalocele CC

Q01.1 Nasofrontal encephalocele CC

Q01.2 Occipital encephalocele CC

Q01.8 Encephalocele of other sites CC

Q01.9 Encephalocele, unspecified CC

Q02 Microcephaly

INCLUDES hydromicrocephaly
- micrencephalon

EXCLUDES 1 *Meckel-Gruber syndrome (Q61.9)*

✓4th **Q03 Congenital hydrocephalus**

INCLUDES hydrocephalus in newborn

EXCLUDES 1 *Arnold-Chiari syndrome, type II (Q07.0-)*
- *acquired hydrocephalus (G91.-)*
- *hydrocephalus due to congenital toxoplasmosis (P37.1)*
- *hydrocephalus with spina bifida (Q05.0-Q05.4)*

Q03.0 Malformations of aqueduct of Sylvius
- Anomaly of aqueduct of Sylvius
- Obstruction of aqueduct of Sylvius, congenital
- Stenosis of aqueduct of Sylvius

Q03.1 Atresia of foramina of Magendie and Luschka
- Dandy-Walker syndrome

Q03.8 Other congenital hydrocephalus

Q03.9 Congenital hydrocephalus, unspecified

✓4th **Q04 Other congenital malformations of brain**

EXCLUDES 1 *cyclopia (Q87.0)*
- *macrocephaly (Q75.3)*

CC Excl: For MCC codes in category Q04, unless otherwise noted: See code: Q01

Q04.0 Congenital malformations of corpus callosum MCC
- Agenesis of corpus callosum

Q04.1 Arhinencephaly MCC

Q04.2 Holoprosencephaly MCC

Q04.3 Other reduction deformities of brain MCC
- Absence of part of brain
- Agenesis of part of brain
- Agyria
- Aplasia of part of brain
- Hydranencephaly
- Hypoplasia of part of brain
- Lissencephaly
- Microgyria
- Pachygyria

EXCLUDES 1 *congenital malformations of corpus callosum (Q04.0)*

Q04.4 Septo-optic dysplasia of brain CC

CC Excl: Q04.4-Q04.8

Q04.5 Megalencephaly CC

CC Excl: See code: Q04.4

Q04.6 Congenital cerebral cysts CC
- Porencephaly
- Schizencephaly

EXCLUDES 1 *acquired porencephalic cyst (G93.0)*

CC Excl: See code: Q04.4

Q04.8 Other specified congenital malformations of brain CC
- Arnold-Chiari syndrome, type IV
- Macrogyria

CC Excl: See code: Q04.4

Q04.9 Congenital malformation of brain, unspecified
- Congenital anomaly NOS of brain
- Congenital deformity NOS of brain
- Congenital disease or lesion NOS of brain
- Multiple anomalies NOS of brain, congenital

✓4th **Q05 Spina bifida**
- Hydromeningocele (spinal)
- Meningocele (spinal)
- Meningomyelocele
- Myelocele
- Myelomeningocele
- Rachischisis
- Spina bifida (aperta)(cystica)
- Syringomyelocele

Use additional code for any associated paraplegia (paraparesis) (G82.2-)

EXCLUDES 1 *Arnold-Chiari syndrome, type II (Q07.0-)*
- *spina bifida occulta (Q76.0)*

CC Excl: For CC codes in category Q05, unless otherwise noted: E78.71-E78.72, G90.1, Q05.0-Q06.1, Q06.3, Q06.8-Q07.9, Q87.1-Q87.89, Q89.7-Q89.8, Q99.2

Q05.0 Cervical spina bifida with hydrocephalus CC

Q05.1 Thoracic spina bifida with hydrocephalus CC
- Dorsal spina bifida with hydrocephalus
- Thoracolumbar spina bifida with hydrocephalus

Q05.2 Lumbar spina bifida with hydrocephalus CC
- Lumbosacral spina bifida with hydrocephalus

Q05.3 Sacral spina bifida with hydrocephalus CC

Q05.4 Unspecified spina bifida with hydrocephalus CC

Q05.5 Cervical spina bifida without hydrocephalus

Q05.6 Thoracic spina bifida without hydrocephalus
- Dorsal spina bifida NOS
- Thoracolumbar spina bifida NOS

Q05.7 Lumbar spina bifida without hydrocephalus
- Lumbosacral spina bifida NOS

Q05.8 Sacral spina bifida without hydrocephalus

Q05.9 Spina bifida, unspecified

✓4th **Q06 Other congenital malformations of spinal cord**

Q06.0 Amyelia

Q06.1 Hypoplasia and dysplasia of spinal cord
- Atelomyelia
- Myelatelia
- Myelodysplasia of spinal cord

Q06.2 Diastematomyelia

Q06.3 Other congenital cauda equina malformations

Q06.4 Hydromyelia
- Hydrorachis

Q06.8 Other specified congenital malformations of spinal cord

Q06.9 Congenital malformation of spinal cord, unspecified
- Congenital anomaly NOS of spinal cord
- Congenital deformity NOS of spinal cord
- Congenital disease or lesion NOS of spinal cord

Q07 Other congenital malformations of nervous system

EXCLUDES 2 *congenital central alveolar hypoventilation syndrome (G47.35)*
familial dysautonomia [Riley-Day] (G90.1)
neurofibromatosis (nonmalignant) (Q85.0-)

CC Excl: For CC codes in category Q07, unless otherwise noted:
See code: Q05.0

Q07.0 Arnold-Chiari syndrome
Arnold-Chiari syndrome, type II
EXCLUDES 1 *Arnold-Chiari syndrome, type III (Q01.-)*
Arnold-Chiari syndrome, type IV (Q04.8)

Q07.00 Arnold-Chiari syndrome without spina bifida or hydrocephalus

Q07.01 Arnold-Chiari syndrome with spina bifida

Q07.02 Arnold-Chiari syndrome with hydrocephalus CC

Q07.03 Arnold-Chiari syndrome with spina bifida and hydrocephalus CC

Q07.8 Other specified congenital malformations of nervous system
Agenesis of nerve
Displacement of brachial plexus
Jaw-winking syndrome
Marcus Gunn's syndrome

Q07.9 Congenital malformation of nervous system, unspecified
Congenital anomaly NOS of nervous system
Congenital deformity NOS of nervous system
Congenital disease or lesion NOS of nervous system

Congenital malformations of eye, ear, face and neck (Q10-Q18)

EXCLUDES 2 *cleft lip and cleft palate (Q35-Q37)*
congenital malformation of cervical spine (Q05.0, Q05.5, Q67.5, Q76.0-Q76.4)
congenital malformation of larynx (Q31.-)
congenital malformation of lip NEC (Q38.0)
congenital malformation of nose (Q30.-)
congenital malformation of parathyroid gland (Q89.2)
congenital malformation of thyroid gland (Q89.2)

Q10 Congenital malformations of eyelid, lacrimal apparatus and orbit

EXCLUDES 1 *cryptophthalmos NOS (Q11.2)*
cryptophthalmos syndrome (Q87.0)

Q10.0 Congenital ptosis

Q10.1 Congenital ectropion

Q10.2 Congenital entropion

Q10.3 Other congenital malformations of eyelid
Ablepharon
Blepharophimosis, congenital
Coloboma of eyelid
Congenital absence or agenesis of cilia
Congenital absence or agenesis of eyelid
Congenital accessory eyelid
Congenital accessory eye muscle
Congenital malformation of eyelid NOS

Q10.4 Absence and agenesis of lacrimal apparatus
Congenital absence of punctum lacrimale

Q10.5 Congenital stenosis and stricture of lacrimal duct

Q10.6 Other congenital malformations of lacrimal apparatus
Congenital malformation of lacrimal apparatus NOS

Q10.7 Congenital malformation of orbit

Q11 Anophthalmos, microphthalmos and macrophthalmos

Q11.0 Cystic eyeball

Q11.1 Other anophthalmos
Anophthalmos NOS
Agenesis of eye
Aplasia of eye

Q11.2 Microphthalmos
Cryptophthalmos NOS
Dysplasia of eye
Hypoplasia of eye
Rudimentary eye
EXCLUDES 1 *cryptophthalmos syndrome (Q87.0)*

Q11.3 Macrophthalmos
EXCLUDES 1 *macrophthalmos in congenital glaucoma (Q15.0)*

Q12 Congenital lens malformations

Q12.0 Congenital cataract

Q12.1 Congenital displaced lens

Q12.2 Coloboma of lens

Q12.3 Congenital aphakia

Q12.4 Spherophakia

Q12.8 Other congenital lens malformations
Microphakia

Q12.9 Congenital lens malformation, unspecified

Q13 Congenital malformations of anterior segment of eye

Q13.0 Coloboma of iris
Coloboma NOS

Q13.1 Absence of iris
Aniridia
Use additional code for associated glaucoma (H42)

Q13.2 Other congenital malformations of iris
Anisocoria, congenital
Atresia of pupil
Congenital malformation of iris NOS
Corectopia

Q13.3 Congenital corneal opacity

Q13.4 Other congenital corneal malformations
Congenital malformation of cornea NOS
Microcornea
Peter's anomaly

Q13.5 Blue sclera

Q13.8 Other congenital malformations of anterior segment of eye

Q13.81 Rieger's anomaly
Use additional code for associated glaucoma (H42)

Q13.89 Other congenital malformations of anterior segment of eye

Q13.9 Congenital malformation of anterior segment of eye, unspecified

Q14 Congenital malformations of posterior segment of eye

EXCLUDES 2 *optic nerve hypoplasia (H47.03-)*

Q14.0 Congenital malformation of vitreous humor
Congenital vitreous opacity

Q14.1 Congenital malformation of retina
Congenital retinal aneurysm

Q14.2 Congenital malformation of optic disc
Coloboma of optic disc

Q14.3 Congenital malformation of choroid

Q14.8 Other congenital malformations of posterior segment of eye
Coloboma of the fundus

Q14.9 Congenital malformation of posterior segment of eye, unspecified

Q15 Other congenital malformations of eye

EXCLUDES 1 *congenital nystagmus (H55.01)*
ocular albinism (E70.31-)
optic nerve hypoplasia (H47.03-)
retinitis pigmentosa (H35.52)

Q15.0 Congenital glaucoma
Axenfeld's anomaly
Buphthalmos
Glaucoma of childhood
Glaucoma of newborn
Hydrophthalmos
Keratoglobus, congenital, with glaucoma
Macrocornea with glaucoma
Macrophthalmos in congenital glaucoma
Megalocornea with glaucoma

Q15.8 Other specified congenital malformations of eye

Q15.9 Congenital malformation of eye, unspecified
Congenital anomaly of eye
Congenital deformity of eye

Q16 Congenital malformations of ear causing impairment of hearing

EXCLUDES 1 *congenital deafness (H90.-)*

Q16.0 Congenital absence of (ear) auricle

Q16.1 Congenital absence, atresia and stricture of auditory canal (external)
Congenital atresia or stricture of osseous meatus

Q16.2 Absence of eustachian tube

Q16.3 Congenital malformation of ear ossicles
Congenital fusion of ear ossicles

Q16.4 Other congenital malformations of middle ear
Congenital malformation of middle ear NOS

Q16.5 Congenital malformation of inner ear
Congenital anomaly of membranous labyrinth
Congenital anomaly of organ of Corti

Q16.9 Congenital malformation of ear causing impairment of hearing, unspecified
Congenital absence of ear NOS

Q17 Other congenital malformations of ear ✓4th

EXCLUDES 1 *congenital malformations of ear with impairment of hearing (Q16.Ø- Q16.9)*
preauricular sinus (Q18.1)

Q17.Ø Accessory auricle
Accessory tragus
Polyotia
Preauricular appendage or tag
Supernumerary ear
Supernumerary lobule

Q17.1 Macrotia

Q17.2 Microtia

Q17.3 Other misshapen ear
Pointed ear

Q17.4 Misplaced ear
Low-set ears
EXCLUDES 1 *cervical auricle (Q18.2)*

Q17.5 Prominent ear
Bat ear

Q17.8 Other specified congenital malformations of ear
Congenital absence of lobe of ear

Q17.9 Congenital malformation of ear, unspecified
Congenital anomaly of ear NOS

Q18 Other congenital malformations of face and neck ✓4th

EXCLUDES 1 *cleft lip and cleft palate (Q35-Q37)*
conditions classified to Q67.Ø-Q67.4
congenital malformations of skull and face bones (Q75.-)
cyclopia (Q87.Ø)
dentofacial anomalies [including malocclusion] (M26.-)
malformation syndromes affecting facial appearance (Q87.Ø)
persistent thyroglossal duct (Q89.2)

Q18.Ø Sinus, fistula and cyst of branchial cleft
Branchial vestige

Q18.1 Preauricular sinus and cyst
Fistula of auricle, congenital
Cervicoaural fistula

Q18.2 Other branchial cleft malformations
Branchial cleft malformation NOS
Cervical auricle
Otocephaly

Q18.3 Webbing of neck
Pterygium colli

Q18.4 Macrostomia

Q18.5 Microstomia

Q18.6 Macrocheilia
Hypertrophy of lip, congenital

Q18.7 Microcheilia

Q18.8 Other specified congenital malformations of face and neck
Medial cyst of face and neck
Medial fistula of face and neck
Medial sinus of face and neck

Q18.9 Congenital malformation of face and neck, unspecified
Congenital anomaly NOS of face and neck

Congenital malformations of the circulatory system (Q2Ø-Q28)

Q2Ø Congenital malformations of cardiac chambers and connections ✓4th

EXCLUDES 1 *dextrocardia with situs inversus (Q89.3)*
mirror-image atrial arrangement with situs inversus (Q89.3)

CC Excl: For CC/MCC codes in category Q2Ø, unless otherwise noted: E78.71-E78.72, I23.Ø-I23.3, I23.6-I23.8, I51.Ø, P29.3, Q2Ø.Ø-Q21.9, Q23.8-Q23.9, Q24.8-Q24.9, Q27.3Ø, Q27.4, Q28.Ø-Q28.1, Q28.8-Q28.9, Q87.1-Q87.89, Q89.7-Q89.8, Q99.2

Q2Ø.Ø Common arterial trunk MCC
Persistent truncus arteriosus
EXCLUDES 1 *aortic septal defect (Q21.4)*

Q2Ø.1 Double outlet right ventricle MCC
Taussig-Bing syndrome

Q2Ø.2 Double outlet left ventricle MCC

Q2Ø.3 Discordant ventriculoarterial connection MCC
Dextrotransposition of aorta
Transposition of great vessels (complete)

Q2Ø.4 Double inlet ventricle MCC
Common ventricle
Cor triloculare biatriatum
Single ventricle

Q2Ø.5 Discordant atrioventricular connection CC
Corrected transposition
Levotransposition
Ventricular inversion

Q2Ø.6 Isomerism of atrial appendages
Isomerism of atrial appendages with asplenia or polysplenia

Q2Ø.8 Other congenital malformations of cardiac chambers and connections
Cor binoculare

Q2Ø.9 Congenital malformation of cardiac chambers and connections, unspecified

Q21 Congenital malformations of cardiac septa ✓4th

EXCLUDES 1 *acquired cardiac septal defect (I51.Ø)*

CC Excl: For CC/MCC codes in category Q 21, unless otherwise noted: See code Q2Ø.Ø

Q21.Ø Ventricular septal defect CC
Roger's disease

Q21.1 Atrial septal defect CC
Coronary sinus defect
Patent or persistent foramen ovale
Patent or persistent ostium secundum defect (type II)
Patent or persistent sinus venosus defect
CC Excl: E78.71-E78.72, I23.Ø-I23.3, I23.6-I23.8, I51.Ø, I51.3, Q2Ø.Ø-Q2Ø.9, Q21.1-Q21.9, Q23.8-Q23.9, Q24.8-Q24.9, Q27.3Ø, Q27.4, Q28.Ø-Q28.1, Q28.8-Q28.9, Q87.2-Q87.3, Q87.5-Q87.89, Q89.7-Q89.8

Q21.2 Atrioventricular septal defect CC
Common atrioventricular canal
Endocardial cushion defect
Ostium primum atrial septal defect (type I)

Q21.3 Tetralogy of Fallot MCC
Ventricular septal defect with pulmonary stenosis or atresia, dextroposition of aorta and hypertrophy of right ventricle.

Q21.4 Aortopulmonary septal defect
Aortic septal defect
Aortopulmonary window

Q21.8 Other congenital malformations of cardiac septa
Eisenmenger's defect
Pentalogy of Fallot
EXCLUDES 1 *Eisenmenger's complex (I27.8)*
Eisenmenger's syndrome (I27.8)

Q21.9 Congenital malformation of cardiac septum, unspecified
Septal (heart) defect NOS

Q22 Congenital malformations of pulmonary and tricuspid valves ✓4th

Q22.Ø Pulmonary valve atresia MCC
CC Excl: E78.71-E78.72, P29.3, Q2Ø.9, Q22.Ø-Q22.3, Q23.8-Q23.9, Q24.8-Q24.9, Q27.3Ø, Q27.4, Q28.Ø-Q28.1, Q28.8-Q28.9, Q87.1-Q87.89, Q89.7-Q89.8, Q99.2

Q22.1 Congenital pulmonary valve stenosis CC
CC Excl: See code: Q22.Ø

Q22.2 Congenital pulmonary valve insufficiency CC
Congenital pulmonary valve regurgitation
CC Excl: E78.71-E78.72, Q2Ø.9, Q22.Ø-Q22.3, Q23.8-Q23.9, Q24.8-Q24.9, Q27.3Ø, Q27.4, Q28.Ø-Q28.1, Q28.8-Q28.9, Q87.2-Q87.3, Q87.5-Q87.89, Q89.7-Q89.8

Q22.3 Other congenital malformations of pulmonary valve CC
Congenital malformation of pulmonary valve NOS
Supernumerary cusps of pulmonary valve
CC Excl: See code: Q22.2

Q22.4 Congenital tricuspid stenosis MCC
Congenital tricuspid atresia
CC Excl: E78.71-E78.72, P29.3, Q2Ø.9, Q22.4-Q23.9, Q24.8-Q24.9, Q27.3Ø, Q27.4, Q28.Ø-Q28.1, Q28.8-Q28.9, Q87.1-Q87.89, Q89.7-Q89.8, Q99.2

Q22.5 Ebstein's anomaly MCC
CC Excl: See code: Q22.4

Q22.6 Hypoplastic right heart syndrome MCC
CC Excl: See code: Q22.4

Q22.8 Other congenital malformations of tricuspid valve MCC
CC Excl: See code: Q22.4

Q22.9 Congenital malformation of tricuspid valve, unspecified MCC
CC Excl: See code: Q22.4

Q23 Congenital malformations of aortic and mitral valves

CC Excl: For CC/MCC codes in category Q23, unless otherwise noted: See code: Q22.4

Q23.0 Congenital stenosis of aortic valve CC
Congenital aortic atresia
Congenital aortic stenosis NOS
EXCLUDES 1 *congenital stenosis of aortic valve in hypoplastic left heart syndrome (Q23.4)*
congenital subaortic stenosis (Q24.4)
supravalvular aortic stenosis (congenital) (Q25.3)

Q23.1 Congenital insufficiency of aortic valve CC
Bicuspid aortic valve
Congenital aortic insufficiency

Q23.2 Congenital mitral stenosis CC
Congenital mitral atresia

Q23.3 Congenital mitral insufficiency CC

Q23.4 Hypoplastic left heart syndrome MCC

Q23.8 Other congenital malformations of aortic and mitral valves

Q23.9 Congenital malformation of aortic and mitral valves, unspecified

Q24 Other congenital malformations of heart
EXCLUDES 1 *endocardial fibroelastosis (I42.4)*

Q24.0 Dextrocardia CC
EXCLUDES 1 *dextrocardia with situs inversus (Q89.3)*
isomerism of atrial appendages (with asplenia or polysplenia) (Q20.6)
mirror-image atrial arrangement with situs inversus (Q89.3)
CC Excl: E78.71-E78.72, Q20.9, Q23.8-Q24.4, Q24.8-Q24.9, Q27.30, Q27.4, Q28.0-Q28.1, Q28.8-Q28.9, Q87.2-Q87.3, Q87.5-Q87.89, Q89.7-Q89.8

Q24.1 Levocardia CC
CC Excl: See code: Q24.0

Q24.2 Cor triatriatum MCC
CC Excl: E78.71-E78.72, P29.3, Q20.9, Q23.8-Q23.9, Q24.2-Q24.4, Q24.8-Q24.9, Q27.30, Q27.4, Q28.0-Q28.1, Q28.8-Q28.9, Q87.1-Q87.89, Q89.7-Q89.8, Q99.2

Q24.3 Pulmonary infundibular stenosis CC
Subvalvular pulmonic stenosis
CC Excl: See code: Q24.2

Q24.4 Congenital subaortic stenosis MCC
CC Excl: See code: Q24.2

Q24.5 Malformation of coronary vessels CC
Congenital coronary (artery) aneurysm
CC Excl: Q20.9-Q23.9, Q24.5, Q24.8-Q24.9

Q24.6 Congenital heart block MCC
CC Excl: E78.71-E78.72, P29.3, Q20.9, Q23.8-Q23.9, Q24.6-Q24.9, Q27.30, Q27.4, Q28.0-Q28.1, Q28.8-Q28.9, Q87.1-Q87.89, Q89.7-Q89.8, Q99.2

Q24.8 Other specified congenital malformations of heart
Congenital diverticulum of left ventricle
Congenital malformation of myocardium
Congenital malformation of pericardium
Malposition of heart
Uhl's disease

Q24.9 Congenital malformation of heart, unspecified
Congenital anomaly of heart
Congenital disease of heart

Q25 Congenital malformations of great arteries

Q25.0 Patent ductus arteriosus CC
Patent ductus Botallo
Persistent ductus arteriosus
CC Excl: Q25.0, Q27.30, Q27.4, Q28.0-Q28.1, Q28.8

Q25.1 Coarctation of aorta CC
Coarctation of aorta (preductal) (postductal)
CC Excl: E78.71-E78.72, Q25.1-Q25.3, Q27.30, Q27.4, Q28.0-Q28.1, Q28.8-Q28.9, Q87.2-Q87.3, Q87.5-Q87.89, Q89.7-Q89.8

Q25.2 Atresia of aorta CC
CC Excl: E78.71-E78.72, P29.3, Q25.1-Q25.3, Q27.30, Q27.4, Q28.0-Q28.1, Q28.8-Q28.9, Q87.1-Q87.89, Q89.7-Q89.8, Q99.2

Q25.3 Supravalvular aortic stenosis CC
EXCLUDES 1 *congenital aortic stenosis NOS (Q23.0)*
congenital stenosis of aortic valve (Q23.0)
CC Excl: See code: Q25.2

Q25.4 Other congenital malformations of aorta CC
Absence of aorta
Aneurysm of sinus of Valsalva (ruptured)
Aplasia of aorta
Congenital aneurysm of aorta
Congenital malformations of aorta
Congenital dilatation of aorta
Double aortic arch [vascular ring of aorta]
Hypoplasia of aorta
Persistent convolutions of aortic arch
Persistent right aortic arch
EXCLUDES 1 *hypoplasia of aorta in hypoplastic left heart syndrome (Q23.4)*
CC Excl: E78.71-E78.72, Q25.1-Q25.4, Q25.8-Q25.9, Q27.30, Q27.4, Q28.0-Q28.1, Q28.8-Q28.9, Q87.2-Q87.3, Q87.5-Q87.89, Q89.7-Q89.8

Q25.5 Atresia of pulmonary artery MCC
CC Excl: Q25.5-Q25.79, Q27.30, Q27.4, Q28.0-Q28.1, Q28.8-Q28.9

Q25.6 Stenosis of pulmonary artery MCC
Supravalvular pulmonary stenosis
CC Excl: See code: Q25.5

Q25.7 Other congenital malformations of pulmonary artery

CC Excl: For CC codes in subcategory Q25.7, unless otherwise noted: See code: Q25.5

Q25.71 Coarctation of pulmonary artery MCC

Q25.72 Congenital pulmonary arteriovenous malformation MCC
Congenital pulmonary arteriovenous aneurysm

Q25.79 Other congenital malformations of pulmonary artery MCC
Aberrant pulmonary artery
Agenesis of pulmonary artery
Congenital aneurysm of pulmonary artery
Congenital anomaly of pulmonary artery
Hypoplasia of pulmonary artery

Q25.8 Other congenital malformations of other great arteries CC
CC Excl: See code: Q25.4

Q25.9 Congenital malformation of great arteries, unspecified CC
CC Excl: See code: Q25.4

Q26 Congenital malformations of great veins

Q26.0 Congenital stenosis of vena cava CC
Congenital stenosis of vena cava (inferior)(superior)
CC Excl: Q26.0-Q26.1, Q26.8, Q27.30, Q27.4, Q28.0-Q28.1, Q28.8-Q28.9

Q26.1 Persistent left superior vena cava CC
CC Excl: See code: Q26.0

Q26.2 Total anomalous pulmonary venous connection CC
Total anomalous pulmonary venous return [TAPVR], subdiaphragmatic
Total anomalous pulmonary venous return [TAPVR], supradiaphragmatic
CC Excl: Q26.2, Q27.30, Q27.4, Q28.0-Q28.1, Q28.8-Q28.9

Q26.3 Partial anomalous pulmonary venous connection CC
Partial anomalous pulmonary venous return
CC Excl: Q26.3-Q26.4, Q27.30, Q27.4, Q28.0-Q28.1, Q28.8-Q28.9

Q26.4 Anomalous pulmonary venous connection, unspecified CC
CC Excl: See code: Q26.3

Q26.5 Anomalous portal venous connection

Q26.6 Portal vein-hepatic artery fistula

Q26.8 Other congenital malformations of great veins CC
Absence of vena cava (inferior) (superior)
Azygos continuation of inferior vena cava
Persistent left posterior cardinal vein
Scimitar syndrome
CC Excl: See code: Q26.0

Q26.9 Congenital malformation of great vein, unspecified CC
Congenital anomaly of vena cava (inferior) (superior) NOS
CC Excl: Q26.9-Q27.30, Q27.4, Q28.0-Q28.1, Q28.8-Q28.9

Q27 Other congenital malformations of peripheral vascular system
EXCLUDES 2 *anomalies of cerebral and precerebral vessels (Q28.0-Q28.3)*
anomalies of coronary vessels (Q24.5)
anomalies of pulmonary artery (Q25.5-Q25.7)
congenital retinal aneurysm (Q14.1)
hemangioma and lymphangioma (D18.-)

Q27.0 Congenital absence and hypoplasia of umbilical artery
Single umbilical artery

Q27.1 Congenital renal artery stenosis

Q27.2 Other congenital malformations of renal artery
Congenital malformation of renal artery NOS
Multiple renal arteries

DRAFT

✓5th **Q27.3 Arteriovenous malformation (peripheral)**
Arteriovenous aneurysm
EXCLUDES 1 *acquired arteriovenous aneurysm (I77.0)*
EXCLUDES 2 *arteriovenous malformation of cerebral vessels (Q28.2)*
arteriovenous malformation of precerebral vessels (Q28.0)

Q27.30 Arteriovenous malformation, site unspecified CC
CC Excl: Q20.0-Q20.8, Q21.0-Q21.9, Q27.30, Q27.4, Q28.0-Q28.1, Q28.8

Q27.31 Arteriovenous malformation of vessel of upper limb

Q27.32 Arteriovenous malformation of vessel of lower limb

Q27.33 Arteriovenous malformation of digestive system vessel

Q27.34 Arteriovenous malformation of renal vessel

Q27.39 Arteriovenous malformation, other site

Q27.4 Congenital phlebectasia CC
CC Excl: See code: Q27.30

Q27.8 Other specified congenital malformations of peripheral vascular system
Absence of peripheral vascular system
Atresia of peripheral vascular system
Congenital aneurysm (peripheral)
Congenital stricture, artery
Congenital varix
EXCLUDES 1 *arteriovenous malformation (Q27.3-)*

Q27.9 Congenital malformation of peripheral vascular system, unspecified
Anomaly of artery or vein NOS

✓4th **Q28 Other congenital malformations of circulatory system**
EXCLUDES 1 *congenital aneurysm NOS (Q27.8)*
congenital coronary aneurysm (Q24.5)
ruptured cerebral arteriovenous malformation (I60.8)
ruptured malformation of precerebral vessels (I72.0)
EXCLUDES 2 *congenital peripheral aneurysm (Q27.8)*
congenital pulmonary aneurysm (Q25.79)
congenital retinal aneurysm (Q14.1)

CC Excl: For CC/MCC codes in category Q28, unless otherwise noted: See code: Q27.30

Q28.0 Arteriovenous malformation of precerebral vessels CC
Congenital arteriovenous precerebral aneurysm (nonruptured)

Q28.1 Other malformations of precerebral vessels CC
Congenital malformation of precerebral vessels NOS
Congenital precerebral aneurysm (nonruptured)

Q28.2 Arteriovenous malformation of cerebral vessels MCC
Arteriovenous malformation of brain NOS
Congenital arteriovenous cerebral aneurysm (nonruptured)
CC Excl: Q27.30, Q27.4, Q28.0-Q28.9

Q28.3 Other malformations of cerebral vessels MCC
Congenital cerebral aneurysm (nonruptured)
Congenital malformation of cerebral vessels NOS
Developmental venous anomaly
CC Excl: See code: Q28.2

Q28.8 Other specified congenital malformations of circulatory system CC
Congenital aneurysm, specified site NEC
Spinal vessel anomaly
CC Excl: Q20.0-Q20.8, Q21.0-Q21.9, Q27.30, Q27.4, Q28.0-Q28.1, Q28.8

Q28.9 Congenital malformation of circulatory system, unspecified CC
CC Excl: Q20.0-Q28.9

Congenital malformations of the respiratory system (Q30-Q34)

✓4th **Q30 Congenital malformations of nose**
EXCLUDES 1 *congenital deviation of nasal septum (Q67.4)*

Q30.0 Choanal atresia
Atresia of nares (anterior) (posterior)
Congenital stenosis of nares (anterior) (posterior)

Q30.1 Agenesis and underdevelopment of nose
Congenital absent of nose

Q30.2 Fissured, notched and cleft nose

Q30.3 Congenital perforated nasal septum

Q30.8 Other congenital malformations of nose
Accessory nose
Congenital anomaly of nasal sinus wall

Q30.9 Congenital malformation of nose, unspecified

✓4th **Q31 Congenital malformations of larynx**
EXCLUDES 1 *congenital laryngeal stridor NOS (P28.89)*

CC Excl: For CC codes in category Q31, unless otherwise noted: J39.8, J45.990, J98.09, Q31.1-Q32.4, Q34.0-Q34.9

Q31.0 Web of larynx
Glottic web of larynx
Subglottic web of larynx
Web of larynx NOS

Q31.1 Congenital subglottic stenosis CC

Q31.2 Laryngeal hypoplasia CC

Q31.3 Laryngocele CC

Q31.5 Congenital laryngomalacia CC

Q31.8 Other congenital malformations of larynx CC
Absence of larynx
Agenesis of larynx
Atresia of larynx
Congenital cleft thyroid cartilage
Congenital fissure of epiglottis
Congenital stenosis of larynx NEC
Posterior cleft of cricoid cartilage

Q31.9 Congenital malformation of larynx, unspecified CC

✓4th **Q32 Congenital malformations of trachea and bronchus**
EXCLUDES 1 *congenital bronchiectasis (Q33.4)*

CC Excl: For CC codes in category Q32, unless otherwise noted: See code: Q31

Q32.0 Congenital tracheomalacia CC

Q32.1 Other congenital malformations of trachea CC
Atresia of trachea
Congenital anomaly of tracheal cartilage
Congenital dilatation of trachea
Congenital malformation of trachea
Congenital stenosis of trachea
Congenital tracheocele

Q32.2 Congenital bronchomalacia CC

Q32.3 Congenital stenosis of bronchus CC

Q32.4 Other congenital malformations of bronchus CC
Absence of bronchus
Agenesis of bronchus
Atresia of bronchus
Congenital diverticulum of bronchus
Congenital malformation of bronchus NOS

✓4th **Q33 Congenital malformations of lung**

CC Excl: For CC/MCC codes in category Q33, unless otherwise noted: Q33.0-Q34.9

Q33.0 Congenital cystic lung CC
Congenital cystic lung disease
Congenital honeycomb lung
Congenital polycystic lung disease
EXCLUDES 1 *cystic fibrosis (E84.0)*
cystic lung disease, acquired or unspecified (J98.4)

Q33.1 Accessory lobe of lung
Azygos lobe (fissured), lung

Q33.2 Sequestration of lung MCC

Q33.3 Agenesis of lung MCC
Congenital absence of lung (lobe)

Q33.4 Congenital bronchiectasis CC
CC Excl: J44.9, J47.0-J47.9, J68.1, J68.4-J68.9, Q33.4

Q33.5 Ectopic tissue in lung

Q33.6 Congenital hypoplasia and dysplasia of lung MCC
EXCLUDES 1 *pulmonary hypoplasia associated with short gestation (P28.0)*
CC Excl: Q33.0-Q34.9

Q33.8 Other congenital malformations of lung

Q33.9 Congenital malformation of lung, unspecified

✓4th **Q34 Other congenital malformations of respiratory system**
EXCLUDES 2 *congenital central alveolar hypoventilation syndrome (G47.35)*

Q34.0 Anomaly of pleura

Q34.1 Congenital cyst of mediastinum

Q34.8 Other specified congenital malformations of respiratory system
Atresia of nasopharynx

Q34.9 Congenital malformation of respiratory system, unspecified
Congenital absence of respiratory system
Congenital anomaly of respiratory system NOS

Cleft lip and cleft palate (Q35-Q37)

Use additional code to identify associated malformation of the nose (Q30.2)

EXCLUDES 1 *Robin's syndrome (Q87.0)*

Q35 Cleft palate

INCLUDES fissure of palate
palatoschisis

EXCLUDES 1 *cleft palate with cleft lip (Q37.-)*

Q35.1 Cleft hard palate

Q35.3 Cleft soft palate

Q35.5 Cleft hard palate with cleft soft palate

Q35.7 Cleft uvula

Q35.9 Cleft palate, unspecified
Cleft palate NOS

Q36 Cleft lip
Cheiloschisis
Congenital fissure of lip
Harelip
Labium leporinum

EXCLUDES 1 *cleft lip with cleft palate (Q37.-)*

Q36.0 Cleft lip, bilateral

Q36.1 Cleft lip, median

Q36.9 Cleft lip, unilateral
Cleft lip NOS

Q37 Cleft palate with cleft lip
Cheilopalatoschisis

Q37.0 Cleft hard palate with bilateral cleft lip

Q37.1 Cleft hard palate with unilateral cleft lip
Cleft hard palate with cleft lip NOS

Q37.2 Cleft soft palate with bilateral cleft lip

Q37.3 Cleft soft palate with unilateral cleft lip
Cleft soft palate with cleft lip NOS

Q37.4 Cleft hard and soft palate with bilateral cleft lip

Q37.5 Cleft hard and soft palate with unilateral cleft lip
Cleft hard and soft palate with cleft lip NOS

Q37.8 Unspecified cleft palate with bilateral cleft lip

Q37.9 Unspecified cleft palate with unilateral cleft lip
Cleft palate with cleft lip NOS

Other congenital malformations of the digestive system (Q38-Q45)

Q38 Other congenital malformations of tongue, mouth and pharynx

EXCLUDES 1 *dentofacial anomalies (M26.-)*
macrostomia (Q18.4)
microstomia (Q18.5)

Q38.0 Congenital malformations of lips, not elsewhere classified
Congenital fistula of lip
Congenital malformation of lip NOS
Van der Woude's syndrome

EXCLUDES 1 *cleft lip (Q36.-)*
cleft lip with cleft palate (Q37.-)
macrocheilia (Q18.6)
microcheilia (Q18.7)

Q38.1 Ankyloglossia
Tongue tie

Q38.2 Macroglossia
Congenital hypertrophy of tongue

Q38.3 Other congenital malformations of tongue
Aglossia
Bifid tongue
Congenital adhesion of tongue
Congenital fissure of tongue
Congenital malformation of tongue NOS
Double tongue
Hypoglossia
Hypoplasia of tongue
Microglossia

Q38.4 Congenital malformations of salivary glands and ducts
Atresia of salivary glands and ducts
Congenital absence of salivary glands and ducts
Congenital accessory salivary glands and ducts
Congenital fistula of salivary gland

Q38.5 Congenital malformations of palate, not elsewhere classified
Congenital absence of uvula
Congenital malformation of palate NOS
Congenital high arched palate

EXCLUDES 1 *cleft palate (Q35.-)*
cleft palate with cleft lip (Q37.-)

Q38.6 Other congenital malformations of mouth
Congenital malformation of mouth NOS

Q38.7 Congenital pharyngeal pouch
Congenital diverticulum of pharynx

EXCLUDES 1 *pharyngeal pouch syndrome (D82.1)*

Q38.8 Other congenital malformations of pharynx
Congenital malformation of pharynx NOS
Imperforate pharynx

Q39 Congenital malformations of esophagus

CC Excl: For CC/MCC codes in category Q39, unless otherwise noted: Q39.0-Q39.9, Q45.8-Q45.9

Q39.0 Atresia of esophagus without fistula MCC
Atresia of esophagus NOS

Q39.1 Atresia of esophagus with tracheo-esophageal fistula MCC
Atresia of esophagus with broncho-esophageal fistula

Q39.2 Congenital tracheo-esophageal fistula without atresia MCC
Congenital tracheo-esophageal fistula NOS

Q39.3 Congenital stenosis and stricture of esophagus MCC

Q39.4 Esophageal web MCC

Q39.5 Congenital dilatation of esophagus CC
Congenital cardiospasm
CC Excl: Q39.5-Q39.9, Q45.8-Q45.9

Q39.6 Congenital diverticulum of esophagus CC
Congenital esophageal pouch
CC Excl: See code: Q39.5

Q39.8 Other congenital malformations of esophagus CC
Congenital absence of esophagus
Congenital displacement of esophagus
Congenital duplication of esophagus
CC Excl: See code: Q39.5

Q39.9 Congenital malformation of esophagus, unspecified CC
CC Excl: See code: Q39.5

Q40 Other congenital malformations of upper alimentary tract

Q40.0 Congenital hypertrophic pyloric stenosis
Congenital or infantile constriction
Congenital or infantile hypertrophy
Congenital or infantile spasm
Congenital or infantile stenosis
Congenital or infantile stricture

Q40.1 Congenital hiatus hernia
Congenital displacement of cardia through esophageal hiatus

EXCLUDES 1 *congenital diaphragmatic hernia (Q79.0)*

Q40.2 Other specified congenital malformations of stomach
Congenital displacement of stomach
Congenital diverticulum of stomach
Congenital hourglass stomach
Congenital duplication of stomach
Megalogastria
Microgastria

Q40.3 Congenital malformation of stomach, unspecified

Q40.8 Other specified congenital malformations of upper alimentary tract

Q40.9 Congenital malformation of upper alimentary tract, unspecified
Congenital anomaly of upper alimentary tract
Congenital deformity of upper alimentary tract

Q41 Congenital absence, atresia and stenosis of small intestine
Congenital obstruction, occlusion or stricture of small intestine or intestine NOS

EXCLUDES 1 *cystic fibrosis with intestinal manifestation (E84.11)*
meconium ileus NOS (without cystic fibrosis) (P76.0)

CC Excl: For CC codes in category Q41, unless otherwise noted: Q41.0-Q41.9, Q45.8-Q45.9

Q41.0 Congenital absence, atresia and stenosis of duodenum CC

Q41.1 Congenital absence, atresia and stenosis of jejunum CC
Apple peel syndrome
Imperforate jejunum

Q41.2 Congenital absence, atresia and stenosis of ileum CC

Q41.8 Congenital absence, atresia and stenosis of other specified parts of small intestine CC

Q41.9 Congenital absence, atresia and stenosis of small intestine, part unspecified CC
Congenital absence, atresia and stenosis of intestine NOS

Q42 Congenital absence, atresia and stenosis of large intestine
Congenital obstruction, occlusion and stricture of large intestine

CC Excl: For CC codes in category Q42, unless otherwise noted: Q42.0-Q42.9, Q45.8-Q45.9

Q42.0 Congenital absence, atresia and stenosis of rectum with fistula CC

Q42.1 Congenital absence, atresia and stenosis of rectum without fistula CC
Imperforate rectum

Q42.2 Congenital absence, atresia and stenosis of anus with fistula CC

Q42.3 Congenital absence, atresia and stenosis of anus without fistula CC
Imperforate anus

Q42.8 Congenital absence, atresia and stenosis of other parts of large intestine CC

Q42.9 Congenital absence, atresia and stenosis of large intestine, part unspecified CC

Q43 Other congenital malformations of intestine

CC Excl: For CC codes in category Q43, unless otherwise noted: Q41.0-Q43.9

Q43.0 Meckel's diverticulum (displaced) (hypertrophic)
Persistent omphalomesenteric duct
Persistent vitelline duct

Q43.1 Hirschsprung's disease CC
Aganglionosis
Congenital (aganglionic) megacolon
CC Excl: Q43.1-Q43.2, Q45.8-Q45.9

Q43.2 Other congenital functional disorders of colon CC
Congenital dilatation of colon
CC Excl: See code: Q43.1

Q43.3 Congenital malformations of intestinal fixation CC
Congenital omental, anomalous adhesions [bands]
Congenital peritoneal adhesions [bands]
Incomplete rotation of cecum and colon
Insufficient rotation of cecum and colon
Jackson's membrane
Malrotation of colon
Rotation failure of cecum and colon
Universal mesentery
CC Excl: Q43.3-Q43.9

Q43.4 Duplication of intestine CC

Q43.5 Ectopic anus CC

Q43.6 Congenital fistula of rectum and anus CC
EXCLUDES 1 *congenital fistula of anus with absence, atresia and stenosis (Q42.2)*
congenital fistula of rectum with absence, atresia and stenosis (Q42.0)
congenital rectovaginal fistula (Q52.2)
congenital urethrorectal fistula (Q64.73)
pilonidal fistula or sinus (L05.-)

Q43.7 Persistent cloaca CC
Cloaca NOS

Q43.8 Other specified congenital malformations of intestine CC
Congenital blind loop syndrome
Congenital diverticulitis, colon
Congenital diverticulum, intestine
Dolichocolon
Megaloappendix
Megaloduodenum
Microcolon
Transposition of appendix
Transposition of colon
Transposition of intestine
AHA: 2013, 2Q, 31

Q43.9 Congenital malformation of intestine, unspecified CC

Q44 Congenital malformations of gallbladder, bile ducts and liver

CC Excl: For CC/MCC codes in category Q44, unless otherwise noted: Q44.0-Q44.7

Q44.0 Agenesis, aplasia and hypoplasia of gallbladder CC
Congenital absence of gallbladder

Q44.1 Other congenital malformations of gallbladder CC
Congenital malformation of gallbladder NOS
Intrahepatic gallbladder

Q44.2 Atresia of bile ducts MCC
CC Excl: Q44.2-Q44.3, Q45.8-Q45.9

Q44.3 Congenital stenosis and stricture of bile ducts MCC
CC Excl: See code: Q44.2

Q44.4 Choledochal cyst CC

Q44.5 Other congenital malformations of bile ducts CC
Accessory hepatic duct
Biliary duct duplication
Congenital malformation of bile duct NOS
Cystic duct duplication

Q44.6 Cystic disease of liver CC
Fibrocystic disease of liver
CC Excl: Q44.0-Q44.1, Q44.4-Q44.7

Q44.7 Other congenital malformations of liver CC
Accessory liver
Alagille's syndrome
Congenital absence of liver
Congenital hepatomegaly
Congenital malformation of liver NOS

Q45 Other congenital malformations of digestive system
EXCLUDES 2 *congenital diaphragmatic hernia (Q79.0)*
congenital hiatus hernia (Q40.1)

CC Excl: For CC/MCC codes in category Q45, unless otherwise noted: Q45.0-Q45.9

Q45.0 Agenesis, aplasia and hypoplasia of pancreas CC
Congenital absence of pancreas

Q45.1 Annular pancreas CC

Q45.2 Congenital pancreatic cyst CC

Q45.3 Other congenital malformations of pancreas and pancreatic duct CC
Accessory pancreas
Congenital malformation of pancreas or pancreatic duct NOS
EXCLUDES 1 *congenital diabetes mellitus (E10.-)*
cystic fibrosis (E84.0-E84.9)
fibrocystic disease of pancreas (E84.-)
neonatal diabetes mellitus (P70.2)

Q45.8 Other specified congenital malformations of digestive system
Absence (complete) (partial) of alimentary tract NOS
Duplication of digestive system
Malposition, congenital of digestive system

Q45.9 Congenital malformation of digestive system, unspecified
Congenital anomaly of digestive system
Congenital deformity of digestive system

Congenital malformations of genital organs (Q50-Q56)

EXCLUDES 1 *androgen insensitivity syndrome (E34.5-)*
syndromes associated with anomalies in the number and form of chromosomes (Q90-Q99)

Q50 Congenital malformations of ovaries, fallopian tubes and broad ligaments

Q50.0 Congenital absence of ovary
EXCLUDES 1 *Turner's syndrome (Q96.-)*

Q50.01 Congenital absence of ovary, unilateral ♀

Q50.02 Congenital absence of ovary, bilateral ♀

Q50.1 Developmental ovarian cyst ♀

Q50.2 Congenital torsion of ovary ♀

Q50.3 Other congenital malformations of ovary

Q50.31 Accessory ovary ♀

Q50.32 Ovarian streak ♀
46, XX with streak gonads

Q50.39 Other congenital malformation of ovary ♀
Congenital malformation of ovary NOS

Q50.4 Embryonic cyst of fallopian tube ♀
Fimbrial cyst

Q50.5 Embryonic cyst of broad ligament ♀
Epoophoron cyst
Parovarian cyst

Q50.6 Other congenital malformations of fallopian tube and broad ligament ♀
Absence of fallopian tube and broad ligament
Accessory fallopian tube and broad ligament
Atresia of fallopian tube and broad ligament
Congenital malformation of fallopian tube or broad ligament NOS

Q51 Congenital malformations of uterus and cervix

Q51.0 Agenesis and aplasia of uterus ♀
Congenital absence of uterus

✓5th **Q51.1 Doubling of uterus with doubling of cervix and vagina**

Q51.1Ø Doubling of uterus with doubling of cervix and vagina without obstruction ♀
Doubling of uterus with doubling of cervix and vagina NOS

Q51.11 Doubling of uterus with doubling of cervix and vagina with obstruction ♀

Q51.2 Other doubling of uterus ♀
Doubling of uterus NOS
Septate uterus, complete or partial

Q51.3 Bicornate uterus ♀
Bicornate uterus, complete or partial

Q51.4 Unicornate uterus ♀
Unicornate uterus with or without a separate uterine horn
Uterus with only one functioning horn

Q51.5 Agenesis and aplasia of cervix ♀
Congenital absence of cervix

Q51.6 Embryonic cyst of cervix ♀

Q51.7 Congenital fistulae between uterus and digestive and urinary tracts ♀

✓5th **Q51.8 Other congenital malformations of uterus and cervix**

✓6th **Q51.81 Other congenital malformations of uterus**

Q51.81Ø Arcuate uterus ♀
Arcuatus uterus

Q51.811 Hypoplasia of uterus ♀

Q51.818 Other congenital malformations of uterus ♀
Müllerian anomaly of uterus NEC

✓6th **Q51.82 Other congenital malformations of cervix**

Q51.82Ø Cervical duplication ♀

Q51.821 Hypoplasia of cervix ♀

Q51.828 Other congenital malformations of cervix ♀

Q51.9 Congenital malformation of uterus and cervix, unspecified ♀

✓4th **Q52 Other congenital malformations of female genitalia**

Q52.Ø Congenital absence of vagina ♀
Vaginal agenesis, total or partial

✓5th **Q52.1 Doubling of vagina**
EXCLUDES 1 *doubling of vagina with doubling of uterus and cervix (Q51.1-)*

Q52.1Ø Doubling of vagina, unspecified ♀
Septate vagina NOS

Q52.11 Transverse vaginal septum ♀

Q52.12 Longitudinal vaginal septum ♀
Longitudinal vaginal septum with or without obstruction

Q52.2 Congenital rectovaginal fistula ♀
EXCLUDES 1 *cloaca (Q43.7)*

Q52.3 Imperforate hymen ♀

Q52.4 Other congenital malformations of vagina ♀
Canal of Nuck cyst, congenital
Congenital malformation of vagina NOS
Embryonic vaginal cyst
Gartner's duct cyst

Q52.5 Fusion of labia ♀

Q52.6 Congenital malformation of clitoris ♀

✓5th **Q52.7 Other and unspecified congenital malformations of vulva**

Q52.7Ø Unspecified congenital malformations of vulva ♀
Congenital malformation of vulva NOS

Q52.71 Congenital absence of vulva ♀

Q52.79 Other congenital malformations of vulva ♀
Congenital cyst of vulva

Q52.8 Other specified congenital malformations of female genitalia ♀

Q52.9 Congenital malformation of female genitalia, unspecified ♀

✓4th **Q53 Undescended and ectopic testicle**

✓5th **Q53.Ø Ectopic testis**

Q53.ØØ Ectopic testis, unspecified ♂

Q53.Ø1 Ectopic testis, unilateral ♂

Q53.Ø2 Ectopic testes, bilateral ♂

✓5th **Q53.1 Undescended testicle, unilateral**

Q53.1Ø Unspecified undescended testicle, unilateral ♂

Q53.11 Abdominal testis, unilateral ♂

Q53.12 Ectopic perineal testis, unilateral ♂

✓5th **Q53.2 Undescended testicle, bilateral**

Q53.2Ø Undescended testicle, unspecified, bilateral ♂

Q53.21 Abdominal testis, bilateral ♂

Q53.22 Ectopic perineal testis, bilateral ♂

Q53.9 Undescended testicle, unspecified ♂
Cryptorchism NOS

✓4th **Q54 Hypospadias**
EXCLUDES 1 *epispadias (Q64.Ø)*

Q54.Ø Hypospadias, balanic ♂
Hypospadias, coronal
Hypospadias, glandular

Q54.1 Hypospadias, penile ♂

Q54.2 Hypospadias, penoscrotal ♂

Q54.3 Hypospadias, perineal ♂

Q54.4 Congenital chordee ♂
Chordee without hypospadias

Q54.8 Other hypospadias ♂
Hypospadias with intersex state

Q54.9 Hypospadias, unspecified ♂

✓4th **Q55 Other congenital malformations of male genital organs**
EXCLUDES 1 *congenital hydrocele (P83.5)*
hypospadias (Q54.-)

Q55.Ø Absence and aplasia of testis ♂
Monorchism

Q55.1 Hypoplasia of testis and scrotum ♂
Fusion of testes

✓5th **Q55.2 Other and unspecified congenital malformations of testis and scrotum**

Q55.2Ø Unspecified congenital malformations of testis and scrotum ♂
Congenital malformation of testis or scrotum NOS

Q55.21 Polyorchism ♂

Q55.22 Retractile testis ♂

Q55.23 Scrotal transposition ♂

Q55.29 Other congenital malformations of testis and scrotum ♂

Q55.3 Atresia of vas deferens ♂
Code first any associated cystic fibrosis (E84.-)

Q55.4 Other congenital malformations of vas deferens, epididymis, seminal vesicles and prostate ♂
Absence or aplasia of prostate
Absence or aplasia of spermatic cord
Congenital malformation of vas deferens, epididymis, seminal vesicles or prostate NOS

Q55.5 Congenital absence and aplasia of penis ♂

✓5th **Q55.6 Other congenital malformations of penis**

Q55.61 Curvature of penis (lateral) ♂

Q55.62 Hypoplasia of penis ♂
Micropenis

Q55.63 Congenital torsion of penis ♂
EXCLUDES 1 *acquired torsion of penis (N48.82)*

Q55.64 Hidden penis ♂
Buried penis
Concealed penis
EXCLUDES 1 *acquired buried penis (N48.83)*

Q55.69 Other congenital malformation of penis ♂
Congenital malformation of penis NOS

Q55.7 Congenital vasocutaneous fistula ♂

Q55.8 Other specified congenital malformations of male genital organs ♂

Q55.9 Congenital malformation of male genital organ, unspecified ♂
Congenital anomaly of male genital organ
Congenital deformity of male genital organ

✓4th **Q56 Indeterminate sex and pseudohermaphroditism**
EXCLUDES 1 *46, XX true hermaphrodite (Q99.1)*
androgen insensitivity syndrome (E34.5-)
chimera 46, XX/46, XY true hermaphrodite (Q99.Ø)
female pseudohermaphroditism with adrenocortical disorder (E25.-)
pseudohermaphroditism with specified chromosomal anomaly (Q96-Q99)
pure gonadal dysgenesis (Q99.1)

Q56.Ø Hermaphroditism, not elsewhere classified
Ovotestis

Q56.1 Male pseudohermaphroditism, not elsewhere classified ♂
46, XY with streak gonads
Male pseudohermaphroditism NOS

Q56.2 Female pseudohermaphroditism, not elsewhere classified ♀
Female pseudohermaphroditism NOS

Q56.3 Pseudohermaphroditism, unspecified

Q56.4 Indeterminate sex, unspecified
Ambiguous genitalia

Congenital malformations of the urinary system (Q60-Q64)

✓4th **Q60 Renal agenesis and other reduction defects of kidney**
Congenital absence of kidney
Congenital atrophy of kidney
Infantile atrophy of kidney

CC Excl: For CC codes in category Q60, unless otherwise noted: N13.9, Q60.0-Q60.6

Q60.0 Renal agenesis, unilateral CC
Q60.1 Renal agenesis, bilateral CC
Q60.2 Renal agenesis, unspecified CC
Q60.3 Renal hypoplasia, unilateral CC
Q60.4 Renal hypoplasia, bilateral CC
Q60.5 Renal hypoplasia, unspecified CC
Q60.6 Potter's syndrome CC

✓4th **Q61 Cystic kidney disease**
EXCLUDES 1 *acquired cyst of kidney (N28.1)*
Potter's syndrome (Q60.6)

✓5th **Q61.0 Congenital renal cyst**

Q61.00 Congenital renal cyst, unspecified CC
Cyst of kidney NOS (congenital)
CC Excl: N13.9, Q61.00, Q61.9

Q61.01 Congenital single renal cyst CC
CC Excl: N13.9, Q61.01

Q61.02 Congenital multiple renal cysts CC
CC Excl: N13.9, Q61.02, Q61.5-Q61.8

✓5th **Q61.1 Polycystic kidney, infantile type**
Polycystic kidney, autosomal recessive

Q61.11 Cystic dilatation of collecting ducts CC
CC Excl: N13.9, Q61.11-Q61.3

Q61.19 Other polycystic kidney, infantile type CC
CC Excl: See code: Q61.11

Q61.2 Polycystic kidney, adult type CC
Polycystic kidney, autosomal dominant
CC Excl: See code: Q61.11

Q61.3 Polycystic kidney, unspecified CC
CC Excl: See code: Q61.11

Q61.4 Renal dysplasia CC
Multicystic dysplastic kidney
Multicystic kidney (development)
Multicystic kidney disease
Multicystic renal dysplasia
EXCLUDES 1 *polycystic kidney disease (Q61.11-Q61.3)*
CC Excl: N13.9, Q61.4

Q61.5 Medullary cystic kidney CC
Nephronopthisis
Sponge kidney NOS
CC Excl: See code: Q61.02

Q61.8 Other cystic kidney diseases CC
Fibrocystic kidney
Fibrocystic renal degeneration or disease
CC Excl: See code: Q61.02

Q61.9 Cystic kidney disease, unspecified CC
Meckel-Gruber syndrome
CC Excl: See code: Q61.00

✓4th **Q62 Congenital obstructive defects of renal pelvis and congenital malformations of ureter**

CC Excl: For CC codes in category Q62, unless otherwise noted: N13.9, Q62.0-Q62.2, Q62.39

Q62.0 Congenital hydronephrosis CC

✓5th **Q62.1 Congenital occlusion of ureter**
Atresia and stenosis of ureter

Q62.10 Congenital occlusion of ureter, unspecified CC
Q62.11 Congenital occlusion of ureteropelvic junction CC
Q62.12 Congenital occlusion of ureterovesical orifice CC

Q62.2 Congenital megaureter CC
Congenital dilatation of ureter

✓5th **Q62.3 Other obstructive defects of renal pelvis and ureter**

Q62.31 Congenital ureterocele, orthotopic CC
Q62.32 Cecoureterocele CC
Ectopic ureterocele
Q62.39 Other obstructive defects of renal pelvis and ureter CC
Ureteropelvic junction obstruction NOS

Q62.4 Agenesis of ureter
Congenital absence ureter

Q62.5 Duplication of ureter
Accessory ureter
Double ureter

✓5th **Q62.6 Malposition of ureter**

Q62.60 Malposition of ureter, unspecified
Q62.61 Deviation of ureter
Q62.62 Displacement of ureter
Q62.63 Anomalous implantation of ureter
Ectopia of ureter
Ectopic ureter
Q62.69 Other malposition of ureter

Q62.7 Congenital vesico-uretero-renal reflux

Q62.8 Other congenital malformations of ureter
Anomaly of ureter NOS

✓4th **Q63 Other congenital malformations of kidney**
EXCLUDES 1 *congenital nephrotic syndrome (N04.-)*

Q63.0 Accessory kidney

Q63.1 Lobulated, fused and horseshoe kidney

Q63.2 Ectopic kidney
Congenital displaced kidney
Malrotation of kidney

Q63.3 Hyperplastic and giant kidney
Compensatory hypertrophy of kidney

Q63.8 Other specified congenital malformations of kidney
Congenital renal calculi

Q63.9 Congenital malformation of kidney, unspecified

✓4th **Q64 Other congenital malformations of urinary system**

Q64.0 Epispadias ♂
EXCLUDES 1 *hypospadias (Q54.-)*

✓5th **Q64.1 Exstrophy of urinary bladder**

CC Excl: For CC codes in subcategory Q64.1, unless otherwise noted: N13.9, Q64.10-Q64.19, Q64.8-Q64.9

Q64.10 Exstrophy of urinary bladder, unspecified CC
Ectopia vesicae
Q64.11 Supravesical fissure of urinary bladder CC
Q64.12 Cloacal extrophy of urinary bladder CC
Q64.19 Other exstrophy of urinary bladder CC
Extroversion of bladder

Q64.2 Congenital posterior urethral valves CC
CC Excl: N13.9, Q64.2-Q64.39, Q64.8-Q64.9

✓5th **Q64.3 Other atresia and stenosis of urethra and bladder neck**

CC Excl: For CC codes in subcategory Q64.3, unless otherwise noted: See code: Q64.2

Q64.31 Congenital bladder neck obstruction CC
Congenital obstruction of vesicourethral orifice
Q64.32 Congenital stricture of urethra CC
Q64.33 Congenital stricture of urinary meatus CC
Q64.39 Other atresia and stenosis of urethra and bladder neck CC
Atresia and stenosis of urethra and bladder neck NOS

Q64.4 Malformation of urachus
Cyst of urachus
Patent urachus
Prolapse of urachus

Q64.5 Congenital absence of bladder and urethra

Q64.6 Congenital diverticulum of bladder

✓5th **Q64.7 Other and unspecified congenital malformations of bladder and urethra**
EXCLUDES 1 *congenital prolapse of bladder (mucosa) (Q79.4)*

Q64.70 Unspecified congenital malformation of bladder and urethra
Malformation of bladder or urethra NOS
Q64.71 Congenital prolapse of urethra
Q64.72 Congenital prolapse of urinary meatus

Q64.73 Congenital urethrorectal fistula
Q64.74 Double urethra
Q64.75 Double urinary meatus
Q64.79 Other congenital malformations of bladder and urethra
Q64.8 Other specified congenital malformations of urinary system
Q64.9 Congenital malformation of urinary system, unspecified
Congenital anomaly NOS of urinary system
Congenital deformity NOS of urinary system

Congenital malformations and deformations of the musculoskeletal system (Q65-Q79)

✓4th **Q65 Congenital deformities of hip**
EXCLUDES 1 *clicking hip (R29.4)*
✓5th **Q65.0 Congenital dislocation of hip, unilateral**
Q65.00 Congenital dislocation of unspecified hip, unilateral
Q65.01 Congenital dislocation of right hip, unilateral
Q65.02 Congenital dislocation of left hip, unilateral
Q65.1 Congenital dislocation of hip, bilateral
Q65.2 Congenital dislocation of hip, unspecified
✓5th **Q65.3 Congenital partial dislocation of hip, unilateral**
Q65.30 Congenital partial dislocation of unspecified hip, unilateral
Q65.31 Congenital partial dislocation of right hip, unilateral
Q65.32 Congenital partial dislocation of left hip, unilateral
Q65.4 Congenital partial dislocation of hip, bilateral
Q65.5 Congenital partial dislocation of hip, unspecified
Q65.6 Congenital unstable hip
Congenital dislocatable hip
✓5th **Q65.8 Other congenital deformities of hip**
Q65.81 Congenital coxa valga
Q65.82 Congenital coxa vara
Q65.89 Other specified congenital deformities of hip
Anteversion of femoral neck
Congenital acetabular dysplasia
Q65.9 Congenital deformity of hip, unspecified

✓4th **Q66 Congenital deformities of feet**
EXCLUDES 1 *reduction defects of feet (Q72.-)*
valgus deformities (acquired) (M21.0-)
varus deformities (acquired) (M21.1-)
Q66.0 Congenital talipes equinovarus
Q66.1 Congenital talipes calcaneovarus
Q66.2 Congenital metatarsus (primus) varus
Q66.3 Other congenital varus deformities of feet
Hallux varus, congenital
Q66.4 Congenital talipes calcaneovalgus
✓5th **Q66.5 Congenital pes planus**
Congenital flat foot
Congenital rigid flat foot
Congenital spastic (everted) flat foot
EXCLUDES 1 *pes planus, acquired (M21.4)*
Q66.50 Congenital pes planus, unspecified foot
Q66.51 Congenital pes planus, right foot
Q66.52 Congenital pes planus, left foot
Q66.6 Other congenital valgus deformities of feet
Congenital metatarsus valgus
Q66.7 Congenital pes cavus
✓5th **Q66.8 Other congenital deformities of feet**
Q66.80 Congenital vertical talus deformity, unspecified foot
Q66.81 Congenital vertical talus deformity, right foot
Q66.82 Congenital vertical talus deformity, left foot
Q66.89 Other specified congenital deformities of feet
Congenital asymmetric talipes
Congenital clubfoot NOS
Congenital talipes NOS
Congenital tarsal coalition
Hammer toe, congenital
Q66.9 Congenital deformity of feet, unspecified

✓4th **Q67 Congenital musculoskeletal deformities of head, face, spine and chest**
EXCLUDES 1 *congenital malformation syndromes classified to Q87-*
Potter's syndrome (Q60.6)
Q67.0 Congenital facial asymmetry
Q67.1 Congenital compression facies
Q67.2 Dolichocephaly
Q67.3 Plagiocephaly
Q67.4 Other congenital deformities of skull, face and jaw
Congenital depressions in skull
Congenital hemifacial atrophy or hypertrophy
Deviation of nasal septum, congenital
Squashed or bent nose, congenital
EXCLUDES 1 *dentofacial anomalies [including malocclusion] (M26.-)*
syphilitic saddle nose (A50.5)
Q67.5 Congenital deformity of spine CC
Congenital postural scoliosis
Congenital scoliosis NOS
EXCLUDES 1 *infantile idiopathic scoliosis (M41.0)*
scoliosis due to congenital bony malformation (Q76.3)
CC Excl: Q67.5, Q76.3, Q76.425-Q76.429
Q67.6 Pectus excavatum
Congenital funnel chest
Q67.7 Pectus carinatum
Congenital pigeon chest
Q67.8 Other congenital deformities of chest CC
Congenital deformity of chest wall NOS
CC Excl: Q67.6-Q67.8, Q68.1, Q74.3

✓4th **Q68 Other congenital musculoskeletal deformities**
EXCLUDES 1 *reduction defects of limb(s) (Q71-Q73)*
EXCLUDES 2 *congenital myotonic chondrodystrophy (G71.13)*
Q68.0 Congenital deformity of sternocleidomastoid muscle
Congenital contracture of sternocleidomastoid (muscle)
Congenital (sternomastoid) torticollis
Sternomastoid tumor (congenital)
Q68.1 Congenital deformity of finger(s) and hand CC
Congenital clubfinger
Spade-like hand (congenital)
CC Excl: See code: Q67.8
Q68.2 Congenital deformity of knee
Congenital dislocation of knee
Congenital genu recurvatum
Q68.3 Congenital bowing of femur
EXCLUDES 1 *anteversion of femur (neck) (Q65.89)*
Q68.4 Congenital bowing of tibia and fibula
Q68.5 Congenital bowing of long bones of leg, unspecified
Q68.6 Discoid meniscus
Q68.8 Other specified congenital musculoskeletal deformities
Congenital deformity of clavicle
Congenital deformity of elbow
Congenital deformity of forearm
Congenital deformity of scapula
Congenital deformity of wrist
Congenital dislocation of elbow
Congenital dislocation of shoulder
Congenital dislocation of wrist

✓4th **Q69 Polydactyly**
Q69.0 Accessory finger(s)
Q69.1 Accessory thumb(s)
Q69.2 Accessory toe(s)
Accessory hallux
Q69.9 Polydactyly, unspecified
Supernumerary digit(s) NOS

✓4th **Q70 Syndactyly**
✓5th **Q70.0 Fused fingers**
Complex syndactyly of fingers with synostosis
Q70.00 Fused fingers, unspecified hand
Q70.01 Fused fingers, right hand
Q70.02 Fused fingers, left hand
Q70.03 Fused fingers, bilateral
✓5th **Q70.1 Webbed fingers**
Simple syndactyly of fingers without synostosis
Q70.10 Webbed fingers, unspecified hand
Q70.11 Webbed fingers, right hand
Q70.12 Webbed fingers, left hand
Q70.13 Webbed fingers, bilateral
✓5th **Q70.2 Fused toes**
Complex syndactyly of toes with synostosis
Q70.20 Fused toes, unspecified foot
Q70.21 Fused toes, right foot
Q70.22 Fused toes, left foot

Q70.23 Fused toes, bilateral

Q70.3 Webbed toes
Simple syndactyly of toes without synostosis
- Q70.30 Webbed toes, unspecified foot
- Q70.31 Webbed toes, right foot
- Q70.32 Webbed toes, left foot
- Q70.33 Webbed toes, bilateral

Q70.4 Polysyndactyly, unspecified
EXCLUDES1 *specified syndactyly of hand and feet—code to specified conditions (Q70.0-Q70.3-)*

Q70.9 Syndactyly, unspecified
Symphalangy NOS

Q71 Reduction defects of upper limb

Q71.0 Congenital complete absence of upper limb
- Q71.00 Congenital complete absence of unspecified upper limb
- Q71.01 Congenital complete absence of right upper limb
- Q71.02 Congenital complete absence of left upper limb
- Q71.03 Congenital complete absence of upper limb, bilateral

Q71.1 Congenital absence of upper arm and forearm with hand present
- Q71.10 Congenital absence of unspecified upper arm and forearm with hand present
- Q71.11 Congenital absence of right upper arm and forearm with hand present
- Q71.12 Congenital absence of left upper arm and forearm with hand present
- Q71.13 Congenital absence of upper arm and forearm with hand present, bilateral

Q71.2 Congenital absence of both forearm and hand
- Q71.20 Congenital absence of both forearm and hand, unspecified upper limb
- Q71.21 Congenital absence of both forearm and hand, right upper limb
- Q71.22 Congenital absence of both forearm and hand, left upper limb
- Q71.23 Congenital absence of both forearm and hand, bilateral

Q71.3 Congenital absence of hand and finger
- Q71.30 Congenital absence of unspecified hand and finger
- Q71.31 Congenital absence of right hand and finger
- Q71.32 Congenital absence of left hand and finger
- Q71.33 Congenital absence of hand and finger, bilateral

Q71.4 Longitudinal reduction defect of radius
Clubhand (congenital)
Radial clubhand
- Q71.40 Longitudinal reduction defect of unspecified radius
- Q71.41 Longitudinal reduction defect of right radius
- Q71.42 Longitudinal reduction defect of left radius
- Q71.43 Longitudinal reduction defect of radius, bilateral

Q71.5 Longitudinal reduction defect of ulna
- Q71.50 Longitudinal reduction defect of unspecified ulna
- Q71.51 Longitudinal reduction defect of right ulna
- Q71.52 Longitudinal reduction defect of left ulna
- Q71.53 Longitudinal reduction defect of ulna, bilateral

Q71.6 Lobster-claw hand
- Q71.60 Lobster-claw hand, unspecified hand
- Q71.61 Lobster-claw right hand
- Q71.62 Lobster-claw left hand
- Q71.63 Lobster-claw hand, bilateral

Q71.8 Other reduction defects of upper limb

Q71.81 Congenital shortening of upper limb
- Q71.811 Congenital shortening of right upper limb
- Q71.812 Congenital shortening of left upper limb
- Q71.813 Congenital shortening of upper limb, bilateral
- Q71.819 Congenital shortening of unspecified upper limb

Q71.89 Other reduction defects of upper limb
- Q71.891 Other reduction defects of right upper limb
- Q71.892 Other reduction defects of left upper limb
- Q71.893 Other reduction defects of upper limb, bilateral
- Q71.899 Other reduction defects of unspecified upper limb

Q71.9 Unspecified reduction defect of upper limb
- Q71.90 Unspecified reduction defect of unspecified upper limb
- Q71.91 Unspecified reduction defect of right upper limb
- Q71.92 Unspecified reduction defect of left upper limb
- Q71.93 Unspecified reduction defect of upper limb, bilateral

Q72 Reduction defects of lower limb

Q72.0 Congenital complete absence of lower limb
- Q72.00 Congenital complete absence of unspecified lower limb
- Q72.01 Congenital complete absence of right lower limb
- Q72.02 Congenital complete absence of left lower limb
- Q72.03 Congenital complete absence of lower limb, bilateral

Q72.1 Congenital absence of thigh and lower leg with foot present
- Q72.10 Congenital absence of unspecified thigh and lower leg with foot present
- Q72.11 Congenital absence of right thigh and lower leg with foot present
- Q72.12 Congenital absence of left thigh and lower leg with foot present
- Q72.13 Congenital absence of thigh and lower leg with foot present, bilateral

Q72.2 Congenital absence of both lower leg and foot
- Q72.20 Congenital absence of both lower leg and foot, unspecified lower limb
- Q72.21 Congenital absence of both lower leg and foot, right lower limb
- Q72.22 Congenital absence of both lower leg and foot, left lower limb
- Q72.23 Congenital absence of both lower leg and foot, bilateral

Q72.3 Congenital absence of foot and toe(s)
- Q72.30 Congenital absence of unspecified foot and toe(s)
- Q72.31 Congenital absence of right foot and toe(s)
- Q72.32 Congenital absence of left foot and toe(s)
- Q72.33 Congenital absence of foot and toe(s), bilateral

Q72.4 Longitudinal reduction defect of femur
Proximal femoral focal deficiency
- Q72.40 Longitudinal reduction defect of unspecified femur
- Q72.41 Longitudinal reduction defect of right femur
- Q72.42 Longitudinal reduction defect of left femur
- Q72.43 Longitudinal reduction defect of femur, bilateral

Q72.5 Longitudinal reduction defect of tibia
- Q72.50 Longitudinal reduction defect of unspecified tibia
- Q72.51 Longitudinal reduction defect of right tibia
- Q72.52 Longitudinal reduction defect of left tibia
- Q72.53 Longitudinal reduction defect of tibia, bilateral

Q72.6 Longitudinal reduction defect of fibula
- Q72.60 Longitudinal reduction defect of unspecified fibula
- Q72.61 Longitudinal reduction defect of right fibula
- Q72.62 Longitudinal reduction defect of left fibula
- Q72.63 Longitudinal reduction defect of fibula, bilateral

Q72.7 Split foot
- Q72.70 Split foot, unspecified lower limb
- Q72.71 Split foot, right lower limb
- Q72.72 Split foot, left lower limb
- Q72.73 Split foot, bilateral

Q72.8 Other reduction defects of lower limb

Q72.81 Congenital shortening of lower limb
- Q72.811 Congenital shortening of right lower limb
- Q72.812 Congenital shortening of left lower limb
- Q72.813 Congenital shortening of lower limb, bilateral
- Q72.819 Congenital shortening of unspecified lower limb

Q72.89 Other reduction defects of lower limb
- Q72.891 Other reduction defects of right lower limb

Q72.892 Other reduction defects of left lower limb

Q72.893 Other reduction defects of lower limb, bilateral

Q72.899 Other reduction defects of unspecified lower limb

✓5th **Q72.9 Unspecified reduction defect of lower limb**

Q72.90 Unspecified reduction defect of unspecified lower limb

Q72.91 Unspecified reduction defect of right lower limb

Q72.92 Unspecified reduction defect of left lower limb

Q72.93 Unspecified reduction defect of lower limb, bilateral

✓4th **Q73 Reduction defects of unspecified limb**

Q73.0 Congenital absence of unspecified limb(s)
Amelia NOS

Q73.1 Phocomelia, unspecified limb(s)
Phocomelia NOS

Q73.8 Other reduction defects of unspecified limb(s)
Longitudinal reduction deformity of unspecified limb(s)
Ectromelia of limb NOS
Hemimelia of limb NOS
Reduction defect of limb NOS

✓4th **Q74 Other congenital malformations of limb(s)**
EXCLUDES 1 *polydactyly (Q69.-)*
reduction defect of limb (Q71-Q73)
syndactyly (Q70.-)

Q74.0 Other congenital malformations of upper limb(s), including shoulder girdle
Accessory carpal bones
Cleidocranial dysostosis
Congenital pseudarthrosis of clavicle
Macrodactylia (fingers)
Madelung's deformity
Radioulnar synostosis
Sprengel's deformity
Triphalangeal thumb

Q74.1 Congenital malformation of knee
Congenital absence of patella
Congenital dislocation of patella
Congenital genu valgum
Congenital genu varum
Rudimentary patella
EXCLUDES 1 *congenital dislocation of knee (Q68.2)*
congenital genu recurvatum (Q68.2)
nail patella syndrome (Q87.2)

Q74.2 Other congenital malformations of lower limb(s), including pelvic girdle
Congenital fusion of sacroiliac joint
Congenital malformation of ankle joint
Congenital malformation of sacroiliac joint
EXCLUDES 1 *anteversion of femur (neck) (Q65.89)*

Q74.3 Arthrogryposis multiplex congenita CC
CC Excl: Q67.5, Q76.3, Q76.425-Q76.429

Q74.8 Other specified congenital malformations of limb(s)

Q74.9 Unspecified congenital malformation of limb(s)
Congenital anomaly of limb(s) NOS

✓4th **Q75 Other congenital malformations of skull and face bones**
EXCLUDES 1 *congenital malformation of face NOS (Q18.-)*
congenital malformation syndromes classified to Q87.-
dentofacial anomalies [including malocclusion] (M26.-)
musculoskeletal deformities of head and face (Q67.0-Q67.4)
skull defects associated with congenital anomalies of brain such as:
anencephaly (Q00.0)
encephalocele (Q01.-)
hydrocephalus (Q03.-)
microcephaly (Q02)

Q75.0 Craniosynostosis
Acrocephaly
Imperfect fusion of skull
Oxycephaly
Trigonocephaly

Q75.1 Craniofacial dysostosis
Crouzon's disease

Q75.2 Hypertelorism

Q75.3 Macrocephaly

Q75.4 Mandibulofacial dysostosis
Franceschetti syndrome
Treacher Collins syndrome

Q75.5 Oculomandibular dysostosis

Q75.8 Other specified congenital malformations of skull and face bones
Absence of skull bone, congenital
Congenital deformity of forehead
Platybasia

Q75.9 Congenital malformation of skull and face bones, unspecified
Congenital anomaly of face bones NOS
Congenital anomaly of skull NOS

✓4th **Q76 Congenital malformations of spine and bony thorax**
EXCLUDES 1 *congenital musculoskeletal deformities of spine and chest (Q67.5-Q67.8)*

Q76.0 Spina bifida occulta
EXCLUDES 1 *meningocele (spinal) (Q05.-)*
spina bifida (aperta) (cystica) (Q05.-)

Q76.1 Klippel-Feil syndrome
Cervical fusion syndrome

Q76.2 Congenital spondylolisthesis
Congenital spondylolysis
EXCLUDES 1 *spondylolisthesis (acquired) (M43.1-)*
spondylolysis (acquired) (M43.0-)

Q76.3 Congenital scoliosis due to congenital bony malformation CC
Hemivertebra fusion or failure of segmentation with scoliosis
CC Excl: See code: Q67.5

✓5th **Q76.4 Other congenital malformations of spine, not associated with scoliosis**

CC Excl: For CC codes in subcategory Q76.4, unless otherwise noted: Q67.5, Q76.3, Q76.425-Q76.429

✓6th **Q76.41 Congenital kyphosis**

Q76.411 Congenital kyphosis, occipito-atlanto-axial region

Q76.412 Congenital kyphosis, cervical region

Q76.413 Congenital kyphosis, cervicothoracic region

Q76.414 Congenital kyphosis, thoracic region

Q76.415 Congenital kyphosis, thoracolumbar region

Q76.419 Congenital kyphosis, unspecified region

✓6th **Q76.42 Congenital lordosis**

Q76.425 Congenital lordosis, thoracolumbar region CC

Q76.426 Congenital lordosis, lumbar region CC

Q76.427 Congenital lordosis, lumbosacral region CC

Q76.428 Congenital lordosis, sacral and sacrococcygeal region CC

Q76.429 Congenital lordosis, unspecified region CC

Q76.49 Other congenital malformations of spine, not associated with scoliosis
Congenital absence of vertebra NOS
Congenital fusion of spine NOS
Congenital malformation of lumbosacral (joint) (region) NOS
Congenital malformation of spine NOS
Hemivertebra NOS
Malformation of spine NOS
Platyspondylisis NOS
Supernumerary vertebra NOS

Q76.5 Cervical rib
Supernumerary rib in cervical region

Q76.6 Other congenital malformations of ribs CC
Accessory rib
Congenital absence of rib
Congenital fusion of ribs
Congenital malformation of ribs NOS
EXCLUDES 1 *short rib syndrome (Q77.2)*
CC Excl: Q76.5-Q76.9, Q77.2

Q76.7 Congenital malformation of sternum CC
Congenital absence of sternum
Sternum bifidum
CC Excl: See code: Q76.6

Q76.8 Other congenital malformations of bony thorax CC
CC Excl: See code: Q76.6

Q76.9 Congenital malformation of bony thorax, unspecified CC
CC Excl: See code: Q76.6b

Q77 Osteochondrodysplasia with defects of growth of tubular bones and spine
EXCLUDES 1 *mucopolysaccharidosis (E76.0-E76.3)*
EXCLUDES 2 *congenital myotonic chondrodystrophy (G71.13)*

Q77.0 Achondrogenesis
Hypochondrogenesis

Q77.1 Thanatophoric short stature

Q77.2 Short rib syndrome CC
Asphyxiating thoracic dysplasia [Jeune]
CC Excl: Q76.5-Q76.9, Q77.2

Q77.3 Chondrodysplasia punctata
EXCLUDES 1 *Rhizomelic chondrodysplasia punctata (E71.43)*

Q77.4 Achondroplasia
Hypochondroplasia
Osteosclerosis congenita

Q77.5 Diastrophic dysplasia

Q77.6 Chondroectodermal dysplasia
Ellis-van Creveld syndrome

Q77.7 Spondyloepiphyseal dysplasia

Q77.8 Other osteochondrodysplasia with defects of growth of tubular bones and spine

Q77.9 Osteochondrodysplasia with defects of growth of tubular bones and spine, unspecified

✓4th **Q78 Other osteochondrodysplasias**
EXCLUDES 2 *congenital myotonic chondrodystrophy (G71.13)*

Q78.0 Osteogenesis imperfecta CC
Fragilitas ossium
Osteopsathyrosis
CC Excl: Q77.3, Q77.6, Q78.0-Q78.3, Q78.5-Q78.9

Q78.1 Polyostotic fibrous dysplasia
Albright(-McCune)(-Sternberg) syndrome

Q78.2 Osteopetrosis CC
Albers-Schönberg syndrome
Osteosclerosis NOS
CC Excl: See code: Q78.0

Q78.3 Progressive diaphyseal dysplasia
Camurati-Engelmann syndrome

Q78.4 Enchondromatosis
Maffucci's syndrome
Ollier's disease

Q78.5 Metaphyseal dysplasia
Pyle's syndrome

Q78.6 Multiple congenital exostoses
Diaphyseal aclasis

Q78.8 Other specified osteochondrodysplasias
Osteopoikilosis

Q78.9 Osteochondrodysplasia, unspecified
Chondrodystrophy NOS
Osteodystrophy NOS

✓4th **Q79 Congenital malformations of musculoskeletal system, not elsewhere classified**
EXCLUDES 2 *congenital (sternomastoid) torticollis (Q68.0)*

CC Excl: For CC/MCC codes in category Q79, unless otherwise noted: Q79.2-Q79.59

Q79.0 Congenital diaphragmatic hernia MCC
EXCLUDES 1 *congenital hiatus hernia (Q40.1)*
CC Excl: Q40.1-Q79.1

Q79.1 Other congenital malformations of diaphragm MCC
Absence of diaphragm
Congenital malformation of diaphragm NOS
Eventration of diaphragm
CC Excl: See code: Q79.0

Q79.2 Exomphalos MCC
Omphalocele
EXCLUDES 1 *umbilical hernia (K42.-)*

Q79.3 Gastroschisis MCC

Q79.4 Prune belly syndrome MCC
Congenital prolapse of bladder mucosa
Eagle-Barrett syndrome

✓5th **Q79.5 Other congenital malformations of abdominal wall**
EXCLUDES 1 *umbilical hernia (K42.-)*

Q79.51 Congenital hernia of bladder MCC

Q79.59 Other congenital malformations of abdominal wall MCC

Q79.6 Ehlers-Danlos syndrome CC
CC Excl: Q79.6

Q79.8 Other congenital malformations of musculoskeletal system
Absence of muscle
Absence of tendon
Accessory muscle
Amyotrophia congenita
Congenital constricting bands
Congenital shortening of tendon
Poland syndrome

Q79.9 Congenital malformation of musculoskeletal system, unspecified
Congenital anomaly of musculoskeletal system NOS
Congenital deformity of musculoskeletal system NOS

Other congenital malformations (Q80-Q89)

✓4th **Q80 Congenital ichthyosis**
EXCLUDES 1 *Refsum's disease (G60.1)*

Q80.0 Ichthyosis vulgaris

Q80.1 X-linked ichthyosis

Q80.2 Lamellar ichthyosis
Collodion baby

Q80.3 Congenital bullous ichthyosiform erythroderma

Q80.4 Harlequin fetus

Q80.8 Other congenital ichthyosis

Q80.9 Congenital ichthyosis, unspecified

✓4th **Q81 Epidermolysis bullosa**

Q81.0 Epidermolysis bullosa simplex
EXCLUDES 1 *Cockayne's syndrome (Q87.1)*

Q81.1 Epidermolysis bullosa letalis
Herlitz' syndrome

Q81.2 Epidermolysis bullosa dystrophica

Q81.8 Other epidermolysis bullosa

Q81.9 Epidermolysis bullosa, unspecified

✓4th **Q82 Other congenital malformations of skin**
EXCLUDES 1 *acrodermatitis enteropathica (E83.2)*
congenital erythropoietic porphyria (E80.0)
pilonidal cyst or sinus (L05.-)
Sturge-Weber (-Dimitri) syndrome (Q85.8)

Q82.0 Hereditary lymphedema

Q82.1 Xeroderma pigmentosum

Q82.2 Mastocytosis
Urticaria pigmentosa
EXCLUDES 1 *malignant mastocytosis (C96.2)*

Q82.3 Incontinentia pigmenti

Q82.4 Ectodermal dysplasia (anhidrotic)
EXCLUDES 1 *Ellis-van Creveld syndrome (Q77.6)*

Q82.5 Congenital non-neoplastic nevus
Birthmark NOS
Flammeus Nevus
Portwine Nevus
Sanguineous Nevus
Strawberry Nevus
Vascular Nevus NOS
Verrucous Nevus
EXCLUDES 2 *araneus nevus (I78.1)*
café au lait spots (L81.3)
lentigo (L81.4)
melanocytic nevus (D22.-)
nevus NOS (D22.-)
pigmented nevus (D22.-)
spider nevus (I78.1)
stellar nevus (I78.1)

Q82.8 Other specified congenital malformations of skin
Abnormal palmar creases
Accessory skin tags
Benign familial pemphigus [Hailey-Hailey]
Congenital poikiloderma
Cutis laxa (hyperelastica)
Dermatoglyphic anomalies
Inherited keratosis palmaris et plantaris
Keratosis follicularis [Darier-White]
EXCLUDES 1 *Ehlers-Danlos syndrome (Q79.6)*

Q82.9 Congenital malformation of skin, unspecified

✓4th **Q83 Congenital malformations of breast**
EXCLUDES 2 *absence of pectoral muscle (Q79.8)*
hypoplasia of breast (N64.82)
micromastia (N64.82)

Q83.0 Congenital absence of breast with absent nipple

Q83.1 Accessory breast
Supernumerary breast

Q83.2 Absent nipple

Q83.3 Accessory nipple
Supernumerary nipple

Q83.8 Other congenital malformations of breast

Q83.9 Congenital malformation of breast, unspecified

✓4th Q84 Other congenital malformations of integument

Q84.0 Congenital alopecia
Congenital atrichosis

Q84.1 Congenital morphological disturbances of hair, not elsewhere classified
Beaded hair
Monilethrix
Pili annulati
EXCLUDES 1 *Menkes' kinky hair syndrome (E83.0)*

Q84.2 Other congenital malformations of hair
Congenital hypertrichosis
Congenital malformation of hair NOS
Persistent lanugo

Q84.3 Anonychia
EXCLUDES 1 *nail patella syndrome (Q87.2)*

Q84.4 Congenital leukonychia

Q84.5 Enlarged and hypertrophic nails
Congenital onychauxis
Pachyonychia

Q84.6 Other congenital malformations of nails
Congenital clubnail
Congenital koilonychia
Congenital malformation of nail NOS

Q84.8 Other specified congenital malformations of integument
Aplasia cutis congenita

Q84.9 Congenital malformation of integument, unspecified
Congenital anomaly of integument NOS
Congenital deformity of integument NOS

✓4th Q85 Phakomatoses, not elsewhere classified
EXCLUDES 1 *ataxia telangiectasia [Louis-Bar] (G11.3)*
familial dysautonomia [Riley-Day] (G90.1)

✓5th Q85.0 Neurofibromatosis (nonmalignant)

Q85.00 Neurofibromatosis, unspecified

Q85.01 Neurofibromatosis, type 1
Von Recklinghausen disease

Q85.02 Neurofibromatosis, type 2
Acoustic neurofibromatosis

Q85.03 Schwannomatosis

Q85.09 Other neurofibromatosis

Q85.1 Tuberous sclerosis CC
Bourneville's disease
Epiloia
CC Excl: Q85.1-Q85.9, Q89.7, Q89.9

Q85.8 Other phakomatoses, not elsewhere classified CC
Peutz-Jeghers Syndrome
Sturge-Weber(-Dimitri) syndrome
von Hippel-Lindau syndrome
EXCLUDES 1 *Meckel-Gruber syndrome (Q61.9)*
CC Excl: Q85.8-Q85.9, Q89.9

Q85.9 Phakomatosis, unspecified CC
Hamartosis NOS
CC Excl: See code: Q85.8

✓4th Q86 Congenital malformation syndromes due to known exogenous causes, not elsewhere classified
EXCLUDES 2 *iodine-deficiency-related hypothyroidism (E00-E02)*
nonteratogenic effects of substances transmitted via placenta or breast milk (P04.-)

Q86.0 Fetal alcohol syndrome (dysmorphic) N

Q86.1 Fetal hydantoin syndrome
Meadow's syndrome

Q86.2 Dysmorphism due to warfarin

Q86.8 Other congenital malformation syndromes due to known exogenous causes

✓4th Q87 Other specified congenital malformation syndromes affecting multiple systems
Use additional code(s) to identify all associated manifestations

Q87.0 Congenital malformation syndromes predominantly affecting facial appearance
Acrocephalopolysyndactyly
Acrocephalosyndactyly [Apert]
Cryptophthalmos syndrome
Cyclopia
Goldenhar syndrome
Moebius syndrome
Oro-facial-digital syndrome
Robin syndrome
Whistling face

Q87.1 Congenital malformation syndromes predominantly associated with short stature CC
Aarskog syndrome
Cockayne syndrome
De Lange syndrome
Dubowitz syndrome
Noonan syndrome
Prader-Willi syndrome
Robinow-Silverman-Smith syndrome
Russell-Silver syndrome
Seckel syndrome
EXCLUDES 1 *Ellis-van Creveld syndrome (Q77.6)*
Smith-Lemli-Opitz syndrome (E78.72)
CC Excl: E78.71-E78.72, Q85.8-Q85.9, Q87.1-Q87.89, Q89.7-Q89.9, Q99.2

Q87.2 Congenital malformation syndromes predominantly involving limbs CC
Holt-Oram syndrome
Klippel-Trenaunay-Weber syndrome
Nail patella syndrome
Rubinstein-Taybi syndrome
Sirenomelia syndrome
Thrombocytopenia with absent radius [TAR] syndrome
VATER syndrome
CC Excl: E78.71-E78.72, Q87.1-Q87.89, Q89.8, Q99.2

Q87.3 Congenital malformation syndromes involving early overgrowth CC
Beckwith-Wiedemann syndrome
Sotos syndrome
Weaver syndrome
CC Excl: See code: Q87.2

✓5th Q87.4 Marfan's syndrome

CC Excl: For CC codes in subcategory Q87.4, unless otherwise noted: See code: Q87.1

Q87.40 Marfan's syndrome, unspecified CC

✓6th Q87.41 Marfan's syndrome with cardiovascular manifestations

Q87.410 Marfan's syndrome with aortic dilation CC

Q87.418 Marfan's syndrome with other cardiovascular manifestations CC

Q87.42 Marfan's syndrome with ocular manifestations CC

Q87.43 Marfan's syndrome with skeletal manifestation CC

Q87.5 Other congenital malformation syndromes with other skeletal changes CC
CC Excl: See code: Q87.2

✓5th Q87.8 Other specified congenital malformation syndromes, not elsewhere classified
EXCLUDES 1 *Zellweger syndrome (E71.510)*

Q87.81 Alport syndrome CC
Use additional code to identify stage of chronic kidney disease (N18.1-N18.6)
CC Excl: See code: Q87.2

Q87.89 Other specified congenital malformation syndromes, not elsewhere classified CC
Laurence-Moon (-Bardet)-Biedl syndrome
CC Excl: See code: Q87.2

✓4th Q89 Other congenital malformations, not elsewhere classified

✓5th Q89.0 Congenital absence and malformations of spleen
EXCLUDES 1 *isomerism of atrial appendages (with asplenia or polysplenia) (Q20.6)*

Q89.01 Asplenia (congenital) CC
CC Excl: Q89.01-Q89.09, Q89.9

Q89.09 Congenital malformations of spleen CC
Congenital splenomegaly
CC Excl: See code: Q89.01

Q89.1 Congenital malformations of adrenal gland
EXCLUDES 1 *adrenogenital disorders (E25.-)*
congenital adrenal hyperplasia (E25.Ø)

Q89.2 Congenital malformations of other endocrine glands
Congenital malformation of parathyroid or thyroid gland
Persistent thyroglossal duct
Thyroglossal cyst
EXCLUDES 1 *congenital goiter (EØ3.Ø)*
congenital hypothyroidism (EØ3.1)

Q89.3 Situs inversus CC
Dextrocardia with situs inversus
Mirror-image atrial arrangement with situs inversus
Situs inversus or transversus abdominalis
Situs inversus or transversus thoracis
Transposition of abdominal viscera
Transposition of thoracic viscera
EXCLUDES 1 *dextrocardia NOS (Q24.Ø)*
CC Excl: Q89.3, Q89.7, Q89.9

Q89.4 Conjoined twins MCC
Craniopagus
Dicephaly
Pygopagus
Thoracopagus
CC Excl: Q89.4-Q89.7, Q89.9

Q89.7 Multiple congenital malformations, not elsewhere classified CC
Multiple congenital anomalies NOS
Multiple congenital deformities NOS
EXCLUDES 1 *congenital malformation syndromes affecting multiple systems (Q87.-)*
CC Excl: See code: Q89.3

Q89.8 Other specified congenital malformations CC
Use additional code(s) to identify all associated manifestations
CC Excl: E78.71-E78.72, Q87.1-Q87.89, Q89.8, Q99.2

Q89.9 Congenital malformation, unspecified
Congenital anomaly NOS
Congenital deformity NOS

Chromosomal abnormalities, not elsewhere classified (Q9Ø-Q99)

EXCLUDES 2 *mitochondrial metabolic disorders (E88.4-)*

✓4th Q9Ø Down syndrome
Use additional code(s) to identify any associated physical conditions and degree of intellectual disabilities (F7Ø-F79)

Q9Ø.Ø Trisomy 21, nonmosaicism (meiotic nondisjunction)
Q9Ø.1 Trisomy 21, mosaicism (mitotic nondisjunction)
Q9Ø.2 Trisomy 21, translocation
Q9Ø.9 Down syndrome, unspecified
Trisomy 21 NOS

✓4th Q91 Trisomy 18 and Trisomy 13

CC Excl: For CC codes in category Q91, unless otherwise noted: Q9Ø.Ø-Q99.1, Q99.8-Q99.9

Q91.Ø Trisomy 18, nonmosaicism (meiotic nondisjunction) CC
Q91.1 Trisomy 18, mosaicism (mitotic nondisjunction) CC
Q91.2 Trisomy 18, translocation CC
Q91.3 Trisomy 18, unspecified CC
Q91.4 Trisomy 13, nonmosaicism (meiotic nondisjunction) CC
Q91.5 Trisomy 13, mosaicism (mitotic nondisjunction) CC
Q91.6 Trisomy 13, translocation CC
Q91.7 Trisomy 13, unspecified CC

✓4th Q92 Other trisomies and partial trisomies of the autosomes, not elsewhere classified
INCLUDES unbalanced translocations and insertions
EXCLUDES 1 *trisomies of chromosomes 13, 18, 21 (Q9Ø-Q91)*

Q92.Ø Whole chromosome trisomy, nonmosaicism (meiotic nondisjunction)
Q92.1 Whole chromosome trisomy, mosaicism (mitotic nondisjunction)
Q92.2 Partial trisomy
Less than whole arm duplicated
Whole arm or more duplicated
EXCLUDES 1 *partial trisomy due to unbalanced translocation (Q92.5)*

Q92.5 Duplications with other complex rearrangements
Partial trisomy due to unbalanced translocations
Code also any associated deletions due to unbalanced translocations, inversions and insertions (Q93.7)

✓5th Q92.6 Marker chromosomes
Trisomies due to dicentrics
Trisomies due to extra rings
Trisomies due to isochromosomes
Individual with marker heterochromatin

Q92.61 Marker chromosomes in normal individual
Q92.62 Marker chromosomes in abnormal individual

Q92.7 Triploidy and polyploidy
Q92.8 Other specified trisomies and partial trisomies of autosomes
Duplications identified by fluorescence in situ hybridization (FISH)
Duplications identified by in situ hybridization (ISH)
Duplications seen only at prometaphase
Q92.9 Trisomy and partial trisomy of autosomes, unspecified

✓4th Q93 Monosomies and deletions from the autosomes, not elsewhere classified

CC Excl: For CC/MCC codes in category Q93, unless otherwise noted: Q9Ø.Ø-Q93.2, Q93.4, Q93.81-Q93.88, Q95.Ø-Q99.1, Q99.8-Q99.9

Q93.Ø Whole chromosome monosomy, nonmosaicism (meiotic nondisjunction)
Q93.1 Whole chromosome monosomy, mosaicism (mitotic nondisjunction)
Q93.2 Chromosome replaced with ring, dicentric or isochromosome
Q93.3 Deletion of short arm of chromosome 4 CC
Wolff-Hirschorn syndrome
Q93.4 Deletion of short arm of chromosome 5 CC
Cri-du-chat syndrome
CC Excl: Q9Ø.Ø-Q93.3, Q93.5-Q99.1, Q99.8-Q99.9
Q93.5 Other deletions of part of a chromosome CC
Angelman syndrome
Q93.7 Deletions with other complex rearrangements CC
Deletions due to unbalanced translocations, inversions and insertions
Code also any associated duplications due to unbalanced translocations, inversions and insertions (Q92.5)

✓5th Q93.8 Other deletions from the autosomes
Q93.81 Velo-cardio-facial syndrome MCC
Deletion 22q11.2
CC Excl: Q9Ø.Ø-Q93.7, Q93.88-Q99.1, Q99.8-Q99.9
Q93.88 Other microdeletions CC
Miller-Dieker syndrome
Smith-Magenis syndrome
CC Excl: Q9Ø.Ø-Q93.81, Q93.89-Q99.1, Q99.8-Q99.9
Q93.89 Other deletions from the autosomes CC
Deletions identified by fluorescence in situ hybridization (FISH)
Deletions identified by in situ hybridization (ISH)
Deletions seen only at prometaphase

Q93.9 Deletion from autosomes, unspecified CC

✓4th Q95 Balanced rearrangements and structural markers, not elsewhere classified
INCLUDES Robertsonian and balanced reciprocal translocations and insertions

Q95.Ø Balanced translocation and insertion in normal individual
Q95.1 Chromosome inversion in normal individual
Q95.2 Balanced autosomal rearrangement in abnormal individual
Q95.3 Balanced sex/autosomal rearrangement in abnormal individual
Q95.5 Individual with autosomal fragile site
Q95.8 Other balanced rearrangements and structural markers
Q95.9 Balanced rearrangement and structural marker, unspecified

✓4th Q96 Turner's syndrome
EXCLUDES 1 *Noonan syndrome (Q87.1)*

Q96.Ø Karyotype 45, X ♀
Q96.1 Karyotype 46, X iso (Xq) ♀
Karyotype 46, isochromosome Xq
Q96.2 Karyotype 46, X with abnormal sex chromosome, except iso (Xq) ♀
Karyotype 46, X with abnormal sex chromosome, except isochromosome Xq
Q96.3 Mosaicism, 45, X/46, XX or XY ♀
Q96.4 Mosaicism, 45, X/other cell line(s) with abnormal sex chromosome ♀
Q96.8 Other variants of Turner's syndrome ♀
Q96.9 Turner's syndrome, unspecified ♀

4th Q97 Other sex chromosome abnormalities, female phenotype, not elsewhere classified

EXCLUDES 1 *Turner's syndrome (Q96.-)*

Q97.0 Karyotype 47, XXX ♀

Q97.1 Female with more than three X chromosomes ♀

Q97.2 Mosaicism, lines with various numbers of X chromosomes ♀

Q97.3 Female with 46, XY karyotype ♀

Q97.8 Other specified sex chromosome abnormalities, female phenotype ♀

Q97.9 Sex chromosome abnormality, female phenotype, unspecified ♀

4th Q98 Other sex chromosome abnormalities, male phenotype, not elsewhere classified

Q98.0 Klinefelter syndrome karyotype 47, XXY ♂

Q98.1 Klinefelter syndrome, male with more than two X chromosomes ♂

Q98.3 Other male with 46, XX karyotype ♂

Q98.4 Klinefelter syndrome, unspecified ♂

Q98.5 Karyotype 47, XYY

Q98.6 Male with structurally abnormal sex chromosome ♂

Q98.7 Male with sex chromosome mosaicism ♂

Q98.8 Other specified sex chromosome abnormalities, male phenotype ♂

Q98.9 Sex chromosome abnormality, male phenotype, unspecified ♂

4th Q99 Other chromosome abnormalities, not elsewhere classified

Q99.0 Chimera 46, XX/46, XY

Chimera 46, XX/46, XY true hermaphrodite

Q99.1 46, XX true hermaphrodite

46, XX with streak gonads
46, XY with streak gonads
Pure gonadal dysgenesis

Q99.2 Fragile X chromosome

Fragile X syndrome

Q99.8 Other specified chromosome abnormalities

Q99.9 Chromosomal abnormality, unspecified

Chapter 18. Symptoms, Signs and Abnormal Clinical and Laboratory Findings, Not Elsewhere Classified (R00-R99)

NOTE This chapter includes symptoms, signs, abnormal results of clinical or other investigative procedures, and ill-defined conditions regarding which no diagnosis classifiable elsewhere is recorded.

Signs and symptoms that point rather definitely to a given diagnosis have been assigned to a category in other chapters of the classification. In general, categories in this chapter include the less well-defined conditions and symptoms that, without the necessary study of the case to establish a final diagnosis, point perhaps equally to two or more diseases or to two or more systems of the body. Practically all categories in the chapter could be designated "not otherwise specified", "unknown etiology" or "transient". The Alphabetical Index should be consulted to determine which symptoms and signs are to be allocated here and which to other chapters. The residual subcategories, numbered .8, are generally provided for other relevant symptoms that cannot be allocated elsewhere in the classification.

The conditions and signs or symptoms included in categories R00-R94 consist of:

(a) cases for which no more specific diagnosis can be made even after all the facts bearing on the case have been investigated;
(b) signs or symptoms existing at the time of initial encounter that proved to be transient and whose causes could not be determined;
(c) provisional diagnosis in a patient who failed to return for further investigation or care;
(d) cases referred elsewhere for investigation or treatment before the diagnosis was made;
(e) cases in which a more precise diagnosis was not available for any other reason;
(f) certain symptoms, for which supplementary information is provided, that represent important problems in medical care in their own right.

EXCLUDES 2 *abnormal findings on antenatal screening of mother (O28.-)*
certain conditions originating in the perinatal period (P04-P96)
signs and symptoms classified in the body system chapters
signs and symptoms of breast (N63, N64.5)

This chapter contains the following blocks:

R00-R09	Symptoms and signs involving the circulatory and respiratory systems
R10-R19	Symptoms and signs involving the digestive system and abdomen
R20-R23	Symptoms and signs involving the skin and subcutaneous tissue
R25-R29	Symptoms and signs involving the nervous and musculoskeletal systems
R30-R39	Symptoms and signs involving the genitourinary system
R40-R46	Symptoms and signs involving cognition, perception, emotional state and behavior
R47-R49	Symptoms and signs involving speech and voice
R50-R69	General symptoms and signs
R70-R79	Abnormal findings on examination of blood, without diagnosis
R80-R82	Abnormal findings on examination of urine, without diagnosis
R83-R89	Abnormal findings on examination of other body fluids, substances and tissues, without diagnosis
R90-R94	Abnormal findings on diagnostic imaging and in function studies, without diagnosis
R97	Abnormal tumor markers
R99	Ill-defined and unknown cause of mortality

Symptoms and signs involving the circulatory and respiratory systems (R00-R09)

✓4th **R00 Abnormalities of heart beat**
EXCLUDES 1 *abnormalities originating in the perinatal period (P29.1-)*
specified arrhythmias (I47-I49)

R00.0 Tachycardia, unspecified
Rapid heart beat
Sinoauricular tachycardia NOS
Sinus [sinusal] tachycardia NOS
EXCLUDES 1 *neonatal tachycardia (P29.11)*
paroxysmal tachycardia (I47.-)

R00.1 Bradycardia, unspecified
Sinoatrial bradycardia
Sinus bradycardia
Slow heart beat
Vagal bradycardia
Use additional code for adverse effect, if applicable, to identify drug (T36-T50 with fifth or sixth character 5)
EXCLUDES 1 *neonatal bradycardia (P29.12)*

R00.2 Palpitations
Awareness of heart beat

R00.8 Other abnormalities of heart beat

R00.9 Unspecified abnormalities of heart beat

✓4th **R01 Cardiac murmurs and other cardiac sounds**
EXCLUDES 1 *cardiac murmurs and sounds originating in the perinatal period (P29.8)*

R01.0 Benign and innocent cardiac murmurs
Functional cardiac murmur

R01.1 Cardiac murmur, unspecified
Cardiac bruit NOS
Heart murmur NOS

R01.2 Other cardiac sounds
Cardiac dullness, increased or decreased
Precordial friction

✓4th **R03 Abnormal blood-pressure reading, without diagnosis**

13 **R03.0 Elevated blood-pressure reading, without diagnosis of hypertension**
NOTE This category is to be used to record an episode of elevated blood pressure in a patient in whom no formal diagnosis of hypertension has been made, or as an isolated incidental finding.

R03.1 Nonspecific low blood-pressure reading
EXCLUDES 1 *hypotension (I95.-)*
maternal hypotension syndrome (O26.5-)
neurogenic orthostatic hypotension (G90.3)

✓4th **R04 Hemorrhage from respiratory passages**

CC Excl: For CC codes in category Q93, unless otherwise noted:
R04.2-R04.9, R09.3, R68.13

R04.0 Epistaxis
Hemorrhage from nose
Nosebleed

R04.1 Hemorrhage from throat
EXCLUDES 2 *hemoptysis (R04.2)*

R04.2 Hemoptysis CC
Blood-stained sputum
Cough with hemorrhage
AHA: 2013, 4Q, 118

✓5th **R04.8 Hemorrhage from other sites in respiratory passages**

R04.81 Acute idiopathic pulmonary hemorrhage in infants CC P
AIPHI
Acute idiopathic hemorrhage in infants over 28 days old
EXCLUDES 1 *perinatal pulmonary hemorrhage (P26.-)*
von Willebrand's disease (D68.0)

R04.89 Hemorrhage from other sites in respiratory passages CC
Pulmonary hemorrhage NOS

R04.9 Hemorrhage from respiratory passages, unspecified CC

R05 Cough
EXCLUDES 1 *cough with hemorrhage (R04.2)*
smoker's cough (J41.0)

✓4th **R06 Abnormalities of breathing**
EXCLUDES 1 *acute respiratory distress syndrome (J80)*
respiratory arrest (R09.2)
respiratory arrest of newborn (P28.81)
respiratory distress syndrome of newborn (P22.-)
respiratory failure (J96.-)
respiratory failure of newborn (P28.5)

✓5th **R06.0 Dyspnea**
EXCLUDES 1 *tachypnea NOS (R06.82)*
transient tachypnea of newborn (P22.1)

R06.00 Dyspnea, unspecified
R06.01 Orthopnea
R06.02 Shortness of breath
R06.09 Other forms of dyspnea

13 Questionable admission when used as PDx.

R06.1 Stridor
EXCLUDES 1 *congenital laryngeal stridor (P28.89)*
laryngismus (stridulus) (J38.5)

R06.2 Wheezing
EXCLUDES 1 *asthma (J45.-)*

R06.3 Periodic breathing CC
Cheyne-Stokes breathing
CC Excl: J22, J80, J96.00-J96.92, J98.8-J98.9, R06.3, R06.81, R09.2

R06.4 Hyperventilation
EXCLUDES 1 *psychogenic hyperventilation (F45.8)*

R06.5 Mouth breathing
EXCLUDES 2 *dry mouth NOS (R68.2)*

R06.6 Hiccough
EXCLUDES 1 *psychogenic hiccough (F45.8)*

R06.7 Sneezing

5th **R06.8 Other abnormalities of breathing**

R06.81 Apnea, not elsewhere classified
Apnea NOS
EXCLUDES 1 *apnea (of) newborn (P28.4)*
sleep apnea (G47.3-)
sleep apnea of newborn (primary) (P28.3)

R06.82 Tachypnea, not elsewhere classified
Tachypnea NOS
EXCLUDES 1 *transitory tachypnea of newborn (P22.1)*

R06.83 Snoring

R06.89 Other abnormalities of breathing
Breath-holding (spells)
Sighing

R06.9 Unspecified abnormalities of breathing

4th **R07 Pain in throat and chest**
EXCLUDES 1 *epidemic myalgia (B33.0)*
EXCLUDES 2 *jaw pain (R68.84)*
pain in breast (N64.4)

R07.0 Pain in throat
EXCLUDES 1 *chronic sore throat (J31.2)*
sore throat (acute) NOS (J02.9)
EXCLUDES 2 *dysphagia (R13.1-)*
pain in neck (M54.2)

R07.1 Chest pain on breathing
Painful respiration

R07.2 Precordial pain

5th **R07.8 Other chest pain**

R07.81 Pleurodynia
Pleurodynia NOS
EXCLUDES 1 *epidemic pleurodynia (B33.0)*

R07.82 Intercostal pain

R07.89 Other chest pain
Anterior chest-wall pain NOS

R07.9 Chest pain, unspecified

4th **R09 Other symptoms and signs involving the circulatory and respiratory system**
EXCLUDES 1 *acute respiratory distress syndrome (J80)*
respiratory arrest of newborn (P28.81)
respiratory distress syndrome of newborn (P22.0)
respiratory failure (J96.-)
respiratory failure of newborn (P28.5)

5th **R09.0 Asphyxia and hypoxemia**
EXCLUDES 1 *asphyxia due to carbon monoxide (T58.-)*
asphyxia due to foreign body in respiratory tract (T17.-)
birth (intrauterine) asphyxia (P84)
hypercapnia (R06.4)
hyperventilation (R06.4)
traumatic asphyxia (T71.-)

R09.01 Asphyxia CC
CC Excl: G89.0-G89.4, J80, J96.00-J96.92, R09.01-R09.02, R09.2, R41.0-R41.3, R41.82, R41.9, R44.8-R44.9, R45.83-R45.84, R46.0-R46.89, R52, R68.0-R68.19, R68.81-R68.83, R68.89-R69

R09.02 Hypoxemia

R09.1 Pleurisy
EXCLUDES 1 *pleurisy with effusion (J90)*

10 **R09.2 Respiratory arrest** MCC
Cardiorespiratory failure
EXCLUDES 1 *cardiac arrest (I46.-)*
respiratory arrest of newborn (P28.81)
respiratory distress of newborn (P22.0)
respiratory failure (J96.-)
respiratory failure of newborn (P28.5)
respiratory insufficiency (R06.89)
respiratory insufficiency of newborn (P28.5)
CC Excl: See code: R09.01

R09.3 Abnormal sputum
Abnormal amount of sputum
Abnormal color of sputum
Abnormal odor of sputum
Excessive sputum
EXCLUDES 1 *blood-stained sputum (R04.2)*

5th **R09.8 Other specified symptoms and signs involving the circulatory and respiratory systems**

R09.81 Nasal congestion

R09.82 Postnasal drip

R09.89 Other specified symptoms and signs involving the circulatory and respiratory systems
Abnormal chest percussion
Bruit (arterial)
Chest tympany
Choking sensation
Feeling of foreign body in throat
Friction sounds in chest
Rales
Weak pulse
EXCLUDES 2 *foreign body in throat (T17.2-)*
wheezing (R06.2)

Symptoms and signs involving the digestive system and abdomen (R10-R19)

EXCLUDES 1 *congenital or infantile pylorospasm (Q40.0)*
gastrointestinal hemorrhage (K92.0-K92.2)
intestinal obstruction (K56.-)
newborn gastrointestinal hemorrhage (P54.0-P54.3)
newborn intestinal obstruction (P76.-)
pylorospasm (K31.3)
signs and symptoms involving the urinary system (R30-R39)
symptoms referable to female genital organs (N94.-)
symptoms referable to male genital organs male (N48-N50)

4th **R10 Abdominal and pelvic pain**
EXCLUDES 1 *renal colic (N23)*
EXCLUDES 2 *dorsalgia (M54.-)*
flatulence and related conditions (R14.-)

R10.0 Acute abdomen
Severe abdominal pain (generalized) (with abdominal rigidity)
EXCLUDES 1 *abdominal rigidity NOS (R19.3)*
generalized abdominal pain NOS (R10.84)
localized abdominal pain (R10.1-R10.3-)

5th **R10.1 Pain localized to upper abdomen**

R10.10 Upper abdominal pain, unspecified

R10.11 Right upper quadrant pain

R10.12 Left upper quadrant pain

R10.13 Epigastric pain
Dyspepsia
EXCLUDES 1 *functional dyspepsia (K30)*

R10.2 Pelvic and perineal pain
EXCLUDES 1 *vulvodynia (N94.81)*

5th **R10.3 Pain localized to other parts of lower abdomen**

R10.30 Lower abdominal pain, unspecified

R10.31 Right lower quadrant pain

R10.32 Left lower quadrant pain

R10.33 Periumbilical pain

5th **R10.8 Other abdominal pain**

6th **R10.81 Abdominal tenderness**
Abdominal tenderness NOS

R10.811 Right upper quadrant abdominal tenderness

R10.812 Left upper quadrant abdominal tenderness

R10.813 Right lower quadrant abdominal tenderness

10 MCC only if patient is discharged alive.

R10.814 Left lower quadrant abdominal tenderness
R10.815 Periumbilic abdominal tenderness
R10.816 Epigastric abdominal tenderness
R10.817 Generalized abdominal tenderness
R10.819 Abdominal tenderness, unspecified site

✓6th R10.82 Rebound abdominal tenderness
R10.821 Right upper quadrant rebound abdominal tenderness
R10.822 Left upper quadrant rebound abdominal tenderness
R10.823 Right lower quadrant rebound abdominal tenderness
R10.824 Left lower quadrant rebound abdominal tenderness
R10.825 Periumbilic rebound abdominal tenderness
R10.826 Epigastric rebound abdominal tenderness
R10.827 Generalized rebound abdominal tenderness
R10.829 Rebound abdominal tenderness, unspecified site

R10.83 Colic P
Colic NOS
Infantile colic
EXCLUDES 1 *colic in adult and child over 12 months old (R10.84)*

R10.84 Generalized abdominal pain
EXCLUDES 1 *generalized abdominal pain associated with acute abdomen (R10.0)*

R10.9 Unspecified abdominal pain

✓4th R11 Nausea and vomiting
EXCLUDES 1 *cyclical vomiting associated with migraine (G43.A-)*
excessive vomiting in pregnancy (O21.-)
hematemesis (K92.0)
neonatal hematemesis (P54.0)
newborn vomiting (P92.0-)
psychogenic vomiting (F50.8)
vomiting associated with bulimia nervosa (F50.2)
vomiting following gastrointestinal surgery (K91.0)

R11.0 Nausea
Nausea NOS
Nausea without vomiting

✓5th R11.1 Vomiting
R11.10 Vomiting, unspecified
Vomiting NOS
R11.11 Vomiting without nausea
R11.12 Projectile vomiting
R11.13 Vomiting of fecal matter
R11.14 Bilious vomiting
Bilious emesis

R11.2 Nausea with vomiting, unspecified
Persistent nausea with vomiting NOS

R12 Heartburn
EXCLUDES 1 *dyspepsia NOS (R10.13)*
functional dyspepsia (K30)

✓4th R13 Aphagia and dysphagia
R13.0 Aphagia
Inability to swallow
EXCLUDES 1 *psychogenic aphagia (F50.9)*

✓5th R13.1 Dysphagia
Code first, if applicable, dysphagia following cerebrovascular disease (I69. with final characters -91)
EXCLUDES 1 *psychogenic dysphagia (F45.8)*
R13.10 Dysphagia, unspecified
Difficulty in swallowing NOS
R13.11 Dysphagia, oral phase
R13.12 Dysphagia, oropharyngeal phase
R13.13 Dysphagia, pharyngeal phase
R13.14 Dysphagia, pharyngoesophageal phase
R13.19 Other dysphagia
Cervical dysphagia
Neurogenic dysphagia

✓4th R14 Flatulence and related conditions
EXCLUDES 1 *psychogenic aerophagy (F45.8)*

R14.0 Abdominal distension (gaseous)
Bloating
Tympanites (abdominal) (intestinal)
R14.1 Gas pain
R14.2 Eructation
R14.3 Flatulence

✓4th R15 Fecal incontinence
Encopresis NOS
EXCLUDES 1 *fecal incontinence of nonorganic origin (F98.1)*

R15.0 Incomplete defecation
EXCLUDES 1 *constipation (K59.0-)*
fecal impaction (K56.41)
R15.1 Fecal smearing
Fecal soiling
R15.2 Fecal urgency
R15.9 Full incontinence of feces
Fecal incontinence NOS

✓4th R16 Hepatomegaly and splenomegaly, not elsewhere classified
R16.0 Hepatomegaly, not elsewhere classified
Hepatomegaly NOS
R16.1 Splenomegaly, not elsewhere classified
Splenomegaly NOS
R16.2 Hepatomegaly with splenomegaly, not elsewhere classified
Hepatosplenomegaly NOS

R17 Unspecified jaundice CC
EXCLUDES 1 *neonatal jaundice (P55, P57-P59)*
CC Excl: P57.8-P59.9, R17, R23.8-R23.9

✓4th R18 Ascites
INCLUDES fluid in peritoneal cavity
EXCLUDES 1 *ascites in alcoholic cirrhosis (K70.31)*
ascites in alcoholic hepatitis (K70.11)
ascites in toxic liver disease with chronic active hepatitis (K71.51)

R18.0 Malignant ascites CC
Code first malignancy, such as:
malignant neoplasm of ovary (C56.-)
secondary malignant neoplasm of retroperitoneum and peritoneum (C78.6)
CC Excl: G89.0-G89.4, R18.0-R19.09, R19.30-R19.37, R41.0-R41.3, R41.82, R41.9, R44.8-R44.9, R45.83-R45.84, R46.0-R46.89, R52, R68.0-R68.19, R68.81-R68.83, R68.89-R69

R18.8 Other ascites CC
Ascites NOS
Peritoneal effusion (chronic)
CC Excl: See code: R18.0

✓4th R19 Other symptoms and signs involving the digestive system and abdomen
EXCLUDES 1 *acute abdomen (R10.0)*

✓5th R19.0 Intra-abdominal and pelvic swelling, mass and lump
EXCLUDES 1 *abdominal distension (gaseous) (R14.-)*
ascites (R18.-)
R19.00 Intra-abdominal and pelvic swelling, mass and lump, unspecified site
R19.01 Right upper quadrant abdominal swelling, mass and lump
R19.02 Left upper quadrant abdominal swelling, mass and lump
R19.03 Right lower quadrant abdominal swelling, mass and lump
R19.04 Left lower quadrant abdominal swelling, mass and lump
R19.05 Periumbilic swelling, mass or lump
Diffuse or generalized umbilical swelling or mass
R19.06 Epigastric swelling, mass or lump
R19.07 Generalized intra-abdominal and pelvic swelling, mass and lump
Diffuse or generalized intra-abdominal swelling or mass NOS
Diffuse or generalized pelvic swelling or mass NOS
R19.09 Other intra-abdominal and pelvic swelling, mass and lump

✓5th R19.1 Abnormal bowel sounds
R19.11 Absent bowel sounds
R19.12 Hyperactive bowel sounds

R19.15 Other **abnormal bowel sounds**
Abnormal bowel sounds NOS

R19.2 Visible peristalsis
Hyperperistalsis

✓5th **R19.3 Abdominal rigidity**
EXCLUDES 1 *abdominal rigidity with severe abdominal pain (R1Ø.Ø)*

R19.3Ø Abdominal rigidity, unspecified site
R19.31 Right upper quadrant abdominal rigidity
R19.32 Left upper quadrant abdominal rigidity
R19.33 Right lower quadrant abdominal rigidity
R19.34 Left lower quadrant abdominal rigidity
R19.35 Periumbilic abdominal rigidity
R19.36 Epigastric abdominal rigidity
R19.37 Generalized abdominal rigidity

R19.4 Change in bowel habit
EXCLUDES 1 *constipation (K59.Ø-)*
functional diarrhea (K59.1)

R19.5 Other fecal abnormalities
Abnormal stool color
Bulky stools
Mucus in stools
Occult blood in feces
Occult blood in stools
EXCLUDES 1 *melena (K92.1)*
neonatal melena (P54.1)

R19.6 Halitosis

R19.7 Diarrhea, unspecified
Diarrhea NOS
EXCLUDES 1 *functional diarrhea (K59.1)*
neonatal diarrhea (P78.3)
psychogenic diarrhea (F45.8)

R19.8 Other specified symptoms and signs involving the digestive system and abdomen

Symptoms and signs involving the skin and subcutaneous tissue (R2Ø-R23)

EXCLUDES 2 *symptoms relating to breast (N64.4-N64.5)*

✓4th **R2Ø Disturbances of skin sensation**
EXCLUDES 1 *dissociative anesthesia and sensory loss (F44.6)*
psychogenic disturbances (F45.8)

R2Ø.Ø Anesthesia of skin
R2Ø.1 Hypoesthesia of skin
R2Ø.2 Paresthesia of skin
Formication
Pins and needles
Tingling skin
EXCLUDES 1 *acroparesthesia (I73.8)*
R2Ø.3 Hyperesthesia
R2Ø.8 Other disturbances of skin sensation
R2Ø.9 Unspecified disturbances of skin sensation

R21 Rash and other nonspecific skin eruption
Rash NOS
EXCLUDES 1 *specified type of rash—code to condition*
vesicular eruption (R23.8)

✓4th **R22 Localized swelling, mass and lump of skin and subcutaneous tissue**
Subcutaneous nodules (localized)(superficial)
EXCLUDES 1 *abnormal findings on diagnostic imaging (R9Ø-R93)*
edema (R6Ø.-)
enlarged lymph nodes (R59.-)
localized adiposity (E65)
swelling of joint (M25.4-)

R22.Ø Localized swelling, mass and lump, head
R22.1 Localized swelling, mass and lump, neck
R22.2 Localized swelling, mass and lump, trunk
EXCLUDES 1 *intra-abdominal or pelvic mass and lump (R19.Ø-)*
intra-abdominal or pelvic swelling (R19.Ø-)
EXCLUDES 2 *breast mass and lump (N63)*

✓5th **R22.3 Localized swelling, mass and lump, upper limb**
R22.3Ø Localized swelling, mass and lump, unspecified upper limb
R22.31 Localized swelling, mass and lump, right upper limb
R22.32 Localized swelling, mass and lump, left upper limb
R22.33 Localized swelling, mass and lump, upper limb, bilateral

✓5th **R22.4 Localized swelling, mass and lump, lower limb**
R22.4Ø Localized swelling, mass and lump, unspecified lower limb
R22.41 Localized swelling, mass and lump, right lower limb
R22.42 Localized swelling, mass and lump, left lower limb
R22.43 Localized swelling, mass and lump, lower limb, bilateral

R22.9 Localized swelling, mass and lump, unspecified

✓4th **R23 Other skin changes**

R23.Ø Cyanosis
EXCLUDES 1 *acrocyanosis (I73.8)*
cyanotic attacks of newborn (P28.2)

R23.1 Pallor
Clammy skin

R23.2 Flushing
Excessive blushing
Code first, if applicable, menopausal and female climacteric states (N95.1)

R23.3 Spontaneous ecchymoses
Petechiae
EXCLUDES 1 *ecchymoses of newborn (P54.5)*
purpura (D69.-)

R23.4 Changes in skin texture
Desquamation of skin
Induration of skin
Scaling of skin
EXCLUDES 1 *epidermal thickening NOS (L85.9)*

R23.8 Other skin changes
R23.9 Unspecified skin changes

Symptoms and signs involving the nervous and musculoskeletal systems (R25-R29)

✓4th **R25 Abnormal involuntary movements**
EXCLUDES 1 *specific movement disorders (G2Ø-G26)*
stereotyped movement disorders (F98.4)
tic disorders (F95.-)

R25.Ø Abnormal head movements
R25.1 Tremor, unspecified
EXCLUDES 1 *chorea NOS (G25.5)*
essential tremor (G25.Ø)
hysterical tremor (F44.4)
intention tremor (G25.2)

R25.2 Cramp and spasm
EXCLUDES 2 *carpopedal spasm (R29.Ø)*
charley-horse (M62.831)
infantile spasms (G4Ø.4-)
muscle spasm of back (M62.83Ø)
muscle spasm of calf (M62.831)

R25.3 Fasciculation
Twitching NOS
R25.8 Other abnormal involuntary movements
R25.9 Unspecified abnormal involuntary movements

✓4th **R26 Abnormalities of gait and mobility**
EXCLUDES 1 *ataxia NOS (R27.Ø)*
hereditary ataxia (G11.-)
locomotor (syphilitic) ataxia (A52.11)
immobility syndrome (paraplegic) (M62.3)

R26.Ø Ataxic gait
Staggering gait
R26.1 Paralytic gait
Spastic gait
R26.2 Difficulty in walking, not elsewhere classified
EXCLUDES 1 *falling (R29.6)*
unsteadiness on feet (R26.81)

✓5th **R26.8 Other abnormalities of gait and mobility**
R26.81 Unsteadiness on feet
R26.89 Other abnormalities of gait and mobility

R26.9 Unspecified abnormalities of gait and mobility

✓4th **R27 Other lack of coordination**
EXCLUDES 1 *ataxic gait (R26.Ø)*
hereditary ataxia (G11.-)
vertigo NOS (R42)

R27.Ø Ataxia, unspecified
EXCLUDES 1 *ataxia following cerebrovascular disease (I69. with final characters -93)*

R27.8 Other lack of coordination

R27.9 Unspecified lack of coordination

✓4th **R29 Other symptoms and signs involving the nervous and musculoskeletal systems**

R29.0 Tetany CC
Carpopedal spasm
EXCLUDES 1 *hysterical tetany (F44.5)*
neonatal tetany (P71.3)
parathyroid tetany (E20.9)
post-thyroidectomy tetany (E89.2)
CC Excl: A33, A35, G10-G11.2, G11.4, G20-G25.79, G25.82-G26, G32.81, G80.3, G81.10-G81.14, G89.0-G89.4, G90.3, R29.0, R41.0-R41.3, R41.82, R41.9, R44.8-R44.9, R45.83-R45.84, R46.0-R46.89, R52, R68.0-R68.19, R68.81-R68.83, R68.89-R69

R29.1 Meningismus CC
CC Excl: R29.1, R29.810

R29.2 Abnormal reflex
EXCLUDES 2 *abnormal pupillary reflex (H57.0)*
hyperactive gag reflex (J39.2)
vasovagal reaction or syncope (R55)

R29.3 Abnormal posture

R29.4 Clicking hip
EXCLUDES 1 *congenital deformities of hip (Q65.-)*

R29.5 Transient paralysis CC
Code first any associated spinal cord injury (S14.0, S14.1-, S24.0, S24.1-, S34.0-, S34.1-)
EXCLUDES 1 *transient ischemic attack (G45.9)*
CC Excl: R29.5, R29.810

R29.6 Repeated falls
Falling
Tendency to fall
EXCLUDES 2 *at risk for falling (Z91.81)*
history of falling (Z91.81)

✓5th **R29.8 Other symptoms and signs involving the nervous and musculoskeletal systems**

✓6th **R29.81 Other symptoms and signs involving the nervous system**

R29.810 Facial weakness
Facial droop
EXCLUDES 1 *Bell's palsy (G51.0)*
facial weakness following cerebrovascular disease (I69. with final characters -92)

R29.818 Other symptoms and signs involving the nervous system

✓6th **R29.89 Other symptoms and signs involving the musculoskeletal system**
EXCLUDES 2 *pain in limb (M79.6-)*

R29.890 Loss of height
EXCLUDES 1 *osteoporosis (M80-M81)*

R29.891 Ocular torticollis
EXCLUDES 1 *congenital (sternomastoid) torticollis Q68.0*
psychogenic torticollis (F45.8)
spasmodic torticollis (G24.3)
torticollis due to birth injury (P15.8)
torticollis NOS M43.6

R29.898 Other symptoms and signs involving the musculoskeletal system

✓5th **R29.9 Unspecified symptoms and signs involving the nervous and musculoskeletal systems**

R29.90 Unspecified symptoms and signs involving the nervous system

R29.91 Unspecified symptoms and signs involving the musculoskeletal system

Symptoms and signs involving the genitourinary system (R30-R39)

✓4th **R30 Pain associated with micturition**
EXCLUDES 1 *psychogenic pain associated with micturition (F45.8)*

R30.0 Dysuria
Strangury

R30.1 Vesical tenesmus

R30.9 Painful micturition, unspecified
Painful urination NOS

✓4th **R31 Hematuria**
EXCLUDES 1 *hematuria included with underlying conditions, such as:*
acute cystitis with hematuria (N30.01)
recurrent and persistent hematuria in glomerular diseases (N02.-)

R31.0 Gross hematuria

R31.1 Benign essential microscopic hematuria

R31.2 Other microscopic hematuria

R31.9 Hematuria, unspecified

R32 Unspecified urinary incontinence
Enuresis NOS
EXCLUDES 1 *functional urinary incontinence (R39.81)*
nonorganic enuresis (F98.0)
stress incontinence and other specified urinary incontinence (N39.3-N39.4-)
urinary incontinence associated with cognitive impairment (R39.81)

✓4th **R33 Retention of urine**
EXCLUDES 1 *psychogenic retention of urine (F45.8)*

R33.0 Drug induced retention of urine
Use additional code for adverse effect, if applicable, to identify drug (T36-T50 with fifth or sixth character 5)

R33.8 Other retention of urine
Code first, if applicable, any causal condition, such as:
enlarged prostate (N40.1)

R33.9 Retention of urine, unspecified

R34 Anuria and oliguria
EXCLUDES 1 *anuria and oliguria complicating abortion or ectopic or molar pregnancy (O00-O07, O08.4)*
anuria and oliguria complicating pregnancy (O26.83-)
anuria and oliguria complicating the puerperium (O90.4)

✓4th **R35 Polyuria**
Code first, if applicable, any causal condition, such as:
enlarged prostate (N40.1)
EXCLUDES 1 *psychogenic polyuria (F45.8)*

R35.0 Frequency of micturition

R35.1 Nocturia

R35.8 Other polyuria
Polyuria NOS

✓4th **R36 Urethral discharge**

R36.0 Urethral discharge without blood

R36.1 Hematospermia ♂

R36.9 Urethral discharge, unspecified
Penile discharge NOS
Urethrorrhea

R37 Sexual dysfunction, unspecified

✓4th **R39 Other and unspecified symptoms and signs involving the genitourinary system**

R39.0 Extravasation of urine CC
CC Excl: R30.1, R39.0, R39.2-R39.9

✓5th **R39.1 Other difficulties with micturition**
Code first, if applicable, any causal condition, such as:
enlarged prostate (N40.1)

R39.11 Hesitancy of micturition

R39.12 Poor urinary stream
Weak urinary steam

R39.13 Splitting of urinary stream

R39.14 Feeling of incomplete bladder emptying

R39.15 Urgency of urination
EXCLUDES 1 *urge incontinence (N39.41, N39.46)*

R39.16 Straining to void

R39.19 Other difficulties with micturition

R39.2 Extrarenal uremia
Prerenal uremia
EXCLUDES 1 *uremia NOS (N19)*

✓5th **R39.8 Other symptoms and signs involving the genitourinary system**

R39.81 Functional urinary incontinence
Urinary incontinence due to cognitive impairment, or severe physical disability or immobility
EXCLUDES 1 *stress incontinence and other specified urinary incontinence (N39.3-N39.4-)*
urinary incontinence NOS (R32)

R39.89 **Other symptoms and signs involving the genitourinary system**

R39.9 **Unspecified symptoms and signs involving the genitourinary system**

Symptoms and signs involving cognition, perception, emotional state and behavior (R40-R46)

EXCLUDES 1 *symptoms and signs constituting part of a pattern of mental disorder (F01-F99)*

4th **R40 Somnolence, stupor and coma**

EXCLUDES 1 *neonatal coma (P91.5)*
somnolence, stupor and coma in diabetes (E08-E13)
somnolence, stupor and coma in hepatic failure (K72.-)
somnolence, stupor and coma in hypoglycemia (nondiabetic) (E15)

R40.0 Somnolence
Drowsiness
EXCLUDES 1 *coma (R40.2-)*

R40.1 Stupor
Catatonic stupor
Semicoma
EXCLUDES 1 *catatonic schizophrenia (F20.2)*
coma (R40.2-)
depressive stupor (F31-F33)
dissociative stupor (F44.2)
manic stupor (F30.2)

5th **R40.2 Coma**
Code first any associated:
fracture of skull (S02.-)
intracranial injury (S06.-)
NOTE One code from subcategories R40.21-R40.23 is required to complete the coma scale
AHA: 2014, 1Q, 19

CC Excl: For MCC codes in subcategory R40.2, unless otherwise noted: B15.0-B19.9, E03.5, E08.00-E08.59, E08.618-E09.59, E09.618-E10.59, E10.618-E10.649, E10.69-E11.59, E11.618-E11.649, E11.69-E13.59, E13.618-E16.2, E89.1, G32.89, G89.0-G89.4, G93.81-G93.9, G96.8-G96.9, G98.0-G98.8, G99.8, I60.00-I62.9, K72.91, R40.0-R40.2124, R40.2210-R40.2224, R40.2310-R40.2324, R40.2340-R40.2344, R40.3-R41.3, R41.82, R41.9-R42, R44.8-R44.9, R45.83-R45.84, R46.0-R46.89, R52, R55, R68.0-R68.19, R68.81-R68.83, R68.89-R69, S02.0XX-S02.19X with 7th character [A, B], S02.91X-S02.91X with 7th character [A, B], S06.0X0-S06.9X9 with 7th character A

R40.20 Unspecified coma MCC
Coma NOS
Unconsciousness NOS

6th **R40.21 Coma scale, eyes open**

The following appropriate 7th character is to be added to subcategory R40.21-.
0 unspecified time
1 in the field [EMT or ambulance]
2 at arrival to emergency department
3 at hospital admission
4 24 hours or more after hospital admission

7th **R40.211 Coma scale, eyes open, never** MCC
7th **R40.212 Coma scale, eyes open, to pain** MCC
7th **R40.213 Coma scale, eyes open, to sound**
7th **R40.214 Coma scale, eyes open, spontaneous**

6th **R40.22 Coma scale, best verbal response**

The following appropriate 7th character is to be added to subcategory R40.22-.
0 unspecified time
1 in the field [EMT or ambulance]
2 at arrival to emergency department
3 at hospital admission
4 24 hours or more after hospital admission

7th **R40.221 Coma scale, best verbal response, none** MCC
7th **R40.222 Coma scale, best verbal response, incomprehensible words** MCC
7th **R40.223 Coma scale, best verbal response, inappropriate words**
7th **R40.224 Coma scale, best verbal response, confused conversation**
7th **R40.225 Coma scale, best verbal response, oriented**

6th **R40.23 Coma scale, best motor response**

The following appropriate 7th character is to be added to subcategory R40.23-.
0 unspecified time
1 in the field [EMT or ambulance]
2 at arrival to emergency department
3 at hospital admission
4 24 hours or more after hospital admission

7th **R40.231 Coma scale, best motor response, none** MCC
7th **R40.232 Coma scale, best motor response, extension** MCC
7th **R40.233 Coma scale, best motor response, abnormal**
7th **R40.234 Coma scale, best motor response, flexion withdrawal** MCC
7th **R40.235 Coma scale, best motor response, localizes pain**
7th **R40.236 Coma scale, best motor response, obeys commands**

6th **R40.24 Glasgow coma scale, total score**
Use codes R40.21- through R40.23- only when the individual score(s) are documented

R40.241 Glasgow coma scale score 13-15
R40.242 Glasgow coma scale score 9-12
R40.243 Glasgow coma scale score 3-8
R40.244 Other coma, without documented Glasgow coma scale score, or with partial score reported

R40.3 Persistent vegetative state CC
CC Excl: See code: R40.2

R40.4 Transient alteration of awareness

4th **R41 Other symptoms and signs involving cognitive functions and awareness**

EXCLUDES 1 *dissociative [conversion] disorders (F44.-)*
mild cognitive impairment, so stated (G31.84)

R41.0 Disorientation, unspecified
Confusion NOS
Delirium NOS

R41.1 Anterograde amnesia

R41.2 Retrograde amnesia

R41.3 Other amnesia
Amnesia NOS
Memory loss NOS
EXCLUDES 1 *amnestic disorder due to known physiologic condition (F04)*
amnestic syndrome due to psychoactive substance use (F10-F19 with 5th character .6)
mild memory disturbance due to known physiological condition (F06.8)
transient global amnesia (G45.4)

R41.4 Neurologic neglect syndrome CC
Asomatognosia
Hemi-akinesia
Hemi-inattention
Hemispatial neglect
Left-sided neglect
Sensory neglect
Visuospatial neglect
EXCLUDES 1 *visuospatial deficit (R41.842)*
CC Excl: R29.3, R29.6-R29.890, R29.90-R29.91, R41.4

5th **R41.8 Other symptoms and signs involving cognitive functions and awareness**

R41.81 Age-related cognitive decline A
Senility NOS

R41.82 Altered mental status, unspecified
Change in mental status NOS
EXCLUDES 1 *altered level of consciousness (R40.-)*
altered mental status due to known condition—code to condition
delirium NOS (R41.0)
AHA: 2012, 4Q, 97

R41.83 Borderline intellectual functioning
IQ level 71 to 84
EXCLUDES 1 *intellectual disabilities (F70-F79)*

R41.84 Other specified cognitive deficit
R41.840 Attention and concentration deficit
EXCLUDES 1 *attention-deficit hyperactivity disorders (F90.-)*
R41.841 Cognitive communication deficit
R41.842 Visuospatial deficit
R41.843 Psychomotor deficit
R41.844 Frontal lobe and executive function deficit
R41.89 Other symptoms and signs involving cognitive functions and awareness
Anosognosia
R41.9 Unspecified symptoms and signs involving cognitive functions and awareness

R42 Dizziness and giddiness
Light-headedness
Vertigo NOS
EXCLUDES 1 *vertiginous syndromes (H81.-)*
vertigo from infrasound (T75.23)

R43 Disturbances of smell and taste
R43.0 Anosmia
R43.1 Parosmia
R43.2 Parageusia
R43.8 Other disturbances of smell and taste
Mixed disturbance of smell and taste
R43.9 Unspecified disturbances of smell and taste

R44 Other symptoms and signs involving general sensations and perceptions
EXCLUDES 1 *alcoholic hallucinations (F1.5)*
hallucinations in drug psychosis (F11-F19 with .5)
hallucinations in mood disorders with psychotic symptoms (F30.2, F31.5, F32.3, F33.3)
hallucinations in schizophrenia, schizotypal and delusional disorders (F20-F29)
EXCLUDES 2 *disturbances of skin sensation (R20.-)*

CC Excl: For CC codes in category R44, unless otherwise noted: G89.0-G89.4, R41.0-R41.3, R41.82, R41.9-R42, R44.0, R44.2-R44.9, R45.83-R45.84, R46.0-R46.89, R52, R68.0-R68.19, R68.81-R68.83, R68.89-R69

R44.0 Auditory hallucinations CC
R44.1 Visual hallucinations
R44.2 Other hallucinations CC
R44.3 Hallucinations, unspecified CC
R44.8 Other symptoms and signs involving general sensations and perceptions
R44.9 Unspecified symptoms and signs involving general sensations and perceptions

R45 Symptoms and signs involving emotional state
R45.0 Nervousness
Nervous tension
R45.1 Restlessness and agitation
R45.2 Unhappiness
R45.3 Demoralization and apathy
EXCLUDES 1 *anhedonia (R45.84)*
R45.4 Irritability and anger
R45.5 Hostility
R45.6 Violent behavior
R45.7 State of emotional shock and stress, unspecified
R45.8 Other symptoms and signs involving emotional state
R45.81 Low self-esteem
R45.82 Worries
R45.83 Excessive crying of child, adolescent or adult
EXCLUDES 1 *excessive crying of infant (baby) R68.11*
R45.84 Anhedonia
R45.85 Homicidal and suicidal ideations
EXCLUDES 1 *suicide attempt (T14.91)*
R45.850 Homicidal ideations
R45.851 Suicidal ideations CC
CC Excl: F05
R45.86 Emotional lability
R45.87 Impulsiveness
R45.89 Other symptoms and signs involving emotional state

R46 Symptoms and signs involving appearance and behavior
EXCLUDES 1 *appearance and behavior in schizophrenia, schizotypal and delusional disorders (F20-F29)*
mental and behavioral disorders (F01-F99)
R46.0 Very low level of personal hygiene
R46.1 Bizarre personal appearance
R46.2 Strange and inexplicable behavior
R46.3 Overactivity
R46.4 Slowness and poor responsiveness
EXCLUDES 1 *stupor (R40.1)*
R46.5 Suspiciousness and marked evasiveness
R46.6 Undue concern and preoccupation with stressful events
R46.7 Verbosity and circumstantial detail obscuring reason for contact
R46.8 Other symptoms and signs involving appearance and behavior
R46.81 Obsessive-compulsive behavior
EXCLUDES 1 *obsessive-compulsive disorder (F42)*
R46.89 Other symptoms and signs involving appearance and behavior

Symptoms and signs involving speech and voice (R47-R49)

R47 Speech disturbances, not elsewhere classified
EXCLUDES 1 *autism (F84.0)*
cluttering (F80.81)
specific developmental disorders of speech and language (F80.-)
stuttering (F80.81)
R47.0 Dysphasia and aphasia
R47.01 Aphasia CC
EXCLUDES 1 *aphasia following cerebrovascular disease (I69. with final characters -20)*
progressive isolated aphasia (G31.01)
CC Excl: F80.1, F80.81, I62.00-I66.9, R47.01-R47.9, R49.0-R49.9
R47.02 Dysphasia
EXCLUDES 1 *dysphasia following cerebrovascular disease (I69. with final characters -21)*
R47.1 Dysarthria and anarthria
EXCLUDES 1 *dysarthria following cerebrovascular disease (I69. with final characters -22)*
R47.8 Other speech disturbances
EXCLUDES 1 *dysarthria following cerebrovascular disease (I69. with final characters -28)*
R47.81 Slurred speech
R47.82 Fluency disorder in conditions classified elsewhere
Stuttering in conditions classified elsewhere
Code first underlying disease or condition, such as:
Parkinson's disease (G20)
EXCLUDES 1 *adult onset fluency disorder (F98.5)*
childhood onset fluency disorder (F80.81)
fluency disorder (stuttering) following cerebrovascular disease (I69. with final characters-23)
R47.89 Other speech disturbances
R47.9 Unspecified speech disturbances

R48 Dyslexia and other symbolic dysfunctions, not elsewhere classified
EXCLUDES 1 *specific developmental disorders of scholastic skills (F81.-)*
R48.0 Dyslexia and alexia
R48.1 Agnosia
Astereognosia (astereognosis)
Autotopagnosia
EXCLUDES 1 *visual object agnosia (R48.3)*
R48.2 Apraxia
EXCLUDES 1 *apraxia following cerebrovascular disease (I69. with final characters -90)*
R48.3 Visual agnosia
Prosopagnosia
Simultanagnosia (asimultagnosia)
R48.8 Other symbolic dysfunctions
Acalculia
Agraphia
R48.9 Unspecified symbolic dysfunctions

✓4th **R49 Voice and resonance disorders**
EXCLUDES 1 *psychogenic voice and resonance disorders (F44.4)*

R49.Ø Dysphonia
Hoarseness

R49.1 Aphonia
Loss of voice

✓5th **R49.2 Hypernasality and hyponasality**

R49.21 Hypernasality

R49.22 Hyponasality

R49.8 Other voice and resonance disorders

R49.9 Unspecified voice and resonance disorder
Change in voice NOS
Resonance disorder NOS

General symptoms and signs (R5Ø-R69)

✓4th **R5Ø Fever of other and unknown origin**
EXCLUDES 1 *chills without fever (R68.83)*
febrile convulsions (R56.Ø-)
fever of unknown origin during labor (O75.2)
fever of unknown origin in newborn (P81.9)
hypothermia due to illness (R68.Ø)
malignant hyperthermia due to anesthesia (T88.3)
puerperal pyrexia NOS (O86.4)

R5Ø.2 Drug induced fever
Use additional code for adverse effect, if applicable, to identify drug (T36-T5Ø with fifth or sixth character 5)
EXCLUDES 1 *postvaccination (postimmunization) fever (R5Ø.83)*

✓5th **R5Ø.8 Other specified fever**

R5Ø.81 Fever presenting with conditions classified elsewhere
Code first underlying condition when associated fever is present, such as with:
leukemia (C91-C95)
neutropenia (D7Ø.-)
sickle-cell disease (D57.-)

R5Ø.82 Postprocedural fever
EXCLUDES 1 *postprocedural infection (T81.4)*
posttransfusion fever (R5Ø.84)
postvaccination (postimmunization) fever (R5Ø.83)

R5Ø.83 Postvaccination fever
Postimmunization fever

R5Ø.84 Febrile nonhemolytic transfusion reaction
FNHTR
Posttransfusion fever

R5Ø.9 Fever, unspecified
Fever NOS
Fever of unknown origin [FUO]
Fever with chills
Fever with rigors
Hyperpyrexia NOS
Persistent fever
Pyrexia NOS

R51 Headache
Facial pain NOS
EXCLUDES 1 *atypical face pain (G5Ø.1)*
migraine and other headache syndromes (G43-G44)
trigeminal neuralgia (G5Ø.Ø)

R52 Pain, unspecified
Acute pain NOS
Generalized pain NOS
Pain NOS
EXCLUDES 1 *acute and chronic pain, not elsewhere classified (G89.-)*
localized pain, unspecified type—code to pain by site, such as:
abdomen pain (R1Ø.-)
back pain (M54.9)
breast pain (N64.4)
chest pain (RØ7.1-RØ7.9)
ear pain (H92.Ø-)
eye pain (H57.1)
headache (R51)
joint pain (M25.5-)
limb pain (M79.6-)
lumbar region pain (M54.5)
pelvic and perineal pain (R1Ø.2)
renal colic (N23)
shoulder pain (M25.51-)
spine pain (M54.-)
throat pain (RØ7.Ø)
tongue pain (K14.6)
tooth pain (KØ8.8)
pain disorders exclusively related to psychological factors (F45.41)

✓4th **R53 Malaise and fatigue**

R53.Ø Neoplastic (malignant) related fatigue
Code first associated neoplasm

R53.1 Weakness
Asthenia NOS
EXCLUDES 1 *age-related weakness (R54)*
muscle weakness (M62.8-)
senile asthenia (R54)

R53.2 Functional quadriplegia MCC
Complete immobility due to severe physical disability or frailty
EXCLUDES 1 *frailty NOS (R54)*
hysterical paralysis (F44.4)
immobility syndrome (M62.3)
neurologic quadriplegia (G82.5-)
quadriplegia (G82.5Ø)
CC Excl: EØ8.4Ø-EØ8.49, EØ8.618-EØ8.638, EØ8.649-EØ8.8, EØ9.4Ø-EØ9.49, EØ9.618-EØ9.638, EØ9.649-EØ9.8, E1Ø.4Ø-E1Ø.49, E1Ø.618-E1Ø.638, E1Ø.649, E1Ø.69-E1Ø.8, E11.4Ø-E11.49, E11.618-E11.638, E11.649, E11.69-E11.8, E13.4Ø-E13.49, E13.618-E13.638, E13.649-E13.8, GØ4.1, G32.89, G8Ø.Ø-G8Ø.2, G8Ø.4-G83.9, G9Ø.1, G93.81, G93.89-G93.9, G96.8-G96.9, G98.Ø-G98.8, G99.8, QØ6.Ø-QØ6.1, QØ6.3, QØ6.8-QØ6.9, QØ7.8-QØ7.9, R53.2

✓5th **R53.8 Other malaise and fatigue**
EXCLUDES 1 *combat exhaustion and fatigue (F43.Ø)*
congenital debility (P96.9)
exhaustion and fatigue due to depressive episode (F32.-)
exhaustion and fatigue due to excessive exertion (T73.3)
exhaustion and fatigue due to exposure (T73.2)
exhaustion and fatigue due to heat (T67.-)
exhaustion and fatigue due to pregnancy (O26.8-)
exhaustion and fatigue due to recurrent depressive episode (F33)
exhaustion and fatigue due to senile debility (R54)

R53.81 Other malaise
Chronic debility
Debility NOS
General physical deterioration
Malaise NOS
Nervous debility
EXCLUDES 1 *age-related physical debility (R54)*

R53.82 Chronic fatigue, unspecified
Chronic fatigue syndrome NOS
EXCLUDES 1 *postviral fatigue syndrome (G93.3)*

R53.83 Other fatigue
Fatigue NOS
Lack of energy
Lethargy
Tiredness

R54 Age-related physical debility A
Frailty
Old age
Senescence
Senile asthenia
Senile debility
EXCLUDES 1 *age-related cognitive decline (R41.81)*
senile psychosis (FØ3)
senility NOS (R41.81)

R55 Syncope and collapse
Blackout
Fainting
Vasovagal attack
EXCLUDES 1 *cardiogenic shock (R57.Ø)*
carotid sinus syncope (G9Ø.Ø1)
heat syncope (T67.1)
neurocirculatory asthenia (F45.8)
neurogenic orthostatic hypotension (G9Ø.3)
orthostatic hypotension (I95.1)
postprocedural shock (T81.1-)
psychogenic syncope (F48.8)
shock NOS (R57.9)
shock complicating or following abortion or ectopic or molar pregnancy (OØØ-OØ7, OØ8.3)
shock complicating or following labor and delivery (O75.1)
Stokes-Adams attack (I45.9)
unconsciousness NOS (R4Ø.2-)

✓4th **R56 Convulsions, not elsewhere classified**
EXCLUDES 1 *dissociative convulsions and seizures (F44.5)*
epileptic convulsions and seizures (G4Ø.-)
newborn convulsions and seizures (P9Ø)

✓5th **R56.Ø Febrile convulsions**

R56.ØØ Simple febrile convulsions CC
Febrile convulsion NOS
Febrile seizure NOS
CC Excl: G32.89, G4Ø.ØØ1-G4Ø.919, G89.Ø-G89.4, G93.81, G93.89-G93.9, G96.8-G96.9, G98.Ø-G98.8, G99.8, P9Ø, P91.8-P91.9, R41.Ø-R41.3, R41.82, R41.9, R44.8-R44.9,

R45.83-R45.84, R46.0-R46.89, R52, R56.00-R56.9, R68.0-R68.19, R68.81-R68.83, R68.89-R69

R56.01 Complex febrile convulsions CC
Atypical febrile seizure
Complex febrile seizure
Complicated febrile seizure
EXCLUDES 1 *status epilepticus (G40.901)*
CC Excl: See code: R56.00

R56.1 Post traumatic seizures CC
EXCLUDES 1 *post traumatic epilepsy (G40.-)*
CC Excl: E08.40-E08.49, E09.40-E09.49, E10.40-E10.49, E11.40-E11.49, E13.40-E13.49, G32.89, G40.001-G40.509, G40.801-G40.804, G40.811-G40.814, G40.821-G40.B19, G93.81, G93.89-G93.9, G96.8-G96.9, G98.0-G98.8, G99.8, R56.1

R56.9 Unspecified convulsions
Convulsion disorder
Fit NOS
Recurrent convulsions
Seizure(s) (convulsive) NOS

✓4th **R57 Shock, not elsewhere classified**
EXCLUDES 1 *anaphylactic shock NOS (T78.2)*
anaphylactic reaction or shock due to adverse food reaction (T78.0-)
anaphylactic shock due to adverse effect of correct drug or medicament properly administered (T88.6)
anaphylactic shock due to serum (T80.5-)
anesthetic shock (T88.3)
electric shock (T75.4)
obstetric shock (O75.1)
postprocedural shock (T81.1-)
psychic shock (F43.0)
septic shock (R65.21)
shock complicating or following ectopic or molar pregnancy (O00-O07, O08.3)
shock due to lightning (T75.01)
traumatic shock (T79.4)
toxic shock syndrome (A48.3)

CC Excl: For CC/MCC codes in category R57, unless otherwise noted: G89.0-G89.4, R09.89, R41.0-R41.3, R41.82, R41.9, R44.8-R44.9, R45.83-R45.84, R46.0-R46.89, R52, R57.0-R57.9, R65.21-R68.19, R68.81-R68.83, R68.89-R69

10 **R57.0 Cardiogenic shock** MCC
10 **R57.1 Hypovolemic shock** MCC
10 **R57.8 Other shock** MCC
R57.9 Shock, unspecified CC
Failure of peripheral circulation NOS

R58 Hemorrhage, not elsewhere classified
Hemorrhage NOS
EXCLUDES 1 *hemorrhage included with underlying conditions, such as:*
acute duodenal ulcer with hemorrhage (K26.0)
acute gastritis with bleeding (K29.01)
ulcerative enterocolitis with rectal bleeding (K51.01)

✓4th **R59 Enlarged lymph nodes**
INCLUDES swollen glands
EXCLUDES 1 *acute lymphadenitis (L04.-)*
chronic lymphadenitis (I88.1)
lymphadenitis NOS (I88.9)
mesenteric (acute) (chronic) lymphadenitis (I88.0)

R59.0 Localized enlarged lymph nodes
R59.1 Generalized enlarged lymph nodes
Lymphadenopathy NOS
R59.9 Enlarged lymph nodes, unspecified

✓4th **R60 Edema, not elsewhere classified**
EXCLUDES 1 *angioneurotic edema (T78.3)*
ascites (R18.-)
cerebral edema (G93.6)
cerebral edema due to birth injury (P11.0)
edema of larynx (J38.4)
edema of nasopharynx (J39.2)
edema of pharynx (J39.2)
gestational edema (O12.0-)
hereditary edema (Q82.0)
hydrops fetalis NOS (P83.2)
hydrothorax (J94.8)
nutritional edema (E40-E46)
hydrops fetalis NOS (P83.2)
newborn edema (P83.3)
pulmonary edema (J81.-)

R60.0 Localized edema
R60.1 Generalized edema
R60.9 Edema, unspecified
Fluid retention NOS

R61 Generalized hyperhidrosis
Excessive sweating
Night sweats
Secondary hyperhidrosis
Code first, if applicable, menopausal and female climacteric states (N95.1)
EXCLUDES 1 *focal (primary) (secondary) hyperhidrosis (L74.5-)*
Frey's syndrome (L74.52)
localized (primary) (secondary) hyperhidrosis (L74.5-)

✓4th **R62 Lack of expected normal physiological development in childhood and adults**
EXCLUDES 1 *delayed puberty (E30.0)*
gonadal dysgenesis (Q99.1)
hypopituitarism (E23.0)

R62.0 Delayed milestone in childhood P
Delayed attainment of expected physiological developmental stage
Late talker
Late walker

✓5th **R62.5 Other and unspecified lack of expected normal physiological development in childhood**
EXCLUDES 1 *HIV disease resulting in failure to thrive (B20)*
physical retardation due to malnutrition (E45)

R62.50 Unspecified lack of expected normal physiological development in childhood P
Infantilism NOS

R62.51 Failure to thrive (child) P
Failure to gain weight
EXCLUDES 1 *failure to thrive in child under 28 days old (P92.6)*

R62.52 Short stature (child) P
Lack of growth
Physical retardation
Short stature NOS
EXCLUDES 1 *short stature due to endocrine disorder (E34.3)*

R62.59 Other lack of expected normal physiological development in childhood P

R62.7 Adult failure to thrive A

✓4th **R63 Symptoms and signs concerning food and fluid intake**
EXCLUDES 1 *bulimia NOS (F50.2)*
eating disorders of nonorganic origin (F50.-)
malnutrition (E40-E46)

R63.0 Anorexia
Loss of appetite
EXCLUDES 1 *anorexia nervosa (F50.0-)*
loss of appetite of nonorganic origin (F50.8)

R63.1 Polydipsia
Excessive thirst

R63.2 Polyphagia
Excessive eating
Hyperalimentation NOS

R63.3 Feeding difficulties
Feeding problem (elderly) (infant) NOS
EXCLUDES 1 *feeding problems of newborn (P92.-)*
infant feeding disorder of nonorganic origin (F98.2-)

R63.4 Abnormal weight loss

R63.5 Abnormal weight gain
EXCLUDES 1 *excessive weight gain in pregnancy (O26.0-)*
obesity (E66.-)

R63.6 Underweight
Use additional code to identify body mass index (BMI), if known (Z68.-)
EXCLUDES 1 *abnormal weight loss (R63.4)*
anorexia nervosa (F50.0-)
malnutrition (E40-E46)

R63.8 Other symptoms and signs concerning food and fluid intake

R64 Cachexia CC
Wasting syndrome
Code first underlying condition, if known
EXCLUDES 1 *abnormal weight loss (R63.4)*
nutritional marasmus (E41)
CC Excl: G89.0-G89.4, R41.0-R41.3, R41.82, R41.9, R44.8-R44.9, R45.83-R45.84, R46.0-R46.89, R52, R64, R68.0-R68.19, R68.81-R68.83, R68.89-R69

10 MCC = only if patient is discharged alive.

R65 Symptoms and signs specifically associated with systemic inflammation and infection

CC Excl: For CC/MCC codes in category R65, unless otherwise noted: A02.1, A20.7, A22.7, A26.7, A32.7, A39.2-A39.4, A40.0-A40.1, A40.8-A41.9, A42.7, A48.2-A48.4, A48.8-A49.9, A54.86, B00.7, B37.7, B92, B94.2-B96.89, R65.10-R65.20, M00.011-M00.012, M00.021-M00.022, M00.031-M00.032, M00.041-M00.042, M00.051-M00.052, M00.061-M00.062, M00.071-M00.072, Z16.10-Z16.39

R65.1 Systemic inflammatory response syndrome [SIRS] of non-infectious origin

Code first underlying condition, such as:
heatstroke (T67.0)
injury and trauma (S00-T88)

EXCLUDES 1 *sepsis—code to infection*
severe sepsis (R65.2)

R65.10 Systemic inflammatory response syndrome [SIRS] of non-infectious origin without acute organ dysfunction CC

Systemic inflammatory response syndrome (SIRS) NOS

R65.11 Systemic inflammatory response syndrome [SIRS] of non-infectious origin with acute organ dysfunction MCC

Use additional code to identify specific acute organ dysfunction, such as:
acute kidney failure (N17.-)
acute respiratory failure (J96.0-)
critical illness myopathy (G72.81)
critical illness polyneuropathy (G62.81)
disseminated intravascular coagulopathy [DIC] (D65)
encephalopathy (metabolic) (septic) (G93.41)
hepatic failure (K72.0-)

R65.2 Severe sepsis

Infection with associated acute organ dysfunction
Sepsis with acute organ dysfunction
Sepsis with multiple organ dysfunction
Systemic inflammatory response syndrome due to infectious process with acute organ dysfunction

Code first underlying infection, such as:
infection following a procedure (T81.4)
infections following infusion, transfusion and therapeutic injection (T80.2-)
puerperal sepsis (O85)
sepsis following complete or unspecified spontaneous abortion (O03.87)
sepsis following ectopic and molar pregnancy (O08.82)
sepsis following incomplete spontaneous abortion (O03.37)
sepsis following (induced) termination of pregnancy (O04.87)
sepsis NOS (A41.9)

Use additional code to identify specific acute organ dysfunction, such as:
acute kidney failure (N17.-)
acute respiratory failure (J96.0-)
critical illness myopathy (G72.81)
critical illness polyneuropathy (G62.81)
disseminated intravascular coagulopathy [DIC] (D65)
encephalopathy (metabolic) (septic) (G93.41)
hepatic failure (K72.0-)

R65.20 Severe sepsis without septic shock MCC

Severe sepsis NOS
AHA: 2013, 4Q, 119

R65.21 Severe sepsis with septic shock PDx MCC MCC

CC Excl: G89.0-G89.4, R09.89, R41.0-R41.3, R41.82, R41.9, R44.8-R44.9, R45.83-R45.84, R46.0-R46.89, R52, R57.0-R57.9, R65.21-R68.19, R68.81-R68.83, R68.89-R69

R68 Other general symptoms and signs

R68.0 Hypothermia, not associated with low environmental temperature

EXCLUDES 1 *hypothermia due to anesthesia (T88.51)*
hypothermia due to low environmental temperature (T68)
hypothermia NOS (accidental) (T68)
newborn hypothermia (P80.-)

R68.1 Nonspecific symptoms peculiar to infancy

EXCLUDES 1 *colic, infantile (R10.83)*
neonatal cerebral irritability (P91.3)
teething syndrome (K00.7)

R68.11 Excessive crying of infant (baby) P

EXCLUDES 1 *excessive crying of child, adolescent, or adult (R45.83)*

R68.12 Fussy infant (baby) P

Irritable infant

R68.13 Apparent life threatening event in infant [ALTE] P

Apparent life threatening event in newborn
Code first confirmed diagnosis, if known
Use additional code(s) for associated signs and symptoms if no confirmed diagnosis established, or if signs and symptoms are not associated routinely with confirmed diagnosis, or provide additional information for cause of ALTE

R68.19 Other nonspecific symptoms peculiar to infancy P

R68.2 Dry mouth, unspecified

EXCLUDES 1 *dry mouth due to dehydration (E86.0)*
dry mouth due to sicca syndrome [Sjögren] (M35.0-)
salivary gland hyposecretion (K11.7)

R68.3 Clubbing of fingers

Clubbing of nails

EXCLUDES 1 *congenital clubfinger (Q68.1)*

R68.8 Other general symptoms and signs

R68.81 Early satiety

R68.82 Decreased libido A

Decreased sexual desire

R68.83 Chills (without fever)

Chills NOS

EXCLUDES 1 *chills with fever (R50.9)*

R68.84 Jaw pain

Mandibular pain
Maxilla pain

EXCLUDES 1 *temporomandibular joint arthralgia (M26.62)*

R68.89 Other general symptoms and signs

R69 Illness, unspecified

Unknown and unspecified cases of morbidity

Abnormal findings on examination of blood, without diagnosis (R70-R79)

EXCLUDES 1 *abnormalities (of)(on):*
abnormal findings on antenatal screening of mother (O28.-)
coagulation hemorrhagic disorders (D65-D68)
lipids (E78.-)
platelets and thrombocytes (D69.-)
white blood cells classified elsewhere (D70-D72)
diagnostic abnormal findings classified elsewhere—see Alphabetical Index
hemorrhagic and hematological disorders of newborn (P50-P61)

R70 Elevated erythrocyte sedimentation rate and abnormality of plasma viscosity

R70.0 Elevated erythrocyte sedimentation rate

R70.1 Abnormal plasma viscosity

R71 Abnormality of red blood cells

EXCLUDES 1 *anemias (D50-D64)*
anemia of premature infant (P61.2)
benign (familial) polycythemia (D75.0)
congenital anemias (P61.2-P61.4)
newborn anemia due to isoimmunization (P55.-)
polycythemia neonatorum (P61.1)
polycythemia NOS (D75.1)
polycythemia vera (D45)
secondary polycythemia (D75.1)

R71.0 Precipitous drop in hematocrit CC

Drop (precipitous) in hemoglobin
Drop in hematocrit
CC Excl: D62, D64.4-D64.9

R71.8 Other abnormality of red blood cells

Abnormal red-cell morphology NOS
Abnormal red-cell volume NOS
Anisocytosis
Poikilocytosis

R73 Elevated blood glucose level

EXCLUDES 1 *diabetes mellitus (E08-E13)*
diabetes mellitus in pregnancy, childbirth and the puerperium (O24.-)
neonatal disorders (P70.0-P70.2)
postsurgical hypoinsulinemia (E89.1)

R73.0 Abnormal glucose

EXCLUDES 1 *abnormal glucose in pregnancy (O99.81-)*
diabetes mellitus (E08-E13)
dysmetabolic syndrome X (E88.81)
gestational diabetes (O24.4-)
glycosuria (R81)
hypoglycemia (E16.2)

R73.01 Impaired fasting glucose

Elevated fasting glucose

R73.02 Impaired glucose tolerance (oral)
Elevated glucose tolerance

R73.09 Other abnormal glucose
Abnormal glucose NOS
Abnormal non-fasting glucose tolerance
Latent diabetes
Prediabetes

R73.9 Hyperglycemia, unspecified

✓4th **R74 Abnormal serum enzyme levels**

R74.0 Nonspecific elevation of levels of transaminase and lactic acid dehydrogenase [LDH]

R74.8 Abnormal levels of other serum enzymes
Abnormal level of acid phosphatase
Abnormal level of alkaline phosphatase
Abnormal level of amylase
Abnormal level of lipase [triacylglycerol lipase]

R74.9 Abnormal serum enzyme level, unspecified

R75 Inconclusive laboratory evidence of human immunodeficiency virus [HIV]
Nonconclusive HIV-test finding in infants
EXCLUDES 1 *asymptomatic human immunodeficiency virus [HIV] infection status (Z21)*
human immunodeficiency virus [HIV] disease (B20)

✓4th **R76 Other abnormal immunological findings in serum**

R76.0 Raised antibody titer
EXCLUDES 1 *isoimmunization in pregnancy (O36.0-O36.1)*
isoimmunization affecting newborn (P55.-)

✓5th **R76.1 Nonspecific reaction to test for tuberculosis**

R76.11 Nonspecific reaction to tuberculin skin test without active tuberculosis
Abnormal result of Mantoux test
PPD positive
Tuberculin (skin test) positive
Tuberculin (skin test) reactor
EXCLUDES 1 *nonspecific reaction to cell mediated immunity measurement of gamma interferon antigen response without active tuberculosis (R76.12)*

R76.12 Nonspecific reaction to cell mediated immunity measurement of gamma interferon antigen response without active tuberculosis
Nonspecific reaction to QuantiFERON-TB test (QFT) without active tuberculosis
EXCLUDES 1 *nonspecific reaction to tuberculin skin test without active tuberculosis (R76.11)*
positive tuberculin skin test (R76.11)

R76.8 Other specified abnormal immunological findings in serum
Raised level of immunoglobulins NOS

R76.9 Abnormal immunological finding in serum, unspecified

✓4th **R77 Other abnormalities of plasma proteins**
EXCLUDES 1 *disorders of plasma-protein metabolism (E88.0)*

R77.0 Abnormality of albumin

R77.1 Abnormality of globulin
Hyperglobulinemia NOS

R77.2 Abnormality of alphafetoprotein

R77.8 Other specified abnormalities of plasma proteins

R77.9 Abnormality of plasma protein, unspecified

✓4th **R78 Findings of drugs and other substances, not normally found in blood**
Use additional code to identify any retained foreign body, if applicable (Z18.-)
EXCLUDES 1 *mental or behavioral disorders due to psychoactive substance use (F10-F19)*

R78.0 Finding of alcohol in blood
Use additional external cause code (Y90.-), for detail regarding alcohol level

R78.1 Finding of opiate drug in blood

R78.2 Finding of cocaine in blood

R78.3 Finding of hallucinogen in blood

R78.4 Finding of other drugs of addictive potential in blood

R78.5 Finding of other psychotropic drug in blood

R78.6 Finding of steroid agent in blood

✓5th **R78.7 Finding of abnormal level of heavy metals in blood**

R78.71 Abnormal lead level in blood
EXCLUDES 1 *lead poisoning (T56.0-)*

R78.79 Finding of abnormal level of heavy metals in blood

✓5th **R78.8 Finding of other specified substances, not normally found in blood**

R78.81 Bacteremia CC
EXCLUDES 1 *sepsis—code to specified infection (A00-B99)*
CC Excl: B34.9, E07.81, G89.0-G89.4, R41.0-R41.3, R41.82, R41.9, R44.8-R44.9, R45.83-R45.84, R46.0-R46.89, R52, R68.0-R68.19, R68.81-R68.83, R68.89-R69, R70.1, R77.0-R77.9, R78.1-R78.6, R78.81, R78.9, R79.1-R79.89, R97.2

R78.89 Finding of other specified substances, not normally found in blood
Finding of abnormal level of lithium in blood

R78.9 Finding of unspecified substance, not normally found in blood

✓4th **R79 Other abnormal findings of blood chemistry**
Use additional code to identify any retained foreign body, if applicable (Z18.-)
EXCLUDES 1 *abnormality of fluid, electrolyte or acid-base balance (E86-E87)*
asymptomatic hyperuricemia (E79.0)
hyperglycemia NOS (R73.9)
hypoglycemia NOS (E16.2)
neonatal hypoglycemia (P70.3-P70.4)
specific findings indicating disorder of amino-acid metabolism (E70-E72)
specific findings indicating disorder of carbohydrate metabolism (E73-E74)
specific findings indicating disorder of lipid metabolism (E75.-)

R79.0 Abnormal level of blood mineral
Abnormal blood level of cobalt
Abnormal blood level of copper
Abnormal blood level of iron
Abnormal blood level of magnesium
Abnormal blood level of mineral NEC
Abnormal blood level of zinc
EXCLUDES 1 *abnormal level of lithium (R78.89)*
disorders of mineral metabolism (E83.-)
neonatal hypomagnesemia (P71.2)
nutritional mineral deficiency (E58-E61)

R79.1 Abnormal coagulation profile
Abnormal or prolonged bleeding time
Abnormal or prolonged coagulation time
Abnormal or prolonged partial thromboplastin time [PTT]
Abnormal or prolonged prothrombin time [PT]
EXCLUDES 1 *coagulation defects (D68.-)*

✓5th **R79.8 Other specified abnormal findings of blood chemistry**

R79.81 Abnormal blood-gas level

R79.82 Elevated C-reactive protein [CRP]

R79.89 Other specified abnormal findings of blood chemistry

R79.9 Abnormal finding of blood chemistry, unspecified

Abnormal findings on examination of urine, without diagnosis (R80-R82)

EXCLUDES 1 *abnormal findings on antenatal screening of mother (O28.-)*
diagnostic abnormal findings classified elsewhere—see Alphabetical Index
specific findings indicating disorder of amino-acid metabolism (E70-E72)

✓4th **R80 Proteinuria**
EXCLUDES 1 *gestational proteinuria (O12.1-)*

R80.0 Isolated proteinuria
Idiopathic proteinuria
EXCLUDES 1 *isolated proteinuria with specific morphological lesion (N06.-)*

R80.1 Persistent proteinuria, unspecified

R80.2 Orthostatic proteinuria, unspecified
Postural proteinuria

R80.3 Bence Jones proteinuria

R80.8 Other proteinuria

R80.9 Proteinuria, unspecified
Albuminuria NOS

R81 Glycosuria
EXCLUDES 1 *renal glycosuria (E74.8)*

✓4th R82 Other and unspecified abnormal findings in urine
Chromoabnormalities in urine
Use additional code to identify any retained foreign body, if applicable (Z18.-)
EXCLUDES 2 *hematuria (R31.-)*

R82.0 Chyluria CC
EXCLUDES 1 *filarial chyluria (B74.-)*
CC Excl: G89.0-G89.4, R41.0-R41.3, R41.82, R41.9, R44.8-R44.9, R45.83-R45.84, R46.0-R46.89, R52, R68.0-R68.19, R68.81-R68.83, R68.89-R69, R82.0, R82.5-R82.99

R82.1 Myoglobinuria CC
CC Excl: G89.0-G89.4, R41.0-R41.3, R41.82, R41.9, R44.8-R44.9, R45.83-R45.84, R46.0-R46.89, R52, R68.0-R68.19, R68.81-R68.83, R68.89-R69, R82.1, R82.3, R82.5-R82.99

R82.2 Biliuria

R82.3 Hemoglobinuria
EXCLUDES 1 *hemoglobinuria due to hemolysis from external causes NEC (D59.6)*
hemoglobinuria due to paroxysmal nocturnal [Marchiafava-Micheli] (D59.5)

R82.4 Acetonuria
Ketonuria

R82.5 Elevated urine levels of drugs, medicaments and biological substances
Elevated urine levels of catecholamines
Elevated urine levels of indoleacetic acid
Elevated urine levels of 17-ketosteroids
Elevated urine levels of steroids

R82.6 Abnormal urine levels of substances chiefly nonmedicinal as to source
Abnormal urine level of heavy metals

R82.7 Abnormal findings on microbiological examination of urine
Positive culture findings of urine
EXCLUDES 1 *colonization status (Z22.-)*

R82.8 Abnormal findings on cytological and histological examination of urine

✓5th R82.9 Other and unspecified abnormal findings in urine

R82.90 Unspecified abnormal findings in urine

R82.91 Other chromoabnormalities of urine
Chromoconversion (dipstick)
Idiopathic dipstick converts positive for blood with no cellular forms in sediment
EXCLUDES 1 *hemoglobinuria (R82.3)*
myoglobinuria (R82.1)

R82.99 Other abnormal findings in urine
Cells and casts in urine
Crystalluria
Melanuria

Abnormal findings on examination of other body fluids, substances and tissues, without diagnosis (R83-R89)

EXCLUDES 1 *abnormal findings on antenatal screening of mother (O28.-)*
diagnostic abnormal findings classified elsewhere—see Alphabetical Index
EXCLUDES 2 *abnormal findings on examination of blood, without diagnosis (R70-R79)*
abnormal findings on examination of urine, without diagnosis (R80-R82)
abnormal tumor markers (R97.-)

✓4th R83 Abnormal findings in cerebrospinal fluid

R83.0 Abnormal level of enzymes in cerebrospinal fluid

R83.1 Abnormal level of hormones in cerebrospinal fluid

R83.2 Abnormal level of other drugs, medicaments and biological substances in cerebrospinal fluid

R83.3 Abnormal level of substances chiefly nonmedicinal as to source in cerebrospinal fluid

R83.4 Abnormal immunological findings in cerebrospinal fluid

R83.5 Abnormal microbiological findings in cerebrospinal fluid
Positive culture findings in cerebrospinal fluid
EXCLUDES 1 *colonization status (Z22.-)*

R83.6 Abnormal cytological findings in cerebrospinal fluid

R83.8 Other abnormal findings in cerebrospinal fluid
Abnormal chromosomal findings in cerebrospinal fluid

R83.9 Unspecified abnormal finding in cerebrospinal fluid

✓4th R84 Abnormal findings in specimens from respiratory organs and thorax
Abnormal findings in bronchial washings
Abnormal findings in nasal secretions
Abnormal findings in pleural fluid
Abnormal findings in sputum
Abnormal findings in throat scrapings
EXCLUDES 1 *blood-stained sputum (R04.2)*

R84.0 Abnormal level of enzymes in specimens from respiratory organs and thorax

R84.1 Abnormal level of hormones in specimens from respiratory organs and thorax

R84.2 Abnormal level of other drugs, medicaments and biological substances in specimens from respiratory organs and thorax

R84.3 Abnormal level of substances chiefly nonmedicinal as to source in specimens from respiratory organs and thorax

R84.4 Abnormal immunological findings in specimens from respiratory organs and thorax

R84.5 Abnormal microbiological findings in specimens from respiratory organs and thorax
Positive culture findings in specimens from respiratory organs and thorax
EXCLUDES 1 *colonization status (Z22.-)*

R84.6 Abnormal cytological findings in specimens from respiratory organs and thorax

R84.7 Abnormal histological findings in specimens from respiratory organs and thorax

R84.8 Other abnormal findings in specimens from respiratory organs and thorax
Abnormal chromosomal findings in specimens from respiratory organs and thorax

R84.9 Unspecified abnormal finding in specimens from respiratory organs and thorax

✓4th R85 Abnormal findings in specimens from digestive organs and abdominal cavity
INCLUDES abnormal findings in peritoneal fluid
abnormal findings in saliva
EXCLUDES 1 *cloudy peritoneal dialysis effluent (R88.0)*
fecal abnormalities (R19.5)

R85.0 Abnormal level of enzymes in specimens from digestive organs and abdominal cavity

R85.1 Abnormal level of hormones in specimens from digestive organs and abdominal cavity

R85.2 Abnormal level of other drugs, medicaments and biological substances in specimens from digestive organs and abdominal cavity

R85.3 Abnormal level of substances chiefly nonmedicinal as to source in specimens from digestive organs and abdominal cavity

R85.4 Abnormal immunological findings in specimens from digestive organs and abdominal cavity

R85.5 Abnormal microbiological findings in specimens from digestive organs and abdominal cavity
Positive culture findings in specimens from digestive organs and abdominal cavity
EXCLUDES 1 *colonization status (Z22.-)*

✓5th **R85.6 Abnormal cytological findings in specimens from digestive organs and abdominal cavity**

✓6th **R85.61 Abnormal cytologic smear of anus**

EXCLUDES 1 *abnormal cytological findings in specimens from other digestive organs and abdominal cavity (R85.69)*
anal intraepithelial neoplasia I [AIN I] (K62.82)
anal intraepithelial neoplasia II [AIN II] (K62.82)
anal intraepithelial neoplasia III [AIN III] (DØ1.3)
carcinoma in situ of anus (histologically confirmed) (DØ1.3)
dysplasia (mild) (moderate) of anus (histologically confirmed) (K62.82)
severe dysplasia of anus (histologically confirmed) (DØ1.3)

EXCLUDES 2 *anal high risk human papillomavirus (HPV) DNA test positive (R85.81)*
anal low risk human papillomavirus (HPV) DNA test positive (R85.82)

R85.61Ø Atypical squamous cells of undetermined significance on cytologic smear of anus [ASC-US]

R85.611 Atypical squamous cells cannot exclude high grade squamous intraepithelial lesion on cytologic smear of anus [ASC-H]

R85.612 Low grade squamous intraepithelial lesion on cytologic smear of anus [LGSIL]

R85.613 High grade squamous intraepithelial lesion on cytologic smear of anus [HGSIL]

R85.614 Cytologic evidence of malignancy on smear of anus

R85.615 Unsatisfactory cytologic smear of anus
Inadequate sample of cytologic smear of anus

R85.616 Satisfactory anal smear but lacking transformation zone

R85.618 Other abnormal cytological findings on specimens from anus

R85.619 Unspecified abnormal cytological findings in specimens from anus
Abnormal anal cytology NOS
Atypical glandular cells of anus NOS

R85.69 Abnormal cytological findings in specimens from other digestive organs and abdominal cavity

R85.7 Abnormal histological findings in specimens from digestive organs and abdominal cavity

✓5th **R85.8 Other abnormal findings in specimens from digestive organs and abdominal cavity**

R85.81 Anal high risk human papillomavirus [HPV] DNA test positive

EXCLUDES 1 *anogenital warts due to human papillomavirus (HPV) (A63.Ø)*
condyloma acuminatum (A63.Ø)

R85.82 Anal low risk human papillomavirus [HPV] DNA test positive
Use additional code for associated human papillomavirus (B97.7)

R85.89 Other abnormal findings in specimens from digestive organs and abdominal cavity
Abnormal chromosomal findings in specimens from digestive organs and abdominal cavity

R85.9 Unspecified abnormal finding in specimens from digestive organs and abdominal cavity

✓4th **R86 Abnormal findings in specimens from male genital organs**

INCLUDES abnormal findings in prostatic secretions
abnormal findings in semen, seminal fluid
abnormal spermatozoa

EXCLUDES 1 *azoospermia (N46.Ø-)*
oligospermia (N46.1-)

R86.Ø Abnormal level of enzymes in specimens from male genital organs ♂

R86.1 Abnormal level of hormones in specimens from male genital organs ♂

R86.2 Abnormal level of other drugs, medicaments and biological substances in specimens from male genital organs ♂

R86.3 Abnormal level of substances chiefly nonmedicinal as to source in specimens from male genital organs ♂

R86.4 Abnormal immunological findings in specimens from male genital organs ♂

R86.5 Abnormal microbiological findings in specimens from male genital organs ♂
Positive culture findings in specimens from male genital organs

EXCLUDES 1 *colonization status (Z22.-)*

R86.6 Abnormal cytological findings in specimens from male genital organs ♂

R86.7 Abnormal histological findings in specimens from male genital organs ♂

R86.8 Other abnormal findings in specimens from male genital organs ♂
Abnormal chromosomal findings in specimens from male genital organs

R86.9 Unspecified abnormal finding in specimens from male genital organs ♂

✓4th **R87 Abnormal findings in specimens from female genital organs**
Abnormal findings in secretion and smears from cervix uteri
Abnormal findings in secretion and smears from vagina
Abnormal findings in secretion and smears from vulva

R87.Ø Abnormal level of enzymes in specimens from female genital organs ♀

R87.1 Abnormal level of hormones in specimens from female genital organs ♀

R87.2 Abnormal level of other drugs, medicaments and biological substances in specimens from female genital organs ♀

R87.3 Abnormal level of substances chiefly nonmedicinal as to source in specimens from female genital organs ♀

R87.4 Abnormal immunological findings in specimens from female genital organs ♀

R87.5 Abnormal microbiological findings in specimens from female genital organs ♀
Positive culture findings in specimens from female genital organs

EXCLUDES 1 *colonization status (Z22.-)*

✓5th **R87.6 Abnormal cytological findings in specimens from female genital organs**

✓6th **R87.61 Abnormal cytological findings in specimens from cervix uteri**

EXCLUDES 1 *abnormal cytological findings in specimens from other female genital organs (R87.69)*
abnormal cytological findings in specimens from vagina (R87.62-)
carcinoma in situ of cervix uteri (histologically confirmed) (DØ6.-)
cervical intraepithelial neoplasia I [CIN I] (N87.Ø)
cervical intraepithelial neoplasia II [CIN II] (N87.1)
cervical intraepithelial neoplasia III [CIN III] (DØ6.-)
dysplasia (mild) (moderate) of cervix uteri (histologically confirmed) (N87.-)
severe dysplasia of cervix uteri (histologically confirmed) (DØ6.-)

EXCLUDES 2 *cervical high risk human papillomavirus (HPV) DNA test positive (R87.81Ø)*
cervical low risk human papillomavirus (HPV) DNA test positive (R87.82Ø)

R87.61Ø Atypical squamous cells of undetermined significance on cytologic smear of cervix [ASC-US] ♀

R87.611 Atypical squamous cells cannot exclude high grade squamous intraepithelial lesion on cytologic smear of cervix [ASC-H] ♀

R87.612 Low grade squamous intraepithelial lesion on cytologic smear of cervix [LGSIL] ♀

R87.613 High grade squamous intraepithelial lesion on cytologic smear of cervix [HGSIL] ♀

R87.614 Cytologic evidence of malignancy on smear of cervix ♀

R87.615 Unsatisfactory cytologic smear of cervix ♀
Inadequate sample of cytologic smear of cervix

R87.616 Satisfactory cervical smear but lacking transformation zone ♀

R87.618 Other abnormal cytological findings on specimens from cervix uteri ♀

R87.619 Unspecified abnormal cytological findings in specimens from cervix uteri ♀
- Abnormal cervical cytology NOS
- Abnormal Papanicolaou smear of cervix NOS
- Abnormal thin preparation smear of cervix NOS
- Atypical endocervical cells of cervix NOS
- Atypical endometrial cells of cervix NOS
- Atypical glandular cells of cervix NOS

✓6th **R87.62 Abnormal cytological findings in specimens from vagina**

Use additional code to identify acquired absence of uterus and cervix, if applicable (Z90.71-)

EXCLUDES 1 *abnormal cytological findings in specimens from cervix uteri (R87.61-)*
abnormal cytological findings in specimens from other female genital organs (R87.69)
carcinoma in situ of vagina (histologically confirmed) (D07.2)
dysplasia (mild) (moderate) of vagina (histologically confirmed) (N89.-)
severe dysplasia of vagina (histologically confirmed) (D07.2)
vaginal intraepithelial neoplasia I [VAIN I] (N89.0)
vaginal intraepithelial neoplasia II [VAIN II] (N89.1)
vaginal intraepithelial neoplasia III [VAIN III] (D07.2)

EXCLUDES 2 *vaginal high risk human papillomavirus (HPV) DNA test positive (R87.811)*
vaginal low risk human papillomavirus (HPV) DNA test positive (R87.821)

R87.620 Atypical squamous cells of undetermined significance on cytologic smear of vagina [ASC-US] ♀

R87.621 Atypical squamous cells cannot exclude high grade squamous intraepithelial lesion on cytologic smear of vagina [ASC-H] ♀

R87.622 Low grade squamous intraepithelial lesion on cytologic smear of vagina [LGSIL] ♀

R87.623 High grade squamous intraepithelial lesion on cytologic smear of vagina [HGSIL] ♀

R87.624 Cytologic evidence of malignancy on smear of vagina ♀

R87.625 Unsatisfactory cytologic smear of vagina ♀
- Inadequate sample of cytologic smear of vagina

R87.628 Other abnormal cytological findings on specimens from vagina ♀

R87.629 Unspecified abnormal cytological findings in specimens from vagina ♀
- Abnormal Papanicolaou smear of vagina NOS
- Abnormal thin preparation smear of vagina NOS
- Abnormal vaginal cytology NOS
- Atypical endocervical cells of vagina NOS
- Atypical endometrial cells of vagina NOS
- Atypical glandular cells of vagina NOS

R87.69 Abnormal cytological findings in specimens from other female genital organs ♀
- Abnormal cytological findings in specimens from female genital organs NOS

EXCLUDES 1 *dysplasia of vulva (histologically confirmed) (N90.0-N90.3)*

R87.7 Abnormal histological findings in specimens from female genital organs ♀

EXCLUDES 1 *carcinoma in situ (histologically confirmed) of female genital organs (D06-D07.3)*
cervical intraepithelial neoplasia I [CIN I] (N87.0)
cervical intraepithelial neoplasia II [CIN II] (N87.1)
cervical intraepithelial neoplasia III [CIN III] (D06.-)
dysplasia (mild) (moderate) of cervix uteri (histologically confirmed) (N87.-)
dysplasia (mild) (moderate) of vagina (histologically confirmed) (N89.-)
severe dysplasia of cervix uteri (histologically confirmed) (D06.-)
severe dysplasia of vagina (histologically confirmed) (D07.2)
vaginal intraepithelial neoplasia I [VAIN I] (N89.0)
vaginal intraepithelial neoplasia II [VAIN II] (N89.1)
vaginal intraepithelial neoplasia III [VAIN III] (D07.2)

✓5th **R87.8 Other abnormal findings in specimens from female genital organs**

✓6th **R87.81 High risk human papillomavirus [HPV] DNA test positive from female genital organs**

EXCLUDES 1 *anogenital warts due to human papillomavirus (HPV) (A63.0)*
condyloma acuminatum (A63.0)

R87.810 Cervical high risk human papillomavirus [HPV] DNA test positive ♀

R87.811 Vaginal high risk human papillomavirus [HPV] DNA test positive ♀

✓6th **R87.82 Low risk human papillomavirus [HPV] DNA test positive from female genital organs**

Use additional code for associated human papillomavirus (B97.7)

R87.820 Cervical low risk human papillomavirus [HPV] DNA test positive ♀

R87.821 Vaginal low risk human papillomavirus [HPV] DNA test positive ♀

R87.89 Other abnormal findings in specimens from female genital organs ♀
- Abnormal chromosomal findings in specimens from female genital organs

R87.9 Unspecified abnormal finding in specimens from female genital organs ♀

✓4th **R88 Abnormal findings in other body fluids and substances**

R88.0 Cloudy (hemodialysis) (peritoneal) dialysis effluent

R88.8 Abnormal findings in other body fluids and substances

✓4th **R89 Abnormal findings in specimens from other organs, systems and tissues**

INCLUDES abnormal findings in nipple discharge
abnormal findings in synovial fluid
abnormal findings in wound secretions

R89.0 Abnormal level of enzymes in specimens from other organs, systems and tissues

R89.1 Abnormal level of hormones in specimens from other organs, systems and tissues

R89.2 Abnormal level of other drugs, medicaments and biological substances in specimens from other organs, systems and tissues

R89.3 Abnormal level of substances chiefly nonmedicinal as to source in specimens from other organs, systems and tissues

R89.4 Abnormal immunological findings in specimens from other organs, systems and tissues

R89.5 Abnormal microbiological findings in specimens from other organs, systems and tissues
- Positive culture findings in specimens from other organs, systems and tissues

EXCLUDES 1 *colonization status (Z22.-)*

R89.6 Abnormal cytological findings in specimens from other organs, systems and tissues

R89.7 Abnormal histological findings in specimens from other organs, systems and tissues

R89.8 Other abnormal findings in specimens from other organs, systems and tissues
- Abnormal chromosomal findings in specimens from other organs, systems and tissues

R89.9 Unspecified abnormal finding in specimens from other organs, systems and tissues

Abnormal findings on diagnostic imaging and in function studies, without diagnosis (R90-R94)

INCLUDES nonspecific abnormal findings on diagnostic imaging by computerized axial tomography [CAT scan]
nonspecific abnormal findings on diagnostic imaging by magnetic resonance imaging [MRI][NMR]
nonspecific abnormal findings on diagnostic imaging by positron emission tomography [PET scan]
nonspecific abnormal findings on diagnostic imaging by thermography
nonspecific abnormal findings on diagnostic imaging by ultrasound [echogram]
nonspecific abnormal findings on diagnostic imaging by X-ray examination

EXCLUDES 1 *abnormal findings on antenatal screening of mother (O28.-)*
diagnostic abnormal findings classified elsewhere—see Alphabetical Index

R90 Abnormal findings on diagnostic imaging of central nervous system

R90.0 Intracranial space-occupying lesion found on diagnostic imaging of central nervous system

R90.8 Other abnormal findings on diagnostic imaging of central nervous system

R90.81 Abnormal echoencephalogram

R90.82 White matter disease, unspecified

R90.89 Other abnormal findings on diagnostic imaging of central nervous system
Other cerebrovascular abnormality found on diagnostic imaging of central nervous system

R91 Abnormal findings on diagnostic imaging of lung

R91.1 Solitary pulmonary nodule
Coin lesion lung
Solitary pulmonary nodule, subsegmental branch of the bronchial tree

R91.8 Other nonspecific abnormal finding of lung field
Lung mass NOS found on diagnostic imaging of lung
Pulmonary infiltrate NOS
Shadow, lung

R92 Abnormal and inconclusive findings on diagnostic imaging of breast

R92.0 Mammographic microcalcification found on diagnostic imaging of breast
EXCLUDES 2 *mammographic calcification (calculus) found on diagnostic imaging of breast (R92.1)*

R92.1 Mammographic calcification found on diagnostic imaging of breast
Mammographic calculus found on diagnostic imaging of breast

R92.2 Inconclusive mammogram
Dense breasts NOS
Inconclusive mammogram NEC
Inconclusive mammography due to dense breasts
Inconclusive mammography NEC

R92.8 Other abnormal and inconclusive findings on diagnostic imaging of breast

R93 Abnormal findings on diagnostic imaging of other body structures

R93.0 Abnormal findings on diagnostic imaging of skull and head, not elsewhere classified
EXCLUDES 1 *intracranial space-occupying lesion found on diagnostic imaging (R90.0)*

R93.1 Abnormal findings on diagnostic imaging of heart and coronary circulation
Abnormal echocardiogram NOS
Abnormal heart shadow

R93.2 Abnormal findings on diagnostic imaging of liver and biliary tract
Nonvisualization of gallbladder

R93.3 Abnormal findings on diagnostic imaging of other parts of digestive tract

R93.4 Abnormal findings on diagnostic imaging of urinary organs
Filling defect of bladder found on diagnostic imaging
Filling defect of kidney found on diagnostic imaging
Filling defect of ureter found on diagnostic imaging
EXCLUDES 1 *hypertrophy of kidney (N28.81)*

R93.5 Abnormal findings on diagnostic imaging of other abdominal regions, including retroperitoneum

R93.6 Abnormal findings on diagnostic imaging of limbs
EXCLUDES 2 *abnormal finding in skin and subcutaneous tissue (R93.8)*

R93.7 Abnormal findings on diagnostic imaging of other parts of musculoskeletal system
EXCLUDES 2 *abnormal findings on diagnostic imaging of skull (R93.0)*

R93.8 Abnormal findings on diagnostic imaging of other specified body structures
Abnormal finding by radioisotope localization of placenta
Abnormal radiological finding in skin and subcutaneous tissue
Mediastinal shift

R93.9 Diagnostic imaging inconclusive due to excess body fat of patient

R94 Abnormal results of function studies
INCLUDES abnormal results of radionuclide [radioisotope] uptake studies
abnormal results of scintigraphy

R94.0 Abnormal results of function studies of central nervous system

R94.01 Abnormal electroencephalogram [EEG]

R94.02 Abnormal brain scan

R94.09 Abnormal results of other function studies of central nervous system

R94.1 Abnormal results of function studies of peripheral nervous system and special senses

R94.11 Abnormal results of function studies of eye

R94.110 Abnormal electro-oculogram [EOG]

R94.111 Abnormal electroretinogram [ERG]
Abnormal retinal function study

R94.112 Abnormal visually evoked potential [VEP]

R94.113 Abnormal oculomotor study

R94.118 Abnormal results of other function studies of eye

R94.12 Abnormal results of function studies of ear and other special senses

R94.120 Abnormal auditory function study

R94.121 Abnormal vestibular function study

R94.128 Abnormal results of other function studies of ear and other special senses

R94.13 Abnormal results of function studies of peripheral nervous system

R94.130 Abnormal response to nerve stimulation, unspecified

R94.131 Abnormal electromyogram [EMG]
EXCLUDES 1 *electromyogram of eye (R94.113)*

R94.138 Abnormal results of other function studies of peripheral nervous system

R94.2 Abnormal results of pulmonary function studies
Reduced ventilatory capacity
Reduced vital capacity

R94.3 Abnormal results of cardiovascular function studies

R94.30 Abnormal result of cardiovascular function study, unspecified

R94.31 Abnormal electrocardiogram [ECG] [EKG]
EXCLUDES 1 *long QT syndrome (I45.81)*

R94.39 Abnormal result of other cardiovascular function study
Abnormal electrophysiological intracardiac studies
Abnormal phonocardiogram
Abnormal vectorcardiogram

R94.4 Abnormal results of kidney function studies
Abnormal renal function test

R94.5 Abnormal results of liver function studies

R94.6 Abnormal results of thyroid function studies

R94.7 Abnormal results of other endocrine function studies
EXCLUDES 2 *abnormal glucose (R73.0-)*

R94.8 Abnormal results of function studies of other organs and systems
Abnormal basal metabolic rate [BMR]
Abnormal bladder function test
Abnormal splenic function test

Abnormal tumor markers (R97)

✓4th **R97 Abnormal tumor markers**
Elevated tumor associated antigens [TAA]
Elevated tumor specific antigens [TSA]

R97.0 Elevated carcinoembryonic antigen [CEA]

R97.1 Elevated cancer antigen 125 [CA 125] ♀

13 **R97.2 Elevated prostate specific antigen [PSA]** A ♂

R97.8 Other abnormal tumor markers

Ill-defined and unknown cause of mortality (R99)

R99 Ill-defined and unknown cause of mortality
Death (unexplained) NOS
Unspecified cause of mortality

13 Questionable admission when used as PDx.

Chapter 19. Injury, Poisoning and Certain Other Consequences of External Causes (S00-T88)

NOTE Use secondary code(s) from Chapter 20, External causes of morbidity, to indicate cause of injury. Codes within the T section that include the external cause do not require an additional external cause code.

Use additional code to identify any retained foreign body, if applicable (Z18.-)

EXCLUDES1 *birth trauma (P10-P15)*
obstetric trauma (O70-O71)

NOTE The chapter uses the S-section for coding different types of injuries related to single body regions and the T-section to cover injuries to unspecified body regions as well as poisoning and certain other consequences of external causes.

This chapter contains the following blocks:

S00-S09	Injuries to the head
S10-S19	Injuries to the neck
S20-S29	Injuries to the thorax
S30-S39	Injuries to the abdomen, lower back, lumbar spine, pelvis and external genitals
S40-S49	Injuries to the shoulder and upper arm
S50-S59	Injuries to the elbow and forearm
S60-S69	Injuries to the wrist, hand and fingers
S70-S79	Injuries to the hip and thigh
S80-S89	Injuries to the knee and lower leg
S90-S99	Injuries to the ankle and foot
T07	Injuries involving multiple body regions
T14	Injury of unspecified body region
T15-T19	Effects of foreign body entering through natural orifice
T20-T25	Burns and corrosions of external body surface, specified by site
T26-T28	Burns and corrosions confined to eye and internal organs
T30-T32	Burns and corrosions of multiple and unspecified body regions
T33-T34	Frostbite
T36-T50	Poisoning by, adverse effect of and underdosing of drugs, medicaments and biological substances
T51-T65	Toxic effects of substances chiefly nonmedicinal as to source
T66-T78	Other and unspecified effects of external causes
T79	Certain early complications of trauma
T80-T88	Complications of surgical and medical care, not elsewhere classified

Injuries to the head (S00-S09)

INCLUDES injuries of ear
injuries of eye
injuries of face [any part]
injuries of gum
injuries of jaw
injuries of oral cavity
injuries of palate
injuries of periocular area
injuries of scalp
injuries of temporomandibular joint area
injuries of tongue
injuries of tooth

Code also for any associated infection

EXCLUDES2 *burns and corrosions (T20-T32)*
effects of foreign body in ear (T16)
effects of foreign body in larynx (T17.3)
effects of foreign body in mouth NOS (T18.0)
effects of foreign body in nose (T17.0-T17.1)
effects of foreign body in pharynx (T17.2)
effects of foreign body on external eye (T15.-)
frostbite (T33-T34)
insect bite or sting, venomous (T63.4)

✓4th **S00 Superficial injury of head**

EXCLUDES1 *diffuse cerebral contusion (S06.2-)*
focal cerebral contusion (S06.3-)
injury of eye and orbit (S05.-)
open wound of head (S01.-)

The appropriate 7th is to be added to each code from category S00.
A initial encounter
D subsequent encounter
S sequela

✓5th **S00.0 Superficial injury of scalp**
✓x7th **S00.00 Unspecified superficial injury of scalp**
✓x7th **S00.01 Abrasion of scalp**
✓x7th **S00.02 Blister (nonthermal) of scalp**
✓x7th **S00.03 Contusion of scalp**
Bruise of scalp
Hematoma of scalp
✓x7th **S00.04 External constriction of part of scalp**
✓x7th **S00.05 Superficial foreign body of scalp**
Splinter in the scalp
✓x7th **S00.06 Insect bite (nonvenomous) of scalp**
✓x7th **S00.07 Other superficial bite of scalp**
EXCLUDES1 *open bite of scalp (S01.05)*

✓5th **S00.1 Contusion of eyelid and periocular area**
Black eye
EXCLUDES2 *contusion of eyeball and orbital tissues (S05.1)*
✓x7th **S00.10 Contusion of unspecified eyelid and periocular area**
✓x7th **S00.11 Contusion of right eyelid and periocular area**
✓x7th **S00.12 Contusion of left eyelid and periocular area**

✓5th **S00.2 Other and unspecified superficial injuries of eyelid and periocular area**
EXCLUDES2 *superficial injury of conjunctiva and cornea (S05.0-)*
✓6th **S00.20 Unspecified superficial injury of eyelid and periocular area**
✓7th **S00.201 Unspecified superficial injury of right eyelid and periocular area**
✓7th **S00.202 Unspecified superficial injury of left eyelid and periocular area**
✓7th **S00.209 Unspecified superficial injury of unspecified eyelid and periocular area**
✓6th **S00.21 Abrasion of eyelid and periocular area**
✓7th **S00.211 Abrasion of right eyelid and periocular area**
✓7th **S00.212 Abrasion of left eyelid and periocular area**
✓7th **S00.219 Abrasion of unspecified eyelid and periocular area**
✓6th **S00.22 Blister (nonthermal) of eyelid and periocular area**
✓7th **S00.221 Blister (nonthermal) of right eyelid and periocular area**
✓7th **S00.222 Blister (nonthermal) of left eyelid and periocular area**
✓7th **S00.229 Blister (nonthermal) of unspecified eyelid and periocular area**
✓6th **S00.24 External constriction of eyelid and periocular area**
✓7th **S00.241 External constriction of right eyelid and periocular area**
✓7th **S00.242 External constriction of left eyelid and periocular area**
✓7th **S00.249 External constriction of unspecified eyelid and periocular area**
✓6th **S00.25 Superficial foreign body of eyelid and periocular area**
Splinter of eyelid and periocular area
EXCLUDES2 *retained foreign body in eyelid (H02.81-)*
✓7th **S00.251 Superficial foreign body of right eyelid and periocular area**
✓7th **S00.252 Superficial foreign body of left eyelid and periocular area**
✓7th **S00.259 Superficial foreign body of unspecified eyelid and periocular area**
✓6th **S00.26 Insect bite (nonvenomous) of eyelid and periocular area**
✓7th **S00.261 Insect bite (nonvenomous) of right eyelid and periocular area**
✓7th **S00.262 Insect bite (nonvenomous) of left eyelid and periocular area**
✓7th **S00.269 Insect bite (nonvenomous) of unspecified eyelid and periocular area**
✓6th **S00.27 Other superficial bite of eyelid and periocular area**
EXCLUDES1 *open bite of eyelid and periocular area (S01.15)*
✓7th **S00.271 Other superficial bite of right eyelid and periocular area**
✓7th **S00.272 Other superficial bite of left eyelid and periocular area**
✓7th **S00.279 Other superficial bite of unspecified eyelid and periocular area**

✓5th **S00.3 Superficial injury of nose**
✓x7th **S00.30 Unspecified superficial injury of nose**
✓x7th **S00.31 Abrasion of nose**

√x7th **S00.32 Blister (nonthermal) of nose**

√x7th **S00.33 Contusion of nose**
Bruise of nose
Hematoma of nose

√x7th **S00.34 External constriction of nose**

√x7th **S00.35 Superficial foreign body of nose**
Splinter in the nose

√x7th **S00.36 Insect bite (nonvenomous) of nose**

√x7th **S00.37 Other superficial bite of nose**
EXCLUDES 1 *open bite of nose (S01.25)*

√5th **S00.4 Superficial injury of ear**

√6th **S00.40 Unspecified superficial injury of ear**

√7th **S00.401 Unspecified superficial injury of right ear**

√7th **S00.402 Unspecified superficial injury of left ear**

√7th **S00.409 Unspecified superficial injury of unspecified ear**

√6th **S00.41 Abrasion of ear**

√7th **S00.411 Abrasion of right ear**

√7th **S00.412 Abrasion of left ear**

√7th **S00.419 Abrasion of unspecified ear**

√6th **S00.42 Blister (nonthermal) of ear**

√7th **S00.421 Blister (nonthermal) of right ear**

√7th **S00.422 Blister (nonthermal) of left ear**

√7th **S00.429 Blister (nonthermal) of unspecified ear**

√6th **S00.43 Contusion of ear**
Bruise of ear
Hematoma of ear

√7th **S00.431 Contusion of right ear**

√7th **S00.432 Contusion of left ear**

√7th **S00.439 Contusion of unspecified ear**

√6th **S00.44 External constriction of ear**

√7th **S00.441 External constriction of right ear**

√7th **S00.442 External constriction of left ear**

√7th **S00.449 External constriction of unspecified ear**

√6th **S00.45 Superficial foreign body of ear**
Splinter in the ear

√7th **S00.451 Superficial foreign body of right ear**

√7th **S00.452 Superficial foreign body of left ear**

√7th **S00.459 Superficial foreign body of unspecified ear**

√6th **S00.46 Insect bite (nonvenomous) of ear**

√7th **S00.461 Insect bite (nonvenomous) of right ear**

√7th **S00.462 Insect bite (nonvenomous) of left ear**

√7th **S00.469 Insect bite (nonvenomous) of unspecified ear**

√6th **S00.47 Other superficial bite of ear**
EXCLUDES 1 *open bite of ear (S01.35)*

√7th **S00.471 Other superficial bite of right ear**

√7th **S00.472 Other superficial bite of left ear**

√7th **S00.479 Other superficial bite of unspecified ear**

√5th **S00.5 Superficial injury of lip and oral cavity**

√6th **S00.50 Unspecified superficial injury of lip and oral cavity**

√7th **S00.501 Unspecified superficial injury of lip**

√7th **S00.502 Unspecified superficial injury of oral cavity**

√6th **S00.51 Abrasion of lip and oral cavity**

√7th **S00.511 Abrasion of lip**

√7th **S00.512 Abrasion of oral cavity**

√6th **S00.52 Blister (nonthermal) of lip and oral cavity**

√7th **S00.521 Blister (nonthermal) of lip**

√7th **S00.522 Blister (nonthermal) of oral cavity**

√6th **S00.53 Contusion of lip and oral cavity**

√7th **S00.531 Contusion of lip**
Bruise of lip
Hematoma of oral cavity

√7th **S00.532 Contusion of oral cavity**
Bruise of lip
Hematoma of oral cavity

√6th **S00.54 External constriction of lip and oral cavity**

√7th **S00.541 External constriction of lip**

√7th **S00.542 External constriction of oral cavity**

√6th **S00.55 Superficial foreign body of lip and oral cavity**

√7th **S00.551 Superficial foreign body of lip**
Splinter of lip and oral cavity

√7th **S00.552 Superficial foreign body of oral cavity**
Splinter of lip and oral cavity

√6th **S00.56 Insect bite (nonvenomous) of lip and oral cavity**

√7th **S00.561 Insect bite (nonvenomous) of lip**

√7th **S00.562 Insect bite (nonvenomous) of oral cavity**

√6th **S00.57 Other superficial bite of lip and oral cavity**

√7th **S00.571 Other superficial bite of lip**
EXCLUDES 1 *open bite of lip (S01.551)*

√7th **S00.572 Other superficial bite of oral cavity**
EXCLUDES 1 *open bite of oral cavity (S01.552)*

√5th **S00.8 Superficial injury of other parts of head**

√x7th **S00.80 Unspecified superficial injury of other part of head**

√x7th **S00.81 Abrasion of other part of head**

√x7th **S00.82 Blister (nonthermal) of other part of head**

√x7th **S00.83 Contusion of other part of head**
Bruise of other part of head
Hematoma of other part of head

√x7th **S00.84 External constriction of other part of head**

√x7th **S00.85 Superficial foreign body of other part of head**
Splinter in other part of head

√x7th **S00.86 Insect bite (nonvenomous) of other part of head**

√x7th **S00.87 Other superficial bite of other part of head**
EXCLUDES 1 *open bite of other part of head (S01.85)*

√5th **S00.9 Superficial injury of unspecified part of head**

√x7th **S00.90 Unspecified superficial injury of unspecified part of head**

√x7th **S00.91 Abrasion of unspecified part of head**

√x7th **S00.92 Blister (nonthermal) of unspecified part of head**

√x7th **S00.93 Contusion of unspecified part of head**
Bruise of head
Hematoma of head

√x7th **S00.94 External constriction of unspecified part of head**

√x7th **S00.95 Superficial foreign body of unspecified part of head**
Splinter of head

√x7th **S00.96 Insect bite (nonvenomous) of unspecified part of head**

√x7th **S00.97 Other superficial bite of unspecified part of head**
EXCLUDES 1 *open bite of head (S01.95)*

√4th **S01 Open wound of head**

Code also any associated:
injury of cranial nerve (S04.-)
injury of muscle and tendon of head (S09.1-)
intracranial injury (S06.-)
wound infection

EXCLUDES 1 *open skull fracture (S02- with 7th B)*

EXCLUDES 2 *injury of eye and orbit (S05.-)*
traumatic amputation of part of head (S08.-)

The appropriate 7th is to be added to each code from category S01.
A initial encounter
D subsequent encounter
S sequela

√5th **S01.0 Open wound of scalp**
EXCLUDES 1 *avulsion of scalp (S08.0)*

√x7th **S01.00 Unspecified open wound of scalp**

√x7th **S01.01 Laceration without foreign body of scalp**

√x7th **S01.02 Laceration with foreign body of scalp**

√x7th **S01.03 Puncture wound without foreign body of scalp**

√x7th **S01.04 Puncture wound with foreign body of scalp**

√x7th **S01.05 Open bite of scalp**
Bite of scalp NOS
EXCLUDES 1 *superficial bite of scalp (S00.06, S00.07-)*

S01.1 Open wound of eyelid and periocular area
Open wound of eyelid and periocular area with or without involvement of lacrimal passages

CC Excl: For CC codes in subcategory S01.1, unless otherwise noted: CC with 7th character A: S01.101-S01.159 with 7th A, S05.20X-S05.8X9 with 7th A, S05.91X-S05.92X with 7th A, S38.3XXA, T14.8-T14.91, T79.A0X-T79.9XX with 7th A

S01.10 Unspecified open wound of eyelid and periocular area
- **S01.101 Unspecified open wound of right eyelid and periocular area** CC
- **S01.102 Unspecified open wound of left eyelid and periocular area** CC
- **S01.109 Unspecified open wound of unspecified eyelid and periocular area** CC

S01.11 Laceration without foreign body of eyelid and periocular area
- **S01.111 Laceration without foreign body of right eyelid and periocular area**
- **S01.112 Laceration without foreign body of left eyelid and periocular area**
- **S01.119 Laceration without foreign body of unspecified eyelid and periocular area**

S01.12 Laceration with foreign body of eyelid and periocular area
- **S01.121 Laceration with foreign body of right eyelid and periocular area**
- **S01.122 Laceration with foreign body of left eyelid and periocular area**
- **S01.129 Laceration with foreign body of unspecified eyelid and periocular area**

S01.13 Puncture wound without foreign body of eyelid and periocular area
- **S01.131 Puncture wound without foreign body of right eyelid and periocular area**
- **S01.132 Puncture wound without foreign body of left eyelid and periocular area**
- **S01.139 Puncture wound without foreign body of unspecified eyelid and periocular area**

S01.14 Puncture wound with foreign body of eyelid and periocular area
- **S01.141 Puncture wound with foreign body of right eyelid and periocular area**
- **S01.142 Puncture wound with foreign body of left eyelid and periocular area**
- **S01.149 Puncture wound with foreign body of unspecified eyelid and periocular area**

S01.15 Open bite of eyelid and periocular area
Bite of eyelid and periocular area NOS
EXCLUDES 1 *superficial bite of eyelid and periocular area (S00.26, S00.27)*
- **S01.151 Open bite of right eyelid and periocular area**
- **S01.152 Open bite of left eyelid and periocular area**
- **S01.159 Open bite of unspecified eyelid and periocular area**

S01.2 Open wound of nose
- **S01.20 Unspecified open wound of nose**
- **S01.21 Laceration without foreign body of nose**
- **S01.22 Laceration with foreign body of nose**
- **S01.23 Puncture wound without foreign body of nose**
- **S01.24 Puncture wound with foreign body of nose**
- **S01.25 Open bite of nose**
  Bite of nose NOS
  EXCLUDES 1 *superficial bite of nose (S00.36, S00.37)*

S01.3 Open wound of ear

S01.30 Unspecified open wound of ear
- **S01.301 Unspecified open wound of right ear**
- **S01.302 Unspecified open wound of left ear**
- **S01.309 Unspecified open wound of unspecified ear**

S01.31 Laceration without foreign body of ear
- **S01.311 Laceration without foreign body of right ear**
- **S01.312 Laceration without foreign body of left ear**
- **S01.319 Laceration without foreign body of unspecified ear**

S01.32 Laceration with foreign body of ear
- **S01.321 Laceration with foreign body of right ear**
- **S01.322 Laceration with foreign body of left ear**
- **S01.329 Laceration with foreign body of unspecified ear**

S01.33 Puncture wound without foreign body of ear
- **S01.331 Puncture wound without foreign body of right ear**
- **S01.332 Puncture wound without foreign body of left ear**
- **S01.339 Puncture wound without foreign body of unspecified ear**

S01.34 Puncture wound with foreign body of ear
- **S01.341 Puncture wound with foreign body of right ear**
- **S01.342 Puncture wound with foreign body of left ear**
- **S01.349 Puncture wound with foreign body of unspecified ear**

S01.35 Open bite of ear
Bite of ear NOS
EXCLUDES 1 *superficial bite of ear (S00.46, S00.47)*
- **S01.351 Open bite of right ear**
- **S01.352 Open bite of left ear**
- **S01.359 Open bite of unspecified ear**

S01.4 Open wound of cheek and temporomandibular area

S01.40 Unspecified open wound of cheek and temporomandibular area
- **S01.401 Unspecified open wound of right cheek and temporomandibular area**
- **S01.402 Unspecified open wound of left cheek and temporomandibular area**
- **S01.409 Unspecified open wound of unspecified cheek and temporomandibular area**

S01.41 Laceration without foreign body of cheek and temporomandibular area
- **S01.411 Laceration without foreign body of right cheek and temporomandibular area**
- **S01.412 Laceration without foreign body of left cheek and temporomandibular area**
- **S01.419 Laceration without foreign body of unspecified cheek and temporomandibular area**

S01.42 Laceration with foreign body of cheek and temporomandibular area
- **S01.421 Laceration with foreign body of right cheek and temporomandibular area**
- **S01.422 Laceration with foreign body of left cheek and temporomandibular area**
- **S01.429 Laceration with foreign body of unspecified cheek and temporomandibular area**

S01.43 Puncture wound without foreign body of cheek and temporomandibular area
- **S01.431 Puncture wound without foreign body of right cheek and temporomandibular area**
- **S01.432 Puncture wound without foreign body of left cheek and temporomandibular area**
- **S01.439 Puncture wound without foreign body of unspecified cheek and temporomandibular area**

S01.44 Puncture wound with foreign body of cheek and temporomandibular area
- **S01.441 Puncture wound with foreign body of right cheek and temporomandibular area**
- **S01.442 Puncture wound with foreign body of left cheek and temporomandibular area**

✓7th **SØ1.449 Puncture wound with foreign body of unspecified cheek and temporomandibular area**

✓6th **SØ1.45 Open bite of cheek and temporomandibular area**
Bite of cheek and temporomandibular area NOS
EXCLUDES 2 *superficial bite of cheek and temporomandibular area (SØØ.86, SØØ.87)*

✓7th **SØ1.451 Open bite of right cheek and temporomandibular area**

✓7th **SØ1.452 Open bite of left cheek and temporomandibular area**

✓7th **SØ1.459 Open bite of unspecified cheek and temporomandibular area**

✓5th **SØ1.5 Open wound of lip and oral cavity**
EXCLUDES 2 *tooth dislocation (SØ3.2)*
tooth fracture (SØ2.5)

✓6th **SØ1.5Ø Unspecified open wound of lip and oral cavity**

✓7th **SØ1.5Ø1 Unspecified open wound of lip**

✓7th **SØ1.5Ø2 Unspecified open wound of oral cavity**

✓6th **SØ1.51 Laceration of lip and oral cavity without foreign body**

✓7th **SØ1.511 Laceration without foreign body of lip**

✓7th **SØ1.512 Laceration without foreign body of oral cavity**

✓6th **SØ1.52 Laceration of lip and oral cavity with foreign body**

✓7th **SØ1.521 Laceration with foreign body of lip**

✓7th **SØ1.522 Laceration with foreign body of oral cavity**

✓6th **SØ1.53 Puncture wound of lip and oral cavity without foreign body**

✓7th **SØ1.531 Puncture wound without foreign body of lip**

✓7th **SØ1.532 Puncture wound without foreign body of oral cavity**

✓6th **SØ1.54 Puncture wound of lip and oral cavity with foreign body**

✓7th **SØ1.541 Puncture wound with foreign body of lip**

✓7th **SØ1.542 Puncture wound with foreign body of oral cavity**

✓6th **SØ1.55 Open bite of lip and oral cavity**

✓7th **SØ1.551 Open bite of lip**
Bite of lip NOS
EXCLUDES 1 *superficial bite of lip (SØØ.571)*

✓7th **SØ1.552 Open bite of oral cavity**
Bite of oral cavity NOS
EXCLUDES 1 *superficial bite of oral cavity (SØØ.572)*

✓5th **SØ1.8 Open wound of other parts of head**

✓x7th **SØ1.8Ø Unspecified open wound of other part of head**

✓x7th **SØ1.81 Laceration without foreign body of other part of head**

✓x7th **SØ1.82 Laceration with foreign body of other part of head**

✓x7th **SØ1.83 Puncture wound without foreign body of other part of head**

✓x7th **SØ1.84 Puncture wound with foreign body of other part of head**

✓x7th **SØ1.85 Open bite of other part of head**
Bite of other part of head NOS
EXCLUDES 1 *superficial bite of other part of head (SØØ.85)*

✓5th **SØ1.9 Open wound of unspecified part of head**

✓x7th **SØ1.9Ø Unspecified open wound of unspecified part of head**

✓x7th **SØ1.91 Laceration without foreign body of unspecified part of head**

✓x7th **SØ1.92 Laceration with foreign body of unspecified part of head**

✓x7th **SØ1.93 Puncture wound without foreign body of unspecified part of head**

✓x7th **SØ1.94 Puncture wound with foreign body of unspecified part of head**

✓x7th **SØ1.95 Open bite of unspecified part of head**
Bite of head NOS
EXCLUDES 1 *superficial bite of head NOS (SØØ.97)*

✓4th **SØ2 Fracture of skull and facial bones**
NOTE A fracture not indicated as open or closed should be coded to closed.
Code also any associated intracranial injury (SØ6.-).

The appropriate 7th is to be added to each code from category SØ2.
A initial encounter for closed fracture
B initial encounter for open fracture
D subsequent encounter for fracture with routine healing
G subsequent encounter for fracture with delayed healing
K subsequent encounter for fracture with nonunion
S sequela

7 ✓x7th **SØ2.Ø Fracture of vault of skull** MCC CC
Fracture of frontal bone
Fracture of parietal bone

CC Excl: For CC/MCC codes in subcategory SØ2.Ø, unless otherwise noted: CC with 7th character A or MCC with 7th character B: SØ1.9ØX-SØ2.92X with 7th A, SØ6.ØXØ-SØ7.9XX with 7th A, SØ8.89X-SØ9.19X with 7th A, SØ9.8XX-SØ9.9ØX with 7th A, SØ9.92X-SØ9.93X with 7th A, S16.8XX-S19.9XX with 7th A, S38.3XX with 7th A, T14.8-T14.91, T79.AØX-T79.9XX with 7th A
CC with 7th character K: M8Ø.ØØX-M84.68X with 7th [K, P], SØ2.ØXX-SØ2.92X with 7th K, S12.ØØØ-S12.691 with 7th K, S22.ØØØ-S22.9XX with 7th K, S32.ØØØ-S32.9XX with 7th K, S42.ØØ1-S42.92X with 7th [K, P], S49.ØØ1-S49.199 with 7th [K, P], S52.ØØ1-S52.92X with 7th [K, M, N, P, Q, R], S59.ØØ1-S59.299 with 7th [K, P], S62.ØØ1-S62.92X with 7th [K, P], S72.ØØ1-S72.92X with 7th [K, M, N, P, Q, R], S79.ØØ1-S79.199 with 7th [K, P], S82.ØØ1-S82.92X with 7th [K, M, N, P, Q, R], S89.ØØ1-S89.399 with 7th [K, P], S92.ØØ1-S92.919 with 7th [K, P]

✓5th **SØ2.1 Fracture of base of skull**
EXCLUDES 1 *orbit NOS (SØ2.8)*
EXCLUDES 2 *orbital floor (SØ2.3-)*

CC Excl: For CC codes in subcategory SØ2.1, unless otherwise noted: CC with 7th character A or MCC with 7th character B: SØ1.9ØX-SØ2.92X with 7th A, SØ6.ØXØ-SØ7.9XX with 7th A, SØ8.89X-SØ9.19X with 7th A, SØ9.8XX-SØ9.9ØX with 7th A, SØ9.92X-SØ9.93X with 7th A, S16.8XX-S19.9XX with 7th A, S38.3XXA, T14.8-T14.91, T79.AØX-T79.9XX with 7th A
CC with 7th character K: M8Ø.ØØX-M84.68X with 7th [K, P], SØ2.ØXX-SØ2.92X with 7th K, S12.ØØØ-S12.691 with 7th K, S22.ØØØ-S22.9XX with 7th K, S32.ØØØ-S32.9XX with 7th K, S42.ØØ1-S42.92X with 7th [K, P], S49.ØØ1-S49.199 with 7th [K, P], S52.ØØ1-S52.92X with 7th [K, M, N, P, Q, R], S59.ØØ1-S59.299 with 7th [K, P], S62.ØØ1-S62.92X with 7th [K, P], S72.ØØ1-S72.92X with 7th [K, M, N, P, Q, R], S79.ØØ1-S79.199 with 7th [K, P], S82.ØØ1-S82.92X with 7th [K, M, N, P, Q, R], S89.ØØ1-S89.399 with 7th [K, P], S92.ØØ1-S92.919 with 7th [K, P]

7 ✓x7th **SØ2.1Ø Unspecified fracture of base of skull** MCC CC

✓6th **SØ2.11 Fracture of occiput**

7 ✓7th **SØ2.11Ø Type I occipital condyle fracture** MCC CC

7 ✓7th **SØ2.111 Type II occipital condyle fracture** MCC CC

7 ✓7th **SØ2.112 Type III occipital condyle fracture** MCC CC

7 ✓7th **SØ2.113 Unspecified occipital condyle fracture** MCC CC

7 ✓7th **SØ2.118 Other fracture of occiput** MCC CC

7 ✓7th **SØ2.119 Unspecified fracture of occiput** MCC CC

7 ✓x7th **SØ2.19 Other fracture of base of skull** MCC CC
Fracture of anterior fossa of base of skull
Fracture of ethmoid sinus
Fracture of frontal sinus
Fracture of middle fossa of base of skull
Fracture of orbital roof
Fracture of posterior fossa of base of skull
Fracture of sphenoid
Fracture of temporal bone

7 HAC = Initial encounter only (7th character A, B or C) and not POA.

7 √x7th **S02.2 Fracture of nasal bones** CC

CC Excl: CC with 7th character B: S01.90X-S02.92X with 7th A, S06.0X0-S07.9XX with 7th A, S08.89-S09.19X with 7th A, S09.8XX-S09.90X with 7th A, S09.92X-S09.93X with 7th A, S16.8XX-S19.9XX with 7th A, S38.3XXA, T14.8-T14.91, T79.A0X-T79.9XX with 7th A
CC Excl: CC with 7th character K: M80.00X-M84.68X with 7th [K, P], S02.0XX-S02.92X with 7th K, S12.000-S12.691 with 7th K, S22.000-S22.9XX with 7th K, S32.000-S32.9XX with 7th K, S42.001-S42.92X with 7th [K, P], S49.001-S49.199 with 7th [K, P], S52.001-S52.92X with 7th [K, M, N, P, Q, R], S59.001-S59.299 with 7th [K, P], S62.001-S62.92X with 7th [K, P], S72.001-S72.92X with 7th [K, M, N, P, Q, R], S79.001-S79.199 with 7th [K, P], S82.001-S82.92X with 7th [K, M, N, P, Q, R], S89.001-S89.399 with 7th [K, P], S92.001-S92.919 with 7th [K, P]

7 √x7th **S02.3 Fracture of orbital floor** CC

EXCLUDES 1 *orbit NOS (S02.8)*
EXCLUDES 2 *orbital roof (S02.1-)*

CC Excl: CC with 7th character A or B: S01.90X-S02.92X with 7th A, S06.0X0-S07.9XX with 7th A, S08.89X-S09.19X with 7th A, S09.8XX-S09.90X with 7th A, S09.92X-S09.93X with 7th A, S16.8XX-S19.9XX with 7th A, S38.3XXA, T14.8-T14.91, T79.A0X-T79.9XX with 7th A
CC with 7th character K: M80.00X-M84.68X with 7th [K, P], S02.0XX-S02.92X with 7th K, S12.000-S12.691 with 7th K, S22.000-S22.9XX with 7th K, S32.000-S32.9XX with 7th K, S42.001-S42.92X with 7th [K, P], S49.001-S49.199 with 7th [K, P], S52.001-S52.92X with 7th [K, M, N, P, Q, R], S59.001-S59.299 with 7th [K, P], S62.001-S62.92X with 7th [K, P], S72.001-S72.92X with 7th [K, M, N, P, Q, R], S79.001-S79.199 with 7th [K, P], S82.001-S82.92X with 7th [K, M, N, P, Q, R], S89.001-S89.399 with 7th [K, P], S92.001-S92.919 with 7th [K, P]

√5th **S02.4 Fracture of malar, maxillary and zygoma bones**

Fracture of superior maxilla
Fracture of upper jaw (bone)
Fracture of zygomatic process of temporal bone

CC Excl: For CC codes in subcategory S02.4, unless otherwise noted: CC with 7th character A or B: S01.90X-S03.0XX with 7th A, S06.0X0-S07.9XX with 7th A, S08.89X-S09.19X with 7th A, S09.8XX-S09.90X with 7th A, S09.92X-S09.93X with 7th A, S16.8XX-S19.9XX with 7th A, S38.3XA, T14.8-T14.91, T79.A0X-T79.9XX with 7th A
CC with 7th character K: M80.00X-M84.68X with 7th [K, P], S02.0XX-S02.92X with 7th K, S12.000-S12.691 with 7th K, S22.000-S22.9XX with 7th K, S32.000-S32.9XX with 7th K, S42.001-S42.92X with 7th [K, P], S49.001-S49.199 with 7th [K, P], S52.001-S52.92X with 7th [K, M, N, P, Q, R], S59.001-S59.299 with 7th [K, P], S62.001-S62.92X with 7th [K, P], S72.001-S72.92X with 7th [K, M, N, P, Q, R], S79.001-S79.199 with 7th [K, P], S82.001-S82.92X with 7th [K, M, N, P, Q, R], S89.001-S89.399 with 7th [K, P], S92.001-S92.919 with 7th [K, P]

√6th **S02.40 Fracture of malar, maxillary and zygoma bones, unspecified**

7 √7th **S02.400 Malar fracture unspecified** CC
7 √7th **S02.401 Maxillary fracture, unspecified** CC
7 √7th **S02.402 Zygomatic fracture, unspecified** CC

√6th **S02.41 LeFort fracture**

7 √7th **S02.411 LeFort I fracture** CC
7 √7th **S02.412 LeFort II fracture** CC
7 √7th **S02.413 LeFort III fracture** CC

7 √x7th **S02.42 Fracture of alveolus of maxilla** CC

CC Excl: CC with 7th character A or B: S01.90X-S02.92X with 7th A, S06.0X0-S07.9XX with 7th A, S08.89X-S09.19X with 7th A, S09.8XX-S09.90X with 7th A, S09.92X-S09.93X with 7th A, S16.8XX-S19.9XX with 7th A, S38.3XXA, T14.8-T14.91, T79.A0X-T79.9XX with 7th A
CC with 7th character K: M80.00X-M84.68X with 7th [K, P], S02.0XX-S02.92X with 7th K, S12.000-S12.691 with 7th K, S22.000-S22.9XX with 7th K, S32.000-S32.9XX with 7th K, S42.001-S42.92X with 7th [K, P], S49.001-S49.199 with 7th [K, P], S52.001-S52.92X with 7th [K, M, N, P, Q, R], S59.001-S59.299 with 7th [K, P], S62.001-S62.92X with 7th [K, P], S72.001-S72.92X with 7th [K, M, N, P, Q, R], S79.001-S79.199 with 7th [K, P], S82.001-S82.92X with 7th [K, M, N, P, Q, R], S89.001-S89.399 with 7th [K, P], S92.001-S92.919 with 7th [K, P]

√x7th **S02.5 Fracture of tooth (traumatic)** CC

Broken tooth

EXCLUDES 1 *cracked tooth (nontraumatic) (K03.81)*

CC Excl: CC with 7th character K: See Code: S02.42

√5th **S02.6 Fracture of mandible**

Fracture of lower jaw (bone)

CC Excl: For CC codes in subcategory S02.6, unless otherwise noted: CC with 7th character A or B: S01.90X-S03.0XX with 7th A, S06.0X0-S07.9XX with 7th A, S08.89-S09.19X with 7th A, S09.8XX-S09.90X with 7th A, S09.92X-S09.93X with 7th A, S16.8XX-S19.9XX with 7th A, S38.3XXA, T14.8-T14.91, T79.A0X-T79.9XX with 7th A
CC with 7th character K: M80.00X-M84.68X with 7th [K, P], S02.0XX-S02.92X with 7th K, S12.000-S12.691 with 7th K, S22.000-S22.9XX with 7th K, S32.000-S32.9XX with 7th K, S42.001-S42.92X with 7th [K, P], S49.001-S49.199 with 7th [K, P], S52.001-S52.92X with 7th [K, M, N, P, Q, R], S59.001-S59.299 with 7th [K, P], S62.001-S62.92X with 7th [K, P], S72.001-S72.92X with 7th [K, M, N, P, Q, R], S79.001-S79.199 with 7th [K, P], S82.001-S82.92X with 7th [K, M, N, P, Q, R], S89.001-S89.399 with 7th [K, P], S92.001-S92.919 with 7th [K, P]

√6th **S02.60 Fracture of mandible, unspecified**

7 √7th **S02.600 Fracture of unspecified part of body of mandible** CC
7 √7th **S02.609 Fracture of mandible, unspecified** CC

7 √x7th **S02.61 Fracture of condylar process of mandible** CC
7 √x7th **S02.62 Fracture of subcondylar process of mandible** CC
7 √x7th **S02.63 Fracture of coronoid process of mandible** CC
7 √x7th **S02.64 Fracture of ramus of mandible** CC
7 √x7th **S02.65 Fracture of angle of mandible** CC
7 √x7th **S02.66 Fracture of symphysis of mandible** CC
7 √x7th **S02.67 Fracture of alveolus of mandible** CC
7 √x7th **S02.69 Fracture of mandible of other specified site** CC

7 √x7th **S02.8 Fractures of other specified skull and facial bones** CC

Fracture of orbit NOS
Fracture of palate

EXCLUDES 1 *fracture of orbital floor (S02.3-)*
fracture of orbital roof (S02.1-)

CC Excl: CC with 7th character A or B: S01.90X-S02.92X with 7th A, S06.0X0-S07.9XX with 7th A, S08.89-S09.19X with 7th A, S09.8XX-S09.90X with 7th A, S09.92X-S09.93X with 7th A, S16.8XX-S19.9XX with 7th A, S38.3XXA, T14.8-T14.91, T79.A0X-T79.9XX with 7th A
CC with 7th character K: M80.00X-M84.68X with 7th [K, P], S02.0XX-S02.92X with 7th K, S12.000-S12.691 with 7th K, S22.000-S22.9XX with 7th K, S32.000-S32.9XX with 7th K, S42.001-S42.92X with 7th [K, P], S49.001-S49.199 with 7th [K, P], S52.001-S52.92X with 7th [K, M, N, P, Q, R], S59.001-S59.299 with 7th [K, P], S62.001-S62.92X with 7th [K, P], S72.001-S72.92X with 7th [K, M, N, P, Q, R], S79.001-S79.199 with 7th [K, P], S82.001-S82.92X with 7th [K, M, N, P, Q, R], S89.001-S89.399 with 7th [K, P], S92.001-S92.919 with 7th [K, P]

√5th **S02.9 Fracture of unspecified skull and facial bones**

CC Excl: For CC codes in subcategory S02.9, unless otherwise noted: CC with 7th character A or MCC with 7th character B: S01.90X-S02.92X with 7th A, S06.0X0-S07.9XXwith 7th A, S08.89X-S09.19X with 7th A, S09.8XX-S09.90X with 7th A, S09.92X-S09.93X with 7th A, S16.8XX-S19.9XX with 7th A, S38.3XXA, T14.8-T14.91, T79.A0X-T79.9XX with 7th A
CC with 7th character K: M80.00X-M84.68X with 7th [K, P], S02.0XX-S02.92X with 7th K, S12.000-S12.691 with 7th K, S22.000-S22.9XX with 7th K, S32.000-S32.9XX with 7th K, S42.001-S42.92X with 7th [K, P], S49.001-S49.199 with 7th [K, P], S52.001-S52.92X with 7th [K, M, N, P, Q, R], S59.001-S59.299 with 7th [K, P], S62.001-S62.92X with 7th [K, P], S72.001-S72.92X with 7th [K, M, N, P, Q, R], S79.001-S79.199 with 7th [K, P], S82.001-S82.92X with 7th [K, M, N, P, Q, R], S89.001-S89.399 with 7th [K, P], S92.001-S92.919 with 7th [K, P]

7 √x7th **S02.91 Unspecified fracture of skull** MCC CC
7 √x7th **S02.92 Unspecified fracture of facial bones** CC

7 HAC = Initial encounter only (7th character A, B or C) and not POA.

S03 Dislocation and sprain of joints and ligaments of head

INCLUDES avulsion of joint (capsule) or ligament of head
laceration of cartilage, joint (capsule) or ligament of head
sprain of cartilage, joint (capsule) or ligament of head
traumatic hemarthrosis of joint or ligament of head
traumatic rupture of joint or ligament of head
traumatic subluxation of joint or ligament of head
traumatic tear of joint or ligament of head

Code also any associated open wound

EXCLUDES 2 *strain of muscle or tendon of head (S09.1)*

The appropriate 7th is to be added to each code from category S03.
A initial encounter
D subsequent encounter
S sequela

S03.0 Dislocation of jaw
Dislocation of jaw (cartilage) (meniscus)
Dislocation of mandible
Dislocation of temporomandibular (joint)

S03.1 Dislocation of septal cartilage of nose

S03.2 Dislocation of tooth

S03.4 Sprain of jaw
Sprain of temporomandibular (joint) (ligament)

S03.8 Sprain of joints and ligaments of other parts of head

S03.9 Sprain of joints and ligaments of unspecified parts of head

S04 Injury of cranial nerve

The selection of side should be based on the side of the body being affected

Code first any associated intracranial injury (S06.-)

Code also any associated:
open wound of head (S01.-)
skull fracture (S02.-)

The appropriate 7th is to be added to each code from category S04.
A initial encounter
D subsequent encounter
S sequela

S04.0 Injury of optic nerve and pathways
Use additional code to identify any visual field defect or blindness (H53.4-, H54)

CC Excl: For CC codes in subcategory S04.0, unless otherwise noted: CC with 7th character A: S04.011-S04.9XX with 7th A

S04.01 Injury of optic nerve
Injury of 2nd cranial nerve

S04.011 Injury of optic nerve, right eye CC

S04.012 Injury of optic nerve, left eye CC

S04.019 Injury of optic nerve, unspecified eye CC
Injury of optic nerve NOS

S04.02 Injury of optic chiasm CC

S04.03 Injury of optic tract and pathways
Injury of optic radiation

S04.031 Injury of optic tract and pathways, right eye CC

S04.032 Injury of optic tract and pathways, left eye CC

S04.039 Injury of optic tract and pathways, unspecified eye CC
Injury of optic tract and pathways NOS

S04.04 Injury of visual cortex

S04.041 Injury of visual cortex, right eye CC

S04.042 Injury of visual cortex, left eye CC

S04.049 Injury of visual cortex, unspecified eye CC
Injury of visual cortex NOS

S04.1 Injury of oculomotor nerve
Injury of 3rd cranial nerve

CC Excl: For CC codes in subcategory S04.1, unless otherwise noted: CC with 7th character A: S04.10X-S04.12X with 7th A, S04.811-S04.9XX with 7th A

S04.10 Injury of oculomotor nerve, unspecified side CC

S04.11 Injury of oculomotor nerve, right side CC

S04.12 Injury of oculomotor nerve, left side CC

S04.2 Injury of trochlear nerve
Injury of 4th cranial nerve

CC Excl: For CC codes in subcategory S04.2, unless otherwise noted: CC with 7th character A: S04.20X-S04.22X with 7th A, S04.811-S04.9XX with 7th A

S04.20 Injury of trochlear nerve, unspecified side CC

S04.21 Injury of trochlear nerve, right side CC

S04.22 Injury of trochlear nerve, left side CC

S04.3 Injury of trigeminal nerve
Injury of 5th cranial nerve

CC Excl: For CC codes in subcategory S04.3, unless otherwise noted: CC with 7th character A: S04.30X-S04.32X with 7th A, S04.811-S04.9XX with 7th A

S04.30 Injury of trigeminal nerve, unspecified side CC

S04.31 Injury of trigeminal nerve, right side CC

S04.32 Injury of trigeminal nerve, left side CC

S04.4 Injury of abducent nerve
Injury of 6th cranial nerve

CC Excl: For CC codes in subcategory S04.4, unless otherwise noted: CC with 7th character A: S04.40X-S04.42X with 7th A, S04.811-S04.9XX with 7th A

S04.40 Injury of abducent nerve, unspecified side CC

S04.41 Injury of abducent nerve, right side CC

S04.42 Injury of abducent nerve, left side CC

S04.5 Injury of facial nerve
Injury of 7th cranial nerve

CC Excl: For CC codes in subcategory S04.5, unless otherwise noted: CC with 7th character A: S04.50X-S04.52X with 7th A, S04.811-S04.9XX with 7th A

S04.50 Injury of facial nerve, unspecified side CC

S04.51 Injury of facial nerve, right side CC

S04.52 Injury of facial nerve, left side CC

S04.6 Injury of acoustic nerve
Injury of auditory nerve
Injury of 8th cranial nerve

CC Excl: For CC codes in subcategory S04.6, unless otherwise noted: CC with 7th character A: S04.60X-S04.62X with 7th A, S04.811-S04.9XX with 7th A

S04.60 Injury of acoustic nerve, unspecified side CC

S04.61 Injury of acoustic nerve, right side CC

S04.62 Injury of acoustic nerve, left side CC

S04.7 Injury of accessory nerve
Injury of 11th cranial nerve

CC Excl: For CC codes in subcategory S04.7 unless otherwise noted: S04.70X-S04.9XX with 7th A

S04.70 Injury of accessory nerve, unspecified side CC

S04.71 Injury of accessory nerve, right side CC

S04.72 Injury of accessory nerve, left side CC

S04.8 Injury of other cranial nerves

CC Excl: For CC codes in subcategory S04.8, unless otherwise noted: CC with 7th character A: S04.811-S04.9XX with 7th A

S04.81 Injury of olfactory [1st] nerve

S04.811 Injury of olfactory [1st] nerve, right side CC

S04.812 Injury of olfactory [1st] nerve, left side CC

S04.819 Injury of olfactory [1st] nerve, unspecified side CC

S04.89 Injury of other cranial nerves
Injury of vagus [10th] nerve

S04.891 Injury of other cranial nerves, right side CC

S04.892 Injury of other cranial nerves, left side CC

S04.899 Injury of other cranial nerves, unspecified side CC

S04.9 Injury of unspecified cranial nerve CC
CC Excl: CC with 7th character A: S04.8[1,9][1,2,9]A, S04.9XXA

S05 Injury of eye and orbit
Open wound of eye and orbit
EXCLUDES 2 *2nd cranial [optic] nerve injury (S04.0-)*
3rd cranial [oculomotor] nerve injury (S04.1-)
open wound of eyelid and periocular area (S01.1-)
orbital bone fracture (S02.1-, S02.3-, S02.8-)
superficial injury of eyelid (S00.1-S00.2)

The appropriate 7th is to be added to each code from category S05.
A initial encounter
D subsequent encounter
S sequela

CC Excl: For CC codes in category S05, unless otherwise noted: CC with 7th character A: S01.101-S01.159 with 7th A, S05.20X-S05.8X9 with 7th A, S05.91X-S05.92X with 7th A, S38.3XXA, T14.8-T14.91, T79.A0X-T79.9XX with 7th A

S05.0 Injury of conjunctiva and corneal abrasion without foreign body
EXCLUDES 1 *foreign body in conjunctival sac (T15.1)*
foreign body in cornea (T15.0)

S05.00 Injury of conjunctiva and corneal abrasion without foreign body, unspecified eye
S05.01 Injury of conjunctiva and corneal abrasion without foreign body, right eye
S05.02 Injury of conjunctiva and corneal abrasion without foreign body, left eye

S05.1 Contusion of eyeball and orbital tissues
Traumatic hyphema
EXCLUDES 2 *black eye NOS (S00.1)*
contusion of eyelid and periocular area (S00.1)

S05.10 Contusion of eyeball and orbital tissues, unspecified eye
S05.11 Contusion of eyeball and orbital tissues, right eye
S05.12 Contusion of eyeball and orbital tissues, left eye

S05.2 Ocular laceration and rupture with prolapse or loss of intraocular tissue
S05.20 Ocular laceration and rupture with prolapse or loss of intraocular tissue, unspecified eye CC
S05.21 Ocular laceration and rupture with prolapse or loss of intraocular tissue, right eye CC
S05.22 Ocular laceration and rupture with prolapse or loss of intraocular tissue, left eye CC

S05.3 Ocular laceration without prolapse or loss of intraocular tissue
Laceration of eye NOS
S05.30 Ocular laceration without prolapse or loss of intraocular tissue, unspecified eye CC
S05.31 Ocular laceration without prolapse or loss of intraocular tissue, right eye CC
S05.32 Ocular laceration without prolapse or loss of intraocular tissue, left eye CC

S05.4 Penetrating wound of orbit with or without foreign body
EXCLUDES 2 *retained (old) foreign body following penetrating wound in orbit (H05.5-)*
S05.40 Penetrating wound of orbit with or without foreign body, unspecified eye CC
S05.41 Penetrating wound of orbit with or without foreign body, right eye CC
S05.42 Penetrating wound of orbit with or without foreign body, left eye CC

S05.5 Penetrating wound with foreign body of eyeball
EXCLUDES 2 *retained (old) intraocular foreign body (H44.6-, H44.7)*

CC Excl: CC with 7th character A: S01.101-S01.159 with 7th A, S05.20X-S05.8X9 with 7th A, S05.91X-S05.92X with 7th A, S38.3XXA, T14.8-T14.91, T79.8XX-T79.9XX with 7th A

S05.50 Penetrating wound with foreign body of unspecified eyeball CC
S05.51 Penetrating wound with foreign body of right eyeball CC
S05.52 Penetrating wound with foreign body of left eyeball CC

S05.6 Penetrating wound without foreign body of eyeball
Ocular penetration NOS
S05.60 Penetrating wound without foreign body of unspecified eyeball
S05.61 Penetrating wound without foreign body of right eyeball
S05.62 Penetrating wound without foreign body of left eyeball

S05.7 Avulsion of eye
Traumatic enucleation
S05.70 Avulsion of unspecified eye CC
S05.71 Avulsion of right eye CC
S05.72 Avulsion of left eye CC

S05.8 Other injuries of eye and orbit
Lacrimal duct injury
S05.8X Other injuries of eye and orbit
S05.8X1 Other injuries of right eye and orbit CC
S05.8X2 Other injuries of left eye and orbit CC
S05.8X9 Other injuries of unspecified eye and orbit CC

S05.9 Unspecified injury of eye and orbit
Injury of eye NOS
S05.90 Unspecified injury of unspecified eye and orbit
S05.91 Unspecified injury of right eye and orbit CC
S05.92 Unspecified injury of left eye and orbit CC

S06 Intracranial injury
Traumatic brain injury
Code also any associated:
open wound of head (S01.-)
skull fracture (S02.-)
EXCLUDES 1 *head injury NOS (S09.90)*

The appropriate 7th is to be added to each code from category S06.
A initial encounter
D subsequent encounter
S sequela

For CC/MCC codes in category S06, unless otherwise noted: CC or MCC as indicated with 7th A: S01.90X-S02.92X with 7th A, S06.0X0-S07.9XX with 7th A, S08.89X-S09.19X with 7th A, S09.8X-S09.90X with 7th A, S09.92X-S09.93X with 7th A, S16.8XX-S19.9XX with 7th A, S38.3XXA, T14.8-T14.91, T79.A0X-T79.9XX with 7th A

S06.0 Concussion
Commotio cerebri
EXCLUDES 1 *concussion with other intracranial injuries classified in category S06—code to specified intracranial injury*

S06.0X Concussion
S06.0X0 Concussion without loss of consciousness
7 **S06.0X1 Concussion with loss of consciousness of 30 minutes or less** CC
7 **S06.0X2 Concussion with loss of consciousness of 31 minutes to 59 minutes** CC
7 **S06.0X3 Concussion with loss of consciousness of 1 hour to 5 hours 59 minutes** CC
7 **S06.0X4 Concussion with loss of consciousness of 6 hours to 24 hours** CC
7 **S06.0X5 Concussion with loss of consciousness greater than 24 hours with return to pre-existing conscious level** CC
7 **S06.0X6 Concussion with loss of consciousness greater than 24 hours without return to pre-existing conscious level with patient surviving** MCC
7 **S06.0X7 Concussion with loss of consciousness of any duration with death due to brain injury prior to regaining consciousness** CC
7 **S06.0X8 Concussion with loss of consciousness of any duration with death due to other cause prior to regaining consciousness** CC
7 **S06.0X9 Concussion with loss of consciousness of unspecified duration** CC
Concussion NOS

7 HAC = Initial encounter only (7th character A, B or C) and not POA.

√5th **S06.1 Traumatic cerebral edema**
Diffuse traumatic cerebral edema
Focal traumatic cerebral edema

√6th **S06.1X Traumatic cerebral edema**

√7th **S06.1X0 Traumatic cerebral edema without loss of consciousness** PDx MCC MCC
CC Excl: CC with 7th character A: G93.6, G93.82

7 √7th **S06.1X1 Traumatic cerebral edema with loss of consciousness of 30 minutes or less** PDx MCC MCC

7 √7th **S06.1X2 Traumatic cerebral edema with loss of consciousness of 31 minutes to 59 minutes** PDx MCC MCC

7 √7th **S06.1X3 Traumatic cerebral edema with loss of consciousness of 1 hour to 5 hours 59 minutes** PDx MCC MCC

7 √7th **S06.1X4 Traumatic cerebral edema with loss of consciousness of 6 hours to 24 hours** PDx MCC MCC

7 √7th **S06.1X5 Traumatic cerebral edema with loss of consciousness greater than 24 hours with return to pre-existing conscious level** PDx MCC MCC

7 √7th **S06.1X6 Traumatic cerebral edema with loss of consciousness greater than 24 hours without return to pre-existing conscious level with patient surviving** PDx MCC MCC

7 √7th **S06.1X7 Traumatic cerebral edema with loss of consciousness of any duration with death due to brain injury prior to regaining consciousness** PDx MCC MCC

7 √7th **S06.1X8 Traumatic cerebral edema with loss of consciousness of any duration with death due to other cause prior to regaining consciousness** PDx MCC MCC

7 √7th **S06.1X9 Traumatic cerebral edema with loss of consciousness of unspecified duration** PDx MCC MCC
Traumatic cerebral edema NOS
CC Excl: CC with 7th character A: G93.6, G93.82, S01.90X-S02.92X with 7th A, S06.0X0-S07.9X with 7th A, S08.89X-S09.19X with 7th A, S09.8XX-S09.90X with 7th A, S09.92X-S09.93XA, S16.8XX-S19.9XX with 7th A, S38.3XXA, T14.8-T14.91, T79.A0X-T79.9XX with 7th A

√5th **S06.2 Diffuse traumatic brain injury**
Diffuse axonal brain injury
EXCLUDES 1 *traumatic diffuse cerebral edema (S06.1X-)*

√6th **S06.2X Diffuse traumatic brain injury**

√7th **S06.2X0 Diffuse traumatic brain injury without loss of consciousness**

7 √7th **S06.2X1 Diffuse traumatic brain injury with loss of consciousness of 30 minutes or less** CC

7 √7th **S06.2X2 Diffuse traumatic brain injury with loss of consciousness of 31 minutes to 59 minutes** CC

7 √7th **S06.2X3 Diffuse traumatic brain injury with loss of consciousness of 1 hour to 5 hours 59 minutes** CC

7 √7th **S06.2X4 Diffuse traumatic brain injury with loss of consciousness of 6 hours to 24 hours** CC

7 √7th **S06.2X5 Diffuse traumatic brain injury with loss of consciousness greater than 24 hours with return to pre-existing conscious levels** CC

7 √7th **S06.2X6 Diffuse traumatic brain injury with loss of consciousness greater than 24 hours without return to pre-existing conscious level with patient surviving** MCC

7 √7th **S06.2X7 Diffuse traumatic brain injury with loss of consciousness of any duration with death due to brain injury prior to regaining consciousness** MCC

7 √7th **S06.2X8 Diffuse traumatic brain injury with loss of consciousness of any duration with death due to other cause prior to regaining consciousness** MCC

7 √7th **S06.2X9 Diffuse traumatic brain injury with loss of consciousness of unspecified duration** CC
Diffuse traumatic brain injury NOS

√5th **S06.3 Focal traumatic brain injury**
EXCLUDES 1 *any condition classifiable to S06.4-S06.6*
focal cerebral edema (S06.1)

√6th **S06.30 Unspecified focal traumatic brain injury**

√7th **S06.300 Unspecified focal traumatic brain injury without loss of consciousness**

7 √7th **S06.301 Unspecified focal traumatic brain injury with loss of consciousness of 30 minutes or less** CC

7 √7th **S06.302 Unspecified focal traumatic brain injury with loss of consciousness of 31 minutes to 59 minutes** CC

7 √7th **S06.303 Unspecified focal traumatic brain injury with loss of consciousness of 1 hour to 5 hours 59 minutes** CC

7 √7th **S06.304 Unspecified focal traumatic brain injury with loss of consciousness of 6 hours to 24 hours** CC

7 √7th **S06.305 Unspecified focal traumatic brain injury with loss of consciousness greater than 24 hours with return to pre-existing conscious level** CC

7 √7th **S06.306 Unspecified focal traumatic brain injury with loss of consciousness greater than 24 hours without return to pre-existing conscious level with patient surviving** MCC

7 √7th **S06.307 Unspecified focal traumatic brain injury with loss of consciousness of any duration with death due to brain injury prior to regaining consciousness** MCC

7 √7th **S06.308 Unspecified focal traumatic brain injury with loss of consciousness of any duration with death due to other cause prior to regaining consciousness** MCC

7 √7th **S06.309 Unspecified focal traumatic brain injury with loss of consciousness of unspecified duration** CC
Unspecified focal traumatic brain injury NOS

√6th **S06.31 Contusion and laceration of right cerebrum**

7 √7th **S06.310 Contusion and laceration of right cerebrum without loss of consciousness** MCC

7 √7th **S06.311 Contusion and laceration of right cerebrum with loss of consciousness of 30 minutes or less** MCC

7 √7th **S06.312 Contusion and laceration of right cerebrum with loss of consciousness of 31 minutes to 59 minutes** MCC

7 √7th **S06.313 Contusion and laceration of right cerebrum with loss of consciousness of 1 hour to 5 hours 59 minutes** MCC

7 √7th **S06.314 Contusion and laceration of right cerebrum with loss of consciousness of 6 hours to 24 hours** MCC

7 √7th **S06.315 Contusion and laceration of right cerebrum with loss of consciousness greater than 24 hours with return to pre-existing conscious level** MCC

7 √7th **S06.316 Contusion and laceration of right cerebrum with loss of consciousness greater than 24 hours without return to pre-existing conscious level with patient surviving** MCC

7 HAC = Initial encounter only (7th character A, B or C) and not POA.

7 ✓7th **S06.317 Contusion and laceration of right cerebrum with loss of consciousness of any duration with death due to brain injury prior to regaining consciousness** MCC

7 ✓7th **S06.318 Contusion and laceration of right cerebrum with loss of consciousness of any duration with death due to other cause prior to regaining consciousness** MCC

7 ✓7th **S06.319 Contusion and laceration of right cerebrum with loss of consciousness of unspecified duration** MCC
Contusion and laceration of right cerebrum NOS

✓6th **S06.32 Contusion and laceration of left cerebrum**

7 ✓7th **S06.320 Contusion and laceration of left cerebrum without loss of consciousness** MCC

7 ✓7th **S06.321 Contusion and laceration of left cerebrum with loss of consciousness of 30 minutes or less** MCC

7 ✓7th **S06.322 Contusion and laceration of left cerebrum with loss of consciousness of 31 minutes to 59 minutes** MCC

7 ✓7th **S06.323 Contusion and laceration of left cerebrum with loss of consciousness of 1 hour to 5 hours 59 minutes** MCC

7 ✓7th **S06.324 Contusion and laceration of left cerebrum with loss of consciousness of 6 hours to 24 hours** MCC

7 ✓7th **S06.325 Contusion and laceration of left cerebrum with loss of consciousness greater than 24 hours with return to pre-existing conscious level** MCC

7 ✓7th **S06.326 Contusion and laceration of left cerebrum with loss of consciousness greater than 24 hours without return to pre-existing conscious level with patient surviving** MCC

7 ✓7th **S06.327 Contusion and laceration of left cerebrum with loss of consciousness of any duration with death due to brain injury prior to regaining consciousness** MCC

7 ✓7th **S06.328 Contusion and laceration of left cerebrum with loss of consciousness of any duration with death due to other cause prior to regaining consciousness** MCC

7 ✓7th **S06.329 Contusion and laceration of left cerebrum with loss of consciousness of unspecified duration** MCC
Contusion and laceration of left cerebrum NOS

✓6th **S06.33 Contusion and laceration of cerebrum, unspecified**

7 ✓7th **S06.330 Contusion and laceration of cerebrum, unspecified, without loss of consciousness** MCC

7 ✓7th **S06.331 Contusion and laceration of cerebrum, unspecified, with loss of consciousness of 30 minutes or less** MCC

7 ✓7th **S06.332 Contusion and laceration of cerebrum, unspecified, with loss of consciousness of 31 minutes to 59 minutes** MCC

7 ✓7th **S06.333 Contusion and laceration of cerebrum, unspecified, with loss of consciousness of 1 hour to 5 hours 59 minutes** MCC

7 ✓7th **S06.334 Contusion and laceration of cerebrum, unspecified, with loss of consciousness of 6 hours to 24 hours** MCC

7 ✓7th **S06.335 Contusion and laceration of cerebrum, unspecified, with loss of consciousness greater than 24 hours with return to pre-existing conscious level** MCC

7 ✓7th **S06.336 Contusion and laceration of cerebrum, unspecified, with loss of consciousness greater than 24 hours without return to pre-existing conscious level with patient surviving** MCC

7 ✓7th **S06.337 Contusion and laceration of cerebrum, unspecified, with loss of consciousness of any duration with death due to brain injury prior to regaining consciousness** MCC

7 ✓7th **S06.338 Contusion and laceration of cerebrum, unspecified, with loss of consciousness of any duration with death due to other cause prior to regaining consciousness** MCC

7 ✓7th **S06.339 Contusion and laceration of cerebrum, unspecified, with loss of consciousness of unspecified duration** MCC
Contusion and laceration of cerebrum NOS

✓6th **S06.34 Traumatic hemorrhage of right cerebrum**
Traumatic intracerebral hemorrhage and hematoma of right cerebrum

7 ✓7th **S06.340 Traumatic hemorrhage of right cerebrum without loss of consciousness** MCC

7 ✓7th **S06.341 Traumatic hemorrhage of right cerebrum with loss of consciousness of 30 minutes or less** MCC

7 ✓7th **S06.342 Traumatic hemorrhage of right cerebrum with loss of consciousness of 31 minutes to 59 minutes** MCC

7 ✓7th **S06.343 Traumatic hemorrhage of right cerebrum with loss of consciousness of 1 hours to 5 hours 59 minutes** MCC

7 ✓7th **S06.344 Traumatic hemorrhage of right cerebrum with loss of consciousness of 6 hours to 24 hours** MCC

7 ✓7th **S06.345 Traumatic hemorrhage of right cerebrum with loss of consciousness greater than 24 hours with return to pre-existing conscious level** MCC

7 ✓7th **S06.346 Traumatic hemorrhage of right cerebrum with loss of consciousness greater than 24 hours without return to pre-existing conscious level with patient surviving** MCC

7 ✓7th **S06.347 Traumatic hemorrhage of right cerebrum with loss of consciousness of any duration with death due to brain injury prior to regaining consciousness** MCC

7 ✓7th **S06.348 Traumatic hemorrhage of right cerebrum with loss of consciousness of any duration with death due to other cause prior to regaining consciousness** MCC

7 ✓7th **S06.349 Traumatic hemorrhage of right cerebrum with loss of consciousness of unspecified duration** MCC
Traumatic hemorrhage of right cerebrum NOS

✓6th **S06.35 Traumatic hemorrhage of left cerebrum**
Traumatic intracerebral hemorrhage and hematoma of left cerebrum

7 ✓7th **S06.350 Traumatic hemorrhage of left cerebrum without loss of consciousness** MCC

7 ✓7th **S06.351 Traumatic hemorrhage of left cerebrum with loss of consciousness of 30 minutes or less** MCC

7 ✓7th **S06.352 Traumatic hemorrhage of left cerebrum with loss of consciousness of 31 minutes to 59 minutes** MCC

7 ✓7th **S06.353 Traumatic hemorrhage of left cerebrum with loss of consciousness of 1 hours to 5 hours 59 minutes** MCC

7 ✓7th **S06.354 Traumatic hemorrhage of left cerebrum with loss of consciousness of 6 hours to 24 hours** MCC

7 ✓7th **S06.355 Traumatic hemorrhage of left cerebrum with loss of consciousness greater than 24 hours with return to pre-existing conscious level** MCC

7 HAC = Initial encounter only (7th character A, B or C) and not POA.

7 ✓7th **SØ6.356 Traumatic hemorrhage of left cerebrum with loss of consciousness greater than 24 hours without return to pre-existing conscious level with patient surviving** MCC

7 ✓7th **SØ6.357 Traumatic hemorrhage of left cerebrum with loss of consciousness of any duration with death due to brain injury prior to regaining consciousness** MCC

7 ✓7th **SØ6.358 Traumatic hemorrhage of left cerebrum with loss of consciousness of any duration with death due to other cause prior to regaining consciousness** MCC

7 ✓7th **SØ6.359 Traumatic hemorrhage of left cerebrum with loss of consciousness of unspecified duration** MCC
Traumatic hemorrhage of left cerebrum NOS

✓6th **SØ6.36 Traumatic hemorrhage of cerebrum, unspecified**
Traumatic intracerebral hemorrhage and hematoma, unspecified

7 ✓7th **SØ6.36Ø Traumatic hemorrhage of cerebrum, unspecified, without loss of consciousness** MCC

7 ✓7th **SØ6.361 Traumatic hemorrhage of cerebrum, unspecified, with loss of consciousness of 3Ø minutes or less** MCC

7 ✓7th **SØ6.362 Traumatic hemorrhage of cerebrum, unspecified, with loss of consciousness of 31 minutes to 59 minutes** MCC

7 ✓7th **SØ6.363 Traumatic hemorrhage of cerebrum, unspecified, with loss of consciousness of 1 hours to 5 hours 59 minutes** MCC

7 ✓7th **SØ6.364 Traumatic hemorrhage of cerebrum, unspecified, with loss of consciousness of 6 hours to 24 hours** MCC

7 ✓7th **SØ6.365 Traumatic hemorrhage of cerebrum, unspecified, with loss of consciousness greater than 24 hours with return to pre-existing conscious level** MCC

7 ✓7th **SØ6.366 Traumatic hemorrhage of cerebrum, unspecified, with loss of consciousness greater than 24 hours without return to pre-existing conscious level with patient surviving** MCC

7 ✓7th **SØ6.367 Traumatic hemorrhage of cerebrum, unspecified, with loss of consciousness of any duration with death due to brain injury prior to regaining consciousness** MCC

7 ✓7th **SØ6.368 Traumatic hemorrhage of cerebrum, unspecified, with loss of consciousness of any duration with death due to other cause prior to regaining consciousness** MCC

7 ✓7th **SØ6.369 Traumatic hemorrhage of cerebrum, unspecified, with loss of consciousness of unspecified duration** MCC
Traumatic hemorrhage of cerebrum NOS

✓6th **SØ6.37 Contusion, laceration, and hemorrhage of cerebellum**

7 ✓7th **SØ6.37Ø Contusion, laceration, and hemorrhage of cerebellum without loss of consciousness** MCC
CC Excl: No Excl

7 ✓7th **SØ6.371 Contusion, laceration, and hemorrhage of cerebellum with loss of consciousness of 3Ø minutes or less** CC

7 ✓7th **SØ6.372 Contusion, laceration, and hemorrhage of cerebellum with loss of consciousness of 31 minutes to 59 minutes** CC

7 ✓7th **SØ6.373 Contusion, laceration, and hemorrhage of cerebellum with loss of consciousness of 1 hour to 5 hours 59 minutes** CC

7 ✓7th **SØ6.374 Contusion, laceration, and hemorrhage of cerebellum with loss of consciousness of 6 hours to 24 hours** CC

7 ✓7th **SØ6.375 Contusion, laceration, and hemorrhage of cerebellum with loss of consciousness greater than 24 hours with return to pre-existing conscious level** CC

7 ✓7th **SØ6.376 Contusion, laceration, and hemorrhage of cerebellum with loss of consciousness greater than 24 hours without return to pre-existing conscious level with patient surviving** MCC

7 ✓7th **SØ6.377 Contusion, laceration, and hemorrhage of cerebellum with loss of consciousness of any duration with death due to brain injury prior to regaining consciousness** MCC

7 ✓7th **SØ6.378 Contusion, laceration, and hemorrhage of cerebellum with loss of consciousness of any duration with death due to other cause prior to regaining consciousness** MCC

7 ✓7th **SØ6.379 Contusion, laceration, and hemorrhage of cerebellum with loss of consciousness of unspecified duration** CC
Contusion, laceration, and hemorrhage of cerebellum NOS

✓6th **SØ6.38 Contusion, laceration, and hemorrhage of brainstem**

7 ✓7th **SØ6.38Ø Contusion, laceration, and hemorrhage of brainstem without loss of consciousness** MCC
CC Excl: No Excl

7 ✓7th **SØ6.381 Contusion, laceration, and hemorrhage of brainstem with loss of consciousness of 3Ø minutes or less** CC

7 ✓7th **SØ6.382 Contusion, laceration, and hemorrhage of brainstem with loss of consciousness of 31 minutes to 59 minutes** CC

7 ✓7th **SØ6.383 Contusion, laceration, and hemorrhage of brainstem with loss of consciousness of 1 hour to 5 hours 59 minutes** CC

7 ✓7th **SØ6.384 Contusion, laceration, and hemorrhage of brainstem with loss of consciousness of 6 hours to 24 hours** CC

7 ✓7th **SØ6.385 Contusion, laceration, and hemorrhage of brainstem with loss of consciousness greater than 24 hours with return to pre-existing conscious level** CC

7 ✓7th **SØ6.386 Contusion, laceration, and hemorrhage of brainstem with loss of consciousness greater than 24 hours without return to pre-existing conscious level with patient surviving** MCC

7 ✓7th **SØ6.387 Contusion, laceration, and hemorrhage of brainstem with loss of consciousness of any duration with death due to brain injury prior to regaining consciousness** MCC

7 ✓7th **SØ6.388 Contusion, laceration, and hemorrhage of brainstem with loss of consciousness of any duration with death due to other cause prior to regaining consciousness** MCC

7 ✓7th **SØ6.389 Contusion, laceration, and hemorrhage of brainstem with loss of consciousness of unspecified duration** CC
Contusion, laceration, and hemorrhage of brainstem NOS

✓5th **SØ6.4 Epidural hemorrhage**
Extradural hemorrhage NOS
Extradural hemorrhage (traumatic)

✓6th **SØ6.4X Epidural hemorrhage**

7 ✓7th **SØ6.4XØ Epidural hemorrhage without loss of consciousness** MCC

7 HAC = Initial encounter only (7th character A, B or C) and not POA.

7 ✓7th **S06.4X1 Epidural hemorrhage with loss of consciousness of 30 minutes or less** MCC

7 ✓7th **S06.4X2 Epidural hemorrhage with loss of consciousness of 31 minutes to 59 minutes** MCC

7 ✓7th **S06.4X3 Epidural hemorrhage with loss of consciousness of 1 hour to 5 hours 59 minutes** MCC

7 ✓7th **S06.4X4 Epidural hemorrhage with loss of consciousness of 6 hours to 24 hours** MCC

7 ✓7th **S06.4X5 Epidural hemorrhage with loss of consciousness greater than 24 hours with return to pre-existing conscious level** MCC

7 ✓7th **S06.4X6 Epidural hemorrhage with loss of consciousness greater than 24 hours without return to pre-existing conscious level with patient surviving** MCC

7 ✓7th **S06.4X7 Epidural hemorrhage with loss of consciousness of any duration with death due to brain injury prior to regaining consciousness** MCC

7 ✓7th **S06.4X8 Epidural hemorrhage with loss of consciousness of any duration with death due to other causes prior to regaining consciousness** MCC

7 ✓7th **S06.4X9 Epidural hemorrhage with loss of consciousness of unspecified duration** MCC
Epidural hemorrhage NOS

✓5th **S06.5 Traumatic subdural hemorrhage**

✓6th **S06.5X Traumatic subdural hemorrhage**

7 ✓7th **S06.5X0 Traumatic subdural hemorrhage without loss of consciousness** MCC

7 ✓7th **S06.5X1 Traumatic subdural hemorrhage with loss of consciousness of 30 minutes or less** MCC

7 ✓7th **S06.5X2 Traumatic subdural hemorrhage with loss of consciousness of 31 minutes to 59 minutes** MCC

7 ✓7th **S06.5X3 Traumatic subdural hemorrhage with loss of consciousness of 1 hour to 5 hours 59 minutes** MCC

7 ✓7th **S06.5X4 Traumatic subdural hemorrhage with loss of consciousness of 6 hours to 24 hours** MCC

7 ✓7th **S06.5X5 Traumatic subdural hemorrhage with loss of consciousness greater than 24 hours with return to pre-existing conscious level** MCC

7 ✓7th **S06.5X6 Traumatic subdural hemorrhage with loss of consciousness greater than 24 hours without return to pre-existing conscious level with patient surviving** MCC

7 ✓7th **S06.5X7 Traumatic subdural hemorrhage with loss of consciousness of any duration with death due to brain injury before regaining consciousness** MCC

7 ✓7th **S06.5X8 Traumatic subdural hemorrhage with loss of consciousness of any duration with death due to other cause before regaining consciousness** MCC

7 ✓7th **S06.5X9 Traumatic subdural hemorrhage with loss of consciousness of unspecified duration** MCC
Traumatic subdural hemorrhage NOS

✓5th **S06.6 Traumatic subarachnoid hemorrhage**

✓6th **S06.6X Traumatic subarachnoid hemorrhage**

7 ✓7th **S06.6X0 Traumatic subarachnoid hemorrhage without loss of consciousness** MCC

7 ✓7th **S06.6X1 Traumatic subarachnoid hemorrhage with loss of consciousness of 30 minutes or less** MCC

7 ✓7th **S06.6X2 Traumatic subarachnoid hemorrhagewith loss of consciousness of 31 minutes to 59 minutes** MCC

7 ✓7th **S06.6X3 Traumatic subarachnoid hemorrhage with loss of consciousness of 1 hour to 5 hours 59 minutes** MCC

7 ✓7th **S06.6X4 Traumatic subarachnoid hemorrhage with loss of consciousness of 6 hours to 24 hours** MCC

7 ✓7th **S06.6X5 Traumatic subarachnoid hemorrhage with loss of consciousness greater than 24 hours with return to pre-existing conscious level** MCC

7 ✓7th **S06.6X6 Traumatic subarachnoid hemorrhage with loss of consciousness greater than 24 hours without return to pre-existing conscious level with patient surviving** MCC

7 ✓7th **S06.6X7 Traumatic subarachnoid hemorrhage with loss of consciousness of any duration with death due to brain injury prior to regaining consciousness** MCC

7 ✓7th **S06.6X8 Traumatic subarachnoid hemorrhage with loss of consciousness of any duration with death due to other cause prior to regaining consciousness** MCC

7 ✓7th **S06.6X9 Traumatic subarachnoid hemorrhage with loss of consciousness of unspecified duration** MCC
Traumatic subarachnoid hemorrhage NOS

✓5th **S06.8 Other specified intracranial injuries**

✓6th **S06.81 Injury of right internal carotid artery, intracranial portion, not elsewhere classified**

✓7th **S06.810 Injury of right internal carotid artery, intracranial portion, not elsewhere classified without loss of consciousness**

7 ✓7th **S06.811 Injury of right internal carotid artery, intracranial portion, not elsewhere classified with loss of consciousness of 30 minutes or less** CC

7 ✓7th **S06.812 Injury of right internal carotid artery, intracranial portion, not elsewhere classified with loss of consciousness of 31 minutes to 59 minutes** CC

7 ✓7th **S06.813 Injury of right internal carotid artery, intracranial portion, not elsewhere classified with loss of consciousness of 1 hour to 5 hours 59 minutes** CC

7 ✓7th **S06.814 Injury of right internal carotid artery, intracranial portion, not elsewhere classified with loss of consciousness of 6 hours to 24 hours** CC

7 ✓7th **S06.815 Injury of right internal carotid artery, intracranial portion, not elsewhere classified with loss of consciousness greater than 24 hours with return to pre-existing conscious level** CC

7 ✓7th **S06.816 Injury of right internal carotid artery, intracranial portion, not elsewhere classified with loss of consciousness greater than 24 hours without return to pre-existing conscious level with patient surviving** MCC

7 ✓7th **S06.817 Injury of right internal carotid artery, intracranial portion, not elsewhere classified with loss of consciousness of any duration with death due to brain injury prior to regaining consciousness** MCC

7 ✓7th **S06.818 Injury of right internal carotid artery, intracranial portion, not elsewhere classified with loss of consciousness of any duration with death due to other cause prior to regaining consciousness** MCC

7 ✓7th **S06.819 Injury of right internal carotid artery, intracranial portion, not elsewhere classified with loss of consciousness of unspecified duration** CC
Injury of right internal carotid artery, intracranial portion, not elsewhere classified NOS

7 HAC = Initial encounter only (7th character A, B or C) and not POA.

✓6th **SØ6.82 Injury of left internal carotid artery, intracranial portion, not elsewhere classified**

✓7th **SØ6.82Ø Injury of left internal carotid artery, intracranial portion, not elsewhere classified without loss of consciousness**

7 ✓7th **SØ6.821 Injury of left internal carotid artery, intracranial portion, not elsewhere classified with loss of consciousness of 3Ø minutes or less** CC

7 ✓7th **SØ6.822 Injury of left internal carotid artery, intracranial portion, not elsewhere classified with loss of consciousness of 31 minutes to 59 minutes** CC

7 ✓7th **SØ6.823 Injury of left internal carotid artery, intracranial portion, not elsewhere classified with loss of consciousness of 1 hour to 5 hours 59 minutes** CC

7 ✓7th **SØ6.824 Injury of left internal carotid artery, intracranial portion, not elsewhere classified with loss of consciousness of 6 hours to 24 hours** CC

7 ✓7th **SØ6.825 Injury of left internal carotid artery, intracranial portion, not elsewhere classified with loss of consciousness greater than 24 hours with return to pre-existing conscious level** CC

7 ✓7th **SØ6.826 Injury of left internal carotid artery, intracranial portion, not elsewhere classified with loss of consciousness greater than 24 hours without return to pre-existing conscious level with patient surviving** MCC

7 ✓7th **SØ6.827 Injury of left internal carotid artery, intracranial portion, not elsewhere classified with loss of consciousness of any duration with death due to brain injury prior to regaining consciousness** MCC

7 ✓7th **SØ6.828 Injury of left internal carotid artery, intracranial portion, not elsewhere classified with loss of consciousness of any duration with death due to other cause prior to regaining consciousness** MCC

7 ✓7th **SØ6.829 Injury of left internal carotid artery, intracranial portion, not elsewhere classified with loss of consciousness of unspecified duration** CC

Injury of left internal carotid artery, intracranial portion, not elsewhere classified NOS

✓6th **SØ6.89 Other specified intracranial injury**

✓7th **SØ6.89Ø Other specified intracranial injury without loss of consciousness**

7 ✓7th **SØ6.891 Other specified intracranial injury with loss of consciousness of 3Ø minutes or less** CC

7 ✓7th **SØ6.892 Other specified intracranial injury with loss of consciousness of 31 minutes to 59 minutes** CC

7 ✓7th **SØ6.893 Other specified intracranial injury with loss of consciousness of 1 hour to 5 hours 59 minutes** CC

7 ✓7th **SØ6.894 Other specified intracranial injury with loss of consciousness of 6 hours to 24 hours** CC

7 ✓7th **SØ6.895 Other specified intracranial injury with loss of consciousness greater than 24 hours with return to pre-existing conscious level** CC

7 ✓7th **SØ6.896 Other specified intracranial injury with loss of consciousness greater than 24 hours without return to pre-existing conscious level with patient surviving** MCC

7 ✓7th **SØ6.897 Other specified intracranial injury with loss of consciousness of any duration with death due to brain injury prior to regaining consciousness** MCC

7 ✓7th **SØ6.898 Other specified intracranial injury with loss of consciousness of any duration with death due to other cause prior to regaining consciousness** MCC

7 ✓7th **SØ6.899 Other specified intracranial injury with loss of consciousness of unspecified duration** CC

✓5th **SØ6.9 Unspecified intracranial injury**

Brain injury NOS
Head injury NOS with loss of consciousness

EXCLUDES 1 *head injury NOS (SØ9.9Ø)*

✓6th **SØ6.9X Unspecified intracranial injury**

✓7th **SØ6.9XØ Unspecified intracranial injury without loss of consciousness**

7 ✓7th **SØ6.9X1 Unspecified intracranial injury with loss of consciousness of 3Ø minutes or less** CC

7 ✓7th **SØ6.9X2 Unspecified intracranial injury with loss of consciousness of 31 minutes to 59 minutes** CC

7 ✓7th **SØ6.9X3 Unspecified intracranial injury with loss of consciousness of 1 hour to 5 hours 59 minutes** CC

7 ✓7th **SØ6.9X4 Unspecified intracranial injury with loss of consciousness of 6 hours to 24 hours** CC

7 ✓7th **SØ6.9X5 Unspecified intracranial injury with loss of consciousness greater than 24 hours with return to pre-existing conscious level** CC

7 ✓7th **SØ6.9X6 Unspecified intracranial injury with loss of consciousness greater than 24 hours without return to pre-existing conscious level with patient surviving** MCC

7 ✓7th **SØ6.9X7 Unspecified intracranial injury with loss of consciousness of any duration with death due to brain injury prior to regaining consciousness** MCC

7 ✓7th **SØ6.9X8 Unspecified intracranial injury with loss of consciousness of any duration with death due to other cause prior to regaining consciousness** MCC

7 ✓7th **SØ6.9X9 Unspecified intracranial injury with loss of consciousness of unspecified duration** CC

✓4th **SØ7 Crushing injury of head**

Use additional code for all associated injuries, such as:
intracranial injuries (SØ6.-)
skull fractures (SØ2.-)

The appropriate 7th is to be added to each code from category SØ7.
A initial encounter
D subsequent encounter
S sequela

For CC/MCC codes in category SØ7, unless otherwise noted: CC with 7th character A: SØ1.9ØX-SØ2.92X with 7th A, SØ7.ØXX-SØ7.9XX with 7th A, SØ8.89X-SØ9.19X with 7th A, SØ9.8XX-SØ9.9ØX with 7th A, SØ9.92X-SØ9.93X with 7th A, S16.8XX-S19.9XX with 7th A, T14.8-T14.91, T79.AØX-T79.9XX with 7th A

7 ✓x7th **SØ7.Ø Crushing injury of face** CC

7 ✓x7th **SØ7.1 Crushing injury of skull** CC

7 ✓x7th **SØ7.8 Crushing injury of other parts of head** CC

7 ✓x7th **SØ7.9 Crushing injury of head, part unspecified** CC

✓4th **SØ8 Avulsion and traumatic amputation of part of head**

NOTE An amputation not identified as partial or complete should be coded to complete

The appropriate 7th is to be added to each code from category SØ8.
A initial encounter
D subsequent encounter
S sequela

✓x7th **SØ8.Ø Avulsion of scalp**

✓5th **SØ8.1 Traumatic amputation of ear**

7 HAC = Initial encounter only (7th character A, B or C) and not POA.

S08.11 **Complete traumatic amputation of ear**
S08.111 **Complete traumatic amputation of right ear**
S08.112 **Complete traumatic amputation of left ear**
S08.119 **Complete traumatic amputation of unspecified ear**
S08.12 **Partial traumatic amputation of ear**
S08.121 **Partial traumatic amputation of right ear**
S08.122 **Partial traumatic amputation of left ear**
S08.129 **Partial traumatic amputation of unspecified ear**
S08.8 **Traumatic amputation of other parts of head**
S08.81 **Traumatic amputation of nose**
S08.811 **Complete traumatic amputation of nose**
S08.812 **Partial traumatic amputation of nose**
S08.89 **Traumatic amputation of other parts of head**

S09 Other and unspecified injuries of head

The appropriate 7th is to be added to each code from category S09.
A initial encounter
D subsequent encounter
S sequela

S09.0 **Injury of blood vessels of head, not elsewhere classified** CC
EXCLUDES 1 *injury of cerebral blood vessels (S06.-)*
injury of precerebral blood vessels (S15.-)
CC Excl: CC with 7th character A: S09.0XX with 7th A, S15.101-S15.199 with 7th A, S15.8XX-S15.9XX with 7th A, T14.8-T14.91, T79.A0X-T79.9XX with 7th A
S09.1 **Injury of muscle and tendon of head**
Code also any associated open wound (S01.-)
EXCLUDES 2 *sprain to joints and ligament of head (S03.9)*
S09.10 **Unspecified injury of muscle and tendon of head**
Injury of muscle and tendon of head NOS
S09.11 **Strain of muscle and tendon of head**
S09.12 **Laceration of muscle and tendon of head**
S09.19 **Other specified injury of muscle and tendon of head**
S09.2 **Traumatic rupture of ear drum**
EXCLUDES 1 *traumatic rupture of ear drum due to blast injury (S09.31-)*

CC Excl: For CC codes in subcategory S09.2, unless otherwise noted: CC with 7th character A: S01.301-S01.359 with 7th A, S08.111-S08.129 with 7th A, S09.20X-S09.399 with 7th A, S09.91XA, S38.3XXA, T14.8-T14.91, T79.8XX-T79.9XX with 7th A

S09.20 **Traumatic rupture of unspecified ear drum** CC
S09.21 **Traumatic rupture of right ear drum** CC
S09.22 **Traumatic rupture of left ear drum** CC
S09.3 **Other specified and unspecified injury of middle and inner ear**
EXCLUDES 1 *injury to ear NOS (S09.91-)*
EXCLUDES 2 *injury to external ear (S00.4-, S01.3-, S08.1-)*

CC Excl: For CC codes in subcategory S09.3, unless otherwise noted: CC with 7th character A: S01.301-S01.359 with 7th A, S08.111-S08.129 with 7th A, S09.20X-S09.399 with 7th A, S09.91X with 7th A, S38.3XXA, T14.8-T14.91, T79.8XX-T79.9XX with 7th A

S09.30 **Unspecified injury of middle and inner ear**
S09.301 **Unspecified injury of right middle and inner ear** CC
S09.302 **Unspecified injury of left middle and inner ear** CC
S09.309 **Unspecified injury of unspecified middle and inner ear** CC
S09.31 **Primary blast injury of ear**
Blast injury of ear NOS
S09.311 **Primary blast injury of right ear** CC
S09.312 **Primary blast injury of left ear** CC
S09.313 **Primary blast injury of ear, bilateral** CC
S09.319 **Primary blast injury of unspecified ear** CC
S09.39 **Other specified injury of middle and inner ear**
Secondary blast injury to ear
S09.391 **Other specified injury of right middle and inner ear** CC
S09.392 **Other specified injury of left middle and inner ear** CC
S09.399 **Other specified injury of unspecified middle and inner ear** CC
S09.8 **Other specified injuries of head** CC
CC Excl: No excl
S09.9 **Unspecified injury of face and head**
S09.90 **Unspecified injury of head**
Head injury NOS
EXCLUDES 1 *brain injury NOS (S06.9-)*
head injury NOS with loss of consciousness (S06.9-)
intracranial injury NOS (S06.9-)
S09.91 **Unspecified injury of ear**
Injury of ear NOS
S09.92 **Unspecified injury of nose**
Injury of nose NOS
S09.93 **Unspecified injury of face**
Injury of face NOS

Injuries to the neck (S10-S19)

INCLUDES injuries of nape
injuries of supraclavicular region
injuries of throat
EXCLUDES 2 *burns and corrosions (T20-T32)*
effects of foreign body in esophagus (T18.1)
effects of foreign body in larynx (T17.3)
effects of foreign body in pharynx (T17.2)
effects of foreign body in trachea (T17.4)
frostbite (T33-T34)
insect bite or sting, venomous (T63.4)

S10 Superficial injury of neck

The appropriate 7th is to be added to each code from category S10.
A initial encounter
D subsequent encounter
S sequela

S10.0 **Contusion of throat**
Contusion of cervical esophagus
Contusion of larynx
Contusion of pharynx
Contusion of trachea
S10.1 **Other and unspecified superficial injuries of throat**
S10.10 **Unspecified superficial injuries of throat**
S10.11 **Abrasion of throat**
S10.12 **Blister (nonthermal) of throat**
S10.14 **External constriction of part of throat**
S10.15 **Superficial foreign body of throat**
Splinter in the throat
S10.16 **Insect bite (nonvenomous) of throat**
S10.17 **Other superficial bite of throat**
EXCLUDES 1 *open bite of throat (S11.85)*
S10.8 **Superficial injury of other specified parts of neck**
S10.80 **Unspecified superficial injury of other specified part of neck**
S10.81 **Abrasion of other specified part of neck**
S10.82 **Blister (nonthermal) of other specified part of neck**
S10.83 **Contusion of other specified part of neck**
S10.84 **External constriction of other specified part of neck**
S10.85 **Superficial foreign body of other specified part of neck**
Splinter in other specified part of neck
S10.86 **Insect bite of other specified part of neck**
S10.87 **Other superficial bite of other specified part of neck**
EXCLUDES 1 *open bite of other specified parts of neck (S11.85)*
S10.9 **Superficial injury of unspecified part of neck**
S10.90 **Unspecified superficial injury of unspecified part of neck**
S10.91 **Abrasion of unspecified part of neck**
S10.92 **Blister (nonthermal) of unspecified part of neck**
S10.93 **Contusion of unspecified part of neck**
S10.94 **External constriction of unspecified part of neck**

✓x7th **S10.95 Superficial foreign body of unspecified part of neck**
✓x7th **S10.96 Insect bite of unspecified part of neck**
✓x7th **S10.97 Other superficial bite of unspecified part of neck**

✓4th **S11 Open wound of neck**
Code also any associated:
spinal cord injury (S14.0, S14.1-)
wound infection
EXCLUDES 2 *open fracture of vertebra (S12- with 7th B)*

The appropriate 7th is to be added to each code from category S11.
A initial encounter
D subsequent encounter
S sequela

✓5th **S11.0 Open wound of larynx and trachea**

CC Excl: For MCC codes in subcategory S11.0, unless otherwise noted: MCC with 7th character A: S11.011-S11.039 with 7th A, S11.80X-S11.95X with 7th A, S13.4XXA, S13.8XXA, S16.1XX-S16.2XX with 7th A, S38.3XXA, T14.8-T14.91, T79.A0X-T79.9XX with 7th A

✓6th **S11.01 Open wound of larynx**
EXCLUDES 2 *open wound of vocal cord (S11.03)*
✓7th **S11.011 Laceration without foreign body of larynx** MCC
✓7th **S11.012 Laceration with foreign body of larynx** MCC
✓7th **S11.013 Puncture wound without foreign body of larynx** MCC
✓7th **S11.014 Puncture wound with foreign body of larynx** MCC
✓7th **S11.015 Open bite of larynx** MCC
Bite of larynx NOS
✓7th **S11.019 Unspecified open wound of larynx** MCC

✓6th **S11.02 Open wound of trachea**
Open wound of cervical trachea
Open wound of trachea NOS
EXCLUDES 2 *open wound of thoracic trachea (S27.5-)*
✓7th **S11.021 Laceration without foreign body of trachea** MCC
✓7th **S11.022 Laceration with foreign body of trachea** MCC
✓7th **S11.023 Puncture wound without foreign body of trachea** MCC
✓7th **S11.024 Puncture wound with foreign body of trachea** MCC
✓7th **S11.025 Open bite of trachea** MCC
Bite of trachea NOS
✓7th **S11.029 Unspecified open wound of trachea** MCC

✓6th **S11.03 Open wound of vocal cord**
✓7th **S11.031 Laceration without foreign body of vocal cord** MCC
✓7th **S11.032 Laceration with foreign body of vocal cord** MCC
✓7th **S11.033 Puncture wound without foreign body of vocal cord** MCC
✓7th **S11.034 Puncture wound with foreign body of vocal cord** MCC
✓7th **S11.035 Open bite of vocal cord** MCC
Bite of vocal cord NOS
✓7th **S11.039 Unspecified open wound of vocal cord** MCC

✓5th **S11.1 Open wound of thyroid gland**

CC Excl: For CC codes in subcategory S11.0, unless otherwise noted: CC with 7th character A: S11.10X-S11.15X with 7th A, S11.80X-S11.95X with 7th A, S13.4XXA, S13.8XXA, S16.1XX-S16.2XX with 7th A, S38.3XXA, T14.8-T14.91, T79.8XX-T79.9XX with 7th A

✓x7th **S11.10 Unspecified open wound of thyroid gland** CC
✓x7th **S11.11 Laceration without foreign body of thyroid gland** CC
✓x7th **S11.12 Laceration with foreign body of thyroid gland** CC
CC Excl: CC with 7th character A: S11.10-S11.15 with 7th A, S11.80-S11.95 with 7th A, S13.4XXA, S13.8XXA, S16.1X-S16.2X with 7th A, S38.3XXA, T14.8-T14.91, T79.A0X-T79.9XX with 7th A
✓x7th **S11.13 Puncture wound without foreign body of thyroid gland** CC
✓x7th **S11.14 Puncture wound with foreign body of thyroid gland** CC
CC Excl: See code: S11.12
✓x7th **S11.15 Open bite of thyroid gland** CC
Bite of thyroid gland NOS

✓5th **S11.2 Open wound of pharynx and cervical esophagus**
EXCLUDES 1 *open wound of esophagus NOS (S27.8-)*
✓x7th **S11.20 Unspecified open wound of pharynx and cervical esophagus** CC

CC Excl: For CC codes in subcategory S11.2, unless otherwise noted: CC with 7th character A: S11.20X-S11.95X with 7th A, S13.4XXA, S13.8XXA, S16.1XX-S16.2XX with 7th A, S38.3XXA, T14.8-T14.91, T79.8XX-T79.9XX with 7th A

✓x7th **S11.21 Laceration without foreign body of pharynx and cervical esophagus** CC
✓x7th **S11.22 Laceration with foreign body of pharynx and cervical esophagus** CC
CC Excl: CC with 7th character A: S11.20X-S11.95X with 7th A, S13.4XXA, S13.8XXA, S16.1XX-S16.2XX with 7th A, S38.3XXA, T14.8-T14.91, T79.A0X-T79.9XX with 7th A
✓x7th **S11.23 Puncture wound without foreign body of pharynx and cervical esophagus** CC
✓x7th **S11.24 Puncture wound with foreign body of pharynx and cervical esophagus** CC
CC Excl: CC with 7th character A: See Code: S11.22
✓x7th **S11.25 Open bite of pharynx and cervical esophagus** CC
Bite of pharynx and cervical esophagus NOS

✓5th **S11.8 Open wound of other specified parts of neck**
✓x7th **S11.80 Unspecified open wound of other specified part of neck**
✓x7th **S11.81 Laceration without foreign body of other specified part of neck**
✓x7th **S11.82 Laceration with foreign body of other specified part of neck**
✓x7th **S11.83 Puncture wound without foreign body of other specified part of neck**
✓x7th **S11.84 Puncture wound with foreign body of other specified part of neck**
✓x7th **S11.85 Open bite of other specified part of neck**
Bite of other specified part of neck NOS
EXCLUDES 1 *superficial bite of other specified part of neck (S10.87)*
✓x7th **S11.89 Other open wound of other specified part of neck**

✓5th **S11.9 Open wound of unspecified part of neck**
✓x7th **S11.90 Unspecified open wound of unspecified part of neck**
✓x7th **S11.91 Laceration without foreign body of unspecified part of neck**
✓x7th **S11.92 Laceration with foreign body of unspecified part of neck**
✓x7th **S11.93 Puncture wound without foreign body of unspecified part of neck**
✓x7th **S11.94 Puncture wound with foreign body of unspecified part of neck**
✓x7th **S11.95 Open bite of unspecified part of neck**
Bite of neck NOS
EXCLUDES 1 *superficial bite of neck (S10.97)*

✓4th **S12 Fracture of cervical vertebra and other parts of neck**

NOTE A fracture not indicated as nondisplaced or displaced should be classified to displaced.
A fracture not indicated as open or closed should be coded to closed.

INCLUDES fracture of cervical neural arch
fracture of cervical spine
fracture of cervical spinous process
fracture of cervical transverse process
fracture of cervical vertebral arch
fracture of neck

Code first any associated cervical spinal cord injury (S14.0, S14.1-)

The appropriate 7th is to be added to all codes from subcategories S12.0-S12.6.
- A initial encounter for closed fracture
- B initial encounter for open fracture
- D subsequent encounter for fracture with routine healing
- G subsequent encounter for fracture with delayed healing
- K subsequent encounter for fracture with nonunion
- S sequela

For CC/MCC codes in subcategory S12.0, unless otherwise noted: CC with 7th character A or MCC with 7th character B: M48.40X-M48.58X with 7th S, M80.08XS, M80.88XS, M84.350XS, M84.454S, M84.550S, M84.58XS, M84.650S, M99.10-M99.11, M99.15-M99.17, M99.19, S03.8XX-S03.9XX with 7th A, S12.000-S13.4XX with 7th [A, B, S], S13.8XX-S14.159 with 7th A, S16.1XXA, S22.000-S22.9XX with 7th S, S23.20X-S23.29X with 7th A, S23.9XXA, S24.109A, S24.119A, S24.139A, S24.149A, S24.159A, S29.001-S29.019 with 7th A, S29.091-S29.9XX with 7th A, S32.000-S32.9XX with 7th S, S33.30X-S33.39X with 7th A, S33.9XXA, S38.1XXA, S38.3XX-S39.013 with 7th A, S39.091-S39.94X with 7th A, T14.8-T14.91, T79.A0X-T79.9XX with 7th A

CC with 7th character K: M80.00X-M84.68X with 7th [K, P], S02.0XX-S02.92X with 7th K, S12.000-S12.691 with 7th K, S22.000-S22.9XX with 7th K, S32.000-S32.9XX with 7th K, S42.001-S42.92X with 7th [K, P], S49.001-S49.199 with 7th [K, P], S52.001-S52.92X with 7th [K, M, N, P, Q, R], S59.001-S59.299 with 7th [K, P], S62.001-S62.92X with 7th [K, P], S72.001-S72.92X with 7th [K, M, N, P, Q, R], S79.001-S79.199 with 7th [K, P], S82.001-S82.92X with 7th [K, M, N, P, Q, R], S89.001-S89.399 with 7th [K, P], S92.001-S92.919 with 7th [K, P]

✓5th **S12.0 Fracture of first cervical vertebra**
Atlas

✓6th **S12.00 Unspecified fracture of first cervical vertebra**
- 7 ✓7th **S12.000 Unspecified displaced fracture of first cervical vertebra** MCC CC
- 7 ✓7th **S12.001 Unspecified nondisplaced fracture of first cervical vertebra** MCC CC

7 ✓x7th **S12.01 Stable burst fracture of first cervical vertebra** MCC CC

7 ✓x7th **S12.02 Unstable burst fracture of first cervical vertebra** MCC CC

✓6th **S12.03 Posterior arch fracture of first cervical vertebra**
- 7 ✓7th **S12.030 Displaced posterior arch fracture of first cervical vertebra** MCC CC
- 7 ✓7th **S12.031 Nondisplaced posterior arch fracture of first cervical vertebra** MCC CC

✓6th **S12.04 Lateral mass fracture of first cervical vertebra**
- 7 ✓7th **S12.040 Displaced lateral mass fracture of first cervical vertebra** MCC CC
- 7 ✓7th **S12.041 Nondisplaced lateral mass fracture of first cervical vertebra** MCC CC

✓6th **S12.09 Other fracture of first cervical vertebra**
- 7 ✓7th **S12.090 Other displaced fracture of first cervical vertebra** MCC CC
- 7 ✓7th **S12.091 Other nondisplaced fracture of first cervical vertebra** MCC CC

✓5th **S12.1 Fracture of second cervical vertebra**
Axis

✓6th **S12.10 Unspecified fracture of second cervical vertebra**
- 7 ✓7th **S12.100 Unspecified displaced fracture of second cervical vertebra** MCC CC
- 7 ✓7th **S12.101 Unspecified nondisplaced fracture of second cervical vertebra** MCC CC

✓6th **S12.11 Type II dens fracture**
- 7 ✓7th **S12.110 Anterior displaced Type II dens fracture** MCC CC
- 7 ✓7th **S12.111 Posterior displaced Type II dens fracture** MCC CC
- 7 ✓7th **S12.112 Nondisplaced Type II dens fracture** MCC CC

✓6th **S12.12 Other dens fracture**
- 7 ✓7th **S12.120 Other displaced dens fracture** MCC CC
- 7 ✓7th **S12.121 Other nondisplaced dens fracture** MCC CC

✓6th **S12.13 Unspecified traumatic spondylolisthesis of second cervical vertebra**
- 7 ✓7th **S12.130 Unspecified traumatic displaced spondylolisthesis of second cervical vertebra** MCC CC
- 7 ✓7th **S12.131 Unspecified traumatic nondisplaced spondylolisthesis of second cervical vertebra** MCC CC

7 ✓x7th **S12.14 Type III traumatic spondylolisthesis of second cervical vertebra** MCC CC

✓6th **S12.15 Other traumatic spondylolisthesis of second cervical vertebra**
- 7 ✓7th **S12.150 Other traumatic displaced spondylolisthesis of second cervical vertebra** MCC CC
- 7 ✓7th **S12.151 Other traumatic nondisplaced spondylolisthesis of second cervical vertebra** MCC CC

✓6th **S12.19 Other fracture of second cervical vertebra**
- 7 ✓7th **S12.190 Other displaced fracture of second cervical vertebra** MCC CC
- 7 ✓7th **S12.191 Other nondisplaced fracture of second cervical vertebra** MCC CC

✓5th **S12.2 Fracture of third cervical vertebra**

✓6th **S12.20 Unspecified fracture of third cervical vertebra**
- 7 ✓7th **S12.200 Unspecified displaced fracture of third cervical vertebra** MCC CC
- 7 ✓7th **S12.201 Unspecified nondisplaced fracture of third cervical vertebra** MCC CC

✓6th **S12.23 Unspecified traumatic spondylolisthesis of third cervical vertebra**
- 7 ✓7th **S12.230 Unspecified traumatic displaced spondylolisthesis of third cervical vertebra** MCC CC
- 7 ✓7th **S12.231 Unspecified traumatic nondisplaced spondylolisthesis of third cervical vertebra** MCC CC

7 ✓x7th **S12.24 Type III traumatic spondylolisthesis of third cervical vertebra** MCC CC

✓6th **S12.25 Other traumatic spondylolisthesis of third cervical vertebra**
- 7 ✓7th **S12.250 Other traumatic displaced spondylolisthesis of third cervical vertebra** MCC CC
- 7 ✓7th **S12.251 Other traumatic nondisplaced spondylolisthesis of third cervical vertebra** MCC CC

✓6th **S12.29 Other fracture of third cervical vertebra**
- 7 ✓7th **S12.290 Other displaced fracture of third cervical vertebra** MCC CC
- 7 ✓7th **S12.291 Other nondisplaced fracture of third cervical vertebra** MCC CC

✓5th **S12.3 Fracture of fourth cervical vertebra**

✓6th **S12.30 Unspecified fracture of fourth cervical vertebra**
- 7 ✓7th **S12.300 Unspecified displaced fracture of fourth cervical vertebra** MCC CC
- 7 ✓7th **S12.301 Unspecified nondisplaced fracture of fourth cervical vertebra** MCC CC

✓6th **S12.33 Unspecified traumatic spondylolisthesis of fourth cervical vertebra**
- 7 ✓7th **S12.330 Unspecified traumatic displaced spondylolisthesis of fourth cervical vertebra** MCC CC
- 7 ✓7th **S12.331 Unspecified traumatic nondisplacedspondylolisthesis of fourth cervical vertebra** MCC CC

7 ✓x7th **S12.34 Type III traumatic spondylolisthesis of fourth cervical vertebra** MCC CC

7 HAC = Initial encounter only (7th character A, B or C) and not POA.

✓6th **S12.35 Other traumatic spondylolisthesis of fourth cervical vertebra**
7 ✓7th **S12.350 Other traumatic displaced spondylolisthesis of fourth cervical vertebra** MCC CC
7 ✓7th **S12.351 Other traumatic nondisplaced spondylolisthesis of fourth cervical vertebra** MCC CC

✓6th **S12.39 Other fracture of fourth cervical vertebra**
7 ✓7th **S12.390 Other displaced fracture of fourth cervical vertebra** MCC CC
7 ✓7th **S12.391 Other nondisplaced fracture of fourth cervical vertebra** MCC CC

✓5th **S12.4 Fracture of fifth cervical vertebra**
✓6th **S12.40 Unspecified fracture of fifth cervical vertebra**
7 ✓7th **S12.400 Unspecified displaced fracture of fifth cervical vertebra** MCC CC
7 ✓7th **S12.401 Unspecified nondisplaced fracture of fifth cervical vertebra** MCC CC

✓6th **S12.43 Unspecified traumatic spondylolisthesis of fifth cervical vertebra**
7 ✓7th **S12.430 Unspecified traumatic displaced spondylolisthesis of fifth cervical vertebra** MCC CC
7 ✓7th **S12.431 Unspecified traumatic nondisplacedspondylolisthesis of fifth cervical vertebra** MCC CC

7 ✓x7th **S12.44 Type III traumatic spondylolisthesis of fifth cervical vertebra** MCC CC

✓6th **S12.45 Other traumatic spondylolisthesis of fifth cervical vertebra**
7 ✓7th **S12.450 Other traumatic displaced spondylolisthesis of fifth cervical vertebra** MCC CC
7 ✓7th **S12.451 Other traumatic nondisplaced spondylolisthesis of fifth cervical vertebra** MCC CC

✓6th **S12.49 Other fracture of fifth cervical vertebra**
7 ✓7th **S12.490 Other displaced fracture of fifth cervical vertebra** MCC CC
7 ✓7th **S12.491 Other nondisplaced fracture of fifth cervical vertebra** MCC CC

✓5th **S12.5 Fracture of sixth cervical vertebra**
✓6th **S12.50 Unspecified fracture of sixth cervical vertebra**
7 ✓7th **S12.500 Unspecified displaced fracture of sixth cervical vertebra** MCC CC
7 ✓7th **S12.501 Unspecified nondisplaced fracture of sixth cervical vertebra** MCC CC

✓6th **S12.53 Unspecified traumatic spondylolisthesis of sixth cervical vertebra**
7 ✓7th **S12.530 Unspecified traumatic displaced spondylolisthesis of sixth cervical vertebra** MCC CC
7 ✓7th **S12.531 Unspecified traumatic nondisplaced spondylolisthesis of sixth cervical vertebra** MCC CC

7 ✓x7th **S12.54 Type III traumatic spondylolisthesis of sixth cervical vertebra** MCC CC

✓6th **S12.55 Other traumatic spondylolisthesis of sixth cervical vertebra**
7 ✓7th **S12.550 Other traumatic displaced spondylolisthesis of sixth cervical vertebra** MCC CC
7 ✓7th **S12.551 Other traumatic nondisplaced spondylolisthesis of sixth cervical vertebra** MCC CC

✓6th **S12.59 Other fracture of sixth cervical vertebra**
7 ✓7th **S12.590 Other displaced fracture of sixth cervical vertebra** MCC CC
7 ✓7th **S12.591 Other nondisplaced fracture of sixth cervical vertebra** MCC CC

✓5th **S12.6 Fracture of seventh cervical vertebra**
✓6th **S12.60 Unspecified fracture of seventh cervical vertebra**
7 ✓7th **S12.600 Unspecified displaced fracture of seventh cervical vertebra** MCC CC
7 ✓7th **S12.601 Unspecified nondisplaced fracture of seventh cervical vertebra** MCC CC

✓6th **S12.63 Unspecified traumatic spondylolisthesis of seventh cervical vertebra**
7 ✓7th **S12.630 Unspecified traumatic displaced spondylolisthesis of seventh cervical vertebra** MCC CC
7 ✓7th **S12.631 Unspecified traumatic nondisplaced spondylolisthesis of seventh cervical vertebra** MCC CC

7 ✓x7th **S12.64 Type III traumatic spondylolisthesis of seventh cervical vertebra** MCC CC

✓6th **S12.65 Other traumatic spondylolisthesis of seventh cervical vertebra**
7 ✓7th **S12.650 Other traumatic displaced spondylolisthesis of seventh cervical vertebra** MCC CC
7 ✓7th **S12.651 Other traumatic nondisplaced spondylolisthesis of seventh cervical vertebra** MCC CC

✓6th **S12.69 Other fracture of seventh cervical vertebra**
7 ✓7th **S12.690 Other displaced fracture of seventh cervical vertebra** MCC CC
7 ✓7th **S12.691 Other nondisplaced fracture of seventh cervical vertebra** MCC CC

7 ✓x7th **S12.8 Fracture of other parts of neck** MCC
Hyoid bone
Larynx
Thyroid cartilage
Trachea

The appropriate 7th is to be added to code S12.8.
A initial encounter
D subsequent encounter
S sequela

CC Excl: MCC with 7th character A: SØ3.8XX-SØ3.9XX with 7th A, S12.8XX with 7th A, S29.Ø11-S29.Ø19 with 7th A, S38.3XX-S39.Ø13 with 7th A, T14.8-T14.91, T79.AØX-T79.9XX with 7th A

7 ✓x7th **S12.9 Fracture of neck, unspecified** CC
Fracture of cervical spine NOS
Fracture of cervical vertebra NOS
Fracture of neck NOS

The appropriate 7th is to be added to code S12.9.
A initial encounter
D subsequent encounter
S sequela

CC Excl: M48.4ØX-M48.58X with 7th S, M8Ø.Ø8XS, M8Ø.88XS, M84.35ØS, M84.454S, M84.55ØS, M84.58XS, M84.65ØS, M99.1Ø-M99.11, M99.15-M99.17, M99.19, SØ3.8XX-SØ3.9XX with 7th A, S12.ØØØ-S13.4XX with 7th [A, B, S], S13.8XX-S14.159 with 7th A, S16.1XXA, S22.ØØØ-S22.9XX with 7th S, S23.2ØX-S23.29X with 7th A, S23.9XXA, S24.1Ø9A, S24.119A, S24.139A, S24.149A, S24.159A, S29.ØØ1-S29.Ø19 with 7th A, S29.Ø91-S29.9XX with 7th A, S32.ØØØ-S32.9XX with 7th S, S33.3ØX-S33.39X with 7th A, S33.9XXA, S38.1XXA, S38.3XX-S39.Ø13 with 7th A, S39.Ø91-S39.94X with 7th A, T14.8-T14.91, T79.AØX-T79.9XX with 7th A

✓4th **S13 Dislocation and sprain of joints and ligaments at neck level**
INCLUDES avulsion of joint or ligament at neck level
laceration of cartilage, joint or ligament at neck level
sprain of cartilage, joint or ligament at neck level
traumatic hemarthrosis of joint or ligament at neck level
traumatic rupture of joint or ligament at neck level
traumatic subluxation of joint or ligament at neck level
traumatic tear of joint or ligament at neck level

Code also any associated open wound
EXCLUDES 2 *strain of muscle or tendon at neck level (S16.1)*

The appropriate 7th is to be added to each code from category S13.
A initial encounter
D subsequent encounter
S sequela

7 HAC = Initial encounter only (7th character A, B or C) and not POA.

7 √x7th **S13.0 Traumatic rupture of cervical intervertebral disc** CC
EXCLUDES 1 *rupture or displacement (nontraumatic) of cervical intervertebral disc NOS (M50.-)*
CC Excl: CC with 7th character A: M99.10-M99.11, S03.8XX-S03.9XX with 7th A, S12.000-S12.691 with 7th [A, B], S12.9XX-S13.4XX with 7th A, S13.8XXA, S14.0XX-S14.108 with 7th A, S14.111-S14.118 with 7th A, S14.121-S14.128 with 7th A, S14.131-S14.138 with 7th A, S14.141-S14.148 with 7th A, S14.151-S14.158 with 7th A, S16.1XXA, S29.011-S29.019 with 7th A, S38.3XX-S39.013 with 7th A, T14.8-T14.91, T79.A0X-T79.9XX with 7th A

√5th **S13.1 Subluxation and dislocation of cervical vertebrae**
Code also any associated:
open wound of neck (S11.-)
spinal cord injury (S14.1-)
EXCLUDES 2 *fracture of cervical vertebrae (S12.0--S12.3-)*

√6th **S13.10 Subluxation and dislocation of unspecified cervical vertebrae**
7 √7th **S13.100 Subluxation of unspecified cervical vertebrae** CC
7 √7th **S13.101 Dislocation of unspecified cervical vertebrae** CC

√6th **S13.11 Subluxation and dislocation of C0/C1 cervical vertebrae**
Subluxation and dislocation of atlantooccipital joint
Subluxation and dislocation of atloidooccipital joint
Subluxation and dislocation of occipitoatloid joint
7 √7th **S13.110 Subluxation of C0/C1 cervical vertebrae** CC
7 √7th **S13.111 Dislocation of C0/C1 cervical vertebrae** CC

√6th **S13.12 Subluxation and dislocation of C1/C2 cervical vertebrae**
Subluxation and dislocation of atlantoaxial joint
7 √7th **S13.120 Subluxation of C1/C2 cervical vertebrae** CC
7 √7th **S13.121 Dislocation of C1/C2 cervical vertebrae** CC

√6th **S13.13 Subluxation and dislocation of C2/C3 cervical vertebrae**
7 √7th **S13.130 Subluxation of C2/C3 cervical vertebrae** CC
7 √7th **S13.131 Dislocation of C2/C3 cervical vertebrae** CC

√6th **S13.14 Subluxation and dislocation of C3/C4 cervical vertebrae**
7 √7th **S13.140 Subluxation of C3/C4 cervical vertebrae** CC
7 √7th **S13.141 Dislocation of C3/C4 cervical vertebrae** CC

√6th **S13.15 Subluxation and dislocation of C4/C5 cervical vertebrae**
7 √7th **S13.150 Subluxation of C4/C5 cervical vertebrae** CC
7 √7th **S13.151 Dislocation of C4/C5 cervical vertebrae** CC

√6th **S13.16 Subluxation and dislocation of C5/C6 cervical vertebrae**
7 √7th **S13.160 Subluxation of C5/C6 cervical vertebrae** CC
7 √7th **S13.161 Dislocation of C5/C6 cervical vertebrae** CC

√6th **S13.17 Subluxation and dislocation of C6/C7 cervical vertebrae**
7 √7th **S13.170 Subluxation of C6/C7 cervical vertebrae** CC
7 √7th **S13.171 Dislocation of C6/C7 cervical vertebrae** CC

√6th **S13.18 Subluxation and dislocation of C7/T1 cervical vertebrae**
7 √7th **S13.180 Subluxation of C7/T1 cervical vertebrae** CC
7 √7th **S13.181 Dislocation of C7/T1 cervical vertebrae** CC

√5th **S13.2 Dislocation of other and unspecified parts of neck**
7 **S13.20 Dislocation of unspecified parts of neck** CC
7 **S13.29 Dislocation of other parts of neck** CC

√x7th **S13.4 Sprain of ligaments of cervical spine**
Sprain of anterior longitudinal (ligament), cervical
Sprain of atlanto-axial (joints)
Sprain of atlanto-occipital (joints)
Whiplash injury of cervical spine

√x7th **S13.5 Sprain of thyroid region**
Sprain of cricoarytenoid (joint) (ligament)
Sprain of cricothyroid (joint) (ligament)
Sprain of thyroid cartilage

√x7th **S13.8 Sprain of joints and ligaments of other parts of neck**
√x7th **S13.9 Sprain of joints and ligaments of unspecified parts of neck**

√4th **S14 Injury of nerves and spinal cord at neck level**
NOTE Code to highest level of cervical cord injury.
Code also any associated:
fracture of cervical vertebra (S12.0- – S12.6-)
open wound of neck (S11.-)
transient paralysis (R29.5)

The appropriate 7th is to be added to each code from category S14.
A initial encounter
D subsequent encounter
S sequela

CC Excl: For MCC codes in category S14, unless otherwise noted: MCC with 7th character A: M48.40X-M48.58X with 7th S, M80.08XS, M80.88XS, M84.350S, M84.454S, M84.550S, M84.58XS, M84.650S, M99.10-M99.11, M99.15-M99.17, M99.19, S12.000-S13.29X with 7th [A, B, S], S13.9XX-S14.159 with 7th A, S22.000-S22.9XX with 7th S, S23.20X-S23.29X with 7th A, S23.9XA, S24.109XA, S24.119A, S24.139A, S24.149A, S24.159A, S29.001-S29.009 with 7th A, S29.091-S29.9XX with 7th A, S32.000-S32.9XX with 7th S, S33.30X-S33.39X with 7th A, S33.9XXA, S38.1XA, S39.001-S39.003 with 7th A, S39.091-S39.94X with 7th A, T14.8-T14.91, T79.A0X-T79.9XX with 7th A

√x7th **S14.0 Concussion and edema of cervical spinal cord** MCC
√5th **S14.1 Other and unspecified injuries of cervical spinal cord**
√6th **S14.10 Unspecified injury of cervical spinal cord**
7 √7th **S14.101 Unspecified injury at C1 level of cervical spinal cord** MCC
7 √7th **S14.102 Unspecified injury at C2 level of cervical spinal cord** MCC
7 √7th **S14.103 Unspecified injury at C3 level of cervical spinal cord** MCC
7 √7th **S14.104 Unspecified injury at C4 level of cervical spinal cord** MCC
7 √7th **S14.105 Unspecified injury at C5 level of cervical spinal cord** MCC
7 √7th **S14.106 Unspecified injury at C6 level of cervical spinal cord** MCC
7 √7th **S14.107 Unspecified injury at C7 level of cervical spinal cord** MCC
√7th **S14.108 Unspecified injury at C8 level of cervical spinal cord** MCC
7 √7th **S14.109 Unspecified injury at unspecified level of cervical spinal cord**
Injury of cervical spinal cord NOS
CC Excl: No excl

√6th **S14.11 Complete lesion of cervical spinal cord**
7 √7th **S14.111 Complete lesion at C1 level of cervical spinal cord** MCC
7 √7th **S14.112 Complete lesion at C2 level of cervical spinal cord** MCC
7 √7th **S14.113 Complete lesion at C3 level of cervical spinal cord** MCC
7 √7th **S14.114 Complete lesion at C4 level of cervical spinal cord** MCC
7 √7th **S14.115 Complete lesion at C5 level of cervical spinal cord** MCC
7 √7th **S14.116 Complete lesion at C6 level of cervical spinal cord** MCC
7 √7th **S14.117 Complete lesion at C7 level of cervical spinal cord** MCC
√7th **S14.118 Complete lesion at C8 level of cervical spinal cord** MCC
√7th **S14.119 Complete lesion at unspecified level of cervical spinal cord**

7 HAC = Initial encounter only (7th character A, B or C) and not POA.

- ✓6th **S14.12 Central cord syndrome of cervical spinal cord**
  - 7 ✓7th **S14.121 Central cord syndrome at C1 level of cervical spinal cord** MCC
  - 7 ✓7th **S14.122 Central cord syndrome at C2 level of cervical spinal cord** MCC
  - 7 ✓7th **S14.123 Central cord syndrome at C3 level of cervical spinal cord** MCC
  - 7 ✓7th **S14.124 Central cord syndrome at C4 level of cervical spinal cord** MCC
  - 7 ✓7th **S14.125 Central cord syndrome at C5 level of cervical spinal cord** MCC
  - 7 ✓7th **S14.126 Central cord syndrome at C6 level of cervical spinal cord** MCC
  - 7 ✓7th **S14.127 Central cord syndrome at C7 level of cervical spinal cord** MCC
  - ✓7th **S14.128 Central cord syndrome at C8 level of cervical spinal cord** MCC
  - ✓7th **S14.129 Central cord syndrome at unspecified level of cervical spinal cord**
- ✓6th **S14.13 Anterior cord syndrome of cervical spinal cord**
  - 7 ✓7th **S14.131 Anterior cord syndrome at C1 level of cervical spinal cord** MCC
  - 7 ✓7th **S14.132 Anterior cord syndrome at C2 level of cervical spinal cord** MCC
  - 7 ✓7th **S14.133 Anterior cord syndrome at C3 level of cervical spinal cord** MCC
  - 7 ✓7th **S14.134 Anterior cord syndrome at C4 level of cervical spinal cord** MCC
  - 7 ✓7th **S14.135 Anterior cord syndrome at C5 level of cervical spinal cord** MCC
  - 7 ✓7th **S14.136 Anterior cord syndrome at C6 level of cervical spinal cord** MCC
  - 7 ✓7th **S14.137 Anterior cord syndrome at C7 level of cervical spinal cord** MCC
  - ✓7th **S14.138 Anterior cord syndrome at C8 level of cervical spinal cord** MCC
  - ✓7th **S14.139 Anterior cord syndrome at unspecified level of cervical spinal cord**
- ✓6th **S14.14 Brown-Séquard syndrome of cervical spinal cord**
  - ✓7th **S14.141 Brown-Séquard syndrome at C1 level of cervical spinal cord** MCC
  - ✓7th **S14.142 Brown-Séquard syndrome at C2 level of cervical spinal cord** MCC
  - ✓7th **S14.143 Brown-Séquard syndrome at C3 level of cervical spinal cord** MCC
  - ✓7th **S14.144 Brown-Séquard syndrome at C4 level of cervical spinal cord** MCC
  - ✓7th **S14.145 Brown-Séquard syndrome at C5 level of cervical spinal cord** MCC
  - ✓7th **S14.146 Brown-Séquard syndrome at C6 level of cervical spinal cord** MCC
  - ✓7th **S14.147 Brown-Séquard syndrome at C7 level of cervical spinal cord** MCC
  - ✓7th **S14.148 Brown-Séquard syndrome at C8 level of cervical spinal cord** MCC
  - ✓7th **S14.149 Brown-Séquard syndrome at unspecified level of cervical spinal cord**
- ✓6th **S14.15 Other incomplete lesions of cervical spinal cord**
  - Incomplete lesion of cervical spinal cord NOS
  - Posterior cord syndrome of cervical spinal cord
  - 7 ✓7th **S14.151 Other incomplete lesion at C1 level of cervical spinal cord** MCC
  - 7 ✓7th **S14.152 Other incomplete lesion at C2 level of cervical spinal cord** MCC
  - 7 ✓7th **S14.153 Other incomplete lesion at C3 level of cervical spinal cord** MCC
  - 7 ✓7th **S14.154 Other incomplete lesion at C4 level of cervical spinal cord** MCC
  - 7 ✓7th **S14.155 Other incomplete lesion at C5 level of cervical spinal cord** MCC
  - 7 ✓7th **S14.156 Other incomplete lesion at C6 level of cervical spinal cord** MCC
  - 7 ✓7th **S14.157 Other incomplete lesion at C7 level of cervical spinal cord** MCC
  - ✓7th **S14.158 Other incomplete lesion at C8 level of cervical spinal cord** MCC
  - ✓7th **S14.159 Other incomplete lesion at unspecified level of cervical spinal cord**
- ✓x7th **S14.2 Injury of nerve root of cervical spine**
- ✓x7th **S14.3 Injury of brachial plexus**
- ✓x7th **S14.4 Injury of peripheral nerves of neck**
- ✓x7th **S14.5 Injury of cervical sympathetic nerves**
- ✓x7th **S14.8 Injury of other specified nerves of neck**
- ✓x7th **S14.9 Injury of unspecified nerves of neck**

✓4th S15 Injury of blood vessels at neck level

Code also any associated open wound (S11.-)

> The appropriate 7th is to be added to each code from category S15.
> A initial encounter
> D subsequent encounter
> S sequela

- ✓5th **S15.0 Injury of carotid artery of neck**
  - Injury of carotid artery (common) (external) (internal, extracranial portion)
  - Injury of carotid artery NOS
  - EXCLUDES 1 *injury of internal carotid artery, intracranial portion (S06.8)*

  > **CC Excl: For CC codes in subcategory S15, unless otherwise noted: CC with 7th character A:** S09.0XXA, S15.009A, S15.029A, S15.099-S15.199 with 7th A, S15.8XX-S15.9XX with 7th A, T14.8-T14.91, T79.A0X-T79.9XX with 7th A

  - ✓6th **S15.00 Unspecified injury of carotid artery**
    - ✓7th **S15.001 Unspecified injury of right carotid artery** CC
    - ✓7th **S15.002 Unspecified injury of left carotid artery** CC
    - ✓7th **S15.009 Unspecified injury of unspecified carotid artery** CC
  - ✓6th **S15.01 Minor laceration of carotid artery**
    - Incomplete transection of carotid artery
    - Laceration of carotid artery NOS
    - Superficial laceration of carotid artery
    - ✓7th **S15.011 Minor laceration of right carotid artery** CC
    - ✓7th **S15.012 Minor laceration of left carotid artery** CC
    - ✓7th **S15.019 Minor laceration of unspecified carotid artery** CC
  - ✓6th **S15.02 Major laceration of carotid artery**
    - Complete transection of carotid artery
    - Traumatic rupture of carotid artery
    - ✓7th **S15.021 Major laceration of right carotid artery** CC
    - ✓7th **S15.022 Major laceration of left carotid artery** CC
    - ✓7th **S15.029 Major laceration of unspecified carotid artery** CC
  - ✓6th **S15.09 Other specified injury of carotid artery**
    - ✓7th **S15.091 Other specified injury of right carotid artery** CC
    - ✓7th **S15.092 Other specified injury of left carotid artery** CC
    - ✓7th **S15.099 Other specified injury of unspecified carotid artery** CC
- ✓5th **S15.1 Injury of vertebral artery**

  > **CC Excl: For CC codes in subcategory S15.1, unless otherwise noted: CC with 7th character A:** S09.0XXA, S15.101-S15.199 with 7th A, S15.8XX-S15.9XX with 7th A, T14.8-T14.91, T79.A0X-T79.9XX with 7th A

  - ✓6th **S15.10 Unspecified injury of vertebral artery**
    - ✓7th **S15.101 Unspecified injury of right vertebral artery** CC
    - ✓7th **S15.102 Unspecified injury of left vertebral artery** CC
    - ✓7th **S15.109 Unspecified injury of unspecified vertebral artery** CC

7 HAC = Initial encounter only (7th character A, B or C) and not POA.

✓6th **S15.11 Minor laceration of vertebral artery**
Incomplete transection of vertebral artery
Laceration of vertebral artery NOS
Superficial laceration of vertebral artery

✓7th **S15.111 Minor laceration of right vertebral artery** CC
✓7th **S15.112 Minor laceration of left vertebral artery** CC
✓7th **S15.119 Minor laceration of unspecified vertebral artery** CC

✓6th **S15.12 Major laceration of vertebral artery**
Complete transection of vertebral artery
Traumatic rupture of vertebral artery

✓7th **S15.121 Major laceration of right vertebral artery** CC
✓7th **S15.122 Major laceration of left vertebral artery** CC
✓7th **S15.129 Major laceration of unspecified vertebral artery** CC

✓6th **S15.19 Other specified injury of vertebral artery**
✓7th **S15.191 Other specified injury of right vertebral artery** CC
✓7th **S15.192 Other specified injury of left vertebral artery** CC
✓7th **S15.199 Other specified injury of unspecified vertebral artery** CC

✓5th **S15.2 Injury of external jugular vein**

CC Excl: For CC codes in subcategory S15.2, unless otherwise noted: See code: S15.1

✓6th **S15.20 Unspecified injury of external jugular vein**
✓7th **S15.201 Unspecified injury of right external jugular vein** CC
✓7th **S15.202 Unspecified injury of left external jugular vein** CC
✓7th **S15.209 Unspecified injury of unspecified external jugular vein** CC

✓6th **S15.21 Minor laceration of external jugular vein**
Incomplete transection of external jugular vein
Laceration of external jugular vein NOS
Superficial laceration of external jugular vein

✓7th **S15.211 Minor laceration of right external jugular vein** CC
✓7th **S15.212 Minor laceration of left external jugular vein** CC
✓7th **S15.219 Minor laceration of unspecified external jugular vein** CC

✓6th **S15.22 Major laceration of external jugular vein**
Complete transection of external jugular vein
Traumatic rupture of external jugular vein

✓7th **S15.221 Major laceration of right external jugular vein** CC
✓7th **S15.222 Major laceration of left external jugular vein** CC
✓7th **S15.229 Major laceration of unspecified external jugular vein** CC

✓6th **S15.29 Other specified injury of external jugular vein**
✓7th **S15.291 Other specified injury of right external jugular vein** CC
✓7th **S15.292 Other specified injury of left external jugular vein** CC
✓7th **S15.299 Other specified injury of unspecified external jugular vein** CC

✓5th **S15.3 Injury of internal jugular vein**

CC Excl: For CC codes in subcategory S15.3, unless otherwise noted: See code: S15.1

✓6th **S15.30 Unspecified injury of internal jugular vein**
✓7th **S15.301 Unspecified injury of right internal jugular vein** CC
✓7th **S15.302 Unspecified injury of left internal jugular vein** CC
✓7th **S15.309 Unspecified injury of unspecified internal jugular vein** CC

✓6th **S15.31 Minor laceration of internal jugular vein**
Incomplete transection of internal jugular vein
Laceration of internal jugular vein NOS
Superficial laceration of internal jugular vein

✓7th **S15.311 Minor laceration of right internal jugular vein** CC
✓7th **S15.312 Minor laceration of left internal jugular vein** CC
✓7th **S15.319 Minor laceration of unspecified internal jugular vein** CC

✓6th **S15.32 Major laceration of internal jugular vein**
Complete transection of internal jugular vein
Traumatic rupture of internal jugular vein

✓7th **S15.321 Major laceration of right internal jugular vein** CC
✓7th **S15.322 Major laceration of left internal jugular vein** CC
✓7th **S15.329 Major laceration of unspecified internal jugular vein** CC

✓6th **S15.39 Other specified injury of internal jugular vein**
✓7th **S15.391 Other specified injury of right internal jugular vein** CC
✓7th **S15.392 Other specified injury of left internal jugular vein** CC
✓7th **S15.399 Other specified injury of unspecified internal jugular vein** CC

✓x7th **S15.8 Injury of other specified blood vessels at neck level** CC
CC Excl: See code: S15.1

✓x7th **S15.9 Injury of unspecified blood vessel at neck level** CC
CC Excl: See code: S15.1

✓4th **S16 Injury of muscle, fascia and tendon at neck level**
Code also any associated open wound (S11.-)
EXCLUDES 2 *sprain of joint or ligament at neck level (S13.9)*

The appropriate 7th is to be added to each code from category S16.
A initial encounter
D subsequent encounter
S sequela

✓x7th **S16.1 Strain of muscle, fascia and tendon at neck level**
✓x7th **S16.2 Laceration of muscle, fascia and tendon at neck level**
✓x7th **S16.8 Other specified injury of muscle, fascia and tendon at neck level**
✓x7th **S16.9 Unspecified injury of muscle, fascia and tendon at neck level**

✓4th **S17 Crushing injury of neck**
Use additional code for all associated injuries, such as:
injury of blood vessels (S15.-)
open wound of neck (S11.-)
spinal cord injury (S14.0, S14.1-)
vertebral fracture (S12.0- – S12.3-)

The appropriate 7th is to be added to each code from category S17.
A initial encounter
D subsequent encounter
S sequela

CC Excl: For CC codes in category S17, unless otherwise noted:
CC with 7th character A: S01.90X-S02.92X with 7th A, S07.0XX-S07.9XX with 7th A, S08.89X-S09.19X with 7th A, S09.8XX-S09.90X with 7th A, S09.92X-S09.93X with 7th A, S16.8XX-S19.9XX with 7th A, T14.8-T14.91, T79.A0X-T79.9XX with 7th A

7 ✓x7th **S17.0 Crushing injury of larynx and trachea** CC
7 ✓x7th **S17.8 Crushing injury of other specified parts of neck** CC
7 ✓x7th **S17.9 Crushing injury of neck, part unspecified** CC

✓4th **S19 Other specified and unspecified injuries of neck**

The appropriate 7th is to be added to each code from category S19.
A initial encounter
D subsequent encounter
S sequela

✓5th **S19.8 Other specified injuries of neck**
✓x7th **S19.80 Other specified injuries of unspecified part of neck**
✓x7th **S19.81 Other specified injuries of larynx**

7 HAC = Initial encounter only (7th character A, B or C) and not POA.

✓x7th **S19.82 Other specified injuries of cervical trachea**
EXCLUDES 2 *other specified injury of thoracic trachea (S27.5-)*

✓x7th **S19.83 Other specified injuries of vocal cord**

✓x7th **S19.84 Other specified injuries of thyroid gland**

✓x7th **S19.85 Other specified injuries of pharynx and cervical esophagus**

✓x7th **S19.89 Other specified injuries of other specified part of neck**

✓x7th **S19.9 Unspecified injury of neck**

Injuries to the thorax (S20-S29)

INCLUDES injuries of breast
injuries of chest (wall)
injuries of interscapular area

EXCLUDES 2 *burns and corrosions (T20-T32)*
effects of foreign body in bronchus (T17.5)
effects of foreign body in esophagus (T18.1)
effects of foreign body in lung (T17.8)
effects of foreign body in trachea (T17.4)
frostbite (T33-T34)
injuries of axilla
injuries of clavicle
injuries of scapular region
injuries of shoulder
insect bite or sting, venomous (T63.4)

✓4th **S20 Superficial injury of thorax**

The appropriate 7th is to be added to each code from category S20.
A initial encounter
D subsequent encounter
S sequela

✓5th **S20.0 Contusion of breast**

✓x7th **S20.00 Contusion of breast, unspecified breast**

✓x7th **S20.01 Contusion of right breast**

✓x7th **S20.02 Contusion of left breast**

✓5th **S20.1 Other and unspecified superficial injuries of breast**

✓6th **S20.10 Unspecified superficial injuries of breast**

✓7th **S20.101 Unspecified superficial injuries of breast, right breast**

✓7th **S20.102 Unspecified superficial injuries of breast, left breast**

✓7th **S20.109 Unspecified superficial injuries of breast, unspecified breast**

✓6th **S20.11 Abrasion of breast**

✓7th **S20.111 Abrasion of breast, right breast**

✓7th **S20.112 Abrasion of breast, left breast**

✓7th **S20.119 Abrasion of breast, unspecified breast**

✓6th **S20.12 Blister (nonthermal) of breast**

✓7th **S20.121 Blister (nonthermal) of breast, right breast**

✓7th **S20.122 Blister (nonthermal) of breast, left breast**

✓7th **S20.129 Blister (nonthermal) of breast, unspecified breast**

✓6th **S20.14 External constriction of part of breast**

✓7th **S20.141 External constriction of part of breast, right breast**

✓7th **S20.142 External constriction of part of breast, left breast**

✓7th **S20.149 External constriction of part of breast, unspecified breast**

✓6th **S20.15 Superficial foreign body of breast**
Splinter in the breast

✓7th **S20.151 Superficial foreign body of breast, right breast**

✓7th **S20.152 Superficial foreign body of breast, left breast**

✓7th **S20.159 Superficial foreign body of breast, unspecified breast**

✓6th **S20.16 Insect bite (nonvenomous) of breast**

✓7th **S20.161 Insect bite (nonvenomous) of breast, right breast**

✓7th **S20.162 Insect bite (nonvenomous) of breast, left breast**

✓7th **S20.169 Insect bite (nonvenomous) of breast, unspecified breast**

✓6th **S20.17 Other superficial bite of breast**
EXCLUDES 1 *open bite of breast (S21.05-)*

✓7th **S20.171 Other superficial bite of breast, right breast**

✓7th **S20.172 Other superficial bite of breast, left breast**

✓7th **S20.179 Other superficial bite of breast, unspecified breast**

✓5th **S20.2 Contusion of thorax**

✓x7th **S20.20 Contusion of thorax, unspecified**

✓6th **S20.21 Contusion of front wall of thorax**

✓7th **S20.211 Contusion of right front wall of thorax**

✓7th **S20.212 Contusion of left front wall of thorax**

✓7th **S20.219 Contusion of unspecified front wall of thorax**

✓6th **S20.22 Contusion of back wall of thorax**

✓7th **S20.221 Contusion of right back wall of thorax**

✓7th **S20.222 Contusion of left back wall of thorax**

✓7th **S20.229 Contusion of unspecified back wall of thorax**

✓5th **S20.3 Other and unspecified superficial injuries of front wall of thorax**

✓6th **S20.30 Unspecified superficial injuries of front wall of thorax**

✓7th **S20.301 Unspecified superficial injuries of right front wall of thorax**

✓7th **S20.302 Unspecified superficial injuries of left front wall of thorax**

✓7th **S20.309 Unspecified superficial injuries of unspecified front wall of thorax**

✓6th **S20.31 Abrasion of front wall of thorax**

✓7th **S20.311 Abrasion of right front wall of thorax**

✓7th **S20.312 Abrasion of left front wall of thorax**

✓7th **S20.319 Abrasion of unspecified front wall of thorax**

✓6th **S20.32 Blister (nonthermal) of front wall of thorax**

✓7th **S20.321 Blister (nonthermal) of right front wall of thorax**

✓7th **S20.322 Blister (nonthermal) of left front wall of thorax**

✓7th **S20.329 Blister (nonthermal) of unspecified front wall of thorax**

✓6th **S20.34 External constriction of front wall of thorax**

✓7th **S20.341 External constriction of right front wall of thorax**

✓7th **S20.342 External constriction of left front wall of thorax**

✓7th **S20.349 External constriction of unspecified front wall of thorax**

✓6th **S20.35 Superficial foreign body of front wall of thorax**
Splinter in front wall of thorax

✓7th **S20.351 Superficial foreign body of right front wall of thorax**

✓7th **S20.352 Superficial foreign body of left front wall of thorax**

✓7th **S20.359 Superficial foreign body of unspecified front wall of thorax**

✓6th **S20.36 Insect bite (nonvenomous) of front wall of thorax**

✓7th **S20.361 Insect bite (nonvenomous) of right front wall of thorax**

✓7th **S20.362 Insect bite (nonvenomous) of left front wall of thorax**

✓7th **S20.369 Insect bite (nonvenomous) of unspecified front wall of thorax**

✓6th **S20.37 Other superficial bite of front wall of thorax**
EXCLUDES 1 *open bite of front wall of thorax (S21.14)*

✓7th **S20.371 Other superficial bite of right front wall of thorax**

✓7th **S20.372 Other superficial bite of left front wall of thorax**

✓7th **S20.379 Other superficial bite of unspecified front wall of thorax**

✓5th **S20.4 Other and unspecified superficial injuries of back wall of thorax**

✓6th **S20.40 Unspecified superficial injuries of back wall of thorax**

✓7th **S20.401 Unspecified superficial injuries of right back wall of thorax**

✓7th **S20.402 Unspecified superficial injuries of left back wall of thorax**

✓7th **S20.409 Unspecified superficial injuries of unspecified back wall of thorax**

✓6th **S20.41 Abrasion of back wall of thorax**

✓7th **S20.411 Abrasion of right back wall of thorax**

✓7th **S20.412 Abrasion of left back wall of thorax**

✓7th **S20.419 Abrasion of unspecified back wall of thorax**

✓6th **S20.42 Blister (nonthermal) of back wall of thorax**

✓7th **S20.421 Blister (nonthermal) of right back wall of thorax**

✓7th **S20.422 Blister (nonthermal) of left back wall of thorax**

✓7th **S20.429 Blister (nonthermal) of unspecified back wall of thorax**

✓6th **S20.44 External constriction of back wall of thorax**

✓7th **S20.441 External constriction of right back wall of thorax**

✓7th **S20.442 External constriction of left back wall of thorax**

✓7th **S20.449 External constriction of unspecified back wall of thorax**

✓6th **S20.45 Superficial foreign body of back wall of thorax**

Splinter of back wall of thorax

✓7th **S20.451 Superficial foreign body of right back wall of thorax**

✓7th **S20.452 Superficial foreign body of left back wall of thorax**

✓7th **S20.459 Superficial foreign body of unspecified back wall of thorax**

✓6th **S20.46 Insect bite (nonvenomous) of back wall of thorax**

✓7th **S20.461 Insect bite (nonvenomous) of right back wall of thorax**

✓7th **S20.462 Insect bite (nonvenomous) of left back wall of thorax**

✓7th **S20.469 Insect bite (nonvenomous) of unspecified back wall of thorax**

✓6th **S20.47 Other superficial bite of back wall of thorax**

EXCLUDES 1 *open bite of back wall of thorax (S21.24)*

✓7th **S20.471 Other superficial bite of right back wall of thorax**

✓7th **S20.472 Other superficial bite of left back wall of thorax**

✓7th **S20.479 Other superficial bite of unspecified back wall of thorax**

✓5th **S20.9 Superficial injury of unspecified parts of thorax**

EXCLUDES 1 *contusion of thorax NOS (S20.20)*

✓x7th **S20.90 Unspecified superficial injury of unspecified parts of thorax**

Superficial injury of thoracic wall NOS

✓x7th **S20.91 Abrasion of unspecified parts of thorax**

✓x7th **S20.92 Blister (nonthermal) of unspecified parts of thorax**

✓x7th **S20.94 External constriction of unspecified parts of thorax**

✓x7th **S20.95 Superficial foreign body of unspecified parts of thorax**

Splinter in thorax NOS

✓x7th **S20.96 Insect bite (nonvenomous) of unspecified parts of thorax**

✓x7th **S20.97 Other superficial bite of unspecified parts of thorax**

EXCLUDES 1 *open bite of thorax NOS (S21.95)*

✓4th **S21 Open wound of thorax**

Code also any associated injury, such as:

- injury of heart (S26.-)
- injury of intrathoracic organs (S27.-)
- rib fracture (S22.3-, S22.4-)
- spinal cord injury (S24.0-, S24.1-)
- traumatic hemopneumothorax (S27.3)
- traumatic hemothorax (S27.1)
- traumatic pneumothorax (S27.0)
- wound infection

EXCLUDES 1 *traumatic amputation (partial) of thorax (S28.1)*

The appropriate 7th is to be added to each code from category S21.

A initial encounter
D subsequent encounter
S sequela

✓5th **S21.0 Open wound of breast**

✓6th **S21.00 Unspecified open wound of breast**

✓7th **S21.001 Unspecified open wound of right breast**

✓7th **S21.002 Unspecified open wound of left breast**

✓7th **S21.009 Unspecified open wound of unspecified breast**

✓6th **S21.01 Laceration without foreign body of breast**

✓7th **S21.011 Laceration without foreign body of right breast**

✓7th **S21.012 Laceration without foreign body of left breast**

✓7th **S21.019 Laceration without foreign body of unspecified breast**

✓6th **S21.02 Laceration with foreign body of breast**

✓7th **S21.021 Laceration with foreign body of right breast**

✓7th **S21.022 Laceration with foreign body of left breast**

✓7th **S21.029 Laceration with foreign body of unspecified breast**

✓6th **S21.03 Puncture wound without foreign body of breast**

✓7th **S21.031 Puncture wound without foreign body of right breast**

✓7th **S21.032 Puncture wound without foreign body of left breast**

✓7th **S21.039 Puncture wound without foreign body of unspecified breast**

✓6th **S21.04 Puncture wound with foreign body of breast**

✓7th **S21.041 Puncture wound with foreign body of right breast**

✓7th **S21.042 Puncture wound with foreign body of left breast**

✓7th **S21.049 Puncture wound with foreign body of unspecified breast**

✓6th **S21.05 Open bite of breast**

Bite of breast NOS

EXCLUDES 1 *superficial bite of breast (S20.17)*

✓7th **S21.051 Open bite of right breast**

✓7th **S21.052 Open bite of left breast**

✓7th **S21.059 Open bite of unspecified breast**

✓5th **S21.1 Open wound of front wall of thorax without penetration into thoracic cavity**

Open wound of chest without penetration into thoracic cavity

CC Excl: For CC codes in subcategory S21.1, unless otherwise noted: CC with 7th character A: S21.101-S21.159 with 7th A, S21.301-S21.95 with 7th A, S23.3XXA, S23.8XXA, S27.50X-S27.69X with 7th A, S27.892-S27.9XX with 7th A, S28.1XXA, S29.021A, S29.029A, S38.3XXA, T14.8-T14.91, T79.7XX-T79.9XX with 7th A

✓6th **S21.10 Unspecified open wound of front wall of thorax without penetration into thoracic cavity**

✓7th **S21.101 Unspecified open wound of right front wall of thorax without penetration into thoracic cavity** CC

✓7th **S21.102 Unspecified open wound of left front wall of thorax without penetration into thoracic cavity** CC

✓7th **S21.109 Unspecified open wound of unspecified front wall of thorax without penetration into thoracic cavity** CC

6th **S21.11** **Laceration without foreign body of front wall of thorax without penetration into thoracic cavity**

7th **S21.111** **Laceration without foreign body of right front wall of thorax without penetration into thoracic cavity** CC

7th **S21.112** **Laceration without foreign body of left front wall of thorax without penetration into thoracic cavity** CC

7th **S21.119** **Laceration without foreign body of unspecified front wall of thorax without penetration into thoracic cavity** CC

6th **S21.12** **Laceration with foreign body of front wall of thorax without penetration into thoracic cavity**

7th **S21.121** **Laceration with foreign body of right front wall of thorax without penetration into thoracic cavity** CC

7th **S21.122** **Laceration with foreign body of left front wall of thorax without penetration into thoracic cavity** CC

7th **S21.129** **Laceration with foreign body of unspecified front wall of thorax without penetration into thoracic cavity** CC

6th **S21.13** **Puncture wound without foreign body of front wall of thorax without penetration into thoracic cavity**

7th **S21.131** **Puncture wound without foreign body of right front wall of thorax without penetration into thoracic cavity** CC

7th **S21.132** **Puncture wound without foreign body of left front wall of thorax without penetration into thoracic cavity** CC

7th **S21.139** **Puncture wound without foreign body of unspecified front wall of thorax without penetration into thoracic cavity** CC

6th **S21.14** **Puncture wound with foreign body of front wall of thorax without penetration into thoracic cavity**

7th **S21.141** **Puncture wound with foreign body of right front wall of thorax without penetration into thoracic cavity** CC

7th **S21.142** **Puncture wound with foreign body of left front wall of thorax without penetration into thoracic cavity** CC

7th **S21.149** **Puncture wound with foreign body of unspecified front wall of thorax without penetration into thoracic cavity** CC

6th **S21.15** **Open bite of front wall of thorax without penetration into thoracic cavity**

Bite of front wall of thorax NOS

EXCLUDES 1 *superficial bite of front wall of thorax (S20.37)*

7th **S21.151** **Open bite of right front wall of thorax without penetration into thoracic cavity** CC

7th **S21.152** **Open bite of left front wall of thorax without penetration into thoracic cavity** CC

7th **S21.159** **Open bite of unspecified front wall of thorax without penetration into thoracic cavity** CC

5th **S21.2** **Open wound of back wall of thorax without penetration into thoracic cavity**

6th **S21.20** **Unspecified open wound of back wall of thorax without penetration into thoracic cavity**

7th **S21.201** **Unspecified open wound of right back wall of thorax without penetration into thoracic cavity**

7th **S21.202** **Unspecified open wound of left back wall of thorax without penetration into thoracic cavity**

7th **S21.209** **Unspecified open wound of unspecified back wall of thorax without penetration into thoracic cavity**

6th **S21.21** **Laceration without foreign body of back wall of thorax without penetration into thoracic cavity**

7th **S21.211** **Laceration without foreign body of right back wall of thorax without penetration into thoracic cavity**

7th **S21.212** **Laceration without foreign body of left back wall of thorax without penetration into thoracic cavity**

7th **S21.219** **Laceration without foreign body of unspecified back wall of thorax without penetration into thoracic cavity**

6th **S21.22** **Laceration with foreign body of back wall of thorax without penetration into thoracic cavity**

7th **S21.221** **Laceration with foreign body of right back wall of thorax without penetration into thoracic cavity**

7th **S21.222** **Laceration with foreign body of left back wall of thorax without penetration into thoracic cavity**

7th **S21.229** **Laceration with foreign body of unspecified back wall of thorax without penetration into thoracic cavity**

6th **S21.23** **Puncture wound without foreign body of back wall of thorax without penetration into thoracic cavity**

7th **S21.231** **Puncture wound without foreign body of right back wall of thorax without penetration into thoracic cavity**

7th **S21.232** **Puncture wound without foreign body of left back wall of thorax without penetration into thoracic cavity**

7th **S21.239** **Puncture wound without foreign body of unspecified back wall of thorax without penetration into thoracic cavity**

6th **S21.24** **Puncture wound with foreign body of back wall of thorax without penetration into thoracic cavity**

7th **S21.241** **Puncture wound with foreign body of right back wall of thorax without penetration into thoracic cavity**

7th **S21.242** **Puncture wound with foreign body of left back wall of thorax without penetration into thoracic cavity**

7th **S21.249** **Puncture wound with foreign body of unspecified back wall of thorax without penetration into thoracic cavity**

6th **S21.25** **Open bite of back wall of thorax without penetration into thoracic cavity**

Bite of back wall of thorax NOS

EXCLUDES 1 *superficial bite of back wall of thorax (S20.47)*

7th **S21.251** **Open bite of right back wall of thorax without penetration into thoracic cavity**

7th **S21.252** **Open bite of left back wall of thorax without penetration into thoracic cavity**

7th **S21.259** **Open bite of unspecified back wall of thorax without penetration into thoracic cavity**

5th **S21.3** **Open wound of front wall of thorax with penetration into thoracic cavity**

Open wound of chest with penetration into thoracic cavity

CC Excl: For MCC codes in subcategory S21.1, unless otherwise noted: MCC with 7th character A: S21.101-S21.159 with 7th A, S21.301-S21.95X with 7th A, S27.50X-S27.69X with 7th A, S27.892-S27.9XX with 7th A, S28.1XXA, S29.021A, S29.029A, S38.3XXA, T14.8-T14.91, T79.7XX-T79.9XX with 7th A

6th **S21.30** **Unspecified open wound of front wall of thorax with penetration into thoracic cavity**

7th **S21.301** **Unspecified open wound of right front wall of thorax with penetration into thoracic cavity** MCC

7th **S21.302** **Unspecified open wound of left front wall of thorax with penetration into thoracic cavity** MCC

7th **S21.309** **Unspecified open wound of unspecified front wall of thorax with penetration into thoracic cavity** MCC

CC Excl: S21.101-S21.159 with 7th A, S21.301-S21.95 with 7th A, S27.0XX-S27.309 with 7th A, S27.329A, S27.339A, S27.409 with 7th A, S27.50X-S27.803 with 7th A, S27.892-S27.9XX with 7th A, S28.1XXA, S29.021A, S29.029A, S38.3XXA, T14.8-T14.91, T79.7XX-T79.9XX with 7th A

6th **S21.31** **Laceration without foreign body of front wall of thorax with penetration into thoracic cavity**

7th **S21.311** **Laceration without foreign body of right front wall of thorax with penetration into thoracic cavity** MCC

✓7th S21.312 Laceration without foreign body of left front wall of thorax with penetration into thoracic cavity MCC

✓7th S21.319 Laceration without foreign body of unspecified front wall of thorax with penetration into thoracic cavity MCC

✓6th S21.32 Laceration with foreign body of front wall of thorax with penetration into thoracic cavity

✓7th S21.321 Laceration with foreign body of right front wall of thorax with penetration into thoracic cavity MCC

✓7th S21.322 Laceration with foreign body of left front wall of thorax with penetration into thoracic cavity MCC

✓7th S21.329 Laceration with foreign body of unspecified front wall of thorax with penetration into thoracic cavity MCC

✓6th S21.33 Puncture wound without foreign body of front wall of thorax with penetration into thoracic cavity

✓7th S21.331 Puncture wound without foreign body of right front wall of thorax with penetration into thoracic cavity MCC

✓7th S21.332 Puncture wound without foreign body of left front wall of thorax with penetration into thoracic cavity MCC

✓7th S21.339 Puncture wound without foreign body of unspecified front wall of thorax with penetration into thoracic cavity MCC

✓6th S21.34 Puncture wound with foreign body of front wall of thorax with penetration into thoracic cavity

✓7th S21.341 Puncture wound with foreign body of right front wall of thorax with penetration into thoracic cavity MCC

✓7th S21.342 Puncture wound with foreign body of left front wall of thorax with penetration into thoracic cavity MCC

✓7th S21.349 Puncture wound with foreign body of unspecified front wall of thorax with penetration into thoracic cavity MCC

✓6th S21.35 Open bite of front wall of thorax with penetration into thoracic cavity

EXCLUDES 1 *superficial bite of front wall of thorax (S20.37)*

✓7th S21.351 Open bite of right front wall of thorax with penetration into thoracic cavity MCC

✓7th S21.352 Open bite of left front wall of thorax with penetration into thoracic cavity MCC

✓7th S21.359 Open bite of unspecified front wall of thorax with penetration into thoracic cavity MCC

✓5th S21.4 Open wound of back wall of thorax with penetration into thoracic cavity

CC Excl: For MCC codes in subcategory S21.4, unless otherwise noted: MCC with 7th character A: See code: S21.3

✓6th S21.40 Unspecified open wound of back wall of thorax with penetration into thoracic cavity

✓7th S21.401 Unspecified open wound of right back wall of thorax with penetration into thoracic cavity MCC

✓7th S21.402 Unspecified open wound of left back wall of thorax with penetration into thoracic cavity MCC

✓7th S21.409 Unspecified open wound of unspecified back wall of thorax with penetration into thoracic cavity MCC

✓6th S21.41 Laceration without foreign body of back wall of thorax with penetration into thoracic cavity

✓7th S21.411 Laceration without foreign body of right back wall of thorax with penetration into thoracic cavity MCC

✓7th S21.412 Laceration without foreign body of left back wall of thorax with penetration into thoracic cavity MCC

✓7th S21.419 Laceration without foreign body of unspecified back wall of thorax with penetration into thoracic cavity MCC

✓6th S21.42 Laceration with foreign body of back wall of thorax with penetration into thoracic cavity

✓7th S21.421 Laceration with foreign body of right back wall of thorax with penetration into thoracic cavity MCC

✓7th S21.422 Laceration with foreign body of left back wall of thorax with penetration into thoracic cavity MCC

✓7th S21.429 Laceration with foreign body of unspecified back wall of thorax with penetration into thoracic cavity MCC

✓6th S21.43 Puncture wound without foreign body of back wall of thorax with penetration into thoracic cavity

✓7th S21.431 Puncture wound without foreign body of right back wall of thorax with penetration into thoracic cavity MCC

✓7th S21.432 Puncture wound without foreign body of left back wall of thorax with penetration into thoracic cavity MCC

✓7th S21.439 Puncture wound without foreign body of unspecified back wall of thorax with penetration into thoracic cavity MCC

✓6th S21.44 Puncture wound with foreign body of back wall of thorax with penetration into thoracic cavity

✓7th S21.441 Puncture wound with foreign body of right back wall of thorax with penetration into thoracic cavity MCC

✓7th S21.442 Puncture wound with foreign body of left back wall of thorax with penetration into thoracic cavity MCC

✓7th S21.449 Puncture wound with foreign body of unspecified back wall of thorax with penetration into thoracic cavity MCC

✓6th S21.45 Open bite of back wall of thorax with penetration into thoracic cavity

Bite of back wall of thorax NOS

EXCLUDES 1 *superficial bite of back wall of thorax (S20.47)*

✓7th S21.451 Open bite of right back wall of thorax with penetration into thoracic cavity MCC

✓7th S21.452 Open bite of left back wall of thorax with penetration into thoracic cavity MCC

✓7th S21.459 Open bite of unspecified back wall of thorax with penetration into thoracic cavity MCC

✓5th S21.9 Open wound of unspecified part of thorax

Open wound of thoracic wall NOS

CC Excl: For CC codes in subcategory S21.9, unless otherwise noted: CC with 7th character A: S21.101-S21.159 with 7th A, S21.301-S21.95X with 7th A, S23.3XXA, S23.8XXA, S27.50X-S27.69X with 7th A, S27.892-S27.9XX with 7th A, S28.1XXA, S29.021A, S29.029A, S38.3XXA, T14.8-T14.91, T79.7XX-T79.9XX with 7th A

✓x7th S21.90 Unspecified open wound of unspecified part of thorax CC

✓x7th S21.91 Laceration without foreign body of unspecified part of thorax CC

✓x7th S21.92 Laceration with foreign body of unspecified part of thorax CC

✓x7th S21.93 Puncture wound without foreign body of unspecified part of thorax CC

✓x7th S21.94 Puncture wound with foreign body of unspecified part of thorax CC

✓x7th S21.95 Open bite of unspecified part of thorax CC

EXCLUDES 1 *superficial bite of thorax (S20.97)*

✓4th S22 Fracture of rib(s), sternum and thoracic spine

NOTE A fracture not indicated as nondisplaced or displaced should be coded to displaced.
A fracture not indicated as open or closed should be coded to closed.

INCLUDES fracture of thoracic neural arch
fracture of thoracic spinous process
fracture of thoracic transverse process
fracture of thoracic vertebra
fracture of thoracic vertebral arch

Code first any associated:
injury of intrathoracic organ (S27.-)
spinal cord injury (S24.0-, S24.1-)

EXCLUDES 1 *transection of thorax (S28.1)*

EXCLUDES 2 *fracture of clavicle (S42.0-)*
fracture of scapula (S42.1-)

The appropriate 7th is to be added to each code from category S22.
A initial encounter for closed fracture
B initial encounter for open fracture
D subsequent encounter for fracture with routine healing
G subsequent encounter for fracture with delayed healing
K subsequent encounter for fracture with nonunion
S sequela

✓5th S22.0 Fracture of thoracic vertebra

CC Excl: For CC/MCC codes in subcategory S22.0, unless otherwise noted: CC with 7th character A or MCC with 7th character B: M48.40X-M48.58X with 7th S, M80.08XS, M80.88XS, M84.350S, M84.454S, M84.550S, M84.58S, M84.650S, M99.12, M99.15-M99.17, M99.19, S03.8XX-S03.9XX with 7th A, S12.000-S12.9XX with 7th S, S13.9XXA, S14.109A, S14.119A, S14.129 A, S14.139A, S14.149A, S14.159A, S22.000-S23.3XX with 7th [A, B, S], S23.8XX-S24.159 with 7th A, S29.001-S29.019 with 7th A, S29.091-S29.9XX with 7th A, S32.000-S32.9XX with 7th S, S33.30X-S33.39X with 7th A, S33.9XA, S38.1XXA, S38.3XX-S39.013 with 7th A, S39.091-S39.94X with 7th A, T14.8-T14.91, T79.A0X-T79.9XX with 7th A

CC with 7th character K: M80.00X-M84.68X with 7th [K, P], S02.0XX-S02.92X with 7th K, S12.000-S12.691 with 7th K, S22.000-S22.9XX with 7th K, S32.000-S32.9XX with 7th K, S42.001-S42.92X with 7th [K, P], S49.001-S49.199 with 7th [K, P], S52.001-S52.92X with 7th [K, M, N, P, Q, R], S59.001-S59.299 with 7th [K, P], S62.001-S62.92X with 7th [K, P], S72.001-S72.92X with 7th [K, M, N, P, Q, R], S79.001-S79.199 with 7th [K, P], S82.001-S82.92X with 7th [K, M, N, P, Q, R], S89.001-S89.399 with 7th [K, P], S92.001-S92.919 with 7th [K, P]

✓6th S22.00 Fracture of unspecified thoracic vertebra
- 7 ✓7th **S22.000 Wedge compression fracture of unspecified thoracic vertebra** MCC CC
- 7 ✓7th **S22.001 Stable burst fracture of unspecified thoracic vertebra** MCC CC
- 7 ✓7th **S22.002 Unstable burst fracture of unspecified thoracic vertebra** MCC CC
- 7 ✓7th **S22.008 Other fracture of unspecified thoracic vertebra** MCC CC
- 7 ✓7th **S22.009 Unspecified fracture of unspecified thoracic vertebra** MCC CC

✓6th S22.01 Fracture of first thoracic vertebra
- 7 ✓7th **S22.010 Wedge compression fracture of first thoracic vertebra** MCC CC
- 7 ✓7th **S22.011 Stable burst fracture of first thoracic vertebra** MCC CC
- 7 ✓7th **S22.012 Unstable burst fracture of first thoracic vertebra** MCC CC
- 7 ✓7th **S22.018 Other fracture of first thoracic vertebra** MCC CC
- 7 ✓7th **S22.019 Unspecified fracture of first thoracic vertebra** MCC CC

✓6th S22.02 Fracture of second thoracic vertebra
- 7 ✓7th **S22.020 Wedge compression fracture of second thoracic vertebra** MCC CC
- 7 ✓7th **S22.021 Stable burst fracture of second thoracic vertebra** MCC CC
- 7 ✓7th **S22.022 Unstable burst fracture of second thoracic vertebra** MCC CC
- 7 ✓7th **S22.028 Other fracture of second thoracic vertebra** MCC CC
- 7 ✓7th **S22.029 Unspecified fracture of second thoracic vertebra** MCC CC

✓6th S22.03 Fracture of third thoracic vertebra
- 7 ✓7th **S22.030 Wedge compression fracture of third thoracic vertebra** MCC CC
- 7 ✓7th **S22.031 Stable burst fracture of third thoracic vertebra** MCC CC
- 7 ✓7th **S22.032 Unstable burst fracture of third thoracic vertebra** MCC CC
- 7 ✓7th **S22.038 Other fracture of third thoracic vertebra** MCC CC
- 7 ✓7th **S22.039 Unspecified fracture of third thoracic vertebra** MCC CC

✓6th S22.04 Fracture of fourth thoracic vertebra
- 7 ✓7th **S22.040 Wedge compression fracture of fourth thoracic vertebra** MCC CC
- 7 ✓7th **S22.041 Stable burst fracture of fourth thoracic vertebra** MCC CC
- 7 ✓7th **S22.042 Unstable burst fracture of fourth thoracic vertebra** MCC CC
- 7 ✓7th **S22.048 Other fracture of fourth thoracic vertebra** MCC CC
- 7 ✓7th **S22.049 Unspecified fracture of fourth thoracic vertebra** MCC CC

✓6th S22.05 Fracture of T5-T6 vertebra
- 7 ✓7th **S22.050 Wedge compression fracture of T5-T6 vertebra** MCC CC
- 7 ✓7th **S22.051 Stable burst fracture of T5-T6 vertebra** MCC CC
- 7 ✓7th **S22.052 Unstable burst fracture of T5-T6 vertebra** MCC CC
- 7 ✓7th **S22.058 Other fracture of T5-T6 vertebra** MCC CC
- 7 ✓7th **S22.059 Unspecified fracture of T5-T6 vertebra** MCC CC

✓6th S22.06 Fracture of T7-T8 vertebra
- 7 ✓7th **S22.060 Wedge compression fracture of T7-T8 vertebra** MCC CC
- 7 ✓7th **S22.061 Stable burst fracture of T7-T8 vertebra** MCC CC
- 7 ✓7th **S22.062 Unstable burst fracture of T7-T8 vertebra** MCC CC
- 7 ✓7th **S22.068 Other fracture of T7-T8 thoracic vertebra** MCC CC
- 7 ✓7th **S22.069 Unspecified fracture of T7-T8 vertebra** MCC CC

✓6th S22.07 Fracture of T9-T10 vertebra
- 7 ✓7th **S22.070 Wedge compression fracture of T9-T10 vertebra** MCC CC
- 7 ✓7th **S22.071 Stable burst fracture of T9-T10 vertebra** MCC CC
- 7 ✓7th **S22.072 Unstable burst fracture of T9-T10 vertebra** MCC CC
- 7 ✓7th **S22.078 Other fracture of T9-T10 vertebra** MCC CC
- 7 ✓7th **S22.079 Unspecified fracture of T9-T10 vertebra** MCC CC

✓6th S22.08 Fracture of T11-T12 vertebra
- 7 ✓7th **S22.080 Wedge compression fracture of T11-T12 vertebra** MCC CC
- 7 ✓7th **S22.081 Stable burst fracture of T11-T12 vertebra** MCC CC
- 7 ✓7th **S22.082 Unstable burst fracture of T11-T12 vertebra** MCC CC
- 7 ✓7th **S22.088 Other fracture of T11-T12 vertebra** MCC CC
- 7 ✓7th **S22.089 Unspecified fracture of T11-T12 vertebra** MCC CC

7 HAC = Initial encounter only (7th character A, B or C) and not POA.

√5th **S22.2 Fracture of sternum**

CC Excl: For CC/MCC codes in subcategory S22.2, unless otherwise noted: CC with 7th character A or MCC with 7th character B: S03.8XX-S03.9XX with 7th A, S22.20X-S22.24X with 7th [A, B], S22.5XX-S22.5XX with 7th [A, B], S29.011-S29.019 with 7th A, S38.3XX-S39.013 with 7th A, T14.8-T14.91, T79.A0X-T79.9XX with 7th A
CC with 7th character K: M80.00X-M84.68X with 7th [K, P], S02.0XX-S02.92X with 7th K, S12.000-S12.691 with 7th K, S22.000-S22.9XX with 7th K, S32.000-S32.9XX with 7th K, S42.001-S42.92X with 7th [K, P], S49.001-S49.199 with 7th [K, P], S52.001-S52.92X with 7th [K, M, N, P, Q, R], S59.001-S59.299 with 7th [K, P], S62.001-S62.92X with 7th [K, P], S72.001-S72.92X with 7th [K, M, N, P, Q, R], S79.001-S79.199 with 7th [K, P], S82.001-S82.92X with 7th [K, M, N, P, Q, R], S89.001-S89.399 with 7th [K, P], S92.001-S92.919 with 7th [K, P]

7 √x7th **S22.20 Unspecified fracture of sternum** MCC CC
7 √x7th **S22.21 Fracture of manubrium** MCC CC
7 √x7th **S22.22 Fracture of body of sternum** MCC CC
7 √x7th **S22.23 Sternal manubrial dissociation** MCC CC
7 √x7th **S22.24 Fracture of xiphoid process** MCC CC

√5th **S22.3 Fracture of one rib**

CC Excl: For CC/MCC codes in subcategory S22.3, unless otherwise noted: CC with 7th character A or MCC with 7th character B: S03.8XX-S03.9XXwith 7th A, S22.20X-S22.5XX with 7th [A, B], S29.011-S29.019 with 7th A, S38.3XX-S39.013 with 7th A, T14.8-T14.91, T79.A0X-T79.9XX with 7th A
CC with 7th character K: M80.00X-M84.68X with 7th [K, P], S02.0XX-S02.92X with 7th K, S12.000-S12.691 with 7th K, S22.000-S22.9XX with 7th K, S32.000-S32.9XX with 7th K, S42.001-S42.92X with 7th [K, P], S49.001-S49.199 with 7th [K, P], S52.001-S52.92X with 7th [K, M, N, P, Q, R], S59.001-S59.299 with 7th [K, P], S62.001-S62.92X with 7th [K, P], S72.001-S72.92X with 7th [K, M, N, P, Q, R], S79.001-S79.199 with 7th [K, P], S82.001-S82.92X with 7th [K, M, N, P, Q, R], S89.001-S89.399 with 7th [K, P], S92.001-S92.919 with 7th [K, P]

7 √x7th **S22.31 Fracture of one rib, right side** MCC CC
7 √x7th **S22.32 Fracture of one rib, left side** MCC CC
7 √x7th **S22.39 Fracture of one rib, unspecified side** MCC CC

√5th **S22.4 Multiple fractures of ribs**
Fractures of two or more ribs
EXCLUDES 1 *flail chest (S22.5-)*

CC Excl: For CC/MCC codes in subcategory S22.4, unless otherwise noted: CC with 7th character A or MCC with 7th character B: S03.8XX-S03.9XX with 7th A, S22.31X-S22.5XX with 7th [A, B], S29.011-S29.019 with 7th A, S38.3XX-S39.013 with 7th A, T14.8-T14.91, T79.A0X-T79.9XX with 7th A
CC with 7th character K: M80.00X-M84.68X with 7th [K, P], S02.0XX-S02.92X with 7th K, S12.000-S12.691 with 7th K, S22.000-S22.9XX with 7th K, S32.000-S32.9XX with 7th K, S42.001-S42.92X with 7th [K, P], S49.001-S49.199 with 7th [K, P], S52.001-S52.92X with 7th [K, M, N, P, Q, R], S59.001-S59.299 with 7th [K, P], S62.001-S62.92X with 7th [K, P], S72.001-S72.92X with 7th [K, M, N, P, Q, R], S79.001-S79.199 with 7th [K, P], S82.001-S82.92X with 7th [K, M, N, P, Q, R], S89.001-S89.399 with 7th [K, P], S92.001-S92.919 with 7th [K, P]

7 √x7th **S22.41 Multiple fractures of ribs, right side** MCC CC
7 √x7th **S22.42 Multiple fractures of ribs, left side** MCC CC
7 √x7th **S22.43 Multiple fractures of ribs, bilateral** MCC CC
7 √x7th **S22.49 Multiple fractures of ribs, unspecified side** MCC CC
CC Excl: No excl for codes with 7th B

7 √x7th **S22.5 Flail chest** MCC CC

CC Excl: For CC/MCC codes in subcategory S22.5, unless otherwise noted: CC with 7th character A or MCC with 7th character B: S03.8XX-S03.9XX with 7th A, S22.20X-S22.5XX with 7th [A, B], S29.011-S29.019 with 7th A, S38.3XX-S39.013 with 7th A, T14.8-T14.91, T79.A0X-T79.9XX with 7th A
CC with 7th character K: M80.00X-M80.88X[K,P], M84.30X-M84.68X[K,P], S02.0X-S02.92X[K], S12.000-S12.691[K], S22.000-S22.9X[K], S32.0[0-4][0-2,8-9]K, S32.050K

7 √x7th **S22.9 Fracture of bony thorax, part unspecified** MCC CC

CC Excl: For CC/MCC codes in subcategory S22.9, unless otherwise noted: CC with 7th character A or MCC with 7th character B: M80.00X-M80.01X9 with 7th A, M80.041-M80.049 with 7th A, M80.80X-M80.819 with 7th A, M80.841-M80.849 with 7th A, M84.40X-M84.419 with 7th A, M84.441-M84.446 with 7th A, M84.454A, M84.474-M84.519 with 7th A, M84.541-M84.550 with 7th A, M84.574-M84.576 with 7th A, M84.60X-M84.619 with 7th A, M84.641-M84.650 with 7th A, M84.674-M84.68X with 7th A, S03.8XX-S03.9XX with 7th A, S22.9XX-S22.9XX with 7th [A, B], S29.011-S29.019 with 7th A, S32.301-S32.811 with 7th [A, B], S32.89X-S32.9XX with 7th [A, B], S33.4XXA, S33.6XX-S33.8XX with 7th A, S38.3XX-S39.013 with 7th A, S73.001-S73.199 with 7th A, S76.001-S76.019 with 7th A, S76.091-S76.119 with 7th A, S76.191-S76.219 with 7th A, S76.291-S76.319 with 7th A, S76.391-S76.819 with 7th A, S76.891-S76.919 with 7th A, S76.991-S76.999 with 7th A, S79.811-S79.929 with 7th A, T14.8-T14.91, T79.A9X-T79.9XX with 7th A
CC with 7th character K: M80.00X-M84.68X with 7th [K, P], S02.0XX-S02.92X with 7th K, S12.000-S12.691 with 7th K, S22.000-S22.9XX with 7th K, S32.000-S32.9XX with 7th K, S42.001-S42.92X with 7th [K, P], S49.001-S49.199 with 7th [K, P], S52.001-S52.92X with 7th [K, M, N, P, Q, R], S59.001-S59.299 with 7th [K, P], S62.001-S62.92X with 7th [K, P], S72.001-S72.92X with 7th [K, M, N, P, Q, R], S79.001-S79.199 with 7th [K, P], S82.001-S82.92X with 7th [K, M, N, P, Q, R], S89.001-S89.399 with 7th [K, P], S92.001-S92.919 with 7th [K, P]

√4th **S23 Dislocation and sprain of joints and ligaments of thorax**
INCLUDES avulsion of joint or ligament of thorax
laceration of cartilage, joint or ligament of thorax
sprain of cartilage, joint or ligament of thorax
traumatic hemarthrosis of joint or ligament of thorax
traumatic rupture of joint or ligament of thorax
traumatic subluxation of joint or ligament of thorax
traumatic tear of joint or ligament of thorax
Code also any associated open wound
EXCLUDES 2 *dislocation, sprain of sternoclavicular joint (S43.2, S43.6)*
strain of muscle or tendon of thorax (S29.01-)

The appropriate 7th is to be added to each code from category S23.
A initial encounter
D subsequent encounter
S sequela

√x7th **S23.0 Traumatic rupture of thoracic intervertebral disc**
EXCLUDES 1 *rupture or displacement (nontraumatic) of thoracic intervertebral disc NOS (M51- with fifth character 4)*

√5th **S23.1 Subluxation and dislocation of thoracic vertebra**
Code also any associated
open wound of thorax (S21.-)
spinal cord injury (S24.0-, S24.1-)
EXCLUDES 2 *fracture of thoracic vertebrae (S22.0-)*

√6th **S23.10 Subluxation and dislocation of unspecified thoracic vertebra**
√7th **S23.100 Subluxation of unspecified thoracic vertebra**
√7th **S23.101 Dislocation of unspecified thoracic vertebra**

√6th **S23.11 Subluxation and dislocation of T1/T2 thoracic vertebra**
√7th **S23.110 Subluxation of T1/T2 thoracic vertebra**
√7th **S23.111 Dislocation of T1/T2 thoracic vertebra**

√6th **S23.12 Subluxation and dislocation of T2/T3-T3/T4 thoracic vertebra**
√7th **S23.120 Subluxation of T2/T3 thoracic vertebra**
√7th **S23.121 Dislocation of T2/T3 thoracic vertebra**
√7th **S23.122 Subluxation of T3/T4 thoracic vertebra**
√7th **S23.123 Dislocation of T3/T4 thoracic vertebra**

√6th **S23.13 Subluxation and dislocation of T4/T5-T5/T6 thoracic vertebra**
√7th **S23.130 Subluxation of T4/T5 thoracic vertebra**
√7th **S23.131 Dislocation of T4/T5 thoracic vertebra**
√7th **S23.132 Subluxation of T5/T6 thoracic vertebra**
√7th **S23.133 Dislocation of T5/T6 thoracic vertebra**

7 HAC = Initial encounter only (7th character A, B or C) and not POA.

✓6th **S23.14** **Subluxation and dislocation of T6/T7-T7/T8 thoracic vertebra**
- ✓7th **S23.14Ø** **Subluxation of T6/T7 thoracic vertebra**
- ✓7th **S23.141** **Dislocation of T6/T7 thoracic vertebra**
- ✓7th **S23.142** **Subluxation of T7/T8 thoracic vertebra**
- ✓7th **S23.143** **Dislocation of T7/T8 thoracic vertebra**

✓6th **S23.15** **Subluxation and dislocation of T8/T9-T9/T1Ø thoracic vertebra**
- ✓7th **S23.15Ø** **Subluxation of T8/T9 thoracic vertebra**
- ✓7th **S23.151** **Dislocation of T8/T9 thoracic vertebra**
- ✓7th **S23.152** **Subluxation of T9/T1Ø thoracic vertebra**
- ✓7th **S23.153** **Dislocation of T9/T1Ø thoracic vertebra**

✓6th **S23.16** **Subluxation and dislocation of T1Ø/T11-T11/T12 thoracic vertebra**
- ✓7th **S23.16Ø** **Subluxation of T1Ø/T11 thoracic vertebra**
- ✓7th **S23.161** **Dislocation of T1Ø/T11 thoracic vertebra**
- ✓7th **S23.162** **Subluxation of T11/T12 thoracic vertebra**
- ✓7th **S23.163** **Dislocation of T11/T12 thoracic vertebra**

✓6th **S23.17** **Subluxation and dislocation of T12/L1 thoracic vertebra**
- ✓7th **S23.17Ø** **Subluxation of T12/L1 thoracic vertebra**
- ✓7th **S23.171** **Dislocation of T12/L1 thoracic vertebra**

✓5th **S23.2** **Dislocation of other and unspecified parts of thorax**
- ✓x7th **S23.2Ø** **Dislocation of unspecified part of thorax**
- ✓x7th **S23.29** **Dislocation of other parts of thorax**

✓x7th **S23.3** **Sprain of ligaments of thoracic spine**

✓5th **S23.4** **Sprain of ribs and sternum**
- ✓x7th **S23.41** **Sprain of ribs**
- ✓6th **S23.42** **Sprain of sternum**
  - ✓7th **S23.42Ø** **Sprain of sternoclavicular (joint) (ligament)**
  - ✓7th **S23.421** **Sprain of chondrosternal joint**
  - ✓7th **S23.428** **Other sprain of sternum**
  - ✓7th **S23.429** **Unspecified sprain of sternum**

✓x7th **S23.8** **Sprain of other specified parts of thorax**

✓x7th **S23.9** **Sprain of unspecified parts of thorax**

✓4th S24 Injury of nerves and spinal cord at thorax level

NOTE Code to highest level of thoracic spinal cord injury.
Injuries to the spinal cord (S24.Ø and S24.1) refer to the cord level and not bone level injury, and can affect nerve roots at and below the level given.

Code also any associated:
- fracture of thoracic vertebra (S22.Ø-)
- open wound of thorax (S21.-)
- transient paralysis (R29.5)

EXCLUDES 2 *injury of brachial plexus (S14.3)*

The appropriate 7th is to be added to each code from category S24.
- A initial encounter
- D subsequent encounter
- S sequela

CC Excl: For MCC codes in category S24 unless otherwise noted: MCC with 7th character A: M48.4ØX-M48.58X with 7th S, M8Ø.Ø8XS, M8Ø.88XS, M84.35ØS, M84.454S, M84.55ØS, M84.58S, M84.65ØS, M99.15-M99.17, M99.19, S12.ØØØ-S12.9XX with 7th S, S13.9XXA, S14.1Ø9A, S14.119A, S14.129A, S14.139A, S14.149A, S14.159A, S22.ØØØ-S22.9XX with 7th S, S23.2ØX-S23.29X with 7th A, S23.9XX-S24.159 with 7th A, S29.ØØ1-S29.ØØ9 with 7th A, S29.Ø91-S29.9XX with 7th A, S32.ØØØ-S32.9XX with 7th S, S33.3ØX-S33.39X with 7th A, S33.9XXA, S38.1XXA, S39.ØØ1-S39.ØØ3 with 7th A, S39.Ø91-S39.94X with 7th A, T14.8-T14.91, T79.AØX-T79.9XX with 7th A

✓x7th **S24.Ø** **Concussion and edema of thoracic spinal cord** MCC

✓5th **S24.1** **Other and unspecified injuries of thoracic spinal cord**
- ✓6th **S24.1Ø** **Unspecified injury of thoracic spinal cord**
  - 7 ✓7th **S24.1Ø1** **Unspecified injury at T1 level of thoracic spinal cord** MCC
  - 7 ✓7th **S24.1Ø2** **Unspecified injury at T2-T6 level of thoracic spinal cord** MCC
  - 7 ✓7th **S24.1Ø3** **Unspecified injury at T7-T1Ø level of thoracic spinal cord** MCC
  - 7 ✓7th **S24.1Ø4** **Unspecified injury at T11-T12 level thoracic spinal cord** MCC
  - 7 ✓7th **S24.1Ø9** **Unspecified injury at unspecified level of thoracic spinal cord**
    Injury of thoracic spinal cord NOS
    CC Excl: No excl
- ✓6th **S24.11** **Complete lesion of thoracic spinal cord**
  - 7 ✓7th **S24.111** **Complete lesion at T1 level of thoracic spinal cord** MCC
  - 7 ✓7th **S24.112** **Complete lesion at T2-T6 level of thoracic spinal cord** MCC
  - 7 ✓7th **S24.113** **Complete lesion at T7-T1Ø level of thoracic spinal cord** MCC
  - 7 ✓7th **S24.114** **Complete lesion at T11-T12 level of thoracic spinal cord** MCC
  - ✓7th **S24.119** **Complete lesion at unspecified level of thoracic spinal cord**
- ✓6th **S24.13** **Anterior cord syndrome of thoracic spinal cord**
  - 7 ✓7th **S24.131** **Anterior cord syndrome at T1 level of thoracic spinal cord** MCC
  - 7 ✓7th **S24.132** **Anterior cord syndrome at T2-T6 level of thoracic spinal cord** MCC
  - 7 ✓7th **S24.133** **Anterior cord syndrome at T7-T1Ø level of thoracic spinal cord** MCC
  - 7 ✓7th **S24.134** **Anterior cord syndrome at T11-T12 level of thoracic spinal cord** MCC
  - ✓7th **S24.139** **Anterior cord syndrome at unspecified level of thoracic spinal cord**
- ✓6th **S24.14** **Brown-Séquard syndrome of thoracic spinal cord**
  - ✓7th **S24.141** **Brown-Séquard syndrome at T1 level of thoracic spinal cord** MCC
  - ✓7th **S24.142** **Brown-Séquard syndrome at T2-T6 level of thoracic spinal cord** MCC
  - ✓7th **S24.143** **Brown-Séquard syndrome at T7-T1Ø level of thoracic spinal cord** MCC
  - ✓7th **S24.144** **Brown-Séquard syndrome at T11-T12 level of thoracic spinal cord** MCC
  - ✓7th **S24.149** **Brown-Séquard syndrome at unspecified level of thoracic spinal cord**
- ✓6th **S24.15** **Other incomplete lesions of thoracic spinal cord**
  Incomplete lesion of thoracic spinal cord NOS
  Posterior cord syndrome of thoracic spinal cord
  - 7 ✓7th **S24.151** **Other incomplete lesion at T1 level of thoracic spinal cord** MCC
  - 7 ✓7th **S24.152** **Other incomplete lesion at T2-T6 level of thoracic spinal cord** MCC
  - 7 ✓7th **S24.153** **Other incomplete lesion at T7-T1Ø level of thoracic spinal cord** MCC
  - 7 ✓7th **S24.154** **Other incomplete lesion at T11-T12 level of thoracic spinal cord** MCC
  - ✓7th **S24.159** **Other incomplete lesion at unspecified level of thoracic spinal cord**

✓x7th **S24.2** **Injury of nerve root of thoracic spine**

✓x7th **S24.3** **Injury of peripheral nerves of thorax**

✓x7th **S24.4** **Injury of thoracic sympathetic nervous system**
- Injury of cardiac plexus
- Injury of esophageal plexus
- Injury of pulmonary plexus
- Injury of stellate ganglion
- Injury of thoracic sympathetic ganglion

✓x7th **S24.8** **Injury of other specified nerves of thorax**

✓x7th **S24.9** **Injury of unspecified nerve of thorax**

✓4th S25 Injury of blood vessels of thorax

Code also any associated open wound (S21.-)

The appropriate 7th is to be added to each code from category S25.
- A initial encounter
- D subsequent encounter
- S sequela

✓5th **S25.Ø** **Injury of thoracic aorta**
Injury of aorta NOS

CC Excl: For MCC codes in subcategory S25.Ø, unless otherwise noted: MCC with 7th character A: S25.ØØX-S25.Ø9X with 7th A, T14.8-T14.91, T79.AØX-T79.9XX with 7th AA

---

7 HAC = Initial encounter only (7th character A, B or C) and not POA.

√x7th **S25.00 Unspecified injury of thoracic aorta** MCC

√x7th **S25.01 Minor laceration of thoracic aorta** MCC
Incomplete transection of thoracic aorta
Laceration of thoracic aorta NOS
Superficial laceration of thoracic aorta

√x7th **S25.02 Major laceration of thoracic aorta** MCC
Complete transection of thoracic aorta
Traumatic rupture of thoracic aorta

√x7th **S25.09 Other specified injury of thoracic aorta** MCC

√5th **S25.1 Injury of innominate or subclavian artery**

CC Excl: For MCC codes in subcategory S25.1, unless otherwise noted: MCC with 7th character A: S25.101-S25.199 with 7th A, T14.8-T14.91, T79.A0X-T79.9XX with 7th A

√6th **S25.10 Unspecified injury of innominate or subclavian artery**

√7th **S25.101 Unspecified injury of right innominate or subclavian artery** MCC

√7th **S25.102 Unspecified injury of left innominate or subclavian artery** MCC

√7th **S25.109 Unspecified injury of unspecified innominate or subclavian artery** MCC

√6th **S25.11 Minor laceration of innominate or subclavian artery**
Incomplete transection of innominate or subclavian artery
Laceration of innominate or subclavian artery NOS
Superficial laceration of innominate or subclavian artery

√7th **S25.111 Minor laceration of right innominate or subclavian artery** MCC

√7th **S25.112 Minor laceration of left innominate or subclavian artery** MCC

√7th **S25.119 Minor laceration of unspecified innominate or subclavian artery** MCC

√6th **S25.12 Major laceration of innominate or subclavian artery**
Complete transection of innominate or subclavian artery
Traumatic rupture of innominate or subclavian artery

√7th **S25.121 Major laceration of right innominate or subclavian artery** MCC

√7th **S25.122 Major laceration of left innominate or subclavian artery** MCC

√7th **S25.129 Major laceration of unspecified innominate or subclavian artery** MCC

√6th **S25.19 Other specified injury of innominate or subclavian artery**

√7th **S25.191 Other specified injury of right innominate or subclavian artery** MCC

√7th **S25.192 Other specified injury of left innominate or subclavian artery** MCC

√7th **S25.199 Other specified injury of unspecified innominate or subclavian artery** MCC

√5th **S25.2 Injury of superior vena cava**
Injury of vena cava NOS

CC Excl: For MCC codes in subcategory S25.2, unless otherwise noted: MCC with 7th character A: S25.20X-S25.29X with 7th A, T14.8-T14.91, T79.A0X-T79.9XX with 7th A

√x7th **S25.20 Unspecified injury of superior vena cava** MCC

√x7th **S25.21 Minor laceration of superior vena cava** MCC
Incomplete transection of superior vena cava
Laceration of superior vena cava NOS
Superficial laceration of superior vena cava

√x7th **S25.22 Major laceration of superior vena cava** MCC
Complete transection of superior vena cava
Traumatic rupture of superior vena cava

√x7th **S25.29 Other specified injury of superior vena cava** MCC

√5th **S25.3 Injury of innominate or subclavian vein**

CC Excl: For MCC codes in subcategory S25.3, unless otherwise noted: MCC with 7th character A: S25.301-S25.399 with 7th A, T14.8-T14.91, T79.A0X-T79.9XX with 7th A

√6th **S25.30 Unspecified injury of innominate or subclavian vein**

√7th **S25.301 Unspecified injury of right innominate or subclavian vein** MCC

√7th **S25.302 Unspecified injury of left innominate or subclavian vein** MCC

√7th **S25.309 Unspecified injury of unspecified innominate or subclavian vein** MCC

√6th **S25.31 Minor laceration of innominate or subclavian vein**
Incomplete transection of innominate or subclavian vein
Laceration of innominate or subclavian vein NOS
Superficial laceration of innominate or subclavian vein

√7th **S25.311 Minor laceration of right innominate or subclavian vein** MCC

√7th **S25.312 Minor laceration of left innominate or subclavian vein** MCC

√7th **S25.319 Minor laceration of unspecified innominate or subclavian vein** MCC

√6th **S25.32 Major laceration of innominate or subclavian vein**
Complete transection of innominate or subclavian vein
Traumatic rupture of innominate or subclavian vein

√7th **S25.321 Major laceration of right innominate or subclavian vein** MCC

√7th **S25.322 Major laceration of left innominate or subclavian vein** MCC

√7th **S25.329 Major laceration of unspecified innominate or subclavian vein** MCC

√6th **S25.39 Other specified injury of innominate or subclavian vein**

√7th **S25.391 Other specified injury of right innominate or subclavian vein** MCC

√7th **S25.392 Other specified injury of left innominate or subclavian vein** MCC

√7th **S25.399 Other specified injury of unspecified innominate or subclavian vein** MCC

√5th **S25.4 Injury of pulmonary blood vessels**

CC Excl: For CC/MCC codes in subcategory S25.4, unless otherwise noted: MCC with 7th character A: S25.401-S25.499 with 7th A, T14.8-T14.91, T79.A0X-T79.9XX with 7th A

√6th **S25.40 Unspecified injury of pulmonary blood vessels**

√7th **S25.401 Unspecified injury of right pulmonary blood vessels** MCC

√7th **S25.402 Unspecified injury of left pulmonary blood vessels** MCC

√7th **S25.409 Unspecified injury of unspecified pulmonary blood vessels** MCC

√6th **S25.41 Minor laceration of pulmonary blood vessels**
Incomplete transection of pulmonary blood vessels
Laceration of pulmonary blood vessels NOS
Superficial laceration of pulmonary blood vessels

√7th **S25.411 Minor laceration of right pulmonary blood vessels** MCC

√7th **S25.412 Minor laceration of left pulmonary blood vessels** MCC

√7th **S25.419 Minor laceration of unspecified pulmonary blood vessels** MCC

√6th **S25.42 Major laceration of pulmonary blood vessels**
Complete transection of pulmonary blood vessels
Traumatic rupture of pulmonary blood vessels

√7th **S25.421 Major laceration of right pulmonary blood vessels** MCC

√7th **S25.422 Major laceration of left pulmonary blood vessels** MCC

√7th **S25.429 Major laceration of unspecified pulmonary blood vessels** MCC

√6th **S25.49 Other specified injury of pulmonary blood vessels**

√7th **S25.491 Other specified injury of right pulmonary blood vessels** MCC

√7th **S25.492 Other specified injury of left pulmonary blood vessels** MCC

√7th **S25.499 Other specified injury of unspecified pulmonary blood vessels** MCC

✓5th **S25.5 Injury of intercostal blood vessels**

> **CC Excl: For CC codes in subcategory S25.5, unless otherwise noted: CC with 7th character A:** S25.501-S25.899 with 7th A

✓6th **S25.50 Unspecified injury of intercostal blood vessels**

✓7th **S25.501 Unspecified injury of intercostal blood vessels, right side** CC

✓7th **S25.502 Unspecified injury of intercostal blood vessels, left side** CC

✓7th **S25.509 Unspecified injury of intercostal blood vessels, unspecified side** CC

✓6th **S25.51 Laceration of intercostal blood vessels**

✓7th **S25.511 Laceration of intercostal blood vessels, right side** CC

✓7th **S25.512 Laceration of intercostal blood vessels, left side** CC

✓7th **S25.519 Laceration of intercostal blood vessels, unspecified side** CC

✓6th **S25.59 Other specified injury of intercostal blood vessels**

✓7th **S25.591 Other specified injury of intercostal blood vessels, right side** CC

✓7th **S25.592 Other specified injury of intercostal blood vessels, left side** CC

✓7th **S25.599 Other specified injury of intercostal blood vessels, unspecified side** CC

✓5th **S25.8 Injury of other blood vessels of thorax**
Injury of azygos vein
Injury of mammary artery or vein

> **CC Excl: For CC codes in subcategory S25.8, unless otherwise noted: CC with 7th character A:** S25.00X-S25.99X with 7th A

✓6th **S25.80 Unspecified injury of other blood vessels of thorax**

✓7th **S25.801 Unspecified injury of other blood vessels of thorax, right side** CC

✓7th **S25.802 Unspecified injury of other blood vessels of thorax, left side** CC

✓7th **S25.809 Unspecified injury of other blood vessels of thorax, unspecified side** CC

✓6th **S25.81 Laceration of other blood vessels of thorax**

✓7th **S25.811 Laceration of other blood vessels of thorax, right side** CC

✓7th **S25.812 Laceration of other blood vessels of thorax, left side** CC

✓7th **S25.819 Laceration of other blood vessels of thorax, unspecified side** CC

✓6th **S25.89 Other specified injury of other blood vessels of thorax**

✓7th **S25.891 Other specified injury of other blood vessels of thorax, right side** CC

✓7th **S25.892 Other specified injury of other blood vessels of thorax, left side** CC

✓7th **S25.899 Other specified injury of other blood vessels of thorax, unspecified side** CC

✓5th **S25.9 Injury of unspecified blood vessel of thorax**

> **CC Excl: For CC codes in subcategory S25.9, unless otherwise noted:** See code: S25.8

✓x7th **S25.90 Unspecified injury of unspecified blood vessel of thorax** CC

✓x7th **S25.91 Laceration of unspecified blood vessel of thorax** CC

✓x7th **S25.99 Other specified injury of unspecified blood vessel of thorax** CC

✓4th **S26 Injury of heart**

Code also any associated:
- open wound of thorax (S21.-)
- traumatic hemopneumothorax (S27.2)
- traumatic hemothorax (S27.1)
- traumatic pneumothorax (S27.0)

> The appropriate 7th is to be added to each code from category S26.
> A initial encounter
> D subsequent encounter
> S sequela

✓5th **S26.0 Injury of heart with hemopericardium**

✓x7th **S26.00 Unspecified injury of heart with hemopericardium** CC
CC Excl: CC with 7th character A: S21.301-S21.459 with 7th A, S26.00X-S26.99X with 7th A, S27.50X-S27.69X with 7th A, S27.892-S27.9XX with 7th A, T14.8-T14.91

✓x7th **S26.01 Contusion of heart with hemopericardium** CC
CC Excl: CC with 7th character A: S21.101-S21.159 with 7th A, S21.301-S21.95X with 7th A, S26.00X-S26.99X with 7th A, S27.50X-S27.69X with 7th A, S27.892-S27.9XX with 7th A, S28.1XXA, S29.021A, S29.029A, S38.3XXA, T14.8-T14.91, T79.7XX-T79.9XX with 7th A

✓6th **S26.02 Laceration of heart with hemopericardium**

✓7th **S26.020 Mild laceration of heart with hemopericardium** MCC
Laceration of heart without penetration of heart chamber
CC Excl: See code: S26.01

✓7th **S26.021 Moderate laceration of heart with hemopericardium** MCC
Laceration of heart with penetration of heart chamber
CC Excl: See code: S26.01

✓7th **S26.022 Major laceration of heart with hemopericardium** MCC
Laceration of heart with penetration of multiple heart chambers
CC Excl: See code: S26.01

✓x7th **S26.09 Other injury of heart with hemopericardium** CC
CC Excl: CC with 7th character A: S21.301-S21.459 with 7th A, S26.00X-S26.99X with 7th A, S27.50X-S27.69X with 7th A, S27.892-S27.9X with 7th A, T14.8-T14.91

✓5th **S26.1 Injury of heart without hemopericardium**

✓x7th **S26.10 Unspecified injury of heart without hemopericardium** CC
CC Excl: See code: S26.09

✓x7th **S26.11 Contusion of heart without hemopericardium** CC
CC Excl: CC with 7th character A: S21.101-S21.159 with 7th A, S21.301-S21.95X with 7th A, S26.00X-S26.99X with 7th A, S27.50X-S27.69X with 7th A, S27.892-S27.9XX with 7th A, S28.1XXA, S29.021A, S29.029A, S38.3XXA, T14.8-T14.91, T79.7XX-T79.9XX with 7th A

✓x7th **S26.12 Laceration of heart without hemopericardium** MCC CC
CC Excl: MCC with 7 th character A: See code: S26.11

✓x7th **S26.19 Other injury of heart without hemopericardium** CC
CC Excl: CC with 7th character A: S21.301-S21.459 with 7th A, S26.00X-S26.99X with 7th A, S27.50X-S27.69X with 7th A, S27.892-S27.9XX with 7th A, T14.8-T14.91

✓5th **S26.9 Injury of heart, unspecified with or without hemopericardium**

✓x7th **S26.90 Unspecified injury of heart, unspecified with or without hemopericardium** CC
CC Excl: See code: S26.19

✓x7th **S26.91 Contusion of heart, unspecified with or without hemopericardium** CC
CC Excl: CC with 7th character A: S21.101-S21.159 with 7th A, S21.301-S21.95 with 7th A, S26.00X-S26.99X with 7th A, S27.50X-S27.69X with 7th A, S27.892-S27.9XX with 7th A, S28.1XX with 7th A, S29.021 with 7th A, S29.029A, S38.3XX with 7th A, T14.8-T14.91, T79.7XX-T79.9XX with 7th A

✓x7th **S26.92 Laceration of heart, unspecified with or without hemopericardium** MCC
Laceration of heart NOS
CC Excl: See code: S26.91

✓x7th **S26.99 Other injury of heart, unspecified with or without hemopericardium** CC
CC Excl: CC with 7th character A: S21.301-S21.459 with 7th A, S26.00X-S26.99X with 7th A, S27.50X-S27.69X with 7th A, S27.892-S27.9X with 7th A, T14.8-T14.91

S27 Injury of other and unspecified intrathoracic organs
Code also any associated open wound of thorax (S21.-)
EXCLUDES 2 *injury of cervical esophagus (S10-S19)*
injury of trachea (cervical) (S10-S19)

The appropriate 7th is to be added to each code from category S27.
A initial encounter
D subsequent encounter
S sequela

S27.0 Traumatic pneumothorax CC
EXCLUDES 1 *spontaneous pneumothorax (J93.-)*
CC Excl: CC with 7th character A: S21.101-S21.159 with 7th A, S21.301-S21.95X with 7th A, S27.0XX-S27.399 with 7th A, S27.50X-S27.69X with 7th A, S27.892-S27.9XXA, S28.1XXA, S29.021A, S29.029A, S38.3XXA, T14.8-T14.91, T79.7XX-T79.9XX with 7th A

S27.1 Traumatic hemothorax MCC
CC Excl: MCC with 7th character A: See code: S27.0

S27.2 Traumatic hemopneumothorax MCC
CC Excl: MCC with 7th character A: See code: S27.0

S27.3 Other and unspecified injuries of lung

CC Excl: For CC codes in subcategory S27.3, unless otherwise noted: CC with 7th character A: S21.101-S21.159 with 7th A, S21.301-S21.95X with 7th A, S27.301-S27.399 with 7th A, S27.50X-S27.69X with 7th A, S27.892-S27.9XX with 7th A, S28.1XXA, S29.021A, S29.029A, S38.3XXA, T14.8-T14.91, T79.7XX-T79.9XX with 7th A

S27.30 Unspecified injury of lung
S27.301 Unspecified injury of lung, unilateral CC
S27.302 Unspecified injury of lung, bilateral CC
S27.309 Unspecified injury of lung, unspecified CC

S27.31 Primary blast injury of lung
Blast injury of lung NOS
S27.311 Primary blast injury of lung, unilateral CC
S27.312 Primary blast injury of lung, bilateral CC
S27.319 Primary blast injury of lung, unspecified CC

S27.32 Contusion of lung
S27.321 Contusion of lung, unilateral CC
S27.322 Contusion of lung, bilateral CC
S27.329 Contusion of lung, unspecified CC

S27.33 Laceration of lung
S27.331 Laceration of lung, unilateral MCC
CC Excl: MCC with 7th character A: S21.101-S21.159 with 7th A, S21.301-S21.95X with 7th A, S27.301-S27.399 with 7th A, S27.50X-S27.69X with 7th A, S27.892-S27.9XX with 7th A, S28.1XXA, S29.021A, S29.029A, S38.3XXA, T14.8-T14.91, T79.7XX-T79.9XX with 7th AA
S27.332 Laceration of lung, bilateral MCC
CC Excl: See code: S27.331
S27.339 Laceration of lung, unspecified MCC
CC Excl: See code: S27.331

S27.39 Other injuries of lung
Secondary blast injury of lung
S27.391 Other injuries of lung, unilateral CC
S27.392 Other injuries of lung, bilateral CC
S27.399 Other injuries of lung, unspecified CC

S27.4 Injury of bronchus

CC Excl: For MCC codes in subcategory S27.4, unless otherwise noted: MCC with 7th character A: S21.101-S21.159 with 7th A, S21.301-S21.95X with 7th A, S27.401-S27.69X with 7th A, S27.892-S27.9XX with 7th A, S28.1XXA, S29.021XA, S29.029XA, S38.3XXA, T14.8-T14.91, T79.7XX-T79.9XX with 7th A

S27.40 Unspecified injury of bronchus
S27.401 Unspecified injury of bronchus, unilateral MCC
S27.402 Unspecified injury of bronchus, bilateral MCC
S27.409 Unspecified injury of bronchus, unspecified MCC

S27.41 Primary blast injury of bronchus
Blast injury of bronchus NOS
S27.411 Primary blast injury of bronchus, unilateral MCC
S27.412 Primary blast injury of bronchus, bilateral MCC
S27.419 Primary blast injury of bronchus, unspecified MCC

S27.42 Contusion of bronchus
S27.421 Contusion of bronchus, unilateral MCC
S27.422 Contusion of bronchus, bilateral MCC
S27.429 Contusion of bronchus, unspecified MCC

S27.43 Laceration of bronchus
S27.431 Laceration of bronchus, unilateral MCC
S27.432 Laceration of bronchus, bilateral MCC
S27.439 Laceration of bronchus, unspecified MCC

S27.49 Other injury of bronchus
Secondary blast injury of bronchus
S27.491 Other injury of bronchus, unilateral MCC
S27.492 Other injury of bronchus, bilateral MCC
S27.499 Other injury of bronchus, unspecified MCC

S27.5 Injury of thoracic trachea

CC Excl: For CC codes in subcategory S27.5, unless otherwise noted: CC with 7th character A: S21.101-S21.159 with 7th A, S21.301-S21.95X with 7th A, S27.50X-S27.69X with 7th A, S27.892-S27.9XX with 7th A, S28.1XXA, S29.021 with 7th A, S29.029A, S38.3XXA, T14.8-T14.91, T79.7XX-T79.9XX with 7th A

S27.50 Unspecified injury of thoracic trachea CC
S27.51 Primary blast injury of thoracic trachea CC
Blast injury of thoracic trachea NOS
S27.52 Contusion of thoracic trachea CC
S27.53 Laceration of thoracic trachea CC
S27.59 Other injury of thoracic trachea CC
Secondary blast injury of thoracic trachea

S27.6 Injury of pleura

CC Excl: For CC codes in subcategory S27.6, unless otherwise noted: See code: S27.5

S27.60 Unspecified injury of pleura CC
S27.63 Laceration of pleura CC
S27.69 Other injury of pleura CC

S27.8 Injury of other specified intrathoracic organs

S27.80 Injury of diaphragm

CC Excl: For CC/MCC codes in subcategory S27.80, unless otherwise noted: CC with 7th character A: S21.101-S21.159 with 7th A, S21.301-S21.95 with 7th A, S27.50X-S27.809 with 7th A, S27.892-S27.9XX with 7th A, S28.1XXA, S29.021A, S29.029A, S38.3XXA, T14.8-T14.91, T79.7XX-T79.9XX with 7th A

S27.802 Contusion of diaphragm CC
S27.803 Laceration of diaphragm CC
S27.808 Other injury of diaphragm CC
S27.809 Unspecified injury of diaphragm CC

S27.81 Injury of esophagus (thoracic part)
S27.812 Contusion of esophagus (thoracic part) MCC
CC Excl: MCC with 7th character A: S21.101-S21.159 with 7th A, S21.301-S21.95 with 7th A, S27.50X-S27.69X with 7th A, S27.812-S27.9XX with 7th A, S28.1XXA, S29.021A, S29.029A, S38.3XXA, T14.8-T14.91, T79.7XX-T79.9XX with 7th A
S27.813 Laceration of esophagus (thoracic part) MCC
CC Excl: See code: S27.812
S27.818 Other injury of esophagus (thoracic part) MCC
CC Excl: See code: S27.812
S27.819 Unspecified injury of esophagus (thoracic part) MCC
CC Excl: See code: S27.812

S27.89 Injury of other specified intrathoracic organs
Injury of lymphatic thoracic duct
Injury of thymus gland

CC Excl: For CC codes in subcategory S27.89, unless otherwise noted: CC with 7th character A: S21.101-S21.159 with 7th A, S21.301-S21.95X with 7th A, S27.50X-S27.69X with 7th A, S27.892-S27.9XX with 7th A, S28.1XXA, S29.021A, S29.029A, S38.3XXA, T14.8-T14.91, T79.7XX-T79.9XX with 7th A

S27.892 Contusion of other specified intrathoracic organs CC

S27.893 Laceration of other specified intrathoracic organs CC

S27.898 Other injury of other specified intrathoracic organs CC

S27.899 Unspecified injury of other specified intrathoracic organs CC

S27.9 Injury of unspecified intrathoracic organ CC
CC Excl: CC with 7th character A: S21.101-S21.159 with 7th A, S21.301-S21.95X with 7th A, S27.50X-S27.69X with 7th A, S27.892-S27.9XX with 7th A, S28.1XXA, S29.021A, S29.029A, S38.3XXA, T14.8-T14.91, T79.7XX-T79.9XX with 7th A

S28 Crushing injury of thorax, and traumatic amputation of part of thorax

The appropriate 7th is to be added to each code from category S28.
A initial encounter
D subsequent encounter
S sequela

S28.0 Crushed chest
Use additional code for all associated injuries
EXCLUDES 1 *flail chest (S22.5)*

S28.1 Traumatic amputation (partial) of part of thorax, except breast CC
CC Excl: CC with 7th character A: S21.101-S21.159 with 7th A, S21.301-S21.95X with 7th A, S23.3XA, S23.8XA, S27.50X-S27.69X with 7th A, S27.892-S27.9XX with 7th A, S28.1XXA, S29.021A, S29.029A, S38.3XXA, T14.8-T14.91, T79.7XX-T79.9XX with 7th A

S28.2 Traumatic amputation of breast

S28.21 Complete traumatic amputation of breast
Traumatic amputation of breast NOS

S28.211 Complete traumatic amputation of right breast

S28.212 Complete traumatic amputation of left breast

S28.219 Complete traumatic amputation of unspecified breast

S28.22 Partial traumatic amputation of breast

S28.221 Partial traumatic amputation of right breast

S28.222 Partial traumatic amputation of left breast

S28.229 Partial traumatic amputation of unspecified breast

S29 Other and unspecified injuries of thorax
Code also any associated open wound (S21.-)

The appropriate 7th is to be added to each code from category S29.
A initial encounter
D subsequent encounter
S sequela

S29.0 Injury of muscle and tendon at thorax level

S29.00 Unspecified injury of muscle and tendon of thorax

S29.001 Unspecified injury of muscle and tendon of front wall of thorax

S29.002 Unspecified injury of muscle and tendon of back wall of thorax

S29.009 Unspecified injury of muscle and tendon of unspecified wall of thorax

S29.01 Strain of muscle and tendon of thorax

S29.011 Strain of muscle and tendon of front wall of thorax

S29.012 Strain of muscle and tendon of back wall of thorax

S29.019 Strain of muscle and tendon of unspecified wall of thorax

S29.02 Laceration of muscle and tendon of thorax

S29.021 Laceration of muscle and tendon of front wall of thorax CC
CC Excl: See code: S28.1

S29.022 Laceration of muscle and tendon of back wall of thorax

S29.029 Laceration of muscle and tendon of unspecified wall of thorax CC
CC Excl: See code: S28.1

S29.09 Other injury of muscle and tendon of thorax

S29.091 Other injury of muscle and tendon of front wall of thorax

S29.092 Other injury of muscle and tendon of back wall of thorax

S29.099 Other injury of muscle and tendon of unspecified wall of thorax

S29.8 Other specified injuries of thorax

S29.9 Unspecified injury of thorax

Injuries to the abdomen, lower back, lumbar spine, pelvis and external genitals (S30-S39)

INCLUDES injuries to the abdominal wall
injuries to the anus
injuries to the buttock
injuries to the external genitalia
injuries to the flank
injuries to the groin

EXCLUDES 2 *burns and corrosions (T20-T32)*
effects of foreign body in anus and rectum (T18.5)
effects of foreign body in genitourinary tract (T19.-)
effects of foreign body in stomach, small intestine and colon (T18.2-T18.4)
frostbite (T33-T34)
insect bite or sting, venomous (T63.4)

S30 Superficial injury of abdomen, lower back, pelvis and external genitals
EXCLUDES 2 *superficial injury of hip (S70.-)*

The appropriate 7th is to be added to each code from category S30.
A initial encounter
D subsequent encounter
S sequela

S30.0 Contusion of lower back and pelvis
Contusion of buttock

S30.1 Contusion of abdominal wall
Contusion of flank
Contusion of groin

S30.2 Contusion of external genital organs

S30.20 Contusion of unspecified external genital organ

S30.201 Contusion of unspecified external genital organ, male ♂

S30.202 Contusion of unspecified external genital organ, female ♀

S30.21 Contusion of penis ♂

S30.22 Contusion of scrotum and testes ♂

S30.23 Contusion of vagina and vulva ♀

S30.3 Contusion of anus

S30.8 Other superficial injuries of abdomen, lower back, pelvis and external genitals

S30.81 Abrasion of abdomen, lower back, pelvis and external genitals

S30.810 Abrasion of lower back and pelvis

S30.811 Abrasion of abdominal wall

S30.812 Abrasion of penis ♂

S30.813 Abrasion of scrotum and testes ♂

S30.814 Abrasion of vagina and vulva ♀

S30.815 Abrasion of unspecified external genital organs, male ♂

S30.816 Abrasion of unspecified external genital organs, female ♀

S30.817 Abrasion of anus

S30.82 **Blister (nonthermal) of abdomen, lower back, pelvis and external genitals**
- S30.820 **Blister (nonthermal) of lower back and pelvis**
- S30.821 **Blister (nonthermal) of abdominal wall**
- S30.822 **Blister (nonthermal) of penis** ♂
- S30.823 **Blister (nonthermal) of scrotum and testes** ♂
- S30.824 **Blister (nonthermal) of vagina and vulva** ♀
- S30.825 **Blister (nonthermal) of unspecified external genital organs, male** ♂
- S30.826 **Blister (nonthermal) of unspecified external genital organs, female** ♀
- S30.827 **Blister (nonthermal) of anus**

S30.84 **External constriction of abdomen, lower back, pelvis and external genitals**
- S30.840 **External constriction of lower back and pelvis**
- S30.841 **External constriction of abdominal wall**
- S30.842 **External constriction of penis** ♂
  Hair tourniquet syndrome of penis
  Use additional cause code to identify the constricting item (W49.0-)
- S30.843 **External constriction of scrotum and testes** ♂
- S30.844 **External constriction of vagina and vulva** ♀
- S30.845 **External constriction of unspecified external genital organs, male** ♂
- S30.846 **External constriction of unspecified external genital organs, female** ♀

S30.85 **Superficial foreign body of abdomen, lower back, pelvis and external genitals**
Splinter in the abdomen, lower back, pelvis and external genitals
- S30.850 **Superficial foreign body of lower back and pelvis**
- S30.851 **Superficial foreign body of abdominal wall**
- S30.852 **Superficial foreign body of penis** ♂
- S30.853 **Superficial foreign body of scrotum and testes** ♂
- S30.854 **Superficial foreign body of vagina and vulva** ♀
- S30.855 **Superficial foreign body of unspecified external genital organs, male** ♂
- S30.856 **Superficial foreign body of unspecified external genital organs, female** ♀
- S30.857 **Superficial foreign body of anus**

S30.86 **Insect bite (nonvenomous) of abdomen, lower back, pelvis and external genitals**
- S30.860 **Insect bite (nonvenomous) of lower back and pelvis**
- S30.861 **Insect bite (nonvenomous) of abdominal wall**
- S30.862 **Insect bite (nonvenomous) of penis** ♂
- S30.863 **Insect bite (nonvenomous) of scrotum and testes** ♂
- S30.864 **Insect bite (nonvenomous) of vagina and vulva** ♀
- S30.865 **Insect bite (nonvenomous) of unspecified external genital organs, male** ♂
- S30.866 **Insect bite (nonvenomous) of unspecified external genital organs, female** ♀
- S30.867 **Insect bite (nonvenomous) of anus**

S30.87 **Other superficial bite of abdomen, lower back, pelvis and external genitals**
EXCLUDES 1 *open bite of abdomen, lower back, pelvis and external genitals (S31.05, S31.15, S31.25, S31.35, S31.45, S31.55)*
- S30.870 **Other superficial bite of lower back and pelvis**
- S30.871 **Other superficial bite of abdominal wall**
- S30.872 **Other superficial bite of penis** ♂
- S30.873 **Other superficial bite of scrotum and testes** ♂
- S30.874 **Other superficial bite of vagina and vulva** ♀
- S30.875 **Other superficial bite of unspecified external genital organs, male** ♂
- S30.876 **Other superficial bite of unspecified external genital organs, female** ♀
- S30.877 **Other superficial bite of anus**

S30.9 **Unspecified superficial injury of abdomen, lower back, pelvis and external genitals**
- S30.91 **Unspecified superficial injury of lower back and pelvis**
- S30.92 **Unspecified superficial injury of abdominal wall**
- S30.93 **Unspecified superficial injury of penis** ♂
- S30.94 **Unspecified superficial injury of scrotum and testes** ♂
- S30.95 **Unspecified superficial injury of vagina and vulva** ♀
- S30.96 **Unspecified superficial injury of unspecified external genital organs, male** ♂
- S30.97 **Unspecified superficial injury of unspecified external genital organs, female** ♀
- S30.98 **Unspecified superficial injury of anus**

S31 Open wound of abdomen, lower back, pelvis and external genitals

Code also any associated:
- spinal cord injury (S24.0, S24.1-, S34.0-, S34.1-)
- wound infection

EXCLUDES 1 *traumatic amputation of part of abdomen, lower back and pelvis (S38.2-, S38.3)*

EXCLUDES 2 *open wound of hip (S71.00-S71.02)*
open fracture of pelvis (S32.1- – S32.9 with 7th B)

The appropriate 7th is to be added to each code from category S31.
- A initial encounter
- D subsequent encounter
- S sequela

S31.0 **Open wound of lower back and pelvis**

S31.00 **Unspecified open wound of lower back and pelvis**
- S31.000 **Unspecified open wound of lower back and pelvis without penetration into retroperitoneum**
  Unspecified open wound of lower back and pelvis NOS
- S31.001 **Unspecified open wound of lower back and pelvis with penetration into retroperitoneum** MCC
  CC Excl: CC with 7th character A: S31.001A, S31.011A, S31.021, S31.031A, S31.041A, S31.051-S31.159 with 7th A, S31.600-S31.659 with 7th A, S31.831-S31.839 with 7th A, S36.81X-S36.99X with 7th A, S38.3XX-S39.023 with 7th A, T14.8-T14.91, T79.A0X-T79.9XX with 7th A

S31.01 **Laceration without foreign body of lower back and pelvis**
- S31.010 **Laceration without foreign body of lower back and pelvis without penetration into retroperitoneum**
  Laceration without foreign body of lower back and pelvis NOS
- S31.011 **Laceration without foreign body of lower back and pelvis with penetration into retroperitoneum** MCC
  CC Excl: See code: S30.001

S31.02 **Laceration with foreign body of lower back and pelvis**
- S31.020 **Laceration with foreign body of lower back and pelvis without penetration into retroperitoneum**
  Laceration with foreign body of lower back and pelvis NOS

7th **S31.021 Laceration with foreign body of lower back and pelvis with penetration into retroperitoneum** MCC
CC Excl: See code: S30.001

6th **S31.03 Puncture wound without foreign body of lower back and pelvis**

7th **S31.030 Puncture wound without foreign body of lower back and pelvis without penetration into retroperitoneum**
Puncture wound without foreign body of lower back and pelvis NOS

7th **S31.031 Puncture wound without foreign body of lower back and pelvis with penetration into retroperitoneum** MCC
CC Excl: See code: S30.001

6th **S31.04 Puncture wound with foreign body of lower back and pelvis**

7th **S31.040 Puncture wound with foreign body of lower back and pelvis without penetration into retroperitoneum**
Puncture wound with foreign body of lower back and pelvis NOS

7th **S31.041 Puncture wound with foreign body of lower back and pelvis with penetration into retroperitoneum** MCC
CC Excl: See code: S30.001

6th **S31.05 Open bite of lower back and pelvis**
Bite of lower back and pelvis NOS
EXCLUDES 1 *superficial bite of lower back and pelvis (S30.860, S30.870)*

7th **S31.050 Open bite of lower back and pelvis without penetration into retroperitoneum**
Open bite of lower back and pelvis NOS

7th **S31.051 Open bite of lower back and pelvis with penetration into retroperitoneum** MCC
CC Excl: See code: S30.001

5th **S31.1 Open wound of abdominal wall without penetration into peritoneal cavity**
Open wound of abdominal wall NOS
EXCLUDES 2 *open wound of abdominal wall with penetration into peritoneal cavity (S31.6-)*

6th **S31.10 Unspecified open wound of abdominal wall without penetration into peritoneal cavity**

7th **S31.100 Unspecified open wound of abdominal wall, right upper quadrant without penetration into peritoneal cavity**

7th **S31.101 Unspecified open wound of abdominal wall, left upper quadrant without penetration into peritoneal cavity**

7th **S31.102 Unspecified open wound of abdominal wall, epigastric region without penetration into peritoneal cavity**

7th **S31.103 Unspecified open wound of abdominal wall, right lower quadrant without penetration into peritoneal cavity**

7th **S31.104 Unspecified open wound of abdominal wall, left lower quadrant without penetration into peritoneal cavity**

7th **S31.105 Unspecified open wound of abdominal wall, periumbilic region without penetration into peritoneal cavity**

7th **S31.109 Unspecified open wound of abdominal wall, unspecified quadrant without penetration into peritoneal cavity**
Unspecified open wound of abdominal wall NOS

6th **S31.11 Laceration without foreign body of abdominal wall without penetration into peritoneal cavity**

7th **S31.110 Laceration without foreign body of abdominal wall, right upper quadrant without penetration into peritoneal cavity**

7th **S31.111 Laceration without foreign body of abdominal wall, left upper quadrant without penetration into peritoneal cavity**

7th **S31.112 Laceration without foreign body of abdominal wall, epigastric region without penetration into peritoneal cavity**

7th **S31.113 Laceration without foreign body of abdominal wall, right lower quadrant without penetration into peritoneal cavity**

7th **S31.114 Laceration without foreign body of abdominal wall, left lower quadrant without penetration into peritoneal cavity**

7th **S31.115 Laceration without foreign body of abdominal wall, periumbilic region without penetration into peritoneal cavity**

7th **S31.119 Laceration without foreign body of abdominal wall, unspecified quadrant without penetration into peritoneal cavity**

6th **S31.12 Laceration with foreign body of abdominal wall without penetration into peritoneal cavity**

7th **S31.120 Laceration of abdominal wall with foreign body, right upper quadrant without penetration into peritoneal cavity**

7th **S31.121 Laceration of abdominal wall with foreign body, left upper quadrant without penetration into peritoneal cavity**

7th **S31.122 Laceration of abdominal wall with foreign body, epigastric region without penetration into peritoneal cavity**

7th **S31.123 Laceration of abdominal wall with foreign body, right lower quadrant without penetration into peritoneal cavity**

7th **S31.124 Laceration of abdominal wall with foreign body, left lower quadrant without penetration into peritoneal cavity**

7th **S31.125 Laceration of abdominal wall with foreign body, periumbilic region without penetration into peritoneal cavity**

7th **S31.129 Laceration of abdominal wall with foreign body, unspecified quadrant without penetration into peritoneal cavity**

6th **S31.13 Puncture wound of abdominal wall without foreign body without penetration into peritoneal cavity**

7th **S31.130 Puncture wound of abdominal wall without foreign body, right upper quadrant without penetration into peritoneal cavity**

7th **S31.131 Puncture wound of abdominal wall without foreign body, left upper quadrant without penetration into peritoneal cavity**

7th **S31.132 Puncture wound of abdominal wall without foreign body, epigastric region without penetration into peritoneal cavity**

7th **S31.133 Puncture wound of abdominal wall without foreign body, right lower quadrant without penetration into peritoneal cavity**

7th **S31.134 Puncture wound of abdominal wall without foreign body, left lower quadrant without penetration into peritoneal cavity**

7th **S31.135 Puncture wound of abdominal wall without foreign body, periumbilic region without penetration into peritoneal cavity**

7th **S31.139 Puncture wound of abdominal wall without foreign body, unspecified quadrant without penetration into peritoneal cavity**

6th **S31.14 Puncture wound of abdominal wall with foreign body without penetration into peritoneal cavity**

7th **S31.140 Puncture wound of abdominal wall with foreign body, right upper quadrant without penetration into peritoneal cavity**

7th **S31.141 Puncture wound of abdominal wall with foreign body, left upper quadrant without penetration into peritoneal cavity**

7th **S31.142 Puncture wound of abdominal wall with foreign body, epigastric region without penetration into peritoneal cavity**

7th **S31.143 Puncture wound of abdominal wall with foreign body, right lower quadrant without penetration into peritoneal cavity**

7th **S31.144 Puncture wound of abdominal wall with foreign body, left lower quadrant without penetration into peritoneal cavity**

7th **S31.145 Puncture wound of abdominal wall with foreign body, periumbilic region without penetration into peritoneal cavity**

✓7th S31.149 **Puncture wound of abdominal wall with foreign body, unspecified quadrant without penetration into peritoneal cavity**

✓6th S31.15 **Open bite of abdominal wall without penetration into peritoneal cavity**
Bite of abdominal wall NOS
EXCLUDES 1 *superficial bite of abdominal wall (S30.871)*

✓7th S31.150 **Open bite of abdominal wall, right upper quadrant without penetration into peritoneal cavity**

✓7th S31.151 **Open bite of abdominal wall, left upper quadrant without penetration into peritoneal cavity**

✓7th S31.152 **Open bite of abdominal wall, epigastric region without penetration into peritoneal cavity**

✓7th S31.153 **Open bite of abdominal wall, right lower quadrant without penetration into peritoneal cavity**

✓7th S31.154 **Open bite of abdominal wall, left lower quadrant without penetration into peritoneal cavity**

✓7th S31.155 **Open bite of abdominal wall, periumbilic region without penetration into peritoneal cavity**

✓7th S31.159 **Open bite of abdominal wall, unspecified quadrant without penetration into peritoneal cavity**

✓5th S31.2 **Open wound of penis**

✓x7th S31.20 **Unspecified open wound of penis** ♂

✓x7th S31.21 **Laceration without foreign body of penis** ♂

✓x7th S31.22 **Laceration with foreign body of penis** ♂

✓x7th S31.23 **Puncture wound without foreign body of penis** ♂

✓x7th S31.24 **Puncture wound with foreign body of penis** ♂

✓x7th S31.25 **Open bite of penis** ♂
Bite of penis NOS
EXCLUDES 1 *superficial bite of penis (S30.862, S30.872)*

✓5th S31.3 **Open wound of scrotum and testes**

✓x7th S31.30 **Unspecified open wound of scrotum and testes** ♂

✓x7th S31.31 **Laceration without foreign body of scrotum and testes** ♂

✓x7th S31.32 **Laceration with foreign body of scrotum and testes** ♂

✓x7th S31.33 **Puncture wound without foreign body of scrotum and testes** ♂

✓x7th S31.34 **Puncture wound with foreign body of scrotum and testes** ♂

✓x7th S31.35 **Open bite of scrotum and testes** ♂
Bite of scrotum and testes NOS
EXCLUDES 1 *superficial bite of scrotum and testes (S30.863, S30.873)*

✓5th S31.4 **Open wound of vagina and vulva**
EXCLUDES 1 *injury to vagina and vulva during delivery (O70-, O71.4)*

✓x7th S31.40 **Unspecified open wound of vagina and vulva** ♀

✓x7th S31.41 **Laceration without foreign body of vagina and vulva** ♀

✓x7th S31.42 **Laceration with foreign body of vagina and vulva** ♀

✓x7th S31.43 **Puncture wound without foreign body of vagina and vulva** ♀

✓x7th S31.44 **Puncture wound with foreign body of vagina and vulva** ♀

✓x7th S31.45 **Open bite of vagina and vulva** ♀
Bite of vagina and vulva NOS
EXCLUDES 1 *superficial bite of vagina and vulva (S30.864, S30.874)*

✓5th S31.5 **Open wound of unspecified external genital organs**
EXCLUDES 1 *traumatic amputation of external genital organs (S38.21, S38.22)*

✓6th S31.50 **Unspecified open wound of unspecified external genital organs**

✓7th S31.501 **Unspecified open wound of unspecified external genital organs, male** ♂

✓7th S31.502 **Unspecified open wound of unspecified external genital organs, female** ♀

✓6th S31.51 **Laceration without foreign body of unspecified external genital organs**

✓7th S31.511 **Laceration without foreign body of unspecified external genital organs, male** ♂

✓7th S31.512 **Laceration without foreign body of unspecified external genital organs, female** ♀

✓6th S31.52 **Laceration with foreign body of unspecified external genital organs**

✓7th S31.521 **Laceration with foreign body of unspecified external genital organs, male** ♂

✓7th S31.522 **Laceration with foreign body of unspecified external genital organs, female** ♀

✓6th S31.53 **Puncture wound without foreign body of unspecified external genital organs**

✓7th S31.531 **Puncture wound without foreign body of unspecified external genital organs, male** ♂

✓7th S31.532 **Puncture wound without foreign body of unspecified external genital organs, female** ♀

✓6th S31.54 **Puncture wound with foreign body of unspecified external genital organs**

✓7th S31.541 **Puncture wound with foreign body of unspecified external genital organs, male** ♂

✓7th S31.542 **Puncture wound with foreign body of unspecified external genital organs, female** ♀

✓6th S31.55 **Open bite of unspecified external genital organs**
Bite of unspecified external genital organs NOS
EXCLUDES 1 *superficial bite of unspecified external genital organs (S30.865, S30.866, S30.875, S30.876)*

✓7th S31.551 **Open bite of unspecified external genital organs, male** ♂

✓7th S31.552 **Open bite of unspecified external genital organs, female** ♀

✓5th S31.6 **Open wound of abdominal wall with penetration into peritoneal cavity**

CC Excl: For MCC codes in category S31.6, unless otherwise noted: MCC with 7th character A: S31.001A, S31.011A, S31.021, S31.031A, S31.041A, S31.051-S31.159 with 7th A, S31.600-S31.659 with 7th A, S31.831-S31.839 with 7th A, S36.81X-S36.99X with 7th A, S38.3XX-S39.023 with 7th A, T14.8-T14.91, T79.A0X-T79.9XX with 7th A

✓6th S31.60 **Unspecified open wound of abdominal wall with penetration into peritoneal cavity**

✓7th S31.600 **Unspecified open wound of abdominal wall, right upper quadrant with penetration into peritoneal cavity** MCC

✓7th S31.601 **Unspecified open wound of abdominal wall, left upper quadrant with penetration into peritoneal cavity** MCC

✓7th S31.602 **Unspecified open wound of abdominal wall, epigastric region with penetration into peritoneal cavity** MCC

✓7th S31.603 **Unspecified open wound of abdominal wall, right lower quadrant with penetration into peritoneal cavity** MCC

✓7th S31.604 **Unspecified open wound of abdominal wall, left lower quadrant with penetration into peritoneal cavity** MCC

✓7th S31.605 **Unspecified open wound of abdominal wall, periumbilic region with penetration into peritoneal cavity** MCC

✓7th S31.609 **Unspecified open wound of abdominal wall, unspecified quadrant with penetration into peritoneal cavity** MCC

✓6th S31.61 **Laceration without foreign body of abdominal wall with penetration into peritoneal cavity**

✓7th S31.610 **Laceration without foreign body of abdominal wall, right upper quadrant with penetration into peritoneal cavity** MCC

- 7th S31.611 Laceration without foreign body of abdominal wall, left upper quadrant with penetration into peritoneal cavity MCC
- 7th S31.612 Laceration without foreign body of abdominal wall, epigastric region with penetration into peritoneal cavity MCC
- 7th S31.613 Laceration without foreign body of abdominal wall, right lower quadrant with penetration into peritoneal cavity MCC
- 7th S31.614 Laceration without foreign body of abdominal wall, left lower quadrant with penetration into peritoneal cavity MCC
- 7th S31.615 Laceration without foreign body of abdominal wall, periumbilic region with penetration into peritoneal cavity MCC
- 7th S31.619 Laceration without foreign body of abdominal wall, unspecified quadrant with penetration into peritoneal cavity MCC

6th **S31.62 Laceration with foreign body of abdominal wall with penetration into peritoneal cavity**

- 7th S31.620 Laceration with foreign body of abdominal wall, right upper quadrant with penetration into peritoneal cavity MCC
- 7th S31.621 Laceration with foreign body of abdominal wall, left upper quadrant with penetration into peritoneal cavity MCC
- 7th S31.622 Laceration with foreign body of abdominal wall, epigastric region with penetration into peritoneal cavity MCC
- 7th S31.623 Laceration with foreign body of abdominal wall, right lower quadrant with penetration into peritoneal cavity MCC
- 7th S31.624 Laceration with foreign body of abdominal wall, left lower quadrant with penetration into peritoneal cavity MCC
- 7th S31.625 Laceration with foreign body of abdominal wall, periumbilic region with penetration into peritoneal cavity MCC
- 7th S31.629 Laceration with foreign body of abdominal wall, unspecified quadrant with penetration into peritoneal cavity MCC

6th **S31.63 Puncture wound without foreign body of abdominal wall with penetration into peritoneal cavity**

- 7th S31.630 Puncture wound without foreign body of abdominal wall, right upper quadrant with penetration into peritoneal cavity MCC
- 7th S31.631 Puncture wound without foreign body of abdominal wall, left upper quadrant with penetration into peritoneal cavity MCC
- 7th S31.632 Puncture wound without foreign body of abdominal wall, epigastric region with penetration into peritoneal cavity MCC
- 7th S31.633 Puncture wound without foreign body of abdominal wall, right lower quadrant with penetration into peritoneal cavity MCC
- 7th S31.634 Puncture wound without foreign body of abdominal wall, left lower quadrant with penetration into peritoneal cavity MCC
- 7th S31.635 Puncture wound without foreign body of abdominal wall, periumbilic region with penetration into peritoneal cavity MCC
- 7th S31.639 Puncture wound without foreign body of abdominal wall, unspecified quadrant with penetration into peritoneal cavity MCC

6th **S31.64 Puncture wound with foreign body of abdominal wall with penetration into peritoneal cavity**

- 7th S31.640 Puncture wound with foreign body of abdominal wall, right upper quadrant with penetration into peritoneal cavity MCC
- 7th S31.641 Puncture wound with foreign body of abdominal wall, left upper quadrant with penetration into peritoneal cavity MCC
- 7th S31.642 Puncture wound with foreign body of abdominal wall, epigastric region with penetration into peritoneal cavity MCC
- 7th S31.643 Puncture wound with foreign body of abdominal wall, right lower quadrant with penetration into peritoneal cavity MCC
- 7th S31.644 Puncture wound with foreign body of abdominal wall, left lower quadrant with penetration into peritoneal cavity MCC
- 7th S31.645 Puncture wound with foreign body of abdominal wall, periumbilic region with penetration into peritoneal cavity MCC
- 7th S31.649 Puncture wound with foreign body of abdominal wall, unspecified quadrant with penetration into peritoneal cavity MCC

6th **S31.65 Open bite of abdominal wall with penetration into peritoneal cavity**

EXCLUDES 1 *superficial bite of abdominal wall (S30.861, S30.871)*

- 7th S31.650 Open bite of abdominal wall, right upper quadrant with penetration into peritoneal cavity MCC
- 7th S31.651 Open bite of abdominal wall, left upper quadrant with penetration into peritoneal cavity MCC
- 7th S31.652 Open bite of abdominal wall, epigastric region with penetration into peritoneal cavity MCC
- 7th S31.653 Open bite of abdominal wall, right lower quadrant with penetration into peritoneal cavity MCC
- 7th S31.654 Open bite of abdominal wall, left lower quadrant with penetration into peritoneal cavity MCC
- 7th S31.655 Open bite of abdominal wall, periumbilic region with penetration into peritoneal cavity MCC
- 7th S31.659 Open bite of abdominal wall, unspecified quadrant with penetration into peritoneal cavity MCC

5th **S31.8 Open wound of other parts of abdomen, lower back and pelvis**

6th **S31.80 Open wound of unspecified buttock**

- 7th S31.801 Laceration without foreign body of unspecified buttock
- 7th S31.802 Laceration with foreign body of unspecified buttock
- 7th S31.803 Puncture wound without foreign body of unspecified buttock
- 7th S31.804 Puncture wound with foreign body of unspecified buttock
- 7th S31.805 Open bite of unspecified buttock
  - Bite of buttock NOS
  - EXCLUDES 1 *superficial bite of buttock (S30.870)*
- 7th S31.809 Unspecified open wound of unspecified buttock

6th **S31.81 Open wound of right buttock**

- 7th S31.811 Laceration without foreign body of right buttock
- 7th S31.812 Laceration with foreign body of right buttock
- 7th S31.813 Puncture wound without foreign body of right buttock
- 7th S31.814 Puncture wound with foreign body of right buttock
- 7th S31.815 Open bite of right buttock
  - Bite of right buttock NOS
  - EXCLUDES 1 *superficial bite of buttock (S30.870)*
- 7th S31.819 Unspecified open wound of right buttock

6th **S31.82 Open wound of left buttock**

- 7th S31.821 Laceration without foreign body of left buttock
- 7th S31.822 Laceration with foreign body of left buttock

S31.823 Puncture wound without foreign body of left buttock
S31.824 Puncture wound with foreign body of left buttock
S31.825 Open bite of left buttock
Bite of left buttock NOS
EXCLUDES 1 *superficial bite of buttock (S30.870)*
S31.829 Unspecified open wound of left buttock
S31.83 Open wound of anus
S31.831 Laceration without foreign body of anus
S31.832 Laceration with foreign body of anus
S31.833 Puncture wound without foreign body of anus
S31.834 Puncture wound with foreign body of anus
S31.835 Open bite of anus
Bite of anus NOS
EXCLUDES 1 *superficial bite of anus (S30.877)*
S31.839 Unspecified open wound of anus

S32 Fracture of lumbar spine and pelvis

NOTE A fracture not indicated as displaced or nondisplaced should be coded to displaced.
A fracture not indicated as opened or closed should be coded to closed.

INCLUDES fracture of lumbosacral neural arch
fracture of lumbosacral spinous process
fracture of lumbosacral transverse process
fracture of lumbosacral vertebra
fracture of lumbosacral vertebral arch

Code first any associated spinal cord and spinal nerve injury (S34.-)
EXCLUDES 1 *transection of abdomen (S38.3)*
EXCLUDES 2 *fracture of hip NOS (S72.0-)*
AHA: 2012, 4Q, 93

The appropriate 7th is to be added to each code from category S32.
A initial encounter for closed fracture
B initial encounter for open fracture
D subsequent encounter for fracture with routine healing
G subsequent encounter for fracture with delayed healing
K subsequent encounter for fracture with nonunion
S sequela

S32.0 Fracture of lumbar vertebra
Fracture of lumbar spine NOS

CC Excl: For CC/MCC codes in subcategory S32.0, unless otherwise noted: CC with 7th character A or MCC with 7th character B: M48.40X-M48.58X with 7th S, M80.08XS, M80.88XS, M84.350S, M84.454S, M84.550S, M84.58XS, M84.650S, M99.13, M99.15-M99.17, M99.19, S03.8XX-S03.9XX with 7th A, S12.000-S12.9XX with 7th S, S13.9XXA, S14.109A, S14.119A, S14.129A, S14.139A, S14.149A, S14.159A, S22.000-S22.9XX with 7th S, S23.20X-S23.29X with 7th A, S23.9XXA, S24.109A, S24.119A, S24.139A, S24.149A, S24.159A, S29.001-S29.019 with 7th A, S29.091-S29.9XX with 7th A, S32.000-S33.39X with 7th [A, B, S], S33.5XXA, S33.9XX-S34.01X with 7th A, S34.101-S34.129 with 7th A, S38.1XXA, S38.3XX-S39.013 with 7th A, S39.091-S39.94X with 7th A, T14.8-T14.91, T79.A0X-T79.9XX with 7th A

CC with 7th character K: M80.00X-M84.68X with 7th [K, P], S02.0XX-S02.92X with 7th K, S12.000-S12.691 with 7th K, S22.000-S22.9XX with 7th K, S32.000-S32.9XX with 7th K, S42.001-S42.92X with 7th [K, P], S49.001-S49.199 with 7th [K, P], S52.001-S52.92X with 7th [K, M, N, P, Q, R], S59.001-S59.299 with 7th [K, P], S62.001-S62.92X with 7th [K, P], S72.001-S72.92X with 7th [K, M, N, P, Q, R], S79.001-S79.199 with 7th [K, P], S82.001-S82.92X with 7th [K, M, N, P, Q, R], S89.001-S89.399 with 7th [K, P], S92.001-S92.919 with 7th [K, P]

S32.00 Fracture of unspecified lumbar vertebra
7 S32.000 Wedge compression fracture of unspecified lumbar vertebra MCC CC
7 S32.001 Stable burst fracture of unspecified lumbar vertebra MCC CC
7 S32.002 Unstable burst fracture of unspecified lumbar vertebra MCC CC
7 S32.008 Other fracture of unspecified lumbar vertebra MCC CC
7 S32.009 Unspecified fracture of unspecified lumbar vertebra MCC CC

S32.01 Fracture of first lumbar vertebra
7 S32.010 Wedge compression fracture of first lumbar vertebra MCC CC
7 S32.011 Stable burst fracture of first lumbar vertebra MCC CC
7 S32.012 Unstable burst fracture of first lumbar vertebra MCC CC
7 S32.018 Other fracture of first lumbar vertebra MCC CC
7 S32.019 Unspecified fracture of first lumbar vertebra MCC CC

S32.02 Fracture of second lumbar vertebra
7 S32.020 Wedge compression fracture of second lumbar vertebra MCC CC
7 S32.021 Stable burst fracture of second lumbar vertebra MCC CC
7 S32.022 Unstable burst fracture of second lumbar vertebra MCC CC
7 S32.028 Other fracture of second lumbar vertebra MCC CC
7 S32.029 Unspecified fracture of second lumbar vertebra MCC CC

S32.03 Fracture of third lumbar vertebra
7 S32.030 Wedge compression fracture of third lumbar vertebra MCC CC
7 S32.031 Stable burst fracture of third lumbar vertebra MCC CC
7 S32.032 Unstable burst fracture of third lumbar vertebra MCC CC
7 S32.038 Other fracture of third lumbar vertebra MCC CC
7 S32.039 Unspecified fracture of third lumbar vertebra MCC CC

S32.04 Fracture of fourth lumbar vertebra
7 S32.040 Wedge compression fracture of fourth lumbar vertebra MCC CC
7 S32.041 Stable burst fracture of fourth lumbar vertebra MCC CC
7 S32.042 Unstable burst fracture of fourth lumbar vertebra MCC CC
7 S32.048 Other fracture of fourth lumbar vertebra MCC CC
7 S32.049 Unspecified fracture of fourth lumbar vertebra MCC CC

S32.05 Fracture of fifth lumbar vertebra
7 S32.050 Wedge compression fracture of fifth lumbar vertebra MCC CC
7 S32.051 Stable burst fracture of fifth lumbar vertebra MCC CC
7 S32.052 Unstable burst fracture of fifth lumbar vertebra MCC CC
7 S32.058 Other fracture of fifth lumbar vertebra MCC CC
7 S32.059 Unspecified fracture of fifth lumbar vertebra MCC CC

7 HAC = Initial encounter only (7th character A, B or C) and not POA.

✓5th **S32.1 Fracture of sacrum**

NOTE For vertical fractures, code to most medial fracture extension.
Use two codes if both a vertical and transverse fracture are present.

Code also any associated fracture of pelvic ring (S32.8-)

CC Excl: For CC/MCC codes in subcategory S32.1, unless otherwise noted: CC with 7th character A or MCC with 7th character B: M48.40X-M48.58X with 7th S, M80.08XS, M80.88XS, M84.350S, M84.454S, M84.550S, M84.58XS, M84.650S, M99.14-M99.17, M99.19, S03.8XX-S03.9XX with 7th A, S12.000-S12.9XX with 7th S, S13.9XXA, S14.109A, S14.119, S14.129A, S14.139A, S14.149 A, S14.159A, S22.000-S22.9XX with 7th S, S23.20X-S23.29X with 7th A, S23.9XXA, S24.109A, S24.119A, S24.139A, S24.149 A, S24.159A, S29.001-S29.019 with 7th A, S29.091-S29.9XX with 7th A, S32.000-S32.9XX with 7th S, S33.2XX-S33.4XX with 7th A, S33.6XX-S34.02X with 7th A, S34.131-S34.139 with 7th A, S34.3XX with 7th A, S38.1XX with 7th A, S38.3XX-S39.013 with 7th A, S39.091-S39.94X A, T14.8-T14.91, T79.A0X-T79.9XX with 7th A

CC with 7th character K: M80.00X-M84.68X with 7th [K, P], S02.0XX-S02.92X with 7th K, S12.000-S12.691 with 7th K, S22.000-S22.9XX with 7th K, S32.000-S32.9XX with 7th K, S42.001-S42.92X with 7th [K, P], S49.001-S49.199 with 7th [K, P], S52.001-S52.92X with 7th [K, M, N, P, Q, R], S59.001-S59.299 with 7th [K, P], S62.001-S62.92X with 7th [K, P], S72.001-S72.92X with 7th [K, M, N, P, Q, R], S79.001-S79.199 with 7th [K, P], S82.001-S82.92X with 7th [K, M, N, P, Q, R], S89.001-S89.399 with 7th [K, P], S92.001-S92.919 with 7th [K, P]

7 ✓x7th **S32.10 Unspecified fracture of sacrum** MCC CC

✓6th **S32.11 Zone I fracture of sacrum**
Vertical sacral ala fracture of sacrum

7 ✓7th **S32.110 Nondisplaced Zone I fracture of sacrum** MCC CC

7 ✓7th **S32.111 Minimally displaced Zone I fracture of sacrum** MCC CC

7 ✓7th **S32.112 Severely displaced Zone I fracture of sacrum** MCC CC

7 ✓7th **S32.119 Unspecified Zone I fracture of sacrum** MCC CC

✓6th **S32.12 Zone II fracture of sacrum**
Vertical foraminal region fracture of sacrum

7 ✓7th **S32.120 Nondisplaced Zone II fracture of sacrum** MCC CC

7 ✓7th **S32.121 Minimally displaced Zone II fracture of sacrum** MCC CC

7 ✓7th **S32.122 Severely displaced Zone II fracture of sacrum** MCC CC

7 ✓7th **S32.129 Unspecified Zone II fracture of sacrum** MCC CC

✓6th **S32.13 Zone III fracture of sacrum**
Vertical fracture into spinal canal region of sacrum

7 ✓7th **S32.130 Nondisplaced Zone III fracture of sacrum** MCC CC

7 ✓7th **S32.131 Minimally displaced Zone III fracture of sacrum** MCC CC

7 ✓7th **S32.132 Severely displaced Zone III fracture of sacrum** MCC CC

7 ✓7th **S32.139 Unspecified Zone III fracture of sacrum** MCC CC

7 ✓x7th **S32.14 Type 1 fracture of sacrum** MCC CC
Transverse flexion fracture of sacrum without displacement

7 ✓x7th **S32.15 Type 2 fracture of sacrum** MCC CC
Transverse flexion fracture of sacrum with posterior displacement

7 ✓x7th **S32.16 Type 3 fracture of sacrum** MCC CC
Transverse extension fracture of sacrum with anterior displacement

7 ✓x7th **S32.17 Type 4 fracture of sacrum** MCC CC
Transverse segmental comminution of upper sacrum

7 ✓x7th **S32.19 Other fracture of sacrum** MCC CC

7 ✓x7th **S32.2 Fracture of coccyx** MCC CC
CC Excl: See code: S32.1

✓5th **S32.3 Fracture of ilium**

EXCLUDES 1 *fracture of ilium with associated disruption of pelvic ring (S32.8-)*

CC Excl: For CC/MCC codes in subcategory S32.3, unless otherwise noted: CC with 7th character A: M80.00X-M80.019 with 7th A, M80.041-M80.049 with 7th A, M80.80X-M80.819 with 7th A, M80.841-M80.849 with 7th A, M84.40X-M84.419 with 7th A, M84.441-M84.446 with 7th A, M84.454 with 7th A, M84.474-M84.519 with 7th A, M84.541-M84.550 with 7th A, M84.574-M84.576 with 7th A, M84.60X-M84.619 with 7th A, M84.641-M84.650 with 7th A, M84.674-M84.68X with 7th A, S03.8XX-S03.9XX with 7th A, S22.9XX-S22.9XX with 7th [A, B], S29.011-S29.019 with 7th A, S32.301-S32.811 with 7th [A, B], S32.89X-S32.9XX with 7th [A, B], S33.4XX with 7th A, S33.6XX-S33.8XX with 7th A, S38.3XX-S39.013 with 7th A, S73.001-S73.199 with 7th A, S76.001-S76.019 with 7th A, S76.091-S76.119 with 7th A, S76.191-S76.219 with 7th A, S76.291-S76.319 with 7th A, S76.391-S76.819 with 7th A, S76.891-S76.919 with 7th A, S76.991-S76.999 with 7th A, S79.811-S79.929 with 7th A, T14.8-T14.91, T79.A9X-T79.9XX with 7th A

MCC with 7th character B: M48.40X-M48.58X with 7th A, M80.00X-M84.68X with 7th A, S03.8XX-S03.9XX with 7th A, S22.9XX-S22.9XX with 7th [A, B], S29.011-S29.019 with 7th A, S32.301-S32.399 with 7th [A, B], S32.810-S32.811 with 7th [A, B], S32.89X-S32.9XX with 7th [A, B], S33.4XX with 7th A, S33.6XX-S33.8XX with 7th A, S38.3XX-S39.013 with 7th A, S73.001-S73.199 with 7th A, S76.001-S76.019 with 7th A, S76.091-S76.119 with 7th A, S76.191-S76.219 with 7th A, S76.291-S76.319 with 7th A, S76.391-S76.819 with 7th A, S76.891-S76.919 with 7th A, S76.991-S76.999 with 7th A, S79.811-S79.929 with 7th A, T14.8-T14.91, T79.A0X-T79.9XX with 7th A

CC with 7th character K: M80.00X-M84.68X with 7th [K, P], S02.0XX-S02.92X with 7th K, S12.000-S12.691 with 7th K, S22.000-S22.9XX with 7th K, S32.000-S32.9XX with 7th K, S42.001-S42.92X with 7th [K, P], S49.001-S49.199 with 7th [K, P], S52.001-S52.92X with 7th [K, M, N, P, Q, R], S59.001-S59.299 with 7th [K, P], S62.001-S62.92X with 7th [K, P], S72.001-S72.92X with 7th [K, M, N, P, Q, R], S79.001-S79.199 with 7th [K, P], S82.001-S82.92X with 7th [K, M, N, P, Q, R], S89.001-S89.399 with 7th [K, P], S92.001-S92.919 with 7th [K, P]

✓6th **S32.30 Unspecified fracture of ilium**

7 ✓7th **S32.301 Unspecified fracture of right ilium** MCC CC

7 ✓7th **S32.302 Unspecified fracture of left ilium** MCC CC

7 ✓7th **S32.309 Unspecified fracture of unspecified ilium** MCC CC

✓6th **S32.31 Avulsion fracture of ilium**

7 ✓7th **S32.311 Displaced avulsion fracture of right ilium** MCC CC

7 ✓7th **S32.312 Displaced avulsion fracture of left ilium** MCC CC

7 ✓7th **S32.313 Displaced avulsion fracture of unspecified ilium** MCC CC

7 ✓7th **S32.314 Nondisplaced avulsion fracture of right ilium** MCC CC

7 ✓7th **S32.315 Nondisplaced avulsion fracture of left ilium** MCC CC

7 ✓7th **S32.316 Nondisplaced avulsion fracture of unspecified ilium** MCC CC

✓6th **S32.39 Other fracture of ilium**

7 ✓7th **S32.391 Other fracture of right ilium** MCC CC

7 ✓7th **S32.392 Other fracture of left ilium** MCC CC

7 ✓7th **S32.399 Other fracture of unspecified ilium** MCC CC

7 HAC = Initial encounter only (7th character A, B or C) and not POA.

✓5th **S32.4 Fracture of acetabulum**

Code also any associated fracture of pelvic ring (S32.8-)

CC Excl: For CC/MCC codes in subcategory S32.4, unless otherwise noted: MCC with 7th character A: M48.40X-M48.58X with 7th A, M80.00X-M84.68X with 7th A, S03.8XX-S03.9XX with 7th A, S22.9XX-S22.9XX with 7th [A, B], S29.011-S29.019 with 7th A, S32.401-S32.499 with 7th [A, B], S32.810-S32.811 with 7th [A, B], S32.89X-S32.9XX with 7th [A, B], S33.4XX with 7th A, S33.6XX-S33.8XX with 7th A, S38.3XX-S39.013 with 7th A, S73.001-S73.199 with 7th A, S76.001-S76.019 with 7th A, S76.091-S76.119 with 7th A, S76.191-S76.219 with 7th A, S76.291-S76.319 with 7th A, S76.391-S76.819 with 7th A, S76.891-S76.919 with 7th A, S76.991-S76.999 with 7th A, S79.811-S79.929 with 7th A, T14.8-T14.91, T79.A0X-T79.9XX with 7th A

MCC with 7th character B: S03.8XX-S03.9XX with 7th A, S22.9XX-S22.9XX with 7th [A, B], S29.011-S29.019 with 7th A, S32.401-S32.499 with 7th [A, B], S32.810-S32.811 with 7th [A, B], S32.89X-S32.9XX with 7th [A, B], S33.4XX with 7th A, S33.6XX-S33.8XX with 7th A, S38.3XX-S39.013 with 7th A, S73.001-S73.199 with 7th A, S76.001-S76.019 with 7th A, S76.091-S76.119 with 7th A, S76.191-S76.219 with 7th A, S76.291-S76.319 with 7th A, S76.391-S76.819 with 7th A, S76.891-S76.919 with 7th A, S76.991-S76.999 with 7th A, S79.811-S79.929 with 7th A, T14.8-T14.91, T79.A0X-T79.9XX with 7th A

CC with 7th character K: M80.00X-M84.68X with 7th [K, P], S02.0XX-S02.92X with 7th K, S12.000-S12.691 with 7th K, S22.000-S22.9XX with 7th K, S32.000-S32.9XX with 7th K, S42.001-S42.92X with 7th [K, P], S49.001-S49.199 with 7th [K, P], S52.001-S52.92X with 7th [K, M, N, P, Q, R], S59.001-S59.299 with 7th [K, P], S62.001-S62.92X with 7th [K, P], S72.001-S72.92X with 7th [K, M, N, P, Q, R], S79.001-S79.199 with 7th [K, P], S82.001-S82.92X with 7th [K, M, N, P, Q, R], S89.001-S89.399 with 7th [K, P], S92.001-S92.919 with 7th [K, P]

✓6th **S32.40 Unspecified fracture of acetabulum**
- 7 ✓7th **S32.401 Unspecified fracture of right acetabulum** MCC CC
- 7 ✓7th **S32.402 Unspecified fracture of left acetabulum** MCC CC
- 7 ✓7th **S32.409 Unspecified fracture of unspecified acetabulum** MCC CC

✓6th **S32.41 Fracture of anterior wall of acetabulum**
- 7 ✓7th **S32.411 Displaced fracture of anterior wall of right acetabulum** MCC CC
- 7 ✓7th **S32.412 Displaced fracture of anterior wall of left acetabulum** MCC CC
- 7 ✓7th **S32.413 Displaced fracture of anterior wall of unspecified acetabulum** MCC CC
- 7 ✓7th **S32.414 Nondisplaced fracture of anterior wall of right acetabulum** MCC CC
- 7 ✓7th **S32.415 Nondisplaced fracture of anterior wall of left acetabulum** MCC CC
- 7 ✓7th **S32.416 Nondisplaced fracture of anterior wall of unspecified acetabulum** MCC CC

✓6th **S32.42 Fracture of posterior wall of acetabulum**
- 7 ✓7th **S32.421 Displaced fracture of posterior wall of right acetabulum** MCC CC
- 7 ✓7th **S32.422 Displaced fracture of posterior wall of left acetabulum** MCC CC
- 7 ✓7th **S32.423 Displaced fracture of posterior wall of unspecified acetabulum** MCC CC
- 7 ✓7th **S32.424 Nondisplaced fracture of posterior wall of right acetabulum** MCC CC
- 7 ✓7th **S32.425 Nondisplaced fracture of posterior wall of left acetabulum** MCC CC
- 7 ✓7th **S32.426 Nondisplaced fracture of posterior wall of unspecified acetabulum** MCC CC

✓6th **S32.43 Fracture of anterior column [iliopubic] of acetabulum**
- 7 ✓7th **S32.431 Displaced fracture of anterior column [iliopubic] of right acetabulum** MCC CC
- 7 ✓7th **S32.432 Displaced fracture of anterior column [iliopubic] of left acetabulum** MCC CC
- 7 ✓7th **S32.433 Displaced fracture of anterior column [iliopubic] of unspecified acetabulum** MCC CC
- 7 ✓7th **S32.434 Nondisplaced fracture of anterior column [iliopubic] of right acetabulum** MCC CC
- 7 ✓7th **S32.435 Nondisplaced fracture of anterior column [iliopubic] of left acetabulum** MCC CC
- 7 ✓7th **S32.436 Nondisplaced fracture of anterior column [iliopubic] of unspecified acetabulum** MCC CC

✓6th **S32.44 Fracture of posterior column [ilioischial] of acetabulum**
- 7 ✓7th **S32.441 Displaced fracture of posterior column [ilioischial] of right acetabulum** MCC CC
- 7 ✓7th **S32.442 Displaced fracture of posterior column [ilioischial] of left acetabulum** MCC CC
- 7 ✓7th **S32.443 Displaced fracture of posterior column [ilioischial] of unspecified acetabulum** MCC CC
- 7 ✓7th **S32.444 Nondisplaced fracture of posterior column [ilioischial] of right acetabulum** MCC CC
- 7 ✓7th **S32.445 Nondisplaced fracture of posterior column [ilioischial] of left acetabulum** MCC CC
- 7 ✓7th **S32.446 Nondisplaced fracture of posterior column [ilioischial] of unspecified acetabulum** MCC CC

✓6th **S32.45 Transverse fracture of acetabulum**
- 7 ✓7th **S32.451 Displaced transverse fracture of right acetabulum** MCC CC
- 7 ✓7th **S32.452 Displaced transverse fracture of left acetabulum** MCC CC
- 7 ✓7th **S32.453 Displaced transverse fracture of unspecified acetabulum** MCC CC
- 7 ✓7th **S32.454 Nondisplaced transverse fracture of right acetabulum** MCC CC
- 7 ✓7th **S32.455 Nondisplaced transverse fracture of left acetabulum** MCC CC
- 7 ✓7th **S32.456 Nondisplaced transverse fracture of unspecified acetabulum** MCC CC

✓6th **S32.46 Associated transverse-posterior fracture of acetabulum**
- 7 ✓7th **S32.461 Displaced associated transverse-posterior fracture of right acetabulum** MCC CC
- 7 ✓7th **S32.462 Displaced associated transverse-posterior fracture of left acetabulum** MCC CC
- 7 ✓7th **S32.463 Displaced associated transverse-posterior fracture of unspecified acetabulum** MCC CC
- 7 ✓7th **S32.464 Nondisplaced associated transverse-posterior fracture of right acetabulum** MCC CC
- 7 ✓7th **S32.465 Nondisplaced associated transverse-posterior fracture of left acetabulum** MCC CC
- 7 ✓7th **S32.466 Nondisplaced associated transverse-posterior fracture of unspecified acetabulum** MCC CC

✓6th **S32.47 Fracture of medial wall of acetabulum**
- 7 ✓7th **S32.471 Displaced fracture of medial wall of right acetabulum** MCC CC
- 7 ✓7th **S32.472 Displaced fracture of medial wall of left acetabulum** MCC CC
- 7 ✓7th **S32.473 Displaced fracture of medial wall of unspecified acetabulum** MCC CC
- 7 ✓7th **S32.474 Nondisplaced fracture of medial wall of right acetabulum** MCC CC
- 7 ✓7th **S32.475 Nondisplaced fracture of medial wall of left acetabulum** MCC CC
- 7 ✓7th **S32.476 Nondisplaced fracture of medial wall of unspecified acetabulum** MCC CC

7 HAC = Initial encounter only (7th character A, B or C) and not POA.

✓6th **S32.48 Dome fracture of acetabulum**

7 ✓7th **S32.481 Displaced dome fracture of right acetabulum** MCC CC

7 ✓7th **S32.482 Displaced dome fracture of left acetabulum** MCC CC

7 ✓7th **S32.483 Displaced dome fracture of unspecified acetabulum** MCC CC

7 ✓7th **S32.484 Nondisplaced dome fracture of right acetabulum** MCC CC

7 ✓7th **S32.485 Nondisplaced dome fracture of left acetabulum** MCC CC

7 ✓7th **S32.486 Nondisplaced dome fracture of unspecified acetabulum** MCC CC

✓6th **S32.49 Other specified fracture of acetabulum**

7 ✓7th **S32.491 Other specified fracture of right acetabulum** MCC CC

7 ✓7th **S32.492 Other specified fracture of left acetabulum** MCC CC

7 ✓7th **S32.499 Other specified fracture of unspecified acetabulum** MCC CC

✓5th **S32.5 Fracture of pubis**

EXCLUDES1 *fracture of pubis with associated disruption of pelvic ring (S32.8-)*

CC Excl: For CC/MCC codes in subcategory S32.5, unless otherwise noted: CC with 7th character A or MCC with 7th character B: M48.40X-M48.58X with 7th A, M80.00X-M84.68X with 7th A, S03.8XX-S03.9XX with 7th A, S22.9XX-S22.9XX with 7th [A, B], S29.011-S29.019 with 7th A, S32.501-S32.599 with 7th [A, B], S32.810-S32.811 with 7th [A, B], S32.89X-S32.9XX with 7th [A, B], S33.4XXA, S33.6XX-S33.8XX with 7th A, S38.3X-S39.013 with 7th A, S73.001-S73.199 with 7th A, S76.001-S76.019 with 7th A, S76.091-S76.119 with 7th A, S76.191-S76.219 A, S76.291-S76.319 with 7th A, S76.391-S76.819 with 7th A, S76.891-S76.919 with 7th A, S76.991-S76.999 with 7th A, S79.811-S79.929 with 7th A, T14.8-T14.91, T79.A0X-T79.9XX with 7th A

CC with 7th character K: M80.00X-M84.68X with 7th [K, P], S02.0XX-S02.92X with 7th K, S12.000-S12.691 with 7th K, S22.000-S22.9XX with 7th K, S32.000-S32.9XX with 7th K, S42.001-S42.92X with 7th [K, P], S49.001-S49.199 with 7th [K, P], S52.001-S52.92X with 7th [K, M, N, P, Q, R], S59.001-S59.299 with 7th [K, P], S62.001-S62.92X with 7th [K, P], S72.001-S72.92X with 7th [K, M, N, P, Q, R], S79.001-S79.199 with 7th [K, P], S82.001-S82.92X with 7th [K, M, N, P, Q, R], S89.001-S89.399 with 7th [K, P], S92.001-S92.919 with 7th [K, P]

✓6th **S32.50 Unspecified fracture of pubis**

7 ✓7th **S32.501 Unspecified fracture of right pubis** MCC CC

7 ✓7th **S32.502 Unspecified fracture of left pubis** MCC CC

7 ✓7th **S32.509 Unspecified fracture of unspecified pubis** MCC CC

✓6th **S32.51 Fracture of superior rim of pubis**

7 ✓7th **S32.511 Fracture of superior rim of right pubis** MCC CC

7 ✓7th **S32.512 Fracture of superior rim of left pubis** MCC CC

7 ✓7th **S32.519 Fracture of superior rim of unspecified pubis** MCC CC

✓6th **S32.59 Other specified fracture of pubis**

7 ✓7th **S32.591 Other specified fracture of right pubis** MCC CC

7 ✓7th **S32.592 Other specified fracture of left pubis** MCC CC

7 ✓7th **S32.599 Other specified fracture of unspecified pubis** MCC CC

✓5th **S32.6 Fracture of ischium**

EXCLUDES1 *fracture of ischium with associated disruption of pelvic ring (S32.8-)*

CC Excl: For CC/MCC codes in subcategory S32.6, unless otherwise noted: CC with 7th character A: S32.601-S32.699 with 7th A

MCC with 7th character B: M48.40X-M48.58X with 7th A, M80.00X-M84.68X with 7th A, S03.8XX-S03.9XX with 7th A, S22.9XX-S22.9XX with 7th [A, B], S29.011-S29.019 with 7th A, S32.601-S32.811 with 7th [A, B], S32.89X-S32.9XX with 7th [A, B], S33.4XX with 7th A, S33.6XX-S33.8XX with 7th A, S38.3XX-S39.013 with 7th A, S73.001-S73.199 with 7th A, S76.001-S76.019 with 7th A, S76.091-S76.119 with 7th A, S76.191-S76.219 with 7th A, S76.291-S76.319 with 7th A, S76.391-S76.819 with 7th A, S76.891-S76.919 with 7th A, S76.991-S76.999 with 7th A, S79.811-S79.929 with 7th A, T14.8-T14.91, T79.A0X-T79.9XX with 7th A

CC with 7th character K: M80.00X-M84.68X with 7th [K, P], S02.0XX-S02.92X with 7th K, S12.000-S12.691 with 7th K, S22.000-S22.9XX with 7th K, S32.000-S32.9XX with 7th K, S42.001-S42.92X with 7th [K, P], S49.001-S49.199 with 7th [K, P], S52.001-S52.92X with 7th [K, M, N, P, Q, R], S59.001-S59.299 with 7th [K, P], S62.001-S62.92X with 7th [K, P], S72.001-S72.92X with 7th [K, M, N, P, Q, R], S79.001-S79.199 with 7th [K, P], S82.001-S82.92X with 7th [K, M, N, P, Q, R], S89.001-S89.399 with 7th [K, P], S92.001-S92.919 with 7th [K, P]

✓6th **S32.60 Unspecified fracture of ischium**

7 ✓7th **S32.601 Unspecified fracture of right ischium** MCC CC

7 ✓7th **S32.602 Unspecified fracture of left ischium** MCC CC

7 ✓7th **S32.609 Unspecified fracture of unspecified ischium** MCC CC

✓6th **S32.61 Avulsion fracture of ischium**

7 ✓7th **S32.611 Displaced avulsion fracture of right ischium** MCC CC

7 ✓7th **S32.612 Displaced avulsion fracture of left ischium** MCC CC

7 ✓7th **S32.613 Displaced avulsion fracture of unspecified ischium** MCC CC

7 ✓7th **S32.614 Nondisplaced avulsion fracture of right ischium** MCC CC

7 ✓7th **S32.615 Nondisplaced avulsion fracture of left ischium** MCC CC

7 ✓7th **S32.616 Nondisplaced avulsion fracture of unspecified ischium** MCC CC

✓6th **S32.69 Other specified fracture of ischium**

7 ✓7th **S32.691 Other specified fracture of right ischium** MCC CC

7 ✓7th **S32.692 Other specified fracture of left ischium** MCC CC

7 ✓7th **S32.699 Other specified fracture of unspecified ischium** MCC CC

✓5th **S32.8 Fracture of other parts of pelvis**

Code also any associated:
- fracture of acetabulum (S32.4-)
- sacral fracture (S32.1-)

7 HAC = Initial encounter only (7th character A, B or C) and not POA.

S32.81 Multiple fractures of pelvis with disruption of pelvic ring
Multiple pelvic fractures with disruption of pelvic circle

CC Excl: For CC/MCC codes in subcategory S32.81, unless otherwise noted: CC with 7th character A or MCC with 7th character B: M48.40X-M48.58X with 7th A, M80.00X-M84.68X with 7th A, S03.8XX-S03.9XX with 7th A, S22.9XX-S22.9XX with 7th [A, B], S29.011-S29.019 with 7th A, S32.301-S32.811 with 7th [A, B], S32.89X-S32.9XX with 7th [A, B], S33.4XX with 7th A, S33.6XX-S33.8XX with 7th A, S38.3XX-S39.013 with 7th A, S73.001-S73.199 with 7th A, S76.001-S76.019 with 7th A, S76.091-S76.119 with 7th A, S76.191-S76.219 with 7th A, S76.291-S76.319 with 7th A, S76.391-S76.819 with 7th A, S76.891-S76.919 with 7th A, S76.991-S76.999 with 7th A, S79.811-S79.929 with 7th A, T14.8-T14.91, T79.A0X-T79.9XX with 7th A
CC with 7th character K: M80.00X-M84.68X with 7th [K, P], S02.0XX-S02.92X with 7th K, S12.000-S12.691 with 7th K, S22.000-S22.9XX with 7th K, S32.000-S32.9XX with 7th K, S42.001-S42.92X with 7th [K, P], S49.001-S49.199 with 7th [K, P], S52.001-S52.92X with 7th [K, M, N, P, Q, R], S59.001-S59.299 with 7th [K, P], S62.001-S62.92X with 7th [K, P], S72.001-S72.92X with 7th [K, M, N, P, Q, R], S79.001-S79.199 with 7th [K, P], S82.001-S82.92X with 7th [K, M, N, P, Q, R], S89.001-S89.399 with 7th [K, P], S92.001-S92.919 with 7th [K, P]

7 **S32.810 Multiple fractures of pelvis with stable disruption of pelvic ring** MCC CC

7 **S32.811 Multiple fractures of pelvis with unstable disruption of pelvic ring** MCC CC

7 **S32.82 Multiple fractures of pelvis without disruption of pelvic ring** MCC CC
Multiple pelvic fractures without disruption of pelvic circle
CC Excl: CC with 7th character A or MCC with 7th character B: S32.89 with 7th A
CC with 7th character K: M80.00X-M84.68X with 7th [K, P], S02.0XX-S02.92X with 7th K, S12.000-S12.691 with 7th K, S22.000-S22.9XX with 7th K, S32.000-S32.9XX with 7th K, S42.001-S42.92X with 7th [K, P], S49.001-S49.199 with 7th [K, P], S52.001-S52.92X with 7th [K, M, N, P, Q, R], S59.001-S59.299 with 7th [K, P], S62.001-S62.92X with 7th [K, P], S72.001-S72.92X with 7th [K, M, N, P, Q, R], S79.001-S79.199 with 7th [K, P], S82.001-S82.92X with 7th [K, M, N, P, Q, R], S89.001-S89.399 with 7th [K, P], S92.001-S92.919 with 7th [K, P]

7 **S32.89 Fracture of other parts of pelvis** MCC CC
CC Excl: CC with 7th character A or MCC with 7th character B: M48.40X-M48.58X with 7th A, M80.00X-M84.68X with 7th A, S03.8XX-S03.9XX with 7th A, S22.9XX-S22.9XX with 7th [A, B], S29.011-S29.019 with 7th A, S32.301-S32.9XX with 7th [A, B], S33.4XX with 7th A, S33.6XX-S33.8XX with 7th A, S38.3X-S39.013 with 7th A, S73.001-S73.199 with 7th A, S76.001-S76.019 with 7th A, S76.091-S76.119 with 7th A, S76.191-S76.219 with 7th A, S76.291-S76.319 with 7th A, S76.391-S76.819 with 7th A, S76.891-S76.919 with 7th A, S76.991-S76.999 with 7th A, S79.811-S79.929 with 7th A, T14.8-T14.91, T79.A0X-T79.9XX with 7th A
CC with 7th character K: M80.00X-M84.68X with 7th [K, P], S02.0XX-S02.92X with 7th K, S12.000-S12.691 with 7th K, S22.000-S22.9XX with 7th K, S32.000-S32.9XX with 7th K, S42.001-S42.92X with 7th [K, P], S49.001-S49.199 with 7th [K, P], S52.001-S52.92X with 7th [K, M, N, P, Q, R], S59.001-S59.299 with 7th [K, P], S62.001-S62.92X with 7th [K, P], S72.001-S72.92X with 7th [K, M, N, P, Q, R], S79.001-S79.199 with 7th [K, P], S82.001-S82.92X with 7th [K, M, N, P, Q, R], S89.001-S89.399 with 7th [K, P], S92.001-S92.919 with 7th [K, P]

7 **S32.9 Fracture of unspecified parts of lumbosacral spine and pelvis** MCC CC
Fracture of lumbosacral spine NOS
Fracture of pelvis NOS
AHA: 2012, 4Q, 93
CC Excl: See code: S82.81

7 HAC = Initial encounter only (7th character A, B or C) and not POA.

S33 Dislocation and sprain of joints and ligaments of lumbar spine and pelvis

INCLUDES avulsion of joint or ligament of lumbar spine and pelvis
laceration of cartilage, joint or ligament of lumbar spine and pelvis
sprain of cartilage, joint or ligament of lumbar spine and pelvis
traumatic hemarthrosis of joint or ligament of lumbar spine and pelvis
traumatic rupture of joint or ligament of lumbar spine and pelvis
traumatic subluxation of joint or ligament of lumbar spine and pelvis
traumatic tear of joint or ligament of lumbar spine and pelvis

Code also any associated open wound

EXCLUDES 1 *nontraumatic rupture or displacement of lumbar intervertebral disc NOS (M51.-)*
obstetric damage to pelvic joints and ligaments (O71.6)

EXCLUDES 2 *dislocation and sprain of joints and ligaments of hip (S73.-)*
strain of muscle of lower back and pelvis (S39.01-)

The appropriate 7th is to be added to each code from category S33.
A initial encounter
D subsequent encounter
S sequela

S33.0 Traumatic rupture of lumbar intervertebral disc
EXCLUDES 1 *rupture or displacement (nontraumatic) of lumbar intervertebral disc NOS (M51- with fifth character 6)*

S33.1 Subluxation and dislocation of lumbar vertebra
Code also any associated:
open wound of abdomen, lower back and pelvis (S31)
spinal cord injury (S24.0, S24.1-, S34.0-, S34.1-)
EXCLUDES 2 *fracture of lumbar vertebrae (S32.0-)*

S33.10 Subluxation and dislocation of unspecified lumbar vertebra
S33.100 Subluxation of unspecified lumbar vertebra
S33.101 Dislocation of unspecified lumbar vertebra

S33.11 Subluxation and dislocation of L1/L2 lumbar vertebra
S33.110 Subluxation of L1/L2 lumbar vertebra
S33.111 Dislocation of L1/L2 lumbar vertebra

S33.12 Subluxation and dislocation of L2/L3 lumbar vertebra
S33.120 Subluxation of L2/L3 lumbar vertebra
S33.121 Dislocation of L2/L3 lumbar vertebra

S33.13 Subluxation and dislocation of L3/L4 lumbar vertebra
S33.130 Subluxation of L3/L4 lumbar vertebra
S33.131 Dislocation of L3/L4 lumbar vertebra

S33.14 Subluxation and dislocation of L4/L5 lumbar vertebra
S33.140 Subluxation of L4/L5 lumbar vertebra
S33.141 Dislocation of L4/L5 lumbar vertebra

S33.2 Dislocation of sacroiliac and sacrococcygeal joint

S33.3 Dislocation of other and unspecified parts of lumbar spine and pelvis
S33.30 Dislocation of unspecified parts of lumbar spine and pelvis
S33.39 Dislocation of other parts of lumbar spine and pelvis

S33.4 Traumatic rupture of symphysis pubis
S33.5 Sprain of ligaments of lumbar spine
S33.6 Sprain of sacroiliac joint
S33.8 Sprain of other parts of lumbar spine and pelvis
S33.9 Sprain of unspecified parts of lumbar spine and pelvis

S34 Injury of lumbar and sacral spinal cord and nerves at abdomen, lower back and pelvis level (4th)

NOTE Code to highest level of lumbar cord injury.
Injuries to the spinal cord (S34.0 and S34.1) refer to the cord level and not bone level injury, and can affect nerve roots at and below the level given.

Code also any associated:
fracture of vertebra (S22.0-, S32.0-)
open wound of abdomen, lower back and pelvis (S31.-)
transient paralysis (R29.5)

The appropriate 7th is to be added to each code from category S34.
A initial encounter
D subsequent encounter
S sequela

S34.0 Concussion and edema of lumbar and sacral spinal cord (5th)

S34.01 Concussion and edema of lumbar spinal cord (x7th) MCC
CC Excl: MCC with 7th character A: M48.40X-M48.58X with 7th S, M80.08XS, M80.88XS, M84.350S, M84.454S, M84.550S, M84.58XS, M84.650S, M99.15-M99.17, M99.19, S12.000-S12.9XX with 7th S, S13.9XXA, S14.109A, S14.119A, S14.129A, S14.139A, S14.149A, S14.159A, S22.000-S22.9X with 7th S, S23.20X-S23.29X with 7th A, S23.9XXA, S24.109A, S24.119A, S24.139A, S24.149A, S24.159A, S29.001-S29.009 with 7th A, S29.091-S29.9XX with 7th A, S32.000-S32.9XX with 7th S, S33.30X-S33.39X with 7th A, S33.9XX-S34.01X with 7th A, S34.101-S34.129 with 7th A, S38.1XA, S39.001-S39.003 with 7th A, S39.091-S39.94X with 7th A, T14.8-T14.91, T79.A0X-T79.9XX with 7th A

S34.02 Concussion and edema of sacral spinal cord (x7th) MCC
Concussion and edema of conus medullaris
CC Excl: MCC with 7th character A: M48.40X-M48.58X with 7th S, M80.08XS, M80.88XS, M84.350S, M84.454S, M84.550S, M84.58XS, M84.650S, M99.15-M99.17, M99.19, S12.000-S12.9XX with 7th S, S13.9XXA, S14.109A, S14.119A, S14.129A, S14.139A, S14.149A, S14.159A, S22.000-S22.9XX with 7th S, S23.20X-S23.29X with 7th A, S23.9XA, S24.109A, S24.119A, S24.139A, S24.149A, S24.159A, S29.001-S29.009 with 7th A, S29.091-S29.9XX with 7th A, S32.000-S32.9XX with 7th S, S33.30X-S33.39X with 7th A, S33.9XX-S34.02X with 7th A, S34.131-S34.139 with 7th A, S34.3XA, S38.1XA, S39.001-S39.003 with 7th A, S39.091-S39.94X with 7th A, T14.8-T14.91, T79.A0X-T79.9XX with 7th A

S34.1 Other and unspecified injury of lumbar and sacral spinal cord (5th)

S34.10 Unspecified injury to lumbar spinal cord (6th)

CC Excl: For MCC codes in subcategory S34.10, unless otherwise noted: MCC with 7th character A: M48.40X-M48.58X with 7th S, M80.08XS, M80.88XS, M84.350S, M84.454S, M84.550S, M84.58XS, M84.650S, M99.15-M99.17, M99.19, S12.000-S12.9XX with 7th S, S13.9XXA, S14.109A, S14.119A, S14.129A, S14.139A, S14.149A, S14.159A, S22.000-S22.9XX with 7th S, S23.20X-S23.29X with 7th A, S23.9XA, S24.109A, S24.119A, S24.139A, S24.149A, S24.159A, S29.001-S29.009 with 7th A, S29.091-S29.9XX with 7th A, S32.000-S32.9XX with 7th S, S33.30X-S33.39X with 7th A, S33.9XX-S34.01X with 7th A, S34.101-S34.129 with 7th A, S38.1XA, S39.001-S39.003 with 7th A, S39.091-S39.94X with 7th A, T14.8-T14.91, T79.A0X-T79.9XX with 7th A

7 **S34.101 Unspecified injury to L1 level of lumbar spinal cord** (7th) MCC
7 **S34.102 Unspecified injury to L2 level of lumbar spinal cord** (7th) MCC
7 **S34.103 Unspecified injury to L3 level of lumbar spinal cord** (7th) MCC
7 **S34.104 Unspecified injury to L4 level of lumbar spinal cord** (7th) MCC
7 **S34.105 Unspecified injury to L5 level of lumbar spinal cord** (7th) MCC
7 **S34.109 Unspecified injury to unspecified level of lumbar spinal cord** (7th) MCC

S34.11 Complete lesion of lumbar spinal cord (6th)

CC Excl: For MCC codes in subcategory S34.11, unless otherwise noted: See code: S34.10

7 **S34.111 Complete lesion of L1 level of lumbar spinal cord** (7th) MCC
7 **S34.112 Complete lesion of L2 level of lumbar spinal cord** (7th) MCC
7 **S34.113 Complete lesion of L3 level of lumbar spinal cord** (7th) MCC
7 **S34.114 Complete lesion of L4 level of lumbar spinal cord** (7th) MCC
7 **S34.115 Complete lesion of L5 level of lumbar spinal cord** (7th) MCC
7 **S34.119 Complete lesion of unspecified level of lumbar spinal cord** (7th) MCC

S34.12 Incomplete lesion of lumbar spinal cord (6th)

CC Excl: For MCC codes in subcategory S34.12, unless otherwise noted: See code: S34.10

7 **S34.121 Incomplete lesion of L1 level of lumbar spinal cord** (7th) MCC
7 **S34.122 Incomplete lesion of L2 level of lumbar spinal cord** (7th) MCC
7 **S34.123 Incomplete lesion of L3 level of lumbar spinal cord** (7th) MCC
7 **S34.124 Incomplete lesion of L4 level of lumbar spinal cord** (7th) MCC
7 **S34.125 Incomplete lesion of L5 level of lumbar spinal cord** (7th) MCC
7 **S34.129 Incomplete lesion of unspecified level of lumbar spinal cord** (7th) MCC

S34.13 Other and unspecified injury to sacral spinal cord (6th)
Other injury to conus medullaris

CC Excl: For MCC codes in subcategory S34.13, unless otherwise noted: MCC with 7th character A: M48.40X-M48.58X with 7th S, M80.08XS, M80.88XS, M84.350S, M84.454S, M84.550S, M84.58XS, M84.650S, M99.15-M99.17, M99.19, S12.000-S12.9XX with 7th S, S13.9XXA, S14.109A, S14.119A, S14.129A, S14.139A, S14.149A, S14.159A, S22.000-S22.9XX with 7th S, S23.20X-S23.29X with 7th A, S23.9XXA, S24.109A, S24.119A, S24.139A, S24.149A, S24.159A, S29.001-S29.009 with 7th A, S29.091-S29.9XX with 7th A, S32.000-S32.9XX with 7th S, S33.30X-S33.39X with 7th A, S33.9XX-S34.02X with 7th A, S34.131-S34.139 with 7th A, S34.3XXA, S38.1XXA, S39.001-S39.003 with 7th A, S39.091-S39.94X with 7th A, T14.8-T14.91, T79.A0X-T79.9XX with 7th A

7 **S34.131 Complete lesion of sacral spinal cord** (7th) MCC
Complete lesion of conus medullaris

7 **S34.132 Incomplete lesion of sacral spinal cord** (7th) MCC
Incomplete lesion of conus medullaris

7 **S34.139 Unspecified injury to sacral spinal cord** (7th) MCC
Unspecified injury of conus medullaris

S34.2 Injury of nerve root of lumbar and sacral spine (5th)
S34.21 Injury of nerve root of lumbar spine (x7th)
S34.22 Injury of nerve root of sacral spine (x7th)

7 **S34.3 Injury of cauda equina** (x7th) MCC
CC Excl: See code: S34.13

S34.4 Injury of lumbosacral plexus (x7th)

S34.5 Injury of lumbar, sacral and pelvic sympathetic nerves (x7th)
Injury of celiac ganglion or plexus
Injury of hypogastric plexus
Injury of mesenteric plexus (inferior) (superior)
Injury of splanchnic nerve

S34.6 Injury of peripheral nerve(s) at abdomen, lower back and pelvis level (x7th)

S34.8 Injury of other nerves at abdomen, lower back and pelvis level (x7th)

S34.9 Injury of unspecified nerves at abdomen, lower back and pelvis level (x7th)

7 HAC = Initial encounter only (7th character A, B or C) and not POA.

S35 Injury of blood vessels at abdomen, lower back and pelvis level
Code also any associated open wound (S31.-)

The appropriate 7th is to be added to each code from category S35.
A initial encounter
D subsequent encounter
S sequela

S35.0 Injury of abdominal aorta
EXCLUDES 1 *injury of aorta NOS (S25.0)*

CC Excl: For MCC codes in subcategory S35.0, unless otherwise noted: MCC with 7th character A: S35.00X-S35.09X with 7th A, S35.8X1-S35.99X with 7th A, T14.8-T14.91, T79.A0X-T79.9XX with 7th A

S35.00 Unspecified **injury of abdominal aorta** MCC
S35.01 Minor laceration **of abdominal aorta** MCC
Incomplete transection of abdominal aorta
Laceration of abdominal aorta NOS
Superficial laceration of abdominal aorta
S35.02 Major laceration **of abdominal aorta** MCC
Complete transection of abdominal aorta
Traumatic rupture of abdominal aorta
S35.09 Other **injury of abdominal aorta** MCC

S35.1 Injury of inferior vena cava
Injury of hepatic vein
EXCLUDES 1 *injury of vena cava NOS (S25.2)*

CC Excl: For MCC codes in subcategory S35.1, unless otherwise noted: MCC with 7th character A: S35.10X-S35.19X with 7th A, S35.8X1-S35.99X with 7th A, T14.8-T14.91, T79.A0X-T79.9XX with 7th A

S35.10 Unspecified **injury of inferior vena cava** MCC
S35.11 Minor laceration **of inferior vena cava** MCC
Incomplete transection of inferior vena cava
Laceration of inferior vena cava NOS
Superficial laceration of inferior vena cava
S35.12 Major laceration **of inferior vena cava** MCC
Complete transection of inferior vena cava
Traumatic rupture of inferior vena cava
S35.19 Other **injury of inferior vena cava** MCC

S35.2 Injury of celiac or mesenteric artery and branches

S35.21 Injury of celiac artery

CC Excl: For MCC codes in subcategory S35.21, unless otherwise noted: MCC with 7th character A: S35.211-S35.219 with 7th A, S35.8X1-S35.99X with 7th A, T14.8-T14.91, T79.A0X-T79.9XX with 7th A

S35.211 Minor laceration **of celiac artery** MCC
Incomplete transection of celiac artery
Laceration of celiac artery NOS
Superficial laceration of celiac artery
S35.212 Major laceration **of celiac artery** MCC
Complete transection of celiac artery
Traumatic rupture of celiac artery
S35.218 Other **injury of celiac artery** MCC
S35.219 Unspecified **injury of celiac artery** MCC

S35.22 Injury of superior mesenteric artery

CC Excl: For MCC codes in subcategory S35.22, unless otherwise noted: MCC with 7th character A: S35.221-S35.229 with 7th A, S35.8X1-S35.99X with 7th A, T14.8-T14.91, T79.A0X-T79.9XX with 7th A

S35.221 Minor laceration **of superior mesenteric artery** MCC
Incomplete transection of superior mesenteric artery
Laceration of superior mesenteric artery NOS
Superficial laceration of superior mesenteric artery
S35.222 Major laceration **of superior mesenteric artery** MCC
Complete transection of superior mesenteric artery
Traumatic rupture of superior mesenteric artery
S35.228 Other **injury of superior mesenteric artery** MCC
S35.229 Unspecified **injury of superior mesenteric artery** MCC

S35.23 Injury of inferior mesenteric artery

CC Excl: For MCC codes in subcategory S35.23, unless otherwise noted: MCC with 7th character A: S35.231-S35.239 with 7th A, S35.8X1-S35.99X with 7th A, T14.8-T14.91, T79.A0X-T79.9XX with 7th A

S35.231 Minor laceration **of inferior mesenteric artery** MCC
Incomplete transection of inferior mesenteric artery
Laceration of inferior mesenteric artery NOS
Superficial laceration of inferior mesenteric artery
S35.232 Major laceration **of inferior mesenteric artery** MCC
Complete transection of inferior mesenteric artery
Traumatic rupture of inferior mesenteric artery
S35.238 Other **injury of inferior mesenteric artery** MCC
S35.239 Unspecified **injury of inferior mesenteric artery** MCC

S35.29 Injury of branches of celiac and mesenteric artery MCC
Injury of gastric artery
Injury of gastroduodenal artery
Injury of hepatic artery
Injury of splenic artery
S35.291 Minor laceration **of branches of celiac and mesenteric artery** MCC
Incomplete transection of branches of celiac and mesenteric artery
Laceration of branches of celiac and mesenteric artery NOS
Superficial laceration of branches of celiac and mesenteric artery
CC Excl: MCC with 7th character A: S35.291A, S35.8X1-S35.99X with 7th A, T14.8-T14.91, T79.A0X with 7th A, T79.A3X-T79.9XX with 7th A
S35.292 Major laceration **of branches of celiac and mesenteric artery** MCC
Complete transection of branches of celiac and mesenteric artery
Traumatic rupture of branches of celiac and mesenteric artery
CC Excl: MCC with 7th character A: S35.292-S35.298 with 7th A, S35.8X1-S35.99X with 7th A, T14.8-T14.91, T79.A0X-T79.9XX with 7th A
S35.298 Other **injury of branches of celiac and mesenteric artery** MCC
CC Excl: See code: S35.292
S35.299 Unspecified **injury of branches of celiac and mesenteric artery** MCC
CC Excl: MCC with 7th character A: S35.299A, S35.8X1-S35.99X with 7th A, T14.8-T14.91, T79.A0X-T79.9XX with 7th A

S35.3 Injury of portal or splenic vein and branches

S35.31 Injury of portal vein

CC Excl: For MCC codes in subcategory S35.31, unless otherwise noted: MCC with 7th character A: S35.311-S35.319 with 7th A, S35.8X1-S35.99X with 7th A, T14.8-T14.91, T79.A0X-T79.9XX with 7th A

S35.311 Laceration **of portal vein** MCC
S35.318 Other **specified injury of portal vein** MCC
S35.319 Unspecified **injury of portal vein** MCC

S35.32 Injury of splenic vein

CC Excl: For MCC codes in subcategory S35.32, unless otherwise noted: MCC with 7th character A: S35.321-S35.329 with 7th A, S35.8X1-S35.99X with 7th A, T14.8-T14.91, T79.A0X-T79.9XX with 7th A

S35.321 Laceration **of splenic vein** MCC
S35.328 Other **specified injury of splenic vein** MCC

Injury, Poisoning and Certain Other Consequences of External Causes S35–S35.328

✓7th S35.329 Unspecified injury of splenic vein MCC

✓6th S35.33 Injury of superior mesenteric vein

CC Excl: For MCC codes in subcategory S35.33, unless otherwise noted: MCC with 7th character A: S35.331-S35.339 with 7th A, S35.8X1-S35.99X with 7th A, T14.8-T14.91, T79.AØX-T79.9XX with 7th A

✓7th S35.331 Laceration of superior mesenteric vein MCC

✓7th S35.338 Other specified injury of superior mesenteric vein MCC

✓7th S35.339 Unspecified injury of superior mesenteric vein MCC

✓6th S35.34 Injury of inferior mesenteric vein

CC Excl: For MCC codes in subcategory S35.34, unless otherwise noted: MCC with 7th character A: S35.341-S35.349 with 7th A, S35.8X1-S35.99X with 7th A, T14.8-T14.91, T79.AØX-T79.9XX with 7th A

✓7th S35.341 Laceration of inferior mesenteric vein MCC

✓7th S35.348 Other specified injury of inferior mesenteric vein MCC

✓7th S35.349 Unspecified injury of inferior mesenteric vein MCC

✓5th S35.4 Injury of renal blood vessels

✓6th S35.40 Unspecified injury of renal blood vessel

✓7th S35.401 Unspecified injury of right renal artery MCC
CC Excl: MCC with 7th character A: S35.401-S35.403 with 7th A, S35.411-S35.413 with 7th A, S35.491-S35.493 with 7th A, S35.8X1-S35.99X with 7th A, T14.8-T14.91, T79.AØX-T79.9XX with 7th A

✓7th S35.402 Unspecified injury of left renal artery MCC
CC Excl: See code: S35.401

✓7th S35.403 Unspecified injury of unspecified renal artery MCC
CC Excl: See code: S35.401

✓7th S35.404 Unspecified injury of right renal vein MCC
CC Excl: MCC with 7th character A: S35.404-S35.406 with 7th A, S35.414-S35.416 with 7th A, S35.494-S35.496 with 7th A, S35.8X1-S35.99X with 7th A, T14.8-T14.91, T79.AØX-T79.9XX with 7th A

✓7th S35.405 Unspecified injury of left renal vein MCC
CC Excl: See code: S35.404

✓7th S35.406 Unspecified injury of unspecified renal vein MCC
CC Excl: See code: S35.404

✓6th S35.41 Laceration of renal blood vessel

✓7th S35.411 Laceration of right renal artery MCC
CC Excl: MCC with 7th character A: S35.401-S35.403 with 7th A, S35.411-S35.413 with 7th A, S35.491-S35.493 with 7th A, S35.8X1-S35.99X with 7th A, T14.8-T14.91, T79.AØX-T79.9XX with 7th A

✓7th S35.412 Laceration of left renal artery MCC
CC Excl: See code: S35.411

✓7th S35.413 Laceration of unspecified renal artery MCC
CC Excl: See code: S35.411

✓7th S35.414 Laceration of right renal vein MCC
CC Excl: MCC with 7th character A: S35.404-S35.406 with 7th A, S35.414-S35.416 with 7th A, S35.494-S35.496 with 7th A, S35.8X1-S35.99X with 7th A, T14.8-T14.91, T79.AØX-T79.9XX with 7th A

✓7th S35.415 Laceration of left renal vein MCC
CC Excl: See code: S35.414

✓7th S35.416 Laceration of unspecified renal vein MCC
CC Excl: See code: S35.414

✓6th S35.49 Other specified injury of renal blood vessel

✓7th S35.491 Other specified injury of right renal artery MCC
CC Excl: MCC with 7th character A: S35.401-S35.403 with 7th A, S35.411-S35.413 with 7th A, S35.491-S35.493 with 7th A, S35.8X1-S35.99X with 7th A, T14.8-T14.91, T79.AØX-T79.9XX with 7th A

✓7th S35.492 Other specified injury of left renal artery MCC
CC Excl: See code: S35.491

✓7th S35.493 Other specified injury of unspecified renal artery MCC
CC Excl: See code: S35.491

✓7th S35.494 Other specified injury of right renal vein MCC
CC Excl: MCC with 7th character A: S35.404-S35.406 with 7th A, S35.414-S35.416 with 7th A, S35.494-S35.496 with 7th A, S35.8X1-S35.99X with 7th A, T14.8-T14.91, T79.AØX-T79.9XX with 7th A

✓7th S35.495 Other specified injury of left renal vein MCC
CC Excl: See code: S35.494

✓7th S35.496 Other specified injury of unspecified renal vein MCC
CC Excl: See code: S35.494

✓5th S35.5 Injury of iliac blood vessels

✓x7th S35.50 Injury of unspecified iliac blood vessel(s) MCC
CC Excl: MCC with 7th character A: S35.50X-S35.516 with 7th A, S35.59X-S35.99X with 7th A, T14.8-T14.91, T79.AØX-T79.9XX with 7th A

✓6th S35.51 Injury of iliac artery or vein
Injury of hypogastric artery or vein

✓7th S35.511 Injury of right iliac artery MCC
CC Excl: MCC with 7th character A: S35.50X-S35.513 with 7th A, S35.59X-S35.99X with 7th A, T14.8-T14.91, T79.AØX-T79.9XX with 7th A

✓7th S35.512 Injury of left iliac artery MCC
CC Excl: See code: S35.511

✓7th S35.513 Injury of unspecified iliac artery MCC
CC Excl: See code: S35.511

✓7th S35.514 Injury of right iliac vein MCC
CC Excl: MCC with 7th character A: S35.50X-S35.516 with 7th A, S35.59X-S35.99X with 7th A, T14.8-T14.91, T79.AØX-T79.9XX with 7th A

✓7th S35.515 Injury of left iliac vein MCC
CC Excl: See code: S35.514

✓7th S35.516 Injury of unspecified iliac vein MCC
CC Excl: See code: S35.514

✓6th S35.53 Injury of uterine artery or vein

✓7th S35.531 Injury of right uterine artery CC ♀
CC Excl: CC with 7th character A: S35.50X with 7th A, S35.531-S35.99X with 7th A, T14.8-T14.91, T79.AØX with 7th A, T79.A3X-T79.9XX with 7th A

✓7th S35.532 Injury of left uterine artery CC ♀
CC Excl: See code: S35.531

✓7th S35.533 Injury of unspecified uterine artery CC ♀
CC Excl: See code: S35.531

✓7th S35.534 Injury of right uterine vein CC ♀
CC Excl: MCC with 7th character A: S35.50X with 7th A, S35.534-S35.99X with 7th A, T14.8-T14.91, T79.AØX with 7th A, T79.A3X-T79.9XX with 7th A

✓7th S35.535 Injury of left uterine vein CC ♀
CC Excl: See code: S35.534

✓7th S35.536 Injury of unspecified uterine vein CC ♀
CC Excl: See code: S35.534

✓x7th S35.59 Injury of other iliac blood vessels MCC
CC Excl: MCC with 7th character A: S35.50X-S35.516 with 7th A, S35.59X-S35.99X with 7th A, T14.8-T14.91, T79.AØX-T79.9XX with 7th A

✓5th S35.8 Injury of other blood vessels at abdomen, lower back and pelvis level
Injury of ovarian artery or vein

✓6th S35.8X Injury of other blood vessels at abdomen, lower back and pelvis level

CC Excl: For CC codes in subcategory S35.8X, unless otherwise noted: CC with 7th character A: S35.8X1-S35.99X with 7th A, T14.8-T14.91, T79.AØX with 7th A, T79.A3X-T79.9XX with 7th A

✓7th S35.8X1 Laceration of other blood vessels at abdomen, lower back and pelvis level CC

✓7th S35.8X8 Other specified injury of other blood vessels at abdomen, lower back and pelvis level CC

√7th **S35.8X9 Unspecified injury of other blood vessels at abdomen, lower back and pelvis level** CC

√5th **S35.9 Injury of unspecified blood vessel at abdomen, lower back and pelvis level**

CC Excl: For CC codes in subcategory S35.9: CC with 7th character A: S35.00-S35.99X with 7th A, T14.8-T14.91, T79.A0X with 7th A, T79.A3X-T79.9XX with 7th A

√x7th **S35.90 Unspecified injury of unspecified blood vessel at abdomen, lower back and pelvis level** CC

√x7th **S35.91 Laceration of unspecified blood vessel at abdomen, lower back and pelvis level** CC

√x7th **S35.99 Other specified injury of unspecified blood vessel at abdomen, lower back and pelvis level** CC

√4th **S36 Injury of intra-abdominal organs**

Code also any associated open wound (S31.-)

The appropriate 7th is to be added to each code from category S36.
- A initial encounter
- D subsequent encounter
- S sequela

√5th **S36.0 Injury of spleen**

CC Excl: For CC/MCC codes in subcategory S36.0, unless otherwise noted: CC or MCC as indicated with 7th A: S31.001A, S31.011A, S31.021A, S31.031A, S31.041A, S31.051-S31.159 with 7th A, S31.600-S31.659 with 7th A, S31.831-S31.839 with 7th A, S36.00X-S36.09X with 7th A, S36.81X-S36.99X with 7th A, S38.3XX-S39.023 with 7th A, T14.8-T14.91, T79.A0X-T79.9XX with 7th A

√x7th **S36.00 Unspecified injury of spleen** CC

√6th **S36.02 Contusion of spleen**

√7th **S36.020 Minor contusion of spleen** CC
Contusion of spleen less than 2 cm

√7th **S36.021 Major contusion of spleen** CC
Contusion of spleen greater than 2 cm

√7th **S36.029 Unspecified contusion of spleen** CC

√6th **S36.03 Laceration of spleen**

√7th **S36.030 Superficial (capsular) laceration of spleen** CC
Laceration of spleen less than 1cm
Minor laceration of spleen

√7th **S36.031 Moderate laceration of spleen** MCC
Laceration of spleen 1 to 3 cm

√7th **S36.032 Major laceration of spleen** MCC
Avulsion of spleen
Laceration of spleen greater than 3 cm
Massive laceration of spleen
Multiple moderate lacerations of spleen
Stellate laceration of spleen

√7th **S36.039 Unspecified laceration of spleen** CC

√x7th **S36.09 Other injury of spleen** CC

√5th **S36.1 Injury of liver and gallbladder and bile duct**

√6th **S36.11 Injury of liver**

CC Excl: For CC/MCC codes in subcategory S36.11, unless otherwise noted: CC or MCC as indicated with 7th A: S31.001A, S31.011A, S31.021A, S31.031A, S31.041A, S31.051-S31.159 with 7th A, S31.600-S31.659 with 7th A, S31.831-S31.839 with 7th A, S36.112-S36.119 with 7th A, S36.81X-S36.99X with 7th A, S38.3XX-S39.023 with 7th A, T14.8-T14.91, T79.A0X-T79.9XX with 7th A

√7th **S36.112 Contusion of liver** CC

√7th **S36.113 Laceration of liver, unspecified degree** CC

√7th **S36.114 Minor laceration of liver** CC
Laceration involving capsule only, or, without significant involvement of hepatic parenchyma [i.e., less than 1cm deep]

√7th **S36.115 Moderate laceration of liver** MCC
Laceration involving parenchyma but without major disruption of parenchyma [i.e., less than 10 cm long and less than 3 cm deep]

√7th **S36.116 Major laceration of liver** MCC
Laceration with significant disruption of hepatic parenchyma [i.e., greater than 10 cm long and 3 cm deep]
Multiple moderate lacerations, with or without hematoma
Stellate laceration of liver

√7th **S36.118 Other injury of liver** CC

√7th **S36.119 Unspecified injury of liver** CC

√6th **S36.12 Injury of gallbladder**

CC Excl: For CC codes in subcategory S36.12, unless otherwise noted: CC with 7th character A: S31.001A, S31.011A, S31.021A, S31.031A, S31.041A, S31.051-S31.159 with 7th A, S31.600-S31.659 with 7th A, S31.831-S31.839 with 7th A, S36.122-S36.13X with 7th A, S36.81X-S36.99X with 7th A, S38.3XX-S39.023 with 7th A, T14.8-T14.91, T79.A0X-T79.9XX with 7th A

√7th **S36.122 Contusion of gallbladder** CC

√7th **S36.123 Laceration of gallbladder** CC

√7th **S36.128 Other injury of gallbladder** CC

√7th **S36.129 Unspecified injury of gallbladder** CC

√x7th **S36.13 Injury of bile duct** CC
CC Excl: See code: S36.12

√5th **S36.2 Injury of pancreas**

CC Excl: For CC codes in subcategory S36.2, unless otherwise noted: CC with 7th character A: M79.A3, S31.001A, S31.011A, S31.021A, S31.031A, S31.041A, S31.051-S31.159 with 7th A, S31.600-S31.659 with 7th A, S31.831-S31.839 with 7th A, S36.200-S36.299 with 7th A, S36.81X-S36.99X with 7th A, S38.3XX-S39.023 with 7th A, T14.8-T14.91, T79.A3X-T79.9XX with 7th A

√6th **S36.20 Unspecified injury of pancreas**

√7th **S36.200 Unspecified injury of head of pancreas** CC

√7th **S36.201 Unspecified injury of body of pancreas** CC

√7th **S36.202 Unspecified injury of tail of pancreas** CC

√7th **S36.209 Unspecified injury of unspecified part of pancreas** CC

√6th **S36.22 Contusion of pancreas**

√7th **S36.220 Contusion of head of pancreas** CC

√7th **S36.221 Contusion of body of pancreas** CC

√7th **S36.222 Contusion of tail of pancreas** CC

√7th **S36.229 Contusion of unspecified part of pancreas** CC

√6th **S36.23 Laceration of pancreas, unspecified degree**

√7th **S36.230 Laceration of head of pancreas, unspecified degree** CC

√7th **S36.231 Laceration of body of pancreas, unspecified degree** CC

√7th **S36.232 Laceration of tail of pancreas, unspecified degree** CC

√7th **S36.239 Laceration of unspecified part of pancreas, unspecified degree** CC

√6th **S36.24 Minor laceration of pancreas**

√7th **S36.240 Minor laceration of head of pancreas** CC

√7th **S36.241 Minor laceration of body of pancreas** CC

√7th **S36.242 Minor laceration of tail of pancreas** CC

√7th **S36.249 Minor laceration of unspecified part of pancreas** CC

√6th **S36.25 Moderate laceration of pancreas**

√7th **S36.250 Moderate laceration of head of pancreas** CC

√7th **S36.251 Moderate laceration of body of pancreas** CC

√7th **S36.252 Moderate laceration of tail of pancreas** CC

√7th **S36.259 Moderate laceration of unspecified part of pancreas** CC

√6th **S36.26 Major laceration of pancreas**

√7th **S36.260 Major laceration of head of pancreas** CC

√7th **S36.261 Major laceration of body of pancreas** CC

√7th **S36.262 Major laceration of tail of pancreas** CC

√7th **S36.269 Major laceration of unspecified part of pancreas** CC

✓6th **S36.29 Other injury of pancreas**
- ✓7th **S36.290 Other injury of head of pancreas** CC
- ✓7th **S36.291 Other injury of body of pancreas** CC
- ✓7th **S36.292 Other injury of tail of pancreas** CC
- ✓7th **S36.299 Other injury of unspecified part of pancreas** CC

✓5th **S36.3 Injury of stomach**

CC Excl: For CC codes in subcategory S36.3, unless otherwise noted: CC with 7th character A: M79.A3, S31.001A, S31.011A, S31.021A, S31.031A, S31.041A, S31.051-S31.159 with 7th A, S31.600-S31.659 with 7th A, S31.831-S31.839 with 7th A, S36.30X-S36.39X with 7th A, S36.81X-S36.99X with 7th A, S38.3XX-S39.023 with 7th A, T14.8-T14.91, T79.A3X-T79.9XX with 7th A

- ✓x7th **S36.30 Unspecified injury of stomach** CC
- ✓x7th **S36.32 Contusion of stomach** CC
- ✓x7th **S36.33 Laceration of stomach** CC
- ✓x7th **S36.39 Other injury of stomach** CC

✓5th **S36.4 Injury of small intestine**

CC Excl: For CC codes in subcategory S36.4, unless otherwise noted: CC with 7th character A: M79.A3, S31.001A, S31.011A, S31.021A, S31.031A, S31.041A, S31.051-S31.159 with 7th A, S31.600-S31.659 with 7th A, S31.831-S31.839 with 7th A, S36.400-S36.499 with 7th A, S36.81X-S36.99X with 7th A, S38.3XX-S39.023 with 7th A, T14.8-T14.91, T79.A3X-T79.9XX with 7th A

✓6th **S36.40 Unspecified injury of small intestine**
- ✓7th **S36.400 Unspecified injury of duodenum** CC
- ✓7th **S36.408 Unspecified injury of other part of small intestine** CC
- ✓7th **S36.409 Unspecified injury of unspecified part of small intestine** CC

✓6th **S36.41 Primary blast injury of small intestine**
Blast injury of small intestine NOS
- ✓7th **S36.410 Primary blast injury of duodenum** CC
- ✓7th **S36.418 Primary blast injury of other part of small intestine** CC
- ✓7th **S36.419 Primary blast injury of unspecified part of small intestine** CC

✓6th **S36.42 Contusion of small intestine**
- ✓7th **S36.420 Contusion of duodenum** CC
- ✓7th **S36.428 Contusion of other part of small intestine** CC
- ✓7th **S36.429 Contusion of unspecified part of small intestine** CC

✓6th **S36.43 Laceration of small intestine**
- ✓7th **S36.430 Laceration of duodenum** CC
- ✓7th **S36.438 Laceration of other part of small intestine** CC
- ✓7th **S36.439 Laceration of unspecified part of small intestine** CC

✓6th **S36.49 Other injury of small intestine**
- ✓7th **S36.490 Other injury of duodenum** CC
- ✓7th **S36.498 Other injury of other part of small intestine** CC
- ✓7th **S36.499 Other injury of unspecified part of small intestine** CC

✓5th **S36.5 Injury of colon**

EXCLUDES 2 *injury of rectum (S36.6-)*

CC Excl: For CC/MCC codes in subcategory S36.5, unless otherwise noted: CC with 7th character A: M79.A3, S31.001A, S31.011A, S31.021A, S31.031A, S31.041A, S31.051-S31.159 with 7th A, S31.600-S31.659 with 7th A, S31.831-S31.839 with 7th A, S36.500-S36.99X with 7th A, S38.3XX-S39.023 with 7th A, T14.8-T14.91, T79.A3X-T79.9XX with 7th A

✓6th **S36.50 Unspecified injury of colon**
- ✓7th **S36.500 Unspecified injury of ascending [right] colon** CC
- ✓7th **S36.501 Unspecified injury of transverse colon** CC
- ✓7th **S36.502 Unspecified injury of descending [left] colon** CC
- ✓7th **S36.503 Unspecified injury of sigmoid colon** CC
- ✓7th **S36.508 Unspecified injury of other part of colon** CC
- ✓7th **S36.509 Unspecified injury of unspecified part of colon** CC

✓6th **S36.51 Primary blast injury of colon**
Blast injury of colon NOS
- ✓7th **S36.510 Primary blast injury of ascending [right] colon** CC
- ✓7th **S36.511 Primary blast injury of transverse colon** CC
- ✓7th **S36.512 Primary blast injury of descending [left] colon** CC
- ✓7th **S36.513 Primary blast injury of sigmoid colon** CC
- ✓7th **S36.518 Primary blast injury of other part of colon** CC
- ✓7th **S36.519 Primary blast injury of unspecified part of colon** CC

✓6th **S36.52 Contusion of colon**
- ✓7th **S36.520 Contusion of ascending [right] colon** CC
- ✓7th **S36.521 Contusion of transverse colon** CC
- ✓7th **S36.522 Contusion of descending [left] colon** CC
- ✓7th **S36.523 Contusion of sigmoid colon** CC
- ✓7th **S36.528 Contusion of other part of colon** CC
- ✓7th **S36.529 Contusion of unspecified part of colon** CC

✓6th **S36.53 Laceration of colon**
- ✓7th **S36.530 Laceration of ascending [right] colon** CC
- ✓7th **S36.531 Laceration of transverse colon** CC
- ✓7th **S36.532 Laceration of descending [left] colon** CC
- ✓7th **S36.533 Laceration of sigmoid colon** CC
- ✓7th **S36.538 Laceration of other part of colon** CC
- ✓7th **S36.539 Laceration of unspecified part of colon** CC

✓6th **S36.59 Other injury of colon**
Secondary blast injury of colon
- ✓7th **S36.590 Other injury of ascending [right] colon** CC
- ✓7th **S36.591 Other injury of transverse colon** CC
- ✓7th **S36.592 Other injury of descending [left] colon** CC
- ✓7th **S36.593 Other injury of sigmoid colon** CC
- ✓7th **S36.598 Other injury of other part of colon** CC
- ✓7th **S36.599 Other injury of unspecified part of colon** CC

✓5th **S36.6 Injury of rectum**

CC Excl: For CC codes in subcategory S36.6, unless otherwise noted: CC with 7th character A: See Code: S86.5

- ✓x7th **S36.60 Unspecified injury of rectum** CC
- ✓x7th **S36.61 Primary blast injury of rectum** CC
  Blast injury of rectum NOS
- ✓x7th **S36.62 Contusion of rectum** CC
- ✓x7th **S36.63 Laceration of rectum** CC
- ✓x7th **S36.69 Other injury of rectum** CC
  Secondary blast injury of rectum

✓5th **S36.8 Injury of other intra-abdominal organs**

CC Excl: For CC codes in subcategory S36.8, unless otherwise noted: CC with 7th character A: S31.001A, S31.011A, S31.021A, S31.031A, S31.041A, S31.051-S31.159 with 7th A, S31.600-S31.659 with 7th A, S31.831-S31.839 with 7th A, S36.81X-S36.99X with 7th A, S38.3XX-S39.023 with 7th A, T14.8-T14.91, T79.A0X-T79.9XX with 7th A

- ✓x7th **S36.81 Injury of peritoneum** CC

✓6th **S36.89 Injury of other intra-abdominal organs**
Injury of retroperitoneum
- ✓7th **S36.892 Contusion of other intra-abdominal organs** CC
- ✓7th **S36.893 Laceration of other intra-abdominal organs** CC
- ✓7th **S36.898 Other injury of other intra-abdominal organs** CC
- ✓7th **S36.899 Unspecified injury of other intra-abdominal organs** CC

DRAFT

S36.9 Injury of unspecified intra-abdominal organ

CC Excl: For CC codes in subcategory S36.9, unless otherwise noted: CC with 7th character A: See Code: S36.8

- **S36.90** Unspecified injury of unspecified intra-abdominal organ CC
- **S36.92** Contusion of unspecified intra-abdominal organ CC
- **S36.93** Laceration of unspecified intra-abdominal organ CC
- **S36.99** Other injury of unspecified intra-abdominal organ CC

S37 Injury of urinary and pelvic organs

Code also any associated open wound (S31.-)

EXCLUDES 1 *obstetric trauma to pelvic organs (O71.-)*

EXCLUDES 2 *injury of peritoneum (S36.81)*
injury of retroperitoneum (S36.89-)

The appropriate 7th is to be added to each code from category S37.
A initial encounter
D subsequent encounter
S sequela

S37.0 Injury of kidney

EXCLUDES 2 *acute kidney injury (nontraumatic) (N17.9)*

CC Excl: For CC/MCC codes in subcategory S37.0, unless otherwise noted: CC or MCC as indicated with 7th A: S31.001A, S31.011A, S31.021A, S31.031A, S31.041A, S31.051-S31.159 with 7th A, S31.600-S31.659 with 7th A, S31.831-S31.839 with 7th A, S36.81X-S37.099 with 7th A, S38.3XX-S39.023 with 7th A, T14.8-T14.91, T79.A0X-T79.9XX with 7th A

S37.00 Unspecified injury of kidney
- **S37.001** Unspecified injury of right kidney CC
- **S37.002** Unspecified injury of left kidney CC
- **S37.009** Unspecified injury of unspecified kidney CC

S37.01 Minor contusion of kidney
Contusion of kidney less than 2 cm
Contusion of kidney NOS
- **S37.011** Minor contusion of right kidney CC
- **S37.012** Minor contusion of left kidney CC
- **S37.019** Minor contusion of unspecified kidney CC

S37.02 Major contusion of kidney
Contusion of kidney greater than 2 cm
- **S37.021** Major contusion of right kidney CC
- **S37.022** Major contusion of left kidney CC
- **S37.029** Major contusion of unspecified kidney CC

S37.03 Laceration of kidney, unspecified degree
- **S37.031** Laceration of right kidney, unspecified degree CC
- **S37.032** Laceration of left kidney, unspecified degree CC
- **S37.039** Laceration of unspecified kidney, unspecified degree CC

S37.04 Minor laceration of kidney
Laceration of kidney less than 1 cm
- **S37.041** Minor laceration of right kidney CC
- **S37.042** Minor laceration of left kidney CC
- **S37.049** Minor laceration of unspecified kidney CC

S37.05 Moderate laceration of kidney
Laceration of kidney 1 to 3 cm
- **S37.051** Moderate laceration of right kidney CC
- **S37.052** Moderate laceration of left kidney CC
- **S37.059** Moderate laceration of unspecified kidney CC

S37.06 Major laceration of kidney
Avulsion of kidney
Laceration of kidney greater than 3 cm
Massive laceration of kidney
Multiple moderate lacerations of kidney
Stellate laceration of kidney
- **S37.061** Major laceration of right kidney MCC
- **S37.062** Major laceration of left kidney MCC
- **S37.069** Major laceration of unspecified kidney MCC

S37.09 Other injury of kidney
- **S37.091** Other injury of right kidney MCC
- **S37.092** Other injury of left kidney MCC
- **S37.099** Other injury of unspecified kidney MCC

S37.1 Injury of ureter

CC Excl: For CC codes in subcategory S37.1, unless otherwise noted: CC with 7th character A: S31.001A, S31.011A, S31.021A, S31.031A, S31.041A, S31.051-S31.159 with 7th A, S31.600-S31.659 with 7th A, S31.831-S31.839 with 7th A, S36.81X-S37.099 with 7th A, S38.3XX-S39.023 with 7th A, T14.8-T14.91, T79.A0X-T79.9XX with 7th A

- **S37.10** Unspecified injury of ureter CC
- **S37.12** Contusion of ureter CC
- **S37.13** Laceration of ureter CC
- **S37.19** Other injury of ureter CC

S37.2 Injury of bladder

CC Excl: For CC codes in subcategory S37.2, unless otherwise noted: CC with 7th character A: S31.001A, S31.011A, S31.021A, S31.031A, S31.041A, S31.051-S31.159 with 7th A, S31.600-S31.659 with 7th A, S31.831-S31.839 with 7th A, S36.81X-S36.99X with 7th A, S37.20-S37.599 with 7th A, S37.822-S37.99 with 7th A, S38.3XX-S39.023 with 7th A, T14.8-T14.91, T79.A0X-T79.9XX with 7th A

- **S37.20** Unspecified injury of bladder CC
- **S37.22** Contusion of bladder CC
- **S37.23** Laceration of bladder CC
- **S37.29** Other injury of bladder CC

S37.3 Injury of urethra

CC Excl: For CC codes in subcategory S37.3, unless otherwise noted: See code: S37.2

- **S37.30** Unspecified injury of urethra CC
- **S37.32** Contusion of urethra CC
- **S37.33** Laceration of urethra CC
- **S37.39** Other injury of urethra CC

S37.4 Injury of ovary

S37.40 Unspecified injury of ovary
- **S37.401** Unspecified injury of ovary, unilateral ♀
- **S37.402** Unspecified injury of ovary, bilateral ♀
- **S37.409** Unspecified injury of ovary, unspecified ♀

S37.42 Contusion of ovary
- **S37.421** Contusion of ovary, unilateral ♀
- **S37.422** Contusion of ovary, bilateral ♀
- **S37.429** Contusion of ovary, unspecified ♀

S37.43 Laceration of ovary
- **S37.431** Laceration of ovary, unilateral ♀
- **S37.432** Laceration of ovary, bilateral ♀
- **S37.439** Laceration of ovary, unspecified ♀

S37.49 Other injury of ovary
- **S37.491** Other injury of ovary, unilateral ♀
- **S37.492** Other injury of ovary, bilateral ♀
- **S37.499** Other injury of ovary, unspecified ♀

S37.5 Injury of fallopian tube

S37.50 Unspecified injury of fallopian tube
- **S37.501** Unspecified injury of fallopian tube, unilateral ♀
- **S37.502** Unspecified injury of fallopian tube, bilateral ♀
- **S37.509** Unspecified injury of fallopian tube, unspecified ♀

S37.51 Primary blast injury of fallopian tube
Blast injury of fallopian tube NOS
- **S37.511** Primary blast injury of fallopian tube, unilateral ♀
- **S37.512** Primary blast injury of fallopian tube, bilateral ♀
- **S37.519** Primary blast injury of fallopian tube, unspecified ♀

√6th S37.52 Contusion of fallopian tube
- √7th S37.521 Contusion of fallopian tube, unilateral ♀
- √7th S37.522 Contusion of fallopian tube, bilateral ♀
- √7th S37.529 Contusion of fallopian tube, unspecified ♀

√6th S37.53 Laceration of fallopian tube
- √7th S37.531 Laceration of fallopian tube, unilateral ♀
- √7th S37.532 Laceration of fallopian tube, bilateral ♀
- √7th S37.539 Laceration of fallopian tube, unspecified ♀

√6th S37.59 Other injury of fallopian tube
Secondary blast injury of fallopian tube
- √7th S37.591 Other injury of fallopian tube, unilateral ♀
- √7th S37.592 Other injury of fallopian tube, bilateral ♀
- √7th S37.599 Other injury of fallopian tube, unspecified ♀

√5th **S37.6 Injury of uterus**
EXCLUDES 1 *injury to gravid uterus (O9A.2-)*
injury to uterus during delivery (O71.-)

CC Excl: For CC codes in subcategory S37.6, unless otherwise noted: CC with 7th character A: S31.001A, S31.011A, S31.021A, S31.031A, S31.041A, S31.051-S31.159 with 7th A, S31.600-S31.659 with 7th A, S31.831-S31.839 with 7th A, S36.81X-S36.99X with 7th A, S37.401-S37.69X with 7th A, S37.822-S37.99X with 7th A, S38.3XX-S39.023 with 7th A, T14.8-T14.91, T79.A0X-T79.9XX with 7th A

- √x7th S37.60 Unspecified injury of uterus CC ♀
- √x7th S37.62 Contusion of uterus CC ♀
- √x7th S37.63 Laceration of uterus CC ♀
- √x7th S37.69 Other injury of uterus CC ♀

√5th **S37.8 Injury of other urinary and pelvic organs**

√6th S37.81 Injury of adrenal gland

CC Excl: For CC codes in subcategory S37.81, unless otherwise noted: CC with 7th character A: S31.001A, S31.011A, S31.021A, S31.031A, S31.041A, S31.051-S31.159 with 7th A, S31.600-S31.659 with 7th A, S31.831-S31.839 with 7th A, S36.81X-S36.99X with 7th A, S37.812-S37.819 with 7th A, S38.3XX-S39.023 with 7th A, T14.8-T14.91, T79.A0X-T79.9XX with 7th A

- √7th S37.812 Contusion of adrenal gland CC
- √7th S37.813 Laceration of adrenal gland CC
- √7th S37.818 Other injury of adrenal gland CC
- √7th S37.819 Unspecified injury of adrenal gland CC

√6th S37.82 Injury of prostate
- √7th S37.822 Contusion of prostate ♂
- √7th S37.823 Laceration of prostate ♂
- √7th S37.828 Other injury of prostate ♂
- √7th S37.829 Unspecified injury of prostate ♂

√6th S37.89 Injury of other urinary and pelvic organ

CC Excl: For CC codes in subcategory S37.89, unless otherwise noted: CC with 7th character A: S31.001A, S31.011A, S31.021A, S31.031A, S31.041A, S31.051-S31.159 with 7th A, S31.600-S31.659 with 7th A, S31.831-S31.839 with 7th A, S36.81X-S36.99X with 7th A, S37.401-S37.599 with 7th A, S37.822-S37.99X with 7th A, S38.3X-S39.023 with 7th A, T14.8-T14.91, T79.A0X-T79.9XX with 7th A

- √7th S37.892 Contusion of other urinary and pelvic organ CC
- √7th S37.893 Laceration of other urinary and pelvic organ CC
- √7th S37.898 Other injury of other urinary and pelvic organ CC
- √7th S37.899 Unspecified injury of other urinary and pelvic organ CC

√5th **S37.9 Injury of unspecified urinary and pelvic organ**

CC Excl: For CC codes in subcategory S37.9, unless otherwise noted: CC with 7th character A: See code: S37.89

- √x7th S37.90 Unspecified injury of unspecified urinary and pelvic organ CC
- √x7th S37.92 Contusion of unspecified urinary and pelvic organ CC
- √x7th S37.93 Laceration of unspecified urinary and pelvic organ CC
- √x7th S37.99 Other injury of unspecified urinary and pelvic organ CC

√4th **S38 Crushing injury and traumatic amputation of abdomen, lower back, pelvis and external genitals**
NOTE An amputation not identified as partial or complete should be coded to complete.

The appropriate 7th is to be added to each code from category S38.
- A initial encounter
- D subsequent encounter
- S sequela

√5th **S38.0 Crushing injury of external genital organs**
Use additional code for any associated injuries

√6th S38.00 Crushing injury of unspecified external genital organs
- √7th S38.001 Crushing injury of unspecified external genital organs, male ♂
- √7th S38.002 Crushing injury of unspecified external genital organs, female ♀

- √x7th S38.01 Crushing injury of penis ♂
- √x7th S38.02 Crushing injury of scrotum and testis ♂
- √x7th S38.03 Crushing injury of vulva ♀

√x7th **S38.1 Crushing injury of abdomen, lower back, and pelvis**
Use additional code for all associated injuries, such as:
fracture of thoracic or lumbar spine and pelvis (S22.0-, S32-)
injury to intra-abdominal organs (S36.-)
injury to urinary and pelvic organs (S37.-)
open wound of abdominal wall (S31.-)
spinal cord injury (S34.0, S34.1-)
EXCLUDES 2 *crushing injury of external genital organs (S38.0-)*

√5th **S38.2 Traumatic amputation of external genital organs**

√6th S38.21 Traumatic amputation of female external genital organs
Traumatic amputation of clitoris
Traumatic amputation of labium (majus) (minus)
Traumatic amputation of vulva
- √7th S38.211 Complete traumatic amputation of female external genital organs ♀
- √7th S38.212 Partial traumatic amputation of female external genital organs ♀

√6th S38.22 Traumatic amputation of penis
- √7th S38.221 Complete traumatic amputation of penis ♂
- √7th S38.222 Partial traumatic amputation of penis ♂

√6th S38.23 Traumatic amputation of scrotum and testis
- √7th S38.231 Complete traumatic amputation of scrotum and testis ♂
- √7th S38.232 Partial traumatic amputation of scrotum and testis ♂

√x7th **S38.3 Transection (partial) of abdomen**

√4th **S39 Other and unspecified injuries of abdomen, lower back, pelvis and external genitals**
Code also any associated open wound (S31.-)
EXCLUDES 2 *sprain of joints and ligaments of lumbar spine and pelvis (S33.-)*

The appropriate 7th is to be added to each code from category S39.
- A initial encounter
- D subsequent encounter
- S sequela

√5th **S39.0 Injury of muscle, fascia and tendon of abdomen, lower back and pelvis**

√6th S39.00 Unspecified injury of muscle, fascia and tendon of abdomen, lower back and pelvis
- √7th S39.001 Unspecified injury of muscle, fascia and tendon of abdomen
- √7th S39.002 Unspecified injury of muscle, fascia and tendon of lower back
- √7th S39.003 Unspecified injury of muscle, fascia and tendon of pelvis

- ✓6th S39.01 Strain of muscle, fascia and tendon of abdomen, lower back and pelvis
  - ✓7th S39.011 Strain of muscle, fascia and tendon of abdomen
  - ✓7th S39.012 Strain of muscle, fascia and tendon of lower back
  - ✓7th S39.013 Strain of muscle, fascia and tendon of pelvis
- ✓6th S39.02 Laceration of muscle, fascia and tendon of abdomen, lower back and pelvis
  - ✓7th S39.021 Laceration of muscle, fascia and tendon of abdomen
  - ✓7th S39.022 Laceration of muscle, fascia and tendon of lower back
  - ✓7th S39.023 Laceration of muscle, fascia and tendon of pelvis
- ✓6th S39.09 Other injury of muscle, fascia and tendon of abdomen, lower back and pelvis
  - ✓7th S39.091 Other injury of muscle, fascia and tendon of abdomen
  - ✓7th S39.092 Other injury of muscle, fascia and tendon of lower back
  - ✓7th S39.093 Other injury of muscle, fascia and tendon of pelvis

✓5th S39.8 Other specified injuries of abdomen, lower back, pelvis and external genitals
- ✓x7th S39.81 Other specified injuries of abdomen
- ✓x7th S39.82 Other specified injuries of lower back
- ✓x7th S39.83 Other specified injuries of pelvis
- ✓6th S39.84 Other specified injuries of external genitals
  - ✓7th S39.840 Fracture of corpus cavernosum penis ♂
  - ✓7th S39.848 Other specified injuries of external genitals

✓5th S39.9 Unspecified injury of abdomen, lower back, pelvis and external genitals
- ✓x7th S39.91 Unspecified injury of abdomen
- ✓x7th S39.92 Unspecified injury of lower back
- ✓x7th S39.93 Unspecified injury of pelvis
- ✓x7th S39.94 Unspecified injury of external genitals

Injuries to the shoulder and upper arm (S40-S49)

INCLUDES injuries of axilla
injuries of scapular region

EXCLUDES 2 *burns and corrosions (T20-T32)*
frostbite (T33-T34)
injuries of elbow (S50-S59)
insect bite or sting, venomous (T63.4)

✓4th S40 Superficial injury of shoulder and upper arm

The appropriate 7th is to be added to each code from category S40.
A initial encounter
D subsequent encounter
S sequela

✓5th S40.0 Contusion of shoulder and upper arm
- ✓6th S40.01 Contusion of shoulder
  - ✓7th S40.011 Contusion of right shoulder
  - ✓7th S40.012 Contusion of left shoulder
  - ✓7th S40.019 Contusion of unspecified shoulder
- ✓6th S40.02 Contusion of upper arm
  - ✓7th S40.021 Contusion of right upper arm
  - ✓7th S40.022 Contusion of left upper arm
  - ✓7th S40.029 Contusion of unspecified upper arm

✓5th S40.2 Other superficial injuries of shoulder
- ✓6th S40.21 Abrasion of shoulder
  - ✓7th S40.211 Abrasion of right shoulder
  - ✓7th S40.212 Abrasion of left shoulder
  - ✓7th S40.219 Abrasion of unspecified shoulder
- ✓6th S40.22 Blister (nonthermal) of shoulder
  - ✓7th S40.221 Blister (nonthermal) of right shoulder
  - ✓7th S40.222 Blister (nonthermal) of left shoulder
  - ✓7th S40.229 Blister (nonthermal) of unspecified shoulder
- ✓6th S40.24 External constriction of shoulder
  - ✓7th S40.241 External constriction of right shoulder
  - ✓7th S40.242 External constriction of left shoulder
  - ✓7th S40.249 External constriction of unspecified shoulder
- ✓6th S40.25 Superficial foreign body of shoulder
  Splinter in the shoulder
  - ✓7th S40.251 Superficial foreign body of right shoulder
  - ✓7th S40.252 Superficial foreign body of left shoulder
  - ✓7th S40.259 Superficial foreign body of unspecified shoulder
- ✓6th S40.26 Insect bite (nonvenomous) of shoulder
  - ✓7th S40.261 Insect bite (nonvenomous) of right shoulder
  - ✓7th S40.262 Insect bite (nonvenomous) of left shoulder
  - ✓7th S40.269 Insect bite (nonvenomous) of unspecified shoulder
- ✓6th S40.27 Other superficial bite of shoulder
  EXCLUDES 1 *open bite of shoulder (S41.05)*
  - ✓7th S40.271 Other superficial bite of right shoulder
  - ✓7th S40.272 Other superficial bite of left shoulder
  - ✓7th S40.279 Other superficial bite of unspecified shoulder

✓5th S40.8 Other superficial injuries of upper arm
- ✓6th S40.81 Abrasion of upper arm
  - ✓7th S40.811 Abrasion of right upper arm
  - ✓7th S40.812 Abrasion of left upper arm
  - ✓7th S40.819 Abrasion of unspecified upper arm
- ✓6th S40.82 Blister (nonthermal) of upper arm
  - ✓7th S40.821 Blister (nonthermal) of right upper arm
  - ✓7th S40.822 Blister (nonthermal) of left upper arm
  - ✓7th S40.829 Blister (nonthermal) of unspecified upper arm
- ✓6th S40.84 External constriction of upper arm
  - ✓7th S40.841 External constriction of right upper arm
  - ✓7th S40.842 External constriction of left upper arm
  - ✓7th S40.849 External constriction of unspecified upper arm
- ✓6th S40.85 Superficial foreign body of upper arm
  Splinter in the upper arm
  - ✓7th S40.851 Superficial foreign body of right upper arm
  - ✓7th S40.852 Superficial foreign body of left upper arm
  - ✓7th S40.859 Superficial foreign body of unspecified upper arm
- ✓6th S40.86 Insect bite (nonvenomous) of upper arm
  - ✓7th S40.861 Insect bite (nonvenomous) of right upper arm
  - ✓7th S40.862 Insect bite (nonvenomous) of left upper arm
  - ✓7th S40.869 Insect bite (nonvenomous) of unspecified upper arm
- ✓6th S40.87 Other superficial bite of upper arm
  EXCLUDES 1 *open bite of upper arm (S41.14)*
  EXCLUDES 2 *other superficial bite of shoulder (S40.27-)*
  - ✓7th S40.871 Other superficial bite of right upper arm
  - ✓7th S40.872 Other superficial bite of left upper arm
  - ✓7th S40.879 Other superficial bite of unspecified upper arm

✓5th S40.9 Unspecified superficial injury of shoulder and upper arm
- ✓6th S40.91 Unspecified superficial injury of shoulder
  - ✓7th S40.911 Unspecified superficial injury of right shoulder
  - ✓7th S40.912 Unspecified superficial injury of left shoulder
  - ✓7th S40.919 Unspecified superficial injury of unspecified shoulder
- ✓6th S40.92 Unspecified superficial injury of upper arm
  - ✓7th S40.921 Unspecified superficial injury of right upper arm

7th **S40.922 Unspecified superficial injury of left upper arm**

7th **S40.929 Unspecified superficial injury of unspecified upper arm**

4th **S41 Open wound of shoulder and upper arm**

Code also any associated wound infection

EXCLUDES 1 *traumatic amputation of shoulder and upper arm (S48.-)*

EXCLUDES 2 *open fracture of shoulder and upper arm (S42.- with 7th chractrer B or C)*

The appropriate 7th is to be added to each code from category S41.
- A initial encounter
- D subsequent encounter
- S sequela

5th **S41.0 Open wound of shoulder**

6th **S41.00 Unspecified open wound of shoulder**

7th **S41.001 Unspecified open wound of right shoulder**

7th **S41.002 Unspecified open wound of left shoulder**

7th **S41.009 Unspecified open wound of unspecified shoulder**

6th **S41.01 Laceration without foreign body of shoulder**

7th **S41.011 Laceration without foreign body of right shoulder**

7th **S41.012 Laceration without foreign body of left shoulder**

7th **S41.019 Laceration without foreign body of unspecified shoulder**

6th **S41.02 Laceration with foreign body of shoulder**

7th **S41.021 Laceration with foreign body of right shoulder**

7th **S41.022 Laceration with foreign body of left shoulder**

7th **S41.029 Laceration with foreign body of unspecified shoulder**

6th **S41.03 Puncture wound without foreign body of shoulder**

7th **S41.031 Puncture wound without foreign body of right shoulder**

7th **S41.032 Puncture wound without foreign body of left shoulder**

7th **S41.039 Puncture wound without foreign body of unspecified shoulder**

6th **S41.04 Puncture wound with foreign body of shoulder**

7th **S41.041 Puncture wound with foreign body of right shoulder**

7th **S41.042 Puncture wound with foreign body of left shoulder**

7th **S41.049 Puncture wound with foreign body of unspecified shoulder**

6th **S41.05 Open bite of shoulder**

Bite of shoulder NOS

EXCLUDES 1 *superficial bite of shoulder (S40.27)*

7th **S41.051 Open bite of right shoulder**

7th **S41.052 Open bite of left shoulder**

7th **S41.059 Open bite of unspecified shoulder**

5th **S41.1 Open wound of upper arm**

6th **S41.10 Unspecified open wound of upper arm**

7th **S41.101 Unspecified open wound of right upper arm**

7th **S41.102 Unspecified open wound of left upper arm**

7th **S41.109 Unspecified open wound of unspecified upper arm**

6th **S41.11 Laceration without foreign body of upper arm**

7th **S41.111 Laceration without foreign body of right upper arm**

7th **S41.112 Laceration without foreign body of left upper arm**

7th **S41.119 Laceration without foreign body of unspecified upper arm**

6th **S41.12 Laceration with foreign body of upper arm**

7th **S41.121 Laceration with foreign body of right upper arm**

7th **S41.122 Laceration with foreign body of left upper arm**

7th **S41.129 Laceration with foreign body of unspecified upper arm**

6th **S41.13 Puncture wound without foreign body of upper arm**

7th **S41.131 Puncture wound without foreign body of right upper arm**

7th **S41.132 Puncture wound without foreign body of left upper arm**

7th **S41.139 Puncture wound without foreign body of unspecified upper arm**

6th **S41.14 Puncture wound with foreign body of upper arm**

7th **S41.141 Puncture wound with foreign body of right upper arm**

7th **S41.142 Puncture wound with foreign body of left upper arm**

7th **S41.149 Puncture wound with foreign body of unspecified upper arm**

6th **S41.15 Open bite of upper arm**

Bite of upper arm NOS

EXCLUDES 1 *superficial bite of upper arm (S40.87)*

7th **S41.151 Open bite of right upper arm**

7th **S41.152 Open bite of left upper arm**

7th **S41.159 Open bite of unspecified upper arm**

4th **S42 Fracture of shoulder and upper arm**

NOTE A fracture not indicated as displaced or nondisplaced should be coded to displaced.
A fracture not indicated as open or closed should be coded to closed.

EXCLUDES 1 *traumatic amputation of shoulder and upper arm (S48.-)*

The appropriate 7th is to be added to all codes from category S42 [unless otherwise indicated].
- A initial encounter for closed fracture
- B initial encounter for open fracture
- D subsequent encounter for fracture with routine healing
- G subsequent encounter for fracture with delayed healing
- K subsequent encounter for fracture with nonunion
- P subsequent encounter for fracture with malunion
- S sequela

5th **S42.0 Fracture of clavicle**

CC Excl: For CC/MCC codes in subcategory S42.0, unless otherwise noted: CC with 7th character B: S42.001-S42.036 with 7th [A, B], S62.90XB
CC with 7th character K or P: M80.00X-M84.68X with 7th [K, P], S02.0XX-S02.92X with 7th K, S12.000-S12.691 with 7th K, S22.000-S22.9XX with 7th K, S32.000-S32.9XX with 7th K, S42.001-S42.92X with 7th [K, P], S49.001-S49.199 with 7th [K, P], S52.001-S52.92X with 7th [K, M, N, P, Q, R], S59.001-S59.299 with 7th [K, P], S62.001-S62.92X with 7th [K, P], S72.001-S72.92X with 7th [K, M, N, P, Q, R], S79.001-S79.199 with 7th [K, P], S82.001-S82.92X with 7th [K, M, N, P, Q, R], S89.001-S89.399 with 7th [K, P], S92.001-S92.919 with 7th [K, P]

6th **S42.00 Fracture of unspecified part of clavicle**

7 7th **S42.001 Fracture of unspecified part of right clavicle** CC

7 7th **S42.002 Fracture of unspecified part of left clavicle** CC

7 7th **S42.009 Fracture of unspecified part of unspecified clavicle** CC

AHA: 2012, 4Q, 93

6th **S42.01 Fracture of sternal end of clavicle**

7 7th **S42.011 Anterior displaced fracture of sternal end of right clavicle** CC

7 7th **S42.012 Anterior displaced fracture of sternal end of left clavicle** CC

7 7th **S42.013 Anterior displaced fracture of sternal end of unspecified clavicle** CC

Displaced fracture of sternal end of clavicle NOS

7 7th **S42.014 Posterior displaced fracture of sternal end of right clavicle** CC

7 7th **S42.015 Posterior displaced fracture of sternal end of left clavicle** CC

7 7th **S42.016 Posterior displaced fracture of sternal end of unspecified clavicle** CC

7 HAC = Initial encounter only (7th character A, B or C) and not POA.

7 ✓7th S42.017 Nondisplaced fracture of sternal end of right clavicle CC
7 ✓7th S42.018 Nondisplaced fracture of sternal end of left clavicle CC
7 ✓7th S42.019 Nondisplaced fracture of sternal end of unspecified clavicle CC

✓6th S42.02 Fracture of shaft of clavicle
7 ✓7th S42.021 Displaced fracture of shaft of right clavicle CC
7 ✓7th S42.022 Displaced fracture of shaft of left clavicle CC
7 ✓7th S42.023 Displaced fracture of shaft of unspecified clavicle CC
7 ✓7th S42.024 Nondisplaced fracture of shaft of right clavicle CC
7 ✓7th S42.025 Nondisplaced fracture of shaft of left clavicle CC
7 ✓7th S42.026 Nondisplaced fracture of shaft of unspecified clavicle CC

✓6th S42.03 Fracture of lateral end of clavicle
Fracture of acromial end of clavicle
7 ✓7th S42.031 Displaced fracture of lateral end of right clavicle CC
7 ✓7th S42.032 Displaced fracture of lateral end of left clavicle CC
7 ✓7th S42.033 Displaced fracture of lateral end of unspecified clavicle CC
7 ✓7th S42.034 Nondisplaced fracture of lateral end of right clavicle CC
7 ✓7th S42.035 Nondisplaced fracture of lateral end of left clavicle CC
7 ✓7th S42.036 Nondisplaced fracture of lateral end of unspecified clavicle CC

✓5th S42.1 Fracture of scapula

CC Excl: For CC/MCC codes in subcatagory S42.1, unless otherwise noted: S42.101-S42.199 with 7th [A, B], S62.90XB
CC with 7th character K or P: M80.00X-M84.68X with 7th [K, P], S02.0XX-S02.92X with 7th K, S12.000-S12.691 with 7th K, S22.000-S22.9XX with 7th K, S32.000-S32.9XX with 7th K, S42.001-S42.92X with 7th [K, P], S49.001-S49.199 with 7th [K, P], S52.001-S52.92X with 7th [K, M, N, P, Q, R], S59.001-S59.299 with 7th [K, P], S62.001-S62.92X with 7th [K, P], S72.001-S72.92X with 7th [K, M, N, P, Q, R], S79.001-S79.199 with 7th [K, P], S82.001-S82.92X with 7th [K, M, N, P, Q, R], S89.001-S89.399 with 7th [K, P], S92.001-S92.919 with 7th [K, P]

✓6th S42.10 Fracture of unspecified part of scapula
7 ✓7th S42.101 Fracture of unspecified part of scapula, right shoulder CC
7 ✓7th S42.102 Fracture of unspecified part of scapula, left shoulder CC
7 ✓7th S42.109 Fracture of unspecified part of scapula, unspecified shoulder CC

✓6th S42.11 Fracture of body of scapula
7 ✓7th S42.111 Displaced fracture of body of scapula, right shoulder CC
7 ✓7th S42.112 Displaced fracture of body of scapula, left shoulder CC
7 ✓7th S42.113 Displaced fracture of body of scapula, unspecified shoulder CC
7 ✓7th S42.114 Nondisplaced fracture of body of scapula, right shoulder CC
7 ✓7th S42.115 Nondisplaced fracture of body of scapula, left shoulder CC
7 ✓7th S42.116 Nondisplaced fracture of body of scapula, unspecified shoulder CC

✓6th S42.12 Fracture of acromial process
7 ✓7th S42.121 Displaced fracture of acromial process, right shoulder CC
7 ✓7th S42.122 Displaced fracture of acromial process, left shoulder CC
7 ✓7th S42.123 Displaced fracture of acromial process, unspecified shoulder CC
7 ✓7th S42.124 Nondisplaced fracture of acromial process, right shoulder CC
7 ✓7th S42.125 Nondisplaced fracture of acromial process, left shoulder CC
7 ✓7th S42.126 Nondisplaced fracture of acromial process, unspecified shoulder CC

✓6th S42.13 Fracture of coracoid process
7 ✓7th S42.131 Displaced fracture of coracoid process, right shoulder CC
7 ✓7th S42.132 Displaced fracture of coracoid process, left shoulder CC
7 ✓7th S42.133 Displaced fracture of coracoid process, unspecified shoulder CC
7 ✓7th S42.134 Nondisplaced fracture of coracoid process, right shoulder CC
7 ✓7th S42.135 Nondisplaced fracture of coracoid process, left shoulder CC
7 ✓7th S42.136 Nondisplaced fracture of coracoid process, unspecified shoulder CC

✓6th S42.14 Fracture of glenoid cavity of scapula
7 ✓7th S42.141 Displaced fracture of glenoid cavity of scapula, right shoulder CC
7 ✓7th S42.142 Displaced fracture of glenoid cavity of scapula, left shoulder CC
7 ✓7th S42.143 Displaced fracture of glenoid cavity of scapula, unspecified shoulder CC
7 ✓7th S42.144 Nondisplaced fracture of glenoid cavity of scapula, right shoulder CC
7 ✓7th S42.145 Nondisplaced fracture of glenoid cavity of scapula, left shoulder CC
7 ✓7th S42.146 Nondisplaced fracture of glenoid cavity of scapula, unspecified shoulder CC

✓6th S42.15 Fracture of neck of scapula
7 ✓7th S42.151 Displaced fracture of neck of scapula, right shoulder CC
7 ✓7th S42.152 Displaced fracture of neck of scapula, left shoulder CC
7 ✓7th S42.153 Displaced fracture of neck of scapula, unspecified shoulder CC
7 ✓7th S42.154 Nondisplaced fracture of neck of scapula, right shoulder CC
7 ✓7th S42.155 Nondisplaced fracture of neck of scapula, left shoulder CC
7 ✓7th S42.156 Nondisplaced fracture of neck of scapula, unspecified shoulder CC

✓6th S42.19 Fracture of other part of scapula
7 ✓7th S42.191 Fracture of other part of scapula, right shoulder CC
7 ✓7th S42.192 Fracture of other part of scapula, left shoulder CC
7 ✓7th S42.199 Fracture of other part of scapula, unspecified shoulder CC

7 HAC = Initial encounter only (7th character A, B or C) and not POA.

5th **S42.2 Fracture of upper end of humerus**
Fracture of proximal end of humerus
EXCLUDES 2 *fracture of shaft of humerus (S42.3-)*
physeal fracture of upper end of humerus (S49.0-)

6th **S42.20 Unspecified fracture of upper end of humerus**

7 7th **S42.201 Unspecified fracture of upper end of right humerus** MCC CC
CC Excl: CC with 7th character A: S42.201-S42.271 with 7th [A, B], S42.279-S42.311 with 7th A, S42.319-S42.481 with 7th A, S42.489-S42.92X with 7th A, S49.001 with 7th A, S49.009-S49.011 with 7th A, S49.019-S49.021 with 7th A, S49.029-S49.031 with 7th A, S49.039-S49.041 with 7th A, S49.049-S49.091 with 7th A, S49.099-S49.101 with 7th A, S49.109-S49.111 with 7th A, S49.119-S49.121 with 7th A, S49.129-S49.131 with 7th A, S49.139-S49.141 with 7th A, S49.149-S49.191 with 7th A, S49.199A
MCC with 7th character B: S42.201-S42.266 with 7th B, S42.291-S42.92X with 7th B, S49.101-S49.199 with 7th A, S62.90XB
CC with 7th character K or P: M80.00X-M84.68X with 7th [K, P], S02.0XX-S02.92X with 7th K, S12.000-S12.691 with 7th K, S22.000-S22.9XX with 7th K, S32.000-S32.9XX with 7th K, S42.001-S42.92X with 7th [K, P], S49.001-S49.199 with 7th [K, P], S52.001-S52.92X with 7th [K, M, N, P, Q, R], S59.001-S59.299 with 7th [K, P], S62.001-S62.92X with 7th [K, P], S72.001-S72.92X with 7th [K, M, N, P, Q, R], S79.001-S79.199 with 7th [K, P], S82.001-S82.92X with 7th [K, M, N, P, Q, R], S89.001-S89.399 with 7th [K, P], S92.001-S92.919 with 7th [K, P]

7 7th **S42.202 Unspecified fracture of upper end of left humerus** MCC CC
CC Excl: CC with 7th character A: S42.201-S42.266 with 7th B, S42.272-S42.309 with 7th A, S42.312-S42.476 with 7th A, S42.482-S42.92X with 7th A, S49.002-S49.009 with 7th A, S49.012-S49.019 with 7th A, S49.022-S49.029 with 7th A, S49.032-S49.039 with 7th A, S49.042-S49.049 with 7th A, S49.092-S49.099 with 7th A, S49.102-S49.109 with 7th A, S49.112-S49.119 with 7th A, S49.122-S49.129 with 7th A, S49.132-S49.139 with 7th A, S49.142-S49.149 with 7th A, S49.192-S49.199 with 7th A
MCC with 7th character B: MCC Excl: S42.201-S42.266 with 7th B, S42.291-S42.92X with 7th B, S49.101-S49.199 with 7th A, S62.90XB
CC with 7th character K or P: CC Excl: M80.00X-M84.68X with 7th [K, P], S02.0XX-S02.92X with 7th K, S12.000-S12.691 with 7th K, S22.000-S22.9XX with 7th K, S32.000-S32.9XX with 7th K, S42.001-S42.92X with 7th [K, P], S49.001-S49.199 with 7th [K, P], S52.001-S52.92X with 7th [K, M, N, P, Q, R], S59.001-S59.299 with 7th [K, P], S62.001-S62.92X with 7th [K, P], S72.001-S72.92X with 7th [K, M, N, P, Q, R], S79.001-S79.199 with 7th [K, P], S82.001-S82.92X with 7th [K, M, N, P, Q, R], S89.001-S89.399 with 7th [K, P], S92.001-S92.919 with 7th [K, P]

7 7th **S42.209 Unspecified fracture of upper end of unspecified humerus** MCC CC
CC Excl: CC with 7th character A: S42.201-S42.92X with 7th [A, B], S49.001-S49.199 with 7th A
MCC with 7th character B: S42.201-S42.266 with 7th B, S42.291-S42.92X with 7th B, S49.101-S49.199 with 7th A, S62.90XB
CC with 7th character K or P: M80.00X-M84.68X with 7th [K, P], S02.0XX-S02.92X with 7th K, S12.000-S12.691 with 7th K, S22.000-S22.9XX with 7th K, S32.000-S32.9XX with 7th K, S42.001-S42.92X with 7th [K, P], S49.001-S49.199 with 7th [K, P], S52.001-S52.92X with 7th [K, M, N, P, Q, R], S59.001-S59.299 with 7th [K, P], S62.001-S62.92X with 7th [K, P], S72.001-S72.92X with 7th [K, M, N, P, Q, R], S79.001-S79.199 with 7th [K, P], S82.001-S82.92X with 7th [K, M, N, P, Q, R], S89.001-S89.399 with 7th [K, P], S92.001-S92.919 with 7th [K, P]

6th **S42.21 Unspecified fracture of surgical neck of humerus**
Fracture of neck of humerus NOS

7 7th **S42.211 Unspecified displaced fracture of surgical neck of right humerus** MCC CC
CC Excl: See code: S42.201

7 7th **S42.212 Unspecified displaced fracture of surgical neck of left humerus** MCC CC
CC Excl: See code: S42.202

7 7th **S42.213 Unspecified displaced fracture of surgical neck of unspecified humerus** MCC CC
CC Excl: See code: S42.209

7 7th **S42.214 Unspecified nondisplaced fracture of surgical neck of right humerus** MCC CC
CC Excl: See code: S42.201

7 7th **S42.215 Unspecified nondisplaced fracture of surgical neck of left humerus** MCC CC
CC Excl: See code: S42.202

7 7th **S42.216 Unspecified nondisplaced fracture of surgical neck of unspecified humerus** MCC CC
CC Excl: See code: S42.209

6th **S42.22 2-part fracture of surgical neck of humerus**

7 7th **S42.221 2-part displaced fracture of surgical neck of right humerus** MCC CC
CC Excl: See code: S42.201

7 7th **S42.222 2-part displaced fracture of surgical neck of left humerus** MCC CC
CC Excl: See code: S42.202

7 7th **S42.223 2-part displaced fracture of surgical neck of unspecified humerus** MCC CC
CC Excl: See code: S42.209

7 7th **S42.224 2-part nondisplaced fracture of surgical neck of right humerus** MCC CC
CC Excl: See code: S42.201

7 7th **S42.225 2-part nondisplaced fracture of surgical neck of left humerus** MCC CC
CC Excl: See code: S42.202

7 7th **S42.226 2-part nondisplaced fracture of surgical neck of unspecified humerus** MCC CC
CC Excl: See code: S42.209

6th **S42.23 3-part fracture of surgical neck of humerus**

7 7th **S42.231 3-part fracture of surgical neck of right humerus** MCC CC
CC Excl: See code: S42.201

7 7th **S42.232 3-part fracture of surgical neck of left humerus** MCC CC
CC Excl: See code: S42.202

7 7th **S42.239 3-part fracture of surgical neck of unspecified humerus** MCC CC
CC Excl: See code: S42.209

6th **S42.24 4-part fracture of surgical neck of humerus**

7 7th **S42.241 4-part fracture of surgical neck of right humerus** MCC CC
CC Excl: See code: S42.201

7 7th **S42.242 4-part fracture of surgical neck of left humerus** MCC CC
CC Excl: See code: S42.202

7 7th **S42.249 4-part fracture of surgical neck of unspecified humerus** MCC CC
CC Excl: See code: S42.209

6th **S42.25 Fracture of greater tuberosity of humerus**

7 7th **S42.251 Displaced fracture of greater tuberosity of right humerus** MCC CC
CC Excl: See code: S42.201

7 7th **S42.252 Displaced fracture of greater tuberosity of left humerus** MCC CC
CC Excl: See code: S42.202

7 7th **S42.253 Displaced fracture of greater tuberosity of unspecified humerus** MCC CC
CC Excl: See code: S42.209

7 7th **S42.254 Nondisplaced fracture of greater tuberosity of right humerus** MCC CC
CC Excl: See code: S42.201

7 HAC = Initial encounter only (7th character A, B or C) and not POA.

7 ✓7th **S42.255 Nondisplaced fracture of greater tuberosity of left humerus** MCC CC
CC Excl: See code: S42.202

7 ✓7th **S42.256 Nondisplaced fracture of greater tuberosity of unspecified humerus** MCC CC
CC Excl: See code: S42.209

✓6th **S42.26 Fracture of lesser tuberosity of humerus**

7 ✓7th **S42.261 Displaced fracture of lesser tuberosity of right humerus** MCC CC
CC Excl: See code: S42.201

7 ✓7th **S42.262 Displaced fracture of lesser tuberosity of left humerus** MCC CC
CC Excl: See code: S42.202

7 ✓7th **S42.263 Displaced fracture of lesser tuberosity of unspecified humerus** MCC CC
CC Excl: See code: S42.209

7 ✓7th **S42.264 Nondisplaced fracture of lesser tuberosity of right humerus** MCC CC
CC Excl: See code: S42.201

7 ✓7th **S42.265 Nondisplaced fracture of lesser tuberosity of left humerus** MCC CC
CC Excl: See code: S42.202

7 ✓7th **S42.266 Nondisplaced fracture of lesser tuberosity of unspecified humerus** MCC CC
CC Excl: See code: S42.209

✓6th **S42.27 Torus fracture of upper end of humerus**

The appropriate 7th is to be added to all codes in subcategory S42.27.
- A initial encounter for closed fracture
- D subsequent encounter for fracture with routine healing
- G subsequent encounter for fracture with delayed healing
- K subsequent encounter for fracture with nonunion
- P subsequent encounter for fracture with malunion
- S sequela

7 ✓7th **S42.271 Torus fracture of upper end of right humerus** CC
CC Excl: See code: S42.201

7 ✓7th **S42.272 Torus fracture of upper end of left humerus** CC
CC Excl: See code: S42.202

7 ✓7th **S42.279 Torus fracture of upper end of unspecified humerus** CC
CC Excl: See code: S42.209

✓6th **S42.29 Other fracture of upper end of humerus**
Fracture of anatomical neck of humerus
Fracture of articular head of humerus

7 ✓7th **S42.291 Other displaced fracture of upper end of right humerus** MCC CC
CC Excl: See code: S42.201

7 ✓7th **S42.292 Other displaced fracture of upper end of left humerus** MCC CC
CC Excl: See code: S42.202

7 ✓7th **S42.293 Other displaced fracture of upper end of unspecified humerus** MCC CC
CC Excl: See code: S42.209

7 ✓7th **S42.294 Other nondisplaced fracture of upper end of right humerus** MCC CC
CC Excl: See code: S42.201

7 ✓7th **S42.295 Other nondisplaced fracture of upper end of left humerus** MCC CC
CC Excl: See code: S42.202

7 ✓7th **S42.296 Other nondisplaced fracture of upper end of unspecified humerus** MCC CC
CC Excl: See code: S42.209

✓5th **S42.3 Fracture of shaft of humerus**
Fracture of humerus NOS
Fracture of upper arm NOS
EXCLUDES 2 *physeal fractures of upper end of humerus (S49.0-)*
physeal fractures of lower end of humerus (S49.1-)

✓6th **S42.30 Unspecified fracture of shaft of humerus**

7 ✓7th **S42.301 Unspecified fracture of shaft of humerus, right arm** MCC CC
CC Excl: See code: S42.201

7 ✓7th **S42.302 Unspecified fracture of shaft of humerus, left arm** MCC CC
CC Excl: See code: S42.202

7 ✓7th **S42.309 Unspecified fracture of shaft of humerus, unspecified arm** MCC CC
CC Excl: See code: S42.209

✓6th **S42.31 Greenstick fracture of shaft of humerus**

The appropriate 7th is to be added to all codes in subcategory S42.31.
- A initial encounter for closed fracture
- D subsequent encounter for fracture with routine healing
- G subsequent encounter for fracture with delayed healing
- K subsequent encounter for fracture with nonunion
- P subsequent encounter for fracture with malunion
- S sequela

7 ✓7th **S42.311 Greenstick fracture of shaft of humerus, right arm** CC
CC Excl: **CC with 7th character A:** S42.311A, S42.319-S42.321 with 7th A, S42.323-S42.324 with 7th A, S42.326-S42.331 with 7th A, S42.333-S42.334 with 7th A, S42.336-S42.341 with 7th A, S42.343-S42.344 with 7th A, S42.346-S42.351 with 7th A, S42.353-S42.354 with 7th A, S42.356-S42.361 with 7th A, S42.363-S42.364 with 7th A, S42.366-S42.391 with 7th A, S42.399A
CC with 7th character K or P: M80.00X-M84.68X with 7th [K, P], S02.0XX-S02.92X with 7th K, S12.000-S12.691 with 7th K, S22.000-S22.9XX with 7th K, S32.000-S32.9XX with 7th K, S42.001-S42.92X with 7th [K, P], S49.001-S49.199 with 7th [K, P], S52.001-S52.92X with 7th [K, M, N, P, Q, R], S59.001-S59.299 with 7th [K, P], S62.001-S62.92X with 7th [K, P], S72.001-S72.92X with 7th [K, M, N, P, Q, R], S79.001-S79.199 with 7th [K, P], S82.001-S82.92X with 7th [K, M, N, P, Q, R], S89.001-S89.399 with 7th [K, P], S92.001-S92.919 with 7th [K, P]

7 ✓7th **S42.312 Greenstick fracture of shaft of humerus, left arm** CC
CC Excl: **CC with 7th character A:** S42.312-S42.319 with 7th A, S42.322-S42.323 with 7th A, S42.325-S42.326 with 7th A, S42.332-S42.333 with 7th A, S42.335-S42.336 with 7th A, S42.342-S42.343 with 7th A, S42.345-S42.346 with 7th A, S42.352-S42.353 with 7th A, S42.355-S42.356 with 7th A, S42.362-S42.363 with 7th A, S42.365-S42.366 with 7th A, S42.392-S42.399 with 7th A
CC with 7th character K or P: M80.00X-M84.68X with 7th [K, P], S02.0XX-S02.92X with 7th K, S12.000-S12.691 with 7th K, S22.000-S22.9XX with 7th K, S32.000-S32.9XX with 7th K, S42.001-S42.92X with 7th [K, P], S49.001-S49.199 with 7th [K, P], S52.001-S52.92X with 7th [K, M, N, P, Q, R], S59.001-S59.299 with 7th [K, P], S62.001-S62.92X with 7th [K, P], S72.001-S72.92X with 7th [K, M, N, P, Q, R], S79.001-S79.199 with 7th [K, P], S82.001-S82.92X with 7th [K, M, N, P, Q, R], S89.001-S89.399 with 7th [K, P], S92.001-S92.919 with 7th [K, P]

7 ✓7th **S42.319 Greenstick fracture of shaft of humerus, unspecified arm** CC
CC Excl: **CC with 7th character A:** S42.311-S42.399 with 7th A
CC with 7th character K or P: M80.00X-M84.68X with 7th [K, P], S02.0XX-S02.92X with 7th K, S12.000-S12.691 with 7th K, S22.000-S22.9XX with 7th K, S32.000-S32.9XX with 7th K, S42.001-S42.92X with 7th [K, P], S49.001-S49.199 with 7th [K, P], S52.001-S52.92X with 7th [K, M, N, P, Q, R], S59.001-S59.299 with 7th [K, P], S62.001-S62.92X with 7th [K, P], S72.001-S72.92X with 7th [K, M, N, P, Q, R], S79.001-S79.199 with 7th [K, P], S82.001-S82.92X with 7th [K, M, N, P, Q, R], S89.001-S89.399 with 7th [K, P], S92.001-S92.919 with 7th [K, P]

7 HAC = Initial encounter only (7th character A, B or C) and not POA.

✓6th S42.32 Transverse fracture of shaft of humerus

7 ✓7th **S42.321 Displaced transverse fracture of shaft of humerus, right arm** MCC CC

CC Excl: CC with 7th character A: S42.311 with 7th A, S42.319-S42.321 with 7th A, S42.323-S42.324 with 7th A, S42.326-S42.331 with 7th A, S42.333-S42.334 with 7th A, S42.336-S42.341 with 7th A, S42.343-S42.344 with 7th A, S42.346-S42.351 with 7th A, S42.353-S42.354 with 7th A, S42.356-S42.361 with 7th A, S42.363-S42.364 with 7th A, S42.366-S42.391 with 7th A, S42.399A
MCC with 7th character B: S42.201-S42.266 with 7th B, S42.291-S42.92X with 7th B, S49.101-S49.199 with 7th A, S62.90XB
CC with 7th character K or P: M80.00X-M84.68X with 7th [K, P], S02.0XX-S02.92X with 7th K, S12.000-S12.691 with 7th K, S22.000-S22.9XX with 7th K, S32.000-S32.9XX with 7th K, S42.001-S42.92X with 7th [K, P], S49.001-S49.199 with 7th [K, P], S52.001-S52.92X with 7th [K, M, N, P, Q, R], S59.001-S59.299 with 7th [K, P], S62.001-S62.92X with 7th [K, P], S72.001-S72.92X with 7th [K, M, N, P, Q, R], S79.001-S79.199 with 7th [K, P], S82.001-S82.92X with 7th [K, M, N, P, Q, R], S89.001-S89.399 with 7th [K, P], S92.001-S92.919 with 7th [K, P]

7 ✓7th **S42.322 Displaced transverse fracture of shaft of humerus, left arm** MCC CC

CC Excl: CC with 7th character A: S42.312-S42.319 with 7th A, S42.322-S42.323 with 7th A, S42.325-S42.326 with 7th A, S42.332-S42.333 with 7th A, S42.335-S42.336 with 7th A, S42.342-S42.343 with 7th A, S42.345-S42.346 with 7th A, S42.352-S42.353 with 7th A, S42.355-S42.356 with 7th A, S42.362-S42.363 with 7th A, S42.365-S42.366 with 7th A, S42.392-S42.399 with 7th A
MCC with 7th character B: S42.201-S42.266 with 7th B, S42.291-S42.92X with 7th B, S49.101-S49.199 with 7th A, S62.90XB
CC with 7th character K or P: M80.00X-M84.68X with 7th [K, P], S02.0XX-S02.92X with 7th K, S12.000-S12.691 with 7th K, S22.000-S22.9XX with 7th K, S32.000-S32.9XX with 7th K, S42.001-S42.92X with 7th [K, P], S49.001-S49.199 with 7th [K, P], S52.001-S52.92X with 7th [K, M, N, P, Q, R], S59.001-S59.299 with 7th [K, P], S62.001-S62.92X with 7th [K, P], S72.001-S72.92X with 7th [K, M, N, P, Q, R], S79.001-S79.199 with 7th [K, P], S82.001-S82.92X with 7th [K, M, N, P, Q, R], S89.001-S89.399 with 7th [K, P], S92.001-S92.919 with 7th [K, P]

7 ✓7th **S42.323 Displaced transverse fracture of shaft of humerus, unspecified arm** MCC CC

CC Excl: CC with 7th character A: S42.311-S42.399 with 7th A
MCC with 7th character B: S42.201-S42.266 with 7th B, S42.291-S42.92X with 7th B, S49.101-S49.199 with 7th A, S62.90XB

7 ✓7th **S42.324 Nondisplaced transverse fracture of shaft of humerus, right arm** MCC CC
CC Excl: See code: S42.321

7 ✓7th **S42.325 Nondisplaced transverse fracture of shaft of humerus, left arm** MCC CC
CC Excl: See code: S42.322

7 ✓7th **S42.326 Nondisplaced transverse fracture of shaft of humerus, unspecified arm** MCC CC
CC Excl: See code: S42.323

✓6th S42.33 Oblique fracture of shaft of humerus

7 ✓7th **S42.331 Displaced oblique fracture of shaft of humerus, right arm** MCC CC
CC Excl: See code: S42.321

7 ✓7th **S42.332 Displaced oblique fracture of shaft of humerus, left arm** MCC CC
CC Excl: See code: S42.322

7 ✓7th **S42.333 Displaced oblique fracture of shaft of humerus, unspecified arm** MCC CC
CC Excl: See code: S42.323

7 ✓7th **S42.334 Nondisplaced oblique fracture of shaft of humerus, right arm** MCC CC
CC Excl: See code: S42.321

7 ✓7th **S42.335 Nondisplaced oblique fracture of shaft of humerus, left arm** MCC CC
CC Excl: See code: S42.322

7 ✓7th **S42.336 Nondisplaced oblique fracture of shaft of humerus, unspecified arm** MCC CC
CC Excl: See code: S42.323

✓6th S42.34 Spiral fracture of shaft of humerus

7 ✓7th **S42.341 Displaced spiral fracture of shaft of humerus, right arm** MCC CC
CC Excl: See code: S42.321

7 ✓7th **S42.342 Displaced spiral fracture of shaft of humerus, left arm** MCC CC
CC Excl: See code: S42.322

7 ✓7th **S42.343 Displaced spiral fracture of shaft of humerus, unspecified arm** MCC CC
CC Excl: See code: S42.323

7 ✓7th **S42.344 Nondisplaced spiral fracture of shaft of humerus, right arm** MCC CC
CC Excl: See code: S42.321

7 ✓7th **S42.345 Nondisplaced spiral fracture of shaft of humerus, left arm** MCC CC
CC Excl: See code: S42.322

7 ✓7th **S42.346 Nondisplaced spiral fracture of shaft of humerus, unspecified arm** MCC CC
CC Excl: See code: S42.323

✓6th S42.35 Comminuted fracture of shaft of humerus

7 ✓7th **S42.351 Displaced comminuted fracture of shaft of humerus, right arm** MCC CC
CC Excl: See code: S42.321

7 ✓7th **S42.352 Displaced comminuted fracture of shaft of humerus, left arm** MCC CC
CC Excl: See code: S42.322

7 ✓7th **S42.353 Displaced comminuted fracture of shaft of humerus, unspecified arm** MCC CC
CC Excl: See code: S42.323

7 ✓7th **S42.354 Nondisplaced comminuted fracture of shaft of humerus, right arm** MCC CC
CC Excl: See code: S42.321

7 ✓7th **S42.355 Nondisplaced comminuted fracture of shaft of humerus, left arm** MCC CC
CC Excl: See code: S42.322

7 ✓7th **S42.356 Nondisplaced comminuted fracture of shaft of humerus, unspecified arm** MCC CC
CC Excl: See code: S42.323

✓6th S42.36 Segmental fracture of shaft of humerus

7 ✓7th **S42.361 Displaced segmental fracture of shaft of humerus, right arm** MCC CC
CC Excl: See code: S42.321

7 ✓7th **S42.362 Displaced segmental fracture of shaft of humerus, left arm** MCC CC
CC Excl: See code: S42.322

7 ✓7th **S42.363 Displaced segmental fracture of shaft of humerus, unspecified arm** MCC CC
CC Excl: See code: S42.323

7 ✓7th **S42.364 Nondisplaced segmental fracture of shaft of humerus, right arm** MCC CC
CC Excl: See code: S42.321

7 ✓7th **S42.365 Nondisplaced segmental fracture of shaft of humerus, left arm** MCC CC
CC Excl: See code: S42.322

7 ✓7th **S42.366 Nondisplaced segmental fracture of shaft of humerus, unspecified arm** MCC CC
CC Excl: See code: S42.323

✓6th S42.39 Other fracture of shaft of humerus

7 ✓7th **S42.391 Other fracture of shaft of right humerus** MCC CC
CC Excl: See code: S42.321

7 ✓7th **S42.392 Other fracture of shaft of left humerus** MCC CC
CC Excl: See code: S42.322

7 ✓7th **S42.399 Other fracture of shaft of unspecified humerus** MCC CC
CC Excl: See code: S42.323

7 HAC = Initial encounter only (7th character A, B or C) and not POA.

✓5th **S42.4 Fracture of lower end of humerus**
Fracture of distal end of humerus
EXCLUDES 2 *fracture of shaft of humerus (S42.3-)*
physeal fracture of lower end of humerus (S49.1-)

✓6th **S42.40 Unspecified fracture of lower end of humerus**
Fracture of elbow NOS

7 ✓7th **S42.401 Unspecified fracture of lower end of right humerus** MCC CC
CC Excl: CC with 7th character A: S42.201-S42.271 with 7th [A, B], S42.279-S42.311 with 7th A, S42.319-S42.481 with 7th A, S42.489-S42.92X with 7th A, S49.001A, S49.009-S49.011 with 7th A, S49.019-S49.021 with 7th A, S49.029-S49.031 with 7th A, S49.039-S49.041 with 7th A, S49.049-S49.091 with 7th A, S49.099-S49.101 with 7th A, S49.109-S49.111 with 7th A, S49.119-S49.121 with 7th A, S49.129-S49.131 with 7th A, S49.139-S49.141 with 7th A, S49.149-S49.191 with 7th A, S49.199A
MCC with 7th character B: S42.201-S42.266 with 7th B, S42.291-S42.92X with 7th B, S49.101-S49.199 with 7th A, S62.9XB
CC with 7th character K or P: M80.00X-M84.68X with 7th [K, P], S02.0XX-S02.92X with 7th K, S12.000-S12.691 with 7th K, S22.000-S22.9XX with 7th K, S32.000-S32.9XX with 7th K, S42.001-S42.92X with 7th [K, P], S49.001-S49.199 with 7th [K, P], S52.001-S52.92X with 7th [K, M, N, P, Q, R], S59.001-S59.299 with 7th [K, P], S62.001-S62.92X with 7th [K, P], S72.001-S72.92X with 7th [K, M, N, P, Q, R], S79.001-S79.199 with 7th [K, P], S82.001-S82.92X with 7th [K, M, N, P, Q, R], S89.001-S89.399 with 7th [K, P], S92.001-S92.919 with 7th [K, P]

7 ✓7th **S42.402 Unspecified fracture of lower end of left humerus** MCC CC
CC Excl: CC with 7th character A: S42.201-S42.266 with 7th B, S42.272-S42.309 with 7th A, S42.312-S42.476 with 7th A, S42.482-S42.92X with 7th A, S49.002-S49.009 with 7th A, S49.012-S49.019 with 7th A, S49.022-S49.029 with 7th A, S49.032-S49.039 with 7th A, S49.042-S49.049 with 7th A, S49.092-S49.099 with 7th A, S49.102-S49.109 with 7th A, S49.112-S49.119 with 7th A, S49.122-S49.129 with 7th A, S49.132-S49.139 with 7th A, S49.142-S49.149 with 7th A, S49.192-S49.199 with 7th A
MCC with 7th character B: S42.201-S42.266 with 7th B, S42.291-S42.92X with 7th B, S49.101-S49.199 with 7th A, S62.90XB
CC with 7th character K or P: M80.00X-M84.68X with 7th [K, P], S02.0XX-S02.92X with 7th K, S12.000-S12.691 with 7th K, S22.000-S22.9XX with 7th K, S32.000-S32.9XX with 7th K, S42.001-S42.92X with 7th [K, P], S49.001-S49.199 with 7th [K, P], S52.001-S52.92X with 7th [K, M, N, P, Q, R], S59.001-S59.299 with 7th [K, P], S62.001-S62.92X with 7th [K, P], S72.001-S72.92X with 7th [K, M, N, P, Q, R], S79.001-S79.199 with 7th [K, P], S82.001-S82.92X with 7th [K, M, N, P, Q, R], S89.001-S89.399 with 7th [K, P], S92.001-S92.919 with 7th [K, P]

7 ✓7th **S42.409 Unspecified fracture of lower end of unspecified humerus** MCC CC
CC Excl: CC with 7th character A: S42.201-S42.92X with 7th [A, B], S49.001-S49.199 with 7th A
MCC with 7th character B: S42.201-S42.266 with 7th B, S42.291-S42.92X with 7th B, S49.101-S49.199 with 7th A, S62.90XB
CC with 7th character K or P: M80.00X-M84.68X with 7th [K, P], S02.0XX-S02.92X with 7th K, S12.000-S12.691 with 7th K, S22.000-S22.9XX with 7th K, S32.000-S32.9XX with 7th K, S42.001-S42.92X with 7th [K, P], S49.001-S49.199 with 7th [K, P], S52.001-S52.92X with 7th [K, M, N, P, Q, R], S59.001-S59.299 with 7th [K, P], S62.001-S62.92X with 7th [K, P], S72.001-S72.92X with 7th [K, M, N, P, Q, R], S79.001-S79.199 with 7th [K, P], S82.001-S82.92X with 7th [K, M, N, P, Q, R], S89.001-S89.399 with 7th [K, P], S92.001-S92.919 with 7th [K, P]

✓6th **S42.41 Simple supracondylar fracture without intercondylar fracture of humerus**

7 ✓7th **S42.411 Displaced simple supracondylar fracture without intercondylar fracture of right humerus** MCC CC
CC Excl: See code: S42.401

7 ✓7th **S42.412 Displaced simple supracondylar fracture without intercondylar fracture of left humerus** MCC CC
CC Excl: See code: S42.402

7 ✓7th **S42.413 Displaced simple supracondylar fracture without intercondylar fracture of unspecified humerus** MCC CC
CC Excl: See code: S42.409

7 ✓7th **S42.414 Nondisplaced simple supracondylar fracture without intercondylar fracture of right humerus** MCC CC
CC Excl: See code: S42.401

7 ✓7th **S42.415 Nondisplaced simple supracondylar fracture without intercondylar fracture of left humerus** MCC CC
CC Excl: See code: S42.402

7 ✓7th **S42.416 Nondisplaced simple supracondylar fracture without intercondylar fracture of unspecified humerus** MCC CC
CC Excl: See code: S42.409

✓6th **S42.42 Comminuted supracondylar fracture without intercondylar fracture of humerus**

7 ✓7th **S42.421 Displaced comminuted supracondylar fracture without intercondylar fracture of right humerus** MCC CC
CC Excl: See code: S42.401

7 ✓7th **S42.422 Displaced comminuted supracondylar fracture without intercondylar fracture of left humerus** MCC CC
CC Excl: See code: S42.402

7 ✓7th **S42.423 Displaced comminuted supracondylar fracture without intercondylar fracture of unspecified humerus** MCC CC
CC Excl: See code: S42.409

7 ✓7th **S42.424 Nondisplaced comminuted supracondylar fracture without intercondylar fracture of right humerus** MCC CC
CC Excl: See code: S42.401

7 ✓7th **S42.425 Nondisplaced comminuted supracondylar fracture without intercondylar fracture of left humerus** MCC CC
CC Excl: See code: S42.402

7 ✓7th **S42.426 Nondisplaced comminuted supracondylar fracture without intercondylar fracture of unspecified humerus** MCC CC
CC Excl: See code: S42.409

✓6th **S42.43 Fracture (avulsion) of lateral epicondyle of humerus**

7 ✓7th **S42.431 Displaced fracture (avulsion) of lateral epicondyle of right humerus** MCC CC
CC Excl: See code: S42.401

7 ✓7th **S42.432 Displaced fracture (avulsion) of lateral epicondyle of left humerus** MCC CC
CC Excl: See code: S42.402

7 ✓7th **S42.433 Displaced fracture (avulsion) of lateral epicondyle of unspecified humerus** MCC CC
CC Excl: See code: S42.409

7 ✓7th **S42.434 Nondisplaced fracture (avulsion) of lateral epicondyle of right humerus** MCC CC
CC Excl: See code: S42.401

7 ✓7th **S42.435 Nondisplaced fracture (avulsion) of lateral epicondyle of left humerus** MCC CC
CC Excl: See code: S42.402

7 HAC = Initial encounter only (7th character A, B or C) and not POA.

7 ✓7th **S42.436 Nondisplaced fracture (avulsion) of lateral epicondyle of unspecified humerus** MCC CC
CC Excl: See code: S42.4Ø9

✓6th **S42.44 Fracture (avulsion) of medial epicondyle of humerus**

7 ✓7th **S42.441 Displaced fracture (avulsion) of medial epicondyle of right humerus** MCC CC
CC Excl: See code: S42.4Ø1

7 ✓7th **S42.442 Displaced fracture (avulsion) of medial epicondyle of left humerus** MCC CC
CC Excl: See code: S42.4Ø2

7 ✓7th **S42.443 Displaced fracture (avulsion) of medial epicondyle of unspecified humerus** MCC CC
CC Excl: See code: S42.4Ø9

7 ✓7th **S42.444 Nondisplaced fracture (avulsion) of medial epicondyle of right humerus** MCC CC
CC Excl: See code: S42.4Ø1

7 ✓7th **S42.445 Nondisplaced fracture (avulsion) of medial epicondyle of left humerus** MCC CC
CC Excl: See code: S42.4Ø2

7 ✓7th **S42.446 Nondisplaced fracture (avulsion) medial epicondyle of unspecified of humerus** MCC CC
CC Excl: See code: S42.4Ø9

7 ✓7th **S42.447 Incarcerated fracture (avulsion) of medial epicondyle of right humerus** MCC CC
CC Excl: See code: S42.4Ø1

7 ✓7th **S42.448 Incarcerated fracture (avulsion) of medial epicondyle of left humerus** MCC CC
CC Excl: See code: S42.4Ø2

7 ✓7th **S42.449 Incarcerated fracture (avulsion) of medial epicondyle of unspecified humerus** MCC CC
CC Excl: See code: S42.4Ø9

✓6th **S42.45 Fracture of lateral condyle of humerus**
Fracture of capitellum of humerus

7 ✓7th **S42.451 Displaced fracture of lateral condyle of right humerus** MCC CC
CC Excl: See code: S42.4Ø1

7 ✓7th **S42.452 Displaced fracture of lateral condyle of left humerus** MCC CC
CC Excl: See code: S42.4Ø2

7 ✓7th **S42.453 Displaced fracture of lateral condyle of unspecified humerus** MCC CC
CC Excl: See code: S42.4Ø9

7 ✓7th **S42.454 Nondisplaced fracture of lateral condyle of right humerus** MCC CC
CC Excl: See code: S42.4Ø1

7 ✓7th **S42.455 Nondisplaced fracture of lateral condyle of left humerus** MCC CC
CC Excl: See code: S42.4Ø2

7 ✓7th **S42.456 Nondisplaced fracture of lateral condyle of unspecified humerus** MCC CC
CC Excl: See code: S42.4Ø9

✓6th **S42.46 Fracture of medial condyle of humerus**
Trochlea fracture of humerus

7 ✓7th **S42.461 Displaced fracture of medial condyle of right humerus** MCC CC
CC Excl: See code: S42.4Ø1

7 ✓7th **S42.462 Displaced fracture of medial condyle of left humerus** MCC CC
CC Excl: See code: S42.4Ø2

7 ✓7th **S42.463 Displaced fracture of medial condyle of unspecified humerus** MCC CC
CC Excl: See code: S42.4Ø9

7 ✓7th **S42.464 Nondisplaced fracture of medial condyle of right humerus** MCC CC
CC Excl: See code: S42.4Ø1

7 ✓7th **S42.465 Nondisplaced fracture of medial condyle of left humerus** MCC CC
CC Excl: See code: S42.4Ø2

7 ✓7th **S42.466 Nondisplaced fracture of medial condyle of unspecified humerus** MCC CC
CC Excl: See code: S42.4Ø9

✓6th **S42.47 Transcondylar fracture of humerus**

7 ✓7th **S42.471 Displaced transcondylar fracture of right humerus** MCC CC
CC Excl: See code: S42.4Ø1

7 ✓7th **S42.472 Displaced transcondylar fracture of left humerus** MCC CC
CC Excl: See code: S42.4Ø2

7 ✓7th **S42.473 Displaced transcondylar fracture of unspecified humerus** MCC CC
CC Excl: See code: S42.4Ø9

7 ✓7th **S42.474 Nondisplaced transcondylar fracture of right humerus** MCC CC
CC Excl: See code: S42.4Ø1

7 ✓7th **S42.475 Nondisplaced transcondylar fracture of left humerus** MCC CC
CC Excl: See code: S42.4Ø2

7 ✓7th **S42.476 Nondisplaced transcondylar fracture of unspecified humerus** MCC CC
CC Excl: See code: S42.4Ø9

✓6th **S42.48 Torus fracture of lower end of humerus**

The appropriate 7th is to be added to all codes in subcategory S42.48.

- A initial encounter for closed fracture
- D subsequent encounter for fracture with routine healing
- G subsequent encounter for fracture with delayed healing
- K subsequent encounter for fracture with nonunion
- P subsequent encounter for fracture with malunion
- S sequela

7 ✓7th **S42.481 Torus fracture of lower end of right humerus** CC
CC Excl: CC with 7th character A: S42.2Ø1-S42.271 with 7th [A, B], S42.279-S42.311 with 7th A, S42.319-S42.481 with 7th A, S42.489-S42.92X with 7th A, S49.ØØ1A, S49.ØØ9-S49.Ø11 with 7th A, S49.Ø19-S49.Ø21 with 7th A, S49.Ø29-S49.Ø31 with 7th A, S49.Ø39-S49.Ø41 with 7th A, S49.Ø49-S49.Ø91 with 7th A, S49.Ø99-S49.1Ø1 with 7th A, S49.1Ø9-S49.111 with 7th A, S49.119-S49.121 with 7th A, S49.129-S49.131 with 7th A, S49.139-S49.141 with 7th A, S49.149-S49.191 with 7th A, S49.199A
CC Excl: with 7th K or P: M8Ø.ØØX-M84.68X with 7th [K, P], SØ2.ØXX-SØ2.92X with 7th K, S12.ØØØ-S12.691 with 7th K, S22.ØØØ-S22.9XX with 7th K, S32.ØØØ-S32.9XX with 7th K, S42.ØØ1-S42.92X with 7th [K, P], S49.ØØ1-S49.199 with 7th [K, P], S52.ØØ1-S52.92X with 7th [K, M, N, P, Q, R], S59.ØØ1-S59.299 with 7th [K, P], S62.ØØ1-S62.92X with 7th [K, P], S72.ØØ1-S72.92X with 7th [K, M, N, P, Q, R], S79.ØØ1-S79.199 with 7th [K, P], S82.ØØ1-S82.92X with 7th [K, M, N, P, Q, R], S89.ØØ1-S89.399 with 7th [K, P], S92.ØØ1-S92.919 with 7th [K, P]

7 ✓7th **S42.482 Torus fracture of lower end of left humerus** CC
CC Excl: CC with 7th character A: S42.2Ø1-S42.266 with 7th B, S42.272-S42.3Ø9 with 7th A, S42.312-S42.476 with 7th A, S42.482-S42.92X with 7th A, S49.ØØ2-S49.ØØ9 with 7th A, S49.Ø12-S49.Ø19 with 7th A, S49.Ø22-S49.Ø29 with 7th A, S49.Ø32-S49.Ø39 with 7th A, S49.Ø42-S49.Ø49 with 7th A, S49.Ø92-S49.Ø99 with 7th A, S49.1Ø2-S49.1Ø9 with 7th A, S49.112-S49.119 with 7th A, S49.122-S49.129 with 7th A, S49.132-S49.139 with 7th A, S49.142-S49.149 with 7th A, S49.192-S49.199 with 7th A
CC Excl: with 7th K or P: M8Ø.ØØX-M84.68X with 7th [K, P], SØ2.ØXX-SØ2.92X with 7th K, S12.ØØØ-S12.691 with 7th K, S22.ØØØ-S22.9XX with 7th K, S32.ØØØ-S32.9XX with 7th K, S42.ØØ1-S42.92X with 7th [K, P], S49.ØØ1-S49.199 with 7th [K, P], S52.ØØ1-S52.92X with 7th [K, M, N, P, Q, R], S59.ØØ1-S59.299 with 7th [K, P], S62.ØØ1-S62.92X with 7th [K, P], S72.ØØ1-S72.92X with 7th [K, M, N, P, Q, R], S79.ØØ1-S79.199 with 7th [K, P], S82.ØØ1-S82.92X with 7th [K, M, N, P, Q, R],

7 HAC = Initial encounter only (7th character A, B or C) and not POA.

N Newborn: Ø P Pediatric: Ø-17 M Maternity: 12-55 A Adult: 15-124 MCC Major CC Condition PDx MCC PDx acts as own MCC CC CC Condition PDx CC PDx acts as own CC

S89.001-S89.399 with 7th [K, P], S92.001-S92.919 with 7th [K, P]

7 ✓7th **S42.489 Torus fracture of lower end of unspecified humerus** CC
CC Excl: CC with 7th character A: S42.201-S42.92X with 7th [A, B], S49.001-S49.199 with 7th A
CC Excl: CC with 7th character K or P: M80.00X-M84.68X with 7th [K, P], S02.0XX-S02.92X with 7th K, S12.000-S12.691 with 7th K, S22.000-S22.9XX with 7th K, S32.000-S32.9XX with 7th K, S42.001-S42.92X with 7th [K, P], S49.001-S49.199 with 7th [K, P], S52.001-S52.92X with 7th [K, M, N, P, Q, R], S59.001-S59.299 with 7th [K, P], S62.001-S62.92X with 7th [K, P], S72.001-S72.92X with 7th [K, M, N, P, Q, R], S79.001-S79.199 with 7th [K, P], S82.001-S82.92X with 7th [K, M, N, P, Q, R], S89.001-S89.399 with 7th [K, P], S92.001-S92.919 with 7th [K, P]

✓6th **S42.49 Other fracture of lower end of humerus**

7 ✓7th **S42.491 Other displaced fracture of lower end of right humerus** MCC CC
CC Excl: See code: S42.401

7 ✓7th **S42.492 Other displaced fracture of lower end of left humerus** MCC CC
CC Excl: See code: S42.402

7 ✓7th **S42.493 Other displaced fracture of lower end of unspecified humerus** MCC CC
CC Excl: See code: S42.409

7 ✓7th **S42.494 Other nondisplaced fracture of lower end of right humerus** MCC CC
CC Excl: See code: S42.401

7 ✓7th **S42.495 Other nondisplaced fracture of lower end of left humerus** MCC CC
CC Excl: See code: S42.402

7 ✓7th **S42.496 Other nondisplaced fracture of lower end of unspecified humerus** MCC CC
CC Excl: See code: S42.409

✓5th **S42.9 Fracture of shoulder girdle, part unspecified**
Fracture of shoulder NOS

7 ✓x7th **S42.90 Fracture of unspecified shoulder girdle, part unspecified** MCC CC
CC Excl: See code: S42.409

7 ✓x7th **S42.91 Fracture of right shoulder girdle, part unspecified** MCC CC
CC Excl: See code: S42.409

7 ✓x7th **S42.92 Fracture of left shoulder girdle, part unspecified** MCC CC
CC Excl: See code: S42.409

✓4th **S43 Dislocation and sprain of joints and ligaments of shoulder girdle**

INCLUDES avulsion of joint or ligament of shoulder girdle
laceration of cartilage, joint or ligament of shoulder girdle
sprain of cartilage, joint or ligament of shoulder girdle
traumatic hemarthrosis of joint or ligament of shoulder girdle
traumatic rupture of joint or ligament of shoulder girdle
traumatic subluxation of joint or ligament of shoulder girdle
traumatic tear of joint or ligament of shoulder girdle

Code also any associated open wound

EXCLUDES 2 *strain of muscle, fascia and tendon of shoulder and upper arm (S46.-)*

The appropriate 7th is to be added to each code from category S43.
A initial encounter
D subsequent encounter
S sequela

✓5th **S43.0 Subluxation and dislocation of shoulder joint**
Dislocation of glenohumeral joint
Subluxation of glenohumeral joint

✓6th **S43.00 Unspecified subluxation and dislocation of shoulder joint**
Dislocation of humerus NOS
Subluxation of humerus NOS

✓7th **S43.001 Unspecified subluxation of right shoulder joint**

✓7th **S43.002 Unspecified subluxation of left shoulder joint**

✓7th **S43.003 Unspecified subluxation of unspecified shoulder joint**

✓7th **S43.004 Unspecified dislocation of right shoulder joint**

✓7th **S43.005 Unspecified dislocation of left shoulder joint**

✓7th **S43.006 Unspecified dislocation of unspecified shoulder joint**

✓6th **S43.01 Anterior subluxation and dislocation of humerus**

✓7th **S43.011 Anterior subluxation of right humerus**

✓7th **S43.012 Anterior subluxation of left humerus**

✓7th **S43.013 Anterior subluxation of unspecified humerus**

✓7th **S43.014 Anterior dislocation of right humerus**

✓7th **S43.015 Anterior dislocation of left humerus**

✓7th **S43.016 Anterior dislocation of unspecified humerus**

✓6th **S43.02 Posterior subluxation and dislocation of humerus**

✓7th **S43.021 Posterior subluxation of right humerus**

✓7th **S43.022 Posterior subluxation of left humerus**

✓7th **S43.023 Posterior subluxation of unspecified humerus**

✓7th **S43.024 Posterior dislocation of right humerus**

✓7th **S43.025 Posterior dislocation of left humerus**

✓7th **S43.026 Posterior dislocation of unspecified humerus**

✓6th **S43.03 Inferior subluxation and dislocation of humerus**

✓7th **S43.031 Inferior subluxation of right humerus**

✓7th **S43.032 Inferior subluxation of left humerus**

✓7th **S43.033 Inferior subluxation of unspecified humerus**

✓7th **S43.034 Inferior dislocation of right humerus**

✓7th **S43.035 Inferior dislocation of left humerus**

✓7th **S43.036 Inferior dislocation of unspecified humerus**

✓6th **S43.08 Other subluxation and dislocation of shoulder joint**

✓7th **S43.081 Other subluxation of right shoulder joint**

✓7th **S43.082 Other subluxation of left shoulder joint**

✓7th **S43.083 Other subluxation of unspecified shoulder joint**

✓7th **S43.084 Other dislocation of right shoulder joint**

✓7th **S43.085 Other dislocation of left shoulder joint**

✓7th **S43.086 Other dislocation of unspecified shoulder joint**

✓5th **S43.1 Subluxation and dislocation of acromioclavicular joint**

✓6th **S43.10 Unspecified dislocation of acromioclavicular joint**

✓7th **S43.101 Unspecified dislocation of right acromioclavicular joint**

✓7th **S43.102 Unspecified dislocation of left acromioclavicular joint**

✓7th **S43.109 Unspecified dislocation of unspecified acromioclavicular joint**

✓6th **S43.11 Subluxation of acromioclavicular joint**

✓7th **S43.111 Subluxation of right acromioclavicular joint**

✓7th **S43.112 Subluxation of left acromioclavicular joint**

✓7th **S43.119 Subluxation of unspecified acromioclavicular joint**

✓6th **S43.12 Dislocation of acromioclavicular joint, 100%-200% displacement**

✓7th **S43.121 Dislocation of right acromioclavicular joint, 100%-200% displacement**

✓7th **S43.122 Dislocation of left acromioclavicular joint, 100%-200% displacement**

✓7th **S43.129 Dislocation of unspecified acromioclavicular joint, 100%-200% displacement**

✓6th **S43.13 Dislocation of acromioclavicular joint, greater than 200% displacement**

✓7th **S43.131 Dislocation of right acromioclavicular joint, greater than 200% displacement**

✓7th **S43.132 Dislocation of left acromioclavicular joint, greater than 200% displacement**

7 HAC = Initial encounter only (7th character A, B or C) and not POA.

Injury, Poisoning and Certain Other Consequences of External Causes S42.489–S43.132

7th **S43.139** **Dislocation of unspecified acromioclavicular joint, greater than 200% displacement**

6th **S43.14** **Inferior dislocation of acromioclavicular joint**

7th **S43.141** **Inferior dislocation of right acromioclavicular joint**

7th **S43.142** **Inferior dislocation of left acromioclavicular joint**

7th **S43.149** **Inferior dislocation of unspecified acromioclavicular joint**

6th **S43.15** **Posterior dislocation of acromioclavicular joint**

7th **S43.151** **Posterior dislocation of right acromioclavicular joint**

7th **S43.152** **Posterior dislocation of left acromioclavicular joint**

7th **S43.159** **Posterior dislocation of unspecified acromioclavicular joint**

5th **S43.2** **Subluxation and dislocation of sternoclavicular joint**

6th **S43.20** **Unspecified subluxation and dislocation of sternoclavicular joint**

7 7th **S43.201** **Unspecified subluxation of right sternoclavicular joint** CC

CC Excl: CC with 7th character A: M99.18, S43.201 with 7th A, S43.203-S43.204 with 7th A, S43.206-S43.211 with 7th A, S43.213-S43.214 with 7th A, S43.216-S43.221 with 7th A, S43.223-S43.224 with 7th A, S43.226A

7 7th **S43.202** **Unspecified subluxation of left sternoclavicular joint** CC

CC Excl: CC with 7th character A: M99.18, S43.202-S43.203 with 7th A, S43.205-S43.206 with 7th A, S43.212-S43.213 with 7th A, S43.215-S43.216 with 7th A, S43.222-S43.223 with 7th A, S43.225-S43.226 with 7th A

7 7th **S43.203** **Unspecified subluxation of unspecified sternoclavicular joint** CC

CC Excl: CC with 7th character A: M99.18, S43.201-S43.226 with 7th A

7 7th **S43.204** **Unspecified dislocation of right sternoclavicular joint** CC

CC Excl: See code: S43.201

7 7th **S43.205** **Unspecified dislocation of left sternoclavicular joint** CC

CC Excl: See code: S43.202

7 7th **S43.206** **Unspecified dislocation of unspecified sternoclavicular joint** CC

CC Excl: See code: S43.203

6th **S43.21** **Anterior subluxation and dislocation of sternoclavicular joint**

7 7th **S43.211** **Anterior subluxation of right sternoclavicular joint** CC

CC Excl: See code: S43.201

7 7th **S43.212** **Anterior subluxation of left sternoclavicular joint** CC

CC Excl: See code: S43.202

7 7th **S43.213** **Anterior subluxation of unspecified sternoclavicular joint** CC

CC Excl: See code: S43.203

7 7th **S43.214** **Anterior dislocation of right sternoclavicular joint** CC

CC Excl: See code: S43.201

7 7th **S43.215** **Anterior dislocation of left sternoclavicular joint** CC

CC Excl: See code: S43.202

7 7th **S43.216** **Anterior dislocation of unspecified sternoclavicular joint** CC

CC Excl: See code: S43.203

6th **S43.22** **Posterior subluxation and dislocation of sternoclavicular joint**

7 7th **S43.221** **Posterior subluxation of right sternoclavicular joint** CC

CC Excl: See code: S43.201

7 7th **S43.222** **Posterior subluxation of left sternoclavicular joint** CC

CC Excl: See code: S43.202

7 7th **S43.223** **Posterior subluxation of unspecified sternoclavicular joint** CC

CC Excl: See code: S43.203

7 7th **S43.224** **Posterior dislocation of right sternoclavicular joint** CC

CC Excl: See code: S43.201

7 7th **S43.225** **Posterior dislocation of left sternoclavicular joint** CC

CC Excl: See code: S43.202

7 7th **S43.226** **Posterior dislocation of unspecified sternoclavicular joint** CC

CC Excl: See code: S43.203

5th **S43.3** **Subluxation and dislocation of other and unspecified parts of shoulder girdle**

6th **S43.30** **Subluxation and dislocation of unspecified parts of shoulder girdle**

Dislocation of shoulder girdle NOS
Subluxation of shoulder girdle NOS

7th **S43.301** **Subluxation of unspecified parts of right shoulder girdle**

7th **S43.302** **Subluxation of unspecified parts of left shoulder girdle**

7th **S43.303** **Subluxation of unspecified parts of unspecified shoulder girdle**

7th **S43.304** **Dislocation of unspecified parts of right shoulder girdle**

7th **S43.305** **Dislocation of unspecified parts of left shoulder girdle**

7th **S43.306** **Dislocation of unspecified parts of unspecified shoulder girdle**

6th **S43.31** **Subluxation and dislocation of scapula**

7th **S43.311** **Subluxation of right scapula**

7th **S43.312** **Subluxation of left scapula**

7th **S43.313** **Subluxation of unspecified scapula**

7th **S43.314** **Dislocation of right scapula**

7th **S43.315** **Dislocation of left scapula**

7th **S43.316** **Dislocation of unspecified scapula**

6th **S43.39** **Subluxation and dislocation of other parts of shoulder girdle**

7th **S43.391** **Subluxation of other parts of right shoulder girdle**

7th **S43.392** **Subluxation of other parts of left shoulder girdle**

7th **S43.393** **Subluxation of other parts of unspecified shoulder girdle**

7th **S43.394** **Dislocation of other parts of right shoulder girdle**

7th **S43.395** **Dislocation of other parts of left shoulder girdle**

7th **S43.396** **Dislocation of other parts of unspecified shoulder girdle**

5th **S43.4** **Sprain of shoulder joint**

6th **S43.40** **Unspecified sprain of shoulder joint**

7th **S43.401** **Unspecified sprain of right shoulder joint**

7th **S43.402** **Unspecified sprain of left shoulder joint**

7th **S43.409** **Unspecified sprain of unspecified shoulder joint**

6th **S43.41** **Sprain of coracohumeral (ligament)**

7th **S43.411** **Sprain of right coracohumeral (ligament)**

7th **S43.412** **Sprain of left coracohumeral (ligament)**

7th **S43.419** **Sprain of unspecified coracohumeral (ligament)**

6th **S43.42** **Sprain of rotator cuff capsule**

EXCLUDES 1 *rotator cuff syndrome (complete) (incomplete), not specified as traumatic (M75.1-)*

EXCLUDES 2 *injury of tendon of rotator cuff (S46.0-)*

7th **S43.421** **Sprain of right rotator cuff capsule**

7th **S43.422** **Sprain of left rotator cuff capsule**

7th **S43.429** **Sprain of unspecified rotator cuff capsule**

6th **S43.43** **Superior glenoid labrum lesion**

SLAP lesion

7th **S43.431** **Superior glenoid labrum lesion of right shoulder**

7th **S43.432** **Superior glenoid labrum lesion of left shoulder**

7 HAC = Initial encounter only (7th character A, B or C) and not POA.

✓7th **S43.439 Superior glenoid labrum lesion of unspecified shoulder**

✓6th **S43.49 Other sprain of shoulder joint**

✓7th **S43.491 Other sprain of right shoulder joint**

✓7th **S43.492 Other sprain of left shoulder joint**

✓7th **S43.499 Other sprain of unspecified shoulder joint**

✓5th **S43.5 Sprain of acromioclavicular joint**

Sprain of acromioclavicular ligament

✓x7th **S43.50 Sprain of unspecified acromioclavicular joint**

✓x7th **S43.51 Sprain of right acromioclavicular joint**

✓x7th **S43.52 Sprain of left acromioclavicular joint**

✓5th **S43.6 Sprain of sternoclavicular joint**

✓x7th **S43.60 Sprain of unspecified sternoclavicular joint**

✓x7th **S43.61 Sprain of right sternoclavicular joint**

✓x7th **S43.62 Sprain of left sternoclavicular joint**

✓5th **S43.8 Sprain of other specified parts of shoulder girdle**

✓x7th **S43.80 Sprain of other specified parts of unspecified shoulder girdle**

✓x7th **S43.81 Sprain of other specified parts of right shoulder girdle**

✓x7th **S43.82 Sprain of other specified parts of left shoulder girdle**

✓5th **S43.9 Sprain of unspecified parts of shoulder girdle**

✓x7th **S43.90 Sprain of unspecified parts of unspecified shoulder girdle**

Sprain of shoulder girdle NOS

✓x7th **S43.91 Sprain of unspecified parts of right shoulder girdle**

✓x7th **S43.92 Sprain of unspecified parts of left shoulder girdle**

✓4th S44 Injury of nerves at shoulder and upper arm level

Code also any associated open wound (S41.-)

EXCLUDES 2 *injury of brachial plexus (S14.3-)*

The appropriate 7th is to be added to each code from category S44.
A initial encounter
D subsequent encounter
S sequela

✓5th **S44.0 Injury of ulnar nerve at upper arm level**

EXCLUDES 1 *ulnar nerve NOS (S54.0)*

✓x7th **S44.00 Injury of ulnar nerve at upper arm level, unspecified arm**

✓x7th **S44.01 Injury of ulnar nerve at upper arm level, right arm**

✓x7th **S44.02 Injury of ulnar nerve at upper arm level, left arm**

✓5th **S44.1 Injury of median nerve at upper arm level**

EXCLUDES 1 *median nerve NOS (S54.1)*

✓x7th **S44.10 Injury of median nerve at upper arm level, unspecified arm**

✓x7th **S44.11 Injury of median nerve at upper arm level, right arm**

✓x7th **S44.12 Injury of median nerve at upper arm level, left arm**

✓5th **S44.2 Injury of radial nerve at upper arm level**

EXCLUDES 1 *radial nerve NOS (S54.2)*

✓x7th **S44.20 Injury of radial nerve at upper arm level, unspecified arm**

✓x7th **S44.21 Injury of radial nerve at upper arm level, right arm**

✓x7th **S44.22 Injury of radial nerve at upper arm level, left arm**

✓5th **S44.3 Injury of axillary nerve**

✓x7th **S44.30 Injury of axillary nerve, unspecified arm**

✓x7th **S44.31 Injury of axillary nerve, right arm**

✓x7th **S44.32 Injury of axillary nerve, left arm**

✓5th **S44.4 Injury of musculocutaneous nerve**

✓x7th **S44.40 Injury of musculocutaneous nerve, unspecified arm**

✓x7th **S44.41 Injury of musculocutaneous nerve, right arm**

✓x7th **S44.42 Injury of musculocutaneous nerve, left arm**

✓5th **S44.5 Injury of cutaneous sensory nerve at shoulder and upper arm level**

✓x7th **S44.50 Injury of cutaneous sensory nerve at shoulder and upper arm level, unspecified arm**

✓x7th **S44.51 Injury of cutaneous sensory nerve at shoulder and upper arm level, right arm**

✓x7th **S44.52 Injury of cutaneous sensory nerve at shoulder and upper arm level, left arm**

✓5th **S44.8 Injury of other nerves at shoulder and upper arm level**

✓6th **S44.8X Injury of other nerves at shoulder and upper arm level**

✓7th **S44.8X1 Injury of other nerves at shoulder and upper arm level, right arm**

✓7th **S44.8X2 Injury of other nerves at shoulder and upper arm level, left arm**

✓7th **S44.8X9 Injury of other nerves at shoulder and upper arm level, unspecified arm**

✓5th **S44.9 Injury of unspecified nerve at shoulder and upper arm level**

✓x7th **S44.90 Injury of unspecified nerve at shoulder and upper arm level, unspecified arm**

✓x7th **S44.91 Injury of unspecified nerve at shoulder and upper arm level, right arm**

✓x7th **S44.92 Injury of unspecified nerve at shoulder and upper arm level, left arm**

✓4th S45 Injury of blood vessels at shoulder and upper arm level

Code also any associated open wound (S41.-)

EXCLUDES 2 *injury of subclavian artery (S25.1)*
injury of subclavian vein (S25.3)

The appropriate 7th is to be added to each code from category S45.
A initial encounter
D subsequent encounter
S sequela

✓5th **S45.0 Injury of axillary artery**

✓6th **S45.00 Unspecified injury of axillary artery**

✓7th **S45.001 Unspecified injury of axillary artery, right side** MCC

CC Excl: MCC with 7th character A: S45.001A, S45.009-S45.011 with 7th A, S45.019-S45.091 with 7th A, S45.099A, S45.301A, S45.309-S45.311 with 7th A, S45.319-S45.391 with 7th A, S45.399-S45.801 with 7th A, S45.809-S45.811 with 7th A, S45.819-S45.891 with 7th A, S45.899-S45.901 with 7th A, S45.909-S45.911 with 7th A, S45.919-S45.991 with 7th A, S45.999A, S55.201A, S55.209-S55.211 with 7th A, S55.219-S55.291 with 7th A, S55.299-S55.801 with 7th A, S55.809-S55.811 with 7th A, S55.819-S55.891 with 7th A, S55.899-S55.901 with 7th A, S55.909-S55.911 with 7th A, S55.919-S55.991 with 7th A, S55.999A, S65.801A, S65.809-S65.811 with 7th A, S65.819-S65.891 with 7th A, S65.899-S65.901 with 7th A, S65.909-S65.911 with 7th A, S65.919-S65.991 with 7th A, S65.999A

✓7th **S45.002 Unspecified injury of axillary artery, left side** MCC

CC Excl: MCC with 7th character A: S45.002-S45.009 with 7th A, S45.012-S45.019 with 7th A, S45.092-S45.099 with 7th A, S45.302-S45.309 with 7th A, S45.312-S45.319 with 7th A, S45.392-S45.399 with 7th A, S45.802-S45.809 with 7th A, S45.812-S45.819 with 7th A, S45.892-S45.899 with 7th A, S45.902-S45.909 with 7th A, S45.912-S45.919 with 7th A, S45.992-S45.999 with 7th A, S55.202-S55.209 with 7th A, S55.212-S55.219 with 7th A, S55.292-S55.299 with 7th A, S55.802-S55.809 with 7th A, S55.812-S55.819 with 7th A, S55.892-S55.899 with 7th A, S55.902-S55.909 with 7th A, S55.912-S55.919 with 7th A, S55.992-S55.999 with 7th A, S65.802-S65.809 with 7th A, S65.812-S65.819 with 7th A, S65.892-S65.899 with 7th A, S65.902-S65.909 with 7th A, S65.912-S65.919 with 7th A, S65.992-S65.999 with 7th A

✓7th **S45.009 Unspecified injury of axillary artery, unspecified side** MCC

CC Excl: MCC with 7th character A: S45.001-S45.099 with 7th A, S45.301-S45.999 with 7th A, S55.201-S55.999 with 7th A, S65.801-S65.999 with 7th A

✓6th **S45.Ø1 Laceration of axillary artery**

✓7th **S45.Ø11 Laceration of axillary artery, right side** MCC

CC Excl: MCC with 7th character A: S45.ØØ1A, S45.ØØ9-S45.Ø11 with 7th A, S45.Ø19-S45.Ø91 with 7th A, S45.Ø99A, S45.3Ø1A, S45.3Ø9-S45.311 with 7th A, S45.319-S45.391 with 7th A, S45.399-S45.8Ø1 with 7th A, S45.8Ø9-S45.811 with 7th A, S45.819-S45.891 with 7th A, S45.899-S45.9Ø1 with 7th A, S45.9Ø9-S45.911 with 7th A, S45.919-S45.991 with 7th A, S45.999A, S55.2Ø1A, S55.2Ø9-S55.211 with 7th A, S55.219-S55.291 with 7th A, S55.299-S55.8Ø1 with 7th A, S55.8Ø9-S55.811 with 7th A, S55.819-S55.891 with 7th A, S55.899-S55.9Ø1 with 7th A, S55.9Ø9-S55.911 with 7th A, S55.919-S55.991 with 7th A, S55.999 with 7th A, S65.8Ø1A, S65.8Ø9-S65.811 with 7th A, S65.819-S65.891 with 7th A, S65.899-S65.9Ø1 with 7th A, S65.9Ø9-S65.911 with 7th A, S65.919-S65.991 with 7th A, S65.999A

✓7th **S45.Ø12 Laceration of axillary artery, left side** MCC

CC Excl: MCC with 7th character A: S45.ØØ2-S45.ØØ9 with 7th A, S45.Ø12-S45.Ø19 with 7th A, S45.Ø92-S45.Ø99 with 7th A, S45.3Ø2-S45.3Ø9 with 7th A, S45.312-S45.319 with 7th A, S45.392-S45.399 with 7th A, S45.8Ø2-S45.8Ø9 with 7th A, S45.812-S45.819 with 7th A, S45.892-S45.899 with 7th A, S45.9Ø2-S45.9Ø9 with 7th A, S45.912-S45.919 with 7th A, S45.992-S45.999 with 7th A, S55.2Ø2-S55.2Ø9 with 7th A, S55.212-S55.219 with 7th A, S55.292-S55.299 with 7th A, S55.8Ø2-S55.8Ø9 with 7th A, S55.812-S55.819 with 7th A, S55.892-S55.899 with 7th A, S55.9Ø2-S55.9Ø9 with 7th A, S55.912-S55.919 with 7th A, S55.992-S55.999 with 7th A, S65.8Ø2-S65.8Ø9 with 7th A, S65.812-S65.819 with 7th A, S65.892-S65.899 with 7th A, S65.9Ø2-S65.9Ø9 with 7th A, S65.912-S65.919 with 7th A, S65.992-S65.999 with 7th A

✓7th **S45.Ø19 Laceration of axillary artery, unspecified side** MCC

CC Excl: MCC with 7th character A: S45.ØØ1-S45.Ø99 with 7th A, S45.3Ø1-S45.999 with 7th A, S55.2Ø1-S55.999 with 7th A, S65.8Ø1-S65.999 with 7th A

✓6th **S45.Ø9 Other specified injury of axillary artery**

✓7th **S45.Ø91 Other specified injury of axillary artery, right side** MCC

CC Excl: MCC with 7th character A: S45.ØØ1A, S45.ØØ9-S45.Ø11 with 7th A, S45.Ø19-S45.Ø91 with 7th A, S45.Ø99A, S45.3Ø1A, S45.3Ø9-S45.311 with 7th A, S45.319-S45.391 with 7th A, S45.399-S45.8Ø1 with 7th A, S45.8Ø9-S45.811 with 7th A, S45.819-S45.891 with 7th A, S45.899-S45.9Ø1 with 7th A, S45.9Ø9-S45.911 with 7th A, S45.919-S45.991 with 7th A, S45.999A, S55.2Ø1A, S55.2Ø9-S55.211 with 7th A, S55.219-S55.291 with 7th A, S55.299-S55.8Ø1 with 7th A, S55.8Ø9-S55.811 with 7th A, S55.819-S55.891 with 7th A, S55.899-S55.9Ø1 with 7th A, S55.9Ø9-S55.911 with 7th A, S55.919-S55.991 with 7th A, S55.999A, S65.8Ø1A, S65.8Ø9-S65.811 with 7th A, S65.819-S65.891 with 7th A, S65.899-S65.9Ø1 with 7th A, S65.9Ø9-S65.911 with 7th A, S65.919-S65.991 with 7th A, S65.999A

✓7th **S45.Ø92 Other specified injury of axillary artery, left side** MCC

CC Excl: MCC with 7th character A: S45.ØØ2-S45.ØØ9 with 7th A, S45.Ø12-S45.Ø19 with 7th A, S45.Ø92-S45.Ø99 with 7th A, S45.3Ø2-S45.3Ø9 with 7th A, S45.312-S45.319 with 7th A, S45.392-S45.399 with 7th A, S45.8Ø2-S45.8Ø9 with 7th A, S45.812-S45.819 with 7th A, S45.892-S45.899 with 7th A, S45.9Ø2-S45.9Ø9 with 7th A, S45.912-S45.919 with 7th A, S45.992-S45.999 with 7th A, S55.2Ø2-S55.2Ø9 with 7th A, S55.212-S55.219 with 7th A, S55.292-S55.299 with 7th A, S55.8Ø2-S55.8Ø9 with 7th A, S55.812-S55.819 with 7th A, S55.892-S55.899 with 7th A, S55.9Ø2-S55.9Ø9 with 7th A, S55.912-S55.919 with 7th A, S55.992-S55.999 with 7th A, S65.8Ø2-S65.8Ø9 with 7th A, S65.812-S65.819 with 7th A, S65.892-S65.899 with 7th A, S65.9Ø2-S65.9Ø9 with 7th A, S65.912-S65.919 with 7th A, S65.992-S65.999 with 7th A

✓7th **S45.Ø99 Other specified injury of axillary artery, unspecified side** MCC

CC Excl:MCC with 7th character A: S45.ØØ1-S45.Ø99 with 7th A, S45.3Ø1-S45.999 with 7th A, S55.2Ø1-S55.999 with 7th A, S65.8Ø1-S65.999 with 7th A

✓5th **S45.1 Injury of brachial artery**

✓6th **S45.1Ø Unspecified injury of brachial artery**

✓7th **S45.1Ø1 Unspecified injury of brachial artery, right side** CC

CC Excl: CC with 7th character A: S45.1Ø1 with 7th A, S45.1Ø9-S45.111 with 7th A, S45.119-S45.191 with 7th A, S45.199-S45.2Ø1 with 7th A, S45.2Ø9-S45.211 with 7th A, S45.219-S45.291 with 7th A, S45.299-S45.3Ø1 with 7th A, S45.3Ø9-S45.311 with 7th A, S45.319-S45.391 with 7th A, S45.399-S45.8Ø1 with 7th A, S45.8Ø9-S45.811 with 7th A, S45.819-S45.891 with 7th A, S45.899-S45.9Ø1 with 7th A, S45.9Ø9-S45.911 with 7th A, S45.919-S45.991 with 7th A, S45.999 with 7th A, S55.2Ø1 with 7th A, S55.2Ø9-S55.211 with 7th A, S55.219-S55.291 with 7th A, S55.299-S55.8Ø1 with 7th A, S55.8Ø9-S55.811 with 7th A, S55.819-S55.891 with 7th A, S55.899-S55.9Ø1 with 7th A, S55.9Ø9-S55.911 with 7th A, S55.919-S55.991 with 7th A, S55.999 with 7th A, S65.8Ø1 with 7th A, S65.8Ø9-S65.811 with 7th A, S65.819-S65.891 with 7th A, S65.899-S65.9Ø1 with 7th A, S65.9Ø9-S65.911 with 7th A, S65.919-S65.991 with 7th A, S65.999A

✓7th **S45.1Ø2 Unspecified injury of brachial artery, left side** CC

CC Excl: CC with 7th character A: S45.1Ø2-S45.1Ø9 with 7th A, S45.112-S45.119 with 7th A, S45.192-S45.199 with 7th A, S45.2Ø2-S45.2Ø9 with 7th A, S45.212-S45.219 with 7th A, S45.292-S45.299 with 7th A, S45.3Ø2-S45.3Ø9 with 7th A, S45.312-S45.319 with 7th A, S45.392-S45.399 with 7th A, S45.8Ø2-S45.8Ø9 with 7th A, S45.812-S45.819 with 7th A, S45.892-S45.899 with 7th A, S45.9Ø2-S45.9Ø9 with 7th A, S45.912-S45.919 with 7th A, S45.992-S45.999 with 7th A, S55.2Ø2-S55.2Ø9 with 7th A, S55.212-S55.219 with 7th A, S55.292-S55.299 with 7th A, S55.8Ø2-S55.8Ø9 with 7th A, S55.812-S55.819 with 7th A, S55.892-S55.899 with 7th A, S55.9Ø2-S55.9Ø9 with 7th A, S55.912-S55.919 with 7th A, S55.992-S55.999 with 7th A, S65.8Ø2-S65.8Ø9 with 7th A, S65.812-S65.819 with 7th A, S65.892-S65.899 with 7th A, S65.9Ø2-S65.9Ø9 with 7th A, S65.912-S65.919 with 7th A, S65.992-S65.999 with 7th A

✓7th **S45.1Ø9 Unspecified injury of brachial artery, unspecified side** CC

CC Excl: CC with 7th character A: S45.1Ø1-S45.999 with 7th A, S55.2Ø1-S55.999 with 7th A, S65.8Ø1-S65.999 with 7th A

✓6th **S45.11 Laceration of brachial artery**

✓7th **S45.111 Laceration of brachial artery, right side** CC
CC Excl: See code: S45.101

✓7th **S45.112 Laceration of brachial artery, left side** CC
CC Excl: See code: S45.102

✓7th **S45.119 Laceration of brachial artery, unspecified side** CC
CC Excl: See code: S45.109

✓6th **S45.19 Other specified injury of brachial artery**

✓7th **S45.191 Other specified injury of brachial artery, right side** CC
CC Excl: See code: S45.101

✓7th **S45.192 Other specified injury of brachial artery, left side** CC
CC Excl: See code: S45.102

✓7th **S45.199 Other specified injury of brachial artery, unspecified side** CC
CC Excl: See code: S45.109

✓5th **S45.2 Injury of axillary or brachial vein**

✓6th **S45.20 Unspecified injury of axillary or brachial vein**

✓7th **S45.201 Unspecified injury of axillary or brachial vein, right side** CC
CC Excl: See code: S45.101

✓7th **S45.202 Unspecified injury of axillary or brachial vein, left side** CC
CC Excl: See code: S45.102

✓7th **S45.209 Unspecified injury of axillary or brachial vein, unspecified side** CC
CC Excl: See code: S45.109

✓6th **S45.21 Laceration of axillary or brachial vein**

✓7th **S45.211 Laceration of axillary or brachial vein, right side** CC
CC Excl: See code: S45.101

✓7th **S45.212 Laceration of axillary or brachial vein, left side** CC
CC Excl: See code: S45.102

✓7th **S45.219 Laceration of axillary or brachial vein, unspecified side** CC
CC Excl: See code: S45.109

✓6th **S45.29 Other specified injury of axillary or brachial vein**

✓7th **S45.291 Other specified injury of axillary or brachial vein, right side** CC
CC Excl: See code: S45.101

✓7th **S45.292 Other specified injury of axillary or brachial vein, left side** CC
CC Excl: See code: S45.102

✓7th **S45.299 Other specified injury of axillary or brachial vein, unspecified side** CC
CC Excl: See code: S45.109

✓5th **S45.3 Injury of superficial vein at shoulder and upper arm level**

✓6th **S45.30 Unspecified injury of superficial vein at shoulder and upper arm level**

✓7th **S45.301 Unspecified injury of superficial vein at shoulder and upper arm level, right arm** CC
CC Excl: CC with 7th character A: S45.301A, S45.309-S45.311 with 7th A, S45.319-S45.391 with 7th A, S45.399-S45.801 with 7th A, S45.809-S45.811 with 7th A, S45.819-S45.891 with 7th A, S45.899-S45.901 with 7th A, S45.909-S45.911 with 7th A, S45.919-S45.991 with 7th A, S45.999 with 7th A, S55.001A, S55.009-S55.011 with 7th A, S55.019-S55.091 with 7th A, S55.099 with 7th A, S55.201 with 7th A, S55.209-S55.211 with 7th A, S55.219-S55.291 with 7th A, S55.299-S55.801 with 7th A, S55.809-S55.811 with 7th A, S55.819-S55.891 with 7th A, S55.899-S55.901 with 7th A, S55.909-S55.911 with 7th A, S55.919-S55.991 with 7th A, S55.999 with 7th A, S65.001 with 7th A, S65.009-S65.011 with 7th A, S65.019-S65.091 with 7th A, S65.099 with 7th A, S65.201 with 7th A, S65.209-S65.211 with 7th A, S65.219-S65.291 with 7th A, S65.299-S65.301 with 7th A, S65.309-S65.311 with 7th A, S65.319-S65.391 with 7th A, S65.399-S65.401 with 7th A, S65.409-S65.411 with 7th A, S65.419-S65.491 with 7th A, S65.499-S65.500 with 7th A, S65.502 with 7th A, S65.504 with 7th A, S65.506 with 7th A, S65.508-S65.510 with 7th A, S65.512 with 7th A, S65.514 with 7th A, S65.516 with 7th A, S65.518-S65.590A, S65.592A, S65.594 A, S65.596A, S65.598-S65.801 with 7th A, S65.809-S65.811 with 7th A, S65.819-S65.891 with 7th A, S65.899-S65.901 with 7th A, S65.909-S65.911 with 7th A, S65.919-S65.991 with 7th A, S65.999A

✓7th **S45.302 Unspecified injury of superficial vein at shoulder and upper arm level, left arm** CC
CC Excl: CC with 7th character A: S45.302-S45.309 with 7th A, S45.312-S45.319 with 7th A, S45.392-S45.399 with 7th A, S45.802-S45.809 with 7th A, S45.812-S45.819 with 7th A, S45.892-S45.899 with 7th A, S45.902-S45.909 with 7th A, S45.912-S45.919 with 7th A, S45.992-S45.999 with 7th A, S55.002-S55.009 with 7th A, S55.012-S55.019 with 7th A, S55.092-S55.099 with 7th A, S55.202-S55.209 with 7th A, S55.212-S55.219 with 7th A, S55.292-S55.299 with 7th A, S55.802-S55.809 with 7th A, S55.812-S55.819 with 7th A, S55.892-S55.899 with 7th A, S55.902-S55.909 with 7th A, S55.912-S55.919 with 7th A, S55.992-S55.999 with 7th A, S65.002-S65.009 with 7th A, S65.012-S65.019 with 7th A, S65.092-S65.099 with 7th A, S65.202-S65.209 with 7th A, S65.212-S65.219 with 7th A, S65.292-S65.299 with 7th A, S65.302-S65.309 with 7th A, S65.312-S65.319 with 7th A, S65.392-S65.399 with 7th A, S65.402-S65.409 with 7th A, S65.412-S65.419 with 7th A, S65.492-S65.499 with 7th A, S65.501A, S65.503A, S65.505A, S65.507-S65.509 with 7th A, S65.511A, S65.513A, S65.515 A, S65.517-S65.519 with 7th A, S65.591A, S65.593 A, S65.595A, S65.597-S65.599 with 7th A, S65.802-S65.809 with 7th A, S65.812-S65.819 with 7th A, S65.892-S65.899 with 7th A, S65.902-S65.909 with 7th A, S65.912-S65.919 with 7th A, S65.992-S65.999 with 7th A

✓7th **S45.309 Unspecified injury of superficial vein at shoulder and upper arm level, unspecified arm** CC
CC Excl: CC with 7th character A: S45.301-S45.999 with 7th A, S55.001-S55.099 with 7th A, S55.201-S55.999 with 7th A, S65.001-S65.099 with 7th A, S65.201-S65.999 A

✓6th **S45.31 Laceration of superficial vein at shoulder and upper arm level**

✓7th **S45.311 Laceration of superficial vein at shoulder and upper arm level, right arm** CC
CC Excl: See code: S45.301

√7th **S45.312 Laceration of superficial vein at shoulder and upper arm level, left arm** CC
CC Excl: See code: S45.302

√7th **S45.319 Laceration of superficial vein at shoulder and upper arm level, unspecified arm** CC
CC Excl: See code: S45.309

√6th **S45.39 Other specified injury of superficial vein at shoulder and upper arm level**

√7th **S45.391 Other specified injury of superficial vein at shoulder and upper arm level, right arm** CC
CC Excl: See code: S45.301

√7th **S45.392 Other specified injury of superficial vein at shoulder and upper arm level, left arm** CC
CC Excl: See code: S45.302

√7th **S45.399 Other specified injury of superficial vein at shoulder and upper arm level, unspecified arm** CC
CC Excl: See code: S45.309

√5th **S45.8 Injury of other specified blood vessels at shoulder and upper arm level**

√6th **S45.80 Unspecified injury of other specified blood vessels at shoulder and upper arm level**

√7th **S45.801 Unspecified injury of other specified blood vessels at shoulder and upper arm level, right arm** CC
CC Excl: See code: S45.301

√7th **S45.802 Unspecified injury of other specified blood vessels at shoulder and upper arm level, left arm** CC
CC Excl: See code: S45.302

√7th **S45.809 Unspecified injury of other specified blood vessels at shoulder and upper arm level, unspecified arm** CC
CC Excl: See code: S45.309

√6th **S45.81 Laceration of other specified blood vessels at shoulder and upper arm level**

√7th **S45.811 Laceration of other specified blood vessels at shoulder and upper arm level, right arm** CC
CC Excl: See code: S45.301

√7th **S45.812 Laceration of other specified blood vessels at shoulder and upper arm level, left arm** CC
CC Excl: See code: S45.302

√7th **S45.819 Laceration of other specified blood vessels at shoulder and upper arm level, unspecified arm** CC
CC Excl: See code: S45.309

√6th **S45.89 Other specified injury of other specified blood vessels at shoulder and upper arm level**

√7th **S45.891 Other specified injury of other specified blood vessels at shoulder and upper arm level, right arm** CC
CC Excl: See code: S45.301

√7th **S45.892 Other specified injury of other specified blood vessels at shoulder and upper arm level, left arm** CC
CC Excl: See code: S45.302

√7th **S45.899 Other specified injury of other specified blood vessels at shoulder and upper arm level, unspecified arm** CC
CC Excl: See code: S45.309

√5th **S45.9 Injury of unspecified blood vessel at shoulder and upper arm level**

√6th **S45.90 Unspecified injury of unspecified blood vessel at shoulder and upper arm level**

√7th **S45.901 Unspecified injury of unspecified blood vessel at shoulder and upper arm level, right arm** CC
CC Excl: See code: S45.301

√7th **S45.902 Unspecified injury of unspecified blood vessel at shoulder and upper arm level, left arm** CC
CC Excl: See code: S45.302

√7th **S45.909 Unspecified injury of unspecified blood vessel at shoulder and upper arm level, unspecified arm** CC
CC Excl: See code: S45.309

√6th **S45.91 Laceration of unspecified blood vessel at shoulder and upper arm level**

√7th **S45.911 Laceration of unspecified blood vessel at shoulder and upper arm level, right arm** CC
CC Excl: See code: S45.301

√7th **S45.912 Laceration of unspecified blood vessel at shoulder and upper arm level, left arm** CC
CC Excl: See code: S45.302

√7th **S45.919 Laceration of unspecified blood vessel at shoulder and upper arm level, unspecified arm** CC
CC Excl: See code: S45.309

√6th **S45.99 Other specified injury of unspecified blood vessel at shoulder and upper arm level**

√7th **S45.991 Other specified injury of unspecified blood vessel at shoulder and upper arm level, right arm** CC
CC Excl: See code: S45.301

√7th **S45.992 Other specified injury of unspecified blood vessel at shoulder and upper arm level, left arm** CC
CC Excl: See code: S45.302

√7th **S45.999 Other specified injury of unspecified blood vessel at shoulder and upper arm level, unspecified arm** CC
CC Excl: See code: S45.309

√4th **S46 Injury of muscle, fascia and tendon at shoulder and upper arm level**

Code also any associated open wound (S41.-)

EXCLUDES 2 *injury of muscle, fascia and tendon at elbow (S56.-)*
sprain of joints and ligaments of shoulder girdle (S43.9)

The appropriate 7th is to be added to each code from category S46.
A initial encounter
D subsequent encounter
S sequela

√5th **S46.0 Injury of muscle(s) and tendon(s) of the rotator cuff of shoulder**

CC Excl: For CC codes in subcategory S46.0, unless otherwise noted: CC with 7th character A: S41.001A, S41.009-S41.011 with 7th A, S41.019-S41.021 with 7th A, S41.029-S41.031 with 7th A, S41.039-S41.041 with 7th A, S41.049-S41.051 with 7th A, S41.059-S41.101 with 7th A, S41.109-S41.111 with 7th A, S41.119-S41.121 with 7th A, S41.129-S41.131 with 7th A, S41.139-S41.141 with 7th A, S41.149-S41.151 with 7th A, S41.159 A, S46.021A, S46.029A, S46.121A, S46.129A, S46.221A, S46.229A, S46.321A, S46.329A, S46.821A, S46.829A, S46.921A, S46.929A

√6th **S46.00 Unspecified injury of muscle(s) and tendon(s) of the rotator cuff of shoulder**

√7th **S46.001 Unspecified injury of muscle(s) and tendon(s) of the rotator cuff of right shoulder**

√7th **S46.002 Unspecified injury of muscle(s) and tendon(s) of the rotator cuff of left shoulder**

√7th **S46.009 Unspecified injury of muscle(s) and tendon(s) of the rotator cuff of unspecified shoulder**

√6th **S46.01 Strain of muscle(s) and tendon(s) of the rotator cuff of shoulder**

√7th **S46.011 Strain of muscle(s) and tendon(s) of the rotator cuff of right shoulder**

√7th **S46.012 Strain of muscle(s) and tendon(s) of the rotator cuff of left shoulder**

√7th **S46.019 Strain of muscle(s) and tendon(s) of the rotator cuff of unspecified shoulder**

√6th **S46.02 Laceration of muscle(s) and tendon(s) of the rotator cuff of shoulder**

√7th **S46.021 Laceration of muscle(s) and tendon(s) of the rotator cuff of right shoulder** CC

√7th **S46.022 Laceration of muscle(s) and tendon(s) of the rotator cuff of left shoulder** CC

√7th **S46.029 Laceration of muscle(s) and tendon(s) of the rotator cuff of unspecified shoulder** CC

6th S46.09 Other injury of muscle(s) and tendon(s) of the rotator cuff of shoulder
7th S46.091 Other injury of muscle(s) and tendon(s) of the rotator cuff of right shoulder
7th S46.092 Other injury of muscle(s) and tendon(s) of the rotator cuff of left shoulder
7th S46.099 Other injury of muscle(s) and tendon(s) of the rotator cuff of unspecified shoulder
5th S46.1 Injury of muscle, fascia and tendon of long head of biceps
6th S46.10 Unspecified injury of muscle, fascia and tendon of long head of biceps
7th S46.101 Unspecified injury of muscle, fascia and tendon of long head of biceps, right arm
7th S46.102 Unspecified injury of muscle, fascia and tendon of long head of biceps, left arm
7th S46.109 Unspecified injury of muscle, fascia and tendon of long head of biceps, unspecified arm
6th S46.11 Strain of muscle, fascia and tendon of long head of biceps
7th S46.111 Strain of muscle, fascia and tendon of long head of biceps, right arm
7th S46.112 Strain of muscle, fascia and tendon of long head of biceps, left arm
7th S46.119 Strain of muscle, fascia and tendon of long head of biceps, unspecified arm
6th S46.12 Laceration of muscle, fascia and tendon of long head of biceps
7th S46.121 Laceration of muscle, fascia and tendon of long head of biceps, right arm CC
CC Excl: CC with 7th character A: S41.001A, S41.009-S41.011 with 7th A, S41.019-S41.021 with 7th A, S41.029-S41.031 with 7th A, S41.039-S41.041 with 7th A, S41.049-S41.051 with 7th A, S41.059-S41.101 with 7th A, S41.109-S41.111 with 7th A, S41.119-S41.121 with 7th A, S41.129-S41.131 with 7th A, S41.139-S41.141 with 7th A, S41.149-S41.151 with 7th A, S41.159A, S46.021A, S46.029A, S46.121A, S46.129A, S46.221A, S46.229 A, S46.321A, S46.329A, S46.821A, S46.829A, S46.921A, S46.929A
7th S46.122 Laceration of muscle, fascia and tendon of long head of biceps, left arm CC
CC Excl: CC with 7th character A: S41.002-S41.009 with 7th A, S41.012-S41.019 with 7th A, S41.022-S41.029 with 7th A, S41.032-S41.039 with 7th A, S41.042-S41.049 with 7th A, S41.052-S41.059 with 7th A, S41.102-S41.109 with 7th A, S41.112-S41.119 with 7th A, S41.122-S41.129 with 7th A, S41.132-S41.139 with 7th A, S41.142-S41.149 with 7th A, S41.152-S41.159 with 7th A, S46.022-S46.029 with 7th A, S46.122-S46.129 with 7th A, S46.222-S46.229 with 7th A, S46.322-S46.329 with 7th A, S46.822-S46.829 with 7th A, S46.922-S46.929 with 7th A
7th S46.129 Laceration of muscle, fascia and tendon of long head of biceps, unspecified arm CC
CC Excl: CC with 7th character A: S41.001-S41.159 with 7th A, S46.021-S46.029 with 7th A, S46.121-S46.129 with 7th A, S46.221-S46.229 with 7th A, S46.321-S46.329 with 7th A, S46.821-S46.829 with 7th A, S46.921-S46.929 with 7th A
6th S46.19 Other injury of muscle, fascia and tendon of long head of biceps
7th S46.191 Other injury of muscle, fascia and tendon of long head of biceps, right arm
7th S46.192 Other injury of muscle, fascia and tendon of long head of biceps, left arm
7th S46.199 Other injury of muscle, fascia and tendon of long head of biceps, unspecified arm
5th S46.2 Injury of muscle, fascia and tendon of other parts of biceps
6th S46.20 Unspecified injury of muscle, fascia and tendon of other parts of biceps
7th S46.201 Unspecified injury of muscle, fascia and tendon of other parts of biceps, right arm
7th S46.202 Unspecified injury of muscle, fascia and tendon of other parts of biceps, left arm
7th S46.209 Unspecified injury of muscle, fascia and tendon of other parts of biceps, unspecified arm
6th S46.21 Strain of muscle, fascia and tendon of other parts of biceps
7th S46.211 Strain of muscle, fascia and tendon of other parts of biceps, right arm
7th S46.212 Strain of muscle, fascia and tendon of other parts of biceps, left arm
7th S46.219 Strain of muscle, fascia and tendon of other parts of biceps, unspecified arm
6th S46.22 Laceration of muscle, fascia and tendon of other parts of biceps
7th S46.221 Laceration of muscle, fascia and tendon of other parts of biceps, right arm CC
CC Excl: CC with 7th character A: See code: S46.121
7th S46.222 Laceration of muscle, fascia and tendon of other parts of biceps, left arm CC
CC Excl: CC with 7th character A: See code: S46.122
7th S46.229 Laceration of muscle, fascia and tendon of other parts of biceps, unspecified arm CC
CC Excl: CC with 7th character A: See code: S46.129
6th S46.29 Other injury of muscle, fascia and tendon of other parts of biceps
7th S46.291 Other injury of muscle, fascia and tendon of other parts of biceps, right arm
7th S46.292 Other injury of muscle, fascia and tendon of other parts of biceps, left arm
7th S46.299 Other injury of muscle, fascia and tendon of other parts of biceps, unspecified arm
5th S46.3 Injury of muscle, fascia and tendon of triceps
6th S46.30 Unspecified injury of muscle, fascia and tendon of triceps
7th S46.301 Unspecified injury of muscle, fascia and tendon of triceps, right arm
7th S46.302 Unspecified injury of muscle, fascia and tendon of triceps, left arm
7th S46.309 Unspecified injury of muscle, fascia and tendon of triceps, unspecified arm
6th S46.31 Strain of muscle, fascia and tendon of triceps
7th S46.311 Strain of muscle, fascia and tendon of triceps, right arm
7th S46.312 Strain of muscle, fascia and tendon of triceps, left arm
7th S46.319 Strain of muscle, fascia and tendon of triceps, unspecified arm
6th S46.32 Laceration of muscle, fascia and tendon of triceps
7th S46.321 Laceration of muscle, fascia and tendon of triceps, right arm CC
CC Excl: CC with 7th character A: See code: S46.121
7th S46.322 Laceration of muscle, fascia and tendon of triceps, left arm CC
CC Excl: CC with 7th character A: See code: S46.122
7th S46.329 Laceration of muscle, fascia and tendon of triceps, unspecified arm CC
CC Excl: CC with 7th character A: See code: S46.129
6th S46.39 Other injury of muscle, fascia and tendon of triceps
7th S46.391 Other injury of muscle, fascia and tendon of triceps, right arm
7th S46.392 Other injury of muscle, fascia and tendon of triceps, left arm
7th S46.399 Other injury of muscle, fascia and tendon of triceps, unspecified arm

√5th **S46.8 Injury of other muscles, fascia and tendons at shoulder and upper arm level**

√6th **S46.8Ø Unspecified injury of other muscles, fascia and tendons at shoulder and upper arm level**

√7th **S46.8Ø1 Unspecified injury of other muscles, fascia and tendons at shoulder and upper arm level, right arm**

√7th **S46.8Ø2 Unspecified injury of other muscles, fascia and tendons at shoulder and upper arm level, left arm**

√7th **S46.8Ø9 Unspecified injury of other muscles, fascia and tendons at shoulder and upper arm level, unspecified arm**

√6th **S46.81 Strain of other muscles, fascia and tendons at shoulder and upper arm level**

√7th **S46.811 Strain of other muscles, fascia and tendons at shoulder and upper arm level, right arm**

√7th **S46.812 Strain of other muscles, fascia and tendons at shoulder and upper arm level, left arm**

√7th **S46.819 Strain of other muscles, fascia and tendons at shoulder and upper arm level, unspecified arm**

√6th **S46.82 Laceration of other muscles, fascia and tendons at shoulder and upper arm level**

√7th **S46.821 Laceration of other muscles, fascia and tendons at shoulder and upper arm level, right arm** CC
CC Excl: CC with 7th character A: See code: S46.121

√7th **S46.822 Laceration of other muscles, fascia and tendons at shoulder and upper arm level, left arm** CC
CC Excl: CC with 7th character A: See code: S46.122

√7th **S46.829 Laceration of other muscles, fascia and tendons at shoulder and upper arm level, unspecified arm** CC
CC Excl: CC with 7th character A: See code: S46.129

√6th **S46.89 Other injury of other muscles, fascia and tendons at shoulder and upper arm level**

√7th **S46.891 Other injury of other muscles, fascia and tendons at shoulder and upper arm level, right arm**

√7th **S46.892 Other injury of other muscles, fascia and tendons at shoulder and upper arm level, left arm**

√7th **S46.899 Other injury of other muscles, fascia and tendons at shoulder and upper arm level, unspecified arm**

√5th **S46.9 Injury of unspecified muscle, fascia and tendon at shoulder and upper arm level**

√6th **S46.9Ø Unspecified injury of unspecified muscle, fascia and tendon at shoulder and upper arm level**

√7th **S46.9Ø1 Unspecified injury of unspecified muscle, fascia and tendon at shoulder and upper arm level, right arm**

√7th **S46.9Ø2 Unspecified injury of unspecified muscle, fascia and tendon at shoulder and upper arm level, left arm**

√7th **S46.9Ø9 Unspecified injury of unspecified muscle, fascia and tendon at shoulder and upper arm level, unspecified arm**

√6th **S46.91 Strain of unspecified muscle, fascia and tendon at shoulder and upper arm level**

√7th **S46.911 Strain of unspecified muscle, fascia and tendon at shoulder and upper arm level, right arm**

√7th **S46.912 Strain of unspecified muscle, fascia and tendon at shoulder and upper arm level, left arm**

√7th **S46.919 Strain of unspecified muscle, fascia and tendon at shoulder and upper arm level, unspecified arm**

√6th **S46.92 Laceration of unspecified muscle, fascia and tendon at shoulder and upper arm level**

√7th **S46.921 Laceration of unspecified muscle, fascia and tendon at shoulder and upper arm level, right arm** CC
CC Excl: CC with 7th character A: See code: S46.121

√7th **S46.922 Laceration of unspecified muscle, fascia and tendon at shoulder and upper arm level, left arm** CC
CC Excl: CC with 7th character A: See code: S46.122

√7th **S46.929 Laceration of unspecified muscle, fascia and tendon at shoulder and upper arm level, unspecified arm** CC
CC Excl: CC with 7th character A: See code: S46.129

√6th **S46.99 Other injury of unspecified muscle, fascia and tendon at shoulder and upper arm level**

√7th **S46.991 Other injury of unspecified muscle, fascia and tendon at shoulder and upper arm level, right arm**

√7th **S46.992 Other injury of unspecified muscle, fascia and tendon at shoulder and upper arm level, left arm**

√7th **S46.999 Other injury of unspecified muscle, fascia and tendon at shoulder and upper arm level, unspecified arm**

√4th **S47 Crushing injury of shoulder and upper arm**

Use additional code for all associated injuries

EXCLUDES 2 *crushing injury of elbow (S57.Ø-)*

The appropriate 7th is to be added to each code from category S47.
A initial encounter
D subsequent encounter
S sequela

√x7th **S47.1 Crushing injury of right shoulder and upper arm**

√x7th **S47.2 Crushing injury of left shoulder and upper arm**

√x7th **S47.9 Crushing injury of shoulder and upper arm, unspecified arm**

√4th **S48 Traumatic amputation of shoulder and upper arm**

NOTE An amputation not identified as partial or complete should be coded to complete.

EXCLUDES 1 *traumatic amputation at elbow level (S58.Ø)*

The appropriate 7th is to be added to each code from category S48.
A initial encounter
D subsequent encounter
S sequela

√5th **S48.Ø Traumatic amputation at shoulder joint**

√6th **S48.Ø1 Complete traumatic amputation at shoulder joint**

√7th **S48.Ø11 Complete traumatic amputation at right shoulder joint** CC
CC Excl: CC with 7th character A: S41.ØØ1A, S41.ØØ9-S41.Ø11 with 7th A, S41.Ø19-S41.Ø21 with 7th A, S41.Ø29-S41.Ø31 with 7th A, S41.Ø39-S41.Ø41 with 7th A, S41.Ø49-S41.Ø51 with 7th A, S41.Ø59-S41.1Ø1 with 7th A, S41.1Ø9-S41.111 with 7th A, S41.119-S41.121 with 7th A, S41.129-S41.131 with 7th A, S41.139-S41.141 with 7th A, S41.149-S41.151 with 7th A, S41.159A, S46.Ø21A, S46.Ø29A, S46.121A, S46.129A, S46.221 A, S46.229 A, S46.321A, S46.329A, S46.821A, S46.829A, S46.921A, S46.929A, S48.Ø11 A, S48.Ø19-S48.Ø21 with 7th A, S48.Ø29-S48.111 with 7th A, S48.119-S48.121 with 7th A, S48.129-S48.911 with 7th A, S48.919-S48.921 with 7th A, S48.929A, S51.ØØ1A, S51.ØØ9-S51.Ø11 with 7th A, S51.Ø19-S51.Ø21 with 7th A, S51.Ø29-S51.Ø31 with 7th A, S51.Ø39-S51.Ø41 with 7th A, S51.Ø49-S51.Ø51 with 7th A, S51.Ø59-S51.8Ø1 with 7th A, S51.8Ø9-S51.811 with 7th A, S51.819-S51.821 with 7th A, S51.829-S51.831 with 7th A, S51.839-S51.841 with 7th A, S51.849-S51.851 with 7th A, S51.859 with 7th A, S56.Ø21A, S56.Ø29A, S56.121A, S56.123A, S56.125A, S56.127A, S56.129A, S56.221A, S56.229A, S56.321A, S56.329A, S56.421A, S56.423A, S56.425A, S56.427A, S56.429A, S56.521A, S56.529A, S56.821A, S56.829A,

S56.921A, S56.929A, S58.011A, S58.019-S58.021 with 7th A, S58.029-S58.111 with 7th A, S58.119-S58.121 with 7th A, S58.129-S58.911 with 7th A, S58.919-S58.921 with 7th A, S58.929A, S61.001A, S61.009-S61.011 with 7th A, S61.019-S61.021 with 7th A, S61.029-S61.031 with 7th A, S61.039-S61.041 with 7th A, S61.049-S61.051 with 7th A, S61.059-S61.101 with 7th A, S61.109-S61.111 with 7th A, S61.119-S61.121 with 7th A, S61.129-S61.131 with 7th A, S61.139-S61.141 with 7th A, S61.149-S61.151 with 7th A, S61.159-S61.200 with 7th A, S61.202A, S61.204A, S61.206A, S61.208-S61.210 with 7th A, S61.212A, S61.214A, S61.216A, S61.218-S61.220 with 7th A, S61.222A, S61.224A, S61.226A, S61.228-S61.230 with 7th A, S61.232A, S61.234A, S61.236 A, S61.238-S61.240 with 7th A, S61.242A, S61.244A, S61.246A, S61.248-S61.250 with 7th A, S61.252A, S61.254A, S61.256A, S61.258-S61.300 with 7th A, S61.302A, S61.304A, S61.306A, S61.308-S61.310 with 7th A, S61.312A, S61.314A, S61.316A, S61.318-S61.320 with 7th A, S61.322A, S61.324 A, S61.326A, S61.328-S61.330 with 7th A, S61.332A, S61.334A, S61.336A, S61.338-S61.340 with 7th A, S61.342 A, S61.344A, S61.346A, S61.348-S61.350 with 7th A, S61.352A, S61.354A, S61.356A, S61.358-S61.401 with 7th A, S61.409-S61.411 with 7th A, S61.419-S61.421 with 7th A, S61.429-S61.431 with 7th A, S61.439-S61.441 with 7th A, S61.449-S61.451 with 7th A, S61.459-S61.501 with 7th A, S61.509-S61.511 with 7th A, S61.519-S61.521 with 7th A, S61.529-S61.531 with 7th A, S61.539-S61.541 with 7th A, S61.549-S61.551 with 7th A, S61.559A, S66.021A, S66.029A, S66.120A, S66.122A, S66.124A, S66.126A, S66.128-S66.129 with 7th A, S66.221A, S66.229A, S66.320A, S66.322A, S66.324A, S66.326A, S66.328-S66.329 with 7th A, S66.421A, S66.429A, S66.520A, S66.522A, S66.524A, S66.526A, S66.528-S66.529 with 7th A, S66.821A, S66.829A, S66.921A, S66.929A, S68.011A, S68.019-S68.021 with 7th A, S68.029-S68.110 with 7th A, S68.112A, S68.114A, S68.116A, S68.118-S68.120 with 7th A, S68.122A, S68.124A, S68.126 A, S68.128-S68.411 with 7th A, S68.419-S68.421 with 7th A, S68.429-S68.511 with 7th A, S68.519-S68.521 with 7th A, S68.529-S68.610 with 7th A, S68.612A, S68.614A, S68.616A, S68.618-S68.620 with 7th A, S68.622A, S68.624A, S68.626A, S68.628-S68.711 with 7th A, S68.719-S68.721 with 7th A, S68.729A, T14.8-T14.91, T79.A0X-T79.9XX with 7th A

✓7th **S48.012 Complete traumatic amputation at left shoulder joint** CC

CC Excl: CC with 7th character A: S41.002-S41.009 with 7th A, S41.012-S41.019 with 7th A, S41.022-S41.029 with 7th A, S41.032-S41.039 with 7th A, S41.042-S41.049 with 7th A, S41.052-S41.059 with 7th A, S41.102-S41.109 with 7th A, S41.112-S41.119 with 7th A, S41.122-S41.129 with 7th A, S41.132-S41.139 with 7th A, S41.142-S41.149 with 7th A, S41.152-S41.159 with 7th A, S46.022-S46.029 with 7th A, S46.122-S46.129 with 7th A, S46.222-S46.229 with 7th A, S46.322-S46.329 with 7th A, S46.822-S46.829 with 7th A, S46.922-S46.929 with 7th A, S48.012-S48.019 with 7th A, S48.022-S48.029 with 7th A, S48.112-S48.119 with 7th A, S48.122-S48.129 with 7th A, S48.912-S48.919 with 7th A, S48.922-S48.929 with 7th A, S51.002-S51.009 with 7th A, S51.012-S51.019 with 7th A, S51.022-S51.029 with 7th A, S51.032-S51.039 with 7th A, S51.042-S51.049 with 7th A, S51.052-S51.059 with 7th A, S51.802-S51.809 with 7th A, S51.812-S51.819 with 7th A, S51.822-S51.829 with 7th A, S51.832-S51.839 with 7th A, S51.842-S51.849 with 7th A, S51.852-S51.859 with 7th A, S56.022-S56.029A, S56.122A, S56.124A, S56.126A, S56.128-S56.129 with 7th A, S56.222-S56.229 with 7th A, S56.322-S56.329 with 7th A, S56.422A, S56.424A, S56.426 A, S56.428-S56.429 with 7th A, S56.522-S56.529 with 7th A, S56.822-S56.829 with 7th A, S56.922-S56.929 with 7th A, S58.012-S58.019 with 7th A, S58.022-S58.029 with 7th A, S58.112-S58.119 with 7th A, S58.122-S58.129 with 7th A, S58.912-S58.919 with 7th A, S58.922-S58.929 with 7th A, S61.002-S61.009 with 7th A, S61.012-S61.019 with 7th A, S61.022-S61.029 with 7th A, S61.032-S61.039 with 7th A, S61.042-S61.049 with 7th A, S61.052-S61.059 with 7th A, S61.102-S61.109 with 7th A, S61.112-S61.119 with 7th A, S61.122-S61.129 with 7th A, S61.132-S61.139 with 7th A, S61.142-S61.149 with 7th A, S61.152-S61.159 with 7th A, S61.201 with 7th A, S61.203A, S61.205A, S61.207-S61.209 with 7th A, S61.211A, S61.213A, S61.215A, S61.217-S61.219 with 7th A, S61.221A, S61.223A, S61.225A, S61.227-S61.229 with 7th A, S61.231A, S61.233A, S61.235A, S61.237-S61.239 with 7th A, S61.241A, S61.243A, S61.245A, S61.247-S61.249 with 7th A, S61.251A, S61.253A, S61.255A, S61.257-S61.259 with 7th A, S61.301A, S61.303A, S61.305A, S61.307-S61.309 with 7th A, S61.311A, S61.313A, S61.315A, S61.317-S61.319 with 7th A, S61.321A, S61.323A, S61.325A, S61.327-S61.329 with 7th A, S61.331A, S61.333A, S61.335A, S61.337-S61.339 with 7th A, S61.341 with 7th A, S61.343A, S61.345A, S61.347-S61.349 with 7th A, S61.351A, S61.353A, S61.355A, S61.357-S61.359 with 7th A, S61.402-S61.409 with 7th A, S61.412-S61.419 with 7th A, S61.422-S61.429 with 7th A, S61.432-S61.439 with 7th A, S61.442-S61.449 with 7th A, S61.452-S61.459 with 7th A, S61.502-S61.509 with 7th A, S61.512-S61.519 with 7th A, S61.522-S61.529 with 7th A, S61.532-S61.539 with 7th A, S61.542-S61.549 with 7th A, S61.552-S61.559 with 7th A, S66.022-S66.029 with 7th A, S66.121A, S66.123A, S66.125A, S66.127-S66.129 with 7th A, S66.222-S66.229 with 7th A, S66.321A, S66.323A, S66.325A, S66.327-S66.329 with 7th A, S66.422-S66.429 with 7th A, S66.521A, S66.523A, S66.525A, S66.527-S66.529 with 7th A, S66.822-S66.829 with 7th A, S66.922-S66.929 with 7th A, S68.012-S68.019 with 7th A, S68.022-S68.029 with 7th A, S68.111A, S68.113A, S68.115A, S68.117-S68.119 with 7th A, S68.121 A, S68.123A, S68.125A, S68.127-S68.129 with 7th A, S68.412-S68.419A, S68.422-S68.429 with 7th A, S68.512-S68.519 with 7th A, S68.522-S68.529 with 7th A, S68.611A, S68.613A, S68.615 with 7th A, S68.617-S68.619 with 7th A, S68.621A, S68.623A, S68.625A, S68.627-S68.629 with 7th A, S68.712-S68.719 with 7th A, S68.722-S68.729 with 7th A, T14.8-T14.91, T79.A0X-T79.9XX with 7th A

✓7th **S48.019 Complete traumatic amputation at unspecified shoulder joint** CC

CC Excl: CC with 7th character A: S41.001-S41.159 with 7th A, S46.021-S46.029 with 7th A, S46.121-S46.129 with 7th A, S46.221-S46.229 with 7th A, S46.321-S46.329 with 7th A, S46.821-S46.829 with 7th A, S46.921-S46.929 with 7th A, S48.011-S48.929 with 7th A, S51.001-S51.859 with 7th A, S56.021-S56.029 with 7th A, S56.121-S56.129 with 7th A, S56.221-S56.229 with 7th A, S56.321-S56.329 with 7th A, S56.421-S56.429 with 7th A, S56.521-S56.529 with 7th A, S56.821-S56.829 with 7th A, S56.921-S56.929 with 7th A, S58.011-S58.929 with 7th A, S61.001-S61.559 with 7th A, S66.021-S66.029 with 7th A, S66.120-S66.129 with 7th A, S66.221-S66.229 with 7th A, S66.320-S66.329 with 7th A, S66.421-S66.429 with 7th A, S66.520-S66.529 with 7th A, S66.821-S66.829 with 7th A, S66.921-S66.929 with 7th A, S68.011-S68.729 with 7th A, T14.8-T14.91, T79.A0X-T79.9XX with 7th A

✓6th **S48.02 Partial traumatic amputation at shoulder joint**

✓7th **S48.021 Partial traumatic amputation at right shoulder joint** CC

CC Excl: CC with 7th character A: See code: S48.011

✓7th **S48.022 Partial traumatic amputation at left shoulder joint** CC
CC Excl: CC with 7th character A: See code: S48.012

✓7th **S48.029 Partial traumatic amputation at unspecified shoulder joint** CC
CC Excl: CC with 7th character A: See code: S48.019

✓5th **S48.1 Traumatic amputation at level between shoulder and elbow**

✓6th **S48.11 Complete traumatic amputation at level between shoulder and elbow**

✓7th **S48.111 Complete traumatic amputation at level between right shoulder and elbow** CC
CC Excl: CC with 7th character A: See code: S48.011

✓7th **S48.112 Complete traumatic amputation at level between left shoulder and elbow** CC
CC Excl: CC with 7th character A: See code: S48.012

✓7th **S48.119 Complete traumatic amputation at level between unspecified shoulder and elbow** CC
CC Excl: CC with 7th character A: See code: S48.019

✓6th **S48.12 Partial traumatic amputation at level between shoulder and elbow**

✓7th **S48.121 Partial traumatic amputation at level between right shoulder and elbow**

✓7th **S48.122 Partial traumatic amputation at level between left shoulder and elbow**

✓7th **S48.129 Partial traumatic amputation at level between unspecified shoulder and elbow**

✓5th **S48.9 Traumatic amputation of shoulder and upper arm, level unspecified**

✓6th **S48.91 Complete traumatic amputation of shoulder and upper arm, level unspecified**

✓7th **S48.911 Complete traumatic amputation of right shoulder and upper arm, level unspecified** CC
CC Excl: CC with 7th character A: See code: S48.011

✓7th **S48.912 Complete traumatic amputation of left shoulder and upper arm, level unspecified** CC
CC Excl: CC with 7th character A: See code: S48.012

✓7th **S48.919 Complete traumatic amputation of unspecified shoulder and upper arm, level unspecified** CC
CC Excl: CC with 7th character A: See code: S48.019

✓6th **S48.92 Partial traumatic amputation of shoulder and upper arm, level unspecified**

✓7th **S48.921 Partial traumatic amputation of right shoulder and upper arm, level unspecified** CC
CC Excl: CC with 7th character A: See code: S48.011

✓7th **S48.922 Partial traumatic amputation of left shoulder and upper arm, level unspecified** CC
CC Excl: CC with 7th character A: See code: S48.012

✓7th **S48.929 Partial traumatic amputation of unspecified shoulder and upper arm, level unspecified** CC
CC Excl: CC with 7th character A: See code: S48.019

✓4th **S49 Other and unspecified injuries of shoulder and upper arm**

The appropriate 7th is to be added to each code from subcategories S49.0 and S49.1.
- A initial encounter for closed fracture
- D subsequent encounter for fracture with routine healing
- G subsequent encounter for fracture with delayed healing
- K subsequent encounter for fracture with nonunion
- P subsequent encounter for fracture with malunion
- S sequela

✓5th **S49.0 Physeal fracture of upper end of humerus**

✓6th **S49.00 Unspecified physeal fracture of upper end of humerus**

7 ✓7th **S49.001 Unspecified physeal fracture of upper end of humerus, right arm** CC
CC Excl: CC with 7th character A: S42.201-S42.271 with 7th [A, B], S42.279-S42.311 with 7th A, S42.319-S42.481 with 7th A, S42.489-S42.92X with 7th A, S49.001A, S49.009-S49.011 with 7th A, S49.019-S49.021 with 7th A, S49.029-S49.031 with 7th A, S49.039-S49.041 with 7th A, S49.049-S49.091 with 7th A, S49.099-S49.101 with 7th A, S49.109-S49.111 with 7th A, S49.119-S49.121 with 7th A, S49.129-S49.131 with 7th A, S49.139-S49.141 A, S49.149-S49.191 with 7th A, S49.199A
CC with 7th character K or P: M80.00X-M84.68X with 7th [K, P], S02.0XX-S02.92X with 7th K, S12.000-S12.691 with 7th K, S22.000-S22.9XX with 7th K, S32.000-S32.9XX with 7th K, S42.001-S42.92X with 7th [K, P], S49.001-S49.199 with 7th [K, P], S52.001-S52.92X with 7th [K, M, N, P, Q, R], S59.001-S59.299 with 7th [K, P], S62.001-S62.92X with 7th [K, P], S72.001-S72.92X with 7th [K, M, N, P, Q, R], S79.001-S79.199 with 7th [K, P], S82.001-S82.92X with 7th [K, M, N, P, Q, R], S89.001-S89.399 with 7th [K, P], S92.001-S92.919 with 7th [K, P]

7 ✓7th **S49.002 Unspecified physeal fracture of upper end of humerus, left arm** CC
CC Excl: CC with 7th character A: S42.201-S42.266 with 7th B, S42.272-S42.309 with 7th A, S42.312-S42.476 with 7th A, S42.482-S42.92X with 7th A, S49.002-S49.009 with 7th A, S49.012-S49.019 with 7th A, S49.022-S49.029 with 7th A, S49.032-S49.039 with 7th A, S49.042-S49.049 with 7th A, S49.092-S49.099 with 7th A, S49.102-S49.109 with 7th A, S49.112-S49.119 with 7th A, S49.122-S49.129 with 7th A, S49.132-S49.139 with 7th A, S49.142-S49.149 with 7th A, S49.192-S49.199 with 7th A
CC with 7th character K or P: M80.00X-M84.68X with 7th [K, P], S02.0XX-S02.92X with 7th K, S12.000-S12.691 with 7th K, S22.000-S22.9XX with 7th K, S32.000-S32.9XX with 7th K, S42.001-S42.92X with 7th [K, P], S49.001-S49.199 with 7th [K, P], S52.001-S52.92X with 7th [K, M, N, P, Q, R], S59.001-S59.299 with 7th [K, P], S62.001-S62.92X with 7th [K, P], S72.001-S72.92X with 7th [K, M, N, P, Q, R], S79.001-S79.199 with 7th [K, P], S82.001-S82.92X with 7th [K, M, N, P, Q, R], S89.001-S89.399 with 7th [K, P], S92.001-S92.919 with 7th [K, P]

7 ✓7th **S49.009 Unspecified physeal fracture of upper end of humerus, unspecified arm** CC
CC Excl: CC with 7th character A: S42.201-S42.92X with 7th [A, B], S49.001-S49.199 with 7th A
CC with 7th character K or P: M80.00X-M84.68X with 7th [K, P], S02.0XX-S02.92X with 7th K, S12.000-S12.691 with 7th K, S22.000-S22.9XX with 7th K, S32.000-S32.9XX with 7th K, S42.001-S42.92X with 7th [K, P], S49.001-S49.199 with 7th [K, P], S52.001-S52.92X with 7th [K, M, N, P, Q, R], S59.001-S59.299 with 7th [K, P], S62.001-S62.92X with 7th [K, P], S72.001-S72.92X with 7th [K, M, N, P, Q, R], S79.001-S79.199 with 7th [K, P], S82.001-S82.92X with 7th [K, M, N, P, Q, R], S89.001-S89.399 with 7th [K, P], S92.001-S92.919 with 7th [K, P]

7 HAC = Initial encounter only (7th character A, B or C) and not POA.

✓6th **S49.01 Salter-Harris Type I physeal fracture of upper end of humerus**

7 ✓7th **S49.011 Salter-Harris Type I physeal fracture of upper end of humerus, right arm** CC
CC Excl: See code: S49.001

7 ✓7th **S49.012 Salter-Harris Type I physeal fracture of upper end of humerus, left arm** CC
CC Excl: See code: S49.002

7 ✓7th **S49.019 Salter-Harris Type I physeal fracture of upper end of humerus, unspecified arm** CC
CC Excl: See code: S49.009

✓6th **S49.02 Salter-Harris Type II physeal fracture of upper end of humerus**

7 ✓7th **S49.021 Salter-Harris Type II physeal fracture of upper end of humerus, right arm** CC
CC Excl: See code: S49.001

7 ✓7th **S49.022 Salter-Harris Type II physeal fracture of upper end of humerus, left arm** CC
CC Excl: See code: S49.002

7 ✓7th **S49.029 Salter-Harris Type II physeal fracture of upper end of humerus, unspecified arm** CC
CC Excl: See code: S49.009

✓6th **S49.03 Salter-Harris Type III physeal fracture of upper end of humerus**

7 ✓7th **S49.031 Salter Harris Type III physeal fracture of upper end of humerus, right arm** CC
CC Excl: See code: S49.001

7 ✓7th **S49.032 Salter Harris Type III physeal fracture of upper end of humerus, left arm** CC
CC Excl: See code: S49.002

7 ✓7th **S49.039 Salter Harris Type III physeal fracture of upper end of humerus, unspecified arm** CC
CC Excl: See code: S49.009

✓6th **S49.04 Salter-Harris Type IV physeal fracture of upper end of humerus**

7 ✓7th **S49.041 Salter-Harris Type IV physeal fracture of upper end of humerus, right arm** CC
CC Excl: See code: S49.001

7 ✓7th **S49.042 Salter-Harris Type IV physeal fracture of upper end of humerus, left arm** CC
CC Excl: See code: S49.002

7 ✓7th **S49.049 Salter-Harris Type IV physeal fracture of upper end of humerus, unspecified arm** CC
CC Excl: See code: S49.009

✓6th **S49.09 Other physeal fracture of upper end of humerus**

7 ✓7th **S49.091 Other physeal fracture of upper end of humerus, right arm** CC
CC Excl: See code: S49.001

7 ✓7th **S49.092 Other physeal fracture of upper end of humerus, left arm** CC
CC Excl: See code: S49.002

7 ✓7th **S49.099 Other physeal fracture of upper end of humerus, unspecified arm** CC
CC Excl: See code: S49.009

✓5th **S49.1 Physeal fracture of lower end of humerus**

✓6th **S49.10 Unspecified physeal fracture of lower end of humerus**

7 ✓7th **S49.101 Unspecified physeal fracture of lower end of humerus, right arm** CC
CC Excl: See code: S49.001

7 ✓7th **S49.102 Unspecified physeal fracture of lower end of humerus, left arm** CC
CC Excl: See code: S49.002

7 ✓7th **S49.109 Unspecified physeal fracture of lower end of humerus, unspecified arm** CC
CC Excl: See code: S49.009

✓6th **S49.11 Salter-Harris Type I physeal fracture of lower end of humerus**

7 ✓7th **S49.111 Salter-Harris Type I physeal fracture of lower end of humerus, right arm** CC
CC Excl: See code: S49.001

7 ✓7th **S49.112 Salter-Harris Type I physeal fracture of lower end of humerus, left arm** CC
CC Excl: See code: S49.002

7 ✓7th **S49.119 Salter-Harris Type I physeal fracture of lower end of humerus, unspecified arm** CC
CC Excl: See code: S49.009

✓6th **S49.12 Salter-Harris Type II physeal fracture of lower end of humerus**

7 ✓7th **S49.121 Salter-Harris Type II physeal fracture of lower end of humerus, right arm** CC
CC Excl: See code: S49.001

7 ✓7th **S49.122 Salter-Harris Type II physeal fracture of lower end of humerus, left arm** CC
CC Excl: See code: S49.002

7 ✓7th **S49.129 Salter-Harris Type II physeal fracture of lower end of humerus, unspecified arm** CC
CC Excl: See code: S49.009

✓6th **S49.13 Salter Harris Type III physeal fracture of lower end of humerus**

7 ✓7th **S49.131 Salter Harris Type III physeal fracture of lower end of humerus, right arm** CC
CC Excl: See code: S49.001

7 ✓7th **S49.132 Salter Harris Type III physeal fracture of lower end of humerus, left arm** CC
CC Excl: See code: S49.002

7 ✓7th **S49.139 Salter Harris Type III physeal fracture of lower end of humerus, unspecified arm** CC
CC Excl: See code: S49.009

✓6th **S49.14 Salter-Harris Type IV physeal fracture of lower end of humerus**

7 ✓7th **S49.141 Salter-Harris Type IV physeal fracture of lower end of humerus, right arm** CC
CC Excl: See code: S49.001

7 ✓7th **S49.142 Salter-Harris Type IV physeal fracture of lower end of humerus, left arm** CC
CC Excl: See code: S49.002

7 ✓7th **S49.149 Salter-Harris Type IV physeal fracture of lower end of humerus, unspecified arm** CC
CC Excl: See code: S49.009

✓6th **S49.19 Other physeal fracture of lower end of humerus**

7 ✓7th **S49.191 Other physeal fracture of lower end of humerus, right arm** CC
CC Excl: See code: S49.001

7 ✓7th **S49.192 Other physeal fracture of lower end of humerus, left arm** CC
CC Excl: See code: S49.002

7 ✓7th **S49.199 Other physeal fracture of lower end of humerus, unspecified arm** CC
CC Excl: See code: S49.009

✓5th **S49.8 Other specified injuries of shoulder and upper arm**

The appropriate 7th is to be added to each code in subcategory S49.8.
A initial encounter
D subsequent encounter
S sequela

✓x7th **S49.80 Other specified injuries of shoulder and upper arm, unspecified arm**

✓x7th **S49.81 Other specified injuries of right shoulder and upper arm**

✓x7th **S49.82 Other specified injuries of left shoulder and upper arm**

✓5th **S49.9 Unspecified injury of shoulder and upper arm**

The appropriate 7th is to be added to each code in subcategory S49.9.
A initial encounter
D subsequent encounter
S sequela

✓x7th **S49.90 Unspecified injury of shoulder and upper arm, unspecified arm**

✓x7th **S49.91 Unspecified injury of right shoulder and upper arm**

✓x7th **S49.92 Unspecified injury of left shoulder and upper arm**

7 HAC = Initial encounter only (7th character A, B or C) and not POA.

Injuries to the elbow and forearm (S50-S59)

EXCLUDES 2 *burns and corrosions (T20-T32)*
frostbite (T33-T34)
injuries of wrist and hand (S60-S69)
insect bite or sting, venomous (T63.4)

4th S50 Superficial injury of elbow and forearm

EXCLUDES 2 *superficial injury of wrist and hand (S60.-)*

The appropriate 7th is to be added to each code from category S50.
A initial encounter
D subsequent encounter
S sequela

- 5th **S50.0 Contusion of elbow**
  - x7th **S50.00 Contusion of unspecified elbow**
  - x7th **S50.01 Contusion of right elbow**
  - x7th **S50.02 Contusion of left elbow**
- 5th **S50.1 Contusion of forearm**
  - x7th **S50.10 Contusion of unspecified forearm**
  - x7th **S50.11 Contusion of right forearm**
  - x7th **S50.12 Contusion of left forearm**
- 5th **S50.3 Other superficial injuries of elbow**
  - 6th **S50.31 Abrasion of elbow**
    - 7th **S50.311 Abrasion of right elbow**
    - 7th **S50.312 Abrasion of left elbow**
    - 7th **S50.319 Abrasion of unspecified elbow**
  - 6th **S50.32 Blister (nonthermal) of elbow**
    - 7th **S50.321 Blister (nonthermal) of right elbow**
    - 7th **S50.322 Blister (nonthermal) of left elbow**
    - 7th **S50.329 Blister (nonthermal) of unspecified elbow**
  - 6th **S50.34 External constriction of elbow**
    - 7th **S50.341 External constriction of right elbow**
    - 7th **S50.342 External constriction of left elbow**
    - 7th **S50.349 External constriction of unspecified elbow**
  - 6th **S50.35 Superficial foreign body of elbow**
    Splinter in the elbow
    - 7th **S50.351 Superficial foreign body of right elbow**
    - 7th **S50.352 Superficial foreign body of left elbow**
    - 7th **S50.359 Superficial foreign body of unspecified elbow**
  - 6th **S50.36 Insect bite (nonvenomous) of elbow**
    - 7th **S50.361 Insect bite (nonvenomous) of right elbow**
    - 7th **S50.362 Insect bite (nonvenomous) of left elbow**
    - 7th **S50.369 Insect bite (nonvenomous) of unspecified elbow**
  - 6th **S50.37 Other superficial bite of elbow**
    EXCLUDES 1 *open bite of elbow (S51.04)*
    - 7th **S50.371 Other superficial bite of right elbow**
    - 7th **S50.372 Other superficial bite of left elbow**
    - 7th **S50.379 Other superficial bite of unspecified elbow**
- 5th **S50.8 Other superficial injuries of forearm**
  - 6th **S50.81 Abrasion of forearm**
    - 7th **S50.811 Abrasion of right forearm**
    - 7th **S50.812 Abrasion of left forearm**
    - 7th **S50.819 Abrasion of unspecified forearm**
  - 6th **S50.82 Blister (nonthermal) of forearm**
    - 7th **S50.821 Blister (nonthermal) of right forearm**
    - 7th **S50.822 Blister (nonthermal) of left forearm**
    - 7th **S50.829 Blister (nonthermal) of unspecified forearm**
  - 6th **S50.84 External constriction of forearm**
    - 7th **S50.841 External constriction of right forearm**
    - 7th **S50.842 External constriction of left forearm**
    - 7th **S50.849 External constriction of unspecified forearm**
  - 6th **S50.85 Superficial foreign body of forearm**
    Splinter in the forearm
    - 7th **S50.851 Superficial foreign body of right forearm**
    - 7th **S50.852 Superficial foreign body of left forearm**
    - 7th **S50.859 Superficial foreign body of unspecified forearm**
  - 6th **S50.86 Insect bite (nonvenomous) of forearm**
    - 7th **S50.861 Insect bite (nonvenomous) of right forearm**
    - 7th **S50.862 Insect bite (nonvenomous) of left forearm**
    - 7th **S50.869 Insect bite (nonvenomous) of unspecified forearm**
  - 6th **S50.87 Other superficial bite of forearm**
    EXCLUDES 1 *open bite of forearm (S51.84)*
    - 7th **S50.871 Other superficial bite of right forearm**
    - 7th **S50.872 Other superficial bite of left forearm**
    - 7th **S50.879 Other superficial bite of unspecified forearm**
- 5th **S50.9 Unspecified superficial injury of elbow and forearm**
  - 6th **S50.90 Unspecified superficial injury of elbow**
    - 7th **S50.901 Unspecified superficial injury of right elbow**
    - 7th **S50.902 Unspecified superficial injury of left elbow**
    - 7th **S50.909 Unspecified superficial injury of unspecified elbow**
  - 6th **S50.91 Unspecified superficial injury of forearm**
    - 7th **S50.911 Unspecified superficial injury of right forearm**
    - 7th **S50.912 Unspecified superficial injury of left forearm**
    - 7th **S50.919 Unspecified superficial injury of unspecified forearm**

4th S51 Open wound of elbow and forearm

Code also any associated wound infection

EXCLUDES 1 *open fracture of elbow and forearm (S52- with open fracture 7th character)*
traumatic amputation of elbow and forearm (S58.-)

EXCLUDES 2 *open wound of wrist and hand (S61.-)*

The appropriate 7th is to be added to each code from category S51.
A initial encounter
D subsequent encounter
S sequela

- 5th **S51.0 Open wound of elbow**
  - 6th **S51.00 Unspecified open wound of elbow**
    - 7th **S51.001 Unspecified open wound of right elbow**
      AHA: 2012, 4Q, 108
    - 7th **S51.002 Unspecified open wound of left elbow**
    - 7th **S51.009 Unspecified open wound of unspecified elbow**
      Open wound of elbow NOS
  - 6th **S51.01 Laceration without foreign body of elbow**
    - 7th **S51.011 Laceration without foreign body of right elbow**
    - 7th **S51.012 Laceration without foreign body of left elbow**
    - 7th **S51.019 Laceration without foreign body of unspecified elbow**
  - 6th **S51.02 Laceration with foreign body of elbow**
    - 7th **S51.021 Laceration with foreign body of right elbow**
    - 7th **S51.022 Laceration with foreign body of left elbow**
    - 7th **S51.029 Laceration with foreign body of unspecified elbow**
  - 6th **S51.03 Puncture wound without foreign body of elbow**
    - 7th **S51.031 Puncture wound without foreign body of right elbow**
    - 7th **S51.032 Puncture wound without foreign body of left elbow**
    - 7th **S51.039 Puncture wound without foreign body of unspecified elbow**
  - 6th **S51.04 Puncture wound with foreign body of elbow**
    - 7th **S51.041 Puncture wound with foreign body of right elbow**
    - 7th **S51.042 Puncture wound with foreign body of left elbow**

S51.049 **Puncture wound with foreign body of unspecified elbow**

S51.05 Open bite of elbow
Bite of elbow NOS
EXCLUDES 1 *superficial bite of elbow (S50.36, S50.37)*

S51.051 **Open bite, right elbow**
S51.052 **Open bite, left elbow**
S51.059 **Open bite, unspecified elbow**

S51.8 **Open wound of forearm**
EXCLUDES 2 *open wound of elbow (S51.0-)*

S51.80 Unspecified open wound of forearm
S51.801 **Unspecified open wound of right forearm**
S51.802 **Unspecified open wound of left forearm**
S51.809 **Unspecified open wound of unspecified forearm**
Open wound of forearm NOS

S51.81 Laceration without foreign body of forearm
S51.811 **Laceration without foreign body of right forearm**
S51.812 **Laceration without foreign body of left forearm**
S51.819 **Laceration without foreign body of unspecified forearm**

S51.82 Laceration with foreign body of forearm
S51.821 **Laceration with foreign body of right forearm**
S51.822 **Laceration with foreign body of left forearm**
S51.829 **Laceration with foreign body of unspecified forearm**

S51.83 Puncture wound without foreign body of forearm
S51.831 **Puncture wound without foreign body of right forearm**
S51.832 **Puncture wound without foreign body of left forearm**
S51.839 **Puncture wound without foreign body of unspecified forearm**

S51.84 Puncture wound with foreign body of forearm
S51.841 **Puncture wound with foreign body of right forearm**
S51.842 **Puncture wound with foreign body of left forearm**
S51.849 **Puncture wound with foreign body of unspecified forearm**

S51.85 Open bite of forearm
Bite of forearm NOS
EXCLUDES 1 *superficial bite of forearm (S50.86, S50.87)*

S51.851 **Open bite of right forearm**
S51.852 **Open bite of left forearm**
S51.859 **Open bite of unspecified forearm**

S52 Fracture of forearm

NOTE A fracture not indicated as displaced or nondisplaced should be coded to displaced.
A fracture not indicated as open or closed should be coded to closed.
The open fracture designations are based on the Gustilo open fracture classification.

EXCLUDES 1 *traumatic amputation of forearm (S58.-)*
EXCLUDES 2 *fracture at wrist and hand level (S62.-)*

The appropriate 7th is to be added to all codes from category S52 [unless otherwise indicated].
- A initial encounter for closed fracture
- B initial encounter for open fracture type I or II
  initial encounter for open fracture NOS
- C initial encounter for open fracture type IIIA, IIIB, or IIIC
- D subsequent encounter for closed fracture with routine healing
- E subsequent encounter for open fracture type I or II with routine healing
- F subsequent encounter for open fracture type IIIA, IIIB, or IIIC with routine healing
- G subsequent encounter for closed fracture with delayed healing
- H subsequent encounter for open fracture type I or II with delayed healing
- J subsequent encounter for open fracture type IIIA, IIIB, or IIIC with delayed healing
- K subsequent encounter for closed fracture with nonunion
- M subsequent encounter for open fracture type I or II with nonunion
- N subsequent encounter for open fracture type IIIA, IIIB, or IIIC with nonunion
- P subsequent encounter for closed fracture with malunion
- Q subsequent encounter for open fracture type I or II with malunion
- R subsequent encounter for open fracture type IIIA, IIIB, or IIIC with malunion
- S sequela

S52.0 **Fracture of upper end of ulna**
Fracture of proximal end of ulna
EXCLUDES 2 *fracture of elbow NOS (S42.40-)*
fractures of shaft of ulna (S52.2-)

S52.00 Unspecified fracture of upper end of ulna
CC Excl: For CC/MCC codes in subcatagory S52.00:
MCC with 7th character B or C: S52.001-S52.009 with 7th [B, C], S52.021-S52.109 with 7th [B, C], S52.121-S52.516 with 7th [B, C], S52.531-S52.616 with 7th [A, B, C], S52.691-S52.92X with 7th [A, B, C], S59.001-S59.099 with 7th A, S59.201-S59.299 with 7th A, S62.90XB
CC with 7th character K, M, N, P, Q, or R: M80.00X-M84.68X with 7th [K, P], S02.0XX-S02.92X with 7th K, S12.000-S12.691 with 7th K, S22.000-S22.9XX with 7th K, S32.000-S32.9XX with 7th K, S42.001-S42.92X with 7th [K, P], S49.001-S49.199 with 7th [K, P], S52.001-S52.92X with 7th [K, M, N, P, Q, R], S59.001-S59.299 with 7th [K, P], S62.001-S62.92X with 7th [K, P], S72.001-S72.92X with 7th [K, M, N, P, Q, R], S79.001-S79.199 with 7th [K, P], S82.001-S82.92X with 7th [K, M, N, P, Q, R], S89.001-S89.399 with 7th [K, P], S92.001-S92.919 with 7th [K, P]

7 S52.001 **Unspecified fracture of upper end of right ulna** MCC CC
7 S52.002 **Unspecified fracture of upper end of left ulna** MCC CC
7 S52.009 **Unspecified fracture of upper end of unspecified ulna** MCC CC

7 HAC = Initial encounter only (7th character A, B or C) and not POA.

✓6th **S52.01 Torus fracture of upper end of ulna**

The appropriate 7th is to be added to all codes in subcategory S52.01.
- A initial encounter for closed fracture
- D subsequent encounter for fracture with routine healing
- G subsequent encounter for fracture with delayed healing
- K subsequent encounter for fracture with nonunion
- P subsequent encounter for fracture with malunion
- S sequela

7 ✓7th **S52.011 Torus fracture of upper end of right ulna** CC

CC Excl: CC with 7th character A: S52.001-S52.011 with 7th [A, B, C], S52.019-S52.111 with 7th A, S52.119-S52.211 with 7th A, S52.219-S52.311 with 7th A, S52.319-S52.521 with 7th A, S52.529-S52.621 with 7th A, S52.629-S52.92X with 7th A, S59.001A, S59.009-S59.011 with 7th A, S59.019-S59.021 with 7th A, S59.029-S59.031 with 7th A, S59.039-S59.041 with 7th A, S59.049-S59.091 with 7th A, S59.099-S59.101 with 7th A, S59.109-S59.111 with 7th A, S59.119-S59.121 with 7th A, S59.129-S59.131 with 7th A, S59.139-S59.141 with 7th A, S59.149-S59.191 with 7th A, S59.199-S59.201 with 7th A, S59.209-S59.211 with 7th A, S59.219-S59.221 with 7th A, S59.229-S59.231 with 7th A, S59.239-S59.241 with 7th A, S59.249-S59.291 with 7th A, S59.299A

CC with 7th character K or P: M80.00X-M84.68X with 7th [K, P], S02.0XX-S02.92X with 7th K, S12.000-S12.691 with 7th K, S22.000-S22.9XX with 7th K, S32.000-S32.9XX with 7th K, S42.001-S42.92X with 7th [K, P], S49.001-S49.199 with 7th [K, P], S52.001-S52.92X with 7th [K, M, N, P, Q, R], S59.001-S59.299 with 7th [K, P], S62.001-S62.92X with 7th [K, P], S72.001-S72.92X with 7th [K, M, N, P, Q, R], S79.001-S79.199 with 7th [K, P], S82.001-S82.92X with 7th [K, M, N, P, Q, R], S89.001-S89.399 with 7th [K, P], S92.001-S92.919 with 7th [K, P]

7 ✓7th **S52.012 Torus fracture of upper end of left ulna** CC

CC Excl: CC with 7th character A: S52.001-S52.009 with 7th [B, C], S52.012-S52.109 with 7th A, S52.112-S52.209 with 7th A, S52.212-S52.309 with 7th A, S52.312-S52.516 with 7th A, S52.522-S52.616 with 7th A, S52.622-S52.92X with 7th A, S59.002-S59.009 with 7th A, S59.012-S59.019 with 7th A, S59.022-S59.029 with 7th A, S59.032-S59.039 with 7th A, S59.042-S59.049 with 7th A, S59.092-S59.099 with 7th A, S59.102-S59.109 with 7th A, S59.112-S59.119 with 7th A, S59.122-S59.129 with 7th A, S59.132-S59.139 with 7th A, S59.142-S59.149 with 7th A, S59.192-S59.199 with 7th A, S59.202-S59.209 with 7th A, S59.212-S59.219 with 7th A, S59.222-S59.229 with 7th A, S59.232-S59.239 with 7th A, S59.242-S59.249 with 7th A, S59.292-S59.299 with 7th A

CC with 7th character K or P: M80.00X-M84.68X with 7th [K, P], S02.0XX-S02.92X with 7th K, S12.000-S12.691 with 7th K, S22.000-S22.9XX with 7th K, S32.000-S32.9XX with 7th K, S42.001-S42.92X with 7th [K, P], S49.001-S49.199 with 7th [K, P], S52.001-S52.92X with 7th [K, M, N, P, Q, R], S59.001-S59.299 with 7th [K, P], S62.001-S62.92X with 7th [K, P], S72.001-S72.92X with 7th [K, M, N, P, Q, R], S79.001-S79.199 with 7th [K, P], S82.001-S82.92X with 7th [K, M, N, P, Q, R], S89.001-S89.399 with 7th [K, P], S92.001-S92.919 with 7th [K, P]

7 ✓7th **S52.019 Torus fracture of upper end of unspecified ulna** CC

CC Excl: CC with 7th character A: S52.001-S52.92X with 7th [A, B, C], S59.001-S59.299 with 7th A

CC with 7th character K or P: M80.00X-M84.68X with 7th [K, P], S02.0XX-S02.92X with 7th K, S12.000-S12.691 with 7th K, S22.000-S22.9XX with 7th K, S32.000-S32.9XX with 7th K, S42.001-S42.92X with 7th [K, P], S49.001-S49.199 with 7th [K, P], S52.001-S52.92X with 7th [K, M, N, P, Q, R], S59.001-S59.299 with 7th [K, P], S62.001-S62.92X with 7th [K, P], S72.001-S72.92X with 7th [K, M, N, P, Q, R], S79.001-S79.199 with 7th [K, P], S82.001-S82.92X with 7th [K, M, N, P, Q, R], S89.001-S89.399 with 7th [K, P], S92.001-S92.919 with 7th [K, P]

✓6th **S52.02 Fracture of olecranon process without intraarticular extension of ulna**

CC Excl: For CC/MCC codes in subcatagory S52.02,unless otherwise noted: MCC with 7th character B or C: S52.001-S52.009 with 7th [B, C], S52.021-S52.109 with 7th [B, C], S52.121-S52.516 with 7th [B, C], S52.531-S52.616 with 7th [B, C], S52.691-S52.92X with 7th [A, B, C], S59.001-S59.099 with 7th A, S59.201-S59.299 with 7th A, S62.90XB

CC with 7th character K, M, N, P, Q, or R: M80.00X-M84.68X with 7th [K, P], S02.0XX-S02.92X with 7th K, S12.000-S12.691 with 7th K, S22.000-S22.9XX with 7th K, S32.000-S32.9XX with 7th K, S42.001-S42.92X with 7th [K, P], S49.001-S49.199 with 7th [K, P], S52.001-S52.92X with 7th [K, M, N, P, Q, R], S59.001-S59.299 with 7th [K, P], S62.001-S62.92X with 7th [K, P], S72.001-S72.92X with 7th [K, M, N, P, Q, R], S79.001-S79.199 with 7th [K, P], S82.001-S82.92X with 7th [K, M, N, P, Q, R], S89.001-S89.399 with 7th [K, P], S92.001-S92.919 with 7th [K, P]

7 ✓7th **S52.021 Displaced fracture of olecranon process without intraarticular extension of right ulna** MCC CC

7 ✓7th **S52.022 Displaced fracture of olecranon process without intraarticular extension of left ulna** MCC CC

7 ✓7th **S52.023 Displaced fracture of olecranon process without intraarticular extension of unspecified ulna** MCC CC

7 ✓7th **S52.024 Nondisplaced fracture of olecranon process without intraarticular extension of right ulna** MCC CC

7 ✓7th **S52.025 Nondisplaced fracture of olecranon process without intraarticular extension of left ulna** MCC CC

7 ✓7th **S52.026 Nondisplaced fracture of olecranon process without intraarticular extension of unspecified ulna** MCC CC

✓6th **S52.03 Fracture of olecranon process with intraarticular extension of ulna**

CC Excl: For CC/MCC codes in subcatagory S52.03, unless otherwise noted: MCC with 7th character B or C: S52.001-S52.009 with 7th [B, C], S52.021-S52.109 with 7th [B, C], S52.121-S52.516 with 7th [B, C], S52.531-S52.616 with 7th [B, C], S52.691-S52.92 with 7th [A, B, C], S59.001-S59.099 with 7th A, S59.201-S59.299 with 7th A, S62.90X with 7th B

CC with 7th character K, M, N, P, Q, or R: M80.00X-M84.68X with 7th [K, P], S02.0XX-S02.92X with 7th K, S12.000-S12.691 with 7th K, S22.000-S22.9XX with 7th K, S32.000-S32.9XX with 7th K, S42.001-S42.92X with 7th [K, P], S49.001-S49.199 with 7th [K, P], S52.001-S52.92X with 7th [K, M, N, P, Q, R], S59.001-S59.299 with 7th [K, P], S62.001-S62.92X with 7th [K, P], S72.001-S72.92X with 7th [K, M, N, P, Q, R], S79.001-S79.199 with 7th [K, P], S82.001-S82.92X with 7th [K, M, N, P, Q, R], S89.001-S89.399 with 7th [K, P], S92.001-S92.919 with 7th [K, P]

7 ✓7th **S52.031 Displaced fracture of olecranon process with intraarticular extension of right ulna** MCC CC

7 HAC = Initial encounter only (7th character A, B or C) and not POA.

7 ✓7th **S52.032 Displaced fracture of olecranon process with intraarticular extension of left ulna** MCC CC

7 ✓7th **S52.033 Displaced fracture of olecranon process with intraarticular extension of unspecified ulna** MCC CC

7 ✓7th **S52.034 Nondisplaced fracture of olecranon process with intraarticular extension of right ulna** MCC CC

7 ✓7th **S52.035 Nondisplaced fracture of olecranon process with intraarticular extension of left ulna** MCC CC

7 ✓7th **S52.036 Nondisplaced fracture of olecranon process with intraarticular extension of unspecified ulna** MCC CC

✓6th **S52.04 Fracture of coronoid process of ulna**

CC Excl: For CC/MCC codes in subcatagory S52.04, unless otherwise noted: MCC with 7th character B or C: S52.001-S52.009 with 7th [B, C], S52.021-S52.109 with 7th [B, C], S52.121-S52.516 with 7th [B, C], S52.531-S52.616 with 7th [A, B, C], S52.691-S52.92X with 7th [A, B, C], S59.001-S59.099 with 7th A, S59.201-S59.299 with 7th A, S62.90XB
CC with 7th character K, M, N, P, Q, or R: M80.00X-M84.68X with 7th [K, P], S02.0XX-S02.92X with 7th K, S12.000-S12.691 with 7th K, S22.000-S22.9XX with 7th K, S32.000-S32.9XX with 7th K, S42.001-S42.92X with 7th [K, P], S49.001-S49.199 with 7th [K, P], S52.001-S52.92X with 7th [K, M, N, P, Q, R], S59.001-S59.299 with 7th [K, P], S62.001-S62.92X with 7th [K, P], S72.001-S72.92X with 7th [K, M, N, P, Q, R], S79.001-S79.199 with 7th [K, P], S82.001-S82.92X with 7th [K, M, N, P, Q, R], S89.001-S89.399 with 7th [K, P], S92.001-S92.919 with 7th [K, P]

7 ✓7th **S52.041 Displaced fracture of coronoid process of right ulna** MCC CC

7 ✓7th **S52.042 Displaced fracture of coronoid process of left ulna** MCC CC

7 ✓7th **S52.043 Displaced fracture of coronoid process of unspecified ulna** MCC CC

7 ✓7th **S52.044 Nondisplaced fracture of coronoid process of right ulna** MCC CC

7 ✓7th **S52.045 Nondisplaced fracture of coronoid process of left ulna** MCC CC

7 ✓7th **S52.046 Nondisplaced fracture of coronoid process of unspecified ulna** MCC CC

✓6th **S52.09 Other fracture of upper end of ulna**

CC Excl: For CC/MCC codes in subcatagory S52.09, unless otherwise noted: MCC with 7th character B or C: S52.001-S52.009 with 7th [B, C], S52.021-S52.109 with 7th [B, C], S52.121-S52.516 with 7th [B, C], S52.531-S52.616 with 7th [A, B, C], S52.691-S52.92X with 7th [A, B, C], S59.001-S59.099 with 7th A, S59.201-S59.299 with 7th A, S62.90XB
CC with 7th character K, M, N, P, Q, or R: M80.00X-M84.68X with 7th [K, P], S02.0XX-S02.92X with 7th K, S12.000-S12.691 with 7th K, S22.000-S22.9XX with 7th K, S32.000-S32.9XX with 7th K, S42.001-S42.92X with 7th [K, P], S49.001-S49.199 with 7th [K, P], S52.001-S52.92X with 7th [K, M, N, P, Q, R], S59.001-S59.299 with 7th [K, P], S62.001-S62.92X with 7th [K, P], S72.001-S72.92X with 7th [K, M, N, P, Q, R], S79.001-S79.199 with 7th [K, P], S82.001-S82.92X with 7th [K, M, N, P, Q, R], S89.001-S89.399 with 7th [K, P], S92.001-S92.919 with 7th [K, P]

7 ✓7th **S52.091 Other fracture of upper end of right ulna** MCC CC

7 ✓7th **S52.092 Other fracture of upper end of left ulna** MCC CC

7 ✓7th **S52.099 Other fracture of upper end of unspecified ulna** MCC CC

✓5th **S52.1 Fracture of upper end of radius**
Fracture of proximal end of radius
EXCLUDES 2 *physeal fractures of upper end of radius (S59.2-)*
fracture of shaft of radius (S52.3-)

✓6th **S52.10 Unspecified fracture of upper end of radius**

CC Excl: For CC/MCC codes in subcatagory S52.10, unless otherwise noted: MCC with 7th character B or C: S52.001-S52.009 with 7th [B, C], S52.021-S52.109 with 7th [B, C], S52.121-S52.516 with 7th [B, C], S52.531-S52.616 with 7th [A, B, C], S52.691-S52.92X with 7th [A, B, C], S59.001-S59.099 with 7th A, S59.201-S59.299 with 7th A, S62.90XB
CC with 7th character K, M, N, P, Q, or R: M80.00X-M84.68X with 7th [K, P], S02.0XX-S02.92X with 7th K, S12.000-S12.691 with 7th K, S22.000-S22.9XX with 7th K, S32.000-S32.9XX with 7th K, S42.001-S42.92X with 7th [K, P], S49.001-S49.199 with 7th [K, P], S52.001-S52.92X with 7th [K, M, N, P, Q, R], S59.001-S59.299 with 7th [K, P], S62.001-S62.92X with 7th [K, P], S72.001-S72.92X with 7th [K, M, N, P, Q, R], S79.001-S79.199 with 7th [K, P], S82.001-S82.92X with 7th [K, M, N, P, Q, R], S89.001-S89.399 with 7th [K, P], S92.001-S92.919 with 7th [K, P]

7 ✓7th **S52.101 Unspecified fracture of upper end of right radius** MCC CC

7 ✓7th **S52.102 Unspecified fracture of upper end of left radius** MCC CC

7 ✓7th **S52.109 Unspecified fracture of upper end of unspecified radius** MCC CC

✓6th **S52.11 Torus fracture of upper end of radius**

The appropriate 7th is to be added to all codes in subcategory S52.11.
- A initial encounter for closed fracture
- D subsequent encounter for fracture with routine healing
- G subsequent encounter for fracture with delayed healing
- K subsequent encounter for fracture with nonunion
- P subsequent encounter for fracture with malunion
- S sequela

7 ✓7th **S52.111 Torus fracture of upper end of right radius** CC

CC Excl: CC with 7th character A: S52.001-S52.011 with 7th [A, B, C], S52.019-S52.111 with 7th A, S52.119-S52.211 with 7th A, S52.219-S52.311 with 7th A, S52.319-S52.521 with 7th A, S52.529-S52.621 with 7th A, S52.629-S52.92X with 7th A, S59.001 with 7th A, S59.009-S59.011 with 7th A, S59.019-S59.021 with 7th A, S59.029-S59.031 with 7th A, S59.039-S59.041 with 7th A, S59.049-S59.091 with 7th A, S59.099-S59.101 with 7th A, S59.109-S59.111 with 7th A, S59.119-S59.121 with 7th A, S59.129-S59.131 with 7th A, S59.139-S59.141 with 7th A, S59.149-S59.191 with 7th A, S59.199-S59.201 with 7th A, S59.209-S59.211 with 7th A, S59.219-S59.221 with 7th A, S59.229-S59.231 with 7th A, S59.239-S59.241 with 7th A, S59.249-S59.291 with 7th A, S59.299A
CC with 7th character K, P: M80.00X-M84.68X with 7th [K, P], S02.0XX-S02.92X with 7th K, S12.000-S12.691 with 7th K, S22.000-S22.9XX with 7th K, S32.000-S32.9XX with 7th K, S42.001-S42.92X with 7th [K, P], S49.001-S49.199 with 7th [K, P], S52.001-S52.92X with 7th [K, M, N, P, Q, R], S59.001-S59.299 with 7th [K, P], S62.001-S62.92X with 7th [K, P], S72.001-S72.92X with 7th [K, M, N, P, Q, R], S79.001-S79.199 with 7th [K, P], S82.001-S82.92X with 7th [K, M, N, P, Q, R], S89.001-S89.399 with 7th [K, P], S92.001-S92.919 with 7th [K, P]

7 HAC = Initial encounter only (7th character A, B or C) and not POA.

7 ✓7th **S52.112 Torus fracture of upper end of left radius** CC

CC Excl: CC with 7th character A: S52.001-S52.009 with 7th [B, C], S52.012-S52.109 with 7th A, S52.112-S52.209 with 7th A, S52.212-S52.309 with 7th A, S52.312-S52.516 with 7th A, S52.522-S52.616 with 7th A, S52.622-S52.92X with 7th A, S59.002-S59.009 with 7th A, S59.012-S59.019 with 7th A, S59.022-S59.029 with 7th A, S59.032-S59.039 with 7th A, S59.042-S59.049 with 7th A, S59.092-S59.099 with 7th A, S59.102-S59.109 with 7th A, S59.112-S59.119 with 7th A, S59.122-S59.129 with 7th A, S59.132-S59.139 with 7th A, S59.142-S59.149 with 7th A, S59.192-S59.199 with 7th A, S59.202-S59.209 with 7th A, S59.212-S59.219 with 7th A, S59.222-S59.229 with 7th A, S59.232-S59.239 with 7th A, S59.242-S59.249 with 7th A, S59.292-S59.299 with 7th A

CC with 7th character K or P: M80.00X-M84.68X with 7th [K, P], S02.0XX-S02.92X with 7th K, S12.000-S12.691 with 7th K, S22.000-S22.9XX with 7th K, S32.000-S32.9XX with 7th K, S42.001-S42.92X with 7th [K, P], S49.001-S49.199 with 7th [K, P], S52.001-S52.92X with 7th [K, M, N, P, Q, R], S59.001-S59.299 with 7th [K, P], S62.001-S62.92X with 7th [K, P], S72.001-S72.92X with 7th [K, M, N, P, Q, R], S79.001-S79.199 with 7th [K, P], S82.001-S82.92X with 7th [K, M, N, P, Q, R], S89.001-S89.399 with 7th [K, P], S92.001-S92.919 with 7th [K, P]

✓7th **S52.119 Torus fracture of upper end of unspecified radius** CC

CC Excl: CC with 7th character A: S52.001-S52.92X with 7th [A, B, C], S59.001-S59.299 with 7th A

CC Excl: CC with 7th character K or P: M80.00X-M84.68X with 7th [K, P], S02.0XX-S02.92X with 7th K, S12.000-S12.691 with 7th K, S22.000-S22.9XX with 7th K, S32.000-S32.9XX with 7th K, S42.001-S42.92X with 7th [K, P], S49.001-S49.199 with 7th [K, P], S52.001-S52.92X with 7th [K, M, N, P, Q, R], S59.001-S59.299 with 7th [K, P], S62.001-S62.92X with 7th [K, P], S72.001-S72.92X with 7th [K, M, N, P, Q, R], S79.001-S79.199 with 7th [K, P], S82.001-S82.92X with 7th [K, M, N, P, Q, R], S89.001-S89.399 with 7th [K, P], S92.001-S92.919 with 7th [K, P]

✓6th **S52.12 Fracture of head of radius**

CC Excl: For CC/MCC codes in subcatagory S52.12: See code: S52.10

7 ✓7th **S52.121 Displaced fracture of head of right radius** MCC CC

7 ✓7th **S52.122 Displaced fracture of head of left radius** MCC CC

7 ✓7th **S52.123 Displaced fracture of head of unspecified radius** MCC CC

7 ✓7th **S52.124 Nondisplaced fracture of head of right radius** MCC CC

7 ✓7th **S52.125 Nondisplaced fracture of head of left radius** MCC CC

7 ✓7th **S52.126 Nondisplaced fracture of head of unspecified radius** MCC CC

✓6th **S52.13 Fracture of neck of radius**

CC Excl: For CC/MCC codes in subcatagory S52.12: See code: S52.10

7 ✓7th **S52.131 Displaced fracture of neck of right radius** MCC CC

7 ✓7th **S52.132 Displaced fracture of neck of left radius** MCC CC

7 ✓7th **S52.133 Displaced fracture of neck of unspecified radius** MCC CC

7 ✓7th **S52.134 Nondisplaced fracture of neck of right radius** MCC CC

7 ✓7th **S52.135 Nondisplaced fracture of neck of left radius** MCC CC

7 ✓7th **S52.136 Nondisplaced fracture of neck of unspecified radius** MCC CC

✓6th **S52.18 Other fracture of upper end of radius**

CC Excl: For CC/MCC codes in subcatagory S52.12: See code: S52.10

7 ✓7th **S52.181 Other fracture of upper end of right radius** MCC CC

7 ✓7th **S52.182 Other fracture of upper end of left radius** MCC CC

7 ✓7th **S52.189 Other fracture of upper end of unspecified radius** MCC CC

✓5th **S52.2 Fracture of shaft of ulna**

✓6th **S52.20 Unspecified fracture of shaft of ulna**

Fracture of ulna NOS

7 ✓7th **S52.201 Unspecified fracture of shaft of right ulna** MCC CC

CC Excl: CC with 7th character A: S52.001-S52.011 with 7th [A, B, C], S52.019-S52.111 with 7th A, S52.119-S52.211 with 7th A, S52.219-S52.311 with 7th A, S52.319-S52.521 with 7th A, S52.529-S52.621 with 7th A, S52.629-S52.92X with 7th A, S59.001A, S59.009-S59.011 with 7th A, S59.019-S59.021 with 7th A, S59.029-S59.031 with 7th A, S59.039-S59.041 with 7th A, S59.049-S59.091 with 7th A, S59.099-S59.101 with 7th A, S59.109-S59.111 with 7th A, S59.119-S59.121 with 7th A, S59.129-S59.131 with 7th A, S59.139-S59.141 with 7th A, S59.149-S59.191 with 7th A, S59.199-S59.201 with 7th A, S59.209-S59.211 with 7th A, S59.219-S59.221 with 7th A, S59.229-S59.231 with 7th A, S59.239-S59.241 with 7th A, S59.249-S59.291 with 7th A, S59.299A

MCC with 7th character B or C: S52.001-S52.009 with 7th [B, C], S52.021-S52.109 with 7th [B, C], S52.121-S52.516 with 7th [B, C], S52.531-S52.616 with 7th [A, B, C], S52.691-S52.92X with 7th [A, B, C], S59.001-S59.099 with 7th A, S59.201-S59.299 with 7th A, S62.90XB

MCC with 7th character K, M, N, P, Q or R: M80.00X-M84.68X with 7th [K, P], S02.0XX-S02.92X with 7th K, S12.000-S12.691 with 7th K, S22.000-S22.9XX with 7th K, S32.000-S32.9XX with 7th K, S42.001-S42.92X with 7th [K, P], S49.001-S49.199 with 7th [K, P], S52.001-S52.92X with 7th [K, M, N, P, Q, R], S59.001-S59.299 with 7th [K, P], S62.001-S62.92X with 7th [K, P], S72.001-S72.92X with 7th [K, M, N, P, Q, R], S79.001-S79.199 with 7th [K, P], S82.001-S82.92X with 7th [K, M, N, P, Q, R], S89.001-S89.399 with 7th [K, P], S92.001-S92.919 with 7th [K, P]

7 ✓7th **S52.202 Unspecified fracture of shaft of left ulna** MCC CC

CC Excl: CC with 7th character A: S52.001-S52.009 with 7th [B, C], S52.012-S52.109 with 7th A, S52.112-S52.209 with 7th A, S52.212-S52.309 with 7th A, S52.312-S52.516 with 7th A, S52.522-S52.616 with 7th A, S52.622-S52.92X with 7th A, S59.002-S59.009 with 7th A, S59.012-S59.019 with 7th A, S59.022-S59.029 with 7th A, S59.032-S59.039 with 7th A, S59.042-S59.049 with 7th A, S59.092-S59.099 with 7th A, S59.102-S59.109 with 7th A, S59.112-S59.119 with 7th A, S59.122-S59.129 with 7th A, S59.132-S59.139 with 7th A, S59.142-S59.149 with 7th A, S59.192-S59.199 with 7th A, S59.202-S59.209 with 7th A, S59.212-S59.219 with 7th A, S59.222-S59.229 with 7th A, S59.232-S59.239 with 7th A, S59.242-S59.249 with 7th A, S59.292-S59.299 with 7th A

MCC with 7th character B or C: S52.001-S52.009 with 7th [B, C], S52.021-S52.109 with 7th [B, C], S52.121-S52.516 with 7th [B, C], S52.531-S52.616 with 7th [A, B, C], S52.691-S52.92X with 7th [A, B, C], S59.001-S59.099 with 7th A, S59.201-S59.299 with 7th A, S62.90X with 7th B

MCC with 7th character K, M, N, P, Q or R: M80.00X-M84.68X with 7th [K, P], S02.0XX-S02.92X with 7th K, S12.000-S12.691 with 7th K, S22.000-S22.9XX with 7th K, S32.000-S32.9XX with 7th K, S42.001-S42.92X with 7th [K, P], S49.001-S49.199 with 7th [K, P], S52.001-S52.92X with 7th [K, M, N, P, Q, R], S59.001-S59.299 with 7th [K, P], S62.001-

7 HAC = Initial encounter only (7th character A, B or C) and not POA.

S62.92X with 7th [K, P], S72.001-S72.92X with 7th [K, M, N, P, Q, R], S79.001-S79.199 with 7th [K, P], S82.001-S82.92X with 7th [K, M, N, P, Q, R], S89.001-S89.399 with 7th [K, P], S92.001-S92.919 with 7th [K, P]

7 ✓7th **S52.209 Unspecified fracture of shaft of unspecified ulna** MCC CC
CC Excl: CC with 7th character A: S52.001-S52.92X with 7th [A, B, C], S59.001-S59.299 with 7th A
MCC with 7th character B or C: S52.001-S52.009 with 7th [B, C], S52.021-S52.109 with 7th [B, C], S52.121-S52.516 with 7th [B, C], S52.531-S52.616 with 7th [A, B, C], S52.691-S52.92X with 7th [A, B, C], S59.001-S59.099 with 7th A, S59.201-S59.299 with 7th A, S62.90XB
MCC with 7th character K, M, N, P, Q or R: M80.00X-M84.68X with 7th [K, P], S02.0XX-S02.92X with 7th K, S12.000-S12.691 with 7th K, S22.000-S22.9XX with 7th K, S32.000-S32.9XX with 7th K, S42.001-S42.92X with 7th [K, P], S49.001-S49.199 with 7th [K, P], S52.001-S52.92X with 7th [K, M, N, P, Q, R], S59.001-S59.299 with 7th [K, P], S62.001-S62.92X with 7th [K, P], S72.001-S72.92X with 7th [K, M, N, P, Q, R], S79.001-S79.199 with 7th [K, P], S82.001-S82.92X with 7th [K, M, N, P, Q, R], S89.001-S89.399 with 7th [K, P], S92.001-S92.919 with 7th [K, P]

✓6th **S52.21 Greenstick fracture of shaft of ulna**

The appropriate 7th is to be added to all codes in subcategory S52.21.
- A initial encounter for closed fracture
- D subsequent encounter for fracture with routine healing
- G subsequent encounter for fracture with delayed healing
- K subsequent encounter for fracture with nonunion
- P subsequent encounter for fracture with malunion
- S sequela

7 ✓7th **S52.211 Greenstick fracture of shaft of right ulna** CC
CC Excl: CC with 7th character A: S52.001-S52.011 with 7th [A, B, C], S52.019-S52.111 with 7th A, S52.119-S52.211 with 7th A, S52.219-S52.311 with 7th A, S52.319-S52.521 with 7th A, S52.529-S52.621 with 7th A, S52.629-S52.92X with 7th A, S59.001 with 7th A, S59.009-S59.011 with 7th A, S59.019-S59.021 with 7th A, S59.029-S59.031 with 7th A, S59.039-S59.041 with 7th A, S59.049-S59.091 with 7th A, S59.099-S59.101 with 7th A, S59.109-S59.111 with 7th A, S59.119-S59.121 with 7th A, S59.129-S59.131 with 7th A, S59.139-S59.141 with 7th A, S59.149-S59.191 with 7th A, S59.199-S59.201 with 7th A, S59.209-S59.211 with 7th A, S59.219-S59.221 with 7th A, S59.229-S59.231 with 7th A, S59.239-S59.241 with 7th A, S59.249-S59.291 with 7th A, S59.299A
CC with 7th character K or P: M80.00X-M84.68X with 7th [K, P], S02.0XX-S02.92X with 7th K, S12.000-S12.691 with 7th K, S22.000-S22.9XX with 7th K, S32.000-S32.9XX with 7th K, S42.001-S42.92X with 7th [K, P], S49.001-S49.199 with 7th [K, P], S52.001-S52.92X with 7th [K, M, N, P, Q, R], S59.001-S59.299 with 7th [K, P], S62.001-S62.92X with 7th [K, P], S72.001-S72.92X with 7th [K, M, N, P, Q, R], S79.001-S79.199 with 7th [K, P], S82.001-S82.92X with 7th [K, M, N, P, Q, R], S89.001-S89.399 with 7th [K, P], S92.001-S92.919 with 7th [K, P]

7 ✓7th **S52.212 Greenstick fracture of shaft of left ulna** CC
CC Excl: CC with 7th character A: S52.001-S52.009 with 7th [B, C], S52.012-S52.109 with 7th A, S52.112-S52.209 with 7th A, S52.212-S52.309 with 7th A, S52.312-S52.516 with 7th A, S52.522-S52.616 with 7th A, S52.622-S52.92X with 7th A, S59.002-S59.009 with 7th A, S59.012-S59.019 with 7th A, S59.022-S59.029 with 7th A, S59.032-S59.039 with 7th A, S59.042-S59.049 with 7th A, S59.092-S59.099 with 7th A, S59.102-S59.109 with 7th A, S59.112-S59.119 with 7th A, S59.122-S59.129 with 7th A, S59.132-S59.139 with 7th A, S59.142-S59.149 with 7th A, S59.192-S59.199 with 7th A, S59.202-S59.209 with 7th A, S59.212-S59.219 with 7th A, S59.222-S59.229 with 7th A, S59.232-S59.239 with 7th A, S59.242-S59.249 with 7th A, S59.292-S59.299 with 7th A
CC with 7th character K or P: M80.00X-M84.68X with 7th [K, P], S02.0XX-S02.92X with 7th K, S12.000-S12.691 with 7th K, S22.000-S22.9XX with 7th K, S32.000-S32.9XX with 7th K, S42.001-S42.92X with 7th [K, P], S49.001-S49.199 with 7th [K, P], S52.001-S52.92X with 7th [K, M, N, P, Q, R], S59.001-S59.299 with 7th [K, P], S62.001-S62.92X with 7th [K, P], S72.001-S72.92X with 7th [K, M, N, P, Q, R], S79.001-S79.199 with 7th [K, P], S82.001-S82.92X with 7th [K, M, N, P, Q, R], S89.001-S89.399 with 7th [K, P], S92.001-S92.919 with 7th [K, P]

7 ✓7th **S52.219 Greenstick fracture of shaft of unspecified ulna** CC
CC Excl: CC with 7th character A: S52.001-S52.92X with 7th [A, B, C], S59.001-S59.299 with 7th A
CC with 7th character K or P: M80.00X-M84.68X with 7th [K, P], S02.0XX-S02.92X with 7th K, S12.000-S12.691 with 7th K, S22.000-S22.9XX with 7th K, S32.000-S32.9XX with 7th K, S42.001-S42.92X with 7th [K, P], S49.001-S49.199 with 7th [K, P], S52.001-S52.92X with 7th [K, M, N, P, Q, R], S59.001-S59.299 with 7th [K, P], S62.001-S62.92X with 7th [K, P], S72.001-S72.92X with 7th [K, M, N, P, Q, R], S79.001-S79.199 with 7th [K, P], S82.001-S82.92X with 7th [K, M, N, P, Q, R], S89.001-S89.399 with 7th [K, P], S92.001-S92.919 with 7th [K, P]

✓6th **S52.22 Transverse fracture of shaft of ulna**

7 ✓7th **S52.221 Displaced transverse fracture of shaft of right ulna** MCC CC
CC Excl: See code: S52.201

7 ✓7th **S52.222 Displaced transverse fracture of shaft of left ulna** MCC CC
CC Excl: See code: S52.202

7 ✓7th **S52.223 Displaced transverse fracture of shaft of unspecified ulna** MCC CC
CC Excl: See code: S52.209

7 ✓7th **S52.224 Nondisplaced transverse fracture of shaft of right ulna** MCC CC
CC Excl: See code: S52.201

7 ✓7th **S52.225 Nondisplaced transverse fracture of shaft of left ulna** MCC CC
CC Excl: See code: S52.202

7 ✓7th **S52.226 Nondisplaced transverse fracture of shaft of unspecified ulna** MCC CC
CC Excl: See code: S52.209

✓6th **S52.23 Oblique fracture of shaft of ulna**

7 ✓7th **S52.231 Displaced oblique fracture of shaft of right ulna** MCC CC
CC Excl: See code: S52.201

7 ✓7th **S52.232 Displaced oblique fracture of shaft of left ulna** MCC CC
CC Excl: See code: S52.202

7 ✓7th **S52.233 Displaced oblique fracture of shaft of unspecified ulna** MCC CC
CC Excl: See code: S52.209

7 ✓7th **S52.234 Nondisplaced oblique fracture of shaft of right ulna** MCC CC
CC Excl: See code: S52.201

7 HAC = Initial encounter only (7th character A, B or C) and not POA.

7 ✓7th **S52.235 Nondisplaced oblique fracture of shaft of left ulna** MCC CC
CC Excl: See code: S52.2Ø2

7 ✓7th **S52.236 Nondisplaced oblique fracture of shaft of unspecified ulna** MCC CC
CC Excl: See code: S52.2Ø9

✓6th **S52.24 Spiral fracture of shaft of ulna**

7 ✓7th **S52.241 Displaced spiral fracture of shaft of ulna, right arm** MCC CC
CC Excl: See code: S52.2Ø1

7 ✓7th **S52.242 Displaced spiral fracture of shaft of ulna, left arm** MCC CC
CC Excl: See code: S52.2Ø2

7 ✓7th **S52.243 Displaced spiral fracture of shaft of ulna, unspecified arm** MCC CC
CC Excl: See code: S52.2Ø9

7 ✓7th **S52.244 Nondisplaced spiral fracture of shaft of ulna, right arm** MCC CC
CC Excl: See code: S52.2Ø1

7 ✓7th **S52.245 Nondisplaced spiral fracture of shaft of ulna, left arm** MCC CC
CC Excl: See code: S52.2Ø2

7 ✓7th **S52.246 Nondisplaced spiral fracture of shaft of ulna, unspecified arm** MCC CC
CC Excl: See code: S52.2Ø9

✓6th **S52.25 Comminuted fracture of shaft of ulna**

7 ✓7th **S52.251 Displaced comminuted fracture of shaft of ulna, right arm** MCC CC
CC Excl: See code: S52.2Ø1

7 ✓7th **S52.252 Displaced comminuted fracture of shaft of ulna, left arm** MCC CC
CC Excl: See code: S52.2Ø2

7 ✓7th **S52.253 Displaced comminuted fracture of shaft of ulna, unspecified arm** MCC CC
CC Excl: See code: S52.2Ø9

7 ✓7th **S52.254 Nondisplaced comminuted fracture of shaft of ulna, right arm** MCC CC
CC Excl: See code: S52.2Ø1

7 ✓7th **S52.255 Nondisplaced comminuted fracture of shaft of ulna, left arm** MCC CC
CC Excl: See code: S52.2Ø2

7 ✓7th **S52.256 Nondisplaced comminuted fracture of shaft of ulna, unspecified arm** MCC CC
CC Excl: See code: S52.2Ø9

✓6th **S52.26 Segmental fracture of shaft of ulna**

7 ✓7th **S52.261 Displaced segmental fracture of shaft of ulna, right arm** MCC CC
CC Excl: See code: S52.2Ø1

7 ✓7th **S52.262 Displaced segmental fracture of shaft of ulna, left arm** MCC CC
CC Excl: See code: S52.2Ø2

7 ✓7th **S52.263 Displaced segmental fracture of shaft of ulna, unspecified arm** MCC CC
CC Excl: See code: S52.2Ø9

7 ✓7th **S52.264 Nondisplaced segmental fracture of shaft of ulna, right arm** MCC CC
CC Excl: See code: S52.2Ø1

7 ✓7th **S52.265 Nondisplaced segmental fracture of shaft of ulna, left arm** MCC CC
CC Excl: See code: S52.2Ø2

7 ✓7th **S52.266 Nondisplaced segmental fracture of shaft of ulna, unspecified arm** MCC CC
CC Excl: See code: S52.2Ø9

✓6th **S52.27 Monteggia's fracture of ulna**
Fracture of upper shaft of ulna with dislocation of radial head

7 ✓7th **S52.271 Monteggia's fracture of right ulna** MCC CC
CC Excl: See code: S52.2Ø1

7 ✓7th **S52.272 Monteggia's fracture of left ulna** MCC CC
CC Excl: See code: S52.2Ø2

7 ✓7th **S52.279 Monteggia's fracture of unspecified ulna** MCC CC
CC Excl: See code: S52.2Ø9

✓6th **S52.28 Bent bone of ulna**

7 ✓7th **S52.281 Bent bone of right ulna** MCC CC
CC Excl: See code: S52.2Ø1

7 ✓7th **S52.282 Bent bone of left ulna** MCC CC
CC Excl: See code: S52.2Ø2

7 ✓7th **S52.283 Bent bone of unspecified ulna** MCC CC
CC Excl: See code: S52.2Ø9

✓6th **S52.29 Other fracture of shaft of ulna**

7 ✓7th **S52.291 Other fracture of shaft of right ulna** MCC CC
CC Excl: See code: S52.2Ø1

7 ✓7th **S52.292 Other fracture of shaft of left ulna** MCC CC
CC Excl: See code: S52.2Ø2

7 ✓7th **S52.299 Other fracture of shaft of unspecified ulna** MCC CC
CC Excl: See code: S52.2Ø9

✓5th **S52.3 Fracture of shaft of radius**

✓6th **S52.3Ø Unspecified fracture of shaft of radius**

7 ✓7th **S52.3Ø1 Unspecified fracture of shaft of right radius** MCC CC
CC Excl: See Code: S52.2Ø1

7 ✓7th **S52.3Ø2 Unspecified fracture of shaft of left radius** MCC CC
CC Excl: See Code: S52.2Ø2

7 ✓7th **S52.3Ø9 Unspecified fracture of shaft of unspecified radius** MCC CC
CC Excl: See Code: S52.2Ø9

✓6th **S52.31 Greenstick fracture of shaft of radius**

The appropriate 7th is to be added to all codes in subcategory S52.31.
A initial encounter for closed fracture
D subsequent encounter for fracture with routine healing
G subsequent encounter for fracture with delayed healing
K subsequent encounter for fracture with nonunion
P subsequent encounter for fracture with malunion
S sequela

7 ✓7th **S52.311 Greenstick fracture of shaft of radius, right arm** CC
CC Excl: CC with 7th character A: S52.ØØ1-S52.Ø11 with 7th [A, B, C], S52.Ø19-S52.111 with 7th A, S52.119-S52.211 with 7th A, S52.219-S52.311 with 7th A, S52.319-S52.521 with 7th A, S52.529-S52.621 with 7th A, S52.629-S52.92X with 7th A, S59.ØØ1 with 7th A, S59.ØØ9-S59.Ø11 with 7th A, S59.Ø19-S59.Ø21 with 7th A, S59.Ø29-S59.Ø31 with 7th A, S59.Ø39-S59.Ø41 with 7th A, S59.Ø49-S59.Ø91 with 7th A, S59.Ø99-S59.1Ø1 with 7th A, S59.1Ø9-S59.111 with 7th A, S59.119-S59.121 with 7th A, S59.129-S59.131 with 7th A, S59.139-S59.141 with 7th A, S59.149-S59.191 with 7th A, S59.199-S59.2Ø1 with 7th A, S59.2Ø9-S59.211 with 7th A, S59.219-S59.221 with 7th A, S59.229-S59.231 with 7th A, S59.239-S59.241 with 7th A, S59.249-S59.291 with 7th A, S59.299A
CC with 7th character K or P: M8Ø.ØØX-M84.68X with 7th [K, P], SØ2.ØXX-SØ2.92X with 7th K, S12.ØØØ-S12.691 with 7th K, S22.ØØØ-S22.9XX with 7th K, S32.ØØØ-S32.9XX with 7th K, S42.ØØ1-S42.92X with 7th [K, P], S49.ØØ1-S49.199 with 7th [K, P], S52.ØØ1-S52.92X with 7th [K, M, N, P, Q, R], S59.ØØ1-S59.299 with 7th [K, P], S62.ØØ1-S62.92X with 7th [K, P], S72.ØØ1-S72.92X with 7th [K, M, N, P, Q, R], S79.ØØ1-S79.199 with 7th [K, P], S82.ØØ1-S82.92X with 7th [K, M, N, P, Q, R], S89.ØØ1-S89.399 with 7th [K, P], S92.ØØ1-S92.919 with 7th [K, P]

7 HAC = Initial encounter only (7th character A, B or C) and not POA.

7 ✓7th **S52.312** **Greenstick fracture of shaft of radius, left arm** CC
CC Excl: CC with 7th character A: S52.001-S52.009 with 7th [B, C], S52.012-S52.109 with 7th A, S52.112-S52.209 with 7th A, S52.212-S52.309 with 7th A, S52.312-S52.516 with 7th A, S52.522-S52.616 with 7th A, S52.622-S52.92X with 7th A, S59.002-S59.009 with 7th A, S59.012-S59.019 with 7th A, S59.022-S59.029 with 7th A, S59.032-S59.039 with 7th A, S59.042-S59.049 with 7th A, S59.092-S59.099 with 7th A, S59.102-S59.109 with 7th A, S59.112-S59.119 with 7th A, S59.122-S59.129 with 7th A, S59.132-S59.139 with 7th A, S59.142-S59.149 with 7th A, S59.192-S59.199 with 7th A, S59.202-S59.209 with 7th A, S59.212-S59.219 with 7th A, S59.222-S59.229 with 7th A, S59.232-S59.239 with 7th A, S59.242-S59.249 with 7th A, S59.292-S59.299 with 7th A
CC with 7th character K or P: M80.00X-M84.68X with 7th [K, P], S02.0XX-S02.92X with 7th K, S12.000-S12.691 with 7th K, S22.000-S22.9XX with 7th K, S32.000-S32.9XX with 7th K, S42.001-S42.92X with 7th [K, P], S49.001-S49.199 with 7th [K, P], S52.001-S52.92X with 7th [K, M, N, P, Q, R], S59.001-S59.299 with 7th [K, P], S62.001-S62.92X with 7th [K, P], S72.001-S72.92X with 7th [K, M, N, P, Q, R], S79.001-S79.199 with 7th [K, P], S82.001-S82.92X with 7th [K, M, N, P, Q, R], S89.001-S89.399 with 7th [K, P], S92.001-S92.919 with 7th [K, P]

7 ✓7th **S52.319** **Greenstick fracture of shaft of radius, unspecified arm** CC
CC Excl: CC with 7th character A: S52.001-S52.92X with 7th [A, B, C], S59.001-S59.299 with 7th A
CC with 7th character K or P: M80.00X-M84.68X with 7th [K, P], S02.0XX-S02.92X with 7th K, S12.000-S12.691 with 7th K, S22.000-S22.9XX with 7th K, S32.000-S32.9XX with 7th K, S42.001-S42.92X with 7th [K, P], S49.001-S49.199 with 7th [K, P], S52.001-S52.92X with 7th [K, M, N, P, Q, R], S59.001-S59.299 with 7th [K, P], S62.001-S62.92X with 7th [K, P], S72.001-S72.92X with 7th [K, M, N, P, Q, R], S79.001-S79.199 with 7th [K, P], S82.001-S82.92X with 7th [K, M, N, P, Q, R], S89.001-S89.399 with 7th [K, P], S92.001-S92.919 with 7th [K, P

✓6th **S52.32** **Transverse fracture of shaft of radius**

7 ✓7th **S52.321** **Displaced transverse fracture of shaft of right radius** MCC CC
CC Excl: See code: S52.201

7 ✓7th **S52.322** **Displaced transverse fracture of shaft of left radius** MCC CC
CC Excl: See code: S52.202

7 ✓7th **S52.323** **Displaced transverse fracture of shaft of unspecified radius** MCC CC
CC Excl: See code: S52.209

7 ✓7th **S52.324** **Nondisplaced transverse fracture of shaft of right radius** MCC CC
CC Excl: See code: S52.201

7 ✓7th **S52.325** **Nondisplaced transverse fracture of shaft of left radius** MCC CC
CC Excl: See code: S52.202

7 ✓7th **S52.326** **Nondisplaced transverse fracture of shaft of unspecified radius** MCC CC
CC Excl: See code: S52.209

✓6th **S52.33** **Oblique fracture of shaft of radius**

7 ✓7th **S52.331** **Displaced oblique fracture of shaft of right radius** MCC CC
CC Excl: See code: S52.201

7 ✓7th **S52.332** **Displaced oblique fracture of shaft of left radius** MCC CC
CC Excl: See code: S52.202

7 ✓7th **S52.333** **Displaced oblique fracture of shaft of unspecified radius** MCC CC
CC Excl: See code: S52.209

7 ✓7th **S52.334** **Nondisplaced oblique fracture of shaft of right radius** MCC CC
CC Excl: See code: S52.201

7 ✓7th **S52.335** **Nondisplaced oblique fracture of shaft of left radius** MCC CC
CC Excl: See code: S52.202

7 ✓7th **S52.336** **Nondisplaced oblique fracture of shaft of unspecified radius** MCC CC
CC Excl: See code: S52.209

✓6th **S52.34** **Spiral fracture of shaft of radius**

7 ✓7th **S52.341** **Displaced spiral fracture of shaft of radius, right arm** MCC CC
CC Excl: See code: S52.201

7 ✓7th **S52.342** **Displaced spiral fracture of shaft of radius, left arm** MCC CC
CC Excl: See code: S52.202

7 ✓7th **S52.343** **Displaced spiral fracture of shaft of radius, unspecified arm** MCC CC
CC Excl: See code: S52.209

7 ✓7th **S52.344** **Nondisplaced spiral fracture of shaft of radius, right arm** MCC CC
CC Excl: See code: S52.201

7 ✓7th **S52.345** **Nondisplaced spiral fracture of shaft of radius, left arm** MCC CC
CC Excl: See code: S52.202

7 ✓7th **S52.346** **Nondisplaced spiral fracture of shaft of radius, unspecified arm** MCC CC
CC Excl: See code: S52.209

✓6th **S52.35** **Comminuted fracture of shaft of radius**

7 ✓7th **S52.351** **Displaced comminuted fracture of shaft of radius, right arm** MCC CC
CC Excl: See code: S52.201

7 ✓7th **S52.352** **Displaced comminuted fracture of shaft of radius, left arm** MCC CC
CC Excl: See code: S52.202

7 ✓7th **S52.353** **Displaced comminuted fracture sof haft of radius, unspecified arm** MCC CC
CC Excl: See code: S52.209

7 ✓7th **S52.354** **Nondisplaced comminuted fracture of shaft of radius, right arm** MCC CC
CC Excl: See code: S52.201

7 ✓7th **S52.355** **Nondisplaced comminuted fracture of shaft of radius, left arm** MCC CC
CC Excl: See code: S52.202

7 ✓7th **S52.356** **Nondisplaced comminuted fracture of shaft of radius, unspecified arm** MCC CC
CC Excl: See code: S52.209

✓6th **S52.36** **Segmental fracture of shaft of radius**

7 ✓7th **S52.361** **Displaced segmental fracture of shaft of radius, right arm** MCC CC
CC Excl: See code: S52.201

7 ✓7th **S52.362** **Displaced segmental fracture of shaft of radius, left arm** MCC CC
CC Excl: See code: S52.202

7 ✓7th **S52.363** **Displaced segmental fracture of shaft of radius, unspecified arm** MCC CC
CC Excl: See code: S52.209

7 ✓7th **S52.364** **Nondisplaced segmental fracture of shaft of radius, right arm** MCC CC
CC Excl: See code: S52.201

7 ✓7th **S52.365** **Nondisplaced segmental fracture of shaft of radius, left arm** MCC CC
CC Excl: See code: S52.202

7 ✓7th **S52.366** **Nondisplaced segmental fracture of shaft of radius, unspecified arm** MCC CC
CC Excl: See code: S52.209

✓6th **S52.37** **Galeazzi's fracture**
Fracture of lower shaft of radius with radioulnar joint dislocation

7 ✓7th **S52.371** **Galeazzi's fracture of right radius** MCC CC
CC Excl: See code: S52.201

7 ✓7th **S52.372** **Galeazzi's fracture of left radius** MCC CC
CC Excl: See code: S52.202

7 ✓7th **S52.379** **Galeazzi's fracture of unspecified radius** MCC CC
CC Excl: See code: S52.209

7 HAC = Initial encounter only (7th character A, B or C) and not POA.

√6th **S52.38 Bent bone of radius**

7 √7th **S52.381 Bent bone of right radius** MCC CC
CC Excl: See code: S52.201

7 √7th **S52.382 Bent bone of left radius** MCC CC
CC Excl: See code: S52.202

7 √7th **S52.389 Bent bone of unspecified radius** MCC CC
CC Excl: See code: S52.209

√6th **S52.39 Other fracture of shaft of radius**

7 √7th **S52.391 Other fracture of shaft of radius, right arm** MCC CC
CC Excl: See code: S52.201

7 √7th **S52.392 Other fracture of shaft of radius, left arm** MCC CC
CC Excl: See code: S52.202

7 √7th **S52.399 Other fracture of shaft of radius, unspecified arm** MCC CC
CC Excl: See code: S52.209

√5th **S52.5 Fracture of lower end of radius**
Fracture of distal end of radius
EXCLUDES 2 *physeal fractures of lower end of radius (S59.2-)*

√6th **S52.50 Unspecified fracture of the lower end of radius**

7 √7th **S52.501 Unspecified fracture of the lower end of right radius** MCC CC
CC Excl: See code: S52.201

7 √7th **S52.502 Unspecified fracture of the lower end of left radius** MCC CC
CC Excl: See code: S52.202

7 √7th **S52.509 Unspecified fracture of the lower end of unspecified radius** MCC CC
CC Excl: See code: S52.209

√6th **S52.51 Fracture of radial styloid process**

7 √7th **S52.511 Displaced fracture of right radial styloid process** MCC CC
CC Excl: See code: S52.201

7 √7th **S52.512 Displaced fracture of left radial styloid process** MCC CC
CC Excl: See code: S52.202

7 √7th **S52.513 Displaced fracture of unspecified radial styloid process** MCC CC
CC Excl: See code: S52.209

7 √7th **S52.514 Nondisplaced fracture of right radial styloid process** MCC CC
CC Excl: See code: S52.201

7 √7th **S52.515 Nondisplaced fracture of left radial styloid process** MCC CC
CC Excl: See code: S52.202

7 √7th **S52.516 Nondisplaced fracture of unspecified radial styloid process** MCC CC
CC Excl: See code: S52.209

√6th **S52.52 Torus fracture of lower end of radius**

The appropriate 7th is to be added to all codes in subcategory S52.52.

A	initial encounter for closed fracture
D	subsequent encounter for fracture with routine healing
G	subsequent encounter for fracture with delayed healing
K	subsequent encounter for fracture with nonunion
P	subsequent encounter for fracture with malunion
S	sequela

7 √7th **S52.521 Torus fracture of lower end of right radius** CC
CC Excl: CC with 7th character A: S52.001-S52.011 with 7th [A, B, C], S52.019-S52.111 with 7th A, S52.119-S52.211 with 7th A, S52.219-S52.311 with 7th A, S52.319-S52.521 with 7th A, S52.529-S52.621 with 7th A, S52.629-S52.92X with 7th A, S59.001 with 7th A, S59.009-S59.011 with 7th A, S59.019-S59.021 with 7th A, S59.029-S59.031 with 7th A, S59.039-S59.041 with 7th A, S59.049-S59.091 with 7th A, S59.099-S59.101 with 7th A, S59.109-S59.111 with 7th A, S59.119-S59.121 with 7th A, S59.129-S59.131 with 7th A, S59.139-S59.141 with 7th A, S59.149-S59.191 with 7th A, S59.199-S59.201 with 7th A, S59.209-S59.211 with 7th A, S59.219-S59.221 with 7th A, S59.229-S59.231 with 7th A, S59.239-S59.241 with 7th A, S59.249-S59.291 with 7th A, S59.299A
CC with 7th character K or P: M80.00X-M84.68X with 7th [K, P], S02.0XX-S02.92X with 7th K, S12.000-S12.691 with 7th K, S22.000-S22.9XX with 7th K, S32.000-S32.9XX with 7th K, S42.001-S42.92X with 7th [K, P], S49.001-S49.199 with 7th [K, P], S52.001-S52.92X with 7th [K, M, N, P, Q, R], S59.001-S59.299 with 7th [K, P], S62.001-S62.92X with 7th [K, P], S72.001-S72.92X with 7th [K, M, N, P, Q, R], S79.001-S79.199 with 7th [K, P], S82.001-S82.92X with 7th [K, M, N, P, Q, R], S89.001-S89.399 with 7th [K, P], S92.001-S92.919 with 7th [K, P]

7 √7th **S52.522 Torus fracture of lower end of left radius** CC
CC Excl: CC with 7th character A: S52.001-S52.009 with 7th [B, C], S52.012-S52.109 with 7th A, S52.112-S52.209 with 7th A, S52.212-S52.309 with 7th A, S52.312-S52.516 with 7th A, S52.522-S52.616 with 7th A, S52.622-S52.92X with 7th A, S59.002-S59.009 with 7th A, S59.012-S59.019 with 7th A, S59.022-S59.029 with 7th A, S59.032-S59.039 with 7th A, S59.042-S59.049 with 7th A, S59.092-S59.099 with 7th A, S59.102-S59.109 with 7th A, S59.112-S59.119 with 7th A, S59.122-S59.129 with 7th A, S59.132-S59.139 with 7th A, S59.142-S59.149 with 7th A, S59.192-S59.199 with 7th A, S59.202-S59.209 with 7th A, S59.212-S59.219 with 7th A, S59.222-S59.229 with 7th A, S59.232-S59.239 with 7th A, S59.242-S59.249 with 7th A, S59.292-S59.299 with 7th A
CC with 7th character K or P: M80.00X-M84.68X with 7th [K, P], S02.0XX-S02.92X with 7th K, S12.000-S12.691 with 7th K, S22.000-S22.9XX with 7th K, S32.000-S32.9XX with 7th K, S42.001-S42.92X with 7th [K, P], S49.001-S49.199 with 7th [K, P], S52.001-S52.92X with 7th [K, M, N, P, Q, R], S59.001-S59.299 with 7th [K, P], S62.001-S62.92X with 7th [K, P], S72.001-S72.92X with 7th [K, M, N, P, Q, R], S79.001-S79.199 with 7th [K, P], S82.001-S82.92X with 7th [K, M, N, P, Q, R], S89.001-S89.399 with 7th [K, P], S92.001-S92.919 with 7th [K, P]

7 √7th **S52.529 Torus fracture of lower end of unspecified radius** CC
CC Excl: See code: S52.209

√6th **S52.53 Colles' fracture**

7 √7th **S52.531 Colles' fracture of right radius** MCC CC
CC Excl: See code: S52.201

7 √7th **S52.532 Colles' fracture of left radius** MCC CC
CC Excl: See code: S52.202

7 √7th **S52.539 Colles' fracture of unspecified radius** MCC CC
CC Excl: See code: S52.209

√6th **S52.54 Smith's fracture**

7 √7th **S52.541 Smith's fracture of right radius** MCC CC
CC Excl: See code: S52.201

7 √7th **S52.542 Smith's fracture of left radius** MCC CC
CC Excl: See code: S52.202

7 √7th **S52.549 Smith's fracture of unspecified radius** MCC CC
CC Excl: See code: S52.209

√6th **S52.55 Other extraarticular fracture of lower end of radius**

7 √7th **S52.551 Other extraarticular fracture of lower end of right radius** MCC CC
CC Excl: See code: S52.201

7 √7th **S52.552 Other extraarticular fracture of lower end of left radius** MCC CC
CC Excl: See code: S52.202

7 √7th **S52.559 Other extraarticular fracture of lower end of unspecified radius** MCC CC
CC Excl: See code: S52.209

√6th **S52.56 Barton's fracture**

7 √7th **S52.561 Barton's fracture of right radius** MCC CC
CC Excl: See code: S52.201

7 √7th **S52.562 Barton's fracture of left radius** MCC CC
CC Excl: See code: S52.202

7 HAC = Initial encounter only (7th character A, B or C) and not POA.

7 ✓7th **S52.569 Barton's fracture of unspecified radius** MCC CC
CC Excl: See code: S52.209

✓6th **S52.57 Other intraarticular fracture of lower end of radius**

7 ✓7th **S52.571 Other intraarticular fracture of lower end of right radius** MCC CC
CC Excl: See code: S52.201

7 ✓7th **S52.572 Other intraarticular fracture of lower end of left radius** MCC CC
CC Excl: See code: S52.202

7 ✓7th **S52.579 Other intraarticular fracture of lower end of unspecified radius** MCC CC
CC Excl: See code: S52.209

✓6th **S52.59 Other fractures of lower end of radius**

7 ✓7th **S52.591 Other fractures of lower end of right radius** MCC CC
CC Excl: See code: S52.201

7 ✓7th **S52.592 Other fractures of lower end of left radius** MCC CC
CC Excl: See code: S52.202

7 ✓7th **S52.599 Other fractures of lower end of unspecified radius** MCC CC
CC Excl: See code: S52.209

✓5th **S52.6 Fracture of lower end of ulna**

✓6th **S52.60 Unspecified fracture of lower end of ulna**

7 ✓7th **S52.601 Unspecified fracture of lower end of right ulna** MCC CC
CC Excl: See code: S52.201

7 ✓7th **S52.602 Unspecified fracture of lower end of left ulna** MCC CC
CC Excl: See code: S52.202

7 ✓7th **S52.609 Unspecified fracture of lower end of unspecified ulna** MCC CC
CC Excl: See code: S52.209

✓6th **S52.61 Fracture of ulna styloid process**

7 ✓7th **S52.611 Displaced fracture of right ulna styloid process** MCC CC
CC Excl: See code: S52.201

7 ✓7th **S52.612 Displaced fracture of left ulna styloid process** MCC CC
CC Excl: See code: S52.202

7 ✓7th **S52.613 Displaced fracture of unspecified ulna styloid process** MCC CC
CC Excl: See code: S52.209

7 ✓7th **S52.614 Nondisplaced fracture of right ulna styloid process** MCC CC
CC Excl: See code: S52.201

7 ✓7th **S52.615 Nondisplaced fracture of left ulna styloid process** MCC CC
CC Excl: See code: S52.202

7 ✓7th **S52.616 Nondisplaced fracture of unspecified ulna styloid process** MCC CC
CC Excl: See code: S52.209

✓6th **S52.62 Torus fracture of lower end of ulna**

The appropriate 7th is to be added to all codes in subcategory S52.62.

- A initial encounter for closed fracture
- D subsequent encounter for fracture with routine healing
- G subsequent encounter for fracture with delayed healing
- K subsequent encounter for fracture with nonunion
- P subsequent encounter for fracture with malunion
- S sequela

7 ✓7th **S52.621 Torus fracture of lower end of right ulna** CC
CC Excl: CC with 7th character A: S52.001-S52.011 with 7th [A, B, C], S52.019-S52.111 with 7th A, S52.119-S52.211 with 7th A, S52.219-S52.311 with 7th A, S52.319-S52.521 with 7th A, S52.529-S52.621 with 7th A, S52.629-S52.92X with 7th A, S59.001 with 7th A, S59.009-S59.011 with 7th A, S59.019-S59.021 with 7th A, S59.029-S59.031 with 7th A, S59.039-S59.041 with 7th A, S59.049-S59.091 with 7th A, S59.099-S59.101 with 7th A, S59.109-S59.111 with 7th A, S59.119-S59.121 with 7th A, S59.129-S59.131 with 7th A, S59.139-S59.141 with 7th A, S59.149-S59.191 with 7th A, S59.199-S59.201 with 7th A, S59.209-S59.211 with 7th A, S59.219-S59.221 with 7th A, S59.229-S59.231 with 7th A, S59.239-S59.241 with 7th A, S59.249-S59.291 with 7th A, S59.299A
CC with 7th character K or P: M80.00X-M84.68X with 7th [K, P], S02.0XX-S02.92X with 7th K, S12.000-S12.691 with 7th K, S22.000-S22.9XX with 7th K, S32.000-S32.9XX with 7th K, S42.001-S42.92X with 7th [K, P], S49.001-S49.199 with 7th [K, P], S52.001-S52.92X with 7th [K, M, N, P, Q, R], S59.001-S59.299 with 7th [K, P], S62.001-S62.92X with 7th [K, P], S72.001-S72.92X with 7th [K, M, N, P, Q, R], S79.001-S79.199 with 7th [K, P], S82.001-S82.92X with 7th [K, M, N, P, Q, R], S89.001-S89.399 with 7th [K, P], S92.001-S92.919 with 7th [K, P]

7 ✓7th **S52.622 Torus fracture of lower end of left ulna** CC
CC Excl: CC with 7th character A: S52.001-S52.009 with 7th [B, C], S52.012-S52.109 with 7th A, S52.112-S52.209 with 7th A, S52.212-S52.309 with 7th A, S52.312-S52.516 with 7th A, S52.522-S52.616 with 7th A, S52.622-S52.92X with 7th A, S59.002-S59.009 with 7th A, S59.012-S59.019 with 7th A, S59.022-S59.029 with 7th A, S59.032-S59.039 with 7th A, S59.042-S59.049 with 7th A, S59.092-S59.099 with 7th A, S59.102-S59.109 with 7th A, S59.112-S59.119 with 7th A, S59.122-S59.129 with 7th A, S59.132-S59.139 with 7th A, S59.142-S59.149 with 7th A, S59.192-S59.199 with 7th A, S59.202-S59.209 with 7th A, S59.212-S59.219 with 7th A, S59.222-S59.229 with 7th A, S59.232-S59.239 with 7th A, S59.242-S59.249 with 7th A, S59.292-S59.299 with 7th A
CC with 7th character K or P: M80.00X-M84.68X with 7th [K, P], S02.0XX-S02.92X with 7th K, S12.000-S12.691 with 7th K, S22.000-S22.9XX with 7th K, S32.000-S32.9XX with 7th K, S42.001-S42.92X with 7th [K, P], S49.001-S49.199 with 7th [K, P], S52.001-S52.92X with 7th [K, M, N, P, Q, R], S59.001-S59.299 with 7th [K, P], S62.001-S62.92X with 7th [K, P], S72.001-S72.92X with 7th [K, M, N, P, Q, R], S79.001-S79.199 with 7th [K, P], S82.001-S82.92X with 7th [K, M, N, P, Q, R], S89.001-S89.399 with 7th [K, P], S92.001-S92.919 with 7th [K, P]

7 ✓7th **S52.629 Torus fracture of lower end of unspecified ulna** CC
CC Excl: CC with 7th character A: S52.001-S52.92X with 7th [A, B, C], S59.001-S59.299 with 7th A
CC with 7th character K or P: M80.00X-M84.68X with 7th [K, P], S02.0XX-S02.92X with 7th K, S12.000-S12.691 with 7th K, S22.000-S22.9XX with 7th K, S32.000-S32.9XX with 7th K, S42.001-S42.92X with 7th [K, P], S49.001-S49.199 with 7th [K, P], S52.001-S52.92X with 7th [K, M, N, P, Q, R], S59.001-S59.299 with 7th [K, P], S62.001-S62.92X with 7th [K, P], S72.001-S72.92X with 7th [K, M, N, P, Q, R], S79.001-S79.199 with 7th [K, P], S82.001-S82.92X with 7th [K, M, N, P, Q, R], S89.001-S89.399 with 7th [K, P], S92.001-S92.919 with 7th [K, P]

✓6th **S52.69 Other fracture of lower end of ulna**

7 ✓7th **S52.691 Other fracture of lower end of right ulna** MCC CC
CC Excl: See code: S52.201

7 HAC = Initial encounter only (7th character A, B or C) and not POA.

7 ✓7th **S52.692 Other fracture of lower end of left ulna** MCC CC
CC Excl: See code: S52.202

7 ✓7th **S52.699 Other fracture of lower end of unspecified ulna** MCC CC
CC Excl: See code: S52.209

✓5th **S52.9 Unspecified fracture of forearm**

7 ✓x7th **S52.90 Unspecified fracture of unspecified forearm** MCC CC
CC Excl: CC with 7th character A: S52.001-S52.92X with 7th [A, B, C], S59.001-S59.299 with 7th A
MCC with 7th character B or C: S52.001-S52.009 with 7th [B, C], S52.021-S52.109 with 7th [B, C], S52.121-S52.516 with 7th [B, C], S52.531-S52.616 with 7th [A, B, C], S52.691-S52.92X with 7th [A, B, C], S59.001-S59.099 with 7th A, S59.201-S59.299 with 7th A, S62.90XB
CC with 7th character K, M, N, P, Q or R: M80.00X-M84.68X with 7th [K, P], S02.0XX-S02.92X with 7th K, S12.000-S12.691 with 7th K, S22.000-S22.9XX with 7th K, S32.000-S32.9XX with 7th K, S42.001-S42.92X with 7th [K, P], S49.001-S49.199 with 7th [K, P], S52.001-S52.92X with 7th [K, M, N, P, Q, R], S59.001-S59.299 with 7th [K, P], S62.001-S62.92X with 7th [K, P], S72.001-S72.92X with 7th [K, M, N, P, Q, R], S79.001-S79.199 with 7th [K, P], S82.001-S82.92X with 7th [K, M, N, P, Q, R], S89.001-S89.399 with 7th [K, P], S92.001-S92.919 with 7th [K, P]

7 ✓x7th **S52.91 Unspecified fracture of right forearm** MCC CC
CC Excl: See code: S52.90

7 ✓x7th **S52.92 Unspecified fracture of left forearm** MCC CC
CC Excl: See code: S52.90

✓4th **S53 Dislocation and sprain of joints and ligaments of elbow**

INCLUDES avulsion of joint or ligament of elbow
laceration of cartilage, joint or ligament of elbow
sprain of cartilage, joint or ligament of elbow
traumatic hemarthrosis of joint or ligament of elbow
traumatic rupture of joint or ligament of elbow
traumatic subluxation of joint or ligament of elbow
traumatic tear of joint or ligament of elbow

Code also any associated open wound

EXCLUDES 2 *strain of muscle, fascia and tendon at forearm level (S56.-)*

The appropriate 7th is to be added to each code from category S53.
A initial encounter
D subsequent encounter
S sequela

✓5th **S53.0 Subluxation and dislocation of radial head**
Dislocation of radiohumeral joint
Subluxation of radiohumeral joint
EXCLUDES 1 *Monteggia's fracture-dislocation (S52.27-)*

✓6th **S53.00 Unspecified subluxation and dislocation of radial head**
✓7th **S53.001 Unspecified subluxation of right radial head**
✓7th **S53.002 Unspecified subluxation of left radial head**
✓7th **S53.003 Unspecified subluxation of unspecified radial head**
✓7th **S53.004 Unspecified dislocation of right radial head**
✓7th **S53.005 Unspecified dislocation of left radial head**
✓7th **S53.006 Unspecified dislocation of unspecified radial head**

✓6th **S53.01 Anterior subluxation and dislocation of radial head**
Anteriomedial subluxation and dislocation of radial head
✓7th **S53.011 Anterior subluxation of right radial head**
✓7th **S53.012 Anterior subluxation of left radial head**
✓7th **S53.013 Anterior subluxation of unspecified radial head**
✓7th **S53.014 Anterior dislocation of right radial head**
✓7th **S53.015 Anterior dislocation of left radial head**
✓7th **S53.016 Anterior dislocation of unspecified radial head**

✓6th **S53.02 Posterior subluxation and dislocation of radial head**
Posteriolateral subluxation and dislocation of radial head
✓7th **S53.021 Posterior subluxation of right radial head**
✓7th **S53.022 Posterior subluxation of left radial head**
✓7th **S53.023 Posterior subluxation of unspecified radial head**
✓7th **S53.024 Posterior dislocation of right radial head**
✓7th **S53.025 Posterior dislocation of left radial head**
✓7th **S53.026 Posterior dislocation of unspecified radial head**

✓6th **S53.03 Nursemaid's elbow**
✓7th **S53.031 Nursemaid's elbow, right elbow**
✓7th **S53.032 Nursemaid's elbow, left elbow**
✓7th **S53.033 Nursemaid's elbow, unspecified elbow**

✓6th **S53.09 Other subluxation and dislocation of radial head**
✓7th **S53.091 Other subluxation of right radial head**
✓7th **S53.092 Other subluxation of left radial head**
✓7th **S53.093 Other subluxation of unspecified radial head**
✓7th **S53.094 Other dislocation of right radial head**
✓7th **S53.095 Other dislocation of left radial head**
✓7th **S53.096 Other dislocation of unspecified radial head**

✓5th **S53.1 Subluxation and dislocation of ulnohumeral joint**
Subluxation and dislocation of elbow NOS
EXCLUDES 1 *dislocation of radial head alone (S53.0-)*

✓6th **S53.10 Unspecified subluxation and dislocation of ulnohumeral joint**
✓7th **S53.101 Unspecified subluxation of right ulnohumeral joint**
✓7th **S53.102 Unspecified subluxation of left ulnohumeral joint**
✓7th **S53.103 Unspecified subluxation of unspecified ulnohumeral joint**
✓7th **S53.104 Unspecified dislocation of right ulnohumeral joint**
✓7th **S53.105 Unspecified dislocation of left ulnohumeral joint**
✓7th **S53.106 Unspecified dislocation of unspecified ulnohumeral joint**

✓6th **S53.11 Anterior subluxation and dislocation of ulnohumeral joint**
✓7th **S53.111 Anterior subluxation of right ulnohumeral joint**
✓7th **S53.112 Anterior subluxation of left ulnohumeral joint**
✓7th **S53.113 Anterior subluxation of unspecified ulnohumeral joint**
✓7th **S53.114 Anterior dislocation of right ulnohumeral joint**
AHA: 2012, 4Q, 108
✓7th **S53.115 Anterior dislocation of left ulnohumeral joint**
✓7th **S53.116 Anterior dislocation of unspecified ulnohumeral joint**

✓6th **S53.12 Posterior subluxation and dislocation of ulnohumeral joint**
✓7th **S53.121 Posterior subluxation of right ulnohumeral joint**
✓7th **S53.122 Posterior subluxation of left ulnohumeral joint**
✓7th **S53.123 Posterior subluxation of unspecified ulnohumeral joint**
✓7th **S53.124 Posterior dislocation of right ulnohumeral joint**
✓7th **S53.125 Posterior dislocation of left ulnohumeral joint**
✓7th **S53.126 Posterior dislocation of unspecified ulnohumeral joint**

✓6th **S53.13 Medial subluxation and dislocation of ulnohumeral joint**
✓7th **S53.131 Medial subluxation of right ulnohumeral joint**
✓7th **S53.132 Medial subluxation of left ulnohumeral joint**
✓7th **S53.133 Medial subluxation of unspecified ulnohumeral joint**

7 HAC = Initial encounter only (7th character A, B or C) and not POA.

✓7th S53.134 Medial dislocation of right ulnohumeral joint
✓7th S53.135 Medial dislocation of left ulnohumeral joint
✓7th S53.136 Medial dislocation of unspecified ulnohumeral joint
✓6th S53.14 Lateral subluxation and dislocation of ulnohumeral joint
✓7th S53.141 Lateral subluxation of right ulnohumeral joint
✓7th S53.142 Lateral subluxation of left ulnohumeral joint
✓7th S53.143 Lateral subluxation of unspecified ulnohumeral joint
✓7th S53.144 Lateral dislocation of right ulnohumeral joint
✓7th S53.145 Lateral dislocation of left ulnohumeral joint
✓7th S53.146 Lateral dislocation of unspecified ulnohumeral joint
✓6th S53.19 Other subluxation and dislocation of ulnohumeral joint
✓7th S53.191 Other subluxation of right ulnohumeral joint
✓7th S53.192 Other subluxation of left ulnohumeral joint
✓7th S53.193 Other subluxation of unspecified ulnohumeral joint
✓7th S53.194 Other dislocation of right ulnohumeral joint
✓7th S53.195 Other dislocation of left ulnohumeral joint
✓7th S53.196 Other dislocation of unspecified ulnohumeral joint
✓5th S53.2 Traumatic rupture of radial collateral ligament
EXCLUDES 1 *sprain of radial collateral ligament NOS (S53.43-)*
✓x7th S53.20 Traumatic rupture of unspecified radial collateral ligament
✓x7th S53.21 Traumatic rupture of right radial collateral ligament
✓x7th S53.22 Traumatic rupture of left radial collateral ligament
✓5th S53.3 Traumatic rupture of ulnar collateral ligament
EXCLUDES 1 *sprain of ulnar collateral ligament (S53.44-)*
✓x7th S53.30 Traumatic rupture of unspecified ulnar collateral ligament
✓x7th S53.31 Traumatic rupture of right ulnar collateral ligament
✓x7th S53.32 Traumatic rupture of left ulnar collateral ligament
✓5th S53.4 Sprain of elbow
EXCLUDES 2 *traumatic rupture of radial collateral ligament (S53.2-)*
traumatic rupture of ulnar collateral ligament (S53.3-)
✓6th S53.40 Unspecified sprain of elbow
✓7th S53.401 Unspecified sprain of right elbow
✓7th S53.402 Unspecified sprain of left elbow
✓7th S53.409 Unspecified sprain of unspecified elbow
Sprain of elbow NOS
✓6th S53.41 Radiohumeral (joint) sprain
✓7th S53.411 Radiohumeral (joint) sprain of right elbow
✓7th S53.412 Radiohumeral (joint) sprain of left elbow
✓7th S53.419 Radiohumeral (joint) sprain of unspecified elbow
✓6th S53.42 Ulnohumeral (joint) sprain
✓7th S53.421 Ulnohumeral (joint) sprain of right elbow
✓7th S53.422 Ulnohumeral (joint) sprain of left elbow
✓7th S53.429 Ulnohumeral (joint) sprain of unspecified elbow
✓6th S53.43 Radial collateral ligament sprain
✓7th S53.431 Radial collateral ligament sprain of right elbow
✓7th S53.432 Radial collateral ligament sprain of left elbow
✓7th S53.439 Radial collateral ligament sprain of unspecified elbow
✓6th S53.44 Ulnar collateral ligament sprain
✓7th S53.441 Ulnar collateral ligament sprain of right elbow
✓7th S53.442 Ulnar collateral ligament sprain of left elbow
✓7th S53.449 Ulnar collateral ligament sprain of unspecified elbow
✓6th S53.49 Other sprain of elbow
✓7th S53.491 Other sprain of right elbow
✓7th S53.492 Other sprain of left elbow
✓7th S53.499 Other sprain of unspecified elbow

✓4th **S54 Injury of nerves at forearm level**
Code also any associated open wound (S51.-)
EXCLUDES 2 *injury of nerves at wrist and hand level (S64.-)*

The appropriate 7th is to be added to each code from category S54.
A initial encounter
D subsequent encounter
S sequela

✓5th S54.0 Injury of ulnar nerve at forearm level
Injury of ulnar nerve NOS
✓x7th S54.00 Injury of ulnar nerve at forearm level, unspecified arm
✓x7th S54.01 Injury of ulnar nerve at forearm level, right arm
✓x7th S54.02 Injury of ulnar nerve at forearm level, left arm
✓5th S54.1 Injury of median nerve at forearm level
Injury of median nerve NOS
✓x7th S54.10 Injury of median nerve at forearm level, unspecified arm
✓x7th S54.11 Injury of median nerve at forearm level, right arm
✓x7th S54.12 Injury of median nerve at forearm level, left arm
✓5th S54.2 Injury of radial nerve at forearm level
Injury of radial nerve NOS
✓x7th S54.20 Injury of radial nerve at forearm level, unspecified arm
✓x7th S54.21 Injury of radial nerve at forearm level, right arm
✓x7th S54.22 Injury of radial nerve at forearm level, left arm
✓5th S54.3 Injury of cutaneous sensory nerve at forearm level
✓x7th S54.30 Injury of cutaneous sensory nerve at forearm level, unspecified arm
✓x7th S54.31 Injury of cutaneous sensory nerve at forearm level, right arm
✓x7th S54.32 Injury of cutaneous sensory nerve at forearm level, left arm
✓5th S54.8 Injury of other nerves at forearm level
✓6th S54.8X Unspecified injury of other nerves at forearm level
✓7th S54.8X1 Unspecified injury of other nerves at forearm level, right arm
✓7th S54.8X2 Unspecified injury of other nerves at forearm level, left arm
✓7th S54.8X9 Unspecified injury of other nerves at forearm level, unspecified arm
✓5th S54.9 Injury of unspecified nerve at forearm level
✓x7th S54.90 Injury of unspecified nerve at forearm level, unspecified arm
✓x7th S54.91 Injury of unspecified nerve at forearm level, right arm
✓x7th S54.92 Injury of unspecified nerve at forearm level, left arm

S55 Injury of blood vessels at forearm level

Code also any associated open wound (S51.-)

EXCLUDES 2 *injury of blood vessels at wrist and hand level (S65.-)*
injury of brachial vessels (S45.1-S45.2)

The appropriate 7th is to be added to each code from category S55.
- A initial encounter
- D subsequent encounter
- S sequela

S55.0 Injury of ulnar artery at forearm level

S55.00 Unspecified injury of ulnar artery at forearm level

S55.001 Unspecified injury of ulnar artery at forearm level, right arm CC
CC Excl: CC with 7th character A: S45.301A, S45.309-S45.311 with 7th A, S45.319-S45.391 with 7th A, S45.399-S45.801 with 7th A, S45.809-S45.811 with 7th A, S45.819-S45.891 with 7th A, S45.899-S45.901 with 7th A, S45.909-S45.911 with 7th A, S45.919-S45.991 with 7th A, S45.999 with 7th A, S55.001A, S55.009-S55.011 with 7th A, S55.019-S55.091 with 7th A, S55.099 A, S55.201 with 7th A, S55.209-S55.211 with 7th A, S55.219-S55.291 with 7th A, S55.299-S55.801 with 7th A, S55.809-S55.811 with 7th A, S55.819-S55.891 with 7th A, S55.899-S55.901 with 7th A, S55.909-S55.911 with 7th A, S55.919-S55.991 with 7th A, S55.999 with 7th A, S65.001 with 7th A, S65.009-S65.011 with 7th A, S65.019-S65.091 with 7th A, S65.099A, S65.801A, S65.809-S65.811 with 7th A, S65.819-S65.891 with 7th A, S65.899-S65.901 with 7th A, S65.909-S65.911 with 7th A, S65.919-S65.991 with 7th A, S65.999A

S55.002 Unspecified injury of ulnar artery at forearm level, left arm CC
CC Excl: CC with 7th character A: S45.302-S45.309 with 7th A, S45.312-S45.319 with 7th A, S45.392-S45.399 with 7th A, S45.802-S45.809 with 7th A, S45.812-S45.819 with 7th A, S45.892-S45.899 with 7th A, S45.902-S45.909 with 7th A, S45.912-S45.919 with 7th A, S45.992-S45.999 with 7th A, S55.002-S55.009 with 7th A, S55.012-S55.019 with 7th A, S55.092-S55.099 with 7th A, S55.202-S55.209 with 7th A, S55.212-S55.219 with 7th A, S55.292-S55.299 with 7th A, S55.802-S55.809 with 7th A, S55.812-S55.819 with 7th A, S55.892-S55.899 with 7th A, S55.902-S55.909 with 7th A, S55.912-S55.919 with 7th A, S55.992-S55.999 with 7th A, S65.002-S65.009 with 7th A, S65.012-S65.019 with 7th A, S65.092-S65.099 with 7th A, S65.802-S65.809 with 7th A, S65.812-S65.819 with 7th A, S65.892-S65.899 with 7th A, S65.902-S65.909 with 7th A, S65.912-S65.919 with 7th A, S65.992-S65.999 with 7th A

S55.009 Unspecified injury of ulnar artery at forearm level, unspecified arm CC
CC Excl: CC with 7th character A: S45.301-S45.999 with 7th A, S55.001-S55.099 with 7th A, S55.201-S55.999 with 7th A, S65.001-S65.099 with 7th A, S65.801-S65.999 with 7th A

S55.01 Laceration of ulnar artery at forearm level

S55.011 Laceration of ulnar artery at forearm level, right arm CC
CC Excl: See code: S55.001

S55.012 Laceration of ulnar artery at forearm level, left arm CC
CC Excl: See code: S55.002

S55.019 Laceration of ulnar artery at forearm level, unspecified arm CC
CC Excl: See code: S55.009

S55.09 Other specified injury of ulnar artery at forearm level

S55.091 Other specified injury of ulnar artery at forearm level, right arm CC
CC Excl: See code: S55.001

S55.092 Other specified injury of ulnar artery at forearm level, left arm CC
CC Excl: See code: S55.002

S55.099 Other specified injury of ulnar artery at forearm level, unspecified arm CC
CC Excl: See code: S55.009

S55.1 Injury of radial artery at forearm level

S55.10 Unspecified injury of radial artery at forearm level

S55.101 Unspecified injury of radial artery at forearm level, right arm CC
CC Excl: CC with 7th character A: S45.301 with 7th A, S45.309-S45.311 with 7th A, S45.319-S45.391 with 7th A, S45.399-S45.801 with 7th A, S45.809-S45.811 with 7th A, S45.819-S45.891 with 7th A, S45.899-S45.901 with 7th A, S45.909-S45.911 with 7th A, S45.919-S45.991 with 7th A, S45.999 with 7th A, S55.101 with 7th A, S55.109-S55.111 with 7th A, S55.119-S55.191 with 7th A, S55.199-S55.201 with 7th A, S55.209-S55.211 with 7th A, S55.219-S55.291 with 7th A, S55.299-S55.801 with 7th A, S55.809-S55.811 with 7th A, S55.819-S55.891 with 7th A, S55.899-S55.901 with 7th A, S55.909-S55.911 with 7th A, S55.919-S55.991 with 7th A, S55.999 with 7th A, S65.101 with 7th A, S65.109-S65.111 with 7th A, S65.119-S65.191 with 7th A, S65.199 with 7th A, S65.801 with 7th A, S65.809-S65.811 with 7th A, S65.819-S65.891 with 7th A, S65.899-S65.901 with 7th A, S65.909-S65.911 with 7th A, S65.919-S65.991 with 7th A, S65.999A

S55.102 Unspecified injury of radial artery at forearm level, left arm CC
CC Excl: CC with 7th character A: S45.302-S45.309 with 7th A, S45.312-S45.319 with 7th A, S45.392-S45.399 with 7th A, S45.802-S45.809 with 7th A, S45.812-S45.819 with 7th A, S45.892-S45.899 with 7th A, S45.902-S45.909 with 7th A, S45.912-S45.919 with 7th A, S45.992-S45.999 with 7th A, S55.102-S55.109 with 7th A, S55.112-S55.119 with 7th A, S55.192-S55.199 with 7th A, S55.202-S55.209 with 7th A, S55.212-S55.219 with 7th A, S55.292-S55.299 with 7th A, S55.802-S55.809 with 7th A, S55.812-S55.819 with 7th A, S55.892-S55.899 with 7th A, S55.902-S55.909 with 7th A, S55.912-S55.919 with 7th A, S55.992-S55.999 with 7th A, S65.102-S65.109 with 7th A, S65.112-S65.119 with 7th A, S65.192-S65.199 with 7th A, S65.802-S65.809 with 7th A, S65.812-S65.819 with 7th A, S65.892-S65.899 with 7th A, S65.902-S65.909 with 7th A, S65.912-S65.919 with 7th A, S65.992-S65.999 with 7th A

S55.109 Unspecified injury of radial artery at forearm level, unspecified arm CC
CC Excl: CC with 7th character A: S45.301-S45.999 with 7th A, S55.101-S55.999 with 7th A, S65.101-S65.199 with 7th A, S65.801-S65.999 with 7th A

S55.11 Laceration of radial artery at forearm level

S55.111 Laceration of radial artery at forearm level, right arm CC
CC Excl: See code: S55.101

S55.112 Laceration of radial artery at forearm level, left arm CC
CC Excl: See code: S55.102

S55.119 Laceration of radial artery at forearm level, unspecified arm CC
CC Excl: See code: S55.109

S55.19 Other specified injury of radial artery at forearm level

S55.191 Other specified injury of radial artery at forearm level, right arm CC
CC Excl: See code: S55.101

S55.192 Other specified injury of radial artery at forearm level, left arm CC
CC Excl: See code: S55.102

S55.199 Other specified injury of radial artery at forearm level, unspecified arm CC
CC Excl: See code: S55.109

S55.2 Injury of vein at forearm level

S55.20 Unspecified injury of vein at forearm level

S55.201 Unspecified injury of vein at forearm level, right arm CC
CC Excl: CC with 7th character A: S45.301A, S45.309-S45.311 with 7th A, S45.319-S45.391 with 7th A, S45.399-S45.801 with 7th A, S45.809-S45.811 with 7th A, S45.819-S45.891 with 7th A, S45.899-S45.901 with 7th A, S45.909-S45.911 with 7th A, S45.919-S45.991 with 7th A, S45.999 with 7th A, S55.001 with 7th A, S55.009-S55.011 with 7th A, S55.019-S55.091 with 7th A, S55.099A, S55.201A, S55.209-S55.211 with 7th A, S55.219-S55.291 with 7th A, S55.299-S55.801 with 7th A, S55.809-S55.811 with 7th A, S55.819-S55.891 with 7th A, S55.899-S55.901 with 7th A, S55.909-S55.911 with 7th A, S55.919-S55.991 with 7th A, S55.999A, S65.001 A, S65.009-S65.011 with 7th A, S65.019-S65.091 with 7th A, S65.099A, S65.201A, S65.209-S65.211 with 7th A, S65.219-S65.291 with 7th A, S65.299-S65.301 with 7th A, S65.309-S65.311 with 7th A, S65.319-S65.391 with 7th A, S65.399-S65.401 with 7th A, S65.409-S65.411 with 7th A, S65.419-S65.491 with 7th A, S65.499-S65.500A, S65.502A, S65.504A, S65.506A, S65.508-S65.510 with 7th A, S65.512A, S65.514A, S65.516A, S65.518-S65.590 with 7th A, S65.592A, S65.594A, S65.596A, S65.598-S65.801 with 7th A, S65.809-S65.811 with 7th A, S65.819-S65.891 with 7th A, S65.899-S65.901 with 7th A, S65.909-S65.911 with 7th A, S65.919-S65.991 with 7th A, S65.999A

S55.202 Unspecified injury of vein at forearm level, left arm CC
CC Excl: CC with 7th character A: S45.302-S45.309 with 7th A, S45.312-S45.319 with 7th A, S45.392-S45.399 with 7th A, S45.802-S45.809 with 7th A, S45.812-S45.819 with 7th A, S45.892-S45.899 with 7th A, S45.902-S45.909 with 7th A, S45.912-S45.919 with 7th A, S45.992-S45.999 with 7th A, S55.002-S55.009 with 7th A, S55.012-S55.019 with 7th A, S55.092-S55.099 with 7th A, S55.202-S55.209 with 7th A, S55.212-S55.219 with 7th A, S55.292-S55.299 with 7th A, S55.802-S55.809 with 7th A, S55.812-S55.819 with 7th A, S55.892-S55.899 with 7th A, S55.902-S55.909 with 7th A, S55.912-S55.919 with 7th A, S55.992-S55.999 with 7th A, S65.002-S65.009 with 7th A, S65.012-S65.019 with 7th A, S65.092-S65.099 with 7th A, S65.202-S65.209 with 7th A, S65.212-S65.219 with 7th A, S65.292-S65.299 with 7th A, S65.302-S65.309 with 7th A, S65.312-S65.319 with 7th A, S65.392-S65.399 with 7th A, S65.402-S65.409 with 7th A, S65.412-S65.419 with 7th A, S65.492-S65.499 with 7th A, S65.501 with 7th A, S65.503 with 7th A, S65.505 with 7th A, S65.507-S65.509 with 7th A, S65.511 with 7th A, S65.513 with 7th A, S65.515 with 7th A, S65.517-S65.519 with 7th A, S65.591 with 7th A, S65.593 with 7th A, S65.595 with 7th A, S65.597-S65.599 with 7th A, S65.802-S65.809 with 7th A, S65.812-S65.819 with 7th A, S65.892-S65.899 with 7th A, S65.902-S65.909 with 7th A, S65.912-S65.919 with 7th A, S65.992-S65.999 with 7th A

S55.209 Unspecified injury of vein at forearm level, unspecified arm CC
CC Excl: CC with 7th character A: S45.301-S45.999 with 7th A, S55.001-S55.099 with 7th A, S55.201-S55.999 with 7th A, S65.001-S65.099 with 7th A, S65.201-S65.999 with 7th A

S55.21 Laceration of vein at forearm level

S55.211 Laceration of vein at forearm level, right arm CC
CC Excl: See code: S55.201

S55.212 Laceration of vein at forearm level, left arm CC
CC Excl: See code: S55.202

S55.219 Laceration of vein at forearm level, unspecified arm CC
CC Excl: See code: S55.209

S55.29 Other specified injury of vein at forearm level

S55.291 Other specified injury of vein at forearm level, right arm CC
CC Excl: See code: S55.201

S55.292 Other specified injury of vein at forearm level, left arm CC
CC Excl: See code: S55.202

S55.299 Other specified injury of vein at forearm level, unspecified arm CC
CC Excl: See code: S55.209

S55.8 Injury of other blood vessels at forearm level

S55.80 Unspecified injury of other blood vessels at forearm level

S55.801 Unspecified injury of other blood vessels at forearm level, right arm CC
CC Excl: See code: S55.201

S55.802 Unspecified injury of other blood vessels at forearm level, left arm CC
CC Excl: See code: S55.202

S55.809 Unspecified injury of other blood vessels at forearm level, unspecified arm CC
CC Excl: See code: S55.209

S55.81 Laceration of other blood vessels at forearm level

S55.811 Laceration of other blood vessels at forearm level, right arm CC
CC Excl: See code: S55.201

S55.812 Laceration of other blood vessels at forearm level, left arm CC
CC Excl: See code: S55.202

S55.819 Laceration of other blood vessels at forearm level, unspecified arm CC
CC Excl: See code: S55.209

S55.89 Other specified injury of other blood vessels at forearm level

S55.891 Other specified injury of other blood vessels at forearm level, right arm CC
CC Excl: See code: S55.201

S55.892 Other specified injury of other blood vessels at forearm level, left arm CC
CC Excl: See code: S55.202

S55.899 Other specified injury of other blood vessels at forearm level, unspecified arm CC
CC Excl: See code: S55.209

S55.9 Injury of unspecified blood vessel at forearm level

S55.90 Unspecified injury of unspecified blood vessel at forearm level

S55.901 Unspecified injury of unspecified blood vessel at forearm level, right arm CC
CC Excl: See code: S55.201

S55.902 Unspecified injury of unspecified blood vessel at forearm level, left arm CC
CC Excl: See code: S55.202

S55.909 Unspecified injury of unspecified blood vessel at forearm level, unspecified arm CC
CC Excl: See code: S55.209

S55.91 Laceration of unspecified blood vessel at forearm level

S55.911 Laceration of unspecified blood vessel at forearm level, right arm CC
CC Excl: See code: S55.201

S55.912 Laceration of unspecified blood vessel at forearm level, left arm CC
CC Excl: See code: S55.202

S55.919 Laceration of unspecified blood vessel at forearm level, unspecified arm CC
CC Excl: See code: S55.209

S55.99 Other specified injury of unspecified blood vessel at forearm level

S55.991 Other specified injury of unspecified blood vessel at forearm level, right arm CC
CC Excl: See code: S55.201

✓7th **S55.992 Other specified injury of unspecified blood vessel at forearm level, left arm** CC
- **CC Excl:** See code: S55.202

✓7th **S55.999 Other specified injury of unspecified blood vessel at forearm level, unspecified arm** CC
- **CC Excl:** See code: S55.209

✓4th **S56 Injury of muscle, fascia and tendon at forearm level**

Code also any associated open wound (S51.-)

EXCLUDES 2 *injury of muscle, fascia and tendon at or below wrist (S66.-)*
sprain of joints and ligaments of elbow (S53.4-)

The appropriate 7th is to be added to each code from category S56.
- A initial encounter
- D subsequent encounter
- S sequela

✓5th **S56.0 Injury of flexor muscle, fascia and tendon of thumb at forearm level**

✓6th **S56.00 Unspecified injury of flexor muscle, fascia and tendon of thumb at forearm level**

✓7th **S56.001 Unspecified injury of flexor muscle, fascia and tendon of right thumb at forearm level**

✓7th **S56.002 Unspecified injury of flexor muscle, fascia and tendon of left thumb at forearm level**

✓7th **S56.009 Unspecified injury of flexor muscle, fascia and tendon of unspecified thumb at forearm level**

✓6th **S56.01 Strain of flexor muscle, fascia and tendon of thumb at forearm level**

✓7th **S56.011 Strain of flexor muscle, fascia and tendon of right thumb at forearm level**

✓7th **S56.012 Strain of flexor muscle, fascia and tendon of left thumb at forearm level**

✓7th **S56.019 Strain of flexor muscle, fascia and tendon of unspecified thumb at forearm level**

✓6th **S56.02 Laceration of flexor muscle, fascia and tendon of thumb at forearm level**

✓7th **S56.021 Laceration of flexor muscle, fascia and tendon of right thumb at forearm level** CC
- **CC Excl: CC with 7th character A:** S51.001A, S51.009-S51.011 with 7th A, S51.019-S51.021 with 7th A, S51.029-S51.031 with 7th A, S51.039-S51.041 with 7th A, S51.049-S51.051 with 7th A, S51.059-S51.801 with 7th A, S51.809-S51.811 with 7th A, S51.819-S51.821 with 7th A, S51.829-S51.831 with 7th A, S51.839-S51.841 with 7th A, S51.849-S51.851 with 7th A, S51.859A, S56.021A, S56.029 A, S56.121A, S56.123A, S56.125A, S56.127A, S56.129 A, S56.221 A, S56.229A, S56.321A, S56.329A, S56.421A, S56.423A, S56.425A, S56.427A, S56.429A, S56.521A, S56.529A, S56.821A, S56.829A, S56.921 A, S56.929A, S61.501A, S61.509-S61.511 with 7th A, S61.519-S61.521 with 7th A, S61.529-S61.531 with 7th A, S61.539-S61.541 with 7th A, S61.549-S61.551 with 7th A, S61.559A

✓7th **S56.022 Laceration of flexor muscle, fascia and tendon of left thumb at forearm level** CC
- **CC Excl: CC with 7th character A:** S51.002-S51.009 with 7th A, S51.012-S51.019 with 7th A, S51.022-S51.029 with 7th A, S51.032-S51.039 with 7th A, S51.042-S51.049 with 7th A, S51.052-S51.059 with 7th A, S51.802-S51.809 with 7th A, S51.812-S51.819 with 7th A, S51.822-S51.829 with 7th A, S51.832-S51.839 with 7th A, S51.842-S51.849 with 7th A, S51.852-S51.859 with 7th A, S56.022-S56.029 with 7th A, S56.122A, S56.124A, S56.126A, S56.128-S56.129 with 7th A, S56.222-S56.229 with 7th A, S56.322-S56.329 with 7th A, S56.422A, S56.424 A, S56.426A, S56.428-S56.429 with 7th A, S56.522-S56.529 with 7th A, S56.822-S56.829 with 7th A, S56.922-S56.929 with 7th A, S61.502-S61.509 with 7th A, S61.512-S61.519 with 7th A, S61.522-S61.529 with 7th A, S61.532-S61.539 with 7th A, S61.542-S61.549 with 7th A, S61.552-S61.559 with 7th A

✓7th **S56.029 Laceration of flexor muscle, fascia and tendon of unspecified thumb at forearm level** CC
- **CC Excl: CC with 7th character A:** S51.001-S51.859 with 7th A, S56.021-S56.029 with 7th A, S56.121-S56.129 with 7th A, S56.221-S56.229 with 7th A, S56.321-S56.329 with 7th A, S56.421-S56.429 with 7th A, S56.521-S56.529 with 7th A, S56.821-S56.829 with 7th A, S56.921-S56.929 with 7th A, S61.501-S61.559 with 7th A

✓6th **S56.09 Other injury of flexor muscle, fascia and tendon of thumb at forearm level**

✓7th **S56.091 Other injury of flexor muscle, fascia and tendon of right thumb at forearm level**

✓7th **S56.092 Other injury of flexor muscle, fascia and tendon of left thumb at forearm level**

✓7th **S56.099 Other injury of flexor muscle, fascia and tendon of unspecified thumb at forearm level**

✓5th **S56.1 Injury of flexor muscle, fascia and tendon of other and unspecified finger at forearm level**

✓6th **S56.10 Unspecified injury of flexor muscle, fascia and tendon of other and unspecified finger at forearm level**

✓7th **S56.101 Unspecified injury of flexor muscle, fascia and tendon of right index finger at forearm level**

✓7th **S56.102 Unspecified injury of flexor muscle, fascia and tendon of left index finger at forearm level**

✓7th **S56.103 Unspecified injury of flexor muscle, fascia and tendon of right middle finger at forearm level**

✓7th **S56.104 Unspecified injury of flexor muscle, fascia and tendon of left middle finger at forearm level**

✓7th **S56.105 Unspecified injury of flexor muscle, fascia and tendon of right ring finger at forearm level**

✓7th **S56.106 Unspecified injury of flexor muscle, fascia and tendon of left ring finger at forearm level**

✓7th **S56.107 Unspecified injury of flexor muscle, fascia and tendon of right little finger at forearm level**

✓7th **S56.108 Unspecified injury of flexor muscle, fascia and tendon of left little finger at forearm level**

✓7th **S56.109 Unspecified injury of flexor muscle, fascia and tendon of unspecified finger at forearm level**

✓6th **S56.11 Strain of flexor muscle, fascia and tendon of other and unspecified finger at forearm level**

✓7th **S56.111 Strain of flexor muscle, fascia and tendon of right index finger at forearm level**

✓7th **S56.112 Strain of flexor muscle, fascia and tendon of left index finger at forearm level**

✓7th **S56.113 Strain of flexor muscle, fascia and tendon of right middle finger at forearm level**

✓7th **S56.114 Strain of flexor muscle, fascia and tendon of left middle finger at forearm level**

✓7th **S56.115 Strain of flexor muscle, fascia and tendon of right ring finger at forearm level**

✓7th **S56.116 Strain of flexor muscle, fascia and tendon of left ring finger at forearm level**

✓7th **S56.117 Strain of flexor muscle, fascia and tendon of right little finger at forearm level**

✓7th **S56.118 Strain of flexor muscle, fascia and tendon of left little finger at forearm level**

✓7th **S56.119 Strain of flexor muscle, fascia and tendon of finger of unspecified finger at forearm level**

✓6th **S56.12 Laceration of flexor muscle, fascia and tendon of other and unspecified finger at forearm level**

✓7th **S56.121 Laceration of flexor muscle, fascia and tendon of right index finger at forearm level** CC
- **CC Excl:** See code: S56.021

✓7th S56.122 Laceration of flexor muscle, fascia and tendon of left index finger at forearm level CC
CC Excl: See code: S56.022

✓7th S56.123 Laceration of flexor muscle, fascia and tendon of right middle finger at forearm level CC
CC Excl: See code: S56.021

✓7th S56.124 Laceration of flexor muscle, fascia and tendon of left middle finger at forearm level CC
CC Excl: See code: S56.022

✓7th S56.125 Laceration of flexor muscle, fascia and tendon of right ring finger at forearm level CC
CC Excl: See code: S56.021

✓7th S56.126 Laceration of flexor muscle, fascia and tendon of left ring finger at forearm level CC
CC Excl: See code: S56.022

✓7th S56.127 Laceration of flexor muscle, fascia and tendon of right little finger at forearm level CC
CC Excl: See code: S56.021

✓7th S56.128 Laceration of flexor muscle, fascia and tendon of left little finger at forearm level CC
CC Excl: See code: S56.022

✓7th S56.129 Laceration of flexor muscle, fascia and tendon of unspecified finger at forearm level CC
CC Excl: See code: S56.029

✓6th S56.19 Other injury of flexor muscle, fascia and tendon of other and unspecified finger at forearm level

✓7th S56.191 Other injury of flexor muscle, fascia and tendon of right index finger at forearm level

✓7th S56.192 Other injury of flexor muscle, fascia and tendon of left index finger at forearm level

✓7th S56.193 Other injury of flexor muscle, fascia and tendon of right middle finger at forearm level

✓7th S56.194 Other injury of flexor muscle, fascia and tendon of left middle finger at forearm level

✓7th S56.195 Other injury of flexor muscle, fascia and tendon of right ring finger at forearm level

✓7th S56.196 Other injury of flexor muscle, fascia and tendon of left ring finger at forearm level

✓7th S56.197 Other injury of flexor muscle, fascia and tendon of right little finger at forearm level

✓7th S56.198 Other injury of flexor muscle, fascia and tendon of left little finger at forearm level

✓7th S56.199 Other injury of flexor muscle, fascia and tendon of unspecified finger at forearm level

✓5th S56.2 Injury of other flexor muscle, fascia and tendon at forearm level

✓6th S56.20 Unspecified injury of other flexor muscle, fascia and tendon at forearm level

✓7th S56.201 Unspecified injury of other flexor muscle, fascia and tendon at forearm level, right arm

✓7th S56.202 Unspecified injury of other flexor muscle, fascia and tendon at forearm level, left arm

✓7th S56.209 Unspecified injury of other flexor muscle, fascia and tendon at forearm level, unspecified arm

✓6th S56.21 Strain of other flexor muscle, fascia and tendon at forearm level

✓7th S56.211 Strain of other flexor muscle, fascia and tendon at forearm level, right arm

✓7th S56.212 Strain of other flexor muscle, fascia and tendon at forearm level, left arm

✓7th S56.219 Strain of other flexor muscle, fascia and tendon at forearm level, unspecified arm

✓6th S56.22 Laceration of other flexor muscle, fascia and tendon at forearm level

✓7th S56.221 Laceration of other flexor muscle, fascia and tendon at forearm level, right arm CC
CC Excl: See code: S56.021

✓7th S56.222 Laceration of other flexor muscle, fascia and tendon at forearm level, left arm CC
CC Excl: See code: S56.022

✓7th S56.229 Laceration of other flexor muscle, fascia and tendon at forearm level, unspecified arm CC
CC Excl: See code: S56.029

✓6th S56.29 Other injury of other flexor muscle, fascia and tendon at forearm level

✓7th S56.291 Other injury of other flexor muscle, fascia and tendon at forearm level, right arm

✓7th S56.292 Other injury of other flexor muscle, fascia and tendon at forearm level, left arm

✓7th S56.299 Other injury of other flexor muscle, fascia and tendon at forearm level, unspecified arm

✓5th S56.3 Injury of extensor or abductor muscles, fascia and tendons of thumb at forearm level

✓6th S56.30 Unspecified injury of extensor or abductor muscles, fascia and tendons of thumb at forearm level

✓7th S56.301 Unspecified injury of extensor or abductor muscles, fascia and tendons of right thumb at forearm level

✓7th S56.302 Unspecified injury of extensor or abductor muscles, fascia and tendons of left thumb at forearm level

✓7th S56.309 Unspecified injury of extensor or abductor muscles, fascia and tendons of unspecified thumb at forearm level

✓6th S56.31 Strain of extensor or abductor muscles, fascia and tendons of thumb at forearm level

✓7th S56.311 Strain of extensor or abductor muscles, fascia and tendons of right thumb at forearm level

✓7th S56.312 Strain of extensor or abductor muscles, fascia and tendons of left thumb at forearm level

✓7th S56.319 Strain of extensor or abductor muscles, fascia and tendons of unspecified thumb at forearm level

✓6th S56.32 Laceration of extensor or abductor muscles, fascia and tendons of thumb at forearm level

✓7th S56.321 Laceration of extensor or abductor muscles, fascia and tendons of right thumb at forearm level CC
CC Excl: See code: S56.021

✓7th S56.322 Laceration of extensor or abductor muscles, fascia and tendons of left thumb at forearm level CC
CC Excl: See code: S56.022

✓7th S56.329 Laceration of extensor or abductor muscles, fascia and tendons of unspecified thumb at forearm level CC
CC Excl: See code: S56.029

✓6th S56.39 Other injury of extensor or abductor muscles, fascia and tendons of thumb at forearm level

✓7th S56.391 Other injury of extensor or abductor muscles, fascia and tendons of right thumb at forearm level

✓7th S56.392 Other injury of extensor or abductor muscles, fascia and tendons of left thumb at forearm level

✓7th S56.399 Other injury of extensor or abductor muscles, fascia and tendons of unspecified thumb at forearm level

✓5th S56.4 Injury of extensor muscle, fascia and tendon of other and unspecified finger at forearm level

✓6th S56.40 Unspecified injury of extensor muscle, fascia and tendon of other and unspecified finger at forearm level

7th **S56.401** Unspecified injury of extensor muscle, fascia and tendon of right index finger at forearm level

7th **S56.402** Unspecified injury of extensor muscle, fascia and tendon of left index finger at forearm level

7th **S56.403** Unspecified injury of extensor muscle, fascia and tendon of right middle finger at forearm level

7th **S56.404** Unspecified injury of extensor muscle, fascia and tendon of left middle finger at forearm level

7th **S56.405** Unspecified injury of extensor muscle, fascia and tendon of right ring finger at forearm level

7th **S56.406** Unspecified injury of extensor muscle, fascia and tendon of left ring finger at forearm level

7th **S56.407** Unspecified injury of extensor muscle, fascia and tendon of right little finger at forearm level

7th **S56.408** Unspecified injury of extensor muscle, fascia and tendon of left little finger at forearm level

7th **S56.409** Unspecified injury of extensor muscle, fascia and tendon of unspecified finger at forearm level

6th **S56.41** Strain of extensor muscle, fascia and tendon of other and unspecified finger at forearm level

7th **S56.411** Strain of extensor muscle, fascia and tendon of right index finger at forearm level

7th **S56.412** Strain of extensor muscle, fascia and tendon of left index finger at forearm level

7th **S56.413** Strain of extensor muscle, fascia and tendon of right middle finger at forearm level

7th **S56.414** Strain of extensor muscle, fascia and tendon of left middle finger at forearm level

7th **S56.415** Strain of extensor muscle, fascia and tendon of right ring finger at forearm level

7th **S56.416** Strain of extensor muscle, fascia and tendon of left ring finger at forearm level

7th **S56.417** Strain of extensor muscle, fascia and tendon of right little finger at forearm level

7th **S56.418** Strain of extensor muscle, fascia and tendon of left little finger at forearm level

7th **S56.419** Strain of extensor muscle, fascia and tendon of finger, unspecified finger at forearm level

6th **S56.42** Laceration of extensor muscle, fascia and tendon of other and unspecified finger at forearm level

7th **S56.421** Laceration of extensor muscle, fascia and tendon of right index finger at forearm level CC
CC Excl: See code: S56.021

7th **S56.422** Laceration of extensor muscle, fascia and tendon of left index finger at forearm level CC
CC Excl: See code: S56.022

7th **S56.423** Laceration of extensor muscle, fascia and tendon of right middle finger at forearm level CC
CC Excl: See code: S56.021

7th **S56.424** Laceration of extensor muscle, fascia and tendon of left middle finger at forearm level CC
CC Excl: See code: S56.022

7th **S56.425** Laceration of extensor muscle, fascia and tendon of right ring finger at forearm level CC
CC Excl: See code: S56.021

7th **S56.426** Laceration of extensor muscle, fascia and tendon of left ring finger at forearm level CC
CC Excl: See code: S56.022

7th **S56.427** Laceration of extensor muscle, fascia and tendon of right little finger at forearm level CC
CC Excl: See code: S56.021

7th **S56.428** Laceration of extensor muscle, fascia and tendon of left little finger at forearm level CC
CC Excl: See code: S56.022

7th **S56.429** Laceration of extensor muscle, fascia and tendon of unspecified finger at forearm level CC
CC Excl: See code: S56.029

6th **S56.49** Other injury of extensor muscle, fascia and tendon of other and unspecified finger at forearm level

7th **S56.491** Other injury of extensor muscle, fascia and tendon of right index finger at forearm level

7th **S56.492** Other injury of extensor muscle, fascia and tendon of left index finger at forearm level

7th **S56.493** Other injury of extensor muscle, fascia and tendon of right middle finger at forearm level

7th **S56.494** Other injury of extensor muscle, fascia and tendon of left middle finger at forearm level

7th **S56.495** Other injury of extensor muscle, fascia and tendon of right ring finger at forearm level

7th **S56.496** Other injury of extensor muscle, fascia and tendon of left ring finger at forearm level

7th **S56.497** Other injury of extensor muscle, fascia and tendon of right little finger at forearm level

7th **S56.498** Other injury of extensor muscle, fascia and tendon of left little finger at forearm level

7th **S56.499** Other injury of extensor muscle, fascia and tendon of unspecified finger at forearm level

5th **S56.5** Injury of other extensor muscle, fascia and tendon at forearm level

6th **S56.50** Unspecified injury of other extensor muscle, fascia and tendon at forearm level

7th **S56.501** Unspecified injury of other extensor muscle, fascia and tendon at forearm level, right arm

7th **S56.502** Unspecified injury of other extensor muscle, fascia and tendon at forearm level, left arm

7th **S56.509** Unspecified injury of other extensor muscle, fascia and tendon at forearm level, unspecified arm

6th **S56.51** Strain of other extensor muscle, fascia and tendon at forearm level

7th **S56.511** Strain of other extensor muscle, fascia and tendon at forearm level, right arm

7th **S56.512** Strain of other extensor muscle, fascia and tendon at forearm level, left arm

7th **S56.519** Strain of other extensor muscle, fascia and tendon at forearm level, unspecified arm

6th **S56.52** Laceration of other extensor muscle, fascia and tendon at forearm level

7th **S56.521** Laceration of other extensor muscle, fascia and tendon at forearm level, right arm CC
CC Excl: See code: S56.021

7th **S56.522** Laceration of other extensor muscle, fascia and tendon at forearm level, left arm CC
CC Excl: See code: S56.022

7th **S56.529** Laceration of other extensor muscle, fascia and tendon at forearm level, unspecified arm CC
CC Excl: See code: S56.029

6th **S56.59** Other injury of other extensor muscle, fascia and tendon at forearm level

7th **S56.591** Other injury of other extensor muscle, fascia and tendon at forearm level, right arm

7th S56.592 **Other injury of other extensor muscle, fascia and tendon at forearm level, left arm**

7th S56.599 **Other injury of other extensor muscle, fascia and tendon at forearm level, unspecified arm**

5th **S56.8 Injury of other muscles, fascia and tendons at forearm level**

6th **S56.8Ø Unspecified injury of other muscles, fascia and tendons at forearm level**

7th S56.8Ø1 **Unspecified injury of other muscles, fascia and tendons at forearm level, right arm**

7th S56.8Ø2 **Unspecified injury of other muscles, fascia and tendons at forearm level, left arm**

7th S56.8Ø9 **Unspecified injury of other muscles, fascia and tendons at forearm level, unspecified arm**

6th **S56.81 Strain of other muscles, fascia and tendons at forearm level**

7th S56.811 **Strain of other muscles, fascia and tendons at forearm level, right arm**

7th S56.812 **Strain of other muscles, fascia and tendons at forearm level, left arm**

7th S56.819 **Strain of other muscles, fascia and tendons at forearm level, unspecified arm**

6th **S56.82 Laceration of other muscles, fascia and tendons at forearm level**

7th S56.821 **Laceration of other muscles, fascia and tendons at forearm level, right arm** CC
CC Excl: See code: S56.Ø21

7th S56.822 **Laceration of other muscles, fascia and tendons at forearm level, left arm** CC
CC Excl: See code: S56.Ø22

7th S56.829 **Laceration of other muscles, fascia and tendons at forearm level, unspecified arm** CC
CC Excl: See code: S56.Ø29

6th **S56.89 Other injury of other muscles, fascia and tendons at forearm level**

7th S56.891 **Other injury of other muscles, fascia and tendons at forearm level, right arm**

7th S56.892 **Other injury of other muscles, fascia and tendons at forearm level, left arm**

7th S56.899 **Other injury of other muscles, fascia and tendons at forearm level, unspecified arm**

5th **S56.9 Injury of unspecified muscles, fascia and tendons at forearm level**

6th **S56.9Ø Unspecified injury of unspecified muscles, fascia and tendons at forearm level**

7th S56.9Ø1 **Unspecified injury of unspecified muscles, fascia and tendons at forearm level, right arm**

7th S56.9Ø2 **Unspecified injury of unspecified muscles, fascia and tendons at forearm level, left arm**

7th S56.9Ø9 **Unspecified injury of unspecified muscles, fascia and tendons at forearm level, unspecified arm**

6th **S56.91 Strain of unspecified muscles, fascia and tendons at forearm level**

7th S56.911 **Strain of unspecified muscles, fascia and tendons at forearm level, right arm**

7th S56.912 **Strain of unspecified muscles, fascia and tendons at forearm level, left arm**

7th S56.919 **Strain of unspecified muscles, fascia and tendons at forearm level, unspecified arm**

6th **S56.92 Laceration of unspecified muscles, fascia and tendons at forearm level**

7th S56.921 **Laceration of unspecified muscles, fascia and tendons at forearm level, right arm** CC
CC Excl: See code: S56.Ø21

7th S56.922 **Laceration of unspecified muscles, fascia and tendons at forearm level, left arm** CC
CC Excl: See code: S56.Ø22

7th S56.929 **Laceration of unspecified muscles, fascia and tendons at forearm level, unspecified arm** CC
CC Excl: See code: S56.Ø29

6th **S56.99 Other injury of unspecified muscles, fascia and tendons at forearm level**

7th S56.991 **Other injury of unspecified muscles, fascia and tendons at forearm level, right arm**

7th S56.992 **Other injury of unspecified muscles, fascia and tendons at forearm level, left arm**

7th S56.999 **Other injury of unspecified muscles, fascia and tendons at forearm level, unspecified arm**

4th **S57 Crushing injury of elbow and forearm**

Use additional code(s) for all associated injuries

EXCLUDES 2 *crushing injury of wrist and hand (S67.-)*

The appropriate 7th is to be added to each code from category S57.
A initial encounter
D subsequent encounter
S sequela

5th **S57.Ø Crushing injury of elbow**

x7th **S57.ØØ Crushing injury of unspecified elbow**

x7th **S57.Ø1 Crushing injury of right elbow**

x7th **S57.Ø2 Crushing injury of left elbow**

5th **S57.8 Crushing injury of forearm**

x7th **S57.8Ø Crushing injury of unspecified forearm**

x7th **S57.81 Crushing injury of right forearm**

x7th **S57.82 Crushing injury of left forearm**

4th **S58 Traumatic amputation of elbow and forearm**

NOTE An amputation not identified as partial or complete should be coded to complete.

EXCLUDES 1 *traumatic amputation of wrist and hand (S68.-)*

The appropriate 7th is to be added to each code from category S58.
A initial encounter
D subsequent encounter
S sequela

5th **S58.Ø Traumatic amputation at elbow level**

6th **S58.Ø1 Complete traumatic amputation at elbow level**

7th **S58.Ø11 Complete traumatic amputation at elbow level, right arm** CC
CC Excl: CC with 7th character A: S41.ØØ1 with 7th A, S41.ØØ9-S41.Ø11 with 7th A, S41.Ø19-S41.Ø21 with 7th A, S41.Ø29-S41.Ø31 with 7th A, S41.Ø39-S41.Ø41 with 7th A, S41.Ø49-S41.Ø51 with 7th A, S41.Ø59-S41.1Ø1 with 7th A, S41.1Ø9-S41.111 with 7th A, S41.119-S41.121 with 7th A, S41.129-S41.131 with 7th A, S41.139-S41.141 with 7th A, S41.149-S41.151 with 7th A, S41.159A, S46.Ø21A, S46.Ø29A, S46.121A, S46.129A, S46.221A, S46.229A, S46.321A, S46.329A, S46.821A, S46.829A, S46.921A, S46.929A, S48.Ø11A, S48.Ø19-S48.Ø21 with 7th A, S48.Ø29-S48.111 with 7th A, S48.119-S48.121 with 7th A, S48.129-S48.911 with 7th A, S48.919-S48.921 with 7th A, S48.929A, S51.ØØ1A, S51.ØØ9-S51.Ø11 with 7th A, S51.Ø19-S51.Ø21 with 7th A, S51.Ø29-S51.Ø31 with 7th A, S51.Ø39-S51.Ø41 with 7th A, S51.Ø49-S51.Ø51 with 7th A, S51.Ø59-S51.8Ø1 with 7th A, S51.8Ø9-S51.811 with 7th A, S51.819-S51.821 with 7th A, S51.829-S51.831 with 7th A, S51.839-S51.841 with 7th A, S51.849-S51.851 with 7th A, S51.859A, S56.Ø21A, S56.Ø29A, S56.121A, S56.123A, S56.125A, S56.127A, S56.129A, S56.221A, S56.229A, S56.321A, S56.329A, S56.421A, S56.423A, S56.425 with 7th A, S56.427 with 7th A, S56.429 with 7th A, S56.521 with 7th A, S56.529 with 7th A, S56.821 with 7th A, S56.829 with 7th A, S56.921 with 7th A, S56.929 with 7th A, S58.Ø11 with 7th A, S58.Ø19-S58.Ø21 with 7th A, S58.Ø29-S58.111 with 7th A, S58.119-S58.121 with 7th A, S58.129-S58.911 with 7th A, S58.919-S58.921 with 7th A, S58.929 with 7th A, S61.ØØ1 with 7th A, S61.ØØ9-S61.Ø11 with 7th A, S61.Ø19-S61.Ø21 with 7th A, S61.Ø29-S61.Ø31 with 7th A, S61.Ø39-S61.Ø41 with

7th A, S61.Ø49-S61.Ø51 with 7th A, S61.Ø59-S61.1Ø1 with 7th A, S61.1Ø9-S61.111 with 7th A, S61.119-S61.121 with 7th A, S61.129-S61.131 with 7th A, S61.139-S61.141 with 7th A, S61.149-S61.151 with 7th A, S61.159-S61.2ØØ with 7th A, S61.2Ø2 with 7th A, S61.2Ø4 with 7th A, S61.2Ø6 with 7th A, S61.2Ø8-S61.21Ø with 7th A, S61.212 with 7th A, S61.214 with 7th A, S61.216 with 7th A, S61.218-S61.22Ø with 7th A, S61.222 with 7th A, S61.224 with 7th A, S61.226 with 7th A, S61.228-S61.23Ø with 7th A, S61.232 with 7th A, S61.234 with 7th A, S61.236 with 7th A, S61.238-S61.24Ø with 7th A, S61.242 with 7th A, S61.244 with 7th A, S61.246 with 7th A, S61.248-S61.25Ø with 7th A, S61.252 with 7th A, S61.254 with 7th A, S61.256 with 7th A, S61.258-S61.3ØØ with 7th A, S61.3Ø2 with 7th A, S61.3Ø4 with 7th A, S61.3Ø6 with 7th A, S61.3Ø8-S61.31Ø with 7th A, S61.312 with 7th A, S61.314 with 7th A, S61.316 with 7th A, S61.318-S61.32Ø with 7th A, S61.322 with 7th A, S61.324 with 7th A, S61.326 with 7th A, S61.328-S61.33Ø with 7th A, S61.332 with 7th A, S61.334 with 7th A, S61.336 with 7th A, S61.338-S61.34Ø with 7th A, S61.342 with 7th A, S61.344 with 7th A, S61.346 with 7th A, S61.348-S61.35Ø with 7th A, S61.352 with 7th A, S61.354 with 7th A, S61.356 with 7th A, S61.358-S61.4Ø1 with 7th A, S61.4Ø9-S61.411 with 7th A, S61.419-S61.421 with 7th A, S61.429-S61.431 with 7th A, S61.439-S61.441 with 7th A, S61.449-S61.451 with 7th A, S61.459-S61.5Ø1 with 7th A, S61.5Ø9-S61.511 with 7th A, S61.519-S61.521 with 7th A, S61.529-S61.531 with 7th A, S61.539-S61.541 with 7th A, S61.549-S61.551 with 7th A, S61.559 with 7th A, S66.Ø21 with 7th A, S66.Ø29 with 7th A, S66.12Ø with 7th A, S66.122 with 7th A, S66.124 with 7th A, S66.126 with 7th A, S66.128-S66.129 with 7th A, S66.221 with 7th A, S66.229 with 7th A, S66.32Ø with 7th A, S66.322 with 7th A, S66.324 with 7th A, S66.326 with 7th A, S66.328-S66.329 with 7th A, S66.421 with 7th A, S66.429 with 7th A, S66.52Ø with 7th A, S66.522 with 7th A, S66.524 with 7th A, S66.526 with 7th A, S66.528-S66.529 with 7th A, S66.821 with 7th A, S66.829 with 7th A, S66.921 with 7th A, S66.929 with 7th A, S68.Ø11 with 7th A, S68.Ø19-S68.Ø21 with 7th A, S68.Ø29-S68.11Ø with 7th A, S68.112 with 7th A, S68.114 with 7th A, S68.116 with 7th A, S68.118-S68.12Ø with 7th A, S68.122 with 7th A, S68.124 with 7th A, S68.126 with 7th A, S68.128-S68.411 with 7th A, S68.419-S68.421 with 7th A, S68.429-S68.511 with 7th A, S68.519-S68.521 with 7th A, S68.529-S68.61Ø with 7th A, S68.612 with 7th A, S68.614 with 7th A, S68.616 with 7th A, S68.618-S68.62Ø with 7th A, S68.622A, S68.624A, S68.626A, S68.628-S68.711 with 7th A, S68.719-S68.721 with 7th A, S68.729A, T14.8-T14.91, T79.AØX-T79.9XX with 7th A

✓7th **S58.Ø12 Complete traumatic amputation at elbow level, left arm** CC

CC Excl: CC with 7th character A: S41.ØØ2-S41.ØØ9 with 7th A, S41.Ø12-S41.Ø19 with 7th A, S41.Ø22-S41.Ø29 with 7th A, S41.Ø32-S41.Ø39 with 7th A, S41.Ø42-S41.Ø49 with 7th A, S41.Ø52-S41.Ø59 with 7th A, S41.1Ø2-S41.1Ø9 with 7th A, S41.112-S41.119 with 7th A, S41.122-S41.129 with 7th A, S41.132-S41.139 with 7th A, S41.142-S41.149 with 7th A, S41.152-S41.159 with 7th A, S46.Ø22-S46.Ø29 with 7th A, S46.122-S46.129 with 7th A, S46.222-S46.229 with 7th A, S46.322-S46.329 with 7th A, S46.822-S46.829 with 7th A, S46.922-S46.929 with 7th A, S48.Ø12-S48.Ø19 with 7th A, S48.Ø22-S48.Ø29 with 7th A, S48.112-S48.119 with 7th A, S48.122-S48.129 with 7th A, S48.912-S48.919 with 7th A, S48.922-S48.929 with 7th A, S51.ØØ2-S51.ØØ9 with 7th A, S51.Ø12-S51.Ø19 with 7th A, S51.Ø22-S51.Ø29 with 7th A, S51.Ø32-S51.Ø39 with 7th A, S51.Ø42-S51.Ø49 with 7th A, S51.Ø52-S51.Ø59 with 7th A, S51.8Ø2-S51.8Ø9 with 7th A, S51.812-S51.819 with 7th A, S51.822-S51.829 with 7th A, S51.832-S51.839 with 7th A, S51.842-S51.849 with 7th A, S51.852-S51.859 with 7th A, S56.Ø22-S56.Ø29 with 7th A, S56.122A, S56.124A, S56.126A, S56.128-S56.129 with 7th A, S56.222-S56.229 with 7th A, S56.322-S56.329 with 7th A, S56.422 with 7th A, S56.424A, S56.426A, S56.428-S56.429 with 7th A, S56.522-S56.529 with 7th A, S56.822-S56.829 with 7th A, S56.922-S56.929 with 7th A, S58.Ø12-S58.Ø19 with 7th A, S58.Ø22-S58.Ø29 with 7th A, S58.112-S58.119 with 7th A, S58.122-S58.129 with 7th A, S58.912-S58.919 with 7th A, S58.922-S58.929 with 7th A, S61.ØØ2-S61.ØØ9 with 7th A, S61.Ø12-S61.Ø19 with 7th A, S61.Ø22-S61.Ø29 with 7th A, S61.Ø32-S61.Ø39 with 7th A, S61.Ø42-S61.Ø49 with 7th A, S61.Ø52-S61.Ø59 with 7th A, S61.1Ø2-S61.1Ø9 with 7th A, S61.112-S61.119 with 7th A, S61.122-S61.129 with 7th A, S61.132-S61.139 with 7th A, S61.142-S61.149 with 7th A, S61.152-S61.159 with 7th A, S61.2Ø1A, S61.2Ø3A, S61.2Ø5A, S61.2Ø7-S61.2Ø9 with 7th A, S61.211A, S61.213A, S61.215A, S61.217-S61.219 with 7th A, S61.221A, S61.223A, S61.225A, S61.227-S61.229 with 7th A, S61.231A, S61.233A, S61.235A, S61.237-S61.239 with 7th A, S61.241A, S61.243A, S61.245A, S61.247-S61.249 with 7th A, S61.251A, S61.253A, S61.255 with 7th A, S61.257-S61.259 with 7th A, S61.3Ø1A, S61.3Ø3A, S61.3Ø5A, S61.3Ø7-S61.3Ø9 with 7th A, S61.311A, S61.313A, S61.315A, S61.317-S61.319A, S61.321A, S61.323A, S61.325A, S61.327-S61.329 with 7th A, S61.331A, S61.333A, S61.335 with 7th A, S61.337-S61.339 with 7th A, S61.341A, S61.343A, S61.345A, S61.347-S61.349 with 7th A, S61.351A, S61.353A, S61.355A, S61.357-S61.359 with 7th A, S61.4Ø2-S61.4Ø9 with 7th A, S61.412-S61.419 with 7th A, S61.422-S61.429 with 7th A, S61.432-S61.439 with 7th A, S61.442-S61.449 with 7th A, S61.452-S61.459 with 7th A, S61.5Ø2-S61.5Ø9 with 7th A, S61.512-S61.519 with 7th A, S61.522-S61.529 with 7th A, S61.532-S61.539 with 7th A, S61.542-S61.549 with 7th A, S61.552-S61.559 with 7th A, S66.Ø22-S66.Ø29 with 7th A, S66.121 character A, S66.123A, S66.125A, S66.127-S66.129 with 7th A, S66.222-S66.229 with 7th A, S66.321A, S66.323A, S66.325A, S66.327-S66.329 with 7th A, S66.422-S66.429 with 7th A, S66.521A, S66.523A, S66.525A, S66.527-S66.529 with 7th A, S66.822-S66.829 with 7th A, S66.922-S66.929 with 7th A, S68.Ø12-S68.Ø19 with 7th A, S68.Ø22-S68.Ø29 with 7th A, S68.111A, S68.113A, S68.115A, S68.117-S68.119A, S68.121A, S68.123A, S68.125A, S68.127-S68.129 with 7th A, S68.412-S68.419 with 7th A, S68.422-S68.429 with 7th A, S68.512-S68.519 with 7th A, S68.522-S68.529 with 7th A, S68.611A, S68.613 , S68.615A, S68.617-S68.619 with 7th A, S68.621A, S68.623A, S68.625A, S68.627-S68.629 with 7th A, S68.712-S68.719 with 7th A, S68.722-S68.729 with 7th A, T14.8-T14.91, T79.AØX-T79.9XX with 7th A

✓7th **S58.Ø19 Complete traumatic amputation at elbow level, unspecified arm** CC

CC Excl: CC with 7th character A: S41.ØØ1-S41.159 with 7th A, S46.Ø21-S46.Ø29 with 7th A, S46.121-S46.129 with 7th A, S46.221-S46.229 with 7th A, S46.321-S46.329 with 7th A, S46.821-S46.829 with 7th A, S46.921-S46.929 with 7th A, S48.Ø11-S48.929 with 7th A, S51.ØØ1-S51.859 with 7th A, S56.Ø21-S56.Ø29 with 7th A, S56.121-S56.129 with 7th A, S56.221-S56.229 with 7th A, S56.321-S56.329 with 7th A, S56.421-S56.429 with 7th A, S56.521-S56.529 with 7th A, S56.821-S56.829 with 7th A, S56.921-S56.929 with 7th A, S58.Ø11-S58.929 with 7th A, S61.ØØ1-S61.559 with 7th A, S66.Ø21-S66.Ø29 with 7th A, S66.12Ø-S66.129 with 7th A, S66.221-S66.229 with 7th A, S66.32Ø-S66.329 with 7th A, S66.421-S66.429 with 7th A, S66.52Ø-S66.529 with 7th A, S66.821-S66.829 with 7th A, S66.921-S66.929 with 7th A, S68.Ø11-S68.729 with 7th A, T14.8-T14.91, T79.AØX-T79.9XX with 7th A

√6th **S58.02 Partial traumatic amputation at elbow level**

√7th **S58.021 Partial traumatic amputation at elbow level, right arm** CC
CC Excl: See code: S58.011

√7th **S58.022 Partial traumatic amputation at elbow level, left arm** CC
CC Excl: See code: S58.012

√7th **S58.029 Partial traumatic amputation at elbow level, unspecified arm** CC
CC Excl: See code: S58.019

√5th **S58.1 Traumatic amputation at level between elbow and wrist**

√6th **S58.11 Complete traumatic amputation at level between elbow and wrist**

√7th **S58.111 Complete traumatic amputation at level between elbow and wrist, right arm** CC
CC Excl: See code: S58.011

√7th **S58.112 Complete traumatic amputation at level between elbow and wrist, left arm** CC
CC Excl: See code: S58.012

√7th **S58.119 Complete traumatic amputation at level between elbow and wrist, unspecified arm** CC
CC Excl: See code: S58.019

√6th **S58.12 Partial traumatic amputation at level between elbow and wrist**

√7th **S58.121 Partial traumatic amputation at level between elbow and wrist, right arm** CC
CC Excl: See code: S58.011

√7th **S58.122 Partial traumatic amputation at level between elbow and wrist, left arm** CC
CC Excl: See code: S58.012

√7th **S58.129 Partial traumatic amputation at level between elbow and wrist, unspecified arm** CC
CC Excl: See code: S58.019

√5th **S58.9 Traumatic amputation of forearm, level unspecified**
EXCLUDES 1 *traumatic amputation of wrist (S68.-)*

√6th **S58.91 Complete traumatic amputation of forearm, level unspecified**

√7th **S58.911 Complete traumatic amputation of right forearm, level unspecified** CC
CC Excl: See code: S58.011

√7th **S58.912 Complete traumatic amputation of left forearm, level unspecified** CC
CC Excl: See code: S58.012

√7th **S58.919 Complete traumatic amputation of unspecified forearm, level unspecified** CC
CC Excl: See code: S58.019

√6th **S58.92 Partial traumatic amputation of forearm, level unspecified**

√7th **S58.921 Partial traumatic amputation of right forearm, level unspecified**

√7th **S58.922 Partial traumatic amputation of left forearm, level unspecified**

√7th **S58.929 Partial traumatic amputation of unspecified forearm, level unspecified**

√4th **S59 Other and unspecified injuries of elbow and forearm**
EXCLUDES 2 *other and unspecified injuries of wrist and hand (S69.-)*

The appropriate 7th is to be added to each code from subcategories S59.0, S59.1, and S59.2.
- A initial encounter for closed fracture
- D subsequent encounter for fracture with routine healing
- G subsequent encounter for fracture with delayed healing
- K subsequent encounter for fracture with nonunion
- P subsequent encounter for fracture with malunion
- S sequela

√5th **S59.0 Physeal fracture of lower end of ulna**

√6th **S59.00 Unspecified physeal fracture of lower end of ulna**

7 √7th **S59.001 Unspecified physeal fracture of lower end of ulna, right arm** CC
CC Excl: CC with 7th character A: S52.001-S52.011 with 7th [A, B, C], S52.019-S52.111 with 7th A, S52.119-S52.211 with 7th A, S52.219-S52.311 with 7th A, S52.319-S52.521 with 7th A, S52.529-S52.621 with 7th A, S52.629-S52.92X with 7th A, S59.001A, S59.009-S59.011 with 7th A, S59.019-S59.021 with 7th A, S59.029-S59.031 with 7th A, S59.039-S59.041 with 7th A, S59.049-S59.091 with 7th A, S59.099-S59.101 with 7th A, S59.109-S59.111 with 7th A, S59.119-S59.121 with 7th A, S59.129-S59.131 with 7th A, S59.139-S59.141 with 7th A, S59.149-S59.191 with 7th A, S59.199-S59.201 with 7th A, S59.209-S59.211 with 7th A, S59.219-S59.221 with 7th A, S59.229-S59.231 with 7th A, S59.239-S59.241 with 7th A, S59.249-S59.291 with 7th A, S59.299A
CC with 7th character K or P: M80.00X-M84.68X with 7th [K, P], S02.0XX-S02.92X with 7th K, S12.000-S12.691 with 7th K, S22.000-S22.9XX with 7th K, S32.000-S32.9XX with 7th K, S42.001-S42.92X with 7th [K, P], S49.001-S49.199 with 7th [K, P], S52.001-S52.92X with 7th [K, M, N, P, Q, R], S59.001-S59.299 with 7th [K, P], S62.001-S62.92X with 7th [K, P], S72.001-S72.92X with 7th [K, M, N, P, Q, R], S79.001-S79.199 with 7th [K, P], S82.001-S82.92X with 7th [K, M, N, P, Q, R], S89.001-S89.399 with 7th [K, P], S92.001-S92.919 with 7th [K, P]

7 √7th **S59.002 Unspecified physeal fracture of lower end of ulna, left arm** CC
CC Excl: CC with 7th character A: S52.001-S52.009 with 7th [B, C], S52.012-S52.109 with 7th A, S52.112-S52.209 with 7th A, S52.212-S52.309 with 7th A, S52.312-S52.516 with 7th A, S52.522-S52.616 with 7th A, S52.622-S52.92X with 7th A, S59.002-S59.009 with 7th A, S59.012-S59.019 with 7th A, S59.022-S59.029 with 7th A, S59.032-S59.039 with 7th A, S59.042-S59.049 with 7th A, S59.092-S59.099 with 7th A, S59.102-S59.109 with 7th A, S59.112-S59.119 with 7th A, S59.122-S59.129 with 7th A, S59.132-S59.139 with 7th A, S59.142-S59.149 with 7th A, S59.192-S59.199 with 7th A, S59.202-S59.209 with 7th A, S59.212-S59.219 with 7th A, S59.222-S59.229 with 7th A, S59.232-S59.239 with 7th A, S59.242-S59.249 with 7th A, S59.292-S59.299 with 7th A
CC with 7th character K or P: M80.00X-M84.68X with 7th [K, P], S02.0XX-S02.92X with 7th K, S12.000-S12.691 with 7th K, S22.000-S22.9XX with 7th K, S32.000-S32.9XX with 7th K, S42.001-S42.92X with 7th [K, P], S49.001-S49.199 with 7th [K, P], S52.001-S52.92X with 7th [K, M, N, P, Q, R], S59.001-S59.299 with 7th [K, P], S62.001-S62.92X with 7th [K, P], S72.001-S72.92X with 7th [K, M, N, P, Q, R], S79.001-S79.199 with 7th [K, P], S82.001-S82.92X with 7th [K, M, N, P, Q, R], S89.001-S89.399 with 7th [K, P], S92.001-S92.919 with 7th [K, P]

7 √7th **S59.009 Unspecified physeal fracture of lower end of ulna, unspecified arm** CC
CC Excl: CC with 7th character A: S52.001-S52.92X with 7th [A, B, C], S59.001-S59.299 with 7th A
CC with 7th character K or P: M80.00X-M84.68X with 7th [K, P], S02.0XX-S02.92X with 7th K, S12.000-S12.691 with 7th K, S22.000-S22.9XX with 7th K, S32.000-S32.9XX with 7th K, S42.001-S42.92X with 7th [K, P], S49.001-S49.199 with 7th [K, P], S52.001-S52.92X with 7th [K, M, N, P, Q, R], S59.001-S59.299 with 7th [K, P], S62.001-S62.92X with 7th [K, P], S72.001-S72.92X with 7th [K, M, N, P, Q, R], S79.001-S79.199 with 7th [K, P], S82.001-S82.92X with 7th [K, M, N, P, Q, R], S89.001-S89.399 with 7th [K, P], S92.001-S92.919 with 7th [K, P]

√6th **S59.01 Salter-Harris Type I physeal fracture of lower end of ulna**

7 √7th **S59.011 Salter-Harris Type I physeal fracture of lower end of ulna, right arm** CC
CC Excl: See code: S59.001

7 HAC = Initial encounter only (7th character A, B or C) and not POA.

7 ✓7th **S59.Ø12 Salter-Harris Type I physeal fracture of lower end of ulna, left arm** CC
CC Excl: See code: S59.ØØ2

7 ✓7th **S59.Ø19 Salter-Harris Type I physeal fracture of lower end of ulna, unspecified arm** CC
CC Excl: See code: S59.ØØ9

✓6th **S59.Ø2 Salter-Harris Type II physeal fracture of lower end of ulna**

7 ✓7th **S59.Ø21 Salter-Harris Type II physeal fracture of lower end of ulna, right arm** CC
CC Excl: See code: S59.ØØ1

7 ✓7th **S59.Ø22 Salter-Harris Type II physeal fracture of lower end of ulna, left arm** CC
CC Excl: See code: S59.ØØ2

7 ✓7th **S59.Ø29 Salter-Harris Type II physeal fracture of lower end of ulna, unspecified arm** CC
CC Excl: See code: S59.ØØ9

✓6th **S59.Ø3 Salter-Harris Type III physeal fracture of lower end of ulna**

7 ✓7th **S59.Ø31 Salter-Harris Type III physeal fracture of lower end of ulna, right arm** CC
CC Excl: See code: S59.ØØ1

7 ✓7th **S59.Ø32 Salter-Harris Type III physeal fracture of lower end of ulna, left arm** CC
CC Excl: See code: S59.ØØ2

7 ✓7th **S59.Ø39 Salter-Harris Type III physeal fracture of lower end of ulna, unspecified arm** CC
CC Excl: See code: S59.ØØ9

✓6th **S59.Ø4 Salter-Harris Type IV physeal fracture of lower end of ulna**

7 ✓7th **S59.Ø41 Salter-Harris Type IV physeal fracture of lower end of ulna, right arm** CC
CC Excl: See code: S59.ØØ1

7 ✓7th **S59.Ø42 Salter-Harris Type IV physeal fracture of lower end of ulna, left arm** CC
CC Excl: See code: S59.ØØ2

7 ✓7th **S59.Ø49 Salter-Harris Type IV physeal fracture of lower end of ulna, unspecified arm** CC
CC Excl: See code: S59.ØØ9

✓6th **S59.Ø9 Other physeal fracture of lower end of ulna**

7 ✓7th **S59.Ø91 Other physeal fracture of lower end of ulna, right arm** CC
CC Excl: See code: S59.ØØ1

7 ✓7th **S59.Ø92 Other physeal fracture of lower end of ulna, left arm** CC
CC Excl: See code: S59.ØØ2

7 ✓7th **S59.Ø99 Other physeal fracture of lower end of ulna, unspecified arm** CC
CC Excl: See code: S59.ØØ9

✓5th **S59.1 Physeal fracture of upper end of radius**

CC Excl: For CC/MCC codes in subcategory S59.1 with 7th K or P: See Code: S59.ØØ9

✓6th **S59.1Ø Unspecified physeal fracture of upper end of radius**

✓7th **S59.1Ø1 Unspecified physeal fracture of upper end of radius, right arm** CC

✓7th **S59.1Ø2 Unspecified physeal fracture of upper end of radius, left arm** CC

✓7th **S59.1Ø9 Unspecified physeal fracture of upper end of radius, unspecified arm** CC

✓6th **S59.11 Salter-Harris Type I physeal fracture of upper end of radius**

✓7th **S59.111 Salter-Harris Type I physeal fracture of upper end of radius, right arm** CC

✓7th **S59.112 Salter-Harris Type I physeal fracture of upper end of radius, left arm** CC

✓7th **S59.119 Salter-Harris Type I physeal fracture of upper end of radius, unspecified arm** CC

✓6th **S59.12 Salter-Harris Type II physeal fracture of upper end of radius**

✓7th **S59.121 Salter-Harris Type II physeal fracture of upper end of radius, right arm** CC

✓7th **S59.122 Salter-Harris Type II physeal fracture of upper end of radius, left arm** CC

✓7th **S59.129 Salter-Harris Type II physeal fracture of upper end of radius, unspecified arm** CC

✓6th **S59.13 Salter-Harris Type III physeal fracture of upper end of radius**

✓7th **S59.131 Salter-Harris Type III physeal fracture of upper end of radius, right arm** CC

✓7th **S59.132 Salter-Harris Type III physeal fracture of upper end of radius, left arm** CC

✓7th **S59.139 Salter-Harris Type III physeal fracture of upper end of radius, unspecified arm** CC

✓6th **S59.14 Salter-Harris Type IV physeal fracture of upper end of radius**

✓7th **S59.141 Salter-Harris Type IV physeal fracture of upper end of radius, right arm** CC

✓7th **S59.142 Salter-Harris Type IV physeal fracture of upper end of radius, left arm** CC

✓7th **S59.149 Salter-Harris Type IV physeal fracture of upper end of radius, unspecified arm** CC

✓6th **S59.19 Other physeal fracture of upper end of radius**

✓7th **S59.191 Other physeal fracture of upper end of radius, right arm** CC

✓7th **S59.192 Other physeal fracture of upper end of radius, left arm** CC

✓7th **S59.199 Other physeal fracture of upper end of radius, unspecified arm** CC

✓5th **S59.2 Physeal fracture of lower end of radius**

✓6th **S59.2Ø Unspecified physeal fracture of lower end of radius**

7 ✓7th **S59.2Ø1 Unspecified physeal fracture of lower end of radius, right arm** CC
CC Excl: CC with 7th character A: S52.ØØ1-S52.Ø11 with 7th [A, B, C], S52.Ø19-S52.111 with 7th A, S52.119-S52.211 with 7th A, S52.219-S52.311 with 7th A, S52.319-S52.521 with 7th A, S52.529-S52.621 with 7th A, S52.629-S52.92X with 7th A, S59.ØØ1A, S59.ØØ9-S59.Ø11 with 7th A, S59.Ø19-S59.Ø21 with 7th A, S59.Ø29-S59.Ø31 with 7th A, S59.Ø39-S59.Ø41 with 7th A, S59.Ø49-S59.Ø91 with 7th A, S59.Ø99-S59.1Ø1 with 7th A, S59.1Ø9-S59.111 with 7th A, S59.119-S59.121 with 7th A, S59.129-S59.131 with 7th A, S59.139-S59.141 with 7th A, S59.149-S59.191 with 7th A, S59.199-S59.2Ø1 with 7th A, S59.2Ø9-S59.211 with 7th A, S59.219-S59.221 with 7th A, S59.229-S59.231 with 7th A, S59.239-S59.241 with 7th A, S59.249-S59.291 with 7th A, S59.299A
CC with 7th character K or P: M8Ø.ØØX-M84.68X with 7th [K, P], SØ2.ØXX-SØ2.92X with 7th K, S12.ØØØ-S12.691 with 7th K, S22.ØØØ-S22.9XX with 7th K, S32.ØØØ-S32.9XX with 7th K, S42.ØØ1-S42.92X with 7th [K, P], S49.ØØ1-S49.199 with 7th [K, P], S52.ØØ1-S52.92X with 7th [K, M, N, P, Q, R], S59.ØØ1-S59.299 with 7th [K, P], S62.ØØ1-S62.92X with 7th [K, P], S72.ØØ1-S72.92X with 7th [K, M, N, P, Q, R], S79.ØØ1-S79.199 with 7th [K, P], S82.ØØ1-S82.92X with 7th [K, M, N, P, Q, R], S89.ØØ1-S89.399 with 7th [K, P], S92.ØØ1-S92.919 with 7th [K, P]

7 ✓7th **S59.2Ø2 Unspecified physeal fracture of lower end of radius, left arm** CC
CC Excl: CC with 7th character A: S52.ØØ1-S52.ØØ9 with 7th [B, C], S52.Ø12-S52.1Ø9 with 7th A, S52.112-S52.2Ø9 with 7th A, S52.212-S52.3Ø9 with 7th A, S52.312-S52.516 with 7th A, S52.522-S52.616 with 7th A, S52.622-S52.92X with 7th A, S59.ØØ2-S59.ØØ9 with 7th A, S59.Ø12-S59.Ø19 with 7th A, S59.Ø22-S59.Ø29 with 7th A, S59.Ø32-S59.Ø39 with 7th A, S59.Ø42-S59.Ø49 with 7th A, S59.Ø92-S59.Ø99 with 7th A, S59.1Ø2-S59.1Ø9 with 7th A, S59.112-S59.119 with 7th A, S59.122-S59.129 with 7th A, S59.132-S59.139 with 7th A, S59.142-S59.149 with 7th A, S59.192-S59.199 with 7th A, S59.2Ø2-S59.2Ø9 with 7th A, S59.212-S59.219 with 7th A, S59.222-S59.229 with 7th A, S59.232-S59.239 with 7th A, S59.242-S59.249 with 7th A, S59.292-S59.299 with 7th A
CC with 7th character K or P: M8Ø.ØØX-M84.68X with 7th [K, P], SØ2.ØXX-SØ2.92X with 7th K, S12.ØØØ-S12.691 with 7th K, S22.ØØØ-S22.9XX with 7th K, S32.ØØØ-S32.9XX with 7th K, S42.ØØ1-S42.92X with 7th [K, P], S49.ØØ1-S49.199 with 7th [K, P],

7 HAC = Initial encounter only (7th character A, B or C) and not POA.

S52.001-S52.92X with 7th [K, M, N, P, Q, R], S59.001-S59.299 with 7th [K, P], S62.001-S62.92X with 7th [K, P], S72.001-S72.92X with 7th [K, M, N, P, Q, R], S79.001-S79.199 with 7th [K, P], S82.001-S82.92X with 7th [K, M, N, P, Q, R], S89.001-S89.399 with 7th [K, P], S92.001-S92.919 with 7th [K, P]

7 ✓7th **S59.209 Unspecified physeal fracture of lower end of radius, unspecified arm** CC
CC Excl: CC with 7th character A: S52.001-S52.92X with 7th [A, B, C], S59.001-S59.299 with 7th A
CC with 7th character K or P: M80.00X-M84.68X with 7th [K, P], S02.0XX-S02.92X with 7th K, S12.000-S12.691 with 7th K, S22.000-S22.9XX with 7th K, S32.000-S32.9XX with 7th K, S42.001-S42.92X with 7th [K, P], S49.001-S49.199 with 7th [K, P], S52.001-S52.92X with 7th [K, M, N, P, Q, R], S59.001-S59.299 with 7th [K, P], S62.001-S62.92X with 7th [K, P], S72.001-S72.92X with 7th [K, M, N, P, Q, R], S79.001-S79.199 with 7th [K, P], S82.001-S82.92X with 7th [K, M, N, P, Q, R], S89.001-S89.399 with 7th [K, P], S92.001-S92.919 with 7th [K, P]

✓6th **S59.21 Salter-Harris Type I physeal fracture of lower end of radius**

7 ✓7th **S59.211 Salter-Harris Type I physeal fracture of lower end of radius, right arm** CC
CC Excl: See code: S59.201

7 ✓7th **S59.212 Salter-Harris Type I physeal fracture of lower end of radius, left arm** CC
CC Excl: See code: S59.202

7 ✓7th **S59.219 Salter-Harris Type I physeal fracture of lower end of radius, unspecified arm** CC
CC Excl: See code: S59.209

✓6th **S59.22 Salter-Harris Type II physeal fracture of lower end of radius**

7 ✓7th **S59.221 Salter-Harris Type II physeal fracture of lower end of radius, right arm** CC
CC Excl: See code: S59.201

7 ✓7th **S59.222 Salter-Harris Type II physeal fracture of lower end of radius, left arm** CC
CC Excl: See code: S59.202

7 ✓7th **S59.229 Salter-Harris Type II physeal fracture of lower end of radius, unspecified arm** CC
CC Excl: See code: S59.209

✓6th **S59.23 Salter-Harris Type III physeal fracture of lower end of radius**

7 ✓7th **S59.231 Salter-Harris Type III physeal fracture of lower end of radius, right arm** CC
CC Excl: See code: S59.201

7 ✓7th **S59.232 Salter-Harris Type III physeal fracture of lower end of radius, left arm** CC
CC Excl: See code: S59.202

7 ✓7th **S59.239 Salter-Harris Type III physeal fracture of lower end of radius, unspecified arm** CC
CC Excl: See code: S59.209

✓6th **S59.24 Salter-Harris Type IV physeal fracture of lower end of radius**

7 ✓7th **S59.241 Salter-Harris Type IV physeal fracture of lower end of radius, right arm** CC
CC Excl: See code: S59.201

7 ✓7th **S59.242 Salter-Harris Type IV physeal fracture of lower end of radius, left arm** CC
CC Excl: See code: S59.202

7 ✓7th **S59.249 Salter-Harris Type IV physeal fracture of lower end of radius, unspecified arm** CC
CC Excl: See code: S59.209

✓6th **S59.29 Other physeal fracture of lower end of radius**

7 ✓7th **S59.291 Other physeal fracture of lower end of radius, right arm** CC
CC Excl: See code: S59.201

7 ✓7th **S59.292 Other physeal fracture of lower end of radius, left arm** CC
CC Excl: See code: S59.202

7 ✓7th **S59.299 Other physeal fracture of lower end of radius, unspecified arm** CC
CC Excl: See code: S59.209

✓5th **S59.8 Other specified injuries of elbow and forearm**

The appropriate 7th is to be added to each code in subcategory S59.8.
A initial encounter
D subsequent encounter
S sequela

✓6th **S59.80 Other specified injuries of elbow**
✓7th **S59.801 Other specified injuries of right elbow**
✓7th **S59.802 Other specified injuries of left elbow**
✓7th **S59.809 Other specified injuries of unspecified elbow**

✓6th **S59.81 Other specified injuries of forearm**
✓7th **S59.811 Other specified injuries right forearm**
✓7th **S59.812 Other specified injuries left forearm**
✓7th **S59.819 Other specified injuries unspecified forearm**

✓5th **S59.9 Unspecified injury of elbow and forearm**

The appropriate 7th is to be added to each code in subcategory S59.9.
A initial encounter
D subsequent encounter
S sequela

✓6th **S59.90 Unspecified injury of elbow**
✓7th **S59.901 Unspecified injury of right elbow**
✓7th **S59.902 Unspecified injury of left elbow**
✓7th **S59.909 Unspecified injury of unspecified elbow**

✓6th **S59.91 Unspecified injury of forearm**
✓7th **S59.911 Unspecified injury of right forearm**
✓7th **S59.912 Unspecified injury of left forearm**
✓7th **S59.919 Unspecified injury of unspecified forearm**

Injuries to the wrist, hand and fingers (S60-S69)

EXCLUDES 2 *burns and corrosions (T20-T32)*
frostbite (T33-T34)
insect bite or sting, venomous (T63.4)

✓4th **S60 Superficial injury of wrist, hand and fingers**

The appropriate 7th is to be added to each code from category S60.
A initial encounter
D subsequent encounter
S sequela

✓5th **S60.0 Contusion of finger without damage to nail**
EXCLUDES 1 *contusion involving nail (matrix) (S60.1)*

✓x7th **S60.00 Contusion of unspecified finger without damage to nail**
Contusion of finger(s) NOS

✓6th **S60.01 Contusion of thumb without damage to nail**
✓7th **S60.011 Contusion of right thumb without damage to nail**
✓7th **S60.012 Contusion of left thumb without damage to nail**
✓7th **S60.019 Contusion of unspecified thumb without damage to nail**

✓6th **S60.02 Contusion of index finger without damage to nail**
✓7th **S60.021 Contusion of right index finger without damage to nail**
✓7th **S60.022 Contusion of left index finger without damage to nail**
✓7th **S60.029 Contusion of unspecified index finger without damage to nail**

✓6th **S60.03 Contusion of middle finger without damage to nail**
✓7th **S60.031 Contusion of right middle finger without damage to nail**
✓7th **S60.032 Contusion of left middle finger without damage to nail**
✓7th **S60.039 Contusion of unspecified middle finger without damage to nail**

7 HAC = Initial encounter only (7th character A, B or C) and not POA.

√6th **S60.04 Contusion of ring finger without damage to nail**
- √7th **S60.041 Contusion of right ring finger without damage to nail**
- √7th **S60.042 Contusion of left ring finger without damage to nail**
- √7th **S60.049 Contusion of unspecified ring finger without damage to nail**

√6th **S60.05 Contusion of little finger without damage to nail**
- √7th **S60.051 Contusion of right little finger without damage to nail**
- √7th **S60.052 Contusion of left little finger without damage to nail**
- √7th **S60.059 Contusion of unspecified little finger without damage to nail**

√5th **S60.1 Contusion of finger with damage to nail**

√x7th **S60.10 Contusion of unspecified finger with damage to nail**

√6th **S60.11 Contusion of thumb with damage to nail**
- √7th **S60.111 Contusion of right thumb with damage to nail**
- √7th **S60.112 Contusion of left thumb with damage to nail**
- √7th **S60.119 Contusion of unspecified thumb with damage to nail**

√6th **S60.12 Contusion of index finger with damage to nail**
- √7th **S60.121 Contusion of right index finger with damage to nail**
- √7th **S60.122 Contusion of left index finger with damage to nail**
- √7th **S60.129 Contusion of unspecified index finger with damage to nail**

√6th **S60.13 Contusion of middle finger with damage to nail**
- √7th **S60.131 Contusion of right middle finger with damage to nail**
- √7th **S60.132 Contusion of left middle finger with damage to nail**
- √7th **S60.139 Contusion of unspecified middle finger with damage to nail**

√6th **S60.14 Contusion of ring finger with damage to nail**
- √7th **S60.141 Contusion of right ring finger with damage to nail**
- √7th **S60.142 Contusion of left ring finger with damage to nail**
- √7th **S60.149 Contusion of unspecified ring finger with damage to nail**

√6th **S60.15 Contusion of little finger with damage to nail**
- √7th **S60.151 Contusion of right little finger with damage to nail**
- √7th **S60.152 Contusion of left little finger with damage to nail**
- √7th **S60.159 Contusion of unspecified little finger with damage to nail**

√5th **S60.2 Contusion of wrist and hand**

EXCLUDES 2 *contusion of fingers (S60.0-, S60.1-)*

√6th **S60.21 Contusion of wrist**
- √7th **S60.211 Contusion of right wrist**
- √7th **S60.212 Contusion of left wrist**
- √7th **S60.219 Contusion of unspecified wrist**

√6th **S60.22 Contusion of hand**
- √7th **S60.221 Contusion of right hand**
- √7th **S60.222 Contusion of left hand**
- √7th **S60.229 Contusion of unspecified hand**

√5th **S60.3 Other superficial injuries of thumb**

√6th **S60.31 Abrasion of thumb**
- √7th **S60.311 Abrasion of right thumb**
- √7th **S60.312 Abrasion of left thumb**
- √7th **S60.319 Abrasion of unspecified thumb**

√6th **S60.32 Blister (nonthermal) of thumb**
- √7th **S60.321 Blister (nonthermal) of right thumb**
- √7th **S60.322 Blister (nonthermal) of left thumb**
- √7th **S60.329 Blister (nonthermal) of unspecified thumb**

√6th **S60.34 External constriction of thumb**

Hair tourniquet syndrome of thumb

Use additional cause code to identify the constricting item (W49.0-)
- √7th **S60.341 External constriction of right thumb**
- √7th **S60.342 External constriction of left thumb**
- √7th **S60.349 External constriction of unspecified thumb**

√6th **S60.35 Superficial foreign body of thumb**

Splinter in the thumb
- √7th **S60.351 Superficial foreign body of right thumb**
- √7th **S60.352 Superficial foreign body of left thumb**
- √7th **S60.359 Superficial foreign body of unspecified thumb**

√6th **S60.36 Insect bite (nonvenomous) of thumb**
- √7th **S60.361 Insect bite (nonvenomous) of right thumb**
- √7th **S60.362 Insect bite (nonvenomous) of left thumb**
- √7th **S60.369 Insect bite (nonvenomous) of unspecified thumb**

√6th **S60.37 Other superficial bite of thumb**

EXCLUDES 1 *open bite of thumb (S61.05-, S61.15-)*
- √7th **S60.371 Other superficial bite of right thumb**
- √7th **S60.372 Other superficial bite of left thumb**
- √7th **S60.379 Other superficial bite of unspecified thumb**

√6th **S60.39 Other superficial injuries of thumb**
- √7th **S60.391 Other superficial injuries of right thumb**
- √7th **S60.392 Other superficial injuries of left thumb**
- √7th **S60.399 Other superficial injuries of unspecified thumb**

√5th **S60.4 Other superficial injuries of other fingers**

√6th **S60.41 Abrasion of fingers**
- √7th **S60.410 Abrasion of right index finger**
- √7th **S60.411 Abrasion of left index finger**
- √7th **S60.412 Abrasion of right middle finger**
- √7th **S60.413 Abrasion of left middle finger**
- √7th **S60.414 Abrasion of right ring finger**
- √7th **S60.415 Abrasion of left ring finger**
- √7th **S60.416 Abrasion of right little finger**
- √7th **S60.417 Abrasion of left little finger**
- √7th **S60.418 Abrasion of other finger**
  Abrasion of specified finger with unspecified laterality
- √7th **S60.419 Abrasion of unspecified finger**

√6th **S60.42 Blister (nonthermal) of fingers**
- √7th **S60.420 Blister (nonthermal) of right index finger**
- √7th **S60.421 Blister (nonthermal) of left index finger**
- √7th **S60.422 Blister (nonthermal) of right middle finger**
- √7th **S60.423 Blister (nonthermal) of left middle finger**
- √7th **S60.424 Blister (nonthermal) of right ring finger**
- √7th **S60.425 Blister (nonthermal) of left ring finger**
- √7th **S60.426 Blister (nonthermal) of right little finger**
- √7th **S60.427 Blister (nonthermal) of left little finger**
- √7th **S60.428 Blister (nonthermal) of other finger**
  Blister (nonthermal) of specified finger with unspecified laterality
- √7th **S60.429 Blister (nonthermal) of unspecified finger**

√6th **S60.44 External constriction of fingers**

Hair tourniquet syndrome of finger

Use additional cause code to identify the constricting item (W49.0-)
- √7th **S60.440 External constriction of right index finger**
- √7th **S60.441 External constriction of left index finger**
- √7th **S60.442 External constriction of right middle finger**
- √7th **S60.443 External constriction of left middle finger**
- √7th **S60.444 External constriction of right ring finger**
- √7th **S60.445 External constriction of left ring finger**
- √7th **S60.446 External constriction of right little finger**
- √7th **S60.447 External constriction of left little finger**

✓7th **S60.448 External constriction of other finger**
External constriction of specified finger with unspecified laterality

✓7th **S60.449 External constriction of unspecified finger**

✓6th **S60.45 Superficial foreign body of fingers**
Splinter in the finger(s)

✓7th **S60.450 Superficial foreign body of right index finger**

✓7th **S60.451 Superficial foreign body of left index finger**

✓7th **S60.452 Superficial foreign body of right middle finger**

✓7th **S60.453 Superficial foreign body of left middle finger**

✓7th **S60.454 Superficial foreign body of right ring finger**

✓7th **S60.455 Superficial foreign body of left ring finger**

✓7th **S60.456 Superficial foreign body of right little finger**

✓7th **S60.457 Superficial foreign body of left little finger**

✓7th **S60.458 Superficial foreign body of other finger**
Superficial foreign body of specified finger with unspecified laterality

✓7th **S60.459 Superficial foreign body of unspecified finger**

✓6th **S60.46 Insect bite (nonvenomous) of fingers**

✓7th **S60.460 Insect bite (nonvenomous) of right index finger**

✓7th **S60.461 Insect bite (nonvenomous) of left index finger**

✓7th **S60.462 Insect bite (nonvenomous) of right middle finger**

✓7th **S60.463 Insect bite (nonvenomous) of left middle finger**

✓7th **S60.464 Insect bite (nonvenomous) of right ring finger**

✓7th **S60.465 Insect bite (nonvenomous) of left ring finger**

✓7th **S60.466 Insect bite (nonvenomous) of right little finger**

✓7th **S60.467 Insect bite (nonvenomous) of left little finger**

✓7th **S60.468 Insect bite (nonvenomous) of other finger**
Insect bite (nonvenomous) of specified finger with unspecified laterality

✓7th **S60.469 Insect bite (nonvenomous) of unspecified finger**

✓6th **S60.47 Other superficial bite of fingers**
EXCLUDES 1 *open bite of fingers (S61.25-, S61.35-)*

✓7th **S60.470 Other superficial bite of right index finger**

✓7th **S60.471 Other superficial bite of left index finger**

✓7th **S60.472 Other superficial bite of right middle finger**

✓7th **S60.473 Other superficial bite of left middle finger**

✓7th **S60.474 Other superficial bite of right ring finger**

✓7th **S60.475 Other superficial bite of left ring finger**

✓7th **S60.476 Other superficial bite of right little finger**

✓7th **S60.477 Other superficial bite of left little finger**

✓7th **S60.478 Other superficial bite of other finger**
Other superficial bite of specified finger with xc vunspecified laterality

✓7th **S60.479 Other superficial bite of unspecified finger**

✓5th **S60.5 Other superficial injuries of hand**
EXCLUDES 2 *superficial injuries of fingers (S60.3-, S60.4-)*

✓6th **S60.51 Abrasion of hand**

✓7th **S60.511 Abrasion of right hand**

✓7th **S60.512 Abrasion of left hand**

✓7th **S60.519 Abrasion of unspecified hand**

✓6th **S60.52 Blister (nonthermal) of hand**

✓7th **S60.521 Blister (nonthermal) of right hand**

✓7th **S60.522 Blister (nonthermal) of left hand**

✓7th **S60.529 Blister (nonthermal) of unspecified hand**

✓6th **S60.54 External constriction of hand**

✓7th **S60.541 External constriction of right hand**

✓7th **S60.542 External constriction of left hand**

✓7th **S60.549 External constriction of unspecified hand**

✓6th **S60.55 Superficial foreign body of hand**
Splinter in the hand

✓7th **S60.551 Superficial foreign body of right hand**

✓7th **S60.552 Superficial foreign body of left hand**

✓7th **S60.559 Superficial foreign body of unspecified hand**

✓6th **S60.56 Insect bite (nonvenomous) of hand**

✓7th **S60.561 Insect bite (nonvenomous) of right hand**

✓7th **S60.562 Insect bite (nonvenomous) of left hand**

✓7th **S60.569 Insect bite (nonvenomous) of unspecified hand**

✓6th **S60.57 Other superficial bite of hand**
EXCLUDES 1 *open bite of hand (S61.45-)*

✓7th **S60.571 Other superficial bite of hand of right hand**

✓7th **S60.572 Other superficial bite of hand of left hand**

✓7th **S60.579 Other superficial bite of hand of unspecified hand**

✓5th **S60.8 Other superficial injuries of wrist**

✓6th **S60.81 Abrasion of wrist**

✓7th **S60.811 Abrasion of right wrist**

✓7th **S60.812 Abrasion of left wrist**

✓7th **S60.819 Abrasion of unspecified wrist**

✓6th **S60.82 Blister (nonthermal) of wrist**

✓7th **S60.821 Blister (nonthermal) of right wrist**

✓7th **S60.822 Blister (nonthermal) of left wrist**

✓7th **S60.829 Blister (nonthermal) of unspecified wrist**

✓6th **S60.84 External constriction of wrist**

✓7th **S60.841 External constriction of right wrist**

✓7th **S60.842 External constriction of left wrist**

✓7th **S60.849 External constriction of unspecified wrist**

✓6th **S60.85 Superficial foreign body of wrist**
Splinter in the wrist

✓7th **S60.851 Superficial foreign body of right wrist**

✓7th **S60.852 Superficial foreign body of left wrist**

✓7th **S60.859 Superficial foreign body of unspecified wrist**

✓6th **S60.86 Insect bite (nonvenomous) of wrist**

✓7th **S60.861 Insect bite (nonvenomous) of right wrist**

✓7th **S60.862 Insect bite (nonvenomous) of left wrist**

✓7th **S60.869 Insect bite (nonvenomous) of unspecified wrist**

✓6th **S60.87 Other superficial bite of wrist**
EXCLUDES 1 *open bite of wrist (S61.55)*

✓7th **S60.871 Other superficial bite of right wrist**

✓7th **S60.872 Other superficial bite of left wrist**

✓7th **S60.879 Other superficial bite of unspecified wrist**

✓5th **S60.9 Unspecified superficial injury of wrist, hand and fingers**

✓6th **S60.91 Unspecified superficial injury of wrist**

✓7th **S60.911 Unspecified superficial injury of right wrist**

✓7th **S60.912 Unspecified superficial injury of left wrist**

✓7th **S60.919 Unspecified superficial injury of unspecified wrist**

✓6th **S60.92 Unspecified superficial injury of hand**

✓7th **S60.921 Unspecified superficial injury of right hand**

✓7th **S60.922 Unspecified superficial injury of left hand**

✓7th **S60.929 Unspecified superficial injury of unspecified hand**

✓6th **S60.93 Unspecified superficial injury of thumb**

✓7th **S60.931 Unspecified superficial injury of right thumb**

✓7th **S60.932 Unspecified superficial injury of left thumb**

√7th **S60.939** Unspecified superficial injury of unspecified thumb

√6th **S60.94** Unspecified superficial injury of other fingers

√7th **S60.940** Unspecified superficial injury of right index finger

√7th **S60.941** Unspecified superficial injury of left index finger

√7th **S60.942** Unspecified superficial injury of right middle finger

√7th **S60.943** Unspecified superficial injury of left middle finger

√7th **S60.944** Unspecified superficial injury of right ring finger

√7th **S60.945** Unspecified superficial injury of left ring finger

√7th **S60.946** Unspecified superficial injury of right little finger

√7th **S60.947** Unspecified superficial injury of left little finger

√7th **S60.948** Unspecified superficial injury of other finger
Unspecified superficial injury of specified finger with unspecified laterality

√7th **S60.949** Unspecified superficial injury of unspecified finger

√4th **S61 Open wound of wrist, hand and fingers**
Code also any associated wound infection
EXCLUDES 1 *open fracture of wrist, hand and finger (S62- with 7th character B)*
traumatic amputation of wrist and hand (S68.-)

The appropriate 7th is to be added to each code from category S61.
A initial encounter
D subsequent encounter
S sequela

√5th **S61.0** Open wound of thumb without damage to nail
EXCLUDES 1 *open wound of thumb with damage to nail (S61.1-)*

√6th **S61.00** Unspecified open wound of thumb without damage to nail

√7th **S61.001** Unspecified open wound of right thumb without damage to nail

√7th **S61.002** Unspecified open wound of left thumb without damage to nail

√7th **S61.009** Unspecified open wound of unspecified thumb without damage to nail

√6th **S61.01** Laceration without foreign body of thumb without damage to nail

√7th **S61.011** Laceration without foreign body of right thumb without damage to nail

√7th **S61.012** Laceration without foreign body of left thumb without damage to nail

√7th **S61.019** Laceration without foreign body of unspecified thumb without damage to nail

√6th **S61.02** Laceration with foreign body of thumb without damage to nail

√7th **S61.021** Laceration with foreign body of right thumb without damage to nail

√7th **S61.022** Laceration with foreign body of left thumb without damage to nail

√7th **S61.029** Laceration with foreign body of unspecified thumb without damage to nail

√6th **S61.03** Puncture wound without foreign body of thumb without damage to nail

√7th **S61.031** Puncture wound without foreign body of right thumb without damage to nail

√7th **S61.032** Puncture wound without foreign body of left thumb without damage to nail

√7th **S61.039** Puncture wound without foreign body of unspecified thumb without damage to nail

√6th **S61.04** Puncture wound with foreign body of thumb without damage to nail

√7th **S61.041** Puncture wound with foreign body of right thumb without damage to nail

√7th **S61.042** Puncture wound with foreign body of left thumb without damage to nail

√7th **S61.049** Puncture wound with foreign body of unspecified thumb without damage to nail

√6th **S61.05** Open bite of thumb without damage to nail
Bite of thumb NOS
EXCLUDES 1 *superficial bite of thumb (S60.36-, S60.37-)*

√7th **S61.051** Open bite of right thumb without damage to nail

√7th **S61.052** Open bite of left thumb without damage to nail

√7th **S61.059** Open bite of unspecified thumb without damage to nail

√5th **S61.1** Open wound of thumb with damage to nail

√6th **S61.10** Unspecified open wound of thumb with damage to nail

√7th **S61.101** Unspecified open wound of right thumb with damage to nail

√7th **S61.102** Unspecified open wound of left thumb with damage to nail

√7th **S61.109** Unspecified open wound of unspecified thumb with damage to nail

√6th **S61.11** Laceration without foreign body of thumb with damage to nail

√7th **S61.111** Laceration without foreign body of right thumb with damage to nail

√7th **S61.112** Laceration without foreign body of left thumb with damage to nail

√7th **S61.119** Laceration without foreign body of unspecified thumb with damage to nail

√6th **S61.12** Laceration with foreign body of thumb with damage to nail

√7th **S61.121** Laceration with foreign body of right thumb with damage to nail

√7th **S61.122** Laceration with foreign body of left thumb with damage to nail

√7th **S61.129** Laceration with foreign body of unspecified thumb with damage to nail

√6th **S61.13** Puncture wound without foreign body of thumb with damage to nail

√7th **S61.131** Puncture wound without foreign body of right thumb with damage to nail

√7th **S61.132** Puncture wound without foreign body of left thumb with damage to nail

√7th **S61.139** Puncture wound without foreign body of unspecified thumb with damage to nail

√6th **S61.14** Puncture wound with foreign body of thumb with damage to nail

√7th **S61.141** Puncture wound with foreign body of right thumb with damage to nail

√7th **S61.142** Puncture wound with foreign body of left thumb with damage to nail

√7th **S61.149** Puncture wound with foreign body of unspecified thumb with damage to nail

√6th **S61.15** Open bite of thumb with damage to nail
Bite of thumb with damage to nail NOS
EXCLUDES 1 *superficial bite of thumb (S60.36-, S60.37-)*

√7th **S61.151** Open bite of right thumb with damage to nail

√7th **S61.152** Open bite of left thumb with damage to nail

√7th **S61.159** Open bite of unspecified thumb with damage to nail

√5th **S61.2** Open wound of other finger without damage to nail
EXCLUDES 1 *open wound of finger involving nail (matrix) (S61.3-)*
EXCLUDES 2 *open wound of thumb without damage to nail (S61.0-)*

√6th **S61.20** Unspecified open wound of other finger without damage to nail

√7th **S61.200** Unspecified open wound of right index finger without damage to nail

√7th **S61.201** Unspecified open wound of left index finger without damage to nail

√7th **S61.202** Unspecified open wound of right middle finger without damage to nail

✓7th **S61.203 Unspecified open wound of left middle finger without damage to nail**

✓7th **S61.204 Unspecified open wound of right ring finger without damage to nail**

✓7th **S61.205 Unspecified open wound of left ring finger without damage to nail**

✓7th **S61.206 Unspecified open wound of right little finger without damage to nail**

✓7th **S61.207 Unspecified open wound of left little finger without damage to nail**

✓7th **S61.208 Unspecified open wound of other finger without damage to nail**
Unspecified open wound of specified finger with unspecified laterality without damage to nail

✓7th **S61.209 Unspecified open wound of unspecified finger without damage to nail**

✓6th **S61.21 Laceration without foreign body of finger without damage to nail**

✓7th **S61.210 Laceration without foreign body of right index finger without damage to nail**

✓7th **S61.211 Laceration without foreign body of left index finger without damage to nail**

✓7th **S61.212 Laceration without foreign body of right middle finger without damage to nail**

✓7th **S61.213 Laceration without foreign body of left middle finger without damage to nail**

✓7th **S61.214 Laceration without foreign body of right ring finger without damage to nail**

✓7th **S61.215 Laceration without foreign body of left ring finger without damage to nail**

✓7th **S61.216 Laceration without foreign body of right little finger without damage to nail**

✓7th **S61.217 Laceration without foreign body of left little finger without damage to nail**

✓7th **S61.218 Laceration without foreign body of other finger without damage to nail**
Laceration without foreign body of specified finger with unspecified laterality without damage to nail

✓7th **S61.219 Laceration without foreign body of unspecified finger without damage to nail**

✓6th **S61.22 Laceration with foreign body of finger without damage to nail**

✓7th **S61.220 Laceration with foreign body of right index finger without damage to nail**

✓7th **S61.221 Laceration with foreign body of left index finger without damage to nail**

✓7th **S61.222 Laceration with foreign body of right middle finger without damage to nail**

✓7th **S61.223 Laceration with foreign body of left middle finger without damage to nail**

✓7th **S61.224 Laceration with foreign body of right ring finger without damage to nail**

✓7th **S61.225 Laceration with foreign body of left ring finger without damage to nail**

✓7th **S61.226 Laceration with foreign body of right little finger without damage to nail**

✓7th **S61.227 Laceration with foreign body of left little finger without damage to nail**

✓7th **S61.228 Laceration with foreign body of other finger without damage to nail**
Laceration with foreign body of specified finger with unspecified laterality without damage to nail

✓7th **S61.229 Laceration with foreign body of unspecified finger without damage to nail**

✓6th **S61.23 Puncture wound without foreign body of finger without damage to nail**

✓7th **S61.230 Puncture wound without foreign body of right index finger without damage to nail**

✓7th **S61.231 Puncture wound without foreign body of left index finger without damage to nail**

✓7th **S61.232 Puncture wound without foreign body of right middle finger without damage to nail**

✓7th **S61.233 Puncture wound without foreign body of left middle finger without damage to nail**

✓7th **S61.234 Puncture wound without foreign body of right ring finger without damage to nail**

✓7th **S61.235 Puncture wound without foreign body of left ring finger without damage to nail**

✓7th **S61.236 Puncture wound without foreign body of right little finger without damage to nail**

✓7th **S61.237 Puncture wound without foreign body of left little finger without damage to nail**

✓7th **S61.238 Puncture wound without foreign body of other finger without damage to nail**
Puncture wound without foreign body of specified finger with unspecified laterality without damage to nail

✓7th **S61.239 Puncture wound without foreign body of unspecified finger without damage to nail**

✓6th **S61.24 Puncture wound with foreign body of finger without damage to nail**

✓7th **S61.240 Puncture wound with foreign body of right index finger without damage to nail**

✓7th **S61.241 Puncture wound with foreign body of left index finger without damage to nail**

✓7th **S61.242 Puncture wound with foreign body of right middle finger without damage to nail**

✓7th **S61.243 Puncture wound with foreign body of left middle finger without damage to nail**

✓7th **S61.244 Puncture wound with foreign body of right ring finger without damage to nail**

✓7th **S61.245 Puncture wound with foreign body of left ring finger without damage to nail**

✓7th **S61.246 Puncture wound with foreign body of right little finger without damage to nail**

✓7th **S61.247 Puncture wound with foreign body of left little finger without damage to nail**

✓7th **S61.248 Puncture wound with foreign body of other finger without damage to nail**
Puncture wound with foreign body of specified finger with unspecified laterality without damage to nail

✓7th **S61.249 Puncture wound with foreign body of unspecified finger without damage to nail**

✓6th **S61.25 Open bite of finger without damage to nail**
Bite of finger without damage to nail NOS
EXCLUDES1 *superficial bite of finger (S60.46-, S60.47-)*

✓7th **S61.250 Open bite of right index finger without damage to nail**

✓7th **S61.251 Open bite of left index finger without damage to nail**

✓7th **S61.252 Open bite of right middle finger without damage to nail**

✓7th **S61.253 Open bite of left middle finger without damage to nail**

✓7th **S61.254 Open bite of right ring finger without damage to nail**

✓7th **S61.255 Open bite of left ring finger without damage to nail**

✓7th **S61.256 Open bite of right little finger without damage to nail**

✓7th **S61.257 Open bite of left little finger without damage to nail**

✓7th **S61.258 Open bite of other finger without damage to nail**
Open bite of specified finger with unspecified laterality without damage to nail

✓7th **S61.259 Open bite of unspecified finger without damage to nail**

✓5th **S61.3 Open wound of other finger with damage to nail**

✓6th **S61.30 Unspecified open wound of finger with damage to nail**

✓7th **S61.300 Unspecified open wound of right index finger with damage to nail**

✓7th **S61.301 Unspecified open wound of left index finger with damage to nail**

7th S61.302 **Unspecified open wound of right middle finger with damage to nail**

7th S61.303 **Unspecified open wound of left middle finger with damage to nail**

7th S61.304 **Unspecified open wound of right ring finger with damage to nail**

7th S61.305 **Unspecified open wound of left ring finger with damage to nail**

7th S61.306 **Unspecified open wound of right little finger with damage to nail**

7th S61.307 **Unspecified open wound of left little finger with damage to nail**

7th S61.308 **Unspecified open wound of other finger with damage to nail**
Unspecified open wound of specified finger with unspecified laterality with damage to nail

7th S61.309 **Unspecified open wound of unspecified finger with damage to nail**

6th S61.31 **Laceration without foreign body of finger with damage to nail**

7th S61.310 **Laceration without foreign body of right index finger with damage to nail**

7th S61.311 **Laceration without foreign body of left index finger with damage to nail**

7th S61.312 **Laceration without foreign body of right middle finger with damage to nail**

7th S61.313 **Laceration without foreign body of left middle finger with damage to nail**

7th S61.314 **Laceration without foreign body of right ring finger with damage to nail**

7th S61.315 **Laceration without foreign body of left ring finger with damage to nail**

7th S61.316 **Laceration without foreign body of right little finger with damage to nail**

7th S61.317 **Laceration without foreign body of left little finger with damage to nail**

7th S61.318 **Laceration without foreign body of other finger with damage to nail**
Laceration without foreign body of specified finger with unspecified laterality with damage to nail

7th S61.319 **Laceration without foreign body of unspecified finger with damage to nail**

6th S61.32 **Laceration with foreign body of finger with damage to nail**

7th S61.320 **Laceration with foreign body of right index finger with damage to nail**

7th S61.321 **Laceration with foreign body of left index finger with damage to nail**

7th S61.322 **Laceration with foreign body of right middle finger with damage to nail**

7th S61.323 **Laceration with foreign body of left middle finger with damage to nail**

7th S61.324 **Laceration with foreign body of right ring finger with damage to nail**

7th S61.325 **Laceration with foreign body of left ring finger with damage to nail**

7th S61.326 **Laceration with foreign body of right little finger with damage to nail**

7th S61.327 **Laceration with foreign body of left little finger with damage to nail**

7th S61.328 **Laceration with foreign body of other finger with damage to nail**
Laceration with foreign body of specified finger with unspecified laterality with damage to nail

7th S61.329 **Laceration with foreign body of unspecified finger with damage to nail**

6th S61.33 **Puncture wound without foreign body of finger with damage to nail**

7th S61.330 **Puncture wound without foreign body of right index finger with damage to nail**

7th S61.331 **Puncture wound without foreign body of left index finger with damage to nail**

7th S61.332 **Puncture wound without foreign body of right middle finger with damage to nail**

7th S61.333 **Puncture wound without foreign body of left middle finger with damage to nail**

7th S61.334 **Puncture wound without foreign body of right ring finger with damage to nail**

7th S61.335 **Puncture wound without foreign body of left ring finger with damage to nail**

7th S61.336 **Puncture wound without foreign body of right little finger with damage to nail**

7th S61.337 **Puncture wound without foreign body of left little finger with damage to nail**

7th S61.338 **Puncture wound without foreign body of other finger with damage to nail**
Puncture wound without foreign body of specified finger with unspecified laterality with damage to nail

7th S61.339 **Puncture wound without foreign body of unspecified finger with damage to nail**

6th S61.34 **Puncture wound with foreign body of finger with damage to nail**

7th S61.340 **Puncture wound with foreign body of right index finger with damage to nail**

7th S61.341 **Puncture wound with foreign body of left index finger with damage to nail**

7th S61.342 **Puncture wound with foreign body of right middle finger with damage to nail**

7th S61.343 **Puncture wound with foreign body of left middle finger with damage to nail**

7th S61.344 **Puncture wound with foreign body of right ring finger with damage to nail**

7th S61.345 **Puncture wound with foreign body of left ring finger with damage to nail**

7th S61.346 **Puncture wound with foreign body of right little finger with damage to nail**

7th S61.347 **Puncture wound with foreign body of left little finger with damage to nail**

7th S61.348 **Puncture wound with foreign body of other finger with damage to nail**
Puncture wound with foreign body of specified finger with unspecified laterality with damage to nail

7th S61.349 **Puncture wound with foreign body of unspecified finger with damage to nail**

6th S61.35 **Open bite of finger with damage to nail**
Bite of finger with damage to nail NOS
EXCLUDES 1 *superficial bite of finger (S60.46-, S60.47-)*

7th S61.350 **Open bite of right index finger with damage to nail**

7th S61.351 **Open bite of left index finger with damage to nail**

7th S61.352 **Open bite of right middle finger with damage to nail**

7th S61.353 **Open bite of left middle finger with damage to nail**

7th S61.354 **Open bite of right ring finger with damage to nail**

7th S61.355 **Open bite of left ring finger with damage to nail**

7th S61.356 **Open bite of right little finger with damage to nail**

7th S61.357 **Open bite of left little finger with damage to nail**

7th S61.358 **Open bite of other finger with damage to nail**
Open bite of specified finger with unspecified laterality with damage to nail

7th S61.359 **Open bite of unspecified finger with damage to nail**

5th S61.4 **Open wound of hand**

6th S61.40 **Unspecified open wound of hand**

7th S61.401 **Unspecified open wound of right hand**

7th S61.402 **Unspecified open wound of left hand**

7th S61.409 **Unspecified open wound of unspecified hand**

6th S61.41 **Laceration without foreign body of hand**
- 7th S61.411 **Laceration without foreign body of right hand**
- 7th S61.412 **Laceration without foreign body of left hand**
- 7th S61.419 **Laceration without foreign body of unspecified hand**

6th S61.42 **Laceration with foreign body of hand**
- 7th S61.421 **Laceration with foreign body of right hand**
- 7th S61.422 **Laceration with foreign body of left hand**
- 7th S61.429 **Laceration with foreign body of unspecified hand**

6th S61.43 **Puncture wound without foreign body of hand**
- 7th S61.431 **Puncture wound without foreign body of right hand**
- 7th S61.432 **Puncture wound without foreign body of left hand**
- 7th S61.439 **Puncture wound without foreign body of unspecified hand**

6th S61.44 **Puncture wound with foreign body of hand**
- 7th S61.441 **Puncture wound with foreign body of right hand**
- 7th S61.442 **Puncture wound with foreign body of left hand**
- 7th S61.449 **Puncture wound with foreign body of unspecified hand**

6th S61.45 **Open bite of hand**

Bite of hand NOS

EXCLUDES 1 *superficial bite of hand (S60.56-, S60.57-)*
- 7th S61.451 **Open bite of right hand**
- 7th S61.452 **Open bite of left hand**
- 7th S61.459 **Open bite of unspecified hand**

5th S61.5 **Open wound of wrist**

6th S61.50 **Unspecified open wound of wrist**
- 7th S61.501 **Unspecified open wound of right wrist**
- 7th S61.502 **Unspecified open wound of left wrist**
- 7th S61.509 **Unspecified open wound of unspecified wrist**

6th S61.51 **Laceration without foreign body of wrist**
- 7th S61.511 **Laceration without foreign body of right wrist**
- 7th S61.512 **Laceration without foreign body of left wrist**
- 7th S61.519 **Laceration without foreign body of unspecified wrist**

6th S61.52 **Laceration with foreign body of wrist**
- 7th S61.521 **Laceration with foreign body of right wrist**
- 7th S61.522 **Laceration with foreign body of left wrist**
- 7th S61.529 **Laceration with foreign body of unspecified wrist**

6th S61.53 **Puncture wound without foreign body of wrist**
- 7th S61.531 **Puncture wound without foreign body of right wrist**
- 7th S61.532 **Puncture wound without foreign body of left wrist**
- 7th S61.539 **Puncture wound without foreign body of unspecified wrist**

6th S61.54 **Puncture wound with foreign body of wrist**
- 7th S61.541 **Puncture wound with foreign body of right wrist**
- 7th S61.542 **Puncture wound with foreign body of left wrist**
- 7th S61.549 **Puncture wound with foreign body of unspecified wrist**

6th S61.55 **Open bite of wrist**

Bite of wrist NOS

EXCLUDES 1 *superficial bite of wrist (S60.86-, S60.87-)*
- 7th S61.551 **Open bite of right wrist**
- 7th S61.552 **Open bite of left wrist**
- 7th S61.559 **Open bite of unspecified wrist**

4th **S62 Fracture at wrist and hand level**

NOTE A fracture not indicated as displaced or nondisplaced should be coded to displaced.
A fracture not indicated as open or closed should be coded to closed.

EXCLUDES 1 *traumatic amputation of wrist and hand (S68.-)*

EXCLUDES 2 *fracture of distal parts of ulna and radius (S52.-)*

The appropriate 7th is to be added to each code from category S62.
- A initial encounter for closed fracture
- B initial encounter for open fracture
- D subsequent encounter for fracture with routine healing
- G subsequent encounter for fracture with delayed healing
- K subsequent encounter for fracture with nonunion
- P subsequent encounter for fracture with malunion
- S sequela

5th S62.0 **Fracture of navicular [scaphoid] bone of wrist**

CC Excl: For CC codes in subcategory S62.0, unless otherwise noted: CC with 7th character B: S62.001-S62.186 with 7th [A, B]

CC with 7th character K or P: M80.00X-M84.68X with 7th [K, P], S02.0XX-S02.92X with 7th K, S12.000-S12.691 with 7th K, S22.000-S22.9XX with 7th K, S32.000-S32.9XX with 7th K, S42.001-S42.92X with 7th [K, P], S49.001-S49.199 with 7th [K, P], S52.001-S52.92X with 7th [K, M, N, P, Q, R], S59.001-S59.299 with 7th [K, P], S62.001-S62.92X with 7th [K, P], S72.001-S72.92X with 7th [K, M, N, P, Q, R], S79.001-S79.199 with 7th [K, P], S82.001-S82.92X with 7th [K, M, N, P, Q, R], S89.001-S89.399 with 7th [K, P], S92.001-S92.919 with 7th [K, P]

6th S62.00 **Unspecified fracture of navicular [scaphoid] bone of wrist**
- 7 7th S62.001 **Unspecified fracture of navicular [scaphoid] bone of right wrist** CC
- 7 7th S62.002 **Unspecified fracture of navicular [scaphoid] bone of left wrist** CC
  AHA: 2012, 4Q, 106
- 7 7th S62.009 **Unspecified fracture of navicular [scaphoid] bone of unspecified wrist** CC

6th S62.01 **Fracture of distal pole of navicular [scaphoid] bone of wrist**

Fracture of volar tuberosity of navicular [scaphoid] bone of wrist
- 7 7th S62.011 **Displaced fracture of distal pole of navicular [scaphoid] bone of right wrist** CC
- 7 7th S62.012 **Displaced fracture of distal pole of navicular [scaphoid] bone of left wrist** CC
- 7 7th S62.013 **Displaced fracture of distal pole of navicular [scaphoid] bone of unspecified wrist** CC
- 7 7th S62.014 **Nondisplaced fracture of distal pole of navicular [scaphoid] bone of right wrist** CC
- 7 7th S62.015 **Nondisplaced fracture of distal pole of navicular [scaphoid] bone of left wrist** CC
- 7 7th S62.016 **Nondisplaced fracture of distal pole of navicular [scaphoid] bone of unspecified wrist** CC

6th S62.02 **Fracture of middle third of navicular [scaphoid] bone of wrist**
- 7 7th S62.021 **Displaced fracture of middle third of navicular [scaphoid] bone of right wrist** CC
- 7 7th S62.022 **Displaced fracture of middle third of navicular [scaphoid] bone of left wrist** CC
- 7 7th S62.023 **Displaced fracture of middle third of navicular [scaphoid] bone of unspecified wrist** CC
- 7 7th S62.024 **Nondisplaced fracture of middle third of navicular [scaphoid] bone of right wrist** CC
- 7 7th S62.025 **Nondisplaced fracture of middle third of navicular [scaphoid] bone of left wrist** CC
- 7 7th S62.026 **Nondisplaced fracture of middle third of navicular [scaphoid] bone of unspecified wrist** CC

7 HAC = Initial encounter only (7th character A, B or C) and not POA.

6th S62.03 Fracture of proximal third of navicular [scaphoid] bone of wrist
- 7 7th **S62.031 Displaced fracture of proximal third of navicular [scaphoid] bone of right wrist** CC
- 7 7th **S62.032 Displaced fracture of proximal third of navicular [scaphoid] bone of left wrist** CC
- 7 7th **S62.033 Displaced fracture of proximal third of navicular [scaphoid] bone of unspecified wrist** CC
- 7 7th **S62.034 Nondisplaced fracture of proximal third of navicular [scaphoid] bone of right wrist** CC
- 7 7th **S62.035 Nondisplaced fracture of proximal third of navicular [scaphoid] bone of left wrist** CC
- 7 7th **S62.036 Nondisplaced fracture of proximal third of navicular [scaphoid] bone of unspecified wrist** CC

5th S62.1 Fracture of other and unspecified carpal bone(s)

EXCLUDES 2 *fracture of scaphoid of wrist (S62.0-)*

S62.1 CC Excl: For CC codes in subcategory S62.1, unless otherwise noted: See code: S62.0

6th S62.10 Fracture of unspecified carpal bone

Fracture of wrist NOS
- 7 7th **S62.101 Fracture of unspecified carpal bone, right wrist** CC
- 7 7th **S62.102 Fracture of unspecified carpal bone, left wrist** CC
  AHA: 2012, 4Q, 95
- 7 7th **S62.109 Fracture of unspecified carpal bone, unspecified wrist** CC

6th S62.11 Fracture of triquetrum [cuneiform] bone of wrist
- 7 7th **S62.111 Displaced fracture of triquetrum [cuneiform] bone, right wrist** CC
- 7 7th **S62.112 Displaced fracture of triquetrum [cuneiform] bone, left wrist** CC
- 7 7th **S62.113 Displaced fracture of triquetrum [cuneiform] bone, unspecified wrist** CC
- 7 7th **S62.114 Nondisplaced fracture of triquetrum [cuneiform] bone, right wrist** CC
- 7 7th **S62.115 Nondisplaced fracture of triquetrum [cuneiform] bone, left wrist** CC
- 7 7th **S62.116 Nondisplaced fracture of triquetrum [cuneiform] bone, unspecified wrist** CC

6th S62.12 Fracture of lunate [semilunar]
- 7 7th **S62.121 Displaced fracture of lunate [semilunar], right wrist** CC
- 7 7th **S62.122 Displaced fracture of lunate [semilunar], left wrist** CC
- 7 7th **S62.123 Displaced fracture of lunate [semilunar], unspecified wrist** CC
- 7 7th **S62.124 Nondisplaced fracture of lunate [semilunar], right wrist** CC
- 7 7th **S62.125 Nondisplaced fracture of lunate [semilunar], left wrist** CC
- 7 7th **S62.126 Nondisplaced fracture of lunate [semilunar], unspecified wrist** CC

6th S62.13 Fracture of capitate [os magnum] bone
- 7 7th **S62.131 Displaced fracture of capitate [os magnum] bone, right wrist** CC
- 7 7th **S62.132 Displaced fracture of capitate [os magnum] bone, left wrist** CC
- 7 7th **S62.133 Displaced fracture of capitate [os magnum] bone, unspecified wrist** CC
- 7 7th **S62.134 Nondisplaced fracture of capitate [os magnum] bone, right wrist** CC
- 7 7th **S62.135 Nondisplaced fracture of capitate [os magnum] bone, left wrist** CC
- 7 7th **S62.136 Nondisplaced fracture of capitate [os magnum] bone, unspecified wrist** CC

6th S62.14 Fracture of body of hamate [unciform] bone

Fracture of hamate [unciform] bone NOS
- 7 7th **S62.141 Displaced fracture of body of hamate [unciform] bone, right wrist** CC
- 7 7th **S62.142 Displaced fracture of body of hamate [unciform] bone, left wrist** CC
- 7 7th **S62.143 Displaced fracture of body of hamate [unciform] bone, unspecified wrist** CC
- 7 7th **S62.144 Nondisplaced fracture of body of hamate [unciform] bone, right wrist** CC
- 7 7th **S62.145 Nondisplaced fracture of body of hamate [unciform] bone, left wrist** CC
- 7 7th **S62.146 Nondisplaced fracture of body of hamate [unciform] bone, unspecified wrist** CC

6th S62.15 Fracture of hook process of hamate [unciform] bone

Fracture of unciform process of hamate [unciform] bone
- 7 7th **S62.151 Displaced fracture of hook process of hamate [unciform] bone, right wrist** CC
- 7 7th **S62.152 Displaced fracture of hook process of hamate [unciform] bone, left wrist** CC
- 7 7th **S62.153 Displaced fracture of hook process of hamate [unciform] bone, unspecified wrist** CC
- 7 7th **S62.154 Nondisplaced fracture of hook process of hamate [unciform] bone, right wrist** CC
- 7 7th **S62.155 Nondisplaced fracture of hook process of hamate [unciform] bone, left wrist** CC
- 7 7th **S62.156 Nondisplaced fracture of hook process of hamate [unciform] bone, unspecified wrist** CC

6th S62.16 Fracture of pisiform
- 7 7th **S62.161 Displaced fracture of pisiform, right wrist** CC
- 7 7th **S62.162 Displaced fracture of pisiform, left wrist** CC
- 7 7th **S62.163 Displaced fracture of pisiform, unspecified wrist** CC
- 7 7th **S62.164 Nondisplaced fracture of pisiform, right wrist** CC
- 7 7th **S62.165 Nondisplaced fracture of pisiform, left wrist** CC
- 7 7th **S62.166 Nondisplaced fracture of pisiform, unspecified wrist** CC

6th S62.17 Fracture of trapezium [larger multangular]
- 7 7th **S62.171 Displaced fracture of trapezium [larger multangular], right wrist** CC
- 7 7th **S62.172 Displaced fracture of trapezium [larger multangular], left wrist** CC
- 7 7th **S62.173 Displaced fracture of trapezium [larger multangular], unspecified wrist** CC
- 7 7th **S62.174 Nondisplaced fracture of trapezium [larger multangular], right wrist** CC
- 7 7th **S62.175 Nondisplaced fracture of trapezium [larger multangular], left wrist** CC
- 7 7th **S62.176 Nondisplaced fracture of trapezium [larger multangular], unspecified wrist** CC

6th S62.18 Fracture of trapezoid [smaller multangular]
- 7 7th **S62.181 Displaced fracture of trapezoid [smaller multangular], right wrist** CC
- 7 7th **S62.182 Displaced fracture of trapezoid [smaller multangular], left wrist** CC
- 7 7th **S62.183 Displaced fracture of trapezoid [smaller multangular], unspecified wrist** CC
- 7 7th **S62.184 Nondisplaced fracture of trapezoid [smaller multangular], right wrist** CC
- 7 7th **S62.185 Nondisplaced fracture of trapezoid [smaller multangular], left wrist** CC
- 7 7th **S62.186 Nondisplaced fracture of trapezoid [smaller multangular], unspecified wrist** CC

7 HAC = Initial encounter only (7th character A, B or C) and not POA.

S62.2 Fracture of first metacarpal bone

S62.2 CC Excl: For CC codes in subcategory S62.2, unless otherwise noted: CC with 7th character B: S62.201-S62.399 with 7th [A, B], S62.90X with 7th A
CC with 7th character K or P: M80.00X-M84.68X with 7th [K, P], S02.0XX-S02.92X with 7th K, S12.000-S12.691 with 7th K, S22.000-S22.9XX with 7th K, S32.000-S32.9XX with 7th K, S42.001-S42.92X with 7th [K, P], S49.001-S49.199 with 7th [K, P], S52.001-S52.92X with 7th [K, M, N, P, Q, R], S59.001-S59.299 with 7th [K, P], S62.001-S62.92X with 7th [K, P], S72.001-S72.92X with 7th [K, M, N, P, Q, R], S79.001-S79.199 with 7th [K, P], S82.001-S82.92X with 7th [K, M, N, P, Q, R], S89.001-S89.399 with 7th [K, P], S92.001-S92.919 with 7th [K, P]

S62.20 Unspecified fracture of first metacarpal bone
- 7 S62.201 Unspecified fracture of first metacarpal bone, right hand CC
- 7 S62.202 Unspecified fracture of first metacarpal bone, left hand CC
- 7 S62.209 Unspecified fracture of first metacarpal bone, unspecified hand CC

S62.21 Bennett's fracture
- 7 S62.211 Bennett's fracture, right hand CC
- 7 S62.212 Bennett's fracture, left hand CC
- 7 S62.213 Bennett's fracture, unspecified hand CC

S62.22 Rolando's fracture
- 7 S62.221 Displaced Rolando's fracture, right hand CC
- 7 S62.222 Displaced Rolando's fracture, left hand CC
- 7 S62.223 Displaced Rolando's fracture, unspecified hand CC
- 7 S62.224 Nondisplaced Rolando's fracture, right hand CC
- 7 S62.225 Nondisplaced Rolando's fracture, left hand CC
- 7 S62.226 Nondisplaced Rolando's fracture, unspecified hand CC

S62.23 Other fracture of base of first metacarpal bone
- 7 S62.231 Other displaced fracture of base of first metacarpal bone, right hand CC
- 7 S62.232 Other displaced fracture of base of first metacarpal bone, left hand CC
- 7 S62.233 Other displaced fracture of base of first metacarpal bone, unspecified hand CC
- 7 S62.234 Other nondisplaced fracture of base of first metacarpal bone, right hand CC
- 7 S62.235 Other nondisplaced fracture of base of first metacarpal bone, left hand CC
- 7 S62.236 Other nondisplaced fracture of base of first metacarpal bone, unspecified hand CC

S62.24 Fracture of shaft of first metacarpal bone
- 7 S62.241 Displaced fracture of shaft of first metacarpal bone, right hand CC
- 7 S62.242 Displaced fracture of shaft of first metacarpal bone, left hand CC
- 7 S62.243 Displaced fracture of shaft of first metacarpal bone, unspecified hand CC
- 7 S62.244 Nondisplaced fracture of shaft of first metacarpal bone, right hand CC
- 7 S62.245 Nondisplaced fracture of shaft of first metacarpal bone, left hand CC
- 7 S62.246 Nondisplaced fracture of shaft of first metacarpal bone, unspecified hand CC

S62.25 Fracture of neck of first metacarpal bone
- 7 S62.251 Displaced fracture of neck of first metacarpal bone, right hand CC
- 7 S62.252 Displaced fracture of neck of first metacarpal bone, left hand CC
- 7 S62.253 Displaced fracture of neck of first metacarpal bone, unspecified hand CC
- 7 S62.254 Nondisplaced fracture of neck of first metacarpal bone, right hand CC
- 7 S62.255 Nondisplaced fracture of neck of first metacarpal bone, left hand CC
- 7 S62.256 Nondisplaced fracture of neck of first metacarpal bone, unspecified hand CC

S62.29 Other fracture of first metacarpal bone
- 7 S62.291 Other fracture of first metacarpal bone, right hand CC
- 7 S62.292 Other fracture of first metacarpal bone, left hand CC
- 7 S62.299 Other fracture of first metacarpal bone, unspecified hand CC

S62.3 Fracture of other and unspecified metacarpal bone

EXCLUDES 2 *fracture of first metacarpal bone (S62.2-)*

CC Excl: For CC codes in subcategory S62.3, unless otherwise noted: See code: S62.2

S62.30 Unspecified fracture of other metacarpal bone
- 7 S62.300 Unspecified fracture of second metacarpal bone, right hand CC
- 7 S62.301 Unspecified fracture of second metacarpal bone, left hand CC
- 7 S62.302 Unspecified fracture of third metacarpal bone, right hand CC
- 7 S62.303 Unspecified fracture of third metacarpal bone, left hand CC
- 7 S62.304 Unspecified fracture of fourth metacarpal bone, right hand CC
- 7 S62.305 Unspecified fracture of fourth metacarpal bone, left hand CC
- 7 S62.306 Unspecified fracture of fifth metacarpal bone, right hand CC
- 7 S62.307 Unspecified fracture of fifth metacarpal bone, left hand CC
- 7 S62.308 Unspecified fracture of other metacarpal bone CC
  Unspecified fracture of specified metacarpal bone with unspecified laterality
- 7 S62.309 Unspecified fracture of unspecified metacarpal bone CC

S62.31 Displaced fracture of base of other metacarpal bone
- 7 S62.310 Displaced fracture of base of second metacarpal bone, right hand CC
- 7 S62.311 Displaced fracture of base of second metacarpal bone, left hand CC
- 7 S62.312 Displaced fracture of base of third metacarpal bone, right hand CC
- 7 S62.313 Displaced fracture of base of third metacarpal bone, left hand CC
- 7 S62.314 Displaced fracture of base of fourth metacarpal bone, right hand CC
- 7 S62.315 Displaced fracture of base of fourth metacarpal bone, left hand CC
- 7 S62.316 Displaced fracture of base of fifth metacarpal bone, right hand CC
- 7 S62.317 Displaced fracture of base of fifth metacarpal bone, left hand CC
- 7 S62.318 Displaced fracture of base of other metacarpal bone CC
  Displaced fracture of base of specified metacarpal bone with unspecified laterality
- 7 S62.319 Displaced fracture of base of unspecified metacarpal bone CC

S62.32 Displaced fracture of shaft of other metacarpal bone
- 7 S62.320 Displaced fracture of shaft of second metacarpal bone, right hand CC
- 7 S62.321 Displaced fracture of shaft of second metacarpal bone, left hand CC
- 7 S62.322 Displaced fracture of shaft of third metacarpal bone, right hand CC
- 7 S62.323 Displaced fracture of shaft of third metacarpal bone, left hand CC
- 7 S62.324 Displaced fracture of shaft of fourth metacarpal bone, right hand CC

7 HAC = Initial encounter only (7th character A, B or C) and not POA.

7 ✓7th **S62.325 Displaced fracture of shaft of fourth metacarpal bone, left hand** CC
7 ✓7th **S62.326 Displaced fracture of shaft of fifth metacarpal bone, right hand** CC
7 ✓7th **S62.327 Displaced fracture of shaft of fifth metacarpal bone, left hand** CC
7 ✓7th **S62.328 Displaced fracture of shaft of other metacarpal bone** CC
Displaced fracture of shaft of specified metacarpal bone with unspecified laterality
7 ✓7th **S62.329 Displaced fracture of shaft of unspecified metacarpal bone** CC

✓6th **S62.33 Displaced fracture of neck of other metacarpal bone**
7 ✓7th **S62.33Ø Displaced fracture of neck of second metacarpal bone, right hand** CC
7 ✓7th **S62.331 Displaced fracture of neck of second metacarpal bone, left hand** CC
7 ✓7th **S62.332 Displaced fracture of neck of third metacarpal bone, right hand** CC
7 ✓7th **S62.333 Displaced fracture of neck of third metacarpal bone, left hand** CC
7 ✓7th **S62.334 Displaced fracture of neck of fourth metacarpal bone, right hand** CC
7 ✓7th **S62.335 Displaced fracture of neck of fourth metacarpal bone, left hand** CC
7 ✓7th **S62.336 Displaced fracture of neck of fifth metacarpal bone, right hand** CC
7 ✓7th **S62.337 Displaced fracture of neck of fifth metacarpal bone, left hand** CC
7 ✓7th **S62.338 Displaced fracture of neck of other metacarpal bone** CC
Displaced fracture of neck of specified metacarpal bone with unspecified laterality
7 ✓7th **S62.339 Displaced fracture of neck of unspecified metacarpal bone** CC

✓6th **S62.34 Nondisplaced fracture of base of other metacarpal bone**
7 ✓7th **S62.34Ø Nondisplaced fracture of base of second metacarpal bone, right hand** CC
7 ✓7th **S62.341 Nondisplaced fracture of base of second metacarpal bone, left hand** CC
7 ✓7th **S62.342 Nondisplaced fracture of base of third metacarpal bone, right hand** CC
7 ✓7th **S62.343 Nondisplaced fracture of base of third metacarpal bone, left hand** CC
7 ✓7th **S62.344 Nondisplaced fracture of base of fourth metacarpal bone, right hand** CC
7 ✓7th **S62.345 Nondisplaced fracture of base of fourth metacarpal bone, left hand** CC
7 ✓7th **S62.346 Nondisplaced fracture of base of fifth metacarpal bone, right hand** CC
7 ✓7th **S62.347 Nondisplaced fracture of base of fifth metacarpal bone, left hand** CC
7 ✓7th **S62.348 Nondisplaced fracture of base of other metacarpal bone** CC
Nondisplaced fracture of base of specified metacarpal bone with unspecified laterality
7 ✓7th **S62.349 Nondisplaced fracture of base of unspecified metacarpal bone** CC

✓6th **S62.35 Nondisplaced fracture of shaft of other metacarpal bone**
7 ✓7th **S62.35Ø Nondisplaced fracture of shaft of second metacarpal bone, right hand** CC
7 ✓7th **S62.351 Nondisplaced fracture of shaft of second metacarpal bone, left hand** CC
7 ✓7th **S62.352 Nondisplaced fracture of shaft of third metacarpal bone, right hand** CC
7 ✓7th **S62.353 Nondisplaced fracture of shaft of third metacarpal bone, left hand** CC
7 ✓7th **S62.354 Nondisplaced fracture of shaft of fourth metacarpal bone, right hand** CC
7 ✓7th **S62.355 Nondisplaced fracture of shaft of fourth metacarpal bone, left hand** CC
7 ✓7th **S62.356 Nondisplaced fracture of shaft of fifth metacarpal bone, right hand** CC
7 ✓7th **S62.357 Nondisplaced fracture of shaft of fifth metacarpal bone, left hand** CC
7 ✓7th **S62.358 Nondisplaced fracture of shaft of other metacarpal bone** CC
Nondisplaced fracture of shaft of specified metacarpal bone with unspecified laterality
7 ✓7th **S62.359 Nondisplaced fracture of shaft of unspecified metacarpal bone** CC

✓6th **S62.36 Nondisplaced fracture of neck of other metacarpal bone**
7 ✓7th **S62.36Ø Nondisplaced fracture of neck of second metacarpal bone, right hand** CC
7 ✓7th **S62.361 Nondisplaced fracture of neck of second metacarpal bone, left hand** CC
7 ✓7th **S62.362 Nondisplaced fracture of neck of third metacarpal bone, right hand** CC
7 ✓7th **S62.363 Nondisplaced fracture of neck of third metacarpal bone, left hand** CC
7 ✓7th **S62.364 Nondisplaced fracture of neck of fourth metacarpal bone, right hand** CC
7 ✓7th **S62.365 Nondisplaced fracture of neck of fourth metacarpal bone, left hand** CC
7 ✓7th **S62.366 Nondisplaced fracture of neck of fifth metacarpal bone, right hand** CC
7 ✓7th **S62.367 Nondisplaced fracture of neck of fifth metacarpal bone, left hand** CC
7 ✓7th **S62.368 Nondisplaced fracture of neck of other metacarpal bone** CC
Nondisplaced fracture of neck of specified metacarpal bone with unspecified laterality
7 ✓7th **S62.369 Nondisplaced fracture of neck of unspecified metacarpal bone** CC

✓6th **S62.39 Other fracture of other metacarpal bone**
7 ✓7th **S62.39Ø Other fracture of second metacarpal bone, right hand** CC
7 ✓7th **S62.391 Other fracture of second metacarpal bone, left hand** CC
7 ✓7th **S62.392 Other fracture of third metacarpal bone, right hand** CC
7 ✓7th **S62.393 Other fracture of third metacarpal bone, left hand** CC
7 ✓7th **S62.394 Other fracture of fourth metacarpal bone, right hand** CC
7 ✓7th **S62.395 Other fracture of fourth metacarpal bone, left hand** CC
7 ✓7th **S62.396 Other fracture of fifth metacarpal bone, right hand** CC
7 ✓7th **S62.397 Other fracture of fifth metacarpal bone, left hand** CC
7 ✓7th **S62.398 Other fracture of other metacarpal bone** CC
Other fracture of specified metacarpal bone with unspecified laterality
7 ✓7th **S62.399 Other fracture of unspecified metacarpal bone** CC

✓5th **S62.5 Fracture of thumb**

CC Excl: For CC codes in subcategory S62.5, unless otherwise noted: CC CC with 7th character B: S62.5Ø1-S62.92X with 7th [A, B]

CC CC with 7th character K or P: M8Ø.ØØX-M84.68X with 7th [K, P], SØ2.ØXX-SØ2.92X with 7th K, S12.ØØØ-S12.691 with 7th K, S22.ØØØ-S22.9XX with 7th K, S32.ØØØ-S32.9XX with 7th K, S42.ØØ1-S42.92X with 7th [K, P], S49.ØØ1-S49.199 with 7th [K, P], S52.ØØ1-S52.92X with 7th [K, M, N, P, Q, R], S59.ØØ1-S59.299 with 7th [K, P], S62.ØØ1-S62.92X with 7th [K, P], S72.ØØ1-S72.92X with 7th [K, M, N, P, Q, R], S79.ØØ1-S79.199 with 7th [K, P], S82.ØØ1-S82.92X with 7th [K, M, N, P, Q, R], S89.ØØ1-S89.399 with 7th [K, P], S92.ØØ1-S92.919 with 7th [K, P]

✓6th **S62.5Ø Fracture of unspecified phalanx of thumb**
7 ✓7th **S62.5Ø1 Fracture of unspecified phalanx of right thumb** CC
7 ✓7th **S62.5Ø2 Fracture of unspecified phalanx of left thumb** CC

7 HAC = Initial encounter only (7th character A, B or C) and not POA.

7 ✓7th S62.509 Fracture of unspecified phalanx of unspecified thumb CC

✓6th S62.51 Fracture of proximal phalanx of thumb

7 ✓7th S62.511 Displaced fracture of proximal phalanx of right thumb CC

7 ✓7th S62.512 Displaced fracture of proximal phalanx of left thumb CC

7 ✓7th S62.513 Displaced fracture of proximal phalanx of unspecified thumb CC

7 ✓7th S62.514 Nondisplaced fracture of proximal phalanx of right thumb CC

7 ✓7th S62.515 Nondisplaced fracture of proximal phalanx of left thumb CC

7 ✓7th S62.516 Nondisplaced fracture of proximal phalanx of unspecified thumb CC

✓6th S62.52 Fracture of distal phalanx of thumb

7 ✓7th S62.521 Displaced fracture of distal phalanx of right thumb CC

7 ✓7th S62.522 Displaced fracture of distal phalanx of left thumb CC

7 ✓7th S62.523 Displaced fracture of distal phalanx of unspecified thumb CC

7 ✓7th S62.524 Nondisplaced fracture of distal phalanx of right thumb CC

7 ✓7th S62.525 Nondisplaced fracture of distal phalanx of left thumb CC

7 ✓7th S62.526 Nondisplaced fracture of distal phalanx of unspecified thumb CC

✓5th S62.6 Fracture of other and unspecified finger(s)

EXCLUDES 2 *fracture of thumb (S62.5-)*

CC Excl: For CC codes in subcategory S62.6, unless otherwise noted: See code: S62.2

✓6th S62.60 Fracture of unspecified phalanx of finger

7 ✓7th S62.600 Fracture of unspecified phalanx of right index finger CC

7 ✓7th S62.601 Fracture of unspecified phalanx of left index finger CC

7 ✓7th S62.602 Fracture of unspecified phalanx of right middle finger CC

7 ✓7th S62.603 Fracture of unspecified phalanx of left middle finger CC

7 ✓7th S62.604 Fracture of unspecified phalanx of right ring finger CC

7 ✓7th S62.605 Fracture of unspecified phalanx of left ring finger CC

7 ✓7th S62.606 Fracture of unspecified phalanx of right little finger CC

7 ✓7th S62.607 Fracture of unspecified phalanx of left little finger CC

7 ✓7th S62.608 Fracture of unspecified phalanx of other finger CC

Fracture of unspecified phalanx of specified finger with unspecified laterality

7 ✓7th S62.609 Fracture of unspecified phalanx of unspecified finger CC

✓6th S62.61 Displaced fracture of proximal phalanx of finger

7 ✓7th S62.610 Displaced fracture of proximal phalanx of right index finger CC

7 ✓7th S62.611 Displaced fracture of proximal phalanx of left index finger CC

7 ✓7th S62.612 Displaced fracture of proximal phalanx of right middle finger CC

7 ✓7th S62.613 Displaced fracture of proximal phalanx of left middle finger CC

7 ✓7th S62.614 Displaced fracture of proximal phalanx of right ring finger CC

7 ✓7th S62.615 Displaced fracture of proximal phalanx of left ring finger CC

7 ✓7th S62.616 Displaced fracture of proximal phalanx of right little finger CC

7 ✓7th S62.617 Displaced fracture of proximal phalanx of left little finger CC

7 ✓7th S62.618 Displaced fracture of proximal phalanx of other finger CC

Displaced fracture of proximal phalanx of specified finger with unspecified laterality

7 ✓7th S62.619 Displaced fracture of proximal phalanx of unspecified finger CC

✓6th S62.62 Displaced fracture of medial phalanx of finger

7 ✓7th S62.620 Displaced fracture of medial phalanx of right index finger CC

7 ✓7th S62.621 Displaced fracture of medial phalanx of left index finger CC

7 ✓7th S62.622 Displaced fracture of medial phalanx of right middle finger CC

7 ✓7th S62.623 Displaced fracture of medial phalanx of left middle finger CC

7 ✓7th S62.624 Displaced fracture of medial phalanx of right ring finger CC

7 ✓7th S62.625 Displaced fracture of medial phalanx of left ring finger CC

7 ✓7th S62.626 Displaced fracture of medial phalanx of right little finger CC

7 ✓7th S62.627 Displaced fracture of medial phalanx of left little finger CC

7 ✓7th S62.628 Displaced fracture of medial phalanx of other finger CC

Displaced fracture of medial phalanx of specified finger with unspecified laterality

7 ✓7th S62.629 Displaced fracture of medial phalanx of unspecified finger CC

✓6th S62.63 Displaced fracture of distal phalanx of finger

7 ✓7th S62.630 Displaced fracture of distal phalanx of right index finger CC

7 ✓7th S62.631 Displaced fracture of distal phalanx of left index finger CC

7 ✓7th S62.632 Displaced fracture of distal phalanx of right middle finger CC

7 ✓7th S62.633 Displaced fracture of distal phalanx of left middle finger CC

7 ✓7th S62.634 Displaced fracture of distal phalanx of right ring finger CC

7 ✓7th S62.635 Displaced fracture of distal phalanx of left ring finger CC

7 ✓7th S62.636 Displaced fracture of distal phalanx of right little finger CC

7 ✓7th S62.637 Displaced fracture of distal phalanx of left little finger CC

7 ✓7th S62.638 Displaced fracture of distal phalanx of other finger CC

Displaced fracture of distal phalanx of specified finger with unspecified laterality

7 ✓7th S62.639 Displaced fracture of distal phalanx of unspecified finger CC

✓6th S62.64 Nondisplaced fracture of proximal phalanx of finger

7 ✓7th S62.640 Nondisplaced fracture of proximal phalanx of right index finger CC

7 ✓7th S62.641 Nondisplaced fracture of proximal phalanx of left index finger CC

7 ✓7th S62.642 Nondisplaced fracture of proximal phalanx of right middle finger CC

7 ✓7th S62.643 Nondisplaced fracture of proximal phalanx of left middle finger CC

7 ✓7th S62.644 Nondisplaced fracture of proximal phalanx of right ring finger CC

7 ✓7th S62.645 Nondisplaced fracture of proximal phalanx of left ring finger CC

7 ✓7th S62.646 Nondisplaced fracture of proximal phalanx of right little finger CC

7 ✓7th S62.647 Nondisplaced fracture of proximal phalanx of left little finger CC

7 HAC = Initial encounter only (7th character A, B or C) and not POA.

7 ✓7th **S62.648 Nondisplaced fracture of proximal phalanx of other finger** CC
Nondisplaced fracture of proximal phalanx of specified finger with unspecified laterality

7 ✓7th **S62.649 Nondisplaced fracture of proximal phalanx of unspecified finger** CC

✓6th **S62.65 Nondisplaced fracture of medial phalanx of finger**

7 ✓7th **S62.65Ø Nondisplaced fracture of medial phalanx of right index finger** CC

7 ✓7th **S62.651 Nondisplaced fracture of medial phalanx of left index finger** CC

7 ✓7th **S62.652 Nondisplaced fracture of medial phalanx of right middle finger** CC

7 ✓7th **S62.653 Nondisplaced fracture of medial phalanx of left middle finger** CC

7 ✓7th **S62.654 Nondisplaced fracture of medial phalanx of right ring finger** CC

7 ✓7th **S62.655 Nondisplaced fracture of medial phalanx of left ring finger** CC

7 ✓7th **S62.656 Nondisplaced fracture of medial phalanx of right little finger** CC

7 ✓7th **S62.657 Nondisplaced fracture of medial phalanx of left little finger** CC

7 ✓7th **S62.658 Nondisplaced fracture of medial phalanx of other finger** CC
Nondisplaced fracture of medial phalanx of specified finger with unspecified laterality

7 ✓7th **S62.659 Nondisplaced fracture of medial phalanx of unspecified finger** CC

✓6th **S62.66 Nondisplaced fracture of distal phalanx of finger**

7 ✓7th **S62.66Ø Nondisplaced fracture of distal phalanx of right index finger** CC

7 ✓7th **S62.661 Nondisplaced fracture of distal phalanx of left index finger** CC

7 ✓7th **S62.662 Nondisplaced fracture of distal phalanx of right middle finger** CC

7 ✓7th **S62.663 Nondisplaced fracture of distal phalanx of left middle finger** CC

7 ✓7th **S62.664 Nondisplaced fracture of distal phalanx of right ring finger** CC

7 ✓7th **S62.665 Nondisplaced fracture of distal phalanx of left ring finger** CC

7 ✓7th **S62.666 Nondisplaced fracture of distal phalanx of right little finger** CC

7 ✓7th **S62.667 Nondisplaced fracture of distal phalanx of left little finger** CC

7 ✓7th **S62.668 Nondisplaced fracture of distal phalanx of other finger** CC
Nondisplaced fracture of distal phalanx of specified finger with unspecified laterality

7 ✓7th **S62.669 Nondisplaced fracture of distal phalanx of unspecified finger** CC

✓5th **S62.9 Unspecified fracture of wrist and hand**

7 ✓x7th **S62.9Ø Unspecified fracture of unspecified wrist and hand** CC
CC Excl: CC CC with 7th character B: S42.2Ø1-S42.92X with 7th [A, B], S49.ØØ1-S49.199 with 7th A, S52.ØØ1-S52.ØØ9 with 7th [A, B, C], S52.Ø21-S52.1Ø9 with 7th [A, B, C], S52.121-S52.516 with 7th [A, B, C], S52.531-S52.616 with 7th [A, B, C], S52.691-S52.92X with 7th [A, B, C], S59.ØØ1-S59.299 with 7th A, S62.ØØ1-S62.92X with 7th [A, B]
CC CC with 7th character K or P: M8Ø.ØØX-M84.68X with 7th [K, P], SØ2.ØXX-SØ2.92X with 7th K, S12.ØØØ-S12.691 with 7th K, S22.ØØØ-S22.9XX with 7th K, S32.ØØØ-S32.9XX with 7th K, S42.ØØ1-S42.92X with 7th [K, P], S49.ØØ1-S49.199 with 7th [K, P], S52.ØØ1-S52.92X with 7th [K, M, N, P, Q, R], S59.ØØ1-S59.299 with 7th [K, P], S62.ØØ1-S62.92X with 7th [K, P], S72.ØØ1-S72.92X with 7th [K, M, N, P, Q, R], S79.ØØ1-S79.199 with 7th [K, P], S82.ØØ1-S82.92X with 7th [K, M, N, P, Q, R], S89.ØØ1-S89.399 with 7th [K, P], S92.ØØ1-S92.919 with 7th [K, P]

7 ✓x7th **S62.91 Unspecified fracture of right wrist and hand** CC
CC Excl: CC CC with 7th character B: S62.5Ø1-S62.92X with 7th [A, B]
CC CC with 7th character K or P: M8Ø.ØØX-M84.68X with 7th [K, P], SØ2.ØXX-SØ2.92X with 7th K, S12.ØØØ-S12.691 with 7th K, S22.ØØØ-S22.9XX with 7th K, S32.ØØØ-S32.9XX with 7th K, S42.ØØ1-S42.92X with 7th [K, P], S49.ØØ1-S49.199 with 7th [K, P], S52.ØØ1-S52.92X with 7th [K, M, N, P, Q, R], S59.ØØ1-S59.299 with 7th [K, P], S62.ØØ1-S62.92X with 7th [K, P], S72.ØØ1-S72.92X with 7th [K, M, N, P, Q, R], S79.ØØ1-S79.199 with 7th [K, P], S82.ØØ1-S82.92X with 7th [K, M, N, P, Q, R], S89.ØØ1-S89.399 with 7th [K, P], S92.ØØ1-S92.919 with 7th [K, P]

7 ✓x7th **S62.92 Unspecified fracture of left wrist and hand** CC
CC Excl: See code: S62.91

✓4th **S63 Dislocation and sprain of joints and ligaments at wrist and hand level**

INCLUDES avulsion of joint or ligament at wrist and hand level
laceration of cartilage, joint or ligament at wrist and hand level
sprain of cartilage, joint or ligament at wrist and hand level
traumatic hemarthrosis of joint or ligament at wrist and hand level
traumatic rupture of joint or ligament at wrist and hand level
traumatic subluxation of joint or ligament at wrist and hand level
traumatic tear of joint or ligament at wrist and hand level

Code also any associated open wound

EXCLUDES 2 *strain of muscle, fascia and tendon of wrist and hand (S66.-)*

The appropriate 7th character is to be added to each code from category S63.
A initial encounter
D subsequent encounter
S sequela

✓5th **S63.Ø Subluxation and dislocation of wrist and hand joints**

✓6th **S63.ØØ Unspecified subluxation and dislocation of wrist and hand**
Dislocation of carpal bone NOS
Dislocation of distal end of radius NOS
Subluxation of carpal bone NOS
Subluxation of distal end of radius NOS

✓7th **S63.ØØ1 Unspecified subluxation of right wrist and hand**

✓7th **S63.ØØ2 Unspecified subluxation of left wrist and hand**

✓7th **S63.ØØ3 Unspecified subluxation of unspecified wrist and hand**

✓7th **S63.ØØ4 Unspecified dislocation of right wrist and hand**

✓7th **S63.ØØ5 Unspecified dislocation of left wrist and hand**

✓7th **S63.ØØ6 Unspecified dislocation of unspecified wrist and hand**

✓6th **S63.Ø1 Subluxation and dislocation of distal radioulnar joint**

✓7th **S63.Ø11 Subluxation of distal radioulnar joint of right wrist**

✓7th **S63.Ø12 Subluxation of distal radioulnar joint of left wrist**

✓7th **S63.Ø13 Subluxation of distal radioulnar joint of unspecified wrist**

✓7th **S63.Ø14 Dislocation of distal radioulnar joint of right wrist**

✓7th **S63.Ø15 Dislocation of distal radioulnar joint of left wrist**

✓7th **S63.Ø16 Dislocation of distal radioulnar joint of unspecified wrist**

✓6th **S63.Ø2 Subluxation and dislocation of radiocarpal joint**

✓7th **S63.Ø21 Subluxation of radiocarpal joint of right wrist**

✓7th **S63.Ø22 Subluxation of radiocarpal joint of left wrist**

✓7th **S63.Ø23 Subluxation of radiocarpal joint of unspecified wrist**

✓7th **S63.Ø24 Dislocation of radiocarpal joint of right wrist**

7 HAC = Initial encounter only (7th character A, B or C) and not POA.

✓7th **S63.025** Dislocation of radiocarpal joint of left wrist
✓7th **S63.026** Dislocation of radiocarpal joint of unspecified wrist

✓6th **S63.03** Subluxation and dislocation of midcarpal joint
✓7th **S63.031** Subluxation of midcarpal joint of right wrist
✓7th **S63.032** Subluxation of midcarpal joint of left wrist
✓7th **S63.033** Subluxation of midcarpal joint of unspecified wrist
✓7th **S63.034** Dislocation of midcarpal joint of right wrist
✓7th **S63.035** Dislocation of midcarpal joint of left wrist
✓7th **S63.036** Dislocation of midcarpal joint of unspecified wrist

✓6th **S63.04** Subluxation and dislocation of carpometacarpal joint of thumb
EXCLUDES 2 *interphalangeal subluxation and dislocation of thumb (S63.1-)*
✓7th **S63.041** Subluxation of carpometacarpal joint of right thumb
✓7th **S63.042** Subluxation of carpometacarpal joint of left thumb
✓7th **S63.043** Subluxation of carpometacarpal joint of unspecified thumb
✓7th **S63.044** Dislocation of carpometacarpal joint of right thumb
✓7th **S63.045** Dislocation of carpometacarpal joint of left thumb
✓7th **S63.046** Dislocation of carpometacarpal joint of unspecified thumb

✓6th **S63.05** Subluxation and dislocation of other carpometacarpal joint
EXCLUDES 2 *subluxation and dislocation of carpometacarpal joint of thumb (S63.04-)*
✓7th **S63.051** Subluxation of other carpometacarpal joint of right hand
✓7th **S63.052** Subluxation of other carpometacarpal joint of left hand
✓7th **S63.053** Subluxation of other carpometacarpal joint of unspecified hand
✓7th **S63.054** Dislocation of other carpometacarpal joint of right hand
✓7th **S63.055** Dislocation of other carpometacarpal joint of left hand
✓7th **S63.056** Dislocation of other carpometacarpal joint of unspecified hand

✓6th **S63.06** Subluxation and dislocation of metacarpal (bone), proximal end
✓7th **S63.061** Subluxation of metacarpal (bone), proximal end of right hand
✓7th **S63.062** Subluxation of metacarpal (bone), proximal end of left hand
✓7th **S63.063** Subluxation of metacarpal (bone), proximal end of unspecified hand
✓7th **S63.064** Dislocation of metacarpal (bone), proximal end of right hand
✓7th **S63.065** Dislocation of metacarpal (bone), proximal end of left hand
✓7th **S63.066** Dislocation of metacarpal (bone), proximal end of unspecified hand

✓6th **S63.07** Subluxation and dislocation of distal end of ulna
✓7th **S63.071** Subluxation of distal end of right ulna
✓7th **S63.072** Subluxation of distal end of left ulna
✓7th **S63.073** Subluxation of distal end of unspecified ulna
✓7th **S63.074** Dislocation of distal end of right ulna
✓7th **S63.075** Dislocation of distal end of left ulna
✓7th **S63.076** Dislocation of distal end of unspecified ulna

✓6th **S63.09** Other subluxation and dislocation of wrist and hand
✓7th **S63.091** Other subluxation of right wrist and hand
✓7th **S63.092** Other subluxation of left wrist and hand
✓7th **S63.093** Other subluxation of unspecified wrist and hand
✓7th **S63.094** Other dislocation of right wrist and hand
✓7th **S63.095** Other dislocation of left wrist and hand
✓7th **S63.096** Other dislocation of unspecified wrist and hand

✓5th **S63.1** Subluxation and dislocation of thumb

✓6th **S63.10** Unspecified subluxation and dislocation of thumb
✓7th **S63.101** Unspecified subluxation of right thumb
✓7th **S63.102** Unspecified subluxation of left thumb
✓7th **S63.103** Unspecified subluxation of unspecified thumb
✓7th **S63.104** Unspecified dislocation of right thumb
✓7th **S63.105** Unspecified dislocation of left thumb
✓7th **S63.106** Unspecified dislocation of unspecified thumb

✓6th **S63.11** Subluxation and dislocation of metacarpophalangeal joint of thumb
✓7th **S63.111** Subluxation of metacarpophalangeal joint of right thumb
✓7th **S63.112** Subluxation of metacarpophalangeal joint of left thumb
✓7th **S63.113** Subluxation of metacarpophalangeal joint of unspecified thumb
✓7th **S63.114** Dislocation of metacarpophalangeal joint of right thumb
✓7th **S63.115** Dislocation of metacarpophalangeal joint of left thumb
✓7th **S63.116** Dislocation of metacarpophalangeal joint of unspecified thumb

✓6th **S63.12** Subluxation and dislocation of unspecified interphalangeal joint of thumb
✓7th **S63.121** Subluxation of unspecified interphalangeal joint of right thumb
✓7th **S63.122** Subluxation of unspecified interphalangeal joint of left thumb
✓7th **S63.123** Subluxation of unspecified interphalangeal joint of unspecified thumb
✓7th **S63.124** Dislocation of unspecified interphalangeal joint of right thumb
✓7th **S63.125** Dislocation of unspecified interphalangeal joint of left thumb
✓7th **S63.126** Dislocation of unspecified interphalangeal joint of unspecified thumb

✓6th **S63.13** Subluxation and dislocation of proximal interphalangeal joint of thumb
✓7th **S63.131** Subluxation of proximal interphalangeal joint of right thumb
✓7th **S63.132** Subluxation of proximal interphalangeal joint of left thumb
✓7th **S63.133** Subluxation of proximal interphalangeal joint of unspecified thumb
✓7th **S63.134** Dislocation of proximal interphalangeal joint of right thumb
✓7th **S63.135** Dislocation of proximal interphalangeal joint of left thumb
✓7th **S63.136** Dislocation of proximal interphalangeal joint of unspecified thumb

✓6th **S63.14** Subluxation and dislocation of distal interphalangeal joint of thumb
✓7th **S63.141** Subluxation of distal interphalangeal joint of right thumb
✓7th **S63.142** Subluxation of distal interphalangeal joint of left thumb
✓7th **S63.143** Subluxation of distal interphalangeal joint of unspecified thumb
✓7th **S63.144** Dislocation of distal interphalangeal joint of right thumb
✓7th **S63.145** Dislocation of distal interphalangeal joint of left thumb
✓7th **S63.146** Dislocation of distal interphalangeal joint of unspecified thumb

Injury, Poisoning and Certain Other Consequences of External Causes S63.025–S63.146

✓5th **S63.2 Subluxation and dislocation of other finger(s)**
EXCLUDES 2 *subluxation and dislocation of thumb (S63.1-)*

✓6th **S63.20 Unspecified subluxation of other finger**
✓7th **S63.200 Unspecified subluxation of right index finger**
✓7th **S63.201 Unspecified subluxation of left index finger**
✓7th **S63.202 Unspecified subluxation of right middle finger**
✓7th **S63.203 Unspecified subluxation of left middle finger**
✓7th **S63.204 Unspecified subluxation of right ring finger**
✓7th **S63.205 Unspecified subluxation of left ring finger**
✓7th **S63.206 Unspecified subluxation of right little finger**
✓7th **S63.207 Unspecified subluxation of left little finger**
✓7th **S63.208 Unspecified subluxation of other finger**
Unspecified subluxation of specified finger with unspecified laterality
✓7th **S63.209 Unspecified subluxation of unspecified finger**

✓6th **S63.21 Subluxation of metacarpophalangeal joint of finger**
✓7th **S63.210 Subluxation of metacarpophalangeal joint of right index finger**
✓7th **S63.211 Subluxation of metacarpophalangeal joint of left index finger**
✓7th **S63.212 Subluxation of metacarpophalangeal joint of right middle finger**
✓7th **S63.213 Subluxation of metacarpophalangeal joint of left middle finger**
✓7th **S63.214 Subluxation of metacarpophalangeal joint of right ring finger**
✓7th **S63.215 Subluxation of metacarpophalangeal joint of left ring finger**
✓7th **S63.216 Subluxation of metacarpophalangeal joint of right little finger**
✓7th **S63.217 Subluxation of metacarpophalangeal joint of left little finger**
✓7th **S63.218 Subluxation of metacarpophalangeal joint of other finger**
Subluxation of metacarpophalangeal joint of specified finger with unspecified laterality
✓7th **S63.219 Subluxation of metacarpophalangeal joint of unspecified finger**

✓6th **S63.22 Subluxation of unspecified interphalangeal joint of finger**
✓7th **S63.220 Subluxation of unspecified interphalangeal joint of right index finger**
✓7th **S63.221 Subluxation of unspecified interphalangeal joint of left index finger**
✓7th **S63.222 Subluxation of unspecified interphalangeal joint of right middle finger**
✓7th **S63.223 Subluxation of unspecified interphalangeal joint of left middle finger**
✓7th **S63.224 Subluxation of unspecified interphalangeal joint of right ring finger**
✓7th **S63.225 Subluxation of unspecified interphalangeal joint of left ring finger**
✓7th **S63.226 Subluxation of unspecified interphalangeal joint of right little finger**
✓7th **S63.227 Subluxation of unspecified interphalangeal joint of left little finger**
✓7th **S63.228 Subluxation of unspecified interphalangeal joint of other finger**
Subluxation of unspecified interphalangeal joint of specified finger with unspecified laterality
✓7th **S63.229 Subluxation of unspecified interphalangeal joint of unspecified finger**

✓6th **S63.23 Subluxation of proximal interphalangeal joint of finger**
✓7th **S63.230 Subluxation of proximal interphalangeal joint of right index finger**
✓7th **S63.231 Subluxation of proximal interphalangeal joint of left index finger**
✓7th **S63.232 Subluxation of proximal interphalangeal joint of right middle finger**
✓7th **S63.233 Subluxation of proximal interphalangeal joint of left middle finger**
✓7th **S63.234 Subluxation of proximal interphalangeal joint of right ring finger**
✓7th **S63.235 Subluxation of proximal interphalangeal joint of left ring finger**
✓7th **S63.236 Subluxation of proximal interphalangeal joint of right little finger**
✓7th **S63.237 Subluxation of proximal interphalangeal joint of left little finger**
✓7th **S63.238 Subluxation of proximal interphalangeal joint of other finger**
Subluxation of proximal interphalangeal joint of specified finger with unspecified laterality
✓7th **S63.239 Subluxation of proximal interphalangeal joint of unspecified finger**

✓6th **S63.24 Subluxation of distal interphalangeal joint of finger**
✓7th **S63.240 Subluxation of distal interphalangeal joint of right index finger**
✓7th **S63.241 Subluxation of distal interphalangeal joint of left index finger**
✓7th **S63.242 Subluxation of distal interphalangeal joint of right middle finger**
✓7th **S63.243 Subluxation of distal interphalangeal joint of left middle finger**
✓7th **S63.244 Subluxation of distal interphalangeal joint of right ring finger**
✓7th **S63.245 Subluxation of distal interphalangeal joint of left ring finger**
✓7th **S63.246 Subluxation of distal interphalangeal joint of right little finger**
✓7th **S63.247 Subluxation of distal interphalangeal joint of left little finger**
✓7th **S63.248 Subluxation of distal interphalangeal joint of other finger**
Subluxation of distal interphalangeal joint of specified finger with unspecified laterality
✓7th **S63.249 Subluxation of distal interphalangeal joint of unspecified finger**

✓6th **S63.25 Unspecified dislocation of other finger**
✓7th **S63.250 Unspecified dislocation of right index finger**
✓7th **S63.251 Unspecified dislocation of left index finger**
✓7th **S63.252 Unspecified dislocation of right middle finger**
✓7th **S63.253 Unspecified dislocation of left middle finger**
✓7th **S63.254 Unspecified dislocation of right ring finger**
✓7th **S63.255 Unspecified dislocation of left ring finger**
✓7th **S63.256 Unspecified dislocation of right little finger**
✓7th **S63.257 Unspecified dislocation of left little finger**
✓7th **S63.258 Unspecified dislocation of other finger**
Unspecified dislocation of specified finger with unspecified laterality
✓7th **S63.259 Unspecified dislocation of unspecified finger**
Unspecified dislocation of specified finger with unspecified laterality

✓6th **S63.26 Dislocation of metacarpophalangeal joint of finger**
✓7th **S63.260 Dislocation of metacarpophalangeal joint of right index finger**
✓7th **S63.261 Dislocation of metacarpophalangeal joint of left index finger**
✓7th **S63.262 Dislocation of metacarpophalangeal joint of right middle finger**
✓7th **S63.263 Dislocation of metacarpophalangeal joint of left middle finger**
✓7th **S63.264 Dislocation of metacarpophalangeal joint of right ring finger**

✓7th **S63.265 Dislocation of metacarpophalangeal joint of left ring finger**

✓7th **S63.266 Dislocation of metacarpophalangeal joint of right little finger**

✓7th **S63.267 Dislocation of metacarpophalangeal joint of left little finger**

✓7th **S63.268 Dislocation of metacarpophalangeal joint of other finger**

Dislocation of metacarpophalangeal joint of specified finger with unspecified laterality

✓7th **S63.269 Dislocation of metacarpophalangeal joint of unspecified finger**

✓6th **S63.27 Dislocation of unspecified interphalangeal joint of finger**

✓7th **S63.270 Dislocation of unspecified interphalangeal joint of right index finger**

✓7th **S63.271 Dislocation of unspecified interphalangeal joint of left index finger**

✓7th **S63.272 Dislocation of unspecified interphalangeal joint of right middle finger**

✓7th **S63.273 Dislocation of unspecified interphalangeal joint of left middle finger**

✓7th **S63.274 Dislocation of unspecified interphalangeal joint of right ring finger**

✓7th **S63.275 Dislocation of unspecified interphalangeal joint of left ring finger**

✓7th **S63.276 Dislocation of unspecified interphalangeal joint of right little finger**

✓7th **S63.277 Dislocation of unspecified interphalangeal joint of left little finger**

✓7th **S63.278 Dislocation of unspecified interphalangeal joint of other finger**

Dislocation of unspecified interphalangeal joint of specified finger with unspecified laterality

✓7th **S63.279 Dislocation of unspecified interphalangeal joint of unspecified finger**

Dislocation of unspecified interphalangeal joint of specified finger without specified laterality

✓6th **S63.28 Dislocation of proximal interphalangeal joint of finger**

✓7th **S63.280 Dislocation of proximal interphalangeal joint of right index finger**

✓7th **S63.281 Dislocation of proximal interphalangeal joint of left index finger**

✓7th **S63.282 Dislocation of proximal interphalangeal joint of right middle finger**

✓7th **S63.283 Dislocation of proximal interphalangeal joint of left middle finger**

✓7th **S63.284 Dislocation of proximal interphalangeal joint of right ring finger**

✓7th **S63.285 Dislocation of proximal interphalangeal joint of left ring finger**

✓7th **S63.286 Dislocation of proximal interphalangeal joint of right little finger**

✓7th **S63.287 Dislocation of proximal interphalangeal joint of left little finger**

✓7th **S63.288 Dislocation of proximal interphalangeal joint of other finger**

Dislocation of proximal interphalangeal joint of specified finger with unspecified laterality

✓7th **S63.289 Dislocation of proximal interphalangeal joint of unspecified finger**

✓6th **S63.29 Dislocation of distal interphalangeal joint of finger**

✓7th **S63.290 Dislocation of distal interphalangeal joint of right index finger**

✓7th **S63.291 Dislocation of distal interphalangeal joint of left index finger**

✓7th **S63.292 Dislocation of distal interphalangeal joint of right middle finger**

✓7th **S63.293 Dislocation of distal interphalangeal joint of left middle finger**

✓7th **S63.294 Dislocation of distal interphalangeal joint of right ring finger**

✓7th **S63.295 Dislocation of distal interphalangeal joint of left ring finger**

✓7th **S63.296 Dislocation of distal interphalangeal joint of right little finger**

✓7th **S63.297 Dislocation of distal interphalangeal joint of left little finger**

✓7th **S63.298 Dislocation of distal interphalangeal joint of other finger**

Dislocation of distal interphalangeal joint of specified finger with unspecified laterality

✓7th **S63.299 Dislocation of distal interphalangeal joint of unspecified finger**

✓5th **S63.3 Traumatic rupture of ligament of wrist**

✓6th **S63.30 Traumatic rupture of unspecified ligament of wrist**

✓7th **S63.301 Traumatic rupture of unspecified ligament of right wrist**

✓7th **S63.302 Traumatic rupture of unspecified ligament of left wrist**

✓7th **S63.309 Traumatic rupture of unspecified ligament of unspecified wrist**

✓6th **S63.31 Traumatic rupture of collateral ligament of wrist**

✓7th **S63.311 Traumatic rupture of collateral ligament of right wrist**

✓7th **S63.312 Traumatic rupture of collateral ligament of left wrist**

✓7th **S63.319 Traumatic rupture of collateral ligament of unspecified wrist**

✓6th **S63.32 Traumatic rupture of radiocarpal ligament**

✓7th **S63.321 Traumatic rupture of right radiocarpal ligament**

✓7th **S63.322 Traumatic rupture of left radiocarpal ligament**

✓7th **S63.329 Traumatic rupture of unspecified radiocarpal ligament**

✓6th **S63.33 Traumatic rupture of ulnocarpal (palmar) ligament**

✓7th **S63.331 Traumatic rupture of right ulnocarpal (palmar) ligament**

✓7th **S63.332 Traumatic rupture of left ulnocarpal (palmar) ligament**

✓7th **S63.339 Traumatic rupture of unspecified ulnocarpal (palmar) ligament**

✓6th **S63.39 Traumatic rupture of other ligament of wrist**

✓7th **S63.391 Traumatic rupture of other ligament of right wrist**

✓7th **S63.392 Traumatic rupture of other ligament of left wrist**

✓7th **S63.399 Traumatic rupture of other ligament of unspecified wrist**

✓5th **S63.4 Traumatic rupture of ligament of finger at metacarpophalangeal and interphalangeal joint(s)**

✓6th **S63.40 Traumatic rupture of unspecified ligament of finger at metacarpophalangeal and interphalangeal joint**

✓7th **S63.400 Traumatic rupture of unspecified ligament of right index finger at metacarpophalangeal and interphalangeal joint**

✓7th **S63.401 Traumatic rupture of unspecified ligament of left index finger at metacarpophalangeal and interphalangeal joint**

✓7th **S63.402 Traumatic rupture of unspecified ligament of right middle finger at metacarpophalangeal and interphalangeal joint**

✓7th **S63.403 Traumatic rupture of unspecified ligament of left middle finger at metacarpophalangeal and interphalangeal joint**

✓7th **S63.404 Traumatic rupture of unspecified ligament of right ring finger at metacarpophalangeal and interphalangeal joint**

√7th **S63.405 Traumatic rupture of unspecified ligament of left ring finger at metacarpophalangeal and interphalangeal joint**

√7th **S63.406 Traumatic rupture of unspecified ligament of right little finger at metacarpophalangeal and interphalangeal joint**

√7th **S63.407 Traumatic rupture of unspecified ligament of left little finger at metacarpophalangeal and interphalangeal joint**

√7th **S63.408 Traumatic rupture of unspecified ligament of other finger at metacarpophalangeal and interphalangeal joint**
Traumatic rupture of unspecified ligament of specified finger with unspecified laterality at metacarpophalangeal and interphalangeal joint

√7th **S63.409 Traumatic rupture of unspecified ligament of unspecified finger at metacarpophalangeal and interphalangeal joint**

√6th **S63.41 Traumatic rupture of collateral ligament of finger at metacarpophalangeal and interphalangeal joint**

√7th **S63.410 Traumatic rupture of collateral ligament of right index finger at metacarpophalangeal and interphalangeal joint**

√7th **S63.411 Traumatic rupture of collateral ligament of left index finger at metacarpophalangeal and interphalangeal joint**

√7th **S63.412 Traumatic rupture of collateral ligament of right middle finger at metacarpophalangeal and interphalangeal joint**

√7th **S63.413 Traumatic rupture of collateral ligament of left middle finger at metacarpophalangeal and interphalangeal joint**

√7th **S63.414 Traumatic rupture of collateral ligament of right ring finger at metacarpophalangeal and interphalangeal joint**

√7th **S63.415 Traumatic rupture of collateral ligament of left ring finger at metacarpophalangeal and interphalangeal joint**

√7th **S63.416 Traumatic rupture of collateral ligament of right little finger at metacarpophalangeal and interphalangeal joint**

√7th **S63.417 Traumatic rupture of collateral ligament of left little finger at metacarpophalangeal and interphalangeal joint**

√7th **S63.418 Traumatic rupture of collateral ligament of other finger at metacarpophalangeal and interphalangeal joint**
Traumatic rupture of collateral ligament of specified finger with unspecified laterality at metacarpophalangeal and interphalangeal joint

√7th **S63.419 Traumatic rupture of collateral ligament of unspecified finger at metacarpophalangeal and interphalangeal joint**

√6th **S63.42 Traumatic rupture of palmar ligament of finger at metacarpophalangeal and interphalangeal joint**

√7th **S63.420 Traumatic rupture of palmar ligament of right index finger at metacarpophalangeal and interphalangeal joint**

√7th **S63.421 Traumatic rupture of palmar ligament of left index finger at metacarpophalangeal and interphalangeal joint**

√7th **S63.422 Traumatic rupture of palmar ligament of right middle finger at metacarpophalangeal and interphalangeal joint**

√7th **S63.423 Traumatic rupture of palmar ligament of left middle finger at metacarpophalangeal and interphalangeal joint**

√7th **S63.424 Traumatic rupture of palmar ligament of right ring finger at metacarpophalangeal and interphalangeal joint**

√7th **S63.425 Traumatic rupture of palmar ligament of left ring finger at metacarpophalangeal and interphalangeal joint**

√7th **S63.426 Traumatic rupture of palmar ligament of right little finger at metacarpophalangeal and interphalangeal joint**

√7th **S63.427 Traumatic rupture of palmar ligament of left little finger at metacarpophalangeal and interphalangeal joint**

√7th **S63.428 Traumatic rupture of palmar ligament of other finger at metacarpophalangeal and interphalangeal joint**
Traumatic rupture of palmar ligament of specified finger with unspecified laterality at metacarpophalangeal and interphalangeal joint

√7th **S63.429 Traumatic rupture of palmar ligament of unspecified finger at metacarpophalangeal and interphalangeal joint**

√6th **S63.43 Traumatic rupture of volar plate of finger at metacarpophalangeal and interphalangeal joint**

√7th **S63.430 Traumatic rupture of volar plate of right index finger at metacarpophalangeal and interphalangeal joint**

√7th **S63.431 Traumatic rupture of volar plate of left index finger at metacarpophalangeal and interphalangeal joint**

√7th **S63.432 Traumatic rupture of volar plate of right middle finger at metacarpophalangeal and interphalangeal joint**

√7th **S63.433 Traumatic rupture of volar plate of left middle finger at metacarpophalangeal and interphalangeal joint**

√7th **S63.434 Traumatic rupture of volar plate of right ring finger at metacarpophalangeal and interphalangeal joint**

√7th **S63.435 Traumatic rupture of volar plate of left ring finger at metacarpophalangeal and interphalangeal joint**

√7th **S63.436 Traumatic rupture of volar plate of right little finger at metacarpophalangeal and interphalangeal joint**

√7th **S63.437 Traumatic rupture of volar plate of left little finger at metacarpophalangeal and interphalangeal joint**

√7th **S63.438 Traumatic rupture of volar plate of other finger at metacarpophalangeal and interphalangeal joint**
Traumatic rupture of volar plate of specified finger with unspecified laterality at metacarpophalangeal and interphalangeal joint

√7th **S63.439 Traumatic rupture of volar plate of unspecified finger at metacarpophalangeal and interphalangeal joint**

√6th **S63.49 Traumatic rupture of other ligament of finger at metacarpophalangeal and interphalangeal joint**

√7th **S63.490 Traumatic rupture of other ligament of right index finger at metacarpophalangeal and interphalangeal joint**

√7th **S63.491 Traumatic rupture of other ligament of left index finger at metacarpophalangeal and interphalangeal joint**

√7th **S63.492 Traumatic rupture of other ligament of right middle finger at metacarpophalangeal and interphalangeal joint**

S63.493 Traumatic rupture of other ligament of left middle finger at metacarpophalangeal and interphalangeal joint
S63.494 Traumatic rupture of other ligament of right ring finger at metacarpophalangeal and interphalangeal joint
S63.495 Traumatic rupture of other ligament of left ring finger at metacarpophalangeal and interphalangeal joint
S63.496 Traumatic rupture of other ligament of right little finger at metacarpophalangeal and interphalangeal joint
S63.497 Traumatic rupture of other ligament of left little finger at metacarpophalangeal and interphalangeal joint
S63.498 Traumatic rupture of other ligament of other finger at metacarpophalangeal and interphalangeal joint
Traumatic rupture of ligament of specified finger with unspecified laterality at metacarpophalangeal and interphalangeal joint
S63.499 Traumatic rupture of other ligament of unspecified finger at metacarpophalangeal and interphalangeal joint

S63.5 Other and unspecified sprain of wrist
S63.50 Unspecified sprain of wrist
S63.501 Unspecified sprain of right wrist
S63.502 Unspecified sprain of left wrist
S63.509 Unspecified sprain of unspecified wrist
S63.51 Sprain of carpal (joint)
S63.511 Sprain of carpal joint of right wrist
S63.512 Sprain of carpal joint of left wrist
S63.519 Sprain of carpal joint of unspecified wrist
S63.52 Sprain of radiocarpal joint
EXCLUDES 1 *traumatic rupture of radiocarpal ligament (S63.32-)*
S63.521 Sprain of radiocarpal joint of right wrist
S63.522 Sprain of radiocarpal joint of left wrist
S63.529 Sprain of radiocarpal joint of unspecified wrist
S63.59 Other specified sprain of wrist
S63.591 Other specified sprain of right wrist
S63.592 Other specified sprain of left wrist
S63.599 Other specified sprain of unspecified wrist

S63.6 Other and unspecified sprain of finger(s)
EXCLUDES 1 *traumatic rupture of ligament of finger at metacarpophalangeal and interphalangeal joint(s) (S63.4-)*
S63.60 Unspecified sprain of thumb
S63.601 Unspecified sprain of right thumb
S63.602 Unspecified sprain of left thumb
S63.609 Unspecified sprain of unspecified thumb
S63.61 Unspecified sprain of other and unspecified finger(s)
S63.610 Unspecified sprain of right index finger
S63.611 Unspecified sprain of left index finger
S63.612 Unspecified sprain of right middle finger
S63.613 Unspecified sprain of left middle finger
S63.614 Unspecified sprain of right ring finger
S63.615 Unspecified sprain of left ring finger
S63.616 Unspecified sprain of right little finger
S63.617 Unspecified sprain of left little finger
S63.618 Unspecified sprain of other finger
Unspecified sprain of specified finger with unspecified laterality
S63.619 Unspecified sprain of unspecified finger
S63.62 Sprain of interphalangeal joint of thumb
S63.621 Sprain of interphalangeal joint of right thumb
S63.622 Sprain of interphalangeal joint of left thumb
S63.629 Sprain of interphalangeal joint of unspecified thumb
S63.63 Sprain of interphalangeal joint of other and unspecified finger(s)
S63.630 Sprain of interphalangeal joint of right index finger
S63.631 Sprain of interphalangeal joint of left index finger
S63.632 Sprain of interphalangeal joint of right middle finger
S63.633 Sprain of interphalangeal joint of left middle finger
S63.634 Sprain of interphalangeal joint of right ring finger
S63.635 Sprain of interphalangeal joint of left ring finger
S63.636 Sprain of interphalangeal joint of right little finger
S63.637 Sprain of interphalangeal joint of left little finger
S63.638 Sprain of interphalangeal joint of other finger
S63.639 Sprain of interphalangeal joint of unspecified finger
S63.64 Sprain of metacarpophalangeal joint of thumb
S63.641 Sprain of metacarpophalangeal joint of right thumb
S63.642 Sprain of metacarpophalangeal joint of left thumb
S63.649 Sprain of metacarpophalangeal joint of unspecified thumb
S63.65 Sprain of metacarpophalangeal joint of other and unspecified finger(s)
S63.650 Sprain of metacarpophalangeal joint of right index finger
S63.651 Sprain of metacarpophalangeal joint of left index finger
S63.652 Sprain of metacarpophalangeal joint of right middle finger
S63.653 Sprain of metacarpophalangeal joint of left middle finger
S63.654 Sprain of metacarpophalangeal joint of right ring finger
S63.655 Sprain of metacarpophalangeal joint of left ring finger
S63.656 Sprain of metacarpophalangeal joint of right little finger
S63.657 Sprain of metacarpophalangeal joint of left little finger
S63.658 Sprain of metacarpophalangeal joint of other finger
Sprain of metacarpophalangeal joint of specified finger with unspecified laterality
S63.659 Sprain of metacarpophalangeal joint of unspecified finger
S63.68 Other sprain of thumb
S63.681 Other sprain of right thumb
S63.682 Other sprain of left thumb
S63.689 Other sprain of unspecified thumb
S63.69 Other sprain of other and unspecified finger(s)
S63.690 Other sprain of right index finger
S63.691 Other sprain of left index finger
S63.692 Other sprain of right middle finger
S63.693 Other sprain of left middle finger
S63.694 Other sprain of right ring finger
S63.695 Other sprain of left ring finger
S63.696 Other sprain of right little finger
S63.697 Other sprain of left little finger
S63.698 Other sprain of other finger
Other sprain of specified finger with unspecified laterality
S63.699 Other sprain of unspecified finger

5th S63.8 Sprain of other part of wrist and hand
6th S63.8X Sprain of other part of wrist and hand
7th S63.8X1 Sprain of other part of right wrist and hand
7th S63.8X2 Sprain of other part of left wrist and hand
7th S63.8X9 Sprain of other part of unspecified wrist and hand
5th S63.9 Sprain of unspecified part of wrist and hand
x7th S63.90 Sprain of unspecified part of unspecified wrist and hand
x7th S63.91 Sprain of unspecified part of right wrist and hand
x7th S63.92 Sprain of unspecified part of left wrist and hand

4th **S64 Injury of nerves at wrist and hand level**
Code also any associated open wound (S61.-)

The appropriate 7th character is to be added to each code from category S64.
A initial encounter
D subsequent encounter
S sequela

5th S64.0 Injury of ulnar nerve at wrist and hand level
x7th S64.00 Injury of ulnar nerve at wrist and hand level of unspecified arm
x7th S64.01 Injury of ulnar nerve at wrist and hand level of right arm
x7th S64.02 Injury of ulnar nerve at wrist and hand level of left arm
5th S64.1 Injury of median nerve at wrist and hand level
x7th S64.10 Injury of median nerve at wrist and hand level of unspecified arm
x7th S64.11 Injury of median nerve at wrist and hand level of right arm
x7th S64.12 Injury of median nerve at wrist and hand level of left arm
5th S64.2 Injury of radial nerve at wrist and hand level
x7th S64.20 Injury of radial nerve at wrist and hand level of unspecified arm
x7th S64.21 Injury of radial nerve at wrist and hand level of right arm
x7th S64.22 Injury of radial nerve at wrist and hand level of left arm
5th S64.3 Injury of digital nerve of thumb
x7th S64.30 Injury of digital nerve of unspecified thumb
x7th S64.31 Injury of digital nerve of right thumb
x7th S64.32 Injury of digital nerve of left thumb
5th S64.4 Injury of digital nerve of other and unspecified finger
x7th S64.40 Injury of digital nerve of unspecified finger
6th S64.49 Injury of digital nerve of other finger
7th S64.490 Injury of digital nerve of right index finger
7th S64.491 Injury of digital nerve of left index finger
7th S64.492 Injury of digital nerve of right middle finger
7th S64.493 Injury of digital nerve of left middle finger
7th S64.494 Injury of digital nerve of right ring finger
7th S64.495 Injury of digital nerve of left ring finger
7th S64.496 Injury of digital nerve of right little finger
7th S64.497 Injury of digital nerve of left little finger
7th S64.498 Injury of digital nerve of other finger
Injury of digital nerve of specified finger with unspecified laterality
5th S64.8 Injury of other nerves at wrist and hand level
6th S64.8X Injury of other nerves at wrist and hand level
7th S64.8X1 Injury of other nerves at wrist and hand level of right arm
7th S64.8X2 Injury of other nerves at wrist and hand level of left arm
7th S64.8X9 Injury of other nerves at wrist and hand level of unspecified arm
5th S64.9 Injury of unspecified nerve at wrist and hand level
x7th S64.90 Injury of unspecified nerve at wrist and hand level of unspecified arm
x7th S64.91 Injury of unspecified nerve at wrist and hand level of right arm
x7th S64.92 Injury of unspecified nerve at wrist and hand level of left arm

4th **S65 Injury of blood vessels at wrist and hand level**
Code also any associated open wound (S61.-)

The appropriate 7th character is to be added to each code from category S65.
A initial encounter
D subsequent encounter
S sequela

5th S65.0 Injury of ulnar artery at wrist and hand level
6th S65.00 Unspecified injury of ulnar artery at wrist and hand level
7th S65.001 Unspecified injury of ulnar artery at wrist and hand level of right arm CC
CC Excl: CC CC with 7th character A: S45.301A, S45.309-S45.311 with 7th A, S45.319-S45.391 with 7th A, S45.399-S45.801 with 7th A, S45.809-S45.811 with 7th A, S45.819-S45.891 with 7th A, S45.899-S45.901 with 7th A, S45.909-S45.911 with 7th A, S45.919-S45.991 with 7th A, S45.999A, S55.001A, S55.009-S55.011 with 7th A, S55.019-S55.091 with 7th A, S55.099A, S55.201A, S55.209-S55.211 with 7th A, S55.219-S55.291 with 7th A, S55.299-S55.801 with 7th A, S55.809-S55.811 with 7th A, S55.819-S55.891 with 7th A, S55.899-S55.901 with 7th A, S55.909-S55.911 with 7th A, S55.919-S55.991 with 7th A, S55.999A, S65.001A, S65.009-S65.011 with 7th A, S65.019-S65.091 with 7th A, S65.099A, S65.801A, S65.809-S65.811 with 7th A, S65.819-S65.891 with 7th A, S65.899-S65.901 with 7th A, S65.909-S65.911 with 7th A, S65.919-S65.991 with 7th A, S65.999A
7th S65.002 Unspecified injury of ulnar artery at wrist and hand level of left arm CC
CC Excl: CC CC with 7th character A: S45.302-S45.309 with 7th A, S45.312-S45.319 with 7th A, S45.392-S45.399 with 7th A, S45.802-S45.809 with 7th A, S45.812-S45.819 with 7th A, S45.892-S45.899 with 7th A, S45.902-S45.909 with 7th A, S45.912-S45.919 with 7th A, S45.992-S45.999 with 7th A, S55.002-S55.009 with 7th A, S55.012-S55.019 with 7th A, S55.092-S55.099 with 7th A, S55.202-S55.209 with 7th A, S55.212-S55.219 with 7th A, S55.292-S55.299 with 7th A, S55.802-S55.809 with 7th A, S55.812-S55.819 with 7th A, S55.892-S55.899 with 7th A, S55.902-S55.909 with 7th A, S55.912-S55.919 with 7th A, S55.992-S55.999 with 7th A, S65.002-S65.009 with 7th A, S65.012-S65.019 with 7th A, S65.092-S65.099 with 7th A, S65.802-S65.809 with 7th A, S65.812-S65.819 with 7th A, S65.892-S65.899 with 7th A, S65.902-S65.909 with 7th A, S65.912-S65.919 with 7th A, S65.992-S65.999 with 7th A
7th S65.009 Unspecified injury of ulnar artery at wrist and hand level of unspecified arm CC
CC Excl: CC CC with 7th character A: S45.301-S45.999 with 7th A, S55.001-S55.099 with 7th A, S55.201-S55.999 with 7th A, S65.001-S65.099 with 7th A, S65.801-S65.999 with 7th A
6th S65.01 Laceration of ulnar artery at wrist and hand level
7th S65.011 Laceration of ulnar artery at wrist and hand level of right arm CC
CC Excl: CC CC with 7th character A: See code: S65.001
7th S65.012 Laceration of ulnar artery at wrist and hand level of left arm CC
CC Excl: CC CC with 7th character A: See code: S65.002
7th S65.019 Laceration of ulnar artery at wrist and hand level of unspecified arm CC
CC Excl: CC CC with 7th character A: See code: S65.009

✓6th **S65.09** **Other specified injury of ulnar artery at wrist and hand level**

✓7th **S65.091** **Other specified injury of ulnar artery at wrist and hand level of right arm** CC
CC Excl: CC CC with 7th character A: See code: S65.001

✓7th **S65.092** **Other specified injury of ulnar artery at wrist and hand level of left arm** CC
CC Excl: CC CC with 7th character A: See code: S65.002

✓7th **S65.099** **Other specified injury of ulnar artery at wrist and hand level of unspecified arm** CC
CC Excl: CC CC with 7th character A: See code: S65.009

✓5th **S65.1** **Injury of radial artery at wrist and hand level**

✓6th **S65.10** **Unspecified injury of radial artery at wrist and hand level**

✓7th **S65.101** **Unspecified injury of radial artery at wrist and hand level of right arm** CC
CC Excl: CC CC with 7th character A: S45.301 A, S45.309-S45.311 with 7th A, S45.319-S45.391 with 7th A, S45.399-S45.801 with 7th A, S45.809-S45.811 with 7th A, S45.819-S45.891 with 7th A, S45.899-S45.901 with 7th A, S45.909-S45.911 with 7th A, S45.919-S45.991 with 7th A, S45.999A, S55.101A, S55.109-S55.111 with 7th A, S55.119-S55.191 with 7th A, S55.199-S55.201 with 7th A, S55.209-S55.211 with 7th A, S55.219-S55.291 with 7th A, S55.299-S55.801 with 7th A, S55.809-S55.811 with 7th A, S55.819-S55.891 with 7th A, S55.899-S55.901 with 7th A, S55.909-S55.911 with 7th A, S55.919-S55.991 with 7th A, S55.999A, S65.101A, S65.109-S65.111 with 7th A, S65.119-S65.191 with 7th A, S65.199A, S65.801 with 7th A, S65.809-S65.811 with 7th A, S65.819-S65.891 with 7th A, S65.899-S65.901 with 7th A, S65.909-S65.911 with 7th A, S65.919-S65.991 with 7th A, S65.999A

✓7th **S65.102** **Unspecified injury of radial artery at wrist and hand level of left arm** CC
CC Excl: CC CC with 7th character A: S45.302-S45.309 with 7th A, S45.312-S45.319 with 7th A, S45.392-S45.399 with 7th A, S45.802-S45.809 with 7th A, S45.812-S45.819 with 7th A, S45.892-S45.899 with 7th A, S45.902-S45.909 with 7th A, S45.912-S45.919 with 7th A, S45.992-S45.999 with 7th A, S55.102-S55.109 with 7th A, S55.112-S55.119 with 7th A, S55.192-S55.199 with 7th A, S55.202-S55.209 with 7th A, S55.212-S55.219 with 7th A, S55.292-S55.299 with 7th A, S55.802-S55.809 with 7th A, S55.812-S55.819 with 7th A, S55.892-S55.899 with 7th A, S55.902-S55.909 with 7th A, S55.912-S55.919 with 7th A, S55.992-S55.999 with 7th A, S65.102-S65.109 with 7th A, S65.112-S65.119 with 7th A, S65.192-S65.199 with 7th A, S65.802-S65.809 with 7th A, S65.812-S65.819 with 7th A, S65.892-S65.899 with 7th A, S65.902-S65.909 with 7th A, S65.912-S65.919 with 7th A, S65.992-S65.999 with 7th A

✓7th **S65.109** **Unspecified injury of radial artery at wrist and hand level of unspecified arm** CC
CC Excl: CC CC with 7th character A: S45.301-S45.301-S45.999 with 7th A, S55.101-S55.999 with 7th A, S65.101-S65.199 with 7th A, S65.801-S65.999 with 7th A

✓6th **S65.11** **Laceration of radial artery at wrist and hand level**

✓7th **S65.111** **Laceration of radial artery at wrist and hand level of right arm** CC
CC Excl: CC CC with 7th character A: See code: S65.101

✓7th **S65.112** **Laceration of radial artery at wrist and hand level of left arm** CC
CC Excl: CC CC with 7th character A: See code: S65.102

✓7th **S65.119** **Laceration of radial artery at wrist and hand level of unspecified arm** CC
CC Excl: CC CC with 7th character A: See code: S65.109

✓6th **S65.19** **Other specified injury of radial artery at wrist and hand level**

✓7th **S65.191** **Other specified injury of radial artery at wrist and hand level of right arm** CC
CC Excl: CC CC with 7th character A: See code: S65.101

✓7th **S65.192** **Other specified injury of radial artery at wrist and hand level of left arm** CC
CC Excl: CC CC with 7th character A: See code: S65.102

✓7th **S65.199** **Other specified injury of radial artery at wrist and hand level of unspecified arm** CC
CC Excl: CC CC with 7th character A: See code: S65.109

✓5th **S65.2** **Injury of superficial palmar arch**

✓6th **S65.20** **Unspecified injury of superficial palmar arch**

✓7th **S65.201** **Unspecified injury of superficial palmar arch of right hand** CC
CC Excl: CC CC with 7th character A: S45.301A, S45.309-S45.311 with 7th A, S45.319-S45.391 with 7th A, S45.399-S45.801 with 7th A, S45.809-S45.811 with 7th A, S45.819-S45.891 with 7th A, S45.899-S45.901 with 7th A, S45.909-S45.911 with 7th A, S45.919-S45.991 with 7th A, S45.999A, S55.201A, S55.209-S55.211 with 7th A, S55.219-S55.291 with 7th A, S55.299-S55.801 with 7th A, S55.809-S55.811 with 7th A, S55.819-S55.891 with 7th A, S55.899-S55.901 with 7th A, S55.909-S55.911 with 7th A, S55.919-S55.991 with 7th A, S55.999A, S65.201A, S65.209-S65.211 with 7th A, S65.219-S65.291 with 7th A, S65.299-S65.301 with 7th A, S65.309-S65.311 with 7th A, S65.319-S65.391 with 7th A, S65.399A, S65.801A, S65.809-S65.811 with 7th A, S65.819-S65.891 with 7th A, S65.899-S65.901 with 7th A, S65.909-S65.911 with 7th A, S65.919-S65.991 with 7th A, S65.999A

✓7th **S65.202** **Unspecified injury of superficial palmar arch of left hand** CC
CC Excl: CC CC with 7th character A: S45.302-S45.309 with 7th A, S45.312-S45.319 with 7th A, S45.392-S45.399 with 7th A, S45.802-S45.809 with 7th A, S45.812-S45.819 with 7th A, S45.892-S45.899 with 7th A, S45.902-S45.909 with 7th A, S45.912-S45.919 with 7th A, S45.992-S45.999 with 7th A, S55.202-S55.209 with 7th A, S55.212-S55.219 with 7th A, S55.292-S55.299 with 7th A, S55.802-S55.809 with 7th A, S55.812-S55.819 with 7th A, S55.892-S55.899 with 7th A, S55.902-S55.909 with 7th A, S55.912-S55.919 with 7th A, S55.992-S55.999 with 7th A, S65.202-S65.209 with 7th A, S65.212-S65.219 with 7th A, S65.292-S65.299 with 7th A, S65.302-S65.309 with 7th A, S65.312-S65.319 with 7th A, S65.392-S65.399 with 7th A, S65.802-S65.809 with 7th A, S65.812-S65.819 with 7th A, S65.892-S65.899 with 7th A, S65.902-S65.909 with 7th A, S65.912-S65.919 with 7th A, S65.992-S65.999 with 7th A

✓7th **S65.209** **Unspecified injury of superficial palmar arch of unspecified hand** CC
CC Excl: CC CC with 7th character A: S45.301-S45.999 with 7th A, S55.201-S55.999 with 7th A, S65.201-S65.399 with 7th A, S65.801-S65.999 with 7th A

✓6th **S65.21** **Laceration of superficial palmar arch**

✓7th **S65.211** **Laceration of superficial palmar arch of right hand** CC
CC Excl: CC CC with 7th character A: See code: S65.201

✓7th **S65.212** **Laceration of superficial palmar arch of left hand** CC
CC Excl: CC CC with 7th character A: See code: S65.202

✓7th **S65.219** **Laceration of superficial palmar arch of unspecified hand** CC
CC Excl: CC CC with 7th character A: See code: S65.209

✓6th **S65.29 Other specified injury of superficial palmar arch**

✓7th **S65.291 Other specified injury of superficial palmar arch of right hand** CC
CC Excl: CC CC with 7th character A: See code: S65.2Ø1

✓7th **S65.292 Other specified injury of superficial palmar arch of left hand** CC
CC Excl: CC CC with 7th character A: See code: S65.2Ø2

✓7th **S65.299 Other specified injury of superficial palmar arch of unspecified hand** CC
CC Excl: CC CC with 7th character A: See code: S65.2Ø9

✓5th **S65.3 Injury of deep palmar arch**

✓6th **S65.3Ø Unspecified injury of deep palmar arch**

✓7th **S65.3Ø1 Unspecified injury of deep palmar arch of right hand** CC
CC Excl: CC CC with 7th character A: See code: S65.2Ø1

✓7th **S65.3Ø2 Unspecified injury of deep palmar arch of left hand** CC
CC Excl: CC CC with 7th character A: See code: S65.2Ø2

✓7th **S65.3Ø9 Unspecified injury of deep palmar arch of unspecified hand** CC
CC Excl: CC CC with 7th character A: See code: S65.2Ø9

✓6th **S65.31 Laceration of deep palmar arch**

✓7th **S65.311 Laceration of deep palmar arch of right hand** CC
CC Excl: CC CC with 7th character A: See code: S65.2Ø1

✓7th **S65.312 Laceration of deep palmar arch of left hand** CC
CC Excl: CC CC with 7th character A: See code: S65.2Ø2

✓7th **S65.319 Laceration of deep palmar arch of unspecified hand** CC
CC Excl: CC with 7th character A: See code: S65.2Ø9

✓6th **S65.39 Other specified injury of deep palmar arch**

✓7th **S65.391 Other specified injury of deep palmar arch of right hand** CC
CC Excl: CC with 7th character A: See code: S65.2Ø1

✓7th **S65.392 Other specified injury of deep palmar arch of left hand** CC
CC Excl: CC with 7th character A: See code: S65.2Ø2

✓7th **S65.399 Other specified injury of deep palmar arch of unspecified hand** CC
CC Excl: CC with 7th character A: See code: S65.2Ø9

✓5th **S65.4 Injury of blood vessel of thumb**

✓6th **S65.4Ø Unspecified injury of blood vessel of thumb**

✓7th **S65.4Ø1 Unspecified injury of blood vessel of right thumb** CC
CC Excl: CC with 7th character A: S45.3Ø1A, S45.3Ø9-S45.311 with 7th A, S45.319-S45.391 with 7th A, S45.399-S45.8Ø1 with 7th A, S45.8Ø9-S45.811 with 7th A, S45.819-S45.891 with 7th A, S45.899-S45.9Ø1 with 7th A, S45.9Ø9-S45.911 with 7th A, S45.919-S45.991 with 7th A, S45.999A, S55.2Ø1A, S55.2Ø9-S55.211 with 7th A, S55.219-S55.291 with 7th A, S55.299-S55.8Ø1 with 7th A, S55.8Ø9-S55.811 with 7th A, S55.819-S55.891 with 7th A, S55.899-S55.9Ø1 with 7th A, S55.9Ø9-S55.911 with 7th A, S55.919-S55.991 with 7th A, S55.999A, S65.4Ø1A, S65.4Ø9-S65.411 with 7th A, S65.419-S65.491 with 7th A, S65.499-S65.5ØØ with 7th A, S65.5Ø2 A, S65.5Ø4A, S65.5Ø6A, S65.5Ø8-S65.51Ø with 7th A, S65.512A, S65.514A, S65.516A, S65.518-S65.59Ø with 7th A, S65.592A, S65.594A, S65.596 A, S65.598-S65.8Ø1 with 7th A, S65.8Ø9-S65.811 with 7th A, S65.819-S65.891 with 7th A, S65.899-S65.9Ø1 with 7th A, S65.9Ø9-S65.911 with 7th A, S65.919-S65.991 with 7th A, S65.999A

✓7th **S65.4Ø2 Unspecified injury of blood vessel of left thumb** CC
CC Excl: CC with 7th character A: S45.3Ø2-S45.3Ø9 with 7th A, S45.312-S45.319 with 7th A, S45.392-S45.399 with 7th A, S45.8Ø2-S45.8Ø9 with 7th A, S45.812-S45.819 with 7th A, S45.892-S45.899 with 7th A, S45.9Ø2-S45.9Ø9 with 7th A, S45.912-S45.919 with 7th A, S45.992-S45.999 with 7th A, S55.2Ø2-S55.2Ø9 with 7th A, S55.212-S55.219 with 7th A, S55.292-S55.299 with 7th A, S55.8Ø2-S55.8Ø9 with 7th A, S55.812-S55.819 with 7th A, S55.892-S55.899 with 7th A, S55.9Ø2-S55.9Ø9 with 7th A, S55.912-S55.919 with 7th A, S55.992-S55.999 with 7th A, S65.4Ø2-S65.4Ø9 with 7th A, S65.412-S65.419 with 7th A, S65.492-S65.499 with 7th A, S65.5Ø1A, S65.5Ø3A, S65.5Ø5A, S65.5Ø7-S65.5Ø9 with 7th A, S65.511A, S65.513A, S65.515A, S65.517-S65.519 with 7th A, S65.591A, S65.593A, S65.595A, S65.597-S65.599 with 7th A, S65.8Ø2-S65.8Ø9 with 7th A, S65.812-S65.819 with 7th A, S65.892-S65.899 with 7th A, S65.9Ø2-S65.9Ø9 with 7th A, S65.912-S65.919 with 7th A, S65.992-S65.999 with 7th A

✓7th **S65.4Ø9 Unspecified injury of blood vessel of unspecified thumb** CC
CC Excl: CC with 7th character A: S45.3Ø1-S45.999 with 7th A, S55.2Ø1-S55.999 with 7th A, S65.4Ø1-S65.999 with 7th A

✓6th **S65.41 Laceration of blood vessel of thumb**

✓7th **S65.411 Laceration of blood vessel of right thumb** CC
CC Excl: CC with 7th character A: See code: S65.4Ø1

✓7th **S65.412 Laceration of blood vessel of left thumb** CC
CC Excl: CC with 7th character A: See code: S65.4Ø2

✓7th **S65.419 Laceration of blood vessel of unspecified thumb** CC
CC Excl: CC with 7th character A: See code: S65.4Ø9

✓6th **S65.49 Other specified injury of blood vessel of thumb**

✓7th **S65.491 Other specified injury of blood vessel of right thumb** CC
CC Excl: CC with 7th character A: See code: S65.4Ø1

✓7th **S65.492 Other specified injury of blood vessel of left thumb** CC
CC Excl: CC with 7th character A: See code: S65.4Ø2

✓7th **S65.499 Other specified injury of blood vessel of unspecified thumb** CC
CC Excl: CC with 7th character A: See code: S65.4Ø9

✓5th **S65.5 Injury of blood vessel of other and unspecified finger**

✓6th **S65.5Ø Unspecified injury of blood vessel of other and unspecified finger**

✓7th **S65.5ØØ Unspecified injury of blood vessel of right index finger** CC
CC Excl: CC with 7th character A: See code: S65.4Ø1

✓7th **S65.5Ø1 Unspecified injury of blood vessel of left index finger** CC
CC Excl: CC with 7th character A: See code: S65.4Ø2

✓7th **S65.5Ø2 Unspecified injury of blood vessel of right middle finger** CC
CC Excl: CC with 7th character A: See code: S65.4Ø1

✓7th **S65.5Ø3 Unspecified injury of blood vessel of left middle finger** CC
CC Excl: CC with 7th character A: See code: S65.4Ø2

✓7th **S65.5Ø4 Unspecified injury of blood vessel of right ring finger** CC
CC Excl: CC with 7th character A: See code: S65.4Ø1

✓7th **S65.5Ø5 Unspecified injury of blood vessel of left ring finger** CC
CC Excl: CC with 7th character A: See code: S65.4Ø2

√7th **S65.506 Unspecified injury of blood vessel of right little finger** CC
CC Excl: CC with 7th character A: See code: S65.401

√7th **S65.507 Unspecified injury of blood vessel of left little finger** CC
CC Excl: CC with 7th character A: See code: S65.402

√7th **S65.508 Unspecified injury of blood vessel of other finger** CC
Unspecified injury of blood vessel of specified finger with unspecified laterality
CC Excl: CC with 7th character A: See code: S65.409

√7th **S65.509 Unspecified injury of blood vessel of unspecified finger** CC
CC Excl: CC with 7th character A: See code: S65.409

√6th **S65.51 Laceration of blood vessel of other and unspecified finger**

√7th **S65.510 Laceration of blood vessel of right index finger** CC
CC Excl: CC with 7th character A: See code: S65.401

√7th **S65.511 Laceration of blood vessel of left index finger** CC
CC Excl: CC with 7th character A: See code: S65.402

√7th **S65.512 Laceration of blood vessel of right middle finger** CC
CC Excl: CC with 7th character A: See code: S65.401

√7th **S65.513 Laceration of blood vessel of left middle finger** CC
CC Excl: CC with 7th character A: See code: S65.402

√7th **S65.514 Laceration of blood vessel of right ring finger** CC
CC Excl: CC with 7th character A: See code: S65.401

√7th **S65.515 Laceration of blood vessel of left ring finger** CC
CC Excl: CC with 7th character A: See code: S65.402

√7th **S65.516 Laceration of blood vessel of right little finger** CC
CC Excl: CC with 7th character A: See code: S65.401

√7th **S65.517 Laceration of blood vessel of left little finger** CC
CC Excl: CC with 7th character A: See code: S65.402

√7th **S65.518 Laceration of blood vessel of other finger** CC
Laceration of blood vessel of specified finger with unspecified laterality
CC Excl: CC with 7th character A: See code: S65.409

√7th **S65.519 Laceration of blood vessel of unspecified finger** CC
CC Excl: CC with 7th character A: See code: S65.409

√6th **S65.59 Other specified injury of blood vessel of other and unspecified finger**

√7th **S65.590 Other specified injury of blood vessel of right index finger** CC
CC Excl: CC with 7th character A: See code: S65.401

√7th **S65.591 Other specified injury of blood vessel of left index finger** CC
CC Excl: CC with 7th character A: See code: S65.402

√7th **S65.592 Other specified injury of blood vessel of right middle finger** CC
CC Excl: CC with 7th character A: See code: S65.401

√7th **S65.593 Other specified injury of blood vessel of left middle finger** CC
CC Excl: CC with 7th character A: See code: S65.402

√7th **S65.594 Other specified injury of blood vessel of right ring finger** CC
CC Excl: CC with 7th character A: See code: S65.401

√7th **S65.595 Other specified injury of blood vessel of left ring finger** CC
CC Excl: CC with 7th character A: See code: S65.402

√7th **S65.596 Other specified injury of blood vessel of right little finger** CC
CC Excl: CC with 7th character A: See code: S65.401

√7th **S65.597 Other specified injury of blood vessel of left little finger** CC
CC Excl: CC with 7th character A: See code: S65.402

√7th **S65.598 Other specified injury of blood vessel of other finger** CC
Other specified injury of blood vessel of specified finger with unspecified laterality
CC Excl: CC with 7th character A: See code: S65.409

√7th **S65.599 Other specified injury of blood vessel of unspecified finger** CC
CC Excl: CC with 7th character A: See code: S65.409

√5th **S65.8 Injury of other blood vessels at wrist and hand level**

√6th **S65.80 Unspecified injury of other blood vessels at wrist and hand level**

√7th **S65.801 Unspecified injury of other blood vessels at wrist and hand level of right arm** CC
CC Excl: CC with 7th character A: S45.301A, S45.309-S45.311 with 7th A, S45.319-S45.391 with 7th A, S45.399-S45.801 with 7th A, S45.809-S45.811 with 7th A, S45.819-S45.891 with 7th A, S45.899-S45.901 with 7th A, S45.909-S45.911 with 7th A, S45.919-S45.991 with 7th A, S45.999A, S55.001A, S55.009-S55.011 with 7th A, S55.019-S55.091 with 7th A, S55.099A, S55.201A, S55.209-S55.211 with 7th A, S55.219-S55.291 with 7th A, S55.299-S55.801 with 7th A, S55.809-S55.811 with 7th A, S55.819-S55.891 with 7th A, S55.899-S55.901 with 7th A, S55.909-S55.911 with 7th A, S55.919-S55.991 with 7th A, S55.999A, S65.001A, S65.009-S65.011 with 7th A, S65.019-S65.091 with 7th A, S65.099A, S65.201A, S65.209-S65.211 with 7th A, S65.219-S65.291 with 7th A, S65.299-S65.301 with 7th A, S65.309-S65.311 with 7th A, S65.319-S65.391 with 7th A, S65.399-S65.401 with 7th A, S65.409-S65.411 with 7th A, S65.419-S65.491 with 7th A, S65.499-S65.500 with 7th A, S65.502A, S65.504A, S65.506A, S65.508-S65.510 with 7th A, S65.512A, S65.514A, S65.516A, S65.518-S65.590 with 7th A, S65.592A, S65.594A, S65.596A, S65.598-S65.801 with 7th A, S65.809-S65.811 with 7th A, S65.819-S65.891 with 7th A, S65.899-S65.901 with 7th A, S65.909-S65.911 with 7th A, S65.919-S65.991 with 7th A, S65.999 with 7th A

7th **S65.802 Unspecified injury of other blood vessels at wrist and hand level of left arm** CC
CC Excl: CC with 7th character A: S45.302-S45.309 with 7th A, S45.312-S45.319 with 7th A, S45.392-S45.399 with 7th A, S45.802-S45.809 with 7th A, S45.812-S45.819 with 7th A, S45.892-S45.899 with 7th A, S45.902-S45.909 with 7th A, S45.912-S45.919 with 7th A, S45.992-S45.999 with 7th A, S55.002-S55.009 with 7th A, S55.012-S55.019 with 7th A, S55.092-S55.099 with 7th A, S55.202-S55.209 with 7th A, S55.212-S55.219 with 7th A, S55.292-S55.299 with 7th A, S55.802-S55.809 with 7th A, S55.812-S55.819 with 7th A, S55.892-S55.899 with 7th A, S55.902-S55.909 with 7th A, S55.912-S55.919 with 7th A, S55.992-S55.999 with 7th A, S65.002-S65.009 with 7th A, S65.012-S65.019 with 7th A, S65.092-S65.099 with 7th A, S65.202-S65.209 with 7th A, S65.212-S65.219 with 7th A, S65.292-S65.299 with 7th A, S65.302-S65.309 with 7th A, S65.312-S65.319 with 7th A, S65.392-S65.399 with 7th A, S65.402-S65.409 with 7th A, S65.412-S65.419 with 7th A, S65.492-S65.499 with 7th A, S65.501A, S65.503A, S65.505A, S65.507-S65.509 with 7th A, S65.511A, S65.513A, S65.515A, S65.517-S65.519 with 7th A, S65.591A, S65.593A, S65.595A, S65.597-S65.599 with 7th A, S65.802-S65.809 with 7th A, S65.812-S65.819 with 7th A, S65.892-S65.899 with 7th A, S65.902-S65.909 with 7th A, S65.912-S65.919 with 7th A, S65.992-S65.999 with 7th A

7th **S65.809 Unspecified injury of other blood vessels at wrist and hand level of unspecified arm** CC
CC Excl: CC with 7th character A: S45.301-S45.999 with 7th A, S55.001-S55.099 with 7th A, S55.201-S55.999 with 7th A, S65.001-S65.099 with 7th A, S65.201-S65.999 with 7th A

6th **S65.81 Laceration of other blood vessels at wrist and hand level**

7th **S65.811 Laceration of other blood vessels at wrist and hand level of right arm** CC
CC Excl: CC with 7th character A: See code: S65.801

7th **S65.812 Laceration of other blood vessels at wrist and hand level of left arm** CC
CC Excl: CC with 7th character A: See code: S65.802

7th **S65.819 Laceration of other blood vessels at wrist and hand level of unspecified arm** CC
CC Excl: CC with 7th character A: See code: S65.809

6th **S65.89 Other specified injury of other blood vessels at wrist and hand level**

7th **S65.891 Other specified injury of other blood vessels at wrist and hand level of right arm** CC
CC Excl: CC with 7th character A: See code: S65.801

7th **S65.892 Other specified injury of other blood vessels at wrist and hand level of left arm** CC
CC Excl: CC with 7th character A: See code: S65.802

7th **S65.899 Other specified injury of other blood vessels at wrist and hand level of unspecified arm** CC
CC Excl: CC with 7th character A: See code: S65.809

5th **S65.9 Injury of unspecified blood vessel at wrist and hand level**

6th **S65.90 Unspecified injury of unspecified blood vessel at wrist and hand level**

7th **S65.901 Unspecified injury of unspecified blood vessel at wrist and hand level of right arm** CC
CC Excl: CC with 7th character A: See code: S65.801

7th **S65.902 Unspecified injury of unspecified blood vessel at wrist and hand level of left arm** CC
CC Excl: CC with 7th character A: See code: S65.802

7th **S65.909 Unspecified injury of unspecified blood vessel at wrist and hand level of unspecified arm** CC
CC Excl: CC with 7th character A: See code: S65.809

6th **S65.91 Laceration of unspecified blood vessel at wrist and hand level**

7th **S65.911 Laceration of unspecified blood vessel at wrist and hand level of right arm** CC
CC Excl: CC with 7th character A: See code: S65.801

7th **S65.912 Laceration of unspecified blood vessel at wrist and hand level of left arm** CC
CC Excl: CC with 7th character A: See code: S65.802

7th **S65.919 Laceration of unspecified blood vessel at wrist and hand level of unspecified arm** CC
CC Excl: CC with 7th character A: See code: S65.809

6th **S65.99 Other specified injury of unspecified blood vessel at wrist and hand level**

7th **S65.991 Other specified injury of unspecified blood vessel at wrist and hand of right arm** CC
CC Excl: CC with 7th character A: See code: S65.801

7th **S65.992 Other specified injury of unspecified blood vessel at wrist and hand of left arm** CC
CC Excl: CC with 7th character A: See code: S65.802

7th **S65.999 Other specified injury of unspecified blood vessel at wrist and hand of unspecified arm** CC
CC Excl: CC with 7th character A: See code: S65.809

4th **S66 Injury of muscle, fascia and tendon at wrist and hand level**
Code also any associated open wound (S61.-)
EXCLUDES 2 *sprain of joints and ligaments of wrist and hand (S63.-)*

The appropriate 7th character is to be added to each code from category S66.
A initial encounter
D subsequent encounter
S sequela

5th **S66.0 Injury of long flexor muscle, fascia and tendon of thumb at wrist and hand level**

6th **S66.00 Unspecified injury of long flexor muscle, fascia and tendon of thumb at wrist and hand level**

7th **S66.001 Unspecified injury of long flexor muscle, fascia and tendon of right thumb at wrist and hand level**

7th **S66.002 Unspecified injury of long flexor muscle, fascia and tendon of left thumb at wrist and hand level**

7th **S66.009 Unspecified injury of long flexor muscle, fascia and tendon of unspecified thumb at wrist and hand level**

6th **S66.01 Strain of long flexor muscle, fascia and tendon of thumb at wrist and hand level**

7th **S66.011 Strain of long flexor muscle, fascia and tendon of right thumb at wrist and hand level**

7th **S66.012 Strain of long flexor muscle, fascia and tendon of left thumb at wrist and hand level**

7th **S66.019 Strain of long flexor muscle, fascia and tendon of unspecified thumb at wrist and hand level**

S66.02 Laceration of long flexor muscle, fascia and tendon of thumb at wrist and hand level

S66.021 Laceration of long flexor muscle, fascia and tendon of right thumb at wrist and hand level CC
CC Excl: CC with 7th character A: S61.401A, S61.409-S61.411 with 7th A, S61.419-S61.421 with 7th A, S61.429-S61.431 with 7th A, S61.439-S61.441 with 7th A, S61.449-S61.451 with 7th A, S61.459A, S66.021A, S66.029A, S66.120A, S66.122A, S66.124A, S66.126A, S66.128-S66.129 with 7th A, S66.221A, S66.229A, S66.320A, S66.322A, S66.324A, S66.326A, S66.328-S66.329 with 7th A, S66.421A, S66.429A, S66.520A, S66.522A, S66.524A, S66.526A, S66.528-S66.529 with 7th A, S66.821A, S66.829A, S66.921A, S66.929 with 7th A

S66.022 Laceration of long flexor muscle, fascia and tendon of left thumb at wrist and hand level CC
CC Excl: CC with 7th character A: S61.402-S61.409 with 7th A, S61.412-S61.419 with 7th A, S61.422-S61.429 with 7th A, S61.432-S61.439 with 7th A, S61.442-S61.449 with 7th A, S61.452-S61.459 with 7th A, S66.022-S66.029 with 7th A, S66.121A, S66.123A, S66.125A, S66.127-S66.129 with 7th A, S66.222-S66.229 with 7th A, S66.321A, S66.323A, S66.325A, S66.327-S66.329 with 7th A, S66.422-S66.429 with 7th A, S66.521A, S66.523A, S66.525A, S66.527-S66.529 with 7th A, S66.822-S66.829 with 7th A, S66.922-S66.929 with 7th A

S66.029 Laceration of long flexor muscle, fascia and tendon of unspecified thumb at wrist and hand level CC
CC Excl: CC with 7th character A: S61.401-S61.459 with 7th A, S66.021-S66.029 with 7th A, S66.120-S66.129 with 7th A, S66.221-S66.229 with 7th A, S66.320-S66.329 with 7th A, S66.421-S66.429 with 7th A, S66.520-S66.529 with 7th A, S66.821-S66.829 with 7th A, S66.921-S66.929 with 7th A

S66.09 Other specified injury of long flexor muscle, fascia and tendon of thumb at wrist and hand level

S66.091 Other specified injury of long flexor muscle, fascia and tendon of right thumb at wrist and hand level

S66.092 Other specified injury of long flexor muscle, fascia and tendon of left thumb at wrist and hand level

S66.099 Other specified injury of long flexor muscle, fascia and tendon of unspecified thumb at wrist and hand level

S66.1 Injury of flexor muscle, fascia and tendon of other and unspecified finger at wrist and hand level

EXCLUDES 2 *Injury of long flexor muscle, fascia and tendon of thumb at wrist and hand level (S66.0-)*

S66.10 Unspecified injury of flexor muscle, fascia and tendon of other and unspecified finger at wrist and hand level

S66.100 Unspecified injury of flexor muscle, fascia and tendon of right index finger at wrist and hand level

S66.101 Unspecified injury of flexor muscle, fascia and tendon of left index finger at wrist and hand level

S66.102 Unspecified injury of flexor muscle, fascia and tendon of right middle finger at wrist and hand level

S66.103 Unspecified injury of flexor muscle, fascia and tendon of left middle finger at wrist and hand level

S66.104 Unspecified injury of flexor muscle, fascia and tendon of right ring finger at wrist and hand level

S66.105 Unspecified injury of flexor muscle, fascia and tendon of left ring finger at wrist and hand level

S66.106 Unspecified injury of flexor muscle, fascia and tendon of right little finger at wrist and hand level

S66.107 Unspecified injury of flexor muscle, fascia and tendon of left little finger at wrist and hand level

S66.108 Unspecified injury of flexor muscle, fascia and tendon of other finger at wrist and hand level
Unspecified injury of flexor muscle, fascia and tendon of specified finger with unspecified laterality at wrist and hand level

S66.109 Unspecified injury of flexor muscle, fascia and tendon of unspecified finger at wrist and hand level

S66.11 Strain of flexor muscle, fascia and tendon of other and unspecified finger at wrist and hand level

S66.110 Strain of flexor muscle, fascia and tendon of right index finger at wrist and hand level

S66.111 Strain of flexor muscle, fascia and tendon of left index finger at wrist and hand level

S66.112 Strain of flexor muscle, fascia and tendon of right middle finger at wrist and hand level

S66.113 Strain of flexor muscle, fascia and tendon of left middle finger at wrist and hand level

S66.114 Strain of flexor muscle, fascia and tendon of right ring finger at wrist and hand level

S66.115 Strain of flexor muscle, fascia and tendon of left ring finger at wrist and hand level

S66.116 Strain of flexor muscle, fascia and tendon of right little finger at wrist and hand level

S66.117 Strain of flexor muscle, fascia and tendon of left little finger at wrist and hand level

S66.118 Strain of flexor muscle, fascia and tendon of other finger at wrist and hand level
Strain of flexor muscle, fascia and tendon of specified finger with unspecified laterality at wrist and hand level

S66.119 Strain of flexor muscle, fascia and tendon of unspecified finger at wrist and hand level

S66.12 Laceration of flexor muscle, fascia and tendon of other and unspecified finger at wrist and hand level

S66.120 Laceration of flexor muscle, fascia and tendon of right index finger at wrist and hand level CC
CC Excl: CC with 7th character A: See code: S66.021

S66.121 Laceration of flexor muscle, fascia and tendon of left index finger at wrist and hand level CC
CC Excl: CC with 7th character A: See code: S66.022

S66.122 Laceration of flexor muscle, fascia and tendon of right middle finger at wrist and hand level CC
CC Excl: CC with 7th character A: See code: S66.021

S66.123 Laceration of flexor muscle, fascia and tendon of left middle finger at wrist and hand level CC
CC Excl: CC with 7th character A: See code: S66.022

S66.124 Laceration of flexor muscle, fascia and tendon of right ring finger at wrist and hand level CC
CC Excl: CC with 7th character A: See code: S66.021

S66.125 Laceration of flexor muscle, fascia and tendon of left ring finger at wrist and hand level CC
CC Excl: CC with 7th character A: See code: S66.022

S66.126 Laceration of flexor muscle, fascia and tendon of right little finger at wrist and hand level CC
CC Excl: CC with 7th character A: See code: S66.021

DRAFT

7th **S66.127 Laceration of flexor muscle, fascia and tendon of left little finger at wrist and hand level** CC
CC Excl: CC with 7th character A: See code: S66.022

7th **S66.128 Laceration of flexor muscle, fascia and tendon of other finger at wrist and hand level** CC
Laceration of flexor muscle, fascia and tendon of specified finger with unspecified laterality at wrist and hand level
CC Excl: CC with 7th character A: See code: S66.029

7th **S66.129 Laceration of flexor muscle, fascia and tendon of unspecified finger at wrist and hand level** CC
CC Excl: CC with 7th character A: See code: S66.029

6th **S66.19 Other injury of flexor muscle, fascia and tendon of other and unspecified finger at wrist and hand level**

7th **S66.190 Other injury of flexor muscle, fascia and tendon of right index finger at wrist and hand level**

7th **S66.191 Other injury of flexor muscle, fascia and tendon of left index finger at wrist and hand level**

7th **S66.192 Other injury of flexor muscle, fascia and tendon of right middle finger at wrist and hand level**

7th **S66.193 Other injury of flexor muscle, fascia and tendon of left middle finger at wrist and hand level**

7th **S66.194 Other injury of flexor muscle, fascia and tendon of right ring finger at wrist and hand level**

7th **S66.195 Other injury of flexor muscle, fascia and tendon of left ring finger at wrist and hand level**

7th **S66.196 Other injury of flexor muscle, fascia and tendon of right little finger at wrist and hand level**

7th **S66.197 Other injury of flexor muscle, fascia and tendon of left little finger at wrist and hand level**

7th **S66.198 Other injury of flexor muscle, fascia and tendon of other finger at wrist and hand level**
Other injury of flexor muscle, fascia and tendon of specified finger with unspecified laterality at wrist and hand level

7th **S66.199 Other injury of flexor muscle, fascia and tendon of unspecified finger at wrist and hand level**

5th **S66.2 Injury of extensor muscle, fascia and tendon of thumb at wrist and hand level**

6th **S66.20 Unspecified injury of extensor muscle, fascia and tendon of thumb at wrist and hand level**

7th **S66.201 Unspecified injury of extensor muscle, fascia and tendon of right thumb at wrist and hand level**

7th **S66.202 Unspecified injury of extensor muscle, fascia and tendon of left thumb at wrist and hand level**

7th **S66.209 Unspecified injury of extensor muscle, fascia and tendon of unspecified thumb at wrist and hand level**

6th **S66.21 Strain of extensor muscle, fascia and tendon of thumb at wrist and hand level**

7th **S66.211 Strain of extensor muscle, fascia and tendon of right thumb at wrist and hand level**

7th **S66.212 Strain of extensor muscle, fascia and tendon of left thumb at wrist and hand level**

7th **S66.219 Strain of extensor muscle, fascia and tendon of unspecified thumb at wrist and hand level**

6th **S66.22 Laceration of extensor muscle, fascia and tendon of thumb at wrist and hand level**

7th **S66.221 Laceration of extensor muscle, fascia and tendon of right thumb at wrist and hand level** CC
CC Excl: CC with 7th character A: See code: S66.021

7th **S66.222 Laceration of extensor muscle, fascia and tendon of left thumb at wrist and hand level** CC
CC Excl: CC with 7th character A: See code: S66.022

7th **S66.229 Laceration of extensor muscle, fascia and tendon of unspecified thumb at wrist and hand level** CC
CC Excl: CC with 7th character A: See code: S66.029

6th **S66.29 Other specified injury of extensor muscle, fascia and tendon of thumb at wrist and hand level**

7th **S66.291 Other specified injury of extensor muscle, fascia and tendon of right thumb at wrist and hand level**

7th **S66.292 Other specified injury of extensor muscle, fascia and tendon of left thumb at wrist and hand level**

7th **S66.299 Other specified injury of extensor muscle, fascia and tendon of unspecified thumb at wrist and hand level**

5th **S66.3 Injury of extensor muscle, fascia and tendon of other and unspecified finger at wrist and hand level**
EXCLUDES 2 *Injury of extensor muscle, fascia and tendon of thumb at wrist and hand level (S66.2-)*

6th **S66.30 Unspecified injury of extensor muscle, fascia and tendon of other and unspecified finger at wrist and hand level**

7th **S66.300 Unspecified injury of extensor muscle, fascia and tendon of right index finger at wrist and hand level**

7th **S66.301 Unspecified injury of extensor muscle, fascia and tendon of left index finger at wrist and hand level**

7th **S66.302 Unspecified injury of extensor muscle, fascia and tendon of right middle finger at wrist and hand level**

7th **S66.303 Unspecified injury of extensor muscle, fascia and tendon of left middle finger at wrist and hand level**

7th **S66.304 Unspecified injury of extensor muscle, fascia and tendon of right ring finger at wrist and hand level**

7th **S66.305 Unspecified injury of extensor muscle, fascia and tendon of left ring finger at wrist and hand level**

7th **S66.306 Unspecified injury of extensor muscle, fascia and tendon of right little finger at wrist and hand level**

7th **S66.307 Unspecified injury of extensor muscle, fascia and tendon of left little finger at wrist and hand level**

7th **S66.308 Unspecified injury of extensor muscle, fascia and tendon of other finger at wrist and hand level**
Unspecified injury of extensor muscle, fascia and tendon of specified finger with unspecified laterality at wrist and hand level

7th **S66.309 Unspecified injury of extensor muscle, fascia and tendon of unspecified finger at wrist and hand level**

6th **S66.31 Strain of extensor muscle, fascia and tendon of other and unspecified finger at wrist and hand level**

7th **S66.310 Strain of extensor muscle, fascia and tendon of right index finger at wrist and hand level**

7th **S66.311 Strain of extensor muscle, fascia and tendon of left index finger at wrist and hand level**

7th **S66.312 Strain of extensor muscle, fascia and tendon of right middle finger at wrist and hand level**

S66.313 Strain of extensor muscle, fascia and tendon of left middle finger at wrist and hand level

S66.314 Strain of extensor muscle, fascia and tendon of right ring finger at wrist and hand level

S66.315 Strain of extensor muscle, fascia and tendon of left ring finger at wrist and hand level

S66.316 Strain of extensor muscle, fascia and tendon of right little finger at wrist and hand level

S66.317 Strain of extensor muscle, fascia and tendon of left little finger at wrist and hand level

S66.318 Strain of extensor muscle, fascia and tendon of other finger at wrist and hand level

Strain of extensor muscle, fascia and tendon of specified finger with unspecified laterality at wrist and hand level

S66.319 Strain of extensor muscle, fascia and tendon of unspecified finger at wrist and hand level

S66.32 Laceration of extensor muscle, fascia and tendon of other and unspecified finger at wrist and hand level

S66.320 Laceration of extensor muscle, fascia and tendon of right index finger at wrist and hand level CC

CC Excl: CC with 7th character A: See code: S66.021

S66.321 Laceration of extensor muscle, fascia and tendon of left index finger at wrist and hand level CC

CC Excl: CC with 7th character A: See code: S66.022

S66.322 Laceration of extensor muscle, fascia and tendon of right middle finger at wrist and hand level CC

CC Excl: CC with 7th character A: See code: S66.021

S66.323 Laceration of extensor muscle, fascia and tendon of left middle finger at wrist and hand level CC

CC Excl: CC with 7th character A: See code: S66.022

S66.324 Laceration of extensor muscle, fascia and tendon of right ring finger at wrist and hand level CC

CC Excl: CC with 7th character A: See code: S66.021

S66.325 Laceration of extensor muscle, fascia and tendon of left ring finger at wrist and hand level CC

CC Excl: CC with 7th character A: See code: S66.022

S66.326 Laceration of extensor muscle, fascia and tendon of right little finger at wrist and hand level CC

CC Excl: CC with 7th character A: See code: S66.021

S66.327 Laceration of extensor muscle, fascia and tendon of left little finger at wrist and hand level CC

CC Excl: CC with 7th character A: See code: S66.022

S66.328 Laceration of extensor muscle, fascia and tendon of other finger at wrist and hand level CC

Laceration of extensor muscle, fascia and tendon of specified finger with unspecified laterality at wrist and hand level

CC Excl: CC with 7th character A: See code: S66.029

S66.329 Laceration of extensor muscle, fascia and tendon of unspecified finger at wrist and hand level CC

CC Excl: CC with 7th character A: See code: S66.029

S66.39 Other injury of extensor muscle, fascia and tendon of other and unspecified finger at wrist and hand level

S66.390 Other injury of extensor muscle, fascia and tendon of right index finger at wrist and hand level

S66.391 Other injury of extensor muscle, fascia and tendon of left index finger at wrist and hand level

S66.392 Other injury of extensor muscle, fascia and tendon of right middle finger at wrist and hand level

S66.393 Other injury of extensor muscle, fascia and tendon of left middle finger at wrist and hand level

S66.394 Other injury of extensor muscle, fascia and tendon of right ring finger at wrist and hand level

S66.395 Other injury of extensor muscle, fascia and tendon of left ring finger at wrist and hand level

S66.396 Other injury of extensor muscle, fascia and tendon of right little finger at wrist and hand level

S66.397 Other injury of extensor muscle, fascia and tendon of left little finger at wrist and hand level

S66.398 Other injury of extensor muscle, fascia and tendon of other finger at wrist and hand level

Other injury of extensor muscle, fascia and tendon of specified finger with unspecified laterality at wrist and hand level

S66.399 Other injury of extensor muscle, fascia and tendon of unspecified finger at wrist and hand level

S66.4 Injury of intrinsic muscle, fascia and tendon of thumb at wrist and hand level

S66.40 Unspecified injury of intrinsic muscle, fascia and tendon of thumb at wrist and hand level

S66.401 Unspecified injury of intrinsic muscle, fascia and tendon of right thumb at wrist and hand level

S66.402 Unspecified injury of intrinsic muscle, fascia and tendon of left thumb at wrist and hand level

S66.409 Unspecified injury of intrinsic muscle, fascia and tendon of unspecified thumb at wrist and hand level

S66.41 Strain of intrinsic muscle, fascia and tendon of thumb at wrist and hand level

S66.411 Strain of intrinsic muscle, fascia and tendon of right thumb at wrist and hand level

S66.412 Strain of intrinsic muscle, fascia and tendon of left thumb at wrist and hand level

S66.419 Strain of intrinsic muscle, fascia and tendon of unspecified thumb at wrist and hand level

S66.42 Laceration of intrinsic muscle, fascia and tendon of thumb at wrist and hand level

S66.421 Laceration of intrinsic muscle, fascia and tendon of right thumb at wrist and hand level CC

CC Excl: CC with 7th character A: See code: S66.021

S66.422 Laceration of intrinsic muscle, fascia and tendon of left thumb at wrist and hand level CC

CC Excl: CC with 7th character A: See code: S66.022

S66.429 Laceration of intrinsic muscle, fascia and tendon of unspecified thumb at wrist and hand level CC

CC Excl: CC with 7th character A: See code: S66.029

S66.49 **Other specified injury of intrinsic muscle, fascia and tendon of thumb at wrist and hand level**

- **S66.491** **Other specified injury of intrinsic muscle, fascia and tendon of right thumb at wrist and hand level**
- **S66.492** **Other specified injury of intrinsic muscle, fascia and tendon of left thumb at wrist and hand level**
- **S66.499** **Other specified injury of intrinsic muscle, fascia and tendon of unspecified thumb at wrist and hand level**

S66.5 **Injury of intrinsic muscle, fascia and tendon of other and unspecified finger at wrist and hand level**

EXCLUDES 2 *injury of intrinsic muscle, fascia and tendon of thumb at wrist and hand level (S66.4-)*

S66.50 **Unspecified injury of intrinsic muscle, fascia and tendon of other and unspecified finger at wrist and hand level**

- **S66.500** **Unspecified injury of intrinsic muscle, fascia and tendon of right index finger at wrist and hand level**
- **S66.501** **Unspecified injury of intrinsic muscle, fascia and tendon of left index finger at wrist and hand level**
- **S66.502** **Unspecified injury of intrinsic muscle, fascia and tendon of right middle finger at wrist and hand level**
- **S66.503** **Unspecified injury of intrinsic muscle, fascia and tendon of left middle finger at wrist and hand level**
- **S66.504** **Unspecified injury of intrinsic muscle, fascia and tendon of right ring finger at wrist and hand level**
- **S66.505** **Unspecified injury of intrinsic muscle, fascia and tendon of left ring finger at wrist and hand level**
- **S66.506** **Unspecified injury of intrinsic muscle, fascia and tendon of right little finger at wrist and hand level**
- **S66.507** **Unspecified injury of intrinsic muscle, fascia and tendon of left little finger at wrist and hand level**
- **S66.508** **Unspecified injury of intrinsic muscle, fascia and tendon of other finger at wrist and hand level**
  Unspecified injury of intrinsic muscle, fascia and tendon of specified finger with unspecified laterality at wrist and hand level
- **S66.509** **Unspecified injury of intrinsic muscle, fascia and tendon of unspecified finger at wrist and hand level**

S66.51 **Strain of intrinsic muscle, fascia and tendon of other and unspecified finger at wrist and hand level**

- **S66.510** **Strain of intrinsic muscle, fascia and tendon of right index finger at wrist and hand level**
- **S66.511** **Strain of intrinsic muscle, fascia and tendon of left index finger at wrist and hand level**
- **S66.512** **Strain of intrinsic muscle, fascia and tendon of right middle finger at wrist and hand level**
- **S66.513** **Strain of intrinsic muscle, fascia and tendon of left middle finger at wrist and hand level**
- **S66.514** **Strain of intrinsic muscle, fascia and tendon of right ring finger at wrist and hand level**
- **S66.515** **Strain of intrinsic muscle, fascia and tendon of left ring finger at wrist and hand level**
- **S66.516** **Strain of intrinsic muscle, fascia and tendon of right little finger at wrist and hand level**
- **S66.517** **Strain of intrinsic muscle, fascia and tendon of left little finger at wrist and hand level**
- **S66.518** **Strain of intrinsic muscle, fascia and tendon of other finger at wrist and hand level**
  Strain of intrinsic muscle, fascia and tendon of specified finger with unspecified laterality at wrist and hand level
- **S66.519** **Strain of intrinsic muscle, fascia and tendon of unspecified finger at wrist and hand level**

S66.52 **Laceration of intrinsic muscle, fascia and tendon of other and unspecified finger at wrist and hand level**

- **S66.520** **Laceration of intrinsic muscle, fascia and tendon of right index finger at wrist and hand level** CC
  CC Excl: CC with 7th character A: See code: S66.021
- **S66.521** **Laceration of intrinsic muscle, fascia and tendon of left index finger at wrist and hand level** CC
  CC Excl: CC with 7th character A: See code: S66.022
- **S66.522** **Laceration of intrinsic muscle, fascia and tendon of right middle finger at wrist and hand level** CC
  CC Excl: CC with 7th character A: See code: S66.021
- **S66.523** **Laceration of intrinsic muscle, fascia and tendon of left middle finger at wrist and hand level** CC
  CC Excl: CC with 7th character A: See code: S66.022
- **S66.524** **Laceration of intrinsic muscle, fascia and tendon of right ring finger at wrist and hand level** CC
  CC Excl: CC with 7th character A: See code: S66.021
- **S66.525** **Laceration of intrinsic muscle, fascia and tendon of left ring finger at wrist and hand level** CC
  CC Excl: CC with 7th character A: See code: S66.022
- **S66.526** **Laceration of intrinsic muscle, fascia and tendon of right little finger at wrist and hand level** CC
  CC Excl: CC with 7th character A: See code: S66.021
- **S66.527** **Laceration of intrinsic muscle, fascia and tendon of left little finger at wrist and hand level** CC
  CC Excl: CC with 7th character A: See code: S66.022
- **S66.528** **Laceration of intrinsic muscle, fascia and tendon of other finger at wrist and hand level** CC
  Laceration of intrinsic muscle, fascia and tendon of specified finger with unspecified laterality at wrist and hand level
  CC Excl: CC with 7th character A: See code: S66.029
- **S66.529** **Laceration of intrinsic muscle, fascia and tendon of unspecified finger at wrist and hand level** CC
  CC Excl: CC with 7th character A: See code: S66.029

S66.59 **Other injury of intrinsic muscle, fascia and tendon of other and unspecified finger at wrist and hand level**

- **S66.590** **Other injury of intrinsic muscle, fascia and tendon of right index finger at wrist and hand level**
- **S66.591** **Other injury of intrinsic muscle, fascia and tendon of left index finger at wrist and hand level**
- **S66.592** **Other injury of intrinsic muscle, fascia and tendon of right middle finger at wrist and hand level**
- **S66.593** **Other injury of intrinsic muscle, fascia and tendon of left middle finger at wrist and hand level**
- **S66.594** **Other injury of intrinsic muscle, fascia and tendon of right ring finger at wrist and hand level**

✓7th **S66.595 Other injury of intrinsic muscle, fascia and tendon of left ring finger at wrist and hand level**

✓7th **S66.596 Other injury of intrinsic muscle, fascia and tendon of right little finger at wrist and hand level**

✓7th **S66.597 Other injury of intrinsic muscle, fascia and tendon of left little finger at wrist and hand level**

✓7th **S66.598 Other injury of intrinsic muscle, fascia and tendon of other finger at wrist and hand level**
Other injury of intrinsic muscle, fascia and tendon of specified finger with unspecified laterality at wrist and hand level

✓7th **S66.599 Other injury of intrinsic muscle, fascia and tendon of unspecified finger at wrist and hand level**

✓5th **S66.8 Injury of other specified muscles, fascia and tendons at wrist and hand level**

✓6th **S66.80 Unspecified injury of other specified muscles, fascia and tendons at wrist and hand level**

✓7th **S66.801 Unspecified injury of other specified muscles, fascia and tendons at wrist and hand level, right hand**

✓7th **S66.802 Unspecified injury of other specified muscles, fascia and tendons at wrist and hand level, left hand**

✓7th **S66.809 Unspecified injury of other specified muscles, fascia and tendons at wrist and hand level, unspecified hand**

✓6th **S66.81 Strain of other specified muscles, fascia and tendons at wrist and hand level**

✓7th **S66.811 Strain of other specified muscles, fascia and tendons at wrist and hand level, right hand**

✓7th **S66.812 Strain of other specified muscles, fascia and tendons at wrist and hand level, left hand**

✓7th **S66.819 Strain of other specified muscles, fascia and tendons at wrist and hand level, unspecified hand**

✓6th **S66.82 Laceration of other specified muscles, fascia and tendons at wrist and hand level**

✓7th **S66.821 Laceration of other specified muscles, fascia and tendons at wrist and hand level, right hand** CC
CC Excl: CC with 7th character A: See code: S66.021

✓7th **S66.822 Laceration of other specified muscles, fascia and tendons at wrist and hand level, left hand** CC
CC Excl: CC with 7th character A: See code: S66.022

✓7th **S66.829 Laceration of other specified muscles, fascia and tendons at wrist and hand level, unspecified hand** CC
CC Excl: CC with 7th character A: See code: S66.029

✓6th **S66.89 Other injury of other specified muscles, fascia and tendons at wrist and hand level**

✓7th **S66.891 Other injury of other specified muscles, fascia and tendons at wrist and hand level, right hand**

✓7th **S66.892 Other injury of other specified muscles, fascia and tendons at wrist and hand level, left hand**

✓7th **S66.899 Other injury of other specified muscles, fascia and tendons at wrist and hand level, unspecified hand**

✓5th **S66.9 Injury of unspecified muscle, fascia and tendon at wrist and hand level**

✓6th **S66.90 Unspecified injury of unspecified muscle, fascia and tendon at wrist and hand level**

✓7th **S66.901 Unspecified injury of unspecified muscle, fascia and tendon at wrist and hand level, right hand**

✓7th **S66.902 Unspecified injury of unspecified muscle, fascia and tendon at wrist and hand level, left hand**

✓7th **S66.909 Unspecified injury of unspecified muscle, fascia and tendon at wrist and hand level, unspecified hand**

✓6th **S66.91 Strain of unspecified muscle, fascia and tendon at wrist and hand level**

✓7th **S66.911 Strain of unspecified muscle, fascia and tendon at wrist and hand level, right hand**

✓7th **S66.912 Strain of unspecified muscle, fascia and tendon at wrist and hand level, left hand**

✓7th **S66.919 Strain of unspecified muscle, fascia and tendon at wrist and hand level, unspecified hand**

✓6th **S66.92 Laceration of unspecified muscle, fascia and tendon at wrist and hand level**

✓7th **S66.921 Laceration of unspecified muscle, fascia and tendon at wrist and hand level, right hand** CC
CC Excl: CC with 7th character A: See code: S66.021

✓7th **S66.922 Laceration of unspecified muscle, fascia and tendon at wrist and hand level, left hand** CC
CC Excl: CC with 7th character A: See code: S66.022

✓7th **S66.929 Laceration of unspecified muscle, fascia and tendon at wrist and hand level, unspecified hand** CC
CC Excl: CC with 7th character A: See code: S66.029

✓6th **S66.99 Other injury of unspecified muscle, fascia and tendon at wrist and hand level**

✓7th **S66.991 Other injury of unspecified muscle, fascia and tendon at wrist and hand level, right hand**

✓7th **S66.992 Other injury of unspecified muscle, fascia and tendon at wrist and hand level, left hand**

✓7th **S66.999 Other injury of unspecified muscle, fascia and tendon at wrist and hand level, unspecified hand**

✓4th **S67 Crushing injury of wrist, hand and fingers**
Use additional code for all associated injuries, such as:
fracture of wrist and hand (S62.-)
open wound of wrist and hand (S61.-)

The appropriate 7th character is to be added to each code from category S67.
A initial encounter
D subsequent encounter
S sequela

✓5th **S67.0 Crushing injury of thumb**

✓x7th **S67.00 Crushing injury of unspecified thumb**

✓x7th **S67.01 Crushing injury of right thumb**

✓x7th **S67.02 Crushing injury of left thumb**

✓5th **S67.1 Crushing injury of other and unspecified finger(s)**
EXCLUDES 2 *crushing injury of thumb (S67.0-)*

✓x7th **S67.10 Crushing injury of unspecified finger(s)**

✓6th **S67.19 Crushing injury of other finger(s)**

✓7th **S67.190 Crushing injury of right index finger**

✓7th **S67.191 Crushing injury of left index finger**

✓7th **S67.192 Crushing injury of right middle finger**

✓7th **S67.193 Crushing injury of left middle finger**

✓7th **S67.194 Crushing injury of right ring finger**

✓7th **S67.195 Crushing injury of left ring finger**

✓7th **S67.196 Crushing injury of right little finger**

✓7th **S67.197 Crushing injury of left little finger**

✓7th **S67.198 Crushing injury of other finger**
Crushing injury of specified finger with unspecified laterality

✓5th **S67.2 Crushing injury of hand**
EXCLUDES 2 *crushing injury of fingers (S67.1-)*
crushing injury of thumb (S67.0-)

✓x7th **S67.20 Crushing injury of unspecified hand**

Injury, Poisoning and Certain Other Consequences of External Causes S66.595–S67.20

✓x7th **S67.21 Crushing injury of right hand**

✓x7th **S67.22 Crushing injury of left hand**

✓5th **S67.3 Crushing injury of wrist**

✓x7th **S67.30 Crushing injury of unspecified wrist**

✓x7th **S67.31 Crushing injury of right wrist**

✓x7th **S67.32 Crushing injury of left wrist**

✓5th **S67.4 Crushing injury of wrist and hand**

EXCLUDES 1 *crushing injury of hand alone (S67.2-)*
crushing injury of wrist alone (S67.3-)

EXCLUDES 2 *crushing injury of fingers (S67.1-)*
crushing injury of thumb (S67.0-)

✓x7th **S67.40 Crushing injury of unspecified wrist and hand**

✓x7th **S67.41 Crushing injury of right wrist and hand**

✓x7th **S67.42 Crushing injury of left wrist and hand**

✓5th **S67.9 Crushing injury of unspecified part(s) of wrist, hand and fingers**

✓x7th **S67.90 Crushing injury of unspecified part(s) of unspecified wrist, hand and fingers**

✓x7th **S67.91 Crushing injury of unspecified part(s) of right wrist, hand and fingers**

✓x7th **S67.92 Crushing injury of unspecified part(s) of left wrist, hand and fingers**

✓4th **S68 Traumatic amputation of wrist, hand and fingers**

NOTE An amputation not identified as partial or complete should be coded to complete.

The appropriate 7th character is to be added to each code from category S68.
A initial encounter
D subsequent encounter
S sequela

✓5th **S68.0 Traumatic metacarpophalangeal amputation of thumb**
Traumatic amputation of thumb NOS

✓6th **S68.01 Complete traumatic metacarpophalangeal amputation of thumb**

✓7th **S68.011 Complete traumatic metacarpophalangeal amputation of right thumb**

✓7th **S68.012 Complete traumatic metacarpophalangeal amputation of left thumb**

✓7th **S68.019 Complete traumatic metacarpophalangeal amputation of unspecified thumb**

✓6th **S68.02 Partial traumatic metacarpophalangeal amputation of thumb**

✓7th **S68.021 Partial traumatic metacarpophalangeal amputation of right thumb**

✓7th **S68.022 Partial traumatic metacarpophalangeal amputation of left thumb**

✓7th **S68.029 Partial traumatic metacarpophalangeal amputation of unspecified thumb**

✓5th **S68.1 Traumatic metacarpophalangeal amputation of other and unspecified finger**
Traumatic amputation of finger NOS

EXCLUDES 2 *traumatic metacarpophalangeal amputation of thumb (S68.0-)*

✓6th **S68.11 Complete traumatic metacarpophalangeal amputation of other and unspecified finger**

✓7th **S68.110 Complete traumatic metacarpophalangeal amputation of right index finger**

✓7th **S68.111 Complete traumatic metacarpophalangeal amputation of left index finger**

✓7th **S68.112 Complete traumatic metacarpophalangeal amputation of right middle finger**

✓7th **S68.113 Complete traumatic metacarpophalangeal amputation of left middle finger**

✓7th **S68.114 Complete traumatic metacarpophalangeal amputation of right ring finger**

✓7th **S68.115 Complete traumatic metacarpophalangeal amputation of left ring finger**

✓7th **S68.116 Complete traumatic metacarpophalangeal amputation of right little finger**

✓7th **S68.117 Complete traumatic metacarpophalangeal amputation of left little finger**

✓7th **S68.118 Complete traumatic metacarpophalangeal amputation of other finger**
Complete traumatic metacarpophalangeal amputation of specified finger with unspecified laterality

✓7th **S68.119 Complete traumatic metacarpophalangeal amputation of unspecified finger**

✓6th **S68.12 Partial traumatic metacarpophalangeal amputation of other and unspecified finger**

✓7th **S68.120 Partial traumatic metacarpophalangeal amputation of right index finger**

✓7th **S68.121 Partial traumatic metacarpophalangeal amputation of left index finger**

✓7th **S68.122 Partial traumatic metacarpophalangeal amputation of right middle finger**

✓7th **S68.123 Partial traumatic metacarpophalangeal amputation of left middle finger**

✓7th **S68.124 Partial traumatic metacarpophalangeal amputation of right ring finger**

✓7th **S68.125 Partial traumatic metacarpophalangeal amputation of left ring finger**

✓7th **S68.126 Partial traumatic metacarpophalangeal amputation of right little finger**

✓7th **S68.127 Partial traumatic metacarpophalangeal amputation of left little finger**

✓7th **S68.128 Partial traumatic metacarpophalangeal amputation of other finger**
Partial traumatic metacarpophalangeal amputation of specified finger with unspecified laterality

✓7th **S68.129 Partial traumatic metacarpophalangeal amputation of unspecified finger**

✓5th **S68.4 Traumatic amputation of hand at wrist level**
Traumatic amputation of hand NOS
Traumatic amputation of wrist

✓6th **S68.41 Complete traumatic amputation of hand at wrist level**

✓7th **S68.411 Complete traumatic amputation of right hand at wrist level** CC

CC Excl: CC with 7th character A: S41.001A, S41.009-S41.011 with 7th A, S41.019-S41.021 with 7th A, S41.029-S41.031 with 7th A, S41.039-S41.041 with 7th A, S41.049-S41.051 with 7th A, S41.059-S41.101 with 7th A, S41.109-S41.111 with 7th A, S41.119-S41.121 with 7th A, S41.129-S41.131 with 7th A, S41.139-S41.141 with 7th A, S41.149-S41.151 with 7th A, S41.159A, S46.021A, S46.029A, S46.121A, S46.129A, S46.221A, S46.229A, S46.321A, S46.329A, S46.821A, S46.829A, S46.921A, S46.929 A, S48.011A, S48.019-S48.021 with 7th A, S48.029-S48.111 with 7th A, S48.119-S48.121 with 7th A, S48.129-S48.911 with 7th A, S48.919-S48.921 with 7th A, S48.929A, S51.001A, S51.009-S51.011 with 7th A, S51.019-S51.021 with 7th A, S51.029-S51.031 with 7th A, S51.039-S51.041 with 7th A, S51.049-S51.051 with 7th A, S51.059-S51.801 with 7th A, S51.809-S51.811 with 7th A, S51.819-S51.821 with 7th A, S51.829-S51.831 with 7th A, S51.839-S51.841 with 7th A, S51.849-S51.851A, S51.859A, S56.021A, S56.029A, S56.121A, S56.123A, S56.125A, S56.127A, S56.129A, S56.221A, S56.229A, S56.321A, S56.329A, S56.421A, S56.423A, S56.425A, S56.427A, S56.429A, S56.521A, S56.529A, S56.821A, S56.829 with 7th A, S56.921 with 7th A, S56.929 with 7th A, S58.011 with 7th A, S58.019-S58.021 with 7th A, S58.029-S58.111 with 7th A, S58.119-S58.121 with 7th A, S58.129-S58.911 with 7th A, S58.919-S58.921 with 7th A, S58.929 with 7th A, S61.001 with 7th A, S61.009-S61.011 with 7th A, S61.019-S61.021 with 7th A, S61.029-S61.031 with 7th A, S61.039-S61.041 with

7th A, S61.Ø49-S61.Ø51 with 7th A, S61.Ø59-S61.1Ø1 with 7th A, S61.1Ø9-S61.111 with 7th A, S61.119-S61.121 with 7th A, S61.129-S61.131 with 7th A, S61.139-S61.141 with 7th A, S61.149-S61.151 with 7th A, S61.159-S61.2ØØ with 7th A, S61.2Ø2A, S61.2Ø4A, S61.2Ø6A, S61.2Ø8-S61.21Ø with 7th A, S61.212A, S61.214A, S61.216A, S61.218-S61.22Ø with 7th A, S61.222A, S61.224A, S61.226A, S61.228-S61.23Ø with 7th A, S61.232A, S61.234A, S61.236A, S61.238-S61.24Ø with 7th A, S61.242A, S61.244A, S61.246A, S61.248-S61.25Ø with 7th A, S61.252A, S61.254A, S61.256A, S61.258-S61.3ØØA, S61.3Ø2A, S61.3Ø4A, S61.3Ø6A, S61.3Ø8-S61.31Ø with 7th A, S61.312A, S61.314A, S61.316A, S61.318-S61.32Ø with 7th A, S61.322A, S61.324A, S61.326A, S61.328-S61.33Ø with 7th A, S61.332A, S61.334A, S61.336A, S61.338-S61.34Ø with 7th A, S61.342A, S61.344A, S61.346A, S61.348-S61.35Ø with 7th A, S61.352A, S61.354A, S61.356A, S61.358-S61.4Ø1 with 7th A, S61.4Ø9-S61.411 with 7th A, S61.419-S61.421 with 7th A, S61.429-S61.431 with 7th A, S61.439-S61.441 with 7th A, S61.449-S61.451 with 7th A, S61.459-S61.5Ø1 with 7th A, S61.5Ø9-S61.511 with 7th A, S61.519-S61.521 with 7th A, S61.529-S61.531 with 7th A, S61.539-S61.541 with 7th A, S61.549-S61.551 with 7th A, S61.559A, S66.Ø21A, S66.Ø29A, S66.12ØA, S66.122A, S66.124A, S66.126A, S66.128-S66.129 with 7th A, S66.221A, S66.229A, S66.32ØA, S66.322A, S66.324A, S66.326A, S66.328-S66.329 with 7th A, S66.421A, S66.429A, S66.52ØA, S66.522A, S66.524A, S66.526A, S66.528-S66.529 with 7th A, S66.821A, S66.829A, S66.921A, S66.929A, S68.Ø11A, S68.Ø19-S68.Ø21 with 7th A, S68.Ø29-S68.11Ø with 7th A, S68.112A, S68.114A, S68.116A, S68.118-S68.12Ø with 7th A, S68.122A, S68.124A, S68.126A, S68.128-S68.411 with 7th A, S68.419-S68.421 with 7th A, S68.429-S68.511 with 7th A, S68.519-S68.521 with 7th A, S68.529-S68.61Ø with 7th A, S68.612A, S68.614A, S68.616A, S68.618-S68.62Ø with 7th A, S68.622A, S68.624A, S68.626A, S68.628-S68.711 with 7th A, S68.719-S68.721 with 7th A, S68.729A, T14.8-T14.91, T79.AØX-T79.9XX with 7th A

✓7th **S68.412 Complete traumatic amputation of left hand at wrist level** CC

CC Excl: CC with 7th character A: S41.ØØ2-S41.ØØ9 with 7th A, S41.Ø12-S41.Ø19 with 7th A, S41.Ø22-S41.Ø29 with 7th A, S41.Ø32-S41.Ø39 with 7th A, S41.Ø42-S41.Ø49 with 7th A, S41.Ø52-S41.Ø59 with 7th A, S41.1Ø2-S41.1Ø9 with 7th A, S41.112-S41.119 with 7th A, S41.122-S41.129 with 7th A, S41.132-S41.139 with 7th A, S41.142-S41.149 with 7th A, S41.152-S41.159 with 7th A, S46.Ø22-S46.Ø29 with 7th A, S46.122-S46.129 with 7th A, S46.222-S46.229 with 7th A, S46.322-S46.329 with 7th A, S46.822-S46.829 with 7th A, S46.922-S46.929 with 7th A, S48.Ø12-S48.Ø19 with 7th A, S48.Ø22-S48.Ø29 with 7th A, S48.112-S48.119 with 7th A, S48.122-S48.129 with 7th A, S48.912-S48.919 with 7th A, S48.922-S48.929 with 7th A, S51.ØØ2-S51.ØØ9 with 7th A, S51.Ø12-S51.Ø19 with 7th A, S51.Ø22-S51.Ø29 with 7th A, S51.Ø32-S51.Ø39 with 7th A, S51.Ø42-S51.Ø49 with 7th A, S51.Ø52-S51.Ø59 with 7th A, S51.8Ø2-S51.8Ø9 with 7th A, S51.812-S51.819 with 7th A, S51.822-S51.829 with 7th A, S51.832-S51.839 with 7th A, S51.842-S51.849 with 7th A, S51.852-S51.859 with 7th A, S56.Ø22-S56.Ø29 with 7th A, S56.122A, S56.124 A, S56.126A, S56.128-S56.129 with 7th A, S56.222-S56.229 with 7th A, S56.322-S56.329 with 7th A, S56.422A, S56.424A, S56.426A, S56.428-S56.429 with 7th A, S56.522-S56.529 with 7th A, S56.822-S56.829 with 7th A, S56.922-S56.929 with 7th A, S58.Ø12-S58.Ø19 with 7th A, S58.Ø22-S58.Ø29 with 7th A, S58.112-S58.119 with 7th A, S58.122-S58.129 with 7th A, S58.912-S58.919 with 7th A, S58.922-S58.929 with 7th A, S61.ØØ2-S61.ØØ9 with 7th A, S61.Ø12-S61.Ø19 with 7th A, S61.Ø22-S61.Ø29 with 7th A, S61.Ø32-S61.Ø39 with 7th A, S61.Ø42-S61.Ø49 with 7th A, S61.Ø52-S61.Ø59 with 7th A, S61.1Ø2-S61.1Ø9 with 7th A, S61.112-S61.119 with 7th A, S61.122-S61.129 with 7th A, S61.132-S61.139 with 7th A, S61.142-S61.149 with 7th A, S61.152-S61.159 with 7th A, S61.2Ø1A, S61.2Ø3A, S61.2Ø5A, S61.2Ø7-S61.2Ø9 with 7th A, S61.211A, S61.213A, S61.215A, S61.217-S61.219 with 7th A, S61.221A, S61.223A, S61.225A, S61.227-S61.229 with 7th A, S61.231A, S61.233A, S61.235A, S61.237-S61.239 with 7th A, S61.241A, S61.243A, S61.245 A, S61.247-S61.249 with 7th A, S61.251A, S61.253 A, S61.255A, S61.257-S61.259 with 7th A, S61.3Ø1 A, S61.3Ø3A, S61.3Ø5A, S61.3Ø7-S61.3Ø9 with 7th A, S61.311A, S61.313A, S61.315A, S61.317-S61.319 with 7th A, S61.321A, S61.323A, S61.325 A, S61.327-S61.329 with 7th A, S61.331A, S61.333A, S61.335A, S61.337-S61.339 with 7th A, S61.341A, S61.343A, S61.345A, S61.347-S61.349 with 7th A, S61.351A, S61.353A, S61.355A, S61.357-S61.359 with 7th A, S61.4Ø2-S61.4Ø9 with 7th A, S61.412-S61.419 with 7th A, S61.422-S61.429 with 7th A, S61.432-S61.439 with 7th A, S61.442-S61.449 with 7th A, S61.452-S61.459 with 7th A, S61.5Ø2-S61.5Ø9 with 7th A, S61.512-S61.519 with 7th A, S61.522-S61.529 with 7th A, S61.532-S61.539 with 7th A, S61.542-S61.549 with 7th A, S61.552-S61.559 with 7th A, S66.Ø22-S66.Ø29 with 7th A, S66.121A, S66.123A, S66.125A, S66.127-S66.129 with 7th A, S66.222-S66.229 with 7th A, S66.321A, S66.323A, S66.325A, S66.327-S66.329 with 7th A, S66.422-S66.429 with 7th A, S66.521A, S66.523A, S66.525A, S66.527-S66.529 with 7th A, S66.822-S66.829 with 7th A, S66.922-S66.929 with 7th A, S68.Ø12-S68.Ø19 with 7th A, S68.Ø22-S68.Ø29 with 7th A, S68.111A, S68.113A, S68.115A, S68.117-S68.119 with 7th A, S68.121A, S68.123A, S68.125A, S68.127-S68.129 with 7th A, S68.412-S68.419 with 7th A, S68.422-S68.429 with 7th A, S68.512-S68.519 with 7th A, S68.522-S68.529 with 7th A, S68.611A, S68.613A, S68.615A, S68.617-S68.619 with 7th A, S68.621A, S68.623A, S68.625A, S68.627-S68.629 with 7th A, S68.712-S68.719 with 7th A, S68.722-S68.729 with 7th A, T14.8-T14.91, T79.AØX-T79.9XX with 7th A

✓7th **S68.419 Complete traumatic amputation of unspecified hand at wrist level** CC

CC Excl: CC with 7th character A: S41.ØØ1-S41.159 with 7th A, S46.Ø21-S46.Ø29 with 7th A, S46.121-S46.129 with 7th A, S46.221-S46.229 with 7th A, S46.321-S46.329 with 7th A, S46.821-S46.829 with 7th A, S46.921-S46.929 with 7th A, S48.Ø11-S48.929 with 7th A, S51.ØØ1-S51.859 with 7th A, S56.Ø21-S56.Ø29 with 7th A, S56.121-S56.129 with 7th A, S56.221-S56.229 with 7th A, S56.321-S56.329 with 7th A, S56.421-S56.429 with 7th A, S56.521-S56.529 with 7th A, S56.821-S56.829 with 7th A, S56.921-S56.929 with 7th A, S58.Ø11-S58.929 with 7th A, S61.ØØ1-S61.559 with 7th A, S66.Ø21-S66.Ø29 with 7th A, S66.12Ø-S66.129 with 7th A, S66.221-S66.229 with 7th A, S66.32Ø-S66.329 with 7th A, S66.421-S66.429 with 7th A, S66.52Ø-S66.529 with 7th A, S66.821-S66.829 with 7th A, S66.921-S66.929 with 7th A, S68.Ø11-S68.729 with 7th A, T14.8-T14.91, T79.AØX-T79.9XX with 7th A

✓6th **S68.42 Partial traumatic amputation of hand at wrist level**

✓7th **S68.421 Partial traumatic amputation of right hand at wrist level** CC

CC Excl: CC with 7th character A: See code: S68.411

✓7th **S68.422 Partial traumatic amputation of left hand at wrist level** CC

CC Excl: CC with 7th character A: See code: S68.412

✓7th **S68.429 Partial traumatic amputation of unspecified hand at wrist level** CC

CC Excl: CC with 7th character A: See code: S68.419

S68.5 Traumatic transphalangeal amputation of thumb

Traumatic interphalangeal joint amputation of thumb

6th S68.51 Complete traumatic transphalangeal amputation of thumb
- 7th S68.511 Complete traumatic transphalangeal amputation of right thumb
- 7th S68.512 Complete traumatic transphalangeal amputation of left thumb
- 7th S68.519 Complete traumatic transphalangeal amputation of unspecified thumb

6th S68.52 Partial traumatic transphalangeal amputation of thumb
- 7th S68.521 Partial traumatic transphalangeal amputation of right thumb
- 7th S68.522 Partial traumatic transphalangeal amputation of left thumb
- 7th S68.529 Partial traumatic transphalangeal amputation of unspecified thumb

5th S68.6 Traumatic transphalangeal amputation of other and unspecified finger

6th S68.61 Complete traumatic transphalangeal amputation of other and unspecified finger(s)
- 7th S68.610 Complete traumatic transphalangeal amputation of right index finger
- 7th S68.611 Complete traumatic transphalangeal amputation of left index finger
- 7th S68.612 Complete traumatic transphalangeal amputation of right middle finger
- 7th S68.613 Complete traumatic transphalangeal amputation of left middle finger
- 7th S68.614 Complete traumatic transphalangeal amputation of right ring finger
- 7th S68.615 Complete traumatic transphalangeal amputation of left ring finger
- 7th S68.616 Complete traumatic transphalangeal amputation of right little finger
- 7th S68.617 Complete traumatic transphalangeal amputation of left little finger
- 7th S68.618 Complete traumatic transphalangeal amputation of other finger
  Complete traumatic transphalangeal amputation of specified finger with unspecified laterality
- 7th S68.619 Complete traumatic transphalangeal amputation of unspecified finger

6th S68.62 Partial traumatic transphalangeal amputation of other and unspecified finger
- 7th S68.620 Partial traumatic transphalangeal amputation of right index finger
- 7th S68.621 Partial traumatic transphalangeal amputation of left index finger
- 7th S68.622 Partial traumatic transphalangeal amputation of right middle finger
- 7th S68.623 Partial traumatic transphalangeal amputation of left middle finger
- 7th S68.624 Partial traumatic transphalangeal amputation of right ring finger
- 7th S68.625 Partial traumatic transphalangeal amputation of left ring finger
- 7th S68.626 Partial traumatic transphalangeal amputation of right little finger
- 7th S68.627 Partial traumatic transphalangeal amputation of left little finger
- 7th S68.628 Partial traumatic transphalangeal amputation of other finger
  Partial traumatic transphalangeal amputation of specified finger with unspecified laterality
- 7th S68.629 Partial traumatic transphalangeal amputation of unspecified finger

5th S68.7 Traumatic transmetacarpal amputation of hand

6th S68.71 Complete traumatic transmetacarpal amputation of hand
- 7th S68.711 Complete traumatic transmetacarpal amputation of right hand CC
  CC Excl: CC with 7th character A: See code: S68.411
- 7th S68.712 Complete traumatic transmetacarpal amputation of left hand CC
  CC Excl: CC with 7th character A: See code: S68.412
- 7th S68.719 Complete traumatic transmetacarpal amputation of unspecified hand CC
  CC Excl: CC with 7th character A: See code: S68.419

6th S68.72 Partial traumatic transmetacarpal amputation of hand
- 7th S68.721 Partial traumatic transmetacarpal amputation of right hand CC
  CC Excl: CC with 7th character A: See code: S68.411
- 7th S68.722 Partial traumatic transmetacarpal amputation of left hand CC
  CC Excl: CC with 7th character A: See code: S68.412
- 7th S68.729 Partial traumatic transmetacarpal amputation of unspecified hand CC
  CC Excl: CC with 7th character A: See code: S68.419

4th **S69 Other and unspecified injuries of wrist, hand and finger(s)**

The appropriate 7th character is to be added to each code from category S69.
A initial encounter
D subsequent encounter
S sequela

5th S69.8 Other specified injuries of wrist, hand and finger(s)
- x7th S69.80 Other specified injuries of unspecified wrist, hand and finger(s)
- x7th S69.81 Other specified injuries of right wrist, hand and finger(s)
- x7th S69.82 Other specified injuries of left wrist, hand and finger(s)

5th S69.9 Unspecified injury of wrist, hand and finger(s)
- x7th S69.90 Unspecified injury of unspecified wrist, hand and finger(s)
- x7th S69.91 Unspecified injury of right wrist, hand and finger(s)
- x7th S69.92 Unspecified injury of left wrist, hand and finger(s)

Injuries to the hip and thigh (S70-S79)

EXCLUDES 2 *burns and corrosions (T20-T32)*
frostbite (T33-T34)
snake bite (T63.0-)
venomous insect bite or sting (T63.4-)

4th **S70 Superficial injury of hip and thigh**

The appropriate 7th character is to be added to each code from category S70.
A initial encounter
D subsequent encounter
S sequela

5th S70.0 Contusion of hip
- x7th S70.00 Contusion of unspecified hip
- x7th S70.01 Contusion of right hip
- x7th S70.02 Contusion of left hip

5th S70.1 Contusion of thigh
- x7th S70.10 Contusion of unspecified thigh
- x7th S70.11 Contusion of right thigh
- x7th S70.12 Contusion of left thigh

5th S70.2 Other superficial injuries of hip

6th S70.21 Abrasion of hip
- 7th S70.211 Abrasion, right hip
- 7th S70.212 Abrasion, left hip
- 7th S70.219 Abrasion, unspecified hip

6th S70.22 Blister (nonthermal) of hip
- 7th S70.221 Blister (nonthermal), right hip
- 7th S70.222 Blister (nonthermal), left hip
- 7th S70.229 Blister (nonthermal), unspecified hip

6th S70.24 External constriction of hip
- 7th S70.241 External constriction, right hip
- 7th S70.242 External constriction, left hip
- 7th S70.249 External constriction, unspecified hip

✓6th S70.25 Superficial foreign body of hip
Splinter in the hip
✓7th S70.251 Superficial foreign body, right hip
✓7th S70.252 Superficial foreign body, left hip
✓7th S70.259 Superficial foreign body, unspecified hip
✓6th S70.26 Insect bite (nonvenomous) of hip
✓7th S70.261 Insect bite (nonvenomous), right hip
✓7th S70.262 Insect bite (nonvenomous), left hip
✓7th S70.269 Insect bite (nonvenomous), unspecified hip
✓6th S70.27 Other superficial bite of hip
EXCLUDES 1 *open bite of hip (S71.05-)*
✓7th S70.271 Other superficial bite of hip, right hip
✓7th S70.272 Other superficial bite of hip, left hip
✓7th S70.279 Other superficial bite of hip, unspecified hip
✓5th S70.3 Other superficial injuries of thigh
✓6th S70.31 Abrasion of thigh
✓7th S70.311 Abrasion, right thigh
✓7th S70.312 Abrasion, left thigh
✓7th S70.319 Abrasion, unspecified thigh
✓6th S70.32 Blister (nonthermal) of thigh
✓7th S70.321 Blister (nonthermal), right thigh
✓7th S70.322 Blister (nonthermal), left thigh
✓7th S70.329 Blister (nonthermal), unspecified thigh
✓6th S70.34 External constriction of thigh
✓7th S70.341 External constriction, right thigh
✓7th S70.342 External constriction, left thigh
✓7th S70.349 External constriction, unspecified thigh
✓6th S70.35 Superficial foreign body of thigh
Splinter in the thigh
✓7th S70.351 Superficial foreign body, right thigh
✓7th S70.352 Superficial foreign body, left thigh
✓7th S70.359 Superficial foreign body, unspecified thigh
✓6th S70.36 Insect bite (nonvenomous) of thigh
✓7th S70.361 Insect bite (nonvenomous), right thigh
✓7th S70.362 Insect bite (nonvenomous), left thigh
✓7th S70.369 Insect bite (nonvenomous), unspecified thigh
✓6th S70.37 Other superficial bite of thigh
EXCLUDES 1 *open bite of thigh (S71.15)*
✓7th S70.371 Other superficial bite of right thigh
✓7th S70.372 Other superficial bite of left thigh
✓7th S70.379 Other superficial bite of unspecified thigh
✓5th S70.9 Unspecified superficial injury of hip and thigh
✓6th S70.91 Unspecified superficial injury of hip
✓7th S70.911 Unspecified superficial injury of right hip
✓7th S70.912 Unspecified superficial injury of left hip
✓7th S70.919 Unspecified superficial injury of unspecified hip
✓6th S70.92 Unspecified superficial injury of thigh
✓7th S70.921 Unspecified superficial injury of right thigh
✓7th S70.922 Unspecified superficial injury of left thigh
✓7th S70.929 Unspecified superficial injury of unspecified thigh

✓4th **S71 Open wound of hip and thigh**
Code also any associated wound infection
EXCLUDES 1 *open fracture of hip and thigh (S72.-)*
traumatic amputation of hip and thigh (S78.-)
EXCLUDES 2 *bite of venomous animal (T63.-)*
open wound of ankle, foot and toes (S91.-)
open wound of knee and lower leg (S81.-)

The appropriate 7th character is to be added to each code from category S71.
A initial encounter
D subsequent encounter
S sequela

✓5th S71.0 Open wound of hip
✓6th S71.00 Unspecified open wound of hip
✓7th S71.001 Unspecified open wound, right hip
✓7th S71.002 Unspecified open wound, left hip
✓7th S71.009 Unspecified open wound, unspecified hip
✓6th S71.01 Laceration without foreign body of hip
✓7th S71.011 Laceration without foreign body, right hip
✓7th S71.012 Laceration without foreign body, left hip
✓7th S71.019 Laceration without foreign body, unspecified hip
✓6th S71.02 Laceration with foreign body of hip
✓7th S71.021 Laceration with foreign body, right hip
✓7th S71.022 Laceration with foreign body, left hip
✓7th S71.029 Laceration with foreign body, unspecified hip
✓6th S71.03 Puncture wound without foreign body of hip
✓7th S71.031 Puncture wound without foreign body, right hip
✓7th S71.032 Puncture wound without foreign body, left hip
✓7th S71.039 Puncture wound without foreign body, unspecified hip
✓6th S71.04 Puncture wound with foreign body of hip
✓7th S71.041 Puncture wound with foreign body, right hip
✓7th S71.042 Puncture wound with foreign body, left hip
✓7th S71.049 Puncture wound with foreign body, unspecified hip
✓6th S71.05 Open bite of hip
Bite of hip NOS
EXCLUDES 1 *superficial bite of hip (S70.26, S70.27)*
✓7th S71.051 Open bite, right hip
✓7th S71.052 Open bite, left hip
✓7th S71.059 Open bite, unspecified hip
✓5th S71.1 Open wound of thigh
✓6th S71.10 Unspecified open wound of thigh
✓7th S71.101 Unspecified open wound, right thigh
✓7th S71.102 Unspecified open wound, left thigh
✓7th S71.109 Unspecified open wound, unspecified thigh
✓6th S71.11 Laceration without foreign body of thigh
✓7th S71.111 Laceration without foreign body, right thigh
✓7th S71.112 Laceration without foreign body, left thigh
✓7th S71.119 Laceration without foreign body, unspecified thigh
✓6th S71.12 Laceration with foreign body of thigh
✓7th S71.121 Laceration with foreign body, right thigh
✓7th S71.122 Laceration with foreign body, left thigh
✓7th S71.129 Laceration with foreign body, unspecified thigh
✓6th S71.13 Puncture wound without foreign body of thigh
✓7th S71.131 Puncture wound without foreign body, right thigh
✓7th S71.132 Puncture wound without foreign body, left thigh
✓7th S71.139 Puncture wound without foreign body, unspecified thigh
✓6th S71.14 Puncture wound with foreign body of thigh
✓7th S71.141 Puncture wound with foreign body, right thigh
✓7th S71.142 Puncture wound with foreign body, left thigh
✓7th S71.149 Puncture wound with foreign body, unspecified thigh
✓6th S71.15 Open bite of thigh
Bite of thigh NOS
EXCLUDES 1 *superficial bite of thigh (S70.37-)*
✓7th S71.151 Open bite, right thigh
✓7th S71.152 Open bite, left thigh

✓7th **S71.159 Open bite, unspecified thigh**

✓4th **S72 Fracture of femur**

NOTE A fracture not indicated as displaced or nondisplaced should be coded to displaced.
The open fracture designations are based on the Gustilo open fracture classification A fracture not indicated as open or closed should be coded to closed.

EXCLUDES 1 *traumatic amputation of hip and thigh (S78.-)*

EXCLUDES 2 *fracture of foot (S92.-)*
fracture of lower leg and ankle (S82.-)
periprosthetic fracture of prosthetic implant of hip (T84.040, T84.041)

AHA: 2013, 4Q, 128

The appropriate 7th character is to be added to all codes from category S72 [unless otherwise indicated].

A initial encounter for closed fracture
B initial encounter for open fracture type I or II
  initial encounter for open fracture NOS
C initial encounter for open fracture type IIIA, IIIB, or IIIC
D subsequent encounter for closed fracture with routine healing
E subsequent encounter for open fracture type I or II with routine healing
F subsequent encounter for open fracture type IIIA, IIIB, or IIIC with routine healing
G subsequent encounter for closed fracture with delayed healing
H subsequent encounter for open fracture type I or II with delayed healing
J subsequent encounter for open fracture type IIIA, IIIB, or IIIC with delayed healing
K subsequent encounter for closed fracture with nonunion
M subsequent encounter for open fracture type I or II with nonunion
N subsequent encounter for open fracture type IIIA, IIIB, or IIIC with nonunion
P subsequent encounter for closed fracture with malunion
Q subsequent encounter for open fracture type I or II with malunion
R subsequent encounter for open fracture type IIIA, IIIB, or IIIC with malunion
S sequela

✓5th **S72.0 Fracture of head and neck of femur**

EXCLUDES 2 *physeal fracture of upper end of femur (S79.0-)*

✓6th **S72.00 Fracture of unspecified part of neck of femur**
Fracture of hip NOS
Fracture of neck of femur NOS

7 ✓7th **S72.001 Fracture of unspecified part of neck of right femur** MCC CC
CC Excl: MCC with 7th A: M48.40X-M48.58X with 7th A, M80.00X-M84.68X with 7th A, S03.8XX-S03.9XX with 7th A, S29.011-S29.019 with 7th A, S38.3XX-S39.013 with 7th A, S72.001-S72.471 with 7th [A, B, C], S72.479-S72.92X with 7th A, S73.101A, S73.109-S73.111 with 7th A, S73.119-S73.121 with 7th A, S73.129-S73.191 with 7th A, S73.199A, S76.001A, S76.009-S76.011 with 7th A, S76.019A, S76.091A, S76.099-S76.101 with 7th A, S76.109-S76.111 with 7th A, S76.119A, S76.191A, S76.199-S76.201 with 7th A, S76.209-S76.211 with 7th A, S76.219A, S76.291A, S76.299-S76.301 with 7th A, S76.309-S76.311 with 7th A, S76.319A, S76.391A, S76.399-S76.801 with 7th A, S76.809-S76.811 with 7th A, S76.819A, S76.891A, S76.899-S76.901 with 7th A, S76.909-S76.911 with 7th A, S76.919A, S76.991A, S76.999A, S79.001A, S79.009-S79.011 with 7th A, S79.019-S79.091 with 7th A, S79.099-S79.101 with 7th A, S79.109-S79.111 with 7th A, S79.119-S79.121 with 7th A, S79.129-S79.131 with 7th A, S79.139-S79.141 with 7th A, S79.149-S79.191 with 7th A, S79.199-S79.811 with 7th A, S79.819-S79.821 with 7th A, S79.829-S79.911 with 7th A, S79.919-S79.921 with 7th A, S79.929A, S82.90X-S82.92X with 7th [A, B, C], T14.8-T14.91, T79.A0X-T79.9XX with 7th A
MCC with 7th B or C: M48.40X-M48.58X with 7th A, M80.00X-M84.68X with 7th A, S03.8XX-S03.9XX with 7th A, S29.011-S29.019 with 7th A, S38.3XX-S39.013 with 7th A, S72.001-S72.92X with 7th [A, B, C], S73.101-S73.199 with 7th A, S76.001-S76.019 with 7th A, S76.091-S76.119 with 7th A, S76.191-S76.219 with 7th A, S76.291-S76.319 with 7th A, S76.391-S76.819 with 7th A, S76.891-S76.919 with 7th A, S76.991-S76.999 with 7th A, S79.001-S79.929 with 7th A, S82.90X-S82.92X with 7th [A, B, C], T14.8-T14.91, T79.A0X-T79.9XX with 7th A
CC with 7th character K, M, N, P, Q or R: M80.00X-M84.68X with 7th [K, P], S02.0XX-S02.92X with 7th K, S12.000-S12.691 with 7th K, S22.000-S22.9XX with 7th K, S32.000-S32.9XX with 7th K, S42.001-S42.92X with 7th [K, P], S49.001-S49.199 with 7th [K, P], S52.001-S52.92X with 7th [K, M, N, P, Q, R], S59.001-S59.299 with 7th [K, P], S62.001-S62.92X with 7th [K, P], S72.001-S72.92X with 7th [K, M, N, P, Q, R], S79.001-S79.199 with 7th [K, P], S82.001-S82.92X with 7th [K, M, N, P, Q, R], S89.001-S89.399 with 7th [K, P], S92.001-S92.919 with 7th [K, P]

7 ✓7th **S72.002 Fracture of unspecified part of neck of left femur** MCC CC
CC Excl: MCC with 7th A: M48.40X-M48.58X with 7th A, M80.00X-M84.68X with 7th A, S03.8XX-S03.9XX with 7th A, S29.011-S29.019 with 7th A, S38.3XX-S39.013 with 7th A, S72.001-S72.466 with 7th [B, C], S72.472-S72.92X with 7th A, S73.102-S73.109 with 7th A, S73.112-S73.119 with 7th A, S73.122-S73.129 with 7th A, S73.192-S73.199 with 7th A, S76.002-S76.009 with 7th A, S76.012-S76.019 with 7th A, S76.092-S76.099 with 7th A, S76.102-S76.109 with 7th A, S76.112-S76.119 with 7th A, S76.192-S76.199 with 7th A, S76.202-S76.209 with 7th A, S76.212-S76.219 with 7th A, S76.292-S76.299 with 7th A, S76.302-S76.309 with 7th A, S76.312-S76.319 with 7th A, S76.392-S76.399 with 7th A, S76.802-S76.809 with 7th A, S76.812-S76.819 with 7th A, S76.892-S76.899 with 7th A, S76.902-S76.909 with 7th A, S76.912-S76.919 with 7th A, S76.992-S76.999 with 7th A, S79.002-S79.009 with 7th A, S79.012-S79.019 with 7th A, S79.092-S79.099 with 7th A, S79.102-S79.109 with 7th A, S79.112-S79.119 with 7th A, S79.122-S79.129 with 7th A, S79.132-S79.139 with 7th A, S79.142-S79.149 with 7th A, S79.192-S79.199 with 7th A, S79.812-S79.819 with 7th A, S79.822-S79.829 with 7th A, S79.912-S79.919 with 7th A, S79.922-S79.929 with 7th A, S82.90-S82.92 with 7th [A, B, C], T14.8-T14.91, T79.A0X-T79.9XX with 7th A
MCC with 7th B or C: M48.40X-M48.58X with 7th A, M80.00X-M84.68X with 7th A, S03.8XX-S03.9XX with 7th A, S29.011-S29.019 with 7th A, S38.3XX-S39.013 with 7th A, S72.001-S72.92X with 7th [A, B, C], S73.101-S73.199 with 7th A, S76.001-S76.019 with 7th A, S76.091-S76.119 with 7th A, S76.191-S76.219 with 7th A, S76.291-S76.319 with 7th A, S76.391-S76.819 with 7th A, S76.891-S76.919 with 7th A, S76.991-S76.999 with 7th A, S79.001-S79.929 with 7th A, S82.90X-S82.92X with 7th [A, B, C], T14.8-T14.91, T79.A0X-T79.9XX with 7th A
CC with 7th character K, M, N, P, Q or R: M80.00X-M84.68X with 7th [K, P], S02.0XX-S02.92X with 7th K, S12.000-S12.691 with 7th K, S22.000-S22.9XX with 7th K, S32.000-S32.9XX with 7th K, S42.001-S42.92X with 7th [K, P], S49.001-S49.199 with 7th [K, P], S52.001-S52.92X with 7th [K, M, N, P, Q, R], S59.001-S59.299 with 7th [K, P], S62.001-S62.92X with 7th [K, P], S72.001-S72.92X with 7th [K, M, N, P, Q, R], S79.001-S79.199 with 7th [K, P], S82.001-S82.92X with 7th [K, M, N, P, Q, R], S89.001-S89.399 with 7th [K, P], S92.001-S92.919 with 7th [K, P]

7 HAC = Initial encounter only (7th character A, B or C) and not POA.

7 ✓7th **S72.009 Fracture of unspecified part of neck of unspecified femur** MCC CC
CC Excl: MCC with 7th A, B or C: M48.40X-M48.58X with 7th A, M80.00X-M84.68X with 7th A, S03.8XX-S03.9X with 7th A, S29.011-S29.019 with 7th A, S38.3XX-S39.013 with 7th A, S72.001-S72.92X with 7th [A, B, C], S73.101-S73.199 with 7th A, S76.001-S76.019 with 7th A, S76.091-S76.119 with 7th A, S76.191-S76.219 with 7th A, S76.291-S76.319 with 7th A, S76.391-S76.819 with 7th A, S76.891-S76.919 with 7th A, S76.991-S76.999 with 7th A, S79.001-S79.929 with 7th A, S82.90X-S82.92X with 7th [A, B, C], T14.8-T14.91, T79.A0X-T79.9XX with 7th A **CC with 7th character K, M, N, P, Q or R:** M80.00X-M84.68X with 7th [K, P], S02.0XX-S02.92X with 7th K, S12.000-S12.691 with 7th K, S22.000-S22.9XX with 7th K, S32.000-S32.9XX with 7th K, S42.001-S42.92X with 7th [K, P], S49.001-S49.199 with 7th [K, P], S52.001-S52.92X with 7th [K, M, N, P, Q, R], S59.001-S59.299 with 7th [K, P], S62.001-S62.92X with 7th [K, P], S72.001-S72.92X with 7th [K, M, N, P, Q, R], S79.001-S79.199 with 7th [K, P], S82.001-S82.92X with 7th [K, M, N, P, Q, R], S89.001-S89.399 with 7th [K, P], S92.001-S92.919 with 7th [K, P]

✓6th **S72.01 Unspecified intracapsular fracture of femur**
Subcapital fracture of femur

7 ✓7th **S72.011 Unspecified intracapsular fracture of right femur** MCC CC
CC Excl: See code: S72.001

7 ✓7th **S72.012 Unspecified intracapsular fracture of left femur** MCC CC
CC Excl: See code: S72.002

7 ✓7th **S72.019 Unspecified intracapsular fracture of unspecified femur** MCC CC
CC Excl: See code: S72.009

✓6th **S72.02 Fracture of epiphysis (separation) (upper) of femur**
Transepiphyseal fracture of femur
EXCLUDES 1 *capital femoral epiphyseal fracture (pediatric) of femur (S79.01-)*
Salter-Harris Type I physeal fracture of upper end of femur (S79.01-)

7 ✓7th **S72.021 Displaced fracture of epiphysis (separation) (upper) of right femur** MCC CC
CC Excl: See code: S72.001

7 ✓7th **S72.022 Displaced fracture of epiphysis (separation) (upper) of left femur** MCC CC
CC Excl: See code: S72.002

7 ✓7th **S72.023 Displaced fracture of epiphysis (separation) (upper) of unspecified femur** MCC CC
CC Excl: See code: S72.009

7 ✓7th **S72.024 Nondisplaced fracture of epiphysis (separation) (upper) of right femur** MCC CC
CC Excl: See code: S72.001

7 ✓7th **S72.025 Nondisplaced fracture of epiphysis (separation) (upper) of left femur** MCC CC
CC Excl: See code: S72.002

7 ✓7th **S72.026 Nondisplaced fracture of epiphysis (separation) (upper) of unspecified femur** MCC CC
CC Excl: See code: S72.009

✓6th **S72.03 Midcervical fracture of femur**
Transcervical fracture of femur NOS

7 ✓7th **S72.031 Displaced midcervical fracture of right femur** MCC CC
CC Excl: See code: S72.001

7 ✓7th **S72.032 Displaced midcervical fracture of left femur** MCC CC
CC Excl: See code: S72.002

7 ✓7th **S72.033 Displaced midcervical fracture of unspecified femur** MCC CC
CC Excl: See code: S72.009

7 ✓7th **S72.034 Nondisplaced midcervical fracture of right femur** MCC CC
CC Excl: See code: S72.001

7 ✓7th **S72.035 Nondisplaced midcervical fracture of left femur** MCC CC
CC Excl: See code: S72.002

7 ✓7th **S72.036 Nondisplaced midcervical fracture of unspecified femur** MCC CC
CC Excl: See code: S72.009

✓6th **S72.04 Fracture of base of neck of femur**
Cervicotrochanteric fracture of femur

7 ✓7th **S72.041 Displaced fracture of base of neck of right femur** MCC CC
CC Excl: See code: S72.001

7 ✓7th **S72.042 Displaced fracture of base of neck of left femur** MCC CC
CC Excl: See code: S72.002

7 ✓7th **S72.043 Displaced fracture of base of neck of unspecified femur** MCC CC
CC Excl: See code: S72.009

7 ✓7th **S72.044 Nondisplaced fracture of base of neck of right femur** MCC CC
CC Excl: See code: S72.001

7 ✓7th **S72.045 Nondisplaced fracture of base of neck of left femur** MCC CC
CC Excl: See code: S72.002

7 ✓7th **S72.046 Nondisplaced fracture of base of neck of unspecified femur** MCC CC
CC Excl: See code: S72.009

✓6th **S72.05 Unspecified fracture of head of femur**
Fracture of head of femur NOS

7 ✓7th **S72.051 Unspecified fracture of head of right femur** MCC CC
CC Excl: See code: S72.001

7 ✓7th **S72.052 Unspecified fracture of head of left femur** MCC CC
CC Excl: See code: S72.002

7 ✓7th **S72.059 Unspecified fracture of head of unspecified femur** MCC CC
CC Excl: See code: S72.009

✓6th **S72.06 Articular fracture of head of femur**

7 ✓7th **S72.061 Displaced articular fracture of head of right femur** MCC CC
CC Excl: See code: S72.001

7 ✓7th **S72.062 Displaced articular fracture of head of left femur** MCC CC
CC Excl: See code: S72.002

7 ✓7th **S72.063 Displaced articular fracture of head of unspecified femur** MCC CC
CC Excl: See code: S72.009

7 ✓7th **S72.064 Nondisplaced articular fracture of head of right femur** MCC CC
CC Excl: See code: S72.001

7 ✓7th **S72.065 Nondisplaced articular fracture of head of left femur** MCC CC
CC Excl: See code: S72.002

7 ✓7th **S72.066 Nondisplaced articular fracture of head of unspecified femur** MCC CC
CC Excl: See code: S72.009

✓6th **S72.09 Other fracture of head and neck of femur**

7 ✓7th **S72.091 Other fracture of head and neck of right femur** MCC CC
CC Excl: See code: S72.001

7 ✓7th **S72.092 Other fracture of head and neck of left femur** MCC CC
CC Excl: See code: S72.002

7 ✓7th **S72.099 Other fracture of head and neck of unspecified femur** MCC CC
CC Excl: See code: S72.009

✓5th **S72.1 Pertrochanteric fracture**

✓6th **S72.10 Unspecified trochanteric fracture of femur**
Fracture of trochanter NOS

7 ✓7th **S72.101 Unspecified trochanteric fracture of right femur** MCC CC
CC Excl: See code: S72.001

7 ✓7th **S72.102 Unspecified trochanteric fracture of left femur** MCC CC
CC Excl: See code: S72.002

7 ✓7th **S72.109 Unspecified trochanteric fracture of unspecified femur** MCC CC
CC Excl: See code: S72.009

7 HAC = Initial encounter only (7th character A, B or C) and not POA.

✓6th **S72.11 Fracture of greater trochanter of femur**
- 7 ✓7th **S72.111 Displaced fracture of greater trochanter of right femur** MCC CC
  CC Excl: See code: S72.001
- 7 ✓7th **S72.112 Displaced fracture of greater trochanter of left femur** MCC CC
  CC Excl: See code: S72.002
- 7 ✓7th **S72.113 Displaced fracture of greater trochanter of unspecified femur** MCC CC
  CC Excl: See code: S72.009
- 7 ✓7th **S72.114 Nondisplaced fracture of greater trochanter of right femur** MCC CC
  CC Excl: See code: S72.001
- 7 ✓7th **S72.115 Nondisplaced fracture of greater trochanter of left femur** MCC CC
  CC Excl: See code: S72.002
- 7 ✓7th **S72.116 Nondisplaced fracture of greater trochanter of unspecified femur** MCC CC
  CC Excl: See code: S72.009

✓6th **S72.12 Fracture of lesser trochanter of femur**
- 7 ✓7th **S72.121 Displaced fracture of lesser trochanter of right femur** MCC CC
  CC Excl: See code: S72.001
- 7 ✓7th **S72.122 Displaced fracture of lesser trochanter of left femur** MCC CC
  CC Excl: See code: S72.002
- 7 ✓7th **S72.123 Displaced fracture of lesser trochanter of unspecified femur** MCC CC
  CC Excl: See code: S72.009
- 7 ✓7th **S72.124 Nondisplaced fracture of lesser trochanter of right femur** MCC CC
  CC Excl: See code: S72.001
- 7 ✓7th **S72.125 Nondisplaced fracture of lesser trochanter of left femur** MCC CC
  CC Excl: See code: S72.002
- 7 ✓7th **S72.126 Nondisplaced fracture of lesser trochanter of unspecified femur** MCC CC
  CC Excl: See code: S72.009

✓6th **S72.13 Apophyseal fracture of femur**
EXCLUDES 1 *chronic (nontraumatic) slipped upper femoral epiphysis (M93.0-)*
- 7 ✓7th **S72.131 Displaced apophyseal fracture of right femur** MCC CC
  CC Excl: See code: S72.001
- 7 ✓7th **S72.132 Displaced apophyseal fracture of left femur** MCC CC
  CC Excl: See code: S72.002
- 7 ✓7th **S72.133 Displaced apophyseal fracture of unspecified femur** MCC CC
  CC Excl: See code: S72.009
- 7 ✓7th **S72.134 Nondisplaced apophyseal fracture of right femur** MCC CC
  CC Excl: See code: S72.001
- 7 ✓7th **S72.135 Nondisplaced apophyseal fractureof left femur** MCC CC
  CC Excl: See code: S72.002
- 7 ✓7th **S72.136 Nondisplaced apophyseal fracture of unspecified femur** MCC CC
  CC Excl: See code: S72.009

✓6th **S72.14 Intertrochanteric fracture of femur**
- 7 ✓7th **S72.141 Displaced intertrochanteric fracture of right femur** MCC CC
  CC Excl: See code: S72.001
- 7 ✓7th **S72.142 Displaced intertrochanteric fracture of left femur** MCC CC
  CC Excl: See code: S72.002
- 7 ✓7th **S72.143 Displaced intertrochanteric fracture of unspecified femur** MCC CC
  CC Excl: See code: S72.009
- 7 ✓7th **S72.144 Nondisplaced intertrochanteric fracture of right femur** MCC CC
  CC Excl: See code: S72.001
- 7 ✓7th **S72.145 Nondisplaced intertrochanteric fracture of left femur** MCC CC
  CC Excl: See code: S72.002
- 7 ✓7th **S72.146 Nondisplaced intertrochanteric fracture of unspecified femur** MCC CC
  CC Excl: See code: S72.009

✓5th **S72.2 Subtrochanteric fracture of femur**
- 7 ✓x7th **S72.21 Displaced subtrochanteric fracture of right femur** MCC CC
  CC Excl: See code: S72.001
- 7 ✓x7th **S72.22 Displaced subtrochanteric fracture of left femur** MCC CC
  CC Excl: See code: S72.002
- 7 ✓x7th **S72.23 Displaced subtrochanteric fracture of unspecified femur** MCC CC
  CC Excl: See code: S72.009
- 7 ✓x7th **S72.24 Nondisplaced subtrochanteric fracture of right femur** MCC CC
  CC Excl: See code: S72.001
- 7 ✓x7th **S72.25 Nondisplaced subtrochanteric fracture of left femur** MCC CC
  CC Excl: See code: S72.002
- 7 ✓x7th **S72.26 Nondisplaced subtrochanteric fracture of unspecified femur** MCC CC
  CC Excl: See code: S72.009

✓5th **S72.3 Fracture of shaft of femur**

✓6th **S72.30 Unspecified fracture of shaft of femur**
- 7 ✓7th **S72.301 Unspecified fracture of shaft of right femur** MCC CC
  CC Excl: See code: S72.001
- 7 ✓7th **S72.302 Unspecified fracture of shaft of left femur** MCC CC
  CC Excl: See code: S72.002
- 7 ✓7th **S72.309 Unspecified fracture of shaft of unspecified femur** MCC CC
  CC Excl: See code: S72.009

✓6th **S72.32 Transverse fracture of shaft of femur**
- 7 ✓7th **S72.321 Displaced transverse fracture of shaft of right femur** MCC CC
  CC Excl: See code: S72.001
- 7 ✓7th **S72.322 Displaced transverse fracture of shaft of left femur** MCC CC
  CC Excl: See code: S72.002
- 7 ✓7th **S72.323 Displaced transverse fracture of shaft of unspecified femur** MCC CC
  CC Excl: See code: S72.009
- 7 ✓7th **S72.324 Nondisplaced transverse fracture of shaft of right femur** MCC CC
  CC Excl: See code: S72.001
- 7 ✓7th **S72.325 Nondisplaced transverse fracture of shaft of left femur** MCC CC
  CC Excl: See code: S72.002
- 7 ✓7th **S72.326 Nondisplaced transverse fracture of shaft of unspecified femur** MCC CC
  CC Excl: See code: S72.009

✓6th **S72.33 Oblique fracture of shaft of femur**
- 7 ✓7th **S72.331 Displaced oblique fracture of shaft of right femur** MCC CC
  CC Excl: See code: S72.001
- 7 ✓7th **S72.332 Displaced oblique fracture of shaft of left femur** MCC CC
  CC Excl: See code: S72.002
- 7 ✓7th **S72.333 Displaced oblique fracture of shaft of unspecified femur** MCC CC
  CC Excl: See code: S72.009
- 7 ✓7th **S72.334 Nondisplaced oblique fracture of shaft of right femur** MCC CC
  CC Excl: See code: S72.001
- 7 ✓7th **S72.335 Nondisplaced oblique fracture of shaft of left femur** MCC CC
  CC Excl: See code: S72.002
- 7 ✓7th **S72.336 Nondisplaced oblique fracture of shaft of unspecified femur** MCC CC
  CC Excl: See code: S72.009

✓6th **S72.34 Spiral fracture of shaft of femur**
- 7 ✓7th **S72.341 Displaced spiral fracture of shaft of right femur** MCC CC
  CC Excl: See code: S72.001
- 7 ✓7th **S72.342 Displaced spiral fracture of shaft of left femur** MCC CC
  CC Excl: See code: S72.002

7 HAC = Initial encounter only (7th character A, B or C) and not POA.

7 ✓7th **S72.343** **Displaced spiral fracture of shaft of unspecified femur** MCC CC
CC Excl: See code: S72.009

7 ✓7th **S72.344** **Nondisplaced spiral fracture of shaft of right femur** MCC CC
CC Excl: See code: S72.001

7 ✓7th **S72.345** **Nondisplaced spiral fracture of shaft of left femur** MCC CC
CC Excl: See code: S72.002

7 ✓7th **S72.346** **Nondisplaced spiral fracture of shaft of unspecified femur** MCC CC
CC Excl: See code: S72.009

✓6th **S72.35** **Comminuted fracture of shaft of femur**

7 ✓7th **S72.351** **Displaced comminuted fracture of shaft of right femur** MCC CC
CC Excl: See code: S72.001

7 ✓7th **S72.352** **Displaced comminuted fracture of shaft of left femur** MCC CC
CC Excl: See code: S72.002

7 ✓7th **S72.353** **Displaced comminuted fracture of shaft of unspecified femur** MCC CC
CC Excl: See code: S72.009

7 ✓7th **S72.354** **Nondisplaced comminuted fracture of shaft of right femur** MCC CC
CC Excl: See code: S72.001

7 ✓7th **S72.355** **Nondisplaced comminuted fracture of shaft of left femur** MCC CC
CC Excl: See code: S72.002

7 ✓7th **S72.356** **Nondisplaced comminuted fracture of shaft of unspecified femur** MCC CC
CC Excl: See code: S72.009

✓6th **S72.36** **Segmental fracture of shaft of femur**

7 ✓7th **S72.361** **Displaced segmental fracture of shaft of right femur** MCC CC
CC Excl: See code: S72.001

7 ✓7th **S72.362** **Displaced segmental fracture of shaft of left femur** MCC CC
CC Excl: See code: S72.002

7 ✓7th **S72.363** **Displaced segmental fracture of shaft of unspecified femur** MCC CC
CC Excl: See code: S72.009

7 ✓7th **S72.364** **Nondisplaced segmental fracture of shaft of right femur** MCC CC
CC Excl: See code: S72.001

7 ✓7th **S72.365** **Nondisplaced segmental fracture of shaft of left femur** MCC CC
CC Excl: See code: S72.002

7 ✓7th **S72.366** **Nondisplaced segmental fracture of shaft of unspecified femur** MCC CC
CC Excl: See code: S72.009

✓6th **S72.39** **Other fracture of shaft of femur**

7 ✓7th **S72.391** **Other fracture of shaft of right femur** MCC CC
CC Excl: See code: S72.001

7 ✓7th **S72.392** **Other fracture of shaft of left femur** MCC CC
CC Excl: See code: S72.002

7 ✓7th **S72.399** **Other fracture of shaft of unspecified femur** MCC CC
CC Excl: See code: S72.009

✓5th **S72.4** **Fracture of lower end of femur**
Fracture of distal end of femur
EXCLUDES 2 *fracture of shaft of femur (S72.3-)*
physeal fracture of lower end of femur (S79.1-)

✓6th **S72.40** **Unspecified fracture of lower end of femur**

7 ✓7th **S72.401** **Unspecified fracture of lower end of right femur** MCC CC
CC Excl: CC with 7th character A: M80.00X-M80.019 with 7th A, M80.041-M80.059 with 7th A, M80.80X-M80.819 with 7th A, M80.841-M80.859 with 7th A, M84.40X-M84.419 with 7th A, M84.441-M84.459 with 7th A, M84.474-M84.519 with 7th A, M84.541-M84.559 with 7th A, M84.574-M84.576 with 7th A, M84.60X-M84.619 with 7th A, M84.641-M84.659 with 7th A, M84.674-M84.68X with 7th A, S03.8XX-S03.9XX with 7th A, S29.011-S29.019 with 7th A, S38.3XX-S39.013 with 7th A, S72.001-S72.471 with 7th [A, B, C], S72.479-S72.92X with 7th A, S73.101A, S73.109-S73.111 with 7th A, S73.119-S73.121 with 7th A, S73.129-S73.191 with 7th A, S73.199A, S76.001A, S76.009-S76.011 with 7th A, S76.019A, S76.091A, S76.099-S76.101 with 7th A, S76.109-S76.111 with 7th A, S76.119A, S76.191A, S76.199-S76.201 with 7th A, S76.209-S76.211 with 7th A, S76.219 with 7th A, S76.291A, S76.299-S76.301 with 7th A, S76.309-S76.311 with 7th A, S76.319A, S76.391A, S76.399-S76.801 with 7th A, S76.809-S76.811 with 7th A, S76.819A, S76.891A, S76.899-S76.901 with 7th A, S76.909-S76.911 with 7th A, S76.919A, S76.991A, S76.999A, S79.001A, S79.009-S79.011 with 7th A, S79.019-S79.091 with 7th A, S79.099-S79.101 with 7th A, S79.109-S79.111 with 7th A, S79.119-S79.121 with 7th A, S79.129-S79.131 with 7th A, S79.139-S79.141 with 7th A, S79.149-S79.191 with 7th A, S79.199-S79.811 with 7th A, S79.819-S79.821 with 7th A, S79.829-S79.911 with 7th A, S79.919-S79.921 with 7th A, S79.929 A, S82.90-S82.92X with 7th [A, B, C], T14.8-T14.91, T79.A9X-T79.9XX with 7th A
MCC with 7th B or C: M80.00X-M80.019 with 7th A, M80.041-M80.059 with 7th A, M80.80X-M80.819 with 7th A, M80.841-M80.859 with 7th A, M84.40X-M84.419 with 7th A, M84.441-M84.459 with 7th A, M84.474-M84.519 with 7th A, M84.541-M84.559 with 7th A, M84.574-M84.576 with 7th A, M84.60X-M84.619 with 7th A, M84.641-M84.659 with 7th A, M84.674-M84.68X with 7th A, S03.8XX-S03.9XX with 7th A, S29.011-S29.019 with 7th A, S38.3XX-S39.013 with 7th A, S72.001-S72.92X with 7th [A, B, C], S73.101-S73.199 with 7th A, S76.001-S76.019 with 7th A, S76.091-S76.119 with 7th A, S76.191-S76.219 with 7th A, S76.291-S76.319 with 7th A, S76.391-S76.819 with 7th A, S76.891-S76.919 with 7th A, S76.991-S76.999 with 7th A, S79.001-S79.929 with 7th A, S82.90X-S82.92X with 7th [A, B, C], T14.8-T14.91, T79.A9X-T79.9XX with 7th A
CC with 7th character K, M, N, P, Q or R: M80.00X-M84.68X with 7th [K, P], S02.0XX-S02.92X with 7th K, S12.000-S12.691 with 7th K, S22.000-S22.9XX with 7th K, S32.000-S32.9XX with 7th K, S42.001-S42.92X with 7th [K, P], S49.001-S49.199 with 7th [K, P], S52.001-S52.92X with 7th [K, M, N, P, Q, R], S59.001-S59.299 with 7th [K, P], S62.001-S62.92X with 7th [K, P], S72.001-S72.92X with 7th [K, M, N, P, Q, R], S79.001-S79.199 with 7th [K, P], S82.001-S82.92X with 7th [K, M, N, P, Q, R], S89.001-S89.399 with 7th [K, P], S92.001-S92.919 with 7th [K, P]

7 HAC = Initial encounter only (7th character A, B or C) and not POA.

7 ✓7th S72.4Ø2 **Unspecified fracture of lower end of left femur** MCC CC

CC Excl: CC with 7th character A: M8Ø.ØØX-M8Ø.Ø19 with 7th A, M8Ø.Ø41-M8Ø.Ø59 with 7th A, M8Ø.8ØX-M8Ø.819 with 7th A, M8Ø.841-M8Ø.859 with 7th A, M84.4ØX-M84.419 with 7th A, M84.441-M84.459 with 7th A, M84.474-M84.519 with 7th A, M84.541-M84.559 with 7th A, M84.574-M84.576 with 7th A, M84.6ØX-M84.619 with 7th A, M84.641-M84.659 with 7th A, M84.674-M84.68 with 7th A, SØ3.8XX-SØ3.9XX with 7th A, S29.Ø11-S29.Ø19 with 7th A, S38.3XX-S39.Ø13 with 7th A, S72.ØØ1-S72.466 with 7th [B, C], S72.472-S72.92X with 7th A, S73.1Ø2-S73.1Ø9 with 7th A, S73.112-S73.119 with 7th A, S73.122-S73.129 with 7th A, S73.192-S73.199 with 7th A, S76.ØØ2-S76.ØØ9 with 7th A, S76.Ø12-S76.Ø19 with 7th A, S76.Ø92-S76.Ø99 with 7th A, S76.1Ø2-S76.1Ø9 with 7th A, S76.112-S76.119 with 7th A, S76.192-S76.199 with 7th A, S76.2Ø2-S76.2Ø9 with 7th A, S76.212-S76.219 with 7th A, S76.292-S76.299 with 7th A, S76.3Ø2-S76.3Ø9 with 7th A, S76.312-S76.319 with 7th A, S76.392-S76.399 with 7th A, S76.8Ø2-S76.8Ø9 with 7th A, S76.812-S76.819 with 7th A, S76.892-S76.899 with 7th A, S76.9Ø2-S76.9Ø9 with 7th A, S76.912-S76.919 with 7th A, S76.992-S76.999 with 7th A, S79.ØØ2-S79.ØØ9 with 7th A, S79.Ø12-S79.Ø19 with 7th A, S79.Ø92-S79.Ø99 with 7th A, S79.1Ø2-S79.1Ø9 with 7th A, S79.112-S79.119 with 7th A, S79.122-S79.129 with 7th A, S79.132-S79.139 with 7th A, S79.142-S79.149 with 7th A, S79.192-S79.199 with 7th A, S79.812-S79.819 with 7th A, S79.822-S79.829 with 7th A, S79.912-S79.919 with 7th A, S79.922-S79.929 with 7th A, S82.9ØX-S82.92X with 7th [A, B, C], T14.8-T14.91, T79.A9X-T79.9XX with 7th A

MCC with 7th B or C: M8Ø.ØØX-M8Ø.Ø19 with 7th A, M8Ø.Ø41-M8Ø.Ø59 with 7th A, M8Ø.8ØX-M8Ø.819 with 7th A, M8Ø.841-M8Ø.859 with 7th A, M84.4ØX-M84.419 with 7th A, M84.441-M84.459 with 7th A, M84.474-M84.519 with 7th A, M84.541-M84.559 with 7th A, M84.574-M84.576 with 7th A, M84.6ØX-M84.619 with 7th A, M84.641-M84.659 with 7th A, M84.674-M84.68X with 7th A, SØ3.8XX-SØ3.9XX with 7th A, S29.Ø11-S29.Ø19 with 7th A, S38.3XX-S39.Ø13 with 7th A, S72.ØØ1-S72.92X with 7th [A, B, C], S73.1Ø1-S73.199 with 7th A, S76.ØØ1-S76.Ø19 with 7th A, S76.Ø91-S76.119 with 7th A, S76.191-S76.219 with 7th A, S76.291-S76.319 with 7th A, S76.391-S76.819 with 7th A, S76.891-S76.919 with 7th A, S76.991-S76.999 with 7th A, S79.ØØ1-S79.929 with 7th A, S82.9Ø-S82.92X with 7th [A, B, C], T14.8-T14.91, T79.A9X-T79.9XX with 7th A

CC with 7th character K, M, N, P, Q or R: M8Ø.ØØX-M84.68X with 7th [K, P], SØ2.ØXX-SØ2.92X with 7th K, S12.ØØØ-S12.691 with 7th K, S22.ØØØ-S22.9XX with 7th K, S32.ØØØ-S32.9XX with 7th K, S42.ØØ1-S42.92X with 7th [K, P], S49.ØØ1-S49.199 with 7th [K, P], S52.ØØ1-S52.92X with 7th [K, M, N, P, Q, R], S59.ØØ1-S59.299 with 7th [K, P], S62.ØØ1-S62.92X with 7th [K, P], S72.ØØ1-S72.92X with 7th [K, M, N, P, Q, R], S79.ØØ1-S79.199 with 7th [K, P], S82.ØØ1-S82.92X with 7th [K, M, N, P, Q, R], S89.ØØ1-S89.399 with 7th [K, P], S92.ØØ1-S92.919 with 7th [K, P]

7 ✓7th S72.4Ø9 **Unspecified fracture of lower end of unspecified femur** MCC CC

CC Excl: CC with 7th character A, MCC with 7th B or C: M8Ø.ØØX-M8Ø.Ø19 with 7th A, M8Ø.Ø41-M8Ø.Ø59 with 7th A, M8Ø.8ØX-M8Ø.819 with 7th A, M8Ø.841-M8Ø.859 with 7th A, M84.4ØX-M84.419 with 7th A, M84.441-M84.459 with 7th A, M84.474-M84.519 with 7th A, M84.541-M84.559 with 7th A, M84.574-M84.576 with 7th A, M84.6ØX-M84.619 with 7th A, M84.641-M84.659 with 7th A, M84.674-M84.68 with 7th A, SØ3.8XX-SØ3.9XX with 7th A, S29.Ø11-S29.Ø19 with 7th A, S38.3XX-S39.Ø13 with 7th A, S72.ØØ1-S72.92X with 7th [A, B, C], S73.1Ø1-S73.199 with 7th A, S76.ØØ1-S76.Ø19 with 7th A, S76.Ø91-S76.119 with 7th A, S76.191-S76.219 with 7th A, S76.291-S76.319 with 7th A, S76.391-S76.819 with 7th A, S76.891-S76.919 with 7th A, S76.991-S76.999 with 7th A, S79.ØØ1-S79.929 with 7th A, S82.9ØX-S82.92X with 7th [A, B, C], T14.8-T14.91, T79.A9X-T79.9XX with 7th A

CC with 7th character K, M, N, P, Q or R: M8Ø.ØØX-M84.68X with 7th [K, P], SØ2.ØXX-SØ2.92X with 7th K, S12.ØØØ-S12.691 with 7th K, S22.ØØØ-S22.9XX with 7th K, S32.ØØØ-S32.9XX with 7th K, S42.ØØ1-S42.92X with 7th [K, P], S49.ØØ1-S49.199 with 7th [K, P], S52.ØØ1-S52.92X with 7th [K, M, N, P, Q, R], S59.ØØ1-S59.299 with 7th [K, P], S62.ØØ1-S62.92X with 7th [K, P], S72.ØØ1-S72.92X with 7th [K, M, N, P, Q, R], S79.ØØ1-S79.199 with 7th [K, P], S82.ØØ1-S82.92X with 7th [K, M, N, P, Q, R], S89.ØØ1-S89.399 with 7th [K, P], S92.ØØ1-S92.919 with 7th [K, P]

✓6th **S72.41 Unspecified condyle fracture of lower end of femur**

Condyle fracture of femur NOS

7 ✓7th S72.411 **Displaced unspecified condyle fracture of lower end of right femur** MCC CC
CC Excl: See code: S72.4Ø1

7 ✓7th S72.412 **Displaced unspecified condyle fracture of lower end of left femur** MCC CC
CC Excl: See code: S72.4Ø2

7 ✓7th S72.413 **Displaced unspecified condyle fracture of lower end of unspecified femur** MCC CC
CC Excl: See code: S72.4Ø9

7 ✓7th S72.414 **Nondisplaced unspecified condyle fracture of lower end of right femur** MCC CC
CC Excl: See code: S72.4Ø1

7 ✓7th S72.415 **Nondisplaced unspecified condyle fracture of lower end of left femur** MCC CC
CC Excl: See code: S72.4Ø2

7 ✓7th S72.416 **Nondisplaced unspecified condyle fracture of lower end of unspecified femur** MCC CC
CC Excl: See code: S72.4Ø9

✓6th **S72.42 Fracture of lateral condyle of femur**

7 ✓7th S72.421 **Displaced fracture of lateral condyle of right femur** MCC CC
CC Excl: See code: S72.4Ø1

7 ✓7th S72.422 **Displaced fracture of lateral condyle of left femur** MCC CC
CC Excl: See code: S72.4Ø2

7 ✓7th S72.423 **Displaced fracture of lateral condyle of unspecified femur** MCC CC
CC Excl: See code: S72.4Ø9

7 ✓7th S72.424 **Nondisplaced fracture of lateral condyle of right femur** MCC CC
CC Excl: See code: S72.4Ø1

7 ✓7th S72.425 **Nondisplaced fracture of lateral condyle of left femur** MCC CC
CC Excl: See code: S72.4Ø2

7 ✓7th S72.426 **Nondisplaced fracture of lateral condyle of unspecified femur** MCC CC
CC Excl: See code: S72.4Ø9

7 HAC = Initial encounter only (7th character A, B or C) and not POA.

✓6th **S72.43 Fracture of medial condyle of femur**

7 ✓7th **S72.431 Displaced fracture of medial condyle of right femur** MCC CC
CC Excl: See code: S72.401

7 ✓7th **S72.432 Displaced fracture of medial condyle of left femur** MCC CC
CC Excl: See code: S72.402

7 ✓7th **S72.433 Displaced fracture of medial condyle of unspecified femur** MCC CC
CC Excl: See code: S72.409

7 ✓7th **S72.434 Nondisplaced fracture of medial condyle of right femur** MCC CC
CC Excl: See code: S72.401

7 ✓7th **S72.435 Nondisplaced fracture of medial condyle of left femur** MCC CC
CC Excl: See code: S72.402

7 ✓7th **S72.436 Nondisplaced fracture of medial condyle of unspecified femur** MCC CC
CC Excl: See code: S72.409

✓6th **S72.44 Fracture of lower epiphysis (separation) of femur**
EXCLUDES1 *Salter-Harris Type I physeal fracture of lower end of femur (S79.11-)*

7 ✓7th **S72.441 Displaced fracture of lower epiphysis (separation) of right femur** MCC CC
CC Excl: See code: S72.401

7 ✓7th **S72.442 Displaced fracture of lower epiphysis (separation) of left femur** MCC CC
CC Excl: See code: S72.402

7 ✓7th **S72.443 Displaced fracture of lower epiphysis (separation) of unspecified femur** MCC CC
CC Excl: See code: S72.409

7 ✓7th **S72.444 Nondisplaced fracture of lower epiphysis (separation) of right femur** MCC CC
CC Excl: See code: S72.401

7 ✓7th **S72.445 Nondisplaced fracture of lower epiphysis (separation) of left femur** MCC CC
CC Excl: See code: S72.402

7 ✓7th **S72.446 Nondisplaced fracture of lower epiphysis (separation) of unspecified femur** MCC CC
CC Excl: See code: S72.409

✓6th **S72.45 Supracondylar fracture without intracondylar extension of lower end of femur**
Supracondylar fracture of lower end of femur NOS
EXCLUDES1 *supracondylar fracture with intracondylar extension of lower end of femur (S72.46-)*

7 ✓7th **S72.451 Displaced supracondylar fracture without intracondylar extension of lower end of right femur** MCC CC
CC Excl: See code: S72.401

7 ✓7th **S72.452 Displaced supracondylar fracture without intracondylar extension of lower end of left femur** MCC CC
CC Excl: See code: S72.402

7 ✓7th **S72.453 Displaced supracondylar fracture without intracondylar extension of lower end of unspecified femur** MCC CC
CC Excl: See code: S72.409

7 ✓7th **S72.454 Nondisplaced supracondylar fracture without intracondylar extension of lower end of right femur** MCC CC
CC Excl: See code: S72.401

7 ✓7th **S72.455 Nondisplaced supracondylar fracture without intracondylar extension of lower end of left femur** MCC CC
CC Excl: See code: S72.402

7 ✓7th **S72.456 Nondisplaced supracondylar fracture without intracondylar extension of lower end of unspecified femur** MCC CC
CC Excl: See code: S72.409

✓6th **S72.46 Supracondylar fracture with intracondylar extension of lower end of femur**
EXCLUDES1 *supracondylar fracture without intracondylar extension of lower end of femur (S72.45-)*

7 ✓7th **S72.461 Displaced supracondylar fracture with intracondylar extension of lower end of right femur** MCC CC
CC Excl: See code: S72.401

7 ✓7th **S72.462 Displaced supracondylar fracture with intracondylar extension of lower end of left femur** MCC CC
CC Excl: See code: S72.402

7 ✓7th **S72.463 Displaced supracondylar fracture with intracondylar extension of lower end of unspecified femur** MCC CC
CC Excl: See code: S72.409

7 ✓7th **S72.464 Nondisplaced supracondylar fracture with intracondylar extension of lower end of right femur** MCC CC
CC Excl: See code: S72.401

7 ✓7th **S72.465 Nondisplaced supracondylar fracture with intracondylar extension of lower end of left femur** MCC CC
CC Excl: See code: S72.402

7 ✓7th **S72.466 Nondisplaced supracondylar fracture with intracondylar extension of lower end of unspecified femur** MCC CC
CC Excl: See code: S72.409

✓6th **S72.47 Torus fracture of lower end of femur**

The appropriate 7th character is to be added to all codes in subcategory S72.47.
A initial encounter for closed fracture
D subsequent encounter for fracture with routine healing
G subsequent encounter for fracture with delayed healing
K subsequent encounter for fracture with nonunion
P subsequent encounter for fracture with malunion
S sequela

7 ✓7th **S72.471 Torus fracture of lower end of right femur** CC
CC Excl: CC with 7th character A: M80.00X-M80.019 with 7th A, M80.041-M80.059 with 7th A, M80.80X-M80.819 with 7th A, M80.841-M80.859 with 7th A, M84.40X-M84.419 with 7th A, M84.441-M84.459 with 7th A, M84.474-M84.519 with 7th A, M84.541-M84.559 with 7th A, M84.574-M84.576 with 7th A, M84.60X-M84.619 with 7th A, M84.641-M84.659 with 7th A, M84.674-M84.68X with 7th A, S03.8XX-S03.9XX with 7th A, S29.011-S29.019 with 7th A, S38.3X-S39.013 with 7th A, S72.001-S72.471 with 7th [A, B, C], S72.479-S72.92X with 7th A, S73.101 with 7th A, S73.109-S73.111 with 7th A, S73.119-S73.121 with 7th A, S73.129-S73.191 with 7th A, S73.199 with 7th A, S76.001 with 7th A, S76.009-S76.011 with 7th A, S76.019A, S76.091A, S76.099-S76.101 with 7th A, S76.109-S76.111 with 7th A, S76.119A, S76.191A, S76.199-S76.201 with 7th A, S76.209-S76.211 with 7th A, S76.219A, S76.291 A, S76.299-S76.301 with 7th A, S76.309-S76.311 with 7th A, S76.319A, S76.391A, S76.399-S76.801 with 7th A, S76.809-S76.811 with 7th A, S76.819A, S76.891A, S76.899-S76.901 with 7th A, S76.909-S76.911 with 7th A, S76.919A, S76.991A, S76.999A, S79.001A, S79.009-S79.011 with 7th A, S79.019-S79.091 with 7th A, S79.099-S79.101 with 7th A, S79.109-S79.111 with 7th A, S79.119-S79.121 with 7th A, S79.129-S79.131 with 7th A, S79.139-S79.141 with 7th A, S79.149-S79.191 with 7th A, S79.199-S79.811 with 7th A, S79.819-S79.821 with 7th A, S79.829-S79.911 with 7th A, S79.919-S79.921 with 7th A, S79.929A, S82.90X-S82.92X with 7th [A, B, C], T14.8-T14.91, T79.A9X-T79.9XX with 7th A

7 HAC = Initial encounter only (7th character A, B or C) and not POA.

CC Excl: CC with 7th character K or P: M80.00X-M84.68X with 7th [K, P], S02.0XX-S02.92X with 7th K, S12.000-S12.691 with 7th K, S22.000-S22.9XX with 7th K, S32.000-S32.9XX with 7th K, S42.001-S42.92X with 7th [K, P], S49.001-S49.199 with 7th [K, P], S52.001-S52.92X with 7th [K, M, N, P, Q, R], S59.001-S59.299 with 7th [K, P], S62.001-S62.92X with 7th [K, P], S72.001-S72.92X with 7th [K, M, N, P, Q, R], S79.001-S79.199 with 7th [K, P], S82.001-S82.92X with 7th [K, M, N, P, Q, R], S89.001-S89.399 with 7th [K, P], S92.001-S92.919 with 7th [K, P]

7 ✓7th **S72.472 Torus fracture of lower end of left femur** CC

CC Excl: CC with 7th character A: M80.00X-M80.019 with 7th A, M80.041-M80.059 with 7th A, M80.80X-M80.819 with 7th A, M80.841-M80.859 with 7th A, M84.40X-M84.419 with 7th A, M84.441-M84.459 with 7th A, M84.474-M84.519 with 7th A, M84.541-M84.559 with 7th A, M84.574-M84.576 with 7th A, M84.60X-M84.619 with 7th A, M84.641-M84.659 with 7th A, M84.674-M84.68 with 7th A, S03.8XX-S03.9XX with 7th A, S29.011-S29.019 with 7th A, S38.3XX-S39.013 with 7th A, S72.001-S72.466 with 7th [B, C], S72.472-S72.92X with 7th A, S73.102-S73.109 with 7th A, S73.112-S73.119 with 7th A, S73.122-S73.129 with 7th A, S73.192-S73.199 with 7th A, S76.002-S76.009 with 7th A, S76.012-S76.019 with 7th A, S76.092-S76.099 with 7th A, S76.102-S76.109 with 7th A, S76.112-S76.119 with 7th A, S76.192-S76.199 with 7th A, S76.202-S76.209 with 7th A, S76.212-S76.219 with 7th A, S76.292-S76.299 with 7th A, S76.302-S76.309 with 7th A, S76.312-S76.319 with 7th A, S76.392-S76.399 with 7th A, S76.802-S76.809 with 7th A, S76.812-S76.819 with 7th A, S76.892-S76.899 with 7th A, S76.902-S76.909 with 7th A, S76.912-S76.919 with 7th A, S76.992-S76.999 with 7th A, S79.002-S79.009 with 7th A, S79.012-S79.019 with 7th A, S79.092-S79.099 with 7th A, S79.102-S79.109 with 7th A, S79.112-S79.119 with 7th A, S79.122-S79.129 with 7th A, S79.132-S79.139 with 7th A, S79.142-S79.149 with 7th A, S79.192-S79.199 with 7th A, S79.812-S79.819 with 7th A, S79.822-S79.829 with 7th A, S79.912-S79.919 with 7th A, S79.922-S79.929 with 7th A, S82.90X-S82.92X with 7th [A, B, C], T14.8-T14.91, T79.A9X-T79.9XX with 7th A

CC Excl: CC with 7th character K or P: M80.00X-M84.68X with 7th [K, P], S02.0XX-S02.92X with 7th K, S12.000-S12.691 with 7th K, S22.000-S22.9XX with 7th K, S32.000-S32.9XX with 7th K, S42.001-S42.92X with 7th [K, P], S49.001-S49.199 with 7th [K, P], S52.001-S52.92X with 7th [K, M, N, P, Q, R], S59.001-S59.299 with 7th [K, P], S62.001-S62.92X with 7th [K, P], S72.001-S72.92X with 7th [K, M, N, P, Q, R], S79.001-S79.199 with 7th [K, P], S82.001-S82.92X with 7th [K, M, N, P, Q, R], S89.001-S89.399 with 7th [K, P], S92.001-S92.919 with 7th [K, P]

7 ✓7th **S72.479 Torus fracture of lower end of unspecified femur** CC

CC Excl: CC with 7th character A: M80.00X-M80.019 with 7th A, M80.041-M80.059 with 7th A, M80.80X-M80.819 with 7th A, M80.841-M80.859 with 7th A, M84.40X-M84.419 with 7th A, M84.441-M84.459 with 7th A, M84.474-M84.519 with 7th A, M84.541-M84.559 with 7th A, M84.574-M84.576 with 7th A, M84.60X-M84.619 with 7th A, M84.641-M84.659 with 7th A, M84.674-M84.68X with 7th A, S03.8XX-S03.9XX with 7th A, S29.011-S29.019 with 7th A, S38.3XX-S39.013 with 7th A, S72.001-S72.471 with 7th [A, B, C], S72.479-S72.92X with 7th A, S73.101A, S73.109-S73.111 with 7th A, S73.119-S73.121 with 7th A, S73.129-S73.191 with 7th A, S73.199A, S76.001A, S76.009-S76.011 with 7th A, S76.019A, S76.091A, S76.099-S76.101 with 7th A, S76.109-S76.111 with 7th A, S76.119A, S76.191A, S76.199-S76.201 with 7th A, S76.209-S76.211 with 7th A, S76.219A, S76.291A, S76.299-S76.301 with 7th A, S76.309-S76.311 with 7th A, S76.319A, S76.391A, S76.399-S76.801 with 7th A, S76.809-S76.811 with 7th A, S76.819A, S76.891A, S76.899-S76.901 with 7th A, S76.909-S76.911 with 7th A, S76.919A, S76.991A, S76.999A, S79.001A, S79.009-S79.011 with 7th A, S79.019-S79.091 with 7th A, S79.099-S79.101 with 7th A, S79.109-S79.111 with 7th A, S79.119-S79.121 with 7th A, S79.129-S79.131 with 7th A, S79.139-S79.141 with 7th A, S79.149-S79.191 with 7th A, S79.199-S79.811 with 7th A, S79.819-S79.821 with 7th A, S79.829-S79.911 with 7th A, S79.919-S79.921 with 7th A, S79.929A, S82.90X-S82.92X with 7th [A, B, C], T14.8-T14.91, T79.A9X-T79.9XX with 7th A

CC with 7th character K or P: M80.00X-M84.68X with 7th [K, P], S02.0XX-S02.92X with 7th K, S12.000-S12.691 with 7th K, S22.000-S22.9XX with 7th K, S32.000-S32.9XX with 7th K, S42.001-S42.92X with 7th [K, P], S49.001-S49.199 with 7th [K, P], S52.001-S52.92X with 7th [K, M, N, P, Q, R], S59.001-S59.299 with 7th [K, P], S62.001-S62.92X with 7th [K, P], S72.001-S72.92X with 7th [K, M, N, P, Q, R], S79.001-S79.199 with 7th [K, P], S82.001-S82.92X with 7th [K, M, N, P, Q, R], S89.001-S89.399 with 7th [K, P], S92.001-S92.919 with 7th [K, P]

✓6th **S72.49 Other fracture of lower end of femur**

7 ✓7th **S72.491 Other fracture of lower end of right femur** MCC CC

CC Excl: CC for codes with 7th A: M80.00X-M80.019 with 7th A, M80.041-M80.059 with 7th A, M80.80X-M80.819 with 7th A, M80.841-M80.859 with 7th A, M84.40X-M84.419 with 7th A, M84.441-M84.459 with 7th A, M84.474-M84.519 with 7th A, M84.541-M84.559 with 7th A, M84.574-M84.576 with 7th A, M84.60X-M84.619 with 7th A, M84.641-M84.659 with 7th A, M84.674-M84.68 with 7th A, S03.8XX-S03.9XX with 7th A, S29.011-S29.019 with 7th A, S38.3XX-S39.013 with 7th A, S72.001-S72.471 with 7th [A, B, C], S72.479-S72.92X with 7th A, S73.101 with 7th A, S73.109-S73.111 with 7th A, S73.119-S73.121 with 7th A, S73.129-S73.191 with 7th A, S73.199A, S76.001A, S76.009-S76.011 with 7th A, S76.019A, S76.091A, S76.099-S76.101 with 7th A, S76.109-S76.111 with 7th A, S76.119 A, S76.191A, S76.199-S76.201 with 7th A, S76.209-S76.211 with 7th A, S76.219A, S76.291A, S76.299-S76.301 with 7th A, S76.309-S76.311 with 7th A, S76.319A, S76.391A, S76.399-S76.801 with 7th A, S76.809-S76.811 with 7th A, S76.819A, S76.891A, S76.899-S76.901 with 7th A, S76.909-S76.911 with 7th A, S76.919A, S76.991A, S76.999A, S79.001A, S79.009-S79.011 with 7th A, S79.019-S79.091 with 7th A, S79.099-S79.101 with 7th A, S79.109-S79.111 with 7th A, S79.119-S79.121 with 7th A, S79.129-S79.131 with 7th A, S79.139-S79.141 with 7th A, S79.149-S79.191 with 7th A, S79.199-S79.811 with 7th A, S79.819-

7 HAC = Initial encounter only (7th character A, B or C) and not POA.

S79.821 with 7th A, S79.829-S79.911 with 7th A, S79.919-S79.921 with 7th A, S79.929A, S82.90-S82.92 with 7th [A, B, C], T14.8-T14.91, T79.A9X-T79.9XX with 7th A

MCC for codes with 7th B or C: M80.00X-M80.019 with 7th A, M80.041-M80.059 with 7th A, M80.80X-M80.819 with 7th A, M80.841-M80.859 with 7th A, M84.40X-M84.419 with 7th A, M84.441-M84.459 with 7th A, M84.474-M84.519 with 7th A, M84.541-M84.559 with 7th A, M84.574-M84.576 with 7th A, M84.60X-M84.619 with 7th A, M84.641-M84.659 with 7th A, M84.674-M84.68 with 7th A, S03.8XX-S03.9XX with 7th A, S29.011-S29.019 with 7th A, S38.3XX-S39.013 with 7th A, S72.491-S72.499 with 7th [B, C], S73.101-S73.199 with 7th A, S76.001-S76.019 with 7th A, S76.091-S76.119 with 7th A, S76.191-S76.219 with 7th A, S76.291-S76.319 with 7th A, S76.391-S76.819 with 7th A, S76.891-S76.919 with 7th A, S76.991-S76.999 with 7th A, S79.811-S79.929 with 7th A, S82.001-S82.099 with 7th [A, B, C], S82.90X-S82.92X with 7th [A, B, C], T14.8-T14.91, T79.A9X-T79.9XX with 7th A

CC for codes with 7th K, M, N, P, Q or R: M80.00X-M84.68X with 7th [K, P], S02.0XX-S02.92X with 7th K, S12.000-S12.691 with 7th K, S22.000-S22.9XX with 7th K, S32.000-S32.9XX with 7th K, S42.001-S42.92X with 7th [K, P], S49.001-S49.199 with 7th [K, P], S52.001-S52.92X with 7th [K, M, N, P, Q, R], S59.001-S59.299 with 7th [K, P], S62.001-S62.92X with 7th [K, P], S72.001-S72.92X with 7th [K, M, N, P, Q, R], S79.001-S79.199 with 7th [K, P], S82.001-S82.92X with 7th [K, M, N, P, Q, R], S89.001-S89.399 with 7th [K, P], S92.001-S92.919 with 7th [K, P]

7 ✓7th **S72.492 Other fracture of lower end of left femur** MCC CC

CC Excl: CC for codes with 7th A: M80.00X-M80.019 with 7th A, M80.041-M80.059 with 7th A, M80.80X-M80.819 with 7th A, M80.841-M80.859 with 7th A, M84.40X-M84.419 with 7th A, M84.441-M84.459 with 7th A, M84.474-M84.519 with 7th A, M84.541-M84.559 with 7th A, M84.574-M84.576 with 7th A, M84.60X-M84.619 with 7th A, M84.641-M84.659 with 7th A, M84.674-M84.68 with 7th A, S03.8XX-S03.9XX with 7th A, S29.011-S29.019 with 7th A, S38.3XX-S39.013 with 7th A, S72.001-S72.466 with 7th [B, C], S72.472-S72.92X with 7th A, S73.102-S73.109 with 7th A, S73.112-S73.119 with 7th A, S73.122-S73.129 with 7th A, S73.192-S73.199 with 7th A, S76.002-S76.009 with 7th A, S76.012-S76.019 with 7th A, S76.092-S76.099 with 7th A, S76.102-S76.109 with 7th A, S76.112-S76.119 with 7th A, S76.192-S76.199 with 7th A, S76.202-S76.209 with 7th A, S76.212-S76.219 with 7th A, S76.292-S76.299 with 7th A, S76.302-S76.309 with 7th A, S76.312-S76.319 with 7th A, S76.392-S76.399 with 7th A, S76.802-S76.809 with 7th A, S76.812-S76.819 with 7th A, S76.892-S76.899 with 7th A, S76.902-S76.909 with 7th A, S76.912-S76.919 with 7th A, S76.992-S76.999 with 7th A, S79.002-S79.009 with 7th A, S79.012-S79.019 with 7th A, S79.092-S79.099 with 7th A, S79.102-S79.109 with 7th A, S79.112-S79.119 with 7th A, S79.122-S79.129 with 7th A, S79.132-S79.139 with 7th A, S79.142-S79.149 with 7th A, S79.192-S79.199 with 7th A, S79.812-S79.819 with 7th A, S79.822-S79.829 with 7th A, S79.912-S79.919 with 7th A, S79.922-S79.929 with 7th A, S82.90X-S82.92X with 7th [A, B, C], T14.8-T14.91, T79.A9X-T79.9XX with 7th A

MCC for codes with 7th B or C: M80.00X-M80.019 with 7th A, M80.041-M80.059 with 7th A, M80.80X-M80.819 with 7th A, M80.841-M80.859 with 7th A, M84.40X-M84.419 with 7th A, M84.441-M84.459 with 7th A, M84.474-M84.519 with 7th A, M84.541-M84.559 with 7th A, M84.574-M84.576 with 7th A, M84.60X-M84.619 with 7th A, M84.641-M84.659 with 7th A, M84.674-M84.68 with 7th A, S03.8XX-S03.9XX with 7th A, S29.011-S29.019 with 7th A, S38.3X-S39.013 with 7th A, S72.491-S72.499 with 7th [B, C], S73.101-S73.199 with 7th A, S76.001-S76.019 with 7th A, S76.091-S76.119 with 7th A, S76.191-S76.219 with 7th A, S76.291-S76.319 with 7th A, S76.391-S76.819 with 7th A, S76.891-S76.919 with 7th A, S76.991-S76.999 with 7th A, S79.811-S79.929 with 7th A, S82.001-S82.099 with 7th [A, B, C], S82.90X-S82.92X with 7th [A, B, C], T14.8-T14.91, T79.A9X-T79.9XX with 7th A

CC for codes with 7th K, M, N, P, Q or R: M80.00X-M84.68 with 7th [K, P], S02.0XX-S02.92X with 7th K, S12.000-S12.691 with 7th K, S22.000-S22.9XX with 7th K, S32.000-S32.9XX with 7th K, S42.001-S42.92X with 7th [K, P], S49.001-S49.199 with 7th [K, P], S52.001-S52.92X with 7th [K, M, N, P, Q, R], S59.001-S59.299 with 7th [K, P], S62.001-S62.92X with 7th [K, P], S72.001-S72.92X with 7th [K, M, N, P, Q, R], S79.001-S79.199 with 7th [K, P], S82.001-S82.92X with 7th [K, M, N, P, Q, R], S89.001-S89.399 with 7th [K, P], S92.001-S92.919 with 7th [K, P]

7 ✓7th **S72.499 Other fracture of lower end of unspecified femur** MCC CC

CC Excl: CC for codes with 7th A: M80.00X-M80.019 with 7th A, M80.041-M80.059 with 7th A, M80.80X-M80.819 with 7th A, M80.841-M80.859 with 7th A, M84.40X-M84.419 with 7th A, M84.441-M84.459 with 7th A, M84.474-M84.519 with 7th A, M84.541-M84.559 with 7th A, M84.574-M84.576 with 7th A, M84.60X-M84.619 with 7th A, M84.641-M84.659 with 7th A, M84.674-M84.68 with 7th A, S03.8XX-S03.9XX with 7th A, S29.011-S29.019 with 7th A, S38.3XX-S39.013 with 7th A, S72.001-S72.92X with 7th [A, B, C], S73.101-S73.199 with 7th A, S76.001-S76.019 with 7th A, S76.091-S76.119 with 7th A, S76.191-S76.219 with 7th A, S76.291-S76.319 with 7th A, S76.391-S76.819 with 7th A, S76.891-S76.919 with 7th A, S76.991-S76.999 with 7th A, S79.001-S79.929 with 7th A, S82.90X-S82.92X with 7th [A, B, C], T14.8-T14.91, T79.A9X-T79.9XX with 7th A

MCC for codes with 7th B or C: M80.00X-M80.019 with 7th A, M80.041-M80.059 with 7th A, M80.80X-M80.819 with 7th A, M80.841-M80.859 with 7th A, M84.40X-M84.419 with 7th A, M84.441-M84.459 with 7th A, M84.474-M84.519 with 7th A, M84.541-M84.559 with 7th A, M84.574-M84.576 with 7th A, M84.60X-M84.619 with 7th A, M84.641-M84.659 with 7th A, M84.674-M84.68X with 7th A, S03.8XX-S03.9XX with 7th A, S29.011-S29.019 with 7th A, S38.3XX-S39.013 with 7th A, S72.491-S72.499 with 7th [B, C], S73.101-S73.199 with 7th A, S76.001-S76.019 with 7th A, S76.091-S76.119 with 7th A, S76.191-S76.219 with 7th A, S76.291-S76.319 with 7th A, S76.391-S76.819 with 7th A, S76.891-S76.919 with 7th A, S76.991-S76.999 with 7th A, S79.811-S79.929 with 7th A, S82.001-S82.099 with 7th [A, B, C], S82.90X-S82.92X with 7th [A, B, C], T14.8-T14.91, T79.A9X-T79.9XX with 7th A

CC for codes with 7th K, M, N, P, Q or R: M80.00X-M84.68X with 7th [K, P], S02.0XX-S02.92X with 7th K, S12.000-S12.691 with 7th K, S22.000-S22.9XX with 7th K, S32.000-S32.9XX with 7th K, S42.001-S42.92X with 7th [K, P], S49.001-S49.199 with 7th [K, P], S52.001-S52.92X with 7th [K, M, N, P, Q, R], S59.001-S59.299 with 7th [K, P], S62.001-S62.92X with 7th [K, P], S72.001-S72.92X with 7th [K, M, N, P, Q, R], S79.001-S79.199 with 7th [K, P], S82.001-S82.92X with 7th [K, M, N, P, Q, R], S89.001-S89.399 with 7th [K, P], S92.001-S92.919 with 7th [K, P]

7 HAC = Initial encounter only (7th character A, B or C) and not POA.

5th S72.8 Other fracture of femur

6th S72.8X Other fracture of femur

CC Excl: For CC/MCC codes in subcategory S72.8X, unless otherwise noted: MCC with 7th A,B or C: M48.40X-M48.58X with 7th A, M80.00X-M84.68X with 7th A, S03.8XX-S03.9XX with 7th A, S29.011-S29.019 with 7th A, S38.3XX-S39.013 with 7th A, S72.001-S72.92X with 7th [A, B, C], S73.101-S73.199 with 7th A, S76.001-S76.019 with 7th A, S76.091-S76.119 with 7th A, S76.191-S76.219 with 7th A, S76.291-S76.319 with 7th A, S76.391-S76.819 with 7th A, S76.891-S76.919 with 7th A, S76.991-S76.999 with 7th A, S79.001-S79.929 with 7th A, S82.90X-S82.92X with 7th [A, B, C], T14.8-T14.91, T79.A0X-T79.9XX with 7th A

CC with 7th character K, M, N, P, Q or R: M80.00X-M84.68X with 7th [K, P], S02.0XX-S02.92X with 7th K, S12.000-S12.691 with 7th K, S22.000-S22.9XX with 7th K, S32.000-S32.9XX with 7th K, S42.001-S42.92X with 7th [K, P], S49.001-S49.199 with 7th [K, P], S52.001-S52.92X with 7th [K, M, N, P, Q, R], S59.001-S59.299 with 7th [K, P], S62.001-S62.92X with 7th [K, P], S72.001-S72.92X with 7th [K, M, N, P, Q, R], S79.001-S79.199 with 7th [K, P], S82.001-S82.92X with 7th [K, M, N, P, Q, R], S89.001-S89.399 with 7th [K, P], S92.001-S92.919 with 7th [K, P]K

7 7th **S72.8X1 Other fracture of right femur** MCC CC

7 7th **S72.8X2 Other fracture of left femur** MCC CC

7 7th **S72.8X9 Other fracture of unspecified femur** MCC CC

5th S72.9 Unspecified fracture of femur

Fracture of thigh NOS

Fracture of upper leg NOS

EXCLUDES1 *fracture of hip NOS (S72.00-, S72.01-)*

7 x7th **S72.90 Unspecified fracture of unspecified femur** MCC CC

AHA: 2012, 4Q, 93

CC Excl: See code: S72.8X

7 x7th **S72.91 Unspecified fracture of right femur** MCC CC

CC Excl: See code: S72.8X

7 x7th **S72.92 Unspecified fracture of left femur** MCC CC

CC Excl: See code: S72.8X

4th S73 Dislocation and sprain of joint and ligaments of hip

INCLUDES avulsion of joint or ligament of hip
laceration of cartilage, joint or ligament of hip
sprain of cartilage, joint or ligament of hip
traumatic hemarthrosis of joint or ligament of hip
traumatic rupture of joint or ligament of hip
traumatic subluxation of joint or ligament of hip
traumatic tear of joint or ligament of hip

Code also any associated open wound

EXCLUDES2 *strain of muscle, fascia and tendon of hip and thigh (S76.-)*

The appropriate 7th character is to be added to each code from category S73.

A initial encounter
D subsequent encounter
S sequela

5th S73.0 Subluxation and dislocation of hip

EXCLUDES2 *dislocation and subluxation of hip prosthesis (T84.020, T84.021)*

6th S73.00 Unspecified subluxation and dislocation of hip

Dislocation of hip NOS

Subluxation of hip NOS

7 7th **S73.001 Unspecified subluxation of right hip** CC

CC Excl: CC with 7th character A: M99.16-M99.17, M99.19, S33.30X-S33.39X with 7th A, S73.001A, S73.003-S73.004 with 7th A, S73.006A, S73.041A, S73.043-S73.044 with 7th A, S73.046A

7 7th **S73.002 Unspecified subluxation of left hip** CC

CC Excl: CC with 7th character A: M99.16-M99.17, M99.19, S33.30X-S33.39X with 7th A, S73.002-S73.003 with 7th A, S73.005-S73.006 with 7th A, S73.042-S73.043 with 7th A, S73.045-S73.046 with 7th A

7 7th **S73.003 Unspecified subluxation of unspecified hip** CC

CC Excl: CC with 7th character A: M99.16-M99.17, M99.19, S33.30X-S33.39X with 7th A, S73.001-S73.006 with 7th A, S73.041-S73.046 with 7th A

7 7th **S73.004 Unspecified dislocation of right hip** CC

CC Excl: See code: S73.001

7 7th **S73.005 Unspecified dislocation of left hip** CC

CC Excl: See code: S73.002

7 7th **S73.006 Unspecified dislocation of unspecified hip** CC

CC Excl: See code: S73.003

6th S73.01 Posterior subluxation and dislocation of hip

7 7th **S73.011 Posterior subluxation of right hip** CC

CC Excl: CC with 7th character A: M99.16-M99.17, M99.19, S33.30X-S33.39X with 7th A, S73.011 with 7th A, S73.013-S73.014 with 7th A, S73.016 with 7th A

7 7th **S73.012 Posterior subluxation of left hip** CC

CC Excl: CC with 7th character A: M99.16-M99.17, M99.19, S33.30X-S33.39X with 7th A, S73.012-S73.013 with 7th A, S73.015-S73.016 with 7th A

7 7th **S73.013 Posterior subluxation of unspecified hip** CC

CC Excl: CC with 7th character A:M99.16-M99.17, M99.19, S33.30X-S33.39X with 7th A, S73.011-S73.016 with 7th A

7 7th **S73.014 Posterior dislocation of right hip** CC

CC Excl: See code: S73.011

7 7th **S73.015 Posterior dislocation of left hip** CC

CC Excl: See code: S73.012

7 7th **S73.016 Posterior dislocation of unspecified hip** CC

CC Excl: See code: S73.013

6th S73.02 Obturator subluxation and dislocation of hip

7 7th **S73.021 Obturator subluxation of right hip** CC

CC Excl: CC with 7th character A: M99.16-M99.17, M99.19, S33.30X-S33.39X with 7th A, S73.021A, S73.023-S73.024 with 7th A, S73.026A

7 7th **S73.022 Obturator subluxation of left hip** CC

CC Excl: CC with 7th character A: M99.16-M99.17, M99.19, S33.30X-S33.39X with 7th A, S73.022-S73.023 with 7th A, S73.025-S73.026 with 7th A

7 7th **S73.023 Obturator subluxation of unspecified hip** CC

CC Excl: CC with 7th character A: M99.16-M99.17, M99.19, S33.30X-S33.39X with 7th A, S73.021-S73.026 with 7th A

7 7th **S73.024 Obturator dislocation of right hip** CC

CC Excl: See code: S73.021

7 7th **S73.025 Obturator dislocation of left hip** CC

CC Excl: See code: S73.022

7 7th **S73.026 Obturator dislocation of unspecified hip** CC

CC Excl: See code: S73.023

6th S73.03 Other anterior dislocation of hip

7 7th **S73.031 Other anterior subluxation of right hip** CC

CC Excl: CC with 7th character A: M99.16-M99.17, M99.19, S33.30X-S33.39X with 7th A, S73.031A, S73.033-S73.034 with 7th A, S73.036A

7 7th **S73.032 Other anterior subluxation of left hip** CC

CC Excl: CC with 7th character AM99.16-M99.17, M99.19, S33.30X-S33.39X with 7th A, S73.032-S73.033 with 7th A, S73.035-S73.036 with 7th A

7 7th **S73.033 Other anterior subluxation of unspecified hip** CC

CC Excl: CC with 7th character A: M99.16-M99.17, M99.19, S33.30X-S33.39X with 7th A, S73.031-S73.036 with 7th A

7 7th **S73.034 Other anterior dislocation of right hip** CC

CC Excl: See code: S73.031

7 7th **S73.035 Other anterior dislocation of left hip** CC

CC Excl: See code: S73.032

7 7th **S73.036 Other anterior dislocation of unspecified hip** CC

CC Excl: See code: S73.033

6th S73.04 Central dislocation of hip

7 HAC = Initial encounter only (7th character A, B or C) and not POA.

7 ✓7th **S73.041 Central subluxation of right hip** CC
CC Excl: See code: S73.001

7 ✓7th **S73.042 Central subluxation of left hip** CC
CC Excl: See code: S73.002

7 ✓7th **S73.043 Central subluxation of unspecified hip** CC
CC Excl: See code: S73.003

7 ✓7th **S73.044 Central dislocation of right hip** CC
CC Excl: See code: S73.001

7 ✓7th **S73.045 Central dislocation of left hip** CC
CC Excl: See code: S73.002

7 ✓7th **S73.046 Central dislocation of unspecified hip** CC
CC Excl: See code: S73.003

✓5th **S73.1 Sprain of hip**

✓6th **S73.10 Unspecified sprain of hip**
- ✓7th **S73.101 Unspecified sprain of right hip**
- ✓7th **S73.102 Unspecified sprain of left hip**
- ✓7th **S73.109 Unspecified sprain of unspecified hip**

✓6th **S73.11 Iliofemoral ligament sprain of hip**
- ✓7th **S73.111 Iliofemoral ligament sprain of right hip**
- ✓7th **S73.112 Iliofemoral ligament sprain of left hip**
- ✓7th **S73.119 Iliofemoral ligament sprain of unspecified hip**

✓6th **S73.12 Ischiocapsular (ligament) sprain of hip**
- ✓7th **S73.121 Ischiocapsular ligament sprain of right hip**
- ✓7th **S73.122 Ischiocapsular ligament sprain of left hip**
- ✓7th **S73.129 Ischiocapsular ligament sprain of unspecified hip**

✓6th **S73.19 Other sprain of hip**
- ✓7th **S73.191 Other sprain of right hip**
- ✓7th **S73.192 Other sprain of left hip**
- ✓7th **S73.199 Other sprain of unspecified hip**

✓4th S74 Injury of nerves at hip and thigh level

Code also any associated open wound (S71.-)

EXCLUDES 2 *injury of nerves at ankle and foot level (S94.-)*
injury of nerves at lower leg level (S84.-)

> The appropriate 7th character is to be added to each code from category S74.
> A initial encounter
> D subsequent encounter
> S sequela

✓5th **S74.0 Injury of sciatic nerve at hip and thigh level**
- ✓x7th **S74.00 Injury of sciatic nerve at hip and thigh level, unspecified leg**
- ✓x7th **S74.01 Injury of sciatic nerve at hip and thigh level, right leg**
- ✓x7th **S74.02 Injury of sciatic nerve at hip and thigh level, left leg**

✓5th **S74.1 Injury of femoral nerve at hip and thigh level**
- ✓x7th **S74.10 Injury of femoral nerve at hip and thigh level, unspecified leg**
- ✓x7th **S74.11 Injury of femoral nerve at hip and thigh level, right leg**
- ✓x7th **S74.12 Injury of femoral nerve at hip and thigh level, left leg**

✓5th **S74.2 Injury of cutaneous sensory nerve at hip and thigh level**
- ✓x7th **S74.20 Injury of cutaneous sensory nerve at hip and thigh level, unspecified leg**
- ✓x7th **S74.21 Injury of cutaneous sensory nerve at hip and high level, right leg**
- ✓x7th **S74.22 Injury of cutaneous sensory nerve at hip and thigh level, left leg**

✓5th **S74.8 Injury of other nerves at hip and thigh level**

✓6th **S74.8X Injury of other nerves at hip and thigh level**
- ✓7th **S74.8X1 Injury of other nerves at hip and thigh level, right leg**
- ✓7th **S74.8X2 Injury of other nerves at hip and thigh level, left leg**
- ✓7th **S74.8X9 Injury of other nerves at hip and thigh level, unspecified leg**

✓5th **S74.9 Injury of unspecified nerve at hip and thigh level**
- ✓x7th **S74.90 Injury of unspecified nerve at hip and thigh level, unspecified leg**
- ✓x7th **S74.91 Injury of unspecified nerve at hip and thigh level, right leg**
- ✓x7th **S74.92 Injury of unspecified nerve at hip and thigh level, left leg**

✓4th S75 Injury of blood vessels at hip and thigh level

Code also any associated open wound (S71.-)

EXCLUDES 2 *injury of blood vessels at lower leg level (S85.-)*
injury of popliteal artery (S85.0)

> The appropriate 7th character is to be added to each code from category S75.
> A initial encounter
> D subsequent encounter
> S sequela

✓5th **S75.0 Injury of femoral artery**

✓6th **S75.00 Unspecified injury of femoral artery**

✓7th **S75.001 Unspecified injury of femoral artery, right leg** MCC
CC Excl: MCC with 7th A: S75.001A, S75.009-S75.011 with 7th A, S75.019-S75.021 with 7th A, S75.029-S75.091 with 7th A, S75.099 A, S75.801A, S75.809-S75.811 with 7th A, S75.819-S75.891 with 7th A, S75.899-S75.901 with 7th A, S75.909-S75.911 with 7th A, S75.919-S75.991 with 7th A, S75.999A, S85.201A, S85.209-S85.211 with 7th A, S85.219-S85.291 with 7th A, S85.299A, S85.801A, S85.809-S85.811 with 7th A, S85.819-S85.891 with 7th A, S85.899-S85.901 with 7th A, S85.909-S85.911 with 7th A, S85.919-S85.991 with 7th A, S85.999A, S95.001A, S95.009-S95.011 with 7th A, S95.019-S95.091 with 7th A, S95.099A, S95.201A, S95.209-S95.211 with 7th A, S95.219-S95.291 with 7th A, S95.299-S95.801 with 7th A, S95.809-S95.811 with 7th A, S95.819-S95.891 with 7th A, S95.899-S95.901 with 7th A, S95.909-S95.911 with 7th A, S95.919-S95.991 with 7th A, S95.999A

✓7th **S75.002 Unspecified injury of femoral artery, left leg** MCC
CC Excl: MCC with 7th A: S75.002-S75.009 with 7th A, S75.012-S75.019 with 7th A, S75.022-S75.029 with 7th A, S75.092-S75.099 with 7th A, S75.802-S75.809 with 7th A, S75.812-S75.819 with 7th A, S75.892-S75.899 with 7th A, S75.902-S75.909 with 7th A, S75.912-S75.919 with 7th A, S75.992-S75.999 with 7th A, S85.202-S85.209 with 7th A, S85.212-S85.219 with 7th A, S85.292-S85.299 with 7th A, S85.802-S85.809 with 7th A, S85.812-S85.819 with 7th A, S85.892-S85.899 with 7th A, S85.902-S85.909 with 7th A, S85.912-S85.919 with 7th A, S85.992-S85.999 with 7th A, S95.002-S95.009 with 7th A, S95.012-S95.019 with 7th A, S95.092-S95.099 with 7th A, S95.202-S95.209 with 7th A, S95.212-S95.219 with 7th A, S95.292-S95.299 with 7th A, S95.802-S95.809 with 7th A, S95.812-S95.819 with 7th A, S95.892-S95.899 with 7th A, S95.902-S95.909 with 7th A, S95.912-S95.919 with 7th A, S95.992-S95.999 with 7th A

✓7th **S75.009 Unspecified injury of femoral artery, unspecified leg** MCC
CC Excl: MCC with 7th A: S75.001-S75.099 with 7th A, S75.801-S75.999 with 7th A, S85.201-S85.299 with 7th A, S85.801-S85.999 with 7th A, S95.001-S95.099 with 7th A, S95.201-S95.999 with 7th A

✓6th **S75.01 Minor laceration of femoral artery**
Incomplete transection of femoral artery
Laceration of femoral artery NOS
Superficial laceration of femoral artery

✓7th **S75.011 Minor laceration of femoral artery, right leg** MCC
CC Excl: See code: S75.001

✓7th **S75.012 Minor laceration of femoral artery, left leg** MCC
CC Excl: See code: S75.002

7 HAC = Initial encounter only (7th character A, B or C) and not POA.

S75.019 Minor laceration of femoral artery, unspecified leg MCC
CC Excl: See code: S75.009

S75.02 Major laceration of femoral artery
Complete transection of femoral artery
Traumatic rupture of femoral artery

S75.021 Major laceration of femoral artery, right leg MCC
CC Excl: See code: S75.001

S75.022 Major laceration of femoral artery, left leg MCC
CC Excl: See code: S75.002

S75.029 Major laceration of femoral artery, unspecified leg MCC
CC Excl: See code: S75.009

S75.09 Other specified injury of femoral artery

S75.091 Other specified injury of femoral artery, right leg MCC
CC Excl: See code: S75.001

S75.092 Other specified injury of femoral artery, left leg MCC
CC Excl: See code: S75.002

S75.099 Other specified injury of femoral artery, unspecified leg MCC
CC Excl: See code: S75.009

S75.1 Injury of femoral vein at hip and thigh level

S75.10 Unspecified injury of femoral vein at hip and thigh level

S75.101 Unspecified injury of femoral vein at hip and thigh level, right leg MCC
CC Excl: MCC with 7th A: S75.101A, S75.109-S75.111 with 7th A, S75.119-S75.121 with 7th A, S75.129-S75.191 with 7th A, S75.199A, S75.801A, S75.809-S75.811 with 7th A, S75.819-S75.891 with 7th A, S75.899-S75.901 with 7th A, S75.909-S75.911 with 7th A, S75.919-S75.991 with 7th A, S75.999 with 7th A, S85.201A, S85.209-S85.211 with 7th A, S85.219-S85.291 with 7th A, S85.299A, S85.801A, S85.809-S85.811 with 7th A, S85.819-S85.891 with 7th A, S85.899-S85.901 with 7th A, S85.909-S85.911 with 7th A, S85.919-S85.991 with 7th A, S85.999A, S95.001A, S95.009-S95.011 with 7th A, S95.019-S95.091 with 7th A, S95.099A, S95.201A, S95.209-S95.211 with 7th A, S95.219-S95.291 with 7th A, S95.299-S95.801 with 7th A, S95.809-S95.811 with 7th A, S95.819-S95.891 with 7th A, S95.899-S95.901 with 7th A, S95.909-S95.911 with 7th A, S95.919-S95.991 with 7th A, S95.999A

S75.102 Unspecified injury of femoral vein at hip and thigh level, left leg MCC
CC Excl: MCC with 7th A: S75.102-S75.109 with 7th A, S75.112-S75.119 with 7th A, S75.122-S75.129 with 7th A, S75.192-S75.199 with 7th A, S75.802-S75.809 with 7th A, S75.812-S75.819 with 7th A, S75.892-S75.899 with 7th A, S75.902-S75.909 with 7th A, S75.912-S75.919 with 7th A, S75.992-S75.999 with 7th A, S85.202-S85.209 with 7th A, S85.212-S85.219 with 7th A, S85.292-S85.299 with 7th A, S85.802-S85.809 with 7th A, S85.812-S85.819 with 7th A, S85.892-S85.899 with 7th A, S85.902-S85.909 with 7th A, S85.912-S85.919 with 7th A, S85.992-S85.999 with 7th A, S95.002-S95.009 with 7th A, S95.012-S95.019 with 7th A, S95.092-S95.099 with 7th A, S95.202-S95.209 with 7th A, S95.212-S95.219 with 7th A, S95.292-S95.299 with 7th A, S95.802-S95.809 with 7th A, S95.812-S95.819 with 7th A, S95.892-S95.899 with 7th A, S95.902-S95.909 with 7th A, S95.912-S95.919 with 7th A, S95.992-S95.999 with 7th A

S75.109 Unspecified injury of femoral vein at hip and thigh level, unspecified leg MCC
CC Excl: MCC with 7th A: S75.101-S75.199 with 7th A, S75.801-S75.999 with 7th A, S85.201-S85.299 with 7th A, S85.801-S85.999 with 7th A, S95.001-S95.099 with 7th A, S95.201-S95.999 with 7th A

S75.11 Minor laceration of femoral vein at hip and thigh level
Incomplete transection of femoral vein at hip and thigh level
Laceration of femoral vein at hip and thigh level NOS
Superficial laceration of femoral vein at hip and thigh level

S75.111 Minor laceration of femoral vein at hip and thigh level, right leg MCC
CC Excl: See code: S75.101

S75.112 Minor laceration of femoral vein at hip and thigh level, left leg MCC
CC Excl: See code: S75.102

S75.119 Minor laceration of femoral vein at hip and thigh level, unspecified leg MCC
CC Excl: See code: S75.109

S75.12 Major laceration of femoral vein at hip and thigh level
Complete transection of femoral vein at hip and thigh level
Traumatic rupture of femoral vein at hip and thigh level

S75.121 Major laceration of femoral vein at hip and thigh level, right leg MCC
CC Excl: See code: S75.101

S75.122 Major laceration of femoral vein at hip and thigh level, left leg MCC
CC Excl: See code: S75.102

S75.129 Major laceration of femoral vein at hip and thigh level, unspecified leg MCC
CC Excl: See code: S75.109

S75.19 Other specified injury of femoral vein at hip and thigh level

S75.191 Other specified injury of femoral vein at hip and thigh level, right leg MCC
CC Excl: See code: S75.101

S75.192 Other specified injury of femoral vein at hip and thigh level, left leg MCC
CC Excl: See code: S75.102

S75.199 Other specified injury of femoral vein at hip and thigh level, unspecified leg MCC
CC Excl: See code: S75.109

S75.2 Injury of greater saphenous vein at hip and thigh level
EXCLUDES 1 *greater saphenous vein NOS (S85.3)*

S75.20 Unspecified injury of greater saphenous vein at hip and thigh level

S75.201 Unspecified injury of greater saphenous vein at hip and thigh level, right leg CC
CC Excl: CC with 7th character A: S75.201A, S75.209-S75.211 with 7th A, S75.219-S75.221 with 7th A, S75.229-S75.291 with 7th A, S75.299-S75.801 with 7th A, S75.809-S75.811 with 7th A, S75.819-S75.891 with 7th A, S75.899-S75.901 with 7th A, S75.909-S75.911 with 7th A, S75.919-S75.991 with 7th A, S75.999A, S85.201A, S85.209-S85.211 with 7th A, S85.219-S85.291 with 7th A, S85.299-S85.301 with 7th A, S85.309-S85.311 with 7th A, S85.319-S85.391 with 7th A, S85.399-S85.401 with 7th A, S85.409-S85.411 with 7th A, S85.419-S85.491 with 7th A, S85.499A, S85.801A, S85.809-S85.811 with 7th A, S85.819-S85.891 with 7th A, S85.899-S85.901 with 7th A, S85.909-S85.911 with 7th A, S85.919-S85.991 with 7th A, S85.999A, S95.001A, S95.009-S95.011 with 7th A, S95.019-S95.091 with 7th A, S95.099A, S95.201A, S95.209-S95.211 with 7th A, S95.219-S95.291 with 7th A, S95.299-S95.801 with 7th A, S95.809-S95.811 with 7th A, S95.819-S95.891 with 7th A, S95.899-S95.901 with 7th A, S95.909-S95.911 with 7th A, S95.919-S95.991 with 7th A, S95.999A

S75.202 Unspecified injury of greater saphenous vein at hip and thigh level, left leg CC
CC Excl: CC with 7th character A: S75.202-S75.209 with 7th A, S75.212-S75.219 with 7th A, S75.222-S75.229 with 7th A, S75.292-S75.299 with 7th A, S75.802-S75.809 with 7th A, S75.812-S75.819 with 7th A, S75.892-S75.899 with 7th A, S75.902-S75.909 with 7th A, S75.912-S75.919 with 7th A, S75.992-S75.999 with 7th A, S85.202-S85.209 with

7th A, S85.212-S85.219 with 7th A, S85.292-S85.299 with 7th A, S85.302-S85.309 with 7th A, S85.312-S85.319 with 7th A, S85.392-S85.399 with 7th A, S85.402-S85.409 with 7th A, S85.412-S85.419 with 7th A, S85.492-S85.499 with 7th A, S85.802-S85.809 with 7th A, S85.812-S85.819 with 7th A, S85.892-S85.899 with 7th A, S85.902-S85.909 with 7th A, S85.912-S85.919 with 7th A, S85.992-S85.999 with 7th A, S95.002-S95.009 with 7th A, S95.012-S95.019 with 7th A, S95.092-S95.099 with 7th A, S95.202-S95.209 with 7th A, S95.212-S95.219 with 7th A, S95.292-S95.299 with 7th A, S95.802-S95.809 with 7th A, S95.812-S95.819 with 7th A, S95.892-S95.899 with 7th A, S95.902-S95.909 with 7th A, S95.912-S95.919 with 7th A, S95.992-S95.999 with 7th A

✓7th **S75.209 Unspecified injury of greater saphenous vein at hip and thigh level, unspecified leg** CC
CC Excl: CC with 7th character A: S75.201-S75.999 with 7th A, S85.201-S85.499 with 7th A, S85.801-S85.999 with 7th A, S95.001-S95.099 with 7th A, S95.201-S95.999 with 7th A

✓6th **S75.21 Minor laceration of greater saphenous vein at hip and thigh level**
Incomplete transection of greater saphenous vein at hip and thigh level
Laceration of greater saphenous vein at hip and thigh level NOS
Superficial laceration of greater saphenous vein at hip and thigh level

✓7th **S75.211 Minor laceration of greater saphenous vein at hip and thigh level, right leg** CC
CC Excl: See code: S75.201

✓7th **S75.212 Minor laceration of greater saphenous vein at hip and thigh level, left leg** CC
CC Excl: See code: S75.202

✓7th **S75.219 Minor laceration of greater saphenous vein at hip and thigh level, unspecified leg** CC
CC Excl: See code: S75.209

✓6th **S75.22 Major laceration of greater saphenous vein at hip and thigh level**
Complete transection of greater saphenous vein at hip and thigh level
Traumatic rupture of greater saphenous vein at hip and thigh level

✓7th **S75.221 Major laceration of greater saphenous vein at hip and thigh level, right leg** CC
CC Excl: See code: S75.201

✓7th **S75.222 Major laceration of greater saphenous vein at hip and thigh level, left leg** CC
CC Excl: See code: S75.202

✓7th **S75.229 Major laceration of greater saphenous vein at hip and thigh level, unspecified leg** CC
CC Excl: See code: S75.209

✓6th **S75.29 Other specified injury of greater saphenous vein at hip and thigh level**

✓7th **S75.291 Other specified injury of greater saphenous vein at hip and thigh level, right leg** CC
CC Excl: See code: S75.201

✓7th **S75.292 Other specified injury of greater saphenous vein at hip and thigh level, left leg** CC
CC Excl: See code: S75.202

✓7th **S75.299 Other specified injury of greater saphenous vein at hip and thigh level, unspecified leg** CC
CC Excl: See code: S75.209

✓5th **S75.8 Injury of other blood vessels at hip and thigh level**

✓6th **S75.80 Unspecified injury of other blood vessels at hip and thigh level**

✓7th **S75.801 Unspecified injury of other blood vessels at hip and thigh level, right leg** CC
CC Excl: CC with 7th character A: M79.A21-M79.A29, S75.001 with 7th A, S75.009-S75.011 with 7th A, S75.019-S75.021 with 7th A, S75.029-S75.091 with 7th A, S75.099-S75.101 with 7th A, S75.109-S75.111 with 7th A, S75.119-S75.121 with 7th A, S75.129-S75.191 with 7th A, S75.199-S75.201 with 7th A, S75.209-S75.211 with 7th A, S75.219-S75.221 with 7th A, S75.229-S75.291 with 7th A, S75.299-S75.801 with 7th A, S75.809-S75.811 with 7th A, S75.819-S75.891 with 7th A, S75.899-S75.901 with 7th A, S75.909-S75.911 with 7th A, S75.919-S75.991 with 7th A, S75.999A, S85.001A, S85.009-S85.011 with 7th A, S85.019-S85.091 with 7th A, S85.099-S85.101 with 7th A, S85.109-S85.111 with 7th A, S85.119-S85.121 with 7th A, S85.129-S85.131 with 7th A, S85.139-S85.141 with 7th A, S85.149-S85.151 with 7th A, S85.159-S85.161 with 7th A, S85.169-S85.171 with 7th A, S85.179-S85.181 with 7th A, S85.189-S85.201 with 7th A, S85.209-S85.211 with 7th A, S85.219-S85.291 with 7th A, S85.299-S85.301 with 7th A, S85.309-S85.311 with 7th A, S85.319-S85.391 with 7th A, S85.399-S85.401 with 7th A, S85.409-S85.411 with 7th A, S85.419-S85.491 with 7th A, S85.499-S85.501 with 7th A, S85.509-S85.511 with 7th A, S85.519-S85.591 with 7th A, S85.599-S85.801 with 7th A, S85.809-S85.811 with 7th A, S85.819-S85.891 with 7th A, S85.899-S85.901 with 7th A, S85.909-S85.911 with 7th A, S85.919-S85.991 with 7th A, S85.999A, S95.001A, S95.009-S95.011 with 7th A, S95.019-S95.091 with 7th A, S95.099-S95.101 with 7th A, S95.109-S95.111 with 7th A, S95.119-S95.191 with 7th A, S95.199-S95.201 with 7th A, S95.209-S95.211 with 7th A, S95.219-S95.291 with 7th A, S95.299-S95.801 with 7th A, S95.809-S95.811 with 7th A, S95.819-S95.891 with 7th A, S95.899-S95.901 with 7th A, S95.909-S95.911 with 7th A, S95.919-S95.991 with 7th A, S95.999A

✓7th **S75.802 Unspecified injury of other blood vessels at hip and thigh level, left leg** CC
CC Excl: CC with 7th character A: M79.A21-M79.A29, S75.002-S75.009 with 7th A, S75.012-S75.019 with 7th A, S75.022-S75.029 with 7th A, S75.092-S75.099 with 7th A, S75.102-S75.109 with 7th A, S75.112-S75.119 with 7th A, S75.122-S75.129 with 7th A, S75.192-S75.199 with 7th A, S75.202-S75.209 with 7th A, S75.212-S75.219 with 7th A, S75.222-S75.229 with 7th A, S75.292-S75.299 with 7th A, S75.802-S75.809 with 7th A, S75.812-S75.819 with 7th A, S75.892-S75.899 with 7th A, S75.902-S75.909 with 7th A, S75.912-S75.919 with 7th A, S75.992-S75.999 with 7th A, S85.002-S85.009 with 7th A, S85.012-S85.019 with 7th A, S85.092-S85.099 with 7th A, S85.102-S85.109 with 7th A, S85.112-S85.119 with 7th A, S85.122-S85.129 with 7th A, S85.132-S85.139 with 7th A, S85.142-S85.149 with 7th A, S85.152-S85.159 with 7th A, S85.162-S85.169 with 7th A, S85.172-S85.179 with 7th A, S85.182-S85.189 with 7th A, S85.202-S85.209 with 7th A, S85.212-S85.219 with 7th A, S85.292-S85.299 with 7th A, S85.302-S85.309 with 7th A, S85.312-S85.319 with 7th A, S85.392-S85.399 with 7th A, S85.402-S85.409 with 7th A, S85.412-S85.419 with 7th A, S85.492-S85.499 with 7th A, S85.502-S85.509 with 7th A, S85.512-S85.519 with 7th A, S85.592-S85.599 with 7th A, S85.802-S85.809 with 7th A, S85.812-S85.819 with 7th A, S85.892-S85.899 with 7th A, S85.902-S85.909 with 7th A, S85.912-S85.919 with 7th A, S85.992-S85.999 with 7th A, S95.002-S95.009 with 7th A, S95.012-S95.019 with 7th A, S95.092-S95.099 with 7th A, S95.102-S95.109 with 7th A, S95.112-S95.119 with 7th A, S95.192-S95.199 with 7th A, S95.202-S95.209 with 7th A, S95.212-S95.219 with 7th A, S95.292-S95.299 with 7th A, S95.802-S95.809 with 7th A, S95.812-S95.819 with 7th A, S95.892-S95.899 with 7th A, S95.902-S95.909 with 7th A, S95.912-S95.919 with 7th A, S95.992-S95.999 with 7th A

✓7th **S75.809 Unspecified injury of other blood vessels at hip and thigh level, unspecified leg** CC
CC Excl: CC with 7th character A: M79.A21-M79.A29, S75.001-S75.999 with 7th A, S85.001-S85.999 with 7th A, S95.001-S95.999 with 7th A

✓6th **S75.81 Laceration of other blood vessels at hip and thigh level**

✓7th **S75.811 Laceration of other blood vessels at hip and thigh level, right leg** CC
CC Excl: See code: S75.801

✓7th **S75.812 Laceration of other blood vessels at hip and thigh level, left leg** CC
CC Excl: See code: S75.802

✓7th **S75.819 Laceration of other blood vessels at hip and thigh level, unspecified leg** CC
CC Excl: See code: S75.809

✓6th **S75.89 Other specified injury of other blood vessels at hip and thigh level**

✓7th **S75.891 Other specified injury of other blood vessels at hip and thigh level, right leg** CC
CC Excl: See code: S75.801

✓7th **S75.892 Other specified injury of other blood vessels at hip and thigh level, left leg** CC
CC Excl: See code: S75.802

✓7th **S75.899 Other specified injury of other blood vessels at hip and thigh level, unspecified leg** CC
CC Excl: See code: S75.809

✓5th **S75.9 Injury of unspecified blood vessel at hip and thigh level**

✓6th **S75.90 Unspecified injury of unspecified blood vessel at hip and thigh level**

✓7th **S75.901 Unspecified injury of unspecified blood vessel at hip and thigh level, right leg** CC
CC Excl: See code: S75.801

✓7th **S75.902 Unspecified injury of unspecified blood vessel at hip and thigh level, left leg** CC
CC Excl: See code: S75.802

✓7th **S75.909 Unspecified injury of unspecified blood vessel at hip and thigh level, unspecified leg** CC
CC Excl: See code: S75.809

✓6th **S75.91 Laceration of unspecified blood vessel at hip and thigh level**

✓7th **S75.911 Laceration of unspecified blood vessel at hip and thigh level, right leg** CC
CC Excl: See code: S75.801

✓7th **S75.912 Laceration of unspecified blood vessel at hip and thigh level, left leg** CC
CC Excl: See code: S75.802

✓7th **S75.919 Laceration of unspecified blood vessel at hip and thigh level, unspecified leg** CC
CC Excl: See code: S75.809

✓6th **S75.99 Other specified injury of unspecified blood vessel at hip and thigh level**

✓7th **S75.991 Other specified injury of unspecified blood vessel at hip and thigh level, right leg** CC
CC Excl: See code: S75.801

✓7th **S75.992 Other specified injury of unspecified blood vessel at hip and thigh level, left leg** CC
CC Excl: See code: S75.802

✓7th **S75.999 Other specified injury of unspecified blood vessel at hip and thigh level, unspecified leg** CC
CC Excl: See code: S75.809

✓4th **S76 Injury of muscle, fascia and tendon at hip and thigh level**

Code also any associated open wound (S71.-)

EXCLUDES 2 *injury of muscle, fascia and tendon at lower leg level (S86)*
sprain of joint and ligament of hip (S73.1)

The appropriate 7th character is to be added to each code from category S76.
A initial encounter
D subsequent encounter
S sequela

✓5th **S76.0 Injury of muscle, fascia and tendon of hip**

✓6th **S76.00 Unspecified injury of muscle, fascia and tendon of hip**

✓7th **S76.001 Unspecified injury of muscle, fascia and tendon of right hip**

✓7th **S76.002 Unspecified injury of muscle, fascia and tendon of left hip**

✓7th **S76.009 Unspecified injury of muscle, fascia and tendon of unspecified hip**

✓6th **S76.01 Strain of muscle, fascia and tendon of hip**

✓7th **S76.011 Strain of muscle, fascia and tendon of right hip**

✓7th **S76.012 Strain of muscle, fascia and tendon of left hip**

✓7th **S76.019 Strain of muscle, fascia and tendon of unspecified hip**

✓6th **S76.02 Laceration of muscle, fascia and tendon of hip**

✓7th **S76.021 Laceration of muscle, fascia and tendon of right hip** CC
CC Excl: CC with 7th character A: S71.001A, S71.009-S71.011 with 7th A, S71.019-S71.021 with 7th A, S71.029-S71.031 with 7th A, S71.039-S71.041 with 7th A, S71.049-S71.051 with 7th A, S71.059-S71.101 with 7th A, S71.109-S71.111 with 7th A, S71.119-S71.121 with 7th A, S71.129-S71.131 with 7th A, S71.139-S71.141 with 7th A, S71.149-S71.151 with 7th A, S71.159 with 7th A, S76.021 with 7th A, S76.029A, S76.121A, S76.129A, S76.221A, S76.229A, S76.321 A, S76.329A, S76.821A, S76.829A, S76.921A, S76.929A

✓7th **S76.022 Laceration of muscle, fascia and tendon of left hip** CC
CC Excl: CC with 7th character A: S71.002-S71.009 with 7th A, S71.012-S71.019 with 7th A, S71.022-S71.029 with 7th A, S71.032-S71.039 with 7th A, S71.042-S71.049 with 7th A, S71.052-S71.059 with 7th A, S71.102-S71.109 with 7th A, S71.112-S71.119 with 7th A, S71.122-S71.129 with 7th A, S71.132-S71.139 with 7th A, S71.142-S71.149 with 7th A, S71.152-S71.159 with 7th A, S76.022-S76.029 with 7th A, S76.122-S76.129 with 7th A, S76.222-S76.229 with 7th A, S76.322-S76.329 with 7th A, S76.822-S76.829 with 7th A, S76.922-S76.929 with 7th A

✓7th **S76.029 Laceration of muscle, fascia and tendon of unspecified hip** CC
CC Excl: CC with 7th character A: S71.001-S71.159 with 7th A, S76.021-S76.029 with 7th A, S76.121-S76.129 with 7th A, S76.221-S76.229 with 7th A, S76.321-S76.329 with 7th A, S76.821-S76.829 with 7th A, S76.921-S76.929 with 7th A

✓6th **S76.09 Other specified injury of muscle, fascia and tendon of hip**

✓7th **S76.091 Other specified injury of muscle, fascia and tendon of right hip**

✓7th **S76.092 Other specified injury of muscle, fascia and tendon of left hip**

✓7th **S76.099 Other specified injury of muscle, fascia and tendon of unspecified hip**

✓5th **S76.1 Injury of quadriceps muscle, fascia and tendon**

Injury of patellar ligament (tendon)

✓6th **S76.10 Unspecified injury of quadriceps muscle, fascia and tendon**

✓7th **S76.101 Unspecified injury of right quadriceps muscle, fascia and tendon**

✓7th **S76.102 Unspecified injury of left quadriceps muscle, fascia and tendon**

✓7th **S76.109 Unspecified injury of unspecified quadriceps muscle, fascia and tendon**

✓6th **S76.11 Strain of quadriceps muscle, fascia and tendon**

✓7th **S76.111 Strain of right quadriceps muscle, fascia and tendon**

✓7th **S76.112 Strain of left quadriceps muscle, fascia and tendon**

✓7th **S76.119 Strain of unspecified quadriceps muscle, fascia and tendon**

✓6th **S76.12 Laceration of quadriceps muscle, fascia and tendon**

✓7th **S76.121 Laceration of right quadriceps muscle, fascia and tendon** CC
CC Excl: See code: S76.021

✓7th **S76.122 Laceration of left quadriceps muscle, fascia and tendon** CC
CC Excl: See code: S76.022

S76.129 Laceration of unspecified quadriceps muscle, fascia and tendon CC
CC Excl: See code: S76.029

S76.19 Other specified injury of quadriceps muscle, fascia and tendon

S76.191 Other specified injury of right quadriceps muscle, fascia and tendon

S76.192 Other specified injury of left quadriceps muscle, fascia and tendon

S76.199 Other specified injury of unspecified quadriceps muscle, fascia and tendon

S76.2 Injury of adductor muscle, fascia and tendon of thigh

S76.20 Unspecified injury of adductor muscle, fascia and tendon of thigh

S76.201 Unspecified injury of adductor muscle, fascia and tendon of right thigh

S76.202 Unspecified injury of adductor muscle, fascia and tendon of left thigh

S76.209 Unspecified injury of adductor muscle, fascia and tendon of unspecified thigh

S76.21 Strain of adductor muscle, fascia and tendon of thigh

S76.211 Strain of adductor muscle, fascia and tendon of right thigh

S76.212 Strain of adductor muscle, fascia and tendon of left thigh

S76.219 Strain of adductor muscle, fascia and tendon of unspecified thigh

S76.22 Laceration of adductor muscle, fascia and tendon of thigh

S76.221 Laceration of adductor muscle, fascia and tendon of right thigh CC
CC Excl: See code: S76.021

S76.222 Laceration of adductor muscle, fascia and tendon of left thigh CC
CC Excl: See code: S76.022

S76.229 Laceration of adductor muscle, fascia and tendon of unspecified thigh CC
CC Excl: See code: S76.029

S76.29 Other injury of adductor muscle, fascia and tendon of thigh

S76.291 Other injury of adductor muscle, fascia and tendon of right thigh

S76.292 Other injury of adductor muscle, fascia and tendon of left thigh

S76.299 Other injury of adductor muscle, fascia and tendon of unspecified thigh

S76.3 Injury of muscle, fascia and tendon of the posterior muscle group at thigh level

S76.30 Unspecified injury of muscle, fascia and tendon of the posterior muscle group at thigh level

S76.301 Unspecified injury of muscle, fascia and tendon of the posterior muscle group at thigh level, right thigh

S76.302 Unspecified injury of muscle, fascia and tendon of the posterior muscle group at thigh level, left thigh

S76.309 Unspecified injury of muscle, fascia and tendon of the posterior muscle group at thigh level, unspecified thigh

S76.31 Strain of muscle, fascia and tendon of the posterior muscle group at thigh level

S76.311 Strain of muscle, fascia and tendon of the posterior muscle group at thigh level, right thigh

S76.312 Strain of muscle, fascia and tendon of the posterior muscle group at thigh level, left thigh

S76.319 Strain of muscle, fascia and tendon of the posterior muscle group at thigh level, unspecified thigh

S76.32 Laceration of muscle, fascia and tendon of the posterior muscle group at thigh level

S76.321 Laceration of muscle, fascia and tendon of the posterior muscle group at thigh level, right thigh CC
CC Excl: See code: S76.021

S76.322 Laceration of muscle, fascia and tendon of the posterior muscle group at thigh level, left thigh CC
CC Excl: See code: S76.022

S76.329 Laceration of muscle, fascia and tendon of the posterior muscle group at thigh level, unspecified thigh CC
CC Excl: See code: S76.029

S76.39 Other specified injury of muscle, fascia and tendon of the posterior muscle group at thigh level

S76.391 Other specified injury of muscle, fascia and tendon of the posterior muscle group at thigh level, right thigh

S76.392 Other specified injury of muscle, fascia and tendon of the posterior muscle group at thigh level, left thigh

S76.399 Other specified injury of muscle, fascia and tendon of the posterior muscle group at thigh level, unspecified thigh

S76.8 Injury of other specified muscles, fascia and tendons at thigh level

S76.80 Unspecified injury of other specified muscles, fascia and tendons at thigh level

S76.801 Unspecified injury of other specified muscles, fascia and tendons at thigh level, right thigh

S76.802 Unspecified injury of other specified muscles, fascia and tendons at thigh level, left thigh

S76.809 Unspecified injury of other specified muscles, fascia and tendons at thigh level, unspecified thigh

S76.81 Strain of other specified muscles, fascia and tendons at thigh level

S76.811 Strain of other specified muscles, fascia and tendons at thigh level, right thigh

S76.812 Strain of other specified muscles, fascia and tendons at thigh level, left thigh

S76.819 Strain of other specified muscles, fascia and tendons at thigh level, unspecified thigh

S76.82 Laceration of other specified muscles, fascia and tendons at thigh level

S76.821 Laceration of other specified muscles, fascia and tendons at thigh level, right thigh CC
CC Excl: See code: S76.021

S76.822 Laceration of other specified muscles, fascia and tendons at thigh level, left thigh CC
CC Excl: See code: S76.022

S76.829 Laceration of other specified muscles, fascia and tendons at thigh level, unspecified thigh CC
CC Excl: See code: S76.029

S76.89 Other injury of other specified muscles, fascia and tendons at thigh level

S76.891 Other injury of other specified muscles, fascia and tendons at thigh level, right thigh

S76.892 Other injury of other specified muscles, fascia and tendons at thigh level, left thigh

S76.899 Other injury of other specified muscles, fascia and tendons at thigh level, unspecified thigh

S76.9 Injury of unspecified muscles, fascia and tendons at thigh level

S76.90 Unspecified injury of unspecified muscles, fascia and tendons at thigh level

S76.901 Unspecified injury of unspecified muscles, fascia and tendons at thigh level, right thigh

S76.902 Unspecified injury of unspecified muscles, fascia and tendons at thigh level, left thigh

S76.909 Unspecified injury of unspecified muscles, fascia and tendons at thigh level, unspecified thigh

Injury, Poisoning and Certain Other Consequences of External Causes S76.129–S76.909

√6th **S76.91 Strain of unspecified muscles, fascia and tendons at thigh level**

√7th **S76.911 Strain of unspecified muscles, fascia and tendons at thigh level, right thigh**

√7th **S76.912 Strain of unspecified muscles, fascia and tendons at thigh level, left thigh**

√7th **S76.919 Strain of unspecified muscles, fascia and tendons at thigh level, unspecified thigh**

√6th **S76.92 Laceration of unspecified muscles, fascia and tendons at thigh level**

√7th **S76.921 Laceration of unspecified muscles, fascia and tendons at thigh level, right thigh** CC
CC Excl: See code: S76.Ø21

√7th **S76.922 Laceration of unspecified muscles, fascia and tendons at thigh level, left thigh** CC
CC Excl: See code: S76.Ø22

√7th **S76.929 Laceration of unspecified muscles, fascia and tendons at thigh level, unspecified thigh** CC
CC Excl: See code: S76.Ø29

√6th **S76.99 Other specified injury of unspecified muscles, fascia and tendons at thigh level**

√7th **S76.991 Other specified injury of unspecified muscles, fascia and tendons at thigh level, right thigh**

√7th **S76.992 Other specified injury of unspecified muscles, fascia and tendons at thigh level, left thigh**

√7th **S76.999 Other specified injury of unspecified muscles, fascia and tendons at thigh level, unspecified thigh**

√4th **S77 Crushing injury of hip and thigh**

Use additional code(s) for all associated injuries

EXCLUDES 2 *crushing injury of ankle and foot (S97.-)*
crushing injury of lower leg (S87.-)

The appropriate 7th character is to be added to each code from category S77.
A initial encounter
D subsequent encounter
S sequela

√5th **S77.Ø Crushing injury of hip**

CC Excl: For CC codes in subcategory S77.Ø, unless otherwise noted: CC with 7th character A: S77.ØØX-S77.Ø2X with 7th A, S77.2ØX-S77.22X with 7th A

7 √x7th **S77.ØØ Crushing injury of unspecified hip** CC

7 √x7th **S77.Ø1 Crushing injury of right hip** CC

7 √x7th **S77.Ø2 Crushing injury of left hip** CC

√5th **S77.1 Crushing injury of thigh**

CC Excl: For CC codes in subcategory S77.1, unless otherwise noted: CC with 7th character A: S77.ØØX-S77.Ø2X with 7th A, S77.2ØX-S77.22X with 7th A

7 √x7th **S77.1Ø Crushing injury of unspecified thigh** CC

7 √x7th **S77.11 Crushing injury of right thigh** CC

7 √x7th **S77.12 Crushing injury of left thigh** CC

√5th **S77.2 Crushing injury of hip with thigh**

√x7th **S77.2Ø Crushing injury of unspecified hip with thigh**

√x7th **S77.21 Crushing injury of right hip with thigh**

√x7th **S77.22 Crushing injury of left hip with thigh**

√4th **S78 Traumatic amputation of hip and thigh**

NOTE An amputation not identified as partial or complete should be coded to complete.

EXCLUDES 1 *traumatic amputation of knee (S88.Ø-)*

The appropriate 7th character is to be added to each code from category S78.
A initial encounter
D subsequent encounter
S sequela

√5th **S78.Ø Traumatic amputation at hip joint**

√6th **S78.Ø1 Complete traumatic amputation at hip joint**

7 HAC = Initial encounter only (7th character A, B or C) and not POA.

√7th **S78.Ø11 Complete traumatic amputation at right hip joint** CC
CC Excl: CC with 7th character A: S71.ØØ1A, S71.ØØ9-S71.Ø11 with 7th A, S71.Ø19-S71.Ø21 with 7th A, S71.Ø29-S71.Ø31 with 7th A, S71.Ø39-S71.Ø41 with 7th A, S71.Ø49-S71.Ø51 with 7th A, S71.Ø59-S71.1Ø1 with 7th A, S71.1Ø9-S71.111 with 7th A, S71.119-S71.121 with 7th A, S71.129-S71.131 with 7th A, S71.139-S71.141 with 7th A, S71.149-S71.151 with 7th A, S71.159A, S76.Ø21A, S76.Ø29A, S76.121A, S76.129A, S76.221 A, S76.229A, S76.321A, S76.329A, S76.821A, S76.829A, S76.921A, S76.929A, S78.Ø11A, S78.Ø19-S78.Ø21 with 7th A, S78.Ø29-S78.111 with 7th A, S78.119-S78.121 with 7th A, S78.129-S78.911 with 7th A, S78.919-S78.921 with 7th A, S78.929A, S81.ØØ1A, S81.ØØ9-S81.Ø11 with 7th A, S81.Ø19-S81.Ø21 with 7th A, S81.Ø29-S81.Ø31 with 7th A, S81.Ø39-S81.Ø41 with 7th A, S81.Ø49-S81.Ø51 with 7th A, S81.Ø59-S81.8Ø1 with 7th A, S81.8Ø9-S81.811 with 7th A, S81.819-S81.821 with 7th A, S81.829-S81.831 with 7th A, S81.839-S81.841 with 7th A, S81.849-S81.851 with 7th A, S81.859A, S98.129-S98.131 with 7th A, S98.139-S98.141 with 7th A, S98.149-S98.211 with 7th A, S98.219-S98.221 with 7th A, S98.229-S98.311 with 7th A, S98.319-S98.321 with 7th A, S98.329-S98.911 with 7th A, S98.919-S98.921 with 7th A, S98.929 A, T14.8-T14.91, T79.AØX-T79.9XX with 7th A

√7th **S78.Ø12 Complete traumatic amputation at left hip joint** CC
CC Excl: CC with 7th character A: S71.ØØ2-S71.ØØ9 with 7th A, S71.Ø12-S71.Ø19 with 7th A, S71.Ø22-S71.Ø29 with 7th A, S71.Ø32-S71.Ø39 with 7th A, S71.Ø42-S71.Ø49 with 7th A, S71.Ø52-S71.Ø59 with 7th A, S71.1Ø2-S71.1Ø9 with 7th A, S71.112-S71.119 with 7th A, S71.122-S71.129 with 7th A, S71.132-S71.139 with 7th A, S71.142-S71.149 with 7th A, S71.152-S71.159 with 7th A, S76.Ø22-S76.Ø29 with 7th A, S76.122-S76.129 with 7th A, S76.222-S76.229 with 7th A, S76.322-S76.329 with 7th A, S76.822-S76.829 with 7th A, S76.922-S76.929 with 7th A, S78.Ø12-S78.Ø19 with 7th A, S78.Ø22-S78.Ø29 with 7th A, S78.112-S78.119 with 7th A, S78.122-S78.129 with 7th A, S78.912-S78.919 with 7th A, S78.922-S78.929 with 7th A, S81.ØØ2-S81.ØØ9 with 7th A, S81.Ø12-S81.Ø19 with 7th A, S81.Ø22-S81.Ø29 with 7th A, S81.Ø32-S81.Ø39 with 7th A, S81.Ø42-S81.Ø49 with 7th A, S81.Ø52-S81.Ø59 with 7th A, S81.8Ø2-S81.8Ø9 with 7th A, S81.812-S81.819 with 7th A, S81.822-S81.829 with 7th A, S81.832-S81.839 with 7th A, S81.842-S81.849 with 7th A, S81.852-S81.859 with 7th A, S86.Ø22-S86.Ø29 with 7th A, S86.122-S86.129 with 7th A, S86.222-S86.229 with 7th A, S86.322-S86.329 with 7th A, S86.822-S86.829 with 7th A, S86.922-S86.929 with 7th A, S88.Ø12-S88.Ø19 with 7th A, S88.Ø22-S88.Ø29 with 7th A, S88.112-S88.119 with 7th A, S88.122-S88.129 with 7th A, S88.912-S88.919 with 7th A, S88.922-S88.929 with 7th A, S91.ØØ2-S91.ØØ9 with 7th A, S91.Ø12-S91.Ø19 with 7th A, S91.Ø22-S91.Ø29 with 7th A, S91.Ø32-S91.Ø39 with 7th A, S91.Ø42-S91.Ø49 with 7th A, S91.Ø52-S91.Ø59 with 7th A, S91.1Ø2-S91.1Ø3 with 7th A, S91.1Ø5-S91.1Ø9 with 7th A, S91.112-S91.113 with 7th A, S91.115-S91.119 with 7th A, S91.122-S91.123 with 7th A, S91.125-S91.129 with 7th A, S91.132-S91.133 with 7th A, S91.135-S91.139 with 7th A, S91.142-S91.143 with 7th A, S91.145-S91.149 with 7th A, S91.152-S91.153 with 7th A, S91.155-S91.159 with 7th A, S91.2Ø2-S91.2Ø3 with 7th A, S91.2Ø5-S91.2Ø9 with 7th A, S91.212-S91.213 with 7th A, S91.215-S91.219 with 7th A, S91.222-S91.223 with 7th A, S91.225-S91.229 with 7th A, S91.232-S91.233 with 7th A, S91.235-S91.239 with 7th A, S91.242-S91.243 with 7th A, S91.245-S91.249 with 7th A, S91.252-S91.253 with 7th A, S91.255-S91.259 with 7th A, S91.3Ø2-S91.3Ø9 with 7th A, S91.312-S91.319 with 7th A, S91.322-S91.329 with 7th A, S91.332-

S91.339 with 7th A, S91.342-S91.349 with 7th A, S91.352-S91.359 with 7th A, S96.022-S96.029 with 7th A, S96.122-S96.129 with 7th A, S96.222-S96.229 with 7th A, S96.822-S96.829 with 7th A, S96.922-S96.929 with 7th A, S98.012-S98.019 with 7th A, S98.022-S98.029 with 7th A, S98.112-S98.119 with 7th A, S98.122-S98.129 with 7th A, S98.132-S98.139 with 7th A, S98.142-S98.149 with 7th A, S98.212-S98.219 with 7th A, S98.222-S98.229 with 7th A, S98.312-S98.319 with 7th A, S98.322-S98.329 with 7th A, S98.912-S98.919 with 7th A, S98.922-S98.929 with 7th A, T14.8-T14.91, T79.A0X-T79.9XX with 7th A

√7th **S78.019 Complete traumatic amputation at unspecified hip joint** CC
CC Excl: CC with 7th character A: S71.001-S71.159 with 7th A, S76.021-S76.029 with 7th A, S76.121-S76.129 with 7th A, S76.221-S76.229 with 7th A, S76.321-S76.329 with 7th A, S76.821-S76.829 with 7th A, S76.921-S76.929 with 7th A, S78.011-S78.929 with 7th A, S81.001-S81.859 with 7th A, S86.021-S86.029 with 7th A, S86.121-S86.129 with 7th A, S86.221-S86.229 with 7th A, S86.321-S86.329 with 7th A, S86.821-S86.829 with 7th A, S86.921-S86.929 with 7th A, S88.011-S88.929 with 7th A, S91.001-S91.359 with 7th A, S96.021-S96.029 with 7th A, S96.121-S96.129 with 7th A, S96.221-S96.229 with 7th A, S96.821-S96.829 with 7th A, S96.921-S96.929 with 7th A, S98.011-S98.929 with 7th A, T14.8-T14.91, T79.A0X-T79.9XX with 7th A

√6th **S78.02 Partial traumatic amputation at hip joint**

√7th **S78.021 Partial traumatic amputation at right hip joint** CC
CC Excl: See code: S78.011

√7th **S78.022 Partial traumatic amputation at left hip joint** CC
CC Excl: See code: S78.012

√7th **S78.029 Partial traumatic amputation at unspecified hip joint** CC
CC Excl: See code: S78.019

√5th **S78.1 Traumatic amputation at level between hip and knee**
EXCLUDES 1 *traumatic amputation of knee (S88.0-)*

√6th **S78.11 Complete traumatic amputation at level between hip and knee**

√7th **S78.111 Complete traumatic amputation at level between right hip and knee** CC
CC Excl: See code: S78.011

√7th **S78.112 Complete traumatic amputation at level between left hip and knee** CC
CC Excl: See code: S78.012

√7th **S78.119 Complete traumatic amputation at level between unspecified hip and knee** CC
CC Excl: See code: S78.019

√6th **S78.12 Partial traumatic amputation at level between hip and knee**

√7th **S78.121 Partial traumatic amputation at level between right hip and knee** CC
CC Excl: See code: S78.011

√7th **S78.122 Partial traumatic amputation at level between left hip and knee** CC
CC Excl: See code: S78.012

√7th **S78.129 Partial traumatic amputation at level between unspecified hip and knee** CC
CC Excl: See code: S78.019

√5th **S78.9 Traumatic amputation of hip and thigh, level unspecified**

√6th **S78.91 Complete traumatic amputation of hip and thigh, level unspecified**

√7th **S78.911 Complete traumatic amputation of right hip and thigh, level unspecified** CC
CC Excl: See code: S78.011

√7th **S78.912 Complete traumatic amputation of left hip and thigh, level unspecified** CC
CC Excl: See code: S78.012

√7th **S78.919 Complete traumatic amputation of unspecified hip and thigh, level unspecified** CC
CC Excl: See code: S78.019

√6th **S78.92 Partial traumatic amputation of hip and thigh, level unspecified**

√7th **S78.921 Partial traumatic amputation of right hip and thigh, level unspecified** CC
CC Excl: See code: S78.011

√7th **S78.922 Partial traumatic amputation of left hip and thigh, level unspecified** CC
CC Excl: See code: S78.012

√7th **S78.929 Partial traumatic amputation of unspecified hip and thigh, level unspecified** CC
CC Excl: See code: S78.019

√4th **S79 Other and unspecified injuries of hip and thigh**

√5th **S79.0 Physeal fracture of upper end of femur**

NOTE A fracture not indicated as open or closed should be coded to closed.

EXCLUDES 1 *apophyseal fracture of upper end of femur (S72.13-)*
nontraumatic slipped upper femoral epiphysis (M93.0-)

The appropriate 7th character is to be added to each code from subcategory S79.0.
- A initial encounter for closed fracture
- D subsequent encounter for fracture with routine healing
- G subsequent encounter for fracture with delayed healing
- K subsequent encounter for fracture with nonunion
- P subsequent encounter for fracture with malunion
- S sequela

√6th **S79.00 Unspecified physeal fracture of upper end of femur**

7 √7th **S79.001 Unspecified physeal fracture of upper end of right femur** MCC CC
CC Excl: MCC with 7th A: M48.40X-M48.58X with 7th A, M80.00X-M84.68X with 7th A, S03.8XX-S03.9XX with 7th A, S29.011-S29.019 with 7th A, S38.3XX-S39.013 with 7th A, S72.001-S72.471 with 7th [A, B, C], S72.479-S72.92X with 7th A, S73.101A, S73.109-S73.111 with 7th A, S73.119-S73.121 with 7th A, S73.129-S73.191 with 7th A, S73.199A, S76.001 A, S76.009-S76.011 with 7th A, S76.019A, S76.091A, S76.099-S76.101 with 7th A, S76.109-S76.111 with 7th A, S76.119A, S76.191A, S76.199-S76.201 with 7th A, S76.209-S76.211 with 7th A, S76.219A, S76.291A, S76.299-S76.301 with 7th A, S76.309-S76.311 with 7th A, S76.319A, S76.391A, S76.399-S76.801 with 7th A, S76.809-S76.811 with 7th A, S76.819 A, S76.891A, S76.899-S76.901 with 7th A, S76.909-S76.911 with 7th A, S76.919A, S76.991A, S76.999A, S79.001A, S79.009-S79.011 with 7th A, S79.019-S79.091 with 7th A, S79.099-S79.101 with 7th A, S79.109-S79.111 with 7th A, S79.119-S79.121 with 7th A, S79.129-S79.131 with 7th A, S79.139-S79.141 with 7th A, S79.149-S79.191 with 7th A, S79.199-S79.811 with 7th A, S79.819-S79.821 with 7th A, S79.829-S79.911 with 7th A, S79.919-S79.921 with 7th A, S79.929 with 7th A, S82.90X-S82.92X with 7th [A, B, C], T14.8-T14.91, T79.A0X-T79.9XX with 7th A
CC Excl: CC with 7th character K or P: M80.00X-M84.68X with 7th [K, P], S02.0XX-S02.92X with 7th K, S12.000-S12.691 with 7th K, S22.000-S22.9XX with 7th K, S32.000-S32.9XX with 7th K, S42.001-S42.92X with 7th [K, P], S49.001-S49.199 with 7th [K, P], S52.001-S52.92X with 7th [K, M, N, P, Q, R], S59.001-S59.299 with 7th [K, P], S62.001-S62.92X with 7th [K, P], S72.001-S72.92X with 7th [K, M, N, P, Q, R], S79.001-S79.199 with 7th [K, P], S82.001-S82.92X with 7th [K, M, N, P, Q, R], S89.001-S89.399 with 7th [K, P], S92.001-S92.919 with 7th [K, P]

7 HAC = Initial encounter only (7th character A, B or C) and not POA.

7 ✓7th **S79.002 Unspecified physeal fracture of upper end of left femur** MCC CC
CC Excl: MCC with 7th A: M48.40X-M48.58X with 7th A, M80.00X-M84.68X with 7th A, S03.8XX-S03.9XX with 7th A, S29.011-S29.019 with 7th A, S38.3XX-S39.013 with 7th A, S72.001-S72.466 with 7th [B, C], S72.472-S72.92X with 7th A, S73.102-S73.109 with 7th A, S73.112-S73.119 with 7th A, S73.122-S73.129 with 7th A, S73.192-S73.199 with 7th A, S76.002-S76.009 with 7th A, S76.012-S76.019 with 7th A, S76.092-S76.099 with 7th A, S76.102-S76.109 with 7th A, S76.112-S76.119 with 7th A, S76.192-S76.199 with 7th A, S76.202-S76.209 with 7th A, S76.212-S76.219 with 7th A, S76.292-S76.299 with 7th A, S76.302-S76.309 with 7th A, S76.312-S76.319 with 7th A, S76.392-S76.399 with 7th A, S76.802-S76.809 with 7th A, S76.812-S76.819 with 7th A, S76.892-S76.899 with 7th A, S76.902-S76.909 with 7th A, S76.912-S76.919 with 7th A, S76.992-S76.999 with 7th A, S79.002-S79.009 with 7th A, S79.012-S79.019 with 7th A, S79.092-S79.099 with 7th A, S79.102-S79.109 with 7th A, S79.112-S79.119 with 7th A, S79.122-S79.129 with 7th A, S79.132-S79.139 with 7th A, S79.142-S79.149 with 7th A, S79.192-S79.199 with 7th A, S79.812-S79.819 with 7th A, S79.822-S79.829 with 7th A, S79.912-S79.919 with 7th A, S79.922-S79.929 with 7th A, S82.90X-S82.92X with 7th [A, B, C], T14.8-T14.91, T79.A0X-T79.9XX with 7th A
CC Excl: CC with 7th character K or P: M80.00X-M84.68X with 7th [K, P], S02.0XX-S02.92X with 7th K, S12.000-S12.691 with 7th K, S22.000-S22.9XX with 7th K, S32.000-S32.9XX with 7th K, S42.001-S42.92X with 7th [K, P], S49.001-S49.199 with 7th [K, P], S52.001-S52.92X with 7th [K, M, N, P, Q, R], S59.001-S59.299 with 7th [K, P], S62.001-S62.92X with 7th [K, P], S72.001-S72.92X with 7th [K, M, N, P, Q, R], S79.001-S79.199 with 7th [K, P], S82.001-S82.92X with 7th [K, M, N, P, Q, R], S89.001-S89.399 with 7th [K, P], S92.001-S92.919 with 7th [K, P]

7 ✓7th **S79.009 Unspecified physeal fracture of upper end of unspecified femur** MCC CC
CC Excl: MCC with 7th A: M48.40X-M48.58X with 7th A, M80.00X-M84.68X with 7th A, S03.8XX-S03.9XX with 7th A, S29.011-S29.019 with 7th A, S38.3XX-S39.013 with 7th A, S72.001-S72.92X with 7th [A, B, C], S73.101-S73.199 with 7th A, S76.001-S76.019 with 7th A, S76.091-S76.119 with 7th A, S76.191-S76.219 with 7th A, S76.291-S76.319 with 7th A, S76.391-S76.819 with 7th A, S76.891-S76.919 with 7th A, S76.991-S76.999 with 7th A, S79.001-S79.929 with 7th A, S82.90X-S82.92X with 7th [A, B, C], T14.8-T14.91, T79.A0X-T79.9XX with 7th A
CC Excl: CC with 7th character K or P: M80.00X-M84.68X with 7th [K, P], S02.0XX-S02.92X with 7th K, S12.000-S12.691 with 7th K, S22.000-S22.9XX with 7th K, S32.000-S32.9XX with 7th K, S42.001-S42.92X with 7th [K, P], S49.001-S49.199 with 7th [K, P], S52.001-S52.92X with 7th [K, M, N, P, Q, R], S59.001-S59.299 with 7th [K, P], S62.001-S62.92X with 7th [K, P], S72.001-S72.92X with 7th [K, M, N, P, Q, R], S79.001-S79.199 with 7th [K, P], S82.001-S82.92X with 7th [K, M, N, P, Q, R], S89.001-S89.399 with 7th [K, P], S92.001-S92.919 with 7th [K, P]

✓6th **S79.01 Salter-Harris Type I physeal fracture of upper end of femur**
Acute on chronic slipped capital femoral epiphysis (traumatic)
Acute slipped capital femoral epiphysis (traumatic)
Capital femoral epiphyseal fracture
EXCLUDES 1 *chronic slipped upper femoral epiphysis (nontraumatic) (M93.02-)*

7 ✓7th **S79.011 Salter-Harris Type I physeal fracture of upper end of right femur** MCC CC
CC Excl: See code: S79.001

7 ✓7th **S79.012 Salter-Harris Type I physeal fracture of upper end of left femur** MCC CC
CC Excl: See code: S79.002

7 ✓7th **S79.019 Salter-Harris Type I physeal fracture of upper end of unspecified femur** MCC CC
CC Excl: See code: S79.009

✓6th **S79.09 Other physeal fracture of upper end of femur**

7 ✓7th **S79.091 Other physeal fracture of upper end of right femur** MCC CC
CC Excl: See code: S79.001

7 ✓7th **S79.092 Other physeal fracture of upper end of left femur** MCC CC
CC Excl: See code: S79.002

7 ✓7th **S79.099 Other physeal fracture of upper end of unspecified femur** MCC CC
CC Excl: See code: S79.009

✓5th **S79.1 Physeal fracture of lower end of femur**
NOTE A fracture not indicated as open or closed should be coded to closed.

The appropriate 7th character is to be added to each code from subcategory S79.1.

A	initial encounter for closed fracture
D	subsequent encounter for fracture with routine healing
G	subsequent encounter for fracture with delayed healing
K	subsequent encounter for fracture with nonunion
P	subsequent encounter for fracture with malunion
S	sequela

✓6th **S79.10 Unspecified physeal fracture of lower end of femur**

7 ✓7th **S79.101 Unspecified physeal fracture of lower end of right femur** CC
CC Excl: CC with 7th character A: M80.00X-M80.019 with 7th A, M80.041-M80.059 with 7th A, M80.80X-M80.819 with 7th A, M80.841-M80.859 with 7th A, M84.40X-M84.419 with 7th A, M84.441-M84.459 with 7th A, M84.474-M84.519 with 7th A, M84.541-M84.559 with 7th A, M84.574-M84.576 with 7th A, M84.60X-M84.619 with 7th A, M84.641-M84.659 with 7th A, M84.674-M84.68X with 7th A, S03.8XX-S03.9XX with 7th A, S29.011-S29.019 with 7th A, S38.3XX-S39.013 with 7th A, S72.001-S72.471 with 7th [A, B, C], S72.479-S72.92X with 7th A, S73.101A, S73.109-S73.111 with 7th A, S73.119-S73.121 with 7th A, S73.129-S73.191 with 7th A, S73.199A, S76.001A, S76.009-S76.011 with 7th A, S76.019A, S76.091A, S76.099-S76.101 with 7th A, S76.109-S76.111 with 7th A, S76.119 with 7th A, S76.191A, S76.199-S76.201 with 7th A, S76.209-S76.211 with 7th A, S76.219A, S76.291A, S76.299-S76.301 with 7th A, S76.309-S76.311 with 7th A, S76.319A, S76.391A, S76.399-S76.801 with 7th A, S76.809-S76.811 with 7th A, S76.819 with 7th A, S76.891A, S76.899-S76.901 with 7th A, S76.909-S76.911 with 7th A, S76.919A, S76.991A, S76.999A, S79.001A, S79.009-S79.011 with 7th A, S79.019-S79.091 with 7th A, S79.099-S79.101 with 7th A, S79.109-S79.111 with 7th A, S79.119-S79.121 with 7th A, S79.129-S79.131 with 7th A, S79.139-S79.141 with 7th A, S79.149-S79.191 with 7th A, S79.199-S79.811 with 7th A, S79.819-S79.821 with 7th A, S79.829-S79.911 with 7th A, S79.919-S79.921 with 7th A, S79.929 with 7th A, S82.90X-S82.92X with 7th [A, B, C], T14.8-T14.91, T79.A9X-T79.9XX with 7th A
CC Excl: CC with 7th character K or P: M80.00X-M84.68 with 7th [K, P], S02.0XX-S02.92X with 7th K, S12.000-S12.691 with 7th K, S22.000-S22.9XX with 7th K, S32.000-S32.9XX with 7th K, S42.001-S42.92X with 7th [K, P], S49.001-S49.199 with 7th [K, P], S52.001-S52.92X with 7th [K, M, N, P, Q, R], S59.001-S59.299 with 7th [K, P], S62.001-S62.92X with 7th [K, P], S72.001-S72.92X with 7th [K, M, N, P, Q, R], S79.001-S79.199 with 7th [K, P], S82.001-S82.92X with 7th [K, M, N, P, Q, R], S89.001-S89.399 with 7th [K, P], S92.001-S92.919 with 7th [K, P]

7 HAC = Initial encounter only (7th character A, B or C) and not POA.

7 ✓7th **S79.102** **Unspecified physeal fracture of lower end of left femur** CC

CC Excl: CC with 7th character A: M80.00X-M80.019 with 7th A, M80.041-M80.059 with 7th A, M80.80X-M80.819 with 7th A, M80.841-M80.859 with 7th A, M84.40X-M84.419 with 7th A, M84.441-M84.459 with 7th A, M84.474-M84.519 with 7th A, M84.541-M84.559 with 7th A, M84.574-M84.576 with 7th A, M84.60X-M84.619 with 7th A, M84.641-M84.659 with 7th A, M84.674-M84.68X with 7th A, S03.8XX-S03.9XX with 7th A, S29.011-S29.019 with 7th A, S38.3XX-S39.013 with 7th A, S72.001-S72.466 with 7th [B, C], S72.472-S72.92 with 7th A, S73.102-S73.109 with 7th A, S73.112-S73.119 with 7th A, S73.122-S73.129 with 7th A, S73.192-S73.199 with 7th A, S76.002-S76.009 with 7th A, S76.012-S76.019 with 7th A, S76.092-S76.099 with 7th A, S76.102-S76.109 with 7th A, S76.112-S76.119 with 7th A, S76.192-S76.199 with 7th A, S76.202-S76.209 with 7th A, S76.212-S76.219 with 7th A, S76.292-S76.299 with 7th A, S76.302-S76.309 with 7th A, S76.312-S76.319 with 7th A, S76.392-S76.399 with 7th A, S76.802-S76.809 with 7th A, S76.812-S76.819 with 7th A, S76.892-S76.899 with 7th A, S76.902-S76.909 with 7th A, S76.912-S76.919 with 7th A, S76.992-S76.999 with 7th A, S79.002-S79.009 with 7th A, S79.012-S79.019 with 7th A, S79.092-S79.099 with 7th A, S79.102-S79.109 with 7th A, S79.112-S79.119 with 7th A, S79.122-S79.129 with 7th A, S79.132-S79.139 with 7th A, S79.142-S79.149 with 7th A, S79.192-S79.199 with 7th A, S79.812-S79.819 with 7th A, S79.822-S79.829 with 7th A, S79.912-S79.919 with 7th A, S79.922-S79.929 with 7th A, S82.90X-S82.92X with 7th [A, B, C], T14.8-T14.91, T79.A9X-T79.9XX with 7th A

CC Excl: CC with 7th character K or P: M80.00X-M84.68X with 7th [K, P], S02.0XX-S02.92X with 7th K, S12.000-S12.691 with 7th K, S22.000-S22.9XX with 7th K, S32.000-S32.9XX with 7th K, S42.001-S42.92X with 7th [K, P], S49.001-S49.199 with 7th [K, P], S52.001-S52.92X with 7th [K, M, N, P, Q, R], S59.001-S59.299 with 7th [K, P], S62.001-S62.92X with 7th [K, P], S72.001-S72.92X with 7th [K, M, N, P, Q, R], S79.001-S79.199 with 7th [K, P], S82.001-S82.92X with 7th [K, M, N, P, Q, R], S89.001-S89.399 with 7th [K, P], S92.001-S92.919 with 7th [K, P]

7 ✓7th **S79.109** **Unspecified physeal fracture of lower end of unspecified femur** CC

CC Excl: CC with 7th character A: M80.00X-M80.019 with 7th A, M80.041-M80.059 with 7th A, M80.80X-M80.819 with 7th A, M80.841-M80.859 with 7th A, M84.40X-M84.419 with 7th A, M84.441-M84.459 with 7th A, M84.474-M84.519 with 7th A, M84.541-M84.559 with 7th A, M84.574-M84.576 with 7th A, M84.60X-M84.619 with 7th A, M84.641-M84.659 with 7th A, M84.674-M84.68X with 7th A, S03.8XX-S03.9XX with 7th A, S29.011-S29.019 with 7th A, S38.3XX-S39.013 with 7th A, S72.001-S72.92 with 7th [A, B, C], S73.101-S73.199 with 7th A, S76.001-S76.019 with 7th A, S76.091-S76.119 with 7th A, S76.191-S76.219 with 7th A, S76.291-S76.319 with 7th A, S76.391-S76.819 with 7th A, S76.891-S76.919 with 7th A, S76.991-S76.999 with 7th A, S79.001-S79.929 with 7th A, S82.90X-S82.92X with 7th [A, B, C], T14.8-T14.91, T79.A9X-T79.9XX with 7th A

CC Excl: CC with 7th character K or P: M80.00X-M84.68 with 7th [K, P], S02.0XX-S02.92X with 7th K, S12.000-S12.691 with 7th K, S22.000-S22.9XX with 7th K, S32.000-S32.9XX with 7th K, S42.001-S42.92X with 7th [K, P], S49.001-S49.199 with 7th [K, P], S52.001-S52.92X with 7th [K, M, N, P, Q, R], S59.001-S59.299 with 7th [K, P], S62.001-S62.92X with 7th [K, P], S72.001-S72.92X with 7th [K, M, N, P, Q, R], S79.001-S79.199 with 7th [K, P], S82.001-S82.92X with 7th [K, M, N, P, Q, R], S89.001-S89.399 with 7th [K, P], S92.001-S92.919 with 7th [K, P]

✓6th **S79.11** **Salter-Harris Type I physeal fracture of lower end of femur**

7 ✓7th **S79.111** **Salter-Harris Type I physeal fracture of lower end of right femur** CC
CC Excl: See code: S79.101

7 ✓7th **S79.112** **Salter-Harris Type I physeal fracture of lower end of left femur** CC
CC Excl: See code: S79.102

7 ✓7th **S79.119** **Salter-Harris Type I physeal fracture of lower end of unspecified femur** CC
CC Excl: See code: S79.109

✓6th **S79.12** **Salter-Harris Type II physeal fracture of lower end of femur**

7 ✓7th **S79.121** **Salter-Harris Type II physeal fracture of lower end of right femur** CC
CC Excl: See code: S79.101

7 ✓7th **S79.122** **Salter-Harris Type II physeal fracture of lower end of left femur** CC
CC Excl: See code: S79.102

7 ✓7th **S79.129** **Salter-Harris Type II physeal fracture of lower end of unspecified femur** CC
CC Excl: See code: S79.109

✓6th **S79.13** **Salter-Harris Type III physeal fracture of lower end of femur**

7 ✓7th **S79.131** **Salter-Harris Type III physeal fracture of lower end of right femur** CC
CC Excl: See code: S79.101

7 ✓7th **S79.132** **Salter-Harris Type III physeal fracture of lower end of left femur** CC
CC Excl: See code: S79.102

7 ✓7th **S79.139** **Salter-Harris Type III physeal fracture of lower end of unspecified femur** CC
CC Excl: See code: S79.109

✓6th **S79.14** **Salter-Harris Type IV physeal fracture of lower end of femur**

7 ✓7th **S79.141** **Salter-Harris Type IV physeal fracture of lower end of right femur** CC
CC Excl: See code: S79.101

7 ✓7th **S79.142** **Salter-Harris Type IV physeal fracture of lower end of left femur** CC
CC Excl: See code: S79.102

7 ✓7th **S79.149** **Salter-Harris Type IV physeal fracture of lower end of unspecified femur** CC
CC Excl: See code: S79.109

✓6th **S79.19** **Other physeal fracture of lower end of femur**

7 ✓7th **S79.191** **Other physeal fracture of lower end of right femur** CC
CC Excl: See code: S79.101

7 ✓7th **S79.192** **Other physeal fracture of lower end of left femur** CC
CC Excl: See code: S79.102

7 ✓7th **S79.199** **Other physeal fracture of lower end of unspecified femur** CC
CC Excl: See code: S79.109

✓5th **S79.8** **Other specified injuries of hip and thigh**

The appropriate 7th character is to be added to each code in subcategory S79.8.
A initial encounter
D subsequent encounter
S sequela

✓6th **S79.81** **Other specified injuries of hip**

✓7th **S79.811** **Other specified injuries of right hip**

✓7th **S79.812** **Other specified injuries of left hip**

✓7th **S79.819** **Other specified injuries of unspecified hip**

✓6th **S79.82** **Other specified injuries of thigh**

✓7th **S79.821** **Other specified injuries of right thigh**

✓7th **S79.822** **Other specified injuries of left thigh**

✓7th **S79.829** **Other specified injuries of unspecified thigh**

7 HAC = Initial encounter only (7th character A, B or C) and not POA.

✓5th **S79.9 Unspecified injury of hip and thigh**

The appropriate 7th character is to be added to each code in subcategory S79.9.
A initial encounter
D subsequent encounter
S sequela

✓6th **S79.91 Unspecified injury of hip**
✓7th **S79.911 Unspecified injury of right hip**
✓7th **S79.912 Unspecified injury of left hip**
✓7th **S79.919 Unspecified injury of unspecified hip**
✓6th **S79.92 Unspecified injury of thigh**
✓7th **S79.921 Unspecified injury of right thigh**
✓7th **S79.922 Unspecified injury of left thigh**
✓7th **S79.929 Unspecified injury of unspecified thigh**

Injuries to the knee and lower leg (S80-S89)

EXCLUDES 2 *burns and corrosions (T20-T32)*
frostbite (T33-T34)
injuries of ankle and foot, except fracture of ankle and malleolus (S90-S99)
insect bite or sting, venomous (T63.4)

✓4th **S80 Superficial injury of knee and lower leg**
EXCLUDES 2 *superficial injury of ankle and foot (S90.-)*

The appropriate 7th character is to be added to each code from category S80.
A initial encounter
D subsequent encounter
S sequela

✓5th **S80.0 Contusion of knee**
✓x7th **S80.00 Contusion of unspecified knee**
✓x7th **S80.01 Contusion of right knee**
✓x7th **S80.02 Contusion of left knee**
✓5th **S80.1 Contusion of lower leg**
✓x7th **S80.10 Contusion of unspecified lower leg**
✓x7th **S80.11 Contusion of right lower leg**
✓x7th **S80.12 Contusion of left lower leg**
✓5th **S80.2 Other superficial injuries of knee**
✓6th **S80.21 Abrasion of knee**
✓7th **S80.211 Abrasion, right knee**
✓7th **S80.212 Abrasion, left knee**
✓7th **S80.219 Abrasion, unspecified knee**
✓6th **S80.22 Blister (nonthermal) of knee**
✓7th **S80.221 Blister (nonthermal), right knee**
✓7th **S80.222 Blister (nonthermal), left knee**
✓7th **S80.229 Blister (nonthermal), unspecified knee**
✓6th **S80.24 External constriction of knee**
✓7th **S80.241 External constriction, right knee**
✓7th **S80.242 External constriction, left knee**
✓7th **S80.249 External constriction, unspecified knee**
✓6th **S80.25 Superficial foreign body of knee**
Splinter in the knee
✓7th **S80.251 Superficial foreign body, right knee**
✓7th **S80.252 Superficial foreign body, left knee**
✓7th **S80.259 Superficial foreign body, unspecified knee**
✓6th **S80.26 Insect bite (nonvenomous) of knee**
✓7th **S80.261 Insect bite (nonvenomous), right knee**
✓7th **S80.262 Insect bite (nonvenomous), left knee**
✓7th **S80.269 Insect bite (nonvenomous), unspecified knee**
✓6th **S80.27 Other superficial bite of knee**
EXCLUDES 1 *open bite of knee (S81.05-)*
✓7th **S80.271 Other superficial bite of right knee**
✓7th **S80.272 Other superficial bite of left knee**
✓7th **S80.279 Other superficial bite of unspecified knee**
✓5th **S80.8 Other superficial injuries of lower leg**
✓6th **S80.81 Abrasion of lower leg**
✓7th **S80.811 Abrasion, right lower leg**
✓7th **S80.812 Abrasion, left lower leg**
✓7th **S80.819 Abrasion, unspecified lower leg**
✓6th **S80.82 Blister (nonthermal) of lower leg**
✓7th **S80.821 Blister (nonthermal), right lower leg**
✓7th **S80.822 Blister (nonthermal), left lower leg**
✓7th **S80.829 Blister (nonthermal), unspecified lower leg**
✓6th **S80.84 External constriction of lower leg**
✓7th **S80.841 External constriction, right lower leg**
✓7th **S80.842 External constriction, left lower leg**
✓7th **S80.849 External constriction, unspecified lower leg**
✓6th **S80.85 Superficial foreign body of lower leg**
Splinter in the lower leg
✓7th **S80.851 Superficial foreign body, right lower leg**
✓7th **S80.852 Superficial foreign body, left lower leg**
✓7th **S80.859 Superficial foreign body, unspecified lower leg**
✓6th **S80.86 Insect bite (nonvenomous) of lower leg**
✓7th **S80.861 Insect bite (nonvenomous), right lower leg**
✓7th **S80.862 Insect bite (nonvenomous), left lower leg**
✓7th **S80.869 Insect bite (nonvenomous), unspecified lower leg**
✓6th **S80.87 Other superficial bite of lower leg**
EXCLUDES 1 *open bite of lower leg (S81.85-)*
✓7th **S80.871 Other superficial bite, right lower leg**
✓7th **S80.872 Other superficial bite, left lower leg**
✓7th **S80.879 Other superficial bite, unspecified lower leg**
✓5th **S80.9 Unspecified superficial injury of knee and lower leg**
✓6th **S80.91 Unspecified superficial injury of knee**
✓7th **S80.911 Unspecified superficial injury of right knee**
✓7th **S80.912 Unspecified superficial injury of left knee**
✓7th **S80.919 Unspecified superficial injury of unspecified knee**
✓6th **S80.92 Unspecified superficial injury of lower leg**
✓7th **S80.921 Unspecified superficial injury of right lower leg**
✓7th **S80.922 Unspecified superficial injury of left lower leg**
✓7th **S80.929 Unspecified superficial injury of unspecified lower leg**

✓4th **S81 Open wound of knee and lower leg**
Code also any associated wound infection
EXCLUDES 1 *open fracture of knee and lower leg (S82.-)*
traumatic amputation of lower leg (S88.-)
EXCLUDES 2 *open wound of ankle and foot (S91.-)*

The appropriate 7th character is to be added to each code from category S81.
A initial encounter
D subsequent encounter
S sequela

✓5th **S81.0 Open wound of knee**
✓6th **S81.00 Unspecified open wound of knee**
✓7th **S81.001 Unspecified open wound, right knee**
✓7th **S81.002 Unspecified open wound, left knee**
✓7th **S81.009 Unspecified open wound, unspecified knee**
✓6th **S81.01 Laceration without foreign body of knee**
✓7th **S81.011 Laceration without foreign body, right knee**
✓7th **S81.012 Laceration without foreign body, left knee**
✓7th **S81.019 Laceration without foreign body, unspecified knee**
✓6th **S81.02 Laceration with foreign body of knee**
✓7th **S81.021 Laceration with foreign body, right knee**
✓7th **S81.022 Laceration with foreign body, left knee**
✓7th **S81.029 Laceration with foreign body, unspecified knee**
✓6th **S81.03 Puncture wound without foreign body of knee**
✓7th **S81.031 Puncture wound without foreign body, right knee**

S81.032 Puncture wound without foreign body, left knee

S81.039 Puncture wound without foreign body, unspecified knee

S81.04 Puncture wound with foreign body of knee

S81.041 Puncture wound with foreign body, right knee

S81.042 Puncture wound with foreign body, left knee

S81.049 Puncture wound with foreign body, unspecified knee

S81.05 Open bite of knee

Bite of knee NOS

EXCLUDES 1 *superficial bite of knee (S80.27-)*

S81.051 Open bite, right knee

S81.052 Open bite, left knee

S81.059 Open bite, unspecified knee

S81.8 Open wound of lower leg

S81.80 Unspecified open wound of lower leg

S81.801 Unspecified open wound, right lower leg

S81.802 Unspecified open wound, left lower leg

S81.809 Unspecified open wound, unspecified lower leg

S81.81 Laceration without foreign body of lower leg

S81.811 Laceration without foreign body, right lower leg

S81.812 Laceration without foreign body, left lower leg

S81.819 Laceration without foreign body, unspecified lower leg

S81.82 Laceration with foreign body of lower leg

S81.821 Laceration with foreign body, right lower leg

S81.822 Laceration with foreign body, left lower leg

S81.829 Laceration with foreign body, unspecified lower leg

S81.83 Puncture wound without foreign body of lower leg

S81.831 Puncture wound without foreign body, right lower leg

S81.832 Puncture wound without foreign body, left lower leg

S81.839 Puncture wound without foreign body, unspecified lower leg

S81.84 Puncture wound with foreign body of lower leg

S81.841 Puncture wound with foreign body, right lower leg

S81.842 Puncture wound with foreign body, left lower leg

S81.849 Puncture wound with foreign body, unspecified lower leg

S81.85 Open bite of lower leg

Bite of lower leg NOS

EXCLUDES 1 *superficial bite of lower leg (S80.86-, S80.87-)*

S81.851 Open bite, right lower leg

S81.852 Open bite, left lower leg

S81.859 Open bite, unspecified lower leg

S82 Fracture of lower leg, including ankle

NOTE A fracture not indicated as displaced or nondisplaced should be coded to displaced.

A fracture not designated as open or closed should be coded to closed.

The open fracture designations are based on the Gustilo open fracture classification.

INCLUDES fracture of malleolus

EXCLUDES 1 *traumatic amputation of lower leg (S88.-)*

EXCLUDES 2 *fracture of foot, except ankle (S92.-)*

periprosthetic fracture of prosthetic implant of knee (T84.042, T84.043)

The appropriate 7th character is to be added to all codes from category S82 [unless otherwise indicated].

- A initial encounter for closed fracture
- B initial encounter for open fracture type I or II
  initial encounter for open fracture NOS
- C initial encounter for open fracture type IIIA, IIIB, or IIIC
- D subsequent encounter for closed fracture with routine healing
- E subsequent encounter for open fracture type I or II with routine healing
- F subsequent encounter for open fracture type IIIA, IIIB, or IIIC with routine healing
- G subsequent encounter for closed fracture with delayed healing
- H subsequent encounter for open fracture type I or II with delayed healing
- J subsequent encounter for open fracture type IIIA, IIIB or IIIC with delayed healing
- K subsequent encounter for closed fracture with nonunion
- M subsequent encounter for open fracture type I or II with nonunion
- N subsequent encounter for open fracture type IIIA, IIIB or IIIC with nonunion
- P subsequent encounter for closed fracture with malunion
- Q subsequent encounter for open fracture type I or II with malunion
- R subsequent encounter for open fracture type IIIA, IIIB or IIIC with malunion
- S sequela

S82.0 Fracture of patella

Knee cap

S82.00 Unspecified fracture of patella

7 S82.001 Unspecified fracture of right patella CC

CC Excl: CC with 7th character A: S82.001-S82.099 with 7th [A, B, C]

CC with 7th character B or C: M80.00X-M80.019 with 7th A, M80.041-M80.049 with 7th A, M80.80X-M80.819 with 7th A, M80.841-M80.849 with 7th A, M84.40X-M84.419 with 7th A, M84.441-M84.446 with 7th A, M84.454 with 7th A, M84.474-M84.519 with 7th A, M84.541-M84.550 with 7th A, M84.574-M84.576 with 7th A, M84.60X-M84.619 with 7th A, M84.641-M84.650 with 7th A, M84.674-M84.68X with 7th A, S03.8XX-S03.9XX with 7th A, S29.011-S29.019 with 7th A, S38.3XX-S39.013 with 7th A, S73.101-S73.199 with 7th A, S76.001-S76.019 with 7th A, S76.091-S76.119 with 7th A, S76.191-S76.219 with 7th A, S76.291-S76.319 with 7th A, S76.391-S76.819 with 7th A, S76.891-S76.919 with 7th A, S76.991-S76.999 with 7th A, S79.811-S79.929 with 7th A, S82.001-S82.156 with 7th [B, C], S82.191-S82.299 with 7th [A, B, C], S82.401-S82.499 with 7th [A, B, C], S82.831-S82.839 with 7th [A, B, C], S82.861-S82.866 with 7th [A, B, C], S82.90X-S82.92X with 7th [A, B, C], S89.001-S89.099 with 7th A, S89.201-S89.299 with 7th A, T14.8-T14.91, T79.A9X-T79.9XX with 7th A

CC Excl: CC with 7th character K, M, N, P, Q or R: M80.00X-M84.68 with 7th [K, P], S02.0XX-S02.92X with 7th K, S12.000-S12.691 with 7th K, S22.000-S22.9XX with 7th K, S32.000-S32.9XX with 7th K, S42.001-S42.92X with 7th [K, P], S49.001-S49.199 with 7th [K, P], S52.001-S52.92X with 7th [K, M, N, P, Q, R], S59.001-S59.299 with 7th [K, P], S62.001-S62.92X with 7th [K, P], S72.001-S72.92X with 7th [K, M, N, P, Q, R], S79.001-S79.199 with 7th [K, P], S82.001-S82.92X with 7th [K, M, N, P, Q, R], S89.001-S89.399 with 7th [K, P], S92.001-S92.919 with 7th [K, P]

7 HAC = Initial encounter only (7th character A, B or C) and not POA.

7 ✓7th **S82.002 Unspecified fracture of left patella** CC
CC Excl: CC with 7th character A: S82.001-S82.099 with 7th [B, C]
CC with 7th character B or C: M80.00X-M80.019 with 7th A, M80.041-M80.049 with 7th A, M80.80X-M80.819 with 7th A, M80.841-M80.849 with 7th A, M84.40X-M84.419 with 7th A, M84.441-M84.446 with 7th A, M84.454 with 7th A, M84.474-M84.519 with 7th A, M84.541-M84.550 with 7th A, M84.574-M84.576 with 7th A, M84.60X-M84.619 with 7th A, M84.641-M84.650 with 7th A, M84.674-M84.68 with 7th A, S03.8XX-S03.9XX with 7th A, S29.011-S29.019 with 7th A, S38.3X-S39.013 with 7th A, S73.101-S73.199 with 7th A, S76.001-S76.019 with 7th A, S76.091-S76.119 with 7th A, S76.191-S76.219 with 7th A, S76.291-S76.319 with 7th A, S76.391-S76.819 with 7th A, S76.891-S76.919 with 7th A, S76.991-S76.999 with 7th A, S79.811-S79.929 with 7th A, S82.001-S82.156 with 7th [B, C], S82.191-S82.299 with 7th [A, B, C], S82.401-S82.499 with 7th [A, B, C], S82.831-S82.839 with 7th [A, B, C], S82.861-S82.866 with 7th [A, B, C], S82.90X-S82.92X with 7th [A, B, C], S89.001-S89.099 with 7th A, S89.201-S89.299 with 7th A, T14.8-T14.91, T79.A9X-T79.9XX with 7th A
CC Excl: CC with 7th character K, M, N, P, Q or R: M80.00X-M84.68X with 7th [K, P], S02.0XX-S02.92X with 7th K, S12.000-S12.691 with 7th K, S22.000-S22.9XX with 7th K, S32.000-S32.9XX with 7th K, S42.001-S42.92X with 7th [K, P], S49.001-S49.199 with 7th [K, P], S52.001-S52.92X with 7th [K, M, N, P, Q, R], S59.001-S59.299 with 7th [K, P], S62.001-S62.92X with 7th [K, P], S72.001-S72.92X with 7th [K, M, N, P, Q, R], S79.001-S79.199 with 7th [K, P], S82.001-S82.92X with 7th [K, M, N, P, Q, R], S89.001-S89.399 with 7th [K, P], S92.001-S92.919 with 7th [K, P]

7 ✓7th **S82.009 Unspecified fracture of unspecified patella** CC
CC Excl: CC with 7th character A: S82.001-S82.099 with 7th [A, B, C]
CC with 7th character B or C: M80.00X-M80.019 with 7th A, M80.041-M80.049 with 7th A, M80.80X-M80.819 with 7th A, M80.841-M80.849 with 7th A, M84.40X-M84.419 with 7th A, M84.441-M84.446 with 7th A, M84.454 with 7th A, M84.474-M84.519 with 7th A, M84.541-M84.550 with 7th A, M84.574-M84.576 with 7th A, M84.60X-M84.619 with 7th A, M84.641-M84.650 with 7th A, M84.674-M84.68X with 7th A, S03.8XX-S03.9XX with 7th A, S29.011-S29.019 with 7th A, S38.3XX-S39.013 with 7th A, S73.101-S73.199 with 7th A, S76.001-S76.019 with 7th A, S76.091-S76.119 with 7th A, S76.191-S76.219 with 7th A, S76.291-S76.319 with 7th A, S76.391-S76.819 with 7th A, S76.891-S76.919 with 7th A, S76.991-S76.999 with 7th A, S79.811-S79.929 with 7th A, S82.001-S82.156 with 7th [B, C], S82.191-S82.299 with 7th [A, B, C], S82.401-S82.499 with 7th [A, B, C], S82.831-S82.839 with 7th [A, B, C], S82.861-S82.866 with 7th [A, B, C], S82.90X-S82.92X with 7th [A, B, C], S89.001-S89.099 with 7th A, S89.201-S89.299 with 7th A, T14.8-T14.91, T79.A9X-T79.9XX with 7th A
CC Excl: CC with 7th character K, M, N, P, Q or R: M80.00X-M84.68 with 7th [K, P], S02.0XX-S02.92X with 7th K, S12.000-S12.691 with 7th K, S22.000-S22.9XX with 7th K, S32.000-S32.9XX with 7th K, S42.001-S42.92X with 7th [K, P], S49.001-S49.199 with 7th [K, P], S52.001-S52.92X with 7th [K, M, N, P, Q, R], S59.001-S59.299 with 7th [K, P], S62.001-S62.92X with 7th [K, P], S72.001-S72.92X with 7th [K, M, N, P, Q, R], S79.001-S79.199 with 7th [K, P], S82.001-S82.92X with 7th [K, M, N, P, Q, R], S89.001-S89.399 with 7th [K, P], S92.001-S92.919 with 7th [K, P]

✓6th **S82.01 Osteochondral fracture of patella**

7 ✓7th **S82.011 Displaced osteochondral fracture of right patella** CC
CC Excl: See code: S82.001

7 ✓7th **S82.012 Displaced osteochondral fracture of left patella** CC
CC Excl: See code: S82.002

7 ✓7th **S82.013 Displaced osteochondral fracture of unspecified patella** CC
CC Excl: See code: S82.009

7 ✓7th **S82.014 Nondisplaced osteochondral fracture of right patella** CC
CC Excl: See code: S82.001

7 ✓7th **S82.015 Nondisplaced osteochondral fracture of left patella** CC
CC Excl: See code: S82.002

7 ✓7th **S82.016 Nondisplaced osteochondral fracture of unspecified patella** CC
CC Excl: See code: S82.009

✓6th **S82.02 Longitudinal fracture of patella**

7 ✓7th **S82.021 Displaced longitudinal fracture of right patella** CC
CC Excl: See code: S82.001

7 ✓7th **S82.022 Displaced longitudinal fracture of left patella** CC
CC Excl: See code: S82.002

7 ✓7th **S82.023 Displaced longitudinal fracture of unspecified patella** CC
CC Excl: See code: S82.009

7 ✓7th **S82.024 Nondisplaced longitudinal fracture of right patella** CC
CC Excl: See code: S82.001

7 ✓7th **S82.025 Nondisplaced longitudinal fracture of left patella** CC
CC Excl: See code: S82.002

7 ✓7th **S82.026 Nondisplaced longitudinal fracture of unspecified patella** CC
CC Excl: See code: S82.009

✓6th **S82.03 Transverse fracture of patella**

7 ✓7th **S82.031 Displaced transverse fracture of right patella** CC
CC Excl: See code: S82.001

7 ✓7th **S82.032 Displaced transverse fracture of left patella** CC
CC Excl: See code: S82.002

7 ✓7th **S82.033 Displaced transverse fracture of unspecified patella** CC
CC Excl: See code: S82.009

7 ✓7th **S82.034 Nondisplaced transverse fracture of right patella** CC
CC Excl: See code: S82.001

7 ✓7th **S82.035 Nondisplaced transverse fracture of left patella** CC
CC Excl: See code: S82.002

7 ✓7th **S82.036 Nondisplaced transverse fracture of unspecified patella** CC
CC Excl: See code: S82.009

✓6th **S82.04 Comminuted fracture of patella**

7 ✓7th **S82.041 Displaced comminuted fracture of right patella** CC
CC Excl: See code: S82.001

7 ✓7th **S82.042 Displaced comminuted fracture of left patella** CC
CC Excl: See code: S82.002

7 ✓7th **S82.043 Displaced comminuted fracture of unspecified patella** CC
CC Excl: See code: S82.009

7 ✓7th **S82.044 Nondisplaced comminuted fracture of right patella** CC
CC Excl: See code: S82.001

7 ✓7th **S82.045 Nondisplaced comminuted fracture of left patella** CC
CC Excl: See code: S82.002

7 ✓7th **S82.046 Nondisplaced comminuted fracture of unspecified patella** CC
CC Excl: See code: S82.009

✓6th **S82.09 Other fracture of patella**

7 ✓7th **S82.091 Other fracture of right patella** CC
CC Excl: See code: S82.001

7 ✓7th **S82.092 Other fracture of left patella** CC
CC Excl: See code: S82.002

7 ✓7th **S82.099 Other fracture of unspecified patella** CC
CC Excl: See code: S82.009

7 HAC = Initial encounter only (7th character A, B or C) and not POA.

S82.1 Fracture of upper end of tibia
Fracture of proximal end of tibia
EXCLUDES 2 *fracture of shaft of tibia (S82.2-)*
physeal fracture of upper end of tibia (S89.0-)

S82.10 Unspecified fracture of upper end of tibia

7 **S82.101 Unspecified fracture of upper end of right tibia** MCC CC

CC Excl: CC with 7th character A: M80.00X-M80.019 with 7th A, M80.041-M80.049 with 7th A, M80.061-M80.079 with 7th A, M80.80X-M80.819 with 7th A, M80.841-M80.849 with 7th A, M80.861-M80.879 with 7th A, M84.40X-M84.419 with 7th A, M84.441-M84.446 with 7th A, M84.454 with 7th A, M84.461-M84.519 with 7th A, M84.541-M84.550 with 7th A, M84.561-M84.576 with 7th A, M84.60X-M84.619 with 7th A, M84.641-M84.650 with 7th A, M84.661-M84.68X with 7th A, S03.8XX-S03.9XX with 7th A, S29.011-S29.019 with 7th A, S38.3XX-S39.013 with 7th A, S73.101A, S73.109-S73.111 with 7th A, S73.119-S73.121 with 7th A, S73.129-S73.191 with 7th A, S73.199A, S76.001A, S76.009-S76.011 with 7th A, S76.019A, S76.091A, S76.099-S76.101 with 7th A, S76.109-S76.111 with 7th A, S76.119A, S76.191A, S76.199-S76.201 with 7th A, S76.209-S76.211 with 7th A, S76.219A, S76.291A, S76.299-S76.301 with 7th A, S76.309-S76.311 with 7th A, S76.319A, S76.391A, S76.399-S76.801 with 7th A, S76.809-S76.811 with 7th A, S76.819A, S76.891A, S76.899-S76.901 with 7th A, S76.909-S76.911 with 7th A, S76.919A, S76.991A, S76.999A, S79.811A, S79.819-S79.821 with 7th A, S79.829-S79.911 with 7th A, S79.919-S79.921 with 7th A, S79.929A, S82.101-S82.156 with 7th [A, B, C], S82.191-S82.299 with 7th [A, B, C], S82.401-S82.499 with 7th [A, B, C], S82.831-S82.839 with 7th [A, B, C], S82.861-S82.866 with 7th [A, B, C], S82.90X-S82.92X with 7th [A, B, C], S89.001A, S89.009-S89.011 with 7th A, S89.019-S89.021 with 7th A, S89.029-S89.031 with 7th A, S89.039-S89.041 with 7th A, S89.049-S89.091 with 7th A, S89.099A, S89.201A, S89.209-S89.211 with 7th A, S89.219-S89.221 with 7th A, S89.229-S89.291 with 7th A, S89.299A, T14.8-T14.91, T79.A9X-T79.9XX with 7th A

MCC with 7th B or C: M80.00X-M80.019 with 7th A, M80.041-M80.049 with 7th A, M80.061-M80.079 with 7th A, M80.80X-M80.819 with 7th A, M80.841-M80.849 with 7th A, M80.861-M80.879 with 7th A, M84.40X-M84.419 with 7th A, M84.441-M84.446 with 7th A, M84.454 with 7th A, M84.461-M84.519 with 7th A, M84.541-M84.550 with 7th A, M84.561-M84.576 with 7th A, M84.60X-M84.619 with 7th A, M84.641-M84.650 with 7th A, M84.661-M84.68X with 7th A, S03.8XX-S03.9XX with 7th A, S29.011-S29.019 with 7th A, S38.3X-S39.013 with 7th A, S73.101-S73.199 with 7th A, S76.001-S76.019 with 7th A, S76.091-S76.119 with 7th A, S76.191-S76.219 with 7th A, S76.291-S76.319 with 7th A, S76.391-S76.819 with 7th A, S76.891-S76.919 with 7th A, S76.991-S76.999 with 7th A, S79.811-S79.929 with 7th A, S82.101-S82.156 with 7th [A, B, C], S82.191-S82.299 with 7th [A, B, C], S82.401-S82.499 with 7th [A, B, C], S82.831-S82.839 with 7th [A, B, C], S82.861-S82.866 with 7th [A, B, C], S82.90X-S82.92X with 7th [A, B, C], S89.001-S89.099 with 7th A, S89.201-S89.299 with 7th A, T14.8-T14.91, T79.A9X-T79.9XX with 7th A

CC with 7th character K, M, N, P, Q or R: M80.00X-M84.68X with 7th [K, P], S02.0XX-S02.92X with 7th K, S12.000-S12.691 with 7th K, S22.000-S22.9XX with 7th K, S32.000-S32.9XX with 7th K, S42.001-S42.92X with 7th [K, P], S49.001-S49.199 with 7th [K, P], S52.001-S52.92X with 7th [K, M, N, P, Q, R], S59.001-S59.299 with 7th [K, P], S62.001-S62.92X with 7th [K, P], S72.001-S72.92X with 7th [K, M, N, P, Q, R], S79.001-S79.199 with 7th [K, P], S82.001-S82.92X with 7th [K, M, N, P, Q, R], S89.001-S89.399 with 7th [K, P], S92.001-S92.919 with 7th [K, P]

7 **S82.102 Unspecified fracture of upper end of left tibia** MCC CC

CC Excl: CC with 7th character A: M80.00X-M80.019 with 7th A, M80.041-M80.049 with 7th A, M80.061-M80.079 with 7th A, M80.80X-M80.819 with 7th A, M80.841-M80.849 with 7th A, M80.861-M80.879 with 7th A, M84.40X-M84.419 with 7th A, M84.441-M84.446 with 7th A, M84.454 with 7th A, M84.461-M84.519 with 7th A, M84.541-M84.550 with 7th A, M84.561-M84.576 with 7th A, M84.60X-M84.619 with 7th A, M84.641-M84.650 with 7th A, M84.661-M84.68 with 7th A, S03.8XX-S03.9XX with 7th A, S29.011-S29.019 with 7th A, S38.3XX-S39.013 with 7th A, S73.102-S73.109 with 7th A, S73.112-S73.119 with 7th A, S73.122-S73.129 with 7th A, S73.192-S73.199 with 7th A, S76.002-S76.009 with 7th A, S76.012-S76.019 with 7th A, S76.092-S76.099 with 7th A, S76.102-S76.109 with 7th A, S76.112-S76.119 with 7th A, S76.192-S76.199 with 7th A, S76.202-S76.209 with 7th A, S76.212-S76.219 with 7th A, S76.292-S76.299 with 7th A, S76.302-S76.309 with 7th A, S76.312-S76.319 with 7th A, S76.392-S76.399 with 7th A, S76.802-S76.809 with 7th A, S76.812-S76.819 with 7th A, S76.892-S76.899 with 7th A, S76.902-S76.909 with 7th A, S76.912-S76.919 with 7th A, S76.992-S76.999 with 7th A, S79.812-S79.819 with 7th A, S79.822-S79.829 with 7th A, S79.912-S79.919 with 7th A, S79.922-S79.929 with 7th A, S82.101-S82.156 with 7th [B, C], S82.191-S82.299 with 7th [B, C], S82.401-S82.499 with 7th [B, C], S82.831-S82.839 with 7th [B, C], S82.861-S82.866 with 7th [B, C], S82.90X-S82.92X with 7th [A, B, C], S89.002-S89.009 with 7th A, S89.012-S89.019 with 7th A, S89.022-S89.029 with 7th A, S89.032-S89.039 with 7th A, S89.042-S89.049 with 7th A, S89.092-S89.099 with 7th A, S89.202-S89.209 with 7th A, S89.212-S89.219 with 7th A, S89.222-S89.229 with 7th A, S89.292-S89.299 with 7th A, T14.8-T14.91, T79.A9X-T79.9XX with 7th A

CC with 7th character K, M, N, P, Q or R: M80.00X-M84.68 with 7th [K, P], S02.0XX-S02.92X with 7th K, S12.000-S12.691 with 7th K, S22.000-S22.9XX with 7th K, S32.000-S32.9XX with 7th K, S42.001-S42.92X with 7th [K, P], S49.001-S49.199 with 7th [K, P], S52.001-S52.92X with 7th [K, M, N, P, Q, R], S59.001-S59.299 with 7th [K, P], S62.001-S62.92X with 7th [K, P], S72.001-S72.92X with 7th [K, M, N, P, Q, R], S79.001-S79.199 with 7th [K, P], S82.001-S82.92X with 7th [K, M, N, P, Q, R], S89.001-S89.399 with 7th [K, P], S92.001-S92.919 with 7th [K, P]

7 HAC = Initial encounter only (7th character A, B or C) and not POA.

7 7th **S82.109 Unspecified fracture of upper end of unspecified tibia** MCC CC
CC Excl: CC with 7th character A: M80.00X-M80.019 with 7th A, M80.041-M80.049 with 7th A, M80.061-M80.079 with 7th A, M80.80X-M80.819 with 7th A, M80.841-M80.849 with 7th A, M80.861-M80.879 with 7th A, M84.40X-M84.419 with 7th A, M84.441-M84.446 with 7th A, M84.454 with 7th A, M84.461-M84.519 with 7th A, M84.541-M84.550 with 7th A, M84.561-M84.576 with 7th A, M84.60X-M84.619 with 7th A, M84.641-M84.650 with 7th A, M84.661-M84.68 with 7th A, S03.8XX-S03.9XX with 7th A, S29.011-S29.019 with 7th A, S38.3XX-S39.013 with 7th A, S73.101-S73.199 with 7th A, S76.001-S76.019 with 7th A, S76.091-S76.119 with 7th A, S76.191-S76.219 with 7th A, S76.291-S76.319 with 7th A, S76.391-S76.819 with 7th A, S76.891-S76.919 with 7th A, S76.991-S76.999 with 7th A, S79.811-S79.929 with 7th A, S82.101-S82.156 with 7th [A, B, C], S82.191-S82.299 with 7th [A, B, C], S82.401-S82.499 with 7th [A, B, C], S82.831-S82.839 with 7th [A, B, C], S82.861-S82.866 with 7th [A, B, C], S82.90X-S82.92X with 7th [A, B, C], S89.001-S89.099 with 7th A, S89.201-S89.299 with 7th A, T14.8-T14.91, T79.A9X-T79.9XX with 7th A
CC with 7th character K, M, N, P, Q or R: M80.00X-M84.68 with 7th [K, P], S02.0XX-S02.92X with 7th K, S12.000-S12.691 with 7th K, S22.000-S22.9XX with 7th K, S32.000-S32.9XX with 7th K, S42.001-S42.92X with 7th [K, P], S49.001-S49.199 with 7th [K, P], S52.001-S52.92X with 7th [K, M, N, P, Q, R], S59.001-S59.299 with 7th [K, P], S62.001-S62.92X with 7th [K, P], S72.001-S72.92X with 7th [K, M, N, P, Q, R], S79.001-S79.199 with 7th [K, P], S82.001-S82.92X with 7th [K, M, N, P, Q, R], S89.001-S89.399 with 7th [K, P], S92.001-S92.919 with 7th [K, P]

6th **S82.11 Fracture of tibial spine**

7 7th **S82.111 Displaced fracture of right tibial spine** MCC CC
CC Excl: See code: S82.101

7 7th **S82.112 Displaced fracture of left tibial spine** MCC CC
CC Excl: See code: S82.102

7 7th **S82.113 Displaced fracture of unspecified tibial spine** MCC CC
CC Excl: See code: S82.109

7 7th **S82.114 Nondisplaced fracture of right tibial spine** MCC CC
CC Excl: See code: S82.101

7 7th **S82.115 Nondisplaced fracture of left tibial spine** MCC CC
CC Excl: See code: S82.102

7 7th **S82.116 Nondisplaced fracture of unspecified tibial spine** MCC CC
CC Excl: See code: S82.109

6th **S82.12 Fracture of lateral condyle of tibia**

7 7th **S82.121 Displaced fracture of lateral condyle of right tibia** MCC CC
CC Excl: See code: S82.101

7 7th **S82.122 Displaced fracture of lateral condyle of left tibia** MCC CC
CC Excl: See code: S82.102

7 7th **S82.123 Displaced fracture of lateral condyle of unspecified tibia** MCC CC
CC Excl: See code: S82.109

7 7th **S82.124 Nondisplaced fracture of lateral condyle of right tibia** MCC CC
CC Excl: See code: S82.101

7 7th **S82.125 Nondisplaced fracture of lateral condyle of left tibia** MCC CC
CC Excl: See code: S82.102

7 7th **S82.126 Nondisplaced fracture of lateral condyle of unspecified tibia** MCC CC
CC Excl: See code: S82.109

6th **S82.13 Fracture of medial condyle of tibia**

7 7th **S82.131 Displaced fracture of medial condyle of right tibia** MCC CC
CC Excl: See code: S82.101

7 7th **S82.132 Displaced fracture of medial condyle of left tibia** MCC CC
CC Excl: See code: S82.102

7 7th **S82.133 Displaced fracture of medial condyle of unspecified tibia** MCC CC
CC Excl: See code: S82.109

7 7th **S82.134 Nondisplaced fracture of medial condyle of right tibia** MCC CC
CC Excl: See code: S82.101

7 7th **S82.135 Nondisplaced fracture of medial condyle of left tibia** MCC CC
CC Excl: See code: S82.102

7 7th **S82.136 Nondisplaced fracture of medial condyle of unspecified tibia** MCC CC
CC Excl: See code: S82.109

6th **S82.14 Bicondylar fracture of tibia**
Fracture of tibial plateau NOS

7 7th **S82.141 Displaced bicondylar fracture of right tibia** MCC CC
CC Excl: See code: S82.101

7 7th **S82.142 Displaced bicondylar fracture of left tibia** MCC CC
CC Excl: See code: S82.102

7 7th **S82.143 Displaced bicondylar fracture of unspecified tibia** MCC CC
CC Excl: See code: S82.109

7 7th **S82.144 Nondisplaced bicondylar fracture of right tibia** MCC CC
CC Excl: See code: S82.101

7 7th **S82.145 Nondisplaced bicondylar fracture of left tibia** MCC CC
CC Excl: See code: S82.102

7 7th **S82.146 Nondisplaced bicondylar fracture of unspecified tibia** MCC CC
CC Excl: See code: S82.109

6th **S82.15 Fracture of tibial tuberosity**

7 7th **S82.151 Displaced fracture of right tibial tuberosity** MCC CC
CC Excl: See code: S82.101

7 7th **S82.152 Displaced fracture of left tibial tuberosity** MCC CC
CC Excl: See code: S82.102

7 7th **S82.153 Displaced fracture of unspecified tibial tuberosity** MCC CC
CC Excl: See code: S82.109

7 7th **S82.154 Nondisplaced fracture of right tibial tuberosity** MCC CC
CC Excl: See code: S82.101

7 7th **S82.155 Nondisplaced fracture of left tibial tuberosity** MCC CC
CC Excl: See code: S82.102

7 7th **S82.156 Nondisplaced fracture of unspecified tibial tuberosity** MCC CC
CC Excl: See code: S82.109

6th **S82.16 Torus fracture of upper end of tibia**

The appropriate 7th character is to be added to all codes in subcategory S82.16.
A initial encounter for closed fracture
D subsequent encounter for fracture with routine healing
G subsequent encounter for fracture with delayed healing
K subsequent encounter for fracture with nonunion
P subsequent encounter for fracture with malunion
S sequela

7 HAC = Initial encounter only (7th character A, B or C) and not POA.

7 ✓7th **S82.161 Torus fracture of upper end of right tibia** CC
CC Excl: CC with 7th character A: S82.101-S82.161 with 7th [A, B, C], S82.169-S82.299 with 7th A, S82.311A, S82.319A, S82.401-S82.811 with 7th [A, B, C], S82.819-S82.821 with 7th A, S82.829-S82.839 with 7th A, S82.861-S82.866 with 7th [A, B, C], S89.001A, S89.009-S89.011 with 7th A, S89.019-S89.021 with 7th A, S89.029-S89.031 with 7th A, S89.039-S89.041 with 7th A, S89.049-S89.091 with 7th A, S89.099A, S89.201A, S89.209-S89.211 with 7th A, S89.219-S89.221 with 7th A, S89.229-S89.291 with 7th A, S89.299A
CC with 7th character K or P: M80.00X-M84.68X with 7th [K, P], S02.0XX-S02.92X with 7th K, S12.000-S12.691 with 7th K, S22.000-S22.9XX with 7th K, S32.000-S32.9XX with 7th K, S42.001-S42.92Xwith 7th [K, P], S49.001-S49.199 with 7th [K, P], S52.001-S52.92X with 7th [K, M, N, P, Q, R], S59.001-S59.299 with 7th [K, P], S62.001-S62.92X with 7th [K, P], S72.001-S72.92X with 7th [K, M, N, P, Q, R], S79.001-S79.199 with 7th [K, P], S82.001-S82.92X with 7th [K, M, N, P, Q, R], S89.001-S89.399 with 7th [K, P], S92.001-S92.919 with 7th [K, P]

7 ✓7th **S82.162 Torus fracture of upper end of left tibia** CC
CC Excl: CC with 7th character A: S82.101-S82.156 with 7th [B, C], S82.162-S82.299 with 7th A, S82.312-S82.319 with 7th A, S82.401-S82.499 with 7th [B, C], S82.812-S82.819 with 7th A, S82.822-S82.839 with 7th A, S82.861-S82.866 with 7th [B, C], S89.002-S89.009 with 7th A, S89.012-S89.019 with 7th A, S89.022-S89.029 with 7th A, S89.032-S89.039 with 7th A, S89.042-S89.049 with 7th A, S89.092-S89.099 with 7th A, S89.202-S89.209 with 7th A, S89.212-S89.219 with 7th A, S89.222-S89.229 with 7th A, S89.292-S89.299 with 7th A
CC with 7th character K or P: M80.00X-M84.68X with 7th [K, P], S02.0XX-S02.92X with 7th K, S12.000-S12.691 with 7th K, S22.000-S22.9XX with 7th K, S32.000-S32.9XX with 7th K, S42.001-S42.92X with 7th [K, P], S49.001-S49.199 with 7th [K, P], S52.001-S52.92X with 7th [K, M, N, P, Q, R], S59.001-S59.299 with 7th [K, P], S62.001-S62.92X with 7th [K, P], S72.001-S72.92X with 7th [K, M, N, P, Q, R], S79.001-S79.199 with 7th [K, P], S82.001-S82.92X with 7th [K, M, N, P, Q, R], S89.001-S89.399 with 7th [K, P], S92.001-S92.919 with 7th [K, P]

7 ✓7th **S82.169 Torus fracture of upper end of unspecified tibia** CC
CC Excl: CC with 7th character A: S82.101-S82.299 with 7th [A, B, C], S82.311-S82.319 with 7th A, S82.401-S82.839 with 7th [A, B, C], S82.861-S82.866 with 7th [A, B, C], S89.001-S89.099 with 7th A, S89.201-S89.299 with 7th A
CC with 7th character K or P: M80.00X-M84.68X with 7th [K, P], S02.0XX-S02.92X with 7th K, S12.000-S12.691 with 7th K, S22.000-S22.9XX with 7th K, S32.000-S32.9XX with 7th K, S42.001-S42.92X with 7th [K, P], S49.001-S49.199 with 7th [K, P], S52.001-S52.92X with 7th [K, M, N, P, Q, R], S59.001-S59.299 with 7th [K, P], S62.001-S62.92X with 7th [K, P], S72.001-S72.92X with 7th [K, M, N, P, Q, R], S79.001-S79.199 with 7th [K, P], S82.001-S82.92X with 7th [K, M, N, P, Q, R], S89.001-S89.399 with 7th [K, P], S92.001-S92.919 with 7th [K, P]

✓6th **S82.19 Other fracture of upper end of tibia**

7 ✓7th **S82.191 Other fracture of upper end of right tibia** MCC CC
CC Excl: See code: S82.101

7 ✓7th **S82.192 Other fracture of upper end of left tibia** MCC CC
CC Excl: See code: S82.102

7 ✓7th **S82.199 Other fracture of upper end of unspecified tibia** MCC CC
CC Excl: See code: S82.109

✓5th **S82.2 Fracture of shaft of tibia**

✓6th **S82.20 Unspecified fracture of shaft of tibia**
Fracture of tibia NOS

7 ✓7th **S82.201 Unspecified fracture of shaft of right tibia** MCC CC
CC Excl: CC with 7th character A: M80.00X-M80.019 with 7th A, M80.041-M80.049 with 7th A, M80.061-M80.079 with 7th A, M80.80X-M80.819 with 7th A, M80.841-M80.849 with 7th A, M80.861-M80.879 with 7th A, M84.40X-M84.419 with 7th A, M84.441-M84.446 with 7th A, M84.454 with 7th A, M84.461-M84.519 with 7th A, M84.541-M84.550 with 7th A, M84.561-M84.576 with 7th A, M84.60X-M84.619 with 7th A, M84.641-M84.650 with 7th A, M84.661-M84.68 with 7th A, S03.8XX-S03.9XX with 7th A, S29.011-S29.019 with 7th A, S38.3XX-S39.013 with 7th A, S73.101A, S73.109-S73.111 with 7th A, S73.119-S73.121 with 7th A, S73.129-S73.191 with 7th A, S73.199A, S76.001A, S76.009-S76.011 with 7th A, S76.019A, S76.091A, S76.099-S76.101 with 7th A, S76.109-S76.111 with 7th A, S76.119A, S76.191A, S76.199-S76.201 with 7th A, S76.209-S76.211 with 7th A, S76.219A, S76.291A, S76.299-S76.301 with 7th A, S76.309-S76.311 with 7th A, S76.319A, S76.391A, S76.399-S76.801 with 7th A, S76.809-S76.811 with 7th A, S76.819A, S76.891A, S76.899-S76.901 with 7th A, S76.909-S76.911 with 7th A, S76.919A, S76.991A, S76.999A, S79.811 A, S79.819-S79.821 with 7th A, S79.829-S79.911 with 7th A, S79.919-S79.921 with 7th A, S79.929A, S82.101-S82.161 with 7th [A, B, C], S82.169-S82.299 with 7th A, S82.311 with 7th A, S82.319 with 7th A, S82.401-S82.811 with 7th [A, B, C], S82.819-S82.821 with 7th A, S82.829-S82.839 with 7th A, S82.861-S82.866 with 7th [A, B, C], S82.90X-S82.92X with 7th [A, B, C], S89.001A, S89.009-S89.011 with 7th A, S89.019-S89.021 with 7th A, S89.029-S89.031 with 7th A, S89.039-S89.041 with 7th A, S89.049-S89.091 with 7th A, S89.099A, S89.201A, S89.209-S89.211 with 7th A, S89.219-S89.221 with 7th A, S89.229-S89.291 with 7th A, S89.299A, T14.8-T14.91, T79.A9X-T79.9XX with 7th A
MCC with 7th B or C: M80.00X-M80.019 with 7th A, M80.041-M80.049 with 7th A, M80.061-M80.079 with 7th A, M80.80X-M80.819 with 7th A, M80.841-M80.849 with 7th A, M80.861-M80.879 with 7th A, M84.40X-M84.419 with 7th A, M84.441-M84.446 with 7th A, M84.454 with 7th A, M84.461-M84.519 with 7th A, M84.541-M84.550 with 7th A, M84.561-M84.576 with 7th A, M84.60X-M84.619 with 7th A, M84.641-M84.650 with 7th A, M84.661-M84.68 with 7th A, S03.8X-S03.9X with 7th A, S29.011-S29.019 with 7th A, S38.3XX-S39.013 with 7th A, S73.101-S73.199 with 7th A, S76.001-S76.019 with 7th A, S76.091-S76.119 with 7th A, S76.191-S76.219 with 7th A, S76.291-S76.319 with 7th A, S76.391-S76.819 with 7th A, S76.891-S76.919 with 7th A, S76.991-S76.999 with 7th A, S79.811-S79.929 with 7th A, S82.101-S82.156 with 7th [A, B, C], S82.191-S82.299 with 7th [A, B, C], S82.401-S82.499 with 7th [A, B, C], S82.831-S82.839 with 7th [A, B, C], S82.861-S82.866 with 7th [A, B, C], S82.90X-S82.92X with 7th [A, B, C], S89.001-S89.099 with 7th A, S89.201-S89.299 with 7th A, T14.8-T14.91, T79.A9X-T79.9XX with 7th A
CC with 7th character K, M, N, P, Q or R: M80.00X-M84.68X with 7th [K, P], S02.0XX-S02.92X with 7th K, S12.000-S12.691 with 7th K, S22.000-S22.9XX with 7th K, S32.000-S32.9XX with 7th K, S42.001-S42.92X with 7th [K, P], S49.001-S49.199 with 7th [K, P], S52.001-S52.92X with 7th [K, M, N, P, Q, R], S59.001-S59.299 with 7th [K, P], S62.001-S62.92X with 7th [K, P], S72.001-S72.92X with 7th [K, M, N, P, Q, R], S79.001-S79.199 with 7th [K, P], S82.001-S82.92X with 7th [K, M, N, P, Q, R], S89.001-S89.399 with 7th [K, P], S92.001-S92.919 with 7th [K, P]

7 HAC = Initial encounter only (7th character A, B or C) and not POA.

7 ✓7th **S82.202** **Unspecified fracture of shaft of left tibia** MCC CC
CC Excl: See code: S82.192

7 ✓7th **S82.209** **Unspecified fracture of shaft of unspecified tibia** MCC CC
CC Excl: See code: S82.199

✓6th **S82.22** **Transverse fracture of shaft of tibia**

7 ✓7th **S82.221** **Displaced transverse fracture of shaft of right tibia** MCC CC
CC Excl: See code: S82.191

7 ✓7th **S82.222** **Displaced transverse fracture of shaft of left tibia** MCC CC
CC Excl: See code: S82.192

7 ✓7th **S82.223** **Displaced transverse fracture of shaft of unspecified tibia** MCC CC
CC Excl: See code: S82.199

7 ✓7th **S82.224** **Nondisplaced transverse fracture of shaft of right tibia** MCC CC
CC Excl: See code: S82.191

7 ✓7th **S82.225** **Nondisplaced transverse fracture of shaft of left tibia** MCC CC
CC Excl: See code: S82.192

7 ✓7th **S82.226** **Nondisplaced transverse fracture of shaft of unspecified tibia** MCC CC
CC Excl: See code: S82.199

✓6th **S82.23** **Oblique fracture of shaft of tibia**

7 ✓7th **S82.231** **Displaced oblique fracture of shaft of right tibia** MCC CC
CC Excl: See code: S82.191

7 ✓7th **S82.232** **Displaced oblique fracture of shaft of left tibia** MCC CC
CC Excl: See code: S82.192

7 ✓7th **S82.233** **Displaced oblique fracture of shaft of unspecified tibia** MCC CC
CC Excl: See code: S82.199

7 ✓7th **S82.234** **Nondisplaced oblique fracture of shaft of right tibia** MCC CC
CC Excl: See code: S82.191

7 ✓7th **S82.235** **Nondisplaced oblique fracture of shaft of left tibia** MCC CC
CC Excl: See code: S82.192

7 ✓7th **S82.236** **Nondisplaced oblique fracture of shaft of unspecified tibia** MCC CC
CC Excl: See code: S82.199

✓6th **S82.24** **Spiral fracture of shaft of tibia**
Toddler fracture

7 ✓7th **S82.241** **Displaced spiral fracture of shaft of right tibia** MCC CC
CC Excl: See code: S82.191

7 ✓7th **S82.242** **Displaced spiral fracture of shaft of left tibia** MCC CC
CC Excl: See code: S82.192

7 ✓7th **S82.243** **Displaced spiral fracture of shaft of unspecified tibia** MCC CC
CC Excl: See code: S82.199

7 ✓7th **S82.244** **Nondisplaced spiral fracture of shaft of right tibia** MCC CC
CC Excl: See code: S82.191

7 ✓7th **S82.245** **Nondisplaced spiral fracture of shaft of left tibia** MCC CC
CC Excl: See code: S82.192

7 ✓7th **S82.246** **Nondisplaced spiral fracture of shaft of unspecified tibia** MCC CC
CC Excl: See code: S82.199

✓6th **S82.25** **Comminuted fracture of shaft of tibia**

7 ✓7th **S82.251** **Displaced comminuted fracture of shaft of right tibia** MCC CC
CC Excl: See code: S82.191

7 ✓7th **S82.252** **Displaced comminuted fracture of shaft of left tibia** MCC CC
CC Excl: See code: S82.192

7 ✓7th **S82.253** **Displaced comminuted fracture of shaft of unspecified tibia** MCC CC
CC Excl: See code: S82.199

7 ✓7th **S82.254** **Nondisplaced comminuted fracture of shaft of right tibia** MCC CC
CC Excl: See code: S82.191

7 ✓7th **S82.255** **Nondisplaced comminuted fracture of shaft of left tibia** MCC CC
CC Excl: See code: S82.192

7 ✓7th **S82.256** **Nondisplaced comminuted fracture of shaft of unspecified tibia** MCC CC
CC Excl: See code: S82.199

✓6th **S82.26** **Segmental fracture of shaft of tibia**

7 ✓7th **S82.261** **Displaced segmental fracture of shaft of right tibia** MCC CC
CC Excl: See code: S82.191

7 ✓7th **S82.262** **Displaced segmental fracture of shaft of left tibia** MCC CC
CC Excl: See code: S82.192

7 ✓7th **S82.263** **Displaced segmental fracture of shaft of unspecified tibia** MCC CC
CC Excl: See code: S82.199

7 ✓7th **S82.264** **Nondisplaced segmental fracture of shaft of right tibia** MCC CC
CC Excl: See code: S82.191

7 ✓7th **S82.265** **Nondisplaced segmental fracture of shaft of left tibia** MCC CC
CC Excl: See code: S82.192

7 ✓7th **S82.266** **Nondisplaced segmental fracture of shaft of unspecified tibia** MCC CC
CC Excl: See code: S82.199

✓6th **S82.29** **Other fracture of shaft of tibia**

7 ✓7th **S82.291** **Other fracture of shaft of right tibia** MCC CC
CC Excl: See code: S82.191

7 ✓7th **S82.292** **Other fracture of shaft of left tibia** MCC CC
CC Excl: See code: S82.192

7 ✓7th **S82.299** **Other fracture of shaft of unspecified tibia** MCC CC
CC Excl: See code: S82.199

✓5th **S82.3** **Fracture of lower end of tibia**

EXCLUDES 1 *bimalleolar fracture of lower leg (S82.84-)*
fracture of medial malleolus alone (S82.5-)
Maisonneuve's fracture (S82.86-)
pilon fracture of distal tibia (S82.87-)
trimalleolar fractures of lower leg (S82.85-)

✓6th **S82.30** **Unspecified fracture of lower end of tibia**

CC Excl: For CC codes in subcategory S82.30, unless otherwise noted: CC with 7th character B or C: M80.00X-M80.019 with 7th A, M80.041-M80.049 with 7th A, M80.061-M80.079 with 7th A, M80.80X-M80.819 with 7th A, M80.841-M80.849 with 7th A, M80.861-M80.879 with 7th A, M84.40X-M84.419 with 7th A, M84.441-M84.446 with 7th A, M84.454 with 7th A, M84.461-M84.519 with 7th A, M84.541-M84.550 with 7th A, M84.561-M84.576 with 7th A, M84.60X-M84.619 with 7th A, M84.641-M84.650 with 7th A, M84.661-M84.68 with 7th A, S03.8XX-S03.9XX with 7th A, S29.011-S29.019 with 7th A, S38.3XX-S39.013 with 7th A, S73.101-S73.199 with 7th A, S76.001-S76.019 with 7th A, S76.091-S76.119 with 7th A, S76.191-S76.219 with 7th A, S76.291-S76.319 with 7th A, S76.391-S76.819 with 7th A, S76.891-S76.919 with 7th A, S76.991-S76.999 with 7th A, S79.811-S79.929 with 7th A, S82.301-S82.309 with 7th [A, B, C], S82.391-S82.399 with 7th [A, B, C], S82.51X-S82.66X with 7th [B, C], S82.841-S82.856 with 7th [A, B, C], S82.871-S82.92X with 7th [B, C], S89.101-S89.199 with 7th A, S89.301-S89.399 with 7th A, T14.8-T14.91, T79.A9X-T79.9XX with 7th A

CC with 7th character K, M, N, P, Q or R: M80.00X-M84.68X with 7th [K, P], S02.0XX-S02.92X with 7th K, S12.000-S12.691 with 7th K, S22.000-S22.9XX with 7th K, S32.000-S32.9XX with 7th K, S42.001-S42.92X with 7th [K, P], S49.001-S49.199 with 7th [K, P], S52.001-S52.92X with 7th [K, M, N, P, Q, R], S59.001-S59.299 with 7th [K, P], S62.001-S62.92X with 7th [K, P], S72.001-S72.92X with 7th [K, M, N, P, Q, R], S79.001-S79.199 with 7th [K, P], S82.001-S82.92X with 7th [K, M, N, P, Q, R], S89.001-S89.399 with 7th [K, P], S92.001-S92.919 with 7th [K, P]

7 ✓7th **S82.301** **Unspecified fracture of lower end of right tibia** CC

7 HAC = Initial encounter only (7th character A, B or C) and not POA.

7 ✓7th **S82.302** **Unspecified fracture of lower end of left tibia** CC

7 ✓7th **S82.309** **Unspecified fracture of lower end of unspecified tibia** CC

✓6th **S82.31** **Torus fracture of lower end of tibia**

The appropriate 7th character is to be added to all codes in subcategory S82.31.
- A initial encounter for closed fracture
- D subsequent encounter for fracture with routine healing
- G subsequent encounter for fracture with delayed healing
- K subsequent encounter for fracture with nonunion
- P subsequent encounter for fracture with malunion
- S sequela

7 ✓7th **S82.311** **Torus fracture of lower end of right tibia** CC

CC Excl: CC with 7th character A: S82.101-S82.161 with 7th [A, B, C], S82.169-S82.299 with 7th A, S82.311 with 7th A, S82.319 with 7th A, S82.401-S82.811 with 7th [A, B, C], S82.819-S82.821 with 7th A, S82.829-S82.839 with 7th A, S82.861-S82.866 with 7th [A, B, C], S89.001 with 7th A, S89.009-S89.011 with 7th A, S89.019-S89.021 with 7th A, S89.029-S89.031 with 7th A, S89.039-S89.041 with 7th A, S89.049-S89.091 with 7th A, S89.099A, S89.201A, S89.209-S89.211 with 7th A, S89.219-S89.221 with 7th A, S89.229-S89.291 with 7th A, S89.299A
CC with 7th character K or P: M80.00X-M84.68X with 7th [K, P], S02.0XX-S02.92X with 7th K, S12.000-S12.691 with 7th K, S22.000-S22.9XX with 7th K, S32.000-S32.9XX with 7th K, S42.001-S42.92X with 7th [K, P], S49.001-S49.199 with 7th [K, P], S52.001-S52.92X with 7th [K, M, N, P, Q, R], S59.001-S59.299 with 7th [K, P], S62.001-S62.92X with 7th [K, P], S72.001-S72.92X with 7th [K, M, N, P, Q, R], S79.001-S79.199 with 7th [K, P], S82.001-S82.92X with 7th [K, M, N, P, Q, R], S89.001-S89.399 with 7th [K, P], S92.001-S92.919 with 7th [K, P]

7 ✓7th **S82.312** **Torus fracture of lower end of left tibia** CC

CC Excl: CC with 7th character A: S82.101-S82.156 with 7th [B, C], S82.162-S82.299 with 7th A, S82.312-S82.319 with 7th A, S82.401-S82.499 with 7th [B, C], S82.812-S82.819 with 7th A, S82.822-S82.839 with 7th A, S82.861-S82.866 with 7th [B, C], S89.002-S89.009 with 7th A, S89.012-S89.019 with 7th A, S89.022-S89.029 with 7th A, S89.032-S89.039 with 7th A, S89.042-S89.049 with 7th A, S89.092-S89.099 with 7th A, S89.202-S89.209 with 7th A, S89.212-S89.219 with 7th A, S89.222-S89.229 with 7th A, S89.292-S89.299 with 7th A
CC with 7th character K or P: M80.00X-M84.68X with 7th [K, P], S02.0XX-S02.92X with 7th K, S12.000-S12.691 with 7th K, S22.000-S22.9XX with 7th K, S32.000-S32.9XX with 7th K, S42.001-S42.92X with 7th [K, P], S49.001-S49.199 with 7th [K, P], S52.001-S52.92X with 7th [K, M, N, P, Q, R], S59.001-S59.299 with 7th [K, P], S62.001-S62.92X with 7th [K, P], S72.001-S72.92X with 7th [K, M, N, P, Q, R], S79.001-S79.199 with 7th [K, P], S82.001-S82.92X with 7th [K, M, N, P, Q, R], S89.001-S89.399 with 7th [K, P], S92.001-S92.919 with 7th [K, P]

7 ✓7th **S82.319** **Torus fracture of lower end of unspecified tibia** CC

CC Excl: CC with 7th character A: S82.101-S82.299 with 7th [A, B, C], S82.311-S82.319 with 7th A, S82.401-S82.839 with 7th [A, B, C], S82.861-S82.866 with 7th [A, B, C], S89.001-S89.099 with 7th A, S89.201-S89.299 with 7th A
CC with 7th character K or P: M80.00X-M84.68X with 7th [K, P], S02.0XX-S02.92X with 7th K, S12.000-S12.691 with 7th K, S22.000-S22.9XX with 7th K, S32.000-S32.9XX with 7th K, S42.001-S42.92X with 7th [K, P], S49.001-S49.199 with 7th [K, P], S52.001-S52.92X with 7th [K, M, N, P, Q, R], S59.001-S59.299 with 7th [K, P], S62.001-S62.92X with 7th [K, P], S72.001-S72.92X with 7th [K, M, N, P, Q, R], S79.001-S79.199 with 7th [K, P], S82.001-S82.92X with 7th [K, M, N, P, Q, R], S89.001-S89.399 with 7th [K, P], S92.001-S92.919 with 7th [K, P]

✓6th **S82.39** **Other fracture of lower end of tibia**

CC Excl: For CC codes in subcategory S82.39, unless otherwise noted: See code: S82.30

7 ✓7th **S82.391** **Other fracture of lower end of right tibia** CC

7 ✓7th **S82.392** **Other fracture of lower end of left tibia** CC

7 ✓7th **S82.399** **Other fracture of lower end of unspecified tibia** CC

✓5th **S82.4** **Fracture of shaft of fibula**

EXCLUDES 2 *fracture of lateral malleolus alone (S82.6-)*

CC Excl: For CC codes in subcategory S82.4, unless otherwise noted: MCC for codes with 7th B or C: M80.00X-M80.019 with 7th A, M80.041-M80.049 with 7th A, M80.061-M80.079 with 7th A, M80.80X-M80.819 with 7th A, M80.841-M80.849 with 7th A, M80.861-M80.879 with 7th A, M84.40X-M84.419 with 7th A, M84.441-M84.446 with 7th A, M84.454 with 7th A, M84.461-M84.519 with 7th A, M84.541-M84.550 with 7th A, M84.561-M84.576 with 7th A, M84.60X-M84.619 with 7th A, M84.641-M84.650 with 7th A, M84.661-M84.68 with 7th A, S03.8XX-S03.9XX with 7th A, S29.011-S29.019 with 7th A, S38.3XX-S39.013 with 7th A, S73.101-S73.199 with 7th A, S76.001-S76.019 with 7th A, S76.091-S76.119 with 7th A, S76.191-S76.219 with 7th A, S76.291-S76.319 with 7th A, S76.391-S76.819 with 7th A, S76.891-S76.919 with 7th A, S76.991-S76.999 with 7th A, S79.811-S79.929 with 7th A, S82.101-S82.156 with 7th [A, B, C], S82.191-S82.299 with 7th [A, B, C], S82.401-S82.499 with 7th [A, B, C], S82.831-S82.839 with 7th [A, B, C], S82.861-S82.866 with 7th [A, B, C], S82.90X-S82.92X with 7th [A, B, C], S89.001-S89.099 with 7th A, S89.201-S89.299 with 7th A, T14.8-T14.91, T79.A9X-T79.9XX with 7th A
CC with 7th character K, M, N, P, Q or R: M80.00X-M84.68X with 7th [K, P], S02.0XX-S02.92X with 7th K, S12.000-S12.691 with 7th K, S22.000-S22.9XX with 7th K, S32.000-S32.9XX with 7th K, S42.001-S42.92X with 7th [K, P], S49.001-S49.199 with 7th [K, P], S52.001-S52.92X with 7th [K, M, N, P, Q, R], S59.001-S59.299 with 7th [K, P], S62.001-S62.92X with 7th [K, P], S72.001-S72.92X with 7th [K, M, N, P, Q, R], S79.001-S79.199 with 7th [K, P], S82.001-S82.92X with 7th [K, M, N, P, Q, R], S89.001-S89.399 with 7th [K, P], S92.001-S92.919 with 7th [K, P]

✓6th **S82.40** **Unspecified fracture of shaft of fibula**

7 ✓7th **S82.401** **Unspecified fracture of shaft of right fibula** MCC CC

7 ✓7th **S82.402** **Unspecified fracture of shaft of left fibula** MCC CC

7 ✓7th **S82.409** **Unspecified fracture of shaft of unspecified fibula** MCC CC

✓6th **S82.42** **Transverse fracture of shaft of fibula**

7 ✓7th **S82.421** **Displaced transverse fracture of shaft of right fibula** MCC CC

7 ✓7th **S82.422** **Displaced transverse fracture of shaft of left fibula** MCC CC

7 ✓7th **S82.423** **Displaced transverse fracture of shaft of unspecified fibula** MCC CC

7 ✓7th **S82.424** **Nondisplaced transverse fracture of shaft of right fibula** MCC CC

7 ✓7th **S82.425** **Nondisplaced transverse fracture of shaft of left fibula** MCC CC

7 HAC = Initial encounter only (7th character A, B or C) and not POA.

7 ✓7th **S82.426 Nondisplaced transverse fracture of shaft of unspecified fibula** MCC CC

✓6th **S82.43 Oblique fracture of shaft of fibula**

7 ✓7th **S82.431 Displaced oblique fracture of shaft of right fibula** MCC CC

7 ✓7th **S82.432 Displaced oblique fracture of shaft of left fibula** MCC CC

7 ✓7th **S82.433 Displaced oblique fracture of shaft of unspecified fibula** MCC CC

7 ✓7th **S82.434 Nondisplaced oblique fracture of shaft of right fibula** MCC CC

7 ✓7th **S82.435 Nondisplaced oblique fracture of shaft of left fibula** MCC CC

7 ✓7th **S82.436 Nondisplaced oblique fracture of shaft of unspecified fibula** MCC CC

✓6th **S82.44 Spiral fracture of shaft of fibula**

7 ✓7th **S82.441 Displaced spiral fracture of shaft of right fibula** MCC CC

7 ✓7th **S82.442 Displaced spiral fracture of shaft of left fibula** MCC CC

7 ✓7th **S82.443 Displaced spiral fracture of shaft of unspecified fibula** MCC CC

7 ✓7th **S82.444 Nondisplaced spiral fracture of shaft of right fibula** MCC CC

7 ✓7th **S82.445 Nondisplaced spiral fracture of shaft of left fibula** MCC CC

7 ✓7th **S82.446 Nondisplaced spiral fracture of sahft of unspecified fibula** MCC CC

✓6th **S82.45 Comminuted fracture of shaft of fibula**

7 ✓7th **S82.451 Displaced comminuted fracture of shaft of right fibula** MCC CC

7 ✓7th **S82.452 Displaced comminuted fracture of shaft of left fibula** MCC CC

7 ✓7th **S82.453 Displaced comminuted fracture of shaft of unspecified fibula** MCC CC

7 ✓7th **S82.454 Nondisplaced comminuted fracture of shaft of right fibula** MCC CC

7 ✓7th **S82.455 Nondisplaced comminuted fracture of shaft of left fibula** MCC CC

7 ✓7th **S82.456 Nondisplaced comminuted fracture of shaft of unspecified fibula** MCC CC

✓6th **S82.46 Segmental fracture of shaft of fibula**

7 ✓7th **S82.461 Displaced segmental fracture of shaft of right fibula** MCC CC

7 ✓7th **S82.462 Displaced segmental fracture of shaft of left fibula** MCC CC

7 ✓7th **S82.463 Displaced segmental fracture of shaft of unspecified fibula** MCC CC

7 ✓7th **S82.464 Nondisplaced segmental fracture of shaft of right fibula** MCC CC

7 ✓7th **S82.465 Nondisplaced segmental fracture of shaft of left fibula** MCC CC

7 ✓7th **S82.466 Nondisplaced segmental fracture of shaft of unspecified fibula** MCC CC

✓6th **S82.49 Other fracture of shaft of fibula**

7 ✓7th **S82.491 Other fracture of shaft of right fibula** MCC CC

7 ✓7th **S82.492 Other fracture of shaft of left fibula** MCC CC

7 ✓7th **S82.499 Other fracture of shaft of unspecified fibula** MCC CC

✓5th **S82.5 Fracture of medial malleolus**

EXCLUDES 1 *pilon fracture of distal tibia (S82.87-)*
Salter-Harris type III of lower end of tibia (S89.13-)
Salter-Harris type IV of lower end of tibia (S89.14-)

CC Excl: For CC codes in subcategory S82.5, unless otherwise noted: CC with 7th character B or C: M8Ø.ØØX-M8Ø.Ø19 with 7th A, M8Ø.Ø41-M8Ø.Ø49 with 7th A, M8Ø.Ø61-M8Ø.Ø79 with 7th A, M8Ø.8ØX-M8Ø.819 with 7th A, M8Ø.841-M8Ø.849 with 7th A, M8Ø.861-M8Ø.879 with 7th A, M84.4ØX-M84.419 with 7th A, M84.441-M84.446 with 7th A, M84.454 with 7th A, M84.461-M84.519 with 7th A, M84.541-M84.55Ø with 7th A, M84.561-M84.576 with 7th A, M84.6ØX-M84.619 with 7th A, M84.641-M84.65Ø with 7th A, M84.661-M84.68X with 7th A, SØ3.8XX-SØ3.9XX with 7th A, S29.Ø11-S29.Ø19 with 7th A, S38.3XX-S39.Ø13 with 7th A, S73.1Ø1-S73.199 with 7th A, S76.ØØ1-S76.Ø19 with 7th A, S76.Ø91-S76.119 with 7th A, S76.191-S76.219 with 7th A, S76.291-S76.319 with 7th A, S76.391-S76.819 with 7th A, S76.891-S76.919 with 7th A, S76.991-S76.999 with 7th A, S79.811-S79.929 with 7th A, S82.3Ø1-S82.3Ø9 with 7th [A, B, C], S82.391-S82.399 with 7th [A, B, C], S82.51X-S82.66X with 7th [B, C], S82.841-S82.856 with 7th [A, B, C], S82.871-S82.92X with 7th [B, C], S89.1Ø1-S89.199 with 7th A, S89.3Ø1-S89.399 with 7th A, T14.8-T14.91, T79.A9X-T79.9XX with 7th A **CC with 7th character K, M, N, P, Q or R:** M8Ø.ØØX-M84.68X with 7th [K, P], SØ2.ØXX-SØ2.92X with 7th K, S12.ØØØ-S12.691 with 7th K, S22.ØØØ-S22.9XX with 7th K, S32.ØØØ-S32.9XX with 7th K, S42.ØØ1-S42.92X with 7th [K, P], S49.ØØ1-S49.199 with 7th [K, P], S52.ØØ1-S52.92X with 7th [K, M, N, P, Q, R], S59.ØØ1-S59.299 with 7th [K, P], S62.ØØ1-S62.92X with 7th [K, P], S72.ØØ1-S72.92X with 7th [K, M, N, P, Q, R], S79.ØØ1-S79.199 with 7th [K, P], S82.ØØ1-S82.92X with 7th [K, M, N, P, Q, R], S89.ØØ1-S89.399 with 7th [K, P], S92.ØØ1-S92.919 with 7th [K, P]

7 ✓x7th **S82.51 Displaced fracture of medial malleolus of right tibia** CC

7 ✓x7th **S82.52 Displaced fracture of medial malleolus of left tibia** CC

7 ✓x7th **S82.53 Displaced fracture of medial malleolus of unspecified tibia** CC

7 ✓x7th **S82.54 Nondisplaced fracture of medial malleolus of right tibia** CC

7 ✓x7th **S82.55 Nondisplaced fracture of medial malleolus of left tibia** CC

7 ✓x7th **S82.56 Nondisplaced fracture of medial malleolus of unspecified tibia** CC

✓5th **S82.6 Fracture of lateral malleolus**

EXCLUDES 1 *pilon fracture of distal tibia (S82.87-)*

CC Excl: For CC codes in subcategory S82.5, unless otherwise noted: CC with 7th character B or C: M8Ø.ØØX-M8Ø.Ø19 with 7th A, M8Ø.Ø41-M8Ø.Ø49 with 7th A, M8Ø.Ø61-M8Ø.Ø79 with 7th A, M8Ø.8ØX-M8Ø.819 with 7th A, M8Ø.841-M8Ø.849 with 7th A, M8Ø.861-M8Ø.879 with 7th A, M84.4ØX-M84.419 with 7th A, M84.441-M84.446 with 7th A, M84.454 with 7th A, M84.461-M84.519 with 7th A, M84.541-M84.55Ø with 7th A, M84.561-M84.576 with 7th A, M84.6ØX-M84.619 with 7th A, M84.641-M84.65Ø with 7th A, M84.661-M84.68X with 7th A, SØ3.8XX-SØ3.9XX with 7th A, S29.Ø11-S29.Ø19 with 7th A, S38.3XX-S39.Ø13 with 7th A, S73.1Ø1-S73.199 with 7th A, S76.ØØ1-S76.Ø19 with 7th A, S76.Ø91-S76.119 with 7th A, S76.191-S76.219 with 7th A, S76.291-S76.319 with 7th A, S76.391-S76.819 with 7th A, S76.891-S76.919 with 7th A, S76.991-S76.999 with 7th A, S79.811-S79.929 with 7th A, S82.3Ø1-S82.3Ø9 with 7th [A, B, C], S82.391-S82.399 with 7th [A, B, C], S82.51X-S82.66X with 7th [B, C], S82.841-S82.856 with 7th [A, B, C], S82.871-S82.92X with 7th [B, C], S89.1Ø1-S89.199 with 7th A, S89.3Ø1-S89.399 with 7th A, T14.8-T14.91, T79.A9X-T79.9XX with 7th A **CC with 7th character K, M, N, P, Q or R:** M8Ø.ØØX-M84.68X with 7th [K, P], SØ2.ØXX-SØ2.92X with 7th K, S12.ØØØ-S12.691 with 7th K, S22.ØØØ-S22.9XX with 7th K, S32.ØØØ-S32.9XX with 7th K, S42.ØØ1-S42.92X with 7th [K, P], S49.ØØ1-S49.199 with 7th [K, P], S52.ØØ1-S52.92X with 7th [K, M, N, P, Q, R], S59.ØØ1-S59.299 with 7th [K, P], S62.ØØ1-S62.92X with 7th [K, P], S72.ØØ1-S72.92X with 7th [K, M, N, P, Q, R], S79.ØØ1-S79.199 with 7th [K, P], S82.ØØ1-S82.92X with 7th [K, M, N, P, Q, R], S89.ØØ1-S89.399 with 7th [K, P], S92.ØØ1-S92.919 with 7th [K, P]

7 ✓x7th **S82.61 Displaced fracture of lateral malleolus of right fibula** CC

7 ✓x7th **S82.62 Displaced fracture of lateral malleolus of left fibula** CC

7 HAC = Initial encounter only (7th character A, B or C) and not POA.

7 ✓x7th **S82.63 Displaced fracture of lateral malleolus of unspecified fibula** CC

7 ✓x7th **S82.64 Nondisplaced fracture of lateral malleolus of right fibula** CC

7 ✓x7th **S82.65 Nondisplaced fracture of lateral malleolus of left fibula** CC

7 ✓x7th **S82.66 Nondisplaced fracture of lateral malleolus of unspecified fibula** CC

✓5th **S82.8 Other fractures of lower leg**

✓6th **S82.81 Torus fracture of upper end of fibula**

The appropriate 7th character is to be added to all codes in subcategory S82.81.
- A initial encounter for closed fracture
- D subsequent encounter for fracture with routine healing
- G subsequent encounter for fracture with delayed healing
- K subsequent encounter for fracture wit nonunion
- P subsequent encounter for fracture with malunion
- S sequela

CC Excl: For codes in subcatgory S82.81, unless otherwise noted: CC with 7th character K or P: See code S82.6

✓7th **S82.811 Torus fracture of upper end of right fibula** CC

✓7th **S82.812 Torus fracture of upper end of left fibula** CC

✓7th **S82.819 Torus fracture of upper end of unspecified fibula** CC

✓6th **S82.82 Torus fracture of lower end of fibula**

The appropriate 7th character is to be added to all codes in subcategory S82.82.
- A initial encounter for closed fracture
- D subsequent encounter for fracture with routine healing
- G subsequent encounter for fracture with delayed healing
- K subsequent encounter for fracture with nonunion
- P subsequent encounter for fracture with malunion
- S sequela

CC Excl: For codes in subcatgory S82.82, unless otherwise noted: CC with 7th character K or P: See code: S82.6

✓7th **S82.821 Torus fracture of lower end of right fibula** CC

✓7th **S82.822 Torus fracture of lower end of left fibula** CC

✓7th **S82.829 Torus fracture of lower end of unspecified fibula** CC

✓6th **S82.83 Other fracture of upper and lower end of fibula**

CC Excl: For codes in subcatgory S82.83, unless otherwise noted: MCC with 7th B or C: M80.00X-M80.019 with 7th A, M80.041-M80.049 with 7th A, M80.061-M80.079 with 7th A, M80.80X-M80.819 with 7th A, M80.841-M80.849 with 7th A, M80.861-M80.879 with 7th A, M84.40X-M84.419 with 7th A, M84.441-M84.446 with 7th A, M84.454 with 7th A, M84.461-M84.519 with 7th A, M84.541-M84.550 with 7th A, M84.561-M84.576 with 7th A, M84.60X-M84.619 with 7th A, M84.641-M84.650 with 7th A, M84.661-M84.68X with 7th A, S03.8XX-S03.9XX with 7th A, S29.011-S29.019 with 7th A, S38.3XX-S39.013 with 7th A, S73.101-S73.199 with 7th A, S76.001-S76.019 with 7th A, S76.091-S76.119 with 7th A, S76.191-S76.219 with 7th A, S76.291-S76.319 with 7th A, S76.391-S76.819 with 7th A, S76.891-S76.919 with 7th A, S76.991-S76.999 with 7th A, S79.811-S79.929 with 7th A, S82.101-S82.156 with 7th [A, B, C], S82.191-S82.299 with 7th [A, B, C], S82.401-S82.499 with 7th [A, B, C], S82.831-S82.839 with 7th [A, B, C], S82.861-S82.866 with 7th [A, B, C], S82.90X-S82.92X with 7th [A, B, C], S89.001-S89.099 with 7th A, S89.201-S89.299 with 7th A, T14.8-T14.91, T79.A9X-T79.9XX with 7th A
CC with 7th character K, M, N, P, Q or R: M80.00X-M84.68X with 7th [K, P], S02.0XX-S02.92X with 7th K, S12.000-S12.691 with 7th K, S22.000-S22.9XX with 7th K, S32.000-S32.9XX with 7th K, S42.001-S42.92X with 7th [K, P], S49.001-S49.199 with 7th [K, P], S52.001-S52.92X with 7th [K, M, N, P, Q, R], S59.001-S59.299 with 7th [K, P], S62.001-S62.92X with 7th [K, P], S72.001-S72.92X with 7th [K, M, N, P, Q, R], S79.001-S79.199 with 7th [K, P], S82.001-S82.92X with 7th [K, M, N, P, Q, R], S89.001-S89.399 with 7th [K, P], S92.001-S92.919 with 7th [K, P]

7 ✓7th **S82.831 Other fracture of upper and lower end of right fibula** MCC CC

7 ✓7th **S82.832 Other fracture of upper and lower end of left fibula** MCC CC

7 ✓7th **S82.839 Other fracture of upper and lower end of unspecified fibula** MCC CC

✓6th **S82.84 Bimalleolar fracture of lower leg**

CC Excl: For codes in subcatgory S82.84, unless otherwise noted: CC with 7th character B or C: M80.00X-M80.019 with 7th A, M80.041-M80.049 with 7th A, M80.061-M80.079 with 7th A, M80.80X-M80.819 with 7th A, M80.841-M80.849 with 7th A, M80.861-M80.879 with 7th A, M84.40X-M84.419 with 7th A, M84.441-M84.446 with 7th A, M84.454 with 7th A, M84.461-M84.519 with 7th A, M84.541-M84.550 with 7th A, M84.561-M84.576 with 7th A, M84.60X-M84.619 with 7th A, M84.641-M84.650 with 7th A, M84.661-M84.68 with 7th A, S03.8XX-S03.9XX with 7th A, S29.011-S29.019 with 7th A, S38.3XX-S39.013 with 7th A, S73.101-S73.199 with 7th A, S76.001-S76.019 with 7th A, S76.091-S76.119 with 7th A, S76.191-S76.219 with 7th A, S76.291-S76.319 with 7th A, S76.391-S76.819 with 7th A, S76.891-S76.919 with 7th A, S76.991-S76.999 with 7th A, S79.811-S79.929 with 7th A, S82.301-S82.309 with 7th [A, B, C], S82.391-S82.399 with 7th [A, B, C], S82.51X-S82.66X with 7th [B, C], S82.841-S82.856 with 7th [A, B, C], S82.871-S82.92X with 7th [B, C], S89.101-S89.199 with 7th A, S89.301-S89.399 with 7th A, T14.8-T14.91, T79.A9X-T79.9XX with 7th A
CC with 7th character K, M, N, P, Q or R: M80.00X-M84.68X with 7th [K, P], S02.0XX-S02.92X with 7th K, S12.000-S12.691 with 7th K, S22.000-S22.9XX with 7th K, S32.000-S32.9XX with 7th K, S42.001-S42.92X with 7th [K, P], S49.001-S49.199 with 7th [K, P], S52.001-S52.92X with 7th [K, M, N, P, Q, R], S59.001-S59.299 with 7th [K, P], S62.001-S62.92X with 7th [K, P], S72.001-S72.92X with 7th [K, M, N, P, Q, R], S79.001-S79.199 with 7th [K, P], S82.001-S82.92X with 7th [K, M, N, P, Q, R], S89.001-S89.399 with 7th [K, P], S92.001-S92.919 with 7th [K, P]

7 ✓7th **S82.841 Displaced bimalleolar fracture of right lower leg** CC

7 ✓7th **S82.842 Displaced bimalleolar fracture of left lower leg** CC

7 ✓7th **S82.843 Displaced bimalleolar fracture of unspecified lower leg** CC

7 ✓7th **S82.844 Nondisplaced bimalleolar fracture of right lower leg** CC

7 HAC = Initial encounter only (7th character A, B or C) and not POA.

7 ✓7th **S82.845** **Nondisplaced bimalleolar fracture of left lower leg** CC

7 ✓7th **S82.846** **Nondisplaced bimalleolar fracture of unspecified lower leg** CC

✓6th **S82.85** **Trimalleolar fracture of lower leg**

CC Excl: For codes in subcatgory S82.85, unless otherwise noted: See code: S82.84

7 ✓7th **S82.851** **Displaced trimalleolar fracture of right lower leg** CC

7 ✓7th **S82.852** **Displaced trimalleolar fracture of left lower leg** CC

7 ✓7th **S82.853** **Displaced trimalleolar fracture of unspecified lower leg** CC

7 ✓7th **S82.854** **Nondisplaced trimalleolar fracture of right lower leg** CC

7 ✓7th **S82.855** **Nondisplaced trimalleolar fracture of left lower leg** CC

7 ✓7th **S82.856** **Nondisplaced trimalleolar fracture of unspecified lower leg** CC

✓6th **S82.86** **Maisonneuve's fracture**

CC Excl: For codes in subcatgory S82.86, unless otherwise noted: See code: S82.84

7 ✓7th **S82.861** **Displaced Maisonneuve's fracture of right leg** MCC CC

7 ✓7th **S82.862** **Displaced Maisonneuve's fracture of left leg** MCC CC

7 ✓7th **S82.863** **Displaced Maisonneuve's fracture of unspecified leg** MCC CC

7 ✓7th **S82.864** **Nondisplaced Maisonneuve's fracture of right leg** MCC CC

7 ✓7th **S82.865** **Nondisplaced Maisonneuve's fracture of left leg** MCC CC

7 ✓7th **S82.866** **Nondisplaced Maisonneuve's fracture of unspecified leg** MCC CC

✓6th **S82.87** **Pilon fracture of tibia**

CC Excl: For codes in subcatgory S82.87, unless otherwise noted: See code: S82.85

7 ✓7th **S82.871** **Displaced pilon fracture of right tibia** CC

7 ✓7th **S82.872** **Displaced pilon fracture of left tibia** CC

7 ✓7th **S82.873** **Displaced pilon fracture of unspecified tibia** CC

7 ✓7th **S82.874** **Nondisplaced pilon fracture of right tibia** CC

7 ✓7th **S82.875** **Nondisplaced pilon fracture of left tibia** CC

7 ✓7th **S82.876** **Nondisplaced pilon fracture of unspecified tibia** CC

✓6th **S82.89** **Other fractures of lower leg**

Fracture of ankle NOS

CC Excl: For codes in subcatgory S82.89, unless otherwise noted: See code: S82.84

7 ✓7th **S82.891** **Other fracture of right lower leg** CC

7 ✓7th **S82.892** **Other fracture of left lower leg** CC

7 ✓7th **S82.899** **Other fracture of unspecified lower leg** CC

✓5th **S82.9** **Unspecified fracture of lower leg**

CC Excl: For codes in subcatgory S82.9, unless otherwise noted: CC with 7th character B or C: See code: S82.84

7 ✓x7th **S82.90** **Unspecified fracture of unspecified lower leg** CC

7 ✓x7th **S82.91** **Unspecified fracture of right lower leg** CC

7 ✓x7th **S82.92** **Unspecified fracture of left lower leg** CC

✓4th **S83** **Dislocation and sprain of joints and ligaments of knee**

INCLUDES avulsion of joint or ligament of knee
laceration of cartilage, joint or ligament of knee
sprain of cartilage, joint or ligament of knee
traumatic hemarthrosis of joint or ligament of knee
traumatic rupture of joint or ligament of knee
traumatic subluxation of joint or ligament of knee
traumatic tear of joint or ligament of knee

Code also any associated open wound

EXCLUDES 1 *derangement of patella (M22.Ø-M22.3)*
injury of patellar ligament (tendon) (S76.1-)
internal derangement of knee (M23.-)
old dislocation of knee (M24.36)
pathological dislocation of knee (M24.36)
recurrent dislocation of knee (M22.Ø)

EXCLUDES 2 *strain of muscle, fascia and tendon of lower leg (S86.-)*

The appropriate 7th character is to be added to each code from category S83.
A initial encounter
D subsequent encounter
S sequela

✓5th **S83.Ø** **Subluxation and dislocation of patella**

✓6th **S83.ØØ** **Unspecified subluxation and dislocation of patella**

✓7th **S83.ØØ1** **Unspecified subluxation of right patella**

✓7th **S83.ØØ2** **Unspecified subluxation of left patella**

✓7th **S83.ØØ3** **Unspecified subluxation of unspecified patella**

✓7th **S83.ØØ4** **Unspecified dislocation of right patella**

✓7th **S83.ØØ5** **Unspecified dislocation of left patella**

✓7th **S83.ØØ6** **Unspecified dislocation of unspecified patella**

✓6th **S83.Ø1** **Lateral subluxation and dislocation of patella**

✓7th **S83.Ø11** **Lateral subluxation of right patella**

✓7th **S83.Ø12** **Lateral subluxation of left patella**

✓7th **S83.Ø13** **Lateral subluxation of unspecified patella**

✓7th **S83.Ø14** **Lateral dislocation of right patella**

✓7th **S83.Ø15** **Lateral dislocation of left patella**

✓7th **S83.Ø16** **Lateral dislocation of unspecified patella**

✓6th **S83.Ø9** **Other subluxation and dislocation of patella**

✓7th **S83.Ø91** **Other subluxation of right patella**

✓7th **S83.Ø92** **Other subluxation of left patella**

✓7th **S83.Ø93** **Other subluxation of unspecified patella**

✓7th **S83.Ø94** **Other dislocation of right patella**

✓7th **S83.Ø95** **Other dislocation of left patella**

✓7th **S83.Ø96** **Other dislocation of unspecified patella**

✓5th **S83.1** **Subluxation and dislocation of knee**

EXCLUDES 2 *instability of knee prosthesis (T84.Ø22, T84.Ø23)*

✓6th **S83.1Ø** **Unspecified subluxation and dislocation of knee**

✓7th **S83.1Ø1** **Unspecified subluxation of right knee**

✓7th **S83.1Ø2** **Unspecified subluxation of left knee**

✓7th **S83.1Ø3** **Unspecified subluxation of unspecified knee**

✓7th **S83.1Ø4** **Unspecified dislocation of right knee**

✓7th **S83.1Ø5** **Unspecified dislocation of left knee**

✓7th **S83.1Ø6** **Unspecified dislocation of unspecified knee**

✓6th **S83.11** **Anterior subluxation and dislocation of proximal end of tibia**

Posterior subluxation and dislocation of distal end of femur

✓7th **S83.111** **Anterior subluxation of proximal end of tibia, right knee**

✓7th **S83.112** **Anterior subluxation of proximal end of tibia, left knee**

✓7th **S83.113** **Anterior subluxation of proximal end of tibia, unspecified knee**

✓7th **S83.114** **Anterior dislocation of proximal end of tibia, right knee**

✓7th **S83.115** **Anterior dislocation of proximal end of tibia, left knee**

✓7th **S83.116** **Anterior dislocation of proximal end of tibia, unspecified knee**

7 HAC = Initial encounter only (7th character A, B or C) and not POA.

- ✓6th **S83.12** Posterior subluxation and dislocation of proximal end of tibia
  - Anterior dislocation of distal end of femur
  - ✓7th **S83.121** Posterior subluxation of proximal end of tibia, right knee
  - ✓7th **S83.122** Posterior subluxation of proximal end of tibia, left knee
  - ✓7th **S83.123** Posterior subluxation of proximal end of tibia, unspecified knee
  - ✓7th **S83.124** Posterior dislocation of proximal end of tibia, right knee
  - ✓7th **S83.125** Posterior dislocation of proximal end of tibia, left knee
  - ✓7th **S83.126** Posterior dislocation of proximal end of tibia, unspecified knee
- ✓6th **S83.13** Medial subluxation and dislocation of proximal end of tibia
  - ✓7th **S83.131** Medial subluxation of proximal end of tibia, right knee
  - ✓7th **S83.132** Medial subluxation of proximal end of tibia, left knee
  - ✓7th **S83.133** Medial subluxation of proximal end of tibia, unspecified knee
  - ✓7th **S83.134** Medial dislocation of proximal end of tibia, right knee
  - ✓7th **S83.135** Medial dislocation of proximal end of tibia, left knee
  - ✓7th **S83.136** Medial dislocation of proximal end of tibia, unspecified knee
- ✓6th **S83.14** Lateral subluxation and dislocation of proximal end of tibia
  - ✓7th **S83.141** Lateral subluxation of proximal end of tibia, right knee
  - ✓7th **S83.142** Lateral subluxation of proximal end of tibia, left knee
  - ✓7th **S83.143** Lateral subluxation of proximal end of tibia, unspecified knee
  - ✓7th **S83.144** Lateral dislocation of proximal end of tibia, right knee
  - ✓7th **S83.145** Lateral dislocation of proximal end of tibia, left knee
  - ✓7th **S83.146** Lateral dislocation of proximal end of tibia, unspecified knee
- ✓6th **S83.19** Other subluxation and dislocation of knee
  - ✓7th **S83.191** Other subluxation of right knee
  - ✓7th **S83.192** Other subluxation of left knee
  - ✓7th **S83.193** Other subluxation of unspecified knee
  - ✓7th **S83.194** Other dislocation of right knee
  - ✓7th **S83.195** Other dislocation of left knee
  - ✓7th **S83.196** Other dislocation of unspecified knee

✓5th **S83.2** Tear of meniscus, current injury

EXCLUDES 1 *old bucket-handle tear (M23.2)*

- ✓6th **S83.20** Tear of unspecified meniscus, current injury
  - Tear of meniscus of knee NOS
  - ✓7th **S83.200** Bucket-handle tear of unspecified meniscus, current injury, right knee
  - ✓7th **S83.201** Bucket-handle tear of unspecified meniscus, current injury, left knee
  - ✓7th **S83.202** Bucket-handle tear of unspecified meniscus, current injury, unspecified knee
  - ✓7th **S83.203** Other tear of unspecified meniscus, current injury, right knee
  - ✓7th **S83.204** Other tear of unspecified meniscus, current injury, left knee
  - ✓7th **S83.205** Other tear of unspecified meniscus, current injury, unspecified knee
  - ✓7th **S83.206** Unspecified tear of unspecified meniscus, current injury, right knee
  - ✓7th **S83.207** Unspecified tear of unspecified meniscus, current injury, left knee
  - ✓7th **S83.209** Unspecified tear of unspecified meniscus, current injury, unspecified knee
- ✓6th **S83.21** Bucket-handle tear of medial meniscus, current injury
  - ✓7th **S83.211** Bucket-handle tear of medial meniscus, current injury, right knee
  - ✓7th **S83.212** Bucket-handle tear of medial meniscus, current injury, left knee
  - ✓7th **S83.219** Bucket-handle tear of medial meniscus, current injury, unspecified knee
- ✓6th **S83.22** Peripheral tear of medial meniscus, current injury
  - ✓7th **S83.221** Peripheral tear of medial meniscus, current injury, right knee
  - ✓7th **S83.222** Peripheral tear of medial meniscus, current injury, left knee
  - ✓7th **S83.229** Peripheral tear of medial meniscus, current injury, unspecified knee
- ✓6th **S83.23** Complex tear of medial meniscus, current injury
  - ✓7th **S83.231** Complex tear of medial meniscus, current injury, right knee
  - ✓7th **S83.232** Complex tear of medial meniscus, current injury, left knee
  - ✓7th **S83.239** Complex tear of medial meniscus, current injury, unspecified knee
- ✓6th **S83.24** Other tear of medial meniscus, current injury
  - ✓7th **S83.241** Other tear of medial meniscus, current injury, right knee
  - ✓7th **S83.242** Other tear of medial meniscus, current injury, left knee
  - ✓7th **S83.249** Other tear of medial meniscus, current injury, unspecified knee
- ✓6th **S83.25** Bucket-handle tear of lateral meniscus, current injury
  - ✓7th **S83.251** Bucket-handle tear of lateral meniscus, current injury, right knee
  - ✓7th **S83.252** Bucket-handle tear of lateral meniscus, current injury, left knee
  - ✓7th **S83.259** Bucket-handle tear of lateral meniscus, current injury, unspecified knee
- ✓6th **S83.26** Peripheral tear of lateral meniscus, current injury
  - ✓7th **S83.261** Peripheral tear of lateral meniscus, current injury, right knee
  - ✓7th **S83.262** Peripheral tear of lateral meniscus, current injury, left knee
  - ✓7th **S83.269** Peripheral tear of lateral meniscus, current injury, unspecified knee
- ✓6th **S83.27** Complex tear of lateral meniscus, current injury
  - ✓7th **S83.271** Complex tear of lateral meniscus, current injury, right knee
  - ✓7th **S83.272** Complex tear of lateral meniscus, current injury, left knee
  - ✓7th **S83.279** Complex tear of lateral meniscus, current injury, unspecified knee
- ✓6th **S83.28** Other tear of lateral meniscus, current injury
  - ✓7th **S83.281** Other tear of lateral meniscus, current injury, right knee
  - ✓7th **S83.282** Other tear of lateral meniscus, current injury, left knee
  - ✓7th **S83.289** Other tear of lateral meniscus, current injury, unspecified knee

✓5th **S83.3** Tear of articular cartilage of knee, current

- ✓x7th **S83.30** Tear of articular cartilage of unspecified knee, current
- ✓x7th **S83.31** Tear of articular cartilage of right knee, current
- ✓x7th **S83.32** Tear of articular cartilage of left knee, current

✓5th **S83.4** Sprain of collateral ligament of knee

- ✓6th **S83.40** Sprain of unspecified collateral ligament of knee
  - ✓7th **S83.401** Sprain of unspecified collateral ligament of right knee
  - ✓7th **S83.402** Sprain of unspecified collateral ligament of left knee
  - ✓7th **S83.409** Sprain of unspecified collateral ligament of unspecified knee

✓6th **S83.41 Sprain of medial collateral ligament of knee**
Sprain of tibial collateral ligament
✓7th **S83.411 Sprain of medial collateral ligament of right knee**
✓7th **S83.412 Sprain of medial collateral ligament of left knee**
✓7th **S83.419 Sprain of medial collateral ligament of unspecified knee**

✓6th **S83.42 Sprain of lateral collateral ligament of knee**
Sprain of fibular collateral ligament
✓7th **S83.421 Sprain of lateral collateral ligament of right knee**
✓7th **S83.422 Sprain of lateral collateral ligament of left knee**
✓7th **S83.429 Sprain of lateral collateral ligament of unspecified knee**

✓5th **S83.5 Sprain of cruciate ligament of knee**
✓6th **S83.50 Sprain of unspecified cruciate ligament of knee**
✓7th **S83.501 Sprain of unspecified cruciate ligament of right knee**
✓7th **S83.502 Sprain of unspecified cruciate ligament of left knee**
✓7th **S83.509 Sprain of unspecified cruciate ligament of unspecified knee**
✓6th **S83.51 Sprain of anterior cruciate ligament of knee**
✓7th **S83.511 Sprain of anterior cruciate ligament of right knee**
✓7th **S83.512 Sprain of anterior cruciate ligament of left knee**
✓7th **S83.519 Sprain of anterior cruciate ligament of unspecified knee**
✓6th **S83.52 Sprain of posterior cruciate ligament of knee**
✓7th **S83.521 Sprain of posterior cruciate ligament of right knee**
✓7th **S83.522 Sprain of posterior cruciate ligament of left knee**
✓7th **S83.529 Sprain of posterior cruciate ligament of unspecified knee**

✓5th **S83.6 Sprain of the superior tibiofibular joint and ligament**
✓x7th **S83.60 Sprain of the superior tibiofibular joint and ligament, unspecified knee**
✓x7th **S83.61 Sprain of the superior tibiofibular joint and ligament, right knee**
✓x7th **S83.62 Sprain of the superior tibiofibular joint and ligament, left knee**

✓5th **S83.8 Sprain of other specified parts of knee**
✓6th **S83.8X Sprain of other specified parts of knee**
✓7th **S83.8X1 Sprain of other specified parts of right knee**
✓7th **S83.8X2 Sprain of other specified parts of left knee**
✓7th **S83.8X9 Sprain of other specified parts of unspecified knee**

✓5th **S83.9 Sprain of unspecified site of knee**
✓x7th **S83.90 Sprain of unspecified site of unspecified knee**
✓x7th **S83.91 Sprain of unspecified site of right knee**
✓x7th **S83.92 Sprain of unspecified site of left knee**

✓4th **S84 Injury of nerves at lower leg level**
Code also any associated open wound (S81.-)
EXCLUDES 2 *injury of nerves at ankle and foot level (S94.-)*

The appropriate 7th character is to be added to each code from category S84.
A initial encounter
D subsequent encounter
S sequela

✓5th **S84.0 Injury of tibial nerve at lower leg level**
✓x7th **S84.00 Injury of tibial nerve at lower leg level, unspecified leg**
✓x7th **S84.01 Injury of tibial nerve at lower leg level, right leg**
✓x7th **S84.02 Injury of tibial nerve at lower leg level, left leg**

✓5th **S84.1 Injury of peroneal nerve at lower leg level**
✓x7th **S84.10 Injury of peroneal nerve at lower leg level, unspecified leg**
✓x7th **S84.11 Injury of peroneal nerve at lower leg level, right leg**
✓x7th **S84.12 Injury of peroneal nerve at lower leg level, left leg**

✓5th **S84.2 Injury of cutaneous sensory nerve at lower leg level**
✓x7th **S84.20 Injury of cutaneous sensory nerve at lower leg level, unspecified leg**
✓x7th **S84.21 Injury of cutaneous sensory nerve at lower leg level, right leg**
✓x7th **S84.22 Injury of cutaneous sensory nerve at lower leg level, left leg**

✓5th **S84.8 Injury of other nerves at lower leg level**
✓6th **S84.80 Injury of other nerves at lower leg level**
✓7th **S84.801 Injury of other nerves at lower leg level, right leg**
✓7th **S84.802 Injury of other nerves at lower leg level, left leg**
✓7th **S84.809 Injury of other nerves at lower leg level, unspecified leg**

✓5th **S84.9 Injury of unspecified nerve at lower leg level**
✓x7th **S84.90 Injury of unspecified nerve at lower leg level, unspecified leg**
✓x7th **S84.91 Injury of unspecified nerve at lower leg level, right leg**
✓x7th **S84.92 Injury of unspecified nerve at lower leg level, left leg**

✓4th **S85 Injury of blood vessels at lower leg level**
Code also any associated open wound (S81.-)
EXCLUDES 2 *injury of blood vessels at ankle and foot level (S95.-)*

The appropriate 7th character is to be added to each code from category S85.
A initial encounter
D subsequent encounter
S sequela

✓5th **S85.0 Injury of popliteal artery**
✓6th **S85.00 Unspecified injury of popliteal artery**
✓7th **S85.001 Unspecified injury of popliteal artery, right leg** MCC
CC Excl: MCC with 7th character A: S75.801 with 7th A, S75.809-S75.811 with 7th A, S75.819-S75.891 with 7th A, S75.899-S75.901 with 7th A, S75.909-S75.911 with 7th A, S75.919-S75.991 with 7th A, S75.999A, S85.001A, S85.009-S85.011 with 7th A, S85.019-S85.091 with 7th A, S85.099A, S85.201A, S85.209-S85.211 with 7th A, S85.219-S85.291 with 7th A, S85.299A, S85.801A, S85.809-S85.811 with 7th A, S85.819-S85.891 with 7th A, S85.899-S85.901 with 7th A, S85.909-S85.911 with 7th A, S85.919-S85.991 with 7th A, S85.999A, S95.001A, S95.009-S95.011 with 7th A, S95.019-S95.091 with 7th A, S95.099A, S95.201A, S95.209-S95.211 with 7th A, S95.219-S95.291 with 7th A, S95.299-S95.801 with 7th A, S95.809-S95.811 with 7th A, S95.819-S95.891 with 7th A, S95.899-S95.901 with 7th A, S95.909-S95.911 with 7th A, S95.919-S95.991 with 7th A, S95.999 with 7th A
✓7th **S85.002 Unspecified injury of popliteal artery, left leg** MCC
CC Excl: MCC with 7th character A: S75.802-S75.809 with 7th A, S75.812-S75.819 with 7th A, S75.892-S75.899 with 7th A, S75.902-S75.909 with 7th A, S75.912-S75.919 with 7th A, S75.992-S75.999 with 7th A, S85.002-S85.009 with 7th A, S85.012-S85.019 with 7th A, S85.092-S85.099 with 7th A, S85.202-S85.209 with 7th A, S85.212-S85.219 with 7th A, S85.292-S85.299 with 7th A, S85.802-S85.809 with 7th A, S85.812-S85.819 with 7th A, S85.892-S85.899 with 7th A, S85.902-S85.909 with 7th A, S85.912-S85.919 with 7th A, S85.992-S85.999 with 7th A, S95.002-S95.009 with 7th A, S95.012-S95.019 with 7th A, S95.092-S95.099 with 7th A, S95.202-S95.209 with 7th A, S95.212-S95.219 with 7th A, S95.292-S95.299 with 7th A, S95.802-S95.809 with 7th A, S95.812-S95.819 with 7th A, S95.892-S95.899 with 7th A, S95.902-S95.909 with 7th A, S95.912-S95.919 with 7th A, S95.992-S95.999 with 7th A

7th **S85.009 Unspecified injury of popliteal artery, unspecified leg** MCC
CC Excl: MCC with 7th character A: S75.801-S75.999 with 7th A, S85.001-S85.099 with 7th A, S85.201-S85.299 with 7th A, S85.801-S85.999 with 7th A, S95.001-S95.099 with 7th A, S95.201-S95.999 with 7th A

6th **S85.01 Laceration of popliteal artery**

7th **S85.011 Laceration of popliteal artery, right leg** MCC
CC Excl: See code: S85.001

7th **S85.012 Laceration of popliteal artery, left leg** MCC
CC Excl: See code: S85.002

7th **S85.019 Laceration of popliteal artery, unspecified leg** MCC
CC Excl: See code: S85.009

6th **S85.09 Other specified injury of popliteal artery**

7th **S85.091 Other specified injury of popliteal artery, right leg** MCC
CC Excl: See code: S85.001

7th **S85.092 Other specified injury of popliteal artery, left leg** MCC
CC Excl: See code: S85.002

7th **S85.099 Other specified injury of popliteal artery, unspecified leg** MCC
CC Excl: See code: S85.009

5th **S85.1 Injury of tibial artery**

6th **S85.10 Unspecified injury of unspecified tibial artery**
Injury of tibial artery NOS

7th **S85.101 Unspecified injury of unspecified tibial artery, right leg** CC
CC Excl: CC with 7th character A: S75.801 with 7th A, S75.809-S75.811 with 7th A, S75.819-S75.891 with 7th A, S75.899-S75.901 with 7th A, S75.909-S75.911 with 7th A, S75.919-S75.991 with 7th A, S75.999A, S85.101A, S85.109-S85.111 with 7th A, S85.119-S85.121 with 7th A, S85.129A, S85.201A, S85.209-S85.211 with 7th A, S85.219-S85.291 with 7th A, S85.299 with 7th A, S85.801A, S85.809-S85.811 with 7th A, S85.819-S85.891 with 7th A, S85.899-S85.901 with 7th A, S85.909-S85.911 with 7th A, S85.919-S85.991 with 7th A, S85.999A, S95.001A, S95.009-S95.011 with 7th A, S95.019-S95.091 with 7th A, S95.099A, S95.201A, S95.209-S95.211 with 7th A, S95.219-S95.291 with 7th A, S95.299-S95.801 with 7th A, S95.809-S95.811 with 7th A, S95.819-S95.891 with 7th A, S95.899-S95.901 with 7th A, S95.909-S95.911 with 7th A, S95.919-S95.991 with 7th A, S95.999

7th **S85.102 Unspecified injury of unspecified tibial artery, left leg** CC
CC Excl: CC with 7th character A: S75.802-S75.809 with 7th A, S75.812-S75.819 with 7th A, S75.892-S75.899 with 7th A, S75.902-S75.909 with 7th A, S75.912-S75.919 with 7th A, S75.992-S75.999 with 7th A, S85.102-S85.109 with 7th A, S85.112-S85.119 with 7th A, S85.122-S85.129 with 7th A, S85.202-S85.209 with 7th A, S85.212-S85.219 with 7th A, S85.292-S85.299 with 7th A, S85.802-S85.809 with 7th A, S85.812-S85.819 with 7th A, S85.892-S85.899 with 7th A, S85.902-S85.909 with 7th A, S85.912-S85.919 with 7th A, S85.992-S85.999 with 7th A, S95.002-S95.009 with 7th A, S95.012-S95.019 with 7th A, S95.092-S95.099 with 7th A, S95.202-S95.209 with 7th A, S95.212-S95.219 with 7th A, S95.292-S95.299 with 7th A, S95.802-S95.809 with 7th A, S95.812-S95.819 with 7th A, S95.892-S95.899 with 7th A, S95.902-S95.909 with 7th A, S95.912-S95.919 with 7th A, S95.992-S95.999 with 7th A

7th **S85.109 Unspecified injury of unspecified tibial artery, unspecified leg** CC
CC Excl: CC with 7th character A: S75.801-S75.999 with 7th A, S85.101-S85.129 with 7th A, S85.201-S85.299 with 7th A, S85.801-S85.999 with 7th A, S95.001-S95.099 with 7th A, S95.201-S95.999 with 7th A

6th **S85.11 Laceration of unspecified tibial artery**

7th **S85.111 Laceration of unspecified tibial artery, right leg** CC
CC Excl: See code: S85.101

7th **S85.112 Laceration of unspecified tibial artery, left leg** CC
CC Excl: See code: S85.102

7th **S85.119 Laceration of unspecified tibial artery, unspecified leg** CC
CC Excl: See code: S85.109

6th **S85.12 Other specified injury of unspecified tibial artery**

7th **S85.121 Other specified injury of unspecified tibial artery, right leg** CC
CC Excl: See code: S85.101

7th **S85.122 Other specified injury of unspecified tibial artery, left leg** CC
CC Excl: See code: S85.102

7th **S85.129 Other specified injury of unspecified tibial artery, unspecified leg** CC
CC Excl: See code: S85.109

6th **S85.13 Unspecified injury of anterior tibial artery**

7th **S85.131 Unspecified injury of anterior tibial artery, right leg** CC
CC Excl: CC with 7th character A: S75.801 with 7th A, S75.809-S75.811 with 7th A, S75.819-S75.891 with 7th A, S75.899-S75.901 with 7th A, S75.909-S75.911 with 7th A, S75.919-S75.991 with 7th A, S75.999A, S85.131A, S85.139-S85.141 with 7th A, S85.149-S85.151 with 7th A, S85.159A, S85.201A, S85.209-S85.211 with 7th A, S85.219-S85.291 with 7th A, S85.299A, S85.801A, S85.809-S85.811 with 7th A, S85.819-S85.891 with 7th A, S85.899-S85.901 with 7th A, S85.909-S85.911 with 7th A, S85.919-S85.991 with 7th A, S85.999A, S95.001A, S95.009-S95.011 with 7th A, S95.019-S95.091 with 7th A, S95.099A, S95.201A, S95.209-S95.211 with 7th A, S95.219-S95.291 with 7th A, S95.299-S95.801 with 7th A, S95.809-S95.811 with 7th A, S95.819-S95.891 with 7th A, S95.899-S95.901 with 7th A, S95.909-S95.911 with 7th A, S95.919-S95.991 with 7th A, S95.999 with 7th A

7th **S85.132 Unspecified injury of anterior tibial artery, left leg** CC
CC Excl: CC with 7th character A: S75.802-S75.809 with 7th A, S75.812-S75.819 with 7th A, S75.892-S75.899 with 7th A, S75.902-S75.909 with 7th A, S75.912-S75.919 with 7th A, S75.992-S75.999 with 7th A, S85.132-S85.139 with 7th A, S85.142-S85.149 with 7th A, S85.152-S85.159 with 7th A, S85.202-S85.209 with 7th A, S85.212-S85.219 with 7th A, S85.292-S85.299 with 7th A, S85.802-S85.809 with 7th A, S85.812-S85.819 with 7th A, S85.892-S85.899 with 7th A, S85.902-S85.909 with 7th A, S85.912-S85.919 with 7th A, S85.992-S85.999 with 7th A, S95.002-S95.009 with 7th A, S95.012-S95.019 with 7th A, S95.092-S95.099 with 7th A, S95.202-S95.209 with 7th A, S95.212-S95.219 with 7th A, S95.292-S95.299 with 7th A, S95.802-S95.809 with 7th A, S95.812-S95.819 with 7th A, S95.892-S95.899 with 7th A, S95.902-S95.909 with 7th A, S95.912-S95.919 with 7th A, S95.992-S95.999 with 7th A

7th **S85.139 Unspecified injury of anterior tibial artery, unspecified leg** CC
CC Excl: CC with 7th character A: S75.801-S75.999 with 7th A, S85.131-S85.159 with 7th A, S85.201-S85.299 with 7th A, S85.801-S85.999 with 7th A, S95.001-S95.099 with 7th A, S95.201-S95.999 with 7th A

6th **S85.14 Laceration of anterior tibial artery**

7th **S85.141 Laceration of anterior tibial artery, right leg** CC
CC Excl: See code: S85.131

7th **S85.142 Laceration of anterior tibial artery, left leg** CC
CC Excl: See code: S85.132

7th **S85.149 Laceration of anterior tibial artery, unspecified leg** CC
CC Excl: See code: S85.139

6th **S85.15 Other specified injury of anterior tibial artery**

7th **S85.151 Other specified injury of anterior tibial artery, right leg** CC
CC Excl: See code: S85.131

7th **S85.152 Other specified injury of anterior tibial artery, left leg** CC
CC Excl: See code: S85.132

7th **S85.159 Other specified injury of anterior tibial artery, unspecified leg** CC
CC Excl: See code: S85.139

6th **S85.16 Unspecified injury of posterior tibial artery**

7th **S85.161 Unspecified injury of posterior tibial artery, right leg** CC
CC Excl: CC with 7th character A: S75.801 with 7th A, S75.809-S75.811 with 7th A, S75.819-S75.891 with 7th A, S75.899-S75.901 with 7th A, S75.909-S75.911 with 7th A, S75.919-S75.991 with 7th A, S75.999 with 7th A, S85.161 with 7th A, S85.169-S85.171 with 7th A, S85.179-S85.181 with 7th A, S85.189-S85.201 with 7th A, S85.209-S85.211 with 7th A, S85.219-S85.291 with 7th A, S85.299A, S85.801A, S85.809-S85.811 with 7th A, S85.819-S85.891 with 7th A, S85.899-S85.901 with 7th A, S85.909-S85.911 with 7th A, S85.919-S85.991 with 7th A, S85.999A, S95.001A, S95.009-S95.011 with 7th A, S95.019-S95.091 with 7th A, S95.099A, S95.201A, S95.209-S95.211 with 7th A, S95.219-S95.291 with 7th A, S95.299-S95.801 with 7th A, S95.809-S95.811 with 7th A, S95.819-S95.891 with 7th A, S95.899-S95.901 with 7th A, S95.909-S95.911 with 7th A, S95.919-S95.991 with 7th A, S95.999 with 7th A

7th **S85.162 Unspecified injury of posterior tibial artery, left leg** CC
CC Excl: CC with 7th character A: S75.802-S75.809 with 7th A, S75.812-S75.819 with 7th A, S75.892-S75.899 with 7th A, S75.902-S75.909 with 7th A, S75.912-S75.919 with 7th A, S75.992-S75.999 with 7th A, S85.162-S85.169 with 7th A, S85.172-S85.179 with 7th A, S85.182-S85.189 with 7th A, S85.202-S85.209 with 7th A, S85.212-S85.219 with 7th A, S85.292-S85.299 with 7th A, S85.802-S85.809 with 7th A, S85.812-S85.819 with 7th A, S85.892-S85.899 with 7th A, S85.902-S85.909 with 7th A, S85.912-S85.919 with 7th A, S85.992-S85.999 with 7th A, S95.002-S95.009 with 7th A, S95.012-S95.019 with 7th A, S95.092-S95.099 with 7th A, S95.202-S95.209 with 7th A, S95.212-S95.219 with 7th A, S95.292-S95.299 with 7th A, S95.802-S95.809 with 7th A, S95.812-S95.819 with 7th A, S95.892-S95.899 with 7th A, S95.902-S95.909 with 7th A, S95.912-S95.919 with 7th A, S95.992-S95.999 with 7th A

7th **S85.169 Unspecified injury of posterior tibial artery, unspecified leg** CC
CC Excl: CC with 7th character A: S75.801-S75.999 with 7th A, S85.161-S85.299 with 7th A, S85.801-S85.999 with 7th A, S95.001-S95.099 with 7th A, S95.201-S95.999 with 7th A

6th **S85.17 Laceration of posterior tibial artery**

7th **S85.171 Laceration of posterior tibial artery, right leg** CC
CC Excl: See code: S85.161

7th **S85.172 Laceration of posterior tibial artery, left leg** CC
CC Excl: See code: S85.162

7th **S85.179 Laceration of posterior tibial artery, unspecified leg** CC
CC Excl: See code: S85.169

6th **S85.18 Other specified injury of posterior tibial artery**

7th **S85.181 Other specified injury of posterior tibial artery, right leg** CC
CC Excl: See code: S85.161

7th **S85.182 Other specified injury of posterior tibial artery, left leg** CC
CC Excl: See code: S85.162

7th **S85.189 Other specified injury of posterior tibial artery, unspecified leg** CC
CC Excl: See code: S85.169

5th **S85.2 Injury of peroneal artery**

6th **S85.20 Unspecified injury of peroneal artery**

7th **S85.201 Unspecified injury of peroneal artery, right leg** CC
CC Excl: CC with 7th character A: M79.A21-M79.A29, S75.001 with 7th A, S75.009-S75.011 with 7th A, S75.019-S75.021 with 7th A, S75.029-S75.091 with 7th A, S75.099-S75.101 with 7th A, S75.109-S75.111 with 7th A, S75.119-S75.121 with 7th A, S75.129-S75.191 with 7th A, S75.199-S75.201 with 7th A, S75.209-S75.211 with 7th A, S75.219-S75.221 with 7th A, S75.229-S75.291 with 7th A, S75.299-S75.801 with 7th A, S75.809-S75.811 with 7th A, S75.819-S75.891 with 7th A, S75.899-S75.901 with 7th A, S75.909-S75.911 with 7th A, S75.919-S75.991 with 7th A, S75.999A, S85.001A, S85.009-S85.011 with 7th A, S85.019-S85.091 with 7th A, S85.099-S85.101 with 7th A, S85.109-S85.111 with 7th A, S85.119-S85.121 with 7th A, S85.129-S85.131 with 7th A, S85.139-S85.141 with 7th A, S85.149-S85.151 with 7th A, S85.159-S85.161 with 7th A, S85.169-S85.171 with 7th A, S85.179-S85.181 with 7th A, S85.189-S85.201 with 7th A, S85.209-S85.211 with 7th A, S85.219-S85.291 with 7th A, S85.299-S85.301 with 7th A, S85.309-S85.311 with 7th A, S85.319-S85.391 with 7th A, S85.399-S85.401 with 7th A, S85.409-S85.411 with 7th A, S85.419-S85.491 with 7th A, S85.499-S85.501 with 7th A, S85.509-S85.511 with 7th A, S85.519-S85.591 with 7th A, S85.599-S85.801 with 7th A, S85.809-S85.811 with 7th A, S85.819-S85.891 with 7th A, S85.899-S85.901 with 7th A, S85.909-S85.911 with 7th A, S85.919-S85.991 with 7th A, S85.999 with 7th A, S95.001 with 7th A, S95.009-S95.011 with 7th A, S95.019-S95.091 with 7th A, S95.099-S95.101 with 7th A, S95.109-S95.111 with 7th A, S95.119-S95.191 with 7th A, S95.199-S95.201 with 7th A, S95.209-S95.211 with 7th A, S95.219-S95.291 with 7th A, S95.299-S95.801 with 7th A, S95.809-S95.811 with 7th A, S95.819-S95.891 with 7th A, S95.899-S95.901 with 7th A, S95.909-S95.911 with 7th A, S95.919-S95.991 with 7th A, S95.999 with 7th A

S85.202 Unspecified injury of peroneal artery, left leg (7th) CC
CC Excl: CC with 7th character A: M79.A21-M79.A29, S75.002-S75.009 with 7th A, S75.012-S75.019 with 7th A, S75.022-S75.029 with 7th A, S75.092-S75.099 with 7th A, S75.102-S75.109 with 7th A, S75.112-S75.119 with 7th A, S75.122-S75.129 with 7th A, S75.192-S75.199 with 7th A, S75.202-S75.209 with 7th A, S75.212-S75.219 with 7th A, S75.222-S75.229 with 7th A, S75.292-S75.299 with 7th A,S75.802-S75.809 with 7th A, S75.812-S75.819 with 7th A, S75.892-S75.899 with 7th A, S75.902-S75.909 with 7th A, S75.912-S75.919 with 7th A, S75.992-S75.999A, S85.002-S85.009 with 7th A, S85.012-S85.019 with 7th A, S85.092-S85.099 with 7th A, S85.102-S85.109 with 7th A, S85.112-S85.119 with 7th A, S85.122-S85.129 with 7th A, S85.132-S85.139 with 7th A, S85.142-S85.149 with 7th A, S85.152-S85.159 with 7th A, S85.162-S85.169 with 7th A, S85.172-S85.179 with 7th A, S85.182-S85.189 with 7th A, S85.202-S85.209 with 7th A, S85.212-S85.219 with 7th A, S85.292-S85.299 with 7th A, S85.302-S85.309 with 7th A, S85.312-S85.319 with 7th A, S85.392-S85.399 with 7th A, S85.402-S85.409 with 7th A, S85.412-S85.419 with 7th A, S85.492-S85.499 with 7th A, S85.502-S85.509 with 7th A, S85.512-S85.519 with 7th A, S85.592-S85.599 with 7th A, S85.802-S85.809 with 7th A, S85.812-S85.819 with 7th A, S85.892-S85.899 with 7th A, S85.902-S85.909 with 7th A, S85.912-S85.919 with 7th A, S85.992-S85.999 with 7th A, S95.002-S95.009 with 7th A, S95.012-S95.019 with 7th A, S95.092-S95.099 with 7th A, S95.102-S95.109 with 7th A, S95.112-S95.119 with 7th A, S95.192-S95.199 with 7th A, S95.202-S95.209 with 7th A, S95.212-S95.219 with 7th A, S95.292-S95.299 with 7th A, S95.802-S95.809 with 7th A, S95.812-S95.819 with 7th A, S95.892-S95.899 with 7th A, S95.902-S95.909 with 7th A, S95.912-S95.919 with 7th A, S95.992-S95.999 with 7th A

S85.209 Unspecified injury of peroneal artery, unspecified leg (7th) CC
CC Excl: CC with 7th character A: M79.A21-M79.A29, S75.001-S75.999 with 7th A, S85.001-S85.999 with 7th A, S95.001-S95.999 with 7th A

S85.21 Laceration of peroneal artery (6th)

S85.211 Laceration of peroneal artery, right leg (7th) CC
CC Excl: See code: S85.201

S85.212 Laceration of peroneal artery, left leg (7th) CC
CC Excl: See code: S85.202

S85.219 Laceration of peroneal artery, unspecified leg (7th) CC
CC Excl: See code: S85.209

S85.29 Other specified injury of peroneal artery (6th)

S85.291 Other specified injury of peroneal artery, right leg (7th) CC
CC Excl: See code: S85.201

S85.292 Other specified injury of peroneal artery, left leg (7th) CC
CC Excl: See code: S85.202

S85.299 Other specified injury of peroneal artery, unspecified leg (7th) CC
CC Excl: See code: S85.209

S85.3 Injury of greater saphenous vein at lower leg level (5th)
Injury of greater saphenous vein NOS
Injury of saphenous vein NOS

S85.30 Unspecified injury of greater saphenous vein at lower leg level (6th)

S85.301 Unspecified injury of greater saphenous vein at lower leg level, right leg (7th) CC
CC Excl: CC with 7th character A: S75.201 with 7th A, S75.209-S75.211 with 7th A, S75.219-S75.221 with 7th A, S75.229-S75.291 with 7th A, S75.299-S75.801 with 7th A, S75.809-S75.811 with 7th A, S75.819-S75.891 with 7th A, S75.899-S75.901 with 7th A, S75.909-S75.911 with 7th A, S75.919-S75.991 with 7th A, S75.999A, S85.201A, S85.209-S85.211 with 7th A, S85.219-S85.291 with 7th A, S85.299-S85.301 with 7th A, S85.309-S85.311 with 7th A, S85.319-S85.391 with 7th A, S85.399-S85.401 with 7th A, S85.409-S85.411 with 7th A, S85.419-S85.491 with 7th A, S85.499 with 7th A, S85.801 with 7th A, S85.809-S85.811 with 7th A, S85.819-S85.891 with 7th A, S85.899-S85.901 with 7th A, S85.909-S85.911 with 7th A, S85.919-S85.991 with 7th A, S85.999A, S95.001A, S95.009-S95.011 with 7th A, S95.019-S95.091 with 7th A, S95.099A, S95.201A, S95.209-S95.211 with 7th A, S95.219-S95.291 with 7th A, S95.299-S95.801 with 7th A, S95.809-S95.811 with 7th A, S95.819-S95.891 with 7th A, S95.899-S95.901 with 7th A, S95.909-S95.911 with 7th A, S95.919-S95.991 with 7th A, S95.999 with 7th A

S85.302 Unspecified injury of greater saphenous vein at lower leg level, left leg (7th) CC
CC Excl: CC with 7th character A: S75.202-S75.209 with 7th A, S75.212-S75.219 with 7th A, S75.222-S75.229 with 7th A, S75.292-S75.299 with 7th A, S75.802-S75.809 with 7th A, S75.812-S75.819 with 7th A, S75.892-S75.899 with 7th A, S75.902-S75.909 with 7th A, S75.912-S75.919 with 7th A, S75.992-S75.999 with 7th A, S85.202-S85.209 with 7th A, S85.212-S85.219 with 7th A, S85.292-S85.299 with 7th A, S85.302-S85.309 with 7th A, S85.312-S85.319 with 7th A, S85.392-S85.399 with 7th A, S85.402-S85.409 with 7th A, S85.412-S85.419 with 7th A, S85.492-S85.499 with 7th A, S85.802-S85.809 with 7th A, S85.812-S85.819 with 7th A, S85.892-S85.899 with 7th A, S85.902-S85.909 with 7th A, S85.912-S85.919 with 7th A, S85.992-S85.999 with 7th A, S95.002-S95.009 with 7th A, S95.012-S95.019 with 7th A, S95.092-S95.099 with 7th A, S95.202-S95.209 with 7th A, S95.212-S95.219 with 7th A, S95.292-S95.299 with 7th A, S95.802-S95.809 with 7th A, S95.812-S95.819 with 7th A, S95.892-S95.899 with 7th A, S95.902-S95.909 with 7th A, S95.912-S95.919 with 7th A, S95.992-S95.999 with 7th A

S85.309 Unspecified injury of greater saphenous vein at lower leg level, unspecified leg (7th) CC
CC Excl: CC with 7th character A: S75.201-S75.999 with 7th A, S85.201-S85.499 with 7th A, S85.801-S85.999 with 7th A, S95.001-S95.099 with 7th A, S95.201-S95.999 with 7th A

S85.31 Laceration of greater saphenous vein at lower leg level (6th)

S85.311 Laceration of greater saphenous vein at lower leg level, right leg (7th) CC
CC Excl: See code: S85.301

S85.312 Laceration of greater saphenous vein at lower leg level, left leg (7th) CC
CC Excl: See code: S85.302

S85.319 Laceration of greater saphenous vein at lower leg level, unspecified leg (7th) CC
CC Excl: See code: S85.309

✓6th **S85.39 Other specified injury of greater saphenous vein at lower leg level**

✓7th **S85.391 Other specified injury of greater saphenous vein at lower leg level, right leg** CC
CC Excl: See code: S85.301

✓7th **S85.392 Other specified injury of greater saphenous vein at lower leg level, left leg** CC
CC Excl: See code: S85.302

✓7th **S85.399 Other specified injury of greater saphenous vein at lower leg level, unspecified leg** CC
CC Excl: See code: S85.309

✓5th **S85.4 Injury of lesser saphenous vein at lower leg level**

✓6th **S85.40 Unspecified injury of lesser saphenous vein at lower leg level**

✓7th **S85.401 Unspecified injury of lesser saphenous vein at lower leg level, right leg** CC
CC Excl: See code: S85.301

✓7th **S85.402 Unspecified injury of lesser saphenous vein at lower leg level, left leg** CC
CC Excl: See code: S85.302

✓7th **S85.409 Unspecified injury of lesser saphenous vein at lower leg level, unspecified leg** CC
CC Excl: See code: S85.309

✓6th **S85.41 Laceration of lesser saphenous vein at lower leg level**

✓7th **S85.411 Laceration of lesser saphenous vein at lower leg level, right leg** CC
CC Excl: See code: S85.301

✓7th **S85.412 Laceration of lesser saphenous vein at lower leg level, left leg** CC
CC Excl: See code: S85.302

✓7th **S85.419 Laceration of lesser saphenous vein at lower leg level, unspecified leg** CC
CC Excl: See code: S85.309

✓6th **S85.49 Other specified injury of lesser saphenous vein at lower leg level**

✓7th **S85.491 Other specified injury of lesser saphenous vein at lower leg level, right leg** CC
CC Excl: See code: S85.301

✓7th **S85.492 Other specified injury of lesser saphenous vein at lower leg level, left leg** CC
CC Excl: See code: S85.302

✓7th **S85.499 Other specified injury of lesser saphenous vein at lower leg level, unspecified leg** CC
CC Excl: See code: S85.309

✓5th **S85.5 Injury of popliteal vein**

✓6th **S85.50 Unspecified injury of popliteal vein**

✓7th **S85.501 Unspecified injury of popliteal vein, right leg** MCC
CC Excl: MCC with 7th A: S75.801 with 7th A, S75.809-S75.811 with 7th A, S75.819-S75.891 with 7th A, S75.899-S75.901 with 7th A, S75.909-S75.911 with 7th A, S75.919-S75.991 with 7th A, S75.999 with 7th A, S85.201 with 7th A, S85.209-S85.211 with 7th A, S85.219-S85.291 with 7th A, S85.299A, S85.501A, S85.509-S85.511 with 7th A, S85.519-S85.591 with 7th A, S85.599-S85.801 with 7th A, S85.809-S85.811 with 7th A, S85.819-S85.891 with 7th A, S85.899-S85.901 with 7th A, S85.909-S85.911 with 7th A, S85.919-S85.991 with 7th A, S85.999A, S95.001A, S95.009-S95.011 with 7th A, S95.019-S95.091 with 7th A, S95.099 with 7th A, S95.201 with 7th A, S95.209-S95.211 with 7th A, S95.219-S95.291 with 7th A, S95.299-S95.801 with 7th A, S95.809-S95.811 with 7th A, S95.819-S95.891 with 7th A, S95.899-S95.901 with 7th A, S95.909-S95.911 with 7th A, S95.919-S95.991 with 7th A, S95.999 with 7th A

✓7th **S85.502 Unspecified injury of popliteal vein, left leg** MCC
CC Excl: MCC with 7th A: S75.802-S75.809 with 7th A, S75.812-S75.819 with 7th A, S75.892-S75.899 with 7th A, S75.902-S75.909 with 7th A, S75.912-S75.919 with 7th A, S75.992-S75.999 with 7th A, S85.202-S85.209 with 7th A, S85.212-S85.219 with 7th A, S85.292-S85.299 with 7th A, S85.502-S85.509 with 7th A, S85.512-S85.519 with 7th A, S85.592-S85.599 with 7th A, S85.802-S85.809 with 7th A, S85.812-S85.819 with 7th A, S85.892-S85.899 with 7th A, S85.902-S85.909 with 7th A, S85.912-S85.919 with 7th A, S85.992-S85.999 with 7th A, S95.002-S95.009 with 7th A, S95.012-S95.019 with 7th A, S95.092-S95.099 with 7th A, S95.202-S95.209 with 7th A, S95.212-S95.219 with 7th A, S95.292-S95.299 with 7th A, S95.802-S95.809 with 7th A, S95.812-S95.819 with 7th A, S95.892-S95.899 with 7th A, S95.902-S95.909 with 7th A, S95.912-S95.919 with 7th A, S95.992-S95.999 with 7th A

✓7th **S85.509 Unspecified injury of popliteal vein, unspecified leg** MCC
CC Excl: MCC with 7th A: S75.801-S75.999 with 7th A, S85.201-S85.299 with 7th A, S85.501-S85.999 with 7th A, S95.001-S95.099 with 7th A, S95.201-S95.999 with 7th A

✓6th **S85.51 Laceration of popliteal vein**

✓7th **S85.511 Laceration of popliteal vein, right leg** MCC
CC Excl: See code: S85.501

✓7th **S85.512 Laceration of popliteal vein, left leg** MCC
CC Excl: See code: S85.502

✓7th **S85.519 Laceration of popliteal vein, unspecified leg** MCC
CC Excl: See code: S85.509

✓6th **S85.59 Other specified injury of popliteal vein**

✓7th **S85.591 Other specified injury of popliteal vein, right leg** MCC
CC Excl: See code: S85.501

✓7th **S85.592 Other specified injury of popliteal vein, left leg** MCC
CC Excl: See code: S85.502

✓7th **S85.599 Other specified injury of popliteal vein, unspecified leg** MCC
CC Excl: See code: S85.509

✓5th **S85.8 Injury of other blood vessels at lower leg level**

✓6th **S85.80 Unspecified injury of other blood vessels at lower leg level**

✓7th **S85.801 Unspecified injury of other blood vessels at lower leg level, right leg** CC
CC Excl: CC with 7th character A: See code: S85.501

✓7th **S85.802 Unspecified injury of other blood vessels at lower leg level, left leg** CC
CC Excl: CC with 7th character A: See code: S85.502

✓7th **S85.809 Unspecified injury of other blood vessels at lower leg level, unspecified leg** CC
CC Excl: CC with 7th character A: See code: S85.509

✓6th **S85.81 Laceration of other blood vessels at lower leg level**

✓7th **S85.811 Laceration of other blood vessels at lower leg level, right leg** CC
CC Excl: CC with 7th character A: See code: S85.501

✓7th **S85.812 Laceration of other blood vessels at lower leg level, left leg** CC
CC Excl: CC with 7th character A: See code: S85.502

✓7th **S85.819 Laceration of other blood vessels at lower leg level, unspecified leg** CC
CC Excl: CC with 7th character A: See code: S85.509

√6th **S85.89 Other specified injury of other blood vessels at lower leg level**

√7th **S85.891 Other specified injury of other blood vessels at lower leg level, right leg** CC
CC Excl: CC with 7th character A: See code: S85.501

√7th **S85.892 Other specified injury of other blood vessels at lower leg level, left leg** CC
CC Excl: CC with 7th character A: See code: S85.502

√7th **S85.899 Other specified injury of other blood vessels at lower leg level, unspecified leg** CC
CC Excl: CC with 7th character A: See code: S85.509

√5th **S85.9 Injury of unspecified blood vessel at lower leg level**

√6th **S85.90 Unspecified injury of unspecified blood vessel at lower leg level**

√7th **S85.901 Unspecified injury of unspecified blood vessel at lower leg level, right leg** CC
CC Excl: See code: S85.501

√7th **S85.902 Unspecified injury of unspecified blood vessel at lower leg level, left leg** CC
CC Excl: See code: S85.502

√7th **S85.909 Unspecified injury of unspecified blood vessel at lower leg level, unspecified leg** CC
CC Excl: See code: S85.509

√6th **S85.91 Laceration of unspecified blood vessel at lower leg level**

√7th **S85.911 Laceration of unspecified blood vessel at lower leg level, right leg** CC
CC Excl: See code: S85.501

√7th **S85.912 Laceration of unspecified blood vessel at lower leg level, left leg** CC
CC Excl: See code: S85.502

√7th **S85.919 Laceration of unspecified blood vessel at lower leg level, unspecified leg** CC
CC Excl: See code: S85.509

√6th **S85.99 Other specified injury of unspecified blood vessel at lower leg level**

√7th **S85.991 Other specified injury of unspecified blood vessel at lower leg level, right leg** CC
CC Excl: See code: S85.501

√7th **S85.992 Other specified injury of unspecified blood vessel at lower leg level, left leg** CC
CC Excl: See code: S85.502

√7th **S85.999 Other specified injury of unspecified blood vessel at lower leg level, unspecified leg** CC
CC Excl: See code: S85.509

√4th **S86 Injury of muscle, fascia and tendon at lower leg level**

Code also any associated open wound (S81.-)

EXCLUDES 2 *injury of muscle, fascia and tendon at ankle (S96.-)*
injury of patellar ligament (tendon) (S76.1-)
sprain of joints and ligaments of knee (S83.-)

The appropriate 7th character is to be added to each code from category S86.
A initial encounter
D subsequent encounter
S sequela

√5th **S86.0 Injury of Achilles tendon**

√6th **S86.00 Unspecified injury of Achilles tendon**

√7th **S86.001 Unspecified injury of right Achilles tendon**

√7th **S86.002 Unspecified injury of left Achilles tendon**

√7th **S86.009 Unspecified injury of unspecified Achilles tendon**

√6th **S86.01 Strain of Achilles tendon**

√7th **S86.011 Strain of right Achilles tendon**

√7th **S86.012 Strain of left Achilles tendon**

√7th **S86.019 Strain of unspecified Achilles tendon**

√6th **S86.02 Laceration of Achilles tendon**

√7th **S86.021 Laceration of right Achilles tendon** CC
CC Excl: CC with 7th character A: S81.001 with 7th A, S81.009-S81.011 with 7th A, S81.019-S81.021 with 7th A, S81.029-S81.031 with 7th A, S81.039-S81.041 with 7th A, S81.049-S81.051 with 7th A, S81.059-S81.801 with 7th A, S81.809-S81.811 with 7th A, S81.819-S81.821 with 7th A, S81.829-S81.831 with 7th A, S81.839-S81.841 with 7th A, S81.849-S81.851 with 7th A, S81.859A, S86.021A, S86.029A, S86.121A, S86.129A, S86.221A, S86.229A, S86.321A, S86.329A, S86.821A, S86.829A, S86.921A, S86.929A, S91.001A, S91.009-S91.011 with 7th A, S91.019-S91.021 with 7th A, S91.029-S91.031 with 7th A, S91.039-S91.041 with 7th A, S91.049-S91.051 with 7th A, S91.059A, S96.021A, S96.029A, S96.121A, S96.129A, S96.221A, S96.229A, S96.821A, S96.829A, S96.921A, S96.929A

√7th **S86.022 Laceration of left Achilles tendon** CC
CC Excl: CC with 7th character A: S81.002-S81.009 with 7th A, S81.012-S81.019 with 7th A, S81.022-S81.029 with 7th A, S81.032-S81.039 with 7th A, S81.042-S81.049 with 7th A, S81.052-S81.059 with 7th A, S81.802-S81.809 with 7th A, S81.812-S81.819 with 7th A, S81.822-S81.829 with 7th A, S81.832-S81.839 with 7th A, S81.842-S81.849 with 7th A, S81.852-S81.859 with 7th A, S86.022-S86.029 with 7th A, S86.122-S86.129 with 7th A, S86.222-S86.229 with 7th A, S86.322-S86.329 with 7th A, S86.822-S86.829 with 7th A, S86.922-S86.929 with 7th A, S91.002-S91.009 with 7th A, S91.012-S91.019 with 7th A, S91.022-S91.029 with 7th A, S91.032-S91.039 with 7th A, S91.042-S91.049 with 7th A, S91.052-S91.059 with 7th A, S96.022-S96.029 with 7th A, S96.122-S96.129 with 7th A, S96.222-S96.229 with 7th A, S96.822-S96.829 with 7th A, S96.922-S96.929 with 7th A

√7th **S86.029 Laceration of unspecified Achilles tendon** CC
CC Excl: CC with 7th character A: S81.001-S81.859 with 7th A, S86.021-S86.029 with 7th A, S86.121-S86.129 with 7th A, S86.221-S86.229 with 7th A, S86.321-S86.329 with 7th A, S86.821-S86.829 with 7th A, S86.921-S86.929 with 7th A, S91.001-S91.059 with 7th A, S96.021-S96.029 with 7th A, S96.121-S96.129 with 7th A, S96.221-S96.229 with 7th A, S96.821-S96.829 with 7th A, S96.921-S96.929 with 7th A

√6th **S86.09 Other specified injury of Achilles tendon**

√7th **S86.091 Other specified injury of right Achilles tendon**

√7th **S86.092 Other specified injury of left Achilles tendon**

√7th **S86.099 Other specified injury of unspecified Achilles tendon**

√5th **S86.1 Injury of other muscle(s) and tendon(s) of posterior muscle group at lower leg level**

√6th **S86.10 Unspecified injury of other muscle(s) and tendon(s) of posterior muscle group at lower leg level**

√7th **S86.101 Unspecified injury of other muscle(s) and tendon(s) of posterior muscle group at lower leg level, right leg**

√7th **S86.102 Unspecified injury of other muscle(s) and tendon(s) of posterior muscle group at lower leg level, left leg**

√7th **S86.109 Unspecified injury of other muscle(s) and tendon(s) of posterior muscle group at lower leg level, unspecified leg**

√6th **S86.11 Strain of other muscle(s) and tendon(s) of posterior muscle group at lower leg level**

√7th **S86.111 Strain of other muscle(s) and tendon(s) of posterior muscle group at lower leg level, right leg**

√7th **S86.112 Strain of other muscle(s) and tendon(s) of posterior muscle group at lower leg level, left leg**

7th **S86.119 Strain of other muscle(s) and tendon(s) of posterior muscle group at lower leg level, unspecified leg**

6th **S86.12 Laceration of other muscle(s) and tendon(s) of posterior muscle group at lower leg level**

7th **S86.121 Laceration of other muscle(s) and tendon(s) of posterior muscle group at lower leg level, right leg** CC
CC Excl: See code: S86.021

7th **S86.122 Laceration of other muscle(s) and tendon(s) of posterior muscle group at lower leg level, left leg** CC
CC Excl: See code: S86.022

7th **S86.129 Laceration of other muscle(s) and tendon(s) of posterior muscle group at lower leg level, unspecified leg** CC
CC Excl: See code: S86.029

6th **S86.19 Other injury of other muscle(s) and tendon(s) of posterior muscle group at lower leg level**

7th **S86.191 Other injury of other muscle(s) and tendon(s) of posterior muscle group at lower leg level, right leg**

7th **S86.192 Other injury of other muscle(s) and tendon(s) of posterior muscle group at lower leg level, left leg**

7th **S86.199 Other injury of other muscle(s) and tendon(s) of posterior muscle group at lower leg level, unspecified leg**

5th **S86.2 Injury of muscle(s) and tendon(s) of anterior muscle group at lower leg level**

6th **S86.20 Unspecified injury of muscle(s) and tendon(s) of anterior muscle group at lower leg level**

7th **S86.201 Unspecified injury of muscle(s) and tendon(s) of anterior muscle group at lower leg level, right leg**

7th **S86.202 Unspecified injury of muscle(s) and tendon(s) of anterior muscle group at lower leg level, left leg**

7th **S86.209 Unspecified injury of muscle(s) and tendon(s) of anterior muscle group at lower leg level, unspecified leg**

6th **S86.21 Strain of muscle(s) and tendon(s) of anterior muscle group at lower leg level**

7th **S86.211 Strain of muscle(s) and tendon(s) of anterior muscle group at lower leg level, right leg**

7th **S86.212 Strain of muscle(s) and tendon(s) of anterior muscle group at lower leg level, left leg**

7th **S86.219 Strain of muscle(s) and tendon(s) of anterior muscle group at lower leg level, unspecified leg**

6th **S86.22 Laceration of muscle(s) and tendon(s) of anterior muscle group at lower leg level**

7th **S86.221 Laceration of muscle(s) and tendon(s) of anterior muscle group at lower leg level, right leg** CC
CC Excl: See code: S86.021

7th **S86.222 Laceration of muscle(s) and tendon(s) of anterior muscle group at lower leg level, left leg** CC
CC Excl: See code: S86.022

7th **S86.229 Laceration of muscle(s) and tendon(s) of anterior muscle group at lower leg level, unspecified leg** CC
CC Excl: See code: S86.029

6th **S86.29 Other injury of muscle(s) and tendon(s) of anterior muscle group at lower leg level**

7th **S86.291 Other injury of muscle(s) and tendon(s) of anterior muscle group at lower leg level, right leg**

7th **S86.292 Other injury of muscle(s) and tendon(s) of anterior muscle group at lower leg level, left leg**

7th **S86.299 Other injury of muscle(s) and tendon(s) of anterior muscle group at lower leg level, unspecified leg**

5th **S86.3 Injury of muscle(s) and tendon(s) of peroneal muscle group at lower leg level**

6th **S86.30 Unspecified injury of muscle(s) and tendon(s) of peroneal muscle group at lower leg level**

7th **S86.301 Unspecified injury of muscle(s) and tendon(s) of peroneal muscle group at lower leg level, right leg**

7th **S86.302 Unspecified injury of muscle(s) and tendon(s) of peroneal muscle group at lower leg level, left leg**

7th **S86.309 Unspecified injury of muscle(s) and tendon(s) of peroneal muscle group at lower leg level, unspecified leg**

6th **S86.31 Strain of muscle(s) and tendon(s) of peroneal muscle group at lower leg level**

7th **S86.311 Strain of muscle(s) and tendon(s) of peroneal muscle group at lower leg level, right leg**

7th **S86.312 Strain of muscle(s) and tendon(s) of peroneal muscle group at lower leg level, left leg**

7th **S86.319 Strain of muscle(s) and tendon(s) of peroneal muscle group at lower leg level, unspecified leg**

6th **S86.32 Laceration of muscle(s) and tendon(s) of peroneal muscle group at lower leg level**

7th **S86.321 Laceration of muscle(s) and tendon(s) of peroneal muscle group at lower leg level, right leg** CC
CC Excl: See code: S86.021

7th **S86.322 Laceration of muscle(s) and tendon(s) of peroneal muscle group at lower leg level, left leg** CC
CC Excl: See code: S86.022

7th **S86.329 Laceration of muscle(s) and tendon(s) of peroneal muscle group at lower leg level, unspecified leg** CC
CC Excl: See code: S86.029

6th **S86.39 Other injury of muscle(s) and tendon(s) of peroneal muscle group at lower leg level**

7th **S86.391 Other injury of muscle(s) and tendon(s) of peroneal muscle group at lower leg level, right leg**

7th **S86.392 Other injury of muscle(s) and tendon(s) of peroneal muscle group at lower leg level, left leg**

7th **S86.399 Other injury of muscle(s) and tendon(s) of peroneal muscle group at lower leg level, unspecified leg**

5th **S86.8 Injury of other muscles and tendons at lower leg level**

6th **S86.80 Unspecified injury of other muscles and tendons at lower leg level**

7th **S86.801 Unspecified injury of other muscle(s) and tendon(s) at lower leg level, right leg**

7th **S86.802 Unspecified injury of other muscle(s) and tendon(s) at lower leg level, left leg**

7th **S86.809 Unspecified injury of other muscle(s) and tendon(s) at lower leg level, unspecified leg**

6th **S86.81 Strain of other muscles and tendons at lower leg level**

7th **S86.811 Strain of other muscle(s) and tendon(s) at lower leg level, right leg**

7th **S86.812 Strain of other muscle(s) and tendon(s) at lower leg level, left leg**

7th **S86.819 Strain of other muscle(s) and tendon(s) at lower leg level, unspecified leg**

6th **S86.82 Laceration of other muscles and tendons at lower leg level**

7th **S86.821 Laceration of other muscle(s) and tendon(s) at lower leg level, right leg** CC
CC Excl: See code: S86.021

7th **S86.822 Laceration of other muscle(s) and tendon(s) at lower leg level, left leg** CC
CC Excl: See code: S86.022

✓7th **S86.829 Laceration of other muscle(s) and tendon(s) at lower leg level, unspecified leg** CC
CC Excl: See code: S86.029

✓6th **S86.89 Other injury of other muscles and tendons at lower leg level**

✓7th **S86.891 Other injury of other muscle(s) and tendon(s) at lower leg level, right leg**

✓7th **S86.892 Other injury of other muscle(s) and tendon(s) at lower leg level, left leg**

✓7th **S86.899 Other injury of other muscle(s) and tendon(s) at lower leg level, unspecified leg**

✓5th **S86.9 Injury of unspecified muscle and tendon at lower leg level**

✓6th **S86.90 Unspecified injury of unspecified muscle and tendon at lower leg level**

✓7th **S86.901 Unspecified injury of unspecified muscle(s) and tendon(s) at lower leg level, right leg**

✓7th **S86.902 Unspecified injury of unspecified muscle(s) and tendon(s) at lower leg level, left leg**

✓7th **S86.909 Unspecified injury of unspecified muscle(s) and tendon(s) at lower leg level, unspecified leg**

✓6th **S86.91 Strain of unspecified muscle and tendon at lower leg level**

✓7th **S86.911 Strain of unspecified muscle(s) and tendon(s) at lower leg level, right leg**

✓7th **S86.912 Strain of unspecified muscle(s) and tendon(s) at lower leg level, left leg**

✓7th **S86.919 Strain of unspecified muscle(s) and tendon(s) at lower leg level, unspecified leg**

✓6th **S86.92 Laceration of unspecified muscle and tendon at lower leg level**

✓7th **S86.921 Laceration of unspecified muscle(s) and tendon(s) at lower leg level, right leg** CC
CC Excl: See code: S86.021

✓7th **S86.922 Laceration of unspecified muscle(s) and tendon(s) at lower leg level, left leg** CC
CC Excl: See code: S86.022

✓7th **S86.929 Laceration of unspecified muscle(s) and tendon(s) at lower leg level, unspecified leg** CC
CC Excl: See code: S86.029

✓6th **S86.99 Other injury of unspecified muscle and tendon at lower leg level**

✓7th **S86.991 Other injury of unspecified muscle(s) and tendon(s) at lower leg level, right leg**

✓7th **S86.992 Other injury of unspecified muscle(s) and tendon(s) at lower leg level, left leg**

✓7th **S86.999 Other injury of unspecified muscle(s) and tendon(s) at lower leg level, unspecified leg**

✓4th **S87 Crushing injury of lower leg**

Use additional code(s) for all associated injuries

EXCLUDES 2 *crushing injury of ankle and foot (S97.-)*

The appropriate 7th character is to be added to each code from category S87.
A initial encounter
D subsequent encounter
S sequela

✓5th **S87.0 Crushing injury of knee**

✓x7th **S87.00 Crushing injury of unspecified knee**

✓x7th **S87.01 Crushing injury of right knee**

✓x7th **S87.02 Crushing injury of left knee**

✓5th **S87.8 Crushing injury of lower leg**

✓x7th **S87.80 Crushing injury of unspecified lower leg**

✓x7th **S87.81 Crushing injury of right lower leg**

✓x7th **S87.82 Crushing injury of left lower leg**

✓4th **S88 Traumatic amputation of lower leg**

NOTE An amputation not identified as partial or complete should be coded to complete.

EXCLUDES 1 *traumatic amputation of ankle and foot (S98.-)*

The appropriate 7th character is to be added to each code from category S88.
A initial encounter
D subsequent encounter
S sequela

✓5th **S88.0 Traumatic amputation at knee level**

✓6th **S88.01 Complete traumatic amputation at knee level**

✓7th **S88.011 Complete traumatic amputation at knee level, right lower leg** CC
CC Excl: CC with 7th character A: S71.001 with 7th A, S71.009-S71.011 with 7th A, S71.019-S71.021 with 7th A, S71.029-S71.031 with 7th A, S71.039-S71.041 with 7th A, S71.049-S71.051 with 7th A, S71.059-S71.101 with 7th A, S71.109-S71.111 with 7th A, S71.119-S71.121 with 7th A, S71.129-S71.131 with 7th A, S71.139-S71.141 with 7th A, S71.149-S71.151 with 7th A, S71.159A, S76.021A, S76.029A, S76.121 A, S76.129A, S76.221A, S76.229A, S76.321A, S76.329A, S76.821A, S76.829A, S76.921A, S76.929A, S78.011A, S78.019-S78.021 with 7th A, S78.029-S78.111 with 7th A, S78.119-S78.121 with 7th A, S78.129-S78.911 with 7th A, S78.919-S78.921 with 7th A, S78.929A, S81.001A, S81.009-S81.011 with 7th A, S81.019-S81.021 with 7th A, S81.029-S81.031 with 7th A, S81.039-S81.041 with 7th A, S81.049-S81.051 with 7th A, S81.059-S81.801 with 7th A, S81.809-S81.811 with 7th A, S81.819-S81.821 with 7th A, S81.829-S81.831 with 7th A, S81.839-S81.841 with 7th A, S81.849-S81.851 with 7th A, S81.859 with 7th A, S86.021A, S86.029A, S86.121A, S86.129A, S86.221A, S86.229A, S86.321A, S86.329A, S86.821A, S86.829A, S86.921A, S86.929A, S88.011A, S88.019-S88.021 with 7th A, S88.029-S88.111 with 7th A, S88.119-S88.121 with 7th A, S88.129-S88.911 with 7th A, S88.919-S88.921 with 7th A, S88.929A, S91.001A, S91.009-S91.011 with 7th A, S91.019-S91.021 with 7th A, S91.029-S91.031 with 7th A, S91.039-S91.041 with 7th A, S91.049-S91.051 with 7th A, S91.059-S91.101 with 7th A, S91.103-S91.104 with 7th A, S91.106-S91.111 with 7th A, S91.113-S91.114 with 7th A, S91.116-S91.121 with 7th A, S91.123-S91.124 with 7th A, S91.126-S91.131 with 7th A, S91.133-S91.134 with 7th A, S91.136-S91.141 with 7th A, S91.143-S91.144 with 7th A, S91.146-S91.151 with 7th A, S91.153-S91.154 with 7th A, S91.156-S91.201 with 7th A, S91.203-S91.204 with 7th A, S91.206-S91.211 with 7th A, S91.213-S91.214 with 7th A, S91.216-S91.221 with 7th A, S91.223-S91.224 with 7th A, S91.226-S91.231 with 7th A, S91.233-S91.234 with 7th A, S91.236-S91.241 with 7th A, S91.243-S91.244 with 7th A, S91.246-S91.251 with 7th A, S91.253-S91.254 with 7th A, S91.256-S91.301 with 7th A, S91.309-S91.311 with 7th A, S91.319-S91.321 with 7th A, S91.329-S91.331 with 7th A, S91.339-S91.341 with 7th A, S91.349-S91.351 with 7th A, S91.359A, S96.021A, S96.029A, S96.121A, S96.129A, S96.221A, S96.229A, S96.821A, S96.829A, S96.921A, S96.929A, S98.011A, S98.019-S98.021 with 7th A, S98.029-S98.111 with 7th A, S98.119-S98.121 with 7th A, S98.122-S98.129 with 7th A, S98.131-S98.139 with 7th A, S98.142-S98.149 with 7th A, S98.212-S98.219 with 7th A, S98.222-S98.229 with 7th A, S98.312-S98.319 with 7th A, S98.322-S98.329 with 7th A, S98.912-S98.919 with 7th A, S98.922-S98.929 with 7th A, T14.8-T14.91, T79.A0X-T79.9XX with 7th A

7th **S88.Ø12 Complete traumatic amputation at knee level, left lower leg** CC
CC Excl: CC with 7th character A: S71.ØØ2-S71.ØØ9 with 7th A, S71.Ø12-S71.Ø19 with 7th A, S71.Ø22-S71.Ø29 with 7th A, S71.Ø32-S71.Ø39 with 7th A, S71.Ø42-S71.Ø49 with 7th A, S71.Ø52-S71.Ø59 with 7th A, S71.1Ø2-S71.1Ø9 with 7th A, S71.112-S71.119 with 7th A, S71.122-S71.129 with 7th A, S71.132-S71.139 with 7th A, S71.142-S71.149 with 7th A, S71.152-S71.159 with 7th A, S76.Ø22-S76.Ø29 with 7th A, S76.122-S76.129 with 7th A, S76.222-S76.229 with 7th A, S76.322-S76.329 with 7th A, S76.822-S76.829 with 7th A, S76.922-S76.929 with 7th A, S78.Ø12-S78.Ø19 with 7th A, S78.Ø22-S78.Ø29 with 7th A, S78.112-S78.119 with 7th A, S78.122-S78.129 with 7th A, S78.912-S78.919 with 7th A, S78.922-S78.929 with 7th A, S81.ØØ2-S81.ØØ9 with 7th A, S81.Ø12-S81.Ø19 with 7th A, S81.Ø22-S81.Ø29 with 7th A, S81.Ø32-S81.Ø39 with 7th A, S81.Ø42-S81.Ø49 with 7th A, S81.Ø52-S81.Ø59 with 7th A, S81.8Ø2-S81.8Ø9 with 7th A, S81.812-S81.819 with 7th A, S81.822-S81.829 with 7th A, S81.832-S81.839 with 7th A, S81.842-S81.849 with 7th A, S81.852-S81.859 with 7th A, S86.Ø22-S86.Ø29 with 7th A, S86.122-S86.129 with 7th A, S86.222-S86.229 with 7th A, S86.322-S86.329 with 7th A, S86.822-S86.829 with 7th A, S86.922-S86.929 with 7th A, S88.Ø12-S88.Ø19 with 7th A, S88.Ø22-S88.Ø29 with 7th A, S88.112-S88.119 with 7th A, S88.122-S88.129 with 7th A, S88.912-S88.919 with 7th A, S88.922-S88.929 with 7th A, S91.ØØ2-S91.ØØ9 with 7th A, S91.Ø12-S91.Ø19 with 7th A, S91.Ø22-S91.Ø29 with 7th A, S91.Ø32-S91.Ø39 with 7th A, S91.Ø42-S91.Ø49 with 7th A, S91.Ø52-S91.Ø59 with 7th A, S91.1Ø2-S91.1Ø3 with 7th A, S91.1Ø5-S91.1Ø9 with 7th A, S91.112-S91.113 with 7th A, S91.115-S91.119 with 7th A, S91.122-S91.123 with 7th A, S91.125-S91.129 with 7th A, S91.132-S91.133 with 7th A, S91.135-S91.139 with 7th A, S91.142-S91.143 with 7th A, S91.145-S91.149 with 7th A, S91.152-S91.153 with 7th A, S91.155-S91.159 with 7th A, S91.2Ø2-S91.2Ø3 with 7th A, S91.2Ø5-S91.2Ø9 with 7th A, S91.212-S91.213 with 7th A, S91.215-S91.219 with 7th A, S91.222-S91.223 with 7th A, S91.225-S91.229 with 7th A, S91.232-S91.233 with 7th A, S91.235-S91.239 with 7th A, S91.242-S91.243 with 7th A, S91.245-S91.249 with 7th A, S91.252-S91.253 with 7th A, S91.255-S91.259 with 7th A, S91.3Ø2-S91.3Ø9 with 7th A, S91.312-S91.319 with 7th A, S91.322-S91.329 with 7th A, S91.332-S91.339 with 7th A, S91.342-S91.349 with 7th A, S91.352-S91.359 with 7th A, S96.Ø22-S96.Ø29 with 7th A, S96.122-S96.129 with 7th A, S96.222-S96.229 with 7th A, S96.822-S96.829 with 7th A, S96.922-S96.929 with 7th A, S98.Ø12-S98.Ø19 with 7th A, S98.Ø22-S98.Ø29 with 7th A, S98.112-S98.119 with 7th A, S98.122-S98.129 with 7th A, S98.132-S98.139 with 7th A, S98.142-S98.149 with 7th A, S98.212-S98.219 with 7th A, S98.222-S98.229 with 7th A, S98.312-S98.319 with 7th A, S98.322-S98.329 with 7th A, S98.912-S98.919 with 7th A, S98.922-S98.929 with 7th A, T14.8-T14.91, T79.AØX-T79.9XX with 7th A

7th **S88.Ø19 Complete traumatic amputation at knee level, unspecified lower leg** CC
CC Excl: CC with 7th character A: S71.ØØ1-S71.159 with 7th A, S76.Ø21-S76.Ø29 with 7th A, S76.121-S76.129 with 7th A, S76.221-S76.229 with 7th A, S76.321-S76.329 with 7th A, S76.821-S76.829 with 7th A, S76.921-S76.929 with 7th A, S78.Ø11-S78.929 with 7th A, S81.ØØ1-S81.859 with 7th A, S86.Ø21-S86.Ø29 with 7th A, S86.121-S86.129 with 7th A, S86.221-S86.229 with 7th A, S86.321-S86.329 with 7th A, S86.821-S86.829 with 7th A, S86.921-S86.929 with 7th A, S88.Ø11-S88.929 with 7th A, S91.ØØ1-S91.359 with 7th A, S96.Ø21-S96.Ø29 with 7th A, S96.121-S96.129 with 7th A, S96.221-S96.229 with 7th A, S96.821-S96.829 with 7th A, S96.921-S96.929 with 7th A, S98.Ø11-S98.929 with 7th A, T14.8-T14.91, T79.AØX-T79.9XX with 7th A

6th **S88.Ø2 Partial traumatic amputation at knee level**

7th **S88.Ø21 Partial traumatic amputation at knee level, right lower leg** CC
CC Excl: See code: S88.Ø11

7th **S88.Ø22 Partial traumatic amputation at knee level, left lower leg** CC
CC Excl: See code: S88.Ø12

7th **S88.Ø29 Partial traumatic amputation at knee level, unspecified lower leg** CC
CC Excl: See code: S88.Ø19

5th **S88.1 Traumatic amputation at level between knee and ankle**

6th **S88.11 Complete traumatic amputation at level between knee and ankle**

7th **S88.111 Complete traumatic amputation at levelbetween knee and ankle, right lower leg** CC
CC Excl: See code: S88.Ø11

7th **S88.112 Complete traumatic amputation at level between knee and ankle, left lower leg** CC
CC Excl: See code: S88.Ø12

7th **S88.119 Complete traumatic amputation at level between knee and ankle, unspecified lower leg** CC
CC Excl: See code: S88.Ø19

6th **S88.12 Partial traumatic amputation at level between knee and ankle**

7th **S88.121 Partial traumatic amputation at level between knee and ankle, right lower leg** CC
CC Excl: See code: S88.Ø11

7th **S88.122 Partial traumatic amputation at levelbetween knee and ankle, left lower leg** CC
CC Excl: See code: S88.Ø12

7th **S88.129 Partial traumatic amputation at level between knee and ankle, unspecified lower leg** CC
CC Excl: See code: S88.Ø19

5th **S88.9 Traumatic amputation of lower leg, level unspecified**

6th **S88.91 Complete traumatic amputation of lower leg, level unspecified**

7th **S88.911 Complete traumatic amputation of right lower leg, level unspecified** CC
CC Excl: See code: S88.Ø11

7th **S88.912 Complete traumatic amputation of left lower leg, level unspecified** CC
CC Excl: See code: S88.Ø12

7th **S88.919 Complete traumatic amputation of unspecified lower leg, level unspecified** CC
CC Excl: See code: S88.Ø19

6th **S88.92 Partial traumatic amputation of lower leg, level unspecified**

7th **S88.921 Partial traumatic amputation of right lower leg, level unspecified** CC
CC Excl: See code: S88.Ø11

7th **S88.922 Partial traumatic amputation of left lower leg, level unspecified** CC
CC Excl: See code: S88.Ø12

7th **S88.929 Partial traumatic amputation of unspecified lower leg, level unspecified** CC
CC Excl: See code: S88.Ø19

✓4th S89 Other and unspecified injuries of lower leg

NOTE A fracture not indicated as open or closed should be coded to closed.

EXCLUDES 2 *other and unspecified injuries of ankle and foot (S99.-)*

The appropriate 7th character is to be added to each code from subcategories S89.0, S89.1, S89.2, and S89.3.

- A initial encounter for closed fracture
- D subsequent encounter for fracture with routine healing
- G subsequent encounter for fracture with delayed healing
- K subsequent encounter for fracture with nonunion
- P subsequent encounter for fracture with malunion
- S sequela

✓5th S89.0 Physeal fracture of upper end of tibia

✓6th S89.00 Unspecified physeal fracture of upper end of tibia

7 ✓7th **S89.001 Unspecified physeal fracture of upper end of right tibia** CC

CC Excl: CC with 7th character A: M80.00X-M80.019 with 7th A, M80.041-M80.049 with 7th A, M80.061-M80.079 with 7th A, M80.80X-M80.819 with 7th A, M80.841-M80.849 with 7th A, M80.861-M80.879 with 7th A, M84.40X-M84.419 with 7th A, M84.441-M84.446 with 7th A, M84.454 with 7th A, M84.461-M84.519 with 7th A, M84.541-M84.550 with 7th A, M84.561-M84.576 with 7th A, M84.60X-M84.619 with 7th A, M84.641-M84.650 with 7th A, M84.661-M84.68X with 7th A, S03.8XX-S03.9XX with 7th A, S29.011-S29.019 with 7th A, S38.3XX-S39.013 with 7th A, S73.101A, S73.109-S73.111 with 7th A, S73.119-S73.121 with 7th A, S73.129-S73.191 with 7th A, S73.199A, S76.001A, S76.009-S76.011 with 7th A, S76.019A, S76.091A, S76.099-S76.101 with 7th A, S76.109-S76.111 with 7th A, S76.119A, S76.191A, S76.199-S76.201 with 7th A, S76.209-S76.211 with 7th A, S76.219A, S76.291A, S76.299-S76.301 with 7th A, S76.309-S76.311 with 7th A, S76.319A, S76.391A, S76.399-S76.801 with 7th A, S76.809-S76.811 with 7th A, S76.819A, S76.891A, S76.899-S76.901 with 7th A, S76.909-S76.911 with 7th A, S76.919A, S76.991A, S76.999A, S79.811A, S79.819-S79.821 with 7th A, S79.829-S79.911 with 7th A, S79.919-S79.921 with 7th A, S79.929A, S82.101-S82.156 with 7th [A, B, C], S82.191-S82.299 with 7th [A, B, C], S82.401-S82.499 with 7th [A, B, C], S82.831-S82.839 with 7th [A, B, C], S82.861-S82.866 with 7th [A, B, C], S82.90X-S82.92X with 7th [A, B, C], S89.001 with 7th A, S89.009-S89.011 with 7th A, S89.019-S89.021 with 7th A, S89.029-S89.031 with 7th A, S89.039-S89.041 with 7th A, S89.049-S89.091 with 7th A, S89.099A, S89.201A, S89.209-S89.211 with 7th A, S89.219-S89.221 with 7th A, S89.229-S89.291 with 7th A, S89.299A, T14.8-T14.91, T79.A9X-T79.9XX with 7th A

CC with 7th character K or P: M80.00X-M84.68X with 7th [K, P], S02.0XX-S02.92X with 7th K, S12.000-S12.691 with 7th K, S22.000-S22.9XX with 7th K, S32.000-S32.9XX with 7th K, S42.001-S42.92X with 7th [K, P], S49.001-S49.199 with 7th [K, P], S52.001-S52.92X with 7th [K, M, N, P, Q, R], S59.001-S59.299 with 7th [K, P], S62.001-S62.92X with 7th [K, P], S72.001-S72.92X with 7th [K, M, N, P, Q, R], S79.001-S79.199 with 7th [K, P], S82.001-S82.92X with 7th [K, M, N, P, Q, R], S89.001-S89.399 with 7th [K, P], S92.001-S92.919 with 7th [K, P]

7 ✓7th **S89.002 Unspecified physeal fracture of upper end of left tibia** CC

CC Excl: CC with 7th character A: M80.00X-M80.019 with 7th A, M80.041-M80.049 with 7th A, M80.061-M80.079 with 7th A, M80.80X-M80.819 with 7th A, M80.841-M80.849 with 7th A, M80.861-M80.879 with 7th A, M84.40X-M84.419 with 7th A, M84.441-M84.446 with 7th A, M84.454 with 7th A, M84.461-M84.519 with 7th A, M84.541-M84.550 with 7th A, M84.561-M84.576 with 7th A, M84.60X-M84.619 with 7th A, M84.641-M84.650 with 7th A, M84.661-M84.68X with 7th A, S03.8XX-S03.9XX with 7th A, S29.011-S29.019 with 7th A, S38.3XX-S39.013 with 7th A, S73.102-S73.109 with 7th A, S73.112-S73.119 with 7th A, S73.122-S73.129 with 7th A, S73.192-S73.199 with 7th A, S76.002-S76.009 with 7th A, S76.012-S76.019 with 7th A, S76.092-S76.099 with 7th A, S76.102-S76.109 with 7th A, S76.112-S76.119 with 7th A, S76.192-S76.199 with 7th A, S76.202-S76.209 with 7th A, S76.212-S76.219 with 7th A, S76.292-S76.299 with 7th A, S76.302-S76.309 with 7th A, S76.312-S76.319 with 7th A, S76.392-S76.399 with 7th A, S76.802-S76.809 with 7th A, S76.812-S76.819 with 7th A, S76.892-S76.899 with 7th A, S76.902-S76.909 with 7th A, S76.912-S76.919 with 7th A, S76.992-S76.999 with 7th A, S79.812-S79.819 with 7th A, S79.822-S79.829 with 7th A, S79.912-S79.919 with 7th A, S79.922-S79.929 with 7th A, S82.101-S82.156 with 7th [B, C], S82.191-S82.299 with 7th [B, C], S82.401-S82.499 with 7th [B, C], S82.831-S82.839 with 7th [B, C], S82.861-S82.866 with 7th [B, C], S82.90X-S82.92X with 7th [A, B, C], S89.002-S89.009 with 7th A, S89.012-S89.019 with 7th A, S89.022-S89.029 with 7th A, S89.032-S89.039 with 7th A, S89.042-S89.049 with 7th A, S89.092-S89.099 with 7th A, S89.202-S89.209 with 7th A, S89.212-S89.219 with 7th A, S89.222-S89.229 with 7th A, S89.292-S89.299 with 7th A, T14.8-T14.91, T79.A9X-T79.9XX with 7th A

CC with 7th character K or P: M80.00X-M84.68X with 7th [K, P], S02.0XX-S02.92X with 7th K, S12.000-S12.691 with 7th K, S22.000-S22.9XX with 7th K, S32.000-S32.9XX with 7th K, S42.001-S42.92X with 7th [K, P], S49.001-S49.199 with 7th [K, P], S52.001-S52.92X with 7th [K, M, N, P, Q, R], S59.001-S59.299 with 7th [K, P], S62.001-S62.92X with 7th [K, P], S72.001-S72.92X with 7th [K, M, N, P, Q, R], S79.001-S79.199 with 7th [K, P], S82.001-S82.92X with 7th [K, M, N, P, Q, R], S89.001-S89.399 with 7th [K, P], S92.001-S92.919 with 7th [K, P]

7 HAC = Initial encounter only (7th character A, B or C) and not POA.

7 7th **S89.009 Unspecified physeal fracture of upper end of unspecified tibia** CC
CC Excl: CC with 7th character A: M80.00X-M80.019 with 7th A, M80.041-M80.049 with 7th A, M80.061-M80.079 with 7th A, M80.80X-M80.819 with 7th A, M80.841-M80.849 with 7th A, M80.861-M80.879 with 7th A, M84.40X-M84.419 with 7th A, M84.441-M84.446 with 7th A, M84.454 with 7th A, M84.461-M84.519 with 7th A, M84.541-M84.550 with 7th A, M84.561-M84.576 with 7th A, M84.60X-M84.619 with 7th A, M84.641-M84.650 with 7th A, M84.661-M84.68X with 7th A, S03.8XX-S03.9XX with 7th A, S29.011-S29.019 with 7th A, S38.3XX-S39.013 with 7th A, S73.101-S73.199 with 7th A, S76.001-S76.019 with 7th A, S76.091-S76.119 with 7th A, S76.191-S76.219 with 7th A, S76.291-S76.319 with 7th A, S76.391-S76.819 with 7th A, S76.891-S76.919 with 7th A, S76.991-S76.999 with 7th A, S79.811-S79.929 with 7th A, S82.101-S82.156 with 7th [A, B, C], S82.191-S82.299 with 7th [A, B, C], S82.401-S82.499 with 7th [A, B, C], S82.831-S82.839 with 7th [A, B, C], S82.861-S82.866 with 7th [A, B, C], S82.90X-S82.92X with 7th [A, B, C], S89.001-S89.099 with 7th A, S89.201-S89.299 with 7th A, T14.8-T14.91, T79.A9X-T79.9XX with 7th A
CC with 7th character K or P: M80.00X-M84.68X with 7th [K, P], S02.0XX-S02.92X with 7th K, S12.000-S12.691 with 7th K, S22.000-S22.9XX with 7th K, S32.000-S32.9XX with 7th K, S42.001-S42.92X with 7th [K, P], S49.001-S49.199 with 7th [K, P], S52.001-S52.92X with 7th [K, M, N, P, Q, R], S59.001-S59.299 with 7th [K, P], S62.001-S62.92X with 7th [K, P], S72.001-S72.92X with 7th [K, M, N, P, Q, R], S79.001-S79.199 with 7th [K, P], S82.001-S82.92X with 7th [K, M, N, P, Q, R], S89.001-S89.399 with 7th [K, P], S92.001-S92.919 with 7th [K, P]

6th **S89.01 Salter-Harris Type I physeal fracture of upper end of tibia**

7 7th **S89.011 Salter-Harris Type I physeal fracture of upper end of right tibia** CC
CC Excl: See code: S89.001

7 7th **S89.012 Salter-Harris Type I physeal fracture of upper end of left tibia** CC
CC Excl: See code: S89.002

7 7th **S89.019 Salter-Harris Type I physeal fracture of upper end of unspecified tibia** CC
CC Excl: See code: S89.009

6th **S89.02 Salter-Harris Type II physeal fracture of upper end of tibia**

7 7th **S89.021 Salter-Harris Type II physeal fracture of upper end of right tibia** CC
CC Excl: See code: S89.001

7 7th **S89.022 Salter-Harris Type II physeal fracture of upper end of left tibia** CC
CC Excl: See code: S89.002

7 7th **S89.029 Salter-Harris Type II physeal fracture of upper end of unspecified tibia** CC
CC Excl: See code: S89.009

6th **S89.03 Salter-Harris Type III physeal fracture of upper end of tibia**

7 7th **S89.031 Salter-Harris Type III physeal fracture of upper end of right tibia** CC
CC Excl: See code: S89.001

7 7th **S89.032 Salter-Harris Type III physeal fracture of upper end of left tibia** CC
CC Excl: See code: S89.002

7 7th **S89.039 Salter-Harris Type III physeal fracture of upper end of unspecified tibia** CC
CC Excl: See code: S89.009

6th **S89.04 Salter-Harris Type IV physeal fracture of upper end of tibia**

7 7th **S89.041 Salter-Harris Type IV physeal fracture of upper end of right tibia** CC
CC Excl: See code: S89.001

7 7th **S89.042 Salter-Harris Type IV physeal fracture of upper end of left tibia** CC
CC Excl: See code: S89.002

7 7th **S89.049 Salter-Harris Type IV physeal fracture of upper end of unspecified tibia** CC
CC Excl: See code: S89.009

6th **S89.09 Other physeal fracture of upper end of tibia**

7 7th **S89.091 Other physeal fracture of upper end of right tibia** CC
CC Excl: See code: S89.001

7 7th **S89.092 Other physeal fracture of upper end of left tibia** CC
CC Excl: See code: S89.002

7 7th **S89.099 Other physeal fracture of upper end of unspecified tibia** CC
CC Excl: See code: S89.009

5th **S89.1 Physeal fracture of lower end of tibia**

CC Excl: For CC codes in subcategory S89.1, unless otherwise noted: CC with 7th character K or P: M80.00X-M80.019 with 7th A, M80.041-M80.049 with 7th A, M80.061-M80.079 with 7th A, M80.80X-M80.819 with 7th A, M80.841-M80.849 with 7th A, M80.861-M80.879 with 7th A, M84.40X-M84.419 with 7th A, M84.441-M84.446 with 7th A, M84.454 with 7th A, M84.461-M84.519 with 7th A, M84.541-M84.550 with 7th A, M84.561-M84.576 with 7th A, M84.60X-M84.619 with 7th A, M84.641-M84.650 with 7th A, M84.661-M84.68X with 7th A, S03.8XX-S03.9XX with 7th A, S29.011-S29.019 with 7th A, S38.3XX-S39.013 with 7th A, S73.101-S73.199 with 7th A, S76.001-S76.019 with 7th A, S76.091-S76.119 with 7th A, S76.191-S76.219 with 7th A, S76.291-S76.319 with 7th A, S76.391-S76.819 with 7th A, S76.891-S76.919 with 7th A, S76.991-S76.999 with 7th A, S79.811-S79.929 with 7th A, S82.101-S82.156 with 7th [A, B, C], S82.191-S82.299 with 7th [A, B, C], S82.401-S82.499 with 7th [A, B, C], S82.831-S82.839 with 7th [A, B, C], S82.861-S82.866 with 7th [A, B, C], S82.90X-S82.92X with 7th [A, B, C], S89.001-S89.099 with 7th A, S89.201-S89.299 with 7th A, T14.8-T14.91, T79.A9X-T79.9XX with 7th A

6th **S89.10 Unspecified physeal fracture of lower end of tibia**

7th **S89.101 Unspecified physeal fracture of lower end of right tibia** CC

7th **S89.102 Unspecified physeal fracture of lower end of left tibia** CC

7th **S89.109 Unspecified physeal fracture of lower end of unspecified tibia** CC

6th **S89.11 Salter-Harris Type I physeal fracture of ower end of tibia**

7th **S89.111 Salter-Harris Type I physeal fracture of lower end of right tibia** CC

7th **S89.112 Salter-Harris Type I physeal fracture oflower end of left tibia** CC

7th **S89.119 Salter-Harris Type I physeal fracture of lower end of unspecified tibia** CC

6th **S89.12 Salter-Harris Type II physeal fracture of lower end of tibia**

7th **S89.121 Salter-Harris Type II physeal fracture of lower end of right tibia** CC

7th **S89.122 Salter-Harris Type II physeal fracture of lower end of left tibia** CC

7th **S89.129 Salter-Harris Type II physeal fracture of lower end of unspecified tibia** CC

6th **S89.13 Salter-Harris Type III physeal fracture of lower end of tibia**
EXCLUDES1 *fracture of medial malleolus (adult) (S82.5-)*

7th **S89.131 Salter-Harris Type III physeal fracture of lower end of right tibia** CC

7th **S89.132 Salter-Harris Type III physeal fracture of lower end of left tibia** CC

7th **S89.139 Salter-Harris Type III physeal fracture of lower end of unspecified tibia** CC

6th **S89.14 Salter-Harris Type IV physeal fracture of lower end of tibia**
EXCLUDES1 *fracture of medial malleolus (adult) (S82.5-)*

7th **S89.141 Salter-Harris Type IV physeal fracture oflower end of right tibia** CC

7th **S89.142 Salter-Harris Type IV physeal fracture of lower end of left tibia** CC

7th **S89.149 Salter-Harris Type IV physeal fracture of lower end of unspecified tibia** CC

7 HAC = Initial encounter only (7th character A, B or C) and not POA.

✓6th **S89.19 Other physeal fracture of lower end of tibia**
✓7th **S89.191 Other physeal fracture of lower end of right tibia** CC
✓7th **S89.192 Other physeal fracture of lower end of left tibia** CC
✓7th **S89.199 Other physeal fracture of lower end of unspecified tibia** CC

✓5th **S89.2 Physeal fracture of upper end of fibula**

CC Excl: For CC codes in subcategory S89.2, unless otherwise noted: See code: S89.1

✓6th **S89.20 Unspecified physeal fracture of upper end of fibula**
✓7th **S89.201 Unspecified physeal fracture of upper end of right fibula** CC
✓7th **S89.202 Unspecified physeal fracture of upper end of left fibula** CC
✓7th **S89.209 Unspecified physeal fracture of upper end of unspecified fibula** CC

✓6th **S89.21 Salter-Harris Type I physeal fracture of upper end of fibula**
✓7th **S89.211 Salter-Harris Type I physeal fracture of upper end of right fibula** CC
✓7th **S89.212 Salter-Harris Type I physeal fracture of upper end of left fibula** CC
✓7th **S89.219 Salter-Harris Type I physeal fracture of upper end of unspecified fibula** CC

✓6th **S89.22 Salter-Harris Type II physeal fracture of upper end of fibula**
✓7th **S89.221 Salter-Harris Type II physeal fracture of upper end of right fibula** CC
✓7th **S89.222 Salter-Harris Type II physeal fracture of upper end of left fibula** CC
✓7th **S89.229 Salter-Harris Type II physeal fracture of upper end of unspecified fibula** CC

✓6th **S89.29 Other physeal fracture of upper end of fibula**
✓7th **S89.291 Other physeal fracture of upper end of right fibula** CC
✓7th **S89.292 Other physeal fracture of upper end of left fibula** CC
✓7th **S89.299 Other physeal fracture of upper end of unspecified fibula** CC

✓5th **S89.3 Physeal fracture of lower end of fibula**

CC Excl: For CC codes in subcategory S89.3, unless otherwise noted: See code: S89.1

✓6th **S89.30 Unspecified physeal fracture of lower end of fibula**
✓7th **S89.301 Unspecified physeal fracture of lower end of right fibula** CC
✓7th **S89.302 Unspecified physeal fracture of lower end of left fibula** CC
✓7th **S89.309 Unspecified physeal fracture of lower end of unspecified fibula** CC

✓6th **S89.31 Salter-Harris Type I physeal fracture of lower end of fibula**
✓7th **S89.311 Salter-Harris Type I physeal fracture of lower end of right fibula** CC
✓7th **S89.312 Salter-Harris Type I physeal fracture of lower end of left fibula** CC
✓7th **S89.319 Salter-Harris Type I physeal fracture of lower end of unspecified fibula** CC

✓6th **S89.32 Salter-Harris Type II physeal fracture of lower end of fibula**
✓7th **S89.321 Salter-Harris Type II physeal fracture of lower end of right fibula** CC
✓7th **S89.322 Salter-Harris Type II physeal fracture of lower end of left fibula** CC
✓7th **S89.329 Salter-Harris Type II physeal fracture of lower end of unspecified fibula** CC

✓6th **S89.39 Other physeal fracture of lower end of fibula**
✓7th **S89.391 Other physeal fracture of lower end of right fibula** CC
✓7th **S89.392 Other physeal fracture of lower end of left fibula** CC
✓7th **S89.399 Other physeal fracture of lower end of unspecified fibula** CC

✓5th **S89.8 Other specified injuries of lower leg**

The appropriate 7th character is to be added to each code in subcategory S89.8.
A initial encounter
D subsequent encounter
S sequela

✓x7th **S89.80 Other specified injuries of unspecified lower leg**
✓x7th **S89.81 Other specified injuries of right lower leg**
✓x7th **S89.82 Other specified injuries of left lower leg**

✓5th **S89.9 Unspecified injury of lower leg**

The appropriate 7th character is to be added to each code in subcategory S89.9.
A initial encounter
D subsequent encounter
S sequela

✓x7th **S89.90 Unspecified injury of unspecified lower leg**
✓x7th **S89.91 Unspecified injury of right lower leg**
✓x7th **S89.92 Unspecified injury of left lower leg**

Injuries to the ankle and foot (S90-S99)

EXCLUDES 2 *burns and corrosions (T20-T32)*
fracture of ankle and malleolus (S82.-)
frostbite (T33-T34)
insect bite or sting, venomous (T63.4)

✓4th **S90 Superficial injury of ankle, foot and toes**

The appropriate 7th character is to be added to each code from category S90.
A initial encounter
D subsequent encounter
S sequela

✓5th **S90.0 Contusion of ankle**
✓x7th **S90.00 Contusion of unspecified ankle**
✓x7th **S90.01 Contusion of right ankle**
✓x7th **S90.02 Contusion of left ankle**

✓5th **S90.1 Contusion of toe without damage to nail**
✓6th **S90.11 Contusion of great toe without damage to nail**
✓7th **S90.111 Contusion of right great toe without damage to nail**
✓7th **S90.112 Contusion of left great toe without damage to nail**
✓7th **S90.119 Contusion of unspecified great toe without damage to nail**
✓6th **S90.12 Contusion of lesser toe without damage to nail**
✓7th **S90.121 Contusion of right lesser toe(s) without damage to nail**
✓7th **S90.122 Contusion of left lesser toe(s) without damage to nail**
✓7th **S90.129 Contusion of unspecified lesser toe(s) without damage to nail**
Contusion of toe NOS

✓5th **S90.2 Contusion of toe with damage to nail**
✓6th **S90.21 Contusion of great toe with damage to nail**
✓7th **S90.211 Contusion of right great toe with damage to nail**
✓7th **S90.212 Contusion of left great toe with damage to nail**
✓7th **S90.219 Contusion of unspecified great toe with damage to nail**
✓6th **S90.22 Contusion of lesser toe with damage to nail**
✓7th **S90.221 Contusion of right lesser toe(s) with damage to nail**
✓7th **S90.222 Contusion of left lesser toe(s) with damage to nail**
✓7th **S90.229 Contusion of unspecified lesser toe(s) with damage to nail**

✓5th **S90.3 Contusion of foot**
EXCLUDES 2 *contusion of toes (S90.1-, S90.2-)*
✓x7th **S90.30 Contusion of unspecified foot**
Contusion of foot NOS
✓x7th **S90.31 Contusion of right foot**
✓x7th **S90.32 Contusion of left foot**

5th S90.4 Other superficial injuries of toe
- 6th S90.41 Abrasion of toe
  - 7th S90.411 Abrasion, right great toe
  - 7th S90.412 Abrasion, left great toe
  - 7th S90.413 Abrasion, unspecified great toe
  - 7th S90.414 Abrasion, right lesser toe(s)
  - 7th S90.415 Abrasion, left lesser toe(s)
  - 7th S90.416 Abrasion, unspecified lesser toe(s)
- 6th S90.42 Blister (nonthermal) of toe
  - 7th S90.421 Blister (nonthermal), right great toe
  - 7th S90.422 Blister (nonthermal), left great toe
  - 7th S90.423 Blister (nonthermal), unspecified great toe
  - 7th S90.424 Blister (nonthermal), right lesser toe(s)
  - 7th S90.425 Blister (nonthermal), left lesser toe(s)
  - 7th S90.426 Blister (nonthermal), unspecified lesser toe(s)
- 6th S90.44 External constriction of toe
  Hair tourniquet syndrome of toe
  - 7th S90.441 External constriction, right great toe
  - 7th S90.442 External constriction, left great toe
  - 7th S90.443 External constriction, unspecified great toe
  - 7th S90.444 External constriction, right lesser toe(s)
  - 7th S90.445 External constriction, left lesser toe(s)
  - 7th S90.446 External constriction, unspecified lesser toe(s)
- 6th S90.45 Superficial foreign body of toe
  Splinter in the toe
  - 7th S90.451 Superficial foreign body, right great toe
  - 7th S90.452 Superficial foreign body, left great toe
  - 7th S90.453 Superficial foreign body, unspecified great toe
  - 7th S90.454 Superficial foreign body, right lesser toe(s)
  - 7th S90.455 Superficial foreign body, left lesser toe(s)
  - 7th S90.456 Superficial foreign body, unspecified lesser toe(s)
- 6th S90.46 Insect bite (nonvenomous) of toe
  - 7th S90.461 Insect bite (nonvenomous), right great toe
  - 7th S90.462 Insect bite (nonvenomous), left great toe
  - 7th S90.463 Insect bite (nonvenomous), unspecified great toe
  - 7th S90.464 Insect bite (nonvenomous), right lesser toe(s)
  - 7th S90.465 Insect bite (nonvenomous), left lesser toe(s)
  - 7th S90.466 Insect bite (nonvenomous), unspecified lesser toe(s)
- 6th S90.47 Other superficial bite of toe
  EXCLUDES 1 *open bite of toe (S91.15-, S91.25-)*
  - 7th S90.471 Other superficial bite of right great toe
  - 7th S90.472 Other superficial bite of left great toe
  - 7th S90.473 Other superficial bite of unspecified great toe
  - 7th S90.474 Other superficial bite of right lesser toe(s)
  - 7th S90.475 Other superficial bite of left lesser toe(s)
  - 7th S90.476 Other superficial bite of unspecified lesser toe(s)

5th S90.5 Other superficial injuries of ankle
- 6th S90.51 Abrasion of ankle
  - 7th S90.511 Abrasion, right ankle
  - 7th S90.512 Abrasion, left ankle
  - 7th S90.519 Abrasion, unspecified ankle
- 6th S90.52 Blister (nonthermal) of ankle
  - 7th S90.521 Blister (nonthermal), right ankle
  - 7th S90.522 Blister (nonthermal), left ankle
  - 7th S90.529 Blister (nonthermal), unspecified ankle
- 6th S90.54 External constriction of ankle
  - 7th S90.541 External constriction, right ankle
  - 7th S90.542 External constriction, left ankle
  - 7th S90.549 External constriction, unspecified ankle
- 6th S90.55 Superficial foreign body of ankle
  Splinter in the ankle
  - 7th S90.551 Superficial foreign body, right ankle
  - 7th S90.552 Superficial foreign body, left ankle
  - 7th S90.559 Superficial foreign body, unspecified ankle
- 6th S90.56 Insect bite (nonvenomous) of ankle
  - 7th S90.561 Insect bite (nonvenomous), right ankle
  - 7th S90.562 Insect bite (nonvenomous), left ankle
  - 7th S90.569 Insect bite (nonvenomous), unspecified ankle
- 6th S90.57 Other superficial bite of ankle
  EXCLUDES 1 *open bite of ankle (S91.05-)*
  - 7th S90.571 Other superficial bite of ankle, right ankle
  - 7th S90.572 Other superficial bite of ankle, left ankle
  - 7th S90.579 Other superficial bite of ankle, unspecified ankle

5th S90.8 Other superficial injuries of foot
- 6th S90.81 Abrasion of foot
  - 7th S90.811 Abrasion, right foot
  - 7th S90.812 Abrasion, left foot
  - 7th S90.819 Abrasion, unspecified foot
- 6th S90.82 Blister (nonthermal) of foot
  - 7th S90.821 Blister (nonthermal), right foot
  - 7th S90.822 Blister (nonthermal), left foot
  - 7th S90.829 Blister (nonthermal), unspecified foot
- 6th S90.84 External constriction of foot
  - 7th S90.841 External constriction, right foot
  - 7th S90.842 External constriction, left foot
  - 7th S90.849 External constriction, unspecified foot
- 6th S90.85 Superficial foreign body of foot
  Splinter in the foot
  - 7th S90.851 Superficial foreign body, right foot
  - 7th S90.852 Superficial foreign body, left foot
  - 7th S90.859 Superficial foreign body, unspecified foot
- 6th S90.86 Insect bite (nonvenomous) of foot
  - 7th S90.861 Insect bite (nonvenomous), right foot
  - 7th S90.862 Insect bite (nonvenomous), left foot
  - 7th S90.869 Insect bite (nonvenomous), unspecified foot
- 6th S90.87 Other superficial bite of foot
  EXCLUDES 1 *open bite of foot (S91.35-)*
  - 7th S90.871 Other superficial bite of right foot
  - 7th S90.872 Other superficial bite of left foot
  - 7th S90.879 Other superficial bite of unspecified foot

5th S90.9 Unspecified superficial injury of ankle, foot and toe
- 6th S90.91 Unspecified superficial injury of ankle
  - 7th S90.911 Unspecified superficial injury of right ankle
  - 7th S90.912 Unspecified superficial injury of left ankle
  - 7th S90.919 Unspecified superficial injury of unspecified ankle
- 6th S90.92 Unspecified superficial injury of foot
  - 7th S90.921 Unspecified superficial injury of right foot
  - 7th S90.922 Unspecified superficial injury of left foot
  - 7th S90.929 Unspecified superficial injury of unspecified foot
- 6th S90.93 Unspecified superficial injury of toes
  - 7th S90.931 Unspecified superficial injury of right great toe
  - 7th S90.932 Unspecified superficial injury of left great toe
  - 7th S90.933 Unspecified superficial injury of unspecified great toe
  - 7th S90.934 Unspecified superficial injury of right lesser toe(s)
  - 7th S90.935 Unspecified superficial injury of left lesser toe(s)

S90.936 Unspecified superficial injury of unspecified lesser toe(s)

S91 Open wound of ankle, foot and toes

Code also any associated wound infection

EXCLUDES 1 *open fracture of ankle, foot and toes (S92-with 7th B)*
traumatic amputation of ankle and foot (S98.-)

The appropriate 7th character is to be added to each code from category S91.
- A initial encounter
- D subsequent encounter
- S sequela

S91.0 Open wound of ankle
- **S91.00 Unspecified open wound of ankle**
  - S91.001 Unspecified open wound, right ankle
  - S91.002 Unspecified open wound, left ankle
  - S91.009 Unspecified open wound, unspecified ankle
- **S91.01 Laceration without foreign body of ankle**
  - S91.011 Laceration without foreign body, right ankle
  - S91.012 Laceration without foreign body, left ankle
  - S91.019 Laceration without foreign body, unspecified ankle
- **S91.02 Laceration with foreign body of ankle**
  - S91.021 Laceration with foreign body, right ankle
  - S91.022 Laceration with foreign body, left ankle
  - S91.029 Laceration with foreign body, unspecified ankle
- **S91.03 Puncture wound without foreign body of ankle**
  - S91.031 Puncture wound without foreign body, right ankle
  - S91.032 Puncture wound without foreign body, left ankle
  - S91.039 Puncture wound without foreign body, unspecified ankle
- **S91.04 Puncture wound with foreign body of ankle**
  - S91.041 Puncture wound with foreign body, right ankle
  - S91.042 Puncture wound with foreign body, left ankle
  - S91.049 Puncture wound with foreign body, unspecified ankle
- **S91.05 Open bite of ankle**

  EXCLUDES 1 *superficial bite of ankle (S90.56-, S90.57-)*
  - S91.051 Open bite, right ankle
  - S91.052 Open bite, left ankle
  - S91.059 Open bite, unspecified ankle

S91.1 Open wound of toe without damage to nail
- **S91.10 Unspecified open wound of toe without damage to nail**
  - S91.101 Unspecified open wound of right great toe without damage to nail
  - S91.102 Unspecified open wound of left great toe without damage to nail
  - S91.103 Unspecified open wound of unspecified great toe without damage to nail
  - S91.104 Unspecified open wound of right lesser toe(s) without damage to nail
  - S91.105 Unspecified open wound of left lesser toe(s) without damage to nail
  - S91.106 Unspecified open wound of unspecified lesser toe(s) without damage to nail
  - S91.109 Unspecified open wound of unspecified toe(s) without damage to nail
- **S91.11 Laceration without foreign body of toe without damage to nail**
  - S91.111 Laceration without foreign body of right great toe without damage to nail
  - S91.112 Laceration without foreign body of left great toe without damage to nail
  - S91.113 Laceration without foreign body of unspecified great toe without damage to nail
  - S91.114 Laceration without foreign body of right lesser toe(s) without damage to nail
  - S91.115 Laceration without foreign body of left lesser toe(s) without damage to nail
  - S91.116 Laceration without foreign body of unspecified lesser toe(s) without damage to nail
  - S91.119 Laceration without foreign body of unspecified toe without damage to nail
- **S91.12 Laceration with foreign body of toe without damage to nail**
  - S91.121 Laceration with foreign body of right great toe without damage to nail
  - S91.122 Laceration with foreign body of left great toe without damage to nail
  - S91.123 Laceration with foreign body of unspecified great toe without damage to nail
  - S91.124 Laceration with foreign body of right lesser toe(s) without damage to nail
  - S91.125 Laceration with foreign body of left lesser toe(s) without damage to nail
  - S91.126 Laceration with foreign body of unspecified lesser toe(s) without damage to nail
  - S91.129 Laceration with foreign body of unspecified toe(s) without damage to nail
- **S91.13 Puncture wound without foreign body of toe without damage to nail**
  - S91.131 Puncture wound without foreign body of right great toe without damage to nail
  - S91.132 Puncture wound without foreign body of left great toe without damage to nail
  - S91.133 Puncture wound without foreign body of unspecified great toe without damage to nail
  - S91.134 Puncture wound without foreign body of right lesser toe(s) without damage to nail
  - S91.135 Puncture wound without foreign body of left lesser toe(s) without damage to nail
  - S91.136 Puncture wound without foreign body of unspecified lesser toe(s) without damage to nail
  - S91.139 Puncture wound without foreign body of unspecified toe(s) without damage to nail
- **S91.14 Puncture wound with foreign body of toe without damage to nail**
  - S91.141 Puncture wound with foreign body of right great toe without damage to nail
  - S91.142 Puncture wound with foreign body of left great toe without damage to nail
  - S91.143 Puncture wound with foreign body of unspecified great toe without damage to nail
  - S91.144 Puncture wound with foreign body of right lesser toe(s) without damage to nail
  - S91.145 Puncture wound with foreign body of left lesser toe(s) without damage to nail
  - S91.146 Puncture wound with foreign body of unspecified lesser toe(s) without damage to nail
  - S91.149 Puncture wound with foreign body of unspecified toe(s) without damage to nail
- **S91.15 Open bite of toe without damage to nail**

  Bite of toe NOS

  EXCLUDES 1 *superficial bite of toe (S90.46-, S90.47-)*
  - S91.151 Open bite of right great toe without damage to nail
  - S91.152 Open bite of left great toe without damage to nail
  - S91.153 Open bite of unspecified great toe without damage to nail
  - S91.154 Open bite of right lesser toe(s) without damage to nail

7th S91.155 Open bite of left lesser toe(s) without damage to nail
7th S91.156 Open bite of unspecified lesser toe(s) without damage to nail
7th S91.159 Open bite of unspecified toe(s) without damage to nail

5th S91.2 Open wound of toe with damage to nail
6th S91.20 Unspecified open wound of toe with damage to nail
7th S91.201 Unspecified open wound of right great toe with damage to nail
7th S91.202 Unspecified open wound of left great toe with damage to nail
7th S91.203 Unspecified open wound of unspecified great toe with damage to nail
7th S91.204 Unspecified open wound of right lesser toe(s) with damage to nail
7th S91.205 Unspecified open wound of left lesser toe(s) with damage to nail
7th S91.206 Unspecified open wound of unspecified lesser toe(s) with damage to nail
7th S91.209 Unspecified open wound of unspecified toe(s) with damage to nail

6th S91.21 Laceration without foreign body of toe with damage to nail
7th S91.211 Laceration without foreign body of right great toe with damage to nail
7th S91.212 Laceration without foreign body of left great toe with damage to nail
7th S91.213 Laceration without foreign body of unspecified great toe with damage to nail
7th S91.214 Laceration without foreign body of right lesser toe(s) with damage to nail
7th S91.215 Laceration without foreign body of left lesser toe(s) with damage to nail
7th S91.216 Laceration without foreign body of unspecified lesser toe(s) with damage to nail
7th S91.219 Laceration without foreign body of unspecified toe(s) with damage to nail

6th S91.22 Laceration with foreign body of toe with damage to nail
7th S91.221 Laceration with foreign body of right great toe with damage to nail
7th S91.222 Laceration with foreign body of left great toe with damage to nail
7th S91.223 Laceration with foreign body of unspecified great toe with damage to nail
7th S91.224 Laceration with foreign body of right lesser toe(s) with damage to nail
7th S91.225 Laceration with foreign body of left lesser toe(s) with damage to nail
7th S91.226 Laceration with foreign body of unspecified lesser toe(s) with damage to nail
7th S91.229 Laceration with foreign body of unspecified toe(s) with damage to nail

6th S91.23 Puncture wound without foreign body of toe with damage to nail
7th S91.231 Puncture wound without foreign body of right great toe with damage to nail
7th S91.232 Puncture wound without foreign body of left great toe with damage to nail
7th S91.233 Puncture wound without foreign body of unspecified great toe with damage to nail
7th S91.234 Puncture wound without foreign body of right lesser toe(s) with damage to nail
7th S91.235 Puncture wound without foreign body of left lesser toe(s) with damage to nail
7th S91.236 Puncture wound without foreign body of unspecified lesser toe(s) with damage to nail
7th S91.239 Puncture wound without foreign body of unspecified toe(s) with damage to nail

6th S91.24 Puncture wound with foreign body of toe with damage to nail
7th S91.241 Puncture wound with foreign body of right great toe with damage to nail
7th S91.242 Puncture wound with foreign body of left great toe with damage to nail
7th S91.243 Puncture wound with foreign body of unspecified great toe with damage to nail
7th S91.244 Puncture wound with foreign body of right lesser toe(s) with damage to nail
7th S91.245 Puncture wound with foreign body of left lesser toe(s) with damage to nail
7th S91.246 Puncture wound with foreign body of unspecified lesser toe(s) with damage to nail
7th S91.249 Puncture wound with foreign body of unspecified toe(s) with damage to nail

6th S91.25 Open bite of toe with damage to nail
Bite of toe with damage to nail NOS
EXCLUDES1 *superficial bite of toe (S90.46-, S90.47-)*
7th S91.251 Open bite of right great toe with damage to nail
7th S91.252 Open bite of left great toe with damage to nail
7th S91.253 Open bite of unspecified great toe with damage to nail
7th S91.254 Open bite of right lesser toe(s) with damage to nail
7th S91.255 Open bite of left lesser toe(s) with damage to nail
7th S91.256 Open bite of unspecified lesser toe(s) with damage to nail
7th S91.259 Open bite of unspecified toe(s) with damage to nail

5th S91.3 Open wound of foot
6th S91.30 Unspecified open wound of foot
7th S91.301 Unspecified open wound, right foot
7th S91.302 Unspecified open wound, left foot
7th S91.309 Unspecified open wound, unspecified foot

6th S91.31 Laceration without foreign body of foot
7th S91.311 Laceration without foreign body, right foot
7th S91.312 Laceration without foreign body, left foot
7th S91.319 Laceration without foreign body, unspecified foot

6th S91.32 Laceration with foreign body of foot
7th S91.321 Laceration with foreign body, right foot
7th S91.322 Laceration with foreign body, left foot
7th S91.329 Laceration with foreign body, unspecified foot

6th S91.33 Puncture wound without foreign body of foot
7th S91.331 Puncture wound without foreign body, right foot
7th S91.332 Puncture wound without foreign body, left foot
7th S91.339 Puncture wound without foreign body, unspecified foot

6th S91.34 Puncture wound with foreign body of foot
7th S91.341 Puncture wound with foreign body, right foot
7th S91.342 Puncture wound with foreign body, left foot
7th S91.349 Puncture wound with foreign body, unspecified foot

6th S91.35 Open bite of foot
EXCLUDES1 *superficial bite of foot (S90.86-, S90.87-)*
7th S91.351 Open bite, right foot
7th S91.352 Open bite, left foot
7th S91.359 Open bite, unspecified foot

√4th S92 Fracture of foot and toe, except ankle

NOTE A fracture not indicated as displaced or nondisplaced should be coded to displaced.
A fracture not indicated as open or closed should be coded to closed.

EXCLUDES 1 *traumatic amputation of ankle and foot (S98.-)*

EXCLUDES 2 *fracture of ankle (S82.-)*
fracture of malleolus (S82.-)

The appropriate 7th character is to be added to each code from category S92.
- A initial encounter for closed fracture
- B initial encounter for open fracture
- D subsequent encounter for fracture with routine healing
- G subsequent encounter for fracture with delayed healing
- K subsequent encounter for fracture with nonunion
- P subsequent encounter for fracture with malunion
- S sequela

√5th S92.0 Fracture of calcaneus
Heel bone
Os calcis

CC Excl: For CC codes in subcategory S92.0, unless otherwise noted: CC with 7th character B: M80.00X-M80.019 with 7th A, M80.041-M80.049 with 7th A, M80.061-M80.079 with 7th A, M80.80X-M80.819 with 7th A, M80.841-M80.849 with 7th A, M80.861-M80.879 with 7th A, M84.40X-M84.419 with 7th A, M84.441-M84.446 with 7th A, M84.454 with 7th A, M84.461-M84.519 with 7th A, M84.541-M84.550 with 7th A, M84.561-M84.576 with 7th A, M84.60X-M84.619 with 7th A, M84.641-M84.650 with 7th A, M84.661-M84.68X with 7th A, S03.8XX-S03.9XX with 7th A, S29.011-S29.019 with 7th A, S38.3XX-S39.013 with 7th A, S73.101-S73.199 with 7th A, S76.001-S76.019 with 7th A, S76.091-S76.119 with 7th A, S76.191-S76.219 with 7th A, S76.291-S76.319 with 7th A, S76.391-S76.819 with 7th A, S76.891-S76.919 with 7th A, S76.991-S76.999 with 7th A, S79.811-S79.929 with 7th A, S82.90X-S82.92X with 7th [A, B, C], S92.001-S92.356 with 7th B, S92.901-S92.909 with 7th [A, B], T14.8-T14.91, T79.A9X-T79.9XX with 7th A

CC with 7th character K or P: M80.00X-M84.68X with 7th [K, P], S02.0XX-S02.92X with 7th K, S12.000-S12.691 with 7th K, S22.000-S22.9XX with 7th K, S32.000-S32.9XX with 7th K, S42.001-S42.92X with 7th [K, P], S49.001-S49.199 with 7th [K, P], S52.001-S52.92X with 7th [K, M, N, P, Q, R], S59.001-S59.299 with 7th [K, P], S62.001-S62.92X with 7th [K, P], S72.001-S72.92X with 7th [K, M, N, P, Q, R], S79.001-S79.199 with 7th [K, P], S82.001-S82.92X with 7th [K, M, N, P, Q, R], S89.001-S89.399 with 7th [K, P], S92.001-S92.919 with 7th [K, P]

√6th S92.00 Unspecified fracture of calcaneus
- 7 √7th **S92.001 Unspecified fracture of right calcaneus** CC
- 7 √7th **S92.002 Unspecified fracture of left calcaneus** CC
- 7 √7th **S92.009 Unspecified fracture of unspecified calcaneus** CC

√6th S92.01 Fracture of body of calcaneus
- 7 √7th **S92.011 Displaced fracture of body of right calcaneus** CC
- 7 √7th **S92.012 Displaced fracture of body of left calcaneus** CC
- 7 √7th **S92.013 Displaced fracture of body of unspecified calcaneus** CC
- 7 √7th **S92.014 Nondisplaced fracture of body of right calcaneus** CC
- 7 √7th **S92.015 Nondisplaced fracture of body of left calcaneus** CC
- 7 √7th **S92.016 Nondisplaced fracture of body of unspecified calcaneus** CC

√6th S92.02 Fracture of anterior process of calcaneus
- 7 √7th **S92.021 Displaced fracture of anterior process of right calcaneus** CC
- 7 √7th **S92.022 Displaced fracture of anterior process of left calcaneus** CC
- 7 √7th **S92.023 Displaced fracture of anterior process of unspecified calcaneus** CC
- 7 √7th **S92.024 Nondisplaced fracture of anterior process of right calcaneus** CC
- 7 √7th **S92.025 Nondisplaced fracture of anterior process of left calcaneus** CC
- 7 √7th **S92.026 Nondisplaced fracture of anterior process of unspecified calcaneus** CC

√6th S92.03 Avulsion fracture of tuberosity of calcaneus
- 7 √7th **S92.031 Displaced avulsion fracture of tuberosity of right calcaneus** CC
- 7 √7th **S92.032 Displaced avulsion fracture of tuberosity of left calcaneus** CC
- 7 √7th **S92.033 Displaced avulsion fracture of tuberosity of unspecified calcaneus** CC
- 7 √7th **S92.034 Nondisplaced avulsion fracture of tuberosity of right calcaneus** CC
- 7 √7th **S92.035 Nondisplaced avulsion fracture of tuberosity of left calcaneus** CC
- 7 √7th **S92.036 Nondisplaced avulsion fracture of tuberosity of unspecified calcaneus** CC

√6th S92.04 Other fracture of tuberosity of calcaneus
- 7 √7th **S92.041 Displaced other fracture of tuberosity of right calcaneus** CC
- 7 √7th **S92.042 Displaced other fracture of tuberosity of left calcaneus** CC
- 7 √7th **S92.043 Displaced other fracture of tuberosity of unspecified calcaneus** CC
- 7 √7th **S92.044 Nondisplaced other fracture of tuberosity of right calcaneus** CC
- 7 √7th **S92.045 Nondisplaced other fracture of tuberosity of left calcaneus** CC
- 7 √7th **S92.046 Nondisplaced other fracture of tuberosity of unspecified calcaneus** CC

√6th S92.05 Other extraarticular fracture of calcaneus
- 7 √7th **S92.051 Displaced other extraarticular fracture of right calcaneus** CC
- 7 √7th **S92.052 Displaced other extraarticular fracture of left calcaneus** CC
- 7 √7th **S92.053 Displaced other extraarticular fracture of unspecified calcaneus** CC
- 7 √7th **S92.054 Nondisplaced other extraarticular fracture of right calcaneus** CC
- 7 √7th **S92.055 Nondisplaced other extraarticular fracture of left calcaneus** CC
- 7 √7th **S92.056 Nondisplaced other extraarticular fracture of unspecified calcaneus** CC

√6th S92.06 Intraarticular fracture of calcaneus
- 7 √7th **S92.061 Displaced intraarticular fracture of right calcaneus** CC
- 7 √7th **S92.062 Displaced intraarticular fracture of left calcaneus** CC
- 7 √7th **S92.063 Displaced intraarticular fracture of unspecified calcaneus** CC
- 7 √7th **S92.064 Nondisplaced intraarticular fracture of right calcaneus** CC
- 7 √7th **S92.065 Nondisplaced intraarticular fracture of left calcaneus** CC
- 7 √7th **S92.066 Nondisplaced intraarticular fracture of unspecified calcaneus** CC

7 HAC = Initial encounter only (7th character A, B or C) and not POA.

✓5th S92.1 Fracture of talus
Astragalus

CC Excl: For CC codes in subcategory S92.1, unless otherwise noted: CC with 7th character B: M80.00X-M80.019 with 7th A, M80.041-M80.049 with 7th A, M80.80X-M80.819 with 7th A, M80.841-M80.849 with 7th A, M84.40X-M84.419 with 7th A, M84.441-M84.446 with 7th A, M84.454 with 7th A, M84.474-M84.519 with 7th A, M84.541-M84.550 with 7th A, M84.574-M84.576 with 7th A, M84.60X-M84.619 with 7th A, M84.641-M84.650 with 7th A, M84.674-M84.68X with 7th A, S03.8XX-S03.9XX with 7th A, S29.011-S29.019 with 7th A, S38.3XX-S39.013 with 7th A, S73.101-S73.199 with 7th A, S76.001-S76.019 with 7th A, S76.091-S76.119 with 7th A, S76.191-S76.219 with 7th A, S76.291-S76.319 with 7th A, S76.391-S76.819 with 7th A, S76.891-S76.919 with 7th A, S76.991-S76.999 with 7th A, S79.811-S79.929 with 7th A, S82.90X-S82.92X with 7th [A, B, C], S92.001-S92.356 with 7th B, S92.901-S92.909 with 7th [A, B], T14.8-T14.91, T79.A9X-T79.9XX with 7th A

CC with 7th character K or P: M80.00X-M84.68X with 7th [K, P], S02.0XX-S02.92X with 7th K, S12.000-S12.691 with 7th K, S22.000-S22.9XX with 7th K, S32.000-S32.9XX with 7th K, S42.001-S42.92X with 7th [K, P], S49.001-S49.199 with 7th [K, P], S52.001-S52.92X with 7th [K, M, N, P, Q, R], S59.001-S59.299 with 7th [K, P], S62.001-S62.92X with 7th [K, P], S72.001-S72.92X with 7th [K, M, N, P, Q, R], S79.001-S79.199 with 7th [K, P], S82.001-S82.92X with 7th [K, M, N, P, Q, R], S89.001-S89.399 with 7th [K, P], S92.001-S92.919 with 7th [K, P]

✓6th S92.10 Unspecified fracture of talus
- 7 ✓7th **S92.101** Unspecified fracture of right talus CC
- 7 ✓7th **S92.102** Unspecified fracture of left talus CC
- 7 ✓7th **S92.109** Unspecified fracture of unspecified talus CC

✓6th S92.11 Fracture of neck of talus
- 7 ✓7th **S92.111** Displaced fracture of neck of right talus CC
- 7 ✓7th **S92.112** Displaced fracture of neck of left talus CC
- 7 ✓7th **S92.113** Displaced fracture of neck of unspecified talus CC
- 7 ✓7th **S92.114** Nondisplaced fracture of neck of right talus CC
- 7 ✓7th **S92.115** Nondisplaced fracture of neck of left talus CC
- 7 ✓7th **S92.116** Nondisplaced fracture of neck of unspecified talus CC

✓6th S92.12 Fracture of body of talus
- 7 ✓7th **S92.121** Displaced fracture of body of right talus CC
- 7 ✓7th **S92.122** Displaced fracture of body of left talus CC
- 7 ✓7th **S92.123** Displaced fracture of body of unspecified talus CC
- 7 ✓7th **S92.124** Nondisplaced fracture of body of right talus CC
- 7 ✓7th **S92.125** Nondisplaced fracture of body of left talus CC
- 7 ✓7th **S92.126** Nondisplaced fracture of body of unspecified talus CC

✓6th S92.13 Fracture of posterior process of talus
- 7 ✓7th **S92.131** Displaced fracture of posterior process of right talus CC
- 7 ✓7th **S92.132** Displaced fracture of posterior process of left talus CC
- 7 ✓7th **S92.133** Displaced fracture of posterior process of unspecified talus CC
- 7 ✓7th **S92.134** Nondisplaced fracture of posterior process of right talus CC
- 7 ✓7th **S92.135** Nondisplaced fracture of posterior process of left talus CC
- 7 ✓7th **S92.136** Nondisplaced fracture of posterior process of unspecified talus CC

✓6th S92.14 Dome fracture of talus
EXCLUDES 1 *osteochondritis dissecans (M93.2)*
- 7 ✓7th **S92.141** Displaced dome fracture of right talus CC
- 7 ✓7th **S92.142** Displaced dome fracture of left talus CC
- 7 ✓7th **S92.143** Displaced dome fracture of unspecified talus CC
- 7 ✓7th **S92.144** Nondisplaced dome fracture of right talus CC
- 7 ✓7th **S92.145** Nondisplaced dome fracture of left talus CC
- 7 ✓7th **S92.146** Nondisplaced dome fracture of unspecified talus CC

✓6th S92.15 Avulsion fracture (chip fracture) of talus
- 7 ✓7th **S92.151** Displaced avulsion fracture (chip fracture) of right talus CC
- 7 ✓7th **S92.152** Displaced avulsion fracture (chip fracture) of left talus CC
- 7 ✓7th **S92.153** Displaced avulsion fracture (chip fracture) of unspecified talus CC
- 7 ✓7th **S92.154** Nondisplaced avulsion fracture (chip fracture) of right talus CC
- 7 ✓7th **S92.155** Nondisplaced avulsion fracture (chip fracture) of left talus CC
- 7 ✓7th **S92.156** Nondisplaced avulsion fracture (chip fracture) of unspecified talus CC

✓6th S92.19 Other fracture of talus
- 7 ✓7th **S92.191** Other fracture of right talus CC
- 7 ✓7th **S92.192** Other fracture of left talus CC
- 7 ✓7th **S92.199** Other fracture of unspecified talus CC

✓5th S92.2 Fracture of other and unspecified tarsal bone(s)

CC Excl: For CC codes in subcategory S92.2, unless otherwise noted: CC with 7th character B: S92.001-S92.919 with 7th [A, B]

CC with 7th character K or P: M80.00X-M84.68X with 7th [K, P], S02.0XX-S02.92X with 7th K, S12.000-S12.691 with 7th K, S22.000-S22.9XX with 7th K, S32.000-S32.9XX with 7th K, S42.001-S42.92X with 7th [K, P], S49.001-S49.199 with 7th [K, P], S52.001-S52.92X with 7th [K, M, N, P, Q, R], S59.001-S59.299 with 7th [K, P], S62.001-S62.92X with 7th [K, P], S72.001-S72.92X with 7th [K, M, N, P, Q, R], S79.001-S79.199 with 7th [K, P], S82.001-S82.92X with 7th [K, M, N, P, Q, R], S89.001-S89.399 with 7th [K, P], S92.001-S92.919 with 7th [K, P]

✓6th S92.20 Fracture of unspecified tarsal bone(s)
- 7 ✓7th **S92.201** Fracture of unspecified tarsal bone(s) of right foot CC
- 7 ✓7th **S92.202** Fracture of unspecified tarsal bone(s) of left foot CC
- 7 ✓7th **S92.209** Fracture of unspecified tarsal bone(s) of unspecified foot CC

✓6th S92.21 Fracture of cuboid bone
- 7 ✓7th **S92.211** Displaced fracture of cuboid bone of right foot CC
- 7 ✓7th **S92.212** Displaced fracture of cuboid bone of left foot CC
- 7 ✓7th **S92.213** Displaced fracture of cuboid bone of unspecified foot CC
- 7 ✓7th **S92.214** Nondisplaced fracture of cuboid bone of right foot CC
- 7 ✓7th **S92.215** Nondisplaced fracture of cuboid bone of left foot CC
- 7 ✓7th **S92.216** Nondisplaced fracture of cuboid bone of unspecified foot CC

✓6th S92.22 Fracture of lateral cuneiform
- 7 ✓7th **S92.221** Displaced fracture of lateral cuneiform of right foot CC
- 7 ✓7th **S92.222** Displaced fracture of lateral cuneiform of left foot CC
- 7 ✓7th **S92.223** Displaced fracture of lateral cuneiform of unspecified foot CC
- 7 ✓7th **S92.224** Nondisplaced fracture of lateral cuneiform of right foot CC
- 7 ✓7th **S92.225** Nondisplaced fracture of lateral cuneiform of left foot CC
- 7 ✓7th **S92.226** Nondisplaced fracture of lateral cuneiform of unspecified foot CC

✓6th S92.23 Fracture of intermediate cuneiform
- 7 ✓7th **S92.231** Displaced fracture of intermediate cuneiform of right foot CC

7 HAC = Initial encounter only (7th character A, B or C) and not POA.

7 ✓7th S92.232 Displaced fracture of intermediate cuneiform of left foot CC

7 ✓7th S92.233 Displaced fracture of intermediate cuneiform of unspecified foot CC

7 ✓7th S92.234 Nondisplaced fracture of intermediate cuneiform of right foot CC

7 ✓7th S92.235 Nondisplaced fracture of intermediate cuneiform of left foot CC

7 ✓7th S92.236 Nondisplaced fracture of intermediate cuneiform of unspecified foot CC

✓6th S92.24 Fracture of medial cuneiform

7 ✓7th S92.241 Displaced fracture of medial cuneiform of right foot CC

7 ✓7th S92.242 Displaced fracture of medial cuneiform of left foot CC

7 ✓7th S92.243 Displaced fracture of medial cuneiform of unspecified foot CC

7 ✓7th S92.244 Nondisplaced fracture of medial cuneiform of right foot CC

7 ✓7th S92.245 Nondisplaced fracture of medial cuneiform of left foot CC

7 ✓7th S92.246 Nondisplaced fracture of medial cuneiform of unspecified foot CC

✓6th S92.25 Fracture of navicular [scaphoid] of foot

7 ✓7th S92.251 Displaced fracture of navicular [scaphoid] of right foot CC

7 ✓7th S92.252 Displaced fracture of navicular [scaphoid] of left foot CC

7 ✓7th S92.253 Displaced fracture of navicular [scaphoid] of unspecified foot CC

7 ✓7th S92.254 Nondisplaced fracture of navicular [scaphoid] of right foot CC

7 ✓7th S92.255 Nondisplaced fracture of navicular [scaphoid] of left foot CC

7 ✓7th S92.256 Nondisplaced fracture of navicular [scaphoid] of unspecified foot CC

✓5th S92.3 Fracture of metatarsal bone(s)

CC Excl: For CC codes in subcategory S92.3, unless otherwise noted: See code: S92.2

✓6th S92.30 Fracture of unspecified metatarsal bone(s)

7 ✓7th S92.301 Fracture of unspecified metatarsal bone(s), right foot CC

7 ✓7th S92.302 Fracture of unspecified metatarsal bone(s), left foot CC

7 ✓7th S92.309 Fracture of unspecified metatarsal bone(s), unspecified foot CC

✓6th S92.31 Fracture of first metatarsal bone

7 ✓7th S92.311 Displaced fracture of first metatarsal bone, right foot CC

7 ✓7th S92.312 Displaced fracture of first metatarsal bone, left foot CC

7 ✓7th S92.313 Displaced fracture of first metatarsal bone, unspecified foot CC

7 ✓7th S92.314 Nondisplaced fracture of first metatarsal bone, right foot CC

7 ✓7th S92.315 Nondisplaced fracture of first metatarsal bone, left foot CC

7 ✓7th S92.316 Nondisplaced fracture of first metatarsal bone, unspecified foot CC

✓6th S92.32 Fracture of second metatarsal bone

7 ✓7th S92.321 Displaced fracture of second metatarsal bone, right foot CC

7 ✓7th S92.322 Displaced fracture of second metatarsal bone, left foot CC

7 ✓7th S92.323 Displaced fracture of second metatarsal bone, unspecified foot CC

7 ✓7th S92.324 Nondisplaced fracture of second metatarsal bone, right foot CC

7 ✓7th S92.325 Nondisplaced fracture of second metatarsal bone, left foot CC

7 ✓7th S92.326 Nondisplaced fracture of second metatarsal bone, unspecified foot CC

✓6th S92.33 Fracture of third metatarsal bone

7 ✓7th S92.331 Displaced fracture of third metatarsal bone, right foot CC

7 ✓7th S92.332 Displaced fracture of third metatarsal bone, left foot CC

7 ✓7th S92.333 Displaced fracture of third metatarsal bone, unspecified foot CC

7 ✓7th S92.334 Nondisplaced fracture of third metatarsal bone, right foot CC

7 ✓7th S92.335 Nondisplaced fracture of third metatarsal bone, left foot CC

7 ✓7th S92.336 Nondisplaced fracture of third metatarsal bone, unspecified foot CC

✓6th S92.34 Fracture of fourth metatarsal bone

7 ✓7th S92.341 Displaced fracture of fourth metatarsal bone, right foot CC

7 ✓7th S92.342 Displaced fracture of fourth metatarsal bone, left foot CC

7 ✓7th S92.343 Displaced fracture of fourth metatarsal bone, unspecified foot CC

7 ✓7th S92.344 Nondisplaced fracture of fourth metatarsal bone, right foot CC

7 ✓7th S92.345 Nondisplaced fracture of fourth metatarsal bone, left foot CC

7 ✓7th S92.346 Nondisplaced fracture of fourth metatarsal bone, unspecified foot CC

✓6th S92.35 Fracture of fifth metatarsal bone

7 ✓7th S92.351 Displaced fracture of fifth metatarsal bone, right foot CC

7 ✓7th S92.352 Displaced fracture of fifth metatarsal bone, left foot CC

7 ✓7th S92.353 Displaced fracture of fifth metatarsal bone, unspecified foot CC

7 ✓7th S92.354 Nondisplaced fracture of fifth metatarsal bone, right foot CC

7 ✓7th S92.355 Nondisplaced fracture of fifth metatarsal bone, left foot CC

7 ✓7th S92.356 Nondisplaced fracture of fifth metatarsal bone, unspecified foot CC

✓5th S92.4 Fracture of great toe

CC Excl: For CC codes in subcategory S92.4, unless otherwise noted: CC with 7th character K or P: M80.00X-M84.68X with 7th [K, P], S02.0XX-S02.92X with 7th K, S12.000-S12.691 with 7th K, S22.000-S22.9XX with 7th K, S32.000-S32.9XX with 7th K, S42.001-S42.92X with 7th [K, P], S49.001-S49.199 with 7th [K, P], S52.001-S52.92X with 7th [K, M, N, P, Q, R], S59.001-S59.299 with 7th [K, P], S62.001-S62.92X with 7th [K, P], S72.001-S72.92X with 7th [K, M, N, P, Q, R], S79.001-S79.199 with 7th [K, P], S82.001-S82.92X with 7th [K, M, N, P, Q, R], S89.001-S89.399 with 7th [K, P], S92.001-S92.919 with 7th [K, P]

✓6th S92.40 Unspecified fracture of great toe

✓7th S92.401 Displaced unspecified fracture of right great toe CC

✓7th S92.402 Displaced unspecified fracture of left great toe CC

✓7th S92.403 Displaced unspecified fracture of unspecified great toe CC

✓7th S92.404 Nondisplaced unspecified fracture of right great toe CC

✓7th S92.405 Nondisplaced unspecified fracture of left great toe CC

✓7th S92.406 Nondisplaced unspecified fracture of unspecified great toe CC

✓6th S92.41 Fracture of proximal phalanx of great toe

✓7th S92.411 Displaced fracture of proximal phalanx of right great toe CC

✓7th S92.412 Displaced fracture of proximal phalanx of left great toe CC

✓7th S92.413 Displaced fracture of proximal phalanx of unspecified great toe CC

✓7th S92.414 Nondisplaced fracture of proximal phalanx of right great toe CC

✓7th S92.415 Nondisplaced fracture of proximal phalanx of left great toe CC

7 HAC = Initial encounter only (7th character A, B or C) and not POA.

7th S92.416 Nondisplaced fracture of proximal phalanx of unspecified great toe CC

6th S92.42 Fracture of distal phalanx of great toe

7th S92.421 Displaced fracture of distal phalanx of right great toe CC

7th S92.422 Displaced fracture of distal phalanx of left great toe CC

7th S92.423 Displaced fracture of distal phalanx of unspecified great toe CC

7th S92.424 Nondisplaced fracture of distal phalanx of right great toe CC

7th S92.425 Nondisplaced fracture of distal phalanx of left great toe CC

7th S92.426 Nondisplaced fracture of distal phalanx of unspecified great toe CC

6th S92.49 Other fracture of great toe

7th S92.491 Other fracture of right great toe CC

7th S92.492 Other fracture of left great toe CC

7th S92.499 Other fracture of unspecified great toe CC

5th S92.5 Fracture of lesser toe(s)

CC Excl: For CC codes in subcategory S92.5, unless otherwise noted: See code: S92.4

6th S92.50 Unspecified fracture of lesser toe(s)

7th S92.501 Displaced unspecified fracture of right lesser toe(s) CC

7th S92.502 Displaced unspecified fracture of left lesser toe(s) CC

7th S92.503 Displaced unspecified fracture of unspecified lesser toe(s) CC

7th S92.504 Nondisplaced unspecified fracture of right lesser toe(s) CC

7th S92.505 Nondisplaced unspecified fracture of left lesser toe(s) CC

7th S92.506 Nondisplaced unspecified fracture of unspecified lesser toe(s) CC

6th S92.51 Fracture of proximal phalanx of lesser toe(s)

7th S92.511 Displaced fracture of proximal phalanx of right lesser toe(s) CC

7th S92.512 Displaced fracture of proximal phalanx of left lesser toe(s) CC

7th S92.513 Displaced fracture of proximal phalanx of unspecified lesser toe(s) CC

7th S92.514 Nondisplaced fracture of proximal phalanx of right lesser toe(s) CC

7th S92.515 Nondisplaced fracture of proximal phalanx of left lesser toe(s) CC

7th S92.516 Nondisplaced fracture of proximal phalanx of unspecified lesser toe(s) CC

6th S92.52 Fracture of medial phalanx of lesser toe(s)

7th S92.521 Displaced fracture of medial phalanx of right lesser toe(s) CC

7th S92.522 Displaced fracture of medial phalanx of left lesser toe(s) CC

7th S92.523 Displaced fracture of medial phalanx of unspecified lesser toe(s) CC

7th S92.524 Nondisplaced fracture of medial phalanx of right lesser toe(s) CC

7th S92.525 Nondisplaced fracture of medial phalanx of left lesser toe(s) CC

7th S92.526 Nondisplaced fracture of medial phalanx of unspecified lesser toe(s) CC

6th S92.53 Fracture of distal phalanx of lesser toe(s)

7th S92.531 Displaced fracture of distal phalanx of right lesser toe(s) CC

7th S92.532 Displaced fracture of distal phalanx of left lesser toe(s) CC

7th S92.533 Displaced fracture of distal phalanx of unspecified lesser toe(s) CC

7th S92.534 Nondisplaced fracture of distal phalanx of right lesser toe(s) CC

7th S92.535 Nondisplaced fracture of distal phalanx of left lesser toe(s) CC

7th S92.536 Nondisplaced fracture of distal phalanx of unspecified lesser toe(s) CC

6th S92.59 Other fracture of lesser toe(s)

7th S92.591 Other fracture of right lesser toe(s) CC

7th S92.592 Other fracture of left lesser toe(s) CC

7th S92.599 Other fracture of unspecified lesser toe(s) CC

5th S92.9 Unspecified fracture of foot and toe

6th S92.90 Unspecified fracture of foot

CC Excl: For CC codes in subcategory S92.90, unless otherwise noted: CC with 7th character B: S92.001-S92.919 with 7th [A, B]
CC with 7th character K or P: M80.00X-M84.68X with 7th [K, P], S02.0XX-S02.92X with 7th K, S12.000-S12.691 with 7th K, S22.000-S22.9XX with 7th K, S32.000-S32.9XX with 7th K, S42.001-S42.92X with 7th [K, P], S49.001-S49.199 with 7th [K, P], S52.001-S52.92X with 7th [K, M, N, P, Q, R], S59.001-S59.299 with 7th [K, P], S62.001-S62.92X with 7th [K, P], S72.001-S72.92X with 7th [K, M, N, P, Q, R], S79.001-S79.199 with 7th [K, P], S82.001-S82.92X with 7th [K, M, N, P, Q, R], S89.001-S89.399 with 7th [K, P], S92.001-S92.919 with 7th [K, P]

7 7th S92.901 Unspecified fracture of right foot CC

7 7th S92.902 Unspecified fracture of left foot CC

7 7th S92.909 Unspecified fracture of unspecified foot CC

6th S92.91 Unspecified fracture of toe

CC Excl: For CC codes in subcategory S92.91, unless otherwise noted: See code: S92.90

7th S92.911 Unspecified fracture of right toe(s) CC

7th S92.912 Unspecified fracture of left toe(s) CC

7th S92.919 Unspecified fracture of unspecified toe(s) CC

4th S93 Dislocation and sprain of joints and ligaments at ankle, foot and toe level

INCLUDES avulsion of joint or ligament of ankle, foot and toe
laceration of cartilage, joint or ligament of ankle, foot and toe
sprain of cartilage, joint or ligament of ankle, foot and toe
traumatic hemarthrosis of joint or ligament of ankle, foot and toe
traumatic rupture of joint or ligament of ankle, foot and toe
traumatic subluxation of joint or ligament of ankle, foot and toe
traumatic tear of joint or ligament of ankle, foot and toe

Code also any associated open wound

EXCLUDES 2 *strain of muscle and tendon of ankle and foot (S96.-)*

The appropriate 7th character is to be added to each code from category S93.
A initial encounter
D subsequent encounter
S sequela

5th S93.0 Subluxation and dislocation of ankle joint
Subluxation and dislocation of astragalus
Subluxation and dislocation of fibula, lower end
Subluxation and dislocation of talus
Subluxation and dislocation of tibia, lower end

x7th S93.01 Subluxation of right ankle joint

x7th S93.02 Subluxation of left ankle joint

x7th S93.03 Subluxation of unspecified ankle joint

x7th S93.04 Dislocation of right ankle joint

x7th S93.05 Dislocation of left ankle joint

x7th S93.06 Dislocation of unspecified ankle joint

5th S93.1 Subluxation and dislocation of toe

6th S93.10 Unspecified subluxation and dislocation of toe
Dislocation of toe NOS
Subluxation of toe NOS

7th S93.101 Unspecified subluxation of right toe(s)

7th S93.102 Unspecified subluxation of left toe(s)

7th S93.103 Unspecified subluxation of unspecified toe(s)

7th S93.104 Unspecified dislocation of right toe(s)

7th S93.105 Unspecified dislocation of left toe(s)

7 HAC = Initial encounter only (7th character A, B or C) and not POA.

S93.106 Unspecified dislocation of unspecified toe(s)

S93.11 Dislocation of interphalangeal joint
- S93.111 Dislocation of interphalangeal joint of right great toe
- S93.112 Dislocation of interphalangeal joint of left great toe
- S93.113 Dislocation of interphalangeal joint of unspecified great toe
- S93.114 Dislocation of interphalangeal joint of right lesser toe(s)
- S93.115 Dislocation of interphalangeal joint of left lesser toe(s)
- S93.116 Dislocation of interphalangeal joint of unspecified lesser toe(s)
- S93.119 Dislocation of interphalangeal joint of unspecified toe(s)

S93.12 Dislocation of metatarsophalangeal joint
- S93.121 Dislocation of metatarsophalangeal joint of right great toe
- S93.122 Dislocation of metatarsophalangeal joint of left great toe
- S93.123 Dislocation of metatarsophalangeal joint of unspecified great toe
- S93.124 Dislocation of metatarsophalangeal joint of right lesser toe(s)
- S93.125 Dislocation of metatarsophalangeal joint of left lesser toe(s)
- S93.126 Dislocation of metatarsophalangeal joint of unspecified lesser toe(s)
- S93.129 Dislocation of metatarsophalangeal joint of unspecified toe(s)

S93.13 Subluxation of interphalangeal joint
- S93.131 Subluxation of interphalangeal joint of right great toe
- S93.132 Subluxation of interphalangeal joint of left great toe
- S93.133 Subluxation of interphalangeal joint of unspecified great toe
- S93.134 Subluxation of interphalangeal joint of right lesser toe(s)
- S93.135 Subluxation of interphalangeal joint of left lesser toe(s)
- S93.136 Subluxation of interphalangeal joint of unspecified lesser toe(s)
- S93.139 Subluxation of interphalangeal joint of unspecified toe(s)

S93.14 Subluxation of metatarsophalangeal joint
- S93.141 Subluxation of metatarsophalangeal joint of right great toe
- S93.142 Subluxation of metatarsophalangeal joint of left great toe
- S93.143 Subluxation of metatarsophalangeal joint of unspecified great toe
- S93.144 Subluxation of metatarsophalangeal joint of right lesser toe(s)
- S93.145 Subluxation of metatarsophalangeal joint of left lesser toe(s)
- S93.146 Subluxation of metatarsophalangeal joint of unspecified lesser toe(s)
- S93.149 Subluxation of metatarsophalangeal joint of unspecified toe(s)

S93.3 Subluxation and dislocation of foot

EXCLUDES 2 *dislocation of toe (S93.1-)*

S93.30 Unspecified subluxation and dislocation of foot
Dislocation of foot NOS
Subluxation of foot NOS
- S93.301 Unspecified subluxation of right foot
- S93.302 Unspecified subluxation of left foot
- S93.303 Unspecified subluxation of unspecified foot
- S93.304 Unspecified dislocation of right foot
- S93.305 Unspecified dislocation of left foot
- S93.306 Unspecified dislocation of unspecified foot

S93.31 Subluxation and dislocation of tarsal joint
- S93.311 Subluxation of tarsal joint of right foot
- S93.312 Subluxation of tarsal joint of left foot
- S93.313 Subluxation of tarsal joint of unspecified foot
- S93.314 Dislocation of tarsal joint of right foot
- S93.315 Dislocation of tarsal joint of left foot
- S93.316 Dislocation of tarsal joint of unspecified foot

S93.32 Subluxation and dislocation of tarsometatarsal joint
- S93.321 Subluxation of tarsometatarsal joint of right foot
- S93.322 Subluxation of tarsometatarsal joint of left foot
- S93.323 Subluxation of tarsometatarsal joint of unspecified foot
- S93.324 Dislocation of tarsometatarsal joint of right foot
- S93.325 Dislocation of tarsometatarsal joint of left foot
- S93.326 Dislocation of tarsometatarsal joint of unspecified foot

S93.33 Other subluxation and dislocation of foot
- S93.331 Other subluxation of right foot
- S93.332 Other subluxation of left foot
- S93.333 Other subluxation of unspecified foot
- S93.334 Other dislocation of right foot
- S93.335 Other dislocation of left foot
- S93.336 Other dislocation of unspecified foot

S93.4 Sprain of ankle

EXCLUDES 2 *injury of Achilles tendon (S86.0-)*

S93.40 Sprain of unspecified ligament of ankle
Sprain of ankle NOS
Sprained ankle NOS
- S93.401 Sprain of unspecified ligament of right ankle
- S93.402 Sprain of unspecified ligament of left ankle
- S93.409 Sprain of unspecified ligament of unspecified ankle

S93.41 Sprain of calcaneofibular ligament
- S93.411 Sprain of calcaneofibular ligament of right ankle
- S93.412 Sprain of calcaneofibular ligament of left ankle
- S93.419 Sprain of calcaneofibular ligament of unspecified ankle

S93.42 Sprain of deltoid ligament
- S93.421 Sprain of deltoid ligament of right ankle
- S93.422 Sprain of deltoid ligament of left ankle
- S93.429 Sprain of deltoid ligament of unspecified ankle

S93.43 Sprain of tibiofibular ligament
- S93.431 Sprain of tibiofibular ligament of right ankle
- S93.432 Sprain of tibiofibular ligament of left ankle
- S93.439 Sprain of tibiofibular ligament of unspecified ankle

S93.49 Sprain of other ligament of ankle
Sprain of internal collateral ligament
Sprain of talofibular ligament
- S93.491 Sprain of other ligament of right ankle
- S93.492 Sprain of other ligament of left ankle
- S93.499 Sprain of other ligament of unspecified ankle

S93.5 Sprain of toe

S93.50 Unspecified sprain of toe
- S93.501 Unspecified sprain of right great toe
- S93.502 Unspecified sprain of left great toe

✓7th S93.503 Unspecified sprain of unspecified great toe
✓7th S93.504 Unspecified sprain of right lesser toe(s)
✓7th S93.505 Unspecified sprain of left lesser toe(s)
✓7th S93.506 Unspecified sprain of unspecified lesser toe(s)
✓7th S93.509 Unspecified sprain of unspecified toe(s)

✓6th **S93.51 Sprain of interphalangeal joint of toe**
✓7th S93.511 Sprain of interphalangeal joint of right great toe
✓7th S93.512 Sprain of interphalangeal joint of left great toe
✓7th S93.513 Sprain of interphalangeal joint of unspecified great toe
✓7th S93.514 Sprain of interphalangeal joint of right lesser toe(s)
✓7th S93.515 Sprain of interphalangeal joint of left lesser toe(s)
✓7th S93.516 Sprain of interphalangeal joint of unspecified lesser toe(s)
✓7th S93.519 Sprain of interphalangeal joint of unspecified toe(s)

✓6th **S93.52 Sprain of metatarsophalangeal joint of toe**
✓7th S93.521 Sprain of metatarsophalangeal joint of right great toe
✓7th S93.522 Sprain of metatarsophalangeal joint of left great toe
✓7th S93.523 Sprain of metatarsophalangeal joint of unspecified great toe
✓7th S93.524 Sprain of metatarsophalangeal joint of right lesser toe(s)
✓7th S93.525 Sprain of metatarsophalangeal joint of left lesser toe(s)
✓7th S93.526 Sprain of metatarsophalangeal joint of unspecified lesser toe(s)
✓7th S93.529 Sprain of metatarsophalangeal joint of unspecified toe(s)

✓5th **S93.6 Sprain of foot**
EXCLUDES 2 *sprain of metatarsophalangeal joint of toe (S93.52-)*
sprain of toe (S93.5-)

✓6th **S93.60 Unspecified sprain of foot**
✓7th S93.601 Unspecified sprain of right foot
✓7th S93.602 Unspecified sprain of left foot
✓7th S93.609 Unspecified sprain of unspecified foot

✓6th **S93.61 Sprain of tarsal ligament of foot**
✓7th S93.611 Sprain of tarsal ligament of right foot
✓7th S93.612 Sprain of tarsal ligament of left foot
✓7th S93.619 Sprain of tarsal ligament of unspecified foot

✓6th **S93.62 Sprain of tarsometatarsal ligament of foot**
✓7th S93.621 Sprain of tarsometatarsal ligament of right foot
✓7th S93.622 Sprain of tarsometatarsal ligament of left foot
✓7th S93.629 Sprain of tarsometatarsal ligament of unspecified foot

✓6th **S93.69 Other sprain of foot**
✓7th S93.691 Other sprain of right foot
✓7th S93.692 Other sprain of left foot
✓7th S93.699 Other sprain of unspecified foot

✓4th S94 Injury of nerves at ankle and foot level

Code also any associated open wound (S91.-)

The appropriate 7th character is to be added to each code from category S94.
A initial encounter
D subsequent encounter
S sequela

✓5th **S94.0 Injury of lateral plantar nerve**
✓x7th S94.00 Injury of lateral plantar nerve, unspecified leg
✓x7th S94.01 Injury of lateral plantar nerve, right leg
✓x7th S94.02 Injury of lateral plantar nerve, left leg

✓5th **S94.1 Injury of medial plantar nerve**
✓x7th S94.10 Injury of medial plantar nerve, unspecified leg
✓x7th S94.11 Injury of medial plantar nerve, right leg
✓x7th S94.12 Injury of medial plantar nerve, left leg

✓5th **S94.2 Injury of deep peroneal nerve at ankle and foot level**
Injury of terminal, lateral branch of deep peroneal nerve
✓x7th S94.20 Injury of deep peroneal nerve at ankle and foot level, unspecified leg
✓x7th S94.21 Injury of deep peroneal nerve at ankle and foot level, right leg
✓x7th S94.22 Injury of deep peroneal nerve at ankle and foot level, left leg

✓5th **S94.3 Injury of cutaneous sensory nerve at ankle and foot level**
✓x7th S94.30 Injury of cutaneous sensory nerve at ankle and foot level, unspecified leg
✓x7th S94.31 Injury of cutaneous sensory nerve at ankle and foot level, right leg
✓x7th S94.32 Injury of cutaneous sensory nerve at ankle and foot level, left leg

✓5th **S94.8 Injury of other nerves at ankle and foot level**
✓6th **S94.8X Injury of other nerves at ankle and foot level**
✓7th S94.8X1 Injury of other nerves at ankle and foot level, right leg
✓7th S94.8X2 Injury of other nerves at ankle and foot level, left leg
✓7th S94.8X9 Injury of other nerves at ankle and foot level, unspecified leg

✓5th **S94.9 Injury of unspecified nerve at ankle and foot level**
✓x7th S94.90 Injury of unspecified nerve at ankle and foot level, unspecified leg
✓x7th S94.91 Injury of unspecified nerve at ankle and foot level, right leg
✓x7th S94.92 Injury of unspecified nerve at ankle and foot level, left leg

✓4th S95 Injury of blood vessels at ankle and foot level

Code also any associated open wound (S91.-)
EXCLUDES 2 *injury of posterior tibial artery and vein (S85.1-, S85.8-)*

The appropriate 7th character is to be added to each code from category S95.
A initial encounter
D subsequent encounter
S sequela

✓5th **S95.0 Injury of dorsal artery of foot**
✓6th **S95.00 Unspecified injury of dorsal artery of foot**
✓7th S95.001 Unspecified injury of dorsal artery of right foot CC
CC Excl: CC with 7th character A: M79.A21-M79.A29, S75.001 with 7th A, S75.009-S75.011 with 7th A, S75.019-S75.021 with 7th A, S75.029-S75.091 with 7th A, S75.099-S75.101 with 7th A, S75.109-S75.111 with 7th A, S75.119-S75.121 with 7th A, S75.129-S75.191 with 7th A, S75.199-S75.201 with 7th A, S75.209-S75.211 with 7th A, S75.219-S75.221 with 7th A, S75.229-S75.291 with 7th A, S75.299-S75.801 with 7th A, S75.809-S75.811 with 7th A, S75.819-S75.891 with 7th A, S75.899-S75.901 with 7th A, S75.909-S75.911 with 7th A, S75.919-S75.991 with 7th A, S75.999A, S85.001A, S85.009-S85.011 with 7th A, S85.019-S85.091 with 7th A, S85.099-S85.101 with 7th A, S85.109-S85.111 with 7th A, S85.119-S85.121 with

7th A, S85.129-S85.131 with 7th A, S85.139-S85.141 with 7th A, S85.149-S85.151 with 7th A, S85.159-S85.161 with 7th A, S85.169-S85.171 with 7th A, S85.179-S85.181 with 7th A, S85.189-S85.201 with 7th A, S85.209-S85.211 with 7th A, S85.219-S85.291 with 7th A, S85.299-S85.301 with 7th A, S85.309-S85.311 with 7th A, S85.319-S85.391 with 7th A, S85.399-S85.401 with 7th A, S85.409-S85.411 with 7th A, S85.419-S85.491 with 7th A, S85.499-S85.501 with 7th A, S85.509-S85.511 with 7th A, S85.519-S85.591 with 7th A, S85.599-S85.801 with 7th A, S85.809-S85.811 with 7th A, S85.819-S85.891 with 7th A, S85.899-S85.901 with 7th A, S85.909-S85.911 with 7th A, S85.919-S85.991 with 7th A, S85.999A, S95.001A, S95.009-S95.011 with 7th A, S95.019-S95.091 with 7th A, S95.099-S95.101 with 7th A, S95.109-S95.111 with 7th A, S95.119-S95.191 with 7th A, S95.199-S95.201 with 7th A, S95.209-S95.211 with 7th A, S95.219-S95.291 with 7th A, S95.299-S95.801 with 7th A, S95.809-S95.811 with 7th A, S95.819-S95.891 with 7th A, S95.899-S95.901 with 7th A, S95.909-S95.911 with 7th A, S95.919-S95.991 with 7th A, S95.999A

✓7th **S95.002** **Unspecified injury of dorsal artery of left foot** CC

CC Excl: CC with 7th character A: M79.A21-M79.A29, S75.002-S75.009 with 7th A, S75.012-S75.019 with 7th A, S75.022-S75.029 with 7th A, S75.092-S75.099 with 7th A, S75.102-S75.109 with 7th A, S75.112-S75.119 with 7th A, S75.122-S75.129 with 7th A, S75.192-S75.199 with 7th A, S75.202-S75.209 with 7th A, S75.212-S75.219 with 7th A, S75.222-S75.229 with 7th A, S75.292-S75.299 with 7th A, S75.802-S75.809 with 7th A, S75.812-S75.819 with 7th A, S75.892-S75.899 with 7th A, S75.902-S75.909 with 7th A, S75.912-S75.919 with 7th A, S75.992-S75.999 with 7th A, S85.002-S85.009 with 7th A, S85.012-S85.019 with 7th A, S85.092-S85.099 with 7th A, S85.102-S85.109 with 7th A, S85.112-S85.119 with 7th A, S85.122-S85.129 with 7th A, S85.132-S85.139 with 7th A, S85.142-S85.149 with 7th A, S85.152-S85.159 with 7th A, S85.162-S85.169 with 7th A, S85.172-S85.179 with 7th A, S85.182-S85.189 with 7th A, S85.202-S85.209 with 7th A, S85.212-S85.219 with 7th A, S85.292-S85.299 with 7th A, S85.302-S85.309 with 7th A, S85.312-S85.319 with 7th A, S85.392-S85.399 with 7th A, S85.402-S85.409 with 7th A, S85.412-S85.419 with 7th A, S85.492-S85.499 with 7th A, S85.502-S85.509 with 7th A, S85.512-S85.519 with 7th A, S85.592-S85.599 with 7th A, S85.802-S85.809 with 7th A, S85.812-S85.819 with 7th A, S85.892-S85.899 with 7th A, S85.902-S85.909 with 7th A, S85.912-S85.919 with 7th A, S85.992-S85.999 with 7th A, S95.002-S95.009 with 7th A, S95.012-S95.019 with 7th A, S95.092-S95.099 with 7th A, S95.102-S95.109 with 7th A, S95.112-S95.119 with 7th A, S95.192-S95.199 with 7th A, S95.202-S95.209 with 7th A, S95.212-S95.219 with 7th A, S95.292-S95.299 with 7th A, S95.802-S95.809 with 7th A, S95.812-S95.819 with 7th A, S95.892-S95.899 with 7th A, S95.902-S95.909 with 7th A, S95.912-S95.919 with 7th A, S95.992-S95.999 with 7th A

✓7th **S95.009** **Unspecified injury of dorsal artery of unspecified foot** CC

CC Excl: CC with 7th character A: M79.A21-M79.A29, S75.001-S75.999 with 7th A, S85.001-S85.999 with 7th A, S95.001-S95.999 with 7th A

✓6th **S95.01** **Laceration of dorsal artery of foot**

✓7th **S95.011** **Laceration of dorsal artery of right foot** CC

CC Excl: M79.A21-M79.A29, S75.001 with 7th A, S75.009-S75.011 with 7th A, S75.019-S75.021 with 7th A, S75.029-S75.091 with 7th A, S75.099-S75.101 with 7th A, S75.109-S75.111 with 7th A, S75.119-S75.121 with 7th A, S75.129-S75.191 with 7th A, S75.199-S75.201 with 7th A, S75.209-S75.211 with 7th A, S75.219-S75.221 with 7th A, S75.229-S75.291 with 7th A, S75.299-S75.801 with 7th A, S75.809-S75.811 with 7th A, S75.819-S75.891 with 7th A, S75.899-S75.901 with 7th A, S75.909-S75.911 with 7th A, S75.919-S75.991 with 7th A, S75.999 with 7th A, S85.001 with 7th A, S85.009-S85.011 with 7th A, S85.019-S85.091 with 7th A, S85.099-S85.101 with 7th A, S85.109-S85.111 with 7th A, S85.119-S85.121 with 7th A, S85.129-S85.131 with 7th A, S85.139-S85.141 with 7th A, S85.149-S85.151 with 7th A, S85.159-S85.161 with 7th A, S85.169-S85.171 with 7th A, S85.179-S85.181 with 7th A, S85.189-S85.201 with 7th A, S85.209-S85.211 with 7th A, S85.219-S85.291 with 7th A, S85.299-S85.301 with 7th A, S85.309-S85.311 with 7th A, S85.319-S85.391 with 7th A, S85.399-S85.401 with 7th A, S85.409-S85.411 with 7th A, S85.419-S85.491 with 7th A, S85.499-S85.501 with 7th A, S85.509-S85.511 with 7th A, S85.519-S85.591 with 7th A, S85.599-S85.801 with 7th A, S85.809-S85.811 with 7th A, S85.819-S85.891 with 7th A, S85.899-S85.901 with 7th A, S85.909-S85.911 with 7th A, S85.919-S85.991 with 7th A, S85.999A, S95.001A, S95.009-S95.011 with 7th A, S95.019-S95.091 with 7th A, S95.099-S95.101 with 7th A, S95.109-S95.111 with 7th A, S95.119-S95.191 with 7th A, S95.199-S95.201 with 7th A, S95.209-S95.211 with 7th A, S95.219-S95.291 with 7th A, S95.299-S95.801 with 7th A, S95.809-S95.811 with 7th A, S95.819-S95.891 with 7th A, S95.899-S95.901 with 7th A, S95.909-S95.911 with 7th A, S95.919-S95.991 with 7th A, S95.999 with 7th A

✓7th **S95.012** **Laceration of dorsal artery of left foot** CC

CC Excl: M79.A21-M79.A29, S75.002-S75.009 with 7th A, S75.012-S75.019 with 7th A, S75.022-S75.029 with 7th A, S75.092-S75.099 with 7th A, S75.102-S75.109 with 7th A, S75.112-S75.119 with 7th A, S75.122-S75.129 with 7th A, S75.192-S75.199 with 7th A, S75.202-S75.209 with 7th A, S75.212-S75.219 with 7th A, S75.222-S75.229 with 7th A, S75.292-S75.299 with 7th A, S75.802-S75.809 with 7th A, S75.812-S75.819 with 7th A, S75.892-S75.899 with 7th A, S75.902-S75.909 with 7th A, S75.912-S75.919 with 7th A, S75.992-S75.999 with 7th A, S85.002-S85.009 with 7th A, S85.012-S85.019 with 7th A, S85.092-S85.099 with 7th A, S85.102-S85.109 with 7th A, S85.112-S85.119 with 7th A, S85.122-S85.129 with 7th A, S85.132-S85.139 with 7th A, S85.142-S85.149 with 7th A, S85.152-S85.159 with 7th A, S85.162-S85.169 with 7th A, S85.172-S85.179 with 7th A, S85.182-S85.189 with 7th A, S85.202-S85.209 with 7th A, S85.212-S85.219 with 7th A, S85.292-S85.299 with 7th A, S85.302-S85.309 with 7th A, S85.312-S85.319 with 7th A, S85.392-S85.399 with 7th A, S85.402-S85.409 with 7th A, S85.412-S85.419 with 7th A, S85.492-S85.499 with 7th A, S85.502-S85.509 with 7th A, S85.512-S85.519 with 7th A, S85.592-S85.599 with 7th A, S85.802-S85.809 with 7th A, S85.812-S85.819 with 7th A, S85.892-S85.899 with 7th A, S85.902-S85.909 with 7th A, S85.912-S85.919 with 7th A, S85.992-S85.999 with 7th A, S95.002-S95.009 with 7th A, S95.012-S95.019 with 7th A, S95.092-S95.099 with 7th A, S95.102-S95.109 with 7th A, S95.112-S95.119 with 7th A, S95.192-S95.199 with 7th A, S95.202-S95.209 with 7th A, S95.212-S95.219 with 7th A, S95.292-S95.299 with 7th A, S95.802-S95.809 with 7th A, S95.812-S95.819 with 7th A, S95.892-S95.899 with 7th A, S95.902-S95.909 with 7th A, S95.912-S95.919 with 7th A, S95.992-S95.999 with 7th A

√7th **S95.Ø19 Laceration of dorsal artery of unspecified foot** CC
CC Excl: M79.A21-M79.A29, S75.ØØ1-S75.999 with 7th A, S85.ØØ1-S85.999 with 7th A, S95.ØØ1-S95.999 with 7th A

√6th **S95.Ø9 Other specified injury of dorsal artery of foot**

√7th **S95.Ø91 Other specified injury of dorsal artery of right foot** CC
CC Excl: See code: S95.ØØ1

√7th **S95.Ø92 Other specified injury of dorsal artery of left foot** CC
CC Excl: See code: S95.ØØ2

√7th **S95.Ø99 Other specified injury of dorsal artery of unspecified foot** CC
CC Excl: See code: S95.ØØ9

√5th **S95.1 Injury of plantar artery of foot**

√6th **S95.1Ø Unspecified injury of plantar artery of foot**

√7th **S95.1Ø1 Unspecified injury of plantar artery of right foot** CC
CC Excl: CC with 7th character A: S75.8Ø1 with 7th A, S75.8Ø9-S75.811 with 7th A, S75.819-S75.891 with 7th A, S75.899-S75.9Ø1 with 7th A, S75.9Ø9-S75.911 with 7th A, S75.919-S75.991 with 7th A, S75.999 with 7th A, S85.2Ø1 with 7th A, S85.2Ø9-S85.211 with 7th A, S85.219-S85.291 with 7th A, S85.299 with 7th A, S85.8Ø1 with 7th A, S85.8Ø9-S85.811 with 7th A, S85.819-S85.891 with 7th A, S85.899-S85.9Ø1 with 7th A, S85.9Ø9-S85.911 with 7th A, S85.919-S85.991 with 7th A, S85.999 with 7th A, S95.ØØ1 with 7th A, S95.ØØ9-S95.Ø11 with 7th A, S95.Ø19-S95.Ø91 with 7th A, S95.Ø99-S95.1Ø1 with 7th A, S95.1Ø9-S95.111 with 7th A, S95.119-S95.191 with 7th A, S95.199-S95.2Ø1 with 7th A, S95.2Ø9-S95.211 with 7th A, S95.219-S95.291 with 7th A, S95.299-S95.8Ø1 with 7th A, S95.8Ø9-S95.811 with 7th A, S95.819-S95.891 with 7th A, S95.899-S95.9Ø1 with 7th A, S95.9Ø9-S95.911 with 7th A, S95.919-S95.991 with 7th A, S95.999 with 7th A

√7th **S95.1Ø2 Unspecified injury of plantar artery of left foot** CC
CC Excl: CC with 7th character A: S75.8Ø2-S75.8Ø9 with 7th A, S75.812-S75.819 with 7th A, S75.892-S75.899 with 7th A, S75.9Ø2-S75.9Ø9 with 7th A, S75.912-S75.919 with 7th A, S75.992-S75.999 with 7th A, S85.2Ø2-S85.2Ø9 with 7th A, S85.212-S85.219 with 7th A, S85.292-S85.299 with 7th A, S85.8Ø2-S85.8Ø9 with 7th A, S85.812-S85.819 with 7th A, S85.892-S85.899 with 7th A, S85.9Ø2-S85.9Ø9 with 7th A, S85.912-S85.919 with 7th A, S85.992-S85.999 with 7th A, S95.ØØ2-S95.ØØ9 with 7th A, S95.Ø12-S95.Ø19 with 7th A, S95.Ø92-S95.Ø99 with 7th A, S95.1Ø2-S95.1Ø9 with 7th A, S95.112-S95.119 with 7th A, S95.192-S95.199 with 7th A, S95.2Ø2-S95.2Ø9 with 7th A, S95.212-S95.219 with 7th A, S95.292-S95.299 with 7th A, S95.8Ø2-S95.8Ø9 with 7th A, S95.812-S95.819 with 7th A, S95.892-S95.899 with 7th A, S95.9Ø2-S95.9Ø9 with 7th A, S95.912-S95.919 with 7th A, S95.992-S95.999 with 7th A

√7th **S95.1Ø9 Unspecified injury of plantar artery of unspecified foot** CC
CC Excl: CC with 7th character A: S75.8Ø1-S75.999 with 7th A, S85.2Ø1-S85.299 with 7th A, S85.8Ø1-S85.999 with 7th A, S95.ØØ1-S95.999 with 7th A

√6th **S95.11 Laceration of plantar artery of foot**

√7th **S95.111 Laceration of plantar artery of right foot** CC
CC Excl: See code: S95.1Ø1

√7th **S95.112 Laceration of plantar artery of left foot** CC
CC Excl: See code: S95.1Ø2

√7th **S95.119 Laceration of plantar artery of unspecified foot** CC
CC Excl: See code: S95.1Ø9

√6th **S95.19 Other specified injury of plantar artery of foot**

√7th **S95.191 Other specified injury of plantar artery of right foot** CC
CC Excl: See code: S95.1Ø1

√7th **S95.192 Other specified injury of plantar artery of left foot** CC
CC Excl: See code: S95.1Ø2

√7th **S95.199 Other specified injury of plantar artery of unspecified foot** CC
CC Excl: See code: S95.1Ø9

√5th **S95.2 Injury of dorsal vein of foot**

√6th **S95.2Ø Unspecified injury of dorsal vein of foot**

√7th **S95.2Ø1 Unspecified injury of dorsal vein of right foot** CC
CC Excl: See code: S95.ØØ1

√7th **S95.2Ø2 Unspecified injury of dorsal vein of left foot** CC
CC Excl: See code: S95.ØØ2

√7th **S95.2Ø9 Unspecified injury of dorsal vein of unspecified foot** CC
CC Excl: See code: S95.ØØ9

√6th **S95.21 Laceration of dorsal vein of foot**

√7th **S95.211 Laceration of dorsal vein of right foot** CC
CC Excl: See code: S95.ØØ1

√7th **S95.212 Laceration of dorsal vein of left foot** CC
CC Excl: See code: S95.ØØ2

√7th **S95.219 Laceration of dorsal vein of unspecified foot** CC
CC Excl: See code: S95.ØØ9

√6th **S95.29 Other specified injury of dorsal vein of foot**

√7th **S95.291 Other specified injury of dorsal vein of right foot** CC
CC Excl: See code: S95.ØØ1

√7th **S95.292 Other specified injury of dorsal vein of left foot** CC
CC Excl: See code: S95.ØØ2

√7th **S95.299 Other specified injury of dorsal vein of unspecified foot** CC
CC Excl: See code: S95.ØØ9

√5th **S95.8 Injury of other blood vessels at ankle and foot level**

√6th **S95.8Ø Unspecified injury of other blood vessels at ankle and foot level**

√7th **S95.8Ø1 Unspecified injury of other blood vessels at ankle and foot level, right leg** CC
CC Excl: See code: S95.ØØ1

√7th **S95.8Ø2 Unspecified injury of other blood vessels at ankle and foot level, left leg** CC
CC Excl: See code: S95.ØØ2

√7th **S95.8Ø9 Unspecified injury of other blood vessels at ankle and foot level, unspecified leg** CC
CC Excl: See code: S95.ØØ9

√6th **S95.81 Laceration of other blood vessels at ankle and foot level**

√7th **S95.811 Laceration of other blood vessels at ankle and foot level, right leg** CC
CC Excl: See code: S95.ØØ1

√7th **S95.812 Laceration of other blood vessels at ankle and foot level, left leg** CC
CC Excl: See code: S95.ØØ2

√7th **S95.819 Laceration of other blood vessels at ankle and foot level, unspecified leg** CC
CC Excl: See code: S95.ØØ9

√6th **S95.89 Other specified injury of other blood vessels at ankle and foot level**

√7th **S95.891 Other specified injury of other blood vessels at ankle and foot level, right leg** CC
CC Excl: See code: S95.ØØ1

√7th **S95.892 Other specified injury of other blood vessels at ankle and foot level, left leg** CC
CC Excl: See code: S95.ØØ2

√7th **S95.899 Other specified injury of other blood vessels at ankle and foot level, unspecified leg** CC
CC Excl: See code: S95.ØØ9

✓5th **S95.9 Injury of unspecified blood vessel at ankle and foot level**

✓6th **S95.9Ø Unspecified injury of unspecified blood vessel at ankle and foot level**

✓7th **S95.9Ø1 Unspecified injury of unspecified blood vessel at ankle and foot level, right leg** CC
CC Excl: See code: S95.ØØ1

✓7th **S95.9Ø2 Unspecified injury of unspecified blood vessel at ankle and foot level, left leg** CC
CC Excl: See code: S95.ØØ2

✓7th **S95.9Ø9 Unspecified injury of unspecified blood vessel at ankle and foot level, unspecified leg** CC
CC Excl: See code: S95.ØØ9

✓6th **S95.91 Laceration of unspecified blood vessel at ankle and foot level**

✓7th **S95.911 Laceration of unspecified blood vessel at ankle and foot level, right leg** CC
CC Excl: See code: S95.ØØ1

✓7th **S95.912 Laceration of unspecified blood vessel at ankle and foot level, left leg** CC
CC Excl: See code: S95.ØØ2

✓7th **S95.919 Laceration of unspecified blood vessel at ankle and foot level, unspecified leg** CC
CC Excl: See code: S95.ØØ9

✓6th **S95.99 Other specified injury of unspecified blood vessel at ankle and foot level**

✓7th **S95.991 Other specified injury of unspecified blood vessel at ankle and foot level, right leg** CC
CC Excl: See code: S95.ØØ1

✓7th **S95.992 Other specified injury of unspecified blood vessel at ankle and foot level, left leg** CC
CC Excl: See code: S95.ØØ2

✓7th **S95.999 Other specified injury of unspecified blood vessel at ankle and foot level, unspecified leg** CC
CC Excl: See code: S95.ØØ9

✓4th **S96 Injury of muscle and tendon at ankle and foot level**

Code also any associated open wound (S91.-)

EXCLUDES 2 *injury of Achilles tendon (S86.Ø-)*
sprain of joints and ligaments of ankle and foot (S93.-)

The appropriate 7th character is to be added to each code from category S96.
A initial encounter
D subsequent encounter
S sequela

✓5th **S96.Ø Injury of muscle and tendon of long flexor muscle of toe at ankle and foot level**

✓6th **S96.ØØ Unspecified injury of muscle and tendon of long flexor muscle of toe at ankle and foot level**

✓7th **S96.ØØ1 Unspecified injury of muscle and tendon of long flexor muscle of toe at ankle and foot level, right foot**

✓7th **S96.ØØ2 Unspecified injury of muscle and tendon of long flexor muscle of toe at ankle and foot level, left foot**

✓7th **S96.ØØ9 Unspecified injury of muscle and tendon of long flexor muscle of toe at ankle and foot level, unspecified foot**

✓6th **S96.Ø1 Strain of muscle and tendon of long flexor muscle of toe at ankle and foot level**

✓7th **S96.Ø11 Strain of muscle and tendon of long flexor muscle of toe at ankle and foot level, right foot**

✓7th **S96.Ø12 Strain of muscle and tendon of long flexor muscle of toe at ankle and foot level, left foot**

✓7th **S96.Ø19 Strain of muscle and tendon of long flexor muscle of toe at ankle and foot level, unspecified foot**

✓6th **S96.Ø2 Laceration of muscle and tendon of long flexor muscle of toe at ankle and foot level**

✓7th **S96.Ø21 Laceration of muscle and tendon of long flexor muscle of toe at ankle and foot level, right foot** CC
CC Excl: CC with 7th character A: S81.ØØ1A, S81.ØØ9-S81.Ø11 with 7th A, S81.Ø19-S81.Ø21 with 7th A, S81.Ø29-S81.Ø31 with 7th A, S81.Ø39-S81.Ø41 with 7th A, S81.Ø49-S81.Ø51 with 7th A, S81.Ø59-S81.8Ø1 with 7th A, S81.8Ø9-S81.811 with 7th A, S81.819-S81.821 with 7th A, S81.829-S81.831 with 7th A, S81.839-S81.841 with 7th A, S81.849-S81.851 with 7th A, S81.859A, S86.Ø21 A, S86.Ø29 with 7th A, S86.121A, S86.129A, S86.221A, S86.229A, S86.321A, S86.329A, S86.821A, S86.829A, S86.921A, S86.929A, S91.ØØ1A, S91.ØØ9-S91.Ø11 with 7th A, S91.Ø19-S91.Ø21 with 7th A, S91.Ø29-S91.Ø31 with 7th A, S91.Ø39-S91.Ø41 with 7th A, S91.Ø49-S91.Ø51 with 7th A, S91.Ø59A, S96.Ø21A, S96.Ø29A, S96.121A, S96.129A, S96.221A, S96.229A, S96.821A, S96.829A, S96.921A, S96.929A

✓7th **S96.Ø22 Laceration of muscle and tendon of long flexor muscle of toe at ankle and foot level, left foot** CC
CC Excl: CC with 7th character A: S81.ØØ2-S81.ØØ9 with 7th A, S81.Ø12-S81.Ø19 with 7th A, S81.Ø22-S81.Ø29 with 7th A, S81.Ø32-S81.Ø39 with 7th A, S81.Ø42-S81.Ø49 with 7th A, S81.Ø52-S81.Ø59 with 7th A, S81.8Ø2-S81.8Ø9 with 7th A, S81.812-S81.819 with 7th A, S81.822-S81.829 with 7th A, S81.832-S81.839 with 7th A, S81.842-S81.849 with 7th A, S81.852-S81.859 with 7th A, S86.Ø22-S86.Ø29 with 7th A, S86.122-S86.129 with 7th A, S86.222-S86.229 with 7th A, S86.322-S86.329 with 7th A, S86.822-S86.829 with 7th A, S86.922-S86.929 with 7th A, S91.ØØ2-S91.ØØ9 with 7th A, S91.Ø12-S91.Ø19 with 7th A, S91.Ø22-S91.Ø29 with 7th A, S91.Ø32-S91.Ø39 with 7th A, S91.Ø42-S91.Ø49 with 7th A, S91.Ø52-S91.Ø59 with 7th A, S96.Ø22-S96.Ø29 with 7th A, S96.122-S96.129 with 7th A, S96.222-S96.229 with 7th A, S96.822-S96.829 with 7th A, S96.922-S96.929 with 7th A

✓7th **S96.Ø29 Laceration of muscle and tendon of long flexor muscle of toe at ankle and foot level, unspecified foot** CC
CC Excl: CC with 7th character A: S81.ØØ1-S81.859 with 7th A, S86.Ø21-S86.Ø29 with 7th A, S86.121-S86.129 with 7th A, S86.221-S86.229 with 7th A, S86.321-S86.329 with 7th A, S86.821-S86.829 with 7th A, S86.921-S86.929 with 7th A, S91.ØØ1-S91.Ø59 with 7th A, S96.Ø21-S96.Ø29 with 7th A, S96.121-S96.129 with 7th A, S96.221-S96.229 with 7th A, S96.821-S96.829 with 7th A, S96.921-S96.929 with 7th A

✓6th **S96.Ø9 Other injury of muscle and tendon of long flexor muscle of toe at ankle and foot level**

✓7th **S96.Ø91 Other injury of muscle and tendon of long flexor muscle of toe at ankle and foot level, right foot**

✓7th **S96.Ø92 Other injury of muscle and tendon of long flexor muscle of toe at ankle and foot level, left foot**

✓7th **S96.Ø99 Other injury of muscle and tendon of long flexor muscle of toe at ankle and foot level, unspecified foot**

✓5th **S96.1 Injury of muscle and tendon of long extensor muscle of toe at ankle and foot level**

✓6th **S96.1Ø Unspecified injury of muscle and tendon of long extensor muscle of toe at ankle and foot level**

✓7th **S96.1Ø1 Unspecified injury of muscle and tendon of long extensor muscle of toe at ankle and foot level, right foot**

✓7th **S96.1Ø2 Unspecified injury of muscle and tendon of long extensor muscle of toe at ankle and foot level, left foot**

✓7th **S96.1Ø9 Unspecified injury of muscle and tendon of long extensor muscle of toe at ankle and foot level, unspecified foot**

✓6th S96.11 Strain of muscle and tendon of long extensor muscle of toe at ankle and foot level

✓7th S96.111 Strain of muscle and tendon of long extensor muscle of toe at ankle and foot level, right foot

✓7th S96.112 Strain of muscle and tendon of long extensor muscle of toe at ankle and foot level, left foot

✓7th S96.119 Strain of muscle and tendon of long extensor muscle of toe at ankle and foot level, unspecified foot

✓6th S96.12 Laceration of muscle and tendon of long extensor muscle of toe at ankle and foot level

✓7th S96.121 Laceration of muscle and tendon of long extensor muscle of toe at ankle and foot level, right foot CC
CC Excl: See code: S95.021

✓7th S96.122 Laceration of muscle and tendon of long extensor muscle of toe at ankle and foot level, left foot CC
CC Excl: See code: S95.022

✓7th S96.129 Laceration of muscle and tendon of long extensor muscle of toe at ankle and foot level, unspecified foot CC
CC Excl: See code: S95.029

✓6th S96.19 Other specified injury of muscle and tendon of long extensor muscle of toe at ankle and foot level

✓7th S96.191 Other specified injury of muscle and tendon of long extensor muscle of toe at ankle and foot level, right foot

✓7th S96.192 Other specified injury of muscle and tendon of long extensor muscle of toe at ankle and foot level, left foot

✓7th S96.199 Other specified injury of muscle and tendon of long extensor muscle of toe at ankle and foot level, unspecified foot

✓5th S96.2 Injury of intrinsic muscle and tendon at ankle and foot level

✓6th S96.20 Unspecified injury of intrinsic muscle and tendon at ankle and foot level

✓7th S96.201 Unspecified injury of intrinsic muscle and tendon at ankle and foot level, right foot

✓7th S96.202 Unspecified injury of intrinsic muscle and tendon at ankle and foot level, left foot

✓7th S96.209 Unspecified injury of intrinsic muscle and tendon at ankle and foot level, unspecified foot

✓6th S96.21 Strain of intrinsic muscle and tendon at ankle and foot level

✓7th S96.211 Strain of intrinsic muscle and tendon at ankle and foot level, right foot

✓7th S96.212 Strain of intrinsic muscle and tendon at ankle and foot level, left foot

✓7th S96.219 Strain of intrinsic muscle and tendon at ankle and foot level, unspecified foot

✓6th S96.22 Laceration of intrinsic muscle and tendon at ankle and foot level

✓7th S96.221 Laceration of intrinsic muscle and tendon at ankle and foot level, right foot CC
CC Excl: See code: S95.021

✓7th S96.222 Laceration of intrinsic muscle and tendon at ankle and foot level, left foot CC
CC Excl: See code: S95.022

✓7th S96.229 Laceration of intrinsic muscle and tendon at ankle and foot level, unspecified foot CC
CC Excl: See code: S95.029

✓6th S96.29 Other specified injury of intrinsic muscle and tendon at ankle and foot level

✓7th S96.291 Other specified injury of intrinsic muscle and tendon at ankle and foot level, right foot

✓7th S96.292 Other specified injury of intrinsic muscle and tendon at ankle and foot level, left foot

✓7th S96.299 Other specified injury of intrinsic muscle and tendon at ankle and foot level, unspecified foot

✓5th S96.8 Injury of other specified muscles and tendons at ankle and foot level

✓6th S96.80 Unspecified injury of other specified muscles and tendons at ankle and foot level

✓7th S96.801 Unspecified injury of other specified muscles and tendons at ankle and foot level, right foot

✓7th S96.802 Unspecified injury of other specified muscles and tendons at ankle and foot level, left foot

✓7th S96.809 Unspecified injury of other specified muscles and tendons at ankle and foot level, unspecified foot

✓6th S96.81 Strain of other specified muscles and tendons at ankle and foot level

✓7th S96.811 Strain of other specified muscles and tendons at ankle and foot level, right foot

✓7th S96.812 Strain of other specified muscles and tendons at ankle and foot level, left foot

✓7th S96.819 Strain of other specified muscles and tendons at ankle and foot level, unspecified foot

✓6th S96.82 Laceration of other specified muscles and tendons at ankle and foot level

✓7th S96.821 Laceration of other specified muscles and tendons at ankle and foot level, right foot CC
CC Excl: See code: S95.021

✓7th S96.822 Laceration of other specified muscles and tendons at ankle and foot level, left foot CC
CC Excl: See code: S95.022

✓7th S96.829 Laceration of other specified muscles and tendons at ankle and foot level, unspecified foot CC
CC Excl: See code: S95.029

✓6th S96.89 Other specified injury of other specified muscles and tendons at ankle and foot level

✓7th S96.891 Other specified injury of other specified muscles and tendons at ankle and foot level, right foot

✓7th S96.892 Other specified injury of other specified muscles and tendons at ankle and foot level, left foot

✓7th S96.899 Other specified injury of other specified muscles and tendons at ankle and foot level, unspecified foot

✓5th S96.9 Injury of unspecified muscle and tendon at ankle and foot level

✓6th S96.90 Unspecified injury of unspecified muscle and tendon at ankle and foot level

✓7th S96.901 Unspecified injury of unspecified muscle and tendon at ankle and foot level, right foot

✓7th S96.902 Unspecified injury of unspecified muscle and tendon at ankle and foot level, left foot

✓7th S96.909 Unspecified injury of unspecified muscle and tendon at ankle and foot level, unspecified foot

✓6th S96.91 Strain of unspecified muscle and tendon at ankle and foot level

✓7th S96.911 Strain of unspecified muscle and tendon at ankle and foot level, right foot

✓7th S96.912 Strain of unspecified muscle and tendon at ankle and foot level, left foot

✓7th S96.919 Strain of unspecified muscle and tendon at ankle and foot level, unspecified foot

√6th **S96.92 Laceration of unspecified muscle and tendon at ankle and foot level**

√7th **S96.921 Laceration of unspecified muscle and tendon at ankle and foot level, right foot** CC
CC Excl: See code: S95.Ø21

√7th **S96.922 Laceration of unspecified muscle and tendon at ankle and foot level, left foot** CC
CC Excl: See code: S95.Ø22

√7th **S96.929 Laceration of unspecified muscle and tendon at ankle and foot level, unspecified foot** CC
CC Excl: See code: S95.Ø29

√6th **S96.99 Other specified injury of unspecified muscle and tendon at ankle and foot level**

√7th **S96.991 Other specified injury of unspecified muscle and tendon at ankle and foot level, right foot**

√7th **S96.992 Other specified injury of unspecified muscle and tendon at ankle and foot level, left foot**

√7th **S96.999 Other specified injury of unspecified muscle and tendon at ankle and foot level, unspecified foot**

√4th **S97 Crushing injury of ankle and foot**
Use additional code(s) for all associated injuries

The appropriate 7th character is to be added to each code from category S97.
A initial encounter
D subsequent encounter
S sequela

√5th **S97.Ø Crushing injury of ankle**

√x7th **S97.ØØ Crushing injury of unspecified ankle**

√x7th **S97.Ø1 Crushing injury of right ankle**

√x7th **S97.Ø2 Crushing injury of left ankle**

√5th **S97.1 Crushing injury of toe**

√6th **S97.1Ø Crushing injury of unspecified toe(s)**

√7th **S97.1Ø1 Crushing injury of unspecified right toe(s)**

√7th **S97.1Ø2 Crushing injury of unspecified left toe(s)**

√7th **S97.1Ø9 Crushing injury of unspecified toe(s)**
Crushing injury of toe NOS

√6th **S97.11 Crushing injury of great toe**

√7th **S97.111 Crushing injury of right great toe**

√7th **S97.112 Crushing injury of left great toe**

√7th **S97.119 Crushing injury of unspecified great toe**

√6th **S97.12 Crushing injury of lesser toe(s)**

√7th **S97.121 Crushing injury of right lesser toe(s)**

√7th **S97.122 Crushing injury of left lesser toe(s)**

√7th **S97.129 Crushing injury of unspecified lesser toe(s)**

√5th **S97.8 Crushing injury of foot**

√x7th **S97.8Ø Crushing injury of unspecified foot**
Crushing injury of foot NOS

√x7th **S97.81 Crushing injury of right foot**

√x7th **S97.82 Crushing injury of left foot**

√4th **S98 Traumatic amputation of ankle and foot**
An amputation not identified as partial or complete should be coded to complete

The appropriate 7th character is to be added to each code from category S98.
A initial encounter
D subsequent encounter
S sequela

√5th **S98.Ø Traumatic amputation of foot at ankle level**

√6th **S98.Ø1 Complete traumatic amputation of foot at ankle level**

√7th **S98.Ø11 Complete traumatic amputation of right foot at ankle level** CC
CC Excl: CC with 7th character A: S71.ØØ1 with 7th A, S71.ØØ9-S71.Ø11 with 7th A, S71.Ø19-S71.Ø21 with 7th A, S71.Ø29-S71.Ø31 with 7th A, S71.Ø39-S71.Ø41 with 7th A, S71.Ø49-S71.Ø51 with 7th A, S71.Ø59-S71.1Ø1 with 7th A, S71.1Ø9-S71.111 with 7th A, S71.119-S71.121 with 7th A, S71.129-S71.131 with 7th A, S71.139-S71.141 with 7th A, S71.149-S71.151 with 7th A, S71.159 with 7th A, S76.Ø21 with 7th A, S76.Ø29 with 7th A, S76.121 with 7th A, S76.129 with 7th A, S76.221 with 7th A, S76.229 with 7th A, S76.321 with 7th A, S76.329 with 7th A, S76.821 with 7th A, S76.829 with 7th A, S76.921 with 7th A, S76.929 with 7th A, S78.Ø11 with 7th A, S78.Ø19-S78.Ø21 with 7th A, S78.Ø29-S78.111 with 7th A, S78.119-S78.121 with 7th A, S78.129-S78.911 with 7th A, S78.919-S78.921 with 7th A, S78.929 with 7th A, S81.ØØ1 with 7th A, S81.ØØ9-S81.Ø11 with 7th A, S81.Ø19-S81.Ø21 with 7th A, S81.Ø29-S81.Ø31 with 7th A, S81.Ø39-S81.Ø41 with 7th A, S81.Ø49-S81.Ø51 with 7th A, S81.Ø59-S81.8Ø1 with 7th A, S81.8Ø9-S81.811 with 7th A, S81.819-S81.821 with 7th A, S81.829-S81.831 with 7th A, S81.839-S81.841 with 7th A, S81.849-S81.851 with 7th A, S81.859 with 7th A, S86.Ø21 with 7th A, S86.Ø29 with 7th A, S86.121 with 7th A, S86.129 with 7th A, S86.221 with 7th A, S86.229 with 7th A, S86.321 with 7th A, S86.329 with 7th A, S86.821 with 7th A, S86.829 with 7th A, S86.921 with 7th A, S86.929 with 7th A, S88.Ø11 with 7th A, S88.Ø19-S88.Ø21 with 7th A, S88.Ø29-S88.111 with 7th A, S88.119-S88.121 with 7th A, S88.129-S88.911 with 7th A, S88.919-S88.921 with 7th A, S88.929 with 7th A, S91.ØØ1 with 7th A, S91.ØØ9-S91.Ø11 with 7th A, S91.Ø19-S91.Ø21 with 7th A, S91.Ø29-S91.Ø31 with 7th A, S91.Ø39-S91.Ø41 with 7th A, S91.Ø49-S91.Ø51 with 7th A, S91.Ø59-S91.1Ø1 with 7th A, S91.1Ø3-S91.1Ø4 with 7th A, S91.1Ø6-S91.111 with 7th A, S91.113-S91.114 with 7th A, S91.116-S91.121 with 7th A, S91.123-S91.124 with 7th A, S91.126-S91.131 with 7th A, S91.133-S91.134 with 7th A, S91.136-S91.141 with 7th A, S91.143-S91.144 with 7th A, S91.146-S91.151 with 7th A, S91.153-S91.154 with 7th A, S91.156-S91.2Ø1 with 7th A, S91.2Ø3-S91.2Ø4 with 7th A, S91.2Ø6-S91.211 with 7th A, S91.213-S91.214 with 7th A, S91.216-S91.221 with 7th A, S91.223-S91.224 with 7th A, S91.226-S91.231 with 7th A, S91.233-S91.234 with 7th A, S91.236-S91.241 with 7th A, S91.243-S91.244 with 7th A, S91.246-S91.251 with 7th A, S91.253-S91.254 with 7th A, S91.256-S91.3Ø1 with 7th A, S91.3Ø9-S91.311 with 7th A, S91.319-S91.321 with 7th A, S91.329-S91.331 with 7th A, S91.339-S91.341 with 7th A, S91.349-S91.351 with 7th A, S91.359 with 7th A, S96.Ø21 with 7th A, S96.Ø29 with 7th A, S96.121 with 7th A, S96.129 with 7th A, S96.221 with 7th A, S96.229 with 7th A, S96.821 with 7th A, S96.829 with 7th A, S96.921 with 7th A, S96.929 with 7th A, S98.Ø11 with 7th A, S98.Ø19-S98.Ø21 with 7th A, S98.Ø29-S98.111 with 7th A, S98.119-S98.121 with 7th A

✓7th **S98.Ø12 Complete traumatic amputation of left foot at ankle level** CC
CC Excl: CC with 7th character A: S71.ØØ2-S71.ØØ9 with 7th A, S71.Ø12-S71.Ø19 with 7th A, S71.Ø22-S71.Ø29 with 7th A, S71.Ø32-S71.Ø39 with 7th A, S71.Ø42-S71.Ø49 with 7th A, S71.Ø52-S71.Ø59 with 7th A, S71.1Ø2-S71.1Ø9 with 7th A, S71.112-S71.119 with 7th A, S71.122-S71.129 with 7th A, S71.132-S71.139 with 7th A, S71.142-S71.149 with 7th A, S71.152-S71.159 with 7th A, S76.Ø22-S76.Ø29 with 7th A, S76.122-S76.129 with 7th A, S76.222-S76.229 with 7th A, S76.322-S76.329 with 7th A, S76.822-S76.829 with 7th A, S76.922-S76.929 with 7th A, S78.Ø12-S78.Ø19 with 7th A, S78.Ø22-S78.Ø29 with 7th A, S78.112-S78.119 with 7th A, S78.122-S78.129 with 7th A, S78.912-S78.919 with 7th A, S78.922-S78.929 with 7th A, S81.ØØ2-S81.ØØ9 with 7th A, S81.Ø12-S81.Ø19 with 7th A, S81.Ø22-S81.Ø29 with 7th A, S81.Ø32-S81.Ø39 with 7th A, S81.Ø42-S81.Ø49 with 7th A, S81.Ø52-S81.Ø59 with 7th A, S81.8Ø2-S81.8Ø9 with 7th A, S81.812-S81.819 with 7th A, S81.822-S81.829 with 7th A, S81.832-S81.839 with 7th A, S81.842-S81.849 with 7th A, S81.852-S81.859 with 7th A, S86.Ø22-S86.Ø29 with 7th A, S86.122-S86.129 with 7th A, S86.222-S86.229 with 7th A, S86.322-S86.329 with 7th A, S86.822-S86.829 with 7th A, S86.922-S86.929 with 7th A, S88.Ø12-S88.Ø19 with 7th A, S88.Ø22-S88.Ø29 with 7th A, S88.112-S88.119 with 7th A, S88.122-S88.129 with 7th A, S88.912-S88.919 with 7th A, S88.922-S88.929 with 7th A, S91.ØØ2-S91.ØØ9 with 7th A, S91.Ø12-S91.Ø19 with 7th A, S91.Ø22-S91.Ø29 with 7th A, S91.Ø32-S91.Ø39 with 7th A, S91.Ø42-S91.Ø49 with 7th A, S91.Ø52-S91.Ø59 with 7th A, S91.1Ø2-S91.1Ø3 with 7th A, S91.1Ø5-S91.1Ø9 with 7th A, S91.112-S91.113 with 7th A, S91.115-S91.119 with 7th A, S91.122-S91.123 with 7th A, S91.125-S91.129 with 7th A, S91.132-S91.133 with 7th A, S91.135-S91.139 with 7th A, S91.142-S91.143 with 7th A, S91.145-S91.149 with 7th A, S91.152-S91.153 with 7th A, S91.155-S91.159 with 7th A, S91.2Ø2-S91.2Ø3 with 7th A, S91.2Ø5-S91.2Ø9 with 7th A, S91.212-S91.213 with 7th A, S91.215-S91.219 with 7th A, S91.222-S91.223 with 7th A, S91.225-S91.229 with 7th A, S91.232-S91.233 with 7th A, S91.235-S91.239 with 7th A, S91.242-S91.243 with 7th A, S91.245-S91.249 with 7th A, S91.252-S91.253 with 7th A, S91.255-S91.259 with 7th A, S91.3Ø2-S91.3Ø9 with 7th A, S91.312-S91.319 with 7th A, S91.322-S91.329 with 7th A, S91.332-S91.339 with 7th A, S91.342-S91.349 with 7th A, S91.352-S91.359 with 7th A, S96.Ø22-S96.Ø29 with 7th A, S96.122-S96.129 with 7th A, S96.222-S96.229 with 7th A, S96.822-S96.829 with 7th A, S96.922-S96.929 with 7th A, S98.Ø12-S98.Ø19 with 7th A, S98.Ø22-S98.Ø29 with 7th A, S98.112-S98.119 with 7th A, S98.122-S98.129 with 7th A, S98.132-S98.139 with 7th A, S98.142-S98.149 with 7th A, S98.212-S98.219 with 7th A, S98.222-S98.229 with 7th A, S98.312-S98.319 with 7th A, S98.322-S98.329 with 7th A, S98.912-S98.919 with 7th A, S98.922-S98.929 with 7th A, T14.8-T14.91, T79.AØX-T79.9XX with 7th A

✓7th **S98.Ø19 Complete traumatic amputation of unspecified foot at ankle level** CC
CC Excl: CC with 7th character A: S71.ØØ1-S71.159 with 7th A, S76.Ø21-S76.Ø29 with 7th A, S76.121-S76.129 with 7th A, S76.221-S76.229 with 7th A, S76.321-S76.329 with 7th A, S76.821-S76.829 with 7th A, S76.921-S76.929 with 7th A, S78.Ø11-S78.929 with 7th A, S81.ØØ1-S81.859 with 7th A, S86.Ø21-S86.Ø29 with 7th A, S86.121-S86.129 with 7th A, S86.221-S86.229 with 7th A, S86.321-S86.329 with 7th A, S86.821-S86.829 with 7th A, S86.921-S86.929 with 7th A, S88.Ø11-S88.929 with 7th A, S91.ØØ1-S91.359 with 7th A, S96.Ø21-S96.Ø29 with 7th A, S96.121-S96.129 with 7th A, S96.221-S96.229 with 7th A, S96.821-S96.829 with 7th A, S96.921-S96.929 with 7th A, S98.Ø11-S98.929 with 7th A, T14.8-T14.91, T79.AØX-T79.9XX with 7th A

✓6th **S98.Ø2 Partial traumatic amputation of foot at ankle level**

✓7th **S98.Ø21 Partial traumatic amputation of right foot at ankle level** CC
CC Excl: See code: S98.Ø11

✓7th **S98.Ø22 Partial traumatic amputation of left foot at ankle level** CC
CC Excl: See code: S98.Ø12

✓7th **S98.Ø29 Partial traumatic amputation of unspecified foot at ankle level** CC
CC Excl: See code: S98.Ø19

✓5th **S98.1 Traumatic amputation of one toe**

✓6th **S98.11 Complete traumatic amputation of great toe**

✓7th **S98.111 Complete traumatic amputation of right great toe**

✓7th **S98.112 Complete traumatic amputation of left great toe**

✓7th **S98.119 Complete traumatic amputation of unspecified great toe**

✓6th **S98.12 Partial traumatic amputation of great toe**

✓7th **S98.121 Partial traumatic amputation of right great toe**

✓7th **S98.122 Partial traumatic amputation of left great toe**

✓7th **S98.129 Partial traumatic amputation of unspecified great toe**

✓6th **S98.13 Complete traumatic amputation of one lesser toe**
Traumatic amputation of toe NOS

✓7th **S98.131 Complete traumatic amputation of one right lesser toe**

✓7th **S98.132 Complete traumatic amputation of one left lesser toe**

✓7th **S98.139 Complete traumatic amputation of one unspecified lesser toe**

✓6th **S98.14 Partial traumatic amputation of one lesser toe**

✓7th **S98.141 Partial traumatic amputation of one right lesser toe**

✓7th **S98.142 Partial traumatic amputation of one left lesser toe**

✓7th **S98.149 Partial traumatic amputation of one unspecified lesser toe**

✓5th **S98.2 Traumatic amputation of two or more lesser toes**

✓6th **S98.21 Complete traumatic amputation of two or more lesser toes**

✓7th **S98.211 Complete traumatic amputation of two or more right lesser toes**

✓7th **S98.212 Complete traumatic amputation of two or more left lesser toes**

✓7th **S98.219 Complete traumatic amputation of two or more unspecified lesser toes**

✓6th **S98.22 Partial traumatic amputation of two or more lesser toes**

✓7th **S98.221 Partial traumatic amputation of two or more right lesser toes**

✓7th **S98.222 Partial traumatic amputation of two or more left lesser toes**

✓7th **S98.229 Partial traumatic amputation of two or more unspecified lesser toes**

✓5th **S98.3 Traumatic amputation of midfoot**

✓6th **S98.31 Complete traumatic amputation of midfoot**

✓7th **S98.311 Complete traumatic amputation of right midfoot** CC
CC Excl: See code: S98.Ø11

✓7th **S98.312 Complete traumatic amputation of left midfoot** CC
CC Excl: See code: S98.Ø12

✓7th **S98.319 Complete traumatic amputation of unspecified midfoot** CC
CC Excl: See code: S98.Ø19

✓6th **S98.32 Partial traumatic amputation of midfoot**

✓7th **S98.321 Partial traumatic amputation of right midfoot** CC
CC Excl: See code: S98.Ø11

✓7th **S98.322 Partial traumatic amputation of left midfoot** CC
CC Excl: See code: S98.Ø12

✓7th **S98.329 Partial traumatic amputation of unspecified midfoot** CC
CC Excl: See code: S98.019

✓5th **S98.9 Traumatic amputation of foot, level unspecified**

✓6th **S98.91 Complete traumatic amputation of foot, level unspecified**

✓7th **S98.911 Complete traumatic amputation of right foot, level unspecified** CC
CC Excl: See code: S98.011

✓7th **S98.912 Complete traumatic amputation of left foot, level unspecified** CC
CC Excl: See code: S98.012

✓7th **S98.919 Complete traumatic amputation of unspecified foot, level unspecified** CC
CC Excl: See code: S98.019

✓6th **S98.92 Partial traumatic amputation of foot, level unspecified**

✓7th **S98.921 Partial traumatic amputation of right foot, level unspecified** CC
CC Excl: See code: S98.011

✓7th **S98.922 Partial traumatic amputation of left foot, level unspecified** CC
CC Excl: See code: S98.012

✓7th **S98.929 Partial traumatic amputation of unspecified foot, level unspecified** CC
CC Excl: See code: S98.019

✓4th **S99 Other and unspecified injuries of ankle and foot**

The appropriate 7th character is to be added to each code from category S99.
A initial encounter
D subsequent encounter
S sequela

✓5th **S99.8 Other specified injuries of ankle and foot**

✓6th **S99.81 Other specified injuries of ankle**

✓7th **S99.811 Other specified injuries of right ankle**

✓7th **S99.812 Other specified injuries of left ankle**

✓7th **S99.819 Other specified injuries of unspecified ankle**

✓6th **S99.82 Other specified injuries of foot**

✓7th **S99.821 Other specified injuries of right foot**

✓7th **S99.822 Other specified injuries of left foot**

✓7th **S99.829 Other specified injuries of unspecified foot**

✓5th **S99.9 Unspecified injury of ankle and foot**

✓6th **S99.91 Unspecified injury of ankle**

✓7th **S99.911 Unspecified injury of right ankle**

✓7th **S99.912 Unspecified injury of left ankle**

✓7th **S99.919 Unspecified injury of unspecified ankle**

✓6th **S99.92 Unspecified injury of foot**

✓7th **S99.921 Unspecified injury of right foot**

✓7th **S99.922 Unspecified injury of left foot**

✓7th **S99.929 Unspecified injury of unspecified foot**

Injury, Poisoning And Certain Other Consequences Of External Causes (T07-T88)

Injuries involving multiple body regions (T07)

EXCLUDES 1 *burns and corrosions (T20-T32)*
frostbite (T33-T34)
insect bite or sting, venomous (T63.4)
sunburn (L55.-)

T07 Unspecified multiple injuries
EXCLUDES 1 *injury NOS (T14)*

Injury of unspecified body region (T14)

✓4th **T14 Injury of unspecified body region**
EXCLUDES 1 *multiple unspecified injuries (T07)*

T14.8 Other injury of unspecified body region
Abrasion NOS
Contusion NOS
Crush injury NOS
Fracture NOS
Skin injury NOS
Vascular injury NOS

✓5th **T14.9 Unspecified injury**

T14.90 Injury, unspecified
Injury NOS

T14.91 Suicide attempt
Attempted suicide NOS

Effects of foreign body entering through natural orifice (T15-T19)

EXCLUDES 2 *foreign body accidentally left in operation wound (T81.5-)*
foreign body in penetrating wound—See open wound by body region
residual foreign body in soft tissue (M79.5)
splinter, without open wound—See superficial injury by body region

✓4th **T15 Foreign body on external eye**
EXCLUDES 2 *foreign body in penetrating wound of orbit and eye ball (S05.4-, S05.5-)*
open wound of eyelid and periocular area (S01.1-)
retained foreign body in eyelid (H02.8-)
retained (old) foreign body in penetrating wound of orbit and eye ball (H05.5-, H44.6-, H44.7-)
superficial foreign body of eyelid and periocular area (S00.25-)

The appropriate 7th character is to be added to each code from category T15.
A initial encounter
D subsequent encounter
S sequela

✓5th **T15.0 Foreign body in cornea**

✓x7th **T15.00 Foreign body in cornea, unspecified eye**

✓x7th **T15.01 Foreign body in cornea, right eye**

✓x7th **T15.02 Foreign body in cornea, left eye**

✓5th **T15.1 Foreign body in conjunctival sac**

✓x7th **T15.10 Foreign body in conjunctival sac, unspecified eye**

✓x7th **T15.11 Foreign body in conjunctival sac, right eye**

✓x7th **T15.12 Foreign body in conjunctival sac, left eye**

✓5th **T15.8 Foreign body in other and multiple parts of external eye**
Foreign body in lacrimal punctum

✓x7th **T15.80 Foreign body in other and multiple parts of external eye, unspecified eye**

✓x7th **T15.81 Foreign body in other and multiple parts of external eye, right eye**

✓x7th **T15.82 Foreign body in other and multiple parts of external eye, left eye**

✓5th **T15.9 Foreign body on external eye, part unspecified**

✓x7th **T15.90 Foreign body on external eye, part unspecified, unspecified eye**

✓x7th **T15.91 Foreign body on external eye, part unspecified, right eye**

✓x7th **T15.92 Foreign body on external eye, part unspecified, left eye**

✓4th **T16 Foreign body in ear**
Foreign body in auditory canal

The appropriate 7th character is to be added to each code from category T16.
A initial encounter
D subsequent encounter
S sequela

✓x7th **T16.1 Foreign body in right ear**

- T16.2 **Foreign body in left ear**
- T16.9 **Foreign body in ear, unspecified ear**

T17 Foreign body in respiratory tract

> The appropriate 7th character is to be added to each code from category T17.
> A initial encounter
> D subsequent encounter
> S sequela

- T17.0 **Foreign body in nasal sinus**
- T17.1 **Foreign body in nostril**
  Foreign body in nose NOS
- T17.2 **Foreign body in pharynx**
  Foreign body in nasopharynx
  Foreign body in throat NOS
  - T17.20 **Unspecified foreign body in pharynx**
    - T17.200 **Unspecified foreign body in pharynx causing asphyxiation**
    - T17.208 **Unspecified foreign body in pharynx causing other injury**
  - T17.21 **Gastric contents in pharynx**
    Aspiration of gastric contents into pharynx
    Vomitus in pharynx
    - T17.210 **Gastric contents in pharynx causing asphyxiation**
    - T17.218 **Gastric contents in pharynx causing other injury**
  - T17.22 **Food in pharynx**
    Bones in pharynx
    Seeds in pharynx
    - T17.220 **Food in pharynx causing asphyxiation**
    - T17.228 **Food in pharynx causing other injury**
  - T17.29 **Other foreign object in pharynx**
    - T17.290 **Other foreign object in pharynx causing asphyxiation**
    - T17.298 **Other foreign object in pharynx causing other injury**
- T17.3 **Foreign body in larynx**
  - T17.30 **Unspecified foreign body in larynx**
    - T17.300 **Unspecified foreign body in larynx causing asphyxiation**
    - T17.308 **Unspecified foreign body in larynx causing other injury**
  - T17.31 **Gastric contents in larynx**
    Aspiration of gastric contents into larynx
    Vomitus in larynx
    - T17.310 **Gastric contents in larynx causing asphyxiation**
    - T17.318 **Gastric contents in larynx causing other injury**
  - T17.32 **Food in larynx**
    Bones in larynx
    Seeds in larynx
    - T17.320 **Food in larynx causing asphyxiation**
    - T17.328 **Food in larynx causing other injury**
  - T17.39 **Other foreign object in larynx**
    - T17.390 **Other foreign object in larynx causing asphyxiation**
    - T17.398 **Other foreign object in larynx causing other injury**
- T17.4 **Foreign body in trachea**

  > **CC Excl: For CC codes in subcategory T17.4: CC with 7th character A, unless otherwise noted:** T17.400-T17.498 with 7th A

  - T17.40 **Unspecified foreign body in trachea**
    - T17.400 **Unspecified foreign body in trachea causing asphyxiation** CC
    - T17.408 **Unspecified foreign body in trachea causing other injury** CC
  - T17.41 **Gastric contents in trachea**
    Aspiration of gastric contents into trachea
    Vomitus in trachea
    - T17.410 **Gastric contents in trachea causing asphyxiation** CC
    - T17.418 **Gastric contents in trachea causing other injury** CC
  - T17.42 **Food in trachea**
    Bones in trachea
    Seeds in trachea
    - T17.420 **Food in trachea causing asphyxiation** CC
    - T17.428 **Food in trachea causing other injury** CC
  - T17.49 **Other foreign object in trachea**
    - T17.490 **Other foreign object in trachea causing asphyxiation** CC
    - T17.498 **Other foreign object in trachea causing other injury** CC
- T17.5 **Foreign body in bronchus**

  > **CC Excl: For CC codes in subcategory T17.5: CC with 7th character A, unless otherwise noted:** T17.400-T17.998 with 7th A

  - T17.50 **Unspecified foreign body in bronchus**
    - T17.500 **Unspecified foreign body in bronchus causing asphyxiation** CC
    - T17.508 **Unspecified foreign body in bronchus causing other injury** CC
  - T17.51 **Gastric contents in bronchus**
    Aspiration of gastric contents into bronchus
    Vomitus in bronchus
    - T17.510 **Gastric contents in bronchus causing asphyxiation** CC
    - T17.518 **Gastric contents in bronchus causing other injury** CC
  - T17.52 **Food in bronchus**
    Bones in bronchus
    Seeds in bronchus
    - T17.520 **Food in bronchus causing asphyxiation** CC
    - T17.528 **Food in bronchus causing other injury** CC
  - T17.59 **Other foreign object in bronchus**
    - T17.590 **Other foreign object in bronchus causing asphyxiation** CC
    - T17.598 **Other foreign object in bronchus causing other injury** CC
- T17.8 **Foreign body in other parts of respiratory tract**
  Foreign body in bronchioles
  Foreign body in lung

  > **CC Excl: For CC codes in subcategory T17.8: CC with 7th character A, unless otherwise noted:** See code: T17.5

  - T17.80 **Unspecified foreign body in other parts of respiratory tract**
    - T17.800 **Unspecified foreign body in other parts of respiratory tract causing asphyxiation** CC
    - T17.808 **Unspecified foreign body in other parts of respiratory tract causing other injury** CC
  - T17.81 **Gastric contents in other parts of respiratory tract**
    Aspiration of gastric contents into other parts of respiratory tract
    Vomitus in other parts of respiratory tract
    - T17.810 **Gastric contents in other parts of respiratory tract causing asphyxiation** CC
    - T17.818 **Gastric contents in other parts of respiratory tract causing other injury** CC
  - T17.82 **Food in other parts of respiratory tract**
    Bones in other parts of respiratory tract
    Seeds in other parts of respiratory tract
    - T17.820 **Food in other parts of respiratory tract causing asphyxiation** CC
    - T17.828 **Food in other parts of respiratory tract causing other injury** CC
  - T17.89 **Other foreign object in other parts of respiratory tract**
    - T17.890 **Other foreign object in other parts of respiratory tract causing asphyxiation** CC
    - T17.898 **Other foreign object in other parts of respiratory tract causing other injury** CC
- T17.9 **Foreign body in respiratory tract, part unspecified**
  - T17.90 **Unspecified foreign body in respiratory tract, part unspecified**
    - T17.900 **Unspecified foreign body in respiratory tract, part unspecified causing asphyxiation**

✓7th **T17.908 Unspecified foreign body in respiratory tract, part unspecified causing other injury**

✓6th **T17.91 Gastric contents in respiratory tract, part unspecified**
Aspiration of gastric contents into respiratory tract, part unspecified
Vomitus in trachea respiratory tract, part unspecified

✓7th **T17.910 Gastric contents in respiratory tract, part unspecified causing asphyxiation**

✓7th **T17.918 Gastric contents in respiratory tract, part unspecified causing other injury**

✓6th **T17.92 Food in respiratory tract, part unspecified**
Bones in respiratory tract, part unspecified
Seeds in respiratory tract, part unspecified

✓7th **T17.920 Food in respiratory tract, part unspecified causing asphyxiation**

✓7th **T17.928 Food in respiratory tract, part unspecified causing other injury**

✓6th **T17.99 Other foreign object in respiratory tract, part unspecified**

✓7th **T17.990 Other foreign object in respiratory tract, part unspecified in causing asphyxiation**

✓7th **T17.998 Other foreign object in respiratory tract, part unspecified causing other injury**

✓4th **T18 Foreign body in alimentary tract**
EXCLUDES 2 *foreign body in pharynx (T17.2-)*

The appropriate 7th character is to be added to each code from category T18.
A initial encounter
D subsequent encounter
S sequela

✓x7th **T18.0 Foreign body in mouth**

✓5th **T18.1 Foreign body in esophagus**
EXCLUDES 2 *foreign body in respiratory tract (T17.-)*

✓6th **T18.10 Unspecified foreign body in esophagus**

✓7th **T18.100 Unspecified foreign body in esophagus causing compression of trachea**
Unspecified foreign body in esophagus causing obstruction of respiration

✓7th **T18.108 Unspecified foreign body in esophagus causing other injury**

✓6th **T18.11 Gastric contents in esophagus**
Vomitus in esophagus

✓7th **T18.110 Gastric contents in esophagus causing compression of trachea**
Gastric contents in esophagus causing obstruction of respiration

✓7th **T18.118 Gastric contents in esophagus causing other injury**

✓6th **T18.12 Food in esophagus**
Bones in esophagus Seeds in esophagus

✓7th **T18.120 Food in esophagus causing compression of trachea**
Food in esophagus causing obstruction of respiration

✓7th **T18.128 Food in esophagus causing other injury**

✓6th **T18.19 Other foreign object in esophagus**

✓7th **T18.190 Other foreign object in esophagus causing compression of trachea**
Other foreign body in esophagus causing obstruction of respiration

✓7th **T18.198 Other foreign object in esophagus causing other injury**

✓x7th **T18.2 Foreign body in stomach**

✓x7th **T18.3 Foreign body in small intestine**

✓x7th **T18.4 Foreign body in colon**

✓x7th **T18.5 Foreign body in anus and rectum**
Foreign body in rectosigmoid (junction)

✓x7th **T18.8 Foreign body in other parts of alimentary tract**

✓x7th **T18.9 Foreign body of alimentary tract, part unspecified**
Foreign body in digestive system NOS
Swallowed foreign body NOS

✓4th **T19 Foreign body in genitourinary tract**
EXCLUDES 2 *complications due to implanted mesh (T83.7-)*
mechanical complications of contraceptive device (intrauterine) (vaginal) (T83.3-)
presence of contraceptive device (intrauterine) (vaginal) (Z97.5)

The appropriate 7th character is to be added to each code from category T19.
A initial encounter
D subsequent encounter
S sequela

✓x7th **T19.0 Foreign body in urethra**

✓x7th **T19.1 Foreign body in bladder**

✓x7th **T19.2 Foreign body in vulva and vagina** ♀

✓x7th **T19.3 Foreign body in uterus** ♀

✓x7th **T19.4 Foreign body in penis** ♂

✓x7th **T19.8 Foreign body in other parts of genitourinary tract**

✓x7th **T19.9 Foreign body in genitourinary tract, part unspecified**

Burns and corrosions (T20-T32)

INCLUDES burns (thermal) from electrical heating appliances
burns (thermal) from electricity
burns (thermal) from flame
burns (thermal) from friction
burns (thermal) from hot air and hot gases
burns (thermal) from hot objects
burns (thermal) from lightning
burns (thermal) from radiation
chemical burn [corrosion] (external) (internal)
scalds

EXCLUDES 2 *erythema [dermatitis] ab igne (L59.0)*
radiation-related disorders of the skin and subcutaneous tissue (L55-L59)
sunburn (L55.-)

Burns and corrosions of external body surface, specified by site (T20-T25)

INCLUDES burns and corrosions of first degree [erythema]
burns and corrosions of second degree [blisters] [epidermal loss]
burns and corrosions of third degree [deep necrosis of underlying tissue] [full-thickness skin loss]

Use additional code from category T31 or T32 to identify extent of body surface involved

✓4th **T20 Burn and corrosion of head, face, and neck**
EXCLUDES 2 *burn and corrosion of ear drum (T28.41, T28.91)*
burn and corrosion of eye and adnexa (T26.-)
burn and corrosion of mouth and pharynx (T28.0)

The appropriate 7th character is to be added to each code from category T20.
A initial encounter
D subsequent encounter
S sequela

✓5th **T20.0 Burn of unspecified degree of head, face, and neck**
Use additional external cause code to identify the source, place and intent of the burn (X00-X19, X75-X77, X96-X98, Y92)

✓x7th **T20.00 Burn of unspecified degree of head, face, and neck, unspecified site**

✓6th **T20.01 Burn of unspecified degree of ear [any part, except ear drum]**
EXCLUDES 2 *burn of ear drum (T28.41-)*

✓7th **T20.011 Burn of unspecified degree of right ear [any part, except ear drum]**

✓7th **T20.012 Burn of unspecified degree of left ear [any part, except ear drum]**

✓7th **T20.019 Burn of unspecified degree of unspecified ear [any part, except ear drum]**

✓x7th **T20.02 Burn of unspecified degree of lip(s)**

✓x7th **T20.03 Burn of unspecified degree of chin**

✓x7th **T20.04 Burn of unspecified degree of nose (septum)**

✓x7th **T20.05 Burn of unspecified degree of scalp [any part]**

✓x7th **T20.06 Burn of unspecified degree of forehead and cheek**

✓x7th **T20.07 Burn of unspecified degree of neck**

✓x7th **T20.09 Burn of unspecified degree of multiple sites of head, face, and neck**

Injury, Poisoning and Certain Other Consequences of External Causes T17.908–T20.09

√5th **T20.1 Burn of first degree of head, face, and neck**
Use additional external cause code to identify the source, place and intent of the burn (X00-X19, X75-X77, X96-X98, Y92)

√x7th **T20.10 Burn of first degree of head, face, and neck, unspecified site**

√6th **T20.11 Burn of first degree of ear [any part, except ear drum]**
EXCLUDES 2 *burn of ear drum (T28.41-)*

√7th **T20.111 Burn of first degree of right ear [any part, except ear drum]**

√7th **T20.112 Burn of first degree of left ear [any part, except ear drum]**

√7th **T20.119 Burn of first degree of unspecified ear [any part, except ear drum]**

√x7th **T20.12 Burn of first degree of lip(s)**

√x7th **T20.13 Burn of first degree of chin**

√x7th **T20.14 Burn of first degree of nose (septum)**

√x7th **T20.15 Burn of first degree of scalp [any part]**

√x7th **T20.16 Burn of first degree of forehead and cheek**

√x7th **T20.17 Burn of first degree of neck**

√x7th **T20.19 Burn of first degree of multiple sites of head, face, and neck**

√5th **T20.2 Burn of second degree of head, face, and neck**
Use additional external cause code to identify the source, place and intent of the burn (X00-X19, X75-X77, X96-X98, Y92)

√x7th **T20.20 Burn of second degree of head, face, and neck, unspecified site**

√6th **T20.21 Burn of second degree of ear [any part, except ear drum]**
EXCLUDES 2 *burn of ear drum (T28.41-)*

√7th **T20.211 Burn of second degree of right ear [any part, except ear drum]**

√7th **T20.212 Burn of second degree of left ear [any part, except ear drum]**

√7th **T20.219 Burn of second degree of unspecified ear [any part, except ear drum]**

√x7th **T20.22 Burn of second degree of lip(s)**

√x7th **T20.23 Burn of second degree of chin**

√x7th **T20.24 Burn of second degree of nose (septum)**

√x7th **T20.25 Burn of second degree of scalp [any part]**

√x7th **T20.26 Burn of second degree of forehead and cheek**

√x7th **T20.27 Burn of second degree of neck**

√x7th **T20.29 Burn of second degree of multiple sites of head, face, and neck**

√5th **T20.3 Burn of third degree of head, face, and neck**
Use additional external cause code to identify the source, place and intent of the burn (X00-X19, X75-X77, X96-X98, Y92)

7 √x7th **T20.30 Burn of third degree of head, face, and neck, unspecified site** CC
CC Excl: CC with 7th character A: T20.30XA, T20.39XA, T20.70XA, T20.79XA

√6th **T20.31 Burn of third degree of ear [any part, except ear drum]**
EXCLUDES 2 *burn of ear drum (T28.41-)*

7 √7th **T20.311 Burn of third degree of right ear [any part, except ear drum]** CC
CC Excl: CC with 7th character A: T20.311-T20.319 with 7th A , T20.39XA, T20.711-T20.719 with 7th A, T20.79XA

7 √7th **T20.312 Burn of third degree of left ear [any part, except ear drum]** CC
CC Excl: See code: T20.311

7 √7th **T20.319 Burn of third degree of unspecified ear [any part, except ear drum]** CC
CC Excl: See code: T20.311

7 √x7th **T20.32 Burn of third degree of lip(s)** CC
CC Excl: CC with 7th character A: T20.32XA,T20.39XA,T20.72XA,T20.79XA

7 √x7th **T20.33 Burn of third degree of chin** CC
CC Excl: CC with 7th character A:T20.33XA,T20.39XA,T20.73XA,T20.79XA

7 √x7th **T20.34 Burn of third degree of nose (septum)** CC
CC Excl: CC with 7th character A: T20.34XA,T20.39XA,T20.74XA,T20.79XA

7 √x7th **T20.35 Burn of third degree of scalp [any part]** CC
CC Excl: CC with 7th character A: T20.35XA,T20.39XA,T20.75XA,T20.79XA

7 √x7th **T20.36 Burn of third degree of forehead and cheek** CC
CC Excl: CC with 7th character A: T20.36XA,T20.39XA,T20.76XA,T20.79XA

7 √x7th **T20.37 Burn of third degree of neck** CC
CC Excl: CC with 7th character A:T20.37XA,T20.39XA,T20.77XA,T20.79XA

7 √x7th **T20.39 Burn of third degree of multiple sites of head, face, and neck** CC
CC Excl: CC with 7th character A:T20.30X-T20.39X with 7th A, T20.70X-T20.79X with 7th A

√5th **T20.4 Corrosion of unspecified degree of head, face, and neck**
Code first (T51-T65) to identify chemical and intent
Use additional external cause code to identify place (Y92)

√x7th **T20.40 Corrosion of unspecified degree of head, face, and neck, unspecified site**

√6th **T20.41 Corrosion of unspecified degree of ear [any part, except ear drum]**
EXCLUDES 2 *corrosion of ear drum (T28.91-)*

√7th **T20.411 Corrosion of unspecified degree of right ear [any part, except ear drum]**

√7th **T20.412 Corrosion of unspecified degree of left ear [any part, except ear drum]**

√7th **T20.419 Corrosion of unspecified degree of unspecified ear [any part, except ear drum]**

√x7th **T20.42 Corrosion of unspecified degree of lip(s)**

√x7th **T20.43 Corrosion of unspecified degree of chin**

√x7th **T20.44 Corrosion of unspecified degree of nose (septum)**

√x7th **T20.45 Corrosion of unspecified degree of scalp [any part]**

√x7th **T20.46 Corrosion of unspecified degree of forehead and cheek**

√x7th **T20.47 Corrosion of unspecified degree of neck**

√x7th **T20.49 Corrosion of unspecified degree of multiple sites of head, face, and neck**

√5th **T20.5 Corrosion of first degree of head, face, and neck**
Code first (T51-T65) to identify chemical and intent
Use additional external cause code to identify place (Y92)

√x7th **T20.50 Corrosion of first degree of head, face, and neck, unspecified site**

√6th **T20.51 Corrosion of first degree of ear [any part, except ear drum]**
EXCLUDES 2 *corrosion of ear drum (T28.91-)*

√7th **T20.511 Corrosion of first degree of right ear [any part, except ear drum]**

√7th **T20.512 Corrosion of first degree of left ear [any part, except ear drum]**

√7th **T20.519 Corrosion of first degree of unspecified ear [any part, except ear drum]**

√x7th **T20.52 Corrosion of first degree of lip(s)**

√x7th **T20.53 Corrosion of first degree of chin**

√x7th **T20.54 Corrosion of first degree of nose (septum)**

√x7th **T20.55 Corrosion of first degree of scalp [any part]**

√x7th **T20.56 Corrosion of first degree of forehead and cheek**

√x7th **T20.57 Corrosion of first degree of neck**

√x7th **T20.59 Corrosion of first degree of multiple sites of head, face, and neck**

√5th **T20.6 Corrosion of second degree of head, face, and neck**
Code first (T51-T65) to identify chemical and intent
Use additional external cause code to identify place (Y92)

√x7th **T20.60 Corrosion of second degree of head, face, and neck, unspecified site**

√6th **T20.61 Corrosion of second degree of ear [any part, except ear drum]**
EXCLUDES 2 *corrosion of ear drum (T28.91-)*

√7th **T20.611 Corrosion of second degree of right ear [any part, except ear drum]**

√7th **T20.612 Corrosion of second degree of left ear [any part, except ear drum]**

√7th **T20.619 Corrosion of second degree of unspecified ear [any part, except ear drum]**

7 HAC = Initial encounter only (7th character A, B or C) and not POA.

✓x7th **T20.62 Corrosion of second degree of lip(s)**

✓x7th **T20.63 Corrosion of second degree of chin**

✓x7th **T20.64 Corrosion of second degree of nose (septum)**

✓x7th **T20.65 Corrosion of second degree of scalp [any part]**

✓x7th **T20.66 Corrosion of second degree of forehead and cheek**

✓x7th **T20.67 Corrosion of second degree of neck**

✓x7th **T20.69 Corrosion of second degree of multiple sites of head, face, and neck**

✓5th **T20.7 Corrosion of third degree of head, face, and neck**
Code first (T51-T65) to identify chemical and intent
Use additional external cause code to identify place (Y92)

7 ✓x7th **T20.70 Corrosion of third degree of head, face, and neck, unspecified site** CC
CC Excl: CC with 7th character A:T20.30XA, T20.39XA, T20.70XA, T20.79XA

✓6th **T20.71 Corrosion of third degree of ear [any part, except ear drum]**
EXCLUDES 2 *corrosion of ear drum (T28.91-)*

7 ✓7th **T20.711 Corrosion of third degree of right ear [any part, except ear drum]** CC
CC Excl: CC with 7th character A: T20.311-T20.319 with 7th A, T20.39XA, T20.711-T20.719 with 7th A, T20.79XA

7 ✓7th **T20.712 Corrosion of third degree of left ear [any part, except ear drum]** CC
CC Excl: See code: T20.711

7 ✓7th **T20.719 Corrosion of third degree of unspecified ear [any part, except ear drum]** CC
CC Excl: See code: T20.711

7 ✓x7th **T20.72 Corrosion of third degree of lip(s)** CC
CC Excl: CC with 7th character A: See code: T20.32

7 ✓x7th **T20.73 Corrosion of third degree of chin** CC
CC Excl: CC with 7th character A: See code: T20.33

7 ✓x7th **T20.74 Corrosion of third degree of nose (septum)** CC
CC Excl: CC with 7th character A: See code: T20.34

7 ✓x7th **T20.75 Corrosion of third degree of scalp [any part]** CC
CC Excl: CC with 7th character A: See code: T20.35

7 ✓x7th **T20.76 Corrosion of third degree of forehead and cheek** CC
CC Excl: CC with 7th character A: See code: T20.36

7 ✓x7th **T20.77 Corrosion of third degree of neck** CC
CC Excl: CC with 7th character A: See code: T20.37

7 ✓x7th **T20.79 Corrosion of third degree of multiple sites of head, face, and neck** CC
CC Excl: CC with 7th character A: See code: T20.39

✓4th **T21 Burn and corrosion of trunk**
Burns and corrosion of hip region
EXCLUDES 2 *burns and corrosion of:*
axilla (T22- with fifth character 4)
scapular region (T22- with fifth character 6)
shoulder (T22.- with fifth character 5)

The appropriate 7th character is to be added to each code from category T21.
A initial encounter
D subsequent encounter
S sequela

✓5th **T21.0 Burn of unspecified degree of trunk**
Use additional external cause code to identify the source, place and intent of the burn (X00-X19, X75-X77, X96-X98, Y92)

✓x7th **T21.00 Burn of unspecified degree of trunk, unspecified site**

✓x7th **T21.01 Burn of unspecified degree of chest wall**
Burn of of unspecified degree of breast

✓x7th **T21.02 Burn of unspecified degree of abdominal wall**
Burn of unspecified degree of flank
Burn of unspecified degree of groin

✓x7th **T21.03 Burn of unspecified degree of upper back**
Burn of unspecified degree of interscapular region

✓x7th **T21.04 Burn of unspecified degree of lower back**

✓x7th **T21.05 Burn of unspecified degree of buttock**
Burn of unspecified degree of anus

✓x7th **T21.06 Burn of unspecified degree of male genital region** ♂
Burn of unspecified degree of penis
Burn of unspecified degree of scrotum
Burn of unspecified degree of testis

✓x7th **T21.07 Burn of unspecified degree of female genital region** ♀
Burn of unspecified degree of labium (majus) (minus)
Burn of unspecified degree of perineum
Burn of unspecified degree of vulva
EXCLUDES 2 *burn of vagina (T28.3)*

✓x7th **T21.09 Burn of unspecified degree of other site of trunk**

✓5th **T21.1 Burn of first degree of trunk**
Use additional external cause code to identify the source, place and intent of the burn (X00-X19, X75-X77, X96-X98, Y92)

✓x7th **T21.10 Burn of first degree of trunk, unspecified site**

✓x7th **T21.11 Burn of first degree of chest wall**
Burn of first degree of breast

✓x7th **T21.12 Burn of first degree of abdominal wall**
Burn of first degree of flank
Burn of first degree of groin

✓x7th **T21.13 Burn of first degree of upper back**
Burn of first degree of interscapular region

✓x7th **T21.14 Burn of first degree of lower back**

✓x7th **T21.15 Burn of first degree of buttock**
Burn of first degree of anus

✓x7th **T21.16 Burn of first degree of male genital region** ♂
Burn of first degree of penis
Burn of first degree of scrotum
Burn of first degree of testis

✓x7th **T21.17 Burn of first degree of female genital region** ♀
Burn of first degree of labium (majus) (minus)
Burn of first degree of perineum
Burn of first degree of vulva
EXCLUDES 2 *burn of vagina (T28.3)*

✓x7th **T21.19 Burn of first degree of other site of trunk**

✓5th **T21.2 Burn of second degree of trunk**
Use additional external cause code to identify the source, place and intent of the burn (X00-X19, X75-X77, X96-X98, Y92)

✓x7th **T21.20 Burn of second degree of trunk, unspecified site**

✓x7th **T21.21 Burn of second degree of chest wall**
Burn of second degree of breast

✓x7th **T21.22 Burn of second degree of abdominal wall**
Burn of second degree of flank
Burn of second degree of groin

✓x7th **T21.23 Burn of second degree of upper back**
Burn of second degree of interscapular region

✓x7th **T21.24 Burn of second degree of lower back**

✓x7th **T21.25 Burn of second degree of buttock**
Burn of second degree of anus

✓x7th **T21.26 Burn of second degree of male genital region** ♂
Burn of second degree of penis
Burn of second degree of scrotum
Burn of second degree of testis

✓x7th **T21.27 Burn of second degree of female genital region** ♀
Burn of second degree of labium (majus) (minus)
Burn of second degree of perineum
Burn of second degree of vulva
EXCLUDES 2 *burn of vagina (T28.3)*

✓x7th **T21.29 Burn of second degree of other site of trunk**

✓5th **T21.3 Burn of third degree of trunk**
Use additional external cause code to identify the source, place and intent of the burn (X00-X19, X75-X77, X96-X98, Y92)

7 ✓x7th **T21.30 Burn of third degree of trunk, unspecified site** CC
CC Excl: CC with 7th character A:
T21.30XA,T21.39XA,T21.70XA,T21.79XA

7 ✓x7th **T21.31 Burn of third degree of chest wall** CC
Burn of third degree of breast
CC Excl: CC with 7th character A:
T21.30XA,T21.31XA,T21.39XA,T21.71XA,T21.79XA

7 ✓x7th **T21.32 Burn of third degree of abdominal wall** CC
Burn of third degree of flank
Burn of third degree of groin
CC Excl: CC with 7th character A:
T21.30XA,T21.32XA,T21.39XA,T21.72XA,T21.79XA

7 ✓x7th **T21.33 Burn of third degree of upper back** CC
Burn of third degree of interscapular region
CC Excl: CC with 7th character A: T2130XA,T2133-T2135 with 7th A, T2139XA, T2170XA,T2173-T2175 with 7th A,T2179XA

7 HAC = Initial encounter only (7th character A, B or C) and not POA.

7 √x7th **T21.34 Burn of third degree of lower back** CC
CC Excl: See code: T21.133

7 √x7th **T21.35 Burn of third degree of buttock** CC
Burn of third degree of anus
CC Excl: See code: T21.133

7 √x7th **T21.36 Burn of third degree of male genital region** CC ♂
Burn of third degree of penis
Burn of third degree of scrotum
Burn of third degree of testis
CC Excl: CC with 7th character A: T21.30XA,T21.36XA,T21.37XA,T21.39XA,T21.70XA,T21.76XA,T21.77XA,T21.79XA

7 √x7th **T21.37 Burn of third degree of female genital region** CC ♀
Burn of third degree of labium (majus) (minus)
Burn of third degree of perineum
Burn of third degree of vulva
EXCLUDES 2 *burn of vagina (T28.3)*
CC Excl: See code: T21.136

7 √x7th **T21.39 Burn of third degree of other site of trunk** CC
CC Excl: CC with 7th character A: T22.30X-T22.312 with 7th A, T22.319A, T22.391-T22.399 with 7th A, T22.70X-T22.719 with 7th A, T22.791-T22.799 with 7th A

√5th **T21.4 Corrosion of unspecified degree of trunk**
Code first (T51-T65) to identify chemical and intent
Use additional external cause code to identify place (Y92)

√x7th **T21.40 Corrosion of unspecified degree of trunk, unspecified site**

√x7th **T21.41 Corrosion of unspecified degree of chest wall**
Corrosion of unspecified degree of breast

√x7th **T21.42 Corrosion of unspecified degree of abdominal wall**
Corrosion of unspecified degree of flank
Corrosion of unspecified degree of groin

√x7th **T21.43 Corrosion of unspecified degree of upper back**
Corrosion of unspecified degree of interscapular region

√x7th **T21.44 Corrosion of unspecified degree of lower back**

√x7th **T21.45 Corrosion of unspecified degree of buttock**
Corrosion of unspecified degree of anus

√x7th **T21.46 Corrosion of unspecified degree of male genital region** ♂
Corrosion of unspecified degree of penis
Corrosion of unspecified degree of scrotum
Corrosion of unspecified degree of testis

√x7th **T21.47 Corrosion of unspecified degree of female genital region** ♀
Corrosion of unspecified degree of labium (majus) (minus)
Corrosion of unspecified degree of perineum
Corrosion of unspecified degree of vulva
EXCLUDES 2 *corrosion of vagina (T28.8)*

√x7th **T21.49 Corrosion of unspecified degree of other site of trunk**

√5th **T21.5 Corrosion of first degree of trunk**
Code first (T51-T65) to identify chemical and intent
Use additional external cause code to identify place (Y92)

√x7th **T21.50 Corrosion of first degree of trunk, unspecified site**

√x7th **T21.51 Corrosion of first degree of chest wall**
Corrosion of first degree of breast

√x7th **T21.52 Corrosion of first degree of abdominal wall**
Corrosion of first degree of flank
Corrosion of first degree of groin

√x7th **T21.53 Corrosion of first degree of upper back**
Corrosion of first degree of interscapular region

√x7th **T21.54 Corrosion of first degree of lower back**

√x7th **T21.55 Corrosion of first degree of buttock**
Corrosion of first degree of anus

√x7th **T21.56 Corrosion of first degree of male genital region** ♂
Corrosion of first degree of penis
Corrosion of first degree of scrotum
Corrosion of first degree of testis

√x7th **T21.57 Corrosion of first degree of female genital region** ♀
Corrosion of first degree of labium (majus) (minus)
Corrosion of first degree of perineum
Corrosion of first degree of vulva
EXCLUDES 2 *corrosion of vagina (T28.8)*

√x7th **T21.59 Corrosion of first degree of other site of trunk**

√5th **T21.6 Corrosion of second degree of trunk**
Code first (T51-T65) to identify chemical and intent
Use additional external cause code to identify place (Y92)

√x7th **T21.60 Corrosion of second degree of trunk, unspecified site**

√x7th **T21.61 Corrosion of second degree of chest wall**
Corrosion of second degree of breast

√x7th **T21.62 Corrosion of second degree of abdominal wall**
Corrosion of second degree of flank
Corrosion of second degree of groin

√x7th **T21.63 Corrosion of second degree of upper back**
Corrosion of second degree of interscapular region

√x7th **T21.64 Corrosion of second degree of lower back**

√x7th **T21.65 Corrosion of second degree of buttock**
Corrosion of second degree of anus

√x7th **T21.66 Corrosion of second degree of male genital region** ♂
Corrosion of second degree of penis
Corrosion of second degree of scrotum
Corrosion of second degree of testis

√x7th **T21.67 Corrosion of second degree of female genital region** ♀
Corrosion of second degree of labium (majus) (minus)
Corrosion of second degree of perineum
Corrosion of second degree of vulva
EXCLUDES 2 *corrosion of vagina (T28.8)*

√x7th **T21.69 Corrosion of second degree of other site of trunk**

√5th **T21.7 Corrosion of third degree of trunk**
Code first (T51-T65) to identify chemical and intent
Use additional external cause code to identify place (Y92)

7 √x7th **T21.70 Corrosion of third degree of trunk, unspecified site** CC
CC Excl: CC with 7th character A: See code: T21.30

7 √x7th **T21.71 Corrosion of third degree of chest wall** CC
Corrosion of third degree of breast
CC Excl: CC with 7th character A: See code: T21.31

7 √x7th **T21.72 Corrosion of third degree of abdominal wall** CC
Corrosion of third degree of flank
Corrosion of third degree of groin
CC Excl: CC with 7th character A: See code: T21.32

7 √x7th **T21.73 Corrosion of third degree of upper back** CC
Corrosion of third degree of interscapular region
CC Excl: CC with 7th character A: See code: T21.33

7 √x7th **T21.74 Corrosion of third degree of lower back** CC
CC Excl: See code: T21.33

7 √x7th **T21.75 Corrosion of third degree of buttock** CC
Corrosion of third degree of anus
CC Excl: See code: T21.33

7 √x7th **T21.76 Corrosion of third degree of male genital region** CC ♂
Corrosion of third degree of penis
Corrosion of third degree of scrotum
Corrosion of third degree of testis
CC Excl: CC with 7th character A: See code: T21.36

7 √x7th **T21.77 Corrosion of third degree of female genital region** CC ♀
Corrosion of third degree of labium (majus) (minus)
Corrosion of third degree of perineum
Corrosion of third degree of vulva
EXCLUDES 2 *corrosion of vagina (T28.8)*
CC Excl: See code: T21.36

7 √x7th **T21.79 Corrosion of third degree of other site of trunk** CC
CC Excl: CC with 7th character A: See code: T21.30

√4th **T22 Burn and corrosion of shoulder and upper limb, except wrist and hand**
EXCLUDES 2 *burn and corrosion of interscapular region (T21.-)*
burn and corrosion of wrist and hand (T23.-)

The appropriate 7th character is to be added to each code from category T22.
A initial encounter
D subsequent encounter
S sequela

√5th **T22.0 Burn of unspecified degree of shoulder and upper limb, except wrist and hand**
Use additional external cause code to identify the source, place and intent of the burn (X00-X19, X75-X77, X96-X98, Y92)

√x7th **T22.00 Burn of unspecified degree of shoulder and upper limb, except wrist and hand, unspecified site**

7 HAC = Initial encounter only (7th character A, B or C) and not POA.

- ✓6th **T22.Ø1 Burn of unspecified degree of forearm**
  - ✓7th **T22.Ø11 Burn of unspecified degree of right forearm**
  - ✓7th **T22.Ø12 Burn of unspecified degree of left forearm**
  - ✓7th **T22.Ø19 Burn of unspecified degree of unspecified forearm**
- ✓6th **T22.Ø2 Burn of unspecified degree of elbow**
  - ✓7th **T22.Ø21 Burn of unspecified degree of right elbow**
  - ✓7th **T22.Ø22 Burn of unspecified degree of left elbow**
  - ✓7th **T22.Ø29 Burn of unspecified degree of unspecified elbow**
- ✓6th **T22.Ø3 Burn of unspecified degree of upper arm**
  - ✓7th **T22.Ø31 Burn of unspecified degree of right upper arm**
  - ✓7th **T22.Ø32 Burn of unspecified degree of left upper arm**
  - ✓7th **T22.Ø39 Burn of unspecified degree of unspecified upper arm**
- ✓6th **T22.Ø4 Burn of unspecified degree of axilla**
  - ✓7th **T22.Ø41 Burn of unspecified degree of right axilla**
  - ✓7th **T22.Ø42 Burn of unspecified degree of left axilla**
  - ✓7th **T22.Ø49 Burn of unspecified degree of unspecified axilla**
- ✓6th **T22.Ø5 Burn of unspecified degree of shoulder**
  - ✓7th **T22.Ø51 Burn of unspecified degree of right shoulder**
  - ✓7th **T22.Ø52 Burn of unspecified degree of left shoulder**
  - ✓7th **T22.Ø59 Burn of unspecified degree of unspecified shoulder**
- ✓6th **T22.Ø6 Burn of unspecified degree of scapular region**
  - ✓7th **T22.Ø61 Burn of unspecified degree of right scapular region**
  - ✓7th **T22.Ø62 Burn of unspecified degree of left scapular region**
  - ✓7th **T22.Ø69 Burn of unspecified degree of unspecified scapular region**
- ✓6th **T22.Ø9 Burn of unspecified degree of multiple sites of shoulder and upper limb, except wrist and hand**
  - ✓7th **T22.Ø91 Burn of unspecified degree of multiple sites of right shoulder and upper limb, except wrist and hand**
  - ✓7th **T22.Ø92 Burn of unspecified degree of multiple sites of left shoulder and upper limb, except wrist and hand**
  - ✓7th **T22.Ø99 Burn of unspecified degree of multiple sites of unspecified shoulder and upper limb, except wrist and hand**

✓5th **T22.1 Burn of first degree of shoulder and upper limb, except wrist and hand**

Use additional external cause code to identify the source, place and intent of the burn (XØØ-X19, X75-X77, X96-X98, Y92)

- ✓x7th **T22.1Ø Burn of first degree of shoulder and upper limb, except wrist and hand, unspecified site**
- ✓6th **T22.11 Burn of first degree of forearm**
  - ✓7th **T22.111 Burn of first degree of right forearm**
  - ✓7th **T22.112 Burn of first degree of left forearm**
  - ✓7th **T22.119 Burn of first degree of unspecified forearm**
- ✓6th **T22.12 Burn of first degree of elbow**
  - ✓7th **T22.121 Burn of first degree of right elbow**
  - ✓7th **T22.122 Burn of first degree of left elbow**
  - ✓7th **T22.129 Burn of first degree of unspecified elbow**
- ✓6th **T22.13 Burn of first degree of upper arm**
  - ✓7th **T22.131 Burn of first degree of right upper arm**
  - ✓7th **T22.132 Burn of first degree of left upper arm**
  - ✓7th **T22.139 Burn of first degree of unspecified upper arm**
- ✓6th **T22.14 Burn of first degree of axilla**
  - ✓7th **T22.141 Burn of first degree of right axilla**
  - ✓7th **T22.142 Burn of first degree of left axilla**
  - ✓7th **T22.149 Burn of first degree of unspecified axilla**
- ✓6th **T22.15 Burn of first degree of shoulder**
  - ✓7th **T22.151 Burn of first degree of right shoulder**
  - ✓7th **T22.152 Burn of first degree of left shoulder**
  - ✓7th **T22.159 Burn of first degree of unspecified shoulder**
- ✓6th **T22.16 Burn of first degree of scapular region**
  - ✓7th **T22.161 Burn of first degree of right scapular region**
  - ✓7th **T22.162 Burn of first degree of left scapular region**
  - ✓7th **T22.169 Burn of first degree of unspecified scapular region**
- ✓6th **T22.19 Burn of first degree of multiple sites of shoulder and upper limb, except wrist and hand**
  - ✓7th **T22.191 Burn of first degree of multiple sites of right shoulder and upper limb, except wrist and hand**
  - ✓7th **T22.192 Burn of first degree of multiple sites of left shoulder and upper limb, except wrist and hand**
  - ✓7th **T22.199 Burn of first degree of multiple sites of unspecified shoulder and upper limb, except wrist and hand**

✓5th **T22.2 Burn of second degree of shoulder and upper limb, except wrist and hand**

Use additional external cause code to identify the source, place and intent of the burn (XØØ-X19, X75-X77, X96-X98, Y92)

- ✓x7th **T22.2Ø Burn of second degree of shoulder and upper limb, except wrist and hand, unspecified site**
- ✓6th **T22.21 Burn of second degree of forearm**
  - ✓7th **T22.211 Burn of second degree of right forearm**
  - ✓7th **T22.212 Burn of second degree of left forearm**
  - ✓7th **T22.219 Burn of second degree of unspecified forearm**
- ✓6th **T22.22 Burn of second degree of elbow**
  - ✓7th **T22.221 Burn of second degree of right elbow**
  - ✓7th **T22.222 Burn of second degree of left elbow**
  - ✓7th **T22.229 Burn of second degree of unspecified elbow**
- ✓6th **T22.23 Burn of second degree of upper arm**
  - ✓7th **T22.231 Burn of second degree of right upper arm**
  - ✓7th **T22.232 Burn of second degree of left upper arm**
  - ✓7th **T22.239 Burn of second degree of unspecified upper arm**
- ✓6th **T22.24 Burn of second degree of axilla**
  - ✓7th **T22.241 Burn of second degree of right axilla**
  - ✓7th **T22.242 Burn of second degree of left axilla**
  - ✓7th **T22.249 Burn of second degree of unspecified axilla**
- ✓6th **T22.25 Burn of second degree of shoulder**
  - ✓7th **T22.251 Burn of second degree of right shoulder**
  - ✓7th **T22.252 Burn of second degree of left shoulder**
  - ✓7th **T22.259 Burn of second degree of unspecified shoulder**
- ✓6th **T22.26 Burn of second degree of scapular region**
  - ✓7th **T22.261 Burn of second degree of right scapular region**
  - ✓7th **T22.262 Burn of second degree of left scapular region**
  - ✓7th **T22.269 Burn of second degree of unspecified scapular region**
- ✓6th **T22.29 Burn of second degree of multiple sites of shoulder and upper limb, except wrist and hand**
  - ✓7th **T22.291 Burn of second degree of multiple sites of right shoulder and upper limb, except wrist and hand**
  - ✓7th **T22.292 Burn of second degree of multiple sites of left shoulder and upper limb, except wrist and hand**
  - ✓7th **T22.299 Burn of second degree of multiple sites of unspecified shoulder and upper limb, except wrist and hand**

✓5th **T22.3 Burn of third degree of shoulder and upper limb, except wrist and hand**
Use additional external cause code to identify the source, place and intent of the burn (X00-X19, X75-X77, X96-X98, Y92)

7 ✓x 7th **T22.30 Burn of third degree of shoulder and upper limb, except wrist and hand, unspecified site** CC
CC Excl: CC with 7th character A: T22.30XA,T22.391-T22.399 with 7th A,T22.70XA,T22.791-T22.799 with 7th A

✓6th **T22.31 Burn of third degree of forearm**

7 ✓7th **T22.311 Burn of third degree of right forearm** CC
CC Excl: CC with 7th character A: T22.30XA,T22.311-T22.319 with 7th A,T22.391-T22.399 with 7th A,T22.70XA,T22.711-T22.719 with 7th A,T22.791-T22.799 with 7th A

7 ✓7th **T22.312 Burn of third degree of left forearm** CC
CC Excl: See code: T22.311

7 ✓7th **T22.319 Burn of third degree of unspecified forearm** CC
CC Excl: See code: T22.311

✓6th **T22.32 Burn of third degree of elbow**

7 ✓7th **T22.321 Burn of third degree of right elbow** CC
CC Excl: CC with 7th character A: T22.30XA,T22.321-T22.329 with 7th A, T22.391-T22.399 with 7th A,T22.70XA,T22.721-T22.729 with 7th A, T22.791-T22.799 with 7th A

7 ✓7th **T22.322 Burn of third degree of left elbow** CC
CC Excl: See code: T22.321

7 ✓7th **T22.329 Burn of third degree of unspecified elbow** CC
CC Excl: See code: T22.321

✓6th **T22.33 Burn of third degree of upper arm**

7 ✓7th **T22.331 Burn of third degree of right upper arm** CC
CC Excl: CC with 7th character A: T22.30XA,T22.331-T22.339 with 7th A, T22.391-T22.399 with 7th A,T22.70XA,T22.731-T22.739 with 7th A, T22.791-T22.799 with 7th A

7 ✓7th **T22.332 Burn of third degree of left upper arm** CC
CC Excl: See code: T22.331

7 ✓7th **T22.339 Burn of third degree of unspecified upper arm** CC
CC Excl: See code: T22.331

✓6th **T22.34 Burn of third degree of axilla**

7 ✓7th **T22.341 Burn of third degree of right axilla** CC
CC Excl: CC with 7th character A: T22.30XA,T22.341-T22.349 with 7th A, T22.391-T22.399 with 7th A,T22.70XA,T22.741-T22.749 with 7th A, T22.791-T22.799 with 7th A

7 ✓7th **T22.342 Burn of third degree of left axilla** CC
CC Excl: See code: T22.341

7 ✓7th **T22.349 Burn of third degree of unspecified axilla** CC
CC Excl: See code: T22.341

✓6th **T22.35 Burn of third degree of shoulder**

7 ✓7th **T22.351 Burn of third degree of right shoulder** CC
CC Excl: CC with 7th character A: T22.30XA,T22.351-T22.359 with 7th A, T22.391-T22.399 with 7th A,T22.70XA,T22.751-T22.759 with 7th A, T22.791-T22.799 with 7th A

7 ✓7th **T22.352 Burn of third degree of left shoulder** CC
CC Excl: See code: T22.351

7 ✓7th **T22.359 Burn of third degree of unspecified shoulder** CC
CC Excl: See code: T22.351

✓6th **T22.36 Burn of third degree of scapular region**

7 ✓7th **T22.361 Burn of third degree of right scapular region** CC
CC Excl: CC with 7th character A: T22.30XA,T22.361-T22.369 with 7th A, T22.391-T22.399 with 7th A,T22.70XA,T22.761-T22.769 with 7th A, T22.791-T22.799 with 7th A

7 ✓7th **T22.362 Burn of third degree of left scapular region** CC
CC Excl: See code: T22.361

7 ✓7th **T22.369 Burn of third degree of unspecified scapular region** CC
CC Excl: See code: T22.361

✓6th **T22.39 Burn of third degree of multiple sites of shoulder and upper limb, except wrist and hand**

7 ✓7th **T22.391 Burn of third degree of multiple sites of right shoulder and upper limb, except wrist and hand** CC
CC Excl: CC with 7th character A: T22.30XA,T22.391-T22.399 with 7th A,T22.70XA,T22.791-T22.799 with 7th A

7 ✓7th **T22.392 Burn of third degree of multiple sites of left shoulder and upper limb, except wrist and hand** CC
CC Excl: See code: T22.391

7 ✓7th **T22.399 Burn of third degree of multiple sites of unspecified shoulder and upper limb, except wrist and hand** CC
CC Excl: See code: T22.391

✓5th **T22.4 Corrosion of unspecified degree of shoulder and upper limb, except wrist and hand**
Code first (T51-T65) to identify chemical and intent
Use additional external cause code to identify place (Y92)

✓x 7th **T22.40 Corrosion of unspecified degree of shoulder and upper limb, except wrist and hand, unspecified site**

✓6th **T22.41 Corrosion of unspecified degree of forearm**

✓7th **T22.411 Corrosion of unspecified degree of right forearm**

✓7th **T22.412 Corrosion of unspecified degree of left forearm**

✓7th **T22.419 Corrosion of unspecified degree of unspecified forearm**

✓6th **T22.42 Corrosion of unspecified degree of elbow**

✓7th **T22.421 Corrosion of unspecified degree of right elbow**

✓7th **T22.422 Corrosion of unspecified degree of left elbow**

✓7th **T22.429 Corrosion of unspecified degree of unspecified elbow**

✓6th **T22.43 Corrosion of unspecified degree of upper arm**

✓7th **T22.431 Corrosion of unspecified degree of right upper arm**

✓7th **T22.432 Corrosion of unspecified degree of left upper arm**

✓7th **T22.439 Corrosion of unspecified degree of unspecified upper arm**

✓6th **T22.44 Corrosion of unspecified degree of axilla**

✓7th **T22.441 Corrosion of unspecified degree of right axilla**

✓7th **T22.442 Corrosion of unspecified degree of left axilla**

✓7th **T22.449 Corrosion of unspecified degree of unspecified axilla**

✓6th **T22.45 Corrosion of unspecified degree of shoulder**

✓7th **T22.451 Corrosion of unspecified degree of right shoulder**

✓7th **T22.452 Corrosion of unspecified degree of left shoulder**

✓7th **T22.459 Corrosion of unspecified degree of unspecified shoulder**

✓6th **T22.46 Corrosion of unspecified degree of scapular region**

✓7th **T22.461 Corrosion of unspecified degree of right scapular region**

✓7th **T22.462 Corrosion of unspecified degree of left scapular region**

✓7th **T22.469 Corrosion of unspecified degree of unspecified scapular region**

✓6th **T22.49 Corrosion of unspecified degree of multiple sites of shoulder and upper limb, except wrist and hand**

✓7th **T22.491 Corrosion of unspecified degree of multiple sites of right shoulder and upper limb, except wrist and hand**

7 HAC = Initial encounter only (7th character A, B or C) and not POA.

✓7th T22.492 Corrosion of unspecified degree of multiple sites of left shoulder and upper limb, except wrist and hand
✓7th T22.499 Corrosion of unspecified degree of multiple sites of unspecified shoulder and upper limb, except wrist and hand

✓5th **T22.5 Corrosion of first degree of shoulder and upper limb, except wrist and hand**
Code first (T51-T65) to identify chemical and intent
Use additional external cause code to identify place (Y92)

✓x7th T22.50 Corrosion of first degree of shoulder and upper limb, except wrist and hand unspecified site
✓6th T22.51 Corrosion of first degree of forearm
✓7th T22.511 Corrosion of first degree of right forearm
✓7th T22.512 Corrosion of first degree of left forearm
✓7th T22.519 Corrosion of first degree of unspecified forearm
✓6th T22.52 Corrosion of first degree of elbow
✓7th T22.521 Corrosion of first degree of right elbow
✓7th T22.522 Corrosion of first degree of left elbow
✓7th T22.529 Corrosion of first degree of unspecified elbow
✓6th T22.53 Corrosion of first degree of upper arm
✓7th T22.531 Corrosion of first degree of right upper arm
✓7th T22.532 Corrosion of first degree of left upper arm
✓7th T22.539 Corrosion of first degree of unspecified upper arm
✓6th T22.54 Corrosion of first degree of axilla
✓7th T22.541 Corrosion of first degree of right axilla
✓7th T22.542 Corrosion of first degree of left axilla
✓7th T22.549 Corrosion of first degree of unspecified axilla
✓6th T22.55 Corrosion of first degree of shoulder
✓7th T22.551 Corrosion of first degree of right shoulder
✓7th T22.552 Corrosion of first degree of left shoulder
✓7th T22.559 Corrosion of first degree of unspecified shoulder
✓6th T22.56 Corrosion of first degree of scapular region
✓7th T22.561 Corrosion of first degree of right scapular region
✓7th T22.562 Corrosion of first degree of left scapular region
✓7th T22.569 Corrosion of first degree of unspecified scapular region
✓6th T22.59 Corrosion of first degree of multiple sites of shoulder and upper limb, except wrist and hand
✓7th T22.591 Corrosion of first degree of multiple sites of right shoulder and upper limb, except wrist and hand
✓7th T22.592 Corrosion of first degree of multiple sites of left shoulder and upper limb, except wrist and hand
✓7th T22.599 Corrosion of first degree of multiple sites of unspecified shoulder and upper limb, except wrist and hand

✓5th **T22.6 Corrosion of second degree of shoulder and upper limb, except wrist and hand**
Code first (T51-T65) to identify chemical and intent
Use additional external cause code to identify place (Y92)

✓x7th T22.60 Corrosion of second degree of shoulder and upper limb, except wrist and hand, unspecified site
✓6th T22.61 Corrosion of second degree of forearm
✓7th T22.611 Corrosion of second degree of right forearm
✓7th T22.612 Corrosion of second degree of left forearm
✓7th T22.619 Corrosion of second degree of unspecified forearm
✓6th T22.62 Corrosion of second degree of elbow
✓7th T22.621 Corrosion of second degree of right elbow
✓7th T22.622 Corrosion of second degree of left elbow
✓7th T22.629 Corrosion of second degree of unspecified elbow
✓6th T22.63 Corrosion of second degree of upper arm
✓7th T22.631 Corrosion of second degree of right upper arm
✓7th T22.632 Corrosion of second degree of left upper arm
✓7th T22.639 Corrosion of second degree of unspecified upper arm
✓6th T22.64 Corrosion of second degree of axilla
✓7th T22.641 Corrosion of second degree of right axilla
✓7th T22.642 Corrosion of second degree of left axilla
✓7th T22.649 Corrosion of second degree of unspecified axilla
✓6th T22.65 Corrosion of second degree of shoulder
✓7th T22.651 Corrosion of second degree of right shoulder
✓7th T22.652 Corrosion of second degree of left shoulder
✓7th T22.659 Corrosion of second degree of unspecified shoulder
✓6th T22.66 Corrosion of second degree of scapular region
✓7th T22.661 Corrosion of second degree of right scapular region
✓7th T22.662 Corrosion of second degree of left scapular region
✓7th T22.669 Corrosion of second degree of unspecified scapular region
✓6th T22.69 Corrosion of second degree of multiple sites of shoulder and upper limb, except wrist and hand
✓7th T22.691 Corrosion of second degree of multiple sites of right shoulder and upper limb, except wrist and hand
✓7th T22.692 Corrosion of second degree of multiple sites of left shoulder and upper limb, except wrist and hand
✓7th T22.699 Corrosion of second degree of multiple sites of unspecified shoulder and upper limb, except wrist and hand

✓5th **T22.7 Corrosion of third degree of shoulder and upper limb, except wrist and hand**
Code first (T51-T65) to identify chemical and intent
Use additional external cause code to identify place (Y92)

7 ✓x7th T22.70 Corrosion of third degree of shoulder and upper limb, except wrist and hand, unspecified site CC
CC Excl: CC with 7th character A: See code: T22.30
✓6th T22.71 Corrosion of third degree of forearm
7 ✓7th T22.711 Corrosion of third degree of right forearm CC
CC Excl: CC with 7th character A: See code: T22.311
7 ✓7th T22.712 Corrosion of third degree of left forearm CC
CC Excl: See code: T22.311
7 ✓7th T22.719 Corrosion of third degree of unspecified forearm CC
CC Excl: See code: T22.311
✓6th T22.72 Corrosion of third degree of elbow
7 ✓7th T22.721 Corrosion of third degree of right elbow CC
CC Excl: CC with 7th character A: See code: T22.321
7 ✓7th T22.722 Corrosion of third degree of left elbow CC
CC Excl: See code: T22.321
7 ✓7th T22.729 Corrosion of third degree of unspecified elbow CC
CC Excl: See code: T22.321
✓6th T22.73 Corrosion of third degree of upper arm
7 ✓7th T22.731 Corrosion of third degree of right upper arm CC
CC Excl: CC with 7th character A: See code: T22.331

7 HAC = Initial encounter only (7th character A, B or C) and not POA.

7 T22.732 **Corrosion of third degree of left upper arm** CC
CC Excl: See code: T22.331

7 T22.739 **Corrosion of third degree of unspecified upper arm** CC
CC Excl: See code: T22.331

T22.74 Corrosion of third degree of axilla

7 T22.741 **Corrosion of third degree of right axilla** CC
CC Excl: CC with 7th character A: See code: T22.341

7 T22.742 **Corrosion of third degree of left axilla** CC
CC Excl: See code: T22.341

7 T22.749 **Corrosion of third degree of unspecified axilla** CC
CC Excl: See code: T22.341

T22.75 Corrosion of third degree of shoulder

7 T22.751 **Corrosion of third degree of right shoulder** CC
CC Excl: CC with 7th character A: See code: T22.351

7 T22.752 **Corrosion of third degree of left shoulder** CC
CC Excl: See code: T22.351

7 T22.759 **Corrosion of third degree of unspecified shoulder** CC
CC Excl: See code: T22.351

T22.76 Corrosion of third degree of scapular region

7 T22.761 **Corrosion of third degree of right scapular region** CC
CC Excl: CC with 7th character A: See code: T22.361

7 T22.762 **Corrosion of third degree of left scapular region** CC
CC Excl: See code: T22.361

7 T22.769 **Corrosion of third degree of unspecified scapular region** CC
CC Excl: See code: T22.361

T22.79 Corrosion of third degree of multiple sites of shoulder and upper limb, except wrist and hand

7 T22.791 **Corrosion of third degree of multiple sites of right shoulder and upper limb, except wrist and hand** CC
CC Excl: CC with 7th character A: See code: T22.391

7 T22.792 **Corrosion of third degree of multiple sites of left shoulder and upper limb, except wrist and hand** CC
CC Excl: See code: T22.391

7 T22.799 **Corrosion of third degree of multiple sites of unspecified shoulder and upper limb, except wrist and hand** CC
CC Excl: See code: T22.391

T23 Burn and corrosion of wrist and hand

The appropriate 7th character is to be added to each code from category T23.
A initial encounter
D subsequent encounter
S sequela

T23.0 Burn of unspecified degree of wrist and hand

Use additional external cause code to identify the source, place and intent of the burn (X00-X19, X75-X77, X96-X98, Y92)

T23.00 Burn of unspecified degree of hand, unspecified site

T23.001 Burn of unspecified degree of right hand, unspecified site

T23.002 Burn of unspecified degree of left hand, unspecified site

T23.009 Burn of unspecified degree of unspecified hand, unspecified site

T23.01 Burn of unspecified degree of thumb (nail)

T23.011 Burn of unspecified degree of right thumb (nail)

T23.012 Burn of unspecified degree of left thumb (nail)

T23.019 Burn of unspecified degree of unspecified thumb (nail)

T23.02 Burn of unspecified degree of single finger (nail) except thumb

T23.021 Burn of unspecified degree of single right finger (nail) except thumb

T23.022 Burn of unspecified degree of single left finger (nail) except thumb

T23.029 Burn of unspecified degree of unspecified single finger (nail) except thumb

T23.03 Burn of unspecified degree of multiple fingers (nail), not including thumb

T23.031 Burn of unspecified degree of multiple right fingers (nail), not including thumb

T23.032 Burn of unspecified degree of multiple left fingers (nail), not including thumb

T23.039 Burn of unspecified degree of unspecified multiple fingers (nail), not including thumb

T23.04 Burn of unspecified degree of multiple fingers (nail), including thumb

T23.041 Burn of unspecified degree of multiple right fingers (nail), including thumb

T23.042 Burn of unspecified degree of multiple left fingers (nail), including thumb

T23.049 Burn of unspecified degree of unspecified multiple fingers (nail), including thumb

T23.05 Burn of unspecified degree of palm

T23.051 Burn of unspecified degree of right palm

T23.052 Burn of unspecified degree of left palm

T23.059 Burn of unspecified degree of unspecified palm

T23.06 Burn of unspecified degree of back of hand

T23.061 Burn of unspecified degree of back of right hand

T23.062 Burn of unspecified degree of back of left hand

T23.069 Burn of unspecified degree of back of unspecified hand

T23.07 Burn of unspecified degree of wrist

T23.071 Burn of unspecified degree of right wrist

T23.072 Burn of unspecified degree of left wrist

T23.079 Burn of unspecified degree of unspecified wrist

T23.09 Burn of unspecified degree of multiple sites of wrist and hand

T23.091 Burn of unspecified degree of multiple sites of right wrist and hand

T23.092 Burn of unspecified degree of multiple sites of left wrist and hand

T23.099 Burn of unspecified degree of multiple sites of unspecified wrist and hand

T23.1 Burn of first degree of wrist and hand

Use additional external cause code to identify the source, place and intent of the burn (X00-X19, X75-X77, X96-X98, Y92)

T23.10 Burn of first degree of hand, unspecified site

T23.101 Burn of first degree of right hand, unspecified site

T23.102 Burn of first degree of left hand, unspecified site

T23.109 Burn of first degree of unspecified hand, unspecified site

T23.11 Burn of first degree of thumb (nail)

T23.111 Burn of first degree of right thumb (nail)

T23.112 Burn of first degree of left thumb (nail)

T23.119 Burn of first degree of unspecified thumb (nail)

T23.12 Burn of first degree of single finger (nail) except thumb

T23.121 Burn of first degree of single right finger (nail) except thumb

T23.122 Burn of first degree of single left finger (nail) except thumb

7 HAC = Initial encounter only (7th character A, B or C) and not POA.

T23.129 Burn of first degree of unspecified single finger (nail) except thumb

T23.13 Burn of first degree of multiple fingers (nail), not including thumb

T23.131 Burn of first degree of multiple right fingers (nail), not including thumb

T23.132 Burn of first degree of multiple left fingers (nail), not including thumb

T23.139 Burn of first degree of unspecified multiple fingers (nail), not including thumb

T23.14 Burn of first degree of multiple fingers (nail), including thumb

T23.141 Burn of first degree of multiple right fingers (nail), including thumb

T23.142 Burn of first degree of multiple left fingers (nail), including thumb

T23.149 Burn of first degree of unspecified multiple fingers (nail), including thumb

T23.15 Burn of first degree of palm

T23.151 Burn of first degree of right palm

T23.152 Burn of first degree of left palm

T23.159 Burn of first degree of unspecified palm

T23.16 Burn of first degree of back of hand

T23.161 Burn of first degree of back of right hand

T23.162 Burn of first degree of back of left hand

T23.169 Burn of first degree of back of unspecified hand

T23.17 Burn of first degree of wrist

T23.171 Burn of first degree of right wrist

T23.172 Burn of first degree of left wrist

T23.179 Burn of first degree of unspecified wrist

T23.19 Burn of first degree of multiple sites of wrist and hand

T23.191 Burn of first degree of multiple sites of right wrist and hand

T23.192 Burn of first degree of multiple sites of left wrist and hand

T23.199 Burn of first degree of multiple sites of unspecified wrist and hand

T23.2 Burn of second degree of wrist and hand

Use additional external cause code to identify the source, place and intent of the burn (X00-X19, X75-X77, X96-X98, Y92)

T23.20 Burn of second degree of hand, unspecified site

T23.201 Burn of second degree of right hand, unspecified site

T23.202 Burn of second degree of left hand, unspecified site

T23.209 Burn of second degree of unspecified hand, unspecified site

T23.21 Burn of second degree of thumb (nail)

T23.211 Burn of second degree of right thumb (nail)

T23.212 Burn of second degree of left thumb (nail)

T23.219 Burn of second degree of unspecified thumb (nail)

T23.22 Burn of second degree of single finger (nail) except thumb

T23.221 Burn of second degree of single right finger (nail) except thumb

T23.222 Burn of second degree of single left finger (nail) except thumb

T23.229 Burn of second degree of unspecified single finger (nail) except thumb

T23.23 Burn of second degree of multiple fingers (nail), not including thumb

T23.231 Burn of second degree of multiple right fingers (nail), not including thumb

T23.232 Burn of second degree of multiple left fingers (nail), not including thumb

T23.239 Burn of second degree of unspecified multiple fingers (nail), not including thumb

T23.24 Burn of second degree of multiple fingers (nail), including thumb

T23.241 Burn of second degree of multiple right fingers (nail), including thumb

T23.242 Burn of second degree of multiple left fingers (nail), including thumb

T23.249 Burn of second degree of unspecified multiple fingers (nail), including thumb

T23.25 Burn of second degree of palm

T23.251 Burn of second degree of right palm

T23.252 Burn of second degree of left palm

T23.259 Burn of second degree of unspecified palm

T23.26 Burn of second degree of back of hand

T23.261 Burn of second degree of back of right hand

T23.262 Burn of second degree of back of left hand

T23.269 Burn of second degree of back of unspecified hand

T23.27 Burn of second degree of wrist

T23.271 Burn of second degree of right wrist

T23.272 Burn of second degree of left wrist

T23.279 Burn of second degree of unspecified wrist

T23.29 Burn of second degree of multiple sites of wrist and hand

T23.291 Burn of second degree of multiple sites of right wrist and hand

T23.292 Burn of second degree of multiple sites of left wrist and hand

T23.299 Burn of second degree of multiple sites of unspecified wrist and hand

T23.3 Burn of third degree of wrist and hand

Use additional external cause code to identify the source, place and intent of the burn (X00-X19, X75-X77, X96-X98, Y92)

T23.30 Burn of third degree of hand, unspecified site

7 T23.301 Burn of third degree of right hand, unspecified site CC

CC Excl: CC with 7th character A: T23.30X-T23.319 with 7th A, T23.391-T23.399 with 7th A, T23.701-T23.719 with 7th A, T23.791-T23.799 with 7th A

7 T23.302 Burn of third degree of left hand, unspecified site CC

CC Excl: See code: T23.301

7 T23.309 Burn of third degree of unspecified hand, unspecified site CC

CC Excl: See code: T23.301

T23.31 Burn of third degree of thumb (nail)

7 T23.311 Burn of third degree of right thumb (nail) CC

CC Excl: CC with 7th character A: T23.301-T23.319 with 7th A, T23.391-T23.399 with 7th A,T23.701-T23.719 with 7th A, T23.791-T23.799 with 7th A

7 T23.312 Burn of third degree of left thumb (nail) CC

CC Excl: See code: T23.311

7 T23.319 Burn of third degree of unspecified thumb (nail) CC

CC Excl: See code: T23.311

T23.32 Burn of third degree of single finger (nail) except thumb

7 T23.321 Burn of third degree of single right finger (nail) except thumb CC

CC Excl: CC with 7th character A: T23.301-T23.309 with 7th A, T23.321-T23.329 with 7th, A T23.391-T23.399 with 7th A, T23.701-T23.709 with 7th A, T23.721-T23.729 with 7th A, T23.791-T23.799 with 7th A

7 HAC = Initial encounter only (7th character A, B or C) and not POA.

7 √7th **T23.322** **Burn of third degree of single left finger (nail) except thumb** CC
CC Excl: See code: T23.321

7 √7th **T23.329** **Burn of third degree of unspecified single finger (nail) except thumb** CC
CC Excl: See code: T23.321

√6th **T23.33** Burn of third degree of multiple fingers (nail), not including thumb

7 √7th **T23.331** **Burn of third degree of multiple right fingers (nail), not including thumb** CC
CC Excl: CC with 7th character A: T23.301-T23.309 with 7th A,T23.331-T23.339 with 7th A,T23.391-T23.399 with 7th A, T23.701-T23.709 with 7th A,T23.731-T23.739 with 7th A,T23.791-T23.799 with 7th A

7 √7th **T23.332** **Burn of third degree of multiple left fingers (nail), not including thumb** CC
CC Excl: See code: T23.331

7 √7th **T23.339** **Burn of third degree of unspecified multiple fingers (nail), not including thumb** CC
CC Excl: See code: T23.331

√6th **T23.34** Burn of third degree of multiple fingers (nail), including thumb

7 √7th **T23.341** **Burn of third degree of multiple right fingers (nail), including thumb** CC
CC Excl: CC with 7th character A: T23.301-T23.309 with 7th A, T23.341-T23.349 with 7th A, T23.391-T23.399 with 7th A, T23.701-T23.709 with 7th A, T23.741-T23.749 with 7th A, T23.791-T23.799 with 7th A

7 √7th **T23.342** **Burn of third degree of multiple left fingers (nail), including thumb** CC
CC Excl: See code: T23.341

7 √7th **T23.349** **Burn of third degree of unspecified multiple fingers (nail), including thumb** CC
CC Excl: See code: T23.341

√6th **T23.35** Burn of third degree of palm

7 √7th **T23.351** **Burn of third degree of right palm** CC
CC Excl: CC with 7th character A: T23.301-T23.309 with 7th A,T23.351-T23.359 with 7th A,T23.391-T23.399 with 7th A, T23.701-T23.709 with 7th A, T23.751-T23.759 with 7th A,T23.791-T23.799 with 7th A

7 √7th **T23.352** **Burn of third degree of left palm** CC
CC Excl: See code: T23.351

7 √7th **T23.359** **Burn of third degree of unspecified palm** CC
CC Excl: See code: T23.351

√6th **T23.36** Burn of third degree of back of hand

7 √7th **T23.361** **Burn of third degree of back of right hand** CC
CC Excl: CC with 7th character A: T23.301-T23.309 with 7th A,T23.361-T23.369 with 7th A,T23.391-T23.399 with 7th A, T23.701-T23.709 with 7th A,T23.761-T23.769 with 7th A,T23.791-T23.799 with 7th A

7 √7th **T23.362** **Burn of third degree of back of left hand** CC
CC Excl: See code: T23.361

7 √7th **T23.369** **Burn of third degree of back of unspecified hand** CC
CC Excl: See code: T23.361

√6th **T23.37** Burn of third degree of wrist

7 √7th **T23.371** **Burn of third degree of right wrist** CC
CC Excl: CC with 7th character A: T23.301-T23.309 with 7th A,T23.371-T23.379 with 7th A, T23.391-T23.399 with 7th A, T23.701-T23.709 with 7th A, T23.771-T23.779 with 7th A, T23.791-T23.799 with 7th A

7 √7th **T23.372** **Burn of third degree of left wrist** CC
CC Excl: See code: T23.371

7 √7th **T23.379** **Burn of third degree of unspecified wrist** CC
CC Excl: See code: T23.371

√6th **T23.39** Burn of third degree of multiple sites of wrist and hand

7 √7th **T23.391** **Burn of third degree of multiple sites of right wrist and hand** CC
CC Excl: See code: T23.301

7 √7th **T23.392** **Burn of third degree of multiple sites of left wrist and hand** CC
CC Excl: See code: T23.301

7 √7th **T23.399** **Burn of third degree of multiple sites of unspecified wrist and hand** CC
CC Excl: See code: T23.301

√5th **T23.4** **Corrosion of unspecified degree of wrist and hand**
Code first (T51-T65) to identify chemical and intent
Use additional external cause code to identify place (Y92)

√6th **T23.40** Corrosion of unspecified degree of hand, unspecified site

√7th **T23.401** **Corrosion of unspecified degree of right hand, unspecified site**

√7th **T23.402** **Corrosion of unspecified degree of left hand, unspecified site**

√7th **T23.409** **Corrosion of unspecified degree of unspecified hand, unspecified site**

√6th **T23.41** Corrosion of unspecified degree of thumb (nail)

√7th **T23.411** **Corrosion of unspecified degree of right thumb (nail)**

√7th **T23.412** **Corrosion of unspecified degree of left thumb (nail)**

√7th **T23.419** **Corrosion of unspecified degree of unspecified thumb (nail)**

√6th **T23.42** Corrosion of unspecified degree of single finger (nail) except thumb

√7th **T23.421** **Corrosion of unspecified degree of single right finger (nail) except thumb**

√7th **T23.422** **Corrosion of unspecified degree of single left finger (nail) except thumb**

√7th **T23.429** **Corrosion of unspecified degree of unspecified single finger (nail) except thumb**

√6th **T23.43** Corrosion of unspecified degree of multiple fingers (nail), not including thumb

√7th **T23.431** **Corrosion of unspecified degree of multiple right fingers (nail), not including thumb**

√7th **T23.432** **Corrosion of unspecified degree of multiple left fingers (nail), not including thumb**

√7th **T23.439** **Corrosion of unspecified degree of unspecified multiple fingers (nail), not including thumb**

√6th **T23.44** Corrosion of unspecified degree of multiple fingers (nail), including thumb

√7th **T23.441** **Corrosion of unspecified degree of multiple right fingers (nail), including thumb**

√7th **T23.442** **Corrosion of unspecified degree of multiple left fingers (nail), including thumb**

√7th **T23.449** **Corrosion of unspecified degree of unspecified multiple fingers (nail), including thumb**

√6th **T23.45** Corrosion of unspecified degree of palm

√7th **T23.451** **Corrosion of unspecified degree of right palm**

√7th **T23.452** **Corrosion of unspecified degree of left palm**

√7th **T23.459** **Corrosion of unspecified degree of unspecified palm**

√6th **T23.46** Corrosion of unspecified degree of back of hand

√7th **T23.461** **Corrosion of unspecified degree of back of right hand**

√7th **T23.462** **Corrosion of unspecified degree of back of left hand**

√7th **T23.469** **Corrosion of unspecified degree of back of unspecified hand**

7 HAC = Initial encounter only (7th character A, B or C) and not POA.

√6th **T23.47** **Corrosion of unspecified degree of wrist**
√7th **T23.471** **Corrosion of unspecified degree of right wrist**
√7th **T23.472** **Corrosion of unspecified degree of left wrist**
√7th **T23.479** **Corrosion of unspecified degree of unspecified wrist**
√6th **T23.49** **Corrosion of unspecified degree of multiple sites of wrist and hand**
√7th **T23.491** **Corrosion of unspecified degree of multiple sites of right wrist and hand**
√7th **T23.492** **Corrosion of unspecified degree of multiple sites of left wrist and hand**
√7th **T23.499** **Corrosion of unspecified degree of multiple sites of unspecified wrist and hand**
√5th **T23.5** **Corrosion of first degree of wrist and hand**
Code first (T51-T65) to identify chemical and intent
Use additional external cause code to identify place (Y92)
√6th **T23.50** **Corrosion of first degree of hand, unspecified site**
√7th **T23.501** **Corrosion of first degree of right hand, unspecified site**
√7th **T23.502** **Corrosion of first degree of left hand, unspecified site**
√7th **T23.509** **Corrosion of first degree of unspecified hand, unspecified site**
√6th **T23.51** **Corrosion of first degree of thumb (nail)**
√7th **T23.511** **Corrosion of first degree of right thumb (nail)**
√7th **T23.512** **Corrosion of first degree of left thumb (nail)**
√7th **T23.519** **Corrosion of first degree of unspecified thumb (nail)**
√6th **T23.52** **Corrosion of first degree of single finger (nail) except thumb**
√7th **T23.521** **Corrosion of first degree of single right finger (nail) except thumb**
√7th **T23.522** **Corrosion of first degree of single left finger (nail) except thumb**
√7th **T23.529** **Corrosion of first degree of unspecified single finger (nail) except thumb**
√6th **T23.53** **Corrosion of first degree of multiple fingers (nail), not including thumb**
√7th **T23.531** **Corrosion of first degree of multiple right fingers (nail), not including thumb**
√7th **T23.532** **Corrosion of first degree of multiple left fingers (nail), not including thumb**
√7th **T23.539** **Corrosion of first degree of unspecified multiple fingers (nail), not including thumb**
√6th **T23.54** **Corrosion of first degree of multiple fingers (nail), including thumb**
√7th **T23.541** **Corrosion of first degree of multiple right fingers (nail), including thumb**
√7th **T23.542** **Corrosion of first degree of multiple left fingers (nail), including thumb**
√7th **T23.549** **Corrosion of first degree of unspecified multiple fingers (nail), including thumb**
√6th **T23.55** **Corrosion of first degree of palm**
√7th **T23.551** **Corrosion of first degree of right palm**
√7th **T23.552** **Corrosion of first degree of left palm**
√7th **T23.559** **Corrosion of first degree of unspecified palm**
√6th **T23.56** **Corrosion of first degree of back of hand**
√7th **T23.561** **Corrosion of first degree of back of right hand**
√7th **T23.562** **Corrosion of first degree of back of left hand**
√7th **T23.569** **Corrosion of first degree of back of unspecified hand**
√6th **T23.57** **Corrosion of first degree of wrist**
√7th **T23.571** **Corrosion of first degree of right wrist**
√7th **T23.572** **Corrosion of first degree of left wrist**
√7th **T23.579** **Corrosion of first degree of unspecified wrist**
√6th **T23.59** **Corrosion of first degree of multiple sites of wrist and hand**
√7th **T23.591** **Corrosion of first degree of multiple sites of right wrist and hand**
√7th **T23.592** **Corrosion of first degree of multiple sites of left wrist and hand**
√7th **T23.599** **Corrosion of first degree of multiple sites of unspecified wrist and hand**
√5th **T23.6** **Corrosion of second degree of wrist and hand**
Code first (T51-T65) to identify chemical and intent
Use additional external cause code to identify place (Y92)
√6th **T23.60** **Corrosion of second degree of hand, unspecified site**
√7th **T23.601** **Corrosion of second degree of right hand, unspecified site**
√7th **T23.602** **Corrosion of second degree of left hand, unspecified site**
√7th **T23.609** **Corrosion of second degree of unspecified hand, unspecified site**
√6th **T23.61** **Corrosion of second degree of thumb (nail)**
√7th **T23.611** **Corrosion of second degree of right thumb (nail)**
√7th **T23.612** **Corrosion of second degree of left thumb (nail)**
√7th **T23.619** **Corrosion of second degree of unspecified thumb (nail)**
√6th **T23.62** **Corrosion of second degree of single finger (nail) except thumb**
√7th **T23.621** **Corrosion of second degree of single right finger (nail) except thumb**
√7th **T23.622** **Corrosion of second degree of single left finger (nail) except thumb**
√7th **T23.629** **Corrosion of second degree of unspecified single finger (nail) except thumb**
√6th **T23.63** **Corrosion of second degree of multiple fingers (nail), not including thumb**
√7th **T23.631** **Corrosion of second degree of multiple right fingers (nail), not including thumb**
√7th **T23.632** **Corrosion of second degree of multiple left fingers (nail), not including thumb**
√7th **T23.639** **Corrosion of second degree of unspecified multiple fingers (nail), not including thumb**
√6th **T23.64** **Corrosion of second degree of multiple fingers (nail), including thumb**
√7th **T23.641** **Corrosion of second degree of multiple right fingers (nail), including thumb**
√7th **T23.642** **Corrosion of second degree of multiple left fingers (nail), including thumb**
√7th **T23.649** **Corrosion of second degree of unspecified multiple fingers (nail), including thumb**
√6th **T23.65** **Corrosion of second degree of palm**
√7th **T23.651** **Corrosion of second degree of right palm**
√7th **T23.652** **Corrosion of second degree of left palm**
√7th **T23.659** **Corrosion of second degree of unspecified palm**
√6th **T23.66** **Corrosion of second degree of back of hand**
√7th **T23.661** **Corrosion of second degree back of right hand**
√7th **T23.662** **Corrosion of second degree back of left hand**
√7th **T23.669** **Corrosion of second degree back of unspecified hand**
√6th **T23.67** **Corrosion of second degree of wrist**
√7th **T23.671** **Corrosion of second degree of right wrist**
√7th **T23.672** **Corrosion of second degree of left wrist**
√7th **T23.679** **Corrosion of second degree of unspecified wrist**
√6th **T23.69** **Corrosion of second degree of multiple sites of wrist and hand**
√7th **T23.691** **Corrosion of second degree of multiple sites of right wrist and hand**

7th T23.692 **Corrosion of second degree of multiple sites of left wrist and hand**

7th T23.699 **Corrosion of second degree of multiple sites of unspecified wrist and hand**

5th **T23.7 Corrosion of third degree of wrist and hand**
Code first (T51-T65) to identify chemical and intent
Use additional external cause code to identify place (Y92)

6th **T23.70 Corrosion of third degree of hand, unspecified site**

7 7th **T23.701 Corrosion of third degree of right hand, unspecified site** CC
CC Excl: CC with 7th character A: T23.301-T23.319 with 7th A, T23.391-T23.399 with 7th A, T23.701-T23.719 with 7th A, T23.791-T23.799 with 7th A

7 7th **T23.702 Corrosion of third degree of left hand, unspecified site** CC
CC Excl: See code: T23.701

7 7th **T23.709 Corrosion of third degree of unspecified hand, unspecified site** CC
CC Excl: See code: T23.701

6th **T23.71 Corrosion of third degree of thumb (nail)**

7 7th **T23.711 Corrosion of third degree of right thumb (nail)** CC
CC Excl: CC with 7th character A: T23.301-T23.319 with 7th A, T23.391-T23.399 with 7th A, T23.701-T23.719 with 7th A, T23.791-T23.799 with 7th A

7 7th **T23.712 Corrosion of third degree of left thumb (nail)** CC
CC Excl: See code: T23.711

7 7th **T23.719 Corrosion of third degree of unspecified thumb (nail)** CC
CC Excl: See code: T23.711

6th **T23.72 Corrosion of third degree of single finger (nail) except thumb**

7 7th **T23.721 Corrosion of third degree of single right finger (nail) except thumb** CC
CC Excl: CC with 7th character A: T23.301-T23.309 with 7th A, T23.321-T23.329 with 7th A, T23.391-T23.399 with 7th A, T23.701-T23.709 with 7th A, T23.721-T23.729 with 7th A, T23.791-T23.799 with 7th A

7 7th **T23.722 Corrosion of third degree of single left finger (nail) except thumb** CC
CC Excl: See code: T23.721

7 7th **T23.729 Corrosion of third degree of unspecified single finger (nail) except thumb** CC
CC Excl: See code: T23.721

6th **T23.73 Corrosion of third degree of multiple fingers (nail), not including thumb**

7 7th **T23.731 Corrosion of third degree of multiple right fingers (nail), not including thumb** CC
CC Excl: CC with 7th character A: T23.301-T23.309 with 7th A, T23.331-T23.339 with 7th A, T23.391-T23.399 with 7th A, T23.701-T23.709 with 7th A, T23.731-T23.739 with 7th A, T23.791-T23.799 with 7th A

7 7th **T23.732 Corrosion of third degree of multiple left fingers (nail), not including thumb** CC
CC Excl: See code: T23.731

7 7th **T23.739 Corrosion of third degree of unspecified multiple fingers (nail), not including thumb** CC
CC Excl: See code: T23.731

6th **T23.74 Corrosion of third degree of multiple fingers (nail), including thumb**

7 7th **T23.741 Corrosion of third degree of multiple right fingers (nail), including thumb** CC
CC Excl: CC with 7th character A: T23.301-T23.309 with 7th A, T23.341-T23.349 with 7th A, T23.391-T23.399 with 7th A, T23.701-T23.709 with 7th A, T23.741-T23.749 with 7th A, T23.791-T23.799 with 7th A

7 7th **T23.742 Corrosion of third degree of multiple left fingers (nail), including thumb** CC
CC Excl: See code: T23.741

7 7th **T23.749 Corrosion of third degree of unspecified multiple fingers (nail), including thumb** CC
CC Excl: See code: T23.741

6th **T23.75 Corrosion of third degree of palm**

7 7th **T23.751 Corrosion of third degree of right palm** CC
CC Excl: CC with 7th character A: T23.301-T23.309 with 7th A, T23.351-T23.359 with 7th A, T23.391-T23.399 with 7th A, T23.701-T23.709 with 7th A, T23.751-T23.759 with 7th A, T23.791-T23.799 with 7th A

7 7th **T23.752 Corrosion of third degree of left palm** CC
CC Excl: See code: T23.751

7 7th **T23.759 Corrosion of third degree of unspecified palm** CC
CC Excl: See code: T23.751

6th **T23.76 Corrosion of third degree of back of hand**

7 7th **T23.761 Corrosion of third degree of back of right hand** CC
CC Excl: CC with 7th character A: T23.301-T23.309 with 7th A, T23.361-T23.369 with 7th A, T23.391-T23.399 with 7th A, T23.701-T23.709 with 7th A, T23.761-T23.769 with 7th A, T23.791-T23.799 with 7th A

7 7th **T23.762 Corrosion of third degree of back of left hand** CC
CC Excl: See code: T23.761

7 7th **T23.769 Corrosion of third degree back of unspecified hand** CC
CC Excl: See code: T23.761

6th **T23.77 Corrosion of third degree of wrist**

7 7th **T23.771 Corrosion of third degree of right wrist** CC
CC Excl: CC with 7th character A: T23.301-T23.309 with 7th A, T23.371-T23.379 with 7th A, T23.391-T23.399 with 7th A, T23.701-T23.709 with 7th A, T23.771-T23.779 with 7th A, T23.791-T23.799 with 7th A

7 7th **T23.772 Corrosion of third degree of left wrist** CC
CC Excl: See code: T23.771

7 7th **T23.779 Corrosion of third degree of unspecified wrist** CC
CC Excl: See code: T23.771

6th **T23.79 Corrosion of third degree of multiple sites of wrist and hand**

7 7th **T23.791 Corrosion of third degree of multiple sites of right wrist and hand** CC
CC Excl: See code: T23.702

7 7th **T23.792 Corrosion of third degree of multiple sites of left wrist and hand** CC
CC Excl: See code: T23.702

7 7th **T23.799 Corrosion of third degree of multiple sites of unspecified wrist and hand** CC
CC Excl: See code: T23.702

4th **T24 Burn and corrosion of lower limb, except ankle and foot**
EXCLUDES 2 *burn and corrosion of ankle and foot (T25.-)*
burn and corrosion of hip region (T21.-)

The appropriate 7th character is to be added to each code from category T24.
A initial encounter
D subsequent encounter
S sequela

5th **T24.0 Burn of unspecified degree of lower limb, except ankle and foot**
Use additional external cause code to identify the source, place and intent of the burn (X00-X19, X75-X77, X96-X98, Y92)

6th **T24.00 Burn of unspecified degree of unspecified site of lower limb, except ankle and foot**

7 HAC = Initial encounter only (7th character A, B or C) and not POA.

T24.001 Burn of unspecified degree of unspecified site of right lower limb, except ankle and foot
T24.002 Burn of unspecified degree of unspecified site of left lower limb, except ankle and foot
T24.009 Burn of unspecified degree of unspecified site of unspecified lower limb, except ankle and foot
T24.01 Burn of unspecified degree of thigh
T24.011 Burn of unspecified degree of right thigh
T24.012 Burn of unspecified degree of left thigh
T24.019 Burn of unspecified degree of unspecified thigh
T24.02 Burn of unspecified degree of knee
T24.021 Burn of unspecified degree of right knee
T24.022 Burn of unspecified degree of left knee
T24.029 Burn of unspecified degree of unspecified knee
T24.03 Burn of unspecified degree of lower leg
T24.031 Burn of unspecified degree of right lower leg
T24.032 Burn of unspecified degree of left lower leg
T24.039 Burn of unspecified degree of unspecified lower leg
T24.09 Burn of unspecified degree of multiple sites of lower limb, except ankle and foot
T24.091 Burn of unspecified degree of multiple sites of right lower limb, except ankle and foot
T24.092 Burn of unspecified degree of multiple sites of left lower limb, except ankle and foot
T24.099 Burn of unspecified degree of multiple sites of unspecified lower limb, except ankle and foot
T24.1 Burn of first degree of lower limb, except ankle and foot
Use additional external cause code to identify the source, place and intent of the burn (X00-X19, X75-X77, X96-X98, Y92)
T24.10 Burn of first degree of unspecified site of lower limb, except ankle and foot
T24.101 Burn of first degree of unspecified site of right lower limb, except ankle and foot
T24.102 Burn of first degree of unspecified site of left lower limb, except ankle and foot
T24.109 Burn of first degree of unspecified site of unspecified lower limb, except ankle and foot
T24.11 Burn of first degree of thigh
T24.111 Burn of first degree of right thigh
T24.112 Burn of first degree of left thigh
T24.119 Burn of first degree of unspecified thigh
T24.12 Burn of first degree of knee
T24.121 Burn of first degree of right knee
T24.122 Burn of first degree of left knee
T24.129 Burn of first degree of unspecified knee
T24.13 Burn of first degree of lower leg
T24.131 Burn of first degree of right lower leg
T24.132 Burn of first degree of left lower leg
T24.139 Burn of first degree of unspecified lower leg
T24.19 Burn of first degree of multiple sites of lower limb, except ankle and foot
T24.191 Burn of first degree of multiple sites of right lower limb, except ankle and foot
T24.192 Burn of first degree of multiple sites of left lower limb, except ankle and foot
T24.199 Burn of first degree of multiple sites of unspecified lower limb, except ankle and foot

T24.2 Burn of second degree of lower limb, except ankle and foot
Use additional external cause code to identify the source, place and intent of the burn (X00-X19, X75-X77, X96-X98, Y92)
T24.20 Burn of second degree of unspecified site of lower limb, except ankle and foot
T24.201 Burn of second degree of unspecified site of right lower limb, except ankle and foot
T24.202 Burn of second degree of unspecified site of left lower limb, except ankle and foot
T24.209 Burn of second degree of unspecified site of unspecified lower limb, except ankle and foot
T24.21 Burn of second degree of thigh
T24.211 Burn of second degree of right thigh
T24.212 Burn of second degree of left thigh
T24.219 Burn of second degree of unspecified thigh
T24.22 Burn of second degree of knee
T24.221 Burn of second degree of right knee
T24.222 Burn of second degree of left knee
T24.229 Burn of second degree of unspecified knee
T24.23 Burn of second degree of lower leg
T24.231 Burn of second degree of right lower leg
T24.232 Burn of second degree of left lower leg
T24.239 Burn of second degree of unspecified lower leg
T24.29 Burn of second degree of multiple sites of lower limb, except ankle and foot
T24.291 Burn of second degree of multiple sites of right lower limb, except ankle and foot
T24.292 Burn of second degree of multiple sites of left lower limb, except ankle and foot
T24.299 Burn of second degree of multiple sites of unspecified lower limb, except ankle and foot
T24.3 Burn of third degree of lower limb, except ankle and foot
Use additional external cause code to identify the source, place and intent of the burn (X00-X19, X75-X77, X96-X98, Y92)
T24.30 Burn of third degree of unspecified site of lower limb, except ankle and foot
7 T24.301 Burn of third degree of unspecified site of right lower limb, except ankle and foot CC
CC Excl: CC with 7th character A: T24.301-T24.309 with 7th A, T24.391-T24.399 with 7th A, T24.701-T24.709 with 7th A, T24.791-T24.799 with 7th A, T25.391-T25.399 with 7th A, T25.791-T25.790 with 7th A
7 T24.302 Burn of third degree of unspecified site of left lower limb, except ankle and foot CC
CC Excl: See code: T24.301
7 T24.309 Burn of third degree of unspecified site of unspecified lower limb, except ankle and foot CC
CC Excl: See code: T24.301
T24.31 Burn of third degree of thigh
7 T24.311 Burn of third degree of right thigh CC
CC Excl: CC with 7th character A: T24.301-T24.309 with 7th A, T24.311-T24.319 with 7th A, T24.391-T24.399 with 7th A, T24.701-T24.709 with 7th A, T24.711-T24.719 with 7th A, T24.791-T24.799 with 7th A, T25.391-T25.399 with 7th A, T25.791-T25.790 with 7th A
7 T24.312 Burn of third degree of left thigh CC
CC Excl: See code: T24.311
7 T24.319 Burn of third degree of unspecified thigh CC
CC Excl: See code: T24.311

7 HAC = Initial encounter only (7th character A, B or C) and not POA.

✓6th **T24.32 Burn of third degree of knee**

7 ✓7th **T24.321 Burn of third degree of right knee** CC
CC Excl: CC with 7th character A: T24.301-T24.309 with 7th A, T24.321-T24.329 with 7th A, T24.391-T24.399 with 7th A, T24.701-T24.709 with 7th A, T24.721-T24.729 with 7th A, T24.791-T24.799 with 7th A, T25.391-T25.399 with 7th A, T25.791-T25.790 with 7th A

7 ✓7th **T24.322 Burn of third degree of left knee** CC
CC Excl: See code: T24.321

7 ✓7th **T24.329 Burn of third degree of unspecified knee** CC
CC Excl: See code: T24.321

✓6th **T24.33 Burn of third degree of lower leg**

7 ✓7th **T24.331 Burn of third degree of right lower leg** CC
CC Excl: CC with 7th character A: T24.301-T24.309 with 7th A, T24.331-T24.339 with 7th A, T24.391-T24.399 with 7th A, T24.701-T24.709 with 7th A, T24.731-T24.739 with 7th A, T24.791-T24.799 with 7th A, T25.391-T25.399 with 7th A, T25.791-T25.790 with 7th A

7 ✓7th **T24.332 Burn of third degree of left lower leg** CC
CC Excl: See code: T24.331

7 ✓7th **T24.339 Burn of third degree of unspecified lower leg** CC
CC Excl: See code: T24.331

✓6th **T24.39 Burn of third degree of multiple sites of lower limb, except ankle and foot**

7 ✓7th **T24.391 Burn of third degree of multiple sites of right lower limb, except ankle and foot** CC
CC Excl: CC with 7th character A: T24.301-T24.309 with 7th A, T24.391-T24.399 with 7th A, T24.701-T24.709 with 7th A, T24.791-T24.799 with 7th A, T25.391-T25.399 with 7th A, T25.791-T25.799 with 7th A

7 ✓7th **T24.392 Burn of third degree of multiple sites of left lower limb, except ankle and foot** CC
CC Excl: See code: T24.301

7 ✓7th **T24.399 Burn of third degree of multiple sites of unspecified lower limb, except ankle and foot** CC
CC Excl: See code: T24.301

✓5th **T24.4 Corrosion of unspecified degree of lower limb, except ankle and foot**
Code first (T51-T65) to identify chemical and intent
Use additional external cause code to identify place (Y92)

✓6th **T24.40 Corrosion of unspecified degree of unspecified site of lower limb, except ankle and foot**

✓7th **T24.401 Corrosion of unspecified degree of unspecified site of right lower limb, except ankle and foot**

✓7th **T24.402 Corrosion of unspecified degree of unspecified site of left lower limb, except ankle and foot**

✓7th **T24.409 Corrosion of unspecified degree of unspecified site of unspecified lower limb, except ankle and foot**

✓6th **T24.41 Corrosion of unspecified degree of thigh**

✓7th **T24.411 Corrosion of unspecified degree of right thigh**

✓7th **T24.412 Corrosion of unspecified degree of left thigh**

✓7th **T24.419 Corrosion of unspecified degree of unspecified thigh**

✓6th **T24.42 Corrosion of unspecified degree of knee**

✓7th **T24.421 Corrosion of unspecified degree of right knee**

✓7th **T24.422 Corrosion of unspecified degree of left knee**

✓7th **T24.429 Corrosion of unspecified degree of unspecified knee**

✓6th **T24.43 Corrosion of unspecified degree of lower leg**

✓7th **T24.431 Corrosion of unspecified degree of right lower leg**

✓7th **T24.432 Corrosion of unspecified degree of left lower leg**

✓7th **T24.439 Corrosion of unspecified degree of unspecified lower leg**

✓6th **T24.49 Corrosion of unspecified degree of multiple sites of lower limb, except ankle and foot**

✓7th **T24.491 Corrosion of unspecified degree of multiple sites of right lower limb, except ankle and foot**

✓7th **T24.492 Corrosion of unspecified degree of multiple sites of left lower limb, except ankle and foot**

✓7th **T24.499 Corrosion of unspecified degree of multiple sites of unspecified lower limb, except ankle and foot**

✓5th **T24.5 Corrosion of first degree of lower limb, except ankle and foot**
Code first (T51-T65) to identify chemical and intent
Use additional external cause code to identify place (Y92)

✓6th **T24.50 Corrosion of first degree of unspecified site of lower limb, except ankle and foot**

✓7th **T24.501 Corrosion of first degree of unspecified site of right lower limb, except ankle and foot**

✓7th **T24.502 Corrosion of first degree of unspecified site of left lower limb, except ankle and foot**

✓7th **T24.509 Corrosion of first degree of unspecified site of unspecified lower limb, except ankle and foot**

✓6th **T24.51 Corrosion of first degree of thigh**

✓7th **T24.511 Corrosion of first degree of right thigh**

✓7th **T24.512 Corrosion of first degree of left thigh**

✓7th **T24.519 Corrosion of first degree of unspecified thigh**

✓6th **T24.52 Corrosion of first degree of knee**

✓7th **T24.521 Corrosion of first degree of right knee**

✓7th **T24.522 Corrosion of first degree of left knee**

✓7th **T24.529 Corrosion of first degree of unspecified knee**

✓6th **T24.53 Corrosion of first degree of lower leg**

✓7th **T24.531 Corrosion of first degree of right lower leg**

✓7th **T24.532 Corrosion of first degree of left lower leg**

✓7th **T24.539 Corrosion of first degree of unspecified lower leg**

✓6th **T24.59 Corrosion of first degree of multiple sites of lower limb, except ankle and foot**

✓7th **T24.591 Corrosion of first degree of multiple sites of right lower limb, except ankle and foot**

✓7th **T24.592 Corrosion of first degree of multiple sites of left lower limb, except ankle and foot**

✓7th **T24.599 Corrosion of first degree of multiple sites of unspecified lower limb, except ankle and foot**

✓5th **T24.6 Corrosion of second degree of lower limb, except ankle and foot**
Code first (T51-T65) to identify chemical and intent
Use additional external cause code to identify place (Y92)

✓6th **T24.60 Corrosion of second degree of unspecified site of lower limb, except ankle and foot**

✓7th **T24.601 Corrosion of second degree of unspecified site of right lower limb, except ankle and foot**

✓7th **T24.602 Corrosion of second degree of unspecified site of left lower limb, except ankle and foot**

✓7th **T24.609 Corrosion of second degree of unspecified site of unspecified lower limb, except ankle and foot**

✓6th **T24.61 Corrosion of second degree of thigh**

✓7th **T24.611 Corrosion of second degree of right thigh**

7 HAC = Initial encounter only (7th character A, B or C) and not POA.

✓7th **T24.612** **Corrosion of second degree of left thigh**

✓7th **T24.619** **Corrosion of second degree of unspecified thigh**

✓6th **T24.62** **Corrosion of second degree of knee**

✓7th **T24.621** **Corrosion of second degree of right knee**

✓7th **T24.622** **Corrosion of second degree of left knee**

✓7th **T24.629** **Corrosion of second degree of unspecified knee**

✓6th **T24.63** **Corrosion of second degree of lower leg**

✓7th **T24.631** **Corrosion of second degree of right lower leg**

✓7th **T24.632** **Corrosion of second degree of left lower leg**

✓7th **T24.639** **Corrosion of second degree of unspecified lower leg**

✓6th **T24.69** **Corrosion of second degree of multiple sites of lower limb, except ankle and foot**

✓7th **T24.691** **Corrosion of second degree of multiple sites of right lower limb, except ankle and foot**

✓7th **T24.692** **Corrosion of second degree of multiple sites of left lower limb, except ankle and foot**

✓7th **T24.699** **Corrosion of second degree of multiple sites of unspecified lower limb, except ankle and foot**

✓5th **T24.7** **Corrosion of third degree of lower limb, except ankle and foot**

Code first (T51-T65) to identify chemical and intent

Use additional external cause code to identify place (Y92)

✓6th **T24.70** **Corrosion of third degree of unspecified site of lower limb, except ankle and foot**

7 ✓7th **T24.701** **Corrosion of third degree of unspecified site of right lower limb, except ankle and foot** CC

CC Excl: CC with 7th character A: See code: T24.301

7 ✓7th **T24.702** **Corrosion of third degree of unspecified site of left lower limb, except ankle and foot** CC

CC Excl: See code: T24.301

7 ✓7th **T24.709** **Corrosion of third degree of unspecified site of unspecified lower limb, except ankle and foot** CC

CC Excl: See code: T24.301

✓6th **T24.71** **Corrosion of third degree of thigh**

7 ✓7th **T24.711** **Corrosion of third degree of right thigh** CC

CC Excl: CC with 7th character A: See code: T24.311

7 ✓7th **T24.712** **Corrosion of third degree of left thigh** CC

CC Excl: See code: T24.311

7 ✓7th **T24.719** **Corrosion of third degree of unspecified thigh** CC

CC Excl: See code: T24.311

✓6th **T24.72** **Corrosion of third degree of knee**

7 ✓7th **T24.721** **Corrosion of third degree of right knee** CC

CC Excl: CC with 7th character A: See code: T24.321

7 ✓7th **T24.722** **Corrosion of third degree of left knee** CC

CC Excl: See code: T24.321

7 ✓7th **T24.729** **Corrosion of third degree of unspecified knee** CC

CC Excl: See code: T24.321

✓6th **T24.73** **Corrosion of third degree of lower leg**

7 ✓7th **T24.731** **Corrosion of third degree of right lower leg** CC

CC Excl: CC with 7th character A: See code: T24.331

7 ✓7th **T24.732** **Corrosion of third degree of left lower leg** CC

CC Excl: See code: T24.331

7 ✓7th **T24.739** **Corrosion of third degree of unspecified lower leg** CC

CC Excl: See code: T24.331

✓6th **T24.79** **Corrosion of third degree of multiple sites of lower limb, except ankle and foot**

7 ✓7th **T24.791** **Corrosion of third degree of multiple sites of right lower limb, except ankle and foot** CC

CC Excl: CC with 7th character A: See code: T24.301

7 ✓7th **T24.792** **Corrosion of third degree of multiple sites of left lower limb, except ankle and foot** CC

CC Excl: See code: T24.301

7 ✓7th **T24.799** **Corrosion of third degree of multiple sites of unspecified lower limb, except ankle and foot** CC

CC Excl: See code: T24.301

✓4th **T25** **Burn and corrosion of ankle and foot**

The appropriate 7th character is to be added to each code from category T25.
A initial encounter
D subsequent encounter
S sequela

✓5th **T25.0** **Burn of unspecified degree of ankle and foot**

Use additional external cause code to identify the source, place and intent of the burn (X00-X19, X75-X77, X96-X98, Y92)

✓6th **T25.01** **Burn of unspecified degree of ankle**

✓7th **T25.011** **Burn of unspecified degree of right ankle**

✓7th **T25.012** **Burn of unspecified degree of left ankle**

✓7th **T25.019** **Burn of unspecified degree of unspecified ankle**

✓6th **T25.02** **Burn of unspecified degree of foot**

EXCLUDES 2 *burn of unspecified degree of toe(s) (nail) (T25.03-)*

✓7th **T25.021** **Burn of unspecified degree of right foot**

✓7th **T25.022** **Burn of unspecified degree of left foot**

✓7th **T25.029** **Burn of unspecified degree of unspecified foot**

✓6th **T25.03** **Burn of unspecified degree of toe(s) (nail)**

✓7th **T25.031** **Burn of unspecified degree of right toe(s) (nail)**

✓7th **T25.032** **Burn of unspecified degree of left toe(s) (nail)**

✓7th **T25.039** **Burn of unspecified degree of unspecified toe(s) (nail)**

✓6th **T25.09** **Burn of unspecified degree of multiple sites of ankle and foot**

✓7th **T25.091** **Burn of unspecified degree of multiple sites of right ankle and foot**

✓7th **T25.092** **Burn of unspecified degree of multiple sites of left ankle and foot**

✓7th **T25.099** **Burn of unspecified degree of multiple sites of unspecified ankle and foot**

✓5th **T25.1** **Burn of first degree of ankle and foot**

Use additional external cause code to identify the source, place and intent of the burn (X00-X19, X75-X77, X96-X98, Y92)

✓6th **T25.11** **Burn of first degree of ankle**

✓7th **T25.111** **Burn of first degree of right ankle**

✓7th **T25.112** **Burn of first degree of left ankle**

✓7th **T25.119** **Burn of first degree of unspecified ankle**

✓6th **T25.12** **Burn of first degree of foot**

EXCLUDES 2 *burn of first degree of toe(s) (nail) (T25.13-)*

✓7th **T25.121** **Burn of first degree of right foot**

✓7th **T25.122** **Burn of first degree of left foot**

✓7th **T25.129** **Burn of first degree of unspecified foot**

✓6th **T25.13** **Burn of first degree of toe(s) (nail)**

✓7th **T25.131** **Burn of first degree of right toe(s) (nail)**

✓7th **T25.132** **Burn of first degree of left toe(s) (nail)**

✓7th **T25.139** **Burn of first degree of unspecified toe(s) (nail)**

✓6th **T25.19** **Burn of first degree of multiple sites of ankle and foot**

✓7th **T25.191** **Burn of first degree of multiple sites of right ankle and foot**

7 HAC = Initial encounter only (7th character A, B or C) and not POA.

✓7th T25.192 **Burn of first degree of multiple sites of left ankle and foot**

✓7th T25.199 **Burn of first degree of multiple sites of unspecified ankle and foot**

✓5th T25.2 **Burn of second degree of ankle and foot**
Use additional external cause code to identify the source, place and intent of the burn (X00-X19, X75-X77, X96-X98, Y92)

✓6th T25.21 **Burn of second degree of ankle**

✓7th T25.211 **Burn of second degree of right ankle**

✓7th T25.212 **Burn of second degree of left ankle**

✓7th T25.219 **Burn of second degree of unspecified ankle**

✓6th T25.22 **Burn of second degree of foot**
EXCLUDES 2 *burn of second degree of toe(s) (nail) (T25.23-)*

✓7th T25.221 **Burn of second degree of right foot**

✓7th T25.222 **Burn of second degree of left foot**

✓7th T25.229 **Burn of second degree of unspecified foot**

✓6th T25.23 **Burn of second degree of toe(s) (nail)**

✓7th T25.231 **Burn of second degree of right toe(s) (nail)**

✓7th T25.232 **Burn of second degree of left toe(s) (nail)**

✓7th T25.239 **Burn of second degree of unspecified toe(s) (nail)**

✓6th T25.29 **Burn of second degree of multiple sites of ankle and foot**

✓7th T25.291 **Burn of second degree of multiple sites of right ankle and foot**

✓7th T25.292 **Burn of second degree of multiple sites of left ankle and foot**

✓7th T25.299 **Burn of second degree of multiple sites of unspecified ankle and foot**

✓5th T25.3 **Burn of third degree of ankle and foot**
Use additional external cause code to identify the source, place and intent of the burn (X00-X19, X75-X77, X96-X98, Y92)

✓6th T25.31 **Burn of third degree of ankle**

7 ✓7th T25.311 **Burn of third degree of right ankle** CC
CC Excl: CC with 7th character A: T24.301-T24.309 with 7th A, T24.391-T24.399 with 7th A, T24.701-T24.709 with 7th A, T24.791-T24.799 with 7th A, T25.311-T25.319 with 7th A, T25.391-T25.399 with 7th A, T25.711-T25.719 with 7th A, T25.791-T25.790 with 7th A

7 ✓7th T25.312 **Burn of third degree of left ankle** CC
CC Excl: See code: T25.311

7 ✓7th T25.319 **Burn of third degree of unspecified ankle** CC
CC Excl: See code: T25.311

✓6th T25.32 **Burn of third degree of foot**
EXCLUDES 2 *burn of third degree of toe(s) (nail) (T25.33-)*

7 ✓7th T25.321 **Burn of third degree of right foot** CC
CC Excl: CC with 7th character A: T24.301-T24.309 with 7th A, T24.391-T24.399 with 7th A, T24.701-T24.709 with 7th A, T24.791-T24.799 with 7th A, T25.321-T25.329 with 7th A, T25.391-T25.399 with 7th A, T25.721-T25.729 with 7th A, T25.791-T25.799 with 7th A

7 ✓7th T25.322 **Burn of third degree of left foot** CC
CC Excl: See code: T25.321

7 ✓7th T25.329 **Burn of third degree of unspecified foot** CC
CC Excl: See code: T25.321

✓6th T25.33 **Burn of third degree of toe(s) (nail)**

7 ✓7th T25.331 **Burn of third degree of right toe(s) (nail)** CC
CC Excl: CC with 7th character A: T24.301-T24.309 with 7th A, T24.391-T24.399 with 7th A, T24.701-T24.709 with 7th A, T24.791-T24.799 with 7th A, T25.331-T25.339 with 7th A, T25.391-T25.399 with 7th A, T25.731-T25.739 with 7th A, T25.791-T25.799 with 7th A

7 ✓7th T25.332 **Burn of third degree of left toe(s) (nail)** CC
CC Excl: See code: T25.331

7 ✓7th T25.339 **Burn of third degree of unspecified toe(s) (nail)** CC
CC Excl: See code: T25.331

✓6th T25.39 **Burn of third degree of multiple sites of ankle and foot**

7 ✓7th T25.391 **Burn of third degree of multiple sites of right ankle and foot** CC
CC Excl: CC with 7th character A: See code: T25.331

7 ✓7th T25.392 **Burn of third degree of multiple sites of left ankle and foot** CC
CC Excl: See code: T25.331

7 ✓7th T25.399 **Burn of third degree of multiple sites of unspecified ankle and foot** CC
CC Excl: See code: T25.331

✓5th T25.4 **Corrosion of unspecified degree of ankle and foot**
Code first (T51-T65) to identify chemical and intent
Use additional external cause code to identify place (Y92)

✓6th T25.41 **Corrosion of unspecified degree of ankle**

✓7th T25.411 **Corrosion of unspecified degree of right ankle**

✓7th T25.412 **Corrosion of unspecified degree of left ankle**

✓7th T25.419 **Corrosion of unspecified degree of unspecified ankle**

✓6th T25.42 **Corrosion of unspecified degree of foot**
EXCLUDES 2 *corrosion of unspecified degree of toe(s) (nail) (T25.43-)*

✓7th T25.421 **Corrosion of unspecified degree of right foot**

✓7th T25.422 **Corrosion of unspecified degree of left foot**

✓7th T25.429 **Corrosion of unspecified degree of unspecified foot**

✓6th T25.43 **Corrosion of unspecified degree of toe(s) (nail)**

✓7th T25.431 **Corrosion of unspecified degree of right toe(s) (nail)**

✓7th T25.432 **Corrosion of unspecified degree of left toe(s) (nail)**

✓7th T25.439 **Corrosion of unspecified degree of unspecified toe(s) (nail)**

✓6th T25.49 **Corrosion of unspecified degree of multiple sites of ankle and foot**

✓7th T25.491 **Corrosion of unspecified degree of multiple sites of right ankle and foot**

✓7th T25.492 **Corrosion of unspecified degree of multiple sites of left ankle and foot**

✓7th T25.499 **Corrosion of unspecified degree of multiple sites of unspecified ankle and foot**

✓5th T25.5 **Corrosion of first degree of ankle and foot**
Code first (T51-T65) to identify chemical and intent
Use additional external cause code to identify place (Y92)

✓6th T25.51 **Corrosion of first degree of ankle**

✓7th T25.511 **Corrosion of first degree of right ankle**

✓7th T25.512 **Corrosion of first degree of left ankle**

✓7th T25.519 **Corrosion of first degree of unspecified ankle**

✓6th T25.52 **Corrosion of first degree of foot**
EXCLUDES 2 *corrosion of first degree of toe(s) (nail) (T25.53-)*

✓7th T25.521 **Corrosion of first degree of right foot**

✓7th T25.522 **Corrosion of first degree of left foot**

✓7th T25.529 **Corrosion of first degree of unspecified foot**

✓6th T25.53 **Corrosion of first degree of toe(s) (nail)**

✓7th T25.531 **Corrosion of first degree of right toe(s) (nail)**

✓7th T25.532 **Corrosion of first degree of left toe(s) (nail)**

✓7th T25.539 **Corrosion of first degree of unspecified toe(s) (nail)**

7 HAC = Initial encounter only (7th character A, B or C) and not POA.

✓6th T25.59 **Corrosion of first degree of multiple sites of ankle and foot**

✓7th T25.591 **Corrosion of first degree of multiple sites of right ankle and foot**

✓7th T25.592 **Corrosion of first degree of multiple sites of left ankle and foot**

✓7th T25.599 **Corrosion of first degree of multiple sites of unspecified ankle and foot**

✓5th T25.6 **Corrosion of second degree of ankle and foot**

Code first (T51-T65) to identify chemical and intent

Use additional external cause code to identify place (Y92)

✓6th T25.61 **Corrosion of second degree of ankle**

✓7th T25.611 **Corrosion of second degree of right ankle**

✓7th T25.612 **Corrosion of second degree of left ankle**

✓7th T25.619 **Corrosion of second degree of unspecified ankle**

✓6th T25.62 **Corrosion of second degree of foot**

EXCLUDES 2 *corrosion of second degree of toe(s) (nail) (T25.63-)*

✓7th T25.621 **Corrosion of second degree of right foot**

✓7th T25.622 **Corrosion of second degree of left foot**

✓7th T25.629 **Corrosion of second degree of unspecified foot**

✓6th T25.63 **Corrosion of second degree of toe(s) (nail)**

✓7th T25.631 **Corrosion of second degree of right toe(s) (nail)**

✓7th T25.632 **Corrosion of second degree of left toe(s) (nail)**

✓7th T25.639 **Corrosion of second degree of unspecified toe(s) (nail)**

✓6th T25.69 **Corrosion of second degree of multiple sites of ankle and foot**

✓7th T25.691 **Corrosion of second degree of right ankle and foot**

✓7th T25.692 **Corrosion of second degree of left ankle and foot**

✓7th T25.699 **Corrosion of second degree of unspecified ankle and foot**

✓5th T25.7 **Corrosion of third degree of ankle and foot**

Code first (T51-T65) to identify chemical and intent

Use additional external cause code to identify place (Y92)

✓6th T25.71 **Corrosion of third degree of ankle**

7 ✓7th T25.711 **Corrosion of third degree of right ankle** CC

CC Excl: CC with 7th character A: T24.301-T24.309 with 7th A, T24.391-T24.399 with 7th A, T24.701-T24.709 with 7th A, T24.791-T24.799 with 7th A, T25.311-T25.319 with 7th A, T25.391-T25.399 with 7th A, T25.711-T25.719 with 7th A, T25.791-T25.799 with 7th A

7 ✓7th T25.712 **Corrosion of third degree of left ankle** CC

CC Excl: See code: T25.711

7 ✓7th T25.719 **Corrosion of third degree of unspecified ankle** CC

CC Excl: See code: T25.711

✓6th T25.72 **Corrosion of third degree of foot**

EXCLUDES 2 *corrosion of third degree of toe(s) (nail) (T25.73-)*

7 ✓7th T25.721 **Corrosion of third degree of right foot** CC

CC Excl: CC with 7th character A: T24.301-T24.309 with 7th A, T24.391-T24.399 with 7th A, T24.701-T24.709 with 7th A, T24.791-T24.799 with 7th A, T25.321-T25.329 with 7th A, T25.391-T25.399 with 7th A, T25.721-T25.729 with 7th A, T25.791-T25.799 with 7th A

7 ✓7th T25.722 **Corrosion of third degree of left foot** CC

CC Excl: See code: T25.721

7 ✓7th T25.729 **Corrosion of third degree of unspecified foot** CC

CC Excl: See code: T25.721

✓6th T25.73 **Corrosion of third degree of toe(s) (nail)**

7 ✓7th T25.731 **Corrosion of third degree of right toe(s) (nail)** CC

CC Excl: CC with 7th character A: T24.301-T24.309 with 7th A, T24.391-T24.399 with 7th A, T24.701-T24.709 with 7th A, T24.791-T24.799 with 7th A, T25.331-T25.399 with 7th A, T25.731-T25.799 with 7th A

7 ✓7th T25.732 **Corrosion of third degree of left toe(s) (nail)** CC

CC Excl: See code: T25.731

7 ✓7th T25.739 **Corrosion of third degree of unspecified toe(s) (nail)** CC

CC Excl: See code: T25.731

✓6th T25.79 **Corrosion of third degree of multiple sites of ankle and foot**

7 ✓7th T25.791 **Corrosion of third degree of multiple sites of right ankle and foot** CC

CC Excl: CC with 7th character A: T24.301-T24.309 with 7th A, T24.391-T24.399 with 7th A, T24.701-T24.709 with 7th A, T24.791-T24.799 with 7th A, T25.391-T25.399 with 7th A, T25.791-T25.799 with 7th A

7 ✓7th T25.792 **Corrosion of third degree of multiple sites of left ankle and foot** CC

CC Excl: See code: T25.791

7 ✓7th T25.799 **Corrosion of third degree of multiple sites of unspecified ankle and foot** CC

CC Excl: See code: T25.791

Burns and corrosions confined to eye and internal organs (T26-T28)

✓4th **T26 Burn and corrosion confined to eye and adnexa**

The appropriate 7th character is to be added to each code from category T26.
A initial encounter
D subsequent encounter
S sequela

✓5th T26.0 **Burn of eyelid and periocular area**

Use additional external cause code to identify the source, place and intent of the burn (X00-X19, X75-X77, X96-X98, Y92)

✓x7th T26.00 **Burn of unspecified eyelid and periocular area**

✓x7th T26.01 **Burn of right eyelid and periocular area**

✓x7th T26.02 **Burn of left eyelid and periocular area**

✓5th T26.1 **Burn of cornea and conjunctival sac**

Use additional external cause code to identify the source, place and intent of the burn (X00-X19, X75-X77, X96-X98, Y92)

✓x7th T26.10 **Burn of cornea and conjunctival sac, unspecified eye**

✓x7th T26.11 **Burn of cornea and conjunctival sac, right eye**

✓x7th T26.12 **Burn of cornea and conjunctival sac, left eye**

✓5th T26.2 **Burn with resulting rupture and destruction of eyeball**

Use additional external cause code to identify the source, place and intent of the burn (X00-X19, X75-X77, X96-X98, Y92)

7 ✓x7th T26.20 **Burn with resulting rupture and destruction of unspecified eyeball** CC

CC Excl: No Excl

7 ✓x7th T26.21 **Burn with resulting rupture and destruction of right eyeball** CC

CC Excl: No Excl

7 ✓x7th T26.22 **Burn with resulting rupture and destruction of left eyeball** CC

CC Excl: No Excl

✓5th T26.3 **Burns of other specified parts of eye and adnexa**

Use additional external cause code to identify the source, place and intent of the burn (X00-X19, X75-X77, X96-X98, Y92)

✓x7th T26.30 **Burns of other specified parts of unspecified eye and adnexa**

✓x7th T26.31 **Burns of other specified parts of right eye and adnexa**

✓x7th T26.32 **Burns of other specified parts of left eye and adnexa**

7 HAC = Initial encounter only (7th character A, B or C) and not POA.

5th T26.4 **Burn of eye and adnexa, part unspecified**
Use additional external cause code to identify the source, place and intent of the burn (X00-X19, X75-X77, X96-X98, Y92)

x7th T26.40 **Burn of unspecified eye and adnexa, part unspecified**

x7th T26.41 **Burn of right eye and adnexa, part unspecified**

x7th T26.42 **Burn of left eye and adnexa, part unspecified**

5th T26.5 **Corrosion of eyelid and periocular area**
Code first (T51-T65) to identify chemical and intent
Use additional external cause code to identify place (Y92)

x7th T26.50 **Corrosion of unspecified eyelid and periocular area**

x7th T26.51 **Corrosion of right eyelid and periocular area**

x7th T26.52 **Corrosion of left eyelid and periocular area**

5th T26.6 **Corrosion of cornea and conjunctival sac**
Code first (T51-T65) to identify chemical and intent
Use additional external cause code to identify place (Y92)

x7th T26.60 **Corrosion of cornea and conjunctival sac, unspecified eye**

x7th T26.61 **Corrosion of cornea and conjunctival sac, right eye**

x7th T26.62 **Corrosion of cornea and conjunctival sac, left eye**

5th T26.7 **Corrosion with resulting rupture and destruction of eyeball**
Code first (T51-T65) to identify chemical and intent
Use additional external cause code to identify place (Y92)

7 x7th T26.70 **Corrosion with resulting rupture and destruction of unspecified eyeball** CC
CC Excl: No Excl

7 x7th T26.71 **Corrosion with resulting rupture and destruction of right eyeball** CC
CC Excl: No Excl

7 x7th T26.72 **Corrosion with resulting rupture and destruction of left eyeball** CC
CC Excl: No Excl

5th T26.8 **Corrosions of other specified parts of eye and adnexa**
Code first (T51-T65) to identify chemical and intent
Use additional external cause code to identify place (Y92)

x7th T26.80 **Corrosions of other specified parts of unspecified eye and adnexa**

x7th T26.81 **Corrosions of other specified parts of right eye and adnexa**

x7th T26.82 **Corrosions of other specified parts of left eye and adnexa**

5th T26.9 **Corrosion of eye and adnexa, part unspecified**
Code first (T51-T65) to identify chemical and intent
Use additional external cause code to identify place (Y92)

x7th T26.90 **Corrosion of unspecified eye and adnexa, part unspecified**

x7th T26.91 **Corrosion of right eye and adnexa, part unspecified**

x7th T26.92 **Corrosion of left eye and adnexa, part unspecified**

4th T27 **Burn and corrosion of respiratory tract**
Use additional external cause code to identify the source and intent of the burn (X00-X19, X75-X77, X96-X98)
Use additional external cause code to identify place (Y92)

The appropriate 7th character is to be added to each code from category T27.
A initial encounter
D subsequent encounter
S sequela

CC Excl: For CC codes in subcategory T27: CC with 7th character A: T27.0XX-T27.7XX with 7th A, T28.3XX-T28.49X with 7th A, T28.8XX-T28.99X with 7th A

7 x7th T27.0 **Burn of larynx and trachea** CC

7 x7th T27.1 **Burn involving larynx and trachea with lung** CC

7 x7th T27.2 **Burn of other parts of respiratory tract** CC
Burn of thoracic cavity

7 x7th T27.3 **Burn of respiratory tract, part unspecified** CC
Code first (T51-T65) to identify chemical and intent for codes T27.4-T27.7

7 x7th T27.4 **Corrosion of larynx and trachea** CC

7 x7th T27.5 **Corrosion involving larynx and trachea with lung** CC

7 x7th T27.6 **Corrosion of other parts of respiratory tract** CC

7 x7th T27.7 **Corrosion of respiratory tract, part unspecified** CC

4th T28 **Burn and corrosion of other internal organs**
Use additional external cause code to identify the source and intent of the burn (X00- X19, X75-X77, X96-X98)
Use additional external cause code to identify place (Y92)

The appropriate 7th character is to be added to each code from category T28.
A initial encounter
D subsequent encounter
S sequela

x7th T28.0 **Burn of mouth and pharynx**

7 x7th T28.1 **Burn of esophagus** CC
CC Excl: CC with 7th character A: T28.1XXA, T28.3XX-T28.49X with 7th A, T28.6XXA, T28.8XX-T28.99X with 7th A

7 x7th T28.2 **Burn of other parts of alimentary tract** CC
CC Excl: CC with 7th character A: T28.2XX-T28.49X with 7th A, T28.7XX-T28.99X with 7th A

x7th T28.3 **Burn of internal genitourinary organs**

5th T28.4 **Burns of other and unspecified internal organs**

x7th T28.40 **Burn of unspecified internal organ**

6th T28.41 **Burn of ear drum**

7th T28.411 **Burn of right ear drum**

7th T28.412 **Burn of left ear drum**

7th T28.419 **Burn of unspecified ear drum**

x7th T28.49 **Burn of other internal organ**
Code first (T51-T65) to identify chemical and intent for T28.5-T28.9-

x7th T28.5 **Corrosion of mouth and pharynx**

7 x7th T28.6 **Corrosion of esophagus** CC
CC Excl: CC with 7th character A: T28.1XXA, T28.3XX-T28.49X with 7th A, T28.6XXA, T28.8XX-T28.99X with 7th A

7 x7th T28.7 **Corrosion of other parts of alimentary tract** CC
CC Excl: CC with 7th character A: T28.2XX-T28.49X with 7th A, T28.7XX-T28.99X with 7th A

x7th T28.8 **Corrosion of internal genitourinary organs**

5th T28.9 **Corrosions of other and unspecified internal organs**

x7th T28.90 **Corrosions of unspecified internal organs**

6th T28.91 **Corrosions of ear drum**

7th T28.911 **Corrosions of right ear drum**

7th T28.912 **Corrosions of left ear drum**

7th T28.919 **Corrosions of unspecified ear drum**

x7th T28.99 **Corrosions of other internal organs**

Burns and corrosions of multiple and unspecified body regions (T30-T32)

4th T30 **Burn and corrosion, body region unspecified**

T30.0 **Burn of unspecified body region, unspecified degree**
NOTE This code is not for inpatient use. Code to specified site and degree of burns.
Burn NOS Multiple burns NOS

T30.4 **Corrosion of unspecified body region, unspecified degree**
NOTE This code is not for inpatient use. Code to specified site and degree of corrosion.
Corrosion NOS Multiple corrosion NOS

4th T31 **Burns classified according to extent of body surface involved**
NOTE This category is to be used as the primary code only when the site of the burn is unspecified. It should be used as a supplementary code with categories T20-T25 when the site is specified.

CC Excl: For CC codes in category T31: CC or MCC as indicated with 7th A, unless otherwise noted: T31.0-T32.99

T31.0 **Burns involving less than 10% of body surface**

5th T31.1 **Burns involving 10-19% of body surface**

T31.10 **Burns involving 10-19% of body surface with 0% to 9% third degree burns** CC
Burns involving 10-19% of body surface NOS

T31.11 **Burns involving 10-19% of body surface with 10-19% third degree burns** CC

5th T31.2 **Burns involving 20-29% of body surface**

T31.20 **Burns involving 20-29% of body surface with 0% to 9% third degree burns** CC
Burns involving 20-29% of body surface NOS

7 HAC = Initial encounter only (7th character A, B or C) and not POA.

T31.21 Burns involving 20-29% of body surface with 10-19% third degree burns MCC

T31.22 Burns involving 20-29% of body surface with 20-29% third degree burns MCC

✓5th T31.3 Burns involving 30-39% of body surface

T31.30 Burns involving 30-39% of body surface with 0% to 9% third degree burns CC
Burns involving 30-39% of body surface NOS

T31.31 Burns involving 30-39% of body surface with 10-19% third degree burns MCC

T31.32 Burns involving 30-39% of body surface with 20-29% third degree burns MCC

T31.33 Burns involving 30-39% of body surface 30-39% third degree burns MCC

✓5th T31.4 Burns involving 40-49% of body surface

T31.40 Burns involving 40-49% of body surface with 0% to 9% third degree burns CC
Burns involving 40-49% of body surface NOS

T31.41 Burns involving 40-49% of body surface with 10-19% third degree burns MCC

T31.42 Burns involving 40-49% of body surface with 20-29% third degree burns MCC

T31.43 Burns involving 40-49% of body surface with 30-39% third degree burns MCC

T31.44 Burns involving 40-49% of body surface with 40-49% third degree burns MCC

✓5th T31.5 Burns involving 50-59% of body surface

T31.50 Burns involving 50-59% of body surface with 0% to 9% third degree burns CC
Burns involving 50-59% of body surface NOS

T31.51 Burns involving 50-59% of body surface with 10-19% third degree burns MCC

T31.52 Burns involving 50-59% of body surface with 20-29% third degree burns MCC

T31.53 Burns involving 50-59% of body surface with 30-39% third degree burns MCC

T31.54 Burns involving 50-59% of body surface with 40-49% third degree burns MCC

T31.55 Burns involving 50-59% of body surface with 50-59% third degree burns MCC

✓5th T31.6 Burns involving 60-69% of body surface

T31.60 Burns involving 60-69% of body surface with 0% to 9% third degree burns CC
Burns involving 60-69% of body surface NOS

T31.61 Burns involving 60-69% of body surface with 10-19% third degree burns MCC

T31.62 Burns involving 60-69% of body surface with 20-29% third degree burns MCC

T31.63 Burns involving 60-69% of body surface with 30-39% third degree burns MCC

T31.64 Burns involving 60-69% of body surface with 40-49% third degree burns MCC

T31.65 Burns involving 60-69% of body surface with 50-59% third degree burns MCC

T31.66 Burns involving 60-69% of body surface with 60-69% third degree burns MCC

✓5th T31.7 Burns involving 70-79% of body surface

T31.70 Burns involving 70-79% of body surface with 0% to 9% third degree burns CC
Burns involving 70-79% of body surface NOS

T31.71 Burns involving 70-79% of body surface with 10-19% third degree burns MCC

T31.72 Burns involving 70-79% of body surface with 20-29% third degree burns MCC

T31.73 Burns involving 70-79% of body surface with 30-39% third degree burns MCC

T31.74 Burns involving 70-79% of body surface with 40-49% third degree burns MCC

T31.75 Burns involving 70-79% of body surface with 50-59% third degree burns MCC

T31.76 Burns involving 70-79% of body surface with 60-69% third degree burns MCC

T31.77 Burns involving 70-79% of body surface with 70-79% third degree burns MCC

✓5th T31.8 Burns involving 80-89% of body surface

T31.80 Burns involving 80-89% of body surface with 0% to 9% third degree burns CC
Burns involving 80-89% of body surface NOS

T31.81 Burns involving 80-89% of body surface with 10-19% third degree burns MCC

T31.82 Burns involving 80-89% of body surface with 20-29% third degree burns MCC

T31.83 Burns involving 80-89% of body surface with 30-39% third degree burns MCC

T31.84 Burns involving 80-89% of body surface with 40-49% third degree burns MCC

T31.85 Burns involving 80-89% of body surface with 50-59% third degree burns MCC

T31.86 Burns involving 80-89% of body surface with 60-69% third degree burns MCC

T31.87 Burns involving 80-89% of body surface with 70-79% third degree burns MCC

T31.88 Burns involving 80-89% of body surface with 80-89% third degree burns MCC

✓5th T31.9 Burns involving 90% or more of body surface

T31.90 Burns involving 90% or more of body surface with 0% to 9% third degree burns CC
Burns involving 90% or more of body surface NOS

T31.91 Burns involving 90% or more of body surface with 10-19% third degree burns MCC

T31.92 Burns involving 90% or more of body surface with 20-29% third degree burns MCC

T31.93 Burns involving 90% or more of body surface with 30-39% third degree burns MCC

T31.94 Burns involving 90% or more of body surface with 40-49% third degree burns MCC

T31.95 Burns involving 90% or more of body surface with 50-59% third degree burns MCC

T31.96 Burns involving 90% or more of body surface with 60-69% third degree burns MCC

T31.97 Burns involving 90% or more of body surface with 70-79% third degree burns MCC

T31.98 Burns involving 90% or more of body surface with 80-89% third degree burns MCC

T31.99 Burns involving 90% or more of body surface with 90% or more third degree burns MCC

✓4th T32 Corrosions classified according to extent of body surface involved

NOTE This category is to be used as the primary code only when the site of the corrosion is unspecified. It may be used as a supplementary code with categories T20-T25 when the site is specified.

CC Excl: For CC/MCC codes in category T32: CC or MCC as indicated with 7th A, unless otherwise noted:
See code: T31

T32.0 Corrosions involving less than 10% of body surface

✓5th T32.1 Corrosions involving 10-19% of body surface

T32.10 Corrosions involving 10-19% of body surface with 0% to 9% third degree corrosion CC
Corrosions involving 10-19% of body surface NOS

T32.11 Corrosions involving 10-19% of body surface with 10-19% third degree corrosion CC

✓5th T32.2 Corrosions involving 20-29% of body surface

T32.20 Corrosions involving 20-29% of body surface with 0% to 9% third degree corrosion CC

T32.21 Corrosions involving 20-29% of body surface with 10-19% third degree corrosion MCC

T32.22 Corrosions involving 20-29% of body surface with 20-29% third degree corrosion MCC

✓5th T32.3 Corrosions involving 30-39% of body surface

T32.30 Corrosions involving 30-39% of body surface with 0% to 9% third degree corrosion CC

T32.31 Corrosions involving 30-39% of body surface with 10-19% third degree corrosion MCC

T32.32 Corrosions involving 30-39% of body surface with 20-29% third degree corrosion MCC

T32.33 Corrosions involving 30-39% of body surface with 30-39% third degree corrosion MCC

✓5th **T32.4 Corrosions involving 4Ø-49% of body surface**

- **T32.4Ø Corrosions involving 4Ø-49% of body surface with Ø% to 9% third degree corrosion** CC
- **T32.41 Corrosions involving 4Ø-49% of body surface with 1Ø-19% third degree corrosion** MCC
- **T32.42 Corrosions involving 4Ø-49% of body surface with 2Ø-29% third degree corrosion** MCC
- **T32.43 Corrosions involving 4Ø-49% of body surface with 3Ø-39% third degree corrosion** MCC
- **T32.44 Corrosions involving 4Ø-49% of body surface with 4Ø-49% third degree corrosion** MCC

✓5th **T32.5 Corrosions involving 5Ø-59% of body surface**

- **T32.5Ø Corrosions involving 5Ø-59% of body surface with Ø% to 9% third degree corrosion** CC
- **T32.51 Corrosions involving 5Ø-59% of body surface with 1Ø-19% third degree corrosion** MCC
- **T32.52 Corrosions involving 5Ø-59% of body surface with 2Ø-29% third degree corrosion** MCC
- **T32.53 Corrosions involving 5Ø-59% of body surface with 3Ø-39% third degree corrosion** MCC
- **T32.54 Corrosions involving 5Ø-59% of body surface with 4Ø-49% third degree corrosion** MCC
- **T32.55 Corrosions involving 5Ø-59% of body surface with 5Ø-59% third degree corrosion** MCC

✓5th **T32.6 Corrosions involving 6Ø-69% of body surface**

- **T32.6Ø Corrosions involving 6Ø-69% of body surface with Ø% to 9% third degree corrosion** CC
- **T32.61 Corrosions involving 6Ø-69% of body surface with 1Ø-19% third degree corrosion** MCC
- **T32.62 Corrosions involving 6Ø-69% of body surface with 2Ø-29% third degree corrosion** MCC
- **T32.63 Corrosions involving 6Ø-69% of body surface with 3Ø-39% third degree corrosion** MCC
- **T32.64 Corrosions involving 6Ø-69% of body surface with 4Ø-49% third degree corrosion** MCC
- **T32.65 Corrosions involving 6Ø-69% of body surface with 5Ø-59% third degree corrosion** MCC
- **T32.66 Corrosions involving 6Ø-69% of body surface with 6Ø-69% third degree corrosion** MCC

✓5th **T32.7 Corrosions involving 7Ø-79% of body surface**

- **T32.7Ø Corrosions involving 7Ø-79% of body surface with Ø% to 9% third degree corrosion** CC
- **T32.71 Corrosions involving 7Ø-79% of body surface with 1Ø-19% third degree corrosion** MCC
- **T32.72 Corrosions involving 7Ø-79% of body surface with 2Ø-29% third degree corrosion** MCC
- **T32.73 Corrosions involving 7Ø-79% of body surface with 3Ø-39% third degree corrosion** MCC
- **T32.74 Corrosions involving 7Ø-79% of body surface with 4Ø-49% third degree corrosion** MCC
- **T32.75 Corrosions involving 7Ø-79% of body surface with 5Ø-59% third degree corrosion** MCC
- **T32.76 Corrosions involving 7Ø-79% of body surface with 6Ø-69% third degree corrosion** MCC
- **T32.77 Corrosions involving 7Ø-79% of body surface with 7Ø-79% third degree corrosion** MCC

✓5th **T32.8 Corrosions involving 8Ø-89% of body surface**

- **T32.8Ø Corrosions involving 8Ø-89% of body surface with Ø% to 9% third degree corrosion** CC
- **T32.81 Corrosions involving 8Ø-89% of body surface with 1Ø-19% third degree corrosion** MCC
- **T32.82 Corrosions involving 8Ø-89% of body surface with 2Ø-29% third degree corrosion** MCC
- **T32.83 Corrosions involving 8Ø-89% of body surface with 3Ø-39% third degree corrosion** MCC
- **T32.84 Corrosions involving 8Ø-89% of body surface with 4Ø-49% third degree corrosion** MCC
- **T32.85 Corrosions involving 8Ø-89% of body surface with 5Ø-59% third degree corrosion** MCC
- **T32.86 Corrosions involving 8Ø-89% of body surface with 6Ø-69% third degree corrosion** MCC
- **T32.87 Corrosions involving 8Ø-89% of body surface with 7Ø-79% third degree corrosion** MCC
- **T32.88 Corrosions involving 8Ø-89% of body surface with 8Ø-89% third degree corrosion** MCC

7 HAC = Initial encounter only (7th character A, B or C) and not POA.

✓5th **T32.9 Corrosions involving 9Ø% or more of body surface**

- **T32.9Ø Corrosions involving 9Ø% or more of body surface with Ø% to 9% third degree corrosion** CC
- **T32.91 Corrosions involving 9Ø% or more of body surface with 1Ø-19% third degree corrosion** MCC
- **T32.92 Corrosions involving 9Ø% or more of body surface with 2Ø-29% third degree corrosion** MCC
- **T32.93 Corrosions involving 9Ø% or more of body surface with 3Ø-39% third degree corrosion** MCC
- **T32.94 Corrosions involving 9Ø% or more of body surface with 4Ø-49% third degree corrosion** MCC
- **T32.95 Corrosions involving 9Ø% or more of body surface with 5Ø-59% third degree corrosion** MCC
- **T32.96 Corrosions involving 9Ø% or more of body surface with 6Ø-69% third degree corrosion** MCC
- **T32.97 Corrosions involving 9Ø% or more of body surface with 7Ø-79% third degree corrosion** MCC
- **T32.98 Corrosions involving 9Ø% or more of body surface with 8Ø-89% third degree corrosion** MCC
- **T32.99 Corrosions involving 9Ø% or more of body surface with 9Ø% or more third degree corrosion** MCC

Frostbite (T33-T34)

EXCLUDES 2 *hypothermia and other effects of reduced temperature (T68, T69-)*

✓4th **T33 Superficial frostbite**

INCLUDES frostbite with partial thickness skin loss

The appropriate 7th character is to be added to each code from category T33.
A initial encounter
D subsequent encounter
S sequela

✓5th **T33.Ø Superficial frostbite of head**

CC Excl: For CC codes in subcategory T33.Ø and T33.1: CC with 7th character A, unless otherwise noted: T33.Ø11-T33.42X with 7th A, T33.6ØX-T33.72X with 7th A, T33.9ØX-T34.42X with 7th A, T34.6ØX-T34.72X with 7th A, T34.9ØX-T34.99X with 7th A

✓6th **T33.Ø1 Superficial frostbite of ear**

- 7 ✓7th **T33.Ø11 Superficial frostbite of right ear** CC
- 7 ✓7th **T33.Ø12 Superficial frostbite of left ear** CC
- 7 ✓7th **T33.Ø19 Superficial frostbite of unspecified ear** CC

7 ✓x7th **T33.Ø2 Superficial frostbite of nose** CC

7 ✓x7th **T33.Ø9 Superficial frostbite of other part of head** CC

7 ✓x7th **T33.1 Superficial frostbite of neck** CC

CC Excl: T33.Ø11-T34.99X with 7th A, T69.Ø21-T69.Ø29 with 7th A

7 ✓x7th **T33.2 Superficial frostbite of thorax** CC

CC Excl: For CC codes in subcategory T33.2: CC with 7th character A, unless otherwise noted: T33.Ø11-T34.99X with 7th A, T69.Ø21-T69.Ø29 with 7th A

7 ✓x7th **T33.3 Superficial frostbite of abdominal wall, lower back and pelvis** CC

CC Excl: See code: T33.2

✓5th **T33.4 Superficial frostbite of arm**

EXCLUDES 2 *superficial frostbite of wrist and hand (T33.5-)*

CC Excl: For CC codes in subcategory T33.4: CC with 7th character A, unless otherwise noted: T33.Ø11-T34.99X with 7th A, T69.Ø21-T69.Ø29 with 7th A

- 7 ✓x7th **T33.4Ø Superficial frostbite of unspecified arm** CC
- 7 ✓x7th **T33.41 Superficial frostbite of right arm** CC
- 7 ✓x7th **T33.42 Superficial frostbite of left arm** CC

✓5th **T33.5 Superficial frostbite of wrist, hand, and fingers**

CC Excl: For CC codes in subcategory T33.5: CC with 7th character A, unless otherwise noted: T33.2XX-T33.72X with 7th A, T33.9ØX-T33.99X with 7th A, T34.2XX-T34.72X with 7th A, T34.9ØX-T34.99X with 7th A

✓6th **T33.51 Superficial frostbite of wrist**

- 7 ✓7th **T33.511 Superficial frostbite of right wrist** CC
- 7 ✓7th **T33.512 Superficial frostbite of left wrist** CC
- 7 ✓7th **T33.519 Superficial frostbite of unspecified wrist** CC

✓6th **T33.52** **Superficial frostbite of hand**
EXCLUDES 2 *superficial frostbite of fingers (T33.53-)*

7 ✓7th **T33.521** **Superficial frostbite of right hand** CC

7 ✓7th **T33.522** **Superficial frostbite of left hand** CC

7 ✓7th **T33.529** **Superficial frostbite of unspecified hand** CC

✓6th **T33.53** **Superficial frostbite of finger(s)**

7 ✓7th **T33.531** **Superficial frostbite of right finger(s)** CC

7 ✓7th **T33.532** **Superficial frostbite of left finger(s)** CC

7 ✓7th **T33.539** **Superficial frostbite of unspecified finger(s)** CC

✓5th **T33.6** **Superficial frostbite of hip and thigh**

CC Excl: For CC codes in subcategory T33.6: CC with 7th character A, unless otherwise noted: T33.Ø11-T34.99X with 7th A, T69.Ø21-T69.Ø29 with 7th A

7 ✓x7th **T33.6Ø** **Superficial frostbite of unspecified hip and thigh** CC

7 ✓x7th **T33.61** **Superficial frostbite of right hip and thigh** CC

7 ✓x7th **T33.62** **Superficial frostbite of left hip and thigh** CC

✓5th **T33.7** **Superficial frostbite of knee and lower leg**

CC Excl: For CC codes in subcategory T33.7: CC with 7th character A, unless otherwise noted: See code: T33.6

EXCLUDES 2 *superficial frostbite of ankle and foot (T33.8-)*

7 ✓x7th **T33.7Ø** **Superficial frostbite of unspecified knee and lower leg** CC

7 ✓x7th **T33.71** **Superficial frostbite of right knee and lower leg** CC

7 ✓x7th **T33.72** **Superficial frostbite of left knee and lower leg** CC

✓5th **T33.8** **Superficial frostbite of ankle, foot, and toe(s)**

CC Excl: For CC codes in subcategory T33.8: CC with 7th character A, unless otherwise noted: T33.2XX-T33.42X with 7th A, T33.6ØX-T33.99X with 7th A, T34.2XX-T34.42X with 7th A, T34.6ØX-T34.99X with 7th A

✓6th **T33.81** **Superficial frostbite of ankle**

7 ✓7th **T33.811** **Superficial frostbite of right ankle** CC

7 ✓7th **T33.812** **Superficial frostbite of left ankle** CC

7 ✓7th **T33.819** **Superficial frostbite of unspecified ankle** CC

✓6th **T33.82** **Superficial frostbite of foot**

7 ✓7th **T33.821** **Superficial frostbite of right foot** CC

7 ✓7th **T33.822** **Superficial frostbite of left foot** CC

7 ✓7th **T33.829** **Superficial frostbite of unspecified foot** CC

✓6th **T33.83** **Superficial frostbite of toe(s)**

7 ✓7th **T33.831** **Superficial frostbite of right toe(s)** CC

7 ✓7th **T33.832** **Superficial frostbite of left toe(s)** CC

7 ✓7th **T33.839** **Superficial frostbite of unspecified toe(s)** CC

✓5th **T33.9** **Superficial frostbite of other and unspecified sites**

CC Excl: For CC codes in subcategory T33.9: CC with 7th character A, unless otherwise noted: T33.Ø11-T34.99X with 7th A, T69.Ø21-T69.Ø29 with 7th A

7 ✓x7th **T33.9Ø** **Superficial frostbite of unspecified sites** CC
Superficial frostbite NOS

7 ✓x7th **T33.99** **Superficial frostbite of other sites** CC
Superficial frostbite of leg NOS
Superficial frostbite of trunk NOS

✓4th T34 Frostbite with tissue necrosis

The appropriate 7th character is to be added to each code from category T34.
A initial encounter
D subsequent encounter
S sequela

✓5th **T34.Ø** **Frostbite with tissue necrosis of head**

CC Excl: For CC codes in subcategory T34.Ø: CC with 7th character A, unless otherwise noted: T33.Ø11-T33.42 with 7th A, T33.6ØX-T33.72X with 7th A, T33.9ØX-T34.42X with 7th A, T34.6ØX-T34.72X with 7th A, T34.9ØX-T34.99X with 7th A

✓6th **T34.Ø1** **Frostbite with tissue necrosis of ear**

7 ✓7th **T34.Ø11** **Frostbite with tissue necrosis of right ear** CC

7 ✓7th **T34.Ø12** **Frostbite with tissue necrosis of left ear** CC

7 ✓7th **T34.Ø19** **Frostbite with tissue necrosis of unspecified ear** CC

7 ✓x7th **T34.Ø2** **Frostbite with tissue necrosis of nose** CC

7 ✓x7th **T34.Ø9** **Frostbite with tissue necrosis of other part of head** CC

7 ✓x7th **T34.1** **Frostbite with tissue necrosis of neck** CC
CC Excl: CC with 7th character A: T33.Ø11-T33.42X with 7th A, T33.6ØX-T33.72X with 7th A, T33.9ØX-T34.42X with 7th A, T34.6ØX-T34.72X with 7th A, T34.9ØX-T34.99X with 7th A

7 ✓x7th **T34.2** **Frostbite with tissue necrosis of thorax** CC
CC Excl: CC with 7th character A: T33.Ø11-T34.99X with 7th A, T69.Ø21-T69.Ø29 with 7th A

7 ✓x7th **T34.3** **Frostbite with tissue necrosis of abdominal wall, lower back and pelvis** CC
CC Excl: CC with 7th character A: See code: T34.2

✓5th **T34.4** **Frostbite with tissue necrosis of arm**
EXCLUDES 2 *frostbite with tissue necrosis of wrist and hand (T34.5-)*

CC Excl: For CC codes in subcategory T34.4: CC with 7th character A, unless otherwise noted: See code: T34.2

7 ✓x7th **T34.4Ø** **Frostbite with tissue necrosis of unspecified arm** CC

7 ✓x7th **T34.41** **Frostbite with tissue necrosis of right arm** CC

7 ✓x7th **T34.42** **Frostbite with tissue necrosis of left arm** CC

✓5th **T34.5** **Frostbite with tissue necrosis of wrist, hand, and finger(s)**

CC Excl: For CC codes in subcategory T34.5: CC with 7th character A, unless otherwise noted: T33.2XX-T33.72X with 7th A, T33.9ØX-T33.99X with 7th A, T34.2XX-T34.72X with 7th A, T34.9ØX-T34.99X with 7th A

✓6th **T34.51** **Frostbite with tissue necrosis of wrist**

7 ✓7th **T34.511** **Frostbite with tissue necrosis of right wrist** CC

7 ✓7th **T34.512** **Frostbite with tissue necrosis of left wrist** CC

7 ✓7th **T34.519** **Frostbite with tissue necrosis of unspecified wrist** CC

✓6th **T34.52** **Frostbite with tissue necrosis of hand**
EXCLUDES 2 *frostbite with tissue necrosis of finger(s) (T34.53-)*

7 ✓7th **T34.521** **Frostbite with tissue necrosis of right hand** CC

7 ✓7th **T34.522** **Frostbite with tissue necrosis of left hand** CC

7 ✓7th **T34.529** **Frostbite with tissue necrosis of unspecified hand** CC

✓6th **T34.53** **Frostbite with tissue necrosis of finger(s)**

7 ✓7th **T34.531** **Frostbite with tissue necrosis of right finger(s)** CC

7 ✓7th **T34.532** **Frostbite with tissue necrosis of left finger(s)** CC

7 ✓7th **T34.539** **Frostbite with tissue necrosis of unspecified finger(s)** CC

✓5th **T34.6** **Frostbite with tissue necrosis of hip and thigh**

CC Excl: For CC codes in subcategory T34.6: CC with 7th character A, unless otherwise noted: T33.Ø11-T34.99X with 7th A, T69.Ø21-T69.Ø29 with 7th A

7 ✓x7th **T34.6Ø** **Frostbite with tissue necrosis of unspecified hip and thigh** CC

7 ✓x7th **T34.61** **Frostbite with tissue necrosis of right hip and thigh** CC

7 ✓x7th **T34.62** **Frostbite with tissue necrosis of left hip and thigh** CC

✓5th **T34.7** **Frostbite with tissue necrosis of knee and lower leg**
EXCLUDES 2 *frostbite with tissue necrosis of ankle and foot (T34.8-)*

CC Excl: For CC codes in subcategory T34.7: CC with 7th character A, unless otherwise noted: See code: T34.6

7 ✓x7th **T34.7Ø** **Frostbite with tissue necrosis of unspecified knee and lower leg** CC

7 ✓x7th **T34.71** **Frostbite with tissue necrosis of right knee and lower leg** CC

7 HAC = Initial encounter only (7th character A, B or C) and not POA.

7 √x7th **T34.72 Frostbite with tissue necrosis of left knee and lower leg** CC

√5th **T34.8 Frostbite with tissue necrosis of ankle, foot, and toe(s)**

CC Excl: For CC codes in subcategory T34.8: CC with 7th character A, unless otherwise noted: T33.2XX-T33.42X with 7th A, T33.60X-T33.99X with 7th A, T34.2XX-T34.42X with 7th A, T34.60X-T34.99X with 7th A

√6th **T34.81 Frostbite with tissue necrosis of ankle**

7 √7th **T34.811 Frostbite with tissue necrosis of right ankle** CC

7 √7th **T34.812 Frostbite with tissue necrosis of left ankle** CC

7 √7th **T34.819 Frostbite with tissue necrosis of unspecified ankle** CC

√6th **T34.82 Frostbite with tissue necrosis of foot**

7 √7th **T34.821 Frostbite with tissue necrosis of right foot** CC

7 √7th **T34.822 Frostbite with tissue necrosis of left foot** CC

7 √7th **T34.829 Frostbite with tissue necrosis of unspecified foot** CC

√6th **T34.83 Frostbite with tissue necrosis of toe(s)**

7 √7th **T34.831 Frostbite with tissue necrosis of right toe(s)** CC

7 √7th **T34.832 Frostbite with tissue necrosis of left toe(s)** CC

7 √7th **T34.839 Frostbite with tissue necrosis of unspecified toe(s)** CC

√5th **T34.9 Frostbite with tissue necrosis of other and unspecified sites**

CC Excl: For CC codes in subcategory T34.9: CC with 7th character A, unless otherwise noted: T33.011-T34.99X with 7th A, T69.021-T69.029 with 7th A

7 √x7th **T34.90 Frostbite with tissue necrosis of unspecified sites** CC

Frostbite with tissue necrosis NOS

7 √x7th **T34.99 Frostbite with tissue necrosis of other sites** CC

Frostbite with tissue necrosis of leg NOS

Frostbite with tissue necrosis of trunk NOS

Poisoning by, adverse effects of and underdosing of drugs, medicaments and biological substances (T36-T50)

INCLUDES adverse effect of correct substance properly administered
poisoning by overdose of substance
poisoning by wrong substance given or taken in error
underdosing by (inadvertently) (deliberately) taking less substance than prescribed or instructed

Code first, for adverse effects, the nature of the adverse effect, such as:
adverse effect NOS (T88.7)
aspirin gastritis (K29.-)
blood disorders (D56-D76)
contact dermatitis (L23-L25)
dermatitis due to substances taken internally (L27.-)
nephropathy (N14.0-N14.2)

NOTE The drug giving rise to the adverse effect should be identified by use of codes from categories T36-T50 with fifth or sixth character 5.

Use additional code(s) to specify:
manifestations of poisoning
underdosing or failure in dosage during medical and surgical care (Y63.6, Y63.8-Y63.9)
underdosing of medication regimen (Z91.12-, Z91.13-)

EXCLUDES 1 *toxic reaction to local anesthesia in pregnancy (O29.3-)*

EXCLUDES 2 *abuse and dependence of psychoactive substances (F10-F19)*
abuse of non-dependence-producing substances (F55.-)
drug reaction and poisoning affecting newborn (P00-P96)
pathological drug intoxication (inebriation) (F10-F19)

√4th **T36 Poisoning by, adverse effect of and underdosing of systemic antibiotics**

EXCLUDES 1 *antineoplastic antibiotics (T45.1-)*
locally applied antibiotic NEC (T49.0)
topically used antibiotic for ear, nose and throat (T49.6)
topically used antibiotic for eye (T49.5)

The appropriate 7th character is to be added to each code from category T36.
A initial encounter
D subsequent encounter
S sequela

√5th **T36.0 Poisoning by, adverse effect of and underdosing of penicillins**

√6th **T36.0X Poisoning by, adverse effect of and underdosing of penicillins**

√7th **T36.0X1 Poisoning by penicillins, accidental (unintentional)**

Poisoning by penicillins NOS

√7th **T36.0X2 Poisoning by penicillins, intentional self-harm**

√7th **T36.0X3 Poisoning by penicillins, assault**

√7th **T36.0X4 Poisoning by penicillins, undetermined**

√7th **T36.0X5 Adverse effect of penicillins**

√7th **T36.0X6 Underdosing of penicillins**

√5th **T36.1 Poisoning by, adverse effect of and underdosing of cephalosporins and other beta-lactam antibiotics**

√6th **T36.1X Poisoning by, adverse effect of and underdosing of cephalosporins and other beta-lactam antibiotics**

√7th **T36.1X1 Poisoning by cephalosporins and other beta-lactam antibiotics, accidental (unintentional)**

Poisoning by cephalosporins and other beta-lactam antibiotics NOS

√7th **T36.1X2 Poisoning by cephalosporins and other beta-lactam antibiotics, intentional self-harm**

√7th **T36.1X3 Poisoning by cephalosporins and other beta-lactam antibiotics, assault**

√7th **T36.1X4 Poisoning by cephalosporins and other beta-lactam antibiotics, undetermined**

√7th **T36.1X5 Adverse effect of cephalosporins and other beta-lactam antibiotics**

√7th **T36.1X6 Underdosing of cephalosporins and other beta-lactam antibiotics**

√5th **T36.2 Poisoning by, adverse effect of and underdosing of chloramphenicol group**

√6th **T36.2X Poisoning by, adverse effect of and underdosing of chloramphenicol group**

√7th **T36.2X1 Poisoning by chloramphenicol group, accidental (unintentional)**

Poisoning by chloramphenicol group NOS

√7th **T36.2X2 Poisoning by chloramphenicol group, intentional self-harm**

√7th **T36.2X3 Poisoning by chloramphenicol group, assault**

√7th **T36.2X4 Poisoning by chloramphenicol group, undetermined**

√7th **T36.2X5 Adverse effect of chloramphenicol group**

√7th **T36.2X6 Underdosing of chloramphenicol group**

√5th **T36.3 Poisoning by, adverse effect of and underdosing of macrolides**

√6th **T36.3X Poisoning by, adverse effect of and underdosing of macrolides**

√7th **T36.3X1 Poisoning by macrolides, accidental (unintentional)**

Poisoning by macrolides NOS

√7th **T36.3X2 Poisoning by macrolides, intentional self-harm**

√7th **T36.3X3 Poisoning by macrolides, assault**

√7th **T36.3X4 Poisoning by macrolides, undetermined**

√7th **T36.3X5 Adverse effect of macrolides**

√7th **T36.3X6 Underdosing of macrolides**

7 HAC = Initial encounter only (7th character A, B or C) and not POA.

T36.4 Poisoning by, adverse effect of and underdosing of tetracyclines
T36.4X Poisoning by, adverse effect of and underdosing of tetracyclines
T36.4X1 Poisoning by tetracyclines, accidental (unintentional)
Poisoning by tetracyclines NOS
T36.4X2 Poisoning by tetracyclines, intentional self-harm
T36.4X3 Poisoning by tetracyclines, assault
T36.4X4 Poisoning by tetracyclines, undetermined
T36.4X5 Adverse effect of tetracyclines
T36.4X6 Underdosing of tetracyclines
T36.5 Poisoning by, adverse effect of and underdosing of aminoglycosides
Poisoning by, adverse effect of and underdosing of streptomycin
T36.5X Poisoning by, adverse effect of and underdosing of aminoglycosides
T36.5X1 Poisoning by aminoglycosides, accidental (unintentional)
Poisoning by aminoglycosides NOS
T36.5X2 Poisoning by aminoglycosides, intentional self-harm
T36.5X3 Poisoning by aminoglycosides, assault
T36.5X4 Poisoning by aminoglycosides, undetermined
T36.5X5 Adverse effect of aminoglycosides
T36.5X6 Underdosing of aminoglycosides
T36.6 Poisoning by, adverse effect of and underdosing of rifampicins
T36.6X Poisoning by, adverse effect of and underdosing of rifampicins
T36.6X1 Poisoning by rifampicins, accidental (unintentional)
Poisoning by rifampicins NOS
T36.6X2 Poisoning by rifampicins, intentional self-harm
T36.6X3 Poisoning by rifampicins, assault
T36.6X4 Poisoning by rifampicins, undetermined
T36.6X5 Adverse effect of rifampicins
T36.6X6 Underdosing of rifampicins
T36.7 Poisoning by, adverse effect of and underdosing of antifungal antibiotics, systemically used
T36.7X Poisoning by, adverse effect of and underdosing of antifungal antibiotics, systemically used
T36.7X1 Poisoning by antifungal antibiotics, systemically used, accidental (unintentional)
Poisoning by antifungal antibiotics, systemically used NOS
T36.7X2 Poisoning by antifungal antibiotics, systemically used, intentional self-harm
T36.7X3 Poisoning by antifungal antibiotics, systemically used, assault
T36.7X4 Poisoning by antifungal antibiotics, systemically used, undetermined
T36.7X5 Adverse effect of antifungal antibiotics, systemically used
T36.7X6 Underdosing of antifungal antibiotics, systemically used
T36.8 Poisoning by, adverse effect of and underdosing of other systemic antibiotics
T36.8X Poisoning by, adverse effect of and underdosing of other systemic antibiotics
T36.8X1 Poisoning by other systemic antibiotics, accidental (unintentional)
Poisoning by other systemic antibiotics NOS
T36.8X2 Poisoning by other systemic antibiotics, intentional self-harm
T36.8X3 Poisoning by other systemic antibiotics, assault
T36.8X4 Poisoning by other systemic antibiotics, undetermined
T36.8X5 Adverse effect of other systemic antibiotics
T36.8X6 Underdosing of other systemic antibiotics
T36.9 Poisoning by, adverse effect of and underdosing of unspecified systemic antibiotic
T36.91 Poisoning by unspecified systemic antibiotic, accidental (unintentional)
Poisoning by systemic antibiotic NOS
T36.92 Poisoning by unspecified systemic antibiotic, intentional self-harm
T36.93 Poisoning by unspecified systemic antibiotic, assault
T36.94 Poisoning by unspecified systemic antibiotic, undetermined
T36.95 Adverse effect of unspecified systemic antibiotic
T36.96 Underdosing of unspecified systemic antibiotic

T37 Poisoning by, adverse effect of and underdosing of other systemic anti- infectives and antiparasitics
EXCLUDES 1 *anti-infectives topically used for ear, nose and throat (T49.6-)*
anti-infectives topically used for eye (T49.5-)
locally applied anti-infectives NEC (T49.Ø-)

The appropriate 7th character is to be added to each code from category T37.
A initial encounter
D subsequent encounter
S sequela

T37.Ø Poisoning by, adverse effect of and underdosing of sulfonamides
T37.ØX Poisoning by, adverse effect of and underdosing of sulfonamides
T37.ØX1 Poisoning by sulfonamides, accidental (unintentional)
Poisoning by sulfonamides NOS
T37.ØX2 Poisoning by sulfonamides, intentional self-harm
T37.ØX3 Poisoning by sulfonamides, assault
T37.ØX4 Poisoning by sulfonamides, undetermined
T37.ØX5 Adverse effect of sulfonamides
T37.ØX6 Underdosing of sulfonamides
T37.1 Poisoning by, adverse effect of and underdosing of antimycobacterial drugs
EXCLUDES 1 *rifampicins (T36.6-)*
streptomycin (T36.5-)
T37.1X Poisoning by, adverse effect of and underdosing of antimycobacterial drugs
T37.1X1 Poisoning by antimycobacterial drugs, accidental (unintentional)
Poisoning by antimycobacterial drugs NOS
T37.1X2 Poisoning by antimycobacterial drugs, intentional self-harm
T37.1X3 Poisoning by antimycobacterial drugs, assault
T37.1X4 Poisoning by antimycobacterial drugs, undetermined
T37.1X5 Adverse effect of antimycobacterial drugs
T37.1X6 Underdosing of antimycobacterial drugs
T37.2 Poisoning by, adverse effect of and underdosing of antimalarials and drugs acting on other blood protozoa
EXCLUDES 1 *hydroxyquinoline derivatives (T37.8-)*
T37.2X Poisoning by, adverse effect of and underdosing of antimalarials and drugs acting on other blood protozoa
T37.2X1 Poisoning by antimalarials and drugs acting on other blood protozoa, accidental (unintentional)
Poisoning by antimalarials and drugs acting on other blood protozoa NOS
T37.2X2 Poisoning by antimalarials and drugs acting on other blood protozoa, intentional self-harm
T37.2X3 Poisoning by antimalarials and drugs acting on other blood protozoa, assault

T37.2X4 Poisoning by antimalarials and drugs acting on other blood protozoa, undetermined

T37.2X5 Adverse effect of antimalarials and drugs acting on other blood protozoa

T37.2X6 Underdosing of antimalarials and drugs acting on other blood protozoa

T37.3 Poisoning by, adverse effect of and underdosing of other antiprotozoal drugs

T37.3X Poisoning by, adverse effect of and underdosing of other antiprotozoal drugs

T37.3X1 Poisoning by other antiprotozoal drugs, accidental (unintentional)
Poisoning by other antiprotozoal drugs NOS

T37.3X2 Poisoning by other antiprotozoal drugs, intentional self-harm

T37.3X3 Poisoning by other antiprotozoal drugs, assault

T37.3X4 Poisoning by other antiprotozoal drugs, undetermined

T37.3X5 Adverse effect of other antiprotozoal drugs

T37.3X6 Underdosing of other antiprotozoal drugs

T37.4 Poisoning by, adverse effect of and underdosing of anthelminthics

T37.4X Poisoning by, adverse effect of and underdosing of anthelminthics

T37.4X1 Poisoning by anthelminthics, accidental (unintentional)
Poisoning by anthelminthics NOS

T37.4X2 Poisoning by anthelminthics, intentional self-harm

T37.4X3 Poisoning by anthelminthics, assault

T37.4X4 Poisoning by anthelminthics, undetermined

T37.4X5 Adverse effect of anthelminthics

T37.4X6 Underdosing of anthelminthics

T37.5 Poisoning by, adverse effect of and underdosing of antiviral drugs
EXCLUDES 1 *amantadine (T42.8-)*
cytarabine (T45.1-)

T37.5X Poisoning by, adverse effect of and underdosing of antiviral drugs

T37.5X1 Poisoning by antiviral drugs, accidental (unintentional)
Poisoning by antiviral drugs NOS

T37.5X2 Poisoning by antiviral drugs, intentional self-harm

T37.5X3 Poisoning by antiviral drugs, assault

T37.5X4 Poisoning by antiviral drugs, undetermined

T37.5X5 Adverse effect of antiviral drugs

T37.5X6 Underdosing of antiviral drugs

T37.8 Poisoning by, adverse effect of and underdosing of other specified systemic anti-infectives and antiparasitics
Poisoning by, adverse effect of and underdosing of hydroxyquinoline derivatives
EXCLUDES 1 *antimalarial drugs (T37.2-)*

T37.8X Poisoning by, adverse effect of and underdosing of other specified systemic anti-infectives and antiparasitics

T37.8X1 Poisoning by other specified systemic anti-infectives and antiparasitics, accidental (unintentional)
Poisoning by other specified systemic anti-infectives and antiparasitics NOS

T37.8X2 Poisoning by other specified systemic anti-infectives and antiparasitics, intentional self-harm

T37.8X3 Poisoning by other specified systemic anti-infectives and antiparasitics, assault

T37.8X4 Poisoning by other specified systemic anti-infectives and antiparasitics, undetermined

T37.8X5 Adverse effect of other specified systemic anti-infectives and antiparasitics

T37.8X6 Underdosing of other specified systemic anti-infectives and antiparasitics

T37.9 Poisoning by, adverse effect of and underdosing of unspecified systemic anti-infective and antiparasitics

T37.91 Poisoning by unspecified systemic anti-infective and antiparasitics, accidental (unintentional)
Poisoning by, adverse effect of and underdosing of systemic anti-infective and antiparasitics NOS

T37.92 Poisoning by unspecified systemic anti-infective and antiparasitics, intentional self-harm

T37.93 Poisoning by unspecified systemic anti-infective and antiparasitics, assault

T37.94 Poisoning by unspecified systemic anti-infective and antiparasitics, undetermined

T37.95 Adverse effect of unspecified systemic anti-infective and antiparasitic

T37.96 Underdosing of unspecified systemic anti-infectives and antiparasitics

T38 Poisoning by, adverse effect of and underdosing of hormones and their synthetic substitutes and antagonists, not elsewhere classified
EXCLUDES 1 *mineralocorticoids and their antagonists (T50.0-)*
oxytocic hormones (T48.0-)
parathyroid hormones and derivatives (T50.9-)

The appropriate 7th character is to be added to each code from category T38.
A initial encounter
D subsequent encounter
S sequela

T38.0 Poisoning by, adverse effect of and underdosing of glucocorticoids and synthetic analogues
EXCLUDES 1 *glucocorticoids, topically used (T49.-)*

T38.0X Poisoning by, adverse effect of and underdosing of glucocorticoids and synthetic analogues

T38.0X1 Poisoning by glucocorticoids and synthetic analogues, accidental (unintentional)
Poisoning by glucocorticoids and synthetic analogues NOS

T38.0X2 Poisoning by glucocorticoids and synthetic analogues, intentional self-harm

T38.0X3 Poisoning by glucocorticoids and synthetic analogues, assault

T38.0X4 Poisoning by glucocorticoids and synthetic analogues, undetermined

T38.0X5 Adverse effect of glucocorticoids and synthetic analogues

T38.0X6 Underdosing of glucocorticoids and synthetic analogues

T38.1 Poisoning by, adverse effect of and underdosing of thyroid hormones and substitutes

T38.1X Poisoning by, adverse effect of and underdosing of thyroid hormones and substitutes

T38.1X1 Poisoning by thyroid hormones and substitutes, accidental (unintentional)
Poisoning by thyroid hormones and substitutes NOS

T38.1X2 Poisoning by thyroid hormones and substitutes, intentional self-harm

T38.1X3 Poisoning by thyroid hormones and substitutes, assault

T38.1X4 Poisoning by thyroid hormones and substitutes, undetermined

T38.1X5 Adverse effect of thyroid hormones and substitutes

T38.1X6 Underdosing of thyroid hormones and substitutes

T38.2 Poisoning by, adverse effect of and underdosing of antithyroid drugs

T38.2X Poisoning by, adverse effect of and underdosing of antithyroid drugs

T38.2X1 Poisoning by antithyroid drugs, accidental (unintentional)
Poisoning by antithyroid drugs NOS

✓7th T38.2X2 **Poisoning by antithyroid drugs, intentional self-harm**
✓7th T38.2X3 **Poisoning by antithyroid drugs, assault**
✓7th T38.2X4 **Poisoning by antithyroid drugs, undetermined**
✓7th T38.2X5 **Adverse effect of antithyroid drugs**
✓7th T38.2X6 **Underdosing of antithyroid drugs**

✓5th T38.3 **Poisoning by, adverse effect of and underdosing of insulin and oral hypoglycemic [antidiabetic] drugs**
✓6th T38.3X **Poisoning by, adverse effect of and underdosing of insulin and oral hypoglycemic [antidiabetic] drugs**
✓7th T38.3X1 **Poisoning by insulin and oral hypoglycemic [antidiabetic] drugs, accidental (unintentional)**
Poisoning by insulin and oral hypoglycemic [antidiabetic] drugs NOS
✓7th T38.3X2 **Poisoning by insulin and oral hypoglycemic [antidiabetic] drugs, intentional self-harm**
✓7th T38.3X3 **Poisoning by insulin and oral hypoglycemic [antidiabetic] drugs, assault**
✓7th T38.3X4 **Poisoning by insulin and oral hypoglycemic [antidiabetic] drugs, undetermined**
✓7th T38.3X5 **Adverse effect of insulin and oral hypoglycemic [antidiabetic] drugs**
✓7th T38.3X6 **Underdosing of insulin and oral hypoglycemic [antidiabetic] drugs**

✓5th T38.4 **Poisoning by, adverse effect of and underdosing of oral contraceptives**
Poisoning by, adverse effect of and underdosing of multiple- and single-ingredient oral contraceptive preparations
✓6th T38.4X **Poisoning by, adverse effect of and underdosing of oral contraceptives**
✓7th T38.4X1 **Poisoning by oral contraceptives, accidental (unintentional)**
Poisoning by oral contraceptives NOS
✓7th T38.4X2 **Poisoning by oral contraceptives, intentional self-harm**
✓7th T38.4X3 **Poisoning by oral contraceptives, assault**
✓7th T38.4X4 **Poisoning by oral contraceptives, undetermined**
✓7th T38.4X5 **Adverse effect of oral contraceptives**
✓7th T38.4X6 **Underdosing of oral contraceptives**

✓5th T38.5 **Poisoning by, adverse effect of and underdosing of other estrogens and progestogens**
Poisoning by, adverse effect of and underdosing of estrogens and progestogens mixtures and substitutes
✓6th T38.5X **Poisoning by, adverse effect of and underdosing of other estrogens and progestogens**
✓7th T38.5X1 **Poisoning by other estrogens and progestogens, accidental (unintentional)**
Poisoning by other estrogens and progestogens NOS
✓7th T38.5X2 **Poisoning by other estrogens and progestogens, intentional self-harm**
✓7th T38.5X3 **Poisoning by other estrogens and progestogens, assault**
✓7th T38.5X4 **Poisoning by other estrogens and progestogens, undetermined**
✓7th T38.5X5 **Adverse effect of other estrogens and progestogens**
✓7th T38.5X6 **Underdosing of other estrogens and progestogens**

✓5th T38.6 **Poisoning by, adverse effect of and underdosing of antigonadotrophins, antiestrogens, antiandrogens, not elsewhere classified**
Poisoning by, adverse effect of and underdosing of tamoxifen
✓6th T38.6X **Poisoning by, adverse effect of and underdosing of antigonadotrophins, antiestrogens, antiandrogens, not elsewhere classified**
✓7th T38.6X1 **Poisoning by antigonadotrophins, antiestrogens, antiandrogens, not elsewhere classified, accidental (unintentional)**
Poisoning by antigonadotrophins, antiestrogens, antiandrogens, not elsewhere classified NOS
✓7th T38.6X2 **Poisoning by antigonadotrophins, antiestrogens, antiandrogens, not elsewhere classified, intentional self-harm**
✓7th T38.6X3 **Poisoning by antigonadotrophins, antiestrogens, antiandrogens, not elsewhere classified, assault**
✓7th T38.6X4 **Poisoning by antigonadotrophins, antiestrogens, antiandrogens, not elsewhere classified, undetermined**
✓7th T38.6X5 **Adverse effect of antigonadotrophins, antiestrogens, antiandrogens, not elsewhere classified**
✓7th T38.6X6 **Underdosing of antigonadotrophins, antiestrogens, antiandrogens, not elsewhere classified**

✓5th T38.7 **Poisoning by, adverse effect of and underdosing of androgens and anabolic congeners**
✓6th T38.7X **Poisoning by, adverse effect of and underdosing of androgens and anabolic congeners**
✓7th T38.7X1 **Poisoning by androgens and anabolic congeners, accidental (unintentional)**
Poisoning by androgens and anabolic congeners NOS
✓7th T38.7X2 **Poisoning by androgens and anabolic congeners, intentional self-harm**
✓7th T38.7X3 **Poisoning by androgens and anabolic congeners, assault**
✓7th T38.7X4 **Poisoning by androgens and anabolic congeners, undetermined**
✓7th T38.7X5 **Adverse effect of androgens and anabolic congeners**
✓7th T38.7X6 **Underdosing of androgens and anabolic congeners**

✓5th T38.8 **Poisoning by, adverse effect of and underdosing of other and unspecified hormones and synthetic substitutes**
✓6th T38.80 **Poisoning by, adverse effect of and underdosing of unspecified hormones and synthetic substitutes**
✓7th T38.801 **Poisoning by unspecified hormones and synthetic substitutes, accidental (unintentional)**
Poisoning by unspecified hormones and synthetic substitutes NOS
✓7th T38.802 **Poisoning by unspecified hormones and synthetic substitutes, intentional self-harm**
✓7th T38.803 **Poisoning by unspecified hormones and synthetic substitutes, assault**
✓7th T38.804 **Poisoning by unspecified hormones and synthetic substitutes, undetermined**
✓7th T38.805 **Adverse effect of unspecified hormones and synthetic substitutes**
✓7th T38.806 **Underdosing of unspecified hormones and synthetic substitutes**
✓6th T38.81 **Poisoning by, adverse effect of and underdosing of anterior pituitary [adenohypophyseal] hormones**
✓7th T38.811 **Poisoning by anterior pituitary [adenohypophyseal] hormones, accidental (unintentional)**
Poisoning by anterior pituitary [adenohypophyseal] hormones NOS
✓7th T38.812 **Poisoning by anterior pituitary [adenohypophyseal] hormones, intentional self-harm**
✓7th T38.813 **Poisoning by anterior pituitary [adenohypophyseal] hormones, assault**
✓7th T38.814 **Poisoning by anterior pituitary [adenohypophyseal] hormones, undetermined**
✓7th T38.815 **Adverse effect of anterior pituitary [adenohypophyseal] hormones**

√7th **T38.816** Underdosing **of anterior pituitary [adenohypophyseal] hormones**

√6th **T38.89** **Poisoning by, adverse effect of and underdosing of** other hormones and synthetic substitutes

√7th **T38.891** **Poisoning by other hormones and synthetic substitutes,** accidental **(unintentional)**
Poisoning by other hormones and synthetic substitutes NOS

√7th **T38.892** **Poisoning by other hormones and synthetic substitutes,** intentional self-harm

√7th **T38.893** **Poisoning by other hormones and synthetic substitutes,** assault

√7th **T38.894** **Poisoning by other hormones and synthetic substitutes,** undetermined

√7th **T38.895** Adverse effect **of other hormones and synthetic substitutes**

√7th **T38.896** Underdosing **of other hormones and synthetic substitutes**

√5th **T38.9** **Poisoning by, adverse effect of and underdosing of other and unspecified hormone antagonists**

√6th **T38.90** **Poisoning by, adverse effect of and underdosing of** unspecified hormone antagonists

√7th **T38.901** **Poisoning by unspecified hormone antagonists,** accidental **(unintentional)**
Poisoning by unspecified hormone antagonists NOS

√7th **T38.902** **Poisoning by unspecified hormone antagonists,** intentional self-harm

√7th **T38.903** **Poisoning by unspecified hormone antagonists,** assault

√7th **T38.904** **Poisoning by unspecified hormone antagonists,** undetermined

√7th **T38.905** Adverse effect **of unspecified hormone antagonists**

√7th **T38.906** Underdosing **of unspecified hormone antagonists**

√6th **T38.99** **Poisoning by, adverse effect of and underdosing of** other hormone antagonists

√7th **T38.991** **Poisoning by other hormone antagonists,** accidental **(unintentional)**
Poisoning by other hormone antagonists NOS

√7th **T38.992** **Poisoning by other hormone antagonists,** intentional self-harm

√7th **T38.993** **Poisoning by other hormone antagonists,** assault

√7th **T38.994** **Poisoning by other hormone antagonists,** undetermined

√7th **T38.995** Adverse effect **of other hormone antagonists**

√7th **T38.996** Underdosing **of other hormone antagonists**

√4th **T39** **Poisoning by, adverse effect of and underdosing of nonopioid analgesics, antipyretics and antirheumatics**

The appropriate 7th character is to be added to each code from category T39.
A initial encounter
D subsequent encounter
S sequela

√5th **T39.0** **Poisoning by, adverse effect of and underdosing of** salicylates

√6th **T39.01** **Poisoning by, adverse effect of and underdosing of** aspirin
Poisoning by, adverse effect of and underdosing of acetylsalicylic acid

√7th **T39.011** **Poisoning by aspirin,** accidental **(unintentional)**

√7th **T39.012** **Poisoning by aspirin,** intentional self-harm

√7th **T39.013** **Poisoning by aspirin,** assault

√7th **T39.014** **Poisoning by aspirin,** undetermined

√7th **T39.015** Adverse effect **of aspirin**

√7th **T39.016** Underdosing **of aspirin**

√6th **T39.09** **Poisoning by, adverse effect of and underdosing of** other salicylates

√7th **T39.091** **Poisoning by salicylates,** accidental **(unintentional)**
Poisoning by salicylates NOS

√7th **T39.092** **Poisoning by salicylates,** intentional self-harm

√7th **T39.093** **Poisoning by salicylates,** assault

√7th **T39.094** **Poisoning by salicylates,** undetermined

√7th **T39.095** Adverse effect **of salicylates**

√7th **T39.096** Underdosing **of salicylates**

√5th **T39.1** **Poisoning by, adverse effect of and underdosing of 4-Aminophenol derivatives**

√6th **T39.1X** **Poisoning by, adverse effect of and underdosing of** 4-Aminophenol derivatives

√7th **T39.1X1** **Poisoning by 4-Aminophenol derivatives,** accidental **(unintentional)**
Poisoning by 4-Aminophenol derivatives NOS

√7th **T39.1X2** **Poisoning by 4-Aminophenol derivatives,** intentional self-harm

√7th **T39.1X3** **Poisoning by 4-Aminophenol derivatives,** assault

√7th **T39.1X4** **Poisoning by 4-Aminophenol derivatives,** undetermined

√7th **T39.1X5** Adverse effect **of 4-Aminophenol derivatives**

√7th **T39.1X6** Underdosing **of 4-Aminophenol derivatives**

√5th **T39.2** **Poisoning by, adverse effect of and underdosing of pyrazolone derivatives**

√6th **T39.2X** **Poisoning by, adverse effect of and underdosing of** pyrazolone derivatives

√7th **T39.2X1** **Poisoning by pyrazolone derivatives,** accidental **(unintentional)**
Poisoning by pyrazolone derivatives NOS

√7th **T39.2X2** **Poisoning by pyrazolone derivatives,** intentional self-harm

√7th **T39.2X3** **Poisoning by pyrazolone derivatives,** assault

√7th **T39.2X4** **Poisoning by pyrazolone derivatives,** undetermined

√7th **T39.2X5** Adverse effect **of pyrazolone derivatives**

√7th **T39.2X6** Underdosing **of pyrazolone derivatives**

√5th **T39.3** **Poisoning by, adverse effect of and underdosing of other nonsteroidal anti-inflammatory drugs [NSAID]**

√6th **T39.31** **Poisoning by, adverse effect of and underdosing of** propionic acid derivatives
Poisoning by, adverse effect of and underdosing of fenoprofen
Poisoning by, adverse effect of and underdosing of flurbiprofen
Poisoning by, adverse effect of and underdosing of ibuprofen
Poisoning by, adverse effect of and underdosing of ketoprofen
Poisoning by, adverse effect of and underdosing of naproxen
Poisoning by, adverse effect of and underdosing of oxaprozin

√7th **T39.311** **Poisoning by propionic acid derivatives,** accidental **(unintentional)**

√7th **T39.312** **Poisoning by propionic acid derivatives,** intentional self-harm

√7th **T39.313** **Poisoning by propionic acid derivatives,** assault

√7th **T39.314** **Poisoning by propionic acid derivatives,** undetermined

√7th **T39.315** Adverse effect **of propionic acid derivatives**

√7th **T39.316** Underdosing **of propionic acid derivatives**

T39.39 **Poisoning by, adverse effect of and underdosing of other nonsteroidal anti-inflammatory drugs [NSAID]**

T39.391 **Poisoning by other nonsteroidal anti-inflammatory drugs [NSAID], accidental (unintentional)**
Poisoning by other nonsteroidal anti-inflammatory drugs NOS

T39.392 **Poisoning by other nonsteroidal anti-inflammatory drugs [NSAID], intentional self-harm**

T39.393 **Poisoning by other nonsteroidal anti-inflammatory drugs [NSAID], assault**

T39.394 **Poisoning by other nonsteroidal anti-inflammatory drugs [NSAID], undetermined**

T39.395 **Adverse effect of other nonsteroidal anti-inflammatory drugs [NSAID]**

T39.396 **Underdosing of other nonsteroidal anti-inflammatory drugs [NSAID]**

T39.4 **Poisoning by, adverse effect of and underdosing of antirheumatics, not elsewhere classified**
EXCLUDES 1 *poisoning by, adverse effect of and underdosing of glucocorticoids (T38.Ø-)*
poisoning by, adverse effect of and underdosing of salicylates (T39.Ø-)

T39.4X **Poisoning by, adverse effect of and underdosing of antirheumatics, not elsewhere classified**

T39.4X1 **Poisoning by antirheumatics, not elsewhere classified, accidental (unintentional)**
Poisoning by antirheumatics, not elsewhere classified NOS

T39.4X2 **Poisoning by antirheumatics, not elsewhere classified, intentional self-harm**

T39.4X3 **Poisoning by antirheumatics, not elsewhere classified, assault**

T39.4X4 **Poisoning by antirheumatics, not elsewhere classified, undetermined**

T39.4X5 **Adverse effect of antirheumatics, not elsewhere classified**

T39.4X6 **Underdosing of antirheumatics, not elsewhere classified**

T39.8 **Poisoning by, adverse effect of and underdosing of other nonopioid analgesics and antipyretics, not elsewhere classified**

T39.8X **Poisoning by, adverse effect of and underdosing of other nonopioid analgesics and antipyretics, not elsewhere classified**

T39.8X1 **Poisoning by other nonopioid analgesics and antipyretics, not elsewhere classified, accidental (unintentional)**
Poisoning by other nonopioid analgesics and antipyretics, not elsewhere classified NOS

T39.8X2 **Poisoning by other nonopioid analgesics and antipyretics, not elsewhere classified, intentional self-harm**

T39.8X3 **Poisoning by other nonopioid analgesics and antipyretics, not elsewhere classified, assault**

T39.8X4 **Poisoning by other nonopioid analgesics and antipyretics, not elsewhere classified, undetermined**

T39.8X5 **Adverse effect of other nonopioid analgesics and antipyretics, not elsewhere classified**

T39.8X6 **Underdosing of other nonopioid analgesics and antipyretics, not elsewhere classified**

T39.9 **Poisoning by, adverse effect of and underdosing of unspecified nonopioid analgesic, antipyretic and antirheumatic**

T39.91 **Poisoning by unspecified nonopioid analgesic, antipyretic and antirheumatic, accidental (unintentional)**
Poisoning by nonopioid analgesic, antipyretic and antirheumatic NOS

T39.92 **Poisoning by unspecified nonopioid analgesic, antipyretic and antirheumatic, intentional self-harm**

T39.93 **Poisoning by unspecified nonopioid analgesic, antipyretic and antirheumatic, assault**

T39.94 **Poisoning by unspecified nonopioid analgesic, antipyretic and antirheumatic, undetermined**

T39.95 **Adverse effect of unspecified nonopioid analgesic, antipyretic and antirheumatic**

T39.96 **Underdosing of unspecified nonopioid analgesic, antipyretic and antirheumatic**

T40 **Poisoning by, adverse effect of and underdosing of narcotics and psychodysleptics [hallucinogens]**
EXCLUDES 2 *drug dependence and related mental and behavioral disorders due to psychoactive substance use (F1Ø-F19-)*

The appropriate 7th character is to be added to each code from category T4Ø.
A initial encounter
D subsequent encounter
S sequela

T40.Ø **Poisoning by, adverse effect of and underdosing of opium**

T40.ØX **Poisoning by, adverse effect of and underdosing of opium**

T40.ØX1 **Poisoning by opium, accidental (unintentional)**
Poisoning by opium NOS

T40.ØX2 **Poisoning by opium, intentional self-harm**

T40.ØX3 **Poisoning by opium, assault**

T40.ØX4 **Poisoning by opium, undetermined**

T40.ØX5 **Adverse effect of opium**

T40.ØX6 **Underdosing of opium**

T40.1 **Poisoning by and adverse effect of heroin**

T40.1X **Poisoning by and adverse effect of heroin**

T40.1X1 **Poisoning by heroin, accidental (unintentional)**
Poisoning by heroin NOS

T40.1X2 **Poisoning by heroin, intentional self-harm**

T40.1X3 **Poisoning by heroin, assault**

T40.1X4 **Poisoning by heroin, undetermined**

T40.2 **Poisoning by, adverse effect of and underdosing of other opioids**

T40.2X **Poisoning by, adverse effect of and underdosing of other opioids**

T40.2X1 **Poisoning by other opioids, accidental (unintentional)**
Poisoning by other opioids NOS

T40.2X2 **Poisoning by other opioids, intentional self-harm**

T40.2X3 **Poisoning by other opioids, assault**

T40.2X4 **Poisoning by other opioids, undetermined**

T40.2X5 **Adverse effect of other opioids**

T40.2X6 **Underdosing of other opioids**

T40.3 **Poisoning by, adverse effect of and underdosing of methadone**

T40.3X **Poisoning by, adverse effect of and underdosing of methadone**

T40.3X1 **Poisoning by methadone, accidental (unintentional)**
Poisoning by methadone NOS

T40.3X2 **Poisoning by methadone, intentional self-harm**

T40.3X3 **Poisoning by methadone, assault**

T40.3X4 **Poisoning by methadone, undetermined**

T40.3X5 **Adverse effect of methadone**

T40.3X6 **Underdosing of methadone**

T40.4 **Poisoning by, adverse effect of and underdosing of other synthetic narcotics**

T40.4X **Poisoning by, adverse effect of and underdosing of other synthetic narcotics**

T40.4X1 **Poisoning by other synthetic narcotics, accidental (unintentional)**
Poisoning by other synthetic narcotics NOS

T40.4X2 **Poisoning by other synthetic narcotics, intentional self-harm**

T40.4X3 Poisoning by other synthetic narcotics, assault

T40.4X4 Poisoning by other synthetic narcotics, undetermined

T40.4X5 Adverse effect of other synthetic narcotics

T40.4X6 Underdosing of other synthetic narcotics

T40.5 Poisoning by, adverse effect of and underdosing of cocaine

T40.5X Poisoning by, adverse effect of and underdosing of cocaine

T40.5X1 Poisoning by cocaine, accidental (unintentional)
Poisoning by cocaine NOS

T40.5X2 Poisoning by cocaine, intentional self-harm

T40.5X3 Poisoning by cocaine, assault

T40.5X4 Poisoning by cocaine, undetermined

T40.5X5 Adverse effect of cocaine

T40.5X6 Underdosing of cocaine

T40.6 Poisoning by, adverse effect of and underdosing of other and unspecified narcotics

T40.60 Poisoning by, adverse effect of and underdosing of unspecified narcotics

T40.601 Poisoning by unspecified narcotics, accidental (unintentional)
Poisoning by narcotics NOS

T40.602 Poisoning by unspecified narcotics, intentional self-harm

T40.603 Poisoning by unspecified narcotics, assault

T40.604 Poisoning by unspecified narcotics, undetermined

T40.605 Adverse effect of unspecified narcotics

T40.606 Underdosing of unspecified narcotics

T40.69 Poisoning by, adverse effect of and underdosing of other narcotics

T40.691 Poisoning by other narcotics, accidental (unintentional)
Poisoning by other narcotics NOS

T40.692 Poisoning by other narcotics, intentional self-harm

T40.693 Poisoning by other narcotics, assault

T40.694 Poisoning by other narcotics, undetermined

T40.695 Adverse effect of other narcotics

T40.696 Underdosing of other narcotics

T40.7 Poisoning by, adverse effect of and underdosing of cannabis (derivatives)

T40.7X Poisoning by, adverse effect of and underdosing of cannabis (derivatives)

T40.7X1 Poisoning by cannabis (derivatives), accidental (unintentional)
Poisoning by cannabis NOS

T40.7X2 Poisoning by cannabis (derivatives), intentional self-harm

T40.7X3 Poisoning by cannabis (derivatives), assault

T40.7X4 Poisoning by cannabis (derivatives), undetermined

T40.7X5 Adverse effect of cannabis (derivatives)

T40.7X6 Underdosing of cannabis (derivatives)

T40.8 Poisoning by and adverse effect of lysergide [LSD]

T40.8X Poisoning by and adverse effect of lysergide [LSD]

T40.8X1 Poisoning by lysergide [LSD], accidental (unintentional)
Poisoning by lysergide [LSD]NOS

T40.8X2 Poisoning by lysergide [LSD], intentional self-harm

T40.8X3 Poisoning by lysergide [LSD], assault

T40.8X4 Poisoning by lysergide [LSD], undetermined

T40.9 Poisoning by, adverse effect of and underdosing of other and unspecified psychodysleptics [hallucinogens]

T40.90 Poisoning by, adverse effect of and underdosing of unspecified psychodysleptics [hallucinogens]

T40.901 Poisoning by unspecified psychodysleptics [hallucinogens], accidental (unintentional)

T40.902 Poisoning by unspecified psychodysleptics [hallucinogens], intentional self-harm

T40.903 Poisoning by unspecified psychodysleptics [hallucinogens], assault

T40.904 Poisoning by unspecified psychodysleptics [hallucinogens], undetermined

T40.905 Adverse effect of unspecified psychodysleptics [hallucinogens]

T40.906 Underdosing of unspecified psychodysleptics

T40.99 Poisoning by, adverse effect of and underdosing of other psychodysleptics [hallucinogens]

T40.991 Poisoning by other psychodysleptics [hallucinogens], accidental (unintentional)
Poisoning by other psychodysleptics [hallucinogens] NOS

T40.992 Poisoning by other psychodysleptics [hallucinogens], intentional self-harm

T40.993 Poisoning by other psychodysleptics [hallucinogens], assault

T40.994 Poisoning by other psychodysleptics [hallucinogens], undetermined

T40.995 Adverse effect of other psychodysleptics [hallucinogens]

T40.996 Underdosing of other psychodysleptics

T41 Poisoning by, adverse effect of and underdosing of anesthetics and therapeutic gases

EXCLUDES 1 *benzodiazepines (T42.4-)*
cocaine (T40.5-)
complications of anesthesia during labor and delivery (O74.-)
complications of anesthesia during pregnancy (O29.-)
complications of anesthesia during the puerperium (O89.-)
opioids (T40.0-T40.2-)

The appropriate 7th character is to be added to each code from category T41.
A initial encounter
D subsequent encounter
S sequela

T41.0 Poisoning by, adverse effect of and underdosing of inhaled anesthetics

EXCLUDES 1 *oxygen (T41.5-)*

T41.0X Poisoning by, adverse effect of and underdosing of inhaled anesthetics

T41.0X1 Poisoning by inhaled anesthetics, accidental (unintentional)
Poisoning by inhaled anesthetics NOS

T41.0X2 Poisoning by inhaled anesthetics, intentional self-harm

T41.0X3 Poisoning by inhaled anesthetics, assault

T41.0X4 Poisoning by inhaled anesthetics, undetermined

T41.0X5 Adverse effect of inhaled anesthetics

T41.0X6 Underdosing of inhaled anesthetics

T41.1 Poisoning by, adverse effect of and underdosing of intravenous anesthetics
Poisoning by, adverse effect of and underdosing of thiobarbiturates

T41.1X Poisoning by, adverse effect of and underdosing of intravenous anesthetics

T41.1X1 Poisoning by intravenous anesthetics, accidental (unintentional)
Poisoning by intravenous anesthetics NOS

T41.1X2 Poisoning by intravenous anesthetics, intentional self-harm

T41.1X3 Poisoning by intravenous anesthetics, assault

T41.1X4 **Poisoning by intravenous anesthetics, undetermined**
T41.1X5 **Adverse effect of intravenous anesthetics**
T41.1X6 **Underdosing of intravenous anesthetics**

T41.2 **Poisoning by, adverse effect of and underdosing of other and unspecified general anesthetics**

T41.20 **Poisoning by, adverse effect of and underdosing of unspecified general anesthetics**
T41.201 **Poisoning by unspecified general anesthetics, accidental (unintentional)**
Poisoning by general anesthetics NOS
T41.202 **Poisoning by unspecified general anesthetics, intentional self-harm**
T41.203 **Poisoning by unspecified general anesthetics, assault**
T41.204 **Poisoning by unspecified general anesthetics, undetermined**
T41.205 **Adverse effect of unspecified general anesthetics**
T41.206 **Underdosing of unspecified general anesthetics**

T41.29 **Poisoning by, adverse effect of and underdosing of other general anesthetics**
T41.291 **Poisoning by other general anesthetics, accidental (unintentional)**
Poisoning by other general anesthetics NOS
T41.292 **Poisoning by other general anesthetics, intentional self-harm**
T41.293 **Poisoning by other general anesthetics, assault**
T41.294 **Poisoning by other general anesthetics, undetermined**
T41.295 **Adverse effect of other general anesthetics**
T41.296 **Underdosing of other general anesthetics**

T41.3 **Poisoning by, adverse effect of and underdosing of local anesthetics**
Cocaine (topical)
EXCLUDES 2 *poisoning by cocaine used as a central nervous system stimulant (T40.5X1-T40.5X4)*

T41.3X **Poisoning by, adverse effect of and underdosing of local anesthetics**
T41.3X1 **Poisoning by local anesthetics, accidental (unintentional)**
Poisoning by local anesthetics NOS
T41.3X2 **Poisoning by local anesthetics, intentional self-harm**
T41.3X3 **Poisoning by local anesthetics, assault**
T41.3X4 **Poisoning by local anesthetics, undetermined**
T41.3X5 **Adverse effect of local anesthetics**
T41.3X6 **Underdosing of local anesthetics**

T41.4 **Poisoning by, adverse effect of and underdosing of unspecified anesthetic**
T41.41 **Poisoning by unspecified anesthetic, accidental (unintentional)**
Poisoning by anesthetic NOS
T41.42 **Poisoning by unspecified anesthetic, intentional self-harm**
T41.43 **Poisoning by unspecified anesthetic, assault**
T41.44 **Poisoning by unspecified anesthetic, undetermined**
T41.45 **Adverse effect of unspecified anesthetic**
T41.46 **Underdosing of unspecified anesthetics**

T41.5 **Poisoning by, adverse effect of and underdosing of therapeutic gases**

T41.5X **Poisoning by, adverse effect of and underdosing of therapeutic gases**
T41.5X1 **Poisoning by therapeutic gases, accidental (unintentional)**
Poisoning by therapeutic gases NOS
T41.5X2 **Poisoning by therapeutic gases, intentional self-harm**
T41.5X3 **Poisoning by therapeutic gases, assault**
T41.5X4 **Poisoning by therapeutic gases, undetermined**
T41.5X5 **Adverse effect of therapeutic gases**
T41.5X6 **Underdosing of therapeutic gases**

T42 Poisoning by, adverse effect of and underdosing of antiepileptic, sedative- hypnotic and antiparkinsonism drugs

EXCLUDES 2 *drug dependence and related mental and behavioral disorders due to psychoactive substance use (F10.- – F19.-)*

The appropriate 7th character is to be added to each code from category T42.
A initial encounter
D subsequent encounter
S sequela

T42.0 **Poisoning by, adverse effect of and underdosing of hydantoin derivatives**

T42.0X **Poisoning by, adverse effect of and underdosing of hydantoin derivatives**
T42.0X1 **Poisoning by hydantoin derivatives, accidental (unintentional)**
Poisoning by hydantoin derivatives NOS
T42.0X2 **Poisoning by hydantoin derivatives, intentional self-harm**
T42.0X3 **Poisoning by hydantoin derivatives, assault**
T42.0X4 **Poisoning by hydantoin derivatives, undetermined**
T42.0X5 **Adverse effect of hydantoin derivatives**
T42.0X6 **Underdosing of hydantoin derivatives**

T42.1 **Poisoning by, adverse effect of and underdosing of iminostilbenes**
Poisoning by, adverse effect of and underdosing of carbamazepine

T42.1X **Poisoning by, adverse effect of and underdosing of iminostilbenes**
T42.1X1 **Poisoning by iminostilbenes, accidental (unintentional)**
Poisoning by iminostilbenes NOS
T42.1X2 **Poisoning by iminostilbenes, intentional self-harm**
T42.1X3 **Poisoning by iminostilbenes, assault**
T42.1X4 **Poisoning by iminostilbenes, undetermined**
T42.1X5 **Adverse effect of iminostilbenes**
T42.1X6 **Underdosing of iminostilbenes**

T42.2 **Poisoning by, adverse effect of and underdosing of succinimides and oxazolidinediones**

T42.2X **Poisoning by, adverse effect of and underdosing of succinimides and oxazolidinediones**
T42.2X1 **Poisoning by succinimides and oxazolidinediones, accidental (unintentional)**
Poisoning by succinimides and oxazolidinediones NOS
T42.2X2 **Poisoning by succinimides and oxazolidinediones, intentional self-harm**
T42.2X3 **Poisoning by succinimides and oxazolidinediones, assault**
T42.2X4 **Poisoning by succinimides and oxazolidinediones, undetermined**
T42.2X5 **Adverse effect of succinimides and oxazolidinediones**
T42.2X6 **Underdosing of succinimides and oxazolidinediones**

T42.3 **Poisoning by, adverse effect of and underdosing of barbiturates**
EXCLUDES 1 *poisoning by, adverse effect of and underdosing of thiobarbiturates (T41.1-)*

T42.3X **Poisoning by, adverse effect of and underdosing of barbiturates**
T42.3X1 **Poisoning by barbiturates, accidental (unintentional)**
Poisoning by barbiturates NOS
T42.3X2 **Poisoning by barbiturates, intentional self-harm**
T42.3X3 **Poisoning by barbiturates, assault**

√7th **T42.3X4 Poisoning by barbiturates, undetermined**

√7th **T42.3X5 Adverse effect of barbiturates**

√7th **T42.3X6 Underdosing of barbiturates**

√5th **T42.4 Poisoning by, adverse effect of and underdosing of benzodiazepines**

√6th **T42.4X Poisoning by, adverse effect of and underdosing of benzodiazepines**

√7th **T42.4X1 Poisoning by benzodiazepines, accidental (unintentional)**
Poisoning by benzodiazepines NOS

√7th **T42.4X2 Poisoning by benzodiazepines, intentional self-harm**

√7th **T42.4X3 Poisoning by benzodiazepines, assault**

√7th **T42.4X4 Poisoning by benzodiazepines, undetermined**

√7th **T42.4X5 Adverse effect of benzodiazepines**

√7th **T42.4X6 Underdosing of benzodiazepines**

√5th **T42.5 Poisoning by, adverse effect of and underdosing of mixed antiepileptics**

√6th **T42.5X Poisoning by, adverse effect of and underdosing of antiepileptics**

√7th **T42.5X1 Poisoning by mixed antiepileptics, accidental (unintentional)**
Poisoning by mixed antiepileptics NOS

√7th **T42.5X2 Poisoning by mixed antiepileptics, intentional self-harm**

√7th **T42.5X3 Poisoning by mixed antiepileptics, assault**

√7th **T42.5X4 Poisoning by mixed antiepileptics, undetermined**

√7th **T42.5X5 Adverse effect of mixed antiepileptics**

√7th **T42.5X6 Underdosing of mixed antiepileptics**

√5th **T42.6 Poisoning by, adverse effect of and underdosing of other antiepileptic and sedative-hypnotic drugs**
Poisoning by, adverse effect of and underdosing of methaqualone
Poisoning by, adverse effect of and underdosing of valproic acid
EXCLUDES 1 *poisoning by, adverse effect of and underdosing of carbamazepine (T42.1-)*

√6th **T42.6X Poisoning by, adverse effect of and underdosing of other antiepileptic and sedative-hypnotic drugs**

√7th **T42.6X1 Poisoning by other antiepileptic and sedative-hypnotic drugs, accidental (unintentional)**
Poisoning by other antiepileptic and sedative-hypnotic drugs NOS

√7th **T42.6X2 Poisoning by other antiepileptic and sedative-hypnotic drugs, intentional self-harm**

√7th **T42.6X3 Poisoning by other antiepileptic and sedative-hypnotic drugs, assault**

√7th **T42.6X4 Poisoning by other antiepileptic and sedative-hypnotic drugs, undetermined**

√7th **T42.6X5 Adverse effect of other antiepileptic and sedative-hypnotic drugs**

√7th **T42.6X6 Underdosing of other antiepileptic and sedative-hypnotic drugs**

√5th **T42.7 Poisoning by, adverse effect of and underdosing of unspecified antiepileptic and sedative-hypnotic drugs**

√x7th **T42.71 Poisoning by unspecified antiepileptic and sedative-hypnotic drugs, accidental (unintentional)**
Poisoning by antiepileptic and sedative-hypnotic drugs NOS

√x7th **T42.72 Poisoning by unspecified antiepileptic and sedative-hypnotic drugs, intentional self-harm**

√x7th **T42.73 Poisoning by unspecified antiepileptic and sedative-hypnotic drugs, assault**

√x7th **T42.74 Poisoning by unspecified antiepileptic and sedative-hypnotic drugs, undetermined**

√x7th **T42.75 Adverse effect of unspecified antiepileptic and sedative-hypnotic drugs**

√x7th **T42.76 Underdosing of unspecified antiepileptic and sedative-hypnotic drugs**

√5th **T42.8 Poisoning by, adverse effect of and underdosing of antiparkinsonism drugs and other central muscle-tone depressants**
Poisoning by, adverse effect of and underdosing of amantadine

√6th **T42.8X Poisoning by, adverse effect of and underdosing of antiparkinsonism drugs and other central muscle-tone depressants**

√7th **T42.8X1 Poisoning by antiparkinsonism drugs and other central muscle-tone depressants, accidental (unintentional)**
Poisoning by antiparkinsonism drugs and other central muscle-tone depressants NOS

√7th **T42.8X2 Poisoning by antiparkinsonism drugs and other central muscle-tone depressants, intentional self-harm**

√7th **T42.8X3 Poisoning by antiparkinsonism drugs and other central muscle-tone depressants, assault**

√7th **T42.8X4 Poisoning by antiparkinsonism drugs and other central muscle-tone depressants, undetermined**

√7th **T42.8X5 Adverse effect of antiparkinsonism drugs and other central muscle-tone depressants**

√7th **T42.8X6 Underdosing of antiparkinsonism drugs and other central muscle-tone depressants**

√4th **T43 Poisoning by, adverse effect of and underdosing of psychotropic drugs, not elsewhere classified**
EXCLUDES 1 *appetite depressants (T50.5-)*
barbiturates (T42.3-)
benzodiazepines (T42.4-)
methaqualone (T42.6-)
psychodysleptics [hallucinogens] (T40.7-T40.9-)
EXCLUDES 2 *drug dependence and related mental and behavioral disorders due to psychoactive substance use (F10.- – F19.-)*

The appropriate 7th character is to be added to each code from category T43.
A initial encounter
D subsequent encounter
S sequela

√5th **T43.0 Poisoning by, adverse effect of and underdosing of tricyclic and tetracyclic antidepressants**

√6th **T43.01 Poisoning by, adverse effect of and underdosing of tricyclic antidepressants**

√7th **T43.011 Poisoning by tricyclic antidepressants, accidental (unintentional)**
Poisoning by tricyclic antidepressants NOS

√7th **T43.012 Poisoning by tricyclic antidepressants, intentional self-harm**

√7th **T43.013 Poisoning by tricyclic antidepressants, assault**

√7th **T43.014 Poisoning by tricyclic antidepressants, undetermined**

√7th **T43.015 Adverse effect of tricyclic antidepressants**

√7th **T43.016 Underdosing of tricyclic antidepressants**

√6th **T43.02 Poisoning by, adverse effect of and underdosing of tetracyclic antidepressants**

√7th **T43.021 Poisoning by tetracyclic antidepressants, accidental (unintentional)**
Poisoning by tetracyclic antidepressants NOS

√7th **T43.022 Poisoning by tetracyclic antidepressants, intentional self-harm**

√7th **T43.023 Poisoning by tetracyclic antidepressants, assault**

√7th **T43.024 Poisoning by tetracyclic antidepressants, undetermined**

√7th **T43.025 Adverse effect of tetracyclic antidepressants**

√7th **T43.026 Underdosing of tetracyclic antidepressants**

T43.1 Poisoning by, adverse effect of and underdosing of monoamine-oxidase-inhibitor antidepressants

T43.1X Poisoning by, adverse effect of and underdosing of monoamine-oxidase-inhibitor antidepressants

T43.1X1 Poisoning by monoamine-oxidase-inhibitor antidepressants, accidental (unintentional)
Poisoning by monoamine-oxidase-inhibitor antidepressants NOS

T43.1X2 Poisoning by monoamine-oxidase-inhibitor antidepressants, intentional self-harm

T43.1X3 Poisoning by monoamine-oxidase-inhibitor antidepressants, assault

T43.1X4 Poisoning by monoamine-oxidase-inhibitor antidepressants, undetermined

T43.1X5 Adverse effect of monoamine-oxidase-inhibitor antidepressants

T43.1X6 Underdosing of monoamine-oxidase-inhibitor antidepressants

T43.2 Poisoning by, adverse effect of and underdosing of other and unspecified antidepressants

T43.20 Poisoning by, adverse effect of and underdosing of unspecified antidepressants

T43.201 Poisoning by unspecified antidepressants, accidental (unintentional)
Poisoning by antidepressants NOS

T43.202 Poisoning by unspecified antidepressants, intentional self-harm

T43.203 Poisoning by unspecified antidepressants, assault

T43.204 Poisoning by unspecified antidepressants, undetermined

T43.205 Adverse effect of unspecified antidepressants

T43.206 Underdosing of unspecified antidepressants

T43.21 Poisoning by, adverse effect of and underdosing of selective serotonin and norepinephrine reuptake inhibitors
Poisoning by, adverse effect of and underdosing of SSNRI antidepressants

T43.211 Poisoning by selective serotonin and norepinephrine reuptake inhibitors, accidental (unintentional)

T43.212 Poisoning by selective serotonin and norepinephrine reuptake inhibitors, intentional self-harm

T43.213 Poisoning by selective serotonin and norepinephrine reuptake inhibitors, assault

T43.214 Poisoning by selective serotonin and norepinephrine reuptake inhibitors, undetermined

T43.215 Adverse effect of selective serotonin and norepinephrine reuptake inhibitors

T43.216 Underdosing of selective serotonin and norepinephrine reuptake inhibitors

T43.22 Poisoning by, adverse effect of and underdosing of selective serotonin reuptake inhibitors
Poisoning by, adverse effect of and underdosing of SSRI antidepressants

T43.221 Poisoning by selective serotonin reuptake inhibitors, accidental (unintentional)

T43.222 Poisoning by selective serotonin reuptake inhibitors, intentional self-harm

T43.223 Poisoning by selective serotonin reuptake inhibitors, assault

T43.224 Poisoning by selective serotonin reuptake inhibitors, undetermined

T43.225 Adverse effect of selective serotonin reuptake inhibitors

T43.226 Underdosing of selective serotonin reuptake inhibitors

T43.29 Poisoning by, adverse effect of and underdosing of other antidepressants

T43.291 Poisoning by other antidepressants, accidental (unintentional)
Poisoning by other antidepressants NOS

T43.292 Poisoning by other antidepressants, intentional self-harm

T43.293 Poisoning by other antidepressants, assault

T43.294 Poisoning by other antidepressants, undetermined

T43.295 Adverse effect of other antidepressants

T43.296 Underdosing of other antidepressants

T43.3 Poisoning by, adverse effect of and underdosing of phenothiazine antipsychotics and neuroleptics

T43.3X Poisoning by, adverse effect of and underdosing of phenothiazine antipsychotics and neuroleptics

T43.3X1 Poisoning by phenothiazine antipsychotics and neuroleptics, accidental (unintentional)
Poisoning by phenothiazine antipsychotics and neuroleptics NOS

T43.3X2 Poisoning by phenothiazine antipsychotics and neuroleptics, intentional self-harm

T43.3X3 Poisoning by phenothiazine antipsychotics and neuroleptics, assault

T43.3X4 Poisoning by phenothiazine antipsychotics and neuroleptics, undetermined

T43.3X5 Adverse effect of phenothiazine antipsychotics and neuroleptics

T43.3X6 Underdosing of phenothiazine antipsychotics and neuroleptics

T43.4 Poisoning by, adverse effect of and underdosing of butyrophenone and thiothixene neuroleptics

T43.4X Poisoning by, adverse effect of and underdosing of butyrophenone and thiothixene neuroleptics

T43.4X1 Poisoning by butyrophenone and thiothixene neuroleptics, accidental (unintentional)
Poisoning by butyrophenone and thiothixene neuroleptics NOS

T43.4X2 Poisoning by butyrophenone and thiothixene neuroleptics, intentional self-harm

T43.4X3 Poisoning by butyrophenone and thiothixene neuroleptics, assault

T43.4X4 Poisoning by butyrophenone and thiothixene neuroleptics, undetermined

T43.4X5 Adverse effect of butyrophenone and thiothixene neuroleptics

T43.4X6 Underdosing of butyrophenone and thiothixene neuroleptics

T43.5 Poisoning by, adverse effect of and underdosing of other and unspecified antipsychotics and neuroleptics
EXCLUDES 1 *poisoning by, adverse effect of and underdosing of rauwolfia (T46.5-)*

T43.50 Poisoning by, adverse effect of and underdosing of unspecified antipsychotics and neuroleptics

T43.501 Poisoning by unspecified antipsychotics and neuroleptics, accidental (unintentional)
Poisoning by antipsychotics and neuroleptics NOS

T43.502 Poisoning by unspecified antipsychotics and neuroleptics, intentional self-harm

T43.503 Poisoning by unspecified antipsychotics and neuroleptics, assault

T43.504 Poisoning by unspecified antipsychotics and neuroleptics, undetermined

T43.505 Adverse effect of unspecified antipsychotics and neuroleptics

T43.506 Underdosing of unspecified antipsychotics and neuroleptics

6th **T43.59 Poisoning by, adverse effect of and underdosing of other antipsychotics and neuroleptics**

7th **T43.591 Poisoning by other antipsychotics and neuroleptics, accidental (unintentional)**
Poisoning by other antipsychotics and neuroleptics NOS

7th **T43.592 Poisoning by other antipsychotics and neuroleptics, intentional self-harm**

7th **T43.593 Poisoning by other antipsychotics and neuroleptics, assault**

7th **T43.594 Poisoning by other antipsychotics and neuroleptics, undetermined**

7th **T43.595 Adverse effect of other antipsychotics and neuroleptics**

7th **T43.596 Underdosing of other antipsychotics and neuroleptics**

5th **T43.6 Poisoning by, adverse effect of and underdosing of psychostimulants**

EXCLUDES 1 *poisoning by, adverse effect of and underdosing of cocaine (T40.5-)*

6th **T43.60 Poisoning by, adverse effect of and underdosing of unspecified psychostimulant**

7th **T43.601 Poisoning by unspecified psychostimulants, accidental (unintentional)**
Poisoning by psychostimulants NOS

7th **T43.602 Poisoning by unspecified psychostimulants, intentional self-harm**

7th **T43.603 Poisoning by unspecified psychostimulants, assault**

7th **T43.604 Poisoning by unspecified psychostimulants, undetermined**

7th **T43.605 Adverse effect of unspecified psychostimulants**

7th **T43.606 Underdosing of unspecified psychostimulants**

6th **T43.61 Poisoning by, adverse effect of and underdosing of caffeine**

7th **T43.611 Poisoning by caffeine, accidental (unintentional)**
Poisoning by caffeine NOS

7th **T43.612 Poisoning by caffeine, intentional self-harm**

7th **T43.613 Poisoning by caffeine, assault**

7th **T43.614 Poisoning by caffeine, undetermined**

7th **T43.615 Adverse effect of caffeine**

7th **T43.616 Underdosing of caffeine**

6th **T43.62 Poisoning by, adverse effect of and underdosing of amphetamines**
Poisoning by, adverse effect of and underdosing of methamphetamines

7th **T43.621 Poisoning by amphetamines, accidental (unintentional)**
Poisoning by amphetamines NOS

7th **T43.622 Poisoning by amphetamines, intentional self-harm**

7th **T43.623 Poisoning by amphetamines, assault**

7th **T43.624 Poisoning by amphetamines, undetermined**

7th **T43.625 Adverse effect of amphetamines**

7th **T43.626 Underdosing of amphetamines**

6th **T43.63 Poisoning by, adverse effect of and underdosing of methylphenidate**

7th **T43.631 Poisoning by methylphenidate, accidental (unintentional)**
Poisoning by methylphenidate NOS

7th **T43.632 Poisoning by methylphenidate, intentional self-harm**

7th **T43.633 Poisoning by methylphenidate, assault**

7th **T43.634 Poisoning by methylphenidate, undetermined**

7th **T43.635 Adverse effect of methylphenidate**

7th **T43.636 Underdosing of methylphenidate**

6th **T43.69 Poisoning by, adverse effect of and underdosing of other psychostimulants**

7th **T43.691 Poisoning by other psychostimulants, accidental (unintentional)**
Poisoning by other psychostimulants NOS

7th **T43.692 Poisoning by other psychostimulants, intentional self-harm**

7th **T43.693 Poisoning by other psychostimulants, assault**

7th **T43.694 Poisoning by other psychostimulants, undetermined**

7th **T43.695 Adverse effect of other psychostimulants**

7th **T43.696 Underdosing of other psychostimulants**

5th **T43.8 Poisoning by, adverse effect of and underdosing of other psychotropic drugs**

6th **T43.8X Poisoning by, adverse effect of and underdosing of other psychotropic drugs**

7th **T43.8X1 Poisoning by other psychotropic drugs, accidental (unintentional)**
Poisoning by other psychotropic drugs NOS

7th **T43.8X2 Poisoning by other psychotropic drugs, intentional self-harm**

7th **T43.8X3 Poisoning by other psychotropic drugs, assault**

7th **T43.8X4 Poisoning by other psychotropic drugs, undetermined**

7th **T43.8X5 Adverse effect of other psychotropic drugs**

7th **T43.8X6 Underdosing of other psychotropic drugs**

5th **T43.9 Poisoning by, adverse effect of and underdosing of unspecified psychotropic drug**

x7th **T43.91 Poisoning by unspecified psychotropic drug, accidental (unintentional)**
Poisoning by psychotropic drug NOS

x7th **T43.92 Poisoning by unspecified psychotropic drug, intentional self-harm**

x7th **T43.93 Poisoning by unspecified psychotropic drug, assault**

x7th **T43.94 Poisoning by unspecified psychotropic drug, undetermined**

x7th **T43.95 Adverse effect of unspecified psychotropic drug**

x7th **T43.96 Underdosing of unspecified psychotropic drug**

4th **T44 Poisoning by, adverse effect of and underdosing of drugs primarily affecting the autonomic nervous system**

The appropriate 7th character is to be added to each code from category T44.
A initial encounter
D subsequent encounter
S sequela

5th **T44.0 Poisoning by, adverse effect of and underdosing of anticholinesterase agents**

6th **T44.0X Poisoning by, adverse effect of and underdosing of anticholinesterase agents**

7th **T44.0X1 Poisoning by anticholinesterase agents, accidental (unintentional)**
Poisoning by anticholinesterase agents NOS

7th **T44.0X2 Poisoning by anticholinesterase agents, intentional self-harm**

7th **T44.0X3 Poisoning by anticholinesterase agents, assault**

7th **T44.0X4 Poisoning by anticholinesterase agents, undetermined**

7th **T44.0X5 Adverse effect of anticholinesterase agents**

7th **T44.0X6 Underdosing of anticholinesterase agents**

5th **T44.1 Poisoning by, adverse effect of and underdosing of other parasympathomimetics [cholinergics]**

6th **T44.1X Poisoning by, adverse effect of and underdosing of other parasympathomimetics [cholinergics]**

7th **T44.1X1 Poisoning by other parasympathomimetics [cholinergics], accidental (unintentional)**
Poisoning by other parasympathomimetics [cholinergics] NOS

√7th T44.1X2 **Poisoning by other parasympathomimetics [cholinergics], intentional self-harm**

√7th T44.1X3 **Poisoning by other parasympathomimetics [cholinergics], assault**

√7th T44.1X4 **Poisoning by other parasympathomimetics [cholinergics], undetermined**

√7th T44.1X5 **Adverse effect of other parasympathomimetics [cholinergics]**

√7th T44.1X6 **Underdosing of other parasympathomimetics**

√5th T44.2 **Poisoning by, adverse effect of and underdosing of ganglionic blocking drugs**

√6th T44.2X **Poisoning by, adverse effect of and underdosing of ganglionic blocking drugs**

√7th T44.2X1 **Poisoning by ganglionic blocking drugs, accidental (unintentional)**
Poisoning by ganglionic blocking drugs NOS

√7th T44.2X2 **Poisoning by ganglionic blocking drugs, intentional self-harm**

√7th T44.2X3 **Poisoning by ganglionic blocking drugs, assault**

√7th T44.2X4 **Poisoning by ganglionic blocking drugs, undetermined**

√7th T44.2X5 **Adverse effect of ganglionic blocking drugs**

√7th T44.2X6 **Underdosing of ganglionic blocking drugs**

T44.3 **Poisoning by, adverse effect of and underdosing of other parasympatholytics [anticholinergics and antimuscarinics] and spasmolytics**
Poisoning by, adverse effect of and underdosing of papaverine

√6th T44.3X **Poisoning by, adverse effect of and underdosing of other parasympatholytics [anticholinergics and antimuscarinics] and spasmolytics**

√7th T44.3X1 **Poisoning by other parasympatholytics [anticholinergics and antimuscarinics] and spasmolytics, accidental (unintentional)**
Poisoning by other parasympatholytics [anticholinergics and antimuscarinics] and spasmolytics NOS

√7th T44.3X2 **Poisoning by other parasympatholytics [anticholinergics and antimuscarinics] and spasmolytics, intentional self-harm**

√7th T44.3X3 **Poisoning by other parasympatholytics [anticholinergics and antimuscarinics] and spasmolytics, assault**

√7th T44.3X4 **Poisoning by other parasympatholytics [anticholinergics and antimuscarinics] and spasmolytics, undetermined**

√7th T44.3X5 **Adverse effect of other parasympatholytics [anticholinergics and antimuscarinics] and spasmolytics**

√7th T44.3X6 **Underdosing of other parasympatholytics [anticholinergics and antimuscarinics] and spasmolytics**

√5th T44.4 **Poisoning by, adverse effect of and underdosing of predominantly alpha-adrenoreceptor agonists**
Poisoning by, adverse effect of and underdosing of metaraminol

√6th T44.4X **Poisoning by, adverse effect of and underdosing of predominantly alpha-adrenoreceptor agonists**

√7th T44.4X1 **Poisoning by predominantly alpha-adrenoreceptor agonists, accidental (unintentional)**
Poisoning by predominantly alpha-adrenoreceptor agonists NOS

√7th T44.4X2 **Poisoning by predominantly alpha-adrenoreceptor agonists, intentional self-harm**

√7th T44.4X3 **Poisoning by predominantly alpha-adrenoreceptor agonists, assault**

√7th T44.4X4 **Poisoning by predominantly alpha-adrenoreceptor agonists, undetermined**

√7th T44.4X5 **Adverse effect of predominantly alpha-adrenoreceptor agonists**

√7th T44.4X6 **Underdosing of predominantly alpha-adrenoreceptor agonists**

√5th T44.5 **Poisoning by, adverse effect of and underdosing of predominantly beta-adrenoreceptor agonists**
EXCLUDES 1 *poisoning by, adverse effect of and underdosing of beta-adrenoreceptor agonists used in asthma therapy (T48.6-)*

√6th T44.5X **Poisoning by, adverse effect of and underdosing of predominantly beta-adrenoreceptor agonists**

√7th T44.5X1 **Poisoning by predominantly beta-adrenoreceptor agonists, accidental (unintentional)**
Poisoning by predominantly beta-adrenoreceptor agonists NOS

√7th T44.5X2 **Poisoning by predominantly beta-adrenoreceptor agonists, intentional self-harm**

√7th T44.5X3 **Poisoning by predominantly beta-adrenoreceptor agonists, assault**

√7th T44.5X4 **Poisoning by predominantly beta-adrenoreceptor agonists, undetermined**

√7th T44.5X5 **Adverse effect of predominantly beta-adrenoreceptor agonists**

√7th T44.5X6 **Underdosing of predominantly beta-adrenoreceptor agonists**

√5th T44.6 **Poisoning by, adverse effect of and underdosing of alpha-adrenoreceptor antagonists**
EXCLUDES 1 *poisoning by, adverse effect of and underdosing of ergot alkaloids (T48.0)*

√6th T44.6X **Poisoning by, adverse effect of and underdosing of alpha-adrenoreceptor antagonists**

√7th T44.6X1 **Poisoning by alpha-adrenoreceptor antagonists, accidental (unintentional)**
Poisoning by alpha-adrenoreceptor antagonists NOS

√7th T44.6X2 **Poisoning by alpha-adrenoreceptor antagonists, intentional self-harm**

√7th T44.6X3 **Poisoning by alpha-adrenoreceptor antagonists, assault**

√7th T44.6X4 **Poisoning by alpha-adrenoreceptor antagonists, undetermined**

√7th T44.6X5 **Adverse effect of alpha-adrenoreceptor antagonists**

√7th T44.6X6 **Underdosing of alpha-adrenoreceptor antagonists**

√5th T44.7 **Poisoning by, adverse effect of and underdosing of beta-adrenoreceptor antagonists**

√6th T44.7X **Poisoning by, adverse effect of and underdosing of beta-adrenoreceptor antagonists**

√7th T44.7X1 **Poisoning by beta-adrenoreceptor antagonists, accidental (unintentional)**
Poisoning by beta-adrenoreceptor antagonists NOS

√7th T44.7X2 **Poisoning by beta-adrenoreceptor antagonists, intentional self-harm**

√7th T44.7X3 **Poisoning by beta-adrenoreceptor antagonists, assault**

√7th T44.7X4 **Poisoning by beta-adrenoreceptor antagonists, undetermined**

√7th T44.7X5 **Adverse effect of beta-adrenoreceptor antagonists**

√7th T44.7X6 **Underdosing of beta-adrenoreceptor antagonists**

√5th T44.8 **Poisoning by, adverse effect of and underdosing of centrally-acting and adrenergic-neuron- blocking agents**
EXCLUDES 1 *poisoning by, adverse effect of and underdosing of clonidine (T46.5)*
poisoning by, adverse effect of and underdosing of guanethidine (T46.5)

√6th T44.8X **Poisoning by, adverse effect of and underdosing of centrally-acting and adrenergic-neuron-blocking agents**

√7th T44.8X1 **Poisoning by centrally-acting and adrenergic-neuron-blocking agents, accidental (unintentional)**
Poisoning by centrally-acting and adrenergic-neuron-blocking agents NOS

√7th **T44.8X2 Poisoning by centrally-acting and adrenergic-neuron-blocking agents, intentional self-harm**

√7th **T44.8X3 Poisoning by centrally-acting and adrenergic-neuron-blocking agents, assault**

√7th **T44.8X4 Poisoning by centrally-acting and adrenergic-neuron-blocking agents, undetermined**

√7th **T44.8X5 Adverse effect of centrally-acting and adrenergic-neuron-blocking agents**

√7th **T44.8X6 Underdosing of centrally-acting and adrenergic-neuron-blocking agents**

√5th **T44.9 Poisoning by, adverse effect of and underdosing of other and unspecified drugs primarily affecting the autonomic nervous system**

Poisoning by, adverse effect of and underdosing of drug stimulating both alpha and beta-adrenoreceptors

√6th **T44.90 Poisoning by, adverse effect of and underdosing of unspecified drugs primarily affecting the autonomic nervous system**

√7th **T44.901 Poisoning by unspecified drugs primarily affecting the autonomic nervous system, accidental (unintentional)**

Poisoning by unspecified drugs primarily affecting the autonomic nervous system NOS

√7th **T44.902 Poisoning by unspecified drugs primarily affecting the autonomic nervous system, intentional self-harm**

√7th **T44.903 Poisoning by unspecified drugs primarily affecting the autonomic nervous system, assault**

√7th **T44.904 Poisoning by unspecified drugs primarily affecting the autonomic nervous system, undetermined**

√7th **T44.905 Adverse effect of unspecified drugs primarily affecting the autonomic nervous system**

√7th **T44.906 Underdosing of unspecified drugs primarily affecting the autonomic nervous system**

√6th **T44.99 Poisoning by, adverse effect of and underdosing of other drugs primarily affecting the autonomic nervous system**

√7th **T44.991 Poisoning by other drug primarily affecting the autonomic nervous system, accidental (unintentional)**

Poisoning by other drugs primarily affecting the autonomic nervous system NOS

√7th **T44.992 Poisoning by other drug primarily affecting the autonomic nervous system, intentional self-harm**

√7th **T44.993 Poisoning by other drug primarily affecting the autonomic nervous system, assault**

√7th **T44.994 Poisoning by other drug primarily affecting the autonomic nervous system, undetermined**

√7th **T44.995 Adverse effect of other drug primarily affecting the autonomic nervous system**

√7th **T44.996 Underdosing of other drug primarily affecting the autonomic nervous system**

√4th **T45 Poisoning by, adverse effect of and underdosing of primarily systemic and hematological agents, not elsewhere classified**

The appropriate 7th character is to be added to each code from category T45.
A initial encounter
D subsequent encounter
S sequela

√5th **T45.0 Poisoning by, adverse effect of and underdosing of antiallergic and antiemetic drugs**

EXCLUDES 1 *poisoning by, adverse effect of and underdosing of phenothiazine-based neuroleptics (T43.3)*

√6th **T45.0X Poisoning by, adverse effect of and underdosing of antiallergic and antiemetic drugs**

√7th **T45.0X1 Poisoning by antiallergic and antiemetic drugs, accidental (unintentional)**

Poisoning by antiallergic and antiemetic drugs NOS

√7th **T45.0X2 Poisoning by antiallergic and antiemetic drugs, intentional self-harm**

√7th **T45.0X3 Poisoning by antiallergic and antiemetic drugs, assault**

√7th **T45.0X4 Poisoning by antiallergic and antiemetic drugs, undetermined**

√7th **T45.0X5 Adverse effect of antiallergic and antiemetic drugs**

√7th **T45.0X6 Underdosing of antiallergic and antiemetic drugs**

√5th **T45.1 Poisoning by, adverse effect of and underdosing of antineoplastic and immunosuppressive drugs**

EXCLUDES 1 *poisoning by, adverse effect of and underdosing of tamoxifen (T38.6)*

√6th **T45.1X Poisoning by, adverse effect of and underdosing of antineoplastic and immunosuppressive drugs**

√7th **T45.1X1 Poisoning by antineoplastic and immunosuppressive drugs, accidental (unintentional)**

Poisoning by antineoplastic and immunosuppressive drugs NOS

√7th **T45.1X2 Poisoning by antineoplastic and immunosuppressive drugs, intentional self-harm**

√7th **T45.1X3 Poisoning by antineoplastic and immunosuppressive drugs, assault**

√7th **T45.1X4 Poisoning by antineoplastic and immunosuppressive drugs, undetermined**

√7th **T45.1X5 Adverse effect of antineoplastic and immunosuppressive drugs**

√7th **T45.1X6 Underdosing of antineoplastic and immunosuppressive drugs**

√5th **T45.2 Poisoning by, adverse effect of and underdosing of vitamins**

EXCLUDES 2 *poisoning by, adverse effect of and underdosing of iron (T45.4)*
poisoning by, adverse effect of and underdosing of nicotinic acid (derivatives) (T46.7)
poisoning by, adverse effect of and underdosing of vitamin K (T45.7)

√6th **T45.2X Poisoning by, adverse effect of and underdosing of vitamins**

√7th **T45.2X1 Poisoning by vitamins, accidental (unintentional)**

Poisoning by vitamins NOS

√7th **T45.2X2 Poisoning by vitamins, intentional self-harm**

√7th **T45.2X3 Poisoning by vitamins, assault**

√7th **T45.2X4 Poisoning by vitamins, undetermined**

√7th **T45.2X5 Adverse effect of vitamins**

√7th **T45.2X6 Underdosing of vitamins**

EXCLUDES 1 *vitamin deficiencies (E50-E56)*

√5th **T45.3 Poisoning by, adverse effect of and underdosing of enzymes**

√6th **T45.3X Poisoning by, adverse effect of and underdosing of enzymes**

√7th **T45.3X1 Poisoning by enzymes, accidental (unintentional)**

Poisoning by enzymes NOS

√7th **T45.3X2 Poisoning by enzymes, intentional self-harm**

√7th **T45.3X3 Poisoning by enzymes, assault**

√7th **T45.3X4 Poisoning by enzymes, undetermined**

√7th **T45.3X5 Adverse effect of enzymes**

√7th **T45.3X6 Underdosing of enzymes**

√5th **T45.4 Poisoning by, adverse effect of and underdosing of iron and its compounds**

√6th **T45.4X Poisoning by, adverse effect of and underdosing of iron and its compounds**

T45.4X1 Poisoning by iron and its compounds, accidental (unintentional)

Poisoning by iron and its compounds NOS

√7th **T45.4X2 Poisoning by iron and its compounds, intentional self-harm**

T45.4X3 Poisoning by iron and its compounds, assault
T45.4X4 Poisoning by iron and its compounds, undetermined
T45.4X5 Adverse effect of iron and its compounds
T45.4X6 Underdosing of iron and its compounds
EXCLUDES 1 *iron deficiency (E61.1)*

T45.5 Poisoning by, adverse effect of and underdosing of anticoagulants and antithrombotic drugs
T45.51 Poisoning by, adverse effect of and underdosing of anticoagulants
T45.511 Poisoning by anticoagulants, accidental (unintentional)
Poisoning by anticoagulants NOS
T45.512 Poisoning by anticoagulants, intentional self-harm
T45.513 Poisoning by anticoagulants, assault
T45.514 Poisoning by anticoagulants, undetermined
T45.515 Adverse effect of anticoagulants
AHA: 2013, 2Q, 34
T45.516 Underdosing of anticoagulants
T45.52 Poisoning by, adverse effect of and underdosing of antithrombotic drugs
Poisoning by, adverse effect of and underdosing of antiplatelet drugs
EXCLUDES 2 *poisoning by, adverse effect of and underdosing of aspirin (T39.01-)*
poisoning by, adverse effect of and underdosing of acetylsalicylic acid (T39.01-)
T45.521 Poisoning by antithrombotic drugs, accidental (unintentional)
Poisoning by antithrombotic drug NOS
T45.522 Poisoning by antithrombotic drugs, intentional self-harm
T45.523 Poisoning by antithrombotic drugs, assault
T45.524 Poisoning by antithrombotic drugs, undetermined
T45.525 Adverse effect of antithrombotic drugs
T45.526 Underdosing of antithrombotic drugs

T45.6 Poisoning by, adverse effect of and underdosing of fibrinolysis-affecting drugs
T45.60 Poisoning by, adverse effect of and underdosing of unspecified fibrinolysis-affecting drugs
T45.601 Poisoning by unspecified fibrinolysis-affecting drugs, accidental (unintentional)
Poisoning by fibrinolysis-affecting drug NOS
T45.602 Poisoning by unspecified fibrinolysis-affecting drugs, intentional self-harm
T45.603 Poisoning by unspecified fibrinolysis-affecting drugs, assault
T45.604 Poisoning by unspecified fibrinolysis-affecting drugs, undetermined
T45.605 Adverse effect of unspecified fibrinolysis-affecting drugs
T45.606 Underdosing of unspecified fibrinolysis-affecting drugs
T45.61 Poisoning by, adverse effect of and underdosing of thrombolytic drugs
T45.611 Poisoning by thrombolytic drug, accidental (unintentional)
Poisoning by thrombolytic drug NOS
T45.612 Poisoning by thrombolytic drug, intentional self-harm
T45.613 Poisoning by thrombolytic drug, assault
T45.614 Poisoning by thrombolytic drug, undetermined
T45.615 Adverse effect of thrombolytic drugs
T45.616 Underdosing of thrombolytic drugs
T45.62 Poisoning by, adverse effect of and underdosing of hemostatic drugs
T45.621 Poisoning by hemostatic drug, accidental (unintentional)
Poisoning by hemostatic drug NOS
T45.622 Poisoning by hemostatic drug, intentional self-harm
T45.623 Poisoning by hemostatic drug, assault
T45.624 Poisoning by hemostatic drug, undetermined
T45.625 Adverse effect of hemostatic drug
T45.626 Underdosing of hemostatic drugs
T45.69 Poisoning by, adverse effect of and underdosing of other fibrinolysis-affecting drugs
T45.691 Poisoning by other fibrinolysis-affecting drugs, accidental (unintentional)
Poisoning by other fibrinolysis-affecting drug NOS
T45.692 Poisoning by other fibrinolysis-affecting drugs, intentional self-harm
T45.693 Poisoning by other fibrinolysis-affecting drugs, assault
T45.694 Poisoning by other fibrinolysis-affecting drugs, undetermined
T45.695 Adverse effect of other fibrinolysis-affecting drugs
T45.696 Underdosing of other fibrinolysis-affecting drugs

T45.7 Poisoning by, adverse effect of and underdosing of anticoagulant antagonists, vitamin K and other coagulants
T45.7X Poisoning by, adverse effect of and underdosing of anticoagulant antagonists, vitamin K and other coagulants
T45.7X1 Poisoning by anticoagulant antagonists, vitamin K and other coagulants, accidental (unintentional)
Poisoning by anticoagulant antagonists, vitamin K and other coagulants NOS
T45.7X2 Poisoning by anticoagulant antagonists, vitamin K and other coagulants, intentional self-harm
T45.7X3 Poisoning by anticoagulant antagonists, vitamin K and other coagulants, assault
T45.7X4 Poisoning by anticoagulant antagonists, vitamin K and other coagulants, undetermined
T45.7X5 Adverse effect of anticoagulant antagonists, vitamin K and other coagulants
T45.7X6 Underdosing of anticoagulant antagonist, vitamin K and other coagulants
EXCLUDES 1 *vitamin K deficiency (E56.1)*

T45.8 Poisoning by, adverse effect of and underdosing of other primarily systemic and hematological agents
Poisoning by, adverse effect of and underdosing of liver preparations and other antianemic agents
Poisoning by, adverse effect of and underdosing of natural blood and blood products
Poisoning by, adverse effect of and underdosing of plasma substitute
EXCLUDES 2 *poisoning by, adverse effect of and underdosing of immunoglobulin (T50.Z1)*
poisoning by, adverse effect of and underdosing of iron (T45.4)
transfusion reactions (T80.-)
T45.8X Poisoning by, adverse effect of and underdosing of other primarily systemic and hematological agents
T45.8X1 Poisoning by other primarily systemic and hematological agents, accidental (unintentional)
Poisoning by other primarily systemic and hematological agents NOS
T45.8X2 Poisoning by other primarily systemic and hematological agents, intentional self-harm
T45.8X3 Poisoning by other primarily systemic and hematological agents, assault
T45.8X4 Poisoning by other primarily systemic and hematological agents, undetermined

√7th T45.8X5 Adverse effect of other primarily systemic and hematological agents

√7th T45.8X6 Underdosing of other primarily systemic and hematological agents

√5th T45.9 Poisoning by, adverse effect of and underdosing of unspecified primarily systemic and hematological agent

√x7th T45.91 Poisoning by unspecified primarily systemic and hematological agent, accidental (unintentional)
Poisoning by primarily systemic and hematological agent NOS

√x7th T45.92 Poisoning by unspecified primarily systemic and hematological agent, intentional self-harm

√x7th T45.93 Poisoning by unspecified primarily systemic and hematological agent, assault

√x7th T45.94 Poisoning by unspecified primarily systemic and hematological agent, undetermined

√x7th T45.95 Adverse effect of unspecified primarily systemic and hematological agent

√x7th T45.96 Underdosing of unspecified primarily systemic and hematological agent

√4th T46 Poisoning by, adverse effect of and underdosing of agents primarily affecting the cardiovascular system
EXCLUDES 1 *poisoning by, adverse effect of and underdosing of metaraminol (T44.4)*

The appropriate 7th character is to be added to each code from category T46.
A initial encounter
D subsequent encounter
S sequela

√5th T46.Ø Poisoning by, adverse effect of and underdosing of cardiac-stimulant glycosides and drugs of similar action

√6th T46.ØX Poisoning by, adverse effect of and underdosing of cardiac-stimulant glycosides and drugs of similar action

√7th T46.ØX1 Poisoning by cardiac-stimulant glycosides and drugs of similar action, accidental (unintentional)
Poisoning by cardiac-stimulant glycosides and drugs of similar action NOS

√7th T46.ØX2 Poisoning by cardiac-stimulant glycosides and drugs of similar action, intentional self-harm

√7th T46.ØX3 Poisoning by cardiac-stimulant glycosides and drugs of similar action, assault

√7th T46.ØX4 Poisoning by cardiac-stimulant glycosides and drugs of similar action, undetermined

√7th T46.ØX5 Adverse effect of cardiac-stimulant glycosides and drugs of similar action

√7th T46.ØX6 Underdosing of cardiac-stimulant glycosides and drugs of similar action

T46.1 Poisoning by, adverse effect of and underdosing of calcium-channel blockers

√6th T46.1X Poisoning by, adverse effect of and underdosing of calcium-channel blockers

√7th T46.1X1 Poisoning by calcium-channel blockers, accidental (unintentional)
Poisoning by calcium-channel blockers NOS

√7th T46.1X2 Poisoning by calcium-channel blockers, intentional self-harm

√7th T46.1X3 Poisoning by calcium-channel blockers, assault

√7th T46.1X4 Poisoning by calcium-channel blockers, undetermined

√7th T46.1X5 Adverse effect of calcium-channel blockers

√7th T46.1X6 Underdosing of calcium-channel blockers

√5th T46.2 Poisoning by, adverse effect of and underdosing of other antidysrhythmic drugs, not elsewhere classified
EXCLUDES 1 *poisoning by, adverse effect of and underdosing of beta-adrenoreceptor antagonists (T44.7-)*

√6th T46.2X Poisoning by, adverse effect of and underdosing of other antidysrhythmic drugs

√7th T46.2X1 Poisoning by other antidysrhythmic drugs, accidental (unintentional)
Poisoning by other antidysrhythmic drugs NOS

√7th T46.2X2 Poisoning by other antidysrhythmic drugs, intentional self-harm

√7th T46.2X3 Poisoning by other antidysrhythmic drugs, assault

√7th T46.2X4 Poisoning by other antidysrhythmic drugs, undetermined

√7th T46.2X5 Adverse effect of other antidysrhythmic drugs

√7th T46.2X6 Underdosing of other antidysrhythmic drugs

√5th T46.3 Poisoning by, adverse effect of and underdosing of coronary vasodilators
Poisoning by, adverse effect of and underdosing of dipyridamole
EXCLUDES 1 *poisoning by, adverse effect of and underdosing of calcium-channel blockers (T46.1)*

√6th T46.3X Poisoning by, adverse effect of and underdosing of coronary vasodilators

√7th T46.3X1 Poisoning by coronary vasodilators, accidental (unintentional)
Poisoning by coronary vasodilators NOS

√7th T46.3X2 Poisoning by coronary vasodilators, intentional self-harm

√7th T46.3X3 Poisoning by coronary vasodilators, assault

√7th T46.3X4 Poisoning by coronary vasodilators, undetermined

√7th T46.3X5 Adverse effect of coronary vasodilators

√7th T46.3X6 Underdosing of coronary vasodilators

√5th T46.4 Poisoning by, adverse effect of and underdosing of angiotensin-converting-enzyme inhibitors

√6th T46.4X Poisoning by, adverse effect of and underdosing of angiotensin-converting-enzyme inhibitors

√7th T46.4X1 Poisoning by angiotensin-converting-enzyme inhibitors, accidental (unintentional)
Poisoning by angiotensin-converting-enzyme inhibitors NOS

√7th T46.4X2 Poisoning by angiotensin-converting-enzyme inhibitors, intentional self-harm

√7th T46.4X3 Poisoning by angiotensin-converting-enzyme inhibitors, assault

√7th T46.4X4 Poisoning by angiotensin-converting-enzyme inhibitors, undetermined

√7th T46.4X5 Adverse effect of angiotensin-converting-enzyme inhibitors

√7th T46.4X6 Underdosing of angiotensin-converting-enzyme inhibitors

√5th T46.5 Poisoning by, adverse effect of and underdosing of other antihypertensive drugs
EXCLUDES 2 *poisoning by, adverse effect of and underdosing of beta-adrenoreceptor antagonists (T44.7)*
poisoning by, adverse effect of and underdosing of calcium-channel blockers (T46.1)
poisoning by, adverse effect of and underdosing of diuretics (T5Ø.Ø-T5Ø.2)

√6th T46.5X Poisoning by, adverse effect of and underdosing of other antihypertensive drugs

√7th T46.5X1 Poisoning by other antihypertensive drugs, accidental (unintentional)
Poisoning by other antihypertensive drugs NOS

√7th T46.5X2 Poisoning by other antihypertensive drugs, intentional self-harm

√7th T46.5X3 Poisoning by other antihypertensive drugs, assault

√7th T46.5X4 Poisoning by other antihypertensive drugs, undetermined

√7th T46.5X5 Adverse effect of other antihypertensive drugs

√7th T46.5X6 Underdosing of other antihypertensive drugs

T46.6 Poisoning by, adverse effect of and underdosing of antihyperlipidemic and antiarteriosclerotic drugs

T46.6X Poisoning by, adverse effect of and underdosing of antihyperlipidemic and antiarteriosclerotic drugs

T46.6X1 Poisoning by antihyperlipidemic and antiarteriosclerotic drugs, accidental (unintentional)
Poisoning by antihyperlipidemic and antiarteriosclerotic drugs NOS

T46.6X2 Poisoning by antihyperlipidemic and antiarteriosclerotic drugs, intentional self-harm

T46.6X3 Poisoning by antihyperlipidemic and antiarteriosclerotic drugs, assault

T46.6X4 Poisoning by antihyperlipidemic and antiarteriosclerotic drugs, undetermined

T46.6X5 Adverse effect of antihyperlipidemic and antiarteriosclerotic drugs

T46.6X6 Underdosing of antihyperlipidemic and antiarteriosclerotic drugs

T46.7 Poisoning by, adverse effect of and underdosing of peripheral vasodilators
Poisoning by, adverse effect of and underdosing of nicotinic acid (derivatives)
EXCLUDES 1 *poisoning by, adverse effect of and underdosing of papaverine (T44.3)*

T46.7X Poisoning by, adverse effect of and underdosing of peripheral vasodilators

T46.7X1 Poisoning by peripheral vasodilators, accidental (unintentional)
Poisoning by peripheral vasodilators NOS

T46.7X2 Poisoning by peripheral vasodilators, intentional self-harm

T46.7X3 Poisoning by peripheral vasodilators, assault

T46.7X4 Poisoning by peripheral vasodilators, undetermined

T46.7X5 Adverse effect of peripheral vasodilators

T46.7X6 Underdosing of peripheral vasodilators

T46.8 Poisoning by, adverse effect of and underdosing of antivaricose drugs, including sclerosing agents

T46.8X Poisoning by, adverse effect of and underdosing of antivaricose drugs, including sclerosing agents

T46.8X1 Poisoning by antivaricose drugs, including sclerosing agents, accidental (unintentional)
Poisoning by antivaricose drugs, including sclerosing agents NOS

T46.8X2 Poisoning by antivaricose drugs, including sclerosing agents, intentional self-harm

T46.8X3 Poisoning by antivaricose drugs, including sclerosing agents, assault

T46.8X4 Poisoning by antivaricose drugs, including sclerosing agents, undetermined

T46.8X5 Adverse effect of antivaricose drugs, including sclerosing agents

T46.8X6 Underdosing of antivaricose drugs, including sclerosing agents

T46.9 Poisoning by, adverse effect of and underdosing of other and unspecified agents primarily affecting the cardiovascular system

T46.90 Poisoning by, adverse effect of and underdosing of unspecified agents primarily affecting the cardiovascular system

T46.901 Poisoning by unspecified agents primarily affecting the cardiovascular system, accidental (unintentional)

T46.902 Poisoning by unspecified agents primarily affecting the cardiovascular system, intentional self-harm

T46.903 Poisoning by unspecified agents primarily affecting the cardiovascular system, assault

T46.904 Poisoning by unspecified agents primarily affecting the cardiovascular system, undetermined

T46.905 Adverse effect of unspecified agents primarily affecting the cardiovascular system

T46.906 Underdosing of unspecified agents primarily affecting the cardiovascular system

T46.99 Poisoning by, adverse effect of and underdosing of other agents primarily affecting the cardiovascular system

T46.991 Poisoning by other agents primarily affecting the cardiovascular system, accidental (unintentional)

T46.992 Poisoning by other agents primarily affecting the cardiovascular system, intentional self-harm

T46.993 Poisoning by other agents primarily affecting the cardiovascular system, assault

T46.994 Poisoning by other agents primarily affecting the cardiovascular system, undetermined

T46.995 Adverse effect of other agents primarily affecting the cardiovascular system

T46.996 Underdosing of other agents primarily affecting the cardiovascular system

T47 Poisoning by, adverse effect of and underdosing of agents primarily affecting the gastrointestinal system

The appropriate 7th character is to be added to each code from category T47.
A initial encounter
D subsequent encounter
S sequela

T47.0 Poisoning by, adverse effect of and underdosing of histamine H2-receptor blockers

T47.0X Poisoning by, adverse effect of and underdosing of histamine H2-receptor blockers

T47.0X1 Poisoning by histamine H2-receptor blockers, accidental (unintentional)
Poisoning by histamine H2-receptor blockers NOS

T47.0X2 Poisoning by histamine H2-receptor blockers, intentional self-harm

T47.0X3 Poisoning by histamine H2-receptor blockers, assault

T47.0X4 Poisoning by histamine H2-receptor blockers, undetermined

T47.0X5 Adverse effect of histamine H2-receptor blockers

T47.0X6 Underdosing of histamine H2-receptor blockers

T47.1 Poisoning by, adverse effect of and underdosing of other antacids and anti-gastric-secretion drugs

T47.1X Poisoning by, adverse effect of and underdosing of other antacids and anti-gastric-secretion drugs

T47.1X1 Poisoning by other antacids and anti-gastric-secretion drugs, accidental (unintentional)
Poisoning by other antacids and anti-gastric-secretion drugs NOS

T47.1X2 Poisoning by other antacids and anti-gastric-secretion drugs, intentional self-harm

T47.1X3 Poisoning by other antacids and anti-gastric-secretion drugs, assault

T47.1X4 Poisoning by other antacids and anti-gastric-secretion drugs, undetermined

T47.1X5 Adverse effect of other antacids and anti-gastric-secretion drugs

T47.1X6 Underdosing of other antacids and anti-gastric-secretion drugs

T47.2 Poisoning by, adverse effect of and underdosing of stimulant laxatives

T47.2X Poisoning by, adverse effect of and underdosing of stimulant laxatives

T47.2X1 Poisoning by stimulant laxatives, accidental (unintentional)
Poisoning by stimulant laxatives NOS

√7th **T47.2X2 Poisoning by stimulant laxatives, intentional self-harm**
√7th **T47.2X3 Poisoning by stimulant laxatives, assault**
√7th **T47.2X4 Poisoning by stimulant laxatives, undetermined**
√7th **T47.2X5 Adverse effect of stimulant laxatives**
√7th **T47.2X6 Underdosing of stimulant laxatives**

√5th **T47.3 Poisoning by, adverse effect of and underdosing of saline and osmotic laxatives**

√6th **T47.3X Poisoning by and adverse effect of saline and osmotic laxatives**

√7th **T47.3X1 Poisoning by saline and osmotic laxatives, accidental (unintentional)**
Poisoning by saline and osmotic laxatives NOS
√7th **T47.3X2 Poisoning by saline and osmotic laxatives, intentional self-harm**
√7th **T47.3X3 Poisoning by saline and osmotic laxatives, assault**
√7th **T47.3X4 Poisoning by saline and osmotic laxatives, undetermined**
√7th **T47.3X5 Adverse effect of saline and osmotic laxatives**
√7th **T47.3X6 Underdosing of saline and osmotic laxatives**

√5th **T47.4 Poisoning by, adverse effect of and underdosing of other laxatives**

√6th **T47.4X Poisoning by, adverse effect of and underdosing of other laxatives**

√7th **T47.4X1 Poisoning by other laxatives, accidental (unintentional)**
Poisoning by other laxatives NOS
√7th **T47.4X2 Poisoning by other laxatives, intentional self-harm**
√7th **T47.4X3 Poisoning by other laxatives, assault**
√7th **T47.4X4 Poisoning by other laxatives, undetermined**
√7th **T47.4X5 Adverse effect of other laxatives**
√7th **T47.4X6 Underdosing of other laxatives**

√5th **T47.5 Poisoning by, adverse effect of and underdosing of digestants**

√6th **T47.5X Poisoning by, adverse effect of and underdosing of digestants**

√7th **T47.5X1 Poisoning by digestants, accidental (unintentional)**
Poisoning by digestants NOS
√7th **T47.5X2 Poisoning by digestants, intentional self-harm**
√7th **T47.5X3 Poisoning by digestants, assault**
√7th **T47.5X4 Poisoning by digestants, undetermined**
√7th **T47.5X5 Adverse effect of digestants**
√7th **T47.5X6 Underdosing of digestants**

√5th **T47.6 Poisoning by, adverse effect of and underdosing of antidiarrheal drugs**

EXCLUDES2 *poisoning by, adverse effect of and underdosing of systemic antibiotics and other anti-infectives (T36-T37)*

√6th **T47.6X Poisoning by, adverse effect of and underdosing of antidiarrheal drugs**

√7th **T47.6X1 Poisoning by antidiarrheal drugs, accidental (unintentional)**
Poisoning by antidiarrheal drugs NOS
√7th **T47.6X2 Poisoning by antidiarrheal drugs, intentional self-harm**
√7th **T47.6X3 Poisoning by antidiarrheal drugs, assault**
√7th **T47.6X4 Poisoning by antidiarrheal drugs, undetermined**
√7th **T47.6X5 Adverse effect of antidiarrheal drugs**
√7th **T47.6X6 Underdosing of antidiarrheal drugs**

√5th **T47.7 Poisoning by, adverse effect of and underdosing of emetics**

√6th **T47.7X Poisoning by, adverse effect of and underdosing of emetics**

√7th **T47.7X1 Poisoning by emetics, accidental (unintentional)**
Poisoning by emetics NOS
√7th **T47.7X2 Poisoning by emetics, intentional self-harm**
√7th **T47.7X3 Poisoning by emetics, assault**
√7th **T47.7X4 Poisoning by emetics, undetermined**
√7th **T47.7X5 Adverse effect of emetics**
√7th **T47.7X6 Underdosing of emetics**

√5th **T47.8 Poisoning by, adverse effect of and underdosing of other agents primarily affecting gastrointestinal system**

√6th **T47.8X Poisoning by, adverse effect of and underdosing of other agents primarily affecting gastrointestinal system**

√7th **T47.8X1 Poisoning by other agents primarily affecting gastrointestinal system, accidental (unintentional)**
Poisoning by other agents primarily affecting gastrointestinal system NOS
√7th **T47.8X2 Poisoning by other agents primarily affecting gastrointestinal system, intentional self-harm**
√7th **T47.8X3 Poisoning by other agents primarily affecting gastrointestinal system, assault**
√7th **T47.8X4 Poisoning by other agents primarily affecting gastrointestinal system, undetermined**
√7th **T47.8X5 Adverse effect of other agents primarily affecting gastrointestinal system**
√7th **T47.8X6 Underdosing of other agents primarily affecting gastrointestinal system**

√5th **T47.9 Poisoning by, adverse effect of and underdosing of unspecified agents primarily affecting the gastrointestinal system**

√x7th **T47.91 Poisoning by unspecified agents primarily affecting the gastrointestinal system, accidental (unintentional)**
Poisoning by agents primarily affecting the gastrointestinal system NOS
√x7th **T47.92 Poisoning by unspecified agents primarily affecting the gastrointestinal system, intentional self-harm**
√x7th **T47.93 Poisoning by unspecified agents primarily affecting the gastrointestinal system, assault**
√x7th **T47.94 Poisoning by unspecified agents primarily affecting the gastrointestinal system, undetermined**
√x7th **T47.95 Adverse effect of unspecified agents primarily affecting the gastrointestinal system**
√x7th **T47.96 Underdosing of unspecified agents primarily affecting the gastrointestinal system**

√4th **T48 Poisoning by, adverse effect of and underdosing of agents primarily acting on smooth and skeletal muscles and the respiratory system**

The appropriate 7th character is to be added to each code from category T48.
A initial encounter
D subsequent encounter
S sequela

√5th **T48.Ø Poisoning by, adverse effect of and underdosing of oxytocic drugs**

EXCLUDES1 *poisoning by, adverse effect of and underdosing of estrogens, progestogens and antagonists (T38.4-T38.6)*

√6th **T48.ØX Poisoning by, adverse effect of and underdosing of oxytocic drugs**

√7th **T48.ØX1 Poisoning by oxytocic drugs, accidental (unintentional)**
Poisoning by oxytocic drugs NOS
√7th **T48.ØX2 Poisoning by oxytocic drugs, intentional self-harm**
√7th **T48.ØX3 Poisoning by oxytocic drugs, assault**
√7th **T48.ØX4 Poisoning by oxytocic drugs, undetermined**
√7th **T48.ØX5 Adverse effect of oxytocic drugs**
√7th **T48.ØX6 Underdosing of oxytocic drugs**

T48.1 Poisoning by, adverse effect of and underdosing of skeletal muscle relaxants [neuromuscular blocking agents]

T48.1X Poisoning by, adverse effect of and underdosing of skeletal muscle relaxants [neuromuscular blocking agents]

T48.1X1 Poisoning by skeletal muscle relaxants [neuromuscular blocking agents], accidental (unintentional)
Poisoning by skeletal muscle relaxants [neuromuscular blocking agents] NOS

T48.1X2 Poisoning by skeletal muscle relaxants [neuromuscular blocking agents], intentional self-harm

T48.1X3 Poisoning by skeletal muscle relaxants [neuromuscular blocking agents], assault

T48.1X4 Poisoning by skeletal muscle relaxants [neuromuscular blocking agents], undetermined

T48.1X5 Adverse effect of skeletal muscle relaxants [neuromuscular blocking agents]

T48.1X6 Underdosing of skeletal muscle relaxants [neuromuscular blocking agents]

T48.2 Poisoning by, adverse effect of and underdosing of other and unspecified drugs acting on muscles

T48.20 Poisoning by, adverse effect of and underdosing of unspecified drugs acting on muscles

T48.201 Poisoning by unspecified drugs acting on muscles, accidental (unintentional)
Poisoning by unspecified drugs acting on muscles NOS

T48.202 Poisoning by unspecified drugs acting on muscles, intentional self-harm

T48.203 Poisoning by unspecified drugs acting on muscles, assault

T48.204 Poisoning by unspecified drugs acting on muscles, undetermined

T48.205 Adverse effect of unspecified drugs acting on muscles

T48.206 Underdosing of unspecified drugs acting on muscles

T48.29 Poisoning by, adverse effect of and underdosing of other drugs acting on muscles

T48.291 Poisoning by other drugs acting on muscles, accidental (unintentional)
Poisoning by other drugs acting on muscles NOS

T48.292 Poisoning by other drugs acting on muscles, intentional self-harm

T48.293 Poisoning by other drugs acting on muscles, assault

T48.294 Poisoning by other drugs acting on muscles, undetermined

T48.295 Adverse effect of other drugs acting on muscles

T48.296 Underdosing of other drugs acting on muscles

T48.3 Poisoning by, adverse effect of and underdosing of antitussives

T48.3X Poisoning by, adverse effect of and underdosing of antitussives

T48.3X1 Poisoning by antitussives, accidental (unintentional)
Poisoning by antitussives NOS

T48.3X2 Poisoning by antitussives, intentional self-harm

T48.3X3 Poisoning by antitussives, assault

T48.3X4 Poisoning by antitussives, undetermined

T48.3X5 Adverse effect of antitussives

T48.3X6 Underdosing of antitussives

T48.4 Poisoning by, adverse effect of and underdosing of expectorants

T48.4X Poisoning by, adverse effect of and underdosing of expectorants

T48.4X1 Poisoning by expectorants, accidental (unintentional)
Poisoning by expectorants NOS

T48.4X2 Poisoning by expectorants, intentional self-harm

T48.4X3 Poisoning by expectorants, assault

T48.4X4 Poisoning by expectorants, undetermined

T48.4X5 Adverse effect of expectorants

T48.4X6 Underdosing of expectorants

T48.5 Poisoning by, adverse effect of and underdosing of other anti-common-cold drugs
Poisoning by, adverse effect of and underdosing of decongestants
EXCLUDES 2 *poisoning by, adverse effect of and underdosing of antipyretics, NEC (T39.9-)*
poisoning by, adverse effect of and underdosing of non-steroidal antiinflammatory drugs (T39.3-)
poisoning by, adverse effect of and underdosing of salicylates (T39.0-)

T48.5X Poisoning by, adverse effect of and underdosing of other anti-common-cold drugs

T48.5X1 Poisoning by other anti-common-cold drugs, accidental (unintentional)
Poisoning by other anti-common-cold drugs NOS

T48.5X2 Poisoning by other anti-common-cold drugs, intentional self-harm

T48.5X3 Poisoning by other anti-common-cold drugs, assault

T48.5X4 Poisoning by other anti-common-cold drugs, undetermined

T48.5X5 Adverse effect of other anti-common-cold drugs

T48.5X6 Underdosing of other anti-common-cold drugs

T48.6 Poisoning by, adverse effect of and underdosing of antiasthmatics, not elsewhere classified
Poisoning by, adverse effect of and underdosing of beta-adrenoreceptor agonists used in asthma therapy
EXCLUDES 1 *poisoning by, adverse effect of and underdosing of anterior pituitary [adenohypophyseal] hormones (T38.8)*
poisoning by, adverse effect of and underdosing of beta-adrenoreceptor agonists not used in asthma therapy (T44.5)

T48.6X Poisoning by, adverse effect of and underdosing of antiasthmatics

T48.6X1 Poisoning by antiasthmatics, accidental (unintentional)
Poisoning by antiasthmatics NOS

T48.6X2 Poisoning by antiasthmatics, intentional self-harm

T48.6X3 Poisoning by antiasthmatics, assault

T48.6X4 Poisoning by antiasthmatics, undetermined

T48.6X5 Adverse effect of antiasthmatics

T48.6X6 Underdosing of antiasthmatics

T48.9 Poisoning by, adverse effect of and underdosing of other and unspecified agents primarily acting on the respiratory system

T48.90 Poisoning by, adverse effect of and underdosing of unspecified agents primarily acting on the respiratory system

T48.901 Poisoning by unspecified agents primarily acting on the respiratory system, accidental (unintentional)

T48.902 Poisoning by unspecified agents primarily acting on the respiratory system, intentional self-harm

T48.903 Poisoning by unspecified agents primarily acting on the respiratory system, assault

T48.904 Poisoning by unspecified agents primarily acting on the respiratory system, undetermined

T48.905 Adverse effect of unspecified agents primarily acting on the respiratory system

T48.906 Underdosing of unspecified agents primarily acting on the respiratory system

T48.99 Poisoning by, adverse effect of and underdosing of other agents primarily acting on the respiratory system

T48.991 Poisoning by other agents primarily acting on the respiratory system, accidental (unintentional)

T48.992 Poisoning by other agents primarily acting on the respiratory system, intentional self-harm

T48.993 Poisoning by other agents primarily acting on the respiratory system, assault

T48.994 Poisoning by other agents primarily acting on the respiratory system, undetermined

T48.995 Adverse effect of other agents primarily acting on the respiratory system

T48.996 Underdosing of other agents primarily acting on the respiratory system

T49 Poisoning by, adverse effect of and underdosing of topical agents primarily affecting skin and mucous membrane and by ophthalmological, otorhinolaryngological and dental drugs

Poisoning by, adverse effect of and underdosing of glucocorticoids, topically used

The appropriate 7th character is to be added to each code from category T49.
A initial encounter
D subsequent encounter
S sequela

T49.0 Poisoning by, adverse effect of and underdosing of local antifungal, anti-infective and anti-inflammatory drugs

T49.0X Poisoning by, adverse effect of and underdosing of local antifungal, anti-infective and anti-inflammatory drugs

T49.0X1 Poisoning by local antifungal, anti-infective and anti-inflammatory drugs, accidental (unintentional)
Poisoning by local antifungal, anti-infective and anti-inflammatory drugs NOS

T49.0X2 Poisoning by local antifungal, anti-infective and anti-inflammatory drugs, intentional self-harm

T49.0X3 Poisoning by local antifungal, anti-infective and anti-inflammatory drugs, assault

T49.0X4 Poisoning by local antifungal, anti-infective and anti-inflammatory drugs, undetermined

T49.0X5 Adverse effect of local antifungal, anti-infective and anti-inflammatory drugs

T49.0X6 Underdosing of local antifungal, anti-infective and anti-inflammatory drugs

T49.1 Poisoning by, adverse effect of and underdosing of antipruritics

T49.1X Poisoning by, adverse effect of and underdosing of antipruritics

T49.1X1 Poisoning by antipruritics, accidental (unintentional)
Poisoning by antipruritics NOS

T49.1X2 Poisoning by antipruritics, intentional self-harm

T49.1X3 Poisoning by antipruritics, assault

T49.1X4 Poisoning by antipruritics, undetermined

T49.1X5 Adverse effect of antipruritics

T49.1X6 Underdosing of antipruritics

T49.2 Poisoning by, adverse effect of and underdosing of local astringents and local detergents

T49.2X Poisoning by, adverse effect of and underdosing of local astringents and local detergents

T49.2X1 Poisoning by local astringents and local detergents, accidental (unintentional)
Poisoning by local astringents and local detergents NOS

T49.2X2 Poisoning by local astringents and local detergents, intentional self-harm

T49.2X3 Poisoning by local astringents and local detergents, assault

T49.2X4 Poisoning by local astringents and local detergents, undetermined

T49.2X5 Adverse effect of local astringents and local detergents

T49.2X6 Underdosing of local astringents and local detergents

T49.3 Poisoning by, adverse effect of and underdosing of emollients, demulcents and protectants

T49.3X Poisoning by, adverse effect of and underdosing of emollients, demulcents and protectants

T49.3X1 Poisoning by emollients, demulcents and protectants, accidental (unintentional)
Poisoning by emollients, demulcents and protectants NOS

T49.3X2 Poisoning by emollients, demulcents and protectants, intentional self-harm

T49.3X3 Poisoning by emollients, demulcents and protectants, assault

T49.3X4 Poisoning by emollients, demulcents and protectants, undetermined

T49.3X5 Adverse effect of emollients, demulcents and protectants

T49.3X6 Underdosing of emollients, demulcents and protectants

T49.4 Poisoning by, adverse effect of and underdosing of keratolytics, keratoplastics, and other hair treatment drugs and preparations

T49.4X Poisoning by, adverse effect of and underdosing of keratolytics, keratoplastics, and other hair treatment drugs and preparations

T49.4X1 Poisoning by keratolytics, keratoplastics, and other hair treatment drugs and preparations, accidental (unintentional)
Poisoning by keratolytics, keratoplastics, and other hair treatment drugs and preparations NOS

T49.4X2 Poisoning by keratolytics, keratoplastics, and other hair treatment drugs and preparations, intentional self-harm

T49.4X3 Poisoning by keratolytics, keratoplastics, and other hair treatment drugs and preparations, assault

T49.4X4 Poisoning by keratolytics, keratoplastics, and other hair treatment drugs and preparations, undetermined

T49.4X5 Adverse effect of keratolytics, keratoplastics, and other hair treatment drugs and preparations

T49.4X6 Underdosing of keratolytics, keratoplastics, and other hair treatment drugs and preparations

T49.5 Poisoning by, adverse effect of and underdosing of ophthalmological drugs and preparations

T49.5X Poisoning by, adverse effect of and underdosing of ophthalmological drugs and preparations

T49.5X1 Poisoning by ophthalmological drugs and preparations, accidental (unintentional)
Poisoning by ophthalmological drugs and preparations NOS

T49.5X2 Poisoning by ophthalmological drugs and preparations, intentional self-harm

T49.5X3 Poisoning by ophthalmological drugs and preparations, assault

T49.5X4 Poisoning by ophthalmological drugs and preparations, undetermined

T49.5X5 Adverse effect of ophthalmological drugs and preparations

T49.5X6 Underdosing of ophthalmological drugs and preparations

T49.6 Poisoning by, adverse effect of and underdosing of otorhinolaryngological drugs and preparations

T49.6X Poisoning by, adverse effect of and underdosing of otorhinolaryngological drugs and preparations

T49.6X1 Poisoning by otorhinolaryngological drugs and preparations, accidental (unintentional)
Poisoning by otorhinolaryngological drugs and preparations NOS

T49.6X2 Poisoning by otorhinolaryngological drugs and preparations, intentional self-harm

T49.6X3 Poisoning by otorhinolaryngological drugs and preparations, assault

T49.6X4 Poisoning by otorhinolaryngological drugs and preparations, undetermined

T49.6X5 Adverse effect of otorhinolaryngological drugs and preparations

T49.6X6 Underdosing of otorhinolaryngological drugs and preparations

T49.7 Poisoning by, adverse effect of and underdosing of dental drugs, topically applied

T49.7X Poisoning by, adverse effect of and underdosing of dental drugs, topically applied

T49.7X1 Poisoning by dental drugs, topically applied, accidental (unintentional)
Poisoning by dental drugs, topically applied NOS

T49.7X2 Poisoning by dental drugs, topically applied, intentional self-harm

T49.7X3 Poisoning by dental drugs, topically applied, assault

T49.7X4 Poisoning by dental drugs, topically applied, undetermined

T49.7X5 Adverse effect of dental drugs, topically applied

T49.7X6 Underdosing of dental drugs, topically applied

T49.8 Poisoning by, adverse effect of and underdosing of other topical agents
Poisoning by, adverse effect of and underdosing of spermicides

T49.8X Poisoning by, adverse effect of and underdosing of other topical agents

T49.8X1 Poisoning by other topical agents, accidental (unintentional)
Poisoning by other topical agents NOS

T49.8X2 Poisoning by other topical agents, intentional self-harm

T49.8X3 Poisoning by other topical agents, assault

T49.8X4 Poisoning by other topical agents, undetermined

T49.8X5 Adverse effect of other topical agents

T49.8X6 Underdosing of other topical agents

T49.9 Poisoning by, adverse effect of and underdosing of unspecified topical agent

T49.91 Poisoning by unspecified topical agent, accidental (unintentional)

T49.92 Poisoning by unspecified topical agent, intentional self-harm

T49.93 Poisoning by unspecified topical agent, assault

T49.94 Poisoning by unspecified topical agent, undetermined

T49.95 Adverse effect of unspecified topical agent

T49.96 Underdosing of unspecified topical agent

T50 Poisoning by, adverse effect of and underdosing of diuretics and other and unspecified drugs, medicaments and biological substances

The appropriate 7th character is to be added to each code from category T50.
A initial encounter
D subsequent encounter
S sequela

T50.0 Poisoning by, adverse effect of and underdosing of mineralocorticoids and their antagonists

T50.0X Poisoning by, adverse effect of and underdosing of mineralocorticoids and their antagonists

T50.0X1 Poisoning by mineralocorticoids and their antagonists, accidental (unintentional)
Poisoning by mineralocorticoids and their antagonists NOS

T50.0X2 Poisoning by mineralocorticoids and their antagonists, intentional self-harm

T50.0X3 Poisoning by mineralocorticoids and their antagonists, assault

T50.0X4 Poisoning by mineralocorticoids and their antagonists, undetermined

T50.0X5 Adverse effect of mineralocorticoids and their antagonists

T50.0X6 Underdosing of mineralocorticoids and their antagonists

T50.1 Poisoning by, adverse effect of and underdosing of loop [high-ceiling] diuretics

T50.1X Poisoning by, adverse effect of and underdosing of loop [high-ceiling] diuretics

T50.1X1 Poisoning by loop [high-ceiling] diuretics, accidental (unintentional)
Poisoning by loop [high-ceiling] diuretics NOS

T50.1X2 Poisoning by loop [high-ceiling] diuretics, intentional self-harm

T50.1X3 Poisoning by loop [high-ceiling] diuretics, assault

T50.1X4 Poisoning by loop [high-ceiling] diuretics, undetermined

T50.1X5 Adverse effect of loop [high-ceiling] diuretics

T50.1X6 Underdosing of loop [high-ceiling] diuretics

T50.2 Poisoning by, adverse effect of and underdosing of carbonic-anhydrase inhibitors, benzothiadiazides and other diuretics
Poisoning by, adverse effect of and underdosing of acetazolamide

T50.2X Poisoning by, adverse effect of and underdosing of carbonic-anhydrase inhibitors, benzothiadiazides and other diuretics

T50.2X1 Poisoning by carbonic-anhydrase inhibitors, benzothiadiazides and other diuretics, accidental (unintentional)
Poisoning by carbonic-anhydrase inhibitors, benzothiadiazides and other diuretics NOS

T50.2X2 Poisoning by carbonic-anhydrase inhibitors, benzothiadiazides and other diuretics, intentional self-harm

T50.2X3 Poisoning by carbonic-anhydrase inhibitors, benzothiadiazides and other diuretics, assault

T50.2X4 Poisoning by carbonic-anhydrase inhibitors, benzothiadiazides and other diuretics, undetermined

T50.2X5 Adverse effect of carbonic-anhydrase inhibitors, benzothiadiazides and other diuretics

T50.2X6 Underdosing of carbonic-anhydrase inhibitors, benzothiadiazides and other diuretics

T50.3 Poisoning by, adverse effect of and underdosing of electrolytic, caloric and water-balance agents
Poisoning by, adverse effect of and underdosing of oral rehydration salts

T50.3X Poisoning by, adverse effect of and underdosing of electrolytic, caloric and water-balance agents

T50.3X1 Poisoning by electrolytic, caloric and water-balance agents, accidental (unintentional)
Poisoning by electrolytic, caloric and water-balance agents NOS

T50.3X2 Poisoning by electrolytic, caloric and water-balance agents, intentional self-harm

T50.3X3 Poisoning by electrolytic, caloric and water-balance agents, assault

T50.3X4 Poisoning by electrolytic, caloric and water-balance agents, undetermined

T50.3X5 Adverse effect of electrolytic, caloric and water-balance agents

T50.3X6 Underdosing of electrolytic, caloric and water-balance agents

5th **T50.4 Poisoning by, adverse effect of and underdosing of drugs affecting uric acid metabolism**
6th **T50.4X Poisoning by, adverse effect of and underdosing of drugs affecting uric acid metabolism**
7th **T50.4X1 Poisoning by drugs affecting uric acid metabolism, accidental (unintentional)**
Poisoning by drugs affecting uric acid metabolism NOS
7th **T50.4X2 Poisoning by drugs affecting uric acid metabolism, intentional self-harm**
7th **T50.4X3 Poisoning by drugs affecting uric acid metabolism, assault**
7th **T50.4X4 Poisoning by drugs affecting uric acid metabolism, undetermined**
7th **T50.4X5 Adverse effect of drugs affecting uric acid metabolism**
7th **T50.4X6 Underdosing of drugs affecting uric acid metabolism**

5th **T50.5 Poisoning by, adverse effect of and underdosing of appetite depressants**
6th **T50.5X Poisoning by, adverse effect of and underdosing of appetite depressants**
7th **T50.5X1 Poisoning by appetite depressants, accidental (unintentional)**
Poisoning by appetite depressants NOS
7th **T50.5X2 Poisoning by appetite depressants, intentional self-harm**
7th **T50.5X3 Poisoning by appetite depressants, assault**
7th **T50.5X4 Poisoning by appetite depressants, undetermined**
7th **T50.5X5 Adverse effect of appetite depressants**
7th **T50.5X6 Underdosing of appetite depressants**

5th **T50.6 Poisoning by, adverse effect of and underdosing of antidotes and chelating agents**
Poisoning by, adverse effect of and underdosing of alcohol deterrents
6th **T50.6X Poisoning by, adverse effect of and underdosing of antidotes and chelating agents**
7th **T50.6X1 Poisoning by antidotes and chelating agents, accidental (unintentional)**
Poisoning by antidotes and chelating agents NOS
7th **T50.6X2 Poisoning by antidotes and chelating agents, intentional self-harm**
7th **T50.6X3 Poisoning by antidotes and chelating agents, assault**
7th **T50.6X4 Poisoning by antidotes and chelating agents, undetermined**
7th **T50.6X5 Adverse effect of antidotes and chelating agents**
7th **T50.6X6 Underdosing of antidotes and chelating agents**

5th **T50.7 Poisoning by, adverse effect of and underdosing of analeptics and opioid receptor antagonists**
6th **T50.7X Poisoning by, adverse effect of and underdosing of analeptics and opioid receptor antagonists**
7th **T50.7X1 Poisoning by analeptics and opioid receptor antagonists, accidental (unintentional)**
Poisoning by analeptics and opioid receptor antagonists NOS
7th **T50.7X2 Poisoning by analeptics and opioid receptor antagonists, intentional self-harm**
7th **T50.7X3 Poisoning by analeptics and opioid receptor antagonists, assault**
7th **T50.7X4 Poisoning by analeptics and opioid receptor antagonists, undetermined**
7th **T50.7X5 Adverse effect of analeptics and opioid receptor antagonists**
7th **T50.7X6 Underdosing of analeptics and opioid receptor antagonists**

5th **T50.8 Poisoning by, adverse effect of and underdosing of diagnostic agents**
6th **T50.8X Poisoning by, adverse effect of and underdosing of diagnostic agents**
7th **T50.8X1 Poisoning by diagnostic agents, accidental (unintentional)**
Poisoning by diagnostic agents NOS
7th **T50.8X2 Poisoning by diagnostic agents, intentional self-harm**
7th **T50.8X3 Poisoning by diagnostic agents, assault**
7th **T50.8X4 Poisoning by diagnostic agents, undetermined**
7th **T50.8X5 Adverse effect of diagnostic agents**
7th **T50.8X6 Underdosing of diagnostic agents**

5th **T50.A Poisoning by, adverse effect of and underdosing of bacterial vaccines**
6th **T50.A1 Poisoning by, adverse effect of and underdosing of pertussis vaccine, including combinations with a pertussis component**
7th **T50.A11 Poisoning by pertussis vaccine, including combinations with a pertussis component, accidental (unintentional)**
7th **T50.A12 Poisoning by pertussis vaccine, including combinations with a pertussis component, intentional self-harm**
7th **T50.A13 Poisoning by pertussis vaccine, including combinations with a pertussis component, assault**
7th **T50.A14 Poisoning by pertussis vaccine, including combinations with a pertussis component, undetermined**
7th **T50.A15 Adverse effect of pertussis vaccine, including combinations with a pertussis component**
7th **T50.A16 Underdosing of pertussis vaccine, including combinations with a pertussis component**
6th **T50.A2 Poisoning by, adverse effect of and underdosing of mixed bacterial vaccines without a pertussis component**
7th **T50.A21 Poisoning by mixed bacterial vaccines without a pertussis component, accidental (unintentional)**
7th **T50.A22 Poisoning by mixed bacterial vaccines without a pertussis component, intentional self-harm**
7th **T50.A23 Poisoning by mixed bacterial vaccines without a pertussis component, assault**
7th **T50.A24 Poisoning by mixed bacterial vaccines without a pertussis component, undetermined**
7th **T50.A25 Adverse effect of mixed bacterial vaccines without a pertussis component**
7th **T50.A26 Underdosing of mixed bacterial vaccines without a pertussis component**
6th **T50.A9 Poisoning by, adverse effect of and underdosing of other bacterial vaccines**
7th **T50.A91 Poisoning by other bacterial vaccines, accidental (unintentional)**
7th **T50.A92 Poisoning by other bacterial vaccines, intentional self-harm**
7th **T50.A93 Poisoning by other bacterial vaccines, assault**
7th **T50.A94 Poisoning by other bacterial vaccines, undetermined**
7th **T50.A95 Adverse effect of other bacterial vaccines**
7th **T50.A96 Underdosing of other bacterial vaccines**

5th **T50.B Poisoning by, adverse effect of and underdosing of viral vaccines**
6th **T50.B1 Poisoning by, adverse effect of and underdosing of smallpox vaccines**
7th **T50.B11 Poisoning by smallpox vaccines, accidental (unintentional)**
7th **T50.B12 Poisoning by smallpox vaccines, intentional self-harm**
7th **T50.B13 Poisoning by smallpox vaccines, assault**

T50.B14 Poisoning by smallpox vaccines, undetermined
T50.B15 Adverse effect of smallpox vaccines
T50.B16 Underdosing of smallpox vaccines
T50.B9 Poisoning by, adverse effect of and underdosing of other viral vaccines
T50.B91 Poisoning by other viral vaccines, accidental (unintentional)
T50.B92 Poisoning by other viral vaccines, intentional self-harm
T50.B93 Poisoning by other viral vaccines, assault
T50.B94 Poisoning by other viral vaccines, undetermined
T50.B95 Adverse effect of other viral vaccines
T50.B96 Underdosing of other viral vaccines
T50.Z Poisoning by, adverse effect of and underdosing of other vaccines and biological substances
T50.Z1 Poisoning by, adverse effect of and underdosing of immunoglobulin
T50.Z11 Poisoning by immunoglobulin, accidental (unintentional)
T50.Z12 Poisoning by immunoglobulin, intentional self-harm
T50.Z13 Poisoning by immunoglobulin, assault
T50.Z14 Poisoning by immunoglobulin, undetermined
T50.Z15 Adverse effect of immunoglobulin
T50.Z16 Underdosing of immunoglobulin
T50.Z9 Poisoning by, adverse effect of and underdosing of other vaccines and biological substances
T50.Z91 Poisoning by other vaccines and biological substances, accidental (unintentional)
T50.Z92 Poisoning by other vaccines and biological substances, intentional self-harm
T50.Z93 Poisoning by other vaccines and biological substances, assault
T50.Z94 Poisoning by other vaccines and biological substances, undetermined
T50.Z95 Adverse effect of other vaccines and biological substances
T50.Z96 Underdosing of other vaccines and biological substances
T50.9 Poisoning by, adverse effect of and underdosing of other and unspecified drugs, medicaments and biological substances
T50.90 Poisoning by, adverse effect of and underdosing of unspecified drugs, medicaments and biological substances
T50.901 Poisoning by unspecified drugs, medicaments and biological substances, accidental (unintentional)
T50.902 Poisoning by unspecified drugs, medicaments and biological substances, intentional self-harm
T50.903 Poisoning by unspecified drugs, medicaments and biological substances, assault
T50.904 Poisoning by unspecified drugs, medicaments and biological substances, undetermined
T50.905 Adverse effect of unspecified drugs, medicaments and biological substances
T50.906 Underdosing of unspecified drugs, medicaments and biological substances
T50.99 Poisoning by, adverse effect of and underdosing of other drugs, medicaments and biological substances
T50.991 Poisoning by other drugs, medicaments and biological substances, accidental (unintentional)
T50.992 Poisoning by other drugs, medicaments and biological substances, intentional self-harm
T50.993 Poisoning by other drugs, medicaments and biological substances, assault
T50.994 Poisoning by other drugs, medicaments and biological substances, undetermined
T50.995 Adverse effect of other drugs, medicaments and biological substances
T50.996 Underdosing of other drugs, medicaments and biological substances

Toxic effects of substances chiefly nonmedicinal as to source (T51-T65)

NOTE When no intent is indicated code to accidental. Undetermined intent is only for use when there is specific documentation in the record that the intent of the toxic effect cannot be determined.

Use additional code(s) for all associated manifestations of toxic effect, such as:
personal history of foreign body fully removed (Z87.821)
respiratory conditions due to external agents (J60-J70)
to identify any retained foreign body, if applicable (Z18.-)

EXCLUDES 1 *contact with and (suspected) exposure to toxic substances (Z77.-)*

T51 Toxic effect of alcohol

The appropriate 7th character is to be added to each code from category T51.
A initial encounter
D subsequent encounter
S sequela

T51.0 Toxic effect of ethanol
Toxic effect of ethyl alcohol
EXCLUDES 2 *acute alcohol intoxication or 'hangover' effects (F10.129, F10.229, F10.929)*
drunkenness (F10.129, F10.229, F10.929)
pathological alcohol intoxication (F10.129, F10.229, F10.929)
T51.0X Toxic effect of ethanol
T51.0X1 Toxic effect of ethanol, accidental (unintentional)
Toxic effect of ethanol NOS
T51.0X2 Toxic effect of ethanol, intentional self-harm
T51.0X3 Toxic effect of ethanol, assault
T51.0X4 Toxic effect of ethanol, undetermined
T51.1 Toxic effect of methanol
Toxic effect of methyl alcohol
T51.1X Toxic effect of methanol
T51.1X1 Toxic effect of methanol, accidental (unintentional)
Toxic effect of methanol NOS
T51.1X2 Toxic effect of methanol, intentional self-harm
T51.1X3 Toxic effect of methanol, assault
T51.1X4 Toxic effect of methanol, undetermined
T51.2 Toxic effect of 2-Propanol
Toxic effect of isopropyl alcohol
T51.2X Toxic effect of 2-Propanol
T51.2X1 Toxic effect of 2-Propanol, accidental (unintentional)
Toxic effect of 2-Propanol NOS
T51.2X2 Toxic effect of 2-Propanol, intentional self-harm
T51.2X3 Toxic effect of 2-Propanol, assault
T51.2X4 Toxic effect of 2-Propanol, undetermined
T51.3 Toxic effect of fusel oil
Toxic effect of amyl alcohol
Toxic effect of butyl [1-butanol] alcohol
Toxic effect of propyl [1-propanol] alcohol
T51.3X Toxic effect of fusel oil
T51.3X1 Toxic effect of fusel oil, accidental (unintentional)
Toxic effect of fusel oil NOS
T51.3X2 Toxic effect of fusel oil, intentional self-harm
T51.3X3 Toxic effect of fusel oil, assault
T51.3X4 Toxic effect of fusel oil, undetermined
T51.8 Toxic effect of other alcohols
T51.8X Toxic effect of other alcohols
T51.8X1 Toxic effect of other alcohols, accidental (unintentional)
Toxic effect of other alcohols NOS

T51.8X2 **Toxic effect of other alcohols, intentional self-harm**
T51.8X3 **Toxic effect of other alcohols, assault**
T51.8X4 **Toxic effect of other alcohols, undetermined**

T51.9 **Toxic effect of unspecified alcohol**
T51.91 **Toxic effect of unspecified alcohol, accidental (unintentional)**
T51.92 **Toxic effect of unspecified alcohol, intentional self-harm**
T51.93 **Toxic effect of unspecified alcohol, assault**
T51.94 **Toxic effect of unspecified alcohol, undetermined**

T52 **Toxic effect of organic solvents**
EXCLUDES 1 *halogen derivatives of aliphatic and aromatic hydrocarbons (T53.-)*

The appropriate 7th character is to be added to each code from category T52.
A initial encounter
D subsequent encounter
S sequela

T52.0 **Toxic effects of petroleum products**
Toxic effects of ether petroleum
Toxic effects of gasoline [petrol]
Toxic effects of kerosene [paraffin oil]
Toxic effects of naphtha petroleum
Toxic effects of paraffin wax
Toxic effects of spirit petroleum

T52.0X **Toxic effects of petroleum products**
T52.0X1 **Toxic effect of petroleum products, accidental (unintentional)**
Toxic effects of petroleum products NOS
T52.0X2 **Toxic effect of petroleum products, intentional self-harm**
T52.0X3 **Toxic effect of petroleum products, assault**
T52.0X4 **Toxic effect of petroleum products, undetermined**

T52.1 **Toxic effects of benzene**
EXCLUDES 1 *homologues of benzene (T52.2)*
nitroderivatives and aminoderivatives of benzene and its homologues (T65.3)

T52.1X **Toxic effects of benzene**
T52.1X1 **Toxic effect of benzene, accidental (unintentional)**
Toxic effects of benzene NOS
T52.1X2 **Toxic effect of benzene, intentional self-harm**
T52.1X3 **Toxic effect of benzene, assault**
T52.1X4 **Toxic effect of benzene, undetermined**

T52.2 **Toxic effects of homologues of benzene**
Toxic effects of toluene [methylbenzene]
Toxic effects of xylene [dimethylbenzene]

T52.2X **Toxic effects of homologues of benzene**
T52.2X1 **Toxic effect of homologues of benzene, accidental (unintentional)**
Toxic effects of homologues of benzene NOS
T52.2X2 **Toxic effect of homologues of benzene, intentional self-harm**
T52.2X3 **Toxic effect of homologues of benzene, assault**
T52.2X4 **Toxic effect of homologues of benzene, undetermined**

T52.3 **Toxic effects of glycols**
T52.3X **Toxic effects of glycols**
T52.3X1 **Toxic effect of glycols, accidental (unintentional)**
Toxic effects of glycols NOS
T52.3X2 **Toxic effect of glycols, intentional self-harm**
T52.3X3 **Toxic effect of glycols, assault**
T52.3X4 **Toxic effect of glycols, undetermined**

T52.4 **Toxic effects of ketones**
T52.4X **Toxic effects of ketones**
T52.4X1 **Toxic effect of ketones, accidental (unintentional)**
Toxic effects of ketones NOS
T52.4X2 **Toxic effect of ketones, intentional self-harm**
T52.4X3 **Toxic effect of ketones, assault**
T52.4X4 **Toxic effect of ketones, undetermined**

T52.8 **Toxic effects of other organic solvents**
T52.8X **Toxic effects of other organic solvents**
T52.8X1 **Toxic effect of other organic solvents, accidental (unintentional)**
Toxic effects of other organic solvents NOS
T52.8X2 **Toxic effect of other organic solvents, intentional self-harm**
T52.8X3 **Toxic effect of other organic solvents, assault**
T52.8X4 **Toxic effect of other organic solvents, undetermined**

T52.9 **Toxic effects of unspecified organic solvent**
T52.91 **Toxic effect of unspecified organic solvent, accidental (unintentional)**
T52.92 **Toxic effect of unspecified organic solvent, intentional self-harm**
T52.93 **Toxic effect of unspecified organic solvent, assault**
T52.94 **Toxic effect of unspecified organic solvent, undetermined**

T53 **Toxic effect of halogen derivatives of aliphatic and aromatic hydrocarbons**

The appropriate 7th character is to be added to each code from category T53.
A initial encounter
D subsequent encounter
S sequela

T53.0 **Toxic effects of carbon tetrachloride**
Toxic effects of tetrachloromethane

T53.0X **Toxic effects of carbon tetrachloride**
T53.0X1 **Toxic effect of carbon tetrachloride, accidental (unintentional)**
Toxic effects of carbon tetrachloride NOS
T53.0X2 **Toxic effect of carbon tetrachloride, intentional self-harm**
T53.0X3 **Toxic effect of carbon tetrachloride, assault**
T53.0X4 **Toxic effect of carbon tetrachloride, undetermined**

T53.1 **Toxic effects of chloroform**
Toxic effects of trichloromethane

T53.1X **Toxic effects of chloroform**
T53.1X1 **Toxic effect of chloroform, accidental (unintentional)**
Toxic effects of chloroform NOS
T53.1X2 **Toxic effect of chloroform, intentional self-harm**
T53.1X3 **Toxic effect of chloroform, assault**
T53.1X4 **Toxic effect of chloroform, undetermined**

T53.2 **Toxic effects of trichloroethylene**
Toxic effects of trichloroethene

T53.2X **Toxic effects of trichloroethylene**
T53.2X1 **Toxic effect of trichloroethylene, accidental (unintentional)**
Toxic effects of trichloroethylene NOS
T53.2X2 **Toxic effect of trichloroethylene, intentional self-harm**
T53.2X3 **Toxic effect of trichloroethylene, assault**
T53.2X4 **Toxic effect of trichloroethylene, undetermined**

✓5th **T53.3 Toxic effects of tetrachloroethylene**
Toxic effects of perchloroethylene
Toxic effect of tetrachloroethene

✓6th **T53.3X Toxic effects of tetrachloroethylene**

✓7th **T53.3X1 Toxic effect of tetrachloroethylene, accidental (unintentional)**
Toxic effects of tetrachloroethylene NOS

✓7th **T53.3X2 Toxic effect of tetrachloroethylene, intentional self-harm**

✓7th **T53.3X3 Toxic effect of tetrachloroethylene, assault**

✓7th **T53.3X4 Toxic effect of tetrachloroethylene, undetermined**

✓5th **T53.4 Toxic effects of dichloromethane**
Toxic effects of methylene chloride

✓6th **T53.4X Toxic effects of dichloromethane**

✓7th **T53.4X1 Toxic effect of dichloromethane, accidental (unintentional)**
Toxic effects of dichloromethane NOS

✓7th **T53.4X2 Toxic effect of dichloromethane, intentional self-harm**

✓7th **T53.4X3 Toxic effect of dichloromethane, assault**

✓7th **T53.4X4 Toxic effect of dichloromethane, undetermined**

✓5th **T53.5 Toxic effects of chlorofluorocarbons**

✓6th **T53.5X Toxic effects of chlorofluorocarbons**

✓7th **T53.5X1 Toxic effect of chlorofluorocarbons, accidental (unintentional)**
Toxic effects of chlorofluorocarbons NOS

✓7th **T53.5X2 Toxic effect of chlorofluorocarbons, intentional self-harm**

✓7th **T53.5X3 Toxic effect of chlorofluorocarbons, assault**

✓7th **T53.5X4 Toxic effect of chlorofluorocarbons, undetermined**

✓5th **T53.6 Toxic effects of other halogen derivatives of aliphatic hydrocarbons**

✓6th **T53.6X Toxic effects of other halogen derivatives of aliphatic hydrocarbons**

✓7th **T53.6X1 Toxic effect of other halogen derivatives of aliphatic hydrocarbons, accidental (unintentional)**
Toxic effects of other halogen derivatives of aliphatic hydrocarbons NOS

✓7th **T53.6X2 Toxic effect of other halogen derivatives of aliphatic hydrocarbons, intentional self-harm**

✓7th **T53.6X3 Toxic effect of other halogen derivatives of aliphatic hydrocarbons, assault**

✓7th **T53.6X4 Toxic effect of other halogen derivatives of aliphatic hydrocarbons, undetermined**

✓5th **T53.7 Toxic effects of other halogen derivatives of aromatic hydrocarbons**

✓6th **T53.7X Toxic effects of other halogen derivatives of aromatic hydrocarbons**

✓7th **T53.7X1 Toxic effect of other halogen derivatives of aromatic hydrocarbons, accidental (unintentional)**
Toxic effects of other halogen derivatives of aromatic hydrocarbons NOS

✓7th **T53.7X2 Toxic effect of other halogen derivatives of aromatic hydrocarbons, intentional self-harm**

✓7th **T53.7X3 Toxic effect of other halogen derivatives of aromatic hydrocarbons, assault**

✓7th **T53.7X4 Toxic effect of other halogen derivatives of aromatic hydrocarbons, undetermined**

✓5th **T53.9 Toxic effects of unspecified halogen derivatives of aliphatic and aromatic hydrocarbons**

✓x7th **T53.91 Toxic effect of unspecified halogen derivatives of aliphatic and aromatic hydrocarbons, accidental (unintentional)**

✓x7th **T53.92 Toxic effect of unspecified halogen derivatives of aliphatic and aromatic hydrocarbons, intentional self-harm**

✓x7th **T53.93 Toxic effect of unspecified halogen derivatives of aliphatic and aromatic hydrocarbons, assault**

✓x7th **T53.94 Toxic effect of unspecified halogen derivatives of aliphatic and aromatic hydrocarbons, undetermined**

✓4th **T54 Toxic effect of corrosive substances**

The appropriate 7th character is to be added to each code from category T54.
A initial encounter
D subsequent encounter
S sequela

✓5th **T54.0 Toxic effects of phenol and phenol homologues**

✓6th **T54.0X Toxic effects of phenol and phenol homologues**

✓7th **T54.0X1 Toxic effect of phenol and phenol homologues, accidental (unintentional)**
Toxic effects of phenol and phenol homologues NOS

✓7th **T54.0X2 Toxic effect of phenol and phenol homologues, intentional self-harm**

✓7th **T54.0X3 Toxic effect of phenol and phenol homologues, assault**

✓7th **T54.0X4 Toxic effect of phenol and phenol homologues, undetermined**

✓5th **T54.1 Toxic effects of other corrosive organic compounds**

✓6th **T54.1X Toxic effects of other corrosive organic compounds**

✓7th **T54.1X1 Toxic effect of other corrosive organic compounds, accidental (unintentional)**
Toxic effects of other corrosive organic compounds NOS

✓7th **T54.1X2 Toxic effect of other corrosive organic compounds, intentional self-harm**

✓7th **T54.1X3 Toxic effect of other corrosive organic compounds, assault**

✓7th **T54.1X4 Toxic effect of other corrosive organic compounds, undetermined**

✓5th **T54.2 Toxic effects of corrosive acids and acid-like substances**
Toxic effects of hydrochloric acid
Toxic effects of sulfuric acid

✓6th **T54.2X Toxic effects of corrosive acids and acid-like substances**

✓7th **T54.2X1 Toxic effect of corrosive acids and acid-like substances, accidental (unintentional)**
Toxic effects of corrosive acids and acid-like substances NOS

✓7th **T54.2X2 Toxic effect of corrosive acids and acid-like substances, intentional self-harm**

✓7th **T54.2X3 Toxic effect of corrosive acids and acid-like substances, assault**

✓7th **T54.2X4 Toxic effect of corrosive acids and acid-like substances, undetermined**

✓5th **T54.3 Toxic effects of corrosive alkalis and alkali-like substances**
Toxic effects of potassium hydroxide
Toxic effects of sodium hydroxide

✓6th **T54.3X Toxic effects of corrosive alkalis and alkali-like substances**

✓7th **T54.3X1 Toxic effect of corrosive alkalis and alkali-like substances, accidental (unintentional)**
Toxic effects of corrosive alkalis and alkali-like substances NOS

✓7th **T54.3X2 Toxic effect of corrosive alkalis and alkali-like substances, intentional self-harm**

✓7th **T54.3X3 Toxic effect of corrosive alkalis and alkali-like substances, assault**

✓7th **T54.3X4 Toxic effect of corrosive alkalis and alkali-like substances, undetermined**

✓5th **T54.9 Toxic effects of unspecified corrosive substance**

✓x7th **T54.91 Toxic effect of unspecified corrosive substance, accidental (unintentional)**

✓x7th **T54.92 Toxic effect of unspecified corrosive substance, intentional self-harm**

✓x7th **T54.93 Toxic effect of unspecified corrosive substance, assault**

✓x7th **T54.94 Toxic effect of unspecified corrosive substance, undetermined**

T55 Toxic effect of soaps and detergents

The appropriate 7th character is to be added to each code from category T55.
A initial encounter
D subsequent encounter
S sequela

T55.Ø Toxic effect of soaps
T55.ØX Toxic effect of soaps
T55.ØX1 Toxic effect of soaps, accidental (unintentional)
Toxic effect of soaps NOS
T55.ØX2 Toxic effect of soaps, intentional self-harm
T55.ØX3 Toxic effect of soaps, assault
T55.ØX4 Toxic effect of soaps, undetermined

T55.1 Toxic effect of detergents
T55.1X Toxic effect of detergents
T55.1X1 Toxic effect of detergents, accidental (unintentional)
Toxic effect of detergents NOS
T55.1X2 Toxic effect of detergents, intentional self-harm
T55.1X3 Toxic effect of detergents, assault
T55.1X4 Toxic effect of detergents, undetermined

T56 Toxic effect of metals

INCLUDES toxic effects of fumes and vapors of metals
toxic effects of metals from all sources, except medicinal substances

Use additional code to identify any retained metal foreign body, if applicable (Z18.Ø-, T18.1-)

EXCLUDES 1 *arsenic and its compounds (T57.Ø)*
manganese and its compounds (T57.2)

The appropriate 7th character is to be added to each code from category T56.
A initial encounter
D subsequent encounter
S sequela

T56.Ø Toxic effects of lead and its compounds
T56.ØX Toxic effects of lead and its compounds
T56.ØX1 Toxic effect of lead and its compounds, accidental (unintentional)
Toxic effects of lead and its compounds NOS
T56.ØX2 Toxic effect of lead and its compounds, intentional self-harm
T56.ØX3 Toxic effect of lead and its compounds, assault
T56.ØX4 Toxic effect of lead and its compounds, undetermined

T56.1 Toxic effects of mercury and its compounds
T56.1X Toxic effects of mercury and its compounds
T56.1X1 Toxic effect of mercury and its compounds, accidental (unintentional)
Toxic effects of mercury and its compounds NOS
T56.1X2 Toxic effect of mercury and its compounds, intentional self-harm
T56.1X3 Toxic effect of mercury and its compounds, assault
T56.1X4 Toxic effect of mercury and its compounds, undetermined

T56.2 Toxic effects of chromium and its compounds
T56.2X Toxic effects of chromium and its compounds
T56.2X1 Toxic effect of chromium and its compounds, accidental (unintentional)
Toxic effects of chromium and its compounds NOS
T56.2X2 Toxic effect of chromium and its compounds, intentional self-harm
T56.2X3 Toxic effect of chromium and its compounds, assault
T56.2X4 Toxic effect of chromium and its compounds, undetermined

T56.3 Toxic effects of cadmium and its compounds
T56.3X Toxic effects of cadmium and its compounds
T56.3X1 Toxic effect of cadmium and its compounds, accidental (unintentional)
Toxic effects of cadmium and its compounds NOS
T56.3X2 Toxic effect of cadmium and its compounds, intentional self-harm
T56.3X3 Toxic effect of cadmium and its compounds, assault
T56.3X4 Toxic effect of cadmium and its compounds, undetermined

T56.4 Toxic effects of copper and its compounds
T56.4X Toxic effects of copper and its compounds
T56.4X1 Toxic effect of copper and its compounds, accidental (unintentional)
Toxic effects of copper and its compounds NOS
T56.4X2 Toxic effect of copper and its compounds, intentional self-harm
T56.4X3 Toxic effect of copper and its compounds, assault
T56.4X4 Toxic effect of copper and its compounds, undetermined

T56.5 Toxic effects of zinc and its compounds
T56.5X Toxic effects of zinc and its compounds
T56.5X1 Toxic effect of zinc and its compounds, accidental (unintentional)
Toxic effects of zinc and its compounds NOS
T56.5X2 Toxic effect of zinc and its compounds, intentional self-harm
T56.5X3 Toxic effect of zinc and its compounds, assault
T56.5X4 Toxic effect of zinc and its compounds, undetermined

T56.6 Toxic effects of tin and its compounds
T56.6X Toxic effects of tin and its compounds
T56.6X1 Toxic effect of tin and its compounds, accidental (unintentional)
Toxic effects of tin and its compounds NOS
T56.6X2 Toxic effect of tin and its compounds, intentional self-harm
T56.6X3 Toxic effect of tin and its compounds, assault
T56.6X4 Toxic effect of tin and its compounds, undetermined

T56.7 Toxic effects of beryllium and its compounds
T56.7X Toxic effects of beryllium and its compounds
T56.7X1 Toxic effect of beryllium and its compounds, accidental (unintentional)
Toxic effects of beryllium and its compounds NOS
T56.7X2 Toxic effect of beryllium and its compounds, intentional self-harm
T56.7X3 Toxic effect of beryllium and its compounds, assault
T56.7X4 Toxic effect of beryllium and its compounds, undetermined

T56.8 Toxic effects of other metals
T56.81 Toxic effect of thallium
T56.811 Toxic effect of thallium, accidental (unintentional)
Toxic effect of thallium NOS
T56.812 Toxic effect of thallium, intentional self-harm
T56.813 Toxic effect of thallium, assault
T56.814 Toxic effect of thallium, undetermined
T56.89 Toxic effects of other metals
T56.891 Toxic effect of other metals, accidental (unintentional)
Toxic effects of other metals NOS
T56.892 Toxic effect of other metals, intentional self-harm
T56.893 Toxic effect of other metals, assault
T56.894 Toxic effect of other metals, undetermined

T56.9 Toxic effects of unspecified metal
- T56.91 Toxic effect of unspecified metal, accidental (unintentional)
- T56.92 Toxic effect of unspecified metal, intentional self-harm
- T56.93 Toxic effect of unspecified metal, assault
- T56.94 Toxic effect of unspecified metal, undetermined

T57 Toxic effect of other inorganic substances

The appropriate 7th character is to be added to each code from category T57.
A initial encounter
D subsequent encounter
S sequela

T57.Ø Toxic effect of arsenic and its compounds
- T57.ØX Toxic effect of arsenic and its compounds
  - T57.ØX1 Toxic effect of arsenic and its compounds, accidental (unintentional)
    Toxic effect of arsenic and its compounds NOS
  - T57.ØX2 Toxic effect of arsenic and its compounds, intentional self-harm
  - T57.ØX3 Toxic effect of arsenic and its compounds, assault
  - T57.ØX4 Toxic effect of arsenic and its compounds, undetermined

T57.1 Toxic effect of phosphorus and its compounds
EXCLUDES 1 *organophosphate insecticides (T6Ø.Ø)*
- T57.1X Toxic effect of phosphorus and its compounds
  - T57.1X1 Toxic effect of phosphorus and its compounds, accidental (unintentional)
    Toxic effect of phosphorus and its compounds NOS
  - T57.1X2 Toxic effect of phosphorus and its compounds, intentional self-harm
  - T57.1X3 Toxic effect of phosphorus and its compounds, assault
  - T57.1X4 Toxic effect of phosphorus and its compounds, undetermined

T57.2 Toxic effect of manganese and its compounds
- T57.2X Toxic effect of manganese and its compounds
  - T57.2X1 Toxic effect of manganese and its compounds, accidental (unintentional)
    Toxic effect of manganese and its compounds NOS
  - T57.2X2 Toxic effect of manganese and its compounds, intentional self-harm
  - T57.2X3 Toxic effect of manganese and its compounds, assault
  - T57.2X4 Toxic effect of manganese and its compounds, undetermined

T57.3 Toxic effect of hydrogen cyanide
- T57.3X Toxic effect of hydrogen cyanide
  - T57.3X1 Toxic effect of hydrogen cyanide, accidental (unintentional)
    Toxic effect of hydrogen cyanide NOS
  - T57.3X2 Toxic effect of hydrogen cyanide, intentional self-harm
  - T57.3X3 Toxic effect of hydrogen cyanide, assault
  - T57.3X4 Toxic effect of hydrogen cyanide, undetermined

T57.8 Toxic effect of other specified inorganic substances
- T57.8X Toxic effect of other specified inorganic substances
  - T57.8X1 Toxic effect of other specified inorganic substances, accidental (unintentional)
    Toxic effect of other specified inorganic substances NOS
  - T57.8X2 Toxic effect of other specified inorganic substances, intentional self-harm
  - T57.8X3 Toxic effect of other specified inorganic substances, assault
  - T57.8X4 Toxic effect of other specified inorganic substances, undetermined

T57.9 Toxic effect of unspecified inorganic substance
- T57.91 Toxic effect of unspecified inorganic substance, accidental (unintentional)
- T57.92 Toxic effect of unspecified inorganic substance, intentional self-harm
- T57.93 Toxic effect of unspecified inorganic substance, assault
- T57.94 Toxic effect of unspecified inorganic substance, undetermined

T58 Toxic effect of carbon monoxide
INCLUDES asphyxiation from carbon monoxide
toxic effect of carbon monoxide from all sources

The appropriate 7th character is to be added to each code from category T58.
A initial encounter
D subsequent encounter
S sequela

T58.Ø Toxic effect of carbon monoxide from motor vehicle exhaust
Toxic effect of exhaust gas from gas engine
Toxic effect of exhaust gas from motor pump
- T58.Ø1 Toxic effect of carbon monoxide from motor vehicle exhaust, accidental (unintentional)
- T58.Ø2 Toxic effect of carbon monoxide from motor vehicle exhaust, intentional self-harm
- T58.Ø3 Toxic effect of carbon monoxide from motor vehicle exhaust, assault
- T58.Ø4 Toxic effect of carbon monoxide from motor vehicle exhaust, undetermined

T58.1 Toxic effect of carbon monoxide from utility gas
Toxic effect of acetylene
Toxic effect of gas NOS used for lighting, heating, cooking
Toxic effect of water gas
- T58.11 Toxic effect of carbon monoxide from utility gas, accidental (unintentional)
- T58.12 Toxic effect of carbon monoxide from utility gas, intentional self-harm
- T58.13 Toxic effect of carbon monoxide from utility gas, assault
- T58.14 Toxic effect of carbon monoxide from utility gas, undetermined

T58.2 Toxic effect of carbon monoxide from incomplete combustion of other domestic fuels
Toxic effect of carbon monoxide from incomplete combustion of coal, coke, kerosene, wood
- T58.2X Toxic effect of carbon monoxide from incomplete combustion of other domestic fuels
  - T58.2X1 Toxic effect of carbon monoxide from incomplete combustion of other domestic fuels, accidental (unintentional)
  - T58.2X2 Toxic effect of carbon monoxide from incomplete combustion of other domestic fuels, intentional self-harm
  - T58.2X3 Toxic effect of carbon monoxide from incomplete combustion of other domestic fuels, assault
  - T58.2X4 Toxic effect of carbon monoxide from incomplete combustion of other domestic fuels, undetermined

T58.8 Toxic effect of carbon monoxide from other source
Toxic effect of carbon monoxide from blast furnace gas
Toxic effect of carbon monoxide from fuels in industrial use
Toxic effect of carbon monoxide from kiln vapor
- T58.8X Toxic effect of carbon monoxide from other source
  - T58.8X1 Toxic effect of carbon monoxide from other source, accidental (unintentional)
  - T58.8X2 Toxic effect of carbon monoxide from other source, intentional self-harm
  - T58.8X3 Toxic effect of carbon monoxide from other source, assault
  - T58.8X4 Toxic effect of carbon monoxide from other source, undetermined

T58.9 Toxic effect of carbon monoxide from unspecified source
- T58.91 Toxic effect of carbon monoxide from unspecified source, accidental (unintentional)

√x7th **T58.92 Toxic effect of carbon monoxide from unspecified source, intentional self-harm**

√x7th **T58.93 Toxic effect of carbon monoxide from unspecified source, assault**

√x7th **T58.94 Toxic effect of carbon monoxide from unspecified source, undetermined**

√4th **T59 Toxic effect of other gases, fumes and vapors**

INCLUDES aerosol propellants

EXCLUDES 1 *chlorofluorocarbons (T53.5)*

The appropriate 7th character is to be added to each code from category T59.
A initial encounter
D subsequent encounter
S sequela

√5th **T59.Ø Toxic effect of nitrogen oxides**

√6th **T59.ØX Toxic effect of nitrogen oxides**

√7th **T59.ØX1 Toxic effect of nitrogen oxides, accidental (unintentional)**
Toxic effect of nitrogen oxides NOS

√7th **T59.ØX2 Toxic effect of nitrogen oxides, intentional self-harm**

√7th **T59.ØX3 Toxic effect of nitrogen oxides, assault**

√7th **T59.ØX4 Toxic effect of nitrogen oxides, undetermined**

√5th **T59.1 Toxic effect of sulfur dioxide**

√6th **T59.1X Toxic effect of sulfur dioxide**

√7th **T59.1X1 Toxic effect of sulfur dioxide, accidental (unintentional)**
Toxic effect of sulfur dioxide NOS

√7th **T59.1X2 Toxic effect of sulfur dioxide, intentional self-harm**

√7th **T59.1X3 Toxic effect of sulfur dioxide, assault**

√7th **T59.1X4 Toxic effect of sulfur dioxide, undetermined**

√5th **T59.2 Toxic effect of formaldehyde**

√6th **T59.2X Toxic effect of formaldehyde**

√7th **T59.2X1 Toxic effect of formaldehyde, accidental (unintentional)**
Toxic effect of formaldehyde NOS

√7th **T59.2X2 Toxic effect of formaldehyde, intentional self-harm**

√7th **T59.2X3 Toxic effect of formaldehyde, assault**

√7th **T59.2X4 Toxic effect of formaldehyde, undetermined**

√5th **T59.3 Toxic effect of lacrimogenic gas**
Toxic effect of tear gas

√6th **T59.3X Toxic effect of lacrimogenic gas**

√7th **T59.3X1 Toxic effect of lacrimogenic gas, accidental (unintentional)**
Toxic effect of lacrimogenic gas NOS

√7th **T59.3X2 Toxic effect of lacrimogenic gas, intentional self-harm**

√7th **T59.3X3 Toxic effect of lacrimogenic gas, assault**

√7th **T59.3X4 Toxic effect of lacrimogenic gas, undetermined**

√5th **T59.4 Toxic effect of chlorine gas**

√6th **T59.4X Toxic effect of chlorine gas**

√7th **T59.4X1 Toxic effect of chlorine gas, accidental (unintentional)**
Toxic effect of chlorine gas NOS

√7th **T59.4X2 Toxic effect of chlorine gas, intentional self-harm**

√7th **T59.4X3 Toxic effect of chlorine gas, assault**

√7th **T59.4X4 Toxic effect of chlorine gas, undetermined**

√5th **T59.5 Toxic effect of fluorine gas and hydrogen fluoride**

√6th **T59.5X Toxic effect of fluorine gas and hydrogen fluoride**

√7th **T59.5X1 Toxic effect of fluorine gas and hydrogen fluoride, accidental (unintentional)**
Toxic effect of fluorine gas and hydrogen fluoride NOS

√7th **T59.5X2 Toxic effect of fluorine gas and hydrogen fluoride, intentional self-harm**

√7th **T59.5X3 Toxic effect of fluorine gas and hydrogen fluoride, assault**

√7th **T59.5X4 Toxic effect of fluorine gas and hydrogen fluoride, undetermined**

√5th **T59.6 Toxic effect of hydrogen sulfide**

√6th **T59.6X Toxic effect of hydrogen sulfide**

√7th **T59.6X1 Toxic effect of hydrogen sulfide, accidental (unintentional)**
Toxic effect of hydrogen sulfide NOS

√7th **T59.6X2 Toxic effect of hydrogen sulfide, intentional self-harm**

√7th **T59.6X3 Toxic effect of hydrogen sulfide, assault**

√7th **T59.6X4 Toxic effect of hydrogen sulfide, undetermined**

√5th **T59.7 Toxic effect of carbon dioxide**

√6th **T59.7X Toxic effect of carbon dioxide**

√7th **T59.7X1 Toxic effect of carbon dioxide, accidental (unintentional)**
Toxic effect of carbon dioxide NOS

√7th **T59.7X2 Toxic effect of carbon dioxide, intentional self-harm**

√7th **T59.7X3 Toxic effect of carbon dioxide, assault**

√7th **T59.7X4 Toxic effect of carbon dioxide, undetermined**

√5th **T59.8 Toxic effect of other specified gases, fumes and vapors**

√6th **T59.81 Toxic effect of smoke**
Smoke inhalation
EXCLUDES 2 *toxic effect of cigarette (tobacco) smoke (T65.22-)*

√7th **T59.811 Toxic effect of smoke, accidental (unintentional)**
Toxic effect of smoke NOS
AHA: 2013, 4Q, 121

√7th **T59.812 Toxic effect of smoke, intentional self-harm**

√7th **T59.813 Toxic effect of smoke, assault**

√7th **T59.814 Toxic effect of smoke, undetermined**

√6th **T59.89 Toxic effect of other specified gases, fumes and vapors**

√7th **T59.891 Toxic effect of other specified gases, fumes and vapors, accidental (unintentional)**

√7th **T59.892 Toxic effect of other specified gases, fumes and vapors, intentional self-harm**

√7th **T59.893 Toxic effect of other specified gases, fumes and vapors, assault**

√7th **T59.894 Toxic effect of other specified gases, fumes and vapors, undetermined**

√5th **T59.9 Toxic effect of unspecified gases, fumes and vapors**

√x7th **T59.91 Toxic effect of unspecified gases, fumes and vapors, accidental (unintentional)**

√x7th **T59.92 Toxic effect of unspecified gases, fumes and vapors, intentional self-harm**

√x7th **T59.93 Toxic effect of unspecified gases, fumes and vapors, assault**

√x7th **T59.94 Toxic effect of unspecified gases, fumes and vapors, undetermined**

√4th **T6Ø Toxic effect of pesticides**

INCLUDES toxic effect of wood preservatives

The appropriate 7th character is to be added to each code from category T6Ø.
A initial encounter
D subsequent encounter
S sequela

√5th **T6Ø.Ø Toxic effect of organophosphate and carbamate insecticides**

√6th **T6Ø.ØX Toxic effect of organophosphate and carbamate insecticides**

√7th **T6Ø.ØX1 Toxic effect of organophosphate and carbamate insecticides, accidental (unintentional)**
Toxic effect of organophosphate and carbamate insecticides NOS

√7th **T6Ø.ØX2 Toxic effect of organophosphate and carbamate insecticides, intentional self-harm**

T60.0X3 Toxic effect of organophosphate and carbamate insecticides, assault

T60.0X4 Toxic effect of organophosphate and carbamate insecticides, undetermined

T60.1 Toxic effect of halogenated insecticides

EXCLUDES 1 *chlorinated hydrocarbon (T53.-)*

T60.1X Toxic effect of halogenated insecticides

T60.1X1 Toxic effect of halogenated insecticides, accidental (unintentional)

Toxic effect of halogenated insecticides NOS

T60.1X2 Toxic effect of halogenated insecticides, intentional self-harm

T60.1X3 Toxic effect of halogenated insecticides, assault

T60.1X4 Toxic effect of halogenated insecticides, undetermined

T60.2 Toxic effect of other insecticides

T60.2X Toxic effect of other insecticides

T60.2X1 Toxic effect of other insecticides, accidental (unintentional)

Toxic effect of other insecticides NOS

T60.2X2 Toxic effect of other insecticides, intentional self-harm

T60.2X3 Toxic effect of other insecticides, assault

T60.2X4 Toxic effect of other insecticides, undetermined

T60.3 Toxic effect of herbicides and fungicides

T60.3X Toxic effect of herbicides and fungicides

T60.3X1 Toxic effect of herbicides and fungicides, accidental (unintentional)

Toxic effect of herbicides and fungicides NOS

T60.3X2 Toxic effect of herbicides and fungicides, intentional self-harm

T60.3X3 Toxic effect of herbicides and fungicides, assault

T60.3X4 Toxic effect of herbicides and fungicides, undetermined

T60.4 Toxic effect of rodenticides

EXCLUDES 1 *strychnine and its salts (T65.1)*
thallium (T56.81-)

T60.4X Toxic effect of rodenticides

T60.4X1 Toxic effect of rodenticides, accidental (unintentional)

Toxic effect of rodenticides NOS

T60.4X2 Toxic effect of rodenticides, intentional self-harm

T60.4X3 Toxic effect of rodenticides, assault

T60.4X4 Toxic effect of rodenticides, undetermined

T60.8 Toxic effect of other pesticides

T60.8X Toxic effect of other pesticides

T60.8X1 Toxic effect of other pesticides, accidental (unintentional)

Toxic effect of other pesticides NOS

T60.8X2 Toxic effect of other pesticides, intentional self-harm

T60.8X3 Toxic effect of other pesticides, assault

T60.8X4 Toxic effect of other pesticides, undetermined

T60.9 Toxic effect of unspecified pesticide

T60.91 Toxic effect of unspecified pesticide, accidental (unintentional)

T60.92 Toxic effect of unspecified pesticide, intentional self-harm

T60.93 Toxic effect of unspecified pesticide, assault

T60.94 Toxic effect of unspecified pesticide, undetermined

T61 Toxic effect of noxious substances eaten as seafood

EXCLUDES 1 *allergic reaction to food, such as:*
anaphylactic reaction or shock due to adverse food reaction (T78.0-)
dermatitis (L23.6, L25.4, L27.2)
gastroenteritis (noninfective) (K52.2)
bacterial foodborne intoxications (A05.-)
toxic effect of aflatoxin and other mycotoxins (T64)
toxic effect of cyanides (T65.0-)
toxic effect of harmful algae bloom (T65.82-)
toxic effect of hydrogen cyanide (T57.3-)
toxic effect of mercury (T56.1-)
toxic effect of red tide (T65.82-)

The appropriate 7th character is to be added to each code from category T61.
A initial encounter
D subsequent encounter
S sequela

T61.0 Ciguatera fish poisoning

T61.01 Ciguatera fish poisoning, accidental (unintentional)

T61.02 Ciguatera fish poisoning, intentional self-harm

T61.03 Ciguatera fish poisoning, assault

T61.04 Ciguatera fish poisoning, undetermined

T61.1 Scombroid fish poisoning

Histamine-like syndrome

T61.11 Scombroid fish poisoning, accidental (unintentional)

T61.12 Scombroid fish poisoning, intentional self-harm

T61.13 Scombroid fish poisoning, assault

T61.14 Scombroid fish poisoning, undetermined

T61.7 Other fish and shellfish poisoning

T61.77 Other fish poisoning

T61.771 Other fish poisoning, accidental (unintentional)

T61.772 Other fish poisoning, intentional self-harm

T61.773 Other fish poisoning, assault

T61.774 Other fish poisoning, undetermined

T61.78 Other shellfish poisoning

T61.781 Other shellfish poisoning, accidental (unintentional)

T61.782 Other shellfish poisoning, intentional self-harm

T61.783 Other shellfish poisoning, assault

T61.784 Other shellfish poisoning, undetermined

T61.8 Toxic effect of other seafood

T61.8X Toxic effect of other seafood

T61.8X1 Toxic effect of other seafood, accidental (unintentional)

T61.8X2 Toxic effect of other seafood, intentional self-harm

T61.8X3 Toxic effect of other seafood, assault

T61.8X4 Toxic effect of other seafood, undetermined

T61.9 Toxic effect of unspecified seafood

T61.91 Toxic effect of unspecified seafood, accidental (unintentional)

T61.92 Toxic effect of unspecified seafood, intentional self-harm

T61.93 Toxic effect of unspecified seafood, assault

T61.94 Toxic effect of unspecified seafood, undetermined

4th T62 Toxic effect of other noxious substances eaten as food

EXCLUDES 1 *allergic reaction to food, such as:*
anaphylactic shock (reaction) due to adverse food reaction (T78.Ø-)
dermatitis (L23.6, L25.4, L27.2)
gastroenteritis (noninfective) (K52.2)
bacterial food borne intoxications (AØ5.-)
toxic effect of aflatoxin and other mycotoxins (T64)
toxic effect of cyanides (T65.Ø-)
toxic effect of hydrogen cyanide (T57.3-)
toxic effect of mercury (T56.1-)

The appropriate 7th character is to be added to each code from category T62.
A initial encounter
D subsequent encounter
S sequela

5th **T62.Ø Toxic effect of ingested mushrooms**
6th **T62.ØX Toxic effect of ingested mushrooms**
7th **T62.ØX1 Toxic effect of ingested mushrooms, accidental (unintentional)**
Toxic effect of ingested mushrooms NOS
7th **T62.ØX2 Toxic effect of ingested mushrooms, intentional self-harm**
7th **T62.ØX3 Toxic effect of ingested mushrooms, assault**
7th **T62.ØX4 Toxic effect of ingested mushrooms, undetermined**

5th **T62.1 Toxic effect of ingested berries**
6th **T62.1X Toxic effect of ingested berries**
7th **T62.1X1 Toxic effect of ingested berries, accidental (unintentional)**
Toxic effect of ingested berries NOS
7th **T62.1X2 Toxic effect of ingested berries, intentional self-harm**
7th **T62.1X3 Toxic effect of ingested berries, assault**
7th **T62.1X4 Toxic effect of ingested berries, undetermined**

5th **T62.2 Toxic effect of other ingested (parts of) plant(s)**
6th **T62.2X Toxic effect of other ingested (parts of) plant(s)**
7th **T62.2X1 Toxic effect of other ingested (parts of) plant(s), accidental (unintentional)**
Toxic effect of other ingested (parts of) plant(s) NOS
7th **T62.2X2 Toxic effect of other ingested (parts of) plant(s), intentional self-harm**
7th **T62.2X3 Toxic effect of other ingested (parts of) plant(s), assault**
7th **T62.2X4 Toxic effect of other ingested (parts of) plant(s), undetermined**

5th **T62.8 Toxic effect of other specified noxious substances eaten as food**
6th **T62.8X Toxic effect of other specified noxious substances eaten as food**
7th **T62.8X1 Toxic effect of other specified noxious substances eaten as food, accidental (unintentional)**
Toxic effect of other specified noxious substances eaten as food NOS
7th **T62.8X2 Toxic effect of other specified noxious substances eaten as food, intentional self-harm**
7th **T62.8X3 Toxic effect of other specified noxious substances eaten as food, assault**
7th **T62.8X4 Toxic effect of other specified noxious substances eaten as food, undetermined**

5th **T62.9 Toxic effect of unspecified noxious substance eaten as food**
x7th **T62.91 Toxic effect of unspecified noxious substance eaten as food, accidental (unintentional)**
Toxic effect of unspecified noxious substance eaten as food NOS
x7th **T62.92 Toxic effect of unspecified noxious substance eaten as food, intentional self-harm**
x7th **T62.93 Toxic effect of unspecified noxious substance eaten as food, assault**
x7th **T62.94 Toxic effect of unspecified noxious substance eaten as food, undetermined**

4th T63 Toxic effect of contact with venomous animals and plants

INCLUDES bite or touch of venomous animal
pricked or stuck by thorn or leaf

EXCLUDES 2 *ingestion of toxic animal or plant (T61.-, T62.-)*

The appropriate 7th character is to be added to each code from category T63.
A initial encounter
D subsequent encounter
S sequela

5th **T63.Ø Toxic effect of snake venom**
6th **T63.ØØ Toxic effect of unspecified snake venom**
7th **T63.ØØ1 Toxic effect of unspecified snake venom, accidental (unintentional)**
Toxic effect of unspecified snake venom NOS
7th **T63.ØØ2 Toxic effect of unspecified snake venom, intentional self-harm**
7th **T63.ØØ3 Toxic effect of unspecified snake venom, assault**
7th **T63.ØØ4 Toxic effect of unspecified snake venom, undetermined**
6th **T63.Ø1 Toxic effect of rattlesnake venom**
7th **T63.Ø11 Toxic effect of rattlesnake venom, accidental (unintentional)**
Toxic effect of rattlesnake venom NOS
7th **T63.Ø12 Toxic effect of rattlesnake venom, intentional self-harm**
7th **T63.Ø13 Toxic effect of rattlesnake venom, assault**
7th **T63.Ø14 Toxic effect of rattlesnake venom, undetermined**
6th **T63.Ø2 Toxic effect of coral snake venom**
7th **T63.Ø21 Toxic effect of coral snake venom, accidental (unintentional)**
Toxic effect of coral snake venom NOS
7th **T63.Ø22 Toxic effect of coral snake venom, intentional self-harm**
7th **T63.Ø23 Toxic effect of coral snake venom, assault**
7th **T63.Ø24 Toxic effect of coral snake venom, undetermined**
6th **T63.Ø3 Toxic effect of taipan venom**
7th **T63.Ø31 Toxic effect of taipan venom, accidental (unintentional)**
Toxic effect of taipan venom NOS
7th **T63.Ø32 Toxic effect of taipan venom, intentional self-harm**
7th **T63.Ø33 Toxic effect of taipan venom, assault**
7th **T63.Ø34 Toxic effect of taipan venom, undetermined**
6th **T63.Ø4 Toxic effect of cobra venom**
7th **T63.Ø41 Toxic effect of cobra venom, accidental (unintentional)**
Toxic effect of cobra venom NOS
7th **T63.Ø42 Toxic effect of cobra venom, intentional self-harm**
7th **T63.Ø43 Toxic effect of cobra venom, assault**
7th **T63.Ø44 Toxic effect of cobra venom, undetermined**
6th **T63.Ø6 Toxic effect of venom of other North and South American snake**
7th **T63.Ø61 Toxic effect of venom of other North and South American snake, accidental (unintentional)**
Toxic effect of venom of other North and South American snake NOS
7th **T63.Ø62 Toxic effect of venom of other North and South American snake, intentional self-harm**
7th **T63.Ø63 Toxic effect of venom of other North and South American snake, assault**
7th **T63.Ø64 Toxic effect of venom of other North and South American snake, undetermined**

√6th T63.07 Toxic effect of venom of other Australian snake
√7th T63.071 Toxic effect of venom of other Australian snake, accidental (unintentional)
Toxic effect of venom of other Australian snake NOS
√7th T63.072 Toxic effect of venom of other Australian snake, intentional self-harm
√7th T63.073 Toxic effect of venom of other Australian snake, assault
√7th T63.074 Toxic effect of venom of other Australian snake, undetermined
√6th T63.08 Toxic effect of venom of other African and Asian snake
√7th T63.081 Toxic effect of venom of other African and Asian snake, accidental (unintentional)
Toxic effect of venom of other African and Asian snake NOS
√7th T63.082 Toxic effect of venom of other African and Asian snake, intentional self-harm
√7th T63.083 Toxic effect of venom of other African and Asian snake, assault
√7th T63.084 Toxic effect of venom of other African and Asian snake, undetermined
√6th T63.09 Toxic effect of venom of other snake
√7th T63.091 Toxic effect of venom of other snake, accidental (unintentional)
Toxic effect of venom of other snake NOS
√7th T63.092 Toxic effect of venom of other snake, intentional self-harm
√7th T63.093 Toxic effect of venom of other snake, assault
√7th T63.094 Toxic effect of venom of other snake, undetermined
√5th T63.1 Toxic effect of venom of other reptiles
√6th T63.11 Toxic effect of venom of gila monster
√7th T63.111 Toxic effect of venom of gila monster, accidental (unintentional)
Toxic effect of venom of gila monster NOS
√7th T63.112 Toxic effect of venom of gila monster, intentional self-harm
√7th T63.113 Toxic effect of venom of gila monster, assault
√7th T63.114 Toxic effect of venom of gila monster, undetermined
√6th T63.12 Toxic effect of venom of other venomous lizard
√7th T63.121 Toxic effect of venom of other venomous lizard, accidental (unintentional)
Toxic effect of venom of other venomous lizard NOS
√7th T63.122 Toxic effect of venom of other venomous lizard, intentional self-harm
√7th T63.123 Toxic effect of venom of other venomous lizard, assault
√7th T63.124 Toxic effect of venom of other venomous lizard, undetermined
√6th T63.19 Toxic effect of venom of other reptiles
√7th T63.191 Toxic effect of venom of other reptiles, accidental (unintentional)
Toxic effect of venom of other reptiles NOS
√7th T63.192 Toxic effect of venom of other reptiles, intentional self-harm
√7th T63.193 Toxic effect of venom of other reptiles, assault
√7th T63.194 Toxic effect of venom of other reptiles, undetermined
√5th T63.2 Toxic effect of venom of scorpion
√6th T63.2X Toxic effect of venom of scorpion
√7th T63.2X1 Toxic effect of venom of scorpion, accidental (unintentional)
Toxic effect of venom of scorpion NOS
√7th T63.2X2 Toxic effect of venom of scorpion, intentional self-harm
√7th T63.2X3 Toxic effect of venom of scorpion, assault
√7th T63.2X4 Toxic effect of venom of scorpion, undetermined
√5th T63.3 Toxic effect of venom of spider
√6th T63.30 Toxic effect of unspecified spider venom
√7th T63.301 Toxic effect of unspecified spider venom, accidental (unintentional)
√7th T63.302 Toxic effect of unspecified spider venom, intentional self-harm
√7th T63.303 Toxic effect of unspecified spider venom, assault
√7th T63.304 Toxic effect of unspecified spider venom, undetermined
√6th T63.31 Toxic effect of venom of black widow spider
√7th T63.311 Toxic effect of venom of black widow spider, accidental (unintentional)
√7th T63.312 Toxic effect of venom of black widow spider, intentional self-harm
√7th T63.313 Toxic effect of venom of black widow spider, assault
√7th T63.314 Toxic effect of venom of black widow spider, undetermined
√6th T63.32 Toxic effect of venom of tarantula
√7th T63.321 Toxic effect of venom of tarantula, accidental (unintentional)
√7th T63.322 Toxic effect of venom of tarantula, intentional self-harm
√7th T63.323 Toxic effect of venom of tarantula, assault
√7th T63.324 Toxic effect of venom of tarantula, undetermined
√6th T63.33 Toxic effect of venom of brown recluse spider
√7th T63.331 Toxic effect of venom of brown recluse spider, accidental (unintentional)
√7th T63.332 Toxic effect of venom of brown recluse spider, intentional self-harm
√7th T63.333 Toxic effect of venom of brown recluse spider, assault
√7th T63.334 Toxic effect of venom of brown recluse spider, undetermined
√6th T63.39 Toxic effect of venom of other spider
√7th T63.391 Toxic effect of venom of other spider, accidental (unintentional)
√7th T63.392 Toxic effect of venom of other spider, intentional self-harm
√7th T63.393 Toxic effect of venom of other spider, assault
√7th T63.394 Toxic effect of venom of other spider, undetermined
√5th T63.4 Toxic effect of venom of other arthropods
√6th T63.41 Toxic effect of venom of centipedes and venomous millipedes
√7th T63.411 Toxic effect of venom of centipedes and venomous millipedes, accidental (unintentional)
√7th T63.412 Toxic effect of venom of centipedes and venomous millipedes, intentional self-harm
√7th T63.413 Toxic effect of venom of centipedes and venomous millipedes, assault
√7th T63.414 Toxic effect of venom of centipedes and venomous millipedes, undetermined
√6th T63.42 Toxic effect of venom of ants
√7th T63.421 Toxic effect of venom of ants, accidental (unintentional)
√7th T63.422 Toxic effect of venom of ants, intentional self-harm
√7th T63.423 Toxic effect of venom of ants, assault
√7th T63.424 Toxic effect of venom of ants, undetermined
√6th T63.43 Toxic effect of venom of caterpillars
√7th T63.431 Toxic effect of venom of caterpillars, accidental (unintentional)
√7th T63.432 Toxic effect of venom of caterpillars, intentional self-harm
√7th T63.433 Toxic effect of venom of caterpillars, assault

Injury, Poisoning and Certain Other Consequences of External Causes T63.07–T63.433

✓7th T63.434 Toxic effect of venom of caterpillars, undetermined

✓6th T63.44 Toxic effect of venom of bees
- ✓7th T63.441 Toxic effect of venom of bees, accidental (unintentional)
- ✓7th T63.442 Toxic effect of venom of bees, intentional self-harm
- ✓7th T63.443 Toxic effect of venom of bees, assault
- ✓7th T63.444 Toxic effect of venom of bees, undetermined

✓6th T63.45 Toxic effect of venom of hornets
- ✓7th T63.451 Toxic effect of venom of hornets, accidental (unintentional)
- ✓7th T63.452 Toxic effect of venom of hornets, intentional self-harm
- ✓7th T63.453 Toxic effect of venom of hornets, assault
- ✓7th T63.454 Toxic effect of venom of hornets, undetermined

✓6th T63.46 Toxic effect of venom of wasps
Toxic effect of yellow jacket
- ✓7th T63.461 Toxic effect of venom of wasps, accidental (unintentional)
- ✓7th T63.462 Toxic effect of venom of wasps, intentional self-harm
- ✓7th T63.463 Toxic effect of venom of wasps, assault
- ✓7th T63.464 Toxic effect of venom of wasps, undetermined

✓6th T63.48 Toxic effect of venom of other arthropod
- ✓7th T63.481 Toxic effect of venom of other arthropod, accidental (unintentional)
- ✓7th T63.482 Toxic effect of venom of other arthropod, intentional self-harm
- ✓7th T63.483 Toxic effect of venom of other arthropod, assault
- ✓7th T63.484 Toxic effect of venom of other arthropod, undetermined

✓5th T63.5 Toxic effect of contact with venomous fish
EXCLUDES 2 *poisoning by ingestion of fish (T61.-)*

✓6th T63.51 Toxic effect of contact with stingray
- ✓7th T63.511 Toxic effect of contact with stingray, accidental (unintentional)
- ✓7th T63.512 Toxic effect of contact with stingray, intentional self-harm
- ✓7th T63.513 Toxic effect of contact with stingray, assault
- ✓7th T63.514 Toxic effect of contact with stingray, undetermined

✓6th T63.59 Toxic effect of contact with other venomous fish
- ✓7th T63.591 Toxic effect of contact with other venomous fish, accidental (unintentional)
- ✓7th T63.592 Toxic effect of contact with other venomous fish, intentional self-harm
- ✓7th T63.593 Toxic effect of contact with other venomous fish, assault
- ✓7th T63.594 Toxic effect of contact with other venomous fish, undetermined

✓5th T63.6 Toxic effect of contact with other venomous marine animals
EXCLUDES 1 *sea-snake venom (T63.09)*
EXCLUDES 2 *poisoning by ingestion of shellfish (T61.78-)*

✓6th T63.61 Toxic effect of contact with Portugese Man-o-war
Toxic effect of contact with bluebottle
- ✓7th T63.611 Toxic effect of contact with Portugese Man-o-war, accidental (unintentional)
- ✓7th T63.612 Toxic effect of contact with Portugese Man-o-war, intentional self-harm
- ✓7th T63.613 Toxic effect of contact with Portugese Man-o-war, assault
- ✓7th T63.614 Toxic effect of contact with Portugese Man-o-war, undetermined

✓6th T63.62 Toxic effect of contact with other jellyfish
- ✓7th T63.621 Toxic effect of contact with other jellyfish, accidental (unintentional)
- ✓7th T63.622 Toxic effect of contact with other jellyfish, intentional self-harm
- ✓7th T63.623 Toxic effect of contact with other jellyfish, assault
- ✓7th T63.624 Toxic effect of contact with other jellyfish, undetermined

✓6th T63.63 Toxic effect of contact with sea anemone
- ✓7th T63.631 Toxic effect of contact with sea anemone, accidental (unintentional)
- ✓7th T63.632 Toxic effect of contact with sea anemone, intentional self-harm
- ✓7th T63.633 Toxic effect of contact with sea anemone, assault
- ✓7th T63.634 Toxic effect of contact with sea anemone, undetermined

✓6th T63.69 Toxic effect of contact with other venomous marine animals
- ✓7th T63.691 Toxic effect of contact with other venomous marine animals, accidental (unintentional)
- ✓7th T63.692 Toxic effect of contact with other venomous marine animals, intentional self-harm
- ✓7th T63.693 Toxic effect of contact with other venomous marine animals, assault
- ✓7th T63.694 Toxic effect of contact with other venomous marine animals, undetermined

✓5th T63.7 Toxic effect of contact with venomous plant

✓6th T63.71 Toxic effect of contact with venomous marine plant
- ✓7th T63.711 Toxic effect of contact with venomous marine plant, accidental (unintentional)
- ✓7th T63.712 Toxic effect of contact with venomous marine plant, intentional self-harm
- ✓7th T63.713 Toxic effect of contact with venomous marine plant, assault
- ✓7th T63.714 Toxic effect of contact with venomous marine plant, undetermined

✓6th T63.79 Toxic effect of contact with other venomous plant
- ✓7th T63.791 Toxic effect of contact with other venomous plant, accidental (unintentional)
- ✓7th T63.792 Toxic effect of contact with other venomous plant, intentional self-harm
- ✓7th T63.793 Toxic effect of contact with other venomous plant, assault
- ✓7th T63.794 Toxic effect of contact with other venomous plant, undetermined

✓5th T63.8 Toxic effect of contact with other venomous animals

✓6th T63.81 Toxic effect of contact with venomous frog
EXCLUDES 1 *contact with nonvenomous frog (W62.0)*
- ✓7th T63.811 Toxic effect of contact with venomous frog, accidental (unintentional)
- ✓7th T63.812 Toxic effect of contact with venomous frog, intentional self-harm
- ✓7th T63.813 Toxic effect of contact with venomous frog, assault
- ✓7th T63.814 Toxic effect of contact with venomous frog, undetermined

✓6th T63.82 Toxic effect of contact with venomous toad
EXCLUDES 1 *contact with nonvenomous toad (W62.1)*
- ✓7th T63.821 Toxic effect of contact with venomous toad, accidental (unintentional)
- ✓7th T63.822 Toxic effect of contact with venomous toad, intentional self-harm
- ✓7th T63.823 Toxic effect of contact with venomous toad, assault
- ✓7th T63.824 Toxic effect of contact with venomous toad, undetermined

✓6th T63.83 Toxic effect of contact with other venomous amphibian
EXCLUDES 1 *contact with nonvenomous amphibian (W62.9)*
- ✓7th T63.831 Toxic effect of contact with other venomous amphibian, accidental (unintentional)

T63.832 Toxic effect of contact with other venomous amphibian, intentional self-harm
T63.833 Toxic effect of contact with other venomous amphibian, assault
T63.834 Toxic effect of contact with other venomous amphibian, undetermined
T63.89 Toxic effect of contact with other venomous animals
T63.891 Toxic effect of contact with other venomous animals, accidental (unintentional)
T63.892 Toxic effect of contact with other venomous animals, intentional self-harm
T63.893 Toxic effect of contact with other venomous animals, assault
T63.894 Toxic effect of contact with other venomous animals, undetermined
T63.9 Toxic effect of contact with unspecified venomous animal
T63.91 Toxic effect of contact with unspecified venomous animal, accidental (unintentional)
T63.92 Toxic effect of contact with unspecified venomous animal, intentional self-harm
T63.93 Toxic effect of contact with unspecified venomous animal, assault
T63.94 Toxic effect of contact with unspecified venomous animal, undetermined

T64 Toxic effect of aflatoxin and other mycotoxin food contaminants

The appropriate 7th character is to be added to each code from category T64.
A initial encounter
D subsequent encounter
S sequela

T64.Ø Toxic effect of aflatoxin
T64.Ø1 Toxic effect of aflatoxin, accidental (unintentional)
T64.Ø2 Toxic effect of aflatoxin, intentional self-harm
T64.Ø3 Toxic effect of aflatoxin, assault
T64.Ø4 Toxic effect of aflatoxin, undetermined
T64.8 Toxic effect of other mycotoxin food contaminants
T64.81 Toxic effect of other mycotoxin food contaminants, accidental (unintentional)
T64.82 Toxic effect of other mycotoxin food contaminants, intentional self-harm
T64.83 Toxic effect of other mycotoxin food contaminants, assault
T64.84 Toxic effect of other mycotoxin food contaminants, undetermined

T65 Toxic effect of other and unspecified substances

The appropriate 7th character is to be added to each code from category T65.
A initial encounter
D subsequent encounter
S sequela

T65.Ø Toxic effect of cyanides
EXCLUDES 1 *hydrogen cyanide (T57.3-)*
T65.ØX Toxic effect of cyanides
T65.ØX1 Toxic effect of cyanides, accidental (unintentional)
Toxic effect of cyanides NOS
T65.ØX2 Toxic effect of cyanides, intentional self-harm
T65.ØX3 Toxic effect of cyanides, assault
T65.ØX4 Toxic effect of cyanides, undetermined
T65.1 Toxic effect of strychnine and its salts
T65.1X Toxic effect of strychnine and its salts
T65.1X1 Toxic effect of strychnine and its salts, accidental (unintentional)
Toxic effect of strychnine and its salts NOS
T65.1X2 Toxic effect of strychnine and its salts, intentional self-harm
T65.1X3 Toxic effect of strychnine and its salts, assault
T65.1X4 Toxic effect of strychnine and its salts, undetermined
T65.2 Toxic effect of tobacco and nicotine
EXCLUDES 2 *nicotine dependence (F17.-)*
T65.21 Toxic effect of chewing tobacco
T65.211 Toxic effect of chewing tobacco, accidental (unintentional)
Toxic effect of chewing tobacco NOS
T65.212 Toxic effect of chewing tobacco, intentional self-harm
T65.213 Toxic effect of chewing tobacco, assault
T65.214 Toxic effect of chewing tobacco, undetermined
T65.22 Toxic effect of tobacco cigarettes
Toxic effect of tobacco smoke
Use additional code for exposure to second hand tobacco smoke (Z57.31, Z77.22)
T65.221 Toxic effect of tobacco cigarettes, accidental (unintentional)
Toxic effect of tobacco cigarettes NOS
T65.222 Toxic effect of tobacco cigarettes, intentional self-harm
T65.223 Toxic effect of tobacco cigarettes, assault
T65.224 Toxic effect of tobacco cigarettes, undetermined
T65.29 Toxic effect of other tobacco and nicotine
T65.291 Toxic effect of other tobacco and nicotine, accidental (unintentional)
Toxic effect of other tobacco and nicotine NOS
T65.292 Toxic effect of other tobacco and nicotine, intentional self-harm
T65.293 Toxic effect of other tobacco and nicotine, assault
T65.294 Toxic effect of other tobacco and nicotine, undetermined
T65.3 Toxic effect of nitroderivatives and aminoderivatives of benzene and its homologues
Toxic effect of anilin [benzenamine]
Toxic effect of nitrobenzene
Toxic effect of trinitrotoluene
T65.3X Toxic effect of nitroderivatives and aminoderivatives of benzene and its homologues
T65.3X1 Toxic effect of nitroderivatives and aminoderivatives of benzene and its homologues, accidental (unintentional)
Toxic effect of nitroderivatives and aminoderivatives of benzene and its homologues NOS
T65.3X2 Toxic effect of nitroderivatives and aminoderivatives of benzene and its homologues, intentional self-harm
T65.3X3 Toxic effect of nitroderivatives and aminoderivatives of benzene and its homologues, assault
T65.3X4 Toxic effect of nitroderivatives and aminoderivatives of benzene and its homologues, undetermined
T65.4 Toxic effect of carbon disulfide
T65.4X Toxic effect of carbon disulfide
T65.4X1 Toxic effect of carbon disulfide, accidental (unintentional)
Toxic effect of carbon disulfide NOS
T65.4X2 Toxic effect of carbon disulfide, intentional self-harm
T65.4X3 Toxic effect of carbon disulfide, assault
T65.4X4 Toxic effect of carbon disulfide, undetermined
T65.5 Toxic effect of nitroglycerin and other nitric acids and esters
Toxic effect of 1,2,3-Propanetriol trinitrate
T65.5X Toxic effect of nitroglycerin and other nitric acids and esters
T65.5X1 Toxic effect of nitroglycerin and other nitric acids and esters, accidental (unintentional)
Toxic effect of nitroglycerin and other nitric acids and esters NOS

T65.5X2 Toxic effect of nitroglycerin and other nitric acids and esters, intentional self-harm

T65.5X3 Toxic effect of nitroglycerin and other nitric acids and esters, assault

T65.5X4 Toxic effect of nitroglycerin and other nitric acids and esters, undetermined

T65.6 Toxic effect of paints and dyes, not elsewhere classified

T65.6X Toxic effect of paints and dyes, not elsewhere classified

T65.6X1 Toxic effect of paints and dyes, not elsewhere classified, accidental (unintentional)
Toxic effect of paints and dyes NOS

T65.6X2 Toxic effect of paints and dyes, not elsewhere classified, intentional self-harm

T65.6X3 Toxic effect of paints and dyes, not elsewhere classified, assault

T65.6X4 Toxic effect of paints and dyes, not elsewhere classified, undetermined

T65.8 Toxic effect of other specified substances

T65.81 Toxic effect of latex

T65.811 Toxic effect of latex, accidental (unintentional)
Toxic effect of latex NOS

T65.812 Toxic effect of latex, intentional self-harm

T65.813 Toxic effect of latex, assault

T65.814 Toxic effect of latex, undetermined

T65.82 Toxic effect of harmful algae and algae toxins
Toxic effect of (harmful) algae bloom NOS
Toxic effect of blue-green algae bloom
Toxic effect of brown tide
Toxic effect of cyanobacteria bloom
Toxic effect of Florida red tide
Toxic effect of pfiesteria piscicida
Toxic effect of red tide

T65.821 Toxic effect of harmful algae and algae toxins, accidental (unintentional)
Toxic effect of harmful algae and algae toxins NOS

T65.822 Toxic effect of harmful algae and algae toxins, intentional self-harm

T65.823 Toxic effect of harmful algae and algae toxins, assault

T65.824 Toxic effect of harmful algae and algae toxins, undetermined

T65.83 Toxic effect of fiberglass

T65.831 Toxic effect of fiberglass, accidental (unintentional)
Toxic effect of fiberglass NOS

T65.832 Toxic effect of fiberglass, intentional self-harm

T65.833 Toxic effect of fiberglass, assault

T65.834 Toxic effect of fiberglass, undetermined

T65.89 Toxic effect of other specified substances

T65.891 Toxic effect of other specified substances, accidental (unintentional)
Toxic effect of other specified substances NOS

T65.892 Toxic effect of other specified substances, intentional self-harm

T65.893 Toxic effect of other specified substances, assault

T65.894 Toxic effect of other specified substances, undetermined

T65.9 Toxic effect of unspecified substance

T65.91 Toxic effect of unspecified substance, accidental (unintentional)
Poisoning NOS

T65.92 Toxic effect of unspecified substance, intentional self-harm

T65.93 Toxic effect of unspecified substance, assault

T65.94 Toxic effect of unspecified substance, undetermined

Other and unspecified effects of external causes (T66-T78)

T66 Radiation sickness, unspecified

EXCLUDES 1 *specified adverse effects of radiation, such as:*
burns (T20-T31)
leukemia (C91-C95)
radiation gastroenteritis and colitis (K52.0)
radiation pneumonitis (J70.0)
radiation related disorders of the skin and subcutaneous tissue (L55-L59)
radiation sunburn (L55.-)

The appropriate 7th character is to be added to code T66.
A initial encounter
D subsequent encounter
S sequela

T67 Effects of heat and light

EXCLUDES 1 *erythema [dermatitis] ab igne (L59.0)*
malignant hyperpyrexia due to anesthesia (T88.3)
radiation-related disorders of the skin and subcutaneous tissue (L55-L59)

EXCLUDES 2 *burns (T20-T31)*
sunburn (L55.-)
sweat disorder due to heat (L74-L75)

The appropriate 7th character is to be added to each code from category T67.
A initial encounter
D subsequent encounter
S sequela

7 **T67.0 Heatstroke and sunstroke** CC
Heat apoplexy
Heat pyrexia
Siriasis
Thermoplegia
Use additional code(s) to identify any associated complications of heatstroke, such as:
coma and stupor (R40.-)
systemic inflammatory response syndrome (R65.1-)
CC Excl: CC with 7th character A:T67.[0-9]XXA

T67.1 Heat syncope
Heat collapse

T67.2 Heat cramp

T67.3 Heat exhaustion, anhydrotic
Heat prostration due to water depletion
EXCLUDES 1 *heat exhaustion due to salt depletion (T67.4)*

T67.4 Heat exhaustion due to salt depletion
Heat prostration due to salt (and water) depletion

T67.5 Heat exhaustion, unspecified
Heat prostration NOS

T67.6 Heat fatigue, transient

T67.7 Heat edema

T67.8 Other effects of heat and light

T67.9 Effect of heat and light, unspecified

T68 Hypothermia
Accidental hypothermia
Hypothermia NOS
Use additional code to identify source of exposure:
exposure to excessive cold of man-made origin (W93)
exposure to excessive cold of natural origin (X31)

EXCLUDES 1 *hypothermia following anesthesia (T88.51)*
hypothermia not associated with low environmental temperature (R68.0)
hypothermia of newborn (P80.-)

EXCLUDES 2 *frostbite (T33-T34)*

The appropriate 7th character is to be added to code T68.
A initial encounter
D subsequent encounter
S sequela

7 HAC = Initial encounter only (7th character A, B or C) and not POA.

T69 Other effects of reduced temperature

Use additional code to identify source of exposure:
exposure to excessive cold of man-made origin (W93)
exposure to excessive cold of natural origin (X31)

EXCLUDES 2 *frostbite (T33-T34)*

The appropriate 7th character is to be added to each code from category T69.
A initial encounter
D subsequent encounter
S sequela

T69.0 Immersion hand and foot

T69.01 Immersion hand

T69.011 Immersion hand, right hand

T69.012 Immersion hand, left hand

T69.019 Immersion hand, unspecified hand

T69.02 Immersion foot

Trench foot

CC Excl: For CC codes in subcategory T69.02: CC with 7th character A, unless otherwise noted: T33.2XX-T33.42X with 7th A, T33.60X-T33.72X with 7th A, T33.90X-T33.99X with 7th A, T34.2XX-T34.42X with 7th A, T34.60X-T34.72X with 7th A, T34.90X-T34.99X with 7th A, T69.021-T69.029 with 7th A

7 **T69.021 Immersion foot, right foot** CC

7 **T69.022 Immersion foot, left foot** CC

7 **T69.029 Immersion foot, unspecified foot** CC

T69.1 Chilblains

T69.8 Other specified effects of reduced temperature

T69.9 Effect of reduced temperature, unspecified

T70 Effects of air pressure and water pressure

The appropriate 7th character is to be added to each code from category T70.
A initial encounter
D subsequent encounter
S sequela

T70.0 Otitic barotrauma

Aero-otitis media
Effects of change in ambient atmospheric pressure or water pressure on ears

T70.1 Sinus barotrauma

Aerosinusitis
Effects of change in ambient atmospheric pressure on sinuses

T70.2 Other and unspecified effects of high altitude

EXCLUDES 2 *polycythemia due to high altitude (D75.1)*

T70.20 Unspecified effects of high altitude

T70.29 Other effects of high altitude

Alpine sickness
Anoxia due to high altitude
Barotrauma NOS
Hypobaropathy
Mountain sickness

7 **T70.3 Caisson disease [decompression sickness]** CC

Compressed-air disease
Diver's palsy or paralysis
CC Excl: CC with 7th character A:T70.3XX-T70.9XX with 7th A

T70.4 Effects of high-pressure fluids

Hydraulic jet injection (industrial)
Pneumatic jet injection (industrial)
Traumatic jet injection (industrial)

T70.8 Other effects of air pressure and water pressure

T70.9 Effect of air pressure and water pressure, unspecified

T71 Asphyxiation

Mechanical suffocation
Traumatic suffocation

EXCLUDES 1 *acute respiratory distress (syndrome) (J80)*
anoxia due to high altitude (T70.2)
asphyxia NOS (R09.01)
asphyxia from carbon monoxide (T58.-)
asphyxia from inhalation of food or foreign body (T17.-)
asphyxia from other gases, fumes and vapors (T59.-)
respiratory distress (syndrome) in newborn (P22.-)

The appropriate 7th character is to be added to each code from category T71.
A initial encounter
D subsequent encounter
S sequela

CC Excl: For CC codes in category T71: CC with 7th character A, unless otherwise noted: T71.111-T71.9XX with 7th A

T71.1 Asphyxiation due to mechanical threat to breathing

Suffocation due to mechanical threat to breathing

T71.11 Asphyxiation due to smothering under pillow

7 **T71.111 Asphyxiation due to smothering under pillow, accidental** CC

Asphyxiation due to smothering under pillow NOS

7 **T71.112 Asphyxiation due to smothering under pillow, intentional self-harm** CC

7 **T71.113 Asphyxiation due to smothering under pillow, assault** CC

7 **T71.114 Asphyxiation due to smothering under pillow, undetermined** CC

T71.12 Asphyxiation due to plastic bag

7 **T71.121 Asphyxiation due to plastic bag, accidental** CC

Asphyxiation due to plastic bag NOS

7 **T71.122 Asphyxiation due to plastic bag, intentional self-harm** CC

7 **T71.123 Asphyxiation due to plastic bag, assault** CC

7 **T71.124 Asphyxiation due to plastic bag, undetermined** CC

T71.13 Asphyxiation due to being trapped in bed linens

7 **T71.131 Asphyxiation due to being trapped in bed linens, accidental** CC

Asphyxiation due to being trapped in bed linens NOS

7 **T71.132 Asphyxiation due to being trapped in bed linens, intentional self-harm** CC

7 **T71.133 Asphyxiation due to being trapped in bed linens, assault** CC

7 **T71.134 Asphyxiation due to being trapped in bed linens, undetermined** CC

T71.14 Asphyxiation due to smothering under another person's body (in bed)

7 **T71.141 Asphyxiation due to smothering under another person's body (in bed), accidental** CC

Asphyxiation due to smothering under another person's body (in bed) NOS

7 **T71.143 Asphyxiation due to smothering under another person's body (in bed), assault** CC

7 **T71.144 Asphyxiation due to smothering under another person's body (in bed), undetermined** CC

T71.15 Asphyxiation due to smothering in furniture

7 **T71.151 Asphyxiation due to smothering in furniture, accidental** CC

Asphyxiation due to smothering in furniture NOS

7 **T71.152 Asphyxiation due to smothering in furniture, intentional self-harm** CC

7 **T71.153 Asphyxiation due to smothering in furniture, assault** CC

7 **T71.154 Asphyxiation due to smothering in furniture, undetermined** CC

DRAFT

7 HAC = Initial encounter only (7th character A, B or C) and not POA.

T71.16 Asphyxiation due to hanging
Hanging by window shade cord
Use additional code for any associated injuries, such as:
crushing injury of neck (S17.-)
fracture of cervical vertebrae (S12.Ø-S12.2-)
open wound of neck (S11.-)

7 **T71.161 Asphyxiation due to hanging, accidental** CC
Asphyxiation due to hanging NOS
Hanging NOS

7 **T71.162 Asphyxiation due to hanging, intentional self-harm** CC

7 **T71.163 Asphyxiation due to hanging, assault** CC

7 **T71.164 Asphyxiation due to hanging, undetermined** CC

T71.19 Asphyxiation due to mechanical threat to breathing due to other causes

7 **T71.191 Asphyxiation due to mechanical threat to breathing due to other causes, accidental** CC
Asphyxiation due to other causes NOS

7 **T71.192 Asphyxiation due to mechanical threat to breathing due to other causes, intentional self-harm** CC

7 **T71.193 Asphyxiation due to mechanical threat to breathing due to other causes, assault** CC

7 **T71.194 Asphyxiation due to mechanical threat to breathing due to other causes, undetermined** CC

T71.2 Asphyxiation due to systemic oxygen deficiency due to low oxygen content in ambient air
Suffocation due to systemic oxygen deficiency due to low oxygen content in ambient air

7 **T71.2Ø Asphyxiation due to systemic oxygen deficiency due to low oxygen content in ambient air due to unspecified cause** CC

7 **T71.21 Asphyxiation due to cave-in or falling earth** CC
Use additional code for any associated cataclysm (X34-X38)

T71.22 Asphyxiation due to being trapped in a car trunk

T71.221 Asphyxiation due to being trapped in a car trunk, accidental CC

T71.222 Asphyxiation due to being trapped in a car trunk, intentional self-harm CC

T71.223 Asphyxiation due to being trapped in a car trunk, assault CC

T71.224 Asphyxiation due to being trapped in a car trunk, undetermined CC

T71.23 Asphyxiation due to being trapped in a (discarded) refrigerator

T71.231 Asphyxiation due to being trapped in a (discarded) refrigerator, accidental CC

T71.232 Asphyxiation due to being trapped in a (discarded) refrigerator, intentional self-harm CC

T71.233 Asphyxiation due to being trapped in a (discarded) refrigerator, assault CC

T71.234 Asphyxiation due to being trapped in a (discarded) refrigerator, undetermined CC

7 **T71.29 Asphyxiation due to being trapped in other low oxygen environment** CC

7 **T71.9 Asphyxiation due to unspecified cause** CC
Suffocation (by strangulation) due to unspecified cause
Suffocation NOS
Systemic oxygen deficiency due to low oxygen content in ambient air due to unspecified cause
Systemic oxygen deficiency due to mechanical threat to breathing due to unspecified cause
Traumatic asphyxia NOS

T73 Effects of other deprivation

The appropriate 7th character is to be added to each code from category T73.
A initial encounter
D subsequent encounter
S sequela

T73.Ø Starvation
Deprivation of food

T73.1 Deprivation of water

T73.2 Exhaustion due to exposure

T73.3 Exhaustion due to excessive exertion
Exhaustion due to overexertion

T73.8 Other effects of deprivation

T73.9 Effect of deprivation, unspecified

T74 Adult and child abuse, neglect and other maltreatment, confirmed
Use additional code, if applicable, to identify any associated current injury
Use additional external cause code to identify perpetrator, if known (YØ7.-)
EXCLUDES 1 *abuse and maltreatment in pregnancy (O9A.3-, O9A.4-, O9A.5-)*
adult and child maltreatment, suspected (T76.-)

The appropriate 7th character is to be added to each code from category T74.
A initial encounter
D subsequent encounter
S sequela

CC Excl: For CC codes in category T74: CC with 7th character A, unless otherwise noted: T74.Ø1X-T74.92X with 7th A, T76.Ø1X-T76.92X with 7th A

T74.Ø Neglect or abandonment, confirmed

T74.Ø1 Adult neglect or abandonment, confirmed CC A

T74.Ø2 Child neglect or abandonment, confirmed CC P

T74.1 Physical abuse, confirmed
EXCLUDES 2 *sexual abuse (T74.2-)*

T74.11 Adult physical abuse, confirmed CC A

T74.12 Child physical abuse, confirmed CC P
EXCLUDES 2 *shaken infant syndrome (T74.4)*

T74.2 Sexual abuse, confirmed
Rape, confirmed
Sexual assault, confirmed

T74.21 Adult sexual abuse, confirmed CC A

T74.22 Child sexual abuse, confirmed CC P

T74.3 Psychological abuse, confirmed

T74.31 Adult psychological abuse, confirmed A

T74.32 Child psychological abuse, confirmed CC P

T74.4 Shaken infant syndrome CC P

T74.9 Unspecified maltreatment, confirmed

T74.91 Unspecified adult maltreatment, confirmed CC A
CC Excl: CC with 7th character A: T74.91X A, T76.91XA

T74.92 Unspecified child maltreatment, confirmed CC P
CC Excl: CC with 7th character A: T74.Ø1X-T74.92X with 7th A, T76.Ø1X-T76.92X with 7th A

T75 Other and unspecified effects of other external causes
EXCLUDES 1 *adverse effects NEC (T78.-)*
EXCLUDES 2 *burns (electric) (T2Ø-T31)*

The appropriate 7th character is to be added to each code from category T75.
A initial encounter
D subsequent encounter
S sequela

T75.Ø Effects of lightning
Struck by lightning

T75.ØØ Unspecified effects of lightning
Struck by lightning NOS

T75.Ø1 Shock due to being struck by lightning

T75.Ø9 Other effects of lightning
Use additional code for other effects of lightning

7 HAC = Initial encounter only (7th character A, B or C) and not POA.

7 √x7th **T75.1 Unspecified effects of drowning and nonfatal submersion** CC
Immersion
EXCLUDES 1 *specified effects of drowning—code to effects*
CC Excl: CC with 7th character A:T75.1XXA

√5th **T75.2 Effects of vibration**
√x7th **T75.20 Unspecified effects of vibration**
√x7th **T75.21 Pneumatic hammer syndrome**
√x7th **T75.22 Traumatic vasospastic syndrome**
√x7th **T75.23 Vertigo from infrasound**
EXCLUDES 1 *vertigo NOS (R42)*
T75.29 Other effects of vibration

√x7th **T75.3 Motion sickness**
Airsickness
Seasickness
Travel sickness
Use additional external cause code to identify vehicle or type of motion (Y92.81-, Y93.5-)

√x7th **T75.4 Electrocution**
Shock from electric current
Shock from electroshock gun (taser)

√5th **T75.8 Other specified effects of external causes**
√x7th **T75.81 Effects of abnormal gravitation [G] forces**
√x7th **T75.82 Effects of weightlessness**
√x7th **T75.89 Other specified effects of external causes**

√4th **T76 Adult and child abuse, neglect and other maltreatment, suspected**
Use additional code, if applicable, to identify any associated current injury
EXCLUDES 1 *adult and child maltreatment, confirmed (T74.-)*
suspected abuse and maltreatment in pregnancy (O9A.3-, O9A.4-, O9A.5-)
suspected adult physical and sexual abuse, ruled out (Z04.71)
suspected adult sexual abused, ruled out (Z04.41)
suspected child physical abuse, ruled out (Z04.72)
suspected child sexual abuse, ruled out (Z04.42)

The appropriate 7th character is to be added to each code from category T76.
A initial encounter
D subsequent encounter
S sequela

CC Excl: For CC codes in category T76: CC with 7th character A, unless otherwise noted: T74.01X-T74.92X with 7th A, T76.01X-T76.92X with 7th A

√5th **T76.0 Neglect or abandonment, suspected**
√x7th **T76.01 Adult neglect or abandonment, suspected** CC A
√x7th **T76.02 Child neglect or abandonment, suspected** CC P

√5th **T76.1 Physical abuse, suspected**
√x7th **T76.11 Adult physical abuse, suspected** CC A
√x7th **T76.12 Child physical abuse, suspected** CC P

√5th **T76.2 Sexual abuse, suspected**
Rape, suspected
Sexual abuse, suspected
EXCLUDES 1 *alleged abuse, ruled out (Z04.7)*
√x7th **T76.21 Adult sexual abuse, suspected** CC A
√x7th **T76.22 Child sexual abuse, suspected** CC P

√5th **T76.3 Psychological abuse, suspected**
√x7th **T76.31 Adult psychological abuse, suspected** A
√x7th **T76.32 Child psychological abuse, suspected** CC P

√5th **T76.9 Unspecified maltreatment, suspected**
√x7th **T76.91 Unspecified adult maltreatment, suspected** CC A
CC Excl: CC with 7th character A: T74.91XA, T76.91XA
√x7th **T76.92 Unspecified child maltreatment, suspected** CC P
CC Excl: CC with 7th character A: T74.01-T74.92 with 7th A, T76.01-T76.92 with 7th A

T78 Adverse effects, not elsewhere classified
EXCLUDES 2 *complications of surgical and medical care NEC (T80-T88)*

The appropriate 7th character is to be added to each code from category T78.
A initial encounter
D subsequent encounter
S sequela

CC Excl: For CC codes in category T78: CC with 7th character A,unless otherwise noted: T78.00X-T78.09X with 7th A

√5th **T78.0 Anaphylactic reaction due to food**
Anaphylactic reaction due to adverse food reaction
Anaphylactic shock or reaction due to nonpoisonous foods
Anaphylactoid reaction due to food
√x7th **T78.00 Anaphylactic reaction due to unspecified food** CC
√x7th **T78.01 Anaphylactic reaction due to peanuts** CC
√x7th **T78.02 Anaphylactic reaction due to shellfish (crustaceans)** CC
√x7th **T78.03 Anaphylactic reaction due to other fish** CC
√x7th **T78.04 Anaphylactic reaction due to fruits and vegetables** CC
√x7th **T78.05 Anaphylactic reaction due to tree nuts and seeds** CC
EXCLUDES 1 *anaphylactic reaction due to peanuts (T78.01)*
√x7th **T78.06 Anaphylactic reaction due to food additives** CC
√x7th **T78.07 Anaphylactic reaction due to milk and dairy products** CC
√x7th **T78.08 Anaphylactic reaction due to eggs** CC
√x7th **T78.09 Anaphylactic reaction due to other food products** CC

√x7th **T78.1 Other adverse food reactions, not elsewhere classified**
Use additional code to identify the type of reaction
EXCLUDES 1 *anaphylactic reaction or shock due to adverse food reaction (T78.0-)*
anaphylactic reaction due to food (T78.0-)
bacterial food borne intoxications (A05.-)
EXCLUDES 2 *allergic and dietetic gastroenteritis and colitis (K52.2)*
allergic rhinitis due to food (J30.5)
dermatitis due to food in contact with skin (L23.6, L24.6, L25.4)
dermatitis due to ingested food (L27.2)

√x7th **T78.2 Anaphylactic shock, unspecified** CC
Allergic shock
Anaphylactic reaction
Anaphylaxis
EXCLUDES 1 *anaphylactic reaction or shock due to adverse effect of correct medicinal substance properly administered (T88.6)*
anaphylactic reaction or shock due to adverse food reaction (T78.0-)
anaphylactic reaction or shock due to serum (T80.5-)

√x7th **T78.3 Angioneurotic edema**
Allergic angioedema
Giant urticaria
Quincke's edema
EXCLUDES 1 *serum urticaria (T80.6-)*
urticaria (L50.-)

√5th **T78.4 Other and unspecified allergy**
EXCLUDES 1 *specified types of allergic reaction such as:*
allergic diarrhea (K52.2)
allergic gastroenteritis and colitis (K52.2)
dermatitis (L23-L25, L27-)
hay fever (J30.1)
√x7th **T78.40 Allergy, unspecified**
Allergic reaction NOS
Hypersensitivity NOS
√x7th **T78.41 Arthus phenomenon**
Arthus reaction
√x7th **T78.49 Other allergy**

√x7th **T78.8 Other adverse effects, not elsewhere classified**

7 HAC = Initial encounter only (7th character A, B or C) and not POA.

Certain early complications of trauma (T79)

✓4th T79 Certain early complications of trauma, not elsewhere classified

EXCLUDES 2 *acute respiratory distress syndrome (J8Ø)*
complications occurring during or following medical procedures (T8Ø-T88)
complications of surgical and medical care NEC (T8Ø-T88)
newborn respiratory distress syndrome (P22.Ø)

The appropriate 7th character is to be added to each code from category T79.
A initial encounter
D subsequent encounter
S sequela

✓x7th T79.Ø Air embolism (traumatic) MCC

EXCLUDES 1 *air embolism complicating abortion or ectopic or molar pregnancy (OØØ-OØ7, OØ8.2)*
air embolism complicating pregnancy, childbirth and the puerperium (O88.Ø)
air embolism following infusion, transfusion, and therapeutic injection (T8Ø.Ø)
air embolism following procedure NEC (T81.7-)

CC Excl: MCC with 7th A: D78.81-D78.89, E36.8, E89.81Ø-E89.89, H59.Ø11-H59.Ø19, H59.Ø31-H59.Ø99, H59.811-H59.89, H95.811-H95.89, I97.3, L76.81-L76.82, M96.89, N98.1-N98.9, T14.8-T14.91, T79.ØXXA, T79.AØX-T8Ø.ØXX with 7th A, T81.82XA, T81.89X-T81.9XX with 7th A

✓x7th T79.1 Fat embolism (traumatic) MCC

EXCLUDES 1 *fat embolism complicating:*
abortion or ectopic or molar pregnancy (OØØ-OØ7, OØ8.2)
pregnancy, childbirth and the puerperium (O88.8)

CC Excl: MCC with 7th A: D78.81-D78.89, E36.8, E89.81Ø-E89.89, H59.Ø11-H59.Ø19, H59.Ø31-H59.Ø99, H59.811-H59.89, H95.811-H95.89, I97.3, L76.81-L76.82, M96.89, N98.1-N98.9, T14.8-T14.91, T79.1XXA, T79.AØX-T79.9XX with 7th A, T81.82XA, T81.89X-T81.9XX with 7th A

✓x7th T79.2 Traumatic secondary and recurrent hemorrhage and seroma CC

CC Excl: CC with 7th character A: D78.81-D78.89, E36.8, E89.81Ø-E89.89, H59.Ø11-H59.Ø19, H59.Ø31-H59.Ø99, H59.811-H59.89, H95.811-H95.89, I97.3, L76.81-L76.82, M96.89, N98.1-N98.9, T14.8-T14.91, T79.2XXA, T79.AØX-T79.9XX with 7th A, T81.82XA, T81.89X-T81.9XX with 7th A

✓x7th T79.4 Traumatic shock MCC

Shock (immediate) (delayed) following injury

EXCLUDES 1 *anaphylactic shock due to adverse food reaction (T78.Ø-)*
anaphylactic shock due to correct medicinal substance properly administered (T88.6)
anaphylactic shock due to serum (T8Ø.5-)
anaphylactic shock NOS (T78.2)
anesthetic shock (T88.2)
electric shock (T75.4)
nontraumatic shock NEC (R57.-)
obstetric shock (O75.1)
postprocedural shock (T81.1-)
septic shock (R65.21)
shock complicating abortion or ectopic or molar pregnancy (OØØ-OØ7, OØ8.3)
shock due to lightning (T75.Ø1)
shock NOS (R57.9)

CC Excl: MCC with 7th A: D78.81-D78.89, E36.8, E89.81Ø-E89.89, H59.Ø11-H59.Ø19, H59.Ø31-H59.Ø99, H59.811-H59.89, H95.811-H95.89, I97.3, L76.81-L76.82, M96.89, N98.1-N98.9, T14.8-T14.91, T79.4XXA, T79.AØX-T79.9XX with 7th A, T81.82XA, T81.89X-T81.9XX with 7th A

✓x7th T79.5 Traumatic anuria MCC

Crush syndrome
Renal failure following crushing

CC Excl: MCC with 7th A: D78.Ø1-D78.Ø2, D78.21-D78.89, E36.Ø1-E36.Ø2, E36.8, E89.81Ø-E89.89, G97.51-G97.52, H59.Ø11-H59.Ø19, H59.Ø31-H59.129, H59.311-H59.329, H59.811-H59.89, H95.21-H95.22, H95.41-H95.89, I97.3-I97.42, I97.61Ø-I97.62, J95.61-J95.62, J95.83Ø-J95.831, K91.61-K91.62, K91.84Ø-K91.841, L76.Ø1-L76.Ø2, L76.21-L76.82, M96.81Ø-M96.811, M96.83Ø-M96.89, N98.1-N98.9, N99.61-N99.62, N99.82Ø-N99.821, T14.8-T14.91, T79.5XXA, T79.AØX-T79.9XX with 7th A, T81.1ØX-T81.19X with 7th A, T81.82XA, T81.89X-T81.9XX with 7th A, T88.2XXA

✓x7th T79.6 Traumatic ischemia of muscle

Traumatic rhabdomyolysis
Volkmann's ischemic contracture

EXCLUDES 2 *anterior tibial syndrome (M76.8)*
compartment syndrome (traumatic) (T79.A-)
nontraumatic ischemia of muscle (M62.2-)

✓x7th T79.7 Traumatic subcutaneous emphysema CC

EXCLUDES 1 *emphysema NOS (J43)*
emphysema (subcutaneous) resulting from a procedure (T81.82)

CC Excl: CC with 7th character A: D78.81-D78.89, E36.8, E89.81Ø-E89.89, H59.Ø11-H59.Ø19, H59.Ø31-H59.Ø99, H59.811-H59.89, H95.811-H95.89, I97.3, L76.81-L76.82, M96.89, N98.1-N98.9, S21.1Ø1-S21.159 with 7th A, S21.3Ø1-S21.95X with 7th A, S27.ØXX-S27.399 with 7th A, S27.5ØX-S27.8Ø9 with 7th A, S27.892-S27.9XX with 7th A, S28.1XXA, S29.Ø21A, S29.Ø29A, T14.8-T14.91, T79.7XX-T79.9XX with 7th A, T81.82A, T81.89X-T81.9XX with 7th A

✓5th T79.A Traumatic compartment syndrome

EXCLUDES 1 *fibromyalgia (M79.7)*
nontraumatic compartment syndrome (M79.A-)
traumatic ischemic infarction of muscle (T79.6)

✓x7th T79.AØ Compartment syndrome, unspecified CC

Compartment syndrome NOS

CC Excl: CC with 7th character A: S31.ØØ1A, S31.Ø11A, S31.Ø21A, S31.Ø31A, S31.Ø41A, S31.Ø51A, S31.6ØØ-S31.659 with 7th A, S36.81X-S36.899 with 7th A

✓6th T79.A1 Traumatic compartment syndrome of upper extremity

Traumatic compartment syndrome of shoulder, arm, forearm, wrist, hand, and fingers

CC Excl: For CC codes in category T79.A1: CC with 7th character A,unless otherwise noted: M7Ø.8Ø-M7Ø.99, M79.81-M79.9, R29.898

✓7th T79.A11 Traumatic compartment syndrome of right upper extremity CC

✓7th T79.A12 Traumatic compartment syndrome of left upper extremity CC

✓7th T79.A19 Traumatic compartment syndrome of unspecified upper extremity CC

✓6th T79.A2 Traumatic compartment syndrome of lower extremity

Traumatic compartment syndrome of hip, buttock, thigh, leg, foot, and toes

CC Excl: For CC codes in category T79.A2 : CC with 7th character A, unless otherwise noted: See code: T79.A1

✓7th T79.A21 Traumatic compartment syndrome of right lower extremity CC

✓7th T79.A22 Traumatic compartment syndrome of left lower extremity CC

✓7th T79.A29 Traumatic compartment syndrome of unspecified lower extremity CC

✓x7th T79.A3 Traumatic compartment syndrome of abdomen CC

CC Excl: CC with 7th character A: S31.ØØ1A, S31.Ø11A, S31.Ø21A, S31.Ø31A, S31.Ø41A, S31.Ø51-S31.159 with 7th A, S31.6ØØ-S31.659 with 7th A, S31.831-S31.839 with 7th A, S36.ØØX-S37.99X with 7th A, S38.3XX-S39.Ø23 with 7th A, T14.8-T14.91, T79.8XX-T79.9XX with 7th A

✓x7th T79.A9 Traumatic compartment syndrome of other sites CC

CC Excl: CC with 7th character A: S31.ØØ1A, S31.Ø11A, S31.Ø21A, S31.Ø31A, S31.Ø41A, S31.Ø51A, S31.6ØØ-S31.659 with 7th A, S36.81X-S36.899 with 7th A

✓x7th T79.8 Other early complications of trauma

✓x7th T79.9 Unspecified early complication of trauma

Complications of surgical and medical care, not elsewhere classified (T8Ø-T88)

Use additional code for adverse effect, if applicable, to identify drug (T36-T5Ø with fifth or sixth character 5)

Use additional code(s) to identify the specified condition resulting from the complication

Use additional code to identify devices involved and details of circumstances (Y62-Y82)

EXCLUDES 2 *any encounters with medical care for postprocedural conditions in which no complications are present, such as:*
artificial opening status (Z93.-)
closure of external stoma (Z43.-)
fitting and adjustment of external prosthetic device (Z44.-)
burns and corrosions from local applications and irradiation (T2Ø-T32)
complications of surgical procedures during pregnancy, childbirth and the puerperium (OØØ-O9A)
mechanical complication of respirator [ventilator] (J95.85Ø)
poisoning and toxic effects of drugs and chemicals (T36-T65 with fifth or sixth character 1-4 or 6)
postprocedural fever (R5Ø.82)
specified complications classified elsewhere, such as:
cerebrospinal fluid leak from spinal puncture (G97.Ø)
colostomy malfunction (K94.Ø-)
disorders of fluid and electrolyte imbalance (E86-E87)
functional disturbances following cardiac surgery (I97.Ø-I97.1)
intraoperative and postprocedural complications of specified body systems (D78.-, E36.-, E89.-, G97.3-, G97.4, H59.3-, H59.-, H95.2-, H95.3, I97.4-, I97.5, J95.6-, J95.7, K91.6-, L76.-, M96.-, N99.-)
ostomy complications (J95.Ø-, K94-, N99.5-)
postgastric surgery syndromes (K91.1)
postlaminectomy syndrome NEC (M96.1)
postmastectomy lymphedema syndrome (I97.2)
postsurgical blind-loop syndrome (K91.2)
ventilator associated pneumonia (J95.851)

√4th **T8Ø Complications following infusion, transfusion and therapeutic injection**

INCLUDES complications following perfusion

EXCLUDES 2 *bone marrow transplant rejection (T86.Ø1)*
febrile nonhemolytic transfusion reaction (R5Ø.84)
fluid overload due to transfusion (E87.71)
posttransfusion purpura (D69.51)
transfusion associated circulatory overload (TACO) (E87.71)
transfusion (red blood cell) associated hemochromatosis (E83.111)
transfusion related acute lung injury (TRALI) (J95.84)

The appropriate 7th character is to be added to each code from category T8Ø.
A initial encounter
D subsequent encounter
S sequela

7 √x7th **T8Ø.Ø Air embolism following infusion, transfusion and therapeutic injection** MCC
CC Excl: MCC with 7th A: T79.ØXXA, T8Ø.ØXXA

√x7th **T8Ø.1 Vascular complications following infusion, transfusion and therapeutic injection** CC
Use additional code to identify the vascular complication
EXCLUDES 2 *extravasation of vesicant agent (T8Ø.81-)*
infiltration of vesicant agent (T8Ø.81-)
postprocedural vascular complications (T81.7-)
vascular complications specified as due to prosthetic devices, implants and grafts (T82.8-, T83.8, T84.8-, T85.8)
CC Excl: CC with 7th character A: T8Ø.1XXA, T8Ø.81Ø-T8Ø.818 with 7th A, T8Ø.9ØXA

√5th **T8Ø.2 Infections following infusion, transfusion and therapeutic injection**
Use additional code to identify the specific infection, such as: sepsis (A41.9)
Use additional code (R65.2-) to identify severe sepsis, if applicable
EXCLUDES 2 *infections specified as due to prosthetic devices, implants and grafts (T82.6-T82.7, T83.5-T83.6, T84.5-T84.7, T85.7)*
postprocedural infections (T81.4)

CC Excl: For CC codes in subcategory T8Ø.2: CC with 7th character A, unless otherwise noted: N98.Ø, T8Ø.211-T8Ø.29X with 7th A, T82.7XXA, T88.ØXXA

√6th **T8Ø.21 Infection due to central venous catheter**

7 √7th **T8Ø.211 Bloodstream infection due to central venous catheter** CC
Catheter-related bloodstream infection (CRBSI) NOS
Central line-associated bloodstream infection (CLABSI)
Bloodstream infection due to Hickman catheter
Bloodstream infection due to peripherally inserted central catheter (PICC)
Bloodstream infection due to portacath (port-a-cath)
Bloodstream infection due to triple lumen catheter
Bloodstream infection due to umbilical venous catheter

7 √7th **T8Ø.212 Local infection due to central venous catheter** CC
Exit or insertion site infection
Local infection due to Hickman catheter
Local infection due to peripherally inserted central catheter (PICC)
Local infection due to portacath (port-a-cath)
Local infection due to triple lumen catheter
Local infection due to umbilical venous catheter
Port or reservoir infection
Tunnel infection

7 √7th **T8Ø.218 Other infection due to central venous catheter** CC
Other central line-associated infection
Other infection due to Hickman catheter
Other infection due to peripherally inserted central catheter (PICC)
Other infection due to portacath (port-a-cath)
Other infection due to triple lumen catheter
Other infection due to umbilical venous catheter

7 √7th **T8Ø.219 Unspecified infection due to central venous catheter** CC
Central line-associated infection NOS
Unspecified infection due to Hickman catheter
Unspecified infection due to peripherally inserted central catheter (PICC)
Unspecified infection due to portacath (port-a-cath)
Unspecified infection due to triple lumen catheter
Unspecified infection due to umbilical venous catheter

√x7th **T8Ø.22 Acute infection following transfusion, infusion, or injection of blood and blood products** CC

√x7th **T8Ø.29 Infection following other infusion, transfusion and therapeutic injection** CC

√5th **T8Ø.3 ABO incompatibility reaction due to transfusion of blood or blood products**
EXCLUDES 1 *minor blood group antigens reactions (Duffy) (E) (K(ell)) (Kidd) (Lewis) (M) (N) (P) (S) (T8Ø.A)*

CC Excl: CC Excl: For CC/MCC codes in subcategory T8Ø.3: CC with 7th character A, unless otherwise noted: T8Ø.3ØX-T8Ø.A9X with 7th A, T8Ø.91Ø-T8Ø.92X with 7th A

7 √x7th **T8Ø.3Ø ABO incompatibility reaction due to transfusion of blood or blood products, unspecified** CC
ABO incompatibility blood transfusion NOS
Reaction to ABO incompatibility from transfusion NOS

√6th **T8Ø.31 ABO incompatibility with hemolytic transfusion reaction**

7 √7th **T8Ø.31Ø ABO incompatibility with acute hemolytic transfusion reaction** CC
ABO incompatibility with hemolytic transfusion reaction less than 24 hours after transfusion
Acute hemolytic transfusion reaction (AHTR) due to ABO incompatibility

7 HAC = Initial encounter only (7th character A, B or C) and not POA.

7 ✓7th **T80.311 ABO incompatibility with delayed hemolytic transfusion reaction** CC
ABO incompatibility with hemolytic transfusion reaction 24 hours or more after transfusion
Delayed hemolytic transfusion reaction (DHTR) due to ABO incompatibility

7 ✓7th **T80.319 ABO incompatibility with hemolytic transfusion reaction, unspecified** CC
ABO incompatibility with hemolytic transfusion reaction at unspecified time after transfusion
Hemolytic transfusion reaction (HTR) due to ABO incompatibility NOS

7 ✓x7th **T80.39 Other ABO incompatibility reaction due to transfusion of blood or blood products** CC
Delayed serologic transfusion reaction (DSTR) from ABO incompatibility
Other ABO incompatible blood transfusion
Other reaction to ABO incompatible blood transfusion

✓x7th **T80.4 Rh incompatibility reaction due to transfusion of blood or blood products**
Reaction due to incompatibility of Rh antigens (C) (c) (D) (E) (e)

CC Excl: For CC/MCC codes in subcategory T80.4: CC with 7th character A, unless otherwise noted: See code: T80.3

✓x7th **T80.40 Rh incompatibility reaction due to transfusion of blood or blood products, unspecified** CC
Reaction due to Rh factor in transfusion NOS
Rh incompatible blood transfusion NOS

✓6th **T80.41 Rh incompatibility with hemolytic transfusion reaction**

✓7th **T80.410 Rh incompatibility with acute hemolytic transfusion reaction** CC
Acute hemolytic transfusion reaction (AHTR) due to Rh incompatibility
Rh incompatibility with hemolytic transfusion reaction less than 24 hours after transfusion

✓7th **T80.411 Rh incompatibility with delayed hemolytic transfusion reaction** CC
Delayed hemolytic transfusion reaction (DHTR) due to Rh incompatibility
Rh incompatibility with hemolytic transfusion reaction 24 hours or more after transfusion

✓7th **T80.419 Rh incompatibility with hemolytic transfusion reaction, unspecified** CC
Hemolytic transfusion reaction (HTR) due to Rh incompatibility NOS
Rh incompatibility with hemolytic transfusion reaction at unspecified time after transfusion

✓x7th **T80.49 Other Rh incompatibility reaction due to transfusion of blood or blood products** CC
Delayed serologic transfusion reaction (DSTR) from Rh incompatibility
Other reaction to Rh incompatible blood transfusion
CC Excl: CC with 7th character A: T80.30X-T80.419 with 7th A, T80.A9XA, T80.910-T80.92X with 7th A

✓5th **T80.A Non-ABO incompatibility reaction due to transfusion of blood or blood products**
Reaction due to incompatibility of minor antigens (Duffy) (Kell) (Kidd) (Lewis) (M) (N) (P) (S)

✓x7th **T80.A0 Non-ABO incompatibility reaction due to transfusion of blood or blood products, unspecified** CC
Non-ABO antigen incompatibility reaction from transfusion NOS
CC Excl: CC with 7th character A, unless otherwise noted: T80.30X-T80.419 with 7th A, T80.A9XA, T80.910-T80.92X with 7th A

✓6th **T80.A1 Non-ABO incompatibility with hemolytic transfusion reaction**

CC Excl: For CC codes in subcategory T80.A1: CC with 7th character A, unless otherwise noted: See code: T80.A0

✓7th **T80.A10 Non-ABO incompatibility with acute hemolytic transfusion reaction** CC
Acute hemolytic transfusion reaction (AHTR) due to non-ABO incompatibility
Non-ABO incompatibility with hemolytic transfusion reaction less than 24 hours after transfusion

✓7th **T80.A11 Non-ABO incompatibility with delayed hemolytic transfusion reaction** CC
Delayed hemolytic transfusion reaction (DHTR) due to non-ABO incompatibility
Non-ABO incompatibility with hemolytic transfusion reaction 24 or more hours after transfusion

✓7th **T80.A19 Non-ABO incompatibility with hemolytic transfusion reaction, unspecified** CC
Hemolytic transfusion reaction (HTR) due to non-ABO incompatibility NOS
Non-ABO incompatibility with hemolytic transfusion reaction at unspecified time after transfusion

✓x7th **T80.A9 Other non-ABO incompatibility reaction due to transfusion of blood or blood products** CC
Delayed serologic transfusion reaction (DSTR) from non-ABO incompatibility
Other reaction to non-ABO incompatible blood transfusion
CC Excl: CC with 7th character A: T80.30X-T80.A9X with 7th A, T80.910-T80.92X with 7th A

✓5th **T80.5 Anaphylactic reaction due to serum**
Allergic shock due to serum
Anaphylactic shock due to serum
Anaphylactoid reaction due to serum
Anaphylaxis due to serum
EXCLUDES 1 *ABO incompatibility reaction due to transfusion of blood or blood products (T80.3-)*
allergic reaction or shock NOS (T78.2)
anaphylactic reaction or shock NOS (T78.2)
anaphylactic reaction or shock due to adverse effect of correct medicinal substance properly administered (T88.6)
other serum reaction (T80.6-)

CC Excl: For CC/MCC codes in subcategory T80.5: CC with 7th character A, unless otherwise noted: T80.51X-T80.69X with 7th A

✓x7th **T80.51 Anaphylactic reaction due to administration of blood and blood products** CC
✓x7th **T80.52 Anaphylactic reaction due to vaccination** CC
✓x7th **T80.59 Anaphylactic reaction due to other serum** CC

✓5th **T80.6 Other serum reactions**
Intoxication by serum
Protein sickness
Serum rash
Serum sickness
Serum urticaria
EXCLUDES 2 *serum hepatitis (B16.-)*

✓x7th **T80.61 Other serum reaction due to administration of blood and blood products** CC
CC Excl: CC with 7th character A: See code: T80.5

✓x7th **T80.62 Other serum reaction due to vaccination** CC
CC Excl: CC with 7th character A: See code: T80.5

✓x7th **T80.69 Other serum reaction due to other serum** CC
CC Excl: CC with 7th character A: T80.61X-T80.69X with 7th A

✓5th **T80.8 Other complications following infusion, transfusion and therapeutic injection**

✓6th **T80.81 Extravasation of vesicant agent**
Infiltration of vesicant agent

✓7th **T80.810 Extravasation of vesicant antineoplastic chemotherapy** CC
Infiltration of vesicant antineoplastic chemotherapy
CC Excl: CC with 7th character A: T80.1XXA, T80.810-T80.818 with 7th A, T80.90XA

✓7th **T80.818 Extravasation of other vesicant agent** CC
Infiltration of other vesicant agent
CC Excl: CC with 7th character A: See code: T81.810

7 HAC = Initial encounter only (7th character A, B or C) and not POA.

√x7th **T8Ø.89 Other complications following infusion, transfusion and therapeutic injection**
Delayed serologic transfusion reaction (DSTR), unspecified incompatibility
Use additional code to identify graft-versus-host reaction, if applicable, (D89.81-)

√5th **T8Ø.9 Unspecified complication following infusion, transfusion and therapeutic injection**

√x7th **T8Ø.9Ø Unspecified complication following infusion and therapeutic injection**

√6th **T8Ø.91 Hemolytic transfusion reaction, unspecified incompatibility**
EXCLUDES 1 *ABO incompatibility with hemolytic transfusion reaction (T8Ø.31-)*
Non-ABO incompatibility with hemolytic transfusion reaction (T8Ø.A1-)
Rh incompatibility with hemolytic transfusion reaction (T8Ø.41-)

CC Excl: For CC codes in subcategory T8Ø.91: CC with 7th character A, unless otherwise noted: T8Ø.3ØX-T8Ø.A9X with 7th A, T8Ø.91Ø-T8Ø.92X with 7th A

√7th **T8Ø.91Ø Acute hemolytic transfusion reaction, unspecified incompatibility** CC

√7th **T8Ø.911 Delayed hemolytic transfusion reaction, unspecified incompatibility** CC

√7th **T8Ø.919 Hemolytic transfusion reaction, unspecified incompatibility, unspecified as acute or delayed** CC
Hemolytic transfusion reaction NOS

√x7th **T8Ø.92 Unspecified transfusion reaction**
Transfusion reaction NOS

√4th **T81 Complications of procedures, not elsewhere classified**
Use additional code for adverse effect, if applicable, to identify drug (T36-T5Ø with fifth or sixth character 5)
EXCLUDES 2 *complications following immunization (T88.Ø-T88.1)*
complications following infusion, transfusion and therapeutic injection (T8Ø.-)
complications of transplanted organs and tissue (T86.-)
specified complications classified elsewhere, such as:
complication of prosthetic devices, implants and grafts (T82-T85)
dermatitis due to drugs and medicaments (L23.3, L24.4, L25.1, L27.Ø-L27.1)
endosseous dental implant failure (M27.6-)
floppy iris syndrome (IFIS) (intraoperative) (H21.81)
intraoperative and postprocedural complications of specific body system (D78.-, E36.-, E89.-, G97.3-, G97.4, H59.3-, H59.-, H95.2-, H95.3, I97.4-, I97.5, J95., K91.-, L76.-, M96.-, N99.-)
ostomy complications (J95.Ø-, K94.-, N99.5-)
plateau iris syndrome (post-iridectomy) (postprocedural) (H21.82)
poisoning and toxic effects of drugs and chemicals (T36-T65 with fifth or sixth character 1-4 or 6)

The appropriate 7th character is to be added to each code from category T81.
A initial encounter
D subsequent encounter
S sequela

√5th **T81.1 Postprocedural shock**
Shock during or resulting from a procedure, not elsewhere classified
EXCLUDES 1 *anaphylactic shock due to correct substance properly administered (T88.6)*
anaphylactic shock due to serum (T8Ø.5-)
anaphylactic shock NOS (T78.2)
anesthetic shock (T88.2)
electric shock (T75.4)
obstetric shock (O75.1)
septic shock (R65.21)
shock following abortion or ectopic or molar pregnancy (OØØ-OØ7, OØ8.3)
traumatic shock (T79.4)

CC Excl: For CC/MCC codes in subcategory T81.1, MCC with 7th A, unless otherwise noted: D78.Ø1-D78.Ø2, D78.21-D78.89, E36.Ø1-E36.Ø2, E36.8, E89.81Ø-E89.89, G97.51-G97.52, H59.Ø11-H59.Ø19, H59.Ø31-H59.129, H59.311-H59.329, H59.811-H59.89, H95.21-H95.22, H95.41-H95.89, I97.3-I97.42, I97.61Ø-I97.62, J95.61-J95.62, J95.83Ø-J95.831, K91.61-K91.62, K91.84Ø-K91.841, L76.Ø1-L76.Ø2, L76.21-L76.82, M96.81Ø-M96.811, M96.83Ø-M96.89, N98.1-N98.9, N99.61-N99.62, N99.82Ø-N99.821, T79.4XXA, T81.1ØX-T81.19X with 7th A, T81.82XA, T81.89X-T81.9XX with 7th A, T88.2XXA

√x7th **T81.1Ø Postprocedural shock unspecified** CC
Collapse NOS during or resulting from a procedure, not elsewhere classified
Postprocedural failure of peripheral circulation
Postprocedural shock NOS

√x7th **T81.11 Postprocedural cardiogenic shock** MCC

12 √x7th **T81.12 Postprocedural septic shock** MCC
Postprocedural endotoxic shock during or resulting from a procedure, not elsewhere classified
Postprocedural gram-negative shock during or resulting from a procedure, not elsewhere classified
Code first underlying infection
Use additional code, to identify any associated acute organ dysfunction, if applicable

√x7th **T81.19 Other postprocedural shock** MCC
Postprocedural hypovolemic shock

√5th **T81.3 Disruption of wound, not elsewhere classified**
Disruption of any suture materials or other closure methods
EXCLUDES 1 *breakdown (mechanical) of permanent sutures (T85.612)*
displacement of permanent sutures (T85.622)
disruption of cesarean delivery wound (O9Ø.Ø)
disruption of perineal obstetric wound (O9Ø.1)
mechanical complication of permanent sutures NEC (T85.692)
AHA: 2Ø14, 1Q, 23

CC Excl: For CC/MCC codes in subcategory T81.3: CC with 7th character A, unless otherwise noted: D78.81-D78.89, E36.8, E89.81Ø-E89.89, H59.Ø11-H59.Ø19, H59.Ø31-H59.Ø99, H59.811-H59.89, H95.811-H95.89, I97.3, L76.81-L76.82, M96.89, N98.1-N98.9, T81.3ØX-T81.33X with 7th A, T81.82A, T81.89X-T81.9XX with 7th A

√x7th **T81.3Ø Disruption of wound, unspecified** CC
Disruption of wound NOS

√x7th **T81.31 Disruption of external operation (surgical) wound, not elsewhere classified** CC
Dehiscence of operation wound NOS
Disruption of operation wound NOS
Disruption or dehiscence of closure of cornea
Disruption or dehiscence of closure of mucosa
Disruption or dehiscence of closure of skin and subcutaneous tissue
Full-thickness skin disruption or dehiscence
Superficial disruption or dehiscence of operation wound
EXCLUDES 1 *dehiscence of amputation stump (T87.81)*

12 Unacceptable PDx = initial encounter only (7th character A).

√x 7th **T81.32 Disruption of internal operation (surgical) wound, not elsewhere classified** CC

Deep disruption or dehiscence of operation wound NOS
Disruption or dehiscence of closure of internal organ or other internal tissue
Disruption or dehiscence of closure of muscle or muscle flap
Disruption or dehiscence of closure of ribs or rib cage
Disruption or dehiscence of closure of skull or craniotomy
Disruption or dehiscence of closure of sternum or sternotomy
Disruption or dehiscence of closure of tendon or ligament
Disruption or dehiscence of closure of superficial or muscular fascia

√x 7th **T81.33 Disruption of traumatic injury wound repair** CC

Disruption or dehiscence of closure of traumatic laceration (external) (internal)

4,6,7,8 √x 7th **T81.4 Infection following a procedure** CC

Intra-abdominal abscess following a procedure
Postprocedural infection, not elsewhere classified
Sepsis following a procedure
Stitch abscess following a procedure
Subphrenic abscess following a procedure
Wound abscess following a procedure
Use additional code to identify infection
Use additional code (R65.2-) to identify severe sepsis, if applicable

EXCLUDES 1 *obstetric surgical wound infection (O86.Ø)*
postprocedural fever NOS (R5Ø.82)
postprocedural retroperitoneal abscess (K68.11)

EXCLUDES 2 *bleb associated endophthalmitis (H59.4-)*
infection due to infusion, transfusion and therapeutic injection (T8Ø.2-)
infection due to prosthetic devices, implants and grafts (T82.6-T82.7, T83.5-T83.6, T84.5-T84.7, T85.7)

AHA: 2Ø14, 1Q, 23

CC Excl: CC with 7th character A: D78.81-D78.89, E36.8, E89.81Ø-E89.89, H59.Ø11-H59.Ø19, H59.Ø31-H59.Ø99, H59.811-H59.89, H95.811-H95.89, I97.3, K68.11, L76.81-L76.82, M96.89, N98.1-N98.9, T81.4XXA, T81.82XA, T81.89X-T81.9XX with 7th A

√5th **T81.5 Complications of foreign body accidentally left in body following procedure**

CC Excl: For CC codes in subcategory T81.5: CC with 7th character A,unless otherwise noted: D78.81-D78.89, E36.8, E89.81Ø-E89.89, H59.Ø11-H59.Ø19, H59.Ø31-H59.Ø99, H59.811-H59.89, H95.811-H95.89, I97.3, L76.81-L76.82, M96.89, N98.1-N98.9, T81.5ØØ-T81.599 with 7th A, T81.82XA, T81.89X-T81.9XX with 7th A

√6th **T81.5Ø Unspecified complication of foreign body accidentally left in body following procedure**

7 √7th **T81.5ØØ Unspecified complication of foreign body accidentally left in body following surgical operation** CC

7 √7th **T81.5Ø1 Unspecified complication of foreign body accidentally left in body following infusion or transfusion** CC

7 √7th **T81.5Ø2 Unspecified complication of foreign body accidentally left in body following kidney dialysis** CC

7 √7th **T81.5Ø3 Unspecified complication of foreign body accidentally left in body following injection or immunization** CC

7 √7th **T81.5Ø4 Unspecified complication of foreign body accidentally left in body following endoscopic examination** CC

7 √7th **T81.5Ø5 Unspecified complication of foreign body accidentally left in body following heart catheterization** CC

7 √7th **T81.5Ø6 Unspecified complication of foreign body accidentally left in body following aspiration, puncture or other catheterization** CC

7 √7th **T81.5Ø7 Unspecified complication of foreign body accidentally left in body following removal of catheter or packing** CC

7 √7th **T81.5Ø8 Unspecified complication of foreign body accidentally left in body following other procedure** CC

7 √7th **T81.5Ø9 Unspecified complication of foreign body accidentally left in body following unspecified procedure** CC

√6th **T81.51 Adhesions due to foreign body accidentally left in body following procedure**

7 √7th **T81.51Ø Adhesions due to foreign body accidentally left in body following surgical operation** CC

7 √7th **T81.511 Adhesions due to foreign body accidentally left in body following infusion or transfusion** CC

7 √7th **T81.512 Adhesions due to foreign body accidentally left in body following kidney dialysis** CC

7 √7th **T81.513 Adhesions due to foreign body accidentally left in body following injection or immunization** CC

7 √7th **T81.514 Adhesions due to foreign body accidentally left in body following endoscopic examination** CC

7 √7th **T81.515 Adhesions due to foreign body accidentally left in body following heart catheterization** CC

7 √7th **T81.516 Adhesions due to foreign body accidentally left in body following aspiration, puncture or other catheterization** CC

7 √7th **T81.517 Adhesions due to foreign body accidentally left in body following removal of catheter or packing** CC

7 √7th **T81.518 Adhesions due to foreign body accidentally left in body following other procedure** CC

7 √7th **T81.519 Adhesions due to foreign body accidentally left in body following unspecified procedure** CC

√6th **T81.52 Obstruction due to foreign body accidentally left in body following procedure**

7 √7th **T81.52Ø Obstruction due to foreign body accidentally left in body following surgical operation** CC

7 √7th **T81.521 Obstruction due to foreign body accidentally left in body following infusion or transfusion** CC

7 √7th **T81.522 Obstruction due to foreign body accidentally left in body following kidney dialysis** CC

7 √7th **T81.523 Obstruction due to foreign body accidentally left in body following injection or immunization** CC

7 √7th **T81.524 Obstruction due to foreign body accidentally left in body following endoscopic examination** CC

7 √7th **T81.525 Obstruction due to foreign body accidentally left in body following heart catheterization** CC

7 √7th **T81.526 Obstruction due to foreign body accidentally left in body following aspiration, puncture or other catheterization** CC

7 √7th **T81.527 Obstruction due to foreign body accidentally left in body following removal of catheter or packing** CC

7 √7th **T81.528 Obstruction due to foreign body accidentally left in body following other procedure** CC

---

4 HAC = as SDx not POA, in combination with PDx E66.Ø1 **AND** one of the following procedure codes: ØD16[Ø,4,8][7,J,K,Z][9,A,B,L] or ØDV64CZ.

6 HAC = as SDx not POA, in combination with one of the following procedure codes: ØRG[Ø,1,2,4,6,7,8,A][Ø,3,4][7,A,J,K,Z][Ø,1,J]; ØRG[E,F,G,H,J,K][Ø,3,4][4,7,J,K,Z]Z; ØRG[L,M][Ø,3,4][4,5,7,J,K,Z]Z; ØRQ[E,F,G,H,J,K,L,M][Ø,3,4,X]ZZ; ØRU[E,F,G,H,J,K,L,M][Ø,3,4][7,J,K]Z; ØSG[Ø,1,3][Ø,3,4][7,A,J,K,Z][Ø,1,J]; ØSG[7,8][Ø,3,4[4,7,J,K,Z]Z.

7 HAC = Initial encounter only (7th character A, B or C) and not POA.

8 HAC = as SDx not POA, in combination with one of the following procedure codes: Ø2H43[J,K,M]Z; Ø2H[6,7]3[J,M]Z; Ø2H[K,L]3JZ; Ø2HN[Ø,3,4][J,M]Z; Ø2PA[Ø,3,4]MZ; Ø2PAXMZ; Ø2WA[Ø,3,4]MZ; ØJH[6,8][Ø,3][4,5,6,7,8,9,P]Z; ØJ[P,W]T[Ø,3]PZ.

7 ✓7th **T81.529 Obstruction due to foreign body accidentally left in body following unspecified procedure** CC

✓6th **T81.53 Perforation due to foreign body accidentally left in body following procedure**

7 ✓7th **T81.530 Perforation due to foreign body accidentally left in body following surgical operation** CC

7 ✓7th **T81.531 Perforation due to foreign body accidentally left in body following infusion or transfusion** CC

7 ✓7th **T81.532 Perforation due to foreign body accidentally left in body following kidney dialysis** CC

7 ✓7th **T81.533 Perforation due to foreign body accidentally left in body following injection or immunization** CC

7 ✓7th **T81.534 Perforation due to foreign body accidentally left in body following endoscopic examination** CC

7 ✓7th **T81.535 Perforation due to foreign body accidentally left in body following heart catheterization** CC

7 ✓7th **T81.536 Perforation due to foreign body accidentally left in body following aspiration, puncture or other catheterization** CC

7 ✓7th **T81.537 Perforation due to foreign body accidentally left in body following removal of catheter or packing** CC

7 ✓7th **T81.538 Perforation due to foreign body accidentally left in body following other procedure** CC

7 ✓7th **T81.539 Perforation due to foreign body accidentally left in body following unspecified procedure** CC

✓6th **T81.59 Other complications of foreign body accidentally left in body following procedure**

EXCLUDES 2 *obstruction or perforation due to prosthetic devices and implants intentionally left in body (T82.Ø-T82.5, T83.Ø-T83.4, T83.7, T84.Ø-T84.4, T85.Ø-T85.6)*

7 ✓7th **T81.59Ø Other complications of foreign body accidentally left in body following surgical operation** CC

7 ✓7th **T81.591 Other complications of foreign body accidentally left in body following infusion or transfusion** CC

7 ✓7th **T81.592 Other complications of foreign body accidentally left in body following kidney dialysis** CC

7 ✓7th **T81.593 Other complications of foreign body accidentally left in body following injection or immunization** CC

7 ✓7th **T81.594 Other complications of foreign body accidentally left in body following endoscopic examination** CC

7 ✓7th **T81.595 Other complications of foreign body accidentally left in body following heart catheterization** CC

7 ✓7th **T81.596 Other complications of foreign body accidentally left in body following aspiration, puncture or other catheterization** CC

7 ✓7th **T81.597 Other complications of foreign body accidentally left in body following removal of catheter or packing** CC

7 ✓7th **T81.598 Other complications of foreign body accidentally left in body following other procedure** CC

7 ✓7th **T81.599 Other complications of foreign body accidentally left in body following unspecified procedure** CC

✓5th **T81.6 Acute reaction to foreign substance accidentally left during a procedure**

EXCLUDES 2 *complications of foreign body accidentally left in body cavity or operation wound following procedure (T81.5-)*

CC Excl: For CC codes in subcategory T81.6: CC with 7th character A, unless otherwise noted: D78.81-D78.89, E36.8, E89.81Ø-E89.89, H59.Ø11-H59.Ø19, H59.Ø31-H59.Ø99, H59.811-H59.89, H95.811-H95.89, I97.3, L76.81-L76.82, M96.89, N98.1-N98.9, T81.6Ø-T81.69 with 7th A, T81.82XA, T81.89X-T81.9XX with 7th A

7 ✓x7th **T81.6Ø Unspecified acute reaction to foreign substance accidentally left during a procedure** CC

7 ✓x7th **T81.61 Aseptic peritonitis due to foreign substance accidentally left during a procedure** CC

Chemical peritonitis

7 ✓x7th **T81.69 Other acute reaction to foreign substance accidentally left during a procedure** CC

✓5th **T81.7 Vascular complications following a procedure, not elsewhere classified**

Air embolism following procedure NEC

Phlebitis or thrombophlebitis resulting from a procedure

EXCLUDES 1 *embolism complicating abortion or ectopic or molar pregnancy (OØØ-OØ7, OØ8.2)*

embolism complicating pregnancy, childbirth and the puerperium (O88.-)

traumatic embolism (T79.Ø)

EXCLUDES 2 *embolism due to prosthetic devices, implants and grafts (T82.8-, T83.8, T84.8-, T85.8)*

embolism following infusion, transfusion and therapeutic injection (T8Ø.Ø)

✓6th **T81.71 Complication of artery following a procedure, not elsewhere classified**

✓7th **T81.71Ø Complication of mesenteric artery following a procedure, not elsewhere classified** CC

CC Excl: CC with 7th character A: D78.81-D78.89, E36.8, E89.81Ø-E89.89, H59.Ø11-H59.Ø19, H59.Ø31-H59.Ø99, H59.811-H59.89, H95.811-H95.89, I97.3, L76.81-L76.82, M96.89, N98.1-N98.9, T81.71Ø-T81.72X with 7th A, T81.82XA, T81.89X-T81.9XX with 7th A

✓7th **T81.711 Complication of renal artery following a procedure, not elsewhere classified** CC

CC Excl: See code: T81.71Ø

✓7th **T81.718 Complication of other artery following a procedure, not elsewhere classified** CC

CC Excl: CC with 7th character A: D78.81-D78.89, E36.8, E89.81Ø-E89.89, H59.Ø11-H59.Ø19, H59.Ø31-H59.Ø99, H59.811-H59.89, H95.811-H95.89, I97.3, L76.81-L76.82, M96.89, N98.1-N98.9, T81.718-T81.72X with 7th A, T81.82XA, T81.89X-T81.9XX with 7th A

✓7th **T81.719 Complication of unspecified artery following a procedure, not elsewhere classified** CC

CC Excl: See code: T81.718

✓x7th **T81.72 Complication of vein following a procedure, not elsewhere classified** CC

CC Excl: See code: T81.718

✓5th **T81.8 Other complications of procedures, not elsewhere classified**

EXCLUDES 2 *hypothermia following anesthesia (T88.51)*

malignant hyperpyrexia due to anesthesia (T88.3)

12 ✓x7th **T81.81 Complication of inhalation therapy**

✓x7th **T81.82 Emphysema (subcutaneous) resulting from a procedure**

✓x7th **T81.83 Persistent postprocedural fistula** CC

CC Excl: CC with 7th character A: D78.81-D78.89, E36.8, E89.81Ø-E89.89, H59.Ø11-H59.Ø19, H59.Ø31-H59.Ø99, H59.811-H59.89, H95.811-H95.89, I97.3, L76.81-L76.82, M96.89, N98.1-N98.9, T81.82X-T81.9XX with 7th A

✓x7th **T81.89 Other complications of procedures, not elsewhere classified**

Use additional code to specify complication, such as: postprocedural delirium (FØ5)

AHA: 2Ø14, 1Q, 23

✓x7th **T81.9 Unspecified complication of procedure**

7 HAC = Initial encounter only (7th character A, B or C) and not POA.

12 Unacceptable PDx = initial encounter only (7th character A).

T82 Complications of cardiac and vascular prosthetic devices, implants and grafts
EXCLUDES 2 *failure and rejection of transplanted organs and tissue (T86.-)*

The appropriate 7th character is to be added to each code from category T82.
A initial encounter
D subsequent encounter
S sequela

T82.0 Mechanical complication of heart valve prosthesis
Mechanical complication of artificial heart valve
EXCLUDES 1 *mechanical complication of biological heart valve graft (T82.22-)*

CC Excl: For CC codes in subcategory T82.0: CC with 7th character A, unless otherwise noted: D78.81-D78.89, E36.8, E89.810-E89.89, H59.011-H59.019, H59.031-H59.099, H59.811-H59.89, H95.811-H95.89, I97.3, L76.81-L76.82, M96.89, N98.1-N98.9, T81.82XA, T81.89X-T82.09X with 7th A

T82.01 Breakdown (mechanical) of heart valve prosthesis CC
T82.02 Displacement of heart valve prosthesis CC
Malposition of heart valve prosthesis
T82.03 Leakage of heart valve prosthesis CC
T82.09 Other mechanical complication of heart valve prosthesis CC
Obstruction (mechanical) of heart valve prosthesis
Perforation of heart valve prosthesis
Protrusion of heart valve prosthesis

T82.1 Mechanical complication of cardiac electronic device

CC Excl: For CC codes in subcategory T82.1: CC with 7th character A, unless otherwise noted: D78.81-D78.89, E36.8, E89.810-E89.89, H59.011-H59.019, H59.031-H59.099, H59.811-H59.89, H95.811-H95.89, I97.3, L76.81-L76.82, M96.89, N98.1-N98.9, T81.82XA, T81.89X-T81.9XX with 7th A, T82.110-T82.111, T82.120, T82.121, T82.190-T82.191 with 7th A

T82.11 Breakdown (mechanical) of cardiac electronic device
T82.110 Breakdown (mechanical) of cardiac electrode CC
T82.111 Breakdown (mechanical) of cardiac pulse generator (battery) CC
T82.118 Breakdown (mechanical) of other cardiac electronic device CC
CC Excl: CC with 7th character A: D78.81-D78.89, E36.8, E89.810-E89.89, H59.011-H59.019, H59.031-H59.099, H59.811-H59.89, H95.811-H95.89, I97.3, L76.81-L76.82, M96.89, N98.1-N98.9, T81.82X, T81.89X-T81.9XX, T82.118, T82.128, T82.198, T82.221-T82.228, T82.512, T82.522, T82.532, T82.592, T82.594, T82.598
T82.119 Breakdown (mechanical) of unspecified cardiac electronic device CC
CC Excl: No Excl

T82.12 Displacement of cardiac electronic device
Malposition of cardiac electronic device
T82.120 Displacement of cardiac electrode CC
T82.121 Displacement of cardiac pulse generator (battery) CC
T82.128 Displacement of other cardiac electronic device CC
CC Excl: See code: T82.118
T82.129 Displacement of unspecified cardiac electronic device CC
CC Excl: No Excl

T82.19 Other mechanical complication of cardiac electronic device
Leakage of cardiac electronic device
Obstruction of cardiac electronic device
Perforation of cardiac electronic device
Protrusion of cardiac electronic device
T82.190 Other mechanical complication of cardiac electrode CC
T82.191 Other mechanical complication of cardiac pulse generator (battery) CC
T82.198 Other mechanical complication of other cardiac electronic device CC
CC Excl: See code: T82.118
T82.199 Other mechanical complication of unspecified cardiac device CC
CC Excl: No Excl

T82.2 Mechanical complication of coronary artery bypass graft and biological heart valve graft
EXCLUDES 1 *mechanical complication of artificial heart valve prosthesis (T82.0-)*

T82.21 Mechanical complication of coronary artery bypass graft)

CC Excl: For CC codes in subcategory T82.21: CC with 7th character A, unless otherwise noted: D78.81-D78.89, E36.8, E89.810-E89.89, H59.011-H59.019, H59.031-H59.099, H59.811-H59.89, H95.811-H95.89, I97.3, L76.81-L76.82, M96.89, N98.1-N98.9, T81.82XA, T81.89X-T81.9XX with 7th A, T82.211-T82.218 with 7th A

T82.211 Breakdown (mechanical) of coronary artery bypass graft CC
T82.212 Displacement of coronary artery bypass graft CC
Malposition of coronary artery bypass graft
T82.213 Leakage of coronary artery bypass graft CC
T82.218 Other mechanical complication of coronary artery bypass graft CC
Obstruction, mechanical of coronary artery bypass graft
Perforation of coronary artery bypass graft
Protrusion of coronary artery bypass graft

T82.22 Mechanical complication of biological heart valve graft)

CC Excl: For CC codes in subcategory T82.22: CC with 7th character A, unless otherwise noted: D78.81-D78.89, E36.8, E89.810-E89.89, H59.011-H59.019, H59.031-H59.099, H59.811-H59.89, H95.811-H95.89, I97.3, L76.81-L76.82, M96.89, N98.1-N98.9, T81.82XA, T81.89X-T81.9XX with 7th A, T82.118A,T82.128A,T82.198A,T82.221-T82.228 with 7th A, T82.512 with 7th A, T82.522 with 7th A, T82.532 with 7th A, T82.592 with 7th A, T82.594 with 7th A, T82.598 with 7th A

T82.221 Breakdown (mechanical) of biological heart valve graft CC
T82.222 Displacement of biological heart valve graft CC
Malposition of biological heart valve graft
T82.223 Leakage of biological heart valve graft CC
T82.228 Other mechanical complication of biological heart valve graft CC
Obstruction of biological heart valve graft
Perforation of biological heart valve graft
Protrusion of biological heart valve graft

T82.3 Mechanical complication of other vascular grafts

CC Excl: For CC codes in subcategory T82.3: CC with 7th character A: D78.81-D78.89, E36.8, E89.810-E89.89, H59.011-H59.019, H59.031-H59.099, H59.811-H59.89, H95.811-H95.89, I97.3, L76.81-L76.82, M96.89, N98.1-N98.9, T81.82XA, T81.89X-T81.9XX with 7th A, T82.310-T82.511 with 7th A, T82.513-T82.518 with 7th A, T82.520-T82.521 with 7th A, T82.523-T82.531 with 7th A, T82.533-T82.538 with 7th A, T82.590-T82.591 with 7th A, T82.593A, T82.595A

T82.31 Breakdown (mechanical) of other vascular grafts
T82.310 Breakdown (mechanical) of aortic (bifurcation) graft (replacement) CC
T82.311 Breakdown (mechanical) of carotid arterial graft (bypass) CC
T82.312 Breakdown (mechanical) of femoral arterial graft (bypass) CC
T82.318 Breakdown (mechanical) of other vascular grafts CC
T82.319 Breakdown (mechanical) of unspecified vascular grafts CC

T82.32 Displacement of other vascular grafts
Malposition of other vascular grafts
T82.320 Displacement of aortic (bifurcation) graft (replacement) CC
T82.321 Displacement of carotid arterial graft (bypass) CC
T82.322 Displacement of femoral arterial graft (bypass) CC

✓7th **T82.328 Displacement of other vascular grafts** CC
✓7th **T82.329 Displacement of unspecified vascular grafts** CC
✓6th **T82.33 Leakage of other vascular grafts**
✓7th **T82.330 Leakage of aortic (bifurcation) graft (replacement)** CC
✓7th **T82.331 Leakage of carotid arterial graft (bypass)** CC
✓7th **T82.332 Leakage of femoral arterial graft (bypass)** CC
✓7th **T82.338 Leakage of other vascular grafts** CC
✓7th **T82.339 Leakage of unspecified vascular graft** CC
✓6th **T82.39 Other mechanical complication of other vascular grafts**
Obstruction (mechanical) of other vascular grafts
Perforation of other vascular grafts
Protrusion of other vascular grafts
✓7th **T82.390 Other mechanical complication of aortic (bifurcation) graft (replacement)** CC
✓7th **T82.391 Other mechanical complication of carotid arterial graft (bypass)** CC
✓7th **T82.392 Other mechanical complication of femoral arterial graft (bypass)** CC
✓7th **T82.398 Other mechanical complication of other vascular grafts** CC
✓7th **T82.399 Other mechanical complication of unspecified vascular grafts** CC
✓5th **T82.4 Mechanical complication of vascular dialysis catheter**
Mechanical complication of hemodialysis catheter
EXCLUDES 1 *mechanical complication of intraperitoneal dialysis catheter (T85.62)*

CC Excl: For CC codes in subcategory T82.4: CC with 7th character A, unless otherwise noted: See code: T82.3

✓x7th **T82.41 Breakdown (mechanical) of vascular dialysis catheter** CC
✓x7th **T82.42 Displacement of vascular dialysis catheter** CC
Malposition of vascular dialysis catheter
✓x7th **T82.43 Leakage of vascular dialysis catheter** CC
✓x7th **T82.49 Other complication of vascular dialysis catheter** CC
Obstruction (mechanical) of vascular dialysis catheter
Perforation of vascular dialysis catheter
Protrusion of vascular dialysis catheter
✓5th **T82.5 Mechanical complication of other cardiac and vascular devices and implants**
EXCLUDES 2 *mechanical complication of epidural and subdural infusion catheter (T85.61)*

CC Excl: For CC codes in subcategory T82.5: CC with 7th character A, unless otherwise noted: D78.81-D78.89, E36.8, E89.810-E89.89, H59.011-H59.019, H59.031-H59.099, H59.811-H59.89, H95.811-H95.89, I97.3, L76.81-L76.82, M96.89, N98.1-N98.9, T81.82XA, T81.89X-T81.9XX with 7th A, T82.310-T82.511 with 7th A, T82.513-T82.518 with 7th A, T82.520-T82.521 with 7th A, T82.523-T82.531 with 7th A, T82.533-T82.538 with 7th A, T82.590-T82.591 with 7th A, T82.593A, T82.595A

✓6th **T82.51 Breakdown (mechanical) of other cardiac and vascular devices and implants**
✓7th **T82.510 Breakdown (mechanical) of surgically created arteriovenous fistula** CC
✓7th **T82.511 Breakdown (mechanical) of surgically created arteriovenous shunt** CC
✓7th **T82.512 Breakdown (mechanical) of artificial heart** CC
CC Excl: CC with 7th character A: D78.81-D78.89, E36.8, E89.810-E89.89, H59.011-H59.019, H59.031-H59.099, H59.811-H59.89, H95.811-H95.89, I97.3, L76.81-L76.82, M96.89, N98.1-N98.9, T81.82XA, T81.89X-T81.9XX with 7th A, T82.118A, T82.128A, T82.198A, T82.221-T82.228 with 7th A, T82.512A, T82.522A, T82.532A, T82.592A, T82.594A, T82.598A
✓7th **T82.513 Breakdown (mechanical) of balloon (counterpulsation) device** CC
✓7th **T82.514 Breakdown (mechanical) of infusion catheter** CC
✓7th **T82.515 Breakdown (mechanical) of umbrella device** CC
✓7th **T82.518 Breakdown (mechanical) of other cardiac and vascular devices and implants** CC
✓7th **T82.519 Breakdown (mechanical) of unspecified cardiac and vascular devices and implants** CC
CC Excl: CC with 7th character A: D78.81-D78.89, E36.8, E89.810-E89.89, H59.011-H59.019, H59.031-H59.099, H59.811-H59.89, H95.811-H95.89, I97.3, L76.81-L76.82, M96.89, N98.1-N98.9, T81.82XA, T81.89X-T81.9XX with 7th A, T82.519A, T82.539A, T82.599-T82.9XX with 7th character A, T85.9XXA
✓6th **T82.52 Displacement of other cardiac and vascular devices and implants**
Malposition of other cardiac and vascular devices and implants
✓7th **T82.520 Displacement of surgically created arteriovenous fistula** CC
✓7th **T82.521 Displacement of surgically created arteriovenous shunt** CC
✓7th **T82.522 Displacement of artificial heart** CC
CC Excl: CC with 7th character A: D78.81-D78.89, E36.8, E89.810-E89.89, H59.011-H59.019, H59.031-H59.099, H59.811-H59.89, H95.811-H95.89, I97.3, L76.81-L76.82, M96.89, N98.1-N98.9, T81.82XA, T81.89X-T81.9XX with 7th A, T82.118A, T82.128A, T82.198A,T82.221-T82.228 with 7th A, T82.512A, T82.522A, T82.532A, T82.592A, T82.594A, T82.598A
✓7th **T82.523 Displacement of balloon (counterpulsation) device** CC
✓7th **T82.524 Displacement of infusion catheter** CC
✓7th **T82.525 Displacement of umbrella device** CC
✓7th **T82.528 Displacement of other cardiac and vascular devices and implants** CC
✓7th **T82.529 Displacement of unspecified cardiac and vascular devices and implants** CC
✓6th **T82.53 Leakage of other cardiac and vascular devices and implants**
✓7th **T82.530 Leakage of surgically created arteriovenous fistula** CC
✓7th **T82.531 Leakage of surgically created arteriovenous shunt** CC
✓7th **T82.532 Leakage of artificial heart** CC
CC Excl: CC with 7th character A: D78.81-D78.89, E36.8, E89.810-E89.89, H59.011-H59.019, H59.031-H59.099, H59.811-H59.89, H95.811-H95.89, I97.3, L76.81-L76.82, M96.89, N98.1-N98.9, T81.82XA, T81.89X-T81.9XX with 7th A, T82.118A, T82.128A, T82.198A, T82.221-T82.228 with 7th A, T82.512A, T82.522A, T82.532A, T82.592A, T82.594A, T82.598A
✓7th **T82.533 Leakage of balloon (counterpulsation) device** CC
✓7th **T82.534 Leakage of infusion catheter** CC
✓7th **T82.535 Leakage of umbrella device** CC
✓7th **T82.538 Leakage of other cardiac and vascular devices and implants** CC
✓7th **T82.539 Leakage of unspecified cardiac and vascular devices and implants** CC
CC Excl: CC with 7th character A: D78.81-D78.89, E36.8, E89.810-E89.89, H59.011-H59.019, H59.031-H59.099, H59.811-H59.89, H95.811-H95.89, I97.3, L76.81-L76.82, M96.89, N98.1-N98.9, T81.82XA, T81.89X-T81.9XX with 7th A, T82.519A, T82.539A, T82.599-T82.9XX with 7th A, T85.9XXA
✓6th **T82.59 Other mechanical complication of other cardiac and vascular devices and implants**
Obstruction (mechanical) of other cardiac and vascular devices and implants
Perforation of other cardiac and vascular devices and implants
Protrusion of other cardiac and vascular devices and implants
✓7th **T82.590 Other mechanical complication of surgically created arteriovenous fistula** CC

√7th **T82.591 Other mechanical complication of surgically created arteriovenous shunt** CC

√7th **T82.592 Other mechanical complication of artificial heart** CC
CC Excl: CC with 7th character A: D78.81-D78.89, E36.8, E89.81Ø-E89.89, H59.Ø11-H59.Ø19, H59.Ø31-H59.Ø99, H59.811-H59.89, H95.811-H95.89, I97.3, L76.81-L76.82, M96.89, N98.1-N98.9, T81.82XA, T81.89X-T81.9XX with 7th A, T82.118A, T82.128A, T82.198A,T82.221-T82.228 with 7th A, T82.512A, T82.522A, T82.532A, T82.592A, T82.594A, T82.598 with 7th A

√7th **T82.593 Other mechanical complication of balloon (counterpulsation) device** CC

√7th **T82.594 Other mechanical complication of infusion catheter** CC
CC Excl: CC with 7th character A: D78.81-D78.89, E36.8, E89.81Ø-E89.89, H59.Ø11-H59.Ø19, H59.Ø31-H59.Ø99, H59.811-H59.89, H95.811-H95.89, I97.3, L76.81-L76.82, M96.89, N98.1-N98.9, T81.82XA, T81.89X-T81.9XX with 7th A, T82.118A, T82.128A, T82.198A, T82.31Ø-T82.511 with 7th A, T82.513-T82.518 with 7th A, T82.52Ø-T82.521 with 7th A, T82.523-T82.531 with 7th A, T82.533-T82.538 with 7th A, T82.59Ø-T82.591 with 7th A, T82.593A, T82.595 with 7th A

√7th **T82.595 Other mechanical complication of umbrella device** CC

√7th **T82.598 Other mechanical complication of other cardiac and vascular devices and implants** CC
CC Excl: CC with 7th character A: D78.81-D78.89, E36.8, E89.81Ø-E89.89, H59.Ø11-H59.Ø19, H59.Ø31-H59.Ø99, H59.811-H59.89, H95.811-H95.89, I97.3, L76.81-L76.82, M96.89, N98.1-N98.9, T81.82XA, T81.89X-T81.9XX with 7th A, T82.118A, T82.128A, T82.198A,T82.221-T82.228 with 7th A, T82.512A, T82.522A, T82.532A, T82.592 A, T82.594A, T82.598A

√7th **T82.599 Other mechanical complication of unspecified cardiac and vascular devices and implants** CC
CC Excl: CC with 7th character A: D78.81-D78.89, E36.8, E89.81Ø-E89.89, H59.Ø11-H59.Ø19, H59.Ø31-H59.Ø99, H59.811-H59.89, H95.811-H95.89, I97.3, L76.81-L76.82, M96.89, N98.1-N98.9, T81.82XA, T81.89X-T81.9XX with 7th A, T82.519A, T82.539A, T82.599-T82.9XX with 7th A, T85.9XXA

8 √x7th **T82.6 Infection and inflammatory reaction due to cardiac valve prosthesis** CC
Use additional code to identify infection
CC Excl: CC with 7th character A: D78.81-D78.89, E36.8, E89.81Ø-E89.89, H59.Ø11-H59.Ø19, H59.Ø31-H59.Ø99, H59.811-H59.89, H95.811-H95.89, I97.3, L76.81-L76.82, M96.89, N98.1-N98.9, T81.82XA, T81.89X-T82.Ø9X with 7th A, T82.11Ø-T82.118 with 7th A, T82.12Ø-T82.128 with 7th A, T82.19Ø-T82.198 with 7th A, T82.211-T82.9XX with 7th A, T85.31Ø-T85.311 with 7th A, T85.32Ø-T85.321 with 7th A, T85.39Ø-T85.391 with 7th A, T85.51Ø-T85.9XX with 7th A, T86.82Ø-T86.829, T86.842-T86.849

8 √x7th **T82.7 Infection and inflammatory reaction due to other cardiac and vascular devices, implants and grafts** CC
Use additional code to identify infection
CC Excl: See code: T82.6

√5th **T82.8 Other specified complications of cardiac and vascular prosthetic devices, implants and grafts**

√6th **T82.81 Embolism of cardiac and vascular prosthetic devices, implants and grafts**

√7th **T82.817 Embolism of cardiac prosthetic devices, implants and grafts** CC
CC Excl: CC with 7th character A: D78.81-D78.89, E36.8, E89.81Ø-E89.89, H59.Ø11-H59.Ø19, H59.Ø31-H59.Ø99, H59.811-H59.89, H95.811-H95.89, I97.3, L76.81-L76.82, M96.89, N98.1-N98.9, T81.82XA, T81.89X-T82.Ø9X with 7th A, T82.11Ø-T82.118 with 7th A, T82.12Ø-T82.128 with 7th A, T82.19Ø-T82.198 with 7th A, T82.221-T82.9XX with 7th A, T85.31Ø-T85.311 with 7th A, T85.32Ø-T85.321 with 7th A, T85.39Ø-T85.391 with 7th A, T85.51Ø-T85.9XX with 7th A, T86.82Ø-T86.829, T86.842-T86.849

√7th **T82.818 Embolism of vascular prosthetic devices, implants and grafts** CC
CC Excl: CC with 7th character A: D78.81-D78.89, E36.8, E89.81Ø-E89.89, H59.Ø11-H59.Ø19, H59.Ø31-H59.Ø99, H59.811-H59.89, H95.811-H95.89, I97.3, L76.81-L76.82, M96.89, N98.1-N98.9, T81.82XA, T81.89X-T82.Ø9X with 7th A, T82.11Ø-T82.118 with 7th A, T82.12Ø-T82.128 with 7th A, T82.19Ø-T82.198 with 7th A, T82.211-T82.9XX with 7th A, T85.31Ø-T85.311 with 7th A, T85.32Ø-T85.321 with 7th A, T85.39Ø-T85.391 with 7th A, T85.51Ø-T85.9XX with 7th A, T86.82Ø-T86.829, T86.842-T86.849

√6th **T82.82 Fibrosis of cardiac and vascular prosthetic devices, implants and grafts**

√7th **T82.827 Fibrosis of cardiac prosthetic devices, implants and grafts** CC
CC Excl: See code: T82.817

√7th **T82.828 Fibrosis of vascular prosthetic devices, implants and grafts** CC
CC Excl: See code: T82.818

√6th **T82.83 Hemorrhage of cardiac and vascular prosthetic devices, implants and grafts**

√7th **T82.837 Hemorrhage of cardiac prosthetic devices, implants and grafts** CC
CC Excl: See code: T82.817

√7th **T82.838 Hemorrhage of vascular prosthetic devices, implants and grafts** CC
CC Excl: See code: T82.818

√6th **T82.84 Pain from cardiac and vascular prosthetic devices, implants and grafts**

√7th **T82.847 Pain from cardiac prosthetic devices, implants and grafts** CC
CC Excl: See code: T82.817

√7th **T82.848 Pain from vascular prosthetic devices, implants and grafts** CC
CC Excl: See code: T82.818

√6th **T82.85 Stenosis of cardiac and vascular prosthetic devices, implants and grafts**

√7th **T82.857 Stenosis of cardiac prosthetic devices, implants and grafts** CC
CC Excl: See code: T82.817

√7th **T82.858 Stenosis of vascular prosthetic devices, implants and grafts** CC
CC Excl: See code: T82.818

√6th **T82.86 Thrombosis of cardiac and vascular prosthetic devices, implants and grafts**

√7th **T82.867 Thrombosis of cardiac prosthetic devices, implants and grafts** CC
CC Excl: See code: T82.817

√7th **T82.868 Thrombosis of vascular prosthetic devices, implants and grafts** CC
CC Excl: See code: T82.818

√6th **T82.89 Other specified complication of cardiac and vascular prosthetic devices, implants and grafts**

√7th **T82.897 Other specified complication of cardiac prosthetic devices, implants and grafts** CC
CC Excl: See code: T82.817

√7th **T82.898 Other specified complication of vascular prosthetic devices, implants and grafts** CC
CC Excl: See code: T82.818

8 HAC = as SDx not POA, in combination with one of the following procedure codes: Ø2H43[J,K,M]Z; Ø2H[6,7]3[J,M]Z; Ø2H[K,L]3JZ; Ø2HN[Ø,3,4][J,M]Z; Ø2PA[Ø,3,4]MZ; Ø2PAXMZ; Ø2WA[Ø,3,4]MZ; ØJH[6,8][Ø,3][4,5,6,7,8,9,P]Z; ØJ[P,W]T[Ø,3]PZ.

√x7th **T82.9 Unspecified complication of cardiac and vascular prosthetic device, implant and graft** CC
CC Excl: See code: T82.817

√4th **T83 Complications of genitourinary prosthetic devices, implants and grafts**
EXCLUDES 2 *failure and rejection of transplanted organs and tissue (T86.-)*

The appropriate 7th character is to be added to each code from category T83.
A initial encounter
D subsequent encounter
S sequela

√5th **T83.0 Mechanical complication of urinary (indwelling) catheter**
EXCLUDES 2 *complications of stoma of urinary tract (N99.5-)*

For CC codes in subcategory T83.0: CC with 7th character A, unless otherwise noted: D78.81-D78.89, E36.8, E89.810-E89.89, H59.011-H59.019, H59.031-H59.099, H59.811-H59.89, H95.811-H95.89, I97.3, L76.81-L76.82, M96.89, N98.1-N98.9, N99.510-N99.518, T81.82XA, T81.89X-T81.9XX with 7th A, T83.010A, T83.020A, T83.030A, T83.090A, T83.110-T83.29X with 7th A, T83.410-T83.718 with 7th A, T83.728-T83.9XX with 7th A

√6th **T83.01 Breakdown (mechanical) of urinary (indwelling) catheter**
√7th **T83.010 Breakdown (mechanical) of cystostomy catheter** CC
√7th **T83.018 Breakdown (mechanical) of other indwelling urethral catheter**

√6th **T83.02 Displacement of urinary (indwelling) catheter**
Malposition of urinary (indwelling) catheter
√7th **T83.020 Displacement of cystostomy catheter** CC
√7th **T83.028 Displacement of other indwelling urethral catheter**

√6th **T83.03 Leakage of urinary (indwelling) catheter**
√7th **T83.030 Leakage of cystostomy catheter** CC
√7th **T83.038 Leakage of other indwelling urethral catheter**

√6th **T83.09 Other mechanical complication of urinary (indwelling) catheter**
Obstruction (mechanical) of urinary (indwelling) catheter
Perforation of urinary (indwelling) catheter
Protrusion of urinary (indwelling) catheter
√7th **T83.090 Other mechanical complication of cystostomy catheter** CC
√7th **T83.098 Other mechanical complication of other indwelling urethral catheter**

√5th **T83.1 Mechanical complication of other urinary devices and implants**

CC Excl: For CC codes in subcategory T83.0: CC with 7th character A, unless otherwise noted: See code: T83.0

√6th **T83.11 Breakdown (mechanical) of other urinary devices and implants**
√7th **T83.110 Breakdown (mechanical) of urinary electronic stimulator device** CC
√7th **T83.111 Breakdown (mechanical) of urinary sphincter implant** CC
√7th **T83.112 Breakdown (mechanical) of urinary stent** CC
√7th **T83.118 Breakdown (mechanical) of other urinary devices and implants** CC

√6th **T83.12 Displacement of other urinary devices and implants**
Malposition of other urinary devices and implants
√7th **T83.120 Displacement of urinary electronic stimulator device** CC
√7th **T83.121 Displacement of urinary sphincter implant** CC
√7th **T83.122 Displacement of urinary stent** CC
√7th **T83.128 Displacement of other urinary devices and implants** CC

√6th **T83.19 Other mechanical complication of other urinary devices and implants**
Leakage of other urinary devices and implants
Obstruction (mechanical) of other urinary devices and implants
Perforation of other urinary devices and implants
Protrusion of other urinary devices and implants
√7th **T83.190 Other mechanical complication of urinary electronic stimulator device** CC
√7th **T83.191 Other mechanical complication of urinary sphincter implant** CC
√7th **T83.192 Other mechanical complication of urinary stent** CC
√7th **T83.198 Other mechanical complication of other urinary devices and implants** CC

√5th **T83.2 Mechanical complication of graft of urinary organ**

CC Excl: For CC codes in subcategory T83.0: CC with 7th character A, unless otherwise noted: See code: T83.0

√x7th **T83.21 Breakdown (mechanical) of graft of urinary organ** CC
√x7th **T83.22 Displacement of graft of urinary organ** CC
Malposition of graft of urinary organ
√x7th **T83.23 Leakage of graft of urinary organ** CC
√x7th **T83.29 Other mechanical complication of graft of urinary organ** CC
Obstruction (mechanical) of graft of urinary organ
Perforation of graft of urinary organ
Protrusion of graft of urinary organ

√5th **T83.3 Mechanical complication of intrauterine contraceptive device**
√x7th **T83.31 Breakdown (mechanical) of intrauterine contraceptive device** ♀
√x7th **T83.32 Displacement of intrauterine contraceptive device** ♀
Malposition of intrauterine contraceptive device
√x7th **T83.39 Other mechanical complication of intrauterine contraceptive device** ♀
Leakage of intrauterine contraceptive device
Obstruction (mechanical) of intrauterine contraceptive device
Perforation of intrauterine contraceptive device
Protrusion of intrauterine contraceptive device

√5th **T83.4 Mechanical complication of other prosthetic devices, implants and grafts of genital tract**

CC Excl: For CC codes in subcategory T83.0: CC with 7th character A, unless otherwise noted: See code: T83.0

√6th **T83.41 Breakdown (mechanical) of other prosthetic devices, implants and grafts of genital tract**
√7th **T83.410 Breakdown (mechanical) of penile (implanted) prosthesis** CC ♂
√7th **T83.418 Breakdown (mechanical) of other prosthetic devices, implants and grafts of genital tract** CC

√6th **T83.42 Displacement of other prosthetic devices, implants and grafts of genital tract**
Malposition of other prosthetic devices, implants and grafts of genital tract
√7th **T83.420 Displacement of penile (implanted) prosthesis** CC ♂
√7th **T83.428 Displacement of other prosthetic devices, implants and grafts of genital tract** CC

√6th **T83.49 Other mechanical complication of other prosthetic devices, implants and grafts of genital tract**
Leakage of other prosthetic devices, implants and grafts of genital tract
Obstruction, mechanical of other prosthetic devices, implants and grafts of genital tract
Perforation of other prosthetic devices, implants and grafts of genital tract
Protrusion of other prosthetic devices, implants and grafts of genital tract
√7th **T83.490 Other mechanical complication of penile (implanted) prosthesis** CC ♂
√7th **T83.498 Other mechanical complication of other prosthetic devices, implants and grafts of genital tract** CC

T83.5 Infection and inflammatory reaction due to prosthetic device, implant and graft in urinary system
Use additional code to identify infection

7 **T83.51 Infection and inflammatory reaction due to indwelling urinary catheter** CC
EXCLUDES 2 *complications of stoma of urinary tract (N99.5-)*
CC Excl: CC with 7th character A: D78.81-D78.89, E36.8, E89.810-E89.89, H59.011-H59.019, H59.031-H59.099, H59.811-H59.89, H95.811-H95.89, I97.3, L76.81-L76.82, M96.89, N39.0, N98.1-N98.9, N99.510-N99.518, T81.82XA, T81.89X-T81.9XX with 7th A, T83.010A, T83.020A, T83.030A, T83.090A, T83.110-T83.29X with 7th A, T83.410-T83.718 with 7th A, T83.728-T83.9XX with 7th A, T85.310-T85.311 with 7th A, T85.320-T85.321 with 7th A, T85.390-T85.391 with 7th A, T85.510-T85.612 with 7th A, T85.614-T85.622 with 7th A, T85.624-T85.692 with 7th A, T85.694-T85.9XX with 7th A, T86.842-T86.849

T83.59 Infection and inflammatory reaction due to prosthetic device, implant and graft in urinary system CC
CC Excl: CC with 7th character A: D78.81-D78.89, E36.8, E89.810-E89.89, H59.011-H59.019, H59.031-H59.099, H59.811-H59.89, H95.811-H95.89, I97.3, L76.81-L76.82, M96.89, N98.1-N98.9, N99.510-N99.518, T81.82XA, T81.89X-T81.9XX with 7th A, T83.010A, T83.020A, T83.030A, T83.090A, T83.110-T83.29X with 7th A, T83.410-T83.718 with 7th A, T83.728-T83.9XX with 7th A, T85.310-T85.311 with 7th A, T85.320-T85.321 with 7th A, T85.390-T85.391 with 7th A, T85.510-T85.9XX with 7th A, T86.820-T86.829, T86.842-T86.849

T83.6 Infection and inflammatory reaction due to prosthetic device, implant and graft in genital tract CC
Use additional code to identify infection
CC Excl: See code: T83.59

T83.7 Complications due to implanted mesh and other prosthetic materials

T83.71 Erosion of implanted mesh and other prosthetic materials to surrounding organ or tissue

T83.711 Erosion of implanted vaginal mesh and other prosthetic materials to surrounding organ or tissue ♀
Erosion of implanted vaginal mesh and other prosthetic materials into pelvic floor muscles

T83.718 Erosion of other implanted mesh and other prosthetic materials to surrounding organ or tissue CC
CC Excl: CC with 7th character A: D78.81-D78.89, E36.8, E89.810-E89.89, H59.011-H59.019, H59.031-H59.099, H59.811-H59.89, H95.811-H95.89, I97.3, L76.81-L76.82, M96.89, N98.1-N98.9, N99.510-N99.518, T81.82XA, T81.89X-T81.9XX with 7th A, T83.010A, T83.020A, T83.030A, T83.090A, T83.110-T83.29X with 7th A, T83.410-T83.718 with 7th A, T83.728-T83.9XX with 7th A

T83.72 Exposure of implanted mesh and other prosthetic materials into surrounding organ or tissue

T83.721 Exposure of implanted vaginal mesh and other prosthetic materials into vagina ♀
Exposure of implanted vaginal mesh and other prosthetic materials through vaginal wall

T83.728 Exposure of other implanted mesh and other prosthetic materials to surrounding organ or tissue CC
CC Excl: See code: T83.718

T83.8 Other specified complications of genitourinary prosthetic devices, implants and grafts

CC Excl: For CC/MCC codes in subcategory T83.8: CC with 7th character A, unless otherwise noted: D78.81-D78.89, E36.8, E89.810-E89.89, H59.011-H59.019, H59.031-H59.099, H59.811-H59.89, H95.811-H95.89, I97.3, L76.81-L76.82, M96.89, N98.1-N98.9, N99.510-N99.518, T81.82XA, T81.89X-T81.9XX with 7th A, T83.010A, T83.020A, T83.030 A, T83.090A, T83.110-T83.29X with 7th A, T83.410-T83.718 with 7th A, T83.728-T83.9XX with 7th A, T85.310-T85.311 with 7th A, T85.320-T85.321 with 7th A, T85.390-T85.391 with 7th A, T85.510-T85.9XX with 7th A, T86.820-T86.829, T86.842-T86.849

T83.81 Embolism of genitourinary prosthetic devices, implants and grafts CC

T83.82 Fibrosis of genitourinary prosthetic devices, implants and grafts CC

T83.83 Hemorrhage of genitourinary prosthetic devices, implants and grafts CC

T83.84 Pain from genitourinary prosthetic devices, implants and grafts CC

T83.85 Stenosis of genitourinary prosthetic devices, implants and grafts CC

T83.86 Thrombosis of genitourinary prosthetic devices, implants and grafts CC

T83.89 Other specified complication of genitourinary prosthetic devices, implants and grafts CC

T83.9 Unspecified complication of genitourinary prosthetic device, implant and graft CC
CC Excl: See code: T83.8

T84 Complications of internal orthopedic prosthetic devices, implants and grafts
EXCLUDES 2 *failure and rejection of transplanted organs and tissues (T86.-)*
fracture of bone following insertion of orthopedic implant, joint prosthesis or bone plate (M96.6)

The appropriate 7th character is to be added to each code from category T84.
A initial encounter
D subsequent encounter
S sequela

T84.0 Mechanical complication of internal joint prosthesis

CC Excl: For CC codes in subcategory T84.0: CC with 7th character A, unless otherwise noted: D78.81-D78.89, E36.8, E89.810-E89.89, H59.011-H59.019, H59.031-H59.099, H59.811-H59.89, H95.811-H95.89, I97.3, L76.81-L76.82, M96.621-M96.69, M96.89, N98.1-N98.9, T81.82XA, T81.89X-T81.9XX with 7th A, T84.010-T84.9XX with 7th A

T84.01 Broken internal joint prosthesis
Breakage (fracture) of prosthetic joint
Broken prosthetic joint implant
EXCLUDES 1 *periprosthetic joint implant fracture (T84.04)*

T84.010 Broken internal right hip prosthesis CC

T84.011 Broken internal left hip prosthesis CC

T84.012 Broken internal right knee prosthesis CC

T84.013 Broken internal left knee prosthesis CC

T84.018 Broken internal joint prosthesis, other site CC
Use additional code to identify the joint (Z96.6-)

T84.019 Broken internal joint prosthesis, unspecified site CC

T84.02 Dislocation of internal joint prosthesis
Instability of internal joint prosthesis
Subluxation of internal joint prosthesis

T84.020 Dislocation of internal right hip prosthesis CC

T84.021 Dislocation of internal left hip prosthesis CC

T84.022 Instability of internal right knee prosthesis CC

T84.023 Instability of internal left knee prosthesis CC

T84.028 Dislocation of other internal joint prosthesis CC
Use additional code to identify the joint (Z96.6-)

7 HAC = Initial encounter only (7th character A, B or C) and not POA.

T84.029 Dislocation of unspecified internal joint prosthesis CC

T84.03 Mechanical loosening of internal prosthetic joint
Aseptic loosening of prosthetic joint

T84.030 Mechanical loosening of internal right hip prosthetic joint CC

T84.031 Mechanical loosening of internal left hip prosthetic joint CC

T84.032 Mechanical loosening of internal right knee prosthetic joint CC

T84.033 Mechanical loosening of internal left knee prosthetic joint CC

T84.038 Mechanical loosening of other internal prosthetic joint CC
Use additional code to identify the joint (Z96.6-)

T84.039 Mechanical loosening of unspecified internal prosthetic joint CC

T84.04 Periprosthetic fracture around internal prosthetic joint
EXCLUDES 2 *breakage (fracture) of prosthetic joint (T84.01)*

T84.040 Periprosthetic fracture around internal prosthetic right hip joint CC

T84.041 Periprosthetic fracture around internal prosthetic left hip joint CC

T84.042 Periprosthetic fracture around internal prosthetic right knee joint CC

T84.043 Periprosthetic fracture around internal prosthetic left knee joint CC

T84.048 Periprosthetic fracture around other internal prosthetic joint CC
Use additional code to identify the joint (Z96.6-)

T84.049 Periprosthetic fracture around unspecified internal prosthetic joint CC

T84.05 Periprosthetic osteolysis of internal prosthetic joint
Use additional code to identify major osseous defect, if applicable (M89.7-)

T84.050 Periprosthetic osteolysis of internal prosthetic right hip joint CC

T84.051 Periprosthetic osteolysis of internal prosthetic left hip joint CC

T84.052 Periprosthetic osteolysis of internal prosthetic right knee joint CC

T84.053 Periprosthetic osteolysis of internal prosthetic left knee joint CC

T84.058 Periprosthetic osteolysis of other internal prosthetic joint CC
Use additional code to identify the joint (Z96.6-)

T84.059 Periprosthetic osteolysis of unspecified internal prosthetic joint CC

T84.06 Wear of articular bearing surface of internal prosthetic joint

T84.060 Wear of articular bearing surface of internal prosthetic right hip joint CC

T84.061 Wear of articular bearing surface of internal prosthetic left hip joint CC

T84.062 Wear of articular bearing surface of internal prosthetic right knee joint CC

T84.063 Wear of articular bearing surface of internal prosthetic left knee joint CC

T84.068 Wear of articular bearing surface of other internal prosthetic joint CC
Use additional code to identify the joint (Z96.6-)

T84.069 Wear of articular bearing surface of unspecified internal prosthetic joint CC

T84.09 Other mechanical complication of internal joint prosthesis
Prosthetic joint implant failure NOS

T84.090 Other mechanical complication of internal right hip prosthesis CC

T84.091 Other mechanical complication of internal left hip prosthesis CC

T84.092 Other mechanical complication of internal right knee prosthesis

T84.093 Other mechanical complication of internal left knee prosthesis CC

T84.098 Other mechanical complication of other internal joint prosthesis CC
Use additional code to identify the joint (Z96.6-)

T84.099 Other mechanical complication of unspecified internal joint prosthesis CC

T84.1 Mechanical complication of internal fixation device of bones of limb
EXCLUDES 2 *mechanical complication of internal fixation device of bones of feet (T84.2-)*
mechanical complication of internal fixation device of bones of fingers (T84.2-)
mechanical complication of internal fixation device of bones of hands (T84.2-)
mechanical complication of internal fixation device of bones of toes (T84.2-)

CC Excl: For CC codes in subcategory T84.1: CC with 7th character A, unless otherwise noted: See code: T84.0

T84.11 Breakdown (mechanical) of internal fixation device of bones of limb

T84.110 Breakdown (mechanical) of internal fixation device of right humerus CC

T84.111 Breakdown (mechanical) of internal fixation device of left humerus CC

T84.112 Breakdown (mechanical) of internal fixation device of bone of right forearm CC

T84.113 Breakdown (mechanical) of internal fixation device of bone of left forearm CC

T84.114 Breakdown (mechanical) of internal fixation device of right femur CC

T84.115 Breakdown (mechanical) of internal fixation device of left femur CC

T84.116 Breakdown (mechanical) of internal fixation device of bone of right lower leg CC

T84.117 Breakdown (mechanical) of internal fixation device of bone of left lower leg CC

T84.119 Breakdown (mechanical) of internal fixation device of unspecified bone of limb CC

T84.12 Displacement of internal fixation device of bones of limb
Malposition of internal fixation device of bones of limb

T84.120 Displacement of internal fixation device of right humerus CC

T84.121 Displacement of internal fixation device of left humerus CC

T84.122 Displacement of internal fixation device of bone of right forearm CC

T84.123 Displacement of internal fixation device of bone of left forearm CC

T84.124 Displacement of internal fixation device of right femur CC

T84.125 Displacement of internal fixation device of left femur CC

T84.126 Displacement of internal fixation device of bone of right lower leg CC

T84.127 Displacement of internal fixation device of bone of left lower leg CC

T84.129 Displacement of internal fixation device of unspecified bone of limb CC

T84.19 Other mechanical complication of internal fixation device of bones of limb
Obstruction (mechanical) of internal fixation device of bones of limb
Perforation of internal fixation device of bones of limb
Protrusion of internal fixation device of bones of limb

T84.190 Other mechanical complication of internal fixation device of right humerus CC

✓7th **T84.191 Other mechanical complication of internal fixation device of left humerus** CC

✓7th **T84.192 Other mechanical complication of internal fixation device of bone of right forearm** CC

✓7th **T84.193 Other mechanical complication of internal fixation device of bone of left forearm** CC

✓7th **T84.194 Other mechanical complication of internal fixation device of right femur** CC

✓7th **T84.195 Other mechanical complication of internal fixation device of left femur** CC

✓7th **T84.196 Other mechanical complication of internal fixation device of bone of right lower leg** CC

✓7th **T84.197 Other mechanical complication of internal fixation device of bone of left lower leg** CC

✓7th **T84.199 Other mechanical complication of internal fixation device of unspecified bone of limb** CC

✓5th **T84.2 Mechanical complication of internal fixation device of other bones**

CC Excl: For CC codes in subcategory T84.2: CC with 7th character A, unless otherwise noted: See code: T84.Ø

✓6th **T84.21 Breakdown (mechanical) of internal fixation device of other bones**

✓7th **T84.21Ø Breakdown (mechanical) of internal fixation device of bones of hand and fingers** CC

✓7th **T84.213 Breakdown (mechanical) of internal fixation device of bones of foot and toes** CC

✓7th **T84.216 Breakdown (mechanical) of internal fixation device of vertebrae** CC

✓7th **T84.218 Breakdown (mechanical) of internal fixation device of other bones** CC

✓6th **T84.22 Displacement of internal fixation device of other bones**

Malposition of internal fixation device of other bones

✓7th **T84.22Ø Displacement of internal fixation device of bones of hand and fingers** CC

✓7th **T84.223 Displacement of internal fixation device of bones of foot and toes** CC

✓7th **T84.226 Displacement of internal fixation device of vertebrae** CC

✓7th **T84.228 Displacement of internal fixation device of other bones** CC

✓6th **T84.29 Other mechanical complication of internal fixation device of other bones**

Obstruction (mechanical) of internal fixation device of other bones
Perforation of internal fixation device of other bones
Protrusion of internal fixation device of other bones

✓7th **T84.29Ø Other mechanical complication of internal fixation device of bones of hand and fingers** CC

✓7th **T84.293 Other mechanical complication of internal fixation device of bones of foot and toes** CC

✓7th **T84.296 Other mechanical complication of internal fixation device of vertebrae** CC

✓7th **T84.298 Other mechanical complication of internal fixation device of other bones** CC

✓5th **T84.3 Mechanical complication of other bone devices, implants and grafts**

EXCLUDES 2 *other complications of bone graft (T86.83-)*

CC Excl: For CC codes in subcategory T84.3: CC with 7th character A, unless otherwise noted: See code: T84.Ø

✓6th **T84.31 Breakdown (mechanical) of other bone devices, implants and grafts**

✓7th **T84.31Ø Breakdown (mechanical) of electronic bone stimulator** CC

✓7th **T84.318 Breakdown (mechanical) of other bone devices, implants and grafts** CC

✓6th **T84.32 Displacement of other bone devices, implants and grafts**

Malposition of other bone devices, implants and grafts

✓7th **T84.32Ø Displacement of electronic bone stimulator** CC

✓7th **T84.328 Displacement of other bone devices, implants and grafts** CC

✓6th **T84.39 Other mechanical complication of other bone devices, implants and grafts**

Obstruction (mechanical) of other bone devices, implants and grafts
Perforation of other bone devices, implants and grafts
Protrusion of other bone devices, implants and grafts

✓7th **T84.39Ø Other mechanical complication of electronic bone stimulator** CC

✓7th **T84.398 Other mechanical complication of other bone devices, implants and grafts** CC

✓5th **T84.4 Mechanical complication of other internal orthopedic devices, implants and grafts**

CC Excl: For CC codes in subcategory T84.4: CC with 7th character A, unless otherwise noted: See code: T84.Ø

✓6th **T84.41 Breakdown (mechanical) of other internal orthopedic devices, implants and grafts**

✓7th **T84.41Ø Breakdown (mechanical) of muscle and tendon graft** CC

✓7th **T84.418 Breakdown (mechanical) of other internal orthopedic devices, implants and grafts** CC

✓6th **T84.42 Displacement of other internal orthopedic devices, implants and grafts**

Malposition of other internal orthopedic devices, implants and grafts

✓7th **T84.42Ø Displacement of muscle and tendon graft** CC

✓7th **T84.428 Displacement of other internal orthopedic devices, implants and grafts** CC

✓6th **T84.49 Other mechanical complication of other internal orthopedic devices, implants and grafts**

Mechanical complication of other internal orthopedic devices, implants and grafts NOS
Obstruction (mechanical) of other internal orthopedic devices, implants and grafts
Perforation of other internal orthopedic devices, implants and grafts
Protrusion of other internal orthopedic devices, implants and grafts

✓7th **T84.49Ø Other mechanical complication of muscle and tendon graft** CC

✓7th **T84.498 Other mechanical complication of other internal orthopedic devices, implants and grafts** CC

✓5th **T84.5 Infection and inflammatory reaction due to internal joint prosthesis**

Use additional code to identify infection

CC Excl: For CC codes in subcategory T84.5: CC with 7th character A, unless otherwise noted: D78.81-D78.89, E36.8, E89.81Ø-E89.89, H59.Ø11-H59.Ø19, H59.Ø31-H59.Ø99, H59.811-H59.89, H95.811-H95.89, I97.3, L76.81-L76.82, M96.621-M96.69, M96.89, N98.1-N98.9, T81.82XA, T81.89X-T81.9XX with 7th A, T84.Ø1Ø-T84.9XX with 7th A, T85.31Ø-T85.311 with 7th A, T85.32Ø-T85.321 with 7th A, T85.39Ø-T85.391 with 7th A, T85.51Ø-T85.9XX with 7th A, T86.82Ø-T86.829, T86.842-T86.849

✓x7th **T84.5Ø Infection and inflammatory reaction due to unspecified internal joint prosthesis** CC

✓x7th **T84.51 Infection and inflammatory reaction due to internal right hip prosthesis** CC

✓x7th **T84.52 Infection and inflammatory reaction due to internal left hip prosthesis** CC

✓x7th **T84.53 Infection and inflammatory reaction due to internal right knee prosthesis** CC

✓x7th **T84.54 Infection and inflammatory reaction due to internal left knee prosthesis** CC

✓x7th **T84.59 Infection and inflammatory reaction due to other internal joint prosthesis** CC

✓5th **T84.6 Infection and inflammatory reaction due to internal fixation device**
Use additional code to identify infection
CC Excl: For CC codes in subcategory T84.6: CC with 7th character A, unless otherwise noted: See code: T84.5

6 ✓x7th **T84.60 Infection and inflammatory reaction due to internal fixation device of unspecified site** CC

✓6th **T84.61 Infection and inflammatory reaction due to internal fixation device of arm**

6 ✓7th **T84.610 Infection and inflammatory reaction due to internal fixation device of right humerus** CC

6 ✓7th **T84.611 Infection and inflammatory reaction due to internal fixation device of left humerus** CC

6 ✓7th **T84.612 Infection and inflammatory reaction due to internal fixation device of right radius** CC

6 ✓7th **T84.613 Infection and inflammatory reaction due to internal fixation device of left radius** CC

6 ✓7th **T84.614 Infection and inflammatory reaction due to internal fixation device of right ulna** CC

6 ✓7th **T84.615 Infection and inflammatory reaction due to internal fixation device of left ulna** CC

6 ✓7th **T84.619 Infection and inflammatory reaction due to internal fixation device of unspecified bone of arm** CC

✓6th **T84.62 Infection and inflammatory reaction due to internal fixation device of leg**

✓7th **T84.620 Infection and inflammatory reaction due to internal fixation device of right femur** CC

✓7th **T84.621 Infection and inflammatory reaction due to internal fixation device of left femur** CC

✓7th **T84.622 Infection and inflammatory reaction due to internal fixation device of right tibia** CC

✓7th **T84.623 Infection and inflammatory reaction due to internal fixation device of left tibia** CC

✓7th **T84.624 Infection and inflammatory reaction due to internal fixation device of right fibula** CC

✓7th **T84.625 Infection and inflammatory reaction due to internal fixation device of left fibula** CC

✓7th **T84.629 Infection and inflammatory reaction due to internal fixation device of unspecified bone of leg** CC

6 ✓x7th **T84.63 Infection and inflammatory reaction due to internal fixation device of spine** CC

6 ✓x7th **T84.69 Infection and inflammatory reaction due to internal fixation device of other site** CC

6 ✓x7th **T84.7 Infection and inflammatory reaction due to other internal orthopedic prosthetic devices, implants and grafts** CC
Use additional code to identify infection
CC Excl: CC with 7th character A: See code: T84.5

✓5th **T84.8 Other specified complications of internal orthopedic prosthetic devices, implants and grafts**
CC Excl: For CC codes in subcategory T84.8: CC with 7th character A, unless otherwise noted: See code: T84.5

✓x7th **T84.81 Embolism due to internal orthopedic prosthetic devices, implants and grafts** CC

✓x7th **T84.82 Fibrosis due to internal orthopedic prosthetic devices, implants and grafts** CC

✓x7th **T84.83 Hemorrhage due to internal orthopedic prosthetic devices, implants and grafts** CC

✓x7th **T84.84 Pain due to internal orthopedic prosthetic devices, implants and grafts** CC

✓x7th **T84.85 Stenosis due to internal orthopedic prosthetic devices, implants and grafts** CC

✓x7th **T84.86 Thrombosis due to internal orthopedic prosthetic devices, implants and grafts** CC

✓x7th **T84.89 Other specified complication of internal orthopedic prosthetic devices, implants and grafts** CC

✓x7th **T84.9 Unspecified complication of internal orthopedic prosthetic device, implant and graft** CC
CC Excl: See code: T84.8

✓4th **T85 Complications of other internal prosthetic devices, implants and grafts**
EXCLUDES 2 *failure and rejection of transplanted organs and tissue (T86.-)*

The appropriate 7th character is to be added to each code from category T85.
A initial encounter
D subsequent encounter
S sequela

✓5th **T85.0 Mechanical complication of ventricular intracranial (communicating) shunt**
CC Excl: For CC codes in subcategory T85.0: CC with 7th character A, unless otherwise noted: D78.81-D78.89, E36.8, E89.810-E89.89, H59.011-H59.019, H59.031-H59.099, H59.811-H59.89, H95.811-H95.89, I97.3, L76.81-L76.82, M96.89, N98.1-N98.9, T81.82XA, T81.89X-T81.9XX with 7th A, T85.01X-T85.199 with 7th A

✓x7th **T85.01 Breakdown (mechanical) of ventricular intracranial (communicating) shunt** CC

✓x7th **T85.02 Displacement of ventricular intracranial (communicating) shunt** CC
Malposition of ventricular intracranial (communicating) shunt

✓x7th **T85.03 Leakage of ventricular intracranial (communicating) shunt** CC

✓x7th **T85.09 Other mechanical complication of ventricular intracranial (communicating) shunt** CC
Obstruction (mechanical) of ventricular intracranial (communicating) shunt
Perforation of ventricular intracranial (communicating) shunt
Protrusion of ventricular intracranial (communicating) shunt

✓5th **T85.1 Mechanical complication of implanted electronic stimulator of nervous system**
CC Excl: For CC codes in subcategory T85.1: CC with 7th character A, unless otherwise noted: See code: T85.0

✓6th **T85.11 Breakdown (mechanical) of implanted electronic stimulator of nervous system**

✓7th **T85.110 Breakdown (mechanical) of implanted electronic neurostimulator (electrode) of brain** CC

✓7th **T85.111 Breakdown (mechanical) of implanted electronic neurostimulator (electrode) of peripheral nerve** CC

✓7th **T85.112 Breakdown (mechanical) of implanted electronic neurostimulator (electrode) of spinal cord** CC

✓7th **T85.118 Breakdown (mechanical) of other implanted electronic stimulator of nervous system** CC

✓6th **T85.12 Displacement of implanted electronic stimulator of nervous system**
Malposition of implanted electronic stimulator of nervous system

✓7th **T85.120 Displacement of implanted electronic neurostimulator (electrode) of brain** CC

✓7th **T85.121 Displacement of implanted electronic neurostimulator (electrode) of peripheral nerve** CC

✓7th **T85.122 Displacement of implanted electronic neurostimulator (electrode) of spinal cord** CC

✓7th **T85.128 Displacement of other implanted electronic stimulator of nervous system** CC

6 HAC = as SDx not POA, in combination with one of the following procedure codes: 0RG[0,1,2,4,6,7,8,A][0,3,4][7,A,J,K,Z][0,1,J]; 0RG[E,F,G,H,J,K][0,3,4][4,7,J,K,Z]Z; 0RG[L,M][0,3,4][4,5,7,J,K,Z]Z; 0RQ[E,F,G,H,J,K,L,M][0,3,4,X]ZZ; 0RU[E,F,G,H,J,K,L,M][0,3,4][7,J,K]Z; 0SG[0,1,3][0,3,4][7,A,J,K,Z][0,1,J]; 0SG[7,8][0,3,4[4,7,J,K,Z]Z.

T85.19 Other mechanical complication of implanted electronic stimulator of nervous system
Leakage of implanted electronic stimulator of nervous system
Obstruction (mechanical) of implanted electronic stimulator of nervous system
Perforation of implanted electronic stimulator of nervous system
Protrusion of implanted electronic stimulator of nervous system

T85.19Ø Other mechanical complication of implanted electronic neurostimulator (electrode) of brain CC
T85.191 Other mechanical complication of implanted electronic neurostimulator (electrode) of peripheral nerve CC
T85.192 Other mechanical complication of implanted electronic neurostimulator (electrode) of spinal cord CC
T85.199 Other mechanical complication of other implanted electronic stimulator of nervous system CC

T85.2 Mechanical complication of intraocular lens
CC Excl: For CC codes in subcategory T85.2: CC with 7th character A, unless otherwise noted: D78.81-D78.89, E89.81Ø-E89.89, H59.Ø11-H59.Ø19, H59.Ø31-H59.Ø99, H59.811-H59.89, H95.811-H95.89, I97.3, M96.89, N98.1-N98.9, T85.21X-T85.29X with 7th A

T85.21 Breakdown (mechanical) of intraocular lens CC
T85.22 Displacement of intraocular lens CC
Malposition of intraocular lens
T85.29 Other mechanical complication of intraocular lens CC
Obstruction (mechanical) of intraocular lens
Perforation of intraocular lens
Protrusion of intraocular lens

T85.3 Mechanical complication of other ocular prosthetic devices, implants and grafts
EXCLUDES 2 *other complications of corneal graft (T86.84-)*
CC Excl: For CC codes in subcategory T85.3: CC with 7th character A, unless otherwise noted: H59.Ø11-H59.Ø19, H59.Ø31-H59.Ø99, H59.811-H59.89, H95.811-H95.89, I97.3, M96.89, N98.1-N98.9, T85.31Ø-T85.311 with 7th A, T85.32Ø-T85.321 with 7th A, T85.39Ø-T85.391 with 7th A, T85.612A, T85.618A, T85.622A, T85.628A, T85.638A, T85.692A, T85.698-T85.9XX with 7th A, T86.842-T86.849

T85.31 Breakdown (mechanical) of other ocular prosthetic devices, implants and grafts
T85.31Ø Breakdown (mechanical) of prosthetic orbit of right eye CC
T85.311 Breakdown (mechanical) of prosthetic orbit of left eye CC
T85.318 Breakdown (mechanical) of other ocular prosthetic devices, implants and grafts
T85.32 Displacement of other ocular prosthetic devices, implants and grafts
Malposition of other ocular prosthetic devices, implants and grafts
T85.32Ø Displacement of prosthetic orbit of right eye CC
T85.321 Displacement of prosthetic orbit of left eye CC
T85.328 Displacement of other ocular prosthetic devices, implants and grafts
T85.39 Other mechanical complication of other ocular prosthetic devices, implants and grafts
Obstruction (mechanical) of other ocular prosthetic devices, implants and grafts
Perforation of other ocular prosthetic devices, implants and grafts
Protrusion of other ocular prosthetic devices, implants and grafts
T85.39Ø Other mechanical complication of prosthetic orbit of right eye CC
T85.391 Other mechanical complication of prosthetic orbit of left eye CC
T85.398 Other mechanical complication of other ocular prosthetic devices, implants and grafts

T85.4 Mechanical complication of breast prosthesis and implant
CC Excl: For CC codes in subcategory T85.4: CC with 7th character A, unless otherwise noted: D78.81-D78.89, E89.81Ø-E89.89, H59.Ø11-H59.Ø19, H59.Ø31-H59.Ø99, H59.811-H59.89, H95.811-H95.89, I97.3, M96.89, N98.1-N98.9, T85.41X-T85.49X with 7th A

T85.41 Breakdown (mechanical) of breast prosthesis and implant CC
T85.42 Displacement of breast prosthesis and implant CC
Malposition of breast prosthesis and implant
T85.43 Leakage of breast prosthesis and implant CC
T85.44 Capsular contracture of breast implant CC
T85.49 Other mechanical complication of breast prosthesis and implant CC
Obstruction (mechanical) of breast prosthesis and implant
Perforation of breast prosthesis and implant
Protrusion of breast prosthesis and implant

T85.5 Mechanical complication of gastrointestinal prosthetic devices, implants and grafts
CC Excl: For CC codes in subcategory T85.5: CC with 7th character A, unless otherwise noted: H95.811-H95.89, I97.3, M96.89, N98.1-N98.9, T85.51Ø-T85.598 with 7th A, T85.612A, T85.618A, T85.622A, T85.628A, T85.638A, T85.692A, T85.698-T85.9XX with 7th A

T85.51 Breakdown (mechanical) of gastrointestinal prosthetic devices, implants and grafts
T85.51Ø Breakdown (mechanical) of bile duct prosthesis CC
T85.511 Breakdown (mechanical) of esophageal anti-reflux device CC
T85.518 Breakdown (mechanical) of other gastrointestinal prosthetic devices, implants and grafts CC
T85.52 Displacement of gastrointestinal prosthetic devices, implants and grafts
Malposition of gastrointestinal prosthetic devices, implants and grafts
T85.52Ø Displacement of bile duct prosthesis CC
T85.521 Displacement of esophageal anti-reflux device CC
T85.528 Displacement of other gastrointestinal prosthetic devices, implants and grafts CC
T85.59 Other mechanical complication of gastrointestinal prosthetic devices, implants and
Obstruction, mechanical of gastrointestinal prosthetic devices, implants and grafts
Perforation of gastrointestinal prosthetic devices, implants and grafts
Protrusion of gastrointestinal prosthetic devices, implants and grafts
T85.59Ø Other mechanical complication of bile duct prosthesis CC
T85.591 Other mechanical complication of esophageal anti-reflux device CC
T85.598 Other mechanical complication of other gastrointestinal prosthetic devices, implants and grafts CC

T85.6 Mechanical complication of other specified internal and external prosthetic devices, implants and grafts
T85.61 Breakdown (mechanical) of other specified internal prosthetic devices, implants and grafts
T85.61Ø Breakdown (mechanical) of epidural and subdural infusion catheter CC
CC Excl: CC with 7th character A: H95.811-H95.89, I97.3, M96.89, N98.1-N98.9, T85.61ØA, T85.612A, T85.618-T85.62Ø with 7th A, T85.622A, T85.628-T85.63Ø with 7th A, T85.638-T85.69Ø with 7th A, T85.692A, T85.698-T85.9XX with 7th A

✓7th **T85.611 Breakdown (mechanical) of intraperitoneal dialysis catheter** CC
EXCLUDES 1 *mechanical complication of vascular dialysis catheter (T82.4-)*
CC Excl: CC with 7th character A: H95.811-H95.89, I97.3, M96.89, N98.1-N98.9, T85.611-T85.612 with 7th A, T85.614-T85.618 with 7th A, T85.621-T85.622 with 7th A, T85.624-T85.628 with 7th A, T85.631-T85.638 with 7th A, T85.691-T85.692 with 7th A, T85.694-T85.9XX with 7th A

✓7th **T85.612 Breakdown (mechanical) of permanent sutures** CC
EXCLUDES 1 *mechanical complication of permanent (wire) suture used in bone repair (T84.1-T84.2)*
CC Excl: CC with 7th character A: D78.81-D78.89, E89.810-E89.89, H59.011-H59.019, H59.031-H59.099, H59.811-H59.89, H95.811-H95.89, I97.3, M96.89, N98.1-N98.9, T85.310-T85.311 with 7th A, T85.320-T85.321 with 7th A, T85.390-T85.391 with 7th A, T85.510-T85.612 with 7th A, T85.614-T85.622 with 7th A, T85.624-T85.692 with 7th A, T85.694-T85.9XX with 7th A, T86.842-T86.849

✓7th **T85.613 Breakdown (mechanical) of artificial skin graft and decellularized allodermis** CC
Failure of artificial skin graft and decellularized allodermis
Non-adherence of artificial skin graft and decellularized allodermis
Poor incorporation of artificial skin graft and decellularized allodermis
Shearing of artificial skin graft and decellularized allodermis
CC Excl: CC with 7th character A: H95.811-H95.89, I97.3, M96.89, N98.1-N98.9, T85.612-T85.613 with 7th A, T85.618A, T85.622-T85.623 with 7th A, T85.628A, T85.638A, T85.692-T85.693 with 7th A, T85.698-T85.9XX with 7th A, T86.820-T86.829

✓7th **T85.614 Breakdown (mechanical) of insulin pump** CC
CC Excl: CC with 7th character A: H95.811-H95.89, I97.3, M96.621-M96.69, M96.89, N98.1-N98.9, N99.510-N99.518, T81.82X with 7th A, T81.89X-T82.09X with 7th A, T82.110-T82.118 with 7th A, T82.120-T82.128 with 7th A, T82.190-T82.198 with 7th A, T82.211-T83.010 with 7th A, T83.020A, T83.030A, T83.090A, T83.110-T83.29X with 7th A, T83.410-T83.718 with 7th A, T83.728-T85.29X with 7th A, T85.41X-T85.49X with 7th A, T85.611-T85.612 with 7th A, T85.614-T85.618 with 7th A, T85.621-T85.622 with 7th A, T85.624-T85.628 with 7th A, T85.631-T85.638 with 7th A, T85.691-T85.692 with 7th A, T85.694-T85.9XX with 7th A, T86.820-T86.829

✓7th **T85.618 Breakdown (mechanical) of other specified internal prosthetic devices, implants and grafts** CC
CC Excl: CC with 7th character A: D78.81-D78.89, E89.810-E89.89, H59.011-H59.019, H59.031-H59.099, H59.811-H59.89, H95.811-H95.89, I97.3, M96.89, N98.1-N98.9, T85.310-T85.311 with 7th A, T85.320-T85.321 with 7th A, T85.390-T85.391 with 7th A, T85.510-T85.612 with 7th A, T85.614-T85.622 with 7th A, T85.624-T85.692 with 7th A, T85.694-T85.9XX with 7th A, T86.842-T86.849

✓6th **T85.62 Displacement of other specified internal prosthetic devices, implants and grafts**
Malposition of other specified internal prosthetic devices, implants and grafts

✓7th **T85.620 Displacement of epidural and subdural infusion catheter** CC
CC Excl: CC with 7th character A: H95.811-H95.89, I97.3, M96.89, N98.1-N98.9, T85.610A, T85.612A, T85.618-T85.620 with 7th A, T85.622A, T85.628-T85.630 with 7th A, T85.638-T85.690 with 7th A, T85.69 A, T85.698-T85.9XX with 7th A

✓7th **T85.621 Displacement of intraperitoneal dialysis catheter** CC
EXCLUDES 1 *mechanical complication of vascular dialysis catheter (T82.4-)*
CC Excl: CC with 7th character A: H95.811-H95.89, I97.3, M96.89, N98.1-N98.9, T85.611-T85.612 with 7th A, T85.614-T85.618 with 7th A, T85.621-T85.622 with 7th A, T85.624-T85.628 with 7th A, T85.631-T85.638 with 7th A, T85.691-T85.692 with 7th A, T85.694-T85.9XX with 7th A

✓7th **T85.622 Displacement of permanent sutures** CC
EXCLUDES 1 *mechanical complication of permanent (wire) suture used in bone repair (T84.1-T84.2)*
CC Excl: CC with 7th character A: D78.81-D78.89, E89.810-E89.89, H59.011-H59.019, H59.031-H59.099, H59.811-H59.89, H95.811-H95.89, I97.3, M96.89, N98.1-N98.9, T85.310-T85.311 with 7th A, T85.320-T85.321 with 7th A, T85.390-T85.391 with 7th A, T85.510-T85.612 with 7th A, T85.614-T85.622 with 7th A, T85.624-T85.692 with 7th A, T85.694-T85.9XX with 7th A, T86.842-T86.849

✓7th **T85.623 Displacement of artificial skin graft and decellularized allodermis** CC
Dislodgement of artificial skin graft and decellularized allodermis
Displacement of artificial skin graft and decellularized allodermis
CC Excl: CC with 7th character A: H95.811-H95.89, I97.3, M96.89, N98.1-N98.9, T85.612-T85.613 with 7th A, T85.618 with 7th A, T85.622-T85.623 with 7th A, T85.628A, T85.638A, T85.692-T85.693 with 7th A, T85.698-T85.9XX with 7th A, T86.820-T86.829

✓7th **T85.624 Displacement of insulin pump** CC
CC Excl: CC with 7th character A: H95.811-H95.89, I97.3, M96.621-M96.69, M96.89, N98.1-N98.9, N99.510-N99.518, T81.82X with 7th A, T81.89X-T82.09X with 7th A, T82.110-T82.118 with 7th A, T82.120-T82.128 with 7th A, T82.190-T82.198 with 7th A, T82.211-T83.010 with 7th A, T83.020A, T83.030 with 7th A, T83.090A, T83.110-T83.29X with 7th A, T83.410-T83.718 with 7th A, T83.728-T85.29X with 7th A, T85.41X-T85.49X with 7th A, T85.611-T85.612 with 7th A, T85.614-T85.618 with 7th A, T85.621-T85.622 with 7th A, T85.624-T85.628 with 7th A, T85.631-T85.638 with 7th A, T85.691-T85.692 with 7th A, T85.694-T85.9XX with 7th A, T86.820-T86.829

T85.628 Displacement of other specified internal prosthetic devices, implants and grafts CC
CC Excl: CC with 7th character A: D78.81-D78.89, E89.810-E89.89, H59.011-H59.019, H59.031-H59.099, H59.811-H59.89, H95.811-H95.89, I97.3, M96.89, N98.1-N98.9, T85.310-T85.311 with 7th A, T85.320-T85.321 with 7th A, T85.390-T85.391 with 7th A, T85.510-T85.612 with 7th A, T85.614-T85.622 with 7th A, T85.624-T85.692 with 7th A, T85.694-T85.9XX with 7th A, T86.842-T86.849

✓6th **T85.63 Leakage of other specified internal prosthetic devices, implants and grafts**

✓7th **T85.630 Leakage of epidural and subdural infusion catheter** CC
CC Excl: CC with 7th character A: See code: T85.620

✓7th **T85.631 Leakage of intraperitoneal dialysis catheter** CC
EXCLUDES 1 *mechanical complication of vascular dialysis catheter (T82.4)*
CC Excl: CC with 7th character A: See code: T85.621

✓7th **T85.633 Leakage of insulin pump** CC
CC Excl: CC with 7th character A: See code: T86.624

7th **T85.638 Leakage of other specified internal prosthetic devices, implants and grafts** CC
CC Excl: CC with 7th character A: See code: T85.628

6th **T85.69 Other mechanical complication of other specified internal prosthetic devices, implants and grafts**
Obstruction, mechanical of other specified internal prosthetic devices, implants and grafts
Perforation of other specified internal prosthetic devices, implants and grafts
Protrusion of other specified internal prosthetic devices, implants and grafts

7th **T85.690 Other mechanical complication of epidural and subdural infusion catheter** CC
CC Excl: CC with 7th character A: See code: T85.620

7th **T85.691 Other mechanical complication of intraperitoneal dialysis catheter** CC
EXCLUDES 1 *mechanical complication of vascular dialysis catheter (T82.4)*
CC Excl: CC with 7th character A: See code: T85.621

T85.692 Other mechanical complication of permanent sutures CC
EXCLUDES 1 *mechanical complication of permanent (wire) suture used in bone repair (T84.1-T84.2)*
CC Excl: CC with 7th character A: See code: T85.622

7th **T85.693 Other mechanical complication of artificial skin graft and decellularized allodermis** CC
CC Excl: CC with 7th character A: See code: T85.623

7th **T85.694 Other mechanical complication of insulin pump** CC
CC Excl: CC with 7th character A: See code: T85.624

7th **T85.698 Other mechanical complication of other specified internal prosthetic devices, implants and grafts** CC
Mechanical complication of nonabsorbable surgical material NOS
CC Excl: CC with 7th character A: See code: T85.628

5th **T85.7 Infection and inflammatory reaction due to other internal prosthetic devices, implants and grafts**
Use additional code to identify infection

x7th **T85.71 Infection and inflammatory reaction due to peritoneal dialysis catheter** CC
CC Excl: CC with 7th character A: See code: T85.628

x7th **T85.72 Infection and inflammatory reaction due to insulin pump** CC
CC Excl: CC with 7th character A: D78.81-D78.89, E36.8, E89.810-E89.89, H59.011-H59.019, H59.031-H59.099, H59.811-H59.89, H95.811-H95.89, I97.3, L76.81-L76.82, M96.621-M96.69, M96.89, N98.1-N98.9, N99.510-N99.518, T81.82XA, T81.89X-T82.09X with 7th A, T82.110-T82.118 with 7th A, T82.120-T82.128 with 7th A, T82.190-T82.198 with 7th A, T82.211-T83.010 with 7th A, T83.020A, T83.030A, T83.090A, T83.110-T83.29X with 7th A, T83.410-T83.718 with 7th A, T83.728-T85.9XX with 7th A, T86.820-T86.829, T86.840-T86.849

x7th **T85.79 Infection and inflammatory reaction due to other internal prosthetic devices, implants and grafts** CC
CC Excl: See code: T85.72

5th **T85.8 Other specified complications of internal prosthetic devices, implants and grafts, not elsewhere classified**

x7th **T85.81 Embolism due to internal prosthetic devices, implants and grafts, not elsewhere classified** CC
CC Excl: See code: T85.72

x7th **T85.82 Fibrosis due to internal prosthetic devices, implants and grafts, not elsewhere classified** CC
CC Excl: See code: T85.72

x7th **T85.83 Hemorrhage due to internal prosthetic devices, implants and grafts, not elsewhere classified** CC
CC Excl: See code: T85.72

x7th **T85.84 Pain due to internal prosthetic devices, implants and grafts, not elsewhere classified** CC
CC Excl: See code: T85.72

x7th **T85.85 Stenosis due to internal prosthetic devices, implants and grafts, not elsewhere classified** CC
CC Excl: See code: T85.72

x7th **T85.86 Thrombosis due to internal prosthetic devices, implants and grafts, not elsewhere classified** CC
CC Excl: See code: T85.72

x7th **T85.89 Other specified complication of internal prosthetic devices, implants and grafts, not elsewhere classified** CC
CC Excl: See code: T85.72

x7th **T85.9 Unspecified complication of internal prosthetic device, implant and graft**
Complication of internal prosthetic device, implant and graft NOS

4th **T86 Complications of transplanted organs and tissue**
Use additional code to identify other transplant complications, such as:
graft-versus-host disease (D89.81-)
malignancy associated with organ transplant (C80.2)
post-transplant lymphoproliferative disorders (PTLD) (D47.Z1)

5th **T86.0 Complications of bone marrow transplant**

CC Excl: For CC codes in subcategory T86.0: CC with 7th character A, unless otherwise noted: D78.81-D78.89, D89.810-D89.813, E89.810-E89.89, H59.011-H59.019, H59.031-H59.099, H59.811-H59.89, H95.811-H95.89, I97.3, M96.89, N98.1-N98.9, T86.00-T86.09

T86.00 Unspecified complication of bone marrow transplant CC
T86.01 Bone marrow transplant rejection CC
T86.02 Bone marrow transplant failure CC
T86.03 Bone marrow transplant infection CC
T86.09 Other complications of bone marrow transplant CC

5th **T86.1 Complications of kidney transplant**

CC Excl: For CC codes in subcategory T86.1: CC with 7th character A, unless otherwise noted: D78.81-D78.89, E89.810-E89.89, H59.011-H59.019, H59.031-H59.099, H59.811-H59.89, H95.811-H95.89, I97.3, M96.89, N98.1-N98.9, T86.10-T86.19

T86.10 Unspecified complication of kidney transplant CC
T86.11 Kidney transplant rejection CC
T86.12 Kidney transplant failure CC
AHA: 2013, 1Q, 24
T86.13 Kidney transplant infection CC
Use additional code to specify infection
T86.19 Other complication of kidney transplant CC

5th **T86.2 Complications of heart transplant**
EXCLUDES 1 *complication of:*
artificial heart device (T82.5)
heart-lung transplant (T86.3)

CC Excl: For CC codes in subcategory T86.2: CC with 7th character A, unless otherwise noted: D78.81-D78.89, E89.810-E89.89, H59.011-H59.019, H59.031-H59.099, H59.811-H59.89, H95.811-H95.89, I97.3, M96.89, N98.1-N98.9, T86.20-T86.39

T86.20 Unspecified complication of heart transplant CC
T86.21 Heart transplant rejection CC
T86.22 Heart transplant failure CC
T86.23 Heart transplant infection CC
Use additional code to specify infection

6th **T86.29 Other complications of heart transplant**
T86.290 Cardiac allograft vasculopathy CC
EXCLUDES 1 *atherosclerosis of coronary arteries (I25.75-, I25.76-, I25.81-)*
T86.298 Other complications of heart transplant CC

5th **T86.3 Complications of heart-lung transplant**

CC Excl: For CC codes in subcategory T86.3: CC with 7th character A, unless otherwise noted: See code: T86.2

T86.30 Unspecified complication of heart-lung transplant PDx CC CC
T86.31 Heart-lung transplant rejection PDx CC CC
T86.32 Heart-lung transplant failure PDx CC CC
T86.33 Heart-lung transplant infection PDx CC CC
Use additional code to specify infection
T86.39 Other complications of heart-lung transplant PDx CC CC

T86.4 Complications of liver transplant

T86.40 Unspecified complication of liver transplant CC

CC Excl: For CC codes in subcategory T86.4: CC with 7th character A, unless otherwise noted: D78.81-D78.89, E89.810-E89.89, H59.011-H59.019, H59.031-H59.099, H59.811-H59.89, H95.811-H95.89, I97.3, M96.89, N98.1-N98.9, T86.40-T86.49

T86.41 Liver transplant rejection CC

T86.42 Liver transplant failure CC

T86.43 Liver transplant infection CC

Use additional code to identify infection, such as: cytomegalovirus (CMV) infection (B25.-)

T86.49 Other complications of liver transplant CC

T86.5 Complications of stem cell transplant CC

Complications from stem cells from peripheral blood
Complications from stem cells from umbilical cord

CC Excl: For CC codes in subcategory T86.5: CC with 7th character A, unless otherwise noted: D78.81-D78.89, E89.810-E89.89, H59.011-H59.019, H59.031-H59.099, H59.811-H59.89, H95.811-H95.89, I97.3, M96.89, N98.1-N98.9, T86.5, T86.830-T86.839

T86.8 Complications of other transplanted organs and tissues

T86.81 Complications of lung transplant

EXCLUDES 1 *complication of heart-lung transplant (T86.3-)*

CC Excl: For CC codes in subcategory T86.81: CC with 7th character A, unless otherwise noted: D78.81-D78.89, E89.810-E89.89, H59.011-H59.019, H59.031-H59.099, H59.811-H59.89, H95.811-H95.89, I97.3, M96.89, N98.1-N98.9, T86.810-T86.819

T86.810 Lung transplant rejection CC

T86.811 Lung transplant failure CC

T86.812 Lung transplant infection CC

Use additional code to specify infection

T86.818 Other complications of lung transplant CC

T86.819 Unspecified complication of lung transplant CC

T86.82 Complications of skin graft (allograft) (autograft)

EXCLUDES 2 *complication of artificial skin graft (T85.693)*

CC Excl: For CC codes in subcategory T86.82: CC with 7th character A, unless otherwise noted: D78.81-D78.89, E89.810-E89.89, H59.011-H59.019, H59.031-H59.099, H59.811-H59.89, H95.811-H95.89, I97.3, M96.89, N98.1-N98.9, T85.613A, T85.623A, T85.693A, T86.820-T86.829

T86.820 Skin graft (allograft) rejection CC

T86.821 Skin graft (allograft) (autograft) failure CC

T86.822 Skin graft (allograft) (autograft) infection CC

Use additional code to specify infection

T86.828 Other complications of skin graft (allograft) (autograft) CC

T86.829 Unspecified complication of skin graft (allograft) (autograft) CC

T86.83 Complications of bone graft

EXCLUDES 2 *mechanical complications of bone graft (T84.3-)*

CC Excl: For CC codes in subcategory T86.83: CC with 7th character A, unless otherwise noted: H95.811-H95.89, I97.3, M96.89, N98.1-N98.9, T86.5, T86.830-T86.839

T86.830 Bone graft rejection CC

T86.831 Bone graft failure CC

T86.832 Bone graft infection CC

Use additional code to specify infection

T86.838 Other complications of bone graft CC

T86.839 Unspecified complication of bone graft CC

T86.84 Complications of corneal transplant

EXCLUDES 2 *mechanical complications of corneal graft (T85.3-)*

T86.840 Corneal transplant rejection CC

CC Excl: CC with 7th character A: H59.011-H59.019, H59.031-H59.099, H59.811-H59.89, H95.811-H95.89, I97.3, M96.89, N98.1-N98.9, T85.318A, T85.328A, T85.398A, T86.840-T86.841

T86.841 Corneal transplant failure CC

CC Excl: See code: T86.840

T86.842 Corneal transplant infection CC

Use additional code to specify infection

CC Excl: CC with 7th character A: H59.011-H59.019, H59.031-H59.099, H59.811-H59.89, H95.811-H95.89, I97.3, M96.621-M96.69, M96.89, N98.1-N98.9, N99.510-N99.518, T81.82XA, T81.89X-T82.09X with 7th A, T82.110-T82.118 with 7th A, T82.120-T82.128 with 7th A, T82.190-T82.198 with 7th A, T82.211-T83.010 with 7th A, T83.020A, T83.030A, T83.090A, T83.110-T83.29X with 7th A, T83.410-T83.718 with 7th A, T83.728-T85.49X with 7th A, T85.612A, T85.618A, T85.622A, T85.628A, T85.638A, T85.692A, T85.698-T85.9XX with 7th A, T86.820-T86.829, T86.840-T86.849

T86.848 Other complications of corneal transplant CC

CC Excl: See code: T86.842

T86.849 Unspecified complication of corneal transplant CC

CC Excl: See code: T86.842

T86.85 Complication of intestine transplant

T86.850 Intestine transplant rejection CC

CC Excl: CC with 7th character A: D47.Z1, D78.81-D78.89, E89.810-E89.89, H59.011-H59.019, H59.031-H59.099, H59.811-H59.89, H95.811-H95.89, I97.3, M96.89, N98.1-N98.9, T86.850-T86.859, T86.90-T86.99

T86.851 Intestine transplant failure CC

CC Excl: See code: T86.850

T86.852 Intestine transplant infection CC

Use additional code to specify infection

CC Excl: See code: T86.850

T86.858 Other complications of intestine transplant CC

CC Excl: See code: T86.850

T86.859 Unspecified complication of intestine transplant CC

CC Excl: See code: T86.850

T86.89 Complications of other transplanted tissue

Transplant failure or rejection of pancreas

T86.890 Other transplanted tissue rejection CC

CC Excl: CC with 7th character A: D78.81-D78.89, E89.810-E89.89, H59.011-H59.019, H59.031-H59.099, H59.811-H59.89, H95.811-H95.89, I97.3, M96.89, N98.1-N98.9, T86.890-T86.899

T86.891 Other transplanted tissue failure CC

CC Excl: See code: T86.890

T86.892 Other transplanted tissue infection CC

Use additional code to specify infection

CC Excl: See code: T86.890

T86.898 Other complications of other transplanted tissue CC

CC Excl: See code: T86.890

T86.899 Unspecified complication of other transplanted tissue CC

CC Excl: See code: T86.890

T86.9 Complication of unspecified transplanted organ and tissue

T86.90 Unspecified complication of unspecified transplanted organ and tissue CC

CC Excl: CC with 7th character A: D47.Z1, D78.81-D78.89, E89.810-E89.89, H59.011-H59.019, H59.031-H59.099, H59.811-H59.89, H95.811-H95.89, I97.3, M96.89, N98.1-N98.9, T86.850-T86.859, T86.90-T86.99

T86.91 Unspecified transplanted organ and tissue rejection CC

CC Excl: See code: T86.90

T86.92 Unspecified transplanted organ and tissue failure CC

CC Excl: See code: T86.90

T86.93 Unspecified transplanted organ and tissue infection CC

Use additional code to specify infection

CC Excl: See code: T86.90

T86.99 Other **complications of unspecified transplanted organ and tissue** CC
CC Excl: See code: T86.90

✓4th **T87 Complications peculiar to reattachment and amputation**

✓5th **T87.0 Complications of reattached (part of)** upper extremity

✓6th **T87.0X Complications of reattached (part of) upper extremity**

> **CC Excl: For CC codes in subcategory T87.0X: CC with 7th character A, unless otherwise noted:** D78.81-D78.89, E36.8, E89.810-E89.89, H59.011-H59.019, H59.031-H59.099, H59.811-H59.89, H95.811-H95.89, I97.3, L76.81-L76.82, M96.89, N98.1-N98.9, T81.82XA, T81.89X-T81.9XX with 7th A, T87.0X1-T87.0X9

T87.0X1 Complications of reattached (part of) right **upper extremity** CC

T87.0X2 Complications of reattached (part of) left **upper extremity** CC

T87.0X9 Complications of reattached (part of) unspecified **upper extremity** CC

✓5th **T87.1 Complications of reattached (part of)** lower extremity

✓6th **T87.1X Complications of reattached (part of) lower extremity**

> **CC Excl: For CC codes in subcategory T87.1X: CC with 7th character A, unless otherwise noted:** D78.81-D78.89, E36.8, E89.810-E89.89, H59.011-H59.019, H59.031-H59.099, H59.811-H59.89, H95.811-H95.89, I97.3, L76.81-L76.82, M96.89, N98.1-N98.9, T81.82XA, T81.89X-T81.9XX with 7th A, T87.1X1-T87.1X9

T87.1X1 Complications of reattached (part of) right **lower extremity** CC

T87.1X2 Complications of reattached (part of) left **lower extremity** CC

T87.1X9 Complications of reattached (part of) unspecified **lower extremity** CC

T87.2 Complications of other reattached **body** part CC
CC Excl: CC with 7th character A: D78.81-D78.89, E36.8, E89.810-E89.89, H59.011-H59.019, H59.031-H59.099, H59.811-H59.89, H95.811-H95.89, I97.3, L76.81-L76.82, M96.89, N98.1-N98.9, T81.82XA, T81.89X-T81.9XX with 7th A, T87.2

✓5th **T87.3** Neuroma **of amputation stump**

T87.30 Neuroma of amputation stump, unspecified **extremity**

T87.31 Neuroma of amputation stump, right upper **extremity**

T87.32 Neuroma of amputation stump, left upper **extremity**

T87.33 Neuroma of amputation stump, right lower **extremity**

T87.34 Neuroma of amputation stump, left lower **extremity**

✓5th **T87.4** Infection **of amputation stump**

> **CC Excl: For CC codes in subcategory T87.4: CC with 7th character A, unless otherwise noted:** D78.81-D78.89, E36.8, E89.810-E89.89, H59.011-H59.019, H59.031-H59.099, H59.811-H59.89, H95.811-H95.89, I97.3, L76.81-L76.82, M96.89, N98.1-N98.9, T81.82XA, T81.89X-T81.9XX with 7th A, T87.40-T87.9

T87.40 Infection of amputation stump, unspecified **extremity** CC

T87.41 Infection of amputation stump, right upper **extremity** CC

T87.42 Infection of amputation stump, left upper **extremity** CC

T87.43 Infection of amputation stump, right lower **extremity** CC

T87.44 Infection of amputation stump, left lower **extremity** CC

✓5th **T87.5** Necrosis **of amputation stump**

T87.50 Necrosis of amputation stump, unspecified **extremity**

T87.51 Necrosis of amputation stump, right upper **extremity**

T87.52 Necrosis of amputation stump, left upper **extremity**

T87.53 Necrosis of amputation stump, right lower **extremity**

T87.54 Necrosis of amputation stump, left lower **extremity**

✓5th **T87.8** Other **complications of amputation stump**

T87.81 Dehiscence **of amputation stump**

T87.89 Other **complications of amputation stump**
Amputation stump contracture
Amputation stump contracture of next proximal joint
Amputation stump flexion
Amputation stump edema
Amputation stump hematoma
EXCLUDES 2 *phantom limb syndrome (G54.6-G54.7)*

T87.9 Unspecified **complications of amputation stump**

✓4th **T88 Other complications of surgical and medical care, not elsewhere classified**

EXCLUDES 2 *complication following infusion, transfusion and therapeutic injection (T80.-)*
complication following procedure NEC (T81.-)
complications of anesthesia in labor and delivery (O74.-)
complications of anesthesia in pregnancy (O29.-)
complications of anesthesia in puerperium (O89.-)
complications of devices, implants and grafts (T82-T85)
complications of obstetric surgery and procedure (O75.4)
dermatitis due to drugs and medicaments (L23.3, L24.4, L25.1, L27.0-L27.1)
poisoning and toxic effects of drugs and chemicals (T36-T65 with fifth or sixth character 1-4 or 6)
specified complications classified elsewhere

> The appropriate 7th character is to be added to each code from category T88.
> A initial encounter
> D subsequent encounter
> S sequela

✓x7th **T88.0 Infection following immunization** CC
Sepsis following immunization
CC Excl: CC with 7th character A: N98.0, T80.211-T80.29X with 7th A, T82.7XXA, T88.0XXA

✓x7th **T88.1 Other complications following immunization, not elsewhere classified** CC
Generalized vaccinia
Rash following immunization
EXCLUDES 1 *vaccinia not from vaccine (B08.011)*
EXCLUDES 2 *anaphylactic shock due to serum (T80.5-)*
other serum reactions (T80.6-)
postimmunization arthropathy (M02.2)
postimmunization encephalitis (G04.02)
postimmunization fever (R50.83)
CC Excl: CC with 7th character A: T88.1X

✓x7th **T88.2 Shock due to anesthesia** CC
Use additional code for adverse effect, if applicable, to identify drug (T41.- with fifth or sixth character 5)
EXCLUDES 1 *complications of anesthesia (in):*
labor and delivery (O74.-)
postprocedural shock NOS (T81.1-)
pregnancy (O29.-)
puerperium (O89.-)
CC Excl: CC with 7th character A: D78.01-D78.02, D78.21-D78.89, E36.01-E36.02, E36.8, E89.810-E89.89, G97.51-G97.52, H59.011-H59.019, H59.031-H59.129, H59.311-H59.329, H59.811-H59.89, H95.21-H95.22, H95.41-H95.89, I97.3-I97.42, I97.610-I97.62, J95.61-J95.62, J95.830-J95.831, K91.61-K91.62, K91.840-K91.841, L76.01-L76.02, L76.21-L76.82, M96.810-M96.811, M96.830-M96.89, N98.1-N98.9, N99.61-N99.62, N99.820-N99.821, T79.4XXA, T81.10X-T81.19X with 7th A, T81.82XA, T81.89X-T81.9XX with 7th A, T88.2XXA

✓x7th **T88.3 Malignant hyperthermia due to anesthesia** CC
Use additional code for adverse effect, if applicable, to identify drug (T41.- with fifth or sixth character 5)
CC Excl: CC with 7th character A: D78.01-D78.02, D78.21-D78.89, E36.01-E36.02, E36.8, E89.810-E89.89, G97.51-G97.52, H59.011-H59.019, H59.031-H59.129, H59.311-H59.329, H59.811-H59.89, H95.21-H95.22, H95.41-H95.89, I97.3-I97.42, I97.610-I97.62, J95.61-J95.62, J95.830-J95.831, K91.61-K91.62, K91.840-K91.841, L76.01-L76.02, L76.21-L76.82, M96.810-M96.811, M96.830-M96.89, N98.1-N98.9, N99.61-N99.62, N99.820-N99.821, T79.4XXA, T81.10X-T81.19X with 7th A, T81.82XA, T81.89X-T81.9XX with 7th A, T88.2XX-T88.3XX with 7th A

12 ✓x7th **T88.4 Failed or difficult intubation**

12 Unacceptable PDx = initial encounter only (7th character A).

√5th **T88.5 Other complications of anesthesia**
Use additional code for adverse effect, if applicable, to identify drug (T41.- with fifth or sixth character 5)

√x7th **T88.51 Hypothermia following anesthesia**

√x7th **T88.52 Failed moderate sedation during procedure**
Failed conscious sedation during procedure
EXCLUDES 2 *personal history of failed moderate sedation (Z92.83)*

√x7th **T88.59 Other complications of anesthesia**

√x7th **T88.6 Anaphylactic reaction due to adverse effect of correct drug or medicament properly administered** CC
Anaphylactic shock due to adverse effect of correct drug or medicament properly administered
Anaphylactoid reaction NOS
Use additional code for adverse effect, if applicable, to identify drug (T41.- with fifth or sixth character 5)
EXCLUDES 1 *anaphylactic reaction due to serum (T80.5-)*
anaphylactic shock or reaction due to adverse food reaction (T78.0-)
CC Excl: CC with 7th character A: T78.00X-T78.09X with 7th A

12 √x7th **T88.7 Unspecified adverse effect of drug or medicament**
Drug hypersensitivity NOS
Drug reaction NOS
Use additional code for adverse effect, if applicable, to identify drug (T41.- with fifth or sixth character 5)
EXCLUDES 1 *specified adverse effects of drugs and medicaments (A00-R94 and T80-T88.6, T88.8)*

12 √x7th **T88.8 Other specified complications of surgical and medical care, not elsewhere classified**
Use additional code to identify the complication

12 √x7th **T88.9 Complication of surgical and medical care, unspecified**

12 Unacceptable PDx = initial encounter only (7th character A).

Chapter 20. External Causes of Morbidity (VØØ-Y99)

NOTE This chapter permits the classification of environmental events and circumstances as the cause of injury, and other adverse effects. Where a code from this section is applicable, it is intended that it shall be used secondary to a code from another chapter of the Classification indicating the nature of the condition. Most often, the condition will be classifiable to Chapter 19, Injury, poisoning and certain other consequences of external causes (SØØ-T88). Other conditions that may be stated to be due to external causes are classified in Chapters I to XVIII. For these conditions, codes from Chapter 2Ø should be used to provide additional information as to the cause of the condition.

This chapter contains the following blocks:

VØØ-VØ9	Pedestrian injured in transport accident
V1Ø-V19	Pedal cycle rider injured in transport accident
V2Ø-V29	Motorcycle rider injured in transport accident
V3Ø-V39	Occupant of three-wheeled motor vehicle injured in transport accident
V4Ø-V49	Car occupant injured in transport accident
V5Ø-V59	Occupant of pick-up truck or van injured in transport accident
V6Ø-V69	Occupant of heavy transport vehicle injured in transport accident
V7Ø-V79	Bus occupant injured in transport accident
V8Ø-V89	Other land transport accidents
V9Ø-V94	Water transport accidents
V95-V97	Air and space transport accidents
V98-V99	Other and unspecified transport accidents
WØØ-X58	Other external causes of accidental injury
WØØ-W19	Slipping, tripping, stumbling and falls
W2Ø-W49	Exposure to inanimate mechanical forces
W5Ø-W64	Exposure to animate mechanical forces
W65-W74	Accidental non-transport drowning and submersion
W85-W99	Exposure to electric current, radiation and extreme ambient air temperature and pressure
XØØ-XØ8	Exposure to smoke, fire and flames
X1Ø-X19	Contact with heat and hot substances
X3Ø-X39	Exposure to forces of nature
X52, X58	Accidental exposure to other specified factors
X71-X83	Intentional self-harm
X92-YØ8	Assault
Y21-Y33	Event of undetermined intent
Y35-Y38	Legal intervention, operations of war, military operations, and terrorism
Y62-Y84	Complications of medical and surgical care
Y62-Y69	Misadventures to patients during surgical and medical care
Y7Ø-Y82	Medical devices associated with adverse incidents in diagnostic and therapeutic use
Y83-Y84	Surgical and other medical procedures as the cause of abnormal reaction of the patient, or of later complication, without mention of misadventure at the time of the procedure
Y9Ø-Y99	Supplementary factors related to causes of morbidity classified elsewhere

Accidents (VØØ-X58)

Transport accidents (VØØ-V99)

Use additional code to identify:
- airbag injury (W22.1)
- type of street or road (Y92.4-)
- use of cellular telephone and other electronic equipment at the time of the transport accident (Y93.C-)

EXCLUDES 1
agricultural vehicles in stationary use or maintenance (W31.-)
assault by crashing of motor vehicle (YØ3.-)
automobile or motor cycle in stationary use or maintenance—code to type of accident
crashing of motor vehicle, undetermined intent (Y32)
intentional self-harm by crashing of motor vehicle (X82)

EXCLUDES 2
transport accidents due to cataclysm (X34-X38)

This section is structured in 12 groups. Those relating to land transport accidents (VØ1-V89) reflect the victim's mode of transport and are subdivided to identify the victim's 'counterpart' or the type of event. The vehicle of which the injured person is an occupant is identified in the first two characters since it is seen as the most important factor to identify for prevention purposes. A transport accident is one in which the vehicle involved must be moving or running or in use for transport purposes at the time of the accident.

Pedestrian injured in transport accident (VØØ-VØ9)

INCLUDES
person changing tire on transport vehicle
person examining engine of vehicle broken down in (on side of) road

EXCLUDES 1
fall due to non-transport collision with other person (WØ3)
pedestrian on foot falling (slipping) on ice and snow (WØØ.-)
struck or bumped by another person (W51)

√4th **VØØ Pedestrian conveyance accident**

Use additional place of occurrence and activity external cause codes, if known (Y92-, Y93-)

EXCLUDES 1
collision with another person without fall (W51)
fall due to person on foot colliding with another person on foot (WØ3)
fall from non-moving wheelchair, nonmotorized scooter and motorized mobility scooter without collision (WØ5.-)
pedestrian (conveyance) collision with other land transport vehicle (VØ1-VØ9)
pedestrian on foot falling (slipping) on ice and snow (WØØ.-)

The appropriate 7th character is to be added to each code from category VØØ.
- A initial encounter
- D subsequent encounter
- S sequela

√5th **VØØ.Ø Pedestrian on foot injured in collision with pedestrian conveyance**

√x7th **VØØ.Ø1 Pedestrian on foot injured in collision with roller-skater**

√x7th **VØØ.Ø2 Pedestrian on foot injured in collision with skateboarder**

√x7th **VØØ.Ø9 Pedestrian on foot injured in collision with other pedestrian conveyance**

√5th **VØØ.1 Rolling-type pedestrian conveyance accident**

EXCLUDES 1
accident with babystroller (VØØ.82-)
accident with motorized mobility scooter (VØØ.83-)
accident with wheelchair (powered) (VØØ.81-)

√6th **VØØ.11 In-line roller-skate accident**

√7th **VØØ.111 Fall from in-line roller-skates**

√7th **VØØ.112 In-line roller-skater colliding with stationary object**

√7th **VØØ.118 Other in-line roller-skate accident**

EXCLUDES 1 *roller-skater collision with other land transport vehicle (VØ1-VØ9 with 5th character 1)*

√6th **VØØ.12 Non-in- line roller-skate accident**

√7th **VØØ.121 Fall from non-in-line roller-skates**

√7th **VØØ.122 Non-in-line roller-skater colliding with stationary object**

√7th **VØØ.128 Other non-in-line roller-skating accident**

EXCLUDES 1 *roller-skater collision with other land transport vehicle (VØ1-VØ9 with 5th character 1)*

√6th **VØØ.13 Skateboard accident**

√7th **VØØ.131 Fall from skateboard**

√7th **VØØ.132 Skateboarder colliding with stationary object**

√7th **VØØ.138 Other skateboard accident**

EXCLUDES 1 *skateboarder collision with other land transport vehicle (VØ1-VØ9 with 5th character 2)*

√6th **VØØ.14 Scooter (nonmotorized) accident**

EXCLUDES 1 *motorscooter accident (V2Ø-V29)*

√7th **VØØ.141 Fall from scooter (nonmotorized)**

√7th **VØØ.142 Scooter (nonmotorized) colliding with stationary object**

√7th **VØØ.148 Other scooter (nonmotorized) accident**

EXCLUDES 1 *scooter (nonmotorized) collision with other land transport vehicle (VØ1-VØ9 with fifth character 9)*

√6th **VØØ.15 Heelies accident**

Rolling shoe
Wheeled shoe
Wheelies accident

√7th **VØØ.151 Fall from heelies**

√7th **VØØ.152 Heelies colliding with stationary object**

√7th **VØØ.158 Other heelies accident**

✓6th **V00.18 Accident on other rolling-type pedestrian conveyance**
- ✓7th **V00.181 Fall from other rolling-type pedestrian conveyance**
- ✓7th **V00.182 Pedestrian on other rolling-type pedestrian conveyance colliding with stationary object**
- ✓7th **V00.188 Other accident on other rolling-type pedestrian conveyance**

✓5th **V00.2 Gliding-type pedestrian conveyance accident**

✓6th **V00.21 Ice-skates accident**
- ✓7th **V00.211 Fall from ice-skates**
- ✓7th **V00.212 Ice-skater colliding with stationary object**
- ✓7th **V00.218 Other ice-skates accident**
  - EXCLUDES 1 *ice-skater collision with other land transport vehicle (V01-V09 with 5th digit 9)*

✓6th **V00.22 Sled accident**
- ✓7th **V00.221 Fall from sled**
- ✓7th **V00.222 Sledder colliding with stationary object**
- ✓7th **V00.228 Other sled accident**
  - EXCLUDES 1 *sled collision with other land transport vehicle (V01-V09 with 5th digit 9)*

✓6th **V00.28 Other gliding-type pedestrian conveyance accident**
- ✓7th **V00.281 Fall from other gliding-type pedestrian conveyance**
- ✓7th **V00.282 Pedestrian on other gliding-type pedestrian conveyance colliding with stationary object**
- ✓7th **V00.288 Other accident on other gliding-type pedestrian conveyance**
  - EXCLUDES 1 *gliding-type pedestrian conveyance collision with other land transport vehicle (V01-V09 with 5th digit 9)*

✓5th **V00.3 Flat-bottomed pedestrian conveyance accident**

✓6th **V00.31 Snowboard accident**
- ✓7th **V00.311 Fall from snowboard**
- ✓7th **V00.312 Snowboarder colliding with stationary object**
- ✓7th **V00.318 Other snowboard accident**
  - EXCLUDES 1 *snowboarder collision with other land transport vehicle (V01-V09 with 5th digit 9)*

✓6th **V00.32 Snow-ski accident**
- ✓7th **V00.321 Fall from snow-skis**
- ✓7th **V00.322 Snow-skier colliding with stationary object**
- ✓7th **V00.328 Other snow-ski accident**
  - EXCLUDES 1 *snow-skier collision with other land transport vehicle (V01-V09 with 5th digit 9)*

✓6th **V00.38 Other flat-bottomed pedestrian conveyance accident**
- ✓7th **V00.381 Fall from other flat-bottomed pedestrian conveyance**
- ✓7th **V00.382 Pedestrian on other flat-bottomed pedestrian conveyance colliding with stationary object**
- ✓7th **V00.388 Other accident on other flat-bottomed pedestrian conveyance**

✓5th **V00.8 Accident on other pedestrian conveyance**

✓6th **V00.81 Accident with wheelchair (powered)**
- ✓7th **V00.811 Fall from moving wheelchair (powered)**
  - EXCLUDES 1 *fall from non-moving wheelchair (W05.0)*
- ✓7th **V00.812 Wheelchair (powered) colliding with stationary object**
- ✓7th **V00.818 Other accident with wheelchair (powered)**

✓6th **V00.82 Accident with babystroller**
- ✓7th **V00.821 Fall from babystroller**
- ✓7th **V00.822 Babystroller colliding with stationary object**
- ✓7th **V00.828 Other accident with babystroller**

✓6th **V00.83 Accident with motorized mobility scooter**
- **V00.831 Fall from motorized mobility scooter**
  - EXCLUDES 1 *fall from non-moving motorized mobility scooter (W05.2)*
- **V00.832 Motorized mobility scooter colliding with stationary object**
- **V00.838 Other accident with motorized mobility scooter**

✓6th **V00.89 Accident on other pedestrian conveyance**
- ✓7th **V00.891 Fall from other pedestrian conveyance**
- ✓7th **V00.892 Pedestrian on other pedestrian conveyance colliding with stationary object**
- ✓7th **V00.898 Other accident on other pedestrian conveyance**
  - EXCLUDES 1 *other pedestrian (conveyance) collision with other land transport vehicle (V01-V09 with 5th digit 9)*

✓4th V01 Pedestrian injured in collision with pedal cycle

The appropriate 7th character is to be added to each code from category V01.
- A initial encounter
- D subsequent encounter
- S sequela

✓5th **V01.0 Pedestrian injured in collision with pedal cycle in nontraffic accident**
- ✓x7th **V01.00 Pedestrian on foot injured in collision with pedal cycle in nontraffic accident**
  - Pedestrian NOS injured in collision with pedal cycle in nontraffic accident
- ✓x7th **V01.01 Pedestrian on roller-skates injured in collision with pedal cycle in nontraffic accident**
- ✓x7th **V01.02 Pedestrian on skateboard injured in collision with pedal cycle in nontraffic accident**
- ✓x7th **V01.09 Pedestrian with other conveyance injured in collision with pedal cycle in nontraffic accident**
  - Pedestrian with babystroller injured in collision with pedal cycle in nontraffic accident
  - Pedestrian on ice-skates injured in collision with pedal cycle in nontraffic accident
  - Pedestrian on nonmotorized scooter injured in collision with pedal cycle in nontraffic accident
  - Pedestrian on sled injured in collision with pedal cycle in nontraffic accident
  - Pedestrian on snowboard injured in collision with pedal cycle in nontraffic accident
  - Pedestrian on snow-skis injured in collision with pedal cycle in nontraffic accident
  - Pedestrian in wheelchair (powered) injured in collision with pedal cycle in nontraffic accident
  - Pedestrian in motorized mobility scooter injured in collision with pedal cycle in nontraffic accident

✓5th **V01.1 Pedestrian injured in collision with pedal cycle in traffic accident**
- ✓x7th **V01.10 Pedestrian on foot injured in collision with pedal cycle in traffic accident**
  - Pedestrian NOS injured in collision with pedal cycle in traffic accident
- ✓x7th **V01.11 Pedestrian on roller-skates injured in collision with pedal cycle in traffic accident**
- ✓x7th **V01.12 Pedestrian on skateboard injured in collision with pedal cycle in traffic accident**

√x7th **V01.19 Pedestrian with other conveyance injured in collision with pedal cycle in traffic accident**
Pedestrian with babystroller injured in collision with pedal cycle in traffic accident
Pedestrian on ice-skates injured in collision with pedal cycle in traffic accident
Pedestrian on nonmotorized scooter injured in collision with pedal cycle in traffic accident
Pedestrian on sled injured in collision with pedal cycle in traffic accident
Pedestrian on snowboard injured in collision with pedal cycle in traffic accident
Pedestrian on snow-skis injured in collision with pedal cycle in traffic accident
Pedestrian in wheelchair (powered) injured in collision with pedal cycle in traffic accident
Pedestrian in motorized mobility scooter injured in collision with pedal cycle in traffic accident

√5th **V01.9 Pedestrian injured in collision with pedal cycle, unspecified whether traffic or nontraffic accident**

√x7th **V01.90 Pedestrian on foot injured in collision with pedal cycle, unspecified whether traffic or nontraffic accident**
Pedestrian NOS injured in collision with pedal cycle, unspecified whether traffic or nontraffic accident

√x7th **V01.91 Pedestrian on roller-skates injured in collision with pedal cycle, unspecified whether traffic or nontraffic accident**

√x7th **V01.92 Pedestrian on skateboard injured in collision with pedal cycle, unspecified whether traffic or nontraffic accident**

√x7th **V01.99 Pedestrian with other conveyance injured in collision with pedal cycle, unspecified whether traffic or nontraffic accident**
Pedestrian with babystroller injured in collision with pedal cycle, unspecified whether traffic or nontraffic accident
Pedestrian on ice-skates injured in collision with pedal cycle unspecified, whether traffic or nontraffic accident
Pedestrian on nonmotorized scooter injured in collision with pedal cycle, unspecified whether traffic or nontraffic accident
Pedestrian on sled injured in collision with pedal cycle unspecified, whether traffic or nontraffic accident
Pedestrian on snowboard injured in collision with pedal cycle, unspecified whether traffic or nontraffic accident
Pedestrian on snow-skis injured in collision with pedal cycle, unspecified whether traffic or nontraffic accident
Pedestrian in wheelchair (powered) injured in collision with pedal cycle, unspecified whether traffic or nontraffic accident
Pedestrian in motorized mobility scooter injured in collision with pedal cycle, unspecified whether traffic or nontraffic accident

√4th **V02 Pedestrian injured in collision with two- or three-wheeled motor vehicle**

The appropriate 7th character is to be added to each code from category V02.
A initial encounter
D subsequent encounter
S sequela

√5th **V02.0 Pedestrian injured in collision with two- or three-wheeled motor vehicle in nontraffic accident**

√x7th **V02.00 Pedestrian on foot injured in collision with two- or three-wheeled motor vehicle in nontraffic accident**
Pedestrian NOS injured in collision with two- or three-wheeled motor vehicle in nontraffic accident

√x7th **V02.01 Pedestrian on roller-skates injured in collision with two- or three-wheeled motor vehicle in nontraffic accident**

√x7th **V02.02 Pedestrian on skateboard injured in collision with two- or three-wheeled motor vehicle in nontraffic accident**

√x7th **V02.09 Pedestrian with other conveyance injured in collision with two- or three-wheeled motor vehicle in nontraffic accident**
Pedestrian with babystroller injured in collision with two- or three-wheeled motor vehicle in nontraffic accident
Pedestrian on ice-skates injured in collision with two- or three-wheeled motor vehicle in nontraffic accident
Pedestrian on nonmotorized scooter injured in collision with two- or three-wheeled motor vehicle in nontraffic accident
Pedestrian on sled injured in collision with two- or three-wheeled motor vehicle in nontraffic accident
Pedestrian on snowboard injured in collision with two- or three-wheeled motor vehicle in nontraffic accident
Pedestrian on snow-skis injured in collision with two- or three-wheeled motor vehicle in nontraffic accident
Pedestrian in wheelchair (powered) injured in collision with two- or three-wheeled motor vehicle in nontraffic accident
Pedestrian in motorized mobility scooter injured in collision with two- or three-wheeled motor vehicle in nontraffic accident

√5th **V02.1 Pedestrian injured in collision with two- or three-wheeled motor vehicle in traffic accident**

√x7th **V02.10 Pedestrian on foot injured in collision with two- or three-wheeled motor vehicle in traffic accident**
Pedestrian NOS injured in collision with two- or three-wheeled motor vehicle in traffic accident

√x7th **V02.11 Pedestrian on roller-skates injured in collision with two- or three-wheeled motor vehicle in traffic accident**

√x7th **V02.12 Pedestrian on skateboard injured in collision with two- or three-wheeled motor vehicle in traffic accident**

√x7th **V02.19 Pedestrian with other conveyance injured in collision with two- or three-wheeled motor vehicle in traffic accident**
Pedestrian with babystroller injured in collision with two- or three-wheeled motor vehicle in traffic accident
Pedestrian on ice-skates injured in collision with two- or three-wheeled motor vehicle in traffic accident
Pedestrian on nonmotorized scooter injured in collision with two- or three-wheeled motor vehicle in traffic accident
Pedestrian on sled injured in collision with two- or three-wheeled motor vehicle in traffic accident
Pedestrian on snowboard injured in collision with two- or three-wheeled motor vehicle in traffic accident
Pedestrian on snow-skis injured in collision with two- or three-wheeled motor vehicle in traffic accident
Pedestrian in wheelchair (powered) injured in collision with two- or three-wheeled motor vehicle in traffic accident
Pedestrian in motorized mobility scooter injured in collision with two- or three-wheeled motor vehicle in traffic accident

√5th **V02.9 Pedestrian injured in collision with two- or three-wheeled motor vehicle, unspecified whether traffic or nontraffic accident**

√x7th **V02.90 Pedestrian on foot injured in collision with two- or three-wheeled motor vehicle, unspecified whether traffic or nontraffic accident**
Pedestrian NOS injured in collision with two- or three-wheeled motor vehicle, unspecified whether traffic or nontraffic accident

√x7th **V02.91 Pedestrian on roller-skates injured in collision with two- or three-wheeled motor vehicle, unspecified whether traffic or nontraffic accident**

√x7th **V02.92 Pedestrian on skateboard injured in collision with two- or three-wheeled motor vehicle, unspecified whether traffic or nontraffic accident**

√x7th **V02.99 Pedestrian with other conveyance injured in collision with two- or three-wheeled motor vehicle, unspecified whether traffic or nontraffic accident**
Pedestrian with babystroller injured in collision with two- or three-wheeled motor vehicle, unspecified whether traffic or nontraffic accident
Pedestrian on ice-skates injured in collision with two- or three-wheeled motor vehicle, unspecified whether traffic or nontraffic accident
Pedestrian on nonmotorized scooter injured in collision with two- or three-wheeled motor vehicle, unspecified whether traffic or nontraffic accident
Pedestrian on sled injured in collision with two- or three-wheeled motor vehicle, unspecified whether traffic or nontraffic accident
Pedestrian on snowboard injured in collision with two- or three-wheeled motor vehicle, unspecified whether traffic or nontraffic accident
Pedestrian on snow-skis injured in collision with two- or three-wheeled motor vehicle, unspecified whether traffic or nontraffic accident
Pedestrian in wheelchair (powered) injured in collision with two- or three-wheeled motor vehicle, unspecified whether traffic or nontraffic accident
Pedestrian in motorized mobility scooter injured in collision with two- or three-wheeled motor vehicle, unspecified whether traffic or nontraffic accident

√4th **V03 Pedestrian injured in collision with car, pick-up truck or van**

The appropriate 7th character is to be added to each code from category V03.
A initial encounter
D subsequent encounter
S sequela

√5th **V03.0 Pedestrian injured in collision with car, pick-up truck or van in nontraffic accident**

√x7th **V03.00 Pedestrian on foot injured in collision with car, pick-up truck or van in nontraffic accident**
Pedestrian NOS injured in collision with car, pick-up truck or van in nontraffic accident

√x7th **V03.01 Pedestrian on roller-skates injured in collision with car, pick-up truck or van in nontraffic accident**

√x7th **V03.02 Pedestrian on skateboard injured in collision with car, pick-up truck or van in nontraffic accident**

√x7th **V03.09 Pedestrian with other conveyance injured in collision with car, pick-up truck or van in nontraffic accident**
Pedestrian with babystroller injured in collision with car, pick-up truck or van in nontraffic accident
Pedestrian on ice-skates injured in collision with car, pick-up truck or van in nontraffic accident
Pedestrian on nonmotorized scooter injured in collision with car, pick-up truck or van in nontraffic accident
Pedestrian on sled injured in collision with car, pick-up truck or van in nontraffic accident
Pedestrian on snowboard injured in collision with car, pick-up truck or van in nontraffic accident
Pedestrian on snow-skis injured in collision with car, pick-up truck or van in nontraffic accident
Pedestrian in wheelchair (powered) injured in collision with car, pick-up truck or van in nontraffic accident
Pedestrian in motorized mobility scooter injured in collision with car, pick-up truck or van in nontraffic accident

√5th **V03.1 Pedestrian injured in collision with car, pick-up truck or van in traffic accident**

√x7th **V03.10 Pedestrian on foot injured in collision with car, pick-up truck or van in traffic accident**
Pedestrian NOS injured in collision with car, pick-up truck or van in traffic accident

√x7th **V03.11 Pedestrian on roller-skates injured in collision with car, pick-up truck or van in traffic accident**

√x7th **V03.12 Pedestrian on skateboard injured in collision with car, pick-up truck or van in traffic accident**

√x7th **V03.19 Pedestrian with other conveyance injured in collision with car, pick-up truck or van in traffic accident**
Pedestrian with babystroller injured in collision with car, pick-up truck or van in traffic accident
Pedestrian on ice-skates injured in collision with car, pick-up truck or van in traffic accident
Pedestrian on nonmotorized scooter injured in collision with car, pick-up truck or van in traffic accident
Pedestrian on sled injured in collision with car, pick-up truck or van in traffic accident
Pedestrian on snowboard injured in collision with car, pick-up truck or van in traffic accident
Pedestrian on snow-skis injured in collision with car, pick-up truck or van in traffic accident
Pedestrian in wheelchair (powered) injured in collision with car, pick-up truck or van in traffic accident
Pedestrian in motorized mobility scooter injured in collision with car, pick-up truck or van in traffic accident

√5th **V03.9 Pedestrian injured in collision with car, pick-up truck or van, unspecified whether traffic or nontraffic accident**

√x7th **V03.90 Pedestrian on foot injured in collision with car, pick-up truck or van, unspecified whether traffic or nontraffic accident**
Pedestrian NOS injured in collision with car, pick-up truck or van, unspecified whether traffic or nontraffic accident

√x7th **V03.91 Pedestrian on roller-skates injured in collision with car, pick-up truck or van, unspecified whether traffic or nontraffic accident**

√x7th **V03.92 Pedestrian on skateboard injured in collision with car, pick-up truck or van, unspecified whether traffic or nontraffic accident**

√x7th **V03.99 Pedestrian with other conveyance injured in collision with car, pick-up truck or van, unspecified whether traffic or nontraffic accident**
Pedestrian with babystroller injured in collision with car, pick-up truck or van, unspecified whether traffic or nontraffic accident
Pedestrian on ice-skates injured in collision with car, pick-up truck or van, unspecified whether traffic or nontraffic accident
Pedestrian on nonmotorized scooter injured in collision with car, pick-up truck or van, unspecified whether traffic or nontraffic accident
Pedestrian on sled injured in collision with car, pick-up truck or van in nontraffic accident
Pedestrian on snowboard injured in collision with car, pick-up truck or van, unspecified whether traffic or nontraffic accident
Pedestrian on snow-skis injured in collision with car, pick-up truck or van, unspecified whether traffic or nontraffic accident
Pedestrian in wheelchair (powered) injured in collision with car, pick-up truck or van, unspecified whether traffic or nontraffic accident
Pedestrian in motorized mobility scooter injured in collision with car, pick-up truck or van, unspecified whether traffic or nontraffic accident

√4th **V04 Pedestrian injured in collision with heavy transport vehicle or bus**

EXCLUDES 1 *pedestrian injured in collision with military vehicle (V09.01, V09.21)*

The appropriate 7th character is to be added to each code from category V04.
A initial encounter
D subsequent encounter
S sequela

√5th **V04.0 Pedestrian injured in collision with heavy transport vehicle or bus in nontraffic accident**

√x7th **V04.00 Pedestrian on foot injured in collision with heavy transport vehicle or bus in nontraffic accident**
Pedestrian NOS injured in collision with heavy transport vehicle or bus in nontraffic accident

√x7th **V04.01 Pedestrian on roller-skates injured in collision with heavy transport vehicle or bus in nontraffic accident**

√x7th **V04.02 Pedestrian on skateboard injured in collision with heavy transport vehicle or bus in nontraffic accident**

√x7th **V04.09 Pedestrian with other conveyance injured in collision with heavy transport vehicle or bus in nontraffic accident**
Pedestrian with babystroller injured in collision with heavy transport vehicle or bus in nontraffic accident
Pedestrian on ice-skates injured in collision with heavy transport vehicle or bus in nontraffic accident
Pedestrian on nonmotorized scooter injured in collision with heavy transport vehicle or bus in nontraffic accident
Pedestrian on sled injured in collision with heavy transport vehicle or bus in nontraffic accident
Pedestrian on snowboard injured in collision with heavy transport vehicle or bus in nontraffic accident
Pedestrian on snow-skis injured in collision with heavy transport vehicle or bus in nontraffic accident
Pedestrian in wheelchair (powered) injured in collision with heavy transport vehicle or bus in nontraffic accident
Pedestrian in motorized mobility scooter injured in collision with heavy transport vehicle or bus in nontraffic accident

√5th **V04.1 Pedestrian injured in collision with heavy transport vehicle or bus in traffic accident**

√x7th **V04.10 Pedestrian on foot injured in collision with heavy transport vehicle or bus in traffic accident**
Pedestrian NOS injured in collision with heavy transport vehicle or bus in traffic accident

√x7th **V04.11 Pedestrian on roller-skates injured in collision with heavy transport vehicle or bus in traffic accident**

√x7th **V04.12 Pedestrian on skateboard injured in collision with heavy transport vehicle or bus in traffic accident**

√x7th **V04.19 Pedestrian with other conveyance injured in collision with heavy transport vehicle or bus in traffic accident**
Pedestrian with babystroller injured in collision with heavy transport vehicle or bus in traffic accident
Pedestrian on ice-skates injured in collision with heavy transport vehicle or bus in traffic accident
Pedestrian on nonmotorized scooter injured in collision with heavy transport vehicle or bus in traffic accident
Pedestrian on sled injured in collision with heavy transport vehicle or bus in traffic accident
Pedestrian on snowboard injured in collision with heavy transport vehicle or bus in traffic accident
Pedestrian on snow-skis injured in collision with heavy transport vehicle or bus in traffic accident
Pedestrian in wheelchair (powered) injured in collision with heavy transport vehicle or bus in traffic accident
Pedestrian in motorized mobility scooter injured in collision with heavy transport vehicle or bus in traffic accident

√5th **V04.9 Pedestrian injured in collision with heavy transport vehicle or bus, unspecified whether traffic or nontraffic accident**

√x7th **V04.90 Pedestrian on foot injured in collision with heavy transport vehicle or bus, unspecified whether traffic or nontraffic accident**
Pedestrian NOS injured in collision with heavy transport vehicle or bus, unspecified whether traffic or nontraffic accident

√x7th **V04.91 Pedestrian on roller-skates injured in collision with heavy transport vehicle or bus, unspecified whether traffic or nontraffic accident**

√x7th **V04.92 Pedestrian on skateboard injured in collision with heavy transport vehicle or bus, unspecified whether traffic or nontraffic accident**

√x7th **V04.99 Pedestrian with other conveyance injured in collision with heavy transport vehicle or bus, unspecified whether traffic or nontraffic accident**
Pedestrian with babystroller injured in collision with heavy transport vehicle or bus, unspecified whether traffic or nontraffic accident
Pedestrian on ice-skates injured in collision with heavy transport vehicle or bus, unspecified whether traffic or nontraffic accident
Pedestrian on nonmotorized scooter injured in collision with heavy transport vehicle or bus, unspecified whether traffic or nontraffic accident
Pedestrian on sled injured in collision with heavy transport vehicle or bus, unspecified whether traffic or nontraffic accident
Pedestrian on snowboard injured in collision with heavy transport vehicle or bus, unspecified whether traffic or nontraffic accident
Pedestrian on snow-skis injured in collision with heavy transport vehicle or bus, unspecified whether traffic or nontraffic accident
Pedestrian in wheelchair (powered) injured in collision with heavy transport vehicle or bus, unspecified whether traffic or nontraffic accident
Pedestrian in motorized mobility scooter injured in collision with heavy transport vehicle or bus, unspecified whether traffic or nontraffic accident

√4th **V05 Pedestrian injured in collision with railway train or railway vehicle**

The appropriate 7th character is to be added to each code from category V05.
A initial encounter
D subsequent encounter
S sequela

√5th **V05.0 Pedestrian injured in collision with railway train or railway vehicle in nontraffic accident**

√x7th **V05.00 Pedestrian on foot injured in collision with railway train or railway vehicle in nontraffic accident**
Pedestrian NOS injured in collision with railway train or railway vehicle in nontraffic accident

√x7th **V05.01 Pedestrian on roller-skates injured in collision with railway train or railway vehicle in nontraffic accident**

√x7th **V05.02 Pedestrian on skateboard injured in collision with railway train or railway vehicle in nontraffic accident**

√x7th **V05.09 Pedestrian with other conveyance injured in collision with railway train or railway vehicle in nontraffic accident**
Pedestrian with babystroller injured in collision with railway train or railway vehicle in nontraffic accident
Pedestrian on ice-skates injured in collision with railway train or railway vehicle in nontraffic accident
Pedestrian on nonmotorized scooter injured in collision with railway train or railway vehicle in nontraffic accident
Pedestrian on sled injured in collision with railway train or railway vehicle in nontraffic accident
Pedestrian on snowboard injured in collision with railway train or railway vehicle in nontraffic accident
Pedestrian on snow-skis injured in collision with railway train or railway vehicle in nontraffic accident
Pedestrian in wheelchair (powered) injured in collision with railway train or railway vehicle in nontraffic accident
Pedestrian in motorized mobility scooter injured in collision with railway train or railway vehicle in nontraffic accident

√5th **V05.1 Pedestrian injured in collision with railway train or railway vehicle in traffic accident**

√x7th **V05.10 Pedestrian on foot injured in collision with railway train or railway vehicle in traffic accident**
Pedestrian NOS injured in collision with railway train or railway vehicle in traffic accident

√x7th **V05.11 Pedestrian on roller-skates injured in collision with railway train or railway vehicle in traffic accident**

√x7th **V05.12 Pedestrian on skateboard injured in collision with railway train or railway vehicle in traffic accident**

√x7th **V05.19 Pedestrian with other conveyance injured in collision with railway train or railway vehicle in traffic accident**
Pedestrian with babystroller injured in collision with railway train or railway vehicle in traffic accident
Pedestrian on ice-skates injured in collision with railway train or railway vehicle in traffic accident
Pedestrian on nonmotorized scooter injured in collision with railway train or railway vehicle in traffic accident
Pedestrian on sled injured in collision with railway train or railway vehicle in traffic accident
Pedestrian on snowboard injured in collision with railway train or railway vehicle in traffic accident
Pedestrian on snow-skis injured in collision with railway train or railway vehicle in traffic accident
Pedestrian in wheelchair (powered) injured in collision with railway train or railway vehicle in traffic accident
Pedestrian in motorized mobility scooter injured in collision with railway train or railway vehicle in traffic accident

√5th **V05.9 Pedestrian injured in collision with railway train or railway vehicle, unspecified whether traffic or nontraffic accident**

√x7th **V05.90 Pedestrian on foot injured in collision with railway train or railway vehicle, unspecified whether traffic or nontraffic accident**
Pedestrian NOS injured in collision with railway train or railway vehicle, unspecified whether traffic or nontraffic accident

√x7th **V05.91 Pedestrian on roller-skates injured in collision with railway train or railway vehicle, unspecified whether traffic or nontraffic accident**

√x7th **V05.92 Pedestrian on skateboard injured in collision with railway train or railway vehicle, unspecified whether traffic or nontraffic accident**

√x7th **V05.99 Pedestrian with other conveyance injured in collision with railway train or railway vehicle, unspecified whether traffic or nontraffic accident**
Pedestrian with babystroller injured in collision with railway train or railway vehicle, unspecified whether traffic or nontraffic
Pedestrian on ice-skates injured in collision with railway train or railway vehicle, unspecified whether traffic or nontraffic
Pedestrian on nonmotorized scooter injured in collision with railway train or railway vehicle, unspecified whether traffic or nontraffic
Pedestrian on sled injured in collision with railway train or railway vehicle, unspecified whether traffic or nontraffic
Pedestrian on snowboard injured in collision with railway train or railway vehicle, unspecified whether traffic or nontraffic
Pedestrian on snow-skis injured in collision with railway train or railway vehicle, unspecified whether traffic or nontraffic
Pedestrian in wheelchair (powered) injured in collision with railway train or railway vehicle, unspecified whether traffic or nontraffic
Pedestrian in motorized mobility scooter injured in collision with railway train or railway vehicle, unspecified whether traffic or nontraffic

√4th **V06 Pedestrian injured in collision with other nonmotor vehicle**
INCLUDES collision with animal-drawn vehicle, animal being ridden, nonpowered streetcar
EXCLUDES 1 *pedestrian injured in collision with pedestrian conveyance (V00.0-)*

The appropriate 7th character is to be added to each code from category V06.
A initial encounter
D subsequent encounter
S sequela

√5th **V06.0 Pedestrian injured in collision with other nonmotor vehicle in nontraffic accident**

√x7th **V06.00 Pedestrian on foot injured in collision with other nonmotor vehicle in nontraffic accident**
Pedestrian NOS injured in collision with other nonmotor vehicle in nontraffic accident

√x7th **V06.01 Pedestrian on roller-skates injured in collision with other nonmotor vehicle in nontraffic accident**

√x7th **V06.02 Pedestrian on skateboard injured in collision with other nonmotor vehicle in nontraffic accident**

√x7th **V06.09 Pedestrian with other conveyance injured in collision with other nonmotor vehicle in nontraffic accident**
Pedestrian with babystroller injured in collision with other nonmotor vehicle in nontraffic accident
Pedestrian on ice-skates injured in collision with other nonmotor vehicle in nontraffic accident
Pedestrian on nonmotorized scooter injured in collision with other nonmotor vehicle in nontraffic accident
Pedestrian on sled injured in collision with other nonmotor vehicle in nontraffic accident
Pedestrian on snowboard injured in collision with other nonmotor vehicle in nontraffic accident
Pedestrian on snow-skis injured in collision with other nonmotor vehicle in nontraffic accident
Pedestrian in wheelchair (powered) injured in collision with other nonmotor vehicle in nontraffic accident
Pedestrian in motorized mobility scooter injured in collision with other nonmotor vehicle in nontraffic accident

√5th **V06.1 Pedestrian injured in collision with other nonmotor vehicle in traffic accident**

√x7th **V06.10 Pedestrian on foot injured in collision with other nonmotor vehicle in traffic accident**
Pedestrian NOS injured in collision with other nonmotor vehicle in traffic accident

√x7th **V06.11 Pedestrian on roller-skates injured in collision with other nonmotor vehicle in traffic accident**

√x7th **V06.12 Pedestrian on skateboard injured in collision with other nonmotor vehicle in traffic accident**

√x7th **V06.19 Pedestrian with other conveyance injured in collision with other nonmotor vehicle in traffic accident**
Pedestrian with babystroller injured in collision with other nonmotor vehicle in nontraffic accident
Pedestrian on ice-skates injured in collision with other nonmotor vehicle in traffic accident
Pedestrian on nonmotorized scooter injured in collision with other nonmotor vehicle in traffic accident
Pedestrian on sled injured in collision with other nonmotor vehicle in traffic accident
Pedestrian on snowboard injured in collision with other nonmotor vehicle in traffic accident
Pedestrian on snow-skis injured in collision with other nonmotor vehicle in traffic accident
Pedestrian in wheelchair (powered) injured in collision with other nonmotor vehicle in traffic accident
Pedestrian in motorized mobility scooter injured in collision with other nonmotor vehicle in traffic accident

√5th **V06.9 Pedestrian injured in collision with other nonmotor vehicle, unspecified whether traffic or nontraffic accident**

√x7th **V06.90 Pedestrian on foot injured in collision with other nonmotor vehicle, unspecified whether traffic or nontraffic accident**
Pedestrian NOS injured in collision with other nonmotor vehicle, unspecified whether traffic or nontraffic accident

√x7th **V06.91 Pedestrian on roller-skates injured in collision with other nonmotor vehicle, unspecified whether traffic or nontraffic accident**

√x7th **V06.92 Pedestrian on skateboard injured in collision with other nonmotor vehicle, unspecified whether traffic or nontraffic accident**

√x7th **V06.99 Pedestrian with other conveyance injured in collision with other nonmotor vehicle, unspecified whether traffic or nontraffic accident**
Pedestrian with babystroller injured in collision with other nonmotor vehicle, unspecified whether traffic or nontraffic accident
Pedestrian on ice-skates injured in collision with other nonmotor vehicle, unspecified whether traffic or nontraffic accident
Pedestrian on nonmotorized scooter injured in collision with other nonmotor vehicle, unspecified whether traffic or nontraffic accident
Pedestrian on sled injured in collision with other nonmotor vehicle, unspecified whether traffic or nontraffic accident
Pedestrian on snowboard injured in collision with other nonmotor vehicle, unspecified whether traffic or nontraffic accident
Pedestrian on snow-skis injured in collision with other nonmotor vehicle, unspecified whether traffic or nontraffic accident
Pedestrian in wheelchair (powered) injured in collision with other nonmotor vehicle, unspecified whether traffic or nontraffic accident
Pedestrian in motorized mobility scooter injured in collision with other nonmotor vehicle, unspecified whether traffic or nontraffic accident

√4th **V09 Pedestrian injured in other and unspecified transport accidents**

The appropriate 7th character is to be added to each code from category V09.
A initial encounter
D subsequent encounter
S sequela

√5th **V09.0 Pedestrian injured in nontraffic accident involving other and unspecified motor vehicles**
√x7th **V09.00 Pedestrian injured in nontraffic accident involving unspecified motor vehicles**
√x7th **V09.01 Pedestrian injured in nontraffic accident involving military vehicle**
√x7th **V09.09 Pedestrian injured in nontraffic accident involving other motor vehicles**
Pedestrian injured in nontraffic accident by special vehicle
√x7th **V09.1 Pedestrian injured in unspecified nontraffic accident**
√5th **V09.2 Pedestrian injured in traffic accident involving other and unspecified motor vehicles**
√x7th **V09.20 Pedestrian injured in traffic accident involving unspecified motor vehicles**
√x7th **V09.21 Pedestrian injured in traffic accident involving military vehicle**
√x7th **V09.29 Pedestrian injured in traffic accident involving other motor vehicles**
√x7th **V09.3 Pedestrian injured in unspecified traffic accident**
√x7th **V09.9 Pedestrian injured in unspecified transport accident**

Pedal cycle rider injured in transport accident (V10-V19)

INCLUDES any non-motorized vehicle, excluding an animal-drawn vehicle, or a sidecar or trailer attached to the pedal cycle
EXCLUDES2 *rupture of pedal cycle tire (W37.0)*

√4th **V10 Pedal cycle rider injured in collision with pedestrian or animal**
EXCLUDES1 *pedal cycle rider collision with animal-drawn vehicle or animal being ridden (V16.-)*

The appropriate 7th character is to be added to each code from category V10.
A initial encounter
D subsequent encounter
S sequela

√x7th **V10.0 Pedal cycle driver injured in collision with pedestrian or animal in nontraffic accident**
√x7th **V10.1 Pedal cycle passenger injured in collision with pedestrian or animal in nontraffic accident**
√x7th **V10.2 Unspecified pedal cyclist injured in collision with pedestrian or animal in nontraffic accident**
√x7th **V10.3 Person boarding or alighting a pedal cycle injured in collision with pedestrian or animal**
√x7th **V10.4 Pedal cycle driver injured in collision with pedestrian or animal in traffic accident**
√x7th **V10.5 Pedal cycle passenger injured in collision with pedestrian or animal in traffic accident**
√x7th **V10.9 Unspecified pedal cyclist injured in collision with pedestrian or animal in traffic accident**

√4th **V11 Pedal cycle rider injured in collision with other pedal cycle**

The appropriate 7th character is to be added to each code from category V11.
A initial encounter
D subsequent encounter
S sequela

√x7th **V11.0 Pedal cycle driver injured in collision with other pedal cycle in nontraffic accident**
√x7th **V11.1 Pedal cycle passenger injured in collision with other pedal cycle in nontraffic accident**
√x7th **V11.2 Unspecified pedal cyclist injured in collision with other pedal cycle in nontraffic accident**
√x7th **V11.3 Person boarding or alighting a pedal cycle injured in collision with other pedal cycle**
√x7th **V11.4 Pedal cycle driver injured in collision with other pedal cycle in traffic accident**
√x7th **V11.5 Pedal cycle passenger injured in collision with other pedal cycle in traffic accident**
√x7th **V11.9 Unspecified pedal cyclist injured in collision with other pedal cycle in traffic accident**

√4th **V12 Pedal cycle rider injured in collision with two- or three-wheeled motor vehicle**

The appropriate 7th character is to be added to each code from category V12.
A initial encounter
D subsequent encounter
S sequela

√x7th **V12.0 Pedal cycle driver injured in collision with two- or three-wheeled motor vehicle in nontraffic accident**
√x7th **V12.1 Pedal cycle passenger injured in collision with two- or three-wheeled motor vehicle in nontraffic accident**
√x7th **V12.2 Unspecified pedal cyclist injured in collision with two- or three-wheeled motor vehicle in nontraffic accident**
√x7th **V12.3 Person boarding or alighting a pedal cycle injured in collision with two- or three-wheeled motor vehicle**
√x7th **V12.4 Pedal cycle driver injured in collision with two- or three-wheeled motor vehicle in traffic accident**
√x7th **V12.5 Pedal cycle passenger injured in collision with two- or three-wheeled motor vehicle in traffic accident**
√x7th **V12.9 Unspecified pedal cyclist injured in collision with two- or three-wheeled motor vehicle in traffic accident**

√4th **V13 Pedal cycle rider injured in collision with car, pick-up truck or van**

The appropriate 7th character is to be added to each code from category V13.
A initial encounter
D subsequent encounter
S sequela

√x7th **V13.0 Pedal cycle driver injured in collision with car, pick-up truck or van in nontraffic accident**
√x7th **V13.1 Pedal cycle passenger injured in collision with car, pick-up truck or van in nontraffic accident**
√x7th **V13.2 Unspecified pedal cyclist injured in collision with car, pick-up truck or van in nontraffic accident**
√x7th **V13.3 Person boarding or alighting a pedal cycle injured in collision with car, pick-up truck or van**
√x7th **V13.4 Pedal cycle driver injured in collision with car, pick-up truck or van in traffic accident**
√x7th **V13.5 Pedal cycle passenger injured in collision with car, pick-up truck or van in traffic accident**
√x7th **V13.9 Unspecified pedal cyclist injured in collision with car, pick-up truck or van in traffic accident**

V14 Pedal cycle rider injured in collision with heavy transport vehicle or bus
EXCLUDES 1 *pedal cycle rider injured in collision with military vehicle (V19.81)*

The appropriate 7th character is to be added to each code from category V14.
A initial encounter
D subsequent encounter
S sequela

V14.0 Pedal cycle driver injured in collision with heavy transport vehicle or bus in nontraffic accident
V14.1 Pedal cycle passenger injured in collision with heavy transport vehicle or bus in nontraffic accident
V14.2 Unspecified pedal cyclist injured in collision with heavy transport vehicle or bus in nontraffic accident
V14.3 Person boarding or alighting a pedal cycle injured in collision with heavy transport vehicle or bus
V14.4 Pedal cycle driver injured in collision with heavy transport vehicle or bus in traffic accident
V14.5 Pedal cycle passenger injured in collision with heavy transport vehicle or bus in traffic accident
V14.9 Unspecified pedal cyclist injured in collision with heavy transport vehicle or bus in traffic accident

V15 Pedal cycle rider injured in collision with railway train or railway vehicle

The appropriate 7th character is to be added to each code from category V15.
A initial encounter
D subsequent encounter
S sequela

V15.0 Pedal cycle driver injured in collision with railway train or railway vehicle in nontraffic accident
V15.1 Pedal cycle passenger injured in collision with railway train or railway vehicle in nontraffic accident
V15.2 Unspecified pedal cyclist injured in collision with railway train or railway vehicle in nontraffic accident
V15.3 Person boarding or alighting a pedal cycle injured in collision with railway train or railway vehicle
V15.4 Pedal cycle driver injured in collision with railway train or railway vehicle in traffic accident
V15.5 Pedal cycle passenger injured in collision with railway train or railway vehicle in traffic accident
V15.9 Unspecified pedal cyclist injured in collision with railway train or railway vehicle in traffic accident

V16 Pedal cycle rider injured in collision with other nonmotor vehicle
INCLUDES collision with animal-drawn vehicle, animal being ridden, streetcar

The appropriate 7th character is to be added to each code from category V16.
A initial encounter
D subsequent encounter
S sequela

V16.0 Pedal cycle driver injured in collision with other nonmotor vehicle in nontraffic accident
V16.1 Pedal cycle passenger injured in collision with other nonmotor vehicle in nontraffic accident
V16.2 Unspecified pedal cyclist injured in collision with other nonmotor vehicle in nontraffic accident
V16.3 Person boarding or alighting a pedal cycle injured in collision with other nonmotor vehicle in nontraffic accident
V16.4 Pedal cycle driver injured in collision with other nonmotor vehicle in traffic accident
V16.5 Pedal cycle passenger injured in collision with other nonmotor vehicle in traffic accident
V16.9 Unspecified pedal cyclist injured in collision with other nonmotor vehicle in traffic accident

V17 Pedal cycle rider injured in collision with fixed or stationary object

The appropriate 7th character is to be added to each code from category V17.
A initial encounter
D subsequent encounter
S sequela

V17.0 Pedal cycle driver injured in collision with fixed or stationary object in nontraffic accident
V17.1 Pedal cycle passenger injured in collision with fixed or stationary object in nontraffic accident
V17.2 Unspecified pedal cyclist injured in collision with fixed or stationary object in nontraffic accident
V17.3 Person boarding or alighting a pedal cycle injured in collision with fixed or stationary object
V17.4 Pedal cycle driver injured in collision with fixed or stationary object in traffic accident
V17.5 Pedal cycle passenger injured in collision with fixed or stationary object in traffic accident
V17.9 Unspecified pedal cyclist injured in collision with fixed or stationary object in traffic accident

V18 Pedal cycle rider injured in noncollision transport accident
INCLUDES fall or thrown from pedal cycle (without antecedent collision)
overturning pedal cycle NOS
overturning pedal cycle without collision

The appropriate 7th character is to be added to each code from category V18.
A initial encounter
D subsequent encounter
S sequela

V18.0 Pedal cycle driver injured in noncollision transport accident in nontraffic accident
V18.1 Pedal cycle passenger injured in noncollision transport accident in nontraffic accident
V18.2 Unspecified pedal cyclist injured in noncollision transport accident in nontraffic accident
V18.3 Person boarding or alighting a pedal cycle injured in noncollision transport accident
V18.4 Pedal cycle driver injured in noncollision transport accident in traffic accident
V18.5 Pedal cycle passenger injured in noncollision transport accident in traffic accident
V18.9 Unspecified pedal cyclist injured in noncollision transport accident in traffic accident

V19 Pedal cycle rider injured in other and unspecified transport accidents

The appropriate 7th character is to be added to each code from category V19.
A initial encounter
D subsequent encounter
S sequela

V19.0 Pedal cycle driver injured in collision with other and unspecified motor vehicles in nontraffic accident
V19.00 Pedal cycle driver injured in collision with unspecified motor vehicles in nontraffic accident
V19.09 Pedal cycle driver injured in collision with other motor vehicles in nontraffic accident
V19.1 Pedal cycle passenger injured in collision with other and unspecified motor vehicles in nontraffic accident
V19.10 Pedal cycle passenger injured in collision with unspecified motor vehicles in nontraffic accident
V19.19 Pedal cycle passenger injured in collision with other motor vehicles in nontraffic accident
V19.2 Unspecified pedal cyclist injured in collision with other and unspecified motor vehicles in nontraffic accident
V19.20 Unspecified pedal cyclist injured in collision with unspecified motor vehicles in nontraffic accident
Pedal cycle collision NOS, nontraffic
V19.29 Unspecified pedal cyclist injured in collision with other motor vehicles in nontraffic accident
V19.3 Pedal cyclist (driver) (passenger) injured in unspecified nontraffic accident
Pedal cycle accident NOS, nontraffic
Pedal cyclist injured in nontraffic accident NOS

√5th **V19.4 Pedal cycle driver injured in collision with other and unspecified motor vehicles in traffic accident**

√x7th **V19.40 Pedal cycle driver injured in collision with unspecified motor vehicles in traffic accident**

√x7th **V19.49 Pedal cycle driver injured in collision with other motor vehicles in traffic accident**

√5th **V19.5 Pedal cycle passenger injured in collision with other and unspecified motor vehicles in traffic accident**

√x7th **V19.50 Pedal cycle passenger injured in collision with unspecified motor vehicles in traffic accident**

√x7th **V19.59 Pedal cycle passenger injured in collision with other motor vehicles in traffic accident**

√5th **V19.6 Unspecified pedal cyclist injured in collision with other and unspecified motor vehicles in traffic accident**

√x7th **V19.60 Unspecified pedal cyclist injured in collision with unspecified motor vehicles in traffic accident**
Pedal cycle collision NOS (traffic)

√x7th **V19.69 Unspecified pedal cyclist injured in collision with other motor vehicles in traffic accident**

√5th **V19.8 Pedal cyclist (driver) (passenger) injured in other specified transport accidents**

√x7th **V19.81 Pedal cyclist (driver) (passenger) injured in transport accident with military vehicle**

√x7th **V19.88 Pedal cyclist (driver) (passenger) injured in other specified transport accidents**

√x7th **V19.9 Pedal cyclist (driver) (passenger) injured in unspecified traffic accident**
Pedal cycle accident NOS

Motorcycle rider injured in transport accident (V20-V29)

INCLUDES moped
motorcycle with sidecar
motorized bicycle
motor scooter

EXCLUDES 1 *three-wheeled motor vehicle (V30-V39)*

√4th **V20 Motorcycle rider injured in collision with pedestrian or animal**

EXCLUDES 1 *motorcycle rider collision with animal-drawn vehicle or animal being ridden (V26.-)*

The appropriate 7th character is to be added to each code from category V20.
A initial encounter
D subsequent encounter
S sequela

√x7th **V20.0 Motorcycle driver injured in collision with pedestrian or animal in nontraffic accident**

√x7th **V20.1 Motorcycle passenger injured in collision with pedestrian or animal in nontraffic accident**

√x7th **V20.2 Unspecified motorcycle rider injured in collision with pedestrian or animal in nontraffic accident**

√x7th **V20.3 Person boarding or alighting a motorcycle injured in collision with pedestrian or animal**

√x7th **V20.4 Motorcycle driver injured in collision with pedestrian or animal in traffic accident**

√x7th **V20.5 Motorcycle passenger injured in collision with pedestrian or animal in traffic accident**

√x7th **V20.9 Unspecified motorcycle rider injured in collision with pedestrian or animal in traffic accident**

√4th **V21 Motorcycle rider injured in collision with pedal cycle**

The appropriate 7th character is to be added to each code from category V21.
A initial encounter
D subsequent encounter
S sequela

√x7th **V21.0 Motorcycle driver injured in collision with pedal cycle in nontraffic accident**

√x7th **V21.1 Motorcycle passenger injured in collision with pedal cycle in nontraffic accident**

√x7th **V21.2 Unspecified motorcycle rider injured in collision with pedal cycle in nontraffic accident**

√x7th **V21.3 Person boarding or alighting a motorcycle injured in collision with pedal cycle**

√x7th **V21.4 Motorcycle driver injured in collision with pedal cycle in traffic accident**

√x7th **V21.5 Motorcycle passenger injured in collision with pedal cycle in traffic accident**

√x7th **V21.9 Unspecified motorcycle rider injured in collision with pedal cycle in traffic accident**

√4th **V22 Motorcycle rider injured in collision with two- or three-wheeled motor vehicle**

The appropriate 7th character is to be added to each code from category V22.
A initial encounter
D subsequent encounter
S sequela

√x7th **V22.0 Motorcycle driver injured in collision with two- or three-wheeled motor vehicle in nontraffic accident**

√x7th **V22.1 Motorcycle passenger injured in collision with two- or three-wheeled motor vehicle in nontraffic accident**

√x7th **V22.2 Unspecified motorcycle rider injured in collision with two- or three-wheeled motor vehicle in nontraffic accident**

√x7th **V22.3 Person boarding or alighting a motorcycle injured in collision with two- or three-wheeled motor vehicle**

√x7th **V22.4 Motorcycle driver injured in collision with two- or three-wheeled motor vehicle in traffic accident**

√x7th **V22.5 Motorcycle passenger injured in collision with two- or three-wheeled motor vehicle in traffic accident**

√x7th **V22.9 Unspecified motorcycle rider injured in collision with two- or three-wheeled motor vehicle in traffic accident**

√4th **V23 Motorcycle rider injured in collision with car, pick-up truck or van**

The appropriate 7th character is to be added to each code from category V23.
A initial encounter
D subsequent encounter
S sequela

√x7th **V23.0 Motorcycle driver injured in collision with car, pick-up truck or van in nontraffic accident**

√x7th **V23.1 Motorcycle passenger injured in collision with car, pick-up truck or van in nontraffic accident**

√x7th **V23.2 Unspecified motorcycle rider injured in collision with car, pick-up truck or van in nontraffic accident**

√x7th **V23.3 Person boarding or alighting a motorcycle injured in collision with car, pick-up truck or van**

√x7th **V23.4 Motorcycle driver injured in collision with car, pick-up truck or van in traffic accident**

√x7th **V23.5 Motorcycle passenger injured in collision with car, pick-up truck or van in traffic accident**

√x7th **V23.9 Unspecified motorcycle rider injured in collision with car, pick-up truck or van in traffic accident**

√4th **V24 Motorcycle rider injured in collision with heavy transport vehicle or bus**

EXCLUDES 1 *motorcycle rider injured in collision with military vehicle (V29.81)*

The appropriate 7th character is to be added to each code from category V24.
A initial encounter
D subsequent encounter
S sequela

√x7th **V24.0 Motorcycle driver injured in collision with heavy transport vehicle or bus in nontraffic accident**

√x7th **V24.1 Motorcycle passenger injured in collision with heavy transport vehicle or bus in nontraffic accident**

√x7th **V24.2 Unspecified motorcycle rider injured in collision with heavy transport vehicle or bus in nontraffic accident**

√x7th **V24.3 Person boarding or alighting a motorcycle injured in collision with heavy transport vehicle or bus**

√x7th **V24.4 Motorcycle driver injured in collision with heavy transport vehicle or bus in traffic accident**

√x7th **V24.5 Motorcycle passenger injured in collision with heavy transport vehicle or bus in traffic accident**

√x7th **V24.9 Unspecified motorcycle rider injured in collision with heavy transport vehicle or bus in traffic accident**

✓4th V25 Motorcycle rider injured in collision with railway train or railway vehicle

> The appropriate 7th character is to be added to each code from category V25.
> A initial encounter
> D subsequent encounter
> S sequela

✓x7th V25.0 Motorcycle driver injured in collision with railway train or railway vehicle in nontraffic accident

✓x7th V25.1 Motorcycle passenger injured in collision with railway train or railway vehicle in nontraffic accident

✓x7th V25.2 Unspecified motorcycle rider injured in collision with railway train or railway vehicle in nontraffic accident

✓x7th V25.3 Person boarding or alighting a motorcycle injured in collision with railway train or railway vehicle

✓x7th V25.4 Motorcycle driver injured in collision with railway train or railway vehicle in traffic accident

✓x7th V25.5 Motorcycle passenger injured in collision with railway train or railway vehicle in traffic accident

✓x7th V25.9 Unspecified motorcycle rider injured in collision with railway train or railway vehicle in traffic accident

✓4th V26 Motorcycle rider injured in collision with other nonmotor vehicle

INCLUDES collision with animal-drawn vehicle, animal being ridden, streetcar

> The appropriate 7th character is to be added to each code from category V26.
> A initial encounter
> D subsequent encounter
> S sequela

✓x7th V26.0 Motorcycle driver injured in collision with other nonmotor vehicle in nontraffic accident

✓x7th V26.1 Motorcycle passenger injured in collision with other nonmotor vehicle in nontraffic accident

✓x7th V26.2 Unspecified motorcycle rider injured in collision with other nonmotor vehicle in nontraffic accident

✓x7th V26.3 Person boarding or alighting a motorcycle injured in collision with other nonmotor vehicle

✓x7th V26.4 Motorcycle driver injured in collision with other nonmotor vehicle in traffic accident

✓x7th V26.5 Motorcycle passenger injured in collision with other nonmotor vehicle in traffic accident

✓x7th V26.9 Unspecified motorcycle rider injured in collision with other nonmotor vehicle in traffic accident

✓4th V27 Motorcycle rider injured in collision with fixed or stationary object

> The appropriate 7th character is to be added to each code from category V27.
> A initial encounter
> D subsequent encounter
> S sequela

✓x7th V27.0 Motorcycle driver injured in collision with fixed or stationary object in nontraffic accident

✓x7th V27.1 Motorcycle passenger injured in collision with fixed or stationary object in nontraffic accident

✓x7th V27.2 Unspecified motorcycle rider injured in collision with fixed or stationary object in nontraffic accident

✓x7th V27.3 Person boarding or alighting a motorcycle injured in collision with fixed or stationary object

✓x7th V27.4 Motorcycle driver injured in collision with fixed or stationary object in traffic accident

✓x7th V27.5 Motorcycle passenger injured in collision with fixed or stationary object in traffic accident

✓x7th V27.9 Unspecified motorcycle rider injured in collision with fixed or stationary object in traffic accident

✓4th V28 Motorcycle rider injured in noncollision transport accident

INCLUDES fall or thrown from motorcycle (without antecedent collision)
overturning motorcycle NOS
overturning motorcycle without collision

> The appropriate 7th character is to be added to each code from category V28.
> A initial encounter
> D subsequent encounter
> S sequela

✓x7th V28.0 Motorcycle driver injured in noncollision transport accident in nontraffic accident

✓x7th V28.1 Motorcycle passenger injured in noncollision transport accident in nontraffic accident

✓x7th V28.2 Unspecified motorcycle rider injured in noncollision transport accident in nontraffic accident

✓x7th V28.3 Person boarding or alighting a motorcycle injured in noncollision transport accident

✓x7th V28.4 Motorcycle driver injured in noncollision transport accident in traffic accident

✓x7th V28.5 Motorcycle passenger injured in noncollision transport accident in traffic accident

✓x7th V28.9 Unspecified motorcycle rider injured in noncollision transport accident in traffic accident

✓4th V29 Motorcycle rider injured in other and unspecified transport accidents

> The appropriate 7th character is to be added to each code from category V29.
> A initial encounter
> D subsequent encounter
> S sequela

✓5th V29.0 Motorcycle driver injured in collision with other and unspecified motor vehicles in nontraffic accident

✓x7th V29.00 Motorcycle driver injured in collision with unspecified motor vehicles in nontraffic accident

✓x7th V29.09 Motorcycle driver injured in collision with other motor vehicles in nontraffic accident

✓5th V29.1 Motorcycle passenger injured in collision with other and unspecified motor vehicles in nontraffic accident

✓x7th V29.10 Motorcycle passenger injured in collision with unspecified motor vehicles in nontraffic accident

✓x7th V29.19 Motorcycle passenger injured in collision with other motor vehicles in nontraffic accident

✓5th V29.2 Unspecified motorcycle rider injured in collision with other and unspecified motor vehicles in nontraffic accident

✓x7th V29.20 Unspecified motorcycle rider injured in collision with unspecified motor vehicles in nontraffic accident

Motorcycle collision NOS, nontraffic

✓x7th V29.29 Unspecified motorcycle rider injured in collision with other motor vehicles in nontraffic accident

✓x7th V29.3 Motorcycle rider (driver) (passenger) injured in unspecified nontraffic accident

Motorcycle accident NOS, nontraffic
Motorcycle rider injured in nontraffic accident NOS

✓5th V29.4 Motorcycle driver injured in collision with other and unspecified motor vehicles in traffic accident

✓x7th V29.40 Motorcycle driver injured in collision with unspecified motor vehicles in traffic accident

✓x7th V29.49 Motorcycle driver injured in collision with other motor vehicles in traffic accident

✓5th V29.5 Motorcycle passenger injured in collision with other and unspecified motor vehicles in traffic accident

✓x7th V29.50 Motorcycle passenger injured in collision with unspecified motor vehicles in traffic accident

✓x7th V29.59 Motorcycle passenger injured in collision with other motor vehicles in traffic accident

✓5th V29.6 Unspecified motorcycle rider injured in collision with other and unspecified motor vehicles in traffic accident

✓x7th V29.60 Unspecified motorcycle rider injured in collision with unspecified motor vehicles in traffic accident

Motorcycle collision NOS (traffic)

✓x7th V29.69 Unspecified motorcycle rider injured in collision with other motor vehicles in traffic accident

✓5th V29.8 Motorcycle rider (driver) (passenger) injured in other specified transport accidents

✓x7th V29.81 Motorcycle rider (driver) (passenger) injured in transport accident with military vehicle

√x7th **V29.88 Motorcycle rider (driver) (passenger) injured in other specified transport accidents**

√x7th **V29.9 Motorcycle rider (driver) (passenger) injured in unspecified traffic accident**
Motorcycle accident NOS

Occupant of three-wheeled motor vehicle injured in transport accident (V30-V39)

INCLUDES motorized tricycle
motorized rickshaw
three-wheeled motor car

EXCLUDES 1 *all-terrain vehicles (V86.-)*
motorcycle with sidecar (V20-V29)
vehicle designed primarily for off-road use (V86.-)

√4th **V30 Occupant of three-wheeled motor vehicle injured in collision with pedestrian or animal**

EXCLUDES 1 *three-wheeled motor vehicle collision with animal-drawn vehicle or animal being ridden (V36.-)*

The appropriate 7th character is to be added to each code from category V30.
A initial encounter
D subsequent encounter
S sequela

√x7th **V30.0 Driver of three-wheeled motor vehicle injured in collision with pedestrian or animal in nontraffic accident**

√x7th **V30.1 Passenger in three-wheeled motor vehicle injured in collision with pedestrian or animal in nontraffic accident**

√x7th **V30.2 Person on outside of three-wheeled motor vehicle injured in collision with pedestrian or animal in nontraffic accident**

√x7th **V30.3 Unspecified occupant of three-wheeled motor vehicle injured in collision with pedestrian or animal in nontraffic accident**

√x7th **V30.4 Person boarding or alighting a three-wheeled motor vehicle injured in collision with pedestrian or animal**

√x7th **V30.5 Driver of three-wheeled motor vehicle injured in collision with pedestrian or animal in traffic accident**

√x7th **V30.6 Passenger in three-wheeled motor vehicle injured in collision with pedestrian or animal in traffic accident**

√x7th **V30.7 Person on outside of three-wheeled motor vehicle injured in collision with pedestrian or animal in traffic accident**

√x7th **V30.9 Unspecified occupant of three-wheeled motor vehicle injured in collision with pedestrian or animal in traffic accident**

√4th **V31 Occupant of three-wheeled motor vehicle injured in collision with pedal cycle**

The appropriate 7th character is to be added to each code from category V31.
A initial encounter
D subsequent encounter
S sequela

√x7th **V31.0 Driver of three-wheeled motor vehicle injured in collision with pedal cycle in nontraffic accident**

√x7th **V31.1 Passenger in three-wheeled motor vehicle injured in collision with pedal cycle in nontraffic accident**

√x7th **V31.2 Person on outside of three-wheeled motor vehicle injured in collision with pedal cycle in nontraffic accident**

√x7th **V31.3 Unspecified occupant of three-wheeled motor vehicle injured in collision with pedal cycle in nontraffic accident**

√x7th **V31.4 Person boarding or alighting a three-wheeled motor vehicle injured in collision with pedal cycle**

√x7th **V31.5 Driver of three-wheeled motor vehicle injured in collision with pedal cycle in traffic accident**

√x7th **V31.6 Passenger in three-wheeled motor vehicle injured in collision with pedal cycle in traffic accident**

√x7th **V31.7 Person on outside of three-wheeled motor vehicle injured in collision with pedal cycle in traffic accident**

√x7th **V31.9 Unspecified occupant of three-wheeled motor vehicle injured in collision with pedal cycle in traffic accident**

√4th **V32 Occupant of three-wheeled motor vehicle injured in collision with two- or three-wheeled motor vehicle**

The appropriate 7th character is to be added to each code from category V32.
A initial encounter
D subsequent encounter
S sequela

√x7th **V32.0 Driver of three-wheeled motor vehicle injured in collision with two- or three-wheeled motor vehicle in nontraffic accident**

√x7th **V32.1 Passenger in three-wheeled motor vehicle injured in collision with two- or three-wheeled motor vehicle in nontraffic accident**

√x7th **V32.2 Person on outside of three-wheeled motor vehicle injured in collision with two- or three-wheeled motor vehicle in nontraffic accident**

√x7th **V32.3 Unspecified occupant of three-wheeled motor vehicle injured in collision with two- or three-wheeled motor vehicle in nontraffic accident**

√x7th **V32.4 Person boarding or alighting a three-wheeled motor vehicle injured in collision with two- or three-wheeled motor vehicle**

√x7th **V32.5 Driver of three-wheeled motor vehicle injured in collision with two- or three-wheeled motor vehicle in traffic accident**

√x7th **V32.6 Passenger in three-wheeled motor vehicle injured in collision with two- or three-wheeled motor vehicle in traffic accident**

√x7th **V32.7 Person on outside of three-wheeled motor vehicle injured in collision with two- or three-wheeled motor vehicle in traffic accident**

√x7th **V32.9 Unspecified occupant of three-wheeled motor vehicle injured in collision with two- or three-wheeled motor vehicle in traffic accident**

√4th **V33 Occupant of three-wheeled motor vehicle injured in collision with car, pick-up truck or van**

The appropriate 7th character is to be added to each code from category V33.
A initial encounter
D subsequent encounter
S sequela

√x7th **V33.0 Driver of three-wheeled motor vehicle injured in collision with car, pick-up truck or van in nontraffic accident**

√x7th **V33.1 Passenger in three-wheeled motor vehicle injured in collision with car, pick-up truck or van in nontraffic accident**

√x7th **V33.2 Person on outside of three-wheeled motor vehicle injured in collision with car, pick-up truck or van in nontraffic accident**

√x7th **V33.3 Unspecified occupant of three-wheeled motor vehicle injured in collision with car, pick-up truck or van in nontraffic accident**

√x7th **V33.4 Person boarding or alighting a three-wheeled motor vehicle injured in collision with car, pick-up truck or van**

√x7th **V33.5 Driver of three-wheeled motor vehicle injured in collision with car, pick-up truck or van in traffic accident**

√x7th **V33.6 Passenger in three-wheeled motor vehicle injured in collision with car, pick-up truck or van in traffic accident**

√x7th **V33.7 Person on outside of three-wheeled motor vehicle injured in collision with car, pick-up truck or van in traffic accident**

√x7th **V33.9 Unspecified occupant of three-wheeled motor vehicle injured in collision with car, pick-up truck or van in traffic accident**

√4th **V34 Occupant of three-wheeled motor vehicle injured in collision with heavy transport vehicle or bus**

EXCLUDES 1 *occupant of three-wheeled motor vehicle injured in collision with military vehicle (V39.81)*

The appropriate 7th character is to be added to each code from category V34.
A initial encounter
D subsequent encounter
S sequela

√x7th **V34.0 Driver of three-wheeled motor vehicle injured in collision with heavy transport vehicle or bus in nontraffic accident**

√x7th **V34.1 Passenger in three-wheeled motor vehicle injured in collision with heavy transport vehicle or bus in nontraffic accident**

√x7th **V34.2 Person on outside of three-wheeled motor vehicle injured in collision with heavy transport vehicle or bus in nontraffic accident**

V34.3 Unspecified **occupant of three-wheeled motor vehicle injured in collision with heavy transport vehicle or bus** in nontraffic accident

V34.4 Person boarding or alighting **a three-wheeled motor vehicle injured in collision with heavy transport vehicle or bus**

V34.5 Driver **of three-wheeled motor vehicle injured in collision with heavy transport vehicle or bus** in traffic accident

V34.6 Passenger **in three-wheeled motor vehicle injured in collision with heavy transport vehicle or bus** in traffic accident

V34.7 Person on outside **of three-wheeled motor vehicle injured in collision with heavy transport vehicle or bus** in traffic accident

V34.9 Unspecified **occupant of three-wheeled motor vehicle injured in collision with heavy transport vehicle or bus** in traffic accident

V35 Occupant of three-wheeled motor vehicle injured in collision with railway train or railway vehicle

The appropriate 7th character is to be added to each code from category V35.
A initial encounter
D subsequent encounter
S sequela

V35.Ø Driver **of three-wheeled motor vehicle injured in collision with railway train or railway vehicle** in nontraffic accident

V35.1 Passenger **in three-wheeled motor vehicle injured in collision with railway train or railway vehicle** in nontraffic accident

V35.2 Person on outside **of three-wheeled motor vehicle injured in collision with railway train or railway vehicle** in nontraffic accident

V35.3 Unspecified **occupant of three-wheeled motor vehicle injured in collision with railway train or railway vehicle** in nontraffic accident

V35.4 Person boarding or alighting **a three-wheeled motor vehicle injured in collision with railway train or railway vehicle**

V35.5 Driver **of three-wheeled motor vehicle injured in collision with railway train or railway vehicle** in traffic accident

V35.6 Passenger **in three-wheeled motor vehicle injured in collision with railway train or railway vehicle** in traffic accident

V35.7 Person on outside **of three-wheeled motor vehicle injured in collision with railway train or railway vehicle** in traffic accident

V35.9 Unspecified **occupant of three-wheeled motor vehicle injured in collision with railway train or railway vehicle** in traffic accident

V36 Occupant of three-wheeled motor vehicle injured in collision with other nonmotor vehicle

INCLUDES collision with animal-drawn vehicle, animal being ridden, streetcar

The appropriate 7th character is to be added to each code from category V36.
A initial encounter
D subsequent encounter
S sequela

V36.Ø Driver **of three-wheeled motor vehicle injured in collision with other nonmotor vehicle** in nontraffic accident

V36.1 Passenger **in three-wheeled motor vehicle injured in collision with other nonmotor vehicle** in nontraffic accident

V36.2 Person on outside **of three-wheeled motor vehicle injured in collision with other nonmotor vehicle** in nontraffic accident

V36.3 Unspecified **occupant of three-wheeled motor vehicle injured in collision with other nonmotor vehicle** in nontraffic accident

V36.4 Person boarding or alighting **a three-wheeled motor vehicle injured in collision with other nonmotor vehicle**

V36.5 Driver **of three-wheeled motor vehicle injured in collision with other nonmotor vehicle** in traffic accident

V36.6 Passenger **in three-wheeled motor vehicle injured in collision with other nonmotor vehicle** in traffic accident

V36.7 Person on outside **of three-wheeled motor vehicle injured in collision with other nonmotor vehicle** in traffic accident

V36.9 Unspecified **occupant of three-wheeled motor vehicle injured in collision with other nonmotor vehicle** in traffic accident

V37 Occupant of three-wheeled motor vehicle injured in collision with fixed or stationary object

The appropriate 7th character is to be added to each code from category V37.
A initial encounter
D subsequent encounter
S sequela

V37.Ø Driver **of three-wheeled motor vehicle injured in collision with fixed or stationary object** in nontraffic accident

V37.1 Passenger **in three-wheeled motor vehicle injured in collision with fixed or stationary object** in nontraffic accident

V37.2 Person on outside **of three-wheeled motor vehicle injured in collision with fixed or stationary object** in nontraffic accident

V37.3 Unspecified **occupant of three-wheeled motor vehicle injured in collision with fixed or stationary object** in nontraffic accident

V37.4 Person boarding or alighting **a three-wheeled motor vehicle injured in collision with fixed or stationary object**

V37.5 Driver **of three-wheeled motor vehicle injured in collision with fixed or stationary object** in traffic accident

V37.6 Passenger **in three-wheeled motor vehicle injured in collision with fixed or stationary object** in traffic accident

V37.7 Person on outside **of three-wheeled motor vehicle injured in collision with fixed or stationary object** in traffic accident

V37.9 Unspecified **occupant of three-wheeled motor vehicle injured in collision with fixed or stationary object** in traffic accident

V38 Occupant of three-wheeled motor vehicle injured in noncollision transport accident

INCLUDES fall or thrown from three-wheeled motor vehicle
overturning of three-wheeled motor vehicle NOS
overturning of three-wheeled motor vehicle without collision

The appropriate 7th character is to be added to each code from category V38.
A initial encounter
D subsequent encounter
S sequela

V38.Ø Driver **of three-wheeled motor vehicle injured in noncollision transport accident** in nontraffic accident

V38.1 Passenger **in three-wheeled motor vehicle injured in noncollision transport accident** in nontraffic accident

V38.2 Person on outside **of three-wheeled motor vehicle injured in noncollision transport accident** in nontraffic accident

V38.3 Unspecified **occupant of three-wheeled motor vehicle injured in noncollision transport accident** in nontraffic accident

V38.4 Person boarding or alighting **a three-wheeled motor vehicle injured in noncollision transport accident**

V38.5 Driver **of three-wheeled motor vehicle injured in noncollision transport accident** in traffic accident

V38.6 Passenger **in three-wheeled motor vehicle injured in noncollision transport accident** in traffic accident

V38.7 Person on outside **of three-wheeled motor vehicle injured in noncollision transport accident** in traffic accident

V38.9 Unspecified **occupant of three-wheeled motor vehicle injured in noncollision transport accident** in traffic accident

V39 Occupant of three-wheeled motor vehicle injured in other and unspecified transport accidents

The appropriate 7th character is to be added to each code from category V39.
A initial encounter
D subsequent encounter
S sequela

V39.Ø Driver **of three-wheeled motor vehicle injured in collision with other and unspecified motor vehicles** in nontraffic accident

V39.ØØ **Driver of three-wheeled motor vehicle injured in collision with** unspecified **motor vehicles in nontraffic accident**

V39.Ø9 **Driver of three-wheeled motor vehicle injured in collision with** other **motor vehicles in nontraffic accident**

√5th **V39.1 Passenger in three-wheeled motor vehicle injured in collision with other and unspecified motor vehicles in nontraffic accident**

√x7th **V39.10 Passenger in three-wheeled motor vehicle injured in collision with unspecified motor vehicles in nontraffic accident**

√x7th **V39.19 Passenger in three-wheeled motor vehicle injured in collision with other motor vehicles in nontraffic accident**

√5th **V39.2 Unspecified occupant of three-wheeled motor vehicle injured in collision with other and unspecified motor vehicles in nontraffic accident**

√x7th **V39.20 Unspecified occupant of three-wheeled motor vehicle injured in collision with unspecified motor vehicles in nontraffic accident**

Collision NOS involving three-wheeled motor vehicle, nontraffic

√x7th **V39.29 Unspecified occupant of three-wheeled motor vehicle injured in collision with other motor vehicles in nontraffic accident**

√x7th **V39.3 Occupant (driver) (passenger) of three-wheeled motor vehicle injured in unspecified nontraffic accident**

Accident NOS involving three-wheeled motor vehicle, nontraffic
Occupant of three-wheeled motor vehicle injured in nontraffic accident NOS

√5th **V39.4 Driver of three-wheeled motor vehicle injured in collision with other and unspecified motor vehicles in traffic accident**

√x7th **V39.40 Driver of three-wheeled motor vehicle injured in collision with unspecified motor vehicles in traffic accident**

√x7th **V39.49 Driver of three-wheeled motor vehicle injured in collision with other motor vehicles in traffic accident**

√5th **V39.5 Passenger in three-wheeled motor vehicle injured in collision with other and unspecified motor vehicles in traffic accident**

√x7th **V39.50 Passenger in three-wheeled motor vehicle injured in collision with unspecified motor vehicles in traffic accident**

√x7th **V39.59 Passenger in three-wheeled motor vehicle injured in collision with other motor vehicles in traffic accident**

√5th **V39.6 Unspecified occupant of three-wheeled motor vehicle injured in collision with other and unspecified motor vehicles in traffic accident**

√x7th **V39.60 Unspecified occupant of three-wheeled motor vehicle injured in collision with unspecified motor vehicles in traffic accident**

Collision NOS involving three-wheeled motor vehicle (traffic)

√x7th **V39.69 Unspecified occupant of three-wheeled motor vehicle injured in collision with other motor vehicles in traffic accident**

√5th **V39.8 Occupant (driver) (passenger) of three-wheeled motor vehicle injured in other specified transport accidents**

√x7th **V39.81 Occupant (driver) (passenger) of three-wheeled motor vehicle injured in transport accident with military vehicle**

√x7th **V39.89 Occupant (driver) (passenger) of three-wheeled motor vehicle injured in other specified transport accidents**

√x7th **V39.9 Occupant (driver) (passenger) of three-wheeled motor vehicle injured in unspecified traffic accident**

Accident NOS involving three-wheeled motor vehicle

Car occupant injured in transport accident (V40-V49)

INCLUDES a four-wheeled motor vehicle designed primarily for carrying passengers
automobile (pulling a trailer or camper)

EXCLUDES 1 *bus (V50-V59)*
minibus (V50-V59)
minivan (V50-V59)
motorcoach (V70-V79)
pick-up truck (V50-V59)
sport utility vehicle (SUV) (V50-V59)

√4th **V40 Car occupant injured in collision with pedestrian or animal**

EXCLUDES 1 *car collision with animal-drawn vehicle or animal being ridden (V46.-)*

The appropriate 7th character is to be added to each code from category V40.
A initial encounter
D subsequent encounter
S sequela

√x7th **V40.0 Car driver injured in collision with pedestrian or animal in nontraffic accident**

√x7th **V40.1 Car passenger injured in collision with pedestrian or animal in nontraffic accident**

√x7th **V40.2 Person on outside of car injured in collision with pedestrian or animal in nontraffic accident**

√x7th **V40.3 Unspecified car occupant injured in collision with pedestrian or animal in nontraffic accident**

√x7th **V40.4 Person boarding or alighting a car injured in collision with pedestrian or animal**

√x7th **V40.5 Car driver injured in collision with pedestrian or animal in traffic accident**

√x7th **V40.6 Car passenger injured in collision with pedestrian or animal in traffic accident**

√x7th **V40.7 Person on outside of car injured in collision with pedestrian or animal in traffic accident**

√x7th **V40.9 Unspecified car occupant injured in collision with pedestrian or animal in traffic accident**

√4th **V41 Car occupant injured in collision with pedal cycle**

The appropriate 7th character is to be added to each code from category V41.
A initial encounter
D subsequent encounter
S sequela

√x7th **V41.0 Car driver injured in collision with pedal cycle in nontraffic accident**

√x7th **V41.1 Car passenger injured in collision with pedal cycle in nontraffic accident**

√x7th **V41.2 Person on outside of car injured in collision with pedal cycle in nontraffic accident**

√x7th **V41.3 Unspecified car occupant injured in collision with pedal cycle in nontraffic accident**

√x7th **V41.4 Person boarding or alighting a car injured in collision with pedal cycle**

√x7th **V41.5 Car driver injured in collision with pedal cycle in traffic accident**

√x7th **V41.6 Car passenger injured in collision with pedal cycle in traffic accident**

√x7th **V41.7 Person on outside of car injured in collision with pedal cycle in traffic accident**

√x7th **V41.9 Unspecified car occupant injured in collision with pedal cycle in traffic accident**

√4th **V42 Car occupant injured in collision with two- or three-wheeled motor vehicle**

The appropriate 7th character is to be added to each code from category V42.
A initial encounter
D subsequent encounter
S sequela

√x7th **V42.0 Car driver injured in collision with two- or three-wheeled motor vehicle in nontraffic accident**

√x7th **V42.1 Car passenger injured in collision with two- or three-wheeled motor vehicle in nontraffic accident**

√x7th **V42.2 Person on outside of car injured in collision with two- or three-wheeled motor vehicle in nontraffic accident**

√x7th **V42.3 Unspecified car occupant injured in collision with two- or three-wheeled motor vehicle in nontraffic accident**

√x7th **V42.4 Person boarding or alighting a car injured in collision with two- or three-wheeled motor vehicle**

√x7th **V42.5 Car driver injured in collision with two- or three-wheeled motor vehicle in traffic accident**

√x7th **V42.6 Car passenger injured in collision with two- or three-wheeled motor vehicle in traffic accident**

√x7th **V42.7 Person on outside of car injured in collision with two- or three-wheeled motor vehicle in traffic accident**

√x7th **V42.9 Unspecified car occupant injured in collision with two- or three-wheeled motor vehicle in traffic accident**

V43 Car occupant injured in collision with car, pick-up truck or van

The appropriate 7th character is to be added to each code from category V43.
A initial encounter
D subsequent encounter
S sequela

V43.0 Car driver injured in collision with car, pick-up truck or van in nontraffic accident
- **V43.01 Car driver injured in collision with sport utility vehicle in nontraffic accident**
- **V43.02 Car driver injured in collision with other type car in nontraffic accident**
- **V43.03 Car driver injured in collision with pick-up truck in nontraffic accident**
- **V43.04 Car driver injured in collision with van in nontraffic accident**

V43.1 Car passenger injured in collision with car, pick-up truck or van in nontraffic accident
- **V43.11 Car passenger injured in collision with sport utility vehicle in nontraffic accident**
- **V43.12 Car passenger injured in collision with other type car in nontraffic accident**
- **V43.13 Car passenger injured in collision with pick-up in nontraffic accident**
- **V43.14 Car passenger injured in collision with van in nontraffic accident**

V43.2 Person on outside of car injured in collision with car, pick-up truck or van in nontraffic accident
- **V43.21 Person on outside of car injured in collision with sport utility vehicle in nontraffic accident**
- **V43.22 Person on outside of car injured in collision with other type car in nontraffic accident**
- **V43.23 Person on outside of car injured in collision with pick-up truck in nontraffic accident**
- **V43.24 Person on outside of car injured in collision with van in nontraffic accident**

V43.3 Unspecified car occupant injured in collision with car, pick-up truck or van in nontraffic accident
- **V43.31 Unspecified car occupant injured in collision with sport utility vehicle in nontraffic accident**
- **V43.32 Unspecified car occupant injured in collision with other type car in nontraffic accident**
- **V43.33 Unspecified car occupant injured in collision with pick-up truck in nontraffic accident**
- **V43.34 Unspecified car occupant injured in collision with van in nontraffic accident**

V43.4 Person boarding or alighting a car injured in collision with car, pick-up truck or van
- **V43.41 Person boarding or alighting a car injured in collision with sport utility vehicle**
- **V43.42 Person boarding or alighting a car injured in collision with other type car**
- **V43.43 Person boarding or alighting a car injured in collision with pick-up truck**
- **V43.44 Person boarding or alighting a car injured in collision with van**

V43.5 Car driver injured in collision with car, pick-up truck or van in traffic accident
- **V43.51 Car driver injured in collision with sport utility vehicle in traffic accident**
- **V43.52 Car driver injured in collision with other type car in traffic accident**
- **V43.53 Car driver injured in collision with pick-up truck in traffic accident**
- **V43.54 Car driver injured in collision with van in traffic accident**

V43.6 Car passenger injured in collision with car, pick-up truck or van in traffic accident
- **V43.61 Car passenger injured in collision with sport utility vehicle in traffic accident**
- **V43.62 Car passenger injured in collision with other type car in traffic accident**
- **V43.63 Car passenger injured in collision with pick-up truck in traffic accident**
- **V43.64 Car passenger injured in collision with van in traffic accident**

V43.7 Person on outside of car injured in collision with car, pick-up truck or van in traffic accident
- **V43.71 Person on outside of car injured in collision with sport utility vehicle in traffic accident**
- **V43.72 Person on outside of car injured in collision with other type car in traffic accident**
- **V43.73 Person on outside of car injured in collision with pick-up truck in traffic accident**
- **V43.74 Person on outside of car injured in collision with van in traffic accident**

V43.9 Unspecified car occupant injured in collision with car, pick-up truck or van in traffic accident
- **V43.91 Unspecified car occupant injured in collision with sport utility vehicle in traffic accident**
- **V43.92 Unspecified car occupant injured in collision with other type car in traffic accident**
- **V43.93 Unspecified car occupant injured in collision with pick-up truck in traffic accident**
- **V43.94 Unspecified car occupant injured in collision with van in traffic accident**

V44 Car occupant injured in collision with heavy transport vehicle or bus

EXCLUDES 1 *car occupant injured in collision with military vehicle (V49.81)*

The appropriate 7th character is to be added to each code from category V44.
A initial encounter
D subsequent encounter
S sequela

- **V44.0 Car driver injured in collision with heavy transport vehicle or bus in nontraffic accident**
- **V44.1 Car passenger injured in collision with heavy transport vehicle or bus in nontraffic accident**
- **V44.2 Person on outside of car injured in collision with heavy transport vehicle or bus in nontraffic accident**
- **V44.3 Unspecified car occupant injured in collision with heavy transport vehicle or bus in nontraffic accident**
- **V44.4 Person boarding or alighting a car injured in collision with heavy transport vehicle or bus**
- **V44.5 Car driver injured in collision with heavy transport vehicle or bus in traffic accident**
- **V44.6 Car passenger injured in collision with heavy transport vehicle or bus in traffic accident**
- **V44.7 Person on outside of car injured in collision with heavy transport vehicle or bus in traffic accident**
- **V44.9 Unspecified car occupant injured in collision with heavy transport vehicle or bus in traffic accident**

V45 Car occupant injured in collision with railway train or railway vehicle

The appropriate 7th character is to be added to each code from category V45.
A initial encounter
D subsequent encounter
S sequela

- **V45.0 Car driver injured in collision with railway train or railway vehicle in nontraffic accident**
- **V45.1 Car passenger injured in collision with railway train or railway vehicle in nontraffic accident**
- **V45.2 Person on outside of car injured in collision with railway train or railway vehicle in nontraffic accident**
- **V45.3 Unspecified car occupant injured in collision with railway train or railway vehicle in nontraffic accident**
- **V45.4 Person boarding or alighting a car injured in collision with railway train or railway vehicle**
- **V45.5 Car driver injured in collision with railway train or railway vehicle in traffic accident**
- **V45.6 Car passenger injured in collision with railway train or railway vehicle in traffic accident**
- **V45.7 Person on outside of car injured in collision with railway train or railway vehicle in traffic accident**
- **V45.9 Unspecified car occupant injured in collision with railway train or railway vehicle in traffic accident**

4th V46 Car occupant injured in collision with other nonmotor vehicle
INCLUDES collision with animal-drawn vehicle, animal being ridden, streetcar

The appropriate 7th character is to be added to each code from category V46.
A initial encounter
D subsequent encounter
S sequela

x7th V46.0 Car driver injured in collision with other nonmotor vehicle in nontraffic accident

x7th V46.1 Car passenger injured in collision with other nonmotor vehicle in nontraffic accident

x7th V46.2 Person on outside of car injured in collision with other nonmotor vehicle in nontraffic accident

x7th V46.3 Unspecified car occupant injured in collision with other nonmotor vehicle in nontraffic accident

x7th V46.4 Person boarding or alighting a car injured in collision with other nonmotor vehicle

x7th V46.5 Car driver injured in collision with other nonmotor vehicle in traffic accident

x7th V46.6 Car passenger injured in collision with other nonmotor vehicle in traffic accident

x7th V46.7 Person on outside of car injured in collision with other nonmotor vehicle in traffic accident

x7th V46.9 Unspecified car occupant injured in collision with other nonmotor vehicle in traffic accident

4th V47 Car occupant injured in collision with fixed or stationary object

The appropriate 7th character is to be added to each code from category V47.
A initial encounter
D subsequent encounter
S sequela

5th V47.0 Car driver injured in collision with fixed or stationary object in nontraffic accident

x7th V47.01 Driver of sport utility vehicle injured in collision with fixed or stationary object in nontraffic accident

x7th V47.02 Driver of other type car injured in collision with fixed or stationary object in nontraffic accident

5th V47.1 Car passenger injured in collision with fixed or stationary object in nontraffic accident

x7th V47.11 Passenger of sport utility vehicle injured in collision with fixed or stationary object in nontraffic accident

x7th V47.12 Passenger of other type car injured in collision with fixed or stationary object in nontraffic accident

x7th V47.2 Person on outside of car injured in collision with fixed or stationary object in nontraffic accident

5th V47.3 Unspecified car occupant injured in collision with fixed or stationary object in nontraffic accident

x7th V47.31 Unspecified occupant of sport utility vehicle injured in collision with fixed or stationary object in nontraffic accident

x7th V47.32 Unspecified occupant of other type car injured in collision with fixed or stationary object in nontraffic accident

x7th V47.4 Person boarding or alighting a car injured in collision with fixed or stationary object

5th V47.5 Car driver injured in collision with fixed or stationary object in traffic accident

x7th V47.51 Driver of sport utility vehicle injured in collision with fixed or stationary object in traffic accident

x7th V47.52 Driver of other type car injured in collision with fixed or stationary object in traffic accident

5th V47.6 Car passenger injured in collision with fixed or stationary object in traffic accident

x7th V47.61 Passenger of sport utility vehicle injured in collision with fixed or stationary object in traffic accident

x7th V47.62 Passenger of other type car injured in collision with fixed or stationary object in traffic accident

x7th V47.7 Person on outside of car injured in collision with fixed or stationary object in traffic accident

5th V47.9 Unspecified car occupant injured in collision with fixed or stationary object in traffic accident

x7th V47.91 Unspecified occupant of sport utility vehicle injured in collision with fixed or stationary object in traffic accident

x7th V47.92 Unspecified occupant of other type car injured in collision with fixed or stationary object in traffic accident

4th V48 Car occupant injured in noncollision transport accident
INCLUDES overturning car NOS
overturning car without collision

The appropriate 7th character is to be added to each code from category V48.
A initial encounter
D subsequent encounter
S sequela

x7th V48.0 Car driver injured in noncollision transport accident in nontraffic accident

x7th V48.1 Car passenger injured in noncollision transport accident in nontraffic accident

x7th V48.2 Person on outside of car injured in noncollision transport accident in nontraffic accident

x7th V48.3 Unspecified car occupant injured in noncollision transport accident in nontraffic accident

x7th V48.4 Person boarding or alighting a car injured in noncollision transport accident

x7th V48.5 Car driver injured in noncollision transport accident in traffic accident

x7th V48.6 Car passenger injured in noncollision transport accident in traffic accident

x7th V48.7 Person on outside of car injured in noncollision transport accident in traffic accident

x7th V48.9 Unspecified car occupant injured in noncollision transport accident in traffic accident

4th V49 Car occupant injured in other and unspecified transport accidents

The appropriate 7th character is to be added to each code from category V49.
A initial encounter
D subsequent encounter
S sequela

5th V49.0 Driver injured in collision with other and unspecified motor vehicles in nontraffic accident

x7th V49.00 Driver injured in collision with unspecified motor vehicles in nontraffic accident

x7th V49.09 Driver injured in collision with other motor vehicles in nontraffic accident

5th V49.1 Passenger injured in collision with other and unspecified motor vehicles in nontraffic accident

x7th V49.10 Passenger injured in collision with unspecified motor vehicles in nontraffic accident

x7th V49.19 Passenger injured in collision with other motor vehicles in nontraffic accident

5th V49.2 Unspecified car occupant injured in collision with other and unspecified motor vehicles in nontraffic accident

x7th V49.20 Unspecified car occupant injured in collision with unspecified motor vehicles in nontraffic accident
Car collision NOS, nontraffic

x7th V49.29 Unspecified car occupant injured in collision with other motor vehicles in nontraffic accident

x7th V49.3 Car occupant (driver) (passenger) injured in unspecified nontraffic accident
Car accident NOS, nontraffic
Car occupant injured in nontraffic accident NOS

5th V49.4 Driver injured in collision with other and unspecified motor vehicles in traffic accident

x7th V49.40 Driver injured in collision with unspecified motor vehicles in traffic accident

x7th V49.49 Driver injured in collision with other motor vehicles in traffic accident

5th V49.5 Passenger injured in collision with other and unspecified motor vehicles in traffic accident

x7th V49.50 Passenger injured in collision with unspecified motor vehicles in traffic accident

x7th V49.59 Passenger injured in collision with other motor vehicles in traffic accident

5th V49.6 Unspecified car occupant injured in collision with other and unspecified motor vehicles in traffic accident

x7th V49.60 Unspecified car occupant injured in collision with unspecified motor vehicles in traffic accident
Car collision NOS (traffic)

√x7th **V49.69 Unspecified car occupant injured in collision with other motor vehicles in traffic accident**

√5th **V49.8 Car occupant (driver) (passenger) injured in other specified transport accidents**

√x7th **V49.81 Car occupant (driver) (passenger) injured in transport accident with military vehicle**

√x7th **V49.88 Car occupant (driver) (passenger) injured in other specified transport accidents**

√x7th **V49.9 Car occupant (driver) (passenger) injured in unspecified traffic accident**

Car accident NOS

Occupant of pick-up truck or van injured in transport accident (V5Ø-V59)

INCLUDES a four or six wheel motor vehicle designed primarily for carrying passengers and property but weighing less than the local limit for classification as a heavy goods vehicle

minibus
minivan
sport utility vehicle (SUV)
truck
van

EXCLUDES 1 *heavy transport vehicle (V6Ø-V69)*

√4th **V5Ø Occupant of pick-up truck or van injured in collision with pedestrian or animal**

EXCLUDES 1 *pick-up truck or van collision with animal-drawn vehicle or animal being ridden (V56.-)*

The appropriate 7th character is to be added to each code from category V5Ø.
A initial encounter
D subsequent encounter
S sequela

√x7th **V5Ø.Ø Driver of pick-up truck or van injured in collision with pedestrian or animal in nontraffic accident**

√x7th **V5Ø.1 Passenger in pick-up truck or van injured in collision with pedestrian or animal in nontraffic accident**

√x7th **V5Ø.2 Person on outside of pick-up truck or van injured in collision with pedestrian or animal in nontraffic accident**

√x7th **V5Ø.3 Unspecified occupant of pick-up truck or van injured in collision with pedestrian or animal in nontraffic accident**

√x7th **V5Ø.4 Person boarding or alighting a pick-up truck or van injured in collision with pedestrian or animal**

√x7th **V5Ø.5 Driver of pick-up truck or van injured in collision with pedestrian or animal in traffic accident**

√x7th **V5Ø.6 Passenger in pick-up truck or van injured in collision with pedestrian or animal in traffic accident**

√x7th **V5Ø.7 Person on outside of pick-up truck or van injured in collision with pedestrian or animal in traffic accident**

√x7th **V5Ø.9 Unspecified occupant of pick-up truck or van injured in collision with pedestrian or animal in traffic accident**

√4th **V51 Occupant of pick-up truck or van injured in collision with pedal cycle**

The appropriate 7th character is to be added to each code from category V51.
A initial encounter
D subsequent encounter
S sequela

√x7th **V51.Ø Driver of pick-up truck or van injured in collision with pedal cycle in nontraffic accident**

√x7th **V51.1 Passenger in pick-up truck or van injured in collision with pedal cycle in nontraffic accident**

√x7th **V51.2 Person on outside of pick-up truck or van injured in collision with pedal cycle in nontraffic accident**

√x7th **V51.3 Unspecified occupant of pick-up truck or van injured in collision with pedal cycle in nontraffic accident**

√x7th **V51.4 Person boarding or alighting a pick-up truck or van injured in collision with pedal cycle**

√x7th **V51.5 Driver of pick-up truck or van injured in collision with pedal cycle in traffic accident**

√x7th **V51.6 Passenger in pick-up truck or van injured in collision with pedal cycle in traffic accident**

√x7th **V51.7 Person on outside of pick-up truck or van injured in collision with pedal cycle in traffic accident**

√x7th **V51.9 Unspecified occupant of pick-up truck or van injured in collision with pedal cycle in traffic accident**

√4th **V52 Occupant of pick-up truck or van injured in collision with two- or three-wheeled motor vehicle**

The appropriate 7th character is to be added to each code from category V52.
A initial encounter
D subsequent encounter
S sequela

√x7th **V52.Ø Driver of pick-up truck or van injured in collision with two- or three-wheeled motor vehicle in nontraffic accident**

√x7th **V52.1 Passenger in pick-up truck or van injured in collision with two- or three-wheeled motor vehicle in nontraffic accident**

√x7th **V52.2 Person on outside of pick-up truck or van injured in collision with two- or three-wheeled motor vehicle in nontraffic accident**

√x7th **V52.3 Unspecified occupant of pick-up truck or van injured in collision with two- or three-wheeled motor vehicle in nontraffic accident**

√x7th **V52.4 Person boarding or alighting a pick-up truck or van injured in collision with two- or three-wheeled motor vehicle**

√x7th **V52.5 Driver of pick-up truck or van injured in collision with two- or three-wheeled motor vehicle in traffic accident**

√x7th **V52.6 Passenger in pick-up truck or van injured in collision with two- or three-wheeled motor vehicle in traffic accident**

√x7th **V52.7 Person on outside of pick-up truck or van injured in collision with two- or three-wheeled motor vehicle in traffic accident**

√x7th **V52.9 Unspecified occupant of pick-up truck or van injured in collision with two- or three-wheeled motor vehicle in traffic accident**

√4th **V53 Occupant of pick-up truck or van injured in collision with car, pick-up truck or van**

The appropriate 7th character is to be added to each code from category V53.
A initial encounter
D subsequent encounter
S sequela

√x7th **V53.Ø Driver of pick-up truck or van injured in collision with car, pick-up truck or van in nontraffic accident**

√x7th **V53.1 Passenger in pick-up truck or van injured in collision with car, pick-up truck or van in nontraffic accident**

√x7th **V53.2 Person on outside of pick-up truck or van injured in collision with car, pick-up truck or van in nontraffic accident**

√x7th **V53.3 Unspecified occupant of pick-up truck or van injured in collision with car, pick-up truck or van in nontraffic accident**

√x7th **V53.4 Person boarding or alighting a pick-up truck or van injured in collision with car, pick-up truck or van**

√x7th **V53.5 Driver of pick-up truck or van injured in collision with car, pick-up truck or van in traffic accident**

√x7th **V53.6 Passenger in pick-up truck or van injured in collision with car, pick-up truck or van in traffic accident**

√x7th **V53.7 Person on outside of pick-up truck or van injured in collision with car, pick-up truck or van in traffic accident**

√x7th **V53.9 Unspecified occupant of pick-up truck or van injured in collision with car, pick-up truck or van in traffic accident**

√4th **V54 Occupant of pick-up truck or van injured in collision with heavy transport vehicle or bus**

EXCLUDES 1 *occupant of pick-up truck or van injured in collision with military vehicle (V59.81)*

The appropriate 7th character is to be added to each code from category V54.
A initial encounter
D subsequent encounter
S sequela

√x7th **V54.Ø Driver of pick-up truck or van injured in collision with heavy transport vehicle or bus in nontraffic accident**

√x7th **V54.1 Passenger in pick-up truck or van injured in collision with heavy transport vehicle or bus in nontraffic accident**

√x7th **V54.2 Person on outside of pick-up truck or van injured in collision with heavy transport vehicle or bus in nontraffic accident**

√x7th **V54.3 Unspecified occupant of pick-up truck or van injured in collision with heavy transport vehicle or bus in nontraffic accident**

√x7th **V54.4 Person boarding or alighting a pick-up truck or van injured in collision with heavy transport vehicle or bus**

√x7th **V54.5** Driver **of pick-up truck or van injured in collision with heavy transport vehicle or bus** in traffic accident

√x7th **V54.6** Passenger **in pick-up truck or van injured in collision with heavy transport vehicle or bus** in traffic accident

√x7th **V54.7** Person on outside **of pick-up truck or van injured in collision with heavy transport vehicle or bus** in traffic accident

√x7th **V54.9** Unspecified **occupant of pick-up truck or van injured in collision with heavy transport vehicle or bus** in traffic accident

√4th **V55 Occupant of pick-up truck or van injured in collision with railway train or railway vehicle**

The appropriate 7th character is to be added to each code from category V55.
A initial encounter
D subsequent encounter
S sequela

√x7th **V55.0** Driver **of pick-up truck or van injured in collision with railway train or railway vehicle** in nontraffic accident

√x7th **V55.1** Passenger **in pick-up truck or van injured in collision with railway train or railway vehicle** in nontraffic accident

√x7th **V55.2** Person on outside **of pick-up truck or van injured in collision with railway train or railway vehicle** in nontraffic accident

√x7th **V55.3** Unspecified **occupant of pick-up truck or van injured in collision with railway train or railway vehicle** in nontraffic accident

√x7th **V55.4** Person boarding or alighting **a pick-up truck or van injured in collision with railway train or railway vehicle**

√x7th **V55.5** Driver **of pick-up truck or van injured in collision with railway train or railway vehicle** in traffic accident

√x7th **V55.6** Passenger **in pick-up truck or van injured in collision with railway train or railway vehicle** in traffic accident

√x7th **V55.7** Person on outside **of pick-up truck or van injured in collision with railway train or railway vehicle** in traffic accident

√x7th **V55.9** Unspecified **occupant of pick-up truck or van injured in collision with railway train or railway vehicle** in traffic accident

√4th **V56 Occupant of pick-up truck or van injured in collision with other nonmotor vehicle**

INCLUDES collision with animal-drawn vehicle, animal being ridden, streetcar

The appropriate 7th character is to be added to each code from category V56.
A initial encounter
D subsequent encounter
S sequela

√x7th **V56.0** Driver **of pick-up truck or van injured in collision with other nonmotor vehicle** in nontraffic accident

√x7th **V56.1** Passenger **in pick-up truck or van injured in collision with other nonmotor vehicle** in nontraffic accident

√x7th **V56.2** Person on outside **of pick-up truck or van injured in collision with other nonmotor vehicle** in nontraffic accident

√x7th **V56.3** Unspecified **occupant of pick-up truck or van injured in collision with other nonmotor vehicle** in nontraffic accident

√x7th **V56.4** Person boarding or alighting **a pick-up truck or van injured in collision with other nonmotor vehicle**

√x7th **V56.5** Driver **of pick-up truck or van injured in collision with other nonmotor vehicle** in traffic accident

√x7th **V56.6** Passenger **in pick-up truck or van injured in collision with other nonmotor vehicle** in traffic accident

√x7th **V56.7** Person on outside **of pick-up truck or van injured in collision with other nonmotor vehicle** in traffic accident

√x7th **V56.9** Unspecified **occupant of pick-up truck or van injured in collision with other nonmotor vehicle** in traffic accident

√4th **V57 Occupant of pick-up truck or van injured in collision with fixed or stationary object**

The appropriate 7th character is to be added to each code from category V57.
A initial encounter
D subsequent encounter
S sequela

√x7th **V57.0** Driver **of pick-up truck or van injured in collision with fixed or stationary object** in nontraffic accident

√x7th **V57.1** Passenger **in pick-up truck or van injured in collision with fixed or stationary object** in nontraffic accident

√x7th **V57.2** Person on outside **of pick-up truck or van injured in collision with fixed or stationary object** in nontraffic accident

√x7th **V57.3** Unspecified **occupant of pick-up truck or van injured in collision with fixed or stationary object** in nontraffic accident

√x7th **V57.4** Person boarding or alighting **a pick-up truck or van injured in collision with fixed or stationary object**

√x7th **V57.5** Driver **of pick-up truck or van injured in collision with fixed or stationary object** in traffic accident

√x7th **V57.6** Passenger **in pick-up truck or van injured in collision with fixed or stationary object** in traffic accident

√x7th **V57.7** Person on outside **of pick-up truck or van injured in collision with fixed or stationary object** in traffic accident

√x7th **V57.9** Unspecified **occupant of pick-up truck or van injured in collision with fixed or stationary object** in traffic accident

√4th **V58 Occupant of pick-up truck or van injured in noncollision transport accident**

INCLUDES overturning pick-up truck or van NOS
overturning pick-up truck or van without collision

The appropriate 7th character is to be added to each code from category V58.
A initial encounter
D subsequent encounter
S sequela

√x7th **V58.0** Driver **of pick-up truck or van injured in noncollision transport accident** in nontraffic accident

√x7th **V58.1** Passenger **in pick-up truck or van injured in noncollision transport accident** in nontraffic accident

√x7th **V58.2** Person on outside **of pick-up truck or van injured in noncollision transport accident** in nontraffic accident

√x7th **V58.3** Unspecified **occupant of pick-up truck or van injured in noncollision transport accident** in nontraffic accident

√x7th **V58.4** Person boarding or alighting **a pick-up truck or van injured in noncollision transport accident**

√x7th **V58.5** Driver **of pick-up truck or van injured in noncollision transport accident** in traffic accident

√x7th **V58.6** Passenger **in pick-up truck or van injured in noncollision transport accident** in traffic accident

√x7th **V58.7** Person on outside **of pick-up truck or van injured in noncollision transport accident** in traffic accident

√x7th **V58.9** Unspecified **occupant of pick-up truck or van injured in noncollision transport accident** in traffic accident

√4th **V59 Occupant of pick-up truck or van injured in other and unspecified transport accidents**

The appropriate 7th character is to be added to each code from category V59.
A initial encounter
D subsequent encounter
S sequela

√5th **V59.0** Driver **of pick-up truck or van injured in collision with other and unspecified motor vehicles** in nontraffic accident

√x7th **V59.00 Driver of pick-up truck or van injured in collision** with unspecified motor vehicles **in nontraffic accident**

√x7th **V59.09 Driver of pick-up truck or van injured in collision** with other motor vehicles **in nontraffic accident**

√5th **V59.1** Passenger **in pick-up truck or van injured in collision with other and unspecified motor vehicles** in nontraffic accident

√x7th **V59.10 Passenger in pick-up truck or van injured in collision** with unspecified motor vehicles **in nontraffic accident**

√x7th **V59.19 Passenger in pick-up truck or van injured in collision** with other motor vehicles **in nontraffic accident**

√5th **V59.2** Unspecified **occupant of pick-up truck or van injured in collision with other and unspecified motor vehicles** in nontraffic accident

√x7th **V59.20 Unspecified occupant of pick-up truck or van injured in collision** with unspecified motor vehicles **in nontraffic accident**

Collision NOS involving pick-up truck or van, nontraffic

√x7th **V59.29 Unspecified occupant of pick-up truck or van injured in collision** with other motor vehicles **in nontraffic accident**

√x7th **V59.3 Occupant (driver) (passenger) of pick-up truck or van injured in unspecified nontraffic accident**
Accident NOS involving pick-up truck or van, nontraffic
Occupant of pick-up truck or van injured in nontraffic accident NOS

√5th **V59.4 Driver of pick-up truck or van injured in collision with other and unspecified motor vehicles in traffic accident**

√x7th **V59.4Ø Driver of pick-up truck or van injured in collision with unspecified motor vehicles in traffic accident**

√x7th **V59.49 Driver of pick-up truck or van injured in collision with other motor vehicles in traffic accident**

√5th **V59.5 Passenger in pick-up truck or van injured in collision with other and unspecified motor vehicles in traffic accident**

√x7th **V59.5Ø Passenger in pick-up truck or van injured in collision with unspecified motor vehicles in traffic accident**

√x7th **V59.59 Passenger in pick-up truck or van injured in collision with other motor vehicles in traffic accident**

√5th **V59.6 Unspecified occupant of pick-up truck or van injured in collision with other and unspecified motor vehicles in traffic accident**

√x7th **V59.6Ø Unspecified occupant of pick-up truck or van injured in collision with unspecified motor vehicles in traffic accident**
Collision NOS involving pick-up truck or van (traffic)

√x7th **V59.69 Unspecified occupant of pick-up truck or van injured in collision with other motor vehicles in traffic accident**

√5th **V59.8 Occupant (driver) (passenger) of pick-up truck or van injured in other specified transport accidents**

√x7th **V59.81 Occupant (driver) (passenger) of pick-up truck or van injured in transport accident with military vehicle**

√x7th **V59.88 Occupant (driver) (passenger) of pick-up truck or van injured in other specified transport accidents**

√x7th **V59.9 Occupant (driver) (passenger) of pick-up truck or van injured in unspecified traffic accident**
Accident NOS involving pick-up truck or van

Occupant of heavy transport vehicle injured in transport accident (V6Ø-V69)

INCLUDES 18 wheeler
armored car
panel truck

EXCLUDES 1 *bus*
motorcoach

√4th **V6Ø Occupant of heavy transport vehicle injured in collision with pedestrian or animal**

EXCLUDES 1 *heavy transport vehicle collision with animal-drawn vehicle or animal being ridden (V66.-)*

The appropriate 7th character is to be added to each code from category V6Ø.
A initial encounter
D subsequent encounter
S sequela

√x7th **V6Ø.Ø Driver of heavy transport vehicle injured in collision with pedestrian or animal in nontraffic accident**

√x7th **V6Ø.1 Passenger in heavy transport vehicle injured in collision with pedestrian or animal in nontraffic accident**

√x7th **V6Ø.2 Person on outside of heavy transport vehicle injured in collision with pedestrian or animal in nontraffic accident**

√x7th **V6Ø.3 Unspecified occupant of heavy transport vehicle injured in collision with pedestrian or animal in nontraffic accident**

√x7th **V6Ø.4 Person boarding or alighting a heavy transport vehicle injured in collision with pedestrian or animal**

√x7th **V6Ø.5 Driver of heavy transport vehicle injured in collision with pedestrian or animal in traffic accident**

√x7th **V6Ø.6 Passenger in heavy transport vehicle injured in collision with pedestrian or animal in traffic accident**

√x7th **V6Ø.7 Person on outside of heavy transport vehicle injured in collision with pedestrian or animal in traffic accident**

√x7th **V6Ø.9 Unspecified occupant of heavy transport vehicle injured in collision with pedestrian or animal in traffic accident**

√4th **V61 Occupant of heavy transport vehicle injured in collision with pedal cycle**

The appropriate 7th character is to be added to each code from category V61.
A initial encounter
D subsequent encounter
S sequela

√x7th **V61.Ø Driver of heavy transport vehicle injured in collision with pedal cycle in nontraffic accident**

√x7th **V61.1 Passenger in heavy transport vehicle injured in collision with pedal cycle in nontraffic accident**

√x7th **V61.2 Person on outside of heavy transport vehicle injured in collision with pedal cycle in nontraffic accident**

√x7th **V61.3 Unspecified occupant of heavy transport vehicle injured in collision with pedal cycle in nontraffic accident**

√x7th **V61.4 Person boarding or alighting a heavy transport vehicle injured in collision with pedal cycle while boarding or alighting**

√x7th **V61.5 Driver of heavy transport vehicle injured in collision with pedal cycle in traffic accident**

√x7th **V61.6 Passenger in heavy transport vehicle injured in collision with pedal cycle in traffic accident**

√x7th **V61.7 Person on outside of heavy transport vehicle injured in collision with pedal cycle in traffic accident**

√x7th **V61.9 Unspecified occupant of heavy transport vehicle injured in collision with pedal cycle in traffic accident**

√4th **V62 Occupant of heavy transport vehicle injured in collision with two- or three-wheeled motor vehicle**

The appropriate 7th character is to be added to each code from category V62.
A initial encounter
D subsequent encounter
S sequela

√x7th **V62.Ø Driver of heavy transport vehicle injured in collision with two- or three-wheeled motor vehicle in nontraffic accident**

√x7th **V62.1 Passenger in heavy transport vehicle injured in collision with two- or three-wheeled motor vehicle in nontraffic accident**

√x7th **V62.2 Person on outside of heavy transport vehicle injured in collision with two- or three-wheeled motor vehicle in nontraffic accident**

√x7th **V62.3 Unspecified occupant of heavy transport vehicle injured in collision with two- or three-wheeled motor vehicle in nontraffic accident**

√x7th **V62.4 Person boarding or alighting a heavy transport vehicle injured in collision with two- or three-wheeled motor vehicle**

√x7th **V62.5 Driver of heavy transport vehicle injured in collision with two- or three-wheeled motor vehicle in traffic accident**

√x7th **V62.6 Passenger in heavy transport vehicle injured in collision with two- or three-wheeled motor vehicle in traffic accident**

√x7th **V62.7 Person on outside of heavy transport vehicle injured in collision with two- or three-wheeled motor vehicle in traffic accident**

√x7th **V62.9 Unspecified occupant of heavy transport vehicle injured in collision with two- or three-wheeled motor vehicle in traffic accident**

√4th **V63 Occupant of heavy transport vehicle injured in collision with car, pick-up truck or van**

The appropriate 7th character is to be added to each code from category V63.
A initial encounter
D subsequent encounter
S sequela

√x7th **V63.Ø Driver of heavy transport vehicle injured in collision with car, pick-up truck or van in nontraffic accident**

√x7th **V63.1 Passenger in heavy transport vehicle injured in collision with car, pick-up truck or van in nontraffic accident**

√x7th **V63.2 Person on outside of heavy transport vehicle injured in collision with car, pick-up truck or van in nontraffic accident**

√x7th **V63.3 Unspecified occupant of heavy transport vehicle injured in collision with car, pick-up truck or van in nontraffic accident**

√x7th **V63.4 Person boarding or alighting a heavy transport vehicle injured in collision with car, pick-up truck or van**

√x7th **V63.5 Driver of heavy transport vehicle injured in collision with car, pick-up truck or van in traffic accident**

√x7th **V63.6** Passenger **in heavy transport vehicle injured in collision with car, pick-up truck or van** in traffic accident

√x7th **V63.7** Person on outside **of heavy transport vehicle injured in collision with car, pick-up truck or van** in traffic accident

√x7th **V63.9** Unspecified **occupant of heavy transport vehicle injured in collision with car, pick-up truck or van** in traffic accident

√4th **V64 Occupant of heavy transport vehicle injured in collision with heavy transport vehicle or bus**

EXCLUDES 1 *occupant of heavy transport vehicle injured in collision with military vehicle (V69.81)*

The appropriate 7th character is to be added to each code from category V64.
A initial encounter
D subsequent encounter
S sequela

√x7th **V64.0** Driver **of heavy transport vehicle injured in collision with heavy transport vehicle or bus** in nontraffic accident

√x7th **V64.1** Passenger **in heavy transport vehicle injured in collision with heavy transport vehicle or bus** in nontraffic accident

√x7th **V64.2** Person on outside **of heavy transport vehicle injured in collision with heavy transport vehicle or bus** in nontraffic accident

√x7th **V64.3** Unspecified **occupant of heavy transport vehicle injured in collision with heavy transport vehicle or bus** in nontraffic accident

√x7th **V64.4** Person boarding or alighting **a heavy transport vehicle injured in collision with heavy transport vehicle or bus while boarding or alighting**

√x7th **V64.5** Driver **of heavy transport vehicle injured in collision with heavy transport vehicle or bus** in traffic accident

√x7th **V64.6** Passenger **in heavy transport vehicle injured in collision with heavy transport vehicle or bus** in traffic accident

√x7th **V64.7** Person on outside **of heavy transport vehicle injured in collision with heavy transport vehicle or bus** in traffic accident

√x7th **V64.9** Unspecified **occupant of heavy transport vehicle injured in collision with heavy transport vehicle or bus** in traffic accident

√4th **V65 Occupant of heavy transport vehicle injured in collision with railway train or railway vehicle**

The appropriate 7th character is to be added to each code from category V65.
A initial encounter
D subsequent encounter
S sequela

√x7th **V65.0** Driver **of heavy transport vehicle injured in collision with railway train or railway vehicle** in nontraffic accident

√x7th **V65.1** Passenger **in heavy transport vehicle injured in collision with railway train or railway vehicle** in nontraffic accident

√x7th **V65.2** Person on outside **of heavy transport vehicle injured in collision with railway train or railway vehicle** in nontraffic accident

√x7th **V65.3** Unspecified **occupant of heavy transport vehicle injured in collision with railway train or railway vehicle** in nontraffic accident

√x7th **V65.4** Person boarding or alighting **a heavy transport vehicle injured in collision with railway train or railway vehicle**

√x7th **V65.5** Driver **of heavy transport vehicle injured in collision with railway train or railway vehicle** in traffic accident

√x7th **V65.6** Passenger **in heavy transport vehicle injured in collision with railway train or railway vehicle** in traffic accident

√x7th **V65.7** Person on outside **of heavy transport vehicle injured in collision with railway train or railway vehicle** in traffic accident

√x7th **V65.9** Unspecified **occupant of heavy transport vehicle injured in collision with railway train or railway vehicle** in traffic accident

√4th **V66 Occupant of heavy transport vehicle injured in collision with other nonmotor vehicle**

INCLUDES collision with animal-drawn vehicle, animal being ridden, streetcar

The appropriate 7th character is to be added to each code from category V66.
A initial encounter
D subsequent encounter
S sequela

√x7th **V66.0** Driver **of heavy transport vehicle injured in collision with other nonmotor vehicle** in nontraffic accident

√x7th **V66.1** Passenger **in heavy transport vehicle injured in collision with other nonmotor vehicle** in nontraffic accident

√x7th **V66.2** Person on outside **of heavy transport vehicle injured in collision with other nonmotor vehicle** in nontraffic accident

√x7th **V66.3** Unspecified **occupant of heavy transport vehicle injured in collision with other nonmotor vehicle** in nontraffic accident

√x7th **V66.4** Person boarding or alighting **a heavy transport vehicle injured in collision with other nonmotor vehicle**

√x7th **V66.5** Driver **of heavy transport vehicle injured in collision with other nonmotor vehicle** in traffic accident

√x7th **V66.6** Passenger **in heavy transport vehicle injured in collision with other nonmotor vehicle** in traffic accident

√x7th **V66.7** Person on outside **of heavy transport vehicle injured in collision with other nonmotor vehicle** in traffic accident

√x7th **V66.9** Unspecified **occupant of heavy transport vehicle injured in collision with other nonmotor vehicle** in traffic accident

√4th **V67 Occupant of heavy transport vehicle injured in collision with fixed or stationary object**

The appropriate 7th character is to be added to each code from category V67.
A initial encounter
D subsequent encounter
S sequela

√x7th **V67.0** Driver **of heavy transport vehicle injured in collision with fixed or stationary object** in nontraffic accident

√x7th **V67.1** Passenger **in heavy transport vehicle injured in collision with fixed or stationary object** in nontraffic accident

√x7th **V67.2** Person on outside **of heavy transport vehicle injured in collision with fixed or stationary object** in nontraffic accident

√x7th **V67.3** Unspecified **occupant of heavy transport vehicle injured in collision with fixed or stationary object** in nontraffic accident

√x7th **V67.4** Person boarding or alighting **a heavy transport vehicle injured in collision with fixed or stationary object**

√x7th **V67.5** Driver **of heavy transport vehicle injured in collision with fixed or stationary object** in traffic accident

√x7th **V67.6** Passenger **in heavy transport vehicle injured in collision with fixed or stationary object** in traffic accident

√x7th **V67.7** Person on outside **of heavy transport vehicle injured in collision with fixed or stationary object** in traffic accident

√x7th **V67.9** Unspecified **occupant of heavy transport vehicle injured in collision with fixed or stationary object** in traffic accident

√4th **V68 Occupant of heavy transport vehicle injured in noncollision transport accident**

INCLUDES overturning heavy transport vehicle NOS
overturning heavy transport vehicle without collision

The appropriate 7th character is to be added to each code from category V68.
A initial encounter
D subsequent encounter
S sequela

√x7th **V68.0** Driver **of heavy transport vehicle injured in noncollision transport accident** in nontraffic accident

√x7th **V68.1** Passenger **in heavy transport vehicle injured in noncollision transport accident** in nontraffic accident

√x7th **V68.2** Person on outside **of heavy transport vehicle injured in noncollision transport accident** in nontraffic accident

√x7th **V68.3** Unspecified **occupant of heavy transport vehicle injured in noncollision transport accident** in nontraffic accident

√x7th **V68.4** Person boarding or alighting **a heavy transport vehicle injured in noncollision transport accident**

√x7th **V68.5** Driver **of heavy transport vehicle injured in noncollision transport accident** in traffic accident

✓x7th **V68.6** Passenger **in heavy transport vehicle injured in noncollision transport accident** in traffic accident

✓x7th **V68.7** Person on outside **of heavy transport vehicle injured in noncollision transport accident** in traffic accident

✓x7th **V68.9** Unspecified **occupant of heavy transport vehicle injured in noncollision transport accident** in traffic accident

✓4th **V69 Occupant of heavy transport vehicle injured in other and unspecified transport accidents**

The appropriate 7th character is to be added to each code from category V69.
A initial encounter
D subsequent encounter
S sequela

✓5th **V69.0** Driver **of heavy transport vehicle injured in collision with other and unspecified motor vehicles** in nontraffic accident

✓x7th **V69.00 Driver of heavy transport vehicle injured in collision** with unspecified motor vehicles **in nontraffic accident**

✓x7th **V69.09 Driver of heavy transport vehicle injured in collision** with other motor vehicles **in nontraffic accident**

✓5th **V69.1** Passenger **in heavy transport vehicle injured in collision with other and unspecified motor vehicles** in nontraffic accident

✓x7th **V69.10 Passenger in heavy transport vehicle injured in collision** with unspecified motor vehicles **in nontraffic accident**

✓x7th **V69.19 Passenger in heavy transport vehicle injured in collision** with other motor vehicles **in nontraffic accident**

✓5th **V69.2** Unspecified **occupant of heavy transport vehicle injured in collision with other and unspecified motor vehicles** in nontraffic accident

✓x7th **V69.20 Unspecified occupant of heavy transport vehicle injured in collision** with unspecified motor vehicles **in nontraffic accident**
Collision NOS involving heavy transport vehicle, nontraffic

✓x7th **V69.29 Unspecified occupant of heavy transport vehicle injured in collision** with other motor vehicles **in nontraffic accident**

✓x7th **V69.3** Occupant **(driver) (passenger) of heavy transport vehicle injured in** unspecified nontraffic accident
Accident NOS involving heavy transport vehicle, nontraffic
Occupant of heavy transport vehicle injured in nontraffic accident NOS

✓5th **V69.4** Driver **of heavy transport vehicle injured in collision with other and unspecified motor vehicles** in traffic accident

✓x7th **V69.40 Driver of heavy transport vehicle injured in collision** with unspecified motor vehicles **in traffic accident**

✓x7th **V69.49 Driver of heavy transport vehicle injured in collision** with other motor vehicles **in traffic accident**

✓5th **V69.5** Passenger **in heavy transport vehicle injured in collision with other and unspecified motor vehicles** in traffic accident

✓x7th **V69.50 Passenger in heavy transport vehicle injured in collision** with unspecified motor vehicles **in traffic accident**

✓x7th **V69.59 Passenger in heavy transport vehicle injured in collision** with other motor vehicles **in traffic accident**

✓5th **V69.6** Unspecified **occupant of heavy transport vehicle injured in collision with other and unspecified motor vehicles** in traffic accident

✓x7th **V69.60 Unspecified occupant of heavy transport vehicle injured in collision** with unspecified motor vehicles **in traffic accident**
Collision NOS involving heavy transport vehicle (traffic)

✓x7th **V69.69 Unspecified occupant of heavy transport vehicle injured in collision** with other motor vehicles **in traffic accident**

✓5th **V69.8** Occupant **(driver) (passenger) of heavy transport vehicle injured in other specified transport accidents**

✓x7th **V69.81 Occupant (driver) (passenger) of heavy transport vehicle injured in transport accidents** with military vehicle

✓x7th **V69.88 Occupant (driver) (passenger) of heavy transport vehicle injured** in other specified transport accidents

✓x7th **V69.9** Occupant **(driver) (passenger) of heavy transport vehicle injured in** unspecified traffic accident
Accident NOS involving heavy transport vehicle

Bus occupant injured in transport accident (V70-V79)

INCLUDES motorcoach
EXCLUDES 1 *minibus (V50-V59)*

✓4th **V70 Bus occupant injured in collision with pedestrian or animal**
EXCLUDES 1 *bus collision with animal-drawn vehicle or animal being ridden (V76.-)*

The appropriate 7th character is to be added to each code from category V70.
A initial encounter
D subsequent encounter
S sequela

✓x7th **V70.0** Driver **of bus injured in collision with pedestrian or animal** in nontraffic accident

✓x7th **V70.1** Passenger **on bus injured in collision with pedestrian or animal** in nontraffic accident

✓x7th **V70.2** Person on outside **of bus injured in collision with pedestrian or animal** in nontraffic accident

✓x7th **V70.3** Unspecified **occupant of bus injured in collision with pedestrian or animal** in nontraffic accident

✓x7th **V70.4** Person boarding or alighting **from bus injured in collision with pedestrian or animal**

✓x7th **V70.5** Driver **of bus injured in collision with pedestrian or animal** in traffic accident

✓x7th **V70.6** Passenger **on bus injured in collision with pedestrian or animal** in traffic accident

✓x7th **V70.7** Person on outside **of bus injured in collision with pedestrian or animal** in traffic accident

✓x7th **V70.9** Unspecified **occupant of bus injured in collision with pedestrian or animal** in traffic accident

✓4th **V71 Bus occupant injured in collision with pedal cycle**

The appropriate 7th character is to be added to each code from category V71.
A initial encounter
D subsequent encounter
S sequela

✓x7th **V71.0** Driver **of bus injured in collision with pedal cycle** in nontraffic accident

✓x7th **V71.1** Passenger **on bus injured in collision with pedal cycle** in nontraffic accident

✓x7th **V71.2** Person on outside **of bus injured in collision with pedal cycle** in nontraffic accident

✓x7th **V71.3** Unspecified **occupant of bus injured in collision with pedal cycle** in nontraffic accident

✓x7th **V71.4** Person boarding or alighting **from bus injured in collision with pedal cycle**

✓x7th **V71.5** Driver **of bus injured in collision with pedal cycle** in traffic accident

✓x7th **V71.6** Passenger **on bus injured in collision with pedal cycle** in traffic accident

✓x7th **V71.7** Person on outside **of bus injured in collision with pedal cycle** in traffic accident

✓x7th **V71.9** Unspecified **occupant of bus injured in collision with pedal cycle** in traffic accident

✓4th **V72 Bus occupant injured in collision with two- or three-wheeled motor vehicle**

The appropriate 7th character is to be added to each code from category V72.
A initial encounter
D subsequent encounter
S sequela

✓x7th **V72.0** Driver **of bus injured in collision with two- or three-wheeled motor vehicle** in nontraffic accident

✓x7th **V72.1** Passenger **on bus injured in collision with two- or three-wheeled motor vehicle** in nontraffic accident

✓x7th **V72.2** Person on outside **of bus injured in collision with two- or three-wheeled motor vehicle** in nontraffic accident

✓x7th **V72.3** Unspecified **occupant of bus injured in collision with two- or three-wheeled motor vehicle** in nontraffic accident

✓x7th **V72.4** Person boarding or alighting **from bus injured in collision with two- or three-wheeled motor vehicle**

✓x7th **V72.5** Driver **of bus injured in collision with two- or three-wheeled motor vehicle** in traffic accident

√x7th **V72.6** Passenger **on bus injured in collision with two- or three-wheeled motor vehicle** in traffic accident

√x7th **V72.7** Person on outside **of bus injured in collision with two- or three-wheeled motor vehicle** in traffic accident

√x7th **V72.9** Unspecified **occupant of bus injured in collision with two- or three-wheeled motor vehicle** in traffic accident

√4th **V73 Bus occupant injured in collision with car, pick-up truck or van**

The appropriate 7th character is to be added to each code from category V73.
A initial encounter
D subsequent encounter
S sequela

√x7th **V73.0** Driver **of bus injured in collision with car, pick-up truck or van** in nontraffic accident

√x7th **V73.1** Passenger **on bus injured in collision with car, pick-up truck or van** in nontraffic accident

√x7th **V73.2** Person on outside **of bus injured in collision with car, pick-up truck or van** in nontraffic accident

√x7th **V73.3** Unspecified **occupant of bus injured in collision with car, pick-up truck or van** in nontraffic accident

√x7th **V73.4** Person boarding or alighting **from bus injured in collision with car, pick-up truck or van**

√x7th **V73.5** Driver **of bus injured in collision with car, pick-up truck or van** in traffic accident

√x7th **V73.6** Passenger **on bus injured in collision with car, pick-up truck or van** in traffic accident

√x7th **V73.7** Person on outside **of bus injured in collision with car, pick-up truck or van** in traffic accident

√x7th **V73.9** Unspecified **occupant of bus injured in collision with car, pick-up truck or van** in traffic accident

√4th **V74 Bus occupant injured in collision with heavy transport vehicle or bus**

EXCLUDES 1 *bus occupant injured in collision with military vehicle (V79.81)*

The appropriate 7th character is to be added to each code from category V74.
A initial encounter
D subsequent encounter
S sequela

√x7th **V74.0** Driver **of bus injured in collision with heavy transport vehicle or bus** in nontraffic accident

√x7th **V74.1** Passenger **on bus injured in collision with heavy transport vehicle or bus** in nontraffic accident

√x7th **V74.2** Person on outside **of bus injured in collision with heavy transport vehicle or bus** in nontraffic accident

√x7th **V74.3** Unspecified **occupant of bus injured in collision with heavy transport vehicle or bus** in nontraffic accident

√x7th **V74.4** Person boarding or alighting **from bus injured in collision with heavy transport vehicle or bus**

√x7th **V74.5** Driver **of bus injured in collision with heavy transport vehicle or bus** in traffic accident

√x7th **V74.6** Passenger **on bus injured in collision with heavy transport vehicle or bus** in traffic accident

√x7th **V74.7** Person on outside **of bus injured in collision with heavy transport vehicle or bus** in traffic accident

√x7th **V74.9** Unspecified **occupant of bus injured in collision with heavy transport vehicle or bus** in traffic accident

√4th **V75 Bus occupant injured in collision with railway train or railway vehicle**

The appropriate 7th character is to be added to each code from category V75.
A initial encounter
D subsequent encounter
S sequela

√x7th **V75.0** Driver **of bus injured in collision with railway train or railway vehicle** in nontraffic accident

√x7th **V75.1** Passenger **on bus injured in collision with railway train or railway vehicle** in nontraffic accident

√x7th **V75.2** Person on outside **of bus injured in collision with railway train or railway vehicle** in nontraffic accident

√x7th **V75.3** Unspecified **occupant of bus injured in collision with railway train or railway vehicle** in nontraffic accident

√x7th **V75.4** Person boarding or alighting **from bus injured in collision with railway train or railway vehicle**

√x7th **V75.5** Driver **of bus injured in collision with railway train or railway vehicle** in traffic accident

√x7th **V75.6** Passenger **on bus injured in collision with railway train or railway vehicle** in traffic accident

√x7th **V75.7** Person **on outside of bus injured in collision with railway train or railway vehicle** in traffic accident

√x7th **V75.9** Unspecified **occupant of bus injured in collision with railway train or railway vehicle** in traffic accident

√4th **V76 Bus occupant injured in collision with other nonmotor vehicle**

INCLUDES collision with animal-drawn vehicle, animal being ridden, streetcar

The appropriate 7th character is to be added to each code from category V76.
A initial encounter
D subsequent encounter
S sequela

√x7th **V76.0** Driver **of bus injured in collision with other nonmotor vehicle** in nontraffic accident

√x7th **V76.1** Passenger **on bus injured in collision with other nonmotor vehicle** in nontraffic accident

√x7th **V76.2** Person on outside **of bus injured in collision with other nonmotor vehicle** in nontraffic accident

√x7th **V76.3** Unspecified **occupant of bus injured in collision with other nonmotor vehicle** in nontraffic accident

√x7th **V76.4** Person boarding or alighting **from bus injured in collision with other nonmotor vehicle**

√x7th **V76.5** Driver **of bus injured in collision with other nonmotor vehicle** in traffic accident

√x7th **V76.6** Passenger **on bus injured in collision with other nonmotor vehicle** in traffic accident

√x7th **V76.7** Person on outside **of bus injured in collision with other nonmotor vehicle** in traffic accident

√x7th **V76.9** Unspecified **occupant of bus injured in collision with other nonmotor vehicle** in traffic accident

√4th **V77 Bus occupant injured in collision with fixed or stationary object**

The appropriate 7th character is to be added to each code from category V77.
A initial encounter
D subsequent encounter
S sequela

√x7th **V77.0** Driver **of bus injured in collision with fixed or stationary object** in nontraffic accident

√x7th **V77.1** Passenger **on bus injured in collision with fixed or stationary object** in nontraffic accident

√x7th **V77.2** Person on outside **of bus injured in collision with fixed or stationary object** in nontraffic accident

√x7th **V77.3** Unspecified **occupant of bus injured in collision with fixed or stationary object** in nontraffic accident

√x7th **V77.4** Person boarding or alighting **from bus injured in collision with fixed or stationary object**

√x7th **V77.5** Driver **of bus injured in collision with fixed or stationary object** in traffic accident

√x7th **V77.6** Passenger **on bus injured in collision with fixed or stationary object** in traffic accident

√x7th **V77.7** Person on outside **of bus injured in collision with fixed or stationary object** in traffic accident

√x7th **V77.9** Unspecified **occupant of bus injured in collision with fixed or stationary object** in traffic accident

√4th **V78 Bus occupant injured in noncollision transport accident**

INCLUDES overturning bus NOS
overturning bus without collision

The appropriate 7th character is to be added to each code from category V78.
A initial encounter
D subsequent encounter
S sequela

√x7th **V78.0** Driver **of bus injured in noncollision transport accident** in nontraffic accident

√x7th **V78.1** Passenger **on bus injured in noncollision transport accident** in nontraffic accident

√x7th **V78.2** Person on outside **of bus injured in noncollision transport accident** in nontraffic accident

DRAFT

√x7th **V78.3** Unspecified **occupant of bus injured in noncollision transport accident** in nontraffic accident

√x7th **V78.4** Person boarding or alighting **from bus injured in noncollision transport accident**

√x7th **V78.5** Driver **of bus injured in noncollision transport accident** in traffic accident

√x7th **V78.6** Passenger **on bus injured in noncollision transport accident** in traffic accident

√x7th **V78.7** Person on outside **of bus injured in noncollision transport accident** in traffic accident

√x7th **V78.9** Unspecified **occupant of bus injured in noncollision transport accident** in traffic accident

√4th **V79 Bus occupant injured in other and unspecified transport accidents**

The appropriate 7th character is to be added to each code from category V79.
A initial encounter
D subsequent encounter
S sequela

√5th **V79.0** Driver **of bus injured in collision with other and unspecified motor vehicles** in nontraffic accident

√x7th **V79.00 Driver of bus injured in collision** with unspecified motor vehicles **in nontraffic accident**

√x7th **V79.09 Driver of bus injured in collision** with other motor vehicles **in nontraffic accident**

√5th **V79.1** Passenger **on bus injured in collision with other and unspecified motor vehicles** in nontraffic accident

√x7th **V79.10 Passenger on bus injured in collision** with unspecified motor vehicles **in nontraffic accident**

√x7th **V79.19 Passenger on bus injured in collision** with other motor vehicles **in nontraffic accident**

√5th **V79.2** Unspecified **bus** occupant **injured in collision with other and unspecified motor vehicles** in nontraffic accident

√x7th **V79.20 Unspecified bus occupant injured in collision** with unspecified motor vehicles **in nontraffic accident**
Bus collision NOS, nontraffic

√x7th **V79.29 Unspecified bus occupant injured in collision** with other motor vehicles **in nontraffic accident**

√x7th **V79.3 Bus** occupant **(driver) (passenger) injured in** unspecified nontraffic accident
Bus accident NOS, nontraffic
Bus occupant injured in nontraffic accident NOS

√5th **V79.4** Driver **of bus injured in collision with other and unspecified motor vehicles** in traffic accident

√x7th **V79.40 Driver of bus injured in collision with** unspecified **motor vehicles in traffic accident**

√x7th **V79.49 Driver of bus injured in collision with** other **motor vehicles in traffic accident**

√5th **V79.5** Passenger **on bus injured in collision with other and unspecified motor vehicles** in traffic accident

√x7th **V79.50 Passenger on bus injured in collision with** unspecified **motor vehicles in traffic accident**

√x7th **V79.59 Passenger on bus injured in collision with** other **motor vehicles in traffic accident**

√5th **V79.6** Unspecified **bus occupant injured in collision with other and unspecified motor vehicles** in traffic accident

√x7th **V79.60 Unspecified bus occupant injured in collision with** unspecified **motor vehicles in traffic accident**
Bus collision NOS (traffic)

√x7th **V79.69 Unspecified bus occupant injured in collision with** other **motor vehicles in traffic accident**

√5th **V79.8 Bus** occupant **(driver) (passenger) injured in** other **specified transport accidents**

√x7th **V79.81 Bus occupant (driver) (passenger) injured in transport accidents** with military vehicle

√x7th **V79.88 Bus occupant (driver) (passenger) injured** in other specified transport accidents

√x7th **V79.9 Bus** occupant **(driver) (passenger) injured in** unspecified traffic accident
Bus accident NOS

Other land transport accidents (V80-V89)

√4th **V80 Animal-rider or occupant of animal-drawn vehicle injured in transport accident**

The appropriate 7th character is to be added to each code from category V80.
A initial encounter
D subsequent encounter
S sequela

√5th **V80.0 Animal-rider or occupant of animal drawn vehicle injured by fall from or being thrown from animal or animal-drawn vehicle in** noncollision accident

√6th **V80.01** Animal-rider **injured by fall from or being thrown from animal in noncollision accident**

√7th **V80.010 Animal-rider injured by fall from or being thrown from** horse **in noncollision accident**

√7th **V80.018 Animal-rider injured by fall from or being thrown from** other animal **in noncollision accident**

√x7th **V80.02** Occupant **of animal-drawn vehicle injured by fall from or being thrown from animal-drawn vehicle in noncollision accident**
Overturning animal-drawn vehicle NOS
Overturning animal-drawn vehicle without collision

√5th **V80.1 Animal-rider or occupant of animal-drawn vehicle injured in collision with** pedestrian or animal
EXCLUDES1 *animal-rider or animal-drawn vehicle collision with animal-drawn vehicle or animal being ridden (V80.7)*

√x7th **V80.11** Animal-rider **injured in collision with pedestrian or animal**

√x7th **V80.12** Occupant **of animal-drawn vehicle injured in collision with pedestrian or animal**

√5th **V80.2 Animal-rider or occupant of animal-drawn vehicle injured in collision with** pedal cycle

√x7th **V80.21** Animal-rider **injured in collision with pedal cycle**

√x7th **V80.22** Occupant **of animal-drawn vehicle injured in collision with pedal cycle**

√5th **V80.3 Animal-rider or occupant of animal-drawn vehicle injured in collision with** two- or three-wheeled motor vehicle

√x7th **V80.31** Animal-rider **injured in collision with two- or three-wheeled motor vehicle**

√x7th **V80.32** Occupant **of animal-drawn vehicle injured in collision with two- or three-wheeled motor vehicle**

√5th **V80.4 Animal-rider or occupant of animal-drawn vehicle injured in collision with** car, pick-up truck, van, heavy transport vehicle or bus
EXCLUDES1 *animal-rider injured in collision with military vehicle (V80.910)*
occupant of animal-drawn vehicle injured in collision with military vehicle (V80.920)

√x7th **V80.41** Animal-rider **injured in collision with car, pick-up truck, van, heavy transport vehicle or bus**

√x7th **V80.42** Occupant **of animal-drawn vehicle injured in collision with car, pick-up truck, van, heavy transport vehicle or bus**

√5th **V80.5 Animal-rider or occupant of animal-drawn vehicle injured in collision with** other **specified** motor vehicle

√x7th **V80.51** Animal-rider **injured in collision with other specified motor vehicle**

√x7th **V80.52** Occupant **of animal-drawn vehicle injured in collision with other specified motor vehicle**

√5th **V80.6 Animal-rider or occupant of animal-drawn vehicle injured in collision with** railway train or railway vehicle

√x7th **V80.61** Animal-rider **injured in collision with railway train or railway vehicle**

√x7th **V80.62** Occupant **of animal-drawn vehicle injured in collision with railway train or railway vehicle**

√5th **V80.7 Animal-rider or occupant of animal-drawn vehicle injured in collision with** other nonmotor vehicles

√6th **V80.71 Animal-rider or occupant of animal-drawn vehicle injured in collision with** animal being ridden

√7th **V80.710** Animal-rider **injured in collision with other animal being ridden**

√7th **V80.711** Occupant **of animal-drawn vehicle injured in collision with animal being ridden**

√6th **V80.72 Animal-rider or occupant of animal-drawn vehicle injured in collision with other animal-drawn vehicle**

√7th **V80.720 Animal-rider injured in collision with animal-drawn vehicle**

√7th **V80.721 Occupant of animal-drawn vehicle injured in collision with other animal-drawn vehicle**

√6th **V80.73 Animal-rider or occupant of animal-drawn vehicle injured in collision with streetcar**

√7th **V80.730 Animal-rider injured in collision with streetcar**

√7th **V80.731 Occupant of animal-drawn vehicle injured in collision with streetcar**

√6th **V80.79 Animal-rider or occupant of animal-drawn vehicle injured in collision with other nonmotor vehicles**

√7th **V80.790 Animal-rider injured in collision with other nonmotor vehicles**

√7th **V80.791 Occupant of animal-drawn vehicle injured in collision with other nonmotor vehicles**

√5th **V80.8 Animal-rider or occupant of animal-drawn vehicle injured in collision with fixed or stationary object**

√x7th **V80.81 Animal-rider injured in collision with fixed or stationary object**

√x7th **V80.82 Occupant of animal-drawn vehicle injured in collision with fixed or stationary object**

√5th **V80.9 Animal-rider or occupant of animal-drawn vehicle injured in other and unspecified transport accidents**

√6th **V80.91 Animal-rider injured in other and unspecified transport accidents**

√7th **V80.910 Animal-rider injured in transport accident with military vehicle**

√7th **V80.918 Animal-rider injured in other transport accident**

√7th **V80.919 Animal-rider injured in unspecified transport accident**
Animal rider accident NOS

√6th **V80.92 Occupant of animal-drawn vehicle injured in other and unspecified transport accidents**

√7th **V80.920 Occupant of animal-drawn vehicle injured in transport accident with military vehicle**

√7th **V80.928 Occupant of animal-drawn vehicle injured in other transport accident**

√7th **V80.929 Occupant of animal-drawn vehicle injured in unspecified transport accident**
Animal-drawn vehicle accident NOS

√4th **V81 Occupant of railway train or railway vehicle injured in transport accident**

INCLUDES derailment of railway train or railway vehicle
person on outside of train

EXCLUDES 1 *streetcar (V82.-)*

The appropriate 7th character is to be added to each code from category V81.
A initial encounter
D subsequent encounter
S sequela

√x7th **V81.0 Occupant of railway train or railway vehicle injured in collision with motor vehicle in nontraffic accident**

EXCLUDES 1 *occupant of railway train or railway vehicle injured due to collision with military vehicle (V81.83)*

√x7th **V81.1 Occupant of railway train or railway vehicle injured in collision with motor vehicle in traffic accident**

EXCLUDES 1 *occupant of railway train or railway vehicle injured due to collision with military vehicle (V81.83)*

√x7th **V81.2 Occupant of railway train or railway vehicle injured in collision with or hit by rolling stock**

√x7th **V81.3 Occupant of railway train or railway vehicle injured in collision with other object**
Railway collision NOS

√x7th **V81.4 Person injured while boarding or alighting from railway train or railway vehicle**

√x7th **V81.5 Occupant of railway train or railway vehicle injured by fall in railway train or railway vehicle**

√x7th **V81.6 Occupant of railway train or railway vehicle injured by fall from railway train or railway vehicle**

√x7th **V81.7 Occupant of railway train or railway vehicle injured in derailment without antecedent collision**

√5th **V81.8 Occupant of railway train or railway vehicle injured in other specified railway accidents**

√x7th **V81.81 Occupant of railway train or railway vehicle injured due to explosion or fire on train**

√x7th **V81.82 Occupant of railway train or railway vehicle injured due to object falling onto train**
Occupant of railway train or railway vehicle injured due to falling earth onto train
Occupant of railway train or railway vehicle injured due to falling rocks onto train
Occupant of railway train or railway vehicle injured due to falling snow onto train
Occupant of railway train or railway vehicle injured due to falling trees onto train

√x7th **V81.83 Occupant of railway train or railway vehicle injured due to collision with military vehicle**

√x7th **V81.89 Occupant of railway train or railway vehicle injured due to other specified railway accident**

√x7th **V81.9 Occupant of railway train or railway vehicle injured in unspecified railway accident**
Railway accident NOS

√4th **V82 Occupant of powered streetcar injured in transport accident**

INCLUDES interurban electric car
person on outside of streetcar
tram (car)
trolley (car)

EXCLUDES 1 *bus (V70-V79)*
motorcoach (V70-V79)
nonpowered streetcar (V76.-)
train (V81.-)

The appropriate 7th character is to be added to each code from category V82.
A initial encounter
D subsequent encounter
S sequela

√x7th **V82.0 Occupant of streetcar injured in collision with motor vehicle in nontraffic accident**

√x7th **V82.1 Occupant of streetcar injured in collision with motor vehicle in traffic accident**

√x7th **V82.2 Occupant of streetcar injured in collision with or hit by rolling stock**

√x7th **V82.3 Occupant of streetcar injured in collision with other object**

EXCLUDES 1 *collision with animal-drawn vehicle or animal being ridden (V82.8)*

√x7th **V82.4 Person injured while boarding or alighting from streetcar**

√x7th **V82.5 Occupant of streetcar injured by fall in streetcar**

EXCLUDES 1 *fall in streetcar:*
while boarding or alighting (V82.4)
with antecedent collision (V82.0-V82.3)

√x7th **V82.6 Occupant of streetcar injured by fall from streetcar**

EXCLUDES 1 *fall from streetcar:*
while boarding or alighting (V82.4)
with antecedent collision (V82.0-V82.3)

√x7th **V82.7 Occupant of streetcar injured in derailment without antecedent collision**

EXCLUDES 1 *occupant of streetcar injured in derailment with antecedent collision (V82.0-V82.3)*

√x7th **V82.8 Occupant of streetcar injured in other specified transport accidents**
Streetcar collision with military vehicle
Streetcar collision with train or nonmotor vehicles

√x7th **V82.9 Occupant of streetcar injured in unspecified traffic accident**
Streetcar accident NOS

V83 Occupant of special vehicle mainly used on industrial premises injured in transport accident

INCLUDES battery-powered airport passenger vehicle
battery-powered truck (baggage) (mail)
coal-car in mine
forklift (truck)
logging car
self-propelled industrial truck
station baggage truck (powered)
tram, truck, or tub (powered) in mine or quarry

EXCLUDES 1 *special construction vehicles (V85.-)*
special industrial vehicle in stationary use or maintenance (W31.-)

The appropriate 7th character is to be added to each code from category V83.
A initial encounter
D subsequent encounter
S sequela

V83.0 Driver of special industrial vehicle injured in traffic accident
V83.1 Passenger of special industrial vehicle injured in traffic accident
V83.2 Person on outside of special industrial vehicle injured in traffic accident
V83.3 Unspecified occupant of special industrial vehicle injured in traffic accident
V83.4 Person injured while boarding or alighting from special industrial vehicle
V83.5 Driver of special industrial vehicle injured in nontraffic accident
V83.6 Passenger of special industrial vehicle injured in nontraffic accident
V83.7 Person on outside of special industrial vehicle injured in nontraffic accident
V83.9 Unspecified occupant of special industrial vehicle injured in nontraffic accident
Special-industrial-vehicle accident NOS

V84 Occupant of special vehicle mainly used in agriculture injured in transport accident

INCLUDES self-propelled farm machinery
tractor (and trailer)

EXCLUDES 1 *animal-powered farm machinery accident (W30.8-)*
contact with combine harvester (W30.0)
special agricultural vehicle in stationary use or maintenance (W30.-)

The appropriate 7th character is to be added to each code from category V84.
A initial encounter
D subsequent encounter
S sequela

V84.0 Driver of special agricultural vehicle injured in traffic accident
V84.1 Passenger of special agricultural vehicle injured in traffic accident
V84.2 Person on outside of special agricultural vehicle injured in traffic accident
V84.3 Unspecified occupant of special agricultural vehicle injured in traffic accident
V84.4 Person injured while boarding or alighting from special agricultural vehicle
V84.5 Driver of special agricultural vehicle injured in nontraffic accident
V84.6 Passenger of special agricultural vehicle injured in nontraffic accident
V84.7 Person on outside of special agricultural vehicle injured in nontraffic accident
V84.9 Unspecified occupant of special agricultural vehicle injured in nontraffic accident
Special-agricultural vehicle accident NOS

V85 Occupant of special construction vehicle injured in transport accident

INCLUDES bulldozer
digger
dump truck
earth-leveller
mechanical shovel
road-roller

EXCLUDES 1 *special industrial vehicle (V83.-)*
special construction vehicle in stationary use or maintenance (W31.-)

The appropriate 7th character is to be added to each code from category V85.
A initial encounter
D subsequent encounter
S sequela

V85.0 Driver of special construction vehicle injured in traffic accident
V85.1 Passenger of special construction vehicle injured in traffic accident
V85.2 Person on outside of special construction vehicle injured in traffic accident
V85.3 Unspecified occupant of special construction vehicle injured in traffic accident
V85.4 Person injured while boarding or alighting from special construction vehicle
V85.5 Driver of special construction vehicle injured in nontraffic accident
V85.6 Passenger of special construction vehicle injured in nontraffic accident
V85.7 Person on outside of special construction vehicle injured in nontraffic accident
V85.9 Unspecified occupant of special construction vehicle injured in nontraffic accident
Special-construction-vehicle accident NOS

V86 Occupant of special all-terrain or other off-road motor vehicle, injured in transport accident

EXCLUDES 1 *special all-terrain vehicle in stationary use or maintenance (W31.-)*
sport-utility vehicle (V50-V59)
three-wheeled motor vehicle designed for on-road use (V30-V39)

The appropriate 7th character is to be added to each code from category V86.
A initial encounter
D subsequent encounter
S sequela

V86.0 Driver of special all-terrain or other off-road motor vehicle injured in traffic accident
V86.01 Driver of ambulance or fire engine injured in traffic accident
V86.02 Driver of snowmobile injured in traffic accident
V86.03 Driver of dune buggy injured in traffic accident
V86.04 Driver of military vehicle injured in traffic accident
V86.09 Driver of other special all-terrain or other off-road motor vehicle injured in traffic accident
Driver of dirt bike injured in traffic accident
Driver of go cart injured in traffic accident
Driver of golf cart injured in traffic accident

V86.1 Passenger of special all-terrain or other off-road motor vehicle injured in traffic accident
V86.11 Passenger of ambulance or fire engine injured in traffic accident
V86.12 Passenger of snowmobile injured in traffic accident
V86.13 Passenger of dune buggy injured in traffic accident
V86.14 Passenger of military vehicle injured in traffic accident
V86.19 Passenger of other special all-terrain or other off-road motor vehicle injured in traffic accident
Passenger of dirt bike injured in traffic accident
Passenger of go cart injured in traffic accident
Passenger of golf cart injured in traffic accident

V86.2 Person on outside of special all-terrain or other off-road motor vehicle injured in traffic accident
V86.21 Person on outside of ambulance or fire engine injured in traffic accident
V86.22 Person on outside of snowmobile injured in traffic accident

√x7th **V86.23 Person on outside of dune buggy injured in traffic accident**

√x7th **V86.24 Person on outside of military vehicle injured in traffic accident**

√x7th **V86.29 Person on outside of other special all-terrain or other off-road motor vehicle injured in traffic accident**

Person on outside of dirt bike injured in traffic accident
Person on outside of go cart in traffic accident
Person on outside of golf cart injured in traffic accident

√5th **V86.3 Unspecified occupant of special all-terrain or other off-road motor vehicle injured in traffic accident**

√x7th **V86.31 Unspecified occupant of ambulance or fire engine injured in traffic accident**

√x7th **V86.32 Unspecified occupant of snowmobile injured in traffic accident**

√x7th **V86.33 Unspecified occupant of dune buggy injured in traffic accident**

√x7th **V86.34 Unspecified occupant of military vehicle injured in traffic accident**

√x7th **V86.39 Unspecified occupant of other special all-terrain or other off-road motor vehicle injured in traffic accident**

Unspecified occupant of dirt bike injured in traffic accident
Unspecified occupant of go cart injured in traffic accident
Unspecified occupant of golf cart injured in traffic accident

√5th **V86.4 Person injured while boarding or alighting from special all-terrain or other off-road motor vehicle**

√x7th **V86.41 Person injured while boarding or alighting from ambulance or fire engine**

√x7th **V86.42 Person injured while boarding or alighting from snowmobile**

√x7th **V86.43 Person injured while boarding or alighting from dune buggy**

√x7th **V86.44 Person injured while boarding or alighting from military vehicle**

√x7th **V86.49 Person injured while boarding or alighting from other special all-terrain or other off-road motor vehicle**

Person injured while boarding or alighting from dirt bike
Person injured while boarding or alighting from go cart
Person injured while boarding or alighting from golf cart

√5th **V86.5 Driver of special all-terrain or other off-road motor vehicle injured in nontraffic accident**

√x7th **V86.51 Driver of ambulance or fire engine injured in nontraffic accident**

√x7th **V86.52 Driver of snowmobile injured in nontraffic accident**

√x7th **V86.53 Driver of dune buggy injured in nontraffic accident**

√x7th **V86.54 Driver of military vehicle injured in nontraffic accident**

√x7th **V86.59 Driver of other special all-terrain or other off-road motor vehicle injured in nontraffic accident**

Driver of dirt bike injured in nontraffic accident
Driver of go cart injured in nontraffic accident
Driver of golf cart injured in nontraffic accident

√5th **V86.6 Passenger of special all-terrain or other off-road motor vehicle injured in nontraffic accident**

√x7th **V86.61 Passenger of ambulance or fire engine injured in nontraffic accident**

√x7th **V86.62 Passenger of snowmobile injured in nontraffic accident**

√x7th **V86.63 Passenger of dune buggy injured in nontraffic accident**

√x7th **V86.64 Passenger of military vehicle injured in nontraffic accident**

√x7th **V86.69 Passenger of other special all-terrain or other off-road motor vehicle injured in nontraffic accident**

Passenger of dirt bike injured in nontraffic accident
Passenger of go cart injured in nontraffic accident
Passenger of golf cart injured in nontraffic accident

√5th **V86.7 Person on outside of special all-terrain or other off-road motor vehicle injured in nontraffic accident**

√x7th **V86.71 Person on outside of ambulance or fire engine injured in nontraffic accident**

√x7th **V86.72 Person on outside of snowmobile injured in nontraffic accident**

√x7th **V86.73 Person on outside of dune buggy injured in nontraffic accident**

√x7th **V86.74 Person on outside of military vehicle injured in nontraffic accident**

√x7th **V86.79 Person on outside of other special all-terrain or other off-road motor vehicles injured in nontraffic accident**

Person on outside of dirt bike injured in nontraffic accident
Person on outside of go cart injured in nontraffic accident
Person on outside of golf cart injured in nontraffic accident

√5th **V86.9 Unspecified occupant of special all-terrain or other off-road motor vehicle injured in nontraffic accident**

√x7th **V86.91 Unspecified occupant of ambulance or fire engine injured in nontraffic accident**

√x7th **V86.92 Unspecified occupant of snowmobile injured in nontraffic accident**

√x7th **V86.93 Unspecified occupant of dune buggy injured in nontraffic accident**

√x7th **V86.94 Unspecified occupant of military vehicle injured in nontraffic accident**

√x7th **V86.99 Unspecified occupant of other special all-terrain or other off-road motor vehicle injured in nontraffic accident**

All-terrain motor-vehicle accident NOS
Off-road motor-vehicle accident NOS
Other motor-vehicle accident NOS
Unspecified occupant of dirt bike injured in nontraffic accident
Unspecified occupant of go cart injured in nontraffic accident
Unspecified occupant of golf cart injured in nontraffic accident

√4th **V87 Traffic accident of specified type but victim's mode of transport unknown**

EXCLUDES1 *collision involving:*
pedal cycle (V10-V19)
pedestrian (V01-V09)

The appropriate 7th character is to be added to each code from category V87.
A initial encounter
D subsequent encounter
S sequela

√x7th **V87.0 Person injured in collision between car and two- or three-wheeled powered vehicle (traffic)**

√x7th **V87.1 Person injured in collision between other motor vehicle and two- or three-wheeled motor vehicle (traffic)**

√x7th **V87.2 Person injured in collision between car and pick-up truck or van (traffic)**

√x7th **V87.3 Person injured in collision between car and bus (traffic)**

√x7th **V87.4 Person injured in collision between car and heavy transport vehicle (traffic)**

√x7th **V87.5 Person injured in collision between heavy transport vehicle and bus (traffic)**

√x7th **V87.6 Person injured in collision between railway train or railway vehicle and car (traffic)**

√x7th **V87.7 Person injured in collision between other specified motor vehicles (traffic)**

√x7th **V87.8 Person injured in other specified noncollision transport accidents involving motor vehicle (traffic)**

√x7th **V87.9 Person injured in other specified (collision)(noncollision) transport accidents involving nonmotor vehicle (traffic)**

√4th **V88 Nontraffic accident of specified type but victim's mode of transport unknown**

EXCLUDES1 *collision involving:*
pedal cycle (V10-V19)
pedestrian (V01-V09)

The appropriate 7th character is to be added to each code from category V88.
A initial encounter
D subsequent encounter
S sequela

√x7th **V88.0 Person injured in collision between car and two- or three-wheeled motor vehicle, nontraffic**

√x7th **V88.1 Person injured in collision between other motor vehicle and two- or three-wheeled motor vehicle, nontraffic**

√x7th **V88.2 Person injured in collision between car and pick-up truck or van, nontraffic**

√x7th **V88.3 Person injured in collision between car and bus, nontraffic**

√x7th **V88.4 Person injured in collision between car and heavy transport vehicle, nontraffic**

√x7th **V88.5 Person injured in collision between heavy transport vehicle and bus, nontraffic**

√x7th **V88.6 Person injured in collision between railway train or railway vehicle and car, nontraffic**

√x7th **V88.7 Person injured in collision between other specified motor vehicle, nontraffic**

√x7th **V88.8 Person injured in other specified noncollision transport accidents involving motor vehicle, nontraffic**

√x7th **V88.9 Person injured in other specified (collision)(noncollision) transport accidents involving nonmotor vehicle, nontraffic**

√4th **V89 Motor- or nonmotor-vehicle accident, type of vehicle unspecified**

The appropriate 7th character is to be added to each code from category V89.
A initial encounter
D subsequent encounter
S sequela

√x7th **V89.0 Person injured in unspecified motor-vehicle accident, nontraffic**
Motor-vehicle accident NOS, nontraffic

√x7th **V89.1 Person injured in unspecified nonmotor-vehicle accident, nontraffic**
Nonmotor-vehicle accident NOS (nontraffic)

√x7th **V89.2 Person injured in unspecified motor-vehicle accident, traffic**
Motor-vehicle accident [MVA] NOS
Road (traffic) accident [RTA] NOS

√x7th **V89.3 Person injured in unspecified nonmotor-vehicle accident, traffic**
Nonmotor-vehicle traffic accident NOS

√x7th **V89.9 Person injured in unspecified vehicle accident**
Collision NOS

Water transport accidents (V90-V94)

√4th **V90 Drowning and submersion due to accident to watercraft**

EXCLUDES 1 *civilian water transport accident involving military watercraft (V94.81-)*
fall into water not from watercraft (W16.-)
military watercraft accident in military or war operations (Y36.0-, Y37.0-)
water-transport-related drowning or submersion without accident to watercraft (V92.-)

The appropriate 7th character is to be added to each code from category V90.
A initial encounter
D subsequent encounter
S sequela

√5th **V90.0 Drowning and submersion due to watercraft overturning**

√x7th **V90.00 Drowning and submersion due to merchant ship overturning**

√x7th **V90.01 Drowning and submersion due to passenger ship overturning**
Drowning and submersion due to Ferry-boat overturning
Drowning and submersion due to Liner overturning

√x7th **V90.02 Drowning and submersion due to fishing boat overturning**

√x7th **V90.03 Drowning and submersion due to other powered watercraft overturning**
Drowning and submersion due to Hovercraft (on open water) overturning
Drowning and submersion due to Jet ski overturning

√x7th **V90.04 Drowning and submersion due to sailboat overturning**

√x7th **V90.05 Drowning and submersion due to canoe or kayak overturning**

√x7th **V90.06 Drowning and submersion due to (nonpowered) inflatable craft overturning**

√x7th **V90.08 Drowning and submersion due to other unpowered watercraft overturning**
Drowning and submersion due to windsurfer overturning

√x7th **V90.09 Drowning and submersion due to unspecified watercraft overturning**
Drowning and submersion due to boat NOS overturning
Drowning and submersion due to ship NOS overturning
Drowning and submersion due to watercraft NOS overturning

√5th **V90.1 Drowning and submersion due to watercraft sinking**

√x7th **V90.10 Drowning and submersion due to merchant ship sinking**

√x7th **V90.11 Drowning and submersion due to passenger ship sinking**
Drowning and submersion due to Ferry-boat sinking
Drowning and submersion due to Liner sinking

√x7th **V90.12 Drowning and submersion due to fishing boat sinking**

√x7th **V90.13 Drowning and submersion due to other powered watercraft sinking**
Drowning and submersion due to Hovercraft (on open water) sinking
Drowning and submersion due to Jet ski sinking

√x7th **V90.14 Drowning and submersion due to sailboat sinking**

√x7th **V90.15 Drowning and submersion due to canoe or kayak sinking**

√x7th **V90.16 Drowning and submersion due to (nonpowered) inflatable craft sinking**

√x7th **V90.18 Drowning and submersion due to other unpowered watercraft sinking**

√x7th **V90.19 Drowning and submersion due to unspecified watercraft sinking**
Drowning and submersion due to boat NOS sinking
Drowning and submersion due to ship NOS sinking
Drowning and submersion due to watercraft NOS sinking

√5th **V90.2 Drowning and submersion due to falling or jumping from burning watercraft**

√x7th **V90.20 Drowning and submersion due to falling or jumping from burning merchant ship**

√x7th **V90.21 Drowning and submersion due to falling or jumping from burning passenger ship**
Drowning and submersion due to falling or jumping from burning Ferry-boat
Drowning and submersion due to falling or jumping from burning Liner

√x7th **V90.22 Drowning and submersion due to falling or jumping from burning fishing boat**

√x7th **V90.23 Drowning and submersion due to falling or jumping from other burning powered watercraft**
Drowning and submersion due to falling and jumping from burning Hovercraft (on open water)
Drowning and submersion due to falling and jumping from burning Jet ski

√x7th **V90.24 Drowning and submersion due to falling or jumping from burning sailboat**

√x7th **V90.25 Drowning and submersion due to falling or jumping from burning canoe or kayak**

√x7th **V90.26 Drowning and submersion due to falling or jumping from burning (nonpowered) inflatable craft**

√x7th **V90.27 Drowning and submersion due to falling or jumping from burning water-skis**

√x7th **V90.28 Drowning and submersion due to falling or jumping from other burning unpowered watercraft**
Drowning and submersion due to falling and jumping from burning surf-board
Drowning and submersion due to falling and jumping from burning windsurfer

√x7th **V90.29 Drowning and submersion due to falling or jumping from unspecified burning watercraft**
Drowning and submersion due to falling or jumping from burning boat NOS
Drowning and submersion due to falling or jumping from burning ship NOS
Drowning and submersion due to falling or jumping from burning watercraft NOS

√5th **V90.3 Drowning and submersion due to falling or jumping from crushed watercraft**

√x7th **V90.30 Drowning and submersion due to falling or jumping from crushed merchant ship**

√x7th **V9Ø.31 Drowning and submersion due to falling or jumping from crushed passenger ship**
Drowning and submersion due to falling and jumping from crushed Ferry boat
Drowning and submersion due to falling and jumping from crushed Liner

√x7th **V9Ø.32 Drowning and submersion due to falling or jumping from crushed fishing boat**

√x7th **V9Ø.33 Drowning and submersion due to falling or jumping from other crushed powered watercraft**
Drowning and submersion due to falling and jumping from crushed Hovercraft
Drowning and submersion due to falling and jumping from crushed Jet ski

√x7th **V9Ø.34 Drowning and submersion due to falling or jumping from crushed sailboat**

√x7th **V9Ø.35 Drowning and submersion due to falling or jumping from crushed canoe or kayak**

√x7th **V9Ø.36 Drowning and submersion due to falling or jumping from crushed (nonpowered) inflatable craft**

√x7th **V9Ø.37 Drowning and submersion due to falling or jumping from crushed water-skis**

√x7th **V9Ø.38 Drowning and submersion due to falling or jumping from other crushed unpowered watercraft**
Drowning and submersion due to falling and jumping from crushed surf-board
Drowning and submersion due to falling and jumping from crushed windsurfer

√x7th **V9Ø.39 Drowning and submersion due to falling or jumping from crushed unspecified watercraft**
Drowning and submersion due to falling and jumping from crushed boat NOS
Drowning and submersion due to falling and jumping from crushed ship NOS
Drowning and submersion due to falling and jumping from crushed watercraft NOS

√5th **V9Ø.8 Drowning and submersion due to other accident to watercraft**

√x7th **V9Ø.8Ø Drowning and submersion due to other accident to merchant ship**

√x7th **V9Ø.81 Drowning and submersion due to other accident to passenger ship**
Drowning and submersion due to other accident to Ferry-boat
Drowning and submersion due to other accident to Liner

√x7th **V9Ø.82 Drowning and submersion due to other accident to fishing boat**

√x7th **V9Ø.83 Drowning and submersion due to other accident to other powered watercraft**
Drowning and submersion due to other accident to Hovercraft (on open water)
Drowning and submersion due to other accident to Jet ski

√x7th **V9Ø.84 Drowning and submersion due to other accident to sailboat**

√x7th **V9Ø.85 Drowning and submersion due to other accident to canoe or kayak**

√x7th **V9Ø.86 Drowning and submersion due to other accident to (nonpowered) inflatable craft**

√x7th **V9Ø.87 Drowning and submersion due to other accident to water-skis**

√x7th **V9Ø.88 Drowning and submersion due to other accident to other unpowered watercraft**
Drowning and submersion due to other accident to surf-board
Drowning and submersion due to other accident to windsurfer

√x7th **V9Ø.89 Drowning and submersion due to other accident to unspecified watercraft**
Drowning and submersion due to other accident to boat NOS
Drowning and submersion due to other accident to ship NOS
Drowning and submersion due to other accident to watercraft NOS

√4th **V91 Other injury due to accident to watercraft**

INCLUDES any injury except drowning and submersion as a result of an accident to watercraft

EXCLUDES 1 *civilian water transport accident involving military watercraft (V94.81-)*
military watercraft accident in military or war operations (Y36, Y37.-)

EXCLUDES 2 *drowning and submersion due to accident to watercraft (V9Ø.-)*

The appropriate 7th character is to be added to each code from category V91.
A initial encounter
D subsequent encounter
S sequela

√5th **V91.Ø Burn due to watercraft on fire**

EXCLUDES 1 *burn from localized fire or explosion on board ship without accident to watercraft (V93.-)*

√x7th **V91.ØØ Burn due to merchant ship on fire**

√x7th **V91.Ø1 Burn due to passenger ship on fire**
Burn due to Ferry-boat on fire
Burn due to Liner on fire

√x7th **V91.Ø2 Burn due to fishing boat on fire**

√x7th **V91.Ø3 Burn due to other powered watercraft on fire**
Burn due to Hovercraft (on open water) on fire
Burn due to Jet ski on fire

√x7th **V91.Ø4 Burn due to sailboat on fire**

√x7th **V91.Ø5 Burn due to canoe or kayak on fire**

√x7th **V91.Ø6 Burn due to (nonpowered) inflatable craft on fire**

√x7th **V91.Ø7 Burn due to water-skis on fire**

√x7th **V91.Ø8 Burn due to other unpowered watercraft on fire**

√x7th **V91.Ø9 Burn due to unspecified watercraft on fire**
Burn due to boat NOS on fire
Burn due to ship NOS on fire
Burn due to watercraft NOS on fire

√5th **V91.1 Crushed between watercraft and other watercraft or other object due to collision**
Crushed by lifeboat after abandoning ship in a collision

NOTE select the specified type of watercraft that the victim was on at the time of the collision

√x7th **V91.1Ø Crushed between merchant ship and other watercraft or other object due to collision**

√x7th **V91.11 Crushed between passenger ship and other watercraft or other object due to collision**
Crushed between Ferry-boat and other watercraft or other object due to collision
Crushed between Liner and other watercraft or other object due to collision

√x7th **V91.12 Crushed between fishing boat and other watercraft or other object due to collision**

√x7th **V91.13 Crushed between other powered watercraft and other watercraft or other object due to collision**
Crushed between Hovercraft (on open water) and other watercraft or other object due to collision
Crushed between Jet ski and other watercraft or other object due to collision

√x7th **V91.14 Crushed between sailboat and other watercraft or other object due to collision**

√x7th **V91.15 Crushed between canoe or kayak and other watercraft or other object due to collision**

√x7th **V91.16 Crushed between (nonpowered) inflatable craft and other watercraft or other object due to collision**

√x7th **V91.18 Crushed between other unpowered watercraft and other watercraft or other object due to collision**
Crushed between surfboard and other watercraft or other object due to collision
Crushed between windsurfer and other watercraft or other object due to collision

√x7th **V91.19 Crushed between unspecified watercraft and other watercraft or other object due to collision**
Crushed between boat NOS and other watercraft or other object due to collision
Crushed between ship NOS and other watercraft or other object due to collision
Crushed between watercraft NOS and other watercraft or other object due to collision

✓5th **V91.2 Fall due to collision between watercraft and other watercraft or other object**
Fall while remaining on watercraft after collision
NOTE Select the specified type of watercraft that the victim was on at the time of the collision.
EXCLUDES 1 *crushed between watercraft and other watercraft and other object due to collision (V91.1-)*
drowning and submersion due to falling from crushed watercraft (V90.3-)

✓x7th **V91.20 Fall due to collision between merchant ship and other watercraft or other object**

✓x7th **V91.21 Fall due to collision between passenger ship and other watercraft or other object**
Fall due to collision between Ferry-boat and other watercraft or other object
Fall due to collision between Liner and other watercraft or other object

✓x7th **V91.22 Fall due to collision between fishing boat and other watercraft or other object**

✓x7th **V91.23 Fall due to collision between other powered watercraft and other watercraft or other object**
Fall due to collision between Hovercraft (on open water) and other watercraft or other object
Fall due to collision between Jet ski and other watercraft or other object

✓x7th **V91.24 Fall due to collision between sailboat and other watercraft or other object**

✓x7th **V91.25 Fall due to collision between canoe or kayak and other watercraft or other object**

✓x7th **V91.26 Fall due to collision between (nonpowered) inflatable craft and other watercraft or other object**

✓x7th **V91.29 Fall due to collision between unspecified watercraft and other watercraft or other object**
Fall due to collision between boat NOS and other watercraft or other object
Fall due to collision between ship NOS and other watercraft or other object
Fall due to collision between watercraft NOS and other watercraft or other object

✓5th **V91.3 Hit or struck by falling object due to accident to watercraft**
Hit or struck by falling object (part of damaged watercraft or other object) after falling or jumping from damaged watercraft
EXCLUDES 2 *drowning or submersion due to fall or jumping from damaged watercraft (V90.2-, V90.3-)*

✓x7th **V91.30 Hit or struck by falling object due to accident to merchant ship**

✓x7th **V91.31 Hit or struck by falling object due to accident to passenger ship**
Hit or struck by falling object due to accident to Ferry-boat
Hit or struck by falling object due to accident to Liner

✓x7th **V91.32 Hit or struck by falling object due to accident to fishing boat**

✓x7th **V91.33 Hit or struck by falling object due to accident to other powered watercraft**
Hit or struck by falling object due to accident to Hovercraft (on open water)
Hit or struck by falling object due to accident to Jet ski

✓x7th **V91.34 Hit or struck by falling object due to accident to sailboat**

✓x7th **V91.35 Hit or struck by falling object due to accident to canoe or kayak**

✓x7th **V91.36 Hit or struck by falling object due to accident to (nonpowered) inflatable craft**

✓x7th **V91.37 Hit or struck by falling object due to accident to water-skis**
Hit by water-skis after jumping off of waterskis

✓x7th **V91.38 Hit or struck by falling object due to accident to other unpowered watercraft**
Hit or struck by surf-board after falling off damaged surf-board
Hit or struck by object after falling off damaged windsurfer

✓x7th **V91.39 Hit or struck by falling object due to accident to unspecified watercraft**
Hit or struck by falling object due to accident to boat NOS
Hit or struck by falling object due to accident to ship NOS
Hit or struck by falling object due to accident to watercraft NOS

✓5th **V91.8 Other injury due to other accident to watercraft**

✓x7th **V91.80 Other injury due to other accident to merchant ship**

✓x7th **V91.81 Other injury due to other accident to passenger ship**
Other injury due to other accident to Ferry-boat
Other injury due to other accident to Liner

✓x7th **V91.82 Other injury due to other accident to fishing boat**

✓x7th **V91.83 Other injury due to other accident to other powered watercraft**
Other injury due to other accident to Hovercraft (on open water)
Other injury due to other accident to Jet ski

✓x7th **V91.84 Other injury due to other accident to sailboat**

✓x7th **V91.85 Other injury due to other accident to canoe or kayak**

✓x7th **V91.86 Other injury due to other accident to (nonpowered) inflatable craft**

✓x7th **V91.87 Other injury due to other accident to water-skis**

✓x7th **V91.88 Other injury due to other accident to other unpowered watercraft**
Other injury due to other accident to surf-board
Other injury due to other accident to windsurfer

✓x7th **V91.89 Other injury due to other accident to unspecified watercraft**
Other injury due to other accident to boat NOS
Other injury due to other accident to ship NOS
Other injury due to other accident to watercraft NOS

✓4th **V92 Drowning and submersion due to accident on board watercraft, without accident to watercraft**
EXCLUDES 1 *civilian water transport accident involving military watercraft (V94.81-)*
drowning or submersion due to accident to watercraft (V90-V91)
drowning or submersion of diver who voluntarily jumps from boat not involved in an accident (W16.711, W16.721)
fall into water without watercraft (W16.-)
military watercraft accident in military or war operations (Y36, Y37)

The appropriate 7th character is to be added to each code from category V92.
A initial encounter
D subsequent encounter
S sequela

✓5th **V92.0 Drowning and submersion due to fall off watercraft**
Drowning and submersion due to fall from gangplank of watercraft
Drowning and submersion due to fall overboard watercraft
EXCLUDES 2 *hitting head on object or bottom of body of water due to fall from watercraft (V94.0-)*

✓x7th **V92.00 Drowning and submersion due to fall off merchant ship**

✓x7th **V92.01 Drowning and submersion due to fall off passenger ship**
Drowning and submersion due to fall off Ferry-boat
Drowning and submersion due to fall off Liner

✓x7th **V92.02 Drowning and submersion due to fall off fishing boat**

✓x7th **V92.03 Drowning and submersion due to fall off other powered watercraft**
Drowning and submersion due to fall off Hovercraft (on open water)
Drowning and submersion due to fall off Jet ski

✓x7th **V92.04 Drowning and submersion due to fall off sailboat**

✓x7th **V92.05 Drowning and submersion due to fall off canoe or kayak**

✓x7th **V92.06 Drowning and submersion due to fall off (nonpowered) inflatable craft**

✓x7th **V92.07 Drowning and submersion due to fall off water-skis**
EXCLUDES 1 *drowning and submersion due to falling off burning water-skis (V90.27)*
drowning and submersion due to falling off crushed water-skis (V90.37)
hit by boat while water-skiing NOS (V94.X)

√x7th **V92.08 Drowning and submersion due to fall off other unpowered watercraft**
Drowning and submersion due to fall off surf-board
Drowning and submersion due to fall off windsurfer
EXCLUDES 1 *drowning and submersion due to fall off burning unpowered watercraft (V90.28)*
drowning and submersion due to fall off crushed unpowered watercraft (V90.38)
drowning and submersion due to fall off damaged unpowered watercraft (V90.88)
drowning and submersion due to rider of nonpowered watercraft being hit by other watercraft (V94.-)
other injury due to rider of nonpowered watercraft being hit by other watercraft (V94.-)

√x7th **V92.09 Drowning and submersion due to fall off unspecified watercraft**
Drowning and submersion due to fall off boat NOS
Drowning and submersion due to fall off ship
Drowning and submersion due to fall off watercraft NOS

√5th **V92.1 Drowning and submersion due to being thrown overboard by motion of watercraft**
EXCLUDES 1 *drowning and submersion due to fall off surf-board (V92.08)*
drowning and submersion due to fall off water-skis (V92.07)
drowning and submersion due to fall off windsurfer (V92.08)

√x7th **V92.10 Drowning and submersion due to being thrown overboard by motion of merchant ship**

√x7th **V92.11 Drowning and submersion due to being thrown overboard by motion of passenger ship**
Drowning and submersion due to being thrown overboard by motion of Ferry-boat
Drowning and submersion due to being thrown overboard by motion of Liner

√x7th **V92.12 Drowning and submersion due to being thrown overboard by motion of fishing boat**

√x7th **V92.13 Drowning and submersion due to being thrown overboard by motion of other powered watercraft**
Drowning and submersion due to being thrown overboard by motion of Hovercraft

√x7th **V92.14 Drowning and submersion due to being thrown overboard by motion of sailboat**

√x7th **V92.15 Drowning and submersion due to being thrown overboard by motion of canoe or kayak**

√x7th **V92.16 Drowning and submersion due to being thrown overboard by motion of (nonpowered) inflatable craft**

√x7th **V92.19 Drowning and submersion due to being thrown overboard by motion of unspecified watercraft**
Drowning and submersion due to being thrown overboard by motion of boat NOS
Drowning and submersion due to being thrown overboard by motion of ship NOS
Drowning and submersion due to being thrown overboard by motion of watercraft NOS

√5th **V92.2 Drowning and submersion due to being washed overboard from watercraft**
Code first any associated cataclysm (X37.0-)

√x7th **V92.20 Drowning and submersion due to being washed overboard from merchant ship**

√x7th **V92.21 Drowning and submersion due to being washed overboard from passenger ship**
Drowning and submersion due to being washed overboard from Ferry-boat
Drowning and submersion due to being washed overboard from Liner

√x7th **V92.22 Drowning and submersion due to being washed overboard from fishing boat**

√x7th **V92.23 Drowning and submersion due to being washed overboard from other powered watercraft**
Drowning and submersion due to being washed overboard from Hovercraft (on open water)
Drowning and submersion due to being washed overboard from Jet ski

√x7th **V92.24 Drowning and submersion due to being washed overboard from sailboat**

√x7th **V92.25 Drowning and submersion due to being washed overboard from canoe or kayak**

√x7th **V92.26 Drowning and submersion due to being washed overboard from (nonpowered) inflatable craft**

√x7th **V92.27 Drowning and submersion due to being washed overboard from water-skis**
EXCLUDES 1 *drowning and submersion due to fall off water-skis (V92.07)*

√x7th **V92.28 Drowning and submersion due to being washed overboard from other unpowered watercraft**
Drowning and submersion due to being washed overboard from surf-board
Drowning and submersion due to being washed overboard from windsurfer

√x7th **V92.29 Drowning and submersion due to being washed overboard from unspecified watercraft**
Drowning and submersion due to being washed overboard from boat NOS
Drowning and submersion due to being washed overboard from ship NOS
Drowning and submersion due to being washed overboard from watercraft NOS

√4th **V93 Other injury due to accident on board watercraft, without accident to watercraft**
EXCLUDES 1 *civilian water transport accident involving military watercraft (V94.81-)*
other injury due to accident to watercraft (V91.-)
military watercraft accident in military or war operations (Y36, Y37.-)
EXCLUDES 2 *drowning and submersion due to accident on board watercraft, without accident to watercraft (V92.-)*

The appropriate 7th character is to be added to each code from category V93.
A initial encounter
D subsequent encounter
S sequela

√5th **V93.0 Burn due to localized fire on board watercraft**
EXCLUDES 1 *burn due to watercraft on fire (V91.0-)*

√x7th **V93.00 Burn due to localized fire on board merchant vessel**

√x7th **V93.01 Burn due to localized fire on board passenger vessel**
Burn due to localized fire on board Ferry-boat
Burn due to localized fire on board Liner

√x7th **V93.02 Burn due to localized fire on board fishing boat**

√x7th **V93.03 Burn due to localized fire on board other powered watercraft**
Burn due to localized fire on board Hovercraft
Burn due to localized fire on board Jet ski

√x7th **V93.04 Burn due to localized fire on board sailboat**

√x7th **V93.09 Burn due to localized fire on board unspecified watercraft**
Burn due to localized fire on board boat NOS
Burn due to localized fire on board ship NOS
Burn due to localized fire on board watercraft NOS

√5th **V93.1 Other burn on board watercraft**
Burn due to source other than fire on board watercraft
EXCLUDES 1 *burn due to watercraft on fire (V91.0-)*

√x7th **V93.10 Other burn on board merchant vessel**

√x7th **V93.11 Other burn on board passenger vessel**
Other burn on board Ferry-boat
Other burn on board Liner

√x7th **V93.12 Other burn on board fishing boat**

√x7th **V93.13 Other burn on board other powered watercraft**
Other burn on board Hovercraft
Other burn on board Jet ski

√x7th **V93.14 Other burn on board sailboat**

√x7th **V93.19 Other burn on board unspecified watercraft**
Other burn on board boat NOS
Other burn on board ship NOS
Other burn on board watercraft NOS

√5th **V93.2 Heat exposure on board watercraft**
EXCLUDES 1 *exposure to man-made heat not aboard watercraft (W92)*
exposure to natural heat while on board watercraft (X30)
exposure to sunlight while on board watercraft (X32)
EXCLUDES 2 *burn due to fire on board watercraft (V93.0-)*

√x7th **V93.20 Heat exposure on board merchant ship**

√x7th **V93.21 Heat exposure on board passenger ship**
Heat exposure on board Ferry-boat
Heat exposure on board Liner

√x7th **V93.22 Heat exposure on board fishing boat**

√x7th **V93.23 Heat exposure on board other powered watercraft**
Heat exposure on board hovercraft

√x7th **V93.24 Heat exposure on board sailboat**

√x7th **V93.29 Heat exposure on board unspecified watercraft**
Heat exposure on board boat NOS
Heat exposure on board ship NOS
Heat exposure on board watercraft NOS

√5th **V93.3 Fall on board watercraft**
EXCLUDES 1 *fall due to collision of watercraft (V91.2-)*

√x7th **V93.3Ø Fall on board merchant ship**

√x7th **V93.31 Fall on board passenger ship**
Fall on board Ferry-boat
Fall on board Liner

√x7th **V93.32 Fall on board fishing boat**

√x7th **V93.33 Fall on board other powered watercraft**
Fall on board Hovercraft (on open water)
Fall on board Jet ski

√x7th **V93.34 Fall on board sailboat**

√x7th **V93.35 Fall on board canoe or kayak**

√x7th **V93.36 Fall on board (nonpowered) inflatable craft**

√x7th **V93.38 Fall on board other unpowered watercraft**

√x7th **V93.39 Fall on board unspecified watercraft**
Fall on board boat NOS
Fall on board ship NOS
Fall on board watercraft NOS

√5th **V93.4 Struck by falling object on board watercraft**
Hit by falling object on board watercraft
EXCLUDES 1 *struck by falling object due to accident to watercraft (V91.3)*

√x7th **V93.4Ø Struck by falling object on merchant ship**

√x7th **V93.41 Struck by falling object on passenger ship**
Struck by falling object on Ferry-boat
Struck by falling object on Liner

√x7th **V93.42 Struck by falling object on fishing boat**

√x7th **V93.43 Struck by falling object on other powered watercraft**
Struck by falling object on Hovercraft

√x7th **V93.44 Struck by falling object on sailboat**

√x7th **V93.48 Struck by falling object on other unpowered watercraft**

√x7th **V93.49 Struck by falling object on unspecified watercraft**

√5th **V93.5 Explosion on board watercraft**
Boiler explosion on steamship
EXCLUDES 2 *fire on board watercraft (V93.Ø-)*

√x7th **V93.5Ø Explosion on board merchant ship**

√x7th **V93.51 Explosion on board passenger ship**
Explosion on board Ferry-boat
Explosion on board Liner

√x7th **V93.52 Explosion on board fishing boat**

√x7th **V93.53 Explosion on board other powered watercraft**
Explosion on board Hovercraft
Explosion on board Jet ski

√x7th **V93.54 Explosion on board sailboat**

√x7th **V93.59 Explosion on board unspecified watercraft**
Explosion on board boat NOS
Explosion on board ship NOS
Explosion on board watercraft NOS

√5th **V93.6 Machinery accident on board watercraft**
EXCLUDES 1 *machinery explosion on board watercraft (V93.4-)*
machinery fire on board watercraft (V93.Ø-)

√x7th **V93.6Ø Machinery accident on board merchant ship**

√x7th **V93.61 Machinery accident on board passenger ship**
Machinery accident on board Ferry-boat
Machinery accident on board Liner

√x7th **V93.62 Machinery accident on board fishing boat**

√x7th **V93.63 Machinery accident on board other powered watercraft**
Machinery accident on board Hovercraft

√x7th **V93.64 Machinery accident on board sailboat**

√x7th **V93.69 Machinery accident on board unspecified watercraft**
Machinery accident on board boat NOS
Machinery accident on board ship NOS
Machinery accident on board watercraft NOS

√5th **V93.8 Other injury due to other accident on board watercraft**
Accidental poisoning by gases or fumes on watercraft

√x7th **V93.8Ø Other injury due to other accident on board merchant ship**

√x7th **V93.81 Other injury due to other accident on board passenger ship**
Other injury due to other accident on board Ferry-boat
Other injury due to other accident on board Liner

√x7th **V93.82 Other injury due to other accident on board fishing boat**

√x7th **V93.83 Other injury due to other accident on board other powered watercraft**
Other injury due to other accident on board Hovercraft
Other injury due to other accident on board Jet ski

√x7th **V93.84 Other injury due to other accident on board sailboat**

√x7th **V93.85 Other injury due to other accident on board canoe or kayak**

√x7th **V93.86 Other injury due to other accident on board (nonpowered) inflatable craft**

√x7th **V93.87 Other injury due to other accident on board water-skis**
Hit or struck by object while waterskiing

√x7th **V93.88 Other injury due to other accident on board other unpowered watercraft**
Hit or struck by object while surfing
Hit or struck by object while on board windsurfer

√x7th **V93.89 Other injury due to other accident on board unspecified watercraft**
Other injury due to other accident on board boat NOS
Other injury due to other accident on board ship NOS
Other injury due to other accident on board watercraft NOS

√4th **V94 Other and unspecified water transport accidents**
EXCLUDES 1 *military watercraft accidents in military or war operations (Y36, Y37)*

The appropriate 7th character is to be added to each code from category V94.
A initial encounter
D subsequent encounter
S sequela

√x7th **V94.Ø Hitting object or bottom of body of water due to fall from watercraft**
EXCLUDES 2 *drowning and submersion due to fall from watercraft (V92.Ø-)*

√5th **V94.1 Bather struck by watercraft**
Swimmer hit by watercraft

√x7th **V94.11 Bather struck by powered watercraft**

√x7th **V94.12 Bather struck by nonpowered watercraft**

√5th **V94.2 Rider of nonpowered watercraft struck by other watercraft**

√x7th **V94.21 Rider of nonpowered watercraft struck by other nonpowered watercraft**
Canoer hit by other nonpowered watercraft
Surfer hit by other nonpowered watercraft
Windsurfer hit by other nonpowered watercraft

√x7th **V94.22 Rider of nonpowered watercraft struck by powered watercraft**
Canoer hit by motorboat
Surfer hit by motorboat
Windsurfer hit by motorboat

√5th **V94.3 Injury to rider of (inflatable) watercraft being pulled behind other watercraft**

√x7th **V94.31 Injury to rider of (inflatable) recreational watercraft being pulled behind other watercraft**
Injury to rider of inner-tube pulled behind motor boat

√x7th **V94.32 Injury to rider of non-recreational watercraft being pulled behind other watercraft**
Injury to occupant of dingy being pulled behind boat or ship
Injury to occupant of life-raft being pulled behind boat or ship

√x7th **V94.4 Injury to barefoot water-skier**
Injury to person being pulled behind boat or ship

√5th **V94.8 Other water transport accident**

√6th **V94.81 Water transport accident involving military watercraft**

√7th **V94.81Ø Civilian watercraft involved in water transport accident with military watercraft**
Passenger on civilian watercraft injured due to accident with military watercraft

√7th **V94.811 Civilian in water injured by military watercraft**

√7th **V94.818 Other water transport accident involving military watercraft**

√x7th **V94.89 Other water transport accident**

√x7th **V94.9 Unspecified water transport accident**
Water transport accident NOS

Air and space transport accidents (V95-V97)

EXCLUDES 1 *military aircraft accidents in military or war operations (Y36, Y37)*

V95 Accident to powered aircraft causing injury to occupant

The appropriate 7th character is to be added to each code from category V95.
A initial encounter
D subsequent encounter
S sequela

V95.0 Helicopter accident injuring occupant
- **V95.00 Unspecified helicopter accident injuring occupant**
- **V95.01 Helicopter crash injuring occupant**
- **V95.02 Forced landing of helicopter injuring occupant**
- **V95.03 Helicopter collision injuring occupant**
  Helicopter collision with any object, fixed, movable or moving
- **V95.04 Helicopter fire injuring occupant**
- **V95.05 Helicopter explosion injuring occupant**
- **V95.09 Other helicopter accident injuring occupant**

V95.1 Ultralight, microlight or powered-glider accident injuring occupant
- **V95.10 Unspecified ultralight, microlight or powered-glider accident injuring occupant**
- **V95.11 Ultralight, microlight or powered-glider crash injuring occupant**
- **V95.12 Forced landing of ultralight, microlight or powered-glider injuring occupant**
- **V95.13 Ultralight, microlight or powered-glider collision injuring occupant**
  Ultralight, microlight or powered-glider collision with any object, fixed, movable or moving
- **V95.14 Ultralight, microlight or powered-glider fire injuring occupant**
- **V95.15 Ultralight, microlight or powered-glider explosion injuring occupant**
- **V95.19 Other ultralight, microlight or powered-glider accident injuring occupant**

V95.2 Other private fixed-wing aircraft accident injuring occupant
- **V95.20 Unspecified accident to other private fixed-wing aircraft, injuring occupant**
- **V95.21 Other private fixed-wing aircraft crash injuring occupant**
- **V95.22 Forced landing of other private fixed-wing aircraft injuring occupant**
- **V95.23 Other private fixed-wing aircraft collision injuring occupant**
  Other private fixed-wing aircraft collision with any object, fixed, movable or moving
- **V95.24 Other private fixed-wing aircraft fire injuring occupant**
- **V95.25 Other private fixed-wing aircraft explosion injuring occupant**
- **V95.29 Other accident to other private fixed-wing aircraft injuring occupant**

V95.3 Commercial fixed-wing aircraft accident injuring occupant
- **V95.30 Unspecified accident to commercial fixed-wing aircraft injuring occupant**
- **V95.31 Commercial fixed-wing aircraft crash injuring occupant**
- **V95.32 Forced landing of commercial fixed-wing aircraft injuring occupant**
- **V95.33 Commercial fixed-wing aircraft collision injuring occupant**
  Commercial fixed-wing aircraft collision with any object, fixed, movable or moving
- **V95.34 Commercial fixed-wing aircraft fire injuring occupant**
- **V95.35 Commercial fixed-wing aircraft explosion injuring occupant**
- **V95.39 Other accident to commercial fixed-wing aircraft injuring occupant**

V95.4 Spacecraft accident injuring occupant
- **V95.40 Unspecified spacecraft accident injuring occupant**
- **V95.41 Spacecraft crash injuring occupant**
- **V95.42 Forced landing of spacecraft injuring occupant**
- **V95.43 Spacecraft collision injuring occupant**
  Spacecraft collision with any object, fixed, moveable or moving
- **V95.44 Spacecraft fire injuring occupant**
- **V95.45 Spacecraft explosion injuring occupant**
- **V95.49 Other spacecraft accident injuring occupant**

V95.8 Other powered aircraft accidents injuring occupant

V95.9 Unspecified aircraft accident injuring occupant
Aircraft accident NOS
Air transport accident NOS

V96 Accident to nonpowered aircraft causing injury to occupant

The appropriate 7th character is to be added to each code from category V96.
A initial encounter
D subsequent encounter
S sequela

V96.0 Balloon accident injuring occupant
- **V96.00 Unspecified balloon accident injuring occupant**
- **V96.01 Balloon crash injuring occupant**
- **V96.02 Forced landing of balloon injuring occupant**
- **V96.03 Balloon collision injuring occupant**
  Balloon collision with any object, fixed, moveable or moving
- **V96.04 Balloon fire injuring occupant**
- **V96.05 Balloon explosion injuring occupant**
- **V96.09 Other balloon accident injuring occupant**

V96.1 Hang-glider accident injuring occupant
- **V96.10 Unspecified hang-glider accident injuring occupant**
- **V96.11 Hang-glider crash injuring occupant**
- **V96.12 Forced landing of hang-glider injuring occupant**
- **V96.13 Hang-glider collision injuring occupant**
  Hang-glider collision with any object, fixed, moveable or moving
- **V96.14 Hang-glider fire injuring occupant**
- **V96.15 Hang-glider explosion injuring occupant**
- **V96.19 Other hang-glider accident injuring occupant**

V96.2 Glider (nonpowered) accident injuring occupant
- **V96.20 Unspecified glider (nonpowered) accident injuring occupant**
- **V96.21 Glider (nonpowered) crash injuring occupant**
- **V96.22 Forced landing of glider (nonpowered) injuring occupant**
- **V96.23 Glider (nonpowered) collision injuring occupant**
  Glider (nonpowered) collision with any object, fixed, moveable or moving
- **V96.24 Glider (nonpowered) fire injuring occupant**
- **V96.25 Glider (nonpowered) explosion injuring occupant**
- **V96.29 Other glider (nonpowered) accident injuring occupant**

V96.8 Other nonpowered-aircraft accidents injuring occupant
Kite carrying a person accident injuring occupant

V96.9 Unspecified nonpowered-aircraft accident injuring occupant
Nonpowered-aircraft accident NOS

V97 Other specified air transport accidents

The appropriate 7th character is to be added to each code from category V97.
A initial encounter
D subsequent encounter
S sequela

V97.0 Occupant of aircraft injured in other specified air transport accidents
Fall in, on or from aircraft in air transport accident
EXCLUDES 1 *accident while boarding or alighting aircraft (V97.1)*

V97.1 Person injured while boarding or alighting from aircraft

V97.2 Parachutist accident
- **V97.21 Parachutist entangled in object**
  Parachutist landing in tree
- **V97.22 Parachutist injured on landing**
- **V97.29 Other parachutist accident**

V97.3 Person on ground injured in air transport accident
- **V97.31 Hit by object falling from aircraft**
  Hit by crashing aircraft
  Injured by aircraft hitting house
  Injured by aircraft hitting car
- **V97.32 Injured by rotating propeller**
- **V97.33 Sucked into jet engine**
- **V97.39 Other injury to person on ground due to air transport accident**

V97.8 Other air transport accidents, not elsewhere classified
EXCLUDES 1 *aircraft accident NOS (V95.9)*
exposure to changes in air pressure during ascent or descent (W94.-)

V97.81 Air transport accident involving military aircraft

V97.810 Civilian aircraft involved in air transport accident with military aircraft
Passenger in civilian aircraft injured due to accident with military aircraft

V97.811 Civilian injured by military aircraft

V97.818 Other air transport accident involving military aircraft

V97.89 Other air transport accidents, not elsewhere classified
Injury from machinery on aircraft

Other and unspecified transport accidents (V98-V99)

EXCLUDES 1 *vehicle accident, type of vehicle unspecified (V89.-)*

V98 Other specified transport accidents

The appropriate 7th character is to be added to each code from category V98.
A initial encounter
D subsequent encounter
S sequela

V98.0 Accident to, on or involving cable-car, not on rails
Caught or dragged by cable-car, not on rails
Fall or jump from cable-car, not on rails
Object thrown from or in cable-car, not on rails

V98.1 Accident to, on or involving land-yacht

V98.2 Accident to, on or involving ice yacht

V98.3 Accident to, on or involving ski lift
Accident to, on or involving ski chair-lift
Accident to, on or involving ski-lift with gondola

V98.8 Other specified transport accidents

V99 Unspecified transport accident

The appropriate 7th character is to be added to code V99.
A initial encounter
D subsequent encounter
S sequela

OTHER EXTERNAL CAUSES OF ACCIDENTAL INJURY (W00-X58)

Slipping, tripping, stumbling and falls (W00-W19)

EXCLUDES 1 *assault involving a fall (Y01-Y02)*
fall from animal (V80.-)
fall (in) (from) machinery (in operation) (W28-W31)
fall (in) (from) transport vehicle (V01-V99)
intentional self-harm involving a fall (X80-X81)
EXCLUDES 2 *at risk for fall (history of fall) Z91.81*
fall (in) (from) burning building (X00.-)
fall into fire (X00-X04, X08-X09)

W00 Fall due to ice and snow
INCLUDES pedestrian on foot falling (slipping) on ice and snow
EXCLUDES 1 *fall on (from) ice and snow involving pedestrian conveyance (V00.-)*
fall from stairs and steps not due to ice and snow (W10.-)

The appropriate 7th character is to be added to each code from category W00.
A initial encounter
D subsequent encounter
S sequela

W00.0 Fall on same level due to ice and snow

W00.1 Fall from stairs and steps due to ice and snow

W00.2 Other fall from one level to another due to ice and snow

W00.9 Unspecified fall due to ice and snow

W01 Fall on same level from slipping, tripping and stumbling
INCLUDES fall on moving sidewalk
EXCLUDES 1 *fall due to bumping (striking) against object (W18.0-)*
fall in shower or bathtub (W18.2-)
fall on same level NOS (W18.30)
fall on same level from slipping, tripping and stumbling due to ice or snow (W00.0)
fall off or from toilet (W18.1-)
slipping, tripping and stumbling NOS (W18.40)
slipping, tripping and stumbling without falling (W18.4-)

The appropriate 7th character is to be added to each code from category W01.
A initial encounter
D subsequent encounter
S sequela

W01.0 Fall on same level from slipping, tripping and stumbling without subsequent striking against object
Falling over animal

W01.1 Fall on same level from slipping, tripping and stumbling with subsequent striking against object

W01.10 Fall on same level from slipping, tripping and stumbling with subsequent striking against unspecified object

W01.11 Fall on same level from slipping, tripping and stumbling with subsequent striking against sharp object

W01.110 Fall on same level from slipping, tripping and stumbling with subsequent striking against sharp glass

W01.111 Fall on same level from slipping, tripping and stumbling with subsequent striking against power tool or machine

W01.118 Fall on same level from slipping, tripping and stumbling with subsequent striking against other sharp object

W01.119 Fall on same level from slipping, tripping and stumbling with subsequent striking against unspecified sharp object

W01.19 Fall on same level from slipping, tripping and stumbling with subsequent striking against other object

W01.190 Fall on same level from slipping, tripping and stumbling with subsequent striking against furniture

W01.198 Fall on same level from slipping, tripping and stumbling with subsequent striking against other object

W03 Other fall on same level due to collision with another person
Fall due to non-transport collision with other person
EXCLUDES 1 *collision with another person without fall (W51)*
crushed or pushed by a crowd or human stampede (W52)
fall involving pedestrian conveyance (V00-V09)
fall due to ice or snow (W00)
fall on same level NOS (W18.30)
AHA: 2012, 4Q, 108

The appropriate 7th character is to be added to code W03.
A initial encounter
D subsequent encounter
S sequela

W04 Fall while being carried or supported by other persons
Accidentally dropped while being carried

The appropriate 7th character is to be added to code W04.
A initial encounter
D subsequent encounter
S sequela

W05 Fall from non-moving wheelchair, nonmotorized scooter and motorized mobility scooter
EXCLUDES 1 *fall from moving motorized mobility scooter (V00.831)*
fall from moving wheelchair (powered) (V00.811)
fall from nonmotorized scooter (V00.141)

The appropriate 7th character is to be added to each code from category W05.
A initial encounter
D subsequent encounter
S sequela

W05.0 Fall from non-moving wheelchair

W05.1 Fall from non-moving nonmotorized scooter

√x7th **WØ5.2 Fall from non-moving motorized mobility scooter**

√x7th **WØ6 Fall from bed**

The appropriate 7th character is to be added to code WØ6.
A initial encounter
D subsequent encounter
S sequela

√x7th **WØ7 Fall from chair**

The appropriate 7th character is to be added to code WØ7.
A initial encounter
D subsequent encounter
S sequela

√x7th **WØ8 Fall from other furniture**

The appropriate 7th character is to be added to code WØ8.
A initial encounter
D subsequent encounter
S sequela

√4th **WØ9 Fall on and from playground equipment**
EXCLUDES 1 *fall involving recreational machinery (W31)*

The appropriate 7th character is to be added to each code from category WØ9.
A initial encounter
D subsequent encounter
S sequela

√x7th **WØ9.Ø Fall on or from playground slide**
√x7th **WØ9.1 Fall from playground swing**
√x7th **WØ9.2 Fall on or from jungle gym**
√x7th **WØ9.8 Fall on or from other playground equipment**

√4th **W1Ø Fall on and from stairs and steps**
EXCLUDES 1 *Fall from stairs and steps due to ice and snow (WØØ.1)*

The appropriate 7th character is to be added to each code from category W1Ø.
A initial encounter
D subsequent encounter
S sequela

√x7th **W1Ø.Ø Fall (on)(from) escalator**
√x7th **W1Ø.1 Fall (on)(from) sidewalk curb**
√x7th **W1Ø.2 Fall (on)(from) incline**
Fall (on) (from) ramp
√x7th **W1Ø.8 Fall (on) (from) other stairs and steps**
√x7th **W1Ø.9 Fall (on) (from) unspecified stairs and steps**

√x7th **W11 Fall on and from ladder**

The appropriate 7th character is to be added code W11.
A initial encounter
D subsequent encounter
S sequela

√x7th **W12 Fall on and from scaffolding**

The appropriate 7th character is to be added code W12.
A initial encounter
D subsequent encounter
S sequela

√4th **W13 Fall from, out of or through building or structure**

The appropriate 7th character is to be added to each code from category W13.
A initial encounter
D subsequent encounter
S sequela

√x7th **W13.Ø Fall from, out of or through balcony**
Fall from, out of or through railing
√x7th **W13.1 Fall from, out of or through bridge**
√x7th **W13.2 Fall from, out of or through roof**
√x7th **W13.3 Fall through floor**
√x7th **W13.4 Fall from, out of or through window**
EXCLUDES 2 *fall with subsequent striking against sharp glass (WØ1.11Ø)*
√x7th **W13.8 Fall from, out of or through other building or structure**
Fall from, out of or through viaduct
Fall from, out of or through wall
Fall from, out of or through flag-pole
√x7th **W13.9 Fall from, out of or through building, not otherwise specified**
EXCLUDES 1 *collapse of a building or structure (W2Ø.-)*
fall or jump from burning building or structure (XØØ.-)

√x7th **W14 Fall from tree**

The appropriate 7th character is to be added to code W14.
A initial encounter
D subsequent encounter
S sequela

√x7th **W15 Fall from cliff**

The appropriate 7th character is to be added to code W15.
A initial encounter
D subsequent encounter
S sequela

√4th **W16 Fall, jump or diving into water**
EXCLUDES 1 *accidental non-watercraft drowning and submersion not involving fall (W65-W74)*
effects of air pressure from diving (W94.-)
fall into water from watercraft (V9Ø-V94)
hitting an object or against bottom when falling from watercraft (V94.Ø)
EXCLUDES 2 *striking or hitting diving board (W21.4)*

The appropriate 7th character is to be added to each code from category W16.
A initial encounter
D subsequent encounter
S sequela

√5th **W16.Ø Fall into swimming pool**
Fall into swimming pool NOS
EXCLUDES 1 *fall into empty swimming pool (W17.3)*
√6th **W16.Ø1 Fall into swimming pool striking water surface**
√7th **W16.Ø11 Fall into swimming pool striking water surface causing drowning and submersion**
EXCLUDES 1 *drowning and submersion while in swimming pool without fall (W67)*
√7th **W16.Ø12 Fall into swimming pool striking water surface causing other injury**
√6th **W16.Ø2 Fall into swimming pool striking bottom**
√7th **W16.Ø21 Fall into swimming pool striking bottom causing drowning and submersion**
EXCLUDES 1 *drowning and submersion while in swimming pool without fall (W67)*
√7th **W16.Ø22 Fall into swimming pool striking bottom causing other injury**
√6th **W16.Ø3 Fall into swimming pool striking wall**
√7th **W16.Ø31 Fall into swimming pool striking wall causing drowning and submersion**
EXCLUDES 1 *drowning and submersion while in swimming pool without fall (W67)*
√7th **W16.Ø32 Fall into swimming pool striking wall causing other injury**

√5th **W16.1 Fall into natural body of water**
Fall into lake
Fall into open sea
Fall into river
Fall into stream
√6th **W16.11 Fall into natural body of water striking water surface**
√7th **W16.111 Fall into natural body of water striking water surface causing drowning and submersion**
EXCLUDES 1 *drowning and submersion while in natural body of water without fall (W69)*
√7th **W16.112 Fall into natural body of water striking water surface causing other injury**
√6th **W16.12 Fall into natural body of water striking bottom**
√7th **W16.121 Fall into natural body of water striking bottom causing drowning and submersion**
EXCLUDES 1 *drowning and submersion while in natural body of water without fall (W69)*
√7th **W16.122 Fall into natural body of water striking bottom causing other injury**

W16.13 Fall into natural body of water striking side
W16.131 Fall into natural body of water striking side causing drowning and submersion
EXCLUDES 1 *drowning and submersion while in natural body of water without fall (W69)*
W16.132 Fall into natural body of water striking side causing other injury
W16.2 Fall in (into) filled bathtub or bucket of water
W16.21 Fall in (into) filled bathtub
EXCLUDES 1 *fall into empty bathtub (W18.2)*
W16.211 Fall in (into) filled bathtub causing drowning and submersion
EXCLUDES 1 *drowning and submersion while in filled bathtub without fall (W65)*
W16.212 Fall in (into) filled bathtub causing other injury
W16.22 Fall in (into) bucket of water
W16.221 Fall in (into) bucket of water causing drowning and submersion
W16.222 Fall in (into) bucket of water causing other injury
W16.3 Fall into other water
Fall into fountain Fall into reservoir
W16.31 Fall into other water striking water surface
W16.311 Fall into other water striking water surface causing drowning and submersion
EXCLUDES 1 *drowning and submersion while in other water without fall (W73)*
W16.312 Fall into other water striking water surface causing other injury
W16.32 Fall into other water striking bottom
W16.321 Fall into other water striking bottom causing drowning and submersion
EXCLUDES 1 *drowning and submersion while in other water without fall (W73)*
W16.322 Fall into other water striking bottom causing other injury
W16.33 Fall into other water striking wall
W16.331 Fall into other water striking wall causing drowning and submersion
EXCLUDES 1 *drowning and submersion while in other water without fall (W73)*
W16.332 Fall into other water striking wall causing other injury
W16.4 Fall into unspecified water
W16.41 Fall into unspecified water causing drowning and submersion
W16.42 Fall into unspecified water causing other injury
W16.5 Jumping or diving into swimming pool
W16.51 Jumping or diving into swimming pool striking water surface
W16.511 Jumping or diving into swimming pool striking water surface causing drowning and submersion
EXCLUDES 1 *drowning and submersion while in swimming pool without jumping or diving (W67)*
W16.512 Jumping or diving into swimming pool striking water surface causing other injury
W16.52 Jumping or diving into swimming pool striking bottom
W16.521 Jumping or diving into swimming pool striking bottom causing drowning and submersion
EXCLUDES 1 *drowning and submersion while in swimming pool without jumping or diving (W67)*
W16.522 Jumping or diving into swimming pool striking bottom causing other injury
W16.53 Jumping or diving into swimming pool striking wall
W16.531 Jumping or diving into swimming pool striking wall causing drowning and submersion
EXCLUDES 1 *drowning and submersion while in swimming pool without jumping or diving (W67)*
W16.532 Jumping or diving into swimming pool striking wall causing other injury
W16.6 Jumping or diving into natural body of water
Jumping or diving into lake
Jumping or diving into open sea
Jumping or diving into river
Jumping or diving into stream
W16.61 Jumping or diving into natural body of water striking water surface
W16.611 Jumping or diving into natural body of water striking water surface causing drowning and submersion
EXCLUDES 1 *drowning and submersion while in natural body of water without jumping or diving (W69)*
W16.612 Jumping or diving into natural body of water striking water surface causing other injury
W16.62 Jumping or diving into natural body of water striking bottom
W16.621 Jumping or diving into natural body of water striking bottom causing drowning and submersion
EXCLUDES 1 *drowning and submersion while in natural body of water without jumping or diving (W69)*
W16.622 Jumping or diving into natural body of water striking bottom causing other injury
W16.7 Jumping or diving from boat
EXCLUDES 1 *Fall from boat into water—see watercraft accident (V90-V94)*
W16.71 Jumping or diving from boat striking water surface
W16.711 Jumping or diving from boat striking water surface causing drowning and submersion
W16.712 Jumping or diving from boat striking water surface causing other injury
W16.72 Jumping or diving from boat striking bottom
W16.721 Jumping or diving from boat striking bottom causing drowning and submersion
W16.722 Jumping or diving from boat striking bottom causing other injury
W16.8 Jumping or diving into other water
Jumping or diving into fountain
Jumping or diving into reservoir
W16.81 Jumping or diving into other water striking water surface
W16.811 Jumping or diving into other water striking water surface causing drowning and submersion
EXCLUDES 1 *drowning and submersion while in other water without jumping or diving (W73)*
W16.812 Jumping or diving into other water striking water surface causing other injury
W16.82 Jumping or diving into other water striking bottom
W16.821 Jumping or diving into other water striking bottom causing drowning and submersion
EXCLUDES 1 *drowning and submersion while in other water without jumping or diving (W73)*
W16.822 Jumping or diving into other water striking bottom causing other injury
W16.83 Jumping or diving into other water striking wall
W16.831 Jumping or diving into other water striking wall causing drowning and submersion
EXCLUDES 1 *drowning and submersion while in other water without jumping or diving (W73)*

√7th **W16.832 Jumping or diving into other water striking wall causing other injury**

√5th **W16.9 Jumping or diving into unspecified water**

√x7th **W16.91 Jumping or diving into unspecified water causing drowning and submersion**

√x7th **W16.92 Jumping or diving into unspecified water causing other injury**

√4th **W17 Other fall from one level to another**

The appropriate 7th character is to be added to each code from category W17.
A initial encounter
D subsequent encounter
S sequela

√x7th **W17.0 Fall into well**

√x7th **W17.1 Fall into storm drain or manhole**

√x7th **W17.2 Fall into hole**
Fall into pit

√x7th **W17.3 Fall into empty swimming pool**
EXCLUDES 1 *fall into filled swimming pool (W16.0-)*

√x7th **W17.4 Fall from dock**

√5th **W17.8 Other fall from one level to another**

√x7th **W17.81 Fall down embankment (hill)**

√x7th **W17.82 Fall from (out of) grocery cart**
Fall due to grocery cart tipping over

√x7th **W17.89 Other fall from one level to another**
Fall from cherry picker
Fall from lifting device
Fall from mobile elevated work platform [MEWP]
Fall from sky lift

√4th **W18 Other slipping, tripping and stumbling and falls**

The appropriate 7th character is to be added to each code from category W18.
A initial encounter
D subsequent encounter
S sequela

√5th **W18.0 Fall due to bumping against object**
Striking against object with subsequent fall
EXCLUDES 1 *fall on same level due to slipping, tripping, or stumbling with subsequent striking against object (W01.1-)*

√x7th **W18.00 Striking against unspecified object with subsequent fall**

√x7th **W18.01 Striking against sports equipment with subsequent fall**

√x7th **W18.02 Striking against glass with subsequent fall**

√x7th **W18.09 Striking against other object with subsequent fall**

√5th **W18.1 Fall from or off toilet**

√x7th **W18.11 Fall from or off toilet without subsequent striking against object**
Fall from (off) toilet NOS

√x7th **W18.12 Fall from or off toilet with subsequent striking against object**

√x7th **W18.2 Fall in (into) shower or empty bathtub**
EXCLUDES 1 *fall in full bathtub causing drowning or submersion (W16.21-)*

√5th **W18.3 Other and unspecified fall on same level**

√x7th **W18.30 Fall on same level, unspecified**

√x7th **W18.31 Fall on same level due to stepping on an object**
Fall on same level due to stepping on an animal
EXCLUDES 1 *slipping, tripping and stumbling without fall due to stepping on animal (W18.41)*

√x7th **W18.39 Other fall on same level**

√5th **W18.4 Slipping, tripping and stumbling without falling**
EXCLUDES 1 *collision with another person without fall (W51)*

√x7th **W18.40 Slipping, tripping and stumbling without falling, unspecified**

√x7th **W18.41 Slipping, tripping and stumbling without falling due to stepping on object**
Slipping, tripping and stumbling without falling due to stepping on animal
EXCLUDES 1 *slipping, tripping and stumbling with fall due to stepping on animal (W18.31)*

√x7th **W18.42 Slipping, tripping and stumbling without falling due to stepping into hole or opening**

√x7th **W18.43 Slipping, tripping and stumbling without falling due to stepping from one level to another**

√x7th **W18.49 Other slipping, tripping and stumbling without falling**

√x7th **W19 Unspecified fall**
Accidental fall NOS
AHA: 2012, 4Q, 95

The appropriate 7th character is to be added to code W19.
A initial encounter
D subsequent encounter
S sequela

Exposure to inanimate mechanical forces (W20-W49)

EXCLUDES 1 *assault (X92-Y08)*
contact or collision with animals or persons (W50-W64)
exposure to inanimate mechanical forces involving military or war operations (Y36-, Y37-)
intentional self-harm (X71-X83)

√4th **W20 Struck by thrown, projected or falling object**
Code first any associated:
cataclysm (X34-X39)
lightning strike (T75.00)
EXCLUDES 1 *falling object in machinery accident (W24, W28-W31)*
falling object in transport accident (V01-V99)
object set in motion by explosion (W35-W40)
object set in motion by firearm (W32-W34)
struck by thrown sports equipment (W21.-)

The appropriate 7th character is to be added to each code from category W20.
A initial encounter
D subsequent encounter
S sequela

√x7th **W20.0 Struck by falling object in cave-in**
EXCLUDES 2 *asphyxiation due to cave-in (T71.21)*

√x7th **W20.1 Struck by object due to collapse of building**
EXCLUDES 1 *struck by object due to collapse of burning building (X00.2, X02.2)*

√x7th **W20.8 Other cause of strike by thrown, projected or falling object**
EXCLUDES 1 *struck by thrown sports equipment (W21.-)*

√4th **W21 Striking against or struck by sports equipment**
EXCLUDES 1 *assault with sports equipment (Y08.0-)*
striking against or struck by sports equipment with subsequent fall (W18.01)

The appropriate 7th character is to be added to each code from category W21.
A initial encounter
D subsequent encounter
S sequela

√5th **W21.0 Struck by hit or thrown ball**

√x7th **W21.00 Struck by hit or thrown ball, unspecified type**

√x7th **W21.01 Struck by football**

√x7th **W21.02 Struck by soccer ball**

√x7th **W21.03 Struck by baseball**

√x7th **W21.04 Struck by golf ball**

√x7th **W21.05 Struck by basketball**

√x7th **W21.06 Struck by volleyball**

√x7th **W21.07 Struck by softball**

√x7th **W21.09 Struck by other hit or thrown ball**

√5th **W21.1 Struck by bat, racquet or club**

√x7th **W21.11 Struck by baseball bat**

√x7th **W21.12 Struck by tennis racquet**

√x7th **W21.13 Struck by golf club**

√x7th **W21.19 Struck by other bat, racquet or club**

√5th **W21.2 Struck by hockey stick or puck**

√6th **W21.21 Struck by hockey stick**

√7th **W21.210 Struck by ice hockey stick**

√7th **W21.211 Struck by field hockey stick**

√6th **W21.22 Struck by hockey puck**

√7th **W21.220 Struck by ice hockey puck**

√7th **W21.221 Struck by field hockey puck**

√5th **W21.3 Struck by sports foot wear**

√x7th **W21.31 Struck by shoe cleats**
Stepped on by shoe cleats

√x7th **W21.32 Struck by skate blades**
Skated over by skate blades
√x7th **W21.39 Struck by other sports foot wear**
√x7th **W21.4 Striking against diving board**
Use additional code for subsequent falling into water, if applicable (W16.-)
√5th **W21.8 Striking against or struck by other sports equipment**
√x7th **W21.81 Striking against or struck by football helmet**
√x7th **W21.89 Striking against or struck by other sports equipment**
√x7th **W21.9 Striking against or struck by unspecified sports equipment**

√4th **W22 Striking against or struck by other objects**
EXCLUDES 1 *striking against or struck by object with subsequent fall (W18.09)*

The appropriate 7th character is to be added to each code from category W22.
A initial encounter
D subsequent encounter
S sequela

√5th **W22.0 Striking against stationary object**
EXCLUDES 1 *striking against stationary sports equipment (W21.8)*
√x7th **W22.01 Walked into wall**
√x7th **W22.02 Walked into lamppost**
√x7th **W22.03 Walked into furniture**
√6th **W22.04 Striking against wall of swimming pool**
√7th **W22.041 Striking against wall of swimming pool causing drowning and submersion**
EXCLUDES 1 *drowning and submersion while swimming without striking against wall (W67)*
√7th **W22.042 Striking against wall of swimming pool causing other injury**
√x7th **W22.09 Striking against other stationary object**
√5th **W22.1 Striking against or struck by automobile airbag**
√x7th **W22.10 Striking against or struck by unspecified automobile airbag**
√x7th **W22.11 Striking against or struck by driver side automobile airbag**
√x7th **W22.12 Striking against or struck by front passenger side automobile airbag**
√x7th **W22.19 Striking against or struck by other automobile airbag**
√x7th **W22.8 Striking against or struck by other objects**
Striking against or struck by object NOS
EXCLUDES 1 *struck by thrown, projected or falling object (W20.-)*

√4th **W23 Caught, crushed, jammed or pinched in or between objects**
EXCLUDES 1 *injury caused by cutting or piercing instruments (W25-W27)*
injury caused by firearms malfunction (W32.1, W33.1-, W34.1-)
injury caused by lifting and transmission devices (W24.-)
injury caused by machinery (W28-W31)
injury caused by nonpowered hand tools (W27.-)
injury caused by transport vehicle being used as a means of transportation (V01-V99)
injury caused by struck by thrown, projected or falling object (W20.-)

The appropriate 7th character is to be added to each code from category W23.
A initial encounter
D subsequent encounter
S sequela

√x7th **W23.0 Caught, crushed, jammed, or pinched between moving objects**
√x7th **W23.1 Caught, crushed, jammed, or pinched between stationary objects**

√4th **W24 Contact with lifting and transmission devices, not elsewhere classified**
EXCLUDES 1 *transport accidents (V01-V99)*

The appropriate 7th character is to be added to each code from category W24.
A initial encounter
D subsequent encounter
S sequela

√x7th **W24.0 Contact with lifting devices, not elsewhere classified**
Contact with chain hoist
Contact with drive belt
Contact with pulley (block)
√x7th **W24.1 Contact with transmission devices, not elsewhere classified**
Contact with transmission belt or cable

√x7th **W25 Contact with sharp glass**
Code first any associated:
injury due to flying glass from explosion or firearm discharge (W32-W40)
transport accident (V00-V99)
EXCLUDES 1 *fall on same level due to slipping, tripping and stumbling with subsequent striking against sharp glass (W01.10)*
striking against sharp glass with subsequent fall (W18.02)

The appropriate 7th character is to be added to code W25.
A initial encounter
D subsequent encounter
S sequela

√4th **W26 Contact with knife, sword or dagger**

The appropriate 7th character is to be added to each code from category W26.
A initial encounter
D subsequent encounter
S sequela

√x7th **W26.0 Contact with knife**
EXCLUDES 1 *contact with electric knife (W29.1)*
√x7th **W26.1 Contact with sword or dagger**

√4th **W27 Contact with nonpowered hand tool**

The appropriate 7th character is to be added to each code from category W27.
A initial encounter
D subsequent encounter
S sequela

√x7th **W27.0 Contact with workbench tool**
Contact with auger
Contact with axe
Contact with chisel
Contact with handsaw
Contact with screwdriver
√x7th **W27.1 Contact with garden tool**
Contact with hoe
Contact with nonpowered lawn mower
Contact with pitchfork
Contact with rake
√x7th **W27.2 Contact with scissors**
√x7th **W27.3 Contact with needle (sewing)**
EXCLUDES 1 *contact with hypodermic needle (W46.-)*
√x7th **W27.4 Contact with kitchen utensil**
Contact with fork
Contact with ice-pick
Contact with can-opener NOS
√x7th **W27.5 Contact with paper-cutter**
√x7th **W27.8 Contact with other nonpowered hand tool**
Contact with nonpowered sewing machine
Contact with shovel

√x7th **W28 Contact with powered lawn mower**
Powered lawn mower (commercial) (residential)
EXCLUDES 1 *contact with nonpowered lawn mower (W27.1)*
EXCLUDES 2 *exposure to electric current (W86.-)*

The appropriate 7th character is to be added to code W28.
A initial encounter
D subsequent encounter
S sequela

√4th **W29 Contact with other powered hand tools and household machinery**
EXCLUDES 1 *contact with commercial machinery (W31.82)*
contact with hot household appliance (X15)
contact with nonpowered hand tool (W27.-)
exposure to electric current (W86)

The appropriate 7th character is to be added to each code from category W29.
A initial encounter
D subsequent encounter
S sequela

√x7th **W29.0 Contact with powered kitchen appliance**
Contact with blender
Contact with can-opener
Contact with garbage disposal
Contact with mixer
√x7th **W29.1 Contact with electric knife**

√x7th **W29.2 Contact with other powered household machinery**
Contact with electric fan
Contact with powered dryer (clothes) (powered) (spin)
Contact with washing-machine
Contact with sewing machine

√x7th **W29.3 Contact with powered garden and outdoor hand tools and machinery**
Contact with chainsaw
Contact with edger
Contact with garden cultivator (tiller)
Contact with hedge trimmer
Contact with other powered garden tool
EXCLUDES 1 *contact with powered lawn mower (W28)*

√x7th **W29.4 Contact with nail gun**

√x7th **W29.8 Contact with other powered powered hand tools and household machinery**
Contact with do-it-yourself tool NOS

√4th **W3Ø Contact with agricultural machinery**
INCLUDES animal-powered farm machine
EXCLUDES 1 *agricultural transport vehicle accident (VØ1-V99)*
explosion of grain store (W4Ø.8)
exposure to electric current (W86.-)

The appropriate 7th character is to be added to each code from category W3Ø.
A initial encounter
D subsequent encounter
S sequela

√x7th **W3Ø.Ø Contact with combine harvester**
Contact with reaper
Contact with thresher

√x7th **W3Ø.1 Contact with power take-off devices (PTO)**

√x7th **W3Ø.2 Contact with hay derrick**

√x7th **W3Ø.3 Contact with grain storage elevator**
EXCLUDES 1 *explosion of grain store (W4Ø.8)*

√5th **W3Ø.8 Contact with other specified agricultural machinery**

√x7th **W3Ø.81 Contact with agricultural transport vehicle in stationary use**
Contact with agricultural transport vehicle under repair, not on public roadway
EXCLUDES 1 *agricultural transport vehicle accident (VØ1-V99)*

√x7th **W3Ø.89 Contact with other specified agricultural machinery**

√x7th **W3Ø.9 Contact with unspecified agricultural machinery**
Contact with farm machinery NOS

√4th **W31 Contact with other and unspecified machinery**
EXCLUDES 1 *contact with agricultural machinery (W3Ø.-)*
contact with machinery in transport under own power or being towed by a vehicle (VØ1-V99)
exposure to electric current (W86)

The appropriate 7th character is to be added to each code from category W31.
A initial encounter
D subsequent encounter
S sequela

√x7th **W31.Ø Contact with mining and earth-drilling machinery**
Contact with bore or drill (land) (seabed)
Contact with shaft hoist
Contact with shaft lift
Contact with undercutter

√x7th **W31.1 Contact with metalworking machines**
Contact with abrasive wheel
Contact with forging machine
Contact with lathe
Contact with mechanical shears
Contact with metal drilling machine
Contact with milling machine
Contact with power press
Contact with rolling-mill
Contact with metal sawing machine

√x7th **W31.2 Contact with powered woodworking and forming machines**
Contact with band saw
Contact with bench saw
Contact with circular saw
Contact with molding machine
Contact with overhead plane
Contact with powered saw
Contact with radial saw
Contact with sander
EXCLUDES 1 *nonpowered woodworking tools (W27.Ø)*

√x7th **W31.3 Contact with prime movers**
Contact with gas turbine
Contact with internal combustion engine
Contact with steam engine
Contact with water driven turbine

√5th **W31.8 Contact with other specified machinery**

√x7th **W31.81 Contact with recreational machinery**
Contact with roller coaster

√x7th **W31.82 Contact with other commercial machinery**
Contact with commercial electric fan
Contact with commercial kitchen appliances
Contact with commercial powered dryer (clothes) (powered) (spin)
Contact with commercial washing-machine
Contact with commercial sewing machine
EXCLUDES 1 *contact with household machinery (W29.-)*
contact with powered lawn mower (W28)

√x7th **W31.83 Contact with special construction vehicle in stationary use**
Contact with special construction vehicle under repair, not on public roadway
EXCLUDES 1 *special construction vehicle accident (VØ1-V99)*

√x7th **W31.89 Contact with other specified machinery**

√x7th **W31.9 Contact with unspecified machinery**
Contact with machinery NOS

√4th **W32 Accidental handgun discharge and malfunction**
INCLUDES accidental discharge and malfunction of gun for single hand use
accidental discharge and malfunction of pistol
accidental discharge and malfunction of revolver
handgun discharge and malfunction NOS
EXCLUDES 1 *accidental airgun discharge and malfunction (W34.Ø1Ø, W34.11Ø)*
accidental BB gun discharge and malfunction (W34.Ø1Ø, W34.11Ø)
accidental pellet gun discharge and malfunction (W34.Ø1Ø, W34.11Ø)
accidental shotgun discharge and malfunction (W33.Ø1, W33.11)
assault by handgun discharge (X93)
handgun discharge involving legal intervention (Y35.Ø-)
handgun discharge involving military or war operations (Y36.4-)
intentional self-harm by handgun discharge (X72)
Very pistol discharge and malfunction (W34.Ø9, W34.19)

The appropriate 7th character is to be added to each code from category W32.
A initial encounter
D subsequent encounter
S sequela

√x7th **W32.Ø Accidental handgun discharge**

√x7th **W32.1 Accidental handgun malfunction**
Injury due to explosion of handgun (parts)
Injury due to malfunction of mechanism or component of handgun
Injury due to recoil of handgun
Powder burn from handgun

√4th **W33 Accidental rifle, shotgun and larger firearm discharge and malfunction**
INCLUDES rifle, shotgun and larger firearm discharge and malfunction NOS
EXCLUDES 1 *accidental airgun discharge and malfunction (W34.Ø1Ø, W34.11Ø)*
accidental BB gun discharge and malfunction (W34.Ø1Ø, W34.11Ø)
accidental handgun discharge and malfunction (W32.-)
accidental pellet gun discharge and malfunction (W34.Ø1Ø, W34.11Ø)
assault by rifle, shotgun and larger firearm discharge (X94)
firearm discharge involving legal intervention (Y35.Ø-)
firearm discharge involving military or war operations (Y36.4-)
intentional self-harm by rifle, shotgun and larger firearm discharge (X73)

The appropriate 7th character is to be added to each code from category W33.
A initial encounter
D subsequent encounter
S sequela

W33.Ø Accidental rifle, shotgun and larger firearm discharge
W33.ØØ Accidental discharge of unspecified larger firearm
Discharge of unspecified larger firearm NOS
W33.Ø1 Accidental discharge of shotgun
Discharge of shotgun NOS
W33.Ø2 Accidental discharge of hunting rifle
Discharge of hunting rifle NOS
W33.Ø3 Accidental discharge of machine gun
Discharge of machine gun NOS
W33.Ø9 Accidental discharge of other larger firearm
Discharge of other larger firearm NOS
W33.1 Accidental rifle, shotgun and larger firearm malfunction
Injury due to explosion of rifle, shotgun and larger firearm (parts)
Injury due to malfunction of mechanism or component of rifle, shotgun and larger firearm
Injury due to piercing, cutting, crushing or pinching due to (by) slide trigger mechanism, scope or other gun part
Injury due to recoil of rifle, shotgun and larger firearm
Powder burn from rifle, shotgun and larger firearm
W33.1Ø Accidental malfunction of unspecified larger firearm
Malfunction of unspecified larger firearm NOS
W33.11 Accidental malfunction of shotgun
Malfunction of shotgun NOS
W33.12 Accidental malfunction of hunting rifle
Malfunction of hunting rifle NOS
W33.13 Accidental malfunction of machine gun
Malfunction of machine gun NOS
W33.19 Accidental malfunction of other larger firearm
Malfunction of other larger firearm NOS

W34 Accidental discharge and malfunction from other and unspecified firearms and guns

The appropriate 7th character is to be added to each code from category W34.
A initial encounter
D subsequent encounter
S sequela

W34.Ø Accidental discharge from other and unspecified firearms and guns
W34.ØØ Accidental discharge from unspecified firearms or gun
Discharge from firearm NOS
Gunshot wound NOS
Shot NOS
W34.Ø1 Accidental discharge of gas, air or spring-operated guns
W34.Ø1Ø Accidental discharge of airgun
Accidental discharge of BB gun
Accidental discharge of pellet gun
W34.Ø11 Accidental discharge of paintball gun
Accidental injury due to paintball discharge
W34.Ø18 Accidental discharge of other gas, air or spring-operated gun
W34.Ø9 Accidental discharge from other specified firearms
Accidental discharge from Very pistol [flare]
W34.1 Accidental malfunction from other and unspecified firearms and guns
W34.1Ø Accidental malfunction from unspecified firearms or gun
Firearm malfunction NOS
W34.11 Accidental malfunction of gas, air or spring-operated guns
W34.11Ø Accidental malfunction of airgun
Accidental malfunction of BB gun
Accidental malfunction of pellet gun
W34.111 Accidental malfunction of paintball gun
Accidental injury due to paintball gun malfunction
W34.118 Accidental malfunction of other gas, air or spring-operated gun
W34.19 Accidental malfunction from other specified firearms
Accidental malfunction from Very pistol [flare]

W35 Explosion and rupture of boiler
EXCLUDES 1 *explosion and rupture of boiler on watercraft (V93.4)*

The appropriate 7th character is to be added to code W35.
A initial encounter
D subsequent encounter
S sequela

W36 Explosion and rupture of gas cylinder

The appropriate 7th character is to be added to each code from category W36.
A initial encounter
D subsequent encounter
S sequela

W36.1 Explosion and rupture of aerosol can
W36.2 Explosion and rupture of air tank
W36.3 Explosion and rupture of pressurized-gas tank
W36.8 Explosion and rupture of other gas cylinder
W36.9 Explosion and rupture of unspecified gas cylinder

W37 Explosion and rupture of pressurized tire, pipe or hose

The appropriate 7th character is to be added to each code from category W37.
A initial encounter
D subsequent encounter
S sequela

W37.Ø Explosion of bicycle tire
W37.8 Explosion and rupture of other pressurized tire, pipe or hose

W38 Explosion and rupture of other specified pressurized devices

The appropriate 7th character is to be added to code W38.
A initial encounter
D subsequent encounter
S sequela

W39 Discharge of firework

The appropriate 7th character is to be added to code W39.
A initial encounter
D subsequent encounter
S sequela

W4Ø Explosion of other materials
EXCLUDES 1 *assault by explosive material (X96)*
explosion involving legal intervention (Y35.1-)
explosion involving military or war operations (Y36.Ø-, Y36.2-)
intentional self-harm by explosive material (X75)

The appropriate 7th character is to be added to each code from category W4Ø.
A initial encounter
D subsequent encounter
S sequela

W4Ø.Ø Explosion of blasting material
Explosion of blasting cap
Explosion of detonator
Explosion of dynamite
Explosion of explosive (any) used in blasting operations
W4Ø.1 Explosion of explosive gases
Explosion of acetylene
Explosion of butane
Explosion of coal gas
Explosion in mine NOS
Explosion of explosive gas
Explosion of fire damp
Explosion of gasoline fumes
Explosion of methane
Explosion of propane
W4Ø.8 Explosion of other specified explosive materials
Explosion in dump NOS
Explosion in factory NOS
Explosion in grain store
Explosion in munitions
EXCLUDES 1 *explosion involving legal intervention (Y35.1-)*
explosion involving military or war operations (Y36.Ø-, Y36.2-)
W4Ø.9 Explosion of unspecified explosive materials
Explosion NOS

W42 Exposure to noise

The appropriate 7th character is to be added to each code from category W42.
A initial encounter
D subsequent encounter
S sequela

W42.Ø Exposure to supersonic waves
W42.9 Exposure to other noise
Exposure to sound waves NOS

W45 Foreign body or object entering through skin

EXCLUDES 2 *contact with hand tools (nonpowered) (powered) (W27-W29)*
contact with knife, sword or dagger (W26.-)
contact with sharp glass (W25.-)
struck by objects (W20-W22)

The appropriate 7th character is to be added to each code from category W45.
A initial encounter
D subsequent encounter
S sequela

W45.0 Nail entering through skin

W45.1 Paper entering through skin
Paper cut

W45.2 Lid of can entering through skin

W45.8 Other foreign body or object entering through skin
Splinter in skin NOS

W46 Contact with hypodermic needle

The appropriate 7th character is to be added to each code from category W46.
A initial encounter
D subsequent encounter
S sequela

W46.0 Contact with hypodermic needle
Hypodermic needle stick NOS

W46.1 Contact with contaminated hypodermic needle

W49 Exposure to other inanimate mechanical forces

INCLUDES exposure to abnormal gravitational [G] forces
exposure to inanimate mechanical forces NEC

EXCLUDES 1 *exposure to inanimate mechanical forces involving military or war operations (Y36.-, Y37.-)*

The appropriate 7th character is to be added to each code from category W49.
A initial encounter
D subsequent encounter
S sequela

W49.0 Item causing external constriction
- **W49.01 Hair causing external constriction**
- **W49.02 String or thread causing external constriction**
- **W49.03 Rubber band causing external constriction**
- **W49.04 Ring or other jewelry causing external constriction**
- **W49.09 Other specified item causing external constriction**

W49.9 Exposure to other inanimate mechanical forces

Exposure to animate mechanical forces (W50-W64)

EXCLUDES 1 *Toxic effect of contact with venomous animals and plants (T63.-)*

W50 Accidental hit, strike, kick, twist, bite or scratch by another person
Hit, strike, kick, twist, bite, or scratch by another person NOS

EXCLUDES 1 *assault by bodily force (Y04)*
struck by objects (W20-W22)

The appropriate 7th character is to be added to each code from category W50.
A initial encounter
D subsequent encounter
S sequela

W50.0 Accidental hit or strike by another person
Hit or strike by another person NOS

W50.1 Accidental kick by another person
Kick by another person NOS

W50.2 Accidental twist by another person
Twist by another person NOS

W50.3 Accidental bite by another person
Human bite
Bite by another person NOS

W50.4 Accidental scratch by another person
Scratch by another person NOS

W51 Accidental striking against or bumped into by another person

EXCLUDES 1 *assault by striking against or bumping into by another person (Y04.2)*
fall due to collision with another person (W03)

The appropriate 7th character is to be added to code W51.
A initial encounter
D subsequent encounter
S sequela

W52 Crushed, pushed or stepped on by crowd or human stampede
Crushed, pushed or stepped on by crowd or human stampede with or without fall

The appropriate 7th character is to be added to code W52.
A initial encounter
D subsequent encounter
S sequela

W53 Contact with rodent

INCLUDES Contact with saliva, feces or urine of rodent

The appropriate 7th character is to be added to each code from category W53.
A initial encounter
D subsequent encounter
S sequela

W53.0 Contact with mouse
- **W53.01 Bitten by mouse**
- **W53.09 Other contact with mouse**

W53.1 Contact with rat
- **W53.11 Bitten by rat**
- **W53.19 Other contact with rat**

W53.2 Contact with squirrel
- **W53.21 Bitten by squirrel**
- **W53.29 Other contact with squirrel**

W53.8 Contact with other rodent
- **W53.81 Bitten by other rodent**
- **W53.89 Other contact with other rodent**

W54 Contact with dog

INCLUDES Contact with saliva, feces or urine of dog

The appropriate 7th character is to be added to each code from category W54.
A initial encounter
D subsequent encounter
S sequela

W54.0 Bitten by dog

W54.1 Struck by dog
Knocked over by dog

W54.8 Other contact with dog

W55 Contact with other mammals

INCLUDES Contact with saliva, feces or urine of mammal

EXCLUDES 1 *animal being ridden—see transport accidents*
bitten or struck by dog (W54)
bitten or struck by rodent (W53.-)
contact with marine mammals (W56.-)

The appropriate 7th character is to be added to each code from category W55.
A initial encounter
D subsequent encounter
S sequela

W55.0 Contact with cat
- **W55.01 Bitten by cat**
- **W55.03 Scratched by cat**
- **W55.09 Other contact with cat**

W55.1 Contact with horse
- **W55.11 Bitten by horse**
- **W55.12 Struck by horse**
- **W55.19 Other contact with horse**

W55.2 Contact with cow
Contact with bull
- **W55.21 Bitten by cow**
- **W55.22 Struck by cow**
  Gored by bull
- **W55.29 Other contact with cow**

W55.3 Contact with other hoof stock
Contact with goats
Contact with sheep
- **W55.31 Bitten by other hoof stock**
- **W55.32 Struck by other hoof stock**
  Gored by goat
  Gored by ram
- **W55.39 Other contact with other hoof stock**

W55.4 Contact with pig
- **W55.41 Bitten by pig**
- **W55.42 Struck by pig**
- **W55.49 Other contact with pig**

W55.5 Contact with raccoon
- **W55.51 Bitten by raccoon**

W55.52 Struck by raccoon
W55.59 Other contact with raccoon

W55.8 Contact with other mammals
W55.81 Bitten by other mammals
W55.82 Struck by other mammals
W55.89 Other contact with other mammals

W56 Contact with nonvenomous marine animal
EXCLUDES 1 *contact with venomous marine animal (T63.-)*

The appropriate 7th character is to be added to each code from category W56.
A initial encounter
D subsequent encounter
S sequela

W56.0 Contact with dolphin
W56.01 Bitten by dolphin
W56.02 Struck by dolphin
W56.09 Other contact with dolphin

W56.1 Contact with sea lion
W56.11 Bitten by sea lion
W56.12 Struck by sea lion
W56.19 Other contact with sea lion

W56.2 Contact with orca
Contact with killer whale
W56.21 Bitten by orca
W56.22 Struck by orca
W56.29 Other contact with orca

W56.3 Contact with other marine mammals
W56.31 Bitten by other marine mammals
W56.32 Struck by other marine mammals
W56.39 Other contact with other marine mammals

W56.4 Contact with shark
W56.41 Bitten by shark
W56.42 Struck by shark
W56.49 Other contact with shark

W56.5 Contact with other fish
W56.51 Bitten by other fish
W56.52 Struck by other fish
W56.59 Other contact with other fish

W56.8 Contact with other nonvenomous marine animals
W56.81 Bitten by other nonvenomous marine animals
W56.82 Struck by other nonvenomous marine animals
W56.89 Other contact with other nonvenomous marine animals

W57 Bitten or stung by nonvenomous insect and other nonvenomous arthropods
EXCLUDES 1 *contact with venomous insects and arthropods (T63.2-, T63.3-, T63.4-)*

The appropriate 7th character is to be added to code W57.
A initial encounter
D subsequent encounter
S sequela

W58 Contact with crocodile or alligator

The appropriate 7th character is to be added to each code from category W58.
A initial encounter
D subsequent encounter
S sequela

W58.0 Contact with alligator
W58.01 Bitten by alligator
W58.02 Struck by alligator
W58.03 Crushed by alligator
W58.09 Other contact with alligator

W58.1 Contact with crocodile
W58.11 Bitten by crocodile
W58.12 Struck by crocodile
W58.13 Crushed by crocodile
W58.19 Other contact with crocodile

W59 Contact with other nonvenomous reptiles
EXCLUDES 1 *contact with venomous reptile (T63.0-, T63.1-)*

The appropriate 7th character is to be added to each code from category W59.
A initial encounter
D subsequent encounter
S sequela

W59.0 Contact with nonvenomous lizards
W59.01 Bitten by nonvenomous lizards
W59.02 Struck by nonvenomous lizards
W59.09 Other contact with nonvenomous lizards
Exposure to nonvenomous lizards

W59.1 Contact with nonvenomous snakes
W59.11 Bitten by nonvenomous snake
W59.12 Struck by nonvenomous snake
W59.13 Crushed by nonvenomous snake
W59.19 Other contact with nonvenomous snake

W59.2 Contact with turtles
EXCLUDES 1 *contact with tortoises (W59.8-)*
W59.21 Bitten by turtle
W59.22 Struck by turtle
W59.29 Other contact with turtle
Exposure to turtles

W59.8 Contact with other nonvenomous reptiles
W59.81 Bitten by other nonvenomous reptiles
W59.82 Struck by other nonvenomous reptiles
W59.83 Crushed by other nonvenomous reptiles
W59.89 Other contact with other nonvenomous reptiles

W60 Contact with nonvenomous plant thorns and spines and sharp leaves
EXCLUDES 1 *contact with venomous plants (T63.7-)*

The appropriate 7th character is to be added to code W60.
A initial encounter
D subsequent encounter
S sequela

W61 Contact with birds (domestic) (wild)
INCLUDES contact with excreta of birds

The appropriate 7th character is to be added to each code from category W61.
A initial encounter
D subsequent encounter
S sequela

W61.0 Contact with parrot
W61.01 Bitten by parrot
W61.02 Struck by parrot
W61.09 Other contact with parrot
Exposure to parrots

W61.1 Contact with macaw
W61.11 Bitten by macaw
W61.12 Struck by macaw
W61.19 Other contact with macaw
Exposure to macaws

W61.2 Contact with other psittacines
W61.21 Bitten by other psittacines
W61.22 Struck by other psittacines
W61.29 Other contact with other psittacines
Exposure to other psittacines

W61.3 Contact with chicken
W61.32 Struck by chicken
W61.33 Pecked by chicken
W61.39 Other contact with chicken
Exposure to chickens

W61.4 Contact with turkey
W61.42 Struck by turkey
W61.43 Pecked by turkey
W61.49 Other contact with turkey

W61.5 Contact with goose
W61.51 Bitten by goose
W61.52 Struck by goose
W61.59 Other contact with goose

W61.6 Contact with duck
W61.61 Bitten by duck
W61.62 Struck by duck
W61.69 Other contact with duck

√5th **W61.9 Contact with other birds**

√x7th **W61.91 Bitten by other birds**

√x7th **W61.92 Struck by other birds**

√x7th **W61.99 Other contact with other birds**

Contact with bird NOS

√4th **W62 Contact with nonvenomous amphibians**

EXCLUDES 1 *contact with venomous amphibians (T63.81-R63.83)*

The appropriate 7th character is to be added to each code from category W62.
A initial encounter
D subsequent encounter
S sequela

√x7th **W62.0 Contact with nonvenomous frogs**

√x7th **W62.1 Contact with nonvenomous toads**

√x7th **W62.9 Contact with other nonvenomous amphibians**

√x7th **W64 Exposure to other animate mechanical forces**

INCLUDES exposure to nonvenomous animal NOS

EXCLUDES 1 *contact with venomous animal (T63.-)*

The appropriate 7th character is to be added to code W64.
A initial encounter
D subsequent encounter
S sequela

Accidental non-transport drowning and submersion (W65-W74)

EXCLUDES 1 *accidental drowning and submersion due to fall into water (W16.-)*
accidental drowning and submersion due to water transport accident (V90.-, V92.-)

EXCLUDES 2 *accidental drowning and submersion due to cataclysm (X34-X39)*

√x7th **W65 Accidental drowning and submersion while in bath-tub**

EXCLUDES 1 *accidental drowning and submersion due to fall in (into) bathtub (W16.211)*

The appropriate 7th character is to be added to code W65.
A initial encounter
D subsequent encounter
S sequela

√x7th **W67 Accidental drowning and submersion while in swimming-pool**

EXCLUDES 1 *accidental drowning and submersion due to fall into swimming pool (W16.011, W16.021, W16.031)*
accidental drowning and submersion due to striking into wall of swimming pool (W22.041)

The appropriate 7th character is to be added to code W67.
A initial encounter
D subsequent encounter
S sequela

√x7th **W69 Accidental drowning and submersion while in natural water**

Accidental drowning and submersion while in lake
Accidental drowning and submersion while in open sea
Accidental drowning and submersion while in river
Accidental drowning and submersion while in stream

EXCLUDES 1 *accidental drowning and submersion due to fall into natural body of water (W16.111, W16.121, W16.131)*

The appropriate 7th character is to be added to code W69.
A initial encounter
D subsequent encounter
S sequela

√x7th **W73 Other specified cause of accidental non-transport drowning and submersion**

Accidental drowning and submersion while in quenching tank
Accidental drowning and submersion while in reservoir

EXCLUDES 1 *accidental drowning and submersion due to fall into other water (W16.311, W16.321, W16.331)*

The appropriate 7th character is to be added to code W73.
A initial encounter
D subsequent encounter
S sequela

√x7th **W74 Unspecified cause of accidental drowning and submersion**

Drowning NOS

The appropriate 7th character is to be added to code W74.
A initial encounter
D subsequent encounter
S sequela

Exposure to electric current, radiation and extreme ambient air temperature and pressure (W85-W99)

EXCLUDES 1 *exposure to:*
failure in dosage of radiation or temperature during surgical and medical care (Y63.2-Y63.5)
lightning (T75.0-)
natural cold (X31)
natural heat (X30)
natural radiation NOS (X39)
radiological procedure and radiotherapy (Y84.2)
sunlight (X32)

√x7th **W85 Exposure to electric transmission lines**

Broken power line

The appropriate 7th character is to be added to code W85.
A initial encounter
D subsequent encounter
S sequela

√4th **W86 Exposure to other specified electric current**

The appropriate 7th character is to be added to each code from category W86.
A initial encounter
D subsequent encounter
S sequela

√x7th **W86.0 Exposure to domestic wiring and appliances**

√x7th **W86.1 Exposure to industrial wiring, appliances and electrical machinery**

Exposure to conductors
Exposure to control apparatus
Exposure to electrical equipment and machinery
Exposure to transformers

√x7th **W86.8 Exposure to other electric current**

Exposure to wiring and appliances in or on farm (not farmhouse)
Exposure to wiring and appliances outdoors
Exposure to wiring and appliances in or on public building
Exposure to wiring and appliances in or on residential institutions
Exposure to wiring and appliances in or on schools

√4th **W88 Exposure to ionizing radiation**

EXCLUDES 1 *exposure to sunlight (X32)*

The appropriate 7th character is to be added to each code from category W88.
A initial encounter
D subsequent encounter
S sequela

√x7th **W88.0 Exposure to X-rays**

√x7th **W88.1 Exposure to radioactive isotopes**

√x7th **W88.8 Exposure to other ionizing radiation**

√4th **W89 Exposure to man-made visible and ultraviolet light**

INCLUDES exposure to welding light (arc)

EXCLUDES 2 *exposure to sunlight (X32)*

The appropriate 7th character is to be added to each code from category W89.
A initial encounter
D subsequent encounter
S sequela

√x7th **W89.0 Exposure to welding light (arc)**

√x7th **W89.1 Exposure to tanning bed**

√x7th **W89.8 Exposure to other man-made visible and ultraviolet light**

√x7th **W89.9 Exposure to unspecified man-made visible and ultraviolet light**

√4th **W90 Exposure to other nonionizing radiation**

EXCLUDES 1 *exposure to sunlight (X32)*

The appropriate 7th character is to be added to each code from category W90.
A initial encounter
D subsequent encounter
S sequela

√x7th **W90.0 Exposure to radiofrequency**

√x7th **W90.1 Exposure to infrared radiation**

√x7th **W90.2 Exposure to laser radiation**

√x7th **W90.8 Exposure to other nonionizing radiation**

√x7th **W92 Exposure to excessive heat of man-made origin**

The appropriate 7th character is to be added to code W92.
A initial encounter
D subsequent encounter
S sequela

√4th **W93 Exposure to excessive cold of man-made origin**

The appropriate 7th character is to be added to each code from category W93.
A initial encounter
D subsequent encounter
S sequela

√5th **W93.0 Contact with or inhalation of dry ice**
√x7th **W93.01 Contact with dry ice**
√x7th **W93.02 Inhalation of dry ice**
√5th **W93.1 Contact with or inhalation of liquid air**
√x7th **W93.11 Contact with liquid air**
Contact with liquid hydrogen
Contact with liquid nitrogen
√x7th **W93.12 Inhalation of liquid air**
Inhalation of liquid hydrogen
Inhalation of liquid nitrogen
√x7th **W93.2 Prolonged exposure in deep freeze unit or refrigerator**
√x7th **W93.8 Exposure to other excessive cold of man-made origin**

√4th **W94 Exposure to high and low air pressure and changes in air pressure**

The appropriate 7th character is to be added to each code from category W94.
A initial encounter
D subsequent encounter
S sequela

√x7th **W94.0 Exposure to prolonged high air pressure**
√5th **W94.1 Exposure to prolonged low air pressure**
√x7th **W94.11 Exposure to residence or prolonged visit at high altitude**
√x7th **W94.12 Exposure to other prolonged low air pressure**
√5th **W94.2 Exposure to rapid changes in air pressure during ascent**
√x7th **W94.21 Exposure to reduction in atmospheric pressure while surfacing from deep-water diving**
√x7th **W94.22 Exposure to reduction in atmospheric pressure while surfacing from underground**
√x7th **W94.23 Exposure to sudden change in air pressure in aircraft during ascent**
√x7th **W94.29 Exposure to other rapid changes in air pressure during ascent**
√5th **W94.3 Exposure to rapid changes in air pressure during descent**
√x7th **W94.31 Exposure to sudden change in air pressure in aircraft during descent**
√x7th **W94.32 Exposure to high air pressure from rapid descent in water**
√x7th **W94.39 Exposure to other rapid changes in air pressure during descent**

√x7th **W99 Exposure to other man-made environmental factors**

The appropriate 7th character is to be added to code W99.
A initial encounter
D subsequent encounter
S sequela

Exposure to smoke, fire and flames (X00-X08)

EXCLUDES 1 *arson (X97)*
EXCLUDES 2 *explosions (W35-W40)*
lightning (T75.0-)
transport accident (V01-V99)

√4th **X00 Exposure to uncontrolled fire in building or structure**
INCLUDES conflagration in building or structure
Code first any associated cataclysm
EXCLUDES 2 *exposure to ignition or melting of nightwear (X05)*
exposure to ignition or melting of other clothing and apparel (X06.-)
exposure to other specified smoke, fire and flames (X08.-)

The appropriate 7th character is to be added to each code from category X00.
A initial encounter
D subsequent encounter
S sequela

√x7th **X00.0 Exposure to flames in uncontrolled fire in building or structure**
√x7th **X00.1 Exposure to smoke in uncontrolled fire in building or structure**
√x7th **X00.2 Injury due to collapse of burning building or structure in uncontrolled fire**
EXCLUDES 1 *injury due to collapse of building not on fire (W20.1)*
√x7th **X00.3 Fall from burning building or structure in uncontrolled fire**
√x7th **X00.4 Hit by object from burning building or structure in uncontrolled fire**
√x7th **X00.5 Jump from burning building or structure in uncontrolled fire**
√x7th **X00.8 Other exposure to uncontrolled fire in building or structure**

√4th **X01 Exposure to uncontrolled fire, not in building or structure**
INCLUDES exposure to forest fire

The appropriate 7th character is to be added to each code from category X01.
A initial encounter
D subsequent encounter
S sequela

√x7th **X01.0 Exposure to flames in uncontrolled fire, not in building or structure**
√x7th **X01.1 Exposure to smoke in uncontrolled fire, not in building or structure**
√x7th **X01.3 Fall due to uncontrolled fire, not in building or structure**
√x7th **X01.4 Hit by object due to uncontrolled fire, not in building or structure**
√x7th **X01.8 Other exposure to uncontrolled fire, not in building or structure**

√4th **X02 Exposure to controlled fire in building or structure**
INCLUDES exposure to fire in fireplace
exposure to fire in stove

The appropriate 7th character is to be added to each code from category X02.
A initial encounter
D subsequent encounter
S sequela

√x7th **X02.0 Exposure to flames in controlled fire in building or structure**
√x7th **X02.1 Exposure to smoke in controlled fire in building or structure**
√x7th **X02.2 Injury due to collapse of burning building or structure in controlled fire**
EXCLUDES 1 *injury due to collapse of building not on fire (W20.1)*
√x7th **X02.3 Fall from burning building or structure in controlled fire**
√x7th **X02.4 Hit by object from burning building or structure in controlled fire**
√x7th **X02.5 Jump from burning building or structure in controlled fire**
√x7th **X02.8 Other exposure to controlled fire in building or structure**

√4th **X03 Exposure to controlled fire, not in building or structure**
INCLUDES exposure to bon fire
exposure to camp-fire
exposure to trash fire

The appropriate 7th character is to be added to each code from category X03.
A initial encounter
D subsequent encounter
S sequela

√x7th **X03.0 Exposure to flames in controlled fire, not in building or structure**
√x7th **X03.1 Exposure to smoke in controlled fire, not in building or structure**
√x7th **X03.3 Fall due to controlled fire, not in building or structure**
√x7th **X03.4 Hit by object due to controlled fire, not in building or structure**
√x7th **X03.8 Other exposure to controlled fire, not in building or structure**

XØ4 Exposure to ignition of highly flammable material
Exposure to ignition of gasoline
Exposure to ignition of kerosene
Exposure to ignition of petrol
EXCLUDES 2 *exposure to ignition or melting of nightwear (XØ5)*
exposure to ignition or melting of other clothing and apparel (XØ6)

The appropriate 7th character is to be added to code XØ4.
A initial encounter
D subsequent encounter
S sequela

XØ5 Exposure to ignition or melting of nightwear
EXCLUDES 2 *exposure to uncontrolled fire in building or structure (XØØ.-)*
exposure to uncontrolled fire, not in building or structure (XØ1.-)
exposure to controlled fire in building or structure (XØ2.-)
exposure to controlled fire, not in building or structure (XØ3.-)
exposure to ignition of highly flammable materials (XØ4.-)

The appropriate 7th character is to be added to code XØ5.
A initial encounter
D subsequent encounter
S sequela

XØ6 Exposure to ignition or melting of other clothing and apparel
EXCLUDES 2 *exposure to uncontrolled fire in building or structure (XØØ.-)*
exposure to uncontrolled fire, not in building or structure (XØ1.-)
exposure to controlled fire in building or structure (XØ2.-)
exposure to controlled fire, not in building or structure (XØ3.-)
exposure to ignition of highly flammable materials (XØ4.-)

The appropriate 7th character is to be added to each code from category XØ6.
A initial encounter
D subsequent encounter
S sequela

XØ6.Ø Exposure to ignition of plastic jewelry
XØ6.1 Exposure to melting of plastic jewelry
XØ6.2 Exposure to ignition of other clothing and apparel
XØ6.3 Exposure to melting of other clothing and apparel

XØ8 Exposure to other specified smoke, fire and flames

The appropriate 7th character is to be added to each code from category XØ8.
A initial encounter
D subsequent encounter
S sequela

XØ8.Ø Exposure to bed fire
Exposure to mattress fire
XØ8.ØØ Exposure to bed fire due to unspecified burning material
XØ8.Ø1 Exposure to bed fire due to burning cigarette
XØ8.Ø9 Exposure to bed fire due to other burning material
XØ8.1 Exposure to sofa fire
XØ8.1Ø Exposure to sofa fire due to unspecified burning material
XØ8.11 Exposure to sofa fire due to burning cigarette
XØ8.19 Exposure to sofa fire due to other burning material
XØ8.2 Exposure to other furniture fire
XØ8.2Ø Exposure to other furniture fire due to unspecified burning material
XØ8.21 Exposure to other furniture fire due to burning cigarette
XØ8.29 Exposure to other furniture fire due to other burning material
XØ8.8 Exposure to other specified smoke, fire and flames

Contact with heat and hot substances (X1Ø-X19)

EXCLUDES 1 *exposure to excessive natural heat (X3Ø)*
exposure to fire and flames (XØØ-XØ9)

X1Ø Contact with hot drinks, food, fats and cooking oils

The appropriate 7th character is to be added to each code from category X1Ø.
A initial encounter
D subsequent encounter
S sequela

X1Ø.Ø Contact with hot drinks
X1Ø.1 Contact with hot food
X1Ø.2 Contact with fats and cooking oils

X11 Contact with hot tap-water
INCLUDES contact with boiling tap-water
contact with boiling water NOS
EXCLUDES 1 *contact with water heated on stove (X12)*

The appropriate 7th character is to be added to each code from category X11.
A initial encounter
D subsequent encounter
S sequela

X11.Ø Contact with hot water in bath or tub
EXCLUDES 1 *contact with running hot water in bath or tub (X11.1)*
X11.1 Contact with running hot water
Contact with hot water running out of hose
Contact with hot water running out of tap
X11.8 Contact with other hot tap-water
Contact with hot water in bucket
Contact with hot tap-water NOS

X12 Contact with other hot fluids
Contact with water heated on stove
EXCLUDES 1 *hot (liquid) metals (X18)*

The appropriate 7th character is to be added to code X12.
A initial encounter
D subsequent encounter
S sequela

X13 Contact with steam and other hot vapors

The appropriate 7th character is to be added to each code from category X13.
A initial encounter
D subsequent encounter
S sequela

X13.Ø Inhalation of steam and other hot vapors
X13.1 Other contact with steam and other hot vapors

X14 Contact with hot air and other hot gases

The appropriate 7th character is to be added to each code from category X14.
A initial encounter
D subsequent encounter
S sequela

X14.Ø Inhalation of hot air and gases
X14.1 Other contact with hot air and other hot gases

X15 Contact with hot household appliances
EXCLUDES 1 *contact with heating appliances (X16)*
contact with powered household appliances (W29.-)
exposure to controlled fire in building or structure due to household appliance (XØ2.8)
exposure to household appliances electrical current (W86.Ø)

The appropriate 7th character is to be added to each code from category X15.
A initial encounter
D subsequent encounter
S sequela

X15.Ø Contact with hot stove (kitchen)
X15.1 Contact with hot toaster
X15.2 Contact with hotplate
X15.3 Contact with hot saucepan or skillet
X15.8 Contact with other hot household appliances
Contact with cooker
Contact with kettle
Contact with light bulbs

X16 Contact with hot heating appliances, radiators and pipes
EXCLUDES 1 *contact with powered appliances (W29.-)*
exposure to controlled fire in building or structure due to appliance (XØ2.8)
exposure to industrial appliances electrical current (W86.1)

The appropriate 7th character is to be added to code X16.
A initial encounter
D subsequent encounter
S sequela

X17 Contact with hot engines, machinery and tools

EXCLUDES 1 *contact with hot heating appliances, radiators and pipes (X16)*
contact with hot household appliances (X15)

The appropriate 7th character is to be added to code X17.
A initial encounter
D subsequent encounter
S sequela

X18 Contact with other hot metals

Contact with liquid metal

The appropriate 7th character is to be added to code X18.
A initial encounter
D subsequent encounter
S sequela

X19 Contact with other heat and hot substances

EXCLUDES 1 *objects that are not normally hot, e.g., an object made hot by a house fire (XØØ-XØ9)*

The appropriate 7th character is to be added to code X19.
A initial encounter
D subsequent encounter
S sequela

Exposure to forces of nature (X3Ø-X39)

X3Ø Exposure to excessive natural heat

Exposure to excessive heat as the cause of sunstroke
Exposure to heat NOS

EXCLUDES 1 *excessive heat of man-made origin (W92)*
exposure to man-made radiation (W89)
exposure to sunlight (X32)
exposure to tanning bed (W89)

The appropriate 7th character is to be added to code X3Ø.
A initial encounter
D subsequent encounter
S sequela

X31 Exposure to excessive natural cold

Excessive cold as the cause of chilblains NOS
Excessive cold as the cause of immersion foot or hand
Exposure to cold NOS
Exposure to weather conditions

EXCLUDES 1 *cold of man-made origin (W93.-)*
contact with or inhalation of dry ice (W93.-)
contact with or inhalation of liquefied gas (W93.-)

The appropriate 7th character is to be added to code X31.
A initial encounter
D subsequent encounter
S sequela

X32 Exposure to sunlight

EXCLUDES 1 *radiation-related disorders of the skin and subcutaneous tissue (L55-L59)*
man-made radiation (tanning bed) (W89)

The appropriate 7th character is to be added to code X32.
A initial encounter
D subsequent encounter
S sequela

X34 Earthquake

EXCLUDES 2 *tidal wave (tsunami) due to earthquake (X37.41)*

The appropriate 7th character is to be added to code X34.
A initial encounter
D subsequent encounter
S sequela

X35 Volcanic eruption

EXCLUDES 2 *tidal wave (tsunami) due to volcanic eruption (X37.41)*

The appropriate 7th character is to be added to code X35.
A initial encounter
D subsequent encounter
S sequela

X36 Avalanche, landslide and other earth movements

INCLUDES victim of mudslide of cataclysmic nature

EXCLUDES 1 *earthquake (X34)*

EXCLUDES 2 *transport accident involving collision with avalanche or landslide not in motion (VØ1-V99)*

The appropriate 7th character is to be added to each code from category X36.
A initial encounter
D subsequent encounter
S sequela

X36.Ø Collapse of dam or man-made structure causing earth movement

X36.1 Avalanche, landslide, or mudslide

X37 Cataclysmic storm

The appropriate 7th character is to be added to each code from category X37.
A initial encounter
D subsequent encounter
S sequela

X37.Ø Hurricane
Storm surge
Typhoon

X37.1 Tornado
Cyclone
Twister

X37.2 Blizzard (snow)(ice)

X37.3 Dust storm

X37.4 Tidalwave

X37.41 Tidal wave due to earthquake or volcanic eruption
Tidal wave NOS
Tsunami

X37.42 Tidal wave due to storm

X37.43 Tidal wave due to landslide

X37.8 Other cataclysmic storms
Cloudburst
Torrential rain

EXCLUDES 2 *flood (X38)*

X37.9 Unspecified cataclysmic storm
Storm NOS

EXCLUDES 1 *collapse of dam or man-made structure causing earth movement (X39.Ø)*

X38 Flood

Flood arising from remote storm
Flood of cataclysmic nature arising from melting snow
Flood resulting directly from storm

EXCLUDES 1 *collapse of dam or man-made structure causing earth movement (X39.Ø)*
tidal wave NOS (X37.41)
tidal wave caused by storm (X37.2)

The appropriate 7th character is to be added to code X38.
A initial encounter
D subsequent encounter
S sequela

X39 Exposure to other forces of nature

The appropriate 7th character is to be added to each code from category X39.
A initial encounter
D subsequent encounter
S sequela

X39.Ø Exposure to natural radiation

EXCLUDES 1 *contact with and (suspected) exposure to radon and other naturally occuring radiation (Z77.122)*
exposure to man-made radiation (W88-W9Ø)
exposure to sunlight (X32)

X39.Ø1 Exposure to radon

X39.Ø8 Exposure to other natural radiation

X39.8 Other exposure to forces of nature

Accidental exposure to other specified factors (X52, X58)

X52 Prolonged stay in weightless environment

Weightlessness in spacecraft (simulator)

The appropriate 7th character is to be added to code X52.
A initial encounter
D subsequent encounter
S sequela

X58 Exposure to other specified factors
Accident NOS
Exposure NOS

The appropriate 7th character is to be added to code X58.
A initial encounter
D subsequent encounter
S sequela

Intentional self-harm (X71-X83)

Purposely self-inflicted injury
Suicide (attempted)

X71 Intentional self-harm by drowning and submersion

The appropriate 7th character is to be added to each code from category X71.
A initial encounter
D subsequent encounter
S sequela

X71.0 Intentional self-harm by drowning and submersion while in bathtub
X71.1 Intentional self-harm by drowning and submersion while in swimming pool
X71.2 Intentional self-harm by drowning and submersion after jump into swimming pool
X71.3 Intentional self-harm by drowning and submersion in natural water
X71.8 Other intentional self-harm by drowning and submersion
X71.9 Intentional self-harm by drowning and submersion, unspecified

X72 Intentional self-harm by handgun discharge
Intentional self-harm by gun for single hand use
Intentional self-harm by pistol
Intentional self-harm by revolver
EXCLUDES 1 *Very pistol (X74.8)*

The appropriate 7th character is to be added to code X72.
A initial encounter
D subsequent encounter
S sequela

X73 Intentional self-harm by rifle, shotgun and larger firearm discharge
EXCLUDES 1 *airgun (X74.01)*

The appropriate 7th character is to be added to each code from category X73.
A initial encounter
D subsequent encounter
S sequela

X73.0 Intentional self-harm by shotgun discharge
X73.1 Intentional self-harm by hunting rifle discharge
X73.2 Intentional self-harm by machine gun discharge
X73.8 Intentional self-harm by other larger firearm discharge
X73.9 Intentional self-harm by unspecified larger firearm discharge

X74 Intentional self-harm by other and unspecified firearm and gun discharge

The appropriate 7th character is to be added to each code from category X74.
A initial encounter
D subsequent encounter
S sequela

X74.0 Intentional self-harm by gas, air or spring-operated guns
X74.01 Intentional self-harm by airgun
Intentional self-harm by BB gun discharge
Intentional self-harm by pellet gun discharge
X74.02 Intentional self-harm by paintball gun
X74.09 Intentional self-harm by other gas, air or spring-operated gun
X74.8 Intentional self-harm by other firearm discharge
Intentional self-harm by Very pistol [flare] discharge
X74.9 Intentional self-harm by unspecified firearm discharge

X75 Intentional self-harm by explosive material

The appropriate 7th character is to be added to code X75.
A initial encounter
D subsequent encounter
S sequela

X76 Intentional self-harm by smoke, fire and flames

The appropriate 7th character is to be added to code X76.
A initial encounter
D subsequent encounter
S sequela

X77 Intentional self-harm by steam, hot vapors and hot objects

The appropriate 7th character is to be added to each code from category X77.
A initial encounter
D subsequent encounter
S sequela

X77.0 Intentional self-harm by steam or hot vapors
X77.1 Intentional self-harm by hot tap water
X77.2 Intentional self-harm by other hot fluids
X77.3 Intentional self-harm by hot household appliances
X77.8 Intentional self-harm by other hot objects
X77.9 Intentional self-harm by unspecified hot objects

X78 Intentional self-harm by sharp object

The appropriate 7th character is to be added to each code from category X78.
A initial encounter
D subsequent encounter
S sequela

X78.0 Intentional self-harm by sharp glass
X78.1 Intentional self-harm by knife
X78.2 Intentional self-harm by sword or dagger
X78.8 Intentional self-harm by other sharp object
X78.9 Intentional self-harm by unspecified sharp object

X79 Intentional self-harm by blunt object

The appropriate 7th character is to be added to code X79.
A initial encounter
D subsequent encounter
S sequela

X80 Intentional self-harm by jumping from a high place
Intentional fall from one level to another

The appropriate 7th character is to be added to code X80.
A initial encounter
D subsequent encounter
S sequela

X81 Intentional self-harm by jumping or lying in front of moving object

The appropriate 7th character is to be added to each code from category X81.
A initial encounter
D subsequent encounter
S sequela

X81.0 Intentional self-harm by jumping or lying in front of motor vehicle
X81.1 Intentional self-harm by jumping or lying in front of (subway) train
X81.8 Intentional self-harm by jumping or lying in front of other moving object

X82 Intentional self-harm by crashing of motor vehicle

The appropriate 7th character is to be added to each code from category X82.
A initial encounter
D subsequent encounter
S sequela

X82.0 Intentional collision of motor vehicle with other motor vehicle
X82.1 Intentional collision of motor vehicle with train
X82.2 Intentional collision of motor vehicle with tree
X82.8 Other intentional self-harm by crashing of motor vehicle

X83 Intentional self-harm by other specified means
EXCLUDES 1 *intentional self-harm by poisoning or contact with toxic substance—see Table of Drugs and Chemicals*

The appropriate 7th character is to be added to each code from category X83.
A initial encounter
D subsequent encounter
S sequela

X83.0 Intentional self-harm by crashing of aircraft
X83.1 Intentional self-harm by electrocution
X83.2 Intentional self-harm by exposure to extremes of cold
X83.8 Intentional self-harm by other specified means

Assault (X92-Y08)

INCLUDES homicide
injuries inflicted by another person with intent to injure or kill, by any means
EXCLUDES 1 *injuries due to legal intervention (Y35.-)*
injuries due to operations of war (Y36.-)
injuries due to terrorism (Y38.-)

X92 Assault by drowning and submersion

The appropriate 7th character is to be added to each code from category X92.
A initial encounter
D subsequent encounter
S sequela

X92.0 Assault by drowning and submersion while in bathtub
X92.1 Assault by drowning and submersion while in swimming pool
X92.2 Assault by drowning and submersion after push into swimming pool
X92.3 Assault by drowning and submersion in natural water
X92.8 Other assault by drowning and submersion
X92.9 Assault by drowning and submersion, unspecified

X93 Assault by handgun discharge
Assault by discharge of gun for single hand use
Assault by discharge of pistol
Assault by discharge of revolver
EXCLUDES 1 *Very pistol (X95.8)*

The appropriate 7th character is to be added to code X93.
A initial encounter
D subsequent encounter
S sequela

X94 Assault by rifle, shotgun and larger firearm discharge
EXCLUDES 1 *airgun (X95.01)*

The appropriate 7th character is to be added to each code from category X94.
A initial encounter
D subsequent encounter
S sequela

X94.0 Assault by shotgun
X94.1 Assault by hunting rifle
X94.2 Assault by machine gun
X94.8 Assault by other larger firearm discharge
X94.9 Assault by unspecified larger firearm discharge

X95 Assault by other and unspecified firearm and gun discharge

The appropriate 7th character is to be added to each code from category X95.
A initial encounter
D subsequent encounter
S sequela

X95.0 Assault by gas, air or spring-operated guns
X95.01 Assault by airgun discharge
Assault by BB gun discharge
Assault by pellet gun discharge
X95.02 Assault by paintball gun discharge
X95.09 Assault by other gas, air or spring-operated gun
X95.8 Assault by other firearm discharge
Assault by Very pistol [flare] discharge
X95.9 Assault by unspecified firearm discharge

X96 Assault by explosive material
EXCLUDES 1 *incendiary device (X97)*
terrorism involving explosive material (Y38.2-)

The appropriate 7th character is to be added to each code from category X96.
A initial encounter
D subsequent encounter
S sequela

X96.0 Assault by antipersonnel bomb
EXCLUDES 1 *antipersonnel bomb use in military or war (Y36.2-)*
X96.1 Assault by gasoline bomb
X96.2 Assault by letter bomb
X96.3 Assault by fertilizer bomb
X96.4 Assault by pipe bomb
X96.8 Assault by other specified explosive
X96.9 Assault by unspecified explosive

X97 Assault by smoke, fire and flames
Assault by arson
Assault by cigarettes
Assault by incendiary device

The appropriate 7th character is to be added to code X97.
A initial encounter
D subsequent encounter
S sequela

X98 Assault by steam, hot vapors and hot objects

The appropriate 7th character is to be added to each code from category X98.
A initial encounter
D subsequent encounter
S sequela

X98.0 Assault by steam or hot vapors
X98.1 Assault by hot tap water
X98.2 Assault by hot fluids
X98.3 Assault by hot household appliances
X98.8 Assault by other hot objects
X98.9 Assault by unspecified hot objects

X99 Assault by sharp object
EXCLUDES 1 *assault by strike by sports equipment (Y08.0-)*

The appropriate 7th character is to be added to each code from category X99.
A initial encounter
D subsequent encounter
S sequela

X99.0 Assault by sharp glass
X99.1 Assault by knife
X99.2 Assault by sword or dagger
X99.8 Assault by other sharp object
X99.9 Assault by unspecified sharp object
Assault by stabbing NOS

Y00 Assault by blunt object
EXCLUDES 1 *assault by strike by sports equipment (Y08.0-)*

The appropriate 7th character is to be added to code Y00.
A initial encounter
D subsequent encounter
S sequela

Y01 Assault by pushing from high place

The appropriate 7th character is to be added to code Y01.
A initial encounter
D subsequent encounter
S sequela

Y02 Assault by pushing or placing victim in front of moving object

The appropriate 7th character is to be added to each code from category Y02.
A initial encounter
D subsequent encounter
S sequela

Y02.0 Assault by pushing or placing victim in front of motor vehicle
Y02.1 Assault by pushing or placing victim in front of (subway) train
Y02.8 Assault by pushing or placing victim in front of other moving object

Y03 Assault by crashing of motor vehicle

The appropriate 7th character is to be added to each code from category Y03.
A initial encounter
D subsequent encounter
S sequela

Y03.0 Assault by being hit or run over by motor vehicle

Y03.8 Other assault by crashing of motor vehicle

Y04 Assault by bodily force

EXCLUDES1 *assault by:*
submersion (X92.-)
use of weapon (X93-X95, X99, Y00)

The appropriate 7th character is to be added to each code from category Y04.
A initial encounter
D subsequent encounter
S sequela

Y04.0 Assault by unarmed brawl or fight

Y04.1 Assault by human bite

Y04.2 Assault by strike against or bumped into by another person

Y04.8 Assault by other bodily force
Assault by bodily force NOS

Y07 Perpetrator of assault, maltreatment and neglect

NOTE Codes from this category are for use only in cases of confirmed abuse (T74.-)
Selection of the correct perpetrator code is based on the relationship between the perpetrator and the victim

INCLUDES perpetrator of abandonment
perpetrator of emotional neglect
perpetrator of mental cruelty
perpetrator of physical abuse
perpetrator of physical neglect
perpetrator of sexual abuse
perpetrator of torture

Y07.0 Spouse or partner, perpetrator of maltreatment and neglect
NOTE Spouse or partner, perpetrator of maltreatment and neglect against spouse or partner

Y07.01 Husband, perpetrator of maltreatment and neglect

Y07.02 Wife, perpetrator of maltreatment and neglect

Y07.03 Male partner, perpetrator of maltreatment and neglect

Y07.04 Female partner, perpetrator of maltreatment and neglect

Y07.1 Parent (adoptive) (biological), perpetrator of maltreatment and neglect

Y07.11 Biological father, perpetrator of maltreatment and neglect

Y07.12 Biological mother, perpetrator of maltreatment and neglect

Y07.13 Adoptive father, perpetrator of maltreatment and neglect

Y07.14 Adoptive mother, perpetrator of maltreatment and neglect

Y07.4 Other family member, perpetrator of maltreatment and neglect

Y07.41 Sibling, perpetrator of maltreatment and neglect
EXCLUDES1 *stepsibling, perpetrator of maltreatment and neglect (Y07.435, Y07.436)*

Y07.410 Brother, perpetrator of maltreatment and neglect

Y07.411 Sister, perpetrator of maltreatment and neglect

Y07.42 Foster parent, perpetrator of maltreatment and neglect

Y07.420 Foster father, perpetrator of maltreatment and neglect

Y07.421 Foster mother, perpetrator of maltreatment and neglect

Y07.43 Stepparent or stepsibling, perpetrator of maltreatment and neglect

Y07.430 Stepfather, perpetrator of maltreatment and neglect

Y07.432 Male friend of parent (co-residing in household), perpetrator of maltreatment and neglect

Y07.433 Stepmother, perpetrator of maltreatment and neglect

Y07.434 Female friend of parent (co-residing in household), perpetrator of maltreatment and neglect

Y07.435 Stepbrother, perpetrator or maltreatment and neglect

Y07.436 Stepsister, perpetrator of maltreatment and neglect

Y07.49 Other family member, perpetrator of maltreatment and neglect

Y07.490 Male cousin, perpetrator of maltreatment and neglect

Y07.491 Female cousin, perpetrator of maltreatment and neglect

Y07.499 Other family member, perpetrator of maltreatment and neglect

Y07.5 Non-family member, perpetrator of maltreatment and neglect

Y07.50 Unspecified non-family member, perpetrator of maltreatment and neglect

Y07.51 Daycare provider, perpetrator of maltreatment and neglect

Y07.510 At-home childcare provider, perpetrator of maltreatment and neglect

Y07.511 Daycare center childcare provider, perpetrator of maltreatment and neglect

Y07.512 At-home adultcare provider, perpetrator of maltreatment and neglect

Y07.513 Adultcare center provider, perpetrator of maltreatment and neglect

Y07.519 Unspecified daycare provider, perpetrator of maltreatment and neglect

Y07.52 Healthcare provider, perpetrator of maltreatment and neglect

Y07.521 Mental health provider, perpetrator of maltreatment and neglect

Y07.528 Other therapist or healthcare provider, perpetrator of maltreatment and neglect
Nurse, perpetrator of maltreatment and neglect
Occupational therapist, perpetrator of maltreatment and neglect
Physical therapist, perpetrator of maltreatment and neglect
Speech therapist, perpetrator of maltreatment and neglect

Y07.529 Unspecified healthcare provider, perpetrator of maltreatment and neglect

Y07.53 Teacher or instructor, perpetrator of maltreatment and neglect
Coach, perpetrator of maltreatment and neglect

Y07.59 Other non-family member, perpetrator of maltreatment and neglect

Y07.9 Unspecified perpetrator of maltreatment and neglect

Y08 Assault by other specified means

The appropriate 7th character is to be added to each code from category Y08.
A initial encounter
D subsequent encounter
S sequela

Y08.0 Assault by strike by sport equipment

Y08.01 Assault by strike by hockey stick

Y08.02 Assault by strike by baseball bat

Y08.09 Assault by strike by other specified type of sport equipment

Y08.8 Assault by other specified means

Y08.81 Assault by crashing of aircraft

Y08.89 Assault by other specified means

Y09 Assault by unspecified means
Assassination (attempted) NOS
Homicide (attempted) NOS
Manslaughter (attempted) NOS
Murder (attempted) NOS

Event of undetermined intent (Y21-Y33)

Undetermined intent is only for use when there is specific documentation in the record that the intent of the injury cannot be determined. If no such documentation is present, code to accidental (unintentional)

Y21 Drowning and submersion, undetermined intent

The appropriate 7th character is to be added to each code from category Y21.
A initial encounter
D subsequent encounter
S sequela

Y21.0 Drowning and submersion while in bathtub, undetermined intent

Y21.1 Drowning and submersion after fall into bathtub, undetermined intent

Y21.2 Drowning and submersion while in swimming pool, undetermined intent

Y21.3 Drowning and submersion after fall into swimming pool, undetermined intent

Y21.4 Drowning and submersion in natural water, undetermined intent

Y21.8 Other drowning and submersion, undetermined intent

Y21.9 Unspecified drowning and submersion, undetermined intent

Y22 Handgun discharge, undetermined intent

Discharge of gun for single hand use, undetermined intent
Discharge of pistol, undetermined intent
Discharge of revolver, undetermined intent
EXCLUDES 2 *Very pistol (Y24.8)*

The appropriate 7th character is to be added to code Y22.
A initial encounter
D subsequent encounter
S sequela

Y23 Rifle, shotgun and larger firearm discharge, undetermined intent

EXCLUDES 2 *airgun (Y24.0)*

The appropriate 7th character is to be added to each code from category Y23.
A initial encounter
D subsequent encounter
S sequela

Y23.0 Shotgun discharge, undetermined intent

Y23.1 Hunting rifle discharge, undetermined intent

Y23.2 Military firearm discharge, undetermined intent

Y23.3 Machine gun discharge, undetermined intent

Y23.8 Other larger firearm discharge, undetermined intent

Y23.9 Unspecified larger firearm discharge, undetermined intent

Y24 Other and unspecified firearm discharge, undetermined intent

The appropriate 7th character is to be added to each code from category Y24.
A initial encounter
D subsequent encounter
S sequela

Y24.0 Airgun discharge, undetermined intent

BB gun discharge, undetermined intent
Pellet gun discharge, undetermined intent

Y24.8 Other firearm discharge, undetermined intent

Paintball gun discharge, undetermined intent
Very pistol [flare] discharge, undetermined intent

Y24.9 Unspecified firearm discharge, undetermined intent

Y25 Contact with explosive material, undetermined intent

The appropriate 7th character is to be added to code Y25.
A initial encounter
D subsequent encounter
S sequela

Y26 Exposure to smoke, fire and flames, undetermined intent

The appropriate 7th character is to be added to code Y26.
A initial encounter
D subsequent encounter
S sequela

Y27 Contact with steam, hot vapors and hot objects, undetermined intent

The appropriate 7th character is to be added to each code from category Y27.
A initial encounter
D subsequent encounter
S sequela

Y27.0 Contact with steam and hot vapors, undetermined intent

Y27.1 Contact with hot tap water, undetermined intent

Y27.2 Contact with hot fluids, undetermined intent

Y27.3 Contact with hot household appliance, undetermined intent

Y27.8 Contact with other hot objects, undetermined intent

Y27.9 Contact with unspecified hot objects, undetermined intent

Y28 Contact with sharp object, undetermined intent

The appropriate 7th character is to be added to each code from category Y28.
A initial encounter
D subsequent encounter
S sequela

Y28.0 Contact with sharp glass, undetermined intent

Y28.1 Contact with knife, undetermined intent

Y28.2 Contact with sword or dagger, undetermined intent

Y28.8 Contact with other sharp object, undetermined intent

Y28.9 Contact with unspecified sharp object, undetermined intent

Y29 Contact with blunt object, undetermined intent

The appropriate 7th character is to be added to code Y29.
A initial encounter
D subsequent encounter
S sequela

Y30 Falling, jumping or pushed from a high place, undetermined intent

Victim falling from one level to another, undetermined intent

The appropriate 7th character is to be added to code Y30.
A initial encounter
D subsequent encounter
S sequela

Y31 Falling, lying or running before or into moving object, undetermined intent

The appropriate 7th character is to be added to code Y31.
A initial encounter
D subsequent encounter
S sequela

Y32 Crashing of motor vehicle, undetermined intent

The appropriate 7th character is to be added to code Y32.
A initial encounter
D subsequent encounter
S sequela

Y33 Other specified events, undetermined intent

The appropriate 7th character is to be added to code Y33.
A initial encounter
D subsequent encounter
S sequela

Legal intervention, operations of war, military operations, and terrorism (Y35-Y38)

Y35 Legal intervention

INCLUDES any injury sustained as a result of an encounter with any law enforcement official, serving in any capacity at the time of the encounter, whether on-duty or off-duty. Includes: injury to law enforcement official, suspect and bystander

The appropriate 7th character is to be added to each code from category Y35.
A initial encounter
D subsequent encounter
S sequela

Y35.0 Legal intervention involving firearm discharge

✓6th **Y35.ØØ Legal intervention involving unspecified firearm discharge**
Legal intervention involving gunshot wound
Legal intervention involving shot NOS

✓7th **Y35.ØØ1 Legal intervention involving unspecified firearm discharge, law enforcement official injured**

✓7th **Y35.ØØ2 Legal intervention involving unspecified firearm discharge, bystander injured**

✓7th **Y35.ØØ3 Legal intervention involving unspecified firearm discharge, suspect injured**

✓6th **Y35.Ø1 Legal intervention involving injury by machine gun**

✓7th **Y35.Ø11 Legal intervention involving injury by machine gun, law enforcement official injured**

✓7th **Y35.Ø12 Legal intervention involving injury by machine gun, bystander injured**

✓7th **Y35.Ø13 Legal intervention involving injury by machine gun, suspect injured**

✓6th **Y35.Ø2 Legal intervention involving injury by handgun**

✓7th **Y35.Ø21 Legal intervention involving injury by handgun, law enforcement official injured**

✓7th **Y35.Ø22 Legal intervention involving injury by handgun, bystander injured**

✓7th **Y35.Ø23 Legal intervention involving injury by handgun, suspect injured**

✓6th **Y35.Ø3 Legal intervention involving injury by rifle pellet**

✓7th **Y35.Ø31 Legal intervention involving injury by rifle pellet, law enforcement official injured**

✓7th **Y35.Ø32 Legal intervention involving injury by rifle pellet, bystander injured**

✓7th **Y35.Ø33 Legal intervention involving injury by rifle pellet, suspect injured**

✓6th **Y35.Ø4 Legal intervention involving injury by rubber bullet**

✓7th **Y35.Ø41 Legal intervention involving injury by rubber bullet, law enforcement official injured**

✓7th **Y35.Ø42 Legal intervention involving injury by rubber bullet, bystander injured**

✓7th **Y35.Ø43 Legal intervention involving injury by rubber bullet, suspect injured**

✓6th **Y35.Ø9 Legal intervention involving other firearm discharge**

✓7th **Y35.Ø91 Legal intervention involving other firearm discharge, law enforcement official injured**

✓7th **Y35.Ø92 Legal intervention involving other firearm discharge, bystander injured**

✓7th **Y35.Ø93 Legal intervention involving other firearm discharge, suspect injured**

✓5th **Y35.1 Legal intervention involving explosives**

✓6th **Y35.1Ø Legal intervention involving unspecified explosives**

✓7th **Y35.1Ø1 Legal intervention involving unspecified explosives, law enforcement official injured**

✓7th **Y35.1Ø2 Legal intervention involving unspecified explosives, bystander injured**

✓7th **Y35.1Ø3 Legal intervention involving unspecified explosives, suspect injured**

✓6th **Y35.11 Legal intervention involving injury by dynamite**

✓7th **Y35.111 Legal intervention involving injury by dynamite, law enforcement official injured**

✓7th **Y35.112 Legal intervention involving injury by dynamite, bystander injured**

✓7th **Y35.113 Legal intervention involving injury by dynamite, suspect injured**

✓6th **Y35.12 Legal intervention involving injury by explosive shell**

✓7th **Y35.121 Legal intervention involving injury by explosive shell, law enforcement official injured**

✓7th **Y35.122 Legal intervention involving injury by explosive shell, bystander injured**

✓7th **Y35.123 Legal intervention involving injury by explosive shell, suspect injured**

✓6th **Y35.19 Legal intervention involving other explosives**
Legal intervention involving injury by grenade
Legal intervention involving injury by mortar bomb

✓7th **Y35.191 Legal intervention involving other explosives, law enforcement official injured**

✓7th **Y35.192 Legal intervention involving other explosives, bystander injured**

✓7th **Y35.193 Legal intervention involving other explosives, suspect injured**

✓5th **Y35.2 Legal intervention involving gas**
Legal intervention involving asphyxiation by gas
Legal intervention involving poisoning by gas

✓6th **Y35.2Ø Legal intervention involving unspecified gas**

✓7th **Y35.2Ø1 Legal intervention involving unspecified gas, law enforcement official injured**

✓7th **Y35.2Ø2 Legal intervention involving unspecified gas, bystander injured**

✓7th **Y35.2Ø3 Legal intervention involving unspecified gas, suspect injured**

✓6th **Y35.21 Legal intervention involving injury by tear gas**

✓7th **Y35.211 Legal intervention involving injury by tear gas, law enforcement official injured**

✓7th **Y35.212 Legal intervention involving injury by tear gas, bystander injured**

✓7th **Y35.213 Legal intervention involving injury by tear gas, suspect injured**

✓6th **Y35.29 Legal intervention involving other gas**

✓7th **Y35.291 Legal intervention involving other gas, law enforcement official injured**

✓7th **Y35.292 Legal intervention involving other gas, bystander injured**

✓7th **Y35.293 Legal intervention involving other gas, suspect injured**

✓5th **Y35.3 Legal intervention involving blunt objects**
Legal intervention involving being hit or struck by blunt object

✓6th **Y35.3Ø Legal intervention involving unspecified blunt objects**

✓7th **Y35.3Ø1 Legal intervention involving unspecified blunt objects, law enforcement official injured**

✓7th **Y35.3Ø2 Legal intervention involving unspecified blunt objects, bystander injured**

✓7th **Y35.3Ø3 Legal intervention involving unspecified blunt objects, suspect injured**

✓6th **Y35.31 Legal intervention involving baton**

✓7th **Y35.311 Legal intervention involving baton, law enforcement official injured**

✓7th **Y35.312 Legal intervention involving baton, bystander injured**

✓7th **Y35.313 Legal intervention involving baton, suspect injured**

✓6th **Y35.39 Legal intervention involving other blunt objects**

✓7th **Y35.391 Legal intervention involving other blunt objects, law enforcement official injured**

✓7th **Y35.392 Legal intervention involving other blunt objects, bystander injured**

✓7th **Y35.393 Legal intervention involving other blunt objects, suspect injured**

✓5th **Y35.4 Legal intervention involving sharp objects**
Legal intervention involving being cut by sharp objects
Legal intervention involving being stabbed by sharp objects

✓6th **Y35.4Ø Legal intervention involving unspecified sharp objects**

✓7th **Y35.4Ø1 Legal intervention involving unspecified sharp objects, law enforcement official injured**

✓7th **Y35.4Ø2 Legal intervention involving unspecified sharp objects, bystander injured**

✓7th **Y35.4Ø3 Legal intervention involving unspecified sharp objects, suspect injured**

✓6th **Y35.41 Legal intervention involving bayonet**

✓7th **Y35.411 Legal intervention involving bayonet, law enforcement official injured**

7th **Y35.412 Legal intervention involving bayonet, bystander injured**

7th **Y35.413 Legal intervention involving bayonet, suspect injured**

6th **Y35.49 Legal intervention involving other sharp objects**

7th **Y35.491 Legal intervention involving other sharp objects, law enforcement official injured**

7th **Y35.492 Legal intervention involving other sharp objects, bystander injured**

7th **Y35.493 Legal intervention involving other sharp objects, suspect injured**

5th **Y35.8 Legal intervention involving other specified means**

6th **Y35.81 Legal intervention involving manhandling**

7th **Y35.811 Legal intervention involving manhandling, law enforcement official injured**

7th **Y35.812 Legal intervention involving manhandling, bystander injured**

7th **Y35.813 Legal intervention involving manhandling, suspect injured**

6th **Y35.89 Legal intervention involving other specified means**

7th **Y35.891 Legal intervention involving other specified means, law enforcement official injured**

7th **Y35.892 Legal intervention involving other specified means, bystander injured**

7th **Y35.893 Legal intervention involving other specified means, suspect injured**

5th **Y35.9 Legal intervention, means unspecified**

x7th **Y35.91 Legal intervention, means unspecified, law enforcement official injured**

x7th **Y35.92 Legal intervention, means unspecified, bystander injured**

x7th **Y35.93 Legal intervention, means unspecified, suspect injured**

4th **Y36 Operations of war**

INCLUDES injuries to military personnel and civilians caused by war, civil insurrection, and peacekeeping missions

EXCLUDES 1 *injury to military personnel occurring during peacetime military operations (Y37.-)*

military vehicles involved in transport accidents with non-military vehicle during peacetime (V09.01, V09.21, V19.81, V29.81, V39.81, V49.81, V59.81, V69.81, V79.81)

The appropriate 7th character is to be added to each code from category Y36.
A initial encounter
D subsequent encounter
S sequela

5th **Y36.0 War operations involving explosion of marine weapons**

6th **Y36.00 War operations involving explosion of unspecified marine weapon**
War operations involving underwater blast NOS

7th **Y36.000 War operations involving explosion of unspecified marine weapon, military personnel**

7th **Y36.001 War operations involving explosion of unspecified marine weapon, civilian**

6th **Y36.01 War operations involving explosion of depth-charge**

7th **Y36.010 War operations involving explosion of depth-charge, military personnel**

7th **Y36.011 War operations involving explosion of depth-charge, civilian**

6th **Y36.02 War operations involving explosion of marine mine**
War operations involving explosion of marine mine, at sea or in harbor

7th **Y36.020 War operations involving explosion of marine mine, military personnel**

7th **Y36.021 War operations involving explosion of marine mine, civilian**

6th **Y36.03 War operations involving explosion of sea-based artillery shell**

7th **Y36.030 War operations involving explosion of sea-based artillery shell, military personnel**

7th **Y36.031 War operations involving explosion of sea-based artillery shell, civilian**

6th **Y36.04 War operations involving explosion of torpedo**

7th **Y36.040 War operations involving explosion of torpedo, military personnel**

7th **Y36.041 War operations involving explosion of torpedo, civilian**

6th **Y36.05 War operations involving accidental detonation of onboard marine weapons**

7th **Y36.050 War operations involving accidental detonation of onboard marine weapons, military personnel**

7th **Y36.051 War operations involving accidental detonation of onboard marine weapons, civilian**

6th **Y36.09 War operations involving explosion of other marine weapons**

7th **Y36.090 War operations involving explosion of other marine weapons, military personnel**

7th **Y36.091 War operations involving explosion of other marine weapons, civilian**

5th **Y36.1 War operations involving destruction of aircraft**

6th **Y36.10 War operations involving unspecified destruction of aircraft**

7th **Y36.100 War operations involving unspecified destruction of aircraft, military personnel**

7th **Y36.101 War operations involving unspecified destruction of aircraft, civilian**

6th **Y36.11 War operations involving destruction of aircraft due to enemy fire or explosives**
War operations involving destruction of aircraft due to air to air missile
War operations involving destruction of aircraft due to explosive placed on aircraft
War operations involving destruction of aircraft due to rocket propelled grenade [RPG]
War operations involving destruction of aircraft due to small arms fire
War operations involving destruction of aircraft due to surface to air missile

7th **Y36.110 War operations involving destruction of aircraft due to enemy fire or explosives, military personnel**

7th **Y36.111 War operations involving destruction of aircraft due to enemy fire or explosives, civilian**

6th **Y36.12 War operations involving destruction of aircraft due to collision with other aircraft**

7th **Y36.120 War operations involving destruction of aircraft due to collision with other aircraft, military personnel**

7th **Y36.121 War operations involving destruction of aircraft due to collision with other aircraft, civilian**

6th **Y36.13 War operations involving destruction of aircraft due to onboard fire**

7th **Y36.130 War operations involving destruction of aircraft due to onboard fire, military personnel**

7th **Y36.131 War operations involving destruction of aircraft due to onboard fire, civilian**

6th **Y36.14 War operations involving destruction of aircraft due to accidental detonation of onboard munitions and explosives**

7th **Y36.140 War operations involving destruction of aircraft due to accidental detonation of onboard munitions and explosives, military personnel**

7th **Y36.141 War operations involving destruction of aircraft due to accidental detonation of onboard munitions and explosives, civilian**

6th **Y36.19 War operations involving other destruction of aircraft**

7th **Y36.190 War operations involving other destruction of aircraft, military personnel**

7th **Y36.191 War operations involving other destruction of aircraft, civilian**

✓5th Y36.2 War operations involving other explosions and fragments

EXCLUDES 1 *war operations involving explosion of aircraft (Y36.1-)*
war operations involving explosion of marine weapons (Y36.0-)
war operations involving explosion of nuclear weapons (Y36.5-)
war operations involving explosion occurring after cessation of hostilities (Y36.8-)

✓6th Y36.20 War operations involving unspecified explosion and fragments
War operations involving air blast NOS
War operations involving blast NOS
War operations involving blast fragments NOS
War operations involving blast wave NOS
War operations involving blast wind NOS
War operations involving explosion NOS
War operations involving explosion of bomb NOS

✓7th Y36.200 War operations involving unspecified explosion and fragments, military personnel

✓7th Y36.201 War operations involving unspecified explosion and fragments, civilian

✓6th Y36.21 War operations involving explosion of aerial bomb

✓7th Y36.210 War operations involving explosion of aerial bomb, military personnel

✓7th Y36.211 War operations involving explosion of aerial bomb, civilian

✓6th Y36.22 War operations involving explosion of guided missile

✓7th Y36.220 War operations involving explosion of guided missile, military personnel

✓7th Y36.221 War operations involving explosion of guided missile, civilian

✓6th Y36.23 War operations involving explosion of improvised explosive device [IED]
War operations involving explosion of person-borne improvised explosive device [IED]
War operations involving explosion of vehicle-borne improvised explosive device [IED]
War operations involving explosion of roadside improvised explosive device [IED]

✓7th Y36.230 War operations involving explosion of improvised explosive device [IED], military personnel

✓7th Y36.231 War operations involving explosion of improvised explosive device [IED], civilian

✓6th Y36.24 War operations involving explosion due to accidental detonation and discharge of own munitions or munitions launch device

✓7th Y36.240 War operations involving explosion due to accidental detonation and discharge of own munitions or munitions launch device, military personnel

✓7th Y36.241 War operations involving explosion due to accidental detonation and discharge of own munitions or munitions launch device, civilian

✓6th Y36.25 War operations involving fragments from munitions

✓7th Y36.250 War operations involving fragments from munitions, military personnel

✓7th Y36.251 War operations involving fragments from munitions, civilian

✓6th Y36.26 War operations involving fragments of improvised explosive device [IED]
War operations involving fragments of person-borne improvised explosive device [IED]
War operations involving fragments of vehicle-borne improvised explosive device [IED]
War operations involving fragments of roadside improvised explosive device [IED]

✓7th Y36.260 War operations involving fragments of improvised explosive device [IED], military personnel

✓7th Y36.261 War operations involving fragments of improvised explosive device [IED], civilian

✓6th Y36.27 War operations involving fragments from weapons

✓7th Y36.270 War operations involving fragments from weapons, military personnel

✓7th Y36.271 War operations involving fragments from weapons, civilian

✓6th Y36.29 War operations involving other explosions and fragments
War operations involving explosion of grenade
War operations involving explosions of land mine
War operations involving shrapnel NOS

✓7th Y36.290 War operations involving other explosions and fragments, military personnel

✓7th Y36.291 War operations involving other explosions and fragments, civilian

✓5th Y36.3 War operations involving fires, conflagrations and hot substances
War operations involving smoke, fumes, and heat from fires, conflagrations and hot substances

EXCLUDES 1 *war operations involving fires and conflagrations aboard military aircraft (Y36.1-)*
war operations involving fires and conflagrations aboard military watercraft (Y36.0-)
war operations involving fires and conflagrations caused indirectly by conventional weapons (Y36.2-)
war operations involving fires and thermal effects of nuclear weapons (Y36.53-)

✓6th Y36.30 War operations involving unspecified fire, conflagration and hot substance

✓7th Y36.300 War operations involving unspecified fire, conflagration and hot substance, military personnel

✓7th Y36.301 War operations involving unspecified fire, conflagration and hot substance, civilian

✓6th Y36.31 War operations involving gasoline bomb
War operations involving incendiary bomb
War operations involving petrol bomb

✓7th Y36.310 War operations involving gasoline bomb, military personnel

✓7th Y36.311 War operations involving gasoline bomb, civilian

✓6th Y36.32 War operations involving incendiary bullet

✓7th Y36.320 War operations involving incendiary bullet, military personnel

✓7th Y36.321 War operations involving incendiary bullet, civilian

✓6th Y36.33 War operations involving flamethrower

✓7th Y36.330 War operations involving flamethrower, military personnel

✓7th Y36.331 War operations involving flamethrower, civilian

✓6th Y36.39 War operations involving other fires, conflagrations and hot substances

✓7th Y36.390 War operations involving other fires, conflagrations and hot substances, military personnel

✓7th Y36.391 War operations involving other fires, conflagrations and hot substances, civilian

✓5th Y36.4 War operations involving firearm discharge and other forms of conventional warfare

✓6th Y36.41 War operations involving rubber bullets

✓7th Y36.410 War operations involving rubber bullets, military personnel

✓7th Y36.411 War operations involving rubber bullets, civilian

✓6th Y36.42 War operations involving firearms pellets

✓7th Y36.420 War operations involving firearms pellets, military personnel

✓7th Y36.421 War operations involving firearms pellets, civilian

✓6th Y36.43 War operations involving other firearms discharge
War operations involving bullets NOS

EXCLUDES 1 *war operations involving munitions fragments (Y36.25-)*
war operations involving incendiary bullets (Y36.32-)

✓7th Y36.430 War operations involving other firearms discharge, military personnel

✓7th **Y36.431 War operations involving other firearms discharge, civilian**

✓6th **Y36.44 War operations involving unarmed hand to hand combat**

EXCLUDES 1 *war operations involving combat using blunt or piercing object (Y36.45-)*
war operations involving intentional restriction of air and airway (Y36.46-)
war operations involving unintentional restriction of air and airway (Y36.47-)

✓7th **Y36.440 War operations involving unarmed hand to hand combat, military personnel**

✓7th **Y36.441 War operations involving unarmed hand to hand combat, civilian**

✓6th **Y36.45 War operations involving combat using blunt or piercing object**

✓7th **Y36.450 War operations involving combat using blunt or piercing object, military personnel**

✓7th **Y36.451 War operations involving combat using blunt or piercing object, civilian**

✓6th **Y36.46 War operations involving intentional restriction of air and airway**

✓7th **Y36.460 War operations involving intentional restriction of air and airway, military personnel**

✓7th **Y36.461 War operations involving intentional restriction of air and airway, civilian**

✓6th **Y36.47 War operations involving unintentional restriction of air and airway**

✓7th **Y36.470 War operations involving unintentional restriction of air and airway, military personnel**

✓7th **Y36.471 War operations involving unintentional restriction of air and airway, civilian**

✓6th **Y36.49 War operations involving other forms of conventional warfare**

✓7th **Y36.490 War operations involving other forms of conventional warfare, military personnel**

✓7th **Y36.491 War operations involving other forms of conventional warfare, civilian**

✓5th **Y36.5 War operations involving nuclear weapons**
War operations involving dirty bomb NOS

✓6th **Y36.50 War operations involving unspecified effect of nuclear weapon**

✓7th **Y36.500 War operations involving unspecified effect of nuclear weapon, military personnel**

✓7th **Y36.501 War operations involving unspecified effect of nuclear weapon, civilian**

✓6th **Y36.51 War operations involving direct blast effect of nuclear weapon**
War operations involving blast pressure of nuclear weapon

✓7th **Y36.510 War operations involving direct blast effect of nuclear weapon, military personnel**

✓7th **Y36.511 War operations involving direct blast effect of nuclear weapon, civilian**

✓6th **Y36.52 War operations involving indirect blast effect of nuclear weapon**
War operations involving being thrown by blast of nuclear weapon
War operations involving being struck or crushed by blast debris of nuclear weapon

✓7th **Y36.520 War operations involving indirect blast effect of nuclear weapon, military personnel**

✓7th **Y36.521 War operations involving indirect blast effect of nuclear weapon, civilian**

✓6th **Y36.53 War operations involving thermal radiation effect of nuclear weapon**
War operations involving direct heat from nuclear weapon
War operation involving fireball effects from nuclear weapon

✓7th **Y36.530 War operations involving thermal radiation effect of nuclear weapon, military personnel**

✓7th **Y36.531 War operations involving thermal radiation effect of nuclear weapon, civilian**

✓6th **Y36.54 War operation involving nuclear radiation effects of nuclear weapon**
War operation involving acute radiation exposure from nuclear weapon
War operation involving exposure to immediate ionizing radiation from nuclear weapon
War operation involving fallout exposure from nuclear weapon
War operation involving secondary effects of nuclear weapons

✓7th **Y36.540 War operation involving nuclear radiation effects of nuclear weapon, military personnel**

✓7th **Y36.541 War operation involving nuclear radiation effects of nuclear weapon, civilian**

✓6th **Y36.59 War operation involving other effects of nuclear weapons**

✓7th **Y36.590 War operation involving other effects of nuclear weapons, military personnel**

✓7th **Y36.591 War operation involving other effects of nuclear weapons, civilian**

✓5th **Y36.6 War operations involving biological weapons**

✓6th **Y36.6X War operations involving biological weapons**

✓7th **Y36.6X0 War operations involving biological weapons, military personnel**

✓7th **Y36.6X1 War operations involving biological weapons, civilian**

✓5th **Y36.7 War operations involving chemical weapons and other forms of unconventional warfare**

EXCLUDES 1 *war operations involving incendiary devices (Y36.3-, Y36.5-)*

✓6th **Y36.7X War operations involving chemical weapons and other forms of unconventional warfare**

✓7th **Y36.7X0 War operations involving chemical weapons and other forms of unconventional warfare, military personnel**

✓7th **Y36.7X1 War operations involving chemical weapons and other forms of unconventional warfare, civilian**

✓5th **Y36.8 War operations occurring after cessation of hostilities**
War operations classifiable to categories Y36.0-Y36.8 but occurring after cessation of hostilities

✓6th **Y36.81 Explosion of mine placed during war operations but exploding after cessation of hostilities**

✓7th **Y36.810 Explosion of mine placed during war operations but exploding after cessation of hostilities, military personnel**

✓7th **Y36.811 Explosion of mine placed during war operations but exploding after cessation of hostilities, civilian**

✓6th **Y36.82 Explosion of bomb placed during war operations but exploding after cessation of hostilities**

✓7th **Y36.820 Explosion of bomb placed during war operations but exploding after cessation of hostilities, military personnel**

✓7th **Y36.821 Explosion of bomb placed during war operations but exploding after cessation of hostilities, civilian**

✓6th **Y36.88 Other war operations occurring after cessation of hostilities**

✓7th **Y36.880 Other war operations occurring after cessation of hostilities, military personnel**

✓7th **Y36.881 Other war operations occurring after cessation of hostilities, civilian**

✓6th **Y36.89 Unspecified war operations occurring after cessation of hostilities**

✓7th **Y36.89Ø Unspecified war operations occurring after cessation of hostilities, military personnel**

✓7th **Y36.891 Unspecified war operations occurring after cessation of hostilities, civilian**

✓5th **Y36.9 Other and unspecified war operations**

✓x7th **Y36.9Ø War operations, unspecified**

✓x7th **Y36.91 War operations involving unspecified weapon of mass destruction [WMD]**

✓x7th **Y36.92 War operations involving friendly fire**

✓4th **Y37 Military operations**

INCLUDES injuries to military personnel and civilians occurring during peacetime on military property and during routine military exercises and operations

EXCLUDES 1 *military aircraft involved in aircraft accident with civilian aircraft (V97.81-)*
military vehicles involved in transport accident with civilian vehicle (VØ9.Ø1, VØ9.21, V19.81, V29.81, V39.81, V49.81, V59.81, V69.81, V79.81)
military watercraft involved in water transport accident with civilian watercraft (V94.81-)
war operations (Y36.-)

The appropriate 7th character is to be added to each code from category Y37.
A initial encounter
D subsequent encounter
S sequela

✓5th **Y37.Ø Military operations involving explosion of marine weapons**

✓6th **Y37.ØØ Military operations involving explosion of unspecified marine weapon**
Military operations involving underwater blast NOS

✓7th **Y37.ØØØ Military operations involving explosion of unspecified marine weapon, military personnel**

✓7th **Y37.ØØ1 Military operations involving explosion of unspecified marine weapon, civilian**

✓6th **Y37.Ø1 Military operations involving explosion of depth-charge**

✓7th **Y37.Ø1Ø Military operations involving explosion of depth-charge, military personnel**

✓7th **Y37.Ø11 Military operations involving explosion of depth-charge, civilian**

✓6th **Y37.Ø2 Military operations involving explosion of marine mine**
Military operations involving explosion of marine mine, at sea or in harbor

✓7th **Y37.Ø2Ø Military operations involving explosion of marine mine, military personnel**

✓7th **Y37.Ø21 Military operations involving explosion of marine mine, civilian**

✓6th **Y37.Ø3 Military operations involving explosion of sea-based artillery shell**

✓7th **Y37.Ø3Ø Military operations involving explosion of sea-based artillery shell, military personnel**

✓7th **Y37.Ø31 Military operations involving explosion of sea-based artillery shell, civilian**

✓6th **Y37.Ø4 Military operations involving explosion of torpedo**

✓7th **Y37.Ø4Ø Military operations involving explosion of torpedo, military personnel**

✓7th **Y37.Ø41 Military operations involving explosion of torpedo, civilian**

✓6th **Y37.Ø5 Military operations involving accidental detonation of onboard marine weapons**

✓7th **Y37.Ø5Ø Military operations involving accidental detonation of onboard marine weapons, military personnel**

✓7th **Y37.Ø51 Military operations involving accidental detonation of onboard marine weapons, civilian**

✓6th **Y37.Ø9 Military operations involving explosion of other marine weapons**

✓7th **Y37.Ø9Ø Military operations involving explosion of other marine weapons, military personnel**

✓7th **Y37.Ø91 Military operations involving explosion of other marine weapons, civilian**

✓5th **Y37.1 Military operations involving destruction of aircraft**

✓6th **Y37.1Ø Military operations involving unspecified destruction of aircraft**

✓7th **Y37.1ØØ Military operations involving unspecified destruction of aircraft, military personnel**

✓7th **Y37.1Ø1 Military operations involving unspecified destruction of aircraft, civilian**

✓6th **Y37.11 Military operations involving destruction of aircraft due to enemy fire or explosives**
Military operations involving destruction of aircraft due to air to air missile
Military operations involving destruction of aircraft due to explosive placed on aircraft
Military operations involving destruction of aircraft due to rocket propelled grenade [RPG]
Military operations involving destruction of aircraft due to small arms fire
Military operations involving destruction of aircraft due to surface to air missile

✓7th **Y37.11Ø Military operations involving destruction of aircraft due to enemy fire or explosives, military personnel**

✓7th **Y37.111 Military operations involving destruction of aircraft due to enemy fire or explosives, civilian**

✓6th **Y37.12 Military operations involving destruction of aircraft due to collision with other aircraft**

✓7th **Y37.12Ø Military operations involving destruction of aircraft due to collision with other aircraft, military personnel**

✓7th **Y37.121 Military operations involving destruction of aircraft due to collision with other aircraft, civilian**

✓6th **Y37.13 Military operations involving destruction of aircraft due to onboard fire**

✓7th **Y37.13Ø Military operations involving destruction of aircraft due to onboard fire, military personnel**

✓7th **Y37.131 Military operations involving destruction of aircraft due to onboard fire, civilian**

✓6th **Y37.14 Military operations involving destruction of aircraft due to accidental detonation of onboard munitions and explosives**

✓7th **Y37.14Ø Military operations involving destruction of aircraft due to accidental detonation of onboard munitions and explosives, military personnel**

✓7th **Y37.141 Military operations involving destruction of aircraft due to accidental detonation of onboard munitions and explosives, civilian**

✓6th **Y37.19 Military operations involving other destruction of aircraft**

✓7th **Y37.19Ø Military operations involving other destruction of aircraft, military personnel**

✓7th **Y37.191 Military operations involving other destruction of aircraft, civilian**

✓5th **Y37.2 Military operations involving other explosions and fragments**

EXCLUDES 1 *military operations involving explosion of aircraft (Y37.1-)*
military operations involving explosion of marine weapons (Y37.Ø-)
military operations involving explosion of nuclear weapons (Y37.5-)

✓6th **Y37.2Ø Military operations involving unspecified explosion and fragments**
Military operations involving air blast NOS
Military operations involving blast NOS
Military operations involving blast fragments NOS
Military operations involving blast wave NOS
Military operations involving blast wind NOS
Military operations involving explosion NOS
Military operations involving explosion of bomb NOS

✓7th **Y37.2ØØ Military operations involving unspecified explosion and fragments, military personnel**

Y37.201 **Military operations involving unspecified explosion and fragments, civilian**

Y37.21 **Military operations involving explosion of aerial bomb**

Y37.210 **Military operations involving explosion of aerial bomb, military personnel**

Y37.211 **Military operations involving explosion of aerial bomb, civilian**

Y37.22 **Military operations involving explosion of guided missile**

Y37.220 **Military operations involving explosion of guided missile, military personnel**

Y37.221 **Military operations involving explosion of guided missile, civilian**

Y37.23 **Military operations involving explosion of improvised explosive device [IED]**
Military operations involving explosion of person-borne improvised explosive device [IED]
Military operations involving explosion of vehicle-borne improvised explosive device [IED]
Military operations involving explosion of roadside improvised explosive device [IED]

Y37.230 **Military operations involving explosion of improvised explosive device [IED], military personnel**

Y37.231 **Military operations involving explosion of improvised explosive device [IED], civilian**

Y37.24 **Military operations involving explosion due to accidental detonation and discharge of own munitions or munitions launch device**

Y37.240 **Military operations involving explosion due to accidental detonation and discharge of own munitions or munitions launch device, military personnel**

Y37.241 **Military operations involving explosion due to accidental detonation and discharge of own munitions or munitions launch device, civilian**

Y37.25 **Military operations involving fragments from munitions**

Y37.250 **Military operations involving fragments from munitions, military personnel**

Y37.251 **Military operations involving fragments from munitions, civilian**

Y37.26 **Military operations involving fragments of improvised explosive device [IED]**
Military operations involving fragments of person-borne improvised explosive device [IED]
Military operations involving fragments of vehicle-borne improvised explosive device [IED]
Military operations involving fragments of roadside improvised explosive device [IED]

Y37.260 **Military operations involving fragments of improvised explosive device [IED], military personnel**

Y37.261 **Military operations involving fragments of improvised explosive device [IED], civilian**

Y37.27 **Military operations involving fragments from weapons**

Y37.270 **Military operations involving fragments from weapons, military personnel**

Y37.271 **Military operations involving fragments from weapons, civilian**

Y37.29 **Military operations involving other explosions and fragments**
Military operations involving explosion of grenade
Military operations involving explosions of land mine
Military operations involving shrapnel NOS

Y37.290 **Military operations involving other explosions and fragments, military personnel**

Y37.291 **Military operations involving other explosions and fragments, civilian**

Y37.3 **Military operations involving fires, conflagrations and hot substances**
Military operations involving smoke, fumes, and heat from fires, conflagrations and hot substances
EXCLUDES 1 *military operations involving fires and conflagrations aboard military aircraft (Y37.1-)*
military operations involving fires and conflagrations aboard military watercraft (Y37.0-)
military operations involving fires and conflagrations caused indirectly by conventional weapons (Y37.2-)
military operations involving fires and thermal effects of nuclear weapons (Y36.53-)

Y37.30 **Military operations involving unspecified fire, conflagration and hot substance**

Y37.300 **Military operations involving unspecified fire, conflagration and hot substance, military personnel**

Y37.301 **Military operations involving unspecified fire, conflagration and hot substance, civilian**

Y37.31 **Military operations involving gasoline bomb**
Military operations involving incendiary bomb
Military operations involving petrol bomb

Y37.310 **Military operations involving gasoline bomb, military personnel**

Y37.311 **Military operations involving gasoline bomb, civilian**

Y37.32 **Military operations involving incendiary bullet**

Y37.320 **Military operations involving incendiary bullet, military personnel**

Y37.321 **Military operations involving incendiary bullet, civilian**

Y37.33 **Military operations involving flamethrower**

Y37.330 **Military operations involving flamethrower, military personnel**

Y37.331 **Military operations involving flamethrower, civilian**

Y37.39 **Military operations involving other fires, conflagrations and hot substances**

Y37.390 **Military operations involving other fires, conflagrations and hot substances, military personnel**

Y37.391 **Military operations involving other fires, conflagrations and hot substances, civilian**

Y37.4 **Military operations involving firearm discharge and other forms of conventional warfare**

Y37.41 **Military operations involving rubber bullets**

Y37.410 **Military operations involving rubber bullets, military personnel**

Y37.411 **Military operations involving rubber bullets, civilian**

Y37.42 **Military operations involving firearms pellets**

Y37.420 **Military operations involving firearms pellets, military personnel**

Y37.421 **Military operations involving firearms pellets, civilian**

Y37.43 **Military operations involving other firearms discharge**
Military operations involving bullets NOS
EXCLUDES 1 *military operations involving munitions fragments (Y37.25-)*
military operations involving incendiary bullets (Y37.32-)

Y37.430 **Military operations involving other firearms discharge, military personnel**

Y37.431 **Military operations involving other firearms discharge, civilian**

Y37.44 **Military operations involving unarmed hand to hand combat**
EXCLUDES 1 *military operations involving combat using blunt or piercing object (Y37.45-)*
military operations involving intentional restriction of air and airway (Y37.46-)
military operations involving unintentional restriction of air and airway (Y37.47-)

✓7th **Y37.440 Military operations involving unarmed hand to hand combat, military personnel**

✓7th **Y37.441 Military operations involving unarmed hand to hand combat, civilian**

✓6th **Y37.45 Military operations involving combat using blunt or piercing object**

✓7th **Y37.450 Military operations involving combat using blunt or piercing object, military personnel**

✓7th **Y37.451 Military operations involving combat using blunt or piercing object, civilian**

✓6th **Y37.46 Military operations involving intentional restriction of air and airway**

✓7th **Y37.460 Military operations involving intentional restriction of air and airway, military personnel**

✓7th **Y37.461 Military operations involving intentional restriction of air and airway, civilian**

✓6th **Y37.47 Military operations involving unintentional restriction of air and airway**

✓7th **Y37.470 Military operations involving unintentional restriction of air and airway, military personnel**

✓7th **Y37.471 Military operations involving unintentional restriction of air and airway, civilian**

✓6th **Y37.49 Military operations involving other forms of conventional warfare**

✓7th **Y37.490 Military operations involving other forms of conventional warfare, military personnel**

✓7th **Y37.491 Military operations involving other forms of conventional warfare, civilian**

✓5th **Y37.5 Military operations involving nuclear weapons**

Military operation involving dirty bomb NOS

✓6th **Y37.50 Military operations involving unspecified effect of nuclear weapon**

✓7th **Y37.500 Military operations involving unspecified effect of nuclear weapon, military personnel**

✓7th **Y37.501 Military operations involving unspecified effect of nuclear weapon, civilian**

✓6th **Y37.51 Military operations involving direct blast effect of nuclear weapon**

Military operations involving blast pressure of nuclear weapon

✓7th **Y37.510 Military operations involving direct blast effect of nuclear weapon, military personnel**

✓7th **Y37.511 Military operations involving direct blast effect of nuclear weapon, civilian**

✓6th **Y37.52 Military operations involving indirect blast effect of nuclear weapon**

Military operations involving being thrown by blast of nuclear weapon

Military operations involving being struck or crushed by blast debris of nuclear weapon

✓7th **Y37.520 Military operations involving indirect blast effect of nuclear weapon, military personnel**

✓7th **Y37.521 Military operations involving indirect blast effect of nuclear weapon, civilian**

✓6th **Y37.53 Military operations involving thermal radiation effect of nuclear weapon**

Military operations involving direct heat from nuclear weapon

Military operation involving fireball effects from nuclear weapon

✓7th **Y37.530 Military operations involving thermal radiation effect of nuclear weapon, military personnel**

✓7th **Y37.531 Military operations involving thermal radiation effect of nuclear weapon, civilian**

✓6th **Y37.54 Military operation involving nuclear radiation effects of nuclear weapon**

Military operation involving acute radiation exposure from nuclear weapon

Military operation involving exposure to immediate ionizing radiation from nuclear weapon

Military operation involving fallout exposure from nuclear weapon

Military operation involving secondary effects of nuclear weapons

✓7th **Y37.540 Military operation involving nuclear radiation effects of nuclear weapon, military personnel**

✓7th **Y37.541 Military operation involving nuclear radiation effects of nuclear weapon, civilian**

✓6th **Y37.59 Military operation involving other effects of nuclear weapons**

✓7th **Y37.590 Military operation involving other effects of nuclear weapons, military personnel**

✓7th **Y37.591 Military operation involving other effects of nuclear weapons, civilian**

✓5th **Y37.6 Military operations involving biological weapons**

✓6th **Y37.6X Military operations involving biological weapons**

✓7th **Y37.6X0 Military operations involving biological weapons, military personnel**

✓7th **Y37.6X1 Military operations involving biological weapons, civilian**

✓5th **Y37.7 Military operations involving chemical weapons and other forms of unconventional warfare**

EXCLUDES 1 *military operations involving incendiary devices (Y36.3-, Y36.5-)*

✓6th **Y37.7X Military operations involving chemical weapons and other forms of unconventional warfare**

✓7th **Y37.7X0 Military operations involving chemical weapons and other forms of unconventional warfare, military personnel**

✓7th **Y37.7X1 Military operations involving chemical weapons and other forms of unconventional warfare, civilian**

✓5th **Y37.9 Other and unspecified military operations**

✓x7th **Y37.90 Military operations, unspecified**

✓x7th **Y37.91 Military operations involving unspecified weapon of mass destruction [WMD]**

✓x7th **Y37.92 Military operations involving friendly fire**

✓4th **Y38 Terrorism**

NOTE These codes are for use to identify injuries resulting from the unlawful use of force or violence against persons or property to intimidate or coerce a Government, the civilian population, or any segment thereof, in furtherance of political or social objective.

Use additional code for place of occurrence (Y92.-)

The appropriate 7th character is to be added to each code from category Y38.
A initial encounter
D subsequent encounter
S sequela

✓5th **Y38.0 Terrorism involving explosion of marine weapons**

Terrorism involving depth-charge

Terrorism involving marine mine

Terrorism involving mine NOS, at sea or in harbor

Terrorism involving sea-based artillery shell

Terrorism involving torpedo

Terrorism involving underwater blast

✓6th **Y38.0X Terrorism involving explosion of marine weapons**

✓7th **Y38.0X1 Terrorism involving explosion of marine weapons, public safety official injured**

✓7th **Y38.0X2 Terrorism involving explosion of marine weapons, civilian injured**

✓7th **Y38.0X3 Terrorism involving explosion of marine weapons, terrorist injured**

Y38.1 **Terrorism involving destruction of aircraft**
Terrorism involving aircraft burned
Terrorism involving aircraft exploded
Terrorism involving aircraft being shot down
Terrorism involving aircraft used as a weapon

Y38.1X **Terrorism involving destruction of aircraft**

Y38.1X1 **Terrorism involving destruction of aircraft, public safety official injured**

Y38.1X2 **Terrorism involving destruction of aircraft, civilian injured**

Y38.1X3 **Terrorism involving destruction of aircraft, terrorist injured**

Y38.2 **Terrorism involving other explosions and fragments**
Terrorism involving antipersonnel (fragments) bomb
Terrorism involving blast NOS
Terrorism involving explosion NOS
Terrorism involving explosion of breech block
Terrorism involving explosion of cannon block
Terrorism involving explosion (fragments) of artillery shell
Terrorism involving explosion (fragments) of bomb
Terrorism involving explosion (fragments) of grenade
Terrorism involving explosion (fragments) of guided missile
Terrorism involving explosion (fragments) of land mine
Terrorism involving explosion of mortar bomb
Terrorism involving explosion of munitions
Terrorism involving explosion (fragments) of rocket
Terrorism involving explosion (fragments) of shell
Terrorism involving shrapnel
Terrorism involving mine NOS, on land

EXCLUDES 1 *terrorism involving explosion of nuclear weapon (Y38.5)*
terrorism involving suicide bomber (Y38.81)

Y38.2X **Terrorism involving other explosions and fragments**

Y38.2X1 **Terrorism involving other explosions and fragments, public safety official injured**

Y38.2X2 **Terrorism involving other explosions and fragments, civilian injured**

Y38.2X3 **Terrorism involving other explosions and fragments, terrorist injured**

Y38.3 **Terrorism involving fires, conflagration and hot substances**
Terrorism involving conflagration NOS
Terrorism involving fire NOS
Terrorism involving petrol bomb

EXCLUDES 1 *terrorism involving fire or heat of nuclear weapon (Y38.5)*

Y38.3X **Terrorism involving fires, conflagration and hot substances**

Y38.3X1 **Terrorism involving fires, conflagration and hot substances, public safety official injured**

Y38.3X2 **Terrorism involving fires, conflagration and hot substances, civilian injured**

Y38.3X3 **Terrorism involving fires, conflagration and hot substances, terrorist injured**

Y38.4 **Terrorism involving firearms**
Terrorism involving carbine bullet
Terrorism involving machine gun bullet
Terrorism involving pellets (shotgun)
Terrorism involving pistol bullet
Terrorism involving rifle bullet
Terrorism involving rubber (rifle) bullet

Y38.4X **Terrorism involving firearms**

Y38.4X1 **Terrorism involving firearms, public safety official injured**

Y38.4X2 **Terrorism involving firearms, civilian injured**

Y38.4X3 **Terrorism involving firearms, terrorist injured**

Y38.5 **Terrorism involving nuclear weapons**
Terrorism involving blast effects of nuclear weapon
Terrorism involving exposure to ionizing radiation from nuclear weapon
Terrorism involving fireball effect of nuclear weapon
Terrorism involving heat from nuclear weapon

Y38.5X **Terrorism involving nuclear weapons**

Y38.5X1 **Terrorism involving nuclear weapons, public safety official injured**

Y38.5X2 **Terrorism involving nuclear weapons, civilian injured**

Y38.5X3 **Terrorism involving nuclear weapons, terrorist injured**

Y38.6 **Terrorism involving biological weapons**
Terrorism involving anthrax
Terrorism involving smallpox
Terrorism involving cholera

Y38.6X **Terrorism involving biological weapons**

Y38.6X1 **Terrorism involving biological weapons, public safety official injured**

Y38.6X2 **Terrorism involving biological weapons, civilian injured**

Y38.6X3 **Terrorism involving biological weapons, terrorist injured**

Y38.7 **Terrorism involving chemical weapons**
Terrorism involving gases, fumes, chemicals
Terrorism involving hydrogen cyanide
Terrorism involving phosgene
Terrorism involving sarin

Y38.7X **Terrorism involving chemical weapons**

Y38.7X1 **Terrorism involving chemical weapons, public safety official injured**

Y38.7X2 **Terrorism involving chemical weapons, civilian injured**

Y38.7X3 **Terrorism involving chemical weapons, terrorist injured**

Y38.8 **Terrorism involving other and unspecified means**

Y38.80 **Terrorism involving unspecified means**
Terrorism NOS

Y38.81 **Terrorism involving suicide bomber**

Y38.811 **Terrorism involving suicide bomber, public safety official injured**

Y38.812 **Terrorism involving suicide bomber, civilian injured**

Y38.89 **Terrorism involving other means**
Terrorism involving drowning and submersion
Terrorism involving lasers
Terrorism involving piercing or stabbing instruments

Y38.891 **Terrorism involving other means, public safety official injured**

Y38.892 **Terrorism involving other means, civilian injured**

Y38.893 **Terrorism involving other means, terrorist injured**

Y38.9 **Terrorism, secondary effects**

NOTE This code is for use to identify injuries occurring subsequent to a terrorist attack, not those that are due to the initial terrorist attack.

Y38.9X **Terrorism, secondary effects**

Y38.9X1 **Terrorism, secondary effects, public safety official injured**

Y38.9X2 **Terrorism, secondary effects, civilian injured**

Complications of medical and surgical care (Y62-Y84)

INCLUDES complications of medical devices
surgical and medical procedures as the cause of abnormal reaction of the patient, or of later complication, without mention of misadventure at the time of the procedure

Misadventures to patients during surgical and medical care (Y62-Y69)

EXCLUDES 2 *breakdown or malfunctioning of medical device (during procedure) (after implantation) (ongoing use) (Y70-Y82)*
surgical and medical procedures as the cause of abnormal reaction of the patient, without mention of misadventure at the time of the procedure (Y83-Y84)

Y62 **Failure of sterile precautions during surgical and medical care**

Y62.0 **Failure of sterile precautions during surgical operation**

Y62.1 **Failure of sterile precautions during infusion or transfusion**

Y62.2 **Failure of sterile precautions during kidney dialysis and other perfusion**

Y62.3 **Failure of sterile precautions during injection or immunization**

Y62.4 **Failure of sterile precautions during endoscopic examination**

Y62.5 **Failure of sterile precautions during heart catheterization**
Y62.6 **Failure of sterile precautions during aspiration, puncture and other catheterization**
Y62.8 **Failure of sterile precautions during other surgical and medical care**
Y62.9 **Failure of sterile precautions during unspecified surgical and medical care**

4th Y63 Failure in dosage during surgical and medical care
EXCLUDES 2 *accidental overdose of drug or wrong drug given in error (T36-T50)*
Y63.0 **Excessive amount of blood or other fluid given during transfusion or infusion**
Y63.1 **Incorrect dilution of fluid used during infusion**
Y63.2 **Overdose of radiation given during therapy**
Y63.3 **Inadvertent exposure of patient to radiation during medical care**
Y63.4 **Failure in dosage in electroshock or insulin-shock therapy**
Y63.5 **Inappropriate temperature in local application and packing**
Y63.6 **Underdosing and nonadministration of necessary drug, medicament or biological substance**
Y63.8 **Failure in dosage during other surgical and medical care**
Y63.9 **Failure in dosage during unspecified surgical and medical care**

4th Y64 Contaminated medical or biological substances
Y64.0 **Contaminated medical or biological substance, transfused or infused**
Y64.1 **Contaminated medical or biological substance, injected or used for immunization**
Y64.8 **Contaminated medical or biological substance administered by other means**
Y64.9 **Contaminated medical or biological substance administered by unspecified means**
Administered contaminated medical or biological substance NOS

4th Y65 Other misadventures during surgical and medical care
Y65.0 **Mismatched blood in transfusion**
Y65.1 **Wrong fluid used in infusion**
Y65.2 **Failure in suture or ligature during surgical operation**
Y65.3 **Endotracheal tube wrongly placed during anesthetic procedure**
Y65.4 **Failure to introduce or to remove other tube or instrument**
5th **Y65.5** **Performance of wrong procedure (operation)**
11 **Y65.51** **Performance of wrong procedure (operation) on correct patient**
Wrong device implanted into correct surgical site
EXCLUDES 1 *performance of correct procedure (operation) on wrong side or body part (Y65.53)*
11 **Y65.52** **Performance of procedure (operation) on patient not scheduled for surgery**
Performance of procedure (operation) intended for another patient
Performance of procedure (operation) on wrong patient
11 **Y65.53** **Performance of correct procedure (operation) on wrong side or body part**
Performance of correct procedure (operation) on wrong side
Performance of correct procedure (operation) on wrong site
Y65.8 **Other specified misadventures during surgical and medical care**

Y66 Nonadministration of surgical and medical care
Premature cessation of surgical and medical care
EXCLUDES 1 *DNR status (Z66)*
palliative care (Z51.5)

Y69 Unspecified misadventure during surgical and medical care

Medical devices associated with adverse incidents in diagnostic and therapeutic use (Y70-Y82)

INCLUDES breakdown or malfunction of medical devices (during use) (after implantation) (ongoing use)
EXCLUDES 1 *misadventure to patients during surgical and medical care, classifiable to (Y62-Y69)*
later complications following use of medical devices without breakdown or malfunctioning of device (Y83-Y84)

4th Y70 Anesthesiology devices associated with adverse incidents
Y70.0 **Diagnostic and monitoring anesthesiology devices associated with adverse incidents**
Y70.1 **Therapeutic (nonsurgical) and rehabilitative anesthesiology devices associated with adverse incidents**
Y70.2 **Prosthetic and other implants, materials and accessory anesthesiology devices associated with adverse incidents**
Y70.3 **Surgical instruments, materials and anesthesiology devices (including sutures) associated with adverse incidents**
Y70.8 **Miscellaneous anesthesiology devices associated with adverse incidents, not elsewhere classified**

4th Y71 Cardiovascular devices associated with adverse incidents
Y71.0 **Diagnostic and monitoring cardiovascular devices associated with adverse incidents**
Y71.1 **Therapeutic (nonsurgical) and rehabilitative cardiovascular devices associated with adverse incidents**
Y71.2 **Prosthetic and other implants, materials and accessory cardiovascular devices associated with adverse incidents**
Y71.3 **Surgical instruments, materials and cardiovascular devices (including sutures) associated with adverse incidents**
Y71.8 **Miscellaneous cardiovascular devices associated with adverse incidents, not elsewhere classified**

4th Y72 Otorhinolaryngological devices associated with adverse incidents
Y72.0 **Diagnostic and monitoring otorhinolaryngological devices associated with adverse incidents**
Y72.1 **Therapeutic (nonsurgical) and rehabilitative otorhinolaryngological devices associated with adverse incidents**
Y72.2 **Prosthetic and other implants, materials and accessory otorhinolaryngological devices associated with adverse incidents**
Y72.3 **Surgical instruments, materials and otorhinolaryngological devices (including sutures) associated with adverse incidents**
Y72.8 **Miscellaneous otorhinolaryngological devices associated with adverse incidents, not elsewhere classified**

4th Y73 Gastroenterology and urology devices associated with adverse incidents
Y73.0 **Diagnostic and monitoring gastroenterology and urology devices associated with adverse incidents**
Y73.1 **Therapeutic (nonsurgical) and rehabilitative gastroenterology and urology devices associated with adverse incidents**
Y73.2 **Prosthetic and other implants, materials and accessory gastroenterology and urology devices associated with adverse incidents**
Y73.3 **Surgical instruments, materials and gastroenterology and urology devices (including sutures) associated with adverse incidents**
Y73.8 **Miscellaneous gastroenterology and urology devices associated with adverse incidents, not elsewhere classified**

4th Y74 General hospital and personal-use devices associated with adverse incidents
Y74.0 **Diagnostic and monitoring general hospital and personal-use devices associated with adverse incidents**
Y74.1 **Therapeutic (nonsurgical) and rehabilitative general hospital and personal-use devices associated with adverse incidents**
Y74.2 **Prosthetic and other implants, materials and accessory general hospital and personal-use devices associated with adverse incidents**
Y74.3 **Surgical instruments, materials and general hospital and personal-use devices (including sutures) associated with adverse incidents**
Y74.8 **Miscellaneous general hospital and personal-use devices associated with adverse incidents, not elsewhere classified**

11 Wrong procedure performed edit applies.

✓4th Y75 Neurological devices associated with adverse incidents

Y75.0 Diagnostic and monitoring neurological devices associated with adverse incidents

Y75.1 Therapeutic (nonsurgical) and rehabilitative neurological devices associated with adverse incidents

Y75.2 Prosthetic and other implants, materials and neurological devices associated with adverse incidents

Y75.3 Surgical instruments, materials and neurological devices (including sutures) associated with adverse incidents

Y75.8 Miscellaneous neurological devices associated with adverse incidents, not elsewhere classified

✓4th Y76 Obstetric and gynecological devices associated with adverse incidents

Y76.0 Diagnostic and monitoring obstetric and gynecological devices associated with adverse incidents ♀

Y76.1 Therapeutic (nonsurgical) and rehabilitative obstetric and gynecological devices associated with adverse incidents ♀

Y76.2 Prosthetic and other implants, materials and accessory obstetric and gynecological devices associated with adverse incidents ♀

Y76.3 Surgical instruments, materials and obstetric and gynecological devices (including sutures) associated with adverse incidents ♀

Y76.8 Miscellaneous obstetric and gynecological devices associated with adverse incidents, not elsewhere classified ♀

✓4th Y77 Ophthalmic devices associated with adverse incidents

Y77.0 Diagnostic and monitoring ophthalmic devices associated with adverse incidents

Y77.1 Therapeutic (nonsurgical) and rehabilitative ophthalmic devices associated with adverse incidents

Y77.2 Prosthetic and other implants, materials and accessory ophthalmic devices associated with adverse incidents

Y77.3 Surgical instruments, materials and ophthalmic devices (including sutures) associated with adverse incidents

Y77.8 Miscellaneous ophthalmic devices associated with adverse incidents, not elsewhere classified

✓4th Y78 Radiological devices associated with adverse incidents

Y78.0 Diagnostic and monitoring radiological devices associated with adverse incidents

Y78.1 Therapeutic (nonsurgical) and rehabilitative radiological devices associated with adverse incidents

Y78.2 Prosthetic and other implants, materials and accessory radiological devices associated with adverse incidents

Y78.3 Surgical instruments, materials and radiological devices (including sutures) associated with adverse incidents

Y78.8 Miscellaneous radiological devices associated with adverse incidents, not elsewhere classified

✓4th Y79 Orthopedic devices associated with adverse incidents

Y79.0 Diagnostic and monitoring orthopedic devices associated with adverse incidents

Y79.1 Therapeutic (nonsurgical) and rehabilitative orthopedic devices associated with adverse incidents

Y79.2 Prosthetic and other implants, materials and accessory orthopedic devices associated with adverse incidents

Y79.3 Surgical instruments, materials and orthopedic devices (including sutures) associated with adverse incidents

Y79.8 Miscellaneous orthopedic devices associated with adverse incidents, not elsewhere classified

✓4th Y80 Physical medicine devices associated with adverse incidents

Y80.0 Diagnostic and monitoring physical medicine devices associated with adverse incidents

Y80.1 Therapeutic (nonsurgical) and rehabilitative physical medicine devices associated with adverse incidents

Y80.2 Prosthetic and other implants, materials and accessory physical medicine devices associated with adverse incidents

Y80.3 Surgical instruments, materials and physical medicine devices (including sutures) associated with adverse incidents

Y80.8 Miscellaneous physical medicine devices associated with adverse incidents, not elsewhere classified

✓4th Y81 General- and plastic-surgery devices associated with adverse incidents

Y81.0 Diagnostic and monitoring general- and plastic-surgery devices associated with adverse incidents

Y81.1 Therapeutic (nonsurgical) and rehabilitative general- and plastic-surgery devices associated with adverse incidents

Y81.2 Prosthetic and other implants, materials and accessory general- and plastic-surgery devices associated with adverse incidents

Y81.3 Surgical instruments, materials and general- and plastic-surgery devices (including sutures) associated with adverse incidents

Y81.8 Miscellaneous general- and plastic-surgery devices associated with adverse incidents, not elsewhere classified

✓4th Y82 Other and unspecified medical devices associated with adverse incidents

Y82.8 Other medical devices associated with adverse incidents

Y82.9 Unspecified medical devices associated with adverse incidents

Surgical and other medical procedures as the cause of abnormal reaction of the patient, or of later complication, without mention of misadventure at the time of the procedure (Y83-Y84)

EXCLUDES 1 *misadventures to patients during surgical and medical care, classifiable to (Y62-Y69)*

✓4th Y83 Surgical operation and other surgical procedures as the cause of abnormal reaction of the patient, or of later complication, without mention of misadventure at the time of the procedure

Y83.0 Surgical operation with transplant of whole organ as the cause of abnormal reaction of the patient, or of later complication, without mention of misadventure at the time of the procedure

Y83.1 Surgical operation with implant of artificial internal device as the cause of abnormal reaction of the patient, or of later complication, without mention of misadventure at the time of the procedure

Y83.2 Surgical operation with anastomosis, bypass or graft as the cause of abnormal reaction of the patient, or of later complication, without mention of misadventure at the time of the procedure

Y83.3 Surgical operation with formation of external stoma as the cause of abnormal reaction of the patient, or of later complication, without mention of misadventure at the time of the procedure

Y83.4 Other reconstructive surgery as the cause of abnormal reaction of the patient, or of later complication, without mention of misadventure at the time of the procedure

Y83.5 Amputation of limb(s) as the cause of abnormal reaction of the patient, or of later complication, without mention of misadventure at the time of the procedure

Y83.6 Removal of other organ (partial) (total) as the cause of abnormal reaction of the patient, or of later complication, without mention of misadventure at the time of the procedure

Y83.8 Other surgical procedures as the cause of abnormal reaction of the patient, or of later complication, without mention of misadventure at the time of the procedure

Y83.9 Surgical procedure, unspecified as the cause of abnormal reaction of the patient, or of later complication, without mention of misadventure at the time of the procedure

✓4th Y84 Other medical procedures as the cause of abnormal reaction of the patient, or of later complication, without mention of misadventure at the time of the procedure

Y84.0 Cardiac catheterization as the cause of abnormal reaction of the patient, or of later complication, without mention of misadventure at the time of the procedure

Y84.1 Kidney dialysis as the cause of abnormal reaction of the patient, or of later complication, without mention of misadventure at the time of the procedure

Y84.2 Radiological procedure and radiotherapy as the cause of abnormal reaction of the patient, or of later complication, without mention of misadventure at the time of the procedure

Y84.3 Shock therapy as the cause of abnormal reaction of the patient, or of later complication, without mention of misadventure at the time of the procedure

Y84.4 Aspiration of fluid as the cause of abnormal reaction of the patient, or of later complication, without mention of misadventure at the time of the procedure

Y84.5 Insertion of gastric or duodenal sound as the cause of abnormal reaction of the patient, or of later complication, without mention of misadventure at the time of the procedure

Y84.6 Urinary catheterization as the cause of abnormal reaction of the patient, or of later complication, without mention of misadventure at the time of the procedure

Y84.7 Blood-sampling as the cause of abnormal reaction of the patient, or of later complication, without mention of misadventure at the time of the procedure

Y84.8 Other medical procedures as the cause of abnormal reaction of the patient, or of later complication, without mention of misadventure at the time of the procedure

Y84.9 Medical procedure, unspecified as the cause of abnormal reaction of the patient, or of later complication, without mention of misadventure at the time of the procedure

Supplementary factors related to causes of morbidity classified elsewhere (Y90-Y99)

NOTE These categories may be used to provide supplementary information concerning causes of morbidity. They are not to be used for single-condition coding.

✓4th Y90 Evidence of alcohol involvement determined by blood alcohol level

Code first any associated alcohol related disorders (F10)

Y90.0 Blood alcohol level of less than 20 mg/100 ml

Y90.1 Blood alcohol level of 20-39 mg/100 ml

Y90.2 Blood alcohol level of 40-59 mg/100 ml

Y90.3 Blood alcohol level of 60-79 mg/100 ml

Y90.4 Blood alcohol level of 80-99 mg/100 ml

Y90.5 Blood alcohol level of 100-119 mg/100 ml

Y90.6 Blood alcohol level of 120-199 mg/100 ml

Y90.7 Blood alcohol level of 200-239 mg/100 ml

Y90.8 Blood alcohol level of 240 mg/100 ml or more

Y90.9 Presence of alcohol in blood, level not specified

✓4th Y92 Place of occurrence of the external cause

The following category is for use, when relevant, to identify the place of occurrence of the external cause. Use in conjunction with an activity code.

Place of occurrence should be recorded only at the initial encounter for treatment

✓5th Y92.0 Non-institutional (private) residence as the place of occurrence of the external cause

EXCLUDES 1 *abandoned or derelict house (Y92.89)*
home under construction but not yet occupied (Y92.6-)
institutional place of residence (Y92.1-)

✓6th Y92.00 Unspecified non-institutional (private) residence as the place of occurrence of the external cause

Y92.000 Kitchen of unspecified non-institutional (private) residence as the place of occurrence of the external cause

Y92.001 Dining room of unspecified non-institutional (private) residence as the place of occurrence of the external cause

Y92.002 Bathroom of unspecified non-institutional (private) residence single-family (private) house as the place of occurrence of the external cause

Y92.003 Bedroom of unspecified non-institutional (private) residence as the place of occurrence of the external cause

Y92.007 Garden or yard of unspecified non-institutional (private) residence as the place of occurrence of the external cause

Y92.008 Other place in unspecified non-institutional (private) residence as the place of occurrence of the external cause

Y92.009 Unspecified place in unspecified non-institutional (private) residence as the place of occurrence of the external cause

Home (NOS) as the place of occurrence of the external cause

✓6th Y92.01 Single-family non-institutional (private) house as the place of occurrence of the external cause

Farmhouse as the place of occurrence of the external cause

EXCLUDES 1 *barn (Y92.71)*
chicken coop or hen house (Y92.72)
farm field (Y92.73)
orchard (Y92.74)
single family mobile home or trailer (Y92.02-)
slaughter house (Y92.86)

Y92.010 Kitchen of single-family (private) house as the place of occurrence of the external cause

Y92.011 Dining room of single-family (private) house as the place of occurrence of the external cause

Y92.012 Bathroom of single-family (private) house as the place of occurrence of the external cause

Y92.013 Bedroom of single-family (private) house as the place of occurrence of the external cause

Y92.014 Private driveway to single-family (private) house as the place of occurrence of the external cause

Y92.015 Private garage of single-family (private) house as the place of occurrence of the external cause

Y92.016 Swimming-pool in single-family (private) house or garden as the place of occurrence of the external cause

Y92.017 Garden or yard in single-family (private) house as the place of occurrence of the external cause

Y92.018 Other place in single-family (private) house as the place of occurrence of the external cause

Y92.019 Unspecified place in single-family (private) house as the place of occurrence of the external cause

✓6th Y92.02 Mobile home as the place of occurrence of the external cause

Y92.020 Kitchen in mobile home as the place of occurrence of the external cause

Y92.021 Dining room in mobile home as the place of occurrence of the external cause

Y92.022 Bathroom in mobile home as the place of occurrence of the external cause

Y92.023 Bedroom in mobile home as the place of occurrence of the external cause

Y92.024 Driveway of mobile home as the place of occurrence of the external cause

Y92.025 Garage of mobile home as the place of occurrence of the external cause

Y92.026 Swimming-pool of mobile home as the place of occurrence of the external cause

Y92.027 Garden or yard of mobile home as the place of occurrence of the external cause

Y92.028 Other place in mobile home as the place of occurrence of the external cause

Y92.029 Unspecified place in mobile home as the place of occurrence of the external cause

✓6th Y92.03 Apartment as the place of occurrence of the external cause

Condominium as the place of occurrence of the external cause

Co-op apartment as the place of occurrence of the external cause

Y92.030 Kitchen in apartment as the place of occurrence of the external cause

Y92.031 Bathroom in apartment as the place of occurrence of the external cause

Y92.032 Bedroom in apartment as the place of occurrence of the external cause

Y92.038 Other place in apartment as the place of occurrence of the external cause

Y92.039 Unspecified place in apartment as the place of occurrence of the external cause

✓6th Y92.04 Boarding-house as the place of occurrence of the external cause

Y92.040 Kitchen in boarding-house as the place of occurrence of the external cause

Y92.041 Bathroom in boarding-house as the place of occurrence of the external cause

Y92.042 Bedroom in boarding-house as the place of occurrence of the external cause

Y92.043 Driveway of boarding-house as the place of occurrence of the external cause

Y92.044 Garage of boarding-house as the place of occurrence of the external cause

Y92.045 Swimming-pool of boarding-house as the place of occurrence of the external cause
Y92.046 Garden or yard of boarding-house as the place of occurrence of the external cause
Y92.048 Other place in boarding-house as the place of occurrence of the external cause
Y92.049 Unspecified place in boarding-house as the place of occurrence of the external cause

✓6th Y92.09 Other non-institutional residence as the place of occurrence of the external cause
Y92.090 Kitchen in other non-institutional residence as the place of occurrence of the external cause
Y92.091 Bathroom in other non-institutional residence as the place of occurrence of the external cause
Y92.092 Bedroom in other non-institutional residence as the place of occurrence of the external cause
Y92.093 Driveway of other non-institutional residence as the place of occurrence of the external cause
Y92.094 Garage of other non-institutional residence as the place of occurrence of the external cause
Y92.095 Swimming-pool of other non-institutional residence as the place of occurrence of the external cause
Y92.096 Garden or yard of other non-institutional residence as the place of occurrence of the external cause
Y92.098 Other place in other non-institutional residence as the place of occurrence of the external cause
Y92.099 Unspecified place in other non-institutional residence as the place of occurrence of the external cause

✓5th Y92.1 Institutional (nonprivate) residence as the place of occurrence of the external cause
Y92.10 Unspecified residential institution as the place of occurrence of the external cause

✓6th Y92.11 Children's home and orphanage as the place of occurrence of the external cause
Y92.110 Kitchen in children's home and orphanage as the place of occurrence of the external cause
Y92.111 Bathroom in children's home and orphanage as the place of occurrence of the external cause
Y92.112 Bedroom in children's home and orphanage as the place of occurrence of the external cause
Y92.113 Driveway of children's home and orphanage as the place of occurrence of the external cause
Y92.114 Garage of children's home and orphanage as the place of occurrence of the external cause
Y92.115 Swimming-pool of children's home and orphanage as the place of occurrence of the external cause
Y92.116 Garden or yard of children's home and orphanage as the place of occurrence of the external cause
Y92.118 Other place in children's home and orphanage as the place of occurrence of the external cause
Y92.119 Unspecified place in children's home and orphanage as the place of occurrence of the external cause

✓6th Y92.12 Nursing home as the place of occurrence of the external cause
Home for the sick as the place of occurrence of the external cause
Hospice as the place of occurrence of the external cause
Y92.120 Kitchen in nursing home as the place of occurrence of the external cause
Y92.121 Bathroom in nursing home as the place of occurrence of the external cause
Y92.122 Bedroom in nursing home as the place of occurrence of the external cause
Y92.123 Driveway of nursing home as the place of occurrence of the external cause
Y92.124 Garage of nursing home as the place of occurrence of the external cause
Y92.125 Swimming-pool of nursing home as the place of occurrence of the external cause
Y92.126 Garden or yard of nursing home as the place of occurrence of the external cause
Y92.128 Other place in nursing home as the place of occurrence of the external cause
Y92.129 Unspecified place in nursing home as the place of occurrence of the external cause

✓6th Y92.13 Military base as the place of occurrence of the external cause
EXCLUDES 1 *military training grounds (Y92.83)*
Y92.130 Kitchen on military base as the place of occurrence of the external cause
Y92.131 Mess hall on military base as the place of occurrence of the external cause
Y92.133 Barracks on military base as the place of occurrence of the external cause
Y92.135 Garage on military base as the place of occurrence of the external cause
Y92.136 Swimming-pool on military base as the place of occurrence of the external cause
Y92.137 Garden or yard on military base as the place of occurrence of the external cause
Y92.138 Other place on military base as the place of occurrence of the external cause
Y92.139 Unspecified place military base as the place of occurrence of the external cause

✓6th Y92.14 Prison as the place of occurrence of the external cause
Y92.140 Kitchen in prison as the place of occurrence of the external cause
Y92.141 Dining room in prison as the place of occurrence of the external cause
Y92.142 Bathroom in prison as the place of occurrence of the external cause
Y92.143 Cell of prison as the place of occurrence of the external cause
Y92.146 Swimming-pool of prison as the place of occurrence of the external cause
Y92.147 Courtyard of prison as the place of occurrence of the external cause
Y92.148 Other place in prison as the place of occurrence of the external cause
Y92.149 Unspecified place in prison as the place of occurrence of the external cause

✓6th Y92.15 Reform school as the place of occurrence of the external cause
Y92.150 Kitchen in reform school as the place of occurrence of the external cause
Y92.151 Dining room in reform school as the place of occurrence of the external cause
Y92.152 Bathroom in reform school as the place of occurrence of the external cause
Y92.153 Bedroom in reform school as the place of occurrence of the external cause
Y92.154 Driveway of reform school as the place of occurrence of the external cause
Y92.155 Garage of reform school as the place of occurrence of the external cause
Y92.156 Swimming-pool of reform school as the place of occurrence of the external cause
Y92.157 Garden or yard of reform school as the place of occurrence of the external cause
Y92.158 Other place in reform school as the place of occurrence of the external cause
Y92.159 Unspecified place in reform school as the place of occurrence of the external cause

✓6th **Y92.16 School dormitory as the place of occurrence of the external cause**
EXCLUDES 1 *reform school as the place of occurrence of the external cause (Y92.15-)*
school buildings and grounds as the place of occurrence of the external cause (Y92.2-)
school sports and athletic areas as the place of occurrence of the external cause (Y92.3-)

Y92.160 Kitchen in school dormitory as the place of occurrence of the external cause

Y92.161 Dining room in school dormitory as the place of occurrence of the external cause

Y92.162 Bathroom in school dormitory as the place of occurrence of the external cause

Y92.163 Bedroom in school dormitory as the place of occurrence of the external cause

Y92.168 Other place in school dormitory as the place of occurrence of the external cause

Y92.169 Unspecified place in school dormitory as the place of occurrence of the external cause

✓6th **Y92.19 Other specified residential institution as the place of occurrence of the external cause**

Y92.190 Kitchen in other specified residential institution as the place of occurrence of the external cause

Y92.191 Dining room in other specified residential institution as the place of occurrence of the external cause

Y92.192 Bathroom in other specified residential institution as the place of occurrence of the external cause

Y92.193 Bedroom in other specified residential institution as the place of occurrence of the external cause

Y92.194 Driveway of other specified residential institution as the place of occurrence of the external cause

Y92.195 Garage of other specified residential institution as the place of occurrence of the external cause

Y92.196 Pool of other specified residential institution as the place of occurrence of the external cause

Y92.197 Garden or yard of other specified residential institution as the place of occurrence of the external cause

Y92.198 Other place in other specified residential institution as the place of occurrence of the external cause

Y92.199 Unspecified place in other specified residential institution as the place of occurrence of the external cause

✓5th **Y92.2 School, other institution and public administrative area as the place of occurrence of the external cause**
Building and adjacent grounds used by the general public or by a particular group of the public
EXCLUDES 1 *building under construction as the place of occurrence of the external cause (Y92.6)*
residential institution as the place of occurrence of the external cause (Y92.1)
school dormitory as the place of occurrence of the external cause (Y92.16-)
sports and athletics area of schools as the place of occurrence of the external cause (Y92.3-)

✓6th **Y92.21 School (private) (public) (state) as the place of occurrence of the external cause**

Y92.210 Daycare center as the place of occurrence of the external cause

Y92.211 Elementary school as the place of occurrence of the external cause
Kindergarten as the place of occurrence of the external cause

Y92.212 Middle school as the place of occurrence of the external cause

Y92.213 High school as the place of occurrence of the external cause
AHA: 2012, 4Q, 108

Y92.214 College as the place of occurrence of the external cause
University as the place of occurrence of the external cause

Y92.215 Trade school as the place of occurrence of the external cause

Y92.218 Other school as the place of occurrence of the external cause

Y92.219 Unspecified school as the place of occurrence of the external cause

Y92.22 Religious institution as the place of occurrence of the external cause
Church as the place of occurrence of the external cause
Mosque as the place of occurrence of the external cause
Synagogue as the place of occurrence of the external cause

✓6th **Y92.23 Hospital as the place of occurrence of the external cause**
EXCLUDES 1 *ambulatory (outpatient) health services establishments (Y92.53-)*
home for the sick as the place of occurrence of the external cause (Y92.12-)
hospice as the place of occurrence of the external cause (Y92.12-)
nursing home as the place of occurrence of the external cause (Y92.12-)

Y92.230 Patient room in hospital as the place of occurrence of the external cause

Y92.231 Patient bathroom in hospital as the place of occurrence of the external cause

Y92.232 Corridor of hospital as the place of occurrence of the external cause

Y92.233 Cafeteria of hospital as the place of occurrence of the external cause

Y92.234 Operating room of hospital as the place of occurrence of the external cause

Y92.238 Other place in hospital as the place of occurrence of the external cause

Y92.239 Unspecified place in hospital as the place of occurrence of the external cause

✓6th **Y92.24 Public administrative building as the place of occurrence of the external cause**

Y92.240 Courthouse as the place of occurrence of the external cause

Y92.241 Library as the place of occurrence of the external cause

Y92.242 Post office as the place of occurrence of the external cause

Y92.243 City hall as the place of occurrence of the external cause

Y92.248 Other public administrative building as the place of occurrence of the external cause

✓6th **Y92.25 Cultural building as the place of occurrence of the external cause**

Y92.250 Art Gallery as the place of occurrence of the external cause

Y92.251 Museum as the place of occurrence of the external cause

Y92.252 Music hall as the place of occurrence of the external cause

Y92.253 Opera house as the place of occurrence of the external cause

Y92.254 Theater (live) as the place of occurrence of the external cause

Y92.258 Other cultural public building as the place of occurrence of the external cause

Y92.26 Movie house or cinema as the place of occurrence of the external cause

Y92.29 Other specified public building as the place of occurrence of the external cause
Assembly hall as the place of occurrence of the external cause
Clubhouse as the place of occurrence of the external cause

Y92.3 Sports and athletics area as the place of occurrence of the external cause

Y92.31 Athletic court as the place of occurrence of the external cause

EXCLUDES 1 *tennis court in private home or garden (Y92.09)*

Y92.310 Basketball court as the place of occurrence of the external cause

Y92.311 Squash court as the place of occurrence of the external cause

Y92.312 Tennis court as the place of occurrence of the external cause

Y92.318 Other athletic court as the place of occurrence of the external cause

Y92.32 Athletic field as the place of occurrence of the external cause

Y92.320 Baseball field as the place of occurrence of the external cause

Y92.321 Football field as the place of occurrence of the external cause

Y92.322 Soccer field as the place of occurrence of the external cause

Y92.328 Other athletic field as the place of occurrence of the external cause

Cricket field as the place of occurrence of the external cause

Hockey field as the place of occurrence of the external cause

Y92.33 Skating rink as the place of occurrence of the external cause

Y92.330 Ice skating rink (indoor) (outdoor) as the place of occurrence of the external cause

Y92.331 Roller skating rink as the place of occurrence of the external cause

Y92.34 Swimming pool (public) as the place of occurrence of the external cause

EXCLUDES 1 *swimming pool in private home or garden (Y92.016)*

Y92.39 Other specified sports and athletic area as the place of occurrence of the external cause

Golf-course as the place of occurrence of the external cause

Gymnasium as the place of occurrence of the external cause

Riding-school as the place of occurrence of the external cause

Stadium as the place of occurrence of the external cause

Y92.4 Street, highway and other paved roadways as the place of occurrence of the external cause

EXCLUDES 1 *private driveway of residence (Y92.014, Y92.024, Y92.043, Y92.093, Y92.113, Y92.123, Y92.154, Y92.194)*

Y92.41 Street and highway as the place of occurrence of the external cause

Y92.410 Unspecified street and highway as the place of occurrence of the external cause

Road NOS as the place of occurrence of the external cause

Y92.411 Interstate highway as the place of occurrence of the external cause

Freeway as the place of occurrence of the external cause

Motorway as the place of occurrence of the external cause

Y92.412 Parkway as the place of occurrence of the external cause

Y92.413 State road as the place of occurrence of the external cause

Y92.414 Local residential or business street as the place of occurrence of the external cause

Y92.415 Exit ramp or entrance ramp of street or highway as the place of occurrence of the external cause

Y92.48 Other paved roadways as the place of occurrence of the external cause

Y92.480 Sidewalk as the place of occurrence of the external cause

Y92.481 Parking lot as the place of occurrence of the external cause

Y92.482 Bike path as the place of occurrence of the external cause

Y92.488 Other paved roadways as the place of occurrence of the external cause

Y92.5 Trade and service area as the place of occurrence of the external cause

EXCLUDES 1 *garage in private home (Y92.015)*
schools and other public administration buildings (Y92.2-)

Y92.51 Private commercial establishments as the place of occurrence of the external cause

Y92.510 Bank as the place of occurrence of the external cause

Y92.511 Restaurant or café as the place of occurrence of the external cause

Y92.512 Supermarket, store or market as the place of occurrence of the external cause

Y92.513 Shop (commercial) as the place of occurrence of the external cause

Y92.52 Service areas as the place of occurrence of the external cause

Y92.520 Airport as the place of occurrence of the external cause

Y92.521 Bus station as the place of occurrence of the external cause

Y92.522 Railway station as the place of occurrence of the external cause

Y92.523 Highway rest stop as the place of occurrence of the external cause

Y92.524 Gas station as the place of occurrence of the external cause

Petroleum station as the place of occurrence of the external cause

Service station as the place of occurrence of the external cause

Y92.53 Ambulatory health services establishments as the place of occurrence of the external cause

Y92.530 Ambulatory surgery center as the place of occurrence of the external cause

Outpatient surgery center, including that connected with a hospital as the place of occurrence of the external cause

Same day surgery center, including that connected with a hospital as the place of occurrence of the external cause

Y92.531 Health care provider office as the place of occurrence of the external cause

Physician office as the place of occurrence of the external cause

Y92.532 Urgent care center as the place of occurrence of the external cause

Y92.538 Other ambulatory health services establishments as the place of occurrence of the external cause

Y92.59 Other trade areas as the place of occurrence of the external cause

Office building as the place of occurrence of the external cause

Casino as the place of occurrence of the external cause

Garage (commercial) as the place of occurrence of the external cause

Hotel as the place of occurrence of the external cause

Radio or television station as the place of occurrence of the external cause

Shopping mall as the place of occurrence of the external cause

Warehouse as the place of occurrence of the external cause

Y92.6 Industrial and construction area as the place of occurrence of the external cause

Y92.61 Building [any] under construction as the place of occurrence of the external cause

Y92.62 Dock or shipyard as the place of occurrence of the external cause

Dockyard as the place of occurrence of the external cause

Dry dock as the place of occurrence of the external cause

Shipyard as the place of occurrence of the external cause

Y92.63 Factory as the place of occurrence of the external cause
Factory building as the place of occurrence of the external cause
Factory premises as the place of occurrence of the external cause
Industrial yard as the place of occurrence of the external cause

Y92.64 Mine or pit as the place of occurrence of the external cause
Mine as the place of occurrence of the external cause

Y92.65 Oil rig as the place of occurrence of the external cause
Pit (coal) (gravel) (sand) as the place of occurrence of the external cause

Y92.69 Other specified industrial and construction area as the place of occurrence of the external cause
Gasworks as the place of occurrence of the external cause
Power-station (coal) (nuclear) (oil) as the place of occurrence of the external cause
Tunnel under construction as the place of occurrence of the external cause
Workshop as the place of occurrence of the external cause

✓5th **Y92.7 Farm as the place of occurrence of the external cause**
Ranch as the place of occurrence of the external cause
EXCLUDES1 *farmhouse and home premises of farm (Y92.Ø1-)*

Y92.71 Barn as the place of occurrence of the external cause

Y92.72 Chicken coop as the place of occurrence of the external cause
Hen house as the place of occurrence of the external cause

Y92.73 Farm field as the place of occurrence of the external cause

Y92.74 Orchard as the place of occurrence of the external cause

Y92.79 Other farm location as the place of occurrence of the external cause

✓5th **Y92.8 Other places as the place of occurrence of the external cause**

✓6th **Y92.81 Transport vehicle as the place of occurrence of the external cause**
EXCLUDES1 *transport accidents (VØØ-V99)*

Y92.81Ø Car as the place of occurrence of the external cause

Y92.811 Bus as the place of occurrence of the external cause

Y92.812 Truck as the place of occurrence of the external cause

Y92.813 Airplane as the place of occurrence of the external cause

Y92.814 Boat as the place of occurrence of the external cause

Y92.815 Train as the place of occurrence of the external cause

Y92.816 Subway car as the place of occurrence of the external cause

Y92.818 Other transport vehicle as the place of occurrence of the external cause

✓6th **Y92.82 Wilderness area**

Y92.82Ø Desert as the place of occurrence of the external cause

Y92.821 Forest as the place of occurrence of the external cause

Y92.828 Other wilderness area as the place of occurrence of the external cause
Swamp as the place of occurrence of the external cause
Mountain as the place of occurrence of the external cause
Marsh as the place of occurrence of the external cause
Prairie as the place of occurrence of the external cause

✓6th **Y92.83 Recreation area as the place of occurrence of the external cause**

Y92.83Ø Public park as the place of occurrence of the external cause

Y92.831 Amusement park as the place of occurrence of the external cause

Y92.832 Beach as the place of occurrence of the external cause
Seashore as the place of occurrence of the external cause

Y92.833 Campsite as the place of occurrence of the external cause

Y92.834 Zoological garden (Zoo) as the place of occurrence of the external cause

Y92.838 Other recreation area as the place of occurrence of the external cause

Y92.84 Military training ground as the place of occurrence of the external cause

Y92.85 Railroad track as the place of occurrence of the external cause

Y92.86 Slaughter house as the place of occurrence of the external cause

Y92.89 Other specified places as the place of occurrence of the external cause
Derelict house as the place of occurrence of the external cause

Y92.9 Unspecified place or not applicable

✓4th **Y93 Activity codes**

NOTE Category Y93 is provided for use to indicate the activity of the person seeking healthcare for an injury or health condition, such as a heart attack while shoveling snow, which resulted from, or was contributed to, by the activity. These codes are appropriate for use for both acute injuries, such as those from chapter 19, and conditions that are due to the long-term, cumulative effects of an activity, such as those from chapter 13. They are also appropriate for use with external cause codes for cause and intent if identifying the activity provides additional information on the event. These codes should be used in conjunction with codes for external cause status (Y99) and place of occurrence (Y92).
This section contains the following broad activity categories:
Y93.Ø Activities involving walking and running
Y93.1 Activities involving water and water craft
Y93.2 Activities involving ice and snow
Y93.3 Activities involving climbing, rappelling, and jumping off
Y93.4 Activities involving dancing and other rhythmic movement
Y93.5 Activities involving other sports and athletics played individually
Y93.6 Activities involving other sports and athletics played as a team or group
Y93.7 Activities involving other specified sports and athletics
Y93.A Activities involving other cardiorespiratory exercise
Y93.B Activities involving other muscle strengthening exercises
Y93.C Activities involving computer technology and electronic devices
Y93.D Activities involving arts and handcrafts
Y93.E Activities involving personal hygiene and interior property and clothing maintenance
Y93.F Activities involving caregiving
Y93.G Activities involving food preparation, cooking and grilling
Y93.H Activities involving exterior property and land maintenance, building and construction
Y93.I Activities involving roller coasters and other types of external motion
Y93.J Activities involving playing musical instrument
Y93.K Activities involving animal care
Y93.8 Activities, other specified
Y93.9 Activity, unspecified

✓5th **Y93.Ø Activities involving walking and running**
EXCLUDES1 *activity, walking an animal (Y93.K1)*
activity, walking or running on a treadmill (Y93.A1)

Y93.Ø1 Activity, walking, marching and hiking
Activity, walking, marching and hiking on level or elevated terrain
EXCLUDES1 *activity, mountain climbing (Y93.31)*

Y93.Ø2 Activity, running

✓5th **Y93.1 Activities involving water and water craft**
EXCLUDES1 *activities involving ice (Y93.2-)*

Y93.11 Activity, swimming

Y93.12 Activity, springboard and platform diving

Y93.13 Activity, water polo

Y93.14 Activity, water aerobics and water exercise

Y93.15 Activity, underwater diving and snorkeling
Activity, SCUBA diving

Y93.16 Activity, rowing, canoeing, kayaking, rafting and tubing
Activity, canoeing, kayaking, rafting and tubing in calm and turbulent water

Y93.17 Activity, water skiing and wake boarding

Y93.18 Activity, surfing, windsurfing and boogie boarding
Activity, water sliding

Y93.19 Activity, other involving water and watercraft
Activity involving water NOS
Activity, parasailing
Activity, water survival training and testing

Y93.2 Activities involving ice and snow
EXCLUDES 1 *activity, shoveling ice and snow (Y93.H1)*

Y93.21 Activity, ice skating
Activity, figure skating (singles) (pairs)
Activity, ice dancing
EXCLUDES 1 *activity, ice hockey (Y93.22)*

Y93.22 Activity, ice hockey

Y93.23 Activity, snow (alpine) (downhill) skiing, snow boarding, sledding, tobogganing and snow tubing
EXCLUDES 1 *activity, cross country skiing (Y93.24)*

Y93.24 Activity, cross country skiing
Activity, nordic skiing

Y93.29 Activity, other involving ice and snow
Activity involving ice and snow NOS

Y93.3 Activities involving climbing, rappelling and jumping off
EXCLUDES 1 *activity, hiking on level or elevated terrain (Y93.01)*
activity, jumping rope (Y93.56)
activity, trampoline jumping (Y93.44)

Y93.31 Activity, mountain climbing, rock climbing and wall climbing

Y93.32 Activity, rappelling

Y93.33 Activity, BASE jumping
Activity, Building, Antenna, Span, Earth jumping

Y93.34 Activity, bungee jumping

Y93.35 Activity, hang gliding

Y93.39 Activity, other involving climbing, rappelling and jumping off

Y93.4 Activities involving dancing and other rhythmic movement
EXCLUDES 1 *activity, martial arts (Y93.75)*

Y93.41 Activity, dancing
AHA: 2012, 4Q, 108

Y93.42 Activity, yoga

Y93.43 Activity, gymnastics
Activity, rhythmic gymnastics
EXCLUDES 1 *activity, trampolining (Y93.44)*

Y93.44 Activity, trampolining

Y93.45 Activity, cheerleading

Y93.49 Activity, other involving dancing and other rhythmic movements

Y93.5 Activities involving other sports and athletics played individually
EXCLUDES 1 *activity, dancing (Y93.41)*
activity, gymnastic (Y93.43)
activity, trampolining (Y93.44)
activity, yoga (Y93.42)

Y93.51 Activity, roller skating (inline) and skateboarding

Y93.52 Activity, horseback riding

Y93.53 Activity, golf

Y93.54 Activity, bowling

Y93.55 Activity, bike riding

Y93.56 Activity, jumping rope

Y93.57 Activity, non-running track and field events
EXCLUDES 1 *activity, running (any form) (Y93.02)*

Y93.59 Activity, other involving other sports and athletics played individually
EXCLUDES 1 *activities involving climbing, rappelling, and jumping (Y93.3-)*
activities involving ice and snow (Y93.2-)
activities involving walking and running (Y93.0-)
activities involving water and watercraft (Y93.1-)

Y93.6 Activities involving other sports and athletics played as a team or group
EXCLUDES 1 *activity, ice hockey (Y93.22)*
activity, water polo (Y93.13)

Y93.61 Activity, American tackle football
Activity, football NOS

Y93.62 Activity, American flag or touch football

Y93.63 Activity, rugby

Y93.64 Activity, baseball
Activity, softball

Y93.65 Activity, lacrosse and field hockey

Y93.66 Activity, soccer

Y93.67 Activity, basketball

Y93.68 Activity, volleyball (beach) (court)

Y93.6A Activity, physical games generally associated with school recess, summer camp and children P
Activity, capture the flag
Activity, dodge ball
Activity, four square
Activity, kickball

Y93.69 Activity, other involving other sports and athletics played as a team or group
Activity, cricket

Y93.7 Activities involving other specified sports and athletics

Y93.71 Activity, boxing

Y93.72 Activity, wrestling

Y93.73 Activity, racquet and hand sports
Activity, handball
Activity, racquetball
Activity, squash
Activity, tennis

Y93.74 Activity, frisbee
Activity, ultimate frisbee

Y93.75 Activity, martial arts
Activity, combatives

Y93.79 Activity, other specified sports and athletics
EXCLUDES 1 *sports and athletics activities specified in categories Y93.0-Y93.6*

Y93.A Activities involving other cardiorespiratory exercise
Activities involving physical training

Y93.A1 Activity, exercise machines primarily for cardiorespiratory conditioning
Activity, elliptical and stepper machines
Activity, stationary bike
Activity, treadmill

Y93.A2 Activity, calisthenics
Activity, jumping jacks
Activity, warm up and cool down

Y93.A3 Activity, aerobic and step exercise

Y93.A4 Activity, circuit training

Y93.A5 Activity, obstacle course
Activity, challenge course
Activity, confidence course

Y93.A6 Activity, grass drills
Activity, guerilla drills

Y93.A9 Activity, other involving cardiorespiratory exercise
EXCLUDES 1 *activities involving cardiorespiratory exercise specified in categories Y93.0-Y93.7*

Y93.B Activities involving other muscle strengthening exercises

Y93.B1 Activity, exercise machines primarily for muscle strengthening

Y93.B2 Activity, push-ups, pull-ups, sit-ups

Y93.B3 Activity, free weights
Activity, barbells
Activity, dumbbells

Y93.B4 Activity, pilates

Y93.B9 Activity, other involving muscle strengthening exercises
EXCLUDES 1 *activities involving muscle strengthening specified in categories Y93.0-Y93.A*

Y93.C Activities involving computer technology and electronic devices
EXCLUDES 1 *activity, electronic musical keyboard or instruments (Y93.J-)*

Y93.C1 Activity, computer keyboarding
Activity, electronic game playing using keyboard or other stationary device

Y93.C2 Activity, hand held interactive electronic device
Activity, cellular telephone and communication device
Activity, electronic game playing using interactive device
EXCLUDES 1 *activity, electronic game playing using keyboard or other stationary device (Y93.C1)*

Y93.C9 Activity, other involving computer technology and electronic devices

Y93.D Activities involving arts and handcrafts
EXCLUDES 1 *activities involving playing musical instrument (Y93.J-)*

Y93.D1 Activity, knitting and crocheting

Y93.D2 Activity, sewing

Y93.D3 Activity, furniture building and finishing
Activity, furniture repair

Y93.D9 Activity, other involving arts and handcrafts

Y93.E Activities involving personal hygiene and interior property and clothing maintenance
EXCLUDES 1 *activities involving cooking and grilling (Y93.G-)*
activities involving exterior property and land maintenance, building and construction (Y93.H-)
activities involving caregiving (Y93.F-)
activity, dishwashing (Y93.G1)
activity, food preparation (Y93.G1)
activity, gardening (Y93.H2)

Y93.E1 Activity, personal bathing and showering

Y93.E2 Activity, laundry

Y93.E3 Activity, vacuuming

Y93.E4 Activity, ironing

Y93.E5 Activity, floor mopping and cleaning

Y93.E6 Activity, residential relocation
Activity, packing up and unpacking involved in moving to a new residence

Y93.E8 Activity, other personal hygiene

Y93.E9 Activity, other interior property and clothing maintenance

Y93.F Activities involving caregiving
Activity involving the provider of caregiving

Y93.F1 Activity, caregiving, bathing

Y93.F2 Activity, caregiving, lifting

Y93.F9 Activity, other caregiving

Y93.G Activities involving food preparation, cooking and grilling

Y93.G1 Activity, food preparation and clean up
Activity, dishwashing

Y93.G2 Activity, grilling and smoking food

Y93.G3 Activity, cooking and baking
Activity, use of stove, oven and microwave oven

Y93.G9 Activity, other involving cooking and grilling

Y93.H Activities involving exterior property and land maintenance, building and construction

Y93.H1 Activity, digging, shoveling and raking
Activity, dirt digging
Activity, raking leaves
Activity, snow shoveling

Y93.H2 Activity, gardening and landscaping
Activity, pruning, trimming shrubs, weeding

Y93.H3 Activity, building and construction

Y93.H9 Activity, other involving exterior property and land maintenance, building and construction

Y93.I Activities involving roller coasters and other types of external motion

Y93.I1 Activity, rollercoaster riding

Y93.I9 Activity, other involving external motion

Y93.J Activities involving playing musical instrument
Activity involving playing electric musical instrument

Y93.J1 Activity, piano playing
Activity, musical keyboard (electronic) playing

Y93.J2 Activity, drum and other percussion instrument playing

Y93.J3 Activity, string instrument playing

Y93.J4 Activity, winds and brass instrument playing

Y93.K Activities involving animal care
EXCLUDES 1 *activity, horseback riding (Y93.52)*

Y93.K1 Activity, walking an animal

Y93.K2 Activity, milking an animal

Y93.K3 Activity, grooming and shearing an animal

Y93.K9 Activity, other involving animal care

Y93.8 Activities, other specified

Y93.81 Activity, refereeing a sports activity

Y93.82 Activity, spectator at an event

Y93.83 Activity, rough housing and horseplay

Y93.84 Activity, sleeping

Y93.89 Activity, other specified

Y93.9 Activity, unspecified

Y95 Nosocomial condition
AHA: 2013, 4Q, 119

Y99 External cause status
NOTE A single code from category Y99 should be used in conjunction with the external cause code(s) assigned to a record to indicate the status of the person at the time the event occurred.

Y99.0 Civilian activity done for income or pay
Civilian activity done for financial or other compensation
EXCLUDES 1 *military activity (Y99.1)*
volunteer activity (Y99.2)

Y99.1 Military activity
EXCLUDES 1 *activity of off duty military personnel (Y99.8)*

Y99.2 Volunteer activity
EXCLUDES 1 *activity of child or other family member assisting in compensated work of other family member (Y99.8)*

Y99.8 Other external cause status
Activity NEC
Activity of child or other family member assisting in compensated work of other family member
Hobby not done for income
Leisure activity
Off-duty activity of military personnel
Recreation or sport not for income or while a student
Student activity
EXCLUDES 1 *civilian activity done for income or compensation (Y99.0)*
military activity (Y99.1)
AHA: 2012, 4Q, 108

Y99.9 Unspecified external cause status

Chapter 21. Factors Influencing Health Status and Contact With Health Services (Z00-Z99)

NOTE Z codes represent reasons for encounters. A corresponding procedure code must accompany a Z code if a procedure is performed. Categories Z00-Z99 are provided for occasions when circumstances other than a disease, injury or external cause classifiable to categories A00-Y89 are recorded as "diagnoses" or "problems". This can arise in two main ways:

(a) When a person who may or may not be sick encounters the health services for some specific purpose, such as to receive limited care or service for a current condition, to donate an organ or tissue, to receive prophylactic vaccination (immunization), or to discuss a problem which is in itself not a disease or injury.

(b) When some circumstance or problem is present which influences the person's health status but is not in itself a current illness or injury.

This chapter contains the following blocks:

Z00-Z13	Persons encountering health services for examinations
Z14-Z15	Genetic carrier and genetic susceptibility to disease
Z16	Resistance to antimicrobial drugs
Z17	Estrogen receptor status
Z18	Retained foreign body fragments
Z20-Z28	Persons with potential health hazards related to communicable diseases
Z30-Z39	Persons encountering health services in circumstances related to reproduction
Z40-Z53	Encounters for other specific health care
Z55-Z65	Persons with potential health hazards related to socioeconomic and psychosocial circumstances
Z66	Do not resuscitate status
Z67	Blood type
Z68	Body mass index (BMI)
Z69-Z76	Persons encountering health services in other circumstances
Z77-Z99	Persons with potential health hazards related to family and personal history and certain conditions influencing health status

Persons encountering health services for examinations (Z00-Z13)

NOTE Nonspecific abnormal findings disclosed at the time of these examinations are classified to categories R70-R94.

EXCLUDES1 *examinations related to pregnancy and reproduction (Z30-Z36, Z39-)*

✓4th **Z00 Encounter for general examination without complaint, suspected or reported diagnosis**

EXCLUDES1 *encounter for examination for administrative purposes (Z02.-)*

EXCLUDES2 *encounter for pre-procedural examinations (Z01.81-)*
special screening examinations (Z11-Z13)

✓5th **Z00.0 Encounter for general adult medical examination**
Encounter for adult periodic examination (annual) (physical) and any associated laboratory and radiologic examinations
EXCLUDES1 *encounter for examination of sign or symptom—code to sign or symptom*
general health check-up of infant or child (Z00.12-)

Z00.00 Encounter for general adult medical examination without abnormal findings A
Encounter for adult health check-up NOS

Z00.01 Encounter for general adult medical examination with abnormal findings A
Use additional code to identify abnormal findings

✓5th **Z00.1 Encounter for newborn, infant and child health examinations**

✓6th **Z00.11 Newborn health examination**
Health check for child under 29 days old
Use additional code to identify any abnormal findings
EXCLUDES1 *health check for child over 28 days old (Z00.12-)*

Z00.110 Health examination for newborn under 8 days old N
Health check for newborn under 8 days old

Z00.111 Health examination for newborn 8 to 28 days old N
Health check for newborn 8 to 28 days old
Newborn weight check

✓6th **Z00.12 Encounter for routine child health examination**
Encounter for development testing of infant or child
Health check (routine) for child over 28 days old
EXCLUDES1 *health check for child under 29 days old (Z00.11-)*
health supervision of foundling or other healthy infant or child (Z76.1-Z76.2)
newborn health examination (Z00.11-)

Z00.121 Encounter for routine child health examination with abnormal findings P
Use additional code to identify abnormal findings

Z00.129 Encounter for routine child health examination without abnormal findings P
Encounter for routine child health examination NOS

Z00.2 Encounter for examination for period of rapid growth in childhood P

Z00.3 Encounter for examination for adolescent development state P
Encounter for puberty development state

Z00.5 Encounter for examination of potential donor of organ and tissue

Z00.6 Encounter for examination for normal comparison and control in clinical research program
Examination of participant or control in clinical research program

✓5th **Z00.7 Encounter for examination for period of delayed growth in childhood**

Z00.70 Encounter for examination for period of delayed growth in childhood without abnormal findings P

Z00.71 Encounter for examination for period of delayed growth in childhood with abnormal findings P
Use additional code to identify abnormal findings

Z00.8 Encounter for other general examination
Encounter for health examination in population surveys

✓4th **Z01 Encounter for other special examination without complaint, suspected or reported diagnosis**

INCLUDES routine examination of specific system

NOTE Codes from category Z01 represent the reason for the encounter. A separate procedure code is required to identify any examinations or procedures performed.

EXCLUDES1 *encounter for examination for administrative purposes (Z02.-)*
encounter for examination for suspected conditions, proven not to exist (Z03.-)
encounter for laboratory and radiologic examinations as a component of general medical examinations (Z00.0-)
encounter for laboratory, radiologic and imaging examinations for sign(s) and symptom(s)—code to the sign(s) or symptom(s)

EXCLUDES2 *screening examinations (Z11-Z13)*

✓5th **Z01.0 Encounter for examination of eyes and vision**
EXCLUDES1 *examination for driving license (Z02.4)*

Z01.00 Encounter for examination of eyes and vision without abnormal findings
Encounter for examination of eyes and vision NOS

Z01.01 Encounter for examination of eyes and vision with abnormal findings
Use additional code to identify abnormal findings

✓5th **Z01.1 Encounter for examination of ears and hearing**

Z01.10 Encounter for examination of ears and hearing without abnormal findings
Encounter for examination of ears and hearing NOS

✓6th **Z01.11 Encounter for examination of ears and hearing with abnormal findings**

Z01.110 Encounter for hearing examination following failed hearing screening

Z01.118 Encounter for examination of ears and hearing with other abnormal findings
Use additional code to identify abnormal findings

Z01.12 Encounter for hearing conservation and treatment

✓5th **Z01.2 Encounter for dental examination and cleaning**

Z01.20 Encounter for dental examination and cleaning without abnormal findings
Encounter for dental examination and cleaning NOS

Z01.21 Encounter for dental examination and cleaning with abnormal findings
Use additional code to identify abnormal findings

✓5th **Z01.3 Encounter for examination of blood pressure**

Z01.30 Encounter for examination of blood pressure without abnormal findings
Encounter for examination of blood pressure NOS

Z01.31 Encounter for examination of blood pressure with abnormal findings
Use additional code to identify abnormal findings

✓5th **Z01.4 Encounter for gynecological examination**
EXCLUDES 2 *pregnancy examination or test (Z32.0-)*
routine examination for contraceptive maintenance (Z30.4-)

✓6th **Z01.41 Encounter for routine gynecological examination**
Encounter for general gynecological examination with or without cervical smear
Encounter for gynecological examination (general) (routine) NOS
Encounter for pelvic examination (annual) (periodic)
Use additional code:
for screening for human papillomavirus, if applicable, (Z11.51)
for screening vaginal pap smear, if applicable (Z12.72)
to identify acquired absence of uterus, if applicable (Z90.71-)
EXCLUDES 1 *gynecologic examination status-post hysterectomy for malignant condition (Z08)*
screening cervical pap smear not a part of a routine gynecological examination (Z12.4)

Z01.411 Encounter for gynecological examination (general) (routine) with abnormal findings ♀

Z01.419 Encounter for gynecological examination (general) (routine) without abnormal findings ♀
Use additional code to identify abnormal findings

Z01.42 Encounter for cervical smear to confirm findings of recent normal smear following initial abnormal smear ♀

✓5th **Z01.8 Encounter for other specified special examinations**

✓6th **Z01.81 Encounter for preprocedural examinations**
Encounter for preoperative examinations
Encounter for radiological and imaging examinations as part of preprocedural examination

Z01.810 Encounter for preprocedural cardiovascular examination

Z01.811 Encounter for preprocedural respiratory examination

Z01.812 Encounter for preprocedural laboratory examination
Blood and urine tests prior to treatment or procedure

Z01.818 Encounter for other preprocedural examination
Encounter for preprocedural examination NOS
Encounter for examinations prior to antineoplastic chemotherapy

Z01.82 Encounter for allergy testing
EXCLUDES 1 *encounter for antibody response examination (Z01.84)*

Z01.83 Encounter for blood typing
Encounter for Rh typing

Z01.84 Encounter for antibody response examination
Encounter for immunity status testing
EXCLUDES 1 *encounter for allergy testing (Z01.82)*

Z01.89 Encounter for other specified special examinations

✓4th **Z02 Encounter for administrative examination**

Z02.0 Encounter for examination for admission to educational institution
Encounter for examination for admission to preschool (education)
Encounter for examination for re-admission to school following illness or medical treatment

Z02.1 Encounter for pre-employment examination

Z02.2 Encounter for examination for admission to residential institution
EXCLUDES 1 *examination for admission to prison (Z02.89)*

Z02.3 Encounter for examination for recruitment to armed forces

Z02.4 Encounter for examination for driving license

Z02.5 Encounter for examination for participation in sport
EXCLUDES 1 *blood-alcohol and blood-drug test (Z02.83)*

Z02.6 Encounter for examination for insurance purposes

✓5th **Z02.7 Encounter for issue of medical certificate**
EXCLUDES 1 *encounter for general medical examination (Z00-Z01, Z02.0-Z02.6, Z02.8-Z02.9)*

Z02.71 Encounter for disability determination
Encounter for issue of medical certificate of incapacity
Encounter for issue of medical certificate of invalidity

Z02.79 Encounter for issue of other medical certificate

✓5th **Z02.8 Encounter for other administrative examinations**

Z02.81 Encounter for paternity testing

Z02.82 Encounter for adoption services

Z02.83 Encounter for blood-alcohol and blood-drug test
Use additional code for findings of alcohol or drugs in blood (R78.-)

Z02.89 Encounter for other administrative examinations
Encounter for examination for admission to prison
Encounter for examination for admission to summer camp
Encounter for immigration examination
Encounter for naturalization examination
Encounter for premarital examination
EXCLUDES 1 *health supervision of foundling or other healthy infant or child (Z76.1-Z76.2)*

Z02.9 Encounter for administrative examinations, unspecified

✓4th **Z03 Encounter for medical observation for suspected diseases and conditions ruled out**

NOTE This category is to be used when a person without a diagnosis is suspected of having an abnormal condition, without signs or symptoms, which requires study, but after examination and observation, is ruled out. This category is also for use for administrative and legal observation status.

EXCLUDES 1 *contact with and (suspected) exposures hazardous to health (Z77.-)*
newborn observation for suspected condition, ruled out (P00-P04)
person with feared complaint in whom no diagnosis is made (Z71.1)
signs or symptoms under study—code to signs or symptoms

Z03.6 Encounter for observation for suspected toxic effect from ingested substance ruled out
Encounter for observation for suspected adverse effect from drug
Encounter for observation for suspected poisoning

✓5th **Z03.7 Encounter for suspected maternal and fetal conditions ruled out**
Encounter for suspected maternal and fetal conditions not found
EXCLUDES 1 *known or suspected fetal anomalies affecting management of mother, not ruled out (O26-, O35-, O36-, O40-, O41-)*

Z03.71 Encounter for suspected problem with amniotic cavity and membrane ruled out M♀
Encounter for suspected oligohydramnios ruled out
Encounter for suspected polyhydramnios ruled out

Z03.72 Encounter for suspected placental problem ruled out M♀

Z03.73 Encounter for suspected fetal anomaly ruled out M♀

Z03.74 Encounter for suspected problem with fetal growth ruled out M♀

Z03.75 Encounter for suspected cervical shortening ruled out M♀

Z03.79 Encounter for other suspected maternal and fetal conditions ruled out M♀

✓5th **Z03.8 Encounter for observation for other suspected diseases and conditions ruled out**

✓6th **Z03.81 Encounter for observation for suspected exposure to biological agents ruled out**

Z03.810 Encounter for observation for suspected exposure to anthrax ruled out

Z03.818 Encounter for observation for suspected exposure to other biological agents ruled out

Z03.89 Encounter for observation for other suspected diseases and conditions ruled out

✓4th Z04 Encounter for examination and observation for other reasons

INCLUDES encounter for examination for medicolegal reasons

NOTE This category is to be used when a person without a diagnosis is suspected of having an abnormal condition, without signs or symptoms, which requires study, but after examination and observation, is ruled-out. This category is also for use for administrative and legal observation status.

Z04.1 Encounter for examination and observation following transport accident

EXCLUDES 1 *encounter for examination and observation following work accident (Z04.2)*

Z04.2 Encounter for examination and observation following work accident

Z04.3 Encounter for examination and observation following other accident

✓5th Z04.4 Encounter for examination and observation following alleged rape

Encounter for examination and observation of victim following alleged rape

Encounter for examination and observation of victim following alleged sexual abuse

Z04.41 Encounter for examination and observation following alleged adult rape A

Suspected adult rape, ruled out

Suspected adult sexual abuse, ruled out

Z04.42 Encounter for examination and observation following alleged child rape P

Suspected child rape, ruled out

Suspected child sexual abuse, ruled out

Z04.6 Encounter for general psychiatric examination, requested by authority

✓5th Z04.7 Encounter for examination and observation following alleged physical abuse

Z04.71 Encounter for examination and observation following alleged adult physical abuse A

Suspected adult physical abuse, ruled out

EXCLUDES 1 *confirmed case of adult physical abuse (T74.-)*

encounter for examination and observation following alleged adult sexual abuse (Z04.41)

suspected case of adult physical abuse, not ruled out (T76.-)

Z04.72 Encounter for examination and observation following alleged child physical abuse P

Suspected child physical abuse, ruled out

EXCLUDES 1 *confirmed case of child physical abuse (T74.-)*

encounter for examination and observation following alleged child sexual abuse (Z04.42)

suspected case of child physical abuse, not ruled out (T76.-)

Z04.8 Encounter for examination and observation for other specified reasons

Encounter for examination and observation for request for expert evidence

Z04.9 Encounter for examination and observation for unspecified reason

Encounter for observation NOS

Z08 Encounter for follow-up examination after completed treatment for malignant neoplasm

Medical surveillance following completed treatment

Use additional code to identify any acquired absence of organs (Z90.-)

Use additional code to identify the personal history of malignant neoplasm (Z85.-)

EXCLUDES 1 *aftercare following medical care (Z43-Z49, Z51)*

Z09 Encounter for follow-up examination after completed treatment for conditions other than malignant neoplasm

Medical surveillance following completed treatment

Use additional code to identify any applicable history of disease code (Z86-, Z87-)

EXCLUDES 1 *aftercare following medical care (Z43-Z49, Z51)*

surveillance of contraception (Z30.4-)

surveillance of prosthetic and other medical devices (Z44-Z46)

✓4th Z11 Encounter for screening for infectious and parasitic diseases

NOTE Screening is the testing for disease or disease precursors in asymptomatic individuals so that early detection and treatment can be provided for those who test positive for the disease.

EXCLUDES 1 *encounter for diagnostic examination—code to sign or symptom*

Z11.0 Encounter for screening for intestinal infectious diseases

Z11.1 Encounter for screening for respiratory tuberculosis

Z11.2 Encounter for screening for other bacterial diseases

Z11.3 Encounter for screening for infections with a predominantly sexual mode of transmission

EXCLUDES 2 *encounter for screening for human immunodeficiency virus [HIV] (Z11.4)*

encounter for screening for human papillomavirus (Z11.51)

Z11.4 Encounter for screening for human immunodeficiency virus [HIV]

✓5th Z11.5 Encounter for screening for other viral diseases

EXCLUDES 2 *encounter for screening for viral intestinal disease (Z11.0)*

Z11.51 Encounter for screening for human papillomavirus (HPV)

Z11.59 Encounter for screening for other viral diseases

Z11.6 Encounter for screening for other protozoal diseases and helminthiases

EXCLUDES 2 *encounter for screening for protozoal intestinal disease (Z11.0)*

Z11.8 Encounter for screening for other infectious and parasitic diseases

Encounter for screening for chlamydia

Encounter for screening for rickettsial

Encounter for screening for spirochetal

Encounter for screening for mycoses

Z11.9 Encounter for screening for infectious and parasitic diseases, unspecified

✓4th Z12 Encounter for screening for malignant neoplasms

NOTE Screening is the testing for disease or disease precursors in asymptomatic individuals so that early detection and treatment can be provided for those who test positive for the disease.

Use additional code to identify any family history of malignant neoplasm (Z80.-)

EXCLUDES 1 *encounter for diagnostic examination—code to sign or symptom*

Z12.0 Encounter for screening for malignant neoplasm of stomach

✓5th Z12.1 Encounter for screening for malignant neoplasm of intestinal tract

Z12.10 Encounter for screening for malignant neoplasm of intestinal tract, unspecified

Z12.11 Encounter for screening for malignant neoplasm of colon

Encounter for screening colonoscopy NOS

Z12.12 Encounter for screening for malignant neoplasm of rectum

Z12.13 Encounter for screening for malignant neoplasm of small intestine

Z12.2 Encounter for screening for malignant neoplasm of respiratory organs

✓5th Z12.3 Encounter for screening for malignant neoplasm of breast

Z12.31 Encounter for screening mammogram for malignant neoplasm of breast

EXCLUDES 1 *inconclusive mammogram (R92.2)*

Z12.39 Encounter for other screening for malignant neoplasm of breast

Z12.4 Encounter for screening for malignant neoplasm of cervix ♀

Encounter for screening pap smear for malignant neoplasm of cervix

EXCLUDES 1 *encounter for screening for human papillomavirus (Z11.51)*

when screening is part of general gynecological examination (Z01.4-)

Z12.5 Encounter for screening for malignant neoplasm of prostate ♂

Z12.6 Encounter for screening for malignant neoplasm of bladder

✓5th **Z12.7 Encounter for screening for malignant neoplasm of other genitourinary organs**

Z12.71 Encounter for screening for malignant neoplasm of testis ♂

Z12.72 Encounter for screening for malignant neoplasm of vagina ♀

Vaginal pap smear status-post hysterectomy for non-malignant condition

Use additional code to identify acquired absence of uterus (Z90.71-)

EXCLUDES 1 *vaginal pap smear status-post hysterectomy for malignant conditions (Z08)*

Z12.73 Encounter for screening for malignant neoplasm of ovary ♀

Z12.79 Encounter for screening for malignant neoplasm of other genitourinary organs

✓5th **Z12.8 Encounter for screening for malignant neoplasm of other sites**

Z12.81 Encounter for screening for malignant neoplasm of oral cavity

Z12.82 Encounter for screening for malignant neoplasm of nervous system

Z12.83 Encounter for screening for malignant neoplasm of skin

Z12.89 Encounter for screening for malignant neoplasm of other sites

Z12.9 Encounter for screening for malignant neoplasm, site unspecified

✓4th **Z13 Encounter for screening for other diseases and disorders**

NOTE Screening is the testing for disease or disease precursors in asymptomatic individuals so that early detection and treatment can be provided for those who test positive for the disease.

EXCLUDES 1 *encounter for diagnostic examination—code to sign or symptom*

Z13.0 Encounter for screening for diseases of the blood and blood-forming organs and certain disorders involving the immune mechanism

Z13.1 Encounter for screening for diabetes mellitus

✓5th **Z13.2 Encounter for screening for nutritional, metabolic and other endocrine disorders**

Z13.21 Encounter for screening for nutritional disorder

✓6th **Z13.22 Encounter for screening for metabolic disorder**

Z13.220 Encounter for screening for lipoid disorders

Encounter for screening for cholesterol level

Encounter for screening for hypercholesterolemia

Encounter for screening for hyperlipidemia

Z13.228 Encounter for screening for other metabolic disorders

Z13.29 Encounter for screening for other suspected endocrine disorder

EXCLUDES 1 *encounter for screening for diabetes mellitus (Z13.1)*

Z13.4 Encounter for screening for certain developmental disorders in childhood P

Encounter for screening for developmental handicaps in early childhood

EXCLUDES 1 *routine development testing of infant or child (Z00.1-)*

Z13.5 Encounter for screening for eye and ear disorders

EXCLUDES 2 *encounter for general hearing examination (Z01.1-)*
encounter for general vision examination (Z01.0-)

Z13.6 Encounter for screening for cardiovascular disorders

✓5th **Z13.7 Encounter for screening for genetic and chromosomal anomalies**

EXCLUDES 1 *genetic testing for procreative management (Z31.4-)*

Z13.71 Encounter for nonprocreative screening for genetic disease carrier status

Z13.79 Encounter for other screening for genetic and chromosomal anomalies

✓5th **Z13.8 Encounter for screening for other specified diseases and disorders**

EXCLUDES 2 *screening for malignant neoplasms (Z12.-)*

✓6th **Z13.81 Encounter for screening for digestive system disorders**

Z13.810 Encounter for screening for upper gastrointestinal disorder

Z13.811 Encounter for screening for lower gastrointestinal disorder

EXCLUDES 1 *encounter for screening for intestinal infectious disease (Z11.0)*

Z13.818 Encounter for screening for other digestive system disorders

✓6th **Z13.82 Encounter for screening for musculoskeletal disorder**

Z13.820 Encounter for screening for osteoporosis

Z13.828 Encounter for screening for other musculoskeletal disorder

Z13.83 Encounter for screening for respiratory disorder NEC

EXCLUDES 1 *encounter for screening for respiratory tuberculosis (Z11.1)*

Z13.84 Encounter for screening for dental disorders

✓6th **Z13.85 Encounter for screening for nervous system disorders**

Z13.850 Encounter for screening for traumatic brain injury

Z13.858 Encounter for screening for other nervous system disorders

Z13.88 Encounter for screening for disorder due to exposure to contaminants

EXCLUDES 1 *those exposed to contaminants without suspected disorders (Z57-Z77-)*

Z13.89 Encounter for screening for other disorder

Encounter for screening for genitourinary disorders

Z13.9 Encounter for screening, unspecified

Genetic carrier and genetic susceptibility to disease (Z14-Z15)

✓4th **Z14 Genetic carrier**

✓5th **Z14.0 Hemophilia A carrier**

Z14.01 Asymptomatic hemophilia A carrier

Z14.02 Symptomatic hemophilia A carrier

Z14.1 Cystic fibrosis carrier

Z14.8 Genetic carrier of other disease

✓4th **Z15 Genetic susceptibility to disease**

Confirmed abnormal gene

Use additional code, if applicable, for any associated family history of the disease (Z80-Z84)

EXCLUDES 1 *chromosomal anomalies (Q90-Q99)*

✓5th **Z15.0 Genetic susceptibility to malignant neoplasm**

Code first, if applicable, any current malignant neoplasm (C00-C75, C81-C96)

Use additional code, if applicable, for any personal history of malignant neoplasm (Z85.-)

Z15.01 Genetic susceptibility to malignant neoplasm of breast

Z15.02 Genetic susceptibility to malignant neoplasm of ovary ♀

Z15.03 Genetic susceptibility to malignant neoplasm of prostate ♂

Z15.04 Genetic susceptibility to malignant neoplasm of endometrium ♀

Z15.09 Genetic susceptibility to other malignant neoplasm

✓5th **Z15.8 Genetic susceptibility to other disease**

Z15.81 Genetic susceptibility to multiple endocrine neoplasia [MEN]

EXCLUDES 1 *multiple endocrine neoplasia [MEN] syndromes (E31.2-)*

Z15.89 Genetic susceptibility to other disease

Resistance to antimicrobial drugs (Z16)

Z16 Resistance to antimicrobial drugs

NOTE The codes in this category are provided for use as additional codes to identify the resistance and non-responsiveness of a condition to antimicrobial drugs.

Code first the infection

EXCLUDES 1 *Methicillin resistant Staphylococcus aureus infection (A49.02)*
Methicillin resistant Staphylococcus aureus infection in diseases classified elsewhere (B95.62)
Methicillin resistant Staphylococcus aureus pneumonia (J15.212)
Sepsis due to Methicillin resistant Staphylococcus aureus (A41.02)

Z16.1 Resistance to beta lactam antibiotics

Z16.10 Resistance to unspecified beta lactam antibiotics

Z16.11 Resistance to penicillins
Resistance to amoxicillin
Resistance to ampicillin

Z16.12 Extended spectrum beta lactamase (ESBL) resistance

Z16.19 Resistance to other specified beta lactam antibiotics
Resistance to cephalosporins

Z16.2 Resistance to other antibiotics

Z16.20 Resistance to unspecified antibiotic
Resistance to antibiotics NOS

Z16.21 Resistance to vancomycin

Z16.22 Resistance to vancomycin related antibiotics

Z16.23 Resistance to quinolones and fluoroquinolones

Z16.24 Resistance to multiple antibiotics

Z16.29 Resistance to other single specified antibiotic
Resistance to aminoglycosides
Resistance to macrolides
Resistance to sulfonamides
Resistance to tetracyclines

Z16.3 Resistance to other antimicrobial drugs

EXCLUDES 1 *resistance to antibiotics (Z16.1-, Z16.2-)*

Z16.30 Resistance to unspecified antimicrobial drugs
Drug resistance NOS

Z16.31 Resistance to antiparasitic drug(s)
Resistance to quinine and related compounds

Z16.32 Resistance to antifungal drug(s)

Z16.33 Resistance to antiviral drug(s)

Z16.34 Resistance to antimycobacterial drug(s)
Resistance to tuberculostatics

Z16.341 Resistance to single antimycobacterial drug
Resistance to antimycobacterial drug NOS

Z16.342 Resistance to multiple antimycobacterial drugs

Z16.35 Resistance to multiple antimicrobial drugs

EXCLUDES 1 *Resistance to multiple antibiotics only (Z16.24)*

Z16.39 Resistance to other specified antimicrobial drug

Estrogen receptor status (Z17)

Z17 Estrogen receptor status

Code first malignant neoplasm of breast (C50.-)

Z17.0 Estrogen receptor positive status [ER+]

Z17.1 Estrogen receptor negative status [ER-]

Retained foreign body fragment (Z18)

Z18 Retained foreign body fragments
Embedded fragment (status)
Embedded splinter (status)
Retained foreign body status

EXCLUDES 1 *artificial joint prosthesis status (Z96.6-)*
foreign body accidentally left during a procedure (T81.5-)
foreign body entering through orifice (T15-T19)
in situ cardiac device (Z95.-)
organ or tissue replaced by means other than transplant (Z96.-, Z97.-)
organ or tissue replaced by transplant (Z94.-)
personal history of retained foreign body fully removed (Z87.821)
superficial foreign body (non-embedded splinter)—code to superficial foreign body, by site

Z18.0 Retained radioactive fragments

Z18.01 Retained depleted uranium fragments

Z18.09 Other retained radioactive fragments
Other retained depleted isotope fragments
Retained nontherapeutic radioactive fragments

Z18.1 Retained metal fragments

EXCLUDES 1 *retained radioactive metal fragments (Z18.01-Z18.09)*

Z18.10 Retained metal fragments, unspecified
Retained metal fragment NOS

Z18.11 Retained magnetic metal fragments

Z18.12 Retained nonmagnetic metal fragments

Z18.2 Retained plastic fragments
Acrylics fragments
Diethylhexylphthalates fragments
Isocyanate fragments

Z18.3 Retained organic fragments

Z18.31 Retained animal quills or spines

Z18.32 Retained tooth

Z18.33 Retained wood fragments

Z18.39 Other retained organic fragments

Z18.8 Other specified retained foreign body

Z18.81 Retained glass fragments

Z18.83 Retained stone or crystalline fragments
Retained concrete or cement fragments

Z18.89 Other specified retained foreign body fragments

Z18.9 Retained foreign body fragments, unspecified material

Persons with potential health hazards related to communicable diseases (Z20-Z28)

Z20 Contact with and (suspected) exposure to communicable diseases

EXCLUDES 1 *carrier of infectious disease (Z22.-)*
diagnosed current infectious or parasitic disease—see Alphabetic Index

EXCLUDES 2 *personal history of infectious and parasitic diseases (Z86.1-)*

Z20.0 Contact with and (suspected) exposure to intestinal infectious diseases

Z20.01 Contact with and (suspected) exposure to intestinal infectious diseases due to Escherichia coli (E. coli)

Z20.09 Contact with and (suspected) exposure to other intestinal infectious diseases

Z20.1 Contact with and (suspected) exposure to tuberculosis

Z20.2 Contact with and (suspected) exposure to infections with a predominantly sexual mode of transmission

Z20.3 Contact with and (suspected) exposure to rabies

Z20.4 Contact with and (suspected) exposure to rubella

Z20.5 Contact with and (suspected) exposure to viral hepatitis

Z20.6 Contact with and (suspected) exposure to human immunodeficiency virus [HIV]

EXCLUDES 1 *asymptomatic human immunodeficiency virus [HIV] HIV infection status (Z21)*

Z20.7 Contact with and (suspected) exposure to pediculosis, acariasis and other infestations

Z20.8 Contact with and (suspected) exposure to other communicable diseases

Z20.81 Contact with and (suspected) exposure to other bacterial communicable diseases

Z20.810 Contact with and (suspected) exposure to anthrax

Z20.811 Contact with and (suspected) exposure to meningococcus

Z20.818 Contact with and (suspected) exposure to other bacterial communicable diseases

Z20.82 Contact with and (suspected) exposure to other viral communicable diseases

Z20.820 Contact with and (suspected) exposure to varicella

Z20.828 Contact with and (suspected) exposure to other viral communicable diseases

Z20.89 Contact with and (suspected) exposure to other communicable diseases

Z20.9 Contact with and (suspected) exposure to unspecified communicable disease

13 Z21 Asymptomatic human immunodeficiency virus [HIV] infection status
HIV positive NOS
Code first human immunodeficiency virus [HIV] disease complicating pregnancy, childbirth and the puerperium, if applicable (O98.7-)
EXCLUDES 1 *acquired immunodeficiency syndrome (B20)*
contact with human immunodeficiency virus [HIV] (Z20.6)
exposure to human immunodeficiency virus [HIV] (Z20.6)
human immunodeficiency virus [HIV] disease (B20)
inconclusive laboratory evidence of human immunodeficiency virus [HIV] (R75)

4th **Z22 Carrier of infectious disease**
Colonization status
Suspected carrier
Z22.0 Carrier of typhoid
Z22.1 Carrier of other intestinal infectious diseases
Z22.2 Carrier of diphtheria
5th **Z22.3 Carrier of other specified bacterial diseases**
Z22.31 Carrier of bacterial disease due to meningococci
6th **Z22.32 Carrier of bacterial disease due to staphylococci**
Z22.321 Carrier or suspected carrier of Methicillin susceptible Staphylococcus aureus
MSSA colonization
Z22.322 Carrier or suspected carrier of Methicillin resistant Staphylococcus aureus
MRSA colonization
6th **Z22.33 Carrier of bacterial disease due to streptococci**
Z22.330 Carrier of Group B streptococcus
Z22.338 Carrier of other streptococcus
Z22.39 Carrier of other specified bacterial diseases
Z22.4 Carrier of infections with a predominantly sexual mode of transmission
5th **Z22.5 Carrier of viral hepatitis**
Z22.50 Carrier of unspecified viral hepatitis
Z22.51 Carrier of viral hepatitis B
Hepatitis B surface antigen [HBsAg] carrier
Z22.52 Carrier of viral hepatitis C
Z22.59 Carrier of other viral hepatitis
Z22.6 Carrier of human T-lymphotropic virus type-1 [HTLV-1] infection
Z22.8 Carrier of other infectious diseases
Z22.9 Carrier of infectious disease, unspecified

Z23 Encounter for immunization
Code first any routine childhood examination
NOTE Procedure codes are required to identify the types of immunizations given

4th **Z28 Immunization not carried out and underimmunization status**
Vaccination not carried out
5th **Z28.0 Immunization not carried out because of contraindication**
Z28.01 Immunization not carried out because of acute illness of patient
Z28.02 Immunization not carried out because of chronic illness or condition of patient
Z28.03 Immunization not carried out because of immune compromised state of patient
Z28.04 Immunization not carried out because of patient allergy to vaccine or component
Z28.09 Immunization not carried out because of other contraindication
Z28.1 Immunization not carried out because of patient decision for reasons of belief or group pressure
Immunization not carried out because of religious belief
5th **Z28.2 Immunization not carried out because of patient decision for other and unspecified reason**
Z28.20 Immunization not carried out because of patient decision for unspecified reason
Z28.21 Immunization not carried out because of patient refusal
Z28.29 Immunization not carried out because of patient decision for other reason
Z28.3 Underimmunization status
Delinquent immunization status
Lapsed immunization schedule status
5th **Z28.8 Immunization not carried out for other reason**
Z28.81 Immunization not carried out due to patient having had the disease
Z28.82 Immunization not carried out because of caregiver refusal
Immunization not carried out because of guardian refusal
Immunization not carried out because of parent refusal
EXCLUDES 1 *immunization not carried out because of caregiver refusal because of religious belief (Z28.1)*
Z28.89 Immunization not carried out for other reason
Z28.9 Immunization not carried out for unspecified reason

Persons encountering health services in circumstances related to reproduction (Z30-Z39)

4th **Z30 Encounter for contraceptive management**
5th **Z30.0 Encounter for general counseling and advice on contraception**
6th **Z30.01 Encounter for initial prescription of contraceptives**
EXCLUDES 1 *encounter for surveillance of contraceptives (Z30.4-)*
Z30.011 Encounter for initial prescription of contraceptive pills ♀
Z30.012 Encounter for prescription of emergency contraception ♀
Encounter for postcoital contraception
Z30.013 Encounter for initial prescription of injectable contraceptive ♀
Z30.014 Encounter for initial prescription of intrauterine contraceptive device ♀
EXCLUDES 1 *encounter for insertion of intrauterine contraceptive device (Z30.430, Z30.432)*
Z30.018 Encounter for initial prescription of other contraceptives ♀
Z30.019 Encounter for initial prescription of contraceptives, unspecified ♀
Z30.02 Counseling and instruction in natural family planning to avoid pregnancy
Z30.09 Encounter for other general counseling and advice on contraception
Encounter for family planning advice NOS
Z30.2 Encounter for sterilization
5th **Z30.4 Encounter for surveillance of contraceptives**
Z30.40 Encounter for surveillance of contraceptives, unspecified
Z30.41 Encounter for surveillance of contraceptive pills ♀
Encounter for repeat prescription for contraceptive pill
Z30.42 Encounter for surveillance of injectable contraceptive ♀
6th **Z30.43 Encounter for surveillance of intrauterine contraceptive device**
Z30.430 Encounter for insertion of intrauterine contraceptive device ♀
Z30.431 Encounter for routine checking of intrauterine contraceptive device ♀
Z30.432 Encounter for removal of intrauterine contraceptive device ♀
Z30.433 Encounter for removal and reinsertion of intrauterine contraceptive device ♀
Encounter for replacement of intrauterine contraceptive device
Z30.49 Encounter for surveillance of other contraceptives ♀
Z30.8 Encounter for other contraceptive management
Encounter for postvasectomy sperm count
Encounter for routine examination for contraceptive maintenance
EXCLUDES 1 *sperm count following sterilization reversal (Z31.42)*
sperm count for fertility testing (Z31.41)

13 Questionable admission when used as PDx.

Z30.9 Encounter for contraceptive management, unspecified

Z31 Encounter for procreative management
EXCLUDES 1 *complications associated with artificial fertilization (N98.-)*
female infertility (N97.-)
male infertility (N46.-)

Z31.0 Encounter for reversal of previous sterilization

Z31.4 Encounter for procreative investigation and testing
EXCLUDES 1 *postvasectomy sperm count (Z30.8)*

Z31.41 Encounter for fertility testing
Encounter for fallopian tube patency testing
Encounter for sperm count for fertility testing

Z31.42 Aftercare following sterilization reversal
Sperm count following sterilization reversal

Z31.43 Encounter for genetic testing of female for procreative management
Use additional code for recurrent pregnancy loss, if applicable (N96, O26.2-)
EXCLUDES 1 *nonprocreative genetic testing (Z13.7-)*

Z31.430 Encounter of female for testing for genetic disease carrier status for procreative management ♀

Z31.438 Encounter for other genetic testing of female for procreative management ♀

Z31.44 Encounter for genetic testing of male for procreative management
EXCLUDES 1 *nonprocreative genetic testing (Z13.7-)*

Z31.440 Encounter of male for testing for genetic disease carrier status for procreative management ♂

Z31.441 Encounter for testing of male partner of patient with recurrent pregnancy loss A♂

Z31.448 Encounter for other genetic testing of male for procreative management A♂

Z31.49 Encounter for other procreative investigation and testing

Z31.5 Encounter for genetic counseling

Z31.6 Encounter for general counseling and advice on procreation

Z31.61 Procreative counseling and advice using natural family planning

Z31.62 Encounter for fertility preservation counseling
Encounter for fertility preservation counseling prior to cancer therapy
Encounter for fertility preservation counseling prior to surgical removal of gonads

Z31.69 Encounter for other general counseling and advice on procreation

Z31.8 Encounter for other procreative management

Z31.81 Encounter for male factor infertility in female patient ♀

Z31.82 Encounter for Rh incompatibility status ♀

Z31.83 Encounter for assisted reproductive fertility procedure cycle ♀
Patient undergoing in vitro fertilization cycle
Use additional code to identify the type of infertility
EXCLUDES 1 *pre-cycle diagnosis and testing—code to reason for encounter*

Z31.84 Encounter for fertility preservation procedure
Encounter for fertility preservation procedure prior to cancer therapy
Encounter for fertility preservation procedure prior to surgical removal of gonads

Z31.89 Encounter for other procreative management

Z31.9 Encounter for procreative management, unspecified

Z32 Encounter for pregnancy test and childbirth and childcare instruction

Z32.0 Encounter for pregnancy test

Z32.00 Encounter for pregnancy test, result unknown ♀
Encounter for pregnancy test NOS

Z32.01 Encounter for pregnancy test, result positive M♀

Z32.02 Encounter for pregnancy test, result negative ♀

Z32.2 Encounter for childbirth instruction

Z32.3 Encounter for childcare instruction
Encounter for prenatal or postpartum childcare instruction

Z33 Pregnant state

Z33.1 Pregnant state, incidental M♀
Pregnant state NOS
EXCLUDES 1 *complications of pregnancy (O00-O9A)*

Z33.2 Encounter for elective termination of pregnancy M♀
EXCLUDES 1 *early fetal death with retention of dead fetus (O02.1)*
late fetal death (O36.4)
spontaneous abortion (O03)

Z34 Encounter for supervision of normal pregnancy
EXCLUDES 1 *any complication of pregnancy (O00-O9A)*
encounter for pregnancy test (Z32.0-)
encounter for supervision of high risk pregnancy (O09.-)

Z34.0 Encounter for supervision of normal first pregnancy

Z34.00 Encounter for supervision of normal first pregnancy, unspecified trimester M♀

Z34.01 Encounter for supervision of normal first pregnancy, first trimester M♀

Z34.02 Encounter for supervision of normal first pregnancy, second trimester M♀

Z34.03 Encounter for supervision of normal first pregnancy, third trimester M♀

Z34.8 Encounter for supervision of other normal pregnancy

Z34.80 Encounter for supervision of other normal pregnancy, unspecified trimester M♀

Z34.81 Encounter for supervision of other normal pregnancy, first trimester M♀

Z34.82 Encounter for supervision of other normal pregnancy, second trimester M♀

Z34.83 Encounter for supervision of other normal pregnancy, third trimester M♀

Z34.9 Encounter for supervision of normal pregnancy, unspecified

Z34.90 Encounter for supervision of normal pregnancy, unspecified, unspecified trimester M♀

Z34.91 Encounter for supervision of normal pregnancy, unspecified, first trimester M♀

Z34.92 Encounter for supervision of normal pregnancy, unspecified, second trimester M♀

Z34.93 Encounter for supervision of normal pregnancy, unspecified, third trimester M♀

Z36 Encounter for antenatal screening of mother M♀
EXCLUDES 1 *abnormal findings on antenatal screening of mother (O28.-)*
diagnostic examination—code to sign or symptom
encounter for suspected maternal and fetal conditions ruled out (Z03.7-)
suspected fetal condition affecting management of pregnancy—code to condition in Chapter 15
EXCLUDES 2 *genetic counseling and testing (Z31.43-, Z31.5)*
routine prenatal care (Z34)

Z3A Weeks of gestation
NOTE Codes from category Z3A are for use, only on the maternal record, to indicate the weeks of gestation of the pregnancy.
Code first complications of pregnancy, childbirth and the puerperium (O00-O9A)
AHA: 2014, 2Q, 9; 2013, 2Q, 33

Z3A.0 Weeks of gestation of pregnancy, unspecified or less than 10 weeks

Z3A.00 Weeks of gestation of pregnancy not specified M♀

Z3A.01 Less than 8 weeks gestation of pregnancy M♀

Z3A.08 8 weeks gestation of pregnancy M♀

Z3A.09 9 weeks gestation of pregnancy M♀

Z3A.1 Weeks of gestation of pregnancy, weeks 10-19

Z3A.10 10 weeks gestation of pregnancy M♀

Z3A.11 11 weeks gestation of pregnancy M♀

Z3A.12 12 weeks gestation of pregnancy M♀

Z3A.13 13 weeks gestation of pregnancy M♀

Z3A.14 14 weeks gestation of pregnancy M♀

Z3A.15 15 weeks gestation of pregnancy M♀

Z3A.16 16 weeks gestation of pregnancy M♀

Z3A.17 17 weeks gestation of pregnancy M♀

Z3A.18 18 weeks gestation of pregnancy M♀

Z3A.19 19 weeks gestation of pregnancy M♀

Z3A.2 Weeks of gestation of pregnancy, weeks 20-29

Z3A.20 20 weeks gestation of pregnancy M♀

Z3A.21 21 weeks gestation of pregnancy M♀

Z3A.22 22 weeks gestation of pregnancy M♀
Z3A.23 23 weeks gestation of pregnancy M♀
Z3A.24 24 weeks gestation of pregnancy M♀
Z3A.25 25 weeks gestation of pregnancy M♀
Z3A.26 26 weeks gestation of pregnancy M♀
Z3A.27 27 weeks gestation of pregnancy M♀
Z3A.28 28 weeks gestation of pregnancy M♀
Z3A.29 29 weeks gestation of pregnancy M♀

✓5th **Z3A.3 Weeks of gestation of pregnancy, weeks 30-39**
Z3A.30 30 weeks gestation of pregnancy M♀
Z3A.31 31 weeks gestation of pregnancy M♀
Z3A.32 32 weeks gestation of pregnancy M♀
Z3A.33 33 weeks gestation of pregnancy M♀
Z3A.34 34 weeks gestation of pregnancy M♀
Z3A.35 35 weeks gestation of pregnancy M♀
Z3A.36 36 weeks gestation of pregnancy M♀
Z3A.37 37 weeks gestation of pregnancy M♀
Z3A.38 38 weeks gestation of pregnancy M♀
Z3A.39 39 weeks gestation of pregnancy M♀

✓5th **Z3A.4 Weeks of gestation of pregnancy, weeks 40 or greater**
Z3A.40 40 weeks gestation of pregnancy M♀
Z3A.41 41 weeks gestation of pregnancy M♀
Z3A.42 42 weeks gestation of pregnancy M♀
Z3A.49 Greater than 42 weeks gestation of pregnancy M♀

✓4th **Z37 Outcome of delivery**
NOTE This category is intended for use as an additional code to identify the outcome of delivery on the mother's record. It is not for use on the newborn record.
EXCLUDES 1 *stillbirth (P95)*

Z37.0 Single live birth M♀
AHA: 2014, 2Q, 9
Z37.1 Single stillbirth M♀
Z37.2 Twins, both liveborn M♀
Z37.3 Twins, one liveborn and one stillborn M♀
Z37.4 Twins, both stillborn M♀
✓5th Z37.5 Other multiple births, all liveborn
Z37.50 Multiple births, unspecified, all liveborn M♀
Z37.51 Triplets, all liveborn M♀
Z37.52 Quadruplets, all liveborn M♀
Z37.53 Quintuplets, all liveborn M♀
Z37.54 Sextuplets, all liveborn M♀
Z37.59 Other multiple births, all liveborn M♀
✓5th Z37.6 Other multiple births, some liveborn
Z37.60 Multiple births, unspecified, some liveborn M♀
Z37.61 Triplets, some liveborn M♀
Z37.62 Quadruplets, some liveborn M♀
Z37.63 Quintuplets, some liveborn M♀
Z37.64 Sextuplets, some liveborn M♀
Z37.69 Other multiple births, some liveborn M♀
Z37.7 Other multiple births, all stillborn M♀
Z37.9 Outcome of delivery, unspecified M♀
Multiple birth NOS
Single birth NOS

✓4th **Z38 Liveborn infants according to place of birth and type of delivery**
NOTE This category is for use as the principal code on the initial record of a newborn baby. It is to be used for the initial birth record only. It is not to be used on the mother's record.

✓5th Z38.0 Single liveborn infant, born in hospital
Single liveborn infant, born in birthing center or other health care facility
Z38.00 Single liveborn infant, delivered vaginally N
Z38.01 Single liveborn infant, delivered by cesarean N
Z38.1 Single liveborn infant, born outside hospital N
Z38.2 Single liveborn infant, unspecified as to place of birth N
Single liveborn infant NOS
✓5th Z38.3 Twin liveborn infant, born in hospital
Z38.30 Twin liveborn infant, delivered vaginally N
Z38.31 Twin liveborn infant, delivered by cesarean N
Z38.4 Twin liveborn infant, born outside hospital N
Z38.5 Twin liveborn infant, unspecified as to place of birth N
✓5th Z38.6 Other multiple liveborn infant, born in hospital
Z38.61 Triplet liveborn infant, delivered vaginally N
Z38.62 Triplet liveborn infant, delivered by cesarean N
Z38.63 Quadruplet liveborn infant, delivered vaginally N
Z38.64 Quadruplet liveborn infant, delivered by cesarean N
Z38.65 Quintuplet liveborn infant, delivered vaginally N
Z38.66 Quintuplet liveborn infant, delivered by cesarean N
Z38.68 Other multiple liveborn infant, delivered vaginally N
Z38.69 Other multiple liveborn infant, delivered by cesarean N
Z38.7 Other multiple liveborn infant, born outside hospital N
Z38.8 Other multiple liveborn infant, unspecified as to place of birth N

✓4th **Z39 Encounter for maternal postpartum care and examination**
Z39.0 Encounter for care and examination of mother immediately after delivery M♀
Care and observation in uncomplicated cases when the delivery occurs outside a healthcare facility
EXCLUDES 1 *care for postpartum complication—see Alphabetic index*
Z39.1 Encounter for care and examination of lactating mother M♀
Encounter for supervision of lactation
EXCLUDES 1 *disorders of lactation (O92.-)*
Z39.2 Encounter for routine postpartum follow-up M♀

Encounters for other specific health care (Z40-Z53)

NOTE Categories Z40-Z53 are intended for use to indicate a reason for care. They may be used for patients who have already been treated for a disease or injury, but who are receiving aftercare or prophylactic care, or care to consolidate the treatment, or to deal with a residual state.
EXCLUDES 2 *follow-up examination for medical surveillance after treatment (Z08-Z09)*

✓4th **Z40 Encounter for prophylactic surgery**
EXCLUDES 1 *organ donations (Z52.-)*
therapeutic organ removal—code to condition
✓5th Z40.0 Encounter for prophylactic surgery for risk factors related to malignant neoplasms
Admission for prophylactic organ removal
Use additional code to identify risk factor
Z40.00 Encounter for prophylactic removal of unspecified organ
Z40.01 Encounter for prophylactic removal of breast
Z40.02 Encounter for prophylactic removal of ovary ♀
Z40.09 Encounter for prophylactic removal of other organ
Z40.8 Encounter for other prophylactic surgery
Z40.9 Encounter for prophylactic surgery, unspecified

✓4th **Z41 Encounter for procedures for purposes other than remedying health state**
Z41.1 Encounter for cosmetic surgery
Encounter for cosmetic breast implant
Encounter for cosmetic procedure
EXCLUDES 1 *encounter for plastic and reconstructive surgery following medical procedure or healed injury (Z42.-)*
encounter for post-mastectomy breast implantation (Z42.1)
Z41.2 Encounter for routine and ritual male circumcision ♂
Z41.3 Encounter for ear piercing
Z41.8 Encounter for other procedures for purposes other than remedying health state
Z41.9 Encounter for procedure for purposes other than remedying health state, unspecified

✓4th **Z42 Encounter for plastic and reconstructive surgery following medical procedure or healed injury**
EXCLUDES 1 *encounter for cosmetic plastic surgery (Z41.1)*
encounter for plastic surgery for treatment of current injury—code to relevent injury
Z42.1 Encounter for breast reconstruction following mastectomy A
EXCLUDES 1 *deformity and disproportion of reconstructed breast (N65.1-)*

Z42.8 **Encounter for other plastic and reconstructive surgery following medical procedure or healed injury**

Z43 Encounter for attention to artificial openings

INCLUDES closure of artificial openings
passage of sounds or bougies through artificial openings
reforming artificial openings
removal of catheter from artificial openings
toilet or cleansing of artificial openings

EXCLUDES 1 *artificial opening status only, without need for care (Z93.-)*
complications of external stoma (J95.Ø-, K94.-, N99.5-)

EXCLUDES 2 *fitting and adjustment of prosthetic and other devices (Z44-Z46)*

Z43.Ø **Encounter for attention to tracheostomy**

Z43.1 **Encounter for attention to gastrostomy** CC
CC Excl: Z43.1

Z43.2 **Encounter for attention to ileostomy**

Z43.3 **Encounter for attention to colostomy**

Z43.4 **Encounter for attention to other artificial openings of digestive tract**

Z43.5 **Encounter for attention to cystostomy**

Z43.6 **Encounter for attention to other artificial openings of urinary tract**
Encounter for attention to nephrostomy
Encounter for attention to ureterostomy
Encounter for attention to urethrostomy

Z43.7 **Encounter for attention to artificial vagina**

Z43.8 **Encounter for attention to other artificial openings**

Z43.9 **Encounter for attention to unspecified artificial opening**

Z44 Encounter for fitting and adjustment of external prosthetic device

INCLUDES removal or replacement of external prosthetic device

EXCLUDES 1 *malfunction or other complications of device—see Alphabetical Index*
presence of prosthetic device (Z97.-)

Z44.Ø **Encounter for fitting and adjustment of artificial arm**

Z44.ØØ **Encounter for fitting and adjustment of unspecified artificial arm**

Z44.ØØ1 **Encounter for fitting and adjustment of unspecified right artificial arm**

Z44.ØØ2 **Encounter for fitting and adjustment of unspecified left artificial arm**

Z44.ØØ9 **Encounter for fitting and adjustment of unspecified artificial arm, unspecified arm**

Z44.Ø1 **Encounter for fitting and adjustment of complete artificial arm**

Z44.Ø11 **Encounter for fitting and adjustment of complete right artificial arm**

Z44.Ø12 **Encounter for fitting and adjustment of complete left artificial arm**

Z44.Ø19 **Encounter for fitting and adjustment of complete artificial arm, unspecified arm**

Z44.Ø2 **Encounter for fitting and adjustment of partial artificial arm**

Z44.Ø21 **Encounter for fitting and adjustment of partial artificial right arm**

Z44.Ø22 **Encounter for fitting and adjustment of partial artificial left arm**

Z44.Ø29 **Encounter for fitting and adjustment of partial artificial arm, unspecified arm**

Z44.1 **Encounter for fitting and adjustment of artificial leg**

Z44.1Ø **Encounter for fitting and adjustment of unspecified artificial leg**

Z44.1Ø1 **Encounter for fitting and adjustment of unspecified right artificial leg**

Z44.1Ø2 **Encounter for fitting and adjustment of unspecified left artificial leg**

Z44.1Ø9 **Encounter for fitting and adjustment of unspecified artificial leg, unspecified leg**

Z44.11 **Encounter for fitting and adjustment of complete artificial leg**

Z44.111 **Encounter for fitting and adjustment of complete right artificial leg**

Z44.112 **Encounter for fitting and adjustment of complete left artificial leg**

Z44.119 **Encounter for fitting and adjustment of complete artificial leg, unspecified leg**

Z44.12 **Encounter for fitting and adjustment of partial artificial leg**

Z44.121 **Encounter for fitting and adjustment of partial artificial right leg**

Z44.122 **Encounter for fitting and adjustment of partial artificial left leg**

Z44.129 **Encounter for fitting and adjustment of partial artificial leg, unspecified leg**

Z44.2 **Encounter for fitting and adjustment of artificial eye**

EXCLUDES 1 *mechanical complication of ocular prosthesis (T85.3)*

Z44.2Ø **Encounter for fitting and adjustment of artificial eye, unspecified**

Z44.21 **Encounter for fitting and adjustment of artificial right eye**

Z44.22 **Encounter for fitting and adjustment of artificial left eye**

Z44.3 **Encounter for fitting and adjustment of external breast prosthesis**

EXCLUDES 1 *complications of breast implant (T85.4-)*
encounter for adjustment or removal of breast implant (Z45.81-)
encounter for initial breast implant insertion for cosmetic breast augmentation (Z41.1)
encounter for breast reconstruction following mastectomy (Z42.1)

Z44.3Ø **Encounter for fitting and adjustment of external breast prosthesis, unspecified breast** ♀

Z44.31 **Encounter for fitting and adjustment of external right breast prosthesis** ♀

Z44.32 **Encounter for fitting and adjustment of external left breast prosthesis** ♀

Z44.8 **Encounter for fitting and adjustment of other external prosthetic devices**

Z44.9 **Encounter for fitting and adjustment of unspecified external prosthetic device**

Z45 Encounter for adjustment and management of implanted device

INCLUDES removal or replacement of implanted device

EXCLUDES 1 *malfunction or other complications of device—see Alphabetical Index*
presence of prosthetic and other devices (Z95-Z97)

EXCLUDES 2 *encounter for fitting and adjustment of non-implanted device (Z46.-)*

Z45.Ø **Encounter for adjustment and management of cardiac device**

Z45.Ø1 **Encounter for adjustment and management of cardiac pacemaker**

EXCLUDES 1 *encounter for adjustment and management of automatic implantable cardiac defibrillator with synchronous cardiac pacemaker (Z45.Ø2)*

[13] Z45.Ø1Ø **Encounter for checking and testing of cardiac pacemaker pulse generator [battery]**
Encounter for replacing cardiac pacemaker pulse generator [battery]

[13] Z45.Ø18 **Encounter for adjustment and management of other part of cardiac pacemaker**

[13] Z45.Ø2 **Encounter for adjustment and management of automatic implantable cardiac defibrillator**
Encounter for adjustment and management of automatic implantable cardiac defibrillator with synchronous cardiac pacemaker

[13] Z45.Ø9 **Encounter for adjustment and management of other cardiac device**

Z45.1 **Encounter for adjustment and management of infusion pump**

Z45.2 **Encounter for adjustment and management of vascular access device**
Encounter for adjustment and management of vascular catheters

EXCLUDES 1 *encounter for adjustment and management of renal dialysis catheter (Z49.Ø1)*

Z45.3 **Encounter for adjustment and management of implanted devices of the special senses**

Z45.31 **Encounter for adjustment and management of implanted visual substitution device**

13 Questionable admission when used as PDx.

6th **Z45.32 Encounter for adjustment and management of implanted hearing device**
EXCLUDES 1 *Encounter for fitting and adjustment of hearing aide (Z46.1)*

Z45.320 Encounter for adjustment and management of bone conduction device

Z45.321 Encounter for adjustment and management of cochlear device

Z45.328 Encounter for adjustment and management of other implanted hearing device

5th **Z45.4 Encounter for adjustment and management of implanted nervous system device**

Z45.41 Encounter for adjustment and management of cerebrospinal fluid drainage device
Encounter for adjustment and management of cerebral ventricular (communicating) shunt

Z45.42 Encounter for adjustment and management of neuropacemaker (brain) (peripheral nerve) (spinal cord)

Z45.49 Encounter for adjustment and management of other implanted nervous system device

5th **Z45.8 Encounter for adjustment and management of other implanted devices**

6th **Z45.81 Encounter for adjustment or removal of breast implant**
Encounter for elective implant exchange (different material) (different size)
Encounter removal of tissue expander without synchronous insertion of permanent implant
EXCLUDES 1 *complications of breast implant (T85.4-)*
encounter for initial breast implant insertion for cosmetic breast augmentation (Z41.1)
encounter for breast reconstruction following mastectomy (Z42.1)

Z45.811 Encounter for adjustment or removal of right breast implant ♀

Z45.812 Encounter for adjustment or removal of left breast implant ♀

Z45.819 Encounter for adjustment or removal of unspecified breast implant ♀

Z45.82 Encounter for adjustment or removal of myringotomy device (stent) (tube)

Z45.89 Encounter for adjustment and management of other implanted devices

Z45.9 Encounter for adjustment and management of unspecified implanted device

4th **Z46 Encounter for fitting and adjustment of other devices**
INCLUDES removal or replacement of other device
EXCLUDES 1 *malfunction or other complications of device—see Alphabetical Index*
EXCLUDES 2 *encounter for fitting and management of implanted devices (Z45.-)*
issue of repeat prescription only (Z76.0)
presence of prosthetic and other devices (Z95-Z97)

Z46.0 Encounter for fitting and adjustment of spectacles and contact lenses

Z46.1 Encounter for fitting and adjustment of hearing aid
EXCLUDES 1 *encounter for adjustment and management of implanted hearing device (Z45.32-)*

Z46.2 Encounter for fitting and adjustment of other devices related to nervous system and special senses
EXCLUDES 2 *encounter for adjustment and management of implanted nervous system device (Z45.4-)*
encounter for adjustment and management of implanted visual substitution device (Z45.31)

Z46.3 Encounter for fitting and adjustment of dental prosthetic device
Encounter for fitting and adjustment of dentures

Z46.4 Encounter for fitting and adjustment of orthodontic device

5th **Z46.5 Encounter for fitting and adjustment of other gastrointestinal appliance and device**
EXCLUDES 1 *encounter for attention to artificial openings of digestive tract (Z43.1-Z43.4)*

Z46.51 Encounter for fitting and adjustment of gastric lap band

Z46.59 Encounter for fitting and adjustment of other gastrointestinal appliance and device

Z46.6 Encounter for fitting and adjustment of urinary device
EXCLUDES 2 *attention to artificial openings of urinary tract (Z43.5, Z43.6)*

5th **Z46.8 Encounter for fitting and adjustment of other specified devices**

Z46.81 Encounter for fitting and adjustment of insulin pump
Encounter for insulin pump instruction and training
Encounter for insulin pump titration

Z46.82 Encounter for fitting and adjustment of non-vascular catheter

Z46.89 Encounter for fitting and adjustment of other specified devices
Encounter for fitting and adjustment of wheelchair

Z46.9 Encounter for fitting and adjustment of unspecified device

4th **Z47 Orthopedic aftercare**
EXCLUDES 1 *aftercare for healing fracture—code to fracture with 7th character D*

Z47.1 Aftercare following joint replacement surgery
Use additional code to identify the joint (Z96.6-)

Z47.2 Encounter for removal of internal fixation device
EXCLUDES 1 *encounter for adjustment of internal fixation device for fracture treatment—code to fracture with appropriate 7th character*
encounter for removal of external fixation device—code to fracture with 7th character D
infection or inflammatory reaction to internal fixation device (T84.6-)
mechanical complication of internal fixation device (T84.1-)

5th **Z47.3 Aftercare following explantation of joint prosthesis**
Aftercare following explantation of joint prosthesis, staged procedure
Encounter for joint prosthesis insertion following prior explantation of joint prosthesis

Z47.31 Aftercare following explantation of shoulder joint prosthesis
EXCLUDES 1 *acquired absence of shoulder joint following prior explantation of shoulder joint prosthesis (Z89.23-)*
shoulder joint prosthesis explantation status (Z89.23-)

Z47.32 Aftercare following explantation of hip joint prosthesis
EXCLUDES 1 *acquired absence of hip joint following prior explantation of hip joint prosthesis (Z89.62-)*
hip joint prosthesis explantation status (Z89.62-)

Z47.33 Aftercare following explantation of knee joint prosthesis
EXCLUDES 1 *acquired absence of knee joint following prior explantation of knee prosthesis (Z89.52-)*
knee joint prosthesis explantation status (Z89.52-)

5th **Z47.8 Encounter for other orthopedic aftercare**

Z47.81 Encounter for orthopedic aftercare following surgical amputation
Use additional code to identify the limb amputated (Z89.-)

Z47.82 Encounter for orthopedic aftercare following scoliosis surgery

Z47.89 Encounter for other orthopedic aftercare

4th **Z48 Encounter for other postprocedural aftercare**
EXCLUDES 1 *encounter for follow-up examination after completed treatment (Z08-Z09)*
EXCLUDES 2 *encounter for attention to artificial openings (Z43.-)*
encounter for fitting and adjustment of prosthetic and other devices (Z44-Z46)

5th **Z48.0 Encounter for attention to dressings, sutures and drains**
EXCLUDES 1 *encounter for planned postprocedural wound closure (Z48.1)*

Z48.00 Encounter for change or removal of nonsurgical wound dressing
Encounter for change or removal of wound dressing NOS

Z48.01 Encounter for change or removal of surgical wound dressing

Z48.02 **Encounter for removal of sutures**
Encounter for removal of staples

Z48.03 **Encounter for change or removal of drains**

Z48.1 **Encounter for planned postprocedural wound closure**
EXCLUDES 1 *encounter for attention to dressings and sutures (Z48.0-)*

✓5th Z48.2 **Encounter for aftercare following organ transplant**

Z48.21 **Encounter for aftercare following heart transplant** PDx CC CC
CC Excl: D47.Z1,T86.20-T86.23,T86.290,T86.298,T86.30-T86.39,T86.850-T86.859,T86.90-T86.99,Z94.1,Z94.3, Z94.89- Z94.9

Z48.22 **Encounter for aftercare following kidney transplant** PDx CC CC
CC Excl: D47.Z1,T86.10-T86.13, T86.19, T86.850-T86.859,T86.90-T86.99,Z94.0,Z94.89-Z94.9

Z48.23 **Encounter for aftercare following liver transplant** PDx CC CC
CC Excl: D47.Z1,T86.40-T86.43,T86.49,T86.850-T86.859,T86.90-T86.99, Z94.4,Z94.89-Z94.9

Z48.24 **Encounter for aftercare following lung transplant** PDx CC CC
CC Excl: D47.Z1, T86.810-T86.819,T86.49,T86.850-T86.859,T86.90-T86.99,Z94.2,Z94.89-Z94.9

✓6th Z48.28 **Encounter for aftercare following multiple organ transplant**

Z48.280 **Encounter for aftercare following heart-lung transplant** PDx CC CC
CC Excl: See Code: Z48.21

Z48.288 **Encounter for aftercare following multiple organ transplant**

✓6th Z48.29 **Encounter for aftercare following other organ transplant**

Z48.290 **Encounter for aftercare following bone marrow transplant** PDx CC CC
CC Excl: D47.Z1, T86.810-T86.813,T86.00-T86.09,T86.850-T86.859,T86.90-T86.99,Z94.9

Z48.298 **Encounter for aftercare following other organ transplant**

Z48.3 **Aftercare following surgery for neoplasm**
Use additional code to identify the neoplasm

✓5th Z48.8 **Encounter for other specified postprocedural aftercare**

✓6th Z48.81 **Encounter for surgical aftercare following surgery on specified body systems**
NOTE These codes identify the body system requiring aftercare. They are for use in conjunction with other aftercare codes to fully explain the aftercare encounter. The condition treated should also be coded if still present.
EXCLUDES 1 *aftercare for injury—code the injury with 7th character D*
aftercare following surgery for neoplasm (Z48.3)
EXCLUDES 2 *aftercare following organ transplant (Z48.2-)*
orthopedic aftercare (Z47.-)

Z48.810 **Encounter for surgical aftercare following surgery on the sense organs**

Z48.811 **Encounter for surgical aftercare following surgery on the nervous system**
EXCLUDES 2 *encounter for surgical aftercare following surgery on the sense organs (Z48.810)*

Z48.812 **Encounter for surgical aftercare following surgery on the circulatory system**
AHA: 2012, 4Q, 96

Z48.813 **Encounter for surgical aftercare following surgery on the respiratory system**

Z48.814 **Encounter for surgical aftercare following surgery on the teeth or oral cavity**

Z48.815 **Encounter for surgical aftercare following surgery on the digestive system**

Z48.816 **Encounter for surgical aftercare following surgery on the genitourinary system**
EXCLUDES 1 *encounter for aftercare following sterilization reversal (Z31.42)*

Z48.817 **Encounter for surgical aftercare following surgery on the skin and subcutaneous tissue**

Z48.89 **Encounter for other specified surgical aftercare**

✓4th Z49 **Encounter for care involving renal dialysis**
Code also associated end stage renal disease (N18.6)

✓5th Z49.0 **Preparatory care for renal dialysis**
Encounter for dialysis instruction and training

Z49.01 **Encounter for fitting and adjustment of extracorporeal dialysis catheter**
Removal or replacement of renal dialysis catheter
Toilet or cleansing of renal dialysis catheter

Z49.02 **Encounter for fitting and adjustment of peritoneal dialysis catheter**

✓5th Z49.3 **Encounter for adequacy testing for dialysis**

Z49.31 **Encounter for adequacy testing for hemodialysis**

Z49.32 **Encounter for adequacy testing for peritoneal dialysis**
Encounter for peritoneal equilibration test

✓4th Z51 **Encounter for other aftercare**
Code also condition requiring care
EXCLUDES 1 *follow-up examination after treatment (Z08-Z09)*

Z51.0 **Encounter for antineoplastic radiation therapy**

✓5th Z51.1 **Encounter for antineoplastic chemotherapy and immunotherapy**
EXCLUDES 2 *encounter for chemotherapy and immunotherapy for nonneoplastic condition—code to condition*

Z51.11 **Encounter for antineoplastic chemotherapy**

Z51.12 **Encounter for antineoplastic immunotherapy**

Z51.5 **Encounter for palliative care**

✓5th Z51.8 **Encounter for other specified aftercare**
EXCLUDES 1 *holiday relief care (Z75.5)*

Z51.81 **Encounter for therapeutic drug level monitoring**
Code also any long-term (current) drug therapy (Z79.-)
EXCLUDES 1 *encounter for blood-drug test for administrative or medicolegal reasons (Z02.83)*

Z51.89 **Encounter for other specified aftercare**
AHA: 2012, 4Q, 95-97

✓4th Z52 **Donors of organs and tissues**
INCLUDES autologous and other living donors
EXCLUDES 1 *cadaveric donor—omit code*
examination of potential donor (Z00.5)
AHA: 2012, 4Q, 99

✓5th Z52.0 **Blood donor**

✓6th Z52.00 **Unspecified blood donor**

Z52.000 **Unspecified donor, whole blood**

Z52.001 **Unspecified donor, stem cells**

Z52.008 **Unspecified donor, other blood**

✓6th Z52.01 **Autologous blood donor**

Z52.010 **Autologous donor, whole blood**

Z52.011 **Autologous donor, stem cells**

Z52.018 **Autologous donor, other blood**

✓6th Z52.09 **Other blood donor**
Volunteer donor

Z52.090 **Other blood donor, whole blood**

Z52.091 **Other blood donor, stem cells**

Z52.098 **Other blood donor, other blood**

✓5th Z52.1 **Skin donor**

Z52.10 **Skin donor, unspecified**

Z52.11 **Skin donor, autologous**

Z52.19 **Skin donor, other**

✓5th Z52.2 **Bone donor**

Z52.20 **Bone donor, unspecified**

Z52.21 **Bone donor, autologous**

Z52.29 **Bone donor, other**

Z52.3 **Bone marrow donor**

Z52.4 **Kidney donor**

Z52.5 **Cornea donor**

Z52.6 **Liver donor**

✓5th Z52.8 **Donor of other specified organs or tissues**

✓6th Z52.81 **Egg (Oocyte) donor**

Z52.810 **Egg (Oocyte) donor under age 35, anonymous recipient** ♀
Egg donor under age 35 NOS

Z52.811 **Egg (Oocyte) donor under age 35, designated recipient** ♀

Z52.812 Egg (Oocyte) donor age 35 and over, anonymous recipient ♀
Egg donor age 35 and over NOS
Z52.813 Egg (Oocyte) donor age 35 and over, designated recipient ♀
Z52.819 Egg (Oocyte) donor, unspecified ♀
Z52.89 Donor of other specified organs or tissues
Z52.9 Donor of unspecified organ or tissue
Donor NOS

Z53 Persons encountering health services for specific procedures and treatment, not carried out
Z53.0 Procedure and treatment not carried out because of contraindication
Z53.01 Procedure and treatment not carried out due to patient smoking
Z53.09 Procedure and treatment not carried out because of other contraindication
Z53.1 Procedure and treatment not carried out because of patient's decision for reasons of belief and group pressure
Z53.2 Procedure and treatment not carried out because of patient's decision for other and unspecified reasons
Z53.20 Procedure and treatment not carried out because of patient's decision for unspecified reasons
Z53.21 Procedure and treatment not carried out due to patient leaving prior to being seen by health care provider
Z53.29 Procedure and treatment not carried out because of patient's decision for other reasons
Z53.8 Procedure and treatment not carried out for other reasons
Z53.9 Procedure and treatment not carried out, unspecified reason

Persons with potential health hazards related to socioeconomic and psychosocial circumstances (Z55-Z65)

Z55 Problems related to education and literacy
EXCLUDES 1 *disorders of psychological development (F80-F89)*
Z55.0 Illiteracy and low-level literacy
Z55.1 Schooling unavailable and unattainable
Z55.2 Failed school examinations
Z55.3 Underachievement in school
Z55.4 Educational maladjustment and discord with teachers and classmates
Z55.8 Other problems related to education and literacy
Problems related to inadequate teaching
Z55.9 Problems related to education and literacy, unspecified
Academic problems NOS

Z56 Problems related to employment and unemployment
EXCLUDES 2 *occupational exposure to risk factors (Z57.-)*
problems related to housing and economic circumstances (Z59.-)
Z56.0 Unemployment, unspecified
Z56.1 Change of job A
Z56.2 Threat of job loss
Z56.3 Stressful work schedule
Z56.4 Discord with boss and workmates
Z56.5 Uncongenial work environment
Difficult conditions at work
Z56.6 Other physical and mental strain related to work
Z56.8 Other problems related to employment
Z56.81 Sexual harassment on the job
Z56.82 Military deployment status
Individual (civilian or military) currently deployed in theater or in support of military war, peacekeeping and humanitarian operations
Z56.89 Other problems related to employment
Z56.9 Unspecified problems related to employment
Occupational problems NOS

Z57 Occupational exposure to risk factors
Z57.0 Occupational exposure to noise
Z57.1 Occupational exposure to radiation
Z57.2 Occupational exposure to dust
Z57.3 Occupational exposure to other air contaminants
Z57.31 Occupational exposure to environmental tobacco smoke
EXCLUDES 2 *exposure to environmental tobacco smoke (Z77.22)*
Z57.39 Occupational exposure to other air contaminants
Z57.4 Occupational exposure to toxic agents in agriculture
Occupational exposure to solids, liquids, gases or vapors in agriculture
Z57.5 Occupational exposure to toxic agents in other industries
Occupational exposure to solids, liquids, gases or vapors in other industries
Z57.6 Occupational exposure to extreme temperature
Z57.7 Occupational exposure to vibration
Z57.8 Occupational exposure to other risk factors
Z57.9 Occupational exposure to unspecified risk factor

Z59 Problems related to housing and economic circumstances
EXCLUDES 2 *problems related to upbringing (Z62.-)*
Z59.0 Homelessness
Z59.1 Inadequate housing
Lack of heating
Restriction of space
Technical defects in home preventing adequate care
Unsatisfactory surroundings
EXCLUDES 1 *problems related to the natural and physical environment (Z77.1-)*
Z59.2 Discord with neighbors, lodgers and landlord
Z59.3 Problems related to living in residential institution
Boarding-school resident
EXCLUDES 1 *institutional upbringing (Z62.2)*
Z59.4 Lack of adequate food and safe drinking water
Inadequate drinking water supply
EXCLUDES 1 *effects of hunger (T73.0)*
inappropriate diet or eating habits (Z72.4)
malnutrition (E40-E46)
Z59.5 Extreme poverty
Z59.6 Low income
Z59.7 Insufficient social insurance and welfare support
Z59.8 Other problems related to housing and economic circumstances
Foreclosure on loan
Isolated dwelling
Problems with creditors
Z59.9 Problem related to housing and economic circumstances, unspecified

Z60 Problems related to social environment
Z60.0 Problems of adjustment to life-cycle transitions
Empty nest syndrome
Phase of life problem
Problem with adjustment to retirement [pension]
Z60.2 Problems related to living alone
Z60.3 Acculturation difficulty
Problem with migration
Problem with social transplantation
Z60.4 Social exclusion and rejection
Exclusion and rejection on the basis of personal characteristics, such as unusual physical appearance, illness or behavior.
EXCLUDES 1 *target of adverse discrimination such as for racial or religious reasons (Z60.5)*
Z60.5 Target of (perceived) adverse discrimination and persecution
EXCLUDES 1 *social exclusion and rejection (Z60.4)*
Z60.8 Other problems related to social environment
Z60.9 Problem related to social environment, unspecified

Z62 Problems related to upbringing
Current and past negative life events in childhood
Current and past problems of a child related to upbringing
EXCLUDES 2 *maltreatment syndrome (T74.-)*
problems related to housing and economic circumstances (Z59.-)
Z62.0 Inadequate parental supervision and control
Z62.1 Parental overprotection
Z62.2 Upbringing away from parents
EXCLUDES 1 *problems with boarding school (Z59.3)*
Z62.21 Child in welfare custody P
Child in care of non-parental family member
Child in foster care
EXCLUDES 2 *problem for parent due to child in welfare custody (Z63.5)*

Z62.22 **Institutional upbringing**
Child living in orphanage or group home
Z62.29 **Other upbringing away from parents**
Z62.3 **Hostility towards and scapegoating of child** P
Z62.6 **Inappropriate (excessive) parental pressure**
✓5th Z62.8 **Other specified problems related to upbringing**
✓6th Z62.81 **Personal history of abuse in childhood**
Z62.810 **Personal history of physical and sexual abuse in childhood**
EXCLUDES 1 *current child physical abuse (T74.12, T76.12)*
current child sexual abuse (T74.22, T76.22)
Z62.811 **Personal history of psychological abuse in childhood**
EXCLUDES 1 *current child psychological abuse (T74.32, T76.32)*
Z62.812 **Personal history of neglect in childhood**
EXCLUDES 1 *current child neglect (T74.02, T76.02)*
Z62.819 **Personal history of unspecified abuse in childhood**
EXCLUDES 1 *current child abuse NOS (T74.92, T76.92)*
✓6th Z62.82 **Parent-child conflict**
Z62.820 **Parent-biological child conflict**
Parent-child problem NOS
Z62.821 **Parent-adopted child conflict**
Z62.822 **Parent-foster child conflict**
✓6th Z62.89 **Other specified problems related to upbringing**
Z62.890 **Parent-child estrangement NEC**
Z62.891 **Sibling rivalry**
Z62.898 **Other specified problems related to upbringing**
Z62.9 **Problem related to upbringing, unspecified**

✓4th **Z63 Other problems related to primary support group, including family circumstances**
EXCLUDES 2 *maltreatment syndrome (T74-, T76)*
parent-child problems (Z62.-)
problems related to negative life events in childhood (Z62.-)
problems related to upbringing (Z62.-)
Z63.0 **Problems in relationship with spouse or partner**
EXCLUDES 1 *counseling for spousal or partner abuse problems (Z69.1)*
counseling related to sexual attitude, behavior, and orientation (Z70.-)
Z63.1 **Problems in relationship with in-laws**
✓5th Z63.3 **Absence of family member**
EXCLUDES 1 *absence of family member due to disappearance and death (Z63.4)*
absence of family member due to separation and divorce (Z63.5)
Z63.31 **Absence of family member due to military deployment**
Individual or family affected by other family member being on military deployment
EXCLUDES 1 *family disruption due to return of family member from military deployment (Z63.71)*
Z63.32 **Other absence of family member**
Z63.4 **Disappearance and death of family member**
Assumed death of family member
Bereavement
AHA: 2014, 1Q, 25
Z63.5 **Disruption of family by separation and divorce**
Marital estrangement
Z63.6 **Dependent relative needing care at home**
✓5th Z63.7 **Other stressful life events affecting family and household**
Z63.71 **Stress on family due to return of family member from military deployment**
Individual or family affected by family member having returned from military deployment (current or past conflict)
Z63.72 **Alcoholism and drug addiction in family**
Z63.79 **Other stressful life events affecting family and household**
Anxiety (normal) about sick person in family
Health problems within family
Ill or disturbed family member
Isolated family
Z63.8 **Other specified problems related to primary support group**
Family discord NOS
Family estrangement NOS
High expressed emotional level within family
Inadequate family support NOS
Inadequate or distorted communication within family
Z63.9 **Problem related to primary support group, unspecified**
Relationship disorder NOS

✓4th **Z64 Problems related to certain psychosocial circumstances**
Z64.0 **Problems related to unwanted pregnancy** M♀
Z64.1 **Problems related to multiparity** ♀
Z64.4 **Discord with counselors**
Discord with probation officer
Discord with social worker

✓4th **Z65 Problems related to other psychosocial circumstances**
Z65.0 **Conviction in civil and criminal proceedings without imprisonment**
Z65.1 **Imprisonment and other incarceration**
Z65.2 **Problems related to release from prison**
Z65.3 **Problems related to other legal circumstances**
Arrest
Child custody or support proceedings
Litigation
Prosecution
Z65.4 **Victim of crime and terrorism**
Victim of torture
Z65.5 **Exposure to disaster, war and other hostilities**
EXCLUDES 1 *target of perceived discrimination or persecution (Z60.5)*
Z65.8 **Other specified problems related to psychosocial circumstances**
Z65.9 **Problem related to unspecified psychosocial circumstances**

Do not resuscitate status (Z66)

Z66 Do not resuscitate
DNR status

Blood type (Z67)

✓4th **Z67 Blood type**
✓5th Z67.1 **Type A blood**
Z67.10 **Type A blood, Rh positive**
Z67.11 **Type A blood, Rh negative**
✓5th Z67.2 **Type B blood**
Z67.20 **Type B blood, Rh positive**
Z67.21 **Type B blood, Rh negative**
✓5th Z67.3 **Type AB blood**
Z67.30 **Type AB blood, Rh positive**
Z67.31 **Type AB blood, Rh negative**
✓5th Z67.4 **Type O blood**
Z67.40 **Type O blood, Rh positive**
Z67.41 **Type O blood, Rh negative**
✓5th Z67.9 **Unspecified blood type**
Z67.90 **Unspecified blood type, Rh positive**
Z67.91 **Unspecified blood type, Rh negative**

Body mass index [BMI] (Z68)

✓4th **Z68 Body mass index [BMI]**
Kilograms per meters squared
NOTE BMI adult codes are for use for persons 21 years of age or older.
BMI pediatric codes are for use for persons 2-20 years of age. These percentiles are based on the growth charts published by the Centers for Disease Control and Prevention (CDC)
Z68.1 **Body mass index [BMI] 19 or less, adult** CC A
CC Excl: E66.01-E66.1,E66.8-E66.9, Z68.1,Z68.20-Z68.39, Z68.1-Z68.54
✓5th Z68.2 **Body mass index [BMI] 20-29, adult**
Z68.20 **Body mass index [BMI] 20.0-20.9, adult** A

Z68.21 **Body mass index [BMI] 21.0-21.9, adult** A
Z68.22 **Body mass index [BMI] 22.0-22.9, adult** A
Z68.23 **Body mass index [BMI] 23.0-23.9, adult** A
Z68.24 **Body mass index [BMI] 24.0-24.9, adult** A
Z68.25 **Body mass index [BMI] 25.0-25.9, adult** A
Z68.26 **Body mass index [BMI] 26.0-26.9, adult** A
Z68.27 **Body mass index [BMI] 27.0-27.9, adult** A
Z68.28 **Body mass index [BMI] 28.0-28.9, adult** A
Z68.29 **Body mass index [BMI] 29.0-29.9, adult** A

✓5th **Z68.3 Body mass index [BMI] 30-39, adult**

Z68.30 **Body mass index [BMI] 30.0-30.9, adult** A
Z68.31 **Body mass index [BMI] 31.0-31.9, adult** A
Z68.32 **Body mass index [BMI] 32.0-32.9, adult** A
Z68.33 **Body mass index [BMI] 33.0-33.9, adult** A
Z68.34 **Body mass index [BMI] 34.0-34.9, adult** A
Z68.35 **Body mass index [BMI] 35.0-35.9, adult** A
Z68.36 **Body mass index [BMI] 36.0-36.9, adult** A
Z68.37 **Body mass index [BMI] 37.0-37.9, adult** A
Z68.38 **Body mass index [BMI] 38.0-38.9, adult** A
Z68.39 **Body mass index [BMI] 39.0-39.9, adult** A

✓5th **Z68.4 Body mass index [BMI] 40 or greater, adult**

CC Excl: For CC codes in subcategory Z68.4: CC with 7th character A, unless otherwise noted: E65-E66.1, E66.8-E66.9, Z68.1-Z68.54

Z68.41 **Body mass index [BMI] 40.0-44.9, adult** CC A
Z68.42 **Body mass index [BMI] 45.0-49.9, adult** CC A
Z68.43 **Body mass index [BMI] 50-59.9, adult** CC A
Z68.44 **Body mass index [BMI] 60.0-69.9, adult** CC A
Z68.45 **Body mass index [BMI] 70 or greater, adult** CC A

✓5th **Z68.5 Body mass index [BMI] pediatric**

Z68.51 **Body mass index [BMI] pediatric, less than 5th percentile for age** P
Z68.52 **Body mass index [BMI] pediatric, 5th percentile to less than 85th percentile for age** P
Z68.53 **Body mass index [BMI] pediatric, 85th percentile to less than 95th percentile for age** P
Z68.54 **Body mass index [BMI] pediatric, greater than or equal to 95th percentile for age** P

Persons encountering health services in other circumstances (Z69-Z76)

✓4th **Z69 Encounter for mental health services for victim and perpetrator of abuse**
Counseling for victims and perpetrators of abuse

✓5th **Z69.0 Encounter for mental health services for child abuse problems**

✓6th **Z69.01 Encounter for mental health services for parental child abuse**

Z69.010 **Encounter for mental health services for victim of parental child abuse** P
Z69.011 **Encounter for mental health services for perpetrator of parental child abuse**
EXCLUDES 1 *encounter for mental health services for non-parental child abuse (Z69.02-)*

✓6th **Z69.02 Encounter for mental health services for non-parental child abuse**

Z69.020 **Encounter for mental health services for victim of non-parental child abuse** P
Z69.021 **Encounter for mental health services for perpetrator of non-parental child abuse**

✓5th **Z69.1 Encounter for mental health services for spousal or partner abuse problems**

Z69.11 **Encounter for mental health services for victim of spousal or partner abuse**
Z69.12 **Encounter for mental health services for perpetrator of spousal or partner abuse**

✓5th **Z69.8 Encounter for mental health services for victim or perpetrator of other abuse**

Z69.81 **Encounter for mental health services for victim of other abuse**
Encounter for rape victim counseling
Z69.82 **Encounter for mental health services for perpetrator of other abuse**

✓4th **Z70 Counseling related to sexual attitude, behavior and orientation**
Encounter for mental health services for sexual attitude, behavior and orientation
EXCLUDES 2 *contraceptive or procreative counseling (Z30-Z31)*

Z70.0 **Counseling related to sexual attitude**
Z70.1 **Counseling related to patient's sexual behavior and orientation**
Patient concerned regarding impotence
Patient concerned regarding non-responsiveness
Patient concerned regarding promiscuity
Patient concerned regarding sexual orientation
Z70.2 **Counseling related to sexual behavior and orientation of third party**
Advice sought regarding sexual behavior and orientation of child
Advice sought regarding sexual behavior and orientation of partner
Advice sought regarding sexual behavior and orientation of spouse
Z70.3 **Counseling related to combined concerns regarding sexual attitude, behavior and orientation**
Z70.8 **Other sex counseling**
Encounter for sex education
Z70.9 **Sex counseling, unspecified**

✓4th **Z71 Persons encountering health services for other counseling and medical advice, not elsewhere classified**
EXCLUDES 2 *contraceptive or procreation counseling (Z30-Z31)*
sex counseling (Z70.-)

Z71.0 **Person encountering health services to consult on behalf of another person**
Person encountering health services to seek advice or treatment for non-attending third party
EXCLUDES 2 *anxiety (normal) about sick person in family (Z63.7)*
expectant (adoptive) parent(s) pre-birth pediatrician visit (Z76.81)
Z71.1 **Person with feared health complaint in whom no diagnosis is made**
Person encountering health services with feared condition which was not demonstrated
Person encountering health services in which problem was normal state
"Worried well"
EXCLUDES 1 *medical observation for suspected diseases and conditions proven not to exist (Z03.-)*
Z71.2 **Person consulting for explanation of examination or test findings**
Z71.3 **Dietary counseling and surveillance**
Use additional code for any associated underlying medical condition
Use additional code to identify body mass index (BMI), if known (Z68.-)

✓5th **Z71.4 Alcohol abuse counseling and surveillance**
Use additional code for alcohol abuse or dependence (F10.-)

Z71.41 **Alcohol abuse counseling and surveillance of alcoholic**
Z71.42 **Counseling for family member of alcoholic**
Counseling for significant other, partner, or friend of alcoholic

✓5th **Z71.5 Drug abuse counseling and surveillance**
Use additional code for drug abuse or dependence (F11-F16, F18-F19)

Z71.51 **Drug abuse counseling and surveillance of drug abuser**
Z71.52 **Counseling for family member of drug abuser**
Counseling for significant other, partner, or friend of drug abuser

Z71.6 **Tobacco abuse counseling**
Use additional code for nicotine dependence (F17.-)
Z71.7 **Human immunodeficiency virus [HIV] counseling**

✓5th **Z71.8 Other specified counseling**
EXCLUDES 2 *counseling for contraception (Z30.0-)*
counseling for genetics (Z31.5)
counseling for procreative management (Z31.6-)

Z71.81 **Spiritual or religious counseling**
Z71.89 **Other specified counseling**

Z71.9 Counseling, unspecified
Encounter for medical advice NOS

Z72 Problems related to lifestyle
EXCLUDES 2 *problems related to life-management difficulty (Z73.-)*
problems related to socioeconomic and psychosocial circumstances (Z55-Z65)

Z72.0 Tobacco use
Tobacco use NOS
EXCLUDES 1 *history of tobacco dependence (Z87.891)*
nicotine dependence (F17.2-)
tobacco dependence (F17.2-)
tobacco use during pregnancy (O99.33-)

Z72.3 Lack of physical exercise

Z72.4 Inappropriate diet and eating habits
EXCLUDES 1 *behavioral eating disorders of infancy or childhood (F98.2- F98.3)*
eating disorders (F50.-)
lack of adequate food (Z59.4)
malnutrition and other nutritional deficiencies (E40-E64)

Z72.5 High risk sexual behavior
Promiscuity
EXCLUDES 1 *paraphilias (F65)*

Z72.51 High risk heterosexual behavior

Z72.52 High risk homosexual behavior

Z72.53 High risk bisexual behavior

Z72.6 Gambling and betting
EXCLUDES 1 *compulsive or pathological gambling (F63.0)*

Z72.8 Other problems related to lifestyle

Z72.81 Antisocial behavior
EXCLUDES 1 *conduct disorders (F91.-)*

Z72.810 Child and adolescent antisocial behavior P
Antisocial behavior (child) (adolescent) without manifest psychiatric disorder
Delinquency NOS
Group delinquency
Offenses in the context of gang membership
Stealing in company with others
Truancy from school

Z72.811 Adult antisocial behavior A
Adult antisocial behavior without manifest psychiatric disorder

Z72.82 Problems related to sleep

Z72.820 Sleep deprivation
Lack of adequate sleep
EXCLUDES 1 *insomnia (G47.0-)*

Z72.821 Inadequate sleep hygiene
Bad sleep habits
Irregular sleep habits
Unhealthy sleep wake schedule
EXCLUDES 1 *insomnia (F51.0-, G47.0-)*

Z72.89 Other problems related to lifestyle
Self-damaging behavior

Z72.9 Problem related to lifestyle, unspecified

Z73 Problems related to life management difficulty
EXCLUDES 2 *problems related to socioeconomic and psychosocial circumstances (Z55-Z65)*

Z73.0 Burn-out

Z73.1 Type A behavior pattern

Z73.2 Lack of relaxation and leisure

Z73.3 Stress, not elsewhere classified
Physical and mental strain NOS
EXCLUDES 1 *stress related to employment or unemployment (Z56.-)*

Z73.4 Inadequate social skills, not elsewhere classified

Z73.5 Social role conflict, not elsewhere classified

Z73.6 Limitation of activities due to disability
EXCLUDES 1 *care-provider dependency (Z74.-)*

Z73.8 Other problems related to life management difficulty

Z73.81 Behavioral insomnia of childhood

Z73.810 Behavioral insomnia of childhood, sleep-onset association type P

Z73.811 Behavioral insomnia of childhood, limit setting type P

Z73.812 Behavioral insomnia of childhood, combined type P

Z73.819 Behavioral insomnia of childhood, unspecified type P

Z73.82 Dual sensory impairment

Z73.89 Other problems related to life management difficulty

Z73.9 Problem related to life management difficulty, unspecified

Z74 Problems related to care provider dependency
EXCLUDES 2 *dependence on enabling machines or devices NEC (Z99.-)*

Z74.0 Reduced mobility

Z74.01 Bed confinement status
Bedridden

Z74.09 Other reduced mobility
Chair ridden
Reduced mobility NOS
EXCLUDES 2 *wheelchair dependence (Z99.3)*

Z74.1 Need for assistance with personal care

Z74.2 Need for assistance at home and no other household member able to render care

Z74.3 Need for continuous supervision

Z74.8 Other problems related to care provider dependency

Z74.9 Problem related to care provider dependency, unspecified

Z75 Problems related to medical facilities and other health care

Z75.0 Medical services not available in home
EXCLUDES 1 *no other household member able to render care (Z74.2)*

Z75.1 Person awaiting admission to adequate facility elsewhere

Z75.2 Other waiting period for investigation and treatment

Z75.3 Unavailability and inaccessibility of health-care facilities
EXCLUDES 1 *bed unavailable (Z75.1)*

Z75.4 Unavailability and inaccessibility of other helping agencies

Z75.5 Holiday relief care

Z75.8 Other problems related to medical facilities and other health care

Z75.9 Unspecified problem related to medical facilities and other health care

Z76 Persons encountering health services in other circumstances

Z76.0 Encounter for issue of repeat prescription
Encounter for issue of repeat prescription for appliance
Encounter for issue of repeat prescription for medicaments
Encounter for issue of repeat prescription for spectacles
EXCLUDES 2 *issue of medical certificate (Z02.7)*
repeat prescription for contraceptive (Z30.4-)

Z76.1 Encounter for health supervision and care of foundling

Z76.2 Encounter for health supervision and care of other healthy infant and child P
Encounter for medical or nursing care or supervision of healthy infant under circumstances such as adverse socioeconomic conditions at home
Encounter for medical or nursing care or supervision of healthy infant under circumstances such as awaiting foster or adoptive placement
Encounter for medical or nursing care or supervision of healthy infant under circumstances such as maternal illness
Encounter for medical or nursing care or supervision of healthy infant under circumstances such as number of children at home preventing or interfering with normal care

Z76.3 Healthy person accompanying sick person

Z76.4 Other boarder to healthcare facility
EXCLUDES 1 *homelessness (Z59.0)*

Z76.5 Malingerer [conscious simulation]
Person feigning illness (with obvious motivation)
EXCLUDES 1 *factitious disorder (F68.1-)*
peregrinating patient (F68.1-)

Z76.8 Persons encountering health services in other specified circumstances

Z76.81 Expectant parent(s) prebirth pediatrician visit
Pre-adoption pediatrician visit for adoptive parent(s)

Z76.82 Awaiting organ transplant status
Patient waiting for organ availability

Z76.89 Persons encountering health services in other specified circumstances
Persons encountering health services NOS
AHA: 2014, 2Q, 10

Persons with potential health hazards related to family and personal history and certain conditions influencing health status (Z77-Z99)

Code also any follow-up examination (Z08-Z09)

Z77 Other contact with and (suspected) exposures hazardous to health
INCLUDES contact with and (suspected) exposures to potential hazards to health
EXCLUDES 2 *contact with and (suspected) exposure to communicable diseases (Z20.-)*
exposure to (parental) (environmental) tobacco smoke in the perinatal period (P96.81)
newborn (suspected to be) affected by noxious substances transmitted via placenta or breast milk (P04.-)
occupational exposure to risk factors (Z57.-)
retained foreign body (Z18.-)
retained foreign body fully removed (Z87.821)
toxic effects of substances chiefly nonmedicinal as to source (T51-T65)

Z77.0 Contact with and (suspected) exposure to hazardous, chiefly nonmedicinal, chemicals

Z77.01 Contact with and (suspected) exposure to hazardous metals
Z77.010 Contact with and (suspected) exposure to arsenic
Z77.011 Contact with and (suspected) exposure to lead
Z77.012 Contact with and (suspected) exposure to uranium
EXCLUDES 1 *retained depleted uranium fragments (Z18.01)*
Z77.018 Contact with and (suspected) exposure to other hazardous metals
Contact with and (suspected) exposure to chromium compounds
Contact with and (suspected) exposure to nickel dust

Z77.02 Contact with and (suspected) exposure to hazardous aromatic compounds
Z77.020 Contact with and (suspected) exposure to aromatic amines
Z77.021 Contact with and (suspected) exposure to benzene
Z77.028 Contact with and (suspected) exposure to other hazardous aromatic compounds
Aromatic dyes NOS
Polycyclic aromatic hydrocarbons

Z77.09 Contact with and (suspected) exposure to other hazardous, chiefly nonmedicinal, chemicals
Z77.090 Contact with and (suspected) exposure to asbestos
Z77.098 Contact with and (suspected) exposure to other hazardous, chiefly nonmedicinal, chemicals
Dyes NOS

Z77.1 Contact with and (suspected) exposure to environmental pollution and hazards in the physical environment

Z77.11 Contact with and (suspected) exposure to environmental pollution
Z77.110 Contact with and (suspected) exposure to air pollution
Z77.111 Contact with and (suspected) exposure to water pollution
Z77.112 Contact with and (suspected) exposure to soil pollution
Z77.118 Contact with and (suspected) exposure to other environmental pollution

Z77.12 Contact with and (suspected) exposure to hazards in the physical environment
Z77.120 Contact with and (suspected) exposure to mold (toxic)
Z77.121 Contact with and (suspected) exposure to harmful algae and algae toxins
Contact with and (suspected) exposure to (harmful) algae bloom NOS
Contact with and (suspected) exposure to blue-green algae bloom
Contact with and (suspected) exposure to brown tide
Contact with and (suspected) exposure to cyanobacteria bloom
Contact with and (suspected) exposure to Florida red tide
Contact with and (suspected) exposure to pfiesteria piscicida
Contact with and (suspected) exposure to red tide
Z77.122 Contact with and (suspected) exposure to noise
Z77.123 Contact with and (suspected) exposure to radon and other naturally occuring radiation
EXCLUDES 2 *radiation exposure as the cause of a confirmed condition (W88-W90, X39.0-)*
radiation sickness NOS (T66)
Z77.128 Contact with and (suspected) exposure to other hazards in the physical environment

Z77.2 Contact with and (suspected) exposure to other hazardous substances
Z77.21 Contact with and (suspected) exposure to potentially hazardous body fluids
Z77.22 Contact with and (suspected) exposure to environmental tobacco smoke (acute) (chronic)
Exposure to second hand tobacco smoke (acute) (chronic)
Passive smoking (acute) (chronic)
EXCLUDES 1 *nicotine dependence (F17.-)*
tobacco use (Z72.0)
EXCLUDES 2 *occupational exposure to environmental tobacco smoke (Z57.31)*
Z77.29 Contact with and (suspected) exposure to other hazardous substances

Z77.9 Other contact with and (suspected) exposures hazardous to health

Z78 Other specified health status
EXCLUDES 2 *asymptomatic human immunodeficiency virus [HIV] infection status (Z21)*
postprocedural status (Z93- Z99)
sex reassignment status (Z87.890)

Z78.0 Asymptomatic menopausal state A ♀
Menopausal state NOS
Postmenopausal status NOS
EXCLUDES 2 *symptomatic menopausal state (N95.1)*

Z78.1 Physical restraint status
EXCLUDES 1 *physical restraint due to a procedure - omit code*

Z78.9 Other specified health status

Z79 Long term (current) drug therapy
INCLUDES long term (current) drug use for prophylactic purposes
Code also any therapeutic drug level monitoring (Z51.81)
EXCLUDES 2 *drug abuse and dependence (F11-F19)*
drug use complicating pregnancy, childbirth, and the puerperium (O99.32-)

Z79.0 Long term (current) use of anticoagulants and antithrombotics/antiplatelets
EXCLUDES 2 *long term (current) use of aspirin (Z79.82)*
Z79.01 Long term (current) use of anticoagulants
Z79.02 Long term (current) use of antithrombotics/antiplatelets

Z79.1 Long term (current) use of non-steroidal anti-inflammatories (NSAID)
EXCLUDES 2 *long term (current) use of aspirin (Z79.82)*

Z79.2 Long term (current) use of antibiotics

Z79.3 Long term (current) use of hormonal contraceptives
Long term (current) use of birth control pill or patch

Z79.4 Long term (current) use of insulin

Z79.5 Long term (current) use of steroids
Z79.51 Long term (current) use of inhaled steroids
Z79.52 Long term (current) use of systemic steroids

Z79.8 Other long term (current) drug therapy

Z79.81 Long term (current) use of agents affecting estrogen receptors and estrogen levels

Code first, if applicable:
- malignant neoplasm of breast (C50.-)
- malignant neoplasm of prostate (C61)

Use additional code, if applicable, to identify:
- estrogen receptor positive status (Z17.0)
- family history of breast cancer (Z80.3)
- genetic susceptibility to malignant neoplasm (cancer) (Z15.0-)
- personal history of breast cancer (Z85.3)
- personal history of prostate cancer (Z85.46)
- postmenopausal status (Z78.0)

EXCLUDES 1 *hormone replacement therapy (postmenopausal) (Z79.890)*

Z79.810 Long term (current) use of selective estrogen receptor modulators (SERMs)
- Long term (current) use of raloxifene (Evista)
- Long term (current) use of tamoxifen (Nolvadex)
- Long term (current) use of toremifene (Fareston)

Z79.811 Long term (current) use of aromatase inhibitors
- Long term (current) use of anastrozole (Arimidex)
- Long term (current) use of exemestane (Aromasin)
- Long term (current) use of letrozole (Femara)

Z79.818 Long term (current) use of other agents affecting estrogen receptors and estrogen levels
- Long term (current) use of estrogen receptor downregulators
- Long term (current) use of fulvestrant (Faslodex)
- Long term (current) use of gonadotropin-releasing hormone (GnRH) agonist
- Long term (current) use of goserelin acetate (Zoladex)
- Long term (current) use of leuprolide acetate (leuprorelin) (Lupron)
- Long term (current) use of megestrol acetate (Megace)

Z79.82 Long term (current) use of aspirin

Z79.83 Long term (current) use of bisphosphonates

Z79.89 Other long term (current) drug therapy

Z79.890 Hormone replacement therapy (postmenopausal) ♀

Z79.891 Long term (current) use of opiate analgesic
- Long term (current) use of methadone for pain management

EXCLUDES 1 *methodone use NOS (F11.2-)*
use of methodone for treatment of heroin addiction (F11.2-)

Z79.899 Other long term (current) drug therapy

Z80 Family history of primary malignant neoplasm

Z80.0 Family history of malignant neoplasm of digestive organs
Conditions classifiable to C15-C26

Z80.1 Family history of malignant neoplasm of trachea, bronchus and lung
Conditions classifiable to C33-C34

Z80.2 Family history of malignant neoplasm of other respiratory and intrathoracic organs
Conditions classifiable to C30-C32, C37-C39

Z80.3 Family history of malignant neoplasm of breast
Conditions classifiable to C50-

Z80.4 Family history of malignant neoplasm of genital organs
Conditions classifiable to C51-C63

Z80.41 Family history of malignant neoplasm of ovary ♀

Z80.42 Family history of malignant neoplasm of prostate ♂

Z80.43 Family history of malignant neoplasm of testis ♂

Z80.49 Family history of malignant neoplasm of other genital organs

Z80.5 Family history of malignant neoplasm of urinary tract
Conditions classifiable to C64-C68

Z80.51 Family history of malignant neoplasm of kidney

Z80.52 Family history of malignant neoplasm of bladder

Z80.59 Family history of malignant neoplasm of other urinary tract organ

Z80.6 Family history of leukemia
Conditions classifiable to C91-C95

Z80.7 Family history of other malignant neoplasms of lymphoid, hematopoietic and related tissues
Conditions classifiable to C81-C90, C96-

Z80.8 Family history of malignant neoplasm of other organs or systems
Conditions classifiable to C00-C14, C40-C49, C69-C79

Z80.9 Family history of malignant neoplasm, unspecified
Conditions classifiable to C80.1

Z81 Family history of mental and behavioral disorders

Z81.0 Family history of intellectual disabilities
Conditions classifiable to F70-F79

Z81.1 Family history of alcohol abuse and dependence
Conditions classifiable to F10-

Z81.2 Family history of tobacco abuse and dependence
Conditions classifiable to F17-

Z81.3 Family history of other psychoactive substance abuse and dependence
Conditions classifiable to F11-F16, F18-F19

Z81.4 Family history of other substance abuse and dependence
Conditions classifiable to F55

Z81.8 Family history of other mental and behavioral disorders
Conditions classifiable elsewhere in F01-F99

Z82 Family history of certain disabilities and chronic diseases (leading to disablement)

Z82.0 Family history of epilepsy and other diseases of the nervous system
Conditions classifiable to G00-G99

Z82.1 Family history of blindness and visual loss
Conditions classifiable to H54-

Z82.2 Family history of deafness and hearing loss
Conditions classifiable to H90-H91

Z82.3 Family history of stroke
Conditions classifiable to I60-I64

Z82.4 Family history of ischemic heart disease and other diseases of the circulatory system
Conditions classifiable to I00-I52, I65-I99

Z82.41 Family history of sudden cardiac death

Z82.49 Family history of ischemic heart disease and other diseases of the circulatory system

Z82.5 Family history of asthma and other chronic lower respiratory diseases
Conditions classifiable to J40-J47

EXCLUDES 2 *family history of other diseases of the respiratory system (Z83.6)*

Z82.6 Family history of arthritis and other diseases of the musculoskeletal system and connective tissue
Conditions classifiable to M00-M99

Z82.61 Family history of arthritis

Z82.62 Family history of osteoporosis

Z82.69 Family history of other diseases of the musculoskeletal system and connective tissue

Z82.7 Family history of congenital malformations, deformations and chromosomal abnormalities
Conditions classifiable to Q00-Q99

Z82.71 Family history of polycystic kidney

Z82.79 Family history of other congenital malformations, deformations and chromosomal abnormalities

Z82.8 Family history of other disabilities and chronic diseases leading to disablement, not elsewhere classified

Z83 Family history of other specific disorders

EXCLUDES 2 *contact with and (suspected) exposure to communicable disease in the family (Z20.-)*

Z83.0 Family history of human immunodeficiency virus [HIV] disease
Conditions classifiable to B20

Z83.1 Family history of other infectious and parasitic diseases
Conditions classifiable to A00-B19, B25-B94, B99

Z83.2 Family history of diseases of the blood and blood-forming organs and certain disorders involving the immune mechanism
Conditions classifiable to D50-D89

Z83.3 **Family history of diabetes mellitus**
Conditions classifiable to EØ8-E13

✓5th **Z83.4** **Family history of other endocrine, nutritional and metabolic diseases**
Conditions classifiable to EØØ-EØ7, E15-E88

Z83.41 **Family history of multiple endocrine neoplasia [MEN] syndrome**

Z83.49 **Family history of other endocrine, nutritional and metabolic diseases**

✓5th **Z83.5** **Family history of eye and ear disorders**

✓6th **Z83.51** **Family history of eye disorders**
Conditions classifiable to HØØ-H53, H55-H59
EXCLUDES 2 *family history of blindness and visual loss (Z82.1)*

Z83.511 **Family history of glaucoma**

Z83.518 **Family history of other specified eye disorder**

Z83.52 **Family history of ear disorders**
Conditions classifiable to H6Ø-H83, H92-H95
EXCLUDES 2 *family history of deafness and hearing loss (Z82.2)*

Z83.6 **Family history of other diseases of the respiratory system**
Conditions classifiable to JØØ-J39, J6Ø-J99
EXCLUDES 2 *family history of asthma and other chronic lower respiratory diseases (Z82.5)*

✓5th **Z83.7** **Family history of diseases of the digestive system**
Conditions classifiable to KØØ-K93

Z83.71 **Family history of colonic polyps**
EXCLUDES 1 *family history of malignant neoplasm of digestive organs (Z8Ø.Ø)*

Z83.79 **Family history of other diseases of the digestive system**

✓4th **Z84** **Family history of other conditions**

Z84.Ø **Family history of diseases of the skin and subcutaneous tissue**
Conditions classifiable to LØØ-L99

Z84.1 **Family history of disorders of kidney and ureter**
Conditions classifiable to NØØ-N29

Z84.2 **Family history of other diseases of the genitourinary system**
Conditions classifiable to N3Ø-N99

Z84.3 **Family history of consanguinity**

✓5th **Z84.8** **Family history of other specified conditions**

Z84.81 **Family history of carrier of genetic disease**

Z84.89 **Family history of other specified conditions**

✓4th **Z85** **Personal history of malignant neoplasm**
Code first any follow-up examination after treatment of malignant neoplasm (ZØ8)
Use additional code to identify:
alcohol use and dependence (F1Ø.-)
exposure to environmental tobacco smoke (Z77.22)
history of tobacco use (Z87.891)
occupational exposure to environmental tobacco smoke (Z57.31)
tobacco dependence (F17.-)
tobacco use (Z72.Ø)
EXCLUDES 2 *personal history of benign neoplasm (Z86.Ø1-)*
personal history of carcinoma-in-situ (Z86.ØØ-)

✓5th **Z85.Ø** **Personal history of malignant neoplasm of digestive organs**

Z85.ØØ **Personal history of malignant neoplasm of unspecified digestive organ**

Z85.Ø1 **Personal history of malignant neoplasm of esophagus**
Conditions classifiable to C15

✓6th **Z85.Ø2** **Personal history of malignant neoplasm of stomach**

Z85.Ø2Ø **Personal history of malignant carcinoid tumor of stomach**
Conditions classifiable to C7A.Ø92

Z85.Ø28 **Personal history of other malignant neoplasm of stomach**
Conditions classifiable to C16

✓6th **Z85.Ø3** **Personal history of malignant neoplasm of large intestine**

Z85.Ø3Ø **Personal history of malignant carcinoid tumor of large intestine**
Conditions classifiable to C7A.Ø22-C7A.Ø25, C7A.Ø29

Z85.Ø38 **Personal history of other malignant neoplasm of large intestine**
Conditions classifiable to C18

✓6th **Z85.Ø4** **Personal history of malignant neoplasm of rectum, rectosigmoid junction, and anus**

Z85.Ø4Ø **Personal history of malignant carcinoid tumor of rectum**
Conditions classifiable to C7A.Ø26

Z85.Ø48 **Personal history of other malignant neoplasm of rectum, rectosigmoid junction, and anus**
Conditions classifiable to C19-C21

Z85.Ø5 **Personal history of malignant neoplasm of liver**
Conditions classifiable to C22

✓6th **Z85.Ø6** **Personal history of malignant neoplasm of small intestine**

Z85.Ø6Ø **Personal history of malignant carcinoid tumor of small intestine**
Conditions classifiable to C7A.Ø1-

Z85.Ø68 **Personal history of other malignant neoplasm of small intestine**
Conditions classifiable to C17

Z85.Ø7 **Personal history of malignant neoplasm of pancreas**
Conditions classifiable to C25

Z85.Ø9 **Personal history of malignant neoplasm of other digestive organs**

✓5th **Z85.1** **Personal history of malignant neoplasm of trachea, bronchus and lung**

✓6th **Z85.11** **Personal history of malignant neoplasm of bronchus and lung**

Z85.11Ø **Personal history of malignant carcinoid tumor of bronchus and lung**
Conditions classifiable to C7A.Ø9Ø

Z85.118 **Personal history of other malignant neoplasm of bronchus and lung**
Conditions classifiable to C34

Z85.12 **Personal history of malignant neoplasm of trachea**
Conditions classifiable to C33

✓5th **Z85.2** **Personal history of malignant neoplasm of other respiratory and intrathoracic organs**

Z85.2Ø **Personal history of malignant neoplasm of unspecified respiratory organ**

Z85.21 **Personal history of malignant neoplasm of larynx**
Conditions classifiable to C32

Z85.22 **Personal history of malignant neoplasm of nasal cavities, middle ear, and accessory sinuses**
Conditions classifiable to C3Ø-C31

✓6th **Z85.23** **Personal history of malignant neoplasm of thymus**

Z85.23Ø **Personal history of malignant carcinoid tumor of thymus**
Conditions classifiable to C7A.Ø91

Z85.238 **Personal history of other malignant neoplasm of thymus**
Conditions classifiable to C37

Z85.29 **Personal history of malignant neoplasm of other respiratory and intrathoracic organs**

Z85.3 **Personal history of malignant neoplasm of breast**
Conditions classifiable to C5Ø-

✓5th **Z85.4** **Personal history of malignant neoplasm of genital organs**
Conditions classifiable to C51-C63

Z85.4Ø **Personal history of malignant neoplasm of unspecified female genital organ** ♀

Z85.41 **Personal history of malignant neoplasm of cervix uteri** ♀

Z85.42 **Personal history of malignant neoplasm of other parts of uterus** ♀

Z85.43 **Personal history of malignant neoplasm of ovary** ♀

Z85.44 **Personal history of malignant neoplasm of other female genital organs** ♀

Z85.45 **Personal history of malignant neoplasm of unspecified male genital organ** ♂

Z85.46 **Personal history of malignant neoplasm of prostate** ♂

Z85.47 **Personal history of malignant neoplasm of testis** ♂

Z85.48 **Personal history of malignant neoplasm of epididymis** ♂

Z85.49 **Personal history of malignant neoplasm of other male genital organs** ♂

✓5th **Z85.5 Personal history of malignant neoplasm of urinary tract**
Conditions classifiable to C64-C68

Z85.50 Personal history of malignant neoplasm of unspecified urinary tract organ

Z85.51 Personal history of malignant neoplasm of bladder

✓6th **Z85.52 Personal history of malignant neoplasm of kidney**
EXCLUDES 1 *personal history of malignant neoplasm of renal pelvis (Z85.53)*

Z85.520 Personal history of malignant carcinoid tumor of kidney
Conditions classifiable to C7A.093

Z85.528 Personal history of other malignant neoplasm of kidney
Conditions classifiable to C64

Z85.53 Personal history of malignant neoplasm of renal pelvis

Z85.54 Personal history of malignant neoplasm of ureter

Z85.59 Personal history of malignant neoplasm of other urinary tract organ

Z85.6 Personal history of leukemia
Conditions classifiable to C91-C95
EXCLUDES 1 *leukemia in remission C91.0-C95.9 with 5th character 1*

✓5th **Z85.7 Personal history of other malignant neoplasms of lymphoid, hematopoietic and related tissues**

Z85.71 Personal history of Hodgkin lymphoma
Conditions classifiable to C81

Z85.72 Personal history of non-Hodgkin lymphomas
Conditions classifiable to C82-C85

Z85.79 Personal history of other malignant neoplasms of lymphoid, hematopoietic and related tissues
Conditions classifiable to C88-C90, C96
EXCLUDES 1 *multiple myeloma in remission (C90.01)*
plasma cell leukemia in remission (C90.11)
plasmacytoma in remission (C90.21)

✓5th **Z85.8 Personal history of malignant neoplasms of other organs and systems**
Conditions classifiable to C00-C14, C40-C49, C69-C79, C7A.098

✓6th **Z85.81 Personal history of malignant neoplasm of lip, oral cavity, and pharynx**

Z85.810 Personal history of malignant neoplasm of tongue

Z85.818 Personal history of malignant neoplasm of other sites of lip, oral cavity, and pharynx

Z85.819 Personal history of malignant neoplasm of unspecified site of lip, oral cavity, and pharynx

✓6th **Z85.82 Personal history of malignant neoplasm of skin**

Z85.820 Personal history of malignant melanoma of skin
Conditions classifiable to C43

Z85.821 Personal history of Merkel cell carcinoma
Conditions classifiable to C4A

Z85.828 Personal history of other malignant neoplasm of skin
Conditions classifiable to C44

✓6th **Z85.83 Personal history of malignant neoplasm of bone and soft tissue**

Z85.830 Personal history of malignant neoplasm of bone

Z85.831 Personal history of malignant neoplasm of soft tissue
EXCLUDES 2 *personal history of malignant neoplasm of skin (Z85.82-)*

✓6th **Z85.84 Personal history of malignant neoplasm of eye and nervous tissue**

Z85.840 Personal history of malignant neoplasm of eye

Z85.841 Personal history of malignant neoplasm of brain

Z85.848 Personal history of malignant neoplasm of other parts of nervous tissue

✓6th **Z85.85 Personal history of malignant neoplasm of endocrine glands**

Z85.850 Personal history of malignant neoplasm of thyroid

Z85.858 Personal history of malignant neoplasm of other endocrine glands

Z85.89 Personal history of malignant neoplasm of other organs and systems

Z85.9 Personal history of malignant neoplasm, unspecified
Conditions classifiable to C7A.00, C80.1

✓4th **Z86 Personal history of certain other diseases**
Code first any follow-up examination after treatment (Z09)

✓5th **Z86.0 Personal history of in-situ and benign neoplasms and neoplasms of uncertain behavior**
EXCLUDES 2 *personal history of malignant neoplasms (Z85.-)*

✓6th **Z86.00 Personal history of in-situ neoplasm**

Z86.000 Personal history of in-situ neoplasm of breast

Z86.001 Personal history of in-situ neoplasm of cervix uteri ♀

Z86.008 Personal history of in-situ neoplasm of other site

✓6th **Z86.01 Personal history of benign neoplasm**

Z86.010 Personal history of colonic polyps

Z86.011 Personal history of benign neoplasm of the brain

Z86.012 Personal history of benign carcinoid tumor

Z86.018 Personal history of other benign neoplasm

Z86.03 Personal history of neoplasm of uncertain behavior

✓5th **Z86.1 Personal history of infectious and parasitic diseases**
Conditions classifiable to A00-B89, B99
EXCLUDES 1 *personal history of infectious diseases specific to a body system*
sequelae of infectious and parasitic diseases (B90-B94)

Z86.11 Personal history of tuberculosis

Z86.12 Personal history of poliomyelitis

Z86.13 Personal history of malaria

Z86.14 Personal history of Methicillin resistant Staphylococcus aureus infection
Personal history of MRSA infection

Z86.19 Personal history of other infectious and parasitic diseases

Z86.2 Personal history of diseases of the blood and blood-forming organs and certain disorders involving the immune mechanism
Conditions classifiable to D50-D89

✓5th **Z86.3 Personal history of endocrine, nutritional and metabolic diseases**
Conditions classifiable to E00-E88

Z86.31 Personal history of diabetic foot ulcer
EXCLUDES 2 *current diabetic foot ulcer (E08.621, E09.621, E10.621, E11.621, E13.621)*

Z86.32 Personal history of gestational diabetes ♀
Personal history of conditions classifiable to O24.4-
EXCLUDES 1 *gestational diabetes mellitus in current pregnancy (O24.4-)*

Z86.39 Personal history of other endocrine, nutritional and metabolic disease

✓5th **Z86.5 Personal history of mental and behavioral disorders**
Conditions classifiable to F40-F59

Z86.51 Personal history of combat and operational stress reaction A

Z86.59 Personal history of other mental and behavioral disorders

✓5th **Z86.6 Personal history of diseases of the nervous system and sense organs**
Conditions classifiable to G00-G99, H00-H95
EXCLUDES 2 *personal history of anaphylactic shock (Z87.892)*

Z86.61 Personal history of infections of the central nervous system
Personal history of encephalitis
Personal history of meningitis

Z86.69 Personal history of other diseases of the nervous system and sense organs

✓5th **Z86.7 Personal history of diseases of the circulatory system**
Conditions classifiable to IØØ-I99
EXCLUDES 2 *old myocardial infarction (I25.2)*
personal history of anaphylactic shock (Z87.892)
postmyocardial infarction syndrome (I24.1)

✓6th **Z86.71 Personal history of venous thrombosis and embolism**
Z86.711 Personal history of pulmonary embolism
Z86.718 Personal history of other venous thrombosis and embolism

Z86.72 Personal history of thrombophlebitis

Z86.73 Personal history of transient ischemic attack (TIA), and cerebral infarction without residual deficits
Personal history of prolonged reversible ischemic neurological deficit (PRIND)
Personal history of stroke NOS without residual deficits
EXCLUDES 1 *personal history of traumatic brain injury (Z87.82Ø)*
sequelae of cerebrovascular disease (I69.-)
AHA: 2Ø12, 4Q, 92

Z86.74 Personal history of sudden cardiac arrest
Personal history of sudden cardiac death successfully resuscitated

Z86.79 Personal history of other diseases of the circulatory system

✓4th **Z87 Personal history of other diseases and conditions**
Code first any follow-up examination after treatment (ZØ9)

✓5th **Z87.Ø Personal history of diseases of the respiratory system**
Conditions classifiable to JØØ-J99
Z87.Ø1 Personal history of pneumonia (recurrent)
Z87.Ø9 Personal history of other diseases of the respiratory system

✓5th **Z87.1 Personal history of diseases of the digestive system**
Conditions classifiable to KØØ-K93
Z87.11 Personal history of peptic ulcer disease
Z87.19 Personal history of other diseases of the digestive system

Z87.2 Personal history of diseases of the skin and subcutaneous tissue
Conditions classifiable to LØØ-L99
EXCLUDES 2 *personal history of diabetic foot ulcer (Z86.31)*

✓5th **Z87.3 Personal history of diseases of the musculoskeletal system and connective tissue**
Conditions classifiable to MØØ-M99
EXCLUDES 2 *personal history of (healed) traumatic fracture (Z87.81)*

✓6th **Z87.31 Personal history of (healed) nontraumatic fracture**
Z87.31Ø Personal history of (healed) osteoporosis fracture
Personal history of (healed) fragility fracture
Personal history of (healed) collapsed vertebra due to osteoporosis
Z87.311 Personal history of (healed) other pathological fracture
Personal history of (healed) collapsed vertebra NOS
EXCLUDES 2 *personal history of osteoporosis fracture (Z87.31Ø)*
Z87.312 Personal history of (healed) stress fracture
Personal history of (healed) fatigue fracture

Z87.39 Personal history of other diseases of the musculoskeletal system and connective tissue

✓5th **Z87.4 Personal history of diseases of genitourinary system**
Conditions classifiable to NØØ-N99

✓6th **Z87.41 Personal history of dysplasia of the female genital tract**
EXCLUDES 1 *personal history of malignant neoplasm of female genital tract (Z85.4Ø-Z85.44)*
Z87.41Ø Personal history of cervical dysplasia ♀
Z87.411 Personal history of vaginal dysplasia ♀
Z87.412 Personal history of vulvar dysplasia ♀

Z87.42 Personal history of other diseases of the female genital tract ♀

✓6th **Z87.43 Personal history of diseases of the male genital organs**
Z87.43Ø Personal history of prostatic dysplasia
EXCLUDES 1 *personal history of malignant neoplasm of prostate (Z85.46)*
Z87.438 Personal history of other diseases of male genital organs

✓6th **Z87.44 Personal history of diseases of the urinary system**
EXCLUDES 1 *personal history of malignant neoplasm of cervix uteri (Z85.41)*
Z87.44Ø Personal history of urinary (tract) infections
Z87.441 Personal history of nephrotic syndrome
Z87.442 Personal history of urinary calculi
Personal history of kidney stones
Z87.448 Personal history of other diseases of urinary system

✓5th **Z87.5 Personal history of complications of pregnancy, childbirth and the puerperium**
Conditions classifiable to OØØ-O9A
EXCLUDES 2 *recurrent pregnancy loss (N96)*
Z87.51 Personal history of pre-term labor ♀
EXCLUDES 1 *current pregnancy with history of pre-term labor (OØ9.21-)*
Z87.59 Personal history of other complications of pregnancy, childbirth and the puerperium ♀
Personal history of trophoblastic disease

✓5th **Z87.7 Personal history of (corrected) congenital malformations**
Conditions classifiable to QØØ-Q89 that have been repaired or corrected
EXCLUDES 1 *congenital malformations that have been partially corrected or repaired but which still require medical treatment—code to condition*
EXCLUDES 2 *other postprocedural states (Z98.-)*
personal history of medical treatment (Z92.-)
presence of cardiac and vascular implants and grafts (Z95.-)
presence of other devices (Z97.-)
presence of other functional implants (Z96.-)
transplanted organ and tissue status (Z94.-)

✓6th **Z87.71 Personal history of (corrected) congenital malformations of genitourinary system**
Z87.71Ø Personal history of (corrected) hypospadias ♂
Z87.718 Personal history of other specified (corrected) congenital malformations of genitourinary system

✓6th **Z87.72 Personal history of (corrected) congenital malformations of nervous system and sense organs**
Z87.72Ø Personal history of (corrected) congenital malformations of eye
Z87.721 Personal history of (corrected) congenital malformations of ear
Z87.728 Personal history of other specified (corrected) congenital malformations of nervous system and sense organs

✓6th **Z87.73 Personal history of (corrected) congenital malformations of digestive system**
Z87.73Ø Personal history of (corrected) cleft lip and palate
Z87.738 Personal history of other specified (corrected) congenital malformations of digestive system

Z87.74 Personal history of (corrected) congenital malformations of heart and circulatory system

Z87.75 Personal history of (corrected) congenital malformations of respiratory system

Z87.76 Personal history of (corrected) congenital malformations of integument, limbs and musculoskeletal system

✓6th **Z87.79 Personal history of other (corrected) congenital malformations**
Z87.79Ø Personal history of (corrected) congenital malformations of face and neck
Z87.798 Personal history of other (corrected) congenital malformations

5th Z87.8 **Personal history of other specified conditions**
EXCLUDES 2 *personal history of self harm (Z91.5)*
Z87.81 **Personal history of (healed) traumatic fracture**
EXCLUDES 2 *personal history of (healed) nontraumatic fracture (Z87.31-)*
6th Z87.82 **Personal history of other (healed) physical injury and trauma**
Conditions classifiable to S00-T88, except traumatic fractures
Z87.820 **Personal history of traumatic brain injury**
EXCLUDES 1 *personal history of transient ischemic attack (TIA), and cerebral infarction without residual deficits (Z86.73)*
Z87.821 **Personal history of retained foreign body fully removed**
Z87.828 **Personal history of other (healed) physical injury and trauma**
6th Z87.89 **Personal history of other specified conditions**
Z87.890 **Personal history of sex reassignment**
Z87.891 **Personal history of nicotine dependence**
EXCLUDES 1 *current nicotine dependence (F17.2-)*
Z87.892 **Personal history of anaphylaxis**
Code also allergy status such as:
allergy status to drugs, medicaments and biological substances (Z88.-)
allergy status, other than to drugs and biological substances (Z91.0-)
Z87.898 **Personal history of other specified conditions**
AHA: 2013, 1Q, 21

4th Z88 **Allergy status to drugs, medicaments and biological substances**
EXCLUDES 2 *allergy status, other than to drugs and biological substances (Z91.0-)*
Z88.0 **Allergy status to penicillin**
Z88.1 **Allergy status to other antibiotic agents status**
Z88.2 **Allergy status to sulfonamides status**
Z88.3 **Allergy status to other anti-infective agents status**
Z88.4 **Allergy status to anesthetic agent status**
Z88.5 **Allergy status to narcotic agent status**
Z88.6 **Allergy status to analgesic agent status**
Z88.7 **Allergy status to serum and vaccine status**
Z88.8 **Allergy status to other drugs, medicaments and biological substances status**
Z88.9 **Allergy status to unspecified drugs, medicaments and biological substances status**

4th Z89 **Acquired absence of limb**
INCLUDES amputation status
postprocedural loss of limb
post-traumatic loss of limb
EXCLUDES 1 *acquired deformities of limbs (M20-M21)*
congenital absence of limbs (Q71-Q73)
5th Z89.0 **Acquired absence of thumb and other finger(s)**
6th Z89.01 **Acquired absence of thumb**
Z89.011 **Acquired absence of right thumb**
Z89.012 **Acquired absence of left thumb**
Z89.019 **Acquired absence of unspecified thumb**
6th Z89.02 **Acquired absence of other finger(s)**
EXCLUDES 2 *acquired absence of thumb (Z89.01-)*
Z89.021 **Acquired absence of right finger(s)**
Z89.022 **Acquired absence of left finger(s)**
Z89.029 **Acquired absence of unspecified finger(s)**
5th Z89.1 **Acquired absence of hand and wrist**
6th Z89.11 **Acquired absence of hand**
Z89.111 **Acquired absence of right hand**
Z89.112 **Acquired absence of left hand**
Z89.119 **Acquired absence of unspecified hand**
6th Z89.12 **Acquired absence of wrist**
Disarticulation at wrist
Z89.121 **Acquired absence of right wrist**
Z89.122 **Acquired absence of left wrist**
Z89.129 **Acquired absence of unspecified wrist**
5th Z89.2 **Acquired absence of upper limb above wrist**
6th Z89.20 **Acquired absence of upper limb, unspecified level**
Z89.201 **Acquired absence of right upper limb, unspecified level**
Z89.202 **Acquired absence of left upper limb, unspecified level**
Z89.209 **Acquired absence of unspecified upper limb, unspecified level**
Acquired absence of arm NOS
6th Z89.21 **Acquired absence of upper limb below elbow**
Z89.211 **Acquired absence of right upper limb below elbow**
Z89.212 **Acquired absence of left upper limb below elbow**
Z89.219 **Acquired absence of unspecified upper limb below elbow**
6th Z89.22 **Acquired absence of upper limb above elbow**
Disarticulation at elbow
Z89.221 **Acquired absence of right upper limb above elbow**
Z89.222 **Acquired absence of left upper limb above elbow**
Z89.229 **Acquired absence of unspecified upper limb above elbow**
6th Z89.23 **Acquired absence of shoulder**
Acquired absence of shoulder joint following explantation of shoulder joint prosthesis, with or without presence of antibiotic-impregnated cement spacer
Z89.231 **Acquired absence of right shoulder**
Z89.232 **Acquired absence of left shoulder**
Z89.239 **Acquired absence of unspecified shoulder**
5th Z89.4 **Acquired absence of toe(s), foot, and ankle**
6th Z89.41 **Acquired absence of great toe**
Z89.411 **Acquired absence of right great toe**
Z89.412 **Acquired absence of left great toe**
Z89.419 **Acquired absence of unspecified great toe**
6th Z89.42 **Acquired absence of other toe(s)**
EXCLUDES 2 *acquired absence of great toe (Z89.41-)*
Z89.421 **Acquired absence of other right toe(s)**
Z89.422 **Acquired absence of other left toe(s)**
Z89.429 **Acquired absence of other toe(s), unspecified side**
6th Z89.43 **Acquired absence of foot**
Z89.431 **Acquired absence of right foot**
Z89.432 **Acquired absence of left foot**
Z89.439 **Acquired absence of unspecified foot**
6th Z89.44 **Acquired absence of ankle**
Disarticulation of ankle
Z89.441 **Acquired absence of right ankle**
Z89.442 **Acquired absence of left ankle**
Z89.449 **Acquired absence of unspecified ankle**
5th Z89.5 **Acquired absence of leg below knee**
6th Z89.51 **Acquired absence of leg below knee**
Z89.511 **Acquired absence of right leg below knee**
Z89.512 **Acquired absence of left leg below knee**
Z89.519 **Acquired absence of unspecified leg below knee**
6th Z89.52 **Acquired absence of knee**
Acquired absence of knee joint following explantation of knee joint prosthesis, with or without presence of antibiotic-impregnated cement spacer
Z89.521 **Acquired absence of right knee**
Z89.522 **Acquired absence of left knee**
Z89.529 **Acquired absence of unspecified knee**
5th Z89.6 **Acquired absence of leg above knee**
6th Z89.61 **Acquired absence of leg above knee**
Acquired absence of leg NOS
Disarticulation at knee
Z89.611 **Acquired absence of right leg above knee**
Z89.612 **Acquired absence of left leg above knee**
Z89.619 **Acquired absence of unspecified leg above knee**

✓6th **Z89.62 Acquired absence of hip**
Acquired absence of hip joint following explantation of hip joint prosthesis, with or without presence of antibiotic-impregnated cement spacer
Disarticulation at hip
Z89.621 Acquired absence of right hip joint
Z89.622 Acquired absence of left hip joint
Z89.629 Acquired absence of unspecified hip joint
Z89.9 Acquired absence of limb, unspecified

✓4th **Z90 Acquired absence of organs, not elsewhere classified**
INCLUDES postprocedural or post-traumatic loss of body part NEC
EXCLUDES 1 *congenital absence—see Alphabetical Index*
EXCLUDES 2 *postprocedural absence of endocrine glands (E89.-)*

✓5th **Z90.0 Acquired absence of part of head and neck**
Z90.01 Acquired absence of eye
Z90.02 Acquired absence of larynx
Z90.09 Acquired absence of other part of head and neck
Acquired absence of nose
EXCLUDES 2 *teeth (K08.1)*

✓5th **Z90.1 Acquired absence of breast and nipple**
Z90.10 Acquired absence of unspecified breast and nipple
Z90.11 Acquired absence of right breast and nipple
Z90.12 Acquired absence of left breast and nipple
Z90.13 Acquired absence of bilateral breasts and nipples
Z90.2 Acquired absence of lung [part of]
Z90.3 Acquired absence of stomach [part of]

✓5th **Z90.4 Acquired absence of other specified parts of digestive tract**
✓6th **Z90.41 Acquired absence of pancreas**
Use additional code to identify any associated:
insulin use (Z79.4)
diabetes mellitus, postpancreatectomy (E13.-)
Z90.410 Acquired total absence of pancreas
Acquired absence of pancreas NOS
Z90.411 Acquired partial absence of pancreas
Z90.49 Acquired absence of other specified parts of digestive tract
Z90.5 Acquired absence of kidney
Z90.6 Acquired absence of other parts of urinary tract
Acquired absence of bladder

✓5th **Z90.7 Acquired absence of genital organ(s)**
EXCLUDES 1 *personal history of sex reassignment (Z87.890)*
EXCLUDES 2 *female genital mutilation status (N90.81-)*
✓6th **Z90.71 Acquired absence of cervix and uterus**
Z90.710 Acquired absence of both cervix and uterus ♀
Acquired absence of uterus NOS
Status post total hysterectomy
Z90.711 Acquired absence of uterus with remaining cervical stump ♀
Status post partial hysterectomy with remaining cervical stump
Z90.712 Acquired absence of cervix with remaining uterus ♀
✓6th **Z90.72 Acquired absence of ovaries**
Z90.721 Acquired absence of ovaries, unilateral ♀
Z90.722 Acquired absence of ovaries, bilateral ♀
Z90.79 Acquired absence of other genital organ(s)

✓5th **Z90.8 Acquired absence of other organs**
Z90.81 Acquired absence of spleen
Z90.89 Acquired absence of other organs

✓4th **Z91 Personal risk factors, not elsewhere classified**
EXCLUDES 2 *contact with and (suspected) exposures hazardous to health (Z77.-)*
exposure to pollution and other problems related to physical environment (Z77.1-)
personal history of physical injury and trauma (Z87.81, Z87.82-)
occupational exposure to risk factors (Z57.-)

✓5th **Z91.0 Allergy status, other than to drugs and biological substances**
EXCLUDES 2 *allergy status to drugs, medicaments, and biological substances (Z88.-)*
✓6th **Z91.01 Food allergy status**
EXCLUDES 2 *food additives allergy status (Z91.02)*
Z91.010 Allergy to peanuts
Z91.011 Allergy to milk products
EXCLUDES 1 *lactose intolerance (E73.-)*
Z91.012 Allergy to eggs
Z91.013 Allergy to seafood
Allergy to shellfish
Allergy to octopus or squid ink
Z91.018 Allergy to other foods
Allergy to nuts other than peanuts
Z91.02 Food additives allergy status
✓6th **Z91.03 Insect allergy status**
Z91.030 Bee allergy status
Z91.038 Other insect allergy status
✓6th **Z91.04 Nonmedicinal substance allergy status**
Z91.040 Latex allergy status
Latex sensitivity status
Z91.041 Radiographic dye allergy status
Allergy status to contrast media used for diagnostic X-ray procedure
Z91.048 Other nonmedicinal substance allergy status
Z91.09 Other allergy status, other than to drugs and biological substances

✓5th **Z91.1 Patient's noncompliance with medical treatment and regimen**
Z91.11 Patient's noncompliance with dietary regimen
✓6th **Z91.12 Patient's intentional underdosing of medication regimen**
Code first underdosing of medication (T36-T50) with fifth or sixth character 6
EXCLUDES 1 *adverse effect of prescribed drug taken as directed—code to adverse effect*
poisoning (overdose)—code to poisoning
Z91.120 Patient's intentional underdosing of medication regimen due to financial hardship
Z91.128 Patient's intentional underdosing of medication regimen for other reason
✓6th **Z91.13 Patient's unintentional underdosing of medication regimen**
Code first underdosing of medication (T36-T50) with fifth or sixth character 6
EXCLUDES 1 *adverse effect of prescribed drug taken as directed—code to adverse effect*
poisoning (overdose)—code to poisoning
Z91.130 Patient's unintentional underdosing of medication regimen due to age-related debility
Z91.138 Patient's unintentional underdosing of medication regimen for other reason
Z91.14 Patient's other noncompliance with medication regimen
Patient's underdosing of medication NOS
Z91.15 Patient's noncompliance with renal dialysis
Z91.19 Patient's noncompliance with other medical treatment and regimen

✓5th **Z91.4 Personal history of psychological trauma, not elsewhere classified**
✓6th **Z91.41 Personal history of adult abuse**
EXCLUDES 2 *personal history of abuse in childhood (Z62.81-)*
Z91.410 Personal history of adult physical and sexual abuse A
EXCLUDES 1 *current adult physical abuse (T74.11, T76.11)*
current adult sexual abuse (T74.21, T76.11)
Z91.411 Personal history of adult psychological abuse A
Z91.412 Personal history of adult neglect A
EXCLUDES 1 *current adult neglect (T74.01, T76.01)*
Z91.419 Personal history of unspecified adult abuse A
Z91.49 Other personal history of psychological trauma, not elsewhere classified
Z91.5 Personal history of self-harm
Personal history of parasuicide
Personal history of self-poisoning
Personal history of suicide attempt

✓5th **Z91.8 Other specified personal risk factors, not elsewhere classified**

Z91.81 History of falling
At risk for falling

Z91.82 Personal history of military deployment A
Individual (civilian or military) with past history of military war, peacekeeping and humanitarian deployment (current or past conflict)
Returned from military deployment

Z91.83 Wandering in diseases classified elsewhere
Code first underlying disorder such as:
Alzheimer's disease (G30.-)
autism or pervasive developmental disorder (F84.-)
intellectual disabilities (F70-F79)
unspecified dementia with behavioral disturbance (F03.9-)

Z91.89 Other specified personal risk factors, not elsewhere classified

✓4th **Z92 Personal history of medical treatment**
EXCLUDES 2 *postprocedural states (Z98.-)*

Z92.0 Personal history of contraception
EXCLUDES 1 *counseling or management of current contraceptive practices (Z30.-)*
long term (current) use of contraception (Z79.3)
presence of (intrauterine) contraceptive device (Z97.5)

✓5th **Z92.2 Personal history of drug therapy**
EXCLUDES 2 *long term (current) drug therapy (Z79.-)*

Z92.21 Personal history of antineoplastic chemotherapy

Z92.22 Personal history of monoclonal drug therapy

Z92.23 Personal history of estrogen therapy

✓6th **Z92.24 Personal history of steroid therapy**

Z92.240 Personal history of inhaled steroid therapy

Z92.241 Personal history of systemic steroid therapy
Personal history of steroid therapy NOS

Z92.25 Personal history of immunosupression therapy
EXCLUDES 2 *personal history of steroid therapy (Z92.24)*

Z92.29 Personal history of other drug therapy

Z92.3 Personal history of irradiation
Personal history of exposure to therapeutic radiation
EXCLUDES 1 *exposure to radiation in the physical environment (Z77.12)*
occupational exposure to radiation (Z57.1)

✓5th **Z92.8 Personal history of other medical treatment**

Z92.81 Personal history of extracorporeal membrane oxygenation (ECMO)

Z92.82 Status post administration of tPA (rtPA) in a different facility within the last 24 hours prior to admission to current facility
Code first condition requiring tPA administration, such as:
acute cerebral infarction (I63.-)
acute myocardial infarction (I21-, I22-)
AHA: 2013, 4Q, 124

Z92.83 Personal history of failed moderate sedation
Personal history of failed conscious sedation
EXCLUDES 2 *failed moderate sedation during procedure (T88.52)*

Z92.89 Personal history of other medical treatment

✓4th **Z93 Artificial opening status**
EXCLUDES 1 *artificial openings requiring attention or management (Z43.-)*
complications of external stoma (J95.0-, K94.-, N99.5-)

Z93.0 Tracheostomy status
AHA: 2013, 4Q, 129

Z93.1 Gastrostomy status

Z93.2 Ileostomy status

Z93.3 Colostomy status

Z93.4 Other artificial openings of gastrointestinal tract status

✓5th **Z93.5 Cystostomy status**

Z93.50 Unspecified cystostomy status

Z93.51 Cutaneous-vesicostomy status

Z93.52 Appendico-vesicostomy status

Z93.59 Other cystostomy status

Z93.6 Other artificial openings of urinary tract status
Nephrostomy status
Ureterostomy status
Urethrostomy status

Z93.8 Other artificial opening status

Z93.9 Artificial opening status, unspecified

✓4th **Z94 Transplanted organ and tissue status**
INCLUDES organ or tissue replaced by heterogenous or homogenous transplant
EXCLUDES 1 *complications of transplanted organ or tissue—see Alphabetical Index*
EXCLUDES 2 *presence of vascular grafts (Z95.-)*

Z94.0 Kidney transplant status CC
CC Excl: D47.Z1, T86.10-T86.13, T86.19, T86.850-T86.859,T86.90-T86.99,Z94.0,Z94.89-Z94.9

Z94.1 Heart transplant status CC
EXCLUDES 1 *artificial heart status (Z95.812)*
heart-valve replacement status (Z95.2-Z95.4)
CC Excl: D47.Z1, T86.20-T86.39, T86.850-T86.859, T86.90-T86.99, Z94.1, Z94.3, Z94.89-Z94.9

Z94.2 Lung transplant status CC
CC Excl: D47.Z1, T86.810-T86.819,T86.850-T86.859,T86.90-T86.99,Z94.2,Z94.89-Z94.9

Z94.3 Heart and lungs transplant status PDx CC CC
CC Excl: See Code: Z94.1

Z94.4 Liver transplant status CC
CC Excl: D47.Z1,T86.40-T86.43,T86.49,T86.850-T86.859,T86.90-T86.99, Z94.4,Z94.89-Z94.9

Z94.5 Skin transplant status
Autogenous skin transplant status

Z94.6 Bone transplant status

Z94.7 Corneal transplant status

✓5th **Z94.8 Other transplanted organ and tissue status**

Z94.81 Bone marrow transplant status CC
CC Excl: D47.Z1, T86.810-T86.813,T86.00-T86.09,T86.850-T86.859,T86.90-T86.99,Z94.9

Z94.82 Intestine transplant status CC
CC Excl: D47.Z1, T86.830-T86.839, T86.90-T86.99, Z94.82, Z94.89-Z94.9

Z94.83 Pancreas transplant status CC
CC Excl: D47.Z1,T86.850-T86.99,Z94.83,Z94.9

Z94.84 Stem cells transplant status CC
CC Excl: D47.Z1,T86.850-T86.859,T86.90-T86.99,Z94.83,Z94.9

Z94.89 Other transplanted organ and tissue status

Z94.9 Transplanted organ and tissue status, unspecified

✓4th **Z95 Presence of cardiac and vascular implants and grafts**
EXCLUDES 1 *complications of cardiac and vascular devices, implants and grafts (T82.-)*

Z95.0 Presence of cardiac pacemaker
EXCLUDES 1 *adjustment or management of cardiac device (Z45.0)*
presence of automatic (implantable) cardiac defibrillator with synchronous cardiac pacemaker (Z95.810)

Z95.1 Presence of aortocoronary bypass graft

Z95.2 Presence of prosthetic heart valve
Presence of heart valve NOS

Z95.3 Presence of xenogenic heart valve

Z95.4 Presence of other heart-valve replacement

Z95.5 Presence of coronary angioplasty implant and graft
EXCLUDES 1 *coronary angioplasty status without implant and graft (Z98.61)*

✓5th **Z95.8 Presence of other cardiac and vascular implants and grafts**

✓6th **Z95.81 Presence of other cardiac implants and grafts**

Z95.810 Presence of automatic (implantable) cardiac defibrillator
Presence of automatic (implantable) cardiac defibrillator with synchronous cardiac pacemaker

Z95.811 Presence of heart assist device CC
CC Excl: D47.Z1, I46.2-I46.9, I49.01, R09.2, R57.0-R57.8, T86.20-T86.39, T86.850-T86.859, T86.90-T86.99, Z94.1, Z94.3, Z95.811-Z95.812

Z95.812 Presence of fully implantable artificial heart CC
CC Excl: See code: Z95.811

Z95.818 Presence of other cardiac implants and grafts

✓6th Z95.82 Presence of other vascular implants and grafts

Z95.820 Peripheral vascular angioplasty status with implants and grafts
EXCLUDES 1 *peripheral vascular angioplasty without implant and graft (Z98.62)*

Z95.828 Presence of other vascular implants and grafts
Presence of intravascular prosthesis NEC

Z95.9 Presence of cardiac and vascular implant and graft, unspecified

✓4th **Z96 Presence of other functional implants**
EXCLUDES 2 *complications of internal prosthetic devices, implants and grafts (T82-T85)*
fitting and adjustment of prosthetic and other devices (Z44-Z46)

Z96.0 Presence of urogenital implants

Z96.1 Presence of intraocular lens
Presence of pseudophakia

✓5th Z96.2 Presence of otological and audiological implants

Z96.20 Presence of otological and audiological implant, unspecified

Z96.21 Cochlear implant status

Z96.22 Myringotomy tube(s) status

Z96.29 Presence of other otological and audiological implants
Presence of bone-conduction hearing device
Presence of eustachian tube stent
Stapes replacement

Z96.3 Presence of artificial larynx

✓5th Z96.4 Presence of endocrine implants

Z96.41 Presence of insulin pump (external) (internal)

Z96.49 Presence of other endocrine implants

Z96.5 Presence of tooth-root and mandibular implants

✓5th Z96.6 Presence of orthopedic joint implants

Z96.60 Presence of unspecified orthopedic joint implant

✓6th Z96.61 Presence of artificial shoulder joint

Z96.611 Presence of right artificial shoulder joint

Z96.612 Presence of left artificial shoulder joint

Z96.619 Presence of unspecified artificial shoulder joint

✓6th Z96.62 Presence of artificial elbow joint

Z96.621 Presence of right artificial elbow joint

Z96.622 Presence of left artificial elbow joint

Z96.629 Presence of unspecified artificial elbow joint

✓6th Z96.63 Presence of artificial wrist joint

Z96.631 Presence of right artificial wrist joint

Z96.632 Presence of left artificial wrist joint

Z96.639 Presence of unspecified artificial wrist joint

✓6th Z96.64 Presence of artificial hip joint
Hip-joint replacement (partial) (total)

Z96.641 Presence of right artificial hip joint

Z96.642 Presence of left artificial hip joint

Z96.643 Presence of artificial hip joint, bilateral

Z96.649 Presence of unspecified artificial hip joint

✓6th Z96.65 Presence of artificial knee joint

Z96.651 Presence of right artificial knee joint

Z96.652 Presence of left artificial knee joint

Z96.653 Presence of artificial knee joint, bilateral

Z96.659 Presence of unspecified artificial knee joint

✓6th Z96.66 Presence of artificial ankle joint

Z96.661 Presence of right artificial ankle joint

Z96.662 Presence of left artificial ankle joint

Z96.669 Presence of unspecified artificial ankle joint

✓6th Z96.69 Presence of other orthopedic joint implants

Z96.691 Finger-joint replacement of right hand

Z96.692 Finger-joint replacement of left hand

Z96.693 Finger-joint replacement, bilateral

Z96.698 Presence of other orthopedic joint implants

Z96.7 Presence of other bone and tendon implants
Presence of skull plate

✓5th Z96.8 Presence of other specified functional implants

Z96.81 Presence of artificial skin

Z96.89 Presence of other specified functional implants

Z96.9 Presence of functional implant, unspecified

✓4th **Z97 Presence of other devices**
EXCLUDES 1 *complications of internal prosthetic devices, implants and grafts (T82-T85)*
fitting and adjustment of prosthetic and other devices (Z44-Z46)
EXCLUDES 2 *presence of cerebrospinal fluid drainage device (Z98.2)*

Z97.0 Presence of artificial eye

✓5th Z97.1 Presence of artificial limb (complete) (partial)

Z97.10 Presence of artificial limb (complete) (partial), unspecified

Z97.11 Presence of artificial right arm (complete) (partial)

Z97.12 Presence of artificial left arm (complete) (partial)

Z97.13 Presence of artificial right leg (complete) (partial)

Z97.14 Presence of artificial left leg (complete) (partial)

Z97.15 Presence of artificial arms, bilateral (complete) (partial)

Z97.16 Presence of artificial legs, bilateral (complete) (partial)

Z97.2 Presence of dental prosthetic device (complete) (partial)
Presence of dentures (complete) (partial)

Z97.3 Presence of spectacles and contact lenses

Z97.4 Presence of external hearing-aid

Z97.5 Presence of (intrauterine) contraceptive device ♀
EXCLUDES 1 *checking, reinsertion or removal of contraceptive device (Z30.43)*

Z97.8 Presence of other specified devices

✓4th **Z98 Other postprocedural states**
EXCLUDES 2 *aftercare (Z43-Z49, Z51)*
follow-up medical care (Z08- Z09)
postprocedural complication—see Alphabetical Index

Z98.0 Intestinal bypass and anastomosis status
EXCLUDES 2 *bariatric surgery status (Z98.84)*
gastric bypass status (Z98.84)
obesity surgery status (Z98.84)

Z98.1 Arthrodesis status

Z98.2 Presence of cerebrospinal fluid drainage device
Presence of CSF shunt

Z98.3 Post therapeutic collapse of lung status
Code first underlying disease

✓5th Z98.4 Cataract extraction status
Use additional code to identify intraocular lens implant status (Z96.1)
EXCLUDES 1 *aphakia (H27.0)*

Z98.41 Cataract extraction status, right eye

Z98.42 Cataract extraction status, left eye

Z98.49 Cataract extraction status, unspecified eye

✓5th Z98.5 Sterilization status
EXCLUDES 1 *female infertility (N97.-)*
male infertility (N46.-)

Z98.51 Tubal ligation status ♀

Z98.52 Vasectomy status A ♂

✓5th Z98.6 Angioplasty status

Z98.61 Coronary angioplasty status
EXCLUDES 1 *coronary angioplasty status with implant and graft (Z95.5)*

Z98.62 Peripheral vascular angioplasty status
EXCLUDES 1 *peripheral vascular angioplasty status with implant and graft (Z95.820)*

✓5th Z98.8 Other specified postprocedural states

✓6th Z98.81 Dental procedure status

Z98.810 Dental sealant status

Z98.811 Dental restoration status
Dental crown status
Dental fillings status

Z98.818 Other dental procedure status

Z98.82 Breast implant status
EXCLUDES 1 *breast implant removal status (Z98.86)*

Z98.83 Filtering (vitreous) bleb after glaucoma surgery status
EXCLUDES 1 *inflammation (infection) of postprocedural bleb (H59.4-)*

Z98.84 Bariatric surgery status
Gastric banding status
Gastric bypass status for obesity
Obesity surgery status
EXCLUDES 1 *bariatric surgery status complicating pregnancy, childbirth, or the puerperium (O99.84)*
EXCLUDES 2 *intestinal bypass and anastomosis status (Z98.0)*

Z98.85 Transplanted organ removal status
Transplanted organ previously removed due to complication, failure, rejection or infection
EXCLUDES 1 *encounter for removal of transplanted organ—code to complication of transplanted organ (T86.-)*

Z98.86 Personal history of breast implant removal

✓6th **Z98.87 Personal history of in utero procedure**

Z98.870 Personal history of in utero procedure during pregnancy ♀
EXCLUDES 2 *complications from in utero procedure for current pregnancy (O35.7)*
supervision of current pregnancy with history of in utero procedure during previous pregnancy (O09.82-)

Z98.871 Personal history of in utero procedure while a fetus

Z98.89 Other specified postprocedural states
Personal history of surgery, not elsewhere classified

✓4th **Z99 Dependence on enabling machines and devices, not elsewhere classified**
EXCLUDES 1 *cardiac pacemaker status (Z95.0)*

Z99.0 Dependence on aspirator

✓5th **Z99.1 Dependence on respirator**
Dependence on ventilator

CC Excl: For CC codes in subcategory Z99.1: CC with 7th character A, unless otherwise noted: J95.850, Z99.0-Z99.12, Z99.81- Z99.89

Z99.11 Dependence on respirator [ventilator] status CC

Z99.12 Encounter for respirator [ventilator] dependence during power failure CC
EXCLUDES 1 *mechanical complication of respirator [ventilator] (J95.850)*

Z99.2 Dependence on renal dialysis
Hemodialysis status
Peritoneal dialysis status
Presence of arteriovenous shunt for dialysis
Renal dialysis status NOS
EXCLUDES 1 *encounter for fitting and adjustment of dialysis catheter (Z49.0-)*
noncompliance with renal dialysis (Z91.15)
AHA: 2013, 4Q, 125

Z99.3 Dependence on wheelchair
Wheelchair confinement status
Code first cause of dependence, such as:
muscular dystrophy (G71.0)
obesity (E66.-)

✓5th **Z99.8 Dependence on other enabling machines and devices**

Z99.81 Dependence on supplemental oxygen
Dependence on long-term oxygen
AHA: 2013, 4Q, 129

Z99.89 Dependence on other enabling machines and devices
Dependence on machine or device NOS

Peripheral Nervous System

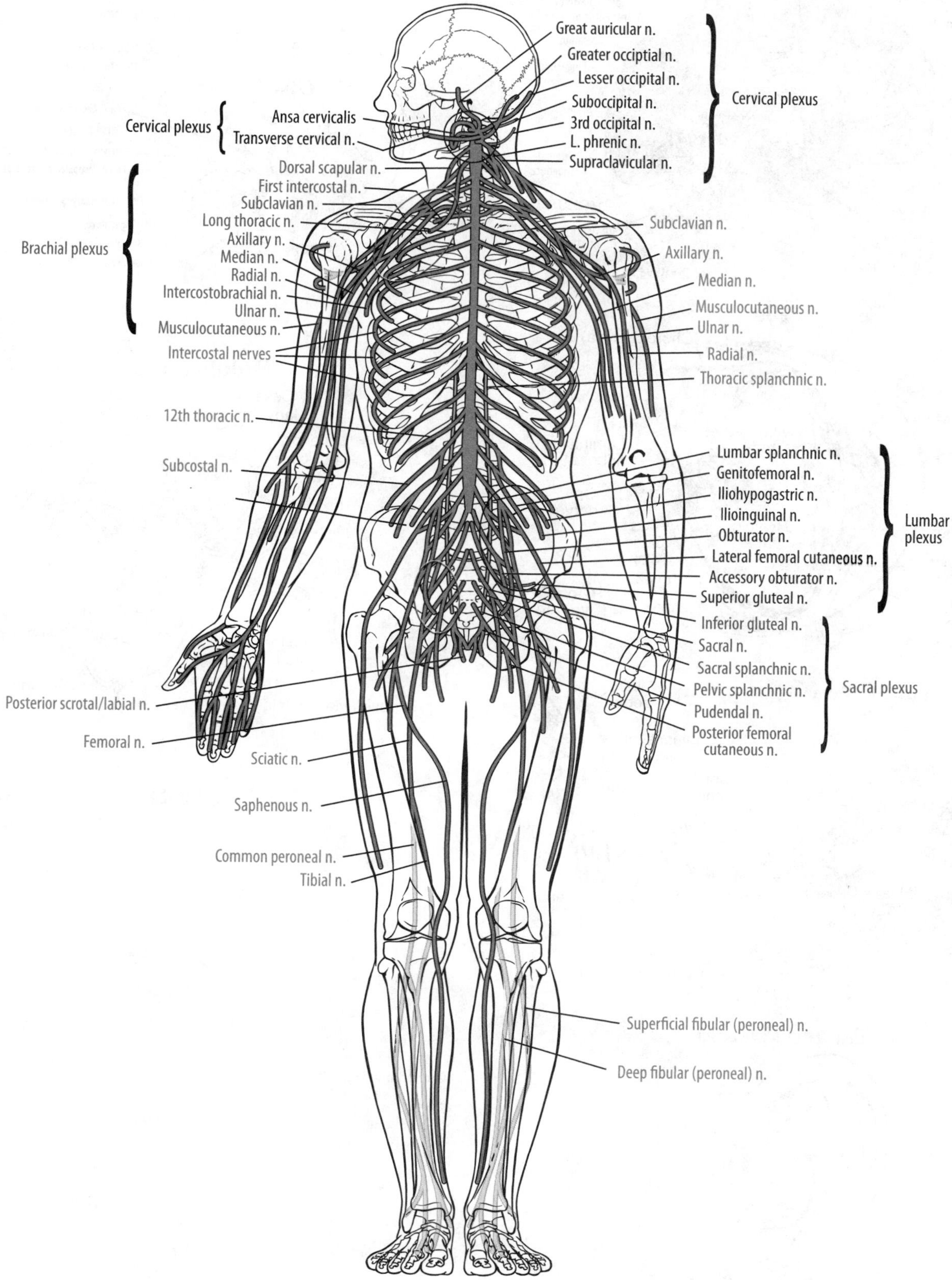

Brain

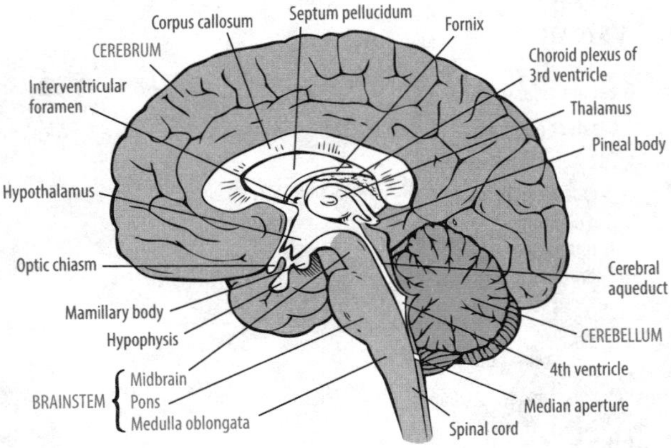

Cranial Nerves

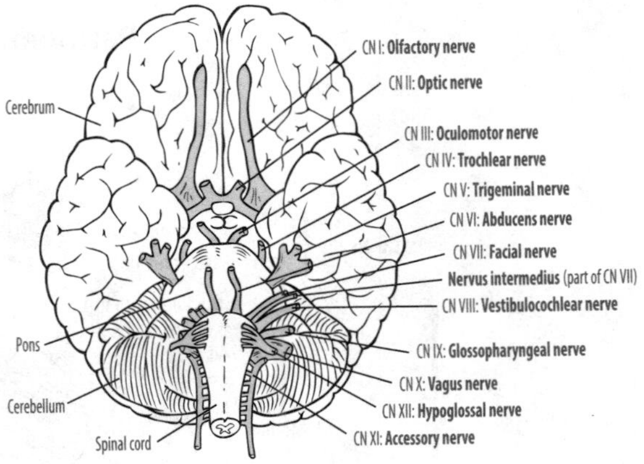

Eye

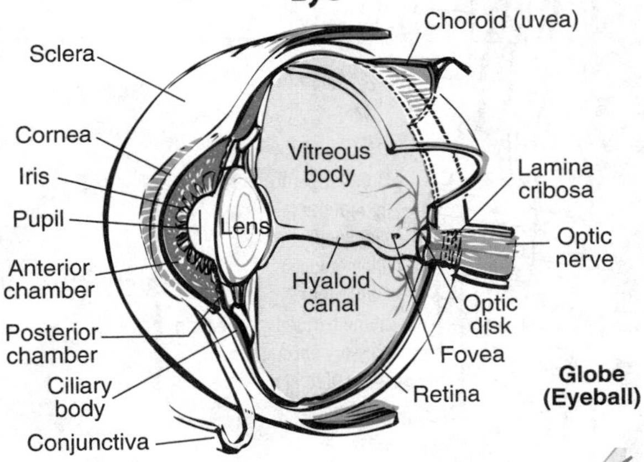

Globe (Eyeball)

Posterior Pole of Globe

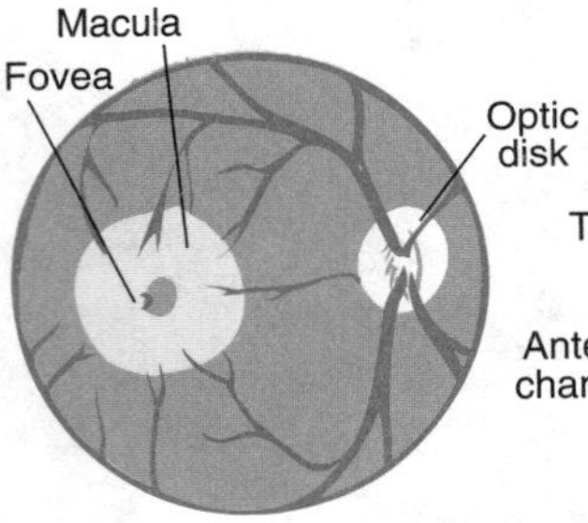

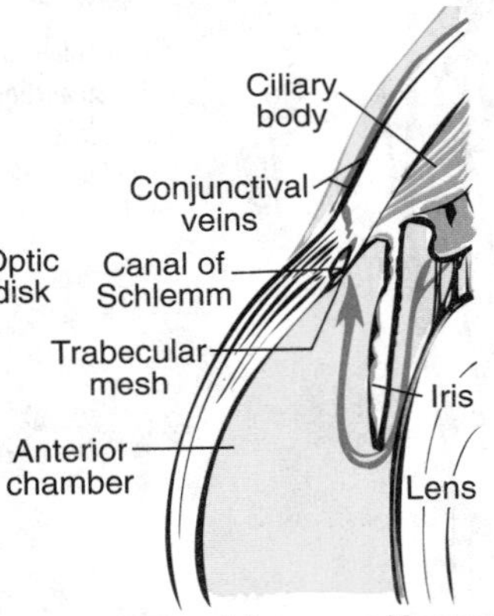

Flow of Aqueous Humor

Middle Ear

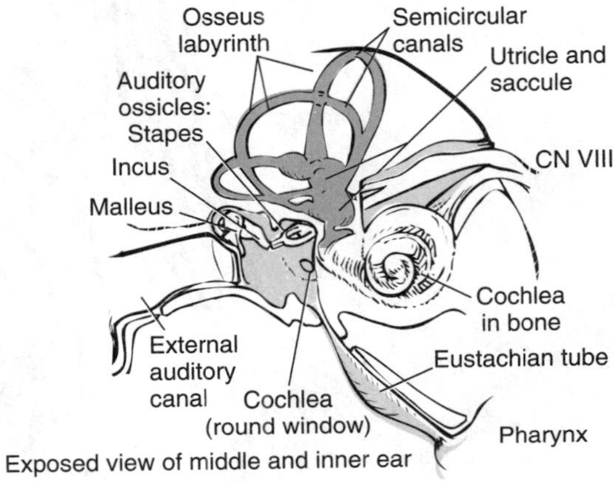

Exposed view of middle and inner ear

Lacrimal System

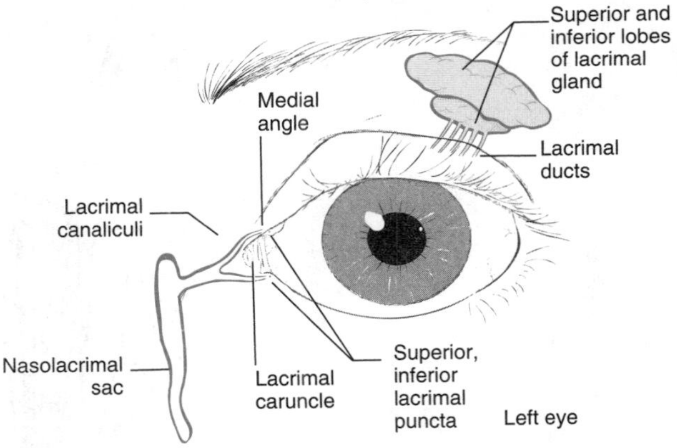

Ear and Mastoid

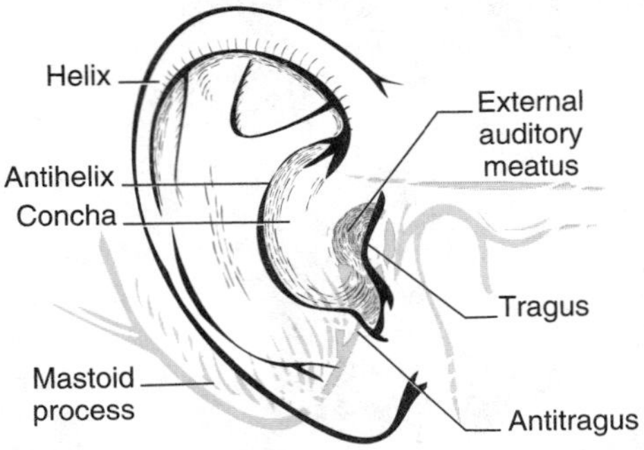

Arteries

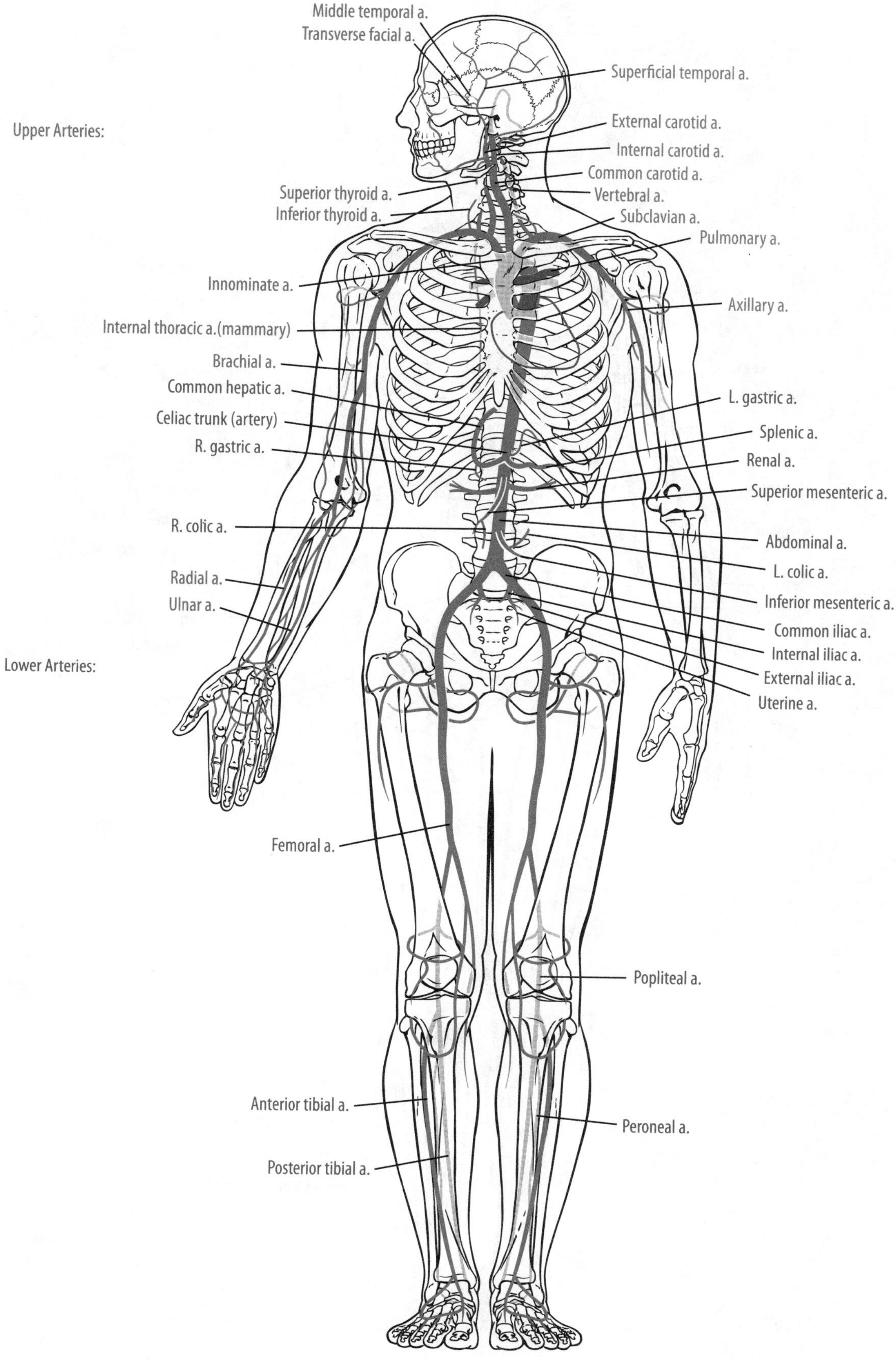
Middle temporal a.
Transverse facial a.
Superficial temporal a.
Upper Arteries:
External carotid a.
Internal carotid a.
Common carotid a.
Superior thyroid a.
Vertebral a.
Inferior thyroid a.
Subclavian a.
Pulmonary a.
Innominate a.
Axillary a.
Internal thoracic a.(mammary)
Brachial a.
Common hepatic a.
L. gastric a.
Celiac trunk (artery)
Splenic a.
R. gastric a.
Renal a.
Superior mesenteric a.
R. colic a.
Abdominal a.
L. colic a.
Radial a.
Inferior mesenteric a.
Ulnar a.
Common iliac a.
Internal iliac a.
Lower Arteries:
External iliac a.
Uterine a.
Femoral a.
Popliteal a.
Anterior tibial a.
Peroneal a.
Posterior tibial a.

Veins

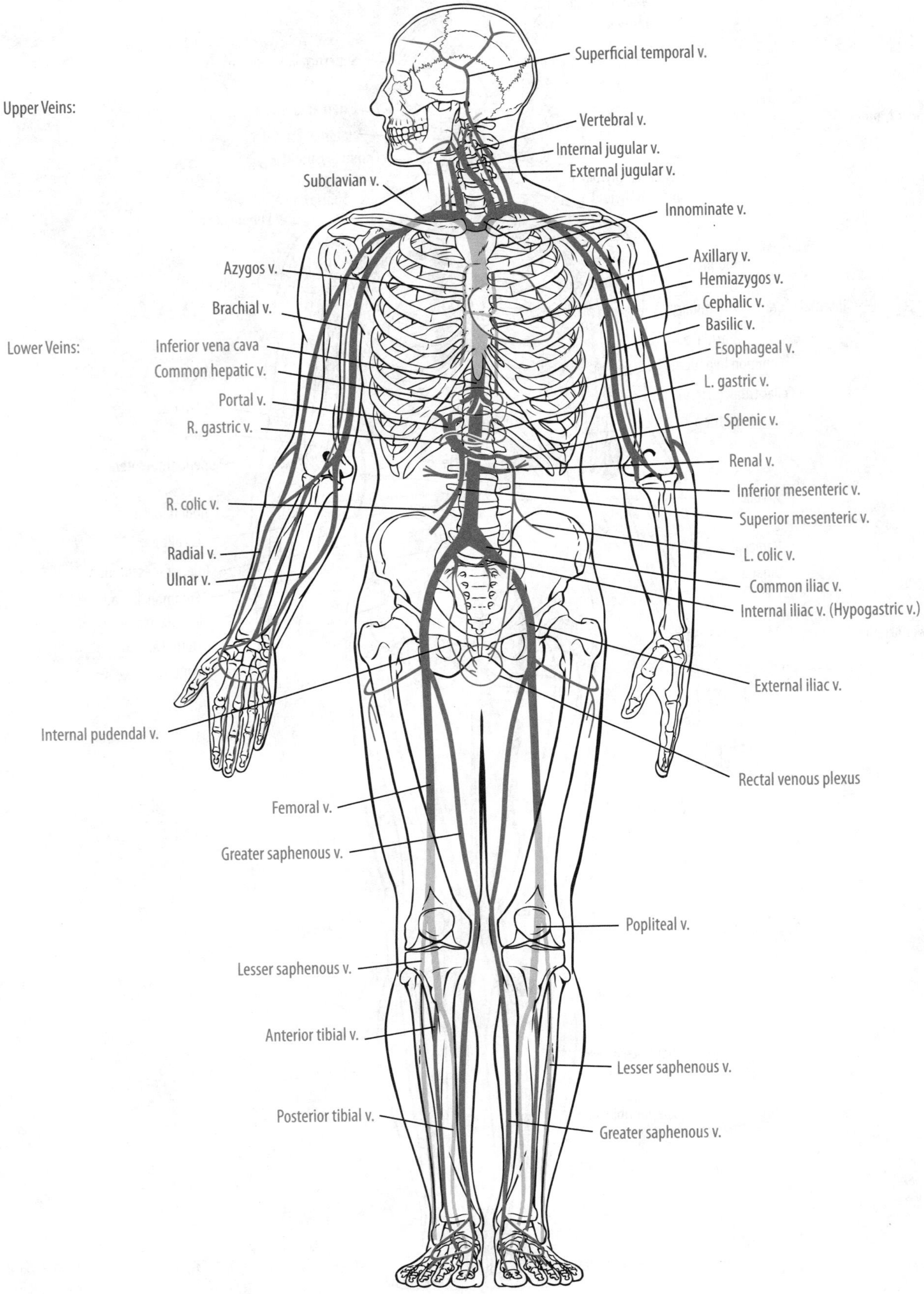
Upper Veins:
Lower Veins:
Superficial temporal v.
Vertebral v.
Internal jugular v.
External jugular v.
Subclavian v.
Innominate v.
Azygos v.
Axillary v.
Hemiazygos v.
Brachial v.
Cephalic v.
Basilic v.
Inferior vena cava
Esophageal v.
Common hepatic v.
L. gastric v.
Portal v.
R. gastric v.
Splenic v.
Renal v.
Inferior mesenteric v.
R. colic v.
Superior mesenteric v.
L. colic v.
Radial v.
Ulnar v.
Common iliac v.
Internal iliac v. (Hypogastric v.)
External iliac v.
Internal pudendal v.
Rectal venous plexus
Femoral v.
Greater saphenous v.
Popliteal v.
Lesser saphenous v.
Anterior tibial v.
Lesser saphenous v.
Posterior tibial v.
Greater saphenous v.

Anatomy of Heart

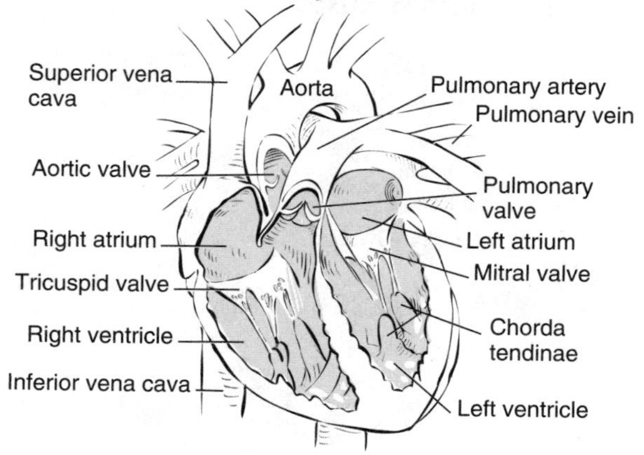

Arteries of Heart

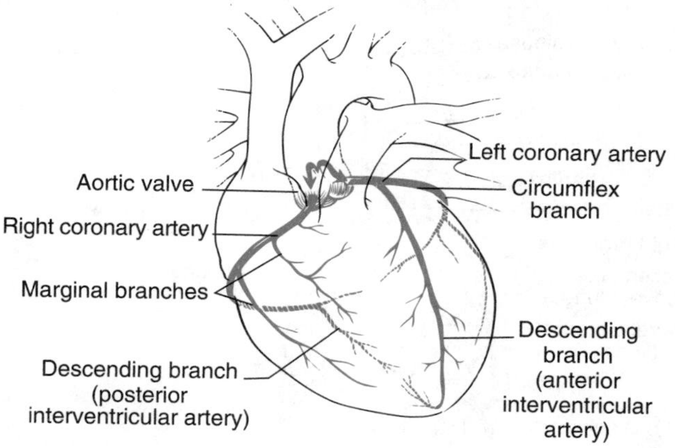

Cerebrovascular Arteries

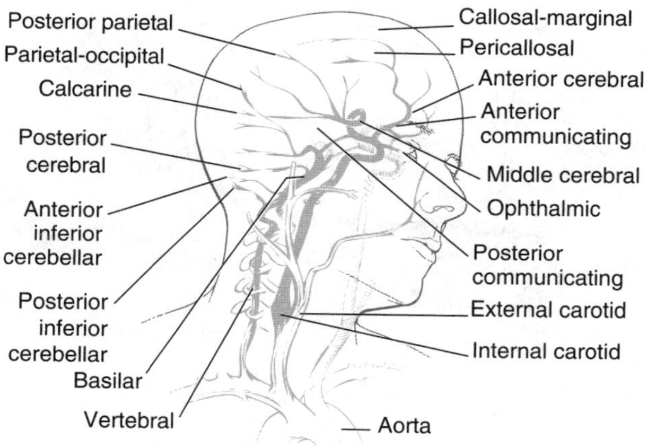

Veins of Head and Neck

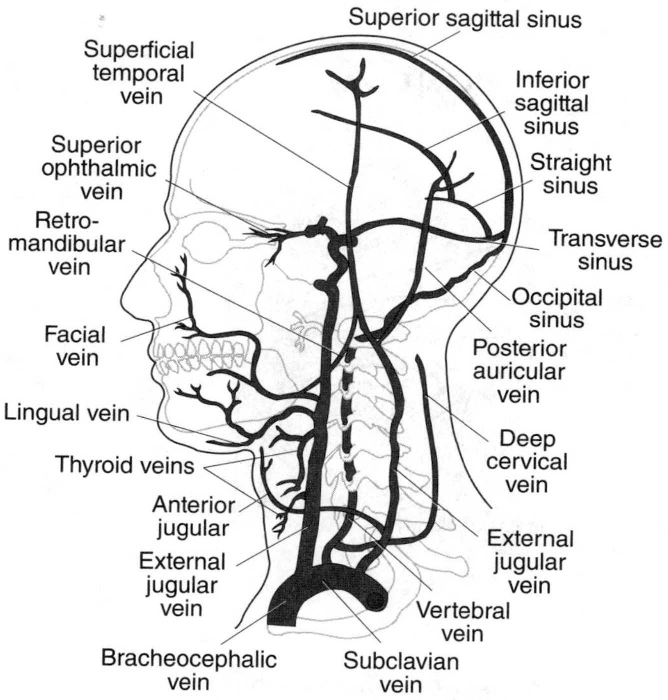

Lymphatic System of Head and Neck

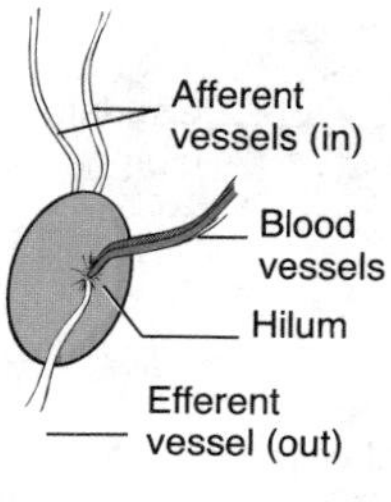

Schematic of lymph node

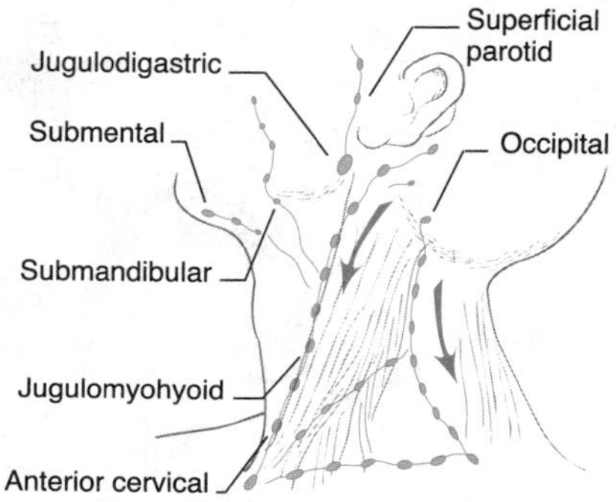

Lymphatic drainage of the head, neck, and face

Lymph Nodes

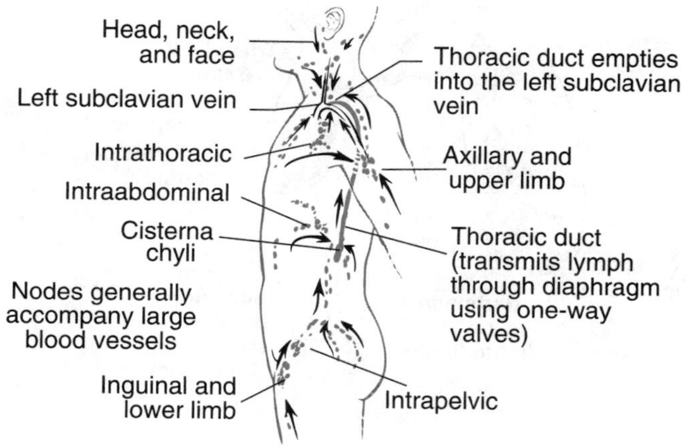

Respiratory System

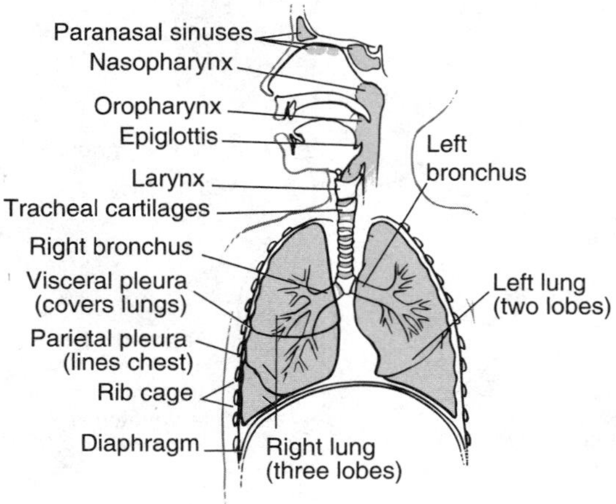

Paranasal Sinuses

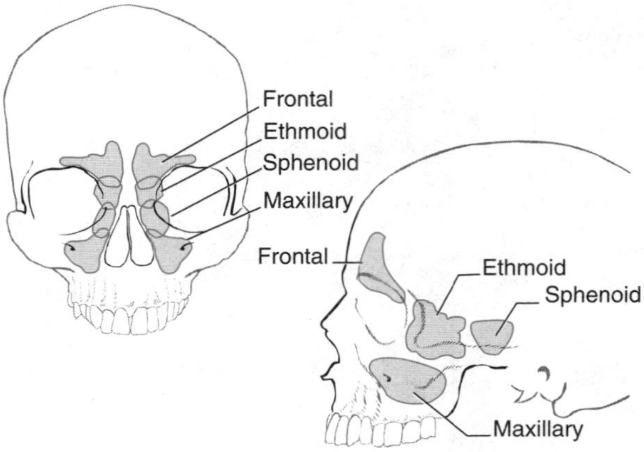

Oral Cavity

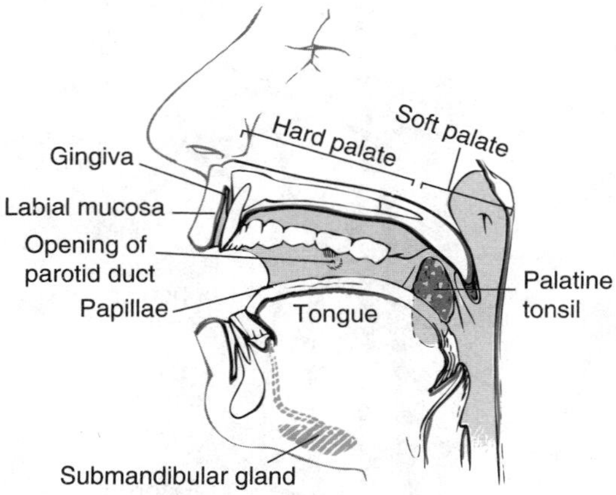

Pancreas

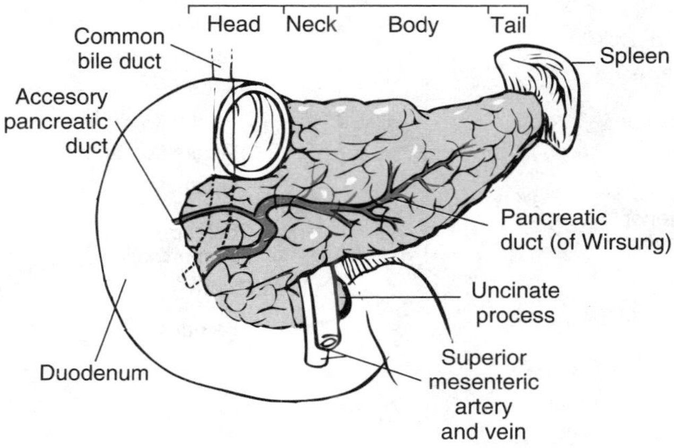

Gallbladder and Bile Ducts

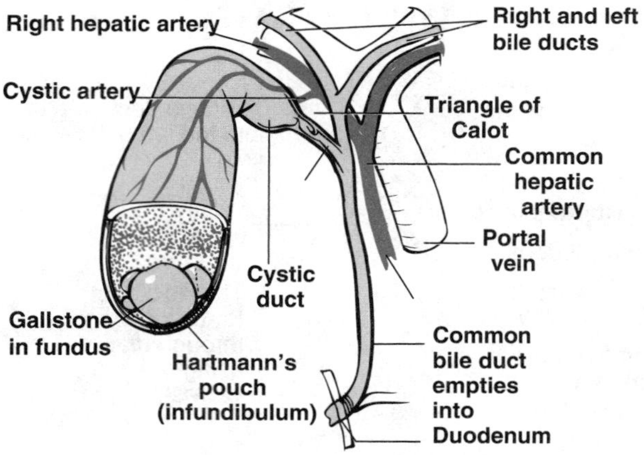

Liver

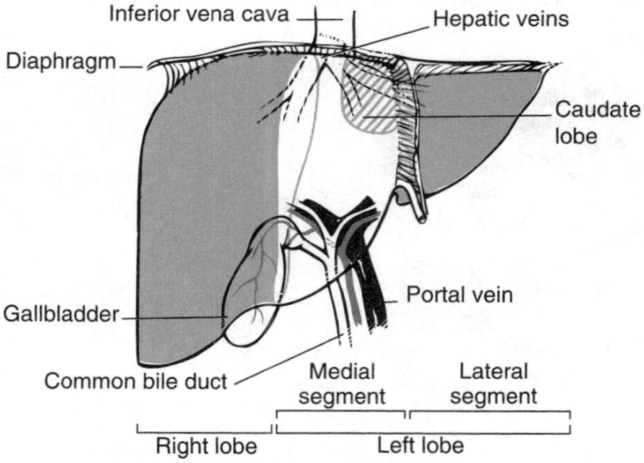

Gastrointestinal System

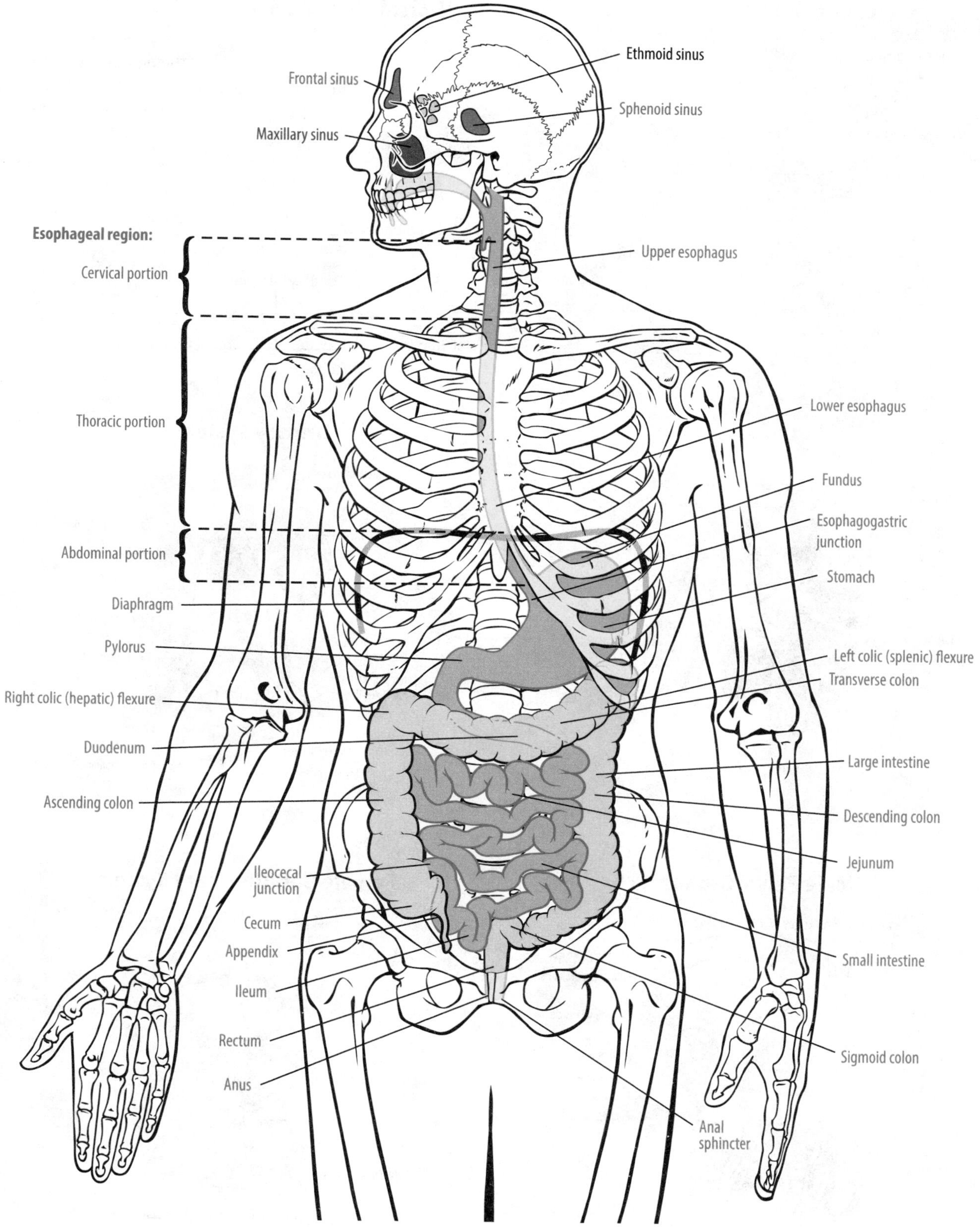

Endocrine System

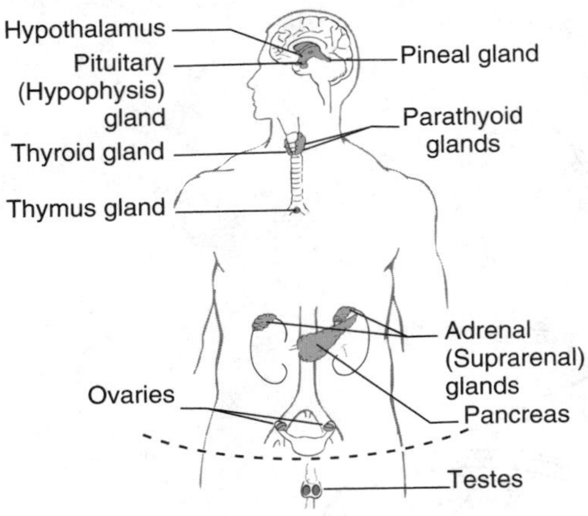

Dorsal View of Parathyroid Gland

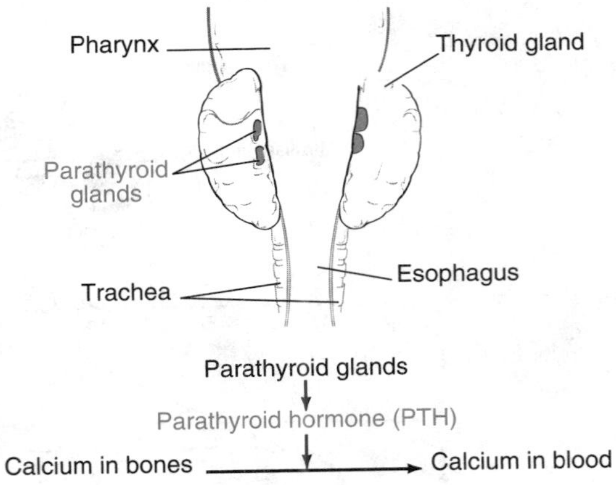

Kidney

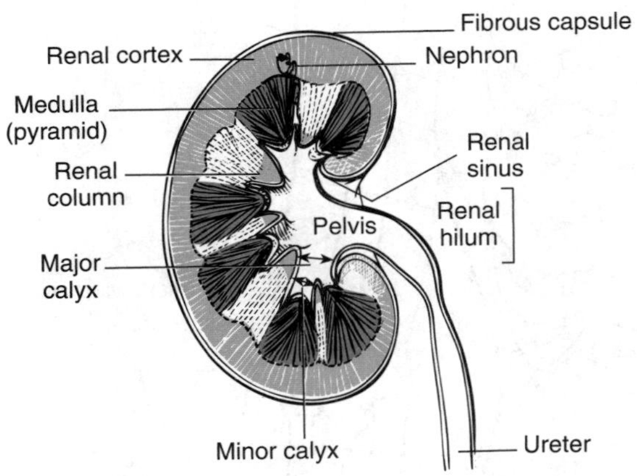

Urinary System

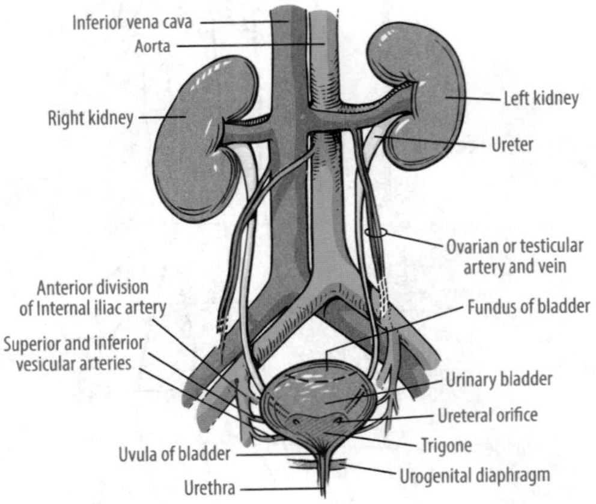

Male Pelvic Organs

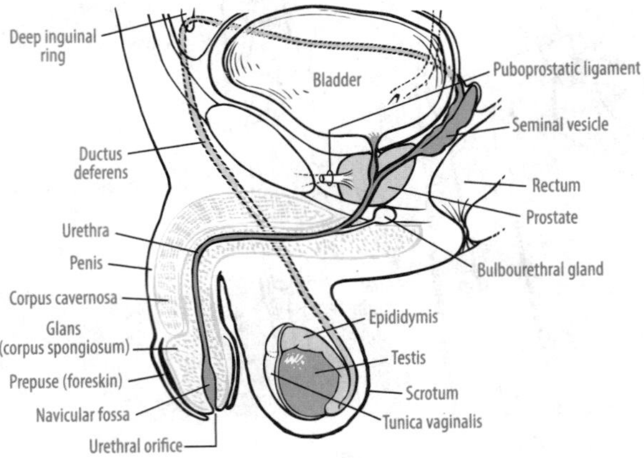

Female Genitourinary System

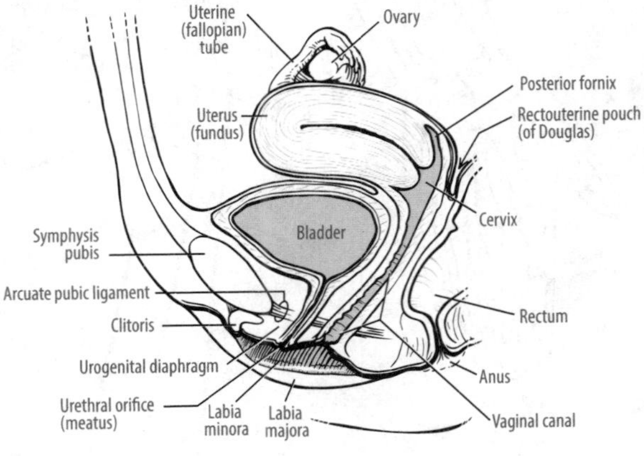

Joints

Shoulder (Anterior View)

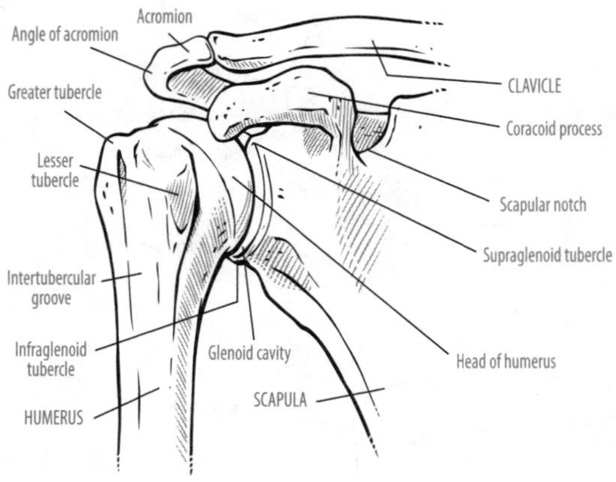

Shoulder (Posterior View)

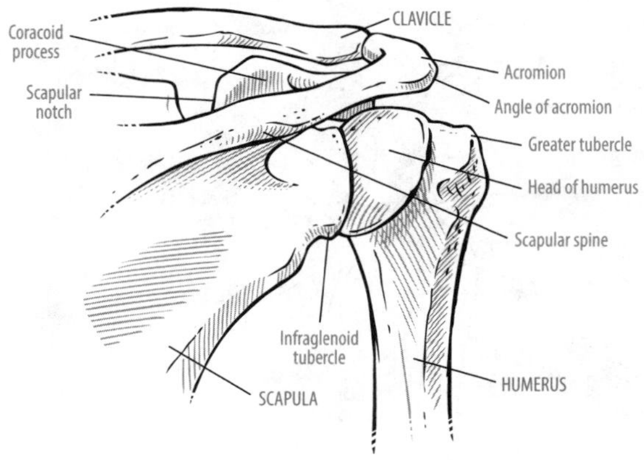

Elbow (Anterior View)

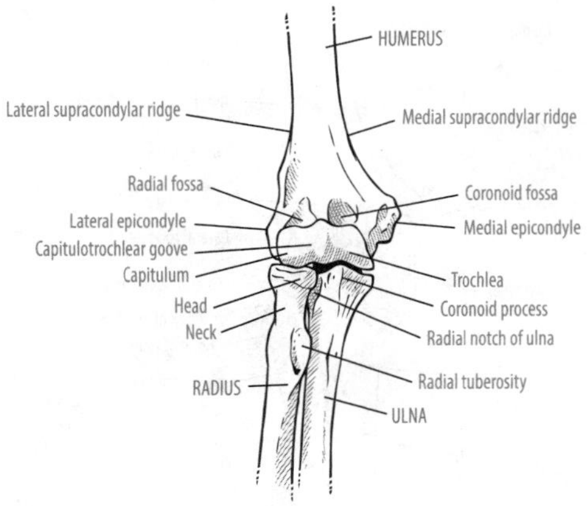

Elbow (Posterior View)

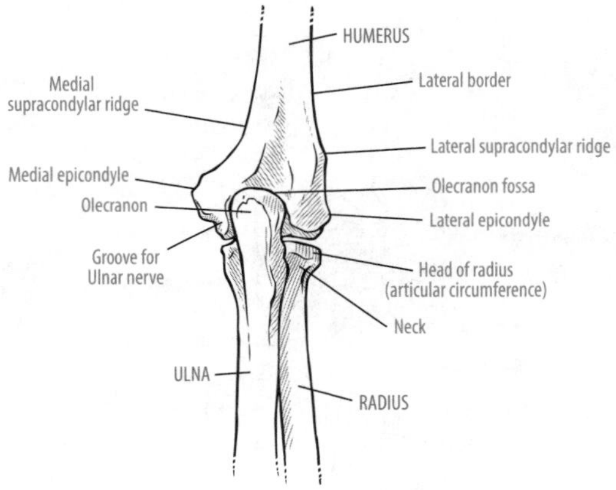

Hand

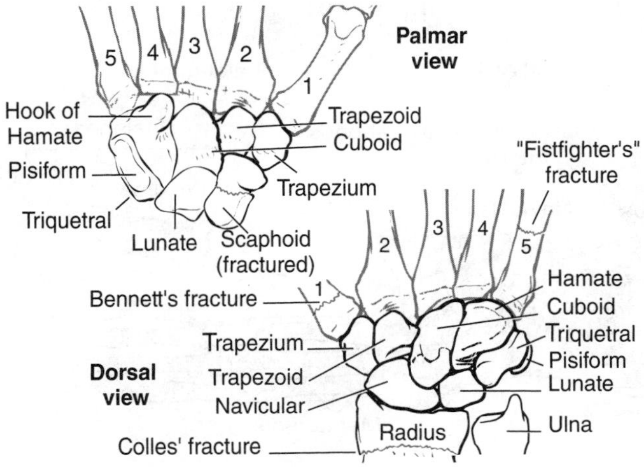

Joints

Hip (Anterior View)

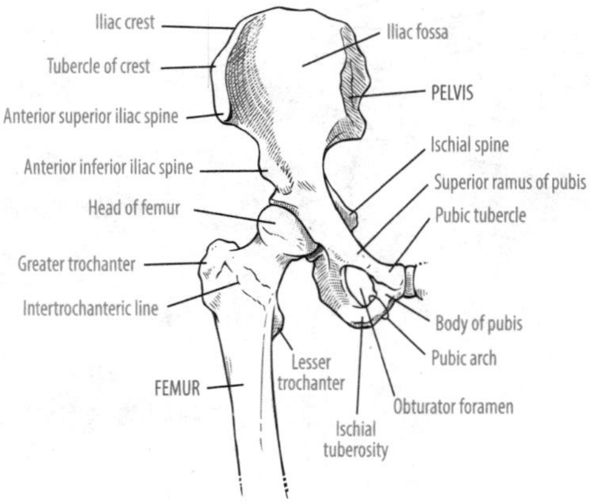

Hip (Posterior View)

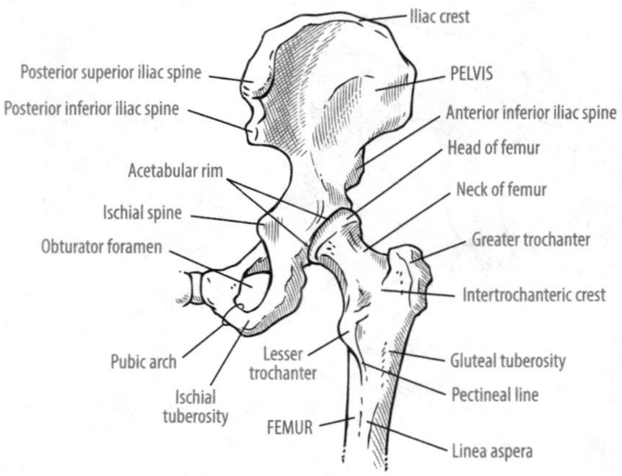

Knee (Anterior View)

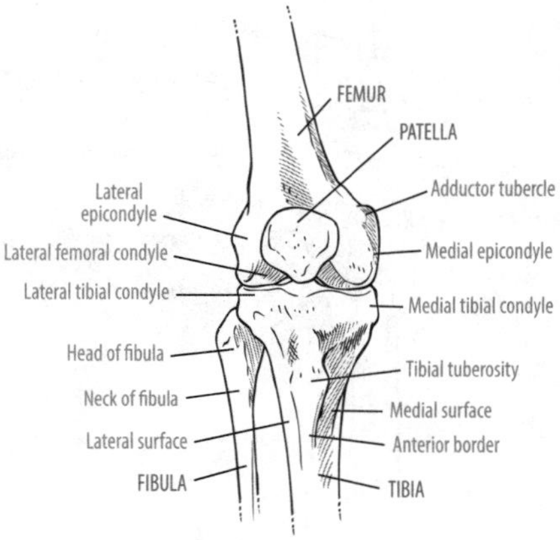

Knee (Posterior View)

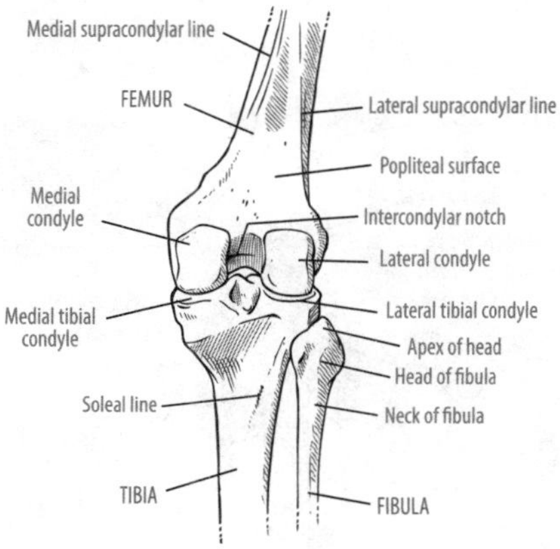

Right Foot

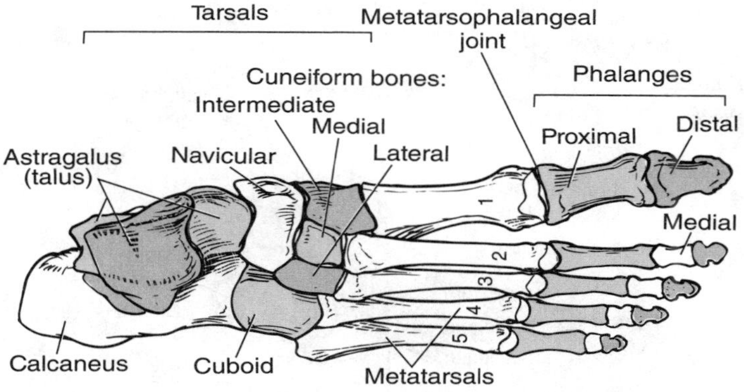

Bones/Joints

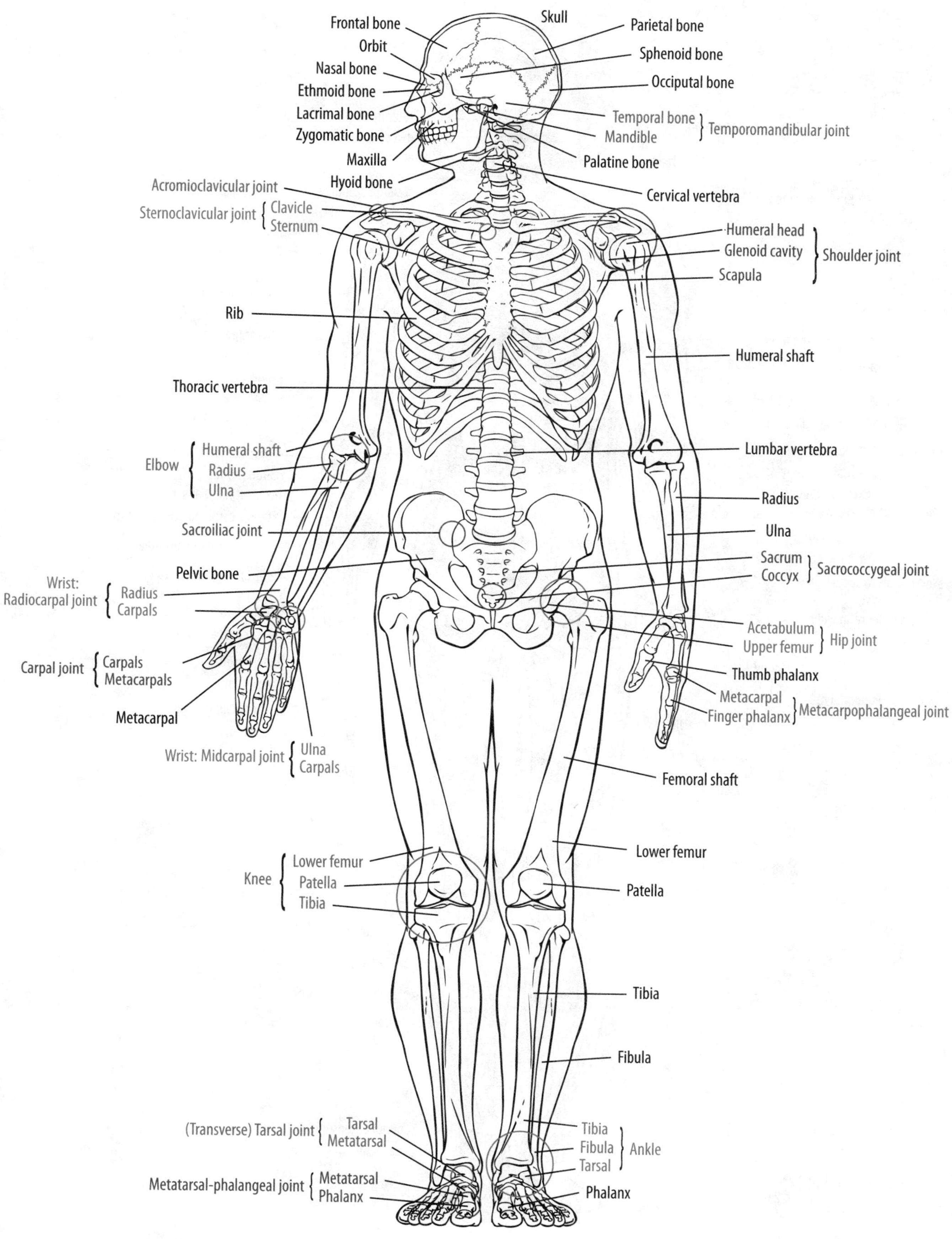

Muscles

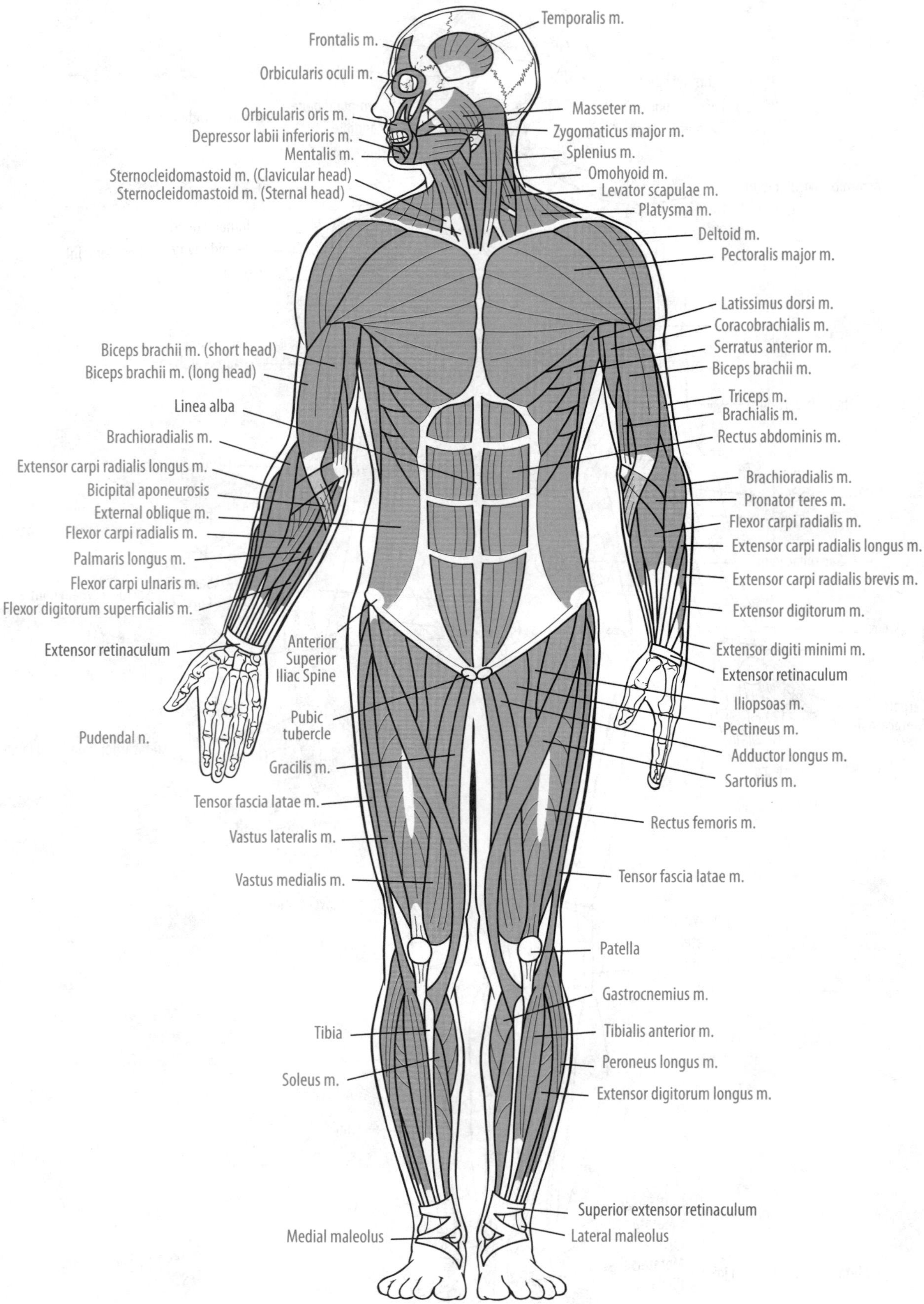
Temporalis m.
Frontalis m.
Orbicularis oculi m.
Orbicularis oris m.
Depressor labii inferioris m.
Mentalis m.
Sternocleidomastoid m. (Clavicular head)
Sternocleidomastoid m. (Sternal head)
Masseter m.
Zygomaticus major m.
Splenius m.
Omohyoid m.
Levator scapulae m.
Platysma m.
Deltoid m.
Pectoralis major m.
Latissimus dorsi m.
Coracobrachialis m.
Serratus anterior m.
Biceps brachii m.
Biceps brachii m. (short head)
Biceps brachii m. (long head)
Linea alba
Triceps m.
Brachialis m.
Rectus abdominis m.
Brachioradialis m.
Extensor carpi radialis longus m.
Bicipital aponeurosis
External oblique m.
Flexor carpi radialis m.
Palmaris longus m.
Flexor carpi ulnaris m.
Flexor digitorum superficialis m.
Brachioradialis m.
Pronator teres m.
Flexor carpi radialis m.
Extensor carpi radialis longus m.
Extensor carpi radialis brevis m.
Extensor digitorum m.
Extensor retinaculum
Anterior Superior Iliac Spine
Extensor digiti minimi m.
Extensor retinaculum
Iliopsoas m.
Pubic tubercle
Pectineus m.
Pudendal n.
Adductor longus m.
Gracilis m.
Sartorius m.
Tensor fascia latae m.
Rectus femoris m.
Vastus lateralis m.
Vastus medialis m.
Tensor fascia latae m.
Patella
Gastrocnemius m.
Tibia
Tibialis anterior m.
Peroneus longus m.
Soleus m.
Extensor digitorum longus m.
Superior extensor retinaculum
Medial maleolus
Lateral maleolus

Notes

Notes